17. PHARMACOKINETICS Important parameters described in the FDA-approved labeling, the majority of which are an average or the approximate values provided in the FDA-approved labeling. Only select parameters are included. Refer to the full prescribing information for more detailed pharmacokinetics information.

18. ABSORPTION The process by which the drug enters the bloodstream and becomes bioavailable; may include time to peak plasma concentration (T_{max}), area under the curve (AUC), peak plasma concentration (C_{max}), and absolute bioavailability.

19. DISTRIBUTION Parameters related to the dispersion and dissemination of the drug through bodily fluids and tissues; may include plasma protein binding and volume of distribution (V_d).

20. METABOLISM Summary of the biotransformation or detoxification of the parent compound into metabolites. Associated enzymes and active metabolites are included if applicable.

21. ELIMINATION Parameters associated with the removal of the drug from the body; may include elimination/terminal half-life ($T_{1/2}$) and percentage eliminated through urine or feces.

NURSING CONSIDERATIONS

22. ASSESSMENT Specific parameters and laboratory tests that the patient must be assessed for or undergo prior to starting treatment with the drug.

23. MONITORING Information used for monitoring patients currently treated with the drug; may include specific lab tests and drug-related or condition-specific information.

24. PATIENT COUNSELING Important treatment information to discuss with the patient.

25. ADMINISTRATION Guidelines for preparing the drug for administration, rate of administration, proper administration technique, and/or compatibility. For more details on the step-by-step administration process, refer to the full prescribing information.

26. STORAGE Instructions for safe storage and disposal of the drug.

1 Drug monographs contain concise information. Not all fields described here are included in every monograph. For more detailed information, please see the full, FDA-approved labeling information.

2 Abbreviations used within monographs are defined in the Abbreviations, Acronyms, and Symbols table on page A1 of the appendix.

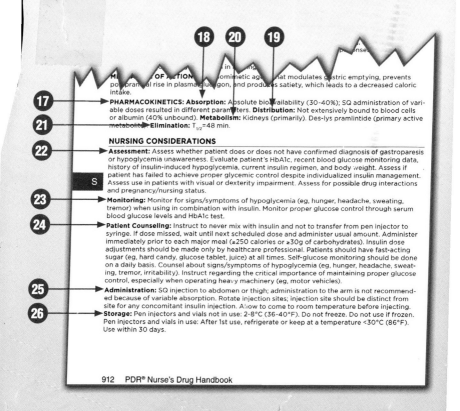

18 20 19

MECHANISM OF ACTION ...mimetic agent that modulates gastric emptying, prevents postprandial rise in plasma glucagon, and produces satiety, which leads to a decreased caloric intake.

17 ➤ **PHARMACOKINETICS: Absorption:** Absolute bioavailability (30-40%); SQ administration of variable doses resulted in different parameters. **Distribution:** Not extensively bound to blood cells or albumin (40% unbound). **Metabolism:** Kidneys (primarily). Des-lys pramlintide (primary active metabolite). **21** ➤ **Elimination:** $T_{1/2}$=48 min.

NURSING CONSIDERATIONS

22 ➤ **Assessment:** Assess whether patient does or does not have confirmed diagnosis of gastroparesis or hypoglycemia unawareness. Evaluate patient's HbA1c, recent blood glucose monitoring data, history of insulin-induced hypoglycemia, current insulin regimen, and body weight. Assess if patient has failed to achieve proper glycemic control despite individualized insulin management. Assess use in patients with visual or dexterity impairment. Assess for possible drug interactions and pregnancy/nursing status.

23 ➤ **Monitoring:** Monitor for signs/symptoms of hypoglycemia (eg, hunger, headache, sweating, tremor) when using in combination with insulin. Monitor proper glucose control through serum blood glucose levels and HbA1c test.

24 ➤ **Patient Counseling:** Instruct to never mix with insulin and not to transfer from pen injector to syringe. If dose missed, wait until next scheduled dose and administer usual amount. Administer immediately prior to each major meal (≥250 calories or ≥30g of carbohydrates). Insulin dose adjustments should be made only by healthcare professional. Patients should have fast-acting sugar (eg, hard candy, glucose tablet, juice) at all times. Self-glucose monitoring should be done on a daily basis. Counsel about signs/symptoms of hypoglycemia (eg, hunger, headache, sweating, tremor, irritability). Instruct regarding the critical importance of maintaining proper glucose control, especially when operating heavy machinery (eg, motor vehicles).

25 ➤ **Administration:** SQ injection to abdomen or thigh; administration to the arm is not recommended because of variable absorption. Rotate injection sites; injection site should be distinct from site for any concomitant insulin injection. Allow to come to room temperature before injecting.

26 ➤ **Storage:** Pen injectors and vials not in use: 2-8°C (36-40°F). Do not freeze. Do not use if frozen. Pen injectors and vials in use: After 1st use, refrigerate or keep at a temperature <30°C (86°F). Use within 30 days.

*FDA/DEA CLASS

OTC: Available over-the-counter.

RX: Requires a prescription.

CII: **HIGH POTENTIAL FOR ABUSE.** Use may lead to severe physical or psychological dependence.

CIII: **POTENTIAL FOR ABUSE.** Use may lead to low-to-moderate physical dependence or high psychological dependence.

CIV: **LOW POTENTIAL FOR ABUSE RELATIVE TO DRUGS OR OTHER SUBSTANCES IN C-III.** Use may lead to limited physical or psychological dependence relative to the drugs or other substances in C-III.

CV: **LOW POTENTIAL FOR ABUSE RELATIVE TO DRUGS OR OTHER SUBSTANCES IN C-IV.** Use may lead to limited physical or psychological dependence relative to the drugs or other substances in C-IV.

---

†FDA USE-IN-PREGNANCY RATINGS

The FDA use-in-pregnancy rating system weighs the degree to which available information has ruled out risk to the fetus against the drug's potential benefit to the patient. The ratings, and the interpretation, are as follows:

CATEGORY	INTERPRETATION
A	**CONTROLLED STUDIES SHOW NO RISK.** Adequate, well-controlled studies in pregnant women have failed to demonstrate a risk to the fetus in the first trimester of pregnancy (and there is no evidence of a risk in later trimesters).
B	**NO EVIDENCE OF RISK IN HUMANS.** Adequate, well-controlled studies in pregnant women are lacking, and animal studies have not shown increased risk of fetal abnormalities. The chance of fetal harm is remote, but remains a possibility.
C	**RISK CANNOT BE RULED OUT.** Adequate, well-controlled human studies are lacking, and animal studies have shown a risk to the fetus. There is a chance of fetal harm if the drug is administered during pregnancy, but the potential benefits may outweigh the potential risk.
D	**POSITIVE EVIDENCE OF RISK.** Studies in humans, or investigational or postmarketing data, have demonstrated fetal risk. Nevertheless, potential benefits from the use of the drug may outweigh the potential risk. For example, the drug may be acceptable if needed in a life-threatening situation or serious disease for which safer drugs cannot be used or are ineffective.
X	**CONTRAINDICATED IN PREGNANCY.** Studies in animals or humans have demonstrated fetal abnormalities or if there is positive evidence of fetal risk based on adverse reaction reports from investigational or marketing experience, or both, and risk of use clearly outweighs any possible benefit.

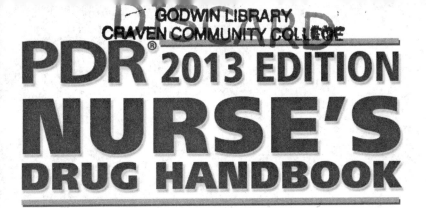

PDR® 2013 EDITION
NURSE'S
DRUG HANDBOOK

THE INFORMATION STANDARD FOR PRESCRIPTION DRUGS AND NURSING CONSIDERATIONS

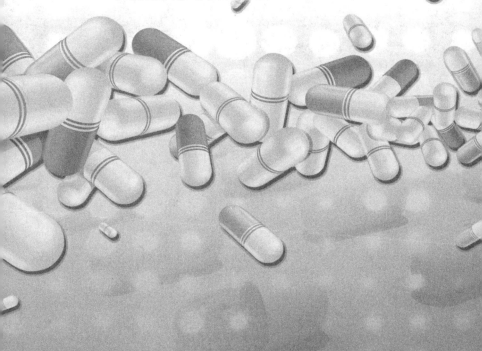

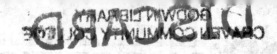

PDR® NURSE'S DRUG HANDBOOK

2013 EDITION

Director, Clinical Services: Sylvia Nashed, PharmD
Senior Manager, Clinical Services: Nermin Shenouda-Kerolous, PharmD
Clinical Database Manager: Christine Sunwoo, PharmD
Senior Drug Information Specialist: Anila Patel, PharmD
Drug Information Specialists: Pauline Lee, PharmD; Kristine Mecca, PharmD
Clinical Editor: Julia Tonelli, MD
Managing Editor: J. Harris Fleming, Jr.
Senior Editor: Wendy S. Kopf
Senior Project Manager: Jennifer Park
Project Manager: Gary Lew
Manager, Art Department: Livio Udina
Senior Director, Operations & Client Services: Stephanie Struble
Associate Director, Manufacturing & Distribution: Thomas Westburgh
Marketing Manager, Product Sales: Brian Triano

PDR NETWORK, LLC

CEO: Edward Fotsch, MD
President: Richard C. Altus
Chief Medical Officer: Steven Merahn, MD
Chief Financial Officer: Dawn Carfora
Chief Technology Officer: David Cheng
Senior Vice President, Publishing & Operations: Valerie Berger
Senior Vice President, Corporate Development, & General Counsel: Andrew Gelman
Senior Vice President, Sales: Jeff Davis
Senior Vice President, Marketing & Product Management: Barbara Senich, BSN, MBA, MPH

ISBN: 978-1-56363-806-0

Printed in Canada

Contents

FOREWORD

The role of nursing professionals in safe medication administration and patient education has never been more crucial—especially as our national healthcare system continues to evolve. The 2011 Institute of Medicine Report on the future of nursing[1] notes that nurses are being called on to practice at the fullest extent of their practice scope. Nurses are central to the goal of ensuring the highest quality healthcare while reducing costs. To accomplish this in the arena of pharmacotherapy and medication administration, nurses must decipher constantly changing information regarding medications, new therapies, and interactions, and rapidly assess patient responses to multiple variables that are important to medication administration. As such, it is vital for each nurse to have a reference that provides accurate and easily accessible drug information. The *PDR® Nurse's Drug Handbook, 2013 Edition* is this reference.

Physicians' Desk Reference® is a well-known and trusted resource for medication information—and *PDR Nurse's Drug Handbook* follows this tradition. This important reference is specifically designed for nurses, with each entry providing the following when applicable: therapeutic class, indications, dosage, how the medication is supplied, contraindications, relevant warnings and precautions, key adverse reactions, interactions, pregnancy category, mechanism of action, pharmacokinetics, and nursing considerations—a special section that features content specific to assessing, monitoring, and counseling patients, as well as administering medications.

The *PDR Nurse's Drug Handbook* is organized to foster quick identification of key drug information, identifying medications by generic and brand names, as well as therapeutic class. Special sections provide important considerations when caring for pregnant or breastfeeding patients, children, and older adults. Other useful resources include a multitude of charts and tables about medications for specific chronic problems such as hypertension, migraine, HIV, hepatitis, and diabetes; immunizations; poison antidotes; lactose-, galactose-, and sugar-free products; cytochrome P450 enzyme inhibitors, substrates, and inducers; and a full-color visual identification guide. New in the 2013 edition are tables providing detailed information about the most commonly used herbal products, obesity guidelines specific to adults and children, screening and diagnosis of gestational diabetes, products for which the FDA has approved Risk Evaluation and Management Strategies (REMS), and a treatment algorithm for tuberculosis.

The *PDR® Nurse's Drug Handbook, 2013 Edition* is an essential reference for enhancing full-scope nursing practice and patient education efforts. Its convenient size and clear layout provide fast access to concise, authoritative drug information, making this book a trusted resource among nurses.

Ivy M. Alexander, PhD, APRN, ANP-BC, FAAN
Professor
Director–Adult-Gerontological, Family, and
  Women's Health NP Specialty
Yale University School of Nursing

1. Committee on the Robert Wood Johnson Foundation Initiative on the Future of Nursing, at the Institute of Medicine. (2011). The Future of Nursing: Leading Change, Advancing Health. The National Academies Press; Washington, DC. Available at: *http://www.nap.edu/catalog.php?record_id=12956*

Concise Drug Monographs

ABELCET

amphotericin B lipid complex (Sigma-Tau)

RX

THERAPEUTIC CLASS: Polyene antifungal

INDICATIONS: Treatment of invasive fungal infections in patients refractory to or intolerant of conventional amphotericin B therapy.

DOSAGE: *Adults:* 5mg/kg given as a single IV infusion at 2.5mg/kg/hr.
Pediatrics: 5mg/kg given as a single IV infusion at 2.5mg/kg/hr.

HOW SUPPLIED: Inj: 5mg/mL

WARNINGS/PRECAUTIONS: Anaphylaxis reported; d/c infusion and do not give further infusions if severe respiratory distress occurs. Administer initial dose under close clinical observation by medically trained personnel. Acute reactions, including fever and chills, may occur 1-2 hrs after starting IV infusion. Frequently monitor SrCr during therapy. Regularly monitor LFTs, serum electrolytes (particularly magnesium and K⁺) and CBC.

ADVERSE REACTIONS: Chills, fever, increased SrCr, multiple organ failure, N/V, hypotension, respiratory failure, dyspnea, sepsis, diarrhea, headache, heart arrest, HTN, hypokalemia.

INTERACTIONS: Antineoplastic agents may enhance potential for renal toxicity, bronchospasm, and hypotension; use with great caution. Corticosteroids and corticotropin may potentiate hypokalemia. Initiation with cyclosporine A within several days of bone marrow ablation may be associated with increased nephrotoxicity. May induce hypokalemia and potentiate digitalis toxicity with digitalis glycosides. May increase flucytosine toxicity; use with caution. Antagonism with imidazole derivatives (eg, miconazole, ketoconazole) reported. Acute pulmonary toxicity reported with leukocyte transfusions; avoid concurrent use. Nephrotoxic agents (eg, aminoglycosides, pentamidine) may enhance the potential for drug-induced renal toxicity; use with caution. Amphotericin B-induced hypokalemia may enhance curariform effect of skeletal muscle relaxants (eg, tubocurarine) due to hypokalemia. Monitor renal and hematologic function with zidovudine.

PREGNANCY: Category B, not for use in nursing.

MECHANISM OF ACTION: Polyene antifungal; binds to sterols in the cell membrane of susceptible fungi, with a resultant change in membrane permeability.

PHARMACOKINETICS: Absorption: C_{max}=1.7µg/mL; AUC=14µg•hr/mL. **Distribution:** V_d=131L/kg. **Elimination:** Urine (0.9%); $T_{1/2}$=173.4 hrs.

NURSING CONSIDERATIONS

Assessment: Assess for previous hypersensitivity to the drug, pregnancy/nursing status, and possible drug interactions.

Monitoring: Monitor clinical condition, cardiac function, renal function, anaphylaxis, severe respiratory distress, and acute reactions. Frequently monitor SrCr. Regularly monitor LFTs, serum electrolytes (particularly magnesium and K⁺) and CBC.

Patient Counseling: Inform of risks and benefits of therapy. Advise to seek medical attention if any adverse reactions occur.

Administration: IV route. Shake the infusion bag q2h if the infusion time exceeds 2 hrs. Refer to PI for preparation of admixture for infusion. Do not dilute with saline sol or mix with other drugs or electrolytes. Do not use an in-line filter. **Storage:** 2-8°C (36-46°F). Protect from light. Do not freeze. Diluted Ready-For-Use Admixture: Stable for up to 48 hrs at 2-8°C (36-46°F) and an additional 6 hrs at room temperature. Do not freeze.

ABILIFY

aripiprazole (Bristol-Myers Squibb/Otsuka America)

RX

Elderly patients with dementia-related psychosis treated with antipsychotic drugs are at an increased risk of death; most deaths appeared to be cardiovascular (CV) (eg, heart failure, sudden death) or infectious (eg, pneumonia) in nature. Not approved for the treatment of patients with dementia-related psychosis. Antidepressants increased the risk of suicidal thinking and behavior (suicidality) in children, adolescents, and young adults in short-term studies with major depressive disorder (MDD) and other psychiatric disorders. Monitor and observe closely for clinical worsening, suicidality, or unusual changes in behavior in patients who are started on antidepressant therapy. Not approved for use in pediatric patients with depression.

OTHER BRAND NAMES: Abilify Discmelt (Bristol-Myers Squibb/Otsuka America)

THERAPEUTIC CLASS: Partial D_2/5HT$_{1A}$ agonist/5HT$_{2A}$ antagonist

INDICATIONS: (PO) Treatment of schizophrenia in adults and adolescents (13-17 yrs). Acute treatment of manic and mixed episodes associated with bipolar I disorder in adults and pediatrics (10-17 yrs). Maintenance treatment of bipolar I disorder, both as monotherapy and adjunct

1

to lithium or valproate in adults. Adjunctive therapy to antidepressants for treatment of MDD in adults. Treatment of irritability associated with autistic disorder in pediatric patients (6-17 yrs). (Inj) Acute treatment of agitation associated with schizophrenia or bipolar disorder, manic or mixed, in adults.

DOSAGE: *Adults:* (PO) Schizophrenia: Initial/Target: 10mg or 15mg qd. Titrate: Should not increase before 2 weeks. Usual: 10-30mg/day. Bipolar Disorder (Monotherapy): Initial/Target: 15mg qd. (Adjunct to Lithium or Valproate): Initial: 10-15mg qd. Target: 15mg qd. Titrate: May increase to 30mg/day based on clinical response. Max: 30mg/day. MDD Adjunct: Initial: 2-5mg/day. Titrate: May adjust dose at increments up to 5mg/day at intervals of no less than 1 week. Usual: 2-15mg/day. Periodically reassess need for maintenance therapy. Oral Sol: May give on mg-per-mg basis up to 25mg. Patients receiving 30mg tabs should receive 25mg of oral sol. (Inj) Schizophrenia or Bipolar Mania: 9.75mg IM. Usual: 5.25-15mg IM. Max: 30mg/day IM or not more frequent than q2h. If clinically indicated, may replace with PO at 10-30mg/day. Refer to PI for dose adjustments when used concomitantly with other medications.
Pediatrics: Schizophrenia (13-17 yrs)/Bipolar Disorder (Monotherapy or Adjunct) (10-17 yrs): Initial: 2mg/day. Titrate: May increase to 5mg/day after 2 days to a target dose of 10mg/day after 2 additional days. Subsequent dose increases should be administered in 5mg increments. Schizophrenia (13-17 yrs): Usual: 10-30mg/day. Irritability Associated with Autistic Disorder (6-17 yrs): Individualize dose. Initial: 2mg/day. Titrate: Increase to 5mg/day. May increase to 10 or 15mg/day if necessary. Dose adjustments of up to 5mg/day should occur gradually at intervals of no less than 1 week. Usual: 5-15mg/day. Periodically reassess need for maint therapy. Oral Sol: May give on mg-per-mg basis up to 25mg. Patients receiving 30mg tabs should receive 25mg of oral sol. Refer to PI for dose adjustments when used concomitantly with other medications.

HOW SUPPLIED: Tab, Disintegrating: (Discmelt) 10mg, 15mg; Tab: 2mg, 5mg, 10mg, 15mg, 20mg, 30mg; Sol: 1mg/mL [150mL]; Inj: 7.5mg/mL

WARNINGS/PRECAUTIONS: Initiate in pediatric patients only after a thorough diagnostic evaluation is conducted and careful consideration given to the risks of therapy. Caution in patients at risk for bipolar disorder; mixed/manic episodes may likely precipitate. Neuroleptic malignant syndrome (NMS) reported; d/c and treat immediately. May develop tardive dyskinesia (TD); consider d/c if this occurs. May cause metabolic changes (hyperglycemia/diabetes mellitus (DM), dyslipidemia, weight gain). Hyperglycemia, in some cases extreme and associated with ketoacidosis or hyperosmolar coma or death reported; monitor for hyperglycemia, and perform FPG testing at the beginning of therapy and periodically in patients at risk for DM. Altered lipids and weight gain reported. May cause orthostatic hypotension; caution with CV disease, cerebrovascular disease, or conditions that predispose to hypotension (eg, dehydration, hypovolemia, and treatment with antihypertensives). Leukopenia, neutropenia, and agranulocytosis reported; d/c at 1st sign of decline in WBC without other causative factors in patients with preexisting low WBC or history of drug-induced leukopenia/neutropenia or if severe neutropenia (absolute neutrophil count <1000/mm^3) develops. Caution with history of seizures or with conditions that lower the seizure threshold. May impair physical/mental abilities. May disrupt body's ability to reduce core body temperature; caution with conditions that may contribute to an elevated core body temperature (eg, strenuous exercise, concomitant medications with anticholinergic activity). Esophageal dysmotility and aspiration may occur; caution in patients at risk for aspiration pneumonia.

ADVERSE REACTIONS: Headache, blurred vision, fatigue, tremor, anxiety, insomnia, N/V, somnolence, constipation, akathisia, extrapyramidal disorder, nasopharyngitis, dizziness, restlessness.

INTERACTIONS: May potentiate effect of antihypertensives. Caution with other centrally acting drugs. Avoid with alcohol. CYP3A4 inducers (eg, carbamazepine) may lower blood levels. CYP3A4 inhibitors (eg, ketoconazole, itraconazole) or 2D6 inhibitors (eg, quinidine, fluoxetine, paroxetine) may increase blood levels. (Inj) Greater intensity of sedation and greater orthostatic hypotension with lorazepam inj; monitor for excessive sedation and orthostatic hypotension with parenteral benzodiazepines.

PREGNANCY: Category C, not for use in nursing.

MECHANISM OF ACTION: Partial $D_2/5HT_{1A}$ agonist/$5HT_{2A}$ antagonist; not established.

PHARMACOKINETICS: Absorption: Absolute bioavailability 87% (Tab), 100% (IM); T_{max}=3-5 hrs (Tab), 1-3 hrs (IM). **Distribution:** V_d=404L or 4.9L/kg (IV); plasma protein binding >99% (IV). **Metabolism:** Hepatic via dehydrogenation (CYP2D6 and CYP3A4), hydroxylation (CYP2D6 and CYP3A4), and N-dealkylation (CYP3A4). Dehydro-aripiprazole (active metabolite). **Elimination:** Urine (25%, <1% unchanged), feces (55%, 18% unchanged); $T_{1/2}$=75 hrs (extensive metabolizers) and 146 hrs (PMs).

NURSING CONSIDERATIONS

Assessment: Assess for history of dementia-related psychosis, MDD, depression, DM, drug hypersensitivity, any other conditions where treatment is cautioned, pregnancy/nursing status, and possible drug interactions. Obtain baseline FPG in patients at risk for DM.

Monitoring: Monitor for clinical worsening, suicidality, unusual changes in behavior, NMS, TD, hyperglycemia, orthostatic hypotension, leukopenia, neutropenia, agranulocytosis, seizures, cognitive/motor impairment, disruption of body temperature, esophageal dysmotility, aspiration, and other possible side effects. Monitor FPG, lipid profile, weight gain, and CBC (in patients with preexisting low WBC or drug-induced leukopenia/neutropenia). In patients with clinically significant neutropenia, monitor for fever or other symptoms or signs of infection. Periodically reassess for continued need for maint treatment.

Patient Counseling: Instruct caregivers and patients to contact physician if signs of agitation, anxiety, panic attacks, insomnia, hostility, aggressiveness, impulsivity, akathisia, hypomania, mania, irritability, worsening of depression, changes in behavior, or suicidal ideation develop. Use caution when operating hazardous machinery. Avoid alcohol use while on therapy. Counsel to avoid overheating and dehydration. Notify physician if become pregnant or intend to become pregnant during therapy and if taking or plan to take any prescription or over-the-counter drugs. Do not breastfeed during therapy. ODT: Inform phenylketonurics that product contains phenylalanine. Instruct not to open blister until ready to administer, not to split tab, and to take without liquid, if possible. Sol: Inform that sol contains sucrose and fructose.

Administration: Oral/IM route. (Inj) Refer to PI for administration instructions. **Storage:** 25°C (77°F); excursions permitted to 15-30°C (59-86°F). Oral Sol: May be used for ≤6 months after opening, not beyond expiration date. Inj: Store in original container; protect from light.

ABRAXANE RX
paclitaxel protein-bound particles (Abraxis)

> Should not be administered to patients with metastatic breast cancer who have baseline neutrophil counts of <1500 cells/mm³. Perform frequent peripheral blood cell counts to monitor occurrence of bone marrow suppression, primarily neutropenia. Do not substitute for or with other paclitaxel formulations.

THERAPEUTIC CLASS: Antimicrotubule agent

INDICATIONS: Treatment of breast cancer after failure of combination chemotherapy for metastatic disease or relapse within 6 months of adjuvant chemotherapy. Prior therapy should have included an anthracycline unless clinically contraindicated.

DOSAGE: *Adults:* Usual: 260mg/m² IV over 30 min q3 weeks. Severe Neutropenia (Neutrophil <500 cells/mm³ for week or longer) or Severe Sensory Neuropathy During Therapy: Reduce dose to 220mg/m² for subsequent courses. For recurrence of severe neutropenia or severe sensory neuropathy, additional dose reduction should be made to 180mg/m². For grade 3 sensory neuropathy, hold treatment until resolution to grade 1 or 2, followed by a dose reduction for all subsequent courses. Moderate Hepatic Impairment (AST <10X ULN and Bilirubin 1.26-2.0X ULN): Usual: 200mg/m² for the 1st course of therapy. Titrate: May adjust dose in subsequent courses based on tolerance. Severe Hepatic Impairment (AST <10X ULN and Bilirubin 2.01-5.0X ULN): Usual: 130mg/m² for the 1st course of therapy. Titrate: May increase to 200mg/m² in subsequent courses based on tolerance. Do not give if AST >10X ULN or bilirubin >5.0X ULN.

HOW SUPPLIED: Inj: 100mg

CONTRAINDICATIONS: Patients with baseline neutrophil counts of <1500 cells/mm³.

WARNINGS/PRECAUTIONS: Bone marrow suppression (primarily neutropenia) is dose-dependent and a dose-limiting toxicity; do not retreat until neutrophils recover to >1500 cells/mm³ and platelets recover to >100,000 cells/mm³. Sensory neuropathy occurs frequently. Caution with hepatic impairment. Contains human albumin; may carry a remote risk for transmission of viral diseases. May cause fetal harm. Men should be advised not to father a child while receiving treatment.

ADVERSE REACTIONS: Alopecia, neutropenia, sensory neuropathy, abnormal ECG, fatigue/asthenia, myalgia/arthralgia, AST elevation, alkaline phosphatase elevation, anemia, nausea, infections, diarrhea.

INTERACTIONS: CYP2C8 and/or CYP3A4 substrates, inducers, or inhibitors may alter pharmacokinetics; caution with medicines known to inhibit (eg, ketoconazole and other imidazole antifungals, erythromycin, fluoxetine, gemfibrozil, cimetidine, ritonavir, saquinavir, indinavir, nelfinavir) or induce (eg, rifampicin, carbamazepine, phenytoin, efavirenz, nevirapine) either CYP2C8 or CYP3A4.

PREGNANCY: Category D, not for use in nursing.

MECHANISM OF ACTION: Antimicrotubule agent; promotes assembly of microtubules from tubulin dimers and stabilizes microtubules by preventing depolymerization. This stability results in inhibition of the normal dynamic reorganization of the microtubule network that is essential for vital interphase and mitotic cellular functions.

PHARMACOKINETICS: Absorption: C_{max}=18,741ng/mL. **Distribution:** V_d=632L/m²; plasma protein binding (89-98%). **Metabolism:** Liver via CYP2C8 to 6α-hydroxypaclitaxel (major metabolite) and CYP3A4 to 3'-*p*-hydroxypaclitaxel and 6α, 3'-*p*-dihydroxypaclitaxel (minor metabolites). **Elimination:** Urine (4% unchanged, <1% metabolites), feces (20%); $T_{1/2}$=27 hrs.

NURSING CONSIDERATIONS

Assessment: Assess for neutrophil count <1500 cells/mm³, previous hypersensitivity reaction to drug, hepatic impairment, pregnancy/nursing status, and possible drug interactions.

Monitoring: Monitor for bone marrow suppression, neutropenia, sensory neuropathy, hypersensitivity reactions, and other adverse reactions. Perform frequent peripheral blood cell counts.

Patient Counseling: Inform that drug may cause fetal harm; advise women of childbearing potential to avoid becoming pregnant. Advise men not to father a child while on therapy. Inform of the risk of low blood cell counts and instruct to contact physician immediately for fever or evidence of infection. Instruct to contact physician for persistent vomiting, diarrhea, signs of dehydration, cough or breathing difficulties, or signs of an allergic reaction. Inform that sensory neuropathy occurs frequently and advise to report to physician any numbness, tingling, pain or weakness involving the extremities. Inform that alopecia, fatigue/asthenia, and myalgia/arthralgia occur frequently with therapy.

Administration: IV route. Refer to PI for preparation and administration precautions and instructions. **Storage:** 20-25°C (68-77°F). Protect from bright light. Reconstituted Sus in the Vial: Use immediately or refrigerate at 2-8°C (36-46°F) for a max of 8 hrs if necessary. Protect from bright light. Reconstituted Sus in Infusion Bag: Use immediately or store at ambient temperature (approximately 25°C) and lighting conditions for up to 4 hrs.

ABSTRAL
fentanyl (Prostrakan)

CII

> Contains fentanyl with abuse liability similar to other opioid analgesics. Must be used only in opioid-tolerant patients. Serious adverse events, including deaths, reported in patients treated with other oral transmucosal fentanyl products. Substitution for any other fentanyl product may result in fatal overdose. Contraindicated for use in opioid non-tolerant patients and management of acute or postoperative pain. Life-threatening respiratory depression in opioid non-tolerant patients reported. Do not convert on a mcg-per-mcg basis from other fentanyl product to Abstral. Keep out of reach of children. Concomitant use with CYP3A4 inhibitors may increase fentanyl plasma concentrations, and may cause fatal respiratory depression. Use only by knowledgeable/skilled Schedule II opioid specialists. Available only through ABSTRAL REMS (Risk Evaluation and Mitigation Strategy) program.

THERAPEUTIC CLASS: Opioid analgesic

INDICATIONS: Management of breakthrough pain in cancer patients ≥18 yrs who are already receiving and are tolerant to around-the-clock opioid therapy for their underlying persistent cancer pain.

DOSAGE: *Adults:* Initial: 100mcg. Maint: If adequate analgesia is obtained within 30 min of 1st 100mcg, continue to treat subsequent episodes of breakthrough pain with this dose. If adequate analgesia not obtained after initiation, use 2nd dose (after 30 min) ud. No more than 2 doses may be used and wait at least 2 hrs before treating another episode of breakthrough pain. Titrate: If adequate analgesia not obtained with the 1st 100mcg dose, continue dose escalation in a stepwise manner over consecutive breakthrough episodes until adequate analgesia with tolerable side effects is achieved. Increase dose by 100mcg multiples up to 400mcg prn. If adequate analgesia not obtained with 400mcg dose, titrate to 600mcg. If adequate analgesia not obtained with a 600mcg dose, titrate to 800mcg. During titration, use multiples of 100mcg tabs and/or 200mcg tabs for any single dose. Do not use >4 tabs at one time. If adequate analgesia not obtained 30 min after use, may repeat the same dose. May use rescue medication ud if adequate analgesia not achieved. Refer to PI for information on dose readjustments and discontinuation of therapy.

HOW SUPPLIED: Tab, SL: 100mcg, 200mcg, 300mcg, 400mcg, 600mcg, 800mcg

CONTRAINDICATIONS: See Boxed Warning.

WARNINGS/PRECAUTIONS: May cause anaphylaxis and hypersensitivity reactions. Caution with chronic obstructive pulmonary disease (COPD) or preexisting medical conditions predisposing to respiratory depression. Extreme caution with evidence of increased intracranial pressure (ICP) or impaired consciousness. May obscure clinical course of head injuries. Caution with bradyarrhythmias. May impair mental and/or physical abilities. Caution with hepatic or renal dysfunction, and in the elderly.

ADVERSE REACTIONS: Respiratory depression, nausea, somnolence, dizziness, headache, constipation, stomatitis, dry mouth, dysgeusia, fatigue, dyspnea, hyperhidrosis.

INTERACTIONS: See Boxed Warning. Concomitant use with other CNS depressants, including other opioids, sedatives or hypnotics, general anesthetics, phenothiazines, tranquilizers, skeletal muscle relaxants, sedating antihistamines, and alcohol may produce increased depressant effects; adjust dose if warranted. May decrease levels and efficacy with CYP3A4 inducers (eg, barbiturates, carbamazepine, glucocorticoids). Withdrawal symptoms may be precipitated with opioid antagonists (eg, naloxone, nalmefene) or mixed agonist/antagonist analgesics (eg, pentazocine, butorphanol). Not recommended with or within 14 days of d/c of MAOIs.

PREGNANCY: Category C, not for use in nursing.

MECHANISM OF ACTION: Opioid analgesic: μ-opioid receptor agonist. Exact mechanism not established. Specific CNS opioid receptors for endogenous compounds have been identified throughout brain and spinal cord and play a role in analgesic effects.

PHARMACOKINETICS: Absorption: Absorbed through the oral mucosa. Administration of various doses led to different parameters. **Distribution:** V_d=4L/kg; plasma protein binding (80-85%). Readily crosses placenta; found in breast milk. **Metabolism:** Liver and intestinal mucosa via CYP3A4; norfentanyl (metabolite). **Elimination:** Urine (<7%, unchanged) (major), feces (1%, unchanged); $T_{1/2}$=5.02 hrs (100mcg), 6.67 hrs (200mcg), 13.5 hrs (400mcg), 10.1 hrs (800mcg).

NURSING CONSIDERATIONS

Assessment: Assess for degree of opioid tolerance, previous opioid dose, level/intensity/type of pain, general condition and medical status, and for conditions where treatment is contraindicated or cautioned. Assess for pregnancy/nursing status, renal/hepatic function, and possible drug interactions.

Monitoring: Monitor for signs/symptoms of respiratory and CNS depression, bradycardia, impairment of mental/physical abilities, abuse/addiction, and hypersensitivity reactions.

Patient Counseling: Inform to notify physician if signs/symptoms of respiratory depression develop. Counsel that therapy may be fatal in children, in individuals for whom it is not prescribed, and who are not opioid tolerant. Counsel on proper administration and disposal. Instruct not to take medication for acute or postoperative pain, pain from injuries, headache, migraine, or any other short-term pain. Instruct to use for the management of breakthrough cancer pain, only if already receiving and are tolerant to around-the-clock opioid therapy. Advise to take as prescribed and not to switch with another fentanyl product. Inform that medication has potential for abuse. Counsel that therapy may impair mental/physical abilities. Advise not to chew, suck, or swallow and not to eat or drink until tab is completely dissolved. In patients with dry mouth, instruct to moisten the buccal mucosa with water before taking the medication.

Administration: Sublingual route. **Storage:** 20-25°C (68-77°F); excursions permitted between 15-30°C (59-86°F). Protect from moisture.

ACANYA   RX
clindamycin phosphate - benzoyl peroxide (Coria Laboratories)

THERAPEUTIC CLASS: Antibacterial/keratolytic

INDICATIONS: Topical treatment of acne vulgaris in patients ≥12 yrs.

DOSAGE: *Adults:* Apply pea-sized amount to face qd.
Pediatrics: ≥12 yrs: Apply pea-sized amount to face qd.

HOW SUPPLIED: Gel: (Clindamycin Phosphate-Benzoyl Peroxide) 1.2%-2.5% [50g]

CONTRAINDICATIONS: History of regional enteritis, ulcerative colitis, or antibiotic-associated colitis.

WARNINGS/PRECAUTIONS: Diarrhea, bloody diarrhea, and colitis (including pseudomembranous colitis) reported; d/c if significant diarrhea occurs. Minimize sun exposure following application. Not for oral, ophthalmic, or intravaginal use. Use for >12 weeks has not been evaluated.

ADVERSE REACTIONS: Erythema, scaling, itching, burning, stinging.

INTERACTIONS: Avoid with topical or oral erythromycin-containing products. Caution with topical acne therapy (eg, peeling, desquamating, or abrasive agents) due to potential cumulative irritancy effects. Caution with other neuromuscular blocking agents. Antiperistaltic agents (eg, opiates, diphenoxylate with atropine) may prolong and/or worsen severe colitis.

PREGNANCY: Category C, not for use in nursing.

MECHANISM OF ACTION: Clindamycin phosphate: Antibacterial; binds to 50S ribosomal subunits of susceptible bacteria and prevents elongation of peptide chains, thereby suppressing bacterial protein synthesis. Benzoyl peroxide: Oxidizing agent; bacteriocidal and keratolytic effects.

NURSING CONSIDERATIONS

Assessment: Assess for history of regional enteritis, ulcerative colitis, or antibiotic-associated colitis, diarrhea, pregnancy/nursing status, and possible drug interactions.

Monitoring: Monitor for erythema, scaling, itching, burning, stinging, allergic reactions, diarrhea, bloody diarrhea, and colitis.

Patient Counseling: Instruct to apply medication as directed and avoid other topical acne products unless directed by physician. Avoid washing of face >2-3x a day and direct contact with mouth, eyes, inside the nose, and all mucous membranes, cuts or open wounds. Instruct to wash hands with soap and water after application. Advise to notify physician if any signs/symptoms of local skin irritation develop. Counsel to minimize exposure to natural and avoid artificial sunlight. Inform that medication may bleach hair or colored fabric. Advise to d/c and notify physician if severe diarrhea, GI discomfort, or allergic reaction occurs. Instruct to keep out of reach of children.

Administration: Topical route. Wash gently with mild soap and pat dry affected areas prior to application. Refer to PI for administration instructions. **Storage:** Prior to Dispensing: 2-8°C (36-46°F). After Dispensing: 25°C (77°F). Do not freeze. Keep container tightly closed.

ACCOLATE
zafirlukast (AstraZeneca)

RX

THERAPEUTIC CLASS: Leukotriene receptor antagonist

INDICATIONS: Prophylaxis and chronic treatment of asthma in patients ≥5 yrs.

DOSAGE: *Adults:* 20mg bid. Take ≥1 hr ac or 2 hrs pc.
Pediatrics: ≥12 yrs: 20mg bid. 5-11 yrs: 10mg bid. Take ≥1 hr ac or 2 hrs pc.

HOW SUPPLIED: Tab: 10mg, 20mg

CONTRAINDICATIONS: Hepatic impairment, including hepatic cirrhosis.

WARNINGS/PRECAUTIONS: Life-threatening hepatic failure reported. Monitor for signs and symptoms of liver dysfunction (eg, right upper quadrant abdominal pain, nausea, fatigue, lethargy, pruritus, jaundice, flu-like symptoms, anorexia, enlarged liver); d/c if liver dysfunction suspected. Monitor LFTs (particularly serum ALT) periodically or if hepatic dysfunction is suspected. Not for reversal of bronchospasm in acute asthma attacks including status asthmaticus. May continue therapy during acute exacerbations of asthma. Systemic eosinophilia, eosinophilic pneumonia, and vasculitis consistent with Churg-Strauss syndrome reported rarely. Neuropsychiatric events (eg, insomnia and depression) reported; carefully evaluate risks and benefits of continuing therapy if such events occur.

ADVERSE REACTIONS: Headache, infection, nausea.

INTERACTIONS: Coadministration with warfarin increases PT time; monitor PT time closely and adjust anticoagulant dose accordingly. Caution with drugs metabolized by CYP2C9 (eg, tolbutamide, phenytoin, carbamazepine). Monitor when coadministered with drugs metabolized by CYP3A4 (eg, dihydropyridine calcium channel blockers, cyclosporine, cisapride). Increased levels with aspirin. Decreased levels with erythromycin and theophylline. May increase theophylline levels. Infections reported were associated with coadministration of inhaled corticosteroids.

PREGNANCY: Category B, not for use in nursing.

MECHANISM OF ACTION: Leukotriene receptor antagonist; selective and competitive receptor antagonist of leukotriene D_4 and E_4, components of slow-reacting substance of anaphylaxis; inhibits bronchoconstriction.

PHARMACOKINETICS: Absorption: Rapid. (Adult) C_{max}=326ng/mL; T_{max}=2 hrs; AUC=1137ng•h/mL. (7-11 yrs) C_{max}=601ng/mL; T_{max}=2.5 hrs; AUC=2027ng•h/mL. (5-6 yrs) C_{max}=756ng/mL; T_{max}=2.1 hrs; AUC=2458ng•h/mL. **Distribution:** V_d= 70L; plasma protein binding (>99%). Found in breast milk. **Metabolism:** Liver, hydroxylation via CYP2C9. **Elimination:** Urine (10%); feces. (Adult) $T_{1/2}$=13.3 hrs.

NURSING CONSIDERATIONS

Assessment: Assess for patient's age, hepatic impairment, hepatic cirrhosis, bronchospasm and acute asthma attacks, drug hypersensitivity, pregnancy/nursing status, and for possible drug interactions. Obtain baseline LFTs.

Monitoring: Monitor for signs/symptoms of liver dysfunction, systemic eosinophilia, eosinophilic pneumonia, vasculitic rash, worsening pulmonary symptoms, cardiac complications, neuropathy, and for neuropsychiatric events. Monitor LFTs periodically.

Patient Counseling: Inform that hepatic dysfunction may occur; seek medical attention if symptoms of hepatic dysfunction (eg, right upper quadrant abdominal pain, nausea, fatigue, lethargy, pruritus, jaundice, flu-like symptoms, anorexia) occur. Advise to take regularly as prescribed, even during symptom-free periods. Inform that it is not a bronchodilator and should not be used to treat acute episodes of asthma. Instruct not to decrease dose or stop taking other anti-asthma medications unless instructed by a physician. Instruct to notify physician if neuropsychiatric events occur. Instruct not to take the medication if breastfeeding; consider alternative anti-asthma medication. Instruct to take drug ≥1 hr ac or 2 hrs pc.

Administration: Oral route. **Storage:** 20-25°C (68-77°F). Protect from light and moisture.

ACCRETROPIN   RX
somatropin (Cangene)

THERAPEUTIC CLASS: Recombinant human growth hormone

INDICATIONS: Treatment of pediatric patients who have growth failure due to inadequate secretion of normal endogenous growth hormone. Treatment of short stature associated with Turner syndrome (TS) in patients whose epiphyses are not closed.

DOSAGE: *Pediatrics:* Individualize dose. Divide into equal daily doses given 6 or 7X/week SQ. Growth Hormone Deficiency: 0.18mg/kg body weight/week to 0.3 mg/kg (0.90 IU/kg) body weight/week. TS: 0.36mg/kg body weight/week.

HOW SUPPLIED: Inj: 5mg/mL (15 IU/mL)

CONTRAINDICATIONS: Closed epiphyses; proliferative or preproliferative diabetic retinopathy; active malignancy (eg, pituitary tumor, progression or recurrence of an underlying intracranial tumor); acute critical illness due to complications following open heart surgery, abdominal surgery, or multiple accidental trauma, or acute respiratory failure; patients with Prader-Willi syndrome (PWS) who are severely obese or have severe respiratory impairment.

WARNINGS/PRECAUTIONS: Increased mortality reported with acute critical illness due to complications following open heart or abdominal surgery, multiple accidental trauma, or with acute respiratory failure; weigh benefits vs risks of continuing therapy in patients who develop acute critical illnesses. Fatalities reported in children with PWS who had severe obesity, history of upper airway obstruction or sleep apnea, or unidentified respiratory tract infection; interrupt treatment if signs develop. Monitor for signs of respiratory infection and weight control with PWS. Not indicated for long-term treatment of growth failure due to genetically confirmed PWS. May decrease insulin sensitivity which may unmask undiagnosed impaired glucose tolerance and overt diabetes mellitus (DM); monitor glucose levels. Monitor for progression or recurrence of underlying disease process in patients with pre-existing tumors or growth hormone deficiency secondary to an intracranial lesion. Intracranial HTN with papilledema, visual changes, headache, N/V reported; perform funduscopic exam before and periodically during treatment; d/c if papilledema occurs. Monitor standard hormonal replacement therapy in patients with hypopituitarism (multiple hormone deficiencies). Undiagnosed/untreated hypothyroidism may prevent optimal response; perform periodic thyroid function tests. Monitor for any malignant transformation of skin lesions. Tissue atrophy may occur if administered at same site over long period; rotate injection site. Slipped capital femoral epiphyses may occur; evaluate carefully with the onset of a limp or complaints of hip or knee pain. Monitor for scoliosis progression. Increased risk of otitis media or other ear disorders in patients with TS. Monitor for cardiovascular (CV) disorders in patients with TS. Allergic reactions may occur.

ADVERSE REACTIONS: Injection site reactions (eg, bruising, erythema, hemorrhage, edema, pain, pruritus, rash, swelling), nausea, headache, fatigue, scoliosis.

INTERACTIONS: May impact cortisol and cortisone metabolism; glucocorticoid replacement therapy may be required for previously undiagnosed, unmasked central (secondary) hypoadrenalism. Use of glucocorticoid replacement therapy for previously diagnosed hypoadrenalism, especially cortisone acetate or prednisone, may require an increase in maintenance or stress doses. Excessive glucocorticoid therapy may attenuate growth- promoting effects; adjust dosage carefully. May alter clearance of compounds metabolized by CYP450 (eg, corticosteroids, sex steroids, anticonvulsants, cyclosporine). May require dosage adjustment of insulin and/or oral hypoglycemic agents. Thyroid replacement therapy may require dosage adjustment.

PREGNANCY: Category C, caution in nursing.

MECHANISM OF ACTION: Human growth hormone; stimulates linear growth in pediatrics. Also demonstrated to stimulate skeletal growth in children, increase the size and number of skeletal muscle cells, increase cellular protein synthesis, modulate carbohydrate metabolism, mobilize lipids, reduce body fat stores, increase plasma fatty acids, and cause Na^+, K^+, and phosphorus retention.

PHARMACOKINETICS: Absorption: Absolute bioavailability (70%), $AUC_{(0-t)}$=238.09ng•h/mL, $AUC_{(0-inf)}$=255.31ng•h/mL, C_{max}=29.49ng/mL, T_{max}=3.5 hrs. **Metabolism:** Liver, kidneys. **Excretion:** $T_{1/2}$=3.63 hrs.

NURSING CONSIDERATIONS

Assessment: Assess for other causes of poor growth (eg, under-nutrition, advanced bone age, hypothyroidism), closed epiphyses, proliferative or preproliferative diabetic retinopathy, active malignancy, DM or impaired glucose tolerance, pregnancy/nursing status, and for possible drug interactions. Assess for pre-existing papilledema by performing funduscopic examination. In patients with TS, assess for presence of otitis media or other ear disorders and for CV disorders.

Monitoring: Monitor for growth/clinical response, malignant transformation of skin lesions, symptoms of slipped capital femoral epiphysis, progression of pre-existing scoliosis, tissue atrophy at the injection site, and for allergic reactions. Monitor glucose levels. Perform thyroid function test and funduscopic examination periodically. In patients with TS, monitor for signs/symptoms of ear disorders (eg, otitis media) and CV disorders. In patients with hypopituitarism (multiple hormone deficiencies), monitor standard hormonal therapy. In patients with PWS, monitor weight and for signs/symptoms of upper airway obstruction or apnea and for respiratory infections. In patients with pre-existing tumors or GH deficiency secondary to an intracranial lesion, monitor for progression or recurrence of underlying disease process.

Patient Counseling: Inform of the potential benefits/risks of therapy. Instruct on proper administration. Advise to seek medical attention if symptoms of an allergic reaction, slipped capital femoral epiphysis (eg, onset of limp, hip or knee pain), or any other adverse reaction occurs.

Administration: SQ route. Do not inject IV. Rotate injection site. Refer to PI for further administration instructions. **Storage:** Unopened Vial: 2-8°C (36-46°F). Avoid freezing and shaking. Opened Vial: 2-8°C (36-46°F); stable up to 14 days. Discard 14 days after first use. Protect from light.

AccuNeb
albuterol sulfate (Dey)

RX

THERAPEUTIC CLASS: Beta$_2$-agonist

INDICATIONS: Relief of bronchospasm in patients 2-12 yrs with asthma (reversible obstructive airway disease).

DOSAGE: *Pediatrics:* 2-12 yrs: Initial: 0.63mg or 1.25mg tid-qid PRN via nebulizer over 5-15 min. Patients 6-12 yrs with more severe asthma (baseline FEV$_1$ <60% predicted), weight >40kg, or patients 11-12 yrs old may achieve better initial response with 1.25mg dose.

HOW SUPPLIED: Sol, Inhalation: 1.25mg/3mL, 0.63mg/3mL

WARNINGS/PRECAUTIONS: Can produce paradoxical bronchospasm; d/c if occurs. Consider adding anti-inflammatory agents (eg, corticosteroids) to adequately control asthma. Re-evaluate patient and treatment regimen if deterioration of asthma observed. Can produce clinically significant cardiovascular (CV) effect (eg, ECG changes); caution with CV disorders (eg, coronary insufficiency, cardiac arrhythmias, HTN). Immediate hypersensitivity reactions reported. Aggravation of pre-existing diabetes mellitus (DM) and ketoacidosis reported with large doses of IV albuterol. May cause hypokalemia. Has not been studied with acute attacks of bronchospasm.

ADVERSE REACTIONS: Asthma exacerbation, otitis media, allergic reaction, gastroenteritis, cold symptoms.

INTERACTIONS: Avoid other short-acting sympathomimetic aerosol bronchodilators and epinephrine. Extreme caution with MAOIs or TCAs, or within 2 weeks of d/c of such agents; action of albuterol may be potentiated. May decrease serum levels of digoxin; monitor levels. May worsen ECG changes and/or hypokalemia caused by non-K$^+$ sparing diuretics (eg, loop/thiazide); caution is advised. Pulmonary effect blocked by β-blockers; caution with cardioselective β-blockers.

PREGNANCY: Category C, not for use in nursing.

MECHANISM OF ACTION: β2-adrenergic agonist; stimulates intracellular adenyl cyclase, which catalyzes conversion of ATP to cAMP to produce relaxation of bronchial smooth muscle.

PHARMACOKINETICS: Absorption: Bioavailability (<20%); (Inh) C$_{max}$=2.1ng/mL, T$_{max}$=0.5 hrs. **Elimination:** Urine; (PO) T$_{1/2}$=5-6 hrs.

NURSING CONSIDERATIONS

Assessment: Assess for previous hypersensitivity to the drug, CV disorders, HTN, DM, pregnancy/nursing status, and possible drug interactions.

Monitoring: Monitor for signs/symptoms of CV effects (measured by pulse rate and BP), worsening of symptoms, paradoxical bronchospasm, deterioration of asthma, hypokalemia, and hypersensitivity reactions.

Patient Counseling: Instruct not to use more frequently than recommended. Advise not to increase dose or frequency without consulting physician. Counsel to seek medical attention if symptoms worsen, if therapy becomes less effective, or if there is need to use the drug more frequently than usual. Inform of the common effects (eg, palpitations, chest pain, rapid HR, tremor, nervousness). Advise not to use if the vial changes color or becomes cloudy. Inform that drug compatibility, clinical efficacy, and safety, when mixed with other drugs in nebulizer, have not been established.

Administration: Inhalation route. Refer to PI for proper administration. **Storage:** 2-25°C (36-77°F). Protect from light and excessive heat. Store in protective foil pouch at all times. Once removed, use within 1 week. Discard if solution not colorless.

ACCUPRIL

RX

quinapril HCl (Parke-Davis)

> D/C if pregnancy is detected. Drugs that act directly on the renin-angiotensin system can cause injury/death to the developing fetus.

THERAPEUTIC CLASS: ACE inhibitor

INDICATIONS: Treatment of HTN alone or in combination with thiazide diuretics. Management of heart failure (HF) as adjunctive therapy when added to conventional therapy including diuretics and/or digitalis.

DOSAGE: *Adults:* HTN: If possible, d/c diuretic 2-3 days prior to therapy. Initial: 10mg or 20mg qd; 5mg qd if with concomitant diuretic with careful monitoring until BP is stabilized. Titrate: May adjust dosage based on BP response at intervals of at least 2 weeks. Usual: 20mg, 40mg, or 80mg/day, given as single dose or in 2 equally divided doses. Max Initial for HTN with Renal Impairment: CrCl >60mL/min: 10mg/day. CrCl 30-60mL/min: 5mg/day. CrCl 10-30mL/min: 2.5mg/day. Elderly: Initial: 10mg qd. Titrate: Adjust to the optimal response. HF: Initial: 5mg bid. Titrate: Adjust weekly until effective dose achieved or hypotension/orthostasis/azotemia prohibits further adjustment. Usual: 20-40mg/day given in 2 equally divided doses. Initial for HF with Renal Impairment: CrCl >30mL/min: 5mg/day. CrCl 10-30mL/min: 2.5mg/day. Give bid in succeeding days if well tolerated. Titrate: Increase dose at weekly intervals based on clinical and hemodynamic response if without excessive hypotension or significant renal deterioration. Elderly: Start at low end of dosing range.

HOW SUPPLIED: Tab: 5mg*, 10mg, 20mg, 40mg *scored

CONTRAINDICATIONS: History of ACE inhibitor-associated angioedema.

WARNINGS/PRECAUTIONS: Less effect on BP and more reports of angioedema in blacks than nonblacks. Angioedema of face, extremities, lips, tongue, glottis, and larynx reported; d/c and administer appropriate therapy if laryngeal stridor or angioedema of the face, tongue, or glottis occurs. Intestinal angioedema reported; monitor for abdominal pain. Patients with history of angioedema unrelated to ACE inhibitor therapy may be at increased risk of angioedema during therapy. Anaphylactoid reactions reported during desensitization with hymenoptera venom, dialysis with high-flux membranes, and LDL apheresis with dextran sulfate absorption. Associated with syndrome that starts with cholestatic jaundice and progresses to fulminant hepatic necrosis, and sometimes death; d/c if jaundice or marked hepatic enzyme elevation occurs. Excessive hypotension sometimes associated with oliguria, azotemia, and rarely acute renal failure, and/or death may occur. Risk factors for excessive hypotension include HF, hyponatremia, high dose diuretic therapy, recent intensive diuresis, dialysis, or severe volume and/or salt depletion; eliminate or reduce the diuretic or cautiously increase salt intake (except with HF) prior to therapy and monitor closely. May cause agranulocytosis and bone marrow depression. May cause renal function changes. May increase BUN and SrCr levels with renal artery stenosis and without renal vascular disease. Risk of hyperkalemia with diabetes mellitus (DM) and renal dysfunction. Persistent nonproductive cough reported. Hypotension may occur with surgery or during anesthesia. Caution in elderly.

ADVERSE REACTIONS: Headache, dizziness, cough.

INTERACTIONS: Hypotension risk and increased BUN and SrCr with diuretics. Coadministration with NSAIDs, including selective cyclooxygenase-2 inhibitors, may decrease antihypertensive effect of ACE inhibitors and may further deteriorate renal function. Decreases tetracycline absorption (possibly due to magnesium content in quinapril); consider interaction with drugs that interact with magnesium. Increased risk of hyperkalemia with K^+-sparing diuretics (eg, spironolactone, amiloride, triamterene), K^+ supplements, or K^+-containing salt substitutes; use caution and monitor serum K^+. May increase lithium levels and risk of toxicity; use caution and monitor serum lithium levels. Nitritoid reactions reported rarely with injectable gold (eg, sodium aurothiomalate).

PREGNANCY: Category D, caution in nursing.

MECHANISM OF ACTION: ACE inhibitor; decreases plasma angiotensin II, which leads to decreased vasopressor activity and decreased aldosterone secretion.

PHARMACOKINETICS: Absorption: T_{max}=1 hr, 2 hrs (quinaprilat). Extent of absorption diminished approximately 25-30% with high-fat meal. **Distribution:** Plasma protein binding (97%); crosses placenta; found in breast milk. **Metabolism:** De-esterification. Quinaprilat (active metabolite). **Elimination:** (IV) Renal (≤96% quinaprilat); $T_{1/2}$=2 hrs.

NURSING CONSIDERATIONS

Assessment: Assess for history of angioedema, hypersensitivity, volume/salt depletion, collagen vascular disease, DM, renal artery stenosis, ischemic heart disease, cerebrovascular disease, renal function, pregnancy/nursing status, and possible drug interactions.

Monitoring: Monitor for signs/symptoms of hypotension, anaphylactoid or hypersensitivity reactions, head/neck and intestinal angioedema, agranulocytosis, neutropenia, bone marrow depression, cholestatic jaundice, fulminant hepatic necrosis, hyperkalemia, and renal dysfunction. Monitor BP, renal function (BUN, SrCr), and WBC periodically in patients with collagen vascular disease and/or renal disease.

Patient Counseling: Inform of pregnancy risks and to notify physician if pregnant/plan to become pregnant as soon as possible. Instruct to d/c therapy and immediately report signs/symptoms of angioedema (eg, swelling of face, extremities, eyes, lips, tongue, difficulty swallowing/breathing). Caution about lightheadedness, especially during the 1st few days of therapy and advise to report to physician. Instruct to d/c and consult physician if syncope occurs. Caution that inadequate fluid intake or excessive perspiration, diarrhea, or vomiting may lead to an excessive fall in BP resulting in lightheadedness or syncope. Instruct to inform physician about therapy if plan to undergo surgery/anesthesia. Instruct to avoid K⁺ supplements or salt substitutes containing K⁺ without consulting physician. Advise to report if symptoms of infection (eg, sore throat, fever) develop.

Administration: Oral route. **Storage:** 15-30°C (59-86°F). Protect from light.

ACCURETIC   RX
quinapril HCl - hydrochlorothiazide (Parke-Davis)

> D/C if pregnancy is detected. Drugs that act directly on the renin-angiotensin system can cause injury/death to the developing fetus.

THERAPEUTIC CLASS: ACE inhibitor/thiazide diuretic

INDICATIONS: Treatment of HTN.

DOSAGE: *Adults:* Use only after failure to achieve desired effect with monotherapy. Not Controlled with Quinapril Monotherapy: Initial: 10mg-12.5mg or 20mg-12.5mg tab qd. Titrate: May increase dose based on clinical response. May increase HCTZ after 2-3 wks. Controlled with HCTZ 25mg/day with Hypokalemia: 10mg-12.5mg or 20mg-12.5mg qd. Replacement Therapy: Adequately treated with 20mg quinapril and 25mg HCTZ without significant electrolye disturbances may switch to 20mg-25mg tab qd. Elderly: Start at low end of dosing range.

HOW SUPPLIED: Tab: (Quinapril-HCTZ) 10mg-12.5mg*, 20mg-12.5mg*, 20mg-25mg *scored

CONTRAINDICATIONS: Anuria, hypersensitivity to other sulfonamide-derived drugs, history of ACE inhibitor-associated angioedema.

WARNINGS/PRECAUTIONS: Not for initial therapy. Caution in elderly. Avoid if CrCl ≤30mL/min. Quinapril: Less effect on BP and more reports of angioedema in blacks than nonblacks. Angioedema of the face, extremities, lips, tongue, glottis, and larynx reported; d/c and administer appropriate therapy. Intestinal angioedema reported; monitor for abdominal pain. Patients with history of angioedema unrelated to ACE inhibitor therapy may be at increased risk of angioedema during therapy. Anaphylactoid reactions reported during desensitization with hymenoptera venom, dialysis with high-flux membranes, and LDL apheresis with dextran sulfate absorption. Associated with syndrome that starts with cholestatic jaundice and progresses to fulminant hepatic necrosis, and sometimes death; d/c if jaundice or marked hepatic enzyme elevation occurs. Symptomatic hypotension sometimes associated with oliguria, azotemia, and rarely acute renal failure, and/or death may occur. Risk factors for symptomatic hypotension include heart failure (HF), hyponatremia, high dose diuretic therapy, recent intensive diuresis, dialysis, or severe volume and/or salt depletion; correct volume/salt depletion prior to therapy and monitor closely. May cause renal function changes. May increase BUN and SrCr levels with renal artery stenosis and without renal vascular disease. May cause agranulocytosis and bone marrow depression. Risk of hyperkalemia with diabetes mellitus (DM) and renal dysfunction. Persistent nonproductive cough reported. Hypotension may occur with surgery or during anesthesia. HCTZ: May precipitate azotemia with renal disease. Caution with liver dysfunction; may precipitate hepatic coma. May exacerbate/activate systemic lupus erythematosus (SLE). May cause idiosyncratic reaction, resulting in acute transient myopia and acute angle-closure glaucoma; d/c rapidly. May increase cholesterol, TG, uric acid levels, and decrease glucose tolerance. Fluid/electrolyte imbalance (hyponatremia, hypokalemia, hypochloremic alkalosis), hypomagnesemia may occur. Dilutional hyponatremia may occur in edematous patients during hot weather; appropriate therapy of water restriction rather than salt administration should be instituted except for life-threatening hyponatremia. Altered parathyroid glands, with hypercalcemia and hypophosphatemia, seen with prolonged therapy. Enhanced effects with postsympathectomy patients.

ADVERSE REACTIONS: Headache, dizziness, cough, increases in SrCr and BUN levels.

INTERACTIONS: Quinapril: Decreases tetracycline absorption (possibly due to magnesium content in quinapril); consider interaction with drugs that interact with magnesium. Increased risk of hyperkalemia with K⁺-sparing diuretics (eg, spironolactone, amiloride, triamterene), K⁺ supplements, or K⁺-containing salt substitutes; use caution and monitor serum K⁺. May increase lithium levels and risk of toxicity; use caution and monitor serum lithium levels. Nitritoid reactions reported rarely with injectable gold (eg, sodium aurothiomalate). Coadministration with NSAIDs, including selective cyclooxygenase-2 inhibitors, may decrease antihypertensive effect of ACE inhibitors and may further deteriorate renal function. HCTZ: May potentiate orthostatic hypotension with alcohol, barbiturates, and narcotics. May need to adjust dose of antidiabetic drugs. Impaired absorption with cholestyramine, colestipol. Corticosteroids and adrenocorticotropic hormone intensify electrolyte depletion. May decrease response to pressor amines. May potentiate action of other antihypertensives, especially ganglionic or peripheral adrenergic-blocking drugs. May increase responsiveness to nondepolarizing skeletal muscle relaxants (eg, tubocurarine). Hypokalemia may sensitize or exaggerate the response of the heart to toxic effects of digitalis.

PREGNANCY: Category D, caution in nursing.

MECHANISM OF ACTION: Quinapril: ACE inhibitor; decreases plasma angiotensin II, which leads to decreased vasopressor activity and decreased aldosterone secretion. HCTZ: Thiazide diuretic; affects renal tubular mechanism of electrolyte reabsorption directly increasing excretion of Na^+ and Cl^-, and indirectly reducing plasma volume.

PHARMACOKINETICS: Absorption: Quinapril: T_{max}=1 hr, 2 hrs (quinaprilat). **Distribution:** Quinapril: Plasma protein binding (97%); crosses placenta; found in breast milk. HCTZ: V_d=3.6-7.8L/kg; plasma protein binding (67.9%); crosses placenta; found in breast milk. **Metabolism:** Quinapril: Deesterification. Quinaprilat (metabolite). **Elimination:** Quinapril: (IV) Renal (≤96% quinaprilat); $T_{1/2}$=2 hrs. HCTZ: Kidney (≥61% unchanged); $T_{1/2}$=4-15 hrs.

NURSING CONSIDERATIONS

Assessment: Assess for anuria, history of angioedema, volume/salt depletion, HF, SLE, and any other conditions where treatment is contraindicated or cautioned. Assess for hypersensitivity to drug or sulfonamides, renal/hepatic function, electrolyte levels, pregnancy/nursing status, and possible drug interactions.

Monitoring: Monitor for angioedema, agranulocytosis, hyperkalemia, anaphylactoid reactions, hypotension, jaundice, sensitivity reactions, SLE, gout, idiosyncratic reaction, myopia, and angle-closure glaucoma. Periodically monitor WBCs in patients with collagen vascular disease and/or renal disease. Monitor serum electrolytes, BP, LFTs, renal function (BUN, SrCr), uric acid levels, and cholesterol/TG levels.

Patient Counseling: Inform of pregnancy risks; notify physician if pregnant/plan to become pregnant as soon as possible. Instruct to d/c therapy and immediately report signs/symptoms of angioedema (eg, swelling of face, eyes, lips, tongue, difficulty breathing). Caution about light-headedness, especially during the 1st days of therapy and advise to report to physician. Instruct to d/c and consult physician if syncope occurs. Caution that inadequate fluid intake or excessive perspiration, diarrhea, or vomiting may lead to an excessive fall in BP resulting in lightheadedness or syncope. Advise to inform physician about therapy if plan to undergo surgery/anesthesia. Instruct to avoid K^+ supplements or salt substitutes containing K^+ without consulting physician. Advise to report if symptoms of infection (eg, sore throat, fever) develop.

Administration: Oral route. **Storage:** 20-25°C (68-77°F).

ACEON

RX

perindopril erbumine (Abbott)

ACE inhibitors can cause death/injury to developing fetus. D/C if pregnancy detected.

THERAPEUTIC CLASS: ACE inhibitor

INDICATIONS: Treatment of essential HTN alone or with other antihypertensives (eg, thiazide diuretics). Treatment of stable coronary artery disease (CAD) to reduce risk of cardiovascular mortality or nonfatal myocardial infarction (MI); may be used with conventional treatment for CAD (eg, antiplatelet, antihypertensive, or lipid-lowering therapy).

DOSAGE: *Adults:* HTN: Initial: 4mg qd. May be titrated PRN to max of 16mg qd. Maint: 4-8mg/day given qd or bid. Elderly: Initial: 4mg/day given qd or bid. Monitor BP and titrate carefully with doses >8mg. Use With Diuretics: Reduce diuretic dose prior to start of treatment. Stable CAD: Initial: 4mg qd for 2 weeks. Maint: 8mg qd if tolerated. Elderly (>70 yrs): Initial: 2mg qd in the 1st week, followed by 4mg qd in the 2nd week. Maint: 8mg qd if tolerated. Renal Impairment: CrCl ≥30mL/min: Initial: 2mg/day. Max: 8mg/day.

HOW SUPPLIED: Tab: 2mg*, 4mg*, 8mg* *scored

CONTRAINDICATIONS: Hereditary or idiopathic angioedema.

WARNINGS/PRECAUTIONS: Not recommended with CrCl <30mL/min. Anaphylactoid reactions and angioedema of the face, extremities, lips, tongue, glottis, or larynx reported; d/c and administer appropriate therapy. Intestinal angioedema reported; monitor for abdominal pain.

Symptomatic hypotension may occur and is most likely with volume/salt depletion. Closely monitor patients at risk for excessive hypotension. May cause agranulocytosis and bone marrow depression, most frequently in renal impairment, especially with collagen vascular disease (eg, systemic lupus erythematosus [SLE] or scleroderma). May cause changes in renal function. Oliguria, progressive azotemia, and rarely, acute renal failure and death may occur with severe congestive heart failure (CHF). May increase BUN and SrCr with renal artery stenosis. May cause hyperkalemia; risk factors include renal insufficiency and diabetes mellitus (DM). Persistent nonproductive cough reported. Rarely, a syndrome of cholestatic jaundice, fulminant necrosis and sometimes death occurs; d/c if jaundice or marked elevations of hepatic enzymes develop. Hypotension may occur with major surgery or during anesthesia.

ADVERSE REACTIONS: Cough, headache, asthenia, dizziness, hypotension, back pain.

INTERACTIONS: Hypotension risk and reduced perindoprilat bioavailability with diuretics. May increase risk of hyperkalemia with K^+-sparing diuretics (eg, spironolactone, amiloride, triamterene), drugs that increase serum K^+ (eg, indomethacin, heparin, cyclosporine), K^+ supplements and/or K^+-containing salt substitutes. May increase lithium levels with lithium toxicity risk; monitor lithium levels. Nitritoid reactions reported with injectable gold (sodium aurothiomalate). Caution with digoxin. May result in deterioration of renal function with NSAIDs including selective cyclooxygenase-2 inhibitors. NSAIDs may also attenuate antihypertensive effect.

PREGNANCY: Category D, caution in nursing.

MECHANISM OF ACTION: ACE inhibitor; inhibits ACE activity resulting in decreased plasma angiotensin II, leading to decreased vasoconstriction, increased plasma renin activity, and decreased aldosterone secretion.

PHARMACOKINETICS: Absorption: Absolute bioavailability (75%, 25% perindoprilat); T_{max}=1 hr, 3-7 hrs (perindoprilat). **Distribution:** Plasma protein binding (60%, 10-20% perindoprilat); crosses placenta. **Metabolism:** Hepatic (extensive); hydrolysis, glucuronidation, cyclization via dehydration. Perindoprilat (active metabolite). **Elimination:** Urine (4-12%, unchanged); $T_{1/2}$=0.8-1 hr, 3-10 hrs (perindoprilat).

NURSING CONSIDERATIONS

Assessment: Assess for hereditary or idiopathic angioedema, volume and/or salt depletion, CHF, renal artery stenosis, ischemic heart disease, cerebrovascular disease, hepatic/renal impairment, DM, collagen vascular disease (eg, SLE), previous hypersensitivity to the drug, pregnancy/nursing status, and possible drug interactions. Obtain baseline BP, BUN, and SrCr.

Monitoring: Monitor for signs/symptoms of anaphylactoid reactions, head/neck/intestinal angioedema, hypotension, agranulocytosis, bone marrow depression, cholestatic jaundice, fulminant hepatic necrosis, hepatic failure, hyperkalemia, persistent nonproductive cough, hypersensitivity reactions, and neutropenia. Monitor hepatic/renal function, BP, BUN, SrCr, and K^+ levels.

Patient Counseling: Inform of potential risks if used during pregnancy. Instruct to d/c and immediately report to physician if any signs/symptoms of angioedema (eg, swelling of the face, extremities, eyes, lips, tongue, hoarseness or difficulty swallowing or breathing) develop. Counsel to report any signs of infection (eg, sore throat, fever) which could be a sign of neutropenia.

Administration: Oral route. **Storage:** 20-25°C (68-77°F). Protect from moisture.

ACETADOTE   RX
acetylcysteine (Cumberland)

THERAPEUTIC CLASS: Acetaminophen antidote

INDICATIONS: Prevent or lessen hepatic injury within 8-10 hrs after ingestion of potentially hepatotoxic dose of acetaminophen (APAP).

DOSAGE: *Adults:* Total Dose: 300mg/kg over 21 hrs. ≥40kg: LD: 150mg/kg IV in 200mL of diluent over 60 min. Second Dose: 50mg/kg in 500mL of diluent over 4 hrs. Third Dose: 100mg/kg in 1000mL of diluent over 16 hrs. >20kg-<40kg: LD: 150mg/kg IV in 100mL of diluent over 60 min. Second Dose: 50mg/kg in 250mL of diluent over 4 hrs. Third Dose: 100mg/kg in 500mL of diluent over 16 hrs. ≤20kg: LD: 150mg/kg IV in 3mL/kg of body weight of diluent over 60 min. Second Dose: 50mg/kg in 7mL/kg of body weight of diluent over 4 hrs. Third Dose: 100mg/kg in 14mL/kg of body weight of diluent over 16 hrs.
Pediatrics: <16 yrs: Total Dose: 300mg/kg over 21 hrs. ≥40kg: LD: 150mg/kg IV in 200mL of diluent over 60 min. Second Dose: 50mg/kg in 500mL of diluent over 4 hrs. Third Dose: 100mg/kg in 1000mL of diluent over 16 hrs. >20kg-<40kg: LD: 150mg/kg IV in 100mL of diluent over 60 min. Second Dose: 50mg/kg in 250mL of diluent over 4 hrs. Third Dose: 100mg/kg in 500mL of diluent over 16 hrs. ≤20kg: LD: 150mg/kg IV in 3mL/kg of body weight of diluent over 60 min. Second Dose: 50mg/kg in 7mL/kg of body weight of diluent over 4 hrs. Third Dose: 100mg/kg in 14mL/kg of body weight of diluent over 16 hrs.

HOW SUPPLIED: Inj: 200mg/mL [30mL]

WARNINGS/PRECAUTIONS: Serious anaphylactoid reactions (eg, rash, hypotension, wheezing, and SOB) reported; interrupt and carefully restart therapy if occur; d/c and consider alternative management if anaphylactoid reaction returns upon reinitiation or increases in severity. Acute flushing and erythema of skin may occur. Caution with asthma or history of bronchospasm. Adjust total volume administered in patients <40kg and for those requiring fluid restriction to avoid fluid overload. May increase plasma levels with hepatic cirrhosis.

ADVERSE REACTIONS: Anaphylactoid reactions, rash, urticaria, pruritus, N/V, tachycardia, facial flushing.

PREGNANCY: Category B, caution in nursing.

MECHANISM OF ACTION: Acetaminophen antidote; protects liver by maintaining or restoring glutathione levels. Also acts as an alternate substrate for conjugation with, and thus detoxification of, the reactive metabolite.

PHARMACOKINETICS: Distribution: V_d=0.47L/kg; plasma protein binding (83%); crosses the placenta. **Metabolism:** May form cysteine, disulfides and conjugates. **Elimination:** $T_{1/2}$=5.6 hrs (adults), 11 hrs (newborns).

NURSING CONSIDERATIONS

Assessment: Assess for previous hypersensitivity to drug, asthma, history of bronchospasm, hepatic impairment, and pregnancy/nursing status. Obtain baseline serum APAP levels, ALT, AST, bilirubin, PT, BUN, blood glucose levels and electrolytes. Determine time of APAP ingestion.

Monitoring: Monitor for anaphylactoid reactions, acute flushing, erythema, fluid overload, hepatic/renal dysfunction, and electrolyte imbalance.

Patient Counseling: Advise to report to the physician any history of sensitivity to the product or history of asthma.

Administration: IV route. **Storage:** 20-25°C (68-77°F). Diluted Sol: Stable at room temperature for 24 hrs.

ACETAMINOPHEN/CODEINE   CIII
codeine phosphate - acetaminophen (Pharmaceutical Associates)

> Associated with cases of acute liver failure, at times resulting in liver transplant and death. Most cases associated with acetaminophen (APAP) doses >4,000mg/day and involved more than one APAP-containing product.

OTHER BRAND NAMES: Tylenol with Codeine (PRICARA)

THERAPEUTIC CLASS: Opioid analgesic

INDICATIONS: (Sol) Relief of mild to moderate pain. (Tab) Relief of mild to moderately severe pain.

DOSAGE: *Adults:* Adjust dose according to severity of pain and response. (Sol) Usual: 15mL PO q4h PRN. (Tab) Usual Range (per dose): 15-60mg codeine; 300-1,000mg APAP. May repeat up to q4h. Max (per 24 hrs): 360mg codeine; 4,000mg APAP.
Pediatrics: Adjust dose according to severity of pain and response. (Sol) Usual: 0.5mg codeine/kg/dose. 7-12 yrs: 10mL PO tid-qid. 3-6 yrs: 5mL PO tid-qid.

HOW SUPPLIED: (APAP-Codeine Phosphate) Sol: (CV) 120mg-12mg/5mL. Tab: (CIII) 300mg-15mg, 300mg-30mg, 300mg-60mg; (Tylenol with Codeine) (#3) 300mg-30mg, (#4) 300mg-60mg

WARNINGS/PRECAUTIONS: Caution in elderly, debilitated, severe renal or hepatic dysfunction, head injuries, elevated intracranial pressure, acute abdominal conditions, hypothyroidism, urethral stricture, Addison's disease, or prostatic hypertrophy. APAP: Increased risk of acute liver failure in patients with underlying liver disease. Hypersensitivity/anaphylaxis reported; d/c if signs/symptoms occur. Codeine: Respiratory depressant effects and elevation of CSF pressure may be markedly enhanced in the presence of head injury or other intracranial lesions. May obscure diagnosis or clinical course of head injuries or acute abdominal conditions. Not for extended use; choose lowest effective dose for the shortest period of time. May be habit-forming and potentially abusable. May increase serum amylase levels. Tylenol with Codeine: Contains sodium metabisulfite; allergic-type reactions including anaphylactic symptoms and life-threatening or less severe asthmatic episodes may occur.

ADVERSE REACTIONS: Acute liver failure, drowsiness, lightheadedness, dizziness, sedation, SOB, N/V.

INTERACTIONS: APAP: Increased risk of acute liver failure with alcohol ingestion. Codeine: Additive CNS depression with other narcotic analgesics, alcohol, general anesthetics, tranquilizers (eg, chlordiazepoxide), sedative-hypnotics, or other CNS depressants.

PREGNANCY: Category C, not for use in nursing.

MECHANISM OF ACTION: Codeine: Narcotic analgesic and antitussive; produces centrally acting analgesic effects. APAP: Nonopiate, nonsalicylate analgesic, and antipyretic; produces peripherally acting analgesic effects.

PHARMACOKINETICS: Absorption: Rapid. **Distribution:** Found in breast milk. Codeine: Crosses placenta. **Metabolism:** APAP: Liver (conjugation). **Elimination:** Codeine: Urine (90%), feces; $T_{1/2}$=2.9 hrs. APAP: Urine (85%); $T_{1/2}$=1.25-3 hrs.

NURSING CONSIDERATIONS

Assessment: Assess for hypersensitivity to other opioids and APAP, hepatic/renal impairment, head injury, intracranial lesions, elevated intracranial pressure, acute abdominal conditions, hypothyroidism, urethral stricture, Addison's disease, prostatic hypertrophy, pregnancy/nursing status, and possible drug interactions.

Monitoring: Monitor for signs/symptoms of hypersensitivity or anaphylaxis, respiratory depression, elevations in CSF pressure, drug abuse, tolerance, and dependence. Monitor serial hepatic/renal function tests in patients with severe hepatic/renal disease.

Patient Counseling: Instruct to d/c and seek medical attention if signs of allergy (eg, rash, difficulty breathing) develop. Instruct patients to not use more than one APAP-containing product. Inform to not take >4000mg/day of APAP, and to seek medical attention if take more than the recommended dose. Advise that medication may impair mental/physical abilities; avoid hazardous tasks (eg, operating machinery/driving). Instruct not to take with alcohol/other CNS depressants. Counsel that drug may be habit-forming and instruct to take ud.

Administration: Oral route. **Storage:** 20-25°C (68-77°F). Protect from light.

ACIPHEX   RX
rabeprazole sodium (Eisai)

THERAPEUTIC CLASS: Proton pump inhibitor

INDICATIONS: Short-term treatment (4-8 weeks) in the healing and symptomatic relief of erosive or ulcerative gastroesophageal reflux disease (GERD). Maintenance of healing and reduction in relapse rates of heartburn symptoms in patients with erosive or ulcerative GERD. Treatment of daytime and nighttime heartburn and other symptoms associated with GERD in patients ≥12 yrs. Short-term treatment (up to 4 weeks) in the healing and symptomatic relief of duodenal ulcers (DU). In combination with amoxicillin and clarithromycin as a 3-drug regimen for the treatment of patients with *Helicobacter pylori* infection and DU disease (active or history within the past 5 yrs) to eradicate *H. pylori* and reduce the risk of DU recurrence. Long-term treatment of pathological hypersecretory conditions, including Zollinger-Ellison syndrome.

DOSAGE: *Adults:* Erosive/Ulcerative GERD: Healing: 20mg qd for 4-8 weeks. Consider for an additional 8 weeks if not healed after 8 weeks of treatment. Maint: 20mg qd. Symptomatic GERD: 20mg qd for 4 weeks. Consider for an additional course if symptoms do not resolve completely after 4 weeks. DU: 20mg qd after am meal for up to 4 weeks. May need additional therapy. *H. pylori* Triple Therapy: 20mg + clarithromycin 500mg + amoxicillin 1000mg, bid (qam and qpm) with food for 7 days. Pathological Hypersecretory Conditions (eg, Zollinger-Ellison syndrome): Initial: 60mg qd. Titrate: Adjust according to need and continue as long as indicated. Max: Up to 100mg qd or 60mg bid. Some have been treated up to 1 yr.
Pediatrics: ≥12 yrs: Symptomatic GERD: 20mg qd for up to 8 weeks.

HOW SUPPLIED: Tab, Delayed-Release: 20mg

WARNINGS/PRECAUTIONS: Symptomatic response does not preclude the presence of gastric malignancy. May increase risk for osteoporosis-related fractures of the hip, wrist, or spine, especially with high-dose and long-term therapy; use lowest dose and shortest duration appropriate to the condition being treated. Hypomagnesemia reported; with prolonged therapy, consider monitoring magnesium levels prior to therapy and periodically. Caution with severe hepatic impairment.

ADVERSE REACTIONS: Headache, flatulence, pain, pharyngitis, diarrhea, N/V, abdominal pain.

INTERACTIONS: May alter absorption of drugs dependent on gastric pH for absorption (eg, ketoconazole, digoxin). May inhibit cyclosporine metabolism. Increased digoxin plasma levels and decreased ketoconazole levels. Monitor for increases in INR and PT with warfarin. Increased levels with combined administration of amoxicillin and clarithromycin. Substantially decreases atazanavir concentrations; concomitant use is not recommended. Caution with digoxin or with drugs that may cause hypomagnesemia (eg, diuretics); consider monitoring magnesium levels prior to therapy and periodically.

PREGNANCY: Category B, not for use in nursing.

MECHANISM OF ACTION: Proton pump inhibitor; suppresses gastric acid secretion by inhibiting the gastric (H⁺, K⁺)-ATPase enzyme at the secretory surface of the gastric parietal cell. Blocks the final step of gastric acid secretion.

PHARMACOKINETICS: Absorption: T_{max}=2-5 hrs; absolute bioavailability (52%). **Distribution:** Plasma protein binding (96.3%). **Metabolism:** Extensive. Liver via CYP3A to sulphone (primary metabolite) and CYP2C19 to desmethyl rabeprazole. Nonenzymatic reduction to thioether compound (primary metabolite). **Elimination:** Urine (90%), feces; $T_{1/2}$=1-2 hrs.

NURSING CONSIDERATIONS

Assessment: Assess for hypersensitivity, hepatic function, osteoporosis, pregnancy/nursing status, and possible drug interactions. Obtain baseline magnesium levels.

Monitoring: Monitor for signs and symptoms of hypersensitivity, hypomagnesemia (eg, tetany, arrhythmia, seizures), and osteoporosis-related fractures of the hip, wrist, or spine. Monitor magnesium levels periodically for prolonged treatment.

Patient Counseling: Instruct to swallow tab whole; do not chew, crush, or split. Advise to immediately report and seek care for any cardiovascular/neurological symptoms (eg, palpitations, dizziness, tetany).

Administration: Oral route. Swallow tab whole; do not chew, crush, or split. **Storage:** 25°C (77°F); excursions permitted to 15-30°C (59-86°F). Protect from moisture.

ACLOVATE   RX
alclometasone dipropionate (PharmaDerm)

THERAPEUTIC CLASS: Corticosteroid

INDICATIONS: Relief of the inflammatory and pruritic manifestations of corticosteroid-responsive dermatoses.

DOSAGE: *Adults:* Apply a thin film to affected area(s) bid-tid; massage gently until medication disappears.
Pediatrics: ≥1 yr: Apply a thin film to affected area(s) bid-tid; massage gently until medication disappears. Max: 3 weeks of therapy.

HOW SUPPLIED: Cre, Oint: 0.05% [15g, 60g]

WARNINGS/PRECAUTIONS: May produce reversible hypothalamic-pituitary-adrenal (HPA) axis suppression, manifestations of Cushing's syndrome, hyperglycemia, and glucosuria. Evaluate for HPA axis suppression when applied to a large surface area or to areas under occlusion. D/C or reduce frequency of application or substitute a less potent corticosteroid if HPA axis suppression is noted. If concomitant skin infections are present or develop, d/c until infection has been controlled. D/C if irritation occurs. Pediatric patients may be more susceptible to systemic toxicity. Allergic contact dermatitis reported. Glucocorticoid insufficiency may occur; may require supplemental systemic corticosteroids. Not for treatment of diaper dermatitis. D/C when control is achieved; reassess if no improvement seen within 2 weeks.

ADVERSE REACTIONS: Itching, burning, erythema, dryness, irritation, papular rash, folliculitis, acneiform eruptions, hypopigmentation, perioral dermatitis, allergic contact dermatitis, secondary infection, skin atrophy, striae.

PREGNANCY: Category C, caution in nursing.

MECHANISM OF ACTION: Corticosteroid; has anti-inflammatory, antipruritic, and vasoconstrictive properties. Anti-inflammatory activity not established. Suspected to act by the induction of phospholipase A_2 inhibitory proteins (lipocortins), which may inhibit the release of arachidonic acid.

PHARMACOKINETICS: Absorption: Percutaneous. **Distribution:** Systemically administered corticosteroids are found in breast milk.

NURSING CONSIDERATIONS

Assessment: Assess for previous hypersensitivity to the drug, dermatological infection, and pregnancy/nursing status.

Monitoring: Monitor for development of skin irritation and infection. Monitor response to treatment, HPA axis suppression (using adrenocorticotropin hormone stimulation, am plasma cortisol, urinary free cortisol test), Cushing's syndrome and other adverse effects if used for long-term treatment.

Patient Counseling: Instruct to use externally and as directed. Instruct to avoid contact with eyes or face, underarms, or groin areas. Instruct not to bandage the treated skin area unless directed by physician. Advise to d/c use when control is achieved and to notify physician if no improvement seen within 2 weeks. Instruct not to apply in diaper areas or to use for any disorder other than for which it was prescribed. Ask to report to physician any signs of local adverse reaction.

Administration: Topical route. Avoid use with occlusive dressing or applying in diaper areas. **Storage:** 2-30°C (36-86°F).

ACTEMRA

RX

tocilizumab (Genentech)

> Increased risk for developing serious infections (eg, active tuberculosis [TB], invasive fungal infections, bacterial/viral infections due to opportunistic pathogens) that may lead to hospitalization or death. Most patients who developed these infections were taking concomitant immunosuppressants (eg, methotrexate [MTX], corticosteroids). If serious infections develop, interrupt treatment until infection is controlled. Test for latent TB prior to and during therapy; initiate latent TB treatment prior to therapy. Consider risks and benefits prior to initiating therapy with chronic or recurrent infections. Monitor for development of signs and symptoms of infection during and after treatment.

THERAPEUTIC CLASS: Interleukin-6 receptor antagonist

INDICATIONS: Treatment of moderate to severe active rheumatoid arthritis (RA) in adults who have had inadequate response to one or more tumor necrosis factor (TNF) antagonist therapies. Treatment of active systemic juvenile idiopathic arthritis (SJIA) in patients ≥2 yrs.

DOSAGE: *Adults:* RA: Monotherapy/With MTX or Other Disease-Modifying Antirheumatic Drugs (DMARDs): Initial: 4mg/kg once q4 weeks as 60-min IV infusion. Titrate: Increase to 8mg/kg based on clinical response. Max: 800mg/infusion. Refer to PI for dose modifications based on liver enzyme abnormalities, absolute neutrophil count (ANC), and platelet count. Do not initiate treatment if ANC <2,000/mm³, platelets <100,000/mm³, or ALT/AST >1.5X ULN. Reduce dose from 8mg/kg to 4mg/kg for management of dose-related laboratory changes (eg, elevated liver enzymes, neutropenia, and thrombocytopenia).
Pediatrics: SJIA: ≥2 yrs: Monotherapy/With MTX: <30kg: 12mg/kg once q2 weeks as a 60-min IV infusion. ≥30kg: 8mg/kg once q2 weeks as 60-min IV infusion. Change in dose should not be made solely on a single visit body weight measurement. Do not initiate treatment if ANC <2,000/mm³, platelets <100,000/mm³, or ALT/AST >1.5X ULN. May interrupt dose for management of dose-related laboratory abnormalities (eg, elevated liver enzymes, neutropenia, and thrombocytopenia).

HOW SUPPLIED: Inj: 20mg/mL [80mg/4mL, 200mg/10mL, 400mg/20mL]

WARNINGS/PRECAUTIONS: Avoid with active infection, including localized infections. Caution in patients with chronic/recurrent infections, who have been exposed to TB, with history of serious/opportunistic infection, who resided or traveled in areas of endemic TB/mycoses, or with underlying conditions that may predispose them to infection. Viral reactivation and herpes zoster exacerbation observed. GI perforation reported; caution in patients at risk for GI perforation. Neutropenia, thrombocytopenia, elevation of liver enzymes, and increase in lipid parameters reported; monitor with appropriate tests q4-8 weeks in RA patients, or at the time of 2nd infusion and q2-4 weeks thereafter in SJIA patients with lipid monitoring same as for RA patients. May increase risk of malignancies. Hypersensitivity reactions (eg, anaphylaxis) reported; d/c immediately and permanently if occurs. Multiple sclerosis (MS) and chronic inflammatory demyelinating polyneuropathy reported rarely in RA studies; caution with preexisting or recent onset demyelinating disorders. Avoid with active hepatic disease or hepatic impairment. Caution in elderly. D/C if ALT or AST >5X ULN, ANC <500/mm³, or platelets <50,000/mm³.

ADVERSE REACTIONS: Infections, upper respiratory tract infections, nasopharyngitis, headache, HTN, increased ALT, dizziness, bronchitis, infusion reaction, neutropenia, thrombocytopenia, diarrhea.

INTERACTIONS: See Boxed Warning. Avoid with live vaccines. May increase metabolism of CYP450 substrates (eg, 1A2, 2B6, 2C9, 2C19, 2D6, 3A4). Upon initiation or d/c of tocilizumab, monitor therapeutic effect (eg, warfarin) or drug concentrations (eg, cyclosporine, theophylline) and adjust dose PRN. Caution with CYP3A4 substrates where decrease in effectiveness is undesirable (eg, oral contraceptives, lovastatin, atorvastatin). Avoid with biological DMARDs (eg, TNF antagonists, IL-1R antagonists, anti-CD20 monoclonal antibodies, and selective co-stimulation modulators) due to increased immunosuppression. GI perforation may develop with NSAIDs, corticosteroids, MTX. Increased frequency and magnitude of transaminase elevations with hepatotoxic drugs (eg, MTX). Decreased exposure of simvastatin, omeprazole, and dextromethorphan.

PREGNANCY: Category C, not for use in nursing.

MECHANISM OF ACTION: Interleukin-6 (IL-6) receptor antagonist; binds specifically to both soluble and membrane-bound IL-6 receptors (sIL-6R and mIL-6R) and inhibits IL-6 mediated signaling through these receptors.

PHARMACOKINETICS: Absorption: Adults: (4mg/kg) C_{max}=88.3mcg/mL; AUC=13,000mcg•h/mL, (8mg/kg) C_{max}=183mcg/mL; AUC=35,000mcg•h/mL. (≥100kg) C_{max}=269mcg/mL; AUC=55,500mcg•h/mL. Pediatrics: (8mg/kg) C_{max}=245mcg/mL; AUC=32,200mcg•h/mL. **Distribution:** V_d=6.4L (adults), 2.54L (pediatrics). **Elimination:** Adults: (4mg/kg) $T_{1/2}$=11 days, (8mg/kg) $T_{1/2}$=13 days. Pediatrics: $T_{1/2}$=23 days.

NURSING CONSIDERATIONS

Assessment: Assess for infections (eg, bacteria, fungi, or viruses), including latent TB. Assess for demyelinating disorders, risk of GI perforation, active hepatic disease or impairment, drug hypersensitivity, pregnancy/nursing status, and for possible drug interactions. Obtain baseline lipid levels, platelet and neutrophil counts.

Monitoring: Monitor for signs/symptoms of TB and infections. Monitor for hypersensitivity reactions, GI perforation, malignancies, and demyelinating disorders (eg, MS, chronic inflammatory demyelinating polyneuropathy). Monitor neutrophil and platelet counts, LFTs, and lipid levels q4-8 weeks in RA patients, or at the time of 2nd infusion and q2-4 weeks thereafter in SJIA patients with lipid monitoring as for RA patients.

Patient Counseling: Advise of the potential risks/benefits of therapy. Inform that therapy may lower resistance to infections and may develop serious GI side effects; instruct to contact physician if symptoms of infection or severe, persistent abdominal pain appears. Inform physician of travel history, especially to places that are endemic for TB/mycoses.

Administration: IV route. See PI for proper administration technique. Do not administer as an IV bolus or push. Inspect for particulate matter and discoloration. **Storage:** 2-8°C (36-46°F). Do not freeze. Protect vials from light; store in original package until time of use. May store fully diluted solutions at room temperature for ≤24 hrs.

ACTIGALL   RX
ursodiol (Watson)

THERAPEUTIC CLASS: Bile acid

INDICATIONS: Indicated for patients with radiolucent, noncalcified gallbladder stones <20mm in diameter in whom elective cholecystectomy would be undertaken if not for the presence of increased surgical risk or for patients who refuse surgery. Prevention of gallstone formation in obese patients experiencing rapid weight loss.

DOSAGE: *Adults:* Gallstone Dissolution: 8-10mg/kg/day given bid-tid. Obtain ultrasound at 6-month intervals for 1 yr. Continue therapy after stones have dissolved and confirm with repeat ultrasound within 1-3 months. Gallstone Prevention: 600mg/day (300mg bid).

HOW SUPPLIED: Cap: 300mg

CONTRAINDICATIONS: Calcified cholesterol stones, radiopaque stones, compelling reasons for cholecystectomy (radiolucent bile pigment stones, unremitting acute cholecystitis, cholangitis, biliary obstruction, gallstone pancreatitis, biliary-gastrointestinal fistula).

WARNINGS/PRECAUTIONS: Monitor SGOT (AST) and SGPT (ALT) at the initiation of therapy and periodically thereafter. Caution in elderly.

ADVERSE REACTIONS: Abdominal pain, constipation, diarrhea, dyspepsia, flatulence, N/V, arthralgia, coughing, viral infection, bronchitis, pharyngitis, back pain, myalgia, headache, sinusitis.

INTERACTIONS: Decreased absorption with bile acid sequestrants and aluminum-based antacids. Estrogens, oral contraceptives, and clofibrate (and perhaps other lipid-lowering drugs) may increase hepatic cholesterol secretion and encourage cholesterol gallstone formation.

PREGNANCY: Category B, caution in nursing.

MECHANISM OF ACTION: Bile acid; suppresses hepatic synthesis, cholesterol secretion, and inhibits intestinal cholesterol absorption; actions combine to change bile from cholesterol-precipitating to cholesterol-solubilizing, resulting in bile conducive to cholesterol stone dissolution.

PHARMACOKINETICS: Absorption: Small bowel (90%). **Metabolism:** Liver (1st pass, conjugation). **Elimination:** Feces.

NURSING CONSIDERATIONS

Assessment: Assess for type of bile pigment stones (calcified cholesterol, radiopaque, radiolucent), unremitting acute cholecystitis, cholangitis, biliary obstruction, gallstone pancreatitis, biliary GI fistula, nursing status, and possible drug interactions. Obtain baseline AST and ALT.

Monitoring: Ultrasound should be taken in 6-month intervals for first year. If appear dissolved, continue therapy and confirm on repeat ultrasound within 1-3 months. If partial dissolution not seen by 12 months, success is greatly reduced. Monitor AST and ALT periodically. Signs/symptoms of hypersensitivity reactions.

Patient Counseling: Seek medical attention if symptoms of hypersensitivity or allergic reactions occur. Advise patient that gallbladder stone dissolution requires months of therapy.

Administration: Oral route. **Storage:** 25°C (77°F); excursions permitted to 15-30°C (59-86°F). Dispense in tight container.

ACTIQ
fentanyl citrate (Cephalon)

> Serious adverse events, including deaths, reported as a result of improper patient selection (eg, use in opioid nontolerant patient) and/or improper dosing. Do not convert patients on a mcg-per-mcg basis from other fentanyl products. Do not substitute for other fentanyl products; may result in fatal overdose. Not indicated for opioid nontolerant patients including those with only PRN prior exposure; life-threatening respiratory depression and deaths may occur. Contraindicated in the management of acute or postoperative pain including headache/migraine. Contains fentanyl, with abuse liability similar to other opioid agonist, legal or illicit. Keep out of reach of children and discard properly. Use only in the care of cancer patients and only by oncologists and pain specialists who are skilled/knowledgeable in the use of Schedule II opioids to treat cancer pain. Concomitant use with moderate and strong CYP3A4 inhibitors may cause fatal respiratory depression. Available only through restrictive distribution program called Actiq REMS (Risk Evaluation Mitigation Strategy) due to risk of misuse, abuse, addiction, and overdose. Prescribing healthcare professionals, outpatients, pharmacies, and distributors must enroll in the program to prescribe, receive, dispense, and distribute.

THERAPEUTIC CLASS: Opioid analgesic

INDICATIONS: Management of breakthrough cancer pain in patients ≥16 yrs with malignancies who are already receiving and are tolerant to around-the-clock opioid therapy.

DOSAGE: *Adults:* ≥16 yrs: Initial: 200mcg (consume over 15 min). Titrate: May take only 1 additional dose of the same strength if breakthrough pain episode is not relieved 15 min after completion of previous dose. Max: 2 doses/breakthrough pain episode; must wait at least 4 hrs before treating another episode of breakthrough pain. May increase to next highest available strength if several breakthrough episodes require >1 unit per pain episode. Repeat titration for each new dose. Prescribe an initial titration supply of six units. Maint: Once titrated to an effective dose, use only 1 unit of the appropriate strength/breakthrough pain episode. Should limit consumption to 4 or few units/day. If >4 breakthrough pain episodes/day are experienced, re-evaluate maint dose (around-the-clock) used for persistent pain. Upon d/c, gradually titrate dose downward.

HOW SUPPLIED: Loz: 200mcg, 400mcg, 600mcg, 800mcg, 1200mcg, 1600mcg

CONTRAINDICATIONS: Opioid nontolerant patients and management of acute or postoperative pain, including headache/migraine and dental pain.

WARNINGS/PRECAUTIONS: Respiratory depression may occur; caution with chronic obstructive pulmonary disease (COPD) or preexisting medical conditions predisposing to respiratory depression. May impair mental and/or physical abilities. Extreme caution with evidence of increased intracranial pressure (ICP) or impaired consciousness. May obscure clinical course of head injuries. Caution with bradyarrhythmias. Anaphylaxis and hypersensitivity reported. Caution with hepatic or renal dysfunction, and in the elderly. Appropriate measures should be taken to limit the incidence of abuse. May cause physical dependence when abruptly d/c therapy; results in withdrawal symptoms. Not use for analgesia during labor/delivery.

ADVERSE REACTIONS: Respiratory depression, circulatory depression, hypotension, shock, N/V, headache, constipation, dizziness, dyspnea, anxiety, somnolence, asthenia, confusion, depression.

INTERACTIONS: See Boxed Warning. Respiratory depression may occur more readily when given with other agents that depress respiration. Increased depressant effects with other CNS depressants (including opioids, sedatives/hypnotics, general anesthetics, phenothiazines, tranquilizers, skeletal muscle relaxants, sedating antihistamines, and alcohol); adjust dose if warranted. Increased levels with strong inhibitors of CYP3A4 (eg, ritonavir, ketoconazole, itraconazole, troleandomycin, clarithromycin, nelfinavir, and nefazodone) or moderate inhibitors (eg, amprenavir, aprepitant, diltiazem, erythromycin, fluconazole, fosamprenavir, and verapamil), resulting in increased depressant effects; increase dosage conservatively. Avoid grapefruit and grapefruit juice. CYP3A4 inducers may have the opposite effect. Not recommended with or within 14 days of d/c of MAOIs.

PREGNANCY: Category C, not for use in nursing.

MECHANISM OF ACTION: Opioid analgesic: μ-opioid receptor agonist. Exact mechanism not established. Specific CNS opioid receptors for endogenous compounds have been identified throughout brain and spinal cord and play a role in analgesic effects.

PHARMACOKINETICS: Absorption: Rapidly absorbed from buccal mucosa; more prolonged absorption of swallowed fentanyl from GI tract. Absolute bioavailability (50%); (200mcg) $C_{max} = 0.39$ng/mL, AUC=102ng/mL•min, $T_{max} = 40$ min; (400mcg) $C_{max} = 0.75$ng/mL, AUC= 243ng/mL•min, $T_{max} = 25$ min; (800mcg) $C_{max} = 1.55$ng/mL, AUC= 573ng/mL•min, $T_{max} = 25$ min; (1600mcg) $C_{max} = 2.51$ng/mL, AUC= 1026ng/mL•min, $T_{max} = 20$ min. **Distribution:** $V_{ss} = 4$L/kg; plasma protein binding (80-85%). Readily crosses placenta; found in breast milk. **Metabolism:** Liver and intestinal mucosa via CYP3A4; norfentanil (metabolite). **Elimination:** Urine (<7%, unchanged) (major), feces (1%, unchanged); $T_{1/2} = 193$ min (200mcg), 386 min (400mcg), 381 min (800mcg), 358 min (1600mcg).

NURSING CONSIDERATIONS

Assessment: Assess for degree of opioid tolerance, previous opioid dose, level of pain intensity, type of pain, patient's general condition and medical status, emotional status, or any other conditions where treatment is contraindicated or cautioned. Assess for history of hypersensitivity, pregnancy/nursing status, renal/hepatic function, and possible drug interactions.

Monitoring: Monitor for signs/symptoms of respiratory and CNS depression, bradycardia, circulatory depression, hypotension, shock, impairment of mental/physical abilities, abuse/addiction, dental decay, and hypersensitivity reactions. Monitor glucose levels with diabetes mellitus.

Patient Counseling: Advise to enroll in Actiq REMS Program. Review the risks, benefits, appropriate use, and sign a patient-prescriber agreement form to confirm understanding. Inform that medication must be kept out of reach of children; may be fatal to child. Seek immediate help if child accidentally consumes medication. Instruct to properly discard partially used units. Counsel about breakthrough pain episodes and advise to notify physician if breakthrough pain is not alleviated or worsens. Inform that medication has potential for abuse. Use may impair mental/physical abilities; use caution if performing hazardous tasks (eg, operating machinery/driving). Notify physician of all concurrently used medications or before taking any other medications. Avoid consumption of grapefruit juice and alcohol. Maintain proper dental hygiene during therapy. Advise diabetics that medication contains approximately 2g sugar/unit. Avoid abrupt withdrawal and instruct not to share medication as it could result in death due to overdose. Counsel on proper administration and disposal. Instruct female patients to notify physician if pregnant or plan to become pregnant.

Administration: Oral route. The lozenge should be sucked, not chewed, and consumed over 15 min. Refer to PI for proper administration. **Storage:** 20-25°C (68-77°F); excursions permitted between 15-30°C (59-86°F). Protect from freezing and moisture. Do not use if blister package has been opened.

ACTIVASE

alteplase (Genentech)

THERAPEUTIC CLASS: Thrombolytic agent

INDICATIONS: Management of acute myocardial infarction (AMI) for the improvement of ventricular function following AMI, the reduction of incidence of congestive heart failure (CHF) and reduction of mortality with AMI. Management of acute ischemic stroke and acute massive pulmonary embolism (PE).

DOSAGE: *Adults:* AMI: Accelerated Infusion: >67kg: 15mg IV bolus, then 50mg over next 30 min, and then 35mg over next 60 min. ≤67kg: 15mg IV bolus, then 0.75mg/kg (max 50mg) over next 30 min, then 0.50mg/kg (max 35mg) over next 60 min. Max: 100mg total dose. 3-hr Infusion: ≥65kg: 60mg in 1st hr (give 6-10mg as IV bolus), then 20mg over 2nd hr, and 20mg over 3rd hr. <65kg: 1.25mg/kg over 3 hrs as described above. Acute Ischemic Stroke: 0.9mg/kg IV over 1 hr (max 90mg total dose). Administer 10% of total dose as IV bolus over 1 min. PE: 100mg IV over 2 hrs. Start heparin at end or immediately after infusion when PTT or thrombin time ≤2X normal.

HOW SUPPLIED: Inj: 50mg, 100mg

CONTRAINDICATIONS: (AMI, PE) Active internal bleeding, history of cerebrovascular accident (CVA), recent intracranial/intraspinal surgery or trauma, intracranial neoplasm, arteriovenous (AV) malformation, aneurysm, bleeding diathesis, severe uncontrolled HTN. (Acute Ischemic Stroke) Active internal bleeding, AV malformation, intracranial neoplasm, history or evidence of intracranial hemorrhage, aneurysm, bleeding diathesis, uncontrolled HTN, subarachnoid hemorrhage at stroke onset. Recent (within 3 months) intracranial or intraspinal surgery, serious head trauma, previous stroke.

WARNINGS/PRECAUTIONS: Weigh benefits/risks with recent major surgery, cerebrovascular disease, recent GI or genitourinary (GU) bleeding, recent trauma, HTN (systolic BP ≥175mmHg and/or diastolic BP >110mmHg), left heart thrombus, acute pericarditis, subacute bacterial endocarditis, hemostatic defects, severe hepatic dysfunction, pregnancy, diabetic hemorrhagic retinopathy or other hemorrhagic ophthalmic conditions, septic thrombophlebitis or occluded AV cannula at a seriously infected site, advanced age or elderly, any other bleeding condition that is difficult to manage. For stroke, also weigh benefits/risks with severe neurological deficit or major early infarct signs on CT. Cholesterol embolism and internal/superficial bleeding reported. Arrhythmias may occur with reperfusion. Avoid IM injection, noncompressible arterial puncture, and internal jugular or subclavian venous puncture. Caution with readministration. D/C therapy if anaphylactoid reaction occurs.

ADVERSE REACTIONS: Bleeding, orolingual angioedema.

INTERACTIONS: Increased risk of bleeding with warfarin, heparin, vitamin K antagonists, drugs that alter platelets (eg, ASA, dipyridamole, abciximab) given before, during, or after alteplase therapy. Orolingual angioedema with ACE inhibitors.

PREGNANCY: Category C, caution in nursing.

MECHANISM OF ACTION: Tissue plasminogen activator (t-PA); serine protease enzyme that has property of fibrin-enhanced conversion of plasminogen to plasmin. Produces limited conversion of plasminogen in absence of fibrin. Binds to fibrin in thrombus and converts entrapped plasminogen to plasmin. Initiates local fibrinolysis with limited systemic proteolysis.

PHARMACOKINETICS: Metabolism: Liver. **Elimination:** $T_{1/2}$=<5 min (initial).

NURSING CONSIDERATIONS

Assessment: In patients with acute MI or PE, assess for presence of active internal bleeding, history of cerebrovascular accident, trauma, aneurysm, known bleeding diathesis, and severe uncontrolled HTN. In patients with acute ischemic stroke, assess for presence or history of hemorrhage, surgery, serious head trauma, previous stroke, uncontrolled HTN, and possible drug interactions.

Monitoring: Monitor for signs/symptoms of bleeding (eg, internal, superficial, surface bleeding), cholesterol embolism (eg, livedo reticularis, "purple toe" syndrome, acute renal failure, gangrenous digits), and for allergic reactions (eg, anaphylactoid reaction, laryngeal edema, orolingual angioedema, rash, urticaria). Monitor BP frequently and arrhythmias with acute MI.

Patient Counseling: Inform about risk of bleeding with medication. Instruct to notify physician if any type of allergic reaction develops during therapy.

Administration: IV route. Reconstitute using appropriate volume of SWFI (without preservatives) to vial. Do not use Bacteriostatic Water for Inj, USP. Reconstitute to a final concentration of 1mg/mL. Reconstitute just prior to use. May further dilute using an equal volume of 0.9% NS or D5W to yield concentration of 0.5mg/mL. Do not add any other medication to infusion solutions containing drug. Discard any unused infusion solution. Do not use if vacuum is not present in 50mg vials. **Storage:** Lyophilized: Controlled room temperature not to exceed 30°C (86°F), or under refrigeration 2-8°C (36-46°F). Protect from excessive exposure to light. Reconstituted: 2-30°C (36-86°F); use within 8 hrs.

ACTIVELLA   RX
norethindrone acetate - estradiol (Novo Nordisk)

Should not be used for the prevention of cardiovascular disease (CVD) or dementia. Increased risk of myocardial infarction (MI), stroke, invasive breast cancer, pulmonary emboli (PE), and deep vein thrombosis (DVT) in postmenopausal women (50-79 yrs of age) reported. Increased risk of developing probable dementia in postmenopausal women ≥65 yrs of age reported. Should be prescribed at the lowest effective doses and for the shortest duration consistent with treatment goals and risks.

THERAPEUTIC CLASS: Estrogen/progestogen combination

INDICATIONS: In women with a uterus, for the treatment of moderate to severe vasomotor symptoms and/or vulvar/vaginal atrophy associated with menopause and for the prevention of postmenopausal osteoporosis.

DOSAGE: *Adults:* 1 tab qd. Re-evaluate treatment need periodically (eg, 3-6 month intervals).

HOW SUPPLIED: Tab: (Estradiol-Norethindrone) 1mg-0.5mg, 0.5mg-0.1mg

CONTRAINDICATIONS: Undiagnosed abnormal genital bleeding, known/suspected/history of breast cancer, known/suspected estrogen-dependent neoplasia, active or history of DVT/PE, active or recent arterial thromboembolic disease (eg, stroke, MI), liver dysfunction or disease, known/suspected pregnancy.

WARNINGS/PRECAUTIONS: Caution in patients with risk factors for arterial vascular disease (eg, HTN, diabetes mellitus [DM], tobacco use, hypercholesterolemia, obesity) and/or venous thromboembolism (eg, personal history or family history of venous thromboembolism, obesity, systemic lupus erythematosus [SLE]). If feasible, d/c at least 4 to 6 weeks before surgery of the type associated with an increased risk of thromboembolism, or during periods of prolonged immobilization. May increase risk of endometrial cancer; perform adequate diagnostic measures, such as endometrial sampling, to rule out malignancy with undiagnosed persistent or recurrent abnormal vaginal bleeding. May increase risk of gallbladder disease requiring surgery and ovarian cancer. May lead to severe hypercalcemia in patients with breast cancer and bone metastases; d/c and take appropriate measures if hypercalcemia occurs. Retinal vascular thrombosis reported; d/c pending examination if sudden partial or complete loss of vision, sudden onset of proptosis, diplopia, migraine, or if examination reveals papilledema or retinal vascular lesions. Consider addition of a progestin to estrogen monotherapy in posthysterectomy for endometriosis. May elevate BP, plasma TG with preexisting hypertriglyceridemia; d/c if pancreatitis occurs. Caution with history of cholestatic jaundice; d/c in case of recurrence. May lead to increase thyroid-binding globulin levels; monitor thyroid function. May cause fluid retention; caution with cardiac/renal dysfunction. Caution with severe hypocalcemia. May exacerbate endometriosis, asthma, DM, epilepsy, migraine, porphyria, SLE, and hepatic hemangiomas; use with caution. May affect certain endocrine and blood components in laboratory tests.

ADVERSE REACTIONS: Back pain, headache, nasopharyngitis, sinusitis, insomnia, upper respiratory tract infection, breast pain, postmenopausal bleeding, vaginal hemorrhage, endometrial thickening, uterine fibroid, pain in extremities, nausea, diarrhea, viral infection.

INTERACTIONS: CYP3A4 inducers (eg, St. John's wort, phenobarbital, carbamazepine, rifampin) may decrease levels, which may decrease therapeutic effects and/or change uterine bleeding profile. CYP3A4 inhibitors (eg, erythromycin, clarithromycin, ketoconazole, itraconazole, ritonavir, grapefruit juice) may increase levels, which may result in side effects. Patients concomitantly receiving thyroid hormone replacement therapy and estrogens may require increased doses of their thyroid replacement therapy.

PREGNANCY: Contraindicated in pregnancy, caution in nursing.

MECHANISM OF ACTION: Estradiol (E_2): Estrogen; binds to nuclear receptors in estrogen-responsive tissues. Circulating estrogens modulate pituitary secretion of the gonadotropins, luteinizing hormone and follicle stimulating hormone, through negative-feedback mechanism. Reduces elevated levels of these hormones in postmenopausal women. Norethindrone: Progestin; binds to specific progesterone receptors that interact with progesterone response elements in target genes. Enhances cellular differentiation and opposing actions of estrogens by decreasing estrogen receptor levels, increasing local metabolism of estrogens to less active metabolites, or inducing gene products that blunt cellular responses to estrogen.

PHARMACOKINETICS: Absorption: E_2: Well-absorbed; T_{max}=5-8 hrs. Norethindrone: Rapid. Oral administration of various doses resulted in different parameters. **Distribution:** E_2: Found in breast milk; sex hormone binding globulin (SHBG) (37%); albumin (61%); unbound (1-2%). Norethindrone: SHBG (36%); albumin (61%). **Metabolism:** E_2: Liver to estrone (metabolite); estriol (major urinary metabolite); enterohepatic recirculation via sulfate and glucuronide conjugation; biliary secretion of conjugates into the intestine; hydrolysis in the gut; reabsorption. Norethindrone: 5α-dihydro-NET, tetrahydro-NET (metabolites). **Elimination:** E_2: Urine (parent compound and metabolites); $T_{1/2}$=12-14 hrs. NET: $T_{1/2}$=8-11 hrs.

NURSING CONSIDERATIONS

Assessment: Assess for presence or history of breast cancer, estrogen-dependent neoplasias, abnormal genital bleeding, active or history of DVT/PE, active or recent arterial thromboembolic disease, liver dysfunction or disease, pregnancy/nursing status, and any other conditions where treatment may be contraindicated or cautioned. Assess use in women ≥65 yrs, and those with asthma, DM, epilepsy, migraines, porphyria, SLE, and hepatic hemangiomas. Assess for possible drug interactions.

Monitoring: Monitor for signs/symptoms of CVD disorders, malignant neoplasms, dementia, gallbladder disease, cholestatic jaundice, hypercalcemia, visual abnormalities, BP elevations, fluid retention, elevations in plasma TG, hypothyroidism, exacerbation of endometriosis or other conditions (eg, asthma, DM, epilepsy, migraine, SLE, and hepatic hemangiomas). Perform periodic monitoring of BP, annual breast exam, thyroid function if on thyroid hormone replacement therapy, and periodic assessment (eg, 3-6 month interval) to determine need for therapy. If abnormal genital bleeding occurs, perform adequate diagnostic measures (eg, endometrial sampling) to rule out malignancies.

Patient Counseling: Counsel that drug is contraindicated in pregnancy. Inform that medication may increase risk of heart attacks, strokes, breast cancer, blood clots, and dementia. Counsel to contact physician for any signs/symptoms of breast lumps, unusual vaginal bleeding dizziness/faintness, changes in speech, severe headaches, chest pain, SOB, leg pain, changes in vision, or vomiting. Advise to have yearly breast exams by a healthcare provider and perform monthly breast self-exams.

Administration: Oral route. **Storage:** 25°C (77°F); excursions permitted to 15-30°C (59-86°F). Protect from light.

ACTONEL
risedronate sodium (Warner Chilcott)

RX

THERAPEUTIC CLASS: Bisphosphonate

INDICATIONS: Treatment and prevention of osteoporosis in postmenopausal women and glucocorticoid-induced osteoporosis in men and women who are either initiating or continuing systemic glucocorticosteroids. Treatment to increase bone mass in men with osteoporosis. Treatment of Paget's disease of bone in men and women.

DOSAGE: *Adults:* Postmenopausal Osteoporosis Prevention/Treatment: 5mg qd, or 35mg once weekly, or 150mg once a month. Glucocorticoid-Induced Osteoporosis Prevention/Treatment: 5mg qd. To Increase Bone Mass in Men with Osteoporosis: 35mg once weekly. Paget's Disease:

30mg qd for 2 months. May retreat after 2 months if relapse occurs, or if treatment fails to normalize serum alkaline phosphatase. Take ≥30 min before 1st food or drink of the day other than water. Swallow tab in upright position with full glass of plain water (6-8 oz). Do not lie down for 30 min after dose.

HOW SUPPLIED: Tab: 5mg, 30mg, 35mg, 150mg

CONTRAINDICATIONS: Hypocalcemia, inability to stand or sit upright for ≥30 min, abnormalities of the esophagus which delay esophageal emptying (eg, stricture or achalasia).

WARNINGS/PRECAUTIONS: May cause local irritation of upper GI mucosa; caution with upper GI problems (eg, Barrett's esophagus, dysphagia, other esophageal diseases, gastritis, duodenitis, or ulcers). D/C if dysphagia, odynophagia, retrosternal pain, or new/worsening heartburn occurs. Gastric and duodenal ulcers reported. Treat hypocalcemia and other disturbances of bone and mineral metabolism before therapy. Osteonecrosis of the jaw (ONJ) reported; d/c for patients requiring invasive dental procedures or consider d/c if ONJ develops. Severe, incapacitating bone, joint, and/or muscle pain reported; d/c if severe symptoms develop. Atypical, low-energy, or low trauma fractures of the femoral shaft reported; consider interrupting therapy. Ascertain sex steroid hormonal status and consider replacement before initiating therapy for the treatment/prevention of glucocorticoid-induced osteoporosis. Avoid with severe renal impairment (CrCl <30mL/min).

ADVERSE REACTIONS: Back pain, arthralgia, abdominal pain, dyspepsia, acute phase reaction, allergic reaction, arthritis, diarrhea, headache, infection, urinary tract infection, bronchitis, HTN, nausea, rash.

INTERACTIONS: Calcium supplements, antacids, or oral medications containing divalent cations (aluminum, magnesium) may interfere with absorption. Risk of ONJ with concomitant corticosteroid or chemotherapy. May interfere with the use of bone-imaging agents. May increase risk of atypical femur fractures with glucocorticoids (eg, prednisone).

PREGNANCY: Category C, not for use in nursing.

MECHANISM OF ACTION: Bisphosphonate; has an affinity for hydroxyapatite crystals in bone and acts as an antiresorptive agent. Inhibits osteoclasts.

PHARMACOKINETICS: Absorption: Upper GI tract; T_{max}=1 hr; absolute bioavailability (0.63%). **Distribution:** V_d=13.8L/kg; plasma protein binding (24%). **Elimination:** Urine (50%), feces (unabsorbed dose); $T_{1/2}$=561 hrs.

NURSING CONSIDERATIONS

Assessment: Assess for hypocalcemia, esophageal abnormalities, upper GI problems or any other conditions where treatment is contraindicated or cautioned, drug hypersensitivity, pregnancy/nursing status and possible drug interactions. Assess sex steroid hormonal status if treatment is for glucocorticoid-induced osteoporosis.

Monitoring: Monitor for signs/symptoms of upper GI disorders (eg, dysphagia, esophagitis, esophageal or gastric ulcers), ONJ, hypersensitivity reactions, and musculoskeletal pain.

Patient Counseling: Instruct to take ≥30 min before 1st food or drink of the day other than water; take in an upright position (while sitting or standing) with a full glass of plain water (6-8 oz.), not to lie down for 30 min after taking medication, and to avoid chewing or sucking tablet. Contact physician if symptoms of esophageal disease develop. Take supplemental calcium and vitamin D if dietary intake is inadequate; take supplement and calcium-, aluminum-, and magnesium-containing medications at a different time of the day than risedronate. Refer to PI for instructions on missed doses.

Administration: Oral route. **Storage:** 20-25°C (68-77°F).

ACTOPLUS MET   RX
metformin HCl - pioglitazone HCl (Takeda)

Thiazolidinediones cause or exacerbate congestive heart failure (CHF) in some patients. After initiation and after dose increases, observe for signs/symptoms of heart failure (HF) and manage accordingly; consider d/c or dose reduction. Not recommended in patients with symptomatic HF. Contraindicated with established New York Heart Association (NYHA) Class III or IV HF. Lactic acidosis may occur due to metformin accumulation (rare); d/c and hospitalize patient immediately if suspected.

OTHER BRAND NAMES: Actoplus Met XR (Takeda)

THERAPEUTIC CLASS: Thiazolidinedione/biguanide

INDICATIONS: Adjunct to diet and exercise to improve glycemic control in adults with type 2 diabetes mellitus (DM) who are already treated with pioglitazone and metformin or who have inadequate glycemic control on pioglitazone or metformin alone.

DOSAGE: *Adults:* Individualize dose. Titrate gradually PRN based on response. Tab: Initial: 15mg-500mg or 15mg-850mg qd or bid with food. Max: 45mg-2550mg/day in divided doses with food.

Tab, Extended-Release: Initial: 15mg-1000mg or 30mg-1000mg qpm with meal. Max: 45mg-2000mg qpm with meal. Elderly: Dose conservatively. Elderly/Debilitated/Malnourished: Do not titrate to max dose.

HOW SUPPLIED: Tab: (Pioglitazone-Metformin) 15mg-500mg, 15mg-850mg; Tab, Extended-Release: (Pioglitazone-Metformin) 15mg-1000mg, 30mg-1000mg

CONTRAINDICATIONS: Established NYHA Class III or IV HF, renal disease/dysfunction (eg, SrCr ≥1.5mg/dL [males], ≥1.4mg/dL [females], or abnormal CrCl), acute or chronic metabolic acidosis including diabetic ketoacidosis with or without coma. Temporarily d/c if undergoing radiologic studies involving intravascular administration of iodinated contrast materials.

WARNINGS/PRECAUTIONS: Check LFTs if hepatic dysfunction symptoms occur. Avoid with active liver disease or if ALT levels >2.5X ULN. Caution with mildly elevated LFTs; monitor LFTs more frequently. D/C if ALT levels remain >3X ULN or if jaundice occurs. Temporarily d/c for any surgical procedure necessitating restricted food/fluid intake; restart after oral intake resumed and renal function is normal. May lose glycemic control with stress; withhold therapy and temporarily administer insulin. Caution in elderly. Pioglitazone: May cause fluid retention. Initiate at lowest dose in patients with systolic HF (NYHA Class II); gradually increase only after several months of therapy with careful monitoring of weight gain, edema, or signs/symptoms of CHF exacerbation. Not for use in type 1 DM. May cause hypoglycemia, weight gain, and decreases in Hgb and Hct. Avoid in patients with active bladder cancer; consider risks vs benefits in patients with a history of bladder cancer. Ovulation in premenopausal anovulatory patients may occur; use adequate contraception. Macular edema reported; refer to an ophthalmologist if visual symptoms develop. Increased incidence of bone fractures reported in females. Metformin: D/C if renal impairment is present or if conditions characterized by hypoxemia occur. May decrease serum vitamin B12 levels; measure hematologic parameters annually. Megaloblastic anemia reported (rare). Increased risk of hypoglycemia in elderly, debilitated/malnourished, adrenal/pituitary insufficiency, and alcohol intoxication.

ADVERSE REACTIONS: Upper respiratory tract infection, diarrhea, nausea, headache, urinary tract infection, sinusitis, dizziness, edema/peripheral edema, weight increased.

INTERACTIONS: See Contraindications. Risk of hypoglycemia with other hypoglycemic agents (eg, sulfonylureas, insulin). (Pioglitazone) Decreased levels of ethinyl estradiol and midazolam. May affect levels of nifedipine ER and atorvastatin calcium. Concomitant use with ketoconazole or atorvastatin calcium may affect pioglitazone levels. Increased exposure with CYP2C8 inhibitors (eg, gemfibrozil). Decreased exposure with CYP2C8 inducers (eg, rifampin). (Metformin) Avoid excessive alcohol intake. May be difficult to recognize hypoglycemia with β-adrenergic blocking drugs. Decreased levels of glyburide and furosemide. Increased levels with furosemide, nifedipine, and cimetidine. May interact with highly protein-bound drugs (eg, salicylates, sulfonamides, chloramphenicol, probenecid). Thiazides, other diuretics, corticosteroids, phenothiazines, thyroid products, estrogens, oral contraceptives, phenytoin, nicotinic acid, sympathomimetics, calcium channel blockers, and isoniazid may cause hyperglycemia and loss of glycemic control. Caution with concomitant medications that may affect renal function or result in significant hemodynamic change or may interfere with the disposition of metformin, such as cationic drugs eliminated by renal tubular secretion (eg, amiloride, digoxin, morphine, procainamide, quinidine, quinine, ranitidine, triamterene, trimethoprim, vancomycin). Hypoglycemia may occur with ethanol.

PREGNANCY: Category C, not for use in nursing.

MECHANISM OF ACTION: Pioglitazone: Thiazolidinedione; insulin-sensitizing agent that acts by enhancing peripheral glucose utilization. Decreases insulin resistance in the periphery and liver, resulting in increased insulin-dependent glucose disposal and decreased hepatic glucose output. Metformin: Biguanide; decreases endogenous hepatic glucose production, decreases intestinal absorption of glucose, and improves insulin sensitivity by increasing peripheral glucose uptake and utilization.

PHARMACOKINETICS: Absorption: Administration of variable doses resulted in different pharmacokinetic parameters. Pioglitazone: T_{max}=Within 2 hrs, 3-4 hrs (with food). Metformin: Absolute bioavailability (50-60%) (immediate-release). **Distribution:** Pioglitazone: V_d=0.63L/kg; plasma protein binding (>99%). Metformin: V_d=654L (immediate-release). **Metabolism:** Pioglitazone: Hydroxylation and oxidation (extensive) via CYP2C8, 3A4, 1A1; M-II and M-IV [hydroxy derivatives], M-III [keto derivative] (active metabolites). **Elimination:** Refer to PI for $T_{1/2}$ values. Pioglitazone: Urine (15-30%), feces. Metformin: Urine (90%).

NURSING CONSIDERATIONS

Assessment: Assess for HF, conditions that increase risk for lactic acidosis, hepatic disease, DM type, diabetic ketoacidosis, bone health, any other conditions where treatment is cautioned or contraindicated, pregnancy/nursing status, and for possible drug interactions. Obtain baseline FPG, HbA1c, LFTs, renal function, and hematological parameters.

Monitoring: Monitor for signs/symptoms of lactic acidosis, HF, edema, weight gain, macular edema, and for bone fractures. Monitor vitamin B12 levels in patients predisposed to developing subnormal levels. Perform regular eye exams and periodic monitoring of FPG, HbA1c, LFTs, hematologic parameters, and renal function.

Patient Counseling: Inform on importance of adherence to dietary instructions, a regular exercise program, and regular testing of blood glucose, HbA1c, LFTs, renal function, and hematologic parameters. Advise to seek medical attention during periods of stress (eg, fever, trauma, infection, or surgery). Explain the risk of lactic acidosis; inform to d/c therapy immediately and notify physician if unexplained hyperventilation, myalgia, malaise, unusual somnolence, or other symptoms occur. Counsel to report unexplained GI symptoms, rapid increase in weight or edema, SOB, N/V, abdominal pain, fatigue, anorexia, or dark urine. Inform to avoid excessive alcohol intake. Counsel females about the use of reliable contraception. Advise about the risk of hypoglycemia, its symptoms and treatment, and conditions that predispose to its development. Instruct to promptly report any sign of macroscopic hematuria or other symptoms such as dysuria or urinary urgency that develop or increase during treatment as these may be due to bladder cancer. Instruct to take drug as prescribed; if dose is missed, inform to take the next dose as prescribed unless directed otherwise by physician. Inform that Actoplus Met XR must be swallowed whole and not chewed, cut, or crushed, and that the inactive ingredients may occasionally be eliminated in the feces as a soft mass that may resemble the original tab.

Administration: Oral route. **Storage:** 25°C (77°F); excursions permitted to 15-30°C (59-86°F). (Tab) Keep container tightly closed. Protect from moisture and humidity. (Tab, Extended-Release) Avoid excessive heat and humidity.

ACTOS   RX
pioglitazone HCl (Takeda)

> Thiazolidinediones cause or exacerbate congestive heart failure (CHF) in some patients. After initiation/dose increases, monitor carefully for signs/symptoms of heart failure (HF) and manage accordingly; consider d/c or dose reduction. Not recommended in patients with symptomatic HF. Contraindicated with established New York Heart Association (NYHA) Class III or IV HF.

THERAPEUTIC CLASS: Thiazolidinedione

INDICATIONS: Adjunct to diet and exercise to improve glycemic control in adults with type 2 diabetes mellitus (DM).

DOSAGE: *Adults:* Without CHF: Initial: 15mg or 30mg qd. With CHF (NYHA Class I or II): Initial: 15mg qd. Titrate: In increments of 15mg. Max: 45mg qd. With Insulin Secretagogue: Reduce dose of insulin secretagogue if hypoglycemia occurs. With Insulin: Decrease insulin dose by 10-25% if hypoglycemia occurs. Further insulin dose adjustment should be individualized based on glycemic response. With Gemfibrozil/Other Strong CYP2C8 Inhibitors: Max: 15mg qd.

HOW SUPPLIED: Tab: 15mg, 30mg, 45mg

CONTRAINDICATIONS: Established NYHA Class III or IV HF.

WARNINGS/PRECAUTIONS: Not for use in treatment of type 1 DM or diabetic ketoacidosis. New onset or worsening of edema reported; caution in patients with edema and in patients at risk for CHF. Fatal and non-fatal hepatic failure reported. Obtain LFTs prior to initiation; caution with liver disease/abnormal LFTs. D/C if ALT >3X ULN; do not restart if cause of abnormal LFTs not established or if ALT remains >3x ULN with total bilirubin >2X ULN without alternative etiologies. May use with caution in patients with lesser ALT elevations or bilirubin and with an alternate probable cause. Increased incidence of bone fractures reported in females. Not for use in patients with active bladder cancer; consider benefits vs risks in patients with a prior history of bladder cancer. Macular edema reported; refer to an ophthalmologist if visual symptoms develop. Ovulation in premenopausal anovulatory patients may occur; use adequate contraception.

ADVERSE REACTIONS: Upper respiratory tract infection, hypoglycemia, edema, headache, cardiac failure, pain in extremity, sinusitis, back pain, myalgia, pharyngitis, chest pain.

INTERACTIONS: Increased exposure and $T_{1/2}$ with CYP2C8 inhibitors (eg, gemfibrozil). Decreased exposure with CYP2C8 inducers (eg, rifampin). Risk of fluid retention and hypoglycemia with insulin and other antidiabetic medications (eg, insulin secretagogues such as sulfonylureas). Increased exposure of digoxin, norethindrone, fexofenadine, ranitidine, theophylline. Decreased exposure of warfarin, ethinyl estradiol, glipizide, metformin, midazolam, nifedipine ER, atorvastatin calcium. Increased exposure with ketoconazole, fexofenadine, nifedipine ER. Decreased exposure with ranitidine, atorvastatin calcium, theophylline.

PREGNANCY: Category C, not for use in nursing.

MECHANISM OF ACTION: Thiazolidinedione; decreases insulin resistance in the periphery and liver resulting in increased insulin-dependent glucose disposal and decreased hepatic glucose output.

PHARMACOKINETICS: **Absorption:** T_{max}=within 2 hrs, 3-4 hrs (with food). **Distribution:** V_d=0.63L/kg; plasma protein binding (>99%). **Metabolism:** Hydroxylation and oxidation (extensive), CYP2C8, CYP3A4; M-III [keto derivative] and M-IV [hydroxyl derivative] (active metabolites). **Elimination:** Urine (15-30%), bile and feces; $T_{1/2}$=3-7 hrs (pioglitazone), 16-24 hrs (metabolites).

NURSING CONSIDERATIONS

Assessment: Assess for previous hypersensitivity, HF, edema, risk factors for developing HF, liver disease, bone health, active/history of bladder cancer, pregnancy/nursing status, and possible drug interactions. Obtain baseline LFTs.

Monitoring: Monitor for signs and symptoms of HF, edema, weight gain, hematological changes (eg, decreases in Hgb, Hct), liver injury, macular edema, and bone fractures. Perform periodic measurements of FPG and HbA1c. Periodically monitor LFTs in patients with liver disease. Perform periodic eye exams.

Patient Counseling: Advise to adhere to dietary instructions and have blood glucose and HbA1c levels tested regularly. Instruct to seek medical advice promptly during periods of stress (eg, fever, trauma, infection, or surgery) and report SOB, rapid increase in weight or edema, or other symptoms of HF to physician. Instruct to d/c and consult physician if unexplained N/V, abdominal pain, anorexia, fatigue, and darkening of urine occurs. Advise to take once daily without regard to meals. If dose is missed, advise to not double the dose the following day. Inform about the risk of hypoglycemia when using with insulin or other antidiabetic medications. Inform that therapy may result in ovulation in some premenopausal anovulatory women; recommend adequate contraception for all premenopausal women.

Administration: Oral route. **Storage:** 25°C (77°F); excursions permitted to 15-30°C (59-86°F). Protect from light, moisture, and humidity.

ACULAR   RX
ketorolac tromethamine (Allergan)

THERAPEUTIC CLASS: NSAID

INDICATIONS: Temporary relief of ocular itching due to seasonal allergic conjunctivitis. Treatment of postoperative inflammation in patients who have undergone cataract extraction.

DOSAGE: *Adults:* Ocular Itching: 1 drop (0.25mg) qid. Postoperative Inflammation: 1 drop to affected eye(s) qid beginning 24 hrs after cataract surgery and continuing through the 1st 2 weeks of the postoperative period.
Pediatrics: ≥3 yrs: Ocular Itching: 1 drop (0.25mg) qid. Postoperative Inflammation: 1 drop to affected eye(s) qid beginning 24 hrs after cataract surgery and continuing through the 1st 2 weeks of the postoperative period.

HOW SUPPLIED: Sol: 0.5% [5mL]

WARNINGS/PRECAUTIONS: Potential for cross-sensitivity to acetylsalicylic acid (ASA), phenylacetic acid derivatives, and other NSAIDs; caution with previous sensitivities to these agents. Increased bleeding of ocular tissues (eg, hyphemas) reported in conjunction with ocular surgery; caution with known bleeding tendencies. May slow or delay healing, or result in keratitis. Continued use may result in epithelial breakdown, corneal thinning, erosion, ulceration, or perforation; these events may be sight-threatening. D/C if corneal epithelial breakdown occurs and monitor for corneal health. Caution with complicated ocular surgeries, corneal denervation, corneal epithelial defects, diabetes mellitus (DM), ocular surface diseases (eg, dry eye syndrome), rheumatoid arthritis (RA), or repeat ocular surgeries within a short period of time. Increased risk for occurrence and severity of corneal adverse events if used for >24 hrs prior to surgery or used beyond 14 days post-surgery.

ADVERSE REACTIONS: Stinging, burning, superficial keratitis, ocular infections, allergic reactions, ocular inflammation/irritation, corneal edema, iritis.

INTERACTIONS: Caution with agents that may prolong bleeding time. Increased potential for healing problems with topical steroids.

PREGNANCY: Category C, caution in nursing.

MECHANISM OF ACTION: NSAID; inhibits prostaglandin biosynthesis.

NURSING CONSIDERATIONS

Assessment: Assess for previous hypersensitivity to the drug or cross-sensitivity to ASA, phenylacetic acid derivatives, and other NSAIDs, bleeding tendencies, complicated or repeated ocular surgeries, corneal denervation, corneal epithelial defects, DM, ocular surface diseases, RA, contact lens use, pregnancy/nursing status, and possible drug interactions.

Monitoring: Monitor for hypersensitivity reactions, wound healing problems, keratitis, increased bleeding of ocular tissues in conjunction with ocular surgery, and evidence of epithelial corneal breakdown.

Patient Counseling: Advise not to administer while wearing contact lenses.

Administration: Intraocular route. **Storage:** 15-25°C (59-77°F). Protect from light.

ACULAR LS   RX
ketorolac tromethamine (Allergan)

OTHER BRAND NAMES: Acular PF (Allergan)

THERAPEUTIC CLASS: NSAID

INDICATIONS: (Acular PF) Reduction of ocular pain and photophobia after incisional refractive surgery. (Acular LS) Reduction of ocular pain and burning/stinging following corneal refractive surgery.

DOSAGE: *Adults:* 1 drop qid post-op PRN for up to 3 days (Acular PF) or 4 days (Acular LS). *Pediatrics:* ≥3 yrs: 1 drop qid post-op PRN for up to 3 days (Acular PF) or 4 days (Acular LS).

HOW SUPPLIED: Sol: (Acular PF) 0.5% [0.4mL, 12ˢ] (PF is preservative free); (Acular LS) 0.4% [5mL]

WARNINGS/PRECAUTIONS: Avoid use with contact lenses. Potential cross-sensitivity to acetyl-salicylic acid, phenylacetic acid derivatives, and other NSAIDs. May increase bleeding of ocular tissue (including hyphemas) in conjunction with ocular surgery. May slow or delay healing. D/C if corneal epithelium breakdown occurs. Caution in known bleeding tendencies, complicated ocular surgeries, corneal denervation, corneal epithelial defects, diabetes mellitus (DM), ocular surface diseases (eg, dry eye syndrome), rheumatoid arthritis, or repeated ocular surgeries within a short period of time. Caution if used >24 hrs prior to surgery and use beyond 14 days post-surgery.

ADVERSE REACTIONS: Transient stinging/burning, allergic reactions, corneal edema, iritis, ocular inflammation/irritation/pain, superficial keratitis, superficial ocular infections.

INTERACTIONS: Concomitant use of topical NSAIDs and topical steroids may increase potential for healing problems. Caution with other medications which may prolong bleeding time.

PREGNANCY: Category C, caution in nursing.

MECHANISM OF ACTION: NSAID; inhibits prostaglandin biosynthesis.

PHARMACOKINETICS: Absorption: C_{max}=960ng/mL.

NURSING CONSIDERATIONS

Assessment: Assess for drug hypersensitivity, cross-sensitivity reactions, bleeding tendencies, complicated ocular surgeries, corneal denervation, corneal epithelial defects, DM, ocular surface disease (dry eye syndrome), rheumatoid arthritis, possible drug interactions.

Monitoring: Monitor for bleeding of ocular tissues (hyphema), healing problems, keratitis, corneal epithelial breakdown, corneal thinning/erosion/ulceration/perforation.

Patient Counseling: Advise not to use while wearing contact lenses. Caution during nursing/late pregnancy. Solution from one Acular PF single-use vial should be used immediately after opening and the remaining contents should be discarded immediately after administration. Avoid contact between tip of vial and any other surface.

Intraocular route. Storage: (Acular PF) 15-30°C (59-86°F), protect from light. (Acular LS) 15-25°C (59-77°F).

ADALAT CC   RX
nifedipine (Bayer Healthcare)

OTHER BRAND NAMES: Nifediac CC (Teva) - Afeditab CR (Watson)

THERAPEUTIC CLASS: Calcium channel blocker (dihydropyridine)

INDICATIONS: Treatment of HTN alone or in combination with other antihypertensive agents.

DOSAGE: *Adults:* Initial: 30mg qd. Titrate: Over 7-14 days. Base upward titration on therapeutic efficacy and safety. Usual: 30-60mg qd. Max: 90mg qd. Elderly: Start at low end of dosing range.

HOW SUPPLIED: Tab, Extended-Release: (Adalat CC) 30mg, 60mg, 90mg, (Afeditab CR) 30mg, 60mg, (Nifediac CC) 30mg, 60mg, 90mg

CONTRAINDICATIONS: (Adalat CC) Concomitant use with strong P450 inducers (eg, rifampin); cardiogenic shock.

WARNINGS/PRECAUTIONS: May cause hypotension; monitor BP initially or with titration. May increase frequency, duration, and/or severity of angina or acute myocardial infarction (MI) with severe obstructive coronary artery disease (CAD) upon starting or at time of dosage increases. May increase risk of congestive heart failure (CHF), especially with tight aortic stenosis or β-blockers. Peripheral edema may occur; rule out peripheral edema caused by left ventricular dysfunction if HTN is complicated by CHF. Transient elevated liver enzymes, cholestasis with or without jaundice, and allergic hepatitis reported (rare). Positive direct Coomb's test reported.

Elevated BUN and SrCr reported with chronic renal insufficiency. Caution with renal/hepatic impairment and in elderly. (Adalat CC) Reduced clearance in cirrhosis. Careful monitoring and dose reduction may be necessary; initiate lowest dose possible. Contains lactose; avoid with hereditary galactose intolerance problems, Lapp lactase deficiency, and glucose-galactose malabsorption. (Nifediac CC [90mg]) Contains tartrazine; may cause allergic type reactions, including bronchial asthma, frequently seen in patients with aspirin hypersensitivity.

ADVERSE REACTIONS: Peripheral edema, headache, flushing, heat sensation, dizziness, fatigue, asthenia, nausea, constipation.

INTERACTIONS: See Contraindications. Impacts exposure with drugs known to either inhibit or induce CYP450 3A4 system. β-blockers may increase risk of CHF, severe hypotension, or angina exacerbation; avoid abrupt β-blocker withdrawal. Caution in patients already taking drugs that are known to lower BP. Possible hypotension with fentanyl. Enhanced hypotensive effect with benazepril and timolol. Increased exposure with CYP3A inhibitors (eg, ketoconazole, erythromycin, grapefruit, nefazodone, fluoxetine, verapamil, amprenavir); monitor BP and consider dose adjustment. Increased exposure with valproic acid; monitor BP and consider dose adjustment. Increased levels with quinidine and diltiazem. Avoid use with strong CYP3A inducers (eg, rifampin, rifabutin, phenobarbital, phenytoin, carbamazepine, St. John's wort). Avoid with grapefruit juice; stop intake ≥3 days prior to therapy. Monitor blood glucose level and consider dose adjustment with acarbose. May increase PT with coumarin anticoagulants. May increase plasma levels of digoxin. Increased plasma levels and absorption of metformin. May increase exposure of tacrolimus; monitor blood levels and consider dose reduction. May decrease doxazosin levels; monitor BP and reduce dose. Increased levels with cimetidine, quinupristin/dalfopristin; monitor BP and reduce dose. Increased plasma concentrations with cisapride. (Adalat CC) May increase the BP-lowering effects of diuretics, PDE5 inhibitors, and α-methyldopa. Coadministration with IV magnesium sulfate in pregnant women may cause excessive fall in BP.

PREGNANCY: Category C, not for use in nursing.

MECHANISM OF ACTION: Calcium channel blocker; inhibits the transmembrane influx of calcium ions into vascular smooth muscle and cardiac muscle. Involves peripheral arterial vasodilation and reduction in peripheral vascular resistance, resulting in reduced arterial blood pressure.

PHARMACOKINETICS: Absorption: Complete; absolute bioavailability (84-89%); C_{max}=115ng/mL (90mg); T_{max}=2.5-5 hrs. **Distribution:** Plasma protein binding (92-98%); found in breast milk. **Metabolism:** Liver via CYP3A4. **Elimination:** Urine (60-80%, metabolite), (<0.1%, unchanged); feces (metabolite); $T_{1/2}$=7 hrs.

NURSING CONSIDERATIONS

Assessment: Assess for severity of HTN, CHF, hepatic/renal impairment, pregnancy/nursing status, drug hypersensitivity, or any other conditions where treatment is contraindicated or cautioned and for possible drug interactions.

Monitoring: Monitor for CHF, hypotension, cholestasis with/without jaundice, allergic hepatitis, peripheral edema, angina, MI, hemolytic anemia, allergic reactions and bronchial asthma. Monitor patients with cirrhosis. Carefully monitor vital signs during initial administration and titration. Monitor LFTs. Monitor BUN and SrCr in patients with chronic renal insufficiency.

Patient Counseling: Inform about potential benefits/risks of therapy. Swallow whole; do not chew, crush, or divide. Take on empty stomach. Do not take with grapefruit juice. Notify physician if pregnant/nursing and if any adverse reactions occur. (Afeditab CR) Advise patients that empty matrix "ghost" (tab) may pass in the stool and that this is normal.

Administration: Oral route. Swallow whole, not bitten or divided. Take on empty stomach. **Storage:** <30°C (86°F). (Nifediac CC): 25°C (77°F); excursions permitted to 15-30°C (59-86°F). Protect from light and moisture.

ADCETRIS

RX

brentuximab vedotin (Seattle Genetics)

| JC virus infection resulting in progressive multifocal leukoencephalopathy (PML) and death may occur. |

THERAPEUTIC CLASS: CD30-directed antibody-drug conjugate

INDICATIONS: Treatment of Hodgkin lymphoma after failure of autologous stem cell transplant (ASCT) or after failure of at least two prior multi-agent chemotherapy regimens in patients who are not ASCT candidates. Treatment of systemic anaplastic large cell lymphoma after failure of at least one prior multi-agent chemotherapy regimen.

DOSAGE: *Adults:* Usual: 1.8mg/kg as IV infusion over 30 min q3 weeks. Continue treatment until max of 16 cycles, disease progression, or unacceptable toxicity. Patients ≥100kg: Calculate based on a weight of 100kg. Peripheral Neuropathy: Use a combination of dose delay and reduction to 1.2mg/kg. Grade 2 or 3 Neuropathy: Hold until neuropathy improves to Grade 1 or baseline, then restart at 1.2mg/kg. Grade 4 Neuropathy: D/C therapy. Neutropenia: Manage by dose delays and reductions. Grade 3 or 4 Neutropenia: Hold until resolution to baseline or Grade 2 or lower. Consider growth factor support for subsequent cycles. Recurrent Grade 4 Neutropenia Despite Growth Factor Support: D/C or reduce dose to 1.2mg/kg.

HOW SUPPLIED: Inj: 50mg

CONTRAINDICATIONS: Concomitant bleomycin due to pulmonary toxicity.

WARNINGS/PRECAUTIONS: Do not administer as IV push or bolus. Peripheral neuropathy (sensory and motor) reported; may require a delay, change in dose, or d/c. Infusion-related reactions, including anaphylaxis reported; d/c and institute appropriate therapy if infusion reaction occurs. Premedicate if experienced a prior infusion-related reaction. Prolonged severe neutropenia may occur; monitor CBC prior to each dose, and monitor frequently with Grade 3 or 4 neutropenia. Tumor lysis syndrome may occur; monitor closely and take appropriate measures. Hold dosing for any suspected case of PML and d/c if diagnosis is confirmed. Stevens-Johnson syndrome (SJS) reported; d/c and administer appropriate therapy if SJS occurs. May cause fetal harm.

ADVERSE REACTIONS: Neutropenia, peripheral sensory neuropathy, anemia, fatigue, upper respiratory tract infection, N/V, pyrexia, diarrhea, rash, thrombocytopenia, pain, abdominal pain, cough.

INTERACTIONS: See Contraindications. May increase exposure of ketoconazole to monomethyl auristatin E (MMAE). Monitor closely for adverse reactions when given concomitantly with strong CYP3A4 inhibitors. Rifampin may decrease exposure to MMAE.

PREGNANCY: Category D, not for nursing.

MECHANISM OF ACTION: CD30-directed antibody drug conjugate (ADC); binds ADC to CD30-expressing cells, followed by internalization of ADC-CD30 complex, and release of MMAE via proteolytic cleavage. Binding of MMAE to tubulin disrupts the microtubule network within the cell, subsequently inducing cell cycle arrest and apoptotic death of the cell.

PHARMACOKINETICS: Absorption: (MMAE) T_{max}=1-3 days. **Distribution:** (MMAE) Plasma protein binding (68-82%); (ADC) V_d=6-10L. **Metabolism:** (MMAE) Via oxidation by CYP3A4/5. **Elimination:** (MMAE) Urine, feces (24%); (ADC) $T_{1/2}$=4-6 days.

NURSING CONSIDERATIONS

Assessment: Assess for history of infusion-related reactions, pregnancy/nursing status, and for possible drug interactions. Assess if tumor is rapidly proliferating and if there is high tumor burden. Obtain CBC.

Monitoring: Monitor for peripheral neuropathy, infusion reactions, tumor lysis syndrome, SJS, and PML. Monitor complete blood counts prior to each dose and perform more frequent monitoring with Grade 3 or 4 neutropenia.

Patient Counseling: Advise to contact physician if symptoms of peripheral neuropathy (eg, numbness/tingling of hands or feet, muscle weakness), an infection (eg, fever ≥100.5°F, chills, cough, pain on urination), or if an infusion reaction (eg, fever, chills, rash, or breathing problems within 24 hours of infusion) occurs. Instruct to immediately report if changes in mood/usual behavior, confusion, thinking problems, loss of memory, changes in vision, speech, or walking, decreased strength or weakness on one side of the body occur. Advise to avoid pregnancy or nursing while receiving therapy and to contact physician immediately if pregnant.

Administration: IV route. Do not mix with, or administer as an infusion with, other medicinal products. Refer to PI for preparation and administration. Use diluted sol immediately. **Storage:** 2-8°C (36-46°F). Protect from light. Reconstituted Sol: Dilute immediately or use within 24 hrs. Do not freeze. Discard any unused portion.

ADCIRCA   RX
tadalafil (Lilly)

THERAPEUTIC CLASS: Phosphodiesterase type 5 inhibitor

INDICATIONS: Treatment of pulmonary arterial hypertension (PAH) (WHO Group I) to improve exercise ability.

DOSAGE: *Adults:* 40mg qd. Mild (CrCl 51-80mL/min) or Moderate (CrCl 31-50mL/min) Renal Impairment/Coadministration in Patients on Ritonavir for ≥1 Week: Initial: 20mg qd. Titrate: May increase to 40mg qd. Mild or Moderate Hepatic Impairment (Child Pugh Class A or B): Initial: 20mg qd. Coadministration of Ritonavir in Patients on Tadalafil: Stop tadalafil ≥24 hrs before ritonavir initiation. After ≥1 week following ritonavir initiation, resume tadalafil at 20mg qd. Titrate: May increase to 40mg qd.

HOW SUPPLIED: Tab: 20mg

CONTRAINDICATIONS: Regular or intermittent use with any form of organic nitrate.

WARNINGS/PRECAUTIONS: Seek immediate medical attention if anginal chest pain, sudden vision loss, decreased or loss of hearing, or erection >4 hrs occurs following use. Transient decrease in BP reported; caution with underlying cardiovascular disease (CVD). Patients with severely impaired autonomic control of BP or left ventricular outflow obstruction may be more sensitive to vasodilatory effects. May worsen cardiovascular (CV) status with pulmonary veno-occlusive disease (PVOD); not recommended with veno-occlusive disease. Avoid use in severe renal impairment (CrCl <30mL/min or on hemodialysis) and hepatic impairment (Child-Pugh Class C). Not recommended with hereditary degenerative retinal disorders (eg, retinal pigmentosa). Non-arteritic anterior ischemic optic neuropathy (NAION) reported. Rare reports of prolonged erections (>4 hrs) and priapism; caution in conditions predisposing to priapism (eg, sickle cell anemia, multiple myeloma, leukemia) or with anatomical deformation of the penis (eg, angulation, cavernosal fibrosis, Peyronie's disease). Assess risk/benefit with bleeding disorders or significant active peptic ulceration.

ADVERSE REACTIONS: Headache, myalgia, nasopharyngitis, flushing, respiratory tract infection, pain in extremity, nausea, back pain, dyspepsia, nasal congestion.

INTERACTIONS: See Contraindications. Additive hypotensive effects with alcohol, α-adrenergic blockers (eg, doxazosin, alfuzosin, tamsulosin), vasodilators, and antihypertensives (eg, amlodipine, angiotensin II receptor blockers, bendroflumethiazide, enalapril, metoprolol). Increased exposure with ritonavir, other HIV protease inhibitors, ketoconazole, and other CYP3A inhibitors. Decreased exposure with rifampin, bosentan, and other CYP3A inducers. Avoid use during initiation of ritonavir. Avoid use with potent CYP3A inhibitors (eg, ketoconazole, itraconazole) and chronic potent CYP3A inducers (eg, rifampin). Increased exposure and levels of ethinyl estradiol. Reduced rate of absorption with antacids (magnesium hydroxide/aluminum hydroxide). Avoid use with Cialis or other PDE5 inhibitors. A small increase in HR seen with theophylline. May increase risk of NAION with smoking.

PREGNANCY: Category B, caution in nursing.

MECHANISM OF ACTION: Phosphodiesterase type 5 (PDE5) inhibitor; increases the concentrations of cGMP, resulting in relaxation of pulmonary vascular smooth muscle cells and vasodilation of the pulmonary vascular bed.

PHARMACOKINETICS: Absorption: T_{max}=2-8 hrs. **Distribution:** V_d=77L; plasma protein binding (94%). **Metabolism:** Via CYP3A to catechol metabolite, which undergoes extensive methylation and glucuronidation; methylcatechol glucuronide (major metabolite). **Elimination:** Feces (61%), Urine (36%); $T_{1/2}$=35 hrs.

NURSING CONSIDERATIONS

Assessment: Assess for CVD, BP, renal/hepatic function, hereditary degenerative retinal disorders, conditions that may predispose to priapism, bleeding disorders, active peptic ulceration, hypersensitivity to drug, nitrite use, pregnancy/nursing status, and possible drug interactions.

Monitoring: Monitor for signs/symptoms of anginal chest pain, vision or hearing loss, pulmonary edema, NAION, prolonged erections >4 hrs, and priapism. Monitor BP.

Patient Counseling: Inform that any use of organic nitrates is contraindicated, may take drug with or without food, and that drug is also marketed as Cialis for erectile dysfunction; instruct to avoid taking Cialis or other PDE5 inhibitors. Advise to seek immediate medical attention if sudden loss of vision in one or both eyes and sudden decrease or loss of hearing develop, or if erection lasts for >4 hrs.

Administration: Oral route. Dividing dose over the course of the day is not recommended.
Storage: 25°C (77°F); excursions permitted to 15-30°C (59-86°F).

ADDERALL
amphetamine salt combo (Shire)

> High potential for abuse; avoid prolonged use. Misuse of amphetamine may cause sudden death and serious cardiovascular adverse events.

THERAPEUTIC CLASS: Sympathomimetic amine

INDICATIONS: Treatment of attention-deficit disorder with hyperactivity (ADHD) and narcolepsy.

DOSAGE: *Adults:* Narcolepsy: Initial: 10mg/day. Titrate: May increase by 10mg/day every week. Usual: 5-60mg/day. Give 1st dose upon awakening, and additional doses q4-6h.
Pediatrics: ADHD: 3-5 yrs: Initial: 2.5mg qd. Titrate: May increase by 2.5mg weekly. ≥6 yrs: 5mg qd-bid. May increase by 5mg weekly. Max (usual): 40mg/day. Narcolepsy: 6-12 yrs: Initial: 5mg/day. May increase by 5mg weekly. ≥12 yrs: Initial: 10mg/day. Titrate: May increase by 10mg/day every week. Usual: 5-60mg/day. Give 1st dose upon awakening, and additional doses q4-6h.

HOW SUPPLIED: Tab: 5mg*, 7.5mg*, 10mg*, 12.5mg*, 15mg*, 20mg*, 30mg* *scored

CONTRAINDICATIONS: Advanced arteriosclerosis, symptomatic cardiovascular (CV) disease, moderate to severe HTN, hyperthyroidism, glaucoma, agitated states, history of drug abuse, during or within 14 days of MAOI use.

WARNINGS/PRECAUTIONS: May exacerbate symptoms of behavior disturbance and thought disorder in psychotic patients. Caution when using stimulants to treat patients with comorbid bipolar disorder because of concern for possible induction of mixed/manic episode in such patients. Stimulants at usual doses can cause treatment emergent psychotic or manic symptoms (eg, hallucinations, delusional thinking, mania) in children and adolescents without prior history of psychotic illness. Aggressive behavior or hostility reported in clinical trials and the postmarketing experience of some medications indicated for the treatment of ADHD. Monitor growth in children. May lower convulsive threshold; d/c in presence of seizures. Visual disturbances reported with stimulant treatment. May exacerbate Tourette's syndrome and phonic or motor tics. Caution with HTN and monitor BP. Interrupt occasionally to determine if patient requires continued therapy. Sudden death reported in children with structural cardiac abnormalities; avoid with known structural cardiac abnormalities or other serious cardiac problems.

ADVERSE REACTIONS: HTN, tachycardia, palpitations, CNS overstimulation, dry mouth, GI disorders, anorexia, impotence, urticaria, rash, angioedema, anaphylaxis, Stevens-Johnson syndrome.

INTERACTIONS: GI acidifying agents (eg, guanethidine, reserpine, glutamic acid, etc.) and urinary acidifying agents (eg, ammonium chloride, etc.) decrease efficacy. MAOIs may cause hypertensive crisis. Potentiated by GI and urinary alkalinizers, propoxyphene overdose. Potentiated effects of both agents with TCAs. May delay absorption of phenytoin, ethosuximide, phenobarbital. Potentiates meperidine, norepinephrine, phenobarbital, phenytoin. Antagonized by haloperidol, chlorpromazine, lithium. Antagonizes adrenergic blockers, antihistamines, antihypertensives, veratrum alkaloids (antihypertensive). Avoid coadministration with alkalinizing agents (eg, antacids).

PREGNANCY: Category C, not for use in nursing.

MECHANISM OF ACTION: CNS stimulant; thought to block reuptake of norepinephrine and dopamine into presynaptic neuron and increase release of these monoamines into extraneuronal space.

PHARMACOKINETICS: Absorption: T_{max}=approximately 3 hrs (fasted). **Metabolism**: CYP2D6 (oxidation): 4-hydroxy-amphetamine and norephedrine. **Elimination**: Urine, $T_{1/2}$=9.77-11 hrs (d-amphetamine), 11.5-13.8 hrs (l-amphetamine).

NURSING CONSIDERATIONS

Assessment: Assess for agitation, glaucoma, tics, family history of Tourette's syndrome, CV conditions (eg, severe HTN, angina pectoris, cardiac abnormalities, arrhythmias, heart failure, recent MI), hyperthyroidism or thyrotoxicosis, bipolar illness, history of drug dependence or alcoholism.

Monitoring: Monitor for cardiac abnormalities, exacerbations of behavior disturbances and thought disorder, bipolar illness, aggression, seizures, and visual disturbances. Periodic monitoring of CBC, differential and platelet count, LFTs. Monitor height and weight in children.

Patient Counseling: Inform about risks of treatment, appropriate use, drug abuse/dependence. Caution while operating machinery/driving.

Administration: Oral route. **Storage**: 20-25°C (68-77°F).

ADDERALL XR `CII`
amphetamine salt combo (Shire)

> High potential for abuse; prolonged use may lead to drug dependence. Misuse may cause sudden death and serious cardiovascular (CV) adverse events.

THERAPEUTIC CLASS: Sympathomimetic amine

INDICATIONS: Treatment of attention-deficit hyperactivity disorder.

DOSAGE: *Adults:* Individualize dose. Amphetamine-Naive/Switching from Another Medication: 20mg qam. Currently on Amphetamine (Immediate-Release [IR]): Switch to ER at the same total daily dose, qd. Titrate at weekly intervals PRN.
Pediatrics: Individualize dose. Currently on Amphetamine (IR): Switch to ER at the same total daily dose, qd. Titrate at weekly intervals PRN. Amphetamine-Naive/Switching from Another Medication: 13-17 yrs: Initial: 10mg qam. Titrate: May increase to 20mg/day after 1 week if symptoms not controlled. 6-12 yrs: Initial: 10mg qam or 5mg qam when lower initial dose is appropriate. Titrate: Adjust daily dosage in increments of 5mg or 10mg at weekly intervals. Max: 30mg/day.

HOW SUPPLIED: Cap, Extended-Release (ER): 5mg, 10mg, 15mg, 20mg, 25mg, 30mg

CONTRAINDICATIONS: Advanced arteriosclerosis, symptomatic CV disease, moderate to severe HTN, hyperthyroidism, glaucoma, agitated states, history of drug abuse, during or within 14 days of MAOI use.

WARNINGS/PRECAUTIONS: Sudden death, stroke, myocardial infarction (MI) reported; avoid with known serious structural cardiac and heart rhythm abnormalities, cardiomyopathy, coronary artery disease, or other serious cardiac problems. May cause modest increase in BP and HR; caution with conditions that could be compromised by BP or HR elevation (eg, preexisting HTN, heart failure, recent MI, or ventricular arrhythmia). Promptly evaluate when symptoms suggestive of cardiac disease develop. May exacerbate symptoms of behavior disturbance and thought disorder in patients with preexisting psychotic disorder. Caution in patients with comorbid bipolar disorder; may cause induction of mixed/manic episode. May cause treatment-emergent psychotic/manic symptoms in children and adolescents without a prior history of psychotic illness or mania; d/c may be appropriate if symptoms occur. Aggressive behavior or hostility reported; monitor for appearance or worsening. May lower convulsive threshold; d/c if seizure develops. Difficulties with accommodation and blurring of vision reported. Exacerbation of motor and phonic tics, and Tourette's syndrome reported. May slow growth rate in children; may need to d/c if patients are not growing or gaining weight as expected. Prescribe or dispense the least amount feasible at one time to minimize possibility of overdosage.

ADVERSE REACTIONS: Dry mouth, loss of appetite, insomnia, headache, abdominal pain, weight loss, emotional lability, agitation, anxiety, N/V, dizziness, tachycardia, nervousness.

INTERACTIONS: See Contraindications. GI acidifying agents (eg, guanethidine, reserpine, glutamic acid hydrochloride, ascorbic acid) and urinary acidifying agents (eg, ammonium chloride, sodium acid phosphate, methenamine salts) may lower blood levels and decrease efficacy. Avoid with GI alkalinizing agents (eg, sodium bicarbonate); may increase absorption. Urinary alkalinizing agents (eg, acetazolamide, some thiazides) may potentiate effects. May reduce CV effects of adrenergic blockers. May counteract sedative effects of antihistamines. May antagonize effect of antihypertensives. May inhibit hypotensive effect of veratrum alkaloids. May delay absorption of phenytoin, ethosuximide, phenobarbital. May enhance activity of TCAs or sympathomimetic agents. May potentiate effects of meperidine. Chlorpromazine and haloperidol may inhibit central stimulant effects. Lithium carbonate may inhibit anorectic and stimulatory effects. May enhance the adrenergic effect of norepinephrine. Use in cases of propoxyphene overdose may potentiate CNS stimulation and cause fatal convulsions. Monitor for changes in clinical effect with proton pump inhibitors. Caution with other sympathomimetic drugs.

PREGNANCY: Category C, not for use in nursing.

MECHANISM OF ACTION: Sympathomimetic amine; mechanism unknown. Thought to block the reuptake of norepinephrine and dopamine into the presynaptic neuron and increase the release of these monoamines into the extraneuronal space.

PHARMACOKINETICS: Absorption: T_{max}=7 hrs. **Distribution:** Found in breast milk. **Metabolism**: CYP2D6 (oxidation); 4-hydroxy-amphetamine and norephedrine (metabolites). **Elimination**: Urine (30-40%); (20mg single dose) d-amphetamine: $T_{1/2}$=10 hrs (adults), 11 hrs (13-17 yrs), 9 hrs (6-12 yrs). l-amphetamine: $T_{1/2}$=13 hrs (adults), 13-14 hrs (13-17 yrs), 11 hrs (6-12 yrs).

NURSING CONSIDERATIONS

Assessment: Assess for psychiatric history (eg, family history of suicide, bipolar disorder, depression, drug abuse, or alcoholism), advanced arteriosclerosis, CV disease, moderate to severe HTN, agitation, glaucoma, tics or Tourette's syndrome, seizure, hyperthyroidism, hypersensitivity or idiosyncratic reactions to other sympathomimetic amines, pregnancy/nursing status, and possible drug interactions.

Monitoring: Monitor for CV abnormalities, exacerbations of behavior disturbances and thought disorder, psychotic or manic symptoms, aggressive behavior, hostility, seizures, visual disturbances, exacerbation of Tourette's syndrome, and for phonic or motor tics exacerbation. Monitor BP and HR. Monitor height and weight in children.

Patient Counseling: Inform about benefits and risks of treatment, appropriate use, and drug abuse/dependence. Advise about serious CV risks (eg, sudden death, MI, stroke, and HTN). Inform that treatment-emergent psychotic or manic symptoms may occur. Advise parents or guardians of pediatric patients that growth should be monitored during treatment. Notify physician if pregnant/planning to become pregnant and to avoid breastfeeding. Instruct to use caution while operating machinery/vehicles.

Administration: Oral route. Take caps whole or sprinkle entire contents on applesauce; do not chew beads. **Storage:** 25°C (77°F); excursions permitted to 15-30°C (59-86°F).

ADENOCARD   RX
adenosine (Astellas)

THERAPEUTIC CLASS: Endogenous nucleoside

INDICATIONS: Conversion to sinus rhythm (SR) of paroxysmal supraventricular tachycardia (PSVT), including that associated with accessory bypass tracts (Wolff-Parkinson-White syndrome).

DOSAGE: *Adults:* Initial: 6mg rapid IV bolus over 1-2 sec. If not converted to SR within 1-2 min, give 12mg rapid IV bolus; may give second 12mg dose if needed. Max: 12mg/dose.
Pediatrics: <50kg: Initial: 0.05-0.1mg/kg rapid IV bolus. If not converted to SR within 1-2 min, give additional bolus doses, incrementally increasing amount by 0.05-0.1mg/kg. Continue process until SR or a max single dose of 0.3mg/kg is used. ≥50kg: Initial: 6mg rapid IV bolus over 1-2 sec. If not converted to SR within 1-2 min, give 12mg rapid IV bolus; may give second 12mg dose if needed. Max: 12mg/dose.

HOW SUPPLIED: Inj: 3mg/mL [2mL, 4mL]

CONTRAINDICATIONS: 2nd- or 3rd-degree atrioventricular (AV) block, and sinus node disease (eg, sinus syndrome or symptomatic bradycardia), except with functioning artificial pacemaker.

WARNINGS/PRECAUTIONS: May produce short-lasting 1st-, 2nd-, 3rd-degree heart block; institute appropriate therapy as needed. Do not give additional doses if high level block develops on 1st dose. Transient or prolonged asystole, respiratory alkalosis, ventricular fibrillation reported. New arrhythmias may appear on ECG at time of conversion. Caution with obstructive lung disease not associated with bronchoconstriction (eg, emphysema, bronchitis). Avoid with bronchoconstriction/bronchospasm (eg, asthma). D/C if severe respiratory difficulties develop. Caution in elderly. Does not convert atrial fibrillation/atrial flutter (A-fib/flutter), or ventricular tachycardia to normal SR. A transient modest slowing of ventricular response may occur immediately following administration in the presence of A-fib/flutter.

ADVERSE REACTIONS: Arrhythmias, facial flushing, dyspnea/SOB, chest pressure, nausea.

INTERACTIONS: Antagonized by methylxanthines (eg, theophylline, caffeine); may need larger dose. Potentiated by nucleoside transport inhibitors (eg, dipyridamole); use lower dose. Potential additive or synergistic depressant effects on the sinoatrial and AV nodes with other cardioactve drugs (eg, β-adrenergic blockers, quinidine, and calcium channel blockers [CCBs]). Caution when used in combination with digoxin/verapamil; ventricular fibrillation reported with digoxin, verapamil, and digitalis. Possible higher degrees of heart block with carbamazepine.

PREGNANCY: Category C, safety in nursing not known.

MECHANISM OF ACTION: Endogenous nucleoside; slows conduction time through AV node, can interrupt reentry pathways through the AV node, and can restore normal sinus rhythm in patients with PSVT, including PSVT associated with Wolff-Parkinson-White syndrome.

PHARMACOKINETICS: Metabolism: Rapid (intracellular); via phosphorylation or deamination. **Elimination:** $T_{1/2}$ =<10 sec (extracellular).

NURSING CONSIDERATIONS

Assessment: Assess for A-fib/flutter, ventricular tachycardia, presence of functioning pacemaker, AV block, sinus node disease, arrhythmias, obstructive lung disease, bronchoconstriction/bronchospasm, hypersensitivity to drug, pregnancy status, and possible drug interactions. Obtain baseline ECG and vital signs.

Monitoring: Monitor for heart block, bradycardia, ventricular fibrillation, asystole, and arrhythmias, respiratory alkalosis/difficulties, or hypersensitivity reactions. Monitor ECG and vital signs.

Patient Counseling: Inform about benefits/risks of therapy. Advise to promptly report any adverse reactions to physician.

Administration: IV route. Administer by rapid IV bolus, either directly into a vein, or given as close to the patient as possible if via IV line. Follow each bolus with a rapid saline flush. Inspect visually for particulate matter and discoloration prior to administration. **Storage:** 15-30°C (59-86°F). Do not refrigerate. Dissolve crystals by warming to room temperature if crystallization occurs. Discard unused portion. Do not break by hand, recap, or purposely bend needles.

ADRENACLICK   RX
epinephrine (Sciele)

THERAPEUTIC CLASS: Sympathomimetic catecholamine

INDICATIONS: Emergency treatment of severe allergic reactions (Type 1) including anaphylaxis to stinging insects (eg, order *Hymenoptera*, which includes bees, wasps, hornets, yellow jackets and fire ants), and biting insects (eg, triatoma, mosquitos), allergen immunotherapy, foods, drugs, diagnostic testing substances (eg, radiocontrast media), and other allergens, as well as anaphylaxis to unknown substances (idiopathic anaphylaxis) or exercise-induced anaphylaxis. For immediate administration with history of anaphylactic reactions.

DOSAGE: *Adults:* 15-30kg: Inject 0.15mg IM/SQ into the anterolateral aspect of the thigh. ≥30kg: Inject 0.3mg IM/SQ into the anterolateral aspect of the thigh.

Pediatrics: 15-30kg: Inject 0.15mg IM/SQ into the anterolateral aspect of the thigh. ≥30kg: Inject 0.3mg IM/SQ into the anterolateral aspect of the thigh.

HOW SUPPLIED: Inj: 1mg/mL [0.15mg, 0.3mg]

WARNINGS/PRECAUTIONS: Avoid injecting into the hands, feet, or buttocks; may result in loss of blood flow if accidentally injected into these areas. Avoid IV use; may result in cerebral hemorrhage due to sharp rise in BP if accidentally injected. Caution with cardiac arrhythmias, coronary artery or heart disease, or HTN. May precipitate/aggravate angina pectoris and produce ventricular arrhythmias in patients with coronary insufficiency or ischemic heart disease. High risk of developing adverse reactions with hyperthyroidism, CV disease, HTN, DM, elderly, and pregnant women. Contains sodium bisulfite; may cause allergic-type reactions including anaphylactic symptoms or life-threatening asthmatic episodes in certain susceptible persons.

ADVERSE REACTIONS: Anxiety, apprehensiveness, restlessness, tremor, weakness, dizziness, sweating, palpitations, pallor, N/V, headache, respiratory difficulties.

INTERACTIONS: Monitor for cardiac arrhythmias with anti-arrhythmics, cardiac glycosides and diuretics. Effects may be potentiated by tricyclic antidepressants, MAOIs, sodium levothyroxine, and certain antihistamines (eg, chlorpheniramine, tripelennamine, diphenhydramine). Cardiostimulating and bronchodilating effects antagonized by β-adrenergic blockers (eg, propranolol). Vasoconstricting and hypertensive effects antagonized by α-adrenergic blockers (eg, phentolamine). Ergot alkaloids and phenothiazines may reverse pressor effects.

PREGNANCY: Category C, caution in nursing.

MECHANISM OF ACTION: Sympathomimetic catecholamine; acts on α-adrenergic receptors by lessening the vasodilation and increasing vascular permeability that occurs during anaphylactic reaction. Acts on β-adrenergic receptors causing bronchial smooth muscle relaxation that helps alleviate bronchospasm, wheezing, and dyspnea that may occur during anaphylaxis.

NURSING CONSIDERATIONS

Assessment: Assess for arrhythmias, coronary artery or organic heart disease, HTN, hyperthyroidism, CV disease, DM, Parkinson's disease, pregnancy/nursing status, and possible drug interactions.

Monitoring: Monitor BP, HR, blood glucose, signs of cerebral hemorrhage, ventricular arrhythmia, HTN, anginal pain, and other adverse reactions.

Patient Counseling: Inform about side effects of therapy (eg, increased pulse rate, sensation of a more forceful heartbeat, palpitations, throbbing headache, pallor, feelings of overstimulation, anxiety, weakness, shakiness, dizziness, or nausea). Avoid injecting into the hands, feet, or buttocks and to avoid IV route. Inform physician if accidental injection occur into these areas. Inspect the solution for particulate matter and discoloration. Inform that patients may develop more severe/persistent effects if with HTN/hyperthyroidism; could experience angina if with coronary artery disease; may increase blood glucose if with diabetes; and may worsen symptoms of Parkinson's disease.

Administration: SQ or IM route. Inject only at the anterolateral aspect of the thigh. **Storage:** 20°-25°C (68°-77°F); excursions permitted to 15°-30°C (59°-86°F). Light sensitive; store in the carrying case provided. Protect from light and freezing. Do not refrigerate. Discard if discolored, cloudy, or has particulate matter. The remaining volume left after the fixed dose should not be further administered and should be discarded.

ADVAIR   RX
fluticasone propionate - salmeterol (GlaxoSmithKline)

> Long-acting β$_2$-adrenergic agonists (LABA), such as salmeterol, increase the risk of asthma-related death. LABAs may increase the risk of asthma-related hospitalization in pediatrics and adolescents. Use only for patients not adequately controlled on a long-term asthma control medication (eg, inhaled corticosteroid) or whose disease severity clearly warrants initiation of treatment with both an inhaled corticosteroid and a LABA. Do not use if asthma is adequately controlled on low- or medium-dose inhaled corticosteroids.

THERAPEUTIC CLASS: Corticosteroid/beta$_2$ agonist

INDICATIONS: Treatment of asthma in patients ≥4 yrs. (250/50) Maintenance treatment of airflow obstruction in patients with chronic obstructive pulmonary disease (COPD), including chronic bronchitis and/or emphysema, and to reduce exacerbations of COPD in patients with history of exacerbations.

DOSAGE: *Adults:* Asthma: Initial: Based upon asthma severity. Usual: 1 inh bid (am/pm q12h). Max: 500/50 bid. Increase to higher strength if response to initial dose is inadequate after 2 weeks. COPD: (250/50): 1 inh bid (am/pm q12h). If asthma symptoms or SOB occurs between doses, use short-acting β$_2$-agonist for immediate relief.
Pediatrics: ≥12 yrs: Asthma: Initial: Based upon asthma severity. Usual: 1 inh bid (am/pm q12h). Max: 500/50 bid. Increase to higher strength if response to initial dose is inadequate after

2 weeks. If asthma symptoms arise between doses, use short-acting β₂-agonist for immediate relief. 4-11 yrs: (100/50): Not Controlled on Inhaled Corticosteroid: 1 inh bid (am/pm q12h).

HOW SUPPLIED: Disk: (Fluticasone Propionate-Salmeterol) (100/50) 100mcg-50mcg/inh, (250/50) 250mcg-50mcg/inh, (500/50) 500mcg-50mcg/inh

CONTRAINDICATIONS: Primary treatment of status asthmaticus or other acute episodes of asthma or COPD where intensive measures are required; severe hypersensitivity to milk proteins.

WARNINGS/PRECAUTIONS: Should not be initiated during rapidly deteriorating or potentially life-threatening episodes of asthma or COPD. Increased use of inhaled, short-acting β2-agonists (SABA) is a marker of deteriorating asthma; re-evaluate and reassess treatment regimen. Should not be used for relief of acute symptoms; use SABA to relieve acute symptoms. Should not be used more often or at higher doses than recommended or in conjunction with other medications containing LABA; cardiovascular (CV) effects and fatalities reported with excessive use. Candida albicans infections of mouth and pharynx reported; treat and/or d/c if needed. Lower respiratory tract infections (eg, pneumonia) reported in patients with COPD. Increased susceptibility to infections (eg, chickenpox, measles), may lead to serious/fatal course; if exposed consider prophylaxis/treatment. Caution with tuberculosis (TB), untreated systemic fungal, bacterial, viral or parasitic infections, and ocular herpes simplex. Deaths due to adrenal insufficiency reported with transfer from systemic to inhaled corticosteroids (ICS); if oral corticosteroids required wean slowly from systemic steroid use after transferring to ICS. Transfer from systemic to inhalation therapy may unmask allergic conditions (eg, rhinitis, conjunctivitis). May produce paradoxical bronchospasm; d/c immediately, treat, and institute alternative therapy. Upper airway symptoms reported. Decreases in bone mineral density (BMD) reported; caution with major risk factors for decreased bone mineral content including chronic use of drugs that can reduce bone mass (eg, anticonvulsants, corticosteroids). May cause reduction in growth velocity in pediatrics. Glaucoma, increased intraocular pressure, cataracts, rare cases of systemic eosinophilic conditions and vasculitis consistent with Churg-Strauss syndrome reported. Observe for systemic corticosteroid effects; if hypercorticism and adrenal suppression appear reduce dose slowly. Immediate hypersensitivity reactions, hypokalemia, and dose-related changes in blood glucose and/or serum K⁺ may occur. ECG changes (eg, flattening of T wave, QTc interval prolongation, and ST segment depression) reported. Caution with CV disorders, convulsive disorders, thyrotoxicosis, hepatic disease, diabetes mellitus, those who are unusually responsive to sympathomimetic amines, and in elderly.

ADVERSE REACTIONS: Upper respiratory tract infection/inflammation, pharyngitis, dysphonia, oral candidiasis, bronchitis, cough, headache, N/V, pneumonia, throat irritation, viral respiratory infection, musculoskeletal pain.

INTERACTIONS: Avoid with strong CYP3A4 inhibitors (eg, ritonavir, atazanavir, clarithromycin, indinavir, itraconazole, nefazodone, nelfinavir, saquinavir, ketoconazole, telithromycin). Avoid use with other medications containing LABAs. Salmeterol: Extreme caution with TCAs or MAOIs, or within 2 weeks of d/c such products. Use with β-blockers may produce severe bronchospasm; if needed, consider cardioselective β-blocker with caution. ECG changes and/or hypokalemia that may result from non-K⁺ sparing diuretics (eg, loop/thiazide diuretics) can be acutely worsened; use with caution. May increase levels, increase HR, and prolong QTc interval with erythromycin. May increase exposure of with ketoconazole; combination may be associated with QTc prolongation. Fluticasone: May increase exposure and reduce cortisol levels with ritonavir and ketoconazole.

PREGNANCY: Category C, not for use in nursing.

MECHANISM OF ACTION: Fluticasone: Corticosteroid with anti-inflammatory activity. Asthma: inhibits multiple cell types (eg, mast cells, eosinophils, basophils, lymphocytes, macrophages, neutrophils) and mediator production or secretion (eg, histamine, eicosanoids, leukotrienes, cytokines) involved in the asthmatic response. COPD: Not well defined. Salmeterol: Selective LABA; stimulates intracellular adenyl cyclase, which catalyzes conversion of ATP to cAMP, producing relaxation of bronchial smooth muscle and inhibits mediator release of immediate hypersensitivity from cells, especially from mast cells.

PHARMACOKINETICS: Absorption: Administration in healthy, asthmatic, and COPD patients resulted in different pharmacokinetic parameters. **Distribution:** Fluticasone: V_d=4.2L/kg; plasma protein binding (91%). Salmeterol: Plasma protein binding (96%). **Metabolism:** Fluticasone: Liver via CYP3A4; 17 β-carboxylic acid derivative (metabolite). Salmeterol: Liver, via CYP3A4 to α-hydroxysalmeterol (metabolite). **Elimination:** Fluticasone: (PO) Urine (<5%); (Inh) $T_{1/2}$=5.6 hrs. Salmeterol (PO): Urine (25%), feces (60%); $T_{1/2}$=5.5 hrs.

NURSING CONSIDERATIONS

Assessment: Assess for hypersensitivity to milk proteins, acute asthma/COPD episodes, status asthmaticus, rapidly deteriorating asthma or COPD, risk factors for decreased bone mineral content, CV disease, convulsive disorder, thyrotoxicosis, DM, history of increased intraocular pressure (IOP), glaucoma, cataracts, active or quiescent pulmonary TB, ocular herpes simplex, untreated systemic infections, hepatic disease, pregnancy/nursing status, and possible drug interactions. Obtain baseline serum K⁺, blood glucose levels, BMD, eye exam, and lung function prior to therapy.

Monitoring: Monitor for localized oral *Candida albicans* infections, upper airway symptoms, worsening or acutely deteriorating asthma, development of glaucoma, increased IOP, CV effects, CNS effects, cataracts, hypercorticism, adrenal suppression, paradoxical bronchospasm, eosinophilic conditions, hypokalemia, hyperglycemia, and hypersensitivity reactions. Monitor ECG changes, BMD, and lung function periodically. Perform periodic eye exams. Monitor growth in pediatric patients. Monitor for lower respiratory tract infections (eg, pneumonia) in patients with COPD.

Patient Counseling: Inform about the risk and benefits of therapy. Advise that medication is not for the relief of acute asthma symptoms or exacerbations of COPD and extra doses should not be used for this purpose. Inform not to d/c unless directed by physician and on administration instructions. Advise to rinse mouth after inhalation and to spit water out; do not swallow water. Instruct to avoid exposure to chickenpox or measles; consult physician if exposed, if existing TB infections or ocular herpes simplex symptoms do not improve or worsen, or if hypersensitivity reactions occur.

Administration: Oral inhalation. Rinse mouth with water without swallowing after inhalation. Refer to PI for further administration instructions. **Storage:** 20-25°C (68-77°F). Keep in a dry place, away from direct heat or sunlight. Discard 1 month after removal from pouch or when indicator reads "0," whichever comes first.

ADVAIR HFA RX

fluticasone propionate - salmeterol (GlaxoSmithKline)

> Long-acting β₂-adrenergic agonists (LABA), such as salmeterol, increase the risk of asthma-related death. LABAs may increase the risk of asthma-related hospitalization in pediatrics and adolescents. Use only for patients not adequately controlled on a long-term asthma control medication (eg, inhaled corticosteroid) or whose disease severity clearly warrants initiation of treatment with both an inhaled corticosteroid and a LABA. Do not use if asthma is adequately controlled on low- or medium-dose inhaled corticosteroids.

THERAPEUTIC CLASS: Corticosteroid/beta₂ agonist

INDICATIONS: Treatment of asthma in patients ≥12 yrs.

DOSAGE: *Adults:* Initial: Based upon patient's current asthma therapy. Usual: 2 inh bid (am/pm q12h). Increase to higher strength if response to initial dose inadequate after 2 weeks. Max: 2 inh of 230/21 bid. If symptoms arise between doses, use an inhaled short-acting β₂-agonist for immediate relief.
Pediatrics: ≥12 yrs: Initial: Based upon patient's current asthma therapy. Usual: 2 inh bid (am/pm q12h). Increase to higher strength if response to initial dose inadequate after 2 weeks. Max: 2 inh of 230/21 bid. If symptoms arise between doses, use an inhaled short-acting β₂-agonist for immediate relief.

HOW SUPPLIED: MDI: (Fluticasone Propionate-Salmeterol) (45/21) 45mcg-21mcg/inh, (115/21) 115mcg-21mcg/inh, (230/21) 230mcg-21mcg/inh [60 inhalations, 120 inhalations]

CONTRAINDICATIONS: Primary treatment of status asthmaticus or other acute episodes of asthma where intensive measures are required.

WARNINGS/PRECAUTIONS: Do not use more often or at higher doses than recommended; fatalities and prolonged QTc interval reported. Deaths due to adrenal insufficiency have occurred during and after transfer from systemic to inhaled corticosteroids. During periods of stress or a severe asthma attack, resume oral corticosteroids in patients who have withdrawn from systemic corticosteroids. Can produce paradoxical bronchospasm; d/c immediately, treat and institute alternative therapy. Immediate hypersensitivity reactions may occur. Upper airway symptoms reported. Cardiovascular (CV) effects may occur; caution with CV disorders. Transferring from systemic corticosteroid therapy may unmask conditions previously suppressed (eg, rhinitis). Increased susceptibility to infections; avoid exposure to chickenpox or measles. Caution with active or quiescent tuberculosis (TB) infection, untreated systemic infections, or ocular herpes simplex. Caution in elderly, patients with convulsive disorder or thyrotoxicosis, hepatic problems, and in those unusually responsive to sympathomimetic amines, diabetes mellitus (DM), and ketoacidosis. Systemic corticosteroid effects may occur; reduce dose slowly if such effects develop. May cause reduction in growth velocity in pediatrics. Long-term use may result in decrease of bone mineral density (BMD), glaucoma, increased intraocular pressure (IOP), and cataracts. Lower respiratory tract infections (eg, pneumonia) reported. Localized *Candida albicans* infection of the pharynx may occur. Significant changes in systolic and/or diastolic BP and pulse rate reported. May cause changes in blood glucose and serum K⁺ levels. Rare cases of eosinophilic conditions (eg, Churg-Strauss syndrome) observed.

ADVERSE REACTIONS: Upper respiratory tract infection, headache, throat irritation, musculoskeletal pain, N/V, menstruation symptoms, muscle pain, dizziness, viral GI infections, hoarseness, GI signs and symptoms, pain, intoxication hangover.

INTERACTIONS: Extreme caution with TCAs or MAOIs, or within 2 weeks of d/c such products. May produce severe bronchospasm in patients with asthma with β-blockers. Caution with cardioselective β-blockers. May increase salmeterol levels, increase heart rate, and prolong QTc interval with erythromycin. Avoid strong CYP3A4 inhibitors (eg, ketoconazole, ritonavir, atazanavir, clarithromycin, indinavir, itraconazole, nefazodone, nelfinavir, saquinavir, telithromycin). Caution with non-K⁺ sparing diuretics (eg, loop or thiazide diuretics); ECG changes, hypokalemia may result. Do not use any additional inhaled LABAs. Increased risk of decreased BMD with tobacco and chronic use of drugs which can reduce bone mass (eg, anticonvulsants, corticosteroids). D/C regular use of oral/inhaled short-acting β₂ agonists at initiation of therapy.

PREGNANCY: Category C, not for use in nursing.

MECHANISM OF ACTION: Fluticasone: Corticosteroid with anti-inflammatory activity; inhibits multiple cell types (eg, mast cells, eosinophils, basophils, lymphocytes, macrophages, neutrophils) and mediator production or secretion (eg, histamine, eicosanoids, leukotrienes, cytokines) involved in the asthmatic response. Salmeterol: LABA; stimulates intracellular adenyl cyclase, which catalyzes conversion of adenosine triphosphate (ATP) to cyclic AMP, producing relaxation of bronchial smooth muscle and inhibits mediator release of immediate hypersensitivity from cells, especially mast cells.

PHARMACOKINETICS: Absorption: Fluticasone: Absolute Bioavailability (5.3%); Salmeterol: C_{max}=150pg/mL. **Distribution:** Fluticasone: V_d=4.2L/kg; plasma protein binding (99%). Salmeterol: Plasma protein binding (96%). **Metabolism:** Fluticasone: Liver, via CYP3A4. Salmeterol: Extensive by hydroxylation. **Elimination:** Fluticasone: Feces (major), urine (<5%); $T_{1/2}$=7.8 hrs. Salmeterol: Feces (60%), urine (25%); $T_{1/2}$=5.5 hrs.

NURSING CONSIDERATIONS

Assessment: Assess for previous hypersensitivity, acute asthma episode, severe asthma, risk factors for decreased bone mineral content, recent trauma or surgery, CVD, convulsive disorder, thyrotoxicosis, DM, history of increased IOP, glaucoma, cataracts, status asthmaticus, active or quiescent pulmonary TB, ocular herpes simplex, untreated systemic infections, hepatic impairment, pregnancy/nursing status, and possible drug interactions. Obtain baseline BMD, eye exam, and lung function prior to therapy.

Monitoring: Monitor for *Candida albicans* infections, upper airway symptoms, worsening or acutely deteriorating asthma, CV effects, development of glaucoma, increased IOP, cataracts, hypercorticism, adrenal suppression, paradoxical bronchospasm, eosinophilic conditions, hypokalemia, hyperglycemia, and for hypersensitivity reactions. Monitor BMD and lung function periodically. Perform periodic eye exams. Monitor growth in pediatric patients.

Patient Counseling: Inform that salmeterol, a component of Advair HFA, increases the risk of asthma-related death. Advise that medication is not for the relief of acute asthma symptoms and extra doses should not be used for this purpose. Inform not to d/c unless directed by physician and on administration instructions. Inform that medication may cause reduction in growth velocity (pediatric) and may also unmask conditions. Instruct to avoid exposure to chickenpox or measles and to seek medical attention if exposed to chickenpox or measles, if existing TB infections or ocular herpes simplex symptoms do not improve or worsen, during periods of stress or severe asthmatic attack, or if adrenal insufficiency, paradoxical bronchospasm, or hypersensitivity reactions occur. Advise to read Medication Guide.

Administration: Oral inhalation. Prime inhaler before 1st use by releasing 4 test sprays into air, away from face, shaking well for 5 sec before each spray. If not used for 4 weeks or dropped, reprime by releasing 2 test sprays into air, away from face, shaking well before each spray. **Storage:** 25°C (77°F); excursions permitted to 15-30°C (59-86°F). Store with mouthpiece down. May cause bursting when exposed to >120°F. Do not puncture, use or store near heat or open flame, or throw container into fire/incinerator.

ADVICOR   RX
niacin - lovastatin (Abbott)

THERAPEUTIC CLASS: HMG-CoA reductase inhibitor/Nicotinic acid

INDICATIONS: As an adjunct to diet, for the treatment of hypercholesterolemia when use of both niacin extended-release and lovastatin is appropriate. Niacin Extended-Release: As adjunct to diet for the treatment of primary hypercholesterolemia and mixed dyslipidemia, as an adjunct for the treatment of hypertriglyceridemia, and for the secondary prevention of cardiovascular events. Lovastatin: Adjunct to diet for the treatment of primary hypercholesterolemia, and for primary and secondary prevention of cardiovascular events. See individual labeling for further details.

DOSAGE: *Adults:* Place on a standard cholesterol-lowering diet before treatment. Individualize dose based on targeted goals for cholesterol, TG, and on patient response. Take qhs with a low-fat snack. Not Currently on Niacin Extended-Release: Initial: 500mg-20mg qhs. Titrate: Niacin Extended-Release: Increase by no more than 500mg qd every 4 weeks. Max: 2000mg-40mg qd. Concomitant Cyclosporine/Danazol: Lovastatin: Initial: 10mg/day. Max: 20mg/day. Concomitant Amiodarone/Verapamil: Lovastatin: Max: 40mg/day. CrCl <30mL/min: Caution with dosage increases >20mg/day of lovastatin. May pretreat with aspirin (ASA) 30 min prior to treatment (up to 325mg) to reduce flushing. D/C for >7 days: Reinstitute at lowest dose. Refer to PI for further dosing information.

HOW SUPPLIED: Tab: (Niacin Extended-Release-Lovastatin) 500mg-20mg, 750mg-20mg, 1000mg-20mg, 1000mg-40mg

CONTRAINDICATIONS: Active liver disease or unexplained persistent elevations in serum transaminases, active peptic ulcer disease (PUD), arterial bleeding, pregnancy, nursing mothers.

WARNINGS/PRECAUTIONS: Do not substitute for equivalent dose of immediate-release (crystalline) niacin or other modified-release (sustained-release or time-release) niacin preparations; severe hepatic toxicity may occur. Caution with history of liver disease or jaundice, hepatobiliary disease, history of peptic ulcer, diabetes, unstable angina or acute phase of myocardial infarction (MI), renal disease/dysfunction. Monitor LFTs prior to therapy, every 6-12 weeks for first 6 months, and periodically thereafter; d/c if transaminase progression, particularly if rises to 3X ULN, or if associated with nausea, fever, and/or malaise. Myopathy and rhabdomyolysis reported. D/C if myopathy diagnosed or suspected and a few days before surgery and when any major acute medical/surgical condition supervenes. Diabetic patients may experience dose-related rise in fasting blood sugar. May increase PT and reduce platelet counts; caution in patients undergoing surgery. May reduce phosphorous levels. Niacin: Elevated uric acid levels reported; caution in patients predisposed to gout. Lovastatin: May elevate creatine phosphokinase. May cause endocrine dysfunction and CNS toxicity.

ADVERSE REACTIONS: Flushing, asthenia, flu syndrome, headache, infection, pain, back pain, diarrhea, N/V, hyperglycemia, myalgia, pruritus, rash, abdominal pain, dyspepsia.

INTERACTIONS: Avoid concomitant fibrates unless benefit outweighs risk. Do not exceed dose of 1000mg-20mg with concomitant cyclosporine, danazol, or fibrates. Antidiabetic agents may need adjustment. Caution with vasoactive drugs (eg, nitrates, calcium channel blockers, adrenergic blockers). Avoid concomitant alcohol and hot drinks; may increase flushing and pruritus. Vitamins or other nutritional supplements containing large doses of niacin or related compounds (eg, nicotinamide) may potentiate adverse effects. Lovastatin: Increased risk of skeletal muscle disorders with potent CYP3A4 inhibitors (eg, cyclosporine, itraconazole, ketoconazole and other azole antifungals, erythromycin, clarithromycin, telithromycin, HIV protease inhibitors, nefazodone, >1 quart/day of grapefruit juice), danazol, fibrates (eg, gemfibrozil), niacin. Do not exceed 20mg/day of lovastatin with concomitant gemfibrozil. Caution with drugs that diminish levels or activity of steroid hormones (eg, ketoconazole, spironolactone, cimetidine). May interact with CYP3A4 substrates. Niacin: May potentiate ganglionic blockers, vasoactive drugs. Decreased clearance with ASA. Binding to bile acid sequestrants (eg, cholestyramine, colestipol) reported; separate administration by 4-6 hrs. Bleeding and/or increased PT reported with concomitant anticoagulants; monitor PT.

PREGNANCY: Category X, not for use in nursing.

MECHANISM OF ACTION: Niacin: Nicotinic acid; mechanism not established. May partially inhibit release of free fatty acids from adipose tissue and increase lipoprotein lipase activity. Decreases hepatic synthesis rate of VLDL-C and LDL-C. Lovastatin: HMG-CoA reductase inhibitor. Inhibits conversion of HMG-CoA to mevalonate. Has LDL-lowering effect by involving both reduction of VLDL-C concentration and induction of the LDL receptor, leading to reduction of production and/or increased catabolism of LDL-C.

PHARMACOKINETICS: Absorption: Niacin: C_{max}=18mcg/mL, T_{max}=5 hrs. Lovastatin: Incomplete, C_{max}=11ng/mL, T_{max}=2 hrs. **Distribution:** Niacin: Plasma protein binding (<20%), found in breast milk. Lovastatin: Plasma protein binding (>95%). **Metabolism:** Niacin: Rapid and extensive. Liver to nicotinamide adenine dinucleotide (NAD) metabolite and other metabolites; conjugation to nicotinuric acid (NUA) (metabolite). Lovastatin: Liver (extensive) via CYP3A4. Lovastatin acid, 6'-hydroxy (active metabolites). **Elimination:** Niacin: Urine (≥60%), (12%, unchanged); $T_{1/2}$=20-48 min. Lovastatin: Urine (10%), feces (83%); $T_{1/2}$=4.5 hrs.

NURSING CONSIDERATIONS

Assessment: Assess for any conditions where treatment is contraindicated or cautioned, pregnancy/nursing status, and for possible drug interactions. Perform LFTs and lipid profile prior to therapy. Attempt to control dyslipidemia with appropriate diet, exercise, and weight reduction in obese patients and treat other underlying medical problems before instituting therapy.

Monitoring: Monitor for signs and symptoms of hepatotoxicity, myopathy (eg, muscle pain, tenderness, weakness), rhabdomyolysis with or without acute renal failure, endocrine dysfunction, CNS toxicity, and for laboratory test interactions. Perform periodic determinations of creatine kinase, phosphorus, glucose, and uric acid levels; platelet counts, and PT. Monitor LFTs every 6-12 weeks during the first 6 months of therapy and periodically thereafter. Perform lipid profile at intervals no less than 4 weeks.

Patient Counseling: Counsel to take at bedtime after a low-fat snack. Inform about risks/benefits of therapy. Advise to avoid alcohol, hot drinks, and spicy foods around time of drug administration to minimize flushing. Counsel to avoid administration with grapefruit juice. Instruct to notify physician if pregnant/nursing. Inform that flushing may occur but should subside after several weeks of therapy and that taking ASA 30 min before administration may minimize it. If awakened at night due to flushing, rise slowly to minimize dizziness/syncope. Advise not to break, crush, or chew, and to swallow whole. Instruct to contact physician if dosing is interrupted for any length of time prior to restarting therapy, taking vitamins or other nutritional supplements, or if unexplained muscle pain, tenderness or weakness, or dizziness occurs. Instruct diabetic patients to contact physician if changes in blood glucose levels occur.

Administration: Oral route. Take qhs with a low-fat snack. Take drug whole; do not break, crush, or chew. Not recommended to take on an empty stomach. **Storage:** 20-25°C (68-77°F).

AFINITOR   RX
everolimus (Novartis)

THERAPEUTIC CLASS: Kinase inhibitor

INDICATIONS: Treatment of progressive neuroendocrine tumors of pancreatic origin (PNET) in adults with unresectable, locally advanced or metastatic disease. Treatment of advanced renal cell carcinoma (RCC) in adults after failure of treatment with sunitinib or sorafenib. Treatment of renal angiomyolipoma and tuberous sclerosis complex (TSC) in adults, not requiring immediate surgery. Treatment of subependymal giant cell astrocytoma (SEGA) associated with TSC in adults and pediatrics (≥3 yrs) who require therapeutic intervention, but are not candidates for curative surgical resection.

DOSAGE: *Adults:* Advanced RCC/PNET/Renal Angiomyolipoma with TSC: Usual: 10mg qd. SEGA: Initial dose based on BSA. ≥2.2m²: 7.5mg qd. 1.3-2.1m²: 5mg qd. 0.5-1.2m²: 2.5mg qd. Refer to PI for therapeutic drug monitoring and for dose modifications with hepatic impairment, severe/intolerable adverse reactions, and concomitant moderate CYP3A4, P-glycoprotein (Pg-P) inhibitors, and strong CYP3A4 inducers. Continue treatment as long as clinical benefit is observed or until unacceptable toxicity occurs.
Pediatrics: ≥3 yrs: SEGA: Initial dose based on BSA. ≥2.2m²: 7.5mg qd. 1.3-2.1m²: 5mg qd. 0.5-1.2m²: 2.5mg qd. Refer to PI for therapeutic drug monitoring and for dose modifications with hepatic impairment, severe/intolerable adverse reactions, and concomitant moderate CYP3A4, Pg-P inhibitors, and strong CYP3A4 inducers. Continue treatment as long as clinical benefit is observed or until unacceptable toxicity occurs.

HOW SUPPLIED: Tab: 2.5mg, 5mg, 7.5mg, 10mg

WARNINGS/PRECAUTIONS: Noninfectious pneumonitis reported; for moderate symptoms, consider interrupting therapy until symptoms resolve and consider corticosteroid use. D/C if symptoms are severe; corticosteroid may be indicated until symptoms resolve. Immunosuppressive properties may predispose patients to localized and systemic infections, including infections with opportunistic pathogens. Treat preexisting invasive fungal infections completely prior to therapy. Institute appropriate treatment if diagnosis of an infection is made and consider interruption or d/c of therapy. Mouth ulcers, stomatitis, and oral mucositis reported. Cases of renal failure observed. Elevated SrCr, proteinuria, hyperglycemia, hyperlipidemia, hypertriglyceridemia, decreased Hgb, lymphocytes, neutrophils, and platelets reported; monitor parameters prior to initiating therapy and periodically thereafter. Not recommended for SEGA patients with severe hepatic impairment. Patients on therapy should avoid close contact with those who have received live vaccines. Fetal harm may occur when administered to a pregnant woman.

ADVERSE REACTIONS: Stomatitis, infections, rash, diarrhea, fatigue, edema, abdominal pain, nausea, fever, headache, upper respiratory tract infection, asthenia, cough, sinusitis, otitis media.

INTERACTIONS: Reduce dose and use with caution in combination with moderate CYP3A4 and/or Pg-P inhibitors (eg, amprenavir, fosamprenavir, aprepitant, erythromycin, fluconazole, verapamil, diltiazem) and avoid use with strong inhibitors of CYP3A4 (eg, ketoconazole, itraconazole, clarithromycin, atazanavir, nefazodone, saquinavir, telithromycin, ritonavir, indinavir, nelfinavir, voriconazole); may increase levels. Strong CYP3A4 inducers (eg, phenytoin, carbamazepine, rifampin, rifabutin, rifapentine, phenobarbital) may decrease levels; avoid use, and if combination cannot be avoided, increase dose of everolimus. Avoid use with St. John's wort; may decrease levels. Avoid use with grapefruit, grapefruit juice, and other foods that are known to inhibit cytochrome P450 and Pg-P activity; may increase everolimus exposures. May increase midazolam and octreotide levels. Avoid use of live vaccines while on therapy.

PREGNANCY: Category D, not for use in nursing.

MECHANISM OF ACTION: Kinase inhibitor; binds to an intracellular protein, FKBP-12, resulting in an inhibitory complex formation with mammalian target of rapamycin complex 1 and leading to inhibition of mammalian target of rapamycin kinase activity. In addition, inhibits the expression of hypoxia-inducible factor and reduces the expression of vascular endothelial growth factor. Reduces cell proliferation, angiogenesis, and glucose uptake.

PHARMACOKINETICS: Absorption: T_{max}=1-2 hrs. **Distribution:** Plasma protein binding (74%). **Metabolism:** CYP3A4 and Pg-P. **Elimination:** Urine (5%), feces (80%); $T_{1/2}$=30 hrs.

NURSING CONSIDERATIONS

Assessment: Assess for hypersensitivity reactions, preexisting fungal infections, pregnancy/nursing status, and possible drug interactions. Assess renal/hepatic function. Obtain FPG, lipid profile, and CBC prior to start of therapy. Consider timing of routine vaccinations in pediatric patients with SEGA prior to therapy.

Monitoring: Monitor for signs/symptoms of hypersensitivity reactions, noninfectious pneumonitis, infections, reactivation of hepatitis B, mouth ulcers, stomatitis, oral mucositis, and other adverse reactions. Monitor renal/hepatic function, FPG, lipid profile, and CBC periodically. For SEGA, evaluate SEGA volume 3 months after initiation and periodically thereafter. Routine therapeutic drug monitoring is recommended.

Patient Counseling: Inform that noninfectious pneumonitis or infections may develop; advise to report new or worsening respiratory symptoms or any signs or symptoms of infection. Inform of the possibility of developing mouth ulcers, stomatitis, oral mucositis, and hepatitis B reactivation. Instruct to use topical treatments and mouthwashes (without alcohol or peroxide) if oral ulceration develops. Inform of the possibility of developing kidney failure and the need to monitor kidney function. Notify healthcare providers of all concomitant medications, including over-the-counter medications and dietary supplements. Advise to avoid the use of live vaccines and close contact with those who have received live vaccines. Advise of risk of fetal harm and to use an effective method of contraception during and for 8 weeks after therapy. Instruct to follow the dosing instructions as directed and if a dose is missed, to take it up to 6 hrs after the time they would normally take it.

Administration: Oral route. Administer at the same time every day, either consistently with food or consistently without food. Swallow tabs whole with a glass of water; do not crush. Disperse tab(s) completely in a glass of water immediately prior to drinking if unable to swallow tab; refer to PI. **Storage:** 25°C (77°F); excursions permitted between 15-30°C (59-86°F). Protect from light and moisture.

AFLURIA

RX

influenza virus vaccine (Merck)

THERAPEUTIC CLASS: Vaccine

INDICATIONS: Active immunization against influenza disease caused by influenza virus subtypes A and B in persons ≥5 yrs.

DOSAGE: *Adults*: Single 0.5mL IM preferably in the deltoid muscle of the upper arm. *Pediatrics*: ≥9 yrs: Single 0.5mL IM. 5-8 yrs: Not Previously Vaccinated/Received Only 1 Dose for the 1st Time Last Season: 0.5mL IM on Day 1, then 0.5 mL IM approximately 4 weeks later. Previously Vaccinated with 2 Doses Last Season/1 Dose ≥2 yrs ago: Single 0.5mL IM. Preferred site is the deltoid muscle of the upper arm.

HOW SUPPLIED: Inj: 0.5mL, 5mL

CONTRAINDICATIONS: Known severe allergic reactions to egg proteins.

WARNINGS/PRECAUTIONS: Increased rates of fever and febrile seizures reported in children predominantly <5 yrs of age; febrile events also reported in children 5 to <9 yrs of age. Guillain-Barre syndrome (GBS) may occur; consider benefits and risks if GBS occurred within 6 weeks of previous influenza vaccination. Appropriate medical treatment and supervision must be available to manage possible anaphylactic reactions. Response may be diminished in immunocompromised individuals. May not protect all recipients.

ADVERSE REACTIONS: Inj-site reactions (pain, redness, swelling, tenderness, erythema, induration), headache, myalgia, malaise, N/V, fever, cough, diarrhea.

INTERACTIONS: Corticosteroids or immunosuppressive therapies may diminish immune response to vaccine.

PREGNANCY: Category B, caution in nursing.

MECHANISM OF ACTION: Vaccine; elicits the formation of antibodies that may protect against influenza virus subtypes A and B.

NURSING CONSIDERATIONS

Assessment: Assess for history of severe allergic reactions to egg proteins, immunosuppression, pregnancy/nursing status, and possible drug interactions. Assess potential benefits and risks if GBS occurred with previous influenza vaccination. Review immunization history for possible vaccine sensitivity and previous vaccination-related adverse reactions.

Monitoring: Monitor for allergic reactions, GBS, and immune response.

Patient Counseling: Inform of potential benefits/risks of vaccination. Inform that vaccination cannot cause influenza but produces antibodies that protect against influenza and that the effect of the vaccine is achieved approximately 3 weeks after vaccination. Advise that annual revaccination is recommended. Instruct to report any adverse reactions to physician.

Administration: IM route. Shake thoroughly before use. Administer at different inj site if to be given at the same time with other injectable vaccine(s). Do not mix with any other vaccine in the same syringe. **Storage:** 2-8°C (36-46°F). Do not freeze. Protect from light. Once stopper has been pierced, discard vial within 28 days.

AGGRASTAT   RX
tirofiban HCl (Medicure)

THERAPEUTIC CLASS: Glycoprotein IIb/IIIa inhibitor

INDICATIONS: In combination with heparin, for treatment of acute coronary syndrome, in patients being medically managed or undergoing percutaneous transluminal coronary angioplasty (PTCA) or atherectomy.

DOSAGE: *Adults:* Initial: 0.4mcg/kg/min IV for 30 min. Maint: 0.1mcg/kg/min IV. Continue through angiography and for 12-24 hrs after angioplasty or atherectomy. CrCl <30mL/min: Administer at half of usual rate of infusion.

HOW SUPPLIED: Inj: 0.05mg/mL

CONTRAINDICATIONS: Active internal bleeding, acute pericarditis, severe HTN, concomitant parenteral GP IIb/IIIa inhibitor, hemorrhagic stroke, aortic dissection, thrombocytopenia with prior exposure. Bleeding diathesis, stroke, major surgical procedure, or severe physical trauma within past 30 days. History of intracranial hemorrhage or neoplasm, arteriovenous malformation, aneurysm.

WARNINGS/PRECAUTIONS: Bleeding reported. Monitor platelets, Hgb, Hct before treatment, within 6 hrs after loading infusion, and daily during therapy. Monitor platelets earlier if previous GP IIb/IIIa inhibitor use. Determine activated partial thromboplastin time (APTT) before and during therapy with heparin. Caution with platelets <150,000/mm³, hemorrhagic retinopathy, chronic hemodialysis patients, femoral access site in percutaneous coronary intervention. When obtaining intravenous access, non-compressible sites (eg, subclavian or jugular veins) should be avoided. Minimize vascular and other trauma. D/C if thrombocytopenia confirmed or if bleeding cannot be controlled by pressure.

ADVERSE REACTIONS: Bleeding, nausea, fever, headache, edema, anaphylaxis.

INTERACTIONS: See Contraindications. Increased bleeding with heparin and ASA. Caution with other drugs that affect hemostasis (eg, warfarin). Increased clearance with levothyroxine or omeprazole.

PREGNANCY: Category B, not for use in nursing.

MECHANISM OF ACTION: Glycoprotein IIb/IIIa inhibitor; reversible antagonist of fibrinogen binding to the GP IIb/IIIa receptor, the major platelet surface receptor involved in platelet aggregation. Inhibits platelet aggregation.

PHARMACOKINETICS: Distribution: V_d=22-42L; plasma protein binding (not highly bound). **Metabolism:** Limited. **Elimination**: Urine (65%), feces (25%); $T_{1/2}$=2 hrs.

NURSING CONSIDERATIONS

Assessment: Assess for presence or history (within previous 30 days) of internal bleeding; history of intracranial hemorrhage/neoplasm, arteriovenous malformation, or aneurysm; history of thrombocytopenia following previous exposure to the medication; history of any stroke; major recent surgical procedure or severe trauma; history, symptoms, or findings of aortic dissection; severe HTN; concomitant use of another parenteral GP IIb/IIIa inhibitor; and acute pericarditis. Assess use in patients with platelet counts <150,000/mm³, presence of hemorrhagic retinopathy, and those on chronic hemodialysis. Assess for drug interactions. Obtain baseline platelet counts, Hgb, Hct, and APTT.

Monitoring: Monitor for signs/symptoms of bleeding, allergic reactions (eg, anaphylaxis), and thrombocytopenia. Monitor platelet counts, Hgb, and Hct within 6 hours of loading infusion, and at least daily thereafter. Monitor APTT for anticoagulant effects of heparin.

Patient Counseling: Counsel to notify physician if allergic reaction (eg, anaphylaxis) or bleeding occurs.
Administration: IV route. Dilute. 1) If using 500mL of 0.9% NS or D5W, withdraw and discard 100mL from bag and replace this volume with 100mL of drug injection from two 50mL vials. 2) If using 250mL of 0.9% NS or D5W, withdraw and discard 50mL from bag and replace this volume with 50mL of drug injection from one 50mL vial. Mix well prior to administration. Refer to PI for proper administration. Any unused solution should be discarded. Do not administer in same line as diazepam. **Storage:** 25°C (77°F) with excursions permitted between 15-30°C (59-86°F). Protect from light. Do not freeze.

AGGRENOX   RX
aspirin - dipyridamole (Boehringer Ingelheim)

THERAPEUTIC CLASS: Platelet aggregation inhibitor
INDICATIONS: To reduce risk of stroke in patients who have had transient ischemia of the brain or completed ischemic stroke due to thrombosis.
DOSAGE: *Adults:* Usual: 1 cap bid (1 in am and 1 in pm). Intolerable Headaches During Initial Treatment: Switch to 1 cap at hs and low-dose aspirin (ASA) in am. Return to usual regimen as soon as possible, usually within 1 week.
HOW SUPPLIED: Cap: (ASA-Dipyridamole Extended-Release) 25mg-200mg
CONTRAINDICATIONS: NSAID allergy, syndrome of asthma, rhinitis, and nasal polyps, and children or teenagers with viral infections.
WARNINGS/PRECAUTIONS: Risk of intracranial hemorrhage reported. Risk of GI side effects (eg, stomach pain, heartburn, N/V, gross GI bleeding, dyspepsia); monitor for signs of ulceration and bleeding. May cause fetal harm; avoid in 3rd trimester of pregnancy. Not interchangeable with individual components of ASA and dipyridamole tabs. ASA: May increase bleeding time; can adversely affect inherited/acquired (liver disease or vitamin K deficiency) bleeding disorders. Avoid with history of active peptic ulcer disease (PUD) and severe hepatic or severe renal (GFR <10mL/min) dysfunction. Bleeding risks reported with alcohol use ($\geq$3 alcoholic drinks/day). May not provide adequate treatment for cardiac indications for stroke/transient ischemic attack patients for whom ASA is indicated to prevent recurrent myocardial infarction or angina pectoris. Dipyridamole: Elevations of hepatic enzymes and hepatic failure reported. Has a vasodilatory effect; may precipitate/aggravate chest pain in patients with underlying coronary artery disease (CAD). May exacerbate preexisting hypotension.
ADVERSE REACTIONS: Headache, dyspepsia, abdominal pain, N/V, diarrhea, fatigue, arthralgia, pain, back pain, GI bleeding, hemorrhage.
INTERACTIONS: Dipyridamole: May increase plasma levels and cardiovascular (CV) effects of adenosine. May counteract effect of cholinesterase inhibitors; potentially aggravating myasthenia gravis. ASA: May decrease effects of angiotensin converting enzyme inhibitors and β-blockers. May lead to high serum concentrations of acetazolamide (and toxicity). Increased risk of bleeding reported with anticoagulants (warfarin [prolongation of both PT and bleeding time], heparin) and NSAIDs. May decrease total concentration of phenytoin. May increase serum valproic acid levels. Decreased effects of diuretics in renal or CV disease. May inhibit renal clearance of methotrexate, leading to bone marrow toxicity (especially in elderly/renal impaired). Decreased renal function with NSAIDs. May increase effectiveness of oral hypoglycemics at moderate doses. May antagonize uricosuric agents (probenecid and sulfinpyrazone).
PREGNANCY: Category D, caution in nursing.
MECHANISM OF ACTION: Dipyridamole: Platelet aggregation inhibitor. Inhibits uptake of adenosine into platelets, endothelial cells, and erythrocytes. ASA: Platelet aggregation inhibitor. Irreversibly inhibits platelet cyclooxygenase and thus inhibits the generation of thromboxane A_2, a powerful inducer of platelet aggregation and vasoconstriction.
PHARMACOKINETICS: Absorption: Dipyridamole: C_{max}=1.98mcg/mL; T_{max}=2 hrs. ASA: C_{max}=319ng/mL; T_{max}=0.63 hrs. **Distribution:** Dipyridamole/ASA: Found in breast milk. Dipyridamole: V_d=92L; plasma protein binding (99%). ASA: V_d=10L; plasma protein binding (concentration-dependent). **Metabolism:** Dipyridamole: Liver (conjugation); monoglucuronide (primary metabolite). ASA: Plasma (hydrolysis) into salicylic acid (metabolite) then liver (conjugation). **Elimination:** Dipyridamole: Feces, urine; $T_{1/2}$=13.6 hrs. ASA: Urine (10% salicylic acid, 75% salicyluric acid); $T_{1/2}$=0.33 hrs, 1.71 hrs (salicylic acid).

NURSING CONSIDERATIONS

Assessment: Assess for NSAID allergy, syndrome of asthma, rhinitis and nasal polyps, renal/hepatic dysfunction, inherited/acquired bleeding disorders, history of active PUD, alcohol use, CAD, hypotension, hypersensitivity, pregnancy/nursing status, and possible drug interactions.

Monitoring: Monitor for signs/symptoms of allergic reactions, GI effects, elevated hepatic enzymes, hepatic failure, and for bleeding. Monitor platelet function (eg, bleeding time).

Patient Counseling: Inform of risk and signs/symptoms of bleeding (eg, occult bleeding). Instruct to notify physician of all medications and supplements being taken, especially drugs that may increase risk of bleeding. Counsel patients who consume ≥3 alcoholic drinks daily about the bleeding risks. Inform that transient headache may occur; notify physician if intolerable headache develops. Inform about signs and symptoms of GI side effects and what steps to take if they occur. Advise to take drug exactly as prescribed; if dose is missed, advise to take next dose on regular schedule and not take a double dose. Inform of potential hazard to fetus if used during pregnancy; notify physician if pregnant/breastfeeding or intend to become pregnant.

Administration: Oral route. Swallow whole; do not chew or crush. **Storage:** 25°C (77°F); excursions permitted to 15-30°C (59-86°F). Protect from excessive moisture.

AGRIFLU   RX
influenza virus vaccine (Novartis)

THERAPEUTIC CLASS: Vaccine

INDICATIONS: Active immunization in persons ≥18 yrs for the prevention of disease caused by influenza virus subtypes A and type B contained in the vaccine.

DOSAGE: *Adults:* 0.5mL IM as a single dose, preferably in the region of deltoid muscle of the upper arm.

HOW SUPPLIED: Inj: 0.5mL

CONTRAINDICATIONS: Known systemic hypersensitivity reactions to egg proteins (eggs or egg products), kanamycin, and neomycin, life-threatening reaction to previous influenza vaccination.

WARNINGS/PRECAUTIONS: Do not inject in the gluteal region or areas where there may be a major nerve trunk. Caution if Guillain-Barre syndrome has occurred within 6 weeks of receipt of prior influenza vaccine. Immunocompromised patients may have a lower immune response than immunocompetent persons. Appropriate medical treatment and supervision must be available to manage possible anaphylactic reactions. Tip caps may contain natural rubber latex which may cause allergic reactions in latex-sensitive individuals. May not protect all recipients.

ADVERSE REACTIONS: Local reaction (pain, induration, swelling, erythema), headache, myalgia, malaise, fatigue, chills, arthralgia, sweating, fever, influenza-like illness.

INTERACTIONS: Immunosuppressive therapies, including corticosteroids, may reduce the immune response to the vaccine.

PREGNANCY: Category B, caution in nursing.

MECHANISM OF ACTION: Vaccine; elicits the formation of antibodies that may protect against influenza virus subtypes A and B.

NURSING CONSIDERATIONS

Assessment: Assess for hypersensitivity reactions to egg proteins, kanamycin, and neomycin. Assess for history of life-threatening reaction to previous influenza vaccination, allergic reaction to latex, immunosuppression, immunization history, pregnancy/nursing status, and for possible drug interactions. Assess potential benefits and risks if Guillain-Barre syndrome occurred with previous influenza vaccination.

Monitoring: Monitor for allergic reactions and for immune response.

Patient Counseling: Advise of potential benefits and risks of immunization. Inform that vaccine contains noninfectious particles and cannot cause influenza. Advise that vaccine is intended to provide protection against illness due to influenza viruses only and cannot protect against other respiratory illnesses. Instruct to report any adverse reaction to physician. Inform that annual vaccination is recommended.

Administration: IM route. Administer at different inj site if to be given at the same time with other injectable vaccine(s). Do not mix with any other vaccine in the same syringe. Allow to reach room temperature and shake before use. **Storage:** 2-8°C (35-46°F). Do not freeze or use if frozen. Protect from light.

ALACORT   RX
hydrocortisone acetate (Crown Laboratories)

OTHER BRAND NAMES: U-cort (Taro)
THERAPEUTIC CLASS: Corticosteroid

INDICATIONS: Relief of the inflammatory and pruritic manifestations of corticosteroid-responsive dermatoses.

DOSAGE: *Adults:* Apply a thin film to affected area(s) bid-qid depending on the severity of the condition.
Pediatrics: Apply a thin film to affected area(s) bid-qid depending on the severity of the condition.

HOW SUPPLIED: Cre: (Alacort) 1% [28.4g, 85.2g]; (U-cort) 1% [28.35g, 85g, 123g]

WARNINGS/PRECAUTIONS: Reversible hypothalamic-pituitary-adrenal (HPA) axis suppression, Cushing's syndrome, hyperglycemia and glucosuria reported with systemic absorption. Application of more potent steroids, use over large areas and with occlusive dressings augment systemic absorption; monitor for HPA axis suppression, d/c, reduce frequency, or substitute less potent steroid if occurs. Signs and symptoms of steroid withdrawal may occur infrequently; may require supplemental systemic corticosteroids. D/C if irritation develops. Use appropriate antifungal or antibacterial agent with dermatological infections. Pediatric patients may be more susceptible to systemic toxicity; Cushing's syndrome, intracranial HTN (eg, bulging fontanelles, headaches, and bilateral papilledema), and adrenal suppression (eg, linear growth retardation, delayed weight gain, low plasma cortisol levels and absence of response to adrenocorticotrophic hormone [ACTH] stimulation). Chronic corticosteroid therapy may interfere with growth and development of children. (Alacort) Not for ophthalmic use. (U-cort) Contains sodium bisulfite; may cause allergic-type reactions in susceptible people; caution with asthmatics. Atrophy of skin and SQ tissues may occur with prolonged use and even with short-term use when used on intertriginous or flexor areas, or on the face.

ADVERSE REACTIONS: HPA suppression, Cushing's syndrome, burning/itching/irritation/dryness at application site, growth retardation, skin atrophy, allergic contact dermatitis, hypertrichosis, maceration of the skin, miliaria, striae, hypopigmentation, folliculitis.

PREGNANCY: Category C, caution in nursing.

MECHANISM OF ACTION: Corticosteroid; possesses anti-inflammatory, antipruritic and vasoconstrictive properties. Mechanism of anti-inflammatory effects has not established.

PHARMACOKINETICS: Absorption: Extent of percutaneous absorption depends on skin integrity, vehicle and use of occlusive dressing. Inflammation and/or other disease processes in the skin increase absorption. **Metabolism:** Liver. **Elimination:** Urine, bile.

NURSING CONSIDERATIONS

Assessment: Assess for dermatological infections, hypersensitivity, surface area, pregnancy/nursing status and possible drug interactions.

Monitoring: Monitor for signs/symptoms of glucocorticoid insufficiency, hyperglycemia, glucosuria, skin irritation, and skin infections (eg, fungal, bacterial). Monitor for HPA-axis suppression by using periodic ACTH stimulation and urinary free cortisol tests in patients applying medication to large surface areas or using occlusive dressings. Monitor for signs/symptoms of systemic toxicity in pediatrics.

Patient Counseling: Instruct patient to use medication as directed by the physician; to avoid contact with the eyes. Advise not to use medication for any disorder other than for which it was prescribed. Do not wrap, cover, or bandage treated skin unless directed by physician. Instruct patients to report adverse reactions. Advise not to use tight-fitting diapers or plastic pants on a child being treated in the diaper area.

Administration: Topical route. Occlusive dressings may be used for psoriasis or recalcitrant conditions; d/c if infection develops. **Storage:** (U-cort) 15-30°C (59-86°F). Protect from freezing. Dispense in tight container.

ALAMAST RX
pemirolast potassium (Vistakon)

THERAPEUTIC CLASS: Mast cell stabilizer

INDICATIONS: Prevention of ocular itching due to allergic conjunctivitis.

DOSAGE: *Adults:* 1-2 drops in each affected eye qid.
Pediatrics: ≥3 yrs: 1-2 drops in each affected eye qid.

HOW SUPPLIED: Sol: 0.1% [10mL]

WARNINGS/PRECAUTIONS: Not for inj or oral use.

ADVERSE REACTIONS: Headache, rhinitis, cold/flu symptoms, ocular burning/discomfort, dry eye, foreign body sensation, allergy, back pain, bronchitis, cough, dysmenorrhea, fever, sinusitis, sneezing/nasal congestion.

PREGNANCY: Category C, caution in nursing.

MECHANISM OF ACTION: Mast cell stabilizer; inhibits type I immediate hypersensitivity reaction, inhibits antigen-induced release of inflammatory mediators (eg, histamine, leukotriene C_4, D_4, E_4) from human mast cell; also inhibits the chemotaxis of eosinophils into ocular tissue and blocks the release of mediators from human eosinophils; prevents calcium influx into mast cells upon antigen stimulation (not established).

PHARMACOKINETICS: Absorption: C_{max}=4.7ng/mL, T_{max}=0.42 hrs. **Elimination:** Urine (10-15%, unchanged); $T_{1/2}$=4.5 hrs.

NURSING CONSIDERATIONS

Assessment: Assess for known drug hypersensitivity.

Monitoring: Monitor for allergy and other adverse reactions.

Patient Counseling: Instruct not to touch dropper tip to eyelids or surrounding areas and not to wear contact lenses if eye is red. Instruct to keep bottle tightly closed when not in use. Inform that drug is not a treatment for contact lens related irritation. Instruct patients who wear soft contact lenses and whose eyes are not red to wait for ≥10 min after instilling before inserting contact lenses.

Administration: Intraocular route. **Storage:** 15-25°C (59-77°F).

ALBUTEROL   RX
albuterol sulfate (Various)

THERAPEUTIC CLASS: Beta$_2$-agonist

INDICATIONS: (Sol) Relief of bronchospasm in patients ≥2 yrs with reversible obstructive airway disease and acute attacks of bronchospasm. (Syrup) Relief of bronchospasm in patients ≥2 yrs with reversible obstructive airway disease. (Tab/ER) Relief of bronchospasm in patients ≥6 yrs with reversible obstructive airway disease.

DOSAGE: *Adults:* (ER) Usual: 4mg or 8mg q12h. If low body weight, start at 4mg q12h and progress to 8mg q12h according to response. Max: 32mg/day in divided doses (q12h). (Sol) Usual: 2.5mg tid-qid by nebulizer. (Syrup/Tab) Initial: 2mg or 4mg tid-qid. Max: 8mg qid as tolerated. Elderly/β-Adrenergic Stimulators Sensitivity: (Syrup/Tab) Initial: 2mg tid-qid. Adjust individually and gradually thereafter. Max: (Tab) 32mg/day. (ER) Refer to PI if switching from PO Albuterol Products.
Pediatrics: >14 yrs: (Syrup) Initial: 2mg or 4mg tid-qid. Max: 8mg qid as tolerated. >12 yrs: (Tab, ER) Usual: 4mg or 8mg q12h. Max: 32mg/day in divided doses (q12h). ≥12 yrs: (0.5% Sol) Usual: 2.5mg tid-qid by nebulizer. (Tab) Initial: 2mg or 4mg tid-qid. Max: 8mg qid as tolerated. 6-14 yrs: (Syrup) Initial: 2mg tid-qid. Max: 24mg/day in divided doses. 6-12 yrs: (ER) Usual: 4mg q12h. Max: 24mg/day in divided doses (q12h). (Tab) Initial: 2mg tid-qid. Max: 24mg/day in divided doses. 2-12 yrs: (0.083% Sol) Usual: ≥15kg: 2.5mg tid-qid by nebulizer. <15kg: Use 0.5% sol if require <2.5mg/dose. (0.5% Sol) Initial: 0.1-0.15mg/kg/dose. Max: 2.5mg tid-qid by nebulizer. Refer to PI for approximate dosing according to body weight. 2-5 yrs: (Syrup) Initial: 0.1mg/kg tid. Initial Max: 2mg tid. Titrate: May increase to 0.2mg/kg tid. Max: 4mg tid. β-Adrenergic Stimulators Sensitivity: (Syrup, Tab) Initial: 2mg tid-qid. Adjust individually and gradually thereafter. Max: ≥12 yrs: (Tab) 32mg/day. (ER) Refer to PI if switching from PO Albuterol Products.

HOW SUPPLIED: Sol, Inhalation: 0.083% [3mL], 0.5% [20mL]; Syrup: 2mg/5mL [4 fl. oz., 8 fl. oz., 16 fl. oz.]; Tab: 2mg*, 4mg*; Tab, Extended-Release (ER): 4mg, 8mg *scored

WARNINGS/PRECAUTIONS: Immediate hypersensitivity reactions reported. Can produce clinically significant cardiovascular (CV) effect (eg, ECG changes) in some patients; caution with CV disorders (eg, coronary insufficiency, cardiac arrhythmias, HTN). Can produce paradoxical bronchospasm; d/c if occurs. Caution with diabetes mellitus (DM), hyperthyroidism, convulsive disorders, and in patients who are unusually responsive to sympathomimetic amines. Aggravation of preexisting DM and ketoacidosis reported with large doses of IV albuterol. May cause transient hypokalemia. Erythema multiforme and Stevens-Johnson syndrome reported with oral administration in children. (0.5% Sol/Syrup/Tab/ER) Consider adding anti-inflammatory agents (eg, corticosteroids) to adequately control asthma. Reevaluate patient and treatment regimen if deterioration of asthma is observed. (ER) Increases in selected serum chemistry and decreases in selected hematologic values reported in adults. (Sol) Fatalities reported with excessive use.

ADVERSE REACTIONS: Tremor, nervousness, headache, tachycardia, dizziness, N/V, palpitations, paradoxical bronchospasm, increased appetite, muscle cramps, excitement.

INTERACTIONS: Not recommended with other sympathomimetic agents. Extreme caution with MAOIs, TCAs, or within 2 weeks of d/c of such agents; action of albuterol may be potentiated. Antagonized by β-blockers; (0.5% Sol/Syrup/Tab/ER) avoid use but if not possible, use cardioselective β-blockers with caution. (0.5% Sol/Syrup/Tab/ER) May decrease serum levels of digoxin; monitor levels. May worsen ECG changes and/or hypokalemia caused by non-K⁺ sparing diuretics (eg, loop/thiazide); caution is advised. (Sol) Avoid epinephrine. (0.5% Sol) Caution with additional adrenergic drugs by any route.

PREGNANCY: Category C, not for use in nursing.

MECHANISM OF ACTION: β_2-adrenergic agonist; stimulates intracellular adenyl cyclase, which catalyzes conversion of adenosine triphosphate to cyclic-3',5'-adenosine monophosphate to produce relaxation of bronchial smooth muscle.

PHARMACOKINETICS: Absorption: (Syrup/Tab) Rapid. C_{max}=18ng/mL, T_{max}=2 hrs. (ER) C_{max}=13.7ng/mL, T_{max}=6 hrs, AUC=134ng•hr/mL. (Sol) C_{max}=2.1ng/mL, T_{max}=0.5 hr. **Elimination:** (Syrup/Tab) Urine (76%), feces (4%); $T_{1/2}$=5 hrs. (ER) $T_{1/2}$=9.3 hrs. (Sol) Urine; $T_{1/2}$=5-6 hrs.

NURSING CONSIDERATIONS

Assessment: Assess for previous hypersensitivity to the drug, CV disorders, HTN, DM, convulsive disorders, hyperthyroidism, pregnancy/nursing status, and possible drug interactions.

Monitoring: Monitor for signs/symptoms of CV effects (measured by pulse rate and BP), worsening of symptoms, paradoxical bronchospasm, destabilization of asthma, hypokalemia, and hypersensitivity reactions.

Patient Counseling: Instruct not to use more frequently than recommended. Advise not to increase dose or frequency without medical consultation. Seek medical attention if symptoms worsen, if therapy becomes less effective, or if there is need to use the drug more frequently than usual. Inform of the common effects (eg, palpitations, chest pain, rapid HR, tremor, nervousness). Inform not to mix with other drugs in nebulizer. (ER) Instruct to swallow tab whole with the aid of liquids and not to chew or crush.

Administration: Oral inhalation/oral route. Refer to PI for proper administration. **Storage:** (Sol) 2-25°C (36-77°F). Protect from light. (Tab/ER) 20-25°C (68-77°F). (Syrup) 2-30°C (36-86°F).

ALCORTIN-A   RX
iodoquinol - hydrocortisone (Primus)

THERAPEUTIC CLASS: Corticosteroid/Anti-infective

INDICATIONS: Possibly effective in contact or atopic dermatitis, impetiginized eczema, nummular eczema, endogenous chronic infectious dermatitis, stasis dermatitis, pyoderma, nuchal eczema and chronic eczematoid otitis externa, acne urticata, localized or disseminated neurodermatitis, lichen simplex chronicus, anogenital pruritus (vulvae, scroti, ani), folliculitis, bacterial dermatoses, mycotic dermatoses (eg, tinea [capitis, cruris, corporis, pedis]), moniliasis, intertrigo.

DOSAGE: *Adults:* Apply to affected area tid-qid or ud.
Pediatrics: ≥12 yrs: Apply to affected area tid-qid or ud.

HOW SUPPLIED: Gel: (Hydrocortisone-Iodoquinol) 2%-1% [2g]

WARNINGS/PRECAUTIONS: For external use only. Keep away from eyes. D/C and institute appropriate therapy if irritation develops. May stain skin, hair, or fabrics. Not for use on infants or under diapers or occlusive dressings. Risk of increased systemic absorption with treatment of extensive areas or use of occlusive dressings; take suitable precautions. Children may absorb larger amounts and be more susceptible to systemic toxicity. Prolonged use may result in overgrowth of nonsusceptible organisms requiring appropriate therapy. Burning, itching, irritation, and dryness reported infrequently. Iodoquinol: May be absorbed through the skin and interfere with thyroid function tests; wait at least 1 month after d/c of therapy to perform tests. Ferric chloride test for phenylketonuria may yield false (+) result if present in the diaper or urine.

ADVERSE REACTIONS: Burning, itching, irritation, dryness, folliculitis, hypertrichosis, acneiform eruptions, hypopigmentation, perioral dermatitis, allergic contact dermatitis, skin maceration, secondary infections, skin atrophy, striae, miliaria.

PREGNANCY: Category C, caution in nursing.

MECHANISM OF ACTION: Hydrocortisone: Corticosteroid; possesses anti-inflammatory, antipruritic, and vasoconstrictive properties. Anti-inflammatory action not established; however, there is a recognizable correlation between vasoconstrictor potency and therapeutic efficacy. Iodoquinol: Anti-infective; possesses both antifungal and antibacterial properties.

PHARMACOKINETICS: Absorption: Hydrocortisone: Percutaneous; inflammation, other disease processes in the skin, and occlusive dressings may increase absorption. **Metabolism:** Glucuronidation. Hydrocortisone: Tetrahydrocortisone and tetrahydrocortisol (metabolites). **Elimination:** Hydrocortisone: Urine. Iodoquinol: (PO) Urine (3-5% glucuronide).

NURSING CONSIDERATIONS

Assessment: Assess for known hypersensitivity to any components of the preparation and pregnancy/nursing status.

Monitoring: Monitor for irritation, development of systemic toxicity in children, and overgrowth of nonsusceptible organisms. If extensive areas are treated or if occlusive dressings are used, monitor for systemic absorption.

Patient Counseling: Instruct parents of pediatric patients not to use tight-fitting diapers or plastic pants on child being treated in diaper area. Counsel to keep medication away from eyes. Instruct to use the medication ud. If irritation develops, counsel to d/c medication and institute appropriate therapy. Inform that medication may cause staining of skin, hair, or fabrics and burning, itching, irritation, or dryness.

Administration: Topical route. **Storage:** 15-30°C (59-86°F). Keep tightly closed.

ALDACTAZIDE   RX
hydrochlorothiazide - spironolactone (G.D. Searle)

> Tumorigenic in chronic toxicity animal studies; avoid unnecessary use. Not for initial therapy of edema or HTN.

THERAPEUTIC CLASS: K⁺-sparing diuretic/thiazide diuretic

INDICATIONS: Management of edematous conditions for patients with congestive heart failure, hepatic cirrhosis with edema/ascites, nephrotic syndrome, and essential HTN. Edema during pregnancy due to pathologic causes.

DOSAGE: *Adults:* Establish by individual titration of components. Edema: Maint: 100mg per component qd or in divided doses. Range: 25-200mg/day per component. HTN: 50-100mg per component qd or in divided doses.

HOW SUPPLIED: Tab: (Spironolactone-HCTZ) 25mg-25mg, 50mg-50mg* *scored

CONTRAINDICATIONS: Acute renal insufficiency, significantly impaired renal excretory function, hyperkalemia, acute or severe hepatic failure, anuria, sulfonamide hypersensitivity.

WARNINGS/PRECAUTIONS: Caution with hepatic dysfunction; may precipitate hepatic coma. Caution with severe renal disease; may precipitate azotemia. May exacerbate/activate systemic lupus erythematosus (SLE). Idiosyncratic reaction, resulting in acute transient myopia and acute angle-closure glaucoma may occur; risk factors include history of sulfonamide or penicillin allergy. Monitor for fluid/electrolyte imbalance (eg, hypomagnesemia, hyponatremia, hypochloremic alkalosis, hypokalemia/hyperkalemia). Obtain ECG if hyperkalemia is suspected; d/c if present. Hypokalemia may develop as a result of profound diuresis, presence of severe cirrhosis, or after prolonged therapy. Hyperchloremic metabolic acidosis reported with decompensated hepatic cirrhosis. Gynecomastia, transient BUN elevation, hypercalcemia, hyperglycemia, hyperuricemia/acute gout precipitation, and sensitivity reactions may occur. Risk of dilutional hyponatremia. Enhanced effects in post-sympathetectomy patient. May increase cholesterol and TG levels. Latent diabetes mellitus (DM) may become manifest. D/C before carrying out parathyroid function test.

ADVERSE REACTIONS: Gastric bleeding, ulceration, gynecomastia, agranulocytosis, fever, urticaria, confusion, ataxia, renal dysfunction, electrolyte disturbances, weakness, irregular menses, amenorrhea, idiosyncratic reactions.

INTERACTIONS: K⁺ supplements, K⁺-sparing diuretics or rich K⁺ diet should not be given concomitantly; hyperkalemia may occur. Extreme caution with NSAIDs (eg, indomethacin), ACE inhibitors; severe hyperkalemia may occur. Alcohol, barbiturates, other antihypertensives, or narcotics may potentiate orthostatic hypotension. Corticosteroids, adrenocorticotropic hormone (ACTH) may intensify electrolyte depletion. Reduced vascular response to norepinephrine, a pressor amine. Increased response to nondepolarizing skeletal muscle relaxants (eg, tubocurarine). Increased levels of digoxin. Hypokalemia may exaggerate effects of digitalis. Avoid with lithium. Dosage adjustment of antidiabetic drugs (eg, oral agents, insulin) may be required. Caution with regional/general anesthesia. Hypokalemia may develop with glucocorticoids, ACTH, or loop diuretics. Dilutional hyponatremia may occur with other diuretics.

PREGNANCY: Category C, not for use in nursing.

MECHANISM OF ACTION: Spironolactone: Aldosterone antagonist; competitively binds to receptors at aldosterone-dependent sodium-potassium exchange site in the distal convoluted renal tubule. HCTZ: Thiazide diuretic and antihypertensive; promotes excretion of sodium and water by inhibiting reabsorption in the cortical diluting segment of the distal renal tubule.

PHARMACOKINETICS: Absorption: Spironolactone: C_{max}=80ng/mL; T_{max}=2.6 hrs. Canrenone: C_{max}=181ng/mL; T_{max}=4.3 hrs. HCTZ: Rapid; T_{max}=1-2 hrs. **Distribution:** Spironolactone: Plasma protein binding (>90%). Canrenone: Found in breast milk. **Metabolism:** Spironolactone: Rapid and extensive. Canrenone (active metabolite). **Elimination:** Spironolactone: Urine (major), bile (minor). $T_{1/2}$=1.4 hrs. Canrenone: $T_{1/2}$=16.5 hrs. HCTZ: Urine. $T_{1/2}$=4-5 hrs.

NURSING CONSIDERATIONS

Assessment: Assess for renal/hepatic impairment, hyperkalemia, pregnancy/nursing status, anuria, possible drug interactions, SLE, DM, drug/sulfonamide/penicillin hypersensitivity, history of allergy or bronchial asthma.

Monitoring: Monitor serum electrolytes, serum K$^+$, TG, cholesterol levels, and renal/hepatic function periodically. Monitor for signs/symptoms of electrolyte imbalance, hyperkalemia, gynecomastia, hyperglycemia, exacerbation or activation of SLE, hyperuricemia or precipitation of gout, hypersensitivity reactions, idiosyncratic reactions, and hepatic/renal impairment.

Patient Counseling: Instruct to avoid K$^+$ supplements and foods containing high levels of K$^+$ including salt substitutes. Inform of pregnancy risks. Advise to seek medical attention if symptoms of electrolyte imbalance (eg, dry mouth, thirst, weakness, lethargy, drowsiness, restlessness, muscle pains/cramps, muscular fatigue, hypotension, oliguria, tachycardia, GI disturbances), hyperkalemia (eg, paresthesia, muscle weakness, fatigue, flaccid paralysis of the extremities, bradycardia, shock), or hypersensitivity reactions occur.

Administration: Oral route. **Storage:** <25°C (77°F).

ALDACTONE   RX
spironolactone (G.D. Searle)

Tumorigenic in chronic toxicity animal studies; avoid unnecessary use.

THERAPEUTIC CLASS: Aldosterone blocker

INDICATIONS: Management of primary hyperaldosteronism (diagnosis, short-term preoperative and long-term maintenance treatment), edematous conditions (for patients with congestive heart failure [CHF], hepatic cirrhosis with edema/ascites, nephrotic syndrome, pathological causes of edema in pregnancy), essential HTN (in combination with other drugs). Treatment and prophylaxis of hypokalemia. In addition to standard therapy in severe heart failure (HF) (New York Heart Association [NYHA] Class III-IV).

DOSAGE: *Adults:* Primary Hyperaldosteronism: (Diagnostic) Long Test: 400mg/day for 3-4 weeks. Short Test: 400mg/day for 4 days. Preoperative: 100-400mg/day. Unsuitable for Surgery: Maint: Lowest effective dose. Edema: Initial: 100mg/day given qd or in divided doses for ≥5 days. Range: 25-200mg/day. May add a second diuretic which acts more proximally in the renal tubule if no adequate diuretic response after 5 days. HTN: Initial: 50-100mg/day given qd or in divided doses for ≥2 weeks. Titrate: Adjust according to response. Diuretic-Induced Hypokalemia: 25-100mg/day. Severe HF (Serum K$^+$ ≤5.0mEq/L, SrCr ≤2.5mg/dL): Initial: 25mg qd. Titrate: May increase to 50mg qd if tolerated or reduce to 25mg qod if not tolerated.

HOW SUPPLIED: Tab: 25mg, 50mg*, 100mg* *scored

CONTRAINDICATIONS: Anuria, acute renal insufficiency, significantly impaired renal excretory function, hyperkalemia.

WARNINGS/PRECAUTIONS: Monitor for fluid/electrolyte imbalance (eg, hypomagnesemia, hyponatremia, hypochloremic alkalosis, hyperkalemia). Caution with hepatic impairment; may precipitate hepatic coma. May cause transient BUN elevation, especially with preexisting renal impairment. Hyperchloremic metabolic acidosis reported with decompensated hepatic cirrhosis. Mild acidosis and gynecomastia may occur. Obtain ECG if hyperkalemia is suspected; d/c if present. May cause/aggravate dilutional hyponatremia.

ADVERSE REACTIONS: Gastric bleeding, ulceration, gynecomastia, agranulocytosis, fever, urticaria, confusion, ataxia, renal dysfunction, irregular menses, postmenopausal bleeding, N/V, diarrhea, cramping.

INTERACTIONS: Avoid with K$^+$-sparing diuretics, K$^+$ supplements (either medication or K$^+$ rich diet), and lithium. Extreme caution with NSAIDs (eg, indomethacin) and angiotensin converting enzyme inhibitors; severe hyperkalemia may occur. Alcohol, barbiturates, or narcotics may potentiate orthostatic hypotension. Corticosteroids and adrenocorticotropic hormone may intensify electrolyte depletion. Reduced vascular response to norepinephrine, a pressor amine; caution with regional/general anesthesia. May increase response to nondepolarizing skeletal muscle relaxants (eg, tubocurarine). Increased levels of digoxin and subsequent digitalis toxicity reported. Dilutional hyponatremia may occur with other diuretics.

PREGNANCY: Category C, not for use in nursing.

MECHANISM OF ACTION: Aldosterone antagonist; competitively binds to receptors at aldosterone-dependent Na$^+$-K$^+$ exchange site in distal convoluted renal tubule, causing increased Na$^+$ and water excretion, and K$^+$ retention.

PHARMACOKINETICS: Absorption: C_{max}=80ng/mL, 181ng/mL (canrenone); T_{max}=2.6 hrs, 4.3 hrs (canrenone). **Distribution:** Plasma protein binding (>90%); found in breast milk (canrenone). **Metabolism:** Rapid and extensive; canrenone (active metabolite). **Elimination:** Urine (major), bile (minor); $T_{1/2}$=1.4 hrs, 16.5 hrs (canrenone).

NURSING CONSIDERATIONS

Assessment: Assess for renal/hepatic function, hyperkalemia, anuria, pregnancy/nursing status, and for possible drug interactions.

Monitoring: Monitor serum K^+, electrolytes, and renal function periodically. Monitor for signs/symptoms of fluid/electrolyte imbalance, dilutional hyponatremia, hyperkalemia, acidosis, gynecomastia, renal/hepatic dysfunction. Monitor for K^+ and creatinine 1 week after initiation/increase dose, monthly for 1st 3 months, then quarterly for a year, and then q6 months with severe HF.

Patient Counseling: Instruct to avoid K^+ supplements and foods containing high levels of K^+, including salt substitutes.

Administration: Oral route. **Storage:** <25°C (77°F).

ALDARA   RX
imiquimod (Graceway)

THERAPEUTIC CLASS: Immune response modifier

INDICATIONS: Topical treatment of nonhyperkeratotic, nonhypertrophic actinic keratoses on face or scalp and biopsy-confirmed, primary superficial basal cell carcinoma (sBCC), with a maximum tumor diameter of 2cm, located on trunk (excluding anogenital skin), neck, or extremities (excluding hands and feet), only when surgical methods are medically less appropriate and follow-up can be assured in immunocompetent adults. Treatment of external genital and perianal warts/condyloma acuminata in patients ≥12 yrs.

DOSAGE: *Adults:* Apply before hs and rub in until no longer visible. Actinic Keratosis: Usual: Apply 2x/week for a full 16 weeks to defined area on face or scalp (but not both concurrently). Wash off after 8 hrs with soap and water. Max: 36 pkts for 16 weeks. External Genital and Perianal Warts/Condyloma: Usual: Apply 3x/week. Use until warts are totally cleared. Wash off after 6-10 hrs with soap and water. May suspend use for several days to manage local reactions. Max: 16 weeks. Do not occlude treatment area. Superficial Basal Cell Carcinoma (sBCC): Apply 5x/week for a full 6 weeks. If tumor diameter is 0.5 to <1cm, use 4mm (10mg) of cre. If tumor is ≥1 to <1.5cm, use 5mm (25mg) of cre. If tumor is ≥1.5 to 2cm, use 7mm (40mg) of cre. Max diameter of tumor: 2cm. Treatment area should include a 1cm margin of skin around the tumor. Wash off after 8 hrs with soap and water. Max: 36 pkts for 6 weeks.
Pediatrics: ≥12 yrs: External Genital and Perianal Warts/Condyloma: Usual: Apply 3x/week before hs. Rub in until no longer visible. Use until warts are totally cleared. Wash off after 6-10 hrs with soap and water. May suspend use for several days to manage local reactions. Max: 16 weeks. Do not occlude treatment area.

HOW SUPPLIED: Cre: 5% [250mg]

WARNINGS/PRECAUTIONS: Not for oral, ophthalmic, or intravaginal use. Not for urethral, intravaginal, cervical, rectal, or intra-anal human papilloma viral disease. Not for repeated use in treatment of actinic keratosis in same area; not for treatment of actinic keratosis on areas of skin >25cm². Not recommended from any previous drug or surgical treament or with sunburn until fully recovered. Not recommended for treatment of basal cell carcinoma (BCC) subtypes, other than sBCC. Avoid or minimize exposure to sunlight. Avoid contact with eyes, lips, nostrils. Caution with inherent sensitivity to sunlight and patients who may have considerable sun exposure. May exacerbate inflammatory skin conditions. Interruption of dosing should be considered, if systemic reactions (eg, flu-like signs/symptoms) or local inflammatory reactions occur. Not effective in pediatrics 2-12 yrs with molluscum contagiosum.

ADVERSE REACTIONS: Application-site reactions, upper respiratory tract infection, sinusitis, headache, squamous cell carcinoma, diarrhea, back pain, rhinitis, lymphadenopathy, influenza-like symptoms.

PREGNANCY: Category C, caution in nursing.

MECHANISM OF ACTION: Immune response modifier; mechanism has not been established. In basal cell carcinoma, suspected to increase infiltration of lymphocytes, dendritic cells, and macrophages into the tumor lesion. In external genital warts, suspected to induce mRNA encoding cytokines, including interferon-α at the treatment site.

PHARMACOKINETICS: Absorption: C_{max}=0.1ng/mL (12.5mg face), 0.2ng/mL (25mg scalp), 3.5ng/mL (75mg hands/arms), 0.4ng/mL (4.6mg average dose). **Elimination:** Urine (0.11% in males, 2.41% in females with 4.6mg average dose), (0.08% in males, 0.15% in females with 75mg dose).

NURSING CONSIDERATIONS

Assessment: Assess for age, preexisting autoimmune conditions, immunosuppression, human papilloma viral disease, basal cell nevus syndrome or xeroderma pigmentosum. For treatment of superficial basal cell carcinoma, assess proper diagnosis (eg, biopsy). Assess use in patients with inherent sensitivity to sunlight, current sunburn, and in pregnancy/nursing.

Monitoring: Monitor for signs/symptoms of local inflammatory reactions (eg, weeping or erosion) and for systemic reactions (eg, flu-like symptoms: malaise, fever, nausea, myalgias, rigors). Monitor for clinical signs of improvement.

Patient Counseling: Inform to wash hands before and after applying cream. Before applying, wash treatment area with mild soap and water and allow area to dry thoroughly. Avoid contact with eyes, lips, and nostrils and exposure to sunlight (including sunlamps) and to use protective clothing (eg, hat) or sunscreen when using medication. May experience local skin reactions and flu-like systemic signs and symptoms during therapy. Advise patients with sunburns not to use the cream until fully recovered. Advise female patients to take special care when applying the cream at the vaginal opening. When using for the treatment of actinic keratosis or superficial basal cell carcinoma, wash the treatment area with mild soap and water 8 hrs following application of the cream. When using for the treatment of external genital warts, wash treatment area with mild soap and water 6-10 hrs following application of cream. Inform that new warts may develop during therapy. May weaken condoms and vaginal diaphragms; concurrent use not recommended.

Administration: Topical route. **Storage:** 4-25°C (39-77°F). Do not freeze.

ALIMTA   RX
pemetrexed (Lilly)

THERAPEUTIC CLASS: Antifolate

INDICATIONS: In combination with cisplatin for the initial treatment of locally advanced, or metastatic nonsquamous non-small cell lung cancer (NSCLC). Maintenance treatment in patients with locally advanced, or metastatic nonsquamous NSCLC whose disease has not progressed after 4 cycles of platinum-based first-line chemotherapy. Single agent for the treatment of patients with locally advanced or metastatic, nonsquamous NSCLC after prior chemotherapy. In combination with cisplatin for the treatment of patients with malignant pleural mesothelioma, whose disease is unresectable or who are otherwise not candidates for curative surgery.

DOSAGE: *Adults:* Premedication: Dexamethasone (or equivalent) 4mg PO bid day before, day of, and day after administration. Give at least five daily doses of folic acid (350-1000mcg) PO during the 7 days prior to first dose. Continue throughout therapy and for 21 days after last dose. Give vitamin B12, 1000mcg, IM once during week preceding first dose and every three cycles thereafter. Combination with Cisplatin: Nonsquamous NSCLC/ Mesothelioma: Usual: 500mg/m² IV infused over 10 min on Day 1 of each 21-day cycle. Give cisplatin 75mg/m² infused over 2 hrs beginning 30 min after the end of administration. Patient should receive appropriate hydration prior to and/or after receiving cisplatin. Single Agent: Nonsquamous NSCLC: Usual: 500mg/m² IV infused over 10 min on Day 1 of each 21-day cycle. Refer to PI for dose adjustments for hematologic, nonhematologic, and neurotoxicities.

HOW SUPPLIED: Inj: 100mg, 500mg

WARNINGS/PRECAUTIONS: Premedicate with folic acid and vitamin B12 as prophylactic measure to reduce hematologic/GI toxicity, and with dexamethasone or its equivalent to reduce the incidence and severity of cutaneous reactions. Bone marrow suppression may occur; myelosuppression is usually the dose-limiting toxicity. Caution with renal/hepatic dysfunction and in elderly. Avoid in patients with CrCl <45mL/min. D/C if hematologic or nonhematologic grade 3 or 4 toxicity after two dose reductions or immediately if grade 3 or 4 neurotoxicity is observed. Do not start new cycle unless CrCl is ≥45mL/min, absolute neutrophil count (ANC) is ≥1500 cells/mm³, and platelet count is ≥100,000 cells/mm³. May cause fetal harm; use effective contraception to prevent pregnancy. Not indicated for the treatment of squamous cell NSCLC.

ADVERSE REACTIONS: Anemia, anorexia, fatigue, leukopenia, N/V, stomatitis, neutropenia, rash/desquamation, thrombocytopenia, constipation, pharyngitis, diarrhea.

INTERACTIONS: Delayed clearance with nephrotoxic or tubularly secreted drugs (eg, probenecid). Reduced clearance with ibuprofen. In patients with mild to moderate renal insufficiency (CrCl 45-79mL/min), caution with NSAIDs; avoid NSAIDs with short elimination half-lives (eg, diclofenac, indomethacin) for a period of 2 days before, the day of, and 2 days following therapy; interrupt dosing of NSAIDs with longer half-lives (eg, meloxicam, nabumetone) for at least 5 days before, the day of, and 2 days following therapy; if concomitant administration is necessary, monitor for toxicity.

PREGNANCY: Category D, not for use in nursing.

MECHANISM OF ACTION: Antifolate; disrupts folate-dependent metabolic processes essential for cell replication. Inhibits thymidylate synthase, dihydrofolate reductase, and glycinamide ribonucleotide formyltransferase.

PHARMACOKINETICS: Distribution: V_d=16.1L; plasma protein binding (81%). **Elimination:** Urine (70-90% unchanged); $T_{1/2}$=3.5 hrs (normal renal function).

NURSING CONSIDERATIONS

Assessment: Assess for renal/hepatic functon, pregnancy/nursing status, drug hypersensitivity, and possible drug interactions. Obtain baseline vital signs, ANC, CBC with platelets, renal function (CrCl), LFTs.

Monitoring: Monitor for signs and symptoms of hematologic/nonhematologic toxicities, bone marrow suppression (eg, neutropenia, thrombocytopenia, anemia), GI toxicity (eg, diarrhea, mucositis), neurotoxicity, cutaneous reactions (eg, rash), hypersensitivity reactions, and other adverse events that may occur. Monitor vital signs, renal function, and CBC with platelet counts. Monitor for nadir and recovery. Perform chemistry test periodically.

Patient Counseling: Inform about benefits and risks of therapy. Instruct to take folic acid and vitamin B12 as prophylactic measures to reduce treatment-related hematological and GI toxicities. Inform about risks of low blood counts and instruct to contact physician if any sign of infection (eg, fever), bleeding, anemia, vomiting, diarrhea, and dehydration occurs. Advise to inform their physician if taking any concomitant prescription or over-the-counter medications (eg, NSAID). Apprise female patients of the potential hazard to fetus; avoid pregnancy and advise to use effective contraceptive measures to prevent pregnancy during treatment.

Administration: IV route. Refer to PI for preparation/administration precautions and preparation for IV administration. **Storage:** Unreconstituted: 25°C (77°F); excursions permitted to 15-30°C (59-86°F). Reconstituted and Infusion Sol: Stable at 2-8°C (36-46°F) or 25°C (77°F) for up to 24 hrs; excursions permitted to 15-30°C (59-86°F). Discard unused portion.

ALINIA   RX
nitazoxanide (Romark)

THERAPEUTIC CLASS: Antiprotozoal agent

INDICATIONS: Treatment of diarrhea caused by *Cryptosporidium parvum* and *Giardia lamblia* in patients ≥1 yr (Sus) and ≥12 yrs (Tab).

DOSAGE: *Adults:* Give for 3 days. (Sus) 25mL q12h; (Tab) 1 tab q12h. Take with food.
Pediatrics: Give for 3 days. 1-3 yrs: 5mL (100mg) q12h. 4-11 yrs: 10mL (200mg) q12h. ≥12 yrs: (Sus) 25mL q12h. (Tab) 1 tab q12h. Take with food.

HOW SUPPLIED: Sus: 100mg/5mL [60mL]; Tab: 500mg.

WARNINGS/PRECAUTIONS: Caution with hepatic and biliary disease, renal disease, and combined renal and hepatic disease. Oral suspension contains 1.48g sucrose/5mL.

ADVERSE REACTIONS: Abdominal pain, diarrhea, headache, nausea (tab), vomiting (sus).

INTERACTIONS: Caution with other highly plasma protein-bound drugs with narrow therapeutic indices, as competition for binding sites may occur (eg, warfarin).

PREGNANCY: Category B; caution in nursing.

MECHANISM OF ACTION: Antiprotozoal agent; interferes with the pyruvate: ferredoxin oxidoreductase (PFOR) enzyme-dependent electron transfer reaction, which is essential to anaerobic energy metabolism.

PHARMACOKINETICS: Absorption: (Tab) (500mg) Tizoxanide: 12-17 yrs: C_{max}=9.1mcg/mL, T_{max}=4 hrs, AUC=39.5mcg•hr/mL; ≥18 yrs: C_{max}=10.6mcg/mL, T_{max}=3 hrs, AUC=41.9mcg•hr/mL. (Sus) Bioavailability (70%); Tizoxanide: 1-3 yrs: (100mg) C_{max}=3.11mcg/mL, T_{max}=3.5 hrs, AUC=11.7mcg•hr/mL; 4-11 yrs: (200mg) C_{max}=3mcg/mL, T_{max}=2 hrs, AUC=13.5mcg•hr/mL. ≥18 yrs: (500mg) C_{max}=5.49mcg/mL, T_{max}=2.5 hrs, AUC= 30.2mcg•hr/mL. ≥18 yrs: (500mg) C_{max}=3.21mcg/mL, T_{max}=4 hrs, AUC= 22.8mcg•hr/mL. **Distribution:** Tizoxanide: Plasma protein binding (>99%). **Metabolism:** Tizoxanide, tizoxanide glucuronide (active metabolites). Conjugation, primarily by glucuronidation. **Elimination:** Nitazoxanide: urine (1/3 of dose), bile and feces (2/3 of the dose). Tizoxanide glucuronide: urine, bile. Tizoxanide: urine, bile, feces. Refer to PI for parameters for active metabolite.

NURSING CONSIDERATIONS

Assessment: Assess for hepatic, renal/biliary impairment, HIV infection, DM, pregnancy/nursing status, and possible drug interactions.

Monitoring: Monitor for abdominal pain, diarrhea, N/V, headache, LFTs, and CBC.

Patient Counseling: Counsel to take exactly as directed. Shake sus well prior to administration. Instruct to report any adverse effects. Advise diabetic patients oral sus contains 1.48g of sucrose/5mL.

Administration: Oral route. Take with food. Reconstitute sus with 48mL of water and keep tightly closed. Shake well before administration. **Storage:** 25°C (77°F); excursions permitted to 15-30°C (59-86°F). Reconstituted sus may be stored for 7 days, after which unused portion should be discarded.

ALOPRIM　　RX
allopurinol sodium (Bioniche)

THERAPEUTIC CLASS: Xanthine oxidase inhibitor

INDICATIONS: Management of elevated serum and urinary uric acid levels in patients with leukemia, lymphoma, and solid tumor malignancies receiving cancer therapy when oral therapy is not tolerated.

DOSAGE: *Adults:* Usual: 200-400mg/m^2/day IV infusion qd or in equally divided infusions every 6, 8, or 12 hrs. Max: 600mg/day. CrCl 10-20mL/min: 200mg/day. CrCl 3-10mL/min: 100mg/day. CrCl <3mL/min: 100mg/day at extended intervals. Elderly: Start at lower end of dosing range. *Pediatrics:* Usual: 200mg/m^2/day IV qd or in divided doses every 6, 8, or 12 hrs.

HOW SUPPLIED: Inj: 500mg

WARNINGS/PRECAUTIONS: D/C at first appearance of hypersensitivity (eg, skin rash or other signs which indicate an allergic reaction); increased risk in patients with decreased renal function. Caution with renal/hepatic impairment or concurrent illnesses affecting renal function such as HTN and diabetes mellitus (DM). Hepatotoxicity may occur; monitor LFTs during early stages of therapy if with pre-existing liver disease. Monitor renal function and uric acid levels; adjust dose if needed. Maintain sufficient fluid intake to yield a daily urinary output ≥2L and maintain neutral/slightly alkaline urine. May impair mental/physical abilities. Drowsiness and bone marrow suppression reported. Caution in elderly.

ADVERSE REACTIONS: Skin rash, eosinophilia, local injection-site reaction, N/V, diarrhea, renal failure/insufficiency.

INTERACTIONS: Inhibits oxidation of mercaptopurine and azathioprine; reduce mercaptopurine and azathioprine dose to 1/3-1/4 of usual dose. Increased frequency of skin rash with ampicillin and amoxicillin. Increased toxicity and risk of hypersensitivity in patients with renal dysfunction with concomitant thiazide diuretics; monitor renal function. Increased risk of hypoglycemia in the presence of renal insufficiency with concomitant chlorpropamide. Enhanced bone marrow suppression when used with cyclophosphamide and other cytotoxic agents among patients with neoplastic disease, except leukemia. May increase cyclosporine levels; monitor cyclosporine levels and adjust dose as required. Decreased inhibition of xanthine oxidase by oxypurinol and increased urinary excretion of uric acid with uricosuric agents. Prolongs half-life of dicumarol; monitor PT with concomitant use.

PREGNANCY: Category C, caution in nursing.

MECHANISM OF ACTION: Xanthine oxidase inhibitor; reduces production of uric acid by inhibiting the biochemical reactions immediately preceding its formation.

PHARMACOKINETICS: Absorption: Absolute bioavailability (100%); C_{max}=1.58µg/mL (100mg), 5.12µg/mL (300mg); T_{max}=0.5 hrs; AUC=1.99 hr•µg/mL (100mg), 7.1 hr•µg/mL (300mg). **Distribution:** V_d=0.84L/kg (100mg), 0.87L/kg (300mg); found in breast milk. **Metabolism:** Oxidative; oxypurinol (active metabolite). **Elimination:** Urine (12% unchanged, 76% as oxypurinol); $T_{1/2}$=(100mg) 1 hr (parent), 24.1 hrs (oxypurinol), (300mg) 1.21 hrs (parent), 23.5 hrs (oxypurinol).

NURSING CONSIDERATIONS

Assessment: Assess for renal/hepatic function, concurrent illnesses affecting renal function (eg, HTN, DM), hypersensitivity reactions (eg, skin rash, Stevens-Johnson syndrome [SJS]), pregnancy/nursing status and possible drug interactions. Obtain serum uric acid to provide correct dosage and schedule.

Monitoring: Monitor for allergic/hypersensitivity reactions (eg, exfoliative, urticarial, purpuric lesions, SJS), generalized vasculitis, hepatotoxicity, drowsiness, bone marrow suppression and fluid intake. Monitor LFTs, serum uric acid, BUN and SrCr.

Patient Counseling: Inform about benefits/risks of therapy. Inform may impair mental/physical abilities. Advise to take sufficient fluid to yield a daily urinary output of at least 2L in adults and the need to maintain a neutral or preferably slightly alkaline urine. Advise to report any adverse events to physician.

Administration: IV infusion. Refer to PI for reconstitution and dilution. Rate of infusion depends on the volume of infusate. Whenever possible, initiate therapy 24-48 hrs before the start of chemotherapy known to cause tumor cell lysis (including adrenocorticosteroids). Do not mix or administer through the same IV port with agents which are incompatible in solution (refer to PI). Begin administration within 10 hrs after reconstitution. **Storage:** 25°C (77°F); excursions permitted to 15-30°C (59-86°F). After dilution, store solution at 20-25°C (68-77°F). Do not refrigerate the reconstituted and/or diluted product.

ALOXI RX

palonosetron HCl (Eisai)

THERAPEUTIC CLASS: 5-HT$_3$ receptor antagonist

INDICATIONS: Prevention of acute and delayed N/V associated with initial and repeat courses of moderately emetogenic cancer chemotherapy and prevention of acute N/V associated with initial and repeat courses of highly emetogenic cancer chemotherapy. Prevention of postoperative nausea and vomiting (PONV) for up to 24 hrs following surgery.

DOSAGE: *Adults:* Prevention of Chemotherapy-Induced N/V: 0.25mg IV single dose over 30 sec. Dosing should occur 30 min before the start of chemotherapy. PONV: 0.075mg IV single dose over 10 sec immediately before induction of anesthesia.

HOW SUPPLIED: Inj: 0.25mg/5mL, 0.075mg/1.5mL

WARNINGS/PRECAUTIONS: Hypersensitivity reactions may occur in patients who have exhibited hypersensitivity to other 5-HT$_3$ receptor antagonists. Routine prophylaxis is not recommended in patients in whom there is little expectation that N/V will occur postoperatively. In patients where N/V must be avoided during the postoperative period, prophylaxis is recommended even when the incidence of PONV is low.

ADVERSE REACTIONS: Headache, constipation, QT prolongation, bradycardia.

PREGNANCY: Category B, not for use in nursing.

MECHANISM OF ACTION: 5-HT$_3$ receptor antagonist; antiemetic and antinauseant.

PHARMACOKINETICS: Absorption: (IV, 3mcg/kg) C_{max}=5.6ng/mL, AUC=35.8ng•hr/mL. **Distribution:** V_d=8.3L/kg; plasma protein binding (62%). **Metabolism:** 50% metabolized via CYP2D6, CYP3A4, CYP1A2; N-oxide-palonosetron and 6-S-hydroxy-palonosetron (primary metabolites). **Elimination:** Urine (80%, 40% unchanged); $T_{1/2}$=40 hrs.

NURSING CONSIDERATIONS

Assessment: Assess for previous hypersensitivity to other 5-HT$_3$ receptor antagonists, risk/possibility of PONV, emetogenicity of chemotherapy, and for pregnancy/nursing status. Obtain baseline vital signs.

Monitoring: Monitor for hypersensitivity reactions, QT interval prolongation, and other adverse events that may occur. Monitor vital signs.

Patient Counseling: Instruct to read patient insert. Advise to report to physician of all medical conditions and infusion-site reactions (eg, pain, redness, swelling).

Administration: IV route. Flush infusion line with normal saline before and after administration. Do not mix with other drugs. Inspect visually for particulate matter and discoloration before administration. **Storage:** 20-25°C (68-77°F); excursions permitted to 15-30°C (59-86°F). Protect from light and freezing.

ALPHAGAN P RX

brimonidine tartrate (Allergan)

THERAPEUTIC CLASS: Selective alpha$_2$ agonist

INDICATIONS: Reduction of elevated intraocular pressure in patients with open-angle glaucoma or ocular HTN.

DOSAGE: *Adults:* 1 drop in affected eye(s) tid (8 hrs apart). Space by at least 5 min if using >1 topical ophthalmic drug.
Pediatrics: ≥2 yrs: 1 drop in affected eye(s) tid (8 hrs apart). Space by at least 5 min if using >1 topical ophthalmic drug.

HOW SUPPLIED: Sol: 0.1%, 0.15% [5mL, 10mL, 15mL]

CONTRAINDICATIONS: Neonates and infants <2 yrs.

WARNINGS/PRECAUTIONS: May potentiate syndromes associated with vascular insufficiency. Caution with severe cardiovascular disease (CVD), depression, cerebral or coronary insufficiency, Raynaud's phenomenon, orthostatic hypotension, or thromboangiitis obliterans. Bacterial keratitis reported with multi-dose containers.

ADVERSE REACTIONS: Allergic conjunctivitis, conjunctival hyperemia, eye pruritus, burning sensation, conjunctival folliculosis, HTN, oral dryness, ocular allergic reaction, visual disturbance, somnolence, decreased alertness.

INTERACTIONS: May potentiate effect with CNS depressants (alcohol, barbiturates, opiates, sedatives, anesthetics). Caution with antihypertensives, cardiac glycosides, and TCAs. May increase systemic side effects (eg, hypotension) with MAOIs; caution is advised.

PREGNANCY: Category B, not for use in nursing.

MECHANISM OF ACTION: Selective α_2 agonist; reduces aqueous humor production and increases uveoscleral outflow.

PHARMACOKINETICS: Absorption: T_{max}=0.5-2.5 hrs. **Metabolism:** Liver (extensive). **Elimination:** (Oral) Urine (74% unchanged and metabolites); $T_{1/2}$=2 hrs.

NURSING CONSIDERATIONS

Assessment: Assess for age, hypersensitivity, severe CVD, depression, cerebral or coronary insufficiency, Raynaud's phenomenon, orthostatic hypotension, or thromboangiitis obliterans, pregnancy/nursing, and possible drug interactions.

Monitoring: Monitor vascular insufficiency, bacterial keratitis, and other adverse reactions.

Patient Counseling: Advise to avoid touching tip of applicator to eye or surrounding areas. Instruct patient to notify physician if they have ocular surgery or develop an intercurrent ocular condition (eg, trauma or infection). Inform patients that fatigue and/or drowsiness may occur; may impair physical or mental abilities. Instruct to space by at least 5 min if using >1 topical ophthalmic drug.

Administration: Ocular route. **Storage:** 15-25°C (59-77°F).

ALREX   RX
loteprednol etabonate (Bausch & Lomb)

THERAPEUTIC CLASS: Corticosteroid

INDICATIONS: Temporary relief of signs and symptoms of seasonal allergic conjunctivitis.

DOSAGE: *Adults:* 1 drop into the affected eye(s) qid.

HOW SUPPLIED: Sus: 0.2% [5mL, 10mL]

CONTRAINDICATIONS: Viral diseases of the cornea and conjunctiva, including epithelial herpes simplex keratitis (dendritic keratitis), vaccinia, and varicella. Mycobacterial infection of the eye and fungal diseases of the ocular structures.

WARNINGS/PRECAUTIONS: Prolonged use may result in glaucoma with optic nerve damage, visual acuity and visual field defects, and posterior subcapsular cataract formation. Caution with glaucoma. Prolonged use may increase the hazard of secondary ocular infections. Caution with diseases causing thinning of the cornea/sclera; perforations may occur. May mask/enhance existing infection in acute purulent conditions of the eye. May prolong the course or exacerbate severity of many viral infections of the eye. Caution with history of herpes simplex virus. Perform eye exam (eg, slit lamp biomicroscopy, fluorescein staining) prior to therapy and renewal of medication order >14 days. Reevaluate if signs/symptoms failed to improve after 2 days. Monitor intraocular pressure (IOP) if used >10 days. Fungal infections of the cornea may develop with long-term use; consider fungal invasion in any persistent corneal ulceration.

ADVERSE REACTIONS: Elevated IOP, abnormal vision/blurring, burning on instillation, chemosis, discharge, dry eyes, epiphora, foreign body sensation, itching, photophobia, headache, rhinitis, pharyngitis.

PREGNANCY: Category C, caution in nursing.

MECHANISM OF ACTION: Corticosteroid; not established. Suspected to act by induction of phospholipase A_2 inhibitory proteins, collectively called lipocortins. Inhibits the inflammatory response to a variety of inciting agents and probably delays or slows healing. Inhibits edema, fibrin deposition, capillary dilation, leukocyte migration, fibroblast proliferation, deposition of collagen, and scar formation associated with inflammation.

PHARMACOKINETICS: Distribution: Found in breast milk (systemic use).

NURSING CONSIDERATIONS

Assessment: Assess for hypersensitivity to the drug, viral diseases of the cornea and conjunctiva (eg, epithelial herpes simplex) [dendritic keratitis]), vaccinia varicella, mycobacterial eye infection, fungal diseases of the ocular structures, glaucoma, diseases causing thinning of the cornea/sclera, acute purulent conditions of the eye, and pregnancy/nursing status. Perform eye exam (eg, slit lamp biomicroscopy, fluorescein staining) prior to therapy.

Monitoring: Monitor for signs and symptoms of glaucoma, optic nerve damage, visual acuity and visual field defects, posterior subcapsular cataracts, sclera/corneal perforations, masking or enhancement of existing infections in acute purulent conditions of the eye, and other adverse reactions. Monitor IOP and perform eye exams.

Patient Counseling: Advise not to touch dropper tip to any surface to avoid contamination. Instruct to contact physician if redness or itching becomes aggravated. Instruct not wear contact lenses if eyes are red. Counsel not to use for contact lens related irritation. Inform that the medication contains benzalkonium chloride that may be absorbed by soft contact lenses. Instruct patients who wear soft contact lenses and whose eyes are not red to wait at least 10 min after administration before wearing contact lenses.

Administration: Ocular route. **Storage:** 15-25°C (59-77°F). Store upright. Do not freeze.

ALSUMA   RX
sumatriptan (King)

THERAPEUTIC CLASS: 5-HT$_{1B/1D}$ agonist

INDICATIONS: Acute treatment of migraine attacks, with or without aura, and acute treatment of cluster headache episodes.

DOSAGE: *Adults:* Usual: 6mg SQ. Max: Two 6mg doses/24 hrs separate by at least 1 hr.

HOW SUPPLIED: Inj: 6mg/0.5mL

CONTRAINDICATIONS: IV administration, ischemic heart disease (eg, angina pectoris, history of myocardial infarction [MI], or documented silent ischemia) or symptoms/findings consistent with ischemic heart disease, coronary vasospasm (eg, Prinzmetal's variant angina), or other significant underlying cardiovascular (CV) disease, cerebrovascular syndromes (eg, stroke, transient ischemic attack), peripheral vascular disease (eg, ischemic bowel disease), uncontrolled HTN, or hemiplegic or basilar migraine, administration of any ergotamine-containing or ergot-type agents (eg, dihydroergotamine or methysergide) or other 5-HT$_1$ agonists (eg, triptan) within 24 hrs.

WARNINGS/PRECAUTIONS: Serious adverse cardiac events (eg, MI, life-threatening arrhythmias), cerebrovascular events, vasospastic reactions (eg, coronary artery vasospasm, peripheral vascular ischemia, colonic ischemia), and hypersensitivity (anaphylaxis/anaphylactoid) reactions reported. Signs and symptoms suggestive of decreased arterial flow should be evaluated for atherosclerosis or predisposition to vasospasm. Evaluate for coronary artery disease (CAD) and its risk factors; administer 1st dose under medical supervision and consider an ECG following administration. Sensations of tightness, pain, pressure and heaviness in the chest, throat, neck, and jaw are common after therapy. Serotonin syndrome may occur; symptoms may include mental status changes, autonomic instability, neuromuscular aberrations, and GI symptoms. Caution with controlled HTN. Elevation in BP, including hypertensive crisis reported. Seizures reported; caution with history of epilepsy or lowered seizure threshold. Corneal opacities may occur. Not recommended for elderly; higher risk for CAD, HTN, and decreased hepatic function.

ADVERSE REACTIONS: Injection-site reactions, tingling, warm/hot sensation, burning sensation, pressure sensation, tight feeling in head, drowsiness/sedation, tightness in chest, flushing, numbness, dizziness/vertigo, weakness, neck pain/stiffness.

INTERACTIONS: See Contraindications. Not recommended with MAO-A inhibitor; reduced sumatriptan clearance. Concomitant ergot-containing drugs may cause prolonged vasospastic reactions. Serotonin syndrome reported when used in combination with SSRIs or serotonin norepinephrine reuptake inhibitors (SNRIs).

PREGNANCY: Category C, caution in nursing.

MECHANISM OF ACTION: Selective 5-HT$_{1B/1D}$ agonist; binds to vascular 5-HT$_1$-type receptors in cranial arteries, basilar artery, and vasculature of isolated dura mater, which causes vasoconstriction.

PHARMACOKINETICS: Absorption: Bioavailability (97%); (Deltoid) C_{max}=74ng/mL; T_{max}=12 min. (Thigh) Manual: C_{max}=61ng/mL. Auto-Injector: C_{max}=52ng/mL. **Distribution:** V_d=50L; plasma protein binding (14%-21%). **Metabolism:** Indole acetic acid (metabolite). **Elimination:** Urine (22%, unchanged; 38%, metabolite); $T_{1/2}$=115 min.

NURSING CONSIDERATIONS

Assessment: Assess for presence/history of ischemic heart disease, CAD and its risk factors (eg, hypercholesterolemia, smoking, obesity, diabetes mellitus), cerebrovascular/peripheral vascular disease, uncontrolled HTN, hemiplegic/basilar migraine, history of epilepsy, pregnancy/nursing status, and possible drug interactions. Establish proper diagnosis of migraine or cluster headache; exclude other potentially serious neurological conditions. Obtain baseline vital signs, weight, CV function, ECG, LFTs.

Monitoring: Monitor for cardiac ischemia; give 1st dose in physician's office or medical facility and obtain ECG after administration for those with CAD risk factors. Monitor for signs/symptoms of cardiac events, colonic ischemia, bloody diarrhea, serotonin syndrome (eg, mental status changes, autonomic instability, neuromuscular aberrations, and/or GI symptoms), hypersensitivity reactions, chest/throat/jaw/neck tightness, seizures, headache, increased BP, and ophthalmic changes. For long-term therapy or with CAD risk factors, perform periodic monitoring of CV function. Monitor vital signs and weight, LFTs.

Patient Counseling: Inform about risks and benefits of therapy, proper use, importance of follow-up, and possible drug interactions. Inform to notify physician if any symptoms such as chest pain, SOB, weakness, or slurring of speech occur, or if pregnant or nursing; not used during pregnancy unless potential benefit outweighs risk to the fetus. Inform about the risk of serotonin syndrome during combined use with SSRIs and SNRIs. Advise on the proper administration techniques and appropriate sites of injection (eg, lateral thigh or upper arms); not to administer via IM/IV.

Administration: SQ route. **Storage:** 25°C; excursions permitted 15-30°C (59-86°F). Protect from light. Do not refrigerate.

ALTABAX RX
retapamulin (GlaxoSmithKline)

THERAPEUTIC CLASS: Pleuromutilin antibacterial

INDICATIONS: Treatment of impetigo due to *Staphylococcus aureus* (methicillin-susceptible isolates only) or *Streptococcus pyogenes,* in patients ≥9 months.

DOSAGE: *Adults*: Apply thin layer to the affected area (up to 100cm² in total area) bid for 5 days. *Pediatrics:* ≥9 months: Apply thin layer to the affected area (up to 2% total BSA) bid for 5 days.

HOW SUPPLIED: Oint: 1% [5g, 10g, 15g, 30g]

WARNINGS/PRECAUTIONS: D/C use, wipe off oint, and institute appropriate alternative therapy in the event of sensitization or severe local irritation. Not intended for PO, intranasal, ophthalmic, or intravaginal use. Has not been evaluated for use on mucosal surfaces; epistaxis reported with use on nasal mucosa. Take appropriate measures if superinfection occurs. Increased risk of development of drug-resistant bacteria if used in the absence of a proven or strongly suspected bacterial infection.

ADVERSE REACTIONS: Application-site irritation and pruritus, headache, diarrhea, nausea, nasopharyngitis, pruritus, fever, eczema, increased creatinine phosphokinase.

INTERACTIONS: PO ketoconazole may increase levels.

PREGNANCY: Category B, caution in nursing.

MECHANISM OF ACTION: Semisynthetic pleuromutilin antibacterial; selectively inhibits bacterial protein synthesis by interacting at a site on the 50S subunit of the bacterial ribosome. The binding site involves ribosomal protein L3 and is in the region of the ribosomal P site and peptidyl transferase center. By virtue of binding to this site, peptidyl transfer is inhibited, P-site interactions are blocked, and the normal formation of active 50S ribosomal subunits is prevented.

PHARMACOKINETICS: Absorption: C_{max}=10.7ng/mL (adults), 18.5ng/mL (pediatrics). **Distribution:** Plasma protein binding (94%). **Metabolism:** Liver (extensive) by mono-oxygenation and N-demethylation via CYP3A4.

NURSING CONSIDERATIONS

Assessment: Assess pregnancy/nursing status and for possible drug interactions.

Monitoring: Monitor for sensitization or severe local irritation, superinfection, and other adverse reactions.

Patient Counseling: Instruct to use medication ud, to wash hands after application (if hands are not the area for treatment), and not to swallow drug or use in the eyes, on the mouth or lips, inside the nose, or inside the female genital area. Inform that treated area may be covered by sterile bandage or gauze dressing if desired. Instruct to use the medication for the full time recommended by physician, even though symptoms may have improved. Advise to notify physician if symptoms do not improve within 3-4 days after starting treatment, and if area of application worsens in irritation, redness, itching, burning, swelling, blistering, or oozing.

Administration: Topical route. **Storage:** 25°C (77°F); excursions permitted to 15-30°C (59-86°F).

ALTACE RX
ramipril (King)

D/C when pregnancy is detected. Drugs that act directly on the renin-angiotensin system can cause injury/death to the developing fetus.

THERAPEUTIC CLASS: ACE inhibitor

INDICATIONS: To reduce risk of myocardial infarction (MI), stroke, and death from cardiovascular (CV) causes in patients ≥55 yrs who are at high risk due to history of coronary artery disease, stroke, peripheral vascular disease, or diabetes with at least one other CV risk factor. Treatment of HTN, alone or with thiazide diuretics. To reduce risk of CV death, heart failure related hospitalization, and progression to severe/resistant heart failure in stable post-acute MI patients who show signs of congestive heart failure (CHF).

DOSAGE: *Adults:* Risk Reduction of MI, Stroke, CV Death: ≥55 yrs: Initial: 2.5mg qd for 1 week. Titrate: Increase to 5mg qd for next 3 weeks, and then increase as tolerated. Maint: 10mg qd. May be given as a divided dose if hypertensive or recently post-MI. HTN: Not Receiving a Diuretic: Initial: 2.5mg qd. Adjust dosage according to BP response. Maint: 2.5-20mg/day given qd or in 2 equally divided doses. May add diuretic if BP not controlled. CrCl ≤40mL/min: Initial: 1.25mg qd. May be titrated upward until BP is controlled. Max: 5mg/day. CHF Post-MI: Initial: 2.5mg bid, or switch to 1.25mg bid if hypotensive. Titrate: If tolerated, may increase to target dose of 5mg bid at 3 week intervals after 1 week of initial dose. CrCl ≤40mL/min: Initial: 1.25mg qd. Titrate: May increase to 1.25mg bid, and up to a max dose of 2.5mg bid depending on response and tolerability. With Renal Artery Stenosis/Volume Depletion (eg, past and current diuretic): Initial: 1.25mg qd. Adjust dosage according to BP response.

HOW SUPPLIED: Cap: 1.25mg, 2.5mg, 5mg, 10mg

CONTRAINDICATIONS: History of ACE inhibitor-associated angioedema.

WARNINGS/PRECAUTIONS: May increase risk of angioedema in patients with history of angioedema unrelated to ACE inhibitor therapy. Angioedema reported; d/c and institute appropriate therapy if laryngeal stridor or angioedema of the face, tongue, or glottis occurs. More reports of angioedema in blacks than nonblacks. Intestinal angioedema reported; monitor for abdominal pain. Anaphylactoid reactions reported during desensitization with hymenoptera venom, dialysis with high-flux membranes, and LDL apheresis with dextran sulfate absorption. Rarely, a syndrome that starts with cholestatic jaundice progressing to fulminant hepatic necrosis and sometimes death reported; d/c if jaundice or marked elevations of hepatic enzymes develop. Renal function changes may occur. Excessive hypotension associated with oliguria or azotemia and rarely, with acute renal failure and death may occur in patients with CHF; closely monitor during 1st 2 weeks of therapy and whenever dose is increased. Increases in BUN and SrCr may occur in patients with renal artery stenosis. Agranulocytosis, pancytopenia, bone marrow depression, and mild reductions in Hgb content, blood cell, or platelet counts may occur; monitor WBCs in patients with collagen vascular disease, especially with renal impairment. Symptomatic hypotension may occur and is most likely in patients with volume and/or salt depletion; correct depletion prior to therapy. Hypotension may occur with surgery or during anesthesia. Hyperkalemia reported; risk factors include renal insufficiency and diabetes mellitus (DM). Persistent nonproductive cough reported.

ADVERSE REACTIONS: Hypotension, cough increased, dizziness, angina pectoris, headache, asthenia, fatigue.

INTERACTIONS: Avoid with telmisartan; increased risk of renal dysfunction. Hypotension risk, and increased BUN and SrCr with diuretics. K⁺-sparing diuretics, K⁺ supplements, and/or K⁺-containing salt substitutes may increase risk of hyperkalemia; use with caution and monitor serum K⁺ frequently. Increased lithium levels and symptoms of lithium toxicity reported; monitor lithium levels. Diuretics may further increase risk of lithium toxicity. Nitritoid reactions (eg, facial flushing, N/V, hypotension) reported rarely with injectable gold (sodium aurothiomalate). NSAIDs, including selective cyclooxygenase-2 inhibitors, may deteriorate renal function and attenuate antihypertensive effect; monitor renal function periodically. Hypoglycemia reported with oral hypoglycemic agents or insulin.

PREGNANCY: Category D, not for use in nursing.

MECHANISM OF ACTION: ACE inhibitor; decreases plasma angiotensin II, which leads to decreased vasopressor activity and aldosterone secretion.

PHARMACOKINETICS: Absorption: Absolute bioavailability (28%, 44% ramiprilat); T_{max}=1 hr, 2-4 hrs (ramiprilat). **Distribution:** Plasma protein binding (73%, 56% ramiprilat); crosses placenta; found in breast milk. **Metabolism:** Cleavage of ester group (liver); ramiprilat (active metabolite). **Elimination:** Urine (60%, <2% unchanged), feces (40%); $T_{1/2}$=>50 hrs (terminal, ramiprilat), 13-17 hrs (multipledose, ramiprilat).

NURSING CONSIDERATIONS

Assessment: Assess for history of angioedema, CHF, renal artery stenosis, collagen vascular disease (eg, systemic lupus erythematosus, scleroderma), volume/salt depletion, DM, hepatic/renal impairment, hypersensitivity to drug, pregnancy/nursing status, and possible drug interactions.

Monitoring: After initial dose, observe for at least 2 hrs and until BP has stabilized for at least an additional hr. Monitor for angioedema, abdominal pain, anaphylactoid reactions, jaundice, hypotension, hyperkalemia, cough, and other adverse effects. Monitor WBCs in patients with collagen vascular disease, especially if with renal impairment. Monitor BP and renal/hepatic function.

Patient Counseling: Advise to d/c and consult physician if any signs/symptoms of angioedema (swelling of the face, eyes, lips, or tongue, or difficulty in breathing), or if syncope occurs. Instruct to immediately report any signs/symptoms of infection. Inform that lightheadedness may occur, especially during 1st days of therapy; report to physician. Inform that inadequate fluid intake or excessive perspiration, diarrhea, or vomiting may lead to excessive fall in BP with same consequences of lightheadedness and possible syncope. Inform about the consequences of exposure during pregnancy in females of childbearing age. Instruct to report pregnancies to physician as soon as possible. Advise not to use salt substitutes containing K⁺ without consulting physician.

Administration: Oral route. Swallow whole. May sprinkle contents on a small amount (about 4 oz.) of applesauce or mix in 4 oz. of water or apple juice. Consume mixture in its entirety.
Storage: 15-30°C (59-86°F). Preprepared Mixtures: Store for up to 24 hrs at room temperature or up to 48 hrs under refrigeration.

ALTOPREV
lovastatin (Shionogi)

RX

THERAPEUTIC CLASS: HMG-CoA reductase inhibitor

INDICATIONS: Adjunct to diet to lower total cholesterol (total-C), LDL-C, apolipoprotein B, and TG, and increase HDL-C in primary hypercholesterolemia (heterozygous familial and non-familial) and mixed dyslipidemia (Fredrickson types IIa and IIb) when the response to diet restricted in saturated fat and cholesterol and to other nonpharmacological measures alone have been inadequate. To slow progression of coronary atherosclerosis in patients with coronary heart disease as part of treatment to lower total-C and LDL-C. To reduce risk of myocardial infarction, unstable angina, and coronary revascularization procedures in patients without symptomatic cardiovascular disease, average to moderately elevated total-C and LDL-C, and below average HDL-C.

DOSAGE: *Adults:* Individualize. Initial: 20, 40, or 60mg qhs. Range: 20-60mg/day. Consider immediate-release lovastatin in patients requiring smaller reductions. Titrate: Adjust at intervals of ≥4 weeks. Elderly (≥65 yrs)/Complicated Medical Conditions (Renal Insufficiency, Diabetes Mellitus [DM]): Initial: 20mg qhs. Severe Renal Insufficiency (CrCl <30mL/min): Caution with increasing doses above 20mg/day. Concomitant Fibrates/Niacin (≥1g/day)/Amiodarone/Verapamil: Max: 20mg/day.

HOW SUPPLIED: Tab: Extended-Release: 20mg, 40mg, 60mg

CONTRAINDICATIONS: Active liver disease/unexplained persistent elevations of serum transaminases, pregnancy, and nursing mothers.

WARNINGS/PRECAUTIONS: Myopathy and rhabdomyolysis with or without acute renal failure secondary to myoglobinuria reported. May increase serum transaminases and creatine phosphokinase levels; consider in differential diagnosis of chest pain. Monitor LFTs prior to therapy, at 6 weeks and 12 weeks after initiation of therapy or elevation of dose, and then periodically thereafter. D/C if AST or ALT ≥3X ULN persists, if myopathy (creatine kinase [CK] level >10X ULN) diagnosed or suspected, and a few days before major surgery. Caution with heavy alcohol use and/or history of liver disease. Caution with dose escalation with complicated medical conditions (eg, renal insufficiency, DM). May cause endocrine dysfunction and CNS toxicity. Lovastatin immediate-release found to be less effective with homozygous familial hypercholesterolemia. Caution in elderly.

ADVERSE REACTIONS: Nausea, abdominal pain, insomnia, dyspepsia, headache, asthenia, myalgia, diarrhea, back pain, flu syndrome, infection, arthralgia, sinusitis.

INTERACTIONS: Increased risk of myopathy/rhabdomyolysis with potent CYP3A4 inhibitors (eg, cyclosporine, itraconazole, ketoconazole, erythromycin, clarithromycin, HIV protease inhibitors, nefazodone, large quantities of grapefruit juice [>1 quart/day]), gemfibrozil, other fibrates, lipid-lowering doses (≥1g/day) of niacin, amiodarone, and verapamil. If concomitant itraconazole, ketoconazole, erythromycin, or clarithromycin unavoidable, suspend lovastatin. Avoid other potent CYP3A4 inhibitors (eg, HIV protease inhibitors, nefazodone, >1 quart/day grapefruit juice) unless benefits outweigh the risk. Do not begin therapy with lovastatin extended-release if taking cyclosporine; consider immediate-release lovastatin; do not exceed lovastatin 20mg/day. Avoid lovastatin doses >20mg/day if used with amiodarone or verapamil. Avoid use with gemfibrozil, other fibrates, or lipid lowering doses of niacin; if necessary, lovastatin dose should not exceed 20mg/day. Monitor PT with anticoagulants (eg, warfarin) before starting lovastatin and during treatment. May interact with other CYP3A4 substrates. Caution with drugs that may decrease the levels or activity of endogenous steroid hormones (eg, ketoconazole, spironolactone, cimetidine).

PREGNANCY: Category X, not for use in nursing.

MECHANISM OF ACTION: HMG-CoA reductase inhibitor; inhibits the conversion of HMG-CoA to mevalonate which is an early step in the biosynthetic pathway for cholesterol. LDL-C-lowering effect involves both reduction of VLDL-C concentration, and induction of the LDL receptor, leading to reduced production and/or increased catabolism of LDL-C.

PHARMACOKINETICS: Absorption: Lovastatin: C_{max}=5.5ng/mL, T_{max}=14.2 hrs, AUC=77ng•hr/mL. Lovastatin acid: C_{max}=5.8ng/mL, T_{max}=11.8 hrs, AUC=87ng•hr/mL. **Distribution:** Plasma protein binding (>95%). Crosses blood-brain/placental barriers. **Metabolism:** Liver (extensive 1st pass), CYP3A4; β-hydroxyacid, 6'-hydroxy derivative, and two additional metabolites (major active metabolites). **Elimination:** Bile.

NURSING CONSIDERATIONS

Assessment: Assess for active/history of liver disease or unexplained persistent elevations in serum transaminases, alcohol use, drug hypersensitivity, pregnancy/nursing status, and for possible drug interactions. Assess lipid profile (total-C, HDL-C, and TG) and LFTs prior to therapy. Assess use in presence of homozygous familial hypercholesterolemia, DM, renal insufficiency.

Monitoring: Monitor for signs/symptoms of myopathy (eg, pain, tenderness, or weakness), rhabdomyolysis, increases in serum transaminases, CNS toxicity, endocrine dysfunction, hypersensitivity reaction, and other adverse reactions. Perform periodic monitoring of cholesterol levels and CK levels. Monitor LFTs (eg, ALT, AST) at 6 and 12 weeks after initiation of therapy and elevation of dose, and periodically thereafter.

Patient Counseling: Inform about risks/benefits of therapy. Advise to report any signs/symptoms of unexplained muscle pain, tenderness, or weakness. Counsel females about risks of use during pregnancy/nursing. Counsel to take at bedtime. Instruct to swallow tab whole and not to chew, crush, or cut.

Administration: Oral route. **Storage:** 20-25°C (68-77°F); excursions permitted to 15-30°C (59-86°F). Avoid excessive heat and humidity.

ALVESCO   RX
ciclesonide (Sunovion)

THERAPEUTIC CLASS: Non-halogenated glucocorticoid

INDICATIONS: Maintenance treatment of asthma as prophylactic therapy in adults and adolescents ≥12 yrs.

DOSAGE: *Adults:* Previous Bronchodilator Alone: Initial: 80mcg bid. Max: 160mcg bid. Previous Inhaled Corticosteroid: Initial: 80mcg bid. Max: 320mcg bid. Previous Oral Corticosteroid: Initial: 320mcg bid. Max: 320mcg bid. Elderly: Start at low end of dosing range. Titrate to the lowest effective dosage after asthma is stable. If inadequate response to initial dose after 4 weeks, may use higher doses.
Pediatrics: ≥12 yrs: Previous Bronchodilator Alone: Initial: 80mcg bid. Max: 160mcg bid. Previous Inhaled Corticosteroid: Initial: 80mcg bid. Max: 320mcg bid. Previous Oral Corticosteroid: Initial: 320mcg bid. Max: 320mcg bid. Titrate to the lowest effective dosage after asthma is stable. If inadequate response to initial dose after 4 weeks, may use higher doses.

HOW SUPPLIED: MDI: 80mcg/actuation, 160mcg/actuation [60 actuations]

CONTRAINDICATIONS: Primary treatment of status asthmaticus or other acute episodes of asthma where intensive measures are required.

WARNINGS/PRECAUTIONS: Localized *Candida albicans* infections of mouth and pharynx may occur; treat accordingly. Not indicated for rapid relief of bronchospasm. Increased susceptibility to infections (eg, chickenpox, measles); avoid exposure in patients who have not had the disease or been properly immunized. Caution with active or quiescent tuberculosis (TB) infections, untreated systemic bacterial, fungal, viral, parasitic infections, or ocular herpes simplex. Caution in patients transferred from systemic to inhaled corticosteroids; deaths due to adrenal insufficiency have occurred and may unmask allergic conditions. Hypercorticism and adrenal suppression may appear with more than recommended doses over prolonged periods of time. May decrease bone mineral density (BMD) with prolonged treatment; monitor those with major risk factors and treat accordingly. May reduce growth velocity in pediatrics. Glaucoma, increased intraocular pressure (IOP), and cataracts reported; monitor closely in patients with change in vision, history of IOP, glaucoma, and/or cataracts. Bronchospasm may occur; d/c use and institute alternative treatment if occur. Caution in elderly.

ADVERSE REACTIONS: Headache, nasopharyngitis, sinusitis, pharyngolaryngeal pain, upper respiratory infection, arthralgia, nasal congestion, pain in extremity, back pain.

INTERACTIONS: Oral ketoconazole may increase levels of the pharmacologically active metabolite des-ciclesonide. Caution with chronic use of drugs that can reduce bone mass (eg, anticonvulsants, oral corticosteroids).

PREGNANCY: Category C, caution in nursing.

MECHANISM OF ACTION: Nonhalogenated glucocorticoid; not established. Exerts anti-inflammatory actions with affinity to glucocorticoid receptor that inhibits activities of multiple cell types (mast cells, eosinophils, basophils, lymphocytes, macrophages, and neutrophils) and mediators (histamine, eicosanoids, leukotrienes, and cytokines) involved in asthmatic response.

PHARMACOKINETICS: **Absorption:** Ciclesonide: Absolute bioavailability (22%). Des-ciclesonide: AUC=2.18ng•hr/mL (multiple dose), C_{max}=1.02ng/mL (single dose), 0.369ng/mL (multiple dose); T_{max}=1.04 hrs. **Distribution:** (IV) V_d=2.9L/kg (ciclesonide), 12.1L/kg (des-ciclesonide); plasma protein binding (≥99%). **Metabolism:** Liver, via CYP3A4, CYP2D6; des-ciclesonide (active metabolite). **Elimination:** (IV) Feces (66%), urine (≤20% des-ciclesonide). $T_{1/2}$=0.71 hrs (ciclesonide), 6-7 hrs (des-ciclesonide).

NURSING CONSIDERATIONS

Assessment: Assess for status asthmaticus, acute episodes of asthma, previous corticosteroid use, risk for decreased bone mineral content, history of glaucoma, increased IOP, and/or cataracts, pregnancy/nursing status, and possible drug interactions.

Monitoring: Monitor for glaucoma, increased IOP, cataracts, visual changes, growth in children, localized infections with *C. albicans*, hypercorticism, adrenal insufficiency, bronchospasm, hypersensitivity, and other adverse events that may occur. Monitor lung function and BMD.

Patient Counseling: Inform patient of the benefits and risks of the treatment. Advise that drug is not a bronchodilator or a rescue medication. Contact physician immediately if deterioration of asthma occurs. Advise to rinse mouth after inhalation. Instruct to use at regular intervals. Inform that maximum benefit may not be seen for ≥4 weeks after starting treatment. Report if symptoms do not improve or if condition worsens; do not increase prescribed dosage. Instruct not to d/c abruptly. Avoid exposure to chickenpox or measles; notify physician immediately if exposed. Inform that drug may worsen existing TB, fungal, bacterial, viral, or parasitic infections, or ocular herpes simplex, and may cause decrease in BMD and growth velocity in children. Instruct to prime drug before using for the 1st time or when not used for >10 days. Instruct on proper administration.

Administration: Inhalation route. Prime pump by actuating 3 times. Refer to PI for further administration instructions. **Storage:** 25°C (77°F); excursions permitted to 15-30°C (59-86°F). Contents under pressure. Do not puncture. Exposure to >49°C (120°F) may cause bursting. Never throw into fire or incinerator.

AMANTADINE   RX
amantadine HCl (Various)

THERAPEUTIC CLASS: Dopamine receptor agonist

INDICATIONS: Prophylaxis and treatment of uncomplicated influenza A infections. Treatment of parkinsonism and drug-induced extrapyramidal reactions.

DOSAGE: *Adults:* Influenza A Virus Prophylaxis/Treatment: 200mg/day as 2 caps/tabs or 4 tsp sol qd, or as 1 cap/tab or 2 tsp sol bid if CNS effects develop. Elderly/Intolerant to 200mg/day: 100mg/day. Refer to PI for commencement/duration of therapy and coadministration with inactivated influenza A vaccine. Parkinsonism: Usual: 100mg bid. Serious Associated Illness/Concomitant High-Dose Antiparkinson Agent: Initial: 100mg qd. Titrate: May increase to 100mg bid after 1 to several weeks. Max: 400mg/day in divided doses. Drug-Induced Extrapyramidal Reactions: Usual: 100mg bid. Max: 300mg/day in divided doses. CrCl 30-50mL/min/1.73m²: 200mg on Day 1, then 100mg qd. CrCl 15-29mL/min/1.73m²: 200mg on Day 1, then 100mg qod. CrCl <15mL/min/1.73m² or Hemodialysis: 200mg q7 days.
Pediatrics: Influenza A Virus Prophylaxis/Treatment: 9-12 yrs: 200mg/day as 1 cap/tab or 2 tsp sol bid. 1-9 yrs: 4.4-8.8mg/kg/day. Max: 150mg/day.

HOW SUPPLIED: Cap: 100mg; Sol: 50mg/5mL; Tab: 100mg

WARNINGS/PRECAUTIONS: May need dose reduction with congestive heart failure (CHF), peripheral edema, orthostatic hypotension, or renal impairment. Deaths reported from overdose. Suicide attempts, impulse control symptoms, and neuroleptic malignant syndrome (NMS) upon dose reduction or withdrawal reported. May exacerbate mental problems in patients with history of psychiatric disorder or substance abuse. May increase seizure activity. May impair mental/physical abilities. Avoid with untreated angle-closure glaucoma. Do not d/c abruptly in Parkinson's disease patients. Caution with liver disease, history of recurrent eczematoid rash, and uncontrolled psychosis or severe psychoneurosis. Monitor for melanomas frequently and regularly. Not shown to prevent complications secondary to influenza-like symptoms or concurrent bacterial infections.

ADVERSE REACTIONS: Nausea, dizziness, insomnia, depression, anxiety, hallucinations, confusion, anorexia, dry mouth, constipation, ataxia, livedo reticularis, peripheral edema, orthostatic hypotension, headache.

INTERACTIONS: Avoid live attenuated influenza vaccine within 2 weeks before or 48 hours after therapy. Caution with neuroleptics and drugs having CNS effects. Triamterene/HCTZ may increase concentration. Quinine or quinidine may reduce renal clearance. Urine acidifying drugs may increase elimination. Anticholinergic agents may potentiate the anticholinergic-like side effects. May worsen tremor in elderly Parkinson's patients with thioridazine.

PREGNANCY: Category C, not for use in nursing.

MECHANISM OF ACTION: Dopamine receptor agonist; not established. Antiviral: Appears to prevent release of infectious viral nucleic acid into host cell by interfering with function of transmembrane domain of viral M2 protein. Also prevents virus assembly during replication. Parkinson's disease: May have direct/indirect effect on dopamine neurons and is a weak, noncompetitive *N*-methyl *D*-aspartate receptor antagonist.

PHARMACOKINETICS: Absorption: Well absorbed. (Cap) C_{max}=0.22mcg/mL, T_{max}=3.3 hrs. (Sol) C_{max}=0.24mcg/mL (single dose), 0.47mcg/mL (multiple dose). (Tab) C_{max}=0.51mcg/mL, T_{max}=2-4 hrs. **Distribution:** V_d=3-8L/kg (IV); plasma protein binding (67%); found in human milk. **Metabolism:** N-acetylation; acetylamantadine (metabolite). **Elimination:** Urine (unchanged); $T_{1/2}$=16 hrs.

NURSING CONSIDERATIONS

Assessment: Assess for CHF, peripheral edema, orthostatic hypotension, history of psychiatric disorders, substance abuse, epilepsy or other "seizures", and recurrent eczematoid rash, untreated angle-closure glaucoma, renal/hepatic impairment, hypersensitivity, pregnancy/nursing status, and possible drug interactions.

Monitoring: Monitor for signs/symptoms of suicide attempt, increased seizure, CNS effects, NMS, impulse control, melanoma, and renal/hepatic function.

Patient Counseling: Advise that blurry vision and/or impaired mental acuity may occur. Instruct to avoid excessive alcohol use, getting up suddenly from sitting or lying position, and taking more than prescribed. Notify physician if mood/mental changes, swelling of extremities, difficulty urinating, SOB, and intense urges occur, no improvement in a few days or drug appears less effective after a few weeks, and suspected that overdose has been taken. Consult physician before discontinuing medication. Instruct Parkinson's disease patients to gradually increase physical activity as symptoms improve.

Administration: Oral route. **Storage:** 20-25°C (68-77°F); (tab) excursions permitted to 15-30°C (59-86°F). (Cap) Protect from moisture.

AMARYL   RX
glimepiride (Sanofi-Aventis)

THERAPEUTIC CLASS: Sulfonylurea (2nd generation)

INDICATIONS: Adjunct to diet and exercise to improve glycemic control in adults with type 2 diabetes mellitus.

DOSAGE: *Adults:* Initial: 1mg or 2mg qd. Titrate: After reaching 2mg qd, may further increase in increments of 1mg or 2mg q1-2 weeks based on glycemic response. Max: 8mg qd. Patients at Increased Risk of Hypoglycemia (eg, elderly or with renal impairment): Initial: 1mg qd. Titrate: Increase conservatively. Max: 8mg qd.

HOW SUPPLIED: Tab: 1mg*, 2mg*, 4mg* *scored

WARNINGS/PRECAUTIONS: May have overlapping drug effect for 1-2 weeks when transferring from longer $T_{1/2}$ sulfonylureas (eg, chlorpropamide); monitor for hypoglycemia. May cause severe hypoglycemia, which may impair mental/physical abilities; caution in patients predisposed to hypoglycemia (eg, elderly, with renal impairment). Hypersensitivity reactions (eg, anaphylaxis, angioedema, Stevens-Johnson syndrome) reported; if suspected, promptly d/c, assess for other causes for the reaction, and institute alternative treatment. May cause hemolytic anemia; caution with glucose-6-phosphate dehydrogenase (G6PD) deficiency and consider use of non-sulfonylurea alternative. Increased risk of cardiovascular mortality reported.

ADVERSE REACTIONS: Dizziness, nausea, asthenia, headache, hypoglycemia, flu syndrome.

INTERACTIONS: Oral antidiabetic medications, pramlintide acetate, insulin, ACE inhibitors, H_2 receptor antagonists, fibrates, propoxyphene, pentoxifylline, somatostatin analogs, anabolic steroids and androgens, cyclophosphamide, phenyramidol, guanethidine, fluconazole, sulfinpyrazone, tetracyclines, clarithromycin, disopyramide, quinolones, and drugs that are highly protein-bound (eg, fluoxetine, NSAIDs, salicylates, sulfonamides, chloramphenicol, coumarins, probenecid, MAOIs) may increase glucose-lowering effect; monitor for hypoglycemia during coadministration and for worsening glycemic control during withdrawal of these drugs. Danazol, glucagon, somatropin, protease inhibitors, atypical antipsychotics (eg, olanzapine, clozapine), barbiturates, diazoxide, laxatives, rifampin, thiazides and other diuretics, corticosteroids, phenothiazines, thyroid hormones, estrogens, oral contraceptives, phenytoin, nicotinic acid, sympathomimetics (eg, epinephrine, albuterol, terbutaline), and isoniazid may reduce glucose-lowering effect; monitor for worsening glycemic control during coadministration and for hypoglycemia during withdrawal of these drugs. β-blockers, clonidine, reserpine, and acute/chronic alcohol intake may potentiate or weaken glucose-lowering effect. Signs of hypoglycemia may be reduced or absent with sympatholytic drugs (eg, β-blockers). Potential interaction leading to severe hypoglycemia reported with oral miconazole. May interact with inhibitors (eg, fluconazole) and inducers (eg, rifampin) of CYP2C9. Aspirin may decrease levels. Propranolol may increase levels. May decrease pharmacodynamic response to warfarin.

PREGNANCY: Category C, not for use in nursing.

MECHANISM OF ACTION: Sulfonylurea (2nd generation); lowers blood glucose by stimulating insulin release from pancreatic β cells.

PHARMACOKINETICS: Absorption: T_{max}=2-3 hrs. **Distribution:** (IV) V_d=8.8L; plasma protein binding (>99.5%). **Metabolism:** Complete by oxidation; cyclohexyl hydroxyl methyl derivative (M1) (via CYP2C9) and carboxyl derivative (M2) (major metabolites). **Elimination:** Urine (60%, 80-90% metabolites), feces (40%, 70% metabolites).

NURSING CONSIDERATIONS

Assessment: Assess for hypersensitivity to drug or sulfonamide derivatives, predisposition to hypoglycemia, autonomic neuropathy, G6PD deficiency, pregnancy/nursing status, and possible drug interactions.

Monitoring: Monitor for hypoglycemia, hypersensitivity reactions, hemolytic anemia, and other adverse reactions.

Patient Counseling: Inform about importance of adhering to dietary instructions, regular exercise program, and regular testing of blood glucose. Inform about potential side effects (eg, hypoglycemia and weight gain). Inform about the symptoms and treatment of hypoglycemia, and the conditions that predispose to it. Inform that ability to concentrate and react may be impaired as a result of hypoglycemia. Advise to inform physician of pregnancy/nursing status.

Administration: Oral route. Administer with breakfast or 1st main meal of the day. **Storage:** 25°C (77°F); excursions permitted to 15-30°C (59-86°F).

AMBIEN   CIV
zolpidem tartrate (Sanofi-Aventis)

THERAPEUTIC CLASS: Imidazopyridine hypnotic

INDICATIONS: Short-term treatment of insomnia characterized by difficulties with sleep initiation.

DOSAGE: *Adults:* Individualize dose. 10mg qhs. Max: 10mg/day. Elderly/Debilitated/Hepatic Insufficiency: 5mg qhs. Adjust dose with other CNS depressants.

HOW SUPPLIED: Tab: 5mg, 10mg

WARNINGS/PRECAUTIONS: Initiate only after careful evaluation; failure of insomnia to remit after 7-10 days of treatment may indicate presence of psychiatric and/or medical illness. Severe anaphylactic/anaphylactoid reactions reported. Abnormal thinking, behavior changes, visual/auditory hallucinations, and complex behaviors (eg, sleep-driving) reported. Worsening of depression, including suicidal thoughts and actions have been reported in depressed patients. Withdrawal symptoms may occur with rapid dose reduction or abrupt d/c. Potential impairment of performance of activities requiring complete mental alertness (eg, operating machinery or driving a motor vehicle) may occur the day following ingestion. Monitor elderly and debilitated patients for impaired motor/cognitive performance and for unusual sensitivity. Caution with hepatic impairment, compromised respiratory function or sleep apnea syndrome, myasthenia gravis, depression, and conditions that could affect metabolism or hemodynamic responses. Closely monitor patients with renal impairment.

ADVERSE REACTIONS: Drowsiness, dizziness, headache, diarrhea, drugged feeling, lethargy, dry mouth, back pain, pharyngitis, sinusitis, allergic reactions.

INTERACTIONS: Consider pharmacology of any CNS-active drug to be used concomitantly. CNS depressants may potentially enhance effects. Avoid use with alcohol. Decreased alertness observed in combination with imipramine/chlorpromazine. Increased $T_{1/2}$ with fluoxetine in females. Increased C_{max} and decreased T_{max} with sertraline in females. Increased exposure with CYP3A inhibitors (itraconazole, ketoconazole). Caution with ketoconazole. Decreased levels with rifampin.

PREGNANCY: Category C, caution in nursing.

MECHANISM OF ACTION: Imidazopyridine, non-benzodiazepine hypnotic; interacts with a GABA-BZ receptor complex and binds the BZ_1 receptor preferentially with a high affinity ratio of the $α_1/α_5$ subunits.

PHARMACOKINETICS: Absorption: Rapid from GI tract. C_{max}=59ng/mL (5mg), 121ng/mL (10mg). T_{max}=1.6 hrs (5mg, 10mg). **Distribution:** Plasma protein binding (92.5%); found in breast milk. **Elimination:** Renal; $T_{1/2}$=2.6 hrs (5mg), 2.5 hrs (10mg).

NURSING CONSIDERATIONS

Assessment: Assess for primary psychiatric and/or medical illness, myasthenia gravis, pre-existing respiratory impairment (sleep apnea syndrome), diseases/conditions that could affect metabolism or hemodynamic responses, depression, hypersensitivity to drug, hepatic/renal impairment, pregnancy/nursing status, possible drug interactions, and history of drug or alcohol addiction or abuse.

Monitoring: Monitor for anaphylactic/anaphylactoid reactions, withdrawal effects, motor/cognitive impairment, abnormal thinking, behavioral changes, complex behaviors, and visual/auditory hallucinations. Monitor patients with hepatic/renal impairment and history of drug or alcohol addiction or abuse.

Patient Counseling: Inform about risks/benefits of use. Instruct to read Medication Guide. Advise to seek medical attention immediately if anaphylactic/anaphylactoid reactions occur. Counsel to take just before bedtime and only when they are able to stay in bed a full night (7-8 hrs) before being active again. Advise not to take with or immediately after a meal. Caution against hazardous tasks (eg, operating machinery/driving); immediately report events such as sleep-driving and other complex behaviors. Advise to report all concomitant medications to the prescriber. Counsel on tolerance, dependence, and withdrawal signs/symptoms. Do not take with alcohol.

Administration: Oral route. **Storage:** 20-25°C (68-77°F).

AMBIEN CR
zolpidem tartrate (Sanofi-Aventis)

CIV

THERAPEUTIC CLASS: Imidazopyridine hypnotic

INDICATIONS: Treatment of insomnia characterized by difficulties with sleep onset and/or sleep maintenance.

DOSAGE: *Adults:* Individualize dose. Usual: 12.5mg qd immediately before hs. Max: 12.5mg/day. Elderly/Debilitated/Hepatic Insufficiency: 6.25mg qd immediately before hs.

HOW SUPPLIED: Tab, Extended-Release: 6.25mg, 12.5mg

WARNINGS/PRECAUTIONS: Failure of insomnia to remit after 7-10 days of treatment may indicate presence of primary psychiatric and/or medical illness; initiate only after careful evaluation. Severe anaphylactic/anaphylactoid reactions reported; do not rechallenge with drug if angioedema develops. Abnormal thinking, behavior changes, visual/auditory hallucinations, and complex behaviors (eg, sleep-driving) reported. Worsening of depression, including suicidal thoughts and actions, reported in primarily depressed patients. Withdrawal symptoms may occur with rapid dose reduction or abrupt d/c. May impair mental/physical abilities. Closely monitor elderly and debilitated patients for impaired motor and/or cognitive performance and unusual sensitivity. Caution with hepatic impairment, compromised respiratory function, sleep apnea syndrome, myasthenia gravis, depression, and conditions that could affect metabolism or hemodynamic responses. Closely monitor patients with renal impairment and history of drug/alcohol addiction or abuse.

ADVERSE REACTIONS: Headache, somnolence, dizziness, anxiety, nausea, influenza, hallucinations, back pain, myalgia, fatigue, disorientation, memory disorder, visual disturbance, nasopharyngitis.

INTERACTIONS: Caution with CNS-active drugs. CNS depressants may potentially enhance effects; consider dose adjustment. Avoid with alcohol. Additive effect of decreased alertness reported with imipramine and chlorpromazine. May decrease levels of imipramine. Fluoxetine may increase half-life. Increased levels and decreased half-life reported with sertraline in females. CYP3A inhibitors (eg, itraconazole, ketoconazole) may increase exposure; use caution and reduce dose with ketoconazole. Rifampin may decrease levels.

PREGNANCY: Category C, caution in nursing.

MECHANISM OF ACTION: Imidazopyridine, non-benzodiazepine hypnotic; interacts with a GABA-BZ receptor complex and preferentially binds the BZ_1 receptor with a high affinity ratio of the α_1/α_5 subunits.

PHARMACOKINETICS: Absorption: Biphasic, rapid from GI tract, then extended; C_{max}=134ng/mL, T_{max}=1.5 hrs, AUC=740ng•hr/mL. **Distribution:** Plasma protein binding (92.5%); found in breast milk. **Elimination:** Renal; $T_{1/2}$=2.8 hrs.

NURSING CONSIDERATIONS

Assessment: Assess for presence of primary psychiatric and/or medical illness, diseases/conditions that could affect metabolism or hemodynamic responses, compromised respiratory function, sleep apnea, myasthenia gravis, depression, history of drug/alcohol addiction or abuse, hypersensitivity to drug, hepatic/renal impairment, pregnancy/nursing status, and possible drug interactions.

Monitoring: Monitor for anaphylactic/anaphylactoid reactions, abnormal thinking, behavioral changes, complex behaviors, visual/auditory hallucinations, worsening of depression, withdrawal effects, motor/cognitive impairment, and other adverse reactions. Monitor patients with hepatic/renal impairment and history of drug/alcohol addiction or abuse.

Patient Counseling: Inform of the benefits, risks and appropriate use of therapy. Advise to immediately seek medical attention if any anaphylactic/anaphylactoid reactions occur. Advise to notify physician of all concomitant medications. Instruct to immediately report events such as sleep-driving and other complex behaviors. Counsel to take drug just before hs and only when able to stay in bed a full night (7-8 hrs) before being active again. Instruct to swallow drug whole and not to divide, crush, or chew. Advise not to take drug with or immediately after a meal, and when drinking alcohol.

Administration: Oral route. **Storage:** 15-25°C (59-77°F); excursions permitted to ≤30°C (86°F).

AMBISOME RX
amphotericin B liposome (Astellas)

THERAPEUTIC CLASS: Polyene antifungal

INDICATIONS: Empirical therapy for presumed fungal infection in febrile, neutropenic patients. Treatment of *Aspergillus, Candida,* or *Cryptococcus* infections refractory to amphotericin B deoxycholate or where renal impairment or unacceptable toxicity precludes its use. Treatment of cryptococcal meningitis in HIV-infected patients. Treatment of visceral leishmaniasis.

DOSAGE: *Adults:* Empirical Therapy: 3mg/kg/day IV. Systemic Infections (*Aspergillus, Candida, Cryptococcus*): 3-5mg/kg/day IV. Cryptococcal Meningitis in HIV: 6mg/kg/day IV. Visceral Leishmaniasis: Immunocompetent: 3mg/kg/day IV on Days 1-5, 14, 21. May repeat course if needed. Immunocompromised: 4mg/kg/day IV on Days 1-5, 10, 17, 24, 31, 38. Infuse over 120 min but may be reduced to 60 min if tolerated.
Pediatrics: 1 month-16 yrs: Empirical Therapy: 3mg/kg/day IV. Systemic Infections (*Aspergillus, Candida, Cryptococcus*): 3-5mg/kg/day IV. Cryptococcal Meningitis in HIV: 6mg/kg/day IV. Visceral Leishmaniasis: Immunocompetent: 3mg/kg/day IV on Days 1-5, 14, 21. May repeat course if needed. Immunocompromised: 4mg/kg/day IV on Days 1-5, 10, 17, 24, 31, 38. Infuse over 120 min but may be reduced to 60 min if tolerated.

HOW SUPPLIED: Inj: 50mg/vial

WARNINGS/PRECAUTIONS: Anaphylaxis reported, d/c all further infusions if severe anaphylactic reaction occurs. Significantly less toxic than amphotericin B deoxycholate.

ADVERSE REACTIONS: Hypokalemia, chills/rigors, SrCr elevation, anemia, N/V, diarrhea, hypomagnesemia, rash, dyspnea, bilirubinemia, BUN increased, headache, abdominal pain.

INTERACTIONS: Concurrent use of antineoplastic agents may potentiate renal toxicity, bronchospasm, hypotension. Corticosteroids and corticotropin may potentiate hypokalemia. May induce hypokalemia and potentiate digitalis toxicity with digitalis glycosides. May increase flucytosine toxicity. Acute pulmonary toxicity reported with leukocyte transfusions. Nephrotoxic drugs enhance potential for renal toxicity. May enhance curariform effect of skeletal muscle relaxants due to hypokalemia. Imidazoles (eg, ketoconazole, miconazole, clotrimazole, fluconazole) may induce fungal resistance; caution with combination therapy, especially in immunocompromised patients.

PREGNANCY: Category B, not for use in nursing.

MECHANISM OF ACTION: Antifungal agent; acts by binding to the sterol component of the cell membrane leading to changes in cell permeability and cell death in susceptible fungi. Also binds to the cholesterol component of the mammalian cell, leading to cytotoxicity.

PHARMACOKINETICS: Absorption: IV administration of variable doses resulted from different pharmacokinetic parameters. **Elimination:** (24-hr dosing interval) $T_{1/2}$=7-10 hrs. (49 days after dosing) $T_{1/2}$=100-153 hrs.

NURSING CONSIDERATIONS

Assessment: Assess hypersensitivity, health status (eg, immunocompetent, immunocompromised), cultures, renal function, pregnancy/nursing status and possible drug interactions.

Monitoring: Monitor for anaphylaxis/severe allergic reaction, infusion reactions (eg, chills, hypotension, hypoxia, rash), renal, hepatic and hematopoietic function, and serum electrolytes (particularly Mg^{2+} and K^+).

Patient Counseling: Advise to seek medical attention if symptoms of acute reaction occur (eg, fevers, chills, respiratory symptoms). Instruct to report all medications being used. Inform that potential risks are involved when used during pregnancy and nursing.

Administration: IV infusion. Infuse over 120 min but may be reduced to 60 min if tolerated. An in-line membrane filter may be used provided the mean pore diameter of the filter is not <1.0 micron. Refer to PI for directions for reconstitution, filtration and dilution. Do not reconstitute with saline or add saline to the reconstituted concentration, or mix with other drugs. Discard partially used vials. **Storage:** Unopened Vials: 25°C (77°F). Reconstituted: 2-8°C (36-46°F) up to 24 hrs. Diluted Product: Injection should commence within 6 hrs of dilution with 5% Dextrose Injection.

AMERGE RX
naratriptan HCl (GlaxoSmithKline)

THERAPEUTIC CLASS: 5-HT$_{1B/1D}$ agonist

INDICATIONS: Acute treatment of migraine with or without aura in adults.

DOSAGE: *Adults:* Individualize dose. Usual: 1mg or 2.5mg taken with fluids. May repeat dose once after 4 hrs if headache returns or with partial response. Max: 5mg/24 hrs. Mild-Moderate Renal/Hepatic Impairment: Initial: Consider a lower dose. Max: 2.5mg/24 hrs. Safety of treating >4 headaches/30 days not known.

HOW SUPPLIED: Tab: 1mg, 2.5mg

CONTRAINDICATIONS: History, symptoms, or signs of ischemic cardiac syndromes (eg, angina pectoris, myocardial infarction [MI], silent myocardial ischemia), cerebrovascular syndromes (eg, strokes, transient ischemic attacks), and peripheral vascular syndromes (eg, ischemic bowel disease). Other significant cardiovascular disease (CVD), uncontrolled HTN, hemiplegic or basilar migraine, severe hepatic/renal impairment, and use within 24 hrs of another 5-HT1 agonists, ergotamine-containing or ergot-type medications (eg, dihydroergotamine, methysergide).

WARNINGS/PRECAUTIONS: Has potential to cause coronary artery vasospasm; do not give with documented ischemic/vasospastic coronary artery disease (CAD). Avoid in patients whom un-recognized CAD is predicted by presence of risk factors (eg, HTN, hypercholesterolemia, smoker, obesity, diabetes, CAD family history, menopause, males >40 yrs) unless with a satisfactory cardiovascular evaluation; administer 1st dose under medical supervision; obtain ECG on the 1st occasion of therapy during the interval immediately following administration. Perform periodic cardiovascular function with long-term intermittent use. Serious adverse cardiac events (eg, acute MI, cardiac rhythm disturbances) reported. Cerebral/subarachnoid hemorrhage, stroke, other cerebrovascular events, vasospastic reactions, and peripheral vascular/colonic ischemia with abdominal pain and bloody diarrhea reported. Serotonin syndrome may occur; symptoms may include mental status changes, autonomic instability, neuromuscular aberrations, and GI symptoms; d/c if serotonin syndrome is suspected. HTN and hypertensive crisis reported rarely. Hypersensitivity reactions may occur. Chest discomfort reported. Evaluate for atherosclerosis or predisposition to vasospasm if signs/symptoms suggestive of decreased arterial flow occurs. Caution with diseases that may alter absorption, metabolism, or excretion of drugs (eg, renal or hepatic dysfunction). Exclude other potentially serious neurological conditions before therapy. Reconsider the diagnosis of migraine before giving a 2nd dose. Overuse of acute migraine drugs may lead to exacerbation of headache. Not recommended in elderly.

ADVERSE REACTIONS: Paresthesias, dizziness, drowsiness, malaise/fatigue, throat and neck symptoms, N/V.

INTERACTIONS: See Contraindications. Serotonin syndrome reported with combined use of an SSRI or SNRI. Increased concentrations with oral contraceptives. Increased clearance with smoking.

PREGNANCY: Category C, caution in nursing.

MECHANISM OF ACTION: Selective 5-HT$_1$ receptor agonist; binds with high affinity to 5-HT$_{1D/1B}$ receptors. Suspected to perform its action by (1) activating 5-HT$_{1D/1B}$ receptors on intracranial blood vessels, including those on arteriovenous anastomoses, leading to vasoconstriction that correlates with migraine relief, or (2) activation of 5-HT$_{1D/1B}$ receptors in the trigeminal system resulting in inhibition of pro-inflammatory neuropeptide release.

PHARMACOKINETICS: Absorption: Well-absorbed; bioavailability (70%); T$_{max}$=2-3 hrs. **Distribution:** V$_d$=170L, plasma protein binding (28-31%). **Metabolism:** Via CYP450 isoenzymes. **Elimination:** Urine (50% unchanged, 30% metabolites); T$_{1/2}$=6 hrs.

NURSING CONSIDERATIONS

Assessment: Confirm diagnosis of migraine before therapy. Assess for CVD, HTN, hemiplegic/basilar migraine, ECG changes, and other conditions where treatment is cautioned or contrain-dicated. Assess hepatic/renal function, pregnancy/nursing status, and possible drug interactions.

Monitoring: Monitor for signs/symptoms of cardiac events (eg, coronary vasospasm, acute MI, arrhythmia, ECG changes, follow-up coronary angiography), cerebrovascular events (eg, hemor-rhage, stroke, transient ischemic attacks), peripheral vascular ischemia, colonic ischemia with bloody diarrhea and abdominal pain, serotonin syndrome (eg, mental status changes, autonomic instability, neuromuscular aberrations and/or GI symptoms), ophthalmic effects, increased BP, anaphylaxis/anaphylactoid reactions, and other adverse reactions.

Patient Counseling: Inform about potential risks of therapy (eg, serotonin syndrome), especially if taken with SSRIs or SNRIs. Instruct to report adverse reactions to physician and to take exactly as directed. Notify if pregnant/nursing or planning to become pregnant.

Administration: Oral route. **Storage:** 20-25°C (68-77°F).

AMEVIVE

alefacept (Astellas)

RX

THERAPEUTIC CLASS: Immunosuppressive agent

INDICATIONS: Moderate to severe chronic plaque psoriasis who are candidates for systemic or phototherapy.

DOSAGE: *Adults:* Usual: 15mg IM once weekly for 12 weeks. May retreat with an additional 12-week course if CD4+ T-lymphocyte counts are within normal range and a 12-week minimum interval has passed since the previous course of treatment.

HOW SUPPLIED: Inj: 15mg

CONTRAINDICATIONS: HIV.

WARNINGS/PRECAUTIONS: Dose-dependent reductions in circulating CD4+ and CD8+ T-lymphocyte counts reported. Do not initiate with CD4+ T-lymphocyte counts below normal. Withhold therapy and institute weekly monitoring if CD4+ T-lymphocyte counts <250 cells/μL; d/c if counts remain <250 cells/μL for 1 month. May increase risk of malignancies; avoid with history of systemic malignancy and caution in high risk patients. May increase risk of infection and reactivate latent, chronic infections; avoid with clinically important infections and caution with chronic infection or history of recurrent infections. D/C if serious infection or malignancy develops. Hypersensitivity reactions (eg, urticaria, angioedema) reported; d/c if anaphylactic or serious allergic reactions occur and initiate appropriate therapy. Liver injury (eg, fatty infiltration, hepatitis) reported; d/c if significant clinical signs of liver injury develop. Caution in elderly. Avoid concurrent phototherapy.

ADVERSE REACTIONS: Lymphopenia, malignancies, serious infections, hypersensitivity reactions, pharyngitis, dizziness, increased cough, nausea, pruritus, myalgia, chills, injection-site reactions, immunogenicity.

INTERACTIONS: Avoid with other immunosuppressive agents. May cause liver failure with concomitant alcohol use.

PREGNANCY: Category B, not for use in nursing.

MECHANISM OF ACTION: Immunosuppressive agent; interferes with lymphocyte activation by specifically binding to the lymphocyte antigen CD2, and inhibiting LFA-3/CD2 interaction. Reduces subsets of CD2+ T lymphocytes (primarily CD45RO+), presumably by bridging between CD2 on target lymphocytes and immunoglobulin Fc receptors on cytotoxic cells, such as natural killer cells. Reduces circulating total CD4+ and CD8+ T-lymphocyte counts.

PHARMACOKINETICS: Absorption: (IM) Bioavailability (63%). **Distribution:** (7.5mg IV) V_d=94mL/kg. **Elimination:** (7.5mg IV) $T_{1/2}$=270 hrs.

NURSING CONSIDERATIONS

Assessment: Assess for HIV infection, hypersensitivity to drug, history of systemic malignancy or risk of malignancy, chronic infections or history of recurrent infection, immunization status, hepatic function, pregnancy/nursing status, and possible drug interactions. Assess for CD4+ T-lymphocyte counts.

Monitoring: Monitor for signs/symptoms of infection during or after a course of therapy. Monitor for new infections, malignancies, hypersensitivity reactions, signs/symptoms of hepatic injury, and other adverse reactions. Monitor CD4+ T-lymphocyte counts q2 weeks throughout the course of the 12-week dosing regimen.

Patient Counseling: Inform about potential risks/benefits of therapy and the need for regular monitoring of WBC counts. Advise that therapy reduces lymphocyte counts and increases chances of infection or malignancy. Report any signs/symptoms of infections, malignancy, or liver injury (eg, N/V, fatigue, jaundice, dark urine) to physician. Notify physician if pregnant/nursing or plan to become pregnant (or within 8 weeks of d/c); encourage to enroll in Pregnancy Registry.

Administration: IM route. Use only under supervision of a physician. **Storage:** 2-8°C (36-46°F). Protect from light, retain in drug/diluent pack until time of use. Discard reconstitute if not used in ≤4 hours.

AMICAR   RX
aminocaproic acid (Xanodyne)

THERAPEUTIC CLASS: Monoamino carboxylic acid anti-fibrinolytic

INDICATIONS: To enhance hemostasis when fibrinolysis contributes to bleeding.

DOSAGE: *Adults:* IV: 16-20mL (4-5g) in 250mL diluent during 1st hr, then 4mL/hr (1g) in 50mL of diluent. PO: 5g during 1st hr, then 5mL (syr) or 1g (tabs) per hr. Continue therapy for 8 hrs or until bleeding is controlled.

HOW SUPPLIED: Inj: 250mg/mL [20mL]; Syrup: 1.25g/5mL; Tab: 500mg*, 1000mg* *scored

CONTRAINDICATIONS: Active intravascular clotting process, disseminated intravascular coagulation without concomitant heparin.

WARNINGS/PRECAUTIONS: Avoid in hematuria of upper urinary tract origin due to risk of intrarenal obstruction from glomerular capillary thrombosis or clots in renal pelvis and ureters. Skeletal muscle weakness with necrosis of muscle fibers reported after prolonged therapy. Consider cardiac muscle damage with skeletal myopathy. Avoid rapid IV infusion. Thrombophlebitis may occur. Contains benzyl alcohol; do not administer to neonates due to risk of fatal "gasping syndrome." Do not administer without a definite diagnosis of hyperfibrinolysis.

ADVERSE REACTIONS: Edema, headache, anaphylactoid reactions, injection-site reactions, pain, bradycardia, hypotension, abdominal pain, diarrhea, N/V, agranulocytosis, increased CPK, confusion, dyspnea, pruritus, tinnitus.

INTERACTIONS: Increased risk of thrombosis with Factor IX complex concentrates, anti-inhibitor coagulant concentrates.

PREGNANCY: Category C, caution in nursing.

MECHANISM OF ACTION: Monoamino carboxylic acid anti-fibrinolytic; fibrinolysis inhibitory effects are exerted principally by inhibition of plasminogen activators and, to a lesser extent, through antiplasmin activity.

PHARMACOKINETICS: Absorption: (PO) C_{max}=164mcg/mL; T_{max}=1.2 hrs. **Distribution:** (PO) V_d=23.1L; (IV) V_d=30L. **Metabolism:** Adipic acid (metabolite). **Elimination:** Renal: Urine (65% unchanged), (11% metabolite); $T_{1/2}$=2 hrs.

NURSING CONSIDERATIONS

Assessment: Assess for evidence of active intravascular clotting, proper diagnosis of hyperfibrinolysis (hyperplasminemia), pregnancy/nursing status, and possible drug interactions. Assess use in presence of hematuria of the upper urinary tract origin.

Monitoring: Monitor for signs/symptoms of subendocardial hemorrhages, fatty degeneration of the myocardium, skeletal muscle weakness with necrosis of muscle fibers (rhabdomyolysis, myoglobinuria, acute renal failure), cardiac muscle damage, thrombophlebitis, and neurological deficits (eg, hydrocephalus, cerebral ischemia, cerebral vasospasm). In patients with upper urinary tract bleeding, monitor for signs/symptoms of intrarenal obstruction (eg, glomerular capillary thrombosis, clots in renal pelvis and ureters). If used in pediatrics, monitor for "gasping syndrome" in neonates. Monitor CPK levels in patients on long-term therapy. Perform periodic monitoring to determine amount of fibrinolysis present.

Patient Counseling: Instruct to contact physician if unusual muscle weakness or pain develops.

Administration: IV or Oral routes. IV: Use compatible intravenous vehicles (eg, Sterile Water for Injection, Sodium Chloride for Injection, 5% Dextrose or Ringer's Injection). Rapid IV administration may induce hypotension, bradycardia, and/or arrhythmias. **Storage:** 15-30°C (59-86°F).

AMIKACIN   RX
amikacin sulfate (Various)

Potential for ototoxicity/nephrotoxicity; reduce dose or d/c on evidence of ototoxicity/nephrotoxicity. Neurotoxicity (eg, vestibular and permanent bilateral auditory ototoxicity) can occur with preexisting renal damage and normal renal function treated at higher doses and/or longer treatment periods than recommended. Neuromuscular blockade, respiratory paralysis reported. Monitor renal and 8th-nerve function and serum amikacin concentration. Increased risk of neuromuscular blockade and respiratory paralysis with anesthetics, neuromuscular blockers (eg, tubocurarine, succinylcholine, decamethonium) or massive transfusions of citrate-anticoagulated blood. Avoid potent diuretics (eg, ethacrynic acid, furosemide) and other neurotoxic, nephrotoxic drugs (eg, bacitracin, cisplatin, amphotericin B, cephaloridine, paromomycin, viomycin, polymyxin B, colistin, vancomycin, aminoglycosides). Safety not established with treatment >14 days.

THERAPEUTIC CLASS: Aminoglycoside

INDICATIONS: Short-term treatment of serious infections due to susceptible strains of gram-negative bacteria. Shown to be effective in bacterial septicemia; respiratory tract, bone/joint, CNS (including meningitis), skin and soft tissue, and intra-abdominal infections; burns and postoperative infections; complicated and recurrent urinary tract infections (UTI) due to susceptible strains of microorganisms; infections caused by gentamicin-and/or tobramycin-resistant strains of Gram-negative organisms; staphylococcal infectons; severe infections such as neonatal sepsis in combination with a penicillin-type drug.

DOSAGE: *Adults:* IM/IV: 15mg/kg/day given q8h or q12h. Max: 15mg/kg/day. Heavier Wt Patients: Max: 1.5g/day. Recurrent Uncomplicated UTI: 250mg bid. Usual Duration: 7-10 days. Renal Impairment: Reduce dose.
Pediatrics: IM/IV: 15mg/kg/day given q8h or q12h. Newborns: LD: 10mg/kg. Maint: 7.5mg/kg q12h. Usual Duration: 7-10 days. D/C therapy if no response after 3-5 days. Renal Impairment: Reduce dose.

HOW SUPPLIED: Inj: 50mg/mL, 250mg/mL

WARNINGS/PRECAUTIONS: May cause fetal harm. Contains sodium metabisulfite; allergic reactions may occur especially in asthmatics. Maintain adequate hydration. Assess kidney function before therapy, then daily. Reduce dose with decreased creatinine clearance and urine specific gravity, increased BUN, creatinine and oliguria. D/C therapy if azotemia increases or if progressive decrease in urinary output occurs. Caution with muscular disorders (eg, myasthenia gravis, parkinsonism); may aggravate muscle weakness.

ADVERSE REACTIONS: Ototoxicity, neuromuscular blockage, nephrotoxicity, skin rash, drug fever, headache, paresthesia, tremor, N/V, arthralgia, anemia, hypotension.

INTERACTIONS: See Boxed Warning. Increased nephrotoxicity with aminoglycosides, antibiotics, cephalosporins. Should not be given concurrently with potent diuretics. Significant mutual inactivation may occur with β-lactams (eg, penicillin, cephalosporins). Cross-allergenicity between aminoglycosides.

PREGNANCY: Category D, not for use in nursing.

MECHANISM OF ACTION: Semisynthetic aminoglycoside antibiotic derived from kanamycin.

PHARMACOKINETICS: Absorption: (IM) Rapid. (IV) C_{max}=38mcg/mL. **Distribution:** V_d=24L; plasma protein binding (0-11%); crosses placenta. **Elimination:** Urine (IM, 91.9-98.2%), (IV, 84-94%); $T_{1/2}$>2 hrs.

NURSING CONSIDERATIONS

Assessment: Assess for pregnancy/nursing status, renal impairment, eighth cranial nerve function, muscular disorders (eg, myasthenia gravis, parkinsonism) and for possible drug interactions. Assess renal function tests prior to and throughout therapy.

Monitoring: Periodic monitoring of urea, creatinine, CrCl, audiometric testing changes, eighth cranial nerve function, serum concentrations of the drug and urine (specific gravity, proteins, presence of cells/casts). Monitor for signs/symptoms of nephrotoxicity, neurotoxicity (vestibular and permanent bilateral auditory ototoxicity, vertigo, numbness, skin tingling, muscle twitches, and convulsions), cochlear damage, neuromuscular blockade, and respiratory paralysis.

Patient Counseling: Inform about potential risks/benefits of therapy and to report signs of ototoxicity (eg, dizziness, vertigo, tinnitus, roaring in the ears, and hearing loss). Notify physician if pregnant/nursing or planning to become pregnant. Inform that drug treats bacterial infections only. Take as prescribed.

Administration: IV, IM route. Obtain pretreatment body weight to calculate correct dosage. Do not physically premix with other drugs; administer separately. Refer to PI for compatibilty and stability in IV fluids. **Storage:** 20-25°C (68-77°F).

AMITIZA   RX
lubiprostone (Sucampo/Takeda)

THERAPEUTIC CLASS: Chloride channel activator

INDICATIONS: Treatment of chronic idiopathic constipation in adults and irritable bowel syndrome with constipation (IBS-C) in women ≥18 yrs.

DOSAGE: *Adults:* Chronic Idiopathic Constipation: 24mcg bid with food and water. Hepatic Dysfunction: Moderate (Child-Pugh Class B): 16mcg bid. Severe (Child-Pugh Class C): 8mcg bid. If dose is tolerated but adequate response not obtained, escalate to full dose with appropriate monitoring. IBS-C: 8mcg bid with food and water. Severe Hepatic Dysfunction (Child-Pugh Class C): 8mcg qd. If dose is tolerated but adequate response not obtained, escalate to full dose with appropriate monitoring.

HOW SUPPLIED: Cap: 8mcg, 24mcg

CONTRAINDICATIONS: Known or suspected mechanical GI obstruction.

WARNINGS/PRECAUTIONS: Use only during pregnancy if benefit justifies the risk to fetus; confirm a negative pregnancy test prior to initiation of therapy and advise complying with effective contraceptive measures. May cause nausea; give with food to reduce symptoms of nausea. May cause diarrhea; avoid in patients with severe diarrhea. Dyspnea reported; resolves within a few hrs after dose but may recur with subsequent doses. Evaluate thoroughly to confirm absence of mechanical GI obstruction prior to initiation.

ADVERSE REACTIONS: N/V, diarrhea, headache, abdominal distention/pain, flatulence, loose stools, dizziness, edema, chest discomfort/pain.

PREGNANCY: Category C, not for use in nursing.

MECHANISM OF ACTION: Chloride channel activator; enhances chloride-rich intestinal fluid secretion, increasing motility in the intestine, thereby facilitating the passage of stool.

PHARMACOKINETICS: Absorption: (M3; active metabolite) C_{max}=41.5pg/mL, T_{max}=1.1 hrs, AUC_{0-t}=57.1pg•hr/mL. **Distribution:** Plasma protein binding (94%). **Metabolism:** Rapid and extensive via carbonyl reductase; M3. **Elimination:** Urine (60%), feces (30%); (M3) $T_{1/2}$=0.9-1.4 hrs.

NURSING CONSIDERATIONS

Assessment: Assess for known or suspected mechanical GI obstruction, severe diarrhea, pregnancy/nursing status, and possible drug interactions. Perform pregnancy test and thorough evaluation to confirm absence of obstruction (if symptoms suggestive of mechanical obstruction) prior to therapy.

Monitoring: Monitor for symptoms of allergic reactions, nausea, dyspnea, severe diarrhea, and other adverse reactions. Assess the need for continued therapy.

Patient Counseling: Advise to take as prescribed, with food and water to reduce symptoms of nausea. Instruct to inform physician if experiencing severe nausea, diarrhea, or dyspnea during treatment. Inform that dyspnea may occur within an hour after 1st dose and resolves within 3 hrs, but may recur with repeat dosing. Advise to swallow caps whole and not to break apart or chew.

Administration: Oral route. **Storage:** 25°C (77°F); excursions permitted to 15-30°C (59-86°F). Protect from extreme temperatures.

AMITRIPTYLINE   RX
amitriptyline HCl (Mylan)

> Antidepressants increased the risk of suicidal thinking and behavior (suicidality) in short-term studies in children, adolescents, and young adults with major depressive disorder (MDD) and other psychiatric disorders. Monitor and observe closely for clinical worsening, suicidality, or unusual changes in behavior in patients who are started on antidepressant therapy. Not approved for use in pediatric patients.

THERAPEUTIC CLASS: Tricyclic antidepressant

INDICATIONS: Relief of symptoms of depression, especially endogenous depression.

DOSAGE: *Adults:* Initiate at low dose and increase gradually according to clinical response and tolerance. Initial: Outpatient: Divided Dose: 75mg/day in divided doses. May increase the late afternoon and/or bedtime doses to a total of 150mg/day. Single Dose: Initial: 50-100mg qhs. May increase by 25mg or 50mg PRN to a total of 150mg/day. Inpatient: Initial: 100mg/day. May increase gradually to 200mg/day PRN. May give as much as 300mg/day. Elderly: May need lower doses. If intolerant to higher doses, give 10mg tid with 20mg qhs. Maint: Usual: 50-100mg qhs. 40mg qhs may be sufficient. Reduce dose to lowest effective dose when satisfactory improvement has been reached. Continue maint ≥3 months to lessen possibility of relapse. Max: 150mg/day (3mg/kg/day for a 50kg patient).
Pediatrics: >12 yrs: Initiate at low dose and increase gradually according to clinical response and tolerance. Intolerant to Higher Doses: 10mg tid and 20mg qhs.

HOW SUPPLIED: Tab: 10mg, 25mg, 50mg, 75mg, 100mg, 150mg

CONTRAINDICATIONS: Use during or within 14 days after d/c of MAOI therapy. Acute recovery phase following myocardial infarction (MI). Concurrent cisapride.

WARNINGS/PRECAUTIONS: Not approved for treatment of bipolar depression. Caution with history of seizures, history of urinary retention, increased intraocular pressure (IOP), or angle-closure glaucoma; may precipitate an attack with angle-closure glaucoma. Caution with cardiovascular diseases (CVD); arrhythmias, sinus tachycardia, and prolongation of the conduction time reported particularly in high doses. Caution with hyperthyroidism and liver dysfunction. MI and stroke reported. Manic depressive, schizophrenic, and paranoid patients may experience increased symptoms of underlying disease; reduction of dose or addition of major tranquilizer (eg, perphenazine) may be given. D/C several days before or during elective surgery. May alter blood glucose levels. May increase hazards associated with electroshock therapy. Caution in elderly.

ADVERSE REACTIONS: MI, stroke, seizure, paralytic ileus, urinary retention, constipation, blurred vision, hyperpyrexia, rash, bone marrow depression, testicular swelling, gynecomastia (male), breast enlargement (female), alopecia, edema.

INTERACTIONS: See Contraindications. May block antihypertensive effects of guanethidine or similarly acting agents. May enhance response to alcohol and the effects of barbiturates and other CNS depressants. May increase levels with CYP2D6 inhibitors (eg, quinidine, cimetidine, phenothiazines, SSRIs such as fluoxetine, sertraline, paroxetine, other antidepressants, propafenone, and flecainide); may require lower doses of either TCA or the other drug. Caution with SSRIs. Allow sufficient time before starting therapy when switching from fluoxetine (eg, ≥5 weeks). Caution with thyroid drugs. Delirium reported with disulfiram and ethchlorvynol. Paralytic ileus reported with anticholinergics. Monitor with sympathomimetics, including local anesthetics with epinephrine. Hyperpyrexia, especially during hot weather, reported with anticholinergics and neuroleptics. Increased plasma levels with cimetidine.

PREGNANCY: Category C, not for use in nursing.

MECHANISM OF ACTION: Tricyclic antidepressant; not established. Inhibits the membrane pump mechanism responsible for uptake of norepinephrine and serotonin in adrenergic and serotonergic neurons.

PHARMACOKINETICS: Absorption: Rapid. **Distribution:** Found in breast milk; crosses the placenta. **Metabolism:** N-demethylation and hydroxylation. **Elimination:** Urine (unchanged and metabolites).

NURSING CONSIDERATIONS

Assessment: Assess for recent MI, bipolar disorder, history of mania, paranoia, seizures, schizophrenia, CVD, hyperthyroidism, IOP, narrow-angle glaucoma, urinary retention, hepatic impairment, hypersensitivity, pregnancy/nursing status, and possible drug interactions.

Monitoring: Monitor for signs/symptoms of clinical worsening (eg, suicidality, unusual changes in behavior), MI, stroke, arrhythmias, sinus tachycardia, prolongation of conduction time, and other adverse reactions. Monitor hepatic/thyroid function and blood glucose levels.

Patient Counseling: Inform patients, families, and caregivers about benefits/risks of therapy. Counsel on appropriate use. Instruct to read Medication Guide and assist in understanding the contents. Instruct to notify physician if clinical worsening, suicidality, unusual changes in behavior, or other adverse reactions occur during treatment or when adjusting the dose. Inform that drug may impair mental/physical abilities.

Administration: Oral route. **Storage:** 20-25°C (68-77°F). Protect from light.

AMNESTEEM   RX
isotretinoin (Genpharm)

> Not for use by females who are or may become pregnant, or if breastfeeding. Birth defects have been documented. Increased risk of spontaneous abortion, and premature births reported. D/C if pregnancy does occur during treatment and should be referred to an obstetrician-gynecologist experienced in reproductive toxicity for evaluation and counseling. Approved for marketing only under special restricted distribution program called iPLEDGE™. Must have 2 negative pregnancy tests. Repeat pregnancy test monthly. Use 2 forms of contraception at least 1 month prior, during, and 1 month following discontinuation. Must fill written prescriptions within 7 days; refills require new prescriptions. Prescriber, dispensing pharmacy, and patient must be registered with iPLEDGE.

OTHER BRAND NAMES: Claravis (Barr) - Sotret (Ranbaxy)

THERAPEUTIC CLASS: Retinoid

INDICATIONS: Severe recalcitrant nodular acne unresponsive to conventional therapy, including systemic antibiotics in female patients who are not pregnant.

DOSAGE: *Adults:* Initial/Usual: 0.5-1mg/kg/day given bid for 15-20 weeks. Max: 2mg/kg/day (for very severe disease with scarring or primary trunk manifestation). Adjust for side effects and disease response. May d/c if nodule count reduced by >70% prior to completion. Repeat only if necessary after 2 months off drug. Take with food.
Pediatrics: ≥12 yrs: Initial/Usual: 0.5-1mg/kg/day given bid for 15-20 weeks. Max: 2mg/kg/day (for very severe disease with scarring or primary trunk manifestation). Adjust for side effects and disease response. May d/c if nodule count reduced by >70% prior to completion. Repeat only if necessary after 2 months off drug. Take with food.

HOW SUPPLIED: Cap: 10mg, 20mg, 40mg, (Claravis, Sortret) 30mg

CONTRAINDICATIONS: Pregnancy, paraben sensitivity (preservative in gelatin cap).

WARNINGS/PRECAUTIONS: Acute pancreatitis, impaired hearing, inflammatory bowel disease, elevated TG and LFTs, hepatotoxicity, premature epiphyseal closure, and hyperostosis reported. May cause depression, psychosis, aggressive and/or violent behaviors, rarely suicidal ideation/attempts and suicide; may need further evaluation after d/c. May cause decreased night vision, and corneal opacities. Associated with pseudotumor cerebri. Check lipids before therapy, and then at intervals until response established (within 4 weeks). D/C if significant decrease in WBC, hearing or visual impairment, abdominal pain, rectal bleeding, or severe diarrhea occurs. May develop musculoskeletal symptoms. Caution with genetic predisposition for age-related osteoporosis, history of childhood osteoporosis, osteomalacia, other bone metabolism disorders (eg, anorexia nervosa). Spontaneous osteoporosis, osteopenia, bone fractures, and delayed fracture healing reported; caution in sports with repetitive impact.

ADVERSE REACTIONS: Cheilitis, dry skin and mucous membranes, conjunctivitis, blood dyscrasias, epistaxis, decreased HDL, elevated cholesterol and TG, elevated blood sugar, arthralgias, back pain, hearing/vision impairment, rash, photosensitivity reactions, psychiatric disorders, abnormal menses, cardiovascular disorders.

INTERACTIONS: Avoid vitamin A. Limit alcohol consumption. Avoid use with tetracyclines; increased incidence of pseudotumor cerebri. Pregnancy reported with oral and injectable/implantable contraceptives. Avoid St. John's wort; may cause breakthrough bleeding with oral contraceptives. Caution with drugs that cause drug-induced osteoporosis/osteomalacia and affect vitamin D metabolism (eg, corticosteroids, phenytoin).

PREGNANCY: Category X, not for use in nursing.

MECHANISM OF ACTION: Retinoid; not established. Suspected to inhibit sebaceous gland function and keratinization.

PHARMACOKINETICS: Absorption: C_{max}=862ng/mL (fed), 301ng/mL (fasted); T_{max}=5.3 hrs (fed), 3.2 hrs (fasted); AUC=10,004ng•hr/mL (fed), 3703ng•hr/mL (fasted). **Distribution:** Plasma protein binding (99.9%). **Metabolism:** Liver via CYP2C8, 2C9, 3A4, and 2B6; 4-*oxo*-isotretinoin, retinoic acid, and 4-*oxo*-retinoic acid (active metabolites). **Elimination:** Urine, feces; $T_{1/2}$=21 hrs (isotretinoin), 24 hrs (4-*oxo*-isotretinoin).

NURSING CONSIDERATIONS

Assessment: Assess that females have had 2 negative pregnancy tests separated by at least 19 days, and are on 2 forms of effective contraception: A primary form (eg, tubal sterilization, partner's vasectomy, intrauterine device, or hormonal) and a secondary form (barrier, vaginal sponge) for at least 1 month prior to administration. Assess for hypersensitivity to parabens, history of psychiatric disorder, depression, risk of hyperlipidemia (eg, DM, obesity, increased alcohol intake, lipid metabolism disorder or family history of such disorder) possible drug interactions and nursing status. Obtain lipid levels profile and LFTs.

Monitoring: Monitor for signs/symptoms of psychiatric disorders (eg, depression, mood disturbances, psychosis, aggression, suicidal ideation), pseudotumor cerebri (eg, papilledema, headache, N/V, visual disturbances), hyperlipidemias (eg, elevated serum TG), acute pancreatitis, hearing impairment, hepatotoxicity, inflammatory bowel disease (regional ileitis), decreased bone mineral density, hyperostosis, premature epiphyseal closure, musculoskeletal symptoms (eg, arthralgia), neutropenia, agranulocytosis, hypersensitivity reactions, visual impairments, corneal opacities, and decreased night vision. Monitor lipid levels and LFTs (weekly or biweekly), glucose levels, and CPK levels until response to drug is established. Monitor that females remain on 2 forms of contraception during therapy and for 1 month following discontinuation.

Patient Counseling: Instruct to read the Medication Guide/iPledge and sign the Patient Information/Informed Consent form. For females of childbearing potential, instruct that 2 forms of contraception are required starting 1 month prior to initiation, during treatment, and for 1 month following discontinuation. Inform that monthly pregnancy tests are required before new prescription is issued. Counsel not to share drug with anyone and not to donate blood during therapy and 1 month following discontinuation. Instruct to take with a meal and swallow capsule with a full glass of liquid. Inform that transient flare of acne may occur when initiating treatment. Notify physician if signs of depression, mood disturbances, psychosis, or aggression occur. Avoid wax epilation and skin resurfacing procedures during therapy and for 6 months following; avoid prolonged exposure to UV rays or sunlight. Inform that decreased tolerance to contact lenses during and after therapy may occur. Inform that musculoskeletal symptoms, transient pain in chest, back pain in pediatrics, arthralgias, neutropenia, agranulocytosis, anaphylactic reactions, allergic vasculitis, purpura or extremities and extraneous involvement may occur.

Administration: Oral route. **Storage:** (Amnesteem) 15-30°C (59-86°F). (Claravis, Sortret) 20-25°C (68-77°F). Protect from light. Keep out of reach of children.

AMOXICILLIN   RX
amoxicillin (Various)

THERAPEUTIC CLASS: Semisynthetic ampicillin derivative

INDICATIONS: Treatment of infections of the ear, nose, throat, genitourinary tract (GU), skin and skin structure (SSSI), lower respiratory tract (LRTI); and acute, uncomplicated gonorrhea (anogenital and urethral infections) due to susceptible (β-lactamase negative) strains of microorganisms. Combination therapy for *Helicobacter pylori* eradication to reduce the risk of duodenal ulcer recurrence.

DOSAGE: *Adults:* Ear/Nose/Throat/SSSI/GU: (Mild/Moderate) 500mg q12h or 250mg q8h. (Severe) 875mg q12h or 500mg q8h. LRTI: 875mg q12h or 500mg q8h. Continue for a minimum of 48 to 72 hrs beyond the time that patient becomes asymptomatic or evidence of bacterial eradication has been obtained. *Streptococcus pyogenes* infections: ≥10 days. Acute Gonorrhea/ Uncomplicated Anogenital and Urethral Infections: 3g as single dose. *H. pylori:* (Dual Therapy) 1g + 30mg lansoprazole, both q8h for 14 days. (Triple Therapy) 1g + 30mg lansoprazole + 500mg clarithromycin, all q12h for 14 days. GFR 10-30mL/min: 250-500mg q12h. GFR<10mL/min: 250-500mg q24h. Hemodialysis: 250-500mg q24h; additional dose during and at end of dialysis. *Pediatrics:* >3 months: ≥40kg: Dose as adult. <40kg: Ear/Nose/Throat/SSSI/GU: (Mild/Moderate) 25mg/kg/day given in divided doses q12h or 20mg/kg/day given in divided doses q8h. (Severe) 45mg/kg/day given in divided doses q12h or 40mg/kg/day given in divided doses q8h. LRTI: 45mg/kg/day given in divided doses q12h or 40mg/kg/day given in divided doses q8h. Continue for a minimum of 48 to 72 hrs beyond the time that patient becomes asymptomatic or evidence of bacterial eradication has been obtained. *S. pyogenes* infections: ≥10 days. Acute Gonorrhea/ Uncomplicated Anogenital and Urethral Infections: Prepubertal: 50mg/kg with 25mg/kg probenecid as single dose (not for <2 yrs). Neonates/Infants: ≤12 weeks: Max: 30mg/kg/day divided q12h.

HOW SUPPLIED: Cap: 250mg, 500mg; Sus: 125mg/5mL [80mL, 100mL, 150mL], 200mg/5mL [50mL, 75mL, 100mL], 250mg/5mL [80mL, 100mL, 150mL], 400mg/5mL [50mL, 75mL, 100mL]; Tab: 500mg, 875mg; Tab, Chewable: 125mg, 250mg

WARNINGS/PRECAUTIONS: Serious, occasionally fatal, hypersensitivity (anaphylactic) reactions reported with penicillin (PCN) therapy; d/c if allergic reaction occurs and institute appropriate therapy. *Clostridium difficile*-associated diarrhea (CDAD) reported. Avoid use with mononucleosis; erythematous skin rash may develop in these patients. May result in bacterial resistance with prolonged use or use in the absence of a proven/suspected bacterial infection or a prophylactic indication; take appropriate measures if superinfection develops. Perform periodic assessment of renal, hepatic, and hematopoietic function with prolonged use. Perform a serologic test for syphilis in all patients with gonorrhea at time of diagnosis, and a follow-up serologic test after 3 months. May result in false-positive urinary glucose tests; glucose tests based on enzymatic glucose oxidase reactions may be used. May cause a transient decrease in plasma concentrations of total conjugated estriol, estriol-glucuronide, conjugated estrone, and estradiol in pregnancy. Caution in elderly.

ADVERSE REACTIONS: N/V, diarrhea, black hairy tongue, pseudomembranous colitis, hypersensitivity reactions, blood dyscrasias, hepatic dysfunction, tooth discoloration.

INTERACTIONS: Decreased renal tubular secretion and increased/prolonged levels with probenecid. May reduce efficacy of combined oral estrogen/progesterone contraceptives. Chloramphenicol, macrolides, sulfonamides, and tetracyclines may interfere with bactericidal effects of PCN.

PREGNANCY: Category B, caution in nursing.

MECHANISM OF ACTION: Ampicillin analog; has broad-spectrum bactericidal activity against susceptible organisms during active multiplication; acts through inhibition of biosynthesis of cell-wall mucopeptide.

PHARMACOKINETICS: Absorption: Rapid. Cap: (250mg) T_{max}=1-2 hrs, C_{max}=3.5-5mcg/mL; (500mg) T_{max}=1-2 hrs, C_{max}=5.5-7.5mcg/mL. Tab: (875mg) C_{max}=13.8mcg/mL, AUC=35.4mcg•hr/mL. Sus: (125mg) T_{max}=1-2 hrs, C_{max}=1.5-3mcg/mL; (250mg) T_{max}=1-2 hrs, C_{max}=3.5-5mcg/mL; (400mg) T_{max}=1 hr, C_{max}=5.92mcg/mL, AUC=17.1mcg•hr/mL. Tab, Chewable: (400mg) T_{max}=1 hr, C_{max}=5.18mcg/mL, AUC=17.9mcg•hr/mL. **Distribution:** Plasma protein binding (20%); found in breast milk. **Elimination:** Urine (60%, unchanged); $T_{1/2}$=61.3 min.

NURSING CONSIDERATIONS

Assessment: Assess for history of allergic reaction to PCNs, cephalosporins, or other allergens, mononucleosis, renal/hepatic function, hematopoietic function, pregnancy/nursing status, and possible drug interactions.

Monitoring: Monitor for serious anaphylactic reactions, erythematous skin rash, development of drug-resistant bacteria or superinfection with mycotic or bacterial pathogens, signs/symptoms of CDAD (may range from mild diarrhea to fatal colitis). Periodically monitor renal, hepatic, and hematopoietic function with prolonged use. Perform serologic test for syphilis at diagnosis of gonorrhea and after 3 months.

Patient Counseling: Inform drug treats bacterial, not viral, infections. Instruct to take exactly as directed; skipping doses or not completing full course may decrease effectiveness and increase likelihood that bacteria will develop resistance. Inform about potential benefits/risks; notify physician if watery/bloody stool (with/without stomach cramps and fever) develops (may occur as late as 2 months after treatment).

Administration: Oral route. Refer to PI for sus preparation. Shake sus well before use. Sus can be added to formula, milk, fruit juice, water, ginger ale or cold drinks; should be taken immediately. **Storage:** 20-25°C (68-77°F). Discard unused sus after 14 days.

AMPHOTEC   RX
amphotericin B lipid complex (InterMune)

THERAPEUTIC CLASS: Polyene antifungal

INDICATIONS: Treatment of invasive aspergillosis in patients where renal impairment or unacceptable toxicity precludes the use of amphotericin B deoxycholate in effective doses, and in patients with invasive aspergillosis where prior amphotericin B deoxycholate therapy has failed.

DOSAGE: *Adults:* Test Dose: Infuse small amount over 15-30 min. Treatment: 3-4mg/kg as required, qd, at infusion rate of 1mg/kg/hr.
Pediatrics: Test Dose: Infuse small amount over 15-30 min. Treatment: 3-4mg/kg as required, qd, at infusion rate of 1mg/kg/hr.

HOW SUPPLIED: Inj: 50mg [20mL], 100mg [50mL]

WARNINGS/PRECAUTIONS: Anaphylaxis reported; administer epinephrine, oxygen, intravenous steroids, and airway management as indicated. D/C if severe respiratory distress occurs; do not give further infusions. Acute infusion-related reactions may occur 1-3 hrs after starting IV infusion; manage by pretreatment with antihistamines and corticosteroids and/or by reducing the rate of infusion and by prompt administration of antihistamines and corticosteroids. Avoid rapid IV infusion. Monitor renal and hepatic function, serum electrolytes, CBC, and PT as medically indicated.

ADVERSE REACTIONS: Chills, fever, tachycardia, N/V, increased creatinine, hypotension, HTN, headache, thrombocytopenia, hypokalemia, hypomagnesemia, hypoxia, abnormal LFTs, dyspnea.

INTERACTIONS: Antineoplastic agents may enhance potential for renal toxicity, bronchospasm, hypotension; use with caution. Corticosteroids and corticotropin may potentiate hypokalemia; monitor serum electrolytes and cardiac function. Cyclosporine and tacrolimus may cause renal toxicity. Concurrent use with digitalis glycosides may induce hypokalemia and may potentiate digitalis toxicity of digitalis glycosides; closely monitor serum K^+ levels. May increase flucytosine toxicity; use with caution. Antagonism with imidazole derivatives (eg, miconazole, ketoconazole) reported. Nephrotoxic agents (eg, aminoglycosides, pentamidine) may enhance the potential for drug-induced renal toxicity; use with caution and intensively monitor renal function. Amphotericin B-induced hypokalemia may enhance curariform effect of skeletal muscle relaxants (eg, tubocurarine) due to hypokalemia; closely monitor serum K^+ levels.

PREGNANCY: Category B, not for use in nursing.

MECHANISM OF ACTION: Polyene antifungal; binds to sterols (primarily ergosterol) in cell membranes of sensitive fungi, with subsequent leakage of intracellular contents and cell death due to changes in membrane permeability. Also binds to cholesterol in mammalian cell membranes, which may account for human toxicity.

PHARMACOKINETICS: Absorption: (3mg/kg/day) AUC=29µg/mL•hr; C_{max}=2.6µg/mL. (4mg/kg/day) AUC=36µg/mL•hr; C_{max}=2.9µg/mL. **Distribution:** V_d=3.8L/kg (3mg/kg/day), 4.1L/kg (4mg/kg/day). **Elimination:** $T_{1/2}$=27.5 hrs (3mg/kg/day), 28.2 hrs (4mg/kg/day).

NURSING CONSIDERATIONS

Assessment: Assess for previous hypersensitivity to the drug, pregnancy/nursing status, and for possible drug interactions. Assess renal function.

Monitoring: Monitor for anaphylaxis, respiratory distress, and acute infusion-related reactions. Monitor renal and hepatic function, serum electrolytes, CBC, and PT. Monitor patients for 30 min after administering the test dose.

Patient Counseling: Inform of risks and benefits of therapy. Advise to seek medical attention if any adverse reactions occur.

Administration: IV route. Refer to PI for further instructions on preparation and administration. **Storage:** Unopened Vials: 15-30°C (59-86°F). Retain in carton until time of use. Reconstituted: 2-8°C (36-46°F). Use within 24 hrs. Do not freeze. Further Diluted with 5% Dextrose for Inj: 2-8°C. Use within 24 hrs. Discard partially used vials.

AMPICILLIN INJECTION   RX
ampicillin sodium (Various)

THERAPEUTIC CLASS: Semisynthetic penicillin derivative

INDICATIONS: Treatment of respiratory tract, urinary tract, and GI infections, bacterial meningitis, septicemia, and endocarditis caused by susceptible strains of microorganisms.

DOSAGE: *Adults:* IM/IV: Respiratory Tract/Soft Tissues: ≥40kg: 250-500mg q6h. <40kg: 25-50mg/kg/day given q6-8h. GI/GU Tract Infections: ≥40kg: 500mg q6h. <40kg: 50mg/kg/day given q6-8h. Urethritis (Caused by *N.gonorrhoeae* in Males): 500mg q8-12h for 2 doses; may retreat if needed. Bacterial Meningitis: 150-200mg/kg/day given q3-4h. Septicemia: 150-200mg/kg/day IV for 3 days, continue with IM q3-4h. Treatment of all infections should be continued for a minimum of 48-72 hrs after becoming asymptomatic or evidence of bacterial eradication has been obtained. Treatment recommended for a minimum of 10 days for Group A β-hemolytic streptococci.
Pediatrics: Bacterial Meningitis: 150-200mg/kg/day given q3-4h. Septicemia: 150-200mg/kg/day IV for 3 days, continue with IM q3-4h. Treatment of all infections should be continued for a minimum of 48-72 hrs after becoming asymptomatic or evidence of bacterial eradication has been obtained. Treatment recommended for a minimum of 10 days for Group A β-hemolytic streptococci.

HOW SUPPLIED: Inj: 125mg, 250mg, 500mg, 1g, 2g, 10g

WARNINGS/PRECAUTIONS: Serious, sometimes fatal, hypersensitivity reactions reported; d/c if occurs. Prior to therapy, assess for previous hypesensitivity reactions to penicillins (PCN), cephalosporins, and other allergens. *Clostridium difficile*-associated diarrhea (CDAD) reported and may range from mild diarrhea to fatal colitis. Avoid in infectious mononucleosis; skin rash reported. May result in bacterial resistance with prolonged use or use in the absence of a proven/ suspected bacterial infection or a prophylactic indication; take appropriate measures if superinfection develops. False-positive glucose reactions reported with Clinitest, Benedict's Solution, or Fehling's solution. Perform periodic assessment of renal, hepatic, and hematopoietic function during prolonged therapy. Rapid direct IV administration may result in convulsive seizures.

ADVERSE REACTIONS: Skin rashes, urticaria, glossitis, N/V, diarrhea, stomatitis, enterocolitis, anemia, thrombocytopenia, eosinophilia, leukopenia, agranulocytosis.

INTERACTIONS: May delay excretion with probenecid. Increased incidence of skin rash with allopurinol.

PREGNANCY: Category B, caution in nursing.

MECHANISM OF ACTION: Penicillin derivative; bactericidal against PCN-susceptible gram-positive organisms and many common gram-negative pathogens.

PHARMACOKINETICS: Distribution: Plasma protein binding (20%), found in breast milk. Penetrates to CSF and brain only if meninges are inflamed. **Elimination:** Urine (unchanged).

NURSING CONSIDERATIONS

Assessment: Assess for proper diagnosis, hypersensitivity to PCNs/cephalosporins or other allergens, infectious mononucleosis, pregnancy/nursing status, and for possible drug interactions.

Monitoring: Monitor for signs/symptoms of hypersensitivity reactions, CDAD, superinfection, and for skin rash. Perform periodic monitoring of renal, hepatic, and hematopoietic function.

Patient Counseling: Inform that drug treats bacterial, not viral, infections. Instruct to take exactly as directed to prevent drug resistance. Instruct to notify physician if pregnant/nursing. Advise to contact physician if watery and bloody stools develop even after 2 or more months after therapy.

Administration: IM/IV routes. Administer within 1 hr after preparation. Administer IV slowly, over at least 10-15 min to avoid convulsive seizures. Refer to PI for information regarding dilution and storage instructions.

AMPICILLIN ORAL   RX
ampicillin (Various)

THERAPEUTIC CLASS: Semisynthetic penicillin derivative

INDICATIONS: Treatment of meningitis and infections of genitourinary (GU) tract (including gonorrhea), respiratory tract, and GI tract caused by susceptible strains of microorganisms.

DOSAGE: *Adults:* GI/GU: 500mg qid in equally spaced doses. Gonorrhea: 3.5g single dose with 1g probenecid. Respiratory: 250mg qid in equally spaced doses. May need larger doses in chronic or severe infections. Treat hemolytic strains of streptococci for ≥10 days. Except for gonorrhea, continue therapy for a minimum of 48-72 hrs after patient becomes asymptomatic or evidence of bacterial eradication has been obtained.
Pediatrics: >20kg: GI/GU: 500mg qid in equally spaced doses. Gonorrhea: 3.5g single dose with 1g probenecid. Respiratory: 250mg qid in equally spaced doses. ≤20kg: GI/GU: 100mg/kg/day total qid, in equally divided and spaced doses. Respiratory: 50mg/kg/day total tid-qid, in equally divided and spaced doses. Do not exceed adult doses. May need larger doses in chronic or severe infections. Treat hemolytic strains of streptococci for ≥10 days. Except for gonorrhea, continue therapy for a minimum of 48-72 hrs after patient becomes asymptomatic or evidence of bacterial eradication has been obtained.

HOW SUPPLIED: Cap: 250mg, 500mg; Sus: 125mg/5mL, 250mg/5mL [100mL, 200mL]

CONTRAINDICATIONS: Infections caused by penicillinase-producing organisms.

WARNINGS/PRECAUTIONS: Serious and fatal hypersensitivity reactions reported with penicillin (PCN) theraphy; anaphylactoid reactions require immediate treatment with epinephrine, oxygen, IV steroids, and airway management. Possible cross-sensitivity with cephalosporins. Pseudomembranous colitis reported; initiate therapeutic measures if diagnosed and consider d/c of treatment. May result in bacterial resistance with prolonged use or use in the absence of a proven/suspected bacterial infection or a prophylactic indication; take appropriate measures if superinfection develops. Give additional parenteral PCN in patients with gonorrhea who also have syphilis. Treatment does not preclude the need for surgical procedures, particularly in staphylococcal infections. May cause false-positive reaction for urinary glucose using copper sulfate tests.

ADVERSE REACTIONS: Stomatitis, N/V, diarrhea, rash, SGOT elevation, agranulocytosis, anemia, eosinophilia, leukopenia, thrombocytopenia, thrombocytopenic purpura, hypersensitivity reactions.

INTERACTIONS: Increased risk of rash with allopurinol. Bacteriostatic antibiotics (eg, chloramphenicol, erythromycins, sulfonamides, or tetracyclines) may interfere with bactericidal activity. May increase breakthrough bleeding with oral contraceptives and decrease oral contraceptive effectiveness. Increased blood levels with probenecid.

PREGNANCY: Category B, not for use in nursing.

MECHANISM OF ACTION: PCN derivative; bactericidal against non-penicillinase-producing gram-positive and gram-negative organisms.

PHARMACOKINETICS: Absorption: Well-absorbed; (500mg Cap) C_{max}=3mcg/mL; (250mg Sus) C_{max}=2.3mcg/mL. **Distribution:** Plasma protein binding (20%); found in breast milk. **Elimination:** Urine (unchanged).

NURSING CONSIDERATIONS

Assessment: Assess for previous hypersensitivity reactions to PCNs, cephalosporins, or other allergens; a history of allergy, asthma, hay fever, or urticaria; pregnancy/nursing status, and possible drug interactions. Conduct susceptibility testing as guide to therapy. Assess for syphilis.

Monitoring: Monitor for hypersensitivity reactions, pseudomembranous colitis, and overgrowth of nonsusceptible organisms. Evaluate renal/hepatic/hematopoietic systems periodically with prolonged therapy. Upon completion, obtain cultures to determine organism eradication. Monitor for masked syphilis; perform follow-up serologic test for each month for 4 months for syphilis in patients without suspected lesions of syphilis.

Patient Counseling: Instruct to notify physician of history of hypersensitivity to PCNs, cephalosporins, or other allergens. Inform diabetics to consult with physician prior to changing diet or dosage of diabetic medication. Inform to take exactly as directed; skipping doses or not completing full course decreases effectiveness and increases bacterial resistance. D/C and notify physician if side effects occur. Inform that therapy only treats bacterial and not viral infections.

Administration: Oral route. Take at least 1/2 hr before or 2 hrs after meals with a full glass of water. Add water to suspension bottle in two portions and shake well after each addition. Refer to PI for directions for reconstitution. **Storage:** 20-25°C (68-77°F). Store reconstituted suspension in a refrigerator; discard unused portion after 14 days.

AMPYRA   RX
dalfampridine (Acorda)

THERAPEUTIC CLASS: Potassium channel blocker

INDICATIONS: Treatment to improve walking in patients with multiple sclerosis (MS).

DOSAGE: *Adults:* 10mg bid (approximately 12 hrs apart). Max recommended dose of 10mg bid should not be exceeded. Do not double dose or take extra if a dose is missed. Take whole; do not divide, crush, chew, or dissolve.

HOW SUPPLIED: Tab, Extended Release: 10mg

CONTRAINDICATIONS: History of seizure, and moderate or severe renal impairment.

WARNINGS/PRECAUTIONS: Increased incidence of seizures has been observed. D/C and do not restart if experience seizure while on treatment. The risk for seizures with mild renal impairment (CrCl 51-80mL/min) is unknown but dalfampridine plasma levels in these patients may approach those seen with 15mg bid, a dose that may increase the risk of seizures. CrCl should be estimated prior to initiating treatment.

ADVERSE REACTIONS: Seizures, urinary tract infection, insomnia, dizziness, headache, nausea, asthenia, multiple sclerosis relapse, paresthesia.

INTERACTIONS: Avoid use with other forms of 4-aminopyridine.

PREGNANCY: Category C, not use for nursing.

MECHANISM OF ACTION: Broad spectrum potassium channel blocker; therapeutic effect has not been fully elucidated. In animal studies it has been shown to increase conduction of action potentials in demyelinated axons through inhibition of potassium channels.

PHARMACOKINETICS: Absorption: Rapid and complete; relative bioavailability (96%); (Tab) C_{max}=17.3-21.6ng/mL (fasted) T_{max}=3-4 hrs (fasted). **Distribution:** V_d=2.6L/kg. **Metabolism:** CYP2E1 (major). **Elimination:** Urine (95.9%); feces (0.5%); $T_{1/2}$=5.2-6.5 hrs.

NURSING CONSIDERATIONS

Assessment: Assess for history of seizures, renal function, concomitant use of 4-aminopyridine, pregnancy/nursing status, and possible drug interactions. Obtain baseline CrCl.

Monitoring: Monitor for seizures, urinary tract infection, headache, dizziness and relapse of multiple sclerosis.

Patient Counseling: Inform that medication may cause seizures, and to d/c use if experience a seizure. Instruct patients to take medication exactly as prescribed. Instruct to take tablet whole; do not crush, chew, or dissolve. Instruct not to take >2 tablets in a 24-hour period and to make sure that there is a 12-hour interval between doses.

Administration: Oral route. **Storage:** 25°C (77°F). Excursions permitted 15-30°C (59-86°F).

AMRIX   RX
cyclobenzaprine HCl (Cephalon)

THERAPEUTIC CLASS: Skeletal muscle relaxant (central-acting)

INDICATIONS: Adjunct to rest and physical therapy to relieve muscle spasm associated with acute, painful musculoskeletal conditions. Use for only short periods of time (up to 2-3 weeks).

DOSAGE: *Adults:* Usual: 15mg qd. Titrate: May increase to 30mg qd if needed. Use for longer than 2-3 weeks not recommended.

HOW SUPPLIED: Cap, Extended-Release: 15mg, 30mg

CONTRAINDICATIONS: MAOI use during or within 14 days. Hyperpyretic crisis seizures and deaths associated with concomitant use of cyclobenzaprine (or drugs structurally similar to TCAs) and MAOIs reported. Acute recovery phase of MI, arrhythmias, heart block conduction disturbances, CHF, hyperthyroidism.

WARNINGS/PRECAUTIONS: Avoid in hepatic impairment and elderly patients. Caution with history of urinary retention, angle-closure glaucoma, increased IOP, and use of anticholinergic medication. May impair mental and/or physical performance.

ADVERSE REACTIONS: Drowsiness, dry mouth, dizziness, somnolence, headache.

INTERACTIONS: Contraindicated with MAOIs. Enhances effects of alcohol, barbiturates and other CNS depressants. TCAs may block antihypertensive action of guanethidine and similar compounds and may enhance seizure risk with tramadol.

PREGNANCY: Category B, caution in nursing.

MECHANISM OF ACTION: Skeletal muscle relaxant; acts primarily within the CNS at brain stem as opposed to spinal cord level, although overlapping action on the latter may contribute to its overall skeletal muscle relaxant activity; suggested to reduce tonic somatic motor activity influencing both gamma and α motor systems.

PHARMACOKINETICS: Absorption: C_{max}=8.3ng/mL, T_{max}=8.1 hrs, AUC=354.1ng•h/mL; see full PI for more detailed information. **Metabolism:** Extensive; via CYP3A4, 1A2, and 2D6 through N-demethylation pathway. **Elimination:** Urine (glucuronides); $T_{1/2}$=33.4 hrs.

NURSING CONSIDERATIONS

Assessment: Assess for hepatic function, history of seizures, hyperthyroidism, urinary retention, angle-closure glaucoma, IOP, recent MI, arrhythmias, heart block, CHF, alcohol intake, pregnancy/nursing status, and possible drug interactions.

Monitoring: Monitor for cardiac arrhythmias, sinus tachycardia, MI, stroke, IOP, CBC, and LFTs.

Patient Counseling: Caution against performing hazardous tasks (eg, operating machinery/driving); avoid alcohol and other CNS depressants. Notify if pregnant/nursing.

Administration: Oral route; take at same time each day. **Storage:** 25°C (77°F); excursions permitted to 15-30°C (59-86°F).

AMTURNIDE   RX
amlodipine - aliskiren - hydrochlorothiazide (Novartis)

> **D/C when pregnancy is detected. Drugs that act directly on the renin-angiotensin system can cause injury/death to the developing fetus.**

THERAPEUTIC CLASS: Renin inhibitor/calcium channel blocker (dihydropyridine)/thiazide diuretic

INDICATIONS: Treatment of HTN.

DOSAGE: *Adults:* Usual: Dose qd. Titrate: May increase after 2 weeks of therapy. Max: 300mg-10mg-25mg. Add-On/Switch Therapy: Use if not adequately controlled with any 2 of the following: aliskiren, dihydropyridine calcium channel blockers, and thiazide diuretics. With dose-limiting adverse reactions to any component on dual therapy, switch to triple therapy at a lower dose of that component. Replacement Therapy: Substitute for individually titrated components.

HOW SUPPLIED: Tab: (Aliskiren-Amlodipine-HCTZ) 150mg-5mg-12.5mg, 300mg-5mg-12.5mg, 300mg-5mg-25mg, 300mg-10mg-12.5mg, 300mg-10mg-25mg

AMTURNIDE

CONTRAINDICATIONS: Anuria, sulfonamide-derived drug hypersensitivity. Concomitant use with angiotensin receptor blockers (ARBs) or ACE inhibitors in patients with diabetes.

WARNINGS/PRECAUTIONS: Not indicated for initial therapy of HTN. In patients with an activated renin-angiotensin-aldosterone system (eg, volume- and/or salt-depleted patients receiving high doses of diuretics), symptomatic hypotension may occur; correct these conditions prior to therapy, or monitor closely. Renal function changes may occur; caution in patients with renal artery stenosis, severe heart failure (HF), post-myocardial infarction (MI), or volume depletion. Monitor renal function periodically and consider withholding or d/c therapy if significant decrease in renal function develops. May cause serum electrolyte abnormalities (eg, hyperkalemia, hypokalemia, hyponatremia, hypomagnesemia); correct hypokalemia and any coexisting hypomagnesemia prior to initiation of therapy and monitor periodically. D/C if hypokalemia is accompanied by clinical signs (eg, muscular weakness, paresis, or ECG alterations). Not studied in patients with heart failure (HF). Monitor calcium levels in patients with hypercalcemia. Aliskiren: Angioedema of the face, extremities, lips, tongue, glottis, and/or larynx reported; d/c therapy and do not readminister. May cause hyperkalemia; monitor serum K⁺ periodically. Amlodipine: Increased frequency, duration/severity of angina, or acute MI rarely reported with dosage initiation or increase, particularly with severe obstructive coronary artery disease (CAD). HCTZ: May cause hypersensitivity reactions and exacerbation or activation of systemic lupus erythematosus (SLE). May precipitate hepatic coma with hepatic dysfunction. May cause idiosyncratic reaction, resulting in acute transient myopia and acute angle-closure glaucoma; d/c as rapidly as possible. May alter glucose tolerance and increase serum cholesterol and TG levels. May cause or exacerbate hyperuricemia and precipitate gout in susceptible patients. May decrease urinary calcium excretion and cause hypercalcemia; monitor levels.

ADVERSE REACTIONS: Peripheral edema, dizziness, headache, hyperkalemia, hypokalemia, nasopharyngitis.

INTERACTIONS: See Contraindications. Concomitant ARBs, ACE inhibitors, or NSAIDs may be at risk of developing renal impairment; avoid with moderate renal impairment (GFR <60mL/min). Aliskiren: Cyclosporine or itraconazole increases levels; avoid concomitant use. May develop hyperkalemia with ARBs, ACE inhibitors, NSAIDs, K⁺ supplements or K⁺-sparing diuretics. Possible interaction with P-glycoprotein inhibitors. NSAIDs, including selective cyclooxygenase-2 inhibitors, may result in deterioration of renal function and attenuation of antihypertensive effect. Amlodipine: May increase simvastatin exposure; limit simvastatin dose to 20mg/day. HCTZ: Potentiation of orthostatic hypotension may occur with alcohol, barbiturates, and narcotics. Dosage adjustment of antidiabetic drugs (insulin or oral hypoglycemic agents) may be required. Ion exchange resins (eg, cholestyramine, colestipol) may reduce exposure; space dosing at least 4 hrs before or 4-6 hrs after the administration of ion exchange resins. May increase responsiveness to skeletal muscle relaxants (eg, curare derivatives). Increased risk of lithium toxicity; avoid concomitant use. Anticholinergic agents (eg, atropine, biperiden) may increase bioavailability. Prokinetic drugs may decrease bioavailability. May reduce renal excretion of cytotoxic agents and enhance myelosuppressive effects. Thiazide-induced hypokalemia/hypomagnesemia may predispose patients to digoxin toxicity.

PREGNANCY: Category D, not for use in nursing.

MECHANISM OF ACTION: Aliskiren: Direct renin inhibitor; decreases plasma renin activity and inhibits conversion of angiotensinogen to angiotensin I. Amlodipine: Dihydropyridine calcium channel blocker; inhibits the transmembrane influx of calcium ions into vascular smooth muscle and cardiac muscle. HCTZ: Thiazide diuretic; has not been established. Affects renal tubular mechanisms of electrolyte reabsorption, directly increasing excretion of Na⁺ and Cl⁻ in approximately equivalent amounts.

PHARMACOKINETICS: Absorption: Aliskiren: Poor; T_{max}=1-2 hrs; bioavailability (2.5%). Amlodipine: Absolute bioavailability (64-90%); T_{max}=6-12 hrs. HCTZ: Absolute bioavailability (70%); T_{max}=1-4 hrs. **Distribution:** Amlodipine: Plasma protein binding (93%). HCTZ: Albumin binding (40-70%). Crosses the placenta; found in breast milk. **Metabolism:** Aliskiren: Via CYP3A4. Amlodipine: Hepatic; extensive. **Elimination:** Aliskiren: Urine (25% parent drug). Amlodipine: Urine (10% parent compound, 60% metabolites), $T_{1/2}$=30-50 hrs. HCTZ: Urine (70% unchanged), $T_{1/2}$=10 hrs.

NURSING CONSIDERATIONS

Assessment: Assess for hepatic/renal impairment, anuria, severe obstructive CAD, angioedema, HF, sulfonamide or penicillin allergy, volume- and/or salt-depletion, history of upper respiratory surgery, allergy or bronchial asthma, SLE, pregnancy/nursing status, and possible drug interactions. Obtain baseline BP.

Monitoring: Monitor for hypersensitivity and anaphylactic reactions, head/neck angioedema, airway obstruction, angina, MI, exacerbation of SLE, idiosyncratic reaction, transient myopia, and acute angle-closure glaucoma. Monitor BP, hepatic function, serum uric acid, BUN, SrCr, and serum electrolytes. Monitor renal function periodically.

Patient Counseling: Counsel women of childbearing age about consequences of exposure during pregnancy; instruct to report pregnancy as soon as possible. Caution that lightheadedness may occur, especially during the 1st days of therapy; report to physician. Advise to d/c treatment and to consult physician if syncope occurs. Caution that inadequate fluid intake, excessive perspiration, diarrhea, or vomiting can lead to excessive fall in BP; leading to lightheadedness and possible syncope. Advise to d/c and immediately report any signs/symptoms of angioedema (eg, swelling of the face, extremities, eyes, lips, tongue, and difficulty swallowing or breathing). Instruct not to use K+ supplements or salt substitutes containing K+ without consulting physician. Instruct to establish a routine pattern for taking medication with regard to meals and inform that high-fat meals decrease absorption substantially.

Administration: Oral route. **Storage:** 25°C (77°F); excursions permitted to 15-30°C (59-86°F). Protect from heat and moisture.

ANAGRELIDE HCL   RX
anagrelide HCl (Various)

OTHER BRAND NAMES: Agrylin (Shire)

THERAPEUTIC CLASS: Platelet-reducing agent

INDICATIONS: Treatment of thrombocythemia, secondary to myeloproliferative disorders, to reduce elevated platelet counts and the risk of thrombosis and to ameliorate associated symptoms (eg, thrombo-hemorrhagic events).

DOSAGE: *Adults:* Initial: 0.5mg qid or 1mg bid for ≥1 week. Titrate: Increase by not more than 0.5mg/day in any 1 week. Max: 10mg/day or 2.5mg/dose. Adjust to lowest effective dose to reduce and maintain platelet count <600,000/μL, and ideally to the normal range. Moderate Hepatic Impairment: Initial: 0.5mg/day for ≥1 week. Titrate: Increase by not more than 0.5mg/day in any 1 week.
Pediatrics: Initial: 0.5mg qd-0.5mg qid. Titrate: Increase by not more than 0.5mg/day in any 1 week. Max: 10mg/day or 2.5mg/dose. Adjust to lowest effective dose to reduce and maintain platelet count <600,000/μL, and ideally to the normal range.

HOW SUPPLIED: Cap: 0.5mg, 1mg, (Agrylin) 0.5mg

CONTRAINDICATIONS: Severe hepatic impairment.

WARNINGS/PRECAUTIONS: Initiate therapy under close medical supervision. Caution with known/suspected heart disease; may cause cardiovascular (CV) effects (eg, vasodilation, tachycardia, palpitations, and congestive heart failure). Perform pretreatment CV exam and monitor during treatment. Caution with mild and moderate hepatic dysfunction; reduce dose in moderate hepatic impairment and monitor for CV effects. Interstitial lung diseases reported. Monitor blood counts (Hgb, WBC) and renal function (SrCr, BUN). Cases of hepatotoxicity (eg, symptomatic ALT and AST elevations and elevation >3X ULN) reported; measure LFTs prior to and during therapy. Fall in standing BP accompanied by dizziness reported. Interruption of treatment may be followed by an increase in platelet count.

ADVERSE REACTIONS: Headache, palpitations, diarrhea, asthenia, edema, N/V, abdominal pain, dizziness, pain, dyspnea, flatulence, fever, peripheral edema, rash (including urticaria).

INTERACTIONS: Aspirin may increase major hemorrhagic events; assess the potential risks and benefits of concomitant use prior to coadministration, particularly in patients with a high-risk profile for hemorrhage. CYP1A2 inhibitors (eg, fluvoxamine) may adversely influence clearance. Potential interaction with CYP1A2 substrates (eg, theophylline). May exacerbate effects of cyclic AMP phosphodiesterase III (PDE III) inhibitors (eg, inotropes: milrinone, enoximone, amrinone, olprinone, cilostazol). Sucralfate may interfere with absorption.

PREGNANCY: Category C, not for use in nursing.

MECHANISM OF ACTION: Platelet-reducing agent; not established. Suspected to reduce platelet production resulting from a decrease in megakaryocyte hypermaturation. Inhibits cyclic AMP PDE III. PDE III inhibitors can also inhibit platelet aggregation.

PHARMACOKINETICS: Metabolism: RL603 and 3-hydroxy anagrelide (major metabolites). **Elimination:** Urine (>70%); $T_{1/2}$=1.3 hrs (0.5mg, fasted).

NURSING CONSIDERATIONS

Assessment: Assess for hepatic impairment, known/suspected heart disease, renal insufficiency, pregnancy/nursing status, and possible drug interactions. Perform CV exam and LFTs.

Monitoring: Monitor for signs/symptoms of CV effects, interstitial lung diseases, and thrombocytopenia. Monitor platelet counts q2 days during 1st week of treatment and at least weekly thereafter until maint dose is reached. Monitor blood counts, renal function, and LFTs.

Patient Counseling: Inform of risks/benefits of therapy. Instruct women of childbearing potential to avoid pregnancy and use contraception during therapy.

Administration: Oral route. **Storage:** 20-25°C (68-77°F). (Agrylin) 25°C (77°F); excursions permitted to 15-30°C (59-86°F). Store in light-resistant container.

ANCOBON   RX
flucytosine (Valeant)

Extreme caution in patients with renal impairment. Monitor hematologic, renal, and hepatic status closely.

THERAPEUTIC CLASS: 5-fluorocytosine antifungal

INDICATIONS: Treatment of serious infections caused by susceptible strains of *Candida* (eg, septicemia, endocarditis, and urinary system infections) and/or *Cryptococcus* (eg, meningitis, pulmonary infections) in combination with amphotericin B.

DOSAGE: *Adults:* Usual: 50-150mg/kg/day in divided doses at 6-hr intervals. Give a few caps at a time over a 15-min period to reduce or avoid N/V. Renal Impairment: Give initial dose at a lower level.

HOW SUPPLIED: Cap: 250mg, 500mg

WARNINGS/PRECAUTIONS: Extreme caution with bone marrow depression and with impaired renal function. Patients with hematologic disease, are being treated with radiation or drugs that depress bone marrow, or have a history of treatment with such drugs or radiation may be more prone to bone marrow depression. Bone marrow toxicity can be irreversible and may lead to death in immunosuppressed patients.

ADVERSE REACTIONS: Myocardial toxicity, chest pain, dyspnea, rash, pruritus, urticaria, photo-sensitivity, nausea, jaundice, renal failure, pyrexia, crystalluria, anemia, leukopenia, eosinophilia.

INTERACTIONS: Inactivated antifungal activity by competitive inhibition with cytosine arabino-side. Drugs that impair glomerular filtration may prolong the biological $T_{1/2}$.

PREGNANCY: Category C, not for use in nursing.

MECHANISM OF ACTION: 5-fluorocytosine antifungal; exerts antifungal activity through the subsequent conversion into several active metabolites, which inhibit protein synthesis by falsely incorporating into fungal RNA or interfere with biosynthesis of fungal DNA through inhibition of enzyme thymidylate synthetase.

PHARMACOKINETICS: Absorption: Rapid and complete; C_{max}=30-40µg/mL; T_{max}=2 hrs. **Distribution:** Plasma protein binding (2.9-4%). Penetrates blood-brain barrier; found in CSF. **Metabolism:** Deamination (by gut bacteria); 5-fluorouracil. α-fluoro-β-ureido-propionic acid (metabolite). **Elimination:** Urine (>90%, 1% metabolite), feces; $T_{1/2}$=2.4-4.8 hrs.

NURSING CONSIDERATIONS

Assessment: Assess for renal impairment, bone marrow depression, immunosuppressed pa-tients, pregnancy/nursing status, and possible drug interactions. Determine serum electrolytes, hematologic, and renal status prior to treatment.

Monitoring: Monitor for adverse reactions. Monitor renal function (using Jaffe reaction) and blood concentrations. Monitor hematologic status (leukocyte and thrombocyte count), hepatic function (alkaline phosphatase, SGOT, and SGPT), and hematopoietic system frequently.

Patient Counseling: Inform of the risks and benefits of therapy. Advise to take a few caps at a time over a 15-min period to reduce or avoid N/V.

Administration: Oral route. **Storage:** 25°C (77°F); excursions permitted to 15-30°C (59-86°F).

ANDRODERM   CIII
testosterone (Watson)

THERAPEUTIC CLASS: Androgen

INDICATIONS: Replacement therapy in adult males for conditions associated with a deficiency or absence of endogenous testosterone (eg, congenital/acquired primary hypogonadism or hypogonadotropic hypogonadism).

DOSAGE: *Adults:* Initial: One 4mg/day system applied nightly for 24 hrs to a clean dry area of the skin on the back, abdomen, upper arms, or thighs. Measure serum testosterone concentra-tions in the early am approximately 2 weeks after starting. If outside the range of 400-930ng/dL, increase daily dose to 6mg (eg, one 4mg/day and one 2mg/day system) or decrease to 2mg (eg, one 2mg/day system), maintaining nightly application. Switching from 2.5mg/day, 5mg/day, or 7.5mg/day patch: Switch to 2mg/day, 4mg/day, or 6mg/day (2mg/day and 4mg/day) systems respectively at the next scheduled dose. Measure early am serum testosterone concentration ap-proximately 2 weeks after switching to ensure proper dosing.

HOW SUPPLIED: Patch: 2mg/24 hrs [60s], 4mg/24 hrs [30s]

CONTRAINDICATIONS: Known/suspected prostate carcinoma or breast carcinoma in men, women who are or may become pregnant, or breastfeeding.

WARNINGS/PRECAUTIONS: Monitor patients with benign prostatic hyperplasia (BPH) for worsening of signs/symptoms of BPH. May increase risk for prostate cancer; evaluate for prostate cancer prior to and during therapy. Increases in Hct and RBC mass may increase risk for thromboembolic events; lower dose or d/c therapy. Suppression of spermatogenesis may occur at large doses. Risk of edema with or without congestive heart failure (CHF) with preexisting cardiac, renal, or hepatic disease. Gynecomastia may develop and may persist. May potentiate sleep apnea, especially with obesity or chronic lung diseases. Changes in serum lipid profile reported; adjust dose or d/c therapy if necessary. Caution in cancer patients at risk of hypercalcemia and associated hypercalciuria. May decrease thyroxine-binding globulin leading to changes in T3 and T4 levels. Not indicated for use in women and children.

ADVERSE REACTIONS: Application-site reactions (pruritus, blistering, erythema, vesicles, burning, induration), back pain prostatic abnormalities, headache, contact dermatitis.

INTERACTIONS: May decrease blood glucose and insulin requirements. May increase fluid retention with adrenocorticotropic hormone or corticosteroids. Changes in anticoagulant activity may occur; frequently monitor INR and PT in patients taking anticoagulants. The rate of complete adherence was lowered with topical administration of 0.1% triamcinolone cream. Pretreatment with triamcinolone ointment formulation may reduce testosterone absorption.

PREGNANCY: Category X, not for use in nursing.

MECHANISM OF ACTION: Endogenous androgen; responsible for normal growth and development of male sex organs and for maintenance of secondary sex characteristics.

PHARMACOKINETICS: Absorption: T_{max}=8 hrs. **Distribution:** Sex hormone binding globulin (SHBG) binding (40%), albumin and plasma protein binding, unbound (2%). **Metabolism:** Estradiol and dihydrotestosterone (major active metabolites). **Elimination:** (IM) Urine (90% glucuronic and sulfuric acid conjugates), feces (6% unconjugated); $T_{1/2}$=10-100 min, $T_{1/2}$=70 min (upon removal).

NURSING CONSIDERATIONS

Assessment: Assess for conditions where treatment is contraindicated, BPH, prostate cancer, cardiac or renal/hepatic disease, obesity, chronic lung disease, and possible drug interactions. Obtain Hct prior to therapy.

Monitoring: Monitor for signs/symptoms of prostate cancer, edema with or without CHF, gynecomastia, sleep apnea, virilization, and worsening of BPH. Monitor Hct, Hgb, prostate specific antigen, serum lipid profile, LFTs, and serum testosterone levels periodically. In cancer patients at risk for hypercalcemia, regularly monitor serum calcium levels. Re-evaluate Hct 3-6 months after start of therapy, then annually.

Patient Counseling: Inform that men with known or suspected prostate/breast cancer should not use androgen therapy. Inform about potential adverse reactions. Instruct to apply ud. Advise not to apply to the scrotum or over a bony prominence, or any part of the body that could be subject to prolonged pressure during sleep or sitting. Advise not to remove during sexual intercourse, nor while taking a shower or bath. Inform that strenuous exercise or excessive perspiration may loosen a patch or cause it to fall off. Advise to avoid swimming or showering until 3 hrs following application. Instruct to use OTC topical hydrocortisone cream after system removal in order to ameliorate mild skin irritation. Advise that applying small amount of 0.1% triamcinolone acetonide cream to skin under the central drug reservoir of patch may reduce incidence and severity of skin irritation. Advise to remove the patch before undergoing MRI. Instruct to apply immediately once removed from pouch and protective liner is removed.

Administration: Transdermal patch system. Apply immediately adhesive side of the system to a clean, dry area of the skin on the back, abdomen, upper arms, or thighs. Rotate application site with an interval of 7 days between applications to the same site. Do not use if the individual pouch seal is broken or damaged. Do not cut patches. Refer to PI for further application instructions. **Storage:** 20-25° (68-77°F). Do not store outside pouch provided.

ANDROGEL
testosterone (Abbott)

> Virilization reported in children secondarily exposed to testosterone gel. Children should avoid contact with unwashed or unclothed application sites in men using testosterone gel. Advise patients to strictly adhere to recommended use instructions.

THERAPEUTIC CLASS: Androgen

INDICATIONS: Replacement therapy in adult males for conditions associated with a deficiency or absence of endogenous testosterone (congenital/acquired primary hypogonadism or hypogonadotropic hypogonadism).

DOSAGE: *Adults:* (1%) Initial: Apply 5g qd, preferably in am, to clean, dry, intact skin of shoulders and upper arms and/or abdomen. Titrate: May increase to 7.5g qd, then 10g qd if serum testosterone is below normal range. May decrease daily dose if serum testosterone exceeds normal range. D/C therapy if serum testosterone consistently exceeds the normal range at a daily dose of 5g. (1.62%) Initial: Apply 40.5mg qd, preferably in am, to shoulders and upper arms. May adjust dose between 20.25mg (minimum) and 81mg (max). Titrate based on the pre-dose am serum testosterone concentration from a single blood draw at approximately 14 days and 28 days after starting or following dose adjustment. Refer to PI for dose adjustments required at each titration step.

HOW SUPPLIED: Gel: 1% [2.5g, 5g pkts; 75g pump]; 1.62% [20.25mg/1.25g]

CONTRAINDICATIONS: Known/suspected prostate carcinoma or breast carcinoma in men, women who are or may become pregnant, or breastfeeding. (1%) Hypersensitivity to alcohol or soy products.

WARNINGS/PRECAUTIONS: Patients with benign prostatic hyperplasia (BPH) may be at increased risk for worsening of signs/symptoms of BPH. May increase risk for prostate cancer; evaluate for prostate cancer prior to and during therapy. May increase prostate specific antigen (PSA) levels. May cause fetal harm. Suppression of spermatogenesis may occur at large doses. Risk of edema with or without congestive heart failure (CHF) with preexisting cardiac, renal, or hepatic disease. Gynecomastia may develop and may persist. May potentiate sleep apnea especially with obesity or chronic lung diseases. Increases in Hct and red blood cell mass may increase risk for thromboembolic events; lower dose or d/c therapy. Changes in serum lipid profile reported; adjust dose or d/c therapy if necessary. Caution in cancer patients at risk of hypercalcemia and associated hypercalciuria. Not indicated for use in women. Gel is flammable; avoid fire, flame, or smoking until the gel has dried. (1.62%) Application site and dose are not interchangeable with other topical testosterone products.

ADVERSE REACTIONS: PSA increase, acne, application-site reactions, prostatic/urinary/testicular disorders, abnormal lab tests, headache, emotional lability, gynecomastia, HTN, nervousness, breast pain, asthenia, decreased libido.

INTERACTIONS: May decrease blood glucose and insulin requirements. May increase fluid retention with adrenocorticotropic hormone or corticosteroids. Changes in anticoagulant activity may occur; frequently monitor INR and PT in patients taking anticoagulants.

PREGNANCY: Category X, not for use in nursing.

MECHANISM OF ACTION: Androgen; responsible for normal growth and development of male sex organs and for maintenance of secondary sex characteristics.

PHARMACOKINETICS: Absorption: (1%) Systemic (10%). **Distribution:** Sex hormone binding globulin (SHBG) binding (40%), albumin and plasma protein binding (58%), unbound (2%). **Metabolism:** Estradiol and dihydrotestosterone (active metabolites). **Elimination:** (IM) Urine (90% glucuronic and sulfuric acid conjugates), feces (6% unconjugated); $T_{1/2}$=10-100 min.

NURSING CONSIDERATIONS

Assessment: Assess for conditions where treatment is contraindicated, BPH, prostate cancer, cardiac or renal/hepatic disease, obesity, chronic lung disease, and possible drug interactions. Obtain Hct prior to therapy. (1%) Assess for hypersensitivity to alcohol or soy products.

Monitoring: Monitor for signs/symptoms of prostate cancer, edema with or without CHF, gynecomastia, sleep apnea, virilization, and worsening of BPH. Monitor Hct, Hgb, PSA, serum lipid profile, LFTs, and serum testosterone levels periodically. In cancer patients at risk for hypercalcemia, regularly monitor serum calcium levels. (1.62%) Reevaluate Hct 3-6 months after start of therapy, then annually.

Patient Counseling: Inform that men with known or suspected prostate/breast cancer should not use androgen therapy. Advise to report signs and symptoms of secondary exposure in children and women to the physician. Instruct to avoid contact with unwashed or unclothed application sites of men. Instruct to apply as directed; wash hands with soap and water after application, cover application site with clothing after gel dries, and wash application site with soap and water prior to direct skin-to-skin contact with others. Inform about possible adverse reactions. Advise to read Medication Guide before therapy and reread each time the prescription is renewed. Inform that drug is flammable. Keep out of reach of children. Inform about importance of adhering to all the recommended monitoring, to report changes in their state of health, and to wait 5 hrs (1%) or 2 hrs (1.62%) before showering or swimming.

Administration: Topical route. Allow application site to dry prior to dressing. Wash hands with soap and water after application. (1%) Do not apply to genitals. Refer to PI for specific dosing guidelines using the multi-dose pump. (1.62%) Do not apply to any other parts of the body (eg, abdomen, genitals). Refer to PI for administration instructions and application sites. **Storage:** (1%) 25°C (77°F); excursions permitted to 15-30°C (59-86°F). (1.62%) 20-25°C (68-77°F); excursions permitted to 15-30°C (59-86°F).

ANGELIQ

RX

estradiol - drospirenone (Bayer Healthcare)

Estrogens increase the risk of endometrial cancer. Perform adequate diagnostic measures, including endometrial sampling, to rule out malignancy with undiagnosed persistent or recurrent abnormal genital bleeding. Should not be used for the prevention of cardiovascular disease (CVD) or dementia. Increased risks of myocardial infarction (MI), stroke, pulmonary embolism (PE), and deep vein thrombosis (DVT) in postmenopausal women (50-79 yrs of age) reported. May increase risk of invasive breast cancer. Increased risk of developing probable dementia in postmenopausal women ≥65 yrs of age reported. Should be prescribed at the lowest effective dose and for the shortest duration consistent with treatment goals and risks.

THERAPEUTIC CLASS: Estrogen/progestogen combination

INDICATIONS: Treatment of moderate to severe vasomotor symptoms and/or vulvar and vaginal atrophy due to menopause in women who have a uterus.

DOSAGE: *Adults:* Moderate to Severe Vasomotor Symptoms: 1 tab (0.25mg-0.5mg or 0.5-1mg) qd. Moderate to Severe Vulvar and Vaginal Atrophy: 1 tab (0.5mg-1mg) qd. Re-evaluate periodically.

HOW SUPPLIED: Tab: (Drospirenone [DSRP]-Estradiol [E2]) 0.25mg-0.5mg, 0.5mg-1mg

CONTRAINDICATIONS: Undiagnosed abnormal genital bleeding, known/suspected/history of breast cancer, known/suspected estrogen-dependent neoplasia, active or history of DVT/PE/ arterial thromboembolic disease (eg, stroke, MI), renal impairment, liver impairment/disease, adrenal insufficiency, protein C, protein S, antithrombin deficiency, or other known thrombophilic disorders; known/suspected pregnancy.

WARNINGS/PRECAUTIONS: D/C immediately if PE, DVT, stroke, or MI occur or are suspected. Caution in patients with risk factors for arterial vascular disease (eg, HTN, diabetes mellitus [DM], tobacco use, hypercholesterolemia, obesity) and/or venous thromboembolism (VTE) (eg, personal/family history of VTE, obesity, systemic lupus erythematosus [SLE]). If feasible, d/c therapy at least 4-6 weeks before surgery of the type associated with increased risk of thromboembolism, or during periods of prolonged immobilization. Potential for hyperkalemia development in high risk patients; contraindicated with conditions that predispose to hyperkalemia. May increase risk of ovarian cancer and gallbladder disease. May lead to severe hypercalcemia in patients with breast cancer and bone metastases; d/c and take appropriate measures if hypercalcemia occurs. Retinal vascular thrombosis reported; d/c pending examination if sudden partial or complete loss of vision, sudden onset of proptosis, diplopia, or migraine occurs. D/C permanently if examination reveals papilledema or retinal vascular lesions. May elevate BP, thyroid binding globulin levels, and plasma TG (with preexisting hypertriglyceridemia); d/c if pancreatitis occurs. Caution with history of cholestatic jaundice associated with past estrogen use or with pregnancy; d/c in case of recurrence. May cause fluid retention; caution with cardiac/renal dysfunction. Caution with hypoparathyroidism; hypocalcemia may occur. May increase possibility of hyponatremia in high-risk patients. May exacerbate symptoms of angioedema in women with hereditary angioedema. May exacerbate endometriosis, asthma, DM, epilepsy, migraine, porphyria, SLE, otosclerosis, chorea minor, and hepatic hemangiomas; use with caution. May affect certain endocrine and blood components in laboratory tests.

ADVERSE REACTIONS: GI and abdominal pain, female genital tract bleeding, headache, breast pain, vulvovaginal fungal infections, nausea.

INTERACTIONS: CYP3A4 inducers (eg, St. John's wort, phenobarbital, carbamazepine, rifampin) may decrease levels which may decrease therapeutic effects and/or change uterine bleeding profile. CYP3A4 inhibitors (eg, erythromycin, clarithromycin, ketoconazole, itraconazole, ritonavir, grapefruit juice) may increase levels which may result in side effects. May increase risk of hyperkalemia with regular intake of other medications that can increase K^+ (eg, NSAIDs, K^+-sparing diuretics, K^+ supplements, ACE inhibitors, angiotensin-II receptor blockers, heparin, aldosterone antagonists). Patients concomitantly receiving thyroid hormone replacement therapy and estrogens may require increased doses of their thyroid replacement therapy. Acute alcohol ingestion may elevate circulating E2 concentrations.

PREGNANCY: Contraindicated in pregnancy, caution in nursing.

MECHANISM OF ACTION: Estrogen/progestogen combination. E2: Binds to nuclear receptors in estrogen-responsive tissues. Modulates pituitary secretion of gonadotropins, luteinizing hormone and follicle stimulating hormone, through negative feedback mechanism. DRSP: Synthetic progestin and spironolactone analog with antimineralocorticoid activity. Possesses anti-androgenic activity. Counters estrogenic effects by decreasing number of nuclear estradiol receptors and suppressing epithelial DNA synthesis in endometrial tissue.

PHARMACOKINETICS: Absorption: (DRSP) Absolute bioavailability (76-85%). Administration of variable doses resulted in different pharmacokinetic parameters. **Distribution:** Found in breast milk. DRSP: V_d=4.2L/kg, serum protein binding (97%). E2: Sex hormone binding globulin (37%); albumin binding (61%). **Metabolism:** DRSP: Extensive; CYP3A4 (minor). E2: Liver to estrone (metabolite); estriol (major urinary metabolite); enterohepatic recirculation via sulfate and

81

glucuronide conjugation in the liver; biliary secretion of conjugates in the intestine; hydrolysis in the gut; reabsorption. **Elimination:** DRSP: Urine (38-47%, glucuronide and sulfate conjugates), feces (17-20%, glucuronide and sulfate conjugates); $T_{1/2}$=36-42 hrs. E2/Estrone: Urine.

NURSING CONSIDERATIONS

Assessment: Assess for undiagnosed abnormal genital bleeding, presence/history of breast cancer, estrogen-dependent neoplasia, arterial thromboembolic disease, pregnancy/nursing status, and any other condition where treatment is cautioned or contraindicated. Assess use in patients ≥65 yrs and those with hypertriglyceridemia, hypothyroidism, hypocalcemia, asthma, DM, epilepsy, migraines or porphyria, SLE, otosclerosis, and hepatic hemangiomas. Assess for possible drug interactions.

Monitoring: Monitor for signs/symptoms of CVD, malignant neoplasms, dementia, gallbladder disease, BP elevations, visual abnormalities, elevations in plasma TG, pancreatitis, cholestatic jaundice, hypothyroidism, fluid retention, hyperkalemia, hyponatremia, and exacerbation of endometriosis and other conditions. Perform annual breast examination; schedule mammography based on patient's age, risk factors, and prior mammogram results. Monitor thyroid function in patients on thyroid hormone replacement therapy. Monitor serum K⁺ levels during 1st month of dosing in patients at risk for hyperkalemia. Perform adequate diagnostic measures (eg, endometrial sampling) in patients with undiagnosed persistent or recurrent genital bleeding. Perform periodic evaluation to determine treatment need.

Patient Counseling: Inform postmenopausal women of the importance of reporting abnormal vaginal bleeding as soon as possible. Advise of possible serious adverse reactions of therapy (eg, CVD, malignant neoplasms, probable dementia) and possible less serious but common adverse reactions (eg, headache, breast pain and tenderness, N/V). Instruct to have yearly breast exams by a healthcare provider and perform monthly self breast exams.

Administration: Oral route. Swallow whole with some liquid irrespective of food. Take at the same time qd. **Storage:** 25°C (77°F); excursions permitted to 15-30°C (59-86°F).

ANGIOMAX   RX
bivalirudin (The Medicines Company)

THERAPEUTIC CLASS: Thrombin inhibitor

INDICATIONS: Adjunct to aspirin (ASA) for anticoagulation in patients with unstable angina undergoing percutaneous transluminal coronary angioplasty (PTCA), with provisional use of glycoprotein IIb/IIIa inhibitor (GPI) undergoing percutaneous coronary intervention (PCI), and patients with, or at risk of, heparin induced thrombocytopenia (HIT)/heparin induced thrombocytopenia and thrombosis syndrome (HITTS) undergoing PCI.

DOSAGE: *Adults:* With ASA (300-325mg/day). Without HIT/HITTS: 0.75mg/kg IV bolus, then 1.75mg/kg/hr infusion for the duration of the PCI/PTCA procedure. Additional bolus of 0.3mg/kg may be given if needed based on activated clotting time which should be performed 5 min after first bolus dose. Consider GPI administration. With HIT/HITTS Undergoing PCI: 0.75mg/kg IV bolus, then 1.75mg/kg/hr infusion for the duration of the procedure. Ongoing Treatment Post Procedure: Continuation of infusion following PCI/PTCA for ≤4 hrs post-procedure is optional. After 4 hrs, if needed, an additional 0.2mg/kg/hr (low-rate infusion) for ≤20 hrs may be initiated. Renal Impairment: CrCl 30-59mL/min: 1.75mg/kg/hr IV infusion. CrCl <30mL/min: Reduce infusion rate to 1mg/kg/hr. Hemodialysis: Reduce infusion rate to 0.25mg/kg/hr. Refer to PI for the dosing table based on weight.

HOW SUPPLIED: Inj: 250mg

CONTRAINDICATIONS: Active major bleeding.

WARNINGS/PRECAUTIONS: Hemorrhage may occur at any site; caution with disease states associated with an increased risk of bleeding. D/C with unexplained fall in BP or Hct. Increased risk of thrombus formation, including fatal outcomes in gamma brachytherapy reported; maintain meticulous catheter technique (with frequent aspiration and flushing, paying special attention to minimize stasis condition within the catheter/vessels). Reduce dose and monitor anticoagulant status in patients with renal impairment.

ADVERSE REACTIONS: Bleeding, back pain, pain, N/V, headache, hypotension, HTN, bradycardia, dyspepsia, urinary retention, insomnia, anxiety, abdominal pain, fever.

INTERACTIONS: Increased risk of major bleeding events with heparin, warfarin, thrombolytics, or GPIs.

PREGNANCY: Category B, caution in nursing.

MECHANISM OF ACTION: Reversible direct thrombin inhibitor; inhibits thrombin by specifically binding both to the catalytic site and to anion-binding exosite of circulating and clot-bound thrombin.

PHARMACOKINETICS: Metabolism: Renal mechanisms and proteolytic cleavage. **Elimination:** $T_{1/2}$=25 min (plasma).

NURSING CONSIDERATIONS

Assessment: Assess for drug hypersensitivity, active major bleeding, renal impairment, with disease states associated with increased risk of bleeding, nursing status, and for possible drug interactions.

Monitoring: Monitor for signs/symptoms of hemorrhage (eg, decreases in BP or Hct), thrombus formation in gamma brachytherapy, and other adverse reactions. For patients with renal impairment, monitor anticoagulant status.

Patient Counseling: Advise to watch for any signs of bleeding/bruising and to report to their physician if these occur. Advise to inform their physician about the use of any other medications including over-the-counter medicines or herbal products prior to therapy.

Administration: IV route. Inspect visually for particulate matter and discoloration prior to administration. Refer to PI for Instructions for Administration. **Storage:** 20-25°C (68-77°F); excursion permitted to 15-30°C. Reconstituted: 2-8°C for ≤24 hrs. Diluted preparation is stable at room temperature for ≤24 hrs. Do not freeze. Discard any unused portion.

ANTARA RX
fenofibrate (Oscient)

THERAPEUTIC CLASS: Fibric acid derivative

INDICATIONS: Adjunct to diet, to reduce elevated LDL-C, Total-C, TG, Apo B, and to increase HDL-C in adult patients with primary hypercholesterolemia or mixed dyslipidemia (Fredrickson Types IIa and IIb). Adjunct to diet, for treatment of hypertriglyceridemia (Fredrickson Types IV and V hyperlipidemia) in adult patients.

DOSAGE: *Adults:* Hypercholesterolemia/Mixed Hyperlipidemia: Initial: 130mg qd. Hypertriglyceridemia: Initial: 43-130mg/day. Titrate: Adjust if needed after repeat lipid levels at 4-8 week intervals. Max: 130mg/day. Renal Dysfunction/Elderly: Initial: 43mg/day. Take without regard to meals.

HOW SUPPLIED: Cap: 43mg, 130mg

CONTRAINDICATIONS: Hepatic or severe renal dysfunction (including primary biliary cirrhosis), unexplained persistent hepatic function abnormality, preexisting gallbladder disease.

WARNINGS/PRECAUTIONS: Hepatocellular, chronic active, and cholestatic hepatitis and cirrhosis (rare) reported. Increases in serum transaminases reported; monitor LFTs regularly; d/c if >3X ULN. May cause cholelithiasis; d/c if gallstones found. May cause myositis, myopathy, or rhabdomyolysis; d/c if myopathy/myositis is suspected or diagnosed or if markedly elevated CPK levels occur. Acute hypersensitivity reactions (rare) and pancreatitis reported. Pulmonary embolus (PE) and deep vein thrombosis (DVT) were observed. Decreased Hgb, Hct, WBCs, thrombocytopenia, and agranulocytosis reported; monitor CBC during first 12 months of therapy. Minimize dose in severe renal impairment. Caution in elderly. Prior to therapy, attempt to control lipid levels with appropriate diet, exercise, and weight loss in obese patients and attempt to control any medical problems (eg, diabetes mellitus [DM]), hypothyroidism) that are contributing to lipid abnormalities. Measure lipid levels prior to therapy and during initial treatment; d/c use if inadequate response after 2 months on maximum recommended dose of 130mg/day.

ADVERSE REACTIONS: Abdominal pain, back pain, headache, abnormal LFTs, respiratory disorder, increased AST,ALT, and creatinine phosphokinase.

INTERACTIONS: Caution with anticoagulants because may potentiate coumarin anticoagulants; reduce anticoagulant dose to maintain desirable INR and PT. Avoid HMG-CoA reductase inhibitors unless benefits outweigh risks. Bile acid sequestrants may impede absorption; take at least 1 hr before or 4-6 hrs after bile acid binding resin. Evaluate benefits/risks with immunosuppressants (eg, cyclosporine) and other nephrotoxic agents. Prior to therapy, d/c or change if possible, medications known to exacerbate hypertriglyceridemia (eg, beta-blockers, thiazides, estrogens). Caution with drugs that are substrates of CYP2C19, CYP2A6, or CYP2C9.

PREGNANCY: Category C, not for use in nursing.

MECHANISM OF ACTION: Fibric acid derivative; activates peroxisome proliferator activated receptor α (PPARα), increasing lipolysis and elimination of triglyceride-rich particles from plasma by activating lipoprotein lipase and reducing production of apoprotein CIII. Decreased triglycerides produces an alteration in the size and composition of LDL particles. LDL particles then have a greater affinity for cholesterol receptors and are catabolized rapidly. Activation of PPARα also induces an increase in the synthesis of apoproteins AI, AII, and HDL cholesterol. Also reduces serum acid uric levels in hyperuricemic and normal individuals by increasing the urinary excretion of uric acid.

PHARMACOKINETICS: Absorption: Well absorbed; T_{max}=4-8 hrs. **Distribution:** Plasma protein binding (99%). **Metabolism:** Rapid, via hydrolysis by esterases to fenofibric acid (active metabolite), conjugation. **Elimination:** Urine (60%), feces (25%); $T_{1/2}$=23 hrs.

NURSING CONSIDERATIONS

Assessment: Assess for renal/hepatic function or primary biliary cirrhosis, preexisting gallbladder disease, pregnancy/nursing status, and for possible drug interactions. Prior to therapy, attempt to control serum lipids with appropriate diet, exercise, and weight loss in obese patients and attempt to control medical problems (eg, DM, hypothyroidism) that are contributing to lipid abnormalities. Measure lipid levels and LFTs prior to therapy.

Monitoring: Monitor for signs/symptoms of myositis, myopathy, and rhabdomyolysis; measure CPK levels if myopathy is suspected. Monitor for signs/symptoms of increases in serum transaminase levels, hepatocellular, chronic active and cholestatic hepatitis; perform periodic monitoring of LFTs. Monitor for signs/symptoms of venothromboembolic disease (eg, PE, DVT), pancreatitis, and for hypersensitivity reactions. Monitor for hematological changes (eg, thrombocytopenia, agranulocytosis); perform periodic monitoring of blood counts. Monitor for signs/symptoms of cholelithiasis; perform gallbladder studies if cholelithiasis is suspected. Perform periodic monitoring of lipid levels.

Patient Counseling: Inform about risks/benefits of therapy. Counsel need to be on a lipid-lowering diet while on therapy. Inform that may be taken without regard to meals. Instruct to promptly report to physician any signs of myopathy (eg, unexplained muscle pain, weakness, or tenderness) particularly if accompanied by malaise and fever. Inform to notify physician if pregnant or nursing.

Administration: Oral route. **Storage:** 25°C (77°F); excursions permitted to 15-30°C (59-86°F).

ANZEMET   RX
dolasetron mesylate (Sanofi-Aventis)

THERAPEUTIC CLASS: 5-HT$_3$ receptor antagonist

INDICATIONS: (Inj) Prevention and treatment of postoperative nausea and/or vomiting (PONV) in patients ≥2 yrs. (Tab) Prevention of N/V associated with moderately emetogenic cancer chemotherapy, including initial and repeat courses, and PONV in patients ≥2 yrs.

DOSAGE: *Adults:* (Inj) Prevention/Treatment of PONV: 12.5mg IV as a single dose 15 min before cessation of anesthesia (prevention) or as soon as N/V presents (treatment). (Tab) Prevention of Cancer Chemotherapy-Induced N/V: 100mg within 1 hr before chemotherapy. Prevention of PONV: 100mg within 2 hrs before surgery. Elderly: Start at lower end of dosing range. *Pediatrics:* 2-16 yrs: (Inj) Prevention/Treatment of PONV: 0.35mg/kg IV as a single dose 15 min before cessation of anesthesia or as soon as N/V presents. Max: 12.5mg. May mix inj sol into apple or apple-grape juice for PO dosing of 1.2mg/kg within 2 hrs before surgery. Max: 100mg. (Tab) Prevention of Cancer Chemotherapy-Induced N/V: 1.8mg/kg within 1 hr before chemotherapy. Max: 100mg. Prevention of PONV: 1.2mg/kg within 2 hrs before surgery. Max: 100mg. May mix inj sol into apple or apple-grape juice for PO dosing if 100mg tab is not appropriate.

HOW SUPPLIED: Inj: 20mg/mL [0.625mL, 5mL, 25mL]; Tab: 50mg, 100mg

CONTRAINDICATIONS: (Inj) Prevention of N/V associated with initial and repeat courses of emetogenic cancer chemotherapy due to dose dependent QT prolongation in adults and pediatrics.

WARNINGS/PRECAUTIONS: May prolong QT interval; avoid with congenital long QT syndrome, correct hypokalemia and hypomagnesemia before administration, and monitor ECG in patients with congestive heart failure (CHF), bradycardia, renal impairment, and in elderly. May cause PR and QRS interval prolongation, 2nd-and 3rd-degree atrioventricular (AV) block, cardiac arrest and serious ventricular arrhythmias; use with caution and monitor ECG in patients with underlying structural heart disease, preexisting conduction system abnormalities, sick sinus syndrome, atrial fibrillation with slow ventricular response, and myocardial ischemia, and avoid with or at risk for complete heart block, unless implanted pacemaker is present. Caution in elderly.

ADVERSE REACTIONS: Headache, dizziness, pain. (Inj) Drowsiness, urinary retention. (Tab) Tachycardia, pruritus, bradycardia, hypotension, fatigue, diarrhea, dyspepsia, fever.

INTERACTIONS: Caution with QT, PR (eg, verapamil), and QRS (eg, flecainide, quinidine) interval prolonging drugs, diuretics with potential for inducing electrolyte abnormalities, antiarrhythmics, cumulative high-dose anthracycline therapy, and drugs that cause hypokalemia or hypomagnesemia. (IV) Atenolol may decrease clearance. (PO) Cimetidine may increase levels. Rifampin may decrease levels.

PREGNANCY: Category B, caution in nursing.

MECHANISM OF ACTION: 5-HT$_3$ receptor antagonist; antiemetic and antinauseant.

PHARMACOKINETICS: Absorption: (Inj) T_{max}=0.6 hr (hydrodolasetron). (Tab) Well-absorbed. Absolute bioavailability (75%); T_{max}=1 hr (hydrodolasetron). **Distribution:** V_d=5.8L/kg (hydrodolasetron); plasma protein binding (69-77%) (hydrodolasetron). **Metabolism:** Complete. Reduction via carbonyl reductase to hydrodolasetron (major metabolite); CYP2D6 (hydroxylation of hydrodolasetron); CYP3A and flavin monooxygenase (N-oxidation of hydrodolasetron). **Elimination:** (Inj) Urine (53%, unchanged hydrodolasetron), feces; $T_{1/2}$=<10 min, 7.3 hrs (hydrodolasetron). (Tab) Urine (61%, unchanged hydrodolasetron), feces; $T_{1/2}$=8.1 hrs (hydrodolasetron). Refer to PI for pharmacokinetic values (hydrodolasetron) in special and targeted patient population.

NURSING CONSIDERATIONS

Assessment: Assess for presence or possibility of cardiac conduction interval prolongation, other conditions where treatment is contraindicated, pregnancy/nursing status, and possible drug interactions.

Monitoring: Monitor ECG in patients with CHF, bradycardia, renal impairment, and those at risk for cardiac conduction interval prolongation. Monitor for torsades de pointes, AV block, ventricular arrhythmias, and cardiac arrest. Monitor serum electrolytes (K^+, magnesium).

Patient Counseling: Inform that drug may cause serious cardiac problems, and to contact physician immediately if HR change is perceived, or lightheadedness or syncopal episode occurs. Instruct to not exceed the recommended dose.

Administration: IV/Oral route. (Inj) Infuse as rapidly as 30 sec, or dilute in a compatible IV sol to 50mL and infuse over ≤15 min. Do not mix with other drugs. Flush the infusion line before and after administration. **Storage:** (Inj) 20-25°C (68-77°F); excursions permitted to 15-30°C (59-86°F). Protect from light. After dilution with compatible IV fluids: Room temperature for 24 hrs or under refrigeration for 48 hrs. After dilution with apple or apple-grape juice: Room temperature ≤2 hrs before use. (Tab) 20-25°C (68-77°F). Protect from light.

APIDRA   RX
insulin glulisine, rdna (Sanofi-Aventis)

OTHER BRAND NAMES: Apidra Solostar (Sanofi-Aventis)

THERAPEUTIC CLASS: Insulin

INDICATIONS: To improve glycemic control in adults and children with diabetes mellitus.

DOSAGE: *Adults:* Individualize dose. Usual Requirement: 0.5-1 U/kg/day. SQ Inj: Give within 15 min ac or within 20 min after starting a meal; use with an intermediate or long-acting insulin. Continuous SQ Insulin Infusion (CSII) by External Pump: Based on total daily insulin dose of the previous regimen. IV Inj: Usual: 05-1 U/mL in infusion systems using polyvinyl chloride (PVC) bags. Hepatic/Renal Impairment: May require dose reduction. *Pediatrics:* ≥4 yrs: Individualize dose. Usual Requirement: 0.5-1 U/kg/day. SQ Inj: Give within 15 min ac or within 20 min after starting a meal; use with an intermediate or long-acting insulin. Continuous SQ Insulin Infusion (CSII) by External Pump: Based on total daily insulin dose of the previous regimen. IV Inj: Usual: 0.05-1 U/mL in infusion systems using PVC bags. Hepatic/Renal Impairment: May require dose reduction.

HOW SUPPLIED: Inj: 100 U/mL [10mL vial]; [3mL, cartridge, SoloStar prefilled pen]

CONTRAINDICATIONS: Episodes of hypoglycemia.

WARNINGS/PRECAUTIONS: Any change in insulin regimen should be made cautiously under medical supervision. Changing from one insulin product to another or changing the insulin strength may result in the need for a change in dosage. May require dose adjustments in patients who change physical activity level or meal plan. Illness, emotional disturbances, or other stresses may alter insulin requirements. Hypoglycemia may occur; caution in patients with hypoglycemia unawareness and patients predisposed to hypoglycemia (eg, pediatric population and patients who fast or have erratic food intake). Hypoglycemia may impair ability to concentrate and react. Severe, life-threatening, generalized allergy including anaphylaxis may occur. Hypokalemia may occur; caution in patients who may be at risk. May be administered IV under medical supervision with close monitoring of blood glucose and serum K^+. Frequent glucose monitoring required in patients with renal/hepatic impairment. Do not mix with insulin preparations other than NPH insulin for SQ inj, or with other insulins for IV or for use in a continuous infusion pump. Malfunction of the insulin pump or infusion set or insulin degradation can rapidly lead to hyperglycemia or ketosis; prompt identification and correction of the cause necessary. Interim SQ inj with the drug may be required if using SQ infusion pump. Train patients using continuous SQ insulin infusion pump to administer by inj; alternate insulin therapy should be available in case of pump failure. Caution in elderly.

ADVERSE REACTIONS: Allergic reactions, infusion-site reactions, lipodystrophy, rash, hypoglycemia, influenza, nasopharyngitis, upper respiratory tract infection, arthralgia, HTN, headache, peripheral edema.

INTERACTIONS: May require dose adjustment and close monitoring with drugs that may increase blood glucose-lowering effect and susceptibility to hypoglycemia (oral antidiabetic products, pramlintide, ACE inhibitors, disopyramide, fibrates, fluoxetine, MAOIs, propoxyphene, pentoxifylline, salicylates, somatostatin analog, sulfonamide antibiotics), drugs that may reduce blood-glucose-lowering effects (corticosteroids, danazol, niacin, diuretics, sympathomimetic agents [eg, epinephrine, albuterol, terbutaline], glucagon, isoniazid, phenothiazine derivatives, somatropin, thyroid hormones, estrogens, progestogens [eg, in oral contraceptives], protease inhibitors, atypical antipsychotics), or drugs that may increase or decrease glucose-lowering effects (β-blockers, clonidine, lithium salts, and alcohol). Pentamidine may cause hypoglycemia, sometimes followed by hyperglycemia. Hypoglycemic signs may be reduced or absent with antiadrenergic drugs (eg, β-blockers, clonidine, guanethidine, and reserpine). Caution with K^+ lowering drugs and drugs sensitive to serum K^+ levels.

PREGNANCY: Category C, caution in nursing.

MECHANISM OF ACTION: Insulin glulisine (rDNA origin); regulates glucose metabolism. Lowers blood glucose by stimulating peripheral glucose uptake by skeletal muscle and fat, and by inhibiting hepatic glucose production.

PHARMACOKINETICS: Absorption: (SQ) Absolute bioavailability (70%); C_{max}=83, 84 µU/mL (0.15, 0.2 U/kg); T_{max}=60, 100 min (0.15, 0.2 U/kg). **Distribution:** (IV) V_d=13L. **Elimination:** (SQ) $T_{1/2}$=42 min, (IV) $T_{1/2}$=13 min.

NURSING CONSIDERATIONS

Assessment: Assess for predisposal to hypoglycemia, risk of hypokalemia, exercise routines, alcohol consumption, hypersensitivity, renal/hepatic function, pregnancy/nursing status, and possible drug interactions. Obtain baseline blood glucose, and HbA1c levels.

Monitoring: Monitor for hypokalemia, lipodystrophy, allergic reactions, hypoglycemia, and other adverse reactions. Monitor blood glucose and HbA1c levels. Monitor glucose and K^+ levels frequently during IV administration.

Patient Counseling: Inform about potential risks and benefits of taking insulin and possible adverse reactions. Counsel on self-management procedures (eg, glucose monitoring, proper inj technique, management of hypoglycemia/hyperglycemia). Instruct on handling of special situations such as intercurrent conditions (eg, illness, stress, emotional disturbance), an inadequate or skipped insulin dose, inadvertent administration of an increased insulin dose, inadequate food intake, and skipped meals. Advise to inform physician if pregnant or are contemplating pregnancy. Instruct to always check the insulin label before each inj to avoid medication errors. Instruct or train on how to use external infusion pump.

Administration: SQ/ IV route. Inject SQ in the abdominal wall, thigh, upper arm. Rotate inj sites. Refer to PI for administration techniques. **Storage:** Unopened: 2-8°C (36-46°F). Open (In-Use): 25°C (77°F). Discard after 28 days. Protect from direct heat and light. Do not refrigerate opened (in-use) cartridge and SoloStar. Discard infusions sets and insulin in the reservoir after 48 hrs of use or after exposure to temperatures >37°C (98.6°F). Prepared Infusion Bags: Room temperature for 48 hrs.

APLENZIN   RX
bupropion hydrobromide (Sanofi-Aventis)

> Antidepressants increased the risk of suicidal thinking and behavior (suicidality) in short-term studies in children, adolescents, and young adults with major depressive disorder (MDD) and other psychiatric disorders. Bupropion is not approved for use in pediatric patients. Not approved for smoking cessation treatment, but bupropion under the name Zyban is approved for this use. Serious neuropsychiatric events, including depression, suicidal ideation, suicide attempt, and complete suicide reported in patients taking bupropion for smoking cessation. Monitor and observe closely for clinical worsening, suicidality, or unusual changes in behavior, and for neuropsychiatric symptoms (eg, behavioral changes, hostility, agitation, depressed mood, and suicide-related events). D/C if psychiatric symptoms observed.

THERAPEUTIC CLASS: Aminoketone

INDICATIONS: Treatment of MDD.

DOSAGE: *Adults:* Initial: 174mg qam. Titrate: If initial dose is tolerated, may increase to 348mg qd as early as day 4 of dosing. There should be an interval of ≥24 hrs between successive doses. Usual: 348mg qam. Max: 522mg/day as single dose if no clinical improvement after several weeks. Maint: Reassess periodically to determine the need for maintenance treatment and the appropriate dose. Switching from Wellbutrin, Wellbutrin SR, or Wellbutrin XL: Give equivalent total daily dose. 522mg bupropion HBr = 450mg bupropion HCl, 348mg bupropion HBr = 300mg bupropion HCl, 174mg bupropion HBr = 150mg bupropion HCl. Mild-Moderate Hepatic Cirrhosis/Renal Impairment: Reduce frequency and/or dose. Severe Hepatic Cirrhosis: Max: 174mg qod.

HOW SUPPLIED: Tab, Extended-Release: 174mg, 348mg, 522mg

CONTRAINDICATIONS: Seizure disorder, bulimia or anorexia nervosa, patients treated with other medications that contain bupropion, use of MAOIs or within 14 days of use, and patients undergoing abrupt d/c of alcohol or sedatives (including benzodiazepines).

WARNINGS/PRECAUTIONS: May precipitate manic episodes in bipolar disorder patients during the depressed phase and may activate latent psychosis in other susceptible patients. Screen for bipolar disorder; not approved for use in treating bipolar depression. Dose-related risk of seizures. D/C and do not restart if seizure occurs. Extreme caution with history of seizures, cranial trauma, or other predisposition(s) toward seizure, and severe hepatic cirrhosis. Caution with hepatic impairment (including mild to moderate hepatic cirrhosis). Potential for hepatotoxicity. Increased restlessness, agitation, anxiety, and insomnia reported after initiation of treatment. Neuropsychiatric signs and symptoms (eg, delusions, hallucinations, psychosis, concentration disturbance, paranoia, confusion) reported. Weight loss/gain reported. Anaphylactoid/anaphylactic reactions and delayed hypersensitivity resembling serum sickness reported. HTN reported; caution with recent history of myocardial infarction (MI) or unstable heart disease.

ADVERSE REACTIONS: Dry mouth, nausea, insomnia, dizziness, pharyngitis, abdominal pain, agitation, anxiety, palpitation, tremor, sweating, tinnitus, myalgia, rash.

INTERACTIONS: See Contraindications. Extreme caution with drugs that lower seizure threshold (eg, antidepressants, antipsychotics, theophylline, systemic steroids); use low initial dose and gradually titrate. Increased seizure risk with excessive alcohol or sedative use; opioids, cocaine, or stimulant addiction; use of OTC stimulants or anorectics, oral hypoglycemics, insulin. Caution with CYP2B6 substrates or inhibitors/inducers (eg, orphenadrine, thiotepa, cyclophosphamide, ticlopidine, clopidogrel). Paroxetine, sertraline, norfluoxetine, fluvoxamine, nelfinavir, ritonavir, and efavirenz inhibited hydroxylation in vitro. Cimetidine increased levels of some active metabolites. Decreased levels with ritonavir or ritonavir/lopinavir and efavirenz; may need to increase bupropion dose but do not exceed max dose. Carbamazepine, phenytoin, and phenobarbital may induce metabolism. Caution with levodopa and amantadine; use low initial doses and gradually titrate. Inhibits CYP2D6; caution with drugs that are metabolized by CYP2D6 (eg, antidepressants, antipsychotics, β-blockers, type 1C antiarrhythmics); use low initial dose of concomitant medication. May reduce efficacy of drugs that require metabolic activation by CYP2D6 to be effective (eg, tamoxifen). Increased citalopram level. Monitor for HTN with nicotine replacement therapy. Minimize or avoid alcohol consumption. Altered PT and/or INR with warfarin.

PREGNANCY: Category C, not for use in nursing.

MECHANISM OF ACTION: Aminoketone antidepressant; not established. Weak inhibitor of the neuronal uptake of norepinephrine and dopamine. Presumed that action is mediated by noradrenergic and/or dopaminergic mechanisms.

PHARMACOKINETICS: Absorption: (348mg) C_{max}=134.3ng/mL; AUC=1409ng•hr/mL; T_{max}=5 hrs, 6 hrs (hydroxybupropion). **Distribution:** Plasma protein binding (84%); found in breast milk. **Metabolism:** Extensive; via hydroxylation (CYP2B6) and reduction of carbonyl group; hydroxybupropion, threohydrobupropion, and erythrohydrobupropion (active metabolites). **Elimination:** Urine (87%), feces (10%), (0.5% unchanged). $T_{1/2}$= 21.3 hrs, 24.3 hrs (hydroxybupropion), 31.1 hrs (erythrohydrobupropion), 50.8 hrs (threohydrobupropion).

NURSING CONSIDERATIONS

Assessment: Assess for bipolar disorder, hepatic/renal function, and conditions where treatment is contraindicated or cautioned, pregnancy/nursing status, and for possible drug interactions.

Monitoring: Monitor for clinical worsening, suicidality, or unusual changes in behavior, seizures, increased restlessness, agitation, anxiety, insomnia, neuropsychiatric signs/symptoms, changes in weight or appetite, anaphylactoid/anaphylactic reactions, delayed hypersensitivity reactions, and HTN.

Patient Counseling: Advise patients and caregivers of need for close observation of clinical worsening and suicidal risks. Inform that Zyban contains the same active ingredient; do not use with Zyban or any other bupropion containing medications. Instruct to d/c and do not restart if experience a seizure while on therapy. Inform that excessive use or abrupt d/c of alcohol or sedatives may alter seizure threshold; advise to minimize or avoid alcohol use. Inform that the drug may impair the ability to perform tasks requiring judgment or motor/cognitive skills; use caution while operating hazardous machinery/driving. Report to physician all prescription or OTC medications being taken. Contact physician if become or intend to be pregnant during therapy. Inform that is is normal to notice something that looks like a tab in the stool.

Administration: Oral route. Swallow tab whole; do not chew, divide, or crush. **Storage:** 25°C (77°F); excursions permitted to 15-30°C (59-86°F).

APOKYN   RX
apomorphine HCl (Ipsen/Tercica)

THERAPEUTIC CLASS: Non-ergoline dopamine agonist

INDICATIONS: Acute, intermittent treatment of hypomobility, "off" episodes ("end-of-dose wearing off" and unpredictable "on/off" episodes) associated with advanced Parkinson's disease.

DOSAGE: *Adults:* Start trimethobenzamide (300mg tid PO) 3 days prior to the initial dose and continue at least during the first 2 months of therapy. Test Dose: 0.2mL (2mg) SQ to patients in an "off" state. Closely monitor BP; do not treat if clinically significant orthostatic hypotension occurs. Initial: 0.2mL (2mg) PRN if test dose is tolerated. Titrate: Increase in increments of 0.1mL (1mg) every few days, if needed, on an outpatient basis. 0.2mL (2mg) Test Dose Tolerated but no Response: Test Dose: 0.4mL (4mg) given at next "off" period (no sooner than 2 hrs after the first test dose). Initial: 0.3mL (3mg) PRN if 0.4mL (4mg) test dose is tolerated. Titrate: Increase in increments of 0.1mL (1mg) every few days, if needed, on an outpatient basis. 0.4mL (4mg) Test Dose not Tolerated: Test Dose: 0.3mL (3mg) during a separate "off" period (no sooner than 2 hrs after the prior test dose). Initial: 0.2mL (2mg) PRN if 0.3mL test dose is tolerated. Titrate: Increase to 0.3mL (3mg) after a few days, if needed; assess efficacy/tolerability; do not increase to 0.4mL on an outpatient basis. Do not give second dose for an "off" period if the first was ineffective. Usual: 0.3-0.6mL (3-6mg) tid. Max: 0.6mL (6mg)/dose. If therapy is interrupted (>1 week), restart at 0.2mL (2mg) and gradually titrate. Renal Impairment: Test Dose/Initial: 0.1mL (1mg) SQ.

HOW SUPPLIED: Inj: 10mg/mL [3mL]

CONTRAINDICATIONS: Concomitant use with $5HT_3$ antagonists (eg, ondansetron, granisetron, dolasetron, palonosetron, alosetron).

WARNINGS/PRECAUTIONS: Avoid IV administration; serious adverse events reported (eg, IV crystallization leading to thrombus formation and pulmonary embolism). N/V, syncope, orthostatic hypotension, falling, and inj-site reactions reported. May prolong the QT interval and potential for proarrhythmic effects; caution with hypokalemia, hypomagnesemia, bradycardia, or genetic predisposition (eg, congenital prolongation of the QT interval). Hallucinations/psychotic-like behavior reported; avoid with major psychotic disorder. Falling asleep during activities of daily living may occur; d/c if daytime sleepiness or episodes of falling asleep develop. May impair mental/physical abilities. Coronary events (eg, angina, myocardial infarction [MI], cardiac ar-rest, sudden death) reported; caution with known cardiovascular (CV)/cerebrovascular disease. Contains sodium metabisulfite; caution with sulfite sensitivity. Potential for abuse. May cause or worsen dyskinesias. Monitor for withdrawal-emergent hyperpyrexia and confusion, fibrotic com-plications (eg, retroperitoneal fibrosis, pulmonary infiltrates, pleural effusion/thickening, cardiac valvulopathy) and melanoma. May cause priapism. Caution with hepatic/renal impairment.

ADVERSE REACTIONS: Yawning, dyskinesia, N/V, somnolence, dizziness, rhinorrhea, hallucina-tions, edema, chest pain, increased sweating, flushing, pallor, postural hypotension, angina.

INTERACTIONS: See Contraindications. Antihypertensives and vasodilators may increase risk of hypotension, MI, serious pneumonia, falls, bone and joint injuries. Dopamine antagonists, such as neuroleptics (eg, phenothiazines, butyrophenones, thioxanthenes) and metoclopramide, may di-minish effectiveness. Caution with drugs that prolong QT/QTc interval. May increase drowsiness with sedating medications. Avoid with alcohol. May significantly reduce levodopa concentration threshold necessary for improved motor response.

PREGNANCY: Category C, not for use in nursing.

MECHANISM OF ACTION: Non-ergoline dopamine agonist; not established, suspected to stimu-late postsynaptic dopamine D_2-type receptors within the caudate-putamen in the brain.

PHARMACOKINETICS: Absorption: Rapid; T_{max}=10-60 min. **Distribution:** V_d=218L. **Metabolism:** Sulfation, N-demethylation, glucuronidation, and oxidation. **Elimination:** $T_{1/2}$=40 min.

NURSING CONSIDERATIONS

Assessment: Assess for hypersensitivity to the drug, sulfite sensitivity, asthma, risk for QT pro-longation, history of psychotic disorders, CV/cerebrovascular disease, dyskinesia, hepatic/renal dysfunction, pregnancy/nursing status, and possible drug interaction. Obtain baseline BP (supine and standing).

Monitoring: Monitor for N/V, syncope, QT/QTc interval prolongation and other proarrhyth-mic effects, hypotension, hallucinations/psychotic-like behavior, coronary/cerebral ischemia, dyskinesia (or exacerbation), hepatic/renal impairment, withdrawal-emergent hyperpyrexia and confusion, fibrotic complications, priapism, drug abuse, and other adverse reactions. Perform periodic skin exams to monitor for melanomas. Monitor BP closely.

Patient Counseling: Inform that medication is intended only for SQ and not IV use. Instruct to take as prescribed. Instruct to rotate the injection site and observe proper aseptic technique. Inform of the potential for hallucination, psychotic-like behavior, hypotension, sedating effects including somnolence, and the possibility of falling asleep. Caution against rising rapidly after sitting or lying down, especially if have been sitting or lying for prolonged periods, and during initiation of treatment. Advise not to drive a car or engage in any other potentially dangerous ac-tivities while on treatment. Advise to notify physician if become pregnant or intend to become pregnant or breastfeed. Advise to avoid alcohol. Advise to inform physician if new or increased gambling urges, increased sexual urges, or other intense urges develop while on treatment.

Administration: SQ route. Storage: 25°C (77°F); excursions permitted to 15-30°C (59-86°F).

APRISO   RX
mesalamine (Salix)

THERAPEUTIC CLASS: 5-Aminosalicylic acid derivative

INDICATIONS: Maint of remission of ulcerative colitis in patients ≥18 yrs.

DOSAGE: *Adults:* 1.5g (4 caps) PO qam.

HOW SUPPLIED: Cap, Extended Release: 0.375g

WARNINGS/PRECAUTIONS: Renal impairment, including minimal change nephropathy, acute and chronic interstitial nephritis, and, rarely, renal failure reported; caution with renal dysfunction or history of renal disease. Evaluate renal function prior to therapy and periodically thereafter. May cause acute intolerance syndrome (eg, acute abdominal pain, cramping, bloody diarrhea); d/c if such syndrome is suspected. Hepatic failure reported in patients with preexisting liver disease; caution with liver disease. Caution with sulfasalazine hypersensitivity and in elderly.

ADVERSE REACTIONS: Headache, diarrhea, upper abdominal pain, nausea, nasopharyngitis, influenza/influenza-like illness, sinusitis.

INTERACTIONS: Avoid with antacids.

PREGNANCY: Category B, caution in nursing.

MECHANISM OF ACTION: 5-aminosalicylic acid derivative; has not been established. Suspected to diminish inflammation by blocking production of arachidonic acid metabolites.

PHARMACOKINETICS: Absorption: (Single dose) T_{max}=4 hrs, C_{max}=2.1μg/mL, AUC_{0-24}=11μg•h/mL, AUC_{0-inf}=14 μg•h/mL. Refer to PI for parameters using multiple doses. **Distribution:** Plasma protein binding (43%); crosses placenta; found in breast milk. **Metabolism:** Liver and intestinal mucosa; N-acetyl-5-aminosalicylic acid (major metabolite). **Elimination:** Urine (2% unchanged; 30% N-acetyl-5-aminosalicylic acid); $T_{1/2}$=9 hrs.

NURSING CONSIDERATIONS

Assessment: Assess for hypersensitivity to sulfasalazine or salicylates, history or known renal/hepatic dysfunction, pregnancy/nursing status, and possible drug interactions. Evaluate renal function prior to initiation of therapy.

Monitoring: Monitor for renal impairment, hepatic failure, acute intolerance syndrome, and hypersensitivity reactions. Perform periodic monitoring of renal function and blood cell counts (in elderly).

Patient Counseling: Inform patients with phenylketonuria that each cap contains aspartame. Instruct not to take with antacids. Instruct to contact a healthcare provider if symptoms of ulcerative colitis worsen.

Administration: Oral route. **Storage:** 20-25°C (68-77°F); excursions permitted between 15-30°C (59-86°F).

APTIVUS   RX
tipranavir (Boehringer Ingelheim)

Both fatal and nonfatal intracranial hemorrhage reported. Clinical hepatitis and hepatic decompensation, including some fatalities, reported. Extra vigilance needed in patients with chronic hepatitis B or hepatitis C coinfection due to increased risk of hepatotoxicity.

THERAPEUTIC CLASS: Protease inhibitor

INDICATIONS: Coadministered with ritonavir for combination antiretroviral treatment of HIV-1 infected patients who are treatment-experienced and infected with HIV-1 strains resistant to >1 protease inhibitor.

DOSAGE: *Adults:* 500mg with 200mg ritonavir bid.
Pediatrics: 2-18 yrs: 14mg/kg with 6mg/kg ritonavir (or 375mg/m² with ritonavir 150mg/m²) bid. Max: 500mg with 200mg ritonavir bid. Intolerance or Toxicity: Decrease dose to 12mg/kg with 5mg/kg ritonavir (or 290mg/m² with ritonavir 115mg/m²) bid. May switch to PO sol if unable to swallow caps.

HOW SUPPLIED: Cap: 250mg; Sol: 100mg/mL [95mL]

CONTRAINDICATIONS: Moderate or severe (Child-Pugh Class B or C) hepatic impairment. Coadministration with drugs that are highly dependent on CYP3A for clearance or are potent CYP3A inducers (eg, amiodarone, bepridil, flecainide, propafenone, quinidine, rifampin, dihydroergotamine, ergonovine, ergotamine, methylergonovine, cisapride, St. John's wort, lovastatin, simvastatin, pimozide, oral midazolam, triazolam, alfuzosin, and sildenafil [for treatment of pulmonary arterial HTN]). Refer to individual monograph for ritonavir.

WARNINGS/PRECAUTIONS: Not recommended for treatment-naive patients. Caution with elevated transaminases, hepatitis B or C coinfection, with mild hepatic impairment (Child-Pugh Class A), with medications known to increase the risk of bleeding (eg, antiplatelet and anticoagulants) or with supplemental high doses of vitamin E, known sulfonamide allergy, patients at risk of increased bleeding from trauma, surgery, or other medical conditions, and in elderly. D/C if signs and symptoms of clinical hepatitis develop. D/C if asymptomatic elevations in AST or ALT >10X the ULN or if asymptomatic elevations in AST or ALT between 5-10X the ULN and increases in total bilirubin >2.5X the ULN occur. Monitor LFTs prior to and during therapy. New onset diabetes mellitus (DM), exacerbation of preexisting DM, hyperglycemia, and diabetic ketoacidosis reported. Increased bleeding in patients with hemophilia type A and B reported; additional factor VIII may be required. Rash (eg, urticarial/maculopapular, possible photosensitivity) accompanied by joint pain/stiffness, throat tightness, and generalized pruritus reported; d/c with severe skin rash. Increased total cholesterol and TG reported; assess lipid levels prior to and during therapy. Possible redistribution/accumulation of body fat. Immune reconstitution syndrome reported with combination therapy. (Sol) Avoid supplemental vitamin E greater than a standard multivitamin as sol contains 116 IU/mL of vitamin E, which is higher than the Reference Daily Intake (adults 30 IU, pediatrics approximately 10 IU). Refer to individual monograph for ritonavir.

ADVERSE REACTIONS: Clinical hepatitis, hepatic decompensation, intracranial hemorrhage, diarrhea, N/V, abdominal pain, pyrexia, fatigue, headache, cough, rash, anemia, weight loss, hypertriglyceridemia, bleeding.

INTERACTIONS: See Contraindications. Not recommended with other protease inhibitors, salmeterol, and fluticasone. Avoid with colchicine in renally/hepatically impaired. May increase levels of SSRIs (eg, fluoxetine, paroxetine, sertraline), atorvastatin, rosuvastatin, trazodone, desipramine, colchicine, bosentan, itraconazole, ketoconazole, clarithromycin, rifabutin, parenteral midazolam, normeperidine, and PDE-5 inhibitors. May decrease levels of abacavir, atazanavir, didanosine, zidovudine, amprenavir, lopinavir, saquinavir, raltegravir, valproic acid, methadone, meperidine, and omeprazole. Fluconazole, enfuvirtide, clarithromycin, atorvastatin, rosuvastatin, and atazanavir may increase levels. Buprenorphine/naloxone, carbamazepine, phenobarbital, and phenytoin may decrease levels. May alter levels of voriconazole, calcium channel blockers, and immunosuppressants. May decrease levels of ethinyl estradiol by 50%; use alternative methods of nonhormonal contraception. Monitor glucose with hypoglycemic agents. Monitor INR with warfarin. (Cap) May produce disulfiram-like reactions with disulfiram or other drugs which produce the reaction (eg, metronidazole). See Prescribing Information for detailed information.

PREGNANCY: Category C, not for use in nursing.

MECHANISM OF ACTION: Protease inhibitor; inhibits virus-specific processing of viral Gag and Gag-Pol polyproteins in HIV-1 infected cells, thus preventing formation of mature virions.

PHARMACOKINETICS: Absorption: Tipranavir/Ritonavir: (Female) C_{max}=94.8μM, T_{max}=2.9 hrs, AUC_{0-12h}=851μM•h; (Male) C_{max}=77.6μM, T_{max}=3.0 hrs, AUC_{0-12h}=710μM•h. **Distribution:** Plasma protein binding (>99.9%). **Metabolism:** Liver via CYP3A4. **Elimination:** Tipranavir/Ritonavir: Feces (82.3%, 79.9% unchanged), urine (4.4%, 0.5% unchanged); $T_{1/2}$=5.5 hrs (females), 6 hrs (males). Refer to Prescribing Information for pediatric parameters by age.

NURSING CONSIDERATIONS

Assessment: Assess for hepatitis B or C infection, hepatic impairment, increased bleeding risk, hemophilia, sulfonamide allergy, DM, pregnancy/nursing status, and possible drug interactions. Determine baseline LFTs and lipid levels. Assess the ability to swallow caps in pediatrics.

Monitoring: Monitor for signs and symptoms of clinical hepatitis, hepatic decompensation, severe skin reaction, DM, intracranial hemorrhage, bleeding, immune reconstitution syndrome, and fat redistribution. Monitor for LFTs and lipid levels periodically during treatment.

Patient Counseling: Inform that therapy is not cure for HIV-1, does not reduce risk of transmission of HIV-1, and that opportunistic infections may develop. Inform that redistribution/accumulation of body fat may occur. Instruct to notify physician if pregnant, planning to become pregnant, or if nursing. Advise to seek medical attention for symptoms of hepatitis (eg, fatigue, malaise, anorexia, nausea), bleeding, and severe skin reaction. Advise to inform physician about all medications, including prescription or nonprescription medications (eg, St. John's wort) before initiating therapy. Instruct to report any history of sulfonamide allergy. Instruct to avoid vitamin E supplements greater than a standard multivitamin when taking PO sol. Instruct to use additional or alternative contraceptive measures for patients taking estrogen-based hormonal contraceptives. Inform that drug must be taken with ritonavir.

Administration: Oral route. Take with meals with ritonavir tabs; take with/without meals with ritonavir caps/sol. **Storage:** Must be used within 60 days after 1st opening the bottle. (Cap) 2-8°C (36-46°F) prior to opening the bottle. After Opening the Bottle: 25°C (77°F); excursions permitted to 15-30°C (59-86°F). (Sol) 25°C (77°F); excursions permitted to 15-30°C (59-86°F). Do not refrigerate or freeze.

ARANESP
darbepoetin alfa (Amgen)

RX

Increased risk of death, myocardial infarction, stroke, venous thromboembolism, thrombosis of vascular access, and tumor progression or occurrence. Use the lowest dose sufficient to reduce the need for RBC transfusions. Chronic Kidney Disease (CKD): Greater risks for death, serious adverse cardiovascular (CV) reactions, and stroke when administered to target Hgb level >11g/dL. Cancer: Shortened overall survival and/or increased risk of tumor progression or recurrence in patients with breast, non-small cell lung, head and neck, lymphoid, and cervical cancers. Must enroll in and comply with the ESA APPRISE Oncology Program to prescribe and/or dispense. Use only for anemia from myelosuppressive chemotherapy. Not indicated for patients receiving myelosuppressive chemotherapy when anticipated outcome is cure. D/C following completion of chemotherapy course.

THERAPEUTIC CLASS: Erythropoiesis stimulator

INDICATIONS: Treatment of anemia due to CKD, including patients on/not on dialysis. Treatment of anemia in patients with non-myeloid malignancies where anemia is due to the effect of concomitant myelosuppressive chemotherapy, and upon initiation, there is a minimum of 2 additional months of planned chemotherapy.

DOSAGE: *Adults:* Initiate when Hgb is <10g/dL (see PI for additional parameters). CKD on Dialysis: Initial: 0.45mcg/kg IV/SQ weekly or 0.75mcg/kg IV/SQ q2 weeks. IV route recommended for hemodialysis patients. CKD not on Dialysis: Initial: 0.45mcg/kg IV/SQ q4 weeks. Titrate: Adjust dose based on Hgb levels; see PI. Conversion from Epoetin Alfa with CKD on Dialysis: See PI. Malignancy: Initial: 2.25mcg/kg SQ weekly or 500mcg SQ q3 weeks until completion of a chemotherapy course. Titrate: Adjust dose based on Hgb levels; see PI.
Pediatrics: >1 year: CKD on Dialysis: Conversion from Epoetin Alfa: See PI.

HOW SUPPLIED: Inj: Prefilled Syringe: 25mcg/0.42mL, 40mcg/0.4mL, 60mcg/0.3mL, 100mcg/0.5mL, 150mcg/0.3mL, 200mcg/0.4mL, 300mcg/0.6mL, 500mcg/mL; Single-dose Vials: 25mcg/mL, 40mcg/mL, 60mcg/mL, 100mcg/mL, 150mcg/0.75mL, 200mcg/mL, 300mcg/mL, 500mcg/mL

CONTRAINDICATIONS: Uncontrolled HTN, pure red cell aplasia (PRCA) that begins after treatment with darbepoetin alfa or other erythropoietin drugs.

WARNINGS/PRECAUTIONS: Not indicated in patients with cancer receiving hormonal agents, biologic products, or radiotherapy, unless also receiving myelosuppressive chemotherapy, and as substitute for RBC transfusions in patients requiring immediate correction of anemia. Correct/exclude other causes of anemia (eg, vitamin deficiency, metabolic/chronic inflammatory conditions, bleeding) prior to therapy. Increased risk of congestive heart failure, deep venous thrombosis undergoing orthopedic procedures, other thromboembolic events, and death in patients undergoing coronary artery bypass surgery. Not approved for reduction of RBC transfusions in patients scheduled for surgical procedures. Hypertensive encephalopathy and seizures reported with CKD. Reduce/withhold therapy if BP becomes difficult to control. PRCA and severe anemia (with or without other cytopenias), with neutralizing antibodies to erythropoietin reported. Withhold and evaluate for neutralizing antibodies to erythropoietin if severe anemia and low reticulocyte count occur; d/c permanently if PRCA develops. Serious allergic reactions may occur; immediately and permanently d/c if it occurs. May require adjustment in dialysis prescriptions and increased anticoagulation with heparin to prevent clotting of extracorporeal circuit during hemodialysis. May cause allergic reaction in latex-sensitive individuals (prefilled syringe).

ADVERSE REACTIONS: HTN, dyspnea, peripheral edema, cough, procedural hypotension, angina pectoris, vascular access complications, fluid overload, abdominal pain, rash/erythema, arteriovenous graft thrombosis, CV/thromboembolic reactions.

PREGNANCY: Category C, caution in nursing.

MECHANISM OF ACTION: Erythropoiesis stimulating protein; stimulates erythropoiesis by the same mechanism as endogenous erythropoietin.

PHARMACOKINETICS: Absorption: Adults with CKD: (SQ on/not on dialysis) Slow; T_{max}=48 hrs; (SQ on dialysis) Bioavailability (37%). Adults with Cancer: (SQ on dialysis) (6.75mcg/kg) T_{max}=71 hrs. **Elimination:** Adults with CKD: $T_{1/2}$=21 hrs (IV on dialysis), 46 hrs (SQ on dialysis), 70 hrs (SQ not on dialysis). Adults with Cancer: $T_{1/2}$=74 hrs (SQ).

NURSING CONSIDERATIONS

Assessment: Assess for uncontrolled HTN, previous hypersensitivity to the drug, latex allergy, causes of anemia, pregnancy/nursing status, and other conditions where treatment is cautioned/contraindicated. Obtain baseline iron status, Hgb levels, transferrin saturation, and serum ferritin.

Monitoring: Monitor for signs/symptoms of an allergic reaction, CV/thromboembolic events, stroke, premonitory neurologic symptoms, PRCA, severe anemia. Monitor Hgb (weekly until stable and then monthly for CKD), BP, iron status, transferrin saturation, and progression or recurrence of tumor in cancer patients. Monitor serum ferritin; supplemental iron is recommended if ferritin is <100mcg/L or serum transferrin saturation is <20%.

Patient Counseling: Inform risks/benefits of therapy, increased risks of mortality, serious CV events, thromboembolic events, stroke, tumor progression/recurrence, and for cancer patients to sign the patient-physician acknowledgment form prior to therapy. Advise of possible side effects of therapy. Instruct to undergo regular BP monitoring, adhere to prescribed antihypertensive regimen, and follow recommended dietary restrictions. Inform of the need to have regular lab tests for Hgb. Advise to contact physician for new-onset neurologic symptoms or change in seizure frequency.

Administration: IV/SQ route. In patients on hemodialysis IV route is recommended. Do not dilute and do not administer in conjunction with other solutions. **Storage:** 2-8°C (36-46°F). Do not freeze or shake. Protect from light.

ARAVA $\qquad$ RX
leflunomide (Sanofi-Aventis)

> Avoid pregnancy during treatment or before completion of drug elimination procedure after treatment. Severe liver injury, including fatal liver failure, reported; not for use with preexisting acute or chronic liver disease, or those with serum ALT >2X ULN before initiating treatment. Caution with other potentially hepatotoxic drugs. Monitor ALT levels at least monthly for 6 months after starting therapy, and thereafter q6-8 weeks. Interrupt therapy if ALT elevation >3X ULN; if leflunomide-induced, start cholestyramine washout and monitor liver tests weekly until normalized. If not leflunomide-induced liver injury, may consider resuming therapy.

THERAPEUTIC CLASS: Pyrimidine synthesis inhibitor

INDICATIONS: Treatment of active rheumatoid arthritis (RA) in adults to reduce signs/symptoms, inhibit structural damage as evidenced by x-ray erosions and joint space narrowing, or to improve physical function.

DOSAGE: *Adults:* LD: 100mg qd for 3 days. Maint: 20mg qd. If not well tolerated, reduce to 10mg qd. Max: 20mg qd.

HOW SUPPLIED: Tab: 10mg, 20mg, 100mg

CONTRAINDICATIONS: Women who are or may become pregnant.

WARNINGS/PRECAUTIONS: Avoid with severe immunodeficiency, bone marrow dysplasia, or severe, uncontrolled infections. May cause immunosuppression, increased susceptibility to infections especially *Pneumocystis jiroveci* pneumonia, tuberculosis (TB), and aspergillosis, or increase risk of malignancy. Rare cases of pancytopenia, agranulocytosis, and thrombocytopenia reported. D/C with evidence of bone marrow suppression. Monitor for hematologic toxicity if switching to another antirheumatic agent with a known potential for hematologic suppression. Serious toxicity (eg, hypersensitivity) and rare cases of Stevens-Johnson syndrome and toxic epidermal necrolysis reported; d/c therapy and drug elimination procedure is recommended if any of these occurs. Cases of peripheral neuropathy and interstitial lung disease reported. New onset or worsening of pulmonary symptoms (eg, cough, dyspnea), with or without associated fever, may be a reason for d/c; consider wash-out procedures if d/c is necessary. Screen for latent TB infection with a tuberculin skin test prior to initiating therapy. Caution in patients with renal impairment. Monitor BP before start of therapy and periodically thereafter. Has uricosuric effect; a separate effect of hypophosphaturia seen in some patients. The safety and effectiveness in pediatrics with polyarticular course juvenile RA have not been fully evaluated.

ADVERSE REACTIONS: Severe liver injury, ALT elevation, diarrhea, respiratory infection, alopecia, headache, nausea, rash, HTN, abnormal liver enzymes, dyspepsia, bronchitis, abdominal/back/GI pain.

INTERACTIONS: See Boxed Warning. Avoid with live vaccines. Decreased plasma levels of M1 (metabolite) with cholestyramine or activated charcoal. Increased levels with rifampin; use with caution. May increase levels of diclofenac, ibuprofen, or tolbutamide. May increase risk of hepatotoxicity with methotrexate or peripheral neuropathy with neurotoxic medications. Increased INR with warfarin (rare). Increased susceptibility to infections with concomitant immunosuppressant therapy.

PREGNANCY: Category X, not for use in nursing.

MECHANISM OF ACTION: Pyrimidine synthesis inhibitor; isoxazole immunomodulatory agent. Inhibits dihydroorotate dehydrogenase and has antiproliferative activity. Has demonstrated an anti-inflammatory effect.

PHARMACOKINETICS: Absorption: T_{max}=6-12 hrs (M1). Oral administration of various doses led to different parameters. **Distribution:** M1: V_d=0.13L/kg; plasma protein binding (>99.3%). **Metabolism:** A77 1726/M1 (primary active metabolite). **Elimination:** Urine (43%), feces (48%). (M1) $T_{1/2}$=2 weeks.

NURSING CONSIDERATIONS

Assessment: Assess for severe immunodeficiency, bone marrow dysplasia, severe uncontrolled infections, hepatic/renal function, comorbid illnesses, latent TB infection, drug hypersensitivity, pregnancy/nursing status, and possible drug interactions. Obtain baseline BP, platelet, WBC count, Hgb, Hct, and ALT levels.

Monitoring: Monitor for signs/symptoms of immunosuppression and opportunistic infections, sepsis, bone marrow suppression, pancytopenia, agranulocytosis, thrombocytopenia, severe liver injury, skin reactions, interstitial lung disease, malignancy, new onset or worsening of pulmonary symptoms, hypersensitivity, and other adverse effects. Monitor BP, platelets, WBC count, Hgb/Hct, and ALT levels monthly for 6 months and q6-8 weeks thereafter. Monitor for hematologic toxicity when switching to another antirheumatic agent with known potential for hematologic suppression. Monitor for bone marrow suppression monthly if used concomitantly with immunosuppressants.

Patient Counseling: Advise women of increased risks of birth defects if used during pregnancy, or if the patient becomes pregnant while the drug has not been completely eliminated from the body. Instruct women of childbearing potential to use reliable form of contraception while on therapy. Advise to notify physician if develop any type of skin rash or mucous membrane lesions, hepatotoxicity (eg, unusual tiredness, abdominal pain, or jaundice), and interstitial lung disease. Advise that lowering of blood counts may develop; instruct to have frequent monitoring and notify physician if symptoms of pancytopenia develop.

Administration: Oral route. **Storage**: 25°C (77°F); excursions permitted to 15-30°C (59-86°F). Protect from light.

ARCALYST   RX
rilonacept (Regeneron)

THERAPEUTIC CLASS: Interleukin-1 receptor antagonist

INDICATIONS: Treatment of cryopyrin-associated periodic syndromes (CAPS), including familial cold autoinflammatory syndrome (FCAS) and Muckle-Wells syndrome (MWS) in adults and children ≥12 yrs.

DOSAGE: *Adults:* ≥18 yrs: LD: 320mg (two 2mL SQ inj of 160mg each given on the same day at 2 different sites). Maint: 160mg/week (single 2mL SQ inj). Do not give more often than once weekly.
Pediatrics: 12-17 yrs: LD: 4.4mg/kg (given as 1 or 2 SQ inj with max single-inj volume of 2mL). Max LD: 320mg. If initial dose is given as 2 inj, give inj on the same day at 2 different sites. Maint: 2.2mg/kg/week. Max Maint Dose: 160mg (single SQ inj up to 2mL). Do not give more often than once weekly.

HOW SUPPLIED: Inj: 220mg

WARNINGS/PRECAUTIONS: May increase risk of infection; d/c if serious infection develops. Do not initiate with active or chronic infection. May increase risk of tuberculosis (TB) or other atypical/opportunistic infections; evaluate and treat possible latent TB infection before initiating therapy. May increase risk of malignancies. All recommended vaccinations (eg, pneumococcal and inactivated influenza vaccine) should be received by patients as appropriate before initiation of therapy. Monitor for changes in lipid profiles. Hypersensitivity reactions reported (rare); d/c and initiate appropriate therapy if occurs.

ADVERSE REACTIONS: Inj-site reactions, upper respiratory tract infection, sinusitis, cough, hypoesthesia, nausea, diarrhea, stomach discomfort, urinary tract infection, *Mycobacterium intracellulare* infection, GI bleeding, colitis, bronchitis, *Streptococcus pneumoniae* meningitis.

INTERACTIONS: Avoid live vaccines. Increased risk of serious infections and neutropenia with tumor necrosis factor (TNF) inhibitors; coadministration not recommended. Not recommended with other interleukin-1 (IL-1) blockers. Monitor effect or concentration of CYP450 substrates with narrow therapeutic index (eg, warfarin); adjust dose PRN.

PREGNANCY: Category C, caution in nursing.

MECHANISM OF ACTION: IL-1 blocker; acts as a soluble decoy receptor that binds IL-1β and prevents its interaction with cell surface receptors. Also binds IL-1α and IL-1 receptor antagonist with reduced affinity.

NURSING CONSIDERATIONS

Assessment: Assess for active or chronic infection, vaccination history, latent TB, pregnancy/nursing status, and possible drug interactions.

Monitoring: Monitor for development of serious infection, malignancies, and hypersensitivity reactions, reactivation of latent TB, and changes in lipid profile.

Patient Counseling: Instruct on aseptic reconstitution, inj technique, preparation, and disposal if to be administered by the patient or caregiver. Inform that inj-site reactions (eg, pain, erythema, swelling, pruritus, bruising, etc) may occur; instruct to notify physician if reaction persists. Advise to avoid injecting at already swollen/red area. Inform that serious/life-threatening infections may occur; instruct to notify physician if an infection develops. Instruct not to take with drugs that block TNF or other IL-1 blockers (eg, anakinra).

Administration: SQ route. Rotate inj sites (eg, abdomen, thigh, upper arm) and do not inject at sites that are bruised, red, tender, or hot. Use each vial for a single dose only. Refer to PI for preparation and administration. **Storage:** 2-8°C (36-46°F). Store inside original carton to protect from light. (Reconstituted Sol) Keep at room temperature and use within 3 hrs of reconstitution. Protect from light.

ARCAPTA NEOHALER   RX
indacaterol (Novartis)

> Long-acting β₂-adrenergic agonists (LABA) may increase the risk of asthma-related death. Not indicated for treatment of asthma.

THERAPEUTIC CLASS: Beta$_2$-agonist

INDICATIONS: Long-term, once-daily maintenance bronchodilator treatment of airflow obstruction in patients with chronic obstructive pulmonary disease (COPD), including chronic bronchitis and/or emphysema.

DOSAGE: *Adults:* 1 inhalation of the contents of 1 cap (75mcg) qd, with Neohaler device.

HOW SUPPLIED: Cap, Inhalation: 75mcg

CONTRAINDICATIONS: Asthma without use of a long-term asthma control medication. Not indicated for treatment of asthma.

WARNINGS/PRECAUTIONS: Not for acutely deteriorating COPD, or relief of acute symptoms (eg, as rescue therapy for treatment of acute episodes of bronchospasm). Cardiovascular (CV) effects and fatalities reported with excessive use; do not use excessively or with other LABA. D/C if paradoxical bronchospasm or CV effects occur. ECG changes reported. Caution with CV disorders (eg, coronary insufficiency, cardiac arrhythmias, HTN), convulsive disorders, thyrotoxicosis, and unusual responsiveness to sympathomimetic amines. Changes in blood glucose and serum potassium may occur.

ADVERSE REACTIONS: Cough, nasopharyngitis, headache, muscle spasm, musculoskeletal pain, edema peripheral, diabetes mellitus (DM), hyperglycemia, sinusitis, upper respiratory tract infection.

INTERACTIONS: Adrenergic drugs may potentiate effects; use with caution. Xanthine derivatives, steroids, or diuretics may potentiate any hypokalemic effect. Hypokalemia and/or ECG changes and/or hypokalemia that may result from non-K⁺ sparing diuretics (eg, loop/thiazide diuretics) can be acutely worsened; use with caution. MAOIs, TCAs, and drugs known to prolong QTc interval may potentiate effect on CV system; use with extreme caution. Drugs that are known to prolong the QTc interval may increase risk of ventricular arrhythmias. Use with β-blockers may block effects and produce severe bronchospasm in COPD patients; if needed, consider cardioselective β-blocker with caution. May result in overdose if used in conjunction with other medications containing LABA. Increased exposure with ketoconazole and increased plasma levels with verapamil, erythromycin, and ritonavir.

PREGNANCY: Category C, caution in nursing.

MECHANISM OF ACTION: Long-acting β$_2$-adrenergic agonist; stimulates intracellular adenyl cyclase, the enzyme that catalyzes the conversion of adenosine triphosphate (ATP) to cyclic 3', 5'-adenosine monophosphate (cyclic monophosphate). Increases cAMP levels causing relaxation of bronchial smooth muscles.

PHARMACOKINETICS: Absorption: Absolute bioavailability (43-45%); T_{max}=15 min. **Distribution:** (IV) V_{dl}=2, 361-2, 557L; plasma protein binding (95.1-96.2%). **Metabolism:** Hydroxylation, glucuronidation, N-dealkylation; CYP3A4, UGT1A1; hydroxylated indacaterol (most prominent metabolite). **Elimination:** Urine (<2%, unchanged), feces (54% unchanged, 23% metabolites); $T_{1/2}$= 45.5-126 hrs.

NURSING CONSIDERATIONS

Assessment: Assess for acute COPD deteriorations, asthma and use of control medication, acute symptoms, CV disorders, convulsive disorders, thyrotoxicosis, unusual responsiveness to sympathomimetic amines, DM, pregnancy/nursing status, and possible drug interactions. Obtain baseline serum K⁺ and blood glucose levels.

Monitoring: Monitor for lung function periodically. Monitor for worsening or acutely deteriorating asthma, CV effects, paradoxical bronchospasm, ECG changes (eg, flattening of the T-wave, QTc interval prolongation, and ST segment depression). Monitor for serum K^+ and glucose levels.

Patient Counseling: Inform the risk and benefits of therapy. Instruct the proper administration of capsules using the inhaler device and not to swallow caps. Caution that inhaler cannot be used more than once a day. Advise to d/c the regular use of SABA, and use them only for the symptomatic relief of acute symptoms. Instruct to notify physician immediately if worsening of symptoms, decreasing effectiveness of inhaled SABA, need for more inhalations than usual inhaled SABA, and significant decrease in lung function, occur. Instruct not to stop therapy without physician's guidance. Inform patients not to use other inhaled medications containing LABA. Inform about the associated adverse effects, such as palpitations, chest pain, rapid heart rate, tremor, or nervousness.

Administration: Oral inhalation route. Refer to PI for proper administration and use. **Storage:** 25°C (77°F); excursion permitted to 15-30°C (59-86°F). Protect from light and moisture.

AREDIA   RX
pamidronate disodium (Novartis)

THERAPEUTIC CLASS: Bisphosphonate

INDICATIONS: Treatment of moderate to severe hypercalcemia in malignancy, with or without bone metastases. Treatment of moderate to severe Paget's disease of the bone. Adjunct to standard antineoplastic therapy for the treatment of osteolytic bone metastases of breast cancer and osteolytic lesions of multiple myeloma.

DOSAGE: *Adults:* Moderate Hypercalcemia: 60-90mg IV single dose over 2-24 hrs. Severe Hypercalcemia: 90mg IV single dose over 2-24 hrs. Retreatment: 7 days should elapse first; retreat at the dose and manner of initial therapy. Paget's disease: 30mg IV qd over 4 hrs for 3 consecutive days. Retreatment: When indicated, retreat at the dose of initial therapy. Osteolytic Bone Lesions of Multiple Myeloma: 90mg IV over 4 hrs once a month. Osteolytic Bone Metastases of Breast Cancer: 90mg IV over 2 hrs every 3-4 weeks. Max: 90mg/single dose for all indications. Give po calcium and vitamin D supplementation to minimize hypocalcemia. Renal Dysfunction with Bone Metastases: Withhold dose if increase of 0.5mg/dL for normal baseline or 1mg/dL for abnormal baseline in SrCr. Resume when SrCr returns to within 10% of baseline. Elderly: Start at lower end of dosing range.

HOW SUPPLIED: Inj: 30mg, 90mg

WARNINGS/PRECAUTIONS: Associated with renal toxicity; assess SrCr prior to each treatment. Focal segmental glomerulosclerosis with or without nephrotic syndrome reported. Avoid use during pregnancy; may cause fetal harm. Asymptomatic cases of hypophosphatemia, hypokalemia, hypomagnesemia, and hypocalcemia reported. Rare cases of symptomatic hypocalcemia (including tetany) reported. Patients with history of thyroid surgery may have relative hypoparathyroidism that may increase the risk for hypocalcemia. Increased risk of renal adverse reactions with renal impairment; monitor renal function. Not recommended in patients with severe renal impairment for treatment of bone metastases. Osteonecrosis of the jaw reported in cancer patients; avoid invasive dental procedures if possible. Severe and occasionally incapacitating bone, joint/and or muscle pain reported. Monitor for 2 weeks post-treatment with preexisting anemia, leukopenia, or thrombocytopenia. Caution in elderly.

ADVERSE REACTIONS: Fever, infusion-site reaction, anorexia, constipation, dyspepsia, N/V, uremia, hypocalcemia, hypokalemia, hypomagnesemia, hypophosphatemia, osteonecrosis of the jaw, myalgia, HTN.

INTERACTIONS: Caution with other potential nephrotoxic drugs. Concurrent use with thalidomide increases risk of renal dysfunction in multiple myeloma.

PREGNANCY: Category D, caution in nursing.

MECHANISM OF ACTION: Bone resorption inhibitor; mechanism not established. Adsorbs to calcium phosphate crystals in bone and may directly block dissolution of this mineral component of bone. Inhibits osteoclast activity that contributes to inhibition of bone resorption.

PHARMACOKINETICS: Elimination: Urine (46%, unchanged); $T_{1/2}$=28 hrs.

NURSING CONSIDERATIONS

Assessment: Assess for hypersensitivity to other biphosphonates, renal impairment (eg, CrCl<30mL/min), history of thyroid surgery, pregnancy/nursing status, and for possible drug interactions. Assess SrCr prior to each treatment. Obtain dental exam with preventive dentistry prior to treatment.

Monitoring: Monitor for signs/symptoms of hypocalcemia, hypophosphatemia, hypokalemia, hypomagnesemia, renal toxicity, osteonecrosis of the jaw, and for musculoskeletal pain. Monitor serum calcium, electrolytes, phosphate, magnesium, and CBC, differential, and Hct/Hgb.

Patient Counseling: Inform of the risks/benefits of therapy.

Administration: IV route. Reconstitution: Add 10mL of Sterile Water for Injection to each vial resulting in a solution of 30mg/10mL or 90mg/10mL. Do not mix with calcium-containing solutions (eg, Ringer's solution); administer in single IV sol and line separate from all other drugs. Refer to PI for method of administration. **Storage:** Do not store >30°C (86°F). Reconstituted: 2-8°C (36-46°F) for ≤24 hrs.

ARGATROBAN   RX
argatroban (Various)

THERAPEUTIC CLASS: Direct thrombin inhibitor

INDICATIONS: Prophylaxis or treatment of thrombosis with heparin-induced thrombocytopenia (HIT). As an anticoagulant in patients with, or at risk for HIT undergoing percutaneous coronary intervention (PCI).

DOSAGE: *Adults:* HIT: Without Hepatic Impairment: Initial: 2mcg/kg/min continuous IV infusion. Check aPTT after 2 hrs. Titrate: Adjust dose until aPTT is 1.5-3X the initial baseline value (not to exceed 100 sec). Max: 10mcg/kg/min. Moderate Hepatic Impairment: Initial: 0.5mcg/kg/min; adjust PRN. PCI: Initial: 25mcg/kg/min and 350mcg/kg IV bolus over 3-5 min. Check activated clotting time (ACT) 5-10 min after bolus dose completed. Proceed with PCI if ACT >300 sec. Titrate: If ACT <300 sec, give additional 150mcg/kg IV bolus and increase infusion to 30mcg/kg/min; check ACT after 5-10 min. If ACT >450 sec, decrease infusion to 15mcg/kg/min; check ACT after 5-10 min. Continue infusion once therapeutic ACT (300-450 sec) achieved. May give additional 150mcg/kg bolus and increase infusion to 40mcg/kg/min in case of dissection, impending abrupt closure, thrombus formation, or inability to achieve/maintain ACT >300 sec. If anticoagulation required after PCI, continue at lower infusion dose (2mcg/kg/min); adjust PRN. Hepatic Impairment: Carefully titrate until desired anticoagulation level is achieved. Refer to PI for tabulated recommended doses and infusion rates in HIT/PCI without hepatic impairment and for instructions for conversion to PO anticoagulant therapy.
Pediatrics: HIT/Heparin-Induced Thrombocytopenia and Thrombosis Syndrome (HITTS): Without Hepatic Impairment: Initial: 0.75mcg/kg/min continuous IV infusion. Check aPTT after 2 hrs. Titrate: May adjust in increments of 0.1-0.25mcg/kg/min until aPTT is 1.5-3X the initial baseline value (not to exceed 100 sec). Hepatic Impairment: Initial: 0.2mcg/kg/min continuous IV infusion. Check aPTT after 2 hrs and adjust dose to achieve target aPTT. Titrate: May adjust in increments of ≤0.05mcg/kg/min until aPTT is 1.5-3X initial baseline (not to exceed 100 sec).

HOW SUPPLIED: Inj: 100mg/mL [2.5mL]; 1mg/mL [50mL, 125mL]

CONTRAINDICATIONS: Overt major bleeding.

WARNINGS/PRECAUTIONS: Hemorrhage may occur; use with extreme caution in conditions with increased danger of hemorrhage (eg, severe HTN, immediately after lumbar puncture, spinal anesthesia, major surgery, bleeding tendencies/disorder, GI lesions). Caution with hepatic impairment; full reversal of anticoagulation may require >4 hrs. Avoid use of high doses in PCI patients with significant hepatic disease or AST/ALT ≥3X ULN.

ADVERSE REACTIONS: Hemorrhage, Hct/Hgb decrease, dyspnea, hypotension, fever, diarrhea, sepsis, cardiac arrest, N/V, ventricular tachycardia, chest pain.

INTERACTIONS: D/C all parenteral anticoagulants before administration; allow sufficient time for heparin's effect on the aPTT to decrease prior to therapy. May result in prolonged PT/INR with warfarin. Antiplatelet agents, thrombolytics, and other anticoagulants may increase risk of bleeding.

PREGNANCY: Category B, not for use in nursing.

MECHANISM OF ACTION: Direct thrombin inhibitor; reversibly binds to thrombin active site. Exerts anticoagulant effects by inhibiting thrombin-catalyzed or thrombin-induced reactions, including fibrin formation; activation of coagulation factors V, VIII, XIII, protein C, and platelet aggregation. Capable of inhibiting both free and clot-associated thrombin.

PHARMACOKINETICS: Distribution: V_d=174mL/Kg; plasma protein binding (54%). **Metabolism:** Liver via hydroxylation and aromatization; CYP3A4/5; M1 (primary metabolite). **Elimination:** Feces (65%, 14% unchanged), urine (22%, 16% unchanged); $T_{1/2}$=39-51 min.

NURSING CONSIDERATIONS

Assessment: Assess for hypersensitivity to the drug, hepatic impairment, overt major bleeding, conditions at risk for a hemorrhagic event (eg, severe HTN, recent lumbar puncture, spinal anesthesia, major surgery, bleeding tendencies, GI lesions), pregnancy/nursing status, and for possible drug interactions. Obtain baseline aPTT and ACT.

Monitoring: Monitor for signs/symptoms of hemorrhagic events (eg, unexplained fall in Hct, decreased in BP) and other adverse reactions. Monitor aPTT 2 hrs after initiation of therapy. Monitor ACT 5-10 min after bolus dosing, after changes in infusion rate, and at the end of PCI procedure, and every 20-30 min during prolonged procedure. Monitor INR when combined with oral anticoagulant therapy.

Patient Counseling: Counsel about the risks and benefits of therapy. Inform of possible adverse reactions (eg, hemorrhage). Instruct to report to physician if pregnant or nursing, if using any products known to affect bleeding, if have a medical history that may increase the risk of bleeding (eg, severe HTN, major surgery), if any bleeding signs/symptoms occur, or if an allergic reaction occurs.

Administration: IV route. Refer to PI for further preparation and administration instructions. **Storage:** Vial: (1mg/mL) 20-25°C (68-77°F). (100mg/mL) 25°C (77°F); with excursions permitted to 15-30°C (59-86°F). Do not freeze. Retain in original carton to protect from light. Diluted Sol: 25°C (77°F) with excursions permitted to 15-30°C (59-86°F) in ambient indoor light stable for 24 hrs; or stable for up to 96 hrs when protected from light at 20-25°C (68-77°F) or at 5°C (41°F). Do not expose to direct sunlight.

ARICEPT   RX
donepezil HCl (Eisai)

THERAPEUTIC CLASS: Acetylcholinesterase inhibitor

INDICATIONS: Treatment of dementia of the Alzheimer's type.

DOSAGE: *Adults:* Take qhs. Mild to Moderate: Initial: 5mg qd. Titrate: May increase to 10mg qd after 4-6 weeks. Usual: 5-10mg qd. Moderate to Severe: Initial: 5mg qd. Titrate: May increase to 10mg qd after 4-6 weeks, then to 23mg qd after at least 3 months. Usual: 10-23mg qd.

HOW SUPPLIED: Tab: 5mg, 10mg, 23mg; Tab, Disintegrating: (ODT) 5mg, 10mg

WARNINGS/PRECAUTIONS: May exaggerate succinylcholine-type muscle relaxation during anesthesia. May have vagotonic effects on sinoatrial (SA) and atrioventricular (AV) nodes, manifesting as bradycardia or heart block. Syncopal episodes reported. May produce diarrhea, N/V; observe closely at initiation of treatment and after dose increases. May increase gastric acid secretion; monitor for active or occult GI bleeding. Caution with increased risk for developing ulcers (eg, history of ulcer disease). May cause weight loss, generalized convulsions, and bladder outflow obstruction. Caution with asthma or obstructive pulmonary disease.

ADVERSE REACTIONS: N/V, diarrhea, insomnia, muscle cramps, fatigue, anorexia, headache, dizziness, weight decrease, infection, HTN, back pain, abnormal dreams, ecchymosis.

INTERACTIONS: Monitor closely for GI bleeding with concurrent NSAID use. Ketoconazole and quinidine, inhibitors of CYP3A4 and CYP2D6, respectively, inhibit metabolism in vitro. Increased concentrations with ketoconazole. Decreased clearance with a known CYP2D6 inhibitor. CYP2D6 and CYP3A4 inducers (eg, phenytoin, carbamazepine, dexamethasone, rifampin, phenobarbital) may increase elimination rate. May interfere with activity of anticholinergic medications. Synergistic effect with neuromuscular blocking agents (eg, succinylcholine) and cholinergic agonists (eg, bethanechol).

PREGNANCY: Category C, caution in nursing.

MECHANISM OF ACTION: Acetylcholinesterase (AChE) inhibitor; may exert effect by increasing acetylcholine concentrations through reversible inhibition of its hydrolysis by AChE.

PHARMACOKINETICS: Absorption: T_{max}=3 hrs (10mg), 8 hrs (23mg). **Distribution:** V_d=12-16L/kg; plasma protein binding (96%). **Metabolism:** Hepatic via CYP2D6 and CYP3A4; glucuronidation. **Elimination:** Urine (57%, 17% unchanged), feces (15%); $T_{1/2}$=70 hrs.

NURSING CONSIDERATIONS

Assessment: Assess for drug hypersensitivity, underlying cardiac conduction abnormalities, risks for developing ulcers, asthma, obstructive pulmonary disease, possible drug interactions, and pregnancy/nursing status.

Monitoring: Monitor for vagotonic effects on SA and AV nodes (eg, bradycardia, heart block), syncopal episodes, diarrhea, N/V, active/occult GI bleeding, weight loss, bladder outflow obstruction, and generalized convulsions.

Patient Counseling: Take qhs without regard to meals. Swallow the 23mg tab whole; do not split, crush or chew. For ODT, dissolve on tongue and follow with water. Caution with NSAID use. Advise that N/V, diarrhea, insomnia, muscle cramps, fatigue, and decreased appetite may occur.

Administration: Oral route. **Storage:** 15-30°C (59-86°F).

ARIMIDEX   RX
anastrozole (AstraZeneca)

THERAPEUTIC CLASS: Nonsteroidal aromatase inhibitor

INDICATIONS: Adjuvant treatment of postmenopausal women with hormone receptor-positive early breast cancer. First-line treatment of postmenopausal women with hormone receptor-positive or hormone receptor-unknown locally advanced or metastatic breast cancer. Treatment of advanced breast cancer in postmenopausal women with disease progression following tamoxifen therapy.

DOSAGE: *Adults:* 1mg qd. Continue until tumor progression with advanced breast cancer.

HOW SUPPLIED: Tab: 1mg

CONTRAINDICATIONS: Pregnancy and premenopausal women.

WARNINGS/PRECAUTIONS: Increased incidence of ischemic cardiovascular (CV) events in patients with preexisting ischemic heart disease reported. May decrease bone mineral density (BMD). May elevate serum cholesterol.

ADVERSE REACTIONS: Hot flashes, asthenia, arthritis, pain, pharyngitis, HTN, depression, N/V, rash, osteoporosis, fractures, headache, bone pain, peripheral edema, dyspnea, pharyngitis.

INTERACTIONS: Avoid with tamoxifen; may decrease plasma levels with tamoxifen. Avoid with estrogen-containing therapies.

PREGNANCY: Category X, not for use in nursing.

MECHANISM OF ACTION: Nonsteroidal aromatase inhibitor; lowers estradiol concentrations and has no detectable effect on formation of adrenal corticosteroids or aldosterone.

PHARMACOKINETICS: Absorption: (Fasted state) Rapid, T_{max}=2 hrs. **Distribution:** Plasma protein binding (40%). **Metabolism:** Liver via N-dealkylation, hydroxylation, and glucuronidation. **Elimination**: Hepatic (85%), renal (10%); $T_{1/2}$=50 hrs.

NURSING CONSIDERATIONS

Assessment: Assess for hypersensitivity to drug, preexisting ischemic cardiac disease, pregnancy/nursing status, menopausal status, hepatic/renal function, and possible drug interactions. Obtain baseline BMD, serum cholesterol.

Monitoring: Monitor BMD, LFTs and cholesterol levels. Monitor for serious side effects and hypersensitivity reactions.

Patient Counseling: Instruct to notify physician if pregnant/nursing or intend to become pregnant. Instruct to report to physician if serious allergic reactions (angioedema) occur. Inform patients with preexisting ischemic heart disease that increased incidence of CV events has been observed. Inform that drug may lower the level of estrogen which may lead to a loss of the mineral content of bones, and might decrease the bone strength leading to increase risk of fractures. Inform that cholesterol levels may increase. Advise not to take drug with tamoxifen.

Administration: Oral route. **Storage:** 20-25°C (68-77°F).

ARIXTRA   RX
fondaparinux sodium (GlaxoSmithKline)

Epidural or spinal hematomas may occur in patients anticoagulated with low molecular weight heparins, heparinoids, or fondaparinux sodium, and who are receiving neuraxial anesthesia or undergoing spinal puncture. These hematomas may result in long-term or permanent paralysis. Increased risk of developing epidural or spinal hematomas in patients using indwelling epidural catheters, concomitant use of other drugs that affect hemostasis (eg, NSAIDs, platelet inhibitors, other anticoagulants), history of traumatic or repeated epidural or spinal puncture, or a history of spinal deformity or spinal surgery. Monitor frequently for signs/symptoms of neurologic impairment; if neurologic compromise noted, urgent treatment is necessary. Consider benefit and risks before neuraxial intervention in patients anticoagulated or to be anticoagulated for thromboprophylaxis.

THERAPEUTIC CLASS: Specific factor Xa inhibitor

INDICATIONS: Prophylaxis of deep vein thrombosis (DVT), which may lead to pulmonary embolism (PE), in patients undergoing hip fracture surgery, including extended prophylaxis, hip replacement surgery, knee replacement surgery, and abdominal surgery who are at risk of thromboembolic complications. Treatment of acute DVT when administered in conjunction with warfarin sodium. Treatment of acute PE when administered in conjunction with warfarin sodium when initial therapy is administered in the hospital.

DOSAGE: *Adults:* DVT Prophylaxis: 2.5mg SQ qd. Administer no earlier than 6-8 hrs post-op for 5-9 days. Hip Fracture Surgery Prophylaxis: Extended prophylaxis ≤24 additional days is recommended. DVT/PE Treatment: <50kg: 5mg SQ qd. 50-100kg: 7.5mg SQ qd. >100kg: 10mg SQ qd. Initiate concomitant treatment with warfarin sodium as soon as possible, usually within 72 hrs. Continue treatment for ≥5 days and until therapeutic oral anticoagulant effect is established (INR=2-3).

HOW SUPPLIED: Inj: 2.5mg/0.5mL, 5mg/0.4mL, 7.5mg/0.6mL, 10mg/0.8mL

CONTRAINDICATIONS: Severe renal impairment (CrCl <30mL/min), active major bleeding, bacterial endocarditis, thrombocytopenia associated with a positive in vitro test for anti-platelet antibody in the presence of fondaparinux sodium, body weight <50kg (for venous thromboembolism [VTE] prophylaxis only).

WARNINGS/PRECAUTIONS: Not for IM injection. Extreme caution in conditions with an increased risk of hemorrhage (eg, congenital or acquired bleeding disorders, active ulcerative and angiodysplastic GI disease, hemorrhagic stroke, uncontrolled arterial HTN, diabetic retinopathy, shortly after brain, spinal, or ophthalmological surgery). Isolated cases of elevated aPTT temporally associated with bleeding events have been reported. Do not administer earlier than 6-8 hrs after surgery; increases risk of major bleeding. Risk of bleeding increases with renal impairment; monitor renal function periodically and d/c if severe renal impairment develops. Do not use for VTE prophylaxis and treatment if CrCl <30mL/min. Caution with CrCl 30-50mL/min. Thrombocytopenia reported; monitor closely. D/C if platelet count falls <100,000/mm³. D/C if unexpected changes in coagulation parameters or major bleeding occurs during therapy. Packaging (needle guard) of the prefilled syringe may cause allergic reaction in latex-sensitive individuals. Caution with moderate hepatic impairment and in elderly.

ADVERSE REACTIONS: Spinal/epidural hematomas, thrombocytopenia, local irritation (inj-site bleeding, rash, pruritus), anemia, insomnia, increased wound drainage, hypokalemia, dizziness, purpura, hypotension, confusion.

INTERACTIONS: See Boxed Warning. Agents that may enhance the risk of hemorrhage should be d/c prior to initiation of therapy unless these agents are essential; if coadministration is necessary, monitor closely for hemorrhage.

PREGNANCY: Category B, caution in nursing.

MECHANISM OF ACTION: Specific factor Xa inhibitor; selectively binds to antithrombin III (ATIII) and potentiates the innate neutralization of Factor Xa by ATIII, thereby interrupting the blood coagulation cascade and inhibiting thrombin formation and thrombus development.

PHARMACOKINETICS: Absorption: Rapid, complete; absolute bioavailability (100%); C_{max}=0.39-0.50mg/L (2.5mg qd), 1.2-1.26mg/L (5mg, 7.5mg, 10mg qd); T_{max}=3 hrs (2.5mg qd). **Distribution:** V_d=7-11L; bound to ATIII (≥94%). **Elimination:** Urine (≤77%, unchanged); $T_{1/2}$=17-21 hrs.

NURSING CONSIDERATIONS

Assessment: Assess for conditions that increase the risk of hemorrhage or any other conditions where treatment is cautioned or contraindicated, hepatic function, latex sensitivity, PE, DVT, pregnancy/nursing status, and for possible drug interactions. Obtain weight and baseline CrCl, aPTT, PT, CBC, SrCr, and stool occult blood test.

Monitoring: Monitor for signs/symptoms of bleeding, thrombocytopenia and other adverse reactions. In patients undergoing neuraxial anesthesia or spinal puncture, monitor for epidural or spinal hematomas and neurologic impairment. Periodically monitor CBC (including platelet count), SrCr, stool occult blood tests, aPTT, CrCl and PT.

Patient Counseling: Instruct on proper administration technique. Counsel on signs and symptoms of possible bleeding. Inform that it may take longer than usual to stop bleeding and may bruise and/or bleed more easily while on therapy. Instruct to report any unusual bleeding, bruising, or signs of thrombocytopenia (eg, rash of dark red spots under the skin). Notify physician or dentist of all prescription and non-prescription medications currently taking. Advise patient that the use of aspirin and other NSAIDs may enhance the risk of hemorrhage. Instruct to watch for signs and symptoms of spinal or epidural hematomas such as tingling, numbness and muscular weakness; contact physician immediately if symptoms occur.

Administration: SQ route. Do not inject IM. Do not mix with other medications or solutions. Do not expel air bubble from syringe before the injection. Administer in fatty tissue, alternating injection sites. Refer to PI for further instructions on administration and preparation. **Storage:** 25°C (77°F); excursions permitted to 15-30°C (59-86°F).

ARMOUR THYROID RX
thyroid (Forest)

THERAPEUTIC CLASS: Thyroid replacement hormone

INDICATIONS: Treatment of hypothyroidism. As a pituitary TSH suppressant in the treatment or prevention of various types of euthyroid goiters. Diagnostic agent in suppression tests to differentiate suspected mild hyperthyroidism or thyroid gland autonomy. Management of thyroid cancer.

DOSAGE: *Adults:* Hypothyroidism: Initial: 30mg qd. Titrate: Increase by 15mg q2-3 weeks. Myxedema with Cardiovascular (CV) Disorder: 15mg qd. Maint: 60-120mg/day. Thyroid Cancer: Higher doses than replacement therapy are required. Myxedema Coma: 400mcg IV levothyroxine sodium (100mcg/mL rapidly) followed by 100-200mcg/day IV. Switch to PO when stable. Thyroid Suppression: 1.56mg/kg/day for 7-10 days. Elderly: Initial: Use lower dose (eg, 15-30mg qd).

Pediatrics: Hypothyroidism: >12 yrs: 1.2-1.8mg/kg/day. 6-12 yrs: 2.4-3mg/kg/day. 1-5 yrs: 3-3.6mg/kg/day. 6-12 months: 3.6-4.8mg/kg/day. 0-6 months: 4.8-6mg/kg/day.

HOW SUPPLIED: Tab: 15mg, 30mg, 60mg, 90mg, 120mg, 180mg*, 240mg, 300mg* *scored

CONTRAINDICATIONS: Untreated thyrotoxicosis; uncorrected adrenal cortical insufficiency.

WARNINGS/PRECAUTIONS: Do not use in the treatment of obesity; larger doses in euthyroid patients can cause serious or even life-threatening toxicity. Caution with cardiovascular disease, DM, diabetes insipidus, elderly, and adrenal cortical insufficiency.

INTERACTIONS: May increase insulin or oral hypoglycemic requirements. Reduced absorption with cholestyramine and colestipol; space dosing by 4-5 hrs. Altered effect of oral anticoagulants; monitor PT/INR. Estrogens increase thyroxine-binding globulin; increase in thyroid dose may be needed. Serious or life-threatening side effects can occur with sympathomimetic amines. Androgens, corticosteroids, estrogens, iodine-containing preparations, and salicylates may interfere with thyroid lab tests.

PREGNANCY: Category A, caution in nursing.

MECHANISM OF ACTION: Thyroid hormone; not established, suspected to enhance oxygen consumption by most body tissues, increase the basal metabolic rate and metabolism of carbohydrates, lipids, and proteins.

PHARMACOKINETICS: Abosrption: (T3) Completely absorbed; T_{max}=4 hrs; (T4) partially absorbed. **Distribution:** Plasma protein binding (>99%), found in breast milk. **Metabolism:** Deiodination in liver, kidneys, other tissues.

NURSING CONSIDERATIONS

Assessment: Assess for diagnosed but uncorrected adrenal cortical insufficiency, untreated thyrotoxicosis, hypersensitivity to any of its active or extraneous constituents, CV system, angina, DM, myxedema coma, and possible drug and test interactions.

Monitoring: Monitor urinary glucose levels in patients with DM, PT in patients receiving anticoagulants, and periodic assessment of thyroid status (TSH suppression test, serum T4 levels, free T4; if TSH is normal, total T4 is low), free T3, T4 signs/symptoms of thyroid hormone toxicity (chest pain, increased pulse rate, palpitations, excessive sweating, heat intolerance, and nervousness), partial hair loss in children.

Patient Counseling: Inform that replacement therapy is to be taken essentially for life, with the exception of cases of transient hypothyroidism, which associated with thyroiditis, and those patients receiving a therapeutical trial of the drug. Report immediately any signs/symptoms of thyroid toxicity.

Administration: Oral route. **Storage:** Store at 15-30°C (59-86°F).

AROMASIN   RX
exemestane (Pharmacia & Upjohn)

THERAPEUTIC CLASS: Aromatase inactivator

INDICATIONS: Adjuvant treatment of postmenopausal women with estrogen-receptor positive early breast cancer who have received 2-3 yrs of tamoxifen and are switched to exemestane for completion of a total of 5 consecutive yrs of adjuvant hormonal therapy. Treatment of advanced breast cancer in postmenopausal women whose disease has progressed following tamoxifen therapy.

DOSAGE: *Adults:* Early/Advanced: 25mg qd after a meal. Concomitant Potent CYP3A4 Inducer (eg, rifampicin, phenytoin): 50mg qd after a meal.

HOW SUPPLIED: Tab: 25mg

CONTRAINDICATIONS: Women who are or may become pregnant, premenopausal women.

WARNINGS/PRECAUTIONS: Lymphocytopenia (CTC grade 3 or 4) reported with advanced breast cancer; most had a preexisting lower grade lymphopenia. Elevations of serum levels of AST, ALT, alkaline phosphatase, and gamma glutamyl transferase >5X ULN (eg, ≥CTC grade 3) have been rarely reported with advanced breast cancer, but appear mostly attributable to the underlying presence of liver and/or bone metastases. Elevations in alkaline phosphatase, bilirubin, and creatinine reported with early breast cancer. Reductions in bone mineral density (BMD) over time reported. The safety of chronic dosing with moderate or severe hepatic or renal impairment has not been studied.

ADVERSE REACTIONS: Hot flashes/flushes, arthralgia, fatigue, N/V, increased sweating, HTN, alopecia, insomnia, headache, pain, depression, anxiety, dyspnea.

INTERACTIONS: Avoid coadministration with estrogen-containing agents. Potent CYP3A4 inducers (eg, rifampicin, phenytoin, carbamazepine, phenobarbital, St. John's wort) may decrease plasma levels.

PREGNANCY: Category X, not for use in nursing.

MECHANISM OF ACTION: Irreversible steroidal aromatase inactivator; acts as false substrate for aromatase enzyme; processed to an intermediate that binds irreversibly to the active site of the enzyme, causing inactivation.

PHARMACOKINETICS: Absorption: Rapid. (Breast cancer) T_{max}=1.2 hrs; AUC=75.4ng•hr/mL. **Distribution:** Plasma protein binding (90%). **Metabolism:** Oxidation and reduction; CYP3A4, aldoketoreductases. **Elimination:** Urine (42%, <1% unchanged), feces (42%); $T_{1/2}$=24 hrs.

NURSING CONSIDERATIONS

Assessment: Assess for preexisting lower grade lymphopenia, liver and/or bone metastases, hypersensitivity, pregnancy/nursing status, and for possible drug interactions.

Monitoring: Monitor for adverse reactions, hematological abnormalities, LFTs, BMD, creatinine and bilirubin levels.

Patient Counseling: Advise that drug is not for use in premenopausal women. Inform not to take concomitant estrogen-containing agents. Counsel that drug lowers estrogen level in the body which may lead to reduction in BMD over time and may increase risk of osteoporosis and fracture.

Administration: Oral route. **Storage:** 25°C (77°F); excursions permitted to 15-30°C (59-86°F).

ARTHROTEC   RX
diclofenac sodium - misoprostol (G.D. Searle)

> Misoprostol can cause abortion, premature birth or birth defects. Uterine rupture reported when used to induce labor or abortion beyond 8th week of pregnancy. Has an abortifacient property and must not be given to others. Should not be taken by pregnant women. Use only in women of childbearing potential if at high risk for gastric or duodenal ulcers or complications with NSAID therapy; must have had a negative serum pregnancy test within 2 weeks before therapy, capable of complying with effective contraceptive measures, has received both oral and written warnings of the hazards of misoprostol, risk of contraceptive failure, the danger to other women of childbearing potential should the drug be taken by mistake, and to begin therapy on 2nd or 3rd day of menstrual period. NSAIDs may increase risk of serious cardiovascular (CV) thrombotic events, myocardial infarction (MI), stroke, and serious GI adverse events including bleeding, ulceration, and perforation of the stomach or intestines. Increased risk of serious GI events in elderly. Contraindicated for the treatment of perioperative pain in the setting of coronary artery bypass graft (CABG) surgery.

THERAPEUTIC CLASS: NSAID/prostaglandin E_1 analogue

INDICATIONS: Treatment of the signs and symptoms of osteoarthritis (OA) or rheumatoid arthritis (RA) in patients at high risk of developing NSAID-induced gastric and duodenal ulcers and their complications.

DOSAGE: *Adults:* OA: 50mg-200mcg tid. RA: 50mg-200mcg tid or qid. OA/RA: If intolerable, may give 50mg-200mcg or 75mg-200mcg bid. May adjust dose and frequency according to individual needs after observing response to initial therapy. Refer to PI for special dosing considerations.

HOW SUPPLIED: Tab: (Diclofenac-Misoprostol) 50mg-200mcg, 75mg-200mcg

CONTRAINDICATIONS: Pregnant women, aspirin (ASA) or other NSAID allergy that precipitates asthma, urticaria, or allergic-type reactions. Treatment of perioperative pain in the setting of CABG.

WARNINGS/PRECAUTIONS: Use lowest effective dose for the shortest duration possible. Not a substitute for corticosteroids or treatment of corticosteroid insufficiency. May lead to onset of new HTN or worsening of preexisting HTN; monitor BP. Fluid retention and edema reported; caution with fluid retention or heart failure (HF). Extreme caution with a prior history of ulcer disease, and/or GI bleeding. May increase risk of GI bleeding with smoking, older age, debilitation, and poor general health status. D/C if a serious GI event occurs. Renal papillary necrosis and other renal injury reported after long-term use. Renal toxicity reported in patients in whom renal prostaglandins have a compensatory role in the maintenance of renal perfusion; caution with impaired renal function, HF, or liver dysfunction. Not recommended for use with advanced renal disease. May cause hepatotoxicity and elevation of transaminases; monitor transaminases periodically. D/C immediately if abnormal liver tests persist or worsen, if clinical signs and/or symptoms consistent with liver disease develop, or if systemic manifestations occur. Anaphylactic reactions may occur; avoid in patients with ASA-triad. May cause serious skin adverse events (eg, exfoliative dermatitis, Stevens-Johnson syndrome [SJS], toxic epidermal necrolysis); d/c if skin rash or hypersensitivity occurs. Anemia may occur; monitor Hgb/Hct if signs/symptoms of anemia develop. May inhibit platelet aggregation and prolong bleeding time; monitor with coagulation disorders. Caution with preexisting asthma. Aseptic meningitis with fever and coma reported. Avoid with hepatic porphyria. Caution in elderly and debilitated patients.

ADVERSE REACTIONS: Abdominal pain, diarrhea, dyspepsia, nausea, flatulence.

INTERACTIONS: Not recommended with magnesium-containing antacids. Diclofenac Sodium: Increased adverse effects with ASA; avoid with ASA. May diminish the antihypertensive effect of ACE inhibitors and increase the risk of renal toxicity. May increase the risk of renal toxicity with diuretics; may reduce the natriuretic effect of furosemide and thiazides. Increased serum potassium with K⁺-sparing diuretics. Loop diuretics and thiazides may have impaired response when given concomitantly with NSAIDs. Synergistic GI bleeding effects when used concomitantly with warfarin. May increase risk of serious GI bleeding when used concomitantly with oral corticosteroids, anticoagulants, or alcohol. May alter response to insulin or oral hypoglycemics. Monitor for digoxin, methotrexate, cyclosporine, phenobarbital, and lithium toxicities. Caution with drugs that are known to be potentially hepatotoxic (eg, antibiotics, anti-epileptics). Voriconazole may increase levels. May minimally interfere with protein binding of prednisolone. Antacids may delay absorption. Misoprostol: Antacids reduce the bioavailability. Magnesium-containing antacids exacerbate misoprostol-associated diarrhea.

PREGNANCY: Category X, caution in nursing.

MECHANISM OF ACTION: Diclofenac: NSAID; not established. May be related to prostaglandin synthetase inhibition. Possesses anti-inflammatory, analgesic, and antipyretic properties. Misoprostol: Synthetic prostaglandin E_1 analogue; has both antisecretory and mucosal protective properties. Inhibits basal and nocturnal gastric acid secretion and acid secretion in response to stimuli (eg, meals, histamine, pentagastrin, coffee).

PHARMACOKINETICS: Absorption: Oral administration of a single dose or multiple doses is similar to pharmacokinetics of two individual components. Refer to PI for further information. **Distribution:** Found in breast milk. Diclofenac: V_d=550mL/kg; plasma protein binding (>99%). Misoprostol: Plasma protein binding (<90%). **Metabolism:** Diclofenac: Glucuronide and sulfate conjugation via CYP2C8, 2C9, 3A4; 4'-hydroxy diclofenac (major metabolite). Misoprostol: Rapid; misoprostol acid (active metabolite). **Elimination:** Diclofenac: Urine (65%), bile (35%); $T_{1/2}$=2 hrs. Misoprostol: Urine (70%); $T_{1/2}$=30 min.

NURSING CONSIDERATIONS

Assessment: Assess for history of hypersensitivity to ASA or other NSAIDs, presence of or risk factors for CV disease, HTN, HF, fluid retention, history of ulcer disease or GI bleeding, and any other conditions where treatment is contraindicated or cautioned. Assess renal/hepatic function, pregnancy/nursing status, and possible drug interactions. Assess use of effective contraceptive measures. Obtain baseline BP and perform pregnancy test 2 weeks prior to therapy,

Monitoring: Monitor for CV thrombotic events, new onset or worsening HTN, fluid retention, GI bleeding, perforation or ulceration, HF, allergic, anaphylactic or skin reactions, renal papillary necrosis or other renal injury/toxicity, hepatotoxicity, systemic manifestations, anemia, prolonged bleeding time, bronchospasm, aseptic meningitis, and porphyria. Monitor BP and renal function. Monitor Hgb/Hct if anemia is suspected. Monitor transaminases within 4-8 weeks after initiating therapy. Periodically monitor CBC and chemistry profile for long-term use. Monitor use of effective contraception.

Patient Counseling: Advise of pregnancy risks; inform women of childbearing potential that they must not be pregnant when therapy is initiated and must use an effective contraception during treatment. Inform that therapy should not be taken by nursing mothers. Instruct not to give medication to other individuals. Instruct to contact physician if signs/symptoms of CV effects (eg, chest pain, SOB, weakness, slurring of speech), GI effects (eg, epigastric pain, dyspepsia, melena, hematemesis), or unexplained weight gain and edema occur. Instruct to contact physician and d/c if signs of skin reactions (eg, rash, blisters, fever, itching) or hepatotoxicity (eg, nausea, fatigue, jaundice) occur. Instruct to seek immediate medical attention if an anaphylactic reaction occurs (eg, breathing difficulty, facial or throat swelling). Instruct to take with meals and avoid the use of magnesium containing antacids. Instruct to swallow tab whole; do not chew, crush, or dissolve.

Administration: Oral route. **Storage:** ≤25°C (77°F), in a dry area.

ARZERRA   RX
ofatumumab (GlaxoSmithKline)

THERAPEUTIC CLASS: Monoclonal antibody/CD20-blocker

INDICATIONS: Treatment of patients with chronic lymphocytic leukemia (CLL) refractory to fludarabine and alemtuzumab.

DOSAGE: *Adults:* 300mg (Dose 1), followed 1 week later by 2,000mg weekly for 7 doses (Doses 2 through 8), followed 4 weeks later by 2,000mg q4 weeks for 4 doses (Doses 9 through 12). Refer to PI for detailed information on infusion rates, dose modifications, and premedication.

HOW SUPPLIED: Inj: 20mg/mL [5mL, 50mL]

WARNINGS/PRECAUTIONS: Do not administer as IV push/bolus. May cause serious infusion reactions; interrupt infusion if reaction develops and institute medical management for severe reactions (eg, angina, myocardial ischemia/infarction, bronchospasm). Not approved with moderate to severe chronic obstructive pulmonary disease (COPD); bronchospasm may develop. Prolonged (≥1 week) severe neutropenia and thrombocytopenia may occur; monitor CBC and platelet counts at regular intervals during therapy and at increased frequency in patients who developed grade 3 or 4 cytopenias. Progressive multifocal leukoencephalopathy (PML) may occur; d/c if PML is suspected and initiate evaluation for PML. Fulminant and fatal hepatitis B virus (HBV) infection and reactivation may occur; screen patients at high risk of HBV infection prior to initiation of therapy. Closely monitor carriers of HBV for clinical and laboratory signs of active HBV infection during treatment and for 6-12 months following last infusion. D/C if viral hepatitis or reactivation of viral hepatitis develops. Obstruction of small intestine may occur; perform diagnostic evaluation if suspected. Do not administer live viral vaccines to patients who have recently received ofatumumab.

ADVERSE REACTIONS: Neutropenia, infusion reactions, pneumonia, pyrexia, cough, diarrhea, bronchitis, dyspnea, infections, anemia, rash, fatigue, back pain, nausea, chills.

PREGNANCY: Category C, caution in nursing.

MECHANISM OF ACTION: IgG1 kappa human monoclonal antibody; binds specifically to extracellular loops of CD20 molecule expressed on normal B lymphocytes and on B-cell CLL. The Fab domain of ofatumumab binds to the CD20 molecule and the Fc domain mediates immune effector functions to result in B-cell lysis in vitro.

PHARMACOKINETICS: Distribution: V_d= 1.7-5.1L. **Elimination**: $T_{1/2}$=14 days (between the 4th and 12th infusions).

NURSING CONSIDERATIONS

Assessment: Assess for COPD, preexisting neurological signs or symptoms, HBV infection, pregnancy/nursing status, and possible drug interactions. Prior to therapy, assess for appropriate premedications.

Monitoring: Monitor for signs/symptoms of infusion reactions, neutropenia, thrombocytopenia, PML, viral hepatitis, intestinal obstruction, and other possible adverse reactions. Monitor CBC and platelet counts at regular intervals during therapy.

Patient Counseling: Instruct to contact physician if signs/symptoms of an infusion reaction (eg, fever, chills, rash, breathing problems), cytopenias (eg, bleeding, easy bruising, petechiae, pallor, worsening weakness, or fatigue), infection (eg, fever, cough), new neurological symptoms (eg, confusion, dizziness, difficulty talking or walking, vision problems), or hepatitis (eg, yellow discoloration of eyes or skin, worsening fatigue) are experienced or if new or worsening abdominal pain or nausea develops. Notify physician if pregnant or nursing. Advise that periodic monitoring of blood counts during therapy is needed. Advise to avoid vaccinations with live viral vaccines.

Administration: IV route. Refer to PI for preparation and administration instructions. **Storage:** Undiluted/Diluted Sol: 2-8°C (36-46°F). Do not freeze. Protect from light. Start infusion within 12 hrs of preparation. Discard prepared sol after 24 hrs.

ASACOL   RX
mesalamine (Warner Chilcott)

OTHER BRAND NAMES: Asacol HD (Warner Chilcott)

THERAPEUTIC CLASS: 5-Aminosalicylic acid derivative

INDICATIONS: (Asacol) Treatment of mildly to moderately active ulcerative colitis and for the maintenance of remission of ulcerative colitis. (Asacol HD) Treatment of moderately active ulcerative colitis.

DOSAGE: *Adults:* (Asacol) Mildly-Moderately Active Ulcerative Colitis: Usual: 2 tabs of 400mg tid for 6 weeks. Maintenance of Remission of Ulcerative Colitis: 1.6g/day in divided doses. (Asacol HD) Moderately Active Ulcerative Colitis: Usual: 2 tabs of 800mg tid for 6 weeks. One Asacol HD 800mg tab has not been shown to be bioequivalent to two Asacol 400mg tabs.

HOW SUPPLIED: Tab, Delayed-Release: (Asacol) 400mg, (Asacol HD) 800mg

WARNINGS/PRECAUTIONS: Renal impairment, including minimal change nephropathy, acute and chronic interstitial nephritis, and, rarely, renal failure, reported; caution with known renal dysfunction or history of renal disease. Evaluate renal function prior to therapy and periodically thereafter. Exacerbation of symptoms of colitis reported. Caution with sulfasalazine hypersensitivity. Patients with pyloric stenosis may have prolonged gastric retention, which could delay mesalamine release in the colon. Hepatic failure reported in patients with preexisting liver disease; caution with liver disease. Caution in elderly.

ADVERSE REACTIONS: Headache, abdominal pain, eructation, pain, nausea, pharyngitis, dizziness, asthenia, diarrhea, back pain, fever, rash, dyspepsia, nasopharyngitis, exacerbation of ulcerative colitis.

PREGNANCY: Category C, caution in nursing.

MECHANISM OF ACTION: 5-aminosalicylic acid derivative; has not been established. Suspected to diminish inflammation by blocking cyclooxygenase and inhibiting prostaglandin production in the colon.

PHARMACOKINETICS: Absorption: (400mg) T_{max}=4-12 hrs. (800mg) T_{max}=10-16 hrs, C_{max} =5mcg/mL, AUC_{tau}=20mcg• h/mL. **Distribution:** Found in breast milk; crosses the placenta. **Metabolism:** Gut mucosal wall and liver via rapid acetylation; N-acetyl-5-aminosalicylic acid (metabolite). **Elimination:** Renally excreted as metabolite. (400mg) $T_{1/2}$=2-15 hrs. (800mg) $T_{1/2}$=12.6 hrs.

NURSING CONSIDERATIONS

Assessment: Assess for hypersensitivity to sulfasalazine or salicylates, history or known renal/hepatic dysfunction, pyloric stenosis, and pregnancy/nursing status. Evaluate renal function prior to initiation.

Monitoring: Monitor for renal impairment including nephropathy, acute and chronic interstitial nephritis, renal/hepatic failure, exacerbation of symptoms of colitis, hypersensitivity reactions. Monitor for prolonged gastric retention if pyloric stenosis exists. Perform periodic monitoring of renal function and blood cell counts (in elderly).

Patient Counseling: Instruct to swallow whole and not to break, cut, or chew tabs. Inform physician if intact, partially intact and/or tablet shells are seen in stool repeatedly. (Asacol) Inform that ulcerative colitis rarely remits completely; risk of relapse can be substantially reduced by continued administration of medication at a maintenance dosage. (Asacol HD) Advise to d/c previous oral mesalamine therapy and follow dosing instructions for Asacol HD if switching therapy. Inform not to substitute 1 Asacol HD tab with 2 Asacol 400mg tab. Instruct to protect tab from moisture; close container tightly and leave any desiccant pouches present in the bottle. Advise pregnant and breastfeeding women, or women of childbearing potential that drug contains dibutyl phthalate, which could possibly cause fetal malformations.

Administration: Oral route. Swallow whole; do not cut, break, or chew. **Storage:** 20-25°C (68-77°F). (Asacol HD) Protect from moisture.

ASCLERA   RX
polidocanol (Merz)

THERAPEUTIC CLASS: Sclerosing Agent

INDICATIONS: To sclerose uncomplicated spider veins (varicose veins ≤1mm in diameter) and uncomplicated reticular veins (varicose veins 1-3mm in diameter) in the lower extremity.

DOSAGE: *Adults:* Spider Veins (Varicose Veins ≤1mm in Diameter): 0.1-0.3mL/inj of 0.5%. Reticular Veins (Varicose Veins 1-3mm in Diameter): 0.1-0.3mL/inj of 1%. Max: 10mL/session. Repeat treatment if extent of varicose veins requires >10mL; separate treatment by 1-2 weeks.

HOW SUPPLIED: Inj: 0.5%, 1% [2mL]

CONTRAINDICATIONS: Acute thromboembolic diseases.

WARNINGS/PRECAUTIONS: Severe allergic reactions, including anaphylactic reactions, reported, more frequently with use of larger volumes (>3mL); minimize dose and be prepared to treat anaphylaxis appropriately. Severe adverse local effects, including tissue necrosis, may occur following extravasation; caution in IV needle placement and use smallest effective volume at each inj site. Apply compression with stocking/bandage after completion of session and have the patient walk for 15-20 min; monitor for anaphylactic/allergic reaction during this period. Avoid intra-arterial and perivascular injections; intra-arterial inj can cause severe necrosis, ischemia, or gangrene and inadvertent perivascular inj can cause pain.

ADVERSE REACTIONS: Inj-site reactions (hematoma, irritation, discoloration, pain, pruritus, warmth, thrombosis), neovascularization.

PREGNANCY: Category C, not for use in nursing.

MECHANISM OF ACTION: Sclerosing agent; locally damages the endothelium of blood vessels, which results in occlusion of vessel.

PHARMACOKINETICS: Elimination: $T_{1/2}$=1.5 hrs.

NURSING CONSIDERATIONS

Assessment: Assess for acute thromboembolic disease, hypersensitivity to drug, and pregnancy/nursing status.

Monitoring: Monitor for anaphylactic/allergic reactions and inj-site reactions.

Patient Counseling: Advise to wear thigh/knee-high compression stockings/support hose on treated legs continuously for 2-3 days and for 2-3 weeks during daytime. Advise to walk for 15-20 min immediately after procedure and daily for the next few days. Advise to avoid heavy exercise, sunbathing, long flights, and hot baths or sauna for 2-3 days after treatment.

Administration: IV route. Refer to PI for administration and compression instructions. **Storage:** 15-30°C (59-86°F). Unopened ampule is stable up to 3 yrs.

ASMANEX
mometasone furoate (Schering)

RX

THERAPEUTIC CLASS: Corticosteroid

INDICATIONS: Maintenance treatment of asthma as prophylactic therapy in patients ≥4 yrs.

DOSAGE: *Adults:* Previous Therapy with Bronchodilators Alone or Inhaled Corticosteroids: Initial: 220mcg qpm. Max: 440mcg qpm or 220mcg bid. Previous Therapy with Oral Corticosteroids: Initial: 440mcg bid. Max: 880mcg/day. Titrate: May need higher dose if inadequate response after 2 weeks. Adjust to lowest effective dose once asthma stability is achieved.
Pediatrics: ≥12 yrs: Previous Therapy with Bronchodilators Alone or Inhaled Corticosteroids: Initial: 220mcg qpm. Max: 440mcg qpm or 220mcg bid. Previous Therapy with Oral Corticosteroids: Initial: 440mcg bid. Max: 880mcg/day. Titrate: May need higher dose if inadequate response after 2 weeks. 4-11 yrs: Initial/Max: 110mcg qpm regardless of prior therapy. Adjust to lowest effective dose once asthma stability is achieved.

HOW SUPPLIED: Twisthaler: 110mcg/actuation, 220mcg/actuation

CONTRAINDICATIONS: Primary treatment of status asthmaticus or other acute episodes of asthma where intensive measures are required. Hypersensitivity to milk proteins.

WARNINGS/PRECAUTIONS: Localized *Candida albicans* infections of the mouth and pharynx reported; treat accordingly. D/C if hypersensitivity reactions occur. Contains small amount of lactose which contains milk proteins; anaphylactic reactions with milk protein allergy reported. Increased susceptibility to infections. Avoid exposure to chickenpox and measles. Caution with active or quiescent tuberculosis (TB) infection, untreated systemic fungal, bacterial, viral, or parasitic infections, or ocular herpes simplex. Deaths due to adrenal insufficiency have occurred with transfer from systemic to inhaled corticosteroids. Wean slowly from systemic corticosteroid therapy. Resume oral corticosteroids during stress or severe asthma attack. Transferring from oral to inhalation therapy may unmask allergic conditions (eg, rhinitis, conjunctivitis, eczema). Monitor for systemic corticosteroid effects such as hypercorticism and adrenal suppression. Prolonged use may result in decrease of bone mineral density (BMD). May cause reduction in growth velocity in pediatrics; monitor growth routinely. Glaucoma, increased intraocular pressure (IOP), and cataracts reported. D/C and institute alternative therapy if bronchospasm occurs after dosing.

ADVERSE REACTIONS: Headache, allergic rhinitis, pharyngitis, upper respiratory tract infection, sinusitis, oral candidiasis, dysmenorrhea, musculoskeletal pain, back pain, dyspepsia, myalgia, abdominal pain, nausea.

INTERACTIONS: Ketoconazole may increase plasma levels. Caution with drugs that reduce bone mass (eg, anticonvulsants and corticosteroids).

PREGNANCY: Category C, caution in nursing.

MECHANISM OF ACTION: Corticosteroid; not established. Shown to have inhibitory effects on multiple cell types (eg, mast cells, eosinophils, neutrophils, macrophages, and lymphocytes) and mediators (eg, histamine, eicosanoids, leukotrienes, and cytokines), involved in inflammatory and asthmatic response.

PHARMACOKINETICS: Absorption: Absolute bioavailability (<1%); C_{max}=94-114pcg/mL; T_{max}=1-2.5 hrs. **Distribution:** (IV) V_d=152L; plasma protein binding (98-99%). **Metabolism:** Liver via CYP3A4. **Elimination:** Feces (74%), urine (8%); $T_{1/2}$=5 hrs.

NURSING CONSIDERATIONS

Assessment: Assess for status asthmaticus, acute asthma episodes, bronchospasm, known hypersensitivity to milk proteins or to any drug component. Assess for risk factors for decreased BMD, history of increased IOP, glaucoma, cataracts, active or quiescent pulmonary TB, ocular herpes simplex, untreated systemic infections, chickenpox, measles, pregnancy/nursing status, and possible drug interactions.

Monitoring: Monitor for localized infections of mouth and pharynx with *Candida albicans*, decreased BMD, chickenpox, measles, asthma instability, growth in pediatrics, development of glaucoma, increased IOP, cataracts, hypercorticism, signs and symptoms of adrenal insufficiency, paradoxical bronchospasm, hypersensitivity reactions, and immunosuppression. Monitor for lung function, β-agonist use, and asthma symptoms during withdrawal of oral corticosteroids.

Patient Counseling: Advise that localized infection with *Candida albicans* may occur in mouth and pharynx; rinse mouth after inhalation. Inform that therapy should not be used to treat status asthmaticus or to relieve acute asthma symptoms. Counsel to d/c if hypersensitivity reactions (eg, rash, pruritus, angioedema, and anaphylactic reactions) occur. Advise to avoid exposure to chickenpox or measles and to seek medical attention if exposed. Inform of potential worsening of existing TB, other infections, or ocular herpes, and that drug may cause systemic corticosteroid effects of hypercorticism and adrenal suppression, may reduce BMD, and may cause reduction in growth rate (pediatrics). Advise to take as directed, to use medication at regular intervals, and to contact physician if symptoms do not improve or if condition worsens. Instruct on proper administration procedures and on when to discard inhaler.

Administration: Oral inhalation. Inhale rapidly and deeply. Rinse mouth after inhalation. Refer to PI for further administration instructions. **Storage:** 25°C (77°F); excursions permitted to 15-30°C (59-86°F). Store in dry place. Discard inhaler 45 days after opening foil pouch or when dose counter reads "00," whichever comes 1st.

ASTELIN   RX
azelastine HCl (Meda)

THERAPEUTIC CLASS: Antihistamine

INDICATIONS: Treatment of the symptoms of seasonal allergic rhinitis (eg, rhinorrhea, sneezing, and nasal pruritus) in patients ≥5 yrs. Treatment of the symptoms of vasomotor rhinitis (eg, rhinorrhea, nasal congestion, and postnasal drip) in patients ≥12 yrs.

DOSAGE: *Adults:* Vasomotor Rhinitis: Usual: 2 sprays/nostril bid. Seasonal Allergic Rhinitis: Usual: 1-2 sprays/nostril bid. Elderly: Start at lower end of dosing range.
Pediatrics: Vasomotor Rhinitis: ≥12 yrs: Usual: 2 sprays/nostril bid. Seasonal Allergic Rhinitis: Usual: ≥12 yrs: 1-2 sprays/nostril bid. 5-11 yrs: 1 spray/nostril bid.

HOW SUPPLIED: Spray: 137mcg/spray [30mL]

WARNINGS/PRECAUTIONS: Occurrence of somnolence reported. Exercise caution when driving a car or operating potentially dangerous machinery; may impair physical/mental abilities. Caution in elderly.

ADVERSE REACTIONS: Bitter taste, headache, somnolence, dysesthesia, rhinitis, epistaxis, sinusitis, nasal burning, pharyngitis, paroxysmal sneezing.

INTERACTIONS: Avoid alcohol or other CNS depressants; additional reductions in alertness and CNS performance impairment may occur. Increased levels of PO azelastine with cimetidine.

PREGNANCY: Category C, caution in nursing.

MECHANISM OF ACTION: Phthalazinone derivative; exhibits histamine H_1-receptor antagonist activity in isolated tissues.

PHARMACOKINETICS: Absorption: T_{max}=2-3 hrs; bioavailability (40%). **Distribution:** V_d=14.5L/kg (PO/IV); plasma protein binding (88%, 97% metabolite). **Metabolism:** Oxidation via CYP450; desmethylazelastine (major metabolite). **Elimination:** (PO) Feces (75%, <10% unchanged); $T_{1/2}$=22 hrs (PO/IV), 54 hrs (PO, metabolite).

NURSING CONSIDERATIONS

Assessment: Assess for known hypersensitivity to the drug, pregnancy/nursing status, and possible drug interactions.

Monitoring: Monitor for somnolence and other adverse reactions.

Patient Counseling: Instruct to use only as prescribed. Instruct to prime the delivery system before initial use and after storage for ≥3 days. Instruct to store the bottle upright at room temperature with pump tightly closed and out of reach of children. Advise to seek professional assistance or contact poison control center in case of accidental ingestion by a young child. Advise to assess individual responses to the drug before engaging in any activity requiring mental alertness (eg, driving a car or operating machinery). Advise against concurrent use with other antihistamines without consulting a physician. Advise that concurrent use with alcohol or other CNS depressants may lead to additional reductions in alertness or CNS performance impairment and to avoid concurrent use. Instruct to consult physician if pregnant/nursing or planning to become pregnant.

Administration: Intranasal route. Avoid spraying in the eyes. Before initial use, the delivery system should be primed with 4 sprays or until a fine mist appears. When ≥3 days have elapsed since the last use, pump should be reprimed with 2 sprays or until a fine mist appears. **Storage:** 20-25°C (68-77F°). Protect from freezing.

ASTEPRO
azelastine HCl (Meda)

THERAPEUTIC CLASS: H_1-antagonist

INDICATIONS: Relief of symptoms of seasonal and perennial allergic rhinitis in patients ≥12 yrs.

DOSAGE: *Adults:* Seasonal allergic rhinitis: (0.1%, 0.15%): 1 or 2 sprays per nostril bid. (0.15%): May be administered as 2 sprays per nostril qd. Perennial allergic rhinitis: (0.15%): 2 sprays per nostril bid. Elderly: Start at the low end of dosing range. *Pediatrics:* ≥12 yrs: Seasonal allergic rhinitis: (0.1%, 0.15%): 1 or 2 sprays per nostril bid. (0.15%): May be administered as 2 sprays per nostril qd. Perennial allergic rhinitis: (0.15%): 2 sprays per nostril bid.

HOW SUPPLIED: Spray: (0.1%) 137mcg; (0.15%) 205.5mcg

WARNINGS/PRECAUTIONS: Somnolence reported. May impair physical/mental abilities. Administer by intranasal route only. Caution in elderly.

ADVERSE REACTIONS: Bitter taste, somnolence, epistaxis, headache, nasal discomfort, fatigue, sneezing.

INTERACTIONS: Avoid concurrent use with alcohol or other CNS depressants; additional reductions in alertness and impairment of CNS performance may occur. Increased levels with cimetidine.

PREGNANCY: Category C, caution in nursing.

MECHANISM OF ACTION: H_1-receptor antagonist; phthalazinone derivative, which exhibits histamine H_1-receptor activity in isolated tissues, animal models, and humans; desmethylazelastine (major metabolite) also possesses H_1-receptor antagonist activity.

PHARMACOKINETICS: Absorption: Bioavailability (40%); (0.1%) C_{max}=200pg/mL; T_{max}=3 hrs; AUC =5122 pg•hr/mL. (0.15%) C_{max}=409pg/mL; T_{max}=4 hrs; AUC=9312pg•hr/mL. Desmethylazelastine: (0.1%) C_{max}=23pg/mL; T_{max}=24 hrs; AUC =2131 pg•hr/mL. (0.15%) C_{max}=38pg/mL; T_{max}=24 hrs; AUC=3824pg•hr/mL. **Distribution:** Plasma protein binding (azelastine, desmethylazelastine [major metabolite]): (88%, 97% respectively); V_d=14.5L/kg. **Metabolism:** Oxidation via CYP450 enzyme system. Desmethylazelastine (major metabolite). **Elimination:** Azelastine: Feces (75%, <10% unchanged); $T_{1/2}$=22-25 hrs. Desmethylazelastine: $T_{1/2}$=52-57 hrs.

NURSING CONSIDERATIONS

Assessment: Assess for hepatic/renal functions, alcohol intake, and possible drug interactions. Assess pregnancy/nursing status.

Monitoring: Monitor for somnolence, bitter taste, epistaxis, headache, nasal discomfort, fatigue, and sneezing.

Patient Counseling: Instruct to use exactly as prescribed. Instruct to use caution while engaging in hazardous activities (eg, operating machinery/driving) that require complete mental alertness and motor coordination. Advise to avoid alcohol or other CNS depressants. Must notify physician if pregnant/nursing or planning to become pregnant. Advise to prime medication before initial spray by releasing 6 sprays or until a fine mist appears. When medication has not been used for ≥3 days, counsel to reprime with 2 sprays or until a fine mist appears. Avoid spraying into eyes. Keep out of the reach of children.

Administration: Intranasal route. **Storage:** 20-25°C (68-77°F). Protect from freezing.

ATACAND
candesartan cilexetil (AstraZeneca)

> **Drugs that act directly on the renin-angiotensin system can cause death/injury to developing fetus during 2nd and 3rd trimesters. D/C if pregnancy detected.**

THERAPEUTIC CLASS: Angiotensin II receptor antagonist

INDICATIONS: Treatment of HTN in adults and children 1-<17 yrs, alone or with other antihypertensive agents. Treatment of heart failure (HF) (New York Heart Association Class II-IV) in adults with left ventricular systolic dysfunction (ejection fraction ≤40%) to reduce cardiovascular death and HF hospitalizations; has an added effect when used with an ACE inhibitor.

DOSAGE: *Adults:* Individualize dose. HTN: Monotherapy Without Volume Depletion: Initial: 16mg qd. Usual: 8-32mg/day given qd-bid. Maximal effects attained within 4-6 weeks. May add diuretic if BP not controlled. Intravascular Volume Depletion/Moderate Hepatic Impairment: Lower initial dose. HF: Initial: 4mg qd. Titrate: Double dose q2 weeks, as tolerated, to target dose of 32mg qd. *Pediatrics:* HTN: Administer qd or divided into 2 equal doses. 6-<17 yrs: <50kg: Initial: 4-8mg. Usual: 2-16mg/day. >50kg: Initial: 8-16mg. Usual: 4-32mg/day. 1-<6 yrs: Initial: 0.20mg/kg (oral sus). Usual: 0.05-0.4mg/kg/day. Adjust according to BP response. Intravascular Volume Depletion: Initiate at a lower dose. Full effect attained within 4 weeks. For children who cannot swallow tab, PO sus may be substituted.

HOW SUPPLIED: Tab: 4mg*, 8mg*, 16mg*, 32mg* *scored

WARNINGS/PRECAUTIONS: Do not give in children <1 yr; may affect the development of immature kidneys. Symptomatic hypotension may occur with activated renin-angiotensin system (eg, volume- and/or salt-depleted patients); correct volume or salt depletion before therapy or monitor closely. Caution when initiating therapy with HF. Hypotension may occur during major surgery. Renal function changes may occur. Oliguria and/or progressive azotemia, with acute renal failure and/or death (rare), may occur in renin-angiotensin-aldosterone system dependent patients (eg, severe HF). May increase SrCr or BUN in patients with renal artery stenosis. May cause hyperkalemia and increase SrCr in patients with HF; monitor serum K$^+$, SrCr, and BP during dose escalation and periodically thereafter. Do not give in pediatrics with GFR <30mL/min/1.73m^2.

ADVERSE REACTIONS: Hypotension, abnormal renal function, hyperkalemia, upper respiratory tract infection, dizziness, back pain.

INTERACTIONS: May deteriorate renal function and attenuate antihypertensive effect with NSAIDs, including selective cyclooxygenase-2 inhibitors; monitor renal function periodically. May increase lithium levels; monitor serum lithium levels carefully. Hypotension may occur with anesthesia. Increased risk of hyperkalemia with ACE inhibitors and K$^+$-sparing diuretics (eg, spironolactone).

PREGNANCY: Category C (1st trimester) and D (2nd and 3rd trimesters), not for use in nursing.

MECHANISM OF ACTION: Angiotensin II receptor antagonist; blocks vasoconstrictor and aldosterone-secreting effects of angiotensin II by selectively blocking binding of angiotensin II to AT$_1$ receptor in many tissues (eg, vascular smooth muscle and adrenal gland).

PHARMACOKINETICS: Absorption: Rapid and complete. Absolute bioavailability (15%); T$_{max}$=3-4 hrs. **Distribution:** V$_d$=0.13L/kg; plasma protein binding (>99%). **Metabolism:** Liver via O-deethylation (minor); candesartan (active metabolite). **Elimination:** Feces (67%), urine (33%; 26%, unchanged); T$_{1/2}$=9 hrs.

NURSING CONSIDERATIONS

Assessment: Assess for hypersensitivity, hepatic/renal function, volume/salt depletion, HF, renal artery stenosis, pregnancy/nursing status, and possible drug interactions.

Monitoring: Monitor for signs/symptoms of hypotension, hypersensitivity reactions, changes in renal function, and other adverse reactions. Monitor serum K$^+$, SrCr, and BP periodically especially in patients with HF.

Patient Counseling: Inform of pregnancy risks. Ask to report pregnancies as soon as possible. Regularly question postmenarche adolescents on changes in menstrual pattern and the possibility of pregnancy.

Administration: Oral route. Take with or without food. Refer to PI for preparation of PO sus. **Storage:** 25°C (77°F); excursions permitted to 15-30°C (59-86°F). Keep container tightly closed. (Sus) <30°C (86°F). Use within 30 days after 1st opening. Do not freeze.

ATACAND HCT   RX
candesartan cilexetil - hydrochlorothiazide (AstraZeneca)

> **D/C when pregnancy is detected. Drugs that act directly on the renin-angiotensin system can cause injury/death to developing fetus.**

THERAPEUTIC CLASS: Angiotensin II receptor antagonist/thiazide diuretic

INDICATIONS: Treatment of HTN.

DOSAGE: *Adults:* BP Not Controlled on 25mg HCTZ qd or Controlled on 25mg HCTZ qd with Hypokalemia: 16mg-12.5mg tab qd. BP Not Controlled on 32mg Candesartan qd: 32mg-12.5mg tab qd; may increase to 32mg-25mg tab qd. Replacement Therapy: Substitute for titrated components.

HOW SUPPLIED: Tab: (Candesartan-HCTZ) 16mg-12.5mg*, 32mg-12.5mg*, 32mg-25mg* *scored

CONTRAINDICATIONS: Anuria, sulfonamide-derived drug hypersensitivity.

WARNINGS/PRECAUTIONS: Not for initial therapy. Not recommended for initial titration with moderate hepatic impairment. Symptomatic hypotension may occur in intravascular volume- or Na$^+$-depleted patients (eg, patients treated vigorously with diuretics or on dialysis); correct these conditions prior to therapy or monitor closely. Not recommended with CrCl ≤30mL/min. Candesartan: Renal function changes may occur. Oliguria and/or progressive azotemia and (rarely) with acute renal failure and/or death may occur in patients whose renal function may depend on the renin-angiotensin-aldosterone system (eg, severe congestive heart failure [CHF]). Increases in SrCr or BUN reported in patients with renal artery stenosis. Hypotension may occur during major surgery and anesthesia. HCTZ: May cause idiosyncratic reaction, resulting in acute transient myopia and acute angle-closure glaucoma; d/c as rapidly as possible. Caution with hepatic impairment or progressive liver disease; may precipitate hepatic coma. May cause hypersensitivity reactions, exacerbation or activation of systemic lupus erythematosus (SLE), hyperuricemia or precipitation of acute gout, hypomagnesemia, and hyperglycemia. Observe for signs of fluid or electrolyte imbalance (eg, hyponatremia, hypochloremic alkalosis, hypokalemia). Enhanced effects in postsympathectomy patient. May increase calcium, cholesterol, and TG levels. D/C before testing for parathyroid function. Caution with severe renal disease; may precipitate azotemia.

ADVERSE REACTIONS: Fetal injury, upper respiratory tract infection, back pain.

INTERACTIONS: May increase levels and risk of lithium toxicity; avoid use. NSAIDs, including selective cyclooxygenase-2 inhibitors, may deteriorate renal function and attenuate the antihypertensive effect. Candesartan: HCTZ: Alcohol, barbiturates, or narcotics may potentiate orthostatic hypotension. Dosage adjustment of antidiabetic drugs (eg, oral hypoglycemic agents, insulin) may be required. Other antihypertensives may cause additive effect or potentiation. Impaired absorption with cholestyramine or colestipol resins. Corticosteroids and adrenocorticotropic hormone may intensify electrolyte depletion, particularly hypokalemia. May decrease response to pressor amines (eg, norepinephrine). May increase responsiveness to nondepolarizing skeletal muscle relaxants (eg, tubocurarine).

PREGNANCY: Category D, not for use in nursing.

MECHANISM OF ACTION: Candesartan: Angiotensin II receptor antagonist; blocks vasoconstrictor and aldosterone-secreting effects of angiotensin II by blocking the binding of angiotensin II to AT_1 receptor in many tissues. HCTZ: Thiazide diuretic; has not been established. Affects renal tubular mechanisms of electrolyte reabsorption, directly increasing excretion of Na^+ and chloride in approximately equivalent amounts.

PHARMACOKINETICS: Absorption: Candesartan: Rapid and complete. Absolute bioavailability (15%); T_{max}=3-4 hrs. **Distribution:** Candesartan: Plasma protein binding (>99%); V_d=0.13L/kg. HCTZ: Crosses placenta; found in breast milk. **Metabolism:** Candesartan: Ester hydrolysis, liver via O-deethylation (minor). **Elimination:** Candesartan: Feces (67%), urine (26% unchanged); $T_{1/2}$=9 hrs. HCTZ: Urine (61% unchanged); $T_{1/2}$=5.6-14.8 hrs.

NURSING CONSIDERATIONS

Assessment: Assess for hypersensitivity to drugs and its components, anuria, sulfonamide-derived drug hypersensitivity, history of penicillin allergy, volume/salt depletion, SLE, diabetes mellitus, CHF, hepatic/renal impairment, postsympathectomy status, renal artery stenosis, pregnancy/nursing status, and possible drug interactions.

Monitoring: Monitor for signs/symptoms of fluid/electrolyte imbalance, exacerbation or activation of SLE, hypotension, hypersensitivity reactions, idiosyncratic reaction, renal function changes, and other adverse reactions. Monitor BP and serum electrolytes periodically.

Patient Counseling: Inform of pregnancy risks; instruct to notify physician if pregnant as soon as possible. Caution that lightheadedness may occur, especially during the 1st days of therapy; instruct to d/c therapy if syncope occurs. Caution that inadequate fluid intake, excessive perspiration, diarrhea, or vomiting may lead to an excessive fall in BP, with the same consequences of lightheadedness and possible syncope. Instruct not to use K^+ supplements or salt substitutes containing K^+ without consulting physician.

Administration: Oral route. **Storage:** 25°C (77°F); excursions permitted to 15-30°C (59-86°F).

ATELVIA   RX
risedronate sodium (Warner Chilcott)

THERAPEUTIC CLASS: Bisphosphonate

INDICATIONS: Treatment of osteoporosis in postmenopausal women.

DOSAGE: *Adults:* 35mg once weekly. Take in am immediately following breakfast. Swallow tab whole in upright position and with at least 4 oz. of plain water. Do not lie down for 30 min after dose. Do not crush, cut, or chew tab.

HOW SUPPLIED: Tab, Delayed-Release: 35mg

CONTRAINDICATIONS: Abnormalities of the esophagus which delay esophageal emptying (eg, stricture, achalasia), inability to stand or sit upright for at least 30 min, hypocalcemia.

WARNINGS/PRECAUTIONS: Should not be given in patients treated with Actonel; contains the same active ingredient. May cause local irritation of the upper GI mucosa; caution with active upper GI problems (eg, Barrett's esophagus, dysphagia, other esophageal diseases, gastritis, duodenitis, or ulcers). D/C if dysphagia, odynophagia, retrosternal pain, or new/worsening heartburn occurs. Gastric and duodenal ulcers reported. Treat hypocalcemia and other disturbances of bone and mineral metabolism before therapy. Osteonecrosis of the jaw (ONJ) reported; d/c for patients requiring invasive dental procedures, or consider d/c if ONJ develops. Severe and occasionally incapacitating bone, joint, and/or muscle pain reported; consider d/c use if severe symptoms develop. Atypical, low-energy, or low trauma fractures of the femoral shaft reported; consider interrupting therapy. Avoid with severe renal impairment (CrCl <30mL/min).

ADVERSE REACTIONS: Diarrhea, abdominal pain, constipation, N/V, dyspepsia, influenza, bronchitis, upper respiratory tract infection, arthralgia, back pain, pain in extremity.

INTERACTIONS: Calcium supplements, antacids, magnesium-based supplements or laxatives, and iron preparations may reduce bioavailability; take at different time of the day. Drugs that raise stomach pH (eg, H_2 blockers, proton pump inhibitors [PPIs], or antacids) may affect enteric coating and thereby reduce bioavailability; avoid concomitant administration with H_2 blockers or PPIs. Upper GI reactions reported with concomitant NSAID use. Risk of ONJ with concomitant corticosteroid/chemotherapy. May interfere with the use of bone-imaging agents. May increase risk of atypical femur fractures with glucocorticoids (eg, prednisone).

PREGNANCY: Category C, not for use in nursing.

MECHANISM OF ACTION: Bisphosphonate; has an affinity for hydroxyapatite crystals in bone and acts as an antiresorptive agent. Inhibits osteoclasts.

PHARMACOKINETICS: Absorption: T_{max}=3 hrs; (immediate release) absolute bioavailability (0.63%). **Distribution:** V_d=13.8L/kg; plasma protein binding (24%). **Elimination:** Urine (50%), feces (unabsorbed dose); $T_{1/2}$=561 hrs.

NURSING CONSIDERATIONS

Assessment: Assess for hypocalcemia, esophageal abnormalities, upper GI problems or any other conditions where treatment is contraindicated/cautioned, drug hypersensitivity, pregnancy/nursing status, and for possible drug interactions.

Monitoring: Monitor for signs/symptoms of upper GI disorders (eg, dysphagia, esophagitis, esophageal, or gastric ulcers), ONJ, atypical femur fracture (eg, unusual hip, groin, or thigh pain), musculoskeletal pain.

Patient Counseling: Inform to pay particular attention to the dosing instructions; advise that benefits may be compromised by failure to take drug accordingly. Instruct to contact physician if symptoms of esophageal disease develop. Counsel to take supplemental calcium and vitamin D if dietary intake is inadequate; advise to take supplement at a different time of the day than risedronate. Advise to consider weight bearing exercises and appropriate lifestyle modifications. Counsel about possible adverse reactions. Instruct that if a dose is missed, take 1 tab on the morning after and to return to original schedule; instruct not to take 2 tabs on the same day.

Administration: Oral route. **Storage:** 20-25°C (68-77°F).

ATIVAN | CIV
lorazepam (Biovail)

THERAPEUTIC CLASS: Benzodiazepine

INDICATIONS: Management of anxiety disorders or for short-term relief of the symptoms of anxiety or anxiety associated with depressive symptoms.

DOSAGE: *Adults:* Individualize dose, frequency, and duration. Anxiety: Initial: 2-3mg/day given bid-tid. Usual: 2-6mg/day in divided doses, largest dose before hs. Daily Dosage Range: 1-10mg/day. Insomnia: 2-4mg qhs. Elderly/Debilitated: Initial: 1-2mg/day in divided doses; adjust PRN and as tolerated. Increase gradually; when higher dosage is indicated, increase pm dose before daytime doses.
Pediatrics: ≥12 yrs: Individualize dose, frequency, and duration. Anxiety: Initial: 2-3mg/day given bid-tid. Usual: 2-6mg/day in divided doses, largest dose before hs. Daily Dosage Range: 1-10mg/day. Insomnia: 2-4mg qhs. Increase gradually; when higher dosage is indicated, increase pm dose before daytime doses.

HOW SUPPLIED: Tab: 0.5mg, 1mg*, 2mg* *scored

CONTRAINDICATIONS: Acute narrow-angle glaucoma.

WARNINGS/PRECAUTIONS: Effectiveness in long-term use (>4 months) has not been assessed; prescribe for short periods only (eg, 2-4 weeks) and periodically reassess usefulness of drug. Preexisting depression may emerge or worsen; not for use with primary depressive disorder or psychosis. May lead to potentially fatal respiratory depression. May impair mental/physical abilities. Potential for abuse and physical/psychological dependence; increased risk with higher doses, longer term use, and in patients with history of alcoholism/drug abuse, or with significant personality disorders. Withdrawal symptoms reported; avoid abrupt d/c. May develop tolerance to sedative effects. Paradoxical reactions reported; d/c if occur. Possible suicide in patients with depression; avoid in such patients without adequate anti-depressant therapy. Caution with compromised respiratory function (eg, chronic obstructive pulmonary disease, sleep apnea syndrome), impaired renal/hepatic function, hepatic encephalopathy, in elderly, and in debilitated patients. Adjust dose with severe hepatic insufficiency; lower doses may be sufficient. Monitor frequently for symptoms of upper GI disease.

ADVERSE REACTIONS: Sedation, dizziness, weakness, unsteadiness.

INTERACTIONS: Increased CNS-depressant effects with other CNS depressants (eg, alcohol, barbiturates, antipsychotics, sedative/hypnotics, anxiolytics, antidepressants, narcotic analgesics, sedative antihistamines, anticonvulsants, anesthetics); may lead to potentially fatal respiratory depression. May produce marked sedation, excessive salivation, hypotension, ataxia, delirium, and respiratory arrest with clozapine. Increased plasma levels with valproate and more rapid onset or prolonged effect with probenecid; reduce dose by 50%. Decreased sedative effects with theophylline or aminophylline.

PREGNANCY: Not for use in pregnancy and nursing.

MECHANISM OF ACTION: Benzodiazepine; has a tranquilizing action on the CNS with no appreciable effect on the respiratory or cardiovascular systems.

PHARMACOKINETICS: Absorption: Readily absorbed. Absolute bioavailability (90%); (2mg) C_{max}=20ng/mL; T_{max}=2 hrs. **Distribution:** Plasma protein binding (85%). **Metabolism:** Glucuronidation. **Elimination:** Urine; $T_{1/2}$=12 hrs (lorazepam), 18 hrs (lorazepam glucuronide).

NURSING CONSIDERATIONS

Assessment: Assess for acute narrow-angle glaucoma, primary depressive disorder, psychosis, history of alcohol/drug abuse, personality disorders, compromised respiratory function, impaired renal/hepatic function, hepatic encephalopathy, previous hypersensitivity to the drug, pregnancy/nursing status, and possible drug interactions.

Monitoring: Monitor for worsening of depression, respiratory depression, physical/psychological dependence, withdrawal symptoms, tolerance, abuse, suicidal thinking, paradoxical reactions, and symptoms of upper GI disease. Reassess usefulness of drug periodically. Monitor elderly/debilitated frequently and addiction-prone individuals carefully. Perform periodic blood counts and LFTs with long-term therapy.

Patient Counseling: Inform that psychological/physical dependence may occur; instruct to consult physician before increasing dose or abruptly d/c drug. Warn not to operate dangerous machinery or motor vehicles and that tolerance for alcohol and other CNS depressants will be diminished.

Administration: Oral route. **Storage:** 25°C (77°F); excursions permitted to 15-30°C (59-86°F).

ATIVAN INJECTION   CIV
lorazepam (Baxter)

THERAPEUTIC CLASS: Benzodiazepine

INDICATIONS: Treatment of status epilepticus and preanesthetic medication in adults.

DOSAGE: *Adults:* ≥18 yrs: Status Epilepticus: 4mg IV (given slowly at 2mg/min); may repeat 1 dose after 10-15 min if seizures recur or fail to cease. Preanesthetic Sedation: Usual: (IM) 0.05mg/kg given at least 2 hrs prior to operation; (IV) 2mg or 0.044mg/kg IV (whichever is smaller) 15-20 min prior to procedure. Max: 4mg IM/IV. Elderly: Start at the low end of the dosing range.

HOW SUPPLIED: Inj: 2mg/mL, 4mg/mL [1mL, 10mL]

CONTRAINDICATIONS: Acute narrow-angle glaucoma, sleep apnea syndrome, severe respiratory insufficiency. Not for intra-arterial injection.

WARNINGS/PRECAUTIONS: May produce heavy sedation; airway obstruction and respiratory depression may occur; ensure airway patency and monitor respiration. May impair mental/physical abilities. Avoid intra-arterial administration. Avoid in patients with hepatic and/or renal failure; caution in patients with hepatic and/or renal impairment. May cause fetal damage during pregnancy. When used for peroral endoscopic procedures; adequate topical/regional anesthesia is recommended to minimize reflex activity. Extreme caution when administering injections to elderly, very ill, or to patients with limited pulmonary reserve as hypoventilation and/or hypoxic cardiac arrest may occur. Paradoxical reaction, propylene glycol toxicity (eg, lactic acidosis, hyperosmolality, hypotension) and polyethylene glycol toxicity (eg, acute tubular necrosis) reported; premature and low birth weight infants as well pediatric patients receiving high-doses may be at higher risk. Pediatric patients may exhibit sensitivity to benzyl alcohol; "gasping syndrome" associated with administration of IV solutions containing benzyl alcohol in neonates. Repeated doses over a prolonged period of time may result in physical and psychological dependence and withdrawal symptoms following abrupt d/c.

ADVERSE REACTIONS: Respiratory depression/failure, hypotension, somnolence, headache, hypoventilation, injection-site reactions (eg, pain, burning, redness), paradoxical excitement.

INTERACTIONS: Additive CNS depression with other CNS depressants (eg, ethyl alcohol, phenothiazines, barbiturates, MAOIs, antidepressants). Increased sedation, hallucinations and irrational behavior with scopolamine. Reduce dose by 50% when given in combination with valproate or probenecid due to decreased clearance. Increased clearance with oral contraceptives. Severe adverse effects with clozapine, loxapine, and haloperidol reported. Prolonged and profound effect with concomitant sedatives, tranquilizers, narcotic analgesics.

PREGNANCY: Category D, not for use in nursing.

MECHANISM OF ACTION: Benzodiazepine; antianxiety, sedative and anticonvulsant effects. Interacts with GABA-benzodiazepine receptor complex in human brain. Exhibits relatively high and specific affinity for its recognition site but does not displace GABA. Attachment to the specific binding site enhances the affinity of GABA for its receptor site on the same receptor complex.

PHARMACOKINETICS: Absorption: Complete, rapid; (IM) C_{max}=48ng/mL, T_{max}=within 3 hrs. **Distribution:** V_d=1.3L/kg, plasma protein binding (91%), crosses blood brain barrier. **Metabolism:** Liver. **Elimination:** Urine (88%), feces (7%), (0.3% unchanged); $T_{1/2}$=14 hrs.

NURSING CONSIDERATIONS

Assessment: Comprehensive review of benefits/risks in status epilepticus. Assess for hypersensitivity to benzodiazepine or its vehicle, acute-angle glaucoma, preexisting respiratory impairment, hepatic/renal impairment, pregnancy/nursing status, and possible drug interactions.

Monitoring: Monitor for respiratory depression, airway obstruction, heavy sedation, drowsiness, excessive sleepiness, hypoglycemia and hyponatremia in status epilepticus, seizures, myoclonus, somnolence, injection-site reactions (eg, pain, burning sensation, and redness), and paradoxical reactions (eg, mania, agitation, psychosis). Signs of toxicity to the vehicle's components (eg, lactic acidosis, hyperosmolarity, hypotension, and acute tubular necrosis). Monitor for hypersensitivity reactions.

Patient Counseling: Inform of risks/benefits. Caution with hazardous tasks (eg, operating machinery/driving). Do not get out of bed unassisted. Avoid alcoholic beverages for at least 24-48 hrs after receiving drug. Advise about potential for physical/psychological dependence and withdrawal symptoms.

Administration: IM/IV route. IV must be diluted with an equal volume of compatible solution. **Storage:** Refrigerate; protect from light.

ATRALIN   RX
tretinoin (Coria Laboratories)

THERAPEUTIC CLASS: Retinoid

INDICATIONS: Treatment of acne vulgaris.

DOSAGE: *Adults:* Apply qd before hs where acne lesions appear; use a thin layer to cover the entire affected area.
Pediatrics: ≥10 yrs: Apply qd before hs where acne lesions appear; use a thin layer to cover the entire affected area.

HOW SUPPLIED: Gel: 0.05% [45g]

WARNINGS/PRECAUTIONS: Keep away from eyes, mouth, paranasal creases, and mucous membranes. Skin may become dry, red, or exfoliated. If degree of irritation warrants, temporarily reduce amount or frequency, or d/c use temporarily or altogether. D/C if sensitivity reaction occurs. Use appropriate moisturizer if mild to moderate skin dryness occurs. Severe irritation on eczematous or sunburned skin reported; use with caution. Minimize exposure to sunlight, including sunlamps. Caution in patients with high level sun exposure. Use sunscreen products (at least SPF 15) and protective clothing over treated areas when exposure to sun cannot be avoided. Extreme weather may increase skin irritation. Caution with known sensitivity or allergy to fish; pruritus or urticaria may develop.

ADVERSE REACTIONS: Dry skin, peeling/scaling/flaking skin, skin burning sensation, erythema.

INTERACTIONS: Caution with topical medications, medicated or abrasive soaps and cleansers, products with strong drying effects, high concentrations of alcohol, astringents, spices, or lime. Caution with topical over-the-counter acne preparations containing benzoyl peroxide, sulfur, resorcinol, or salicylic acid; allow effects of these agents to subside before use.

PREGNANCY: Category C, caution in nursing.

MECHANISM OF ACTION: Retinoic acid derivative; not established. Suspected to decrease cohesiveness of follicular epithelial cells with decreased microcomedo formation; also stimulates mitotic activity and increased turnover of follicular epithelial cells, causing extrusion of the comedones.

PHARMACOKINETICS: Metabolism: 13-cis-retinoic acid and 4-oxo-13-cis-retinoic acid (major metabolites).

NURSING CONSIDERATIONS

Assessment: Assess for drug hypersensitivity, presence of eczematous/sunburned skin, known sensitivity/allergy to fish, history of sun exposure or inherent sensitivity to sun, pregnancy/nursing status, and possible drug interactions.

Monitoring: Monitor for signs/symptoms of skin sensitivity, development of dry/red/exfoliated skin, and other adverse reactions.

Patient Counseling: Instruct to notify physician if planning to become pregnant; advise to d/c if pregnancy is suspected/confirmed. Inform about drying and irritation effects during treatment and to continue treatment if effects are tolerable. Advise to avoid application around the eyes, mouth, paranasal creases, and mucous membranes. Instruct to clean affected areas with appropriate cleanser before application. Advise to use noncomedogenic moisturizers and to avoid drying or irritating products. Inform that cosmetics can be worn while on treatment, but areas should be thoroughly cleansed before treatment. Instruct to avoid direct exposure to sun or sunlamps and to use sunscreen.

Administration: Topical route. **Storage:** 20-25°C (68-77°F); excursions permitted to 15-30°C (59-86°F). Protect from freezing.

ATRIPLA RX
tenofovir disoproxil fumarate - efavirenz - emtricitabine (Bristol-Myers Squibb/Gilead Sciences)

> Lactic acidosis and severe hepatomegaly with steatosis, including fatal cases, reported with the use of nucleoside analogues. Not approved for the treatment of chronic hepatitis B virus (HBV) infection. Severe acute exacerbations of hepatitis B reported in patients coinfected with HBV upon d/c of therapy; closely monitor hepatic function for at least several months. If appropriate, initiation of anti-hepatitis B therapy may be warranted.

THERAPEUTIC CLASS: Non-nucleoside reverse transcriptase inhibitor/nucleoside analogue combination

INDICATIONS: For use alone as a complete regimen or in combination with other antiretroviral agents for the treatment of HIV-1 infection in adults.

DOSAGE: *Adults:* ≥18 yrs: 1 tab qd on empty stomach, hs dosing may improve tolerability of nervous system symptoms.

HOW SUPPLIED: Tab: (Efavirenz-Emtricitabine-Tenofovir Disoproxil Fumarate [TDF]) 600mg-200mg-300mg

CONTRAINDICATIONS: Coadministration with CYP3A substrates for which inhibition of metabolism can potentiate serious and/or life-threatening reactions (eg, voriconazole, dihydroergotamine, ergonovine, ergotamine, methylergonovine, midazolam, triazolam, bepridil, cisapride, pimozide, St. John's wort).

WARNINGS/PRECAUTIONS: Test for presence of chronic HBV prior to treatment. Monitor LFTs before and during treatment. Immune reconstitution syndrome and redistribution/accumulation of body fat reported. Avoid in patients with CrCl <50mL/min. Efavirenz: Serious psychiatric adverse events and CNS symptoms reported; may impair mental/physical abilities. Use adequate contraceptive measures up to 12 weeks after d/c. Skin rash reported; d/c if severe rash associated with blistering, desquamation, mucosal involvement, or fever develops. Caution in patients with history of seizures; convulsions reported. TDF: Caution with liver disease, obesity, prolonged nucleoside exposure; may increase risk of lactic acidosis and severe hepatomegaly; d/c treatment if hepatotoxicity occurs. Renal impairment reported; calculate CrCl prior and during therapy. Decreased bone mineral density (BMD), fractures, and osteomalacia reported. Monitor BMD in patients with history of pathologic bone fracture or are at risk for osteopenia.

ADVERSE REACTIONS: Diarrhea, nausea, fatigue, depression, dizziness, rash, headache, insomnia, anxiety, hematuria, nasopharyngitis, laboratory abnormalities, lactic acidosis, severe hepatomegaly with steatosis.

INTERACTIONS: See Contraindications. Avoid with adefovir dipivoxil, atazanavir, drugs containing same component or lamivudine, saquinavir (alone), posaconazole, or nephrotoxic agents. Potential additive CNS effects with alcohol or psychoactive drugs. May increase levels of didanosine and ritonavir. May decrease levels of amprenavir, lopinavir, saquinavir, sertraline, ketoconazole, itraconazole, clarithromycin, rifabutin, diltiazem or other calcium channel blockers, HMG-CoA reductase inhibitors (eg, atorvastatin, pravastatin, simvastatin), indinavir, maraviroc, anticonvulsants, norelgestromin, levonorgestrel, etonogestrel, immunosuppressants, and methadone. May alter levels of warfarin and substrates of CYP2C9, 2C19, and 3A4. Efavirenz: CYP3A inhibitors or inducers may alter levels. Ritonavir may increase levels. Anticonvulsants and rifampin may decrease levels. TDF/Emtricitabine: Drugs that reduce renal function or compete for active tubular secretion (eg, acyclovir, cidofovir, ganciclovir, valacyclovir, valganciclovir) may increase levels. Lopinavir/ritonavir may increase TDF levels.

PREGNANCY: Category D, not for use in nursing.

MECHANISM OF ACTION: Efavirenz: Non-nucleoside reverse transcriptase inhibitor; noncompetitive inhibition of HIV-1 reverse transcriptase (RT). Emtricitabine: Nucleoside analogue of cytidine; inhibits activity of HIV-1 RT by competing with natural substrate deoxycytidine 5'-triphosphate and incorporating into nascent viral DNA, resulting in chain termination. TDF: Acyclic nucleoside phosphonate diester analogue of adenosine monophosphate; inhibits activity of HIV-1 RT by competing with the natural substrate deoxyadenosine 5'-triphosphate and, after incorporation into the DNA, by DNA chain termination.

PHARMACOKINETICS: Absorption: Efavirenz: C_{max}=12.9μM, T_{max}=3-5 hrs, AUC=184μM•hr. Emtricitabine: Rapid; absolute bioavailability (93%), C_{max}=1.8μg/mL, T_{max}=1-2 hrs, AUC=10μg•hr/mL. TDF: C_{max}=296ng/mL, T_{max}=1 hr, AUC=2287ng•hr/mL, bioavailability (25%). **Distribution:** Efavirenz: Plasma protein binding (99.5-99.75%). Emtricitabine: Plasma protein binding (<4%). TDF: Plasma protein binding (<0.7%). **Metabolism:** Efavirenz: Via CYP3A and CYP2B6. Emtricitabine: (metabolites) 3'-sulfoxide diastereomers; glucuronic acid conjugate. **Elimination:** Efavirenz: Urine (14-34%, mostly metabolites; <1% unchanged), feces (16-61%, mostly unchanged); $T_{1/2}$=52-76 hrs (single dose), 40-55 hrs (multiple doses). Emtricitabine: Urine (86%, 13% metabolites); $T_{1/2}$=10 hrs. TDF: Urine (IV, 70-80% unchanged); $T_{1/2}$=17 hrs.

NURSING CONSIDERATIONS

Assessment: Assess for obesity, prolonged nucleoside exposure, liver dysfunction or risk factors for liver disease, renal impairment, HBV or HCV infection, psychiatric history, history of injection drug use or seizures, hypersensitivity, pregnancy/nursing status, and possible drug interactions. Assess BMD in patients with a history of pathological bone fracture or those at risk for osteopenia. Obtain baseline LFTs, CrCl, serum phosphorus levels, total cholesterol, and TG levels.

Monitoring: Monitor for signs/symptoms of lactic acidosis, severe hepatomegaly with steatosis, psychiatric/nervous system symptoms, new onset/worsening renal impairment, skin rash, decreases in BMD, convulsions, immune reconstitution syndrome (eg, opportunistic infections), and fat redistribution/accumulation. Monitor for acute exacerbations of hepatitis B in patients with coinfection upon d/c of therapy. Monitor CD4+ cell count, HIV-1 RNA levels, LFTs, CrCl, serum phosphorus, total cholesterol, and TG levels. Monitor didanosine-associated adverse effects, anticonvulsants and immunosuppressant levels.

Patient Counseling: Inform that therapy is not a cure for HIV-1, does not reduce transmission of HIV-1, and illnesses associated with HIV-1 may still be experienced. Advise to practice safer sex, use latex or polyurethane condoms, and never to reuse or share needles. Instruct to take on an empty stomach and on a regular dosing schedule. Instruct to contact physician if nausea, vomiting, unusual stomach discomfort, weakness, aggressive behavior, depression, suicide attempts, delusions, paranoia, dizziness, insomnia, impaired concentration, drowsiness, abnormal dreams, or skin rash develops. Advise that fat redistribution/accumulation and decreases in bone mineral density may occur. Counsel to avoid pregnancy while on therapy and up to 12 weeks after d/c; instruct that barrier contraception must always be used in combination with other methods of contraception. Advise to avoid potentially hazardous tasks (eg, driving, operating machinery) if experiencing CNS/psychiatric symptoms or taking alcohol or psychoactive drugs. Advise that severe acute exacerbation of hepatitis B may occur if coinfected. Advise to report use of any prescription, nonprescription medication, or herbal products, particularly St. John's wort.

Administration: Oral route. Take on an empty stomach. **Storage:** 25°C (77°F); excursions permitted to 15-30°C (59-86°F).

ATROVENT HFA   RX
ipratropium bromide (Boehringer Ingelheim)

THERAPEUTIC CLASS: Anticholinergic bronchodilator

INDICATIONS: Maintenance treatment of bronchospasm associated with chronic obstructive pulmonary disease (COPD), including chronic bronchitis and emphysema.

DOSAGE: *Adults:* Initial: 2 inh qid. Max: 12 inh/24 hrs.

HOW SUPPLIED: MDI: 17mcg/inh [12.9g]

CONTRAINDICATIONS: Hypersensitivity to atropine or its derivatives.

WARNINGS/PRECAUTIONS: Not for acute episodes. Immediate hypersensitivity reactions reported. Can produce paradoxical bronchospasm. Caution with narrow-angle glaucoma, prostatic hyperplasia or bladder-neck obstruction.

ADVERSE REACTIONS: Back pain, bronchitis, dyspnea, dizziness, headache, nausea, blurred vision, dry mouth, exacerbation of symptoms.

INTERACTIONS: Avoid coadministration with other anticholinergic-containing drugs.

PREGNANCY: Category B, caution in nursing.

MECHANISM OF ACTION: Anticholinergic; inhibits vagally-mediated reflexes by antagonizing the action of acetylcholine.

PHARMACOKINETICS: Absorption: (4 inh) C_{max}=59pg/mL. **Distribution:** Plasma protein binding (0-9%). **Metabolism:** Partial. **Elimination:** $T_{1/2}$=2 hrs.

NURSING CONSIDERATIONS

Assessment: Assess for hypersensitivity to atropine or its derivatives, narrow-angle glaucoma, prostatic hyperplasia, bladder-neck obstruction, pregnancy/nursing status, and possible drug interactions.

Monitoring: Monitor for urinary retention, mydriasis, GI distress (diarrhea, N/V), paradoxical bronchospasm, and allergic type-reaction (pruritus, angioedema of tongue, lips and face, urticaria, laryngospasm, anaphylaxis).

Patient Counseling: Remind patients to read the Patient Instructions for Use. Advise not to increase the dose or frequency. Not for acute episodes of bronchospasm. Avoid spraying in the eyes. Inform patient that paradoxical bronchospasm, which can be life-threatening, can occur; if occurs d/c use. Seek medical attention if symptoms of precipitation or worsening of narrow-angle glaucoma, mydriasis, increased intraocular pressure, acute eye pain/discomfort, blurring of vision, visual halos or colored images with red eyes from conjunctival and corneal congestion, or allergic/hypersensitivity reactions occur. Contact physician if difficulty in urinating occurs. Instruct patient that priming the medication is essential to ensure proper dosing.

Administration: Oral inhalation. Prime medication before first use with 2 sprays. If not used for >3 days, reprime with 2 sprays. **Storage:** 25°C (77°F); excursions permitted to 15-30°C (59-86°F). Do not puncture, use or store near heat or open flame.

ATROVENT NASAL RX
ipratropium bromide (Boehringer Ingelheim)

THERAPEUTIC CLASS: Anticholinergic

INDICATIONS: (0.03%) Symptomatic relief of rhinorrhea associated with allergic and nonallergic perennial rhinitis in adults and children ≥6 yrs. (0.06%) Symptomatic relief of rhinorrhea associated with the common cold or seasonal allergic rhinitis in adults and children ≥5 yrs.

DOSAGE: *Adults:* (0.03%) Rhinorrhea with Allergic/Nonallergic Perennial Rhinitis: 2 sprays/nostril bid-tid. (0.06%) Rhinorrhea Associated with Common Cold: 2 sprays/nostril tid-qid for ≤4 days. Rhinorrhea Associated with Seasonal Allergic Rhinitis: 2 sprays/nostril qid for ≤3 weeks. *Pediatrics:* (0.03%) ≥6 yrs: Rhinorrhea with Allergic/Nonallergic Perennial Rhinitis: 2 sprays/nostril bid-tid. (0.06%) Rhinorrhea Associated with Common Cold: ≥12 yrs: 2 sprays/nostril tid-qid for ≤4 days. 5-11 yrs: 2 sprays/nostril tid for ≤4 days. ≥5 yrs: Rhinorrhea Associated with Seasonal Allergic Rhinitis: 2 sprays/nostril qid for ≤3 weeks.

HOW SUPPLIED: Spray: (0.03%) 21mcg/spray [31.1g], (0.06%) 42mcg/spray [16.6g]

CONTRAINDICATIONS: Hypersensitivity to atropine or its derivatives.

WARNINGS/PRECAUTIONS: Immediate hypersensitivity reactions reported; d/c at once if reaction occurs and consider alternative treatment. Caution with narrow-angle glaucoma, prostatic hyperplasia, or bladder-neck obstruction, and hepatic or renal insufficiency.

ADVERSE REACTIONS: Epistaxis, pharyngitis, upper respiratory tract infection, nasal dryness, dry mouth/throat, headache, taste perversion.

INTERACTIONS: May produce additive effects with other anticholinergic agents.

PREGNANCY: Category B, caution in nursing.

MECHANISM OF ACTION: Anticholinergic; inhibits vagally-mediated reflexes by antagonizing action of acetylcholine at the cholinergic receptor. Inhibits secretions from serous and seromucous glands lining the nasal mucosa.

PHARMACOKINETICS: Absorption: Bioavailability (<20%). **Distribution:** Plasma protein binding (0-9%). **Metabolism:** Partial; ester hydrolysis products, tropic acid, tropane. **Elimination:** Urine (half of administered dose, unchanged). (IV) $T_{1/2}$=1.6 hrs.

NURSING CONSIDERATIONS

Assessment: Assess for hypersensitivity to atropine or its derivatives, narrow-angle glaucoma, prostatic hyperplasia, bladder-neck obstruction, hepatic/renal insufficiency, pregnancy/nursing status, and possible drug interactions.

Monitoring: Monitor for signs and symptoms of hypersensitivity reactions (eg, urticaria, angioedema, rash, bronchospasm, anaphylaxis, oropharyngeal edema). Monitor visual changes and nasal symptoms.

Patient Counseling: Advise not to alter size of nasal spray opening. Instruct to avoid spraying medication into the eyes. Inform that temporary blurring of vision, precipitation or worsening of narrow-angle glaucoma, mydriasis, increased intraocular pressure, acute eye pain or discomfort, visual halos or colored images in association with red eyes from conjunctival and corneal congestion may occur if medication comes into direct contact with the eyes. Instruct to contact physician if eye pain, blurred vision, excessive nasal dryness, or episodes of nasal bleeding occurs. Caution about engaging in activities requiring balance and visual acuity (eg, driving or operating machines).

Administration: Intranasal route. Prime the nasal spray pump and blow nose to clear nostrils before first use. Refer to PI for proper administration. **Storage:** 25°C (77°F); excursions permitted to 15-30°C (59-86°F). Avoid freezing.

AUGMENTIN RX
clavulanate potassium - amoxicillin (Dr. Reddy's)

THERAPEUTIC CLASS: Aminopenicillin/beta lactamase inhibitor

INDICATIONS: Treatment of lower respiratory tract (LRTI), skin and skin structure, urinary tract infections, otitis media (OM), and sinusitis caused by susceptible strains of microorganisms.

DOSAGE: *Adults:* (Dose based on amoxicillin) Usual: One 500mg tab q12h or one 250mg tab q8h. Severe/Respiratory Tract Infections: One 875mg tab q12h or one 500mg tab q8h. May use 125mg/5mL or 250mg/5mL sus in place of 500mg tab and 200mg/5mL or 400mg/5mL sus in place of 875mg tab. CrCl <30mL/min: Do not give 875mg tab. CrCl 10-30mL/min: 500mg or 250mg q12h. CrCl <10mL/min: 500mg or 250mg q24h. Hemodialysis: 500mg or 250mg q24h; give additional dose during and at end of dialysis.
Pediatrics: (Dose based on amoxicillin) ≥40kg: Use adult dose. ≥12 Weeks: Sinusitis/OM/LRTI/Severe Infections: (Sus/Tab, Chewable) 45mg/kg/day q12h or 40mg/kg/day q8h. Treat OM for 10 days. Less Severe Infections: 25mg/kg/day q12h or 20mg/kg/day q8h. <12 Weeks: 30mg/kg/day divided q12h (use 125mg/5mL sus).

HOW SUPPLIED: (Amoxicillin-Clavulanic acid) Sus: 125-31.25mg/5mL, 250-62.5mg/5mL [75mL, 100mL, 150mL], 200-28.5mg/5mL, 400-57mg/5mL [50mL, 75mL, 100mL]; Tab: 250-125mg, 500-125mg, 875-125mg*; Tab, Chewable: 125-31.25mg, 200-28.5mg, 250-62.5mg, 400-57mg *scored

CONTRAINDICATIONS: History of penicillin (PCN) allergy or amoxicillin clavulanate-associated cholestatic jaundice/hepatic dysfunction.

WARNINGS/PRECAUTIONS: Serious, occasionally fatal, hypersensitivity reactions reported with PCN therapy; d/c if allergic reaction occurs and institute appropriate therapy. *Clostridium difficile*-associated diarrhea (CDAD) reported. Caution with hepatic dysfunction. Monitor renal, hepatic, and hematopoietic functions with prolonged use. May result in bacterial resistance with prolonged use or use in the absence of a proven/suspected bacterial infection or a prophylactic indication; take appropriate measures if superinfection develops. Avoid with mononucleosis. May decrease estrogen levels in pregnant women. Lab test interactions may occur. The 200mg and 400mg chewable tabs and 200mg/5mL and 400mg/5mL sus contain phenylalanine; avoid with phenylketonurics. The 250mg tab and chewable tab are not interchangeable due to unequal clavulanic acid amounts. Do not substitute two 250mg tab for one 500mg tab. (Tab) Caution in elderly.

ADVERSE REACTIONS: Diarrhea/loose stools, N/V, skin rashes, urticaria, vaginitis.

INTERACTIONS: Probenecid may increase levels; coadministration not recommended. Increased PT reported with anticoagulants; may require oral anticoagulant dose adjustment. Allopurinol may increase incidence of rashes. May reduce efficacy of oral contraceptives.

PREGNANCY: Category B, caution in nursing.

MECHANISM OF ACTION: Amoxicillin: Aminopenicillin; semisynthetic antibiotic with broad spectrum of bactericidal activity against gram-positive and gram-negative organisms. Clavulanate: β-lactamase inhibitor; possesses ability to inactivate a wide range of β-lactamase enzymes commonly found in microorganisms resistant to PCN and cephalosporins.

PHARMACOKINETICS: Absorption: Well absorbed. Refer to PI for absorption parameters. **Distribution:** Plasma protein binding: Amoxicillin (18%), clavulanate (25%). Amoxicillin: Found in breast milk. **Elimination:** Amoxicillin: Urine (50-70% unchanged); $T_{1/2}$=1.3 hrs. Clavulanate: Urine (25-40% unchanged); $T_{1/2}$=1 hr.

NURSING CONSIDERATIONS

Assessment: Assess for history of allergic reactions to PCNs, cephalosporins or other allergens, cholestatic jaundice, and hepatic/renal impairment. Assess for infectious mononucleosis, phenylketonuria, pregnancy/nursing status, and possible drug interactions.

Monitoring: Periodically monitor renal, hepatic, and hematopoietic organ functions with prolonged use. Monitor for anaphylactic reactions, development of superinfection, skin rash, and CDAD. Monitor for transient decrease in plasma concentration of total conjugated estriol, estriol-glucuronide, conjugated estrone, and estradiol if given to pregnant women.

Patient Counseling: Instruct to take q8h or q12h with a meal or snack to reduce possibility of GI upset. Advise to consult physician if severe diarrhea or watery/bloody stools occur (even as late as ≥2 months after treatment). Instruct to take ud; skipping doses or not completing the full course of therapy may decrease effectiveness of the drug and increase resistance of bacteria. Instruct to use a dosing spoon or medicine dropper when dosing a child with sus, and rinse them after each use. Instruct to discard any unused medicine. Instruct to shake sus bottle well before each use.

Administration: Oral route. Take at the start of a meal. (Sus) Refer to PI for mixing directions. Shake well before use. **Storage:** ≤25°C (77°F). Refrigerate reconstituted sus; discard after 10 days.

AUGMENTIN ES-600 RX
clavulanate potassium - amoxicillin (Dr. Reddy's)

THERAPEUTIC CLASS: Aminopenicillin/beta lactamase inhibitor

INDICATIONS: Treatment of pediatrics with recurrent or persistent acute otitis media due to susceptible strains of microorganisms.

DOSAGE: *Pediatrics:* ≥3 months (<40kg): (Dose based on amoxicillin) 90mg/kg/day divided q12h for 10 days.

HOW SUPPLIED: Sus: (Amoxicillin-Clavulanic acid) 600mg-42.9mg/5mL [75mL, 125mL, 200mL]

CONTRAINDICATIONS: History of penicillin (PCN) allergy or amoxicillin clavulanate-associated cholestatic jaundice/hepatic dysfunction.

WARNINGS/PRECAUTIONS: Serious, occasionally fatal, hypersensitivity reactions reported with PCN therapy; d/c if allergic reaction occurs and institute appropriate therapy. Pseudomembranous colitis/*Clostridium difficile*-associated diarrhea reported. Caution with hepatic dysfunction. Monitor renal, hepatic, and hematopoietic functions with prolonged use. May result in bacterial resistance with prolonged use or use in the absence of a proven/suspected bacterial infection or a prophylactic indication; take appropriate measures if superinfection develops. Avoid with mononucleosis. Contains phenylalanine. May decrease estrogen levels in pregnant women. Lab test interactions may occur. Do not substitute 200mg/5mL and 400mg/5mL Augmentin sus for Augmentin ES-600.

ADVERSE REACTIONS: Contact dermatitis (diaper rash), diarrhea, vomiting, moniliasis, rash.

INTERACTIONS: Probenecid may increase levels; coadmistration not recommended. Increased PT reported with anticoagulants; may require oral anticoagulant dose adjustment. Allopurinol may increase incidence of rashes. May reduce efficacy of oral contraceptives.

PREGNANCY: Category B, caution in nursing.

MECHANISM OF ACTION: Amoxicillin: Aminopenicillin; semisynthetic antibiotic with broad spectrum of bactericidal activity against gram-positive and gram-negative organisms. Clavulanate: β-lactamase inhibitor; possesses ability to inactivate a wide range of β-lactamase enzymes commonly found in microorganisms resistant to PCN and cephalosporins.

PHARMACOKINETICS: Absorption: Amoxicillin: C_{max}=15.7mcg/mL, T_{max}=2 hrs; AUC=59.8mcg•hr/mL. Clavulanate: C_{max}=1.7mcg/mL, T_{max}=1.1 hrs; AUC=4.0mcg•hr/mL. **Distribution:** Plasma protein binding: Amoxicillin (18%), clavulanate (25%). Amoxicillin: Found in breast milk. **Elimination:** Amoxicillin: Urine (50-70% unchanged); $T_{1/2}$=1.4 hrs. Clavulanate: Urine (25-40% unchanged); $T_{1/2}$=1.1 hrs.

NURSING CONSIDERATIONS

Assessment: Assess for history of allergic reactions to PCNs, cephalosporins or other allergens, cholestatic jaundice, and hepatic dysfunction. Assess for infectious mononucleosis, phenylketonuria, pregnancy/nursing status, and possible drug interactions.

Monitoring: Periodically monitor renal, hepatic, and hematopoietic organ functions with prolonged use. Monitor for anaphylactic reactions, development of superinfection, skin rash, and pseudomembranous colitis. Monitor for transient decrease in plasma concentration of total conjugated estriol, estriol-glucuronide, conjugated estrone, and estradiol if given to pregnant women.

Patient Counseling: Instruct to take q12h with a meal or snack to reduce possibility of GI upset. Advise to consult physician if severe diarrhea or watery/bloody stools occur (even as late as ≥2 months after treatment). Instruct to take ud; skipping doses or not completing the full course of therapy may decrease effectiveness of the drug and increase resistance of bacteria. Instruct to use a dosing spoon or medicine dropper when dosing, and rinse them after each use. Instruct to discard any unused medicine. Instruct to shake sus bottle well before each use.

Administration: Oral route. Take at the start of a meal. Refer to PI for mixing directions. Shake well before use. **Storage:** ≤25°C (77°F). Refrigerate reconstituted sus; discard after 10 days.

AUGMENTIN XR   RX
clavulanate potassium - amoxicillin (Dr. Reddy's)

THERAPEUTIC CLASS: Aminopenicillin/beta lactamase inhibitor

INDICATIONS: Treatment of community-acquired pneumonia (CAP) or acute bacterial sinusitis due to confirmed or suspected β-lactamase-producing pathogens and *Streptococcus pneumoniae* with reduced susceptibility to penicillin (PCN).

DOSAGE: *Adults:* Sinusitis: 2 tabs q12h for 10 days. CAP: 2 tabs q12h for 7-10 days. Take at the start of a meal.
Pediatrics: ≥40kg (Able to swallow tab): Sinusitis: 2 tabs q12h for 10 days. CAP: 2 tabs q12h for 7-10 days. Take at the start of a meal.

HOW SUPPLIED: Tab, Extended-Release: (Amoxicillin-Clavulanic Acid) 1000mg-62.5mg*
*scored

CONTRAINDICATIONS: Severe renal impairment (CrCl <30mL/min), hemodialysis, history of PCN allergy or amoxicillin clavulanate-associated cholestatic jaundice/hepatic dysfunction.

WARNINGS/PRECAUTIONS: Serious, occasionally fatal, hypersensitivity reactions reported with PCN therapy; d/c if allergic reaction occurs and institute appropriate therapy. *Clostridium difficile*-associated diarrhea (CDAD) reported. Caution with hepatic dysfunction. Monitor renal, hepatic, and hematopoietic functions with prolonged use. Avoid with mononucleosis. May result in bacterial resistance with prolonged use or use in the absence of a proven/suspected bacterial infection or a prophylactic indication; take appropriate measures if superinfection develops. May decrease estrogen levels in pregnant women. Lab test interactions may occur.

ADVERSE REACTIONS: Diarrhea, vaginal mycosis, nausea, loose stools.

INTERACTIONS: Probenecid may increase levels; coadministration not recommended. Increased PT/INR reported with oral anticoagulants; may require anticoagulant dose adjustment. Allopurinol may increase incidence of rashes. May reduce efficacy of oral contraceptives.

PREGNANCY: Category B, caution in nursing.

MECHANISM OF ACTION: Amoxicillin: Aminopenicillin; semisynthetic antibiotic with broad spectrum of bactericidal activity against gram-positive and gram-negative organisms. Clavulanate: β-lactamase inhibitor; possesses ability to inactivate a wide range of β-lactamase enzymes commonly found in microorganisms resistant to PCN and cephalosporins.

PHARMACOKINETICS: Absorption: Well-absorbed. Refer to PI for absorption parameters in adults and pediatrics. **Distribution:** Plasma protein binding: Amoxicillin (18%), clavulanate (25%). Amoxicillin: Found in breast milk. **Elimination:** Amoxicillin: Urine (60-80% unchanged); $T_{1/2}$=1.3 hrs. Clavulanate: Urine (30-50% unchanged); $T_{1/2}$=1.0 hrs.

NURSING CONSIDERATIONS

Assessment: Assess for history of allergic reactions to PCNs, cephalosporins or other allergens, cholestatic jaundice, and hepatic/renal impairment. Assess for infectious mononucleosis, pregnancy/nursing status, and possible drug interactions.

Monitoring: Periodically monitor renal, hepatic, and hematopoietic organ functions with prolonged use. Monitor for anaphylactic reactions, hepatic toxicity, cholestatic jaundice, development of superinfection, skin rash, diarrhea, and pseudomembranous colitis/CDAD. Monitor for transient decrease in plasma concentration of total conjugated estriol, estriol-glucuronide, conjugated estrone, and estradiol if given to pregnant women.

Patient Counseling: Instruct to take q12h with a meal or snack to reduce possibility of GI upset. Advise to consult physician if severe diarrhea or watery/bloody stools occur (even as late as ≥2 months after treatment). Instruct to take ud; skipping doses or not completing the full course of therapy may decrease effectiveness of the drug and increase resistance of bacteria. Instruct to discard any unused medicine.

Administration: Oral route. Take at the start of a meal. **Storage:** ≤25°C (77°F).

AVALIDE

RX

irbesartan - hydrochlorothiazide (Sanofi-Aventis)

> **D/C when pregnancy is detected. Drugs that act directly on the renin-angiotensin system can cause injury/death to the developing fetus.**

THERAPEUTIC CLASS: Angiotensin II receptor antagonist/thiazide diuretic

INDICATIONS: Treatment of HTN. May be used in patients whose BP is not adequately controlled on monotherapy. May also be used as initial therapy in patients likely to need multiple drugs to achieve BP goals.

DOSAGE: *Adults:* Initial Therapy: 150mg-12.5mg qd. Titrate: May increase after 1-2 weeks of therapy. Max: 300mg-25mg qd. Add-On Therapy: Use if not controlled on monotherapy with irbesartan or HCTZ. Recommended doses in order of increasing mean effect are 150mg-12.5mg, 300mg-12.5mg, and 300mg-25mg. Replacement Therapy: May substitute for titrated components.

HOW SUPPLIED: Tab: (Irbesartan-HCTZ) 150mg-12.5mg, 300mg-12.5mg

CONTRAINDICATIONS: Anuria, sulfonamide-derived drug hypersensitivity.

WARNINGS/PRECAUTIONS: Not for initial therapy with intravascular volume depletion. Not recommended with severe renal impairment (CrCl ≤30mL/min). Symptomatic hypotension may occur in intravascular volume- or Na^+-depleted patients; correct volume depletion before therapy. Hypokalemia and hyperkalemia reported; monitor serum electrolytes periodically. Irbesartan: May increase BUN and SrCr levels with renal artery stenosis. Oliguria and/or progressive azotemia, and (rarely) acute renal failure and/or death may occur in patients whose renal function is dependent on the renin-angiotensin-aldosterone system activity (eg, severe congestive heart failure [CHF]). HCTZ: May cause hypersensitivity reactions, exacerbation or activation of systemic lupus erythematosus (SLE), hyponatremia, hypomagnesemia, and hyperuricemia or precipitation of frank gout. May alter glucose tolerance and increase cholesterol, TG, and calcium levels. D/C before testing for parathyroid function. May cause idiosyncratic reaction, resulting in transient myopia and acute angle-closure glaucoma; d/c as rapidly as possible. Enhanced effects in postsympathectomy patients. Caution with hepatic impairment or progressive liver disease; may precipitate hepatic coma. May precipitate azotemia with renal disease.

ADVERSE REACTIONS: Dizziness, hypokalemia, fatigue, musculoskeletal pain, influenza, edema, N/V, headache.

INTERACTIONS: NSAIDs, including selective cyclooxygenase-2 inhibitors, may decrease effects of diuretics and angiotensin II receptor antagonists and may further deteriorate renal function. HCTZ: Alcohol, barbiturates, and narcotics may potentiate orthostatic hypotension. Antidiabetic drugs (eg, oral agents, insulin) may require dosage adjustment. Anionic exchange resins (eg, cholestyramine or colestipol) may impair absorption; take at least 1 hr before or 4 hrs after these medications. Additive effect or potentiation with other antihypertensive drugs. Corticosteroids and adrenocorticotropic hormone may intensify electrolyte depletion, particularly hypokalemia. May decrease response to pressor amines (eg, norepinephrine). May increase responsiveness to nondepolarizing skeletal muscle relaxants (eg, tubocurarine). Increased risk of lithium toxicity; avoid concurrent use. Risk of symptomatic hyponatremia with carbamazepine; monitor serum electrolytes. Irbesartan: May increase serum K^+ with K^+-sparing diuretics, K^+ supplements, or salt substitutes containing K^+.

PREGNANCY: Category D, not for use in nursing.

MECHANISM OF ACTION: Irbesartan: Angiotensin II receptor antagonist; blocks the vasoconstrictor and aldosterone-secreting effects of angiotensin II by selectively binding to the AT_1 angiotensin II receptor. HCTZ: Thiazide diuretic; not established. Affects renal tubular mechanisms of electrolyte reabsorption, directly increasing Na^+ and chloride excretion in approximately equivalent amounts, and indirectly reducing plasma volume.

PHARMACOKINETICS: Absorption: Irbesartan: Rapid and complete. Absolute bioavailability (60-80%); T_{max}=1.5-2 hrs. **Distribution:** Irbesartan: V_d=53-93L; plasma protein binding (90%). HCTZ: Crosses placenta; found in breast milk. **Metabolism:** Irbesartan: CYP2C9 (oxidation), glucuronide conjugation. **Elimination:** Irbesartan: Urine (20%), feces; $T_{1/2}$=11-15 hrs. HCTZ: Kidney (≥61% unchanged); $T_{1/2}$=5.6-14.8 hrs.

NURSING CONSIDERATIONS

Assessment: Assess for hypersensitivity to drugs and its components, anuria, sulfonamide-derived drug hypersensitivity, history of penicillin allergy, volume/salt depletion, SLE, CHF, renal/hepatic function, postsympathectomy status, renal artery stenosis, pregnancy/nursing status, and possible drug interactions.

Monitoring: Monitor for hypersensitivity reactions, idiosyncratic reaction, decreased visual acuity, and ocular pain. Monitor BP, serum electrolytes (periodically), and hepatic/renal function.

Patient Counseling: Inform of potential risks if exposure occurs during pregnancy and of treatment options in women planning to become pregnant. Instruct to report pregnancies to physician as soon as possible. Inform that lightheadedness may occur, especially during 1st days of use; d/c and contact physician if fainting occurs. Inform that dehydration, which may occur with excessive sweating, diarrhea, vomiting, and not drinking enough liquids, may lower BP too much and lead to lightheadedness and possibly fainting.

Administration: Oral route. **Storage:** 25°C (77°F); excursions permitted to 15-30°C (59-86°F).

AVANDAMET   RX
metformin HCl - rosiglitazone maleate (GlaxoSmithKline)

Thiazolidinediones cause or exacerbate congestive heart failure (CHF) in some patients. After initiation and dose increases, observe for signs and symptoms of heart failure (HF) and manage accordingly; consider d/c or dose reduction. Not recommended in patients with symptomatic HF. Contraindicated with established New York Heart Association (NYHA) Class III or IV HF. Meta-analysis showed association with increased risk of myocardial infarction (MI). Lactic acidosis reported due to metformin accumulation (rare); d/c if suspected. Available only through a restricted distribution program called AVANDIA-Rosiglitazone Medicines Access Program.

THERAPEUTIC CLASS: Thiazolidinedione/biguanide

INDICATIONS: Adjunct to diet and exercise to improve glycemic control when treatment with both rosiglitazone and metformin is appropriate in adults with type 2 diabetes mellitus (DM) already taking rosiglitazone, or not taking rosiglitazone and unable to achieve glycemic control on other diabetes medication and have decided not to take pioglitazone or pioglitazone-containing products upon consultation.

DOSAGE: *Adults:* Take in divided doses with meals. Initial: Take rosiglitazone component at lowest recommended dose. Switching From Prior Metformin Therapy of 1000mg/day: Initial: 2mg-500mg tab bid. Prior Metformin Therapy of 2000mg/day: Initial: 2mg-1000mg tab bid. Prior Rosiglitazone Therapy of 4mg/day: Initial: 2mg-500mg tab bid. Prior Rosiglitazone Therapy of 8mg/day: 4mg-500mg tab bid. Titrate: May increase by increments of 4mg rosiglitazone and/or 500mg metformin. After increasing metformin, titrate if inadequate after 1-2 weeks. After increasing rosiglitazone, titrate if inadequate after 8-12 weeks. Max: 8mg-2000mg/day. Elderly: Conservative dosing. Elderly/Debilitated/Malnourished: Do not titrate to max dose.

HOW SUPPLIED: Tab: (Rosiglitazone-Metformin) 2mg-500mg, 4mg-500mg, 2mg-1000mg, 4mg-1000mg

CONTRAINDICATIONS: Established NYHA Class III or IV HF, renal disease/dysfunction (SrCr ≥1.5mg/dL [males], ≥1.4mg/dL [females], or abnormal CrCl), acute or chronic metabolic acidosis (eg, diabetic ketoacidosis with or without coma). Temporarily d/c if undergoing radiologic studies involving IV administration of iodinated contrast materials.

WARNINGS/PRECAUTIONS: Initiation with patients experiencing acute coronary event is not recommended; consider d/c during the acute phase. Caution with edema and patients at risk for HF. Avoid with active liver disease or if ALT levels >2.5X ULN. May start or continue therapy with caution if ALT levels ≤2.5X ULN; monitor LFTs periodically. D/C if ALT levels remain >3X ULN or if jaundice occurs. Check LFTs if hepatic dysfunction symptoms occur. May lose glycemic control with stress; withhold therapy and temporarily administer insulin. Caution in elderly. (Metformin) Avoid use in patients ≥80 yrs unless renal function is normal. Elderly, debilitated/malnourished, with adrenal/pituitary insufficiency, or alcohol intoxication may have increased susceptibility to hypoglycemia. (Rosiglitazone) Increased risk of cardiovascular events with CHF NYHA Class I and II. Dose-related edema and weight gain reported. Macular edema reported; refer to an ophthalmologist if visual symptoms develop. Increased incidence of bone fracture; risk appears higher in females than males. May decrease Hgb and Hct. Decreased serum vitamin B12 levels reported. Ovulation in premenopausal anovulatory patients may occur, resulting in an increased risk of pregnancy; adequate contraception should be recommended. Review benefits of continued therapy if menstrual dysfunction occurs.

ADVERSE REACTIONS: CHF, lactic acidosis, upper respiratory tract infection, headache, back pain, fatigue, sinusitis, diarrhea, viral infection, arthralgia, anemia.

INTERACTIONS: See Contraindications. Avoid use with insulin. Metformin: Alcohol may potentiate effect on lactate metabolism. Caution with drugs that may affect renal function or result in significant hemodynamic change or may interfere with the disposition of metformin (eg, cationic drugs eliminated by renal tubular secretion). Hypoglycemia may occur with concomitant use of hypoglycemic agents (eg, sulfonylureas, insulin) or ethanol. May be difficult to recognize hypoglycemia with concomitant use of β-adrenergic blocking drugs. Increased levels with furosemide, nifedipine, cimetidine, and cationic drugs (eg, digoxin, amiloride, procainamide, quinidine, etc.). Observe for loss of glycemic control with thiazides and other diuretics, corticosteroids, phenothiazines, thyroid products, estrogens, oral contraceptives, phenytoin, nicotinic acid, sympathomimetics, calcium channel blockers, and isoniazid. May decrease furosemide levels. Rosiglitazone: Higher incidence of MI with ramipril. Dose-related weight gain and risk of hypoglycemia with other hypoglycemic agents. Increased levels with CYP2C8 inhibitors (eg, gemfibrozil). Decreased levels with CYP2C8 inducers (eg, rifampin).

PREGNANCY: Category C, not for use in nursing.

MECHANISM OF ACTION: Rosiglitazone: Thiazolidinedione; insulin-sensitizing agent that acts by enhancing peripheral glucose utilization. Metformin: Biguanide; decreases hepatic glucose production, decreases intestinal absorption of glucose, and increases peripheral glucose uptake and utilization.

PHARMACOKINETICS: Absorption: Rosiglitazone: Absolute bioavailability (99%). (4mg) $AUC_{0\text{-}inf}$=1442ng•h/mL; C_{max}=242ng/mL; T_{max}=0.95 hr. Metformin: (500mg) Absolute bioavailability (50-60%) (fasted); $AUC_{0\text{-}inf}$=7116ng•h/mL; C_{max}=1106ng/mL; T_{max}=2.97 hrs. **Distribution:** Rosiglitazone: V_d=17.6L; plasma protein binding (99.8%); crosses the placenta. Metformin: (850mg) V_d=654L. **Metabolism:** Rosiglitazone: Extensive by N-demethylation and hydroxylation, then conjugation with sulfate and glucuronic acid; CYP2C8 (major), 2C9 (minor). **Elimination:** Rosiglitazone: Urine (64%), feces (23%); $T_{1/2}$=3-4 hrs. Metformin: Urine (90%); $T_{1/2}$=6.2 hrs (plasma), 17.6 hrs (blood).

NURSING CONSIDERATIONS

Assessment: Assess for renal/hepatic function, CHF, hypoxemia, dehydration, active liver disease, acute coronary event, edema, risk factors for HF, pregnancy/nursing status, and possible drug interactions. Obtain baseline FPG, HbA1c, renal function, LFTs, and hematological parameters.

Monitoring: Monitor for signs/symptoms of lactic acidosis, HF, MI, acute coronary event, edema, weight gain, hepatic function, macular edema, bone fractures, hematologic changes, hypoglycemia, menstrual function. Monitor renal function, especially in elderly, at least annually. Monitor vitamin B12 levels in patients predisposed to develop subnormal vitamin B12 levels. Periodically monitor LFTs, FPG, HbA1c, CBC, bone health, and hematologic parameters. Perform periodic eye exams in DM.

Patient Counseling: Inform about benefits/risks of therapy and must be enrolled in the AVANDIA-Rosiglitazone Medicines Access Program. Inform on importance of adherence to dietary instructions and regular testing of blood glucose, HbA1c, renal function, and hematologic parameters. Advise to d/c and notify physician if unexplained hyperventilation, myalgia, malaise, unusual somnolence, or nonspecific symptoms occur. Immediately report rapid increase in weight or edema, or SOB to physician and to avoid excessive alcohol intake. Inform that the drug is not recommended with symptomatic HF and patients taking insulin.

Administration: Oral route. **Storage:** 25°C (77°F); excursions permitted to 15-30°C (59-86°F).

AVANDARYL RX
rosiglitazone maleate - glimepiride (GlaxoSmithKline)

> Thiazolidinediones cause or exacerbate congestive heart failure (CHF) in some patients. After initiation and dose increases, observe for signs and symptoms of heart failure (HF) and manage accordingly; consider d/c or dose reduction. Not recommended in patients with symptomatic HF. Contraindicated with established New York Heart Association (NYHA) Class III or IV HF. Meta-analysis has shown to be associated with increased risk of myocardial infarction (MI). Available only through a restricted distribution program called AVANDIA-Rosiglitazone Medicines Access Program.

THERAPEUTIC CLASS: Thiazolidinedione/sulfonylurea

INDICATIONS: Adjunct to diet and exercise to improve glycemic control when treatment with both rosiglitazone and glimepiride is appropriate in adults with type 2 diabetes mellitus (DM) already taking rosiglitazone or not taking rosiglitazone and unable to achieve glycemic control on other diabetes medication and have decided not to take pioglitazone or pioglitazone-containing products upon consultation.

DOSAGE: *Adults:* Initial: 4mg-1mg qd with 1st meal of day. Already Treated with Sulfonylurea or Rosiglitazone: Initial: 4mg-2mg qd. Switching from Prior Combination Therapy as Separate Tab: Start with dose of each component already being taken. Switching from Current Rosiglitazone Monotherapy: Increase glimepiride component in no >2mg increments if inadequately controlled after 1-2 weeks. After an increase in glimepiride component, titrate Avandaryl if inadequately controlled after 1-2 weeks. Switching from Current Sulfonylurea Monotherapy: Titrate rosiglitazone component if inadequately controlled after 8-12 weeks. After an increase in rosiglitazone component, titrate Avandaryl if inadequately controlled after 2-3 months. Max: 8mg-4mg/day. Elderly/Debilitated/Malnourished/Renal, Hepatic, or Adrenal Insufficiency: Initial: 4mg-1mg qd. Titrate carefully. Consider dose reduction of glimepiride component if hypoglycemia occurs during up-titration or maintenance.

HOW SUPPLIED: Tab: (Rosiglitazone-Glimepiride) 4mg-1mg, 4mg-2mg, 4mg-4mg, 8mg-2mg, 8mg-4mg

CONTRAINDICATIONS: Established NYHA Class III or IV HF.

WARNINGS/PRECAUTIONS: Avoid with active liver disease or if ALT levels >2.5X ULN. Caution with mildly elevated liver enzymes (ALT levels ≤2.5X ULN). D/C if ALT levels remain >3X ULN on therapy or if jaundice occurs. Check LFTs if hepatic dysfunction symptoms occur. May lose glycemic control with stress; withhold therapy and temporarily administer insulin. (Rosiglitazone) Increased risk of cardiovascular (CV) events with CHF NYHA Class I and II. Initiation with patients experiencing acute coronary event is not recommended; consider d/c during the acute phase. Caution with edema and patients at risk for HF. Edema and weight gain reported. Macular edema reported; refer to an ophthalmologist if visual symptoms develop. Increased incidence of bone fracture; risk appears higher in females than in males. May decrease Hgb and Hct. Ovulation in premenopausal anovulatory patients may occur, resulting in an increased risk of pregnancy; adequate contraception should be recommended. Review benefits of continued therapy if menstrual dysfunction occurs. (Glimepiride) Increased risk of CV mortality. Hypoglycemia may be masked in elderly; risk in debilitated, malnourished, or with adrenal, pituitary, renal or hepatic insufficiency. May elevate liver enzyme levels in rare cases. Hemolytic anemia reported; caution with G6PD deficiency.

ADVERSE REACTIONS: Headache, hypoglycemia, anemia. (Rosiglitazone) CHF, upper respiratory tract infection, nasopharyngitis, HTN, back pain, arthralgia. (Glimepiride) Dizziness, asthenia, nausea.

INTERACTIONS: Severe hypoglycemia with oral miconazole. Avoid use with insulin. Glimepiride: Hypoglycemia may be masked with β-blockers and other sympatholytic agents. Increased hypoglycemia risk with alcohol and use of >1 glucose-lowering drug. Observe for loss of glycemic control with thiazides and other diuretics, corticosteroids, phenothiazines, thyroid products, estrogens, oral contraceptives, phenytoin, nicotinic acid, sympathomimetics, and isoniazid. Hypoglycemic action may be potentiated by certain drugs, including NSAIDs and other drugs that are highly protein bound (eg, salicylates, sulfonamides, chloramphenicol, coumarins, probenecid, MAOIs, and β-blockers). Potential interactions with inhibitors (eg, fluconazole), inducers (eg, rifampicin), other drugs metabolized by CYP2C9 (eg, phenytoin, diclofenac, ibuprofen, naproxen, mefenamic acid). Changes in levels with aspirin and propranolol. Decrease in the pharmacodynamic response to warfarin. Rosiglitazone: Dose-related weight gain with other hypoglycemic agents. Higher incidence of MI with ramipril. Increased levels with CYP2C8 inhibitors (eg, gemfibrozil). Decreased levels with CYP2C8 inducers (eg, rifampin).

PREGNANCY: Category C, not for use in nursing.

MECHANISM OF ACTION: Glimepiride: Sulfonylurea; stimulates insulin release from functional pancreatic β cells. Rosiglitazone: Thiazolidinedione; insulin-sensitizing agent that acts by enhancing peripheral glucose utilization.

PHARMACOKINETICS: Absorption: Glimepiride: Complete; T_{max}=2-3 hrs; (4mg) C_{max}=151ng/mL; $AUC_{(0-inf, 0-t)}$=1052ng•hr/mL, 944ng•hr/mL. Rosiglitazone: Absolute bioavailability (99%); T_{max}=1 hr; (4mg) C_{max}=257ng/mL; $AUC_{(0-inf, 0-t)}$=1259ng•hr/mL, 1231ng•hr/mL. **Distribution:** Glimepiride: Protein binding (>99.5%). Rosiglitazone: V_d=17.6L; plasma protein binding (99.8%); crosses the placenta. **Metabolism:** Glimepiride: Liver (complete) via oxidative biotransformation; cyclohexyl hydroxy methyl (M1) and carboxyl (M2) derivative (major metabolites); CYP2C9. Rosiglitazone: Liver (extensive) via N-demethylation and hydroxylation then conjugation with sulfate and glucuronic acid; CYP2C8 (major), 2C9 (minor). **Elimination:** Glimepiride: Urine (60%, 80-90% major metabolites), feces (40%, 70% major metabolites). Rosiglitazone: Urine (64%), feces (23%); $T_{1/2}$=3-4 hrs.

NURSING CONSIDERATIONS

Assessment: Assess for HF, active liver disease, acute coronary event, edema, G6PD deficiency, premenopausal anovulation, risk factors for HF, pregnancy/nursing status, and for possible drug interactions. Assess baseline renal function, LFTs, CBC, and bone health.

Monitoring: Monitor for adverse events related to fluid retention during dose increases. Periodically monitor LFTs, FPG, HbA1c, CBC, and bone health. Monitor for signs and symptoms of HF, MI, acute coronary event, edema, weight gain, hepatic function, macular edema, bone fractures, hematologic changes, hypoglycemia, hypersensitivity reactions, ovulation in premenopausal anovulatory women, and menstrual function. Perform periodic eye exams. Monitor renal function in elderly.

Patient Counseling: Inform about benefits/risks of therapy and must be enrolled in the AVANDIA-Rosiglitazone Medicines Access Program. Inform about importance of caloric restrictions, weight loss, exercise, and regular testing of blood glucose levels. Advise to immediately report unexplained N/V, anorexia, abdominal pain, fatigue, dark urine, unusual rapid increase in weight or edema, SOB, or other symptoms of HF to physician. Instruct to take drug with 1st meal of the day. Explain to patients and their family members the risks, symptoms, treatment, and conditions that predispose to the development of hypoglycemia.

Administration: Oral route. **Storage:** 25°C (77°F); excursions permitted to 15-30°C (59-86°F).

AVANDIA RX
rosiglitazone maleate (GlaxoSmithKline)

Thiazolidinediones, including rosiglitazone, cause or exacerbate congestive heart failure (CHF) in some patients. After initiation and dose increases, observe for signs and symptoms of heart failure (HF) and manage accordingly; consider d/c or dose reduction. Not recommended in patients with symptomatic HF. Contraindicated with established New York Heart Association (NYHA) Class III or IV HF. Meta-analysis has shown to be associated with increased risk of myocardial infarction (MI). Available only through a restricted distribution program called AVANDIA-Rosiglitazone Medicines Access Program.

THERAPEUTIC CLASS: Thiazolidinedione

INDICATIONS: Adjunct to diet and exercise to improve glycemic control in adults with type 2 diabetes mellitus (DM) who either are already taking rosiglitazone or not already taking rosiglitazone and have inadequate glycemic control on other diabetes medications and have decided not to take pioglitazone upon consultation.

DOSAGE: *Adults:* Initial: 4mg as qd dose or in 2 divided doses. Titrate: May increase to 8mg/day after 8-12 weeks if response to treatment is inadequate. Max: 8mg/day.

HOW SUPPLIED: Tab: 2mg, 4mg, 8mg

CONTRAINDICATIONS: Established NYHA Class III or IV HF.

WARNINGS/PRECAUTIONS: Avoid with type 1 DM or diabetic ketoacidosis. Increased risk of cardiovascular events with CHF NYHA Class I and II. Initiation not recommended if experiencing an acute coronary event; consider d/c therapy during the acute phase. Caution with edema and patients at risk for HF. Edema and weight gain reported. Monitor LFTs prior to initiation of and during therapy. Avoid with active liver disease or if ALT levels >2.5X ULN. Caution if liver enzymes are mildly elevated (ALT levels ≤2.5X ULN). D/C if ALT levels remain >3X ULN while on therapy or if jaundice occurs. Check LFTs if hepatic dysfunction symptoms occur. Macular edema reported; refer to an ophthalmologist if visual symptoms develop. Increased incidence of bone fracture; risk appears higher in females than in males. Decreases in Hgb and Hct reported. Perform periodic measurements of FPG and HbA1c to monitor therapeutic response. May cause ovulation in premenopausal anovulatory patients resulting in an increased risk of pregnancy. Review benefits of continued therapy if menstrual dysfunction occurs.

ADVERSE REACTIONS: CHF, upper respiratory tract infection, headache, back pain, hyperglycemia, fatigue, sinusitis, edema.

INTERACTIONS: Risk of hypoglycemia when used with other hypoglycemic agents. May increase levels with CYP2C8 inhibitors (eg, gemfibrozil). May decrease levels with CYP2C8 inducers (eg, rifampin). Coadministration with insulin is not recommended; may increase risk of CHF and MI. Higher incidence of MI reported with ramipril.

PREGNANCY: Category C, not for use in nursing.

MECHANISM OF ACTION: Thiazolidinedione; improves insulin sensitivity.

PHARMACOKINETICS: Absorption: Administration of variable doses resulted in different parameters. Absolute bioavailability (99%); T_{max}=1 hr. **Distribution:** V_d=17.6L; plasma protein binding (99.8%); crosses the placenta. **Metabolism:** N-demethylation and hydroxylation followed by conjugation (extensive); CYP2C8 (major), 2C9 (minor). **Elimination:** Urine (64%), feces (23%); $T_{1/2}$=3-4 hrs.

NURSING CONSIDERATIONS

Assessment: Assess for CHF or risk factors for HF, symptomatic HF, type 1 DM, diabetic ketoacidosis, presence of an acute coronary event, hepatic dysfunction, edema, pregnancy/nursing status, and possible drug interactions. Assess baseline LFTs, CBC, and bone health.

Monitoring: Monitor for signs/symptoms of HF, MI, edema, weight gain, hepatic dysfunction, macular edema, bone fractures, hematologic changes, ovulation in premenopausal anovulatory women, and menstrual dysfunction. Perform periodic eye exams. Periodically monitor LFTs, fasting blood glucose, HbA1c, CBC and bone health.

Patient Counseling: Advise of risks and benefits of therapy. Inform that drug may be taken with or without food. Inform about importance of caloric restriction, weight loss, exercise, and regular testing of blood glucose levels. Instruct to immediately report to physician any symptoms of HF (eg, rapid increase in weight or edema, SOB) or hepatic dysfunction (eg, anorexia, N/V, dark urine, abdominal pain, fatigue). Inform about risk of hypoglycemia, its symptoms and treatment, and conditions that predispose to its development. Advise that ovulation may occur in some premenopausal anovulatory women and adequate contraception should be used.

Administration: Oral route. **Storage:** 25°C (77°F); excursions permitted to 15-30°C (59-86°F).

AVAPRO   RX

irbesartan (Sanofi-Aventis)

> D/C when pregnancy is detected. Drugs that act directly on the renin-angiotensin system can cause injury/death to developing fetus.

THERAPEUTIC CLASS: Angiotensin II receptor antagonist

INDICATIONS: Treatment of HTN alone or in combination with other antihypertensives. Treatment of diabetic nephropathy with an elevated SrCr and proteinuria (>300mg/day) in patients with type 2 diabetes and HTN.

DOSAGE: *Adults:* HTN: Initial: 150mg qd. Titrate: May increase to 300mg qd. A low dose diuretic may be added if BP is not controlled. Max: 300mg qd. Intravascular Volume/Salt Depletion: Initial: 75mg qd. Nephropathy: Maint: 300mg qd.

HOW SUPPLIED: Tab: 75mg, 150mg, 300mg

WARNINGS/PRECAUTIONS: Symptomatic hypotension may occur in volume- or salt-depleted patients (eg, patients treated vigorously with diuretics or on dialysis); correct volume depletion prior to therapy or use low starting dose. May cause changes in renal function. Oliguria and/or progressive azotemia and (rarely) acute renal failure and/or death may occur in patients whose renal function is dependent on the renin-angiotensin-aldosterone system (eg, severe congestive heart failure [CHF]). Increased SrCr or BUN may occur in patients with renal artery stenosis.

ADVERSE REACTIONS: Hyperkalemia, dizziness, orthostatic dizziness, orthostatic hypotension, fatigue, diarrhea, dyspepsia, heartburn.

INTERACTIONS: CYP2C9 substrates/inhibitors sulphenazole, tolbutamide, and nifedipine significantly inhibited metabolism in vitro. Increased serum K^+ with K^+-sparing diuretics, K^+ supplements, or salt substitutes containing K^+. May deteriorate renal function and attenuate antihypertensive effect with NSAIDs, including selective cyclooxygenase-2 inhibitors; monitor renal function periodically.

PREGNANCY: Category D, not for use in nursing.

MECHANISM OF ACTION: Angiotensin II receptor antagonist; blocks the vasoconstrictor and aldosterone-secreting effects of angiotensin II by selectively binding to the AT_1 angiotensin II receptor.

PHARMACOKINETICS: Absorption: Rapid and complete. Absolute bioavailability (60-80%); T_{max}=1.5-2 hrs. **Distribution:** V_d=53-93L; plasma protein binding (90%). **Metabolism:** CYP2C9 (oxidation), glucuronide conjugation. **Elimination:** Urine (20%), feces; $T_{1/2}$=11-15 hrs.

NURSING CONSIDERATIONS

Assessment: Assess for intravascular volume/salt depletion, renal impairment, CHF, renal artery stenosis, hypersensitivity, pregnancy/nursing status, and possible drug interactions.

Monitoring: Monitor for signs/symptoms of hypotension, hyperkalemia, and other adverse reactions. Monitor BP and renal function periodically.

Patient Counseling: Inform about the consequences of exposure during pregnancy in females of childbearing age. Discuss treatment options with women planning to become pregnant. Instruct to report pregnancies to physician as soon as possible.

Administration: Oral route. **Storage:** 25°C (77°F); excursions permitted to 15-30°C (59-86°F).

AVASTIN   RX

bevacizumab (Genentech)

> Increased incidences of wound healing and surgical complications; d/c at least 28 days prior to elective surgery. Do not initiate for at least 28 days after surgery and until surgical wound is fully healed. Severe or fatal hemorrhage, including hemoptysis, GI bleeding, CNS hemorrhage, epistaxis, and vaginal bleeding have occurred; avoid with serious hemorrhage or recent hemoptysis. D/C with GI perforation or wound dehiscence.

THERAPEUTIC CLASS: Vascular endothelial growth factor (VEGF) inhibitor

INDICATIONS: 1st- or 2nd-line treatment of metastatic colorectal cancer (mCRC) in combination with IV 5-fluorouracil (5-FU)-based chemotherapy. 1st-line treatment of unresectable, locally advanced, recurrent or metastatic non-squamous non-small cell lung cancer (NSCLC) in combination with carboplatin and paclitaxel. Treatment of glioblastoma with progressive disease in adults following prior therapy as a single agent. Treatment of metastatic renal cell carcinoma (mRCC), in combination with interferon alfa.

DOSAGE: *Adults:* Continue treatment until disease progression or unacceptable toxicity. mCRC: In Combination with 5-FU: Usual: 5mg/kg q2 weeks (with bolus-IFL) or 10mg/kg q2 weeks (with

FOLFOX4). NSCLC: Usual: 15mg/kg q3 weeks (with carboplatin and paclitaxel). Glioblastoma: Usual: 10mg/kg q2 weeks. mRCC: Usual: 10mg/kg q2 weeks (with interferon alfa).

HOW SUPPLIED: Inj: 25mg/mL [4mL, 16mL]

WARNINGS/PRECAUTIONS: Serious and fatal non-GI fistula formation (eg, in tracheo-esophageal, bronchopleural, biliary, vaginal, renal, and bladder sites), may occur. Arterial thromboembolic events (eg, cerebral infarction, transient ischemic attacks, myocardial infarction, angina) reported; increased risk with history of arterial thromboembolism, or age >65 yrs. Increased incidence of severe HTN; d/c if hypertensive crisis and hypertensive encephalopathy occurs. D/C if reversible posterior leukoencephalopathy syndrome develops. Monitor for the development or worsening of proteinuria with serial urinalyses by dipstick urine analysis. Suspend therapy if ≥2g proteinuria/24 hrs and resume when proteinuria is <2g/24 hrs. Infusion reactions (eg, HTN, hypertensive crisis with neurologic signs/symptoms, wheezing, oxygen desaturation, Grade 3 hypersensitivity, chest pain, headache, rigors, and diaphoresis) reported; stop infusion if a severe infusion reaction occurs and institute appropriate therapy. Increase the risk of ovarian failure and may impair fertility in reproductive females. Not approved for adjuvant treatment of colorectal cancer. D/C if severe arterial thromboembolic events, fistula involving an internal organ, or if nephrotic syndrome develops. Temporarily suspend for severe HTN that is not controlled with medical management.

ADVERSE REACTIONS: Hemorrhage, wound healing complications, GI perforations, epistaxis, headache, HTN, rhinitis, proteinuria, taste alteration, dry skin, rectal hemorrhage, lacrimation disorder, back pain, exfoliative dermatitis, diarrhea.

INTERACTIONS: May increase thromboembolic events with PO anticoagulants (eg, warfarin). May decrease paclitaxel exposure with paclitaxel/carboplatin.

PREGNANCY: Category C, not for use in nursing.

MECHANISM OF ACTION: VEGF inhibitor; binds vascular endothelial growth factor and prevents interaction with receptors (Flt-1, KDR) on surface of endothelial cells, which leads to endothelial cell proliferation and new blood vessel formation.

PHARMACOKINETICS: Elimination: $T_{1/2}$=20 days.

NURSING CONSIDERATIONS

Assessment: Assess for recent hemoptysis, serious hemorrhage, HTN, proteinuria, nephrotic syndrome, history of arterial thromboembolism, pregnancy/nursing status, and possible drug interactions. Obtain baseline urinalysis and BP. Assess for prior scheduled elective surgery.

Monitoring: Monitor for GI perforation, fistula formation, wound-healing complications, serious hemorrhage, arterial thromboembolic events, hypertensive crisis/encephalopathy, reversible posterior leukoencephalopathy syndrome, proteinuria, nephrotic syndrome, severe infusion reactions, and other adverse reactions. Monitor BP q2-3 weeks and perform serial urinalysis.

Patient Counseling: Inform of pregnancy risks and the need to continue contraception for at least 6 months after therapy. Instruct to immediately seek medical attention if unusual bleeding, high fever, rigors, sudden onset of worsening neurological function, persistent/severe abdominal pain, severe constipation, or vomiting occurs. Inform of increased risk for wound-healing complications, ovarian failure, and arterial thromboembolic events. Advise to undergo BP monitoring and contact physician if BP is elevated.

Administration: IV route. Do not administer as an IV push/bolus; administer only as an IV infusion. 1st Infusion: Give over 90 min. 2nd Infusion: Give over 60 min if 1st infusion is tolerated. Subsequent Infusions: Give over 30 min if 2nd infusion is tolerated. Refer to PI for preparation for administration. **Storage:** 2-8°C (36-46°F). Protect from light. Do not freeze or shake. Diluted Sol: 2-8°C (36-46°F) for up to 8 hrs. Store in the original carton until time of use.

AVELOX   RX
moxifloxacin HCl (Merck)

> Fluoroquinolones are associated with an increased risk of tendinitis and tendon rupture in all ages. Risk is further increased in patients >60 yrs, patients taking corticosteroids, and with kidney, heart, or lung transplants. May exacerbate muscle weakness with myasthenia gravis; avoid in patients with known history of myasthenia gravis.

THERAPEUTIC CLASS: Fluoroquinolone

INDICATIONS: Treatment of acute bacterial sinusitis, acute bacterial exacerbation of chronic bronchitis (ABECB), uncomplicated and complicated skin and skin structure infections (SSSI), community-acquired pneumonia (CAP), complicated intra-abdominal infections, including polymicrobial infections (eg, abscess), caused by susceptible strains of microorganisms in adults ≥18 yrs.

DOSAGE: *Adults:* Sinusitis: 400mg PO/IV q24h for 10 days. ABECB: 400mg PO/IV q24h for 5 days. Uncomplicated SSSI: 400mg PO/IV q24h for 7 days. Complicated SSSI: 400mg PO/

IV q24h for 7-21 days. CAP: 400mg PO/IV q24h for 7-14 days. Complicated Intra-Abdominal Infections: 400mg PO/IV q24h for 5-14 days.

HOW SUPPLIED: Inj: 400mg/250mL; Tab: 400mg

WARNINGS/PRECAUTIONS: D/C if experience pain, swelling, inflammation, or rupture of tendon. May prolong QT interval; avoid with QT interval prolongation or uncorrected hypokalemia. Caution with ongoing proarrhythmic conditions (eg, significant bradycardia, acute myocardial ischemia) and liver cirrhosis. Serious anaphylactic and sometimes fatal reactions reported; d/c if skin rash, jaundice, or hypersensitivity occurs. Convulsions, toxic psychoses, and increased intracranial pressure (including pseudotumor cerebri) reported. May also cause CNS events (eg, dizziness, confusion, hallucinations, depression); d/c if these events occur. Caution with CNS disorders (eg, severe cerebral arteriosclerosis, epilepsy) or risk factors that may predispose to seizures or lower seizure threshold. *Clostridium difficile*-associated diarrhea (CDAD) reported. May result in bacterial resistance with prolonged use or use in the absence of a proven/suspected bacterial infection or a prophylactic indication; take appropriate measures if superinfection develops. Rare cases of sensory or sensorimotor axonal polyneuropathy, resulting in paresthesias, hypoesthesias, dysesthesias, and weakness reported. May cause photosensitivity/phototoxicity reactions; d/c if phototoxicity occurs. Avoid excessive exposure to sun/UV light. Caution in elderly and in patients with hepatic impairment.

ADVERSE REACTIONS: Tendinitis, tendon rupture, nausea, diarrhea, headache, dizziness.

INTERACTIONS: See Boxed Warning. Avoid Class IA (eg, quinidine, procainamide) or Class III (eg, amiodarone, sotalol) antiarrhythmics. Caution with drugs that prolong the QT interval (eg, cisapride, erythromycin, antipsychotics, TCAs). NSAIDs may increase risk of CNS stimulation and convulsions. May enhance anticoagulant effects with warfarin or its derivatives; monitor PT and INR with warfarin or its derivatives. (Tab) Antacids containing aluminum or magnesium, with sucralfate, with metal cations such as iron, with multivitamins containing iron or zinc, or with formulations containing divalent and trivalent cations such as Videx (didanosine) chewable/buffered tabs or the pediatric powder for oral sol, may substantially interfere with the absorption and lower systemic concentrations.

PREGNANCY: Category C, not for use in nursing.

MECHANISM OF ACTION: Fluoroquinolone; inhibits topoisomerase II (DNA gyrase) and topoisomerase IV, which are required for bacterial DNA replication, transcription, repair, and recombination.

PHARMACOKINETICS: Absorption: (PO) well-absorbed; absolute bioavailability (90%). Refer to PI for various parameters. **Distribution:** V_d=1.7-2.7L/kg; plasma protein binding (30-50%); found in breast milk. **Metabolism:** Glucuronide and sulfate conjugation. **Elimination:** Single dose: $T_{1/2}$=11.5-15.6 hrs (PO), 8.2-15.4 hrs (IV). Multiple dose: $T_{1/2}$=12.7 hrs (PO), 14.8 hrs (IV). 45% unchanged; urine (20%), feces (25%).

NURSING CONSIDERATIONS

Assessment: Assess for risk factors for developing tendinitis and tendon rupture, history of myasthenia gravis, drug hypersensitivity, QT interval prolongation, uncorrected hypokalemia, ongoing proarrhythmic conditions, liver cirrhosis, CNS disorders or risk factors that may predispose to seizures or lower seizure threshold, pregnancy/nursing status, and possible drug interactions.

Monitoring: Monitor for ECG changes (eg, QT interval prolongation), signs/symptoms of anaphylactic reactions, ventricular arrhythmia/torsades de pointes, CNS events, drug resistance, CDAD, development of superinfection, peripheral neuropathy, tendon rupture, tendinitis, and photosensitivity/phototoxicity reactions. Monitor for muscle weakness in patients with myasthenia gravis.

Patient Counseling: Instruct to take exactly as directed; skipping doses or not completing full course may decrease effectiveness and increase bacterial resistance. Inform to notify physician if experience pain, swelling, or inflammation of a tendon, or weakness or inability to move joints; rest and refrain from exercise and d/c therapy. Advise to notify physician of any personal or family history of QT prolongation, proarrhythmic conditions, and convulsions. Instruct to d/c and notify physician if an allergic reaction, skin rash, watery and bloody stools, or symptoms of peripheral neuropathy develop. Instruct to notify physician if worsening muscle weakness or breathing problems, palpitations or fainting spells, or sunburn-like reaction occurs, if pregnant/nursing, and all medications and supplements currently being used. Advise to use caution while performing hazardous tasks (eg, operating machinery/driving). Advise to avoid exposure to sunlight and artificial light. (Tab) Inform that may be taken with or without food, to drink fluids liberally, and that antacids, metal cations, and multivitamins should be taken ≥4 hrs before or 8 hrs after.

Administration: Oral, IV routes. (Tab) Administer ≥4 hrs before or 8 hrs after products containing magnesium, aluminum, iron or zinc, including antacids, sucralfate, multivitamins, and Videx (didanosine) chewable/buffered tabs or the pediatric powder for oral sol. May take with or without food; drink fluids liberally. (Inj) Infuse over 60 min. Avoid rapid or bolus IV infusion. Do not add other IV substances, additives, or other medications to inj or infuse simultaneously through same

IV line. Refer to PI for preparation for administration. **Storage:** 25°C (77°F); excursions permitted to 15-30°C (59-86°F). (Tab) Avoid high humidity. (IV) Do not refrigerate.

AVIANE   RX
ethinyl estradiol - levonorgestrel (Barr)

Cigarette smoking increases the risk of serious cardiovascular (CV) side effects. This risk increases with age (>35 yrs) and with heavy smoking (≥15 cigarettes/day). Women who use oral contraceptives should be strongly advised not to smoke.

OTHER BRAND NAMES: Orysthia (Qualitest)

THERAPEUTIC CLASS: Estrogen/progestogen combination

INDICATIONS: Prevention of pregnancy.

DOSAGE: *Adults:* 1 tab qd for 28 days, then repeat. Start 1st Sunday after menses begins or on Day 1 of cycle.
Pediatrics: Postpubertal: 1 tab qd for 28 days, then repeat. Start 1st Sunday after menses begins or on Day 1 of cycle.

HOW SUPPLIED: Tab: (Ethinyl Estradiol-Levonorgestrel) 0.02mg-0.1mg

CONTRAINDICATIONS: Thrombophlebitis or history of deep vein thrombophlebitis, presence or history of thromboembolic disorders, presence or history of cerebrovascular or coronary artery disease, valvular heart disease with thrombogenic complications, thrombogenic rhythm disorders, hereditary or acquired thrombophilias, major surgery with prolonged immobilization, uncontrolled HTN, diabetes mellitus (DM) with vascular involvement, headaches with focal neurological symptoms, presence or history of breast cancer, carcinoma of the endometrium or other known or suspected estrogen-dependent neoplasia, undiagnosed abnormal genital bleeding, cholestatic jaundice of pregnancy or jaundice with prior pill use, hepatic adenomas/carcinomas or active liver disease, known/suspected pregnancy.

WARNINGS/PRECAUTIONS: Increased risk of myocardial infarction (MI), vascular disease, thromboembolism, stroke, hepatic neoplasia, and gallbladder disease. Increased risk of morbidity and mortality with certain inherited/acquired thrombophilias, HTN, hyperlipidemia, obesity, DM, and surgery or trauma with increased risk of thrombosis. D/C at least 4 weeks before and for 2 weeks after elective surgery with increased risk of thromboembolism, and during or following prolonged immobilization. Caution with CV disease risk factors. May develop visual changes with contact lens. Retinal thrombosis reported; d/c if unexplained partial/complete loss of vision or other ophthalmic irregularities develop. May cause glucose intolerance, elevated LDL or other lipid abnormalities, or exacerbate migraine headaches. Caution with history of depression; d/c if symptoms recur or worsen. May cause increased BP and fluid retention; d/c if significant BP elevations occur. Breakthrough bleeding and spotting reported; rule out malignancies or pregnancy. Diarrhea and/or vomiting may reduce hormone absorption, resulting in decreased serum concentrations. Not indicated for use before menarche. May affect certain endocrine, LFTs, and blood components in laboratory tests. Perform periodic history/physical exam; monitor patients with a strong family history of breast cancer.

ADVERSE REACTIONS: N/V, breakthrough bleeding, spotting, amenorrhea, migraine, depression, vaginal candidiasis, edema, weight changes, melasma, breast changes, changes in cervical erosion and secretion, allergic rash.

INTERACTIONS: Reduced effects result in pregnancy or breakthrough bleeding with antibiotics, anticonvulsants, and other drugs that increase the metabolism of contraceptive steroids (eg, rifampin, rifabutin, barbiturates, primidone, phenylbutazone, phenytoin, dexamethasone, carbamazepine, felbamate, oxcarbazepine, topiramate, griseofulvin, modafinil, ampicillin, other penicillins, tetracyclines, St. John's wort). Anti-HIV protease inhibitors may increase or decrease plasma levels. Atorvastatin, ascorbic acid, acetaminophen (APAP), CYP3A4 inhibitors (eg, indinavir, itraconazole, ketoconazole, fluconazole, and troleandomycin) may increase plasma ethinyl estradiol levels. Increased risk of intrahepatic cholestasis with troleandomycin. Increased plasma levels of cyclosporine, prednisolone and other corticosteroids, and theophylline have been reported. Decreased plasma concentrations of APAP and increased clearance of temazepam, salicylic acid, morphine, and clofibric acid have also been reported.

PREGNANCY: Category X, not for use in nursing.

MECHANISM OF ACTION: Estrogen/progestogen oral contraceptive; acts by suppressing gonadotropins and inhibiting ovulation. Also causes changes in cervical mucus (increasing difficulty of sperm entry into uterus) and endometrium (reducing likelihood of implantation).

PHARMACOKINETICS: Absorption: Levonorgestrel: Rapid and complete. Bioavailability (100%); C_{max}=2.8ng/mL (single dose), 6.0ng/mL (multiple doses); T_{max}=1.6 hrs (single dose), 1.5 hrs (multiple doses). Ethinyl Estradiol: Rapid. Bioavailability (38-48%); C_{max}=62pg/mL (single dose), 77pg/mL (multiple doses); T_{max}=1.5 hrs (single dose), 1.3 hrs (multiple doses). **Distribution:** Levonorgestrel: Primarily bound to sex hormone binding globulin (SHBG). Ethinyl estradiol: Plasma protein binding (97%); found in breast milk. **Metabolism:** Levonorgestrel: Reduction, hydroxylation, and conjugation. Ethinyl Estradiol: Hepatic, via CYP3A4 (hydroxylation), methylation, and glucuronidation. **Elimination:** Levonorgestrel: Urine (40-68%), feces (16-48%); $T_{1/2}$=36 hrs. Ethinyl Estradiol: $T_{1/2}$=18 hrs.

NURSING CONSIDERATIONS

Assessment: Assess for current or history of thrombophlebitis or thromboembolic disorders, history of HTN, hyperlipidemia, DM, obesity, breast cancer, and any other conditions where treatment is contraindicated or cautioned. Assess use in patients >35 yrs and heavy smokers (≥15 cigarettes/day). Assess pregnancy/nursing status and for possible drug interactions.

Monitoring: Monitor for signs/symptoms of MI, thromboembolism, stroke, hepatic neoplasia and other adverse effects. Monitor BP with history of HTN, serum glucose levels in DM or prediabetic patients, lipid levels with history of hyperlipidemia, and for signs of worsening depression if with history of the disorder. Monitor liver function and for signs of liver toxicity (eg, jaundice). Refer to an ophthalmologist if ocular changes develop.

Patient Counseling: Inform that the drug does not protect against HIV infection (AIDS) and other sexually transmitted diseases. Counsel about potential adverse effects. Advise to avoid smoking. Instruct to take exactly as directed at intervals not exceeding 24 hrs. Advise about risks of pregnancy if dose is missed; counsel to have a back-up non-hormonal birth control method (eg, condoms, spermicide) at all times. Instruct that if one dose is missed, take as soon as possible and take next pill at regular scheduled time. Inform that spotting, light bleeding, or nausea may occur during the first 1-3 packs of pills; advise not to d/c medication and if symptoms persist, notify physician. D/C if pregnancy is confirmed/suspected.

Administration: Oral route. **Storage:** 20-25°C (68-77°F).

AVINZA
morphine sulfate (King)

CII

> Swallow capsules whole or sprinkle contents on applesauce. Do not crush, chew, or dissolve capsule beads. Avoid alcohol and alcohol-containing medications; consumption of alcohol may result in the rapid release and absorption of potentially fatal dose of morphine.

THERAPEUTIC CLASS: Opioid analgesic

INDICATIONS: Relief of moderate to severe pain requiring continuous opioid therapy for an extended period of time.

DOSAGE: *Adults:* Individualize dose. Conversion from Other Oral Morphine Products: Give total daily dose as a single dose q24h. Conversion from Parenteral Morphine: Initial: Give about 3x the previous daily parenteral requirement. Conversion from Other Parenteral or Oral Non-Morphine Opioids: Initial: Give 1/2 of estimated daily requirement q24h. Supplement with immediate-release (IR) morphine or short-acting analgesics if needed. Titrate: Adjust dose as frequently as qod. Non-Opioid Tolerant: Initial: 30mg q24h. Titrate: Increase by increments ≤30mg every 4 days. The 45, 60, 75, 90, and 120mg caps are for opioid-tolerant patients. Max: 1,600mg/day. Doses >1,600mg/day contain a quantity of fumaric acid, which may cause renal toxicity. Elderly: Start at low end of dosing range.

HOW SUPPLIED: Cap, Extended-Release: 30mg, 45mg, 60mg, 75mg, 90mg, 120mg

CONTRAINDICATIONS: Respiratory depression in the absence of resuscitative equipment, acute or severe bronchial asthma, paralytic ileus.

WARNINGS/PRECAUTIONS: Abuse potential. Extreme caution with chronic obstructive pulmonary disease (COPD), cor pulmonale, decreased respiratory reserve (eg, severe kyphoscoliosis), hypoxia, hypercapnia, pre-existing respiratory depression. May obscure neurologic signs of increased intracranial pressure (ICP) with head injury. May cause orthostatic hypotension, syncope, severe hypotension with depleted blood volume. Caution with circulatory shock, biliary tract disease (eg, acute pancreatitis), severe renal/hepatic insufficiency, Addison's disease, hypothyroidism, prostatic hypertrophy, urethral stricture, elderly or debilitated; consider dose reduction. Caution with CNS depression, toxic psychosis, acute alcoholism, delirium tremens, seizure disorders. Avoid with GI obstruction. Avoid abrupt withdrawal. Tolerance and physical dependence may develop. Potential for severe constipation; use laxatives, stool softeners at onset of therapy. May impair mental/physical abilities. Not for use as a PRN or postoperative analgesic.

ADVERSE REACTIONS: Constipation, N/V, somnolence, dehydration, headache, peripheral edema, diarrhea, abdominal pain, infection, urinary tract infection (UTI), flu syndrome, back pain, rash, insomnia, depression.

INTERACTIONS: See Boxed Warning. Additive effects with alcohol, other opioids, illicit drugs that cause CNS depression. Reduce dose with other CNS depressants (eg, sedatives, hypnotics, general anesthetics, antiemetics, phenothiazines, tranquilizers, alcohol); caution when coadministering. May enhance neuromuscular blocking action of skeletal muscle relaxants and increase risk of respiratory depression. Avoid with mixed agonist/antagonists (eg, pentazocine, nalbuphine, butorphanol) and within 14 days of MAOI use. Risk of precipitating apnea, confusion, muscle twitching reported with cimetidine; monitor for respiratory and CNS depression.

PREGNANCY: Category C, not for use in nursing.

MECHANISM OF ACTION: Opioid analgesic; pure opioid agonist that is relatively selective for μ-receptor but may interact with other opioid receptors at higher doses. Mechanism of analgesic action is unknown. Specific CNS opiate receptors (eg, μ-receptors) and endogenous compounds with morphine-like activity are found throughout brain and spinal cord and are likely to play a role in analgesic effects.

PHARMACOKINETICS: Absorption: C_{max}=18.65ng/mL; AUC=273.25ng/mL•hr. **Distribution:** Plasma protein binding (20-35%), V_d=1-6L/kg, distributed to skeletal muscle, kidneys, liver, GI tract, lung, spleen, and brain. Small quantities cross the blood-brain barrier. Crosses the placenta and found in human breast milk. **Metabolism:** Hepatic conjugation; 3-glucuronide (M3G) (metabolite); 6-glucuronide (M6G) (active metabolite). **Elimination:** Urine (major M3G/M6G, 10% unchanged), feces (7-10%), bile (small); $T_{1/2}$=15 hrs.

NURSING CONSIDERATIONS

Assessment: Assess for degree of opioid tolerance, previous opioid dose, level of pain intensity, type of pain, patient's general condition and medical status, emotional status or any other conditions where treatment is contraindicated or cautioned. Assess for history of hypersensitivity, pregnancy/nursing status, renal/hepatic function, and possible drug interactions.

Monitoring: Monitor for signs/symptoms of respiratory depression, orthostatic hypotension, syncope, drug dependence and tolerance, and withdrawal syndrome (eg, restlessness, lacrimation, rhinorrhea, myalgia, mydriasis). Monitor for signs of increased ICP with head injuries. Monitor for relief of pain and need for IR morphine.

Patient Counseling: Advise that medication should be taken once daily and that it may be taken with/without food. Instruct to swallow whole (not to chew, crush, or dissolve) or open and sprinkle onto small amount of applesauce. Instruct not to consume alcohol during therapy, including Rx/OTC drugs containing alcohol. Notify physician of all concurrent medications and avoid use of other CNS depressants. Caution when performing hazardous tasks (eg, operating machinery/driving). Do not adjust dose or abruptly d/c medication without consulting physician. Advise that medication has potential for abuse. Instruct to keep out of reach of children. Advise to dispose of any unused medication via toilet. Counsel about severe constipation; take appropriate laxatives or stool softeners at start of therapy.

Administration: Oral route. Swallow capsules whole or sprinkle contents on a small amount of applesauce. **Storage:** 25°C (77°F); excursions permitted to 15-30°C (59-86°F). Protect from light and moisture.

AVODART   RX
dutasteride (GlaxoSmithKline)

THERAPEUTIC CLASS: Type I and II 5 alpha-reductase inhibitor (2nd generation)

INDICATIONS: Treatment of symptomatic benign prostatic hyperplasia (BPH) in men with an enlarged prostate, either as monotherapy or in combination with the α-adrenergic antagonist, tamsulosin.

DOSAGE: *Adults:* Monotherapy: 1 cap (0.5mg) qd. With Tamsulosin: 1 cap (0.5mg) qd and tamsulosin 0.4mg qd.

HOW SUPPLIED: Cap: 0.5mg

CONTRAINDICATIONS: Pregnancy, women of childbearing potential, pediatrics.

WARNINGS/PRECAUTIONS: Not approved for the prevention of prostate cancer. May decrease serum prostate specific antigen (PSA) concentration during therapy or in the presence of prostate cancer; establish a new baseline PSA ≥3 months after starting treatment and monitor PSA periodically thereafter. Any confirmed increase from lowest PSA value during treatment may signal presence of prostate cancer. May increase risk of high-grade prostate cancer. Prior to treatment initiation, consider other urological conditions that may cause similar symptoms; BPH and prostate cancer may coexist. Risk to male fetus; cap should not be handled by pregnant women or women who may become pregnant. Avoid donating blood until ≥6 months after last dose. Reduced total sperm count, semen volume, and sperm motility reported.

ADVERSE REACTIONS: Impotence, decreased libido, breast disorders, ejaculation disorders.

INTERACTIONS: Caution with potent, chronic CYP3A4 inhibitors (eg, ritonavir). CYP3A4/5 inhibitors (eg, ritonavir, ketoconazole, verapamil, diltiazem, cimetidine, troleandomycin, ciprofloxacin) may increase levels.

PREGNANCY: Category X, not for use in nursing.

MECHANISM OF ACTION: Selective type I and II 5α-reductase inhibitor; inhibits conversion of testosterone to dihydrotestosterone, the androgen primarily responsible for initial development and subsequent enlargement of the prostate gland.

PHARMACOKINETICS: Absorption: Absolute bioavailability (60%); T_{max}=2-3 hrs. **Distribution:** V_d=300-500L; plasma protein binding (99% albumin, 96.6% α-1 acid glycoprotein). **Metabolism:** Liver (extensive) via CYP3A4, 3A5; 4'-hydroxydutasteride, 1,2-dihydrodutasteride, 6-hydroxy-dutasteride (major active metabolites). **Elimination:** Feces (5% unchanged, 40% metabolites), urine (<1% unchanged); $T_{1/2}$=5 weeks.

NURSING CONSIDERATIONS

Assessment: Assess for urological conditions that may cause similar symptoms, previous hypersensitivity to the drug, and for possible drug interactions.

Monitoring: Monitor for signs/symptoms of prostate cancer and other urological diseases. Obtain new PSA baseline ≥3 months after starting treatment and monitor PSA periodically thereafter.

Patient Counseling: Inform the importance of periodic PSA monitoring. Advise that therapy may increase risk of high-grade prostate cancer. Counsel that drug should not be handled by woman who are pregnant or who could become pregnant due to potential fetal risks; advise to wash area immediately with soap and water if contact is made. Instruct not to donate blood for ≥6 months after last dose.

Administration: Oral route. Swallow whole; do not chew or open. **Storage:** 25°C (77°F); excursions permitted to 15-30°C (59-86°F).

AXERT   RX
almotriptan malate (Ortho-McNeil/Janssen)

THERAPEUTIC CLASS: 5-$HT_{1B/1D}$ agonist

INDICATIONS: Acute treatment of migraine attacks with a history of migraine with or without aura in adults. Acute treatment of migraine headache pain with a history of migraine attacks with or without aura usually lasting ≥4 hrs in adolescents 12-17 yrs.

DOSAGE: *Adults:* Initial: 6.25-12.5mg at onset of headache. May repeat after 2 hrs. Max: 25mg/day. Hepatic/Renal Impairment: 6.25mg at onset of headache. Max: 12.5mg/24 hrs. Elderly: Start at lower end of dosing range.
Pediatrics: 12-17 yrs: Initial: 6.25-12.5mg at onset of headache. May repeat after 2 hrs. Max: 25mg/day. Hepatic/Renal Impairment: 6.25mg at onset of headache. Max: 12.5mg/24 hrs.

HOW SUPPLIED: Tab: 6.25mg, 12.5mg

CONTRAINDICATIONS: Ischemic heart disease, coronary artery vasospasm, other significant cardiovascular disesase, cerebrovascular syndromes (eg, stroke, transient ischemic attacks [TIA]), peripheral vascular disease (eg, ischemic bowel disease), uncontrolled HTN, hemiplegic or basilar migraine. Avoid use within 24 hrs of another 5-HT_1 agonist (eg, triptans) or ergot-amine-containing or ergot-type medications (eg, dihydroergotamine, ergotamine tartrate, methysergide).

WARNINGS/PRECAUTIONS: Confirm diagnosis. Supervise first dose and monitor cardiac function in those at risk of coronary artery disease (CAD) (eg, HTN, hypercholesterolemia, smoker, obesity, diabetes, CAD family history, postmenopausal women, males >40 yrs). Monitor cardiovascular function with long-term intermittent use. May cause vasospastic reactions or cerebrovascular events. Serotonin syndrome symptoms (eg, mental status changes, autonomic instability, neuromuscular aberrations, and GI symptoms) reported. Sensations of tightness, pain, pressure, and heaviness in the precordium, throat, neck, and jaw reported. May bind to melanin in the eye. Caution with renal or hepatic dysfunction. Caution with known hypersensitivity to sulfonamides. Caution in elderly.

ADVERSE REACTIONS: N/V, dizziness, somnolence, headache, paresthesia, coronary artery vasospasm, myocardial infarction, ventricular tachycardia, ventricular fibrillation, transient myocardial ischemia, dry mouth.

INTERACTIONS: See Contraindications. Additive vasospastic reactions with ergotamines. Selective serotonin reuptake inhibitors (SSRIs) may cause weakness, hyperreflexia, and incoordination. Life-threatening serotonin syndrome reported with combined use of SSRIs or serotonin norepinephrine reuptake inhibitors (SNRIs). Clearance may be decreased by MAOIs. Increased levels possible with CYP3A4 inhibitors (eg, ketoconazole).

PREGNANCY: Category C, caution in nursing.

MECHANISM OF ACTION: Selective 5-$HT_{1B/1D}$ receptor agonist; binds with high affinity to 5-$HT_{1B/1D}$ receptors on extracerebral, intracranial blood vessels that become dilated during migraine attack and on nerve terminal in trigeminal system. Activation of these receptors results in cranial nerve constriction, inhibition of neuropeptide release, and reduced transmission in trigeminal pain pathways.

PHARMACOKINETICS: Absorption: Absolute bioavailability (70%); T_{max}=1-3 hrs. **Distribution:** V_d=180-200L; plasma protein binding (35%). **Metabolism:** Monoamine oxidase (MAO)-mediated oxidative deamination and CYP450-mediated oxidation (major pathways), flavin monooxygenase (minor pathway); indoleacetic acid, gamma-aminobutyric acid (inactive metabolites). **Elimination:** Urine (75%, 40% unchanged), feces (13%, unchanged and metabolite); $T_{1/2}$=3-4 hrs.

NURSING CONSIDERATIONS

Assessment: Confirm diagnosis of migraine before therapy. Assess for cluster headache, ischemic heart disease (eg, angina pectoris, Prinzmetal's variant angina, MI or documented silent MI), HTN, hemiplegic or basilar migraine, presence of risk factors (eg, hypercholesterolemia, smoking, obesity, diabetes mellitus), ECG changes, hepatic/renal impairment, hypersensitivity to the drug and to sulfonamides, pregnancy/nursing status, and possible drug interactions.

Monitoring: Administration of 1st dose should be in physician's office or medically staffed and equipped facility as cardiac ischemia may occur in absence of clinical symptoms; ECG should be obtained immediately during interval in those with risk factors. Monitor for signs/symptoms of cardiac events (eg, coronary vasospasm, acute MI, arrhythmia, ECG changes, follow-up coronary angiography), cerebrovascular events (eg, hemorrhage, stroke, TIAs), peripheral vascular ischemia, colonic ischemia with bloody diarrhea and abdominal pain, serotonin syndrome (eg, mental status changes, autonomic instability, neuromuscular aberrations and/or GI symptoms), ophthalmic effects, hypersensitivity reactions, and increased BP.

Patient Counseling: Inform about potential risks (eg, serotonin syndrome manifestations such as confusion, hallucinations, fast heartbeat, fever, sweating, muscle spasm, and diarrhea), especially if taken with SSRIs or SNRIs. Report adverse reactions to physician. Advise to take exactly as directed. Counsel to use caution during hazardous tasks (eg, driving/operating machinery). Notify if pregnant/nursing or planning to become pregnant.

Administration: Oral route. **Storage:** 25°C (77°F); excursions permitted to 15-30°C (59-86°F).

AXIRON
testosterone (Lilly)

Virilization reported in children secondarily exposed to topical testosterone. Children should avoid contact with unwashed or unclothed application sites in men using topical testosterone. Advise patients to strictly adhere to recommended instructions for use.

THERAPEUTIC CLASS: Androgen

INDICATIONS: Replacement therapy in males ≥18 yrs for conditions associated with a deficiency or absence of endogenous testosterone (congenital/acquired primary hypogonadism or hypogonadotropic hypogonadism).

DOSAGE: *Adults:* Initial: Apply 60mg (1 actuation of 30mg to each axilla) qam, to clean, dry, intact skin of axilla. Titrate: May adjust dose based on serum testosterone concentration from a single blood draw 2-8 hrs after application, and at least 14 days after starting treatment or following dose adjustment. If Serum Concentration <300ng/dL: May increase to 90mg or from 90mg to 120mg. If Serum Concentration >1050ng/dL: Decrease from 60mg to 30mg. D/C if consistently >1050ng/dL at lowest qd dose of 30mg. Refer to PI for application techniques.

HOW SUPPLIED: Sol: 30mg/actuation [110mL]

CONTRAINDICATIONS: Known/suspected prostate carcinoma or breast carcinoma in men, women who are or may become pregnant, or nursing mothers.

WARNINGS/PRECAUTIONS: Application site and dose are not interchangeable with other topical testosterone products. Patients with benign prostatic hyperplasia (BPH) may be at increased risk for worsening of signs/symptoms of BPH. May increase risk for prostate cancer; evaluate for prostate cancer before and 3-6 months after initiation of therapy. Increases in Hct and RBC mass may increase risk for thromboembolic events; consider lowering or d/c therapy. Not indicated for use in women. Suppression of spermatogenesis may occur at large doses. Edema with or without congestive heart failure (CHF) may occur in patients with preexisting cardiac, renal, or hepatic disease. Gynecomastia may develop and persist. May potentiate sleep apnea, especially with obesity or chronic lung disease. Changes in serum lipid profile reported; adjust dose or d/c therapy if necessary. Caution in cancer patients at risk of hypercalcemia and associated hypercalciuria. May decrease concentrations of thyroxin-binding globulins, resulting in decreased total T4 and increased resin uptake of T3 and T4. Alcohol-based products are flammable; avoid fire, flame, or smoking until applied dose has dried.

ADVERSE REACTIONS: Application-site irritation, application-site erythema, headache, Hct increase, diarrhea, vomiting, prostate specific antigen (PSA) increase.

INTERACTIONS: May decrease blood glucose and insulin requirements. Changes in anticoagulant activity may occur; frequently monitor INR and PT in patients taking anticoagulants. May increase fluid retention with adrenocorticotropic hormone or corticosteroids.

PREGNANCY: Category X, not for use in nursing.

MECHANISM OF ACTION: Androgen; responsible for normal growth and development of male sex organs and for maintenance of secondary sex characteristics.

PHARMACOKINETICS: Absorption: Systemic. **Metabolism:** Estradiol, dihydrotestosterone (active metabolites). **Elimination:** (IM) Urine (90% glucuronic, sulfuric acid conjugates), feces (6% unconjugated); $T_{1/2}$=10-100 min.

NURSING CONSIDERATIONS

Assessment: Assess for conditions where treatment is contraindicated, prostate cancer, BPH, cardiac or renal/hepatic disease, obesity, chronic lung disease, and possible drug interactions. Assess Hct.

Monitoring: Monitor for signs/symptoms of prostate cancer, worsening of BPH, edema with or without CHF, gynecomastia, and sleep apnea. Periodically monitor Hct, Hgb, PSA, serum lipid profile, and serum testosterone levels. In cancer patients at risk for hypercalcemia, monitor serum calcium levels.

Patient Counseling: Advise to strictly adhere to recommended instructions for use. Inform that men with known or suspected prostate/breast cancer should not use androgen therapy. Advise that children and women should avoid contact with application sites, and to report to physician any signs/symptoms of secondary exposure in these individuals. Instruct to apply only to axilla and not to any other part of the body, to wash hands immediately with soap and water after application, and to cover application site with clothing after waiting 3 min for the solution to dry. Instruct to wash application site with soap and water prior to direct skin-to-skin contact with others, and to immediately wash area of contact if unwashed/unclothed skin comes in direct contact with skin of another person. Inform of possible adverse reactions (eg, changes in urinary habits, breathing disturbances, frequent or persistent erections of the penis, N/V, changes in skin color, or ankle swelling). Inform that antiperspirant or deodorant may be used before applying the medication. Counsel to avoid swimming or washing application site until 2 hrs following application. Advise to avoid splashing in the eyes; instruct to flush thoroughly with water in case of contact and to seek medical advice if irritation persists.

Administration: Topical route. Refer to PI for administration instructions. **Storage:** 25°C (77°F); excursions permitted to 15-30°C (59-86°F).

AZACTAM   RX
aztreonam (Bristol-Myers Squibb)

THERAPEUTIC CLASS: Monobactam

INDICATIONS: Treatment of complicated/uncomplicated urinary tract infections (UTI) (eg, pyelonephritis and initial/recurrent cystitis), lower respiratory tract infections (eg, pneumonia, bronchitis), septicemia, skin and skin-structure infections (eg, postoperative wounds, ulcers, burns), intra-abdominal infections (eg, peritonitis), and gynecologic infections (eg, endometritis, pelvic cellulitis) caused by susceptible gram-negative microorganisms. Adjunct therapy to surgery for management of infections caused by susceptible microorganisms (eg, abscesses, hollow viscus perforation infections, cutaneous infections, infections of serous surfaces). Concurrent initial therapy with other antimicrobial agents before causative organism(s) is known in seriously ill who are also at risk of having gram-positive aerobic/anaerobic infection.

DOSAGE: *Adults:* Individualize dose. UTI: 500mg or 1g IM/IV q8 or 12h. Max: 8g/day. Moderately Severe Systemic Infections: 1 or 2g IM/IV q8 or 12h. Max: 8g/day. Severe Systemic/Life-Threatening Infections/*Pseudomonas aeruginosa* Infection: 2g IV q6 or 8h. Max: 8g/day. Renal Impairment/Elderly: CrCl 10-30mL/min/1.73m²: Initial: 1g or 2g. Maint: 50% of usual dose. CrCl <10mL/min/1.73m²: Initial: 500mg, 1g or 2g. Maint: 25% of initial dose at fixed intervals of 6, 8 or 12 hrs. Serious/Life-Threatening Infections: Give additional 1/8 of initial dose after each hemodialysis session. Administer IV for single doses >1g or with bacterial septicemia, localized parenchymal abscess, peritonitis, or other severe systemic or life-threatening infections. Continue treatment for at least 48 hrs after resolution of symptoms or evident bacterial eradication. *Pediatrics:* 9 months-16 yrs: Individualize dose. Mild-Moderate Infections: 30mg/kg IV q8h. Max: 120mg/kg/day. Moderate-Severe Infections: 30mg/kg IV q6 or 8h. Max: 120mg/kg/day. In patients with cystic fibrosis, higher doses may be warranted. Continue treatment for at least 48 hrs after resolution of symptoms or evident bacterial eradication.

HOW SUPPLIED: Inj: 1g, 2g; 1g/50mL, 2g/50mL [Galaxy].

WARNINGS/PRECAUTIONS: Caution with history of hypersensitivity to other β-lactams (eg, penicillins, cephalosporins, carbapenems); d/c and institute supportive treatment if allergic reaction occurs. *Clostridium difficile*-associated diarrhea (CDAD) reported; d/c if CDAD is suspected or confirmed. Toxic epidermal necrolysis (TEN) reported (rarely) in patients undergoing bone marrow transplant with multiple risk factors (eg, sepsis, radiation therapy, concomitant drugs associated with TEN). May result in bacterial resistance with prolonged use or use in the absence of a proven/suspected bacterial infection or a prophylactic indication; take appropriate measures if superinfection develops. Caution with renal/hepatic impairment and in the elderly.

ADVERSE REACTIONS: ALT/AST elevation, rash, eosinophilia, neutropenia, pain at injection site, increased serum creatinine, thrombocytosis.

INTERACTIONS: Avoid with β-lactamase inducing antibiotics (eg, cefoxitin, imipinem). Potential nephrotoxicity and ototoxicity with aminoglycosides; monitor renal function.

PREGNANCY: Category B, not for use in nursing.

MECHANISM OF ACTION: Monobactam; inhibits bacterial cell wall synthesis due to high affinity of aztreonam for penicillin-binding protein 3 (PBP3).

PHARMACOKINETICS: Absorption: Administration of variable doses resulted in different pharmacokinetic parameters. **Distribution:** Plasma protein binding (56%); V_d=12.6L; crosses placenta; found in breast milk. **Metabolism:** Ring hydrolysis. **Elimination:** Urine (60-70%; unchanged and metabolites), feces (12%; unchanged and metabolites); $T_{1/2}$=1.7 hr.

NURSING CONSIDERATIONS

Assessment: Assess for drug hypersensitivity, hypersensitivity to any allergens, history of hypersensitivity to other β-lactams, hepatic/renal impairment, pregnancy/nursing status, and for possible drug interactions. Assess use in patients undergoing bone marrow transplant with multiple risk factors (eg, sepsis, radiation therapy). Confirm diagnosis of causative organisms.

Monitoring: Monitor for signs/symptoms of hypersensitivity reactions, CDAD, superinfection, TEN in patients undergoing bone marrow transplant, and hepatic/renal function.

Patient Counseling: Inform that therapy should only be used to treat bacterial and not viral infections (eg, common cold). Advise to take exactly as directed. Inform that skipping doses or not completing course of therapy may decrease the effectiveness of treatment and increase the likelihood of drug resistant bacteria. Inform that diarrhea is a common problem caused by therapy and will usually end upon d/c of therapy. Instruct to immediately contact physician if watery and bloody stools (with or without stomach cramps and fever) occur, even as late as two or more months after d/c therapy.

Administration: IM/IV route. Refer to PI for preparation/administration instructions and compatibility information. **Storage:** Room temperature. Avoid excessive heat. (Galaxy) ≤-20°C (-4°F). Thawed solution stable for 14 days at 2-8°C (36-46°F) or 48 hrs at 25°C (77°F). Refer to PI for storage information of diluted/reconstituted solution.

Azasite RX
azithromycin (Inspire)

THERAPEUTIC CLASS: Macrolide

INDICATIONS: Treatment of bacterial conjunctivitis caused by susceptible strains of microorganisms.

DOSAGE: *Adults:* Initial: 1 drop in the affected eye(s) bid, 8-12 hrs apart, for the 1st 2 days, then 1 drop qd for next 5 days.
Pediatrics: ≥1 yr: Initial: 1 drop in the affected eye(s) bid, 8-12 hrs apart, for the 1st 2 days, then 1 drop qd for next 5 days.

HOW SUPPLIED: Sol: 1% [2.5mL]

WARNINGS/PRECAUTIONS: Not for injection. Do not give systemically, inject subconjunctivally, or introduce directly into the anterior chamber of the eye. Serious allergic reactions (eg, angioedema, anaphylaxis) and dermatological reactions (eg, Stevens-Johnson syndrome [SJS] and toxic epidermal necrolysis [TEN]) rarely reported when administered systemically. Overgrowth of non-susceptible organisms (eg, fungi) may occur with prolonged use. D/C and institute alternative therapy if superinfection occurs. Avoid contact lens use.

ADVERSE REACTIONS: Eye irritation, burning, stinging and irritation upon instillation, contact dermatitis, corneal erosion, dry eye, dysgeusia, nasal congestion, ocular discharge, hives, rash, punctate keratitis, sinusitis, facial swelling.

PREGNANCY: Category B, caution in nursing.

MECHANISM OF ACTION: Macrolide; binds to the 50S ribosomal subunit of susceptible microorganisms and interferes with microbial protein synthesis.

NURSING CONSIDERATIONS

Assessment: Assess for hypersensitivity, proper diagnosis of causative bacteria, and pregnancy/nursing status.

Monitoring: Monitor for serious allergic reactions (eg, angioedema, anaphylaxis) and dermatologic reactions (eg, SJS, TEN), superinfection, and other adverse reactions.

Patient Counseling: Advise patients with signs/symptoms of bacterial conjunctivitis to avoid wearing contact lenses. Instruct not to allow applicator tip to touch the eye, fingers, or other sources. Instruct to take exactly as directed. Advise that if doses are skipped or medication is stopped early, treatment effectiveness will be decreased and bacteria may develop resistance. Advise to wash hands thoroughly before instillation. Instruct to d/c and contact physician if signs of allergic reaction occur. Instruct to use medication as prescribed.

Administration: Ocular route. **Storage:** Unopened Bottle: Refrigerate at 2-8°C (36-46°F). Opened Bottle: 2-25°C (36-77°F) for ≤14 days. Discard after 14 days.

Azilect   RX
rasagiline mesylate (Teva)

THERAPEUTIC CLASS: Monoamine oxidase inhibitor (Type B)

INDICATIONS: Treatment of signs and symptoms of idiopathic Parkinson's disease as initial monotherapy and as adjunct therapy to levodopa.

DOSAGE: *Adults:* Monotherapy: 1mg qd. Adjunctive Therapy: Initial: 0.5mg qd. Titrate: May increase to 1mg qd. May reduce dose of concomitant levodopa based on individual response. Concomitant Ciprofloxacin or Other CYP1A2 Inhibitors/Mild Hepatic Impairment: 0.5mg qd.

HOW SUPPLIED: Tab: 0.5mg, 1mg

CONTRAINDICATIONS: Concomitant use with meperidine and within 14 days after d/c rasagiline and starting meperidine. Concomitant use with tramadol, methadone, propoxyphene, dextromethorphan, St. John's wort, cyclobenzaprine, and other MAOIs.

WARNINGS/PRECAUTIONS: Avoid with moderate/severe hepatic impairment. Should not exceed recommended doses due to risks of hypertensive crisis and nonselective MAO inhibition. Avoid food containing very high amounts of tyramine while on therapy; potential for large increases in BP. Monitor for melanomas. May potentiate dopaminergic side effects, cause/exacerbate dyskinesia, cause postural hypotension, and increase incidence of high BP when used as adjunct to levodopa. Hallucinations reported. May cause/exacerbate psychotic-like behavior; avoid in patients with a major psychotic disorder. Symptom complex resembling neuroleptic malignant syndrome reported with rapid dose reduction, withdrawal of, or changes in drugs that increase central dopaminergic tone.

ADVERSE REACTIONS: Headache, arthralgia, dyspepsia, depression, fall, flu syndrome, conjunctivitis, fever, gastroenteritis, rhinitis.

INTERACTIONS: See Contraindications. Severe CNS toxicity reported with antidepressants (eg, SSRIs, serotonin norepinephrine reuptake inhibitors [SNRIs], TCAs, tetracyclic antidepressants, triazolopyridine antidepressants); allow ≥14 days between d/c of therapy and initiation of a SSRI, SNRI, tricyclic, tetracyclic, or triazolopyridine antidepressant. Allow ≥5 weeks between d/c of fluoxetine and initiation of therapy. Levodopa may increase levels. Ciprofloxacin and other CYP1A2 inhibitors may increase levels. Caution with sympathomimetics (eg, nasal, oral, and ophthalmic decongestants, cold remedies). Hypertensive crisis reported with ephedrine. Elevated BP reported with tetrahydrozoline ophthalmic drops.

PREGNANCY: Category C, caution in nursing.

MECHANISM OF ACTION: MAO-B inhibitor; mechanism not established. Suspected to inhibit MAO type B, which causes an increase in extracellular dopamine levels in the striatum, subsequently increasing dopaminergic activity.

PHARMACOKINETICS: Absorption: Rapid. Absolute bioavailability (36%); T_{max}=1 hr. **Distribution:** V_d=87L; plasma protein binding (88-94%). **Metabolism:** Liver via N-dealkylation, hydroxylation; CYP1A2: 1-aminoindan, 3-hydroxy-N-propargyl-1 aminoindan and 3-hydroxy-1-aminoindan. **Elimination:** Urine (62% over 7 days), (<1% unchanged), feces (7% over 7 days); $T_{1/2}$=3 hrs.

NURSING CONSIDERATIONS

Assessment: Assess for hepatic impairment, dyskinesia, major psychotic disorder, pregnancy/nursing status, and possible drug interactions.

Monitoring: Monitor for melanoma, dyskinesia, postural hypotension, HTN, hallucinations, psychotic-like behavior, and other adverse reactions. Perform periodic skin examinations.

Patient Counseling: Instruct to inform physician if taking or planning to take any prescription or over-the-counter (OTC) drugs, especially antidepressants, ciprofloxacin, and OTC cold medications. Advise to avoid foods containing very large amounts of tyramine (eg, aged cheese) and to have periodic skin examinations. Inform of the possibility of developing hallucinations, dyskinesia with concomitant levodopa, and increases in BP. Inform that postural (orthostatic) hypotension; caution against standing up rapidly after sitting or lying down for prolonged periods and at the initiation of treatment. Instruct to take drug as prescribed and not to double dose if a dose is missed. Instruct to contact physician if d/c of therapy is desired, if new or increased gambling urges, sexual urges, or other intense urges develop.

Administration: Oral route. **Storage:** 25°C (77°F); excursions permitted to 15-30°C (59-86°F).

AZMACORT   RX
triamcinolone acetonide (Abbott)

THERAPEUTIC CLASS: Corticosteroid

INDICATIONS: Maintenance treatment of asthma as prophylactic therapy in patients ≥6 yrs; to reduce or eliminate the need for oral corticosteroidal therapy.

DOSAGE: *Adults:* 2 inh (150mcg) tid-qid or 4 inh (300mcg) bid. Severe Asthma: Initial: 12-16 inh/day. Max: 16 inh/day (1200mcg). Rinse mouth after use.
Pediatrics: >12 yrs: 2 inh (150mcg) tid-qid or 4 inh (300mcg) bid. Severe Asthma: Initial: 12-16 inh/day. Max: 16 inh/day (1200mcg). 6-12 yrs: 1-2 inh (75-150mcg) tid-qid or 2-4 (150-300mcg) inh bid. Max: 12 inh/day (900mcg). Rinse mouth after use.

HOW SUPPLIED: MDI: 75mcg/inh [20g]

CONTRAINDICATIONS: Primary treatment of status asthmaticus or other acute asthma attacks.

WARNINGS/PRECAUTIONS: Deaths due to adrenal insufficiency have occurred with transfer from systemic corticosteroids to inhaled corticosteroids. Resume oral corticosteroids during stress or severe asthma attack. Observe for adrenal insufficiency, systemic corticosteroid withdrawal effects, hypercorticoidism and growth suppression (children). More susceptible to infections. Not for acute bronchospasm. D/C if bronchospasm occurs after dosing. Caution with tuberculosis (TB) of respiratory tract; untreated systemic fungal, bacterial, viral or parasitic infections; or ocular herpes simplex. *Candida* infection of mouth and pharynx reported.

ADVERSE REACTIONS: Pharyngitis, sinusitis, headache, flu syndrome.

INTERACTIONS: Caution with prednisone.

PREGNANCY: Category C, caution in nursing.

MECHANISM OF ACTION: Corticosteroid; not established. Inhaled route makes possible to provide local anti-inflammatory activity.

PHARMACOKINETICS: Absorption: T_{max}=1.5-2 hrs. **Distribution:** V_d=99.5L; plasma protein binding (68%). **Elimination:** Urine (40%), feces (60%); $T_{1/2}$=88 min.

NURSING CONSIDERATIONS

Assessment: Assess for concomitant diseases such as status asthmaticus, active or quiescent pulmonary TB, untreated systemic fungal, bacterial, parasitic or viral infections, and possible drug interactions.

Monitoring: Monitor for localized oral infections with *Candida albicans*, body height in children, adrenal insufficiency, paradoxical bronchospasm, and hypersensitivity reactions.

Patient Counseling: Inform not for relief of acute bronchospasm. Advise that drug may unmask allergies (rhinitis, conjunctivitis, eczema). Instruct to track use of drug and dispose canister after 240 actuations since reliable dose delivery not assured after 240 doses. Warn to avoid exposure to chickenpox or measles. Advise to seek medical attention if exposed to chickenpox or measles, symptoms do not improve or worsen, during periods of stress or severe asthmatic attack, paradoxical bronchospasm or hypersensitivity reaction occurs. Counsel to avoid spraying in eyes and shake well before each use.

Administration: Oral inhalation. **Storage:** 20-25°C (68-77°F). Do not puncture, use, or store near heat or open flame; do not freeze.

AZOPT   RX
brinzolamide (Alcon)

THERAPEUTIC CLASS: Carbonic anhydrase inhibitor

INDICATIONS: Treatment of elevated intraocular pressure (IOP) in patients with ocular HTN or open-angle glaucoma.

DOSAGE: *Adults:* 1 drop in the affected eye(s) tid. Space dosing with other topical ophthalmic drugs by at least 10 min.

HOW SUPPLIED: Sus: 1% [5mL, 10mL, 15mL]

WARNINGS/PRECAUTIONS: Systemically absorbed. Rare fatalities have occurred due to severe sulfonamide reactions, including Stevens-Johnson syndrome, toxic epidermal necrolysis, fulminant hepatic necrosis, agranulocytosis, aplastic anemia, and other blood dyscrasias. Sensitization may recur when re-administered. D/C if signs of serious reactions or hypersensitivity occur. Caution with low endothelial cell counts; increased potential for corneal edema. Avoid with severe renal impairment (CrCl <30mL/ min). The preservative used, benzalkonium chloride, may be absorbed by soft contact lenses; contact lenses should be removed during instillation and reinserted 15 min after instillation. Not studied in acute angle-closure glaucoma.

ADVERSE REACTIONS: Blurred vision, taste disturbances, blepharitis, dermatitis, dry eye, foreign body sensation, headache, hyperemia, ocular discharge, ocular discomfort, ocular keratitis, ocular pain, ocular pruritus, rhinitis.

INTERACTIONS: Acid-base alterations reported with oral carbonic anhydrase inhibitors; caution with high-dose salicylates. Potential additive systemic effects with oral carbonic anhydrase inhibitors; coadministration is not recommended.

PREGNANCY: Category C, not for use in nursing.

MECHANISM OF ACTION: Carbonic anhydrase II inhibitor; inhibits aqueous humor formation and reduces elevated intraocular pressure.

PHARMACOKINETICS: Distribution: Plasma protein binding (60%). **Elimination:** Urine (unchanged).

NURSING CONSIDERATIONS

Assessment: Assess for sulfonamide hypersensitivity, low endothelial cell counts, acute angle-closure glaucoma, contact lens use, renal function, pregnancy/nursing status, and possible drug interactions.

Monitoring: Monitor for sulfonamide hypersensitivity reactions. If using chronically, monitor for ocular reactions (eg, conjunctivitis and lid reactions); d/c therapy and evaluate patient if such reactions occur. Monitor for bacterial keratitis if using multiple dose container. Monitor for choroidal detachment following filtration procedures.

Patient Counseling: Advise to d/c and contact physician if any serious or unusual ocular or systemic reactions, or signs of hypersensitivity occur. Inform that temporary blurred vision may occur after dosing; caution with operating machinery or driving motor vehicle. Instruct to avoid touching container tip to the eye or any other surfaces. Instruct to contact physician about the continued use of present multidose container if having ocular surgery or if an intercurrent ocular condition (eg, trauma, infection) develops. Instruct to remove contact lenses during instillation and reinsert 15 min after instillation. Advise that if using >1 topical ophthalmic medication, separate administration by at least 10 min.

Administration: Ocular route. Shake well before use. **Storage:** 4-30°C (39-86°F).

AZOR   RX
olmesartan medoxomil - amlodipine (Daiichi Sankyo)

> D/C when pregnancy is detected. Drugs that act directly on the renin-angiotensin system can cause death/injury to developing fetus.

THERAPEUTIC CLASS: ARB/Calcium channel blocker (dihydropyridine)

INDICATIONS: Treatment of HTN, alone or with other antihypertensive agents. Initial therapy in patients who are likely to need multiple antihypertensive agents to achieve their BP goals.

DOSAGE: *Adults:* Initial: 5mg-20mg qd. Titrate: May increase dose after 1-2 weeks to control BP. Max: 10mg-40mg qd. Replacement Therapy: May substitute for individually titrated components. When substituting for individual components, the dose of 1 or both components may be increased if inadequate BP control. Add-On Therapy: May be used to provide additional BP lowering when not adequately controlled on amlodipine (or another dihydropyridine calcium channel blocker) or olmesartan (or another angiotensin receptor blocker) alone.

HOW SUPPLIED: Tab: (Amlodipine-Olmesartan) 5mg-20mg, 5mg-40mg, 10mg-20mg, 10mg-40mg

WARNINGS/PRECAUTIONS: Avoid initial therapy with hepatic impairment and patients ≥75 yrs. May decrease Hct and Hgb levels. Amlodipine: Acute hypotension reported (rare); caution with severe aortic stenosis. May increase frequency, duration, or severity of angina or acute myocardial infarction (MI) reported with dosage initiation or increase, particularly with severe obstructive coronary artery disease (CAD). May cause hepatic enzyme elevation. Caution with severe hepatic impairment. Olmesartan: Symptomatic hypotension, especially in patients with an activated renin-angiotensin system (eg, volume- and/or salt-depleted patients receiving high doses of diuretics), may occur with treatment initiation; monitor closely. Changes in renal function may occur. Oliguria or progressive azotemia and (rarely) acute renal failure and/or death may occur in patients whose renal function is dependent on the renin-angiotensin-aldosterone system (eg, severe congestive heart failure [CHF]). May increase BUN and SrCr levels with renal artery stenosis. Increase in SrCr and hyperkalemia may occur.

ADVERSE REACTIONS: Edema, hypotension, headache, palpitations, rash, pruritus, urinary frequency, nocturia, dizziness, flushing.

INTERACTIONS: Amlodipine: May increase simvastatin exposure; limit simvastatin dose to 20mg/day. Olmesartan: May deteriorate renal function and attenuate antihypertensive effect with NSAIDs (eg, selective cyclooxygenase-2 inhibitors).

PREGNANCY: Category D, not for use in nursing.

MECHANISM OF ACTION: Amlodipine: Calcium channel receptor blocker (dihydropyridine); inhibits transmembrane influx of calcium ion into vascular smooth muscle and cardiac muscle. Acts directly on vascular smooth muscle to cause a reduction in peripheral vascular resistance and reduction in BP. Olmesartan: Angiotensin II receptor blocker; blocks the vasoconstrictor effects of angiotensin II by selectively blocking the binding of angiotensin II to the AT_1 receptor in vascular smooth muscle.

PHARMACOKINETICS: Absorption: Amlodipine: Absolute bioavailability (64-90%); T_{max}=6-12 hrs. Olmesartan: Absolute bioavailability (26%); T_{max}=1-2 hrs. **Distribution:** Amlodipine: Plasma protein binding (93%). Olmesartan: V_d=17L; plasma protein binding (99%). **Metabolism:** Amlodipine: Liver (extensive). Olmesartan: Ester hydrolysis. **Elimination:** Amlodipine: Urine (10% parent, 60% metabolites); $T_{1/2}$=30-50 hrs. Olmesartan: Urine (35-50%), feces; $T_{1/2}$=13 hrs.

NURSING CONSIDERATIONS

Assessment: Assess for severe obstructive CAD, CHF, severe aortic stenosis, volume-/salt-depletion, renal/hepatic function, pregnancy/nursing status, and possible drug interactions. Obtain baseline BP.

Monitoring: Monitor for signs/symptoms of hypotension, renal/hepatic dysfunction, and other adverse reactions. Monitor for symptoms of angina or MI, particularly in patients with severe obstructive CAD, after dosage initiation or increase. Monitor for decrease in Hct and Hgb, and increase in SrCr, BUN, K^+ levels, and hepatic enzymes.

Patient Counseling: Inform of the consequences of exposure during pregnancy in females of childbearing age and of the treatment options in women planning to become pregnant. Instruct to report pregnancy to the physician as soon as possible.

Administration: Oral route. **Storage:** 25°C (77°F); excursions permitted to 15-30°C (59-86°F).

AZULFIDINE   RX
sulfasalazine (Pharmacia & Upjohn)

THERAPEUTIC CLASS: 5-Aminosalicylic acid derivative/sulfapyridine

INDICATIONS: Treatment of mild to moderate ulcerative colitis. Adjunctive therapy in severe ulcerative colitis. To prolong remission period between acute attacks of ulcerative colitis.

DOSAGE: *Adults:* Initial: 3-4g/day in evenly divided doses with intervals not >8 hrs. May initiate at 1-2g/day to reduce GI intolerance. Maint: 2g/day. When endoscopic examination confirms satisfactory improvement, reduce dose to maint level. If diarrhea recurs, increase dose to previously effective levels. If symptoms of GI intolerance occur after 1st few doses, reduce daily dose in 1/2, then gradually increase over several days. If GI intolerance continues, d/c for 5-7 days, then reintroduce at a lower daily dose. Densensitization: Initial: 50-250mg/day. Double every 4-7 days until desired therapeutic level achieved. D/C if sensitivity recurs.
Pediatrics: ≥6 yrs: Initial: 40-60mg/kg/day divided into 3-6 doses. Maint: 30mg/kg/day divided into 4 doses. When endoscopic examination confirms satisfactory improvement, reduce dose to maint level. If diarrhea recurs, increase dose to previously effective levels. If symptoms of GI intolerance occur after 1st few doses, reduce daily dose in 1/2, then gradually increase over several days. If GI intolerance continues, d/c for 5-7 days, then reintroduce at a lower daily dose. Densensitization: Initial: 50-250mg/day. Double every 4-7 days until desired therapeutic level achieved. D/C if sensitivity recurs.

HOW SUPPLIED: Tab: 500mg* *scored

CONTRAINDICATIONS: Intestinal or urinary obstruction, porphyria.

WARNINGS/PRECAUTIONS: Caution with hepatic/renal impairment, blood dyscrasias, severe allergy, and bronchial asthma. Deaths reported from hypersensitivity reactions, agranulocytosis, aplastic anemia, other blood dyscrasias, renal and liver damage, irreversible neuromuscular and CNS changes, and fibrosing alveolitis. Presence of sore throat, fever, pallor, purpura, or jaundice may be indications of serious blood disorder or hepatotoxicity. Monitor CBC, including differential WBC, and LFTs, at baseline, every 2nd week for 1st 3 months, monthly for next 3 months, and every 3 months thereafter; d/c while awaiting the results of blood tests. Monitor urinalysis and renal function periodically. Oligospermia and infertility reported in males. Maintain adequate fluid intake to prevent crystalluria and stone formation. Monitor patients with glucose-6-phosphate dehydrogenase deficiency for signs of hemolytic anemia. D/C if toxic or hypersensitivity reactions occur. Do not attempt desensitization in patients who have history of agranulocytosis, or who have experienced anaphylactoid reaction with previous sulfasalazine (SSZ).

ADVERSE REACTIONS: Anorexia, headache, N/V, gastric distress, reversible oligospermia.

INTERACTIONS: May reduce absorption of folic acid and digoxin.

PREGNANCY: Category B, caution in nursing.

MECHANISM OF ACTION: 5-aminosalicylic acid (5-ASA) derivative/sulfapyridine (SP); not established. May be related to anti-inflammatory and/or immunomodulatory properties, to its affinity for connective tissue, and/or to relatively high concentration reached in serous fluids, the liver, and intestinal walls.

PHARMACOKINETICS: Absorption: SSZ: Absolute bioavailability (<15%); C_{max}=6µg/mL, T_{max}=6 hrs. SP: Well absorbed from colon. Bioavailability (60%); T_{max}=10 hrs. 5-ASA: Much less well absorbed from GI tract. Bioavailability (10-30%); T_{max}=10 hrs. **Distribution:** Crosses placenta; found in breast milk. SSZ (IV): V_d=7.5L; plasma protein binding (>99.3%). SP (IV): Plasma protein binding (70%). **Metabolism:** Intestinal bacteria and liver to SP and 5-ASA (metabolites). SP: Acetylation to acetylsulfapyridine (metabolite). 5-ASA: Liver and intestine. **Elimination:** Urine, feces. SSZ (IV): $T_{1/2}$=7.6 hrs. SP: $T_{1/2}$=10.4 hrs (fast acetylators), 14.8 hrs (slow acetylators).

NURSING CONSIDERATIONS

Assessment: Assess for intestinal or urinary obstruction, porphyria, hepatic/renal impairment, blood dyscrasias, severe allergy or bronchial asthma, glucose-6-phosphate dehydrogenase deficiency, pregnancy/nursing status, possible drug interactions, and hypersensitivity to the drug, its metabolites, sulfonamides, or salicylates. Obtain baseline CBC, including differential WBC, and LFTs.

Monitoring: Monitor for hypersensitivity reactions, agranulocytosis, aplastic anemia or other blood dyscrasias, renal and liver damage, irreversible neuromuscular and CNS changes, fibrosing alveolitis, signs of hemolytic anemia (in patients with glucose-6-phosphate dehydrogenase deficiency), and response to therapy. Monitor CBC, including differential WBC, and LFTs every 2nd week for 1st 3 months, monthly for next 3 months, and every 3 months thereafter. Monitor urinalysis and renal function periodically. May be useful to monitor serum SP levels; >50µg/mL appears to be associated with an increased incidence of adverse reactions.

Patient Counseling: Inform of the possibility of adverse reactions and of the need for careful medical supervision. Instruct to seek medical attention if sore throat, fever, pallor, purpura, or jaundice occurs. Inform that ulcerative colitis rarely remits completely and that risk of relapse can be substantially reduced by continued administration at a maint dosage. Instruct to take in evenly divided doses, preferably pc. Advise that orange-yellow discoloration of urine or skin may occur.

Administration: Oral route. **Storage:** 25°C (77°F); excursions permitted to 15-30°C (59-86°F).

AZULFIDINE EN   RX
sulfasalazine (Pharmacia & Upjohn)

THERAPEUTIC CLASS: 5-Aminosalicylic acid derivative/sulfapyridine

INDICATIONS: Treatment of mild to moderate ulcerative colitis. Adjunctive therapy in severe ulcerative colitis. To prolong remission period between acute attacks of ulcerative colitis. Treatment of rheumatoid arthritis (RA) and polyarticular-course juvenile RA that has responded inadequately to salicylates or other NSAIDs.

DOSAGE: *Adults:* Ulcerative Colitis: Initial: 3-4g/day in evenly divided doses with intervals not >8 hrs. May initiate at 1-2g/day to reduce GI intolerance. Maint: 2g/day. When endoscopic examination confirms satisfactory improvement, reduce dose to maint level. If diarrhea recurs, increase dose to previously effective levels. If symptoms of GI intolerance occur after 1st few doses, reduce daily dose in 1/2, then gradually increase over several days. If GI intolerance continues, d/c for 5-7 days, then reintroduce at a lower daily dose. RA: Initial: 0.5-1g/day. Maint: 2g/day in 2 evenly divided doses. May increase daily dose to 3g if clinical response after 12 weeks is inadequate. Refer to PI for dosing schedule. Densensitization: Initial: 50-250mg/day. Double every 4-7 days until desired therapeutic level achieved. D/C if sensitivity recurs.
Pediatrics: ≥6 yrs: Ulcerative Colitis: Initial: 40-60mg/kg/day divided into 3-6 doses. Maint: 30mg/kg/day divided into 4 doses. When endoscopic examination confirms satisfactory improvement, reduce dose to maint level. If diarrhea recurs, increase dose to previously effective levels. If symptoms of GI intolerance occur after 1st few doses, reduce daily dose in 1/2, then gradually increase over several days. If GI intolerance continues, d/c for 5-7 days, then reintroduce at a lower daily dose. Juvenile RA: 30-50mg/kg/day in 2 evenly divided doses. To reduce GI effects, initiate with 1/4 to 1/3 of planned maint dose and increase weekly until reaching maint

dose at 1 month. Max: 2g/day. Densensitization: Initial: 50-250mg/day. Double every 4-7 days until desired therapeutic level achieved. D/C if sensitivity recurs.

HOW SUPPLIED: Tab, Delayed-Release: 500mg

CONTRAINDICATIONS: Intestinal or urinary obstruction, porphyria.

WARNINGS/PRECAUTIONS: Caution with hepatic/renal impairment, blood dyscrasias, severe allergy, and bronchial asthma. Deaths reported from hypersensitivity reactions, agranulocytosis, aplastic anemia, other blood dyscrasias, renal and liver damage, irreversible neuromuscular and CNS changes, and fibrosing alveolitis. Presence of sore throat, fever, pallor, purpura, or jaundice may be indications of serious blood disorder or hepatotoxicity. Monitor CBC, including differential WBC, and LFTs, at baseline, every 2nd week for 1st 3 months, monthly for next 3 months, and every 3 months thereafter; d/c while awaiting the results of blood tests. Monitor urinalysis and renal function periodically. Oligospermia and infertility reported in males. Maintain adequate fluid intake to prevent crystalluria and stone formation. Monitor patients with glucose-6-phosphate dehydrogenase deficiency for signs of hemolytic anemia. D/C if toxic or hypersensitivity reactions occur. D/C if toxic or hypersensitivity reactions occur. Do not attempt desensitization in patients who have history of agranulocytosis, or who have experienced anaphylactoid reaction with previous sulfasalazine (SSZ). D/C if tabs passed undisintegrated.

ADVERSE REACTIONS: Anorexia, headache, N/V, gastric distress, reversible oligospermia, dyspepsia, rash, abdominal pain, fever, dizziness, stomatitis, pruritus, abnormal LFTs, leukopenia.

INTERACTIONS: May reduce absorption of folic acid and digoxin. Methotrexate may increase incidence of GI adverse events (especially nausea).

PREGNANCY: Category B, caution in nursing.

MECHANISM OF ACTION: 5-aminosalicylic acid (5-ASA) derivative/sulfapyridine (SP); not established. May be related to the anti-inflammatory and/or immunomodulatory properties, to its affinity for connective tissue, and/or to the relatively high concentration reached in serous fluids, liver, and intestinal walls.

PHARMACOKINETICS: Absorption: SSZ: Absolute bioavailability (<15%); C_{max}=6µg/mL, T_{max}=6 hrs. SP: Well absorbed from colon. Bioavailability (60%); T_{max}=10 hrs. 5-ASA: Much less well absorbed from GI tract. Bioavailability (10-30%); T_{max}=10 hrs. **Distribution:** Crosses placenta; found in breast milk. SSZ (IV): V_d=7.5L; plasma protein binding (>99.3%). SP (IV): Plasma protein binding (70%). **Metabolism:** Intestinal bacteria and liver to SP and 5-ASA (metabolites). SP: Acetylation to acetylsulfapyridine (metabolite). 5-ASA: Liver and intestine. **Elimination:** Urine, feces. SSZ (IV): $T_{1/2}$=7.6 hrs. SP: $T_{1/2}$=10.4 hrs (fast acetylators), 14.8 hrs (slow acetylators).

NURSING CONSIDERATIONS

Assessment: Assess for intestinal or urinary obstruction, porphyria, hepatic/renal impairment, blood dyscrasias, severe allergy or bronchial asthma, glucose-6-phosphate dehydrogenase deficiency, pregnancy/nursing status, possible drug interactions, and hypersensitivity to drug, its metabolites, sulfonamides, or salicylates. Obtain baseline CBC, including differential WBC, and LFTs.

Monitoring: Monitor for hypersensitivity reactions, agranulocytosis, aplastic anemia or other blood dyscrasias, renal and liver damage, irreversible neuromuscular and CNS changes, fibrosing alveolitis, signs of hemolytic anemia (in patients with glucose-6-phosphate dehydrogenase deficiency), and response to therapy. Monitor CBC, including differential WBC, and LFTs every 2nd week for 1st 3 months, monthly for next 3 months, and every 3 months thereafter. Monitor urinalysis and renal function periodically. Monitor if tabs passed undisintegrated. May be useful to monitor serum SP levels; >50µg/mL appears to be associated with an increased incidence of adverse reactions.

Patient Counseling: Inform of the possibility of adverse effects and of the need for careful medical supervision. Instruct to seek medical attention if sore throat, fever, pallor, purpura, or jaundice occurs. Instruct to take in evenly divided doses, preferably pc, and to swallow tabs whole. Advise that orange-yellow discoloration of urine or skin may occur. Inform that ulcerative colitis rarely remits completely and that risk of relapse can be substantially reduced by continued administration at a maint dosage. Inform that RA rarely remits; instruct to follow up with their physicians to determine the need for continued administration.

Administration: Oral route. Swallow tabs whole, preferably pc. **Storage:** 25°C (77°F); excursions permitted to 15-30°C (59-86°F).

BACTRIM   RX
sulfamethoxazole - trimethoprim (AR Scientific)

OTHER BRAND NAMES: Bactrim DS (AR Scientific)
THERAPEUTIC CLASS: Sulfonamide/tetrahydrofolic acid inhibitor

B

INDICATIONS: Treatment of urinary tract infection (UTI), acute otitis media in pediatric patients, acute exacerbations of chronic bronchitis (AECB) in adults, traveler's diarrhea in adults, and for enteritis caused by susceptible strains of microorganisms. Treatment and prophylaxis against *Pneumocystis carinii* pneumonia (PCP) in immunosuppressed and those at increased risk.

DOSAGE: *Adults:* UTI/Shigellosis: 800mg-160mg or 2 tabs of 400mg-80mg q12h for 10-14 days (UTI) or 5 days (Shigellosis). AECB: 800mg-160mg or 2 tabs of 400mg-80mg q12h for 14 days. Traveler's Diarrhea: 800mg-160mg or 2 tabs of 400mg-80mg q12h for 5 days. PCP Treatment: 75-100mg/kg SMX and 15-20mg/kg TMP per 24 hrs given in equally divided doses q6h for 14-21 days. PCP Prophylaxis: 800mg-160mg qd. Renal Impairment: CrCl 15-30mL/min: 1/2 of usual dose. CrCl <15mL/min: Not recommended.
Pediatrics: ≥2 months: UTI/Otitis Media/Shigellosis: 40mg/kg SMX and 8mg/kg TMP per 24 hrs given in 2 divided doses q12h for 10 days (UTI/Otitis Media) or 5 days (Shigellosis). PCP Treatment: 75-100mg/kg SMX and 15-20mg/kg TMP per 24 hrs given in equally divided doses q6h for 14-21 days. PCP Prophylaxis: Usual: 750mg/m^2/day SMX and 150mg/m^2/day TMP given in equally divided doses bid, on 3 consecutive days/week. Max: 1,600mg SMX and 320mg TMP/day. Renal Impairment: CrCl 15-30mL/min: 1/2 of usual dose. CrCl <15mL/min: Not recommended.

HOW SUPPLIED: (Sulfamethoxazole [SMX]-Trimethoprim [TMP]) Tab: 400mg-80mg*; Tab, DS: 800mg-160mg* *scored

CONTRAINDICATIONS: Megaloblastic anemia due to folate deficiency, history of drug-induced immune thrombocytopenia with TMP and/or sulfonamides, pregnancy, nursing, infants <2 months, marked hepatic damage, severe renal insufficiency when renal status cannot be monitored.

WARNINGS/PRECAUTIONS: Stevens-Johnson syndrome (SJS), toxic epidermal necrolysis (TEN), fulminant hepatic necrosis, agranulocytosis, aplastic anemia and other blood dyscrasias may occur; d/c at 1st appearance of skin rash or any sign of adverse reaction. *Clostridium difficile*-associated diarrhea (CDAD) reported. Cough, SOB, and pulmonary infiltrates are hypersensitivity reactions of the respiratory tract that have been reported. Thrombocytopenia reported; usually resolves within a week upon d/c. Monitor CBC frequently; d/c with significant reduction in any formed blood element. Avoid use with group A β-hemolytic streptococcal infections. Hemolysis may occur in glucose-6-phosphate dehydrogenase (G6PD)-deficient patients. Patients with renal dysfunction, liver disease, malnutrition, or those receiving high doses are at risk for hypoglycemia. Hematological changes indicative of folic acid deficiency may occur in elderly patients or in patients with preexisting folic acid deficiency or kidney failure; reversible by folinic acid therapy. Caution with hepatic/renal impairment, possible folate deficiency (eg, elderly, chronic alcoholics, malabsorption syndrome, malnutrition), bronchial asthma and severe allergies. Increased incidence of adverse events reported in AIDS patients; re-evaluate therapy if develops skin rash or any sign of adverse reaction develops. Hyperkalemia reported; caution in patients receiving high doses of TMP, underlying disorders of K$^+$ metabolism and renal insufficiency. Ensure adequate fluid intake and urinary output to prevent crystalluria. Slow acetylators more prone to idiosyncratic reactions to sulfonamides. Caution with porphyria or thyroid dysfunction. May result in bacterial resistance with prolonged use or use in the absence of a proven/suspected bacterial infection or a prophylactic indication; take appropriate measures if superinfection develops.

ADVERSE REACTIONS: N/V, anorexia, allergic skin reactions (eg, rash, urticaria), agranulocytosis, aplastic anemia, SJS, TEN, hepatitis, renal failure, hyperkalemia, aseptic meningitis, arthralgia, convulsions, cough.

INTERACTIONS: Increased incidence of thrombocytopenia with purpura in elderly patients with diuretics (primarily thiazides). May prolong PT with anticoagulant warfarin. May increase the effects of phenytoin and levels of methotrexate and digoxin. Marked but reversible nephrotoxicity reported with cyclosporine in renal transplant recipients. May develop megaloblastic anemia with pyrimethamine >25mg/week. Increased SMX levels with indomethacin. May decrease efficacy of TCAs. Single case of toxic delirium reported with amantadine. Potentiates effects of oral hypoglycemics. May cause hyperkalemia in elderly patients with ACE inhibitors.

PREGNANCY: Category C, not for use in nursing.

MECHANISM OF ACTION: SMX: Sulfonamide; inhibits bacterial synthesis of dyhydrofolic acid by competing with para-aminobenzoic acid (PABA). TMP: Tetrahydrofolic acid inhibitor; blocks the production of tetrahydrofolic acid from dihydrofolic acid by binding to and reversibly inhibiting the required enzyme, dihydrofolate reductase.

PHARMACOKINETICS: Absorption: Rapid; T_{max}=1-4 hrs. **Distribution:** Crosses placenta; found in breast milk. SMX: Plasma protein binding (70%); TMP: Plasma protein binding (44%). **Metabolism:** SMX: N$_4$-acetylation; TMP: 1- and 3-oxides, 3'- and 4'-hydroxy derivatives (principal metabolites). **Elimination:** Urine (84.5% total sulfonamide), (66.8%, free TMP); $T_{1/2}$=10 hrs (SMX), 8-10 hrs (TMP).

NURSING CONSIDERATIONS

Assessment: Assess for hypersensitivity reaction to drug components, history of drug-induced immune thrombocytopenia, documented megaloblastic anemia due to folate deficiency (eg, malabsorption syndrome, group A β-hemolytic streptococcal infections, chronic alcoholic, malnutrition status, elderly, receiving anticonvulsant therapy), hepatic/renal insufficiency, CDAD, severe allergies, bronchial asthma, G6PD deficiency, phenylketonurics, porphyria or thyroid dysfunction, underlying disorders of K$^+$ metabolism, slow acetylators, pregnancy/nursing status, and for possible drug interactions. Obtain baseline CBC.

Monitoring: Monitor for severe allergic reactions (eg, SJS, TEN, fulminant hepatic necrosis, agranulocytosis, aplastic anemia and other blood dyscrasias), thrombocytopenia, CDAD (mild diarrhea to fatal colitis), development of drug resistance, overgrowth of nonsusceptible microorganisms, hypersensitivity reactions of the respiratory tract (eg, cough, SOB, pulmonary infiltrates), kernicterus, hypogylcemia, signs of bone marrow depression after chronic use. Periodically monitor CBC, renal function, LFTs and K$^+$ levels, coagulation time, digoxin levels, and perform urinalysis with careful microscopic exam.

Patient Counseling: Inform about potential benefits/risks of therapy. Inform that drug only treats bacterial, not viral infections (eg, common colds). Instruct to take exactly as directed; skipping doses or not completing full course may decrease effectiveness and increase bacterial resistance. Instruct to notify physician if allergic reaction, watery/bloody diarrhea (with/without stomach cramps and fever) occur (may occur up to ≥2 months after treatment). Counsel to drink adequate fluids to prevent crystalluria and stone formation. Notify physician if pregnant/nursing or planning to become pregnant.

Administration: Oral route. **Storage:** 20-25°C (68-77°F).

BACTROBAN   RX
mupirocin calcium (GlaxoSmithKline)

THERAPEUTIC CLASS: Bacterial protein synthesis inhibitor

INDICATIONS: (Oint) Topical treatment of impetigo due to *Staphylococcus aureus* and *Streptococcus pyogenes*. (Cre) Treatment of secondarily infected traumatic skin lesions (up to 10cm in length or 100cm^2 in area) due to *S. aureus* and *S. pyogenes*.

DOSAGE: *Adults:* Apply a small amount tid to the affected area. May be covered with gauze dressing if desired. Reevaluate if no response within 3-5 days. (Cre) Treat for 10 days.
Pediatrics: (Oint) 2 months-16 yrs/(Cre) 3 months-16 yrs: Apply a small amount tid to the affected area. May be covered with gauze dressing if desired. Reevaluate if no response within 3-5 days. (Cre) Treat for 10 days.

HOW SUPPLIED: Cre: 2% [15g, 30g]; Oint: 2% [22g]

WARNINGS/PRECAUTIONS: Avoid contact with the eyes; not for ophthalmic use. Prolonged use may result in overgrowth of nonsusceptible organism (including fungi). Not for use on mucosal surfaces. D/C and institute appropriate therapy if sensitivity or chemical irritation occurs. (Oint) Contains polyethylene glycol; avoid use in conditions where absorption of large quantities is possible, especially if there is evidence of moderate or severe renal impairment.

ADVERSE REACTIONS: (Cre) Headache, rash, nausea, burning at application site, pruritus, abdominal pain, bleeding secondary to eczema, hives. (Oint) Burning, stinging, pain, itching, rash, nausea, erythema.

PREGNANCY: (Cre) Category B, (Oint) Safety not known in pregnancy; (Oint/Cre) caution in nursing.

MECHANISM OF ACTION: Bacterial protein synthesis inhibitor; inhibits bacterial protein synthesis by reversibly and specifically binding to bacterial isoleucyl transfer-RNA synthetase. Active against a wide range of gram-positive bacteria, including methicillin-resistant *S. aureus*. Also active against certain gram-negative bacteria.

PHARMACOKINETICS: Absorption: (Cre) Minimal skin absorption. **Distribution:** Plasma protein binding (>97%). **Metabolism:** (Cre) Rapid once in systemic circulation. **Elimination:** Urine (metabolite); (IV) T$_{1/2}$=20-40 mins.

NURSING CONSIDERATIONS

Assessment: Assess for hypersensitivity, area of skin infection, and pregnancy/nursing status.

Monitoring: Monitor for sensitivity or chemical irritation of the skin. In patients on prolonged therapy, monitor for possible overgrowth of nonsusceptible microorganisms, including fungi.

Patient Counseling: Instruct to use as prescribed. Inform that medication is for external use only and to avoid contact with eyes. Counsel that treated area can be covered with a gauze dressing. Advise d/c medication and notify physician if any signs of local adverse reactions (eg, irritation, severe itching, or rash) develop. Instruct to notify if no clinical improvement is seen within 3-5 days.

Administration: Topical route. **Storage:** (Cre) ≤25°C (77°F). Do not freeze. (Oint) 20-25°C (68-77°F).

BACTROBAN NASAL RX
mupirocin calcium (GlaxoSmithKline)

THERAPEUTIC CLASS: Bacterial protein synthesis inhibitor

INDICATIONS: Eradication of nasal colonization of methicillin-resistant *Staphylococcus aureus* (MRSA) in adults and healthcare workers in certain institutional settings during outbreaks of MRSA.

DOSAGE: *Adults:* Apply 1/2 of the single-use tube into each nostril bid for 5 days. Spread oint by pressing together and releasing the sides of the nose repetitively for 1 min. Do not reuse tube. *Pediatrics:* ≥12 yrs: Apply 1/2 of the single-use tube into each nostril bid for 5 days. Spread oint by pressing together and releasing the sides of the nose repetitively for 1 min. Do not reuse tube.

HOW SUPPLIED: Oint: 2% [1g pkt]

WARNINGS/PRECAUTIONS: Avoid eyes. D/C if sensitization or irritation occur. May cause super-infection with prolonged use.

ADVERSE REACTIONS: Headache, rhinitis, respiratory disorder, pharyngitis, taste perversion.

INTERACTIONS: Avoid use with other intranasal products.

PREGNANCY: Category B, caution in nursing.

MECHANISM OF ACTION: Antibacterial agent; inhibits protein synthesis by reversibly and specifically binding to bacterial isoleucyl transfer-RNA synthetase.

PHARMACOKINETICS: Absorption: Significant in neonates and premature infants. **Elimination:** Urine.

NURSING CONSIDERATIONS

Assessment: Assess for drug hypersensitivity, high-risk healthcare workers during institutional outbreaks of MRSA, possible drug interactions.

Monitoring: Monitor for sensitization, severe local irritation, tearing, and for overgrowth of non-susceptible microorganisms (eg, fungi).

Patient Counseling: Avoid contact with eyes. Consult physician if sensitization or severe irritation occurs.

Administration: Intranasal route. Apply approximately half of ointment from single-use tube directly into 1 nostril and other half into other nostril; discard tube after using. Press sides of nose together and gently massage after application to spread ointment throughout inside of nostril. **Storage:** 20-25°C (68-77°F); excursions permitted to 15-30°C (59-86°F). Do not refrigerate.

BANZEL RX
rufinamide (Eisai)

THERAPEUTIC CLASS: Triazole derivative

INDICATIONS: Adjunctive treatment of seizures associated with Lennox-Gastaut syndrome in adults and children ≥4 yrs.

DOSAGE: *Adults:* Initial: 400-800mg/day in two equally divided doses. Titrate: May increase by 400-800mg qod until max reached. Max: 3200mg/day. Hemodialysis: Consider dosage adjustment. With Valproate: Initiate dose lower than 400mg/day. Elderly: Start at lower end of dosing range. *Pediatrics:* ≥4 yrs: Initial: 10mg/kg/day in two equally divided doses. Titrate: May increase by 10mg/kg increments qod to target dose of 45mg/kg/day or 3200mg/day, whichever is less, given in two equally divided doses. With Valproate: Initiate dose lower than 10mg/kg/day.

HOW SUPPLIED: Sus: 40mg/mL [460mL]; Tab: 200mg*, 400mg* *scored

CONTRAINDICATIONS: Familial short QT syndrome.

WARNINGS/PRECAUTIONS: May increase risk of suicidal thoughts or behavior; monitor for emergence or worsening of depression, suicidal thoughts or behavior, and/or any unusual changes in mood or behavior. Associated with CNS-related adverse effects (eg, somnolence/fatigue, coordination abnormalities, dizziness, gait disturbances, and ataxia). QT interval shortening and leukopenia reported. Multi-organ hypersensitivity syndrome reported; d/c if suspected and start alternative treatment. Withdraw gradually to minimize risk of precipitating seizures, seizure exacerbation, or status epilepticus. If abrupt d/c is necessary, transition to other antiepileptic drugs should be made under close medical supervision. Not recommended in severe hepatic impairment. Caution with mild to moderate hepatic impairment and elderly.

ADVERSE REACTIONS: Somnolence, N/V, headache, fatigue, dizziness, tremor, nystagmus, nasopharyngitis, decreased appetite, rash, ataxia, diplopia, bronchitis, blurred vision.

INTERACTIONS: Carboxylesterase inducers may increase clearance; carboxylesterase inhibitors may decrease metabolism of rufinamide. Potent CYP450 inducers (eg, carbamazepine, phenytoin, primodone, phenobarbital) may increase clearance and decrease levels of rufinamide. Valproate may reduce clearance and increase levels of rufinamide. May increase phenytoin, phenobarbital, CYP2E1 substrates (eg, chlorzoxazone) levels. May decrease lamotrigine, carbamazepine, CYP3A4 substrates (eg, triazolam), hormonal contraceptives levels. Additional forms of nonhormonal contraception are recommended during coadministration. Caution with other drugs that shorten QT interval.

PREGNANCY: Category C, not for use in nursing.

MECHANISM OF ACTION: Triazole derivative; mechanism not established. Suspected to modulate activity of sodium channels and, in particular, prolongation of the inactive state of the channel. Slows sodium channel recovery from inactivation after prolonged prepulse in cultured cortical neurons, and limited sustained repetitive firing of sodium-dependent action potentials.

PHARMACOKINETICS: Absorption: Well-absorbed, T_{max}=4-6 hrs. **Distribution:** Plasma protein binding (34%); V_d=50L (3200mg/day); likely to be excreted in breast milk. **Metabolism:** Extensive; via carboxylesterase mediated hydrolysis; CYP2E1 (weak inhibitor), CYP3A4 (weak inducer). **Elimination:** Urine (2%, unchanged; 66%, acid metabolite CGP 47292); $T_{1/2}$=6-10 hrs.

NURSING CONSIDERATIONS

Assessment: Assess for familial short QT syndrome, presence or history of depression, hepatic/renal impairment, pregnancy/nursing status, and for possible drug interactions.

Monitoring: Monitor for emergence or worsening of depression, suicidal thoughts, changes in behavior, CNS reactions (eg, somnolence, fatigue, coordination abnormalities, dizziness, gait disturbances, ataxia), QT interval shortening, multi-organ hypersensitivity syndrome, and leukopenia. Upon withdrawal of therapy, monitor for precipitation of seizures, exacerbation of seizures, and status epilepticus.

Patient Counseling: Inform patients, caregivers, and families of increased risk of suicidal thoughts/behavior and to be alert for emergence or worsening of signs/symptoms. Instruct to avoid alcohol and take only as prescribed. May develop somnolence or dizziness. Advise not to drive or operate machinery until gain sufficient experience to gauge whether therapy adversely affects mental and/or motor performance. Encourage to enroll in North American Antiepileptic Drug (NAAED) Pregnancy Registry. Instruct to notify physician if rash associated with fever develops. Advise to take with food; tabs may be taken whole, cut in half, or crushed. Must shake suspension well before every administration.

Administration: Oral route. Take with food. Tab: May administer as whole; half or crushed tab. Sus: Refer to PI for complete instructions. **Storage:** Tab/Sus: 25°C (77°F); excursions permitted to 15-30°C (59-86°F). Tab: Protect from moisture. Sus: Store in an upright position. Use within 90 days of first opening the bottle, discard any remainder.

BARACLUDE

RX

entecavir (Bristol-Myers Squibb)

Lactic acidosis and severe hepatomegaly with steatosis, including fatal cases, have been reported alone or in combination with antiretrovirals. Severe acute exacerbations of hepatitis B reported upon d/c of therapy; closely monitor liver function for at least several months after d/c. If appropriate, may initiate anti-hepatitis B therapy. Limited clinical experience suggests there is a potential for the development of resistance to HIV nucleoside reverse transcriptase inhibitors if entecavir is used to treat chronic hepatitis B virus (HBV) infection in patients with untreated HIV infection. Not recommended for HIV/HBV coinfected patients not receiving highly active antiretroviral therapy (HAART).

THERAPEUTIC CLASS: Guanosine nucleoside analogue

INDICATIONS: Treatment of chronic HBV infection with active viral replication and persistent elevations in serum aminotransferases (ALT/AST) or histologically active disease.

DOSAGE: *Adults:* ≥16 yrs: Compensated Liver Disease: Nucleoside-Treatment-Naive: 0.5mg qd. History of Hepatitis B Viremia While Receiving Lamivudine or Known Lamivudine/Telbivudine Resistance Mutations: 1mg qd. Decompensated Liver Disease: 1mg qd. Take on an empty stomach (at least 2 hrs after a meal and 2 hrs before the next meal). Renal Impairment: Refer to PI for dose modifications.

HOW SUPPLIED: Sol: 0.05mg/mL [210mL]; Tab: 0.5mg, 1mg

WARNINGS/PRECAUTIONS: Reduce dose in renal dysfunction (CrCl <50mL/min), including patients on hemodialysis or continuous ambulatory peritoneal dialysis. May require HIV antibody testing prior to treatment. Caution with known risk factors for liver disease. D/C if lactic acidosis or profound hepatotoxicity occurs. Caution with dose selection in elderly.

ADVERSE REACTIONS: Post-treatment exacerbation of hepatitis B, lactic acidosis, severe hepatomegaly with steatosis, headache, fatigue, dizziness, nausea, ALT/lipase elevation, total bilirubin elevation, hyperglycemia, glycosuria, hematuria.

INTERACTIONS: See Boxed Warning. May increase levels of either entecavir or concomitant drugs that reduce renal function or compete for active tubular secretion; closely monitor for adverse events.

PREGNANCY: Category C, not for use in nursing.

MECHANISM OF ACTION: Guanosine nucleoside analogue; inhibits base priming, reverse transcription of negative strand from pregenomic mRNA, and synthesis of positive strand of HBV DNA.

PHARMACOKINETICS: Absorption: Bioavailability (100%); C_{max}=4.2ng/mL (0.5mg), 8.2ng/mL (1.0mg); T_{max}=0.5-1.5 hrs. Refer to PI for pharmacokinetic parameters in patients with selected degrees of renal function. **Distribution:** Plasma protein binding (13%). **Metabolism:** Hepatic (minor). **Elimination:** Urine (62-73% unchanged); $T_{1/2}$=128-149 hrs.

NURSING CONSIDERATIONS

Assessment: Assess for hepatic/renal impairment, pregnancy/nursing status, other medical conditions, and possible drug interactions. Perform HIV antibody testing and assess CrCl.

Monitoring: Monitor for signs/symptoms of lactic acidosis, hepatotoxicity, and other adverse reactions. Monitor renal function and (after d/c) hepatic function.

Patient Counseling: Advise to remain under care of physician during therapy and report any new symptoms or concurrent medications. Inform that treatment has not been shown to reduce risk of transmission of HBV. Advise to take on an empty stomach (at least 2 hrs after a meal and 2 hrs before the next meal). Instruct to hold dosing spoon in a vertical position and fill gradually to the mark corresponding to prescribed dose for oral sol. Inform that treatment may lower the amount of HBV in the body, lower the ability of HBV to multiply and infect new liver cells, and improve the condition of the liver, but will not cure HBV. Counsel that it is not known whether treatment will reduce risk of liver cancer or cirrhosis. Inform that deterioration of liver disease may occur in some cases if treatment is d/c, and to discuss any change in regimen with physician. Inform that drug may increase the chance of HIV resistance to HIV medication if HIV-infected and not receiving effective HIV treatment.

Administration: Oral route. **Storage:** 25°C (77°F); excursions permitted between 15-30°C (59-86°F). Protect oral sol from light.

BAYER ASPIRIN OTC
aspirin (Bayer Healthcare)

OTHER BRAND NAMES: Bayer Aspirin Children's (Bayer Healthcare) - Bayer Aspirin Regimen with Calcium (Bayer Healthcare) - Bayer Aspirin Regimen (Bayer Healthcare) - Genuine Bayer Aspirin (Bayer Healthcare)

THERAPEUTIC CLASS: Salicylate

INDICATIONS: To reduce the risk of death and nonfatal stroke with previous ischemic stroke or transient ischemia of the brain. To reduce risk of vascular mortality with suspected acute myocardial infarction (MI). To reduce risk of death and nonfatal MI with previous MI or unstable angina. To reduce risk of MI and sudden death in chronic stable angina pectoris. For patients who have undergone revascularization procedures with a preexisting condition for which ASA is indicated. Relief of signs of rheumatoid arthritis (RA), juvenile rheumatoid arthritis (JRA), osteoarthritis (OA), spondyloarthropathies, arthritis, and pleurisy associated with systemic lupus erythematosus (SLE). For minor aches and pains.

DOSAGE: *Adults:* Ischemic Stroke/TIA: 50-325mg qd. Suspected Acute MI: Initial: 160-162.5mg qd as soon as suspect MI. Maint: 160-162.5mg qd for 30 days post-infarction, consider further therapy for prevention/recurrent MI. Prevention or Recurrent MI/Unstable Angina/Chronic Stable Angina: 75-325mg qd. CABG: 325mg qd, start 6 hrs post-surgery. Continue for 1 yr. PTCA: Initial: 325mg, 2 hrs pre-surgery. Maint: 160-325mg qd. Carotid Endarterectomy: 80mg qd to 650mg bid, start pre-surgery. RA: Initial: 3g qd in divided doses. Increase for anti-inflammatory efficacy to 150-300mcg/mL plasma salicylate level. Spondyloarthropathies: Up to 4g/day in divided doses. OA: Up to 3g/day in divided doses. Arthritis/SLE Pleurisy: Initial: 3g/day in divided doses. Increase for anti-inflammatory efficacy to 150-300mcg/mL plasma salicylate level. Pain: 325-650mg q4-6h. Max: 4g/day.
Pediatrics: JRA: Initial: 90-130mg/kg/day in divided doses. Increase for anti-inflammatory efficacy to 150-300mcg/mL plasma salicylate level. Pain: ≥12 yrs: 325-650mg q4-6h. Max: 4g/day.

HOW SUPPLIED: Tab: (Genuine Bayer Aspirin) 325mg; Tab: (Bayer Aspirin Regimen with Calcium) 81mg; Tab, Chewable: (Bayer Aspirin Children's) 81mg; Tab, Delayed-Release: (Bayer Aspirin Regimen) 81mg, 325mg

CONTRAINDICATIONS: NSAID allergy, viral infections in children or teenagers, syndrome of asthma, rhinitis, and nasal polyps.

WARNINGS/PRECAUTIONS: Increased risk of bleeding with heavy alcohol use (≥3 drinks/day). May inhibit platelet function; can adversely affect inherited (hemophilia) or acquired (hepatic disease, vitamin K deficiency) bleeding disorders. Monitor for bleeding and ulceration. Avoid in history of active peptic ulcer, severe renal failure, severe hepatic insufficiency, and sodium restricted diets. Associated with elevated LFTs, BUN, and SrCr; hyperkalemia; proteinuria; and prolonged bleeding time. Avoid 1 week before and during labor.

ADVERSE REACTIONS: Fever, hypothermia, dysrhythmias, hypotension, agitation, cerebral edema, dehydration, hyperkalemia, dyspepsia, GI bleed, hearing loss, tinnitus, problems in pregnancy.

INTERACTIONS: Diminished hypotensive and hyponatremic effects of ACE inhibitors. May increase levels of acetazolamide, valproic acid. Increased bleeding risk with heparin, warfarin. Decreased levels of phenytoin. Decreased hypotensive effects of β-blockers. Decreased diuretic effects with renal or cardiovascular disease. Decreased methotrexate clearance; increased risk of bone marrow toxicity. Avoid NSAIDs. Increased effects of hypoglycemic agents. Antagonizes uricosuric agents.

PREGNANCY: Avoid in 3rd trimester of pregnancy and nursing.

MECHANISM OF ACTION: Provides temporary relief from arthritis pain and arthritis inflammation.

NURSING CONSIDERATIONS

Assessment: Assess for hypersensitivity, stomach problems, bleeding problems, ulcers, history of chickenpox or flu symptoms, and possible drug interactions.

Monitoring: Monitor for Reye's syndrome, allergic reactions include hives, facial swelling, asthma (wheezing) and shock.

Patient Counseling: Instruct to immediately report worsening of any adverse effects.

Administration: Oral route. **Storage:** Room temperature.

BENICAR   RX
olmesartan medoxomil (Daiichi Sankyo)

> D/C when pregnancy is detected. Drugs that act directly on the renin-angiotensin system can cause death/injury to developing fetus.

THERAPEUTIC CLASS: Angiotensin II receptor antagonist

INDICATIONS: Treatment of HTN alone or in combination with other antihypertensives.

DOSAGE: *Adults:* Individualize dose. Monotherapy Without Volume Contraction: Initial: 20mg qd. Titrate: May increase to 40mg qd after 2 weeks if needed. May add diuretic if BP is not controlled. Intravascular Volume Depletion (eg, treated with diuretics, particularly those with impaired renal function): Lower initial dose; monitor closely.
Pediatrics: 6-16 yrs: Individualize dose. ≥35kg: Initial: 20mg qd. Titrate: May increase to 40mg qd after 2 weeks if needed. Max: 40mg qd. 20-<35kg: Initial: 10mg qd. Titrate: May increase to 20mg qd after 2 weeks if needed. Max: 20mg qd. Cannot Swallow Tab: Refer to PI for preparation of sus; same dose as tab.

HOW SUPPLIED: Tab: 5mg, 20mg, 40mg

WARNINGS/PRECAUTIONS: Symptomatic hypotension may occur in volume- and/or salt-depleted patients after treatment initiation; monitor closely. Changes in renal function may occur. Oliguria and/or progressive azotemia and (rarely) acute renal failure and/or death may occur in patients whose renal function is dependent on the renin-angiotensin-aldosterone system (eg, severe congestive heart failure [CHF]). May increase SrCr or BUN levels with renal artery stenosis.

ADVERSE REACTIONS: Dizziness.

INTERACTIONS: May increase risk of symptomatic hypotension with high dose diuretics. NSAIDs (eg, selective cyclooxygenase-2 inhibitors) may attenuate antihypertensive effect and deteriorate renal function.

PREGNANCY: Category D, not for use in nursing.

MECHANISM OF ACTION: Angiotensin II receptor antagonist; blocks vasoconstrictor effects of angiotensin II by selectively blocking binding of angiotensin II to AT_1 receptor in vascular smooth muscle.

PHARMACOKINETICS: Absorption: Rapid. Absolute bioavailability (26%); T_{max}=1-2 hrs. **Distribution:** V_d=17L; plasma protein binding (99%). **Metabolism:** Ester hydrolysis. **Elimination:** Urine (35-50%), feces; $T_{1/2}$=13 hrs.

NURSING CONSIDERATIONS

Assessment: Assess for CHF, renal artery stenosis, volume/salt depletion, renal/hepatic function, pregnancy/nursing status, and possible drug interactions. Obtain baseline BP.

Monitoring: Monitor for signs/symptoms of hypotension, renal/hepatic dysfunction, and other adverse reactions.

Patient Counseling: Inform of the consequences of exposure during pregnancy in females of childbearing age and of the treatment options in women planning to become pregnant. Instruct to report pregnancy to the physician as soon as possible.

Administration: Oral route. Refer to PI for preparation of sus. Shake sus before use. **Storage:** (Tab) 20-25°C (68-77°F). (Sus) 2-8°C (36-46°F) for up to 4 weeks.

BENICAR HCT   RX

olmesartan medoxomil - hydrochlorothiazide (Daiichi Sankyo)

> Drugs that act directly on the renin-angiotensin system can cause death/injury to developing fetus. D/C therapy if pregnancy is detected.

THERAPEUTIC CLASS: Angiotensin II receptor antagonist/thiazide diuretic

INDICATIONS: Treatment of HTN.

DOSAGE: *Adults:* Replacement Therapy: Individualize dose. Combination may be substituted for titrated components. Uncontrolled BP on Olmesartan or HCTZ Alone: Switch to 1 tab qd of combination therapy. Titrate: May increase at intervals of 2-4 weeks. Max: 1 tab/day. Elderly: Start at lower end of dosing range.

HOW SUPPLIED: Tab: (Olmesartan-HCTZ) 20mg-12.5mg, 40mg-12.5mg, 40mg-25mg

CONTRAINDICATIONS: Anuria, sulfonamide-derived drug hypersensitivity.

WARNINGS/PRECAUTIONS: Not indicated for initial therapy of HTN. Symptomatic hypotension may occur in patients with activated renin-angiotensin system (eg, volume- or salt-depleted); correct these conditions prior to therapy and monitor closely. Hypokalemia/hyperkalemia reported. Not recommended with CrCl ≤30mL/min. Caution in elderly. HCTZ: Caution with hepatic impairment or progressive liver disease; may precipitate hepatic coma. May cause hypersensitivity reactions, exacerbation or activation of systemic lupus erythematosus (SLE), hyperuricemia or precipitation of frank gout, hyperglycemia, hypomagnesemia, hypercalcemia, and manifestations of latent diabetes mellitus (DM). May cause idiosyncratic reaction, resulting in acute transient myopia and acute angle-closure glaucoma; d/c as rapidly as possible. Observe for signs of fluid and electrolyte imbalance (eg, hyponatremia, hypochloremic alkalosis, hypokalemia). Hypokalemia may sensitize/exaggerate the response of the heart to toxic effects of digitalis. Hypokalemia may develop, especially with brisk diuresis, severe cirrhosis, or after prolonged therapy. D/C before testing for parathyroid function. Enhanced effects in postsympathectomy patients. D/C or withhold if progressive renal impairment becomes evident. Increased cholesterol, TG levels reported. May precipitate azotemia with renal disease. Olmesartan: Oliguria and/or progressive azotemia and (rarely) acute renal failure and/or death may occur in patients whose renal function is dependent on the renin-angiotensin-aldosterone system (eg, severe congestive heart failure [CHF]). May increase BUN and SrCr levels with renal artery stenosis.

ADVERSE REACTIONS: Dizziness, upper respiratory tract infection, hyperuricemia, nausea.

INTERACTIONS: May decrease effects of diuretics and angiotensin II receptor antagonists and may further deteriorate renal function with NSAIDs, including selective cyclooxygenase-2 inhibitors. HCTZ: May increase risk of lithium toxicity; avoid concurrent use. Alcohol, barbiturates, and narcotics may potentiate orthostatic hypotension. Dose adjustment of antidiabetic drugs (eg, oral agents and insulin) may be required. Additive effect or potentiation with other antihypertensives. Anionic exchange resins (eg, cholestyramine, colestipol) may impair absorption. Corticosteroids and adrenocorticotropic hormone may intensify electrolyte depletion, particularly hypokalemia. May decrease response to pressor amines (eg, norepinephrine). May increase response to nondepolarizing skeletal muscle relaxants (eg, tubocurarine).

PREGNANCY: Category D, not for use in nursing.

MECHANISM OF ACTION: Olmesartan: Angiotensin II receptor antagonist; blocks vasoconstrictor effects of angiotensin II by selectively blocking binding of angiotensin II to AT1 receptor in vascular smooth muscle. HCTZ: Thiazide diuretic; not established. Affects renal tubular mechanism of electrolyte reabsorption, directly increasing excretion of Na^+ and chloride in approximately equivalent amounts.

PHARMACOKINETICS: Absorption: Olmesartan: Rapid; absolute bioavailability (26%); T_{max}=1-2 hrs. **Distribution:** Olmesartan: V_d=17L; plasma protein binding (99%). HCTZ: Crosses placenta; found in breast milk. **Metabolism:** Olmesartan: Ester hydrolysis. **Elimination:** Olmesartan: Urine (35-50%), feces; $T_{1/2}$=13 hrs. HCTZ: Kidney (≥61% unchanged); $T_{1/2}$=5.6-14.8 hrs.

NURSING CONSIDERATIONS

Assessment: Assess for hypersensitivity to drugs and its components, anuria, sulfonamide hypersensitivity, history of penicillin allergy, volume/salt depletion, SLE, DM, CHF, hepatic/renal function, postsympathectomy status, cirrhosis, renal artery stenosis, pregnancy/nursing status, and possible drug interactions. Obtain baseline BP.

Monitoring: Monitor for signs/symptoms of fluid/electrolyte imbalance, exacerbation/activation of SLE, idiosyncratic reaction, latent DM, precipitation of gout, hypersensitivity reactions, and other adverse reactions. Monitor BP, serum electrolytes, renal function, cholesterol, and TG levels periodically.

Patient Counseling: Inform of pregnancy risks and instruct to report pregnancy to their physician immediately. Counsel that lightheadedness may occur especially during the 1st days of therapy; instruct to report to physician. Instruct to d/c therapy and consult physician if syncope occurs. Advise that inadequate fluid intake, excessive perspiration, diarrhea, or vomiting may result in excessive fall in BP, leading to lightheadedness or syncope.

Administration: Oral route. **Storage:** 20-25°C (68-77°F).

BENLYSTA   RX

belimumab (Human Genome Sciences)

THERAPEUTIC CLASS: Monoclonal antibody/BLyS blocker

INDICATIONS: Treatment of adult patients with active, autoantibody-positive, systemic lupus erythematosus who are receiving standard therapy.

DOSAGE: *Adults:* 10mg/kg IV infusion over 1 hr at 2-week intervals for the 1st 3 doses and at 4-week intervals thereafter. Slow or interrupt infusion rate if infusion reaction develops. Consider premedication for prophylaxis against infusion and hypersensitivity reactions.

HOW SUPPLIED: Inj: 120mg [5mL], 400mg [20mL]

WARNINGS/PRECAUTIONS: Deaths reported; etiologies included infection, cardiovascular disease, and suicide. Serious and sometimes fatal infections reported; caution with chronic infections and interrupt treatment if new infection develops. Malignancies, infusion reactions, psychiatric events (eg, depression) reported. Hypersensitivity reactions, including anaphylaxis and death, reported; onset may be delayed; d/c immediately if serious hypersensitivity reactions occur. Caution with history of depression or other serious psychiatric disorders, and in elderly. Women of childbearing potential should use adequate contraception during treatment and for ≥4 months after the final treatment. Not recommended with severe active lupus nephritis or severe active CNS lupus.

ADVERSE REACTIONS: Serious infections, nausea, diarrhea, pyrexia, nasopharyngitis, bronchitis, insomnia, pain in extremity, depression, migraine, pharyngitis, cystitis, leukopenia, viral gastroenteritis.

INTERACTIONS: Not recommended with other biologics or IV cyclophosphamide. Live vaccines should not be given for 30 days before or concurrently; may interfere with the response to immunizations.

PREGNANCY: Category C, not for use in nursing.

MECHANISM OF ACTION: Monoclonal antibody/BLyS blocker; blocks binding of soluble human B lymphocyte stimulator protein (BLyS) to its receptors on B cells. Inhibits survival of B cells, including autoreactive B cells, and reduces differentiation of B cells into immunoglobulin-producing plasma cells.

PHARMACOKINETICS: Absorption: AUC=3083µg•day/mL; C_{max}=313µg/mL. **Distribution:** V_d=5.29L; crosses placenta. **Elimination:** $T_{1/2}$=19.4 days.

NURSING CONSIDERATIONS

Assessment: Assess for chronic infection, history of depression or other serious psychiatric disorders, previous anaphylaxis with the drug, history of multiple drug allergies or significant hypersensitivity, pregnancy/nursing status, and possible drug interactions.

Monitoring: Monitor for infusion and hypersensitivity reactions, infections, malignancy, and psychiatric events.

Patient Counseling: Advise to read Medication Guide before treatment session. Advise that drug may decrease ability to fight infections. Instruct to notify physician if signs or symptoms of infection, allergic reaction, new or worsening depression, suicidal thoughts, or other mood changes develop, and if planning to breastfeed or become pregnant. Inform about signs and symptoms of hypersensitivity reaction and instruct to seek medical care should reaction occur. Advise not to receive live vaccines while on therapy.

Administration: IV route. Reconstitute and dilute prior to administration; refer to PI for preparation and administration instructions. Dilute with 0.9% NaCl only. Do not administer as an IV push or bolus. **Storage:** Unreconstituted/Reconstituted: 2-8°C (36-46°F). Do not freeze. Protect from light and store vials in original carton until use. Avoid exposure to heat. Diluted Sol: 2-8°C (36-46°F) or room temperature. Total time from reconstitution to completion of infusion should not exceed 8 hrs.

BENTYL   RX
dicyclomine HCl (Axcan Scandipharm)

THERAPEUTIC CLASS: Anticholinergic

INDICATIONS: Treatment of functional bowel/irritable bowel syndrome.

DOSAGE: *Adults:* Individualize dose. (PO) Initial: 20mg qid. Titrate: May increase to 40mg qid after 1 week of initial dose, unless side effects limit dose escalation. D/C if efficacy not achieved within 2 weeks or side effects require doses below 80mg/day. (Inj) Initial: 10-20mg IM qid for 1-2 days if unable to take PO medication. Elderly: Start at lower end of dosing range.

HOW SUPPLIED: Cap: 10mg; Inj: 10mg/mL; Syrup: 10mg/5mL; Tab: 20mg

CONTRAINDICATIONS: GI tract obstructive disease, obstructive uropathy, severe ulcerative colitis, reflux esophagitis, glaucoma, myasthenia gravis, unstable cardiovascular status in acute hemorrhage, nursing mothers, infants <6 months of age.

WARNINGS/PRECAUTIONS: Caution in conditions characterized by tachyarrhythmia which may further accelerate heart rate (eg, thyrotoxicosis and congestive heart failure). Caution with coronary heart disease; ischemia and infarction may be worsened. Peripheral effects (eg, dryness of mouth with difficulty in swallowing/talking), CNS signs/symptoms (eg, confusion and disorientation), and psychosis reported. Heat prostration may occur in high environmental temperature; d/c if symptoms occur and institute supportive measures. May impair mental abilities. Avoid with myasthenia gravis except to reduce adverse muscarinic effects of an anticholinesterase. Diarrhea may be the early symptom of intestinal obstruction especially with ileostomy/colostomy patients; treatment would be inappropriate and possibly harmful. Ogilvie's syndrome (colonic pseudo-obstruction) rarely reported. Caution with salmonella dysentery; toxic dilation of intestine and intestinal perforation may occur. Caution with ulcerative colitis; large doses may suppress intestinal motility producing paralytic ileus and precipitate/aggravate serious complication of toxic megacolon. Caution in patients with HTN, fever, autonomic neuropathy, prostatic enlargement, hepatic/renal impairment, and in elderly. Serious respiratory symptoms, seizures, syncope, and death reported in infants. (Inj) For IM use only; inadvertent IV use may result in thrombosis, thrombophlebitis, and inj-site reactions.

ADVERSE REACTIONS: Dry mouth, dizziness, blurred vision, nausea, somnolence, asthenia, nervousness.

INTERACTIONS: May antagonize the effect of antiglaucoma agents and drugs that alter GI motility such as metoclopramide. Avoid concomitant use with corticosteroids in glaucoma patients. Potentiated by amantadine, Class I antiarrhythmics (eg, quinidine), antihistamines, antipsychotics (eg, phenothiazines), benzodiazepines, MAOIs, narcotic analgesics (eg, meperidine), nitrates/nitrites, sympathomimetics, TCAs, and other drugs with anticholinergic activity. Antacids may interfere with absorption; avoid simultaneous use. May affect GI absorption of various drugs by affecting on GI motility, such as slowly dissolving forms of digoxin; increased serum digoxin concentration may result. Antagonized by drugs used to treat achlorhydria and those used to test gastric secretion.

PREGNANCY: Category B, contraindicated in nursing.

MECHANISM OF ACTION: Anticholinergic and antispasmodic agent; relieves smooth muscle spasm of the GI tract, and antagonizes bradykinin- and histamine-induced spasms.

PHARMACOKINETICS: Absorption: Rapid; T_{max}=60-90 mins. **Distribution:** V_d=approximately 3.65L/kg (extensive); found in breast milk. **Elimination:** Urine (79.5%), feces (8.4%); $T_{1/2}$=1.8 hrs.

NURSING CONSIDERATIONS

Assessment: Assess for cardiovascular conditions, myasthenia gravis, glaucoma, intestinal obstructive, psychosis, ulcerative colitis, renal/hepatic dysfunction, pregnancy status, possible drug interactions, or any other conditions where treatment is contraindicated or cautioned.

Monitoring: Monitor for increased HR, worsening of ischemia/infarction, heat prostration, drowsiness, blurred vision, curare-like action, Ogilvie's syndrome, toxic dilation of intestine and intestinal perforation in patients with Salmonella dysentery, paralytic ileus with large doses, urinary retention, hypersensitivity reactions, and other adverse reactions, renal function in elderly.

Patient Counseling: Counsel of proper administration. Advise not to breastfeed while on therapy and not to administer to infants less than 6 months. Instruct to exercise caution while operating machinery/driving. Inform of risk of heat prostration in high environmental temperature; d/c if symptoms occur and consult a physician.

Administration: PO, IM route. Refer to PI for preparation for IM administration. **Storage:** <30°C (86°F). Tab: Avoid exposure to direct sunlight. Syrup: Protect from excessive heat. Inj: Protect from freezing.

BENZACLIN
clindamycin phosphate - benzoyl peroxide (Dermik)

RX

THERAPEUTIC CLASS: Antibacterial/keratolytic

INDICATIONS: Topical treatment of acne vulgaris.

DOSAGE: *Adults:* Wash face and pat dry. Apply bid (am and pm) or ud.
Pediatrics: ≥12 yrs: Wash face and pat dry. Apply bid (am and pm) or ud.

HOW SUPPLIED: Gel: (Clindamycin Phosphate-Benzoyl Peroxide) 10mg-50mg [25g, 35g, 50g]; (Generic) [50g]

CONTRAINDICATIONS: History of regional enteritis, ulcerative colitis (UC), or antibiotic-associated colitis. Hypersensitivity to lincomycin.

WARNINGS/PRECAUTIONS: Severe colitis reported with oral and parenteral clindamycin. Topical use of clindamycin may result in absorption of the antibiotic from the skin surface. Diarrhea, bloody diarrhea, and colitis (including pseudomembranous colitis) reported; d/c if significant diarrhea occurs. Avoid contact with eyes and mucous membranes. May cause an overgrowth of nonsusceptible organisms, including fungi; d/c use and treat appropriately.

ADVERSE REACTIONS: Dry skin, application-site reactions.

INTERACTIONS: Antiperistaltic agents (eg, opiates, diphenoxylate with atropine) may prolong and/or worsen severe colitis. Caution with concomitant topical acne therapy (eg, peeling, desquamating, or abrasive agents) because of possible cumulative irritancy. Avoid erythromycin agents.

PREGNANCY: Category C, not for use in nursing.

MECHANISM OF ACTION: Antibacterial/keratolytic; acts against *Propionibacterium acnes* an organism associated with acne vulgaris.

PHARMACOKINETICS: Absorption: (Benzoyl peroxide) Skin. (Clindamycin Phosphate) Bioavailability (>1%). C_{max}=(1.47-2.77ng/mL, Day 1), (1.43-7.18ng/mL, Day 5). AUC=(2.74-12.86ng•h/mL, Day 1), (11.4-69.7ng•h/mL, Day 5). **Distribution:** Orally and parenterally administered clindamycin has been reported to appear in breast milk. **Metabolism:** (Benzoyl peroxide) Benzoic acid. **Elimination:** (Clindamycin Phosphate) Urine (0.03-0.08%).

NURSING CONSIDERATIONS

Assessment: Assess for hypersensitivity to lincomycin, history of regional enteritis, UC, antibiotic-associated colitis, pregnancy/nursing status and for possible drug interactions.

Monitoring: Monitor for signs/symptoms of diarrhea, bloody diarrhea and colitis (pseudomembranous colitis), overgrowth of nonsusceptible organisms (eg, fungi), local adverse reactions, and allergic reactions. Perform endoscopic exam to diagnose pseudomembranous colitis. Perform stool culture for *Clostridium difficile* and stool assay for *Clostridium difficile* toxin if diarrhea occurs. Perform large bowel endoscopy if severe diarrhea occurs.

Patient Counseling: Counsel to notify physician if diarrhea develops during therapy and up to several weeks after. Advise to use as directed, for external use only, to avoid contact with eyes, inside the nose, mouth, and mucous membranes. Advise not to use any other topical acne preparation unless otherwise directed by physician. Inform that drug may bleach hair or colored fabric. Advise to limit exposure to sunlight and to wear protective clothing. Instruct to contact physician if develop any signs of adverse reactions. Counsel to d/c use if severe allergic symptoms (eg, severe swelling, shortness of breath) develop. Instruct to wash skin gently, then rinse with warm water and pat dry prior to use. Keep out of reach of children.

Administration: Topical route. **Storage:** 25°C (77°F). Do not freeze. Keep tightly closed. Keep out of reach of children. Discard unused product after 3 months.

BENZTROPINE
benztropine mesylate (Various)

RX

OTHER BRAND NAMES: Cogentin (Lundbeck)
THERAPEUTIC CLASS: Anticholinergic

B

INDICATIONS: Adjunct in all forms of parkinsonism. Control of drug-induced extrapyramidal disorders.

DOSAGE: *Adults:* Individualize dose. Titrate: May increase by 0.5mg/day q5-6 days. Idiopathic Parkinsonism: Initial: 0.5-1mg qhs. Postencephalitic Parkinsonism: 2mg/day given in 1 or more doses. Extrapyramidal Disorders: 1-4mg/day given qd-bid. D/C and re-evaluate necessity after 1-2 weeks; may reinstitute if disorders recur. (Inj) Acute Dystonic Reactions: 1-2mg IM/IV. *Pediatrics:* >3 yrs: Individualize dose. Titrate: May increase by 0.5mg/day q5-6 days. Idiopathic Parkinsonism: Initial: 0.5-1mg qhs. Postencephalitic Parkinsonism: 2mg/day given in 1 or more doses. Extrapyramidal Disorders: 1-4mg/day given qd-bid. D/C and re-evaluate necessity after 1-2 weeks; may reinstitute if disorders recur. (Inj) Acute Dystonic Reactions: 1-2mg IM/IV.

HOW SUPPLIED: Inj: 1mg/mL; Tab: 0.5mg*, 1mg*, 2mg* *scored

CONTRAINDICATIONS: Patients <3 yrs.

WARNINGS/PRECAUTIONS: May produce anhidrosis, caution in hot weather. Muscle weakness and dysuria may occur. Caution in pediatrics >3 years of age. Not recommended for tardive dyskinesia (TD). Avoid with angle-closure glaucoma. Caution with CNS disease, mental disorders, tachycardia, prostatic hypertrophy, alcoholics, chronically ill, those exposed to hot environments. May impair mental/physical abilities.

ADVERSE REACTIONS: Tachycardia, paralytic ileus, constipation, N/V, dry mouth, confusion, blurred vision, urinary retention, heat stroke, hyperthermia, fever.

INTERACTIONS: Paralytic ileus, hyperthermia and heat stroke reported with phenothiazines and TCAs. Caution with other atropine-like agents.

PREGNANCY: Safety in pregnancy and nursing not known.

MECHANISM OF ACTION: Anticholinergic agent; controls extrapyramidal symptoms in parkinsonism.

NURSING CONSIDERATIONS

Assessment: Assess for tachycardia, prostatic hypertrophy, anhidrosis, TD. Note other diseases/conditions and drug therapy.

Monitoring: Monitor for tachycardia, prostatic hypertrophy, anhidrosis, hyperthermia, constipation, urinary retention, paralytic ileus, toxic psychosis.

Patient Counseling: Caution during hot weather, especially when given concomitantly with other atropine-like drugs to the chronically ill, alcoholics, those who have CNS disease, and those who do manual labor in a hot environment. Caution while operating machinery/driving.

Administration: IV/IM, Oral route. **Storage:** 15-30°C (59-86°F). Dispense in tightly closed container.

BEPREVE   RX
bepotastine besilate (Ista)

THERAPEUTIC CLASS: H$_1$-antagonist

INDICATIONS: Treatment of itching associated with signs and symptoms of allergic conjunctivitis.

DOSAGE: *Adults:* 1 drop into the affected eye(s) bid.
Pediatrics: >2 yrs: 1 drop into the affected eye(s) bid.

HOW SUPPLIED: Sol: 1.5% [2.5mL, 5mL, 10mL]

WARNINGS/PRECAUTIONS: For topical ophthalmic use only. Not for treatment of contact lens-related irritation. Remove contact lenses prior to instillation and reinsert after 10 min. This product contains benzalkonium chloride.

ADVERSE REACTIONS: Mild taste, eye irritation, headache, and nasopharyngitis.

INTERACTIONS: Low potential for drug interaction via inhibition of CYP3A4, CYP2C9, and CYP2C19. May be absorbed by soft contact lenses because of benzalkonium chloride.

PREGNANCY: Category C, caution in nursing.

MECHANISM OF ACTION: H$_1$ antagonist; antagonizes H$_1$ receptor and inhibits release of histamine from mast cells.

PHARMACOKINETICS: Absorption: T$_{max}$=1-2 hrs. C$_{max}$=7.3 ng/mL. **Distribution:** Plasma protein binding (55%). **Metabolism:** Liver via CYP450 (minimal). **Excretion:** Urine (75-90%, unchanged).

NURSING CONSIDERATIONS

Assessment: Assess for contact lens usage, pregnancy/nursing status.

Monitoring: Monitor for relief of itching associated with signs and symptoms of allergic conjunctivitis.

Patient Counseling: Counsel the patient that therapy is not for the treatment of lens-related irritation and not to wear contact lenses if their eyes are red. Remove lens first prior to instillation and reinsert after 10 min. Advise that solution contains benzalkonium chloride, which may be absorbed by soft lenses. Advise not to touch the dropper's tip to any surface to maintain sterility. Inform that solution is for topical ophthalmic use only.

Administration: Ocular route. **Storage:** 15-25°C (59-77°F).

BESIVANCE   RX
besifloxacin (Bausch & Lomb)

THERAPEUTIC CLASS: Fluoroquinolone

INDICATIONS: Treatment of bacterial conjunctivitis caused by susceptible microorganisms.

DOSAGE: *Adults:* Instill 1 drop in affected eye(s) tid, 4-12 hrs apart for 7 days.
Pediatrics: >1 yr : Instill 1 drop in affected eye(s) tid, 4-12 hrs apart for 7 days.

HOW SUPPLIED: Sus (Ophthalmic): 0.6% [7.5mL]

WARNINGS/PRECAUTIONS: For topical ophthalmic use only; should not be injected subconjuctivally, nor should be introduced directly into the anterior chamber of the eye. May result in overgrowth of non-susceptible organisms (eg, fungi). D/C if superinfection occurs; institute alternative therapy. Avoid contact lenses if signs or symptoms of bacterial conjunctivitis occur, or during the course of therapy.

ADVERSE REACTIONS: Conjunctival redness, blurred vision, eye pain, eye irritation, eye pruritus and headache.

PREGNANCY: Category C, caution in nursing.

MECHANISM OF ACTION: Fluoroquinolone antibacterial; inhibits bacterial DNA gyrase and topoisomerase. May be active against pathogens that are resistant to aminoglycoside, macrolide, and β-lactam antibiotics.

PHARMACOKINETICS: Absorption: C_{max}=0.37ng/mL (Day 1), 0.43ng/mL (Day 6). **Elimination:** $T_{1/2}$=7 hrs.

NURSING CONSIDERATIONS

Assessment: Assess for bacterial conjunctivitis, pregnancy/nursing status.

Monitoring: Monitor for overgrowth of non-susceptible organisms (eg, fungi), superinfection, conjunctival redness, blurring of vision, eye pain, eye irritation, eye pruritus, headache, and hypersensitivity reactions.

Patient Counseling: Advise to avoid contaminating applicator tip with material from the eye, fingers, or other source. D/C if rash or allergic reaction occurs; notify physician immediately. Instruct to take medication exactly as directed. Advise to avoid wearing contact lenses if signs or symptoms of bacterial conjunctivitis occur during the course of therapy. Advise to wash hands thoroughly before use. Instruct to invert closed bottle and shake once before each use. Inform that skipping doses or not completing the therapy may decrease effectiveness and increase likelihood that bacteria may develop resistance.

Administration: Ocular route. Invert closed bottle and shake once before each use. Tilt head back, and gently squeeze bottle to instill one drop into the affected eye. **Storage:** Store at 15-25°C (59-77°F). Protect from light.

BETAGAN   RX
levobunolol HCl (Allergan)

THERAPEUTIC CLASS: Nonselective beta-blocker

INDICATIONS: Treatment of elevated intraocular pressure (IOP) in chronic open-angle glaucoma and ocular hypertension.

DOSAGE: *Adults:* (0.5%) 1-2 drops qd; bid for more severe or uncontrolled glaucoma. (0.25%): 1-2 drops bid.

HOW SUPPLIED: Sol: 0.25% [5mL, 10mL], 0.5% [2mL, 5mL, 10mL, 15mL]

CONTRAINDICATIONS: Bronchial asthma, chronic obstructive pulmonary disease (COPD), overt cardiac failure, sinus bradycardia, 2nd- and 3rd-degree AV block, cardiogenic shock.

WARNINGS/PRECAUTIONS: Caution with cardiac failure, diabetes mellitus (DM), COPD, cerebral insufficiency, pulmonary disease, bronchospastic disease, surgery and hepatic impairment. May mask symptoms of hypoglycemia and thyrotoxicosis. Contains sodium metabisulfite. Follow with a miotic in angle-closure glaucoma. Potentiates muscle weakness (eg, diplopia, ptosis).

B

ADVERSE REACTIONS: Ocular burning, ocular stinging, decreased heart rate, decreased blood pressure.

INTERACTIONS: Mydriasis with epinephrine. Additive effects with catecholamine-depleting drugs (eg, reserpine) and systemic β-blockers. AV conduction disturbance with calcium antagonists and digitalis. Left ventricular failure and hypotension with calcium antagonists. Additive hypotensive effects with phenothiazine-related drugs. Risk of hypoglycemia with insulin and oral hypoglycemic agents.

PREGNANCY: Category C, caution in nursing.

MECHANISM OF ACTION: Noncardioselective β-adrenoceptor blocking agent; equipotent at both $β_1$ and $β_2$ receptors. Responsible for reducing cardiac output, increasing airway resistance, and lowering elevated as well as normal IOP. Presumed to lower IOP through decreasing production of aqueous humor.

PHARMACOKINETICS: Absorption: T_{max}=2 and 6 hrs.

NURSING CONSIDERATIONS

Assessment: Assess for conditions where treatment may be contraindicated or cautioned. Assess for possible sulfite allergy prior to therapy. Assess use in patients who have DM, hyperthyroidism, diminished pulmonary function, cerebrovascular insufficiencies, patients undergoing major elective surgery, and in pregnant/nursing females. Assess that patients with angle-closure glaucoma are not using this drug as monotherapy. Assess for possible drug interactions.

Monitoring: Monitor for signs/symptoms of muscle weakness (eg, diplopia, ptosis), severe respiratory and cardiac reactions, and anaphylactic reactions. Monitor for occurrence of a thyroid storm in patients who have thyrotoxicosis and withdraw abruptly from medication. Monitor for signs/symptoms of acute hypoglycemia with DM.

Patient Counseling: Counsel to notify physician immediately if any signs of anaphylactic reaction, cardiac or respiratory symptoms develop while on medication. Counsel patients with DM medication may mask symptoms of hypoglycemia.

Administration: Ocular route. **Storage:** 15-25°C (59-77°F), protect from light.

BETAPACE   RX
sotalol HCl (Bayer Healthcare)

> To minimize risk of arrhythmia, for a minimum of 3 days, place patients initiated or reinitiated on therapy in a facility that can provide cardiac resuscitation and continuous ECG monitoring. Obtain CrCl before therapy. Not approved for the atrial fibrillation or atrial flutter indication; do not substitute for Betapace AF.

THERAPEUTIC CLASS: Beta-blocker (group II/III antiarrhythmic)

INDICATIONS: Treatment of documented life-threatening ventricular arrhythmias such as sustained ventricular tachycardia.

DOSAGE: *Adults:* Individualize dose. Initial: 80mg bid. Titrate: May increase to 120-160mg bid PRN. Adjust dose gradually, allowing 3 days between dosing increments. Usual: 160-320mg/day in 2-3 divided doses. Refractory Ventricular Arrhythmia Patients: 480-640mg/day; use this dose when benefit outweighs risk. Renal Impairment: CrCl 30-59mL/min: Dose q24h. CrCl 10-29mL/min: Dose q36-48h. CrCl <10mL/min: Individualize dose. May increase dose with renal impairment after ≥5-6 doses. Transfer to Betapace: Withdraw previous antiarrhythmic for a minimum of 2-3 plasma half-lives before initiating Betapace. After d/c of amiodarone, do not initiate Betapace until QT interval is normalized.
Pediatrics: Individualize dose. ≥2 yrs: Initial: 30mg/m² tid. Titrate: Wait ≥36 hrs between dose increases. Guide dose by response, HR, and QTc. Max: 60mg/m². <2 yrs: See dosing chart in PI. Reduce dose or d/c if QTc >550 msec. Renal Impairment: Reduce dose or increase interval. Transfer to Betapace: Withdraw previous antiarrhythmic for a minimum of 2-3 plasma half-lives before initiating Betapace. After d/c of amiodarone, do not initiate Betapace until QT interval is normalized.

HOW SUPPLIED: Tab: 80mg*, 120mg*, 160mg* *scored

CONTRAINDICATIONS: Bronchial asthma, sinus bradycardia, 2nd- and 3rd-degree atrioventricular (AV) block (unless a functioning pacemaker is present), congenital or acquired long QT syndromes, cardiogenic shock, uncontrolled congestive heart failure (CHF).

WARNINGS/PRECAUTIONS: May provoke new or worsen ventricular arrhythmias (eg, sustained ventricular tachycardia or ventricular fibrillation). Torsades de pointes, QT interval prolongation, and new or worsened CHF reported. Anticipate proarrhythmic events upon initiation and every upward dose adjustment. Avoid with hypokalemia, hypomagnesemia, excessive QT interval prolongation (>550 msec). Correct electrolyte imbalances before therapy. Caution with heart failure controlled by digitalis and/or diuretics, left ventricular dysfunction, sick sinus syndrome, renal impairment, renal failure undergoing hemodialysis, and 2 weeks post-myocardial infarction

(MI). Avoid abrupt withdrawal. Avoid in patients with bronchospastic diseases. Impairs ability of heart to respond to adrenergic stimuli, potentially increasing the risks of general anesthesia and surgical procedures; chronically administered therapy should not be routinely withdrawn prior to major surgery. Patients with a history of severe anaphylactic reaction to variety of allergens may be more reactive to repeated challenge and may be unresponsive to usual doses of epinephrine. May mask hypoglycemia, hyperthyroidism symptoms.

ADVERSE REACTIONS: Torsades de pointes, dyspnea, fatigue, dizziness, bradycardia, chest pain, palpitation, asthenia, abnormal ECG, hypotension, headache, light-headedness, edema, N/V.

INTERACTIONS: Avoid with Class Ia (eg, disopyramide, quinidine, procainamide) and Class III (eg, amiodarone) antiarrhythmics. Additive Class II effects with β-blockers. Proarrhythmic events were more common with digoxin. May increase risk of bradycardia with digitalis glycosides. Additive effects on AV conduction or ventricular function and BP with calcium-blocking agents. May produce excessive reduction of resting sympathetic nervous tone with catecholamine-depleting drugs (eg, reserpine and guanethidine). Insulin and antidiabetic agents may need dose adjustment. $β_2$-agonists (eg, salbutamol, terbutaline and isoprenaline) may need dose increase. Potentiates rebound HTN with clonidine withdrawal. Reduced levels with antacids containing aluminum oxide and magnesium hydroxide. Caution with drugs that prolong the QT interval (eg, Class I and III antiarrhythmics, phenothiazines, TCAs, astemizole, bepridil, certain quinolones, and oral macrolides).

PREGNANCY: Category B, not for use in nursing.

MECHANISM OF ACTION: Antiarrhythmic drug (Class II and III properties); has both β-adrenoreceptor-blocking and cardiac action potential duration prolongation antiarrhythmic properties.

PHARMACOKINETICS: Absorption: Bioavailability (90-100%); T_{max}=2.5-4 hrs. **Distribution:** Crosses placenta; found in breast milk. **Elimination:** Urine (unchanged); $T_{1/2}$=12 hrs.

NURSING CONSIDERATIONS

Assessment: Obtain CrCl prior to dosing. Assess for previous evidence of hypersensitivity to drug, bronchial asthma, sinus bradycardia, sick sinus syndrome, 2nd- and 3rd-degree AV block, pacemaker, long QT syndromes, cardiogenic shock, left ventricular dysfunction or uncontrolled CHF, recent MI, ischemic heart disease, hypokalemia or hypomagnesemia, bronchospastic disease, diabetes mellitus, episodes of hypoglycemia, upcoming major surgery, hyperthyroidism, renal impairment, nursing status, and possible drug interactions.

Monitoring: Monitor ECG changes, HR, CrCl, asystole, arrhythmias, signs/symptoms of depressed myocardial contractility and more severe HF, anaphylaxis, bronchospasm, MI, hypotension, masking of hypoglycemia, signs of electrolyte imbalance, and thyrotoxicosis.

Patient Counseling: Advise not to d/c without consulting physician. Inform of benefits/risks of drug. Report any adverse reactions to physician.

Administration: Oral route. Preparation of 5mg/mL Oral Sol: Refer to PI for preparation. **Storage:** 25°C (77°F); excursions permitted to 15-30°C (59-86°F). Sus: Stable for 3 months at controlled room temperature and ambient humidity.

BETAPACE AF   RX
sotalol HCl (Bayer Healthcare)

> To minimize risk of arrhythmia, for a minimum of 3 days, place patients initiated or reinitiated on therapy in a facility that can provide cardiac resuscitation, continuous ECG monitoring, and calculations of CrCl. Do not substitute Betapace for Betapace AF.

THERAPEUTIC CLASS: Beta-blocker (group II/III antiarrhythmic)

INDICATIONS: Maintenance of normal sinus rhythm in patients with symptomatic atrial fibrillation/atrial flutter who are currently in sinus rhythm.

DOSAGE: *Adults:* Individualize dose. Start only if baseline QT interval is ≤450 msec. Initial: 80mg qd (CrCl 40-60mL/min) or bid (CrCl >60mL/min). Monitor QT 2-4 hrs after each dose. Reduce or d/c if QT ≥500 msec. May discharge patient if QT <500 msec after at least 3 days. Alternatively, may increase dose to 120mg bid during hospitalization, and follow for 3 days (follow for 5 or 6 doses if receiving qd doses). If 120mg is inadequate, may increase to 160mg qd or bid depending on CrCl. Maint: Reduce dose if QT interval is ≥520 msec and monitor until QT returns to <520 msec. D/C if QT is ≥520 msec while on 80mg dose. Max: 160mg bid (CrCl >60mL/min). Transfer to Betapace AF: Withdraw previous antiarrhythmic for a minimum of 2-3 plasma half-lives before initiating Betapace AF. After d/c of amiodarone, do not initiate Betapace AF until QT interval is normalized.
Pediatrics: Individualize dose. ≥2 yrs: Initial: 30mg/m² tid. Titrate: Wait ≥36 hrs between dose increases. Guide dose by response, HR, and QTc. Max: 60mg/m². <2 yrs: See dosing chart in

PI. Reduce dose or d/c if QTc >550 msec. Renal Impairment: Reduce dose or increase interval. Transfer to Betapace AF: Withdraw previous antiarrhythmic for a minimum of 2-3 plasma half-lives before initiating Betapace AF. After d/c of amiodarone, do not initiate Betapace AF until QT interval is normalized.

HOW SUPPLIED: Tab: 80mg*, 120mg*, 160mg* *scored

CONTRAINDICATIONS: Sinus bradycardia (<50bpm during waking hrs), sick sinus syndrome or 2nd- or 3rd-degree atrioventricular (AV) block (unless a functioning pacemaker is present), congenital or acquired long QT syndromes, baseline QT interval >450 msec, cardiogenic shock, uncontrolled heart failure (HF), hypokalemia (<4meq/L), CrCl <40mL/min, bronchial asthma.

WARNINGS/PRECAUTIONS: Can cause serious ventricular arrhythmias, primarily torsades de pointes. QT interval prolongation, bradycardia, and new or worsened congestive HF reported. Avoid with hypokalemia, hypomagnesemia; correct electrolyte imbalances before therapy. Caution with HF controlled by digitalis and/or diuretics, sick sinus syndrome, left ventricular dysfunction, renal dysfunction, post-myocardial infarction (MI). Avoid abrupt withdrawal. Avoid in patients with bronchospastic disease. Impairs ability of heart to respond to adrenergic stimuli, potentially increasing the risks of general anesthesia and surgical procedures; chronically administered therapy should not be routinely withdrawn prior to major surgery. Patients with a history of severe anaphylactic reaction to variety of allergens may be more reactive to repeated challenge and may be unresponsive to usual doses of epinephrine. May mask hypoglycemia, hyperthyroidism symptoms.

ADVERSE REACTIONS: Bradycardia, dyspnea, fatigue, QT interval prolongation, abnormal ECG, chest pain, abdominal pain, disturbance rhythm subjective, diarrhea, N/V, hyperhidrosis, dizziness, headache.

INTERACTIONS: Avoid with Class 1a (eg, disopyramide, quinidine, and procainamide) and Class III (eg, amiodarone) antiarrhythmics. Not recommended with drugs that prolong the QT interval (eg, many antiarrhythmics, phenothiazines, TCAs, bepridil, and oral macrolides). Proarrhythmic events more common with digoxin. Increased risk of bradycardia with digitalis glycosides. Additive effects on AV conduction or ventricular function and BP with calcium-blocking agents. May produce excessive reduction of resting sympathetic nervous system tone with catecholamine-depleting drugs (eg, reserpine and guanethidine). Insulin and antidiabetic agents may need adjustment. β_2-agonists (eg, salbutamol, terbutaline, and isoprenaline) may need dose increase. Potentiates rebound HTN with clonidine withdrawal. Reduced levels with antacids containing aluminum oxide and magnesium hydroxide.

PREGNANCY: Category B, not for use in nursing.

MECHANISM OF ACTION: Antiarrhythmic drug (Class II and III properties); has both β-adrenoreceptor blocking and cardiac action potential duration prolongation antiarrhythmic properties.

PHARMACOKINETICS: Absorption: Bioavailability (90-100%); T_{max}=2.5-4 hrs. **Distribution:** Crosses placenta; found in breast milk. **Elimination:** Urine (unchanged); $T_{1/2}$=12 hrs.

NURSING CONSIDERATIONS

Assessment: Obtain CrCl prior to dosing. Assess for sinus bradycardia, sick sinus syndrome, 2nd- and 3rd-degree AV block, pacemaker, long QT syndromes, cardiogenic shock, uncontrolled HF, bronchial asthma, previous evidence of hypersensitivity to drug, recent MI, ischemic heart disease, hypokalemia or hypomagnesemia, bronchospastic disease, diabetes mellitus, episodes of hypoglycemia, upcoming major surgery, hyperthyroidism, renal impairment, nursing status, and possible drug interactions.

Monitoring: Monitor ECG changes, HR, CrCl, asystole, arrhythmias, signs/symptoms of depressed myocardial contractility and more severe HF, anaphylaxis, bronchospasm, MI, hypotension, masking of hypoglycemia, signs of electrolyte imbalance, and thyrotoxicosis.

Patient Counseling: Advise not to d/c therapy without consulting physician. Inform of benefits/risks of drug, to report signs of electrolyte balance (eg, diarrhea, vomiting), and if taking any other medications or over-the-counter drugs. Instruct not to double the next dose if a dose is missed; take next dose at the usual time.

Administration: Oral route. Preparation of 5mg/mL Oral Sol: Refer to PI. **Storage:** 25°C (77°F); excursions permitted to 15-30°C (59-86°F). Sus: Stable for 3 months at controlled room temperature and ambient humidity.

BETIMOL

timolol (Vistakon)

RX

THERAPEUTIC CLASS: Nonselective beta-blocker

INDICATIONS: Treatment of elevated intraocular pressure (IOP) in patients with open-angle glaucoma or ocular hypertension.

DOSAGE: *Adults:* Initial: 1 drop 0.25% bid. May increase to max of 1 drop 0.5% bid. Maint: If adequate control, may try 1 drop 0.25-0.5% qd.

HOW SUPPLIED: Sol: 0.25%, 0.5% [2.5mL, 5mL, 10mL, 15mL]

CONTRAINDICATIONS: Bronchial asthma, history of bronchial asthma, severe chronic obstructive pulmonary disease (COPD), sinus bradycardia, 2nd- or 3rd-degree AV block, overt cardiac failure, cardiogenic shock.

WARNINGS/PRECAUTIONS: Caution with cardiac failure, diabetes mellitus (DM), cerebrovascular insufficiency. Severe cardiac and respiratory reactions reported. May mask symptoms of hypoglycemia and hyperthyroidism. Bacterial keratitis reported with contaminated containers. May reinsert contacts 5 min after applying drops. Avoid with COPD, bronchospastic disease. Not for use alone in angle-closure glaucoma. May potentiate muscle weakness. D/C if cardiac failure develops. Withdrawal before surgery is controversial.

ADVERSE REACTIONS: Burning/stinging on instillation, dry eyes, itching, foreign body sensation, eye discomfort, eyelid erythema, conjunctival injection, headache.

INTERACTIONS: May potentiate systemic β-blockers and catecholamine-depleting drugs (eg, reserpine). Oral/IV calcium antagonists can cause AV conduction disturbances, left ventricular failure, or hypotension. Digitalis can cause additive effects in prolonging AV conduction time. May antagonize epinephrine.

PREGNANCY: Category C, not for use in nursing.

MECHANISM OF ACTION: Nonselective β-adrenergic antagonist; blocks both β_1- and β_2-adrenergic receptors. Thought to reduce IOP through reducing production of aqueous humor.

PHARMACOKINETICS: Elimination: Urine (metabolites); $T_{1/2}$=4 hrs

NURSING CONSIDERATIONS

Assessment: Assess for overt heart failure, cardiogenic shock, sinus bradycardia, 2nd- or 3rd-degree AV block, active or history of bronchial asthma, and severe COPD. Assess use in patients with cerebrovascular insufficiencies, undergoing elective surgery, with diabetes mellitus (DM), with hyperthyroidism, and in pregnant/nursing females. Assess patients with angle-closure glaucoma are not on monotherapy with this drug. Assess for possible drug interactions.

Monitoring: Monitor for signs/symptoms of reduced cerebral blood flow, cardiac failure, muscle weakness, bacterial keratitis when using multi-dose container, severe anaphylactic reactions, and hypoglycemia in patients with DM. Monitor for occurrence of thyroid storm in patients who abruptly withdraw from medication and have thyrotoxicosis.

Patient Counseling: Counsel to immediately notify physician if signs of cardiac, respiratory, or anaphylactic symptoms develop while on medication. Instruct patients with DM that this medication may mask signs of hypoglycemia. To avoid contaminating solution, avoid touching container tip to the eye or surrounding structures. Counsel that if taking concomitant topical ophthalmic medications, to separate dosing by at least 5 min. Instruct patients who wear soft contact lenses to wait at least 5 min after administration before reinserting.

Administration: Ocular route. **Storage:** 15-25°C (59-77°F). Do not freeze. Protect from light.

BETOPTIC S   RX
betaxolol HCl (Alcon)

THERAPEUTIC CLASS: Selective beta$_1$-blocker

INDICATIONS: Treatment of elevated intraocular pressure (IOP) in patients with chronic open-angle glaucoma or ocular HTN.

DOSAGE: *Adults:* Instill 1 drop in affected eyes bid.
Pediatrics: Instill 1 drop in affected eyes bid.

HOW SUPPLIED: Sus: 0.25% [2.5mL, 5mL, 10mL, 15mL]

CONTRAINDICATIONS: Sinus bradycardia, >1st-degree atrioventricular (AV) block, cardiogenic shock, overt cardiac failure.

WARNINGS/PRECAUTIONS: Do not use alone in treating angle-closure glaucoma. Absorbed systemically; severe respiratory/cardiac reactions reported. Caution with history of cardiac failure or heart block, diabetes mellitus, and cerebrovascular insufficiency. D/C on 1st sign of cardiac failure. May mask signs/symptoms of acute hypoglycemia and hyperthyroidism. Avoid abrupt withdrawal; may precipitate thyroid storm. May potentiate muscle weakness consistent with certain myasthenic symptoms. Withdrawal prior to major surgery is controversial. Caution in glaucoma patients with excessive restriction of pulmonary function; asthmatic attacks and pulmonary distress reported. May be more reactive to repeated challenge with history of atopy or severe anaphylactic reaction to variety of allergens; may be unresponsive to usual doses of epinephrine. Bacterial keratitis and choroidal detachment may occur.

ADVERSE REACTIONS: Transient ocular discomfort, blurred vision, corneal punctuate keratitis, foreign body sensation, photophobia, tearing, itching, dryness of eye, erythema, inflammation, discharge, ocular pain, decreased visual acuity, crusty lashes.

INTERACTIONS: Potential additive effects with oral β-blockers and catecholamine-depleting drugs (eg, reserpine). May produce hypotension and/or bradycardia with catecholamine-depleting drugs. Caution with adrenergic psychotropics and in patients receiving insulin or oral hypoglycemic agents. May augment risk of general anesthesia.

PREGNANCY: Category C, caution with nursing.

MECHANISM OF ACTION: Cardioselective (β-1-adrenergic) receptor inhibitor; reduces IOP through a reduction of aqueous production.

NURSING CONSIDERATIONS

Assessment: Assess for conditions where treatment is contraindicated or cautioned, hypersensitivity to the drug, pregnancy/nursing status, and possible drug interactions.

Monitoring: Monitor for signs/symptoms of cardiac/respiratory reactions, cardiac failure, muscle weakness, reduced cerebral blood flow, choroidal detachment, and hypersensitivity reactions. Monitor for development of bacterial keratitis in patients who are using multidose containers.

Patient Counseling: Instruct to avoid allowing tip of dispensing container to contact eye(s) or surrounding structures. Ocular solutions may become contaminated by bacteria that may cause ocular infections. Seek physician's advice if having an ocular surgery or if ocular condition (eg, trauma or infection) develops. Administer ≥10 min apart when receiving concomitant ophthalmic medications.

Administration: Ocular route. May be used alone or in combination with other IOP lowering medications. Refer to PI for administration instructions. Shake well before use. **Storage:** 2-25°C (36-77°F). Store upright.

BEYAZ   RX
levomefolate calcium - drospirenone - ethinyl estradiol (Bayer Healthcare)

> Cigarette smoking increases the risk of serious cardiovascular (CV) events from combination oral contraceptive (COC) use. Risk increases with age (>35 yrs) and with the number of cigarettes smoked. Should not be used by women who are >35 yrs and smoke.

THERAPEUTIC CLASS: Estrogen/progestogen combination

INDICATIONS: Prevention of pregnancy. Treatment of symptoms of premenstrual dysphoric disorder (PMDD). Treatment of moderate acne vulgaris in women ≥14 yrs who have achieved menarche and who desire an oral contraceptive for birth control. To raise folate levels for the purpose of reducing the risk of neural tube defect in a pregnancy conceived while taking the product or shortly after d/c.

DOSAGE: *Adults:* Contraception/Acne/PMDD: 1 tab qd for 28 days, then repeat. Start 1st Sunday after menses begin or 1st day of menses. Take at the same time each day, preferably pm pc or hs. *Pediatrics:* Postpubertal: Contraception/Acne (≥14 yrs)/PMDD: 1 tab qd for 28 days, then repeat. Start 1st Sunday after menses begin or 1st day of menses. Take at the same time each day, preferably pm pc or hs.

HOW SUPPLIED: Tab: (Drospirenone [DRSP]-Ethinyl Estradiol [EE]-Levomefolate calcium) 3mg-0.02mg-0.451mg; Tab: (Levomefolate calcium) 0.451mg

CONTRAINDICATIONS: Renal impairment, adrenal insufficiency, high risk of arterial/venous thrombotic disease (eg, smoking if >35 yrs, history/presence of deep vein thrombosis/pulmonary embolism, cerebrovascular disease, coronary artery disease, thrombogenic valvular or thrombogenic rhythm diseases of the heart [eg, subacute bacterial endocarditis with valvular disease, or atrial fibrillation], inherited/acquired hypercoagulopathies, uncontrolled HTN, diabetes mellitus [DM] with vascular disease, headaches with focal neurological symptoms or migraine with/without aura if >35 yrs), undiagnosed abnormal uterine bleeding, history/presence of breast or other estrogen-/progestin-sensitive cancer, benign/malignant liver tumors, liver disease, pregnancy.

WARNINGS/PRECAUTIONS: Increased risk of venous thromboembolism; greatest risk during the first 6 months of COC use and is present after initially starting COC or restarting the same or different COC. Increased risk of stroke, myocardial infarction (MI), gallbladder disease, and cerebrovascular events. May increase risk of breast cancer, cervical cancer, and intraepithelial neoplasia. Caution in women with cardiovascular disease (CVD) risk factors. D/C if arterial/deep venous thrombotic events, unexplained loss of vision, proptosis, diplopia, papilledema, or retinal vascular lesions occur. D/C at least 4 weeks before and through 2 weeks after major surgery or other surgeries with elevated risk of thromboembolism. Avoid with conditions predisposing to hyperkalemia. Hepatic adenoma and increased risk of hepatocellular carcinoma reported; d/c if jaundice or acute/chronic disturbances of liver function occur. Cholestasis may occur with history of pregnancy-related cholestasis. Increased BP reported; d/c if BP rises significantly.

May decrease glucose tolerance; monitor prediabetic and diabetic patients. Consider alternative contraception with uncontrolled dyslipidemia. May increase risk of pancreatitis in patients with hypertriglyceridemia or family history thereof. May increase frequency/severity of migraine; d/c if new headaches that are recurrent, persistent, or severe develop. Unscheduled bleeding and spotting may occur; rule out pregnancy or malignancies. Caution with history of depression; d/c if depression recurs to serious degree. May change results of laboratory tests (eg, coagulation factors, lipids, glucose tolerance, binding proteins). Folate may mask vitamin B12 deficiency. May induce/exacerbate angioedema in patients with hereditary angioedema. Chloasma may occur; avoid sun exposure or UV radiation. Women who do not breastfeed may start therapy no earlier than 4 weeks postpartum. Not for treatment of premenstrual syndrome.

ADVERSE REACTIONS: Menstrual irregularities, N/V, headache/migraine, breast pain/tenderness, fatigue.

INTERACTIONS: Potential for an increase in serum K⁺ with angiotensin converting enzyme inhibitors, angiotensin II receptor antagonists, K⁺-sparing diuretics, K⁺ supplementation, heparin, aldosterone antagonists, and NSAIDs. Drugs or herbal products that induce certain enzymes, including CYP3A4 (eg, phenytoin, barbiturates, carbamazepine, bosentan, felbamate, griseofulvin, oxcarbazepine, rifampicin, topiramate, and products containing St. John's wort), may reduce drug effectiveness or increase incidence of breakthrough bleeding. Significant changes (increase/decrease) in plasma estrogen and progestin levels reported with HIV/Hepatitis C virus protease inhibitors or non-nucleoside reverse transcriptase inhibitors. Pregnancy reported with antibiotics. Atorvastatin, ascorbic acid, acetaminophen, CYP3A4 inhibitors (eg, itraconazole, ketoconazole) may increase hormone levels. May decrease levels of lamotrigine and reduce seizure control. May need to increase dose of thyroid hormone in patients on thyroid hormone replacement therapy due to increased thyroid binding globulin. May decrease pharmacological effect of antifolate drugs (eg, antiepileptics, methotrexate, or pyrimethamine). Reduced folate levels via inhibition of dihydrofolate reductase enzyme (eg, methotrexate, sulfasalazine), reduced folate absorption (eg, cholestyramine), or unknown mechanism (eg, antiepileptics, such as carbamazepine, phenytoin, phenobarbital, primidone, valproic acid).

PREGNANCY: Contraindicated in pregnancy, not for use in nursing.

MECHANISM OF ACTION: Estrogen/progestogen oral contraceptive; acts by suppressing gonadotropins and inhibits ovulation. Also causes changes in cervical mucus (increasing difficulty of sperm entry into uterus) and endometrium (reducing likelihood of implantation). (Levomefolate calcium) Folate supplementation.

PHARMACOKINETICS: Absorption: DRSP: Absolute bioavailability (76%); (Cycle 1/Day 21) C_{max}=70.3ng/mL; T_{max}=1.5 hrs; AUC=763ng•h/mL. EE: Absolute bioavailability (40%); (Cycle 1/Day 21) C_{max}=45.1pg/mL; T_{max}=1.5 hrs; AUC=220pg•h/mL. Levomefolate: T_{max}=0.5-1.5 hrs. **Distribution:** Found in breast milk; DRSP: V_d=4L/kg; serum protein binding (97%). EE: V_d=4-5L/kg; serum albumin binding (98.5%). **Metabolism:** DRSP: Liver, via CYP3A4 (minor). EE: Hydroxylation (via CYP3A4), conjugation with glucuronide and sulfate. **Elimination:** DRSP: Urine, feces; $T_{1/2}$=30 hrs. EE: Urine, feces; $T_{1/2}$=24 hrs. Levomefolate (L-5-methyl-THF): Urine, feces; $T_{1/2}$=4-5 hrs.

NURSING CONSIDERATIONS

Assessment: Assess for renal impairment, abnormal uterine bleeding, adrenal insufficiency, and known/suspected pregnancy or any other conditions where treatment is cautioned or contraindicated. Assess use in patients who are >35 yrs and heavy smokers (≥15 cigarettes/day), patients with CVD risk factors, predisposition to hyperkalemia, pregnancy-related cholestasis, HTN, DM, uncontrolled dyslipidemia, history/present hypertriglyceridemia, history of depression, hereditary angioedema, and history of chloasma. Assess for possible drug interactions.

Monitoring: Monitor for bleeding irregularities, venous/arterial thrombotic and thromboembolic events (eg, MI, stroke), cervical cancer or intraepithelial neoplasia, retinal vein thrombosis or any other ophthalmic changes, jaundice, acute/chronic disturbances in liver function, new/worsening headaches or migraines, cholestasis with history of pregnancy related cholestasis, and pancreatitis in hypertriglyceridemia. Monitor K⁺ levels, glucose levels in DM or prediabetes, and BP with history of HTN. Perform annual history and physical exam.

Patient Counseling: Inform that drug does not protect against HIV-infection (AIDS) and other sexually transmitted diseases. Counsel to avoid smoking while on treatment. Instruct to take at the same time everyday preferably pm, or hs. Instruct on what to do in the event pills are missed. If breastfeeding, inform that COCs may reduce breast milk production. Inform that amenorrhea may occur and pregnancy should be ruled out if amenorrhea occurs in ≥2 consecutive cycles. Counsel to report if taking folate supplements and advise to maintain folate supplementation upon d/c due to pregnancy. Counsel patient who starts COCs postpartum and has not yet had a period, to use additional method of contraception until drug taken for 7 consecutive days.

Administration: Oral route. **Storage:** 25°C (77°F); excursions permitted to 15-30°C (59-86°F).

B

BIAXIN
clarithromycin (Abbott)

RX

OTHER BRAND NAMES: Biaxin XL (Abbott)

THERAPEUTIC CLASS: Macrolide

INDICATIONS: Treatment of the following mild to moderate infections caused by susceptible strains of microorganisms: (Tab, Sus) Pharyngitis/tonsillitis, acute maxillary sinusitis, acute bacterial exacerbation of chronic bronchitis (ABECB), community-acquired pneumonia (CAP), uncomplicated skin and skin structure infections (SSSI), and disseminated mycobacterial infections in pediatrics and adults. Mycobacterium avium complex (MAC) prophylaxis in advanced HIV in pediatrics and adults. (Pediatrics) Acute otitis media. (Tab) Combination therapy for *Helicobacter pylori* infection with duodenal ulcer disease (active or 5-year history of duodenal ulcer) in adults. (Tab, ER) Acute maxillary sinusitis, CAP, and ABECB in adults.

DOSAGE: *Adults:* (Tab, Sus) Pharyngitis/Tonsillitis: 250mg q12h for 10 days. Sinusitis: 500mg q12h for 14 days. ABECB: 250-500mg q12h for 7-14 days. SSSI/CAP: 250mg q12h for 7-14 days. MAC Prophylaxis/Treatment: 500mg bid. CrCl <30mL/min: Reduce dose by 50%. *H. pylori:* Triple Therapy: 500mg + amoxicillin 1g + omeprazole 20mg, all q12h for 10 days (give additional omeprazole 20mg qd for 18 days with active ulcer); or 500mg + amoxicillin 1g + lansoprazole 30mg, all q12h for 10-14 days. Dual Therapy: 500mg q8h + omeprazole 40mg qd (qam) for 14 days (give additional omeprazole 20mg qd for 14 days with active ulcer); or 500mg q8h or q12h + ranitidine bismuth citrate 400mg q12h for 14 days (give additional ranitidine bismuth citrate 400mg bid for 14 days with active ulcer). (Tab, ER) Sinusitis: 1000mg qd for 14 days. ABECB/ CAP: 1000mg qd for 7 days. CrCl <30mL/min: Reduce dose by 50%.
Pediatrics: ≥6 months: (Tab, Sus) Usual: 15mg/kg/day q12h for 10 days. MAC Prophylaxis/ Treatment: ≥20 months: 7.5mg/kg bid, up to 500mg bid. CrCl <30mL/min: Reduce dose by 50%. Refer to PI for further pediatric dosage guidelines.

HOW SUPPLIED: Sus: 125mg/5mL, 250mg/5mL [50mL, 100mL]; Tab: 250mg, 500mg; Tab, Extended-Release (ER): 500mg

CONTRAINDICATIONS: History of cholestatic jaundice/hepatic dysfunction associated with prior use of clarithromycin. History of QT prolongation or ventricular cardiac arrhythmia, including torsades de pointes. Concomitant use with cisapride, pimozide, astemizole, terfenadine, ergotamine, or dihydroergotamine, and with HMG-CoA reductase inhibitors (statins), lovastatin or simvastatin. Concomitant use with colchicine in patients with renal/hepatic impairment.

WARNINGS/PRECAUTIONS: Avoid in pregnancy except in clinical circumstances where no alternative therapy is appropriate. Hepatic dysfunction including increased liver enzymes, and hepatocellular and/or cholestatic hepatitis, with or without jaundice reported; d/c immediately if hepatitis occurs. *Clostridium difficile*-associated diarrhea (CDAD) reported and may range in severity from mild diarrhea to fatal colitis; d/c if CDAD is suspected or confirmed. Increased risk for QT prolongation; caution with medical conditions associated with increased tendency toward QT prolongation and torsades de pointes. D/C therapy immediately and initiate prompt treatment if severe acute hypersensitivity reactions (eg, Stevens-Johnson syndrome, toxic epidermal necrolysis, drug rash with eosinophilia and systemic symptoms) occur. May result in bacterial resistance with prolonged use or use in the absence of a proven/suspected bacterial infection or a prophylactic indication; take appropriate measures if superinfection develops. May exacerbate symptoms of myasthenia gravis; new onset of symptoms of myasthenic syndrome reported.

ADVERSE REACTIONS: Diarrhea, N/V, abnormal taste, (Tab, Sus) abdominal pain, rash.

INTERACTIONS: See Contraindications. May increase serum theophylline, carbamazepine, omeprazole, digoxin, drugs metabolized by CYP3A, colchicine, saquinavir, and tolterodine levels. Hypotension may occur with calcium channel blockers (CCBs) metabolized by CYP3A4 (eg, verapamil, amlodipine, diltiazem). Risk of serious hemorrhage and significant elevations in INR and PT with warfarin. Rare cases of rhabdomyolysis reported with atorvastatin and rosuvastatin. Ranitidine bismuth citrate is not recommended if CrCl <25mL/min or with history of acute porphyria. Hypotension, bradyarrhythmias, and lactic acidosis observed with verapamil. Increased levels with fluconazole. Avoid doses of >1000mg/day with protease inhibitors. May potentiate oral anticoagulant effects. Caution with other drugs known to be CYP3A enzyme substrates, especially if substrate has a narrow safety margin (eg, carbamazepine) and/or substrate is extensively metabolized by this enzyme. Decreased plasma levels with CYP3A inducers (eg, efavirenz, nevirapine, rifampicin, rifabutin, rifapentine). Concomitant use with phosphodiesterase inhibitors (sildenafil, tadalafil, vardenafil) is not recommended. May increase area under the curve of midazolam; dose adjustments may be necessary and possible prolongation and intensity of effect should be anticipated. Caution and appropriate dose adjustments with alprazolam and triazolam. Somnolence and confusion may occur with concomitant use of triazolam; monitor for additive CNS effects. Reduce dose by 50 or 75% with CrCl 30-60mL/min or <30mL/min if given with atazanavir or ritonavir. Concomitant use with itraconazole may increase levels of itraconazole and clarithromycin. Occurrence of torsades de pointes with quinidine or disopyramide reported;

monitor ECG for QT prolongation during coadministration. Interaction may occur when concomitantly used with cyclosporine, tacrolimus, alfentanil, rifabutin, methylprednisolone, cilostazol, bromocriptine, vinblastine, hexobarbital, phenytoin, or valproate. Significant hypoglycemia may occur with oral hypoglycemic agents (nateglinide, pioglitazone, repaglinide, and rosiglitazone) and/or insulin. (Tab) May decrease levels of zidovudine; separate zidovudine administration by at least 2 hrs.

PREGNANCY: Category C, caution in nursing.

MECHANISM OF ACTION: Semisynthetic macrolide antibiotic; exerts antibacterial action by binding to the 50S ribosomal subunit of susceptible microorganisms resulting in inhibition of protein synthesis. Active against aerobic and anaerobic gram-positive and gram-negative microorganisms.

PHARMACOKINETICS: Absorption: Rapid; (250mg tab) Absolute bioavailability (50%). Administration of variable doses resulted in different parameters. **Metabolism:** 14-OH clarithromycin (primary metabolite). **Elimination:** Urine: 20% (250mg tab), 30% (500mg tab), 40% (250mg sus), 10-15% (14-OH). $T_{1/2}$=3-4 hrs (250mg tab), 5-7 hrs (500mg). 14-OH: $T_{1/2}$=5-6 hrs (250mg), 7-9 hrs (500mg).

NURSING CONSIDERATIONS

Assessment: Assess for history of cholestatic jaundice/hepatic dysfunction associated with prior use of clarithromycin, hepatic/renal impairment, history of QT prolongation, ventricular cardiac arrhythmia, torsades de pointes, myasthenia gravis, pregnancy/nursing status, history of acute porphyria, hypersensitivity to the drug, any of its ingredients, erythromycin, or any of the macrolide antibiotics, and possible drug interactions.

Monitoring: Monitor for development of drug-resistant bacteria, CDAD, hepatitis, acute severe hypersensitivity reactions, myopathy, exacerbation of myasthenia gravis, and other adverse reactions. Monitor for LFTs, INR/PT, and renal/hepatic function.

Patient Counseling: Inform about potential benefits/risks of therapy. Counsel that drug only treats bacterial, not viral, infections. Instruct to take exactly as directed; inform that skipping doses or not completing full course may decrease effectiveness and increase antibiotic resistance. Notify physician if watery/bloody diarrhea (with/without stomach cramps) develop; inform that this may occur up to 2 or more months after treatment. Notify physician if pregnant/nursing and all medications currently taking. (Tab/Sus) Inform that may take with or without food and can be taken with milk. (Sus) Instruct not to refrigerate. (Tab, ER) Instruct to take with food.

Administration: Oral route. (Sus) Refer to PI for constituting instructions. (Tab, ER) Swallow whole with food; do not chew, crush, or break. **Storage:** (250mg tab) 15-30°C (59-86°F). Protect from light. (500mg tab) 20-25°C (68-77°F). (Sus) 15-30°C (59-86°F). Use within 14 days. Do not refrigerate. (Tab, ER) 20-25°C (68-77°F); excursions permitted 15-30°C (59-86°F).

BONIVA   RX
ibandronate sodium (Genentech)

THERAPEUTIC CLASS: Bisphosphonate

INDICATIONS: (Inj) Treatment of osteoporosis in postmenopausal women. (PO) Treatment and prevention of postmenopausal osteoporosis.

DOSAGE: *Adults:* Inj: 3mg IV over 15-30 sec q3 months. PO: 150mg once monthly on the same date each month. Swallow whole with 6-8 oz. water. Do not lie down for 60 min after dose. Take ≥60 min before 1st food, drink (other than water), medication, or supplementation. Must not take 2 tabs within the same week.

HOW SUPPLIED: Inj: 3mg/3mL; Tab: 150mg

CONTRAINDICATIONS: Hypocalcemia. (PO) Inability to stand or sit upright for ≥60 min and abnormalities of the esophagus that delay esophageal emptying (eg, stricture or achalasia).

WARNINGS/PRECAUTIONS: Not recommended in severe renal impairment (CrCl <30mL/min). Osteonecrosis, primarily in the jaw reported; weigh benefit/risk. Caution with risk factors for osteonecrosis of the jaw (ONJ) including dental procedures, cancer diagnosis, and comorbid disorders (eg, anemia, coagulopathy, infection, and preexisting dental disease). Severe, incapacitating bone, joint, and/or muscle pain reported; consider d/c if severe symptoms develop. Treat hypocalcemia and other bone and mineral disturbances prior to therapy; hypocalcemia reported. Atypical, low-energy, or low-trauma fractures of the femoral shaft reported; consider interrupting therapy. (PO) May cause local irritation of upper GI mucosa. Caution with upper GI problems (eg, Barrett's esophagus, dysphagia, esophageal diseases, gastritis, duodenitis or ulcer). D/C if dysphagia, odynophagia, retrosternal pain or new or worsening heartburn develops. Gastric and duodenal ulcers reported. (Inj) Avoid intra-arterial or paravenous inj.

ADVERSE REACTIONS: Acute phase reaction, arthralgia, abdominal pain, headache, dyspepsia, back pain. (Inj) Influenza, nasopharyngitis, constipation, HTN. (PO) Extremity pain, diarrhea.

INTERACTIONS: Caution with risk factors for osteonecrosis (eg, chemotherapy, radiotherapy, corticosteroids). May increase risk of atypical femur fractures with glucocorticoids (eg, prednisone). May interfere with bone-imaging agents. (PO) Products containing calcium and other multivalent cations (eg, aluminum, magnesium, iron) may interfere with absorption. Should be taken ≥60 min before any oral medication. Caution when used concomitantly with NSAIDs or aspirin due to GI irritation. Increased bioavailability with ranitidine.

PREGNANCY: Category C, caution in nursing.

MECHANISM OF ACTION: Bisphosphonate; has affinity for hydroxyapatite, a component of the mineral matrix of the bone. Inhibits osteoclast activity and reduces bone resorption and turnover. In postmenopausal women, it reduces the elevated rate of bone turnover, leading to, on average, net gain in bone mass.

PHARMACOKINETICS: Absorption: (PO) Upper GI tract; T_{max}=0.5-2 hrs. **Distribution:** V_d= ≥90L; Plasma protein binding: PO (90.9-99.5%); IV (86%). **Elimination:** (IV/PO) Kidney (50-60%); (PO) Feces (unabsorbed dose); (PO) (150mg): $T_{1/2}$=37-157 hrs; (IV, 2mg): $T_{1/2}$=4.6-15.3 hrs; (IV, 4mg): $T_{1/2}$=5-25.5 hrs.

NURSING CONSIDERATIONS

Assessment: Assess for any other conditions where treatment is contraindicated or cautioned, pregnancy/nursing status, and possible drug interactions. Obtain baseline serum calcium, CrCl.

Monitoring: Monitor for signs/symptoms of ONJ, musculoskeletal pain, hypocalcemia, atypical femur fracture, and renal function. PO: Monitor for signs/symptoms of upper GI disorders (eg, dysphagia, esophageal disease or ulcer).

Patient Counseling: (PO) Counsel to take ≥60 min before 1st food or drink (other than water) and before taking other oral medication or supplementation. Instruct to swallow whole with full glass of plain water (6-8 oz) while standing or sitting in upright position; avoid lying down for ≥60 min. Inform not to chew or suck medication. Advise to take supplemental calcium and vitamin D if dietary intake is inadequate. Counsel to take tab on the same date each month. If dose is missed and next scheduled dose is >7 days away, instruct to take one tab in the morning following the date it is remembered. If next dose is 1-7 days away, instruct to wait for next scheduled day to take tab. Instruct to d/c treatment and seek medical attention if signs of esophageal irritation develop during therapy. (Inj) Advise patients to take supplemental calcium and vitamin D.

Administration: Oral or IV route. (Inj) Do not mix with calcium-containing solutions or other IV drugs. Inspect visually for particulate matter and discoloration before administration. **Storage:** 25°C (77°F); excursions permitted to 15-30°C (59-86°F).

BOOSTRIX   RX
diphtheria toxoid, reduced - pertussis vaccine acellular, adsorbed - tetanus toxoid
(GlaxoSmithKline)

THERAPEUTIC CLASS: Vaccine/toxoid combination

INDICATIONS: Active booster immunization against tetanus, diphtheria, and pertussis as a single dose in individuals ≥10 yrs.

DOSAGE: *Adults:* 0.5mL IM into the deltoid muscle of the upper arm. Wound Management: May be given as a tetanus prophylaxis if no previous dose of any tetanus toxoid, reduced diphtheria toxoid and acellular pertussis vaccine, adsorbed (Tdap) has been administered.
Pediatrics: ≥10 yrs: 0.5mL IM into the deltoid muscle of the upper arm. Wound Management: May be given as a tetanus prophylaxis if no previous dose of any Tdap has been administered.

HOW SUPPLIED: Inj: 0.5mL

CONTRAINDICATIONS: Encephalopathy (eg, coma, decreased level of consciousness, prolonged seizures) within 7 days of administration of a previous dose of a pertussis antigen-containing vaccine that is not attributable to another identifiable cause.

WARNINGS/PRECAUTIONS: Administer 5 yrs after last dose of recommended series of diphtheria and tetanus toxoids and acellular pertussis vaccine adsorbed (DTaP) and/or tetanus and diphtheria toxoids adsorbed for adult use (Td) vaccine. Tip cap and rubber plunger of prefilled syringe may contain natural latex rubber; allergic reactions may occur in latex-sensitive individuals. May cause brachial neuritis and Guillain-Barre syndrome. Risk of Guillain-Barre syndrome may increase if Guillain-Barre syndrome occurred within 6 weeks of receipt of a prior tetanus toxoid containing vaccine. Syncope may be accompanied by transient neurological signs. Defer vaccination with progressive/unstable neurologic conditions (eg, cerebrovascular events, acute encephalopathic conditions). Avoid if experienced an Arthus-type hypersensitivity reaction following a prior dose of tetanus toxoid-containing vaccine unless at least 10 yrs have elapsed since last dose of tetanus toxoid-containing vaccine. Expected immune response may not be obtained in immunosuppressed persons. Review immunization history for possible vaccine sensitivity and previous vaccination-related adverse reactions; epinephrine and other appropriate agents should be immediately available for control of allergic reactions.

ADVERSE REACTIONS: Inj-site reactions (eg, pain, redness, swelling, increased arm circumference), headache, fatigue, fever, GI symptoms.

INTERACTIONS: Lower post-vaccination geometric mean antibody concentrations (GMCs) to pertactin observed following concomitant administration with meningococcal conjugate vaccine as compared to Boostrix administered first. Lower GMCs for antibodies to the pertussis antigens filamentous hemagglutinin and pertactin observed when concomitantly administered with influenza virus vaccine as compared with Boostrix alone. Immunosuppressive therapies (eg, irradiation, antimetabolites, alkylating agents, cytotoxic drugs, corticosteroids [used in greater than physiologic doses]), may reduce the immune response to vaccine.

PREGNANCY: Category C, caution in nursing.

MECHANISM OF ACTION: Vaccine/toxoid combination; develops neutralizing antibodies to tetanus, diphtheria, and pertussis.

NURSING CONSIDERATIONS

Assessment: Review immunization history, current health/medical status (eg, immunosuppression), and for previous sensitivity/vaccination-related adverse reactions. Assess for history of encephalopathy, latex hypersensitivity, progressive/unstable neurologic conditions, pregnancy/nursing status, and for possible drug interactions.

Monitoring: Monitor for signs and symptoms of Guillain-Barre syndrome, brachial neuritis, allergic reactions, immune response, syncope, neurological signs, and other adverse reactions.

Patient Counseling: Inform about benefits/risks of immunization. Advise about the potential for adverse reactions. Instruct to notify physician if any adverse reactions occur, if pregnant, or plan to become pregnant.

Administration: IM route. Shake well before use. Do not administer SQ, intradermally, or IV. Do not mix with any other vaccine in the same syringe or vial. **Storage:** 2-8°C (36-46°F). Do not freeze; discard if has been frozen.

BOTOX   RX
onabotulinumtoxinA (Allergan)

> Distant spread of toxin effects reported hrs to weeks after inj (eg, asthenia, generalized muscle weakness, diplopia, ptosis, dysphagia, dysphonia, dysarthria, urinary incontinence, breathing difficulties). Swallowing and breathing difficulties can be life-threatening and there have been reports of death. Risk of symptoms is greatest in children treated for spasticity but can also occur in adults. In unapproved uses and approved indications, cases of spread of effect have been reported at doses comparable to those used to treat cervical dystonia and at lower doses.

THERAPEUTIC CLASS: Purified neurotoxin complex

INDICATIONS: Treatment of urinary incontinence due to detrusor overactivity associated with a neurologic condition (eg, spinal cord injury, multiple sclerosis) in adults who have an inadequate response to or are intolerant of an anticholinergic medication. Prophylaxis of headaches in adults with chronic migraine (≥15 days/month with headache lasting ≥4 hrs/day). Treatment of upper limb spasticity in adults, to decrease the severity of increased muscle tone in elbow flexors (biceps), wrist flexors (flexor carpi radialis and flexor carpi ulnaris) and finger flexors (flexor digitorum profundus and flexor digitorum sublimis). Treatment of adults with cervical dystonia, to reduce severity of abnormal head position and neck pain associated with cervical dystonia. Treatment of severe primary axillary hyperhidrosis that is inadequately managed with topical agents. Treatment of strabismus and blepharospasm associated with dystonia, including benign essential blepharospasm or VII nerve disorders in patients ≥12 yrs.

DOSAGE: *Adults:* Detrusor Overactivity: Usual/Max: 200 U/treatment injected into the detrusor muscle. Consider reinjection when clinical effect of previous inj diminishes, but no sooner than 12 weeks from the prior bladder inj. Administer prophylactic antibiotics (except aminoglycosides) 1-3 days pretreatment, on the treatment day, and 1-3 days post-treatment. D/C antiplatelet therapy ≥3 days before inj. Chronic Migraine: Usual: 155 U IM as 0.1mL (5 U)/site. Should be divided across 7 specific head/neck muscle areas. Refer to PI for recommended inj sites and doses. Retreatment Schedule: Every 12 weeks. Upper Limb Spasticity: Individualize dose. Range: 75-360 U divided among selected muscles. Biceps Brachii: 100-200 U divided in 4 sites. Flexor Carpi Radialis/Flexor Carpi Ulnaris: 12.5-50 U in 1 site. Flexor Digitorum Profundus/Flexor Digitorum Sublimis: 30-50 U in 1 site. Max: 50 U/site. May repeat no sooner than 12 weeks after effect of previous inj diminishes. Cervical Dystonia: Individualize dose. Average Dose: 236 U divided among affected muscles. Max: 50 U/site. Primary Axillary Hyperhidrosis: 50 U/axilla intradermally (ID). Repeat inj when clinical effect of previous inj diminishes. Blepharospasm: Initial: 1.25-2.5 U into medial and lateral pre-tarsal orbicularis oculi of the upper lid and into the lateral pre-tarsal orbicularis oculi of the lower lid. May increase up to 2-fold if initial treatment response is insufficient.

Max: 200 U/30 days. Strabismus: Initial: Vertical Muscle and Horizontal Strabismus <20 Prism Diopters: 1.25-2.5 U in any 1 muscle. Horizontal Strabismus of 20-50 Prism Diopters: 2.5-5 U in any 1 muscle. Persistent VI Nerve Palsy of ≥1 Month: 1.25-2.5 U into medial rectus muscle. Max: 25 U/muscle. Dose may be increased up to 2-fold if previous dose resulted in incomplete paralysis of target muscle. Reassess 7-14 days after each inj. Instill several drops of a local anesthetic and an ocular decongestant several min prior to inj. ≥1 Indications: Max Cumulative Dose: 360 U in a 3 month interval. Elderly: Start at lower end of dosing range.

Pediatrics: ≥16 yrs: Cervical Dystonia: Individualize dose. Average Dose: 236 U divided among affected muscles. Max: 50 U/site. ≥12 yrs: Blepharospasm: Initial: 1.25-2.5 U into medial and lateral pre-tarsal orbicularis oculi of the upper lid and into the lateral pre-tarsal orbicularis oculi of the lower lid. May increase up to 2-fold if initial treatment response is insufficient. Max: 200 U/30 days. Strabismus: Initial: Vertical Muscle and Horizontal Strabismus <20 Prism Diopters: 1.25-2.5 U in any 1 muscle. Horizontal Strabismus of 20-50 Prism Diopters: 2.5-5 U in any 1 muscle. Persistent VI Nerve Palsy of ≥1 Month: 1.25-2.5 U into the medial rectus muscle. Max: 25 U/muscle. Dose may be increased up to 2-fold if previous dose resulted in incomplete paralysis of target muscle. Reassess 7-14 days after each inj. Instill several drops of a local anesthetic and an ocular decongestant several min prior to inj.

HOW SUPPLIED: Inj: 100 U, 200 U

CONTRAINDICATIONS: Infection at the proposed inj site(s), intradetrusor inj in patients with detrusor overactivity associated with a neurologic condition who have acute urinary tract infection (UTI), and in patients with acute urinary retention who are not routinely performing clean intermittent self-catheterization.

WARNINGS/PRECAUTIONS: Not interchangeable with other botulinum toxin products; cannot be compared or converted into U of any other botulinum toxin products. Caution when injecting in or near vulnerable anatomic structures; serious adverse events, including fatal outcomes, reported when injected directly into salivary glands, the oro-lingual-pharyngeal region, esophagus, and stomach. Pneumothorax reported following administration near the thorax; caution when injecting in proximity to the lung. Serious and/or immediate hypersensitivity reactions reported; d/c if such reactions occur. Aspiration and death due to severe dysphagia reported. Serious breathing difficulties reported with cervical dystonia. Increased risk of dysphagia reported in patients with smaller neck muscle mass and those who require bilateral inj into the sternocleidomastoid muscles. Inj in levator scapulae may increase risk of upper respiratory infection and dysphagia. Closely monitor patients with peripheral motor neuropathic diseases, amyotrophic lateral sclerosis, or neuromuscular junction disorders, and with patients being treated for upper limb spasticity with compromised respiratory status. Reduced blinking from inj of orbicularis muscle may lead to corneal exposure, persistent epithelial defect, and corneal ulceration; vigorously treat any epithelial defect. Retrobulbar hemorrhages compromising retinal circulation reported. Bronchitis and upper respiratory tract infections (URI) reported in patients being treated for upper limb spasticity. Contains albumin; carries extremely remote risk for transmission of viral diseases and Creutzfeldt-Jakob disease. Autonomic dysreflexia associated with intradetrusor inj may occur. In patients who are not catheterizing, assess post-void residual (PVR) urine volume within 2 weeks post-treatment and periodically as medically appropriate up to 12 weeks; institute catheterization if PVR urine volume >200mL and continue until PVR falls <200mL. Not intended to substitute for usual standard of care rehabilitation regimens. Weakness of hand muscles and blepharoptosis may occur in patients treated for palmar hyperhidrosis and facial hyperhidrosis, respectively. Caution with inflammation at the proposed inj site(s) or when excessive weakness or atrophy is present in the target muscle(s). Caution in elderly.

ADVERSE REACTIONS: UTI, urinary retention, asthenia, muscle weakness, diplopia, ptosis, dysphagia, dysphonia, dysarthria, breathing difficulties, URI, headache, neck pain, musculoskeletal stiffness, fatigue.

INTERACTIONS: Potentiation of toxin effect may occur with aminoglycosides or other agents interfering with neuromuscular transmission (eg, curare-like compounds). Use of anticholinergic drugs after administration may potentiate systemic anticholinergic effects. Excessive neuromuscular weakness may be exacerbated if another botulinum toxin is administered before effects resolve from the previous botulinum toxin inj administration. Use of a muscle relaxant before/after administration may exaggerate excessive weakness.

PREGNANCY: Category C, caution in nursing.

MECHANISM OF ACTION: Purified neurotoxin complex; blocks neuromuscular transmission by binding to acceptor sites on motor or sympathetic nerve terminals, entering the nerve terminals, and inhibiting release of acetylcholine.

NURSING CONSIDERATIONS

Assessment: Assess for infection/inflammation at proposed inj site, weakness/atrophy in target muscle, compromised swallowing or respiratory function, peripheral motor neuropathic diseases, amyotrophic lateral sclerosis, neuromuscular junction disorders, increased risk for dysphagia, VII nerve disorders, potential causes of secondary hyperhidrosis (eg, hyperthyroidism), hypersensitivity, pregnancy/nursing status, and possible drug interactions. In patients undergoing intradetrusor inj, assess for acute UTI and acute urinary retention.

Monitoring: Monitor for spread of toxin effects, hypersensitivity reactions, weakening of neck muscles, swallowing/speech/respiratory disorders, and autonomic dysreflexia (associated with intradetrusor inj). Monitor patients with peripheral motor neuropathic diseases, amyotrophic lateral sclerosis, neuromuscular junction disorders, or compromised respiratory status. In patients with strabismus, monitor for retrobulbar hemorrhage during administration, and for effects of dose by re-examining 7-14 days after inj. Monitor PVR urine volume (in patients who are not catheterizing) within 2 weeks post-treatment and periodically as medically appropriate up to 12 weeks.

Patient Counseling: Advise to seek immediate medical attention if unusual symptoms (eg, swallowing, speaking, or breathing difficulty) develop, or if any existing symptom worsens. Instruct to avoid driving or engaging in other potentially hazardous activities if loss of strength, muscle weakness, blurred vision, or drooping eyelids occurs. Instruct to contact physician if experience difficulties in voiding after bladder inj for urinary incontinence.

Administration: ID/IM routes. Refer to PI for preparation and administration instructions.
Storage: 2-8°C for up to 24 months (200 U) or 36 months (100 U). Reconstituted Sol: 2-8°C; use within 24 hrs.

BOTOX COSMETIC   RX
onabotulinumtoxinA (Allergan)

> Distant spread of toxin effects hours to weeks after inj (eg, asthenia, generalized muscle weakness, diplopia, blurred vision, ptosis, dysphagia, dysphonia, dysarthria, urinary incontinence, breathing difficulties). Swallowing and breathing difficulties can be life-threatening and there have been reports of death. Risk of symptoms is greater in children treated for spasticity than in adults. In unapproved uses and approved indications, cases of spread of effect have occurred at doses comparable to those used to treat cervical dystonia and at lower doses.

THERAPEUTIC CLASS: Purified neurotoxin complex

INDICATIONS: For temporary improvement in appearance of moderate to severe glabellar lines associated with corrugator and/or procerus muscle activity in adults ≤65 years of age.

DOSAGE: *Adults:* ≤65 yrs: Inject a dose of 0.1mL IM into each of five sites, two in each corrugator muscle and one in the procerus muscle for a total dose of 20 U. Intervals should be no more frequent than every 3 months.

HOW SUPPLIED: Inj: 50 U, 100 U

CONTRAINDICATIONS: Infection at proposed injection sites.

WARNINGS/PRECAUTIONS: Not interchangeable with other botulinum toxin products and cannot be compared or converted to other products. Do not exceed dosing recommendations. Caution with peripheral motor neuropathic diseases, amyotrophic lateral sclerosis (ALS), neuromuscular junctional disorders (eg, myasthenia gravis, Lambert-Eaton syndrome); increased risk of dysphagia and respiratory compromise. Hypersensitivity reactions (eg, anaphylaxis, urticaria, soft tissue edema, and dyspnea) reported. Contains albumin; possible risk of transmission of (eg, viruses, Creutzfeldt-Jakob disease). Caution with inflammation at injection sites, excessive weakness or atrophy in target muscles. Injection of the orbicularis muscle may reduce blinking, especially with VII nerve disorders. Reduced blinking can lead to corneal exposure, persistent epithelial defect, and corneal ulceration. Carefully test corneal sensation in eyes previously operated upon, avoid injection into lower lid area to avoid ectropion, and vigorously treat any epithelial defect. Inducing paralysis in one or more extraocular muscles may produce spatial disorientation, double vision, or past pointing; covering affected eye may alleviate symptoms. Caution with inflammatory skin problems at the injection site, marked facial asymmetry, ptosis, excessive dermatochalasis, deep dermal scarring, thick sebaceous skin, or inability to substantially lessen glabellar lines by physically spreading them apart. Cardiovascular system adverse events including arrhythmia and myocardial infarction reported; caution with pre-existing cardiovascular disease (CVD). Needle-related pain and/or anxiety may result in vasovagal responses.

ADVERSE REACTIONS: Asthenia, generalized muscle weakness, diplopia, blurred vision, ptosis, dysphagia, dysphonia, dysarthria, urinary incontinence, breathing difficulties, headache, respiratory infection, flu syndrome, blepharoptosis, nausea.

INTERACTIONS: May be potentiated with aminoglycosides, and agents interfering with neuromuscular transmission (eg, curare-like nondepolarizing blockers, lincosamides, polymyxins, quinidine, magnesium sulfate, anticholinesterases, succinylcholine chloride). Excessive neuromuscular weakness may be exacerbated if another botulinum toxin is administered before effects resolve from the previous botulinum toxin injection.

PREGNANCY: Category C, caution in nursing.

MECHANISM OF ACTION: Purified neurotoxin complex; blocks neuromuscular transmission by binding to acceptor sites on motor nerve terminals, entering the nerve terminals, and inhibiting

B

the release of acetylcholine. Produces partial chemical denervation of the muscle resulting in a localized reduction in muscle activity if injected IM.

NURSING CONSIDERATIONS

Assessment: Assess for breathing or swallowing difficulties, infection at proposed injection site or weakness/atrophy in target muscle, and other conditions where treatment is contraindicated or cautioned. Assess for pregnancy/nursing status and possible drug interactions.

Monitoring: Monitor for spread of toxin effect, breathing difficulties, injection site reactions, and other severe side effects.

Patient Counseling: Provide a copy and review the contents of the FDA-approved Patient Medication Guide with the patient. Advise to inform doctor or pharmacist if they develop any unusual symptoms (including difficulty with swallowing, speaking, or breathing), or if any existing symptom worsens. Counsel to avoid driving a car or engaging in other potentially hazardous activities if loss of strength, muscle weakness, or impaired vision occur.

Administration: IM route. Refer to PI for proper dilution and injection technique. **Storage:** Refrigerate (2-8°C) for up to 36 months for 100 U vial (unopened) or up to 24 months for 50 U vial (unopened). Refrigerate (2-8°C) reconstituted solution and administer within 24 hrs.

BREVIBLOC   RX
esmolol HCl (Baxter)

THERAPEUTIC CLASS: Selective beta₁-blocker

INDICATIONS: For rapid control of ventricular rate in atrial fibrillation or atrial flutter in perioperative, postoperative, or other emergent circumstances. For noncompensatory sinus tachycardia. Treatment of tachycardia and hypertension that occur during induction and tracheal intubation, during surgery, on emergence from anesthesia, and in the postoperative period.

DOSAGE: *Adults:* Supraventricular Tachycardia: Titrate dose based on ventricular rate. Initial Load: 0.5mg/kg over 1 min. Maint: 0.05mg/kg/min for next 4 min. May increase by 0.05mg/kg/min or increased step-wise at intervals of 4 min or more up to 0.2mg/kg/min depending upon the desired response. Rapid Slowing of Ventricular Response: Repeat 0.5mg/kg load over 1 min, then 0.1mg/kg/min for 4 min. If needed, another (final) load of 0.5mg/kg over 1 min, then 0.15mg/kg/min for 4 min up to 0.2mg/kg/min. May continue infusions for as long as 24 hrs. Intraoperative/Postoperative Tachycardia and/or HTN: Immediate Control: Initial: 80mg (approx 1mg/kg) bolus over 30 sec followed by 0.15mg/kg/min prn. May titrate up to 0.3mg/kg/min to maintain desired heart rate and BP. Gradual Control: Initial: 0.5mg/kg over 1 min followed by maintenance infusion of 0.05mg/kg/min for 4 min. Then, may repeat load and follow maintenance infusion increased to 0.1mg/kg/min prn.

HOW SUPPLIED: Inj: 10mg/mL [10mL, 250mL], 20mg/mL [5mL, 100mL]

CONTRAINDICATIONS: Sinus bradycardia, heart block greater than first degree, cardiogenic shock or overt heart failure.

WARNINGS/PRECAUTIONS: Hypotension may occur; monitor BP and reduce dose or d/c if needed. May cause cardiac failure; withdraw at 1st sign of impending cardiac failure. Caution with supraventricular arrhythmias when patient is compromised hemodynamically. Not for HTN associated with hypothermia. Caution in bronchospastic diseases; titrate to lowest possible effective dose and terminate immediately in the event of bronchospasm. Caution in diabetics; may mask tachycardia occuring with hypoglycemia. Caution with renal impairment. Local infusion site reaction may develop; use alternate infusion site; caution should be taken to prevent extravasation. Avoid use of butterfly needles. Use caution when abruptly discontinuing infusions in coronary artery disease patients.

ADVERSE REACTIONS: Hypotension, dizziness, diaphoresis, somnolence, confusion, headache, agitation, bronchospasm, nausea, infusion-site reactions.

INTERACTIONS: Additive effects with catecholamine-depleting agents (eg, reserpine); monitor for evidence of hypotension or marked bradycardia. Levels increased by warfarin or morphine; titrate with caution. May increase digoxin levels; titrate with caution. May prolong effects of succinylcholine; titrate with caution. Caution when using with verapamil in depressed myocardial function; fatal cardiac arrest may occur. Do not use to control supraventricular tachycardia with vasoconstrictive and inotropic agents (eg, dopamine, epinephrine, norepinephrine) because of the danger of blocking cardiac contractility when systemic vascular resistance is high. Patients with a history of severe anaphylactic reaction may be more reactive to repeated challenge and unresponsive to the usual doses of epinephrine used to treat allergic reaction. Caution with supraventricular arrhythmias when patient is taking other drugs that decrease peripheral resistance, myocardial filling/contractility, and/or electrical impulse propagation in the myocardium.

PREGNANCY: Category C, caution in nursing.

MECHANISM OF ACTION: Selective β_1 blocker; inhibits β_1 receptors located chiefly in cardiac muscle, and at higher doses begins to inhibit β_2 receptors located chiefly in the bronchial and vascular musculature.

PHARMACOKINETICS: Distribution: Plasma protein binding (55%). **Metabolism:** Rapid. Through hydrolysis of the ester linkage in red blood cells to methanol and free acid. **Elimination:** Urine (73-88%, <2% unchanged); $T_{1/2}$=9 min (esmolol HCl), 3.7 hrs (acid metabolites).

NURSING CONSIDERATIONS

Assessment: Assess for sinus bradycardia, heart block greater than first degree, cardiogenic shock or overt heart failure, hypotension, HTN associated with hypothermia, bronchospastic disease, diabetes mellitus, renal impairment, and possible drug interactions.

Monitoring: Monitor BP, HR. Monitor for signs/symptoms of impending cardiac failure, hypotension (eg, diaphoresis or dizziness), postoperative tachycardia/HTN, bronchospasm, and masking signs of tachycardia occuring with hypoglycemia.

Patient Counseling: Inform about benefits/risks. Report any adverse reactions to physician.

Administration: IV route. Refer to PI for Directions for Use of Premixed Bag and Ready-to-Use Vials. Prediluted to provide ready-to-use vials. Do not introduce additives to premixed injections.

Storage: 25°C (77°F); excursions permitted to 15-30°C (59-86°F). Protect from freezing. Avoid excessive heat.

BRILINTA   RX
ticagrelor (AstraZeneca)

> May cause significant, sometimes fatal bleeding. Not for use in patients with active pathological bleeding or a history of intracranial hemorrhage. Do not start therapy in patients planning to undergo urgent coronary artery bypass graft surgery (CABG); d/c at least 5 days prior to any surgery when possible. Suspect bleeding in hypotensive patients and who have recently undergone coronary angiography, percutaneous coronary intervention (PCI), CABG, or other surgical procedures. D/C increases the risk of subsequent cardiovascular (CV) events; manage bleeding without d/c of therapy if possible. Maintenance doses of aspirin (ASA) >100mg may reduce effectiveness and should be avoided.

THERAPEUTIC CLASS: Platelet aggregation inhibitor

INDICATIONS: Reduction of rate of thrombotic CV events in patients with acute coronary syndrome (ACS) (unstable angina, non-ST elevation myocardial infarction [MI], or ST elevation MI). Reduction of rate of combined endpoint of CV death, MI, or stroke. Reduction of rate of stent thrombosis in patients treated with PCI.

DOSAGE: *Adults:* Initial: LD: 180mg with ASA (usually 325mg). Maint: 90mg bid with ASA (75-100mg/day). ACS patients who have received LD of clopidogrel may start ticagrelor therapy.

HOW SUPPLIED: Tab: 90mg

CONTRAINDICATIONS: History of intracranial hemorrhage, active pathological bleeding (eg, peptic ulcer, intracranial hemorrhage), severe hepatic impairment.

WARNINGS/PRECAUTIONS: Not studied with moderate hepatic impairment; consider the risks and benefits of therapy. Dyspnea reported; exclude underlying diseases that may require treatment if patient develops new, prolonged, or worsened dyspnea, and continue without interruption if determined to be related to therapy. Avoid interruption of therapy; if temporarily d/c, restart as soon as possible.

ADVERSE REACTIONS: Bleeding, dyspnea, headache, cough, dizziness, nausea, atrial fibrillation, HTN, non-cardiac chest pain, diarrhea, back pain, hypotension, fatigue, chest pain.

INTERACTIONS: See Boxed Warning. Avoid with strong CYP3A inhibitors (eg, atazanavir, clarithromycin, indinavir, itraconazole, ketoconazole, nefazodone, nelfinavir, ritonavir, saquinavir, telithromycin, and voriconazole). Avoid with potent CYP3A inducers (eg, rifampin, dexamethasone, phenytoin, carbamazepine, and phenobarbital). Avoid simvastatin and lovastatin doses >40mg. Monitor digoxin levels with initiation of or any change in therapy. Concomitant use with anticoagulants, fibrinolytic therapy, high doses of ASA, and chronic NSAIDs increase the risk of bleeding.

PREGNANCY: Category C, not for use in nursing.

MECHANISM OF ACTION: Platelet activation and aggregation inhibitor; reversibly interacts with the platelet $P2Y_{12}$ adenosine diphosphate (ADP) receptor to prevent signal transduction and platelet activation.

PHARMACOKINETICS: Absorption: Absolute bioavailability (36%); T_{max}=1.5 hrs, 2.5 hrs (active metabolite). Refer to PI for other pharmacokinetic parameters. **Distribution:** V_d=88L; plasma protein binding (>99%). **Metabolism:** Hepatic via CYP3A4; AR-C124910XX (active metabolite). **Elimination:** Urine (<1%, unchanged and metabolite), biliary; $T_{1/2}$=7 hrs, 9 hrs (active metabolite).

NURSING CONSIDERATIONS

Assessment: Assess for status of patient, history of intracranial hemorrhage, active pathological bleeding, patients at risk of bleeding, severe hepatic impairment, pregnancy/nursing status, and possible drug interactions.

Monitoring: Monitor for bleeding, dyspnea, and other adverse reactions.

Patient Counseling: Inform of the risks and benefits of therapy. Tell patient to take exactly as prescribed and not to d/c therapy without consulting prescribing physician. Inform patients not to exceed the 100mg daily dose of ASA. Inform patients that they may bruise and/or bleed more easily and that bleeding will take longer than usual to stop. Instruct to report to physician any unanticipated, prolonged, or excessive bleeding, or blood in stool or urine, notify physician if taking, or plan to take any prescription or over-the-counter drugs, including dietary supplements. Notify physician or dentist about therapy before scheduling any surgery or dental procedure. Inform patients that shortness of breath may occur; contact doctor if unexpected or severe. Instruct to take 1 tab (the next dose) at its scheduled time if a dose is missed.

Administration: Oral route. **Storage:** 25°C (77°F); excursions permitted to 15-30°C (59-86°F).

BROMDAY   RX
bromfenac (Ista)

THERAPEUTIC CLASS: NSAID

INDICATIONS: Treatment of postoperative inflammation and reduction of ocular pain after cataract surgery.

DOSAGE: *Adults:* 1 drop qd in affected eye(s), start 1 day prior to surgery, the day of surgery and continue for 2 weeks post surgery.

HOW SUPPLIED: Sol: 0.09% [1.7mL]

WARNINGS/PRECAUTIONS: Contains sodium sulfite; may cause allergic-type reactions (eg, anaphylactic symptoms, asthmatic episodes). Sulfite sensitivity is seen more frequently in asthmatics. May slow or delay healing. Potential cross-sensitivity to acetylsalicylic acid, phenylacetic acid derivatives, and other NSAIDs. Caution when treating individuals who previously exhibited sensitivity to these drugs. May increase bleeding of ocular tissues (eg, hyphemas) in conjunction with ocular surgery. Caution in patients with known bleeding tendencies. May result in keratitis. Continued use may lead to sight-threatening epithelial breakdown, corneal thinning, corneal erosion, corneal ulceration, or corneal perforation; d/c if corneal epithelium breakdown occurs. Caution in patients with complicated ocular surgeries, corneal denervation, corneal epithelial defects, diabetes mellitus (DM), ocular surface diseases (eg, dry eye syndrome), rheumatoid arthritis (RA), or repeat ocular surgeries within a short period of time. Increased risk for occurrence and severity of corneal adverse events if used >24 hrs prior to surgery or use beyond 14 days post-surgery. Avoid use with contact lenses. Avoid use during late pregnancy because of the known effects on the fetal cardiovascular system (closure of ductus arteriosus).

ADVERSE REACTIONS: Abnormal sensation in eye, conjunctival hyperemia, eye irritation (burning/stinging), eye pain, eye pruritus, eye redness, headache, iritis.

INTERACTIONS: Concomitant use of topical NSAIDs and topical steroids may increase potential for healing problems. Caution with other medications which may prolong bleeding time.

PREGNANCY: Category C, caution in nursing.

MECHANISM OF ACTION: NSAID; thought to block prostaglandin synthesis by inhibiting cyclooxygenase 1 and 2.

NURSING CONSIDERATIONS

Assessment: Assess for hypersensitivity (eg, sodium sulfite) or cross-sensitivity (eg, ASA) reactions, history of complicated or repeated ocular surgeries, corneal denervation, corneal epithelial defects, DM, ocular surface diseases (eg, dry eye syndrome), RA, bleeding tendencies, pregnancy/nursing status, and possible drug interactions.

Monitoring: Monitor for anaphylactic symptoms, severe asthma attacks, wound-healing problems, keratitis, corneal epithelial breakdown, corneal thinning/erosion/ulceration/perforation, increased bleeding time, and bleeding of ocular tissues (hyphemas) in conjunction with ocular surgery.

Patient Counseling: Advise not to wear contact lenses during therapy. Advise patients of the possibility of slow or delayed healing which may occur while using this product. Advise not to touch the dropper tip to any surface, as this may contaminate the contents. If >1 topical ophthalmic medication is used, instruct to administer 5 min apart.

Administration: Ocular route. May be used in conjunction with other topical ophthalmic medications (eg, α-agonists, β-blockers, carbonic anhydrase inhibitors, cycloplegics, mydriatics). Administer at least 5 min apart. **Storage:** 15-25°C (59-77°F).

BUMETANIDE RX

bumetanide (Various)

THERAPEUTIC CLASS: Loop diuretic

INDICATIONS: Treatment of edema associated with congestive heart failure (CHF), hepatic disease, and renal disease including nephrotic syndrome.

DOSAGE: *Adults:* ≥18 yrs: PO: Usual: 0.5-2mg qd. Maint: May give every other day or every 3-4 days. Max: 10mg/day. IV/IM: Initial: 0.5-1mg over 1-2 min, may repeat every 2-3 hrs for 2-3 doses. Max: 10mg/day. Elderly: Start at low end of dosing range.

HOW SUPPLIED: Inj: 0.25mg/mL; Tab: 0.5mg*, 1mg*, 2mg* *scored

CONTRAINDICATIONS: Anuria, hepatic coma, severe electrolyte depletion.

WARNINGS/PRECAUTIONS: Monitor for volume/electrolyte depletion, hypokalemia, blood dyscrasias, hepatic damage. Elderly are prone to volume/electrolyte depletion. Caution in elderly, hepatic cirrhosis and ascites. Associated with ototoxicity, hypocalcemia, thrombocytopenia, hypomagnesemia, hypokalemia, and hyperuricemia. Hypersensitivity with sulfonamide allergy. D/C if marked increase in BUN or creatinine or if develop oliguria with progressive renal disease.

ADVERSE REACTIONS: Muscle cramps, dizziness, hypotension, headache, nausea, hyperuricemia, hypokalemia, hyponatremia, hyperglycemia, azotemia, increased serum creatinine.

INTERACTIONS: Avoid aminoglycosides, ototoxic and nephrotoxic drugs, indomethacin. Lithium toxicity. Probenecid reduces effects. Potentiates antihypertensives.

PREGNANCY: Category C, not for use in nursing.

MECHANISM OF ACTION: Loop diuretic; inhibits sodium reabsorption in ascending loop of Henle.

PHARMACOKINETICS: Absorption: (IV) T_{max}=15-30 min. (Tab) T_{max}=1-2 hrs. **Distribution:** Plasma protein binding (94-96%). **Metabolism:** Oxidation. **Elimination:** Urine, bile (2%); $T_{1/2}$=1-1.5 hrs.

NURSING CONSIDERATIONS

Assessment: Assess for progressive renal disease, severe electrolyte depletion, anuria, oliguria, risk for vetricular arrhythmia, possible drug interactions, DM, impaired GI absorption, CHF, sulfonamide allergy, and liver disease (hepatic coma).

Monitoring: Periodically monitor serum potassium, serum electrolytes, CBC, blood glucose, and renal function. Monitor for signs/symptoms of ototoxicity, hypersensitivity reactions, hyperuricemia, oliguria, and thrombocytopenia.

Patient Counseling: Advise to seek medical attention if symptoms of ototoxicity, oliguria, hypersensitivity reactions, or thrombocytopenia occur.

Administration: Oral route. **Storage:** IV: 20-25°C (68-77°F). Protect from light. Tab: 15-30°C (59-86°F).

BUPHENYL RX

sodium phenylbutyrate (Ucyclyd Pharma)

THERAPEUTIC CLASS: Urea cycle disorder agent

INDICATIONS: Adjunctive therapy in chronic management of urea cycle disorders involving deficiencies of carbamylphosphate synthetase (CPS), ornithine transcarbamylase (OTC), or argininosuccinic acid synthetase (AS), neonatal-onset deficiency (complete enzymatic deficiency presenting within the first 28 days of life), and late-onset disease (partial enzymatic deficiency, presenting after the first month of life) in patients who have a history of hyperammonemic encephalopathy.

DOSAGE: *Adults:* <20kg: 450-600mg/kg/day. >20kg: 9.9-13g/m²/day. Take in equally divided amounts with each meal or feeding (eg, 3-6 times a day). Powder is for oral use via mouth, gastronomy, or nasogastric tube only. Mix powder with food (solid or liquid) for immediate use. *Pediatrics:* <20kg: 450-600mg/kg/day. >20kg: 9.9-13m²/day. Take in equally divided amounts with meal or feeding (eg, 3-6 times a day). Powder is for oral use via mouth, gastronomy, or nasogastric tube only. Mix powder with food (solid or liquid) for immediate use.

HOW SUPPLIED: Powder: 250g; Tab: 500mg

CONTRAINDICATIONS: Acute hyperammonemia.

WARNINGS/PRECAUTIONS: Caution with congestive heart failure (CHF), hepatic/renal insufficiency, inborn errors of beta oxidation, and sodium retention with edema. Maintain plasma glutamine <1,000μmol/L. Monitor serum phenylbutyrate and its metabolites, phenylacetate, and phenylacetylglutamine periodically. Use of tablets for neonates, infants, and children <20kg is not recommended.

ADVERSE REACTIONS: Amenorrhea/menstrual dysfunction, decreased appetite, body odor, bad taste/taste aversion, hypoalbuminemia, metabolic acidosis/alkalosis, anemia, hyperchloremia, hypophosphatemia, decreased total protein, increased alkaline phosphatase, increased liver transaminase, leukopenia/leukocytosis, thrombocytopenia.

INTERACTIONS: Probenecid may affect renal excretion of conjugated product of sodium phenylbutyrate, including metabolite. Reports of hyperammonemia being induced by haloperidol and valproic acid. Use of corticosteroids may cause the breakdown of body protein and increase plasma ammonia levels.

PREGNANCY: Category C, caution in nursing.

MECHANISM OF ACTION: Prodrug of phenylacetate; decreases elevated plasma ammonia glutamine levels and increases waste nitrogen excretion in the form of phenylacetylglutamine.

PHARMACOKINETICS: Absorption: (Powder/tab) T_{max}=1 hr; C_{max}=195mcg/mL (powder) and 218mcg/mL (tab). Phenylbutyrate: T_{max} = 1.35 hrs; C_{max}=218mcg/mL. Phenylacetate: T_{max}=3.74 hrs; C_{max}=48.5mcg/mL. **Metabolism:** Hepatic and renal. **Elimination:** Renal (80-100%, phenylacetylglutamine). (Powder) $T_{1/2}$=0.76 hrs; (Tab) $T_{1/2}$=0.77 hrs.

NURSING CONSIDERATIONS

Assessment: Assess for acute hyperammonemia, CHF, hepatic/renal insufficiency, inborn errors of beta oxidation, sodium retention with edema, hypersensitivity to drug, pregnancy/nursing status, and possible drug interactions. Assess for plasma levels of ammonia, arginine, branched-chain amino acids, serum proteins, glutamine.

Monitoring: Monitor for adverse reactions and hypersensitivity reactions. Monitor periodically serum phenylbutyrate and its metabolites, phenylacetate and phenylacetylglutamine levels. Monitor urinalysis, blood chemistry profiles, and hematologic tests.

Patient Counseling: Instruct to take drug exactly as prescribed and follow the prescribed diet. If a dose is missed, take as soon as possible that same day. Total daily dose should be taken in equally divided amounts with meals. Inform the physician of other medications being taken and when symptoms of sleepiness and lightheadedness occur.

Administration: Oral route, nasogastric or gastrostomy tube. Powder should be mixed with food (solid or liquid); however, when dissolved in water, it is stable for 1 week at room temperature or refrigerated. **Storage:** 15-30°C (59-86°F). Keep bottle tightly closed.

BUPRENEX   CIII
buprenorphine HCl (Reckitt Benckiser)

THERAPEUTIC CLASS: Opioid analgesic

INDICATIONS: Relief of moderate to severe pain.

DOSAGE: *Adults:* 0.3mg IM/IV q6h PRN. Repeat if needed, 30-60 min after initial dose and then prn. High Risk Patients/Concomitant CNS depressants: Reduce dose by approximately 50%. May use single doses ≤0.6mg IM if not at high risk.
Pediatrics: ≥13 yrs: 0.3mg IM/IV q6h prn. Repeat if needed, 30-60 min after initial dose and then prn. High Risk Patients/Concomitant CNS depressants: Reduce dose by approximately 50%. May use single doses ≤0.6mg IM if not at high risk. 2-12 yrs: 2-6mcg/kg IM/IV q4-6h.

HOW SUPPLIED: Inj: 0.3mg/mL

WARNINGS/PRECAUTIONS: Significant respiratory depression reported; caution with compromised respiratory function. May increase cerebrospinal fluid (CSF) pressure; caution with head injury, intracranial lesions. Caution with debilitated, BPH, biliary tract dysfunction, myxedema, hypothyroidism, urethral stricture, acute alcoholism, Addison's disease, CNS disease, coma, toxic psychoses, delirium tremens, elderly, pediatrics, kyphoscoliosis or hepatic/renal/pulmonary impairment. May impair mental or physical abilities. May precipitate withdrawal in narcotic-dependence. May lead to psychological dependence.

ADVERSE REACTIONS: Sedation, N/V, dizziness, sweating, hypotension, headache, miosis, hypoventilation.

INTERACTIONS: Caution with MAOIs, CNS and respiratory depressants. Respiratory and cardiovascular collapse reported with diazepam. Increased CNS depression with other narcotic analgesics, general anesthetics, antihistamines, benzodiazepines, phenothiazines, other tranquilizers, sedative-hypnotics. Decreased clearance with CYP3A4 inhibitors (eg, macrolides, azole antifungals, protease inhibitors). Increased clearance with CYP3A4 inducers (eg, rifampin, carbamazepine, phenytoin).

PREGNANCY: Category C, not for use in nursing.

MECHANISM OF ACTION: Opioid analgesic; high affinity binding to μ-opiate receptors in CNS. Possesses slow rate of dissociation from its receptor. Also possesses narcotic antagonist activity.

PHARMACOKINETICS: Absorption: T_{max}=1 hr. **Distribution:** Found in breast milk. **Metabolism:** Liver. **Elimination:** $T_{1/2}$=1.2-7.2 hrs.

NURSING CONSIDERATIONS

Assessment: Assess for compromised respiratory function (eg, COPD, hypoxia), head injury, intracranial lesions, age of patient, hepatic/renal function, myxedema or hypothyroidism, adrenal cortical insufficiencies (eg, Addison's disease), CNS depression or coma, toxic psychosis, prostatic hypertrophy or urethral stricture, acute alcoholism, delirium tremens, kyphoscoliosis, biliary tract dysfunction, pregnancy/nursing, and possible drug interactions.

Monitoring: Monitor for signs/symptoms of respiratory depression, CNS depression, elevation of CSF pressure, increased intracholedochal pressure, drug dependence, and withdrawal effects.

Patient Counseling: Inform that medication may impair mental/physicial abilities; use caution when performing dangerous tasks (eg, operating machinery/driving). Advise to notify physician of all medications currently taken. Instruct to avoid use of other CNS depressants and alcohol during therapy. Advise that medication may lead to dependence. Counsel to not exceed prescribed dosage. Advise to avoid abruptly discontinuing medication. Counsel to contact physician if signs/symptoms of respiratory depression develop.

Administration: Deep IM or slow IV route. **Storage:** Avoid excessive heat (over 40°C or 104°F). Protect from prolonged exposure to light.

BUSPIRONE   RX
buspirone HCl (Various)

THERAPEUTIC CLASS: Atypical anxiolytic

INDICATIONS: Management of anxiety disorders or short-term relief of anxiety symptoms.

DOSAGE: *Adults:* Initial: 7.5mg bid. Titrate: May increase by 5mg/day at intervals of 2-3 days, PRN. Usual: 20-30mg/day in divided doses. Max: 60mg/day. With Potent CYP3A4 Inhibitor: Low dose given cautiously.

HOW SUPPLIED: Tab: 5mg*, 7.5 mg*, 10mg*, 15mg*, 30mg* *scored

WARNINGS/PRECAUTIONS: May impair mental/physical abilities. Does not exhibit cross-tolerance with benzodiazepine or other common sedatives/hypnotics; withdraw patients gradually from these agents before starting therapy, especially with chronic CNS depressants. May cause acute and chronic changes in dopamine-mediated neurological function; syndrome of restlessness has been reported shortly after initiation. May interfere with urinary metanephrine/catecholamine assay; d/c therapy for at least 48 hrs prior to undergoing urine collection for catecholamines. Not recommended with severe hepatic/renal impairment. Periodically reassess usefulness of drug if used for extended periods.

ADVERSE REACTIONS: Dizziness, nausea, headache, nervousness, lightheadedness, excitement, drowsiness, fatigue, insomnia, dry mouth.

INTERACTIONS: Elevation of BP with MAOI reported; avoid concomitant use. Avoid with alcohol. Dizziness, headache, and nausea, and increased nordiazepam reported with diazepam. May increase serum concentrations of haloperidol. ALT elevations reported with trazodone. Caution with CNS-active drugs. Diltiazem, verapamil, erythromycin, grapefruit juice, itraconazole, nefazodone, and other CYP3A4 inhibitors (eg, ketoconazole, ritonavir) may increase concentrations; may require dose adjustment. Rifampin and other CYP3A4 inducers (eg, dexamethasone, phenytoin, phenobarbital, carbamazepine), including potent CYP3A4 inducers, may decrease concentrations; may require dose adjustment. Avoid with large amounts of grapefruit juice. May increase levels of nefazodone. Cimetidine may increase levels. Prolonged PT reported with warfarin. May displace less firmly bound drugs like digoxin.

PREGNANCY: Category B, not for use in nursing.

MECHANISM OF ACTION: Atypical anxiolytic; has not been established. Binds with high affinity to serotonin (5-HT1$_A$) receptors and moderate affinity for brain D$_2$-dopamine receptors; may have indirect effects on other neurotransmitter systems.

PHARMACOKINETICS: Absorption: Rapid. C_{max}=1-6ng/mL, T_{max}=40-90 min. **Distribution:** Plasma protein binding (86%). **Metabolism:** Liver (extensive), primarily by oxidation via CYP3A4, and by hyroxylation; 1-pyrimidinylpiperazine (active metabolite). **Elimination:** Urine (29-63%), feces (18-38%); $T_{1/2}$=2-3 hrs.

NURSING CONSIDERATIONS

Assessment: Assess for hypersensitivity to drug, hepatic/renal impairment, pregnancy/nursing status, and possible drug interactions.

Monitoring: Monitor for CNS effects, syndrome of restlessness, and other adverse reactions.

Patient Counseling: Inform physician about any medications, prescription or nonprescription, alcohol, or drugs being taken or plan to take, and if pregnant/breastfeeding, become pregnant, or plan to become pregnant. Advise not to drive a car or operate potentially dangerous machinery until effects have been determined. Avoid drinking large amounts of grapefruit juice. Advise to take in a consistent manner with regard to timing and food.

Administration: Oral route. **Storage:** 20-25°C (68-77°F). (7.5mg) 25°C (77°F); excursions permitted between 15-30°C (59-86°F).

BUTRANS | CIII
buprenorphine (Purdue Pharmaceutical)

> Exercise proper patient selection for around-the-clock therapy. Schedule III controlled substance with potential for abuse; assess for clinical risks for opioid abuse or addiction prior to prescribing opioids. Monitor all patients receiving opioids for signs of misuse, abuse, and addiction. Do not exceed a dose of one 20-mcg/hr buprenorphine transdermal system due to the risk of QTc interval prolongation. Avoid exposing application site and surrounding area to direct external heat sources. Temperature-dependent increases in buprenorphine release from the system may result in a possible overdose and death.

THERAPEUTIC CLASS: Opioid analgesic

INDICATIONS: Management of moderate to severe chronic pain in patients requiring a continuous, around-the-clock opioid analgesic for an extended period of time.

DOSAGE: *Adults:* Individualize dose. Refer to PI for the considerations needed when selecting the initial dose. Conversion from Other Opioids: Refer to PI. Opioid-Naive: Initial: 5mcg/hr. Titrate: Increase to the next higher level after a minimum of 72 hrs. Max: 20mcg/hr. Maint: Use dose with adequate analgesia and tolerable side effects for as long as pain management is necessary. May use immediate-release opioid and non-opioid medications as supplemental analgesia. Periodically reassess continued need for around-the-clock therapy. Patch is intended to be worn for 7 days. Mild to Moderate Hepatic Impairment: Initial: 5mcg/hr. Titrate: Increase to a level that provides adequate analgesia and tolerable side effects, under close supervision. Cessation Therapy: Taper dose gradually until d/c; consider introduction of immediate-release opioid medication.

HOW SUPPLIED: Patch: 5mcg/hr, 10mcg/hr, 20mcg/hr

CONTRAINDICATIONS: Management of acute pain or requirement of opioid analgesia for a short period of time, postoperative pain, mild/intermittent pain. Known or suspected paralytic ileus, severe bronchial asthma or significant respiratory depression.

WARNINGS/PRECAUTIONS: May cause respiratory depression; caution with significant chronic obstructive pulmonary disease or cor pulmonale, other risks of substantially decreased respiratory reserve, hypoxia, hypercapnia, and preexisting respiratory depression. May cause CNS depression. May prolong QTc interval; caution with hypokalemia or clinically unstable cardiac disease. Avoid use with history/family history of long QT syndrome. May cause carbon dioxide retention leading to increased cerebrospinal fluid (CSF) pressure; caution with head injury, intracranial lesions, or other sources of preexisting increased intracranial pressure (ICP). May obscure neurological signs associated with increased ICP with head injuries. May cause severe hypotension/orthostatic hypotension; caution in circulatory shock and in compromised ability to maintain blood pressure. May cause hepatotoxicity; obtain baseline and periodic LFTs in high risk patients. D/C if severe application-site reaction develops. Acute and chronic hypersensitivity reactions including bronchospasm, angioneurotic edema, and anaphylactic shock reported. High temperature increases drug release causing possible overdose and death; avoid exposure of application site and surrounding areas to external heat sources. If fever develops or increases in core temperature due to exertion, monitor for side effects and adjust dose PRN. May impair mental and physical abilities. Caution with history of a seizure disorder, alcoholism, delirium tremens, debilitation, adrenocortical insufficiency, kyphoscoliosis associated with respiratory compromise, myxedema or hypothyroidism, prostatic hypertrophy or urethral stricture, toxic psychosis, or severe impairment of hepatic, pulmonary, or renal function. May cause spasm of the sphincter of Oddi; caution with biliary tract disease. May increase serum amylase. May obscure diagnosis or clinical course of patients with acute abdominal conditions; caution in patients at risk of developing ileus. Not approved for management of addictive disorders.

ADVERSE REACTIONS: Nausea, headache, application-site pruritus/irritation/erythema/rash, dizziness, constipation, somnolence, vomiting, dry mouth, peripheral edema, fatigue, hyperhidrosis.

INTERACTIONS: Concomitant use with other CNS depressants (eg, alcohol, sedatives, anxiolytics, hypnotics, neuroleptics, muscle relaxants, other opioids) may cause respiratory depression, hypotension, profound sedation, or coma. Not recommended for use within 14 days of MAOIs. Avoid use with Class IA antiarrhythmics (eg, quinidine, procainamide, disopyramide) or Class III antiarrhythmics (eg, sotalol, amiodarone, dofetilide). Concurrent use with phenothiazines or other agents may cause hypotension. Concomitant use with certain protease inhibitors (eg, atazanavir, atazanavir/ritonavir) may elevate levels. May interact with CYP3A4 inhibitors depending on route of administration as well as specificity of enzyme inhibition. May reduce efficacy if coadministered with CYP3A4 inducers (eg, phenobarbital, carbamazepine, phenytoin, rifampin). Caution with benzodiazepines; may alter usual ceiling effect on respiratory depression. Concomitant use with skeletal muscle relaxants may enhance neuromuscular blocking action and increase respiratory depression.

PREGNANCY: Category C, not for use in nursing.

MECHANISM OF ACTION: Opioid analgesic; partial agonist at μ-opioid and ORL-1 (nociceptin) receptors, antagonist at kappa opioid receptors, and agonist at delta receptors. Its clinical action results from binding to opioid receptors.

PHARMACOKINETICS: Absorption: (IV) Absolute bioavailability: 15%. (5mcg/hr) C_{max}=176pg/mL, AUC=12087pg•h/mL. (10mcg/hr) C_{max}=191pg/mL, AUC=27035pg•h/mL. (20mcg/hr) C_{max}=471pg/mL, AUC=54294pg•h/mL. **Distribution:** Plasma protein binding (96%); found in breast milk; crosses placenta. (IV) V_d=430L. **Metabolism:** Liver. N-dealkylation and glucuronidation; CYP3A4, UGT1A1, 1A3, 2B7; norbuprenorphine (active metabolite). **Elimination:** $T_{1/2}$=26 hrs; (IM) Feces (70%), urine (27%).

NURSING CONSIDERATIONS

Assessment: Assess for opioid tolerance, level and type of pain, clinical risks for opioid abuse or addiction, hypokalemia, history/family history of long QT syndrome, cardiac/respiratory function, hepatic/renal function, debilitation, hypothyroidism, prostatic hypertrophy, seizures, toxic psychosis, biliary tract dysfunction, fever, pregnancy/nursing status, and for possible drug interactions. Obtain baseline LFTs in high risk patients.

Monitoring: Monitor for signs/symptoms of respiratory depression, CNS depression, elevation of CSF pressure, QTc prolongation, hypotension, hepatotoxicity, seizures, spasm of the sphincter of Oddi, drug addiction and abuse, and level of pain intensity. Monitor LFTs in high risk patients.

Patient Counseling: Advise to wear continuously for 7 days. Educate on proper application, removal, and disposal. Instruct to apply to upper outer arms, upper chest, upper back, or the side of the chest and rotate application site with a minimum of 3 weeks between applications to a previously used site. Advise to apply patch to a hairless or nearly hairless skin site and avoid exposing application site to external heat sources. Instruct that if patch falls off during use, a new patch should be applied to a different skin site. Counsel that medication may impair mental/physical abilities. Advise to notify physician of all medications currently taking and avoid use of other CNS depressants and alcohol during therapy. Warn that medication may lead to dependence and to not exceed prescribed dosage. Advise to avoid abruptly d/c medication. Instruct to contact physician if signs/symptoms of respiratory depression develop. Counsel about pregnancy risks.

Administration: Transdermal patch. Apply immediately after removal from individually sealed pouch. Do not use if the pouch seal is broken, cut, damaged, or changed in any way. Next patch should be applied to a different site. Apply to intact skin on upper outer arm, upper chest, upper back, or the side of the chest. **Storage:** 25°C (77°F); excursions permitted to 15-30°C (59-86°F).

BYDUREON
exenatide (Amylin)

RX

> Increased incidence in thyroid C-cell tumors at clinically relevant exposures in animal studies. It is unknown whether drug causes thyroid C-cell tumors (eg, medullary thyroid carcinoma [MTC]) in humans. Contraindicated in patients with a personal or family history of MTC and with multiple endocrine neoplasia syndrome type 2 (MEN 2). Routine serum calcitonin or thyroid ultrasound monitoring is of uncertain value in patients. Counsel patients on risks and symptoms of thyroid tumors.

THERAPEUTIC CLASS: Incretin mimetic

INDICATIONS: Adjunct to diet and exercise to improve glycemic control in adults with type 2 diabetes mellitus (DM).

DOSAGE: *Adults:* 2mg/dose once q7 days. May change the day of weekly administration PRN as long as the last dose was given ≥3 days before.

HOW SUPPLIED: Inj, Extended-release: 2mg/dose

CONTRAINDICATIONS: Personal/family history of MTC or with MEN 2.

WARNINGS/PRECAUTIONS: Not for IV or IM administration. Not recommended as 1st line therapy with inadequate glycemic control on diet and exercise. Not a substitute for insulin; do not use in type 1 DM or for treatment of diabetic ketoacidosis. Acute pancreatitis reported; observe for signs/symptoms after initiation and d/c if suspected and do not restart if confirmed. Consider other antidiabetic therapies with history of pancreatitis. Refer patient to endocrinologist if serum calcitonin is elevated. Altered renal function, including increased SrCr, renal impairment, worsened chronic renal failure, and acute renal failure reported; avoid with severe renal impairment (CrCl <30mL/min) or end stage renal disease. Caution with renal transplantation and moderate renal impairment (CrCl 30-50mL/min). Avoid with severe GI disease. May develop antibodies; consider alternative antidiabetic therapy if there is worsening glycemic control or failure to achieve targeted glycemic control. Hypersensitivity reactions reported; d/c if occurs. No conclusive evidence of macrovascular risk reduction. Caution in elderly.

ADVERSE REACTIONS: Constipation, diarrhea, dyspepsia, headache, nausea, inj-site nodule, inj-site reaction.

INTERACTIONS: Not recommended with insulin and drugs with same active ingredient (eg, Byetta). Caution with oral medications. May increase INR sometimes associated with bleeding with warfarin; monitor INR more frequently after initiation of therapy. Sulfonylureas or other glucose-independent insulin secretagogues (eg, meglitinides) may increase the risk of hypoglycemia; may require lower dose of sulfonylurea. May alter levels of acetaminophen, digoxin, lovastatin, lisinopril, ethinyl estradiol, and levonorgestrel.

PREGNANCY: Category C, not for use in nursing.

MECHANISM OF ACTION: Glucagon-like peptide-1 receptor agonist; enhances glucose-dependent insulin secretion by the pancreatic β-cell, suppresses inappropriately elevated glucagon secretion, and slows gastric emptying.

PHARMACOKINETICS: Absorption: T_{max}=week 2 and week 6-7. **Distribution:** V_d=28.3L. **Elimination:** Kidney.

NURSING CONSIDERATIONS

Assessment: Assess for MEN 2, type 1 DM, diabetic ketoacidosis, renal impairment, severe GI disease, history of MTC or pancreatitis, pregnancy/nursing status, other conditions where treatment is cautioned or contraindicated, and possible drug interactions.

Monitoring: Monitor for signs/symptoms of acute pancreatitis, hypoglycemia, GI events, immunogenicity, and for hypersensitivity reactions. Monitor renal function, glucose levels, and HbA1c levels.

Patient Counseling: Inform about risks/benefits of therapy and of alternative modes of therapy. Counsel on importance of diabetes self management practices. Report symptoms of thyroid symptoms (eg, lump in the neck, hoarseness, dysphagia, dyspnea). Inform of potential risk for pancreatitis, hypoglycemia, worsening of renal function, and hypersensitivity reactions. D/c therapy and seek medical attention if persistent abdominal pain occurs. Review and reinforce instructions for hypoglycemia management. Inform not to substitute needles or any other components in the tray, and not to reuse or share needles or syringes. Use a different inj site each week when injecting in the same region. If a dose is missed, it should be administered as soon as noticed, provided the regularly scheduled dose is due ≥3 days later but if the next regularly dose is due 1 or 2 days later, do not administer dose and resume with the next regularly scheduled dose. Inform physician if pregnant or intend to become pregnant.

Administration: SQ route. Inject into thigh, abdomen, or upper arm. Administer immediately after powder is suspended in diluent and transferred to syringe. Refer to PI for administration instructions. **Storage:** 2-8°C (36-46°F). May store at room temperature not to exceed 25°C (77°F) for ≤4 weeks. Do not freeze and do not use if product has been frozen. Protect from light.

Bʏᴇᴛᴛᴀ   RX
exenatide (Amylin)

THERAPEUTIC CLASS: Incretin mimetic

INDICATIONS: Adjunct to diet and exercise to improve glycemic control in adults with type 2 diabetes mellitus (DM).

DOSAGE: *Adults:* Initial: 5mcg SQ bid, at anytime within 60 min before am and pm meals (or before the 2 main meals of the day, approximately 6 hrs or more apart). Titrate: May increase to 10mcg bid after 1 month based on clinical response. CrCl 30-50mL/min: Caution when initiating or escalating doses from 5mcg to 10mcg. Elderly: Start at the low end of dosing range.

HOW SUPPLIED: Inj: 5mcg/dose, 10mcg/dose [60-dose prefilled pen]

WARNINGS/PRECAUTIONS: Not a substitute for insulin; do not use in type 1 diabetes or for the treatment of diabetic ketoacidosis. Not studied and not recommmended with prandial insulin. Evaluate dose of insulin if used in combination; consider dose reduction in patients at risk of hypoglycemia. Acute pancreatitis reported; observe for signs and symptoms after initiation and dose increases; d/c if suspected and do not restart if confirmed. Consider other antidiabetic therapies with history of pancreatitis. Altered renal function, including increased SrCr, renal impairment, worsened chronic renal failure, and acute renal failure reported; avoid with severe renal impairment (CrCl <30mL/min) or end stage renal disease. Caution with renal transplantation. Avoid with severe GI disease. May develop antibodies; consider alternative antidiabetic therapy if there is worsening glycemic control or failure to achieve targeted glycemic control.

Hypersensitivity reactions reported; d/c if occurs. No conclusive evidence of macrovascular risk reduction. Caution in elderly.

ADVERSE REACTIONS: N/V, immunogenicity, dyspepsia.

INTERACTIONS: Caution with oral medications with narrow therapeutic index or require rapid GI absorption. Drugs dependent on threshold concentrations for efficacy (eg, contraceptives and antibiotics) should be taken at least 1 hr before inj. May increase INR sometimes associated with bleeding with warfarin; monitor PT more frequently after initiation or alteration of therapy. Sulfonylureas or other glucose-independent insulin secretagogues (eg, meglitinides) may increase the risk of hypoglycemia; may require lower dose of sulfonylurea. May alter levels of acetaminophen, digoxin, lovastatin, lisinopril, ethinyl estradiol, and levonorgestrel.

PREGNANCY: Category C, not for use in nursing.

MECHANISM OF ACTION: Glucagon-like peptide-1 receptor agonist; enhances glucose-dependent insulin secretion by the pancreatic β-cell, suppresses inappropriately elevated glucagon secretion, and slows gastric emptying.

PHARMACOKINETICS: Absorption: C_{max}=211pg/mL (10mcg), AUC=1036pg•h/mL (10mcg), T_{max}=2.1 hrs. **Distribution:** V_d=28.3L. **Elimination:** $T_{1/2}$=2.4 hrs.

NURSING CONSIDERATIONS

Assessment: Assess for type 1 diabetes, diabetic ketoacidosis, history of pancreatitis, renal impairment, severe GI disease, pregnancy/nursing status, and for possible drug interactions.

Monitoring: Monitor for signs/symptoms of acute pancreatitis, hypoglycemia, GI events, immunogenicity, and for hypersensitivity reactions. Monitor renal function, glucose levels, and HbA1c levels.

Patient Counseling: Advise of the potential risks and benefits of therapy. Advise to never share inj pen. Inform about self-management practices (eg, proper storage of drug, inj technique, timing of dosage and concomitant oral drugs, adherence to meal planning, regular physical activity). Inform that pen needles are purchased separately and advise on proper needle selection and disposal. Advise not to reuse needle and not to transfer drug from pen to a syringe or vial. Advise to not to mix with insulin or administer after a meal. Inform that if a dose is missed, treatment regimen should be resumed as prescribed with the next scheduled dose. Inform physician if pregnant or intend to become pregnant. Advise to contact a physician if signs/symptoms suggestive of acute pancreatitis (eg, severe abdominal pain), renal dysfunction, or hypersensitivity develop.

Administration: SQ route. Inject into thigh, abdomen, or upper arm. Refer to PI for further information on administration and preparation. **Storage:** Prior to 1st use: 2-8°C (36-46°F). After 1st use: <25°C (77°F). Do not freeze. Protect from light. Discard pen 30 days after the 1st use.

BYSTOLIC   RX
nebivolol (Forest)

THERAPEUTIC CLASS: Selective beta₁-blocker

INDICATIONS: Treatment of HTN alone or in combination with other antihypertensive agents.

DOSAGE: *Adults:* Individualize dose. Initial: 5mg qd. Titrate: May increase at 2-week intervals. Max: 40mg. Moderate Hepatic Impairment/Severe Renal Impairment (CrCl <30mL/min): Initial: 2.5mg qd; titrate up slowly if needed.

HOW SUPPLIED: Tab: 2.5mg, 5mg, 10mg, 20mg

CONTRAINDICATIONS: Severe bradycardia, heart block >1st degree, cardiogenic shock, decompensated cardiac failure, sick sinus syndrome (unless permanent pacemaker in place), severe hepatic impairment (Child-Pugh >B).

WARNINGS/PRECAUTIONS: Severe exacerbation of angina, myocardial infarction, and ventricular arrhythmias reported in patients with coronary artery disease (CAD) following abrupt d/c; taper over 1-2 weeks when possible. Restart therapy promptly, at least temporarily, if angina worsens or acute coronary insufficiency develops. Avoid with bronchospastic disease. Should generally continue therapy throughout perioperative period. Monitor patients closely with anesthetic agents that depress myocardial function (eg, ether, cyclopropane, trichloroethylene). If d/c therapy prior to major surgery, impaired ability of heart to respond to reflex adrenergic stimuli may augment risks of general anesthesia and surgical procedures. May mask signs/symptoms of hypoglycemia or hyperthyroidism, particularly tachycardia. Abrupt withdrawal may be followed by exacerbation of the symptoms of hyperthyroidism or precipitate a thyroid storm. May precipitate/aggravate symptoms of arterial insufficiency in patients with peripheral vascular disease (PVD). Patients with history of severe anaphylactic reactions to variety of allergens may be more reactive to repeated accidental/diagnostic/therapeutic challenge; may be unresponsive to usual doses of epinephrine. Initiate an α-blocker prior to use of any β-blocker in patients with known/suspected pheochromocytoma. Not recommended with severe hepatic impairment.

ADVERSE REACTIONS: Headache, fatigue, dizziness, diarrhea, nausea.

INTERACTIONS: Avoid with other β-blockers. D/C for several days before gradually tapering clonidine. CYP2D6 inhibitors (eg, quinidine, propafenone, paroxetine, fluoxetine) and cimetidine may increase levels. May decrease levels of sildenafil. Sildenafil may affect levels of nebivolol. May produce excessive reduction of sympathetic activity with catecholamine-depleting drugs (eg, reserpine, guanethidine). May increase risk of bradycardia with digitalis glycosides. May exacerbate effects of myocardial depressants/inhibitors of atrioventricular conduction (eg, antiarrhythmics, certain calcium antagonists). May need to adjust dose with CYP2D6 inducers. May potentiate hypoglycemic effect of insulin and PO hypoglycemics. Monitor ECG and BP with verapamil and diltiazem.

PREGNANCY: Category C, not for use in nursing.

MECHANISM OF ACTION: Selective β_1-blocker; mechanism not established. Possible factors include decreased HR and myocardial contractility, diminution of tonic sympathetic outflow to the periphery from cerebral vasomotor centers, suppression of renin activity, vasodilation, and decreased peripheral vascular resistance.

PHARMACOKINETICS: Absorption: T_{max}=1.5-4 hrs. **Distribution:** Plasma protein binding (98%). **Metabolism:** Glucuronidation, N-dealkylation, and oxidation via CYP2D6. **Elimination:** Urine (38%, extensive metabolizers [EM]), (67%, poor metabolizers [PM]); feces (44%, EM), (13%, PM); $T_{1/2}$=12 hrs (EM), 19 hrs (PM).

NURSING CONSIDERATIONS

Assessment: Assess for CAD, bronchospastic disease, diabetes mellitus, hypoglycemia, hyperthyroidism, PVD, pheochromocytoma, any conditions where treatment is contraindicated, hepatic/renal impairment, pregnancy/nursing status, and possible drug interactions.

Monitoring: Monitor for precipitation/aggravation of arterial insufficiency, hypersensitivity, and other adverse reactions. Monitor BP and serum glucose levels.

Patient Counseling: Inform of the risks and benefits of therapy. Advise to take drug regularly and continuously, as directed, without regard to food. Instruct to take only the next scheduled dose (without doubling it) if a dose is missed, and not to d/c without consulting physician. Advise to consult physician if any difficulty in breathing occurs, or signs/symptoms of worsening congestive heart failure (eg, weight gain, increased SOB, excessive bradycardia) develop. Caution about operating automobiles, using machinery, or engaging in tasks requiring alertness. Caution patients subject to spontaneous hypoglycemia, or diabetic patients receiving insulin or PO hypoglycemics, that the drug may mask some of the manifestations of hypoglycemia, particularly tachycardia.

Administration: Oral route. **Storage:** 20-25°C (68-77°F).

CADUET   RX
atorvastatin calcium - amlodipine besylate (Pfizer)

THERAPEUTIC CLASS: Calcium channel blocker/HMG-CoA reductase inhibitor

INDICATIONS: Amlodipine: Treatment of HTN, chronic stable or vasospastic angina (Prinzmetal's/variant) alone or in combination with other antihypertensives/antianginals. To reduce the risk of hospitalization due to angina and to reduce risk of coronary revascularization procedure in patients with recently documented coronary artery disease (CAD) by angiography and without heart failure or ejection fraction <40%. Atorvastatin: To reduce the risk of myocardial infarction (MI), stroke, revascularization procedures, and angina in adults without clinically evident coronary heart disease (CHD) but with multiple risk factors for CHD. To reduce the risk of MI and stroke in patients with type 2 diabetes, and without clinically evident CHD, but with multiple risk factors for CHD. To reduce the risk of non-fatal MI, fatal and non-fatal stroke, revascularization procedures, hospitalization for congestive heart failure (CHF), and angina in patients with clinically evident CHD. Adjunct to diet to reduce elevated total cholesterol (total-C), LDL-C, TG, and Apo B levels, and to increase HDL-C in primary hypercholesterolemia (heterozygous familial and nonfamilial) and mixed dyslipidemia (Types IIa and IIb). Adjunct to diet for treatment of patients with elevated serum TG levels (Type IV). Treatment of primary dysbetalipoproteinemia (Type III) inadequately responding to diet. Adjunct to other lipid-lowering treatments or if treatments are unavailable, to reduce total-C and LDL-C in homozygous familial hypercholesterolemia. Adjunct to diet to lower total-C, LDL-C, and Apo B in boys and postmenarchal girls, 10-17 yrs of age, with heterozygous familial hypercholesterolemia.

DOSAGE: *Adults:* Individualize dose. (Amlodipine) HTN: Initial: 5mg qd. Titrate over 7-14 days. Adjust dosage according to patient's need. Max: 10mg qd. Small/Fragile/Elderly/Hepatic Insufficiency/Concomitant Antihypertensive: Initial: 2.5mg qd. Chronic Stable Angina/Vasospastic Angina/CAD: Usual: 5-10mg qd. Elderly/Hepatic Insufficiency: Give the lower dose. (Atorvastatin) Hyperlipidemia/Mixed Dyslipidemia: Initial: 10-20mg qd (or 40mg qd for LDL-C reduction >45%). Titrate: Adjust dose as needed at 2-4 week intervals. Usual: 10-80mg qd.

Homozygous Familial Hypercholesterolemia: 10-80mg qd. Concomitant Cyclosporine: Max: 10mg qd. Concomitant Clarithromycin/Itraconazole/Ritonavir plus Saquinavir or Lopinavir: Caution with >20mg; use lowest dose necessary. Replacement Therapy: May substitute for individually titrated components. *Pediatrics:* 10-17 yrs: (Atorvastatin): Individualize dose. Heterozygous Familial Hypercholesterolemia: Initial: 10mg/day. Titrate: Adjust dose at intervals of ≥4 weeks. Max: 20mg/day. 6-17 yrs: (Amlodipine): HTN: Usual: 2.5-5mg qd. Max: 5mg qd.

HOW SUPPLIED: Tab: (Amlodipine-Atorvastatin) 2.5mg-10mg, 2.5mg-20mg, 2.5mg-40mg, 5mg-10mg, 5mg-20mg, 5mg-40mg, 5mg-80mg, 10mg-10mg, 10mg-20mg, 10mg-40mg, 10mg-80mg

CONTRAINDICATIONS: Active liver disease, which may include unexplained persistent elevations in hepatic transaminases, women who are pregnant or may become pregnant, and nursing mothers.

WARNINGS/PRECAUTIONS: Symptomatic hypotension may occur. Atorvastatin: Rare cases of rhabdomyolysis with acute renal failure secondary to myoglobinuria reported. Increased risk of rhabdomyolysis in patients with history of renal impairment. D/C if markedly elevated CPK levels occur or if myopathy is diagnosed or suspected. Temporarily withhold or d/c if acute, serious conditions suggestive of myopathy occur or if with risk factor predisposing to development of renal failure secondary to rhabdomyolysis. May cause biochemical abnormalities of liver function; monitor LFTs prior to therapy, at time of any elevation, and periodically thereafter. Reduce dose or d/c if AST or ALT >3X ULN persists. Increased risk of hemorrhagic stroke in patients with recent stroke or transient ischemic attack (TIA). May blunt adrenal and/or gonadal steroid production. Amlodipine: May cause worsening angina and acute MI after starting or increasing the dose. Not a β-blocker and gives no protection against dangers of abrupt β-blocker withdrawal. Caution in the elderly.

ADVERSE REACTIONS: Headache, edema, palpitations, dizziness, fatigue, flushing, nasopharyngitis, nausea, insomnia, diarrhea, arthralgia, pain in extremities, urinary tract infection, dyspepsia, myalgia.

INTERACTIONS: Amlodipine: Diltiazem may increase systemic exposure in elderly hypertensive patients. Strong inhibitors of CYP3A4 (eg, ketoconazole, itraconazole, ritonavir) may increase plasma concentrations to a greater extent; monitor for symptoms of hypotension and edema with CYP3A4 inhibitors. Monitor BP if coadministered with CYP3A4 inducers. Atorvastatin: Strong CYP3A4 inhibitors (eg, clarithromycin, HIV protease inhibitors, itraconazole) and grapefruit juice (>1.2L/day) may increase levels. Inhibitors of OATP1B1 (eg, cyclosporine) may increase bioavailability. Inducers of CYP3A4 (eg, efavirenz, rifampin) may decrease levels. Coadministration with digoxin may increase digoxin levels. Coadministration with oral contraceptives increases AUC of norethindrone and ethinyl estradiol. Increased risk of myopathy with immunosuppressive drugs, strong CYP3A4 inhibitors, cyclosporine, fibric acid derivatives, erythromycin, clarithromycin, combination of ritonavir plus saquinavir or lopinavir plus ritonavir, lipid-modifying dose of niacin, and azole antifungals. Caution with drugs that decrease levels or activity of endogenous steroid hormones (eg, ketoconazole, spironolactone, cimetidine).

PREGNANCY: Category X, not for use in nursing

MECHANISM OF ACTION: Amlodipine: Dihydropyridine calcium channel blocker; inhibits transmembrane influx of Ca^{2+} ions into vascular smooth muscle and cardiac muscle. Atorvastatin: HMG-CoA reductase inhibitor; inhibits conversion of HMG-CoA to mevalonate (precursor of sterols, including cholesterol).

PHARMACOKINETICS: Absorption: Amlodipine: Absolute bioavailability (64-90%); T_{max}=6-12 hrs. Atorvastatin: Rapid; absolute bioavailability (14%); T_{max}=1-2 hrs. **Distribution:** Amlodipine: Plasma protein binding (93%). Atorvastatin: V_d=381L; plasma protein binding (≥98%). **Metabolism:** Amlodipine: Hepatic (Extensive). Atorvastatin: CYP3A4 (Extensive); ortho- and parahydroxylated derivatives (active metabolites). **Elimination:** Amlodipine: Urine (10% unchanged; 60% metabolites); $T_{1/2}$=30-50 hrs. Atorvastatin: Bile (major), urine (<2%); $T_{1/2}$=14 hrs.

NURSING CONSIDERATIONS

Assessment: Assess for active or history of liver disease, renal impairment, unexplained and persistent elevations in serum transaminase levels, alcohol intake, recent stroke or TIA, heart disease (eg, MI, severe aortic stenosis), severe obstructive CAD, pregnancy/nursing status, and for possible drug interactions. Perform LFTs prior to therapy.

Monitoring: Monitor LFTs at 12 weeks following initiation of therapy and any drug dose elevation, then periodically thereafter. Monitor for signs/symptoms of hypotension, rhabdomyolysis with acute renal failure, hypersensitivity reaction, angina, MI, and myopathy. Monitor lipid profile and CPK levels.

Patient Counseling: Inform about potential risks/benefits of therapy. Instruct to follow standard cholesterol-lowering diet and regular exercise program as appropriate. Advise to seek medical attention if symptoms of hypotension, hypersensitivity reaction, angina, myopathy (eg, unexplained muscle pain, tenderness/weakness, fever, malaise) or other adverse reactions occur.

Instruct to notify physician if pregnant/nursing or planning to become pregnant. Instruct to take as prescribed.

Administration: Oral route. **Storage:** 25°C (77°F); excursions permitted to 15-30°C (59-86°F).

CALAN

RX

verapamil HCl (G.D. Searle)

THERAPEUTIC CLASS: Calcium channel blocker (nondihydropyridine)

INDICATIONS: Treatment of essential HTN and vasospastic, unstable, and chronic stable angina. Control of ventricular rate at rest and during stress in patients with chronic atrial flutter (A-flutter) and/or atrial fibrillation (A-fib), in association with digitalis. Prophylaxis of repetitive paroxysmal supraventricular tachycardia (PSVT).

DOSAGE: *Adults:* Individualize dose by titration. Max: 480mg/day. HTN: Initial (Monotherapy): 80mg tid. Usual: 360-480mg/day. Elderly/Small Stature: Initial: 40mg tid. Upward titration should be based on therapeutic efficacy. Angina: Usual: 80-120mg tid. Patients with Increased Response to Verapamil (eg, Elderly, Decreased Hepatic Function): Initial: 40mg tid. Upward titration should be based on therapeutic efficacy and safety evaluated approximately 8 hrs after dosing. Titrate: May increase at daily (eg, patients with unstable angina) or weekly intervals until optimum response is obtained. A-Fib (Digitalized): Usual: 240-320mg/day given in divided doses tid-qid. PSVT Prophylaxis (Non-Digitalized): Usual: 240-480mg/day given in divided doses tid-qid. Severe Hepatic Dysfunction: Give 30% of normal dose.

HOW SUPPLIED: Tab: 40mg, 80mg*, 120mg* *scored

CONTRAINDICATIONS: Severe left ventricular dysfunction, hypotension or cardiogenic shock, sick sinus syndrome or 2nd/3rd-degree atrioventricular (AV) block (except with functioning ventricular artificial pacemaker), A-fib/flutter with an accessory bypass tract (eg, Wolff-Parkinson-White, Lown-Ganong-Levine syndromes).

WARNINGS/PRECAUTIONS: Has negative inotropic effect; avoid with moderate to severe cardiac failure symptoms or any degree of ventricular dysfunction if taking a β-blocker. Patients with milder ventricular dysfunction should, if possible, be controlled with optimum doses of digitalis and/or diuretics before treatment. May cause congestive heart failure (CHF), pulmonary edema, hypotension, asymptomatic 1st-degree AV block, transient bradycardia, and PR interval prolongation. Marked 1st-degree block or progressive development to 2nd/3rd-degree AV block requires dose reduction, or d/c and institution of appropriate therapy (rare). Elevated transaminases with and without concomitant elevations in alkaline phosphatase and bilirubin reported; periodically monitor LFTs. Hepatocellular injury reported. Sinus bradycardia, 2nd-degree AV block, pulmonary edema, severe hypotension, and sinus arrest reported in patients with hypertrophic cardiomyopathy. Caution with hepatic dysfunction; monitor for abnormal PR interval prolongation or other signs of excessive pharmacologic effects. May decrease neuromuscular transmission in patients with Duchenne's muscular dystrophy and cause worsening of myasthenia gravis; decrease dose with attenuated neuromuscular transmission. Caution with renal dysfunction; monitor for abnormal PR interval prolongation or other signs of overdosage.

ADVERSE REACTIONS: Constipation, dizziness, sinus bradycardia, hypotension, 2nd-degree AV block.

INTERACTIONS: Increased levels with CYP3A4 inhibitors (eg, erythromycin, ritonavir) and grapefruit juice. Decreased levels with CYP3A4 inducers (eg, rifampin). May cause myopathy/rhabdomyolysis with HMG-CoA reductase inhibitors that are CYP3A4 substrates and may increase levels of such drugs; limit dose of simvastatin to 10mg/day or lovastatin to 40mg/day, and may need to lower doses of other CYP3A4 substrates (eg, atorvastatin). Increased bleeding times with aspirin. Additive negative effects on HR, AV conduction, and/or cardiac contractility with β-blockers. Combined therapy with propranolol should usually be avoided in patients with AV conduction abnormalities and depressed left ventricular function. May produce asymptomatic bradycardia with a wandering atrial pacemaker with timolol eye drops. Decreased metoprolol and propranolol clearance and variable effect with atenolol reported. Chronic treatment may increase digoxin levels, which may result in digitalis toxicity. May reduce clearance of digitoxin. Additive effect on lowering BP with other antihypertensives (eg, vasodilators, ACE inhibitors, diuretics, β-blockers). Excessive reduction in BP with agents that attenuate α-adrenergic function (eg, prazosin). Avoid disopyramide within 48 hrs before or 24 hrs after therapy. Additive negative inotropic effects and AV conduction prolongation with flecainide. Avoid quinidine with hypertrophic cardiomyopathy. Reduced or unchanged clearance with cimetidine. Increased sensitivity to effects of lithium when used concomitantly; monitor carefully. May increase carbamazepine, theophylline, cyclosporine, and alcohol levels. Increased clearance with phenobarbital. Reduced oral bioavailability with rifampin. Titrate carefully with inhalation anesthetics to avoid excessive CV depression. May potentiate neuromuscular blockers (curare-like and depolarizing); both agents may need dose reduction. May cause hypotension and bradyarrhythmias with telithromycin. Sinus bradycardia resulting in hospitalization and pacemaker insertion with clonidine; monitor HR. Prolonged recovery from neuromuscular blocking agent vecuronium reported.

PREGNANCY: Category C, not for use in nursing.

MECHANISM OF ACTION: Calcium channel blocker (nondihydropyridine); modulates influx of ionic calcium across cell membrane of arterial smooth muscle, and in conductile and contractile myocardial cells.

PHARMACOKINETICS: Absorption: Bioavailability (20-35%); T_{max}=1-2 hrs. **Distribution:** Plasma protein binding (90%); crosses placental barrier, found in breast milk. **Metabolism:** Liver (extensive); norverapamil (metabolite). **Elimination:** Urine (70% metabolites, 3-4% unchanged), feces ($\geq$16%); $T_{1/2}$=2.8-7.4 hrs (single dose), 4.5-12 hrs (repetitive dose).

NURSING CONSIDERATIONS

Assessment: Assess for cardiac failure symptoms, ventricular dysfunction, hypertrophic cardiomyopathy, hepatic/renal function, Duchenne's muscular dystrophy, attenuated neuromuscular transmission, any conditions where treatment is contraindicated, pregnancy/nursing status, and possible drug interactions.

Monitoring: Monitor for CHF, hypotension, AV block, abnormal PR interval prolongation, and worsening of myasthenia gravis. Periodically monitor LFTs and renal function.

Patient Counseling: Advise to seek medical attention if any adverse reactions occur. Counsel not to breastfeed and to report immediately if pregnant.

Administration: Oral route. **Storage:** 15-25°C (59-77°F). Protect from light.

CALAN SR   RX
verapamil HCl (G.D. Searle)

THERAPEUTIC CLASS: Calcium channel blocker (nondihydropyridine)

INDICATIONS: Management of essential HTN.

DOSAGE: *Adults:* Individualize dose. Initial: 180mg qam. Titrate: If response is inadequate, increase to 240mg qam, then 180mg bid (am and pm) or 240mg qam plus 120mg qpm, then 240mg q12h. Switching from Immediate-Release Calan to Calan SR: Total daily dose in mg may remain the same. Elderly/Small Stature: Initial: 120mg qam. Take with food.

HOW SUPPLIED: Tab, Extended-Release: 120mg, 180mg* , 240mg* *scored

CONTRAINDICATIONS: Severe left ventricular dysfunction, hypotension, cardiogenic shock, sick sinus syndrome or 2nd- or 3rd-degree atrioventricular (AV) block (except with functioning ventricular pacemaker), atrial fibrillation/flutter (A-fib/flutter) with an accessory bypass tract (eg, Wolff-Parkinson-White, Lown-Ganong-Levine syndromes).

WARNINGS/PRECAUTIONS: Avoid with severe left ventricular dysfunction or moderate to severe cardiac failure. May cause hypotension, congestive heart failure (CHF), pulmonary edema, AV block, and transient bradycardia. Transaminase elevation and hepatocellular injury reported; monitor LFTs periodically. Caution with hypertrophic cardiomyopathy and renal/hepatic impairment; monitor carefully. Decreased neuromuscular transmission with Duchenne's muscular dystrophy reported; reduce dose.

ADVERSE REACTIONS: Constipation, dizziness, sinus bradycardia, AV block, nausea, hypotension, headache, edema, CHF, fatigue, dyspnea.

INTERACTIONS: Additive negative effects on HR, AV conduction, and contractility with β-adrenergic blockers; monitor closely, use with caution, and avoid with any degree of ventricular dysfunction. Additive effect on lowering BP with other antihypertensives (eg, vasodilators, angiotensin-converting enzyme inhibitors, diuretics, β-blockers). Coadministration with agents that attenuate α-adrenergic function (eg, prazosin) may excessively reduce BP. May increase digoxin, carbamazepine, theophylline, cyclosporine, and ethanol levels; decrease digoxin dosing and monitor carefully. Avoid disopyramide within 48 hrs before or 24 hrs after therapy. Coadministration with flecainide may result in additive negative inotropic effects, AV conduction prolongation, and effects on myocardial contractility as well as repolarization. Avoid quinidine with hypertrophic cardiomyopathy. Increased sensitivity to effects of lithium; monitor carefully. Increased clearance with phenobarbital. Rifampin may reduce oral bioavailability. May potentiate neuromuscular blockers; both agents may need dose reduction. Careful titration is needed with inhalation anesthetics to avoid excessive cardiovascular depression. Asymptomatic bradycardia reported with timolol eye drops. Decreased metoprolol and propranolol clearance; variable effects on clearance reported with atenolol. Hypotension and bradyarrhythmias observed with concurrent telithromycin. Sinus bradycardia resulting in hospitalization and pacemaker insertion reported with the use of concurrent clonidine; monitor HR.

PREGNANCY: Category C, not for use in nursing.

MECHANISM OF ACTION: Calcium channel blocker; modulates influx of ionic calcium across cell membrane of arterial smooth muscle, and in conductile and contractile myocardial cells. Decreases systemic vascular resistance, usually without orthostatic decreases in BP or reflex tachycardia.

PHARMACOKINETICS: Absorption: (240mg) T_{max}=7.71 hrs, C_{max}=79ng/mL, $AUC_{(0-24\ hr)}$=841ng•hr/mL (fed). T_{max}=5.21 hrs, C_{max}=164ng/mL, $AUC_{(0-24\ hr)}$=1,478ng•hr/mL (fasted). **Distribution:** Plasma protein binding (90%); crosses placenta; found in breast milk. **Metabolism:** Liver (extensive); norverapamil (metabolite). **Elimination:** Urine (70% metabolites, 3-4% unchanged); feces (≥16%).

NURSING CONSIDERATIONS

Assessment: Assess for severe left ventricular dysfunction, Duchenne's muscular dystrophy, cardiac failure, hypotension, sick sinus syndrome, 2nd- or 3rd-degree AV block, A-fib/flutter with accessory bypass tract, hypertrophic cardiomyopathy, hepatic/renal impairment, hypersensitivity, pregnancy/nursing status, and for possible drug interactions.

Monitoring: Monitor for abnormal prolongation of PR-interval, CHF, pulmonary edema, AV block, and transient bradycardia. Monitor LFTs and renal function periodically.

Patient Counseling: Inform of the risks/benefits of therapy. Advise to seek medical attention if severe adverse reactions occur.

Administration: Oral route. **Storage:** 15-25°C (59-77°F). Protect from light and moisture.

CALDOLOR   RX
ibuprofen (Cumberland)

> NSAIDs increase risk of serious cardiovascular (CV) thrombotic events, myocardial infarction (MI), stroke, and serious GI adverse events including bleeding, ulceration, and perforation of the stomach and intestine. Contraindicated for the treatment of perioperative pain in the setting of coronary artery bypass graft (CABG) surgery.

THERAPEUTIC CLASS: NSAID

INDICATIONS: Management of mild to moderate pain and moderate to severe pain as an adjunct to opioid analgesics in adults. For reduction of fever in adults.

DOSAGE: *Adults:* Analgesia: 400-800mg IV q6h PRN. Infusion time must be no less than 30 min. Antipyretic: 400mg IV followed by 400mg q4-6h or 100-200mg q4h prn. Infusion time must be no less than 30 min. Elderly: Start at lower end of dosing range.

HOW SUPPLIED: Inj: 100mg/mL

CONTRAINDICATIONS: Asthma, urticaria, or allergic-type reactions to aspirin or other NSAIDs. Treatment of perioperative pain in the setting of coronary artery bypass graft (CABG) surgery.

WARNINGS/PRECAUTIONS: Severe hepatic reactions (rare) reported (eg, jaundice, fulminant hepatitis, liver necrosis, and hepatic failure); d/c if signs/symptoms of liver disease develop or if systemic manifestations occur. May lead to onset of new HTN or worsening of preexisting HTN; monitor BP closely. Fluid retention and edema reported; caution in patients with fluid retention or heart failure. Caution in patients with considerable dehydration. Renal papillary necrosis and other renal injury reported after long-term use. Caution with impaired renal function, heart failure, liver dysfunction, the elderly and those taking diuretics and ACE inhibitors. Anaphylactoid reactions may occur. May cause serious skin adverse events (eg, exfoliative dermatitis, Stevens-Johnson syndrome [SJS], and toxic epidermal necrolysis [TEN]). Avoid in late pregnancy; may cause premature closure of ductus arteriosis. May mask signs of inflammation and fever. Anemia may occur; with long-term use, monitor Hgb/Hct if signs or symptoms of anemia develop. May inhibit platelet aggregation and prolong bleeding time; monitor with coagulation disorders. Infusion of drug product without dilution may cause hemolysis. Caution with preexisting asthma. Blurred or diminished vision, scotomata, and changes in color vision reported; d/c if such complaints develop. Aseptic meningitis with fever and coma reported in patients on oral ibuprofen therapy. Caution in elderly.

ADVERSE REACTIONS: N/V, flatulence, headache, hemorrhage, dizziness, urinary retention, peripheral edema, anemia, dyspepsia, eosinophilia, hypokalemia, hypoproteinemia, neutropenia.

INTERACTIONS: May increase adverse effects with ASA. Synergistic effects on GI bleeding with warfarin. May decrease natriuretic effect of furosemide and thiazides; monitor for renal failure. May impair therapeutic response to ACE inhibitors, thiazides or loop diuretics. Increase risk of renal effects with diuretics or ACE inhibitors. May increase lithium levels; monitor for toxicity. May enhance methotrexate toxicity; caution when coadministered. Increase GI bleeding with use of oral corticosteroids or anticoagulants and use of alcohol.

PREGNANCY: Category C (prior to 30 weeks' gestation); Category D (starting 30 weeks' gestation), not for use in nursing.

MECHANISM OF ACTION: NSAID; not established. May be related to prostaglandin synthetase inhibition. Possesses anti-inflammatory, analgesic, and antipyretic activity.

PHARMACOKINETICS: Absorption: (400mg) AUC=109.3mcg•h/mL, (800mg) AUC=192.8mcg•h/mL; (400mg) C_{max}=39.2mcg/mL, (800mg) C_{max}=72.6mcg/mL. **Distribution:** Plasma protein binding (>99%). **Elimination:** (400mg) $T_{1/2}$=2.22 hrs, (800mg) $T_{1/2}$= 2.44 hrs.

NURSING CONSIDERATIONS

Assessment: Assess LFTs, CBC and coagulation profile. Assess for history of asthma, urticaria or allergic-type reaction with previous use of NSAIDs, asthma, perioperative pain in setting of CABG surgery, cardiovascular disease (CVD) or risk factors for CVD, HTN, fluid retention or HF, ulcer disease or GI bleeding, coagulation disorders or anticoagulant therapy, renal/hepatic impairment, pregnancy/nursing status, possible drug interactions.

Monitoring: Monitor BP during initiation of therapy and thereafter. Monitor Hgb/Hct, coagulation profiles, LFTs, and renal function. Monitor signs/symptoms of anaphylactic/anaphylactoid reactions, adverse skin events (eg, exfoliative dermatitis, SJS, TEN), eosinophilia, rash, GI bleeding/ulceration and perforation, anemia, CV thrombotic events, MI, stroke, new or worsening HTN, renal toxicity, renal papillary necrosis and other renal injury, ophthalmological effects (blurred or diminished vision, scotomata and changes in color vision) and aseptic meningitis.

Patient Counseling: Counsel about potential CV, GI, hepatotoxic, and skin adverse events, as well as possible weight gain/edema. Inform of the signs of an anaphylactoid reaction; d/c and initiate medical therapy if this occurs. Inform pregnant women starting at 30 weeks' gestation to avoid use of the product. Counsel patients to be well hydrated prior to administration in order to reduce renal adverse reactions.

Administration: IV (infusion) route. Infusion time must be no less than 30 mins. Must be diluted prior to infusion. Refer to PI for preparation and administration. **Storage:** 20-25°C (68-77°F). Diluted solutions are stable for up to 24 hrs at ambient temperature (approximately 20-25°C) and room lighting.

CAMBIA   RX
diclofenac potassium (Kowa)

NSAIDs may cause an increased risk of serious cardiovascular (CV) thrombotic events, myocardial infarction (MI), stroke and serious GI adverse events including bleeding, ulceration, and perforation of the stomach or intestines. Contraindicated for the treatment of perioperative pain in the setting of coronary artery bypass graft (CABG) surgery.

THERAPEUTIC CLASS: NSAID

INDICATIONS: Acute treatment of migraine attacks with or without aura in adults ≥18 yrs.

DOSAGE: *Adults:* Administer 1 packet (50mg) in 1-2 oz. (30-60mL) water. Mix well and drink immediately. Do not use liquids other than water.

HOW SUPPLIED: Powder: 50mg

CONTRAINDICATIONS: Asthma, urticaria, or allergic reactions after taking ASA or other NSAIDs. Treatment of peri-operative pain in the setting of CABG surgery.

WARNINGS/PRECAUTIONS: Not indicated for prophylactic therapy of migraine. Safety and effectiveness not established for cluster headache. May lead to new onset or worsening of preexisting HTN; monitor BP regularly. Elevation of one or more liver tests reported. D/C if abnormal LFTs or renal tests persist or worsen, if clinical signs and/or symptoms consistent with liver disease develop, or if systemic manifestations occur (eg, eosinophilia, rash, abdominal pain, diarrhea, dark urine). Caution with hepatic impairment. Fluid retention and edema reported; caution with fluid retention or heart failure. Caution when initiating treatment with considerable dehydration. Renal papillary necrosis and other renal injury reported after long-term use. Caution with renal/liver dysfunction. Not recommended for use with advanced renal disease; if therapy must be initiated, closely monitor renal function. May cause anaphylactoid reactions, serious skin adverse events (eg, exfoliative dermatitis, Stevens-Johnson syndrome [SJS], and toxic epidermal necrolysis [TEN]). May cause premature closure of ductus arteriosus; avoid in pregnancy starting at 30 weeks' gestation. May mask symptoms of infection (eg, fever, inflammation). Anemia may occur; monitor Hgb/Hct with long-term use. May inhibit platelet aggregation and prolong bleeding time; monitor platelet function in patients with coagulation disorders. Caution with preexisting asthma, phenylketonurics and in the elderly.

ADVERSE REACTIONS: Abdominal pain, constipation, diarrhea, dyspepsia, flatulence, anemia, edema, N/V, dizziness, headache, rashes, heartburn, pruritus, abnormal renal function.

INTERACTIONS: See Contraindications. Caution with concomitant use of potentially hepatotoxic drugs (eg, acetaminophen, certain antibiotics, antiepileptics). Increased adverse effects with ASA. Synergistic effects on GI bleeding with anticoagulants (eg, warfarin). May diminish antihypertensive effect of ACE inhibitors. May reduce natriuretic effect of furosemide and thiazides. May increase lithium levels. May enhance methotrexate toxicity. May increase nephrotoxicity of cyclosporine. May affect pharmacokinetics with CYP2C9 inhibitors.

PREGNANCY: Category C (prior to 30 weeks' gestation) and D (starting at 30 weeks' gestation); not for use in nursing.

MECHANISM OF ACTION: NSAID (benzeneacetic acid derivative); mechanism not completely understood but may be related to prostaglandin synthetase inhibition.

PHARMACOKINETICS: Absorption: Absolute bioavailability (50%). T_{max}=0.25 hr. **Distribution:** V_d=1.3 L/kg; plasma protein binding (>99%). **Metabolism:** Glucoronidation or sulfation via CYP2C8, 2C9, 3A4; 4'-hydroxydiclofenac (major metabolite), 5-hydroxy-, 3'-hydroxy-, 4',5-dihydroxy- and 3'-hydroxy-4'-methoxy diclofenac (minor metabolites). **Elimination:** Urine (65%), bile (35%); $T_{1/2}$=2 hrs.

NURSING CONSIDERATIONS

Assessment: Assess LFTs, renal function, CBC, platelet count and chemistry profile. Assess for asthma, urticaria or allergic-type reactions after taking aspirin or other NSAIDs, risk factors for cardiovascular (CV) disease, GI adverse events, history of ulcer disease, GI bleeding, smoking, alcohol use, health status, preexisting HTN, fluid retention, heart failure, dehydration, renal/liver dysfunction, coagulation disorders, pregnancy/nursing status, and possible drug interactions.

Monitoring: Monitor for signs/symptoms of CV thrombotic events, MI, stroke, GI adverse events (eg, inflammation, bleeding, ulceration, perforation), liver injury, anaphylactoid reactions, serious skin reactions (eg, exfoliative dermatitis, SJS, TEN). Periodic monitoring of BP, LFTs, renal function. CBC with differential and platelet count, coagulation parameters (especially if on anticoagulation therapy or with coagulation disorders).

Patient Counseling: Advise patients to be alert for signs/symptoms of chest pains, shortness of breath, weakness, slurring of speech, GI ulcerations, bleeding, epigastric pain, dyspepsia, melena, hematemesis, anaphylactoid reactions (eg, difficulty breathing, swelling of face or throat), skin rash and blisters, fever, other signs of hypersensitivity (eg, itching) during therapy. Inform about signs/symptoms of hepatotoxicity (eg, nausea, fatigue, lethargy, pruritus, jaundice, right upper quadrant tenderness and flulike symptoms); d/c therapy immediately if any of these occur. Notify healthcare professional if signs/symptoms of unexplained weight gain or edema occur. Advise women to avoid use in late pregnancy. Inform that the product contains aspartame equivalent to phenylalanine 25mg/packet.

Administration: Oral route. Mix packet well with 1-2 ounces of water and drink immediately.
Storage: 25°C (77°F) Excursions permitted from 15-30°C (59-86°F).

CAMPATH   RX
alemtuzumab (Bayer Healthcare)

> Serious, including fatal, pancytopenia/marrow hypoplasia, autoimmune idiopathic thrombocytopenia, and autoimmune hemolytic anemia may occur; single doses >30mg or cumulative doses >90mg/week may increase incidence of pancytopenia. Serious, including fatal, infusion reactions may occur; monitor patients during infusion and withhold therapy for Grade 3/4 infusion reactions. Gradually escalate dose at initiation of therapy and if interrupted for ≥ 7days. Serious, including fatal, bacterial, viral, fungal, and protozoan infections can occur; administer prophylaxis against *Pneumocystis jiroveci* pneumonia (PCP) and herpes virus infections.

THERAPEUTIC CLASS: Monoclonal antibody/CD52-blocker

INDICATIONS: Treatment of B-cell chronic lymphocytic leukemia.

DOSAGE: *Adults:* Administer as IV infusion over 2 hrs. Initial: 3mg IV qd until infusion reactions are ≤Grade 2, then increase to 10mg IV qd. Continue until ≤Grade 2. Increase to maint dose of 30mg (usually takes 3-7 days). Maint: 30mg/day IV 3X/week on alternate days. Max: 30mg single dose or 90mg/week cumulative dose. Total duration of therapy is 12 weeks. Refer to PI for recommended concomitant medications and dose modifications for neutropenia or thrombocytopenia.

HOW SUPPLIED: Inj: 30mg/mL [1mL]

WARNINGS/PRECAUTIONS: Prolonged myelosuppresion, pure red cell/bone marrow aplasia reported; withhold therapy for severe cytopenias and d/c for autoimmune cytopenias or recurrent/persistent severe cytopenias. Severe and prolonged lymphopenias with increased incidence of opportunistic infections reported; administer prophylactic therapy during and for a minimum of 2 months after therapy or until CD4+ count is ≥200 cells/μL. Monitor for cytomegalovirus (CMV) infection during and for ≥2 months after completion of treatment; withhold therapy for serious infections and during CMV infection treatment or confirmed CMV viremia. Administer only irradiated blood products to avoid transfusion-associated graft versus host disease unless emergent circumstances dictate immediate transfusion.

ADVERSE REACTIONS: Cytopenias, infusion reactions, CMV and other infections, immunosuppression, nausea, emesis, abdominal pain, insomnia, anxiety.

INTERACTIONS: Avoid live viral vaccines.

PREGNANCY: Category C, not for use in nursing.

MECHANISM OF ACTION: Monoclonal antibody/CD52-blocker; binds to CD52; proposed action is antibody-dependent cellular-mediated lysis following cell surface binding to the leukemic cells.

PHARMACOKINETICS: Distribution: V_d=0.18L/kg; crosses the placenta. **Elimination:** (1st dose) $T_{1/2}$=11 hrs. (Last dose) $T_{1/2}$=6 days.

NURSING CONSIDERATIONS

Assessment: Assess for pregnancy/nursing status and possible drug interaction. Obtain baseline CBC, CD4+, and platelet count.

Monitoring: Monitor CBC weekly and more frequently if worsening anemia, neutropenia, or thrombocytopenia occurs. Assess CD4+ counts after therapy until recovery to ≥200 cells/µL. Monitor for CMV infections during therapy and for ≥2 months following completion. Monitor for cytopenias, infusion reactions, immunosuppression, infection, and other adverse reactions.

Patient Counseling: Advise to seek medical attention if symptoms of bleeding, easy bruising, petechiae/purpura, pallor, weakness, fatigue, infusion reactions, or infections occur. Counsel patients of the need to take premedications and prophylactic anti-infectives as prescribed. Advise patients that irradiation of blood products is required. Inform to not be immunized with live vaccines if recently treated. Advise patients to use effective contraceptive methods during treatment and ≥6 months following therapy.

Administration: IV infusion. Do not administer as IV push or bolus. Refer to PI for preparation and administration instructions. Do not add or simultaneously infuse other drugs through the same IV line. **Storage:** 2-8°C (36-46°F). Do not freeze. If frozen, thaw at 2-8°C before administration. Protect from direct sunlight. Diluted Sol: 2-8°C or 15-30°C. Use ≤8 hrs. Protect from light.

CAMPRAL   RX
acamprosate calcium (Forest)

THERAPEUTIC CLASS: GABA analog

INDICATIONS: Maintenance of abstinence from alcohol in patients with alcohol dependence who are abstinent at treatment initiation.

DOSAGE: *Adults:* 2 tabs tid. Moderate Renal Impairment (CrCl 30-50mL/min): 1 tab tid.

HOW SUPPLIED: Tab, Delayed Release: 333mg

CONTRAINDICATIONS: Severe renal impairment (CrCl ≤30mL/min).

WARNINGS/PRECAUTIONS: Does not eliminate or diminish withdrawal symptoms. Suicidal events infrequently reported. Caution in elderly and with renal impairment.

ADVERSE REACTIONS: Diarrhea, insomnia, anxiety, nervousness, depression, asthenia, anorexia, pain, flatulence, nausea, dizziness, pruritus, dry mouth, paresthesia, sweating.

INTERACTIONS: Naltrexone may increase levels. Weight gain and weight loss more commonly reported with antidepressants.

PREGNANCY: Category C, caution in nursing.

MECHANISM OF ACTION: Gamma-aminobutyric acid (GABA) analog; not established. Suspected to interact with glutamate and GABA neurotransmitter systems centrally and to remedy the imbalance between neuronal excitation and inhibition caused by chronic alcohol intake.

PHARMACOKINETICS: Absorption: Absolute bioavailability (11%); C_{max}=350ng/mL; T_{max}=3-8 hrs. **Distribution:** (IV) V_d=72-109L (approximately 1L/kg). **Elimination:** Urine (major, unchanged); $T_{1/2}$=20-33 hrs.

NURSING CONSIDERATIONS

Assessment: Assess for renal impairment, hypersensitivity, pregnancy/nursing status, and possible drug interactions.

Monitoring: Monitor for symptoms of depression or suicidality, renal function and other adverse reactions.

Patient Counseling: Instruct to use caution in performing hazardous tasks (operating machinery/driving); may impair judgment, thinking or motor skills. Instruct to notify physician if pregnant/nursing or planning to become pregnant. Advise to continue therapy as directed, even in the event of relapse; remind to discuss any renewed drinking with physician. Advise that therapy has been shown to help maintain abstinence only when used as part of treatment program that includes counseling and support. Family and caregivers should monitor patients being treated for symptoms of depression and suicidality, and should report any of these symptoms to the patient's healthcare provider.

Administration: Oral route. **Storage:** 25°C (77°F); excursions permitted to 15-30°C (59-86°F).

CAMPTOSAR   RX
irinotecan HCl (Pharmacia & Upjohn)

C

Administer only under the supervision of a physician experienced in the use of cancer chemotherapeutic agents. May induce early and/or late forms of diarrhea. Early diarrhea (during or shortly after infusion) may be accompanied by cholinergic symptoms; may be prevented or ameliorated by atropine. Late diarrhea (>24 hrs after administration) can be life-threatening since it may be prolonged, and lead to dehydration, electrolyte imbalance, or sepsis; treat with loperamide. Monitor patients with diarrhea; give fluid/electrolyte replacement if dehydrated or give antibiotics if ileus, fever, or severe neutropenia develop. Interrupt and reduce subsequent doses if severe diarrhea occurs. Severe myelosuppression may occur.

THERAPEUTIC CLASS: Topoisomerase I inhibitor

INDICATIONS: First-line therapy in combination with 5-fluorouracil (5-FU) and leucovorin (LV) for metastatic carcinoma of the colon and rectum, and for patients with metastatic carcinoma of the colon or rectum whose disease has progressed or recurred following initial 5-FU therapy.

DOSAGE: *Adults:* Combination Therapy: Dose of LV should be administered immediately after irinotecan, then 5-FU after LV. Regimen 1 (6-week cycle with bolus 5-FU/LV): 125mg/m^2 IV over 90 min on Days 1, 8, 15, 22. Regimen 2 (6-week cycle with infusional 5-FU/LV): 180mg/m^2 IV over 90 min on Days 1, 15, and 29. Both Regimens: Begin next cycle on Day 43. Refer to PI for doses of 5-FU/LV. Single Therapy: Weekly Regimen: 125mg/m^2 IV over 90 min on Days 1, 8, 15, 22 followed by 2 week rest. Titrate: Dose may be adjusted to as high as 150mg/m^2 or as low as 50mg/m^2 in 25-50mg/m^2 decrements depending upon individual tolerance. Once-Every-3-Week Regimen: 350mg/m^2 IV over 90 min once q3 weeks. Titrate: Dose may be adjusted as low as 200mg/m^2 in 50mg/m^2 decrements depending upon individual tolerance. Refer to PI for Dose Modifications for Combination and Single-agent schedules. All dose modifications should be based on worst preceding toxicity. Reduced UGT1A1 Activity: Consider reducing the starting dose by at least one level for patients known to be homozygous for the UGT1A1*28 allele. Subsequent dose modifications are based on individual tolerance; refer to PI. Elderly (≥70 yrs): Initial: (once-every-3-week regimen) 300mg/m^2.

HOW SUPPLIED: Inj: 20mg/mL [2mL, 5mL]

WARNINGS/PRECAUTIONS: Do not use with the "Mayo Clinic" regimen of 5-FU/LV for 4-5 consecutive days q4 weeks due to increased toxicity. Not for use in patients on dialysis. Transient, severe early diarrhea may occur with symptoms of rhinitis. If late diarrhea occurs after the first treatment, delay subsequent weekly therapy until return of pretreatment bowel function for at least 24 hrs without antidiarrheals; decrease subsequent doses within current cycle if late diarrhea is Grade 2, 3, or 4. Deaths due to sepsis following severe neutropenia reported; temporarily omit therapy if neutropenic fever occurs, or if absolute neutrophil count <1000/mm^3. Increased risk for neutropenia in patients homozygous for the UGT1A1*28 allele; consider reducing initial dose. Severe anaphylactic reactions, colitis/ileus, renal impairment/failure, thromboembolic and interstitial pulmonary disease (IPD) events reported. D/C therapy with IPD and institute treatment if needed. May cause fetal harm. Monitor for extravasation and inflammation at infusion site. Premedicate with antiemetics at least 30 min prior to therapy. Consider prophylactic/therapeutic administration of atropine if cholinergic symptoms develop. Caution with hepatic dysfunction, deficient glucuronidation of bilirubin (eg, Gilbert's syndrome), elderly with comorbidities, previous pelvic/abdominal irradiation. Careful monitoring of WBC with differential, Hgb, and platelets are recommended before each dose. Avoid in severe bone marrow failure, hereditary fructose intolerance, or unresolved bowel obstruction.

ADVERSE REACTIONS: N/V, diarrhea, neutropenia, abdominal pain, anemia, asthenia, mucositis, anorexia, alopecia, fever, pain, constipation, infection, dyspnea, increased bilirubin.

INTERACTIONS: Exacerbated myelosuppression and diarrhea with antineoplastic agents having similar adverse effects. Avoid concurrent irradiation therapy. Possible hyperglycemia and lymphocytopenia with dexamethasone. Avoid vaccination with live vaccines due to risk of serious or fatal infections. Response to killed/inactivated vaccines may be diminished; use with caution. Greater incidence of akathisia reported with prochlorperazine. Laxatives may worsen diarrhea. Consider withholding diuretics with irinotecan therapy. Decreased levels with CYP3A4 inducing anticonvulsants (eg, phenytoin, phenobarbital, and carbamazepine) and St. John's wort reported; d/c at least 2 weeks prior to first cycle. Consider substituting nonenzyme inducing anticonvulsants 2 weeks prior to and during treatment. Increased levels with ketoconazole; d/c ketoconazole at least 1 week prior to and during therapy. Increased systemic exposure of SN-38 with atazanavir sulfate. May prolong neuromuscular blocking effects of suxamethonium and the neuromuscular blockade of nondepolarizing drugs may be antagonized.

PREGNANCY: Category D, not for use in nursing.

MECHANISM OF ACTION: Topoisomerase I inhibitor; binds to topoisomerase I-DNA complex and prevents religation of single-strand breaks induced by the enzyme to relieve torsional strain in DNA.

PHARMACOKINETICS: Absorption: Irinotecan: (125mg/m²); C_{max}=1660ng/mL; AUC_{0-24}=10200ng•h/mL. (340mg/m²); C_{max}=3392ng/mL; AUC_{0-24}=20604ng•h/mL. SN-38: (125mg/m²) C_{max}=26.3ng/mL; AUC_{0-24}=229ng•h/mL. (340mg/m²) C_{max}=56ng/mL; AUC_{0-24}=474ng•h/mL. **Distribution:** Irinotecan: (125mg/m²) V_d=110L/m². (340mg/m²) V_d=234L/m². Plasma protein binding (30-68%). SN-38: Plasma protein binding (95%). **Metabolism:** Liver via carboxyl esterase. SN-38 (active metabolite). **Elimination:** Irinotecan: Urine (11-20%). (125mg/m²) $T_{1/2}$=5.8 hrs. (340mg/m²) $T_{1/2}$=11.7 hrs. SN-38: Urine (<1%). (125mg/m²) $T_{1/2}$=10.4 hrs. (340mg/m²) $T_{1/2}$=21 hrs.

NURSING CONSIDERATIONS

Assessment: Assess for severe bone marrow failure, unresolved bowel obstruction, hereditary fructose intolerance, reduced UDP-glucuronosyl transferase 1A1 activity, pregnancy/nursing status, diabetes mellitus, glucose intolerance, pelvic/abdominal radiation. Assess for deficient glucuronidation of bilirubin (Gilbert's syndrome), possible drug interactions, renal/hepatic function, underlying cardiac disease, preexisting lung disease. Assess use in elderly patients with comorbid conditions. Obtain baseline CBC with platelets.

Monitoring: Monitor for diarrhea, signs/symptoms of neutropenia, neutropenic complications (eg, neutropenic fever), ileus, pulmonary symptoms, inflammation and/or extravasation of infusion site, dehydration, cholinergic symptoms (eg, rhinitis, increased salivation, miosis, lacrimation, diaphoresis) especially when receiving higher doses, infections, and hypersensitivity reactions. For patients with diarrhea, monitor for signs/symptoms of dehydration, electrolyte imbalance, ileus, fever, or severe neutropenia. Monitor WBC with differential, Hgb, platelet count before each dose.

Patient Counseling: Instruct to avoid live vaccines. Inform of pregnancy risks, toxic effects (GI complications). Instruct to have loperamide readily available and to begin treatment of late diarrhea at 1st episode of poorly formed or loose stool or the earliest onset of bowel movement more frequent than normally expected. Seek medical attention if the following occur: diarrhea for first time during treatment; black or bloody stools; unexplained pulmonary symptoms (eg, dyspnea, cough, fever), dehydration (eg, lightheadedness, dizziness, faintness), inability to take fluids by mouth due to N/V, inability to get diarrhea under control within 24 hrs, fever, evidence of infection, toxicity, or anaphylactic reactions. Inform of the potential of dizziness or visual disturbances which may occur within 24 hrs and advise not to drive or operate machinery if these symptoms occur. Alert for the possibility of alopecia.

Administration: IV route. Administer as IV infusion over 90 min. Dilute in D5W or 0.9% NaCl to final concentration range of 0.12-2.8mg/mL. **Storage**: 15-30°C (59-86°F). Protect from light. Keep in the carton until the time of use. Avoid freezing. Refer to PI for storage instructions for reconstituted sol.

CANASA   RX
mesalamine (Aptalis)

THERAPEUTIC CLASS: 5-Aminosalicylic acid derivative

INDICATIONS: Treatment of active ulcerative proctitis.

DOSAGE: *Adults:* Usual: 1000mg rectally qhs. Retain sup for at least 1-3 hrs.

HOW SUPPLIED: Sup: 1000mg

CONTRAINDICATIONS: Hypersensitivity to suppository vehicle (eg, saturated vegetable fatty acid esters).

WARNINGS/PRECAUTIONS: D/C if acute intolerance syndrome characterized by cramping, acute abdominal pain and bloody diarrhea, sometimes fever, headache and a rash develops. Re-evaluate history of sulfasalazine intolerance; if rechallenge is considered, perform under close observation and only if clearly needed. Caution with sulfasalazine hypersensitivity, in elderly, and with patients on concurrent oral products which contain or release mesalamine and with pre-existing renal disease; monitor urinalysis, BUN, and creatinine. Pancolitis, pericarditis (rare) reported.

ADVERSE REACTIONS: Dizziness, headache, flatulence, abdominal pain, diarrhea, nausea.

PREGNANCY: Category B, caution in nursing.

MECHANISM OF ACTION: 5-Aminosalicylic acid derivative; not fully established, anti-inflammatory drug appears to act topically rather than systemically. Postulated to have a role as free radical scavenger or inhibitor of tumor necrosis factor.

PHARMACOKINETICS: Absorption: Variable; C_{max}=361ng/mL. **Metabolism:** Extensively metabolized to N-acetyl-5-ASA (metabolite). **Elimination:** Urine (≤11% unchanged 5-ASA, 3-35% metabolite); $T_{1/2}$=7 hrs.

C

NURSING CONSIDERATIONS

Assessment: Assess for hypersensitivity to drug or suppository vehicle, sulfasalazine allergy, pre-existing renal disease, and possible drug interactions. Obtain baseline renal function (BUN, creatinine, urinalysis).

Monitoring: Monitor for signs/symptoms of pericarditis, acute intolerance syndrome, hypersensitivity, and allergic reactions. Carefully monitor renal function (BUN, creatinine, urinalysis), especially in patients with renal dysfunction and in elderly.

Patient Counseling: Inform that sup may cause stains. Advise to empty rectum before use and not to handle too much. If miss dose, use as soon as possible, unless almost time for next dose. Do not use 2 doses at once. Advise to stop use and seek medical attention if chest pain, cramping, abdominal pain, bloody diarrhea, fever, or rash occur. Advise to inform physician if chest pain or SOB develop. Inform that mild hair loss, worsening colitis, headache, gas or flatulence, and diarrhea may occur.

Administration: Rectal route. Refer to PI for administration instruction. **Storage:** <25°C (77°F). Keep away from direct heat, light, or humidity.

CANCIDAS   RX
caspofungin acetate (Merck)

THERAPEUTIC CLASS: Glucan synthesis inhibitor

INDICATIONS: In adults and pediatric patients (≥3 months) for empirical therapy for presumed fungal infections in febrile, neutropenic patients; treatment of candidemia and the *Candida* infections (intra-abdominal abscesses, peritonitis, and pleural space infections); treatment of esophageal candidiasis; and treatment of invasive aspergillosis in patients who are refractory to or intolerant of other therapies (eg, amphotericin B, lipid formulations of amphotericin B, itraconazole).

DOSAGE: *Adults:* ≥18 yrs: Give by slow IV infusion over approximately 1 hr. Empirical Therapy: 70mg LD on Day 1, followed by 50mg qd thereafter. Continue until resolution of neutropenia. If fungal infection found, treat for a minimum of 14 days; continue for at least 7 days after neutropenia and clinical symptoms resolve. May increase to 70mg/day if 50mg dose is well tolerated but provides inadequate response. Candidemia/Other *Candida* Infections: 70mg LD on Day 1, followed by 50mg qd thereafter. Continue for at least 14 days after the last positive culture. Persistently neutropenic patients may require longer course of therapy. Esophageal Candidiasis: 50mg qd for 7-14 days after symptom resolution. Consider suppressive PO therapy in patients with HIV infections due to risk of relapse. Invasive Aspergillosis: 70mg LD on Day 1, followed by 50mg qd thereafter. Duration of treatment based on severity of underlying disease, recovery from immunosuppression, and clinical response. Moderate Hepatic Impairment (Child-Pugh 7-9): Usual: 35mg qd. May still administer 70mg LD on Day 1 if recommended. Concomitant Rifampin: 70mg qd. Concomitant Nevirapine/Efavirenz/Carbamazepine/Dexamethasone/Phenytoin: May require an increase dose to 70mg qd.
Pediatrics: 3 months-17 yrs: Give by slow IV infusion over approximately 1 hr. Dosing based on the patient's BSA. Usual: 70mg/m² LD on Day 1, followed by 50mg/m² qd thereafter. Max LD/ Maint: 70mg/day. Individualized duration based on indication. May increase to 70mg/m²/ day if 50mg/m²/day dose is well tolerated but provides inadequate response. Concomitant with Inducers of Drug Clearance (eg, Rifampin, Nevirapine, Efavirenz, Carbamazepine, Dexamethasone, Phenytoin): 70mg/m² qd.

HOW SUPPLIED: Inj: 50mg, 70mg

WARNINGS/PRECAUTIONS: Limit concomitant use with cyclosporine to patients for whom potential benefit outweighs potential risk. Monitor patients who develop abnormal liver function tests and evaluate risk/benefit of continuing therapy.

ADVERSE REACTIONS: Pyrexia, chills, hypokalemia, hypotension, diarrhea, increased blood alkaline phosphatase, increased ALT/AST, N/V, abdominal pain, peripheral edema, headache, rash.

INTERACTIONS: Isolated cases of significant hepatic dysfunction, hepatitis, and hepatic failure reported with multiple concomitant medications in patients with serious underlying conditions. Reduced levels of tacrolimus; monitor tacrolimus blood concentrations and adjust tacrolimus dose. Increased levels and transient increase in ALT and AST reported with cyclosporine. Inducers of drug clearance (eg, efavirenz, nevirapine, phenytoin, rifampin, dexamethasone, carbamazepine) may decrease levels.

PREGNANCY: Category C, caution in nursing.

MECHANISM OF ACTION: Glucan synthesis inhibitor; inhibits the synthesis of β (1,3)-D-glucan, an essential component of the cell wall of susceptible *Aspergillus* and *Candida* species.

PHARMACOKINETICS: Absorption: Administration to different age groups resulted in different parameters. **Distribution:** Plasma protein binding (97%). **Metabolism:** Hydrolysis and N-acetylation. **Elimination:** Urine (41%, 1.4% unchanged), feces (35%).

NURSING CONSIDERATIONS

Assessment: Assess for drug hypersensitivity, use in patients who are on concomitant therapy with cyclosporine, hepatic function, pregnancy/nursing status, and possible drug interactions.

Monitoring: Monitor for histamine-related and anaphylaxis reactions (eg, rash, facial swelling, bronchospasm) during administration. Monitor LFTs and CBC.

Patient Counseling: Inform that there have been isolated reports of serious hepatic effects and that therapy can cause hypersensitivity reactions (eg, rash, facial swelling, pruritus, sensation of warmth, or bronchospasm).

Administration: IV route. Not for IV bolus administration. Refer to PI for preparation and reconstitution for administration. **Storage:** 2-8°C (36-46°F). Reconstituted: ≤25°C (≤77°F) for 1 hr prior to preparation of infusion sol. Diluted: ≤25°C (≤77°F) for 24 hrs or 2-8°C (36-46°F) for 48 hrs.

CAPRELSA   RX
vandetanib (AstraZeneca)

> QT interval prolongation, torsades de pointes, and sudden death reported. Avoid with hypocalcemia, hypokalemia, hypomagnesemia, or long QT syndrome. Correct hypocalcemia, hypokalemia and/or hypomagnesemia prior to therapy; monitor periodically. Avoid drugs known to prolong QT interval; if administered, frequent ECG monitoring recommended. Obtain ECG at baseline, at 2-4 weeks, 8-12 weeks after initial therapy, q3 months thereafter, and following any dose reduction for QT prolongation, or any dose interruptions >2 weeks. Only prescribers and pharmacies certified through the restricted distribution program are able to prescribe and dispense this therapy.

THERAPEUTIC CLASS: Kinase inhibitor

INDICATIONS: Treatment of symptomatic or progressive medullary thyroid cancer in patients with unresectable locally advanced or metastatic disease.

DOSAGE: *Adults:* Usual: 300mg PO qd. Continue until no longer benefiting from treatment or until unacceptable toxicity occurs. Corrected QT interval, Fridericia (QTcF) >500ms: Interrupt dosing until QTcF returns <450ms, then resume at 200mg (two 100mg tabs). Common Terminology Criteria for Adverse Events (CTCAE) Grade ≥3 Toxicity: Interrupt dosing until toxicity resolves or improves to Grade 1, resume at 200mg (two 100mg tabs) and then to 100mg. CrCl <50mL/min: Initial: 200mg PO qd.

HOW SUPPLIED: Tab: 100mg, 300mg

CONTRAINDICATIONS: Congenital long QT syndrome.

WARNINGS/PRECAUTIONS: Caution in patients with indolent, asymptomatic or slowly progressing disease. Not recommended with moderate (Child-Pugh B) and severe (Child-Pugh C) hepatic impairment. Do not start therapy with QTcF interval >450ms. Avoid with history of torsades de pointes, bradyarrhythmias, or uncompensated heart failure (HF). D/C therapy if QTcF is >500ms; may resume at a reduced dose if QTcF returns to <450ms. D/C permanently and institute appropriate therapy if severe skin reactions (eg, Steven-Johnson syndrome) develop. If CTCAE ≥grade 3 reactions occur, d/c therapy until improved. Photosensitivity reactions may develop; wear sunscreen and protective clothing during and for 4 months after d/c of treatment. Interstitial lung disease (ILD) or pneumonitis and deaths reported; d/c therapy and institute appropriate therapy if symptoms are severe. Serious hemorrhagic events and ischemic cerebrovascular events observed; d/c if severe. Avoid with recent history of hemoptysis of ≥1/2 tsp of red blood. HF may develop; monitor for signs/symptoms of HF and d/c if necessary. Diarrhea and electrolyte imbalance reported; d/c therapy if severe diarrhea develops. Reduce dose or interrupt therapy if HTN occurs; do not restart therapy if BP is uncontrolled. Reversible posterior leukoencephalopathy syndrome (RPLS) reported; consider d/c therapy. Avoid exposure to crushed tabs.

ADVERSE REACTIONS: Diarrhea, rash, acne, N/V, HTN, headache, fatigue, decreased appetite, abdominal pain, increased ALT, prolong QT interval.

INTERACTIONS: See Boxed Warning. CYP3A4 inducers may alter plasma concentrations. Avoid use with strong CYP3A4 inducers (eg, dexamethasone, phenytoin, carbamazepine, rifampin, rifabutin, rifapentine, phenobarbital), St. John's wort, anti-arrhythmic drugs (eg, amiodarone, disopyramide, procainamide, sotalol, dofetilide) and other drugs that may prolong QT interval (eg, chloroquine, clarithromycin, dolasentron, granisetron, haloperidol, methadone, moxifloxacin, pimozide). May increase dose of thyroid replacement therapy; examine TSH levels and adjust accordingly.

PREGNANCY: Category D, not for use in nursing.

MECHANISM OF ACTION: Kinase inhibitor; inhibits the activity of tyrosine kinases, inhibits endothelial cell migration, proliferation, survival, and new blood vessel formation.

PHARMACOKINETICS: Absorption: Slow; T_{max}=6 hrs. **Distribution:** V_d=7450L; plasma protein binding (90% in vitro). **Metabolism:** Liver via CYP3A4; vandetanib N-oxide and N-desmethyl vandetanib (metabolites). **Elimination:** Urine (25%), feces (44%); $T_{1/2}$=19 days.

NURSING CONSIDERATIONS

Assessment: Assess for congenital long QT syndrome, QTcF interval, history of torsades de pointes or hemoptysis, bradyarrhythmias, uncompensated HF, renal/hepatic function, pregnancy/nursing status, and possible drug interactions. Obtain baseline ECG, serum K⁺/calcium/magnesium, and TSH levels.

Monitoring: Monitor for torsades de pointes, ventricular arrhythmias, skin/photosensitivity reactions, ILD, pneumonitis, hemorrhagic events, HF, diarrhea, electrolyte imbalance, hypothyroidism, HTN, RPLS, cerebrovascular event, visual changes, and other adverse reactions. Monitor ECG, electrolytes, serum K⁺/calcium/magnesium, and TSH levels periodically. Monitor renal/hepatic function.

Patient Counseling: Inform that electrolytes and electrical activity of heartbeat (via ECG) should be monitored regularly during therapy. Inform susceptibility to sunburn and advise to use appropriate sun protection (eg, sunscreen and/or clothing) while on therapy and ≥4 months after d/c. Inform that diarrhea may occur and to use standard anti-diarrheal medications. Instruct to consult physician promptly if skin rash, sudden onset or worsening of breathlessness, persistent cough or fever, persistent or severe diarrhea, seizures, headaches, visual disturbances, confusion or difficulty thinking develops. Advise women of childbearing potential to use effective contraception during therapy and ≥4 months after last dose. Advise to d/c nursing while on therapy. Instruct that tab should not be crushed and to avoid direct contact with skin or mucous membranes.

Administration: Oral route. Do not crush tabs. Missed dose should not be taken if it is <12 hrs before the next dose. Refer to PI for administration details if unable to swallow tabs. **Storage:** 25°C (77°F); excursions permitted to 15-30°C (59-86°F).

CAPTOPRIL

RX

captopril (Various)

> D/C when pregnancy is detected. Drugs that act directly on the renin-angiotensin system can cause injury/death to the developing fetus.

THERAPEUTIC CLASS: ACE inhibitor

INDICATIONS: Treatment of HTN alone or in combination with other antihypertensive agents (especially thiazide-type diuretics), and congestive heart failure (CHF) usually in combination with diuretics and digitalis. To improve survival following myocardial infarction (MI) in clinically stable patients with left ventricular dysfunction and to reduce the incidence of overt heart failure and subsequent hospitalizations for CHF in these patients. Treatment of diabetic nephropathy (proteinuria >500mg/day) in patients with type I insulin-dependent diabetes mellitus and retinopathy.

DOSAGE: *Adults:* Individualize dose. HTN: If possible, d/c previous antihypertensive drug for 1 week prior to therapy. Initial: 25mg bid or tid. Titrate: May increase to 50mg bid-tid after 1-2 weeks. May add a modest dose of thiazide diuretic if BP not controlled after 1-2 weeks at 50mg tid. If further BP reduction required, may increase to 100mg bid or tid and then, if necessary, to 150mg bid or tid (while continuing the diuretic). Usual Range: 25-150mg bid or tid. Max: 450mg/day. Severe HTN: Continue diuretic but d/c other current antihypertensive. Initial: 25mg bid or tid. Titrate: May increase q24h or less under supervision until satisfactory response is obtained or max dose is reached. May add a more potent diuretic (eg, furosemide). CHF: Initial: 25mg tid. Titrate: After a dose of 50mg tid is reached, delay further dose increases for at least 2 weeks to determine satisfactory response. Usual: 50mg-100mg tid. Max: 450mg/day. Diuretic-Treated/Hyponatremic/Hypovolemic Patients: Initial: 6.25mg or 12.5mg tid. Titrate to the usual daily dose within the next several days. Left Ventricular Dysfunction Post-MI: Initial: 6.25mg single dose, then 12.5mg tid. Titrate: Increase to 25mg tid during the next several days. Maint: 50mg tid. Diabetic Nephropathy: Usual: 25mg tid. Significant Renal Impairment: Reduce initial daily dose and titrate slowly (1- to 2-week intervals). Back-titrate slowly after desired therapeutic effect is achieved to determine minimal effective dose.

HOW SUPPLIED: Tab: 12.5mg*, 25mg*, 50mg*, 100mg* *scored

CONTRAINDICATIONS: History of ACE inhibitor-associated angioedema.

WARNINGS/PRECAUTIONS: Anaphylactoid reactions reported during desensitization with hymenoptera venom, dialysis with high-flux membranes, and LDL apheresis with dextran sulfate absorption. Angioedema involving the extremities, face, lips, mucous membranes, tongue, glottis, or larynx reported; administer appropriate therapy if this occurs. Intestinal angioedema reported; monitor for abdominal pain. More reports of angioedema in blacks than non-blacks. Neutropenia/agranulocytosis reported; assess and monitor WBCs in patients with renal disease and collagen vascular disease. D/C if neutropenia (neutrophil count <1000/mm³) occurs. Perform WBC counts if infection suspected. Proteinuria reported. Excessive hypotension rarely seen with HTN. Transient hypotension reported in heart failure patients; initiate therapy under close medical supervision in these patients. Rarely, associated with syndrome of cholestatic jaundice progressing to fulminant hepatic necrosis and death; d/c if jaundice or marked LFTs elevation occur. May increase BUN/SrCr in patients with severe renal artery stenosis or in heart failure patients on long-term treatment. Hyperkalemia and persistent nonproductive cough reported. Risk of decreased coronary perfusion in patients with aortic stenosis. Hypotension may occur with major surgery or during anesthesia. May cause false-positive urine test for acetone.

ADVERSE REACTIONS: Rash, eosinophilia, loss of taste, cough.

INTERACTIONS: NSAIDs, including selective cyclooxygenase-2 inhibitors may deteriorate renal function and attenuate the antihypertensive effect. Risk of hypotension and hyponatremia with diuretics. D/C nitroglycerin, other nitrates (as used for management of angina), or other drugs having vasodilator activity before starting treatment. Antihypertensive agents that cause renin release may augment effect (eg, diuretics, such as thiazides, may activate renin-angiotensin-aldosterone system). Caution with agents affecting sympathetic activity (eg, ganglionic-blocking agents or adrenergic neuron-blocking agents). Additive effect with β-blockers. K⁺-sparing diuretics (eg, spironolactone, triamterene, amiloride), K⁺ supplements, or salt substitutes containing K⁺ may increase serum K⁺ levels; use with caution. Lithium toxicity with lithium; monitor lithium levels. Nitritoid reactions reported with injectable gold. May cause neutropenia with allopurinol.

PREGNANCY: Category D, not for use in nursing.

MECHANISM OF ACTION: ACE inhibitor; not established. Effects appear to result from suppression of renin-angiotensin-aldosterone system. Decreases plasma angiotensin II, which leads to decreased aldosterone secretion.

PHARMACOKINETICS: Absorption: Rapid. T_{max}=1 hr. **Distribution:** Plasma protein binding (25-30%); found in breast milk. **Elimination:** Urine (40-50%, unchanged); $T_{1/2}$=<2 hrs.

NURSING CONSIDERATIONS

Assessment: Assess for history of ACE inhibitor-associated angioedema, risk of excessive hypotension, renal artery stenosis, risk of hyperkalemia, collagen vascular disease, renal function, aortic stenosis, hypersensitivity to drug, pregnancy/nursing status, and possible drug interactions. Obtain baseline WBC and differential count.

Monitoring: Monitor for angioedema, anaphylactoid reactions, hyperkalemia, infection, and cough. Monitor WBC and differential counts q2 weeks for 3 months, then periodically in patients with renal impairment. Monitor BP, LFTs, and renal function.

Patient Counseling: Advise to d/c and immediately report to physician for any signs/symptoms of angioedema (eg, swelling of face, eyes, lips, tongue, larynx and extremities; difficulty swallowing or breathing; hoarseness). Advise to promptly report to physician for any indication of infection (eg, sore throat, fever). Inform that excessive perspiration, dehydration, and other causes of volume depletion (eg, diarrhea, vomiting) may lead to fall in BP. Instruct not to use K⁺-sparing diuretics, K⁺-containing salt substitutes, or K⁺ supplements without consulting physician. Advise against interruption or d/c of medication unless directed by physician. Advise heart failure patients against rapid increases in physical activity. Inform about the consequences of exposure during pregnancy in females of childbearing age. Discuss treatment options with women planning to become pregnant. Instruct to report pregnancies to physician as soon as possible.

Administration: Oral route. Take 1 hr ac. **Storage:** 20-25°C (68-77°F).

CARBAGLU   RX
carglumic acid (Orphan Europe)

THERAPEUTIC CLASS: Carbamoyl Phosphate Synthetase 1

INDICATIONS: Adjunctive therapy in pediatrics and adults for the treatment of acute hyperammonemia due to deficiency of the hepatic enzyme N-acetylglutamate synthase (NAGS). Maintenance therapy in pediatrics and adults for chronic hyperammonemia due to deficiency of NAGS.

DOSAGE: *Adults:* Acute Hyperammonemia: Initial: 100-250mg/kg/day. Titrate dose based on individual plasma ammonia levels and clinical symptoms. Chronic Hyperammonemia: Maint: Usual: <100mg/kg/day. Titrate to target normal plasma ammonia by age. Divide total daily dose into 2-4 doses and round to the nearest 100mg.
Pediatrics: Acute Hyperammonemia: Initial: 100-250mg/kg/day. Titrate dose based on individual plasma ammonia levels and clinical symptoms. Chronic Hyperammonemia: Maint: Usual: <100mg/kg/day. Titrate to target normal plasma ammonia by age. Divide total daily dose into 2-4 doses.

HOW SUPPLIED: Tab: 200mg* *scored

WARNINGS/PRECAUTIONS: Any episode of acute symptomatic hyperammonemia should be treated as a life-threatening emergency; management may require dialysis. Uncontrolled hyperammonemia can rapidly result in brain injury/damage or death; use all therapies necessary to

C

reduce plasma ammonia levels. Monitor plasma ammonia levels, neurological status, laboratory tests, and clinical responses during treatment. Maintain normal range of plasma ammonia levels for age via individual dose adjustment. Protein restriction and hypercaloric intake is recommended during acute hyperammonemic episodes until plasma ammonia levels normalize, then aim for unrestricted protein intake.

ADVERSE REACTIONS: Infection, abdominal pain, anemia, ear infection, diarrhea, vomiting, pyrexia, tonsilitis, headache, nasopharyngitis.

PREGNANCY: Category C, not for use in nursing.

MECHANISM OF ACTION: Carbamoyl phosphate synthetase 1 activator; synthetic analog of N-acetylglutamate (NAG), which acts as a replacement for NAG in NAGS deficiency patients by activating carbamoyl phosphate synthetase 1, the enzyme that converts ammonia into urea.

PHARMACOKINETICS: Absorption: T_{max}=3 hrs. **Distribution:** V_d=2657L. **Metabolism:** Via intestinal bacterial flora. **Elimination:** $T_{1/2}$=5.6 hrs; urine (9%, unchanged), feces (up to 60%, unchanged).

NURSING CONSIDERATIONS

Assessment: Assess for plasma ammonia levels and pregnancy/nursing status.

Monitoring: Monitor plasma ammonia levels, neurological status, laboratory tests, and clinical responses.

Patient Counseling: Inform that tablets should not be swallowed whole or crushed; disperse each tablet in a minimum of 2.5mL of water. Advise to rinse mixing container with additional volumes of water and to swallow contents immediately. Instruct to keep product in a refrigerator before opening and not to refrigerate after 1st opening; advise to discard 1 month after 1st opening. Counsel to keep container tightly closed. Advise that dietary protein may be increased when plasma ammonia levels have normalized. Inform of the most common adverse reactions (eg, vomiting, abdominal pain, pyrexia, tonsillitis, anemia, ear infection, diarrhea, nasopharyngitis, and headache). Advise not to breastfeed.

Administration: Oral and NG route. Disperse tab in water immediately before use. Refer to PI for preparation for PO and NG tube administration. **Storage:** Before Opening: 2-8°C (36-46°F). After Opening: Do not refrigerate, do not store >30°C (86°F). Discard 1 month after 1st opening. Protect from moisture.

CARBATROL   RX
carbamazepine (Shire)

Serious and fatal dermatologic reactions, including toxic epidermal necrolysis (TEN) and Stevens-Johnson syndrome (SJS) reported; increased risk with presence of HLA-B*1502 allele; screen prior to initiation of therapy. Aplastic anemia and agranulocytosis reported. Obtain complete pretreatment hematological testing as a baseline. Consider d/c if evidence of bone marrow depression develops.

THERAPEUTIC CLASS: Carboxamide

INDICATIONS: Treatment of partial seizures with complex symptomatology (psychomotor, temporal lobe), generalized tonic-clonic seizures (grand mal), and mixed seizure patterns of these, or other partial or generalized seizures. Treatment of pain associated with true trigeminal or glossopharyngeal neuralgia.

DOSAGE: *Adults:* Epilepsy: Initial: 200mg bid. Titrate: Increase weekly by ≤200mg/day. Maint: Adjust to minimum effective level, usually 800-1200mg/day. Max: 1600mg/day. Combination Therapy: When added to existing anticonvulsant therapy, may be added gradually while other anticonvulsants are maintained or gradually decreased, except phenytoin, which may be increased. Trigeminal Neuralgia: Initial (Day 1): 200mg qd. Titrate: May increase by ≤200mg/day q12h PRN. Maint: Usual: 400-800mg/day. Attempts to reduce dose to minimum effective level or even to d/c therapy is at least once q3 months. Max: 1200mg/day.
Pediatrics: Epilepsy: >12 yrs: Initial: 200mg bid. Titrate: Increase weekly by ≤200mg/day. Maint: Adjust to minimum effective level, usually 800-1200mg/day. >15 yrs: Max: 1200mg/day. 12-15 yrs: Max: 1000mg/day. <12 yrs: May convert immediate-release dose ≥400mg/day to equal daily dose using bid regimen. Usual: <35mg/kg/day. Max: ≤35mg/kg/day.

HOW SUPPLIED: Cap, Extended-Release: 100mg, 200mg, 300mg

CONTRAINDICATIONS: History of bone marrow depression, MAOI use within 14 days, sensitivity to TCAs (eg, amitriptyline, desipramine, imipramine, protriptyline, nortriptyline), coadministration with nefazodone.

WARNINGS/PRECAUTIONS: Increased risk of suicidal thoughts or behavior reported. May cause fetal harm with pregnancy. Avoid abrupt d/c in patients with seizure disorder; may precipitate status epilepticus. Caution in patients with history of cardiac, hepatic, or renal damage; adverse hematologic reactions to other drugs; interrupted courses of therapy with carbamazepine;

increased intraocular pressure (IOP); and mixed seizure disorder. May cause activation of latent psychosis and, in the elderly, confusion or agitation. Caution with history of liver disease; d/c immediately in cases of aggravated liver dysfunction or active liver disease. Hyponatremia, interference with some pregnancy tests, decreased values of thyroid function tests, renal dysfunction, eye changes, increased total cholesterol, LDL, and HDL reported.

ADVERSE REACTIONS: Dizziness, drowsiness, unsteadiness, N/V, bone marrow depression, congestive heart failure (CHF), aplastic anemia, agranulocytosis, SJS, TEN.

INTERACTIONS: See Contraindications. CYP3A4 and/or epoxide hydrolase inhibitors (eg, azole antifungals, cimetidine, erythromycin, protease inhibitors) may increase plasma level. CYP3A4 inducers (eg, cisplatin, doxorubicin, rifampin) may decrease plasma level. May decrease plasma levels of CYP1A2 and CYP3A4 substrates (eg, acetaminophen, oral contraceptives, trazodone, warfarin). Breakthrough bleeding reported with oral contraceptives. May reduce warfarin's anticoagulant effect. May increase plasma levels of clomipramine HCl and primidone. May increase or decrease plasma level of phenytoin. Increased risk of neurotoxic side effects with lithium. Antimalarial drugs (eg, chloroquine, mefloquine) may antagonize activity. Caution with other centrally acting drugs and alcohol. Coadministration with delavirdine may lead to loss of virologic response and possible resistance to non-nucleoside reverse transcriptase inhibitors (NNRTIs). Hyponatremia and a case of meningitis reported in combination with other drugs. Isolated cases of neuroleptic malignant syndrome reported with psychotropic drugs.

PREGNANCY: Category D, not for use in nursing.

MECHANISM OF ACTION: Anticonvulsant: Reduces polysynaptic response and blocks post-tetanic potentiation. Neuralgia: Depresses thalamic potential and bulbar and polysynaptic reflexes.

PHARMACOKINETICS: Absorption: (Single 200mg dose) C_{max}=1.9µg/mL, 0.11 µg/mL (CBZ-E); T_{max}=19 hrs, 36 hrs (CBZ-E). (Multiple 800mg dose) C_{max}=11µg/mL, 2.2µg/mL (CBZ-E); T_{max}=5.9 hrs, 14 hrs (CBZ-E). **Distribution:** Plasma protein binding (76%), (50% CBZ-E); crosses the placenta; found in breast milk. **Metabolism:** Liver via CYP3A4; carbamazepine-10,11-epoxide (CBZ-E) (active metabolite). **Elimination:** Urine (72%, 3% unchanged), feces (28%); $T_{1/2}$=35-40 hrs (single dose), 12-17 hrs (multiple doses), 34 hrs (CBZ-E).

NURSING CONSIDERATIONS

Assessment: Assess for conditions where treatment is contraindicated or cautioned, pregnancy/nursing status, and possible drug interactions. Perform detailed history and physical exam prior to treatment. Screen for HLA-B*1502 allele in suspected population. Obtain baseline CBC with platelet and reticulocyte counts, serum iron, LFTs, urinalysis, BUN, lipid profile, and eye exam.

Monitoring: Monitor for signs/symptoms of dermatologic reactions, aplastic anemia, agranulocytosis, signs of bone marrow depression, emergence or worsening of depression, suicidal thoughts or behavior, unusual changes in mood or behavior, and liver dysfunction aggravation or active liver disease. Periodically monitor WBC, platelet count, LFTs, urinalysis, BUN, lipid profile, and serum drug levels. Perform periodic eye exams, including slit-lamp exam, funduscopy, and tonometry.

Patient Counseling: Instruct to read Medication Guide prior to taking drug. Report toxic signs/symptoms of potential hematologic problems (eg, fever, sore throat, rash, ulcers in mouth, easy bruising, petechial or purpuric hemorrhage), and emergence of suicidal thoughts or behavior. Use caution while operating machinery/driving. Inform that caps can be opened and contents sprinkled over food (eg, teaspoon of applesauce) if necessary; do not crush or chew. Notify physician if pregnant or intend to become pregnant, and to report the use of any other prescription or nonprescription medication or herbal products. Encourage patients to enroll in North American Antiepileptic Drug (NAAED) Pregnancy Registry by calling 1-888-233-2334 or go to www.aedpregnancyregistry.org.

Administration: Oral route. **Storage:** 25°C (77°F); excursions permitted to 15-30°C (59-86°F). Protect from light and moisture.

CARDENE IV

RX

nicardipine HCl (EKR)

THERAPEUTIC CLASS: Calcium channel blocker (dihydropyridine)

INDICATIONS: Short-term treatment of HTN when PO therapy is not feasible or not desirable.

DOSAGE: *Adults:* Individualize dose. Patients Not Receiving PO Nicardipine: Initial: 5mg/hr IV infusion. Titrate: May increase by 2.5mg/hr q5 min (for rapid titration) to 15 min (for gradual titration). Max: 15mg/hr. Decrease rate to 3mg/hr after BP goal achieved with rapid titration. Equivalent PO Dose to IV Dose: 20mg q8h=0.5mg/hr; 30mg q8h=1.2mg/hr; 40mg q8h=2.2mg/hr. Transition to PO Nicardipine: Give 1st dose 1 hr prior to d/c of infusion. Hepatic Impairment/Reduced Hepatic Blood Flow: Consider lower dosages. Renal Impairment: Titrate gradually. Elderly: Start at low end of dosing range. (Cardene Premixed) Impending Hypotension/

Tachycardia: D/C then restart at 3-5mg/hr when BP has stabilized and adjust to maintain desired BP.

HOW SUPPLIED: Inj: 2.5mg/mL [10mL], 0.1mg/mL [200mL], 0.2mg/mL [200mL]

CONTRAINDICATIONS: Advanced aortic stenosis.

WARNINGS/PRECAUTIONS: May induce or exacerbate angina in coronary artery disease (CAD) patients. Caution with heart failure (HF) or significant left ventricular dysfunction. To reduce possibility of venous thrombosis, phlebitis, local irritation, swelling, extravasation, and occurrence of vascular impairment, administer through large peripheral or central veins. Change IV site q12h to minimize risk of peripheral venous irritation. May occasionally produce symptomatic hypotension or tachycardia. Avoid systemic hypotension when administering in sustained acute cerebral infarction or hemorrhage. Caution in hepatic/renal impairment, reduced hepatic blood flow, and elderly.

ADVERSE REACTIONS: Headache, hypotension, tachycardia, N/V.

INTERACTIONS: Titrate slowly with β-blockers in HF or significant left ventricular dysfunction due to possible negative inotropic effects. Increased nicardipine levels when PO nicardipine is given with cimetidine. Elevated cyclosporine levels reported with PO nicardipine; closely monitor cyclosporine levels and reduce its dose accordingly.

PREGNANCY: Category C, not for use in nursing.

MECHANISM OF ACTION: Calcium channel blocker (dihydropyridine); inhibits transmembrane influx of calcium ions into cardiac muscle and smooth muscles without changing serum calcium concentrations.

PHARMACOKINETICS: Distribution: V_d=8.3L/kg; plasma protein binding (>95%); found in breast milk. **Metabolism:** Liver (extensive). **Elimination:** Urine (49%), feces (43%); $T_{1/2}$=14.4 hrs.

NURSING CONSIDERATIONS

Assessment: Assess for advanced aortic stenosis, HF, CAD, left ventricular dysfunction, sustained acute cerebral infarction or hemorrhage, hepatic/renal impairment, pregnancy/nursing status, and possible drug interactions.

Monitoring: Monitor BP and HR during administration. Monitor for symptomatic hypotension, tachycardia, induction or exacerbation of angina, and hepatic/renal function.

Patient Counseling: Advise to seek medical attention if adverse reactions occur.

Administration: IV route. Refer to PI for preparation and administration instructions. Cardene IV: Dilute before infusion. Cardene Premixed: No further dilution required. **Storage:** 20-25°C (68-77°F). Avoid elevated temperatures. Protect from light. Store in carton until ready to use. Diluted Sol: Stable at room temperature for 24 hrs. Premixed: Protect from freezing.

CARDENE SR   RX
nicardipine HCl (PDL BioPharma)

THERAPEUTIC CLASS: Calcium channel blocker (dihydropyridine)

INDICATIONS: Treatment of hypertension.

DOSAGE: *Adults:* Initial: 30mg bid. Usual: 30-60mg bid. Adjust according to BP response.

HOW SUPPLIED: Cap, Sustained-Release: 30mg, 45mg, 60mg

CONTRAINDICATIONS: Advanced aortic stenosis.

WARNINGS/PRECAUTIONS: Increased angina reported in patients with angina. Caution with congestive heart failure (CHF) when titrating dose. Caution in hepatic/renal impairment, or reduced hepatic blood flow. May cause symptomatic hypotension. Monitor BP during initial administration and dose titration.

ADVERSE REACTIONS: Headache, pedal edema, vasodilation, palpitations, N/V, dizziness, asthenia, postural hypotension, increased urinary frequency, pain, rash, increased sweating.

INTERACTIONS: Increased levels with cimetidine. Elevates cyclosporine levels. With β-blocker withdrawal, gradually reduce over 8-10 days. Monitor digoxin levels. Severe hypotension reported with fentanyl anesthesia.

PREGNANCY: Category C, not for use in nursing.

MECHANISM OF ACTION: Ca^{2+} channel blocker; inhibits transmembrane influx of Ca^{2+} ions into cardiac muscle and smooth muscle without changing serum Ca^{2+} concentration.

PHARMACOKINETICS: Absorption: Complete; bioavailability (35%); C_{max}=13.4ng/mL (30mg), 34.0ng/mL (45mg), 58.4ng/mL (60mg); T_{max}=1-4 hrs. **Distribution:** Plasma protein binding (>95%). **Metabolism:** Liver. **Elimination:** Urine (<1%, intact), feces; $T_{1/2}$=8.6 hrs.

NURSING CONSIDERATIONS

Assessment: Assess for advanced aortic stenosis, CHF, acute cerebral infarction or hemorrhage, liver/renal impairment, pregnancy/nursing status, and possible drug interactions. Obtain baseline BP.

Monitoring: Monitor BP initially and during titration. Monitor for signs/symptoms of angina, hypersensitivity reactions, hypotension, liver/renal dysfunction.

Patient Counseling: Advise to seek medical attention if symptoms of hypotension, angina, or hypersensitivity reactions occur.

Administration: Oral route. **Storage:** 15-30°C (59-86°F); keep in light-resistant container.

CARDIZEM   RX
diltiazem HCl (Biovail)

THERAPEUTIC CLASS: Calcium channel blocker (nondihydropyridine)

INDICATIONS: Management of chronic stable angina and angina due to coronary artery spasm.

DOSAGE: *Adults:* Initial: 30mg qid (before meals and hs). Titrate: Increase gradually (given in divided doses tid-qid) at 1-2 day intervals until optimum response obtained. Usual: 180-360mg/day. Elderly: Start at lower end of dosing range.

HOW SUPPLIED: Tab: 30mg, 60mg*, 90mg*, 120mg* *scored

CONTRAINDICATIONS: Sick sinus syndrome and 2nd- or 3rd-degree AV block (except with functioning ventricular pacemaker); hypotension (<90mmHg systolic); acute myocardial infarction (MI) and pulmonary congestion documented by x-ray on admission.

WARNINGS/PRECAUTIONS: May cause abnormally slow heart rates, particularly in patients with sick sinus syndrome. May cause 2nd- or 3rd-degree AV block. Periods of asystole reported in patients with Prinzmetal's angina. Caution in renal, hepatic, or ventricular dysfunction. Symptomatic hypotension may occur. Elevations in enzymes (eg, alkaline phosphatase, lactate dehydrogenase [LDH], AST, ALT) and other phenomena consistent with acute hepatic injury reported; reversible upon d/c. Monitor LFTs and renal function. Dermatologic reactions (eg, erythema multiforme, exfoliative dermatitis) may occur; d/c if a dermatologic reaction persists. Caution in elderly.

ADVERSE REACTIONS: Edema, headache, nausea, dizziness, rash, asthenia.

INTERACTIONS: May increase levels of propranolol, carbamazepine, quinidine, midazolam, triazolam, lovastatin, simvastatin; monitor closely. Increased levels with cimetidine. Monitor digoxin and cyclosporine levels if used concomitantly. Potentiates depression of cardiac contractility, conductivity, automaticity and vascular dilation with anesthetics. Additive cardiac conduction effects with digitalis or β-blockers. Potential additive effects with agents known to affect cardiac contractility and/or conduction; caution and careful titration warranted. May have significant impact on efficacy and side effect profile with CYP450 3A4 substrates, inducers, and inhibitors. Avoid with CYP3A4 inducers (eg, rifampin). May enhance the effects and increase the toxicity of buspirone. Concomitant use with statins metabolized by CYP3A4 may increase the risk of myopathy and rhabdomyolysis. Sinus bradycardia resulting in hospitalization and pacemaker insertion reported with clonidine; monitor heart rate.

PREGNANCY: Category C, not for use in nursing.

MECHANISM OF ACTION: Calcium channel blocker; inhibits cellular influx of calcium ions during membrane depolarization of cardiac and vascular smooth muscle. Angina Due to Coronary Artery Spasm: A potent dilator of coronary arteries both epicardial and subendocardial; inhibits spontaneous and ergonovine-induced coronary artery spasm. Exertional Angina: Produces increases in exercise tolerance by its ability to reduce myocardial oxygen demand; accomplished via reduction in heart rate and systemic BP.

PHARMACOKINETICS: Absorption: Well absorbed; Absolute bioavailability (40%); T_{max}=2-4 hrs. **Distribution:** Plasma protein binding (70-80%); found in breast milk. **Metabolism:** Liver (extensive). **Elimination:** Urine (2-4%, unchanged), bile. $T_{1/2}$=3-4.5 hrs.

NURSING CONSIDERATIONS

Assessment: Assess for sick sinus syndrome, 2nd- or 3rd-degree AV block, hypotension, acute MI, pulmonary congestion, congestive heart failure (CHF), ventricular dysfunction, hepatic/renal impairment, pregnancy/nursing status, and for possible drug interactions.

Monitoring: Monitor for slow HR, 2nd- or 3rd-degree AV block, hypotension, hepatic injury (eg, increased alkaline phosphatase, increased LDH, increased AST, increased ALT) and for dermatological events (eg, skin eruptions progressing to erythema multiforme and/or exfoliative dermatitis). Monitor liver and renal function regularly.

Patient Counseling: Inform about benefits/risks of therapy. Counsel to report any adverse reactions to physician and to notify physician if pregnant or nursing.

Administration: Oral route. **Storage:** 25°C (77°F); excursions permitted to 15-30°C (59-86°F). Avoid excessive humidity.

CARDIZEM CD

RX

diltiazem HCl (Biovail)

OTHER BRAND NAMES: Cardizem LA (Abbott) - Cartia XT (Watson)

THERAPEUTIC CLASS: Calcium channel blocker (nondihydropyridine)

INDICATIONS: Treatment of HTN used alone or in combination with other antihypertensive medications. Management of chronic stable angina and (CD, Cartia XT) angina due to coronary artery spasm.

DOSAGE: *Adults:* Individualize dose. HTN: (CD, Cartia XT) Initial (Monotherapy): 180-240mg qd. Titrate: Adjust to individual patient needs (schedule accordingly). Usual: 240-360mg qd. Max: 480mg qd. (LA) Initial (Monotherapy): 180-240mg qd (am or hs). Titrate: Adjust to individual patient needs (schedule accordingly). Range: 120-540mg qd. Max: 540mg/day. Angina: (CD, Cartia XT) Initial: 120mg or 180mg qd. Titrate: Adjust to each patient's needs; may be carried out over a 7- to 14-day period when necessary. Max: 480mg qd. (LA) Initial: 180mg qd (am or pm). Titrate: Increase at 1-2 week intervals. Max: 360mg. Elderly: Start at lower end of dosing range.

HOW SUPPLIED: Cap, Extended-Release: (Cardizem CD, Cartia XT) 120mg, 180mg, 240mg, 300mg, (Cardizem CD) 360mg; Tab, Extended-Release: (Cardizem LA) 120mg, 180mg, 240mg, 300mg, 360mg, 420mg

CONTRAINDICATIONS: Sick sinus syndrome and 2nd- or 3rd-degree atrioventricular (AV) block (except with functioning ventricular pacemaker), hypotension (<90mmHg systolic), acute myocardial infarction (MI), and pulmonary congestion documented by x-rays on admission.

WARNINGS/PRECAUTIONS: Prolongs AV node refractory periods without significantly prolonging sinus node recovery time. Periods of asystole reported in a patient with Prinzmetal's angina. Worsening of congestive heart failure reported in patients with preexisting ventricular dysfunction. Symptomatic hypotension may occur. Mild transaminase elevation with or without concomitant alkaline phosphatase and bilirubin elevation reported. Significant enzyme elevations and other phenomena consistent with acute hepatic injury reported in rare instances. Caution with renal/hepatic dysfunction. Dermatologic reactions (eg, erythema multiforme, exfoliative dermatitis) may occur; d/c if such reaction persists. Caution in elderly.

ADVERSE REACTIONS: Dizziness, bradycardia, 1st-degree AV block. (CD, Cartia XT) Headache, edema. (LA) Edema lower limb, fatigue.

INTERACTIONS: May increase levels of propranolol, carbamazepine, quinidine, midazolam, triazolam, buspirone, and lovastatin. Increased levels with cimetidine. Monitor digoxin and cyclosporine levels. Depression of cardiac contractility, conductivity, automaticity, and vascular dilation potentiated with anesthetics. Additive cardiac conduction effects with digitalis or β-blockers. Potential additive effects with agents known to affect cardiac contractility and/or conduction; caution and careful titration warranted. May have significant impact on efficacy and side effect profile with CYP450 3A4 substrates, inducers, and inhibitors. Avoid with CYP3A4 inducers (eg, rifampin). (CD, LA) Sinus bradycardia resulting in hospitalization and pacemaker insertion reported with clonidine; monitor HR. Increased exposure of simvastatin; limit daily doses of both agents. Risk of myopathy and rhabdomyolysis with statins metabolized by CYP3A4 may be increased; monitor closely.

PREGNANCY: Category C, not for use in nursing.

MECHANISM OF ACTION: Calcium channel blocker; inhibits cellular influx of calcium ions during membrane depolarization of cardiac and vascular smooth muscle. HTN: Relaxes vascular smooth muscle resulting in decreased peripheral vascular resistance. Angina: Produces increases in exercise tolerance by its ability to reduce myocardial oxygen demand; accomplished via reduction in HR and systemic BP at submaximal and maximal work loads.

PHARMACOKINETICS: Absorption: Well absorbed. Absolute bioavailability (40%); T_{max}=10-14 hrs (CD, Cartia XT), 11-18 hrs (LA). **Distribution:** Plasma protein binding (70-80%); found in breast milk. **Metabolism:** Liver (extensive). **Elimination:** Urine (2-4%, unchanged), bile. $T_{1/2}$=5-8 hrs (CD, Cartia XT), 6-9 hrs (LA).

NURSING CONSIDERATIONS

Assessment: Assess for sick sinus syndrome, 2nd- or 3rd-degree AV block, hypotension, acute MI and pulmonary congestion, ventricular dysfunction, hepatic/renal impairment, pregnancy/nursing status, and possible drug interactions.

Monitoring: Monitor for bradycardia, AV block, symptomatic hypotension, and dermatological reactions. Perform regular monitoring of liver and renal function.

Patient Counseling: Counsel to report any adverse reactions to physician and to notify physician if pregnant or nursing. Instruct to swallow tab whole; do not chew or crush.

Administration: Oral route. (LA) Swallow whole; do not chew or crush. **Storage:** 25°C (77°F); excursions permitted to 15-30°C (59-86°F) (CD, LA); 20-25°C (68-77°F) (Cartia XT). Avoid excessive humidity and (LA) temperature >30°C (86°F).

CARDURA   RX
doxazosin mesylate (Pfizer)

THERAPEUTIC CLASS: Alpha$_1$-blocker (quinazoline)

INDICATIONS: Treatment of HTN alone or with other antihypertensive agents and/or treatment of both the urinary outflow obstruction and obstructive and irritative symptoms associated with BPH.

DOSAGE: *Adults:* Individualize dose. HTN: Initial: 1mg qd (am or pm). Titrate: Increase stepwise to 2mg, 4mg, 8mg, or 16mg qd PRN based on standing BP response. Dosing Range: 1-16mg qd. BPH: Initial: 1mg qd (am or pm). Titrate: Increase stepwise to 2mg, 4mg, and 8mg in 1-2 week intervals based on urodynamics and BPH symptomatology. Max: 8mg qd.

HOW SUPPLIED: Tab: 1mg*, 2mg*, 4mg*, 8mg* *scored

WARNINGS/PRECAUTIONS: May cause syncope and orthostatic hypotension (eg, dizziness, lightheadedness, vertigo) especially with 1st dose, dose increase, or if therapy is interrupted for more than a few days; restart using initial dosing regimen if therapy was d/c for several days. Rule out prostate cancer prior to therapy. Priapism (rare) and leukopenia/neutropenia reported. Intraoperative floppy iris syndrome observed during cataract surgery. Caution with hepatic dysfunction and elderly.

ADVERSE REACTIONS: Dizziness, headache, fatigue/malaise, somnolence, edema, nausea, rhinitis, vertigo.

INTERACTIONS: Caution with additional antihypertensive agents and drugs known to influence hepatic metabolism. Additive BP-lowering effects and symptomatic hypotension with phosphodiesterase type 5 inhibitors.

PREGNANCY: Category C, caution with nursing.

MECHANISM OF ACTION: Alpha$_1$-blocker; (BPH) antagonizes phenylephrine (α_1-agonist)-induced contractions in prostate; (HTN) competitively antagonizes pressor effects of phenylephrine and systolic pressor effect of norepinephrine.

PHARMACOKINETICS: Absorption: Bioavailability (65%); T_{max}=2-3 hrs. **Distribution:** Plasma protein binding (98%). **Metabolism:** Liver (extensive); O-demethylation or hydroxylation. **Elimination:** Feces (63%, 4.8% unchanged), urine (9%, trace amounts unchanged); $T_{1/2}$=22 hrs.

NURSING CONSIDERATIONS

Assessment: Assess for previous sensitivity to the drug, liver impairment, pregnancy/nursing status, and possible drug interactions. Rule out prostate cancer prior to therapy.

Monitoring: Measure BP periodically particularly 2-6 hrs after the 1st dose and with each increase in dose. Monitor for signs/symptoms of hypotension, priapism, liver dysfunction, hypersensitivity reactions, and other adverse effects.

Patient Counseling: Inform of the possibility of syncope and orthostatic symptoms, especially at initiation of therapy; urge to avoid driving or hazardous tasks for 24 hrs after 1st dose, dose increase, and interruption of therapy when treatment is resumed. Caution to avoid situations where injury could result should syncope occur. Advise to sit or lie down when symptoms of low BP occur. Instruct to report to physician if dizziness, lightheadedness, or palpitations are bothersome. Inform of possibility of priapism; advise to seek medical attention immediately if priapism occurs. Counsel to inform surgeon of drug use prior to cataract surgery.

Administration: Oral route. **Storage:** 25°C (77°F); excursions permitted to 15-30°C (59-86°F).

CARDURA XL   RX
doxazosin mesylate (Pfizer)

THERAPEUTIC CLASS: Alpha$_1$-blocker (quinazoline)

INDICATIONS: Treatment of the signs and symptoms of benign prostatic hyperplasia (BPH).

DOSAGE: *Adults:* Initial: 4mg qd with breakfast. Titrate: May increase to 8mg after 3-4 weeks based on symptomatic response and tolerability. Max: 8mg. If d/c for several days, restart using 4mg qd dose. Switching from Cardura Immediate-Release to Cardura XL: Initial: 4mg qd. Final evening dose of Cardura should not be taken. Concomitant PDE-5 Inhibitors: Initiate phosphodiesterase-5 (PDE-5) inhibitor therapy at the lowest dose.

HOW SUPPLIED: Tab, Extended-Release: 4mg, 8mg

C

WARNINGS/PRECAUTIONS: Postural hypotension with or without symptoms (eg, dizziness) and syncope may develop; caution with symptomatic hypotension or patients who have hypotensive response to other medications. Intraoperative floppy iris syndrome has been observed during cataract surgery in some patients on, or previously treated with, α_1-blockers. Caution with preexisting severe GI narrowing (pathologic or iatrogenic). Prostate cancer causes many of the same symptoms associated with BPH; rule out prostate cancer prior to therapy. Caution with mild or moderate hepatic impairment; avoid with severe hepatic impairment. D/C if symptoms of worsening of or new onset angina pectoris develop.

ADVERSE REACTIONS: Dizziness, asthenia, headache, respiratory tract infection, dyspnea, somnolence, hypotension, postural hypotension.

INTERACTIONS: Caution with potent CYP3A4 inhibitors (eg, atazanavir, clarithromycin, indinavir, itraconazole, ketoconazole, nefazodone, nelfinavir, ritonavir, saquinavir, telithromycin, voriconazole). Additive blood pressure lowering effects and symptomatic hypotension with PDE-5 inhibitor. Caution with drugs known to influence hepatic metabolism. Drugs which reduce GI motility leading to markedly prolonged GI retention times may increase systemic exposure to doxazosin (eg, anticholinergics).

PREGNANCY: Category C, not for use in nursing.

MECHANISM OF ACTION: Alpha$_1$-blocker; antagonizes α_1-agonist-induced contractions, decreasing urethral resistance, which may relieve BPH symptoms and improve urine flow.

PHARMACOKINETICS: Absorption: (4mg) C_{max}=10.1ng/mL, AUC=183ng•hr/mL, T_{max}=8 hrs. (8mg) C_{max}=25.8ng/mL, AUC=472ng•hr/mL, T_{max}=9 hrs. **Distribution:** Plasma protein binding (98%). **Metabolism:** Liver (extensive) via CYP3A4 (major) and CYP2D6, CYP2C19 (minor). **Elimination:** $T_{1/2}$=15-19 hrs.

NURSING CONSIDERATIONS

Assessment: Assess for hepatic impairment, symptomatic hypotension, history of hypotensive response to other medications, severe GI narrowing (chronic constipation), coronary insufficiency, and possible drug interactions. Rule out prostate cancer.

Monitoring: Monitor for signs/symptoms of postural hypotension and new onset or worsening of angina pectoris.

Patient Counseling: Instruct to take with breakfast; swallow whole; do not chew, divide, cut, or crush. Advise that symptoms related to postural hypotension (eg, dizziness, syncope) may occur; caution about driving, operating machinery, and performing hazardous tasks. Caution not to be alarmed if something that looks like a tablet is occasionally noticed in the stool. Instruct to inform ophthalmologist of drug use prior to cataract surgery.

Admininstration: Oral route. **Storage:** 25°C (77°F); excursions permitted to 15-30°C (59-86°F).

CASODEX   RX
bicalutamide (AstraZeneca)

THERAPEUTIC CLASS: Nonsteroidal antiandrogen

INDICATIONS: Treatment of stage D$_2$ metastatic carcinoma of the prostate in combination with a luteinizing hormone-releasing hormone (LHRH) analog.

DOSAGE: *Adults:* Usual: 50mg qd (am or pm) in combination with an LHRH analog. Take at the same time each day and start at the same time as treatment with an LHRH analog.

HOW SUPPLIED: Tab: 50mg

CONTRAINDICATIONS: Women, pregnancy.

WARNINGS/PRECAUTIONS: Cases of death or hospitalization due to severe liver injury (hepatic failure) reported. Hepatitis and marked increases in liver enzymes leading to drug d/c reported; measure serum transaminase levels prior to treatment, at regular intervals for the 1st 4 months, and periodically thereafter. Measure serum ALT immediately if signs/symptoms of liver dysfunction occur; d/c immediately with close follow-up of liver function if jaundice occurs or ALT rises >2X ULN. Reduction in glucose tolerance reported; monitor blood glucose. Regularly assess serum prostate-specific antigen (PSA) to monitor response; evaluate for clinical progression if PSA levels rise during therapy. For patients with objective disease progression with an elevated PSA, consider a treatment period free of antiandrogen, while continuing the LHRH analog. Caution with moderate-severe hepatic impairment; monitor LFTs periodically on long term therapy.

ADVERSE REACTIONS: Pain, hot flashes, HTN, constipation, nausea, diarrhea, anemia, peripheral edema, dizziness, dyspnea, rash, nocturia, hematuria, urinary tract infection, gynecomastia.

INTERACTIONS: Can displace coumarin anticoagulants from binding sites; monitor PT and consider anticoagulant dose adjustment. Caution with CYP3A4 substrates. May increase levels of midazolam.

PREGNANCY: Category X, not for use in nursing.

MECHANISM OF ACTION: Nonsteroidal antiandrogen; inhibits the action of androgens by binding to cytosol androgen receptors in target tissue.

PHARMACOKINETICS: Absorption: Well-absorbed; C_{max}=0.768µg/mL; T_{max}=31.3 hrs. **Distribution:** Plasma protein binding (96%). **Metabolism:** Liver via oxidation and glucuronidation. **Elimination:** Urine, feces; $T_{1/2}$=5.8 days.

NURSING CONSIDERATIONS

Assessment: Assess for drug hypersensitivity, diabetes, hepatic impairment, and possible drug interactions. Measure serum transaminase levels.

Monitoring: Measure serum transaminase levels at regular intervals for the 1st 4 months of treatment, then periodically thereafter. Measure serum ALT for signs/symptoms of liver dysfunction. Monitor LFT in hepatic impaired patients on long term therapy. Regularly monitor serum PSA levels. Monitor for hypersensitivity reactions and blood glucose levels.

Patient Counseling: Advise not to interrupt or stop taking the medication without consulting their physician. Inform that somnolence may occur; advise to use caution when driving or operating machinery. Advise to monitor blood glucose levels while on therapy.

Administration: Oral route. **Storage:** 20-25°C (68-77°F).

CATAFLAM RX
diclofenac potassium (Novartis)

NSAIDs may cause an increased risk of serious cardiovascular (CV) thrombotic events, myocardial infarction (MI), stroke, and serious GI adverse events including bleeding, ulceration, and perforation of the stomach or intestines. Contraindicated for the treatment of perioperative pain in the setting of coronary artery bypass graft (CABG) surgery.

THERAPEUTIC CLASS: NSAID

INDICATIONS: Relief of signs and symptoms of osteoarthritis (OA) and rheumatoid arthritis (RA). Treatment of primary dysmenorrhea and relief of mild to moderate pain.

DOSAGE: *Adults:* OA: 100-150mg/day in divided doses, 50mg bid or tid. RA: 150-200mg/day in divided doses, 50mg tid or qid. Pain/Primary Dysmenorrhea: Initial: 50mg tid or 100mg on 1st dose, then 50mg on subsequent doses.

HOW SUPPLIED: Tab: 50mg

CONTRAINDICATIONS: ASA or other NSAID allergy that precipitates asthma, urticaria, or allergic reactions. Treatment of perioperative pain in the setting of CABG surgery.

WARNINGS/PRECAUTIONS: May lead to onset of new HTN or worsening of preexisting HTN; monitor BP closely. Fluid retention and edema reported; caution in patients with fluid retention or heart failure. Caution with history of ulcer disease or GI bleeding. Caution in patients with considerable dehydration. Renal papillary necrosis and other renal injury reported after long-term use. Caution with impaired renal function, heart failure, liver dysfunction, and the elderly. Not recommended for use with advanced renal disease; if therapy must be initiated, monitor renal function. May cause elevations of LFTs; d/c if liver disease develops or systemic manifestations occur. Anaphylactoid reactions may occur. May cause serious skin adverse events (eg, exfoliative dermatitis, Stevens-Johnson syndrome, toxic epidermal necrolysis). Avoid in late pregnancy; may cause premature closure of ductus arteriosis. Not a substitute for corticosteroids or for the treatment of corticosteroid insufficiency. Anemia may occur; with long-term use, monitor Hgb/Hct if signs or symptoms of anemia develop. May inhibit platelet aggregation and prolong bleeding time; monitor with coagulation disorders. Caution with asthma and avoid with ASA-sensitive asthma.

ADVERSE REACTIONS: Dyspepsia, constipation, diarrhea, GI ulceration/perforation, N/V, flatulence, abnormal renal function, anemia, dizziness, edema, elevated liver enzymes, headache, increased bleeding time, rash, tinnitus.

INTERACTIONS: Avoid use with ASA. May enhance methotrexate toxicity; caution when coadministering. May increase nephrotoxicity of cyclosporine; caution when coadministering. May diminish antihypertensive effect of ACE inhibitors. May reduce natriuretic effect of furosemide and thiazides; monitor for renal failure. May increase lithium levels; monitor for toxicity. Synergistic effects on GI bleeding with warfarin. Caution with hepatotoxic drugs (eg, antibiotics, anti-epileptics). Increase risk for GI bleeding with concomitant oral corticosteroids, anticoagulants, or alcohol. ACE inhibitors and diuretics may increase the risk of overt renal decompensation.

PREGNANCY: Category C, not for use in nursing.

MECHANISM OF ACTION: NSAID (benzeneacetic acid derivative); suspected to inhibit prostaglandin synthetase.

PHARMACOKINETICS: Absorption: Absolute bioavailabilty (55%), T_{max}=1 hr. **Distribution:** V_d=1.3L/kg; serum protein binding (>99%). **Metabolism**: Metabolites: 4'-hydroxy-, 5-hydroxy-,

3'-hydroxy-, 4',5-dihydroxy-, and 3'-hydroxy-4'-methoxy diclofenac. **Elimination:** Urine (65%), bile (35%); $T_{1/2}$=2 hrs.

NURSING CONSIDERATIONS

Assessment: Assess for history of a hypersensitivity reaction to aspirin or other NSAIDS, asthma, cardiovascular disease (eg, preexisting HTN, congestive heart failure) or risk factors for CVD, risk factors for a GI event (eg, prior history of ulcer disease or GI disease, smoking), fluid retention, renal/hepatic dysfunction, coagulation disorders, pregnancy/nursing status, and for possible drug interactions. Assess baseline LFTs, renal function, and CBC.

Monitoring: Monitor for signs/symptoms of CV thrombotic events, new onset or worsening of pre-existing HTN, GI events (eg, inflammation, bleeding, ulceration, perforation), fluid retention and edema, renal effects (eg, renal papillary necrosis), hepatic effects (eg, jaundice, liver necrosis, liver failure), anaphylactoid reactions, skin reactions (eg, exfoliative dermatitis, Stevens-Johnson syndrome, toxic epidermal necrolysis), hematological effects (eg, anemia, prolongation of bleeding time), and for bronchospasm. Monitor BP. Perform periodic monitoring of CBC, renal function, and LFTs.

Patient Counseling: Instruct to seek medical attention for symptoms of hepatotoxicity (eg, nausea, fatigue, jaundice), anaphylactic reactions (eg, difficulty breathing, swelling of the face/throat), rash, CV events (eg, chest pain, SOB, weakness, slurring of speech), or if unexplained weight gain or edema occur. Inform of risks if used during pregnancy.

Administration: Oral route. **Storage:** Do not store above 30°C (86°F). Dispense in tight container.

CATAPRES   RX
clonidine HCl (Boehringer Ingelheim)

OTHER BRAND NAMES: Catapres-TTS (Boehringer Ingelheim)

THERAPEUTIC CLASS: Alpha-adrenergic agonist

INDICATIONS: Treatment of HTN, alone or with other antihypertensives.

DOSAGE: *Adults:* Renal Impairment: Adjust according to the degree of impairment. (Patch) Apply to hairless, intact area of upper outer arm or chest once q7 days. Each new patch should be applied on different skin site from previous location. Initial: Adjust according to individual therapeutic requirements, starting with TTS-1. Titrate: If inadequate reduction in BP after 1-2 weeks, increase dosage by adding another TTS-1 or changing to a larger system. Max: 0.6mg/day. (Tab) Adjust dose according to patient's individual BP response. Initial: 0.1mg bid (am and hs). Maint: May increase by 0.1mg/day at weekly intervals PRN until desired response is achieved. Usual: 0.2-0.6mg/day in divided doses. Max: 2.4mg/day. Elderly: May benefit from lower end of dosing.

HOW SUPPLIED: Patch, Extended-Release (TTS): (TTS-1) 0.1mg, (TTS-2) 0.2mg, (TTS-3) 0.3mg; Tab: 0.1mg, 0.2mg, 0.3mg

WARNINGS/PRECAUTIONS: Avoid abrupt d/c; reduce dose gradually over 2 to 4 days to avoid withdrawal symptoms. Sudden cessation may cause nervousness, agitation, headache, (patch) confusion, and (tab) tremor accompanied or followed by a rapid rise in BP and elevated catecholamine concentrations. Rare instances of hypertensive encephalopathy, cerebrovascular accidents (CVA), and death reported after withdrawal. Substitution to PO may cause generalized skin rash and elicit an allergic reaction if with localized contact sensitization or allergic reaction to clonidine transdermal system. Caution with severe coronary insufficiency, conduction disturbances, recent myocardial infarction (MI), cerebrovascular disease, or chronic renal failure. Monitor BP during surgery; additional measures to control BP should be available. (Tab) Continue to within 4 hrs of surgery and resume as soon as possible thereafter. (Patch) Loss of BP control reported rarely. Do not remove during surgery. Remove before defibrillation or cardioconversion due to the potential risk of altered electrical conductivity, and before undergoing an MRI due to the occurrence of skin burns.

ADVERSE REACTIONS: Dry mouth, drowsiness, dizziness, constipation, sedation, fatigue, headache.

INTERACTIONS: May potentiate CNS depressive effects of alcohol, barbiturates, or other sedating drugs. Hypotensive effect reduced by TCAs; may need to increase clonidine dose. Monitor HR with agents that affect sinus node function or atrioventricular nodal conduction (eg, digitalis, calcium channel blockers, β-blockers). D/C β-blockers several days before the gradual withdrawal of clonidine in patients taking both. Reports of sinus bradycardia and pacemaker insertion with diltiazem or verapamil.

PREGNANCY: Category C, caution in nursing.

MECHANISM OF ACTION: Central acting α-agonist; stimulates α-adrenoreceptors in brain stem, reducing sympathetic outflow from CNS and decreasing peripheral resistance, renal vascular resistance, HR, and BP.

PHARMACOKINETICS: Absorption: (Tab) T_{max}=3-5 hrs. **Distribution:** Found in breast milk. **Metabolism:** Liver. **Elimination:** Urine (40-60%, unchanged); (Tab) $T_{1/2}$=12-16 hrs; (Patch) $T_{1/2}$=12.7 hrs.

NURSING CONSIDERATIONS

Assessment: Assess for severe coronary insufficiency, conduction disturbances, recent MI, cerebrovascular disease, renal impairment, allergic reactions/contact sensitization, pregnancy/ nursing status, and for possible drug interactions.

Monitoring: Monitor BP and renal function periodically. Monitor for withdrawal signs/symptoms (eg, hypertensive encephalopathy, CVA), presence of generalized skin rash, and allergic reactions.

Patient Counseling: Instruct to exercise caution against interruption of therapy without physician's advice. Advise patients who engage in potentially hazardous activities (eg, operating machinery, driving) of a possible sedative effect of the drug. Inform that sedative effect may be increased by concomitant use of alcohol, barbiturates, or other sedating drugs. Inform that medication may cause dryness of eyes; caution with contact lenses. (Patch) Instruct to seek medical attention promptly about possible need to remove patch due to adverse skin reactions. Inform that if patch begins to loosen, place adhesive cover directly over the patch to ensure adhesion for 7 days total. Advise to keep used and unused patch out of reach of children; fold in half with adhesive sides together and discard.

Administration: (Patch) Transdermal route; (Tab) oral route. **Storage:** (Tab) 25°C (77°F); excursions permitted to 15-30°C (59-86°F). (Patch) Below 30°C (86°F).

CAYSTON   RX
aztreonam (Gilead Sciences)

THERAPEUTIC CLASS: Monobactam

INDICATIONS: To improve respiratory symptoms in cystic fibrosis patients with *Pseudomonas aeruginosa*.

DOSAGE: *Adults*: 75mg tid administered via inhalation using an Altera Nebulizer System for 28 days followed by 28 days off therapy. Doses should be taken at least 4 hrs apart. Use bronchodilator before administration. Short-acting Bronchodilator: Give 15 min-4 hrs prior to each dose. Long-acting Bronchodilator: Give 30 min-12 hrs prior to each dose. Order of Administration if Taking Multiple Inhaled Therapies: Bronchodilator, mucolytics, aztreonam.
Pediatrics: ≥7 yrs: 75mg tid via inhalation using an Altera Nebulizer System for 28 days followed by 28 days of therapy. Doses should be taken at least 4 hrs apart. Use bronchodilator before administration. Short-acting Bronchodilator: Give 15 min-4 hrs prior to each dose. Long-acting Bronchodilator: Give 30 min-12 hrs prior to each dose. Order of Administration if Taking Multiple Inhaled Therapies: Bronchodilator, mucolytics, aztreonam.

HOW SUPPLIED: Sol: 75mg/mL

WARNINGS/PRECAUTIONS: Not for IV or IM administration. Severe allergic reactions reported; d/c if an allergic reaction occurs (eg, facial rash, facial swelling, throat tightness). Caution with beta-lactam allergy (eg, penicillins, cephalosporins, carbapenems), cross-reactivity may occur. Bronchospasm reported. Decreases in FEV_1 reported after 28-day treatment cycle; consider baseline FEV_1 prior to therapy and presence of other symptoms when evaluating whether posttreatment changes in FEV_1 are caused by a pulmonary exacerbation. May increase the risk of development of drug-resistant bacteria if given in the absence of known *P. aeruginosa* infection.

ADVERSE REACTIONS: Cough, nasal congestion, wheezing, pharyngolaryngeal pain, pyrexia, chest discomfort, abdominal pain, vomiting, bronchospasm.

PREGNANCY: Category B, safe in nursing.

MECHANISM OF ACTION: Monobactam; binds to penicillin-binding proteins of susceptible bacteria, which leads to inhibition of bacterial cell wall synthesis and death of the cell.

PHARMACOKINETICS: Absorption: C_{max}=0.55mcg/mL, 0.67mcg/mL, 0.65mcg/mL (Days 0, 14, and 28, respectively). **Distribution:** Plasma protein binding (56%); found in breastmilk; crosses the placenta. **Elimination:** Urine (10%, unchanged), feces (12%), $T_{1/2}$=2.1 hrs.

NURSING CONSIDERATIONS

Assessment: Assess for history of beta-lactam allergy and pregnancy/nursing status. Assess baseline FEV_1.

Monitoring: Monitor for signs/symptoms of an allergic reaction (eg, facial rash, facial swelling, throat tightness). Monitor for pulmonary exacerbations following the 28-day treatment cycle. Measure FEV_1.

Patient Counseling: Advise that therapy is for inhalation use only and therapy should only be administered using the Altera Nebulizer System. Reconstitute only with the diluent provided and not mix with other drugs in the nebulizer. Complete full 28-day course of therapy and take as directed, even if feeling better. Inform that if dose is missed, all 3 daily doses should be taken, as long as the doses are at least 4 hrs apart. Advise to use bronchodilator prior to administration and instruct to take medications in the following order: bronchodilator, mucolytics, aztreonam. Contact physician if an allergic reaction develops, new symptoms develop, or if symptoms worsen. Counsel that it should only be used to treat bacterial, not viral infections. Counsel that skipping dose and not completing therapy may decrease effectiveness of the treatment and may increase the likelihood that bacteria will develop resistance to the drug.

Administration: Inhalation route via Altera Nebulizer System. Do not administer with any other nebulizer and do not mix with any other drugs in the nebulizer. Administer immediately after re-constitution. See PI for reconstitution and administration details. **Storage:** 2-8°C (36-46°F). Once removed from refrigerator, store at 25°C (77°F) for up to 28 days. Protect from light.

CEFACLOR　　　　　　　　　　　　　　　　　　RX
cefaclor (Various)

THERAPEUTIC CLASS: Cephalosporin (2nd generation)

INDICATIONS: Treatment of otitis media, pharyngitis, tonsillitis, lower respiratory tract, urinary tract, and skin and skin structure infections caused by susceptible strains of microorganisms.

DOSAGE: *Adults:* Usual: 250mg q8h. Severe Infections/Pneumonia: 500mg q8h. Treat β-hemolytic strep for 10 days.
Pediatrics: ≥1 month: Usual: 20mg/kg/day given q8h. Otitis Media/Serious Infections/Infections Caused by Less Susceptible Organisms: 40mg/kg/day. Max: 1g/day. May administer q12h for otitis media and pharyngitis. Treat β-hemolytic strep for 10 days.

HOW SUPPLIED: Cap: 250mg, 500mg; Sus: 125mg/5mL [75mL, 150mL], 250mg/5mL [75mL, 150mL], 375mg/5mL [50mL, 100mL]

WARNINGS/PRECAUTIONS: Cross-sensitivity to penicillins (PCNs) and other cephalosporins may occur. *Clostridium difficile*-associated diarrhea (CDAD) reported. May result in bacterial resistance with prolonged use or use in the absence of a proven/suspected bacterial infection or a prophylactic indication; take appropriate measures if superinfection develops. Lab test interactions may occur. Caution with markedly impaired renal function, history of GI disease.

ADVERSE REACTIONS: Hypersensitivity reactions, diarrhea, eosinophilia, genital pruritus and vaginitis, serum-sickness-like reactions.

INTERACTIONS: Renal excretion inhibited by probenecid. May potentiate warfarin and other anticoagulants; monitor PT/INR.

PREGNANCY: Category B, caution in nursing.

MECHANISM OF ACTION: Cephalosporin; bactericidal agent, inhibits cell-wall synthesis.

PHARMACOKINETICS: Absorption: Well-absorbed; (Fasting): C_{max}=7mcg/mL (250mg), 13mcg (500mg), 23mcg (1g); T_{max}=30-60 min. **Elimination:** Urine (60-85% unchanged); $T_{1/2}$= 0.6-0.9 hrs.

NURSING CONSIDERATIONS

Assessment: Assess for hypersensitivity reactions to cephalosporins, PCNs and other drugs; pregnancy/nursing status; renal function; and possible drug interactions.

Monitoring: Monitor for anaphylactic reactions, CDAD, superinfection, drug resistance, positive Coombs' test, and increased anticoagulant effect when used concomitantly with anticoagulants.

Patient Counseling: Inform drug only treats bacterial, not viral, infections. Take exactly as directed; skipping doses or not completing full course may decrease effectiveness and increase resistance. Inform about potential benefits/risks. D/C and notify physician if experience allergic reaction or watery/bloody diarrhea (with/without muscle cramps and fever) as late as 2 months after treatment end. Notify if pregnant/nursing.

Administration: Oral route. **Storage:** 20-25°C (68-77°F).

CEFACLOR ER　　　　　　　　　　　　　　　　RX
cefaclor (Various)

THERAPEUTIC CLASS: Cephalosporin (2nd generation)

INDICATIONS: Treatment of the following mild to moderate infections: acute bacterial exacerbations of chronic bronchitis (ABECB), secondary bacterial infections of acute bronchitis, pharyngitis, tonsillitis, and uncomplicated skin and skin structure infections (SSSI) caused by susceptible strains of microorganisms.

DOSAGE: *Adults:* ≥16 yrs: ABECB/Acute Bronchitis: 500mg q12h for 7 days. Pharyngitis/Tonsillitis: 375mg q12h for 10 days. SSSI: 375mg q12h for 7-10 days. Take with meals.

HOW SUPPLIED: Tab, Extended-Release: 500mg

WARNINGS/PRECAUTIONS: Cross-sensitivity among beta-lactam antibiotics reported; caution with penicillin allergy. D/C if allergic reaction occurs and institute appropriate therapy. *Clostridium difficile* associated diarrhea (CDAD) reported. May result in bacterial resistance with prolonged use or use in the absence of a proven/suspected bacterial infection or a prophylactic indication; take appropriate measures if superinfection develops. Lab test interactions may occur.

ADVERSE REACTIONS: Headache, rhinitis, diarrhea, nausea.

INTERACTIONS: Decreased absorption with magnesium or aluminum hydroxide-containing antacids. Renal excretion inhibited by probenecid. Concomitant use with warfarin may increase PT.

PREGNANCY: Category B, caution in nursing.

MECHANISM OF ACTION: Cephalosporin; bactericidal, inhibits cell-wall synthesis.

PHARMACOKINETICS: Absorption: Fed: (375mg) C_{max}=3.7mcg/mL, T_{max}=2.7 hrs, AUC=9.9mcg•hr/mL. (500mg) C_{max}=8.2mcg/mL, T_{max}=2.5 hrs, AUC=18.1mcg•hr/mL. Fasting: (500mg) C_{max}=5.4mcg/mL, T_{max}=1.5 hrs, AUC=14.8mcg•hr/mL. **Distribution:** Found in breast milk. **Elimination:** $T_{1/2}$=1 hr.

NURSING CONSIDERATIONS

Assessment: Assess for hypersensitivity reactions to the drug, cephalosporins, penicillins, and other drugs, pregnancy/nursing status, and possible drug interactions. Perform appropriate culture and susceptibility tests for diagnosis and identification of causative organisms.

Monitoring: Monitor for allergic reactions, CDAD, superinfection, and drug resistance.

Patient Counseling: Take exactly as directed; skipping doses or not completing full course may decrease effectiveness and increase resistance. Inform that diarrhea may occur; usually ends once treatment is completed. Notify physician as soon as possible if watery and bloody stools (with/without stomach cramps and fever) develop, even as late as ≥2 months after taking last dose.

Administration: Oral route. Take with meals (within 1 hr of eating). Do not crush, cut, or chew tab. **Storage:** 20-25°C (68-77°F). Store in a tight, light-resistant container.

CEFADROXIL   RX
cefadroxil monohydrate (Various)

THERAPEUTIC CLASS: Cephalosporin (1st generation)

INDICATIONS: Treatment of urinary tract infections (UTI), skin and skin structure infections (SSSI), pharyngitis and/or tonsillitis caused by susceptible strains of microorganisms.

DOSAGE: *Adults:* Uncomplicated Lower UTI: Usual: 1-2g/day given qd or bid. Other UTI: Usual: 2g/day in divided doses (bid). SSSI: Usual: 1g/day once qd or bid. Group A β-hemolytic Strep Pharyngitis/Tonsillitis: 1g/day given qd or bid for 10 days. CrCl ≤50mL/min: Initial: 1g. Maint: CrCl 25-50mL/min: 500mg q12h; CrCl 10-25mL/min: 500mg q24h; CrCl 0-10mL/min: 500mg q36h.
Pediatrics: UTI/SSSI: Usual: 30mg/kg/day in equally divided doses q12h. Pharyngitis/Tonsillitis/Impetigo: Usual: 30mg/kg/day in a single dose or in equally divided doses q12h. Treat β-hemolytic strep infections for at least 10 days. Refer to PI for daily dosage of PO sus.

HOW SUPPLIED: Cap: 500mg; Sus: 250mg/5mL [50mL, 100mL], 500mg/5mL [50mL, 75mL, 100mL]; Tab: 1g

WARNINGS/PRECAUTIONS: Caution in penicillin (PCN)-sensitive patients; cross-sensitivity among β-lactam antibiotics may occur. D/C if an allergic reaction occurs. Serious acute hypersensitivity reactions may require treatment with epinephrine and other emergency measures. *Clostridium difficile*-associated diarrhea (CDAD) reported. May result in bacterial resistance with prolonged use or use in the absence of a proven/suspected bacterial infection or a prophylactic indication; take appropriate measures if superinfection develops. Caution with renal impairment (CrCl <50mL/min/1.73 m²); monitor prior to and during therapy with known/suspected renal impairment. Caution with history of GI disease (particularly colitis). Lab test interactions may occur. Caution in elderly.

ADVERSE REACTIONS: Diarrhea, allergies, hepatic dysfunction, genital moniliasis, vaginitis, moderate transient neutropenia, fever, toxic epidermal necrolysis, abdominal pain, superinfection, renal dysfunction, toxic nephropathy, aplastic anemia, hemolytic anemia, hemorrhage.

PREGNANCY: Category B, caution in nursing.

MECHANISM OF ACTION: Cephalosporin; bactericidal due to inhibition of cell-wall synthesis.

PHARMACOKINETICS: Absorption: Rapid. C_{max}=16mcg/mL (500mg), 28mcg/mL (1000mg). **Elimination:** Urine (90% unchanged).

NURSING CONSIDERATIONS

Assessment: Assess for history of hypersensitivity to the drug or PCNs, renal impairment, history of GI disease, and pregnancy/nursing status. Initiate culture and susceptibility tests prior to therapy.

Monitoring: Monitor for signs/symptoms of an allergic reaction, CDAD, and superinfection. Monitor renal function (when indicated) and perform culture and susceptibility tests during therapy.

Patient Counseling: Instruct to take exactly ud; skipping doses or not completing full course may decrease effectiveness and increase bacterial resistance. Inform that diarrhea is a common problem and usually ends when antibiotic is d/c. Advise that watery and bloody stools (with or without stomach cramps and fever) may develop even as late as ≥2 months after last dose; notify physician as soon as possible if occurs.

Administration: Oral route. (Sus) Refer to PI for reconstitution directions. Shake well before use. **Storage:** 20-25°C (68-77°F). (Sus) After Reconstitution: Store in refrigerator; discard unused portion after 14 days. Keep container tightly closed.

CEFAZOLIN   RX
cefazolin sodium (Various)

THERAPEUTIC CLASS: Cephalosporin (1st generation)

INDICATIONS: Treatment of respiratory tract, urinary tract (UTI), skin and skin structure, biliary tract, bone and joint, and genital infections, septicemia, and endocarditis caused by susceptible strains of microorganisms. Perioperative prophylaxis for surgical procedures classified as contaminated or potentially contaminated.

DOSAGE: *Adults:* Moderate to Severe Infections: 500mg-1g q6-8h. Mild Gram-Positive Cocci Infection: 250-500mg q8h. Acute, Uncomplicated UTI: 1g q12h. Pneumococcal Pneumonia: 500mg q12h. Severe Life-Threatening Infection (eg, Endocarditis, Septicemia): 1-1.5g q6h; Max: 12g/day (rare). Perioperative Prophylaxis: 1g IV 0.5-1 hr before surgery. For Procedures ≥2 hrs: 500mg-1g IV during surgery. Maint: 500mg-1g IV q6-8h for 24 hrs postop. Continue for 3-5 days post-op for devastating procedures (eg, open-heart surgery, prosthetic arthroplasty). Renal Impairment: CrCl 35-54mL/min or SrCr of 1.6-3mg/dL: Full dose q8h. CrCl 11-34mL/min or SrCr of 3.1-4.5mg/dL: 1/2 usual dose q12h. CrCl ≤10mL/min or SrCr of ≥4.6mg/dL: 1/2 usual dose q18-24h. Apply reduced dosage recommendations after initial LD is given.
Pediatrics: >1 month: Mild to Moderately Severe Infections: 25-50mg/kg/day, given tid or qid. Titrate: May increase to 100mg/kg/day for severe infections. Renal Impairment: CrCl 40-70mL/min: 60% of normal daily dose given in equally divided doses every 12 hrs. CrCl 20-40mL/min: 25% of normal daily dose given in equally divided doses every 12 hrs. CrCl 5-20mL/min: 10% of normal daily dose every 24 hrs. Apply reduced dosage recommendations after initial LD is given.

HOW SUPPLIED: Inj: 500mg, 1g, 10g, 20g

WARNINGS/PRECAUTIONS: Caution with penicillin (PCN) allergy; possible cross-hypersensitivity among β-lactam antibiotics. D/C if an allergic reaction develops. *Clostridium difficile*-associated diarrhea (CDAD) reported. May result in bacterial resistance with prolonged use or use in the absence of a proven/suspected bacterial infection or a prophylactic indication; take appropriate measures if superinfection develops. Seizures may occur if inappropriately high doses are administered to patients with renal impairment. Caution with history of colitis or other GI diseases. Safety in premature infants and neonates not established. Lab test interactions may occur. May cause a fall in prothrombin activity; caution in patients with renal/hepatic impairment or poor nutrional state, patients on protracted course of antimicrobial therapy, and in patients previously stabilized on anticoagulant therapy; monitor PT and administer vitamin K as indicated.

ADVERSE REACTIONS: Diarrhea, oral candidiasis, N/V, stomach cramps, anorexia, allergic reactions, blood dyscrasias, renal failure, transient rise in AST/ALT/BUN/SrCr/alkaline phosphatase, genital and anal pruritus.

INTERACTIONS: Decreased renal tubular secretion with probenecid.

PREGNANCY: Category B, caution in nursing.

MECHANISM OF ACTION: Cephalosporin; inhibits cell wall synthesis.

PHARMACOKINETICS: Absorption: C_{max}=185mcg/mL. **Distribution:** Crosses placenta; found in breast milk. **Elimination:** Urine (unchanged); $T_{1/2}$=1.8 hrs.

NURSING CONSIDERATIONS

Assessment: Assess for hypersensitivity to PCN, renal/hepatic impairment, history of GI disease (eg, colitis), nutritional status, pregnancy/nursing status, and possible drug interactions.

Monitoring: Monitor for signs/symptoms of a hypersensitivity reaction, CDAD, drug resistance or superinfection. Monitor PT in patients at risk of a fall in prothrombin activity. Monitor for seizures in patients with renal dysfunction.

Patient Counseling: Inform drug only treats bacterial, not viral, infections. Instruct to take as directed; skipping doses or not completing full course may decrease effectiveness and increase resistance. Advise to d/c therapy and notify physician if an allergic reaction or diarrhea occurs. Instruct to notify if pregnant/nursing.

Administration: IV route. **Storage:** -20°C (-4°F). Do not force thaw by immersion in water baths or by microwave irridiation. Thawed solution is stable for 30 days under refrigeration 5°C (41°F) and for 48 hrs at 25°C (77°F). Do not refreeze thawed antibiotics.

CEFDINIR   RX
cefdinir (Various)

THERAPEUTIC CLASS: Cephalosporin (3rd generation)

INDICATIONS: Community-acquired pneumonia (CAP), acute exacerbations of chronic bronchitis (AECB), acute maxillary sinusitis, pharyngitis/tonsillitis, and uncomplicated skin and skin structure infections (SSSIs) in adult and adolescent patients. Acute bacterial otitis media, pharyngitis/tonsillitis, and uncomplicated SSSIs in pediatric patients.

DOSAGE: *Adults:* (Cap) SSSI/CAP: 300mg q12h for 10 days. AECB/Pharyngitis/Tonsillitis: 300mg q12h for 5-10 days or 600mg q24h for 10 days. Sinusitis: 300mg q12h or 600mg q24h for 10 days. CrCl <30mL/min: 300mg qd. Hemodialysis: Initial: 300mg or 7mg/kg qod. 300mg or 7mg/kg should be given at end of each hemodialysis session. Usual: 300mg or 7mg/kg qod. *Pediatrics:* (Sus) ≥43 kg: Max dose: 600mg/day. 6 months-12 yrs: Otitis Media/Pharyngitis/Tonsillitis: 7mg/kg q12h for 5-10 days or 14mg/kg q24h for 10 days. Sinusitis: 7mg/kg q12h or 14mg/kg q24h for 10 days. SSSI: 7mg/kg q12h for 10 days. (Cap) ≥13 yrs: CAP/SSSI: 300mg q12h for 10 days. AECB/Pharyngitis/Tonsillitis: 300mg q12h for 5-10 days or 600mg q24h for 10 days. Sinusitis: 300mg q12h or 600mg q24h for 10 days. CrCl <30mL/min/1.73m²: 7mg/kg qd. Max: 300mg qd.

HOW SUPPLIED: Cap: 300mg; Sus: 125mg/5mL, 250mg/5mL [60mL, 100mL]

WARNINGS/PRECAUTIONS: Cross-sensitivity to penicillins (PCNs) and other cephalosporins may occur. D/C use if an allergic reaction occurs. *Clostridium difficile*-associated diarrhea (CDAD) has been reported. May result in bacterial resistance with prolonged use or use in the absence of a proven/suspected bacterial infection or a prophylactic indication; take appropriate measures if superinfection develops. Reduce dose in patients with transient or persistent renal insufficiency (CrCl <30mL/min). Caution in patients with a history of colitis. Sus contains sucrose; caution in diabetes. Lab test abnormalities may occur.

ADVERSE REACTIONS: Diarrhea, vaginal moniliasis, nausea.

INTERACTIONS: Iron-fortified foods, iron supplements, and aluminum- or magnesium-containing antacids reduce absorption; separate doses by 2 hrs. Probenecid inhibits the renal excretion. Reddish stools reported with iron-containing products. Possible interaction between cefdinir and diclofenac.

PREGNANCY: Category B, safe in nursing.

MECHANISM OF ACTION: Extended-spectrum cephalosporin; bactericidal activity from inhibition of cell-wall synthesis.

PHARMACOKINETICS: Absorption: Cap: (300mg) C_{max}=1.6mcg/mL, T_{max}=2.9 hrs, AUC=7.05mcg•hr/mL. (600mg) C_{max}=2.87mcg/mL, T_{max}=3 hrs, AUC=11.1mcg•hr/mL. Sus: (7mg/kg) C_{max}=2.3mcg/mL, T_{max}=2.2 hrs, AUC=8.31mcg•hr/mL. (14mg/kg) C_{max}=3.86mcg/mL, T_{max}=1.8 hrs, AUC=13.4mcg•hr/mL. **Distribution:** V_d=0.35L/kg (adults), 0.67L/kg (pediatrics); plasma protein binding (60-70%). **Elimination:** (300mg) Urine (18.4% unchanged); (600mg) Urine (11.6% unchanged); $T_{1/2}$=1.7 hrs.

NURSING CONSIDERATIONS

Assessment: Assess for allergy to other cephalosporins, PCN, or to other drugs, history of colitis, renal impairment, and for possible drug interactions. Assess for diabetes if planning to use sus formulation. Assess proper diagnosis of causative organisms.

C

Monitoring: Monitor for signs/symptoms of hypersensitivity reactions, CDAD, and for development of a superinfection.

Patient Counseling: Treats bacterial, not viral, infections. Take as directed; skipping doses or not completing full course may decrease effectiveness and increase bacterial resistance. Take 2 hrs before or after antacid or iron supplements. Inform diabetics that sus contains sucrose. Diarrhea may occur; notify physician if watery/bloody stools, superinfection, or hypersensitivity reactions occur.

Administration: Oral route. **Storage:** Cap/Unsuspended Powder: 25°C (77°F); excursions permitted to 15-30°C (59-86°F). Reconstituted Sus: Can be stored at controlled room temperature for 10 days.

CEFEPIME   RX
cefepime HCl (Sandoz)

THERAPEUTIC CLASS: Cephalosporin (4th generation)

INDICATIONS: Treatment of uncomplicated/complicated urinary tract infections (UTI) including pyelonephritis, uncomplicated skin and skin structure infections (SSSI), complicated intra-abdominal infections (in combination with metronidazole), pneumonia (moderate to severe), and empirical therapy for febrile neutropenia caused by susceptible strains of microorganisms.

DOSAGE: *Adults:* When giving IV, infuse over 30 min. Moderate-Severe Pneumonia: 1-2g IV q12h for 10 days. Febrile Neutropenia: 2g IV q8h for 7 days or until neutropenia resolves. Mild-Moderate UTI: 0.5-1g IM/IV q12h for 7-10 days. Severe UTI /Moderate-Severe Uncomplicated SSSI: 2g IV q12h for 10 days. Complicated Intra-Abdominal Infections: 2g IV q12h for 7-10 days. Renal Impairment: Refer to PI for recommended dosing.
Pediatrics: 2 months-16 yrs: ≤40kg: When giving IV, infuse over 30 min. UTI /Uncomplicated SSSI/Pneumonia: 50mg/kg/dose q12h. Severe UTI/Pneumonia/SSSI: Give IV for 10 days. Mild-Moderate UTI: Give IM/IV for 7-10 days. Febrile Neutropenia: 50mg/kg/dose IV q8h for 7 days until neutropenia resolves. Max: Do not exceed the recommended adult dose.

HOW SUPPLIED: Inj: 500mg, 1g, 2g; 1g/50mL, 2g/100mL [Galaxy]

CONTRAINDICATIONS: Hypersensitivity to penicillins (PCNs) or other β-lactam antibiotics.

WARNINGS/PRECAUTIONS: Caution with PCN sensitivity; cross hypersensitivity among β-lactam antibiotics may occur. D/C if an allergic reaction occurs. Caution with renal impairment; maint dose reduction may be needed. Encephalopathy, myoclonus, seizures, and *Clostridium difficile*-associated diarrhea (CDAD) reported. May result in overgrowth of nonsusceptible organisms with prolonged use; take appropriate measures if superinfection develops. Use in the absence of a proven or strongly suspected bacterial infection or prophylactic indication is unlikely to provide benefit and increases the risk of development of drug-resistant bacteria. May cause a fall in prothrombin activity; caution in patients with renal or hepatic impairment, or poor nutritional state, and in patients on a protracted course of antimicrobials. Monitor PT in patients at risk and administer vitamin K as indicated. Positive direct Coombs' tests reported. Caution with history of GI disease, especially colitis. May result a false-positive reaction for glucose in the urine with Clinitest tabs. Caution in elderly.

ADVERSE REACTIONS: Local reactions, rash, diarrhea, positive Coombs' test without hemolysis.

INTERACTIONS: Increased risk of nephrotoxicity and ototoxicity with high doses of aminoglycosides; monitor renal function. Risk of nephrotoxicity with potent diuretics (eg, furosemide).

PREGNANCY: Category B, caution in nursing.

MECHANISM OF ACTION: Cephalosporin (4th generation); bactericidal agent that acts by inhibiting cell wall synthesis.

PHARMACOKINETICS: Absorption: Complete (IM). (IV/IM) Administration of variable doses resulted in different parameters. **Distribution:** V_d=18L; plasma protein binding (20%); found in breastmilk. **Metabolism:** Metabolized to N-methylpyrrolidine (NMP), which is rapidly converted to the N-oxide (NMP-N-oxide). **Elimination:** Urine (85% unchanged, <1% NMP, 6.8% NMP-N-oxide); $T_{1/2}$=2 hrs.

NURSING CONSIDERATIONS

Assessment: Assess for PCN allergy, nutritional status, history of GI disease, renal/hepatic impairment, pregnancy/nursing status, and for possible drug interactions. Document indications for therapy with culture and susceptibility testing.

Monitoring: Monitor for signs/symptoms of hypersensitivity reactions (anaphylaxis), CDAD, superinfection, encephalopathy, myoclonus, and seizures. Monitor PT in patients at risk. Monitor renal function.

Patient Counseling: Inform that drug treats only bacterial, not viral infections (eg, common colds). Instruct to take as directed; inform that skipping doses or not completing full course of therapy may decrease effectiveness and increase the risk of bacterial resistance. Inform patients that diarrhea, encephalopathy, myoclonus, and seizures may occur. Instruct to contact physician if watery/bloody stools (with/without stomach cramps and fever), hypersensitivity reactions, or neurological signs/symptoms (eg, confusion, hallucinations, stupor, or coma) occur.

Administration: IV/IM route. Refer to PI for administration instructions. **Storage:** 2-25°C (36-77°F). Protect from light. (Galaxy) ≤-20°C (-4°F). Thawed solution stable for 7 days at 5°C (41°F) or 24 hrs at 25°C (77°F). Do not refreeze. Refer to PI for storage information of reconstituted solution.

CEFOXITIN   RX
cefoxitin sodium (Various)

THERAPEUTIC CLASS: Cephalosporin (2nd generation)

INDICATIONS: Treatment of lower respiratory tract/urinary tract/intra-abdominal/gynecological/skin and skin structure/bone and joint infections and septicemia caused by susceptible strains of microorganisms. Prophylaxis in patients undergoing uncontaminated GI surgery, abdominal/vaginal hysterectomy, or cesarean section (CS).

DOSAGE: *Adults:* Usual: 1-2g IV q6-8h. Uncomplicated Infections: 1g IV q6-8h. Moderate-Severe Infections: 1g IV q4h or 2g IV q6-8h. Gas Gangrene/Other Infections Requiring Higher Dose: 2g IV q4h or 3g IV q6h. Renal Insufficiency: LD: 1-2g IV. Maint: CrCl 30-50mL/min: 1-2g IV q8-12h. CrCl 10-29mL/min: 1-2g IV q12-24h. CrCl 5-9mL/min: 0.5-1g IV q12-24h. CrCl <5mL/min: 0.5-1g IV q24-48h. Hemodialysis: LD: 1-2g IV after dialysis. Maint: See renal insufficiency doses above. Group A β-Hemolytic Streptococcal Infection: Maintain therapy ≥10 days. Prophylaxis: Uncontaminated GI Surgery/Hysterectomy: 2g IV prior to surgery (1/2-1 hr before initial incision), then 2g IV q6h after 1st dose ≤24 hrs. CS: 2g IV single dose as soon as umbilical cord is clamped, or 2g IV as soon as umbilical cord is clamped, followed by 2g IV at 4 and 8 hrs after initial dose. *Pediatrics:* ≥3 months: 80-160mg/kg/day divided into 4-6 equal doses. Max: 12g/day. Renal Insufficiency: Modify dosage and frequency of dosage consistent with recommendations for adults. Prophylaxis: Uncontaminated GI Surgery/Hysterectomy: 30-40mg/kg IV prior to surgery (1/2-1 hr before initial incision), then 30-40mg/kg IV q6h after 1st dose ≤24 hrs.

HOW SUPPLIED: Inj: 1g, 2g. Also available as a Duplex and Pharmacy Bulk Package; refer to individual PI.

WARNINGS/PRECAUTIONS: Caution with previous hypersensitivity to cephalosporins, penicillins (PCNs), or other drugs. D/C if allergic reaction occurs. *Clostridium difficile*-associated diarrhea (CDAD) reported. May result in bacterial resistance with prolonged use or use in the absence of a proven/suspected bacterial infection or a prophylactic indication; take appropriate measures if superinfection develops. Lab test interactions may occur.

ADVERSE REACTIONS: Thrombophlebitis, rash, pseudomembranous colitis, pruritus, fever, dyspnea, hypotension, diarrhea, blood dyscrasias, elevated LFTs, changes in renal function tests, exacerbation of myasthenia gravis.

INTERACTIONS: Increased nephrotoxicity with aminoglycoside antibiotics.

PREGNANCY: Category B, caution in nursing.

MECHANISM OF ACTION: 2nd-generation cephalosporin; inhibits bacterial cell-wall synthesis.

PHARMACOKINETICS: Distribution: Passes pleural and joint fluids; found in breast milk. **Elimination:** Urine (85% unchanged); $T_{1/2}$=41-59 min.

NURSING CONSIDERATIONS

Assessment: Assess for previous hypersensitivity reactions to cephalosporins, PCNs, or other drugs, renal/hepatic function, GI disease, pregnancy/nursing status, and possible drug interactions. Perform appropriate culture and susceptibility studies to determine susceptible causative organisms.

Monitoring: Periodically monitor renal/hepatic/hematopoietic functions, especially with prolonged therapy. Monitor for CDAD (may range from mild diarrhea to fatal colitis), development of superinfections or drug resistance, allergic reactions (eg, toxic epidermal necrolysis or exfoliative dermatitis), and other adverse reactions. Monitor LFTs.

Patient Counseling: Inform that drug only treats bacterial, not viral infections. Instruct to take exactly as directed; skipping doses or not completing full course may decrease effectiveness and increase resistance. Inform about potential benefits/risks. Advise to notify physician if watery/bloody stools (with/without muscle cramps or fever) occurs even ≥2 months after therapy. Notify if pregnant/nursing.

Administration: IV route. Inspect for particulate matter and discoloration prior to use. Refer to PI for preparation, administration, and compatibility and stability instructions. **Storage:** Dry state at 2-25°C (36-77°F). Avoid >50°C. Reconstituted in vial: Satisfactory potency at room temperature for 6 hrs; <5°C for 1 wk. Diluted Sol: Room temperature for 18 hrs; 48 hrs under refrigeration.

CEFPODOXIME

RX

cefpodoxime proxetil (Various)

THERAPEUTIC CLASS: Cephalosporin (3rd generation)

INDICATIONS: Treatment of mild to moderate infections (acute otitis media, pharyngitis/tonsillitis, community-acquired pneumonia [CAP], acute bacterial exacerbation of chronic bronchitis [ABECB], acute uncomplicated urethral and cervical gonorrhea, acute uncomplicated anorectal infections in women, uncomplicated skin and skin structure infections [SSSI], acute maxillary sinusitis, and uncomplicated urinary tract infections [cystitis]) caused by susceptible strains of microorganisms.

DOSAGE: *Adults:* Pharyngitis/Tonsillitis: 100mg q12h for 5-10 days. CAP: 200mg q12h for 14 days. ABECB: 200mg q12h for 10 days. Uncomplicated Gonorrhea (Men/Women)/Rectal Gonococcal Infections (Women): 200mg single dose. SSSI: 400mg q12h for 7-14 days. Sinusitis: 200mg q12h for 10 days. Cystitis: 100mg q12h for 7 days. CrCl <30mL/min: Increase interval to q24h. Hemodialysis: Dose 3 times weekly after dialysis. Take with food.
Pediatrics: ≥12 yrs: (Susp/Tabs): Pharyngitis/Tonsillitis: 100mg q12h for 5-10 days. CAP: 200mg q12h for 14 days. Uncomplicated Gonorrhea (Men/Women)/Rectal Gonococcal Infections (Women): 200mg single dose. SSSI: 400mg q12h for 7-14 days. Sinusitis: 200mg q12h for 10 days. Cystitis: 100mg q12h for 7 days. (Tabs) ABECB: 200mg q12h for 10 days. 2 months to 12 yrs: (Susp): Otitis media: 5mg/kg (Max 200mg/dose) q12h for 5 days. Pharyngitis/Tonsillitis: 5mg/kg/dose (Max 100mg/dose) q12h for 5-10 days. Sinusitis: 5mg/kg (Max 200mg/dose) for 10 days. CrCl <30mL/min: Increase interval to q24h. Hemodialysis: Dose 3 times weekly after dialysis. Take with food.

HOW SUPPLIED: Sus: 50mg/5mL, 100mg/5mL; Tab: 100mg, 200mg

WARNINGS/PRECAUTIONS: Caution with penicillin (PCN)-sensitive patients; cross hypersensitivity reaction may occur; d/c if an allergic reaction occurs. *Clostridium difficile*-associated diarrhea (CDAD) reported. Pseudomembranous colitis reported. Reduce dose with renal impairment. May result in bacterial resistance with prolonged use or use in the absence of a proven/suspected bacterial infection or a prophylactic indication; take appropriate measures if superinfection develops. Lab test interactions may occur. Oral sus may contain phenylalanine. Tabs may contain tartrazine which may cause an allergic reaction in susceptible individuals.

ADVERSE REACTIONS: Diarrhea, nausea.

INTERACTIONS: Decreased plasma levels and extent of absorption with antacids and H_2-blockers. Delayed peak plasma levels with oral anticholinergics. Probenecid inhibits renal excretion. Closely monitor renal function with nephrotoxic agents. Caution with potent diuretics.

PREGNANCY: Category B, not for use in nursing.

MECHANISM OF ACTION: Cephalosporin; inhibits cell-wall synthesis.

PHARMACOKINETICS: Absorption: C_{max}(100mg)=1.4mcg/mL, (200mg)=2.3mcg/mL, (400mg)=3.9mcg/mL; T_{max}=2-3 hrs. **Distribution:** Plasma protein binding (21-29%), found in breast milk. **Metabolism:** Via desterification; cefpodoxime (active metabolite). **Elimination:** Urine; $T_{1/2}$= 2.09-2.84 hrs.

NURSING CONSIDERATIONS

Assessment: Assess for history of hypersensitivity to cephalosporins/PCNs, renal impairment, pregnancy/nursing status, and for possible drug interactions. Document indications for therapy, culture, and susceptibility testing.

Monitoring: Monitor for signs/symptoms of hypersensitivity reactions, CDAD, pseudomembranous colitis, and for superinfection. Monitor renal function.

Patient Counseling: Inform that drug only treats bacterial, not viral infections. Instruct to take as directed; inform that skipping doses or not completing full course of therapy may decrease effectiveness of immediate treatment and increase resistance to drug. Inform that may experience diarrhea; instruct to contact physician if watery/bloody stools develop.

Administration: Oral route. **Storage:** Sus (Prior to reconstitution)/Tab: 20-25°C (68-77°F). Sus (Following reconstitution) 2-8°C (36-46°F). Shake well before using. Keep tightly closed. May be used for 14 days; discard unused portion after 14 days. (Tab) Protect from excessive moisture.

CEFPROZIL

RX

cefprozil (Various)

THERAPEUTIC CLASS: Cephalosporin (2nd generation)

INDICATIONS: Treatment of mild to moderate pharyngitis/tonsillitis, otitis media, acute sinusitis, secondary bacterial infection of acute bronchitis, acute bacterial exacerbation of chronic bronchitis (ABECB), and uncomplicated skin and skin structure infections (SSSI) caused by susceptible strains of microorganisms.

DOSAGE: *Adults:* Pharyngitis/Tonsillitis: 500mg q24h for 10 days. Acute Sinusitis: 250-500mg q12h for 10 days. ABECB/Acute Bronchitis: 500mg q12h for 10 days. SSSI: 250-500mg q12h or 500mg q24h for 10 days. CrCl <30mL/min: 50% of standard dose.
Pediatrics: ≥13 yrs: Use adult dose. 2-12 yrs: Pharyngitis/Tonsillitis: 7.5mg/kg q12h for 10 days. SSSI: 20mg/kg q24h for 10 days. 6 months-12 yrs: Otitis Media: 15mg/kg q12h for 10 days. Acute Sinusitis: 7.5-15mg/kg q12h for 10 days. Do not exceed adult dose. CrCl <30mL/min: 50% of standard dose.

HOW SUPPLIED: Sus: 125mg/5mL, 250mg/5mL [50mL, 75mL, 100mL]; Tab: 250mg, 500mg

WARNINGS/PRECAUTIONS: Caution with previous hypersensitivity to cephalosporins, penicillins (PCNs), or other drugs; cross-sensitivity may occur with history of PCN allergy. D/C if allergic reaction occurs. *Clostridium difficile*-associated diarrhea (CDAD) reported. May result in bacterial resistance with prolonged use or use in the absence of a proven/suspected bacterial infection or a prophylactic indication; take appropriate measures if superinfection develops. Caution with GI disease, particularly colitis. Caution with renal impairment and elderly. Lab test interactions may occur.

ADVERSE REACTIONS: Diarrhea, N/V, ALT/AST elevation, eosinophilia, genital pruritus, vaginitis, superinfection, diaper rash, dizziness, abdominal pain.

INTERACTIONS: Nephrotoxicity with aminoglycosides reported. Probenecid may increase plasma levels. Caution with potent diuretics.

PREGNANCY: Category B, caution in nursing.

MECHANISM OF ACTION: 2nd-generation cephalosporin; inhibits bacterial cell-wall synthesis.

PHARMACOKINETICS: Absorption: C_{max}=6.1mcg/mL (250mg), 10.5mcg/mL (500mg), 18.3mcg/mL (1g); T_{max}=1.5 hrs (adults), 1-2 hrs (peds). Plasma concentration (peds) at 7.5, 15, and 30mg/kg doses similar to those observed within same time frame in normal adults at 250, 500, and 1000mg doses, respectively. **Distribution:** V_d=0.23L/kg; plasma protein binding (36%); found in breast milk. **Elimination:** Urine (60%); $T_{1/2}$=1.3 hrs (adults), 1.5 hrs (peds).

NURSING CONSIDERATIONS

Assessment: Assess for previous hypersensitivity reactions to PCNs/cephalosporins or other drugs, renal/hepatic function, GI disease, pregnancy/nursing status, and possible drug interactions. Perform appropriate culture and susceptibility studies to determine susceptible causative organisms.

Monitoring: Periodically monitor renal/hepatic/hematopoietic functions. Monitor for CDAD (may range from mild diarrhea to fatal colitis), development of superinfections or drug resistance, allergic reactions, and other adverse reactions.

Patient Counseling: Inform that the oral sus contains phenylalanine. Inform that drug only treats bacterial, not viral infections. Instruct to take exactly as directed; skipping doses or not completing full course may decrease effectiveness and increase resistance. Inform about potential benefits/risks. Notify physician if watery/bloody stools (with/without stomach cramps/fever) occur even ≥2 months after therapy. Notify if pregnant/nursing.

Administration: Oral route. Shake sus well before use. Refer to PI for reconstitution direction.
Storage: Tab/Dry Powder: 20-25°C (68-77°F). Reconstituted Sus: Refrigerate after mixing and discard unused portion after 14 days.

CEFTIN   RX
cefuroxime axetil (GlaxoSmithKline)

THERAPEUTIC CLASS: Cephalosporin (2nd generation)

INDICATIONS: Treatment of the following infections caused by susceptible strains of microorganisms: (Sus/Tab) Pharyngitis/tonsillitis and acute otitis media. (Sus) Impetigo. (Tab) Uncomplicated skin and skin structure infections (SSSI), uncomplicated urinary tract infections (UTI), uncomplicated gonorrhea, early Lyme disease, acute bacterial maxillary sinusitis, acute bacterial exacerbations of chronic bronchitis (ABECB), and secondary bacterial infections of acute bronchitis.

DOSAGE: *Adults:* (Tab) Pharyngitis/Tonsillitis/Sinusitis: 250mg bid for 10 days. ABECB/SSSI: 250-500mg bid for 10 days. Acute Bronchitis: 250-500mg bid for 5-10 days. UTI: 250mg bid for 7-10 days. Gonorrhea: 1000mg single dose. Lyme Disease: 500mg bid for 20 days.
Pediatrics: ≥13 yrs: (Tab) Pharyngitis/Tonsillitis/Sinusitis: 250mg bid for 10 days. ABECB/SSSI: 250-500mg bid for 10 days. Acute Bronchitis: 250-500mg bid for 5-10 days. UTI: 250mg bid for 7-10 days. Gonorrhea: 1000mg single dose. Lyme Disease: 500mg bid for 20 days.
3 months-12 yrs: (Sus) Pharyngitis/Tonsillitis: 20mg/kg/day divided bid for 10 days. Max:

500mg/day. Otitis Media/Sinusitis/Impetigo: 30mg/kg/day divided bid for 10 days. Max: 1000mg/day. (Tab-if can swallow whole) Otitis Media/Sinusitis: 250mg bid for 10 days.

HOW SUPPLIED: Sus: 125mg/5mL [100mL], 250mg/5mL [50mL, 100mL]; Tab: 250mg, 500mg

WARNINGS/PRECAUTIONS: Tabs are not bioequivalent to sus. Caution in patients with previous hypersensitivity to penicillins (PCNs) or other drugs; cross-sensitivity may occur in patients with a history of PCN allergy. D/C if an allergic reaction occurs. Watery, bloody stools (with or without stomach cramps and fever) may develop after starting treatment. *Clostridium difficile*-associated diarrhea (CDAD) reported. May result in bacterial resistance with prolonged use or use in the absence of a proven/suspected bacterial infection or a prophylactic indication; take appropriate measures if superinfection develops. May cause fall in PT; those at risk include patients previously stable on anticoagulants, patients receiving protracted course of antibiotics, patients with renal/hepatic impairment, and in patients with a poor nutritional state. Monitor PT and give vitamin K as needed. Safety and efficacy not established in patients with renal failure. Lab test interactions may occur. (Sus) Contains phenylalanine.

ADVERSE REACTIONS: Diarrhea, N/V, vaginitis, (suspension) dislike of taste, diaper rash.

INTERACTIONS: Probenecid increases plasma levels. Lower bioavailability with drugs that lower gastric acidity. Caution with agents causing adverse effects on renal function (diuretics). May lower estrogen reabsorption and reduce the efficacy of combined oral estrogen/progesterone contraceptives.

PREGNANCY: Category B, not for use in nursing.

MECHANISM OF ACTION: 2nd-generation cephalosporin; binds to essential target proteins and the resultant inhibition of cell-wall synthesis.

PHARMACOKINETICS: Absorption: Absolute bioavailability (37% before food), (52% after food). PO administration of variable doses resulted in different parameters. **Distribution:** Plasma protein binding (50%); found in breast milk. **Metabolism:** Rapid hydrolysis, via nonspecific esterases in the intestinal mucosa and blood. **Elimination:** Urine (50% unchanged).

NURSING CONSIDERATIONS

Assessment: Assess for previous hypersensitivity reactions to cephalosporins/PCNs or other drugs, renal/hepatic impairment, nutritional state, history of colitis, GI malabsorption, pregnancy/nursing status, and for possible drug interactions. For patients planning on using sus formulation, assess for phenylketonuria.

Monitoring: Monitor signs/symptoms of an allergic reaction, CDAD, and superinfection. Monitor PT and renal function.

Patient Counseling: Advise of potential benefits/risks of therapy. Inform that drug only treats bacterial, not viral infections. Instruct to take exactly as directed; skipping doses or not completing full course may decrease effectiveness and increase resistance. Counsel to d/c and notify physician if an allergic reaction or if watery/bloody diarrhea (with/without stomach cramps or fever) develop. Instruct to notify physician if pregnant/nursing. Inform caregivers of pediatric patients that if cannot swallow tab whole, should receive oral sus. Advise that crushed tab, has a strong/persistent bitter taste. Inform that tab may be administered without regard to meals but oral sus must be administered with food.

Administration: Oral route. Tab and sus not bioequivalent and not substitutable on mg-per-mg basis. Refer to PI for reconstitution instructions for sus. Shake sus well before use. **Storage:** Tab: Store at 15-30°C (59-86°F). Sus Powder: Store at 2-30°C (36-86°F). Reconstituted Sus: Store at 2-8°C (36-46°F) in a refrigerator; discard after 10 days.

CEFTRIAXONE   RX
ceftriaxone sodium (Various)

OTHER BRAND NAMES: Rocephin (Roche)

THERAPEUTIC CLASS: Cephalosporin (3rd generation)

INDICATIONS: Treatment of lower respiratory tract infections, skin and skin structure infections (SSSI), bone and joint infections, intra-abdominal infections, urinary tract infections, acute bacterial otitis media, uncomplicated gonorrhea, pelvic inflammatory disease, bacterial septicemia, and meningitis caused by susceptible strains of microorganisms. Surgical prophylaxis during surgical procedures classified as contaminated or potentially contaminated.

DOSAGE: *Adults:* Usual: 1-2g/day IV/IM given qd or bid in equally divided doses depending on the type and severity of infection. Max: 4g/day. Gonorrhea: 250mg IM single dose. Surgical Prophylaxis: 1g IV 1/2-2 hrs before surgery. Continue therapy for ≥2 days after signs and symptoms of infection disappear. Usual duration: 4-14 days; complicated infections may require longer therapy. *Streptococcus pyogenes* Infections: Continue therapy for ≥10 days. Hepatic Dysfunction and Significant Renal Disease: Max: 2g/day.
Pediatrics: SSSI: 50-75mg/kg/day IV/IM given qd or in equally divided doses bid. Max: 2g/day.

Otitis Media: 50mg/kg (up to 1g) IM single dose. Serious Infections: 50-75mg/kg IV/IM given q12h. Max: 2g/day. Meningitis: Initial: 100mg/kg (up to 4g) IV/IM, then 100mg/kg/day IV/IM given qd or in equally divided doses q12h for 7-14 days. Max: 4g/day.

HOW SUPPLIED: Inj: 250mg, 500mg, 1g, 2g; (Rocephin) 500mg, 1g. Also available as a Pharmacy Bulk Package. Refer to individual package insert for more information

CONTRAINDICATIONS: Hyperbilirubinemic neonates (≤28 days), especially if premature; concurrent use of calcium-containing IV solutions used in neonates.

WARNINGS/PRECAUTIONS: Caution in penicillin-sensitive patients and in patients who have demonstrated any form of an allergy, particularly to drugs. Serious acute hypersensitivity reactions may require the use of SQ epinephrine and other emergency measures. Anaphylactic reactions reported. *Clostridium difficile*-associated diarrhea (CDAD) reported. Severe cases of hemolytic anemia reported; d/c until cause is determined. Transient BUN and SrCr elevations may occur. Caution in patients with both hepatic and significant renal disease. Alterations in PT may occur; monitor with impaired vitamin K synthesis or low vitamin K stores during treatment. May result in bacterial resistance with prolonged use or use in the absence of a proven/suspected bacterial infection or a prophylactic indication; take appropriate measures if superinfection develops. Caution with history of GI disease, especially colitis. Gallbladder sonographic abnormalities reported; d/c if gallbladder disease develops. Pancreatitis reported rarely.

ADVERSE REACTIONS: Injection-site reactions (eg, warmth, tightness, induration), eosinophilia, thrombocytosis, AST elevation, ALT elevation.

INTERACTIONS: See Contraindications.

PREGNANCY: Category B, caution in nursing.

MECHANISM OF ACTION: 3rd-generation cephalosporin; bactericidal activity results from inhibition of cell-wall synthesis.

PHARMACOKINETICS: Absorption: (Adults IM) Complete; T_{max}=2-3 hrs. (Pediatrics) Bacterial meningitis: C_{max}=216mcg/mL (50mg/kg IV), 275mcg/mL (75mg/kg IV). Middle ear fluid: C_{max}=35mcg/mL; T_{max}=24 hrs. **Distribution:** Found in breast milk and crosses blood placenta barrier; plasma protein binding (95%) (<25mcg/mL), (85%) (300mcg/mL); (Adults) V_d=5.78-13.5L. (Pediatrics) Bacterial meningitis: V_d=338mL/kg (50mg/kg IV), 373mL/kg (75mg/kg IV). **Elimination:** Urine (33-67%, unchanged), feces. (Adults) $T_{1/2}$=5.8-8.7 hrs. (Pediatrics) Bacterial meningitis: $T_{1/2}$=4.6 hrs (50mg/kg IV), 4.3 hrs (75mg/kg IV); Middle ear fluid: $T_{1/2}$=25 hrs.

NURSING CONSIDERATIONS

Assessment: Assess for hyperbilirubinemic neonates, especially if premature, hypersensitivity to penicillins or other drugs, presence of both hepatic dysfunction and significant renal disease, impaired vitamin K synthesis or low vitamin K stores, history of GI disease (eg, colitis), pregnancy/nursing status, and for possible drug interactions.

Monitoring: Monitor for signs/symptoms of hypersensitivity reactions, CDAD, overgrowth of nonsusceptible organisms (eg, superinfection), gallbladder disease, and pancreatitis. Periodically monitor BUN and SrCr levels. Monitor PT levels in patients with low impaired vitamin K synthesis or in patients with low vitamin K stores (eg, chronic hepatic disease, malnutrition).

Patient Counseling: Inform that therapy only treats bacterial, not viral, infections (eg, common cold). Instruct to take as directed; skipping doses or not completing full course may decrease drug effectiveness and increase risk of bacteria developing resistance. Inform that diarrhea (watery/bloody stools) may be experienced as late as 2 months or more after last dose; contact a physician as soon as possible if this occurs.

Administration: IV/IM route. Incompatible with vancomycin, amsacrine, aminoglycosides, and fluconazole; when administered concomitantly by intermittent IV infusion, give sequentially, with thorough flushing of the intravenous lines between administrations. Avoid physically mixing with or piggybacking with solutions containing antimicrobial drugs. IV infusion should be administered over a period of 30 min. Refer to PI for reconstitution and stability directions. **Storage:** ≤25°C (77°F). Protect from light. Do not refreeze unused portions.

CELEBREX   RX
celecoxib (G.D. Searle)

NSAIDs may cause an increased risk of serious cardiovascular thrombotic events, myocardial infarction (MI), stroke, and serious GI adverse events (eg, bleeding, ulceration, and perforation of stomach/intestines), which may be fatal. Contraindicated for treatment of perioperative pain in the setting of coronary artery bypass graft (CABG) surgery.

THERAPEUTIC CLASS: COX-2 inhibitor

INDICATIONS: Relief of signs and symptoms of osteoarthritis (OA), rheumatoid arthritis (RA), and ankylosing spondylitis (AS). Management of acute pain in adults. Treatment of primary dysmenorrhea. Relief of signs and symptoms of juvenile rheumatoid arthritis (JRA) in patients ≥2 yrs.

DOSAGE: *Adults:* Individualize dose. OA: 200mg qd or 100mg bid. RA: 100-200mg bid. AS: 200mg qd or divided (bid) doses. Titrate: May increase to 400mg/day if no effect observed after 6 weeks. Acute Pain/Primary Dysmenorrhea: Day 1: 400mg initially, then add 200mg if needed. Maint: 200mg bid prn. Moderate Hepatic Impairment: Reduce daily dose by 50%. Poor Metabolizers of CYP2C9 Substrates: Initial: Half the lowest recommended dose. Elderly: <50kg: Initial: Lowest recommended dose.
Pediatrics: JRA: ≥2 yrs: 10-25kg: 50mg bid. >25kg: 100mg bid.

HOW SUPPLIED: Cap: 50mg, 100mg, 200mg, 400mg

CONTRAINDICATIONS: Aspirin (ASA) or other NSAID allergy that precipitates asthma, urticaria, or allergic-type reactions. Allergic-type reactions to sulfonamides. Treatment of perioperative pain in the setting of CABG surgery.

WARNINGS/PRECAUTIONS: May lead to onset of new HTN or worsening of preexisting HTN; monitor BP closely. Fluid retention and edema reported; caution with fluid retention or heart failure (HF). Extreme caution with history of ulcer disease and/or GI bleeding. Rare cases of severe hepatic reactions (eg, jaundice, fatal fulminant hepatitis, liver necrosis, hepatic failure) reported. May cause elevations of LFTs; d/c if liver disease develops or systemic manifestations occur. Renal papillary necrosis and other renal injury reported after long-term use. Anaphylactoid reactions may occur; avoid in patients with ASA-triad. May cause serious skin adverse events (eg, exfoliative dermatitis, Stevens-Johnson syndrome, toxic epidermal necrolysis); d/c at 1st appearance of skin rash or any other sign of hypersensitivity. Avoid in late pregnancy (starting at 30 weeks gestation); may cause premature closure of ductus arteriosus. Not a substitute for corticosteroids or for treatment of corticosteroid insufficiency. Anemia may occur; monitor Hgb/Hct with long-term use. Caution in pediatrics with systemic onset JRA due to risk of disseminated intravascular coagulation. D/C if abnormal liver/renal tests persist or worsen. May diminish utility of diagnostic signs in detecting infectious complications of presumed noninfectious, painful conditions. Use lowest effective dose for the shortest duration possible. Caution in elderly/debilitated patients, poor CYP2C9 metabolizers, and patients with preexisting asthma. Consider alternative management in JRA patients identified to be CYP2C9 poor metabolizers. Not recommended with severe hepatic impairment and severe renal insufficiency. Not a substitute for ASA for cardiovascular prophylaxis.

ADVERSE REACTIONS: Cardiovascular thrombotic events, GI adverse events, headache, HTN, diarrhea, fever, dyspepsia, upper respiratory infection, abdominal pain, N/V, cough, arthralgia, nasopharyngitis, sinusitis.

INTERACTIONS: Caution with CYP2C9 inhibitors. Potential interaction with CYP2D6 substrates. Warfarin or similar agents may increase risk of bleeding complications; monitor anticoagulant activity. May increase lithium levels; monitor closely. May decrease effects of thiazides and loop diuretics. ASA may increase GI complications. May diminish antihypertensive effects of angiotensin converting enzyme (ACE) inhibitors and angiotensin II antagonists. Fluconazole may increase levels. May reduce the natriuretic effect of furosemide and thiazides. Avoid with non-ASA NSAIDs. Oral corticosteroids, anticoagulants, smoking, or alcohol may increase risk of GI bleeding. Diuretics, ACE inhibitors, or angiotensin II antagonists may increase risk of renal toxicity. Aluminum- and magnesium-containing antacids may reduce plasma concentrations.

PREGNANCY: Category C (<30 weeks gestation) and D (≥30 weeks gestation), caution in nursing.

MECHANISM OF ACTION: NSAID; inhibits prostaglandin synthesis primarily via inhibition of cyclooxygenase-2.

PHARMACOKINETICS: Absorption: C_{max}=705ng/mL, T_{max}=2.8 hrs (fasted, 200mg). **Distribution:** V_d=429L (fasted, 200mg); plasma protein binding (97%); found in breast milk. **Metabolism:** CYP2C9. Primary alcohol, carboxylic acid, glucuronide conjugate (metabolites). **Elimination:** Feces (57%), urine (27%); $T_{1/2}$=11.2 hrs (fasted, 200mg).

NURSING CONSIDERATIONS

Assessment: History/presence of cardiovascular disease (CVD), risk factors for CVD, renal/hepatic insufficiency, HTN, peptic ulcer disease, GI bleeding, asthma, ASA/NSAID hypersensitivity, other conditions where treatment is contraindicated/cautioned, pregnancy/nursing status, and possible drug interactions.

Monitoring: Monitor for signs/symptoms of CV thrombotic/serious GI events, new/worsening HTN, fluid retention, edema, renal/hepatic injury, anaphylactoid/hypersensitivity reactions, and other adverse events. Monitor BP, renal function, and LFTs. Periodically monitor CBC and chemistry profile in patients on long-term treatment. Monitor for development of abnormal coagulation tests in patients with systemic onset JRA. Monitor anticoagulant activity in patients on warfarin or similar agents.

Patient Counseling: Advise to seek medical attention if signs/symptoms of cardiovascular events (eg, chest pain, SOB, weakness, slurring of speech), GI ulceration/bleeding (eg, epigastric pain, dyspepsia, melena, hematemesis), hepatotoxicity (eg, nausea, fatigue, pruritus), anaphylactoid reactions (eg, difficulty breathing, swelling of face/ throat), hypersensitivity (eg, rash), weight gain, or edema occur. Inform of pregnancy risks and instruct to avoid use during late pregnancy. **Administration:** Oral route. For patients with difficulty swallowing, contents may be added to applesauce and ingested with water. **Storage:** 25°C (77°F); excursions permitted to 15-30°C (59-86°F). Sprinkled contents on applesauce are stable for up to 6 hrs under 2-8°C (35-45°F).

CELEXA RX
citalopram hbr (Forest)

Antidepressants increased the risk of suicidal thinking and behavior (suicidality) in short-term studies in children, adolescents, and young adults with major depressive disorder (MDD) and other psychiatric disorders. Monitor and observe closely for clinical worsening, suicidality, or unusual changes in behavior in patients who are started on antidepressant therapy. Not approved for use in pediatric patients.

THERAPEUTIC CLASS: Selective serotonin reuptake inhibitor

INDICATIONS: Treatment of depression.

DOSAGE: *Adults:* Initial: 20mg qd. Titrate: Increase dose to 40mg at an interval of no less than 1 week. Max: 40mg/day. Maint: Consider decreasing dose to 20mg/day if adverse reactions are bothersome. D/C of Treatment: Consider resuming previously prescribed dose if intolerable symptoms occur following a decrease in dose or upon d/c of treatment. May continue decreasing the dose subsequently but at a more gradual rate. Elderly (>60 yrs)/Hepatic Impairment/CYP2C19 Poor Metabolizers/Concomitant Cimetidine or Another CYP2C19 Inhibitor: Max: 20mg/day. Pregnancy (3rd Trimester): Consider tapering dose. Switching To/From a MAOI: Allow at least 14 days between d/c of MAOI and initiation of citalopram, or vice versa.

HOW SUPPLIED: Sol: 10mg/5mL [240mL]; Tab: 10mg, 20mg*, 40mg* *scored

CONTRAINDICATIONS: During or within 14 days of d/c of MAOI therapy, concomitant use of pimozide.

WARNINGS/PRECAUTIONS: May cause dose-dependent QTc prolongation which is associated with torsades de pointes, ventricular tachycardia, and sudden death. Avoid in patients with congenital long QT syndrome, bradycardia, hypokalemia or hypomagnesemia, recent acute myocardial infarction (MI), or uncompensated heart failure (HF); monitor ECG if therapy is needed. Correct hypokalemia and/or hypomagnesemia prior to initiation of therapy and monitor periodically. D/C therapy if found to have persistent QTc measurements >500 msec. May precipitate mixed/manic episode in patients at risk for bipolar disorder; screen for risk for bipolar disorder prior to initiating treatment. Not approved for the treatment of bipolar depression. Serotonin syndrome or neuroleptic malignant syndrome (NMS)-like reactions reported. Avoid abrupt d/c; gradually reduce dose whenever possible. May increase the risk of bleeding events. Hyponatremia may occur; caution in elderly and volume-depleted patients. Consider d/c in patients with symptomatic hyponatremia and institute appropriate medical intervention. Activation of mania/hypomania reported; caution with history of mania. Seizures reported; caution with history of seizure disorders. Caution with hepatic impairment and severe renal impairment. May impair mental/physical abilities.

ADVERSE REACTIONS: N/V, dyspepsia, diarrhea, dry mouth, somnolence, insomnia, increased sweating, ejaculation disorder, rhinitis, anxiety, anorexia, tremor, agitation, sinusitis.

INTERACTIONS: See Contraindications. Avoid with SNRIs or tryptophan, other SSRIs, and alcohol. Avoid with other drugs that prolong the QTc interval (class 1A [eg, quinidine, procainamide] or class III [eg, amiodarone, sotalol] antiarrhythmics medications, antipsychotic medications [eg, chlorpromazine, thioridazine], antibiotics [eg, gatifloxacin, moxifloxacin], or any other class of medications known to prolong the QTc interval [eg, pentamidine, levomethadyl acetate, methadone]); monitor ECG if used concomitantly. Caution with other drugs that may affect the serotonergic neurotransmitter systems (eg, triptans, linezolid, lithium, tramadol, or St. John's wort), other centrally acting drugs, TCAs (eg, imipramine), cimetidine, and CYP2C19 inhibitors. Increased risk of bleeding with aspirin, NSAIDs, warfarin, and other drugs that affect coagulation. Rare reports of weakness, hyperreflexia, incoordination with sumatriptan. Possible increased clearance with carbamazepine. May decrease levels of ketoconazole. May increase levels of metoprolol. May cause serotonin syndrome with serotonergic drugs, drugs which impair metabolism of serotonin, or antipsychotics or other dopamine antagonists.

PREGNANCY: Category C, not for use in nursing.

MECHANISM OF ACTION: SSRI; presumed to be linked to potentiation of serotonergic activity in the CNS resulting from its inhibition of CNS neuronal reuptake of serotonin.

PHARMACOKINETICS: **Absorption:** T_{max}=4 hrs, absolute bioavailability (80%). **Distribution:** Plasma protein binding (80%); V_d=12L/kg; found in breast milk. **Metabolism:** Hepatic; N-demethylation via CYP3A4, 2C19; demethylcitalopram (DCT), didemethylcitalopram, citalopram-N-oxide, deaminated proprionic acid derivative (metabolites). **Elimination:** (IV) Urine (10% unchanged, 5% DCT); $T_{1/2}$=35 hrs.

NURSING CONSIDERATIONS

Assessment: Assess for risk for bipolar disorder, history of mania, history of seizures, volume depletion, hypokalemia, hypomagnesemia, bradycardia, recent acute MI, uncompensated HF, hepatic/renal impairment, drug hypersensitivity, congenital long QT syndrome, pregnancy/nursing status, and possible drug interactions. Obtain baseline serum K$^+$ and magnesium measurements for patients being considered for therapy who are at risk for significant electrolyte disturbances.

Monitoring: Monitor for signs/symptoms of clinical worsening (suicidality, unusual changes in behavior), serotonin syndrome/NMS-like reactions, abnormal bleeding, hyponatremia, seizures, cognitive and motor impairment and other adverse reactions. Monitor electrolytes in patients with diseases or conditions that cause hypokalemia or hypomagnesemia. Monitor ECG in patients with cardiac conditions/disorders and in patients on concomitant QTc interval prolonging agents. If therapy is abruptly d/c, monitor for d/c symptoms.

Patient Counseling: Inform about the benefits and risks associated with treatment and counsel on the appropriate use of the drug. Advise to look for emergence of symptoms associated with an increased risk for suicidal thinking/behavior; instruct to report such symptoms, especially if severe, abrupt in onset, or not part of presenting symptoms. Caution against concomitant use with triptans, tramadol, other serotonergic agents, ASA, NSAIDS, warfarin, or other drugs that affect coagulation. Instruct to notify physician if taking or plan to take any prescribed or over-the-counter drugs. Inform that may notice improvement in 1-4 weeks; instruct to continue therapy ud. Caution against hazardous tasks (eg, operating machinery and driving). Instruct to avoid alcohol. Instruct to notify physician if pregnant, intend to become pregnant, or are breastfeeding.

Administration: Oral route. Administer qd, in am or pm. **Storage:** 25°C (77°F); excursions permitted to 15-30°C (59-86°F).

CELLCEPT   RX
mycophenolate mofetil (Genentech)

> Immunosuppression may lead to increased susceptibility to infection and possible development of lymphoma. Only physicians experienced in immunosuppressive therapy and management of renal, cardiac or hepatic transplant patients should use mycophenolate mofetil. Women of childbearing potential must use contraception; use during pregnancy is associated with increased risk of pregnancy loss and congenital malformations.

THERAPEUTIC CLASS: Inosine monophosphate dehydrogenase inhibitor

INDICATIONS: Prophylaxis of organ rejection in allogeneic renal, cardiac, or hepatic transplants; used concomitantly with cyclosporine and corticosteroids.

DOSAGE: *Adults:* Renal Transplant: 1g IV/PO bid. Cardiac Transplant: 1.5g IV/PO bid. Hepatic Transplant: 1g IV bid or 1.5g PO bid. Start PO as soon as possible after transplant. Start IV within 24 hrs after transplant; can continue for up to 14 days. IV infusion should be administered over at least 2 hrs. Switch to oral when tolerated. Give on an empty stomach.
Pediatrics: 3 months-18 yrs: Renal Transplant: (Sus) 600mg/m^2 PO bid. Max: 2g/10mL/day. (Cap) BSA 1.25m^2 to 1.5m^2: 750mg PO bid. (Cap/Tab) BSA >1.5m^2: 1g PO bid.

HOW SUPPLIED: Cap: 250mg; Tab: 500mg; Inj: 500mg/20mL; Sus: 200mg/mL

CONTRAINDICATIONS: (Inj) Hypersensitivity to Polysorbate 80 (TWEEN).

WARNINGS/PRECAUTIONS: Do not administer by rapid or bolus IV injection. Risk of lymphomas and other malignancies, especially of the skin. Limit exposure to sunlight to decrease risk of skin cancer. May cause fetal harm; must have negative serum/urine pregnancy test within 1 week before therapy. Two reliable forms of contraception required before and during therapy, and 6 weeks following d/c. Severe neutropenia reported; if ANC <1.3 x 10^3/μL, d/c or reduce dose. Monitor for bone marrow suppression. Risk of GI ulceration, hemorrhage, and perforation; caution with active digestive system disease. Caution with delayed renal graft function post-transplant. Oral suspension contains phenylalanine; caution with phenylketonurics. Monitor CBC weekly during the 1st month, twice monthly for the 2nd and 3rd months, and then monthly through 1st year. Avoid with rare hereditary deficiency of hypoxanthine-guanine phosphoribosyl-transferase (eg, Lesch-Nyhan and Kelley-Seegmiller syndromes). Increased susceptibility to infections/sepsis. Cases of pure red cell aplasia reported when used with other immunosuppressive agents. Activation of latent viral infections, including progressive multifocal leukoencephalopathy (PML) and BK virus-associated nephropathy (BKVAN), reported; reduce dose in patients who develop evidence of BKVAN or PML. Caution in elderly.

ADVERSE REACTIONS: Infections, diarrhea, leukopenia, sepsis, N/V, HTN, peripheral edema, constipation, pain, abdominal pain, fever, headache, asthenia, insomnia, anemia.

INTERACTIONS: Additive bone marrow suppression with azathioprine; avoid use. Reduced efficacy with drugs that interfere with enterohepatic recirculation (eg, cholestyramine); avoid concomitant use. Avoid live attenuated vaccines. Increased levels of both drugs with acyclovir, ganciclovir. Decreased levels with sevelamer and other calcium-free phosphate binders, magnesium- and aluminum-containing antacids; space dosing. Decreased levels of oral contraceptives;

caution and consider additional birth control. Decreased exposure with rifampin; concomitant use not recommended unless benefit outweighs risk. May decrease levels with ciprofloxacin or amoxicillin plus clavulanic acid. Decreased exposure with combination of norfloxacin and metronidazole; avoid concomitant use. Other drugs that compete for renal tubular secretion may raise levels of both drugs.

PREGNANCY: Category D, not for use in nursing.

MECHANISM OF ACTION: Inosine monophosphate dehydrogenase inhibitor; inhibits the de novo pathway of guanosine nucleotide synthesis without incorporation into DNA.

PHARMACOKINETICS: Absorption: Oral: Rapid and complete, absolute bioavailability (94%). **Distribution:** V_d=3.6L/kg (IV), 4L/kg (oral); plasma protein binding of MPA (97%), MPAG (82%). **Metabolism:** MPA (active metabolite) metabolized by glucuronyl transferase to MPAG, which is converted to MPA via enterohepatic recirculation. **Elimination:** Oral: Urine (93%), feces (6%). Urine: MPA (<1%) and MPAG (87%). MPA: (Oral) $T_{1/2}$=17.9 hrs. (IV) $T_{1/2}$=16.6 hrs. **Pediatrics:** Oral administration in different age groups ranging between 1-18 years results in different pharmacokinetics.

NURSING CONSIDERATIONS

Assessment: Assess for drug hypersensitivity, hepatic/renal impairment, phenylketonuria, hereditary deficiency of hypoxanthin-guanine phosphoribosyl tranferase such as Lesch-Nyhan and Kelley-Seegmiller syndromes, and active digestive disease. Assess vaccination history, pregnancy/nursing status, and possible drug interactions.

Monitoring: Monitor for signs of delayed graft rejection (eg, anemia, thrombocytopenia, and hyperkalemia), neutropenia, lymphomas, skin cancer, GI bleeding/perforation/ulceration, infections (including opportunistic infections, latent viral infections, herpes, sepsis), unexpected bruising, bleeding, or any signs of bone marrow suppression. Monitor CBC weekly during the 1st month, twice monthly for the 2nd and 3rd months, and then monthly through the 1st year. Monitor pregnancy status and enroll patient in the National Transplantation Pregnancy Registry if patient becomes pregnant while on medication.

Patient Counseling: Counsel on importance of following dosage instructions and having periodic laboratory tests. Inform about increased risk of malignancies and infection, and reduced efficacy of concurrent vaccines; notify physician for any signs of infection, bruising, and/or bleeding. Advise to avoid prolonged exposure to sunlight. Not for use in pregnant/nursing women or those planning to become pregnant; inform of need for highly effective contraception before, during, and after therapy. Take on an empty stomach.

Administration: Oral route and slow IV infusion route. Administration of the infusion solution should be within 4 hrs from reconstitution and dilution. **Storage:** 25°C (77°F); excursions permitted to 15-30°C (59-86°F). Constituted Sus: Stable up to 60 days and may be refrigerated at 2-8°C (36-46°F). Do not freeze.

CEPHALEXIN   RX
cephalexin (Various)

OTHER BRAND NAMES: Keflex (Middlebrook)

THERAPEUTIC CLASS: Cephalosporin (1st generation)

INDICATIONS: Treatment of otitis media and skin and skin structure (SSSI), bone, genitourinary tract, and respiratory tract infections caused by susceptible strains of microorganisms.

DOSAGE: *Adults:* Usual: 250mg q6h. Streptococcal Pharyngitis/SSSI/Uncomplicated Cystitis (>15yrs): 500mg q12h. Treat cystitis for 7-14 days. Max: 4g/day.
Pediatrics: Usual: 25-50mg/kg/day in divided doses. Streptococcal Pharyngitis (>1 yr)/SSSI: May divide dose and give q12h. Otitis Media: 75-100mg/kg/day in 4 divided doses. Administer for at least 10 days in β-hemolytic streptococcal infections. In severe infections, the dosage may be doubled.

HOW SUPPLIED: (Keflex) Cap: 250mg, 500mg, 750mg; (Generic) Cap: 250mg, 500mg; Tab: 250mg, 500mg; Sus: 125mg/5mL [60mL, 100mL, 200mL], 250mg/5mL [100mL, 200mL]

WARNINGS/PRECAUTIONS: Caution in penicillin (PCN)-sensitive patients, cross-hypersensivity reactions may occur. Caution in patients with any type of allergy. D/C use if an allergic reaction occurs. *Clostridium difficile*-associated diarrhea (CDAD) reported. May result in bacterial resistance with prolonged use or use in the absence of a proven/suspected bacterial infection or a prophylactic indication; take appropriate measures if superinfection develops. Indicated surgical procedures should be performed in conjunction with antibiotic therapy. Caution in patients with markedly impaired renal function, history of GI disease. May cause a fall in PT; monitor PT in patients at risk (eg, hepatic/renal impairment, protracted course of antimicrobial therapy) and administer vitamin K as indicated. Lab test interactions may occur.

ADVERSE REACTIONS: Diarrhea, allergic reactions, dyspepsia, gastritis, abdominal pain.

INTERACTIONS: Probenecid inhibits excretion. Concomitant use with metformin may increase concentrations of metformin and produce adverse effects; monitor patient closely and adjust dose of metformin accordingly. Patients previously stabilized on anticoagulants may be at risk for a fall in PT; monitor PT and administer vitamin K as indicated.

PREGNANCY: Category B, caution in nursing.

MECHANISM OF ACTION: Cephalosporin; bactericidal due to inhibition of cell-wall synthesis.

PHARMACOKINETICS: Absorption: Rapid; oral administration of variable doses resulted in different parameters. T_{max}=1 hr. **Distribution:** Found in breast milk. **Elimination:** Urine (90% unchanged).

NURSING CONSIDERATIONS

Assessment: Assess for history of hypersensitivity to cephalosporins/PCNs, pregnancy/nursing status, renal impairment, history of GI disease, and for possible drug interactions. Document indications for therapy, culture and susceptibility testing. Perform indicated surgical procedures in conjunction with antibiotic therapy when indicated.

Monitoring: Monitor for signs/symptoms of hypersensitivity reactions (eg, anaphylaxis), CDAD, superinfection, seizures, and aplastic anemia. Monitor renal function, and LDH. Monitor PT in patients at risk for a decrease in PT (eg, hepatic/renal impairement, poor nutritional state, protracted course of antimicrobial therapy).

Patient Counseling: Inform drug only treats bacterial, not viral, infections. Instruct to take exactly as directed; skipping doses or not completing full course may decrease effectiveness and increase bacterial resistance. Inform patient may experience diarrhea. Instruct to contact physician if watery/bloody stools, superinfection, or hypersensitivity reactions occur.

Administration: Oral route. Sus: Refer to label for reconstitution instructions. Shake well before use. **Storage:** 20°-25°C (68°-77°F). Store sus in refrigerator after mixing.

CEREBYX   RX
fosphenytoin sodium (Parke-Davis)

THERAPEUTIC CLASS: Hydantoin

INDICATIONS: Short-term (up to 5 days) parenteral administration when other means of phenytoin administration are unavailable, inappropriate, or less advantageous, including to control general convulsive status epilepticus, prevent or treat seizures during neurosurgery, or as a short-term substitute for oral phenytoin.

DOSAGE: *Adults:* Doses, concentration in dosing solutions, and infusion rates are expressed as phenytoin sodium equivalents (PE). Status Epilepticus: LD: 15-20 PE/kg IV at 100-150mg PE/min then switch to maintenance dose. Non-Emergent Cases: LD: 10-20mg PE/kg IV (max 150mg PE/min) or IM. Maint: Initial: 4-6mg PE/kg/day. May substitute for oral phenytoin sodium at the same total daily dose. Elderly: Lower and less frequent dosing required.

HOW SUPPLIED: Inj: 50mg PE/mL (2mL, 10mL)

CONTRAINDICATIONS: Sinus bradycardia, sino-atrial block, 2nd- and 3rd-degree AV block, Adams-Stokes syndrome.

WARNINGS/PRECAUTIONS: Avoid abrupt d/c. Not for use in absence seizures. Hypotension and severe cardiovascular reactions and fatalities reported especially after IV administration at high doses and rates; continuously monitor ECG, BP, and respiration during and for at least 20 min after IV infusion and monitor phenytoin levels at least 2 hrs after IV infusion or 4 hrs after IM injection. Caution with severe myocardial insufficiency, porphyria, hepatic/renal dysfunction, hypoalbuminemia, elderly, and diabetes. Acute hepatotoxicity, lymphadenopathy, hemopoietic complications, hyperglycemia reported. D/C if rash or acute hepatotoxicity occurs. Severe sensory disturbances (eg, burning, itching, paresthesia) reported. Neonatal postpartum bleeding disorder, congenital malformations, and increased seizure frequency reported with use during pregnancy. Avoid use with seizures caused by hypoglycemia or other metabolic causes. Caution with phosphate restriction because of phosphate load (0.0037mmol phosphate/mg PE).

ADVERSE REACTIONS: Nystagmus, dizziness, pruritus, paresthesia, headache, somnolence, ataxia, tinnitus, stupor, nausea, hypotension, vasodilation, tremor, incoordination, dry mouth.

INTERACTIONS: Increased levels with acute alcohol intake, amiodarone, chloramphenicol, chlordiazepoxide, cimetidine, diazepam, dicumarol, disulfiram, estrogens, ethosuximide, fluoxetine, H_2-antagonists, halothane, isoniazid, methylphenidate, phenothiazines, phenylbutazone, salicylates, succinimides, sulfonamides, tolbutamide, trazodone. Decreased levels with carbamazepine, chronic alcohol abuse, reserpine. Decreases efficacy of anticoagulants, corticosteroids, coumarin, digitoxin, doxycycline, estrogens, furosemide, oral contraceptives, rifampin, quinidine, theophylline, vitamin D. Variable effects (increased or decreased levels) with phenobarbital, valproic acid, and sodium valproate. Caution with drugs highly bound to serum albumin. TCAs may precipitate seizures. May lower folate levels.

PREGNANCY: Category D, not for use in nursing.

MECHANISM OF ACTION: Anticonvulsant; prodrug of phenytoin. Modulates voltage-dependent sodium and calcium channels of neurons, inhibits calcium flux across neuronal membranes, and enhances sodium-potassium ATPase activity of neurons and glial cells.

PHARMACOKINETICS: Absorption: Fosphenytoin is completely converted to phenytoin. (IM) T_{max}=30 min. **Distribution:** Plasma protein binding (95-99%); V_d=4.3-10.8L. **Metabolism:** Phosphatases (conversion to phenytoin); liver (phenytoin metabolism). **Elimination:** Urine (1-5% phenytoin and metabolites); $T_{1/2}$=15 min (fosphenytoin), 12-28.9 hrs (phenytoin).

NURSING CONSIDERATIONS

Assessment: Assess LFTs, renal function, CBC with platelets and differential, hypoalbuminemia, porphyria, cardiac conduction defects, pregnancy status, and phosphate levels. Note other diseases/conditions and drug therapies.

Monitoring: Careful cardiac monitoring is needed when administering IV loading doses. Monitor LFTs, renal function, CBC with differential and platelets, hypersensitivity reactions, myasthenia, pneumonia, and hypokalemia.

Patient Counseling: Instruct patient to call a physician if skin rash develops. Inform patient about the importance of adhering strictly to prescribed dosage regimen and not to abruptly d/c medication. Advise patient of possible risk to fetus during pregnancy. Encourage patients to enroll in North American Antiepileptic Drug (NAAED) Pregnancy Registry by calling 888-233-2334 or go to www.aedpregnancyregistry.org.

Administration: IM/IV route. Should be prescribed in phenytoin sodium equivalent units (PE). Rate of IV administration should not exceed 150mg PE/min. **Storage:** Refrigerate at 2-8°C (36-46°F). Do not store at room temperature for more than 48 hours.

CERVARIX RX
human papillomavirus recombinant vaccine, bivalent (GlaxoSmithKline)

THERAPEUTIC CLASS: Vaccine

INDICATIONS: Prevention of cervical cancer, cervical intraepithelial neoplasia (CIN) Grade 2 or worse and adenocarcinoma *in situ*, and CIN grade 1 caused by oncogenic human papillomavirus (HPV) types 16 and 18 in females 9-25 yrs.

DOSAGE: *Adults:* ≤25 yrs: Give 3 separate doses of 0.5mL IM in deltoid region of the upper arm at 0, 1, and 6 months.
Pediatrics: ≥9 yrs: Give 3 separate doses of 0.5mL IM in deltoid region of the upper arm at 0, 1, and 6 months.

HOW SUPPLIED: Inj: 0.5mL

WARNINGS/PRECAUTIONS: Does not provide protection against disease due to all HPV types or from vaccine and non-vaccine HPV types to which a woman has previously been exposed through sexual activity. May not result in protection in all vaccine recipients. Females should continue to adhere to recommended cervical cancer screening procedures. Syncope sometimes associated with falling, tonic-clonic movements and other seizure-like activity reported; observe for 15 min after administration. Tip cap and rubber plunger of prefilled syringes may contain natural rubber latex; allergic reactions may occur in latex-sensitive individuals. Review immunization history for possible vaccine hypersensitivity and previous vaccination-related adverse reactions. Appropriate treatment and supervision must be available for possible anaphylactic reactions. Immunocompromised individuals may have diminished immune response.

ADVERSE REACTIONS: Local reactions (eg, pain, redness and swelling at the inj site), fatigue, headache, myalgia, GI symptoms, arthralgia, fever, rash, urticaria, nasopharyngitis, influenza.

INTERACTIONS: Immunosuppressive therapies (eg, irradiation, antimetabolites, alkylating agents, cytotoxic drugs, and corticosteroids [used in greater than physiologic doses]), may reduce the immune response to vaccine.

PREGNANCY: Category B, caution in nursing.

MECHANISM OF ACTION: Vaccine; may be mediated by the development of immunoglobulin G-neutralizing antibodies directed against HPV-L1 capsid proteins generated as a result of vaccination.

NURSING CONSIDERATIONS

Assessment: Assess for latex hypersensitivity, immunosuppression, age of patient, pregnancy/nursing status, and possible drug interactions. Review immunization history for possible vaccine sensitivity and previous vaccination-related adverse reactions.

Monitoring: Monitor for syncope, tonic-clonic movements, seizure-like activity, anaphylactic reactions, and other adverse reactions.

Patient Counseling: Advise of the potential benefits and risks associated with vaccination. Inform that vaccine does not substitute for routine cervical cancer screening and advise women who receive the vaccine to continue to undergo cervical screening per standard of care. Counsel that vaccine does not protect against disease from HPV types to which a woman has previously been exposed through sexual activity. Inform that since syncope has been reported following vaccination in young females, observation for 15 min after administration is recommended. Instruct to report any adverse events to physician. Advise to notify physician if pregnant or planning to become pregnant.

Administration: IM route. Shake well before withdrawal and use. Do not administer IV, intradermally, or SQ. Do not mix with any other vaccine in the same syringe or vial. **Storage:** 2-8°C (36-46°F). Do not freeze; discard if has been frozen.

CESAMET
nabilone (Meda)

CII

THERAPEUTIC CLASS: Cannabinoid

INDICATIONS: Treatment of N/V associated with cancer chemotherapy in patients who have failed to respond adequately to conventional antiemetic treatments.

DOSAGE: *Adults:* Night Before Chemotherapy: May give 1 or 2 mg. Day of Chemotherapy: Start with a lower dose 1-3 hrs before the chemotherapy agent. Titrate: Increase PRN; may be given bid or tid during the entire course of each chemotherapy cycle and, PRN, for 48 hrs after the last dose of each cycle. Usual: 1 or 2mg bid. Max: 6mg/day in divided doses tid. Elderly: Start at the low end of dosing range.

HOW SUPPLIED: Cap: 1mg

WARNINGS/PRECAUTIONS: Not intended for use on PRN basis or as 1st antiemetic product prescribed. High potential for abuse. Adverse psychiatric reactions can persist for 48-72 hrs following d/c of treatment. May cause dizziness, drowsiness, euphoria, ataxia, anxiety, disorientation, depression, hallucinations, psychosis, tachycardia, and orthostatic hypotension. May alter mental states; keep patients under adult supervision especially during initial use and dose adjustments. May impair mental/physical abilities. May elevate supine and standing HR and may cause postural hypotension. Caution with HTN, heart disease, elderly, current or previous psychiatric disorders (eg, manic depressive illness, depression, schizophrenia) and history of substance abuse. Caution in pregnant/nursing patients and pediatrics.

ADVERSE REACTIONS: Drowsiness, vertigo, dizziness, dry mouth, euphoria, ataxia, headache, concentration difficulties, dysphoria, sleep/visual disturbance, asthenia, anorexia, depression, hypotension.

INTERACTIONS: Avoid with alcohol, sedatives, hypnotics, or other psychoactive drugs. Additive HTN, tachycardia, and possible cardiotoxicity with sympathomimetics (eg, amphetamines, cocaine). Additive or super-additive tachycardia, and drowsiness with anticholinergics (eg, atropine, scopolamine, antihistamines). Additive tachycardia, HTN, and drowsiness with TCAs (eg, amitriptyline, amoxapine, desipramine). Additive drowsiness and CNS depression with CNS depressants (eg, barbiturates, benzodiazepines, ethanol, lithium, opioids, buspirone, antihistamines, muscle relaxants). May result in hypomanic reaction with disulfiram and fluoxetine in patients who smoked marijuana. May decrease clearance of antipyrine and barbiturates. May increase theophylline metabolism in patients who smoked marijuana/tobacco. Cross-tolerance and mutual potentiation with opioids. Enhanced tetrahydrocannabinol effects with naltrexone. Increase in the positive subjective mood effects of smoked marijuana with alcohol. Impaired psychomotor function with diazepam. May displace highly protein-bound drugs; dose requirement changes may be needed.

PREGNANCY: Category C, not for use in nursing.

MECHANISM OF ACTION: Cannabinoid; interacts with the cannabinoid receptor system, CB (1) receptor, which has been discovered in neural tissues.

PHARMACOKINETICS: Absorption: Complete, C_{max}=2ng/mL, T_{max}=2 hrs. **Distribution:** V_d=12.5L/kg. **Metabolism:** Liver (extensive) via reduction and oxidation; CYP450. **Elimination:** Feces (60%), urine (24%); $T_{1/2}$=2 hrs (identified metabolites), 35 hrs (unidentified metabolites).

NURSING CONSIDERATIONS

Assessment: Assess for history of hypersensitivity to cannabinoids, heart disease, HTN, previous/current psychiatric disorders, history of substance abuse (eg, alcohol abuse/dependence, marijuana use), pregnancy/nursing status, and possible drug interactions.

Monitoring: Monitor for adverse psychiatric reactions or unmasking of symptoms of psychiatric disorders, signs/symptoms of CNS effects (eg, dizziness, drowsiness, euphoria, ataxia, anxiety, disorientation, depression, hallucinations and psychosis), postural hypotension. Monitor BP and

HR. Monitor for signs of excessive use, abuse, and misuse. Monitor for signs and symptoms of hypersensitivity and other adverse reactions.

Patient Counseling: Inform about additive CNS depression effect if taken concomitantly with alcohol or other CNS depressants (eg, benzodiazepines, barbiturates); advise to avoid this combination. Advise not to engage in hazardous activity (eg, operating machinery/driving). Inform of possible mood changes and other adverse behavioral effects that may occur during therapy. Instruct to remain under supervision of responsible adult during treatment.

Administration: Oral route. **Storage:** 25°C (77°F); excursions permitted to 15-30°C (59-86°F).

CHANTIX
varenicline (Pfizer)

RX

Serious neuropsychiatric events including, but not limited to, depression, suicidal ideation, suicide attempt, and completed suicide reported. Some reported cases may be complicated by nicotine withdrawal symptoms in patients who stopped smoking. Monitor for neuropsychiatric symptoms including changes in behavior, hostility, agitation, depressed mood, and suicide-related events. Worsening of preexisting psychiatric illness and completed suicide reported in some patients attempting to quit smoking while on therapy. Advise patients and caregivers that the patient should stop taking therapy and contact a healthcare provider immediately if agitation, hostility, depressed mood, changes in behavior or thinking, suicidal ideation, or suicidal behavior occurs. Safety and efficacy not established in patients with serious psychiatric illness (eg, schizophrenia, bipolar disorder, and major depressive disorder). Weigh risks against benefits of use.

THERAPEUTIC CLASS: Nicotinic Acetylcholine Receptor Agonist

INDICATIONS: Aid to smoking cessation treatment.

DOSAGE: *Adults:* Set quit date and start 1 week before the quit date. Alternatively, may begin therapy and then quit smoking between Days 8 and 35 of treatment. Days 1-3: 0.5mg qd. Days 4-7: 0.5mg bid. Day 8-End of Treatment: 1mg bid. Treat for 12 weeks; additional course of 12 weeks' treatment is recommended after successful completion to ensure long-term abstinence. Make another attempt if failed to quit smoking during the 12 weeks of initial therapy or if relapsed after treatment once factors contributing to failed attempt are identified and addressed. Consider a temporary/permanent dose reduction in patients who cannot tolerate adverse effects. Severe Renal Impairment (CrCl <30mL/min): Initial: 0.5mg qd. Titrate: May titrate PRN to a max dose of 0.5mg bid. End-Stage Renal Disease with Hemodialysis: Max: 0.5mg qd if tolerated.

HOW SUPPLIED: Tab: 0.5mg, 1mg

WARNINGS/PRECAUTIONS: Hypersensitivity reactions including angioedema and rare but serious skin reactions (eg, Stevens-Johnson syndrome, erythema multiforme) reported; d/c if skin rash w/mucosal lesions or any other signs of hypersensitivity develop. Cardiovascular (CV) events (eg, angina pectoris, nonfatal myocardial infarction [MI], nonfatal stroke) reported in patients with stable CV disease. Somnolence, dizziness, loss of consciousness, or difficulty concentrating reported; may impair physical/mental abilities. Consider dose reduction for patients with intolerable nausea. Caution in elderly.

ADVERSE REACTIONS: N/V, headache, insomnia, somnolence, abnormal dreams, flatulence, constipation, dysgeusia, fatigue, upper respiratory tract disorder, abdominal pain, dry mouth, dyspepsia.

INTERACTIONS: Nicotine replacement therapy (transdermal nicotine) may increase incidence of adverse events. Physiological changes resulting from smoking cessation may alter pharmacokinetics or pharmacodynamics of certain drugs (eg, theophylline, warfarin, insulin) for which dosage adjustment may be necessary.

PREGNANCY: Category C, not for use in nursing.

MECHANISM OF ACTION: Nicotinic acetylcholine receptor agonist; binds with high affinity and selectivity at $\alpha 4\beta 2$ neuronal nicotinic acetylcholine receptors. The binding produces agonist activity while simultaneously preventing nicotine binding to these receptors.

PHARMACOKINETICS: Absorption: Complete; bioavailability (90%); T_{max}=3-4 hrs. **Distribution:** Plasma protein binding (≤20%). **Metabolism:** Minimal. **Elimination:** Urine (92% unchanged); $T_{1/2}$=24 hrs.

NURSING CONSIDERATIONS

Assessment: Assess for preexisting psychiatric illness, renal impairment, CV disease, history of hypersensitivity/skin reaction to the drug, pregnancy/nursing status, and for possible drug interactions.

Monitoring: Monitor for neuropsychiatric symptoms (eg, changes in behavior, agitation, depressed mood, suicidal ideation/behavior) or worsening of preexisting psychiatric illness, CV events, nausea, insomnia, skin reactions and for hypersensitivity reactions. Monitor renal function.

C

Patient Counseling: Inform about risks and benefits of treatment. Instruct to notify physician of all prescription and nonprescription medications currently taking, if pregnant or nursing, and if any adverse events occur. Instruct to set a date to quit smoking and initiate treatment 1 week before the quit date. Encourage to continue to attempt to quit even with early lapses after quit day. Provide with educational materials and necessary counseling to support attempt at quitting smoking. Encourage to reveal any history of psychiatric illness prior to treatment. Inform that quitting smoking may be associated with nicotine withdrawal symptoms or exacerbation of preexisting psychiatric illness. Caution about performing hazardous tasks (eg, driving/operating machinery). Inform that may experience vivid, unusual, or strange dreams.

Administration: Oral route. Take pc and with a full glass of water. **Storage:** 25°C (77°F); excursions permitted to 15-30°C (59-86°F).

CHENODAL   RX
chenodiol (Manchester)

THERAPEUTIC CLASS: Bile acid

INDICATIONS: Patients with radiolucent stones in well-opacifying gallbladders, in whom selective surgery would be undertaken except for the presence of increased surgical risk due to systemic disease or age.

DOSAGE: *Adults:* Initial: 250mg bid the first two weeks. Titrate: Increase by 250mg/day each week thereafter until recommended or maximum tolerated dose is reached. Range: 13-16mg/kg/day in two divided doses, am and pm. 45-58kg: 3 tabs/day; 59-75kg: 4 tabs/day; 76-90kg: 5 tabs/day; 91-107kg: 6 tabs/day; 108-125kg: 7 tabs/day. Adjust dose temporarily if diarrhea occurs until symptoms abate. D/C if no response by 18 months.

HOW SUPPLIED: Tab: 250mg

CONTRAINDICATIONS: Presence of known hepatocyte dysfunction or bile ductal abnormalities (eg, intrahepatic cholestasis, primary biliary cirrhosis, sclerosing cholangitis), nonvisualizing gallbladder after two consecutive single doses of dye, radiopaque stones, gallstone complications or compelling reasons for gallbladder surgery including unremitting acute cholecystitis, cholangitis, biliary obstruction, gallstone pancreatitis, or biliary GI fistula.

WARNINGS/PRECAUTIONS: Has the potential to cause hepatotoxicity or may increase rate of need for cholecystectomy. Treatment should be reserved for carefully selected patients and must be accompanied by systemic monitoring for liver function alterations. Will not dissolve radiolucent bile pigment stones. May cause serious hepatic disease and fetal harm. May contribute to colon cancer in susceptible individuals. Use in patient without pre-existing liver disease; monitor for serum aminotransferase to detect drug-induced liver toxicity. D/C if with aminotransferase elevations over 3X ULN, if cholesterol rises above acceptable age-adjusted limit and if there is confirmed dissolution. Caution in patients with history of jaundice. Stone recurrence may occur; maintenance of reduced weight recommended. Safety of use beyond 24 months not established.

ADVERSE REACTIONS: Aminotransferase elevations (mainly SGPT), intrahepatic cholestasis, diarrhea, gastrointestinal side effects, increase in serum total cholesterol and LDL, decrease in WBC count.

INTERACTIONS: May reduce absorption with bile acid sequestering agents (eg, cholestyramine, colestipol) and aluminum-based antacids. Estrogen, oral contraceptive and clofibrate (and perhaps other lipid-lowering drugs) may counteract the effectiveness of chenodiol. May cause unexpected prolongation of PT and hemorrhages with coumarin and its derivatives.

PREGNANCY: Category X, caution in nursing.

MECHANISM OF ACTION: Bile acid; suppresses hepatic synthesis of both cholesterol and cholic acid, gradually replacing the latter and its metabolite, deoxycholic acid in an expanded bile acid pool that contributes to biliary cholesterol desaturation and gradual dissolution of radiolucent cholesterol gallstone.

PHARMACOKINETICS: Absorption: Well absorbed. **Metabolism:** Liver, converted in the colon by bacterial action to lithocholic acid (metabolite). **Elimination:** Lithocholate: Feces (80%).

NURSING CONSIDERATIONS

Assessment: Assess for hepatocyte dysfunction or bile ductal abnormalities or any other diseases or conditions where treatment is contraindicated or cautioned. Assess for pregnancy/nursing status and possible drug interactions. Obtain LFTs (AST/ALT), serum cholesterol and TG levels.

Monitoring: Monitor for patient's weight, increased risk for cholecystectomy and for signs and symptoms of hepatotoxicity, colon cancer or other adverse reactions. Monitor liver function alterations. Monitor serum aminotransferase levels monthly for the first 3 months and every 3 months thereafter during medication. Monitor serum cholesterol at 6-month intervals. Monitor response and/or recurrence with cholecystograms or ultrasonograms at 6-9-month intervals.

Patient Counseling: Counsel on the importance of periodic visits for LFTs and oral cholecystograms (or ultrasonograms) for monitoring stone dissolution. Inform about the symptoms of gallstone complications and advise to notify physician immediately if occurs. Instruct ways to facilitate faithful compliance with the dosage regimen throughout the usual long term of therapy, and on temporary dose reduction if episodes of diarrhea occur. Advise to maintain reduced weight to forestall stone recurrence.

Administration: Oral route. **Storage:** 20-25°C (68-77°F). Dispense in tight container.

CIALIS

tadalafil (Lilly)

RX

THERAPEUTIC CLASS: Phosphodiesterase type 5 inhibitor

INDICATIONS: Treatment of erectile dysfunction (ED), signs and symptoms of benign prostatic hyperplasia (BPH). Treatment of ED and signs and symptoms of BPH.

DOSAGE: *Adults:* PRN Use: ED: Initial: 10mg prior to sexual activity. Titrate: May increase to 20mg or decrease to 5mg based on efficacy and tolerability. Max Dosing Frequency: qd. CrCl 30-50mL/min: Initial: 5mg qd. Max: 10mg/48 hrs. CrCl <30mL/min or Hemodialysis: Max: 5mg/72 hrs. Mild/Moderate Hepatic Impairment: Max: 10mg qd. With Alpha Blockers: Initial: Use lowest recommended dose. With Potent CYP3A4 Inhibitors (eg, ketoconazole, ritonavir): Max: 10mg/72 hrs. Once-Daily Use: ED: Initial: 2.5mg qd. Titrate: May increase to 5mg qd based on individual response. BPH and ED/BPH: 5mg qd. Take at the same time everyday. BPH and ED/BPH with CrCl 30-50mL/min: Initial: 2.5mg. Titrate: May increase to 5mg based on individual response. With Potent CYP3A4 Inhibitors (eg, ketoconazole, ritonavir): Max: 2.5mg.

HOW SUPPLIED: Tab: 2.5mg, 5mg, 10mg, 20mg

CONTRAINDICATIONS: Any form of organic nitrate, either regularly and/or intermittently used.

WARNINGS/PRECAUTIONS: Cardiac risk associated with sexual activity may occur; avoid in men for whom sexual activity is inadvisable due to underlying cardiovascular (CV) status. Avoid with myocardial infarction (within last 90 days), unstable angina or angina occurring during sexual intercourse, NYHA Class 2 or greater heart failure (in the last 6 months), uncontrolled arrhythmias, hypotension (<90/50mmHg), or uncontrolled HTN, and stroke within the last 6 months. Mild systemic vasodilatory properties may result in transient decrease in BP. Increased sensitivity to vasodilatory effect with left ventricular outflow obstruction and severely impaired autonomic control of BP. Prolonged erections (>4 hrs) and priapism reported; caution in conditions predisposing to priapism (eg, sickle cell anemia, multiple myeloma, leukemia), anatomical deformation of the penis (eg, angulation, cavernosal fibrosis, Peyronie's disease). Non-arteritic anterior ischemic optic neuropathy (NAION) rarely reported; d/c if sudden loss of vision is experienced in one or both eyes. Sudden decrease or loss of hearing reported with tinnitus and dizziness; d/c if occurs. Avoid qd use in severe renal impairment (CrCl <30mL/min or on hemodialysis). Avoid use with severe hepatic impairment (Child-Pugh Class C), hereditary degenerative retinal disorders, including retinitis pigmentosa. Caution with mild to moderate hepatic impairment, bleeding disorders, or significant active peptic ulceration. Consider other urological condition that may cause similar symptoms prior to initiating treatment for BPH.

ADVERSE REACTIONS: Headache, dyspepsia, back pain, myalgia, nasal congestion, flushing, limb pain, nasopharyngitis, upper respiratory tract infection, gastroenteritis (viral), influenza, cough, gastroesophageal reflux disease, HTN.

INTERACTIONS: See Contraindications. Avoid concomitant use with nitrates within 48 hrs. Concomitant use not recommended with alpha blockers in BPH. BP lowering effects may be increased with alcohol. Additive hypotensive effects with alpha-adrenergic blockers (eg, doxazosin, alfuzosin, tamsulosin), antihypertensives (eg, amlodipine, angiotensin II receptor blockers, bendrofluazide, enalapril, metoprolol). Increased tadalafil exposure with ritonavir and possibly other HIV protease inhibitors. CYP3A4 inhibitors (eg, ketoconazole, itraconazole, erythromycin, grapefruit juice) may result in increased exposure of tadalafil. CYP3A4 inducers (eg, rifampin, carbamazepine, phenytoin, phenobarbital) may result in decreased tadalafil exposure. Antacids (magnesium hydroxide/aluminum hydroxide) shown to reduce rate of absorption. Avoid concomitant use with Adcirca or other PDE5 inhibitors. A small increase in heart rate seen with theophylline.

PREGNANCY: Category B, not for use in nursing.

MECHANISM OF ACTION: Phosphodiesterase type 5 inhibitor; increases amount of cGMP that causes smooth muscle relaxation and increased blood flow into the corpus cavernosum.

PHARMACOKINETICS: Absorption: T_{max}=2 hrs. **Distribution:** V_d=63L; plasma protein binding (94%). **Metabolism:** Liver, via CYP3A4 to a catechol metabolite, which undergoes extensive methylation and glucuronidation; methylcatechol glucuronide (major metabolite). **Elimination:** Urine (36%), feces (61%); $T_{1/2}$=17.5 hrs.

NURSING CONSIDERATIONS

Assessment: Assess for previous hypersensitivity to drug, CV disease, long QT syndrome, retinitis pigmentosa, bleeding disorders, active peptic ulceration, anatomical deformation of the penis or presence of conditions that would predispose to priapism (eg, sickle cell anemia, multiple myeloma, leukemia), renal/hepatic impairment, contraindications for sexual activity. Assess for potential underlying causes of ED, other urological conditions, and for possible drug interactions.

Monitoring: Monitor for hypersensitivity reactions, decreases in BP, abnormalities in vision (eg, NAION), decrease/loss of hearing, prolonged erection, priapism, and other adverse reactions. Monitor therapeutic effect when used in combination with other drugs.

Patient Counseling: Instruct to seek medical assistance if erection persists >4 hrs. Advise of potential BP-lowering effect of alpha-blockers, other antihypertensive medications, alcohol, and cardiac risk of sexual activity. Counsel about the protective measures necessary to guard against sexually transmitted disease, including HIV. Inform about contraindication with organic nitrates and potential interactions with other medications. Instruct to d/c and seek medical attention if sudden loss of vision or hearing occur. Counsel to take one tab at least 30 min before anticipated sexual activity for PRN use, and approximately the same time qd without regard to timing of sexual activity for qd use. Instruct to not split tab and to take entire dose.

Administration: Oral route. Do not split; entire dose should be taken. **Storage:** 25°C (77°F); excursions permitted to 15-30°C (59-86°F).

CILOXAN   RX
ciprofloxacin HCl (Alcon)

THERAPEUTIC CLASS: Fluoroquinolone

INDICATIONS: Treatment of bacterial conjunctivitis (sol/oint) and corneal ulcers (sol) caused by susceptible strains of microorganisms.

DOSAGE: *Adults:* (Oint) Bacterial Conjunctivitis: Apply 1/2-inch ribbon tid into conjunctival sac for 2 days, then bid for the next 5 days. (Sol) Bacterial Conjunctivitis: Instill 1-2 drops into conjunctival sac q2h while awake for 2 days, then 1-2 drops q4h while awake for the next 5 days. Corneal Ulcer: Instill 2 drops into the affected eye every 15 min for 1st 6 hrs, then 2 drops every 30 min for rest of Day 1, then 2 drops every hr on Day 2, then 2 drops q4h on Days 3-14. May continue treatment after 14 days if re-epithelialization has not occurred.
Pediatrics: (Oint) Bacterial Conjunctivitis: ≥2 yrs: Apply 1/2-inch ribbon tid into conjunctival sac for 2 days, then bid for the next 5 days. (Sol) ≥1 yr: Bacterial Conjunctivitis: Instill 1-2 drops into conjunctival sac q2h while awake for 2 days, then 1-2 drops q4h while awake for the next 5 days. Corneal Ulcer: Instill 2 drops into the affected eye every 15 min for 1st 6 hrs, then 2 drops every 30 min for rest of Day 1, then 2 drops every hr on Day 2, then 2 drops q4h on Days 3-14. May continue treatment after 14 days if re-epithelialization has not occurred.

HOW SUPPLIED: Oint: 0.3% [3.5g]; Sol: 0.3% [2.5mL, 5mL, 10mL]

WARNINGS/PRECAUTIONS: For topical ophthalmic use only; do not inject into eye. Serious and occasionally fatal hypersensitivity (anaphylactic) reactions reported in patients receiving systemic therapy; immediate emergency treatment with epinephrine and other resuscitation measures may be required as clinically indicated. Prolonged use may result in overgrowth of nonsusceptible organisms, including fungi; initiate appropriate therapy if superinfection occurs. D/C at 1st appearance of skin rash or other signs of hypersensitivity reaction. Remove contact lenses before use; avoid wearing contact lenses when signs/symptoms of bacterial conjunctivitis are present. (Oint) May retard corneal healing and cause visual blurring. (Sol) May form a white crystalline precipitate in the superficial portion of the corneal defect.

ADVERSE REACTIONS: Local discomfort, keratopathy, allergic reactions, corneal staining, foreign body sensation. (Oint) Blurred vision, irritation, lid margin hyperemia. (Sol) Local burning, white crystalline precipitate formation, lid margin crusting, conjunctival hyperemia, crystals/scales, itching, bad taste.

INTERACTIONS: Systemic quinolone therapy may increase theophylline levels, interfere with caffeine metabolism, enhance effects of warfarin and its derivatives, and elevate SrCr with cyclosporine.

PREGNANCY: Category C, caution in nursing.

MECHANISM OF ACTION: Fluoroquinolone; bactericidal, interferes with the enzyme DNA gyrase, which is needed for synthesis of bacterial DNA.

PHARMACOKINETICS: Absorption: (Sol) C_{max}=<5ng/mL.

NURSING CONSIDERATIONS

Assessment: Assess for previous hypersensitivity to the drug and other quinolones, use of contact lenses, pregnancy/nursing status, and possible drug interactions.

Monitoring: Monitor for signs/symptoms of hypersensitivity/anaphylactic reactions and other adverse reactions. Monitor for superinfection; examine with magnification (eg, slit lamp biomicroscopy) and fluorescein staining, where appropriate.

Patient Counseling: Instruct to use as prescribed. Instruct not to touch dropper tip to any surface; may contaminate solution. Advise to contact physician if hypersensitivity reaction occurs (eg, rash). Instruct to remove contact lenses before use and not to wear contact lenses if signs/symptoms of bacterial conjunctivitis are present.

Administration: Ocular route. **Storage:** 2-25°C (36-77°F). (Sol) Protect from light.

CIMZIA   RX
certolizumab pegol (UCB)

> Increased risk for developing serious infections (eg, tuberculosis [TB], TB reactivation, invasive fungal infection, bacterial/viral infection, or other opportunistic infections) leading to hospitalization or death. Most patients who developed these infections were taking concomitant immunosuppressants (eg, methotrexate [MTX] or corticosteroids). D/C if serious infection or sepsis develops. Evaluate for latent TB and treat prior to initiation of therapy. Monitor for development of signs and symptoms of infection during and after treatment. Lymphoma and other malignancies reported in children and adolescents. Not indicated for pediatrics.

THERAPEUTIC CLASS: TNF-receptor blocker

INDICATIONS: Reduce signs/symptoms of Crohn's disease and maintain clinical response in adults with moderately to severely active disease who have inadequate response to conventional therapy. Treatment of moderately to severely active rheumatoid arthritis (RA) in adults.

DOSAGE: *Adults:* Crohn's disease: Initial: 400mg (given as 2 SQ inj of 200mg) initially and at Weeks 2 and 4. Maint: 400mg SQ every 4 weeks. RA: Initial: 400mg (given as 2 SQ inj of 200mg) initially and at Weeks 2 and 4, followed by 200mg every other week. Maint: 400mg SQ every 4 weeks. With Concomitant MTX: 200mg SQ every other week.

HOW SUPPLIED: Inj: 200mg/mL [prefilled syringe, single-dose vial]

WARNINGS/PRECAUTIONS: Do not initiate with an active infection. Patients with RA are at a higher risk for lymphoma and leukemia. New onset or worsening of congestive heart failure reported; caution with heart failure and monitor carefully. Hypersensitivity reactions (eg, angioedema, dyspnea, hypotension, rash, serum sickness, urticaria) reported rarely; d/c and institute appropriate therapy if these occur. Increased risk of hepatitis B virus (HBV) reactivation in carriers; if reactivation occurs, d/c and start antiviral therapy. Caution with preexisting or recent onset CNS demyelinating disorders (eg, multiple sclerosis) or peripheral demyelinating disorders (Guillain-Barre syndrome). Rare cases of neurological disorders (eg, seizure disorder, optic neuritis, peripheral neuropathy) reported. Pancytopenia, including aplastic anemia, and significant cytopenia reported; seek medical attention if signs/symptoms of blood dyscrasias/infection develop and d/c for significant hematologic abnormalities. May cause autoantibody formation; d/c if lupus-like syndrome develops. Caution in elderly.

ADVERSE REACTIONS: Infections, upper respiratory infections, rash, urinary tract infections, nasopharyngitis, arthralgia.

INTERACTIONS: See Boxed Warning. Avoid with live/attenuated vaccines, other TNF-blocker therapies, and biological disease-modifying antirheumatic drugs (DMARDs). Increased risk of infection with anakinra, abatacept, rituximab, and natalizumab; avoid combination. Additive hypertensive effects with NSAIDs and corticosteroids.

PREGNANCY: Category B, not for use in nursing.

MECHANISM OF ACTION: TNF-blocker; binds to TNF-α and selectively neutralizes and inhibits its central role in inflammatory processes.

PHARMACOKINETICS: Absorption: T_{max}=54-171 hrs; C_{max}=43-49mcg/mL; bioavailability (80%). **Distribution:** V_d=6-8L. **Elimination:** $T_{1/2}$=14 days.

NURSING CONSIDERATIONS

Assessment: Assess for active/chronic/recurrent infection (eg, TB, HBV), TB exposure, recent travel in areas of endemic TB or endemic mycoses, underlying conditions that may predispose to infection, presence or history of significant hematologic abnormalities, heart failure, neurologic disorders, preexisting or recurrent CNS demyelinating disorders, pregnancy/nursing status, and possible drug interactions. Perform test for latent infection (eg, TB). Perform appropriate screening tests (eg, tuberculin skin test and chest x-ray).

Monitoring: Monitor for signs/symptoms of serious infection (eg, sepsis, pneumonia, TB, invasive fungal infection, HBV infection, neurologic disorders (eg, seizures, optic neuritis, peripheral neuropathy), hematologic reactions (eg, aplastic anemia, pancytopenia, leukopenia, neutropenia, thrombocytopenia), hypersensitivity reactions (eg, angioedema, dyspnea, rash, serum sickness, urticaria), malignancies (eg, lymphoma), lupus-like syndrome, and injection-site reactions. In patients with heart failure, monitor for worsening of symptoms.

C

Patient Counseling: Inform about risks/benefits of therapy. Inform that drug may lower ability to fight infections and discuss the importance of contacting physician if symptoms of infections develop. Counsel about possible risk of lymphoma and other malignancies. Advise to seek medical attention if any severe allergic reactions occur. Instruct to report any signs of new or worsening medical conditions such as heart disease; neurological or autoimmune disorders; bruising, bleeding, pallor, cough, persistent fever, or flu-like symptoms; or if any symptoms of TB, histoplasmosis, or HBV develop. Instruct not to use if cloudy or if foreign particulate matter is present and to discard unused portions of drug remaining in the syringe or vial.

Administration: SQ route. Rotate inj sites; avoid tender, bruised, red, or hard areas of the skin. When a 400mg dose is needed (given as 2 SQ inj of 200mg), inj should occur at separate sites in the thigh or abdomen. Refer to PI for proper reconstitution and administration. **Storage:** 2-8°C (36-46°F). Do not freeze. Protect from light. Once reconstituted, can be stored in vials for up to 24 hrs prior to inj.

CIPRO HC   RX
ciprofloxacin HCl - hydrocortisone (Alcon)

THERAPEUTIC CLASS: Antibacterial/corticosteroid combination

INDICATIONS: Treatment of acute otitis externa in adults and pediatric patients ≥1 year caused by susceptible strains of microorganisms.

DOSAGE: *Adults:* 3 drops into affected ear bid for 7 days.
Pediatrics: ≥1 yr: 3 drops into affected ear bid for 7 days.

HOW SUPPLIED: Sus: (Ciprofloxacin-Hydrocortisone) 0.2%-1% [10mL]

CONTRAINDICATIONS: Perforated tympanic membrane, viral infections of external ear canal including varicella and herpes simplex infections.

WARNINGS/PRECAUTIONS: Not for inj and ophthalmic use. D/C at 1st appearance of skin rash or any other sign of hypersensitivity. Serious and occasionally fatal hypersensitivity (anaphylactic) reactions reported; may require immediate emergency treatment. May result in overgrowth of nonsusceptible organisms (eg, fungi). Reevaluate if no improvement after 1 week.

ADVERSE REACTIONS: Headache, pruritus.

PREGNANCY: Category C, not for use in nursing.

MECHANISM OF ACTION: Ciprofloxacin: Fluoroquinolone antibacterial; bactericidal action results from interference with the enzyme (DNA gyrase), which is needed for the synthesis of bacterial DNA. Hydrocortisone: Corticosteroid; aids in resolution of inflammatory response accompanying bacterial infection.

NURSING CONSIDERATIONS

Assessment: Assess for history of drug hypersensitivity, perforated tympanic membrane, viral infections of external ear canal including varicella and herpes simplex infections, and pregnancy/nursing status.

Monitoring: Monitor for hypersensitivity reactions, overgrowth of nonsusceptible organisms (eg, fungi), and possible adverse reactions.

Patient Counseling: Instruct to d/c immediately and consult physician if rash or allergic reaction occurs. Advise not to use in the eyes. Advise to avoid contaminating the dropper with material from the ear, fingers, or other sources. Counsel to protect product from light. Instruct to shake well before using and to discard unused portion after therapy is completed.

Administration: Otic route. Shake well before use. Warm bottle in hand for 1-2 min to avoid dizziness. Lie with affected ear upward, then instill drops. Maintain position for 30-60 sec and repeat, if necessary, for the opposite ear. **Storage:** Below 25°C (77°F). Avoid freezing. Protect from light. Discard unused portion after therapy is completed.

CIPRO IV   RX
ciprofloxacin (Bayer Healthcare)

> Fluoroquinolones are associated with an increased risk of tendinitis and tendon rupture in all ages. Risk is further increased in patients >60 yrs, patients taking corticosteroids, and with kidney, heart, or lung transplants. May exacerbate muscle weakness with myasthenia gravis; avoid in patients with known history of myasthenia gravis.

THERAPEUTIC CLASS: Fluoroquinolone

INDICATIONS: Treatment of urinary tract infections (UTI), lower respiratory tract infections (LRTI), acute exacerbations of chronic bronchitis, nosocomial pneumonia, skin and skin structure infections (SSSI), bone and joint infections, complicated intra-abdominal infections (in combination with metronidazole), acute sinusitis, chronic bacterial prostatitis, and empirical therapy for febrile neutropenia (in combination with piperacillin sodium) in adults. Treatment of complicated UTI and pyelonephritis in pediatrics 1-17 yrs. To reduce the incidence or progression of post-exposure inhalational anthrax in both adults and pediatrics.

DOSAGE: *Adults:* Infuse as IV over 60 min. UTI: Mild/Moderate: 200mg q12h for 7-14 days. Severe/Complicated: 400mg q12h (or q8h) for 7-14 days. LRTI/SSSI: Mild/Moderate: 400mg q12h for 7-14 days. Severe/Complicated: 400mg q8h for 7-14 days. Nosocomial Pneumonia: 400mg q8h for 10-14 days. Bone and Joint: Mild/Moderate: 400mg q12h for ≥4-6 weeks. Severe/Complicated: 400mg q8h for ≥4-6 weeks. Complicated Intra-Abdominal (with metronidazole): 400mg q12h for 7-14 days. Acute Sinusitis: Mild/Moderate: 400mg q12h for 10 days. Chronic Bacterial Prostatitis: Mild/Moderate: 400mg q12h for 28 days. Febrile Neutropenia (Empirical Therapy): Severe: 400mg q8h (with piperacillin 50mg/kg q4h; Max: 24g/day) for 7-14 days. Inhalational Anthrax (Post-Exposure): 400mg q12h for 60 days. CrCl 5-29mL/min: 200-400mg q18-24h. Refer to PI for conversion of IV to PO dosing.
Pediatrics: Infuse as IV over 60 min. Inhalational Anthrax (Post-Exposure): 10mg/kg q12h for 60 days. Max: 400mg/dose. 1-17 yrs: Complicated UTI/Pyelonephritis: 6-10mg/kg q8h for 10-21 days. Max: 400mg/dose.

HOW SUPPLIED: Inj: 400mg/200mL (0.2%)

CONTRAINDICATIONS: Concomitant administration with tizanidine.

WARNINGS/PRECAUTIONS: D/C if experience pain, swelling, inflammation, or rupture of tendon. Serious and occasionally fatal hypersensitivity reactions reported; d/c if skin rash, jaundice, or hypersensitivity occurs. Convulsions, increased intracranial pressure (including pseudotumor cerebri), toxic psychosis, and other CNS events reported; d/c and institute appropriate measures if CNS events occur. Caution with CNS disorders (eg, severe cerebral arteriosclerosis, epilepsy) or other risk factors that may predispose to seizures or lower the seizure threshold. *Clostridium difficile*-associated diarrhea (CDAD) reported. Rare cases of sensory or sensorimotor axonal polyneuropathy resulting in paresthesias, hypoesthesias, dysesthesias, and weakness reported; d/c if symptoms of neuropathy occur. Increased incidence of musculoskeletal disorders in pediatrics. May prolong QT interval; avoid with known QT interval prolongation or uncorrected hypokalemia. Local site reactions reported. Crystalluria reported; maintain hydration and avoid alkalinity of urine. May cause photosensitivity/phototoxicity reactions; d/c if phototoxicity occurs. Avoid excessive exposure to sun/UV light. Monitor renal, hepatic, and hematopoietic function with prolonged use. May result in bacterial resistance with prolonged use or use in the absence of a proven/suspected bacterial infection or a prophylactic indication; take appropriate measures if superinfection develops. Caution in elderly and in patients with renal/hepatic impairment.

ADVERSE REACTIONS: Tendinitis, tendon rupture, exacerbation of myasthenia gravis, musculoskeletal symptoms, arthralgia, N/V, diarrhea, abdominal pain, neurological events, rhinitis, abnormal LFTs, rash.

INTERACTIONS: See Boxed Warning and Contraindications. May increase levels of CYP1A2 substrates (eg, theophylline, methylxanthines, tizanidine), caffeine- or pentoxifylline-containing products, duloxetine, ropinirole, lidocaine, clozapine, or sildenafil. Increased theophylline levels and its related adverse reactions; if use cannot be avoided, monitor theophylline level and adjust dose. May reduce clearance of caffeine and prolong its $T_{1/2}$. May alter serum levels of phenytoin. Severe hypoglycemia with glyburide. Probenecid may increase levels. Transient SrCr elevations with cyclosporine. May augment effects of oral anticoagulant (eg, warfarin); monitor PT and INR frequently. May increase levels and toxic reactions of methotrexate. High-dose quinolones shown to provoke convulsions with NSAIDs (not aspirin). Avoid with class IA (eg, quinidine, procainamide) and class III (eg, amiodarone, sotalol) antiarrhythmics. Caution with drugs that may lower seizure threshold. Mean serum concentration changes reported with piperacillin sodium 6-8 hrs after end of infusion.

PREGNANCY: Category C, not for use in nursing.

MECHANISM OF ACTION: Fluoroquinolone; inhibits enzymes topoisomerase II (DNA gyrase) and topoisomerase IV (both Type II topoisomerases), which are required for bacterial DNA replication, transcription, repair, and recombination.

PHARMACOKINETICS: Absorption: Absolute bioavailability (PO) (70-80%). Administration of various doses resulted in different parameters. **Distribution:** Plasma protein binding (20-40%); found in breast milk. **Elimination:** Bile (<1%, unchanged), urine (50-70%, unchanged), feces (15%); $T_{1/2}$=5-6 hrs.

NURSING CONSIDERATIONS

Assessment: Assess for risk factors for developing tendinitis and tendon rupture, history of myasthenia gravis, drug hypersensitivity, CNS disorders or other risk factors that may predispose to seizures or lower seizure threshold, QT interval prolongation, uncorrected hypokalemia, renal/hepatic function, pregnancy/nursing status, and possible drug interactions. Obtain baseline culture and susceptibility test.

Monitoring: Monitor for tendinitis or tendon rupture, signs/symptoms of hypersensitivity reactions, development of superinfection, ECG changes (eg, QT interval prolongation), CNS events, CDAD, peripheral neuropathy, musculoskeletal disorders (pediatrics), photosensitivity/phototoxicity reactions, and local site reactions. Periodically assess renal, hepatic and hematopoietic functions (with prolonged use), and repeat culture and susceptibility tests.

Patient Counseling: Inform to notify physician if experience pain, swelling, or inflammation of a tendon, or weakness or inability to move joints; rest and refrain from exercise and d/c therapy. Instruct to notify physician if worsening muscle weakness or breathing problems, sunburn-like reaction or skin eruption occurs, and of all medications and supplements currently being taken. Inform that drug treats only bacterial, not viral, infections. Instruct to take exactly ud; skipping doses or not completing full course may decrease effectiveness and increase bacterial resistance. Instruct to d/c and notify physician if an allergic reaction, skin rash, or symptoms of peripheral neuropathy occur. Advise to avoid exposure to natural or artificial sunlight (tanning beds or UVA/B treatment). Instruct to assess their reaction to therapy before engaging in activities that require mental alertness or coordination. Instruct to notify physician of any history of convulsions. Instruct to inform physician if child has joint-related problems prior to, during or after therapy. Instruct to contact physician as soon as possible if watery and bloody stools (with or without stomach cramps and fever) develop.

Administration: IV route. Refer to PI for preparation, administration, and compatibility instructions. **Storage:** 5-25°C (41-77°F). Protect from light and freezing. Avoid excessive heat. Diluted Sol (0.5-2mg/mL): Stable at room temperature or refrigeration for 14 days.

CIPRO ORAL   RX

ciprofloxacin (Bayer Healthcare)

> Fluoroquinolones are associated with an increased risk of tendinitis and tendon rupture in all ages. Risk is further increased in patients >60 yrs, patients taking corticosteroids, and with kidney, heart, or lung transplants. May exacerbate muscle weakness with myasthenia gravis; avoid in patients with known history of myasthenia gravis.

THERAPEUTIC CLASS: Fluoroquinolone

INDICATIONS: Treatment of urinary tract infections (UTI), acute uncomplicated cystitis in females, chronic bacterial prostatitis, lower respiratory tract infections (LRTI), acute exacerbations of chronic bronchitis, acute sinusitis, skin and skin structure infections (SSSI), bone and joint infections, complicated intra-abdominal infections (in combination with metronidazole), infectious diarrhea, typhoid fever, and uncomplicated cervical and urethral gonorrhea in adults. Treatment of complicated UTI and pyelonephritis in pediatrics 1-17 yrs. To reduce the incidence or progression of post-exposure inhalational anthrax in both adults and pediatrics.

DOSAGE: *Adults:* Acute Uncomplicated UTI: 250mg q12h for 3 days. Mild/Moderate UTI: 250mg q12h for 7-14 days. Severe/Complicated UTI: 500mg q12h for 7-14 days. Chronic Bacterial Prostatitis: Mild/Moderate: 500mg q12h for 28 days. LRTI/SSSI: Mild/Moderate: 500mg q12h for 7-14 days. Severe/Complicated: 750mg q12h for 7-14 days. Acute Sinusitis/Typhoid Fever: Mild/Moderate: 500mg q12h for 10 days. Bone and Joint: Mild/Moderate: 500mg q12h for ≥4-6 weeks. Severe/Complicated: 750mg q12h for ≥4-6 weeks. Complicated Intra-Abdominal (with metronidazole): 500mg q12h for 7-14 days. Infectious Diarrhea: 500mg q12h for 5-7 days. Uncomplicated Urethral/Cervical Gonococcal Infections: 250mg single dose. Inhalational Anthrax (Post-Exposure): 500mg q12h for 60 days. CrCl 30-50mL/min: 250-500mg q12h. CrCl 5-29mL/min: 250-500mg q18h. Hemodialysis/Peritoneal Dialysis: 250-500mg q24h (after dialysis). Refer to PI for conversion of IV to PO dosing.
Pediatrics: Inhalational Anthrax (Post-Exposure): 15mg/kg q12h for 60 days. Max: 500mg/dose. 1-17 yrs: Complicated UTI/Pyelonephritis: 10-20mg/kg q12h for 10-21 days. Max: 750mg/dose.

HOW SUPPLIED: Sus: 250mg/5mL, 500mg/5mL [100mL]; Tab: (HCl) 250mg, 500mg

CONTRAINDICATIONS: Concomitant administration with tizanidine.

WARNINGS/PRECAUTIONS: D/C if experience pain, swelling, inflammation, or rupture of tendon. Serious and occasionally fatal hypersensitivity reactions reported; d/c if skin rash, jaundice, or hypersensitivity occurs. Convulsions, increased intracranial pressure (including pseudotumor cerebri), toxic psychosis, and other CNS events reported; d/c and institute appropriate measures if CNS events occur. Caution with CNS disorders (eg, severe cerebral arteriosclerosis, epilepsy) or other risk factors that may predispose to seizures or lower the seizure threshold. *Clostridium difficile*-associated diarrhea (CDAD) reported. Rare cases of sensory or sensorimotor axonal polyneuropathy resulting in paresthesias, hypoesthesias, dysesthesias, and weakness reported; d/c if symptoms of neuropathy occur. Increased incidence of musculoskeletal disorders in pediatrics. May prolong QT interval; avoid with known QT interval prolongation or uncorrected hypokalemia. May mask or delay symptoms of incubating syphilis if used in high doses for short periods of time to treat gonorrhea; perform serologic test for syphilis at the time of gonorrhea diagnosis and repeat after 3 months of therapy. Crystalluria reported; maintain hydration and avoid alkalinity of urine. May cause photosensitivity/phototoxicity reactions; d/c if phototoxicity occurs. Avoid excessive exposure to sun/UV light. Monitor renal, hepatic, and hematopoietic function with prolonged use. May result in bacterial resistance with prolonged use or use in the absence of a proven/suspected bacterial infection or a prophylactic indication; take appropriate measures if superinfection develops. Caution in elderly and in patients with renal impairment.

ADVERSE REACTIONS: Tendinitis, tendon rupture, exacerbation of myasthenia gravis, musculoskeletal symptoms, arthralgia, N/V, diarrhea, abdominal pain, neurological events, rhinitis, abnormal LFTs, rash.

INTERACTIONS: See Boxed Warning and Contraindications. May increase levels of CYP1A2 substrates (eg, theophylline, methylxanthines, tizanidine), caffeine- or pentoxifylline (oxpentifylline)-containing products, duloxetine, ropinirole, lidocaine, clozapine, or sildenafil. Increased theophylline levels and its related adverse reactions; if use cannot be avoided, monitor theophylline level and adjust dose. May decrease caffeine clearance and inhibit formation of paraxanthine after caffeine administration. Multivalent cation-containing products (eg, magnesium/aluminum antacids, polymeric phosphate binders [eg, sevelamer, lanthanum carbonate], sucralfate, Videx [didanosine] chewable/buffered tab or pediatric powder, other highly buffered drugs, products containing calcium, iron, or zinc) may substantially decrease absorption, resulting in serum and urine levels lower than desired; administer ≥2 hrs before or 6 hrs after these drugs. May alter serum levels of phenytoin. Severe hypoglycemia with glyburide (rare). Probenecid may increase levels. Transient SrCr elevations with cyclosporine. May augment effects of oral anticoagulant (eg, warfarin); monitor PT and INR frequently. May increase levels and toxic reactions of methotrexate. High-dose quinolones shown to provoke convulsions with NSAIDs (not aspirin). Avoid with class IA (eg, quinidine, procainamide) and class III (eg, amiodarone, sotalol) antiarrhythmics. Caution with drugs that may lower seizure threshold. Metoclopramide may significantly accelerate oral absorption. Omeprazole may decrease levels.

PREGNANCY: Category C, not for use in nursing.

MECHANISM OF ACTION: Fluoroquinolone; inhibits enzymes topoisomerase II (DNA gyrase) and topoisomerase IV (both Type II topoisomerases), which are required for bacterial DNA replication, transcription, repair, and recombination.

PHARMACOKINETICS: Absorption: T_{max}=1-2 hrs. (Tab) Rapid, well absorbed. Absolute bioavailability (70%). Administration of various doses resulted in different parameters. **Distribution:** Plasma protein binding (20-40%); found in breast milk. **Elimination:** Urine (40-50%, unchanged), feces (20-35%); $T_{1/2}$=4 hrs.

NURSING CONSIDERATIONS

Assessment: Assess for risk factors for developing tendinitis and tendon rupture, history of myasthenia gravis, drug hypersensitivity, CNS disorders or other risk factors that may predispose to seizures or lower seizure threshold, QT interval prolongation, uncorrected hypokalemia, renal/hepatic function, pregnancy/nursing status, and possible drug interactions. Obtain baseline culture and susceptibility test. Perform serologic test for syphilis in patients with gonorrhea.

Monitoring: Monitor for tendinitis or tendon rupture, signs/symptoms of hypersensitivity reactions, development of superinfection, ECG changes (eg, QT interval prolongation), CNS events, CDAD, peripheral neuropathy, musculoskeletal disorders (pediatrics), and photosensitivity/phototoxicity reactions. Periodically assess renal, hepatic and hematopoietic functions (with prolonged use), and repeat culture and susceptibility tests. Perform follow-up serologic test for syphilis after 3 months.

Patient Counseling: Inform to notify physician if experience pain, swelling, or inflammation of a tendon, or weakness or inability to move joints; rest and refrain from exercise and d/c therapy. Instruct to notify physician if worsening muscle weakness or breathing problems, sunburn-like reaction or skin eruption occurs, and of all medications and supplements currently being taken. Inform that drug treats only bacterial, not viral, infections. Instruct to take exactly ud; skipping doses or not completing full course may decrease effectiveness and increase bacterial resistance. Instruct to take with or without meals, and drink fluids liberally. Instruct to avoid concomitant use with dairy products (like milk or yogurt) or calcium-fortified juices alone. Instruct to d/c and notify physician if an allergic reaction, skin rash, or symptoms of peripheral neuropathy occur. Advise to avoid exposure to natural or artificial sunlight (tanning beds or UVA/B treatment). Instruct to assess their reaction to therapy before engaging in activities that require mental alertness or coordination. Instruct to notify physician of any history of convulsions. Instruct to inform physician if child has joint-related problems prior to, during, or after therapy. Instruct to contact physician as soon as possible if watery and bloody stools (with or without stomach cramps and fever) develop.

Administration: Oral route. Administer ≥2 hrs before or 6 hrs after magnesium/aluminum antacids, polymeric phosphate binders, sucralfate, Videx (didanosine) chewable/buffered tab or pediatric powder for oral sol, other highly buffered drugs, or other products containing calcium, iron, or zinc. **Storage:** Tab/Reconstituted Sol: <30°C (<86°F). Reconstituted Sol: Store for 14 days. Microcapsules and Diluent: <25°C (<77°F). Protect from freezing.

CIPRO XR

RX

ciprofloxacin (Bayer Healthcare)

C

> Fluoroquinolones are associated with an increased risk of tendinitis and tendon rupture in all ages. Risk is further increased in patients >60 yrs, patients taking corticosteroids, and with kidney, heart, or lung transplants. May exacerbate muscle weakness with myasthenia gravis; avoid in patients with known history of myasthenia gravis.

THERAPEUTIC CLASS: Fluoroquinolone

INDICATIONS: Treatment of uncomplicated urinary tract infections (UTI) (acute cystitis), complicated UTI, and acute uncomplicated pyelonephritis caused by susceptible strains of microorganisms.

DOSAGE: *Adults:* Uncomplicated UTI: 500mg q24h for 3 days. Complicated UTI/Acute Uncomplicated Pyelonephritis: 1000mg q24h for 7-14 days. CrCl ≤30mL/min: 500mg qd. Hemodialysis/Peritoneal Dialysis: Give after procedure is completed. Max: 500mg q24h. Continuous Ambulatory Peritoneal Dialysis: Max: 500mg q24h. May switch from ciprofloxacin IV to extended release at discretion of physician.

HOW SUPPLIED: Tab, Extended-Release: 500mg, 1000mg

CONTRAINDICATIONS: Concomitant administration with tizanidine.

WARNINGS/PRECAUTIONS: D/C if experience pain, swelling, inflammation, or rupture of tendon. Serious and occasionally fatal hypersensitivity reactions reported; d/c if skin rash, jaundice, or hypersensitivity occurs. Convulsions, increased intracranial pressure (including pseudotumor cerebri), toxic psychosis, and other CNS events reported; d/c and institute appropriate measures if CNS events occur. Caution with CNS disorders (eg, severe cerebral arteriosclerosis, epilepsy) or other risk factors that may predispose to seizures or lower the seizure threshold. *Clostridium difficile*-associated diarrhea (CDAD) reported. Rare cases of sensory or sensorimotor axonal polyneuropathy resulting in paresthesias, hypoesthesias, dysesthesias, and weakness reported; d/c if symptoms of neuropathy occur. May prolong QT interval; avoid with known QT interval prolongation or uncorrected hypokalemia. Crystalluria reported; maintain hydration and avoid alkalinity of urine. May cause photosensitivity/phototoxicity reactions; d/c if phototoxicity occurs. Avoid excessive exposure to sun/UV light. May result in bacterial resistance with prolonged use or use in the absence of a proven/suspected bacterial infection or a prophylactic indication; take appropriate measures if superinfection develops. Caution in elderly and in patients with renal impairment. Not interchangeable with immediate-release tabs.

ADVERSE REACTIONS: Tendinitis, tendon rupture, exacerbation of myasthenia gravis, N/V, headache, diarrhea, dizziness, vaginal moniliasis, dyspepsia.

INTERACTIONS: See Boxed Warning and Contraindications. May increase levels of CYP1A2 substrates (eg, theophylline, methylxanthines, tizanidine), caffeine- or pentoxifylline (oxpentifylline)-containing products, duloxetine, ropinirole, lidocaine, clozapine, or sildenafil. Increased theophylline levels and its related adverse reactions; if use cannot be avoided, monitor theophylline levels and adjust dose. May decrease caffeine clearance and inhibit formation of paraxanthine after caffeine administration. Multivalent cation-containing products (eg, magnesium/aluminum antacids, polymeric phosphate binders [eg, sevelamer, lanthanum carbonate], sucralfate, Videx [didanosine] chewable/buffered tab or pediatric powder, other highly buffered drugs, products containing calcium, iron, or zinc) may substantially decrease absorption, resulting in serum and urine levels lower than desired; administer ≥2 hrs before or 6 hrs after these drugs. Avoid concomitant administration with dairy products alone, or with calcium-fortified products. May alter serum levels of phenytoin. Severe hypoglycemia with glyburide (rare). Transient SrCr elevations with cyclosporine. May augment effects of oral anticoagulant (eg, warfarin); monitor PT and INR frequently. Probenecid may increase levels. May increase levels and toxic reactions of methotrexate. High-dose quinolones shown to provoke convulsions with NSAIDs (not aspirin). Avoid with class IA (eg, quinidine, procainamide) and Class III (eg, amiodarone, sotalol) antiarrhythmics. Caution with drugs that may lower seizure threshold. Metoclopramide may significantly accelerate oral absorption. Omeprazole may decrease levels.

PREGNANCY: Category C, not for use in nursing.

MECHANISM OF ACTION: Fluoroquinolone; inhibits enzymes topoisomerase II (DNA gyrase) and topoisomerase IV (both Type II topoisomerases), which are required for bacterial DNA replication, transcription, repair, and recombination.

PHARMACOKINETICS: Absorption: (500mg) C_{max}=1.59mg/L; T_{max}=1.5 hrs; AUC_{0-24h}=7.97mg•h/L. (1000mg) C_{max}=3.11mg/L; T_{max}=2 hrs; AUC_{0-24h}=16.83mg•h/L. **Distribution:** V_d=2.1-2.7L/kg (IV); plasma protein binding (20-40%); found in breast milk. **Metabolism:** Oxociprofloxacin (M_1), sulfociprofloxacin (M_2) (primary metabolites). **Elimination:** Urine (35%, unchanged); $T_{1/2}$=6.6 hrs (500mg), 6.31 hrs (1000mg).

NURSING CONSIDERATIONS

Assessment: Assess for risk factors for developing tendinitis and tendon rupture, history of myasthenia gravis, drug hypersensitivity, CNS disorders or other risk factors that may predispose to seizures or lower seizure threshold, QT interval prolongation, uncorrected hypokalemia, renal/hepatic function, pregnancy/nursing status, and possible drug interactions. Obtain baseline culture and susceptibility test.

Monitoring: Monitor for tendinitis or tendon rupture, signs/symptoms of hypersensitivity reactions, development of superinfection, ECG changes (eg, QT interval prolongation), CNS events, CDAD, peripheral neuropathy, and photosensitivity/phototoxicity reactions. Assess renal function and perform periodic culture and susceptibility testing.

Patient Counseling: Inform to notify physician if experience pain, swelling, or inflammation of a tendon, or weakness or inability to move joints; rest and refrain from exercise and d/c therapy. Instruct to notify physician if worsening muscle weakness or breathing problems, sunburn-like reaction or skin eruption occurs, and of all medications and supplements currently being taken. Inform that drug treats only bacterial, not viral, infections. Instruct to take exactly ud; skipping doses or not completing full course may decrease effectiveness and increase bacterial resistance. Instruct to take with or without meals, and drink fluids liberally. Instruct to avoid concomitant use with dairy products (like milk or yogurt) or calcium-fortified juices alone. Counsel to take dose later in the day if missed at the usual time. Advise not to take >1 tab/day if a dose is missed. Instruct to d/c and notify physician if an allergic reaction, skin rash, or symptoms of peripheral neuropathy occur. Advise to avoid exposure to natural or artificial sunlight (tanning beds or UVA/B treatment). Instruct to assess their reaction to therapy before engaging in activities that require mental alertness or coordination. Instruct to notify physician of any history of convulsions. Instruct to contact physician as soon as possible if watery and bloody stools (with or without stomach cramps and fever) develop.

Administration: Oral route. Swallow tab whole; do not split, crush, or chew. Administer ≥2 hrs before or 6 hrs after magnesium/aluminum-containing antacids, sucralfate, (Videx) didanosine chewable/buffered tab or pediatric powder, other highly buffered drugs, or other products containing calcium, iron, or zinc. Space calcium intake (>800mg) by 2 hrs. **Storage:** 25°C (77°F); excursions permitted to 15-30°C (59-86°F).

CIPRODEX   RX
ciprofloxacin HCl - dexamethasone (Alcon)

THERAPEUTIC CLASS: Antibacterial/corticosteroid combination

INDICATIONS: Treatment of acute otitis media in pediatric patients (≥6 months) with tympanostomy tubes and acute otitis externa in pediatric (≥6 months), adult and elderly patients caused by susceptible organisms.

DOSAGE: *Adults:* Acute Otitis Externa: 4 drops into the affected ear(s) bid for 7 days. *Pediatrics:* Acute Otitis Media/Externa: ≥6 months: 4 drops into the affected ear(s) bid for 7 days.

HOW SUPPLIED: Sus: (Ciprofloxacin-Dexamethasone) 0.3%-0.1% [7.5mL]

CONTRAINDICATIONS: Viral infections of external canal including herpes simplex infections.

WARNINGS/PRECAUTIONS: For otic use only; not for inj. D/C at 1st appearance of rash or other sign of hypersensitivity. Serious and occasionally fatal hypersensitivity/anaphylactic reactions reported; may require emergency treatment. May result in overgrowth of nonsusceptible organisms (eg, yeast, fungi); perform culture testing if infection not improved after 1 week. If otorrhea persists after full course therapy, or if ≥2 episodes of otorrhea occur within 6 months, evaluate to exclude underlying condition such as cholesteatoma, foreign body, or tumor.

ADVERSE REACTIONS: Ear discomfort/pain/precipitate/pruritus/debris/congestion, irritability, taste perversion, superimposed ear infection, erythema.

PREGNANCY: Category C, not for use in nursing.

MECHANISM OF ACTION: Ciprofloxacin: Fluoroquinolone antibacterial; bactericidal action results from interference with the enzyme (DNA gyrase), which is needed for the synthesis of bacterial DNA. Dexamethasone: Corticosteroid; aids in resolution of inflammatory response accompanying bacterial infection.

PHARMACOKINETICS: Absorption: Ciprofloxacin: C_{max}=1.39ng/mL; T_{max}=15 min-2 hrs. Dexamethasone: C_{max}=1.14ng/mL; T_{max}=15 min-2 hrs.

NURSING CONSIDERATIONS

Assessment: Assess for history of drug hypersensitivity and viral infection of the external canal, including herpes simplex virus infection, and pregnancy/nursing status.

C

Monitoring: Monitor for anaphylactic reactions, skin rash, overgrowth of nonsusceptible organisms (eg, fungi and yeast), lesions or erosions of cartilage in weight-bearing joints, and other signs of arthropathy.

Patient Counseling: Inform that drug is for otic use only. Instruct to warm bottle in hand for 1-2 min prior to use and shake well before using. Advise to avoid contaminating the tip with material from the ear, fingers, or other sources. Counsel to protect product from light. Instruct to d/c immediately and consult physician if rash or allergic reaction occurs. Instruct to take as prescribed, even if symptoms improve. Advise to discard unused portion after therapy is completed.

Administration: Otic route. Shake well before use. Warm bottle by holding in hand for 1-2 min. Lie with affected ear upward, then instill drops. Maintain position for 60 sec and repeat, if necessary, with opposite ear. **Storage:** 15-30°C (59-86°F). Protect from light; avoid freezing.

CLARINEX RX
desloratadine (Merck)

THERAPEUTIC CLASS: H$_1$-antagonist

INDICATIONS: Relief of nasal and non-nasal symptoms of seasonal allergic rhinitis in patients ≥2 yrs. Relief of nasal and non-nasal symptoms of perennial allergic rhinitis in patients ≥6 months. Symptomatic relief of pruritus and reduction in number and size of hives in patients ≥6 months with chronic idiopathic urticaria.

DOSAGE: *Adults:* 5mg or 10mL qd. Hepatic/Renal Impairment: Initial: 5mg tab qod. *Pediatrics:* ≥12 yrs: 5mg or 10mL qd. 6-11 yrs: 2.5mg RediTab or 5mL qd. 12 months-5 yrs: 2.5mL qd. 6-11 months: 2mL qd.

HOW SUPPLIED: Sol: 0.5mg/mL; Tab: 5mg; Tab, Disintegrating: (RediTabs) 2.5mg, 5mg

WARNINGS/PRECAUTIONS: Hypersensitivity reactions (eg, rash, pruritus, urticaria, edema, dyspnea, anaphylaxis) reported; d/c therapy if any occur and consider alternative treatment. Caution in elderly.

ADVERSE REACTIONS: Pharyngitis, dry mouth, headache, N/V, fatigue, myalgia, fever, diarrhea, cough, upper respiratory tract infection, irritability, somnolence, bronchitis, otitis media.

INTERACTIONS: CYP450 3A4 inhibitors (eg, erythromycin, ketoconazole, azithromycin), fluoxetine, and cimetidine may increase levels.

PREGNANCY: Category C, not for use in nursing.

MECHANISM OF ACTION: Long-acting tricyclic histamine antagonist with selective H$_1$-receptor histamine antagonist activity; inhibits histamine release from human mast cells *in vitro*.

PHARMACOKINETICS: **Absorption:** (5mg tab) T$_{max}$=3 hrs, C$_{max}$=4ng/mL, AUC=56.9ng•hr/mL. **Distribution:** Plasma protein binding (82-87%, 85-89% 3-hydroxydesloratadine); found in breast milk. **Metabolism:** Extensive; 3-hydroxydesloratadine (active metabolite) and glucuronidation pathway. **Elimination:** Urine and feces (87%); T$_{1/2}$=27 hrs.

NURSING CONSIDERATIONS

Assessment: Assess for hypersensitivity to drug, renal/hepatic function, pregnancy/nursing status, and possible drug interactions.

Monitoring: Monitor for hypersensitivity and other adverse reactions.

Patient Counseling: Instruct to take drug as directed; may be taken without regard to meals. Advise not to increase dose or dosing frequency. Inform that RediTabs contain phenylalanine.

Administration: Oral route. (RediTabs) Place on tongue and allow to disintegrate before swallowing. Take immediately after opening the blister. Administer with or without water. (Sol) Administer age-appropriate dose of sol with a measuring dropper or syringe calibrated to deliver 2mL and 2.5mL. **Storage:** 25°C (77°F); excursions permitted to 15-30°C (59-86°F). (Tab) Avoid exposure at ≥30°C (86°F). (Sol) Protect from light.

CLARINEX-D RX
pseudoephedrine sulfate - desloratadine (Merck)

THERAPEUTIC CLASS: H$_1$-antagonist/sympathomimetic amine

INDICATIONS: Relief of nasal and non-nasal symptoms of seasonal allergic rhinitis, including nasal congestion, in adults and adolescents ≥12 yrs.

DOSAGE: *Adults:* (12 Hr) 1 tab bid, approximately 12 hrs apart. (24 Hr) 1 tab qd. *Pediatrics:* ≥12 yrs: (12 Hr) 1 tab bid, approximately 12 hrs apart. (24 Hr) 1 tab qd.

HOW SUPPLIED: Tab, Extended-Release: (Desloratadine-Pseudoephedrine) (12 Hr) 2.5mg-120mg, (24 Hr) 5mg-240mg

CONTRAINDICATIONS: Narrow-angle glaucoma, urinary retention, MAOI therapy or within 14 days of d/c MAOI, severe HTN, severe coronary artery disease (CAD).

WARNINGS/PRECAUTIONS: Avoid in patients with hepatic and/or renal impairment. Caution in elderly. Pseudoephedrine: Cardiovascular (CV) and CNS effects (eg, insomnia, dizziness, weakness, tremor, arrhythmias) reported; caution in patients with CV disorder. CNS stimulation with convulsions and CV collapse with hypotension reported. Caution in patients with diabetes mellitus (DM), hyperthyroidism, prostatic hypertrophy or increased intraocular pressure (IOP); urinary retention and narrow-angle glaucoma may occur. Elderly are more likely to have adverse reactions to sympathomimetic amines. Desloratadine: Hypersensitivity reactions (eg, rash, pruritus, urticaria, edema, dyspnea, anaphylaxis) reported; d/c if any occur and consider alternative treatment.

ADVERSE REACTIONS: Dry mouth, headache, insomnia, fatigue, pharyngitis, somnolence, dizziness, nausea, anorexia, psychomotor hyperactivity, nervousness.

INTERACTIONS: See Contraindications. Pseudoephedrine: Antihypertensive effects of β-adrenergic blocking agents, methyldopa, and reserpine may be reduced; use with caution. May increase ectopic pacemaker activity with concomitant digitalis; use with caution. Desloratadine: CYP450 3A4 inhibitors (eg, ketoconazole, erythromycin, azithromycin), fluoxetine, and cimetidine may increase levels.

PREGNANCY: Category C, not for use in nursing.

MECHANISM OF ACTION: Desloratadine: H_1-receptor antagonist; inhibits histamine release from human mast cells *in vitro*. Pseudoephedrine: Sympathomimetic amine; exerts a decongestant action on nasal mucosa.

PHARMACOKINETICS: Absorption: Desloratadine: (24 Hr) C_{max}=1.79ng/mL; T_{max}=6-7 hrs, AUC=61.1ng•hr/mL. (12 Hr) C_{max}=1.09ng/mL; T_{max}=4-5 hrs, AUC=31.6ng•hr/mL. Pseudoephedrine: (24 Hr) C_{max}=328ng/mL, T_{max}=8-9 hrs, AUC=6438ng•hr/mL. (12 Hr) C_{max}=263ng/mL, T_{max}=6-7 hrs, AUC=4588ng•hr/mL. **Distribution:** Desloratadine: Plasma protein binding (82-87%, 85-89% 3-hydroxydesloratadine); found in breast milk. **Metabolism:** Desloratadine: Extensive, 3-hydroxydesloratadine (active metabolite) and glucuronidation pathway. Pseudoephedrine: Liver (incomplete), through N-demethylation. **Elimination:** Desloratadine: Urine and feces (87%). (24 Hr) $T_{1/2}$=24 hrs, (12 Hr) $T_{1/2}$=27 hrs. Pseudoephedrine: Urine (55-96% unchanged). $T_{1/2}$=3-6 hrs (urinary pH=5), 9-16 hrs (urinary pH=8).

NURSING CONSIDERATIONS

Assessment: Assess for drug hypersensitivity, hepatic/renal impairment, increased IOP, narrow-angle glaucoma, prostatic hypertrophy, urinary retention, CV disorders, HTN, CAD, DM, hyperthyroidism, pregnancy/nursing status, and possible drug interactions (eg, MAOIs).

Monitoring: Monitor for CV and CNS effects (eg, insomnia, dizziness, weakness, tremor, arrhythmias), hypersensitivity reactions, BP, IOP, urinary retention in patients with prostatic hypertrophy, and hepatic/renal function.

Patient Counseling: Inform patients that CV or CNS effects (eg, insomnia, dizziness, tremor, arrhythmias) may occur. Advise not to increase the dose or dosing frequency. Advise not to use other antihistamines and/or decongestants. Advise patients with severe HTN, severe CAD, narrow-angle glaucoma, or urinary retention not to use drug. Instruct patient to swallow tab whole and not to break, crush, or chew tab. Instruct to take without regard to meals.

Administration: Oral route. **Storage:** 25°C (77°F); excursions permitted to 15-30°C (59-86°F). Avoid exposure at ≥30°C (86°F). Protect from excessive moisture. Protect from light.

CLARIPEL   RX
hydroquinone (Stiefel)

THERAPEUTIC CLASS: Depigmentation agent

INDICATIONS: Gradual treatment of ultraviolet induced dyschromia and discoloration resulting from use of oral contraceptives, pregnancy, hormone replacement therapy, or skin trauma.

DOSAGE: *Adults:* Apply bid.
Pediatrics: ≥12 yrs: Apply bid.

HOW SUPPLIED: Cre: 4% [28g, 45g]

WARNINGS/PRECAUTIONS: Avoid sun exposure on bleached skin. Claripel contains sunscreen. May produce unwanted cosmetic effects if not used as directed. Test for skin sensitivity. D/C if no lightening effect after 2 months of therapy, if blue-black skin discoloration occurs, or if itching, vesicle formation, or excessive inflammatory reactions occur. Contains sodium metabisulfite; may cause serious allergic type reactions. Avoid contact with eyes.

ADVERSE REACTIONS: Cutaneous hypersensitivity (contact dermatitis).

PREGNANCY: Category C, caution in nursing.

MECHANISM OF ACTION: Produces a reversible depigmentation of the skin by inhibition of the enzymatic oxidation of tyrosine to 3-(3,4-dihydroxyphenyl) alanine (dopa)[1] and suppression of other melanocyte metabolic processes.

C

NURSING CONSIDERATIONS

Assessment: Test for skin sensitivity prior to treatment.

Monitoring: Monitor allergic-type reactions including anaphylactic symptoms and life-threatening or severe asthmatic episodes in susceptible patients, itching, vesicles and gradual blue-darkening of the skin.

Patient Counseling: Take drug as prescribed and use sunscreen during therapy. D/C drug and contact physician if any signs of allergy occur. Avoid contact with eyes.

Administration: Topical route. **Storage:** 15-30°C (59-86°F).

CLEOCIN   RX
clindamycin (Pharmacia & Upjohn)

> *Clostridium difficile*-associated diarrhea (CDAD) reported and may range in severity from mild diarrhea to fatal colitis. Not for use with nonbacterial infections. CDAD must be considered in all patients with diarrhea following antibiotic use. If CDAD is suspected or confirmed, ongoing antibiotic use not directed against *C. difficile* may need to be d/c. Appropriate fluid and electrolyte management, protein supplementation, antibiotic treatment of *C. difficile* and surgical evaluation may be instituted as clinically indicated.

THERAPEUTIC CLASS: Lincomycin derivative

INDICATIONS: Treatment of serious infections caused by susceptible anaerobes, streptococci, pneumococci, and staphylococci.

DOSAGE: *Adults:* Serious Infection: 150-300mg PO q6h or 600-1200mg/day IM/IV given bid-qid. More Severe Infections: 300-450mg PO q6h or 1200-2700mg/day IM/IV given bid-qid. Life-Threatening Infections: Up to 4800mg/day IV. Max: 600mg per IM injection. Alternatively may administer as a single rapid infusion for the first dose followed by continuous IV infusion; see PI for dosing. Treat β-hemolytic strep for at least 10 days.
Pediatrics: PO: Serious Infections: (Cap) 8-16mg/kg/day given tid-qid or (Sol) 8-12mg/kg/day tid-qid. Severe Infection: (Sol) 13-16mg/kg/day tid-qid. More Severe Infections: (Cap) 16-20mg/kg/day given tid-qid or (Sol) 17-25mg/kg/day tid-qid. ≤10kg: 1/2 tsp (37.5mg) tid should be the minimum recommended dose. IM/IV: 1 month-16 yrs: 20-40mg/kg/day tid-qid; use the higher dose for more severe infections. Alternatively may give 350mg/m²/day for serious infections and 450mg/m²/day for more severe infections. <1 month: 15-20mg/kg/day tid-qid. Treat β-hemolytic strep for at least 10 days.

HOW SUPPLIED: Cap: (HCl) 75mg, 150mg, 300mg; Inj: (Phosphate) 150mg/mL [2mL, 4mL, 6mL, 60mL] 300mg/50mL, 600mg/50mL, 900mg/50mL; Sol: (Palmitate) 75mg/5mL [100mL]

WARNINGS/PRECAUTIONS: Due to association with severe colitis, reserve use for serious infections where less toxic agents are inappropriate. May result in bacterial resistance with prolonged use or use in the absence of a proven/suspected bacterial infection or a prophylactic indication; take appropriate measures if superinfection develops. Not for treatment of meningitis. Caution with patients with liver disease; perform periodic liver enzyme determinations with severe liver disease. Caution with atopic patients, renal disease, history of GI disease (eg, colitis), and the elderly. Perform periodic monitoring of blood counts, hepatic and renal function with long-term use. Do not give injection undiluted as bolus. (75mg/150mg caps) Contains tartrazine, may cause allergic-type reactions. (Inj) Contains benzyl alcohol; associated with "gasping syndrome" in premature infants.

ADVERSE REACTIONS: Abdominal pain, colitis, esophagitis, N/V, diarrhea, maculopapular skin rash, jaundice, pruritus, vaginitis.

INTERACTIONS: Antagonism may occur with erythromycin. May potentiate neuromuscular blockers.

PREGNANCY: Category B, not for use in nursing.

MECHANISM OF ACTION: Lincomycin-derivative antibiotic; inhibits bacterial protein synthesis by binding to the 50s subunit of the ribosome.

PHARMACOKINETICS: Absorption: Cap: Rapid, complete; C_{max}=2.5mcg/mL, T_{max}=45 min. Inj: C_{max}=10.8mcg/mL (Adults, 600mg IV q8h), 9mcg/mL (Adults, 600 mg IM q12h), 10mcg/mL (Peds, 5-7mg/kg IV in 1 hr), 8mcg/mL (Peds, 5-7mg/kg IM); T_{max}=3 hrs (Adults, IM), 1 hr (Peds, IM). **Distribution:** Wide; body fluids, tissues, and bones; found in breast milk. **Elimination:** Cap: Urine (10% unchanged), feces (3.6% unchanged); $T_{1/2}$=2.4 hr. Inj: $T_{1/2}$=3 hrs (Adults), 2.5 hrs (Peds). Sol: $T_{1/2}$=2 hrs.

NURSING CONSIDERATIONS

Assessment: Assess for previous sensitivities to drugs and other allergens, history of GI disease (eg, colitis), renal/hepatic function, pregnancy/nursing status, presence of meningitis, upcoming surgical procedures, and for possible drug interactions. Assess use in atopic patients and in elderly patients with severe illness.

Monitoring: Monitor for CDAD, overgrowth of nonsusceptible organisms, and for anaphylactoid reactions. Monitor for changes in bowel frequency in older patients. When culture and susceptibility information is available, consider modifying antibacterial therapy. If on prolonged therapy, perform periodic liver and kidney function tests and blood counts. Perform periodic liver enzyme determinations in patients with severe liver disease.

Patient Counseling: Inform about potential benefits/risks of use. Inform that therapy only treats bacterial, not viral infections. Instruct to take exactly as directed; skipping doses or not completing full course may decrease effectiveness and increase antibiotic resistance. Instruct to contact physician if an allergic reaction develops. Advise that watery and bloody stools may occur as late as 2 months after therapy. Instruct to notify physician if pregnant/nursing.

Administration: Oral/IM/IV route. See PI for proper preparation and administration. **Storage:** 20-25°C (68-77°F). (Sol) Do not refrigerate the reconstituted solution; stable at room temperature for 2 weeks.

CLEVIPREX   RX
clevidipine (The Medicines Company)

THERAPEUTIC CLASS: Calcium channel blocker (dihydropyridine)

INDICATIONS: Reduction of BP in patients when PO therapy is not feasible or desirable.

DOSAGE: *Adults:* Individualize dose. Give by IV infusion. Initial: 1-2mg/hr. Titrate: May double the dose at 90-second intervals initially. As BP approaches goal, increase in doses should be less than doubling and the time between dose adjustments should be lengthened to every 5-10 minutes. Maint: 4-6mg/hr. Max: 16mg/hr. Due to lipid load restrictions, no more than 1000mL or an average of 21mg/hr of infusion is recommended/24-hr period. Transition to PO Therapy: D/C or titrate downward until PO therapy is established. Consider the lag time of onset of the PO agent's effect when PO antihypertensive is instituted. Continue BP monitoring until desired effect is reached. Elderly: Start at the lower end of dosing range.

HOW SUPPLIED: Inj: 0.5mg/mL [50mL, 100mL]

CONTRAINDICATIONS: Allergies to soybeans, soy products, eggs, or egg products, severe aortic stenosis, defective lipid metabolism such as pathologic hyperlipemia, lipoid nephrosis, or acute pancreatitis if it is accompanied by hyperlipidemia.

WARNINGS/PRECAUTIONS: Systemic hypotension and reflex tachycardia may occur; decrease dose if either occurs. Lipid intake restrictions may be necessary with significant disorders of lipid metabolism; a reduction in the quantity of concurrently administered lipids may be necessary to compensate for the amount of lipid infused as part of the drug's formulation. May produce negative inotropic effects and exacerbation of heart failure (HF); monitor HF patients carefully. Does not reduce HR and does not protect against the effects of abrupt β-blocker withdrawal. Monitor for the possibility of rebound HTN for at least 8 hrs after d/c of infusion in patients who receive prolonged infusions and are not transitioned to other antihypertensive therapies. Caution in elderly.

ADVERSE REACTIONS: Atrial fibrillation, acute renal failure, headache, N/V, hypotension, reflex tachycardia.

PREGNANCY: Category C, safety not known in nursing.

MECHANISM OF ACTION: Calcium channel blocker (dihydropyridine); mediates the influx of calcium during depolarization in arterial smooth muscle and reduces mean arterial blood pressure by decreasing systemic vascular resistance; does not reduce cardiac filling pressure (preload).

PHARMACOKINETICS: Distribution: V_d=0.17L/kg; plasma protein binding (>99.5%). **Metabolism:** Hydrolysis of the ester linkage, glucuronidation or oxidation; carboxylic acid metabolite and formaldehyde (primary metabolites). **Elimination:** Urine (63-74%), feces (7-22%); $T_{1/2}$=15 min.

NURSING CONSIDERATIONS

Assessment: Assess for allergies to soybeans, eggs or soy/egg products, defective lipid metabolism, β-blocker usage, and pregnancy/nursing status. Obtain baseline parameters for BP, HR, and lipid profile.

Monitoring: Monitor for hypotension, reflex tachycardia, rebound HTN, HF exacerbation, and other adverse reactions. Monitor BP and HR during infusion, and until vital signs are stable.

Patient Counseling: Advise patients with underlying HTN that they require continued follow-up for their medical condition, and, if applicable, to continue taking PO antihypertensive medication(s) as directed. Instruct to report any signs of new hypertensive emergency (eg, neurological symptoms, visual changes, evidence of congestive HF) to a healthcare provider immediately.

Administration: IV route. Use aseptic technique. Refer to PI for administration and preparation instructions. **Storage:** 2-8°C (36-46°F). Do not freeze. Leave vials in cartons until use; may be transferred to 25°C (77°F) for a period not to exceed 2 months. Do not return to refrigerated storage after beginning room temperature storage. Discard any unused portion within 12 hrs of stopper puncture.

CLIMARA

RX

estradiol (Bayer Healthcare)

> Estrogens increase the risk of endometrial cancer. Perform adequate diagnostic measures, including endometrial sampling, to rule out malignancy with undiagnosed persistent or recurrent abnormal vaginal bleeding. Should not be used for the prevention of cardiovascular disease or dementia. Increased risk of myocardial infarction (MI), stroke, invasive breast cancer, pulmonary embolism (PE), and deep vein thrombosis (DVT) in postmenopausal women (50-79 yrs of age) reported. Increased risk of developing probable dementia in postmenopausal women ≥65 yrs of age reported. Should be prescribed at the lowest effective dose and for the shortest duration consistent with treatment goals and risks.

THERAPEUTIC CLASS: Estrogen

INDICATIONS: Treatment of moderate to severe vasomotor symptoms and/or vulvar/vaginal atrophy associated with menopause. Treatment of hypoestrogenism due to hypogonadism, castration, or primary ovarian failure. Prevention of postmenopausal osteoporosis.

DOSAGE: *Adults:* Apply 1 patch weekly to lower abdomen or upper area of buttocks (avoid breasts and waistline). Rotate application sites. Vasomotor Symptoms: Initial: 0.025mg/day (6.5cm²) patch once weekly. Titrate: Adjust dose PRN at 3-6 month intervals. Women Currently taking Oral Estrogen: Initiate 1 week after withdrawal of oral therapy or sooner if symptoms reappear in <1 week. Osteoporosis Prevention: Min Effective Dose: 0.025mg/day.

HOW SUPPLIED: Patch: 0.025mg/day, 0.0375mg/day, 0.05mg/day, 0.06mg/day, 0.075mg/day, 0.1mg/day [4ˢ]

CONTRAINDICATIONS: Undiagnosed abnormal genital bleeding, known/suspected/history of breast cancer, known/suspected estrogen-dependent neoplasia, active or history of DVT/PE, active or recent arterial thromboembolic disease (eg, stroke, MI), liver dysfunction or disease, known/suspected pregnancy.

WARNINGS/PRECAUTIONS: Increased risk of cardiovascular (CV) events. Caution in patients with risk factors for arterial vascular disease (eg, HTN, diabetes mellitus [DM], tobacco use, hypercholesterolemia, obesity) and/ or venous thromboembolism (eg, personal history or family history of venous thromboembolism, obesity, systemic lupus erythematosus [SLE]). If feasible, d/c at least 4 to 6 weeks before surgery of the type associated with an increased risk of thromboembolism, or during periods of prolonged immobilization. May increase risk of gallbladder disease. May lead to severe hypercalcemia in patients with breast cancer and bone metastases; d/c and take appropriate measures if hypercalcemia occurs. Retinal vascular thrombosis reported; d/c pending examination if sudden partial or complete loss of vision, sudden onset of proptosis, diplopia, migraine, or if examination reveals papilledema or retinal vascular lesions. Consider addition of a progestin if no hysterectomy. May elevate BP, thyroid binding globulin levels, and plasma TG leading to pancreatitis and other complications. Caution with history of cholestatic jaundice; d/c in case of recurrence. May cause fluid retention; caution with cardiac/renal dysfunction. Caution with severe hypocalcemia. May increase risk of ovarian cancer. May exacerbate endometriosis, asthma, DM, epilepsy, migraine or porphyria, SLE, and hepatic hemangiomas; use with caution. May induce or exacerbate symptoms in women with hereditary angioderma. May affect certain endocrine, LFTs, and blood components in laboratory tests.

ADVERSE REACTIONS: Headache, arthralgia, edema, abdominal pain, flatulence, depression, breast pain, leukorrhea, upper respiratory tract infection, sinusitis, rhinitis, pruritus, nausea, pharyngitis, pain.

INTERACTIONS: CYP3A4 inducers (eg, St. John's wort, phenobarbital, carbamazepine, rifampin) may decrease levels, which may decrease therapeutic effects and/or change uterine bleeding profile. CYP3A4 inhibitors (eg, erythromycin, clarithromycin, ketoconazole, itraconazole, ritonavir, grapefruit juice) may increase levels, which may result in side effects. Patients concomitantly receiving thyroid hormone replacement therapy and estrogens may require increased doses of their thyroid replacement therapy.

PREGNANCY: Contraindicated in pregnancy, caution in nursing.

MECHANISM OF ACTION: Estrogen; binds to nuclear receptors in estrogen-responsive tissues. Circulating estrogen modulates pituitary secretion of gonadotropins, luteinizing hormone, and follicle stimulating hormone, through negative feedback mechanism. Reduces elevated levels of these hormones in postmenopausal women.

PHARMACOKINETICS: Absorption: Transdermal administration of different doses resulted in different parameters. **Distribution:** Largely bound to sex hormone binding globulin and albumin; found in breast milk. **Metabolism:** Liver to estrone (metabolite); estriol (major urinary metabolite); sulfate and glucuronide conjugation (liver), gut hydrolysis; CYP 3A4 (partial metabolism). **Elimination:** Urine.

NURSING CONSIDERATIONS

Assessment: Assess for abnormal genital bleeding, presence or history of breast cancer, estrogen-dependent neoplasias, DVT, PE, active or recent (within past yr) arterial thromboembolic disease, and any other conditions where treatment may be contraindicated or cautioned. Assess use in women ≥65 yrs, nursing patients, and those with DM, asthma, epilepsy, migraines or porphyria, SLE, and hepatic hemangiomas. Assess for possible drug interactions. Assess need for progestin therapy in women who have not had a hysterectomy.

Monitoring: Monitor for signs/symptoms of CV disorders, malignant neoplasms, dementia, gallbladder disease, hypercalcemia, visual abnormalities, increased BP, hypertriglyceridemia, hypothyroidism, fluid retention, cholestatic jaundice, exacerbation of endometriosis, and other conditions. Perform annual mammography, regular monitoring of BP, and periodic evaluation (q3-6 months) to determine need of therapy. Monitor thyroid function if patient on thyroid hormone replacement therapy. In cases of undiagnosed, persistent, or recurrent vaginal bleeding in women with uterus, perform adequate diagnostic measures (eg, endometrial sampling) to rule out malignancies.

Patient Counseling: Inform that medication increases risk for uterine cancer and may increase chances for heart attack, stroke, breast cancer, and blood clots. Advise to contact physician if breast lumps, unusual vaginal bleeding, dizziness or faintness, changes in speech, severe headaches, chest pain, SOB, leg pain, visual changes, or vomiting occur. Inform once in place, transdermal system should not be exposed to sun for prolonged periods of time. Inform that removal of system should be done carefully and slowly to avoid skin irritation and if patch falls off during dosing interval, apply new patch for remainder of the 7-day period. Advise to have yearly breast examinations by a healthcare provider and perform monthly breast self-examinations.

Administration: Topical route. Refer to PI for proper application and removal of the system (patch). **Storage:** Do not store above 30°C (86°F). Do not store unpouched.

CLINDAGEL   RX
clindamycin phosphate (Galderma)

THERAPEUTIC CLASS: Lincomycin derivative

INDICATIONS: Acne vulgaris.

DOSAGE: *Adults:* Apply thin film once daily.
Pediatrics: ≥12 yrs: Apply thin film once daily.

HOW SUPPLIED: Gel: 1% [40mL, 75mL]

CONTRAINDICATIONS: Hypersensitivity to lincomycin. History of regional enteritis, ulcerative colitis, or antibiotic-associated colitis.

WARNINGS/PRECAUTIONS: D/C if significant diarrhea occurs. Caution in atopic individuals.

ADVERSE REACTIONS: Peeling, pruritus, pseudomembranous colitis (rare).

INTERACTIONS: May potentiate neuromuscular blockers.

PREGNANCY: Category B, not for use in nursing.

MECHANISM OF ACTION: Lincomycin derivative; inhibits bacteria protein synthesis at ribosomal level by binding to the 50S ribosomal subunit and affecting the process of peptide chain initiation.

PHARMACOKINETICS: Absorption: C_{max}≤5.5ng/mL. **Distribution:** Orally and parenterally administered clindamycin appears in breast milk. **Excretion:** Urine (<0.4% of total dose).

NURSING CONSIDERATIONS

Assessment: Assess for hypersensitivity to lincomycin, history of regional or ulcerative colitis, antibiotic-associated colitis, nursing status. Assess use in atopic individuals and for possible drug interactions.

Monitoring: Monitor for signs/symptoms of colitis (pseudomembranous colitis), diarrhea, and bloody diarrhea. In patients with diarrhea, consider stool culture for *C. difficile* and stool assay for *C. difficile* toxin. In patients with significant diarrhea, consider large bowel endoscopy.

Patient Counseling: Instruct to notify physician of significant diarrhea during therapy or up to several weeks following end of therapy.

Administration: Topical application. **Storage:** Controlled room temperature, 20-25°C (68-77°F); excursions permitted to 15-30°C (59-86°F). Keep container tightly closed, out of direct sunlight.

C

CLINDESSE RX
clindamycin phosphate (KV Pharm)

THERAPEUTIC CLASS: Lincomycin derivative

INDICATIONS: Treatment of bacterial vaginosis in nonpregnant women.

DOSAGE: *Adults:* Usual: 1 applicatorful once intravaginally at any time of the day.
Pediatrics: Postmenarchal: Usual: 1 applicatorful once intravaginally at any time of the day.

HOW SUPPLIED: Cre: 2% [5g]

CONTRAINDICATIONS: Regional enteritis, ulcerative colitis, or history of *Clostridium difficile*-associated diarrhea (CDAD).

WARNINGS/PRECAUTIONS: Not for ophthalmic, dermal, or oral use. CDAD, ranging from mild diarrhea to fatal colitis reported; d/c therapy if suspected or confirmed and institute appropriate therapy as clinically indicated. Contains mineral oil that may weaken latex or rubber products (eg, condoms or vaginal contraceptive diaphragms); avoid use concurrently or for 5 days following treatment.

ADVERSE REACTIONS: Fungal vaginosis, headache, back pain, constipation, urinary tract infection.

INTERACTIONS: May enhance the action of other neuromuscular blockers with PO or IV clindamycin; use with caution.

PREGNANCY: Category B, not for use in nursing.

MECHANISM OF ACTION: Lincosamide derivative; inhibits bacterial protein synthesis at the level of the bacterial ribosome by binding preferentially to the 50S ribosomal subunit and affecting the process of peptide chain initiation.

PHARMACOKINETICS: Absorption: C_{max}=6.6ng/mL, T_{max}=20 hrs, AUC=175ng/mL·hr. **Distribution:** Found in breast milk (PO/parenteral administration).

NURSING CONSIDERATIONS

Assessment: Assess for history of hypersensitivity to the drug or other lincosamides, regional enteritis, ulcerative colitis, history of CDAD, nursing status, and possible drug interactions.

Monitoring: Monitor for CDAD (mild diarrhea to fatal colitis), hypersensitivity, overgrowth of nonsusceptible organisms in the vagina, and for any possible adverse reactions.

Patient Counseling: Instruct not to engage in vaginal intercourse or use other vaginal products (eg, tampons, douches) during treatment. Inform that medication contains mineral oil that may weaken latex or rubber products, such as condoms or vaginal contraceptive diaphragms; instruct not to use such barrier contraceptives concurrently or for 5 days following treatment. Inform that vaginal fungal infection can occur and may require antifungal drug treatment. Inform that medication contains ingredients that can cause burning and irritation of the eye. Instruct to rinse eye with copious amounts of cool tap water and consult physician if accidental eye contact occurs.

Administration: Intravaginal route. Refer to PI for administration instructions. **Storage:** 20-25°C (68-77°F). Avoid heat >30°C (86°F).

CLONAZEPAM
clonazepam (Various)

OTHER BRAND NAMES: Klonopin (Genentech)

THERAPEUTIC CLASS: Benzodiazepine

INDICATIONS: Adjunct or monotherapy in the treatment of Lennox-Gastaut syndrome, akinetic and myoclonic seizures. May be useful with absence seizures who have failed to respond to succinimides. Treatment of panic disorder with or without agoraphobia.

DOSAGE: *Adults:* Seizure Disorders: Initial: Not to exceed 1.5mg/day divided into three doses. Titrate: May increase in increments of 0.5-1mg q3 days until seizures are controlled or until side effects preclude any further increase. Maint: Individualize dose. Max: 20mg/day. Panic Disorder: Initial: 0.25mg bid. Titrate: Increase to 1mg/day after 3 days; for some, then may increase in increments of 0.125-0.25mg bid q3 days until panic disorder is controlled or until side effects preclude any further increase. Max: 4mg/day. D/C: Decrease by 0.125mg bid q3 days. Elderly: Start at low end of dosing range.
Pediatrics: Seizure Disorders: ≤10 yrs or 30kg: Initial: 0.01-0.03mg/kg/day up to 0.05mg/kg/day given in two or three doses. Titrate: May increase by no more than 0.25-0.5mg q3 days until maintenance dose is reached, unless seizures are controlled or until side effects preclude any further increase. Maint: 0.1-0.2mg/kg/day given tid.

HOW SUPPLIED: Tab: (Klonopin) 0.5mg*, 1mg, 2mg; (Generic) Tab, Disintegrating: (ODT) 0.125mg, 0.25mg, 0.5mg, 1mg, 2mg *scored

CONTRAINDICATIONS: Significant liver disease, untreated open-angle glaucoma, acute narrow-angle glaucoma.

WARNINGS/PRECAUTIONS: May impair mental/physical abilities. May increase risk of suicidal thoughts or behavior; monitor for the emergence of worsening of depression, suicidal thoughts or behavior, and/or any unusual changes in mood or behavior. Caution with use in pregnancy and women of childbearing potential; may increase risk of congential malformations. May increase incidence or precipitate the onset of generalized tonic-clonic seizures; addition of appropriate anticonvulsants or increase in their dosages may be required. Withdrawal symptoms reported after d/c of therapy. Avoid abrupt withdrawal; may precipitate status epilepticus. Caution with renal impairment. May produce an increase in salivation; caution with chronic respiratory diseases. Caution with addiction-prone individuals and elderly. (ODT) Contains phenylalanine.

ADVERSE REACTIONS: Ataxia, drowsiness, coordination abnormal, depression, behavior problems, dizziness, upper respiratory tract infection, memory disturbance, dysmenorrhea, fatigue, influenza, nervousness, sinusitis.

INTERACTIONS: Decreased serum levels with CYP450 inducers (eg, phenytoin, carbamazepine, phenobarbital), and propantheline. Caution with CYP3A inhibitors (eg, oral antifungals). Alcohol, narcotics, barbiturates, nonbarbiturate hypnotics, antianxiety agents, phenothiazines, thioxanthene and butyrophenone antipsychotics, MAOIs, TCAs, other anticonvulsant drugs, and other CNS depressant drugs may potentiate CNS-depressant effects. May produce absence status with valproic acid.

PREGNANCY: Category D, not for use in nursing.

MECHANISM OF ACTION: Benzodiazepine; has not been established. Suspected to enhance activity of gamma aminobutyric acid (GABA), the major inhibitory neurotransmitter in the CNS.

PHARMACOKINETICS: Absorption: Rapid and complete. Absolute bioavailability (90%); T_{max}=1-4 hrs. **Distribution:** Plasma protein binding (85%). **Metabolism:** Liver via CYP450 (including CYP3A4), then acetylation, hydroxylation, and glucuronidation. **Elimination:** Urine (<2% unchanged); $T_{1/2}$=30-40 hrs.

NURSING CONSIDERATIONS

Assessment: Assess for history of sensitivity to benzodiazepines, acute narrow-angle glaucoma, untreated open-angle glaucoma, liver/renal impairment, mental depression, history of drug or alcohol addiction, chronic respiratory diseases, pregnancy/nursing status, and possible drug interactions.

Monitoring: Monitor for CNS depression, emergence or worsening of depression, suicidal thoughts/behavior, unusual changes in mood or behavior, and worsening of seizures. Periodically monitor blood counts and LFTs during prolonged therapy. Upon withdrawal, monitor for withdrawal symptoms and monitor for status epilepticus with abrupt withdrawal.

Patient Counseling: Instruct to take medication as prescribed. Inform that therapy may produce physical and psychological dependence; instruct to consult physician before either increasing the dose or abruptly discontinuing the drug. Caution while operating hazardous machinery including automobiles. Counsel that drug may increase risk of suicidal thoughts/behavior and advise of need to be alert for the emergence/worsening of symptoms of depression, or any unusual changes in mood or behavior. Advise to notify physician if patient becomes pregnant or intends to become pregnant during therapy. Advise not to breastfeed while on therapy. Advise to inform physician if taking, or planning to take any prescription or OTC drugs and to avoid alcohol while on therapy. (ODT) Inform that drug contains phenylalanine.

Administration: Oral route. ODT: 1) Peel back foil on blister. Do not push tablet through foil. 2) Using dry hands, remove tab and place it in mouth. Tab: Swallow whole. **Storage:** 20-25°C (68-77°F). (Klonopin) 25°C (77°F); excursions permitted to 15-30°C (59-86°F).

CLORPRES
clonidine HCl - chlorthalidone (Mylan)

RX

THERAPEUTIC CLASS: Alpha-agonist/monosulfamyl diuretic

INDICATIONS: Treatment of hypertension. Not for initial therapy.

DOSAGE: *Adults:* Determine dose by individual titration. 0.1mg-15mg tab qd-bid. Max: 0.6mg-30mg/day.

HOW SUPPLIED: Tab: (Clonidine-Chlorthalidone) 0.1mg-15mg*, 0.2mg-15mg*, 0.3mg-15mg* *scored

CONTRAINDICATIONS: Anuria, sulfonamide hypersensitivity.

C

WARNINGS/PRECAUTIONS: Caution with severe renal disease, hepatic dysfunction, asthma, severe coronary insufficiency, recent myocardial infarction (MI), cerebrovascular disease. May develop allergic reaction to oral clonidine if sensitive to clonidine patch. Avoid abrupt withdrawal. Continue therapy to within 4 hrs of surgery and resume after. Monitor for fluid/electrolyte imbalance. Hyperuricemia, hypokalemia, hyponatremia, hypochloremic alkalosis, and hyperglycemia may occur.

ADVERSE REACTIONS: Drowsiness, dizziness, constipation, sedation, fatigue, dry mouth, N/V, orthostatic symptoms.

INTERACTIONS: Potentiates other antihypertensives. May increase response to tubocurarine. May decrease arterial response to norepinephrine. Antidiabetic agents may need adjustment. Risk of lithium toxicity. TCAs may reduce effects of clonidine. Amitriptyline may enhance ocular toxicity. Enhanced CNS-depressive effects of alcohol, barbiturates, or other sedatives. Orthostatic hypotension aggravated by alcohol, barbiturates, narcotics. D/C β-blockers several days before the gradual withdrawal of clonidine in patients taking both.

PREGNANCY: (Clonidine) Category C, caution in nursing. (Chlorthalidone) Category B, not for use in nursing.

MECHANISM OF ACTION: Clonidine: Imidazoline derivative; stimulates α-adrenoceptor in brain stem, resulting in reduced sympathetic outflow from CNS and decrease in peripheral resistance, renal vascular resistance, HR, and BP. Chlorthalidone: Monosulfamyl diuretic; increases excretion of Na^+ and Cl^-; decreases extracellular fluid volume, plasma volume, cardiac output, total exchangeable sodium, glomerular filtration rate, and renal plasma flow.

PHARMACOKINETICS: Absorption: Clonidine: T_{max}=3-5 hrs. **Distribution:** Chlorthalidone: Plasma protein binding (75%). **Metabolism:** Clonidine: Liver (50%). **Elimination:** Clonidine: Urine (40-60% unchanged); $T_{1/2}$=12-16 hrs; $T_{1/2}$ in severe renal impairment=41 hrs. Chlorthalidone: Urine (unchanged); $T_{1/2}$=40-60 hrs.

NURSING CONSIDERATIONS

Assessment: Assess for anuria, sulfonamide hypersensitivity, coronary insufficiency, recent MI, cerebrovascular disease, history of allergy or bronchial asthma, systemic lupus erythematosus (SLE), diabetes mellitus, renal/hepatic impairment, pregnancy/nursing status, and possible drug interactions. Perform and obtain serum and urine electrolytes.

Monitoring: Monitor blood pressure. Periodically monitor serum and urine electrolytes, serum PBI level, serum K+ levels, and renal function. Monitor for signs/symptoms of electrolyte imbalance, hypokalemia, possible exacerbation or activation of SLE, hyperglycemia, withdrawal symptoms, hyperuricemia or precipitation of gout, hypersensitivity reactions, renal/hepatic dysfunction.

Patient Counseling: Caution that drug may impair physical/mental abilities. Inform to avoid alcohol. Instruct not to interrupt or d/c therapy without consulting physician. Seek medical attention if symptoms of electrolyte imbalance (dry mouth, thirst, weakness), hypokalemia (thirst, tiredness, restlessness), withdrawal (nervousness, agitation, headaches), or hypersensitivity reactions occur.

Administration: Oral route. **Storage:** 15-30°C (59-86°F). Avoid excessive humidity.

CLOZAPINE RX
clozapine (Various)

Risk of potentially life-threatening agranulocytosis. Reserve use for severely ill patients with schizophrenia unresponsive to standard antipsychotic treatment or for patients with schizophrenia/schizoaffective disorder at risk for re-experiencing suicidal behavior. Obtain baseline WBC count and absolute neutrophil count (ANC) prior to therapy, regularly during treatment, and for ≥4 weeks after d/c. Seizures associated with use and with greater likelihood at higher doses; caution with history of seizures or other predisposing factors. Increased risk of fatal myocarditis, especially during 1st month of therapy; d/c if suspected. Orthostatic hypotension, with or without syncope can occur. Rare reports of profound collapse with respiratory and/or cardiac arrest in patients taking benzodiazepines or any other psychotropic drugs. Elderly patients with dementia-related psychosis treated with antipsychotic drugs are at an increased risk for death. Not approved for the treatment of dementia-related psychosis.

OTHER BRAND NAMES: Clozaril (Novartis)

THERAPEUTIC CLASS: Dibenzapine derivative

INDICATIONS: Management of severely ill schizophrenic patients who fail to respond adequately to standard drug treatment for schizophrenia. Reduction of risk for recurrent suicidal behavior in patients with schizophrenia/schizoaffective disorder who are judged to be at chronic risk for re-experiencing suicidal behavior.

DOSAGE: *Adults:* Treatment-Resistant Schizophrenia: Initial: 12.5mg qd-bid. Titrate: Increase by 25-50mg/day, up to 300-450mg/day by end of 2 weeks, then increase once or twice weekly in increments ≤100mg. Usual: 300-600mg/day on a divided basis. Titrate: May increase to 600-

900mg/day. Max: 900mg/day. Maint: Lowest effective dose. To d/c, gradually reduce dose over 1-2 weeks. Monitor for psychotic and cholinergic rebound symptoms if abrupt d/c (eg, leukopenia). Re-initiation (even with brief interval off clozapine): Start with 12.5mg qd-bid. May titrate more quickly if initial dosing tolerated. Retitrate with extreme caution in cardiac/respiratory arrest with initial dose but was successfully titrated to therapeutic dose. Do not restart if d/c for WBC <2000/mm³ or ANC <1000/mm³. Reduction of Risk of Suicidal Behavior in Schizophrenia/ Schizoaffective Disorder: May follow dosing recommendations for treatment-resistant schizophrenia. Range: 12.5-900mg/day (mean 300mg). To reduce the risk of suicidal behavior in patients who otherwise responded to therapy with another antipsychotic, treat for ≥2 years and then reevaluate. If risk for suicidal behavior is still present, continue treatment and revisit at regular intervals. If no longer at risk of suicidal behavior, d/c treatment. Elderly: Start at lower end of dosing range.

HOW SUPPLIED: Tab: 25mg*, 50mg*, 100mg*; (Clozaril) 25mg*, 100mg* *scored

CONTRAINDICATIONS: Myeloproliferative disorders, uncontrolled epilepsy, paralytic ileus, history of clozapine-induced agranulocytosis or severe granulocytopenia, severe CNS depression, comatose states. Concomitant use with agents having potential to cause agranulocytosis or suppress bone marrow function.

WARNINGS/PRECAUTIONS: QT prolongation, ventricular arrhythmia, torsades de pointes, and cardiac arrest associated with therapy. Caution with cardiovascular disease (CAD), risk for significant electrolyte disturbance (eg, hypokalemia, hypomagnesemia), history or family history of long QT syndrome. Correct electrolyte abnormalities prior to therapy. D/C if QTc interval >500 msec. Hyperglycemia, sometimes with ketoacidosis, hyperosmolar coma, or death, reported. Monitor for worsening of glucose control with diabetes mellitus (DM) and fasting blood glucose (FBG) levels with diabetes risk or symptoms of hyperglycemia. Tachycardia and cardiomyopathy reported. D/C if cardiomyopathy is confirmed unless benefits outweigh risk. Neuroleptic malignant syndrome (NMS), tardive dyskinesia (TD), impaired intestinal peristalsis, deep vein thrombosis (DVT), pulmonary embolism (PE), and ECG changes reported. Fever reported; rule out infection or agranulocytosis. Consider NMS in the presence of high fever. Hepatitis reported. If N/V and/or anorexia develop, perform LFTs. D/C if symptoms of jaundice occur. Has potent anticholinergic effects; caution with prostatic enlargement and narrow-angle glaucoma. May impair mental/physical abilities. Caution with renal, cardiac, hepatic, or pulmonary disease. Increased risk of cerebrovascular adverse events; caution with risk factors for stroke. Obtain WBC and ANC at baseline, then weekly for 1st six months of therapy, then every 2 weeks for next 6 months, and then every 4 weeks thereafter if counts are acceptable (WBC ≥3500/mm³ or ANC ≥2000/mm³). Refer to PI for frequency of monitoring based on stage of therapy, WBC count, and ANC. Avoid treatment if WBC <3500/mm³ or ANC <2000/mm³. D/C treatment and do not rechallenge if WBC <2000/mm³ or ANC <1000/mm³. Interrupt therapy if eosinophilia (>4000/mm³) develops. Caution in elderly.

ADVERSE REACTIONS: Drowsiness, vertigo, headache, tremor, salivation, sweating, dry mouth, visual disturbances, tachycardia, hypotension, syncope, constipation, N/V, weight gain.

INTERACTIONS: See Contraindications and Boxed Warning. Avoid using epinephrine to treat clozapine-induced hypotension. Use with carbamazepine is not recommended. Caution with CNS-active drugs, general anesthesia, alcohol, paroxetine, fluoxetine, fluvoxamine, sertraline, drugs that inhibit clozapine metabolism, inhibitors/inducers or in patients with reduced acitivity of CYP1A2, 2D6, 3A4. Consider reduced dose with paroxetine, fluoxetine, fluvoxamine, and sertraline. Dosage reduction may be needed with drugs metabolized by CYP2D6 (eg, antidepressants, phenothiazines, carbamazepine, Type 1C antiarrhythmics) or that inhibit this enzyme (eg, quinidine). May potentiate hypotensive effects of antihypertensives and anticholinergic effects of atropine-type drugs. CYP450 inducers (eg, phenytoin, tobacco smoke, rifampin) may decrease plasma levels. CYP450 inhibitors (eg, cimetidine, caffeine, citalopram, ciprofloxacin, fluvoxamine, erythromycin) may increase plasma levels. NMS reported with lithium and other CNS-active drugs. May interact with other highly protein-bound drugs. Caution with drugs known to prolong the QTc interval, such as Class 1A antiarrhythmics (eg, quinidine, procainamide), Class III antiarrhythmics (eg, amiodarone, sotalol), certain antipsychotics (eg, ziprasidone, iloperidone, chlorpromazine, thioridazine, mesoridazine, droperidol, pimozide), certain antibiotics (eg, erythromycin, gatifloxacin, moxifloxacin, sparfloxacin), and other drugs known to prolong the QT interval (eg, pentamidine, levomethadyl acetate, methadone, halofantrine, mefloquine, dolasetron mesylate, probucol, and tacrolimus). Caution with drugs that can cause electrolyte imbalance (eg, diuretics)

PREGNANCY: Category B, not for use in nursing.

MECHANISM OF ACTION: Tricyclic dibenzodiazepine derivative; atypical antipsychotic agent. Interferes with binding of dopamine at D_1, D_2, D_3, and D_5 receptors and has a high affinity for D_4 receptor. Also acts as an antagonist at the adrenergic, cholinergic, histaminergic, and serotonergic receptors.

PHARMACOKINETICS: Absorption: C_{max}=319ng/mL; T_{max}=2.5 hrs (100mg bid). **Distribution:** Plasma protein binding (97%). **Metabolism:** Demethylation, hydroxylation, N-oxidation. **Elimination:** Urine (50%), feces (30%); $T_{1/2}$=8 hrs (75mg single dose), $T_{1/2}$=12 hrs (100mg bid).

NURSING CONSIDERATIONS

Assessment: Assess previous course of standard therapy prior to treatment. Assess for my-eloproliferative disorders, uncontrolled epilepsy, paralytic ileus, history of clozapine-induced agranulocytosis or severe granulocytopenia, severe CNS depression or comatose states, history of seizures or other predisposing factors, history or family history of long QT syndrome or QT prolongation, CAD, and other conditions where treatment is cautioned or contraindicated. Assess pregnancy/nursing status and possible drug interactions. Obtain baseline WBC count, ANC, FBG levels in patients at risk for hyperglycemia/DM, serum K+ and magnesium levels.

Monitoring: Monitor for clinical response and need to continue treatment. Monitor for agranu-locytosis, myocarditis, orthostatic hypotension, HF, tachycardia, severe respiratory effects, seizures, flu-like symptoms, infection (eg, pneumonia), eosinophilia, fever, DVT, PE, NMS, TD, impairment of intestinal peristalsis, impairment of mental/physical abilities, and signs/symptoms of hyperglycemia. Monitor WBC counts and ANC during and for ≥4 weeks following d/c or until WBC ≥3500/mm³ and ANC ≥2000/mm³. Check periodic FBG levels if at risk for hyperglycemia/DM and for signs/symptoms of hepatitis while on therapy. Obtain LFTs if patient develops N/V and/or anorexia. Monitor electrolytes periodically.

Patient Counseling: Inform that drug is available only through a program designed to ensure the required blood monitoring schedule. Counsel on risks of treatment (eg, agranulocytosis, seizures, orthostatic hypotension). Inform about signs/symptoms of agranulocytosis; advise to immedi-ately report lethargy, weakness, fever, sore throat, malaise, mucous membrane ulceration, flu-like complaints, or other possible signs of infection. Instruct to avoid potentially hazardous activities (eg, operating machinery, driving). Counsel to notify physician if intending to become pregnant, planning to take any prescription or over-the-counter drugs or alcohol. Advise females to avoid breastfeeding. Advise that drug can be taken with/without food. Inform that if a dose is missed for >2 days, consult physician before restarting medication.

Administration: Oral route. **Storage:** 15-30°C (59-86°F). (Clozaril) ≤30°C (86°F).

COARTEM   RX
lumefantrine - artemether (Novartis)

THERAPEUTIC CLASS: Artemisinin-based combination therapy

INDICATIONS: Treatment of acute, uncomplicated malaria infections due to *Plasmodium falci-parum* in patients ≥5kg.

DOSAGE: *Adults:* >16 yrs: ≥35kg: Initial: 4 tabs as single dose. Maint: 4 tabs again after 8 hrs and then 4 tabs bid (am and pm) for the following 2 days. <35kg: Refer to pediatric dosage.
Pediatrics: 5-<15kg: Initial: 1 tab. Maint: 1 tab again after 8 hrs and then 1 tab bid (am and pm) for the following 2 days. 15-<25kg: Initial: 2 tabs. Maint: 2 tabs again after 8 hrs and then 2 tabs bid for the following 2 days. 25-<35kg: Initial: 3 tabs. Maint: 3 tabs again after 8 hrs and then 3 tabs bid for the following 2 days. ≥35kg: Initial: 4 tabs as single dose. Maint: 4 tabs again after 8 hrs and then 4 tabs bid for the following 2 days.

HOW SUPPLIED: Tab: (Artemether-Lumefantrine) 20mg-120mg* *scored

WARNINGS/PRECAUTIONS: May prolong the QT interval; avoid with congenital prolongation of the QT interval (eg, long QT syndrome) or any other clinical conditions known to prolong the QTc interval (eg, history of symptomatic cardiac arrhythmias with bradycardia or with severe cardiac disease), family history of congenital prolongation of the QT interval or sudden death, known disturbances of electrolyte balance (eg, hypokalemia, hypomagnesemia). Caution with severe renal/hepatic impairment. Not approved for prevention of malaria or for patients with severe or complicated *P. falciparum* malaria. Risk of recrudescence may be greater in patients who remain adverse to food during treatment.

ADVERSE REACTIONS: Headache, abdominal pain, anorexia, dizziness, asthenia, arthralgia, myalgia, pyrexia, cough, N/V, chills, fatigue, splenomegaly, hepatomegaly, sleep disorder.

INTERACTIONS: Avoid with other medications that prolong the QT interval such as class IA (eg, quinidine, procainamide, disopyramide) or class III (eg, amiodarone, sotalol) antiarrhyth-mic agents; antipsychotics (eg, pimozide, ziprasidone); antidepressants; certain antibiotics (eg, macrolide or fluroquinolone antibiotics, imidazole, and triazole antifungal agents); certain non-sedating antihistaminics (eg, terfenadine, astemizole), or cisapride. Avoid concurrent use with medications metabolized by CYP2D6, which also have cardiac effects (eg, flecainide, imipramine, amitriptyline, clomipramine). Avoid coadministration with halofantrine within 1 month of each other due to potential additive effects on the QT interval. Avoid with other antimalarials. May decrease efficacy with mefloquine. Concomitant use with CYP3A4 substrates may decrease substrate concentration and substrate efficacy. May increase levels and potentiate QT prolonga-tion with CYP3A4 inhibitors (eg, ketoconazole, grapefruit juice). Coadministration with CYP3A4 inducers may decrease levels and antimalarial efficacy. May reduce hormonal contraceptives effectiveness. Caution with quinine. Caution with drugs that have a mixed effect on CYP3A4 (eg, antiretroviral drugs).

PREGNANCY: Category C, caution in nursing.

MECHANISM OF ACTION: Artemether: Artemisinin derivative; antimalarial activity attributed to endoperoxide moiety. Lumefantrine: Not established; suspected to inhibit the formation of β-hematin by forming a complex with hemin. Both artemether and lumefantrine inhibit nucleic acid and protein synthesis.

PHARMACOKINETICS: Absorption: T_{max}= 2 hrs (Artemether), 6-8 hrs (Lumefantrine). Refer to PI for additional absorption parameters. **Distribution:** Plasma protein binding (95.4% [Artemether], 47-76% [DHA], 99.7% [Lumefantrine]). **Metabolism:** Artemether: Liver via CYP3A4/5 (Major), CYP2B6, CYP2C9, CYP2C19 (minor); Dihydroartemisinin [DHA] (active metabolite). Lumefantrine: Liver via CYP3A4. **Elimination:** $T_{1/2}$=2 hrs (Artemether and DHA), 3-6 days (Lumefantrine).

NURSING CONSIDERATIONS

Assessment: Assess for severe/complicated *P. falciparum* malaria, hepatic/renal impairment, congenital prolongation of the QT interval (eg, long QT syndrome), symptomatic cardiac arrhythmias with clinically relevant bradycardia or severe cardiac disease, family history of congenital prolongation of the QT interval or sudden death, electrolyte disturbances (eg, hypokalemia, hypomagnesemia), pregnancy/nursing status, and for possible drug interactions. Obtain baseline ECG, serum electrolytes, LFTs, renal function.

Monitoring: Monitor for hepatic/renal impairment, ECG changes (eg, QT interval prolongation), electrolyte imbalance, and other adverse events that may occur. Monitor ECG, serum electrolytes, LFTs, renal function, and for recrudescence of malaria.

Patient Counseling: Inform about risks and benefits of therapy. Instruct to take with food. Inform that if unable to swallow, tab may be crushed and mixed with a small amount of water (1-2 tsp). Inform that administration should be over 3 days for a total of six doses. Counsel about risk for recrudescence of malaria with inadequate food intake. Advise childbearing patients to use an additional nonhormonal method of birth control. Instruct to d/c therapy if hypersensitivity reactions (eg, rash, hives, rapid heart beat, difficulty swallowing/breathing, any swelling suggesting angioedema) or other symptoms of an allergic reaction occur; advise to inform physician if these and other adverse events develop.

Administration: Oral route. Take with food. Resume normal eating as soon as food can be tolerated. If unable to swallow, may crush tabs and mix with small amount of water (eg, 1-2 tsp) in a clean container prior to administration; crushed tab preparation should be followed whenever possible by food/drink (eg, milk, formula, pudding, broth, and porridge). If vomiting occurs within 1-2 hrs of administration, repeat the dose. If vomiting continues, d/c and start alternative antimalarial treatment. **Storage:** 25°C (77°F); excursions permitted to 15-30°C (59-86°F).

COLAZAL   RX
balsalazide disodium (Salix)

THERAPEUTIC CLASS: 5-Aminosalicylic acid derivative

INDICATIONS: Treatment of mild-to-moderate active ulcerative colitis in patients ≥5 yrs.

DOSAGE: *Adults:* 3 caps tid for up to 8 weeks (or 12 weeks if needed). May open cap and sprinkle on applesauce.
Pediatrics: 5-17 yrs: 1 or 3 caps tid for 8 weeks. May open cap and sprinkle on applesauce.

HOW SUPPLIED: Cap: 750mg

WARNINGS/PRECAUTIONS: May exacerbate symptoms of colitis. Prolonged gastric retention with pyloric stenosis. Caution with renal dysfunction or history of renal disease.

ADVERSE REACTIONS: Headache, abdominal pain, diarrhea, N/V, respiratory problems, arthralgia, rhinitis, insomnia, fatigue, rectal bleeding, flatulence, fever, dyspepsia.

INTERACTIONS: Oral antibiotics may interfere with the release of mesalamine in the colon.

PREGNANCY: Category B, caution in nursing.

MECHANISM OF ACTION: Not established; a prodrug enzymatically cleaved in colon to produce mesalamine (5-ASA), an anti-inflammatory drug that acts locally to block production of arachidonic acid metabolites in the colon.

PHARMACOKINETICS: Absorption: Different dosing conditions (fasted, fed, sprinkled) resulted in variable parameters. **Distribution:** Plasma protein binding (≥99%). **Metabolism:** Key metabolites: 5-ASA and N-acetyl-5-ASA. **Elimination:** Urine, feces.

NURSING CONSIDERATIONS

Assessment: Assess for pyloric stenosis, possible drug interactions, history of renal/hepatic disease.

COLCRYS

Monitoring: Monitor renal function, LFTs, and CBC, signs/symptoms of prolonged gastric retention with pyloric stenosis, worsening of colitis symptoms, and hypersensitivity.

Patient Counseling: Inform can take with/without food or sprinkle on applesauce. Teeth and/or tongue may get stained when using sprinkle form with food. Seek medical attention if diagnosed with pyloric stenosis or renal dysfunction, experience worsening of colitis symptoms or hypersensitivity (eg, anaphylaxis, bronchospasm, skin reaction).

Administration: Oral route. **Storage:** 20-25°C (68-77°F); excursions permitted to 15-30°C (59-86°F).

COLCRYS   RX
colchicine (AR Scientific)

THERAPEUTIC CLASS: Miscellaneous gout agent

INDICATIONS: Prophylaxis and treatment of acute gout flares. Treatment of familial Mediterranean fever (FMF) in patients ≥4 yrs.

DOSAGE: *Adults:* Individualize dose. Gout Flare Prophylaxis: >16 yrs: Usual: 0.6mg qd or bid. Max: 1.2mg/day. Severe Renal Impairment: Initial: 0.3mg/day. Titrate: Increase dose with close monitoring. Dialysis: Initial: 0.3mg twice a week. Severe Hepatic Impairment: Consider reducing dose. Gout Flare Treatment: 1.2mg at the 1st sign of the flare followed by 0.6mg 1 hr later. Max: 1.8mg over a 1 hr period. May be administered for treatment of a gout flare during prophylaxis; wait 12 hrs then resume prophylactic dose. Severe Renal/Hepatic Impairment: Do not repeat treatment course more than once every 2 weeks; consider alternate therapy if repeated courses for treatment required. Dialysis: Reduce to 0.6mg single dose. Do not repeat treatment course more than once every 2 weeks. FMF: Usual Range/Max: 1.2-2.4mg/day in 1-2 divided doses. Titrate: Modify dose in increments of 0.3mg/day as needed to control disease or if with intolerable side effects. Mild (CrCl 50-80mL/min) to Moderate (CrCl 30-50mL/min) Renal/Severe Hepatic Impairment: Consider reducing dose. Severe Renal Impairment (CrCl <30mL/min)/Dialysis: Initial: 0.3mg/day. Titrate: Increase dose with close monitoring. Refer to PI for dose modifications for coadministration of interacting drugs.
Pediatrics: FMF: May be given qd or bid. >12 yrs: 1.2-2.4mg/day. 6-12 yrs: 0.9-1.8mg/day. 4-6 yrs: 0.3-1.8mg/day. Mild (CrCl 50-80mL/min) to Moderate (CrCl 30-50mL/min) Renal/Severe Hepatic Impairment: Consider reducing dose. Severe Renal Impairment (CrCl <30mL/min)/Dialysis: Initial: 0.3mg/day. Titrate: Increase dose with close monitoring. Refer to PI for dose modifications for coadministration of interacting drugs.

HOW SUPPLIED: Tab: 0.6mg* *scored

CONTRAINDICATIONS: Concomitant use with P-glycoprotein (P-gp) or strong CYP3A4 inhibitors (this includes all protease inhibitors, except fosamprenavir) in patients with renal/hepatic impairment.

WARNINGS/PRECAUTIONS: Not recommended for pediatric use in prophylaxis or treatment of gout flares. Treatment of gout flare not recommended in patients with renal/hepatic impairment receiving prophylaxis. Not an analgesic medication and should not be used to treat pain from other causes. Fatal overdoses (accidental/intentional), myelosuppression, leukopenia, granulocytopenia, thrombocytopenia, pancytopenia, and aplastic anemia reported. Drug-induced neuromuscular toxicity and rhabdomyolysis reported with chronic use; increased risk with elderly and in patients with renal dysfunction. Caution in elderly and renal/hepatic impairment. D/C if toxicity is suspected.

ADVERSE REACTIONS: Diarrhea, pharyngolaryngeal pain, cramping, abdominal pain, N/V.

INTERACTIONS: See Contraindications. Significant increase in plasma levels reported with moderate (amprenavir, aprepitant, diltiazem, erythromycin, fluconazole, fosamprenavir, grapefruit juice, verapamil) and strong (atazanavir, clarithromycin, darunavir/ritonavir, indinavir, itraconazole, ketoconazole, lopinavir/ritonavir, nefazodone, nelfinavir, ritonavir, saquinavir, telithromycin, tipranavir/ritonavir) CYP3A4 inhibitors, and P-gp inhibitors (cyclosporine, ranolazine); see PI for dose adjustment. Fatal toxicity reported with clarithromycin and cyclosporine. Neuromuscular toxicity reported with diltiazem and verapamil. May potentiate the development of myopathy and rhabdomyolysis when used with HMG-CoA reductase inhibitors (atorvastatin, simvastatin, pravastatin, fluvastatin), gemfibrozil and fibrates, and cyclosporine. Rhabdomyolysis reported with digoxin.

PREGNANCY: Category C, caution in nursing.

MECHANISM OF ACTION: Alkaloid; may interfere with the intracellular assembly of the inflammasome complex in neutrophils and monocytes that mediates activation of interleukin-1β in patients with FMF. Disrupts cytoskeletal functions through inhibition of β-tubulin polymerization into microtubules, consequently preventing the activation, degranulation, and migration of neutrophils thought to mediate some gout symptoms.

PHARMACOKINETICS: Absorption: C_{max}=2.5ng/mL; T_{max}=1-2 hrs; absolute bioavailability (45%). See PI for additional parameters for different doses. **Distribution:** V_d=5-8L/kg; plasma protein binding (39%). Crosses placenta; found in breast milk. **Metabolism:** CYP3A4; demethylation; 2-O-demethylcolchicine and 3-O-demethylcolchicine (primary metabolites). **Elimination:** Urine (40-65%, unchanged); $T_{1/2}$=26.6-31.2 hrs.

NURSING CONSIDERATIONS

Assessment: Assess for renal/hepatic impairment, pregnancy/nursing status, and possible drug interactions. Weigh potential benefits/risks when coadministered with other drugs. Note other diseases/conditions and drug therapies.

Monitoring: Monitor for rhabdomyolysis and signs/symptoms of toxicity (eg, cramping, diarrhea, abdominal pain, N/V). Monitor for blood dyscrasias (myelosupression, leukopenia, granulocytopenia, pancytopenia, agranulocytosis, aplastic anemia, thrombocytopenia).

Patient Counseling: Inform about benefits and risks of therapy. Instruct to take medication as prescribed. If dose is missed for treatment of gout flare, instruct to take missed dose as soon as possible. If dose is missed for treatment of gout flare during prophylaxis, instruct to take missed dose immediately, wait 12 hrs, then resume previous schedule. If dose is missed for prophylaxis without treatment of gout flares or FMF, instruct to take the next dose as soon as possible, then return to normal schedule, and not to double the next dose. Inform that fatal overdoses were reported. Counsel to avoid grapefruit/grapefruit juice consumption during treatment. Inform that bone marrow depression may occur with agranulocytosis, aplastic anemia, and thrombocytopenia. Advise to notify physician of all current medications being taken and before starting any new medications, particularly antibiotics. Advise to d/c drug and notify physician if muscle pain/weakness, and/or tingling/numbness of fingers/toes occur.

Administration: Oral route. **Storage:** 20-25°C (68-77°F). Protect from light.

COLESTID   RX

colestipol HCl (Pharmacia & Upjohn)

THERAPEUTIC CLASS: Bile acid sequestrant

INDICATIONS: Adjunct to diet, to reduce elevated serum total and LDL-C in primary hypercholesterolemia.

DOSAGE: *Adults:* Initial: Tab: 2g qd-bid. Granules: 1 pkt or 1 scoopful qd-bid. Titrate: Tab: Increase by 2g qd or bid at 1- to 2-month intervals. Granules: May increase at an increment of one dose/day (1 pkt or level tsp of granules) at 1- to 2-month intervals. Usual: 2-16g/day (tab) or 1-6 pkts or scoopfuls (granules) qd or in divided doses. Always mix granules with liquid. Take 1 tab at a time and swallow tabs whole with plenty of liquid.

HOW SUPPLIED: Granules: 5g/pkt [30^s 90^s], 5g/scoopful [300g, 500g]; Tab: 1g

WARNINGS/PRECAUTIONS: Exclude secondary causes of hypercholesterolemia and obtain a lipid profile prior to therapy. May interfere with normal fat absorption. Chronic use may increase bleeding tendency due to vitamin K deficiency. Monitor cholesterol and TG based on National Cholesterol Education Program guidelines. May cause hypothyroidism. May produce or worsen constipation. Avoid constipation with symptomatic coronary artery disease. Constipation associated with colestipol may aggravate hemorrhoids. May produce hyperchloremic acidosis with prolonged use. (Granules) Flavored form contains phenylalanine. Always mix granules with water or other fluids before ingesting.

ADVERSE REACTIONS: Constipation, abdominal discomfort, indigestion, musculoskeletal pain, headache, AST elevation, ALT elevation, alkaline phosphatase elevation, headache, chest pain, rash, anorexia, fatigue, tachycardia, SOB.

INTERACTIONS: May interfere with absorption of folic acid, fat-soluble vitamins (eg, A, D, K), oral phosphate supplements, hydrocortisone. May delay or reduce absorption of concomitant oral medication; take other drugs 1 hr before or 4 hrs after colestipol. Reduces absorption of chlorothiazide, tetracycline, furosemide, penicillin G, HCTZ, and gemfibrozil. Caution with digitalis agents, propranolol.

PREGNANCY: Safety in pregnancy not known, caution in nursing.

MECHANISM OF ACTION: Bile acid sequestrant; binds bile acids in the intestine, forming a complex that is excreted in the feces, leading to increased fecal loss of bile acids and increased oxidation of cholesterol to bile acids, a decrease in β lipoprotein or LDL, and a decrease in serum cholesterol levels.

PHARMACOKINETICS: Elimination: Feces.

NURSING CONSIDERATIONS

Assessment: Assess for secondary causes of hypercholesterolemia (eg, hypothyroidism, diabetes mellitus, nephrotic syndrome, dysproteinemia, obstructive liver disease, alcoholism), pre-existing constipation, pregnancy/nursing status, and for possible drug interactions. Determine baseline lipid profile.

Monitoring: Monitor for signs/symptoms of vitamin K deficiency (eg, tendency for bleeding), constipation, hypothyroidism, and for hyperchloremic acidosis. Monitor serum cholesterol, lipoprotein and TG levels.

Patient Counseling: Instruct to take as prescribed. Advise to take other medications at least 1 hr before or 4 hrs after taking colestipol. Inform about benefits/risks of therapy. Instruct to report any adverse reactions to physician. (Tab) Instruct to take tab one at a time, with plenty of water. Counsel not to cut, crush, or chew tab. (Granules) Advise to mix with water or other fluids before ingesting.

Administration: Oral route. **Storage:** 20-25°C (68-77°F).

COMBIGAN RX
timolol maleate - brimonidine tartrate (Allergan)

THERAPEUTIC CLASS: Alpha$_2$-agonist/beta-blocker

INDICATIONS: Reduction of elevated intraocular pressure (IOP) in patients with glaucoma or ocular hypertension who require adjunctive or replacement therapy due to inadequately controlled IOP.

DOSAGE: *Adults:* 1 drop in affected eye(s) bid q12 hrs. Space by at least 5 min if using >1 topical ophthalmic drug.
Pediatrics: ≥2 yrs: 1 drop in affected eye(s) bid q12 hrs. Space by at least 5 min if using >1 topical ophthalmic drug.

HOW SUPPLIED: Sol: (Brimonidine-Timolol) 2mg-5mg/mL [5mL, 10mL]

CONTRAINDICATIONS: Bronchial asthma, history of bronchial asthma, severe chronic obstructive pulmonary disease (COPD), sinus bradycardia, second- or third-degree atrioventricular (AV) block, overt cardiac failure, cardiogenic shock.

WARNINGS/PRECAUTIONS: May potentiate respiratory reactions including asthma. Systemic absorption, leading to adverse reactions (including severe respiratory reactions) may occur. Caution with cardiac failure; d/c at the first sign or symptom of cardiac failure. Avoid with bronchospastic disease, history of bronchospastic disease and/or mild-to-moderate COPD. May potentiate syndromes associated with vascular insufficiency; caution with depression, cerebral or coronary insufficiency, Raynaud's phenomenon, orthostatic hypotension, or thromboangiitis obliterans. May increase reactivity to allergens. May potentiate muscle weakness consistent with certain myasthenic symptoms (eg, diplopia, ptosis, and generalized weakness). May mask signs/symptoms of acute hypoglycemia; caution in patients subject to spontaneous hypoglycemia or diabetic patients receiving insulin or hypoglycemic agents. May mask certain clinical signs of hyperthyroidism (eg, tachycardia); if suspected of developing thyrotoxicosis, manage carefully to avoid abrupt withdrawal that may precipitate a thyroid storm. Bacterial keratitis reported with use of multiple-dose containers of topical ophthalmic products. May impair the ability of the heart to respond to β-adrenergically mediated reflex during surgery; gradual withdrawal of β-blocking agents is recommended.

ADVERSE REACTIONS: Allergic conjunctivitis, conjunctival folliculosis, conjunctival hyperemia, eye pruritus, ocular burning/stinging.

INTERACTIONS: May reduce BP; caution with antihypertensives and/or cardiac glycosides. Monitor for potentially additive effects, both systemic and on IOP with β-blockers; concomitant use of 2 topical β-blocking agents is not recommended. Possible AV conduction disturbances, left ventricular failure, and hypotension may occur with oral or IV calcium antagonists; use with caution and avoid use with impaired cardiac function. Close observation with catecholamine-depleting drugs (eg, reserpine) because of possible additive effects and the production of hypotension and/or marked bradycardia. Possibility of additive or potentiating effect with CNS depressants (eg, alcohol, barbiturates, opiates, sedatives, anesthetics). Concomitant use of β-blockers with digitalis and/or calcium antagonists may have additive effects in prolonging AV-conduction time. Potentiated systemic β-blockade reported with CYP2D6 inhibitors (eg, quinidine, SSRIs) and timolol. May affect the metabolism and uptake of circulating amines with TCAs and/or MAOIs; use with caution with TCAs and MAOIs.

PREGNANCY: Category C, not for use in nursing.

MECHANISM OF ACTION: Decreases elevated IOP. Brimonidine: Selective α-2 adrenergic receptor. Timolol: Nonselective β-blocker.

PHARMACOKINETICS: Absorption: Brimonidine: C_{max}=30pg/mL; T_{max}= 1-4 hrs. Timolol: C_{max}=400pg/mL; T_{max}=1-3 hrs. **Distribution:** Timolol: Plasma protein binding (60%). **Metabolism:** Brimonidine: Liver (extensive). Timolol: Liver (partial). **Elimination:** Brimonidine: $T_{1/2}$=3 hrs. Timolol: $T_{1/2}$=7 hrs.

NURSING CONSIDERATIONS

Assessment: Assess for bronchial asthma, history of bronchial asthma, severe COPD, sinus bradycardia, second- or third-degree AV block, overt cardiac failure, cardiogenic shock, pregnancy/nursing, and possible drug interactions.

Monitoring: Monitor for potentiation of respiratory failure, vascular insufficiency and muscle weakness, increased reactivity to allergens, masking of hypoglycemia symptoms and thyrotoxicosis, bacterial keratitis and other adverse reactions.

Patient Counseling: Inform that ocular infections may occur if handled improperly or if the tip of dispensing container contacts eye or surrounding structure. Inform that serious eye damage and subsequent loss of vision may result from using contaminated solutions. Advise to immediately consult physician concerning continued use of multidose container if undergoing ocular surgery or developed an intercurrent ocular condition. Instruct to space dosing of at least 5 min apart if >1 topical ophthalmic drug is being used. Advise to remove contact lens prior to administration of the solution and may reinsert after 15 min following administration.

Administration: Ocular route. **Storage:** 15-25°C (59-77°F). Protect from light.

COMBIPATCH   RX
norethindrone acetate - estradiol (Novartis)

> Should not be used for prevention of cardiovascular disease (CVD) or dementia. Increased risks of myocardial infarction (MI), stroke, invasive breast cancer, pulmonary embolism (PE), and deep vein thrombosis (DVT) in postmenopausal women (50-79 yrs) reported. Increased risk of developing probable dementia in postmenopausal women ≥65 yrs of age reported. Should be prescribed at the lowest effective dose and for the shortest duration consistent with treatment goals and risks.

THERAPEUTIC CLASS: Estrogen/progestogen combination

INDICATIONS: In women with an intact uterus, for the treatment of moderate to severe vasomotor symptoms and/or vulvar/vaginal atrophy associated with menopause. Treatment of hypoestrogenism due to hypogonadism, castration, or primary ovarian failure.

DOSAGE: *Adults:* Continuous Combined Regimen: Apply 0.05mg-0.14mg patch on lower abdomen. Apply 2X/week during 28-day cycle. Continuous Sequential Regimen: Wear estradiol-only patch for 1st 14 days of 28-day cycle, replace 2X/week. Apply 0.05mg-0.14mg patch on the lower abdomen for remaining 14 days, replace 2X/week. For both regimens, use 0.05mg-0.25mg patch if greater progestin is required. Reevaluate at 3-6 month intervals.

HOW SUPPLIED: Patch: (Estradiol-Norethindrone Acetate) 0.05-0.14mg/day, 0.05-0.25mg/day [8[s], 24[s]]

CONTRAINDICATIONS: Undiagnosed abnormal genital bleeding, known/suspected/history of breast cancer, known/suspected estrogen-dependent neoplasia, active or history of DVT/PE, active or recent arterial thromboembolic disease (eg, stroke, MI), liver dysfunction or disease, known/suspected pregnancy.

WARNINGS/PRECAUTIONS: Increased risk of CV events (eg, MI, stroke), venous thrombosis, and PE; d/c immediately if any of these events occur or are suspected. Caution in patients with risk factors for arterial vascular disease (eg, HTN, diabetes mellitus [DM], tobacco use, hypercholesterolemia, obesity) and/or venous thromboembolism (eg, personal history or family history of venous thromboembolism, obesity, systemic lupus erythematosus [SLE]). If feasible, d/c at least 4 to 6 weeks before surgery of the type associated with an increased risk of thromboembolism or during periods of prolonged immobilization. May increase risk of breast/endometrial cancer and gallbladder disease. May lead to severe hypercalcemia with breast cancer and bone metastases; d/c and take appropriate measures if hypercalcemia occurs. Retinal vascular thrombosis reported; if visual abnormalities or migraine occurs, d/c pending examination. If examination reveals papilledema or retinal vascular lesions, d/c permanently. Consider addition of a progestin if no hysterectomy. May elevate BP, thyroid-binding globulin levels, and plasma TG leading to pancreatitis and other complications. Caution with history of cholestatic jaundice associated with past estrogen use or with pregnancy; d/c in case of recurrence. May cause fluid retention; caution with cardiac/renal dysfunction. Caution with severe hypocalcemia. May increase risk of ovarian cancer. May exacerbate endometriosis, asthma, DM, epilepsy, migraine, porphyria, SLE, and hepatic hemangiomas; use with caution. May affect certain endocrine, LFTs, and blood components in laboratory tests.

ADVERSE REACTIONS: Abdominal pain, back pain, asthenia, flu syndrome, headache, application-site reaction, diarrhea, nausea, nervousness, pharyngitis, respiratory disorder, breast pain, dysmenorrhea, menstrual disorder, vaginitis.

INTERACTIONS: CYP3A4 inducers (eg, St. John's wort, phenobarbital, carbamazepine, rifampin) may decrease levels, which may decrease therapeutic effects and/or change uterine bleeding profile. CYP3A4 inhibitors (eg, erythromycin, clarithromycin, ketoconazole, itraconazole, ritonavir, grapefruit juice) may increase levels, which may result in side effects. Patients concomitantly receiving thyroid hormone replacement therapy and estrogens may require increased doses of their thyroid replacement therapy.

PREGNANCY: Contraindicated in pregnancy, caution in nursing.

MECHANISM OF ACTION: Estrogen/progestogen combination; estrogens act through binding to nuclear receptors in estrogen-responsive tissues. Circulating estrogen modulates pituitary secretion of gonadotropins, luteinizing hormone and follicle stimulating hormone, through negative feedback mechanism. Reduces elevated levels of these hormones in postmenopausal women.

PHARMACOKINETICS: Absorption: Estradiol/Norethindrone: Well-absorbed. Administration of various doses resulted in different parameters. **Distribution:** Estradiol: Largely bound to sex hormone-binding globulin (SHBG) and albumin; found in breast milk. Norethindrone: 90% to SHBG and albumin; found in breast milk. **Metabolism:** Liver, to estrone (metabolite); estriol (major urinary metabolite); sulfate and glucuronide conjugation (liver); gut hydrolysis; CYP3A4 (partial metabolism). Norethindrone: Liver. **Elimination:** Estradiol: Urine (parent compound and metabolites); $T_{1/2}$=2-3 hrs. Norethindrone: $T_{1/2}$=6-8 hrs.

NURSING CONSIDERATIONS

Assessment: Assess for abnormal genital bleeding, presence or history of breast cancer, estrogen-dependent neoplasias, DVT, PE, active or recent (within past yr), arterial thromboembolic disease, and any other conditions where treatment may be contraindicated or cautioned. Assess use in women ≥65 yrs, and those with DM, asthma, epilepsy, migraines or porphyria, SLE, and hepatic hemangiomas. Assess for nursing status, and possible drug/lab interactions. Assess need for progestin therapy in women who have not had a hysterectomy.

Monitoring: Monitor for signs/symptoms of CVD, malignant neoplasms, dementia, gallbladder disease, hypercalcemia, visual abnormalities, increased BP, hypertriglyceridemia, hypothyroidism, fluid retention, cholestatic jaundice, exacerbation of endometriosis, and other conditions. Perform annual mammography, periodic monitoring of BP, and periodic evaluation (every 3-6 months) to determine need of therapy. Monitor thyroid function if patient on thyroid hormone replacement therapy. In cases of undiagnosed, persistent, or recurrent vaginal bleeding in women with uterus, perform adequate diagnostic measures (eg, endometrial sampling) to rule out malignancies.

Patient Counseling: Inform that medication may increase risk for heart attack, stroke, breast cancer, blood clots, and dementia. Counsel to report any breast lumps, unusual vaginal bleeding, dizziness or faintness, changes in speech, chest pain, SOB, leg pain, changes in vision, and vomiting. Counsel that if patch falls off, reapply same patch to different area of lower abdomen or use new patch. Advise not to expose patch to sun for prolonged periods of time.

Administration: Transdermal route. Place on a smooth (fold-free), clean, dry area of the skin on the lower abdomen; avoid application to waistline and to or near the breasts. Rotate sites; allow 1 week interval between same site application. Only 1 system should be worn at any 1 time during the 3- to 4- day dosing interval. Refer to PI for complete instructions on application of the system. **Storage:** Prior to Dispensing: Refrigerated at 2-8°C (36-46°F). After Dispensing: Room temperature <25°C (77°F) for up to 6 months. Do not store in areas where extreme temperatures may occur.

COMBIVENT   RX
ipratropium bromide - albuterol sulfate (Boehringer Ingelheim)

THERAPEUTIC CLASS: Beta$_2$-agonist/anticholinergic

INDICATIONS: Treatment of patients with chronic obstructive pulmonary disease on a regular aerosol bronchodilator who continue to have evidence of bronchospasm and who require a second bronchodilator.

DOSAGE: *Adults:* 2 inh qid. Max: 12 inh/24 hrs.

HOW SUPPLIED: MDI: (Albuterol Sulfate-Ipratropium Bromide) 103mcg-18mcg/inh [14.7g]

CONTRAINDICATIONS: History of hypersensitivity to soya lecithin or related food products (eg, soybean, peanut).

WARNINGS/PRECAUTIONS: Paradoxical bronchospasm reported; d/c if symptoms occur. May produce significant cardiovascular (CV) effects (eg, ECG changes); d/c if symptoms occur. Caution with CV disorders (eg, coronary insufficiency, cardiac arrhythmias, HTN). Rare occurrences of myocardial ischemia reported. Fatalities reported with excessive use of inhaled sympathomimetic drugs in patients with asthma. Immediate hypersensitivity may occur after administration; d/c if occurs. Caution with narrow-angle glaucoma, prostatic hyperplasia, bladder-neck obstruction, convulsive disorders, hyperthyroidism, diabetes mellitus (DM), unusual responsiveness to sympathomimetic amines, and hepatic/renal insufficiency. May produce significant but usually transient hypokalemia.

ADVERSE REACTIONS: Bronchitis, upper respiratory tract infection, headache, dyspnea, cough.

INTERACTIONS: Additive effects with other anticholinergic-containing drugs; use with caution. Increased risk of adverse CV events with sympathomimetic agents; use with caution. Potential worsening of ECG changes and/or hypokalemia with non-K⁺-sparing diuretics (eg, loop or thiazide diuretics); use with caution and consider monitoring K⁺ levels. β-blockers and albuterol inhibit effects of each other; use β-blockers with caution in patients with hyper-reactive airways. Administration with MAOIs or TCAs, or within 2 weeks of d/c of such agents may potentiate the action of albuterol on CV system; use with exterme caution and consider alternative therapy.

PREGNANCY: Category C, not for use in nursing.

MECHANISM OF ACTION: Ipratropium: Anticholinergic bronchodilator; appears to inhibit vagally-mediated reflexes by antagonizing the action of acetylcholine. Prevents the increases in intracellular concentration of calcium which is caused by interaction of acetylcholine with the muscarinic receptors on bronchial smooth muscle. Albuterol: Selective β₂-adrenergic bronchodilator; activates β₂-receptors on airway smooth muscle, leading to activation of adenylyl cyclase and increase of intracellular concentration of cyclic-3',5'-adenosine monophosphate. This leads to activation of protein kinase A, which inhibits phosphorylation of myosin and lowers intracellular ionic calcium concentrations, resulting in relaxation.

PHARMACOKINETICS: Absorption: Ipratropium: Not readily absorbed. Albuterol: Rapid, complete; C_{max}=492pg/mL; T_{max}=3 hrs. **Distribution:** Ipratropium: Plasma protein binding (0-9%). **Metabolism:** Ipratropium: Partial; ester hydrolysis. Albuterol: Conjugation; albuterol 4'-O-sulfate metabolite. **Elimination:** Urine (27.1%, unchanged). Ipratropium: $T_{1/2}$=2 hrs. Albuterol: Urine (30.8%, unchanged).

NURSING CONSIDERATIONS

Assessment: Assess for known history of hypersensitivity to soya lecithin or related food products, CV disorders, narrow-angle glaucoma, prostatic hyperplasia, bladder-neck obstruction, convulsive disorders, hyperthyroidism, DM, unusual responsiveness to sympathomimetic amines, hepatic/renal insufficiency, pregnancy/nursing status, and possible drug interactions.

Monitoring: Monitor serum K⁺, pulse rate, BP, and for signs/symptoms of hypersensitivity reactions, paradoxical bronchospasm, CV effects, unexpected development of severe acute asthmatic crisis, hypoxia, and other adverse reactions.

Patient Counseling: Instruct to use caution to avoid spraying eyes with this product. Advise not to exceed recommended dose or frequency without consulting physician. Instruct to seek immediate medical attention if therapy lessens in effectiveness, symptoms worsen, and/or need to use product more frequently than usual. Counsel to take other inhaled drugs only ud by physician. Instruct to contact physician if pregnant or nursing. Instruct to exercise caution when engaging in activities requiring balance and visual acuity (eg, driving a car, operating appliances/machinery). Advise not to puncture, not to use or store near heat or open flame, and to never throw container into fire or incinerator; exposure to temperature >120°F may cause bursting. Advise to discard canister after using the labeled number of actuations.

Administration: Inhalation route. Shake for ≥10 sec before use. Refer to PI for administration instructions. **Storage:** 25°C (77°F); excursions permitted to 15-30°C (59-86°F). Store canister at room temperature before use and avoid excessive humidity. Do not store near heat or open flame.

COMBIVIR   RX
zidovudine - lamivudine (ViiV Healthcare)

Lactic acidosis and severe hepatomegaly with steatosis, including fatal cases, reported with nucleoside analogues; suspend treatment if lactic acidosis or pronounced hepatotoxicity occurs. Lamivudine: Severe acute exacerbations of hepatitis B reported in patients coinfected with hepatitis B virus (HBV) after d/c of therapy; closely monitor hepatic function for at least several months. If appropriate, initiation of anti-hepatitis B therapy may be warranted. Zidovudine: Associated with hematologic toxicity (eg, neutropenia, anemia), particularly with advanced HIV-1 disease. Symptomatic myopathy associated with prolonged use.

THERAPEUTIC CLASS: Nucleoside reverse transcriptase inhibitor

INDICATIONS: Treatment of HIV-1 infection in combination with other antiretrovirals.

DOSAGE: *Adults:* ≥30kg: CrCl ≥50mL/min: Usual: 1 tab bid.
Pediatrics: ≥30kg: CrCl ≥50mL/min: Usual: 1 tab bid.

HOW SUPPLIED: Tab: (Lamivudine-Zidovudine) 150mg-300mg* *scored

WARNINGS/PRECAUTIONS: Do not use in pediatrics weighing <30 kg, or patients requiring dosage adjustment (eg, renal impairment [CrCl <50mL/min], hepatic impairment, or those experiencing dose-limiting adverse reactions). Caution with history or known risk factors for pancreatitis; d/c if pancreatitis occurs. Immune reconstitution syndrome reported. Autoimmune disorders (eg, Graves' disease, polymyositis, Guillain-Barre syndrome) reported to occur in the setting of immune reconstitution and can occur many months after initiation of treatment. May cause redistribution/accumulation of body fat. Obesity and prolonged nucleoside exposure may be risk factors for lactic acidosis and hepatomegaly with steatosis. Caution with any known risk factors for liver disease and in elderly. Lamivudine: Emergence of lamivudine-resistant HBV reported. Zidovudine: Caution with granulocyte count <1000 cells/mm³ or Hgb <9.5g/dL; monitor blood counts frequently with advanced HIV-1 and periodically with other HIV-1 infected patients. Interrupt therapy if anemia or neutropenia develops.

ADVERSE REACTIONS: Lactic acidosis, severe hepatomegaly with steatosis, myopathy, hematologic toxicities, headache, malaise, fatigue, fever, chills, N/V, diarrhea, anorexia, insomnia, nasal signs and symptoms, cough.

INTERACTIONS: Avoid with other lamivudine-, zidovudine-, and/or emtricitabine-containing products. Lamivudine: Avoid with zalcitabine. Hepatic decompensation may occur in HIV/hepatitis C virus (HCV) coinfected patients receiving interferon-alfa with or without ribavirin. Nelfinavir and trimethoprim/sulfamethoxazole may increase levels. Zidovudine: Avoid with stavudine, doxorubicin, and nucleoside analogues affecting DNA replication (eg, ribavirin). May increase risk of hematologic toxicities with ganciclovir, interferon alfa, ribavirin, bone marrow suppressors, or cytotoxic agents. Atovaquone, fluconazole, methadone, probenecid, and valproic acid may increase levels. Clarithromycin, nelfinavir, rifampin, and ritonavir may decrease levels.

PREGNANCY: Category C, not for use in nursing.

MECHANISM OF ACTION: Nucleoside analogue combination; inhibits reverse transcriptase via DNA chain termination after incorporation of the nucleotide analogue.

PHARMACOKINETICS: Absorption: Lamivudine: Rapid; bioavailability (86%). Zidovudine: Rapid; bioavailability (64%). **Distribution:** Lamivudine: V_d=1.3L/kg; plasma protein binding (<36%); found in breast milk. Zidovudine: V_d=1.6L/kg; plasma protein binding (<38%); crosses the placenta; found in breast milk. **Metabolism:** Lamivudine: Trans-sulfoxide (metabolite). Zidovudine: Hepatic; 3'-azido-3'-deoxy-5'-O-β-D-glucopyranuronosylthymidine (GZDV) (major metabolite). **Elimination:** Lamivudine: (IV) Urine (70% unchanged); $T_{1/2}$=5-7 hrs. Zidovudine: Urine (14% unchanged, 74% GZDV); $T_{1/2}$=0.5-3 hrs.

NURSING CONSIDERATIONS

Assessment: Assess for advanced HIV disease, bone marrow compromise, liver function and risk factors for liver disease, hepatitis B infection, history of pancreatitis and risk factors for its development, renal function, hypersensitivity to drug, pregnancy/nursing status, and possible drug interaction. Obtain baseline weight and CBC.

Monitoring: Monitor signs/symptoms that suggest pancreatitis, lactic acidosis, hepatotoxicity, myopathy and myositis, immune reconstitution syndrome (eg, opportunistic infections), autoimmune disorders, and hypersensitivity reactions. Monitor CBC and renal/hepatic function.

Patient Counseling: Inform about risk for hematologic toxicities and advise on importance of close blood count monitoring while on therapy. Counsel about the possible occurrence of myopathy and myositis with pathological changes during prolonged use and that therapy may cause a rare but serious condition called lactic acidosis with liver enlargement (hepatomegaly). Inform that deterioration of liver disease has occurred in patients coinfected with HBV with treatment d/c. Instruct to discuss with physician any changes in regimen. Caution patients about the use of other medication and instruct to avoid use with other lamivudine-, zidovudine-, and/or emtricitabine-containing products. Inform that hepatic decompensation has been reported in patients coinfected with HCV receiving interferon alfa with or without ribavirin. Inform that fat redistribution/accumulation may occur. Inform that therapy is not a cure for HIV-1 infection and patients may continue to experience illnesses associated with HIV-1. Advise to avoid doing things that can spread HIV-1 infection to others (eg, sharing of needles/inj equipment/personal items that can have blood or body fluids on them, having sex without protection, breastfeeding). Advise to take exactly as prescribed.

Administration: Oral route. **Storage:** 2-30°C (36-86°F).

COMPLERA   RX
tenofovir disoproxil fumarate - rilpivirine - emtricitabine (Gilead)

> Lactic acidosis and severe hepatomegaly with steatosis, including fatal cases, reported with the use of nucleoside analogues. Not approved for the treatment of chronic hepatitis B virus (HBV) infection. Severe acute exacerbations of hepatitis B reported in patients coinfected with HBV upon d/c of therapy; closely monitor hepatic function for at least several months. If appropriate, initiation of anti-hepatitis B therapy may be warranted.

THERAPEUTIC CLASS: Non-nucleoside reverse transcriptase inhibitor/nucleoside analogue combination

INDICATIONS: For use as a complete regimen for the treatment of HIV-1 infection in antiretroviral treatment-naive adults.

DOSAGE: *Adults:* ≥18 yrs: 1 tab qd with meal.

HOW SUPPLIED: Tab: (Emtricitabine-Rilpivirine-Tenofovir Disoproxil Fumarate [TDF]) 200mg-25mg-300mg

CONTRAINDICATIONS: Coadministration with CYP3A inducers or agents that increase gastric pH causing decreased plasma concentrations and resultant loss of virologic response or resistance (eg, carbamazepine, oxcarbazepine, phenobarbital, phenytoin, rifabutin, rifampin, rifapentine, proton pump inhibitors, systemic dexamethasone [more than a single dose], St. John's wort).

WARNINGS/PRECAUTIONS: Fat redistribution/accumulation may occur. Immune reconstitution syndrome reported. Not recommended with CrCl <50mL/min. Caution in elderly. Rilpivirine: Depressive disorders reported; immediate medical evaluation is recommended if severe symptoms occur. TDF: Caution with liver disease, obesity, prolonged nucleoside exposure; may increase risk of lactic acidosis and severe hepatomegaly; d/c treatment if hepatotoxicity occurs. Renal impairment reported; calculate CrCl prior to and during therapy. Decreased bone mineral density (BMD), fractures, and osteomalacia reported; assess BMD with history of pathologic bone fracture or other risk factors for osteoporosis or bone loss.

ADVERSE REACTIONS: Lactic acidosis, nausea, headache, dizziness, depressive disorders, insomnia, abnormal dreams, rash.

INTERACTIONS: See Contraindications. Avoid with concurrent or recent use of nephrotoxic agents, other antiretrovirals, drugs containing any of the same components, lamivudine, or adefovir dipivoxil. Rilpivirine: Caution with drugs that may reduce exposure or drugs with a known risk of torsades de pointes. Decreased levels, loss of virologic response, and possible resistance with CYP3A inducers or drugs increasing gastric pH (eg, antacids, H_2-receptor antagonists [H_2-RAs]). Administer antacids 2 hrs before or 4 hrs after dosing and H_2-RAs 12 hrs before or 4 hrs after dosing. CYP3A inhibitors, azole antifungals, and macrolide antibiotics may increase levels. May decrease levels of ketoconazole and methadone. Emtricitabine and TDF: Drugs that reduce renal function or compete for active tubular secretion (eg, acyclovir, adefovir dipivoxil, cidofovir, ganciclovir, valacyclovir, valganciclovir) may increase levels.

PREGNANCY: Category B, not for use in nursing.

MECHANISM OF ACTION: Emtricitabine: Nucleoside analogue of cytidine; inhibits activity of HIV-1 reverse transcriptase (RT) by competing with natural substrate deoxycytidine 5'-triphosphate and incorporating into nascent viral DNA, resulting in chain termination. Rilpivirine: Non-nucleoside reverse transcriptase inhibitor of HIV-1; inhibits HIV-1 replication by noncompetitive inhibition of HIV-1 RT. TDF: Acyclic nucleoside phosphonate diester analogue of adenosine monophosphate; inhibits activity of HIV-1 RT by competing with the natural substrate deoxyadenosine 5'-triphosphate and, after incorporation into the DNA, by DNA chain termination.

PHARMACOKINETICS: Absorption: Emtricitabine: Absolute bioavailability (93%), C_{max}=1.8μg/mL, T_{max}=1-2 hrs, AUC=10μg•hr/mL. Rilpivirine: C_{max}=80ng/mL, T_{max}=4-5 hrs, AUC=2397ng•hr/mL. TDF: Bioavailability (25%, fasted), C_{max}=0.30μg/mL, T_{max}=1 hr, AUC=2.29μg•hr/mL. **Distribution:** Emtricitabine: Plasma protein binding (<4%). Rilpivirine: Plasma protein binding (99.7%). TDF: Plasma protein binding (<0.7%). **Metabolism:** Emtricitabine: 3'-sulfoxide diastereomers, glucuronic acid conjugate (metabolites). Rilpivirine: Oxidative metabolism by CYP3A system. **Elimination:** Emtricitabine: Feces (14%) urine (86%); $T_{1/2}$=10 hrs. Rilpivirine: Feces (85%, 25% unchanged), urine (6.1%, <1% unchanged); $T_{1/2}$=50 hrs. TDF: Urine (IV, 70-80% unchanged); $T_{1/2}$=17 hrs.

NURSING CONSIDERATIONS

Assessment: Assess for obesity, prolonged nucleoside exposure, liver dysfunction or risk factors for liver disease, renal impairment, HBV infection, pregnancy/nursing status, and possible drug interactions. Assess BMD in patients with a history of pathological bone fracture or those at risk for osteoporosis/bone loss. Obtain baseline CrCl.

Monitoring: Monitor for signs/symptoms of lactic acidosis, severe hepatomegaly with steatosis, depressive symptoms, fat redistribution/accumulation, and immune reconstitution syndrome (eg, opportunistic infections). Monitor clinical and laboratory follow-up for acute exacerbations of hepatitis B in patients coinfected with HBV and HIV-1 upon d/c of therapy. Perform BMD monitoring. Routinely monitor CrCl and also serum phosphorus levels in patients at risk for renal impairment.

Patient Counseling: Inform that it does not cure HIV infection; continuous therapy is necessary to control infection and decrease related illnesses. Advise to practice safe sex and use latex or polyurethane condoms. Instruct never to reuse or share needles. Counsel to take on a regular dosing schedule with meal and avoid missing doses. Inform not to take more or less than the prescribed dose at any one time. Instruct to contact physician if symptoms of lactic acidosis or severe hepatomegaly with steatosis (eg, N/V, unusual stomach discomfort, weakness) occurs. Advise to inform physician if taking any other prescription or nonprescription herbal products (eg, St. John's wort). Instruct to seek medical evaluation if depressive symptoms are experienced and inform physician immediately if symptoms of infection occur.

Administration: Oral route. Take with meal. **Storage:** 25°C (77°F); excursions permitted to 15-30°C (59-86°F).

COMTAN

RX

entacapone (Novartis)

THERAPEUTIC CLASS: COMT inhibitor

INDICATIONS: Adjunct to levodopa/carbidopa to treat patients with idiopathic Parkinson's disease who experience the signs and symptoms of end-of-dose "wearing-off."

DOSAGE: *Adults:* 200mg with each levodopa/carbidopa dose. Max: 1600mg/day. Consider levodopa dose adjustment.

HOW SUPPLIED: Tab: 200mg

WARNINGS/PRECAUTIONS: Orthostatic hypotension/syncope and hallucinations reported. Diarrhea and colitis reported; consider d/c and institute appropriate therapy if prolonged diarrhea is suspected to be related to therapy. May cause and/or exacerbate preexisting dyskinesia. Severe rhabdomyolysis and symptom complex resembling neuroleptic malignant syndrome (NMS) reported. Retroperitoneal fibrosis, pulmonary infiltrates, pleural effusion, and pleural thickening reported. May increase risk of developing melanoma; monitor for melanomas frequently and on regular basis and perform periodic skin exams. Caution with hepatic impairment (eg, biliary obstruction). Rapid withdrawal or abrupt dose reduction may lead to emergence of signs and symptoms of Parkinson's disease, and hyperpyrexia and confusion; when d/c, closely monitor patients and adjust other dopaminergic treatment PRN.

ADVERSE REACTIONS: Dyskinesia, hyperkinesia, hypokinesia, N/V, diarrhea, abdominal pain, urine discoloration, dizziness, constipation, dry mouth, fatigue, dyspnea, back pain.

INTERACTIONS: Avoid with nonselective MAOIs (eg, phenelzine, tranylcypromine). Caution with drugs metabolized by catechol-O-methyltransferase (COMT) (eg, isoproterenol, epinephrine, norepinephrine, dopamine, dobutamine, α-methyldopa, apomorphine, isoetharine, bitolterol); increased HR, possibly arrhythmias, and excessive BP changes may occur. Caution with drugs known to interfere with biliary excretion, glucuronidation, and intestinal β-glucuronidase (eg, probenecid, cholestyramine, some antibiotics [eg, erythromycin, rifampicin, ampicillin, chloramphenicol]). May potentiate dopaminergic side effects of levodopa.

PREGNANCY: Category C, caution in nursing.

MECHANISM OF ACTION: COMT inhibitor; inhibits COMT and alters the plasma pharmacokinetics of levodopa.

PHARMACOKINETICS: Absorption: Rapid, absolute bioavailability (35%); C_{max}=1.2μg/mL, T_{max}=1 hr. **Distribution:** Plasma protein binding (98%); (IV) V_d=20L. **Metabolism:** Isomerization to *cis*-isomer, and direct glucuronidation. **Elimination:** Urine (10%, 0.2% unchanged), feces (90%); $T_{1/2}$=0.4-0.7 hrs (β-phase); $T_{1/2}$=2.4 hrs (gamma-phase).

NURSING CONSIDERATIONS

Assessment: Assess for dyskinesia, biliary obstruction, hepatic function, history of hypotension, hypersensitivity to drug, pregnancy/nursing status, and possible drug interactions.

Monitoring: Monitor for signs/symptoms of orthostatic hypotension, diarrhea, hallucinations, dyskinesia, rhabdomyolysis, a symptom complex resembling NMS, retroperitoneal fibrosis, pulmonary infiltrates, pleural effusion, and pleural thickening. Monitor for melanoma frequently and on a regular basis; perform periodic skin exams.

Patient Counseling: Instruct to take drug only as prescribed. Inform that postural hypotension, hallucinations, nausea, diarrhea, increased dyskinesia, and change in urine color (brownish orange discoloration) may occur. Caution against rising rapidly after sitting or lying down for prolonged periods and during initiation of treatment. Instruct to avoid driving a car or operating other complex machinery until aware of how medication affects mental and/or motor performance. Advise to inform physician if experiencing new or increased gambling urges, sexual urges, or other intense urges while on therapy. Instruct to notify physician if intend to become or are pregnant/nursing.

Administration: Oral route. **Storage:** 25°C (77°F); excursions permitted to 15-30°C (59-86°F).

CONCERTA

CII

methylphenidate HCl (Ortho-McNeil/Janssen)

Caution with history of drug dependence or alcoholism. Marked tolerance and psychological dependence with varying degrees of abnormal behavior may result from chronic abusive use. Frank psychotic episodes may occur. Careful supervision required for withdrawal from abusive use to avoid severe depression. Withdrawal following chronic use may unmask symptoms of underlying disorder that may require follow-up.

THERAPEUTIC CLASS: Sympathomimetic amine

INDICATIONS: Treatment of attention-deficit hyperactivity disorder (ADHD) in patients ≥6-65 yrs.

DOSAGE: *Adults:* ≤65 yrs: Methylphenidate-Naive or Receiving Other Stimulant: Initial: 18mg or 36mg qam. Titrate: May increase by 18mg weekly if optimal response not achieved. Max: 72mg/day. Currently on Methylphenidate: Initial: 18mg qam if previous dose 10-15mg/day; 36mg qam if previous dose 20-30mg/day; 54mg qam if previous dose 30-45mg/day; 72mg qam if previous dose 40-60mg/day. Conversion should not exceed 72mg/day. Titrate: May increase by 18mg weekly if optimal response not achieved. Max: 72mg/day. Reduce dose or d/c if paradoxical aggravation of symptoms or other adverse effects occur. D/C if no improvement after appropriate dosage adjustments over 1 month. Swallow whole with liquids; do not crush, divide, or chew. *Pediatrics:* ≥6 yrs: Methylphenidate-Naive or Receiving Other Stimulant: Initial: 18mg qam. Titrate: May increase by 18mg weekly if optimal response not achieved. Max: 6-12 yrs: 54mg/day; 13-17 yrs: 72mg/day not to exceed 2mg/kg/day. Currently on Methylphenidate: Initial: 18mg qam if previous dose 10-15mg/day; 36mg qam if previous dose 20-30mg/day; 54mg qam if previous dose 30-45mg/day; 72mg qam if previous dose 40-60mg/day. Conversion should not exceed 72mg/day. Titrate: May increase by 18mg weekly if optimal response not achieved. Max: 6-12 yrs: 54mg/day; 13-17 yrs: 72mg/day. Reduce dose or d/c if paradoxical aggravation of symptoms or other adverse effects occur. D/C if no improvement after appropriate dosage adjustments over 1 month. Swallow whole with liquids; do not crush, divide, or chew.

HOW SUPPLIED: Tab, Extended-Release: 18mg, 27mg, 36mg, 54mg

CONTRAINDICATIONS: Patients with marked anxiety, tension, agitation, glaucoma, motor tics or family history or diagnosis of Tourette's syndrome. Treatment with or within a minimum of 14 days following d/c of an MAOI.

WARNINGS/PRECAUTIONS: Sudden death, stroke, and myocardial infarction (MI) reported; avoid with known structural cardiac abnormalities, cardiomyopathy, serious heart abnormalities, coronary artery disease, or other serious cardiac problems. May increase BP and HR; caution with preexisting HTN, heart failure, MI, or ventricular arrhythmias. Promptly evaluate when symptoms suggestive of cardiac disease develop. May exacerbate symptoms of behavior disturbance and thought disorder in psychotic patients. May induce mixed/manic episode in patients with bipolar disorder. Use at usual doses can cause treatment-emergent psychotic or manic symptoms (eg, hallucinations, delusional thinking, mania) without prior history of psychotic illness. Aggressive behavior or hostility reported. May lower convulsive threshold; d/c if seizures develop. May cause long-term suppression of growth in children. Visual disturbances reported. Avoid with preexisting severe GI narrowing (eg, esophageal motility disorders, small bowel inflammatory disease, "short gut" syndrome). Perform periodic monitoring of CBC, differential, and platelet counts during prolonged use.

ADVERSE REACTIONS: Decreased appetite, headache, dry mouth, nausea, insomnia, anxiety, dizziness, decreased weight, irritability, upper abdominal pain, hyperhidrosis, palpitations, tachycardia, depressed mood, nervousness.

INTERACTIONS: See Contraindications. Caution with vasopressor agents; increased blood pressure may result. May inhibit metabolism of coumarin anticoagulants, anticonvulsants (eg, phenobarbital, phenytoin, primidone), and some antidepressants (eg, TCAs, SSRIs).

PREGNANCY: Category C, caution in nursing.

MECHANISM OF ACTION: Sympathomimetic amine; not established. CNS stimulant, thought to block the reuptake of norepinephrine and dopamine into the presynaptic neuron and increase the release of these monoamines into the extraneuronal space.

PHARMACOKINETICS: Absorption: Readily absorbed; (18mg qd dose) C_{max}=3.7ng/mL, AUC=41.8ng•hr/mL; T_{max}=6.8 hrs. **Metabolism:** De-esterification. α-phenyl-piperidine acetic acid (metabolite). **Elimination:** Urine (90%); $T_{1/2}$=3.5 hrs.

NURSING CONSIDERATIONS

Assessment: Assess for history of drug dependence or alcoholism, presence of anxiety, tension, family history or diagnosis of Tourette's syndrome, underlying medical conditions that might be compromised by increased BP or HR, psychotic disorders, seizure disorder, severe GI narrowing, drug hypersensitivity, pregnancy/nursing status, and for possible drug interactions. Perform careful history and physical exam to assess for presence of cardiac disease and psychiatric history. Prior to treatment, adequately screen patients with depressive symptoms to determine risk for bipolar disorder. Obtain baseline CBC, differential and platelet counts. Obtain baseline height/weight in children.

Monitoring: Monitor for cardiac abnormalities, increased BP and HR, cardiac disease symptoms, behavioral disturbances, thought disorder, new psychotic or manic symptoms, aggression, hostility, seizures, and for visual disturbances. In patients suspected of chronic abuse, monitor for marked tolerance or psychological dependence. In patients with bipolar disorder, monitor for mixed/manic episode. Perform periodic monitoring of height and weight in children, CBC, differential and platelet counts.

Patient Counseling: Inform about benefits, risks, and appropriate use of therapy. Instruct to swallow tablet whole with the aid of liquids; do not crush, divide, or chew. Advise to read Medication Guide. Inform that therapy may impair mental/physical abilities; caution with hazardous tasks (eg, operating machinery, driving). Inform that medication contains a nonabsorbable shell and to not be concerned if something that looks like a tablet is seen in the stool.

Administration: Oral route. Administer qam. Swallow whole with liquids; do not crush, divide, or chew. **Storage:** 25°C (77°F); excursions permitted to 15-30°C (59-86°F). Protect from humidity.

COPAXONE

RX

glatiramer acetate (Teva Neuroscience)

THERAPEUTIC CLASS: Immunomodulatory agent

INDICATIONS: Reduce frequency of relapses in patients with relapsing-remitting multiple sclerosis (RRMS), including those who have experienced a first clinical episode and have magnetic resonance imaging (MRI) features consistent with multiple sclerosis (MS).

DOSAGE: *Adults:* 20mg SQ qd.

HOW SUPPLIED: Inj: 20mg/mL [prefilled syringe]

CONTRAINDICATIONS: Hypersensitivity to mannitol.

WARNINGS/PRECAUTIONS: Immediate post-injection reaction (eg, flushing, palpitations, dyspnea, urticaria, anxiety, throat constriction), chest pain, lipoatrophy, and injection-site skin necrosis (rare) reported. May interfere with normal functioning of immune system.

ADVERSE REACTIONS: Injection-site reactions, infection, asthenia, vasodilation, pain, rash, N/V, influenza, dyspnea, chest pain, anxiety, back pain, palpitations, edema.

PREGNANCY: Category B, caution in nursing.

MECHANISM OF ACTION: Immunomodulatory agent; not established. Thought to act by modifying immune processes believed to be responsible for the pathogenesis of MS.

NURSING CONSIDERATIONS

Assessment: Assess for known hypersensitivity, clinical episodes of MS, and pregnancy/nursing status. Perform MRI to assess for features consistent with MS.

Monitoring: Monitor for immediate post-injection reactions, chest pain, lipoatrophy, injection-site necrosis, hypersensitivity, and other adverse reactions.

Patient Counseling: Advise to notify physician if pregnant/nursing or plan to become pregnant. Inform that symptoms (eg, flushing, chest pain, palpitations, anxiety, dyspnea, throat constriction, and urticaria) may occur early or several months after initiation, and are generally transient and self-limiting. Inform that transient chest pain may occur and to seek medical attention if chest pain of unusual duration or intensity occurs. Instruct to follow proper injection technique and rotate injection sites on a daily basis to avoid lipoatrophy and injection-site necrosis. Instruct to use aseptic technique.

Administration: SQ route. Refer to PI for preparation and administration instructions. **Storage:** 2-8°C (36-46°F); excursions permitted to 15-30°C (59-86°F) for up to 1 month. Do not expose to higher temperatures or intense light. Do not freeze.

COPEGUS

RX

ribavirin (Genentech)

Not for monotherapy treatment of chronic hepatitis C (CHC) virus infection. Primary toxicity is hemolytic anemia. Anemia associated with therapy may result in worsening of cardiac disease and lead to fatal and nonfatal myocardial infarctions (MI). Avoid with history of significant or unstable cardiac disease. Contraindicated in women who are pregnant and male partners of pregnant women. Extreme care must be taken to avoid pregnancy during therapy and for 6 months after completion of therapy. Use at least 2 reliable forms of effective contraception during therapy and 6 months after d/c.

THERAPEUTIC CLASS: Nucleoside analogue

INDICATIONS: Treatment of CHC virus infection in combination with Pegasys (peginterferon alfa-2a) in patients ≥5 yrs with compensated liver disease not previously treated with interferon alfa.

DOSAGE: *Adults:* CHC Monoinfection: Individualize dose. Usual: 800-1200mg/day in 2 divided doses. Treat for 24-48 weeks with Pegasys 180mcg once weekly. Genotypes 1 and 4: ≥75kg: 1200mg/day for 48 weeks. <75kg: 1000mg/day for 48 weeks. Genotypes 2 and 3: 800mg/day for 24 weeks. CHC with HIV Coinfection: Usual: 800mg/day. Treat for 48 weeks with Pegasys 180mcg SQ once weekly. D/C if patient fails to demonstrate at least a 2 log$_{10}$ reduction from baseline in HCV RNA by 12 weeks of therapy, or undetectable HCV RNA levels after 24 weeks of therapy. Refer to PI for dose modifications.

Pediatrics: ≥5 yrs: CHC Monoinfection: ≥75kg: 600mg qam and qpm. 60-74kg: 400mg qam and 600mg qpm. 47-59kg: 400mg qam and qpm. 34-46kg: 200mg qam and 400mg qpm. 23-33kg: 200mg qam and qpm. Treat for 24 weeks in genotypes 2/3 or 48 weeks in other genotypes with Pegasys 180mcg/1.73m^2 x BSA SQ once weekly. Max dose of Pegasys: 180mcg/week. Remain on pediatric dosing if reached 18th birthday while receiving therapy. D/C if patient fails to demonstrate at least a 2 log$_{10}$ reduction from baseline in HCV RNA by 12 weeks of therapy, or undetectable HCV RNA levels after 24 weeks of therapy. Refer to PI for dose modifications.

HOW SUPPLIED: Tab: 200mg

CONTRAINDICATIONS: Women who are or may become pregnant and men whose female partners are pregnant, hemoglobinopathies (eg, thalassemia major, sickle cell anemia), and combination with didanosine. When used with Pegasys, refer to the individual monograph.

WARNINGS/PRECAUTIONS: Combination therapy associated with significant adverse reactions (eg, severe depression, suicidal ideation, hemolytic anemia, suppression of bone marrow function, autoimmune/infectious/ophthalmologic/cerebrovascular disorders, pulmonary dysfunction, colitis, pancreatitis, diabetes). Do not start therapy unless obtain a negative pregnancy test prior to therapy. Caution with baseline risk of severe anemia (eg, spherocytosis, history of GI bleeding). Risk of hepatic decompensation and death in CHC patients with cirrhosis. Severe acute hypersensitivity reactions (eg, urticaria, angioedema, bronchoconstriction, and anaphylaxis) and skin reactions reported. D/C with hepatic decompensation, confirmed pancreatitis, severe hypersensitivity, developing signs or symptoms of severe skin reactions, severe adverse reactions, or if laboratory abnormalities develop or if intolerance persists. Pulmonary disorders (eg, dyspnea, pulmonary infiltrates, pneumonitis, pulmonary HTN, pneumonia, sarcoidosis/exacerbation of sarcoidosis, pulmonary function impairment) reported; monitor closely and if appropriate, d/c therapy. Caution with preexisting cardiac disease; d/c if cardiovascular status deteriorates. Delay in height/weight increase reported in pediatric patients. Not for treatment of HIV infection, adenovirus, respiratory syncytial virus, parainfluenza, or influenza infections.

ADVERSE REACTIONS: Hemolytic anemia, fatigue, asthenia, neutropenia, headache, pyrexia, myalgia, irritability, anxiety, nervousness, insomnia, alopecia, rigors, N/V.

INTERACTIONS: See Contraindications. Closely monitor for toxicities (eg, hepatic decompensation) with nucleoside reverse transcriptase inhibitors (NRTIs); consider d/c or reduce dose. May reduce phosphorylation of lamivudine, stavudine, and zidovudine. Severe pancytopenia, bone marrow suppression, and myelotoxicity reported with azathioprine.

PREGNANCY: Category X, not for use in nursing.

MECHANISM OF ACTION: Nucleoside analogue; not established. Has direct antiviral activity in tissue culture against many RNA viruses; increases mutation frequency in the genomes of several RNA viruses and ribavirin triphosphate inhibits HCV polymerase in a biochemical reaction.

PHARMACOKINETICS: Absorption: C$_{max}$=2748ng/mL; T$_{max}$=2 hrs; AUC$_{0-12h}$=25,361ng•hr/mL. **Elimination:** T$_{1/2}$=120-170 hrs.

NURSING CONSIDERATIONS

Assessment: Assess for history of hemoglobinopathies (eg, thalassemia major, sickle cell anemia), autoimmune hepatitis, hepatic decompensation, baseline risk of severe anemia (eg, spherocytosis, history of GI bleeding), history of drug abuse, history of significant or unstable cardiac disease, renal/hepatic/pulmonary function, pulmonary infiltrates, pancreatitis, hypersensitivity, pregnancy (including female partners of male patients), nursing status, and possible drug interactions. Obtain baseline hematological laboratory test (eg, CBC, Hgb, Hct), biochemical laboratory test, ECG with preexisting cardiac abnormalities, thyroid function, and CD4 count in HIV/AIDS patients. Confirm use of ≥2 forms of effective contraception.

Monitoring: Monitor CBC, LFTs, TSH, and ECG periodically. Obtain Hct and Hgb (Weeks 2 and 4, more if needed) and biochemical tests at Week 4. Perform pregnancy testing monthly and for 6 months after d/c (including female partners of male patients). Monitor the use of effective contraception during therapy and for 6 months after d/c. Monitor for severe depression, suicidal ideation, bone marrow suppression, autoimmune/infectious/ophthalmologic/cerebrovascular disorders, colitis, diabetes, pancreatitis, laboratory abnormalities, worsening of cardiac disease, and for hypersensitivity reactions. Monitor clinical status and hepatic/renal/pulmonary function.

Patient Counseling: Counsel on risks/benefits associated with treatment. Inform of pregnancy risks; instruct to use 2 forms of effective contraception during therapy and 6 months post-therapy (including female partners of male patients). Advise to notify physician in the event of pregnancy. Instruct not to drink alcohol; inform that alcohol may exacerbate CHC infection. Inform to take missed doses as soon as possible during the same day; do not double next dose. Inform that appropriate precautions to prevent HCV transmission should be taken. Caution to avoid driving/operating machinery if symptoms of dizziness, confusion, somnolence, or fatigue occur. Counsel to take with food and to keep well-hydrated. Advise that laboratory evaluations are required prior to starting therapy and periodically thereafter.

Administration: Oral route. Take with food. **Storage:** 25°C (77°F); excursions permitted between 15-30°C (59-86°F).

C CORDARONE   RX
amiodarone HCl (Wyeth)

> Use only in patients with the indicated life-threatening arrhythmias because use is accompanied by potentially fatal toxicities, the most important of which is pulmonary toxicity (hypersensitivity pneumonitis or interstitial/alveolar pneumonitis). Liver injury is common, usually mild, and evidenced by abnormal liver enzymes. Overt liver disease may occur, and has been fatal in a few cases. May exacerbate arrhythmia. Significant heart block or sinus bradycardia reported. Patients must be hospitalized while loading dose is given, and a response generally requires at least 1 week, usually 2 or more. Maint dose selection is difficult and may require dosage decrease or d/c of treatment.

THERAPEUTIC CLASS: Class III antiarrhythmic

INDICATIONS: Treatment of documented, life-threatening recurrent ventricular fibrillation and recurrent hemodynamically unstable ventricular tachycardia when these have not responded to documented adequate doses of other available antiarrhythmics or when alternative agents could not be tolerated.

DOSAGE: *Adults:* Give LD in hospital. LD: 800-1600mg/day for 1-3 weeks. Give in divided doses with meals for total daily dose ≥1000mg or if GI intolerance occurs. After control is achieved or with prominent side effects, 600-800mg/day for 1 month. Maint: 400mg/day; up to 600mg/day if needed. May be administered as a single dose, or in patients with severe GI intolerance, as a bid dose. Use lowest effective dose. Take consistently with regard to meals. Elderly: Start at the lower end of dosing range.

HOW SUPPLIED: Tab: 200mg* *scored

CONTRAINDICATIONS: Cardiogenic shock, severe sinus-node dysfunction causing marked sinus bradycardia, 2nd- or 3rd-degree atrioventricular (AV) block, when episodes of bradycardia have caused syncope (except when used with a pacemaker).

WARNINGS/PRECAUTIONS: Pulmonary toxicities reported; d/c and institute steroid therapy if hypersensitivity pneumonitis occurs, or reduce dose if interstitial/alveolar pneumonitis occurs and institute appropriate treatment. In patients with implanted defibrillators or pacemakers, pacing and defibrillation thresholds should be assessed before and during treatment. Can cause either hypo- or hyperthyroidism. Amiodarone-induced hyperthyroidism may result in thyrotoxicosis and/or the possibility of arrhythmia breakthrough or aggravation; consider the possibility of hyperthyroidism if any new signs of arrhythmia appear. D/C or reduce dose if LFTs are >3X normal or doubles in patients with elevated baseline; monitor LFTs regularly. Optic neuropathy and/or optic neuritis usually resulting in visual impairment reported. May cause fetal harm in pregnancy and neonatal hypo- or hyperthyroidism. May develop reversible corneal microdeposits (eg, visual halos, blurred vision), photosensitivity, and peripheral neuropathy (rare). Adult respiratory distress syndrome (ARDS) reported with surgery. Rare occurrences of hypotension reported upon d/c of cardiopulmonary bypass during open-heart surgery. Correct K⁺ or magnesium deficiency before therapy. Caution in elderly.

ADVERSE REACTIONS: Pulmonary toxicity, malaise, fatigue, involuntary movements, abnormal gait, constipation, arrhythmia exacerbation, hepatic injury, tremor, poor coordination, paresthesia, N/V, anorexia, photosensitivity, cardiac heart failure.

INTERACTIONS: Risk of interactions after d/c due to long half-life. May increase sensitivity to myocardial depressant and conduction effects of halogenated inhalation anesthetics. CYP3A4 inhibitors may decrease metabolism and increase serum levels (eg, protease inhibitors, loratadine, cimetidine, trazodone, grapefruit juice). Avoid with grapefruit juice. Initiate added antiarrhythmic drug at a lower than usual dose with monitoring. Monitor for toxicity and serum levels of amiodarone when used with protease inhibitors. QT interval prolongation and torsades de pointes reported with loratadine and trazodone. Caution with loratadine, trazodone, disopyramide, fluoroquinolones, macrolides, azoles; QT prolongation reported. Inhibits P-glycoprotein, CYP1A2, CYP2C9, CYP2D6, CYP3A4 and may increase levels of their substrates. Rhabdomyolysis/myopathy reported with HMG-CoA reductase inhibitors that are CYP3A4 substrates; limit simvastatin dose to 20mg/day, lovastatin to 40mg/day, and lower initial/maint doses of other CYP3A4 substrates (eg, atorvastatin) may be required. Elevated SrCr reported with cyclosporine. May increase levels of cyclosporine, quinidine, procainamide, flecainide, phenytoin, and digoxin. D/C or reduce dose by 50% upon amiodarone initiation. Quinidine and procainamide doses should be reduced by 1/3 if coadministered. Caution with β-blockers and calcium channel blockers. Reduce warfarin dose by 1/3-1/2; monitor PTT closely. Ineffective inhibition of platelet aggregation reported with clopidogrel. CYP3A4 inducers may accelerate metabolism and decrease levels, potentially decreasing efficacy (eg, St. John's wort, rifampin). Fentanyl may cause hypotension, bradycardia, and decreased cardiac output. Sinus bradycardia reported with lidocaine; seizure associated with increased lidocaine concentrations reported with IV amiodarone. Cholestyramine increases enterohepatic elimination and may decrease levels and

$T_{1/2}$. Hemodynamic and electrophysiologic interactions observed with propranolol, diltiazem, and verapamil. May impair metabolism of dextromethorphan, methotrexate, and phenytoin with chronic use (>2 weeks). Antithyroid drugs' action may be delayed in amiodarone-induced thyrotoxicosis. Radioactive iodine is contraindicated with amiodarone-induced hyperthyroidism. Caution with drugs that may induce hypokalemia and/or hypomagnesemia.

PREGNANCY: Category D, not for use in nursing.

MECHANISM OF ACTION: Class III antiarrhythmic; prolongs myocardial cell-action potential duration and refractory period, and causes noncompetitive α- and β-adrenergic inhibition.

PHARMACOKINETICS: Absorption: Slow and variable; T_{max}=3-7 hrs; bioavailability (50%). **Distribution:** V_d=60L/kg; plasma protein binding (96%); crosses the placenta, found in breast milk. **Metabolism:** Liver via CYP3A4, 2C8; desethylamiodarone (DEA) [major metabolite]. **Elimination:** Bile, urine; $T_{1/2}$=58 days, 36 days (DEA).

NURSING CONSIDERATIONS

Assessment: Assess for cardiogenic shock, severe sinus node dysfunction causing marked sinus bradycardia, 2nd- or 3rd-degree AV block, episodes of bradycardia causing syncope (except when used with a pacemaker), life-threatening arrhythmias, renal/hepatic impairment, thyroid function, preexisting pulmonary disease, recent myocardial infarction, hypersensitivity to the drug including iodine, presence of implanted defibrillators or pacemakers, optic neuropathy/ neuritis, pregnancy/nursing status, and possible drug interactions. Assess for failure of prior therapies. Correct hypokalemia and hypomagnesemia prior to initiation. Obtain chest x-ray, pulmonary function tests (including diffusion capacity), and physical exam.

Monitoring: Monitor for pulmonary toxicities and worsened arrhythmia. Perform history, physical exam, and chest x-ray every 3-6 months. Monitor for sinus bradycardia, sinus arrest, and heart block. Monitor for induced hyperthyroidism/thyrotoxicosis, hypothyroidism, hepatic failure, optic neuritis/neuropathy, corneal microdeposits, vision loss, fetal harm, peripheral neuropathy, photosensitivity. Monitor LFTs and thyroid function tests. Peri- and postoperative monitoring for hypotension and ARDS recommended. Monitor patients with severe left ventricular dysfunction. Perform regular ophthalmic examination, including fundoscopy and slit-lamp examination.

Patient Counseling: Inform about benefits/risks, including possibility of vision impairment, thyroid abnormalities, peripheral neuropathy, photosensitivity, and skin discoloration. Advise to report any adverse reactions to physician. Counsel to take as directed and not to take with grapefruit juice. Advise to avoid prolonged sunlight exposure and to use sun-barrier creams or protective clothing. Advise that corneal refractive laser surgery is contraindicated with concurrent use. Notify physician if pregnant/nursing. Advise to take with meals.

Administration: Oral route. **Storage:** 20-25°C (68-77°F). Protect from light.

CORDRAN   RX
flurandrenolide (Aqua)

OTHER BRAND NAMES: Cordran SP (Aqua)

THERAPEUTIC CLASS: Corticosteroid

INDICATIONS: Relief of the inflammatory and pruritic manifestations of corticosteroid-responsive dermatoses. (Tape) May use for relief of particularly dry, scaling localized lesions.

DOSAGE: *Adults:* (Cre) For moist lesions, apply a small quantity and rub gently into affected area bid-tid. May use occlusive dressings for psoriasis or recalcitrant conditions. (Lot) Apply a small quantity and rub gently into affected area bid-tid. (Tape) Replace q12h, but may be left in place for 24 hrs if well tolerated and adheres satisfactorily. May be used at night only and removed during the day when necessary. May use occlusive dressings for psoriasis or recalcitrant conditions. *Pediatrics:* (Cre) For moist lesions, apply a small quantity and rub gently into affected area bid-tid. May use occlusive dressings for psoriasis or recalcitrant conditions. (Lot) Apply a small quantity and rub gently into the affected area bid-tid. (Tape) Replace q12h, but may be left in place for 24 hrs if well tolerated and adheres satisfactorily. May be used at night only and removed during the day when necessary. May use occlusive dressings for psoriasis or recalcitrant conditions. Use least amount effective for condition.

HOW SUPPLIED: Cre (SP): 0.025% [30g, 60g], 0.05% [15g, 30g, 60g]; Lot: 0.05% [15mL, 60mL, 120mL]; Tape: 4mcg/cm² [60cm x 7.5cm, 200cm x 7.5cm]

CONTRAINDICATIONS: (Tape) Not recommended for lesions exuding serum or in intertriginous areas.

WARNINGS/PRECAUTIONS: Systemic absorption may produce reversible hypothalamic pituitary adrenal (HPA) axis suppression, manifestations of Cushing's syndrome, hyperglycemia, and glucosuria. Application of more potent steroids, use over large surface areas, prolonged use, or occlusive dressings may augment systemic absorption. Evaluate periodically for HPA axis suppression if large dose is applied to a large surface area or under an occlusive dressing. D/C or reduce frequency of application or substitute a less potent steroid if HPA axis suppression is noted. HPA axis suppression, Cushing's syndrome, and intracranial HTN reported in children. Steroid withdrawal may occur (infrequent) requiring supplemental systemic corticosteroids. Pediatrics may be more susceptible to systemic toxicity. D/C and institute appropriate therapy if irritation develops. Use appropriate antifungal or antibacterial agent in the presence of dermatologic infections; d/c if favorable response does not occur promptly. (Lot) D/C when control is achieved; reassess if no improvement seen within 2 weeks. Should not be used with occlusive dressings unless directed by a physician.

ADVERSE REACTIONS: Burning, itching, irritation, dryness, folliculitis, hypertrichosis, acneiform eruptions, hypopigmentation, dermatitis, skin maceration, secondary infection, skin atrophy, striae, miliaria.

PREGNANCY: Category C, caution in nursing.

MECHANISM OF ACTION: Corticosteroid; not established. Suspected to stabilize cellular and lysosomal membranes, thereby preventing release of proteolytic enzymes and consequently reducing inflammation.

PHARMACOKINETICS: Absorption: Percutaneous; occlusion, inflammation, and other disease processes in the skin may increase absorption. **Distribution:** Bound to plasma proteins in varying degrees; found in breast milk (systemically administered). **Metabolism:** Liver. **Elimination:** Kidney (major), bile.

NURSING CONSIDERATIONS

Assessment: Assess for age of the patient, hypersensitivity to corticosteroids, dermatological infections, conditions that augment systemic absorption, and pregnancy/nursing status.

Monitoring: Monitor for HPA axis suppression, Cushing's syndrome, hyperglycemia, glucosuria, skin irritation, development of dermatological infections, and hypersensitivity reactions. In patients receiving large doses applied to a large surface area or using occlusive dressings, perform periodic testing for HPA axis suppression using urinary free cortisol and adrenocorticotropic hormone stimulation tests. Monitor for signs/symptoms of steroid withdrawal following d/c. Monitor for systemic toxicity, HPA axis suppression, Cushing's syndrome, and intracranial HTN in pediatric patients.

Patient Counseling: Instruct to use externally, exactly as directed. Counsel to avoid contact with eyes. Advise not to use for any disorder other than that for which it was prescribed. Counsel not to bandage or wrap treated skin unless directed by physician. Advise to report any signs of local adverse reactions to physician. Advise parents of pediatric patients to avoid using tight-fitting diapers or plastic pants on treatment area. (Lot) Advise to avoid using medication on face, underarms, or groin areas unless directed by physician. Advise to notify physician if no improvement seen within 2 weeks. Advise not to use other corticosteroid-containing products without first consulting a physician.

Administration: Topical route. (Lot) Shake well before use. (Tape) Refer to PI for application and replacement of tape. **Storage:** (Cre) 15-30°C (59-86°F). (Lot) 20-25°C (68-77°F); excursions permitted to 15-30°C (59-86°F). (Tape) 20-25°C (68-77°F).

Coreg CR   RX
carvedilol phosphate - carvedilol (GlaxoSmithKline)

OTHER BRAND NAMES: Coreg (GlaxoSmithKline)

THERAPEUTIC CLASS: Alpha₁/Beta-blocker

INDICATIONS: Treatment of mild-to-severe chronic heart failure of ischemic or cardiomyopathic origin. Reduction of cardiovascular mortality in clinically stable patients who have survived the acute phase of a myocardial infarction (MI) and have a left ventricular ejection fraction of ≤40%. Management of essential HTN.

DOSAGE: *Adults:* Individualize dose and take with food. (Tab) Heart Failure: Minimize fluid retention prior to initiation. Initial: 3.125mg bid for 2 weeks. Titrate: May double dose over successive intervals of at least 2 weeks up to 25mg bid as tolerated. Maintain on lower doses if higher doses not tolerated. Max: 50mg bid if >85kg with mild-moderate heart failure. Reduce dose if HR <55 beats/min. HTN: Initial: 6.25mg bid. Titrate: May double dose q7-14 days as tolerated and PRN. Max: 50mg/day. Left Ventricular Dysfunction (LVD) Post-MI: Start if hemodynamically stable and fluid retention has been minimized. Initial: 6.25mg bid. Titrate: May double dose q3-10 days based on tolerability. Target dose: 25mg bid. May begin with 3.125mg bid and/or slow up-titration rate if clinically indicated. Maintain on lower doses if higher doses not tolerated. (Cap, ER) Heart Failure: Minimize fluid retention prior to initiation. Initial: 10mg qd for 2 weeks. Titrate: May double dose over successive intervals of at least 2 weeks up to 80mg qd as tolerated. Maintain on lower doses if higher doses not tolerated. Reduce dose if HR <55 beats/min. HTN: Initial: 20mg qd. Titrate: May double dose q7-14 days as tolerated and PRN. Max: 80mg/day. LVD

Post-MI: Start if hemodynamically stable and fluid retention has been minimized. Initial: 20mg qd. Titrate: May double dose q3-10 days based on tolerability. Target dose: 80mg qd. May begin with 10mg qd and/or slow up-titration if clinically indicated. Maintain on lower doses if higher doses not tolerated. Elderly: Start at a lower dose (40mg) when switching from higher doses of immediate-release; may increase dose after an interval of at least 2 weeks as appropriate.

HOW SUPPLIED: Tab: 3.125mg, 6.25mg, 12.5mg, 25mg; **Cap,** Extended-Release: (Phosphate) 10mg, 20mg, 40mg, 80mg

CONTRAINDICATIONS: Bronchial asthma or related bronchospastic conditions, 2nd- or 3rd-degree atrioventricular (AV) block, sick sinus syndrome, severe bradycardia (without permanent pacemaker), cardiogenic shock, decompensated heart failure requiring IV inotropic therapy, severe hepatic impairment.

WARNINGS/PRECAUTIONS: Severe exacerbation of angina, MI, and ventricular arrhythmias reported with abrupt d/c; whenever possible, d/c over 1-2 weeks. Bradycardia reported. Hypotension, postural hypotension, and syncope reported, most commonly during up-titration period; avoid driving or hazardous tasks. Worsening heart failure or fluid retention may occur during up-titration. May mask signs of hypoglycemia and hyperthyroidism (eg, tachycardia). Caution with pheochromocytoma, peripheral vascular disease, Prinzmetal's variant angina, and in patients with bronchospastic disease who do not respond to, or cannot tolerate, other antihypertensives. Monitor renal function during up-titration in patients with low BP (systolic BP <100mmHg), ischemic heart disease, diffuse vascular disease, and/or underlying renal insufficiency. Chronically administered therapy should not be routinely withdrawn prior to major surgery. Patients with history of severe anaphylactic reaction to variety of allergens may be more reactive to repeated challenge; may be unresponsive to usual doses of epinephrine. Intraoperative floppy iris syndrome (IFIS) observed during cataract surgery.

ADVERSE REACTIONS: Bradycardia, fatigue, hypotension, dizziness, headache, diarrhea, N/V, hyperglycemia, weight increase, increased cough, asthenia, angina pectoris, syncope, edema.

INTERACTIONS: Potentially increased levels with potent CYP2D6 inhibitors (eg, quinidine, fluoxetine, paroxetine, propafenone). Monitor for hypotension and bradycardia with catecholamine-depleting agents (eg, reserpine, MAOIs). BP- and HR-lowering effects potentiated with clonidine. Reduced plasma levels with rifampin. Increased exposure with cimetidine. Conduction disturbances seen with diltiazem; monitor ECG and BP with verapamil and diltiazem. May enhance blood glucose-reducing effect of insulin and oral hypoglycemics; monitor blood glucose. May increase concentration of cyclosporine and digoxin; monitor levels of cyclosporine and digoxin. Caution with anesthetic agents which depress myocardial function (eg, ether, cyclopropane, trichloroethylene). Digitalis glycosides slow AV conduction and decrease HR; concomitant use can increase the risk of bradycardia. Amiodarone or other CYP2C9 inhibitors (eg, fluconazole) may enhance β-blocking properties resulting in further slowing of the HR or cardiac conduction. Additive effects and exaggerated orthostatic component with diuretics.

PREGNANCY: Category C, not for use in nursing.

MECHANISM OF ACTION: Nonselective β-adrenergic and α_1 blocker.

PHARMACOKINETICS: Absorption: (Tab) Rapid and extensive; absolute bioavailability (25-35%). (Cap, ER) T_{max}=5 hrs. **Distribution:** Plasma protein binding (>98%); V_d=115L. **Metabolism:** Extensive by oxidation and glucuronidation; CYP2D6, 2C9 (primary); CYP3A4, 2C19, 1A2, 2E1 (minor). **Elimination:** Urine (<2% unchanged), feces; $T_{1/2}$=7-10 hrs.

NURSING CONSIDERATIONS

Assessment: Assess for coronary artery disease, hypotension, ischemic heart disease, diffuse vascular disease, hyperthyroidism, and any other conditions where treatment is contraindicated or cautioned. Assess for any upcoming surgery, history of serious hypersensitivity reaction, pregnancy/nursing status, and possible drug interactions. Obtain baseline blood glucose levels, LFTs, and renal function.

Monitoring: Monitor for bradycardia, signs/symptoms of cardiac failure, masking of hypoglycemia/hyperthyroidism, withdrawal symptoms, precipitation or aggravation of arterial insufficiency, hypotension, hypersensitivity reactions, and for IFIS during cataract surgery. Monitor blood glucose during initiation/dosage adjustments, and upon d/c of therapy. Monitor LFTs and renal function.

Patient Counseling: Instruct not to d/c therapy without consulting physician. Instruct patients with heart failure to consult physician if signs/symptoms of worsening heart failure occur. Inform that a drop in BP when standing, resulting in dizziness and, rarely, fainting, may occur; advise to sit or lie down if these symptoms occur. Advise to avoid driving or hazardous tasks if experiencing dizziness or fatigue and to notify physician if dizziness or faintness occurs. Inform contact lens wearers that decreased lacrimation may be experienced, diabetic patients to report any changes in blood sugar levels, and to take drug with food. (Cap, ER) Advise not to divide, chew, or crush cap.

Administration: Oral route. Take with food. (Cap, ER) Take in am. Swallow caps whole or may open and sprinkle contents on applesauce; do not chew, crush, or divide. **Storage:** (Tab) <30°C

(86°F). Protect from moisture. (Cap, ER) 25°C (77°F); excursions permitted to 15-30°C (59-86°F).

CORGARD
nadolol (King)

RX

Hypersensitivity to catecholamines observed upon withdrawal; exacerbation of angina and, in some cases, myocardial infarction (MI) reported after abrupt d/c. To d/c chronically administered nadolol, reduce dose gradually over 1-2 weeks and monitor carefully. Following d/c, reinstitute promptly, at least temporarily, and treat if marked worsening of angina or acute coronary insufficiency develops. Advise patients to not interrupt or d/c therapy without physician's advise.

THERAPEUTIC CLASS: Nonselective beta-blocker

INDICATIONS: Long-term management of angina pectoris. Management of HTN; may be used alone or in combination with other antihypertensive agents, especially thiazide type diuretics.

DOSAGE: *Adults:* Individualize dose. Angina Pectoris: Initial: 40mg qd. Titrate: Gradually increase in 40-80mg increments at 3-7 day intervals until optimum response achieved or pronounced slowing of HR occurs. Maint: Usual: 40 or 80mg qd. Doses up to 160 or 240mg qd may be needed. Max: 240mg/day. Reduce gradually over 1-2 weeks when d/c. HTN: Initial: 40mg qd. Titrate: May gradually increase in 40-80mg increments until optimum BP reduction achieved. Maint: Usual: 40 or 80mg qd. Doses up to 240 or 320mg qd may be needed. Renal Impairment: CrCl >50mL/min: Dose q24h. CrCl 31-50mL/min: Dose q24-36h. CrCl 10-30mL/min: Dose q24-48h. CrCl <10mL/min: Dose q40-60h.

HOW SUPPLIED: Tab: 20mg*, 40mg*, 80mg* *scored

CONTRAINDICATIONS: Bronchial asthma, sinus bradycardia and >1st-degree conduction block, cardiogenic shock, overt cardiac failure.

WARNINGS/PRECAUTIONS: May precipitate more severe heart failure in patients with congestive heart failure (CHF) and cause cardiac failure in patients without history of heart failure; caution with history of well compensated HF. Avoid in patients with bronchospastic disease. Impairs ability of heart to respond to adrenergic stimuli, potentially increasing the risks of general anesthesia and surgical procedures; chronically administered therapy should not be routinely withdrawn prior to major surgery. May prevent appearance of signs and symptoms of acute hypoglycemia (eg, tachycardia, BP changes). May mask clinical signs of hyperthyroidism and precipitate thyroid storm with abrupt withdrawal. Caution in patients with renal impairment. Patients with a history of severe anaphylactic reaction to variety of allergens may be more reactive to repeated challenge and may be unresponsive to usual doses of epinephrine.

ADVERSE REACTIONS: Bradycardia, dizziness, fatigue, nausea, diarrhea, anorexia, abdominal discomfort, rash, pruritus, weight gain, blurred vision, peripheral vascular insufficiency, cardiac failure, rhythm/conduction disturbances.

INTERACTIONS: Additive hypotension and/or bradycardia with catecholamine-depleting drugs (eg, reserpine) and digitalis glycosides. Hyperglycemia or hypoglycemia may occur with antidiabetic drugs (oral agents and insulin); adjust doses of antidiabetic agents accordingly. May exaggerate hypotension due to general anesthetics.

PREGNANCY: Category C, not for use in nursing.

MECHANISM OF ACTION: Nonselective β-blocker; not established. Inhibits β_1 and β_2 receptors, inhibiting chronotropic, inotropic, and vasodilator responses to β-adrenergic stimulation.

PHARMACOKINETICS: Absorption: T_{max}=3-4 hrs. **Distribution:** Plasma protein binding (30%); found in breast milk. **Elimination:** Urine (unchanged); $T_{1/2}$=20-24 hrs.

NURSING CONSIDERATIONS

Assessment: Assess for bronchial asthma, sinus bradycardia, atrioventricular block, cardiogenic shock, CHF, bronchospastic disease, coronary artery disease, hyperthyroidism, diabetes mellitus, renal impairment, pregnancy/nursing status, and possible drug interactions.

Monitoring: Monitor for signs/symptoms of CHF, hypoglycemia, thyrotoxicosis, withdrawal symptoms, renal dysfunction, and hypersensitivity reactions. Monitor renal function periodically.

Patient Counseling: Warn against interruption or d/c of therapy without consulting physician. Advise to consult physician at 1st sign/symptom of impending cardiac failure. Inform patient of proper course in the event of an inadvertently missed dose.

Administration: Oral route. **Storage:** 20-25°C (68-77°F). Avoid excessive heat and protect from light.

CORTISPORIN-TC OTIC   RX

hydrocortisone acetate - thonzonium bromide - neomycin sulfate - colistin sulfate

(JHP Pharmaceuticals, LLC)

THERAPEUTIC CLASS: Antibacterial/corticosteroid combination

INDICATIONS: Treatment of superficial bacterial infections of the external auditory canal and infections of mastoidectomy and fenestration cavities, caused by susceptible organisms.

DOSAGE: *Adults:* Instill 5 drops into affected ear tid or qid.
Pediatrics: ≥1 yr: Instill 4 drops into affected ear tid or qid.

HOW SUPPLIED: Sus: (Colistin-Hydrocortisone-Neomycin-Thonzonium bromide) 3mg-10mg-3.3mg-0.5mg/mL [10mL]

CONTRAINDICATIONS: External auditory disorder suspected or due to cutaneous viral infection (eg, herpes simplex virus, varicella zoster virus).

WARNINGS/PRECAUTIONS: Prolonged treatment may result in overgrowth of nonsusceptible organisms or fungi; verify causative organism with culture studies if infection does not improve after a week. Limit therapy to 10 days. Neomycin: Sensorineural hearing loss due to cochlear damage may occur; risk is greater with prolonged use. Caution in patients with perforated tympanic membranes. May cause cutaneous sensitization. Examine periodically for redness with swelling, dry scaling and itching, or failure to heal; d/c if observed. Allergic cross-reactions may occur. Hydrocortisone: Excessive systemic levels of hydrocortisone may reduce number of circulating eosinophils and urinary excretion of 17-hydroxycorticosteroids. D/C if sensitivity or irritation occurs. Do not heat above body temperature to avoid loss of potency.

ADVERSE REACTIONS: Skin sensitization, ototoxicity, allergic skin reactions, burning, itching, irritation, dryness, folliculitis, hypertrichosis, acneiform eruptions, hypopigmentation, perioral dermatitis, maceration of the skin.

PREGNANCY: Category C, caution in nursing.

MECHANISM OF ACTION: Colistin: Polypeptide antibiotic; penetrates into and disrupts bacterial cell membrane. Neomycin sulfate: Aminoglycoside antibiotic; inhibits protein synthesis, disrupting the normal cycle of ribosomal function. Hydrocortisone acetate: Corticosteroid hormone; regulates rate of protein synthesis, controls inflammation, inhibit the body's defense mechanism against infection. Thonzonium bromide: surface active agent; promotes tissue contact by dispersion and penetration of the cellular debris and exudate.

NURSING CONSIDERATIONS

Assessment: Assess for external auditory canal disease (viral/nonviral), perforated tympanic membrane, drug hypersensitivity and pregnancy/nursing status.

Monitoring: Monitor for sensorineural hearing loss, cutaneous sensitization or irritation (eg, redness with swelling, dry scaling, itching). Monitor for persistence of infection >1 week.

Patient Counseling: Instruct regarding proper use; avoid contaminating the dropper. D/C use and contact physician if sensitization or irritation occurs. Counsel on proper application; do not use in the eyes. Instruct to notify physician if pregnant, plan to become pregnant or breastfeeding.

Administration: Otic route. Clean and dry ear canal with sterile cotton before application. Lie down with affected ear upward, instill drops, and maintain position for 5 mins to ensure penetration into ear canal. If preferred, insert cotton wick saturated with suspension into canal; keep moist by adding further solution every 4 hrs and replace wick at least once every 24 hrs. Shake well before using. **Storage:** 20-25°C (68-77°F).

CORVERT   RX

ibutilide fumarate (Pharmacia & Upjohn)

May cause potentially fatal arrhythmias, particularly sustained polymorphic ventricular tachycardia, usually in association with QT prolongation (torsades de pointes), but sometimes without documented QT prolongation. Administer in a setting of continuous ECG monitoring and by personnel trained in identification and treatment of acute ventricular arrhythmias. Patients with atrial fibrillation (A-fib) of >2-3 days' duration must be adequately anticoagulated, generally for ≥2 weeks. Patients should be carefully selected such that the expected benefits of maintaining sinus rhythm outweigh the immediate and maintenance therapy risks.

THERAPEUTIC CLASS: Class III antiarrhythmic

INDICATIONS: For rapid conversion of A-fib or atrial flutter of recent onset to sinus rhythm.

DOSAGE: *Adults:* ≥60kg: 1mg over 10 min. <60kg: 0.01mg/kg over 10 min. If arrhythmia still present within 10 min after the end of the initial infusion, repeat infusion 10 min after completion of 1st infusion. Elderly: Start at lower end of dosing range.

HOW SUPPLIED: Inj: 0.1mg/mL

WARNINGS/PRECAUTIONS: May induce/worsen ventricular arrhythmias. Not recommended in patients who have previously demonstrated polymorphic ventricular tachycardia (eg, torsades de pointes). Anticipate proarrhythmic events. Correct hypokalemia and hypomagnesemia before therapy. Reversible heart block reported. Caution in elderly.

ADVERSE REACTIONS: Sustained/nonsustained polymorphic ventricular tachycardia, nonsustained monomorphic ventricular tachycardia, bundle branch/atrioventricular block, ventricular/supraventricular extrasystoles, hypotension, bradycardia, headache, nausea, HTN, syncope, nodal arrhythmia, congestive heart failure.

INTERACTIONS: Avoid Class IA (eg, disopyramide, quinidine, procainamide) and other Class III (eg, amiodarone, sotalol) antiarrhythmics with or within 4 hrs postinfusion. Increased proarrhythmia potential with drugs that prolong the QT interval (eg, phenothiazines, TCAs, tetracyclic antidepressants, and antihistamine drugs [H$_1$ receptor antagonists]). Caution in patients with elevated or above the usual therapeutic range of plasma digoxin levels.

PREGNANCY: Category C, not for use in nursing.

MECHANISM OF ACTION: Class III antiarrhythmic agent; prolongs atrial and ventricular action potential duration and refractoriness. Delays repolarization by activation of a slow, inward current, rather than blocking outward K$^+$ currents.

PHARMACOKINETICS: Distribution: V$_d$=11L/kg; plasma protein binding (40%). **Metabolism:** Omega-oxidation and β-oxidation. **Elimination:** Urine (82%, 7% unchanged), feces (19%); T$_{1/2}$=6 hrs.

NURSING CONSIDERATIONS

Assessment: Assess for arrhythmia, bradycardia, polymorphic ventricular tachycardia, electrolyte imbalance, renal/hepatic function, pregnancy/nursing status, and for possible drug interactions. Perform ECG. Obtain baseline QT$_c$.

Monitoring: Monitor for worsening of induction of new ventricular arrhythmia, torsades de pointes (polymorphic ventricular tachycardia), and any arrhythmic activity. Monitor ECG continuously for ≥4 hrs following infusion.

Patient Counseling: Inform about benefits/risks of therapy. Instruct to report any adverse reactions to physician.

Administration: IV route. Refer to PI for dilution instructions. **Storage:** Vial: 20-25°C (68-77°F). Admixture: 0.9% NaCl or D5W: Stable at 15-30°C (59-86°F) for 24 hrs; 2-8°C (36-46°F) for 48 hrs in polyvinyl chloride plastic or polyolefin bags.

Cosopt   RX
dorzolamide HCl - timolol maleate (Merck)

THERAPEUTIC CLASS: Carbonic anhydrase inhibitor/nonselective beta-blocker

INDICATIONS: Reduction of elevated intraocular pressure (IOP) in patients with ocular HTN or open-angle glaucoma who are insufficiently responsive to β-blockers.

DOSAGE: *Adults:* 1 drop in the affected eye(s) bid. Space dosing of drugs at least 10 min apart if using >1 topical ophthalmic drug.
Pediatrics: ≥2 yrs: 1 drop in the affected eye(s) bid. Space dosing of drugs at least 10 min apart if using >1 topical ophthalmic drug.

HOW SUPPLIED: Sol: (Dorzolamide Hydrochloride-Timolol Maleate) 2%-0.5% [10mL]

CONTRAINDICATIONS: Bronchial asthma, history of bronchial asthma, severe chronic obstructive pulmonary disease, sinus bradycardia, 2nd- or 3rd-degree atrioventricular (AV) block, overt cardiac failure, cardiogenic shock.

WARNINGS/PRECAUTIONS: Absorbed systemically; severe respiratory/cardiac reactions in patients with asthma and death in association with cardiac failure reported. Rare reports of fatal sulfonamide hypersensitivity reactions reported; d/c if signs of hypersensitivity or other serious reactions occur. Sensitizations may recur if readministered irrespective of the route of administration. May precipitate more severe failure in patients with diminished myocardial contractility; sympathetic stimulation may be essential for support of the circulation. D/C at the first sign/symptom of cardiac failure in patients without a history of cardiac failure. Withdrawal before surgery is controversial. May augment the risk of general anesthesia in surgical procedures. Caution in diabetic patients (especially those with labile diabetes) who are receiving insulin or oral hypoglycemics, hepatic impairment, and patients suspected of developing thyrotoxicosis. May mask symptoms of acute hypoglycemia and hyperthyroidism. Avoid abrupt withdrawal; may precipitate thyroid storm. Not recommended in severe renal impairment (CrCl <30mL/min). May be more reactive to repeated challenge with history of atopy or severe anaphylactic reaction to variety of allergens; may be unresponsive to usual doses of epinephrine. Bacterial keratitis with contaminated containers, and choroidal detachment after filtration procedures reported. May potentiate muscle weakness consistent with certain myasthenic symptoms. Caution in patients with low endothelial cell counts. Local ocular adverse effects (conjunctivitis and lid reactions) reported with chronic administration; d/c and evaluate before restarting therapy. Not studied in patients with acute angle-closure glaucoma.

ADVERSE REACTIONS: Taste perversion, ocular burning/stinging, conjunctival hyperemia, blurred vision, superficial punctate keratitis, eye itching.

INTERACTIONS: Concomitant administration of oral carbonic anhydrase inhibitors and topical β-blockers not recommended. Caution with oral/IV calcium antagonists; avoid coadministration in patients with impaired cardiac function. Potentiated systemic β-blockade with concomitant CYP2D6 inhibitors (eg, quinidine, SSRIs) and oral β-blockers. Possible additive effects and the production of hypotension and/or marked bradycardia with catecholamine-depleting drugs (eg, reserpine); observe patient closely. May have additive effects in prolonging AV conduction time with digitalis and calcium antagonists. Acid-base disturbances reported with oral carbonic anhydrase inhibitors; caution with high-dose salicylates.

PREGNANCY: Category C, not for use in nursing.

MECHANISM OF ACTION: Dorzolamide: Carbonic anhydrase inhibitor; decreases aqueous humor secretion, presumably by slowing formation of bicarbonate ions with subsequent reduction in Na^+ and fluid transport. Timolol: β_1 and β_2 (non-selective) adrenergic receptor blocking agent; decreases elevated IOP by reducing aqueous humor secretion.

PHARMACOKINETICS: Absorption: Timolol: C_{max}=0.46ng/mL. **Distribution:** Dorzolamide: Plasma protein binding (33%). Timolol: Found in breast milk. **Elimination:** Dorzolamide: Urine (unchanged, metabolite).

NURSING CONSIDERATIONS

Assessment: Assess for hypersensitivity, severe renal impairment, acute angle-closure glaucoma, conditions where the treatment is contraindicated or cautioned, pregnancy/nursing status, and for possible drug interactions.

Monitoring: Monitor for improvement in IOP, ocular HTN, serious reactions or hypersensitivity, corneal edema in patients with low endothelial cell counts, conjunctivitis and lid reactions with chronic therapy, and bacterial keratitis with use of multi-dose containers. Monitor serum electrolyte levels and blood pH levels.

Patient Counseling: Instruct to handle solution properly. Instruct not to touch container tip to eye or surrounding structures; may become contaminated. Advise to remove contact lenses prior to administration; may be reinserted 15 min after. Advise to administer at least 10 min apart if using >1 ophthalmic medications. Inform that product contains dorzolamide (a sulfonamide); d/c use and contact physician if serious/unusual reactions, hypersensitivity, or ocular reactions (eg, conjunctivitis, lid reactions) occur. Advise to immediately contact physician concerning use of present multidose container if undergoing ocular surgery or a concomitant ocular condition (eg, trauma, infection) develops.

Administration: Ocular route. Refer to PI for instructions for Use. **Storage:** 15-30°C (59-86°F). Protect from light.

COUMADIN   RX
warfarin sodium (Bristol-Myers Squibb)

> May cause major or fatal bleeding; monitor INR regularly. Drugs, dietary changes, and other factors affect INR levels achieved with therapy. Instruct patients about prevention measures to minimize risk of bleeding and to report signs/symptoms of bleeding.

OTHER BRAND NAMES: Jantoven (Upsher-Smith)

THERAPEUTIC CLASS: Vitamin K-dependent coagulation factor inhibitor

INDICATIONS: Prophylaxis and treatment of venous thrombosis and its extension, pulmonary embolism (PE), and thromboembolic complications associated with atrial fibrillation (A-fib) and/or cardiac valve replacement. To reduce risk of death, recurrent myocardial infarction (MI), and thromboembolic events, such as stroke or systemic embolization after MI.

DOSAGE: *Adults:* Individualize dose and duration of therapy. Adjust dose based on INR and condition being treated. (Coumadin) IV dose is the same as PO dose. CYP2C9 and VKORC1 Genotypes Unknown: Initial: 2-5mg qd. Maintenance: 2-10mg qd. Venous Thromboembolism (including deep vein thrombosis [DVT] and PE)/Non-Valvular A-fib: Target INR 2.5 (INR Range, 2-3). Mechanical/Bioprosthetic Heart Valve: Bileaflet Mechanical Valve/Medtronic Hall Tilting Disk Valve in the Aortic Position with Sinus Rhythm and without Left Atrial Enlargement: Target

INR: 2.5 (INR Range, 2-3). Tilting Disk Valves and Bileaflet Mechanical Valves in the Mitral Position: Target INR: 3 (INR Range, 2.5-3.5). Caged Ball or Caged Disk Valve: Target INR 3 (INR Range, 2.5-3.5). Bioprosthetic Valves in the Mitral Position: Target INR: 2.5 (INR Range, 2-3) for the 1st 3 months after valve insertion. If additional risk factors for thromboembolism present, target INR 2.5 (INR Range, 2-3). Post-MI: INR 2-3 plus low-dose aspirin (ASA) (≤100mg/day) for at least 3 months after MI. Valvular Disease Associated with A-Fib/Mitral Stenosis/Recurrent Systemic Embolism of Unknown Etiology: INR 2-3. Elderly/Debilitated/Asians: Consider lower initial and maintenance doses. Refer to PI for recommended dosing durations, conversion from other anticoagulants (heparin), dosing recommendations with consideration of genotype, and for further dosing instructions.

HOW SUPPLIED: Inj: (Coumadin) 5mg; Tab: (Coumadin, Jantoven) 1mg*, 2mg*, 2.5mg*, 3mg*, 4mg*, 5mg*, 6mg*, 7.5mg*, 10mg* *scored

CONTRAINDICATIONS: Pregnancy except in pregnant women with mechanical heart valves, who are at high risk of thromboembolism. Hemorrhagic tendencies or blood dyscrasias. Recent or contemplated surgery of the CNS, eye, or traumatic surgery resulting in large open surfaces. Bleeding tendencies associated with active ulceration or overt bleeding of GI/genitourinary/respiratory tract, CNS hemorrhage, cerebral aneurysms, dissecting aorta, pericarditis and pericardial effusions, or bacterial endocarditis. Threatened abortion, eclampsia, and preeclampsia. Unsupervised patients with conditions associated with potential high level of noncompliance. Spinal puncture and other diagnostic/therapeutic procedures with potential for uncontrollable bleeding. Major regional, lumbar block anesthesia. Malignant HTN.

WARNINGS/PRECAUTIONS: Has no direct effect on established thrombus, nor does it reverse ischemic tissue damage. Some dental/surgical procedures may need interruption or change in the dose; determine INR immediately prior to procedure. Has a narrow therapeutic range (index) and its action may be affected by endogenous factors, other drugs, and dietary vitamin K; perform periodic INR monitoring. Risk of necrosis and/or gangrene of skin and other tissues; d/c if necrosis occurs and consider alternative therapy. May enhance the release of atheromatous plaque emboli, and systemic atheroemboli and cholesterol microemboli may occur. D/C if distinct syndrome resulting from microemboli to the feet ("purple toes syndrome") occurs. Do not use as initial therapy with heparin-induced thrombocytopenia (HIT) and with heparin-induced thrombocytopenia with thrombosis syndrome (HITTS); limb ischemia, necrosis, and gangrene reported when heparin d/c and warfarin started or continued. Can cause fetal harm in pregnant women. Increased risks of therapy in patients with hepatic impairment, infectious diseases/disturbances of intestinal flora, indwelling catheter, severe/moderate HTN, deficiency in protein C-mediated anticoagulant response, polycythemia vera, vasculitis, diabetes, and those undergoing eye surgery. Caution in elderly and hepatic impairment.

ADVERSE REACTIONS: Hemorrhage, necrosis of the skin and other tissues, systemic atheroemboli, cholesterol microemboli, hypersensitivity/allergic reactions, vasculitis, hepatitis, elevated liver enzymes, N/V, diarrhea, rash, dermatitis, tracheal/tracheobronchial calcifications, chills.

INTERACTIONS: May increase effect (increase INR) with CYP2C9, 1A2, and/or 3A4 inhibitors. May decrease effect (decrease INR) with CYP2C9, 1A2, and/or 3A4 inducers. Increased risk of bleeding with anticoagulants (argatroban, dabigatran, bivalirudin, desirudin, heparin, lepirudin), antiplatelet agents (ASA, cilostazol, clopidogrel, dipyridamole, prasugrel, ticlopidine), NSAIDs (celecoxib, diclofenac, diflunisal, fenoprofen, ibuprofen, indomethacin, ketoprofen, ketorolac, mefenamic acid, naproxen, oxaprozin, piroxicam, sulindac), serotonin reuptake inhibitors (eg, citalopram, desvenlafaxine, duloxetine, escitalopram, fluoxetine, fluvoxamine, milnacipran, paroxetine, sertraline, venlafaxine, vilazodone). Changes in INR reported with antibiotics or antifungals; closely monitor INR when starting or stopping any antibiotics or antifungals. Use caution with botanical (herbal) products. May potentiate anticoagulant effects with some botanicals (eg, garlic and *Ginkgo biloba*). May decrease effects with some botanicals (eg, coenzyme Q10, St. John's wort, ginseng). Some botanicals and foods can interact through CYP450 interactions (eg, echinacea, grapefruit juice, ginkgo, goldenseal, St. John's wort). Cholestatic hepatitis has been associated with coadministration of warfarin and ticlopidine.

PREGNANCY: Category D (with mechanical heart valves) or Category X (for other pregnant populations), caution in nursing.

MECHANISM OF ACTION: Vitamin K-dependent coagulation factor inhibitor; thought to interfere with clotting factor synthesis by inhibition of the C1 subunit of the vitamin K epoxide reductase enzyme complex, thereby reducing the regeneration of vitamin K_1 epoxide.

PHARMACOKINETICS: Absorption: (PO) Complete; T_{max}=4 hrs. **Distribution:** V_d=0.14L/kg; plasma protein binding (99%); crosses placenta. **Metabolism:** Hepatic via CYP2C9, 2C19, 2C8, 2C18, 1A2, 3A4; hydroxylation (major), reduction. **Elimination:** Urine (≤92%, metabolites); $T_{1/2}$=1 week.

NURSING CONSIDERATIONS

Assessment: Assess for risk factors for bleeding (eg, age ≥65 yrs, history of highly variable INR, GI bleeding, HTN, cerebrovascular disease, malignancy, anemia, trauma, renal impairment, certain genetic factors), factors affecting INR (eg, diarrhea, hepatic disorders, poor nutritional state, steatorrhea, vitamin K deficiency, increased vitamin K intake, or hereditary warfarin resistance), pregnancy/nursing status, other conditions where treatment is contraindicated or cautioned, and drug-drug/drug-disease interactions. Assess INR. Obtain platelet counts in patients with HIT or HITTS.

Monitoring: Monitor for signs/symptoms of bleeding, necrosis/gangrene of skin and other tissues, systemic atheroemboli, cholesterol microemboli, "purple toes syndrome," and other adverse reactions. Perform periodic INR testing.

Patient Counseling: Inform physician if they fall often as this may increase risk for complications. Counsel to maintain strict adherence to dosing regimen. Advise not to start or stop other medications, including salicylates (eg, ASA, topical analgesics), over-the-counter drugs, or herbal medications, except on advice of physician. Instruct to inform physician if pregnancy is suspected, to discuss pregnancy planning, or if considering breastfeeding. Counsel to avoid any activity or sport that may result in traumatic injury. Instruct that regular PT tests and visits to physician are required during therapy. Advise patient to carry ID card stating drug is being taken. Instruct to eat a normal, balanced diet to maintain consistent intake of vitamin K and to avoid drastic changes in diet, such as eating large amounts of leafy green vegetables. If dose is missed, advise to take missed dose as soon as possible on the same day, but not to double dose the next day. Advise to immediately report unusual bleeding or symptoms or any serious illness, such as severe diarrhea, infection, or fever. Inform that anticoagulant effects may persist for about 2 to 5 days after d/c.

Administration: (Coumadin, Jantoven) Oral or (Coumadin) IV route. Inj: Reconstitute with 2.7mL sterile water for inj to yield 2mg/mL. Administer as slow bolus inj over 1-2 mins into a peripheral vein. **Storage:** Tab: (Coumadin) 15-30°C (59-86°F). (Jantoven) 20-25°C (68-77°F); excursions permitted 15-30°C (59-86°F). Protect from light and moisture. Inj: (Coumadin) 15-30°C (59-86°F). Protect from light. Use reconstituted sol within 4 hrs. Do not refrigerate. Discard any unused sol.

COVERA-HS   RX
verapamil HCl (G.D. Searle)

THERAPEUTIC CLASS: Calcium channel blocker (nondihydropyridine)

INDICATIONS: Management of HTN and angina.

DOSAGE: *Adults:* Individualize dose by titration. Initial: 180mg qhs. Titrate: If inadequate response with 180mg, increase to 240mg qhs, then 360mg (two 180mg tab) qhs, then 480mg (two 240mg tab) qhs. Severe Hepatic Dysfunction: Give 30% of normal dose. Elderly: Start at lower end of dosing range.

HOW SUPPLIED: Tab, Extended-Release: 180mg, 240mg

CONTRAINDICATIONS: Severe left ventricular dysfunction, hypotension or cardiogenic shock, sick sinus syndrome or 2nd/3rd-degree atrioventricular (AV) block (except with functioning artificial ventricular pacemaker), atrial fibrillation/flutter with an accessory bypass tract.

WARNINGS/PRECAUTIONS: Has negative inotropic effect; avoid with moderate to severe cardiac failure symptoms or any degree of ventricular dysfunction if taking a β-blocker. Patients with milder ventricular dysfunction should, if possible, be controlled with optimum doses of digitalis and/or diuretics before treatment. May cause congestive heart failure (CHF), pulmonary edema, hypotension, asymptomatic 1st-degree AV block, transient bradycardia, and PR interval prolongation. Marked 1st-degree block or progressive development to 2nd/3rd-degree AV block requires dose reduction, or d/c and institution of appropriate therapy (rare). Elevated transaminases with and without concomitant elevations in alkaline phosphatase and bilirubin reported; periodically monitor LFTs. Sinus bradycardia, 2nd-degree AV block, pulmonary edema, severe hypotension, and sinus arrest reported in patients with hypertrophic cardiomyopathy. Caution with preexisting severe GI narrowing. Caution with hepatic dysfunction; monitor for abnormal PR interval prolongation or other signs of excessive pharmacologic effects. May decrease neuromuscular transmission in patients with Duchenne's muscular dystrophy and cause worsening of myasthenia gravis; decrease dose with attenuated neuromuscular transmission. Caution with renal dysfunction; monitor for abnormal PR interval prolongation or other signs of overdosage. Caution in elderly.

ADVERSE REACTIONS: Constipation, dizziness, headache, edema, fatigue, sinus bradycardia, 2nd-degree AV block, upper respiratory infection.

INTERACTIONS: Increased levels with CYP3A4 inhibitors (eg, erythromycin, ritonavir) and grapefruit juice. Decreased levels with CYP3A4 inducers (eg, rifampin). May cause myopathy/rhabdomyolysis with HMG-CoA reductase inhibitors that are CYP3A4 substrates (eg, atorvastatin) and may increase levels of such drugs; limit dose of simvastatin to 10mg/day or lovastatin to 40mg/day. Increased bleeding times with aspirin. Additive negative effects on HR, AV conduction, and/or cardiac contractility with β-blockers. May produce asymptomatic bradycardia with a wandering pacemaker with timolol eye drops. Decreased metoprolol and propranolol clearance while variable effect with atenolol. Chronic treatment may increase digoxin levels, which may

C

result in digitalis toxicity. May reduce clearance of digitoxin. Additive effect on lowering BP with other antihypertensives (eg, vasodilators, ACE inhibitors, diuretics, β-blockers). Excessive reduction in BP with prazosin. Avoid disopyramide within 48 hrs before or 24 hrs after therapy. Additive negative inotropic effects and AV conduction prolongation with flecainide. Avoid quinidine with hypertrophic cardiomyopathy. Reduced or unchanged clearance with cimetidine. Increased sensitivity to effects of lithium when used concomitantly; monitor carefully. May increase carbamazepine, theophylline, cyclosporine, and alcohol levels. Increased clearance with phenobarbital. Reduced oral bioavailability with rifampin. Titrate carefully with inhalation anesthetics to avoid excessive cardiovascular depression. May potentiate neuromuscular blockers (curare-like and depolarizing); both agents may need dose reduction. May cause hypotension and bradyarrhythmias with telithromycin. Sinus bradycardia resulting in hospitalization and pacemaker insertion with clonidine; monitor HR. Prolonged recovery from neuromuscular blocking agent vecuronium reported.

PREGNANCY: Category C, not for use in nursing.

MECHANISM OF ACTION: Calcium channel blocker (nondihydropyridine); selectively inhibits transmembrane influx of ionic calcium into arterial smooth muscle and in conductile and contractile myocardial cells without altering serum calcium concentrations.

PHARMACOKINETICS: Absorption: Administration of variable doses resulted in different pharmacokinetic parameters. T_{max}=11 hrs. (Immediate-release) Bioavailability (33-65%, R-verapamil), (13-34%, S-verapamil). **Distribution:** Plasma protein binding (94% to albumin and 92% to α-1 acid glycoprotein, R-verapamil), (88% to albumin and 86% to α-1 acid glycoprotein, S-verapamil); crosses placenta, found in breast milk. **Metabolism:** Liver (extensive); norverapamil (active metabolite). **Elimination:** Urine (70% metabolites, 3-4% unchanged), feces (≥16%).

NURSING CONSIDERATIONS

Assessment: Assess for cardiac failure symptoms, ventricular dysfunction, preexisting severe GI narrowing, hypertrophic cardiomyopathy, hepatic/renal function, Duchenne's muscular dystrophy, attenuated neuromuscular transmission, any conditions where treatment is contraindicated, pregnancy/nursing status, and possible drug interactions.

Monitoring: Monitor for CHF, hypotension, AV block, abnormal PR interval prolongation, and worsening of myasthenia gravis. Periodically monitor LFTs and renal function.

Patient Counseling: Instruct to swallow tab whole; do not chew, break, or crush. Inform that outer shell of tab does not dissolve; may occasionally be observed in stool. Advise to seek medical attention if any adverse reactions occur. Counsel not to breastfeed and to report immediately if pregnant.

Administration: Oral route. Swallow whole; do not chew, break, or crush. **Storage:** 20-25°C (68-77°F).

COZAAR   RX
losartan potassium (Merck)

> Drugs that act directly on the renin-angiotensin system can cause injury/death to developing fetus during 2nd and 3rd trimesters. D/C when pregnancy is detected.

THERAPEUTIC CLASS: Angiotensin II receptor antagonist

INDICATIONS: Treatment of HTN, alone or with other antihypertensives, including diuretics. Reduce the risk of stroke in patients with HTN and left ventricular hypertrophy (LVH) (may not apply to black patients). Treatment of diabetic nephropathy with an elevated SrCr and proteinuria (urinary albumin to creatinine ratio ≥300mg/g) in patients with type 2 diabetes mellitus (DM) and a history of HTN.

DOSAGE: *Adults:* HTN: Individualize dose. Initial: 50mg qd. Intravascular Volume Depletion/History of Hepatic Impairment: Initial: 25mg qd. Usual Range: 25-100mg/day given qd-bid. HTN with LVH: Initial: 50mg qd. Add HCTZ 12.5mg qd and/or increase losartan to 100mg qd, followed by an increase in HCTZ to 25mg qd based on BP response. Diabetic Nephropathy: Initial: 50mg qd. Titrate: Increase to 100mg qd based on BP response.
Pediatrics: ≥6 yrs: HTN: Initial: 0.7mg/kg qd (up to 50mg total) administered as a tab or sus. Adjust dose according to BP response. Max: 1.4mg/kg/day (or 100mg/day).

HOW SUPPLIED: Tab: 25mg, 50mg*, 100mg *scored

WARNINGS/PRECAUTIONS: Symptomatic hypotension may occur in patients who are intravascularly volume-depleted; correct volume depletion before therapy or start therapy at a lower dose. Hypersensitivity including angioedema reported. Consider dose adjustment with hepatic dysfunction. Changes in renal function reported. Oliguria and/or progressive azotemia and (rarely) acute renal failure and/or death may occur in patients whose renal function is dependent on the renin-angiotensin-aldosterone system (eg, severe congestive heart failure [CHF]). May increase BUN and SrCr levels with renal artery stenosis. Electrolyte imbalances reported with renal impairment, with or without DM. Hyperkalemia reported in type 2 diabetics with proteinuria. Not recommended in pediatrics with GFR <30mL/min/1.73m² and <6 yrs. Dual blockade of the renin-angiotensin-aldosterone system is associated with increased risk of hypotension, syncope, hyperkalemia, and changes in renal function (including acute renal failure); closely monitor BP, renal function, and electrolytes with concomitant ACE inhibitors.

ADVERSE REACTIONS: Dizziness, cough, upper respiratory infection, diarrhea, asthenia/fatigue, chest pain, headache, nausea, hypoglycemia, back pain, sinusitis, nasal congestion, muscle cramp, leg pain.

INTERACTIONS: Rifampin or phenobarbital may decrease levels. Fluconazole may decrease levels of the active metabolite and increase levels of losartan. Cimetidine or erythromycin may increase area under the curve. K⁺-sparing diuretics (eg, spironolactone, triamterene, amiloride), K⁺ supplements, or salt substitutes containing K⁺ may increase serum K⁺. May reduce excretion of lithium; monitor lithium levels. Combination with NSAIDs, including cyclooxygenase-2 inhibitors, may lead to deterioration of renal function and attenuate antihypertensive effect.

PREGNANCY: Category C (1st trimester) and D (2nd and 3rd trimesters), not for use in nursing.

MECHANISM OF ACTION: Angiotensin II receptor antagonist; blocks vasoconstrictor and aldosterone-secreting effects of angiotensin II by selectively blocking the binding of angiotensin II to AT_1 receptor in many tissues (eg, vascular smooth muscle, adrenal gland).

PHARMACOKINETICS: Absorption: Well-absorbed; T_{max}=1 hr, 3-4 hrs (active metabolite). **Distribution:** V_d=34L, 12L (active metabolite); plasma protein binding (98.7%, 99.8% active metabolite). **Metabolism:** Liver via CYP2C9, 3A4; carboxylic acid (active metabolite). **Elimination:** Urine (35%, 4% unchanged, 6% active metabolite), feces (60%); $T_{1/2}$=2 hrs, 6-9 hrs (active metabolite).

NURSING CONSIDERATIONS

Assessment: Assess for volume depletion, CHF, DM, unilateral or bilateral renal artery stenosis, hepatic/renal impairment, history of hypersensitivity, pregnancy/nursing status, and possible drug interactions. Obtain baseline SrCr, BUN, and serum electrolytes.

Monitoring: Monitor BP, serum electrolytes, and renal function periodically. Monitor for signs/symptoms of electrolyte imbalance, hypotension, hypersensitivity reactions, oliguria, azotemia, hyperkalemia, renal/hepatic dysfunction.

Patient Counseling: Inform of pregnancy risks and instruct to report pregnancy to their physician immediately. Instruct patients not to use K⁺ supplements or salt substitutes containing K⁺ without consulting physician. Advise to seek medical attention if symptoms of electrolyte imbalance, hypotension, or hypersensitivity reactions occur.

Administration: Oral route. Refer to PI for preparation of sus. **Storage:** (Tab) 25°C (77°F); excursions permitted to 15-30°C (59-86°F). Protect from light. (Sus) 2-8°C (36-46°F) for up to 4 weeks.

CREON   RX
pancrelipase (Abbott)

THERAPEUTIC CLASS: Pancreatic enzyme supplement

INDICATIONS: Treatment of exocrine pancreatic insufficiency due to cystic fibrosis, chronic pancreatitis, pancreatectomy, or other conditions.

DOSAGE: *Adults:* Individualize dose based on clinical symptoms, degree of steatorrhea present, and fat content of diet. Initial: 500 lipase U/kg/meal. Max: 2,500 lipase U/kg/meal (or ≤10,000 lipase U/kg/day) or <4,000 lipase U/g fat ingested/day. Half of the dose used for an individualized full meal should be given with each snack.
Pediatrics: Individualize dose based on clinical symptoms, degree of steatorrhea present, and fat content of diet. ≥4 yrs: Initial: 500 lipase U/kg/meal. Max: 2,500 lipase U/kg/meal (or ≤10,000 lipase U/kg/day) or <4,000 lipase U/g fat ingested/day. Half of the dose used for an individualized full meal should be given with each snack. >12 months-<4 yrs: Initial: 1,000 lipase U/kg/meal. Max: 2,500 lipase U/kg/meal (or ≤10,000 lipase U/kg/day) or <4,000 lipase U/g fat ingested/day. ≤12 months: 3,000 lipase U/120mL of formula or per breastfeeding.

HOW SUPPLIED: Cap, Delayed-Release: (Amylase-Lipase-Protease) (Creon 1203) 15,000 U-3,000 U-9,500 U; (Creon 1206) 30,000 U-6,000 U-19,000 U; (Creon 1212) 60,000 U-12,000 U-38,000 U; (Creon 1224) 120,000 U-24,000 U-76,000 U

WARNINGS/PRECAUTIONS: Fibrosing colonopathy reported; monitor closely for progression to stricture formation. Caution with doses >2,500 lipase U/kg/meal (or >10,000 lipase U/kg/day); use only if these doses are documented to be effective by 3-day fecal fat measures indicating improvement. Examine patients receiving >6,000 lipase U/kg/meal; immediately decrease dose or titrate dose downward to a lower range. Caution with gout, renal impairment, or hyperuricemia; may increase blood uric acid levels. Should not be crushed or chewed, or mixed in foods with pH >4.5; may disrupt enteric coating of cap and cause early release of enzymes, irritation of oral mucosa, and/or loss of enzyme activity. Ensure that no drug is retained in the mouth. Risk for transmission of viral diseases. Caution with known allergy to proteins of porcine origin; severe allergic reactions reported. Not interchangeable with other pancrelipase products. Should not be mixed directly into formula or breast milk.

ADVERSE REACTIONS: Vomiting, flatulence, abdominal pain, headache, cough, dizziness, frequent bowel movements, abnormal feces, hyperglycemia, hypoglycemia, nasopharyngitis, decreased appetite, irritability.

PREGNANCY: Category C, caution in nursing.

MECHANISM OF ACTION: Pancreatic enzyme supplement; catalyzes the hydrolysis of fats to monoglyceride, glycerol and free fatty acids, proteins into peptides and amino acids, and starches into dextrins and short-chain sugars.

NURSING CONSIDERATIONS

Assessment: Assess for allergy to porcine protein, gout, renal impairment, hyperuricemia, and pregnancy/nursing status.

Monitoring: Monitor for fibrosing colonopathy, stricture formation, oral mucosa irritation, viral diseases, gout, and allergic reactions. Monitor serum uric acid levels and renal function.

Patient Counseling: Instruct to take as prescribed and with food. Advise that total daily dose should not exceed 10,000 lipase U/kg/day unless clinically indicated, especially for those eating multiple snacks and meals per day. Inform to take next dose with next meal/snack ud if a dose is missed; inform that doses should not be doubled. Instruct to swallow intact cap with adequate amounts of liquid at mealtimes. Advise to contact physician immediately if an allergic reaction develops. Inform that doses >6,000 U/kg/meal have been associated with colonic strictures in children <12 yrs. Instruct to notify physician if pregnant/breastfeeding, plan to become pregnant, or if breastfeeding.

Administration: Oral route. Refer to PI for proper administration. **Storage:** ≤25°C (77°F); excursions permitted between 25-40°C (77-104°F) for ≤30 days. Discard if exposed to higher temperature and moisture conditions >70%. Keep tightly closed. Protect from moisture. Store Creon 1203 in original container.

CRESTOR   RX
rosuvastatin calcium (AstraZeneca)

THERAPEUTIC CLASS: HMG-CoA reductase inhibitor

INDICATIONS: Adjunctive therapy to diet to reduce elevated total-C, LDL, ApoB, non-HDL, and TG levels, and to increase HDL in adults with primary hyperlipidemia or mixed dyslipidemia; to reduce total-C, LDL and ApoB levels in adolescents, who are at least 1 yr post-menarche, 10-17 yrs of age with heterozygous familial hypercholesterolemia who fail diet therapy and present with: LDL >190mg/dL or >160mg/dL with a positive family history of premature cardiovascular disease (CVD) or ≥2 other CVD risk factors; for the treatment of hypertriglyceridemia in adults; for the treatment of primary dysbetalipoproteinemia (Type III hyperlipoproteinemia); to slow the progression of atherosclerosis in adults as part of a treatment strategy to lower total-C and LDL to target levels. Adjunctive therapy to other lipid-lowering treatments (eg, LDL apheresis), or alone if such treatments are unavailable, to reduce LDL, total-C, and Apo B in adults with homozygous familial hypercholesterolemia. Reduces risk of myocardial infarction, stroke, and arterial revascularization procedures in individuals with an increased risk of CVD.

DOSAGE: *Adults:* Initial: 10-20mg qd. Dose Range: 5-40mg qd. Use the appropriate starting dose first, and only then titrate according to patient's response and individualized goal of therapy when initiating therapy or switching from another HMG-CoA reductase inhibitor therapy. Adjust dose accordingly when lipid levels are analyzed within 2-4 weeks. Use the 40mg dose only if LDL goal not achieved with 20mg dose. Homozygous Familial Hypercholesterolemia: Initial: 20mg qd. Asian Patients: Initial: 5mg qd. Concomitant Cyclosporine: Max: 5mg qd. Concomitant Lopinavir/Ritonavir or Atazanavir/Ritonavir or Gemfibrozil: Max 10mg qd. Severe Renal Impairment (CrCl <30mL/min/1.73m²) Not on Hemodialysis: Initial: 5mg qd. Max: 10mg qd.
Pediatrics: 10-17 yrs: Individualize dose. Heterozygous Familial Hypercholesterolemia: Usual: 5-20mg/day. Titrate: Adjust dose at intervals of ≥4 weeks. Max: 20mg/day.

HOW SUPPLIED: Tab: 5mg, 10mg, 20mg, 40mg

CONTRAINDICATIONS: Active liver disease, including unexplained persistent elevations of hepatic transaminase levels; women who are pregnant or may become pregnant; nursing women.

WARNINGS/PRECAUTIONS: Myopathy/rhabdomyolysis reported with highest risk at 40mg; predisposing factors for myopathy include age ≥65 yrs, inadequately treated hypothyroidism, and renal impairment. D/C if markedly elevated creatinine kinase (CK) levels occur or myopathy is diagnosed or suspected. Temporarily withhold in any patient with an acute, serious condition indicative of myopathy or predisposing to the development of renal failure secondary to rhabdomyolysis. Increases in serum transaminases reported; perform liver enzyme tests before initiation of therapy, and if signs and symptoms of liver injury occur. Fatal and nonfatal hepatic failure reported; promptly interrupt therapy if serious liver injury with clinical symptoms and/ or hyperbilirubinemia or jaundice occurs, and if an alternate etiology is not found, do not restart therapy. Caution in patients who consume substantial quantities of alcohol and/or have a history of chronic liver disease, severe renal impairment not requiring hemodialysis, Asian patients, and in elderly. Proteinuria and microscopic hematuria observed; consider dose reduction for patients with unexplained persistent proteinuria and/or hematuria. Increases in HbA1c and FPG levels reported.

ADVERSE REACTIONS: Headache, myalgia, nausea, dizziness, arthralgia, constipation, abdominal pain.

INTERACTIONS: Increased risk of myopathy with some other lipid-lowering therapies (fibrates or niacin), gemfibrozil, cyclosporine, lopinavir/ritonavir, or atazanavir/ritonavir. Avoid with gemfibrozil. Caution with coumarin anticoagulants; monitor INR before and frequently during early therapy. May enhance the risk of skeletal muscle effects with ≥1g/day of niacin. Caution with drugs that may decrease levels or activity of endogenous steroid hormones (eg, ketoconazole, spironolactone, cimetidine), protease inhibitors in combination with ritonavir or fenofibrates. May increase levels with cyclosporine, itraconazole, and fluconazole. May decrease levels with aluminum/magnesium hydroxide combination antacid and erythromycin, increase levels of digoxin and oral contraceptive containing ethinyl estradiol and norgestrel, and alter pharmacokinetics of warfarin.

PREGNANCY: Category X, not for use in nursing.

MECHANISM OF ACTION: HMG-CoA reductase inhibitor; produces lipid-modifying effects by increasing the number of hepatic LDL receptors on the cell surface to enhance uptake and catabolism of LDL and by inhibiting hepatic synthesis of VLDL, which reduces the total number of VLDL and LDL particles.

PHARMACOKINETICS: Absorption: Absolute bioavailability (20%); T_{max}=3-5 hrs. **Distribution:** V_d=134L; plasma protein binding (88%). **Metabolism:** CYP2C9; N-desmethyl rosuvastatin (major metabolite). **Elimination:** Feces (90%); $T_{1/2}$=19 hrs.

NURSING CONSIDERATIONS

Assessment: Assess for active or history of liver disease, unexplained persistent elevations in serum transaminases, risk factors for developing myopathy and rhabdomyolysis, history of alcohol consumption, renal impairment, pregnancy/nursing status, and possible drug interactions. Obtain baseline lipid profile, LFTs, and evaluate renal function.

Monitoring: Monitor for signs/symptoms of myopathy/rhabdomyolysis, increases in serum transaminase levels, liver dysfunction, endocrine dysfunction, proteinuria, and hematuria. Monitor lipid levels, CK, and LFTs.

Patient Counseling: Counsel about substances to avoid and to promptly report unexplained muscle pain, tenderness or weakness, particularly if accompanied by malaise or fever, to report any symptoms that may indicate liver injury (eg, fatigue, anorexia, right upper abdominal discomfort, dark urine, or jaundice) to the physician, and to take aluminum and magnesium hydroxide combination antacid at least 2 hrs after administration of medication.

Administration: Oral route. **Storage:** 20-25°C (68-77°F). Protect from moisture.

CRIXIVAN   RX
indinavir sulfate (Merck)

THERAPEUTIC CLASS: Protease inhibitor

INDICATIONS: Treatment of HIV infection in combination with other antiretrovirals.

DOSAGE: *Adults:* Usual: 800mg PO q8h. Take without food but with water 1 hr before or 2 hrs after meals. Mild-Moderate Hepatic Insufficiency/Concomitant Delavirdine, Itraconazole, Ketoconazole: Reduce to 600mg PO q8h. Concomitant Didanosine: Administer at least 1 hr apart. Concomitant Rifabutin: 1g PO q8h (reduce rifabutin dose by 1/2).

HOW SUPPLIED: Cap: 100mg, 200mg, 400mg

CONTRAINDICATIONS: Coadministration with CYP3A4 substrates (eg, pimozide, cisapride, amiodarone, triazolam, oral midazolam, alprazolam, dihydroergotamine, ergonovine, ergotamine, methylergonovine, alfuzosin and sildenafil [for treatment of pulmonary arterial HTN]) for which elevated plasma concentrations potentially cause serious or life-threatening reactions.

WARNINGS/PRECAUTIONS: Nephrolithiasis/urolithiasis reported; temporarily interrupt (eg, 1-3 days) or d/c if signs/symptoms occur. Maintain adequate hydration (1.5L fluid/24 hrs). Acute hemolytic anemia reported; d/c once diagnosis is apparent. Immune reconstitution syndrome, new onset/exacerbation of diabetes mellitus (DM), hyperglycemia, diabetic ketoacidosis,

C

hepatitis including hepatic failure, and indirect hyperbilirubinemia reported. Reduce dose with hepatic insufficiency due to cirrhosis. Tubulointerstitial nephritis with medullary calcification and cortical atrophy reported in patients with asymptomatic severe leukocyturia; monitor frequently with urinalyses. Consider d/c with severe leukocyturia (>100 cells/high power field). Spontaneous bleeding may occur with hemophilia A and B. Body fat redistribution/accumulation (eg, central obesity, dorsocervical fat enlargement, peripheral wasting, facial wasting, breast enlargement, "cushingoid appearance") may develop. May increase myopathy and rhabdomyolysis with HMG-CoA reductase inhibitors. Caution in elderly.

ADVERSE REACTIONS: Nephrolithiasis/urolithiasis, hyperbilirubinemia, abdominal pain, headache, N/V, dizziness, pruritus, diarrhea, back pain.

INTERACTIONS: See Contraindications. Not recommended with lovastatin, simvastatin, rosuvastatin, St. John's wort, salmeterol, fluticasone (with ritonavir), and atazanavir. Avoid colchicine (in renal/hepatic impairment) and rifampin. May increase levels of CYP3A4 substrates, ritonavir, salmeterol, fluticasone, parenteral midazolam, PDE5 inhibitors, saquinavir, antiarrhythmics, trazodone, colchicine, dihydropyridine calcium channel blockers, clarithromycin, bosentan, atorvastatin, immunosuppressants, rifabutin, and benzodiazepine. CYP3A4 inducers, St. John's wort, efavirenz, nevirapine, anticonvulsants, rifabutin, and venlafaxine may decrease levels. CYP3A4 inhibitors, delavirdine, nelfinavir, ritonavir, clarithromycin, itraconazole, and ketoconazole may increase levels.

PREGNANCY: Category C, not for use in nursing.

MECHANISM OF ACTION: Protease inhibitor; binds to protease active site and inhibits enzyme activity hence preventing cleavage of viral polyproteins resulting in the formation of immature noninfectious viral particles.

PHARMACOKINETICS: Absorption: Rapid; C_{max}=12617nM; T_{max}=0.8 hrs; AUC=30691nM•hr. **Distribution:** Plasma protein binding (60%). **Metabolism:** Hepatic via CYP3A4 (major). **Elimination:** Urine (<20%, unchanged); $T_{1/2}$=1.8 hrs.

NURSING CONSIDERATIONS

Assessment: Assess for asymptomatic severe leukocyturia, hemophilia, hepatic/renal dysfunction, DM, hypersensitivity reactions, pregnancy/nursing status, and possible drug interactions.

Monitoring: Monitor for possible indirect hyperbilirubinemia, increase in serum transaminase, immune reconstitution syndrome, signs and symptoms of nephrolithiasis/urolithiasis, hemolytic anemia, hepatitis, hyperglycemia and new onset/exacerbation of DM. Monitor urinalyses frequently with severe leukocyturia and for possible tubulointerstitial nephritis.

Patient Counseling: Inform the drug is not a cure for HIV; opportunistic infections may still occur. Inform that drug therapy has not been shown to reduce the risk of transmitting HIV to others through sexual contact or blood contamination. Instruct not to alter dose or d/c without consulting physician. If dose is missed, instruct to take the next dose at the regularly scheduled time and not to double next dose. Advise to report to physician the use of other Rx, OTC, or herbal products (eg, St. John's wort). Instruct to take without food but with water, other liquid or a light meal and to drink at least 1.5L of liquids in 24 hrs. Inform that redistribution or accumulation of body fat may occur. Inform patients of the increased risk of PDE5 inhibitor-associated adverse events (eg, hypotension, visual changes, priapism) if used concomitantly; report to physician if symptoms occur.

Administration: Oral route. Take without food but with water 1 hr before or 2 hrs after meals. Maintain hydration (1.5L fluid/24 hrs). **Storage:** 15-30°C (59-86°F). Protect from moisture.

CUBICIN   RX
daptomycin (Cubist)

THERAPEUTIC CLASS: Cyclic lipopeptide

INDICATIONS: Susceptible complicated skin and skin structure infections (cSSSI) and *Staphylococcus aureus* bloodstream infections (bacteremia), including right-sided infective endocarditis.

DOSAGE: *Adults:* ≥18 yrs: Administer as IV inj over 2 min or infusion over a 30 min period. cSSSI: 4mg/kg once q24h for 7-14 days. *S. aureus* Bacteremia: 6mg/kg once q24h for 2-6 weeks. Limited safety data for use >28 days. Do not dose more frequently than qd. Renal impairment: CrCl <30mL/min, Hemodialysis, Continuous Ambulatory Peritoneal Dialysis: 4mg/kg (cSSSI) or 6mg/kg (*S. aureus* bacteremia) once q48h.

HOW SUPPLIED: Inj: 500mg [10mL]

WARNINGS/PRECAUTIONS: Anaphylaxis/hypersensitivity reactions reported; d/c and institute appropriate therapy if allergic reaction occurs. Myopathy, CPK elevation and rhabdomyolysis with or without acute renal failure reported. D/C with unexplained signs and symptoms of myopathy and CPK elevations to levels >1000 U/L (-5X ULN), or without symptoms and levels >2000

U/L (≥10X ULN). Eosinophilic pneumonia reported; d/c therapy and treat with systemic steroids if fever, dyspnea with hypoxic respiratory insufficiency, and diffuse pulmonary infiltrates occur. Peripheral neuropathy reported. *Clostridium difficile*-associated diarrhea (CDAD) reported. May result in bacterial resistance with prolonged use or use in the absence of a proven/suspected bacterial infection or a prophylactic indication; take appropriate measures if superinfection develops. Repeat blood cultures for persisting or relapsing *S. aureus* bacteremia/endocarditis or poor clinical response; appropriate surgical intervention and/or change in antibiotic regimen may be required. Not indicated for the treatment of pneumonia and left-sided infective endocarditis due to *S. aureus*. May cause false prolongation of PT and elevation of INR when certain recombinant thromboplastin reagents are utilized for the assay.

ADVERSE REACTIONS: Headache, diarrhea, insomnia, CPK increased, chest pain, abdominal pain, pharyngolaryngeal pain, rash, abnormal LFTs, sepsis, bacteremia, edema, pruritus, sweating increased, HTN.

INTERACTIONS: Concomitant tobramycin increased daptomycin levels and decreased tobramycin levels. Concomitant therapy with agents associated with rhabdomyolysis (eg, HMG-CoA reductase inhibitors) may increase CPK levels; consider temporary d/c.

PREGNANCY: Category B, caution in nursing.

MECHANISM OF ACTION: Cyclic lipopeptide; binds to bacterial membranes and causes a rapid depolarization of membrane potential, causing inhibition of DNA, RNA, and protein synthesis, which results in bacterial cell death.

PHARMACOKINETICS: Absorption: (4mg/kg) C_{max}=57.8μg/mL, AUC=494μg•h/mL (over 30 min); AUC=475μg•h/mL (over 2 min). (6mg/kg) C_{max}=93.9μg/mL, AUC=632μg•h/mL (over 30 min); AUC=701μg•h/mL (over 2 min). Refer to PI for pharmacokinetic parameters with various degrees of renal function. **Distribution:** Plasma protein binding (90-93%); V_d=0.1L/kg. **Elimination:** Urine (78%), feces (5.7%); (4mg/kg over 30 min) $T_{1/2}$=8.1 hrs; (6mg/kg over 30 min) $T_{1/2}$=7.9 hrs.

NURSING CONSIDERATIONS

Assessment: Assess renal function, hypersensitivity to the drug, pregnancy/nursing status and possible drug interactions. Obtain baseline CPK levels. Obtain specimens for microbiological examination to determine pathogen identity and susceptibility.

Monitoring: Monitor renal/hepatic function. Monitor for anaphylaxis or hypersensitivity reactions, development of superinfection, eosinophilic pneumonia, CDAD, rhabdomyolysis, myopathy, muscle pain or weakness particularly of the distal extremities, peripheral neuropathy, and persisting or relapsing *S. aureus* infection or poor clinical response. Monitor CPK levels weekly, and more frequently in patients who received recent prior or concomitant therapy with an HMG-CoA reductase inhibitor or if CPK elevations occur during therapy. Monitor renal function and CPK levels more frequently than once weekly with renal impairment.

Patient Counseling: Instruct to report any previous allergic reactions to the drug. Inform that serious allergic reactions may occur and require immediate treatment. Instruct to report muscle pain or weakness, tingling, numbness, cough, breathlessness or fever. Instruct to notify physician immediately if watery/bloody diarrhea (with or without stomach cramps and fever) develops even as late as 2 months after therapy. Inform that drug is used to treat bacterial, not viral infections (eg, common cold). Administer exactly as directed; skipping doses or not completing full course of therapy may decrease effectiveness and increase likelihood of drug resistance. Notify physician if pregnant/nursing.

Administration: IV route. Refer to PI for instructions on reconstitution and administration. Not compatible with dextrose-containing diluents. Do not add with other IV substances, additives and other medications. **Storage:** 2-8°C (36-46°F). Avoid excessive heat. Reconstituted/Diluted Solution: Stable for 12 hrs at room temperature or ≤48 hrs if refrigerated.

CUTIVATE   RX
fluticasone propionate (PharmaDerm)

THERAPEUTIC CLASS: Corticosteroid

INDICATIONS: (Cre, Oint) Relief of the inflammatory and pruritic manifestations of corticosteroid-responsive dermatoses. Cream may be used with caution in pediatric patients ≥3 months of age. (Lot) Relief of the inflammatory and pruritic manifestations of atopic dermatitis in patients ≥1 yr of age.

DOSAGE: *Adults:* Atopic Dermatitis: (Cre) Apply a thin film to affected areas qd-bid. (Lot) Apply a thin film to affected areas qd. Other Corticosteroid-Responsive Dermatoses: (Cre/Oint) Apply a thin film to affected areas qd. Rub in gently.
Pediatrics: ≥3 months: (Cre) Atopic Dermatitis: Apply a thin film to affected areas qd-bid. Other Corticosteroid-Responsive Dermatoses: Apply a thin film to affected areas bid ≥1 yr: (Lot) Atopic Dermatitis: Apply a thin film to affected areas qd. (Cre, Lot): Rub in gently.

HOW SUPPLIED: Cre: 0.05% [15g, 30g, 60g]; Lot: 0.05% [60mL]; Oint: 0.005% [15g, 30g, 60g].

WARNINGS/PRECAUTIONS: (Cre, Lot, Oint) May produce reversible hypothalamic-pituitary-adrenal (HPA) axis suppression, manifestations of Cushing's syndrome, hyperglycemia and glucosuria; withdraw, reduce frequency, or substitute to a less potent steroid if HPA axis suppression is noted. Glucocorticosteroid insufficiency may occur infrequently, requiring supplemental systemic steroids. May cause local cutaneous adverse reactions; d/c if irritation occurs and institute appropriate therapy. Use appropriate antifungal or antibacterial agent if concomitant skin infections are present/develop; if favorable response does not occur promptly, d/c until infection is controlled. Pediatrics may be more susceptible to systemic toxicity. HPA axis suppression, Cushing's syndrome, linear growth retardation, delayed weight, and intracranial HTN reported in pediatrics. Caution when applied to large surface areas or areas under occlusion. Avoid with preexisting skin atrophy and presence of infection at treatment site. Not for use in rosacea or perioral dermatitis. Avoid occlusive dressings and reevaluate if no improvement within 2 weeks. (Cre, Lot) Contains imidurea excipient which releases formaldehyde as a breakdown product; avoid with hypersensitivity to formaldehyde as it may prevent healing or worsen dermatitis. D/C if control is achieved before 4 weeks. (Lot) Avoid excessive exposure to either natural/artificial sunlight (eg, tanning booths, sun lamps) if applied to exposed portions of the body.

ADVERSE REACTIONS: (Cre) Pruritus, dryness, numbness of fingers, burning, facial telangiectasia. (Oint) Pruritus, burning, hypertrichosis, increased erythema, hives, irritation, lightheadedness. (Lot) Common cold, upper respiratory tract infection, cough, fever, dry skin, stinging at application site.

PREGNANCY: Category C, caution in nursing.

MECHANISM OF ACTION: Corticosteroid; possesses anti-inflammatory, antipruritic, and vasoconstrictive properties. Anti-inflammatory activity not established; suspected to act by the induction of phospholipase A_2 inhibitory proteins (lipocortins). Lipocortins control biosynthesis of potent mediators of inflammation (eg, prostaglandins, leukotrienes) by inhibiting release of common precursor, arachidonic acid.

PHARMACOKINETICS: Absorption: Percutaneous; extent is determined by vehicle, integrity of skin, and use of occlusive dressings. **Distribution:** (IV) V_d=4.2L/kg (1mg); plasma protein binding (91%). Systemically administered corticosteroids are found in breast milk. **Metabolism:** (Oral) Hydrolysis via CYP450 3A4. **Elimination:** (IV) $T_{1/2}$=7.2 hrs (1mg).

NURSING CONSIDERATIONS

Assessment: (Cre, Lot, Oint) Assess for drug hypersensitivity, proper diagnosis, preexisting skin atrophy, presence of skin infection at treatment site, rosacea and perioral dermatitis, pregnancy/nursing status. (Cre, Lot) Assess use in pediatrics.

Monitoring: (Cre, Lot, Oint) Monitor for signs/symptoms of reversible HPA axis suppression, presence of dermatological infections (eg, fungal, bacterial), local cutaneous adverse reactions, and glucocorticosteroid insufficiency after withdrawal of therapy. If applying to a large surface area or if using occlusive dressings, evaluate periodically for evidence of HPA axis suppression by using urinary free cortisol and adrenocorticotropic hormone stimulation tests. (Cre, Lot) Monitor for signs/symptoms of systemic toxicity in pediatrics.

Patient Counseling: (Cre, Lot, Oint) Use as directed and should not be used for any disorder. Advise to avoid contact with eyes. Advise not to bandage, cover, or wrap treated skin, and to avoid using on face, underarms or groin areas unless directed by physician. Advise to contact physician if any signs of local adverse reactions, non-healing/worsening of skin conditions, or no clinical improvement within 2 weeks of therapy occurs. (Cre, Lot) Advise that product is not for treatment of diaper dermatitis and not for application in diaper areas. Report to physician if allergic to formaldehyde. (Lot) Counsel that should not be used longer than 4 weeks. Notify physician if no improvement is seen within 2 weeks. Advise to avoid excessive or unnecessary exposure to either natural/artificial sunlight.

Administration: Topical route. **Storage:** (Cre, Oint) 2-30°C (36-86°F). (Lot) 15-30°C (59-86°F). Do not refrigerate. Keep container tightly sealed.

CYCLOPHOSPHAMIDE   RX
cyclophosphamide (Various)

THERAPEUTIC CLASS: Nitrogen mustard alkylating agent

INDICATIONS: Treatment of malignant lymphomas, Hodgkin's disease, lymphocytic lymphoma (nodular or diffuse), mixed-cell type lymphoma, histiocytic lymphoma, Burkitt's lymphoma, multiple myeloma, chronic lymphocytic leukemia, chronic granulocytic leukemia (ineffective in acute blastic crisis), acute myelogenous and monocytic leukemia, acute lymphoblastic (stem-cell) leukemia in children, mycosis fungoides (advanced disease), neuroblastoma (disseminated disease), ovary adenocarcinoma, retinoblastoma, breast carcinoma. Treatment of selected cases of biopsy proven "minimal change" nephrotic syndrome in children, but not as primary therapy.

DOSAGE: *Adults:* Malignant Diseases (No Hemolytic Deficiency): (IV) Monotherapy: Initial: 40-50mg/kg in divided doses over 2-5 days, or 10-15mg/kg given every 7-10 days, or 3-5mg/kg twice weekly. (PO) Initial/Maint: 1-5mg/kg/day. (IV/PO) Adjust dose according to antitumor activity and/or leukopenia. (IV) Elderly: Start at the lower end of dosing range.

Pediatrics: Malignant Diseases (No Hemolytic Deficiency): (IV) Monotherapy: Initial: 40-50mg/kg in divided doses over 2-5 days, or 10-15mg/kg given every 7-10 days, or 3-5mg/kg twice weekly. (PO) Initial/Maint: 1-5mg/kg/day. (IV/PO) Adjust dose according to antitumor activity and/or leukopenia. Nephrotic Syndrome: (PO) 2.5-3mg/kg/day for 60-90 days.

HOW SUPPLIED: Inj: 500mg, 1g, 2g; Tab: 25mg, 50mg

CONTRAINDICATIONS: Severely depressed bone marrow function.

WARNINGS/PRECAUTIONS: Not indicated for the nephrotic syndrome in adults or for any other renal disease. Second malignancies (eg, urinary bladder, myeloproliferative, lymphoproliferative), cardiac dysfunction, and acute cardiac toxicity reported. May cause fetal harm. May cause sterility in both sexes. Amenorrhea, ovarian fibrosis, azoospermia, and oligospermia reported. Testicular atrophy may occur. Hemorrhagic cystitis may develop; d/c with severe hemorrhagic cystitis. May cause significant suppression of immune response; serious, sometimes fatal, infections may develop in severely immunosuppressed patients. D/C or reduce dose in patients who have/who develop viral, bacterial, fungal, protozoan, or helminthic infections. Anaphylactic reactions reported; possible cross-sensitivity with other alkylating agents reported. Caution with leukopenia, thrombocytopenia, tumor cell infiltration of bone marrow, and hepatic/renal impairment; monitor for possible development of toxicity. May interfere with normal wound healing. (IV) Caution in elderly.

ADVERSE REACTIONS: Impairment of fertility, syndrome of inappropriate antidiuretic hormone secretion, N/V, anorexia, abdominal discomfort/pain, diarrhea, alopecia, leukopenia, thrombocytopenia, hemorrhagic ureteritis, interstitial pneumonitis, malaise, asthenia, renal tubular necrosis.

INTERACTIONS: Chronic administration of high doses of phenobarbital increases metabolism and leukopenic activity. Possible combined drug actions (desirable or undesirable) with other drugs (including other cytotoxic drugs). Caution with previous x-ray therapy or therapy with other cytotoxic agents; may develop toxicity. Potentiates succinylcholine chloride effects and doxorubicin-induced cardiotoxicity. Caution within 10 days of general anesthesia. Adjust dose of both drugs with replacement steroids in adrenalectomized patients.

PREGNANCY: Category D, not for use in nursing.

MECHANISM OF ACTION: Nitrogen mustard alkylating agent; thought to involve cross linking of tumor cell DNA.

PHARMACOKINETICS: Absorption: (PO) Well absorbed; bioavailability (>75%). (IV) T_{max}=2-3 hrs (metabolite). **Distribution:** Plasma protein binding (>60% as metabolites); found in breast milk. **Metabolism:** Liver. **Elimination:** Urine (5-25% unchanged); $T_{1/2}$=3-12 hrs.

NURSING CONSIDERATIONS

Assessment: Assess for drug hypersensitivity, immunosuppression, leukopenia, thrombocytopenia, tumor cell infiltration of bone marrow, previous x-ray therapy, hepatic/renal impairment, pregnancy/nursing status, and possible drug interactions.

Monitoring: Monitor for anaphylactic reactions, second malignancies, cardiac dysfunction, sterility, ovarian fibrosis, amenorrhea, azoospermia, oligospermia, testicular atrophy, infections, toxicity, and other adverse reactions. Monitor hematologic profile (particularly neutrophils and platelets) and urine (for red cells) regularly.

Patient Counseling: Inform of the risks and benefits of therapy. Instruct to take exactly ud. Advise women of childbearing potential to avoid becoming pregnant while on therapy.

Administration: Oral/IV route. (IV) Refer to PI for procedures in preparation, handling, stability, and compatibility of sol. **Storage:** ≤25°C (77°F). (Tab) Excursions permitted up to 30°C (86°F).

CYCLOSET   RX
bromocriptine mesylate (VeroScience)

THERAPEUTIC CLASS: Dopamine receptor agonist

INDICATIONS: Adjunct to diet and exercise to improve glycemic control in adults with type 2 diabetes mellitus (DM).

DOSAGE: *Adults:* Initial: 0.8mg qd within 2 hrs after waking in the am. Titrate: Increase by 0.8mg/week until max dose or maximal tolerated number of tabs (2-6 tabs/day). Usual: 1.6-4.8mg qd. Max: 4.8mg/day. Take with food.

HOW SUPPLIED: Tab: 0.8mg

CONTRAINDICATIONS: Syncopal migraine, nursing women.

WARNINGS/PRECAUTIONS: Hypotension, including orthostatic hypotension, and syncope may occur; assess orthostatic vital signs prior to therapy and monitor periodically. May exacerbate psychotic disorders; avoid with severe psychotic disorders. Somnolence reported; may impair mental/physical abilities. Caution with renal/hepatic impairment. Not for use to treat type 1 DM or diabetic ketoacidosis.

ADVERSE REACTIONS: N/V, rhinitis, headache, asthenia, dizziness, constipation, sinusitis, diarrhea, amblyopia, dyspepsia, infection, anorexia.

INTERACTIONS: Diminished effectiveness of/with dopamine receptor antagonists, such as neuroleptics (eg, phenothiazines, butyrophenones, thioxanthenes) or metoclopramide; concomitant use not recommended. May increase unbound fraction of highly protein-bound therapies (eg, salicylates, sulfonamides, chloramphenicol, and probenecid). Avoid with ergot-related agents within 6 hrs of therapy. Avoid with other dopamine agonists and selective 5-hydroxytryptamine$_{1B}$ agonists (eg, sumatriptan). Caution with strong inhibitors, inducers, or substrates of CYP3A4 (eg, azole antimycotics, HIV protease inhibitors). HTN and tachycardia reported with sympathomimetic agents (eg, phenylpropanolamine, isometheptene) in postpartum women; concomitant use for >10 days is not recommended. Caution with antihypertensives.

PREGNANCY: Category B, contraindicated in nursing.

MECHANISM OF ACTION: Dopamine receptor agonist; mechanism not established.

PHARMACOKINETICS: Absorption: Bioavailability (65-95%), T_{max}=53 min (fasted). **Distribution:** V_d=61L; plasma protein binding (90-96%). **Metabolism:** GI tract and liver (extensive) via CYP3A4. **Excretion:** Bile (major), urine (2-6%); $T_{1/2}$=6 hrs.

NURSING CONSIDERATIONS

Assessment: Assess for previous hypersensitivity to the drug, syncopal migraine, renal/hepatic impairment, psychotic disorders, orthostatic vital signs, pregnancy/nursing status, and possible drug interactions. Obtain baseline FPG and HbA1c.

Monitoring: Monitor blood glucose levels, HbA1c testing, and orthostatic vital signs periodically. Monitor for hypersensitivity reactions, hypoglycemia, DM complications, and exacerbation of psychotic disorder.

Patient Counseling: Counsel about potential risks and benefits of therapy and of alternative therapies. Stress importance of adherence to dietary instructions, regular physical activity, periodic blood glucose monitoring and HbA1c testing, recognition and management of hypoglycemia and hyperglycemia, and assessment for diabetes complications. Caution against operating heavy machinery if symptoms of somnolence occur. Instruct to notify physician if any unusual symptoms develop or if any known symptom persists or worsens. Counsel to seek medical advice when periods of stress occur. Advise to make slow postural changes and avoid situations that could predispose to injury if syncope was to occur.

Administration: Oral route. **Storage:** ≤25°C (77°F).

CYMBALTA RX
duloxetine HCl (Lilly)

> Antidepressants increased the risk of suicidal thinking and behavior (suicidality) in children, adolescents, and young adults in short-term studies of major depressive disorder (MDD) and other psychiatric disorders. Monitor and observe closely for clinical worsening, suicidality, or unusual changes in behavior. Not approved for use in pediatric patients.

THERAPEUTIC CLASS: Serotonin and norepinephrine reuptake inhibitor

INDICATIONS: Treatment of MDD and generalized anxiety disorder (GAD). Management of neuropathic pain associated with diabetic peripheral neuropathy (DPNP). Management of fibromyalgia (FM) and chronic musculoskeletal pain.

DOSAGE: *Adults:* MDD: Initial: 40mg/day (given as 20mg bid) to 60mg/day (given qd or as 30mg bid) or 30mg qd for 1 week before increasing to 60mg qd. Maint: 60mg qd. Reassess periodically to determine need for maint therapy and appropriate dose. Max: 120mg/day. GAD: Initial: 60mg qd or 30mg qd for 1 week before increasing to 60mg qd. Maint: 60-120mg qd. Dose increases to above 60mg qd should be in increments of 30mg qd. Reassess periodically to determine need for maint and appropriate dose. Max: 120mg/day. DPNP: Initial: 60mg qd. May lower starting dose if tolerability is a concern. Consider lower starting dose and gradual increase in renal impairment. Maint: Individualize dose. Treat for up to 12 weeks. Max: 60mg qd. FM: Initial: 60mg qd or 30mg qd for 1 week before increasing to 60mg qd. Maint: Based on patient's response. Max: 60mg qd. Chronic Musculoskeletal Pain: Initial: 60mg qd or 30mg qd for 1 week before increasing to 60mg qd. Maint: 60mg qd for up to 13 weeks. Max: 60mg/day. Elderly: Start at lower end of dosing range. Swallow cap whole.

HOW SUPPLIED: Cap, Delayed-Release: 20mg, 30mg, 60mg

CONTRAINDICATIONS: Concomitant use of MAOIs or use within 14 days of taking an MAOI. Uncontrolled narrow-angle glaucoma.

WARNINGS/PRECAUTIONS: Not approved for use in treating bipolar depression. Hepatic failure (sometimes fatal), cholestatic jaundice with minimal elevation of serum transaminases, and elevated LFTs reported; d/c if jaundice or other evidence of hepatic dysfunction occurs. Avoid with substantial alcohol use or evidence of chronic liver disease and/or hepatic insufficiency. Serotonin syndrome or neuroleptic malignant syndrome (NMS)-like reactions reported; monitor and d/c if signs/symptoms develop. Orthostatic hypotension and syncope reported; consider d/c if orthostatic hypotension and/or syncope develop. May increase risk of bleeding events. Severe skin reactions, including erythema multiforme and Stevens-Johnson syndrome (SJS) may occur; d/c if blisters, peeling rash, mucosal erosions, or if any other signs of hypersensitivity develop. D/C should be gradual. Activation of mania or hypomania reported in patients with MDD. Caution with history of mania and/or seizure disorder. May increase BP; obtain baseline BP and monitor periodically throughout therapy. May cause hyponatremia; volume depletion may increase risk. D/C if symptomatic hyponatremia occurs and institute appropriate management. Urinary hesitation and retention reported. Caution with conditions that may slow gastric emptying, controlled narrow-angle glaucoma, diabetes, and in the elderly; glycemic control may be worsened in patients with diabetes. Avoid in end-stage renal disease/severe renal impairment (CrCl <30mL/min).

ADVERSE REACTIONS: Nausea, dry mouth, constipation, diarrhea, decreased appetite, fatigue, dizziness, somnolence, hyperhidrosis, headache, insomnia, abdominal pain.

INTERACTIONS: See Contraindications. Upon d/c, wait ≥5 days before starting MAOI therapy. Avoid use with thioridazine, CYP1A2 inhibitors (eg, fluvoxamine, cimetidine, some quinolone antibiotics), substantial alcohol use. Increased levels with potent CYP2D6 inhibitors (eg, paroxetine, fluoxetine, quinidine). Caution with drugs metabolized by CYP2D6 having a narrow therapeutic index (eg, TCAs, phenothiazines, type 1C antiarrhythmics), and CNS-acting drugs; consider monitoring TCA plasma levels. May increase free concentrations of highly protein-bound drugs. Potential for interaction with drugs that affect gastric acidity. Caution with serotonergic drugs (eg, triptans, tramadol, linezolid, lithium, or St. John's wort). Avoid with other SSRIs, SNRIs, or serotonin precursors (eg, tryptophan). Coadministration with antipsychotics or other dopamine antagonists may increase risk of serotonin syndrome or NMS-like reactions; d/c if signs/symptoms develop. Caution with NSAIDs, aspirin (ASA), warfarin, or other drugs that affect coagulation due to potential increased risk of bleeding. Greater risk of hypotension with concomitant use of medications that induce orthostatic hypotension (eg, antihypertensives) and potent CYP1A2 inhibitors. Increased risk of hyponatremia with diuretics.

PREGNANCY: Category C, not for use in nursing.

MECHANISM OF ACTION: Selective SNRI; not established. Believed to be related to potentiation of serotonergic and noradrenergic activity in the CNS.

PHARMACOKINETICS: **Absorption:** Well absorbed; T_{max}=6 hrs. **Distribution:** V_d=1640L; plasma protein binding (>90%); found in breast milk. **Metabolism:** Extensive, hepatic via CYP1A2, 2D6; oxidation and conjugation. **Elimination:** Urine (70% metabolites; <1% unchanged), feces (20%); $T_{1/2}$=12 hrs.

NURSING CONSIDERATIONS

Assessment: Assess for bipolar disorder risk, history of mania, chronic liver disease, substantial alcohol use, history of seizures, diseases/conditions that slow gastric emptying (eg, diabetes mellitus), narrow-angle glaucoma, risk factors for hyponatremia, history of urinary retention, hepatic/renal impairment, pregnancy/nursing status, and possible drug interactions. Assess baseline BP, LFTs, BUN, SrCr, and blood glucose.

Monitoring: Monitor for signs/symptoms of clinical worsening (eg, suicidality, unusual changes in behavior), hepatotoxicity, serotonin syndrome or NMS-like reactions, abnormal bleeding, skin reactions, erythema multiforme, SJS, hyponatremia, seizures, orthostatic hypotension, worsened glycemic control, urinary hesitation/retention, mydriasis, and hepatic/renal dysfunction. If abruptly d/c, monitor for symptoms of dizziness, N/V, headache, paresthesia, fatigue, irritability, insomnia, diarrhea, anxiety, and hyperhidrosis. Periodically monitor BP, LFTs, SrCr, and BUN.

Patient Counseling: Inform about benefits/risks of therapy. Counsel to swallow whole, and not to chew, crush, nor open and sprinkle on food or mix with liquids. Advise to avoid alcohol. Instruct to seek medical attention for clinical worsening (eg, suicidal ideation, unusual changes in behavior) and symptoms of serotonin syndrome (with use of triptans, tramadol, or other serotonergic agents). Abnormal bleeding (with use of NSAIDs, ASA, warfarin, or other drugs that affect coagulation), hyponatremia, orthostatic hypotension, syncope, hepatotoxicity, urinary hesitation/retention, seizures, or d/c symptoms (eg, irritability, agitation, dizziness, anxiety, headache, insomnia) may occur. Counsel to immediately seek consult if skin blisters, peeling rash, mouth sores, hives, or any other allergic reactions occur. Advise to inform if taking or plan to take any prescription or OTC medications, if pregnant, intend to become pregnant, or are breastfeeding. Caution with operating hazardous machinery, including automobiles; may impair judgement, thinking, or motor skills. May notice improvement within 1-4 weeks; instruct to continue therapy ud.

Administration: Oral route. Swallow cap whole; do not chew, crush, nor open and sprinkle on food or mix with liquids. **Storage:** 25°C (77°F); excursions permitted to 15-30°C (59-86°F).

CYTOMEL RX
liothyronine sodium (King)

THERAPEUTIC CLASS: Thyroid replacement hormone

INDICATIONS: As replacement or supplemental therapy in patients with hypothyroidism of any etiology, except transient hypothyroidism during the recovery phase of subacute thyroiditis. In the treatment or prevention of various types of euthyroid goiters, including thyroid nodules, and Hashimoto's and multinodular goiter. As diagnostic agent in suppression tests to differentiate mild hyperthyroidism or thyroid gland autonomy.

DOSAGE: *Adults:* Individualize dose. Mild Hypothyroidism: Initial: 25mcg qd. Titrate: May increase by up to 25mcg qd every 1-2 weeks. Maint: 25-75mcg qd. Myxedema: Initial: 5mcg qd. Titrate: May increase by 5-10mcg qd every 1-2 weeks up to 25mcg qd, then increase by 5-25mcg qd every 1-2 weeks until desired response. Maint: 50-100mcg/day. Simple (Non-Toxic) Goiter: Initial: 5mcg/day. Titrate: May increase by 5-10mcg qd every 1-2 weeks up to 25mcg qd, then by 12.5-25mcg qd every 1-2 weeks. Maint: 75mcg qd. Elderly/Angina Pectoris/Coronary Artery Disease: Initial: 5mcg qd. Titrate: Increase by no more than 5mcg qd at 2-week intervals. Switch to Cytomel Tablets from Thyroid, L-Thyroxine or Thyroglobulin: D/C other medication and initiate Cytomel at low dose then increase gradually based on patient response. Thyroid Suppression Therapy: 75-100mcg qd for 7 days. Radioactive iodine uptake is determined before and after administration of the hormone. *Pediatrics:* Congenital Hypothyroidism: Initial: 5mcg qd. Titrate: Increase by 5mcg qd every 3-4 days until desired response achieved. Maint: >3 yrs: 25-75mcg/day. 1-3 yrs: 50mcg qd. <1 yr: 20mcg qd.

HOW SUPPLIED: Tab: 5mcg, 25mcg*, 50mcg* *scored

CONTRAINDICATIONS: Uncorrected adrenal cortical insufficiency and untreated thyrotoxicosis.

WARNINGS/PRECAUTIONS: Do not use in the treatment of obesity; larger doses in euthyroid patients can cause serious or life-threatening toxicity. Caution with cardiovascular (CV) disorders (eg, angina pectoris) and in the elderly; use lower doses. Not for the treatment of male or female infertility unless accompanied by hypothyroidism. Rule out morphological hypogonadism and nephrosis prior to therapy. If hypopituitarism present, adrenal insufficiency must be corrected prior to starting therapy. Caution in myxedematous patients; start at very low dose and increase gradually. Severe and prolonged hypothyroidism can lead to adrenocortical insufficiency; supplement with adrenocortical steroids. May precipitate a hyperthyroid state or aggravate hyperthyroidism. Concurrent use with androgens, corticosteroids, estrogens, oral contraceptives containing estrogens, iodine-containing preparations, and salicylates may interfere with thyroid laboratory tests. May aggravate symptoms of diabetes mellitus (DM) or insipidus (DI) or adrenal cortical insufficiency. Add glucocorticoids with myxedema coma. Excessive doses may cause craniosynostosis in infants.

ADVERSE REACTIONS: Allergic skin reactions (rare).

INTERACTIONS: Coadministration of larger doses with sympathomimetic amines such as those used for their anorectic effects may cause serious or even life-threatening toxicity. Hypothyroidism decreases and hyperthyroidism increases sensitivity to oral anticoagulants; monitor PT. May cause increases in insulin and oral hypoglycemics requirements. Impaired absorption with cholestyramine; space dosing by 4-5 hrs. Estrogens increase thyroxine-binding globulin; increase in thyroid dose may be needed. Increased effects of both agents with TCAs (eg, imipramine). HTN and tachycardia may occur with ketamine. May potentiate digitalis toxicity. Increased adrenergic effects of catecholamines (eg, epinephrine, norepinephrine); caution with coronary artery disease (CAD).

PREGNANCY: Category A, caution in nursing.

MECHANISM OF ACTION: Synthetic thyroid hormone; mechanism not established. Suspected to enhance oxygen consumption by tissues and increase the basal metabolic rate and metabolism of carbohydrates, lipids, and proteins.

PHARMACOKINETICS: Distribution: Minimal amount found in breast milk. **Elimination:** $T_{1/2}$=2.5 days.

NURSING CONSIDERATIONS

Assessment: Assess thyroid status, CV disease (eg, CAD, angina pectoris), DM/DI, adrenal cortical insufficiency, thyrotoxicosis, myxedema, hypogonadism, nephrosis, pregnancy/nursing status, and for possible drug interactions.

Monitoring: Monitor thyroid function periodically. Monitor PT on oral anticoagulants, urinary glucose with DM and renal function. Monitor for signs/symptoms of precipitation of adrenocortical insufficiency, aggravation of DM/DI, hypoglycemia, hyperthyroidism, toxicity, and hypersensitivity reactions.

Patient Counseling: Inform that replacement therapy is taken for life. Warn that partial hair loss may be seen in pediatrics in first few months of therapy. Instruct to seek medical attention if symptoms of toxicity (eg, chest pain, increased HR, palpitations, excessive sweating, heat intolerance, nervousness), hypoglycemia, aggravation of DM/DI, or hypersensitivity reactions occur.

Administration: Oral route. **Storage:** 15-30°C (59-86°F).

DACOGEN   RX
decitabine (Eisai)

THERAPEUTIC CLASS: DNA methyltransferase inhibitor

INDICATIONS: Treatment of myelodysplastic syndromes.

DOSAGE: *Adults:* Treat for a minimum of 4 cycles. May premedicate with standard anti-emetic therapy. Treatment Option 1: 15mg/m^2 by continuous IV infusion over 3 hrs q8h for 3 days. Repeat cycle q6 weeks. Adjust dose based on hematologic recovery and disease progression; see PI. Treatment Option 2: 20mg/m^2 by continuous IV infusion over 1 hr qd for 5 days. Repeat cycle q4 weeks. Myelosuppression: Delay subsequent treatment cycles until hematologic recovery. Following the 1st cycle, do not restart treatment if SrCr ≥2mg/dL, SGPT/total bilirubin ≥2X ULN, and has an active or uncontrolled infection.

HOW SUPPLIED: Inj: 50mg

WARNINGS/PRECAUTIONS: Neutropenia and thrombocytopenia may occur; monitor CBC and platelets periodically (at minimum, before each dosing cycle). Myelosuppression and worsening neutropenia may occur more frequently in the 1st or 2nd treatment cycles; consider early institution of growth factors and/or antimicrobial agents. May cause fetal harm. Avoid pregnancy during and for 1 month after completion of treatment. Men should not father a child during and for 2 months after completion of treatment. Caution with renal and hepatic dysfunction.

ADVERSE REACTIONS: Neutropenia, thrombocytopenia, anemia, fatigue, pyrexia, N/V, cough, petechiae, constipation, diarrhea, hyperglycemia, anorexia, leukopenia, headache, insomnia.

PREGNANCY: Category D, not for use in nursing.

MECHANISM OF ACTION: DNA methyltransferase inhibitor; causes hypomethylation of DNA and cellular differentiation or apoptosis. In rapidly dividing cells, forms covalent adducts with DNA methyltransferase incorporated into DNA.

PHARMACOKINETICS: Absorption: (15mg/m^2) C_{max}= 73.8ng/mL, AUC=163ng•h/mL; (20mg/m^2) C_{max}=147ng/mL, AUC=115ng•h/mL. **Metabolism:** Deamination in liver, granulocytes, intestinal epithelium, and blood. **Elimination:** $T_{1/2}$=0.62 hrs (15mg/m^2), 0.54 hrs (20mg/m^2).

NURSING CONSIDERATIONS

Assessment: Assess CBC and platelets count, renal/hepatic function and pregnancy/nursing status.

Monitoring: Monitor for signs/symptoms of neutropenia, thrombocytopenia, myelosuppression, hypersensitivity reactions, renal/hepatic function, infections and infestations, and other adverse reactions. Monitor CBC and platelet counts prior to each dosing cycle.

Patient Counseling: Advise women to avoid becoming pregnant during and for 1 month after completion of treatment and men not to father a child during and for 2 months after completion of treatment; counsel to use effective contraception. Advise to monitor and report any symptoms of neutropenia, thrombocytopenia, or fever to physician as soon as possible.

Administration: IV route. Refer to PI for instructions for IV administration. **Storage:** Vial: 25°C (77°F); excursions permitted to 15-30°C (59-86°F). Reconstituted Sol: 2-8°C (36-46°F) for up to 7 hrs until administration.

DALIRESP   RX
roflumilast (Forest)

THERAPEUTIC CLASS: Selective phosphodiesterase 4 (PDE4) inhibitor

INDICATIONS: Treatment to reduce the risk of chronic obstructive pulmonary disease (COPD) exacerbations in patients with severe COPD associated with chronic bronchitis and a history of exacerbations.

DOSAGE: *Adults:* Usual: 500mcg/day, with or without food.

HOW SUPPLIED: Tab: 500mcg

CONTRAINDICATIONS: Moderate to severe liver impairment (Child-Pugh B or C).

WARNINGS/PRECAUTIONS: Not a bronchodilator; not indicated for the relief of acute broncho-spasm. Caution with history of depression and/or suicidal thoughts or behavior; psychiatric adverse reactions, including suicidality, reported. Weight loss may occur; monitor weight regularly. Evaluate and consider d/c if unexplained or significant weight loss occurs. Caution with mild hepatic impairment (Child-Pugh A).

ADVERSE REACTIONS: Diarrhea, weight decreased, nausea, headache, backpain, influenza, insomnia, dizziness, decreased appetite.

INTERACTIONS: Concomitant use of strong CYP450 enzyme inducers (eg, rifampicin, phenobarbital, carbamazepine, phenytoin) is not recommended. CYP3A4 inhibitors or dual inhibitors that inhibit CYP3A4 and CYP1A2 simultaneously (eg, erythromycin, ketoconazole, fluvoxamine, enoxacin, cimetidine) and oral contraceptives containing gestodene and ethinyl estradiol may increase systemic exposure, resulting in increased side effects.

PREGNANCY: Category C, not for use in nursing.

MECHANISM OF ACTION: Selective phosphodiesterase 4 (PDE4) inhibitor; specific therapeutic mechanism (s) not well defined; thought to be related to the effects of increased intracellular cyclic AMP in lung cells.

PHARMACOKINETICS: Absorption: Absolute bioavailability (80%); T_{max}=1 hr, 8 hrs (roflumilast N-oxide). **Distribution:** V_d=2.9L/kg; plasma protein binding (99%, 97% roflumilast N-oxide). **Metabolism:** Extensive via Phase 1 (CYP450) and Phase 2 (conjugation) reactions; roflumilast N-oxide (major metabolite). **Elimination:** Urine (70%); $T_{1/2}$=17 hrs, 30 hrs (roflumilast N-oxide).

NURSING CONSIDERATIONS

Assessment: Assess for hepatic impairment, history of depression, suicidal thoughts or behavior, pregnancy/nursing status, and for possible drug interactions.

Monitoring: Monitor for psychiatric events, including suicidality, and for weight loss. Monitor weight regularly.

Patient Counseling: Inform that drug is not a bronchodilator and should not be used for the relief of acute bronchospasm. Advise of the need to be alert for the emergence or worsening of insomnia, anxiety, depression, suicidal thoughts, or other mood changes; instruct to contact physician if such changes occur. Counsel to monitor weight regularly and seek medical attention if unexplained or significant weight loss occurs. Instruct to notify physician if using other Rx or OTC products.

Administration: Oral route. **Storage:** 20-25°C (68-77°F); excursions permitted to 15-30°C (59-86°F).

DANTRIUM   RX
dantrolene sodium (JHP Pharmaceuticals, LLC)

> Has potential for hepatotoxicity. Symptomatic/overt hepatitis and liver dysfunction reported. Risk of hepatic injury greater in females, patients >35 yrs, and patients taking other medications. Monitor hepatic function. D/C if no benefit after 45 days. Lowest possible effective dose should be prescribed.

THERAPEUTIC CLASS: Direct acting skeletal muscle relaxant

INDICATIONS: To control manifestations of clinical spasticity from upper motor neuron disorders (eg, spinal cord injury, stroke, cerebral palsy, multiple sclerosis). Preoperatively to prevent or attenuate development of signs of malignant hyperthermia in known, or strongly suspect, malignant hyperthermia susceptible patients who require anesthesia and/or surgery.

DOSAGE: *Adults:* Chronic Spasticity: Individualize dose. Initial: 25mg qd for 7 days. Titrate: Increase to 25mg tid for 7 days, then 50mg tid for 7 days, then 100mg tid. Max: 100mg qid. If no further benefit at next higher dose, decrease to previous lower dose. Malignant Hyperthermia: Pre-Op: 4-8mg/kg/day given tid-qid for 1-2 days before surgery, with last dose given 3-4 hrs before scheduled surgery with minimum of water. Adjust dose within recommended dose range to avoid incapacitation or excessive GI irritation. Post-Op Following Malignant Hyperthermia Crisis: 4-8mg/kg/day given qid for 1-3 days.
Pediatrics: ≥5 yrs: Chronic Spasticity: Individualize dose. Initial: 0.5mg/kg qd for 7 days. Titrate: Increase to 0.5mg/kg tid for 7 days, then 1mg/kg tid for 7 days, then 2mg/kg tid. Max: 100mg qid. If no further benefit at next higher dose, decrease to previous lower dose.

HOW SUPPLIED: Cap: 25mg, 50mg, 100mg

CONTRAINDICATIONS: Active hepatic disease (eg, hepatitis, cirrhosis); where spasticity is utilized to sustain upright posture and balance in locomotion, or whenever spasticity is utilized to obtain or maintain increased function.

WARNINGS/PRECAUTIONS: Brief withdrawal for 2-4 days may exacerbate manifestations of spasticity. Obtain LFTs at baseline, then periodically thereafter. D/C if LFT abnormalities or jaundice appear. Caution with impaired pulmonary dysfunction (eg, obstructive pulmonary disease), severely impaired cardiac function due to myocardial disease, and history of liver disease/dysfunction.

ADVERSE REACTIONS: Hepatoxicity, hepatitis, liver dysfunction, drowsiness, dizziness, weakness, general malaise, fatigue, diarrhea, hepatitis, tachycardia.

INTERACTIONS: See Boxed Warning. Increased drowsiness with CNS depressants (eg, sedatives, tranquilizers). Caution with estrogens; risk of hepatotoxicity especially in women >35 yrs. Avoid with calcium channel blockers; cardiovascular collapse with concomitant verapamil reported (rare). May potentiate vecuronium-induced neuromuscular block.

PREGNANCY: Category C, not for use in nursing.

MECHANISM OF ACTION: Direct-acting skeletal muscle relaxant; interferes with release of calcium ions from the sarcoplasmic reticulum.

PHARMACOKINETICS: Absorption: Incomplete, slow. **Distribution:** Crosses placenta. **Metabolism:** Hepatic microsomal enzymes; 5-hydroxy and acetamido analog (major metabolites). **Elimination:** Urine; $T_{1/2}$=8.7 hrs.

NURSING CONSIDERATIONS

Assessment: Assess for active hepatic disease, if spasticity is used for upright posture and balance or increased function, history of liver disease/dysfunction, pulmonary dysfunction, impaired cardiac function due to myocardial disease, pregnancy/nursing status, and possible drug interactions. Perform baseline LFTs. Assess use in patients >35 yrs.

Monitoring: Monitor for liver disorders, jaundice, hepatotoxicity, and hepatitis. Monitor LFTs regularly.

Patient Counseling: Inform about risks and benefits of therapy. Caution against performing hazardous tasks (eg, operating machinery/driving). Caution with sunlight exposure; photosensitivity reactions may occur. Inform about other medications being taken. Notify if pregnant/nursing.

Administration: Oral route. **Storage:** <40°C (104°F). Avoid excessive heat.

DANTRIUM IV   RX
dantrolene sodium (Procter & Gamble Pharmaceuticals)

THERAPEUTIC CLASS: Direct acting skeletal muscle relaxant

INDICATIONS: Adjunct management of fulminant hypermetabolism of skeletal muscle characteristic of malignant hyperthermia crises. For pre- and post-operative use to prevent or attenuate development of malignant hyperthermia.

DOSAGE: *Adults:* Malignant Hyperthermia: Initial: Minimum 1mg/kg IV push. Continue until symptoms subside or max cumulative dose 10mg/kg. Pre-Op Malignant Hyperthermia Prophylaxis: 2.5mg/kg 1.25 hrs before anesthesia and infuse over 1 hr. May need additional therapy during anesthesia/surgery if symptoms arise. Post-Op Prophylaxis: Initial: 1mg/kg or more as clinical situation dictates.
Pediatrics: Malignant Hyperthermia: Initial: Minimum 1mg/kg IV push. Continue until symptoms subside or max cumulative dose 10mg/kg.

HOW SUPPLIED: Inj: 20mg

WARNINGS/PRECAUTIONS: Use with supportive therapies to treat malignant hyperthermia. Take steps to prevent extravasation. Fatal and non-fatal hepatic disorders reported. Do not operate automobile or engage hazardous activity for 48 hrs after therapy. Caution at meals on day of administration because difficulty in swallowing/choking reported. Monitor vital signs if receive pre-operatively.

ADVERSE REACTIONS: Loss of grip strength, weakness in legs, drowsiness, dizziness, pulmonary edema, thrombophlebitis, urticaria, erythema.

INTERACTIONS: Plasma protein-binding reduced by warfarin and clofibrate, and increased by tolbutamide. Avoid with calcium channel blockers (CCBs); possible risk of cardiovascular collapse. Caution with tranquilizers. Possible increased metabolism by drugs known to induce hepatic microsomal enzymes. May potentiate vecuronium-induced neuromuscular block.

PREGNANCY: Category C, safety in nursing not known.

MECHANISM OF ACTION: Direct acting skeletal muscle relaxant; interferes with release of calcium ions from sarcoplasmic reticulum.

PHARMACOKINETICS: Distribution: Found in breast milk. **Metabolism:** Hydrolysis and oxidation; 5-hydroxy dantrolene and acetylamino analog (major metabolites). **Elimination:** Urine; $T_{1/2}$=4-8 hrs.

NURSING CONSIDERATIONS

Assessment: Assess for active hepatic disease (hepatitis and cirrhosis), pregnancy/nursing status, and possible drug interactions.

Monitoring: Monitor for vital signs, tissue necrosis, LFTs. Monitor for cardiovascular collapse if given concomitantly with CCBs.

Patient Counseling: Caution against performing hazardous tasks (eg, operating machinery/driving). Inform that at meals, on administration day, choking and difficulty swallowing have been reported. Inform about postop muscle weakness, reduced grip strength, and lightheadedness. Notify if pregnant/nursing.

Administration: IV route. **Storage:** Unreconstituted/Reconstituted Sol: 15-30°C (59-86°F); avoid prolonged light exposure. Reconstituted sol must be protected from direct light and used within 6 hrs after reconstitution.

DAYPRO   RX
oxaprozin (G.D. Searle)

NSAIDs may cause an increased risk of serious cardiovascular (CV) thrombotic events, myocardial infarction (MI), stroke and serious GI adverse events including bleeding, ulceration, and perforation of the stomach or intestines. Contraindicated for the treatment of perioperative pain in the setting of coronary artery bypass graft (CABG) surgery.

THERAPEUTIC CLASS: NSAID

INDICATIONS: Relief of signs and symptoms of osteoarthritis (OA), rheumatoid arthritis (RA), and juvenile rheumatoid arthritis (JRA).

DOSAGE: *Adults:* RA: 1200mg qd. Max: 1800mg/day in divided doses (not to exceed 26mg/kg/day). OA: 1200mg qd, give 600mg qd for low weight or milder disease. Max: 1800mg/day in divided doses (not to exceed 26mg/kg/day). Renal Dysfunction/Hemodialysis: Initial: 600mg qd.
Pediatrics: 6-16yrs: JRA: ≥55kg: 1200mg qd. 32-54kg: 900mg qd. 22-31kg: 600mg qd.

HOW SUPPLIED: Tab: 600mg* *scored

CONTRAINDICATIONS: ASA or other NSAID allergy that precipitates asthma, urticaria, or allergic-type reactions. Treatment of perioperative pain in the setting of CABG surgery.

WARNINGS/PRECAUTIONS: May lead to onset of new HTN or worsening of preexisting HTN; monitor BP during initiation and throughout the course of therapy. Fluid retention and edema reported; caution with fluid retention or heart failure. Renal papillary necrosis and other renal injury reported after long-term use. Not recommended for use with advanced renal disease; if therapy must be initiated, monitor renal function. Anaphylactoid reactions may occur. May cause serious skin adverse events (eg, exfoliative dermatitis, Stevens-Johnson syndrome (SJS), and toxic epidermal necrolysis). Avoid with patients with the aspirin triad (complex symptoms of rhinitis with or without nasal polyps and bronchospasm). Avoid in late pregnancy; may cause premature closure of ductus arteriosus. May cause elevations of LFTs; d/c if liver disease develop or systemic manifestations (eg, eosinophilia, rash) occur. Not a substitute for corticosteroids or for treatment of corticosteroid insufficiency. Caution in elderly. Anemia may occur; with long-term use, monitor Hgb/Hct if signs or symptoms of anemia develop. May inhibit platelet aggregation and prolong bleeding time; monitor with coagulation disorders. Caution with preexisting asthma and avoid with ASA-sensitive asthma. Rash and/or mild photosensitivity reactions reported.

ADVERSE REACTIONS: Edema, abdominal pain/distress, anorexia, diarrhea, dyspepsia, GI ulcers (gastric/duodenal), gross bleeding/perforation, heartburn, liver enzyme elevations, N/V, rash, anemia, CNS inhibition (eg, depression, sedation, somnolence, or confusion), headache.

INTERACTIONS: Avoid use with ASA. May diminish antihypertensive effect of ACE inhibitors. May decrease natriuretic effects of furosemide and thiazide diuretics; monitor for renal failure. May elevate lithium plasma levels; observe for signs of lithium toxicity. May increase methotrexate toxicities. Increased risk of GI bleeding with anticoagulants (eg, warfarin), smoking, alcohol, and oral corticosteroids. Monitor blood glucose in the beginning phase of glyburide and oxaprozin co-therapy. Monitor BP levels when coadministered with β-blockers (eg, metoprolol). Concurrent use with H_2-receptor antagonists (eg, cimetidine or ranitidine) reduced total body clearance of oxaprozin.

PREGNANCY: Category C, not for use in nursing.

MECHANISM OF ACTION: NSAIDs; unknown, suspected to inhibit prostaglandin synthetase.

PHARMACOKINETICS: Absorption: 95% absorbed. **Distribution:** V_d/F=11-17L/70kg; plasma protein binding primarily albumin (99%). **Metabolism:** Liver via oxidation (65%) and glucuronic acid conjugation (35%). **Elimination:** Feces (35%), urine (5% unchanged, 65% as metabolite).

NURSING CONSIDERATIONS

Assessment: Assess for hypersensitivity reaction to ASA or other NSAIDs, history of asthma, CV disease (eg, pre-existing HTN, congestive heart failure) or risk factors for CV disease, risk factors for GI events (eg, prior history of ulcer disease or GI bleeding, ulceration, perforation, smoking), coagulation disorders, pregnancy/nursing status, possible drug interactions, and renal/hepatic dysfunction. Assess use in elderly and debilitated patients. Obtain baseline LFTs, renal function, BP, and CBC.

Monitoring: Monitor CBC, LFTs, renal function, blood glucose, and chemistries periodically. Monitor for signs/symptoms of serious skin side effects, GI events, CV thrombotic events, MI, stroke, HTN, renal/liver dysfunction, and anaphylactoid reaction (difficulty breathing, swelling of face/throat), hematological effects, and bronchospasm.

Patient Counseling: Instruct to read medication guide. Seek medical attention for symptoms of hepatotoxicity (nausea, fatigue, pruritus), anaphylactic reactions (difficulty breathing, swelling of face/throat), hypersensitivity reaction (rash), CV events (chest pain, SOB, weakness, slurring of speech), GI ulceration and bleeding (epigastric pain, dyspepsia, melena, hematemesis), weight gain, and edema. Inform of risks in pregnancy.

Administration: Oral route. **Storage:** 25°C (77°F); excursions permitted to 15-30°C (59-86°F). Protect from light.

DAYTRANA
methylphenidate (Shire)

> Give cautiously to patients with history of drug dependence or alcoholism. Chronic abusive use may lead to marked tolerance and psychological dependence with varying degrees of abnormal behavior. Careful supervision required during withdrawal from abusive use to avoid severe depression. Withdrawal following chronic therapeutic use may unmask symptoms of the underlying disorder that may require follow-up.

THERAPEUTIC CLASS: Sympathomimetic amine

INDICATIONS: Treatment of attention-deficit hyperactivity disorder (ADHD).

DOSAGE: *Adults:* Individualize dose. Apply to hip area 2 hrs before effect is needed and remove 9 hrs after application. Recommended Titration Schedule: Week 1: 10mg/9 hrs. Week 2: 15mg/9 hrs. Week 3: 20mg/9 hrs. Week 4: 30mg/9 hrs.
Pediatrics: ≥6 yrs: Individualize dose. Apply to hip area 2 hrs before effect is needed and remove 9 hrs after application. Recommended Titration Schedule: Week 1: 10mg/9 hrs. Week 2: 15mg/9 hrs. Week 3: 20mg/9 hrs. Week 4: 30mg/9 hrs.

HOW SUPPLIED: Patch: 10mg/9 hrs, 15mg/9 hrs, 20mg/9 hrs, 30mg/9 hrs [30ˢ]

CONTRAINDICATIONS: Patients with marked anxiety, tension, agitation, glaucoma, motor tics or family history or diagnosis of Tourette's syndrome. Treatment with or within a minimum of 14 days following d/c of an MAOI.

WARNINGS/PRECAUTIONS: Sudden death, stroke, myocardial infarction (MI) reported; avoid with known structural cardiac abnormalities or other serious cardiac problems. May increase BP and HR; caution with underlying conditions that may be compromised by increased BP or HR (eg, pre-existing HTN, heart failure, recent myocardial infarction, ventricular arrhythmia). Perform history and physical exam prior to use to assess for cardiac disease; perform prompt cardiac evaluation if cardiac disease symptoms develop during treatment. May exacerbate symptoms of behavior disturbance and thought disorder in psychotic patients. Caution in treating patients with comorbid bipolar disorder because of concern for possible induction of mixed/manic episode. May cause treatment-emergent psychotic or manic symptoms (eg, hallucinations, delusional thinking, mania) in children and adolescents without prior history of psychotic illness at usual doses. Aggressive behavior or hostility reported. May lower convulsive threshold; d/c in the presence of seizures. Monitor growth during treatment in children; consider interrupting treatment if expected height or weight gain does not occur. Difficulties with accommodation and blurred vision reported with stimulant treatment. May lead to contact sensitization; d/c if suspected. Avoid exposing application site to external heat sources (eg, heating pads, electric blankets, heated water beds, etc.). Caution with history of drug dependence or alcoholism.

ADVERSE REACTIONS: Decreased appetite, headache, insomnia, N/V, decreased weight, irritability, tics, affect lability, anorexia, abdominal pain, dizziness.

INTERACTIONS: See Contraindications. Caution with pressor agents. May decrease effectiveness of antihypertensive agents. May inhibit metabolism of coumarin anticoagulants, anticonvulsants (eg, phenobarbital, phenytoin, primidone), some tricyclic drugs (eg, imipramine, clomipramine, desipramine), and SSRIs. Monitor drug levels (or coagulation times with coumarin) and consider dose adjustments with concomitant use. Serious adverse events reported with concomitant clonidine use.

PREGNANCY: Category C, caution in nursing.

MECHANISM OF ACTION: Sympathomimetic amine; CNS stimulant. Suspected to block reuptake of norepinephrine and dopamine into presynaptic neuron and increase release of these monoamines into extraneuronal spaces.

PHARMACOKINETICS: Absorption: Different doses (single and repeated) resulted in different pharmacokinetic parameters. T_{max}=10 hrs (single dose); T_{max}=8 hrs (repeated patch application). **Metabolism:** De-esterification; ritalinic acid (metabolite). **Elimination:** $T_{1/2}$=4-5 hrs (d-methylphenidate); $T_{1/2}$=1.4-2.9 hrs (l-methylphenidate).

NURSING CONSIDERATIONS

Assessment: Assess for history of marked anxiety, tension, agitation, known hypersensitivity to methylphenidate, glaucoma, behavior disturbances, thought disorder, bipolar disorder, depression, family history of suicide, pre-existing structural cardiac abnormalities, psychiatric history, history of seizures or any other conditions where treatment is contraindicated. Assess for presence of cardiac disease and careful history (eg, family history of sudden death or ventricular arrhythmia); perform further cardiac evaluation if findings suggest such disease (eg, ECG). Assess for history of drug dependence or alcoholism.

Monitoring: Monitor periodically for long-term usefulness, possible drug interactions, BP, HR, contact sensitization evidenced by erythema, edema, papules, vesicles, psychotic or manic symptoms such as hallucinations, delusional thinking, mania, confused state, crying, tics, headaches, irritability, anorexia, insomnia, infectious mononucleosis, and viral infection. Monitor for appearance of or worsening aggressive behavior or hostility. Perform follow-up weight and height in children 7-10 yrs. Perform periodic CBC, differential, and platelet counts during prolonged therapy.

Patient Counseling: Counsel about drug abuse/dependence potential. Avoid exposing application site to direct external heat sources while wearing the patch. Apply intact patches only; do not cut patches. Apply patch to a clean, dry site on hip. Site of application must be alternated daily and patch should not be applied to waistline, where tight clothing may rub the patch. Encourage parent/caregiver to use administration chart to monitor application and removal time, and method of disposal. Patient/caregiver should avoid touching adhesive side of patch during application; if touched, wash hands after application. If any swelling or blistering occurs, remove patch and inform physician. Do not apply hydrocortisone or other solutions, creams, ointments, or emollients immediately prior to patch application. Inform of potential side effects (eg, heart-related problems, mental problems); notify physician if any occur. Caution in operating potentially hazardous machinery or vehicles.

Administration: Transdermal route. Apply patch immediately upon removal from protective pouch. If patch does not fully adhere to skin, or is partially or fully detached during wear time, discard patch and apply a new one. Inspect release liner to ensure no adhesive-containing medication has transferred to liner; if adhesive transfer has occurred, discard patch. If a patch is replaced, total recommended wear time for the day should remain 9 hrs. Peel patches off slowly. Patches should not be applied or re-applied with dressings, tape, or other common adhesives. May take patch off earlier if unacceptable duration of appetite loss or insomnia in the evening occurs. **Storage:** 25°C (77°F); excursions permitted to 15-30°C (59-86°F). Do not store patches unpouched; once sealed tray/outer pouch is opened, use within 2 months. Do not refrigerate or freeze patches.

DEMEROL INJECTION `CII`
meperidine HCl (Hospira)

THERAPEUTIC CLASS: Opioid analgesic

INDICATIONS: For relief of moderate to severe pain. For preoperative medication, anesthesia support, and obstetrical analgesia.

DOSAGE: *Adults:* Pain: Usual: 50-150mg IM/SQ q3-4h PRN. Preoperative: Usual: 50-100mg IM/SQ 30-90 min before anesthesia. Anesthesia Support: Use repeated slow IV inj of fractional doses (eg, 10mg/mL) or continuous IV infusion of a more diluted solution (eg, 1mg/mL). Titrate as needed. Obstetrical Analgesia: Usual: 50-100mg IM/SQ when pain is regular, may repeat at 1- to 3-hr intervals. Elderly: Start at lower end of dosage range and observe. With Phenothiazines/Other Tranquilizers: Reduce dose by 25-50%. IM method preferred with repeated use. For IV injection: Reduce dose and administer slowly, preferably using diluted solution.
Pediatrics: Pain: Usual: 0.5-0.8mg/lb IM/SQ, up to 50-150mg, q3-4h prn. Preoperative: Usual: 0.5-1mg/lb IM/SQ, up to 50-100mg, 30-90 min before anesthesia. With Phenothiazines/Other Tranquilizers: Reduce dose by 25-50%. IM method preferred with repeated use. For IV injection: Reduce dose and administer slowly, preferably using diluted solution.

HOW SUPPLIED: Inj: 25mg/mL, 50mg/mL, 75mg/mL, 100mg/mL

CONTRAINDICATIONS: During or within 14 days of MAOI use.

WARNINGS/PRECAUTIONS: May develop tolerance and dependence; abuse potential. Extreme caution with head injury, increased intracranial pressure, intracranial lesions, acute asthmatic attack, chronic obstructive pulmonary disease or cor pulmonale, decreased respiratory reserve, respiratory depression, hypoxia, and hypercapnia. Rapid IV infusion may result in increased adverse reactions. Caution with acute abdominal conditions, atrial flutter, supraventricular tachycardias. May aggravate convulsive disorders. Caution and reduce initial dose with elderly or debilitated, renal/hepatic impairment, hypothyroidism, Addison's disease, prostatic hypertrophy or urethral stricture. Severe hypotension may occur post-op or if depleted blood volume. Orthostatic hypotension may occur. May impair mental/physical abilities. Not for use in pregnancy prior to labor. May produce depression of respiration and psychophysiologic functions in newborns when used as an obstetrical analgesic.

ADVERSE REACTIONS: Lightheadedness, dizziness, sedation, N/V, sweating, respiratory/circulatory depression.

INTERACTIONS: See Contraindications. Caution and reduce dose with other CNS depressants (eg, narcotics, anesthetics, phenothiazines, tranquilizers, sedative-hypnotics, TCAs, alcohol).

PREGNANCY: Safety in pregnancy and nursing not known.

MECHANISM OF ACTION: Narcotic analgesic; produces actions similiar to morphine. Principal actions involve the CNS and organs composed of smooth muscle. Produces analgesic and sedative effects.

PHARMACOKINETICS: Distribution: Crosses placental barrier; found in breast milk.

NURSING CONSIDERATIONS

Assessment: Assess for pain intensity, or any other conditions where treatment is contraindicated or cautioned. Assess for pregnancy/nursing status, renal/hepatic function, and possible drug interactions.

Monitoring: Monitor for signs/symptoms of drug dependence (eg, psychic dependence, physical dependence), respiratory depression, circulatory depression (eg, hypotension), and convulsions.

Patient Counseling: Inform that medication may impair mental/physical abilities; use caution when performing hazardous tasks (eg, operating machinery/driving). Notify physician of all medications currently taking. Avoid using other CNS depressants and alcohol during medication. Advise about potential for dependence upon repeated administration.

Administration: SQ, IM, IV route. SQ route is suitable for occasional use, IM administration is preferred if repeated doses are required. IM injection should be injected well into the body of a large muscle. If IV route is required, dosage should be decreased and injection should be made very slowly, preferably using a diluted solution. Dosage should be adjusted according to severity of pain. **Storage:** 20-25°C (68-77°F).

DENAVIR   RX
penciclovir (Novartis)

THERAPEUTIC CLASS: Nucleoside analogue

INDICATIONS: Treatment of recurrent herpes labialis (cold sores) in adults and children ≥12 yrs.

DOSAGE: *Adults:* Apply q2h while awake for 4 days. Start with earliest sign or symptom. *Pediatrics:* ≥12 yrs: Apply q2h while awake for 4 days. Start with earliest sign or symptom.

HOW SUPPLIED: Cre: 1% [1.5g]

WARNINGS/PRECAUTIONS: Only use on herpes labialis on the lips and face. Avoid mucous membranes or near the eyes. Effectiveness not established in immunocompromised patients.

ADVERSE REACTIONS: Headache, application-site reaction, local anesthesia, taste perversion, rash.

PREGNANCY: Category B, not for use in nursing.

MECHANISM OF ACTION: Antiviral agent; active against herpes simplex virus types 1 (HSV-1) and 2 (HSV-2). Inhibits HSV polymerase competitively with deoxyguanosine triphosphate. Consequently, herpes viral DNA synthesis and replication are selectively inhibited.

NURSING CONSIDERATIONS

Assessment: Assess for severity, signs and symptoms of cold sore, use in pregnancy/nursing.

Monitoring: Monitor lesions for clinical response. If lesions worsen or do not improve, monitor for secondary bacterial infection.

Patient Counseling: Counsel to avoid applying medication in or near eyes. Instruct to wash hands with soap and water after applying product. Advise females to notify physician if they become pregnant or are nursing.

Administration: Topical. **Storage**: 20-25°C (68-77°F).

DEPACON

RX

valproate sodium (Abbott)

Fatal hepatic failure may occur; risk increased in children <2 yrs, especially if on multiple anticonvulsants, with congenital metabolic disorders, severe seizure disorders with mental retardation, and organic brain disease; use with extreme caution and as a sole agent. Serious/fatal hepatotoxicity may be preceded by nonspecific symptoms such as malaise, weakness, lethargy, facial edema, anorexia, and vomiting, or loss of seizure control in patients with epilepsy. Monitor LFTs prior to therapy, frequently during 1st 6 months of treatment and at frequent intervals thereafter. Teratogenic effects (eg, neural tube defects) and life-threatening pancreatitis reported; d/c if pancreatitis diagnosed and initiate appropriate treatment.

THERAPEUTIC CLASS: Valproate compound

INDICATIONS: Alternative when oral administration of valproate products is temporarily not feasible in the following conditions: monotherapy and adjunctive therapy for treatment of simple and complex absence seizures, and complex partial seizures; adjunctive therapy for multiple seizure types that include absence seizures.

DOSAGE: *Adults:* Simple/Complex Absence Seizure: Initial: 15mg/kg/day. Titrate: Increase by 5-10mg/kg/day at weekly intervals until optimal response. Max: 60mg/kg/day. Complex Partial Seizure: Monotherapy/Conversion to Monotherapy/Adjunctive Therapy: Initial: 10-15mg/kg/day. Titrate: Increase by 5-10mg/kg/week until optimal response. Max: 60mg/kg/day. Elderly: Reduce initial dose and titrate slowly. Consider dose reduction or d/c in patients with decreased food or fluid intake and in patients with excessive somnolence. Replacement Therapy: Give equivalent total daily dose as that of oral valproate. Administer as 60 min IV infusion, not >20mg/min. Adjunctive Therapy/Simple/Complex Absence Seizure/Replacement Therapy: If dose >250mg/day, give in divided doses. Not for use >14 days; switch to oral route as soon as clinically feasible.
Pediatrics: ≥2 yrs: Simple/Complex Absence Seizure: Initial: 15mg/kg/day. Titrate: Increase by 5-10mg/kg/day at weekly intervals until optimal response. Max: 60mg/kg/day. ≥10 yrs: Complex Partial Seizure: Monotherapy/Conversion to Monotherapy/Adjunctive Therapy: Initial: 10-15mg/kg/day. Titrate: Increase by 5-10mg/kg/week until optimal response. Max: 60mg/kg/day. Replacement Therapy: Give equivalent total daily dose as that of oral valproate. Administer as 60 min IV infusion, not >20mg/min. Adjunctive Therapy/Simple/Complex Absence Seizure/ Replacement Therapy: If dose >250mg/day, give in divided doses. Not for use >14 days; switch to oral route as soon as clinically feasible.

HOW SUPPLIED: Inj: 100mg/mL [5mL]

CONTRAINDICATIONS: Hepatic disease, significant hepatic dysfunction, known urea cycle disorders (UCD).

WARNINGS/PRECAUTIONS: Caution with hepatic disease; d/c if significant hepatic dysfunction suspected or apparent. Hyperammonemic encephalopathy, sometimes fatal, in UCD patients reported; d/c if it occurs. Prior to therapy, evaluate for UCD in high-risk patients (eg, history of unexplained encephalopathy, coma, etc). Hypothermia and hyperammonemia reported; measure ammonia levels if unexplained lethargy, vomiting, or mental status changes occur. Caution in elderly; monitor for fluid/nutritional intake, dehydration, and somnolence. Dose-related thrombocytopenia and elevated liver enzymes reported; monitor platelet and coagulation parameters prior to therapy, periodically thereafter, and prior to surgery. Altered thyroid function tests and urine ketone tests reported. May stimulate replication of HIV and cytomegalovirus. Avoid abrupt d/c. Developmental delay, autism and/or autism spectrum disorder reported in the offspring of women exposed to valproate during pregnancy. Rare cases of multi-organ hypersensitivity reactions reported; d/c if suspected. May impair mental/physical abilities. Not for prophylaxis of post-traumatic seizures in acute head trauma.

ADVERSE REACTIONS: Hepatotoxicity, teratogenicity, pancreatitis, dizziness, headache, N/V, injection-site pain/reaction, somnolence, chest pain, pain, paresthesia, taste perversion.

INTERACTIONS: Drugs that affect the level of expression of hepatic enzymes (eg, phenytoin, carbamazepine, phenobarbital, primidone) may increase valproate clearance; monitor levels. Concomitant use with aspirin decreases protein binding and metabolism of valproate; use with caution. Carbapenem antibiotics (eg, meropenem, ertapenem, imipenem) may reduce serum valproic concentration to subtherapeutic levels, resulting in loss of seizure control. Rifampin increases oral clearance and may require valproate dosage adjustment. Concomitant use with felbamate leads to an increase in valproate C_{max}. Increased trough plasma levels with chlorpromazine. Reduces the clearance of amitriptyline, nortriptyline, and lorazepam; consider dose reduction of amitriptyline/nortriptyline. Induces metabolism of carbamazepine. Inhibits metabolism of ethosuximide, phenobarbital, and phenytoin; monitor drug serum concentrations and adjust dose appropriately. Breakthrough seizures reported with concomitant valproate and phenytoin use. Inhibits metabolism of diazepam and displaces it from protein binding sites. Administration with clonazepam may induce absence status in patients with absence seizures. Increases $T_{1/2}$ of lamotrigine and serious skin reactions reported with concomitant use; reduce lamotrigine dose.

Concomitant use with topiramate associated with hyperammonemia with/without encephalopathy, and hypothermia. May displace protein-bound drugs (eg, phenytoin, carbamazepine, warfarin, tolbutamide); monitor coagulation tests when coadministered with warfarin. Additive CNS depression with other CNS depressants (eg, alcohol). May decrease clearance of zidovudine in HIV-seropositive patients.

PREGNANCY: Category D, not for use in nursing.

MECHANISM OF ACTION: Anticonvulsant; has not been established. Proposed to increase gamma aminobutyric acid concentrations in the brain.

PHARMACOKINETICS: Absorption: (1000mg single dose) C_{max}=115µg/mL. **Distribution:** V_d=11L/1.73m²; plasma protein binding (81.5%-90%); found in breast milk. **Metabolism:** Liver; glucuronidation, mitochondrial β-oxidation. **Elimination:** Urine (<3% unchanged); $T_{1/2}$=16 hrs.

NURSING CONSIDERATIONS

Assessment: Assess for history of/current liver disease, pancreatitis, UCD, congenital metabolic disorders, organic brain disease, acute head injuries, pregnancy/nursing status, and possible drug interactions. Prior to therapy, evaluate for UCD in high-risk patients (eg, history of unexplained encephalopathy, coma, etc). Perform LFTs, CBC with platelet count and coagulation tests before initiating therapy.

Monitoring: Monitor LFTs, CBC with platelets, coagulation parameters, pancreatitis, hypersensitivity reactions, hypothermia, hyperammonemia, thyroid function tests. Monitor for fluid and nutritional intake, dehydration, somnolence, and other adverse events in the elderly. Perform periodic plasma concentration determinations of valproate and concomitant enzyme-inducing drugs during the early course of therapy.

Patient Counseling: Advise not to engage in hazardous activities (eg, driving/operating machinery) until it is known that they do not become drowsy from the drug. Counsel about signs/symptoms of pancreatitis, hepatotoxicity, and hyperammonemia; notify physician if any symptoms or adverse effects occur. Instruct that a fever associated with other organ system involvement (rash, lymphadenopathy, etc.) may be drug-related and should be reported to physician immediately. Advise to notify physician if pregnant or intend to become pregnant; inform women of childbearing age of potential risks and alternative therapies.

Administration: IV route. Give as a 60-min infusion (not >20mg/min) after diluting with at least 50mL of a compatible diluent. Refer to PI for preparation instructions. **Storage:** 15-30°C (59-86°F). Refer to PI for stability of infusion sol.

DEPAKENE   RX
valproic acid (Abbott)

Fatal hepatic failure may occur, especially in children <2 yrs on multiple anticonvulsants, with congenital metabolic disorders, severe seizure disorders with mental retardation, or organic brain disease. Hepatotoxicity may be preceded by nonspecific symptoms such as malaise, weakness, lethargy, facial edema, anorexia, and vomiting, or loss of seizure control in patients with epilepsy. Monitor LFTs prior to therapy, frequently during 1st 6 months of treatment and at frequent intervals thereafter. Teratogenic effects (eg, neural tube defects), and life-threatening pancreatitis reported; d/c if pancreatitis diagnosed and initiate appropriate treatment.

THERAPEUTIC CLASS: Carboxylic acid derivative

INDICATIONS: Monotherapy and adjunctive therapy for treatment of simple and complex absence seizures, and complex partial seizures. Adjunctive therapy for multiple seizure types, including absence seizures.

DOSAGE: *Adults:* Simple/Complex Absence Seizures: Initial: 15mg/kg/day. Titrate: Increase weekly by 5-10mg/kg/day until optimal response. Max: 60mg/kg/day. If dose >250mg/day, give in divided doses. Complex Partial Seizures: Monotherapy/Conversion to Monotherapy/Adjunctive Therapy: Initial: 10-15mg/kg/day. Titrate: Increase weekly by 5-10mg/kg/week until optimal response. If clinical response has not been achieved, plasma levels should be measured to determine whether they are in usually accepted therapeutic range (50-100µg/mL). Max: 60mg/kg/day. Concomitant anti-epileptic drug (AED) dosage can ordinarily be reduced by approximately 25% q2 weeks starting at initiation of valproic acid or delayed 1-2 weeks if there is concern seizures are likely to occur. Elderly: Reduce initial dose and titrate slowly. Consider dose reduction or d/c in patients with decreased food or fluid intake and in patients with excessive somnolence. GI irritation: May benefit from administration of the drug with food or by slowly building up the dose from an initial low level.
Pediatrics: >2 yrs: Simple/Complex Absence Seizure: Initial: 15mg/kg/day. Titrate: Increase by 5-10mg/kg/day until optimal response. Max: 60 mg/kg/day. If dose >250mg/day, give in divided doses. ≥10 yrs: Complex Partial Seizure: Monotherapy/Conversion to Monotherapy/Adjunctive Therapy: Initial: 10-15mg/kg/day. Titrate: Increase weekly by 5-10mg/kg/week until optimal response. If clinical response has not been achieved, plasma levels should be measured to determine whether they are in usually accepted therapeutic range (50-100µg/mL).

Max: 60mg/kg/day. Concomitant AED dosage can ordinarily be reduced by approximately 25% q2 weeks starting at initiation of valproic acid or delayed 1-2 weeks if there is a concern that seizures are likely to occur. GI irritation: May benefit from administration of the drug with food or by slowly building up the dose from an initial low level.

HOW SUPPLIED: Cap: 250mg; Sol: 250mg/5mL

CONTRAINDICATIONS: Hepatic disease, significant hepatic dysfunction, known urea cycle disorders (UCD).

WARNINGS/PRECAUTIONS: Increased risk of suicidal thoughts or behavior; monitor for emergence or worsening of depression. Hyperammonemic encephalopathy in UCD patients; d/c if this occurs. Prior to therapy, evaluate for UCD in high-risk patients (eg, history of unexplained encephalopathy, coma, etc.). Measure ammonia levels if develop unexplained lethargy, vomiting, or mental status changes. Caution in elderly; monitor for fluid/nutritional intake, dehydration, somnolence. Multi-organ hypersensitivity reactions and hypothermia, with or without hyperammonemia, reported. Monitor platelets and coagulation tests before therapy and periodically thereafter. Elevated liver enzymes and thrombocytopenia may be dose-related. May interfere with urine ketone and thyroid function tests. May impair mental/physical abilities. Caution with history of hepatic disease. May stimulate replication of HIV and CMV. Avoid abrupt d/c.

ADVERSE REACTIONS: Abdominal pain, amblyopia/blurred vision, alopecia, asthenia, diarrhea, diplopia, dizziness, headache, nystagmus, N/V, peripheral edema, somnolence, tremor, thrombocytopenia, weight gain.

INTERACTIONS: Carbapenem antibiotics may reduce serum valproic concentration to subtherapeutic levels, leading to loss of seizure control. Oral clearance increased by rifampin. Concomitant administration with clonazepam may induce absence status in patients with history thereof. Increases $T_{1/2}$ of lamotrigine; may result in serious skin reaction with lamotrigine. Reports of breakthrough seizures with the combination of valproate and phenytoin; monitor levels of both. Concomitant use with ASA decreases protein binding and metabolism of valproate. Reduces the clearance of amitriptyline, nortriptyline, zidovudine, and lorazepam. Induces metabolism of carbamazepine. Displaces protein-bound diazepam and decreases its V_d and clearance. Inhibits metabolism and decreases clearance of ethosuximide. Concomitant use with felbamate leads to an increase in valproate C_{max}. Inhibits the metabolism of phenobarbital. Monitor for neurological toxicity when used with barbiturates. Displaces protein-bound tolbutamide, and warfarin; monitor coagulation tests. Concomitant use with topiramate has been associated with hyperammonemia with or without encephalopathy and hypothermia. Drugs that affect the level of expression of hepatic enzymes (eg, phenytoin, carbamazepine, phenobarbital, primidone) may increase valproate clearance. Additive CNS depression with other CNS depressants (eg, alcohol). Increased plasma level with chlorpromazine.

PREGNANCY: Category D, not for use in nursing.

MECHANISM OF ACTION: Carboxylic acid derivative; has not been established. Activity in epilepsy is proposed to be related to increased GABA concentration in the brain.

PHARMACOKINETICS: Absorption: Depakote:(Tab) T_{max}=4 hrs (fasting), 8 hrs (fed); (Cap) T_{max}=3.3 hrs (fasting), 4.8 hrs (fed). **Distribution:** V_d=11L/1.73m^2; plasma protein binding (10%-18.5%). **Metabolism:** Liver; glucuronidation, mitochondrial β-oxidation. **Elimination:** Urine (<3% unchanged); $T_{1/2}$=9-16 hrs.

NURSING CONSIDERATIONS

Assessment: Assess LFTs, CBC with platelets, pancreatitis, plasma ammonia levels, hepatic dysfunction/disease, pregnancy/nursing status. Note other diseases/conditions and drug therapies. Prior to therapy, evaluate for UCD in high-risk patients (eg, history of unexplained encephalopathy, coma, etc.).

Monitoring: Monitor LFTs (at frequent intervals during first 6 months), CBC with platelets, coagulation parameters, pancreatitis, thyroid function tests, hypersensitivity reactions, hyperammonemia, ketone and thyroid function tests. Monitor for emergence of worsening of depression, suicidal thoughts or behavior, and/or unusual changes in mood or behavior.

Patient Counseling: Counsel to avoid alcohol, sedatives, over-the-counter drugs. Caution while operating machinery/driving. Counsel about signs/symptoms of hepatotoxicity, pancreatitis, and hyperammonemic encephalopathy; notify physician if symptoms or adverse effects occur. Instruct that a fever associated with other organ system involvement (eg, rash, lymphadenopathy, etc.) may be drug-related and should be reported to physician immediately. Notify physician if suicidal thoughts, behavior, or thoughts about self-harm emerge. Advise patients to enroll in the North American Antiepileptic Drug (NAAED) Pregnancy Registry if they become pregnant. To enroll, call 888-233-2334 or go to www.aedpregnancyregistry.org.

Administration: Oral route. Swallow caps whole; do not chew. **Storage:** Cap: 15-25°C (59-77°F). Sol: Below 30°C (86°F).

DEPAKOTE

RX

divalproex sodium (Abbott)

> Fatal hepatic failure may occur, risk increased in children <2 yrs, especially if on multiple anticonvulsants, with congenital metabolic disorders, severe seizure disorders with mental retardation, and organic brain disease; use with extreme caution and as a sole agent. Serious/fatal hepatotoxicity may be preceded by nonspecific symptoms such as malaise, weakness, lethargy, facial edema, anorexia, and vomiting, or loss of seizure control in patients with epilepsy. Monitor LFTs prior to therapy, frequently during 1st 6 months of treatment and at frequent intervals thereafter. Teratogenic effects (eg, neural tube defects) and life-threatening pancreatitis reported; d/c if pancreatitis diagnosed and initiate appropriate treatment.

OTHER BRAND NAMES: Depakote Sprinkle Capsules (Abbott)

THERAPEUTIC CLASS: Valproate compound

INDICATIONS: (Tab, Cap) Monotherapy and adjunctive therapy for complex partial seizures and simple/complex absence seizures; adjunctive therapy for multiple seizure types that include absence seizures. (Tab) Treatment of mania associated with bipolar disorder and migraine prophylaxis.

DOSAGE: *Adults:* (Cap/Tab) Complex Partial Seizures: Monotherapy/Conversion to Monotherapy/Adjunctive Therapy: Initial: 10-15mg/kg/day. Titrate: Increase by 5-10mg/kg/week until optimal response. Max: 60mg/kg/day. Simple/Complex Absence Seizures: Initial: 15mg/kg/day. Titrate: Increase by 5-10mg/kg/day at weekly intervals until seizure control or limiting side effects. Max: 60mg/kg/day. Adjunctive Therapy/Simple/Complex Absence Seizure: If dose >250mg/day, give in divided doses. Elderly: Reduce initial dose and titrate slowly; decrease dose or d/c if decreased food/fluid intake or if excessive somnolence occurs. (Tab) Migraine: Initial: 250mg bid. Max: 1000mg/day. Mania: Initial: 750mg daily in divided doses. Titrate: Increase dose as rapidly as possible to desired clinical effect. Max: 60mg/kg/day.
Pediatrics: (Cap/Tab) ≥10 yrs: Complex Partial Seizures: Monotherapy/Conversion to Monotherapy/Adjunctive Therapy: Initial: 10-15mg/kg/day. Titrate: Increase by 5-10mg/kg/week until optimal response. Max: 60mg/kg/day. Adjunctive Therapy: If dose >250mg/day, give in divided doses. (Tab) ≥16 yrs: Migraine: Initial: 250mg bid. Max: 1000mg/day.

HOW SUPPLIED: Cap, Delayed-Release: (Sprinkle) 125mg; Tab, Delayed-Release: 125mg, 250mg, 500mg

CONTRAINDICATIONS: Hepatic disease, significant hepatic dysfunction, known urea cycle disorders (UCD).

WARNINGS/PRECAUTIONS: Increased risk of suicidal thoughts or behavior; monitor for emergence/worsening of depression, suicidal thoughts or behavior, thoughts of self-harm, and/or any unusual changes in mood or behavior. Hyperammonemic encephalopathy, sometimes fatal, in UCD patients reported; d/c if this occurs. Prior to therapy, evaluate for UCD in high-risk patients (eg, history of unexplained encephalopathy, coma, etc). Hypothermia and hyperammonemia reported; measure ammonia levels if unexplained lethargy, vomiting, or mental status changes occur. Caution with hepatic disease; d/c if significant hepatic dysfunction suspected or apparent. Caution in the elderly; monitor fluid/nutritional intake, dehydration, and somnolence. Dose-related thrombocytopenia and elevated liver enzymes reported. Monitor platelet and coagulation parameters prior to therapy, periodically thereafter, and prior to surgery. Altered thyroid function tests and urine ketone tests reported. May stimulate replication of HIV and cytomegalovirus. Avoid abrupt d/c. Rare cases of multi-organ hypersensitivity reactions and hypothermia reported; d/c if suspected. Developmental delay, autism and/or autism spectrum disorder reported in the offspring of women exposed to valproate during pregnancy. Safety and efficacy for long-term use (eg, >3 weeks) in mania not established. May impair mental/physical abilities.

ADVERSE REACTIONS: Hepatotoxicity, teratogenicity, pancreatitis, diarrhea, N/V, somnolence, dyspepsia, thrombocytopenia, asthenia, abdominal pain, tremor, headache, anorexia, diplopia, blurred vision, dizziness.

INTERACTIONS: Drugs that affect the level of expression of hepatic enzymes (eg, phenytoin, carbamazepine, phenobarbital, primidone) may increase valproate clearance; monitor levels. Concomitant use with aspirin decreases protein binding and inhibits metabolism of valproate; use with caution. Carbapenem antibiotics (eg, ertapenem, imipenem, meropenem) may reduce serum valproic concentrations to subtherapeutic levels, resulting in loss of seizure control. Rifampin increases oral clearance and may require valproate dosage adjustment. Concomitant use with felbamate leads to an increase in valproate C_{max}. Increased trough plasma levels with chlorpromazine. Reduces the clearance of amitriptyline, nortriptyline, and lorazepam; consider dose reduction of amitriptyline/nortriptyline. Induces metabolism of carbamazepine. Inhibits metabolism of ethosuximide, phenobarbital, and phenytoin; monitor drug serum concentrations and adjust dose appropriately. Breakthrough seizures reported with concomitant valproate and phenytoin use. Administration with clonazepam may induce absence status in patients with absence seizures. Inhibits metabolism of diazepam and displaces it from protein binding sites. Increases $T_{1/2}$ of lamotrigine and serious skin reactions reported with concomitant use; reduce lamotrigine dose. Concomitant use with topiramate associated with hyperammonemia, with or without encephalopathy, and hypothermia. May displace protein-bound drugs (eg, phenytoin, carbamazepine, warfarin, tolbutamide); monitor coagulation tests when coadministered with warfarin. Additive CNS depression with other CNS depressants (eg, alcohol). May decrease clearance of zidovudine in HIV-seropositive patients.

PREGNANCY: Category D, not for use in nursing.

MECHANISM OF ACTION: Anticonvulsant; has not been established. Suggested to increase brain concentrations of gamma aminobutyric acid.

PHARMACOKINETICS: Absorption: T_{max}=4-8 hrs (tab), T_{max}=3.3-4.8 hrs (cap). **Distribution:** V_d=11L/1.73m² (total valproate), 92L/1.73m² (free valproate); plasma protein binding (81.5%-90%). Found in breast milk. **Metabolism:** Liver; glucuronidation, mitochondrial β-oxidation. **Elimination:** Urine (<3% unchanged); $T_{1/2}$=9-16 hrs.

NURSING CONSIDERATIONS

Assessment: Assess for history of/current liver disease, pancreatitis, UCD, congenital metabolic disorders, organic brain disease, pregnancy/nursing status, and possible drug interactions. Prior to therapy, evaluate for UCD in high-risk patients (eg, history of unexplained encephalopathy, coma, etc). Perform LFTs, CBC with platelet count and coagulation tests before initiating therapy.

Monitoring: Monitor LFTs, CBC with platelets, coagulation parameters, pancreatitis, hypersensitivity reactions, hypothermia, hyperammonemia, thyroid function tests. Monitor for fluid and nutritional intake, dehydration, somnolence, and other adverse events in the elderly. Perform periodic plasma concentration determinations of valproate and concomitant enzyme-inducing/inhibiting drugs during the early course of therapy.

Patient Counseling: Advise not to engage in hazardous activities (eg, driving/operating machinery) until it is known that they do not become drowsy from the drug. Counsel about signs/symptoms of pancreatitis, hepatotoxicity, and hyperammonemia; advise to notify physician if any symptoms or adverse effects occur. Instruct that a fever associated with other organ system involvement (eg, rash, lymphadenopathy, etc.) may be drug-related and should be reported to physician immediately. Advise to inform physician if depression, suicidal thoughts, behavior, or thoughts about self-harm emerge or worsen. Advise to notify physician if pregnant or plan to become pregnant; encourage to enroll in North American Antiepileptic Drug (NAAED) Pregnancy Registry if become pregnant.

Administration: Oral route. (Cap) May be swallowed whole or contents sprinkled on soft food. Swallow drug/food mixture immediately; avoid chewing. **Storage:** (Cap) Store below 25°C (77°F). (Tab) Store below 30°C (86°F).

DEPAKOTE ER   RX
divalproex sodium (Abbott)

Fatal hepatic failure may occur, risk increased in children <2 yrs, especially if on multiple anticonvulsants, with congenital metabolic disorders, severe seizure disorders with mental retardation, and organic brain disease; use with extreme caution and as a sole agent. Serious/fatal hepatotoxicity may be preceded by nonspecific symptoms such as malaise, weakness, lethargy, facial edema, anorexia, and vomiting, or loss of seizure control in patients with epilepsy. Monitor LFTs prior to therapy, frequently during 1st 6 months of treatment and at frequent intervals thereafter. Teratogenic effects (eg, neural tube defects) and life-threatening pancreatitis reported; d/c if pancreatitis diagnosed and initiate appropriate treatment.

THERAPEUTIC CLASS: Valproate compound

INDICATIONS: Migraine prophylaxis. Treatment of acute manic or mixed episodes associated with bipolar disorder, with or without psychotic features. In adults and children ≥10 years, monotherapy and adjunctive treatment of complex partial seizures, and simple and complex absence seizures; an adjunct for multiple seizure types that include absence seizures.

DOSAGE: *Adults:* Individualize dose. Migraine: Initial: 500mg qd for 1 week. Titrate: Increase to 1000mg qd. Mania: Initial: 25mg/kg/day given qd. Titrate: Rapidly increase dose to achieve clinical effect. Max: 60mg/kg/day. Complex Partial Seizures: Monotherapy/Conversion to Monotherapy/Adjunctive Therapy: Initial: 10-15mg/kg/day. Titrate: Increase by 5-10mg/kg/week until optimal response. Max: 60mg/kg/day. When converting to monotherapy, reduce concomitant antiepilepsy drug by 25% every 2 weeks starting at initiation or delay 1-2 weeks after start of therapy. Simple/Complex Absence Seizures: Initial: 15mg/kg/day. Titrate: Increase weekly by 5-10mg/kg/day until optimal response. Max: 60mg/kg/day. Conversion from Depakote: Administer qd using a dose 8-20% higher than total daily dose of Depakote. Refer to PI for dose conversion. If dose cannot be directly converted, consider increasing to next higher Depakote total daily dose before converting to appropriate total daily Depakote ER dose. Elderly: Reduce initial dose and titrate slowly. Decrease dose or d/c if with decreased food or fluid intake or if excessive somnolence occurs.

Pediatrics: ≥10 yrs: Complex Partial Seizures: Monotherapy/Conversion to Monotherapy/

Adjunctive Therapy: Initial: 10-15mg/kg/day. Titrate: Increase by 5-10mg/kg/week until optimal response. Max: 60mg/kg/day. When converting to monotherapy, reduce concomitant antiepilepsy drug by 25% every 2 weeks starting at initiation or delay 1-2 weeks after start of therapy. Simple/Complex Absence Seizures: Initial: 15mg/kg/day. Titrate: Increase weekly by 5-10mg/kg/day until optimal response. Max: 60mg/kg/day. Conversion from Depakote: Administer qd using a dose 8-20% higher than total daily dose of Depakote. Refer to PI for dose conversion. If dose cannot be directly converted, consider increasing to next higher Depakote total daily dose before converting to appropriate total daily Depakote ER dose.

HOW SUPPLIED: Tab, Extended-Release: 250mg, 500mg

CONTRAINDICATIONS: Hepatic disease, significant hepatic dysfunction, known urea cycle disorders (UCD).

WARNINGS/PRECAUTIONS: Increased risk of suicidal thoughts or behavior reported; monitor for the emergence/worsening of depression, suicidal thoughts or behavior, thoughts of self-harm, and/or any unusual changes in mood or behavior. Hyperammonemic encephalopathy reported in UCD patients; d/c and initiate treatment if symptoms develop. Prior to therapy, evaluate for UCD in high-risk patients (eg, history of unexplained encephalopathy, coma, etc). Measure ammonia levels if unexplained lethargy, vomiting, or mental status changes occur. Caution in the elderly; monitor fluid/nutritional intake, and for dehydration and somnolence. Dose-related thrombocytopenia and elevated liver enzymes reported; monitor LFTs and platelet and coagulation parameters prior to therapy and periodically thereafter. Altered thyroid function tests and urine ketone tests reported. Avoid abrupt d/c. May stimulate replication of HIV and cytomegalovirus. Multi-organ hypersensitivity reactions and hypothermia reported. Developmental delay, autism and/or autism spectrum disorder reported in the offspring of women exposed to valproate during pregnancy.

ADVERSE REACTIONS: N/V, dyspepsia, diarrhea, abdominal pain, asthenia, somnolence, headache, fever, anorexia, infection, dizziness, hepatotoxicity, neural tube defects, pancreatitis.

INTERACTIONS: Drugs that affect the level of expression of hepatic enzymes (eg, phenytoin, carbamazepine, phenobarbital, primidone) may increase valproate clearance. Concomitant use with aspirin decreases protein binding and inhibits metabolism of valproate. Carbapenem antibiotics (eg, ertapenem, imipenem, meropenem) may reduce serum concentrations to subtherapeutic levels, resulting in loss of seizure control. Rifampin increases oral clearance and may require valproate dosage adjustment. Concomitant use with felbamate leads to an increase in valproate C_{max}. Reduces the clearance of amitriptyline, nortriptyline, and lorazepam. Induces metabolism of carbamazepine. Inhibits metabolism of diazepam, ethosuximide, phenobarbital and phenytoin; monitor drug serum concentrations and adjust dose appropriately. Breakthrough seizures reported with concomitant use with phenytoin. Administration with clonazepam may induce absence status in patients with absence seizures. Increases $T_{1/2}$ of lamotrigine; serious skin reactions reported. Concomitant use with topiramate associated with hyperammonemia, with or without encephalopathy, and hypothermia. Increased trough plasma levels reported with chlorpromazine. May displace protein-bound warfarin; monitor coagulation parameters. May decrease clearance of zidovudine in HIV-seropositive patients. May increase concentrations of tolbutamide.

PREGNANCY: Category D, not for use in nursing.

MECHANISM OF ACTION: Anticonvulsant; has not been established. Suggested to increase brain concentrations of gamma aminobutyric acid.

PHARMACOKINETICS: Absorption: Bioavailability (90%); T_{max}=4-17 hrs. **Distribution:** Found in breast milk, CSF. (Free valproate) V_d=92 L/1.73m². (Total valproate) V_d=11 L/1.73m². **Metabolism:** Liver; glucuronidation, mitochondrial β-oxidation. **Elimination:** Urine (<3% unchanged); $T_{1/2}$=9-16 hrs.

NURSING CONSIDERATIONS

Assessment: Assess for hepatic dysfunction, UCD, pancreatitis, history of hypersensitivity, pregnancy/nursing status, other diseases/conditions, and possible drug interactions. Assess LFTs, CBC with platelet counts, and coagulation parameters.

Monitoring: Monitor for hypersensitivity reactions, pancreatitis, hepatotoxicity, hyperammonemia, and hypothermia. Monitor for emergence/worsening of depression, suicidality or unusual changes in behavior. Monitor LFTs, CBC with platelets, and coagulation parameters.

Patient Counseling: Counsel to avoid alcohol, sedatives, and over-the-counter drugs. Advise not to engage in hazardous activities (eg, driving/operating machinery). Counsel about signs/symptoms of pancreatitis, hepatotoxicity, hyperammonemia; advise to notify physician if any symptoms or adverse effects occur. Instruct that a fever associated with other organ system involvement (eg, rash, lymphadenopathy, etc.) may be drug-related and should be reported to physician immediately. Advise to notify physician if depression, suicidal thoughts, behavior, or thoughts about self-harm emerge. Inform to take as prescribed and if dose is missed, take as soon as possible; do not skip or double the dose. Notify physician if pregnant or intend to become pregnant. Encourage patients to enroll in North American Antiepileptic Drug (NAAED) Pregnancy Registry.

Administration: Oral route. Swallow whole; do not crush or chew. **Storage:** 25°C (77°F); excursions permitted to 15-30°C (59-86°F).

DEPO-MEDROL RX
methylprednisolone acetate (Pharmacia & Upjohn)

THERAPEUTIC CLASS: Glucocorticoid

INDICATIONS: Steroid-responsive disorders.

DOSAGE: *Adults:* Local Effect: Rheumatoid/Osteoarthritis: Large Joint: 20-80mg. Medium Joint: 10-40mg. Small Joint: 4-10mg. Administer intra-articularly into synovial space q1-5 weeks or more depending on relief. Ganglion/Tendinitis/Epicondylitis: 4-30mg into cyst/area of greatest tenderness. May repeat if necessary. Dermatologic Conditions: Inject 20-60mg into lesion. Distribute 20-40mg dose by repeated injections into large lesions. Usual: 1-4 injections. Systemic Effect: Substitute for Oral Therapy: IM dose should equal total daily PO methylprednisolone dose q24h. Prolonged Therapy: Administer weekly PO dose as single IM injection. Androgenital Syndrome: 40mg IM q2 weeks. Rheumatoid Arthritis: 40-120mg IM weekly. Dermatologic Lesions: 40-120mg IM weekly for 1-4 weeks. Acute Severe Dermatitis (Poison Ivy): 80-120mg IM single dose. Chronic Contact Dermatitis: May repeat injections q5-10 days. Seborrheic Dermatitis: 80mg IM weekly. Multiple Sclerosis: 160mg/day methylprednisolone for 1 week, then 64mg qod for 1 month. Asthma/Allergic Rhinitis: 80-120mg IM. Elderly: Start at lower end of dosing. *Pediatrics:* Initial: 0.11-1.6mg/kg/day. Individualize dose depending on the severity of disease and response.

HOW SUPPLIED: Inj: 20mg/mL, 40mg/mL, 80mg/mL

CONTRAINDICATIONS: Idiopathic thrombocytopenic purpura (IM preparations), intrathecal administration, premature infants, systemic fungal infections except as an intra-articular injection for localized joint conditions.

WARNINGS/PRECAUTIONS: Contains benzyl alcohol, which is potentially toxic to neural tissue. Excessive amounts of benzyl alcohol have been associated with toxicity, particularly in neonates, and an increased incidence of kernicterus, particularly in small preterm infants. May result in dermal/subdermal changes forming depressions in the skin at the injection site; do not exceed recommended doses. Avoid injection into deltoid muscle or into an infected site or a previously infected joint. Rare instances of anaphylactoid reactions reported. Do not use to treat traumatic brain injury. May cause elevation of BP, salt and water retention, and increased excretion of K$^+$ and Ca^{2+}; dietary salt restriction and K$^+$ supplementation may be necessary. Caution with recent myocardial infarction. HPA axis suppression, Cushing's syndrome, and hyperglycemia reported; monitor prolonged use. Possible increased susceptibility to infections (eg, viral, fungal, protozoan, or helminthic). May exacerbate systemic fungal infections. Latent disease due to certain pathogens may be activated or intercurrent infections exacerbated. Assess for latent or active amebiasis prior to therapy. Caution with known or suspected *Strongyloides*, active or latent tuberculosis (TB), HTN, congestive heart failure (CHF), renal insufficiency, active ocular herpes simplex, osteoporosis, active or latent peptic ulcer, diverticulitis, fresh intestinal anastomoses, and nonspecific ulcerative colitis. Not for use in cerebral malaria and optic neuritis. May produce posterior subcapsular cataracts, glaucoma with possible damage to optic nerves, and enhance the establishment of secondary ocular infections due to bacteria, fungi, or viruses. May elevate intraocular pressure (IOP). Kaposi's sarcoma reported. Chickenpox and measles may have more serious or fatal course. Metabolic clearance is decreased in hypothyroidism and increased in hyperthyroidism. May decrease bone formation and increase bone resorption. Acute myopathy reported with high doses. May elevate creatine kinase levels. Psychic derangements may appear during therapy.

ADVERSE REACTIONS: Anaphylactoid reaction, bradycardia, cardiac arrhythmias, cardiac enlargement, acne, erythema, fluid/sodium retention, abdominal distention, decreased carbohydrate and glucose tolerance, glycosuria, hirsutism, convulsions, depression.

INTERACTIONS: Administration of live or live, attenuated vaccines is contraindicated in patients receiving immunosuppressive doses. Killed or inactivated vaccines may be administered, though response can not be predicted. Use with aminoglutethimide may lead to a loss of corticosteroid-induced adrenal suppression. May develop hypokalemia with K$^+$-depleting agents (eg, amphotericin-B, diuretics). Case reports of cardiac enlargement and CHF reported with concomitant amphotericin-B. Macrolide antibiotics decrease clearance. Anticholinesterase agents may produce severe weakness in patients with myasthenia gravis. Serum concentrations of isoniazid may be decreased. Cholestyramine may increase clearance. Coadministration of digitalis glycosides increases risk of arrhythmias due to hypokalemia. Estrogens (eg, oral contraceptives) may decrease hepatic metabolism leading to increased effects. Hepatic enzyme inducers (eg, barbiturates, phenytoin, carbamazepine, and rifampin) enhance metabolism. Hepatic enzyme inhibitors (eg, ketoconazole, macrolide antibiotics such as erythromycin and troleandomycin) may increase plasma concentrations. Concomitant use with ASA or other NSAIDs increases risks of GI side effects. The clearance of salicylates may be increased. Coadministration with warfarin usually results in inhibition of response to warfarin. Antidiabetic agents may require dosage adjustment. Increased activity of both cyclosporine and corticosteroids when used concomitantly; convulsions reported. Ketoconazole decreases metabolism leading to increased risk of side effects. Acute myopathy observed in patients receiving concomitant therapy with neuromuscular blocking drugs (eg, pancuronium).

PREGNANCY: Category C, not for use in nursing.

MECHANISM OF ACTION: Glucocorticoid; causes profound and varied metabolic effects and modifies the body's immune responses to diverse stimuli.

D

NURSING CONSIDERATIONS

Assessment: Assess for hypersensitivity to drug, unusual stress, systemic fungal infections, current infections, active TB, vaccination history, ulcerative colitis, renal/hepatic insufficiency, septic arthritis/unstable joint, HTN, osteoporosis, myasthenia gravis, thyroid status, psychotic tendencies, and possible drug interactions.

Monitoring: Monitor for anaphylactoid reactions, Cushing's syndrome, hyperglycemia, adrenocortical insufficiency, occurrence of infections, psychic derangement, cataracts, acute myopathy, Kaposi's sarcoma, fluid retention, measurement of serum electrolytes, creatine kinase, thyroid-stimulating hormone, LFTs, IOP, BP, and HR. Monitor urinalysis, blood sugar, weight, ECG for cardiac arrhythmias and bradycardia, chest X-ray, and upper GI X-ray (if ulcer history) regularly during prolonged therapy. Monitor linear growth in pediatrics.

Patient Counseling: Inform that susceptibility to infections may increase. Advise that exposure to chicken pox and measles must be reported immediately. Advise not to d/c abruptly or without medical supervision. Instruct to seek medical advice once fever or signs of infection develops. Warn not to d/c abruptly or without medical supervision.

Administration: IM, intra-articular, or intralesional. **Storage:** 20-25°C (68-77°F).

DEPO-PROVERA   RX
medroxyprogesterone acetate (Pharmacia & Upjohn)

THERAPEUTIC CLASS: Progestogen

INDICATIONS: Adjunct and palliative treatment of inoperable, recurrent, and metastatic endometrial or renal carcinoma.

DOSAGE: *Adults:* Initial: 400-1000mg IM weekly. Maint: 400mg/month if disease stabilizes and/or improves within a few weeks or months.

HOW SUPPLIED: Inj: 400mg/mL [2.5mL]

CONTRAINDICATIONS: Pregnancy, undiagnosed vaginal bleeding, breast malignancy, thrombophlebitis, thromboembolic disorders, cerebral vascular disease, liver dysfunction.

WARNINGS/PRECAUTIONS: Avoid during first 4 months of pregnancy; risk of genital abnormalities in fetuses with exposure. May cause thromboembolic disorders, ocular disorders, fluid retention. Caution with history of depression; d/c if depression recurs to serious degree. Caution with family history of breast cancer or patients with breast nodules. Annual physical exam for all patients, with attention to BP, breasts, abdomen and pelvic organs. May mask the onset of climacteric.

ADVERSE REACTIONS: Menstrual irregularities, nervousness, dizziness, edema, weight and cervical changes, cholestatic jaundice, breast tenderness, galactorrhea, rash, acne, alopecia, hirsutism, depression, pyrexia, fatigue, insomnia, nausea.

INTERACTIONS: Aminoglutethimide may decrease serum levels.

PREGNANCY: Not recommended in pregnancy, caution in nursing.

MECHANISM OF ACTION: Progestogen; inhibits secretion of gonadotropins, preventing follicular maturation and ovulation, resulting in endometrial thinning and producing a contraceptive effect.

PHARMACOKINETICS: Absorption: C_{max}=1-7ng/mL; T_{max}=3 weeks. **Distribution:** Found in breast milk. **Elimination:** $T_{1/2}$=50 days.

NURSING CONSIDERATIONS

Assessment: Physical exam of BP, breast, abdominal, pelvic exam, including cervical cytology and relevant lab tests, with assessment of pregnancy status, vaginal bleeding, history of breast cancer, thromboembolic disorders/active thrombophlebitis and/or cerebrovascular disease, drug hypersensitivity, diabetes mellitus, mental depression, hepatic/renal impairment, and possible drug/lab test interactions.

Monitoring: Monitor for amenorrhea, menstrual irregularity, breast cancer risk, manifestations of thrombotic disorders (eg, thrombophlebitis, pulmonary embolism, cerebrovascular disorders, retinal thrombosis), ocular disorders (eg, partial/complete vision loss, proptosis, diplopia, migraine), anaphylaxis/anaphylactoid reaction, manifestations of fluid retentions, epilepsy,

abdominal pain, weight changes. Lab monitoring of plasma/urinary steroid levels, gonadotropin level, sex hormone-binding globulin level, LFTs, glucose, lipid profile, and coagulation tests.
Patient Counseling: Counsel on risk/benefits. Notify if pregnant/nursing.
Administration: IM route. **Storage:** 20-25°C (68-77°F).

DEPO-PROVERA CONTRACEPTIVE   RX
medroxyprogesterone acetate (Pharmacia & Upjohn)

> May lose significant bone mineral density (BMD); greater with increasing duration of use and may not be completely reversible. Unknown if use during adolescence or early adulthood will reduce peak bone mass and increase risk of osteoporotic fractures in later life. Should not be used as long-term birth control (>2 yrs) unless other birth control methods are considered inadequate.

THERAPEUTIC CLASS: Progestogen

INDICATIONS: Prevention of pregnancy.

DOSAGE: *Adults:* 150mg IM every 3 months (13 weeks) in gluteal or deltoid muscle. Give 1st injection during 1st 5 days of menses; within 1st 5 days postpartum if not nursing; or at 6th postpartum week if exclusively nursing. If >13 weeks between injections, physician should determine that the patient is not pregnant before administering the drug.
Pediatrics: Postpubertal Adolescents: 150mg IM every 3 months (13 weeks) in gluteal or deltoid muscle. Give 1st injection during 1st 5 days of menses; within 1st 5 days postpartum if not nursing; or at 6th postpartum week if exclusively nursing. If >13 weeks between injections, physician should determine that the patient is not pregnant before administering the drug.

HOW SUPPLIED: Inj: 150mg/mL

CONTRAINDICATIONS: Known or suspected pregnancy or as a diagnostic test for pregnancy; undiagnosed vaginal bleeding; known or suspected malignancy of breast; active thrombophlebitis, current or past history of thromboembolic disorders or cerebral vascular disease; significant liver disease.

WARNINGS/PRECAUTIONS: Caution in patients with osteoporosis risk factors (eg, metabolic bone disease, anorexia nervosa, family history of osteoporosis); consider other birth control methods. Serious thrombotic events reported; d/c if thrombosis develops while on therapy. Do not readminister pending examination if with sudden partial or complete loss of vision; sudden onset of proptosis, diplopia, or migraine; or if examination reveals papilledema or retinal vascular lesions. May carry cancer risk (breast and cervix). Monitor women with family history of breast cancer or with breast nodules carefully. Be alert to the possibility of ectopic pregnancy. Anaphylaxis and anaphylactoid reaction reported. D/C if jaundice or acute or chronic disturbances of liver function develop. Convulsion reported. Monitor patients who have a history of depression; do not readminister if depression recurs. May cause disruption of menstrual bleeding patterns (eg, amenorrhea, irregular or unpredictable bleeding/spotting, prolonged spotting/bleeding, heavy bleeding). Rule out organic pathology if abnormal bleeding persists or is severe. May cause weight gain and decrease glucose tolerance; monitor diabetic patients. May cause fluid retention; caution with epilepsy, migraine, asthma, and cardiac/renal dysfunction. Return to fertility after stopping therapy may be delayed. Does not protect against HIV infection and other sexually transmitted diseases (STDs). Annual physical exam recommended for a BP check and for other indicated healthcare. May change the results of some laboratory tests (eg, coagulation factors, lipids, glucose tolerance, binding proteins).

ADVERSE REACTIONS: Menstrual irregularities, weight gain, abdominal pain/discomfort, dizziness, headache, asthenia/fatigue, nervousness, decreased libido, nausea, leg cramps.

INTERACTIONS: May decrease effectiveness with drugs or herbal products that induce enzymes, including CYP3A4, (eg, barbiturates, bosentan, carbamazepine, felbamate, griseofulvin, oxcarbazepine, phenytoin, rifampin, St. John's wort, topiramate) that metabolize contraceptive hormones. Significant changes (increase or decrease) in plasma levels with protease inhibitors or non-nucleoside reverse transcriptase inhibitors. Pregnancy reported with use of antibiotics. Aminoglutethimide may decrease serum levels. May cause a significant loss of BMD; additional risk with risk factors for osteoporosis (eg, chronic alcohol and/or tobacco use, chronic use of drugs that can reduce bone mass, such as anticonvulsants or corticosteroids).

PREGNANCY: Contraindicated in pregnancy; safety in nursing not known.

MECHANISM OF ACTION: Progestogen; inhibits secretion of gonadotropins which, in turn, prevents follicular maturation and ovulation, resulting in endometrial thinning.

PHARMACOKINETICS: Absorption: C_{max}=1-7ng/mL; T_{max}=3 weeks. **Distribution:** Plasma protein binding (86%); found in breast milk. **Metabolism:** Liver (extensive) by P450 enzymes; reduction, loss of the acetyl group and hydroxylation. **Elimination:** Urine; $T_{1/2}$=50 days.

NURSING CONSIDERATIONS

Assessment: Assess for active thrombophlebitis, current/past history of thromboembolic disorders or cerebral vascular disease, malignancy of breast, hypersensitivity reactions, significant liver disease, vaginal bleeding, breast nodules, history of depression, diabetes mellitus (DM), pregnancy/nursing status and possible drug interactions. Assess use in patients with known osteoporosis risk factors (metabolic bone disease, anorexia nervosa, chronic alcohol and/or tobacco use, strong family history of osteoporosis), strong history of breast cancer, epilepsy, migraine, asthma and cardiac/renal dysfunction.

Monitoring: Monitor for thrombosis, loss of vision, proptosis, diplopia, migraine, papilledema, retinal vascular lesions, severe abdominal pain, anaphylaxis or anaphylactoid reactions, jaundice, disturbances in liver function, convulsions, fluid retention, and disruption of menstrual bleeding patterns. Monitor patients with DM. Monitor for recurrence of depression with previous history. Monitor BP and BMD and perform annual physical exam while on therapy. Monitor carefully in women with a strong family history of breast cancer or who have breast nodules.

Patient Counseling: Counsel about risk/benefits of drug. Inform that drug does not protect against HIV infection and other STDs. Advise at the beginning of treatment that their menstrual cycle may be disrupted and that irregular and unpredictable bleeding or spotting results, and that this usually decreases to the point of amenorrhea. Advise to take adequate calcium and vitamin D.

Administration: IM route. Shake vigorously before use. Administer by deep IM injection in the gluteal or deltoid muscle. **Storage:** 20-25°C (68-77°F). Must be stored upright.

DEPO-TESTOSTERONE

testosterone cypionate (Pharmacia & Upjohn)

THERAPEUTIC CLASS: Androgen

INDICATIONS: Testosterone replacement in males with congenital or acquired primary hypogonadism or hypogonadotropic hypogonadism.

DOSAGE: *Adults:* Individualize dose. Give 50-400mg IM deep in the gluteal muscle q2-4 weeks. Consider chronological and skeletal ages in determining initial dose and titration. Adjust according to response and adverse reactions.
Pediatrics: ≥12 yrs: Individualize dose. Give 50-400mg IM deep in the gluteal muscle q2-4 weeks. Consider chronological and skeletal ages in determining initial dose and titration. Adjust according to response and adverse reactions.

HOW SUPPLIED: Inj: 100mg/mL [10mL], 200mg/mL [1mL, 10mL]

CONTRAINDICATIONS: Serious cardiac, hepatic or renal disease. Males with carcinoma of the breast or known or suspected carcinoma of the prostate gland. Women who are or may become pregnant.

WARNINGS/PRECAUTIONS: May cause hypercalcemia in immobilized patients; d/c when occurs. May develop hepatic adenomas, hepatocellular carcinoma, and peliosis hepatis with prolonged use of high doses. Caution in elderly; increased risk of prostatic hypertrophy and prostatic carcinoma. May develop gynecomastia. May accelerate bone maturation without linear growth. D/C with appearance of acute urethral obstruction, priapism, excessive sexual stimulation, or oligospermia; restart at lower doses. Caution with benign prostatic hypertrophy (BPH) and males with delayed puberty. Do not use interchangeably with testosterone propionate, for enhancement of athletic performance, or as IV. Contains benzyl alcohol.

ADVERSE REACTIONS: Gynecomastia, excessive frequency/duration of penile erections, male pattern baldness, increased/decreased libido, oligospermia, hirsutism, acne, nausea, hypercholesterolemia, clotting factor suppression, polycythemia, altered LFTs, priapism, anxiety, depression.

INTERACTIONS: May increase sensitivity to oral anticoagulants. Increased levels of oxyphenbutazone. May decrease insulin requirements in diabetic patients.

PREGNANCY: Category X, not for use in nursing.

MECHANISM OF ACTION: Endogenous androgen; responsible for normal growth and development of male sex organs and for maintenance of secondary sex characteristics.

PHARMACOKINETICS: Metabolism: Liver. **Elimination:** Urine (90%), feces (6%); $T_{1/2}$=8 days.

NURSING CONSIDERATIONS

Assessment: Assess males for known drug hypersensitivity, carcinoma of the breast, known or suspected carcinoma of the prostate gland, cardiac/hepatic/renal disease, delayed puberty, BPH, and possible drug interactions.

Monitoring: Periodically monitor Hgb and Hct. Monitor for signs/symptoms of hypersensitivity reactions, edema with/without congestive heart failure, gynecomastia, and hypercalcemia. Assess bone development q6 months in males with delayed puberty.

Patient Counseling: Instruct to report to physician if N/V, changes in skin color, ankle swelling, or too frequent or persistent penile erections occur.

Administration: IM route. **Storage:** 20-25°C (68-77°F). Protect from light.

DESOXYN **CII**
methamphetamine HCl (Lundbeck)

> High potential for abuse. Administration for prolonged periods of time in obesity may lead to drug dependence and must be avoided. Misuse may cause sudden death and serious cardiovascular adverse events.

THERAPEUTIC CLASS: Sympathomimetic amine

INDICATIONS: Attention-deficit hyperactivity disorder (ADHD). Short-term adjunct to treat exogenous obesity.

DOSAGE: *Adults:* Obesity: 5mg, 1/2 hr before each meal. Do not exceed a few weeks of treatment.
Pediatrics: ADHD: ≥6 yrs: Initial: 5mg qd-bid. Titrate: May be raised in increments of 5mg at weekly intervals until optimum response is achieved. Usual: 20-25mg/day. Total daily dose may be given in two divided doses daily. Obesity: ≥12 yrs: 5mg, 1/2 hr before each meal. Do not exceed a few weeks of treatment.

HOW SUPPLIED: Tab: 5mg

CONTRAINDICATIONS: Advanced arteriosclerosis, symptomatic cardiovascular (CV) disease, moderate to severe HTN, hyperthyroidism, glaucoma, agitated states, history of drug abuse, during or within 14 days of MAOI use.

WARNINGS/PRECAUTIONS: Tolerance to anorectic effect develop within a few weeks; do not exceed recommended dose to increase effect. Sudden death reported in children and adolescents with structural cardiac abnormalities or other serious heart problems. Sudden death, stroke, and myocardial infarction (MI) reported in adults. Avoid use with serious structural abnormalities, cardiomyopathy, serious heart rhythm abnormalities, coronary artery disease, or other serious cardiac problems. May increase BP and HR; caution with underlying medical conditions that might be compromised by increases in BP/HR (eg, preexisting HTN, heart failure, recent MI, ventricular arrhythmia). Patients with symptoms suggestive of cardiac disease (eg, exertional chest pain, unexplained syncope) should undergo prompt cardiac evaluation. May exacerbate behavior disturbance and thought disorder in psychotic patients. Treatment-emergent psychotic or manic symptoms may occur. Aggressive behavior or hostility reported in patients treated for ADHD. May cause growth suppression; monitor growth in children; interrupt therapy if not growing or gaining height/weight. Caution in patients with comorbid bipolar disorder. May lower convulsive threshold and cause blurring of vision and difficulty with accommodation. Do not use to combat fatigue or replace rest. Exacerbation of motor and phonic tics and Tourette's syndrome reported. Prescription should be limited to the smallest feasible amount to minimize overdosage. May cause significant elevation of plasma corticosteroids.

ADVERSE REACTIONS: BP elevation, tachycardia, palpitations, dizziness, dysphoria, overstimulation, insomnia, tremor, diarrhea, constipation, dry mouth, urticaria, impotence, changes in libido, growth suppression in children.

INTERACTIONS: See Contraindications. May alter insulin requirements. May decrease hypotensive effect of guanethidine. Caution with TCAs. Antagonized by phenothiazines.

PREGNANCY: Category C, not for use in nursing.

MECHANISM OF ACTION: Sympathomimetic amine; CNS stimulant: peripheral actions involve elevation of BP, weak bronchodilation, and respiratory stimulant actions. Anorectics/anorexigenics: mechanism not established; suspected to suppress appetite.

PHARMACOKINETICS: Absorption: Rapid. **Metabolism:** Liver; aromatic hydroxylation, N-dealkylation and deamination. **Elimination:** Urine (62%); $T_{1/2}$=4-5 hrs.

NURSING CONSIDERATIONS

Assessment: Assess for glaucoma, agitation, CV conditions, hyperthyroidism, history of drug abuse. Screen for comorbid depressive symptoms, psychiatric history (including family history of suicide, bipolar disorder, depression, psychotic disorder, mania). Assess for history of motor and phonic tics and Tourette's syndrome. Assess pregnancy/nursing status and for possible drug interactions. Assess for history of seizures, diabetes.

Monitoring: Monitor BP and HR. Monitor for cardiac abnormalities, exacerbations of behavior disturbances and thought disorders, aggression or hostility, psychotic or manic symptoms, seizures, and visual disturbances. Monitor growth (height and weight) in children. Interrupt occasionally to determine if patient requires continued therapy.

Patient Counseling: Inform about risks and benefits of treatment, appropriate use, drug abuse/dependence. Advise not to engage in hazardous activities (eg, operating machinery/driving). Avoid late evening doses; insomnia may result. Instruct not to increase dosage unless advised by physician.

Administration: Oral route. **Storage**: Store below 30°C (86°F). Dispense in a tight, light-resistant container.

D

DETROL LA
tolterodine tartrate (Pharmacia & Upjohn)

RX

OTHER BRAND NAMES: Detrol (Pharmacia & Upjohn)

THERAPEUTIC CLASS: Muscarinic antagonist

INDICATIONS: Treatment of overactive bladder with symptoms of urge urinary incontinence, urgency, and frequency.

DOSAGE: *Adults:* (Cap, ER) Usual: 4mg qd. May lower to 2mg qd based on response and tolerability. Mild to Moderate Hepatic Impairment (Child-Pugh Class A or B)/Severe Renal Impairment (CrCl 10-30mL/min)/With Potent CYP3A4 Inhibitors: 2mg qd. (Tab) Initial: 2mg bid. May lower to 1mg bid based on response and tolerability. Significantly Reduced Hepatic/Renal Function/With Potent CYP3A4 Inhibitors: 1mg bid.

HOW SUPPLIED: Cap, Extended-Release (Cap, ER): (Detrol LA) 2mg, 4mg; Tab: (Detrol) 1mg, 2mg

CONTRAINDICATIONS: Urinary retention, gastric retention, uncontrolled narrow-angle glaucoma, hypersensitivity to fesoterodine fumarate extended-release tablets.

WARNINGS/PRECAUTIONS: Anaphylaxis and angioedema requiring hospitalization and emergency treatment have occurred with 1st dose and subsequent doses; d/c and provide appropriate therapy if difficulty in breathing, upper airway obstruction, or fall in BP occurs. Risk of urinary retention in patients with clinically significant bladder outflow obstruction and gastric retention in patients with GI obstructive disorders. Caution with decreased GI motility (eg, intestinal atony), narrow-angle glaucoma, myasthenia gravis, known history of QT prolongation and hepatic/renal dysfunction. (Cap, ER) Not recommended with severe hepatic impairment (Child-Pugh Class C) and CrCl <10mL/min.

ADVERSE REACTIONS: Dry mouth, dizziness, headache, abdominal pain, constipation, diarrhea, dyspepsia, fatigue, somnolence.

INTERACTIONS: May increase levels with fluoxetine (potent CYP2D6 inhibitors) and ketoconazole (potent CYP3A4 inhibitor). Reduce dose with concomitant potent CYP3A4 inhibitors (eg, clarithromycin, ketoconazole, itraconazole, ritonavir). Caution with Class IA (eg, quinidine, procainamide) or Class III (eg, amiodarone, sotalol) antiarrhythmics and cholinesterase inhibitors. (Cap, ER) May increase anticholinergic effects with anticholinergic agents.

PREGNANCY: Category C, not for use in nursing.

MECHANISM OF ACTION: Muscarinic receptor antagonist; competitive antagonist of acetylcholine at postganglionic muscarinic receptors mediating urinary bladder contraction and salivation via cholinergic muscarinic receptors.

PHARMACOKINETICS: Absorption: Administration of variable doses resulted in different parameters. **Distribution:** (IV) V_d=113L; high plasma protein binding. **Metabolism:** Extensive Metabolizers (EM): CYP2D6 (oxidation); 5-hydroxymethyl (active metabolite). Poor Metabolizers (PM): CYP3A4 (dealkylation). **Elimination:** Urine (77% unchanged), feces (17% unchanged). (Tab) EM: $T_{1/2}$=2.2 hrs; PM: $T_{1/2}$=9.6 hrs. (Cap, ER) EM: $T_{1/2}$=6.9 hrs; PM: $T_{1/2}$=18 hrs.

NURSING CONSIDERATIONS

Assessment: Assess for bladder outflow obstruction (urinary retention), GI obstructive disorder (gastric retention), narrow-angle glaucoma, myasthenia gravis, history of QT prolongation, hepatic/renal impairment, pregnancy/nursing status, and possible drug interactions.

Monitoring: Monitor for signs/symptoms of urinary retention, gastric retention, QT prolongation, and hypersensitivity reactions. Monitor renal/hepatic function and HR.

Patient Counseling: Inform patients that drug may produce blurred vision, dizziness, or drowsiness. Advise to exercise caution against potentially dangerous activities until drug effects have been determined. Instruct to notify physician if pregnant/nursing or planning to become pregnant.

Administration: Oral route. (Cap, ER) Take with liquids and swallow whole. **Storage:** Tab: 25°C (77°F). Cap, ER: 20-25°C (68-77°F); excursions permitted to 15-30°C (59-86°F).

DEXAMETHASONE   RX
dexamethasone (Various)

THERAPEUTIC CLASS: Glucocorticoid

INDICATIONS: (PO) Treatment of steroid-responsive disorders. (Inj) Treatment of steroid-responsive disorders when oral therapy is not feasible.

DOSAGE: *Adults:* Individualize for disease and patient response. Withdraw gradually. (Tab) Initial: 0.75-9mg/day PO. Maint: Decrease in small amounts to lowest effective dose. Cushing's Syndrome Test: 1mg PO at 11pm; draw blood at 8 am next morning. Or, 0.5mg PO q6h for 48 hrs; or 2mg (to distinguish if excess pituitary adrenocorticotropic hormone [ACTH] or other causes) PO q6h for 48 hrs; obtain 24-hr urine collections. (Inj) Initial: 0.5-9mg/day IV/IM. Cerebral Edema: Initial: 10mg IV, then 4mg IM q6h until edema subsides. Reduce dose after 2-4 days and gradually d/c over 5-7 days. Palliative Management of Recurrent/Inoperable Brain Tumors: Maint: 2mg IV/PO bid-tid. Acute Allergic Disorders: 4-8mg IM on 1st day, then 1.5mg PO bid for 2 days, then 0.75mg PO bid for 1 day, then 0.75mg PO qd for 2 days. (Inj) Usual: 0.2-9mg. Maint: Decrease in small amounts to lowest effective dose. Intra-Articular/Intralesional/Soft Tissue Injection: Usual: 0.2-6mg once every 3-5 days to once every 2-3 weeks. See PI for Shock Treatment. Take tabs and oral Sol with meals and antacids to prevent peptic ulcer.
Pediatrics: Individualize for disease and patient response. Withdraw gradually. (Tab) Initial: 0.75-9mg/day PO. Maint: Decrease in small amounts to lowest effective dose. Cushing's Syndrome Test: 1mg PO at 11pm; draw blood at 8 am next morning. Or, 0.5mg PO q6h for 48 hrs; or 2mg (to distinguish if excess pituitary ATCH or other causes) PO q6h for 48 hrs; obtain 24-hr urine collections. (Inj) Initial: 0.5-9mg/day IV/IM. Cerebral Edema: Initial: 10mg IV, then 4mg IM q6h until edema subsides. Reduce dose after 2-4 days and gradually d/c over 5-7 days. Palliative Management of Recurrent/Inoperable Brain Tumors: Maint: 2mg IV/PO bid-tid. Acute Allergic Disorders: 4-8mg IM on 1st day, then 1.5mg PO bid for 2 days, then 0.75mg PO bid for 1 day, then 0.75mg PO qd for 2 days. (Inj) Usual: 0.2-9mg. Maint: Decrease in small amounts to lowest effective dose. Intra-Articular/Intralesional/Soft Tissue Injection: Usual: 0.2-6mg once every 3-5 days to once every 2-3 weeks. See PI for shock treatment. Take tabs and oral Sol with meals and antacids to prevent peptic ulcer.

HOW SUPPLIED: Inj: (Dexamethasone Sodium Phosphate) 4mg/mL, 10mg/mL; Sol: (Dexamethasone) 0.5mg/5mL, 1mg/mL; Tab: (Dexamethasone) 0.5mg*, 0.75mg*, 1mg*, 1.5mg*, 2mg*, 4mg*, 6mg* *scored

CONTRAINDICATIONS: Systemic fungal infections.

WARNINGS/PRECAUTIONS: Increase dose before, during, and after stressful situations. Avoid abrupt withdrawal. May mask signs of infection, activate latent amebiasis, elevate BP, cause salt/water retention, increase excretion of potassium and calcium. Prolonged use may produce cataracts, glaucoma, secondary ocular infections. Caution with recent myocardial infarction (MI), ocular herpes simplex, emotional instability, nonspecific ulcerative colitis, diverticulitis, peptic ulcer, renal insufficiency, HTN, osteoporosis, myasthenia gravis, threadworm infection, active tuberculosis (TB). Enhanced effect with hypothyroidism, cirrhosis. Consider prophylactic therapy if exposed to measles or chickenpox. Risk of glaucoma, cataracts, and eye infections. False negative dexamethasone suppression test with indomethacin.

ADVERSE REACTIONS: Fluid/electrolyte disturbances, muscle weakness, osteoporosis, peptic ulcer, pancreatitis, ulcerative esophagitis, impaired wound healing, headache, psychic disturbances, growth suppression (pediatrics), glaucoma, hyperglycemia, weight gain, nausea, malaise.

INTERACTIONS: Caution with ASA. Inducers of CYP3A4 (eg, phenytoin, phenobarbital, carbamazepine, rifampin) and ephedrine enhance clearance; increase steroid dose. Inhibitors of CYP3A4 (ketoconazole, macrolides) may increase plasma levels. Drugs that affect metabolism may interfere with dexamethasone suppression tests. Increased clearance of drugs metabolized by CYP3A4 (eg, indinavir, erythromycin). May increase or decrease phenytoin levels. Ketoconazole may inhibit adrenal corticosteroid synthesis and cause adrenal insufficiency during corticosteroid withdrawal. Antagonizes or potentiates coumarins. Hypokalemia with potassium-depleting diuretics. Live virus vaccines are contraindicated with immunosuppressive doses.

PREGNANCY: Category C, not for use in nursing.

MECHANISM OF ACTION: Adrenocortical steroid; produces anti-inflammatory effects.

PHARMACOKINETICS: Distribution: Found in breast milk. **Metabolism:** Liver; CYP3A4.

NURSING CONSIDERATIONS

Assessment: Assess for hypersensitivity to drug, systemic fungal or current infections, active TB, vaccination, unusual stress, hypothyroidism, hepatic/renal impairment, ulcerative colitis, diverticulitis, peptic ulcer with/without impending perforation, fresh intestinal anastomoses, HTN, recent MI, osteoporosis, myasthenia gravis, unstable joints, septic arthritis, existing psychotic tendencies, and for possible drug interactions (eg, indomethacin).

Monitoring: Monitor for anaphylactoid reactions, appearance/exacerbation of infections, cataracts, fluid retention, psychic derangement, fat embolism, adrenocortical insufficiency. Monitor infants for hypoadrenalism and growth development. Monitor LFTs, thyroid stimulating hormone, PT, glucose, intraocular pressure, BP, and ECG.

Patient Counseling: Inform that susceptibility to infection may increase. Avoid exposure to chickenpox or measles; report immediately if exposed. Advise to restrict dietary sodium and potassium supplements. Counsel not to overuse joint after intra-articular injection, and not to d/c abruptly without medical supervision.

Administration: Oral route. Parenteral: IM, IV, intra-articular, intralesional, and soft-tissue injection. **Storage:** Inj: 20-25°C (68-77°F); excursions permitted to 15-30°C (59-86°F). PO: 20-25°C (68-77°F).

D

DEXEDRINE SPANSULES

CII

dextroamphetamine sulfate (GlaxoSmithKline)

> High potential for abuse. Prolonged use may lead to drug dependence and must be avoided. Misuse may cause sudden death and serious cardiovascular adverse events.

THERAPEUTIC CLASS: Sympathomimetic amine

INDICATIONS: Treatment of attention deficit disorder with hyperactivity (ADHD) in patients 6-16 yrs and narcolepsy.

DOSAGE: *Adults:* Individualize dose. Administer at lowest effective dose. Narcolepsy: Initial: 10mg/day. Titrate: May increase by 10mg/day at weekly intervals until optimal response is obtained. Usual: 5-60mg/day in divided doses. May give once daily. Avoid late-evening doses. *Pediatrics:* Individualize dose. Administer at lowest effective dose. Narcolepsy: ≥12 yrs: Initial: 10mg qd. Titrate: May increase by 10mg/day at weekly intervals until optimal response is obtained. 6-12 yrs: Initial: 5mg qd. Titrate: May increase weekly by 5mg/day until optimal response is obtained. Usual: 5-60mg/day in divided doses. ADHD: ≥6 yrs: Initial: 5mg qd-bid. Titrate: May increase 5mg/day at weekly intervals until optimal response is obtained. Only in rare cases will it be necessary to exceed a total of 40mg/day. May give once daily. Avoid late-evening doses.

HOW SUPPLIED: Cap, Sustained-Release: 5mg, 10mg, 15mg

CONTRAINDICATIONS: Advanced arteriosclerosis, symptomatic cardiovascular disease (CVD), moderate to severe HTN, hyperthyroidism, glaucoma, agitated states, history of drug abuse, during or within 14 days of MAOI use.

WARNINGS/PRECAUTIONS: Sudden death reported in children and adolescents with structural cardiac abnormalities or other serious heart problems. Sudden death, stroke, myocardial infarction (MI) reported in adults. Avoid use with serious structural cardiac abnormalities, cardiomyopathy, serious heart rhythm abnormalities, coronary artery disease (CAD), or other serious cardiac problems. Caution with HTN. Prior to treatment, obtain a careful history and perform physical exam to assess for cardiac disease. May exacerbate symptoms of behavior disturbance and thought disorder in psychotic patients. May induce mixed/manic episode in patients with bipolar disorder. Use at usual doses can cause treatment-emergent psychotic or manic symptoms (eg, hallucinations, delusional thinking, mania) in children and adolescents without prior history of psychotic illness. Monitor for appearance of, or worsening of, aggressive behavior or hostility in patients being treated for ADHD. May cause long-term suppression of growth in children; monitor growth during treatment. May lower seizure threshold; d/c if seizures develop. Visual disturbances (eg, difficulties with accommodation, blurring of vision) reported. May exacerbate motor and phonic tics and Tourette's syndrome.

ADVERSE REACTIONS: Palpitations, tachycardia, BP elevation, CNS overstimulation, restlessness, insomnia, dry mouth, GI disturbances, anorexia, urticaria, impotence.

INTERACTIONS: See Contraindications. GI acidifying agents (eg, guanethidine, reserpine, glutamic acid HCl, ascorbic acid, fruit juices) and urinary acidifying agents (eg, ammonium chloride, sodium acid, phosphate) lower blood levels and efficacy. Increased blood levels and potentiated by GI alkalinizing agents (eg, sodium bicarbonate) and urinary alkalinizing agents (eg, acetazolamide, some thiazides). Potentiates CNS stimulation and fatal convulsions may occur with propoxyphene overdosage. Urinary excretion of amphetamines is increased and efficacy is reduced by acidifying agents used in methenamine therapy. Potentiated effects of both agents with TCAs (eg, desipramine, protriptyline). May delay intestinal absorption of phenytoin, ethosuximide, phenobarbital. Enhanced effect with sympathomimetic agents. Inhibits adrenergic blockers. Counteracts the sedative effect of antihistamines. Antagonizes the hypotensive effect of antihypertensives. Inhibits the central stimulant effect by chlorpromazine, haloperidol, and lithium carbonate. Potentiates the analgesic effect of meperidine. Enhances the adrenergic effect of norepinephrine. Inhibits the hypotensive effect of veratrum alkaloids. Increases plasma levels of corticosteroids.

PREGNANCY: Category C, not for use in nursing.

MECHANISM OF ACTION: Amphetamine; noncatecholamine sympathomimetic amine with CNS stimulant activity. Peripheral actions include elevation of BP, weak bronchodilation, and respiratory stimulant action.

PHARMACOKINETICS: Absorption: (15mg cap) C_{max}=23.5ng/mL; T_{max}=8 hrs. **Distribution:** Found in breast milk. **Elimination:** $T_{1/2}$=12 hrs.

D

NURSING CONSIDERATIONS

Assessment: Assess for cardiovascular conditions (eg, advanced arteriosclerosis, moderate to severe HTN, cardiac structural abnormalities, cardiomyopathy, arrhythmias, heart failure, recent MI, symptomatic CVD), hyperthyroidism, agitation, glaucoma, history of drug abuse, pre-existing psychosis, bipolar disorder, prior history of seizures, pregnancy/nursing status, and possible drug interactions. Assess for presence or family history of Tourette's syndrome.

Monitoring: Monitor for cardiac abnormalities, exacerbations of behavior disturbances and thought disorders, new psychotic or manic symptoms (eg, hallucinations, delusional thinking, mania), seizures, and visual disturbances. Monitor for signs/symptoms of mixed/manic episodes in patients with bipolar disorder. Monitor HR and BP. Monitor for appearance/worsening of aggressive behavior or hostility. Monitor growth in pediatrics.

Patient Counseling: Inform of benefits and risks of treatment. Advise on appropriate use of medication. Instruct that therapy may impair the ability to engage in potentially hazardous activities (eg, operating machinery or vehicles). Inform that late-evening doses should be avoided due to the risk of insomnia. Instruct to read and understand the medication guide. Instruct to notify physician of present or family history of any health conditions.

Administration: Oral route. **Storage:** 20-25°C (68-77°F).

DEXILANT   RX
dexlansoprazole (Takeda)

THERAPEUTIC CLASS: Proton pump inhibitor

INDICATIONS: Healing of all grades of erosive esophagitis (EE) for ≤8 weeks. Maintain healing of EE and relief of heartburn for ≤6 months. Treatment of heartburn associated with symptomatic non-erosive gastroesophageal reflux disease (GERD) for 4 weeks.

DOSAGE: *Adults*: Healing of EE: 60mg qd for ≤8 weeks. Maint: 30mg qd for ≤6 months. Symptomatic Non-Erosive GERD: 30mg qd for 4 weeks. Moderate Hepatic Impairment (Child-Pugh Class B): Max: 30mg qd.

HOW SUPPLIED: Cap, Delayed-Release: 30mg, 60mg

WARNINGS/PRECAUTIONS: Symptomatic response does not preclude the presence of gastric malignancy. May increase risk of osteoporosis-related fractures of the hip, wrist or spine, especially with high-dose and long-term therapy; use lowest dose and shortest duration appropriate to the condition being treated. Hypomagnesemia reported; treatment may require d/c of therapy and monitoring of magnesium levels prior to and periodically during therapy.

ADVERSE REACTIONS: Diarrhea, abdominal pain, N/V, upper respiratory tract infection, flatulence.

INTERACTIONS: Substantially decreases atazanavir concentrations; avoid concurrent use. May alter absorption of other drugs where gastric pH is an important determinant of oral bioavailability (eg, ampicillin esters, digoxin, iron salts, ketoconazole). Monitor for increases in INR and PT with warfarin. May increase whole blood levels of tacrolimus, especially in transplant patients who are intermediate or poor metabolizers of CYP2C19. Caution with digoxin or other drugs that may cause hypomagnesemia (eg, diuretics). May decrease the mean area under the curve (AUC) of the active metabolite of clopidogrel.

PREGNANCY: Category B, not for use in nursing.

MECHANISM OF ACTION: Proton pump inhibitor; suppresses gastric acid secretion by specific inhibition of the (H^+, K^+)-ATPase in the gastric parietal cell. Blocks the final step of acid production.

PHARMACOKINETICS: Absorption: C_{max}=658ng/mL (30mg), 1397ng/mL (60mg); AUC=3275ng•h/mL (30mg), 6529ng•h/mL (60mg). T_{max}=1-2 hrs (1st peak), 4-5 hrs (2nd peak). **Distribution:** V_d=40.3L; plasma protein binding (96.1%-98.8%). **Metabolism:** Liver (extensive) via CYP3A4 (oxidation) and CYP2C19 (hydroxylation). **Elimination:** Urine (50.7%), feces (47.6%); $T_{1/2}$=1-2 hrs.

NURSING CONSIDERATIONS

Assessment: Assess for presence of gastric malignancy, osteoporosis, hepatic impairment, drug hypersensitivity, pregnancy/nursing status, and possible drug interactions. Obtain baseline magnesium levels.

Monitoring: Monitor for signs and symptoms of hypersensitivity, hypomagnesemia, bone fractures, and other adverse reactions. Monitor magnesium levels periodically.

Patient Counseling: Instruct to swallow caps whole or may open caps and sprinkle intact granules on 1 tbsp of applesauce; swallow immediately without chewing (granules should not be chewed). May be taken without regard to food. Inform to watch for signs of allergic reactions as these could be serious and may require d/c. Advise to seek medical help for any cardiovascular/ neurological symptoms, including palpitations, dizziness, seizures, and tetany.

Administration: Oral route. Refer to PI for additional administration instructions. **Storage:** 25°C (77°F); excursions permitted to 15-30°C (59-86°F).

DiaBeta RX
glyburide (Sanofi-Aventis)

THERAPEUTIC CLASS: Sulfonylurea (2nd generation)

INDICATIONS: Adjunct to diet and exercise, to improve glycemic control in adults with type 2 diabetes mellitus (DM).

DOSAGE: *Adults:* Initial: 2.5-5mg qd with breakfast or first main meal; give 1.25mg if sensitive to hypoglycemia. Titrate: Increase by no more than 2.5mg/day at weekly intervals. Maint: 1.25-20mg given qd or in divided doses. May give bid with doses >10mg/day. Max: 20mg/day. Transfer From Other Oral Antidiabetic Agents: Initial: 2.5-5mg/day. Transfer From Maximum Dose of Other Sulfonylureas: Initial: 5mg qd. Switch From Insulin: If <20 U/day: 2.5-5mg qd. If 20-40 U/ day: 5mg qd. If >40 U/day: Decrease insulin dose by 50% and give 5mg qd. Titrate: Progressive withdrawal of insulin and increase by 1.25-2.5mg/day every 2-10 days. Elderly/Debilitated/ Malnourished/Renal or Hepatic Impairment/Adrenal or Pituitary Insufficiency: Initial: 1.25mg qd. Dose conservatively.

HOW SUPPLIED: Tab: 1.25mg*, 2.5mg*, 5mg* *scored

CONTRAINDICATIONS: Diabetic ketoacidosis with or without coma, treatment with bosentan.

WARNINGS/PRECAUTIONS: Increased risk of cardiovascular (CV) mortality. Risk of hypoglycemia, especially with renal and hepatic disease; elderly, debilitated, or malnourished patients; and those with adrenal or pituitary insufficiency. May need to d/c and give insulin with stress (eg, fever, trauma). Secondary failure may occur. Hemolytic anemia may occur in patients with G6PD deficiency; caution during administration.

ADVERSE REACTIONS: Hypoglycemia, cholestatic jaundice, hepatitis, nausea, epigastric fullness, heartburn, allergic skin reactions (eg, pruritus, erythema, urticaria, morbilliform), disulfiram-like reactions (rarely), hyponatremia, LFT abnormalities, photosensitivity reactions, hematologic reactions (eg, leukopenia, agranulocytosis, thrombocytopenia), porphyria, cutanea tarda, blurred vision.

INTERACTIONS: See Contraindications. Potentiate hypoglycemia with alcohol, NSAIDs, miconazole, fluoroquinolones, highly protein-bound drugs, salicylates, sulfonamides, chloramphenicol, probenecid, MAOIs, β-blockers, ACE inhibitors, disopyramide, fluoxetine, and clarithromycin. Risk of hyperglycemia and loss of glucose control with thiazides and other diuretics, corticosteroids, phenothiazines, thyroid products, estrogens, oral contraceptives, phenytoin, nicotinic acid, sympathomimetics, calcium channel blockers, and isoniazid. Increased or decreased coumarin effects. Disulfiram-like reactions (rarely) with alcohol. Elevated liver enzymes reported with bosentan. May increase cyclosporine plasma levels and toxicity. May worsen glucose control with rifampin. β-blockers may mask signs of hypoglycemia.

PREGNANCY: Category C, not for use in nursing.

MECHANISM OF ACTION: Sulfonylurea; acts by stimulating the release of insulin from functioning β-cells in the pancreas.

PHARMACOKINETICS: Absorption: T_{max}=4 hrs. **Distribution:** Plasma protein binding (extensive). **Metabolism:** Hydroxylation. **Elimination:** Bile (50%), urine (50%); $T_{1/2}$=10 hrs.

NURSING CONSIDERATIONS

Assessment: Assess for fasting blood glucose levels, glycosylated Hgb, type 1 DM, CV complications, hypoglycemia risk factors, renal/hepatic impairment, G6PD deficiency, pregnancy/nursing status, and possible drug interactions.

Monitoring: Monitor fasting blood glucose levels regularly and glycosylated Hgb periodically. Monitor GI, dermatologic, hematologic, metabolic, DM complications (eg, diabetic ketoacidosis), hypersensitivity reactions, and blurring of vision.

Patient Counseling: Stress importance of adherence to dietary instructions, regular exercise programs, and regular testing of blood glucose levels. Advise to take with breakfast or first meal. Inform patients for potential risks, advantages, and alternative modes of therapy. Counsel about the risks, symptoms, treatment, and conditions of hypoglycemia.

Administration: Oral route. **Storage:** 25°C (77°F); excursions permitted to 15-30°C (59-86°F).

DIABINESE   RX
chlorpropamide (Pfizer)

THERAPEUTIC CLASS: Sulfonylurea (1st generation)

INDICATIONS: Adjunct to diet and exercise to improve glycemic control in adults with type 2 diabetes mellitus (DM).

DOSAGE: *Adults:* Initial: Mild-Moderately Severe, Middle-Aged, Stable DM: 250mg qd. Switch From Insulin: If <40 U/day: 250mg qd; d/c insulin abruptly. If >40 U/day: 250mg qd; reduce insulin dose by 50% for 1st few days, with subsequent further reductions based on response. Elderly: 100-125mg qd. Titrate: After 5-7 days, adjust dose upward or downward by increments of ≤50-125mg at 3-5 day intervals. Maint: Mild DM: May respond to ≤100mg qd. Moderately Severe DM: 250mg qd. Severe DM: May require 500mg qd. Max: 750mg/day. Switch From Other Oral Hypoglycemic Agents: Start at once; d/c other agents abruptly. Elderly/Debilitated/Malnourished/Renal or Hepatic Impairment: Conservative initial and maint dosing.

HOW SUPPLIED: Tab: 100mg*, 250mg* *scored

CONTRAINDICATIONS: Type 1 DM, diabetic ketoacidosis with or without coma.

WARNINGS/PRECAUTIONS: Increased risk of cardiovascular (CV) mortality reported. May produce severe hypoglycemia particularly with the elderly, debilitated, malnourished, and patients with renal/hepatic, adrenal or pituitary insufficiency; manage with appropriate glucose therapy, and monitor for a minimum of 24-48 hrs. Loss of blood glucose control may occur when exposed to stress (eg, fever, trauma, infection, or surgery); d/c therapy and start insulin. Secondary failure can occur over period of time. Treatment in patients with glucose 6-phosphate dehydrogenase (G6PD) deficiency may lead to hemolytic anemia but is also reported in patients without G6PD deficiency. Caution with G6PD deficiency and consider a non-sulfonylurea alternative therapy. Caution in elderly and while driving or operating machinery. Do not use loading or priming dose.

ADVERSE REACTIONS: Hypoglycemia, pruritus, GI disturbances (N/V, diarrhea, anorexia, hunger), leukopenia, agranulocytosis, thrombocytopenia.

INTERACTIONS: Hypoglycemic effects potentiated by alcohol, NSAIDs, other highly protein-bound drugs, salicylates, sulfonamides, chloramphenicol, probenecid, coumarins, MAOIs, β-blockers, and glucose-lowering drugs. Severe hypoglycemia reported with oral miconazole. β-blockers may mask signs of hypoglycemia. May produce disulfiram-like reaction with alcohol. May cause hyperglycemia and may lead to loss of glycemic control with thiazides and other diuretics, corticosteroids, phenothiazines, thyroid products, estrogens, oral contraceptives, phenytoin, nicotinic acid, sympathomimetics, calcium channel blockers (CCBs), and isoniazid. May prolong the effects of barbiturates; use with caution.

PREGNANCY: Category C, not for use in nursing.

MECHANISM OF ACTION: Sulfonylurea; lowers blood glucose acutely by stimulating the release of insulin from the pancreas.

PHARMACOKINETICS: Absorption: Rapid; T_{max}=2-4 hrs. **Distribution:** Found in breast milk. **Metabolism:** Hydroxylation or hydrolyzation. **Elimination:** Urine (80-90%); $T_{1/2}$=36 hrs.

NURSING CONSIDERATIONS

Assessment: Assess for type 1 DM, diabetic ketoacidosis, drug hypersensitivity, CV risk factors, hyperglycemia, adrenal/pituitary/hepatic/renal insufficiency, debilitated/malnourished condition, G6PD deficiency, pregnancy/nursing status and possible drug interactions.

Monitoring: Monitor blood glucose periodically and glycosylated Hgb. Monitor for hypoglycemia, loss of blood glucose control, hemolytic anemia, and other possible side effects.

Patient Counseling: Inform of the risks and benefits of therapy and of alternative modes of therapy. Inform of importance of adherence to dietary instructions, regular exercise, and of regular testing of blood glucose. Explain the risks, predisposing factors, symptoms, and treatment of hypoglycemia. Discuss about primary and secondary therapy failure. Instruct to promptly notify physician if symptoms of hypoglycemia or other adverse reactions occur.

Administration: Oral route. Take at a single time each am with breakfast. May divide daily dose with GI intolerance. **Storage:** Below 30°C (86°F).

DIAZEPAM INJECTION   CIV
diazepam (Various)

THERAPEUTIC CLASS: Benzodiazepine

INDICATIONS: Management of anxiety disorders or short-term relief of anxiety symptoms. Symptomatic relief of acute alcohol withdrawal symptoms (eg, acute agitation, tremor). Adjunct therapy prior to endoscopic procedures if apprehension, anxiety, or acute stress reactions are present, and to diminish the patient's recall of the procedures. Adjunct therapy for the relief of skeletal muscle spasm due to reflex spasm to local pathology (eg, inflammation of the muscles or joints, or secondary to trauma), spasticity caused by upper motor neuron disorders (eg, cerebral palsy, paraplegia), athetosis; stiff-man syndrome, and tetanus. Adjunct therapy in status epilepticus and severe recurrent convulsive seizures. Premedication for relief of anxiety and tension in patients who are to undergo surgical procedures or prior to cardioversion.

DOSAGE: *Adults:* Individualize dose. Moderate Anxiety: Usual: 2-5mg IM/IV, may repeat in 3-4 hrs. Severe Anxiety: Usual: 5-10mg IM/IV, may repeat in 3-4 hrs. Alcohol Withdrawal: Initial: 10mg IM/IV, then 5-10mg in 3-4 hrs if necessary. Endoscopic Procedures: ≤10mg IV (up to 20mg), or 5-10mg IM 30 min prior to procedure. Muscle Spasm: Initial: 5-10mg IM/IV, then 5-10mg in 3-4 hrs if necessary. For tetanus, larger doses may be required. Status Epilepticus/Severe Recurrent Seizures: Initial: 5-10mg (IV preferred), may be repeated at 10-15 min intervals up to 30mg. May repeat in 2-4 hrs with caution. Preoperative: Usual: 10mg IM. Cardioversion: 5-15mg IV, within 5-10 min prior to procedure. Elderly/Debilitated: Usual: 2-5mg. Titrate: Increase slowly. *Pediatrics:* Individualize dose. Tetanus: ≥5 yrs: Usual: 5-10mg IM/IV repeated q3-4 hrs. >30 days: Usual: 1-2mg IM/IV, slowly, repeated q3-4 hrs PRN. Respiratory assistance should be available. Status Epilepticus/Severe Recurrent Seizures: ≥5 yrs: 1mg (IV preferred, slowly) q2-5 min. Max: 10mg. Repeat in 2-4 hrs if necessary. >30 days-<5 yrs: 0.2-0.5mg (IV preferred, slowly) q2-5 min. Max: 5mg.

HOW SUPPLIED: Inj: 5mg/mL [2mL]

CONTRAINDICATIONS: Acute narrow-angle glaucoma, untreated open-angle glaucoma.

WARNINGS/PRECAUTIONS: To reduce possibility of venous thrombosis, phlebitis, local irritation, swelling, and rarely, vascular impairment, when used IV, inject slowly (taking at least 1 min for each 5mg (1mL) given), do not use small veins (eg, those on the dorsum of hand/wrist). Extreme caution during administration (particularly by IV route) to elderly, very ill patients, and those with limited pulmonary reserve due to possibility of apnea and/or cardiac arrest; resuscitative equipment should be readily available. Avoid in patients in shock, coma, or in acute alcoholic intoxication with depressed vital signs. May impair mental/physical abilities. May precipitate tonic status epilepticus in patients treated with IV for petit mal status or petit mal variant status. May increase risk of congenital malformations during 1st trimester of pregnancy; avoid during this period. Not recommended for obstetrical use. Withdrawal symptoms may occur after d/c; avoid abrupt d/c and follow gradual dosage tapering schedule. Return to seizure activity may occur, due to short-lived effect of drug after IV administration; prepare to readminister drug. Not recommended for maint. Protective measures may be necessary in highly anxious patients with evidence of depression, particularly with suicidal tendencies. Caution with hepatic/renal dysfunction. Increase in cough reflex and laryngospasm may occur with peroral endoscopic procedures; use of topical anesthetic agent and availability of necessary countermeasures are recommended. Monitor addiction-prone individuals (eg, drug addicts or alcoholics).

ADVERSE REACTIONS: Drowsiness, fatigue, ataxia, inj-site venous thrombosis and phlebitis, paradoxical reactions.

INTERACTIONS: Barbiturates, alcohol, or other CNS depressants increases depression with increased risk of apnea; resuscitative equipment should be readily available. Reduce dose of narcotic by at least 1/3 and administer in small increments. Caution with other psychotropic agents or anticonvulsants, particularly with compounds that may potentiate action (eg, phenothiazines, narcotics, barbiturates, MAOIs, antidepressants). May produce hypotension or muscular weakness with narcotics, barbiturates, or alcohol. Tagamet (cimetidine) may delay clearance. Use lower doses (2-5mg) and slow dose increase with other sedatives.

PREGNANCY: Not safe in pregnancy; safety not known in nursing.

MECHANISM OF ACTION: Benzodiazepine; induces calming effect, acts on parts of the limbic system, thalamus, and hypothalamus (animal study).

PHARMACOKINETICS: Distribution: Crosses the placenta.

NURSING CONSIDERATIONS

Assessment: Assess for acute narrow-angle glaucoma, untreated open-angle glaucoma, hypersensitivity to drug, serious illness, limited pulmonary reserve, acute alcoholic intoxication, shock, coma, evidence of depression, suicidal tendencies, chronic lung disease, unstable cardiovascular status, hepatic/renal function, pregnancy/nursing status, and possible drug interactions.

Monitoring: Monitor for apnea, cardiac arrest, return to seizure activity, increased cough reflex and laryngospasm during peroral endoscopic procedures, and other adverse reactions.

Patient Counseling: Instruct to notify physician if pregnant or intend to become pregnant. Instruct to use caution when engaging in hazardous occupation requiring complete mental alertness (eg, operating machinery, driving).

Administration: IM/IV route. (IV) Do not mix or dilute with other sol or drugs in syringe or infusion flask. May inject slowly through the infusion tubing as close as possible to the vein insertion if not feasible to administer directly IV. **Storage:** 20-25°C (68-77°F). Protect from light.

DICLOXACILLIN RX
dicloxacillin sodium (Various)

THERAPEUTIC CLASS: Penicillin (penicillinase-resistant)

INDICATIONS: Treatment of infections caused by penicillinase-producing staphylococci. May be used to initiate therapy in suspected cases of resistant staphylococcal infections prior to the availability of laboratory test results.

DOSAGE: *Adults:* Duration of therapy varies with the type and severity of infection and clinical response. Mild-Moderate Infections: 125mg q6h. Severe Infections: 250mg q6h for at least 14 days. Continue therapy for at least 48 hrs after patient becomes afebrile, asymptomatic, and cultures are negative. Treatment of endocarditis and osteomyelitis may require longer term of therapy. Group A β-hemolytic streptococcal infections should be treated for ≥10 days. May treat concurrently with probenecid if very high serum levels of penicillin are necessary.
Pediatrics: <40kg: Duration of therapy varies with the type and severity of infection and clinical response. Mild-Moderate Infections: 12.5mg/kg/day in equally divided doses q6h. Severe Infections: 25mg/kg/day in equally divided doses q6h for at least 14 days. Continue therapy for at least 48 hrs after patient becomes afebrile, asymptomatic, and cultures are negative. Treatment of endocarditis and osteomyelitis may require longer term of therapy. Group A β-hemolytic streptococcal infections should be treated for ≥10 days. May treat concurrently with probenecid if very high serum levels of penicillin are necessary.

HOW SUPPLIED: Cap: 250mg, 500mg

WARNINGS/PRECAUTIONS: Serious and occasionally fatal hypersensitivity (anaphylactic shock with collapse) reactions reported; initiate only after a comprehensive drug and allergy history has been obtained. Caution with history of allergy and/or asthma. Should not be relied upon in patients with severe illness, N/V, gastric dilatation, cardiospasm, or intestinal hypermotility. May result in bacterial resistance with prolonged use or use in the absence of a proven/suspected bacterial infection or a prophylactic indication; take appropriate measures if superinfection develops. Change to another active agent if culture tests fail to demonstrate the presence of staphylococci. Monitor organ system functions (eg, renal, hepatic, and hematopoietic) periodically with prolonged use. If renal impairment is suspected/known, reduce dose and monitor blood levels. Monitor for possible liver function abnormalities.

ADVERSE REACTIONS: Allergic reactions, N/V, diarrhea, stomatitis, black or hairy tongue, GI irritation.

INTERACTIONS: Tetracycline may antagonize the bactericidal effects; avoid concurrent use. Probenecid may increase and prolong serum levels.

PREGNANCY: Category B, caution in nursing.

MECHANISM OF ACTION: PCN (penicillinase-resistant); exerts bactericidal action against PCN-susceptible microorganisms during state of active multiplication. Inhibits biosynthesis of bacterial cell wall.

PHARMACOKINETICS: Absorption: Rapid, incomplete; C_{max}=10-17mcg/mL; T_{max}=1-1.5 hrs. **Distribution:** Plasma protein binding (97.9%); crosses placenta, found in breast milk. **Elimination:** Urine (unchanged); $T_{1/2}$=0.7 hrs.

NURSING CONSIDERATIONS

Assessment: Assess for drug hypersensitivity, history of allergy/asthma, severe illness, N/V, gastric dilatation, cardiospasm, renal impairment, intestinal hypermotility, pregnancy/nursing status, and possible drug interactions. Obtain bacteriologic studies with susceptibility testing, blood cultures, WBC, and differential cell count prior to therapy.

Monitoring: Monitor for hypersensitivity reactions, development of superinfection, new infection, and renal/hepatic impairment. Monitor organ system function periodically during prolonged therapy. Monitor blood cultures, WBC and differential cell count weekly. Monitor BUN, urinalysis, creatinine, ALT, and AST periodically.

Patient Counseling: Counsel that drug should only be used to treat bacterial, and not viral, infections (eg, common cold). Advise to take exactly ud; inform that skipping doses or not taking full course may decrease effectiveness and increase resistance. Advise not to take drug if with previous allergic reaction to PCN and to inform physician of any allergies or previous allergic reactions to any drugs. Advise to take 1 hr ac or 2 hrs pc. Advise to d/c and notify physician if SOB, wheezing, skin rash, mouth irritation, black tongue, sore throat, N/V, diarrhea, fever, swollen joints, or any unusual bleeding or bruising occurs. Advise to notify physician if taking additional medications, including nonprescription drugs.

Administration: Oral route. **Storage:** 20-25°C (68-77°F).

DIDRONEL   RX
etidronate disodium (Warner Chilcott)

THERAPEUTIC CLASS: Bisphosphonate

INDICATIONS: Treatment of symptomatic Paget's disease of bone and in the prevention and treatment of heterotopic ossification following total hip replacement or due to spinal cord injury.

DOSAGE: *Adults:* Paget's Disease: Initial: 5-10mg/kg/day for ≤6 months or 11-20mg/kg/day for ≤3 months. Doses >10mg/kg/day should be reserved when lower doses are ineffective or there is overriding need to suppress rapid bone turnover or reduce elevated cardiac output. Max: 20mg/kg/day. Retreatment Regimen: Only after an etidronate-free period of 90 days and if evidence of active disease process. Heterotopic Ossification: Total Hip Replacement: 20mg/kg/day for 1 month before and 3 months after surgery. Spinal Cord Injury: 20mg/kg/day for 2 weeks, followed by 10mg/kg/day for 10 weeks. Begin as soon as medically feasible following the injury, preferably prior to evidence of heterotopic ossification.

HOW SUPPLIED: Tab: 400mg* *scored

CONTRAINDICATIONS: Overt osteomalacia, abnormalities of the esophagus which delay esophageal emptying (eg, stricture or achalasia).

WARNINGS/PRECAUTIONS: May cause local irritation of the upper GI mucosa; caution with active upper GI problems (eg, Barrett's esophagus, dysphagia, other esophageal diseases, gastritis, duodenitis, ulcers). Esophageal adverse experiences (eg, esophagitis, esophageal ulcers, esophageal erosions) reported; d/c if dysphagia, odynophagia, retrosternal pain, or new/worsening heartburn develops. Gastric and duodenal ulcers reported. Do not increase dose prematurely in patients with Paget's disease. Maintain adequate nutritional status, particularly calcium and vitamin D. Therapy may need to be withheld in patients with enterocolitis due to diarrhea. Hyperphosphatemia may occur at doses 10-20mg/kg/day. Monitor with renal impairment; reduce dose with decreased GFR. Mild-to-moderate renal function abnormalities may occur. Delay or interrupt treatment in patients with fractures, especially of long bones, until callus is evident. Osteonecrosis of the jaw (ONJ) reported; d/c for patients requiring invasive dental procedures or consider d/c if ONJ develops. Severe, incapacitating bone, joint, and/or muscle pain reported. Monitor radiographically and biochemically, Paget's patients with predominantly lytic lesions to permit termination of therapy if unresponsive. Not for the treatment of osteoporosis. Caution in elderly.

ADVERSE REACTIONS: Diarrhea, nausea, bone pain, alopecia, arthropathy, esophagitis, hypersensitivity reactions, osteomalacia, amnesia, confusion, agranulocytosis, pancytopenia, leukopenia.

INTERACTIONS: Increased PT reported with warfarin; monitor PT. Food, especially food high in calcium (eg, milk, milk products), vitamins with minerals, or antacids which are high in metals (eg, calcium, iron, magnesium, aluminum) should be avoided within 2 hrs of dosing. Caution with risk factors for ONJ (eg, chemotherapy, corticosteroids).

PREGNANCY: Category C, caution with nursing.

MECHANISM OF ACTION: Bisphosphonate; inhibits the formation, growth, and dissolution of hydroxyapatite crystals and their amorphous precursors by chemisorption to calcium phosphate surfaces.

PHARMACOKINETICS: Elimination: Urine (50%), feces; $T_{1/2}$=1-6 hrs.

NURSING CONSIDERATIONS

Assessment: Assess for clinically overt osteomalacia, abnormalities of the esophagus which delay esophageal emptying (eg, stricture, achalasia), active upper GI problems (eg, Barrett's esophagus, dysphagia, other esophageal diseases, gastritis, duodenitis, ulcers), renal impairment, enterocolitis, fractures, upcoming dental procedures, pregnancy/nursing status, and for possible drug interactions.

Monitoring: Monitor for local irritation of the upper GI mucosa, esophageal adverse experiences (eg, esophagitis, esophageal ulcers, esophageal erosions), hyperphosphatemia, ONJ, bone pain, joint pain, and muscle pain. Monitor renal function. In Paget's patients with lytic lesions, monitor radiographically and biochemically to determine if responsive to therapy. Monitor patients with Paget's disease every 3-6 months to assess retreatment.

Patient Counseling: Instruct to notify physician if any adverse reactions occur. Counsel to maintain adequate nutritional status, particularly adequate intake of calcium and vitamin D. Food high in calcium, vitamins with minerals, or antacids which are high in metals (eg, calcium, iron, magnesium, aluminum) should be avoided within 2 hrs of dosing. Dose may be divided if GI discomfort occurs. Drink with full glass (6-8 oz.) of water, and avoid lying down after taking medication. Instruct to notify physician if any adverse reactions occur.

Administration: Oral route. Swallow with full glass (6-8 oz.) of water and avoid lying down after taking the medication. **Storage:** 25°C (77°F); excursions permitted to 15-30°C (59-86°F).

DIFFERIN
adapalene (Galderma)

RX

THERAPEUTIC CLASS: Naphthoic acid derivative (retinoid-like)

INDICATIONS: Topical treatment of acne vulgaris in patients ≥12 yrs.

DOSAGE: *Adults:* (Cre) Apply a thin film enough to cover the entire affected areas of the skin qpm. (0.1% Gel) Apply a thin film enough to cover the affected areas of the skin qhs after washing. (0.3% Gel) Apply a thin film enough to cover the entire face and other affected areas of the skin qpm after washing. Reevaluate if therapeutic results are not noticed after 12 weeks of treatment. (Lot) Apply a thin film to cover the entire face (3-4 actuations of pump) and other affected areas qd after washing.
Pediatrics: ≥12 yrs: (Cre) Apply a thin film enough to cover the entire affected areas of the skin qpm. (0.1% Gel) Apply a thin film enough to cover the affected areas of the skin qhs after washing. (0.3% Gel) Apply a thin film enough to cover the entire face and other affected areas of the skin qpm after washing. Reevaluate if therapeutic results are not noticed after 12 weeks of treatment. (Lot) Apply a thin film to cover the entire face (3-4 actuations of pump) and other affected areas qd after washing.

HOW SUPPLIED: Cre: 0.1% [45g]; Gel: 0.1% [45g, 75g], 0.3% [45g]; Lot: 0.1% [2 oz., 4 oz.]

WARNINGS/PRECAUTIONS: Certain cutaneous signs and symptoms of treatment (eg, erythema, dryness, scaling, burning) may be experienced. Minimize exposure to sunlight including sunlamps; use sunscreen products and protective clothing over treated areas if exposure cannot be avoided. Caution in patients with high levels of sun exposure, and those with inherent sensitivity to sun. Extreme weather (eg, wind, cold) may cause irritation. Avoid contact with the eyes, lips, angles of the nose, and mucous membranes. Avoid application to cuts, abrasions, eczematous or sunburned skin. (Cre/0.3% Gel) A mild transitory sensation of warmth or slight stinging may occur shortly after application. (Cre/0.1% Gel) D/C if reaction suggesting sensitivity or chemical reaction occurs. (0.1% Gel) Avoid in patients with sunburn until fully recovered. Apparent exacerbation of acne may occur. (0.3% Gel) Reactions characterized by symptoms (eg, pruritus, face edema, eyelid edema, and lip swelling) requiring medical treatment reported during postmarketing use. (Cre/0.3% Gel/Lot) Avoid waxing as a depilatory method.

ADVERSE REACTIONS: Skin erythema, scaling, dryness, burning/stinging sensation, (Gel) skin discomfort, (Cre) pruritus.

INTERACTIONS: Caution with preparations containing sulfur, resorcinol, or salicylic acid. (Cre/Gel) Caution with other potentially irritating topical products (eg, medicated/abrasive soaps and cleansers, soaps/cosmetics with strong drying effect, products with high concentrations of alcohol, astringents, spices, or limes); local irritation may be increased. (Lot) Caution with peeling, desquamating, or abrasive agents. Avoid with other potentially irritating topical products (abrasive soaps/cleansers, soaps/cosmetics with strong drying effect, products with high concentrations of alcohol, astringents, spices, or limes).

PREGNANCY: Category C, caution in nursing.

MECHANISM OF ACTION: Naphthoic acid derivative; not established. Binds to specific retinoic acid nuclear receptors and modulates cellular differentiation, keratinization, and inflammatory processes. (Cre/0.1% Gel) Suspected to normalize differentiation of follicular epithelial cells resulting in decreased microcomedone formation.

PHARMACOKINETICS: Absorption: (0.3% Gel) C_{max}=0.553ng/mL, AUC=8.37ng•h/mL. **Elimination:** (Cre/Gel) Bile. (0.3% Gel) $T_{1/2}$=17.2 hrs.

NURSING CONSIDERATIONS

Assessment: Assess for patients with high levels of sun exposure, inherent sensitivity to sun, hypersensitivity to any of the components of the drug, pregnancy/nursing status, and for possible drug interactions.

Monitoring: Monitor for sensitivity or chemical irritation, cutaneous signs/symptoms (eg, erythema, dryness, scaling, burning/stinging, or pruritus), and other adverse reactions.

Patient Counseling: Instruct to avoid exposure to sunlight and sunlamps and use sunscreen/protective clothing over treated areas when exposed. Inform that the drug may cause skin irritation when exposed to wind or cold. Instruct to avoid contact with eyes, lips, angles of the nose, and mucous membranes. Advise not to apply medication to cuts, abrasions, eczematous or sunburned skin. Counsel to avoid use of waxing as depilatory method. Advise to use moisturizers, reduce frequency of application, or d/c use, depending upon severity of side effects. Instruct to use as directed by physician.

Administration: Topical route. Storage: 20-25°C (68-77°F), excursions permitted to 15-30°C (59-86°F). Protect from freezing. (Lot) Do not refrigerate. Protect from light. Keep away from heat. Keep bottle tightly closed.

DIFICID
fidaxomicin (Optimer)

RX

THERAPEUTIC CLASS: Macrolide

INDICATIONS: Treatment of *Clostridium difficile*-associated diarrhea (CDAD) in adults ≥18 yrs.

DOSAGE: *Adults:* ≥18 yrs: Usual: 200mg bid for 10 days.

HOW SUPPLIED: Tab: 200mg

WARNINGS/PRECAUTIONS: Not effective for treatment of systemic infections. May increase the risk of the development of drug-resistant bacteria when prescribed in the absence of a proven or strongly suspected *C. difficile* infection.

ADVERSE REACTIONS: N/V, abdominal pain, GI hemorrhage, anemia, neutropenia.

PREGNANCY: Category B, caution in nursing.

MECHANISM OF ACTION: Macrolide; bactericidal against *C. difficile*, inhibiting RNA synthesis by RNA polymerases.

PHARMACOKINETICS: Absorption: Minimal; refer to PI for other pharmacokinetic parameters. **Metabolism:** Hydrolysis; OP-1118 (active metabolite). **Elimination:** Urine (0.59% OP-1118), feces (>92% fidaxomicin and OP-1118); $T_{1/2}$=11.7 hrs, 11.2 hrs (OP-1118).

NURSING CONSIDERATIONS

Assessment: Assess for CDAD and pregnancy/nursing status.

Monitoring: Monitor for development of drug-resistant bacteria and other adverse reactions.

Patient Counseling: Inform that drug only treats CDAD infections, not other bacterial or viral infections. Instruct to take exactly as directed; inform that skipping doses or not completing full course may decrease effectiveness and increase antibiotic resistance. Advise that may take with or without food.

Administration: Oral route. **Storage:** 20-25°C (68-77°F); excursions permitted 15-30°C (59-86°F).

DIFLUCAN
fluconazole (Pfizer)

RX

THERAPEUTIC CLASS: Azole antifungal

INDICATIONS: Treatment of vaginal, oropharyngeal, and esophageal candidiasis; urinary tract infection (UTI) and peritonitis caused by *Candida*; systemic *Candida* infections (eg, candidemia, disseminated candidiasis, pneumonia); and cryptococcal meningitis. Prophylaxis of candidiasis in patients undergoing bone marrow transplantation who receive cytotoxic chemotherapy and/or radiation therapy.

DOSAGE: *Adults:* Single Dose: Vaginal Candidiasis: 150mg PO. Multiple Dose: IV/PO: Individualize dose. Oropharyngeal Candidiasis: 200mg on 1st day, then 100mg qd for ≥2 weeks. Esophageal Candidiasis: 200mg on 1st day, then 100mg qd for ≥3 weeks and for ≥2 weeks following resolution of symptoms. Max: 400mg/day. Systemic *Candida* Infections: Up to 400mg/day. UTI/Peritonitis: 50-200mg/day. Cryptococcal Meningitis: 400mg on 1st day, then 200mg qd for 10-12 weeks after negative CSF culture. 400mg qd may be used. Suppression of Cryptococcal Meningitis Relapse in AIDS: 200mg qd. Prophylaxis in Bone Marrow Transplant: 400mg qd. Start prophylaxis several days before the anticipated onset of neutropenia in patients who are anticipated to have severe granulocytopenia; continue for 7 days after neutrophil count rises >1000 cells/cu mm. Renal Impairment (Multiple Doses): Initial LD: 50-400mg. Maint: CrCl ≤50mL/min (No Dialysis): Give 50% of recommended dose. Dialysis: Give 100% of recommended dose after each dialysis.
Pediatrics: IV/PO: Individualize dose. Oropharyngeal Candidiasis: 6mg/kg on 1st day, then 3mg/kg qd for ≥2 weeks. Esophageal Candidiasis: 6mg/kg on 1st day, then 3mg/kg qd for ≥3 weeks and for ≥2 weeks following resolution of symptoms. Max: 12mg/kg/day. Systemic *Candida* Infections: 6-12mg/kg/day. Cryptococcal Meningitis: 12mg/kg on 1st day, then 6mg/kg qd for 10-12 weeks after negative CSF culture. 12mg/kg qd may be used. Suppression of Cryptococcal Meningitis Relapse in AIDS: 6mg/kg qd. Renal Impairment (Multiple Doses): Initial LD: 50-400mg. Maint: CrCl ≤50mL/min (No Dialysis): Give 50% of recommended dose. Dialysis: Give 100% of recommended dose after each dialysis.

HOW SUPPLIED: Inj: 200mg/100mL, 400mg/200mL; Sus: 50mg/5mL, 200mg/5mL [35mL]; Tab: 50mg, 100mg, 150mg, 200mg

CONTRAINDICATIONS: Coadministration with terfenadine (with multiple doses ≥400mg of fluconazole), other drugs known to prolong QT interval and which are metabolized via CYP3A4 enzyme (eg, cisapride, astemizole, pimozide, quinidine).

WARNINGS/PRECAUTIONS: Associated with rare cases of serious hepatic toxicity; monitor for more severe hepatic injury if abnormal LFTs develop. D/C if signs and symptoms of liver disease develop. Rare anaphylaxis and exfoliative skin disorders reported; monitor for rash and d/c if lesions progress. Rare cases of QT prolongation and torsades de pointes reported; caution with potentially proarrhythmic conditions. Caution in elderly or with renal/hepatic dysfunction. May impair mental/physical abilities. (Sus) Contains sucrose; avoid with hereditary fructose, glucose/galactose malabsorption, and sucrase-isomaltase deficiency. (Tab) Consider risk vs. benefits of single dose PO tab vs. intravaginal agent therapy for the treatment of vaginal yeast infections.

ADVERSE REACTIONS: Headache, N/V, abdominal pain, diarrhea.

INTERACTIONS: See Contraindications. Avoid use with erythromycin or voriconazole. Risk of increased plasma concentration of other compounds metabolized by CYP2C9 and CYP3A4. Oral hypoglycemics may precipitate clinically significant hypoglycemia; monitor and adjust dose of sulfonylurea. May increase PT with coumarin-type anticoagulants; monitor and adjust dose of warfarin if necessary. May increase levels of phenytoin, voriconazole, cyclosporine, rifabutin, tacrolimus, triazolam, glipizide, glyburide, tolbutamide, theophylline, carbamazepine, dihydro-pyridine calcium channel antagonists, celecoxib, halofantrine, flurbiprofen, racemic ibuprofen, NSAIDs metabolized by CYP2C9, sirolimus, vinca alkaloids, or ethinyl estradiol-, levonorgestrel-, and norethindrone-containing oral contraceptives. Monitor SrCr with cyclosporine. Rifampin may enhance metabolism. May increase levels and psychomotor effects of midazolam; consider dose reduction and monitoring of short-acting benzodiazepines metabolized by CYP450. Cimetidine may decrease levels. HCTZ may increase levels. May reduce clearance of alfentanil, increase effect of amitriptyline or nortriptyline, and increase levels of methadone, saquinavir, or zidovudine; adjust dose if necessary. Greater incidence of abnormally elevated serum transaminases with rifampin, phenytoin, isoniazid, valproic acid, or oral sulfonylureas. Risk of carbamazepine toxicity. May increase serum bilirubin and SrCr with cyclophosphamide. May delay elimination of fentanyl leading to respiratory depression. May increase risk of myopathy and rhabdomyolysis with HMG-CoA reductase inhibitors metabolized through CYP3A4 (eg, atorvastatin and simvastatin) or CYP2C9 (eg, fluvastatin). May inhibit the metabolism of losartan; monitor BP continuously. Acute adrenal cortex insufficiency reported after d/c of long-term fluconazole in liver-transplanted patients treated with prednisone. CNS-related undesirable effects reported with all-trans-retinoid acid.

PREGNANCY: Category C (single 150mg tab for vaginal candidiasis) and D (all other indications), caution in nursing.

MECHANISM OF ACTION: Triazole antifungal; selectively inhibits fungal CYP450 dependent enzyme lanosterol 14-α-demethylase, the enzyme which converts lanosterol to ergosterol. Subsequent loss of normal sterol correlates with accumulation of 14-α-methyl sterols in fungi and may be responsible for its fungistatic activity.

PHARMACOKINETICS: Absorption: (PO) Rapid, almost complete; bioavailability (>90%); C_{max}=6.72µg/mL (fasted, single 400mg dose), T_{max}=1-2 hrs (fasted). **Distribution:** Plasma protein binding (11-12%); found in breast milk. **Elimination:** Urine (80% unchanged, 11% metabolites); $T_{1/2}$=30 hrs (PO, fasted). Refer to PI for pediatric and elderly pharmacokinetic parameters.

NURSING CONSIDERATIONS

Assessment: Assess for clinical diagnosis of fungal infection, AIDS, malignancies, serious underlying medical condition, renal/hepatic impairment, structural heart disease, electrolyte abnormalities, potential proarrhythmic conditions, hypersensitivity, pregnancy/nursing status, and possible drug interactions. (Sus) Assess for hereditary fructose, glucose/galactose malabsorption, and sucrase-isomaltase deficiency.

Monitoring: Monitor for signs/symptoms of liver disease, rash, lesions progression, and other adverse reactions. Monitor LFTs, renal function, and ECG.

Patient Counseling: Inform about risks/benefits of therapy. Advise to notify physician if pregnant/nursing and counsel about potential hazard to the fetus if pregnant or become pregnant. Counsel to d/c if skin lesions progress. Instruct to inform physician of all medications currently taking.

Administration: IV, Oral routes. Max Continuous IV Infusion Rate: 200mg/hr. Refer to PI for proper preparation and administration of each formulation. **Storage:** Tab: <30°C (86°F). Sus: Dry Powder: <30°C (86°F). Reconstituted: 5-30°C (41-86°F); discard unused portion after 2 weeks. Protect from freezing. Inj in Glass Bottles: 5-30°C (41-86°F). Protect from freezing. Inj in Viaflex Plus Plastic Containers: 5-25°C (41-77°F). Brief Exposure: Up to 40°C (104°F). Protect from freezing.

DIGIBIND

RX

digoxin immune fab (ovine) (GlaxoSmithKline)

THERAPEUTIC CLASS: Antidote, digoxin toxicity

INDICATIONS: Treatment of life-threatening digoxin intoxication. Also has been successfully used to treat digitoxin overdose.

DOSAGE: *Adults:* Acute Ingestion of Unknown Amount: Usual: Administer 10 vials, observe response, then additional 10 vials if clinically indicated. Calculation: # vials = total digitalis body load (mg)/0.5mg of digitalis bound per vial. 1 vial will bind approximately 0.5mg of digoxin (or digitoxin). Steady-State Serum Digoxin Concentrations: # of vials = (serum dig conc in ng/mL) x (wt in kg)/100. Steady-State Digitoxin Concentrations: # of vials = (serum digitoxin conc in ng/mL) x (wt in kg)/1000. If toxicity not adequately reversed after several hrs or appears to recur, may need readministration. See PI for details.
Pediatrics: Acute Ingestion of Unknown Amount: Usual: Administer 10 vials, observe response, then additional 10 vials if clinically indicated. Calculation: # vials = total digitalis body load (mg)/0.5mg of digitalis bound per vial. 1 vial will bind approximately 0.5mg of digoxin (or digitoxin). Steady-State Serum Digoxin Concentrations: Dose (mg) = (# vials) (38mg/vial). Steady-State Digitoxin Concentrations: # of vials = (serum digitoxin conc in ng/mL) x (wt in kg)/1000. If toxicity not adequately reversed after several hrs or appears to recur, may need readministration. See PI for details.

HOW SUPPLIED: Inj: 38mg

WARNINGS/PRECAUTIONS: Obtain digoxin level before initiation. Do not overlook possibility of multiple drug overdose. Risk of hypersensitivity is greater with allergies to papain, chymopapain, or other papaya extracts; skin testing may be appropriate for high-risk individuals. K⁺ levels may drop rapidly after administration; monitor closely. Digitalis toxicity may recur with renal dysfunction; caution and monitor closely. Caution with cardiac dysfunction; further deterioration may occur from digoxin withdrawal. Consider additional support with inotropes or vasodilators. Monitor for volume overload in children. D/C if anaphylactoid reaction occurs and treat appropriately.

ADVERSE REACTIONS: Allergic reactions, exacerbation of low cardiac output, congestive heart failure, hypokalemia.

PREGNANCY: Category C, caution in nursing.

MECHANISM OF ACTION: Antidote; digoxin toxicity. Binds to molecules of digoxin, making them unavailable for binding at their site of action on cells.

PHARMACOKINETICS: Elimination: Urine; $T_{1/2}$=15-20 hrs.

NURSING CONSIDERATIONS

Assessment: Assess for serum digoxin or digitoxin concentration, serum electrolytes, hypoxia, acid base disturbances, cardiovascular disease, and renal functions. Note other diseases/conditions and drug therapies.

Monitoring: Monitor for serum potassium concentration, arrhythmias, and renal function.

Patient Counseling: Counsel about adverse effects.

Administration: IV route. Refer to PI for further information. **Storage:** 2-8°C (36-46°F). Unreconstituted vials can be stored at up to 30°C (86°F) for 30 days. Reconstituted vials should be used immediately or refrigerated at 2-8°C (36-46°F) for up to 4 hrs.

DILACOR XR

RX

diltiazem HCl (Watson)

OTHER BRAND NAMES: Diltia XT (Watson)

THERAPEUTIC CLASS: Calcium channel blocker (nondihydropyridine)

INDICATIONS: Treatment of HTN alone or in combination with other antihypertensives. Management of chronic stable angina.

DOSAGE: *Adults:* Individualize dose. Take in am on an empty stomach. HTN: Initial: 180mg or 240mg qd. Titrate: May be adjusted PRN based on antihypertensive effect. Usual: 180-480mg qd. ≥60 yrs: May respond to 120mg qd. Max: 540mg qd. Angina: Initial: 120mg qd. Titrate: Adjust according to patient's needs; may titrate to a dose of up to 480mg qd. May be carried out over a 7- to 14-day period when necessary.

HOW SUPPLIED: Cap, Extended-Release: (Dilacor XR) 240mg; (Diltia XT) 120mg, 180mg, 240mg

CONTRAINDICATIONS: Sick sinus syndrome and 2nd- or 3rd-degree atrioventricular (AV) block (except with functioning ventricular pacemaker), hypotension (<90mmHg systolic), and acute myocardial infarction (MI) and pulmonary congestion documented by x-ray.

D

WARNINGS/PRECAUTIONS: Prolongs AV node refractory periods without significantly prolonging sinus node recovery time. Periods of asystole reported in a patient with Prinzmetal's angina. Worsening of congestive heart failure (CHF) reported in patients with preexisting ventricular dysfunction. Decreases in BP may occasionally result in symptomatic hypotension. Mild transaminase elevation with or without concomitant alkaline phosphatase and bilirubin elevation reported. Significant enzyme elevations and other phenomena consistent with acute hepatic injury reported in rare instances. Caution in renal, hepatic, and preexisting severe GI narrowing (pathologic or iatrogenic). Dermatologic reactions (eg, erythema multiforme, exfoliative dermatitis) may occur; d/c if such reaction persists.

ADVERSE REACTIONS: Rhinitis, pharyngitis, increased cough, asthenia, headache, constipation.

INTERACTIONS: Additive cardiac conduction effects with digitalis or β-blockers. Potential additive effects with agents known to affect cardiac contractility and/or conduction; caution and careful titration warranted. Competitive inhibition of metabolism with agents that undergo biotransformation by CYP450 mixed function oxidase. May require dosage adjustment of similarly metabolized drugs, particularly those of low therapeutic ratio (eg, cyclosporine) when initiating or stopping concomitantly administered diltiazem, especially in patients with renal/hepatic impairment. Increased levels of propranolol and carbamazepine. Increased levels with cimetidine and ranitidine. Monitor digoxin levels. Potentiates depression of cardiac contractility, conductivity, and automaticity as well as vascular dilation with anesthetics. Additive antihypertensive effect when used concomitantly with other antihypertensive agents. Dilacor XR: Sinus bradycardia resulting in hospitalization and pacemaker insertion reported with clonidine; monitor HR. Increased exposure of simvastatin; limit daily doses of both agents. Increased exposure of lovastatin. Risk of myopathy and rhabdomyolysis with statins metabolized by CYP3A4 may be increased; monitor closely.

PREGNANCY: Category C, not for use in nursing.

MECHANISM OF ACTION: Calcium channel blocker; inhibits influx of calcium ions during membrane depolarization of cardiac and vascular smooth muscles. HTN: Relaxation of vascular smooth muscle with resultant decrease in peripheral vascular resistance. Angina: Reduces myocardial oxygen demand via reductions in heart rate and systemic blood pressure at submaximal and maximal work loads.

PHARMACOKINETICS: Absorption: Well absorbed; absolute bioavailability (41%); T_{max}=4-6 hrs. **Distribution:** Plasma protein binding (70-80%); found in breast milk. **Metabolism:** Liver (extensive). Desacetyldiltiazem (major metabolite). **Elimination:** Urine (2-4%, unchanged), bile; $T_{1/2}$=5-10 hrs.

NURSING CONSIDERATIONS

Assessment: Assess for sick sinus syndrome, 2nd- or 3rd-degree AV block, hypotension, acute MI and pulmonary congestion, preexisting impairment of ventricular function, preexisting GI narrowing, renal/hepatic impairment, hypersensitivity to drug, pregnancy/nursing status, and possible drug interactions.

Monitoring: Monitor for bradycardia, AV block, symptomatic hypotension, dermatological reactions, and renal/hepatic function. Monitor laboratory parameters at regular intervals when given over prolonged periods.

Patient Counseling: Instruct to take on empty stomach and swallow cap whole; do not open, chew, or crush.

Administration: Oral route. **Storage:** 20-25°C (68-77°F).

DILANTIN   RX
phenytoin sodium (Parke-Davis)

OTHER BRAND NAMES: Dilantin-125 (Parke-Davis) - Dilantin Infatabs (Parke-Davis)

THERAPEUTIC CLASS: Hydantoin

INDICATIONS: (Cap, Extended-Release [CER], Tab, Chewable [CTB]) Control of generalized tonic-clonic (grand mal) and complex partial (psychomotor, temporal lobe) seizures. Prevention and treatment of seizures during or following neurosurgery. (Sus) Control of tonic-clonic (grand mal) and psychomotor (temporal lobe) seizures.

DOSAGE: *Adults:* Individualize dose. Do not change dose at intervals <7-10 days. (CER) Divided Daily Dosage: Initial: 100mg tid. Maint: 100mg tid-qid. Titrate: May increase up to 200mg tid, if necessary. QD Dosing: May give 300mg qd if seizure is controlled on divided doses of three 100mg cap daily. LD (Clinic/Hospital): 1g in 3 divided doses (400mg, 300mg, 300mg) given 2 hrs apart. Start maint dose 24 hrs after LD. (CTB) Initial: 100mg tid. Maint: 300-400mg/day. Titrate: May increase to 600mg/day, if necessary. May chew or swallow tab whole. Not for qd dosing. (Sus) Initial: 125mg tid. Titrate: May increase to 5 tsp (625mg) daily, if necessary. Determine serum level for optimal dosage adjustment. Elderly: Decrease dose or frequency of dosing.

Pediatrics: Individualize dose. Initial: 5mg/kg/day in two or three equally divided doses. Maint: 4-8mg/kg/day. Max: 300mg/day. >6 yrs: May require the minimum adult dose (300mg/day).

HOW SUPPLIED: CER: 30mg, 100mg; Sus: 125mg/5mL; CTB [Infatabs]: 50mg* *scored

CONTRAINDICATIONS: (Sus) Coadministration with delavirdine.

WARNINGS/PRECAUTIONS: Caution in switching patient from a product formulated with the free acid (eg, Sus, CTB) to a product formulated with the sodium salt (eg, CER) and vice versa. CTB/Sus yield higher plasma levels than CER; dose adjustments and serum level monitoring may be necessary. Avoid abrupt withdrawal; may precipitate status epilepticus. May increase risk of suicidal thoughts/behavior; monitor for worsening of depression and any unusual changes in mood or behavior. Caution with porphyria, hepatic dysfunction, elderly, and gravely ill patients. Bleeding disorder in newborns may occur; give vitamin K to mother before delivery and to neonate after birth. May cause serious skin adverse events (eg, Stevens-Johnson syndrome [SJS], toxic epidermal necrolysis [TEN]); d/c if rash occurs. Chronic use has been associated with decreased bone mineral density (eg, osteoporosis, osteomalacia) and bone fractures. May produce confusional states (eg, delirium, psychosis, encephalopathy, or cerebral dysfunction) at levels above optimal range; reduce dose or d/c if symptoms persist. Avoid use for seizures due to hypoglycemia or other metabolic causes. Not effective for absence (petit mal) seizures. Caution in the interpretation of total phenytoin plasma concentrations with renal/hepatic disease. Avoid use as an alternative therapy in patients positive for HLA-B*1502. Caution with history of hypersensitivity to structurally similar drugs (eg, barbiturates, succinimides, oxazoli-dinediones). Hyperglycemia, hematopoietic complications (eg, thrombocytopenia, leukopenia, granulocytopenia, agranulocytosis, pancytopenia with or without bone marrow suppression), and lymphadenopathy (eg, lymph node hyperplasia, pseudolymphoma, lymphoma, Hodgkin's disease) reported. (Sus) Drug reaction with eosinophilia and systemic symptoms (DRESS)/multiorgan hypersensitivity reported; evaluate immediately if signs and symptoms (eg, rash, fever, lymphadenopathy) are present and d/c if alternative etiology cannot be established. Hepatic injury, including cases of acute hepatic failure, reported; d/c with acute hepatotoxicity. (CTB, CER) Anticonvulsant hypersensitivity syndrome (AHS) (eg, arthralgias, eosinophilia, fever, liver dysfunction, lymphadenopathy, rash) reported.

ADVERSE REACTIONS: Nystagmus, ataxia, slurred speech, decreased coordination, confusion, dizziness, insomnia, transient nervousness, motor twitching, headaches, N/V, constipation, rash, hypersensitivity reactions.

INTERACTIONS: See Contraindications. Increased levels with acute alcohol intake, amiodarone, antiepileptics (eg, felbamate, topiramate, oxcarbazepine), azoles (eg, fluconazole, ketoconazole, itraconazole, voriconazole), chloramphenicol, chlordiazepoxide, cimetidine, diazepam, disulfiram, estrogens, ethosuximide, fluorouracil, fluoxetine, fluvoxamine, H$_2$-antagonists, halothane, isoniazid, methylphenidate, omeprazole, phenothiazines, salicylates, sertraline, succinimides, sulfonamides, ticlopidine, tolbutamide, trazodone, and warfarin. Decreased levels with chronic alcohol abuse, carbamazepine, reserpine, sucralfate. Decreases effects of azoles, corticosteroids, doxycycline, estrogens, furosemide, irinotecan, oral contraceptives, paclitaxel, paroxetine, quinidine, rifampin, sertraline, teniposide, theophylline, vitamin D, and warfarin. Phenobarbital, sodium valproate, valproic acid may increase or decrease levels. May decrease levels of HIV antivirals (eg, amprenavir, efavirenz, Kaletra, indinavir, nelfinavir, ritonavir, saquinavir), and antiepileptics. May increase or decrease levels of phenobarbital, sodium valproate, valproic acid. Calcium antacids decrease absorption; space dosing. Avoid with enteral feeding preparations and/or nutritional supplements. (CTB, CER) Increased levels with phenylbutazone and dicumarol. Decreased effects of coumarin anticoagulants and digitoxin. Moban brand molindone contains calcium ions that interfere with absorption. TCAs may precipitate seizures. (Sus) Decreased levels with ritonavir, nelfinavir.

PREGNANCY: Pregnancy D, not for use in nursing.

MECHANISM OF ACTION: Hydantoin; inhibits seizure activity by promoting Na efflux from neurons, stabilizing threshold against hyperexcitability caused by excessive stimulation of environmental changes capable of reducing membrane sodium gradient. Reduces the maximal activity of the brain stem centers responsible for the tonic phase of the tonic-clonic (grand mal) seizures.

PHARMACOKINETICS: Absorption: (CTB, Sus) T$_{max}$=1.5-3 hrs; (CER) T$_{max}$=4-12 hrs. **Distribution:** Highly protein bound; found in breast milk. **Metabolism:** Liver (hydroxylation). **Elimination:** Bile (inactive metabolite), urine; T$_{1/2}$=22 hrs, (CTB) T$_{1/2}$=14 hrs.

NURSING CONSIDERATIONS

Assessment: Assess the etiology of seizure. Assess for previous hypersensitivity, family history of AHS, immunosuppression, presence of grave illness, impaired hepatic function, porphyria, pregnancy/nursing status, and possible drug interactions.

Monitoring: Monitor for signs/symptoms of skin rash (eg, SJS, TEN), lymphadenopathy, and hyperglycemia in diabetic patients. Monitor for occurrence of confused states (eg, delirium, psychosis, encephalopathy), osteomalacia, and serum levels in pregnant women. Monitor for emergence/worsening of depression, suicidal thoughts, and/or any unusual changes in mood/behavior.

Patient Counseling: Inform of the importance of strictly adhering to prescribed dosage regimen. Caution on use of other drugs or alcoholic beverages without consulting physician. Counsel about the early signs and symptoms of potential hematologic, dermatologic, hypersensitivity, or hepatic reactions and instruct to immediately contact physician if these develop. Instruct to maintain proper dental hygiene while on medication to minimize risk of gingival hyperplasia. Instruct to notify physician if suicidal thoughts or mood/behavior changes emerge. Advise females about dangers of using medication during pregnancy and apprise of the potential harm to fetus. Advise that Infatabs can either be chewed thoroughly before swallowing or swallowed whole. Encourage pregnant patients to enroll in the North American Antiepileptic Drug (NAAED) Pregnancy Registry by calling 1-888-233-2334 or go to www.aedpregnancyregistry.org.

Administration: Oral route. **Storage:** 20-25°C (68-77°F). Protect from moisture. (CER) Preserve in tight, light-resistant containers. (Sus) Protect from freezing and light.

DILAUDID CII

hydromorphone HCl (Purdue Pharma)

> A schedule II opioid agonist with the highest potential for abuse and risk of respiratory depression. Alcohol, other opioids, and CNS depressants (eg, sedative-hypnotics, skeletal muscle relaxants) can potentiate respiratory depressant effects, increasing the risk of adverse outcomes, including death. (HP) A more concentrated sol and for use in opioid-tolerant patients only; do not confuse with standard parenteral formulations of hydromorphone or other opioids as overdose and death could result.

OTHER BRAND NAMES: Dilaudid-HP (Purdue Pharma)

THERAPEUTIC CLASS: Opioid analgesic

INDICATIONS: Management of pain where opioid analgesic is appropriate. (HP) Management of moderate to severe pain in opioid-tolerant patients who require higher doses of opioids.

DOSAGE: *Adults:* Individualize dose. Reassess periodically after the initial dose. (Inj) Opioid-Naive Patients: SQ/IM: Initial: 1-2mg q2-3h PRN. Titrate: Adjust dose according to severity of pain or adverse events, and patient's underlying disease and age. IV: Initial: 0.2-1mg q2-3h given slowly, over at least 2-3 min depending on dose. Titrate: Adjust dose based on response. Elderly/Debilitated: May be lowered to 0.2mg. Hepatic/Renal Impairment: Initial: 25-50% the usual starting dose depending on degree of impairment. (HP) Base starting dose on the prior dose of hydromorphone inj or on the prior dose of an alternate opioid. Refer to PI for Conversion From Prior Opioid. (Tab/Sol): Nonopioid Tolerant: Initial: 2-4mg q4h. Patients Taking Opioids: Initial: Based on prior opioid usage. Refer to PI Conversion From Prior Opioid. (Sol) Usual: 2.5-10mg q3-6h ud. (Tab) Initial: 2-4mg q4-6h. Titrate: May require gradual increase in dose if analgesia is inadequate, as tolerance develops, or pain severity increases. Elderly/Hepatic/Renal Impairment: Start at lower end of dosing range.

HOW SUPPLIED: Inj: 1mg/mL, 2mg/mL, 4mg/mL, (HP) 10mg/mL [1mL, 5mL, 50mL], 250mg; Sol: 1mg/mL [473mL]; Tab: 2mg, 4mg, 8mg* *scored

CONTRAINDICATIONS: Respiratory depression in the absence of resuscitative equipment or (Inj, HP) in unmonitored settings; (Inj, HP) Acute or severe bronchial asthma, patients with or at risk of developing GI obstruction especially paralytic ileus; (HP) Patients who are not opioid tolerant; (PO) status asthmaticus, obstetrical analgesia (labor and delivery).

WARNINGS/PRECAUTIONS: Increased risk of respiratory depression in elderly, debilitated, those suffering from conditions accompanied by hypoxia, hypercapnia; use extreme caution with chronic obstructive pulmonary disease or cor pulmonale, decreased respiratory reserve, or preexisting respiratory depression. May cause neonatal withdrawal syndrome. May exaggerate respiratory depression in the presence of head injuries, intracranial lesions, or a preexisting increase in intracranial pressure (ICP). May obscure clinical course and neurologic signs of increases in ICP with head injury. May cause severe hypotension; caution with circulatory shock. May produce orthostatic hypotension in ambulatory patients. Contains sodium metabisulfite; allergic-type reactions, including anaphylactic symptoms and life-threatening or less severe asthmatic episodes, may occur. May obscure the diagnosis or clinical course in patients with acute abdominal condition. Caution with debilitation, severe pulmonary/hepatic/renal function, myxedema, hypothyroidism, adrenocortical insufficiency (eg, Addison's disease), CNS depression or coma, toxic psychoses, prostatic hypertrophy, urethral stricture, acute alcoholism, delirium tremens, kyphoscoliosis, and in elderly; reduce initial dose. May cause spasm of the sphincter of Oddi; caution with biliary tract disease. Caution in alcoholism and other drug dependencies. May aggravate preexisting convulsions. Administration at very high doses is associated with seizures and myoclonus. No approved use in the management of addiction disorders. May impair mental/physical abilities. Physical dependence and tolerance are common during chronic therapy. Avoid abrupt d/c. (PO) Caution with gallbladder disease or following GI surgery; reduce initial dose. (Inj) Always initiate dosing in opioid-naive patients. (HP) Never administer to opioid-naive patients. Do not use for patients who are not tolerant to the respiratory depressant or sedating effects of opioids.

ADVERSE REACTIONS: Respiratory depression, apnea, cardiac arrest, lightheadedness, dizziness, sedation, N/V, sweating, flushing, dysphoria, euphoria, dry mouth, pruritus.

INTERACTIONS: See Boxed Warning. Use with caution and in reduced dosages with other CNS depressants (eg, general anesthetics, phenothiazines, centrally-acting antiemetics, tranquilizers). May enhance action of neuromuscular blocking agents and produce an increased degree of respiratory depression. May cause severe hypotension with phenothiazines, general anesthetics, or other agents which compromise vasomotor tone. Mixed agonist/antagonist analgesics (eg, pentazocine, nalbuphine, butorphanol, buprenorphine) may reduce analgesia and/or precipitate withdrawal symptoms; use with caution. (PO) Avoid with alcohol. (Inj/HP) MAOIs may potentiate action; allow at least 14 days after d/c treatment with MAOIs before starting therapy. May increase risk of urinary retention and severe constipation leading to paralytic ileus with anticholinergics or other medications with anticholinergic activity. Respiratory depression may develop with other agents that depress respiration.

PREGNANCY: Category C, not for use in nursing.

MECHANISM OF ACTION: Opioid analgesic; mechanism not established. Suspected to bind to specific CNS opiate receptors to produce analgesia.

PHARMACOKINETICS: Absorption: (PO) Rapid. (Tab) Bioavailability (24%); C_{max}=5.5ng, T_{max}=0.74 hrs, AUC=23.7ng•hr/mL. (Sol) C_{max}=5.7ng, T_{max}=0.73 hrs, AUC=24.6ng•hr/mL. **Distribution:** Plasma protein binding (8-19%); V_d=302.9L (IV Bolus); crosses placenta, found in breast milk. **Metabolism:** Liver (extensive) via glucuronidation; hydromorphone-3-glucuronide (metabolite). **Elimination:** Urine; $T_{1/2}$=2.3 hrs (IV), 2.6 hrs (Tab), 2.8 hrs (Sol).

NURSING CONSIDERATIONS

Assessment: Assess for pain intensity, medical status, opioid tolerance, risk factors for abuse/addiction, or any other conditions where treatment is contraindicated or cautioned. Assess for drug hypersensitivity, pregnancy/nursing status, renal/hepatic function, and possible drug interactions.

Monitoring: Monitor for signs/symptoms of respiratory depression, hypotension, increasing airway resistance, apnea, misuse or abuse, addiction, tolerance or dependence, allergic/anaphylactic reactions, asthmatic episodes, hypersensitivity, seizures, myoclonus, alleviation of pain, and other adverse reactions. Monitor BP and cardiac output.

Patient Counseling: Inform that medication may cause serious adverse effects (eg, respiratory depression) if not taken ud. Instruct to report pain and any adverse effects experienced, avoid using other CNS depressants and alcohol, avoid abrupt withdrawal, and not to adjust dose without prescriber's consent. Inform that drug may impair mental/physical abilities; use caution when performing hazardous tasks (eg, operating machinery/driving). Inform pregnant women and women who plan to become pregnant about effects of analgesics and other drugs used on pregnancy. Educate that medication has abuse potential. Advise to keep secure and to dispose of unused tab and inj down the toilet.

Administration: Oral, SQ, IM, IV routes. Refer to PI for safety and handling instructions. (Inj, HP) Refer to PI for administration and reconstitution instructions. **Storage:** Tab/Sol: 25°C (77°F), Inj: 20-25°C (68-77°F); excursions permitted to 15-30° (59-86°F). Protect from light. Diluted Sol: Stable at 25°C for at least 24 hrs; protected from light in most common large-volume parental solutions.

DILTIAZEM INJECTION

RX

diltiazem HCl (Various)

THERAPEUTIC CLASS: Calcium channel blocker (nondihydropyridine)

INDICATIONS: Temporary control of rapid ventricular rate in atrial fibrillation/flutter (A-Fib/Flutter). Rapid conversion of paroxysmal supraventricular tachycardia (PSVT) to sinus rhythm.

DOSAGE: *Adults:* Bolus: 0.25mg/kg IV over 2 min. If no response after 15 min, may give 2nd dose of 0.35mg/kg over 2 min. Continuous Infusion: 0.25-0.35mg/kg IV bolus, then 10mg/hr. Titrate: Increase by 5mg/hr. Max: 15mg/hr and duration up to 24 hrs.

HOW SUPPLIED: Inj: 5mg/mL

CONTRAINDICATIONS: Sick sinus syndrome and 2nd- or 3rd-degree atrioventricular (AV) block (except with functioning pacemaker), severe hypotension, cardiogenic shock, concomitant IV β-blockers or within a few hrs of use, A-Fib/Flutter associated with accessory bypass tract (eg, Wolff-Parkinson-White [WPW] syndrome, short PR syndrome), ventricular tachycardia.

WARNINGS/PRECAUTIONS: Initiate in setting with resuscitation capabilities. Caution if hemodynamically compromised, and renal, hepatic, or ventricular dysfunction. Monitor ECG continuously and BP frequently. Symptomatic hypotension, acute hepatic injury reported. D/C if high-degree

AV block occurs in sinus rhythm or if persistent rash occurs. Ventricular premature beats may be present on conversion of PSVT to sinus rhythm.

ADVERSE REACTIONS: Hypotension, injection-site reactions (eg, itching, burning), vasodilation (flushing), arrhythmias.

INTERACTIONS: See Contraindications. Caution with drugs that decrease peripheral resistance, intravascular volume, myocardial contractility or conduction. Increased area under teh curve (AUC) of midazolam, triazolam, buspirone, quinidine, and lovastatin, which may require a dose adjustment due to increased clinical effects or increased adverse events. Elevates carbamazepine levels, which may result in toxicity. Cyclosporine may need dose adjustment. Potentiates the depression of cardiac contractility, conductivity, automaticity, and vascular dilation with anesthetics. Possible bradycardia, AV block, and contractility depression with oral β-blockers. Possible competitive inhibition of metabolism with drugs metabolized by CYP450. Avoid rifampin. Monitor for excessive slowing of HR and/or AV block with digoxin. Cimetidine increases peak diltiazem plasma levels and AUC.

PREGNANCY: Category C, not for use in nursing.

MECHANISM OF ACTION: Calcium channel blocker; inhibits influx of Ca^{2+} ions during membrane depolarization of cardiac and vascular smooth muscle. Has ability to slow AV nodal conduction time and prolong AV nodal refractoriness, which has therapeutic benefits on supraventricular tachycardia. Decreases peripheral resistance, resulting in decreased systolic and diastolic BP.

PHARMACOKINETICS: Distribution: V_d=305-391L; plasma protein binding (70-80%); found in breast milk. **Metabolism:** Liver (extensive) via CYP450; deacetylation, N-demethylation, O-demethylation, and conjugation; N-monodesmethyldiltiazem and desacetyldiltiazem (major metabolites). **Elimination:** Urine and bile; $T_{1/2}$=3.4 hrs (single IV inj), 4.1-4.9 hrs (constant IV infusion).

NURSING CONSIDERATIONS

Assessment: Assess for sick sinus syndrome and 2nd- or 3rd-degree AV block, presence of functioning pacemaker, severe hypotension, cardiogenic shock, A-fib or A-flutter associated with accessory bypass tract (eg, WPW syndrome, short PR syndrome), ventricular tachycardia, wide complex tachycardia, AMI, CHF, pulmonary congestion documented by x-ray, hypertrophic cardiomyopathy, renal/hepatic impairment, pregnancy/nursing status, and possible drug interactions.

Monitoring: Initiation of therapy should be done in setting with monitoring and resuscitation capabilities, including DC cardioversion/defibrillation. Monitor BP, HR, LFTs, and ECG. Monitor for hemodynamic deterioration, ventricular fibrillation, cardiac conduction abnormalities (eg, 2nd- or 3rd-degree AV block), hypotension, bradycardia, ventricular premature beats, dermatologic events (erythema multiforme/exfoliative dermatitis), and acute hepatic injury.

Patient Counseling: Initiation of therapy should be done in a setting with monitoring and resuscitation capabilities, including DC cardioversion/defibrillation. Inform of risks/benefits; report adverse reactions. Notify if pregnant/nursing.

Administration: IV route. **Storage:** 2-8°C (36-46°F). Do not freeze. Room temperature for up to 1 month. Destroy after 1 month. Diluted Sol: D5W, 0.9% NaCl, or D5W & 0.45% NaCl: Stable at 20-25°C (68-77°F) or 2-8°C (36-46°F) for at least 24 hrs when stored in a glass or polyvinylchloride bag.

DIOVAN   RX
valsartan (Novartis)

D/C when pregnancy is detected. Drugs that act directly on the renin-angiotensin system can cause injury/death to the developing fetus.

THERAPEUTIC CLASS: Angiotensin II receptor antagonist

INDICATIONS: Treatment of HTN alone or in combination with other antihypertensives. Treatment of heart failure (HF) (NYHA Class II-IV). Reduction of cardiovascular mortality in clinically stable patients with left ventricular failure/dysfunction following myocardial infarction (MI).

DOSAGE: *Adults:* HTN: Monotherapy Without Volume Depletion: Initial: 80mg or 160mg qd. Titrate: May increase to a max of 320mg qd or add diuretic. Max: 320mg/day. HF: Initial: 40mg bid. Titrate: May increase to 80mg or 160mg bid (use highest dose tolerated). Consider dose reduction of concomitant diuretics. Max: 320mg/day in divided doses. Post-MI: Initial: 20mg bid as early as 12 hrs after MI. Titrate: May increase to 40mg bid within 7 days, with subsequent titrations to 160mg bid as tolerated. Maint: 160mg bid. Consider decreasing dose if develop symptomatic hypotension or renal dysfunction. May be given with other standard post-MI treatments, including thrombolytics, aspirin, β-blockers, and statins.
Pediatrics: 6-16 yrs: HTN: Initial: 1.3mg/kg qd (up to 40mg total). Adjust dose according to BP response. Max: 2.7mg/kg (up to 160mg) qd. Use of a sus is recommended for children who cannot

swallow tabs, or if calculated dosage does not correspond to available tab strength. Adjust dose accordingly when switching dosage forms; exposure with sus is 1.6X greater than with tab.

HOW SUPPLIED: Tab: 40mg*, 80mg, 160mg, 320mg *scored

WARNINGS/PRECAUTIONS: Symptomatic hypotension may occur in patients with an activated renin-angiotensin system (eg, volume- and/or salt-depleted patients receiving high doses of diuretics); correct this condition before therapy or monitor closely. Caution when initiating therapy in HF or post-MI patients. Caution with hepatic impairment (including biliary obstructive disorders); decreased clearance shown. Changes in renal function may occur in susceptible patients. May increase SrCr/BUN with renal artery stenosis. Oliguria and/or progressive azotemia and (rarely) acute renal failure and/or death, may occur in patients with severe HF patients whose renal function may depend on the renin-angiotensin-aldosterone system activity. Increased BUN, SrCr, and K⁺ may occur in some patients with HF and preexisting renal impairment; dosage reduction and/or d/c may be required. Not recommended for pediatrics <6 yrs.

ADVERSE REACTIONS: Headache, abdominal pain, cough, increased BUN, hyperkalemia, dizziness, hypotension, SrCr elevation, viral infection, fatigue, diarrhea, arthralgia, back pain.

INTERACTIONS: Inhibitors of the hepatic uptake transporter OATP1B1 (rifampin, cyclosporine) or the hepatic efflux transporter MRP2 (ritonavir) may increase exposure. Other agents that block the renin-angiotensin system, K⁺-sparing diuretics (eg, spironolactone, triamterene, amiloride), K⁺ supplements, or salt substitutes containing K⁺ may increase serum K⁺ levels, and in HF patients may increase SrCr. Greater antihypertensive effect with atenolol. NSAIDs, including selective cyclooxygenase-2 inhibitors, may deteriorate renal function; monitor renal function periodically. Antihypertensive effect may be attenuated by NSAIDs.

PREGNANCY: Category D, not for use in nursing.

MECHANISM OF ACTION: Angiotensin II receptor antagonist; blocks vasoconstrictor and aldosterone-secreting effects of angiotensin II by selectively blocking the binding of angiotensin II to the AT_1 receptor in many tissues.

PHARMACOKINETICS: Absorption: Absolute bioavailability (25%); T_{max}=2-4 hrs. **Distribution:** Plasma protein binding (95%); (IV) V_d=17L. **Metabolism:** Valeryl 4-hydroxy valsartan (primary metabolite). **Elimination:** (Sol) Feces (83%), urine (13%). (IV) $T_{1/2}$=6 hrs.

NURSING CONSIDERATIONS

Assessment: Assess for renal/hepatic dysfunction, biliary obstruction, renal artery stenosis, volume/salt depletion, pregnancy/nursing status, and possible drug interactions.

Monitoring: Monitor for signs/symptoms of hypotension and other adverse reactions. Monitor serum K⁺ levels, BP, and renal function.

Patient Counseling: Inform about the consequences of exposure during pregnancy in females of childbearing age. Discuss treatment options with women planning to become pregnant. Instruct to report pregnancies to physician as soon as possible.

Administration: Oral route. Refer to PI for instructions on preparation of oral sus for children. **Storage:** (Tab) 25°C (77°F); excursions permitted to 15-30°C (59-86°F). Protect from moisture. (Sus) <30°C (<86°F) for up to 30 days or at 2-8°C (35-46°F) for up to 75 days.

DIOVAN HCT   RX
valsartan - hydrochlorothiazide (Novartis)

> D/C when pregnancy is detected. Drugs that act directly on the renin-angiotensin system can cause injury/death to the developing fetus.

THERAPEUTIC CLASS: Angiotensin II receptor antagonist/thiazide diuretic

INDICATIONS: Treatment of HTN. May be used in patients whose BP is not adequately controlled on monotherapy. May also be used as initial therapy in patients likely to need multiple drugs to achieve BP goals.

DOSAGE: *Adults:* Initial Therapy: 160mg-12.5mg qd. Titrate: May increase after 1-2 weeks of therapy. Max: 320mg-25mg qd. Add-On Therapy: Use if not adequately controlled with valsartan (or another angiotensin receptor blocker) alone or HCTZ alone. With dose-limiting adverse reactions to either component alone, may switch to valsartan-HCTZ containing a lower dose of that component. Titrate: May increase after 3-4 weeks of therapy if BP uncontrolled. Max: 320mg-25mg. Replacement Therapy: May substitute for titrated components.

HOW SUPPLIED: Tab: (Valsartan-HCTZ) 80mg-12.5mg, 160mg-12.5mg, 160mg-25mg, 320mg-12.5mg, 320mg-25mg

CONTRAINDICATIONS: Anuria, sulfonamide-derived drug hypersensitivity.

WARNINGS/PRECAUTIONS: Not for initial therapy with intravascular volume depletion. Symptomatic hypotension may occur in patients with activated renin-angiotensin system (eg, volume- and/or salt-depleted patients receiving high doses of diuretics); correct these conditions prior to therapy or monitor closely. Renal function changes may occur; caution in patients with renal artery stenosis, chronic kidney disease, severe congestive heart failure, or volume depletion. Monitor renal function periodically and consider withholding or d/c if clinically significant decrease in renal function develops. May cause serum electrolyte abnormalities (eg, hyperkalemia, hypokalemia, hyponatremia, hypomagnesemia); correct hypokalemia and any coexisting hypomagnesemia prior to initiation of therapy and monitor periodically. D/C if hypokalemia is accompanied by clinical signs (eg, muscular weakness, paresis, or ECG alterations). HCTZ: May cause hypersensitivity reactions and exacerbation or activation of systemic lupus erythematosus (SLE). May precipitate hepatic coma with hepatic dyfunction. May cause idiosyncratic reaction, resulting in acute transient myopia and acute angle-closure glaucoma; d/c as rapidly as possible. May alter glucose tolerance and increase serum cholesterol and TG levels. May cause or exacerbate hyperuricemia and precipitate gout in susceptible patients. May decrease urinary calcium excretion and cause elevations of serum calcium; monitor levels.

ADVERSE REACTIONS: Headache, dizziness, BUN elevations, hypokalemia, angioedema, rhabdomyolysis, dry cough, nasopharyngitis.

INTERACTIONS: HCTZ: May increase risk of lithium toxicity; avoid concurrent use. Dosage adjustment of antidiabetic drugs (eg, oral agents, insulin) may be require. May lead to symptomatic hyponatremia with carbamazepine. Ion exchange resins (eg, cholestyramine, colestipol) may reduce exposure; space dosing at least 4 hrs before or 4-6 hrs after the administration of ion exchange resins. Cyclosporine may increase risk of hyperuricemia and gout-type complications. Alcohol, barbiturates, and narcotics may potentiate orthostatic hypotension. May increase responsiveness to skeletal muscle relaxants (eg, curare derivatives). Thiazide-induced hypokalemia or hypomagnesemia may predispose patient to digoxin toxicity. Anticholinergic agents (eg, atropine, biperiden) may increase bioavailability. Prokinetic drugs may decrease bioavailability. May reduce renal excretion and enhance myelosuppressive effects of cytotoxic agents. Valsartan: Greater antihypertensive effect with atenolol. Inhibitors of the hepatic uptake transporter OATP1B1 (rifampin, cyclosporine) or the hepatic efflux transporter MRP2 (ritonavir) may increase exposure. NSAIDs (eg, selective cyclooxygenase-2 inhibitors) may deteriorate renal function including possible acute renal failure, and may attenuate antihypertensive effect.

PREGNANCY: Category D, not for use in nursing.

MECHANISM OF ACTION: Valsartan: Angiotensin II receptor antagonist; blocks vasoconstrictor and aldosterone-secreting effects of angiotensin II by selectively blocking binding of angiotensin II to AT_1 receptor. HCTZ: Thiazide diuretic; has not been established. Affects the renal tubular mechanisms of electrolyte reabsorption, directly increasing excretion of Na^+ and chloride in approximately equivalent amounts.

PHARMACOKINETICS: Absorption: Valsartan: (Cap) Absolute bioavailability (25%); T_{max}=2-4 hrs. HCTZ: Absolute bioavailability (70%); T_{max}=2-5 hrs. **Distribution:** Valsartan: Plasma protein binding (95%); (IV) V_d=17L. HCTZ: Albumin binding (40-70%); crosses placenta; found in breast milk. **Metabolism:** Valsartan: Via CYP2C9; valeryl 4-hydroxy valsartan (primary metabolite). **Elimination:** Valsartan: (Sol) Feces (83%), urine (13%); (IV) $T_{1/2}$=6 hrs. HCTZ: Urine (70% unchanged); $T_{1/2}$=10 hrs.

NURSING CONSIDERATIONS

Assessment: Assess for hypersensitivity to drugs and its components, anuria, sulfonamide-derived drug hypersensitivity, history of penicillin allergy, volume/salt depletion, risk for acute renal failure, SLE, hypokalemia, hypomagnesemia, metabolic disturbances, renal/hepatic function, pregnancy/nursing status, and possible drug interactions.

Monitoring: Monitor for signs/symptoms of hypotension, hypersensitivity reactions, idiosyncratic reaction, metabolic disturbances, decreased visual acuity, and ocular pain. Monitor BP, serum electrolytes, and renal function periodically.

Patient Counseling: Counsel about risks/benefits of therapy and possible adverse effects. Inform of potential risks if exposure occurs during pregnancy and of treatment options in women planning to become pregnant. Instruct to report pregnancies to physician as soon as possible. Caution patients that lightheadedness can occur, especially during 1st days of therapy; instruct to d/c and consult physician if syncope occurs. Caution that inadequate fluid intake, excessive perspiration, diarrhea, and vomiting may lead to an excessive fall in BP with the same consequences of lightheadedness and possible syncope. Advise not to use K^+ supplements or salt substitutes containing K^+ without consulting the physician.

Administration: Oral route. **Storage:** 25°C (77°F); excursions permitted to 15-30°C (59-86°F). Protect from moisture.

DIPHENHYDRAMINE

RX

diphenhydramine HCl (Various)

THERAPEUTIC CLASS: Antihistamine

INDICATIONS: For amelioration of allergic reactions to blood or plasma, in anaphylaxis as an adjunct to epinephrine and other standard measures after the acute symptoms have been controlled, and for other uncomplicated allergic conditions of the immediate type when PO therapy is impossible or contraindicated. For active treatment of motion sickness when PO form is impractical. For parkinsonism when PO therapy is impossible or contraindicated.

DOSAGE: *Adults:* Individualize dose. Usual: 10-50mg IV at a rate ≤25mg/min, or deep IM. May use 100mg if required. Max: 400mg/day.
Pediatrics: Individualize dose. Usual: 5mg/kg/24 hrs or 150mg/m²/24 hrs in 4 divided doses. Administer IV at a rate ≤25mg/min, or deep IM. Max: 300mg/day.

HOW SUPPLIED: Inj: 50mg/mL [1mL]

CONTRAINDICATIONS: Neonates, premature infants, nursing, as a local anesthetic use.

WARNINGS/PRECAUTIONS: Caution with narrow-angle glaucoma, stenosing peptic ulcer, pyloroduodenal obstruction, symptomatic prostatic hypertrophy, or bladder-neck obstruction. May cause hallucinations, convulsions, or death in pediatrics, especially, in overdosage. May produce excitation and may diminish mental alertness in pediatrics. Increased risk of dizziness, sedation, and hypotension in elderly. Caution with a history of bronchial asthma, increased intraocular pressure (IOP), hyperthyroidism, lower respiratory disease (eg, asthma), cardiovascular disease (CVD), or HTN. Local necrosis reported with SQ or intradermal use of IV formulation.

ADVERSE REACTIONS: Sedation, sleepiness, dizziness, disturbed coordination, epigastric distress, thickening of bronchial secretions, drug rash, hypotension, hemolytic anemia, urinary frequency, headache, photosensitivity, agranulocytosis, insomnia, anorexia.

INTERACTIONS: Additive effects with alcohol and other CNS depressants (hypnotics, sedatives, tranquilizers). MAOIs prolong and intensify anticholinergic effects.

PREGNANCY: Category B, contraindicated in nursing.

MECHANISM OF ACTION: Antihistamine; appear to compete with histamine for cell receptor sites on effector cells.

PHARMACOKINETICS: Metabolism: Liver. **Elimination:** Urine.

NURSING CONSIDERATIONS

Assessment: Assess for narrow-angle glaucoma, stenosing peptic ulcer, pyloroduodenal obstruction, prostatic hypertrophy, bladder-neck obstruction, history of bronchial asthma, increased IOP, hyperthyroidism, CVD, lower respiratory disease, HTN, local anesthetic use, nursing status, and possible drug interactions. Assess age of pediatric patients.

Monitoring: Monitor for diminished mental alertness and for other adverse reactions. Monitor for dizziness, sedation, and hypotension in elderly. Monitor for hallucinations and convulsions in pediatric patients.

Patient Counseling: Advise that the drug may cause drowsiness and has an additive effect with alcohol. Warn about engaging in activities requiring mental alertness; inform that therapy may impair physical/mental abilities.

Administration: IV/IM route. **Storage:** 20-25°C (68-77°F); excursions permitted to 15-30°C (59-86°F). Protect from light.

DIVIGEL

RX

estradiol (Upsher-Smith)

> Estrogens increase the risk of endometrial cancer. Perform adequate diagnostic measures (eg, endometrial sampling), to rule out malignancy with undiagnosed persistent or recurring abnormal vaginal bleeding. Should not be used for the prevention of cardiovascular disease or dementia. Increased risk of myocardial infarction (MI), stroke, invasive breast cancer, pulmonary embolism (PE), and deep vein thrombosis (DVT) in postmenopausal women (50-79 yrs) reported. Increased risk of developing probable dementia in postmenopausal women ≥65 yrs of age reported. Should be prescribed at the lowest effective dose and for the shortest duration consistent with treatment goals and risks.

THERAPEUTIC CLASS: Estrogen

INDICATIONS: Treatment of moderate to severe vasomotor symptoms associated with menopause.

DOSAGE: *Adults:* Initial: 0.25g qd applied on skin of right or left upper thigh. Adjust dose based on individual response. Reevaluate periodically.

HOW SUPPLIED: Gel: 0.1% [0.25g, 0.5g, 1g pkts]

CONTRAINDICATIONS: Undiagnosed abnormal genital bleeding, known/suspected/history of breast cancer, known/suspected estrogen-dependent neoplasia, active or history of DVT/PE, active or recent (within past year) arterial thromboembolic disease (eg, stroke, MI), liver dysfunction or disease, known/suspected pregnancy.

WARNINGS/PRECAUTIONS: D/C immediately if stroke, DVT, PE, or MI occur or are suspected. Caution in patients with risk factors for arterial vascular disease (eg, HTN, diabetes mellitus [DM], tobacco use, hypercholesterolemia, obesity) and/or venous thromboembolism (VTE) (eg, personal/family history of VTE, obesity, systemic lupus erythematosus [SLE]). If feasible, d/c at least 4 to 6 weeks before surgery of the type associated with increased risk of thromboembolism, or during periods of prolonged immobilization. May increase risk of breast/ovarian cancer and gallbladder disease. May lead to severe hypercalcemia in patients with breast cancer and bone metastases; d/c and take appropriate measures if occurs. Retinal vascular thrombosis reported; if visual abnormalities or migraine occurs, d/c pending examination. If examination reveals papilledema or retinal vascular lesions, d/c permanently. Consider addition of a progestin if no hysterectomy. May elevate BP, thyroid-binding globulin levels, and plasma TG, leading to pancreatitis and other complications. Caution with history of cholestatic jaundice; d/c in case of recurrence. May cause fluid retention; caution with cardiac/renal dysfunction. Caution with impaired liver function and severe hypocalcemia. May exacerbate endometriosis, asthma, DM, epilepsy, migraine or porphyria, SLE, and hepatic hemangiomas; use with caution. May affect certain endocrine and blood components in laboratory tests.

ADVERSE REACTIONS: Nasopharyngitis, upper respiratory tract infection, vaginal mycosis, breast tenderness, metrorrhagia, headache, nausea, pruritus, abdominal cramps.

INTERACTIONS: CYP3A4 inducers (eg, St. John's wort, phenobarbital, carbamazepine, rifampin) may decrease levels, which may decrease therapeutic effects and/or change uterine bleeding profile. CYP3A4 inhibitors (eg, erythromycin, clarithromycin, ketoconazole, itraconazole, ritonavir, grapefruit juice) may increase levels, which may result in side effects. Patients concomitantly receiving thyroid replacement therapy and estrogens may require increased doses of thyroid hormone.

PREGNANCY: Contraindicated in pregnancy, caution in nursing.

MECHANISM OF ACTION: Estrogen; binds to nuclear receptors in estrogen-responsive tissues. Circulating estrogens modulate pituitary secretion of gonadotropins, luteinizing hormone and follicle-stimulating hormone, through negative feedback mechanism. Reduces elevated levels of these hormones seen in postmenopausal women.

PHARMACOKINETICS: Absorption: Topical administration of variable doses resulted in different parameters. **Distribution:** Largely bound to sex hormone-binding globulin and albumin; found in breast milk. **Metabolism:** Liver to estrone (metabolite), estriol (major urinary metabolite); sulfate and glucuronide conjugation (liver); intestinal hydrolysis; CYP3A4 (partial metabolism). **Elimination:** Urine (parent compound and metabolites); $T_{1/2}$=10 hrs.

NURSING CONSIDERATIONS

Assessment: Assess for undiagnosed abnormal genital bleeding, presence/history of breast cancer, estrogen-dependent neoplasia, DVT, PE, active or recent (within past yr) arterial thromboembolic disease, liver dysfunction, history of cholestatic jaundice, drug hypersensitivity, pregnancy/nursing status, and any other conditions where treatment is contraindicated or cautioned. Assess use in patients ≥65 yrs and those with hypertriglyceridemia, hypothyroidism, hypocalcemia, asthma, DM, epilepsy, migraines or porphyria, or SLE. Assess for possible drug interactions. Assess need for progestin in women who have not had a hysterectomy.

Monitoring: Monitor for signs/symptoms of cardiovascular events, malignant neoplasms, dementia, gallbladder disease, hypercalcemia, visual abnormalities, elevations in plasma TG, pancreatitis, hypothyroidism, fluid retention, exacerbation of endometriosis or other conditions. Perform annual breast exam and regular BP monitoring. Do periodic evaluation (q3 or q6 months) to determine need for continuing therapy. Monitor thyroid function in patients on thyroid replacement therapy. In cases of undiagnosed persistent or recurring abnormal vaginal bleeding in patients with a uterus, perform adequate diagnostic measures (eg, endometrial sampling) to rule out malignancy.

Patient Counseling: Inform that therapy increases risk for uterine cancer and may increase chances of getting a heart attack, stroke, breast cancer, and blood clots. Instruct to contact physician if breast lumps, unusual vaginal bleeding, dizziness or faintness, changes in speech, severe headaches, chest pain, SOB, leg pains, changes in vision, or vomiting occurs. Advise to have yearly breast exams by a physician and to perform monthly self breast exams. Instruct not to apply on the face, breast, irritated skin, or in or around vagina. To avoid skin irritation, advise to apply to left or right upper thigh on alternating days. Instruct to avoid skin contact with others until gel is completely dried and to refrain from washing application site for at least 1 hr after application. Advise to wash hands before and after application. Inform that medication should be applied by patient, or if others need to apply, a disposable plastic glove should be used. Inform that medication contains alcohol; advise to avoid fire, flame, or smoking until applied dose has dried. If a dose is missed and next dosing is <12 hrs away, instruct to wait to apply regular dose at

normal time; if dosing is >12 hrs away, instruct to apply missed dose and resume normal dosing schedule.
Administration: Topical route. **Storage:** 20-25°C (68-77°F); excursions permitted to 15-30°C (59-86°F).

DOBUTAMINE   RX D
dobutamine HCl (Various)

THERAPEUTIC CLASS: Inotropic agent

INDICATIONS: Inotropic support in short-term treatment of cardiac decompensation due to depressed contractility resulting from organic heart disease or from cardiac surgical procedures.

DOSAGE: *Adults:* Initial: 0.5-1mcg/kg/min. Titrate: Adjust rate at intervals of few min and duration based on BP, urine flow, ectopic activity, HR, and when possible, cardiac output, central venous pressure, and/or pulmonary capillary wedge pressure. Elderly: Start at low end of dosing range. Avoid bolus injection (Dextrose). Refer to PI for infusion rate based on patient body weight.
Pediatrics: ≥30kg: (Dextrose) Initial: 0.5-1mcg/kg/min. Titrate: Adjust rate at intervals of few min and duration based on BP, urine flow, ectopic activity, HR, and when possible, cardiac output, central venous pressure, and/or pulmonary capillary wedge pressure. Avoid bolus injection. Refer to PI for infusion rate based on patient body weight.

HOW SUPPLIED: Inj: 12.5mg/mL [20mL, 40mL]; (Dextrose) 250mg/250mL, 250mg/500mL, 500mg/250mL, 500mg/500mL, 1000mg/250mL

CONTRAINDICATIONS: Idiopathic hypertrophic subaortic stenosis (IHSS). (Dextrose) Allergy to corn or corn product.

WARNINGS/PRECAUTIONS: May increase HR or BP, especially systolic pressure; caution with atrial fibrillation (A-fib) and HTN. May precipitate/exacerbate ventricular ectopic activity. Hypersensitivity reactions (eg, skin rash, fever, eosinophilia, bronchospasm) reported. Contains sulfites; caution in asthmatics. Monitor ECG, BP, pulmonary wedge pressure, and cardiac output. Correct hypovolemia prior to infusion. Improvement may not be observed with marked mechanical obstruction (eg, severe valvular aortic stenosis). May decrease serum K⁺ levels. Caution in myocardial infarction (MI) and elderly. (Dextrose) Should not administer through the same administration set as blood; pseudoagglutination or hemolysis may occur. May cause fluid/solute overloading. Avoid bolus administration. Caution with known subclinical or overt diabetes mellitus.

ADVERSE REACTIONS: Increased HR, BP and ventricular ectopic activity, hypotension, infusion-site reactions, nausea, headache, anginal pain, palpitations, SOB, decreased K⁺ levels, nonspecific chest pain, phlebitis.

INTERACTIONS: May reduce effectiveness and increase peripheral vascular resistance with recent administration of β-blockers. May increase cardiac output and lower pulmonary wedge pressure with nitroprusside.

PREGNANCY: Category B, not for use in nursing.

MECHANISM OF ACTION: Direct-acting inotropic agent; stimulates β-receptors of the heart while producing comparatively mild chronotropic, hypertensive, arrhythmogenic, and vasodilative effects.

PHARMACOKINETICS: Absorption: T_{max}=10 min. **Metabolism:** Catechol methylation and conjugation. **Elimination:** Urine (metabolites); $T_{1/2}$=2 min.

NURSING CONSIDERATIONS

Assessment: Assess for sulfite hypersensitivity or previous hypersensitivity to the drug, corn/corn product allergy, asthma, IHSS, A-fib, HTN, ventricular ectopic activity, MI, mechanical obstruction (eg, valvular aortic stenosis), pregnancy/nursing status, and possible drug interactions. Correct hypovolemia prior to treatment.

Monitoring: Closely monitor ECG, BP, urine flow, frequency of ectopic activity, HR, cardiac output, central venous pressure, and pulmonary wedge pressure. Monitor for ventricular tachycardia, hypersensitivity and allergic-type reactions, including anaphylactic symptoms and life-threatening or less severe asthmatic episodes. Monitor serum K⁺ levels.

Patient Counseling: Inform about benefits/risks of therapy. Advise to report any adverse reactions. Instruct to notify physician if pregnant or breastfeeding.

Administration: IV route. Refer to PI for compatibility, preparation, and administration instructions. **Storage:** 15-30°C (59-86°F); (Dextrose) 20-25°C (68-77°F). (VIAFLEX): Avoid excessive heat. Brief exposure to 40°C (104°F) does not adversely affect product. Protect from freezing. Do not remove from overwrap until time of use.

DOCETAXEL

RX

docetaxel (Sandoz)

> Increased treatment-related mortality reported with hepatic dysfunction, high-dose therapy, in non-small cell lung carcinoma (NSCLC) and prior platinum-based chemotherapy with docetaxel at 100mg/m². Avoid if neutrophils <1500 cells/mm³, bilirubin >ULN, or AST/ALT >1.5X ULN with alkaline phosphatase >2.5X ULN; may increase risk for the development of grade 4 neutropenia, febrile neutropenia, infections, severe thrombocytopenia, severe stomatitis, severe skin toxicity, and toxic death. Obtain LFTs before each treatment cycle and frequent blood counts to monitor for neutropenia. Severe hypersensitivity reactions reported with dexamethasone premedication; d/c immediately if rash/erythema, hypotension, bronchospasm, or anaphylaxis occurs. Contraindicated with history of severe hypersensitivity reactions to docetaxel or to drugs formulated with polysorbate 80. Severe fluid retention may occur despite dexamethasone.

OTHER BRAND NAMES: Taxotere (Sanofi-Aventis)

THERAPEUTIC CLASS: Antimicrotubule agent

INDICATIONS: Treatment of locally advanced or metastatic breast cancer (BC) and NSCLC after failure of prior chemotherapy. In combination with doxorubicin and cyclophosphamide for the adjuvant treatment of operable node-positive breast cancer. In combination with cisplatin for treatment of unresectable, locally advanced or metastatic NSCLC who have not previously received chemotherapy for this condition. In combination with prednisone for treatment of androgen-independent (hormone refractory) metastatic prostate cancer (HRPC). In combination with cisplatin and fluorouracil for the treatment of advanced gastric adenocarcinoma (GC), including adenocarcinoma of the gastroesophageal junction, in patients who have not received prior chemotherapy for advanced disease. In combination with cisplatin and fluorouracil for the induction treatment of patients with locally advanced squamous cell carcinoma of the head and neck (SCCHN).

DOSAGE: *Adults:* Premedicate with oral corticosteroids (eg, dexamethasone 8mg bid for 3 days); start 1 day prior to docetaxel (premedication regimen different with HRPC). Premedicate patients receiving cisplatin with antiemetics and provide appropriate hydration. Refer to PI for dosage adjustments during treatment. BC: 60-100mg/m² IV over 1 hr q3 weeks. Adjuvant to Operable Node-Positive BC: 75mg/m² 1 hr after doxorubicin 50mg/m² and cyclophosphamide 500mg/m² q3 weeks for 6 courses. Granulocyte-colony stimulating factor may be given as prophylaxis. NSCLC: After Platinum Therapy Failure: 75mg/m² IV over 1 hr q3 weeks. Chemotherapy-Naive: 75mg/m² IV over 1 hr followed by cisplatin 75mg/m² over 30-60 min q3 weeks. HRPC: 75mg/m² IV over 1 hr q3 weeks with prednisone 5mg bid. Premedicate with PO dexamethasone 8mg at 12 hrs, 3 hrs, and 1 hr before docetaxel. GC: 75mg/m² IV over 1 hr, followed by cisplatin 75mg/m² IV over 1-3 hrs (both on Day 1 only), followed by fluorouracil 750mg/m²/day IV over 24 hrs for 5 days, starting at end of cisplatin infusion. Repeat treatment q3 weeks. SCCHN: Induction Followed by Radiotherapy: 75mg/m² IV over 1 hr, followed by cisplatin 75mg/m² IV over 1 hr, on Day 1, followed by fluorouracil as a continuous IV infusion at 750mg/m²/day for 5 days. Administer q3 weeks for 4 cycles. Induction Followed by Chemoradiotherapy: 75mg/m² IV over 1 hr on Day 1, followed by cisplatin 100mg/m² IV over 30 min to 3 hrs, followed by fluorouracil 1000mg/m²/day as a continuous IV infusion from Day 1 to Day 4. Administer q3 weeks for 3 cycles.

HOW SUPPLIED: Inj: 10mg/mL [2mL, 8mL, 16mL], (Taxotere) 20mg/mL [1mL, 4mL]

CONTRAINDICATIONS: Neutrophils <1500 cells/mm³.

WARNINGS/PRECAUTIONS: Monitor CBC and avoid subsequent cycles until neutrophils recover to level >1500 cells/mm³ and platelets to >100,000 cells/mm³. Monitor from the first dose for possible exacerbation of preexisting effusions. Acute myeloid leukemia or myelodysplasia may occur in adjuvant therapy. Localized erythema of extremities with edema and desquamation, severe asthenia, severe peripheral motor neuropathy reported. Dose adjustment is recommended if severe skin toxicity occurs. Adjust dose or consider d/c if severe neurosensory symptoms (eg, paresthesia, dysesthesia, pain) develop. May cause fetal harm. Caution in elderly.

ADVERSE REACTIONS: Myalgia, alopecia, N/V, diarrhea, nail disorders, skin reactions, fluid retention, thrombocytopenia, anemia, neutropenia, infections, hypersensitivity, neuropathy, constipation.

INTERACTIONS: Avoid with strong CYP3A4 inhibitors (eg, ketoconazole, itraconazole, clarithromycin, atazanavir, indinavir, nefazodone, nelfinavir, ritonavir, saquinavir, telithromycin, and voriconazole). Caution with CYP3A4 inducers, inhibitors, and substrates. Increased exposure with protease inhibitors (eg, ritonavir). Renal insufficiency and renal failure reported; majority of the cases were associated with concomitant nephrotoxic drugs. Rare cases of radiation pneumonitis reported in patients receiving concomitant radiotherapy.

PREGNANCY: Category D, not for use in nursing.

MECHANISM OF ACTION: Antimicrotubule agent; acts by disrupting the microtubular network in cells that is essential for mitotic and interphase cellular functions. Binds to free tubulin and promotes assembly of tubulin into stable microtubules while simultaneously inhibiting their disassembly which results in the inhibition of mitosis in cells.

PHARMACOKINETICS: Distribution: V_d=113L; plasma protein binding (94%). **Metabolism:** CYP3A4. **Elimination:** Urine (6%, within 7 days), feces (75%, within 7 days) (80%, first 48 hrs); $T_{1/2}$=11.1 hrs.

NURSING CONSIDERATIONS

Assessment: Assess for NSCLC, preexisting effusion, hepatic impairment, hypersensitivity/allergy, pregnancy/nursing status, and possible drug interactions. Obtain baseline vital signs, weight, CBC with platelets and differential count, and LFTs.

Monitoring: Monitor for fluid retention, acute myeloid leukemia, hematologic effects, cutaneous reactions, exacerbation of effusions, neurosensory symptoms, hepatic impairment, hypersensitivity reactions, and other adverse effects. Monitor vital signs and weight, CBC with platelets and differential count, and LFTs.

Patient Counseling: Inform about risks and benefits of therapy. Advise that drug may cause fetal harm; avoid becoming pregnant and use effective contraceptives. Explain the significance of oral corticosteroid administration to help facilitate compliance; instruct to report if not compliant. Instruct to report signs of hypersensitivity reactions, fluid retention, myalgia, cutaneous, or neurologic reactions. Counsel about side effects that are associated with the drug. Explain the significance of routine blood cell counts. Instruct to monitor temperature frequently and immediately report any occurrence of fever.

Administration: IV route. Refer to PI for preparation and administration procedures/precautions. **Storage:** 2-25°C (36-77°F). Protect from bright light. After initial puncture, multiple dose vials are stable for 28 days at 2-8°C (36-46°F) and room temperature, with or without protection from light. Reconstituted Sol: 0.9% NaCl or D5W: Stable at 2-25°C (36-77°F) for 4 hrs; use within 4 hrs, including storage and administration. Do not freeze infusion sol.

DOLOPHINE
methadone HCl (Roxane)

`CII`

> Deaths, cardiac and respiratory, reported during initiation and conversion from other opioid agonists. Respiratory depression, QT interval prolongation, and serious arrhythmia (torsades de pointes) observed. Only certified/approved opioid treatment programs can dispense PO methadone for treatment of narcotic addiction. Use as analgesia should be initiated only if benefits outweigh the risks.

THERAPEUTIC CLASS: Opioid analgesic

INDICATIONS: Treatment of moderate to severe pain not responsive to non-narcotic analgesics. For detoxification treatment of opioid addiction (heroin or other morphine-like drugs). For maintenance treatment of opioid addiction (heroin or other morphine-like drugs), in conjunction with appropriate social and medical services.

DOSAGE: *Adults:* Individualize dose. Detoxification: Initial: 20-30mg single dose. Max: 30mg. Evaluate after 2-4 hrs. Give 5-10mg if withdrawal symptoms reappear. Max on 1st day of treatment: 40mg/day. Short-term Detoxification: Titrate to 40mg/day in divided doses. Continue stabilization for 2-3 days, then may decrease every 1-2 days depending on symptoms. Maint: Titrate to a dose at which opioid symptoms are prevented for 24 hrs. Usual: 80-120mg/day. Medically Supervised Withdrawal After Maint Treatment: Reduce dose <10% of established tolerance or maint dose q10-14 days. Pain (Opioid Non-Tolerant): Usual: 2.5-10mg q8-12h slowly titrated to effect. Conversion from Parenteral to PO Methadone: Initial: Use 1:2 dose ratio. See PI for switching to methadone from other chronic opioids.

HOW SUPPLIED: Tab: 5mg*, 10mg* *scored

CONTRAINDICATIONS: In any situation where opioids are contraindicated such as respiratory depression (in the absence of resuscitative equipment or in unmonitored settings), acute bronchial asthma or hypercarbia, and paralytic ileus.

WARNINGS/PRECAUTIONS: Caution with conditions accompanied by hypoxia, hypercapnia, or decreased respiratory reserve. Caution in patients with risk of prolonged QT interval; monitor CV status. Methadone given on fixed-dose schedule should be initiated only if benefits outweigh risks. Respiratory depressant effects and CSF pressure elevation may be markedly exaggerated in the presence of head injury, intracranial lesions, or preexisting increased intracranial pressure (ICP). May obscure diagnosis/clinical course of acute abdominal conditions or the clinical course of head injuries. Patients tolerant to other opioids may be incompletely tolerant to methadone. Deaths reported during conversion from chronic, high dose treatment with other opioid agonists. Drug tolerance, misuse, abuse, diversion, and physical dependence may occur; abstinence syndrome may occur if d/c abruptly in physically dependent patient. Avoid abrupt d/c if chronically administered. Abrupt d/c may lead to opioid withdrawal symptoms. May produce hypotension in patients whose ability to maintain normal BP is compromised. Ineffective in relieving anxiety. Higher and/or more frequent doses for acute pain required in maint patients on stable dose of methadone. Infants born to opioid-dependent mothers may exhibit respiratory difficulties and withdrawal symptoms. Caution in elderly/debilitated, severe hepatic or renal impairment, hypo-thyroidism, Addison's disease, prostatic hypertrophy, or urethral stricture; reduce initial dose.

ADVERSE REACTIONS: Respiratory depression, QT prolongation, arrhythmia, systemic hypoten-sion, lightheadedness, dizziness, sedation, sweating, N/V.

INTERACTIONS: Concomitant use with other opioid analgesics, general anesthesia, phenothi-azines, tranquilizers, sedatives, hypnotics, and other CNS depressants (including alcohol) may cause respiratory depression, hypotension, profound sedation, or coma. Additive effects with alcohol, other opioids, or illicit drugs that cause CNS depression. Deaths reported when abused in conjunction with benzodiazepines. Inhibitors and inducers of CYP3A4, CYP2B6, CYP2C19, CYP2C9, and CYP2D6 may alter metabolism and effects. Opioid antagonists, mixed agonist/an-tagonists, and partial agonists may precipitate withdrawal symptoms. MAOIs may cause severe reactions. Caution with drugs known to prolong QT interval and concomitant medications which may predispose to dysrhythmia. Caution with drugs capable of inducing electrolyte imbalance (eg, diuretics, laxatives, mineralocorticoid hormones). Monitor patients taking medications af-fecting cardiac conduction. Abacavir, amprenavir, efavirenz, nelfinavir, nevirapine, ritonavir, lopi-navir + ritonavir (combination) may increase clearance or decrease levels. May decrease levels of didanosine and stavudine. May increase area under the curve of zidovudine. May increase levels of desipramine.

PREGNANCY: Category C, not for use in nursing.

MECHANISM OF ACTION: Synthetic opioid analgesic; µ-agonist. Produces actions similar to morphine; acts on CNS and organs composed of smooth muscle. May also act as an N-methyl-D-aspartate (NMDA) receptor antagonist.

PHARMACOKINETICS: Absorption: Bioavailability (36-100%); C_{max}=124-1255ng/mL; T_{max}=1-7.5 hrs. **Distribution:** V_d=1.0-8.0L/kg; plasma protein binding (85-90%); found in breast milk. **Metabolism:** Hepatic N-demethylation; CYP3A4, 2B6, 2C19 (major); 2C9; 2D6 (minor). **Elimination:** Urine, feces; $T_{1/2}$=8-59 hrs.

NURSING CONSIDERATIONS

Assessment: Assess for history of acute bronchial asthma or chronic obstructive pulmonary disease, respiratory status, CNS depression, cardiac conduction abnormalities, increased intrac-ranial pressure, acute abdominal conditions, volume depletion, hepatic/renal impairment, or any other conditions where treatment is contraindicated or cautioned. Assess hypersensitivity to drug, pregnancy/nursing status, and for possible drug interactions.

Monitoring: Monitor for signs/symptoms of respiratory depression, QT prolongation and arrhyth-mias, misuse or abuse of medication, physical dependence and tolerance, withdrawal symptoms, elevations in CSF pressure, orthostatic hypotension, and hypersensitivity reactions.

Patient Counseling: Inform that drug may impair mental/physical abilities; instruct to use caution when performing hazardous tasks (eg, operating machinery/driving). Advise that drug may pro-duce orthostatic hypotension. Counsel to avoid use of other CNS depressants and alcohol during therapy. Instruct to seek medical attention if symptoms suggestive of arrhythmia (eg, palpita-tions, dizziness, lightheadedness, syncope) develop. Advise to take drug as prescribed and avoid abrupt withdrawal.

Administration: Oral route. **Storage**: 25°C (77°F); excursions permitted to 15-30°C (59-86°F).

Donnatal   RX

atropine sulfate - hyoscyamine sulfate - scopolamine hydrobromide - phenobarbital (PBM Pharmaceuticals)

OTHER BRAND NAMES: Donnatal Extentabs (PBM Pharmaceuticals)

THERAPEUTIC CLASS: Anticholinergic/barbiturate

INDICATIONS: Adjunct therapy for irritable bowel syndrome (irritable colon, spastic colon, mu-cous colitis), acute enterocolitis, and duodenal ulcers.

DOSAGE: *Adults:* (Elixir/Tab) 1-2 tabs or 5-10mL tid-qid. (Extentabs) 1 tab q8-12h. Hepatic Disease: Use lower doses.
Pediatrics: (Elixir) 45.4kg: 5mL q4h or 7.5mL q6h. 34kg: 3.75mL q4h or 5mL q6h. 22.7kg: 2.5mL q4h or 3.75mL q6h. 13.6kg: 1.5mL q4h or 2mL q6h. 9.1kg: 1mL q4h or 1.5mL q6h. 4.5kg: 0.5mL q4h or 0.75mL q6h. Hepatic Disease: Use lower doses.

HOW SUPPLIED: (Atropine-Hyoscyamine-Phenobarbital-Scopolamine) Elixir: 0.0194mg-0.1037mg-16.2mg-0.0065mg/5mL; Tab: 0.0194mg-0.1037mg-16.2mg-0.0065mg; Tab, Extended-Release: (Extentabs) 0.0582mg-0.3111mg-48.6mg-0.0195mg

CONTRAINDICATIONS: Glaucoma, obstructive uropathy (eg, bladder neck obstruction due to prostatic hypertrophy), obstructive GI disease (achalasia, pyloroduodenal stenosis, etc.), paralytic ileus, intestinal atony in elderly or debilitated, unstable cardiovascular status in acute hemorrhage, severe ulcerative colitis especially if complicated by toxic megacolon, myasthenia gravis, hiatal hernia associated with reflux esophagitis, acute intermittent porphyria, and for patients in whom phenobarbital produces restlessness and/or excitement.

WARNINGS/PRECAUTIONS: Inconclusive whether anticholinergic/antispasmodic drugs aid in duodenal ulcer healing, decrease recurrence rate, or prevent complications. Heat prostration can occur with high environmental temperatures. May be habit forming; caution with history of physical and/or psychological drug dependence. Exercise caution while operating machinery/ driving. Use with caution and lower dosage in patients with hepatic dysfunction. Caution with hepatic/renal disease, autonomic neuropathy, hyperthyroidism, coronary heart disease, congestive heart failure (CHF), arrhythmias, tachycardia, HTN. May delay gastric emptying. Diarrhea may be an early symptom of incomplete intestinal obstruction, especially with ileostomy or colostomy; treatment would be inappropriate. Avoid abrupt withdrawal in patients habituated to barbiturates.

ADVERSE REACTIONS: Xerostomia, urinary hesitancy/retention, blurred vision, tachycardia, mydriasis, cycloplegia, increased ocular tension, loss of taste, headache, nervousness, drowsiness, weakness, dizziness, insomnia, N/V.

INTERACTIONS: Phenobarbital may decrease anticoagulant effects; adjust dose.

PREGNANCY: Category C, caution in nursing.

MECHANISM OF ACTION: Anticholinergic/barbiturate; provides natural belladonna alkaloids in a specific, fixed ratio combined with phenobarbital to provide peripheral anticholinergic/antispasmodic action and mild sedation.

NURSING CONSIDERATIONS

Assessment: Assess for glaucoma, obstructive uropathy (eg, bladder-neck obstruction due to prostatic hypertrophy) obstructive disease of the GIT (achalasia, pyloroduodenal stenosis, etc.) paralytic ileus, intestinal atony, coronary heart disease, CHF, cardiac arrhythmias, tachycardia, HTN, hypersensitivity and for any other conditions where treatment is contraindicated or cautioned. Assess pregnancy/nursing status and possible drug interactions.

Monitoring: Monitor occurrence of heat prostration, drowsiness, blurred vision, HR, constipation, diarrhea, urinary hesitancy/retention, and hypersensitivity reactions.

Patient Counseling: Counsel about possible side effects and to report to a healthcare provider if any occur. Counsel about drug abuse/dependence. Advise not to engage in activities requiring mental alertness, such as operating a motor vehicle or other machinery, and not to perform hazardous work. Advise to avoid high environmental temperatures.

Administration: Oral route. **Storage**: 20-25°C (68-77°F). Protect from light and moisture.

DOPAMINE   RX
dopamine HCl (Various)

OTHER BRAND NAMES: Dopamine HCl and 5% Dextrose (Baxter)

THERAPEUTIC CLASS: Inotropic agent

INDICATIONS: For correction of hemodynamic imbalances present in shock due to MI, trauma, endotoxic septicemia, open-heart surgery, renal failure, and chronic cardiac decompensation. (Dextrose); Hypotension due to inadequate cardiac output.

DOSAGE: *Adults:* Initial: 2-5mcg/kg/min. Use 5mcg/kg/min in seriously ill. Increase in 5-10mcg/kg/min increments, up to 20-50mcg/kg/min. (Dextrose): Avoid bolus administration. Elderly: Start at low end of dosing range. Drug additives should not be made. *Pediatrics:* (Dextrose): Initial: 1-5mcg/kg/min. Max: 15-20mcg/kg/min, occasional ≥50mcg/kg/min.

HOW SUPPLIED: Inj: 40mg/mL, 80mg/mL, 160mg/mL, (Dopamine HCl and Dextrose) 800mcg/mL, 1600mcg/mL, 3200mcg/mL

CONTRAINDICATIONS: Pheochromocytoma, uncorrected tachyarrhythmias or ventricular fibrillation. (Dextrose); Allergy to corn or corn products.

WARNINGS/PRECAUTIONS: Contains sulfites. Monitor BP, urine flow, cardiac output and pulmonary wedge pressure. Correct hypovolemia, hypoxia, hypercapnia, and acidosis prior to use. Reduce infusion rate with increase in diastolic BP/marked decrease in pulse pressure; increase rate if hypotension occurs. D/C if hypotension persists. Reduce dose if increased ectopic beats occurs. Caution with history of occlusive vascular disease (eg, atherosclerosis, arterial embolism, Raynaud's disease, cold injury, diabetic endarteritis, and Buerger's disease); monitor for changes in skin color or temperature. Administer phentolamine if extravasation noted. Avoid abrupt withdrawal. (Dextrose): Do not add to any alkaline diluent solution. Do not administer at the same set as blood; pseudoagglutination or hemolysis may result. May cause fluid overloading. Caution in children and elderly. Avoid bolus administration.

ADVERSE REACTIONS: Tachycardia, palpitation, ventricular arrhythmia (high doses), dyspnea, N/V, headache, anxiety, bradycardia, hypotension, HTN, vasoconstriction.

INTERACTIONS: If treated with MAOIs within 2-3 weeks prior to administration of dopamine, reduce initial dose of dopamine to not greater than 1/10th of usual dose. Potential additive or potentiating effects on urine flow with diuretics. TCAs may potentiate cardiovascular effects of adrenergic agents. Cardiac effects antagonized by β-blockers. Peripheral vasoconstriction antagonized by α-blockers. Butyrophenones (eg, haloperidol) and phenothiazines may suppress renal and mesenteric vasodilation. Extreme caution with cyclopropane or halogenated hydrocarbon anesthetics. Concomitant use with vasopressors, vasoconstricting agents (eg, ergonovine), some oxytocic drugs, and local anesthetics may result in severe HTN. Hypotension and bradycardia reported with phenytoin; consider alternatives.

PREGNANCY: Category C, caution in nursing.

MECHANISM OF ACTION: Catecholamine; produces positive chronotropic and inotropic effects on the myocardium, resulting in increased heart rate and cardiac contractility. Acts directly by exerting an agonist action on β-adrenoreceptor and indirectly by causing release of norepinephrine from storage sites in sympathetic nerve endings.

PHARMACOKINETICS: Metabolism: Liver, kidneys, and plasma via MAO and catechol-O-methyltransferase. **Elimination:** Urine (80%) as homovanillic acid and 3,4-dihydroxyphenylacetic acid.

NURSING CONSIDERATIONS

Assessment: Assess for sulfite hypersensitivity, pheochromocytoma, uncorrected tachyarrhythmias/ventricular fibrillation, history of occlusive vascular disease (eg, atherosclerosis, arterial embolism, Raynaud's disease, cold injury, diabetic endarteritis, and Buerger's disease), pregnancy status, and possible drug interactions. Assess and correct prior to, or concurrently with, administration of therapy for hypovolemia, hypoxia, acidosis, and hypercapnia. Assess pregnancy/nursing status.

Monitoring: Close monitoring of urine flow, cardiac output, BP, and central venous pressure. Monitor for ventricular arrhythmias, decreased pulse pressure, hypotension, extravasation/peripheral ischemia; sloughing and necrosis of the surrounding tissue and allergic-type reactions, including anaphylactic symptoms and life-threatening or less severe asthmatic episodes. In occlusive vascular disease, monitor for changes in color or temperature of skin in extremities.

Patient Counseling: Inform about benefits/risks of therapy.

Administration: IV infusion route. Not for direct IV injection; drug must be diluted before administration to patient. Avoid injection to sodium bicarbonate or other alkaline and/or amphotericin B sol. Refer to PI for stability and compatibility instructions. **Storage:** 20-25°C (68-77°F); excursions permitted to 15-30°C (59-86°F). (Dopamine HCl and Dextrose): Room temperature (25°C [68°F]); excursions permitted to 40°C (77°F). Avoid excessive heat. Protect from freezing.

DORIBAX   RX
doripenem (Ortho-McNeil)

THERAPEUTIC CLASS: Carbapenem

INDICATIONS: Treatment of complicated intra-abdominal and urinary tract infections, including pyelonephritis, caused by susceptible microorganisms.

DOSAGE: *Adults:* ≥18 yrs: 500mg by IV infusion over 1 hr for 5-14 days (intra-abdominal infection) or 10 days (UTI). Renal Impairment: CrCl >50mL/min: No dose adjustment. CrCl 30-50mL/min: 250mg IV (over 1 hr) q8h. CrCl >10 to <30mL/min: 250mg IV (over 1 hr) q12h.

HOW SUPPLIED: Inj: 250mg, 500mg

WARNINGS/PRECAUTIONS: Serious and fatal hypersensitivity (anaphylactic) and serious skin reactions reported. Carefully assess previous reactions to penicillins (PCNs), cephalosporins, other β-lactams, and other allergens; d/c if allergic reaction occurs. *Clostridium difficile*-associated diarrhea (CDAD) reported. May result in bacterial resistance with prolonged use or use in the absence of a proven/suspected bacterial infection or a prophylactic indication; take appropriate measures if superinfection develops. Do not administer via inhalation; pneumonia reported. Caution in elderly. Consider alternative antibacterial therapies in patients receiving valproic acid or sodium valproate due to increased risk of breakthrough seizures.

ADVERSE REACTIONS: Headache, nausea, diarrhea, rash, phlebitis, anemia, pruritus.

INTERACTIONS: May reduce serum valproic acid levels below the therapeutic concentrations, which may increase risk of breakthrough seizures. Probenecid may increase levels by reducing renal clearance of doripenem; avoid coadministration.

PREGNANCY: Category B, caution in nursing.

MECHANISM OF ACTION: Broad-spectrum carbapenem; exerts bactericidal activity by inhibiting bacterial cell wall biosynthesis, resulting in cell death.

PHARMACOKINETICS: Absorption: C_{max}=23mcg/mL, AUC=36.3mcg•hr/mL. **Distribution:** V_d=16.8L; plasma protein binding (8.1%). **Metabolism:** Via dehydropeptidase-1; doripenem-M1 (inactive ring-opened metabolite). **Elimination:** Urine (70% unchanged and 15% metabolites), feces (<1%); $T_{1/2}$=1 hr.

NURSING CONSIDERATIONS

Assessment: Assess for previous hypersensitivity reactions to other carbapenems, cephalosporins, PCNs, or other allergens, renal function, nursing status, and possible drug interactions. Document indications for therapy and culture and susceptibility testing.

Monitoring: Monitor for signs/symptoms of anaphylactoid/hypersensitivity reactions, CDAD, superinfection, cross hyperreactivity, seizures, and other adverse reactions. Monitor for renal function with moderate or severe renal impairment and in elderly.

Patient Counseling: Inform drug only treats bacterial, not viral, infections. Take exactly as directed; inform that skipping doses or not completing full course may decrease effectiveness and increase resistance. Instruct to notify physician if taking valproic acid or if diarrhea, watery/bloody stools, hypersensitivity reactions, seizures, and other adverse reactions occur.

Administration: IV route. Refer to PI for preparation of solutions and storage of constituted solutions. Do not mix with or physically add to solutions containing other drugs. **Storage:** 25°C (77°F); excursions permitted to 15-30°C (59-86°F).

DORYX   RX
doxycycline hyclate (Warner Chilcott)

THERAPEUTIC CLASS: Tetracycline derivative

INDICATIONS: Treatment of the following infections: respiratory tract, urinary tract (UTI), lymphogranuloma venereum, psittacosis (ornithosis), trachoma, nongonococcal urethritis, relapsing fever, Rocky Mountain spotted fever, typhus fever and the typhus group, Q fever, rickettsialpox, tick fevers, inclusion conjunctivitis, tularemia, *Campylobacter fetus* infections, bartonellosis, granuloma inguinale, plague, cholera, brucellosis (in conjuction with streptomycin), anthrax (including inhalational anthrax, post-exposure), *Escherichia coli*, *Enterobacter aerogenes*, *Shigella*, and *Acinetobacter species*. Treatment of uncomplicated urethral/endocervical/rectal infections in adults. When penicillin is contraindicated, treatment of syphilis, yaws, Vincent's infection, actinomycosis, and infections caused by *Clostridium* species. Adjunct therapy for acute intestinal amebiasis and severe acne. Prophylaxis of malaria due to *Plasmodium falciparum* in short-term travelers (<4 months) to areas with chloroquine and/or pyrimethamine-sulfadoxine resistant strains.

DOSAGE: *Adults:* Usual: 100mg q12h on 1st day, followed by 100mg/day (single dose or as 50mg q12h). More Severe Infections (Chronic UTI): 100mg q12h. Streptococcal Infection: Treat for 10 days. Uncomplicated Urethral, Endocervical, or Rectal Infection/Nongonococcal Urethritis: 100mg bid for 7 days. Syphilis (Early): 100mg bid for 14 days. Syphilis (>1 yr): 100mg bid for 28 days. Acute Epididymo-Orchitis: 100mg bid for ≥10 days. Inhalational Anthrax (postexposure): 100mg bid for 60 days. Malaria Prophylaxis: 100mg qd, beginning 1-2 days before travel, continuing daily during travel and for 28 days after departure from malarious area. Elderly: Start at lower end of dosing range.
Pediatrics: >8 yrs: Usual: ≤45kg: 4.4mg/kg in 2 divided doses on 1st day, followed by 2.2mg/kg as a single or 2 divided doses on subsequent days. More Severe Infections: Up to 4.4mg/kg of body weight. >45kg: 100mg q12h on 1st day, followed by: 100mg/day (single dose or as 50mg q12h). Streptococcal Infection: Treat for 10 days. Malaria Prophylaxis: 2mg/kg qd up to 100mg qd, beginning 1-2 days before travel, continuing daily during travel and for 28 days after departure from malarious area. Inhalation Anthrax (post-exposure): <45kg: 2.2mg/kg of body weight po bid for 60 days. ≥45kg: 100mg bid for 60 days.

HOW SUPPLIED: Tab, Delayed-Release: 75mg*, 100mg*, 150mg* *scored

WARNINGS/PRECAUTIONS: May cause permanent discoloration of the teeth if used in last half of pregnancy, infancy or <8 yrs; avoid in this age group except for anthrax. Enamel hypoplasia and *Clostridium difficile*-associated diarrhea (CDAD) reported. Photosensitivity, increased BUN, and false elevations of urinary catecholamines may occur. D/C at first evidence of skin erythema. Bulging fontanels in infants and benign intracranial HTN in adults reported. May decrease fibula growth rate in premature infants, and cause fetal harm during pregnancy. Incision and drainage or other surgical procedures should be performed in conjunction with antibiotic therapy, when indicated. Those using doxycycline as a prophylaxis for malaria may transmit the infection to mosquitoes outside endemic areas. May result in bacterial resistance with prolonged use or use in the absence of a proven/suspected bacterial infection or a prophylactic indication; take appropriate measures if superinfection develops. When coexistent syphilis is suspected, perform dark-field examination before treatment and repeat blood serology monthly for ≥4 months. Caution in elderly.

ADVERSE REACTIONS: Anorexia, N/V, diarrhea, dysphagia, enterocolitis, rash, inflammatory lesions in the anogenital area, exfoliative dermatitis, hemolytic anemia, hypersensitivity reactions.

INTERACTIONS: May depress plasma PT, may require downward adjustment of anticoagulant dose. May interfere with bactericidal action of penicillin; avoid concurrent use. Impaired absorption with bismuth subsalicylate and antacids containing aluminum, calcium or magnesium and iron-containing preparations. Decreased $T_{1/2}$ with barbiturates, carbamazepine, and phenytoin. Fatal renal toxicity with methoxyflurane. May render oral contraceptives less effective.

PREGNANCY: Category D, not for use in nursing.

MECHANISM OF ACTION: Tetracycline; exert bacteriostatic effect by the inhibition of protein synthesis.

PHARMACOKINETICS: Absorption: Complete; C_{max}=2.6mcg/mL; T_{max}=2 hrs. **Distribution:** Found in breast milk. **Metabolism:** Liver. **Elimination:** Urine and feces. $T_{1/2}$=18-22 hrs.

NURSING CONSIDERATIONS

Assessment: Assess for previous hypersensitivity to the drug, pregnancy/nursing status, and possible drug interactions. Document indications for therapy, culture and susceptibility testing. Perform dark-field examinations and blood serology when coexistent syphilis is suspected.

Monitoring: Monitor for hypersensitivity reactions, photosensitivity, skin erythema, superinfection, CDAD, bulging fontanels in infants, and benign intracranial HTN in adults. Perform periodic laboratory evaluation of organ systems (eg, hematopoietic, renal, and hepatic studies) in long term therapy. When coexistent syphilis is suspected, perform blood serology repeated monthly for ≥4 months.

Patient Counseling: Apprise pregnant women of the potential hazard to fetus. Inform that the therapy does not guarantee protection against malaria; use measures that help avoid contact with mosquitoes. Advise to avoid excessive sunlight/UV light and to d/c therapy if phototoxicity occurs. Instruct to avoid food with calcium, take with adequate amount of fluid, take with food or milk if gastric irritation occurs, and may sprinkle contents on spoonful of applesauce to be swallowed without chewing followed by a glass of water. Inform that drug may increase the incidence of vaginal candidiasis. Diarrhea may occur; contact physician if watery/bloody stools develop. Inform that drug only treats bacterial, not viral, infections. Instruct to take exactly as directed, skipping doses or not completing full course may decrease effectiveness and increase resistance. Counsel on malaria prophylaxis to begin therapy 2 days before travel, continue while in the malarious area and for 4 weeks after return.

Administration: Oral route. **Storage:** 25°C (77°F); excursions permitted to 15-30°C (59-86°F). Dispense in tight, light-resistant container.

DOVONEX   RX
calcipotriene (Leo Pharma)

THERAPEUTIC CLASS: Vitamin D3 derivative

INDICATIONS: Treatment of plaque psoriasis.

DOSAGE: *Adults:* Apply a thin layer to the affected skin bid and rub in gently and completely.

HOW SUPPLIED: Cre: 0.005% [60g, 120g]

CONTRAINDICATIONS: Hypercalcemia, evidence of vitamin D toxicity. Do not use on the face.

WARNINGS/PRECAUTIONS: Transient irritation of both lesions and surrounding uninvolved skin may occur; d/c if irritation develops. Reversible elevation of serum calcium reported; d/c until normal calcium levels are restored. Safety and effectiveness in dermatoses other than psoriasis not established. Safety and effectiveness not established in pediatrics; pediatrics are at greater risk than adults of systemic adverse effects when treated with topical medication. For external use only; not for ophthalmic, PO, or intravaginal use.

ADVERSE REACTIONS: Skin irritation, rash, pruritus, dermatitis, worsening of psoriasis.

PREGNANCY: Category C, caution in nursing.

MECHANISM OF ACTION: Vitamin D3 derivative; synthetic analog of vitamin D3.

PHARMACOKINETICS: Metabolism: Liver. **Elimination:** Bile.

NURSING CONSIDERATIONS

Assessment: Assess for history of hypersensitivity to any of the components of the preparation, hypercalcemia, evidence of vitamin D toxicity, and pregnancy/nursing status.

Monitoring: Monitor for serum calcium elevation, irritation, and other adverse reactions.

Patient Counseling: Advise to use drug only ud by the physician. Inform that the medication is for external use only; instruct to avoid contact with face or eyes. Advise to wash hands after application. Counsel that the drug should not be used for any disorder other than for which it was prescribed. Instruct to report any signs of adverse reactions to the physician. Instruct patients who apply medication to the exposed portions of the body to avoid excessive exposure to either natural or artificial sunlight (eg, tanning booths, sun lamps). Instruct to keep out of the reach of children.

Administration: Topical route. Safety and efficacy demonstrated in patients treated for eight weeks. Wash hands thoroughly after use. **Storage:** 15-25°C (59-77°F). Do not freeze.

DOVONEX SCALP RX
calcipotriene (Leo Pharma)

THERAPEUTIC CLASS: Vitamin D$_3$ derivative

INDICATIONS: Topical treatment of chronic, moderately severe psoriasis of the scalp.

DOSAGE: *Adults:* Comb the hair to remove scaly debris. After suitably parting hair, apply only on lesions bid and rub in gently and completely.

HOW SUPPLIED: Sol: 0.005% [60mL]

CONTRAINDICATIONS: Acute psoriatic eruptions, hypercalcemia, evidence of vitamin D toxicity.

WARNINGS/PRECAUTIONS: Avoid contact with the eyes or mucous membranes. D/C if sensitivity reaction occurs or if excessive irritation develops on uninvolved skin areas; transient irritation of both lesions and surrounding uninvolved skin may occur. Reversible elevation of serum calcium reported; d/c until normal calcium levels are restored. Safety and effectiveness in dermatoses other than psoriasis not established. Safety and effectiveness not established in pediatrics; pediatrics are at greater risk than adults of systemic adverse effects when treated with topical medication. For external use only; not for ophthalmic, PO, or intravaginal use.

ADVERSE REACTIONS: Transient burning, stinging, tingling, rash, dry skin, irritation, worsening of psoriasis.

PREGNANCY: Category C, caution in nursing.

MECHANISM OF ACTION: Vitamin D3 derivative; has not been established. Suggests that it is roughly equipotent to the natural vitamin in its effects on proliferation and differentiation of a variety of cell types.

PHARMACOKINETICS: Metabolism: Liver. **Elimination:** Bile.

NURSING CONSIDERATIONS

Assessment: Assess for history of hypersensitivity to any of the components of the preparation, acute psoriatic eruptions, hypercalcemia, evidence of vitamin D toxicity, and pregnancy/nursing status.

Monitoring: Monitor for sensitivity reaction, irritation on uninvolved skin areas, and serum calcium elevation.

Patient Counseling: Advise to use drug only ud by the physician. Inform that the medication is for external use only; instruct to avoid contact with face or eyes. Advise to wash hands after application. Counsel that the drug should not be used for any disorder other than for which it was prescribed. Instruct to report any signs of adverse reactions to the physician. Instruct patients who apply medication to the exposed portions of the body to avoid excessive exposure to either natural or artificial sunlight (eg, tanning booths, sun lamps). Instruct to keep out of the reach of children.

Administration: Topical route. Safety and efficacy demonstrated in patients treated for eight weeks. Avoid application to uninvolved scalp margins. Wash hands thoroughly after use. **Storage:** 15-25°C (59-77°F). Avoid sunlight. Do not freeze. Keep away from open flame.

DOXIL RX
doxorubicin HCl liposome (Janssen)

May lead to cardiac toxicity; include prior use of anthracyclines or anthracenediones in cumulative dose calculations. Myocardial damage may lead to congestive heart failure (CHF) when cumulative dose approaches 550mg/m². Cardiac toxicity may occur at lower cumulative doses with prior mediastinal irradiation or concurrent cyclophosphamide therapy. Acute infusion-associated reactions reported. Severe myelosuppression may occur. Reduce dose with impaired hepatic function. Severe side effects reported with accidental substitution for doxorubicin HCl; do not substitute on mg-per-mg basis.

THERAPEUTIC CLASS: Anthracycline

INDICATIONS: Treatment of ovarian cancer which has progressed or recurred after platinum-based chemotherapy. Treatment of AIDS-related Kaposi's sarcoma (KS) in patients after failure of/intolerance to prior systemic chemotherapy. In combination with bortezomib for the treatment of multiple myeloma (MM) in patients who have not previously received bortezomib and have received at least 1 prior therapy.

DOSAGE: *Adults:* Administer as IV infusion at initial rate of 1mg/min to minimize risk of infusion-related reactions; if no reactions, may increase rate to complete infusion over 1 hr. Ovarian Cancer: 50mg/m^2 IV q4 weeks (for as long as patient tolerates treatment, does not progress, and has no evidence of cardiotoxicity) for a minimum of 4 courses. Consider pretreatment or concomitant antiemetics. KS: 20mg/m^2 IV q3 weeks for as long as responding satisfactorily and tolerating treatment. MM: Give bortezomib 1.3mg/m^2 IV bolus on Days 1, 4, 8, and 11, q3 weeks. Give doxorubicin 30mg/m^2 IV as a 1-hr IV infusion on Day 4 following bortezomib. May treat for up to 8 cycles until disease progression or occurrence of unacceptable toxicity. Hepatic Dysfunction: If serum bilirubin 1.2-3mg/dL, give 50% of normal dose. If serum bilirubin >3mg/dL, give 25% of normal dose. Adjust or delay dose based on toxicities; refer to PI for recommended dose modification guidelines.

HOW SUPPLIED: Inj: 2mg/mL [10mL, 30mL]

CONTRAINDICATIONS: Nursing mothers.

WARNINGS/PRECAUTIONS: Monitor cardiac function. Administer only when benefits outweigh the risks in patients with a history of cardiovascular disease (CVD). Potential for myelosuppression; perform hematological monitoring during use, including WBC, neutrophil, platelet counts, and Hgb/Hct. If hematologic toxicity occurs, dose reduction, delay of therapy, or suspension of therapy may be required. Hand-foot syndrome (HFS) reported; may need to modify dose or d/c. Recall reaction reported after radiotherapy. May cause fetal harm. Avoid extravasation.

ADVERSE REACTIONS: Cardiac toxicity, myelosuppression, neutropenia, anemia, thrombocytopenia, stomatitis, fever, fatigue, N/V, asthenia, rash, acute infusion-related reactions, diarrhea, constipation, hand-foot syndrome.

INTERACTIONS: See Boxed Warning. May potentiate toxicity of other anticancer therapies. May exacerbate cyclophosphamide-induced hemorrhagic cystitis. May enhance hepatotoxicity of 6-mercaptopurine. May increase radiation-induced toxicity of the myocardium, mucosa, skin, and liver. Hematological toxicity may be more severe with agents that cause bone-marrow suppression.

PREGNANCY: Category D, not for use in nursing.

MECHANISM OF ACTION: Anthracycline topoisomerase inhibitor; suspected to bind DNA and inhibit nucleic acid synthesis.

PHARMACOKINETICS: Absorption: (10mg/m^2) C_{max}=4.12µg/mL, AUC=277µg/mL•h. (20mg/m^2) C_{max}=8.34µg/mL, AUC=590µg/mL•h. **Distribution:** (10mg/m^2) V_d=2.83L/m^2; (20mg/m^2) V_d=2.72L/m^2. **Metabolism:** Doxorubicinol (major metabolite). **Elimination:** 1st Phase: $T_{1/2}$=4.7 hrs (10mg/m^2); 5.2 hrs (20mg/m^2). 2nd Phase: $T_{1/2}$=52.3 hrs (10mg/m^2); 55 hrs (20mg/m^2).

NURSING CONSIDERATIONS

Assessment: Assess for history of CVD, hepatic dysfunction, hypersensitivity, pregnancy/nursing status, history of drug/radiotherapy use, and for possible drug interactions. Obtain baseline WBC, neutrophil, platelet counts, Hgb/Hct, and hepatic/cardiac function.

Monitoring: Monitor signs/symptoms of cardiotoxicity, infusion reactions, myelosuppression, radiation recall reaction, extravasation, hand-foot syndrome, and hypersensitivity reactions. Periodically monitor hepatic and cardiac function (endomyocardial biopsy, ECG, multigated radionuclide scan). Complete blood counts, including platelet counts, should be frequently obtained; at least once prior to each dose.

Patient Counseling: Inform that reddish-orange color may appear in urine and other bodily fluids may occur. Advise of pregnancy risks. Instruct to notify physician if symptoms of infusion reaction (eg, flushing, tightness in chest, or throat), HFS (eg, tingling, burning, redness, flaking, bothersome swelling, small blisters), fever of 100.5°F or higher, N/V, tiredness, weakness, rash, mild hair loss, or stomatitis occur.

Administration: IV route. Refer to PI for instructions on handling, preparation, administration, and disposal. **Storage:** Diluted/Undiluted Sol: 2-8°C (36-46°F). Administer diluted sol within 24 hrs. Avoid freezing.

DOXYCYCLINE IV   RX
doxycycline hyclate (Bedford)

THERAPEUTIC CLASS: Tetracycline derivative

INDICATIONS: Treatment of rickettsiae, *Mycoplasma pneumoniae*, psittacosis, ornithosis, lymphogranuloma venereum, granuloma inguinale, relapsing fever, chancroid, *Pasteurella pestis*, *Pasturella tularensis*, *Bartonella bacilliformis*, *Bacteroides* species, *Vibrio comma*, *Vibrio fetus*, *Brucella* species, *Escherichia coli*, *Enterobacter aerogenes*, *Shigella* species, *Mima* species, *Herellea* species, *Haemophilus influenzae*, *Klebsiella* species, *Streptococcus* species, *Diplococcus* *pneumoniae, Staphylococcus aureus,* anthrax, and trachoma. When PCN is contraindicated; treatment of *Neisseria gonorrhoeae, N.meningitis,* syphilis, yaws, *Listeria monocytogenes, Clostridium* species, *Fusobacterium fusiforme,* and *Actinomyces* species. Adjunct therapy for amebiasis.

DOSAGE: *Adults:* Usual: 200mg IV divided qd-bid on Day 1 then 100-200mg/day IV depending on severity, with 200mg administered in 1 or 2 infusions. Primary/Secondary Syphilis: 300mg/day IV for at least 10 days. Inhalational Anthrax (postexposure): 100mg IV bid. Institute oral therapy as soon as possible and continue therapy for a total of 60 days.
Pediatrics: >8 yrs: >100 lbs: Usual: 200mg IV divided qd-bid on Day 1 then 100-200mg/day IV depending on severity, with 200mg administered in 1 or 2 infusions. ≤100 lbs: 2mg/lb IV divided qd-bid on Day 1 then 1-2mg/lb/day IV divided qd-bid depending on severity. Inhalational Anthrax (postexposure): <100 lbs: 1 mg/lb IV bid. Institute oral therapy as soon as possible and continue therapy for total of 60 days.

HOW SUPPLIED: Inj: 100mg

WARNINGS/PRECAUTIONS: *Clostridium difficile*-associated diarrhea (CDAD) reported. May cause fetal harm during pregnancy. Permanent tooth discoloration during tooth development (last half of pregnancy and children <8 yrs) reported; avoid use in this age group except for anthrax treatment. Decreased bone growth in premature infants, bulging fontanels in infants and benign intracranial HTN in adults reported. May increase BUN. Photosensitivity, enamel hypoplasia reported. May result in bacterial resistance with prolonged use or use in the absence of a proven/suspected bacterial infection or a prophylactic indication; take appropriate measures if superinfection develops. Monitor hematopoietic, renal and hepatic labs periodically with long term therapy. When coexistent syphilis is suspected, perform dark-field examination before treatment and repeat blood serology monthly for ≥4 months.

ADVERSE REACTIONS: GI effects, increased BUN, rash, hypersensitivity reactions, hemolytic anemia, thrombocytopenia.

INTERACTIONS: May decrease PT; adjust anticoagulants. Avoid use with bactericidal agents (eg, penicillin).

PREGNANCY: Safety in pregnancy not known; not for use in nursing.

MECHANISM OF ACTION: Tetracycline derivative; thought to inhibit protein synthesis.

PHARMACOKINETICS: Absorption: Readily absorbed; C_{max}=2.5mcg/mL. **Elimination:** $T_{1/2}$=18-22 hrs.

NURSING CONSIDERATIONS

Assessment: Assess pregnancy status, possible drug interactions, and renal impairment. Document indications for therapy, culture, and susceptibility testing. Perform incision and drainage in conjunction with antibiotic therapy when indicated.

Monitoring: Monitor for signs/symptoms of hypersensitivity reactions, photosensitivity, superinfection, CDAD, vaginal candidiasis, benign intracranial HTN, LFTs, renal function, and hematological manifestations. In venereal disease with suspected coexistent syphilis, perform dark field exam before treatment; repeat monthly for 4 months.

Patient Counseling: Inform of pregnancy risks and photosensitivity reactions (d/c at 1st sign of skin erythema). Advise to avoid excessive sunlight/UV light; wear sunscreen or sunblock. Take as directed; skipping doses or not completing full course may decrease effectiveness and increase resistance. Inform may experience diarrhea; contact physician if watery or bloody stools, hypersensitivity reactions, superinfections, photosensitivity, or benign intracranial HTN occurs.

Administration: IV route. **Storage:** Solutions after reconstitution are stable for 8 weeks when stored at -20°C. If product warmed, care should be taken to avoid heating after thawing is complete.

DUETACT   RX
pioglitazone HCl - glimepiride (Takeda)

> Thiazolidinediones may cause or exacerbate congestive heart failure (CHF) in some patients. After initiation, observe for signs/symptoms of heart failure (HF) and manage accordingly or consider d/c therapy. Not recommended in patients with symptomatic HF. Initiation with NYHA Class III or IV HF is contraindicated.

THERAPEUTIC CLASS: Thiazolidinedione/sulfonylurea

INDICATIONS: Adjunct to diet and exercise to improve glycemic control in adults with type 2 diabetes mellitus (DM) already being treated with a thiazolidinedione and a sulfonylurea or who have inadequate glycemic control on a thiazolidinedione alone or sulfonylurea alone.

DOSAGE: *Adults:* Individualize dose. Base starting dose on current regimen of pioglitazone and/ or sulfonylurea. Administer single dose qd with 1st main meal. Current Glimepiride Monotherapy/ Switching from Combination Therapy of Pioglitazone plus Glimepiride as Separate Tabs: Initial: 30mg-2mg or 30mg-4mg qd. Adjust dose after assessing adequacy of therapeutic response.

Current Pioglitazone/Different Sulfonylurea Monotherapy or Switching from Combination Therapy of Pioglitazone plus a Different Sulfonylurea: Initial: 30mg-2mg qd. Adjust dose after assessing adequacy of therapeutic response. Elderly/Debilitated/Malnourished/Renal or Hepatic Insufficiency (ALT ≤2.5X ULN): Initial: 1mg glimepiride prior to prescribing Duetact. Systolic Dysfunction: Give lowest approved dose only after titration from 15-30mg of pioglitazone is safely tolerated. Max: 45mg-8mg. Not given more than once daily at any tab strength.

HOW SUPPLIED: Tab: (Pioglitazone-Glimepiride) 30mg-2mg, 30mg-4mg

CONTRAINDICATIONS: Established NYHA Class III or IV HF; diabetic ketoacidosis with or without coma.

WARNINGS/PRECAUTIONS: Glimepiride: Increased cardiovascular mortality has been reported. May produce severe hypoglycemia; risk may be increased if debilitated, malnourished; with adrenal, pituitary, renal, or hepatic insufficiency; and after severe or prolonged exercise. Hypoglycemia may be masked in elderly patients and in patients taking β-adrenergic blocking drugs or other sympatholytic agents. May lose blood glucose control with stress. Hemolytic anemia reported; caution in patients with glucose-6-phosphate dehydrogenase (G6PD) deficiency and consider alternate non-sulfonylurea treatment. Pioglitazone: Not for use in type 1 DM. Initiation or worsening of edema reported; caution in patients at risk for HF. Weight gain reported. Not for use in patients with active bladder cancer; consider benefits vs risks in patients with prior history of bladder cancer. Ovulation in premenopausal anovulatory patients may occur; use adequate contraception. May decrease Hgb and Hct. Avoid with active liver disease or if ALT levels >2.5X ULN. Hepatitis and hepatic enzyme elevations >3X or more ULN reported and rarely hepatic failure reported. Obtain LFTs if hepatic dysfunction symptoms occur. D/C if ALT remains >3X ULN on therapy or if jaundice occurs. Macular edema reported; refer patients who develop any type of visual symptoms to an ophthalmologist. Increased incidence of bone fractures reported in female patients.

ADVERSE REACTIONS: HF, weight gain, dyspnea, edema, hypoglycemia, upper respiratory tract infection, headache, diarrhea, urinary tract infection, limb pain, nausea.

INTERACTIONS: Pioglitazone: Risk for hypoglycemia if used concomitantly with insulin or oral hypoglycemic agents; may require dose reduction of concomitant agent. Concomitant use with other antidiabetic agents and insulin may cause fluid retention; d/c or reduce pioglitazone dose. May be a weak inducer of CYP3A4 substrates. Increased area under the curve (AUC) levels with CYP2C8 inhibitors (eg, gemfibrozil). Decreased AUC levels with CYP2C8 inducers (eg, rifampin). May affect levels of nifedipine ER and atorvastatin calcium. Concomitant use with ketoconazole or atorvastatin calcium may affect pioglitazone levels. May decrease levels of midazolam and ethinyl estradiol. Glimepiride: Combined use with insulin, metformin, or more than one glucose agent may increase the potential for hypoglycemia. Hypoglycemia more likely to occur when alcohol is ingested. Hypoglycemia may be potentiated with NSAIDs and other drugs that are highly protein bound (eg, salicylates, sulfonamides, chloramphenicol, coumarins, probenecid, MAOIs, β-blockers). Risk of severe hypoglycemia with oral miconazole. Risk of hyperglycemia with thiazides and other diuretics, corticosteroids, phenothiazines, thyroid products, estrogens, oral contraceptives, phenytoin, nicotinic acid, sympathomimetics, and isoniazid. Decreased concentrations with aspirin. Increased C_{max}, AUC, and $T_{1/2}$ with propranolol. May interact with inhibitors (eg, fluconazole) and inducers (eg, rifampicin) of CYP2C9.

PREGNANCY: Category C, not for use in nursing.

MECHANISM OF ACTION: Pioglitazone: Thiazolidinedione; insulin-sensitizing agent acts primarily by enhancing peripheral glucose utilization. Glimepiride: Sulfonylurea; insulin secretagogue that acts primarily by stimulating release of insulin from functioning pancreatic beta cells.

PHARMACOKINETICS: Absorption: Administration of variable doses resulted in different parameters. Glimepiride: Complete. T_{max}=2-3 hrs. Pioglitazone: T_{max}=2 hrs. **Distribution:** Pioglitazone: V_d=0.63L/kg, plasma protein binding (>99%). Glimepiride: (IV) V_d=8.8L, plasma protein binding (>99.5%). **Metabolism:** Pioglitazone: Extensive (hydroxylation & oxidation) via CYP2C8, CYP3A4, CYP1A1. M-II and M-IV (hydroxy derivatives) and M-III (keto derivatives) (active metabolites). Glimepiride: Complete. Oxidative biotransformation via CYP2C9. Cyclohexyl hydroxy methyl derivative (M1), carboxyl derivative (M2) (major metabolites). **Elimination:** Pioglitazone: Urine (15-30%), bile (unchanged), feces (metabolites); $T_{1/2}$=3-7 hrs (pioglitazone), 16-24 hrs (total pioglitazone). Glimepiride: Urine (60%), feces (40%).

NURSING CONSIDERATIONS

Assessment: Assess for diabetic ketoacidosis, HF, type 1 DM, risk factors for HF, history of bladder cancer, premenopausal anovulation, active liver disease, renal insufficiency, G6PD deficiency, drug hypersensitivity, pregnancy/nursing status, and possible drug interactions. Assess LFTs and obtain CBC prior to therapy.

Monitoring: Monitor for signs and symptoms of HF, edema, hypoglycemia, weight gain, decreases in Hgb/Hct, hepatic dysfunction, macular edema, bone fractures, and hemolytic anemia. Perform periodic monitoring of LFTs, FBG, and HbA1c. Perform periodic eye exams.

Patient Counseling: Advise to adhere to dietary instructions and have blood glucose and HbA1c levels tested regularly. Instruct to seek medical advice promptly during periods of stress (eg, fever, trauma, infection, or surgery) and report SOB, rapid increase in weight or edema, or other symptoms of HF to physician. Instruct to d/c and consult physician if unexplained N/V, abdominal pain, anorexia, fatigue, and darkening of urine occurs. Instruct to report any signs of macroscopic hematuria or other symptoms such as dysuria or urinary urgency that develop or increase during treatment. Advise to take a single dose once daily with the first main meal. Inform about the possible increased risk for pregnancy in premenopausal women while on therapy; recommend adequate contraception for all premenopausal women.

Administration: Oral route. **Storage:** 25°C (77°F); excursions permitted to 15-30°C (59-86°F). Protect from moisture and humidity.

DUEXIS RX
famotidine - ibuprofen (Horizon)

May increase risk of serious cardiovascular (CV) thrombotic events, myocardial infarction, stroke, and serious GI adverse reactions (eg, bleeding, ulceration, perforation of stomach/intestines). Contraindicated for treatment of perioperative pain in the setting of coronary artery bypass graft (CABG) surgery.

THERAPEUTIC CLASS: NSAID/H_2-blocker

INDICATIONS: Relief of signs/symptoms of rheumatoid arthritis and osteoarthritis and to decrease the risk of developing upper GI ulcers (eg, gastric/duodenal ulcer) in patients taking ibuprofen for those indications.

DOSAGE: *Adults:* 1 tab tid.

HOW SUPPLIED: Tab: (Ibuprofen-Famotidine) 800mg-26.6mg

CONTRAINDICATIONS: Late stages of pregnancy, treatment of perioperative pain in the setting of CABG surgery, patients who have experienced asthma, urticaria, or allergic reactions after taking aspirin (ASA) or other NSAIDs.

WARNINGS/PRECAUTIONS: Ibuprofen: May lead to onset of new HTN or worsening of pre-existing HTN; monitor BP closely. Fluid retention and edema reported; caution with fluid retention or heart failure (HF). Extreme caution with history of ulcer disease or GI bleeding; consider d/c if serious GI adverse reactions occur. Caution with history of inflammatory bowel disease (ulcerative colitis, Crohn's disease); may exacerbate condition. D/C if active and clinically significant bleeding from any source occurs. Renal papillary necrosis and other renal injury reported with long-term use; d/c if clinical signs (eg, azotemia, HTN, proteinuria) and symptoms consistent with renal disease develop. Anaphylaxis may occur; avoid with ASA-triad. May cause serious skin adverse reactions (eg, exfoliative dermatitis, Steven-Johnson syndrome, toxic epidermal necrolysis); d/c at 1st sign of skin rash/hypersensitivity. Elevations of LFTs and severe hepatic reactions reported; d/c if liver disease develops or systemic manifestations occur. May cause anemia and inhibit platelet aggregation. Avoid with ASA-sensitive patients; caution with preexisting asthma. Aseptic meningitis with fever and coma observed (rare). Not a substitute for corticosteroids or for treatment of corticosteroid insufficiency. May mask inflammation and fever. D/C if visual disturbances occur. Caution in debilitated patients or elderly. Famotidine: CNS adverse effects (eg, seizures, delirium, coma) reported with moderate (CrCl <50mL/min) and severe renal insufficiency (CrCl <10mL/min); avoid with CrCl <50mL/min. Symptomatic response does not preclude presence of gastric malignancy.

ADVERSE REACTIONS: Bleeding/ulceration/perforations of stomach or intestines, nausea, diarrhea, constipation, upper abdominal pain, headache, dyspepsia, upper respiratory tract infection, HTN.

INTERACTIONS: Increased risk of serious GI bleeding with oral corticosteroids, anticoagulants (eg, warfarin), antiplatelet drugs (eg, low-dose ASA), use of alcohol, and SSRIs; use with caution. May diminish effects of angiotensin enzyme inhibitors, furosemide, thiazides; observe closely for signs of renal failure. May increase lithium, methotrexate levels; observe for toxicity. May delay absorption with cholestyramine. Increased risk of adverse events with other NSAIDs, including ASA. Avoid with other ibuprofen-containing products.

PREGNANCY: Category C, not for use in nursing.

MECHANISM OF ACTION: Famotidine: H_2-receptor antagonist; inhibits gastric secretion. Ibuprofen: NSAIDs; has not been established. May be related to prostaglandin synthetase inhibition.

PHARMACOKINETICS: Absorption: Rapid. Famotidine: C_{max}=61ng/mL, T_{max}=2 hrs. Ibuprofen: C_{max}=45ug/mL, T_{max}=1.9 hrs. **Distribution:** Famotidine: Plasma protein binding (15-20%); found in breast milk. **Metabolism:** Famotidine: S-oxide (metabolite). **Elimination:** Famotidine: Urine (25-30%, unchanged); $T_{1/2}$=4 hrs. Ibuprofen: Urine (45-79%, metabolites); $T_{1/2}$=2 hrs.

NURSING CONSIDERATIONS

Assessment: Assess for CABG surgery, cardiovascular disease, and a history of hypersensitivity to ASA or other NSAIDs. Assess for pregnancy/nursing status and for possible drug interactions. Obtain baseline BP, LFTs, CBC, and renal function.

Monitoring: Monitor for signs/symptoms of CV thrombotic events, new onset/worsening of HTN, fluid retention and edema, GI events (eg, bleeding, ulceration, perforation), renal effects (eg, renal papillary necrosis), anaphylactoid reactions, skin reactions, hepatic effects (eg, jaundice, liver necrosis, hepatic failure), and hematological effects. Monitor BP during course of therapy, renal/hepatic function, CBC and chemistry profile periodically, Hgb and Hct for patients on long term treatment.

Patient Counseling: Inform of possible serious CV side effects, GI discomfort, skin reactions. Advise to d/c immediately and contact physician if any type of rash develops. Advise to d/c therapy and seek medical therapy if nephrotoxicity, hepatotoxicity, or anaphylaxis occurs. Advise to report signs/symptoms of unexplained weight gain or edema. Avoid in late pregnancy. Instruct to take tab whole and not to chew, divide, or crush.

Administration: Oral route. **Storage:** 25°C (77°F); excursions permitted to 15-30°C (59-86°F).

DULERA   RX
mometasone furoate - formoterol fumarate dihydrate (Merck)

> Long-acting β₂-adrenergic agonists (LABA), such as formoterol, increase the risk of asthma-related death. LABA increase the risk of asthma-related hospitalization in pediatrics and adolescents. Use only for patients not adequately controlled on a long-term asthma control medication (eg, inhaled corticosteroid) or whose disease severity clearly warrants initiation of treatment with both an inhaled corticosteroid and LABA. Do not use if asthma is adequately controlled on low- or medium-dose inhaled corticosteroids.

THERAPEUTIC CLASS: Corticosteroid/beta₂ agonist

INDICATIONS: Treatment of asthma in patients ≥12 yrs.

DOSAGE: *Adults:* 2 inh bid (am and pm). Max: 2 inh of 200mcg-50mcg bid. Previous Therapy: Inhaled Medium-Dose Corticosteroids: Initial: 2 inh bid of 100mcg-5mcg. Max: 400mcg-20mcg daily. Inhaled High-Dose Corticosteroids: Initial: 2 inh bid of 200mcg-5mcg. Max: 800mcg-20mcg daily. Do not use >2 inh bid of the prescribed strength. May need higher strength if inadequate response after 2 weeks.
Pediatrics: ≥12 yrs: 2 inh bid (am and pm). Max: 2 inh of 200mcg-50mcg bid. Previous Therapy: Inhaled Medium-Dose Corticosteroids: Initial: 2 inh bid of 100mcg-5mcg. Max: 400mcg-20mcg daily. Inhaled High-Dose Corticosteroids: Initial: 2 inh bid of 200mcg-5mcg. Max: 800mcg-20mcg daily. Do not use >2 inh bid of the prescribed strength. May need higher strength if inadequate response after 2 weeks of therapy.

HOW SUPPLIED: MDI: (Mometasone furoate-Formoterol fumarate dihydrate) 100mcg-5mcg, 200mcg-5mcg

CONTRAINDICATIONS: Primary treatment of status asthmaticus or other acute episodes of asthma where intensive measures are required.

WARNINGS/PRECAUTIONS: Do not use if rapidly deteriorating/potentially life-threatening asthma, relief of acute symptoms. D/C regular use of oral/inhaled, short-acting β₂-agonists (SABA) prior to treatment; use only for relief of acute asthma. Cardiovascular (CV) effects and fatalities reported with excessive use; do not use excessively or with other LABA. *Candida albicans* infections of mouth and pharynx reported; treat and/or d/c if needed. Increased susceptibility to infections (eg, chickenpox, measles), may lead to serious/fatal course; avoid exposure. Caution with tuberculosis (TB), untreated systemic fungal, bacterial, viral or parasitic infections, or ocular herpes simplex. Deaths due to adrenal insufficiency reported with transfer from systemic to inhaled corticosteroids (ICS); if oral corticosteroids required wean slowly from systemic steroid. Transfer from systemic to inhalation therapy may unmask allergic conditions (eg, rhinitis). Observe for systemic corticosteroid withdrawal effects. Appearance of hypercorticism and adrenal suppression; reduce dose slowly. Bronchospasm, with immediate increase in wheezing, may occur; d/c immediately. Immediate hypersensitivity reactions may occur. Caution with CV disorders; d/c if CV effects occur. Decreases in bone mineral density (BMD) reported; caution with major risk factors for decreased bone mineral content including chronic use of drugs that can reduce bone mass (eg, anticonvulsants, corticosteroids). May cause reduction in growth velocity in pediatrics. Glaucoma, increased intraocular pressure, and cataracts reported. Caution in elderly and patients with convulsive disorders, thyrotoxicosis, unusual responsiveness to sympathomimetic amines, diabetes mellitus (DM), and ketoacidosis. May cause changes in blood glucose and serum K⁺ levels.

ADVERSE REACTIONS: Nasopharyngitis, sinusitis, headache.

INTERACTIONS: Do not use with other medications containing LABA (eg, salmeterol, formoterol fumarate, arformoterol tartrate); increased risk of CV effects. Caution with ketoconazole, other known strong CYP3A4 inhibitors (eg, ritonavir, clarithromycin, itraconazole, nefazodone), non-K⁺-sparing diuretics (eg, loop or thiazide diuretics). Caution with MAOIs, TCAs, drugs known to prolong QTc interval or within 2 weeks of d/c such products. Mometasone: Increased plasma concentration with oral ketoconazole and increased systemic exposure with CYP3A4 inhibitors. Formoterol: Potentiation of sympathetic effects with additional adrenergic drugs; use with caution. Potentiation of hypokalemic effect with xanthine derivatives and diuretics. Potentiation of CV effect with MAOIs, TCAs, or drugs known to prolong QTc interval. Use with β-blockers may block effects and produce severe bronchospasm in asthma patients; if needed, consider cardioselective β-blocker with caution.

PREGNANCY: Category C, caution in nursing.

MECHANISM OF ACTION: Mometasone furoate: Corticosteroid; not established. Shown to have inhibitory effects on multiple cell types (eg, mast cells, eosinophils, neutrophils, macrophages, and lymphocytes) and mediators (eg, histamine, eicosanoids, leukotrienes, and cytokines) involved in inflammatory and asthmatic response. Formoterol: LABA (β$_2$-agonist); stimulates intracellular adenyl cyclase, which catalyzes conversion of ATP to cAMP, producing relaxation of bronchial smooth muscle and inhibition of release of mediators of immediate hypersensitivity from cells, especially from mast cells.

PHARMACOKINETICS: Absorption: (Asthma Patients) Mometasone: C_{max}=20pg/mL; AUC=170pg•hr/mL; T_{max}=1-2 hrs. Formoterol: C_{max}=22pmol/L; AUC=125pmol•h/L; T_{max}=0.58-1.97 hrs. **Distribution:** Mometasone: V_d=152L (IV); plasma protein binding (98-99%). Formoterol: Plasma protein binding (61-64%). **Metabolism:** Mometasone: Liver (extensive) via CYP3A4. Formoterol: Direct glucuronidation, O-demethylation (via CYP2D6, 2C19, 2C9, 2A6), and conjugation. **Elimination:** Mometasone: Feces (74%); urine (8%); $T_{1/2}$=25 hrs. Formoterol: Urine (6.2-6.8%, unchanged); $T_{1/2}$=9.1-10.8 hrs (single dose), 9-11 hrs (multi-dose).

NURSING CONSIDERATIONS

Assessment: Assess for status asthmaticus, acute asthma episodes, rapidly deteriorating asthma, bronchospasm, known hypersensitivity to any drug component, risk factors for decreased bone mineral content, CV or convulsive disorders, thyrotoxicosis, other condition where treatment is contraindicated or cautioned, pregnancy/nursing status, and possible drug interactions. Obtain baseline BMD, eye exam, and lung function prior to therapy.

Monitoring: Monitor for localized oral *Candida albicans* infections, worsening or acutely deteriorating asthma, development of glaucoma, increased intraocular pressure, cataracts, CV effects, hypercorticism, adrenal suppression, inhalation induced bronchospasm, hypokalemia, hyperglycemia, and hypersensitivity reactions. Monitor BMD and lung function periodically. Perform periodic eye exams. Monitor growth in pediatric patients routinely. Monitor pulse rate, BP, ECG changes, blood glucose and serum K⁺ levels.

Patient Counseling: Inform of the risk and benefits of therapy. Instruct not to use to relieve acute asthma symptoms, if symptoms arise between doses use an inhaled SABA for immediate relief. Instruct to seek medical attention if symptoms worsen, if lung function decreases, or if needs more inhalations of a SABA than usual. If a dose is missed, instruct to take next dose at the same time they normally do. Instruct not to d/c or reduce therapy without physician's guidance.

Administration: Oral inhalational route. After use, rinse mouth with water without swallowing. Refer to PI for proper priming and administration. **Storage:** 20-25°C (68-77°F); excursions permitted to 15-30°C (59-86°F). Do not puncture. Do not use or store near heat or open flame. Discard inhaler when dose counter reads "0".

DUONEB
ipratropium bromide - albuterol sulfate (Dey)

RX

THERAPEUTIC CLASS: Beta₂-agonist/anticholinergic

INDICATIONS: Treatment of bronchospasm associated with chronic obstructive pulmonary disease (COPD) in patients requiring more than one bronchodilator.

DOSAGE: *Adults:* 3mL qid via nebulizer. May give up to 2 additional 3mL doses/day, PRN.

HOW SUPPLIED: Sol, Inhalation: (Ipratropium-Albuterol) 0.5mg-3mg/3mL [30ˢ, 60ˢ]

CONTRAINDICATIONS: Hypersensitivity to atropine and its derivatives.

WARNINGS/PRECAUTIONS: Paradoxical bronchospasm reported; d/c if symptoms occur. Fatalities reported with excessive use of inhaled products containing sympathomimetic amines and with home use of nebulizers. May produce significant cardiovascular (CV) effect (eg, ECG changes); caution with CV disorders (eg, coronary insufficiency, cardiac arrhythmias, HTN). Immediate hypersensitivity reactions reported. Caution with convulsive disorders, hyperthyroidism, diabetes mellitus (DM), narrow-angle glaucoma, prostatic hypertrophy, bladder-neck obstruction, and hepatic/renal insufficiency. Aggravation of preexisting DM and ketoacidosis reported with large doses of IV albuterol. May decrease serum K⁺.

D

ADVERSE REACTIONS: Lung disease, pharyngitis, pain, chest pain, diarrhea, dyspepsia, nausea, leg cramps, bronchitis, pneumonia, urinary tract infection, constipation, voice alterations.

INTERACTIONS: Caution with anticholinergic agents, other sympathomimetic agents, non-potassium sparing diuretics, and MAOIs or TCAs. Additive interactions with anticholinergic agents. Increased risk of adverse CV effects with other sympathomimetics. β-blockers and albuterol inhibit the effect of each other; use β-blockers with caution in patients with hyperreactive airways. Administration with MAOIs or TCAs, or within 2 weeks of d/c of such agents may potentiate the action of albuterol on CV system. ECG changes and/or hypokalemia that may result from non-potassium sparing diuretics (eg, loop or thiazide diuretics) may be worsened with β-agonist-containing drugs.

PREGNANCY: Category C (albuterol) and B (ipratropium), not for use in nursing.

MECHANISM OF ACTION: Albuterol: β_2-adrenergic bronchodilator; stimulates adenyl cyclase, enzyme that catalyzes formation of cyclic-3',5'-adenosine monophosphate (cAMP) and mediates cellular response resulting in relaxation of bronchial smooth muscle. Ipratropium: Anticholinergic bronchodilator; blocks muscarinic receptors of acetylcholine. Prevents the increases in intracellular concentration of cyclic guanosine monophosphate (cGMP), resulting from interaction of acetylcholine with the muscarinic receptors of bronchial smooth muscle.

PHARMACOKINETICS: Absorption: C_{max}=4.65mg/mL; (albuterol) T_{max}=0.8 hrs; AUC=24.2ng•hr/mL. **Distribution:** Ipratropium: Plasma protein binding (0-9%). **Metabolism:** Albuterol: Conjugation; albuterol 4'-O-sulfate (metabolite). Ipratropium: Ester hydrolysis. **Elimination:** $T_{1/2}$=6.7 hrs. Albuterol: Urine (8.4%, unchanged). Ipratropium: Urine (3.9%, unchanged).

NURSING CONSIDERATIONS

Assessment: Assess for history of hypersensitivity to atropine or its derivatives, narrow-angle glaucoma, prostatic hypertrophy, bladder-neck obstruction, convulsive disorders, hyperthyroidism, DM, hepatic/renal insufficiency, CV disorders, pregnancy/nursing status, and possible drug interactions.

Monitoring: Monitor serum K⁺, pulse rate, BP, and for signs/symptoms of hypersensitivity reactions, parodoxical brochospasm, CV effects, anticholinergic effects, and other adverse reactions.

Patient Counseling: Instruct to use caution to avoid exposing their eyes to this product as temporary papillary dilation, blurred vision, eye pain, or precipitation or worsening of narrow-angle glaucoma may occur. Inform that proper nebulizer technique should be assured, particularly if a mask is used. Inform that the action of the drug should last ≤5 hrs. Advise not to exceed recommended dose or frequency without consulting physician. Instruct to seek medical consultation if symptoms worsen. Instruct to contact physician if pregnant or nursing. Instruct to see illustrated Patient's Instruction for Use.

Administration: Oral inhalation. 1) Remove vial and squeeze contents into nebulizer reservoir. 2) Connect nebulizer to mouthpiece and compressor. 3) Place mouthpiece in mouth or put on face mask and turn on compressor. 4) Breathe as calmly as possible through mouth until no more mist is formed (5-15 min). 5) Clean nebulizer. **Storage:** 2-25°C (36-77°F). Protect from light.

DURAGESIC

CII

fentanyl (Ortho-McNeil)

> Contains a schedule II opioid agonist with potential for abuse/diversion and risk of respiratory depression; monitor for signs of misuse, abuse, or addiction. Life-threatening hypoventilation may occur. Avoid in patients <2 yrs. Only for use in patients who are already receiving opioid therapy, opioid-tolerant patients, and those who require a total dose at least equivalent to 25mcg/hr. Contraindicated in patients who are not opioid tolerant, management of acute pain, short-term or PRN treatment; postoperative pain, mild/intermittent pain; use in nonopioid-tolerant patients may lead to fatal respiratory depression. Overestimating the fentanyl transdermal dose when converting patients from another opioid medication can result in fatal overdose with the first dose. Concomitant use with all CYP3A4 inhibitors may increase plasma concentrations and cause fatal respiratory depression. For transdermal use only. Avoid exposing application site to direct external heat source (eg, heating pads, tanning lamps). Potential for temperature-dependent increases in fentanyl release from patch.

THERAPEUTIC CLASS: Opioid analgesic

INDICATIONS: Management of persistent, moderate to severe chronic pain in opioid-tolerant patients that requires continuous, around-the-clock opioid administration for an extended period of time, and cannot be managed by other means, such as nonsteroidal analgesics, opioid combination products, or immediate-release opioids.

DOSAGE: *Adults:* Individualize dose. Determine dose based on opioid tolerance, previous analgesic requirement, and general condition and medical status of the patient. Minimum Initial Dose: 25mcg/hr for 72 hrs. Titrate: Initial dose may be increased after 3 days; further increase in dosage should be made after the higher dose is worn through two applications. Dosage increments may be based on the daily dose of supplementary opioids using the ratio of 45mg/24 hrs of oral morphine to a 12.5mcg/hr increase in dose. Some patients may not achieve adequate analgesia and may require systems to be applied q48h rather than q72h; an increase in dose should first be evaluated prior to changing the interval. Refer to PI for Dose Conversion Guidelines. Elderly/Debilitated/Cachectic/Cardiac Disease/Renal/Hepatic Impairment: Reduce dose. *Pediatrics:* ≥2 yrs: Individualize dose. Determine dose based on opioid tolerance, previous analgesic requirement, and general condition and medical status of the patient. Minimum Initial Dose: 25mcg/hr for 72 hrs. Titrate: Initial dose may be increased after 3 days; further increase in dosage should be made after the higher dose is worn through two applications. Dosage increments may be based on the daily dose of supplementary opioids using the ratio of 45mg/24 hrs of oral morphine to a 12.5mcg/hr increase in dose. Refer to PI for Dose Conversion Guidelines.

D

HOW SUPPLIED: Patch: 12mcg/hr, 25mcg/hr, 50mcg/hr, 75mcg/hr, 100mcg/hr [5ᶺ]

CONTRAINDICATIONS: Opioid nontolerant patients, management of acute pain or in patients who require opioid analgesia for a short period of time, postoperative pain, including use after out-patient/day surgeries (eg, tonsillectomies). Mild/intermittent pain (eg, use as PRN basis), significant respiratory depression especially in unmonitored settings where there is a lack of resuscitative equipment, acute or severe bronchial asthma, diagnosis or suspicion of paralytic ileus.

WARNINGS/PRECAUTIONS: Do not use if seal is broken or patch is cut, damaged, or changed. Monitor patients with serious adverse events for at least 24 hrs after removal. Death and other serious medical problems have occurred from accidental exposure to fentanyl (eg, transfer from adult's body to a child while hugging, accidentally sitting on a patch). May increase risk of respiratory depression in elderly/debilitated patients. Extreme caution with chronic obstructive pulmonary diseases or cor pulmonale, decreased respiratory reserve, hypoxia, hypercapnia, or preexisting respiratory depression; consider alternative non-opioid analgesics or supervise at the lowest effective dose. Avoid with increased intracranial pressure, impaired consciousness, or coma; caution with brain tumors. May obscure clinical course of head injury. May cause bradycardia; caution with bradyarrhythmias. Caution with renal/hepatic impairment. May cause spasm of the sphincter of Oddi; caution with biliary tract disease (eg, acute pancreatitis). May cause increases in serum amylase concentrations. Tolerance and physical dependence may occur. May impair mental/physical abilities. Withdrawal symptoms may occur; gradual downward titration recommended.

ADVERSE REACTIONS: Hypoventilation, headache, fever, N/V, constipation, dry mouth, somnolence, confusion, asthenia, sweating, nervousness, pruritus, apnea, dyspnea.

INTERACTIONS: See Boxed Warning. Concomitant use with CNS depressants (eg, opioids, sedatives, hypnotics, tranquilizers, general anesthetics, phenothiazines, skeletal muscle relaxants, alcohol) may cause respiratory depression, hypotension, profound sedation, or potentially coma; dose of one or both agents should be significantly reduced. Coadministration with CYP3A4 inducers may lead to reduced efficacy of fentanyl. Avoid use within 14 days of an MAOI. Concomitant use with CNS-active drugs requires special patient care and observation.

PREGNANCY: Category C, not for use in nursing.

MECHANISM OF ACTION: Opioid analgesic; interacts predominantly with the opioid μ-receptor in the brain, spinal cord, and other tissues. Exerts principal pharmacological actions on CNS.

PHARMACOKINETICS: Absorption: T_{max}=20-72 hrs. Transdermal administration of variable doses resulted in different parameters. **Distribution:** V_d=6L/kg; found in breast milk; readily crosses placenta. **Metabolism:** Liver via CYP3A4; oxidative N-dealkylation to norfentanyl. **Elimination:** (IV) Urine (75%, <10% unchanged), feces (9%, primarily metabolites); $T_{1/2}$=20-27 hrs.

NURSING CONSIDERATIONS

Assessment: Assess for degree of opioid tolerance, previous opioid dose, level/intensity/type of pain, patient's general condition and medical status, and other conditions where treatment is contraindicated or cautioned. Assess for pregnancy/nursing status, renal/hepatic function, and possible drug interactions.

Monitoring: Monitor for signs/symptoms of respiratory depression, bradycardia, increases in serum amylase levels, abuse, misuse, addiction, and tolerance/physical dependence. Monitor for signs and symptoms of overdose, especially when converting patient from another opioid. Monitor for fever/increase in body temperature and other adverse reactions.

Patient Counseling: Advise that patch contains fentanyl, an opioid pain medicine similar to morphine, hydromorphone, methadone, oxycodone, and oxymorphone. Instruct to wear patch continuously for 72 hrs, and apply patch to different area of intact, nonirritated, and nonirradiated skin on a flat surface (eg, chest, back, flank, upper arm) following removal of previous patch. Advise to place on upper back to decrease chance of removal in pediatric/cognitively impaired patients. Instruct to clean with water and dry skin prior to application; avoid soaps, oils, lotions, or any skin irritants. Instruct to apply immediately upon removal from sealed package and after removal of protective liner. Counsel not use a broken, cut, or damaged patch. Advise never to adjust the dose or the number of patches applied to the skin without instruction from the physician. Instruct to avoid exposing patch to direct external heat sources. Advise to contact physician if fever develops. Advise to fold patch and flush down the toilet following use. Counsel to use caution if performing hazardous tasks (eg, driving, operating machinery) and advise to notify physician of all medications currently taking and to avoid using other CNS depressants and alcohol. Inform that constipation may develop during therapy. Instruct to avoid abrupt withdrawal of medication; taper dose. Inform that medication has high potential for abuse and to keep in secure place; keep patches (new and used) out of reach of children. Instruct that if patch sticks to a person other than the patient, remove patch and wash exposed area with water, and contact physician. Advise women who are pregnant/planning to become pregnant to consult physician prior to initiating/continuing therapy.

Administration: Transdermal patch. Do not use if the pouch seal is broken. Refer to PI for further details on proper application. **Storage:** Up to 25°C (77°F); excursions permitted to 15-30°C (59-86°F). Store in original unopened pouch.

DURAMORPH `CII`
morphine sulfate (Baxter)

> Risk of severe adverse reactions with epidural or intrathecal route; observe patients in an equipped and staffed environment for at least 24 hrs after initial dose. Naloxone inj and resuscitative equipment should be immediately available in case of life-threatening or intolerable side effects and whenever therapy is initiated. Intrathecal dose is usually 1/10 that of epidural dose. Remove any contaminated clothing and rinse affected area with water if accidental dermal exposure occurs. Special measures must be taken to control this product within the hospital/clinic. Do not use if color is darker than pale yellow, discolored in any other way, or contains a precipitate.

THERAPEUTIC CLASS: Opioid analgesic

INDICATIONS: Management of pain unresponsive to non-narcotic analgesics.

DOSAGE: *Adults:* IV: Initial: 2-10mg/70kg body weight. Epidural: Initial: 5mg in lumbar region. Titrate: If inadequate pain relief within 1 hr, increase by 1-2mg. Max: 10mg/24 hrs. Intrathecal: 0.2-1mg single dose in lumbar area. May administer a constant IV infusion of 0.6mg/hr naloxone, for 24 hrs after intrathecal inj.

HOW SUPPLIED: Inj: 0.5mg/mL [10ml], 1mg/mL [10mL]

CONTRAINDICATIONS: Acute bronchial asthma, upper airway obstruction.

WARNINGS/PRECAUTIONS: Not for use in continuous microinfusion devices. Repeated intrathecal inj not recommended. Do not inject intrathecally more than 2mL of the 0.5mg/mL or 1mL of the 1mg/mL. May be habit forming. Rapid IV administration may result in chest wall rigidity. Should be administered by those familiar with respiratory depression management. Epidural or intrathecal administration should be given by or under the direction of a physician experienced in techniques and familiar with patient management problems associated with administration. Severe respiratory depression up to 24 hrs following epidural/intrathecal administration reported. Limit epidural/intrathecal route to lumbar area. Incidence of respiratory depression higher in intrathecal than in epidural use. Seizures may result from high doses; caution with known seizure disorders. High doses of neuraxial morphine may produce myoclonic events. Caution with head injury, increased intracranial pressure, decreased respiratory reserve (eg, emphysema, severe obesity, kyphoscoliosis, paralysis of the phrenic nerve). Caution with epidural route in hepatic/renal dysfunction. Avoid in chronic asthma or in any other chronic pulmonary disorder. Smooth muscle hypertonicity may cause biliary colic. Initiation of neuraxial opiate analgesia associated with micturition disturbances, especially in males with prostatic enlargement. Orthostatic hypotension may occur with reduced circulating blood volume and myocardial dysfunction. Severe hypotension may occur in volume-depleted patients. Infants born to mothers taking morphine may exhibit withdrawal symptoms. Caution in elderly.

ADVERSE REACTIONS: Respiratory depression, convulsions, dysphoric reactions, pruritus, urinary retention, constipation, lumbar puncture-type headache, toxic psychoses.

INTERACTIONS: CNS depressants (eg, alcohol, sedatives, antihistamines, psychotropics) potentiate depressant effects. Neuroleptics may increase risk of respiratory depression. Severe hypotension may occur with phenothiazines or general anesthetics. Monitor for orthostatic hypotension in patients on sympatholytic drugs.

PREGNANCY: Category C, safety in nursing not known.

MECHANISM OF ACTION: Opioid analgesic; analgesic effects are produced via at least 3 areas of the CNS: the periaqueductal-periventricular gray matter, the ventromedial medulla, and the spinal cord. Interacts predominantly with μ-receptors distributed in the brain, spinal cord, and trigeminal nerve.

PHARMACOKINETICS: Absorption: (Epidural): Rapid; C_{max}=33-40ng/mL; T_{max}=10-15 min; (Intrathecal): C_{max}<1-7.8ng/mL; T_{max}=5-10 min. **Distribution:** Plasma protein binding (36%); found in breast milk. (IV) V_d=1.0-4.7L/kg. **Metabolism:** Hepatic glucuronidation. **Elimination:** Urine (2-12% unchanged), feces (10%); (IV, IM) $T_{1/2}$=1.5-4.5 hrs; (epidural) $T_{1/2}$=39-249 min.

NURSING CONSIDERATIONS

Assessment: Assess for level of pain intensity or any other conditions where treatment is contraindicated or cautioned. Assess for history of hypersensitivity, pregnancy/nursing status, renal/hepatic function, and possible drug interactions.

Monitoring: Monitor for signs/symptoms of respiratory depression, myoclonic events, seizures, dysphoric reactions, toxic psychoses, biliary colic, urinary retention, drug abuse/dependence, and other adverse reactions.

Patient Counseling: Inform about risks and benefits of therapy. Inform of adverse reactions that may occur. Instruct to inform physician of other medications taken. Inform that medication has potential for abuse and dependence.

Administration: IV, epidural, or intrathecal route. Proper placement of needle or catheter should be verified before epidural inj. **Storage:** 20-25°C (68-77°F); excursions permitted to 15-30°C (59-86°F). Protect from light. Do not freeze. Do not heat-sterilize.

DUREZOL   RX
difluprednate (Alcon)

THERAPEUTIC CLASS: Corticosteroid

INDICATIONS: Treatment of inflammation and pain associated with ocular surgery.

DOSAGE: *Adults:* 1 drop into affected conjunctival sac of affected eye(s) qid beginning 24 hrs after ocular surgery and continue throughout the first 2 weeks post-op, followed by bid for a week and then taper based on response.

HOW SUPPLIED: Emulsion: 0.05% [5mL]

CONTRAINDICATIONS: Active viral diseases of the cornea and conjunctiva, including epithelial herpes simplex keratitis, vaccinia, varicella, mycobacterial infection of the eye, and fungal disease of ocular structures.

WARNINGS/PRECAUTIONS: Prolonged use may result in glaucoma with optic nerve damage, visual acuity and visual field defects. Caution with glaucoma. Monitor intraocular pressure (IOP) if used ≥10 days. May cause posterior subcapsular cataract formation. Use in cataract surgery may delay healing and increase incidence of bleb formation. Caution with diseases causing thinning of the cornea or sclera; perforations may occur. Perform eye exam (eg, slit lamp biomicroscopy, fluorescein staining) prior to therapy and renewal of medication order >28 days. Prolonged use may suppress host response and increase risk of secondary ocular infections. May mask or enhance existing infection in acute purulent conditions; reevaluate if fail to improve after 2 days. May prolong the course or exacerbate severity of many viral infections; caution with herpes simplex. Fungal infections of the cornea may develop with long-term use; consider fungal invasion in any persistent corneal ulceration. Not for intraocular administration.

ADVERSE REACTIONS: Corneal edema, ciliary and conjunctival hyperemia, eye pain, photophobia, posterior capsular opacification, anterior chamber cells and flare, conjunctival edema, blepharitis, reduced visual acuity, punctate keratitis, eye inflammation, and iritis.

PREGNANCY: Category C, caution in nursing.

MECHANISM OF ACTION: Corticosteroid; Not established. Suspected to induce phospholipase A_2 inhibitory proteins which control the biosynthesis of potent mediators of inflammation such as prostaglandins and leukotrienes.

PHARMACOKINETICS: Absorption: Limited. **Metabolism**: Deacetylation; 6α, 9-difluoroprednisolone 17-butyrate (active metabolite).

NURSING CONSIDERATIONS

Assessment: Assess for active viral diseases of the cornea and conjunctiva, epithelial herpes simplex keratitis, vaccinia, varicella, mycobacterial infection of the eye, fungal disease of ocular structures, glaucoma, optic nerve damage, visual acuity and visual field defects, diseases causing thinning of sclera or cornea, acute purulent conditions and pregnancy/nursing status. Perform eye exam (eg, slit lamp biomicroscopy, fluorescein staining) prior to therapy in certain patients.

Monitoring: Monitor for signs and symptoms of glaucoma, optic nerve damage, visual acuity and visual field defects, subcapsular cataract, ocular/corneal perforations, acute purulent conditions, bacterial, viral, fungal infections. Monitor post-operative cataract patients (eg, delayed healing, bleb formation) and increased risk for secondary ocular infections. Monitor IOP and perform eye exams.

Patient Counseling: Advise not to touch dropper tip to any surface; may contaminate drug. Advise to consult physician when pain develops or if redness, itching, or inflammation becomes aggravated. Instruct not to wear contact lenses during therapy.

Administration: Ocular route. **Storage**: 15-25°C (59-77°F). Do not freeze. Protect from light. Keep bottles in the protective carton when not in use.

DYAZIDE

RX

triamterene - hydrochlorothiazide (GlaxoSmithKline)

> Abnormal elevation of serum K⁺ levels (≥5.5mEq/L) may occur with all K⁺-sparing diuretic combinations. Hyperkalemia is more likely to occur with renal impairment and diabetes (even without evidence of renal impairment), and in elderly or severely ill; monitor serum K⁺ levels at frequent intervals.

THERAPEUTIC CLASS: K⁺-sparing diuretic/thiazide diuretic

INDICATIONS: Treatment of HTN or edema if hypokalemia occur on HCTZ alone, or when a thiazide diuretic is required and cannot risk hypokalemia. May be used alone or as an adjunct to other antihypertensives, such as β-blockers.

DOSAGE: *Adults:* 1-2 caps PO qd.

HOW SUPPLIED: Cap: (HCTZ-Triamterene) 25mg-37.5mg

CONTRAINDICATIONS: Anuria, acute and chronic renal insufficiency or significant renal impairment, sulfonamide hypersensitivity, preexisting elevated serum K⁺ (hyperkalemia), K⁺-sparing agents (eg, spironolactone, amiloride, or other formulations containing triamterene), K⁺ salt substitutes, K⁺ supplements (except with severe hypokalemia).

WARNINGS/PRECAUTIONS: Avoid in severely ill in whom respiratory or metabolic acidosis may occur; if used, frequent evaluations of acid/base balance and serum electrolytes are necessary. May cause idiosyncratic reaction, resulting in acute transient myopia and acute angle-closure glaucoma; d/c as rapidly as possible. Caution with diabetes; may cause hyperglycemia and glycosuria. May manifest diabetes mellitus (DM). Caution with hepatic impairment; may precipitate hepatic coma with severe liver disease. Corrective measures must be taken if hypokalemia develops; d/c and initiate potassium chloride (KCl) supplementation if serious hypokalemia develops (serum K⁺ <3.0 mEq/L). May potentiate electrolyte imbalance with heart failure, renal disease, or cirrhosis of the liver. May cause hypochloremia. Dilutional hyponatremia may occur in edematous patients in hot weather. Caution with history of renal stones. May increase BUN and SrCr. May decrease serum PBI levels. Decreased calcium excretion reported. Changes in parathyroid glands with hypercalcemia and hypophosphatemia reported during prolonged therapy. May interfere with the fluorescent measurement of quinidine.

ADVERSE REACTIONS: Muscle cramps, N/V, pancreatitis, weakness, arrhythmia, impotence, dry mouth, jaundice, paresthesia, renal stones, anaphylaxis, acute renal failure, hyperkalemia, hyponatremia.

INTERACTIONS: See Contraindications. Increased risk of hyperkalemia with ACE inhibitors, blood from blood bank, and low-salt milk. Increased risk of severe hyponatremia with chlorpropamide. Possible interaction resulting in acute renal failure with indomethacin; caution with NSAIDs. Avoid with lithium due to risk of lithium toxicity. Decreased arterial responsiveness to norepinephrine. Amphotericin B, corticosteroids, and corticotropin may intensify electrolyte imbalance, particularly hypokalemia. Adjust dose of antigout drugs to control hyperuricemia and gout. May decrease effect of oral anticoagulants. May alter insulin requirements. Increased paralyzing effects of nondepolarizing muscle relaxants (eg, tubocurarine). Reduced K⁺ levels with chronic or overuse of laxatives or use of exchange resins (eg, sodium polystyrene sulfonate). May reduce effectiveness of methenamine. Potentiated action of other antihypertensive drugs (eg, β-blockers).

PREGNANCY: Category C, not for use in nursing.

MECHANISM OF ACTION: Triamterene: K⁺-sparing diuretic; exerts diuretic effect on distal renal tubules to inhibit the reabsorption of Na in exchange for K⁺ and hydrogen ions. HCTZ: thiazide diuretic; blocks reabsorption of Na and chloride ions and thereby increases the quantity of Na transversing the distal tubule and the volume of water excreted.

PHARMACOKINETICS: Absorption: Well absorbed. Triamterene: C_{max}=46.4ng/mL; T_{max}=1.1 hrs; AUC=148.7ng•hrs/mL. HCTZ: C_{max}=135.1ng/mL; T_{max}=2 hrs; AUC=834ng•hrs/mL. **Distribution:** Crosses placenta; found in breast milk.

NURSING CONSIDERATIONS

Assessment: Assess for anuria, renal/hepatic impairment, sulfonamide hypersensitivity, hyperkalemia, diabetes, history of renal stones, pregnancy/nursing status, and for possible drug interactions. Obtain baseline BUN, SrCr, and serum electrolytes.

Monitoring: Monitor for signs/symptoms of hyperkalemia, hypokalemia, hyperglycemia, hypochloremia, renal stones, and for electrolyte imbalance. Monitor for hepatic coma in patients with severe liver disease. Monitor serum K⁺ levels, BUN, SrCr, and serum electrolytes.

Patient Counseling: Inform about risks/benefits of therapy. Advise to seek medical attention if symptoms of hyperkalemia (eg, paresthesias, muscular weakness, fatigue), hypokalemia, hyperglycemia, renal stones, electrolyte imbalance (eg, dry mouth, thirst, weakness), or hypersensitivity reactions occur.

Administration: Oral route. **Storage:** 20-25°C (68-77°F); excursions permitted to 15-30°C (59-86°F). Protect from light. Dispense in a tight, light-resistant container.

DYNACIN   RX
minocycline HCl (Medicis)

THERAPEUTIC CLASS: Tetracycline derivative

INDICATIONS: Treatment of rocky mountain spotted fever, typhus fever and the typhus group, Q fever, rickettsialpox, tick fevers, respiratory tract infections, lymphogranuloma venereum, psittacosis, trachoma, inclusion conjunctivitis, non-gonococcal urethritis, endocervical or rectal infections in adults, relapsing fever, chancroid, plague, tularemia, cholera, *Campylobacter fetus* infections, brucellosis, bartonellosis, and granuloma inguinale caused by susceptible strains of microorganisms. Treatment of infections caused by gram-negative microorganisms when bacteriologic testing indicates appropriate susceptibility to the drug (eg, respiratory tract and urinary tract infections) and gram-positive microorganisms (eg, upper respiratory tract, skin and skin structure infections). Alternative treatment in certain other infections (eg, uncomplicated urethritis in men, gonococcal infections, syphilis, yaws, listeriosis, anthrax, Vincent's infection, actinomycosis). Adjunctive therapy in acute intestinal amebiasis and severe acne. Treatment of *Mycobacterium marinum* and asymptomatic carriers of *Neisseria meningitidis*.

DOSAGE: *Adults:* Usual: 200mg initially, then 100mg q12h; alternative is 100-200mg initially, then 50mg qid. Uncomplicated Gonococcal Infection (Men, other than urethritis and anorectal infections): 200mg initially, then 100mg q12h for minimum 4 days, with post-therapy cultures within 2-3 days. Uncomplicated Gonococcal Urethritis (Men): 100mg q12h for 5 days. Syphilis: Administer usual dose for 10-15 days. Meningococcal Carrier State: 100mg q12h for 5 days. *Mycobacterium marinum:* 100mg q12h for 6-8 weeks. Uncomplicated urethral, endocervical, or rectal infection: 100mg q12h for at least 7 days. Renal Dysfunction: Reduce dose and/or extend dose intervals. Take with plenty of fluids. Take 1 hr before or 2 hrs after meals.
Pediatrics: >8 yrs: 4mg/kg initially followed by 2mg/kg q12h. Take with plenty of fluids. Taken 1 hr before or 2 hrs after meals.

HOW SUPPLIED: Tab: 50mg, 75mg, 100mg

WARNINGS/PRECAUTIONS: May cause fetal harm during pregnancy. Use during tooth development (eg, last half of pregnancy, infancy, ≤8 yrs) may cause permanent discoloration of the teeth or enamel hypoplasia; avoid use during this period. Bulging fontanels in infants have been associated with use. May decrease bone growth in premature infants. Renal toxicity, hepatotoxicity, photosensitivity, increased BUN, superinfection, pseudotumor cerebri may occur; perform hematopoietic, renal and hepatic monitoring. May impair mental/physical abilities. Not for treatment of meningococcal infections. *Clostridium difficile*-associated diarrhea (CDAD) reported. May result in bacterial resistance with prolonged use or use in the absence of a proven/suspected bacterial infection or a prophylactic indication; take appropriate measures if superinfection develops.

ADVERSE REACTIONS: Anorexia, N/V, diarrhea, dysphagia, enterocolitis, pancreatitis, increased liver enzymes, maculopapular/erythematous rash, exfoliative dermatitis, Stevens-Johnson syndrome, skin and mucous membrane pigmentation, hemolytic anemia, headache.

INTERACTIONS: May require downward adjustments of anticoagulant dosage with concomitant use. May interfere with bactericidal action of penicillin; avoid concurrent use when possible. May decrease efficacy of oral contraceptives. Impaired absorption with antacids containing aluminum, calcium or magnesium and iron-containing products. Fatal renal toxicity with methoxyflurane has been reported.

PREGNANCY: Category D, not for use in nursing.

MECHANISM OF ACTION: Tetracycline derivative; bacteriostatic. Thought to inhibit protein synthesis.

PHARMACOKINETICS: Absorption: Rapid; C_{max}= 758.29ng/mL; T_{max}= 1.71 hrs. **Distribution:** Found in breast milk. **Elimination:** Urine and feces; $T_{1/2}$= 17.03 hrs, (hepatic dysfunction) 11-16 hrs, (renal dysfunction) 18-69 hrs.

NURSING CONSIDERATIONS

Assessment: Assess for renal impairment, meningococcal infection, pregnancy/nursing status and possible drug interactions. Document indications for therapy, culture and susceptibility testing. Perform incision and drainage in conjunction with antibiotic therapy when indicated.

Monitoring: Monitor for signs/symptoms of hypersensitivity reactions, photosensitivity, superinfection, benign intracranial HTN, LFTs, renal function, CBC with platelet and differential count. In venereal disease with coexistent syphilis, conduct serologic test before treatment and after 3 months.

Patient Counseling: Inform of pregnancy risks and photosensitivity reactions (d/c at 1st sign of skin erythema). Avoid excessive sunlight/UV light and wear sunscreen/sunblock. Inform therapy treats bacterial, not viral, infections. Take as directed; skipping doses or not completing full course may decrease effectiveness and increase resistance. Notify physician if hypersensitivity reactions, superinfections, photosensitivity or benign intracranial HTN occur. Inform that concomitant use of tetracyclines may render oral contraceptives less effective.

Administration: Oral route. **Storage:** Store at 20-25°C (68-77°F). Protect from light, moisture and excessive heat.

DynaCirc CR   RX
isradipine (GlaxoSmithKline)

THERAPEUTIC CLASS: Calcium channel blocker (dihydropyridine)

INDICATIONS: Management of HTN alone or concurrently with thiazide-type diuretics.

DOSAGE: *Adults:* Individualize dose. Initial: 5mg qd alone or with a thiazide diuretic. Titrate: May adjust in increments of 5mg/day at 2-4 week intervals. Max: 20mg/day.

HOW SUPPLIED: Tab, Controlled-Release: 5mg, 10mg

WARNINGS/PRECAUTIONS: May produce symptomatic hypotension. Syncope and severe dizziness reported rarely. Caution in patients with congestive heart failure (CHF), especially with concomitant β-blockers. Peripheral edema, usually mild to moderate, may occur. Caution with preexisting severe GI narrowing; obstructive symptoms reported. Caution in elderly. Increased bioavailability in elderly, patients with hepatic functional impairment, and mild renal impairment reported.

ADVERSE REACTIONS: Headache, edema, dizziness, constipation, fatigue, flushing, abdominal discomfort.

INTERACTIONS: May increase levels of propranolol. Fentanyl anesthesia with a β-blocker may cause severe hypotension; increase in volume of circulating fluids may be required.

PREGNANCY: Category C, not for use in nursing.

MECHANISM OF ACTION: Dihydropyridine calcium channel blocker; binds to calcium channels with high affinity and specificity, and inhibits calcium flux into cardiac and smooth muscle.

PHARMACOKINETICS: Absorption: Bioavailability (15-24%), food decreased bioavailability by up to 25%; (10mg) C_{max}=3-4ng/mL; AUC=62-73ng•h/mL. **Distribution:** Plasma protein binding (95%). **Metabolism:** Complete; oxidation, ester cleavage; CYP3A4. **Elimination:** Urine (60-65%), feces (25-30%).

NURSING CONSIDERATIONS

Assessment: Assess for known hypersensitivity, CHF, preexisting severe GI narrowing, pregnancy/nursing status, and possible drug interactions.

Monitoring: Monitor for signs/symptoms of hypotension (eg, syncope and dizziness), peripheral edema, obstructive symptoms, hypersensitivity reactions, and other adverse reactions.

Patient Counseling: Instruct to swallow tab whole and not to chew, divide, or crush tab. Inform that it is normal to occasionally notice a shell resembling a tab in the stool; the medication is contained within a nonabsorbable shell designed to slowly release drug for the body to absorb. Inform of the possible risks and benefits of therapy.

Administration: Oral route. Swallow whole; do not chew, divide, or crush. **Storage:** <30°C (86°F). Protect from moisture and humidity.

Dyrenium   RX
triamterene (WellSpring)

Abnormal elevation of serum K⁺ levels (≥5.5mEq/L) can occur with all K⁺-sparing agents, including triamterene. Hyperkalemia is more likely to occur with renal impairment and diabetes (even without evidence of renal impairment), and in the elderly, or severely ill. Monitor serum K⁺ at frequent intervals.

THERAPEUTIC CLASS: K⁺-sparing diuretic

INDICATIONS: Treatment of edema associated with congestive heart failure (CHF), liver cirrhosis, and nephrotic syndrome. Treatment of steroid induced edema, idiopathic edema, and edema due to secondary hyperaldosteronism.

DOSAGE: *Adults:* Initial: 100mg bid pc. Max: 300mg/day. Titrate dose to the needs of the individual patient.

HOW SUPPLIED: Cap: 50mg, 100mg

CONTRAINDICATIONS: Anuria, severe or progressive kidney disease or dysfunction (except with nephrosis), severe hepatic disease, hyperkalemia, K$^+$ supplements, K$^+$ salts or K$^+$ containing salt substitutes, K$^+$-sparing agents (eg, spironolactone, amiloride hydrochloride).

WARNINGS/PRECAUTIONS: Check ECG if hyperkalemia occurs. Isolated reports of hypersensitivity reactions; monitor for possible occurrence of blood dyscrasias, liver damage, or other idiosyncratic reactions. In cirrhotics with splenomegaly, may contribute to megaloblastosis in cases where folic stores have been depleted; perform periodic blood studies and observe for exacerbation of liver disease. Monitor BUN periodically. Caution with gouty arthritis; may elevate uric acid levels. May aggravate or cause electrolyte imbalances in CHF, renal disease, or cirrhosis. Caution with history of renal stones.

ADVERSE REACTIONS: Hypersensitivity reactions, hyper- or hypokalemia, azotemia, renal stones, jaundice, thrombocytopenia, megaloblastic anemia, N/V, diarrhea, weakness, dizziness.

INTERACTIONS: See Contraindications. Increased risk of hyperkalemia with ACE inhibitors. Indomethacin may cause renal failure; caution with NSAIDs. Risk of lithium toxicity. Hyperkalemia may occur when used concomitantly with blood from blood bank, low-salt milk, or potassium containing medications (eg, parenteral penicillin G potassium). May cause hyperglycemia; adjust antidiabetic agents. Chlorpropamide may increase risk of severe hyponatremia. May potentiate nondepolarizing muscle relaxants, antihypertensives, other diuretics, preanesthetics, and anesthetics.

PREGNANCY: Category C, not for use in nursing.

MECHANISM OF ACTION: K$^+$ sparing diuretic; inhibits reabsorption of Na$^+$ ions in exchange for K$^+$ and H$^+$ ions at segment of distal tubule under control of adrenal mineralocorticoids.

PHARMACOKINETICS: Absorption: Rapid; C$_{max}$=30ng/mL, T$_{max}$=3 hrs. **Distribution:** Plasma protein binding (67%); crosses placental barrier. **Metabolism:** Hydroxytriamterene (metabolite). **Elimination:** Urine (21%).

NURSING CONSIDERATIONS

Assessment: Assess for anuria, CHF, diabetes mellitus, gout, hyperkalemia, history of kidney stones, liver/renal impairment, pregnancy/nursing status, and for possible drug interactions.

Monitoring: Monitor for signs/symptoms of electrolyte imbalance, exacerbation of gout, hypersensitivity reactions (eg, blood dyscrasias, liver damage), and for liver/renal dysfunction. Monitor for signs/symptoms of hyperkalemia and perform ECG if suspected. Monitor BUN, serum K$^+$ levels, and CBC periodically.

Patient Counseling: Advise to take after meals to avoid stomach upset. Inform that if single dose is prescribed, it may be preferable to take in a.m. to minimize frequency of urination during nighttime sleep. Instruct not to take more than prescribed dose at next dosing interval if dose missed. Seek medical attention if symptoms of hyperkalemia, electrolyte imbalance, or hypersensitivity reactions occur.

Administration: Oral route. **Storage:** 25°C (77°F); excursions permitted to 15-30°C (59-86°F). Dispense in tight, light-resistant container.

DYSPORT   RX
abobotulinumtoxinA (Ipsen)

> Distant spread of toxin effects reported hrs to weeks after inj (eg, asthenia, generalized muscle weakness, diplopia, blurred vision, ptosis, dysphagia, dysphonia, dysarthria, urinary incontinence, breathing difficulties). Swallowing and breathing difficulties can be life threatening and there have been reports of death. Risk of symptoms is greatest in children treated for spasticity but can also occur in adults. In unapproved uses and approved indications, cases of spread of effect have been reported at doses comparable to those used to treat cervical dystonia and at lower doses.

THERAPEUTIC CLASS: Purified neurotoxin complex

INDICATIONS: Treatment of adults with cervical dystonia to reduce the severity of abnormal head position and neck pain in both toxin-naive and previously treated patients. For temporary improvement in the appearance of moderate to severe glabellar lines associated with procerus and corrugator muscle activity in adults <65 yrs.

DOSAGE: *Adults:* Initial: Cervical Dystonia: 500 U IM as a divided dose among affected muscles. Titrate: 250 U steps according to response; retreat q12 weeks or longer PRN, based on return of clinical symptoms. Max: 1000 U. Do not retreat in intervals of <12 weeks. Glabellar Lines: 50 U IM in 5 equal aliquots of 10 U each. Do not administer more frequently than q3 months.

HOW SUPPLIED: Inj: 300 U, 500 U

CONTRAINDICATIONS: Allergy to cow's milk protein, infection at the proposed inj site(s).

WARNINGS/PRECAUTIONS: Not interchangeable with other botulinum toxin products; cannot be compared or converted into units of any other botulinum toxin products. Aspiration and death due to severe dysphagia reported. May weaken neck muscles that serve as accessory muscles of ventilation. Serious breathing difficulties, including respiratory failure, reported with cervical dystonia. May require immediate medical attention if swallowing, speech, or respiratory disorders occur. Caution with surgical alterations to facial anatomy, excessive weakness or atrophy in the target muscle(s), marked facial asymmetry, inflammation at the inj site(s), ptosis, excessive dermatochalasis, deep dermal scarring, thick sebaceous skin, or the inability to substantially lessen glabellar lines by physically spreading them apart. Increased incidence of eyelid ptosis with higher doses. Closely monitor patients with peripheral motor neuropathic diseases, amyotrophic lateral sclerosis, neuromuscular junction disorders (eg, myasthenia gravis or Lambert-Eaton syndrome); may increase risk of clinically significant effects including severe dysphagia and respiratory compromise from typical doses. Contains albumin; risk of transmitting viral diseases and Creutzfeldt-Jakob disease. Caution in elderly.

ADVERSE REACTIONS: Asthenia, generalized muscle weakness, diplopia, blurred vision, ptosis, dysphagia, dysphonia, dysarthria, urinary incontinence, breathing difficulties, discomfort at inj site, dry mouth, fatigue, headache, nasopharyngitis.

INTERACTIONS: Potentiation of toxin effect may occur with aminoglycosides or with other agents interfering with neuromuscular transmission (eg, curare-like agents); monitor closely. Use of anticholinergic drugs after administration may potentiate systemic anticholinergic effects. Excessive weakness may be exacerbated if another botulinum toxin is administered before effects resolve from the previous botulinum toxin inj administration. Use of a muscle relaxant before/after administration may exaggerate excessive weakness.

PREGNANCY: Category C, safety not known in nursing.

MECHANISM OF ACTION: Purified neurotoxin type A complex; inhibits release of acetylcholine from peripheral cholinergic nerve endings; produces chemical denervation of the muscle resulting in a localized reduction in muscle activity.

NURSING CONSIDERATIONS

Assessment: Assess for allergy to cow's milk protein, infection/inflammation at proposed inj site(s), preexisting swallowing/breathing difficulties, surgical facial alterations, excessive weakness or atrophy in the target muscle(s), marked facial asymmetry, ptosis, excessive dermatochalasis, deep dermal scarring, thick sebaceous skin, inability to substantially lessen glabellar lines by physically spreading them apart, preexisting neuromuscular disorders, pregnancy/nursing status, and possible drug interactions.

Monitoring: Monitor for spread of the toxin effects, weakening of neck muscles, and swallowing/speech/respiratory disorders. Monitor patients with peripheral motor neuropathic diseases, amyotrophic lateral sclerosis, or neuromuscular junction disorders.

Patient Counseling: Advise to notify physician if any unusual symptoms develop (eg, difficulty with swallowing, speaking, or breathing) or if any known symptom persists or worsens. Instruct to avoid driving or engaging in potentially hazardous activities if loss of strength, muscle weakness, blurred vision, or drooping eyelids occur.

Administration: IM route. Refer to PI for instructions for preparation and administration instructions. Storage: 2-8°C (36-46°F). Protect from light. Reconstituted: Use within 4 hrs. Do not freeze.

EDARBI   RX
azilsartan medoxomil (Takeda)

> Drugs that act directly on the renin-angiotensin system can cause death/injury to developing fetus. D/C therapy if pregnancy is detected.

THERAPEUTIC CLASS: Angiotensin II receptor antagonist

INDICATIONS: Treatment of HTN alone or in combination with other antihypertensives.

DOSAGE: *Adults:* Usual: 80mg qd. With High Dose Diuretics: Initial: 40mg qd. May add other antihypertensives if BP is not controlled with monotherapy.

HOW SUPPLIED: Tab: 40mg, 80mg

WARNINGS/PRECAUTIONS: Symptomatic hypotension may occur in patients with an activated renin-angiotensin system (eg, volume- and/or salt-depleted patients such as those receiving high doses of diuretics); correct this condition prior to therapy or start with 40mg. Changes in renal function may occur. Oliguria or progressive azotemia and (rarely) acute renal failure and death may occur in patients whose renal function is dependent on the renin-angiotensin system (eg, severe congestive heart failure [CHF], renal artery stenosis, volume depletion). May increase SrCr or BUN in patients with renal artery stenosis.

ADVERSE REACTIONS: Dizziness, postural dizziness, diarrhea, nausea, asthenia, fatigue, muscle spasm, cough.

INTERACTIONS: May deteriorate renal function and attenuate antihypertensive effect with NSAIDs, including cyclooxygenase-2 inhibitors; monitor renal function periodically. Increases in SrCr may be larger with chlorthalidone or HCTZ.

PREGNANCY: Category D, not for use in nursing.

MECHANISM OF ACTION: Angiotensin II receptor antagonist; blocks the vasoconstrictor and aldosterone-secreting effects of angiotensin II by selectively blocking the binding of angiotensin II to AT_1 receptor in many tissues, such as vascular smooth muscle, and adrenal glands.

PHARMACOKINETICS: Absorption: Absolute bioavailability (60%); T_{max}=1.5-3 hrs. **Distribution:** V_d=16L; plasma protein binding (>99%). **Metabolism:** Converted to azilsartan (active metabolite) in GI tract via hydrolysis, then in the liver via CYP2C9 by O-dealkylation and decarboxylation. **Elimination:** Urine (42%; 15% azilsartan), feces (55%); $T_{1/2}$=11 hrs.

NURSING CONSIDERATIONS

Assessment: Assess for volume/salt depletion, renal impairment, CHF, renal artery stenosis, pregnancy/nursing status, and possible drug interactions.

Monitoring: Monitor for signs/symptoms of hypotension, renal dysfunction, and other adverse reactions.

Patient Counseling: Inform of pregnancy risks. Instruct to notify physician if pregnant or plan to become pregnant. Advise to seek medical attention if symptoms of hypotension or other adverse events occur. Inform that drug may be taken with/without food.

Administration: Oral route. **Storage:** 25°C (77°F); excursions permitted to 15-30°C (59-86°F). Protect from moisture and light.

EDLUAR
zolpidem tartrate (Meda)

CIV

THERAPEUTIC CLASS: Imidazopyridine hypnotic

INDICATIONS: Short-term treatment of insomnia, characterized by difficulties with sleep initiation.

DOSAGE: *Adults:* Individualize dose. 10mg SL qhs. Max: 10mg/day. Elderly/Debilitated Patients: 5mg SL qhs. Concomitant Use with CNS-Depressant Drugs: Require dose adjustment.

HOW SUPPLIED: Tab, Sublingual: 5mg, 10mg

WARNINGS/PRECAUTIONS: Evaluate for primary psychiatric and/or medical illness if insomnia fails to remit after 7-10 days of treatment. Severe anaphylactic and anaphylactoid reactions reported; do not rechallenge if patient develops reactions. Visual/auditory hallucinations, complex behavior (eg, sleep-driving), abnormal thinking and behavior changes reported. Worsening of depression, including suicidal thoughts and actions have been reported in depressed patients. May impair mental/physical abilities. Caution with conditions that could affect metabolism or hemodynamic responses, sleep apnea, myasthenia gravis, and worsening depression. Signs and symptoms of withdrawal reported with abrupt d/c of sedative/hypnotics. Monitor elderly and debilitated patients for impaired motor and/or cognitive performance.

ADVERSE REACTIONS: Drowsiness, dizziness, diarrhea, headache, drugged feeling, dry mouth, back pain, allergy, sinusitis, pharyngitis.

INTERACTIONS: CNS-active drugs may potentially enhance effects. Additive effects on psychomotor performance with alcohol/chlorpromazine. Decreased alertness observed with imipramine/chlorpromazine. Ketoconazole may enhance sedative effects. May decrease effects with rifampin.

PREGNANCY: Category C, caution in nursing.

MECHANISM OF ACTION: Imidazopyridine, non-benzodiazepine hypnotic; binds to GABA-BZ receptor complex at the a_1/a_5 subunits.

PHARMACOKINETICS: Absorption: Rapid; C_{max}=106ng/mL; T_{max}=82 min. **Distribution:** Plasma protein binding (92.5%). **Elimination:** Renal; (5mg) $T_{1/2}$=2.85 hrs, (10mg) $T_{1/2}$=2.65 hrs.

NURSING CONSIDERATIONS

Assessment: Assess for primary psychiatric and/or medical illness, preexisting respiratory impairment (eg, sleep apnea syndrome), myasthenia gravis, hypersensitivity reactions, hepatic impairment, history of alcohol, pregnancy/nursing status, and possible drug interactions.

Monitoring: Monitor for anaphylactic/anaphylactoid reactions, abnormal thinking, behavioral changes, complex behavior (eg, sleep-driving), hepatic impairment, and those on long-term treatment for drug abuse/dependence.

Patient Counseling: Instruct not to swallow or take with water. Tablet should be placed under the tongue. Should not to be given with or immediately after a meal. Inform to take just before bedtime. Advise not to take with alcohol. Caution against hazardous tasks (eg, driving/operating machinery). Counsel about risks/benefits of use. Seek medical attention if severe anaphylactic and anaphylactoid reactions occur. Notify physician of all concomitant medications and any episodes of sleep-driving or complex behaviors.

Administration: Oral route. Tablet should be placed under the tongue. **Storage:** 20-25°C (68-77°F). Protect from light and moisture.

EDURANT RX
rilpivirine (Tibotec)

THERAPEUTIC CLASS: Non-nucleoside reverse transcriptase inhibitor

INDICATIONS: Treatment of HIV-1 infection in combination with other antiretrovirals in treatment-naive adults.

DOSAGE: *Adults:* 1 tab qd with a meal.

HOW SUPPLIED: Tab: 25mg

CONTRAINDICATIONS: Concomitant use with carbamazepine, oxcarbazepine, phenobarbital, phenytoin, rifabutin, rifampin, rifapentine, proton pump inhibitors, systemic dexamethasone (more than a single dose), St. John's wort.

WARNINGS/PRECAUTIONS: Depressive disorders reported; immediate medical evaluation is recommended if severe symptoms occur. May cause redistribution/accumulation of body fat. Immune reconstitution syndrome reported. Monitor for adverse effects in severe renal impairment or end-stage renal disease. Caution in elderly.

ADVERSE REACTIONS: Increased LFTs (AST, ALT, total bilirubin), increased serum lipids (total cholesterol, LDL), increased SrCr, depressive disorders, insomnia, headache, rash.

INTERACTIONS: See Contraindications. Coadministration with drugs that induce or inhibit CYP3A may affect plasma concentrations or result in loss of virologic response and possible resistance. Not recommended with delavirdine and other non-nucleoside reverse transcriptase inhibitors (NNRTIs). Concomitant didanosine should be given on an empty stomach and at least 2 hrs before or 4 hrs after dosing. Darunavir, lopinavir, and other HIV protease inhibitors boosted with ritonavir or unboosted, azole antifungals (eg, ketoconazole), and macrolide antibiotics may increase levels. Monitor for potential breakthrough fungal infections or use alternatives to macrolides such as azithromycin when necessary. Antacids and H_2-receptor antagonists (H_2-RAs) (eg, famotidine) may decrease levels due to increased gastric pH. Administer antacids at least 2 hrs before or 4 hrs after dosing and H_2-RAs at least 12 hrs before or 4 hrs after dosing. Clinical monitoring recommended when coadministered with methadone maintenance therapy. Caution with drugs with a known risk of torsades de pointes.

PREGNANCY: Category B, not for use in nursing.

MECHANISM OF ACTION: NNRTI; inhibits HIV-1 replication by noncompetitive inhibition of HIV-1 reverse transcriptase.

PHARMACOKINETICS: Absorption: T_{max}=4-5 hrs. Exposure reduced during fasted state. **Distribution:** Plasma protein binding (99.7%). **Metabolism:** Liver via CYP3A oxidation. **Elimination:** Feces (85%, 25% unchanged), urine (6.1%, <1% unchanged); $T_{1/2}$=50 hrs.

NURSING CONSIDERATIONS

Assessment: Assess for severe hepatic or renal impairment, pregnancy/nursing status, and possible drug interactions.

Monitoring: Monitor for depressive disorders, immune reconstitution syndrome (eg, opportunistic infections), and body fat redistribution/accumulation.

Patient Counseling: Inform patient that it does not cure HIV infection; continuous therapy is necessary to control infection and decrease related illness. Precautions should be taken to avoid transmission (eg, safe sex practices, do not reuse or share needles). Inform mothers to avoid nursing to reduce risk of transmission to their baby. Instruct to always take with a meal and at recommended dosing schedules in combination with other antiretrovirals. Patients should seek immediate evaluation for severe depressive symptoms or if a potential opportunistic infection develops. Advise that redistribution or accumulation of body fat may occur.

Administration: Oral route. **Storage:** 25°C (77°F); excursions permitted to 15-30°C (59-86°F). Protect from light.

336 PDR® Nurse's Drug Handbook

EFFEXOR XR
venlafaxine HCl (Wyeth)

RX

THERAPEUTIC CLASS: Serotonin and norepinephrine reuptake inhibitor

INDICATIONS: Treatment of MDD, generalized anxiety disorder (GAD), social anxiety disorder (SAD), and panic disorder (PD).

DOSAGE: *Adults:* MDD/GAD: Initial: 75mg qd, or 37.5mg qd for 4-7 days and then increase to 75mg qd. Titrate: May increase by increments of up to 75mg/day at ≥4-day intervals. Max: 225mg/day. PD: Initial: 37.5mg qd for 7 days. Titrate: May increase by increments of up to 75mg/day at ≥7 day intervals. Max: 225mg/day. SAD: 75mg/day. Switching from Effexor IR Tablets: Give the nearest equivalent dose (mg/day) qd. Individual dose adjustments may be necessary. Hepatic Impairment (Mild-Moderate)/Hemodialysis: Individualize. Reduce total daily dose by 50%. Renal Impairment: Individualize. Reduce total daily dose by 25-50%.

HOW SUPPLIED: Cap, Extended-Release: 37.5mg, 75mg, 150mg

CONTRAINDICATIONS: Concomitant use of MAOIs or use within 14 days of taking an MAOI; allow ≥7 days after stopping drug before starting an MAOI.

WARNINGS/PRECAUTIONS: Avoid abrupt withdrawal; gradually reduce dose and monitor for d/c symptoms. Not approved for use in treating bipolar depression. Serotonin syndrome or neuroleptic malignant syndrome (NMS)-like reactions reported; d/c immediately and initiate supportive symptomatic treatment. May cause sustained increases in BP; consider dose reduction or d/c. Mydriasis reported; monitor patients with increased intraocular pressure (IOP) or those at risk of acute narrow-angle glaucoma. Treatment-emergent nervousness, insomnia, weight loss, anorexia, and activation of mania/hypomania reported. May cause hyponatremia; d/c if with symptomatic hyponatremia and institute appropriate intervention. May increase risk of bleeding events. Elevation of cholesterol levels reported; monitor periodically. Caution with history of mania or seizures, conditions affecting hemodynamic responses or metabolism, conditions that may be compromised by HR increases (eg, hyperthyroidism, heart failure [HF], recent myocardial infarction [MI]), renal/hepatic impairment, and in elderly. Interstitial lung disease and eosinophilic pneumonia reported rarely. D/C if seizures, interstitial lung disease, and eosinophilic pneumonia occur.

ADVERSE REACTIONS: Asthenia, sweating, headache, N/V, constipation, anorexia, dry mouth, dizziness, insomnia, nervousness, somnolence, abnormal ejaculation/orgasm, abnormal dreams, pharyngitis.

INTERACTIONS: See Contraindications. Serotonin syndrome or NMS-like reactions reported when used alone and in combination with serotonergic drugs (eg, triptans), drugs that impair serotonin metabolism, antipsychotics, and dopamine antagonists. Avoid alcohol and tryptophan. Increased risk of bleeding with aspirin (ASA), NSAIDs, warfarin, and other anticoagulants. Caution with cimetidine in elderly, with HTN, and hepatic dysfunction. Altered coagulation effects with warfarin. Decreases clearance of haloperidol. May increase levels of metoprolol, risperidone, and desipramine. Increased levels with cimetidine and ketoconazole. Decreased indinavir levels. May inhibit metabolism of CYP2D6 substrates. Caution with metoprolol, CYP3A4 inhibitors, CYP2D6 inhibitors, CNS-active drugs, and serotonergic drugs (eg, triptans, SSRIs, other serotonin and norepinephrine reuptake inhibitors [SNRIs], linezolid, lithium, tramadol, or St. John's wort). Coadministration with weight-loss agents not recommended. Diuretics may increase risk of hyponatremia.

PREGNANCY: Category C, not for use in nursing.

MECHANISM OF ACTION: SNRI; potentiates neurotransmitter activity in CNS by inhibiting neuronal serotonin and norepinephrine reuptake.

PHARMACOKINETICS: Absorption: Venlafaxine: Well absorbed. Absolute bioavailability (45%), C_{max}=150ng/mL, T_{max}=5.5 hrs. O-desmethylvenlafaxine (ODV) (metabolite): C_{max}=260ng/mL, T_{max}=9 hrs. **Distribution:** Venlafaxine: V_d=7.5L/kg; plasma protein binding (27%). ODV: V_d=5.7L/kg; plasma protein binding (30%); found in breast milk. **Metabolism:** Extensive. Hepatic; ODV (major active metabolite). **Elimination:** Urine (87%, 5% unchanged, 29% unconjugated ODV, 26% conjugated ODV, 27% minor inactive metabolites); Venlafaxine: $T_{1/2}$=5 hrs. ODV: $T_{1/2}$=11 hrs.

NURSING CONSIDERATIONS

Assessment: Assess for bipolar disorder, history of mania and drug abuse, hyperthyroidism, HF, recent MI, history of glaucoma, increased IOP, risk factors for acute narrow-angle glaucoma, preexisting HTN, history of seizures, disease/condition that alters metabolism or hemodynamic response, cholesterol levels, hepatic/renal impairment, drug hypersensitivity, pregnancy/nursing status, and possible drug interactions. Obtain a detailed psychiatric history.

Monitoring: Monitor HR, BP, LFTs, renal function, cholesterol, height and weight, TG and ECG changes. Monitor for signs/symptoms of clinical worsening, suicidality, unusual behavior, serotonin syndrome or NMS-like reactions, mydriasis, severe HTN, lung disease, abnormal bleeding, allergic reactions, hyponatremia, seizures, cognitive/motor impairment, and hepatic/renal dysfunction. If abruptly d/c, monitor for d/c symptoms (eg, dysphoric mood, irritability, agitation). Periodically reevaluate long-term usefulness of therapy.

Patient Counseling: Advise to avoid alcohol. Inform about the risks and benefits associated with treatment. Instruct to read the Medication Guide. Advise to inform physician if taking, or plan to take, any prescription or OTC drugs, including herbal preparations and nutritional supplements, since there is a potential for interactions. Seek medical attention for symptoms of serotonin syndrome, abnormal bleeding (particularly if using NSAIDs or ASA), hyponatremia, mydriasis, severe HTN, lung disease (eg, progressive dyspnea, cough, chest discomfort), activation of mania, seizures, clinical worsening (eg, suicidal ideation, unusual changes in behavior), or d/c symptoms (eg, irritability, agitation, dizziness, anxiety, headache, insomnia). May impair physical/mental abilities. Notify physician if pregnant or breastfeeding or if rash, hives, or related allergic phenomenon develop.

Administration: Oral route. Take with food at same time each day, either in am or pm. Swallow whole with fluid and do not divide, crush, chew, or place in water. May administer by sprinkling contents of cap on spoonful of applesauce; swallow without chewing and follow with glass of water. **Storage:** 20-25°C (68-77°F).

EFFIENT   RX
prasugrel (Daiichi Sankyo/Eli Lilly)

May cause significant, sometimes fatal, bleeding; risk factors include <60kg body weight, propensity to bleed, and concomitant use of medications that may increase bleeding (eg, warfarin, heparin, fibrinolytic therapy, chronic use of NSAIDs). Do not use in patients with active pathological bleeding or history of transient ischemic attacks (TIA) or stroke. Not recommended in patients ≥75 yrs due to increased risk of fatal and intracranial bleeding and uncertain benefit, except in high-risk situations (diabetes or history of prior myocardial infarction [MI]) where the effect appears to be greater and use may be considered. Do not start in patients likely to undergo urgent coronary artery bypass graft surgery (CABG); d/c at least 7 days prior to any surgery when possible. Suspect bleeding in any patient who is hypotensive and has recently undergone coronary angiography, percutaneous coronary intervention (PCI), CABG, or other surgical procedures; if possible, manage bleeding without d/c. Discontinuing particularly in the 1st few weeks after acute coronary syndrome (ACS), increases the risk of subsequent cardiovascular (CV) events.

THERAPEUTIC CLASS: Platelet aggregation inhibitor

INDICATIONS: To reduce the rate of thrombotic CV events (eg, stent thrombosis) in patients with ACS (eg, unstable angina, non-ST-elevation MI, ST-elevation MI) who are to be managed with PCI. To reduce the rate of a combined endpoint of CV death, nonfatal MI, or nonfatal stroke.

DOSAGE: *Adults:* LD: 60mg PO single dose. Maint: 10mg qd. <60kg: Consider lowering the maintenance dose to 5mg qd. Take with aspirin (ASA) (75-325mg/day).

HOW SUPPLIED: Tab: 5mg, 10mg

CONTRAINDICATIONS: Active pathological bleeding (eg, peptic ulcer, intracranial hemorrhage), history of prior TIA or stroke.

WARNINGS/PRECAUTIONS: Withholding a dose will not be useful in managing a bleeding event or the risk of bleeding associated with an invasive procedure. CABG-related bleeding may be treated with blood transfusion; platelet transfusion within 6 hrs of LD or 4 hrs of maint dose may be less effective. D/C if active bleeding, elective surgery, stroke, or TIA occurs. Lapses in therapy should be avoided; if therapy is temporarily d/c because of adverse events, restart as soon as possible. Thrombotic thrombocytopenic purpura (TTP) reported; may occur after a brief exposure (<2 weeks) and requires urgent treatment (eg, plasmapheresis). Hypersensitivity including angioedema reported.

ADVERSE REACTIONS: CABG/non-CABG-related bleeding, HTN, hypercholesterolemia/hyperlipidemia, headache, back pain, dyspnea, nausea, dizziness, cough, hypotension, fatigue, noncardiac chest pain.

INTERACTIONS: See Boxed Warning. Ranitidine or lansoprazole may decrease C_{max} of prasugrel active metabolite. Ketoconazole may decrease C_{max}. ASA may increase bleeding time.

PREGNANCY: Category B, caution in nursing.

MECHANISM OF ACTION: Platelet aggregation inhibitor (thienopyridine class); inhibits platelet activation and aggregation through irreversible binding of its active metabolite to the $P2Y_{12}$ class of ADP receptors on platelets.

PHARMACOKINETICS: Absorption: Rapid; T_{max}=30 min. **Distribution:** V_d=44-68L (active metabolite). **Metabolism:** Hydrolysis; converted to active metabolite via CYP3A4 and CYP2B6 and to a lesser extent by CYP2C9 and CYP2C19. **Elimination:** Urine (68%), feces (27%); $T_{1/2}$=7 hrs (active metabolite).

NURSING CONSIDERATIONS

Assessment: Assess for active pathological bleeding, history of prior TIA or stroke, ACS, concomitant use of medications that may increase bleeding, recent trauma/surgery, recent or recurrent GI bleeding, active peptic ulcer disease, severe hepatic impairment, age, weight, history of hypersensitivity reaction to other thienopyridines, pregnancy/nursing status, and possible drug interactions.

Monitoring: Monitor for bleeding, TTP (eg, thrombocytopenia), hypersensitivity, and other adverse reactions. Monitor for cardiac events in patients who require premature d/c.

Patient Counseling: Inform about the benefits and risks of treatment. Instruct to take exactly as prescribed and not to d/c without consulting the prescribing physician. Inform that they may bruise and/or bleed more easily and that bleeding will take longer than usual to stop. Advise to report to physician any unanticipated, prolonged, or excessive bleeding, or blood in stool or urine. Inform that TTP, a rare but serious condition, has been reported; instruct to seek prompt medical attention if unexplained fever, weakness, extreme skin paleness, purple skin patches, yellowing of the skin or eyes, or neurological changes occur. Inform that hypersensitivity reactions may occur and that patients who have had hypersensitivity reactions to other thienopyridines may experience this as well. Instruct to notify physician or dentist about therapy before scheduling any invasive procedure.

Administration: Oral route. Do not break the tab. **Storage:** 25°C (77°F); excursions permitted to 15-30°C (59-86°F).

EGRIFTA   RX
tesamorelin (EMD Serono)

THERAPEUTIC CLASS: Growth hormone-releasing factor

INDICATIONS: Reduction of excess abdominal fat in HIV-infected patients with lipodystrophy.

DOSAGE: *Adults:* 2mg SQ in the abdomen qd.

HOW SUPPLIED: Inj (powder): 1mg

CONTRAINDICATIONS: Pregnancy, newly diagnosed or recurrent active malignancy, and disruption of hypothalamic-pituitary axis (HPA) due to hypophysectomy, hypopituitarism, pituitary tumor/surgery, head irradiation or head trauma.

WARNINGS/PRECAUTIONS: Carefully consider continuation of treatment in patients who do not show clear efficacy response. Not indicated for weight loss management. Caution with history of non-malignant neoplasms or treated and stable malignancies. Increases serum insulin growth factor-I (IGF-I); monitor IGF-I levels closely and consider d/c with persistent elevations. Fluid retention (eg, edema, arthralgia, carpal tunnel syndrome) may occur. May cause glucose intolerance and diabetes; evaluate glucose status prior to therapy then monitor periodically. May develop or worsen retinopathy in patients with diabetes. Hypersensitivity reactions may occur; d/c treatment immediately when reactions suspected. Rotate site of injection to different areas of abdomen to reduce injection-site reactions (eg, erythema, pruritus, pain, irritation, bruising). Consider d/c in critically ill patients; increased mortality reported in patients with acute critical illness after treatment with growth hormone (GH).

ADVERSE REACTIONS: Arthralgia, pain in extremity, myalgia, injection-site reactions (eg, erythema, pruritus, pain), peripheral edema, paresthesia, hypoesthesia, nausea, rash.

INTERACTIONS: GH may modulate CYP450 mediated antipyrine clearance; caution with CYP450 substrates (eg, corticosteroids, sex steroids, anticonvulsants, cyclosporine). May require an increase in maintenance or stress doses of glucocorticoids particularly in patients taking cortisone acetate and prednisone. Decreased absorption of simvastatin, simvastatin acid, and ritonavir.

PREGNANCY: Category X, not for use in nursing.

MECHANISM OF ACTION: Human Growth Hormone-Releasing Factor (GRF) synthetic analog; acts on pituitary somatotroph cells to stimulate the synthesis and pulsatile release of endogenous GH, which is both anabolic and lipolytic.

PHARMACOKINETICS: Absorption: Absolute bioavailability (<4%, healthy); AUC=634.6pg•h/mL (healthy), 852.8pg•h/mL (HIV-infected); C_{max}=2874.6pg/mL (healthy), 2822.3pg/mL (HIV-infected); T_{max}=0.15 hr (healthy, HIV infected). **Distribution:** V_d=9.4L/kg (healthy), 10.5L/kg (HIV-infected). **Elimination:** $T_{1/2}$=26 min (healthy), 38 min (HIV-infected).

NURSING CONSIDERATIONS

Assessment: Assess for active malignancy, hypersensitivity to tesamorelin and/or mannitol, HPA disruption due to hypophysectomy, hypopituitarism, pituitary tumor/surgery, head irritation or head trauma, history of non-malignant neoplasms or treated and stable malignancies, increased background risk of malignancies, glucose status, acute critical illness, pregnancy/nursing status, and possible drug interactions.

E

Monitoring: Monitor for response, IGF-I levels, HbA1c levels, changes in glucose metabolism, glucose intolerance, diabetes, worsening or development of retinopathy, and hypersensitivity reactions.

Patient Counseling: Advise that treatment may cause transient symptoms consistent with fluid retention (eg, edema, arthralgia, carpal tunnel syndrome) which resolve upon d/c. Seek medical attention and d/c therapy immediately when hypersensitivity reactions occur (eg, rash, urticaria). Advise to rotate the site of injection to different areas of abdomen to reduce incidence of injection site reactions (eg, erythema, pruritus, pain, irritation, bruising). Counsel not to share syringe with another person, even if the needle is changed. Advise women to d/c treatment if pregnant and not to breastfeed; apprise of the potential hazard to the fetus.

Administration: SQ route. Recommended site is the abdomen. Do not inject into scar tissue, bruises, or the navel. Refer to Instructions For Use leaflet for reconstitution procedures. Reconstituted sol (1mg/mL) should be injected immediately. **Storage:** Unreconstituted: 2-8°C (36-46°F). Diluent/Syringes/Needles: 20-25°C (68-77°F). Protect from light. Keep in the original box until use.

ELDEPRYL   RX
selegiline HCl (Somerset)

THERAPEUTIC CLASS: Monoamine oxidase inhibitor (Type B)

INDICATIONS: Adjunct in the management of parkinsonian patients being treated with levodopa/carbidopa who exhibit deterioration in the quality of their response to this therapy.

DOSAGE: *Adults:* 10mg qd as divided doses of 5mg each taken at breakfast and lunch. Max: 10mg/day. May attempt to reduce levodopa/carbidopa after 2-3 days of therapy. Usual reduction of 10-30%; may reduce further with continued therapy.

HOW SUPPLIED: Cap: 5mg; (Generic) Tab: 5mg

CONTRAINDICATIONS: Concomitant meperidine, or other opioids.

WARNINGS/PRECAUTIONS: Selegiline should not be used at doses >10mg/day due to risks associated with nonselective inhibition of MAO. Decrease levodopa/carbidopa by 10-30% to prevent exacerbation of levodopa-associated side effects. Patients with Parkinson's disease have higher risk of melanoma; monitor frequently for melanoma.

ADVERSE REACTIONS: Nausea, dizziness/lightheadedness/fainting, abdominal pain, confusion, hallucinations, dry mouth, vivid dreams, dyskinesias, headache.

INTERACTIONS: See Contraindications. Avoid SSRIs and TCAs; severe toxicity reported. Allow ≥2 weeks between d/c of selegiline and initiation of TCAs or SSRIs. Allow ≥5 weeks between d/c of fluoxetine and initiation of selegiline due to long half-lives of fluoxetine and its active metabolite. Caution with ephedrine and tyramine-containing foods; hypertensive crises/reactions reported.

PREGNANCY: Category C, not for use in nursing.

MECHANISM OF ACTION: MAOI (type B); mechanism not established. Irreversibly inhibits MAO type B (selectivity is dose-dependent) blocking the catabolism of dopamine. May also act through other mechanisms to increase dopaminergic activity.

PHARMACOKINETICS: Absorption: C_{max}=1ng/mL. **Metabolism:** Extensive via gut and liver. N-desmethylselegiline (active metabolite). **Elimination:** $T_{1/2}$=2 hrs (single-dose), 10 hrs (steady-state).

NURSING CONSIDERATIONS

Assessment: Assess pregnancy/nursing status, hypersensitivity, and possible drug interactions.

Monitoring: Monitor for hypersensitivity reactions, adverse effects, hypertensive crisis, hallucinations, myoclonic jerks, intense urges to gamble and for increased sexual urges. Monitor frequently for melanoma. Periodic skin examinations should be performed by qualified individuals (eg, dermatologists).

Patient Counseling: Advise of the possible need to reduce levodopa dosage, not to exceed 10mg/day, and of the risk of using higher daily doses. Inform patients or their families about signs and symptoms of MAOI-induced hypertensive reactions; immediately report severe headache or other atypical/unusual symptoms. Report any intense urges to gamble, increased sexual urges and other intense urges and inability to control these urges. Avoid tyramine-containing foods (eg, cheese), and provide a description of the 'cheese reaction.'

Administration: Oral route. **Storage:** 20-25°C (68-77°F).

ELESTAT

epinastine HCl (Allergan)

THERAPEUTIC CLASS: H$_1$-antagonist

INDICATIONS: Prevention of itching associated with allergic conjunctivitis.

DOSAGE: *Adults:* 1 drop in ou bid. Continue treatment throughout the period of exposure, even when symptoms are absent.
Pediatrics: ≥2 yrs: 1 drop in ou bid. Continue treatment throughout the period of exposure, even when symptoms are absent.

HOW SUPPLIED: Sol: 0.05% [5mL]

WARNINGS/PRECAUTIONS: For topical ophthalmic use only. Avoid allowing tip of dispensing container to contact eye, surrounding structures, fingers, or any other surface to avoid contamination of sol; serious damage to eye and subsequent loss of vision may result from using contaminated sol. Not for treatment of contact lens-related irritation. Remove contact lenses prior to instillation and reinsert after 10 min.

ADVERSE REACTIONS: Burning sensation in the eye, folliculosis, hyperemia, pruritus, infection, headache, rhinitis, sinusitis, increased cough, pharyngitis.

PREGNANCY: Category C, caution in nursing.

MECHANISM OF ACTION: H$_1$-receptor antagonist; antagonizes H$_1$-receptor and inhibits histamine release from the mast cell. Selective for the histamine H$_1$-receptor and has affinity for the histamine H$_2$-receptor and possesses affinity for the α$_1$-α$_2$- and 5-HT$_2$-receptors.

PHARMACOKINETICS: Absorption: C$_{max}$=0.04ng/mL; T$_{max}$=2 hrs. **Distribution:** Plasma protein binding (64%). **Elimination:** (IV) Urine (55%, unchanged), feces (30%); T$_{1/2}$=12 hrs.

NURSING CONSIDERATIONS

Assessment: Assess for drug hypersensitivity, contact lens-related irritation, and pregnancy/nursing status.

Monitoring: Monitor for adverse events such as burning sensation in the eye, folliculosis, hyperemia, pruritus, and infection (cold symptoms and upper respiratory infections).

Patient Counseling: Advise not to touch dropper tip of container to any surface to avoid contamination. Counsel that therapy is not for the treatment of contact lens-related irritation and instruct not to wear contact lenses if the eyes are red. Instruct to remove contact lens prior to instillation and reinsert after 10 min.

Administration: Ocular route. **Storage:** 15-25°C (59-77°F). Keep bottle tightly closed when not in use.

ELIDEL

pimecrolimus (Novartis)

> Rare cases of malignancy (eg, skin and lymphoma) reported with topical calcineurin inhibitors, including pimecrolimus, although causal relationship is not established. Avoid long-term use and application should be limited to areas of involvement with atopic dermatitis. Not indicated for children <2 yrs.

THERAPEUTIC CLASS: Macrolactam ascomycin derivative

INDICATIONS: Second-line therapy for the short-term and noncontinuous chronic treatment of mild to moderate atopic dermatitis in non-immunocompromised patients ≥2 yrs who failed to respond adequately to other topical prescription treatments, or when those treatments are not advisable.

DOSAGE: *Adults:* Apply thin layer to the affected skin bid until signs and symptoms resolve. Reevaluate if signs and symptoms persist beyond 6 weeks.
Pediatrics: ≥2 yrs: Apply thin layer to the affected skin bid until signs and symptoms resolve. Reevaluate if signs and symptoms persist beyond 6 weeks.

HOW SUPPLIED: Cre: 1% [30g, 60g, 100g]

WARNINGS/PRECAUTIONS: Long-term safety, beyond 1 yr of noncontinuous use, has not been established. Avoid with malignant or premalignant skin conditions, Netherton's syndrome, or other skin diseases that may increase the potential for systemic absorption. Avoid in immunocompromised patients. May cause local symptoms, such as skin burning (eg, burning sensation, stinging, soreness) or pruritus and may improve as the lesions of atopic dermatitis resolve. Resolve bacterial or viral infections at treatment sites before starting treatment. Increased risk of varicella zoster virus infection, herpes simplex virus infection, or eczema herpeticum. Skin papilloma/warts reported; consider d/c until complete resolution is achieved if skin papillomas worsen or are unresponsive to conventional treatment. Lymphadenopathy reported; monitor to

E

ensure it resolves. D/C if lymphadenopathy of uncertain etiology or acute infectious mononucleosis occurs. Minimize or avoid natural or artificial sunlight exposure during treatment.

ADVERSE REACTIONS: Application-site burning, application-site reaction, upper respiratory tract infection, headache, nasopharyngitis, influenza, abdominal pain, diarrhea, sore throat, hypersensitivity, pyrexia, cough, rhinitis, N/V.

INTERACTIONS: Caution with CYP3A4 inhibitors (eg, erythromycin, itraconazole, ketoconazole, fluconazole, calcium channel blockers, cimetidine) in patients with widespread and/or erythrodermic disease. Skin flushing associated with alcohol use reported. Increased incidence of impetigo, skin infection, superinfection, rhinitis, and urticaria reported with topical corticosteroid administered sequentially.

PREGNANCY: Category C, not for use in nursing.

MECHANISM OF ACTION: Macrolactam ascomycin derivative; not fully established. Suspected to bind with high affinity to macrophilin-12 (FKBP-12) and inhibit the calcium-dependent phosphatase, calcineurin. Consequently, this inhibits T cell activation by blocking the transcription of early cytokines. In particular, pimecrolimus inhibits at nanomolar concentrations interleukin-2 (IL-2) and interferon gamma (Th1-type) and IL-4 and IL-10 (Th2-type) cytokine synthesis in human T cells. In addition, pimecrolimus prevents the release of inflammatory cytokines and mediators from mast cells in vitro after stimulation by antigen/IgE.

PHARMACOKINETICS: Absorption: C_{max}=1.4ng/mL (adults). **Distribution:** Plasma protein binding (99.5%). **Metabolism:** Liver via CYP3A; O-demethylation (metabolites). **Elimination:** Feces (78.4% metabolites, <1% unchanged).

NURSING CONSIDERATIONS

Assessment: Assess for malignant or premalignant skin conditions (eg, cutaneous-cell lymphoma), Netherton's syndrome or other skin diseases, viral or bacterial skin infections, generalized erythroderma, pregnancy/nursing status, and possible drug interactions.

Monitoring: Monitor for infections (eg, varicella virus infection, herpes simplex virus infection, eczema herpeticum), lymphomas, lymphadenopathy, skin malignancies, local symptoms such as skin burning (eg, burning sensation, stinging, soreness) or pruritus, and other adverse reactions.

Patient Counseling: Instruct to use as prescribed. Inform not to use drug continuously for long periods of time and should be used only on areas of skin with eczema. Advise to d/c medication when signs/symptoms of eczema subside (eg, itching, rash, and redness). Instruct to contact physician if symptoms get worse, a skin infection develops, if burning on skin lasts >1 week or if symptoms do not improve after 6 weeks of treatment. Instruct to wash hands and dry skin before applying cream. Instruct not to bathe, shower, or swim after applying cream. Instruct to avoid natural or artificial sunlight exposure while on therapy. Instruct not to cover treated skin area with bandages, dressings, or wraps. Inform that the medication is for external use only; instruct to avoid contact with eyes, nose, mouth, vagina, or rectum (mucous membranes).

Administration: Topical route. **Storage:** 25°C (77°F); excursions permitted to 15-30°C (59-86°F). Do not freeze.

ELIGARD   RX
leuprolide acetate (Sanofi-Aventis)

THERAPEUTIC CLASS: Synthetic gonadotropin releasing hormone analog

INDICATIONS: Palliative treatment of advanced prostate cancer.

DOSAGE: *Adults:* SQ: 7.5mg monthly or 22.5mg q3 months or 30mg q4 months or 45mg q6 months.

HOW SUPPLIED: Inj: 7.5mg, 22.5mg, 30mg, 45mg

CONTRAINDICATIONS: Women who are or may become pregnant.

WARNINGS/PRECAUTIONS: Transient increase in serum concentrations of testosterone and worsening of symptoms or onset of new signs/symptoms during 1st few weeks of therapy may occur. Closely monitor patients with metastatic vertebral lesions and/or urinary tract obstruction during 1st few weeks of therapy. Cases of ureteral obstruction and/or spinal cord compression reported; institute standard treatment if these complications occur. Suppresses pituitary-gonadal system. Hyperglycemia and increased risk of developing diabetes, myocardial infarction, sudden cardiac death, and stroke reported in men.

ADVERSE REACTIONS: Hot flashes/sweats, inj-site reactions (eg, pain, erythema, bruising), malaise/fatigue, testicular atrophy, weakness, gynecomastia, myalgia, dizziness, decreased libido, clamminess.

PREGNANCY: Category X, not for use in nursing.

MECHANISM OF ACTION: Synthetic gonadotropin releasing hormone analog; inhibits pituitary gonadotropin secretion and suppresses testicular and ovarian steroidogenesis when given continuously.

PHARMACOKINETICS: Absorption: (7.5mg dose; 1st inj) C_{max}=25.3ng/mL, T_{max}=5 hrs. (22.5mg dose; 1st inj, 2nd inj) C_{max}=127ng/mL, 107ng/mL; T_{max}=5 hrs. (30mg dose; 1st inj) C_{max}=150ng/mL, T_{max}=3.3 hrs. (45mg dose; 1st inj, 2nd inj) C_{max}=82ng/mL, 102ng/mL; T_{max}=4.5 hrs. **Distribution:** (IV bolus dose) V_d=27L; plasma protein binding (43-49%). **Metabolism:** Pentapeptide (M-1) metabolite (major metabolite). **Elimination:** (1mg IV bolus dose) $T_{1/2}$=3 hrs.

NURSING CONSIDERATIONS

Assessment: Assess for diabetes, cardiovascular risk factors, hypersensitivity to drug, metastatic vertebral lesions, and urinary tract obstructions.

Monitoring: Monitor for spinal cord compression, ureteral obstruction, suppression of pituitary-gonadal system, and signs/symptoms suggestive of cardiovascular disease development. Periodically monitor blood glucose, HbA1c, and response by measuring serum concentrations of testosterone and prostate specific antigen.

Patient Counseling: Inform that hot flashes may be experienced. Inform that increased bone pain and difficulty in urinating, and onset or aggravation of weakness or paralysis may be experienced during the 1st few weeks of therapy. Notify physician if new or worsened symptoms develop after beginning treatment. Inform about inj-site related adverse reactions (eg, transient burning/stinging, pain, bruising, redness); notify physician if such reactions do not resolve. Contact physician immediately if an allergic reaction develops.

Administration: SQ route. Rotate inj sites. Specific inj location chosen should be an area with sufficient soft or loose SQ tissue; avoid areas with brawny or fibrous SQ tissue or locations that can be rubbed or compressed. Refer to PI for mixing and administration procedures. Allow product to reach room temperature before using. **Storage:** 2-8°C (35.6-46.4°F). Once mixed, discard if not administered within 30 min.

ELLA   RX
ulipristal acetate (Watson)

THERAPEUTIC CLASS: Emergency contraceptive kit

INDICATIONS: Prevention of pregnancy following unprotected intercourse or a known or suspected contraceptive failure.

DOSAGE: *Adults:* 1 tab as soon as possible within 120 hrs (5 days) after unprotected intercourse or a known or suspected contraceptive failure. Consider repeating the dose if vomiting occurs within 3 hrs of intake.
Pediatrics: Postpubertal: 1 tab as soon as possible within 120 hrs (5 days) after unprotected intercourse or a known or suspected contraceptive failure. Consider repeating the dose if vomiting occurs within 3 hrs of intake.

HOW SUPPLIED: Tab: 30mg

CONTRAINDICATIONS: Known or suspected pregnancy.

WARNINGS/PRECAUTIONS: Not for routine use as a contraceptive. Not indicated for termination of existing pregnancy. Exclude pregnancy prior to prescribing; perform pregnancy test if pregnancy cannot be excluded. History of ectopic pregnancy not a contraindication to use. Consider possibility of ectopic pregnancy if lower abdominal pain or pregnancy occurs following use. For occasional use as emergency contraceptive only; should not replace regular method of contraception. Repeated use within the same menstrual cycle not recommended. Rapid return of fertility may occur following treatment; continue or initiate routine contraception as soon as possible following use. After intake, menses sometimes occur earlier or later than expected; rule out pregnancy if menses delayed >1 week. Intermenstrual bleeding reported. Does not protect against HIV infection (AIDS) or other sexually transmitted infections.

ADVERSE REACTIONS: Headache, abdominal/upper abdominal pain, nausea, dysmenorrhea, fatigue, dizziness.

INTERACTIONS: Drugs or herbal products that induce enzymes, including CYP3A4, (eg, barbiturates, bosentan, carbamazepine, felbamate, griseofulvin, oxcarbazepine, phenytoin, rifampin, St. John's wort, topiramate) may decrease plasma concentrations and may decrease effectiveness. CYP3A4 inhibitors (eg, itraconazole, ketoconazole) may increase plasma concentrations. May reduce contraceptive action of regular hormonal contraceptive methods.

PREGNANCY: Category X, not for use in nursing.

MECHANISM OF ACTION: Synthetic progesterone agonist/antagonist; postpones follicular rupture when taken immediately before ovulation is to occur. The likely primary mechanism of action for emergency contraception is inhibition or delay of ovulation; however, alterations to the endometrium that may affect implantation may also contribute to efficacy.

PHARMACOKINETICS: Absorption: C_{max}=176ng/mL, T_{max}=0.9 hr; AUC_{0-t}=548ng•hr/mL. (Monodemethyl-ulipristal acetate) C_{max}=69ng/mL, T_{max}=1 hr; AUC_{0-t}=240ng•hr/mL. **Distribution:** Plasma protein binding (>94%). **Metabolism:** CYP3A4; monodemethyl-ulipristal acetate (active metabolite). **Elimination:** $T_{1/2}$=32.4 hrs. (Monodemethyl-ulipristal acetate) $T_{1/2}$=27 hrs.

NURSING CONSIDERATIONS

Assessment: Assess pregnancy/nursing status and for possible drug interactions.

Monitoring: Monitor for ectopic pregnancy and effect on menstrual cycle.

Patient Counseling: Instruct to take as soon as possible and not >120 hrs after unprotected intercourse or a known or suspected contraceptive failure. Advise not to take if pregnancy is known or suspected; inform that drug is not indicated for termination of an existing pregnancy. Advise to contact healthcare provider immediately if vomiting occurs within 3 hrs of taking the tab or if period is delayed by >1 week beyond expected date. Instruct to seek medical attention if severe lower abdominal pain 3-5 weeks after use is experienced. Advise not to use as routine contraception or repeatedly in the same menstrual cycle. Inform that therapy may reduce contraceptive action of regular hormonal contraceptive methods; instruct to use a reliable barrier method of contraception after using medication, for any subsequent acts of intercourse that occur in that same menstrual cycle. Inform that drug does not protect against HIV infection (AIDS) and other sexually transmitted diseases/infections. Advise not to use if breastfeeding.

Administration: Oral route. Can be taken at any time during the menstrual cycle. **Storage:** 20-25°C (68-77°F). Keep blister in the outer carton in order to protect from light.

ELLENCE   RX
epirubicin HCl (Pfizer)

> Severe local tissue necrosis associated with extravasation during administration. Not for IM/SQ administration. Cardiac toxicity including congestive heart failure (CHF) may occur during or after termination of therapy. Use extreme caution if exceeding cumulative dose of 900mg/m². Increased risk of cardiac toxicity with active or dormant cardiovascular disese (CVD), prior or concomitant radiotherapy to the mediastinal/pericardial area, previous therapy with other anthracyclines or anthracenediones, or concomitant use of other cardiotoxic drugs. Secondary acute myelogenous leukemia (AML) reported in patients with breast cancer treated with anthracyclines. More common occurrence of refractory secondary leukemia when given with DNA-damaging antineoplastics, heavy pretreatment with cytotoxic drugs, or escalated doses of anthracyclines have been escalated. Severe myelosuppression may occur.

THERAPEUTIC CLASS: Anthracycline

INDICATIONS: Adjuvant therapy in patients with evidence of axillary node tumor involvement following resection of primary breast cancer.

DOSAGE: *Adults:* Initial: 100-120mg/m², repeat at 3- to 4-week cycles. May give total dose on Day 1 of each cycle or divide equally on Days 1 and 8 of each cycle. Give prophylactic antibiotic therapy if administered with 120mg/m² regimen. Administer as IV infusion over 15-20 min. Consider pretreatment of antiemetics. Bone Marrow Dysfunction: Consider a lower starting dose (75-90 mg/m²). Hepatic Impairment: Bilirubin 1.2-3mg/dL or AST 2-4X ULN: Give 1/2 of initial dose. Bilirubin >3mg/dL or AST >4X ULN: Give 1/4 of initial dose. Severe Renal Impairment (SrCr >5mg/dL): Consider lower doses. Refer to PI for the recommended regimens of combination chemotherapy and for dose modifications based on toxicities or bone marrow dysfunction.

HOW SUPPLIED: Inj: 2mg/mL [25mL, 100mL]

CONTRAINDICATIONS: Severe myocardial insufficiency, recent myocardial infarction or severe arrhythmias, previous treatment with max cumulative dose of anthracyclines, or anthracenedione hypersensitivity.

WARNINGS/PRECAUTIONS: Administer only under the supervision of qualified physicians experienced in the use of cytotoxic therapy. Resolve acute toxicities of prior cytotoxic treatment before initiation. Inj-related reactions may occur. Excessive rapid administration may cause facial flushing as well as local erythematous streaking along the vein. May suppress bone marrow function as manifested by leukopenia, thrombocytopenia, and anemia. D/C immediately at the 1st sign of impaired left ventricular ejection fraction (LVEF) function. Avoid with severe hepatic impairment. May induce hyperuricemia and tumor-lysis syndrome; hydration, urine alkalinization, and prophylaxis with allopurinol to prevent hyperuricemia may minimize potential complications of tumor-lysis syndrome. Emetogenic; consider prophylactic use of antiemetics before administration to reduce N/V. Thrombophlebitis and thromboembolic phenomena reported. May cause fetal harm during pregnancy. Caution in female patients ≥70 yrs.

ADVERSE REACTIONS: Alopecia, amenorrhea, anemia, anorexia, conjunctivitis, N/V, infection, keratitis, lethargy, leukopenia, mucositis, neutropenia, diarrhea, rash, thrombocytopenia.

INTERACTIONS: See Boxed Warning. Avoid with other cardiotoxic agents unless cardiac function is closely monitored. Monitor cardiac function closely with cardioactive compounds that could cause heart failure (eg, calcium channel blockers). Drugs with the ability to suppress cardiac contractility may increase the risk of cardiotoxicity. Avoid with live vaccines; may diminish response with killed or inactivated vaccines. Cimetidine may increase levels; d/c cimetidine during treatment. May have additive toxicity, especially hematologic and GI effects with other cytotoxic drugs (eg, paclitaxel, docetaxel). May cause severe leukopenia, neutropenia, thrombocytopenia, and anemia with cyclophosphamide and fluorouracil. Changes in hepatic function induced by concomitant therapies may affect metabolism, pharmacokinetics, therapeutic efficacy, and/or toxicity. Administration after previous radiation therapy may induce an inflammatory recall reaction at irradiation site.

PREGNANCY: Category D, not for use in nursing.

MECHANISM OF ACTION: Anthracycline; suspected to bind with DNA and inhibit nucleic acid (DNA and RNA) and protein synthesis.

PHARMACOKINETICS: Absorption: (120mg/m²) C_{max}=9µg/mL, AUC=3.4µg.h/mL. Refer to PI for additional parameters. **Distribution:** Plasma protein binding (77%). **Metabolism:** Liver (extensive and rapid); reduction, conjugation, hydrolytic, and redox process; epirubicinol (metabolite). **Elimination:** Biliary, urine; (120mg/m²)$T_{1/2}$=33.7 hrs.

NURSING CONSIDERATIONS

Assessment: Assess for CVD, acute toxicities, hepatic/renal dysfunction, risk factors for cardiac toxicities, pregnancy/nursing status, possible drug interactions and other conditions where drug is contraindicated or cautioned. Obtain baseline CBC, total bilirubin, AST, creatinine, and cardiac function (LVEF). Assess need for antiemetics.

Monitoring: Monitor for hypersensitivity reaction, CHF, liver dysfunction, cardiotoxicity/toxicity, myelosuppression, hyperuricemia, tumor lysis syndrome, extravasation, facial flushing or local erythematous streaking, and other adverse effects. Monitor LVEF regularly in patients with risk of serious cardiac impairment. Monitor cardiac function with cardioactive compounds that may cause heart failure. Monitor total and differential WBC, RBC, platelet count, creatinine, AST, total bilirubin, and cardiac function before and during each cycle. Monitor serum uric acid, K⁺, calcium, phosphate, and creatinine immediately after initial chemotherapy administration.

Patient Counseling: Inform patients of the expected adverse effects including GI symptoms, alopecia, and potential neutropenic complications. Advise about the risk of leukemia or irreversible myocardial damage. Instruct to seek medical attention if vomiting, dehydration, fever, evidence of infection, symptoms of CHF, or inj-site pain occur. Inform that their urine may appear red for 1-2 days and should not be alarmed. Advise men to use effective contraceptive methods. Counsel that women may develop irreversible amenorrhea or premature menopause.

Administration: IV route. Refer to PI for preparation and administration precautions and techniques. **Storage:** 2-8°C (36-46°F). Sol should be used within 24 hrs after removal from refrigeration. Do not freeze. Protect from light.

ELOCON RX
mometasone furoate (Schering)

THERAPEUTIC CLASS: Corticosteroid

INDICATIONS: Relief of inflammatory and pruritic manifestations of corticosteroid-responsive dermatoses.

DOSAGE: *Adults:* (Lot) Apply a few drops to affected skin qd and massage lightly until the lotion disappears. (Cre/Oint) Apply a thin film to affected skin qd.
Pediatrics: (Lot) ≥12 yrs: Apply a few drops to affected skin qd and massage lightly until the lotion disappears. (Cre/Oint) ≥2 yrs: Apply a thin film to affected skin qd.

HOW SUPPLIED: Cre, Oint: 0.1% [15g, 45g]; Lot: 0.1% [30mL, 60mL]

WARNINGS/PRECAUTIONS: Systemic absorption may produce reversible hypothalamic pituitary adrenal (HPA) axis suppression, manifestations of Cushing's syndrome, hyperglycemia, and glucosuria. Evaluate for HPA axis suppression when applied to a large surface area or to areas under occlusion. D/C or reduce frequency of application or substitute a less potent steroid if HPA axis suppression is noted. D/C and institute appropriate therapy if irritation develops. Use appropriate antifungal or antibacterial agent in the presence of dermatological infections; d/c if favorable response does not occur. Glucocorticosteroid insufficiency may occur (infrequent) requiring supplemental systemic corticosteroids. Pediatric patients may be more susceptible to systemic toxicity. Allergic contact dermatitis reported. HPA axis suppression, Cushing's syndrome, linear growth retardation, delayed weight gain, and intracranial HTN reported in pediatrics. Should not be used with occlusive dressings unless directed by a physician. D/C when control is achieved; reassess if no improvement seen within 2 weeks. Not for use in treatment of diaper dermatitis. Caution in elderly. (Lot) Not recommended in children <12 yrs. (Cre/Oint) May be used in pediatric patients ≥2 yrs.

ADVERSE REACTIONS: Burning, irritation, dryness, secondary infection, acneiform reaction, folliculitis, hypertrichosis, hypopigmentation, perioral dermatitis, allergic contact dermatitis, striae, miliaria.

PREGNANCY: Category C, caution in nursing.

MECHANISM OF ACTION: Corticosteroid; not established. Possesses anti-inflammatory, antipruritic, and vasoconstrictive properties. Suspected to induce phospholipase A_2 inhibitory proteins, lipocortins.

PHARMACOKINETICS: Absorption: Percutaneous; inflammation and other disease processes in the skin may increase absorption. **Distribution:** Found in breast milk (systemically administered).

NURSING CONSIDERATIONS

Assessment: Assess for patient's age, drug hypersensitivity, skin infection, and pregnancy/nursing status.

Monitoring: Monitor for signs/symptoms of systemic toxicity in pediatrics, HPA axis suppression (using adrenocorticotropin hormone stimulation, am plasma cortisol, urinary free cortisol test), glucocorticosteroid insufficiency, Cushing's syndrome, hyperglycemia, glucosuria, skin irritation, allergic contact dermatitis, and skin infections. Monitor for signs of clinical improvement; if no improvement within 2 weeks, reassess diagnosis.

Patient Counseling: Instruct to use externally, exactly as directed. Advise not to use for any disorder other than that for which it was prescribed. Counsel to avoid contact with eyes. Inform not to bandage, cover, or wrap treated skin unless directed by a physician. Advise to report any signs of local adverse reactions to physician. Advise not to use medication for treatment of diaper dermatitis and not to apply to diaper area. Advise to avoid using medication on face, underarms, or groin areas unless directed by physician. Advise to d/c use when control is achieved and to notify physician if no improvement seen within 2 weeks. Advise that other corticosteroid-containing products should not be used without 1st consulting with the physician.

Administration: Topical route. **Storage:** 25°C (77°F); excursions permitted to 15-30°C (59-86°F).

ELOXATIN RX
oxaliplatin (Sanofi-Aventis)

> **Anaphylactic reactions reported and may occur within min of administration. Employ epinephrine, corticosteroids, and antihistamines to alleviate symptoms.**

THERAPEUTIC CLASS: Organoplatinum complex

INDICATIONS: Treatment of advanced colorectal cancer and adjuvant treatment of Stage III colon cancer in patients who have undergone complete resection of the primary tumor in combination with infusional 5-fluorouracil (5-FU) and leucovorin (LV).

DOSAGE: *Adults:* Day 1: 85mg/m² IV simultaneously with LV 200mg/m²; give over 120 min in separate bags using a Y-line; followed by 5-FU 400mg/m² IV bolus over 2-4 min, then 5-FU 600mg/m² as a 22-hr IV infusion. Day 2: LV 200mg/m² IV infusion over 120 min; followed by 5-FU 400mg/m² IV bolus over 2-4 min, then 5-FU 600mg/m² as a 22-hr IV infusion. Repeat cycle q2 weeks. Advanced Colorectal Cancer: Continue treatment until disease progression or unacceptable toxicity. Adjuvant Therapy Stage III Colon Cancer: Treat for 6 months. Dose Modification: Persistent Grade 2 Neurosensory Events: Reduce oxaliplatin to 75mg/m². Persistent Grade 3 Neurosensory Events: Consider d/c. After Recovery From Grade 3/4 GI or Grade 4 Neutropenia or Grade 3/4 Thrombocytopenia: Reduce oxaliplatin to 75mg/m² and 5-FU to 300mg/m² bolus and 500mg/m² 22-hr infusion. Delay next dose until neutrophils ≥1.5 x 10⁹/L and platelets ≥75 x 10⁹/L. Advanced Colorectal Cancer: Persistent Grade 2 Neurosensory Events: Reduce oxaliplatin to 65mg/m². Grade 3 Neurosensory Events: Consider d/c. After Recovery From Grade 3/4 GI or Grade 4 neutropenia or grade 3/4 Thrombocytopenia: Reduce oxaliplatin to 65mg/m² and 5-FU by 20%. Delay next dose until neutrophils ≥1.5 x 10⁹/L and platelets ≥75 x 10⁹/L. Mild-Moderate Renal Impairment: 85mg/m². Severe Renal Impairment: Reduce Initial dose to 65mg/m².

HOW SUPPLIED: Inj: (Concentrate) 5mg/mL [50mg, 100mg, 200mg]; (Powder) 50mg, 100mg

WARNINGS/PRECAUTIONS: Acute, reversible, primarily peripheral and persistent sensory neuropathy reported. Cold may exacerbate acute neurological symptoms; avoid ice for mucositis prophylaxis. May cause persistent, primarily peripheral sensory neuropathy. Potentially fatal pulmonary fibrosis reported. If unexplained respiratory symptoms develop, d/c until interstitial lung disease or pulmonary fibrosis is ruled out. Reversible posterior leukoencephalopathy syndrome (RPLS, also known as PRES, posterior reversible encephalopathy syndrome) and hepatotoxicity observed. Caution and close monitoring with renal impairment.

ADVERSE REACTIONS: Peripheral sensory neuropathy, fatigue, nausea, neutropenia, emesis, diarrhea, thrombocytopenia, anemia, increase in transaminases and alkaline phosphatase, stomatitis, interstitial or other lung diseases.

INTERACTIONS: Increased 5-FU plasma levels with doses of 130mg/m² oxaliplatin dosed q3 weeks; clearance may be decreased with nephrotoxic agents. May prolong PT and INR with anticoagulants.

PREGNANCY: Category D, not for use in nursing.

MECHANISM OF ACTION: Organoplatinum complex; inhibits DNA replication and transcription.

PHARMACOKINETICS: Absorption: C_{max}=0.814mcg/mL. **Distribution:** V_d=440L; plasma protein binding (>90%). **Metabolism:** Rapid, extensive nonenzymatic biotransformation. **Elimination:** Urine (54%), feces (2%); $T_{1/2}$=391 hrs.

NURSING CONSIDERATIONS

Assessment: Assess for preexisting hepatic/renal impairment, hypersensitivity to platinum compounds, pregnancy status, and possible drug interactions.

Monitoring: Monitor LFTs, WBC with differential, Hgb, platelet count, bilirubin, and creatinine periodically and before each dose. Monitor for signs/symptoms of anaphylactic reactions, neuropathy, neurosensory toxicity, portal HTN, RPLS, PRES, liver/renal dysfunction, pulmonary toxicity, and possible adverse effects.

Patient Counseling: Inform of pregnancy risks, expected side effects, particulary its neurologic effects and persistent neurosensory toxicity that may be precipitated by exposure to cold or cold objects. Advise to avoid cold drinks and ice, cover exposed skin prior to exposure to cold temperature or cold objects. Inform of the risk of low blood cell counts and instruct to contact physician immediately if fever, particularly if associated with persistent diarrhea, or evidence of infection develops. Advise to seek medical attention if persistent vomiting, diarrhea, fever, signs of dehydration, cough, breathing difficulties, or signs of allergic reactions occur. Counsel that vision abnormalities may impair ability to drive and use machinery; promptly report any vision problems to physician.

Administration: IV route. Refer to PI for preparation/administration. **Storage:** 25°C (77°F); excursions permitted to 15-30°C (59-86°F). Unreconstituted Powder: Store under normal lighting conditions. Concentrate: Do not freeze and protect from light. Reconstituted Powder/Final Diluted Sol: 2-8°C (36-46°F) for up to 24 hrs. Final Diluted Sol: 20-25°C (68-77°F) for 6 hrs.

EMEND   RX
aprepitant (Merck)

THERAPEUTIC CLASS: Substance P/neurokinin 1 receptor antagonist

INDICATIONS: Prevention of acute and delayed N/V associated with initial and repeat courses of highly emetogenic cancer chemotherapy, including high-dose cisplatin or moderately emetogenic cancer chemotherapy in combination with other antiemetics. Prevention of postoperative nausea and vomiting.

DOSAGE: *Adults:* Prevention of Chemotherapy-Induced N/V: Day 1: 125mg 1 hr prior to chemotherapy. Days 2 and 3: 80mg qam. Regimen should include a corticosteroid and a 5-HT₃ antagonist. Refer to PI for dosing with corticosteroid (dexamethasone) and 5-HT₃ antagonist (ondansetron). Prevention of PONV: 40mg within 3 hrs prior to induction of anesthesia.

HOW SUPPLIED: Cap: 40mg, 80mg, 125mg; BiPack: (two 80mg); TriPack: (one 125mg and two 80mg)

CONTRAINDICATIONS: Concomitant use with pimozide, terfenadine, astemizole, or cisapride.

WARNINGS/PRECAUTIONS: Not recommended for chronic continuous use. Caution with severe hepatic impairment (Child-Pugh score >9).

ADVERSE REACTIONS: Asthenia/fatigue, N/V, constipation, diarrhea, hiccups, anorexia, headache, dehydration, pruritus, dizziness, alopecia, hypotension, pyrexia.

INTERACTIONS: See Contraindications. May increase levels of drugs metabolized by CYP3A4 in dose-dependent manner, including chemotherapeutic agents (eg, docetaxel, paclitaxel, etoposide, irinotecan, ifosfamide, imatinib, vinorelbine, vinblastine, and vincristine) and certain benzodiazepines (eg, midazolam, alprazolam, triazolam). May increase levels of dexamethasone or methylprednisolone. May reduce efficacy of oral contraceptives; use alternative or back-up contraception during treatment and for 1 month after last dose. May induce metabolism of drugs metabolized by CYP2C9 (eg, warfarin, tolbutamide, phenytoin) which may result in lower plasma concentrations of these drugs. May increase levels with CYP3A4 inhibitors; caution with strong inhibitors (eg, ketoconazole, itraconazole, nefazodone, troleandomycin, clarithromycin, ritonavir, nelfinavir, diltiazem) and moderate inhibitors (eg, diltiazem) of CYP3A4. Decreased levels and efficacy reported with strong CYP3A4 inducers (eg, rifampin, carbamazepine, phenytoin).

Concomitant paroxetine may decrease levels of both drugs. Coadministration with warfarin may result in a clinically significant decrease in INR of PT.

PREGNANCY: Category B, not for use in nursing.

MECHANISM OF ACTION: Substance P/neurokinin 1 receptor antagonist; augments the antiemetic activity of the 5-HT$_3$ receptor antagonist ondansetron and the corticosteroid dexamethasone and inhibits both the acute and delayed phases of cisplatin-induced emesis.

PHARMACOKINETICS: Absorption: Fast; (40mg) AUC=7.8mcg•hr/mL, C$_{max}$=0.7mcg/mL, T$_{max}$=3 hrs. **Distribution:** V$_d$=70L; plasma protein binding (>95%); crosses blood-brain barrier. **Metabolism:** Liver (extensive) via CYP3A4 (major), 1A2 (minor), 2C19 (minor). Oxidation. **Elimination:** (100mg IV fosaprepitant) Urine (57%), feces (45%); T$_{1/2}$=9-13 hrs.

NURSING CONSIDERATIONS

Assessment: Assess for history of hypersensitivity reactions to the drug and its components, hepatic impairment, pregnancy/nursing status, and possible drug interactions.

Monitoring: Monitor INR in the 2-week period following therapy (especially at 7-10 days) if on chronic warfarin therapy. Monitor for hypersensitivity reactions and other adverse reactions.

Patient Counseling: Instruct to take drug as prescribed. Instruct to d/c medication and to inform physician immediately if allergic reactions (eg, hives, rash, itching, and difficulty in breathing or swallowing) or severe skin reactions (rare) occur. Advise patients on chronic warfarin therapy to have clotting status closely monitored. Advise to notify physician if using other prescription, OTC, or herbal products. Instruct patients using hormonal contraceptives to use alternative or backup methods of contraception during therapy and for 1 month after the last dose of the medication.

Administration: Oral route. **Storage:** 20-25°C (68-77°F).

EMEND FOR INJECTION RX
fosaprepitant dimeglumine (Merck)

THERAPEUTIC CLASS: Substance P/neurokinin 1 receptor antagonist

INDICATIONS: Prevention of acute and delayed N/V associated with initial and repeat courses of highly emetogenic cancer chemotherapy including high-dose cisplatin or moderately emetogenic cancer chemotherapy in adults in combination with other antiemetics.

DOSAGE: *Adults:* Prevention of N/V Associated with Highly Emetogenic Chemotherapy: 150mg IV infusion over 20-30 min. Prevention of N/V Associated with Highly/Moderately Emetogenic Chemotherapy: 115mg IV infusion over 15 min. Give 30 min prior to chemotherapy on Day 1 only of a single or 3-day dosing regimen. Regimen should include a corticosteroid and a 5-HT$_3$ antagonist. Refer to PI for dosing with corticosteroid (dexamethasone) and 5-HT$_3$ antagonist (ondansetron).

HOW SUPPLIED: Inj (powder): 115mg, 150mg

CONTRAINDICATIONS: Concurrent use with pimozide or cisapride.

WARNINGS/PRECAUTIONS: Immediate hypersensitivity reactions reported; avoid reinitiating infusion if hypersensitivity occurs during 1st-time use. Not recommended for chronic continuous use. Caution with severe hepatic insufficiency (Child-Pugh score >9).

ADVERSE REACTIONS: Infusion-site reactions (erythema, pruritus, pain, induration), BP increased, thrombophlebitis.

INTERACTIONS: See Contraindications. May increase levels of drugs metabolized by CYP3A4, including chemotherapeutic agents (eg, docetaxel, paclitaxel, etoposide, irinotecan, ifosfamide, imatinib, vinorelbine, vinblastine, vincristine), and certain benzodiazepines (eg, midazolam, alprazolam, triazolam). May increase levels of dexamethasone and methylprednisolone; reduce dose of PO dexamethasone/methylprednisolone by 50% and IV methylprednisolone by 25% when given with 115mg fosaprepitant followed by aprepitant. May reduce efficacy of hormonal contraceptives (eg, ethinyl estradiol, norethindrone); use alternative or back-up contraception during treatment and for 1 month after last dose. May decrease levels of warfarin and tolbutamide. May increase levels with CYP3A4 inhibitors; caution with strong inhibitors (eg, ketoconazole, itraconazole, nefazodone, troleandomycin, clarithromycin, ritonavir, nelfinavir, diltiazem) and moderate inhibitors (eg, diltiazem) of CYP3A4. Decreased levels and efficacy reported with strong CYP3A4 inducers (eg, rifampin, carbamazepine, phenytoin). Concomitant paroxetine may decrease levels of both drugs. Coadministration with warfarin may result in a clinically significant decrease in INR of PT.

PREGNANCY: Category B, not for use in nursing.

MECHANISM OF ACTION: Substance P/neurokinin 1 receptor antagonist; prodrug of aprepitant. Augments the antiemetic activity of the 5-HT$_3$ receptor antagonist ondansetron and the corticosteroid dexamethasone and inhibits both the acute and delayed phases of cisplatin-induced emesis.

PHARMACOKINETICS: Absorption: (Aprepitant, given as 150mg IV fosaprepitant) AUC=37.38mcg•hr/mL, C_{max}=4.15mcg/mL; (Given as 115mg IV fosaprepitant) AUC=31.7mcg•hr/mL, C_{max}=3.27mcg/mL. **Distribution:** (Aprepitant) V_d=70L; plasma protein binding (>95%); crosses blood-brain barrier. **Metabolism:** Rapidly converted to aprepitant by liver and extrahepatic tissues. (Aprepitant) CYP3A4 (major), 1A2 and 2C19 (minor) via oxidation. **Elimination:** (100mg IV fosaprepitant) Urine (57%), feces (45%); (Aprepitant) $T_{1/2}$=9-13 hrs.

NURSING CONSIDERATIONS

Assessment: Assess for history of hypersensitivity to drug and its components, hepatic function, pregnancy/nursing status, and possible drug interactions.

Monitoring: Monitor INR in the 2-week period following therapy, (especially at 7-10 days) if on chronic warfarin therapy. Monitor for hypersensitivity reactions and other adverse reactions.

Patient Counseling: Instruct to d/c medication and to inform physician immediately if allergic reactions (eg, hives, rash, itching, red face/skin, difficulty in breathing or swallowing) or severe skin reactions (rare) occur. Advise patients on chronic warfarin therapy to have clotting status closely monitored particularly 7-10 days following initiation with each chemotherapy cycle. Counsel patients on how to care for local reactions and when to seek further evaluation. Advise to notify physician if using other prescription, OTC, or herbal products. Instruct patients using hormonal contraceptives to use alternative or back-up methods of contraception during therapy and for 1 month after the last dose of the medication.

Administration: IV route. Refer to PI for compatibility and preparation. **Storage:** 2-8°C (36-46°F). Reconstituted Sol: Stable for 24 hrs ≤25°C.

EMLA RX
lidocaine - prilocaine (APP Pharmaceuticals)

THERAPEUTIC CLASS: Acetamide local anesthetic

INDICATIONS: Topical anesthetic for use on normal intact skin. Topical anesthetic for genital mucous membranes for superficial minor surgery and as pretreatment for infiltration anesthesia.

DOSAGE: *Adults:* Apply thick layer of cream to intact skin and cover with occlusive dressing. Minor Dermal Procedure: Apply 2.5g over 20-25cm² of skin surface for at least 1 hr. Major Dermal Procedure: Apply 2g/10cm² of skin for 2 hrs. Adult Male Genital Skin: Apply 1g/10cm² of skin surface for 15 min. Female External Genitalia: Apply 5-10g for 5-10 min.
Pediatrics: 7-12 yrs and >20kg: Max: 20g/200cm² for up to 4 hrs. 1-6 yrs and >10kg: Max:10g/100cm² for up to 4 hrs. 3-12 months and >5kg: Max: 2g/20cm² for up to 4 hrs. 0-3 months or <5kg: Max: 1g/10cm² for up to 1 hr. If >3 months and does not meet minimum weight requirement, max dose restricted to corresponding weight.

HOW SUPPLIED: Cre: (Lidocaine-Prilocaine) 2.5%-2.5%

WARNINGS/PRECAUTIONS: Application to larger areas or for longer than recommended times, may result in serious adverse effects. Should not be used where penetration or migration beyond the tympanic membrane into the middle ear is possible. Avoid with congenital or idiopathic methemoglobinemia and infants <12 months receiving treatment with methemoglobin-inducing agents. Very young or patients with glucose-6-phosphate dehydrogenase (G6PD) deficiency are more susceptible to methemoglobinemia. Reports of methemoglobinemia in infants and children following excessive applications. Monitor neonates and infants up to 3 months for Met-Hb levels before, during, and after application. Repeated doses may increase blood levels; caution in patients who may be more susceptible to systemic effects (eg, acutely ill, debilitated, elderly). Avoid eye contact and application to open wounds. Has been shown to inhibit viral and bacterial growth. Caution with severe hepatic disease and in patients with drug sensitivities.

ADVERSE REACTIONS: Erythema, edema, abnormal sensations, paleness (pallor or blanching), altered temperature sensations, burning sensation, itching, rash.

INTERACTIONS: Additive and potentially synergistic toxic effects with Class I antiarrhythmic drugs (eg, tocainide, mexiletine). May have additive cardiac effects with Class III antiarrhythmic drugs (eg, amiodarone, bretylium, sotalol, dofetilide). Avoid drugs associated with drug-induced methemoglobinemia (eg, sulfonamides, acetaminophen, acetanilid, aniline dyes, benzocaine, chloroquine, dapsone, naphthalene, nitrates/nitrites, nitrofurantoin, nitroglycerin, nitroprusside, phenobarbital, phenytoin, primaquine, pamaquine, para-aminosalicylic acid, phenacetin, quinine). Caution with other products containing lidocaine/prilocaine; consider the amount absorbed from all formulations.

PREGNANCY: Category B, caution in nursing.

MECHANISM OF ACTION: Amide-type local anesthetics; stabilizes neuronal membranes by inhibiting ionic fluxes required for initiation and conduction impulses, thereby effecting local anesthetic action.

PHARMACOKINETICS: Absorption: Lidocaine: (3 hrs 400cm^2) C_{max}=0.12mcg/mL, T_{max}=4 hrs; (24 hrs 400cm^2) C_{max}=0.28mcg/mL, T_{max}=10 hrs. Prilocaine: (3 hrs 400cm^2) C_{max}=0.07mcg/mL, T_{max}=4 hrs; (24 hrs 400cm^2) C_{max}=0.14mcg/mL, T_{max}=10 hrs. **Distribution:** (IV) V_d=1.5L/kg (lidocaine), 2.6L/kg (prilocaine); (Cre) plasma protein binding 70% (lidocaine), 55% (prilocaine). Crosses placental and blood-brain barrier; found in breast milk. **Metabolism:** Lidocaine: Liver (rapid); monoethylglycinexylidide and glycinexylidide (active metabolites). Prilocaine: Liver and kidneys by amidases; ortho-toluidine and N-n-propylalanine (metabolites). **Elimination:** (IV) Lidocaine: Urine (>98%); $T_{1/2}$=110 min. Prilocaine: $T_{1/2}$=70 min.

NURSING CONSIDERATIONS

Assessment: Assess for congenital or idiopathic methemoglobinemia, G6PD deficiency, hepatic disease, open wounds, presence of acute illness, presence of debilitation, history of drug sensitivities, pregnancy/nursing status, and for possible drug interactions. In neonates and infants ≤3 months, obtain Met-Hb levels prior to application.

Monitoring: Monitor for signs/symptoms of methemoglobinemia, ototoxicity, local skin reactions and for allergic/anaphylactoid reactions. Monitor Met-Hb levels in neonates and infants ≤3 months during and after application.

Patient Counseling: Inform about potential risks/benefits of drug. Advise to avoid inadvertent trauma to treated area. Instruct not to apply near eyes or on open wounds. Apply as directed by physician. Advise to notify physician if pregnant/nursing or planning to become pregnant. Instruct to remove cream and consult physician if child becomes very dizzy, excessively sleepy, or develops duskiness on the face or lips after application.

Administration: Topical route. Not for ophthalmic use. **Storage:** 20-25°C (68-77°F). Keep tightly closed.

EMSAM   RX
selegiline (Dey)

> Antidepressants increased the risk of suicidal thinking and behavior (suicidality) in short-term studies in children, adolescents, and young adults with major depressive disorder (MDD) and other psychiatric disorders. Monitor and observe closely for clinical worsening, suicidality, or unusual changes in behavior in patients who are started on antidepressant therapy. Not approved for use in pediatric patients.

THERAPEUTIC CLASS: Monoamine oxidase inhibitor (Type B)

INDICATIONS: Treatment of MDD.

DOSAGE: *Adults:* Initial/Target Dose: 6mg/24 hrs. Titrate: May increase in increments of 3mg/24 hrs at intervals ≥2 weeks. Max: 12mg/24 hrs. Elderly: 6mg/24 hrs. Increase dose cautiously.

HOW SUPPLIED: Patch: 6mg/24 hrs, 9mg/24 hrs, 12mg/24 hrs [30^s]

CONTRAINDICATIONS: Pheochromocytoma. Concomitant use with SSRIs (eg, fluoxetine, sertraline, paroxetine), dual SNRIs (eg, venlafaxine, duloxetine), TCAs (eg, imipramine, amitriptyline), bupropion HCl, meperidine, analgesics (eg, tramadol, methadone, propoxyphene), dextromethorphan, St. John's wort, mirtazapine, cyclobenzaprine, oral selegiline or other MAOIs (eg, isocarboxazid, phenelzine, tranylcypromine), carbamazepine, oxcarbazepine, sympathomimetic amines including amphetamines, cold products and weight-reducing preparations that contain vasoconstrictors (eg, pseudoephedrine, phenylephrine, phenylpropanolamine, ephedrine), elective surgery requiring general anesthesia, cocaine or local anesthesia containing sympathomimetic vasoconstrictors, (for patients receiving 9mg/24 hrs and 12mg/24 hrs) high tyramine-containing foods. D/C therapy at least 10 days prior to elective surgery.

WARNINGS/PRECAUTIONS: Not approved for treatment of bipolar depression. Postural hypotension may occur; monitor elderly for postural changes in BP, caution with preexisting orthostasis during dose increases, and consider dose adjustment if orthostatic symptoms occur. Activation of mania/hypomania may occur; caution with history of mania. Caution with disorders or conditions that can produce altered metabolism or hemodynamic responses.

ADVERSE REACTIONS: Headache, diarrhea, dyspepsia, insomnia, dry mouth, pharyngitis, sinusitis, application-site reaction, rash, low systolic BP, orthostatic hypotension, weight change.

INTERACTIONS: See Contraindications. Not recommended with buspirone HCl and alcohol. Approximately 1 week should elapse between d/c of SSRIs, SNRIs, TCAs, other MAOIs, meperidine, analgesics (eg, tramadol, methadone, propoxyphene), dextromethorphan, St. John's wort, mirtazapine, bupropion HCl, buspirone HCl and start of therapy. At least 5 weeks should elapse between d/c of fluoxetine and start of therapy. At least 2 weeks should elapse after d/c of therapy before starting buspirone HCl or any contraindicated drug. Hypertensive crisis can occur with high tyramine-containing foods.

PREGNANCY: Category C, caution in nursing.

MECHANISM OF ACTION: MAOI (Type B); not established. Presumed to be linked to potentiation of monoamine neurotransmitter activity in the CNS resulting from its inhibition of MAO activity.

PHARMACOKINETICS: Absorption: AUC=46.2ng•hr/mL. **Distribution:** Plasma protein binding (90%). **Metabolism:** Extensive via N-dealkylation or N-depropargylation by CYP2B6, CYP2C9, CYP3A4/5 (major), CYP2A6 (minor); N-desmethylselegiline, R(-)-methamphetamine (metabolites). **Elimination:** Urine (10%, 0.1% unchanged), feces (2%); $T_{1/2}$=18-25 hrs (IV).

NURSING CONSIDERATIONS

Assessment: Assess for hypersensitivity to drug, pheochromocytoma, risk of bipolar disorder, history of mania, preexisting orthostasis, diseases/conditions that alter metabolism or hemodynamic response, pregnancy/nursing status, and possible drug interactions.

Monitoring: Monitor for worsening of depression, emergence of suicidal ideation, unusual changes in behavior, hypertensive crisis, postural hypotension, activation of mania/hypomania, and other adverse reactions.

Patient Counseling: Counsel about benefits, risks, and appropriate use of therapy. Advise to report to physician if unusual changes in behavior, worsening of depression, suicidal ideation, or any acute symptoms (eg, severe headache, neck stiffness, heart racing or palpitations) occur. Advise to use caution when performing hazardous tasks (eg, operating machinery/driving). Counsel to avoid alcohol, tyramine-containing foods/supplements/beverages, and any cough medicine containing dextromethorphan, and to notify physician if taking or planning to take any prescription or over-the-counter drugs. Instruct to use exactly as prescribed and avoid exposing application site to external sources of direct heat. Instruct not to cut patch into smaller portions. Advise to change position gradually if lightheaded, faint, or dizzy. Instruct to notify physician if pregnant, intend to become pregnant, or breastfeeding.

Administration: Transdermal route. Apply to dry, intact skin on the upper torso, upper thigh, or outer surface of upper arm. Apply immediately upon removal from the protective pouch. Refer to PI for further instructions. **Storage:** 20-25°C (68-77°F). Do not store outside sealed pouch.

EMTRIVA   RX
emtricitabine (Gilead)

Lactic acidosis and severe hepatomegaly with steatosis, including fatal cases, reported with nucleoside analogues. Not approved for the treatment of chronic hepatitis B virus (HBV) infection. Severe acute exacerbations of hepatitis B reported in patients coinfected with HBV upon d/c of therapy; closely monitor hepatic function for at least several months. If appropriate, initiation of anti-HBV therapy may be warranted.

THERAPEUTIC CLASS: Nucleoside reverse transcriptase inhibitor

INDICATIONS: Treatment of HIV-1 infection in combination with other antiretrovirals.

DOSAGE: *Adults:* ≥18 yrs: Cap: 200mg qd. Renal Impairment: CrCl ≥50mL/min: 200mg q24h. CrCl 30-49mL/min: 200mg q48h. CrCl 15-29mL/min: 200mg q72h. CrCl <15mL/min/Hemodialysis: 200mg q96h. Sol: 240mg (24mL) qd. Renal Impairment: CrCl ≥50mL/min: 240mg q24h. CrCl 30-49mL/min: 120mg (12mL) q24h. CrCl 15-29mL/min: 80mg (8mL) q24h. CrCl <15mL/min/Hemodialysis: 60mg (6mL) q24h. Give dose after dialysis if dosing on day of dialysis.
Pediatrics: 3 months-17 yrs: Cap: >33kg: 200mg qd. Sol: 6mg/kg qd. Max: 240mg (24mL). 0-3 months: Sol: 3mg/kg qd. Renal Impairment: Consider dose reduction and/or increase in dosing interval similar to adjustments for adults.

HOW SUPPLIED: Cap: 200mg; Sol: 10mg/mL [170mL]

WARNINGS/PRECAUTIONS: Obesity and prolonged nucleoside exposure may be risk factors for lactic acidosis and severe hepatomegaly with steatosis. Caution with known risk factors for liver disease; d/c if findings suggestive of lactic acidosis or pronounced hepatotoxicity develop. Prior to treatment, all patients with HIV-1 should be tested for the presence of chronic HBV. Reduce dose with impaired renal function. Redistribution/accumulation of body fat may occur. Immune reconstitution syndrome reported. Autoimmune disorders (eg, Graves' disease, polymyositis, Guillain-Barre syndrome) reported in the setting of immune reconstitution and can occur many months after initiation of treatment. Caution in elderly. Modify dose or dosing interval in patients with creatinine clearance <50mL/min or in patients who require dialysis.

ADVERSE REACTIONS: Lactic acidosis, severe hepatomegaly with steatosis, headache, diarrhea, nausea, fatigue, dizziness, depression, insomnia, abnormal dreams, rash, abdominal pain, asthenia, increased cough, rhinitis.

INTERACTIONS: Avoid with other emtricitabine- or lamivudine-containing products.

PREGNANCY: Category B, not for use in nursing.

MECHANISM OF ACTION: Nucleoside reverse transcriptase inhibitor; inhibits the activity of HIV-1 reverse transcriptase by competing with the natural substrate deoxycytidine 5'-triphosphate and by being incorporated into nascent viral DNA, result in chain termination.

PHARMACOKINETICS: Absorption: Rapid and extensive. T_{max}=1-2 hrs. (Cap) Absolute bioavailability (93%); C_{max}=1.8mcg/mL, AUC=10mcg•hr/mL. Refer to PI for other pharmacokinetic parameters. (Sol) Absolute bioavailability (75%). **Distribution:** Plasma protein binding (<4%). **Metabolism:** Oxidation and conjugation; 3'-sulfoxide diastereomers and 2'-O-glucuronide (metabolites). **Elimination:** Urine (86%), feces (14%); $T_{1/2}$=10 hrs.

NURSING CONSIDERATIONS

Assessment: Assess for obesity, prolonged nucleoside exposure, risk factors for lactic acidosis and liver disease, renal impairment, HBV infection, pregnancy/nursing status, and possible drug interactions.

Monitoring: Monitor for signs/symptoms of lactic acidosis, severe hepatomegaly with steatosis, hepatotoxicity, renal impairment, fat redistribution/accumulation, and immune reconstitution syndrome (eg, opportunistic infections).

Patient Counseling: Inform that therapy is not a cure for HIV-1 infection and may still experience illnesses associated with HIV-1 (eg, opportunistic infections). Counsel that therapy has not been shown to reduce risk of transmission of HIV-1 to others through sexual contact or blood contamination. Instruct to take orally and on a regular dosing schedule. Counsel to d/c drug if symptoms of lactic acidosis/hepatotoxicity (eg, N/V, unusual or unexpected stomach discomfort, weakness) develop.

Administration: Oral route. **Storage:** Cap: 25°C (77°F); excursions permitted to 15-30°C (59-86°F). (Sol) 2-8°C (36-46°F). Use within 3 months if stored at 25°C (77°F); excursions permitted to 15-30°C (59-86°F).

ENABLEX   RX
darifenacin (Warner Chilcott)

THERAPEUTIC CLASS: Muscarinic antagonist

INDICATIONS: Treatment of overactive bladder with symptoms of urge urinary incontinence, urgency, and frequency.

DOSAGE: *Adults:* Initial: 7.5mg qd with water. Titrate: May increase to 15mg qd as early as 2 weeks after starting therapy based on individual response. Moderate Hepatic Impairment (Child-Pugh B)/Concomitant Potent CYP3A4 Inhibitors (eg, ketoconazole, itraconazole, ritonavir, nelfinavir, clarithromycin, nefazodone): Max: 7.5mg/day.

HOW SUPPLIED: Tab, Extended-Release: 7.5mg, 15mg

CONTRAINDICATIONS: Urinary retention, gastric retention, uncontrolled narrow-angle glaucoma, and in patients at risk for these conditions.

WARNINGS/PRECAUTIONS: Not recommended in patients with severe hepatic impairment (Child-Pugh C). Risk of urinary retention; caution with significant bladder outflow obstruction. Risk of gastric retention; caution with GI obstructive disorders. May decrease GI motility; caution with severe constipation, ulcerative colitis, and myasthenia gravis. Caution with moderate hepatic impairment and in patients being treated for narrow-angle glaucoma. Angioedema of the face, lips, tongue, and/or larynx reported. Angioedema with upper airway swelling may be life-threatening; d/c and institute appropriate therapy if involvement of the tongue, hypopharynx, or larynx occurs.

ADVERSE REACTIONS: Dry mouth, constipation, dyspepsia, abdominal pain, nausea, urinary tract infection, headache, flu syndrome.

INTERACTIONS: Pharmacokinetics may be altered by CYP3A4 inducers and CYP2D6/CYP3A4 inhibitors. Caution with medications metabolized by CYP2D6 and which have a narrow therapeutic window (eg, flecainide, thioridazine, TCAs). May increase the frequency and/or severity of dry mouth, constipation, blurred vision, and other anticholinergic pharmacologic effects with other anticholinergic agents. May alter the absorption of some concomitantly administered drugs due to effects on gastrointestinal motility. Increased concentration with cimetidine, erythromycin, fluconazole, or ketoconazole. May increase imipramine and desipramine (imipramine active metabolite) concentrations. Monitor PT with warfarin. May increase digoxin exposure; perform routine therapeutic drug monitoring for digoxin. May increase midazolam exposure. Increased exposure with paroxetine.

PREGNANCY: Category C, caution in nursing.

MECHANISM OF ACTION: Muscarinic receptor antagonist; inhibits cholinergic muscarinic receptors, which mediate contractions of urinary bladder smooth muscle, and stimulation of salivary secretions.

PHARMACOKINETICS: Absorption: Variable doses resulted in different pharmacokinetic parameters in extensive metabolizers and poor metabolizers of CYP2D6. **Distribution:** V_d=163L; plasma protein binding (98%). **Metabolism:** Liver (extensive) via CYP2D6 and 3A4 (monohydroxylation, dihydrobenzofuran ring opening, N-dealkylation). **Elimination:** Urine (60%); feces (40%); unchanged, 3%. $T_{1/2}$=13-19 hrs.

NURSING CONSIDERATIONS

Assessment: Assess for urinary retention, gastric retention, narrow-angle glaucoma and risk for these conditions, bladder outflow obstruction, GI obstructive disorders, severe constipation, ulcerative colitis, myasthenia gravis, hepatic impairment, pregnancy/nursing status, and possible drug interactions.

Monitoring: Monitor for symptoms of urinary retention, gastric retention, decreased GI motility, and for angioedema (face, lips, tongue, hypopharynx, larynx). Monitor therapeutic PT for warfarin and digoxin levels routinely when coadministered.

Patient Counseling: Advise that dizziness or blurred vision may occur; instruct to exercise caution when engaging in potentially dangerous activities. Instruct to take qd with liquid, with/without food. Instruct to swallow whole; advise to not chew, divide, or crush. Inform that symptoms of constipation, urinary retention, heat prostration when used in a hot environment, or angioedema may occur. Advise to d/c therapy and seek medical attention if edema of the tongue or laryngopharynx, or difficulty breathing occurs. Advise to read the patient information leaflet before starting therapy.

Administration: Oral route. **Storage:** 25°C (77°F); excursions permitted to 15-30°C (59-86°F). Protect from light.

ENALAPRIL/HCTZ RX
enalapril maleate - hydrochlorothiazide (Various)

> D/C when pregnancy is detected. Drugs that act directly on the renin-angiotensin system can cause death/injury to developing fetus.

OTHER BRAND NAMES: Vaseretic (Valeant)

THERAPEUTIC CLASS: ACE inhibitor/thiazide diuretic

INDICATIONS: Treatment of HTN.

DOSAGE: *Adults:* Not Controlled with Enalapril/HCTZ Monotherapy: Initial: 5mg-12.5mg or 10mg-25mg qd. Titrate: Increase dose based on clinical response. May increase HCTZ dose after 2-3 weeks. Max: 20mg-50mg qd. Replacement Therapy: May substitute for titrated components. Elderly: Start at lower end of dosing range.

HOW SUPPLIED: Tab: (Enalapril-HCTZ) 5mg-12.5mg, 10mg-25mg, (Vaseretic) 10mg-25mg* *scored

CONTRAINDICATIONS: Hereditary/idiopathic angioedema, anuria, hypersensitivity to other sulfonamide-derived drugs, history of ACE inhibitor-associated angioedema.

WARNINGS/PRECAUTIONS: Not for initial therapy of HTN. Not recommended with CrCl ≤30mL/min/1.73m². Caution in elderly. Enalapril: Excessive hypotension associated with oliguria and/or progressive azotemia, and rarely with acute renal failure and/or death has been observed in congestive heart failure (CHF) patients; monitor closely upon initiation and during 1st 2 weeks of therapy and whenever dose is increased. Head/neck angioedema reported; d/c and administer appropriate therapy. Intestinal angioedema reported; monitor for abdominal pain. More reports of angioedema in blacks than nonblacks. Anaphylactoid reactions reported during desensitization with hymenoptera venom, dialysis with high-flux membranes, and LDL apheresis with dextran sulfate absorption. Neutropenia/agranulocytosis reported; monitor WBCs in patients with collagen vascular disease and renal disease. Rarely, associated with syndrome that starts with cholestatic jaundice and progresses to fulminant hepatic necrosis and (sometimes) death; d/c if jaundice or marked elevations of hepatic enzymes develop. Caution with left ventricular outflow obstruction. May cause changes in renal function. May increase BUN/SrCr in patients with renal artery stenosis or with no preexisting renal vascular disease; monitor renal function during the 1st few weeks of therapy in patients with renal artery stenosis. Hyperkalemia and persistent nonproductive cough reported. Hypotension may occur with major surgery or during anesthesia. HCTZ: May precipitate azotemia in patients with renal disease; caution with severe renal disease. Caution with hepatic impairment or progressive liver disease; may precipitate hepatic coma. Sensitivity reactions may occur. May exacerbate/activate systemic lupus erythematosus (SLE). May cause idiosyncratic reaction, resulting in acute transient myopia and acute angle-closure glaucoma; d/c as rapidly as possible. Observe for signs of fluid or electrolyte imbalance (eg, hyponatremia, hypochloremic alkalosis, hypokalemia). Hyperuricemia, gout precipitation, hyperglycemia, hypomagnesemia, hypercalcemia, and increased cholesterol and TG levels may occur. D/C before testing for parathyroid function. Enhanced effects in postsympathectomy patients.

ADVERSE REACTIONS: Dizziness, cough, fatigue, headache.

INTERACTIONS: NSAIDs, including selective cyclooxygenase-2 inhibitors, may diminish effects of diuretics and ACE inhibitors, and may cause further deterioration of renal function. Increased risk of lithium toxicity; avoid with lithium. Enalapril: Hypotension risk, and increased BUN and SrCr with diuretics. Increased risk of hyperkalemia with K⁺-sparing diuretics, K⁺ supplements, and/or K⁺-containing salt substitutes. Nitritoid reactions reported with injectable gold. HCTZ: Potentiation of orthostatic hypotension may occur with alcohol, barbiturates, and narcotics. Dose adjustment of the antidiabetic drug (oral agents and insulin) may be required. Potentiation may occur with other antihypertensives. Cholestyramine and colestipol resins impair absorption. Corticosteroids and adrenocorticotropic hormone may intensify electrolyte depletion, particularly hypokalemia. May decrease response to pressor amines (eg, norepinephrine). May increase responsiveness to nondepolarizing skeletal muscle relaxants (eg, tubocurarine).

PREGNANCY: Category D, not for use in nursing.

MECHANISM OF ACTION: Enalapril: ACE inhibitor; decreases plasma angiotensin II, which leads to decreased vasopressor activity and decreased aldosterone secretion. HCTZ: Thiazide diuretic; not established. Affects distal renal tubular mechanism of electrolyte reabsorption. Increases excretion of Na⁺ and chloride.

PHARMACOKINETICS: Absorption: Enalapril: T_{max}=1 hr, 3-4 hrs (enalaprilat). **Distribution:** Crosses placenta; found in breast milk. **Metabolism:** Enalapril: Hydrolysis to enalaprilat (active metabolite). **Elimination:** Enalapril: Urine and feces (94% as enalapril or enalaprilat); $T_{1/2}$=11 hrs (enalaprilat). HCTZ: Kidneys (at least 61% unchanged); $T_{1/2}$=5.6-14.8 hrs.

NURSING CONSIDERATIONS

Assessment: Assess for hereditary/idiopathic or history of ACE inhibitor-associated angioedema, anuria, hypersensitivity to drug or sulfonamide-derived drugs, CHF, left ventricular outflow obstruction, collagen vascular disease, SLE, risk factors for hyperkalemia, renal/hepatic function, pregnancy/nursing status, and possible drug interactions.

Monitoring: Monitor for signs/symptoms of angioedema, exacerbation/activation of SLE, idiosyncratic reaction, hyperglycemia, hypercalcemia, hypomagnesemia, hyperuricemia or precipitation of gout, sensitivity reactions, and other adverse reactions. Periodically monitor WBCs in patients with collagen vascular disease and renal disease. Monitor BP, serum electrolytes, renal/hepatic function, and cholesterol/TG levels.

Patient Counseling: Inform about fetal risks if taken during pregnancy and discuss treatment options in women planning to become pregnant; report pregnancy to physician as soon as possible. Instruct to d/c therapy and immediately report any signs/symptoms of angioedema (swelling of the face, extremities, eyes, lips, tongue; difficulty in swallowing or breathing). Instruct to report lightheadedness and to d/c therapy if actual syncope occurs. Inform that excessive perspiration, dehydration, and other causes of volume depletion (eg, diarrhea or vomiting) may lead to an excessive fall in BP. Instruct to avoid salt substitutes containing K⁺ without consulting physician, and to report promptly any signs/symptoms of infection.

Administration: Oral route. **Storage:** Protect from moisture. 20-25°C (68-77°F). (Vaseretic) 25°C (77°F); excursions permitted to 15-30°C (59-86°F).

ENALAPRILAT   RX
enalaprilat (Various)

> ACE inhibitors can cause death/injury to developing fetus during 2nd and 3rd trimesters. D/C therapy if pregnancy detected.

THERAPEUTIC CLASS: ACE inhibitor

INDICATIONS: Treatment of HTN when oral therapy is not practical.

DOSAGE: *Adults:* Administer IV over a 5 min period. Usual: 1.25mg q6h for no longer than 48 hrs. Max: 20mg/day. Concomitant Diuretic: Initial: 0.625mg. May repeat after 1 hr if response is inadequate. May administer an additional dose of 1.25mg at 6 hr intervals. CrCl ≤30mL/min: Initial: 0.625mg. May repeat after 1 hr if response is inadequate. May administer an additional dose of 1.25mg at 6 hr intervals. Risk of Excessive Hypotension: Initial: 0.625mg over 5 min to 1 hr. IV to PO Conversion: Refer to PI.

HOW SUPPLIED: Inj: 1.25mg/mL [1mL, 2mL]

CONTRAINDICATIONS: History of ACE inhibitor-associated angioedema and hereditary or idiopathic angioedema.

WARNINGS/PRECAUTIONS: Excessive hypotension sometimes associated with oliguria or azotemia and (rarely) acute renal failure or death may occur; monitor closely whenever dose is adjusted and/or diuretic increased. May increase risk of angioedema in patients with history of angioedema unrelated to ACE inhibitor therapy. Angioedema of the face, extremities, lips, tongue, glottis, and larynx reported; d/c and administer appropriate therapy if this occurs. Higher incidence of angioedema reported in blacks than nonblacks. Anaphylactoid reactions reported during desensitization with hymenoptera venom, dialysis with high-flux membranes, and LDL apheresis with dextran sulfate absorption. Neutropenia or agranulocytosis and bone marrow depression reported; monitor WBCs in patients with renal disease and collagen vascular disease. Rarely, a syndrome that starts with cholestatic jaundice and progresses to fulminant hepatic necrosis and sometimes death reported; d/c if jaundice or marked elevations of hepatic enzymes develop. Caution with left ventricular outflow obstruction. May cause changes in renal function. Increases in BUN and SrCr reported with renal artery stenosis; monitor renal function during the 1st few weeks of therapy. Increases in BUN and SrCr reported with no preexisting renal vascular disease. Hyperkalemia may occur; risk factors include diabetes mellitus (DM) and renal insufficiency. Persistent nonproductive cough reported. Hypotension may occur with major surgery or during anesthesia; may be corrected by volume expansion.

ADVERSE REACTIONS: Hypotension, headache, nausea, angioedema, myocardial infarction, fatigue, dizziness, fever, rash, constipation, cough.

INTERACTIONS: Hypotension risk with diuretics. May increase BUN and SrCr with diuretics; may require dose reduction and/or d/c of diuretic and/or therapy. May further decrease renal dysfunction with NSAIDs. Increase risk of hyperkalemia with K⁺-sparing diuretics, K⁺-containing salt substitutes or K⁺ supplements. Antihypertensives that cause renin release (eg, thiazides) may augment antihypertensive effect. NSAIDs may diminish antihypertensive effect. Lithium toxicity reported with lithium; monitor serum lithium levels frequently. Nitritoid reactions (eg, facial flushing, N/V, hypotension) reported rarely with injectable gold.

PREGNANCY: Category C (1st trimester) and D (2nd and 3rd trimesters), not for use in nursing.

MECHANISM OF ACTION: ACE inhibitor; inhibition results in decreased plasma angiotensin II, which leads to decreased vasopressor activity and decreased aldosterone secretion.

PHARMACOKINETICS: Absorption: (PO) Poorly absorbed. **Distribution:** Crosses placenta (enalapril), found in breast milk. **Elimination:** (PO) Urine (>90% unchanged), $T_{1/2}$=11 hrs (enalaprilat).

NURSING CONSIDERATIONS

Assessment: Assess for history of angioedema, renal dysfunction/disease, collagen vascular disease, renal artery stenosis, left ventricular outflow obstruction, DM, pregnancy/nursing status, and possible drug interactions. Obtain baseline BP, WBC, serum K⁺ levels, and renal function.

Monitoring: Monitor anaphylactoid reaction, angioedema, hypotension, hypersensitivity, and other adverse reactions. Monitor BP, renal function, WBC, serum K⁺ levels.

Patient Counseling: Inform about the risks and benefits of therapy.

Administration: IV route. Should be administered as slow IV infusion as provided or diluted with up to 50mL of a compatible diluent. Refer to PI for list of compatible diluents. **Storage:** Below 30°C (86°F). (Diluted Sol) Stable for 24 hrs at room temperature.

ENBREL
etanercept (Amgen)

RX

Increased risk for developing serious infections (eg, tuberculosis [TB], TB reactivation, invasive fungal infection, bacterial/viral and other infections due to opportunistic pathogens) that may lead to hospitalization or death. Most patients were taking concomitant immunosuppressants (eg, methotrexate [MTX] or corticosteroids). D/C if serious infection or sepsis develops. Evaluate for latent TB and treat prior to initiation of therapy. Consider empiric antifungal therapy in patients at risk for invasive fungal infection who develop severe systemic illness. Consider risks and benefits prior to therapy with chronic and recurrent infection. Monitor for development of signs and symptoms of infection during and after treatment. Lymphoma and other malignancies reported in children and adolescents.

THERAPEUTIC CLASS: TNF-receptor blocker

INDICATIONS: Reduce signs/symptoms, induce major clinical response, inhibit progression of structural damage, and improve physical function in moderately to severely active rheumatoid arthritis (RA), alone or in combination with MTX. Reduce signs/symptoms, inhibit progression of structural damage of active arthritis, and improve physical function in psoriatic arthritis (PsA), alone or in combination with MTX. Reduce signs/symptoms of moderately to severely active polyarticular juvenile idiopathic arthritis (JIA) in patients ≥2 yrs. Reduce signs/symptoms of active ankylosing spondylitis (AS). Treatment of patients ≥18 yrs with chronic moderate to severe plaque psoriasis (PsO) who are candidates for systemic therapy or phototherapy.

DOSAGE: *Adults*: RA/AS/PsA: 50mg SQ weekly. May continue MTX, glucocorticoids, salicylates, NSAIDs, or analgesics. Max: 50mg/week. PsO: Initial: 50mg SQ twice weekly for 3 months. May begin with 25-50mg/week. Maint: 50mg once weekly.
Pediatrics: ≥2 yrs: JIA: <63kg: 0.8mg/kg SQ weekly. ≥63kg: 50mg SQ weekly. May continue glucocorticoids, NSAIDs, or analgesics.

HOW SUPPLIED: Inj: (MDV) 25mg, (Prefilled Syringe) 25mg, 50mg

E

CONTRAINDICATIONS: Sepsis.

WARNINGS/PRECAUTIONS: Avoid with active infection. New onset/exacerbation of CNS demyelinating disorders (rare), transverse myelitis, optic neuritis, multiple sclerosis, Guillain-Barre syndrome, other peripheral demyelinating neuropathies, and new onset/exacerbation of seizure disorders, reported; caution with preexisting/recent onset CNS or peripheral nervous system demyelinating disorders. Acute and chronic leukemia reported. Melanoma and non-melanoma skin cancer (NMSC) reported; perform periodic skin exams for patients at increased risk. Postmarketing cases of Merkel cell carcinoma reported. New onset/worsening of preexisting heart failure (HF) reported; caution with HF and monitor carefully. Pancytopenia and aplastic anemia reported (rare); caution with history of significant hematologic abnormalities; seek medical attention if blood dyscrasias/infection develop, and consider d/c if significant hematologic abnormalities occur. Closely monitor chronic hepatitis B (HBV) carriers; consider d/c and start antiviral therapy if reactivation occurs. Allergic reactions reported; d/c if anaphylaxis or other serious allergic reaction occurs. Needle cap on prefilled syringe and autoinjector contains dry natural rubber; caution with latex allergy. Pediatric patients should be brought up-to-date with current immunization guidelines prior to therapy. May result in autoantibody formation; d/c if lupus-like syndrome or autoimmune hepatitis develops. May affect host defenses against infections. Caution with moderate to severe alcoholic hepatitis, in patients with comorbid conditions, and in elderly.

ADVERSE REACTIONS: Infections, sepsis, upper respiratory infections, non-upper respiratory infections, injection-site reactions, diarrhea, rash, pruritus, lymphoma, other malignancies.

INTERACTIONS: See Boxed Warning. Avoid with live vaccines. Neutropenia and increased rate of infection observed with anakinra. Increased incidence of serious adverse events (eg, infections) reported with abatacept. Use with antidiabetic agents may cause hypoglycemia. Mild decrease in mean neutrophil count reported with sulfasalazine. Immunosuppressants may increase risk of infection and contribute to HBV reactivation. Avoid with immunosuppressive agents (eg, cyclophosphamide) in patients with Wegener's granulomatosis.

PREGNANCY: Category B, not for use in nursing.

MECHANISM OF ACTION: TNF-receptor blocker; inhibits binding of TNF-α and TNF-β (lymphotoxin alpha [LT-α]) to cell surface TNF-receptors, rendering TNF biologically inactive.

PHARMACOKINETICS: Absorption: Various doses resulted in different parameters. **Elimination:** (25mg) $T_{1/2}$=102 hrs.

NURSING CONSIDERATIONS

Assessment: Assess for sepsis, active/localized/chronic/recurrent infection, TB exposure, recent travel in areas of endemic TB/mycoses, predisposition to infection (eg, diabetes), CNS/peripheral nervous system demyelinating disorders, seizure disorder, HF, hematological abnormalities, latex allergy, alcoholic hepatitis, other medical conditions, pregnancy/nursing status, and possible drug interactions. Assess immunization history in pediatric patients. Test for latent TB and HBV infection.

Monitoring: Monitor for serious infections, sepsis, lymphoma, other malignancies, melanoma, NMSC, CNS/peripheral nervous system demyelinating disorders, hematological abnormalities, hypersensitivity reactions, and other adverse reactions. Periodically evaluate for TB infection. Perform periodic skin examination in patients with increased risk for NMSC. Monitor for active HBV infection during and for several months after therapy.

Patient Counseling: Advise of the possible risks/benefits of therapy. Inform that therapy may lower the ability of immune system to fight infections. Advise to contact physician if signs/symptoms of infection, severe allergic reactions, new/worsening medical conditions, or other adverse reactions develop. Counsel about the risk of lymphoma and other malignancies. Advise latex-sensitive patients that the needle cover contains dry natural rubber, a derivative of latex.

Administration: SQ route. Refer to PI for preparation and administration. **Storage:** 2-8°C (36-46°F). Do not freeze. Prefilled Syringe: Protect from light. Do not shake. Reconstituted Sol: Use within 14 days.

ENGERIX-B $\qquad$ RX
hepatitis B (recombinant) (GlaxoSmithKline)

THERAPEUTIC CLASS: Vaccine

INDICATIONS: Immunization against infection caused by all known hepatitis B virus (HBV) subtypes.

DOSAGE: *Adults:* ≥20 yrs: Primary Immunization: 3-Dose Schedule: 1mL IM at 0, 1, 6 months. Booster: 1mL IM. Hemodialysis: Primary Immunization: 4-Dose Schedule: 2mL IM (given as a single 2-mL dose or two 1-mL doses) at 0, 1, 2, 6 months. Booster: 2mL IM when antibody levels decline <10 mIU/mL. Alternate Schedule: 1mL IM at 0, 1, 2, 12 months. Additional hepatitis B

immune globulin (HBIG) should be given with known or presumed exposure to HBV.
Pediatrics: ≤19 yrs: Primary Immunization: 3-Dose Schedule: 0.5mL IM at 0, 1, 6 months. Booster: 11-19 yrs: 1mL IM. ≤10 yrs: 0.5mL IM. Alternate Schedule: 11-19 yrs: 1mL IM at 0, 1, 6 months or at 0, 1, 2, 12 months. 5-16 yrs: 0.5mL IM at 0, 12, 24 months. ≤10 yrs/Infants Born of HBsAg-Positive Mothers: 0.5mL IM at 0, 1, 2, 12 months. Additional HBIG should be given with known or presumed exposure to HBV.

HOW SUPPLIED: Inj: 10mcg/0.5mL, 20mcg/mL

CONTRAINDICATIONS: History of severe allergic reaction to yeast.

WARNINGS/PRECAUTIONS: Tip cap and rubber plunger of prefilled syringes may contain natural rubber latex; allergic reactions may occur in latex-sensitive individuals. Syncope may occur and can be accompanied by transient neurological signs. Defer vaccine for infants weighing <2000g if mother is documented to be HBsAg negative at the time of infant's birth. Apnea in premature infants following IM administration observed; decisions about when to administer vaccine should be based on consideration of medical status, and the potential benefits and possible risks of vaccination. Review immunization history for possible vaccine sensitivity and previous vaccination-related adverse reactions; appropriate treatment must be available for possible anaphylactic reactions. Delay vaccination with moderate or severe acute febrile illness unless at immediate risk of hepatitis B infection (eg, infants born of HBsAg-positive mothers). Immunocompromised persons may have a diminished immune response to vaccine. May not prevent hepatitis B infection in individuals who had an unrecognized hepatitis B infection at the time of vaccination. May not prevent infection in individuals who do not achieve protective antibody titers.

ADVERSE REACTIONS: Inj-site reactions (soreness, erythema, swelling, induration), fatigue, fever, headache, dizziness.

INTERACTIONS: May diminish immune response with immunosuppressant therapy.

PREGNANCY: Category C, caution in nursing.

MECHANISM OF ACTION: Vaccine; may produce immune response for protection against HBV infection.

NURSING CONSIDERATIONS

Assessment: Assess for hypersensitivity to yeast or latex, moderate or severe acute febrile illness, immunosuppression, unrecognized hepatitis B infection, weight of infants, pregnancy/nursing status, and for possible drug interactions. Review immunization history for possible vaccine sensitivity and previous vaccination-related adverse reactions.

Monitoring: Monitor for allergic reactions, inj-site reactions, syncope, and other adverse reactions. Monitor immune response. Perform annual antibody testing in hemodialysis patients to assess the need for booster doses.

Patient Counseling: Inform vaccine recipients and parents/guardians of the potential benefits/risks of immunization. Inform that vaccine contains noninfectious purified HBsAg and cannot cause hepatitis B infection. Instruct to report any adverse events to the healthcare provider.

Administration: IM route. Do not administer in the gluteal region; anterolateral aspect of the thigh (<1 yr) and deltoid muscle (older children and adults) is the preferred administration site. May give SQ if at risk of hemorrhage (eg, hemophiliacs). Shake well before use. Do not dilute to administer. Do not mix with any other vaccine or product in the same syringe or vial. **Storage:** 2-8°C (36-46°F). Do not freeze; discard if has been frozen.

ENJUVIA   RX
conjugated estrogens (Teva)

> Estrogens increase the risk of endometrial cancer. Perform adequate diagnostic measures, including endometrial sampling, to rule out malignancy with undiagnosed persistent or recurrent abnormal vaginal bleeding. Should not be used for the prevention of cardiovascular disease (CVD) or dementia. Increased risks of myocardial infarction (MI), stroke, invasive breast cancer, pulmonary embolism (PE), and deep vein thrombosis (DVT) in postmenopausal women (50-79 yrs) reported. Increased risk of developing probable dementia in postmenopausal women ≥65 yrs reported. Should be prescribed at the lowest effective dose and for the shortest duration consistent with treatment goals and risks.

THERAPEUTIC CLASS: Estrogen

INDICATIONS: Treatment of moderate to severe vasomotor symptoms associated with menopause. Treatment of moderate to severe vaginal dryness and pain with intercourse, symptoms of vulvar and vaginal atrophy associated with menopause.

DOSAGE: *Adults:* Initial: 0.3mg qd. Adjust dose based on response. Reevaluate treatment need periodically (eg, 3-6 month intervals).

HOW SUPPLIED: Tab: 0.3mg, 0.45mg, 0.625mg, 0.9mg, 1.25mg

CONTRAINDICATIONS: Undiagnosed abnormal genital bleeding, known/suspected/history of breast cancer, known/suspected estrogen-dependent neoplasia, active or history of DVT/PE, active or recent arterial thromboembolic disease (eg, stroke, MI), liver dysfunction or disease, known/suspected pregnancy.

WARNINGS/PRECAUTIONS: Increased risk of CV events; d/c immediately if these occur or are suspected. Caution in patients with risk factors for arterial vascular disease (eg, HTN, diabetes mellitus [DM], tobacco use, hypercholesterolemia, obesity) and/or venous thromboembolism (VTE) (eg, personal/family history of VTE, obesity, systemic lupus erythematosus [SLE]). If feasible, d/c at least 4 to 6 weeks before surgery of the type associated with an increased risk of thromboembolism, or during prolonged immobilization. May increase the risk of gallbladder disease. May lead to severe hypercalcemia in patients with breast cancer and bone metastases; d/c and take appropriate measures if hypercalcemia occurs. Retinal vascular thrombosis reported; d/c pending examination if sudden partial/complete loss of vision, sudden onset of proptosis, diplopia, or migraine occurs, or if examination reveals papilledema or retinal vascular lesions, d/c therapy permanently. Consider addition of a progestin if no hysterectomy. May elevate BP, thyroid-binding globulin levels, plasma TG leading to pancreatitis and other complications. Caution in patients with history of cholestatic jaundice; d/c in case of recurrence. May cause fluid retention; caution with cardiac/renal dysfunction. Caution with severe hypocalcemia. May increase risk of ovarian cancer. May exacerbate endometriosis, asthma, DM, epilepsy, migraine or porphyria, SLE, and hepatic hemangiomas; use with caution. May affect certain endocrine, LFTs, and blood components in laboratory tests.

ADVERSE REACTIONS: Abdominal pain, flu syndrome, headache, pain, flatulence, nausea, dizziness, paresthesia, bronchitis, rhinitis, sinusitis, breast pain, dysmenorrhea, vaginitis.

INTERACTIONS: CYP3A4 inducers (eg, St. John's wort, phenobarbital, carbamazepine, rifampin) may decrease levels, which may decrease therapeutic effects and/or change uterine bleeding profile. CYP3A4 inhibitors (eg, erythromycin, clarithromycin, ketoconazole, itraconazole, ritonavir, grapefruit juice) may increase levels, which may result in side effects. Patients concomitantly receiving thyroid replacement therapy and estrogens may require increased doses of thyroid hormone.

PREGNANCY: Contraindicated in pregnancy, caution in nursing.

MECHANISM OF ACTION: Estrogen; binds to nuclear receptors in estrogen-responsive tissues. Circulating estrogens modulate pituitary secretion of the gonadotropins, luteinizing hormone and follicle-stimulating hormone, through a negative feedback mechanism. Reduces elevated levels of these hormones in postmenopausal women.

PHARMACOKINETICS: Absorption: Refer to PI for conjugated and unconjugated estrogen parameters. **Distribution:** Largely bound to sex hormone-binding globulin and albumin; found in breast milk. **Metabolism:** Liver to estrone (metabolite); estriol (major urinary metabolite); sulfate and glucuronide conjugation (liver), gut hydrolysis; CYP3A4 (partial metabolism). **Elimination:** Urine; $T_{1/2}$=14 hrs (estrone), 11 hrs (equilin).

NURSING CONSIDERATIONS

Assessment: Assess for undiagnosed abnormal genital bleeding, presence/history of breast cancer estrogen-dependent neoplasia, active/history of DVT/PE, active or recent (eg, within past yr) arterial thromboembolic disease (eg, stroke, MI), liver dysfunction/disease, pregnancy/ nursing status, and any other conditions where treatment is contraindicated or cautioned. Assess use in patient ≥65 yrs and in those with preexisting hypertriglyceridemia, history of cholestatic jaundice, presence of hypothyroidism, hypocalcemia, asthma, DM, epilepsy, migraine, porphyria, SLE, presence of hepatic hemangiomas, and for possible drug interactions. Assess need for progestin therapy in patients who have not had a hysterectomy.

Monitoring: Monitor for signs/symptoms of CV disorders (eg, stroke, MI), malignant neoplasms (eg, endometrial, breast/ovarian cancer), dementia, gallbladder disease, hypercalcemia, visual abnormalities, elevations in BP, fluid retention, elevations in serum triglycerides, pancreatitis, hypothyroidism, hypocalcemia, exacerbation of endometriosis and other conditions (eg, asthma, DM, epilepsy, migraine, SLE). Monitor BP. Monitor thyroid function in patients on thyroid replacement therapy. If undiagnosed, persistent, or recurring abnormal vaginal bleeding occurs, perform proper diagnostic testing (eg, endometrial sampling) to rule out malignancy. Perform annual breast exam. Perform periodic monitoring (every 3-6 months) to determine need for therapy.

Patient Counseling: Inform that therapy increases the risk for uterine cancer and may increase the chances of getting a heart attack, stroke, breast cancer, and blood clots. Advise to report breast lumps, unusual vaginal bleeding, dizziness or faintness, changes in speech, severe headaches, chest pain, SOB, leg pains, vision changes, or vomiting. Instruct to notify physician if taking other medications or if planning surgery or prolonged immobilization. Advise to have yearly breast examinations by a physician and to perform monthly breast self-examinations. Instruct that if a dose is missed, take as soon as possible; if almost time for next dose, skip missed dose and return to normal dosing schedule.

Administration: Oral route. **Storage:** 20-25°C (68-77°F).

ENTEREG   RX
alvimopan (GlaxoSmithKline)

THERAPEUTIC CLASS: Opioid antagonist

INDICATIONS: To accelerate time to upper and lower GI recovery following partial large or small bowel resection surgery with primary anastomosis.

DOSAGE: *Adults:* ≥18 yrs: 12mg given 30 min to 5 hrs prior to surgery followed by 12mg bid beginning day after surgery for maximum of 7 days or until discharge. Max: 15 doses.

HOW SUPPLIED: Cap: 12mg

CONTRAINDICATIONS: Therapeutic doses of opioids for >7 consecutive days immediately prior to therapy.

WARNINGS/PRECAUTIONS: Recent exposure to opioids may increase sensitivity to adverse reactions, mainly GI (eg, abdominal pain, N/V, diarrhea) associated with alvimopan; caution in patients receiving >3 doses of opioids within the week prior to surgery. Avoid using in severe hepatic impairment (Child-Pugh Class C), end-stage renal disease, surgery for correction of complete bowel obstruction. Myocardial Infarction (MI) reported in patients treated with opioids for chronic pain. Caution in Japanese patients.

ADVERSE REACTIONS: Anemia, constipation, dyspepsia, flatulence, hypokalemia, back pain, urinary retention.

INTERACTIONS: See Contraindications.

PREGNANCY: Category B, caution in nursing.

MECHANISM OF ACTION: Selective antagonist of μ-opioid receptor; antagonizes the peripheral effects of opioids on GI motility and secretion by competitively binding to GI tract μ-opioid receptors.

PHARMACOKINETICS: Absorption: Absolute bioavailability (6%); T_{max}=2 hrs; C_{max}=10.98ng/mL; AUC_{0-12h}=40.2ng•h/mL; (Metabolite): T_{max}=36 hrs; C_{max}=35.73ng/mL. **Distribution:** V_d=30L. Plasma protein binding (80%, alvimopan; 94%, metabolite). **Elimination:** Renal excretion (35% of total clearance); biliary (primary pathway); $T_{1/2}$=10-17 hrs; (Metabolite): $T_{1/2}$=10-18 hrs.

NURSING CONSIDERATIONS

Assessment: Assess for hepatic/renal impairment, bowel obstruction, history of opioid use, and pregnancy/nursing status, and for possible drug interactions.

Monitoring: Monitor for signs/symptoms of possible side effects when recently exposed to opioids (eg, abdominal pain, N/V, diarrhea) and for MI. Monitor hepatic and renal function.

Patient Counseling: Instruct to disclose long-term or intermittent opioid pain therapy, including any use of opioids in the week prior to receiving therapy. Inform that recent use of opioids may cause adverse reactions primarily those limited to the GI tract (eg, abdominal pain, N/V, diarrhea). Advise that therapy must be administered in a hospital setting for no more than 7 days after bowel resection surgery. Inform that constipation, dyspepsia, and flatulence may occur.

Administration: Oral route. **Storage:** 25°C (77°F); excursions permitted to 15-30°C (59-86°F).

ENTOCORT EC   RX
budesonide (Prometheus)

THERAPEUTIC CLASS: Corticosteroid

INDICATIONS: Treatment of mild to moderate active Crohn's disease of the ileum and/or ascending colon. Maintenance of clinical remission of mild to moderate Crohn's disease of the ileum and/or ascending colon for up to 3 months.

DOSAGE: *Adults:* Usual: 9mg qd, in the am for up to 8 weeks. Recurring Episodes: Repeat therapy for 8 weeks. Maint: 6mg qd for 3 months, then taper to complete cessation. Moderate to Severe Hepatic Insufficiency/Concomitant CYP3A4 Inhibitors: Reduce dose. Swallow whole; do not chew or break.

HOW SUPPLIED: Cap, Delayed-Release: 3mg

WARNINGS/PRECAUTIONS: May reduce response of hypothalamic pituitary adrenal axis to stress. Supplement with systemic glucocorticosteroids if undergoing surgery or other stressful situations. Increased risk of infection; avoid exposure to varicella/varicella zoster and measles. Caution with TB, HTN, diabetes mellitus (DM), osteoporosis, peptic ulcer, glaucoma, cirrhosis, cataracts, family history of DM or glaucoma. Replacement of systemic glucocorticosteroids may unmask allergies. Chronic use may cause hypercorticism and adrenal suppression.

ADVERSE REACTIONS: Headache, respiratory infection, N/V, back pain, dyspepsia, dizziness, abdominal pain, diarrhea, flatulence, sinusitis, viral infection, arthralgia, benign intracranial HTN, signs/symptoms of hypercorticism.

INTERACTIONS: Ketoconazole caused an eight-fold increase of systemic exposure to oral budesonide. Increased levels with CYP3A4 inhibitors (eg, ketoconazole, itraconazole, saquinavir, erythromycin, grapefruit, grapefruit juice); monitor for increased signs and symptoms of hypercorticism and reduce budesonide dose if coadministered.

PREGNANCY: Category C, not for use in nursing.

MECHANISM OF ACTION: Glucocorticosteroid.

PHARMACOKINETICS: Absorption: C_{max}=5nmol/L; T_{max}=30-600 min; AUC=30nmol•hr/L. Bioavailability=9-21%. **Distribution:** V_d=2.2-3.9L/kg; plasma protein binding (85-90%). **Metabolism:** Liver; CYP3A4. **Elimination:** Urine (60%); $T_{1/2}$=2-3.6 hrs.

NURSING CONSIDERATIONS

Assessment: Assess for liver disease, history of chickenpox or measles, TB, HTN, osteoporosis, peptic ulcers, cataracts, history and/or family history of DM or glaucoma and possible drug interactions. Obtain baseline LFTs.

Monitoring: Monitor LFTs periodically and for signs/symptoms of hypercorticism and hypersensitivity reactions.

Patient Counseling: Advise to swallow whole; do not chew or break. Avoid consumption of grapefruit and grapefruit juice during therapy. Take particular care to avoid exposure to chickenpox or measles.

Administration: Oral route. **Storage:** 25° (77°F); excursions permitted to 15-30°C (59-86°F). Keep container tightly closed.

EPIDUO   RX
adapalene - benzoyl peroxide (Galderma)

THERAPEUTIC CLASS: Antibacterial/keratolytic

INDICATIONS: Topical treatment of acne vulgaris in patients ≥12 yrs.

DOSAGE: *Adults:* Apply a pea-sized amount to the affected areas of the face and/or trunk qd after washing.
Pediatrics: ≥12 yrs: Apply a pea-sized amount to the affected areas of the face and/or trunk once qd after washing.

HOW SUPPLIED: Gel: (Adapalene-Benzoyl Peroxide) 0.1%-2.5% [45g]

WARNINGS/PRECAUTIONS: Not for oral, ophthalmic, or intravaginal use. Minimize exposure to sunlight and sunlamps. Extreme weather may increase skin irritation. Avoid contact with eyes, lips, mucous membranes, cuts, abrasions, eczematous, or sunburned skin. Local cutaneous reactions, or irritant and allergic dermatitis may occur; may apply moisturizer, reduce frequency of application, or d/c use. Avoid "waxing" as depilatory method on the treated skin.

ADVERSE REACTIONS: Local cutaneous reactions (eg, erythema, scaling, stinging/burning, dryness), contact dermatitis, skin irritation.

INTERACTIONS: Caution with topical acne therapy, especially with peeling, desquamating, or abrasive agents. Avoid with other potentially irritating topical products (medicated or abrasive soaps and cleansers, soaps and cosmetics that have strong skin-drying effect, and products with high concentrations of alcohol, astringents, spices, or limes).

PREGNANCY: Category C, caution in nursing.

MECHANISM OF ACTION: Adapalene: Naphthoic acid derivative; not established. Binds to specific retinoic acid nuclear receptors. Benzoyl peroxide: Oxidizing agent with bactericidal and keratolytic effects.

PHARMACOKINETICS: Absorption: (Adapalene) C_{max}=0.21ng/mL; AUC_{0-24h}=1.99ng•h/mL. **Excretion:** (Adapalene) Bile. (Benzoyl peroxide) Urine.

NURSING CONSIDERATIONS

Assessment: Assess for sunburned skin, eczema, abrasion, skin cuts, use in pregnancy/nursing, and possible drug interactions.

Monitoring: Monitor for sensitivity or irritation, cutaneous signs/symptoms (eg, erythema, dryness, scaling, burning, stinging, contact dermatitis).

Patient Counseling: Advise to cleanse area with mild or soapless cleanser; pat dry. Avoid contact with eyes, lips, and mucous membranes. Do not use more than the recommended amount. May cause irritation and bleach hair and colored fabric. Minimize exposure to sunlight and sunlamps; use sunscreen and protective clothing.

Administration: Topical route. **Storage:** 25°C; excursions permitted to 15-30°C (59-86°F). Protect from light. Keep away from heat. Keep tube tightly closed.

EPIFOAM
pramoxine HCl - hydrocortisone acetate (Alaven)

RX

THERAPEUTIC CLASS: Corticosteroid/anesthetic

INDICATIONS: Relief of the inflammatory and pruritic manifestations of corticosteroid-responsive dermatoses.

DOSAGE: *Adults:* Apply a small amount to the affected area tid-qid depending on severity of condition. May use occlusive dressings for management of psoriasis or recalcitrant conditions; d/c occlusive dressing if infection develops.
Pediatrics: Apply a small amount to the affected area tid-qid depending on severity of condition. May use occlusive dressings for management of psoriasis or recalcitrant conditions; d/c occlusive dressing if infection develops. Use least amount effective for the condition.

HOW SUPPLIED: Foam: (Hydrocortisone-Pramoxine) 1%-1% [10g]

WARNINGS/PRECAUTIONS: Not for prolonged use. D/C if redness, pain, irritation, or swelling persists. Systemic absorption may produce reversible hypothalamic-pituitary-adrenal (HPA) axis suppression, manifestations of Cushing's syndrome, hyperglycemia, and glucosuria; evaluate periodically for evidence of HPA axis suppression when large dose is applied to large surface areas or under an occlusive dressing. Withdraw treatment, reduce frequency of application, or substitute with a less potent steroid if HPA axis suppression is noted. Application of more potent steroids, use over large surface areas, prolonged use, and the addition of occlusive dressings may augment systemic absorption. Signs and symptoms of steroid withdrawal may occur (infrequent) requiring supplemental systemic corticosteroids. D/C and institute appropriate therapy if irritation occurs. Use appropriate antifungal or antibacterial agent in the presence of dermatological infections; if favorable response does not occur promptly, d/c until infection is controlled. Pediatrics may be more susceptible to systemic toxicity. Chronic therapy may interfere with growth and development of pediatrics.

ADVERSE REACTIONS: Burning, itching, irritation, dryness, folliculitis, hypertrichosis, acneiform eruptions, hypopigmentation, perioral dermatitis, allergic contact dermatitis, maceration, secondary infection, skin atrophy, striae, miliaria.

PREGNANCY: Category C, caution in nursing.

MECHANISM OF ACTION: Hydrocortisone: Corticosteroid; possesses anti-inflammatory, antipruritic, and vasoconstrictive properties. Anti-inflammatory activity not established. Pramoxine: Local anesthetic.

PHARMACOKINETICS: Absorption: Percutaneous; inflammation, other disease processes in the skin, and occlusive dressings may increase absorption. **Distribution:** Plasma protein binding in varying degrees; found in breast milk (systemically administered). **Metabolism:** Liver. **Elimination:** Urine, feces.

NURSING CONSIDERATIONS

Assessment: Assess for previous hypersensitivity to any components of the drug, dermatological infections, and pregnancy/nursing status.

Monitoring: Monitor for signs/symptoms of reversible HPA axis suppression, Cushing's syndrome, hyperglycemia, glucosuria, skin irritation, skin infections, systemic toxicity in pediatrics, hypersensitivity reactions, and other adverse reactions. When large dose is applied to large surface area or under occlusive dressings, monitor for HPA axis suppression by using urinary free cortisol and adrenocorticotropic hormone stimulation tests. Monitor for signs/symptoms of steroid withdrawal following d/c.

Patient Counseling: Instruct to use externally and as directed; instruct to avoid contact with eyes. Advise not to use for any disorder other than for which it was prescribed. Instruct not to bandage, cover, or wrap treated skin, unless directed by physician. Advise to report any signs of local adverse reactions, especially under occlusive dressing. Instruct not to use tight-fitting diapers or plastic pants on a child being treated in the diaper area, as these garments may constitute occlusive dressings.

Administration: Topical route. Shake container vigorously for 5-10 sec before each use. May also dispense a small amount to a pad and apply to affected areas. Rinse container and cap with warm water after use. Do not insert container into vagina or anus. **Storage:** 20-25°C (68-77°F). Store upright. Do not store at temperatures >120°F (49°C). Do not burn or puncture the aerosol container. Do not refrigerate.

EPIPEN
epinephrine (Dey)

RX

OTHER BRAND NAMES: Epipen Jr. (Dey)

THERAPEUTIC CLASS: Sympathomimetic catecholamine

INDICATIONS: Emergency treatment of allergic reactions (Type I), including anaphylaxis to stinging insects (eg, bees, wasps, hornets, yellow jackets, and fire ants) and biting insects (eg, triatoma, mosquitoes), allergen immunotherapy, foods, drugs, diagnostic testing substances (eg, radiocontrast media), and other allergens, as well as idiopathic or exercise-induced anaphylaxis. For immediate administration with history of anaphylactic reactions.

DOSAGE: *Adults:* 15-30kg: 0.15mg (Epipen Jr). ≥30kg: 0.3mg (Epipen). Inject IM/SQ into the anterolateral aspect of the thigh. May repeat with severe anaphylaxis.
Pediatrics: 15-30kg: 0.15mg (Epipen Jr). ≥30kg: 0.3mg (Epipen). Inject IM/SQ into anterolateral aspect of the thigh. May repeat with severe anaphylaxis.

HOW SUPPLIED: Inj: (Epipen Jr) 0.15mg/0.3mL, (Epipen) 0.3mg/0.3mL

WARNINGS/PRECAUTIONS: Intended for immediate self-administration as emergency supportive therapy only and is not a substitute for immediate medical care. Do not inject into buttock; may not provide effective treatment of anaphylaxis. Do not inject into digits, hands, or feet. Not for IV use. Large doses or accidental IV use may cause cerebral hemorrhage due to sharp rise in BP. Contains sodium metabisulfite; may cause allergic-type reactions, including anaphylactic symptoms or life-threatening or less severe asthmatic episodes in certain susceptible persons. Caution in patients with heart disease, including cardiac arrhythmias, coronary artery or organic heart disease, or HTN. More than two sequential doses should only be administered under direct medical supervision. Higher risk of developing adverse reactions with hyperthyroidism, cardiovascular disease (CVD), HTN, diabetes mellitus (DM), in elderly, pregnant women, pediatrics <30kg using Epipen, and pediatrics <15kg using Epipen Jr.

ADVERSE REACTIONS: Palpitations, sweating, N/V, respiratory difficulty, pallor, dizziness, weakness, tremor, headache, apprehensiveness, anxiety, restlessness, arrhythmias (including fatal ventricular fibrillation), angina, cerebral hemorrhage.

INTERACTIONS: Rapidly acting vasodilators can counteract the marked pressor effects of epinephrine. Drugs that sensitize the heart to arrhythmias (eg, digitalis, diuretics, quinidine, or other antiarrhythmics) may precipitate or aggravate angina pectoris as well as produce ventricular arrhythmias. Coadministration with TCAs, MAOIs, levothyroxine sodium, and certain antihistamines, including chlorpheniramine, tripelennamine and diphenhydramine, may lead to potentiation of epinephrine effects. Antagonized cardiostimulating and bronchodilating effects with beta-adrenergic blocking drugs, such as propranolol. Antagonized vasoconstricting and hypertensive effects with alpha-adrenergic blocking drugs such as phentoloamine. Ergot alkaloids may reverse pressor effects.

PREGNANCY: Category C, safety not known in nursing.

MECHANISM OF ACTION: Sympathomimetic catecholamine; acts on α- and β-adrenergic receptors.

NURSING CONSIDERATIONS

Assessment: Assess for heart disease including arrhythmias, coronary artery/organic heart disease, and HTN. Assess for DM, hyperthyroidism, Parkinson's disease, pregnancy/nursing status, and for possible drug interactions.

Monitoring: Monitor for signs/symptoms of angina pectoris, ventricular arrhythmias, cerebral hemorrhage, and for other adverse reactions. Monitor HR and BP. Monitor glucose levels in patients with DM. Monitor for worsening of symptoms in patients with Parkinson's disease.

Patient Counseling: Inform about side effects of therapy (eg, increased pulse rate, sense of forceful heartbeat, palpitations, sweating, n/v, headache, pallor, anxiety, shakiness) and advise to notify physician if any adverse reactions develop. Instruct not to inject into buttock or by IV route. Advise to go to nearest emergency room if accidentally inject self. Advise that epinephrine is not intended as a substitute for immediate medical care.

Administration: IM or SQ route. Inject into the anterolateral aspect of the thigh, through clothing if necessary. **Storage:** 25°C (77°F); excursions permitted to 15-30°C (59-86°F). Protect from light. Do not refrigerate. Discard if discolored or contains a precipitate.

EPIQUIN MICRO   RX
hydroquinone (SkinMedica)

THERAPEUTIC CLASS: Depigmentation agent

INDICATIONS: Gradual treatment of UV-induced dyschromia and discoloration resulting from the use of oral contraceptives, pregnancy, hormone replacement therapy, or skin trauma.

DOSAGE: *Adults/Pediatrics:* >12 yrs: Apply to affected areas bid (am and hs) or ud.

HOW SUPPLIED: Cre: 4% [40g]

WARNINGS/PRECAUTIONS: May produce unwanted cosmetic effects if not used ud. Test for skin sensitivity prior to use; do not use if itching, vesicle formation, or excessive inflammatory response occurs. Avoid contact with eyes. D/C if no lightening effect observed after 2 months of therapy. Avoid sun exposure; use sunscreen (SPF 15 or greater) or protective clothing. Contains Na metabisulfite; may cause serious allergic reactions. D/C if blue-black darkening of the skin occurs. Limit treatment to small areas of the body at one time.

ADVERSE REACTIONS: Hypersensitivity (localized contact dermatitis).

PREGNANCY: Category C, caution in nursing.

MECHANISM OF ACTION: Depigmentation agent; produces a reversible depigmentation of the skin by inhibition of the enzymatic oxidation of tyrosine to 3-(3,4-dihydroxyphenyl) alanine (dopa) and suppresses other melanocyte metabolic processes.

NURSING CONSIDERATIONS

Assessment: Assess for drug hypersensitivity and pregnancy/nursing status.

Monitoring: Monitor for hypersensitivity reactions, blue-black darkening of the skin, and effectiveness for 2 months.

Patient Counseling: Advise to take as prescribed. Instruct to d/c and contact physician if a gradual blue-black darkening of skin occurs. Advise to avoid contact with eyes. Inform that sunscreen is essential during therapy; instruct to avoid exposure to sun and to wear protective clothing.

Administration: Topical route. **Storage:** 25°C (77°F); excursions permitted to 15-30°C (59-86°F).

EPIVIR   RX
lamivudine (ViiV Healthcare)

> Lactic acidosis and severe hepatomegaly with steatosis, including fatal cases, reported with nucleoside analogues; suspend treatment if lactic acidosis or pronounced hepatotoxicity occurs. Severe acute exacerbations of hepatitis B reported in patients coinfected with hepatitis B virus (HBV) upon d/c of therapy; closely monitor hepatic function for at least several months. If appropriate, initiation of anti-hepatitis B therapy may be warranted. Epivir tabs and sol, used to treat HIV-1 infection, contain higher dose of lamivudine than Epivir-HBV tabs and sol, used to treat chronic HBV infection; only use appropriate dosing forms for HIV-1 treatment.

THERAPEUTIC CLASS: Nucleoside reverse transcriptase inhibitor

INDICATIONS: Treatment of HIV-1 infection in combination with other antiretrovirals.

DOSAGE: *Adults:* Usual: 150mg bid or 300mg qd. Renal Impairment (≥30kg): CrCl ≥50mL/min: 150mg bid or 300mg qd. CrCl 30-49mL/min: 150mg qd. CrCl 15-29mL/min: 150mg first dose, then 100mg qd. CrCl 5-14mL/min: 150mg first dose, then 50mg qd. CrCl <5mL/min: 50mg first dose, then 25mg qd. Elderly: Start at the low end of dosing range.
Pediatrics: >16 yrs: Usual: 150mg bid or 300mg qd. 3 months-16 yrs: (Sol) 4mg/kg bid. Max: 150mg bid. (Tab) 14-21kg: 1/2 tab (75mg) in am and pm. >21-<30kg: 1/2 tab (75mg) in am and 1 tab (150mg) in pm. ≥30kg: 1 tab (150mg) in am and pm. Renal Impairment (≥30kg): ≥16 yrs: CrCl ≥50mL/min: 150mg bid or 300mg qd. CrCl 30-49mL/min: 150mg qd. CrCl 15-29mL/min: 150mg first dose, then 100mg qd. CrCl 5-14mL/min: 150mg first dose, then 50mg qd. CrCl <5mL/min: 50mg first dose, then 25mg qd. 3 months-16 yrs: Consider dose reduction and/or increase in dosing interval.

HOW SUPPLIED: Sol: 10mg/mL [240mL]; Tab: 150mg*, 300mg *scored

WARNINGS/PRECAUTIONS: Obesity and prolonged nucleoside exposure may be risk factors for lactic acidosis and severe hepatomegaly with steatosis. Caution with known risk factors for liver disease. Emergence of lamivudine-resistant HBV reported. Caution in pediatric patients with history of prior antiretroviral nucleoside exposure, history of pancreatitis, or other significant risk factors for development of pancreatitis; d/c if pancreatitis develops. Immune reconstitution syndrome reported. Autoimmune disorders (eg, Graves' disease, polymyositis, Guillain-Barre syndrome) reported to occur in the setting of immune reconstitution and can occur many months after initiation of treatment. Redistribution/accumulation of body fat observed. Caution in elderly.

ADVERSE REACTIONS: Headache, malaise, fatigue, N/V, diarrhea, nasal signs/symptoms, neuropathy, insomnia, musculoskeletal pain, cough, fever, dizziness, anorexia/decreased appetite, lactic acidosis, severe hepatomegaly with steatosis.

INTERACTIONS: Avoid with other lamivudine-containing products, emtricitabine-containing products, and zalcitabine. Hepatic decompensation has occurred in HIV/hepatitis C virus coinfected patients receiving interferon-alfa, with or without ribavirin. Trimethoprim/Sulfamethoxazole may increase levels. Possible interaction with drugs whose main route of elimination is active renal secretion via the organic cationic transport system.

PREGNANCY: Category C, not for use in nursing.

MECHANISM OF ACTION: Nucleoside analogue; inhibits HIV-1 reverse transcriptase via DNA chain termination after incorporation of the nucleotide analogue into viral DNA.

PHARMACOKINETICS: Absorption: Rapid; absolute bioavailability (86% tab, 87% sol); C_{max}=1.5mcg/mL; T_{max}=0.9 hrs (fasting), 3.2 hrs (fed). **Distribution:** V_d=1.3L/kg (IV); plasma protein binding (<36%); found in breast milk. **Metabolism:** Trans-sulfoxide (metabolite). **Elimination:** Urine (71% unchanged [IV], 5.2% metabolite [PO]); $T_{1/2}$=5-7 hrs.

NURSING CONSIDERATIONS

Assessment: Assess for impaired hepatic/renal function, risk factors for liver disease, HIV-1 and HBV coinfection, previous hypersensitivity, pregnancy/nursing status, and possible drug interactions. In pediatric patients, assess for a history of prior antiretroviral nucleoside exposure, a history of pancreatitis, or risk factors for pancreatitis.

Monitoring: Monitor for signs/symptoms of pancreatitis, immune reconstitution syndrome (eg, opportunistic infections), fat redistribution, lactic acidosis, severe hepatomegaly with steatosis, hepatitis B exacerbation, hepatic/renal dysfunction, and hypersensitivity reactions. Monitor hepatic function closely for several months in patients with HIV/HBV coinfection who d/c therapy. Monitor CBC.

Patient Counseling: Inform that drug may rarely cause a serious condition called lactic acidosis with liver enlargement. Instruct to discuss any changes in regimen with physician. Instruct not to take concomitantly with emtricitabine- or other lamivudine-containing products and to avoid missing doses. Advise parents or guardians of pediatric patients about signs and symptoms of pancreatitis; instruct to contact physician if any signs/symptoms of pancreatitis develop. Inform that drug is not a cure for HIV-1 infection and that may continue to experience illnesses associated with HIV-1 infection, including opportunistic infections. Counsel that therapy does not reduce risk of HIV transmission through sexual contact or blood contamination. Inform that redistribution or accumulation of body fat may occur. Advise diabetic patients that each 15-mL dose of solution contains 3g of sucrose. Counsel not to share needles, other inj equipment or personal items that can have blood or body fluids on them (eg, toothbrush, razor blades). Instruct no to have any kind of sex without protection. Advise to avoid breastfeeding.

Administration: Oral route. **Storage:** (Tab) 25°C (77°F); excursions permitted to 15-30°C (59-86°F). (Sol) 25°C (77°F). Store in tightly closed bottles.

EPIVIR-HBV   RX
lamivudine (GlaxoSmithKline)

> Lactic acidosis and severe hepatomegaly with steatosis, including fatal cases, reported with nucleoside analogues. Contains a lower dose of lamivudine than Epivir (used to treat HIV). Rapid emergence of HIV resistance is likely if prescribed for hepatitis B in patients with unrecognized/untreated HIV infection. Offer HIV counseling and testing to all patients prior to therapy and periodically thereafter. Severe acute exacerbations of hepatitis B reported upon d/c of therapy; closely monitor hepatic function for at least several months. If appropriate, initiation of anti-hepatitis B therapy may be warranted.

THERAPEUTIC CLASS: Nucleoside reverse transcriptase inhibitor

INDICATIONS: Treatment of chronic hepatitis B (HBV) associated with evidence of hepatitis B viral replication and active liver inflammation.

DOSAGE: *Adults:* CrCl ≥50mL/min: 100mg qd. CrCl 30-49mL/min: 100mg 1st dose, then 50mg qd. CrCl 15-29mL/min: 100mg 1st dose, then 25mg qd. CrCl 5-14mL/min: 35mg 1st dose, then 15mg qd. CrCl <5mL/min: 35mg 1st dose, then 10mg qd. Elderly: Start at lower end of dosing range.
Pediatrics: 2-17 yrs: 3mg/kg qd. Max: 100mg/day. Renal Impairment: Dose reduction should be considered.

HOW SUPPLIED: Sol: 5mg/mL [240mL]; Tab: 100mg

WARNINGS/PRECAUTIONS: Obesity and prolonged nucleoside exposure may be risk factors for lactic acidosis and severe hepatomegaly with steatosis. Caution with known risk factors for liver disease; d/c if findings suggestive of lactic acidosis or pronounced hepatotoxicity. Pancreatitis reported, especially in HIV-infected pediatrics with prior nucleoside exposure. Emergence of resistance-associated HBV mutations reported; monitor ALT and HBV DNA levels during treatment. Use appropriate infant immunizations to prevent neonatal acquisition of HBV. Should only be used when alternative antiviral agent with a higher genetic barrier to resistance is not available/appropriate. Not appropriate for patients dually infected with HBV and HIV. Caution in elderly.

ADVERSE REACTIONS: Lactic acidosis, severe hepatomegaly with steatosis, post-treatment exacerbations of hepatitis, pancreatitis, malaise, fatigue, ear/nose/throat infections, myalgia, abdominal discomfort/pain, diarrhea, headache, N/V.

INTERACTIONS: Avoid with other lamivudine-containing products. Not recommended with zalcitabine. Possible interaction with other drugs whose main route of elimination is active renal secretion via the organic cationic transport system. Trimethoprim/sulfamethoxazole may increase levels.

PREGNANCY: Category C, not for use in nursing.

MECHANISM OF ACTION: Nucleoside reverse transcriptase inhibitors; incorporation of monophosphate form into viral DNA by HBV reverse transcriptase results in DNA termination.

PHARMACOKINETICS: Absorption: Rapid; absolute bioavailability (86% tab, 87% sol); AUC=4.3mcg•hr/mL (single dose), AUC=4.7mcg•hr/mL (repeated daily doses); C_{max}=1.28mcg/mL; T_{max}=0.5-2.0 hrs. Refer to PI for pharmacokinetic parameters in patients with impaired renal/hepatic function. **Distribution:** Plasma protein binding (<36%); V_d=1.3L/kg (IV); found in breast milk. **Metabolism:** Trans-sulfoxide (metabolite). **Elimination:** Urine (unchanged); $T_{1/2}$=5-7 hrs.

NURSING CONSIDERATIONS

Assessment: Assess weight, hepatic/renal function, for nucleoside exposure, risk factors for liver disease, HIV infection, history of pancreatitis, drug hypersensitivity, pregnancy/nursing status, and possible drug interactions. Perform HIV counseling and testing in all patients prior to therapy and periodically thereafter.

Monitoring: Monitor renal/hepatic function, therapeutic response, for signs/symptoms of pancreatitis, lactic acidosis, hepatomegaly with steatosis, emergence of resistant HIV, post-treatment exacerbations of hepatitis, and ALT and HBV DNA levels if emergence of viral mutants is suspected. Monitor hepatic function during and for at least several months after d/c therapy.

Patient Counseling: Advise to discuss any new symptoms or concurrent medications with physician. Inform that drug is not a cure for HBV; long-term benefits and relationship of initial treatment response to outcomes are unknown. Inform that liver disease deterioration may occur upon d/c. Advise to discuss any changes in regimen with physician. Inform that emergence of resistant HBV and worsening of disease can occur; advise to report any new symptoms to physician. Counsel on importance of HIV testing to avoid inappropriate therapy and development of resistant HIV. Instruct not to take concurrently with other lamivudine-containing products. Inform that therapy does not reduce risk of HBV transmission through sexual contact/blood contamination. Inform diabetics that each 20-mL of oral sol contains 4g of sucrose.

Administration: Oral route. **Storage:** Tab: 25°C (77°F); excursions permitted to 15-30°C (59-86°F). Sol: 20-25°C (68-77°F); store in tightly closed bottles.

EPOGEN   RX
epoetin alfa (Amgen)

Increased risk of death, myocardial infarction, stroke, venous thromboembolism, thrombosis of vascular access, and tumor progression or recurrence. Use the lowest dose sufficient to reduce/avoid the need for RBC transfusions. Chronic Kidney Disease (CKD): Greater risks for death, serious cardiovascular (CV) reactions, and stroke when administered to target Hgb level >11g/dL. Cancer: Shortened overall survival and/or increased risk of tumor progression or recurrence in patients with breast, non-small cell lung, head and neck, lymphoid, and cervical cancers. Must enroll in and comply with the ESA APPRISE Oncology Program to prescribe and/or dispense to patients. Use only for anemia from myelosuppressive chemotherapy. Not indicated for patients receiving myelosuppressive chemotherapy when anticipated outcome is cure. D/C following completion of chemotherapy course. Perisurgery: due to increased risk of deep venous thrombosis (DVT), consider DVT prophylaxis.

THERAPEUTIC CLASS: Erythropoiesis stimulator

INDICATIONS: Treatment of anemia due to CKD, including patients on/not on dialysis; anemia due to zidovudine administered at ≤4200mg/week in HIV-infected patients with endogenous serum erythropoietin levels of ≤500 mU/mL; anemic patients with non-myeloid malignancies where anemia is due to the effect of concomitant myelosuppressive chemotherapy, and upon initiation, there is a minimum of 2 additional months of planned chemotherapy. To reduce the need for allogeneic RBC transfusions in patients with perioperative Hgb >10 to ≤13g/dL, who are at high risk for perioperative blood loss from elective, noncardiac, nonvascular surgery.

DOSAGE: *Adults:* Initiate when Hgb is <10g/dL (see PI for additional parameters). CKD on Dialysis: Initial: 50-100 U/kg IV/SQ TIW. CKD not on Dialysis: Initial: 50-100 U/kg IV/SQ TIW.

Titrate: Adjust dose based on Hgb levels; see PI. Zidovudine-Treated HIV Patients: Initial: 100 U/kg IV/SQ TIW. Titrate: Adjust dose based on Hgb levels; see PI. Malignancy: Initial: 150 U/kg SQ TIW or 40,000 U SQ weekly until completion of a chemotherapy course. Titrate: Adjust dose based on Hgb levels; see PI. Surgery Patients: Usual: 300 U/kg/day SQ for 10 days before, on day of, and for 4 days after surgery; or 600 U/kg SQ in 4 doses administered 21, 14, and 7 days before surgery and on the day of surgery. DVT prophylaxis recommended. Individualize dose selection and adjustment for the elderly to achieve/maintain target Hb.

Pediatrics: 5-18 yrs: Malignancy: Initial: 600 U/kg IV weekly until completion of a chemotherapy course. Titrate: Adjust dose based on Hgb levels; see PI. Max: 60,000 U weekly. 1 month-16 yrs: Initiate when Hgb is <10g/dL (see PI for additional parameters). CKD on Dialysis: Initial: 50 U/kg IV/SQ TIW.

HOW SUPPLIED: Inj: Single-dose: 2000 U/mL, 3000 U/mL, 4000 U/mL, 10,000 U/mL, 40,000 U/mL; Multidose: 10,000 U/mL [2mL], 20,000 U/mL [1mL]

CONTRAINDICATIONS: Uncontrolled HTN, pure red cell aplasia (PRCA) that begins after treatment with epoetin alfa or other erythropoietin drugs. Multidose: Neonates, infants, pregnant women, and nursing mothers.

WARNINGS/PRECAUTIONS: Not indicated in patients with cancer receiving hormonal agents, biologic products, or radiotherapy, unless also receiving concomitant myelosuppressive chemotherapy, in patients scheduled for surgery willing to donate autologous blood, in patients undergoing cardiac/vascular surgery, and as substitute for RBC transfusions in patients requiring immediate correction of anemia. Correct/exclude other causes of anemia (eg, vitamin deficiency, metabolic/chronic inflammatory conditions, bleeding) prior to therapy. Increased risk of congestive heart failure, deep venous thrombosis undergoing orthopedic procedures, other thromboembolic events, and death in patients undergoing coronary artery bypass surgery. Hypertensive encephalopathy and seizures reported with CKD. Reduce/withhold therapy if BP becomes difficult to control. PRCA and severe anemia (with or without other cytopenias), with neutralizing antibodies to erythropoietin reported. Withhold and evaluate for neutralizing antibodies to erythropoietin if severe anemia and low reticulocyte count occur; d/c permanently if PRCA develops. Immediately and permanently d/c if serious allergic/anaphylactic reactions occur. Contains albumin; may carry an extremely remote risk for transmission of viral diseases or Creutzfeldt-Jakob disease. May require adjustment in dialysis prescriptions and increased anticoagulation with heparin to prevent clotting of extracorporeal circuit during hemodialysis. Multidose vials contains benzyl alcohol; benzyl alcohol associated with serious adverse events and death, particularly in pediatrics.

ADVERSE REACTIONS: CV/thromboembolic reactions, pyrexia, N/V, HTN, cough, arthralgia, myalgia, pruritus, rash, headache, injection-site pain, stomatitis, dizziness.

PREGNANCY: Category C, caution in nursing.

MECHANISM OF ACTION: Erythropoiesis stimulating protein; stimulates erythropoiesis by the same mechanism as endogenous erythropoietin.

PHARMACOKINETICS: Absorption: Adults and Pediatrics with CKD: (SQ) T_{max}=5-24 hrs. Anemic Cancer Patients: (SQ) T_{max}=5-24 hrs. **Elimination:** Adults and Pediatrics with CKD: (IV) $T_{1/2}$=4-13 hrs. Anemic Cancer Patients: (SQ) $T_{1/2}$=16-67 hrs.

NURSING CONSIDERATIONS

Assessment: Assess for uncontrolled HTN, previous hypersensitivity to the drug, causes of anemia, pregnancy/nursing status, and other conditions where treatment is cautioned/contraindicated. Obtain baseline iron status, Hgb levels, transferrin saturation, and serum ferritin.

Monitoring: Monitor for signs/symptoms of an allergic reaction, CV/thromboembolic events, stroke, premonitory neurologic symptoms, PRCA, severe anemia. Monitor Hgb (weekly until stable and then monthly for CKD), BP, iron status, transferrin saturation, and progression or recurrence of tumor in cancer patients. Monitor serum ferritin; supplemental iron is recommended if ferritin is <100mcg/L or serum transferrin saturation is <20%.

Patient Counseling: Inform risks/benefits of therapy, increased risks of mortality, serious CV events, thromboembolic events, stroke, tumor progression/recurrence, need to have regular laboratory tests for Hgb, and for cancer patients to sign the patient-physician acknowledgment form prior to therapy. Instruct to undergo regular BP monitoring, adhere to prescribed antihypertensive regimen, and follow recommended dietary restrictions. Advise to contact physician for new-onset neurologic symptoms or change in seizure frequency, and other possible side effects of therapy. Inform that risks are associated with benzyl alcohol in neonates, infants, pregnant women, and nursing mothers. Instruct on the importance of proper disposal and caution against reuse of needles, syringes, or drug product.

Administration: IV/SQ route. IV route recommended in hemodialysis patients. Do not dilute and do not mix with other solutions; refer to PI for admixing exceptions. **Storage:** 2-8°C (36-46°F). Do not freeze or shake. Protect from light. Discard unused portions of multidose vials 21 days after initial entry.

EPZICOM

abacavir sulfate - lamivudine (ViiV Healthcare)

> Lactic acidosis and severe hepatomegaly with steatosis, including fatal cases, reported with nucleoside analogues. Abacavir: Serious and sometimes fatal hypersensitivity reactions (multiorgan clinical syndrome) reported; d/c as soon as suspected and never restart therapy with any abacavir-containing product. Patients with HLA-B*5701 allele are at high risk for hypersensitivity; screen for HLA-B*5701 allele prior to therapy. Lamivudine: Severe acute exacerbations of hepatitis B reported in patients coinfected with hepatitis B virus (HBV) upon d/c of therapy; closely monitor hepatic function for at least several months. If appropriate, initiation of anti-hepatitis B therapy may be warranted.

THERAPEUTIC CLASS: Nucleoside reverse transcriptase inhibitor

INDICATIONS: Treatment of HIV-1 infection in combination with other antiretrovirals.

DOSAGE: *Adults:* CrCl ≥50mL/min: 1 tab qd.

HOW SUPPLIED: Tab: (Abacavir Sulfate-Lamivudine) 600mg-300mg

CONTRAINDICATIONS: Hepatic impairment.

WARNINGS/PRECAUTIONS: Obesity and prolonged nucleoside exposure may be risk factors for lactic acidosis and severe hepatomegaly with steatosis. Caution with known risk factors for liver disease; suspend therapy if clinical or laboratory findings suggestive of lactic acidosis or pronounced hepatotoxicity develop. Immune reconstitution syndrome reported. Autoimmune disorders (eg, Grave's disease, polymyositis, Guillain-Barre syndrome) reported to occur in the setting of immune reconstitution and can occur many months after initiation of treatment. Redistribution/accumulation of body fat may occur. Cross-resistance potential with nucleoside reverse transcriptase inhibitors reported. Not recommended with renal impairment (CrCl <50mL/min). Caution in elderly. Abacavir: Increased risk of myocardial infarction (MI) reported; consider the underlying risk of coronary heart disease when prescribing therapy. Lamivudine: Emergence of lamivudine-resistant HBV reported.

ADVERSE REACTIONS: Lactic acidosis, severe hepatomegaly with steatosis, hypersensitivity, insomnia, depression/depressed mood, headache/migraine, fatigue/malaise, dizziness/vertigo, nausea, diarrhea, rash, pyrexia.

INTERACTIONS: Avoid with other abacavir-, lamivudine-, and/or emtricitabine-containing products. Abacavir: Ethanol may decrease elimination causing an increase overall exposure. May increase PO methadone clearance. Lamivudine: Hepatic decompensation may occur in HIV-1/hepatitis C virus (HCV) coinfected patients receiving interferon-alfa with or without ribavirin; closely monitor for treatment-associated toxicities. Trimethoprim/sulfamethoxazole and nelfinavir may increase levels.

PREGNANCY: Category C, not for use in nursing.

MECHANISM OF ACTION: Abacavir: Carbocyclic nucleoside analogue; inhibits HIV-1 reverse transcriptase (RT) activity by competing with natural substrate dGTP and incorporating into viral DNA. Lamivudine: Nucleoside analogue; inhibits RT via DNA chain termination after incorporation of the nucleotide analogue.

PHARMACOKINETICS: Absorption: Rapid. Abacavir: Bioavailability (86%), C_{max}=4.26mcg/mL, AUC=11.95mcg•hr/mL. Lamivudine: Bioavailability (86%), C_{max}=2.04mcg/mL, AUC=8.87mcg•hr/mL. **Distribution:** Abacavir: V_d=0.86L/kg; plasma protein binding (50%). Lamivudine: V_d=1.3L/kg; found in breast milk. **Metabolism:** Abacavir: Via alcohol dehydrogenase and glucuronyl transferase; 5'-carboxylic acid, 5'-glucuronide (metabolites). Lamivudine: Trans-sulfoxide (metabolite). **Elimination:** Abacavir: $T_{1/2}$=1.45 hrs. Lamivudine: Urine (70%, unchanged) (IV); $T_{1/2}$=5-7 hrs.

NURSING CONSIDERATIONS

Assessment: Assess medical history for prior exposure to any abacavir-containing product. Assess for HBV infection, history of hypersensitivity reactions, HLA-B*5701 status, hepatic/renal impairment, risk factors for coronary heart disease and lactic acidosis, pregnancy/nursing status, and possible drug interactions.

Monitoring: Monitor for signs/symptoms of hypersensitivity reactions, lactic acidosis, hepatomegaly with steatosis, immune reconstitution syndrome (eg, opportunistic infections), autoimmune disorders, fat redistribution/accumulation, and MI. Monitor hepatic and renal function. Closely monitor hepatic function for several months after d/c of therapy.

Patient Counseling: Inform patients regarding hypersensitivity reactions with abacavir; instruct to contact physician immediately if symptoms develop and not to restart or replace with any other abacavir-containing products without medical consultation. Inform that the drug may cause a rare but serious condition called lactic acidosis with liver enlargement (hepatomegaly). Inform patients coinfected with HIV-1 and HBV that deterioration of liver disease has occurred in some cases when treatment with lamivudine was d/c; instruct to discuss any changes of regimen with the physician. Inform that hepatic decompensation has occurred in HIV-1/HCV coinfected patients with interferon alfa with or without ribavirin. Inform that redistribution/accumulation of body fat may occur. Advise that drug is not a cure for HIV-1 infection and that illnesses associated with HIV-1 may still be experienced. Advise to avoid doing things that can spread HIV-1 to others (eg, sharing needles/inj equipment/personal items that can have blood or body fluids on them, having sex without protection, breastfeeding). Inform patients to take all HIV medications exactly as prescribed.

Administration: Oral route. **Storage:** 25°C (77°F); excursions permitted to 15-30°C (59-86°F).

EQUETRO   RX

carbamazepine (Validus)

Serious and fatal dermatologic reactions, including toxic epidermal necrolysis (TEN) and Stevens-Johnson syndrome (SJS) reported. Increased risk with presence of HLA-B*1502 allele; screen at risk patients prior to initiating treatment. Aplastic anemia and agranulocytosis reported; obtain complete pretreatment hematological testing as a baseline. Consider d/c if evidence of bone marrow depression develops.

THERAPEUTIC CLASS: Carboxamide

INDICATIONS: Treatment of acute manic and mixed episodes associated with bipolar I disorder.

DOSAGE: *Adults:* Initial: 400mg/day in divided doses, bid. Titrate: Adjust in increments of 200mg/day. Max: 1600mg/day.

HOW SUPPLIED: Cap, Extended-Release: 100mg, 200mg, 300mg

CONTRAINDICATIONS: History of previous bone marrow depression, MAOI use within 14 days, hypersensitivity to TCAs (eg, amitriptyline, desipramine, imipramine, protriptyline, and nortriptyline), coadministration with nefazodone.

WARNINGS/PRECAUTIONS: Increased risk of suicidal thoughts or behavior reported. Avoid abrupt d/c in patients with seizure disorder to avoid precipitating status epilepticus. Mild anticholinergic activity may occur; closely observe patients with increased intraocular pressure (IOP) during therapy. D/C at first sign of rash, unless rash is clearly not drug-related. Caution in patients with history of cardiac/hepatic/renal damage or interrupted courses of therapy with carbamazepine. May activate latent psychosis, and cause confusion/agitation in elderly. May impair physical/mental abilities. May cause fetal harm.

ADVERSE REACTIONS: Dizziness, somnolence, N/V, agranulocytosis, headache, infection, pain, rash, diarrhea, dyspepsia, asthenia, aplastic anemia, amnesia, TEN, SJS.

INTERACTIONS: See Contraindications. CYP3A4 and/or epoxide hydrolase inhibitors (eg, acetazolamide, azole antifungals, cimetidine, clarithromycin, protease inhibitors) may increase plasma levels. CYP3A4 inducers (eg, cisplatin, phenobarbital, rifampin) may decrease plasma levels. May decrease levels of trazodone, CYP1A2 substrates and CYP3A4 substrates (eg, acetaminophen, bupropion, clonazepam, doxycycline, oral contraceptives). May increase plasma levels of clomipramine HCl and primidone. May increase/decrease phenytoin plasma levels. Breakthrough bleeding reported with oral contraceptives. May reduce anticoagulant effect of warfarin. Increased risk of neurotoxic side effects reported with lithium. May reduce thyroid function with other anticonvulsants. Antimalarial drugs (eg, chloroquine, mefloquine) may antagonize carbamazepine activity. Caution with other centrally acting drugs and alcohol. Coadministration with delavirdine may lead to loss of virologic response and possible resistance to Rescriptor or to the class of non-nucleoside reverse transcriptase inhibitors.

PREGNANCY: Category D, not for use in nursing.

MECHANISM OF ACTION: Carboxamide; mechanism has not been established. Modulates sodium and calcium ion channels, receptor-mediated neurotransmitters, and intracellular signaling pathways.

PHARMACOKINETICS: Absorption: C_{max}=1.9mcg/mL (single 200mg dose), 11mcg/mL (multiple 800mg dose), 3.2mcg/mL (400mg dose, fasted), 4.3mcg/mL (400mg dose, fed); T_{max}=19 hrs (single 200mg dose), 5.9 hrs (multiple 800mg dose), 24 hrs (400mg dose, fasted), 14 hrs (400mg dose, fed). **Distribution:** Plasma protein binding (76%); crosses placenta; found in breast milk. **Metabolism:** Liver via CYP3A4; carbamazepine-10,11-epoxide (metabolite). **Elimination:** Urine (72%; 3% unchanged), feces (28%); $T_{1/2}$=35-40 hrs (single dose), 12-17 hrs (multiple doses).

NURSING CONSIDERATIONS

Assessment: Assess for history of cardiac/hepatic/renal damage, increased IOP, previous hematological reaction to other medications, bone marrow depression, hypersensitivity to TCAs, seizure disorders, depression, pregnancy/nursing status, and possible drug interactions. Assess renal function, presence of HLA-B*1502, CBC, reticulocyte count, serum iron levels, LFTs, urinalysis, BUN, and eye exam. Perform detailed history and physical examination.

Monitoring: Monitor for signs/symptoms of dermatological reactions, aplastic anemia, agranulocytosis, suicidal behavior/ideation, depression, mood changes, latent psychosis, bone marrow depression, and confusion/agitation in elderly. Periodically monitor CBC (including reticulocytes), serum iron levels, LFTs, urinalysis, BUN, total cholesterol levels, LDL/HDL levels, thyroid function tests, and serum drug levels. Perform periodic eye exams (eg, slitlamp examination, funduscopy, and tonometry).

Patient Counseling: Inform to take drug as prescribed and to read Medication Guide. Instruct to immediately report signs/symptoms of hematologic disorders (eg, fever, sore throat, rash, mouth ulcers, easy bruising, petechial or purpuric hemorrhage). Advise that drug may increase risk of suicidal thoughts/behavior, and to notify physician if new/worsening depression, unusual behavior/mood changes, suicidal thoughts/behavior, or thoughts of self-harm develop. Inform that drug may cause dizziness and drowsiness, and to observe caution when operating machinery/automobiles or potentially dangerous tasks. Advise to report all medications or herbal products currently being taken. Counsel to avoid alcohol and other sedatives. Instruct not to crush or chew caps; if necessary, caps may be opened and contents sprinkled over food. Advise to notify physician if pregnant or planning to get pregnant; encourage patients to enroll in the North American Antiepileptic Drug (NAAED) Pregnancy Registry.

Administration: Oral route. **Storage:** 25°C (77°F); excursions permitted to 15-30°C (59-86°F). Protect from light and moisture.

ERAXIS   RX
anidulafungin (Pfizer)

THERAPEUTIC CLASS: Echinocandin

INDICATIONS: Treatment of candidemia, and other forms of *Candida* infections (intra-abdominal abscess and peritonitis), esophageal candidiasis.

DOSAGE: *Adults:* Give by IV infusion of ≤1.1mg/min. Candidemia/Other *Candida* Infections (Intra-Abdominal Abscess, and Peritonitis): Usual: 200mg LD on Day 1, followed by 100mg/day dose thereafter. Continue for at least 14 days after last positive culture. Esophageal Candidiasis: Usual: 100mg LD on Day 1, followed by 50mg/day dose thereafter. Treat for a minimum of 14 days and for at least 7 days following resolution of symptoms. Consider suppressive antifungal therapy after a course of treatment in patients with HIV infections due to risk of relapse.

HOW SUPPLIED: Inj: 50mg, 100mg

WARNINGS/PRECAUTIONS: Not for IV bolus inj. LFTs abnormalities reported; monitor for worsening of hepatic function and evaluate for risk/benefit of continuing therapy. Isolated cases of significant hepatic dysfunction, hepatitis, or hepatic failure reported.

ADVERSE REACTIONS: Diarrhea, hypokalemia.

INTERACTIONS: Significant hepatic abnormalities reported with multiple concomitant medications in patients with serious underlying medical conditions. Slight increased levels with cyclosporine.

PREGNANCY: Category C, caution in nursing.

MECHANISM OF ACTION: Echinocandin; inhibits glucan synthase which results in inhibition of the formation of 1,3-β-D-glucan, an essential component of fungal cell walls.

PHARMACOKINETICS: Absorption: Administration of variable doses resulted in different parameters. **Distribution:** V_d=30-50L; plasma protein binding (>99%). **Elimination:** Urine (<1%), feces (30%, <10% intact drug); $T_{1/2}$=40-50 hrs.

NURSING CONSIDERATIONS

Assessment: Assess for hypersensitivity to the drug or other echinocandins, serious underlying medical conditions, hepatic function, pregnancy/nursing status, and possible drug interactions. Obtain specimens for fungal culture and other relevant laboratory studies (eg, histopathology) prior to therapy.

Monitoring: Monitor for hepatic dysfunction, hepatitis or hepatic failure, and other adverse reactions. Monitor LFTs.

Patient Counseling: Counsel about the risks and benefits of therapy.

Administration: IV route. Refer to PI for preparation for administration. **Storage:** 2-8°C (36-46°F). Do not freeze. Reconstituted: Stable for up to 1 hr. Infusion Sol: Administer within 24 hrs of preparation.

ERBITUX

RX

cetuximab (Bristol-Myers Squibb)

THERAPEUTIC CLASS: Epidermal growth factor receptor (EGFR) antagonist

INDICATIONS: In combination with radiation therapy for the initial treatment of locally/regionally advanced SCCHN. In combination with platinum-based therapy with 5-FU for the first-line treatment of recurrent locoregional disease/metastatic SCCHN. As monotherapy for treatment of recurrent/metastatic SCCHN for whom prior platinum-based therapy has failed. In combination with irinotecan for treatment of EGFR-expressing metastatic colorectal cancer in patients who are refractory to irinotecan-based chemotherapy. As monotherapy for EGFR-expressing metastatic colorectal cancer in patients who are intolerant to irinotecan-based regimens or after failure of both irinotecan- and oxaliplatin-based regimens.

DOSAGE: *Adults:* Premedication: H$_1$-antagonist (eg, 50mg diphenhydramine) IV 30-60 min prior to 1st dose. Premedicate for subsequent doses based on clinical judgment and presence/severity of prior infusion reactions. Max Infusion Rate: 10mg/min. SCCHN (With Radiation Therapy/Platinum-Based Therapy with 5-FU): Initial: 400mg/m² IV over 120 min, 1 week prior to initiation of a course of radiation therapy or on the day of initiation of platinum-based therapy with 5-FU. Complete administration 1 hr prior to platinum-based therapy with 5-FU. Maint: 250mg/m² IV over 60 min weekly for duration of radiation therapy (6-7 weeks) or until disease progression or unacceptable toxicity with platinum-based therapy with 5-FU. Complete administration 1 hr prior to radiation therapy/platinum-based therapy with 5-FU. SCCHN (Monotherapy)/Colorectal Cancer (Monotherapy/With Irinotecan): Initial: 400mg/m² IV over 120 min. Maint: 250mg/m² IV over 60 min weekly until disease progression or unacceptable toxicity. Dose Modifications due to Infusion Reactions/Dermatologic Toxicity: Refer to PI.

HOW SUPPLIED: Inj: 2mg/mL [50mL, 100mL]

WARNINGS/PRECAUTIONS: Not recommended for colorectal cancer treatment with KRAS mutations in codon 12 or 13. Caution when used in combination with radiation therapy or platinum-based therapy with 5-FU in head and neck cancer patients with history of coronary artery disease (CAD), congestive heart failure (CHF), or arrhythmias. Interstitial lung disease (ILD) reported; interrupt for acute onset or worsening of pulmonary symptoms and permanently d/c if ILD is confirmed. Dermatologic toxicities (eg, acneiform rash, skin drying/fissuring, paronychial inflammation, infectious sequelae, hypertrichosis) may occur; limit sun exposure during therapy. Hypomagnesemia and electrolyte abnormalities may occur; replete electrolytes as necessary.

ADVERSE REACTIONS: Cutaneous reactions (eg, rash, pruritus, nail changes), headache, diarrhea, infection, infusion reactions, cardiopulmonary arrest, dermatologic toxicity, radiation dermatitis, sepsis, renal failure, ILD, pulmonary embolus.

INTERACTIONS: Serious cardiotoxicity and death observed with radiation therapy and cisplatin with locally advanced SCCHN.

PREGNANCY: Category C, not for use in nursing.

MECHANISM OF ACTION: Epidermal growth factor receptor antagonist (human/mouse chimeric monoclonal antibody); binds specifically to EGFR on both normal and tumor cells and competitively inhibits the binding of epidermal growth factor and other ligands, such as transforming growth factor-α.

PHARMACOKINETICS: Absorption: C$_{max}$=168-235mcg/mL. **Distribution:** V$_d$=2-3L/m²; may cross the placenta. **Elimination:** T$_{1/2}$=112 hrs.

NURSING CONSIDERATIONS

Assessment: Assess for history of CAD, CHF, arrhythmias, pulmonary disorders, and colorectal cancer with mutations. Assess pregnancy/nursing status and possible drug interactions. Obtain baseline serum electrolyte levels (magnesium, K⁺, calcium).

Monitoring: Closely monitor electrolytes (magnesium, K⁺, calcium) during and after drug administration. Periodically monitor for hypomagnesemia, hypocalcemia, and hypokalemia during and for at least 8 weeks after therapy. Monitor for signs/symptoms of acute onset or worsening of pulmonary symptoms, infusion reactions, dermatologic toxicities, and infectious sequelae. Monitor patients for 1 hr after infusion, and for a longer period to confirm resolution of the event in patients requiring treatment for infusion reactions.

Patient Counseling: Advise to report signs and symptoms of infusion reactions (eg, fever, chills, or breathing problems). Inform of pregnancy/nursing risks; advise to use effective contraceptive methods during and for 6 months after therapy for both sexes. Inform that nursing is not recommended during and for 2 months following therapy. Instruct to limit sun exposure (eg, use of sunscreen) during and for 2 months after therapy.

Administration: IV route. Do not administer as IV push or bolus. Administer via infusion pump or syringe pump. Administer through low protein binding 0.22-μm in-line filter. Do not shake or dilute. **Storage:** Vials: 2-8°C (36-46°F). Do not freeze. Infusion Containers: Stable for up to 12 hrs at 2-8°C (36-46°F) and up to 8 hrs at 20-25°C (68-77°F). Discard unused portion of vial.

ERTACZO   RX
sertaconazole nitrate (Ortho-McNeil/Janssen)

THERAPEUTIC CLASS: Azole antifungal

INDICATIONS: Treatment of interdigital tinea pedis in immunocompetent patients ≥12 yrs caused by *Trichophyton rubrum*, *Trichophyton mentagrophytes*, and *Epidermophyton floccosum*.

DOSAGE: *Adults:* Apply to the affected areas between the toes and adjacent areas bid for 4 weeks. Reevaluate if no clinical improvement is seen 2 weeks after the treatment period. *Pediatrics:* ≥12 yrs: Apply to the affected areas between the toes and adjacent areas bid for 4 weeks. Reevaluate if no clinical improvement is seen 2 weeks after the treatment period.

HOW SUPPLIED: Cre: 2% [30g, 60g]

WARNINGS/PRECAUTIONS: Not for ophthalmic, PO, or intravaginal use. D/C and institute appropriate therapy if irritation or sensitivity occurs. Caution in patients sensitive to other imidazole antifungals; cross-reactivity may occur.

ADVERSE REACTIONS: Contact dermatitis, dry skin, burning skin, application-site reaction, skin tenderness, erythema, pruritus, vesiculation, desquamation, hyperpigmentation.

PREGNANCY: Category C, caution in nursing.

MECHANISM OF ACTION: Azole antifungal; not established. Suspected to act primarily by inhibiting CYP450-dependent synthesis of ergosterol, a key component of fungi cell membranes. Lack of ergosterol leads to fungal cell injury through leakage of key constituents in cytoplasm from cell.

NURSING CONSIDERATIONS

Assessment: Assess for hypersensitivity to imidazoles and pregnancy/nursing status. Perform direct microscopic examination of infected superficial epidermal tissue in a sol of potassium hydroxide or by culture on an appropriate medium to confirm diagnosis of the disease.

Monitoring: Monitor for signs/symptoms of skin irritation or sensitivity and other adverse reactions. Monitor for signs of clinical response.

Patient Counseling: Instruct to use the medication ud. Instruct to dry affected area before application and to avoid contact with eyes, mouth, or other mucous membranes. Instruct to wash hands after applying medication and to avoid occlusive dressings on treated site unless directed. Instruct to use medication for fully prescribed treatment time, even if symptoms improve. Advise to contact physician if no clinical improvement or if condition worsens or if signs of irritation, redness, itching, burning, blistering, swelling, or oozing develop from application site. Advise not to use for any disorder other than that for which it was prescribed.

Administration: Topical route. **Storage:** 25°C (77°F); excursions permitted to 15-30°C (59-86°F).

ERY-TAB   RX
erythromycin (Abbott)

THERAPEUTIC CLASS: Macrolide

INDICATIONS: Treatment of mild to moderate upper/lower respiratory tract and skin and skin structure infections, listeriosis, pertussis, diphtheria, erythrasma, intestinal amebiasis, acute pelvic inflammatory disease (PID) (*Neisseria gonorrhoeae*), primary syphilis (if penicillin [PCN] allergy), Legionnaires' disease, chlamydial infections (eg, newborn conjunctivitis, pneumonia of infancy, urogenital infections during pregnancy, or urethral, endocervical, or rectal infections when tetracyclines are contraindicated or not tolerated), and nongonococcal urethritis caused by susceptible strains of microorganisms. Prophylaxis of initial and recurrent attacks of rheumatic fever if PCN allergy.

DOSAGE: *Adults:* Usual: 250mg qid, 333mg q8h or 500mg q12h. Max: 4g/day. Do not take bid when dose is >1g/day. Treat strep infections for at least 10 days. Streptococcal Infection Long-Term Prophylaxis with Rheumatic Fever: 250mg bid. Chlamydial Urogenital Infection During Pregnancy: 500mg qid or 666mg q8h for at least 7 days, or 500mg q12h, 333mg q8h, or 250mg qid for at least 14 days. Urethral/Endocervical/Rectal Chlamydial Infections and Nongonococcal Urethritis: 500mg qid or 666mg q8h for at least 7 days. Primary Syphilis: 30-

40g in divided doses for 10-15 days. Acute PID: 500mg (erythromycin lactobionate) IV q6h for 3 days, then 500mg PO q12h or 333mg q8h for 7 days. Intestinal Amebiasis: 500mg q12h, 333mg q8h, or 250mg q6h for 10-14 days. Pertussis: 40-50mg/kg/day in divided doses for 5-14 days. Legionnaires' disease: 1-4g/day in divided doses.

Pediatrics: Usual: 30-50mg/kg/day in divided doses. Severe Infections: May double dose. Max: 4g/day. Treat strep infections for at least 10 days. Streptococcal Infection Long-Term Prophylaxis with Rheumatic Fever: 250mg bid. Chlamydial Conjunctivitis of Newborns/Chlamydial Pneumonia in Infancy: 12.5mg/kg qid for 2 weeks and 3 weeks, respectively. Intestinal Amebiasis: 30-50mg/kg/day in divided doses for 10-14 days.

HOW SUPPLIED: Tab, Delayed-Release: 250mg, 333mg, 500mg

CONTRAINDICATIONS: Concomitant terfenadine, astemizole, pimozide, or cisapride.

WARNINGS/PRECAUTIONS: Pseudomembranous colitis and hepatic dysfunction reported. Caution with impaired hepatic function. May result in bacterial resistance with prolonged use or use in the absence of a proven/suspected bacterial infection or a prophylactic indication; take appropriate measures if superinfection develops. May aggravate weakness of patients with myasthenia gravis. Erythromycin does not reach adequate concentrations in fetus to prevent congenital syphilis.

ADVERSE REACTIONS: N/V, abdominal pain, diarrhea, anorexia, abnormal LFTs, allergic reactions, superinfection (prolonged use).

INTERACTIONS: See Contraindications. Rhabdomyolysis reported with lovastatin. May increase levels of theophylline, digoxin, drugs metabolized by CYP450 (eg, carbamazepine, cyclosporine, phenytoin, alfentanil, disopyramide, lovastatin, bromocriptine, valproate, etc). Increases effects of oral anticoagulants, triazolam, midazolam. Risk of acute ergot toxicity with ergotamine or dihydroergotamine. May increase Aarea under the curve of sildenafil; consider dose reduction of sildenafil.

PREGNANCY: Category B, caution in nursing.

MECHANISM OF ACTION: Macrolide antibiotic; inhibits protein synthesis by binding 50S ribosomal subunits of susceptible organisms.

PHARMACOKINETICS: Absorption: (PO) Readily absorbed. **Distribution:** Largely bound to plasma proteins. Crosses blood-brain barrier, placenta, and breast milk. Diffuses into most bodily fluids. **Elimination:** Biliary and urinary excretion (<5%).

NURSING CONSIDERATIONS

Assessment: Assess age of patient, conditions such as myasthenia gravis, arrhythmias and hepatic/renal function. Note other diseases/conditions and drug therapies.

Monitoring: Monitor LFTs, renal function, *Clostridium difficile*-associated diarrhea, superinfection, pancreatitis, arrhythmias, and hypersensitivity reactions.

Patient Counseling: Instruct to take exactly as directed; skipping doses or not completing full course may decrease effectiveness and increase bacterial resistance. Instruct to take on empty stomach. Advise to report any adverse effects, lack of response, and prolonged/persistent diarrhea.

Administration: Oral route. **Storage:** 30°C (86°F).

ESTRACE   RX
estradiol (Warner Chilcott)

> Estrogens increase the risk of endometrial cancer. Perform adequate diagnostic measures, including endometrial sampling, to rule out malignancy with undiagnosed persistent or recurrent abnormal vaginal bleeding. Should not be used for the prevention of cardiovascular disease (CVD). Increased risks of myocardial infarction (MI), stroke, invasive breast cancer, pulmonary embolism (PE), and deep vein thrombosis (DVT) in postmenopausal women (50-79 yrs of age) reported. Increased risk of developing probable dementia in postmenopausal women ≥65 yrs of age reported. Should be prescribed at the lowest effective dose and for the shortest duration consistent with treatment goals and risks.

THERAPEUTIC CLASS: Estrogen

INDICATIONS: (Cre/Tab) Treatment of vulvar and vaginal atrophy associated with menopause. (Tab) Treatment of moderate to severe vasomotor symptoms associated with menopause. Treatment of hypoestrogenism due to hypogonadism, castration, or primary ovarian failure. Palliative treatment of metastatic breast cancer and advanced androgen-dependent prostate carcinoma. Prevention of osteoporosis.

DOSAGE: *Adults:* (Cre) Vulvar or Vaginal Atrophy: Initial: 2-4g/day for 1-2 weeks, then gradually decrease to 1/2 initial dose for 1-2 weeks. Maint: 1g 1-3X/week. D/C or taper at 3-6 month intervals. (Tab) Vulvar or Vaginal Atrophy/Vasomotor Symptoms: Initial: 1-2mg/day. Titrate: Adjust PRN to control presenting symptoms. Maint: Minimum effective dose. D/C or taper at 3-6 month intervals. Administer cyclically (eg, 3 weeks on and 1 week off). Hypoestrogenism: Initial:

1-2mg/day. Titrate: Adjust PRN to control presenting symptoms. Maint: Minimum effective dose. Metastatic Breast Cancer: Usual: 10mg tid for at least 3 months. Prostate Carcinoma: Usual: 1-2mg tid. Osteoporosis Prevention: Use lowest effective dose. Reevaluate treatment need periodically (eg, 3-6 month intervals).

HOW SUPPLIED: Cre: 0.1mg/g [42.5g]; Tab: 0.5mg*, 1mg*, 2mg* *scored

CONTRAINDICATIONS: Undiagnosed abnormal genital bleeding, known/suspected/history of breast cancer unless being treated for metastatic disease, known/suspected estrogen-dependent neoplasia, active/history of DVT/PE, active or recent arterial thromboembolic disease (eg, stroke, MI), liver dysfunction or disease, known/suspected pregnancy.

WARNINGS/PRECAUTIONS: Increased risk of CV events; d/c immediately if these occur or are suspected. Caution in patients with risk factors for aterial vascular disease (eg, HTN, diabetes mellitus [DM], tobacco use, hypercholesterolemia, obesity) and/or venous thromboembolism (VTE) (eg, personal/family history of VTE, obesity, systemic lupus erythematosus [SLE]). If feasible, d/c at least 4 to 6 weeks before surgery of the type associated with an increased risk of thromboembolism, or during periods of prolonged immobilization. May increase the risk of gallbladder disease. May lead to severe hypercalcemia in patients with breast cancer and bone metastases; d/c and take appropriate measures if hypercalcemia occurs. Retinal vascular thrombosis reported; d/c pending examination if sudden partial or complete loss of vision, sudden onset of proptosis, diplopia, or migraine occurs, or if examination reveals papilledema or retinal vascular lesions, d/c therapy permanently. Consider addition of a progestin if no hysterectomy. May elevate BP, thyroid-binding globulin levels, and plasma TG leading to pancreatitis and other complications. Caution with history of cholestatic jaundice; d/c in case of recurrence. May cause fluid retention; caution with cardiac/renal dysfunction. Caution with severe hypocalcemia. May increase risk of ovarian cancer. May exacerbate endometriosis, asthma, DM, epilepsy, migraine or porphyria, SLE, and hepatic hemangiomas; use with caution. May affect certain endocrine, LFTs, and blood components in laboratory tests. (Tab) 2mg tab contains tartrazine which may cause allergic-type reactions.

ADVERSE REACTIONS: Altered vaginal bleeding, vaginal candidiasis, breast tenderness/enlargement, galactorrhea, N/V, thrombophlebitis, melasma, abdominal cramps, headache, mental depression, weight changes, edema, altered libido.

INTERACTIONS: CYP3A4 inducers (eg, St. John's wort, phenobarbital, carbamazepine, rifampin) may decrease levels, which may decrease therapeutic effects and/or change uterine bleeding profile. CYP3A4 inhibitors (eg, erythromycin, clarithromycin, ketoconazole, itraconazole, ritonavir, grapefruit juice) may increase levels, which may result in side effects. Patients on thyroid replacement therapy may require higher doses of thyroid hormone.

PREGNANCY: (Cre) Contraindicated in pregnancy, (Tab) Category X; caution in nursing.

MECHANISM OF ACTION: Estrogen; binds to nuclear receptors in estrogen-responsive tissue. Circulating estrogens modulates pituitary secretion of gonadotropins, luteinizing hormone and follicle stimulating hormone, through a negative feedback mechanism. Reduces elevated levels of these hormones in postmenopausal women.

PHARMACOKINETICS: Absorption: (Cre) Absorbed through skin, mucous membranes, and GI tract. **Distribution:** Largely bound to sex hormone-binding globulin and albumin; found in breast milk. **Metabolism:** Liver to estrone (metabolite), estriol (major urinary metabolite); sulfate and glucuronide conjugation (liver); gut hydrolysis; CYP3A4 (partial metabolism). **Elimination:** Urine.

NURSING CONSIDERATIONS

Assessment: Assess for abnormal genital bleeding, presence or history of breast cancer, estrogen-dependent neoplasias, DVT, PE, active or recent (within past yr) arterial thromboembolic disease, pregnancy/nursing status, and any other conditions where treatment may be contraindicated or cautioned. Assess use in women ≥65 yrs, and those with DM, asthma, epilepsy, migraines or porphyria, SLE, and hepatic hemangiomas. Assess for possible drug interactions. Assess need for progestin therapy in women who have not had a hysterectomy.

Monitoring: Monitor for signs/symptoms of CV disorders, malignant neoplasms, dementia, gallbladder disease, hypercalcemia, visual abnormalities, increased BP, hypertriglyceridemia, hypothyroidism, fluid retention, cholestatic jaundice, exacerbation of endometriosis, and other conditions. Perform annual mammography, regular monitoring of BP, and periodic evaluation (q3-6 months) to determine need of therapy. Monitor thyroid function if patient is on thyroid hormone replacement therapy. In cases of undiagnosed, persistent, or recurrent vaginal bleeding in women with a uterus, perform adequate diagnostic measures (eg, endometrial sampling) to rule out malignancies.

Patient Counseling: Inform that therapy may increase the risk for uterine cancer, heart attack, stroke, breast cancer, and blood clots. Instruct to contact physician if breast lumps, unusual vaginal bleeding, dizziness or faintness, changes in speech, severe headaches, chest pain, SOB, leg pain, visual changes, or vomiting occur. Advise to have yearly breast examinations by a healthcare provider and perform monthly breast self-examinations.

Administration: (Cre) Intravaginal route. (Tab) Oral route. **Storage:** (Cre) Room temperature. Protect from temperatures in excess of 40°C (104°F). (Tab) 20-25°C (68-77°F).

ESTRADERM   RX

estradiol (Novartis)

Estrogens increase the risk of endometrial cancer. Perform adequate diagnostic measures, including endometrial sampling, to rule out malignancy with undiagnosed persistent or recurrent abnormal vaginal bleeding. Should not be used for the prevention of cardiovascular disease (CVD) or dementia. Increased risk of myocardial infarction (MI), stroke, invasive breast cancer, pulmonary emboli (PE), and deep vein thrombosis (DVT) in postmenopausal women (50-79 yrs of age) reported. Increased risk of developing probable dementia in postmenopausal women ≥65 yrs of age reported. Should be prescribed at the lowest effective dose and for the shortest duration consistent with treatment goals and risks.

THERAPEUTIC CLASS: Estrogen

INDICATIONS: Treatment of moderate to severe vasomotor symptoms and vulvar/vaginal atrophy associated with menopause. Treatment of hypoestrogenism due to hypogonadism, castration, or primary ovarian failure. Prevention of postmenopausal osteoporosis.

DOSAGE: *Adults:* Vasomotor Symptoms/Vulvar/Vaginal Atrophy: Apply 0.05mg/day 2X weekly. Osteoporosis Prevention: Initial: 0.05mg/day as soon as possible after menopause and adjust dose if necessary. Currently Taking Oral Estrogen: Initiate 1 week after d/c oral hormonal therapy, or sooner if menopausal symptoms reappear in <1 week. May give continuously in patients with no intact uterus or cyclically (3 weeks on, 1 week off) with intact uterus. Reevaluate treatment need periodically (eg, 3-6 months interval).

HOW SUPPLIED: Patch: 0.05mg/day, 0.1mg/day [8s]

CONTRAINDICATIONS: Undiagnosed abnormal genital bleeding, known/suspected/history of breast cancer, known/suspected estrogen-dependent neoplasia, active or history of DVT/PE, active or recent arterial thromboembolic disease (eg, stroke, MI), liver dysfunction or disease, known/suspected pregnancy.

WARNINGS/PRECAUTIONS: D/C immediately if stroke, DVT, PE, or MI occur or are suspected. Caution in patients with risk factors for arterial vascular disease (eg, HTN, diabetes mellitus [DM], tobacco use, hypercholesterolemia, obesity) and/or venous thromboembolism (VTE) (eg, personal history or family history of VTE, obesity, systemic lupus erythematosus [SLE]). If feasible, d/c at least 4 to 6 weeks before surgery of the type associated with an increased risk of thromboembolism, or during periods of prolonged immobilization. May increase risk of breast/ovarian cancer and gallbladder disease. Unopposed estrogens in women with intact uterus has been associated with an increased risk of endometrial cancer. May lead to severe hypercalcemia in patients with breast cancer and bone metastases; d/c and take appropriate measures if hypercalcemia occurs. Retinal vascular thrombosis reported; if sudden partial or complete loss of vision, sudden onset of proptosis, diplopia, migraine occurs, d/c pending examination. If examinations reveal papilledema or retinal vascular lesions, d/c permanently. Consider addition of a progestin if no hysterectomy. May elevate BP, thyroid-binding globulin levels, and plasma TG leading to pancreatitis and other complications. Caution with history of cholestatic jaundice; d/c in case of recurrence. May cause fluid retention; caution with cardiac/renal dysfunction. Caution with impaired liver function and severe hypocalcemia. May exacerbate endometriosis, asthma, DM, epilepsy, migraine, porphyria, SLE, and hepatic hemangiomas; use with caution. May affect certain endocrine and blood components in laboratory tests.

ADVERSE REACTIONS: Altered vaginal bleeding, vaginal candidiasis, breast tenderness/enlargement, N/V, chloasma, melasma, weight changes, VTE, pulmonary embolism, MI, stroke, application-site redness/irritation.

INTERACTIONS: CYP3A4 inducers (eg, St. John's wort, phenobarbital, carbamazepine, rifampin) may decrease levels, which may decrease therapeutic effects and/or changes in uterine bleeding profile. CYP3A4 inhibitors (eg, erythromycin, clarithromycin, ketoconazole, itraconazole, ritonavir, grapefruit juice) may increase levels, which may result in side effects. Patients concomitantly receiving thyroid hormone replacement therapy and estrogens may require increased doses of their thyroid replacement therapy.

PREGNANCY: Contraindicated in pregnancy, caution in nursing.

MECHANISM OF ACTION: Estrogen; binds to nuclear receptors in estrogen-responsive tissues. Circulating estrogen modulates pituitary secretion of gonadotropins, luteinizing hormone and follicle-stimulating hormone, through negative feedback mechanism. Reduces elevated levels of these hormones in postmenopausal women.

PHARMACOKINETICS: Distribution: Largely bound to sex hormone-binding globulin and albumin; found in breast milk. **Metabolism:** Liver to estrone (metabolite); estriol (major urinary metabolite); sulfate and glucuronide conjugation (liver), gut hydrolysis; CYP3A4 (partial metabolism). **Elimination:** Urine (parent compound and metabolites); $T_{1/2}$=1 hr.

NURSING CONSIDERATIONS

Assessment: Assess for undiagnosed abnormal genital bleeding, presence/history of breast cancer, estrogen-dependent neoplasia, active or history of DVT/PE, active or recent (within past yr) arterial thromboembolic disease, liver dysfunction/disease, known/suspected pregnancy, and any other conditions where treatment is contraindicated or cautioned. Assess use in women ≥65 yrs, nursing patients, and those with hypertriglyceridemia, hypothyroidism, DM, asthma, epilepsy, migraine or porphyria, SLE, and hepatic hemangiomas. Assess for possible drug interactions. Assess need for progestin therapy in women who have not had a hysterectomy.

Monitoring: Monitor for signs/symptoms of CVD, malignant neoplasms, dementia, gallbladder disease, hypercalcemia, visual abnormalities, hypertriglyceridemia, pancreatitis, hypothyroidism, fluid retention, cholestatic jaundice, exacerbation of endometriosis and other conditions. Perform annual mammography, regular monitoring of BP, and periodic evaluation (q3-6 months) to determine need of therapy. Monitor thyroid function in patients on thyroid replacement therapy. In case of undiagnosed, persistent, or recurrent vaginal bleeding in women with uterus, perform adequate diagnostic testing measures (eg, endometrial sampling) to rule out malignancy.

Patient Counseling: Inform that therapy may increase the risk for uterine cancer and may increase changes of getting a heart attack, stroke, breast cancer, blood clots, and dementia. Instruct to report to physician any breast lumps, unusual vaginal bleeding, dizziness and faintness, changes in speech, severe headaches, chest pain, SOB, leg pains, changes in vision, or vomiting. Advise to notify physician if pregnant or nursing. Instruct to have annual breast examination by a physician and perform monthly breast self examination. Instruct to place medication system on clean, dry skin on the trunk (including buttocks and abdomen); site should not be exposed to sunlight; area should not be oily, damaged, or irritated; and should not be applied on breasts or waistline. Counsel to rotate application sites with an interval of 1 week, and to apply immediately after opening pouch. Inform that if medication system falls off, reapply same system or apply new system PRN and continue with original treatment schedule.

Administration: Transdermal route. Apply immediately upon removal from the protective pouch. Refer to PI for application instructions. **Storage:** Do not store above 30°C (86°F). Do not store unpouched.

ESTRASORB   RX
estradiol (Graceway)

Estrogens increase the risk of endometrial cancer. Perform adequate diagnostic measures, including endometrial sampling, to rule out malignancy with undiagnosed persistent or recurring abnormal vaginal bleeding. Should not be used for the prevention of cardiovascular disease or dementia. Increased risks of myocardial infarction (MI), stroke, invasive breast cancer, pulmonary emboli (PE), and deep vein thrombosis (DVT) in postmenopausal women (50-79 yrs of age) reported. Increased risk of developing probable dementia in postmenopausal women ≥65 yrs of age reported. Estrogens, with or without progestins, should be prescribed at the lowest effective dose and for the shortest duration consistent with treatment goals and risks.

THERAPEUTIC CLASS: Estrogen

INDICATIONS: Treatment of moderate to severe vasomotor symptoms associated with menopause.

DOSAGE: *Adults:* Apply 2 pouches (0.05 mg/day) qam. Apply 1 pouch to each leg from the upper thigh to the calf. Rub in for 3 min until thoroughly absorbed. Rub any excess remaining on both hands on the buttocks.

HOW SUPPLIED: Emulsion: 2.5mg/g [pouch]

CONTRAINDICATIONS: Undiagnosed abnormal genital bleeding, known/suspected/history of breast cancer, known/suspected estrogen-dependent neoplasia, active or history of DVT/PE, active or recent arterial thromboembolic disease (eg, stroke, MI), liver dysfunction or disease, pregnancy.

WARNINGS/PRECAUTIONS: Limit use to the shortest duration consistent with goals and risks; reevaluate periodically. Increased risk of cardiovascular (CV) events. Caution in patients with risk factors for arterial vascular disease (eg, HTN, diabetes mellitus [DM], tobacco use, hypercholesterolemia, obesity) and/or venous thromboembolism (VTE) (eg, personal history or family history of VTE, obesity, systemic lupus erythematosus [SLE]). If feasible, d/c at least 4 to 6 weeks before surgery of the type associated with an increased risk of thromboembolism, or during periods of prolonged immobilization. May increase risk of gallbladder disease. May lead to severe hypercalcemia in patients with breast cancer and bone metastases; monitor and d/c if hypercalcemia occurs. Retinal vascular thrombosis reported; d/c pending examination if sudden partial or complete loss of vision, sudden onset of proptosis, diplopia, migraine, or if examination reveals papilledema or retinal vascular lesions. Consider addition of a progestin if no hysterectomy. May elevate BP, thyroid-binding globulin levels, and plasma TG leading to pancreatitis and other complications. Caution with history of cholestatic jaundice; d/c in case of recurrence. May cause fluid retention; caution with cardiac/renal dysfunction. Caution with severe hypocalcemia. May increase risk of ovarian cancer. May exacerbate endometriosis, asthma, DM, epilepsy, migraine or porphyria, SLE, and hepatic hemangiomas; use with caution. Should not be used in close proximity to sunscreen application; may increase absorption. May affect certain endocrine, LFTs, and blood components in laboratory tests.

ADVERSE REACTIONS: Headache, infection, breast pain, endometrial disorder, sinusitis, pruritus.

INTERACTIONS: CYP3A4 inducers (eg, St. John's wort, phenobarbital, carbamazepine, rifampin) may decrease levels, which may decrease therapeutic effects and/or change uterine bleeding profile. CYP3A4 inhibitors (eg, erythromycin, clarithromycin, ketoconazole, itraconazole, ritonavir, grapefruit juice) may increase levels, which may result in side effects.

PREGNANCY: Contraindicated in pregnancy, caution in nursing.

MECHANISM OF ACTION: Estrogen; binds to nuclear receptors in estrogen-responsive tissues. Circulating estrogens modulate pituitary secretion of gonadotropins, luteinizing hormone and follicle stimulating hormone, through a negative feedback mechanism. Reduces elevated levels of these hormones in postmenopausal women.

PHARMACOKINETICS: Distribution: Largely bound to sex hormone-binding globulin and albumin; found in breast milk. **Metabolism:** Liver to estrone (metabolite), estriol (major urinary metabolite); sulfate and glucuronide conjugation (liver), gut hydrolysis; CYP 3A4 (partial metabolism). **Excretion:** Urine (parent compound and metabolites).

NURSING CONSIDERATIONS

Assessment: Assess for abnormal genital bleeding, presence or history of breast cancer, estrogen-dependent neoplasias, DVT, PE, active or recent (within past yr) arterial thromboembolic disease, and any other conditions where treatment may be contraindicated or cautioned. Assess use in women ≥65 yrs, and those with DM, asthma, epilepsy, migraines or porphyria, SLE, and hepatic hemangiomas. Assess for possible drug interactions. Assess need for progestin therapy in women who have not had a hysterectomy.

Monitoring: Monitor for signs/symptoms of CV disorders, malignant neoplasms, dementia, gallbladder disease, hypercalcemia, visual abnormalities, increased BP, hypertriglyceridemia, hypothyroidism, fluid retention, cholestatic jaundice, exacerbation of endometriosis and other conditions. Perform annual mammography, regular monitoring of BP, and periodic evaluation (q3-6 months) to determine need for therapy. Monitor thyroid function if patient on thyroid hormone replacement therapy. In cases of undiagnosed, persistent, or recurrent vaginal bleeding in women with uterus, perform adequate diagnostic measures (eg, endometrial sampling) to rule out malignancies.

Patient Counseling: Inform that estrogens increase chances of developing uterine cancer. Instruct to contact physician if breast lumps, unusual vaginal bleeding, dizziness or faintness, changes in speech, severe headaches, chest pain, SOB, leg pains, changes in vision, or vomiting occur. Advise to open medication pouches just prior to use. Instruct to apply in the morning to clean, dry skin of both thighs and calves. Instruct to avoid applying medication to irritated or red skin. Instruct that sunscreen should not be applied to treatment area at same time; may interact with medication. Advise to have yearly breast examinations conducted by a healthcare provider and to perform monthly breast self-examinations.

Administration: Topical route. Refer to PI for instructions on daily application. **Storage:** 20-25°C (68-77°F); excursions permitted to 15-40°C (59-104°F).

ESTROSTEP FE   RX
norethindrone acetate - ferrous fumarate - ethinyl estradiol (Warner Chilcott)

> Cigarette smoking increases the risk of serious cardiovascular (CV) side effects. Risk increases with age (>35 yrs) and with heavy smoking (≥15 cigarettes/day). Women who use oral contraceptives should be strongly advised not to smoke.

THERAPEUTIC CLASS: Estrogen/progestogen combination

INDICATIONS: Prevention of pregnancy. Treatment of moderate acne vulgaris in females ≥15 yrs who want contraception (for at least 6 months), have achieved menarche, and are unresponsive to topical acne agents.

DOSAGE: *Adults:* Contraception/Acne: 1 tab qd for 28 days, then repeat. Start 1st Sunday after menses begins or the 1st day of menses.
Pediatrics: Postpubertal: Contraception/Acne (≥15 yrs): 1 tab qd for 28 days, then repeat. Start 1st Sunday after menses begins or the 1st day of menses.

HOW SUPPLIED: Tab: (Ethinyl Estradiol-Norethindrone) 0.035mg-1mg, 0.030mg-1mg, 0.020mg-1mg; Tab: (Ferrous Fumarate) 75mg

CONTRAINDICATIONS: Thrombophlebitis, thromboembolic disorders, history of deep vein thrombophlebitis or thromboembolic disorders, pregnancy, cerebrovascular disease, coronary artery disease, undiagnosed abnormal genital bleeding, cholestatic jaundice of pregnancy, jaundice with prior pill use, hepatic adenoma or carcinoma, breast carcinoma, carcinoma of the endometrium or other estrogen-dependent neoplasia.

WARNINGS/PRECAUTIONS: Increased risk of myocardial infarction (MI), vascular disease, thromboembolism, stroke, hepatic neoplasia and gallbladder disease. May increase risk of breast and cervical cancer. Benign hepatic adenomas and hepatocellular carcinoma reported; d/c if jaundice develops. Retinal thrombosis reported; d/c if unexplained partial or complete loss of vision, onset of proptosis or diplopia, papilledema, or retinal vascular lesions develops. Should not be used to induce withdrawal bleeding as a test for pregnancy, or to treat threatened or habitual abortion during pregnancy. May cause glucose intolerance; monitor prediabetic and diabetic patients. May cause fluid retention and increase BP; monitor closely with HTN and d/c if significant elevation of BP occurs. May elevate LDL levels or cause other lipid changes. May cause/exacerbate migraine or may develop headache with new pattern. Breakthrough bleeding and spotting reported; rule out malignancy or pregnancy. Perform annual physical exam. Monitor closely with depression and d/c if depression recurs to serious degree. Use before menarche is not indicated. May affect certain endocrine tests, LFTs, and blood components. Does not protect against HIV infection (AIDS) and other sexually transmitted disease (STD).

ADVERSE REACTIONS: Thrombophlebitis, arterial thromboembolism, pulmonary embolism, MI, cerebral hemorrhage, cerebral thrombosis, HTN, gallbladder disease, Hepatic adenomas, benign liver tumors, N/V, breakthrough bleeding, spotting, amenorrhea.

INTERACTIONS: Reduced effects, increased breakthrough bleeding, and menstrual irregularities with rifampin, phenylbutazone and St. John's wort. Increased plasma levels with atorvastatin, ascorbic acid and acetaminophen (APAP). Decreased plasma levels of APAP. Increased clearance of temazepam, salicylic acid, morphine, and clofibric acid. Increased plasma levels of cyclosporine, prednisolone, and theophylline. Pregnancy reported when administered with antimicrobials, such as ampicillin, tetracycline, and griseofulvin. Reduced effects when used with anticonvulsants such as phenobarbital, phenytoin, and carbamazepine.

PREGNANCY: Category X, not for use in nursing.

MECHANISM OF ACTION: Estrogen/progestogen oral contraceptive; acts by suppressing gonadotropins, inhibiting ovulation, and causing other alterations, including changes in the cervical mucus (increasing difficulty of sperm entry into uterus) and the endometrium (reducing likelihood of implantation). Acne: not established; increases sex hormone-binding globulin and decreases free testosterone (reducing androgen stimulation of sebum production).

PHARMACOKINETICS: Absorption: Rapid and complete. Absolute bioavailability: Norethindrone (64%), ethinyl estradiol (43%); T_{max}=1-2 hrs. Refer to PI for dose specific parameters. **Distribution:** V_d=2-4L/kg; plasma protein binding (>95%). Excreted in breast milk. **Metabolism:** Norethindrone: Extensive; reduction, sulfate/glucuronide conjugation. Ethinyl estradiol: Extensive; oxidation via CYP3A4 and conjugation; 2-hydroxy ethinyl estradiol (major metabolite). **Elimination:** Urine, feces. Norethindrone: $T_{1/2}$=13 hrs. Ethinyl estradiol: $T_{1/2}$=19 hrs.

NURSING CONSIDERATIONS

Assessment: Assess for current or history of thrombophlebitis or thromboembolic disorders, cerebrovascular or coronary artery disease, known or suspected carcinoma of the breast, endometrium or other known or suspected estrogen-dependent neoplasia, undiagnosed abnormal genital bleeding, history of cholestatic jaundice of pregnancy or jaundice with previous pill use, hepatic adenomas or carcinomas, known or suspected pregnancy. Assess use in patients >35 yrs who smoke ≥15 cigarettes/day. Assess use in patients with HTN, hyperlipidemias, diabetes mellitus (DM), and obesity. Assess for conditions that might be aggravated by fluid retention, nursing status and for possible drug interactions.

Monitoring: Monitor for venous and arterial thrombotic and thromboembolic events (eg, MI, stroke), hepatic neoplasia, gallbladder disease, ocular lesions, HTN, fluid retention, bleeding irregularities, and onset or exacerbation of headaches or migraines. Monitor blood glucose levels with history of DM or in prediabetic patients, BP with history of HTN, lipid levels with a history of hyperlipidemia. Monitor for signs/symptoms of liver toxicity (eg, jaundice), GI upset (eg, diarrhea, vomiting), and signs of worsening depression with previous history. Refer patients with contact lenses to ophthalmologist if ocular changes develop. Perform annual physical exam.

Patient Counseling: Counsel about possible side effects. Inform that medication does not protect against HIV and other STDs. Avoid smoking while on medication. Advise if spotting, light bleeding, or nausea develops during first 1-3 packs of pills, to continue taking medication, and to notify physician if symptoms do not subside. If N/V or diarrhea occurs, use backup birth control method until physician is contacted. Counsel to go for an annual physical, the appropriate way to use the pack and when to start. Take at the same time every day; if a dose is missed, take as soon as possible, then take next dose at regular time. See PI for detailed notes on administration regarding missed doses.

Administration: Oral route. **Storage:** Do not store above 25°C (77°F). Protect from light. Store tabs inside pouch when not in use.

ETODOLAC

RX

etodolac (Various)

> NSAIDs may increase risk of serious cardiovascular thrombotic events, myocardial infarction (MI), stroke; increased risk with duration of use and with cardiovascular disease (CVD) or risk factors for CVD. Increased risk of serious GI adverse events (eg, bleeding, ulceration, stomach/intestinal perforation) that can be fatal and occur anytime during use without warning symptoms; elderly patients are at a greater risk. Contraindicated for the treatment of perioperative pain in the setting of coronary artery bypass graft (CABG) surgery.

THERAPEUTIC CLASS: NSAID

INDICATIONS: Acute and long-term use in the management of signs and symptoms of osteoarthritis (OA) and rheumatoid arthritis (RA). Management of acute pain.

DOSAGE: *Adults:* ≥18 yrs: Use lowest effective dose for the shortest duration consistent with individual patient treatment goals. After observing the response to initial therapy, adjust dose and frequency based on individual patient's need. Acute Pain: Usual: 200-400mg q6-8h. Max: 1000mg/day. OA/RA: Initial: 300mg bid-tid, or 400mg bid, or 500mg bid. May give a lower dose of 600mg/day for long-term use. Max: 1000mg/day. Elderly: Caution with dose selection.

HOW SUPPLIED: Cap: 200mg, 300mg; Tab: 400mg, 500mg

CONTRAINDICATIONS: History of asthma, urticaria, or other allergic-type reactions with aspirin (ASA) or other NSAIDs. Treatment of perioperative pain in the setting of CABG surgery.

WARNINGS/PRECAUTIONS: Use lowest effective dose for the shortest duration possible. May cause HTN or worsen preexisting HTN; monitor BP closely. Fluid retention and edema reported; caution with fluid retention or heart failure. Extreme caution with prior history of ulcer disease, GI bleeding, or risk factors for GI bleeding (eg, prolonged NSAID therapy, older age, poor general health status); monitor for GI ulceration/bleeding and d/c if serious GI event occurs. Renal papillary necrosis and other renal injury reported after long-term use; increased risk with renal/hepatic impairment, heart failure (HF), and elderly. Caution with preexisting kidney disease. Not recommended for use with advanced renal disease; monitor renal function closely if therapy is initiated. Caution with mild to moderate renal impairment. Anaphylactoid reactions may occur. Avoid with aspirin (ASA)-triad. Caution with asthma and avoid with ASA-sensitive asthma. May cause serious skin adverse events (eg, exfoliative dermatitis, Stevens-Johnson syndrome, toxic epidermal necrolysis); d/c at 1st appearance of skin rash or any other signs of hypersensitivity. Avoid in late pregnancy; may cause premature closure of ductus arteriosus. Not a substitute for corticosteroids or for the treatment of corticosteroid insufficiency; may mask signs of inflammation and fever. May cause elevations of LFTs or severe hepatic reactions (eg, jaundice, fulminant hepatitis, liver necrosis, hepatic failure); d/c if liver disease or systemic manifestations occur, or if abnormal LFTs persist/worsen. Anemia reported; monitor Hgb/Hct if signs or symptoms of anemia develop. May inhibit platelet aggregation and prolong bleeding time; monitor patients with coagulation disorders. Caution in debilitated and elderly (≥65 yrs).

ADVERSE REACTIONS: Dyspepsia, abdominal pain, diarrhea, flatulence, N/V, constipation, anemia, pruritus, rashes, dizziness, increased bleeding time, GI ulcers, heartburn, abnormal renal function.

INTERACTIONS: Not recommended with phenylbutazone and ASA. Increased risk of GI bleeding with oral corticosteroids, anticoagulants, alcohol use, and smoking. May diminish antihypertensive effect of ACE inhibitors. May decrease peak concentration with antacids. May elevate cyclosporine, digoxin, and methotrexate levels. May enhance nephrotoxicity associated with cyclosporine. May enhance methotrexate toxicity; caution with concomitant use. May reduce natriuretic effect of furosemide and thiazides; monitor for signs of renal insufficiency or failure and diuretic efficacy. May impair response with thiazides or loop diuretics. Monitor for signs of lithium toxicity with lithium. Risk of renal toxicity with diuretics and ACE inhibitors. Caution with warfarin; prolonged PT, with or without bleeding, may occur with warfarin.

PREGNANCY: Category C, not for use in nursing.

MECHANISM OF ACTION: NSAID; has not been established. Suspected to inhibit prostaglandin synthetase.

PHARMACOKINETICS: **Absorption:** Well absorbed. Bioavailability (100%); C_{max}=14-37µg/mL, T_{max}=80 min. Administration in various population resulted in different pharmacokinetic parameters. **Distribution:** V_d=390mL/kg; plasma protein binding (>99%). **Metabolism:** Liver (extensive); hydroxylation, glucuronidation; 6-, 7-, and 8- hydroxylated-etodolac, etodolac glucuronide (metabolites). **Elimination:** Urine (1% unchanged, 72% parent drug and metabolites), feces (16%); $T_{1/2}$=6.4 hrs.

NURSING CONSIDERATIONS

Assessment: Assess previous hypersensitivity to the drug, history of asthma, urticaria, or allergic-type reactions with ASA or other NSAIDs, ASA-triad, CVD, risk factors for CVD, HTN, fluid retention, HF, history of ulcer disease, history of/risk factors for GI bleeding, general health status, renal/hepatic impairment, coagulation disorders, pregnancy/nursing status, and possible drug interactions. Obtain baseline CBC and BP.

Monitoring: Monitor for bleeding time, GI bleeding/ulceration/perforation, cardiovascular thrombotic events, MI, HTN, stroke, fluid retention, edema, asthma, hypersensitivity, and other adverse reactions. Monitor for BP, LFTs, and renal function. Monitor for CBC and chemistry profile periodically with long-term use.

Patient Counseling: Inform to seek medical advice if symptoms of CV events, GI ulceration/bleeding, skin/hypersensitivity reactions, unexplained weight gain or edema, hepatotoxicity, or anaphylactoid reactions occur. Instruct to avoid use in late pregnancy.

Administration: Oral route. **Storage:** 20-25°C (68-77°F). (Cap) Protect from moisture. (Tab) Store in original container until ready to use.

E

ETOPOPHOS   RX
etoposide phosphate (Bristol-Myers Squibb)

> **Administer under the supervision of a qualified physician experienced in use of cancer chemotherapeutic agents. Severe myelosuppression with resulting infection or bleeding may occur.**

THERAPEUTIC CLASS: Podophyllotoxin derivative

INDICATIONS: Adjunct therapy for management of refractory testicular tumors. First-line combination therapy for management of small cell lung cancer (SCLC).

DOSAGE: *Adults:* Testicular Cancer: Usual: 50-100mg/m^2/day IV on Days 1-5 to 100mg/m^2/day on Days 1, 3, and 5. SCLC: 35mg/m^2/day IV for 4 days to 50mg/m^2/day for 5 days. Administer at infusion rates 5-210 min. After adequate recovery from any toxicity, repeat course for either therapy at 3-4 week intervals. CrCl 15-50mL/min: 75% of dose.

HOW SUPPLIED: Inj: 100mg

WARNINGS/PRECAUTIONS: Observe for myelosuppression during and after therapy. Withhold therapy if platelet count <50,000/mm^3 or if absolute neutrophil count (ANC) <500/mm^3. Risk of anaphylactic reaction, manifested by chills, fever, tachycardia, bronchospasm, dyspnea, and hypotension reported. Inj-site reactions may occur; monitor infusion site for possible infiltration during administration. May be carcinogenic in humans; acute leukemia with or without a preleukemic phase may occur. Caution with low serum albumin; increased risk of toxicity. May cause fetal harm in pregnancy. D/C or reduce dose if severe reactions occur. Dosage may be modified to account for other myelosuppressive drugs or the effects of prior x-ray or chemotherapy, which may have compromised bone marrow reserve. Do not give by bolus IV inj. Caution in elderly.

ADVERSE REACTIONS: Leukopenia, neutropenia, thrombocytopenia, anemia, constipation, diarrhea, leukopenia, dizziness, alopecia, N/V, mucositis, asthenia/malaise, chills, fever, anorexia.

INTERACTIONS: Caution with drugs known to inhibit phosphatase activities (eg, levamisole hydrochloride). High-dose cyclosporin A reduces clearance and increases exposure of oral etoposide. Prior use of cisplatin may decrease etoposide total body clearance in children. Displaced from protein binding sites by phenylbutazone, sodium salicylate, and aspirin.

PREGNANCY: Category D, not for use in nursing.

MECHANISM OF ACTION: Podophyllotoxin derivative; induces DNA strand breaks by interacting with DNA-topoisomerase II or formation of free radicals.

PHARMACOKINETICS: Absorption: Rapid, complete; Etopophos 150mg/m^2: AUC=168.3μg•hr/mL, C_{max}=20μg/mL. Refer to PI for pharmacokinetic parameters for VePesid, which is similar to Etoposide.

NURSING CONSIDERATIONS

Assessment: Assess for renal function, low serum albumin, pregnancy/nursing status, and possible drug interactions. Obtain platelet, Hgb, and WBC with differential at start of therapy.

Monitoring: Monitor for signs/symptoms of anaphylactic reaction, severe myelosuppression, severe reactions, and renal dysfunction. Monitor for infusion site reactions. Perform periodic CBC prior to each cycle of therapy and at appropriate intervals during and after therapy.

Patient Counseling: Inform of pregnancy risks; avoid pregnancy. Advise to seek medical attention if experience symptoms of severe myelosuppression (infection or bleeding) or anaphylactic reaction (chills, fever, tachycardia, bronchospasm, dyspnea, hypotension).

Administration: IV (infusion) route. Refer to PI for preparation and administration. **Storage:** 2-8°C (36-46°F); protect from light. Reconstituted and diluted vials stable for 7 days at 2-8°C (36-46°F) or 24 hrs at 20-25°C (68-77°F).

EUFLEXXA RX
sodium hyaluronate (Ferring)

THERAPEUTIC CLASS: Hyaluronan

INDICATIONS: Treatment of pain in osteoarthritis of the knee in patients who have failed to respond adequately to conservative nonpharmacologic therapy and simple analgesics (eg, acetaminophen).

DOSAGE: *Adults:* 2mL intra-articularly into affected knee at weekly intervals for 3 weeks.

HOW SUPPLIED: Inj: 1% [2mL]

CONTRAINDICATIONS: Knee joint infections, infections or skin disease in the area of inj site.

WARNINGS/PRECAUTIONS: Mixing with quaternary ammonium salts (eg, benzalkonium chloride) results in precipitate formation; do not administer through a needle previously used with medical sol containing benzalkonium chloride and do not use disinfectants for skin preparation that contain quaternary ammonium salts. Do not inject intravascularly. Patients having repeated exposure have the potential for an immune response. Safety and effectiveness of inj with other intra-articular injectables, or into joints other than the knee have not been established. Remove any joint effusion before injecting. Transient pain/swelling of injected joint may occur.

ADVERSE REACTIONS: Arthralgia, asthenia, eyelid/knee swelling, herpes simplex, herpes zoster, rhinitis, BP increase, upper respiratory tract infection, knee replacement, back/knee/skeletal pain, rash, peptic ulcer.

PREGNANCY: Safety not known in pregnancy/nursing.

MECHANISM OF ACTION: Hyaluronan.

NURSING CONSIDERATIONS

Assessment: Assess for knee joint infections, infections or skin disease in the inj-site area, and joint effusion.

Monitoring: Monitor for pain/swelling of injected joint.

Patient Counseling: Inform that transient pain/swelling of injected joint may occur after inj. Instruct to avoid any strenuous activities or prolonged (>1 hr) weight-bearing activities (eg, jogging, tennis) within 48 hrs following inj.

Administration: Intra-articular route. Use strict aseptic inj procedures. Refer to PI for administration instructions. **Storage:** 2-25°C (36-77°F). Protect from light. Do not freeze.

EVAMIST RX
estradiol (Ther-Rx)

Estrogens increase the risk of endometrial cancer. Perform adequate diagnostic measures, including endometrial sampling, to rule out malignancy with undiagnosed persistent or recurring abnormal vaginal bleeding. Should not be used for the prevention of cardiovascular disease (CVD) or dementia. Increased risk of myocardial infarction (MI), stroke, invasive breast cancer, pulmonary emboli (PE), and deep-vein thrombosis (DVT) in postmenopausal women (50-79 yrs of age) reported. Increased risk of developing probable dementia in postmenopausal women ≥65 yrs of age reported. Should be prescribed at the lowest effective dose for the shortest duration consistent with treatment goals and risks. Breast budding/masses in prepubertal females and gynecomastia and breast masses in prepubertal males following unintentional secondary exposure reported. Ensure that children do not come in contact with the application site. Advise to strictly adhere to recommended instructions for use.

THERAPEUTIC CLASS: Estrogen

INDICATIONS: Treatment of moderate to severe vasomotor symptoms due to menopause.

DOSAGE: *Adults:* Initial: 1 spray qd. Adjust dose based on response. Usual: 1-3 sprays qam to adjacent, non-overlapping areas on the inner surface of the forearm, starting near the elbow. Reevaluate treatment need periodically.

HOW SUPPLIED: Spray: 1.53mg/spray [8.1mL]

CONTRAINDICATIONS: Undiagnosed abnormal genital bleeding, known/suspected/history of breast cancer, known/suspected estrogen-dependent neoplasia, active or history of DVT/PE, active or recent arterial thromboembolic disease (eg, stroke, MI), liver dysfunction or disease, known/suspected pregnancy.

WARNINGS/PRECAUTIONS: Caution in patients with risk factors for arterial vascular disease (eg, HTN, diabetes mellitus [DM], tobacco use, hypercholesterolemia, obesity) and/or venous thromboembolism (VTE) (eg, personal history or family history of VTE, obesity, systemic lupus erythematosus [SLE]). If feasible, d/c at least 4 to 6 weeks before surgery of the type associated with an increased risk of thromboembolism, or during periods of prolonged immobilization. Application site should be covered with clothing if another person may come in contact with the site. Consider d/c if conditions of safe use cannot be met. May increase risk of gallbladder disease and ovarian cancer. May lead to severe hypercalcemia in patients with breast cancer and bone metastases; d/c and take appropriate measures if hypercalcemia occurs. Retinal vascular thrombosis reported; d/c pending examination if sudden partial/complete loss of vision, sudden onset of proptosis, diplopia, or migraine occurs, or if examination reveals papilledema or retinal vascular lesions, d/c therapy permanently. Consider adding a progestin if no hysterectomy. May elevate BP, thyroid-binding globulin levels, and plasma TG with preexisting hypertriglyceridemia; consider d/c if pancreatitis occurs. Caution with history of cholestatic jaundice; d/c in case of recurrence. May cause fluid retention; caution with cardiac/renal dysfunction. Caution with severe hypocalcemia. May exacerbate endometriosis, asthma, DM, epilepsy, migraine, porphyria, SLE, and hepatic hemangiomas. Avoid fire, flame, or smoking until spray has dried. May affect certain endocrine and blood components in laboratory tests.

ADVERSE REACTIONS: Breast tenderness, nipple pain, nausea, nasopharyngitis, back pain, arthralgia, headache.

INTERACTIONS: CYP3A4 inducers (eg, St. John's wort, phenobarbital, carbamazepine, rifampin) may decrease levels, which may decrease therapeutic effects and/or change uterine bleeding profile. CYP3A4 inhibitors (eg, erythromycin, clarithromycin, ketoconazole, itraconazole, ritonavir, grapefruit juice) may increase levels, which may result in side effects. Patients concomitantly receiving thyroid replacement therapy may require increased doses of their thyroid replacement therapy. Decreased absorption with sunscreen applied 1 hr after estradiol application.

PREGNANCY: Contraindicated in pregnancy, not for use in nursing.

MECHANISM OF ACTION: Estrogen; binds to nuclear receptors in estrogen-responsive tissues. Circulating estrogens modulate pituitary secretion of the gonadotropins, luteinizing hormone and follicle-stimulating hormone, through a negative feedback mechanism. Reduces elevated levels of these hormones in postmenopausal women.

PHARMACOKINETICS: Absorption: Topical administration of various doses resulted in different parameters. **Distribution:** Found in breast milk. Largely bound to sex hormone-binding globulin and albumin. **Metabolism:** Liver; estrone (metabolite); estriol (major urinary metabolite); sulfate and glucuronide conjugation (liver), gut hydrolysis; reabsorption. **Elimination:** Urine (parent and metabolites).

NURSING CONSIDERATIONS

Assessment: Assess for presence or history of breast cancer, estrogen-dependent neoplasia, abnormal genital bleeding, active or history of DVT/PE, active or recent (within past yr) arterial thromboembolic disease, pregnancy/nursing status, or any other conditions where treatment is contraindicated or cautioned. Assess use in women ≥65 yrs, and those with DM, asthma, epilepsy, migraines or porphyria, SLE, and hepatic hemangiomas. Assess for possible drug interactions.

Monitoring: Monitor for signs/symptoms of CVD, malignant neoplasms, dementia, gallbladder disease, hypercalcemia, visual abnormalities, BP elevations, fluid retention, elevations in plasma TG, hypothyroidism, pancreatitis, exacerbation of endometriosis and other conditions (eg, asthma, DM, epilepsy, migraines, SLE, hepatic hemangiomas). Periodically monitor BP levels at regular intervals and thyroid function for patients on thyroid replacement therapy. Perform proper diagnostic testing (eg, endometrial sampling) in patients with undiagnosed, persistent, or recurring vaginal bleeding. Perform annual breast exam. Perform periodic evaluation to determine treatment need.

Patient Counseling: Instruct to contact physician if vaginal bleeding develops. Counsel about the possible side effects of therapy (eg, headache, breast pain and tenderness, N/V). Instruct to apply therapy ud and keep children from contacting exposed application site; if direct contact occurs, advise to thoroughly wash contact area with soap and water. Counsel to look for signs of unexpected sexual development (eg, breast mass or increased breast size) in prepubertal children; advise to have children evaluated by a physician if signs of unintentional secondary exposure are noticed and to d/c therapy until cause is identified. Instruct that before applying the 1st dose from a new applicator, the pump should be primed by spraying 3 sprays with cover on. Advise that medication contains alcohol; avoid fire, flame, or smoking until medication is dry. Inform to have yearly breast examinations by a physician and perform monthly breast self-examinations.

Administration: Topical route. Sprays should be allowed to dry for 2 min; do not wash site for 30 min. Should not be applied to skin surfaces other than the forearm. **Storage:** 25°C (77°F); excursions permitted to 15-30°C (59-86°F). Do not freeze.

EVISTA
raloxifene HCl (Lilly)

> Increased risk of deep vein thrombosis (DVT) and pulmonary embolism (PE) reported. Avoid use in women with active or past history of venous thromboembolism (VTE). Increased risk of death due to stroke in postmenopausal women with documented coronary heart disease or at increased risk for major coronary events; consider risk-benefit balance in women at risk for stroke.

THERAPEUTIC CLASS: Selective estrogen receptor modulator

INDICATIONS: Treatment and prevention of osteoporosis in postmenopausal women. Reduction in risk of invasive breast cancer in postmenopausal women with osteoporosis and in postmenopausal women at high risk for invasive breast cancer.

DOSAGE: *Adults:* 60mg qd. May be given at any time of day without regard to meals. Refer to PI for recommendations regarding calcium and vitamin D supplementation.

HOW SUPPLIED: Tab: 60mg

CONTRAINDICATIONS: Nursing, pregnancy, women who may become pregnant, active/past history of VTE (eg, DVT, PE, retinal vein thrombosis).

WARNINGS/PRECAUTIONS: VTE events including superficial venous thrombophlebitis reported; d/c at least 72 hrs prior to and during prolonged immobilization (eg, postsurgical recovery, prolonged bed rest); therapy should only be resumed after fully ambulatory. Caution in women at risk of thromboembolic disease. Should not be used for primary or secondary prevention of cardiovascular disease. Avoid in premenopausal women. Use not adequately studied in women with a history of breast cancer. Not recommended for use in men. May increase levels of triglycerides with preexisting hypertriglyceridemia; monitor serum triglyceride levels in women with history of hypertriglyceridemia. Caution with hepatic impairment or with moderate or severe renal impairment. Monitor for unexplained uterine bleeding and breast abnormalites.

ADVERSE REACTIONS: DVT, pulmonary embolism, vaginal bleeding, hot flashes, leg cramps, arthralgia, infection, flu syndrome, headache, nausea, weight gain, sinusitis, rhinitis, cough increased, peripheral edema.

INTERACTIONS: Cholestyramine may decrease absorption; avoid concomitant administration with cholestyramine and other anion exchange resins. Monitor PT with warfarin and other warfarin derivatives. Caution with other highly protein-bound drugs (eg, diazepam, diazoxide, lidocaine). Avoid concomitant use with systemic estrogens.

PREGNANCY: Category X, contraindicated in nursing.

MECHANISM OF ACTION: Selective estrogen receptor modulator; binds to estrogen receptors. Binding results in activation of estrogenic pathways in some tissues and blockade of estrogenic pathways in others depending on extent of recruitment of coactivators and corepressors to estrogen receptor target gene promotors. Acts as an estrogen agonist in bone. Decreases bone resorption and bone turnover, increases bone mineral density, and decreases fracture incidence.

PHARMACOKINETICS: Absorption: Rapid; absolute bioavailability (2%). Single dose: C_{max}=0.5(ng/mL)/(mg/kg); AUC=27.2(ng•hr/mL)/(mg/kg). Multiple doses: C_{max}=1.36(ng/mL)/(mg/kg); AUC=24.2(ng•hr/mL)/(mg/kg). **Distribution:** V_d=2348L/kg. Plasma protein binding (95%). **Metabolism:** Extensive; glucuronidation; raloxifene-4'-glucuronide, raloxifene-6-glucuronide, raloxifene-6',4'-diglucuronide (metabolites). **Elimination:** Feces (primary), urine (<0.2% unchanged); $T_{1/2}$=27.7 hrs (single dose); $T_{1/2}$=32.5 hrs (multiple doses).

NURSING CONSIDERATIONS

Assessment: Assess for active or history of VTE (eg, DVT, PE, retinal vein thrombosis), cardiovascular disease, risk factors for stroke, history of breast cancer, history of hypertriglyceridemia, prolonged immobilization, renal/hepatic impairment, pregnancy/nursing status, and for possible drug interactions.

Monitoring: Monitor for VTE (eg, DVT, PE, retinal vein thrombosis), stroke, unexplained uterine bleeding, and breast abnormalities. Monitor serum TG with history of hypertriglyceridemia.

Patient Counseling: For osteoporosis treatment/prevention, instruct to take supplemental calcium and/or vitamin D if intake is inadequate. Consider weight-bearing exercise and behavioral modification factors (eg, smoking, excessive alcohol consumption) for osteoporosis treatment/prevention. Advise to d/c therapy at least 72 hrs prior to and during prolonged immobilization. Avoid prolonged restrictions of movement during travel. Counsel that therapy may increase incidence of hot flashes or hot flashes may occur upon initiation of therapy. Inform that regular breast exams and mammography should be done before initiation of therapy and should continue during therapy. Instruct to read the medication guide before starting therapy.

Administration: Oral route. **Storage:** 20-25°C (68-77°F); excursions permitted to 15-30°C (59-86°F).

EVOCLIN
clindamycin phosphate (Stiefel)

RX

THERAPEUTIC CLASS: Lincomycin derivative

INDICATIONS: Topical treatment of acne vulgaris in patients ≥12 yrs.

DOSAGE: *Adults:* Apply to affected areas qd. Use enough to cover the entire affected area. D/C if no improvement after 6-8 weeks or if condition worsens.
Pediatrics: ≥12 yrs: Apply to affected areas qd. Use enough to cover the entire affected area. D/C if no improvement after 6-8 weeks or if condition worsens.

HOW SUPPLIED: Foam: 1% [50g, 100g]

CONTRAINDICATIONS: History of regional enteritis, ulcerative colitis, or antibiotic-associated colitis (including pseudomembranous colitis).

WARNINGS/PRECAUTIONS: Diarrhea, bloody diarrhea, and colitis (including pseudomembranous colitis) reported; d/c if significant diarrhea occurs. May cause irritation; d/c if irritation or dermatitis occurs. Avoid contact with eyes, mouth, lips, other mucous membranes, or areas of broken skin; rinse thoroughly with water if contact occurs. Caution in atopic individuals and when applying to the chest during lactation to avoid accidental ingestion by the infant.

ADVERSE REACTIONS: Diarrhea, bloody diarrhea, colitis, headache, application-site burning.

INTERACTIONS: Antiperistaltic agents (eg, opiates, diphenoxylate with atropine) may prolong and/or worsen severe colitis. Possible antagonism with topical/oral erythromycin-containing products; avoid concomitant use. May enhance the action of other neuromuscular blockers; caution with concomitant use. Caution with concomitant topical acne therapy (eg, peeling, desquamating, or abrasive agents) due to possible cumulative irritancy effect.

PREGNANCY: Category B, not for use in nursing.

MECHANISM OF ACTION: Lincomycin derivative; not established. Binds to the 50S ribosomal subunits of susceptible bacteria and prevents elongation of peptide chains by interfering with peptidyl transfer, thereby suppressing protein synthesis. Shown to have in vitro activity against *Propionibacterium acnes*, which is associated with acne vulgaris.

PHARMACOKINETICS: Distribution: Orally and parenterally administered clindamycin found in breast milk. **Elimination:** Urine (<0.024% unchanged).

NURSING CONSIDERATIONS

Assessment: Assess for history of regional enteritis/ulcerative colitis or antibiotic-associated colitis (including pseudomembranous colitis), pregnancy/nursing status, and possible drug interactions. Assess use in atopic individuals.

Monitoring: Monitor for significant diarrhea, colitis, and irritation/dermatitis. For colitis, perform stool culture and assay for *Clostridium difficile* toxin.

Patient Counseling: Advise to wash skin with mild soap and allow drying before application. Instruct to dispense foam directly into cap or onto cool surface, then apply enough to cover the face. Instruct to wash hands after application, and to avoid contact with eyes, mouth, lips, other mucous membranes, or areas of broken skin; instruct to rinse thoroughly with water if contact occurs. Inform that irritation (eg, erythema, scaling, itching, burning, stinging) may occur; advise to d/c if excessive irritancy or dermatitis occur. Instruct to d/c and contact physician if severe diarrhea or GI discomfort develops. Instruct that medication is flammable; instruct to avoid smoking or contact with fire during and immediately following application.

Administration: Topical route. Not for PO, ophthalmic, or intravaginal use. Wash skin with mild soap and allow to fully dry before application. **Storage:** 20-25°C (68-77°F). Do not expose to heat or store >49°C (120°F). Contents under pressure; do not puncture or incinerate.

EXALGO
hydromorphone HCl (Mallinckrodt)

CII

> Indicated for opioid-tolerant patients only. Contains hydromorphone, a Schedule II controlled substance, that has a high potential for abuse and is subject to misuse, addiction, and criminal diversion. Fatal respiratory depression could occur in nonopioid-tolerant patients. Accidental consumption, especially in children, can result in a fatal overdose. Not indicated for use in the management of acute or postoperative pain and is not intended for use as a PRN analgesic. Swallow whole. Do not break, chew, dissolve, crush, or inject tabs.

THERAPEUTIC CLASS: Opioid analgesic

INDICATIONS: Management of moderate to severe pain in opioid-tolerant patients requiring continuous, around-the-clock opioid analgesia for an extended period of time.

DOSAGE: *Adults:*>17 yrs: Individualize dose. Dose range: 8-64mg. Administer once q24h. Titrate: Not more often than 3-4 days. Increase 25-50% of the current daily dose for each titration step. Titrate dose upward, if >2 doses of rescue medication are needed within 24 hr period for 2 consecutive days. Conversion from intermediate-release hydromorphone: Starting dose equivalent to the patient's total daily oral hydromorphone dose taken qd. Conversion from other oral opioids: Refer to published relative potency information. Administer 50% of the calculated total daily dose every 24 hrs. Conversion from Transdermal Fentanyl: Administer 12mg q24h for each 25mcg/hr of transdermal fentanyl after 18 hrs following the removal of fentanyl transdermal patch. Moderate/Severe Hepatic and Moderate Renal Impairment: Reduce dose; closely monitor during dose titration. Severe Renal Impairment: Consider alternate analgesic. Elderly: Reduce initial dose. Maintenance: Assess the continued need for around-the-clock opioid therapy periodically, particularly with high-dose formulations. Discontinuation: Taper dose gradually, 25-50% every 2 or 3 days down to a dose of 8mg. Refer to PI for standard conversion of total daily (24-hr) dose of previous opioid therapy and for dosing recommendations.

HOW SUPPLIED: Tab, Extended-Release: 8mg, 12mg, 16mg

CONTRAINDICATIONS: Opiod non-tolerant patients. Significant respiratory depression, especially in the absence of resuscitative equipment or in unmonitored settings. Acute or severe bronchial asthma or hypercarbia, known or suspected paralytic ileus, previous surgical procedures and/or underlying disease that would result in narrowed or obstructed GI tract or presence of "blind loops" of the GI tract or GI obstruction.

WARNINGS/PRECAUTIONS: Do not use as a first opioid. May cause respiratory depression; caution with conditions accompanied by hypoxia, hypercapnia, or decreased respiratory reserve such as asthma, chronic obstructive pulmonary disease or cor pulmonale, severe obesity, sleep apnea, myxedema, kyphoscoliosis, or CNS depression. Avoid with head injury, intracranial lesions, or preexisting elevated intracranial pressure (ICP). May obscure neurologic signs of further increases in ICP in patients with head injury. May cause severe hypotension; caution in patients with circulatory shock. May obscure the diagnosis or clinical course in patients with acute abdominal condition. Contains sodium metabisulfite; may cause allergic-type reactions including anaphylactic symptoms and life-threatening or less severe asthmatic episodes. Caution with adrenocortical insufficiency, delirium tremens, hypothyroidism, prostatic hypertrophy or urethral stricture, and toxic psychosis. May aggravate convulsions in patients with convulsive disorders. May increase biliary tract pressure; caution with inflammatory or obstructive bowel disorder, acute pancreatitis secondary to biliary tract disease, and in biliary surgery. May cause mental/physical impairment. Avoid abrupt withdrawal. Tolerance and physical dependence may occur. Caution with elderly/debilitated.

ADVERSE REACTIONS: Constipation, N/V, somnolence, headache, asthenia, dizziness, diarrhea, insomnia, back pain, pruritus, anorexia, peripheral edema, hyperhidrosis, respiratory depression, hypotension, arthralgia, weight loss.

INTERACTIONS: Concomitant use with CNS depressants (eg, other opioids, illicit drugs, sedatives, hypnotics, tranquilizers, general anesthetics, phenothiazines, muscle relaxants, alcohol) may cause respiratory depression, hypotension, profound sedation, or potentially coma. Avoid concomitant use with alcohol. May cause CNS excitation or depression, hypotension, or HTN with MAOIs. Mixed agonist/antagonist analgesics (eg, buprenorphone, nalbuphine, pentazocine, butorphanol) may reduce analgesic effect and/or may precipitate withdrawal symptoms. May increase risk of urinary retention and/or severe constipation, leading to paralytic ileus with anticholinergics or other medications with anticholinergic activity.

PREGNANCY: Category C, not for use in nursing.

MECHANISM OF ACTION: Opioid analgesic; not established. Mediated through opioid-specific receptors located in CNS to produce analgesia.

PHARMACOKINETICS: Absorption: Single dose: (8mg) T_{max}=12 hrs, C_{max}=0.93ng/mL. Refer to PI for pharmacokinetic parameters for different dosage forms. **Distribution:** Plasma protein binding (27%); (IV) V_d=2.9L/kg; crosses placenta, found in breast milk. **Metabolism:** Liver; glucuronidation (extensive); hydromorphone-3-glucuronide (metabolite). **Elimination:** Urine (75%), (7% unchanged); feces (1% unchanged); $T_{1/2}$=11 hrs.

NURSING CONSIDERATIONS

Assessment: Assess for degree of opioid tolerance; level of pain intensity; previous opioid dose; patient's general condition, age, and medical status; risk factors for abuse; or any other conditions where treatment is contraindicated or cautioned. Assess for history of hypersensitivity, pregnancy/nursing status, renal/hepatic function, and possible drug interactions.

Monitoring: Monitor for signs/symptoms of respiratory depression; circulatory depression (eg, hypotension), misuse or abuse, addiction, tolerance or dependence, hypersensitivity, seizures, and for alleviation of pain.

Patient Counseling: Advise to take as directed; swallow whole. Advise that drug is for use only in patients who are already receiving opioid pain medicine. Advise not to change the dose without consulting a healthcare provider. Report episodes of breakthrough pain and adverse experiences occurring during therapy. Advise that certain stomach or intestinal problems such as narrowing of the intestines or previous surgery may be at higher risk of developing a blockage. Contact healthcare provider if GI obstruction symptoms develop such as abdominal pain/distention, severe constipation, or vomiting. May impair mental and/or physical abilities. Advise not to combine other pain medications, sleep aids, or tranquilizers. Avoid abrupt withdrawal. Educate that medication has the potential for abuse. Advise to keep reach out of children and to dispose unused tablets down the toilet.

Administration: Oral route. **Storage:** 25°C (77°F); excursions permitted to 15-30°C (59-86°F).

EXELON   RX
rivastigmine tartrate (Novartis)

THERAPEUTIC CLASS: Acetylcholinesterase inhibitor

INDICATIONS: Treatment of mild to moderate dementia of the Alzheimer's type and mild to moderate dementia associated with Parkinson's disease.

DOSAGE: *Adults:* PO: Alzheimer's Dementia: Initial: 1.5mg bid. Titrate: May increase to 3mg bid after a minimum of 2 weeks, if 1.5mg bid is well tolerated. Subsequent increase to 4.5mg bid and 6mg bid should be attempted after a minimum of 2 weeks at the previous dose. Max: 12mg/day (6mg bid). If not tolerated, d/c therapy for several doses and restart at same or next lower dose. If interrupted longer than several days, reinitiate with lowest daily dose and titrate as above. Dementia Associated with Parkinson's Disease: Initial: 1.5mg bid. Titrate: May subsequently increase to 3mg bid and further to 4.5mg bid and 6mg bid with a minimum of 4 weeks at each dose, based on tolerability. Patch: Alzheimer's Dementia/Dementia Associated with Parkinson's Disease: Initial: Apply 4.6mg/24 hrs patch qd to clean, dry, hairless, intact skin. Titrate: Increase to 9.5mg/24 hrs patch after 4 weeks, if well tolerated. Maint/Max: 9.5mg/24 hrs. If not tolerating, d/c for ≥3 days and restart at the same or next lower dose level. If interrupted >3 days, reinitiate with lowest daily dose and titrate as above. Switching from Cap/PO Sol: Total PO Daily Dose <6mg: Switch to 4.6mg/24 hrs patch. Total PO Daily Dose 6-12mg: Switch to 9.5mg/24 hrs patch. Apply 1st patch on day following last oral dose.

HOW SUPPLIED: Cap: 1.5mg, 3mg, 4.5mg, 6mg; Patch: 4.6mg/24 hrs, 9.5mg/24 hrs [30^s]; Sol: 2mg/mL [120mL]

CONTRAINDICATIONS: Hypersensitivity to carbamate derivatives.

WARNINGS/PRECAUTIONS: Associated with significant GI adverse reactions such as N/V, diarrhea, anorexia, weight loss (at higher than recommended doses with patch); always follow dosing guidelines. Monitor for symptoms of active/occult GI bleeding especially those at increased risk of developing ulcers (eg, history of ulcer disease, receiving NSAIDs). May have vagotonic effect on HR (eg, bradycardia), especially in "sick sinus syndrome" or supraventricular conduction abnormalities. May cause urinary obstruction and seizures. Caution in patients with asthma and obstructive pulmonary disease. May exacerbate or induce extrapyramidal symptoms and impair mental/physical abilities. (PO) Syncopal episodes reported. Worsening of parkinsonian symptoms observed, who were treated with cap. (Patch) Caution with low body weight (<50kg). Should not be applied to a skin area where cre, lot, or powder has recently been applied.

ADVERSE REACTIONS: N/V, anxiety, weight decreased, anorexia, headache, dizziness, fatigue, diarrhea, depression.

INTERACTIONS: May interfere with the activity of anticholinergics. Synergistic effect with succinylcholine, similar neuromuscular blockers, or cholinergic agonists (eg, bethanechol). May exaggerate succinylcholine-type muscle relaxation during anesthesia. Increased clearance with nicotine. (Patch) Avoid with cholinomimetic drugs.

PREGNANCY: Category B, not for use in nursing.

MECHANISM OF ACTION: Reversible cholinesterase inhibitor; not fully established, suspected to enhance cholinergic function by increasing concentration of acetylcholine through reversible inhibition of cholinesterase.

PHARMACOKINETICS: Absorption: Patch: T_{max}=8-16 hrs. PO: Rapid, complete; absolute bioavailability (36%) (3mg); T_{max}=1 hr. **Distribution:** V_d=1.8-2.7L/kg; plasma protein binding (40%). **Metabolism:** Cholinesterase-mediated hydrolysis. **Elimination:** PO: Urine (97%), feces (0.4%); $T_{1/2}$=1.5 hrs. Patch: Urine (>90%, unchanged), feces (<1%); $T_{1/2}$=3 hrs.

NURSING CONSIDERATIONS

Assessment: Assess for drug hypersensitivity, history of ulcer disease, sick sinus syndrome, conduction defects, asthma or obstructive pulmonary disease, urinary obstruction, seizures, pregnancy/nursing status, and possible drug interactions. (Patch) Assess patient's body weight.

Monitoring: Monitor for signs/symptoms of active or occult GI bleeding, hypersensitivity reactions, and other adverse reactions. (Patch) Monitor for body weight, extrapyramidal symptoms, and mental status.

EXFORGE

Patient Counseling: Advise to inform their physician if GI adverse events occurs. Advise that may exacerbate or induce extrapyramidal symptoms (Patch) Inform of the importance of applying the correct dose and correct part of the body. Instruct to wash hands after application, and avoid contact with eyes; do not rub in or apply to area that is red, irritated, cut or to areas where cre, lot, powder has recently been applied; replace q24h and consistent time of day; do not apply new patch to same spot for at least 14 days; can be used while bathing but avoid exposure to external heat sources (eg, excessive sunlight, saunas, solariums) for long periods of time; fold the patch in half and return to its original container after use when discarding. If dose is missed, instruct to apply new patch immediately, then continue scheduled dosage; do not apply 2 patches at once. Advise not to take cap or PO sol or other drugs with cholinergic effect while wearing patch.

Administration: Oral/transdermal route. (PO) Take with meal in am and pm. (Sol) Swallow directly from syringe or mix with small glass of water, cold fruit juice, or soda; stir before drinking. (Patch) Refer to PI for method of administration. **Storage:** 25°C (77°F); excursions permitted to 15-30°C (59-86°F). Sol: Store in upright position and protect from freezing. Store for up to 4 hrs if combined with cold fruit juice or soda. Patch: Keep in sealed pouch until use. Cap: Store in a tight container.

EXFORGE

RX

amlodipine - valsartan (Novartis)

D/C when pregnancy is detected. Drugs that act directly on the renin-angiotensin system can cause injury/death to the developing fetus.

THERAPEUTIC CLASS: ARB/Calcium channel blocker (dihydropyridine)

INDICATIONS: Treatment of HTN. May be used in patients whose BP is not adequately controlled on either monotherapy. May also be used as initial therapy in patients likely to need multiple drugs to achieve their BP goals.

DOSAGE: *Adults:* Initial: 5mg-160mg qd. Titrate: If inadequate control, may increase after 1-2 weeks of therapy. Max: 10mg-320mg qd. Add-On Therapy: May be used if BP not adequately controlled with amlodipine (or another dihydropyridine calcium channel blocker) alone or with valsartan (or another angiotensin II receptor blocker) alone. With dose-limiting adverse reactions to individual component, switch to amlodipine-valsartan containing a lower dose of that component in combination with the other. Titrate: May increase dose if BP remains uncontrolled after 3-4 weeks of therapy. Max: 10mg-320mg qd. Replacement Therapy: May substitute for titrated components. Elderly: Initial: 2.5mg amlodipine. Hepatic/Severe Renal Impairment: Titrate slowly.

HOW SUPPLIED: Tab: (Amlodipine-Valsartan) 5mg-160mg, 10mg-160mg, 5mg-320mg, 10mg-320mg

WARNINGS/PRECAUTIONS: Caution with hepatic impairment (including biliary obstructive disorders), heart failure (HF), recent myocardial infarction (MI), or surgery/dialysis. Amlodipine: Increased frequency, duration or severity of angina, or acute MI rarely reported with dosage initiation or increase, particularly with severe obstructive coronary artery disease (CAD). Caution in elderly and in patients with severe aortic stenosis. Valsartan: Symptomatic hypotension may occur in patients with an activated renin-angiotensin system (eg, volume- and/or salt-depleted patients receiving high doses of diuretics); correct volume depletion before therapy. Oliguria and/or progressive azotemia and (rarely) acute renal failure and/or death may occur in patients with severe HF whose renal function may depend on renin-angiotensin-aldosterone system activity. May increase BUN/SrCr with renal artery stenosis. Increased BUN, SrCr, and K+ reported in some patients with HF; dosage reduction and/or d/c may be required.

ADVERSE REACTIONS: Increased BUN, peripheral edema, nasopharyngitis, upper respiratory tract infection, hyperkalemia, dizziness.

INTERACTIONS: Amlodipine: May increase exposure to simvastatin; limit dose of simvastatin to 20mg daily. Valsartan: Greater antihypertensive effect with atenolol. May deteriorate renal function and attenuate antihypertensive effect with NSAIDs, including selective cyclooxygenase-2 inhibitors; monitor renal function periodically. K+ supplements, K+-sparing diuretics (eg, spironolactone, triamterene, amiloride), or salt substitutes containing K+ may increase SrCr in HF patients and serum K+. Inhibitors of the hepatic uptake transporter OATP1B1 (rifampin, cyclosporine) or the hepatic efflux transporter MRP2 (ritonavir) may increase exposure.

PREGNANCY: Category D, not for use in nursing.

MECHANISM OF ACTION: Amlodipine: Calcium channel blocker (dihydropyridine); inhibits transmembrane influx of calcium ions into vascular smooth muscle and cardiac muscle. Valsartan: Angiotensin II receptor blocker; blocks vasoconstrictor and aldosterone-secreting effects of angiotensin II by selectively blocking binding of angiotensin II to AT_1 receptor.

PHARMACOKINETICS: Absorption: Amlodipine: Absolute bioavailability (64-90%); T_{max}=6-12 hrs, 6-8 hrs (amlodipine-valsartan). Valsartan: Absolute bioavailability (25%); T_{max}=2-4 hrs, 3 hrs (amlodipine-valsartan). **Distribution:** Amlodipine: V_d=21L/kg; plasma protein binding (93%).

Valsartan: (IV) V_d=17L; plasma protein binding (95%). **Metabolism:** Amlodipine: Extensive, liver. Valsartan: Via CYP2C9; valeryl 4-hydroxy valsartan (metabolite). **Elimination:** Amlodipine: Urine (10%, parent compound; 60%, metabolites); $T_{1/2}$=30-50 hrs. Valsartan: (Sol) Feces (83%), urine (13%); (IV) $T_{1/2}$=6 hrs.

NURSING CONSIDERATIONS

Assessment: Assess for volume/salt depletion, HF, recent MI, severe aortic stenosis, severe obstructive CAD, renal/hepatic function, biliary obstruction, renal artery stenosis, pregnancy/nursing status, other conditions where treatment is cautioned, and possible drug interactions.

Monitoring: Monitor for signs/symptoms of hypotension, hyperkalemia, hypersensitivity reactions, renal/hepatic impairment, and symptoms of angina or MI at dosage initiation or increase. Monitor BP and renal function.

Patient Counseling: Counsel about risks/benefits of therapy and possible adverse effects. Inform of consequences of exposure during pregnancy; advise to notify physician if pregnant/plan to become pregnant as soon as possible.

Administration: Oral route. **Storage:** 25°C (77°F); excursions permitted to 15-30°C (59-86°F). Protect from moisture.

E

EXFORGE HCT

RX

amlodipine - valsartan - hydrochlorothiazide (Novartis)

D/C when pregnancy is detected. Drugs that act directly on the renin-angiotensin system can cause injury and death to the developing fetus.

THERAPEUTIC CLASS: ARB/Calcium channel blocker (dihydropyridine)/Thiazide diuretic

INDICATIONS: Treatment of HTN.

DOSAGE: *Adults:* May be given with other antihypertensive agents. Usual: Dose qd. May increase after 2 weeks. Max: 10mg-320mg-25mg qd. Add-On/Switch Therapy: Use if not adequately controlled on any 2 of the following antihypertensive classes: calcium channel blockers, angiotensin receptor blockers, and diuretics. With dose-limiting adverse reactions to any component on dual therapy, switch to triple therapy containing a lower dose of that component. Replacement Therapy: May substitute for individually titrated components.

HOW SUPPLIED: Tab: (Amlodipine-Valsartan-HCTZ) 5mg-160mg-12.5mg, 5mg-160mg-25mg, 10mg-160mg-12.5mg, 10mg-160mg-25mg, 10mg-320mg-25mg

CONTRAINDICATIONS: Anuria, sulfonamide-derived drug hypersensitivity.

WARNINGS/PRECAUTIONS: Not for initial therapy of HTN. Symptomatic hypotension may occur in patients with activated renin-angiotensin system (eg, volume- and/or salt-depleted patients receiving high doses of diuretics); correct these conditions prior to therapy. Not studied in heart failure (HF), recent myocardial infarction (MI), or patients undergoing surgery or dialysis. Renal function changes may occur; caution in patients with renal artery stenosis, chronic kidney disease, severe congestive HF, or volume depletion. Monitor renal function periodically and consider withholding or d/c if clinically significant decrease in renal function develops. Avoid with aortic or mitral stenosis or obstructive hypertrophic cardiomyopathy. Hypokalemia and hyperkalemia reported. Amlodipine: Increased frequency, duration or severity of angina, or acute MI rarely reported with dosage initiation or increase, particularly with severe obstructive coronary artery disease (CAD). Monitor fluid status, electrolytes, renal function, and BP in patients with HF. Valsartan: May increase BUN, SrCr, and K⁺ levels in some patients with HF; dose reduction and/or d/c may be required. HCTZ: May cause hypersensitivity reactions and exacerbation or activation of systemic lupus erythematosus (SLE). May precipitate hepatic coma with hepatic dysfunction or progressive liver disease. May cause idiosyncratic reaction, resulting in acute transient myopia and acute angle-closure glaucoma; d/c as rapidly as possible. May alter glucose tolerance and increase serum cholesterol and TG levels. May cause or exacerbate hyperuricemia and precipitate gout in susceptible patients. May decrease urinary calcium excretion and cause elevations of serum calcium; monitor calcium levels.

ADVERSE REACTIONS: Increased BUN, hypokalemia, dizziness, edema, headache, dyspepsia, fatigue, muscle spasms, back pain, nausea, nasopharyngitis.

INTERACTIONS: Amlodipine: May increase exposure to simvastatin; limit dose of simvastatin to 20mg daily. Valsartan: Greater antihypertensive effect with atenolol. NSAIDs, including selective cyclooxygenase-2 inhibitors may result in deterioration of renal function and attenuation of antihypertensive effect. K⁺ supplements, K⁺-sparing diuretics (eg, spironolactone, triamterene, amiloride), or salt substitutes containing K⁺ may increase SrCr in HF patients and serum K⁺. HCTZ: May increase risk of lithium toxicity; avoid concurrent use. Dosage adjustment of antidiabetic drugs (eg, oral agents, insulin) may be required. May lead to symptomatic hyponatremia with carbamazepine. Ion exchange resins (eg, cholestyramine, colestipol) may reduce exposure; space dosing ≥4 hrs before or 4-6 hrs after the administration of ion exchange resins. Cyclosporine may increase risk of hyperuricemia and gout-type complications. Alcohol, barbiturates, and narcotics may potentiate orthostatic hypotension. May increase responsiveness to skeletal muscle relaxants (eg, curare derivatives). Thiazide-induced hypokalemia or hypomagnesemia may predispose patient to digoxin toxicity. Anticholinergic agents (eg, atropine, biperiden) may increase bioavailability. Prokinetic drugs may decrease bioavailability. May reduce renal excretion and enhance myelosuppressive effects of cytotoxic agents.

PREGNANCY: Category D, not for use in nursing.

MECHANISM OF ACTION: Amlodipine: Calcium channel blocker (dihydropyridine); inhibits transmembrane influx of calcium ions into vascular smooth muscle and cardiac muscle. Valsartan: Angiotensin II receptor blocker; blocks vasoconstrictor and aldosterone-secreting effects of angiotensin II by selectively blocking binding of angiotensin II to AT_1 receptor. HCTZ: Thiazide diuretic; has not been established. Affects the renal tubular mechanisms of electrolyte reabsorption, directly increasing excretion of Na^+ and chloride in approximately equivalent amounts.

PHARMACOKINETICS: Absorption: Amlodipine: Absolute bioavailability (64-90%); T_{max}=6-12 hrs. Valsartan: Absolute bioavailability (25%); T_{max}=2-4 hrs. HCTZ: Absolute bioavailability (70%); T_{max}=2-5 hrs. **Distribution:** Amlodipine: V_d=21L/kg; plasma protein binding (93%). Valsartan: (IV) V_d=17L; plasma protein binding (95%). HCTZ: Plasma protein binding (40-70%). Crosses placenta; found in breast milk. **Metabolism:** Amlodipine: Extensive, liver. Valsartan: Via CYP2C9; valeryl-4-hydroxy valsartan (metabolite). **Elimination:** Amlodipine: Urine (10%, parent; 60%, metabolites); $T_{1/2}$=30-50 hrs. Valsartan: (Sol) Feces (83%), urine (13%); (IV) $T_{1/2}$=6 hrs. HCTZ: Urine (70%, unchanged); $T_{1/2}$=10 hrs.

NURSING CONSIDERATIONS

Assessment: Assess for hypersensitivity to drugs and its components, anuria, sulfonamide-derived drug or penicillin hypersensitivity, history of allergy or bronchial asthma, renal/hepatic function, HF, recent MI, aortic or mitral stenosis, renal artery stenosis, obstructive hypertrophic cardiomyopathy, SLE, volume/salt depletion, electrolyte imbalances, CAD, pregnancy/nursing status, other conditions where treatment is cautioned, and possible drug interactions.

Monitoring: Monitor for signs/symptoms of hypotension, hypersensitivity reactions, idiosyncratic reaction, metabolic disturbances, myopia and angle-closure glaucoma (eg, decreased visual acuity, ocular pain), renal function, symptoms of angina or MI after dosage initiation or increase, fluid or electrolyte imbalance, exacerbation or activation of SLE, hyperglycemia, hyperuricemia or precipitation of gout, and increases in cholesterol and TG. Monitor BP, serum electrolytes, BUN, and SrCr.

Patient Counseling: Counsel about risks/benefits of therapy and possible adverse effects. Inform of consequences of exposure during pregnancy; notify physician if pregnant/plan to become pregnant as soon as possible. Caution about lightheadedness, especially during the 1st days of therapy, and advise to report to physician. Instruct to d/c and consult physician if syncope occurs. Caution that inadequate fluid intake, excessive perspiration, diarrhea, or vomiting may lead to an excessive fall in BP, which may result in lightheadedness or syncope. Instruct to avoid K^+ supplements or salt substitutes containing K^+ without consulting a physician.

Administration: Oral route. **Storage:** 25°C (77°F); excursions permitted to 15-30°C (59-86°F). Protect from moisture.

EXTAVIA   RX
interferon beta-1b (Novartis)

THERAPEUTIC CLASS: Biological response modifier

INDICATIONS: Treatment of relapsing forms of multiple sclerosis to reduce the frequency of clinical exacerbations.

DOSAGE: *Adults:* Initial: 0.0625mg SQ qod. Titrate: Increase over 6 weeks to 0.25mg qod SQ. Refer to PI for dose titration schedule.

HOW SUPPLIED: Inj: 0.3mg

CONTRAINDICATIONS: Hypersensitivity to human albumin.

WARNINGS/PRECAUTIONS: Caution in patients with depression. Increased frequency of depression and suicide reported; consider d/c if depression develops. Inj-site necrosis reported; d/c if multiple lesions occur. Inj-site reactions reported. Anaphylaxis/allergic reactions (eg, dyspnea, bronchospasm, tongue edema, skin rash, urticaria), flu-like symptom complex, leukopenia, and hepatic enzyme elevation (ALT, AST) reported. Contains albumin; risk of viral disease transmission.

ADVERSE REACTIONS: Inj-site reactions/necrosis, flu-like symptom complex, headache, lymphopenia, hypertonia, asthenia, increased liver enzymes, skin disorder, insomnia, abdominal pain, incoordination, neutropenia, leukopenia, lymphadenopathy.

PREGNANCY: Category C, not for use in nursing.

MECHANISM OF ACTION: Biological response modifier; not established. Believed that interferon β-1b receptor binding induces expression of proteins that are responsible for pleiotropic bioactivities. Immunomodulatory effects include the enhancement of suppressor T cell activity, reduction of proinflammatory cytokine production, down-regulation of antigen presentation, and inhibition of lymphocyte trafficking into the CNS.

NURSING CONSIDERATIONS

Assessment: Assess for hypersensitivity to the drug or human albumin, depression, thyroid dysfunction, liver function, myelosuppression, and pregnancy/nursing status.

Monitoring: Monitor for anaphylaxis, depression, suicidal ideation, inj-site reactions, inj-site necrosis, and flu-like symptom complex. Monitor CBC, differential WBC, platelet count, LFTs, and blood chemistry at regular intervals (1, 3, and 6 months) following introduction, then periodically thereafter. Perform thyroid function test every 6 months with history of thyroid dysfunction or as clinically indicated.

Patient Counseling: Inform about potential benefits/risks of therapy. Advise not to change dose or schedule of administration. Inform that depression and suicidal ideation, inj-site reactions, inj-site necrosis, allergic reactions and anaphylaxis may occur; advise to d/c and notify physician if symptoms are experienced. Inform that antipyretics and analgesics are permitted for relief of flu-like symptoms which are common following initiation of therapy. Advise to notify physician if pregnant or become pregnant. Instruct on how to administer therapy.

Administration: SQ route. Rotate inj sites. Refer to PI for reconstitution instructions. **Storage:** 25°C (77°F); excursions permitted to 15-30°C (59-86°F). After reconstitution, if not used immediately, refrigerate and use within 3 hrs. Avoid freezing.

EXTINA   RX
ketoconazole (Stiefel)

THERAPEUTIC CLASS: Azole antifungal

INDICATIONS: Topical treatment of seborrheic dermatitis in immunocompetent patients ≥12 yrs of age.

DOSAGE: *Adults:* Apply to affected area(s) bid for 4 weeks.
Pediatrics: ≥12 yrs: Apply to affected area(s) bid for 4 weeks.

HOW SUPPLIED: Foam: 2% [50g, 100g]

WARNINGS/PRECAUTIONS: Not for ophthalmic, oral, or intravaginal use. Safety and efficacy for the treatment of fungal infections not established. May cause contact sensitization, including photoallergenicity. Contents are flammable; avoid fire, flame, and/or smoking during and immediately following application. Hepatitis, lowered testoterone, and adrenocorticotropic hormone-induced corticosteroid serum levels reported with orally administered ketoconazole; not seen with topical ketoconazole.

ADVERSE REACTIONS: Application-site burning, application-site reactions (eg, dryness, erythema, irritation, paresthesia, pruritus, rash, warmth), photoallergenicity, contact sensitization.

PREGNANCY: Category C, caution in nursing.

MECHANISM OF ACTION: Azole antifungal; not established. Inhibits the synthesis of ergosterol, a key sterol in the cell membrane of *Malassezia furfur*.

PHARMACOKINETICS: Absorption: C_{max}=11ng/mL.

NURSING CONSIDERATIONS

Assessment: Assess pregnancy/nursing status.

Monitoring: Monitor for contact sensitization reactions, and application-site reactions.

Patient Counseling: Instruct to use ud. Instruct to avoid fire, flame and/or smoking during and immediately following application. Instruct not to apply directly to hands; apply to affected areas using the fingertips. Inform that skin irritation, and contact sensitization may occur; instruct to inform a physician if the area show signs of increased irritation, and to report any signs of adverse reactions. Instruct to wash hands after application.

Administration: Topical route. Refer to PI for proper administration techniques. **Storage:** 20-25°C (68-77°F). Do not store under refrigerated conditions or in direct sunlight. Do not expose containers to heat or store at temperatures above 49°C (120°F). Do not puncture and/or incinerate container.

EYLEA

RX

aflibercept (Regeneron)

THERAPEUTIC CLASS: Vascular endothelial growth factor (VEGF) inhibitor

INDICATIONS: Treatment of neovascular (wet) age-related macular degeneration.

DOSAGE: *Adults:* 2mg (0.05mL) by intravitreal inj q4 weeks for the 1st 12 weeks, then q8 weeks thereafter.

HOW SUPPLIED: Inj: 40mg/mL

CONTRAINDICATIONS: Ocular or periocular infections, and active intraocular inflammation.

WARNINGS/PRECAUTIONS: Endophthalmitis or retinal detachments may occur; always use proper aseptic inj technique. Acute increases in intraocular pressure (IOP) noted within 60 min of inj; IOP and perfusion of the optic nerve head should be monitored and managed appropriately. Potential risk of arterial thromboembolic events (ATEs) (eg, nonfatal stroke, nonfatal myocardial infarction, or vascular death).

ADVERSE REACTIONS: Conjunctival hemorrhage/hyperemia, eye pain, cataract, vitreous detachment/floaters, increased IOP, corneal erosion, retinal pigment epithelium detachment, inj-site pain, foreign body sensation in eyes, increased lacrimation.

PREGNANCY: Category C, not for use in nursing.

MECHANISM OF ACTION: VEGF inhibitor; acts as a soluble decoy receptor that binds VEGF-A and placental growth factor, and thereby can inhibit the binding and activation of these cognate VEGF receptors.

PHARMACOKINETICS: Absorption: C_{max}=0.02mcg/mL, T_{max}=1-3 days. **Distribution:** (IV) V_d=6L. **Metabolism:** Proteolysis. **Elimination:** (IV) $T_{1/2}$=5-6 days.

NURSING CONSIDERATIONS

Assessment: Assess for ocular or periocular infections, active intraocular inflammation, hypersensitivity to drug, and pregnancy/nursing status.

Monitoring: Monitor IOP and perfusion of the optic nerve head. Monitor for signs/symptoms of endophthalmitis, retinal detachment, and ATEs.

Patient Counseling: Inform that temporary visual disturbances may be experienced after inj and the associated eye examinations; advise not to drive or use machinery until visual function has recovered sufficiently. Instruct to seek immediate care from an ophthalmologist if eye becomes red, sensitive to light, painful, or develops a change in vision in the days following administration.

Administration: Intravitreal route. Administer under controlled aseptic conditions. Give adequate anesthesia and a topical broad-spectrum microbicide prior to inj. Refer to PI for preparation and administration instructions. **Storage:** 2-8°C (36-46°F). Do not freeze. Protect from light.

FACTIVE

RX

gemifloxacin mesylate (Cornerstone)

Fluoroquinolones are associated with an increased risk of tendinitis and tendon rupture in all ages. Risk is further increased in patients >60 yrs, patients taking corticosteroids, and with kidney, heart, or lung transplants. May exacerbate muscle weakness with myasthenia gravis; avoid in patients with known history of myasthenia gravis.

THERAPEUTIC CLASS: Fluoroquinolone

INDICATIONS: Treatment of community-acquired pneumonia (CAP) and acute bacterial exacerbation of chronic bronchitis (ABECB) caused by susceptible strains of microorganisms.

DOSAGE: *Adults:* ≥18 yrs: ABECB: 320mg qd for 5 days. CAP: 320mg qd for 5 days (*S. pneumoniae, H. influenzae, M. pneumoniae,* or *C. pneumoniae*) or 7 days (multi-drug resistant *S. pneumoniae, K. pneumoniae,* or *M. catarrhalis*). CrCl ≤40mL/min or Dialysis: 160mg q24h.

HOW SUPPLIED: Tab: 320mg

WARNINGS/PRECAUTIONS: D/C if pain, swelling, inflammation, or rupture of a tendon occurs. May prolong QT interval; avoid with history of QTc interval prolongation or uncontrolled electrolyte disorders, and caution with proarrhythmic conditions. Serious and sometimes fatal hypersensitivity reactions reported; d/c if skin rash, jaundice, or any other sign of hypersensitivity appears and institute appropriate therapy. Rare cases of sensory or sensorimotor axonal polyneuropathy resulting in paresthesias, hypoesthesias, dysesthesias, and weakness reported. CNS effects (infrequent) reported; caution with CNS diseases (eg, epilepsy or patients predisposed to convulsions), and d/c if CNS stimulation occurs. Convulsions, toxic psychoses, and increased intracranial pressure (including pseudotumor cerebri) reported. *Clostridium difficile*-associated diarrhea (CDAD) reported; consider d/c if CDAD suspected or confirmed. May cause photosensitivity/phototoxicity reactions; d/c if photosensitivity/phototoxicity occurs. Avoid excessive exposure to source of light. Liver enzyme elevations reported. Caution in elderly and with renal impairment. Maintain adequate hydration. Increased risk of development of drug-resistant bacteria if used in the absence of a strongly suspected bacterial infection.

ADVERSE REACTIONS: Diarrhea, rash, N/V, headache, abdominal pain, dizziness.

INTERACTIONS: See Boxed Warning. Avoid magnesium- or aluminum-containing antacids, ferrous sulfate (iron), Videx (didanosine) chewable/buffered tab or pediatric powder for oral sol, and multivitamin preparations containing zinc or other metal cations, within 3 hrs before or 2 hrs after therapy and sucralfate within 2 hrs of therapy. Calcium carbonate may decrease levels. Reduced levels with oral estrogen/progesterone contraceptive product. Increased levels with cimetidine, omeprazole, probenecid. Avoid Class IA (eg, quinidine, procainamide) or Class III (eg, amiodarone, sotalol) antiarrhythmics. Caution with drugs that prolong the QTc interval (eg, erythromycin, antipsychotics, TCAs). Increased INR or PT and/or clinical episodes of bleeding reported with warfarin or its derivatives.

PREGNANCY: Category C, not for use in nursing.

MECHANISM OF ACTION: Fluoroquinolone; inhibits DNA synthesis through inhibition of both DNA gyrase and topoisomerase IV, which are essential for bacterial growth.

PHARMACOKINETICS: Absorption: Rapid. Absolute bioavailability (71%); AUC=8.36µg•hr/mL, C_{max}=1.61µg/mL, T_{max}=0.5-2 hrs. **Distribution:** V_d=4.18L/kg; plasma protein binding (55-73%). **Metabolism:** Liver. **Elimination:** Feces (61%), urine (36% unchanged); $T_{1/2}$=7 hrs.

NURSING CONSIDERATIONS

Assessment: Assess for hypersensitivity to drug, factors that increase the risk of tendon rupture, history of myasthenia gravis and QTc interval prolongation, uncontrolled electrolyte disorders, proarrhythmic conditions, CNS disease, pregnancy/nursing status, and possible drug interactions. Obtain baseline renal function and LFTs.

Monitoring: Monitor for signs/symptoms of tendinitis or tendon rupture, muscle weakness exacerbation, hypersensitivity and photosensitivity/phototoxicity reactions, peripheral neuropathy, CNS effects, and CDAD. Monitor renal function and LFTs.

Patient Counseling: Instruct to contact physician and advise to rest, refrain from exercise, and d/c therapy if pain, swelling, or inflammation of a tendon, or weakness or inability to move joints occur. Inform that drug may worsen myasthenia gravis symptoms; immediately contact physician if muscle weakness worsens or breathing problems occur. Inform that drug treats bacterial, not viral, infections. Instruct to take drug exactly as directed, swallow whole, drink fluids liberally, and not to skip doses. Instruct to d/c therapy and notify physician if rash or other allergic reaction develops. Counsel to notify physician if watery and bloody stools, palpitations, sunburn-like reaction, or skin eruption occur, and about medications taken concurrently. Instruct not to engage in activities requiring mental alertness and coordination if dizziness occurs, and to minimize or avoid sun/UV light exposure.

Administration: Oral route. Swallow whole with fluids. **Storage:** 25°C (77°F); excursions permitted to 15-30°C (59-86°F). Protect from light.

FAMOTIDINE   RX
famotidine (Various)

OTHER BRAND NAMES: Pepcid Tablet (Merck) - Pepcid Oral Suspension (Salix)

THERAPEUTIC CLASS: H_2-blocker

INDICATIONS: Short-term treatment of active duodenal ulcer (DU), active benign gastric ulcer (GU), gastroesophageal reflux disease (GERD), and esophagitis due to GERD, including erosive or ulcerative disease. Maintenance therapy for DU patients at reduced dosage after the healing of an active ulcer. Treatment of pathological hypersecretory conditions (eg, Zollinger-Ellison syndrome, multiple endocrine adenomas). (Inj) Indicated in some hospitalized patients with pathological hypersecretory conditions or intractable ulcers, or as an alternative to oral dosage forms for short-term use in patients who are unable to take oral medication.

DOSAGE: *Adults:* (PO) DU: Usual: 40mg qhs or 20mg bid for 4-8 weeks. Maint: 20mg qhs. Benign GU: Usual: 40mg qhs. (Inj) Intractable Ulcer: Usual: 20mg IV q12h. (PO) GERD: Usual: 20mg bid for up to 6 weeks. (PO) GERD with Esophagitis: 20-40mg bid for up to 12 weeks. Hypersecretory Conditions: Initial: (PO) 20mg q6h. Max: 160mg q6h. (Inj) Usual: 20mg IV q12h; higher starting dose may be required in some patients. Adjust dose according to individual patient needs and continue as long as indicated. Moderate (CrCl <50mL/min) or Severe (CrCl <10mL/min) Renal Impairment: Reduce to 1/2 dose, or increase dosing interval to q36-48h.
Pediatrics: 1-16 yrs: Peptic Ulcer: Usual: (PO) 0.5mg/kg/day qhs or divided bid. Max: 40mg/day. (Inj) 0.25mg/kg IV over a period not <2 min or as 15-min infusion q12h. Max: 40mg/day. Individualized based on clinical response, gastric pH determination, and endoscopy. GERD with or without Esophagitis: (PO) 1mg/kg/day divided bid. Max: 40mg bid. (Inj) 0.25mg/kg IV over

not <2 min or as 15-min infusion q12h. Max: 40mg/day. Individualized based on clinical response, gastric pH determination, and endoscopy. 3 months-<1 yr: (PO) GERD: 0.5mg/kg bid for up to 8 weeks. <3 months: (PO) GERD: 0.5mg/kg qd for up to 8 weeks. Moderate (CrCl <50mL/min) or Severe (CrCl <10mL/min) Renal Impairment: Reduce to 1/2 dose, or increase dosing interval to q36-48h.

HOW SUPPLIED: Inj: 10mg/mL [2mL, 4mL, 20mL], 20mg/50mL [50mL]; Sus: (Pepcid) 40mg/5mL; Tab: (Pepcid) 20mg, 40mg

WARNINGS/PRECAUTIONS: Symptomatic response to therapy does not preclude presence of gastric malignancy. CNS adverse effects reported with moderate to severe renal insufficiency; may need to prolong dosing intervals or reduce dose. (Inj) For IV use only. Inj from multiple-dose vials contains benzyl alcohol; avoid in neonates and pregnant women. (Tab) Prolonged QT interval reported (very rare) in patients with impaired renal function whose dose interval may not have been adjusted appropriately.

ADVERSE REACTIONS: Headache, dizziness, constipation, diarrhea, agitation.

INTERACTIONS: (PO) Bioavailability may be slightly decreased by antacids.

PREGNANCY: Category B, not for use in nursing.

MECHANISM OF ACTION: Histamine H_2-receptor antagonist; inhibits both acid concentration and volume of gastric secretion.

PHARMACOKINETICS: Absorption: (PO) Incompletely absorbed; bioavailability (40-45%); T_{max}=1-3 hrs. **Distribution:** Plasma protein binding (15-20%); found in breast milk. **Metabolism:** Minimal first-pass metabolism; S-oxide (metabolite). **Elimination:** Renal (65-70%; 25-30% unchanged [PO], 65-70% unchanged [IV]); metabolic (30-35%); $T_{1/2}$=2.5-3.5 hrs. Refer to PI for pediatric parameters.

NURSING CONSIDERATIONS

Assessment: Assess for hypersensitivity to drug and to other H_2-receptor antagonists, renal function, pregnancy/nursing status, and possible drug interactions.

Monitoring: Monitor for renal function, signs/symptoms of hypersensitivity reactions, and other adverse reactions.

Patient Counseling: Inform risks/benefits of therapy. Instruct to contact physician if hypersensitivity or other adverse reactions develop. Inform that antacids may be taken concomitantly. Advise to avoid nursing while on medication. Instruct to shake oral sus vigorously for 5-10 sec prior to each use. Instruct to discard unused constituted sus after 30 days.

Administration: IV and Oral route. May be given with antacids if needed. Refer to PI for directions for preparing oral sus and preparation/stability of inj/premixed inj. **Storage:** (Inj) 2-8°C (36-46°). Bring to room temperature and solubilize if sol freezes. Diluted sol should be refrigerated and used within 48 hrs. (Premixed Inj) 25°C (77°F); avoid exposure to excessive heat; brief exposure to temperatures up to 35°C (95°F) does not adversely affect product. (Tab) Controlled room temperature; preserve in well-closed, light-resistant container. (Sus) 25°C (77°F); excursions permitted to 15-30°C (59-86°F). Protect from freezing. Discard unused sus after 30 days.

FAMVIR   RX
famciclovir (Novartis)

THERAPEUTIC CLASS: Nucleoside analogue

INDICATIONS: Treatment of herpes zoster (shingles) and recurrent herpes labialis (cold sores). Treatment or suppression of recurrent genital herpes. Treatment of recurrent episodes of orolabial/genital herpes in HIV-infected adults.

DOSAGE: *Adults:* Immunocompetent Patients: Herpes Labialis: 1500mg as a single dose; initiate at the 1st sign/symptoms (eg, tingling, itching, burning, pain, or lesion). Genital Herpes: Recurrent Episodes: 1000mg bid for 1 day; initiate at the 1st sign/symptoms. Suppressive Therapy: 250mg bid. Herpes Zoster: 500mg q8h for 7 days; initiate as soon as herpes zoster is diagnosed. HIV-Infected Patients: Recurrent Orolabial/Genital Herpes: 500mg bid for 7 days; initiate at the first sign/symptoms. Refer to PI for dosage recommendations for renal impairment.

HOW SUPPLIED: Tab: 125mg, 250mg, 500mg

WARNINGS/PRECAUTIONS: Acute renal failure reported. Caution in elderly and with renal impairment. Not for use in patients with first episode of genital herpes, with ophthalmic zoster, with immunocompromised patients other than for the treatment of recurrent orolabial or genital herpes in HIV-infected patients, and black/African American patients with recurrent genital herpes.

ADVERSE REACTIONS: Headache, N/V, diarrhea, elevated lipase, ALT elevation, fatigue, flatulence, pruritus, rash, neutropenia, abdominal pain, dysmenorrhea, migraine.

INTERACTIONS: Probenecid or other drugs significantly eliminated by active renal tubular secretion may increase levels. Potential interaction with drugs metabolized by and/or inhibiting aldehyde oxidase may occur. Raloxifene may decrease formation of penciclovir.

PREGNANCY: Category B, not for use in nursing.

MECHANISM OF ACTION: Nucleoside analogue; inhibits HSV-2 DNA polymerase competitively with deoxyguanosine triphosphate, inhibiting herpes viral DNA synthesis and replication.

PHARMACOKINETICS: Absorption: Absolute bioavailability (77% penciclovir); parameters varied for different doses. **Distribution:** V_d=1.08L/kg (IV penciclovir); plasma protein binding (<20% penciclovir). **Metabolism:** Deacetylation and oxidation; famciclovir (prodrug) converted to penciclovir. **Elimination:** Urine (73%), feces (27%); $T_{1/2}$=2.8 hrs (single dose), 2.7 hrs (repeated doses).

NURSING CONSIDERATIONS

Assessment: Assess for renal dysfunction, hypersensitivity to drug, pregnancy/nursing status, and possible drug interactions.

Monitoring: Monitor for acute renal failure and hypersensitivity reactions. Monitor CrCl and maternal-fetal outcomes of pregnant women exposed to the drug.

Patient Counseling: Inform to take exactly as directed. Advise to initiate treatment at earliest signs/symptoms of recurrence of cold sores, at the 1st sign/symptom of recurrent genital herpes if episodic therapy is indicated, and immediately once diagnosed with herpes zoster. Inform that drug is not a cure for cold sores or genital herpes. Instruct not to exceed 1 dose for cold sores. Advise to avoid contact with lesions or intercourse when lesions and/or symptoms are present to avoid infecting partners. Counsel to use safer sex practices. Instruct to refrain from driving or operating machinery if dizziness, somnolence, or confusion, or other CNS disturbances occur. Inform that drug contains lactose; notify physician if with rare genetic problems of galactose intolerance, severe lactase deficiency/glucose-galactose malabsorption, and if pregnant or plan to become pregnant.

Administration: Oral route. **Storage:** 25°C (77°F); excursions permitted to 15-30°C (59-86°F).

FANAPT   RX
iloperidone (Novartis)

> Elderly patients with dementia-related psychosis treated with antipsychotic drugs are at an increased risk of death; most deaths appeared to be cardiovascular (CV) (eg, heart failure, sudden death) or infectious (eg, pneumonia) in nature. Not approved for the treatment of patients with dementia-related psychosis.

THERAPEUTIC CLASS: Benzisoxazole derivative

INDICATIONS: Treatment of adults with schizophrenia.

DOSAGE: *Adults:* Initial: 1mg bid. Titrate: Titrate slowly from low starting dose. Day 2: 2mg bid. Day 3: 4mg bid. Day 4: 6mg bid. Day 5: 8mg bid. Day 6: 10mg bid. Day 7: 12mg bid. Range: 6-12mg bid. Max: 12mg bid (24mg/day). Concomitant Strong CYP2D6/CYP3A4 Inhibitors: Reduce dose by 50%. Increase to previous iloperidone dose upon withdrawal of CYP2D6/CYP3A4 inhibitors. Poor CYP2D6 Metabolizers: Reduce dose by 50%. Maint: Responding patients may continue beyond acute response; periodically reassess need for maintenance treatment. Reinitiation of Treatment: Follow initial titration schedule if have had an interval off for >3 days. Switching From Other Antipsychotics: Minimize overlapping period of antipsychotics.

HOW SUPPLIED: Tab: 1mg, 2mg, 4mg, 6mg, 8mg, 10mg, 12mg

WARNINGS/PRECAUTIONS: Avoid with hepatic impairment. QT prolongation reported; avoid with congenital long QT syndrome, history of cardiac arrhythmias, or history of significant CV illnesses. Obtain baseline measurements and periodically monitor K^+ and magnesium levels in patients at risk of electrolyte disturbances. D/C if persistent QTc measurements >500 msec occur. Risk of tardive dyskinesia (TD), especially in the elderly; consider d/c if signs/symptoms develop. Neuroleptic malignant syndrome (NMS) reported; d/c and treat immediately. May cause metabolic changes (hyperglycemia, dyslipidemia, weight gain) that may increase CV and cerebrovascular risk. Hyperglycemia, in some cases extreme and associated with ketoacidosis or hyperosmolar coma or death reported; monitor for worsening of glucose control, and perform FPG testing at the beginning of therapy and periodically in patients at risk for diabetes mellitus (DM). Undesirable alterations in lipids and weight gain reported. Caution with history of seizures or conditions that lower seizure threshold. May induce orthostatic hypotension; caution with cardiovascular disease (CVD), cerebrovascular disease, or conditions that predispose to hypotension. Leukopenia, neutropenia, and agranulocytosis reported; d/c in cases of severe neutropenia (absolute neutrophil count <1000/mm³). Monitor CBC and d/c at 1st sign of decline in WBC if with preexisting low WBC count or history of drug-induced leukopenia/neutropenia. May elevate prolactin levels. May disrupt body's ability to reduce core body temperature; caution in conditions that may elevate body core temperature. Esophageal dysmotility and aspiration reported; caution in patients at risk of aspiration pneumonia. Closely supervise high-risk patients for suicide attempt. Priapism reported. May impair mental/physical abilities.

ADVERSE REACTIONS: Dizziness, somnolence, tachycardia, nausea, dry mouth, weight gain, nasal congestion, diarrhea, fatigue, extrapyramidal disorder, orthostatic hypotension, nasopharyngitis, arthralgia, tremor.

INTERACTIONS: May increase levels with concomitant use of CYP3A4 (eg, ketoconazole, clarithromycin) or CYP2D6 (eg, fluoxetine, paroxetine) inhibitors; concomitant use may augment effect on QTc interval. May increase total exposure of dextromethorphan with concomitant use. Avoid with Class IA (eg, quinidine, procainamide) or Class III (eg, amiodarone, sotalol) antiarrhythmics, antipsychotics (eg, chlorpromazine, thioridazine), antibiotics (eg, gatifloxacin, moxifloxacin), or other drugs known to prolong QTc interval (eg, pentamidine, levomethadyl acetate, methadone). Caution with other centrally acting drugs and alcohol. May potentiate effects of antihypertensive agents. Concomitant use with medications with anticholinergic activity may contribute to an elevation in core body temperature.

PREGNANCY: Category C, not for use in nursing.

MECHANISM OF ACTION: Piperidinyl-benzisoxazole derivative; not established. Proposed to be mediated through a combination of dopamine type 2 (D_2) and serotonin type 2 (5-HT_2) antagonisms.

PHARMACOKINETICS: Absorption: Well absorbed; T_{max}=2-4 hrs. **Distribution:** V_d=1340-2800L; plasma protein binding (95%). **Metabolism:** Liver via carbonyl reduction, hydroxylation (CYP2D6), O-demethylation (CYP3A4); P88, P95 (major metabolites). **Elimination:** Urine (58.2% in extensive metabolizers [EM], 45.1% in poor metabolizers [PM]), feces (19.9% [EM], 22.1% [PM]); $T_{1/2}$= 18 hrs (EM), 33 hrs (PM).

NURSING CONSIDERATIONS

Assessment: Assess for known hypersensitivity to the drug, dementia-related psychosis, hepatic impairment, DM, risk factors for DM, CVD, cerebrovascular disease, conditions that predispose to hypotension, history of clinically significant low WBCs or drug-induced leukopenia/neutropenia, history of seizures, risk for aspiration pneumonia, risk for suicide, pregnancy/nursing status, and possible drug interactions. Obtain baseline FPG in patients with DM and risk factors for DM. Perform baseline CBC, orthostatic vital signs, serum K+ and magnesium levels.

Monitoring: Monitor for TD, NMS, priapism, extrapyramidal symptoms, cerebrovascular events, CVD, esophageal dysmotility, aspiration, orthostatic hypotension, body temperature lability, seizures, QT prolongation, suicide attempts, and cognitive/motor impairment. Monitor for signs of hyperglycemia; periodically monitor FPG levels in patients with DM or at risk for DM. Monitor for weight gain. Monitor for signs/symptoms of leukopenia, neutropenia, and agranulocytosis; frequently monitor CBC in patients with risk factors for leukopenia/neutropenia. Monitor serum K+ and magnesium levels, and orthostatic vital signs.

Patient Counseling: Advise to inform physician immediately if feeling faint, lose consciousness or have heart palpitations. Counsel to avoid drugs that cause QT interval prolongation and inform physician if taking or plan to take any drug (prescription or over-the-counter drugs). Inform about the signs/symptoms of NMS, hyperglycemia, and DM. Counsel that weight gain may occur during treatment. Advise of risk of orthostatic hypotension particularly at time of initiating/re-initiating treatment, or increasing dose. Inform that the drug may impair judgment, thinking, or motor skills; advise to use caution against driving or operating hazardous machinery. Instruct to notify physician if pregnant or intend to become pregnant. Advise not to breastfeed. Instruct to avoid alcohol. Counsel about appropriate care to avoid overheating and dehydration.

Administration: Oral route. **Storage:** 25°C (77°F); excursions permitted to 15-30°C (59-86°F). Protect from light and moisture.

FASLODEX   **RX**
fulvestrant (AstraZeneca)

THERAPEUTIC CLASS: Estrogen receptor antagonist

INDICATIONS: Treatment of hormone receptor positive metastatic breast cancer in postmenopausal women with disease progression following antiestrogen therapy.

DOSAGE: *Adults:* Usual: 500mg IM into buttocks slowly (1-2 min/inj) as two 5-mL inj, one in each buttock. Moderate Hepatic Impairment (Child-Pugh Class B): Usual: 250mg IM into buttock slowly (1-2 min) as one 5-mL inj. Administer on Days 1, 15, 29, and once monthly thereafter.

HOW SUPPLIED: Inj: 50mg/mL [5mL]

WARNINGS/PRECAUTIONS: Caution with bleeding diatheses and thrombocytopenia. Not studied in severe hepatic impairment (Child-Pugh Class C). May cause fetal harm during pregnancy.

ADVERSE REACTIONS: Inj-site pain, headache, back pain, diarrhea, N/V, bone pain, fatigue, pain in extremity, asthenia, hot flash, anorexia, musculoskeletal pain, cough, dyspnea.

INTERACTIONS: Caution with anticoagulant use.

PREGNANCY: Category D, not for use in nursing.

MECHANISM OF ACTION: Estrogen receptor antagonist; binds to estrogen receptor (ER) and downregulates ER protein in human breast cancer cells.

PHARMACOKINETICS: Absorption: (Single dose) C_{max}=25.1ng/mL; AUC=11,400ng•hr/mL. (Multiple dose) C_{max}=28ng/mL; AUC=13,100ng•hr/mL. **Distribution:** V_d=3-5L/kg; plasma protein binding (99%). **Metabolism:** CYP3A4 (oxidation), aromatic hydroxylation, conjugation. **Elimination:** Feces (90%), urine (<1%); $T_{1/2}$=40 days.

NURSING CONSIDERATIONS

Assessment: Assess for hypersensitivity to drug, pregnancy/nursing status, bleeding diatheses, thrombocytopenia, hepatic impairment, and possible drug interactions.

Monitoring: Monitor for inj-site reactions, hepatic impairment, and other adverse reactions.

Patient Counseling: Inform to avoid pregnancy and breastfeeding while taking drug. Counsel on side effects and symptoms of an allergic reaction; instruct to seek medical attention if any develop.

Administration: IM route. Refer to PI for further administration instructions. **Storage:** 2-8°C (36-46°F). Protect from light. Store in original carton until time of use.

FAZACLO   RX
clozapine (Azur)

> Risk of potentially life-threatening agranulocytosis. Reserve use for severely ill patients with schizophrenia unresponsive to standard antipsychotic treatment or for patients with schizophrenia/schizoaffective disorder at risk for re-experiencing suicidal behavior. Obtain baseline WBC count and absolute neutrophil count (ANC) prior to therapy, regularly during treatment, and for at least 4 weeks after d/c. Seizures associated with use and with greater likelihood at higher doses; caution with history of seizures or other predisposing factors. Increased risk of fatal myocarditis, especially during 1st month of therapy; d/c if suspected. Orthostatic hypotension, with or without syncope can occur. Rare reports of profound collapse with respiratory and/or cardiac arrest in patients taking benzodiazepines or any other psychotropic drugs. Elderly patients with dementia-related psychosis treated with atypical antipsychotic drugs are at an increased risk for death. Not approved for the treatment of dementia-related psychosis.

THERAPEUTIC CLASS: Dibenzapine derivative

INDICATIONS: Management of severely ill schizophrenic patients who fail to respond adequately to standard drug treatment for schizophrenia. Reduction of risk for recurrent suicidal behavior in patients with schizophrenia/schizoaffective disorder who are judged to be at chronic risk for re-experiencing suicidal behavior.

DOSAGE: *Adults:* Treatment-Resistant Schizophrenia: Initial: 12.5mg qd-bid. Titrate: Increase by 25-50mg/day, up to 300-450mg/day by end of 2 weeks; then increase by no more than once or twice weekly in increments not to exceed 100mg. Usual: 300-600mg/day given on a divided basis. Titrate: May increase to 600-900mg/day. Max: 900mg/day. Maint: Lowest effective dos. To d/c, gradually reduce dose over 1-2 weeks. Monitor for psychotic and cholinergic rebound symptoms if abrupt d/c warranted (eg, leukopenia). Reinitiation (even with brief interval off clozapine): Start with 12.5mg qd-bid; may titrate more quickly if initial dosing tolerated. Do not restart if d/c for WBC <2000/mm³ or absolute neutrophil count (ANC) <1000/mm³. Reduction of Risk of Recurrent Suicidal Behavior in Schizophrenia/Schizoaffective Disorder: May follow dosing recommendations for treatment-resistant schizophrenia or schizoaffective disorder. Range: 12.5-900mg/day (mean 300mg). Refer to PI for recommendations to reduce the risk of recurrent suicidal behavior who previously responded to treatment with another antipsychotic medication.

HOW SUPPLIED: Tab, Disintegrating: 12.5mg, 25mg, 100mg, 150mg, 200mg

CONTRAINDICATIONS: Myeloproliferative disorders, uncontrolled epilepsy, paralytic ileus, history of clozapine-induced agranulocytosis or severe granulocytopenia, severe CNS depression, comatose states. Concomitant use with agents with potential to cause agranulocytosis or suppress bone marrow function.

WARNINGS/PRECAUTIONS: QT prolongation, ventricular arrhythmia, torsades de pointes, cardiac arrest and sudden death may occur. Caution with history or family history of long QT syndrome, history of or other conditions that may increase risk for QT prolongation, recent acute myocardial infarction, uncompensated heart failure (HF), cardiac arrhythmia, cardiovascular disease (CVD), risk for significant electrolyte disturbance (eg, hypokalemia, hypomagnesemia). D/C if QTc interval >500 msec. Hyperglycemia, sometimes with ketoacidosis, hyperosmolar coma or death, reported. Monitor for worsening of glucose control with diabetes mellitus (DM) and fasting blood glucose (FBG) levels with diabetes risk or symptoms of hyperglycemia. Tachycardia and cardiomyopathy reported. D/C if cardiomyopathy is confirmed unless benefits outweigh risk. Neuroleptic malignant syndrome (NMS), tardive dyskinesia (TD), impaired intestinal peristalsis, deep-vein thrombosis, pulmonary embolism, and ECG changes reported. Fever reported; rule out infection or agranulocytosis. Consider NMS in the presence of high fever. Hepatitis reported. If N/V and/or anorexia develop, perform LFTs. D/C if symptoms of jaundice occur. Has potent anticholinergic effects; caution with prostatic enlargement and narrow-angle glaucoma. May impair mental/physical abilities. Caution with renal, cardiac, hepatic, or pulmonary disease. Increased risk of cerebrovascular adverse events; caution with risk factors for stroke. Obtain WBC and ANC at baseline, then weekly for 1st six months of therapy, then every 2 weeks for next 6 months, and then every 4 weeks thereafter if counts are acceptable (WBC ≥3500/mm³ or ANC ≥2000/mm³). Refer to PI for frequency of monitoring based on stage of therapy, WBC count and ANC. Avoid treatment if WBC <3500/mm³ or ANC <2000/mm³. D/C treatment and do not rechallenge if WBC <2000/mm³, ANC <1000/mm³. Interrupt therapy if eosinophilia (>4000/mm³) develops. Contains aspartame (of which phenylalanine is a component); caution with phenylketonurics. Not for use in infants. Caution in elderly.

ADVERSE REACTIONS: Agranulocytosis, seizure, myocarditis, orthostatic hypotension, salivation hypersecretion, somnolence, drowsiness/sedation, weight increased, dizziness/vertigo, constipation, insomnia, N/V, dyspepsia.

INTERACTIONS: See Contraindications and Boxed Warning. Avoid using epinephrine to treat clozapine-induced hypotension. Use with carbamazepine is not recommended. Caution with CNS-active drugs, general anesthesia, alcohol, paroxetine, fluoxetine, fluvoxamine, sertraline, or inhibitors/inducers of CYP1A2, 2D6, 3A4. Consider reduced dose with paroxetine, fluoxetine, fluvoxamine, and sertraline. Dosage reduction may be needed with drugs metabolized by CYP2D6 (eg, antidepressants, phenothiazines, carbamazepine, Type 1C antiarrhythmics) or that inhibit this enzyme (eg, quinidine); use with caution. May potentiate hypotensive effects of antihypertensives and anticholinergic effects of atropine-type drugs. CYP450 inducers (eg, phenytoin, tobacco smoke, carbamazepine, rifampin) may decrease plasma levels. CYP450 inhibitors (eg, cimetidine, caffeine, citalopram, ciprofloxacin, fluvoxamine, erythromycin) may increase plasma levels. NMS reported with lithium and other CNS-active drugs. Concurrent psychopharmaceuticals may affect plasma clozapine levels. May interact with other highly protein-bound drugs. Caution with drugs known to prolong the QTc interval such as Class 1A antiarrhythmics (eg, quinidine, procainamide), Class III antiarrhythmics (eg, amiodarone, sotalol), certain antipsychotics (eg, ziprasidone, iloperidone, chlorpromazine, thioridazine, mesoridazine, droperidol, pimozide), certain antibiotics (eg, erythromycin, gatifloxacin, moxifloxacin, sparfloxacin), and other drugs known to prolong the QT interval (e.g., pentamidine, levomethadyl acetate, methadone, halofantrine, mefloquine, dolasetron mesylate, probucol, and tacrolimus). Caution with drugs that can cause electrolyte imbalance (eg, diuretics).

PREGNANCY: Category B, not for use in nursing.

MECHANISM OF ACTION: Tricyclic dibenzodiazepine derivative; atypical antipsychotic agent. Interferes with the binding of dopamine specifically at the D_1, D_2, D_3, and D_5 receptors, and has a high affinity for D_4 receptor. Also acts as an antagonist at the adrenergic, cholinergic, histaminergic, and serotonergic receptors.

PHARMACOKINETICS: Absorption: C_{max}=413ng/mL, T_{max}=2.3 hrs (100mg bid). **Distribution:** Plasma protein binding (97%). **Metabolism:** Demethylation, hydroxylation, N-oxidation. Norclozapine (active metabolite). **Elimination:** Urine (50%), feces (30%); $T_{1/2}$=8 hrs (Single 75mg dose), 12 hrs (100mg bid).

NURSING CONSIDERATIONS

Assessment: Assess previous course of standard therapy prior to treatment. Assess for myeloproliferative disorders, paralytic ileus, history of clozapine-induced agranulocytosis or severe granulocytopenia, severe CNS depression or comatose states, history of seizures or other predisposing factors, pregnancy/nursing status, possible drug interactions, and other conditions where treatment is cautioned or contraindicated. Obtain baseline WBC count and ANC, baseline FBG levels in patients at risk for hyperglycemia/DM, and serum K⁺ and magnesium levels.

Monitoring: Monitor for clinical response and need to continue treatment. Monitor for agranulocytosis, myocarditis, orthostatic hypotension, HF, tachycardia, severe respiratory effects, seizures, flu-like symptoms, infection, eosinophilia, fever, DVT, PE, NMS, TD, intestinal peristalsis impairment, hyperglycemia, or other adverse reactions. Monitor WBC counts and ANC during and for ≥4 weeks following d/c or until WBC ≥3500/mm³ and ANC ≥2000/mm³. Check periodic FBG levels if at risk for hyperglycemia and for signs/symptoms of hepatitis while on therapy. Obtain LFTs if patient develops N/V and/or anorexia. Monitor electrolytes and ECG periodically.

Patient Counseling: Inform that drug is available only through a program designed to ensure the required blood monitoring schedule. Counsel on the significant risks of developing agranulocytosis. Advise to immediately report the appearance of lethargy, weakness, fever, sore throat, malaise, mucous membrane ulceration, flu-like complaints, or other possible signs of infection. Inform patients of the significant risk of seizure during treatment; advise to avoid driving and any other potentially hazardous activity while on treatment. Inform phenylketonuric patients that drugs contain phenylalanine. Advise about the risk of orthostatic hypotension, especially during the period of initial dose titration. Inform that missed dose for >2 days should not restart the medication at the same dosage but should contact the physician's dosing instructions. Notify physician if taking or planning to take any prescription or OTC drugs or alcohol. Instruct to notify physician if become pregnant or intend to become pregnant during therapy. Advise not to breast feed if taking the drug. Advise that tabs should remain in the original package until immediately before use.

Administration: Oral route. Allow to disintegrate in mouth and swallow with saliva or chew if desired. No water needed. **Storage:** 25°C (77°F); excursions permitted to 15-30°C (59-86°F). Protect from moisture.

FELBATOL   RX
felbamate (Meda)

F

> Associated with increased incidence of aplastic anemia; d/c if any evidence of bone marrow depression occurs. Acute liver failure reported. Initiate treatment only in patients without active liver disease and with normal baseline serum transaminases. Obtain baseline and periodic monitoring of AST and ALT; d/c if AST or ALT increased ≥2X ULN or if clinical signs and symptoms suggest liver failure. Monitor blood count and LFTs routinely. Avoid with history of hepatic dysfunction.

THERAPEUTIC CLASS: Dicarbamate anticonvulsant

INDICATIONS: Monotherapy or adjunctive therapy in partial seizures, with and without generalization, in adults with epilepsy. Adjunctive therapy for partial and generalized seizures with Lennox-Gastaut syndrome in children. Use in patients who respond inadequately to alternative treatments and whose epilepsy is so severe that a substantial risk of aplastic anemia and/or liver failure is deemed acceptable.

DOSAGE: *Adults:* Monotherapy: Initial: 1200mg/day in divided doses (tid or qid). Titrate: Increase by 600mg q2 weeks to 2400mg/day based on response and thereafter to 3600mg/day if indicated. Monotherapy Conversion: Initial: 1200mg/day in divided doses (tid or qid) while reducing present antiepileptic drugs (AEDs) (Refer to PI). Titrate: Increase at Week 2 to 2400mg/day and at Week 3 up to 3600mg/day while reducing present AEDs (Refer to PI) . Adjunctive Therapy: 1200mg/day in divided doses (tid or qid) while reducing present AEDs by 20%. Further reductions of AEDs dosage may be needed. Titrate: Increase by 1200mg/day increments at weekly intervals. Max: 3600mg/day. Renal Impairment: Initial/Maint: Reduce by 1/2. Adjunctive Therapy: May need further reductions in daily doses. Elderly: Start at lower end of dosing range. *Pediatrics:* ≥14 yrs: Monotherapy: Initial: 1200mg/day in divided doses (tid or qid). Titrate: Increase by 600mg q2 weeks to 2400mg/day based on response and thereafter to 3600mg/day if indicated. Monotherapy Conversion: Initial: 1200mg/day in divided doses (tid or qid) while reducing present AEDs (Refer to PI). Titrate: Increase at Week 2 to 2400mg/day and at Week 3 up to 3600mg/day while reducing present AEDs (Refer to PI). Adjunctive Therapy: 1200mg/day in divided doses (tid or qid) while reducing present AEDs by 20%. Further reductions of AEDs dosage may be needed. Titrate: Increase by 1200mg/day increments at weekly intervals. Max: 3600mg/day. Renal Impairment: Initial/Maint: Reduce by 1/2. Adjunctive Therapy: May need further reductions in daily doses. 2-14 yrs: Lennox-Gastaut Adjunctive Therapy: Initial: 15mg/kg/day in divided doses (tid or qid) while reducing present AEDs by 20%. Further reductions of AEDs dosage may be needed. Titrate: Increase by 15mg/kg/day increments at weekly intervals to 45mg/kg/day.

HOW SUPPLIED: Sus: 600mg/5mL [8 oz., 32 oz.]; Tab: 400mg*, 600mg* *scored

CONTRAINDICATIONS: History of any blood dyscrasia or hepatic dysfunction.

WARNINGS/PRECAUTIONS: Not for first-line therapy. Avoid abrupt d/c; may increase seizure frequency. Weigh the risk of suicidal thought/behavior with the risk of untreated illness. Increased risk of suicidal thoughts or behavior; monitor for emergence or worsening of depression, suicidal thoughts/behavior, and any unusual changes in mood or behavior. Obtain full hematologic evaluations (eg, blood counts including platelets and reticulocytes) and LFTs before, during and after d/c. Encourage pregnant patients to enroll in North American Antiepileptic Drug (NAAED) Pregnancy Registry. Caution with renal impairment and in elderly.

ADVERSE REACTIONS: Aplastic anemia, acute liver failure, anorexia, upper respiratory tract infection, N/V, headache, fever, somnolence, dizziness, insomnia, fatigue, ataxia, constipation.

INTERACTIONS: Increases plasma concentrations of phenytoin, valproate, carbamazepine epoxide, and phenobarbital. Decreases carbamazepine concentration. Decreased felbamate levels with phenytoin, carbamazepine, and phenobarbital.

PREGNANCY: Category C, safety not known in nursing.

MECHANISM OF ACTION: Anticonvulsant; mechanism not established. Has weak inhibitory effects on gamma-aminobutyric acid receptor binding and benzodiazepine receptor binding. Acts as an antagonist at the strychnine-insensitive glycine recognition site of the N-methyl-D-aspartate receptor-ionophore complex.

PHARMACOKINETICS: Absorption: Well-absorbed. **Distribution:** V_d=756mL/kg (1200mg dose); plasma protein binding (22-25%); found in breast milk. **Metabolism:** Parahydroxyfelbamate,

2-hydroxyfelbamate, felbamate monocarbamate (metabolites). **Elimination:** Urine (90%, 40-50% unchanged); $T_{1/2}$=20-23 hrs.

NURSING CONSIDERATIONS

Assessment: Assess for known hypersensitivity, history of any blood dyscrasia, hepatic/renal function, depression, suicidal thoughts/behavior, pregnancy/nursing status, and possible drug interactions. Obtain baseline CBC (reticulocytes, platelets) and LFTs. Perform full hematologic evaluations prior to therapy.

Monitoring: Monitor for signs/symptoms of hepatic failure, renal impairment, aplastic anemia, bone marrow depression, seizures, emergence or worsening of depression, suicidal thoughts/behavior and any unusual changes in mood or behavior. Monitor LFTs and CBC (platelets, reticulocytes) while on therapy and following treatment. Obtain hematologic evaluations frequently during and after treatment.

Patient Counseling: Inform of the need to obtain written, informed consent prior to therapy. Inform that use of drug is associated with aplastic anemia and hepatic failure. Advise to be alert for signs of infection, bleeding, easy bruising, or signs of anemia (fatigue, weakness, lassitude) and liver dysfunction (jaundice, anorexia, GI complaints, malaise) and to report immediately if any signs or symptoms appear. Advise to follow physician's directives for LFTs before and during therapy.

Administration: Oral route. (Sus) Shake well before using. **Storage:** 20-25°C (68-77°F).

FELODIPINE RX
felodipine (Various)

THERAPEUTIC CLASS: Calcium channel blocker (dihydropyridine)

INDICATIONS: Treatment of hypertension alone or concomitantly with other antihypertensive agents.

DOSAGE: *Adults:* Initial: 5mg qd. Titrate: May increase to 10mg qd or decrease to 2.5mg qd at intervals not <2 weeks depending on patient's response. Range: 2.5-10mg qd. Hepatic dysfunction/Elderly: Initial: 2.5mg qd. Take without food or with a light meal. Swallow whole; do not crush or chew.

HOW SUPPLIED: Tab, Extended-Release: 2.5mg, 5mg, 10mg

WARNINGS/PRECAUTIONS: May cause hypotension and syncope (rare). May lead to reflex tachycardia, which may precipitate angina pectoris. Caution with heart failure or compromised ventricular function. Monitor BP during dose adjustment with hepatic impairment or elderly. Peripheral edema reported. Caution in elderly.

ADVERSE REACTIONS: Peripheral edema, headache, flushing, dizziness, asthenia, dyspepsia, upper respiratory infection.

INTERACTIONS: CYP3A4 inhibitors (eg, itraconazole, ketoconazole, erythromycin, grapefruit juice, cimetidine) may increase plasma levels. Decreased levels with long-term anticonvulsant therapy (eg, phenytoin, carbamazepine, phenobarbital). May increase metoprolol and tacrolimus levels. Caution with β-blockers in patients with heart failure or compromised ventricular function.

PREGNANCY: Category C, not for use in nursing.

MECHANISM OF ACTION: Calcium channel blocker: reversibly competes with nitrendipine and/or other calcium channel blockers for dihydropyridine binding sites and blocks voltage-dependent Ca^{++} currents in vascular smooth muscle.

PHARMACOKINETICS: Absorption: (PO) Complete, systemic bioavailability (20%); T_{max}=2.5-5 hrs. **Distribution:** V_d=10L/kg; plasma protein binding (99%). **Elimination:** Urine (70%), feces (10%); $T_{1/2}$=11-16 hrs (immediate-release).

NURSING CONSIDERATIONS

Assessment: Assess for heart failure, compromised ventricular function, hepatic dysfunction, age, pregnancy/nursing status, and possible drug interactions. Obtain baseline LFTs.

Monitoring: Monitor BP, syncope, angina pectoris, and peripheral edema.

Patient Counseling: Instruct to take tab whole; do not crush or chew. Counsel about adverse side effects; notify physician if any develop. Inform that mild gingival hyperplasia (gum swelling) has been reported; maintain good dental hygiene.

Administration: Oral route. **Storage:** <30°C (86°F). Protect from light.

FEMARA

letrozole (Novartis)

THERAPEUTIC CLASS: Nonsteroidal aromatase inhibitor

INDICATIONS: Adjuvant treatment of postmenopausal women with hormone receptor positive early breast cancer. Extended adjuvant treatment of early breast cancer in postmenopausal women who have received 5 yrs of adjuvant tamoxifen therapy. First-line treatment of postmenopausal women with hormone receptor positive or unknown locally advanced or metastatic breast cancer. Treatment of advanced breast cancer in postmenopausal women with disease progression following antiestrogen therapy.

DOSAGE: *Adults:* 2.5mg qd. Adjuvant Early Breast Cancer: D/C at tumor relapse. Advanced Breast Cancer: Continue until tumor progression is evident. Cirrhosis/Severe Hepatic Dysfunction: Usual: 2.5mg qod.

HOW SUPPLIED: Tab: 2.5mg

CONTRAINDICATIONS: Women who are or may become pregnant. Clinical benefit to premenopausal women with breast cancer has not been demonstrated.

WARNINGS/PRECAUTIONS: May decrease bone mineral density (BMD); bone fractures and osteoporosis reported; consider monitoring BMD. Hypercholesterolemia reported; consider monitoring serum cholesterol levels. Reduce dose by 50% with cirrhosis and severe hepatic impairment. May cause fatigue, dizziness, and somnolence; caution when driving or using machinery. Moderately decreased lymphocyte counts and thrombocytopenia reported.

ADVERSE REACTIONS: Hypercholesterolemia, hot flushes, asthenia, edema, arthralgia, myalgia, headache, dizziness, night sweats, constipation, nausea, sweating increased, bone fractures, weight increased, fatigue.

INTERACTIONS: Reduced plasma levels with tamoxifen.

PREGNANCY: Category X, not for use in nursing.

MECHANISM OF ACTION: Nonsteroidal aromatase inhibitor; inhibits conversion of androgens to estrogens. Inhibits the aromatase enzyme by competitively binding to the heme of cytochrome P450 subunit of the enzyme, resulting in a reduction of estrogen biosynthesis in all tissues.

PHARMACOKINETICS: Absorption: Rapid and complete. **Distribution:** V_d=1.9L/kg. **Metabolism:** Liver via CYP3A4, CYP2A6. **Elimination:** Urine (75% glucuronide of carbinol metabolite, 9% unidentified metabolites, 6% unchanged); $T_{1/2}$=2 days.

NURSING CONSIDERATIONS

Assessment: Assess for premenopausal endocrine status, cirrhosis or hepatic impairment, pregnancy/nursing status, and for possible drug interactions. Obtain baseline BMD and serum cholesterol levels.

Monitoring: Monitor for bone fractures, osteoporosis, fatigue, dizziness, somnolence, decreased lymphocytes, and for thrombocytopenia. Monitor LFTs, BMD, and serum cholesterol levels.

Patient Counseling: Inform that the drug is contraindicated in pregnant women and women of premenopausal endocrine status. Counsel perimenopausal and recently postmenopausal women to use contraception until postmenopausal status is fully established. Advise about possible fatigue, dizziness, and somnolence; caution against operating machinery/driving. Advise that bone mineral density may be monitored while on therapy. Counsel about side effects; instruct to seek medical attention if any develop.

Administration: Oral route. **Storage:** 25°C (77°F); excursions permitted to 15-30°C (59-86°F).

FEMCON FE

ethinyl estradiol - ferrous fumarate - norethindrone (Warner Chilcott)

> Cigarette smoking increases the risk of serious CV side effects from oral contraceptive use. Risk increases with age (>35 yrs) and with heavy smoking (≥15 cigarettes/day). Women who use oral contraceptives should be strongly advised not to smoke.

THERAPEUTIC CLASS: Estrogen/progestogen combination

INDICATIONS: Prevention of pregnancy.

DOSAGE: *Adults:* Take 1 white tab qd for 21 days, followed by 1 brown tab qd for 7 days. Begin next and all subsequent courses of tablets on the same day of the week first course began. Intervals between doses should not exceed 24 hrs. Start first Sunday after menses begin or the first day of menses. Take at the same time each day. Initiate no earlier than Day 28 postpartum in nonlactating mother.
Pediatrics: Postpubertal: Take 1 white tab qd for 21 days, followed by 1 brown tab qd for 7 days.

Begin next and all subsequent courses of tablets on the same day of the week first course began. Intervals between doses should not exceeding 24 hrs. Start first Sunday after menses begin or the first day of menses. Take at the same time each day. Initiate no earlier than Day 28 postpartum in nonlactating mother.

HOW SUPPLIED: Tab, Chewable: (Ethinyl Estradiol-Norethindrone) 0.035mg-0.4mg, Tab: (Ferrous Fumarate) 75mg

CONTRAINDICATIONS: Thrombophlebitis, current or history of thromboembolic disorders, history of deep vein thrombophlebitis (DVT), current or history of cerebral vascular disease (CVD) or coronary artery disease (CAD), valvular heart disease with thrombogenic complications, uncontrolled HTN, diabetes mellitus (DM) with vascular involvement, headaches with focal neurological symptoms such as aura, major surgery with prolonged immobilization, known or suspected breast carcinoma (or personal history), carcinoma of the endometrium or other known or suspected estrogen-dependent neoplasia, undiagnosed abnormal genital bleeding, cholestatic jaundice of pregnancy or jaundice with prior hormonal contraceptive use, hepatic adenomas or carcinoma or active liver disease, and known or suspected pregnancy.

WARNINGS/PRECAUTIONS: Increased risk of venous and arterial thrombotic and thromboembolic events (such as myocardial infarction, thromboembolism, and stroke), vascular disease, hepatic neoplasia, gallbladder disease, and HTN. May increase risk of breast and cervical cancer. Benign hepatic adenomas and hepatocellular carcinoma reported (rare). Retinal thrombosis reported; d/c if unexplained partial or complete loss of vision, onset of proptosis or diplopia, papilledema, or retinal vascular lesions develop. Should not be used to induce withdrawal bleeding as a test for pregnancy, or to treat threatened or habitual abortion during pregnancy. May cause glucose intolerance; monitor prediabetic and diabetic patients. May cause fluid retention and increase BP; monitor closely with HTN and d/c if significant elevation of BP occurs. D/C with onset or exacerbation of migraine or development of headache with new pattern which is persistent, recurrent, and severe. May cause breakthrough bleeding and spotting; if persistent or recurrent rule out malignancy or pregnancy. Ectopic and intrauterine pregnancies may occur with contraceptive failures. Perform annual physical exam. Monitor closely with hyperlipidemias; may elevate LDL and/or plasma TG. Caution with impaired liver function; d/c if jaundice develops. May cause depression; caution with history of depression and d/c if it recurs to serious degree. Visual changes or changes in lens tolerance may develop with contact lens use. Use before menarche is not indicated. May affect certain endocrine tests, LFTs, and blood components. Does not protect AIDS and other sexually transmitted disease.

ADVERSE REACTIONS: N/V, breakthrough bleeding, spotting, amenorrhea, migraine, depression, vaginal candidiasis, edema, weight changes.

INTERACTIONS: Reduced contraceptive effectiveness leading to unintended pregnancy or breakthrough bleeding with some anticonvulsants, other drugs that increase the metabolism of contraceptive steroids (eg, barbiturates, rifampin, phenylbutazone, phenytoin, carbamazepine, felbamate, oxcarbazepine, topiramate, griseofulvin). Contraceptive failure and breakthrough bleeding reported with antibiotics such as ampicillin and tetracyclines. Anti-HIV protease inhibitors may increase or decrease levels. Reduced effectiveness with St. John's wort. Atorvastatin, ascorbic acid, acetaminophen, CYP3A4 inhibitors (eg, itraconazole, ketoconazole) may increase hormone levels. Increased plasma concentrations of cyclosporine, prednisolone, and theophylline. Decreased plasma concentrations of acetaminophen and increased clearance of temazepam, salicylic acid, morphine, and clofibric acid.

PREGNANCY: Category X, not for use in nursing.

MECHANISM OF ACTION: Estrogen/progestogen combination oral contraceptive; acts by suppressing gonadotropins. Primarily inhibits ovulation. Also causes changes in cervical mucus (increases difficulty of sperm entry into uterus) and endometrium (reduces likelihood of implantation).

PHARMACOKINETICS: Absorption: Rapid. Norethindrone: Absolute bioavailability (65%), C_{max}=4210.6pg/mL, T_{max}=1.24 hr, AUC=18034.9pg•h/mL. Ethinyl estradiol: Absolute bioavailability (43%), C_{max}=131.4pg/mL, T_{max}=1.44 hrs, AUC=1065.8pg•h/mL. **Distribution:** V_d=2-4L/kg; Norethindone: Sex hormone-binding globulin (36%), albumin binding (61%). Ethinyl estradiol: Albumin binding (98.5%). **Metabolism:** Norethindone: Reduction, sulfate, glucuronide conjugation. Ethinyl estradiol: CYP3A4, via oxidation (conjugation with sulfate and glucuronide), 2-hydroxy-ethinyl estradiol (primary oxidative metabolite). **Elimination:** Norethindrone: Urine (>50%), feces (20-40%); $T_{1/2}$=8.6 hrs. Ethinyl Estradiol: Urine, feces; $T_{1/2}$=17.1 hrs.

NURSING CONSIDERATIONS

Assessment: Assess for presence or history of breast cancer, estrogen dependent neoplasia, abnormal genital bleeding, active liver disease, and known/suspected pregnancy or any other conditions where treatment is cautioned or contraindicated. Assess use in patients who are >35 yrs and heavy smokers (≥15 cigarettes/day). Assess use with HTN, hyperlipidemias, obesity, DM, or in patients at increased risk for thrombosis and for possible drug interactions.

Monitoring: Monitor bleeding irregularities, thromboembolic events, onset or exacerbation of headaches or migraines, and ectopic pregnancy. Monitor fasting blood glucose levels in DM and prediabetic patients, BP with history of HTN, lipid levels with a history of hyperlipidemia. Monitor for signs of liver dysfunction (eg, jaundice) and signs of depression with previous history. Refer patients with contact lenses to an ophthalmologist if visual changes occur. Perform annual history and physical exam.

Patient Counseling: Advise about possible serious CV and respiratory effects. Inform that medication does not protect against HIV infection (AIDS) and other sexually transmitted diseases. Avoid smoking while on medication. Instruct to take medication at same time each day. Instruct if dose missed, take as soon as possible; take next pill at regularly scheduled time. If patient misses more than one dose, instruct to discuss with a pharmacist or physician, or refer to PI and to use back-up contraception. Inform may have spotting, light bleeding, or stomach upset during first 1-3 packs of pills; advise not to d/c medication and if symptoms persist, notify physician. Vomiting, diarrhea, or concomitant medications may alter efficacy; use backup forms of contraception. Perform regular physical exams.

Administration: Oral route. **Storage:** 25° (77°F); excursions permitted to 15-30°C (59-86°F).

Fentanyl Citrate
fentanyl citrate (Various)

CII

THERAPEUTIC CLASS: Opioid analgesic

INDICATIONS: For analgesic action of short duration during the anesthetic periods, premedication, induction and maintenance, and in the immediate postoperative period (recovery room) as the need arises. For use as a narcotic analgesic supplement in general or regional anesthesia. For administration with a neuroleptic (eg, droperidol inj) as an anesthetic premedication, for the induction of anesthesia, and as an adjunct in the maintenance of general and regional anesthesia. For use as an anesthetic agent with oxygen in selected high-risk patients (eg, those undergoing open heart surgery, certain complicated neurological/orthopedic procedures).

DOSAGE: Adults: Individualize dose. Premedication: 50-100mcg IM 30-60 min prior to surgery. Adjunct to General Anesthesia: Low-Dose: Total Dose: 2mcg/kg for minor surgery. Maint: 2mcg/kg. Moderate Dose: Total Dose: 2-20mcg/kg for major surgery. Maint: 2-20mcg/kg or 25-100mcg IM or IV if surgical stress or lightening of analgesia. High-Dose: Total Dose: 20-50mcg/kg for open heart surgery, complicated neurosurgery, or orthopedic surgery. Maint: 20-50mcg/kg. Additional dosage selected must be individualized, especially if the anticipated remaining operative time is short. Adjunct to Regional Anesthesia: 50-100mcg IM or slow IV over 1-2 min. Postop: 50-100mcg IM, repeat q1-2 hrs PRN. General Anesthetic: 50-100mcg/kg with oxygen and a muscle relaxant. Max: 150mcg/kg. Elderly/Debilitated: Reduce dose.
Pediatrics: 2-12 yrs: Individualize dose. Induction/Maint: 2-3mcg/kg.

HOW SUPPLIED: Inj: 50mcg/mL

WARNINGS/PRECAUTIONS: Administer only by persons specifically trained in the use of IV anesthetics and management of the respiratory effects of potent opioids. An opioid antagonist, resuscitative and intubation equipment, and oxygen should be readily available. Fluids and other countermeasures to manage hypotension should be available when used with tranquilizers. Initial dose reduction recommended with narcotic analgesia for recovery. May cause muscle rigidity, particularly with muscles used for respiration. Adequate facilities should be available for postoperative monitoring and ventilation. May cause euphoria, miosis, bradycardia, and bronchoconstriction. Caution in respiratory depression-susceptible patients (eg, comatose patients with head injury or brain tumor); may obscure the clinical course of patients with head injury. Caution with chronic obstructive pulmonary disease, decreased respiratory reserve, potentially compromised respiration, liver/kidney dysfunction, and cardiac bradyarrhythmias. Monitor vital signs routinely.

ADVERSE REACTIONS: Respiratory depression, apnea, rigidity, bradycardia.

INTERACTIONS: Severe and unpredictable potentiation with MAOIs; appropriate monitoring and availability of vasodilators and β-blockers for HTN treatment is indicated. Additive or potentiating effects with other CNS depressants (eg, barbiturates, tranquilizers, narcotics, general anesthetics); reduce dose of other CNS depressants. Reports of cardiovascular (CV) depression with nitrous oxide. Alteration of respiration with certain forms of conduction anesthesia (eg, spinal anesthesia, some peridural anesthesia). Decreased pulmonary arterial pressure and hypotension, or may increase BP in patients with/without HTN with tranquilizers (eg, droperidol). May cause CV depression with diazepam.

PREGNANCY: Category C, caution with nursing.

MECHANISM OF ACTION: Narcotic analgesic; produces analgesic and sedative effects. Alters respiratory rate and alveolar ventilation, which may last longer than analgesic effects.

PHARMACOKINETICS: Distribution: V_d=4L/kg. **Metabolism:** Liver. **Elimination:** Urine (75%, <10% unchanged), feces (9%); $T_{1/2}$=219 min.

NURSING CONSIDERATIONS

Assessment: Assess level of pain intensity, patient's general condition and medical status, or any other conditions where treatment is contraindicated or cautioned. Assess for history of hypersensitivity, pregnancy/nursing status, renal/hepatic function, and possible drug interactions. Assess use in the elderly and debilitated patient.

Monitoring: Monitor for signs/symptoms of respiratory depression, muscle rigidity, medication abuse, and drug dependence. If given with nitrous oxide, monitor for CV depression. If administered with a tranquilizer, monitor for hypotension and hypovolemia. If combined with a droperidol, monitor for increases in BP; perform ECG monitoring. Perform routine monitoring of vital signs.

Patient Counseling: Advise patient about the benefits and risk of the medication. Instruct to notify physician if any adverse reactions occur.

Administration: IM/IV route. **Storage:** 20-25°C (68-77°F); excursions permitted to 15-30°C (59-86°F). Protect from light.

FENTORA   CII
fentanyl citrate (Cephalon)

> Serious adverse events, including deaths, reported as a result of improper patient selection (eg, use in opioid-nontolerant patient) and/or improper dosing. Do not convert patients on a mcg-per-mcg basis from other fentanyl products. Do not substitute for other fentanyl products; may result in fatal overdose. Not indicated for opioid-nontolerant patients including those with only PRN prior exposure; life-threatening respiratory depression and deaths may occur. Contraindicated in the management of acute or postoperative pain including headache/migraine. Contains fentanyl, with abuse liability similar to other opioid agonist, legal or illicit. Keep out of reach of children and discard properly. Use only in the care of cancer patients and only by oncologists and pain specialists who are skilled/knowledgeable in the use of Schedule II opioids to treat cancer pain. Concomitant use with CYP3A4 inhibitors may cause fatal respiratory depression. Available only through restrictive distribution program called Fentora REMS (Risk Evaluation Mitigation Strategy) due to risk of misuse, abuse, addiction, and overdose. Prescribing healthcare professionals, outpatients, pharmacies, and distributors must enroll in the program to prescribe, receive, dispense, and distribute.

THERAPEUTIC CLASS: Opioid analgesic

INDICATIONS: Management of breakthrough pain in patients with cancer who are already receiving and tolerant to around-the-clock opioid therapy for their underlying persistent cancer pain.

DOSAGE: *Adults:* Breakthrough Pain: Initial: 100mcg. Titration >100mcg: Two 100mcg tabs (one on each side of mouth in buccal cavity) with next breakthrough pain episode. Use two 100mcg tabs on each side of mouth (total of four 100mcg tabs) if dosage is not successful. Max: 2 doses/breakthrough pain episode; must wait at least 4 hrs before treating another episode of breakthrough pain. Titration >400mcg: 200mcg increments. Max: 4 tabs. Maint: Once titrated to an effective dose, use only one tab of the appropriate strength per breakthrough pain episode. May take only one additional dose of the same strength if not relieved after 30 min. Wait at least 4 hrs before treating another breakthrough pain episode. If >4 breakthrough pain episodes/day are experienced, reevaluate maint dose (around-the-clock) used for persistent pain. Refer to PI for information on conversion of dosing from Actiq to Fentora. Hepatic/Renal Impairment/With CYP3A4 Inhibitors: Use with caution & carefully monitor. >65 yrs: Titrate to slightly lower dose.

HOW SUPPLIED: Tab, Buccal: 100mcg, 200mcg, 300mcg, 400mcg, 600mcg, 800mcg

CONTRAINDICATIONS: Opioid-nontolerant patients and management of acute or postoperative pain including headache/migraine, and dental pain.

WARNINGS/PRECAUTIONS: Not bioequivalent with other fentanyl products. May cause respiratory depression; caution with underlying respiratory disorders (eg, chronic obstructive pulmonary disease), elderly, debilitated patients, patients predisposed to respiratory depression or when using large initial doses in opioid-nontolerant patients. May impair physical or mental abilities. Extreme caution in patients who may be susceptible to the intracranial effects of CO_2 retention (eg, evidence of increased intracranial pressure or impaired consciousness). May obscure clinical course of a head injury. Application-site reactions (eg, paresthesia, ulceration, bleeding) reported. Caution in patients with renal/hepatic impairment, bradyarrhythmias, and those at risk for suicide. Appropriate measures should be taken to limit the incidence of abuse (eg, proper assessment of patient, proper prescribing practices, periodic reevaluation of therapy, proper dispensing, and storage). Caution in patients who have higher risk of substance abuse, including patients with bipolar disorder and/or schizophrenia. May cause physical dependence, which results in withdrawal symptoms when abruptly d/c therapy. Not use for analgesia during labor/delivery.

ADVERSE REACTIONS: Application-site reactions (eg, pain, ulcer, irritation), headache, N/V, constipation, dizziness, dyspnea, somnolence, fatigue, anemia, neutropenia, asthenia, abdominal pain, dehydration, peripheral edema, diarrhea.

INTERACTIONS: See Boxed Warning. Respiratory depression and opioid toxicity may occur given with CYP3A4 inhibitors, other agents that depress respiration. Avoid concomitant use with grapefruit or grapefruit juice. Decreased efficacy with CYP3A4 inducers; signs of increased activity of fentanyl citrate should be monitored and adjust dose accordingly. Concomitant use with other CNS depressants, including other opioids, sedatives, hypnotics, general anesthetics, phenothiazines, tranquilizers, skeletal muscle relaxants, sedating antihistamines, potent inhibitors of CYP450 A4 isoform (eg, erythromycin, ketoconazole, certain protease inhibitors), and alcoholic beverages may produce increased depressant effects. Severe and unpredictable potentiation with MAOIs; avoid use within 14 days. Withdrawal may be precipitated through administration of drugs with opioid antagonist activity (eg, naloxone, nalmefene, mixed agonist/antagonist analgesics like pentazocine, butorphanol, buprenorphine, nalbuphine).

PREGNANCY: Category C, not for use in nursing.

MECHANISM OF ACTION: Opioid analgesic: μ-opioid receptor agonist. Exact mechanism not established. Specific CNS opioid receptors for endogenous compounds have been identified throughout brain and spinal cord and play a role in analgesic effects.

PHARMACOKINETICS: Absorption: Readily absorbed. Absolute bioavailability (65%); (400mcg) C_{max}=1.02ng/mL, T_{max}=46.8 min, AUC_{0-inf}=6.48ng•hr/mL. Refer to PI for parameters of dosage variability. **Distribution:** V_d=25.4L/kg; plasma protein binding (80-85%); found in breast milk, readily crosses the placenta. **Metabolism:** Liver and intestinal mucosa via CYP3A4; norfentanyl (metabolite). **Elimination:** Urine (<7% unchanged), feces (1% unchanged).

NURSING CONSIDERATIONS

Assessment: Assess for degree of opioid tolerance, previous opioid dose, level of pain intensity, type of pain, patient's general condition and medical status, emotional status or any other conditions where treatment is contraindicated or cautioned. Assess for history of hypersensitivity, pregnancy/nursing status, renal/hepatic function, and possible drug interactions.

Monitoring: Monitor for signs/symptoms of opioid toxicity, respiratory depression, abuse, addiction, tolerance, physical dependence, application-site reactions, bradycardia, and for suicidality.

Patient Counseling: Advise that patient must be enrolled in Fentora REMS Program; review benefits, appropriate use, and to sign a patient-physician agreement form. Advise to avoid abrupt withdrawal, avoid using other CNS depressants (eg, alcohol), and to use with caution during hazardous tasks (eg, operating machinery/driving). Advise to notify physician if pregnant or plan to become pregnant, and if signs/symptoms of respiratory depression, worsening of breakthrough pain, or other adverse side effects occur. Counsel not to take drug for acute/postoperative/ short-term pain, pain from injuries, or for headache/migraine. Instruct not to chew, suck, swallow, split tablet, not to take more than as prescribed; if not taking on around-the-clock scheduled basis, not to take more than one tablet (unless instructed to titrate). Instruct for proper disposal; drug has potential for abuse. Counsel on proper administration and storage.

Administration: Oral route. Do not open blister package until ready for use. Do not attempt to push tablet through blister card. Place tablet in buccal cavity (above a rear molar, between the upper cheek and gum). Do not attempt to split tablet. Do not suck, chew, or swallow. Leave tablet between cheek and gum until disintegrated (approxiamtely 14-25 min). After 30 min, swallow remnants with glass of water. Alternate sides of the mouth when administering subsequent doses. **Storage:** 20-25°C (68-77°F); excursions permitted to 15-30°C (59-86°F). Protect from freezing and moisture. Should not be stored once it has been removed from blister package. Do not use if blister package has been tampered with. Keep out of reach of children.

FERRLECIT   RX
sodium ferric gluconate complex (Sanofi-Aventis)

THERAPEUTIC CLASS: Hematinic

INDICATIONS: Treatment of iron deficiency anemia in patients ≥6 yrs with chronic kidney disease receiving hemodialysis and receiving supplemental epoetin therapy.

DOSAGE: *Adults:* 10mL (125mg), diluted in 100mL 0.9% NaCl via IV infusion over 1 hr or undiluted as slow IV inj at a rate of up to 12.5mg/min. Most patients will require a minimum cumulative dose of 1g of elemental iron administered over 8 sessions. Elderly: Start at lower end of dosing range. *Pediatrics:* ≥6 yrs: 0.12mL/kg (1.5mg/kg) diluted in 25mL 0.9% NaCl via IV infusion over 1 hr. Max: 125mg/dose.

HOW SUPPLIED: Inj: 62.5mg elemental iron [5mL]

WARNINGS/PRECAUTIONS: Hypersensitivity reactions, which may be life-threatening and fatal, reported; monitor for signs/symptoms ≥30 min during and after administration. May cause hypotension, usually resolving within 1 to 2 hrs. Excessive IV iron therapy may lead to excess storage of iron, possibly causing iatrogenic hemosiderosis. Contains benzyl alcohol which can cause serious adverse events and death in pediatric patients. Caution in elderly.

ADVERSE REACTIONS: Inj-site reactions, chest pain, pain, asthenia, headache, abdominal pain, cramps, dizziness, dyspnea, hypotension, HTN, N/V, diarrhea, pruritus, abnormal erythrocytes.

INTERACTIONS: May reduce absorption of coadministered oral iron products.

PREGNANCY: Category B, caution in nursing.

MECHANISM OF ACTION: Hematinic; used to replete the total body content of iron, which is critical for normal Hgb synthesis to maintain oxygen transport.

PHARMACOKINETICS: Absorption: Administration of variable doses resulted in different pharmacokinetic parameters. **Elimination: Adults:** $T_{1/2}$=1 hr. **Pediatrics:** (1.5mg/kg) $T_{1/2}$=2 hrs; (3mg/kg) $T_{1/2}$=2.5 hrs.

NURSING CONSIDERATIONS

Assessment: Assess for evidence of iron overload, known hypersensitivity, pregnancy/nursing status, and possible drug interactions.

Monitoring: Monitor for signs/symptoms of hypersensitivity reactions, iatrogenic hemosiderosis, and hypotension. Perform periodic monitoring of hematologic/iron parameters (eg, Hgb, Hct, serum ferritin, transferrin saturation).

Patient Counseling: Advise of the risks associated with the treatment. Instruct to report adverse reactions (eg, hypersensitivity/allergic reaction, dizziness, light-headedness, swelling, breathing problems).

Administration: IV route. Do not mix with other medications or add to parenteral nutrition sol for IV infusion. If diluted, use immediately. **Storage:** 20-25°C (68-77°F); excursions permitted to 15-30° (59-86°F). Do not freeze.

FIBRICOR   RX
fenofibric acid (AR Scientific)

THERAPEUTIC CLASS: Fibric acid derivative

INDICATIONS: Adjunctive therapy to diet for treatment of severe hypertriglyceridemia (≥500mg/dL). Adjunctive therapy to diet to reduce elevated LDL-C, total-C, TG, and Apo B, and to increase HDL-C in patients with primary hypercholesterolemia or mixed dyslipidemia.

DOSAGE: *Adults:* Severe Hypertriglyceridemia: Individualize dose. Initial: 35-105mg/day. Titrate: May adjust dose if necessary following repeat lipid determinations at 4-8 week intervals. Max: 105mg qd. Primary Hyperlipidemia/Mixed Dyslipidemia: 105mg/day. Mild to Moderate Renal Impairment: Initial: 35mg qd. Titrate: May increase after evaluation of effects on renal function and lipid levels. Elderly: Dose based on renal function. Consider reducing dose if lipid levels significantly fall below target range. D/C if no adequate response after 2 months of treatment at max dose.

HOW SUPPLIED: Tab: 35mg, 105mg

CONTRAINDICATIONS: Severe renal impairment (including dialysis), active liver disease (including primary biliary cirrhosis and unexplained persistent liver function abnormalities), pre-existing gallbladder disease, and nursing mothers.

WARNINGS/PRECAUTIONS: Increased risk of myopathy and rhabdomyolysis; risk increased with diabetes, renal failure, hypothyroidism, and in elderly. D/C if marked creatinine phosphokinase (CPK) elevation occurs or myopathy/myositis is suspected/diagnosed. Increases in serum transaminases, hepatocellular, chronic active and cholestatic hepatitis, and cirrhosis (rare) reported; periodically monitor LFTs, and d/c therapy if enzyme levels persist >3X the normal limit. Elevations in SrCr reported; monitor renal function in patients with renal impairment or at risk for renal insufficiency. May cause cholelithiasis; d/c if gallstones are found. Acute hypersensitivity reactions and pancreatitis reported. Thrombocytopenia, agranulocytosis, and decreases in Hgb, Hct, and WBCs reported. May cause venothromboembolic disease (eg, pulmonary embolus [PE], deep vein thrombosis [DVT]). D/C or change medications known to exacerbate hypertriglyceridemia (β-blockers, estrogens, thiazides) prior to therapy.

ADVERSE REACTIONS: Abdominal pain, back pain, headache, abnormal liver tests, increased ALT/AST and CPK, respiratory disorder.

INTERACTIONS: Increased risk of rhabdomyolysis with HMG-CoA reductase inhibitors (statins); avoid combination unless benefit outweighs risk. May potentiate anticoagulant effects of coumarin anticoagulants; caution with use, monitor PT/INR frequently, and adjust dose of the anticoagulant. Bile acid-binding resins may bind other drugs given concurrently; space dosing by at least 1 hr before or 4-6 hrs after the bile acid-binding resin. Immunosuppressants (eg, cyclosporine, tacrolimus) may produce nephrotoxicity; consider benefits and risks, and use lowest effective dose. Changes in exposure/levels with atorvastatin, pravastatin, fluvastatin, glimepiride, metformin, rosiglitazone, and efavirenz.

PREGNANCY: Category C, not for use in nursing.

MECHANISM OF ACTION: Fibric acid derivative; activates peroxisome proliferator-activated receptor α. Increases lipolysis and elimination of TG-rich particles from plasma by activating lipoprotein lipase and reducing production of apoprotein C-III (lipoprotein lipase activity inhibitor). Also induces an increase in the synthesis of apoproteins A-I, A-II, and HDL-C.

PHARMACOKINETICS: Absorption: T_{max}=2.5 hrs. **Distribution:** Plasma protein binding (99%). **Metabolism:** Conjugation with glucuronic acid. **Elimination:** Urine; $T_{1/2}$=20 hrs.

NURSING CONSIDERATIONS

Assessment: Assess for renal impairment, active liver disease, pre-existing gallbladder disease, other medical conditions (eg, diabetes, hypothyroidism), hypersensitivity to drug, pregnancy/nursing status, and possible drug interactions.

Monitoring: Monitor for signs/symptoms of myopathy/myositis, rhabdomyolysis; measure CPK levels if myopathy is suspected. Monitor for cholelithiasis, pancreatitis, hypersensitivity reactions, PE, and DVT. Monitor renal function, LFTs, CBC, and lipid levels.

Patient Counseling: Advise of potential benefits and risks of therapy, and medications to be avoided during treatment. Instruct to follow appropriate lipid-modifying diet during therapy, and to take drug qd without regard to food at prescribed dose. Instruct to notify physician of all medications, supplements, and herbal preparations being taken, any changes in medical conditions, development of muscle pain, tenderness, or weakness, and onset of abdominal pain or any other new symptoms.

Administration: Oral route. **Storage:** 20-25°C (68-77°F).

FIORICET WITH CODEINE `CIII`
codeine phosphate - caffeine - butalbital - acetaminophen (Watson)

> Contains butalbital, acetaminophen (APAP), caffeine, and codeine phosphate. Associated with cases of acute liver failure, at times resulting in liver transplant and death. Most cases associated with APAP doses >4000 mg/day and involved more than one APAP-containing product.

THERAPEUTIC CLASS: Barbiturate/analgesic

INDICATIONS: Relief of the symptom complex of tension (or muscle contraction) headache.

DOSAGE: *Adults:* 1 or 2 caps q4h. Max: 6 caps/day. Elderly: Start at lower end of dosing range.

HOW SUPPLIED: Cap: (Butalbital-APAP-Caffeine-Codeine Phosphate) 50mg-325mg-40mg-30mg

CONTRAINDICATIONS: Porphyria.

WARNINGS/PRECAUTIONS: Not for extended use; may be habit-forming and potentially abusable. Hypersensitivity/anaphylaxis reported; d/c if signs/symptoms occur. Respiratory depression and elevation of CSF pressure enhanced with head injury or intracranial lesions. May further obscure the clinical course with head injuries. Caution in elderly, debilitated, severe renal/hepatic impairment, head injuries, elevated intracranial pressure, acute abdominal conditions, hypothyroidism, urethral stricture, Addison's disease, or prostatic hypertrophy. Increased risk of acute liver failure in patients with underlying liver disease. May mask signs of acute abdominal conditions.

ADVERSE REACTIONS: Acute liver failure, drowsiness, lightheadedness, dizziness, sedation, SOB, N/V, abdominal pain, intoxicated feeling.

INTERACTIONS: Enhanced CNS effects with MAOIs. May enhance CNS depressant effects of other narcotic analgesics, alcohol, general anesthetics, tranquilizers, sedative hypnotics, or other CNS depressants. Increased risk of acute liver failure with alcohol ingestion. Coadministration with erythromycin may lead to stomach upset.

PREGNANCY: Category C, not for use in nursing.

MECHANISM OF ACTION: Codeine: Narcotic analgesic and antitussive. Butalbital: Short- to intermediate-acting barbiturate. Caffeine: CNS stimulant. APAP: Nonopiate, nonsalicylate analgesic, and antipyretic. The role each component plays in relief of complex of symptoms, known as tension headache, is incompletely understood.

PHARMACOKINETICS: Absorption: Butalbital: Well absorbed. Caffeine, APAP: Rapid. **Distribution:** Caffeine, codeine: Found in breast milk. Butalbital: Plasma protein binding (45%); found in breast milk, crosses the placenta. **Metabolism:** Caffeine: Liver; 1-methylxanthine, 1-methyluric acid (metabolites). APAP: Liver (glucuronide conjugation). **Elimination:** Codeine: Urine (90%), feces; $T_{1/2}$=2.9 hrs. Butalbital: Urine (59-88% unchanged or metabolites); $T_{1/2}$=35 hrs. Caffeine: Urine (70%, 3% unchanged); $T_{1/2}$=3 hrs. APAP: Urine (85%); $T_{1/2}$=1.25-3 hrs.

NURSING CONSIDERATIONS

Assessment: Assess for porphyria, hypersensitivity or intolerance to any of the drug's ingredients, renal/hepatic impairment, hypothyroidism, urethral stricture, prostatic hypertrophy, pregnancy/nursing status, possible drug interactions or any other conditions in which treatment is cautioned or contraindicated.

Monitoring: Serially monitor LFTs and/or renal function in patients severe hepatic/renal disease. Monitor for improvement in symptoms, drug abuse/dependence, and signs of CNS depression.

Patient Counseling: Instruct to d/c and contact a physician immediately if signs of allergy (eg, rash or difficulty breathing) develop. Instruct patients to not use more than one APAP-containing product. Inform patients to not take >4g/day of APAP and to seek medical attention if the recommended dose is exceeded. May impair mental/physical abilites; advise to use caution during hazardous tasks (eg, driving/operating machinery). Instruct not to take with other CNS depressants or alcohol. May be habit-forming; only take ud.

Administration: Oral route. **Storage**: Below 30°C (86°F); tight container.

FIORINAL   CIII
caffeine - aspirin - butalbital (Watson)

THERAPEUTIC CLASS: Barbiturate/analgesic

INDICATIONS: Relief of the symptom complex of tension (or muscle contraction) headache.

DOSAGE: *Adults:* 1-2 caps q4h. Max: 6 caps/day.

HOW SUPPLIED: Cap: (Butalbital-Aspirin [ASA]-Caffeine) 50mg-325mg-40mg

CONTRAINDICATIONS: Porphyria, peptic ulcer or other serious GI lesions, hemorrhagic diathesis (eg, hemophilia, hypoprothrombinemia, von Willebrand's disease, thrombocytopenia, thrombasthenia and other ill-defined hereditary platelet dysfunctions, severe vitamin K deficiency, severe liver damage). Syndrome of nasal polyps, angioedema, and bronchospastic reactivity to aspirin (ASA) or NSAIDs.

WARNINGS/PRECAUTIONS: Not for extended and repeated use. May be habit-forming. Caution in elderly, debilitated, with severe renal/hepatic impairment, hypothyroidism, urethral stricture, head injuries, elevated intracranial pressure, acute abdominal conditions, Addison's disease, prostatic hypertrophy, presence of peptic ulcer, and coagulation disorders. Therapeutic doses of ASA can lead to anaphylactic shock and severe allergic reactions. Significant bleeding possible with peptic ulcers, GI lesions, or bleeding disorders. Caution in children, including teenagers, with chickenpox or flu. Preoperative ASA may prolong bleeding time.

ADVERSE REACTIONS: Drowsiness, lightheadedness, dizziness, N/V, flatulence.

INTERACTIONS: Caution with anticoagulant therapy; may enhance bleeding. CNS effects enhanced by MAOIs. Additive CNS depression with alcohol, other narcotic analgesics, general anesthetics, tranquilizers (eg, chlordiazepoxide), sedatives/hypnotics, other CNS depressants. May cause hypoglycemia with oral antidiabetic agents and insulin. May cause bone marrow toxicity and blood dyscrasias with 6-mercaptopurine and methotrexate. Increased risk of peptic ulceration and bleeding with NSAIDs. Decreased effects of uricosuric agents (eg, probenecid, sulfinpyrazone). Withdrawal of corticosteroids may cause salicylism with chronic ASA use.

PREGNANCY: Category C, not for use in nursing.

MECHANISM OF ACTION: Butalbital: Short- to intermediate-acting barbiturate. Aspirin: Analgesic, antipyretic, and anti-inflammatory. Caffeine: CNS stimulant. Combines analgesic properties of ASA with anxiolytic and muscle relaxant properties of butalbital.

PHARMACOKINETICS: Absorption: ASA: (650mg dose) T_{max}=40 min, C_{max}=8.8mcg/mL. Butalbital: Well-absorbed; (100mg dose) C_{max}=2020ng/mL, T_{max}=1.5 hrs. Caffeine: Rapid; (80mg dose) C_{max}=1660ng/mL, T_{max}=<1 hr. **Distribution:** ASA: Found in fetal tissue, breast milk; Plasma protein binding (50-80%). Butalbital: Crosses placenta, found in breast milk; Plasma protein binding (45%). Caffeine: Found in fetal tissue, breast milk. **Metabolism:** ASA: Liver; salicyluric acid, phenolic/acyl glucuronides of salicylate, gentisic and gentisuric acid (major metabolites). Caffeine: Liver; 1-methylxanthine and 1-methyluric acid (metabolites). **Elimination:** ASA: Urine; $T_{1/2}$=12 min (ASA), 3 hrs (salicylic acid/total salicylates). Butalbital: Urine (59-88%); $T_{1/2}$=35 hrs. Caffeine: Urine (70%, 3% unchanged); $T_{1/2}$=3 hrs.

NURSING CONSIDERATIONS

Assessment: Assess for previous hypersensitivity to drug, renal/hepatic function, porphyria, peptic ulcer, other serious GI lesions, bleeding disorders, or any other conditions where treatment is cautioned or contraindicated. Assess for pregnancy/nursing status and possible drug interactions.

Monitoring: Serial monitoring of LFTs and/or renal function with severe hepatic/renal disease. Monitor for anaphylactoid/hypersensitivity reactions, drug abuse/dependence and bleeding.

Patient Counseling: Advise not to take if patient has ASA allergy. Instruct to take exactly as prescribed; instruct to avoid coadministration with alcohol or other CNS depressants. Advise to avoid hazardous tasks (eg, operating machinery/driving) while on therapy. Counsel that drug may be habit-forming.

Administration: Oral route. **Storage:** Below 25°C (77°F); tight container. Protect from moisture.

FIORINAL WITH CODEINE `CIII`
codeine phosphate - caffeine - aspirin - butalbital (Watson)

OTHER BRAND NAMES: Ascomp with Codeine (Breckenridge)

THERAPEUTIC CLASS: Barbiturate/analgesic

INDICATIONS: Relief of the symptom complex of tension or muscle contraction headache.

DOSAGE: *Adults:* 1-2 caps q4h PRN. Max: 6 caps/day. Not for extended use. Elderly: Start at low end of dosing range.

HOW SUPPLIED: Cap: (Butalbital-aspirin [ASA]-Caffeine-Codeine) 50mg-325mg-40mg-30mg

CONTRAINDICATIONS: Porphyria, peptic ulcer disease, serious GI lesions, hemorrhagic diathesis (eg, hemophilia, hypoprothrombinemia, von Willbrand's disease, thrombocytopenias, thrombo-asthenia and other ill-defined hereditary platelet dysfunctions, severe vitamin K deficiency and severe liver damage). Syndrome of nasal polyps, angioedema and bronchospastic reactivity to ASA or NSAIDs.

WARNINGS/PRECAUTIONS: May cause anaphylactic shock and other severe allergic reactions. Caution with peptic ulcer, GI lesions and bleeding disorders; significant bleeding may result. Aspirin administered preoperatively may prolong bleeding time. May be habit-forming and potentially abusable. Not for extended use. Respiratory depression and CSF pressure may be enhanced with head injury or intracranial lesions. Caution in elderly, debilitated, severe renal or hepatic impairment, hypothyroidism, urethral stricture, elevated ICP, acute abdominal conditions, Addison's disease, prostatic hypertrophy. Caution in children with chickenpox or flu. Avoid with ASA allergy. Risk of ASA hypersensitivity with nasal polyps and asthma. Ultra-rapid metabolizers may experience overdose symptoms (eg, extreme sleepiness, confusion, or shallow breathing). May impair physical/mental ability.

ADVERSE REACTIONS: Drowsiness, lightheadedness, dizziness, sedation, SOB, N/V, abdominal pain, intoxicated feeling.

INTERACTIONS: CNS effects enhanced by MAOIs. Additive CNS depression with alcohol, other narcotic analgesics, general anesthetics, tranquilizers (eg, chlordiazepoxide), sedatives/hypnotics, other CNS depressants. May enhance effects of anticoagulants. May cause hypoglycemia with oral antidiabetic agents, insulin. May cause bone marrow toxicity, blood dyscrasias with 6-MP and methotrexate. Increased risk of peptic ulceration, bleeding with NSAIDs. Decreased effects of uricosuric agents (eg, probenecid, sulfinpyrazone). Withdrawal of corticosteroids may cause salicylism with chronic ASA use.

PREGNANCY: Category C, not for use in nursing.

MECHANISM OF ACTION: Butalbital: Short- to intermediate-acting barbiturate. ASA: Analgesic, antipyretic, and anti-inflammatory. Caffeine: Stimulates CNS. Codeine: Narcotic analgesic and antitussive. Role each component plays in relief of complex of symptoms known as tension headache is incompletely understood.

PHARMACOKINETICS: Absorption: ASA: C_{max}=8.8mcg/mL, T_{max}=40 mins. Codeine: Readily absorbed; C_{max}=198ng/mL, T_{max}=1 hr. Butalbital: Well-absorbed; C_{max}=2020ng/mL, T_{max}=1.5 hrs. Caffeine: Rapid; C_{max}=1660ng/mL, T_{max}≤1 hr. **Distribution:** ASA: Plasma protein binding (50-80%); found in breast milk. Codeine: Found in breast milk. Butalbital: Plasma protein binding (45%); crosses placenta; found in breast milk. Caffeine: Found in breast milk. **Metabolism:** ASA: Liver; salicyluric acid, phenolic/acyl glucuronides of salicylate, and gentisic and gentisuric acid (major metabolites). Codeine: Glucuronidation. Caffeine: Liver; 1-methylxanthine and 1-methyluric acid. **Elimination:** ASA: Urine; $T_{1/2}$=12 min (ASA), 3 hrs (salicylic acid/total salicylate). Codeine: Urine (90%), feces; $T_{1/2}$=2.9 hrs. Butalbital: Urine (59-88%); $T_{1/2}$=35 hrs. Caffeine: Urine 70% (3% unchanged); $T_{1/2}$=3 hrs.

NURSING CONSIDERATIONS

Assessment: Assess for severity of headache, previous hypersensitivity to drug, renal/hepatic function, or any other conditions where treatment is cautioned or contraindicated. Assess for pregnancy/nursing status, history of drug abuse, and for possible drug interactions.

Monitoring: Serial monitoring of LFTs, renal function tests. Monitor for anaphylactoid reactions, symptoms of CNS depression (eg, drowsiness, confusion, shallow breathing), drug abuse/de-pendence, bleeding, prolonged bleeding time, PT, urinary (glucose, 5-hydroxyindoleactic acid, Gerhardt ketone, VMA, uric acid, diacetic acid, spectrophotometric detection of barbiturates),

Reye's syndrome, serum amylase, FBG, cholesterol, SGOT, protein, and uric acid. Monitor mother-infant pairs and notify doctor about the use of codeine during breastfeeding.

Patient Counseling: Advise not to take if patient has aspirin allergy. Take as prescribed; do not take with alcohol or other CNS depressants. Caution during hazardous tasks (eg, operating machinery/driving). Potential psychological dependence and abuse. Notify if pregnant/nursing or planning to become pregnant. Inform about risks/benefits and to report any adverse reactions to physician.

Administration: Oral route. **Storage:** <25°C (77°F); tight container. Protect form moisture.

FLAGYL

RX

metronidazole (G.D. Searle)

Shown to be carcinogenic in mice and rats. Avoid unnecessary use. Use should be reserved for conditions for which it is indicated.

THERAPEUTIC CLASS: Nitroimidazole

INDICATIONS: Treatment of symptomatic/asymptomatic trichomoniasis, asymptomatic consorts, acute intestinal amebiasis, amebic liver abscess, and anaerobic bacterial infections (following IV metronidazole therapy for serious infections) caused by susceptible strains of microorganisms. Treatment of intra-abdominal, skin and skin structure, bone/joint, CNS, lower respiratory tract, and gynecologic infections, bacterial septicemia, and endocarditis caused by susceptible strains of microorganisms.

DOSAGE: *Adults:* Trichomoniasis (Female/Male): Individualize dose. Seven-Day Treatment: (Cap) 375mg bid or (Tab) 250mg tid for 7 days. One-Day Treatment: (Tab) 2g as single dose or in two divided doses of 1g each given in the same day. If repeat course needed, reconfirm diagnosis and allow 4-6 weeks between courses. Acute Intestinal Amebiasis: 750mg tid for 5-10 days. Amebic Liver Abscess: (Tab) 500mg or (Cap, Tab) 750mg tid for 5-10 days. Anaerobic Bacterial Infection: Usually IV therapy administered initially if serious. Usual: 7.5mg/kg q6h for 7-10 days or longer. Approximately 500mg for a 70-kg adult. Max: 4g/24 hrs. Elderly: Adjust dose based on serum levels. Severe Hepatic Disease: Give lower dose cautiously; monitor levels for toxicity. *Pediatrics:* Amebiasis: 35-50mg/kg/24 hrs in 3 divided doses for 10 days.

HOW SUPPLIED: Cap: 375mg; Tab: 250mg, 500mg

CONTRAINDICATIONS: 1st trimester of pregnancy in patients with trichomoniasis.

WARNINGS/PRECAUTIONS: Convulsive seizures, encephalopathy, aseptic meningitis, optic and peripheral neuropathy; d/c if abnormal neurological signs occur. Caution with Crohn's disease, severe hepatic disease, evidence or history of blood dyscrasias, CNS disease, and with the elderly. Mild leukopenia reported; monitor total and differential leukocyte counts before and after treatment for trichomoniasis and amebiasis. Use in the absence of proven or strongly suspected bacterial infection or prophylactic indication is unlikely to provide benefit and increases the risk of drug-resistant bacteria. Candidiasis may present with more prominent symptoms; treat with candidacidal agents. May interfere with serum chemistry values (eg, AST, ALT, LDH, TG, hexokinase glucose).

ADVERSE REACTIONS: Convulsive seizures, encephalopathy, aseptic meningitis, optic and peripheral neuropathy, N/V, headache, anorexia, unpleasant metallic taste, reversible neutropenia.

INTERACTIONS: Avoid alcohol during and for at least 1 day (Tab) or 3 days (Cap) afterward. Should not be given within 2 weeks of disulfiram; psychotic reactions reported in alcoholic patients who are concurrently using disulfiram. May potentiate anticoagulant effects of warfarin and other oral coumarin anticoagulants; monitor PT. Increased elimination with microsomal liver enzyme inducers (eg, phenytoin, phenobarbital). May impair phenytoin clearance. Half-life increased and clearance decreased by microsomal liver enzyme inhibitors (eg, cimetidine). May increase serum lithium levels.

PREGNANCY: Category B, not for use in nursing.

MECHANISM OF ACTION: Antibacterial and antiprotozoal nitroimidazole; exerts effect in anaerobic environment. Possesses bactericidal, amoebicidal, and trichomonacidal activity.

PHARMACOKINETICS: Absorption: Well absorbed. (Tab) T_{max}=1-2 hrs, C_{max}=(250mg) 6mcg/mL, (500mg) 12mcg/mL, (2000mg) 40mcg/mL. (750mg, Cap) C_{max}=21.4mcg/mL, T_{max}=1.6 hrs, AUC=223mcg•hr/mL. **Distribution:** Plasma protein binding (<20%); found in breast milk; crosses the placenta. **Metabolism:** Liver, via side-chain oxidation and glucuronide conjugation; 1-(β-hydroxyethyl)-2-hydroxymethyl-5-nitroimidazole and 2-methyl-5-nitroimidazole-1-yl-acetic acid (metabolites). **Elimination:** Urine (60-80%), feces (6-15%); $T_{1/2}$=8 hrs.

NURSING CONSIDERATIONS

Assessment: Assess for hepatic impairment, alcohol use, evidence/history of blood dyscrasias, CNS disease, candidiasis infections, Crohn's disease, pregnancy/nursing status, and for possible drug interactions. Obtain LFTs, and total and differential leukocyte count.

Monitoring: Monitor for symptoms of alcohol use (eg, abdominal distress, N/V, flushing, headache), neurologic symptoms (eg, convulsive seizures, encephalopathy, aseptic meningitis, optic and peripheral neuropathy), candidiasis infections, leukopenia, and hypersensitivity reactions. Monitor LFTs, and total and differential leukocyte counts.

Patient Counseling: Instruct to avoid alcohol during and for at least 1 day (Tab) or 3 days (Cap) after therapy. Inform that drug treats bacterial, not viral infections. Instruct to take exactly as directed; inform that skipping doses or not completing full course may decrease effectiveness and increase resistance.

Administration: Oral route. **Storage:** Cap: 15-25°C (59-77°F). Dispense in well-closed container with child-resistant closure. Tab: Below 25°C (77°F). Protect from light.

F

FLAGYL ER RX
metronidazole (G.D. Searle)

> Shown to be carcinogenic in mice and rats; avoid unnecessary use of drug and reserve use for conditions for which it is indicated.

THERAPEUTIC CLASS: Nitroimidazole

INDICATIONS: Treatment of bacterial vaginosis.

DOSAGE: *Adults:* 750mg qd for 7 consecutive days. Severe Hepatic Disease: Cautiously give doses below recommended; monitor plasma levels and for toxicity. Elderly: Adjust dose based on serum levels.

HOW SUPPLIED: Tab, Extended-Release: 750mg

CONTRAINDICATIONS: 1st trimester of pregnancy.

WARNINGS/PRECAUTIONS: Convulsive seizures, encephalopathy, aseptic meningitis, and optic and peripheral neuropathy reported; d/c promptly if abnormal neurologic signs occur. Caution with CNS diseases. Known or previously unrecognized candidiasis may present more prominent symptoms during therapy; treat with candidacidal agent. Use in the absence of proven or strongly suspected bacterial infection or prophylactic indication may increase risk of drug-resistant bacteria. Caution with evidence of or history of blood dyscrasia; mild leukopenia reported. May interfere with certain types of determinations of serum chemistry values.

ADVERSE REACTIONS: Headache, vaginitis, nausea, metallic taste, bacterial infection, influenza-like symptoms, genital pruritus, abdominal pain, dizziness, diarrhea, upper respiratory tract infection, rhinitis, sinusitis, pharyngitis, dysmenorrhea.

INTERACTIONS: Avoid with alcoholic beverages during therapy and for at least 3 days afterward. Psychotic reactions reported with disulfiram in alcoholic patients; avoid in patients who have taken disulfiram within the last 2 weeks. May potentiate anticoagulant effect of warfarin and other oral coumarin anticoagulants, resulting in PT prolongation. Microsomal liver enzyme inducers (eg, phenytoin, phenobarbital) may accelerate elimination, resulting in reduced levels; impaired clearance of phenytoin reported. Microsomal liver enzyme inhibitors (eg, cimetidine) may prolong $T_{1/2}$ and decrease clearance. Increased serum lithium and signs of lithium toxicity reported; obtain serum lithium and SrCr levels several days after beginning treatment.

PREGNANCY: Category B, not for use in nursing.

MECHANISM OF ACTION: Nitroimidazole; exerts effect in an anaerobic environment. Upon entering the organism, drug is reduced by intracellular electron transport proteins. Because of this alteration, a concentration gradient is maintained which promotes the drug's intracellular transport. Presumably, free radicals are formed that, in turn, react with cellular components resulting in death of the microorganism.

PHARMACOKINETICS: Absorption: C_{max}=19.4µg/mL (fed), 12.5µg/mL (fasted); T_{max}=4.6 hrs (fed), 6.8 hrs (fasted); AUC=211µg•hr/mL (fed), 198µg•hr/mL (fasted). **Distribution:** Found in breast milk; crosses the placenta. **Metabolism:** Side-chain oxidation and glucuronide conjugation; 1-(β-hydroxyethyl)-2-hydroxymethyl-5-nitroimidazole and 2-methyl-5-nitroimidazole-1-yl-acetic acid (metabolites). **Elimination:** Urine (60-80%, 20% unchanged), feces (6-15%); $T_{1/2}$=7.4 hrs (fed), 8.7 hrs (fasted).

NURSING CONSIDERATIONS

Assessment: Assess for history of hypersensitivity to drug, CNS diseases, severe hepatic disease, candidiasis, evidence/history of blood dyscrasia, pregnancy/nursing status, and possible drug interactions.

Monitoring: Monitor for abnormal neurologic signs, candidiasis, and other adverse reactions. Monitor total and differential leukocyte counts before and after retreatments. Closely monitor plasma levels and for toxicity in patients with severe hepatic disease or in elderly.

Patient Counseling: Instruct to avoid alcoholic beverages during therapy and for at least 3 days afterward. Inform that drug only treats bacterial, not viral, infections. Instruct to take exactly ud; inform that skipping doses or not completing full course may decrease effectiveness and increase resistance.

Administration: Oral route. Take at least 1 hr ac or 2 hrs pc. **Storage:** 25°C (77°F); excursions permitted to 15-30°C (59-86°F).

FLAGYL IV   RX
metronidazole (Baxter)

Shown to be carcinogenic in mice and rats; reserve use for conditions for which it is indicated.

THERAPEUTIC CLASS: Nitroimidazole

INDICATIONS: Treatment of intra-abdominal (eg, peritonitis, intra-abdominal abscess, liver abscess), skin and skin structure, gynecologic (eg, endometritis, endomyometritis, tubo-ovarian abscess, postsurgical vaginal cuff infection), CNS (eg, meningitis, brain abscess), and lower respiratory tract (eg, pneumonia, empyema, lung abscess) infections, bacterial septicemia, endocarditis, and (as adjunctive therapy) bone and joint infections caused by susceptible strains of microorganisms (anaerobic bacteria). Prophylactic use to reduce incidence of postoperative infection in contaminated or potentially contaminated elective colorectal surgery. Effective against *Bacteroides fragilis* infections resistant to clindamycin, chloramphenicol, and penicillin.

DOSAGE: *Adults:* Anaerobic Infections: LD: 15mg/kg IV infusion over 1 hr (approximately 1g for a 70kg adult). Maint: 7.5mg/kg IV infusion over 1 hr q6h (approximately 500mg for a 70kg adult), starting 6 hrs after LD initiation. Usual Duration: 7-10 days; bone/joint, lower respiratory tract, and endocardium infections may require longer treatment. Max: 4g/24 hrs. Severe Hepatic Disease: Cautiously give doses below recommended; monitor plasma levels and for toxicity. Surgical Prophylaxis: Usual: 15mg/kg IV infusion over 30-60 min and completed 1 hr before surgery, then 7.5mg/kg IV infusion over 30-60 min at 6 and 12 hrs after initial dose. D/C within 12 hrs after surgery. Elderly: Adjust dose based on serum levels.

HOW SUPPLIED: Inj: 5mg/mL [100mL]

WARNINGS/PRECAUTIONS: Encephalopathy, peripheral neuropathy (including optic neuropathy), convulsive seizures, and aseptic meningitis reported; promptly evaluate benefit/risk ratio of continuation of therapy if abnormal neurologic signs/symptoms occur. Caution with severe hepatic disease. May cause Na retention due to Na$^+$ content; caution in patients predisposed to edema. Known or previously unrecognized candidiasis may present more prominent symptoms during therapy; treat with candicidal agent. Use in the absence of proven or strongly suspected bacterial infection or prophylactic indication may increase risk of development of drug-resistant bacteria. Caution with evidence of or history of blood dyscrasias; mild leukopenia reported; monitor total and differential leukocyte counts before and after therapy. May interfere with certain types of determinations of serum chemistry values.

ADVERSE REACTIONS: Convulsive seizures, encephalopathy, aseptic meningitis, optic and peripheral neuropathy.

INTERACTIONS: Avoid with alcoholic beverages. Psychotic reactions reported with disulfiram in alcoholic patients; avoid in patients who have taken disulfiram within the last 2 weeks. May potentiate anticoagulant effect of warfarin and other oral coumarin anticoagulants, resulting in PT prolongation. Microsomal liver enzyme inducers (eg, phenytoin, phenobarbital) may accelerate elimination, resulting in reduced levels; impaired clearance of phenytoin reported. Microsomal liver enzyme inhibitors (eg, cimetidine) may prolong $T_{1/2}$ and decrease clearance. Caution with corticosteroids.

PREGNANCY: Category B, not for use in nursing.

MECHANISM OF ACTION: Nitroimidazole; active *in vitro* against most obligate anaerobes.

PHARMACOKINETICS: Absorption: C_{max}=25mcg/mL. **Distribution:** Plasma protein binding (<20%); found in breast milk; crosses the placenta. **Metabolism:** Side-chain oxidation and glucuronide conjugation; 2-hydroxymethyl metabolite (active). **Elimination:** Urine (60-80%, 20% unchanged), feces (6-15%); $T_{1/2}$=8 hrs.

NURSING CONSIDERATIONS

Assessment: Assess for history of hypersensitivity to drug, severe hepatic disease, predisposition to edema, candidiasis, evidence/history of blood dyscrasia, pregnancy/nursing status, and possible drug interactions. Obtain baseline total and differential leukocyte counts.

Monitoring: Monitor for abnormal neurologic signs/symptoms, Na retention, candidiasis, and other adverse reactions. Monitor total and differential leukocyte counts. Closely monitor plasma levels and for toxicity in patients with severe hepatic disease or in elderly.

Patient Counseling: Inform that drug treats only bacterial, not viral, infections. Instruct to take exactly ud; inform that skipping doses or not completing full course may decrease effectiveness and increase resistance.

Administration: IV route. Administer by slow IV drip infusion (either as continuous or intermittent) only. Do not introduce additives into drug sol. D/C primary sol during infusion if used with a primary IV fluid system. Do not use equipment containing aluminum (eg, needles, cannulae) that would come in contact with drug sol. **Storage:** 15-30°C (59-86°F). Protect from light. Do not remove unit from overwrap until ready for use.

F

FLECTOR   RX
diclofenac epolamine (King)

NSAIDs may cause an increased risk of serious cardiovascular thrombotic events, myocardial infarction (MI), stroke, and serious GI adverse events including bleeding, ulceration, and perforation of the stomach or intestines, which can be fatal. Patients with cardiovascular disease (CVD) or risk factors for CVD may be at greater risk. Elderly patients are at a greater risk for GI events. Contraindicated in the perioperative setting of coronary artery bypass graft (CABG) surgery.

THERAPEUTIC CLASS: NSAID

INDICATIONS: Topical treatment of acute pain due to minor strains, sprains, and contusions.

DOSAGE: *Adults:* Apply 1 patch to most painful area bid.

HOW SUPPLIED: Patch: 180mg (1.3%) [5^s]

CONTRAINDICATIONS: Asthma, urticaria, or allergic-type reactions after taking aspirin (ASA) or other NSAIDs. Treatment of perioperative pain in the setting of CABG surgery. Use on nonintact or damaged skin.

WARNINGS/PRECAUTIONS: Use lowest effective dose for shortest duration possible. Extreme caution in history of ulcer disease/GI bleeding. Cases of severe hepatic reactions reported. May cause elevations of LFTs; d/c if abnormal LFTs/renal tests persist or worsen, liver disease develops, or systemic manifestations occur. May lead to new onset or worsening of preexisting HTN; caution with HTN and monitor BP closely. Fluid retention and edema reported; caution with fluid retention/heart failure. Caution when initiating treatment in patients with dehydration. Renal papillary necrosis and other renal injury reported after long-term use; increased risk in patients with renal/hepatic impairment or heart failure. Not recommended for use with advanced renal disease; if therapy must be initiated, monitor renal function. Anaphylactic reactions may occur; avoid in patients with ASA-triad. May cause serious skin adverse events (eg, exfoliative dermatitis, Stevens-Johnson syndrome [SJS], toxic epidermal necrolysis [TEN]); d/c at 1st appearance of skin rash or any other signs of hypersensitivity. Avoid starting at 30 weeks gestation; may cause premature closure of ductus arteriosus. Cannot replace corticosteroid nor treat corticosteroid insufficiency. May diminish the utility of diagnostic signs in detecting complications of presumed noninfectious, painful conditions. Anemia may occur; monitor Hgb/Hct if signs/symptoms of anemia develop with long-term use. May inhibit platelet aggregation and prolong bleeding time; carefully monitor patients with coagulation disorders. Caution with preexisting asthma and avoid with ASA-sensitive asthma. Avoid contact with eyes and mucosa. Caution in elderly and debilitated patients.

ADVERSE REACTIONS: Application-site reactions, pruritus, GI bleeding/perforation/ulceration, nausea.

INTERACTIONS: Increased adverse effects with ASA; avoid use. May result in higher rate of hemorrhage, more frequent abnormal creatinine, urea, and Hgb with oral NSAIDs; avoid combination unless benefit outweighs risk. May diminish response to ACE inhibitors, thiazides and loop diuretics. Increased risk of renal toxicity with diuretics and ACE inhibitors; monitor for signs of renal failure and diuretic efficacy. May increase lithium levels; monitor for toxicity. May enhance methotrexate toxicity and cyclosporine nephrotoxicity; caution when coadministering. Increased risk of GI bleeding with oral corticosteroids, anticoagulants (eg, warfarin), smoking, and alcohol. Synergistic effects on GI bleeding with anticoagulants (eg, warfarin) reported. Caution with drugs known to be potentially hepatotoxic (eg, acetaminophen [APAP], certain antibiotics, antiepileptics).

PREGNANCY: Category C (<30 weeks gestation) and D (≥30 weeks gestation), not for use in nursing.

MECHANISM OF ACTION: NSAID; not established. Suspected to inhibit prostaglandin synthesis.

PHARMACOKINETICS: Absorption: C_{max}=0.7-6ng/mL, T_{max}=10-20 hrs. **Distribution:** Plasma protein binding (>99%). **Metabolism:** 4'-hydroxy-diclofenac (major) via CYP2C9. **Elimination:** Urine (65%), bile (35%); $T_{1/2}$=12 hrs.

NURSING CONSIDERATIONS

Assessment: Assess for hypersensitivity to ASA or NSAIDs, history of ulcers or GI bleeding, HTN, fluid retention, congestive heart failure, asthma, CVD (or risk factors for CVD), renal/hepatic impairment, pregnancy/nursing status, and for possible drug interactions. Obtain baseline BP.

Monitoring: Monitor BP and renal function. Periodically monitor CBC, LFTs, and chemistry profile. Monitor for signs/symptoms of GI events, CV thrombotic events, liver disease, edema, HTN, anaphylactic reactions, skin rash or other signs of hypersensitivity, and hematologic effects.

Patient Counseling: Instruct only to use on intact skin. Instruct to wash hands after applying, handling, or removing the patch. Instruct not to wear patch during bathing or showering. Instruct to avoid contact with eyes and mucosa; advise to wash out the eye with water or saline immediately and consult physician if irritation persists for >1 hr. Advise to seek medical attention if experience symptoms of hepatotoxicity (nausea, fatigue, lethargy, pruritus, jaundice, right upper quadrant tenderness, flu-like symptoms), anaphylactic reactions (difficulty breathing, swelling of face/throat), skin and hypersensitivity reactions (rash, blisters, fever, itching), CV events (chest pain, SOB, weakness, slurring of speech), GI ulceration and bleeding (epigastric pain, dyspepsia, melena, hematemesis), bronchospasm (wheezing, SOB), weight gain, or edema. Inform of pregnancy risks. Instruct to tape down edges of patch if it begins to peel-off. Instruct to keep out of the reach of children and pets. Advise to avoid coadministration with unprescribed APAP.

Administration: Transdermal route. **Storage:** 25°C (77°F); excursions permitted to 15-30°C (59-86°F). Keep sealed at all times when not in use.

FLEXERIL   RX
cyclobenzaprine HCl (McNeil Consumer)

THERAPEUTIC CLASS: Skeletal muscle relaxant (central-acting)

INDICATIONS: Relief of muscle spasm associated with acute, painful musculoskeletal conditions.

DOSAGE: *Adults:* Usual: 5mg tid. Titrate: May increase to 10mg tid. Mild Hepatic Dysfunction/Elderly: Initial: 5mg qd, then slowly increase. Moderate/Severe Hepatic Dysfunction: Avoid use. Treatment should not exceed 2-3 weeks.
Pediatrics: ≥15 yrs: Usual: 5mg tid. Titrate: May increase to 10mg tid. Mild Hepatic Dysfunction/Elderly: Initial: 5mg qd, then slowly increase. Moderate/Severe Hepatic Dysfunction: Avoid use. Treatment should not exceed 2-3 weeks.

HOW SUPPLIED: Tab: 5mg, 10mg

CONTRAINDICATIONS: Acute recovery phase of myocardial infarction (MI), arrhythmias, heart block or conduction disturbances, congestive heart failure (CHF), hyperthyroidism, MAOI use during or within 14 days.

WARNINGS/PRECAUTIONS: Caution with history of urinary retention, angle-closure glaucoma, increased intraocular pressure (IOP), hepatic dysfunction. Caution in elderly due to increased risk of CNS effects. May produce arrhythmias, sinus tachycardia, and conduction time prolongation. May impair mental/physical abilities.

ADVERSE REACTIONS: Drowsiness, dry mouth, headache, fatigue.

INTERACTIONS: See Contraindications. Enhances effects of alcohol, barbiturates, and other CNS depressants. May block antihypertensive action of guanethidine and similar compounds. May enhance seizure risk with tramadol. Caution with anticholinergic medication.

PREGNANCY: Category B, caution in nursing.

MECHANISM OF ACTION: Centrally acting skeletal muscle relaxant; relieves skeletal muscle spasm of local origin without interfering with muscle function; reduces tonic somatic motor activity by influencing both gamma and α-motor systems.

PHARMACOKINETICS: Absorption: Oral bioavailability (33-55%); C_{max}=25.9ng/mL; AUC=177ng•hr/mL. **Metabolism**: Extensive; through N-demethylation pathway. Via CYP3A4, 1A2, and 2D6. **Elimination**: Urine (glucuronides); $T_{1/2}$=18 hrs.

NURSING CONSIDERATIONS

Assessment: Assess for hepatic impairment, seizures, hyperthyroidism, urinary retention, angle-closure glaucoma, IOP, recent MI, arrhythmias, heart block, CHF, alcohol intake, pregnancy/nursing status, and possible drug interactions (eg, MAOIs if concomitant use or within 14 days after d/c, and anticholinergic medications).

Monitoring: Monitor for cardiac arrhythmias, sinus tachycardia, MI, increased seizure risk, stroke, IOP, CBC, and LFTs.

Patient Counseling: Caution while performing hazardous tasks (eg, operating machinery/driving). Avoid alcohol or other CNS depressants. Notify if pregnant/nursing.

Administration: Oral route. **Storage:** 25°C (77°F); excursions permitted to 15-30°C (59-86°F).

FLOMAX   RX
tamsulosin HCl (Boehringer Ingelheim/Astellas Pharma)

THERAPEUTIC CLASS: Alpha$_1$-antagonist

INDICATIONS: Treatment of signs and symptoms of benign prostatic hyperplasia (BPH).

DOSAGE: *Adults:* Usual: 0.4mg qd, 30 min after same meal each day. Titrate: May increase to 0.8mg qd after 2-4 weeks if response is inadequate. If therapy is d/c or interrupted, restart with 0.4mg qd.

HOW SUPPLIED: Cap: 0.4mg

WARNINGS/PRECAUTIONS: Orthostasis/syncope may occur; caution to avoid situations in which injury could result should syncope occur. May cause priapism, which may lead to permanent impotence if not properly treated. Screen for presence of prostate cancer prior to treatment and at regular intervals afterward. Intraoperative floppy iris syndrome (IFIS) observed during cataract surgery; avoid initiation in patients who are scheduled for cataract surgery. Caution with sulfa allergy; allergic reaction has been rarely reported. Not for treatment of HTN. Not indicated for use in women nor in pediatrics.

ADVERSE REACTIONS: Headache, abnormal ejaculation, rhinitis, dizziness, infection, asthenia, back pain, diarrhea, pharyngitis, cough increased, somnolence, nausea, sinusitis.

INTERACTIONS: Avoid with other α-adrenergic blockers. Caution with cimetidine and warfarin. Avoid with strong inhibitors of CYP3A4 (eg, ketoconazole); may increase plasma exposure. Caution with moderate inhibitors of CYP3A4 (eg, erythromycin), with strong (eg, paroxetine), or moderate (eg, terbinafine) inhibitors of CYP2D6; potential for significant increase in tamsulosin exposure. Caution with PDE5 inhibitors; may cause symptomatic hypotension.

PREGNANCY: Category B, not for use in nursing.

MECHANISM OF ACTION: α$_1$-antagonist; selective blockade of α$_1$ receptors in the prostate results in relaxation of the smooth muscles of the bladder neck and prostate, improving urine flow and reducing symptoms.

PHARMACOKINETICS: Absorption: Complete. Bioavailability (>90%). **Distribution:** (IV) V$_d$=16L. Plasma protein binding (94-99%). **Metabolism:** Liver (extensive); CYP3A4, CYP2D6. **Elimination:** Urine (76%, <10% unchanged), feces (21%); T$_{1/2}$=14-15 hrs, 9-13 hrs (healthy).

NURSING CONSIDERATIONS

Assessment: Assess for BPH, known hypersensitivity, sulfa allergy, and possible drug interactions. Screen for the presence of prostate cancer prior to treatment.

Monitoring: Monitor for signs/symptoms of orthostasis (eg, postural hypotension, dizziness, vertigo), syncope, priapism, prostate cancer, IFIS during cataract surgery, and allergic/hypersensitivity reactions.

Patient Counseling: Inform about the possible occurrence of symptoms related to orthostatic hypotension (eg, dizziness); caution about driving, operating machinery, or performing hazardous tasks. Instruct not to crush or chew cap. Inform of the importance of screening for prostate cancer prior to therapy and at regular intervals afterwards. Advise to inform ophthalmologist of drug use if considering cataract surgery. Advise about the possibility of priapism and to seek immediate medical attention if it occurs.

Administration: Oral route. **Storage:** 25°C (77°F); excursions permitted to 15-30°C (59-86°F).

FLONASE   RX
fluticasone propionate (GlaxoSmithKline)

THERAPEUTIC CLASS: Corticosteroid

INDICATIONS: Management of the nasal symptoms of seasonal and perennial allergic and nonallergic rhinitis in adults and pediatrics ≥4 yrs.

DOSAGE: *Adults:* Initial: 2 sprays per nostril qd or 1 spray per nostril bid. Maint: 1 spray per nostril qd. May dose as 2 sprays per nostril qd PRN for seasonal allergic rhinitis.
Pediatrics: ≥4 yrs: Initial: 1 spray per nostril qd. If inadequate response, may increase to 2 sprays per nostril. Maint: 1 spray per nostril qd. Max: 2 sprays per nostril/day. ≥12 yrs: May dose as 2 sprays per nostril qd PRN for seasonal allergic rhinitis.

HOW SUPPLIED: Spray: 50mcg/spray [16g]

WARNINGS/PRECAUTIONS: Caution with active or quiescent tuberculosis (TB), ocular herpes simplex, or untreated bacterial, fungal, and systemic viral or parasitic infections. Avoid with recent nasal trauma, surgery, or septal ulcers. Risk for more severe/fatal course of infections (eg, chickenpox, measles); avoid exposure in patients who have not had disease or not have been properly immunized. *Candida albicans* infection of nose and pharynx reported (rare). Potential for reduced growth velocity in pediatrics. Hypercorticism and adrenal suppression may appear when used at higher than recommended doses or in susceptible individuals at recommended doses; d/c slowly if such changes occur. Rare hypersensitivity reactions or contact dermatitis may occur. Rare instances of wheezing, nasal septum perforation, cataracts, glaucoma, and increased intraocular pressure (IOP) reported. Avoid spraying in eyes.

ADVERSE REACTIONS: Headache, pharyngitis, epistaxis, nasal burning/irritation, asthma symptoms, N/V, cough.

INTERACTIONS: Levels increased with ketoconazole or other potent CYP3A4 inhibitors. Concomitant inhaled corticosteroids increase risk of hypercorticism and/or hypothalamic-pituitary-adrenal (HPA)-axis suppression. Increased levels with ritonavir; avoid use unless benefit outweighs risk.

PREGNANCY: Category C, caution in nursing.

MECHANISM OF ACTION: Synthetic trifluorinated corticosteroid; not established. Anti-inflammatory agent with wide range of effects on multiple cell types (eg, mast cells, eosinophils, macrophages, and lymphocytes) and mediators (eg, histamine, eicosanoids, leukotrienes, and cytokines) involved in inflammation.

PHARMACOKINETICS: Absorption: Absolute bioavailability (<2%), C_{max}=50pg/mL. **Distribution:** (IV) Plasma protein binding (91%); V_d=4.2L/kg. **Metabolism:** CYP3A4. **Elimination:** (IV) Urine (<5%, metabolite), feces (parent drug, metabolite); $T_{1/2}$=7.8 hrs.

NURSING CONSIDERATIONS

Assessment: Assess for hypersensitivity, TB, infections, ocular herpes simplex, history of recent nasal septal ulcers, nasal surgery/trauma, immunization status, pregnancy/nursing status, and possible drug interactions. May give prophylaxis with varicella zoster immune globulin (VZIG) if exposed to chickenpox, or with pooled IM immunogobulin if exposed to measles.

Monitoring: Monitor for acute adrenal insufficiency, withdrawal symptoms, hypercorticism and/or HPA axis suppression, infections, chickenpox and measles, nasal or pharyngeal *Candida albicans* infections, hypersensitivity or contact dermatitis, wheezing, nasal septum perforation, cataracts, glaucoma, and increased IOP. Monitor growth of pediatric patients routinely.

Patient Counseling: Take as directed at regular intervals and do not increase prescribed dosage. Avoid exposure to chickenpox or measles; consult physician immediately if exposed. Do not spray into eyes. Contact physician if symptoms do not improve or worsen.

Administration: Intranasal route. **Storage:** 4-30°C (39-86°F).

FLOVENT DISKUS   RX
fluticasone propionate (GlaxoSmithKline)

THERAPEUTIC CLASS: Corticosteroid

INDICATIONS: Maintenance treatment of asthma as prophylactic therapy in patients ≥4 yrs and for patients requiring oral corticosteroid therapy for asthma.

DOSAGE: *Adults:* Previous Therapy: Bronchodilator Only: Initial: 100mcg bid. Max: 500mcg bid. Inhaled Corticosteroid: Initial: 100-250mcg bid. Max: 500mcg bid. Oral Corticosteroid: Initial: 500-1000mcg bid. Max: 1000mcg bid. Starting dosages >100mcg bid may be considered for patients with poorer asthma control or previous high-dose inhaled corticosteroid requirement. Reduce PO prednisone no faster than 2.5-5mg/day weekly, beginning at least 1 week after starting therapy. Titrate to the lowest effective dose once asthma stability is achieved.
Pediatrics: ≥12 yrs: Previous Therapy: Bronchodilator Only: Initial: 100mcg bid. Max: 500mcg bid. Inhaled Corticosteroid: Initial: 100-250mcg bid. Max: 500mcg bid. Oral Corticosteroid: Initial: 500-1000mcg bid. Max: 1000mcg bid. 4-11 yrs: Initial: 50mcg bid. Max: 100mcg bid. Starting dosages >100mcg bid may be considered for adolescent patients and >50mcg for patients 4-11 yrs with poorer asthma control or previous high-dose inhaled corticosteroid requirement. Reduce PO prednisone no faster than 2.5-5mg/day weekly, beginning at least 1 week after starting therapy. Titrate to the lowest effective dose once asthma stability is achieved.

HOW SUPPLIED: Disk: 50mcg/inh, 100mcg/inh, 250mcg/inh [60 blisters]

CONTRAINDICATIONS: Primary treatment of status asthmaticus or other acute episodes of asthma where intensive measures are required. Severe hypersensitivity to milk proteins.

WARNINGS/PRECAUTIONS: *Candida albicans* infections of mouth and pharynx reported; treat and/or d/c if needed. Not indicated for rapid relief of bronchospasm or other acute episodes of asthma; may require oral corticosteroids. Increased susceptibility to infections (eg, chickenpox, measles), may lead to serious/fatal course; if exposed, consider prophylaxis/treatment. Caution with tuberculosis (TB), untreated systemic fungal, bacterial, viral or parasitic infections, and ocular herpes simplex. Deaths due to adrenal insufficiency reported with transfer from systemic to inhaled corticosteroids (ICSs); if oral corticosteroids is required, wean slowly from systemic steroid use after transferring to ICS. Transfer from systemic to inhalation therapy may unmask allergic conditions (eg, rhinitis, conjunctivitis). Observe for systemic corticosteroid withdrawal effects; if hypercorticism and adrenal suppression appear reduce dose slowly. Hypersensitivity reactions, including anaphylaxis, angioedema, urticaria, and bronchospasm may occur. Decrease in bone mineral density (BMD) reported; caution with major risk factors for decreased bone mineral content including chronic use of drugs that can reduce bone mass (eg, anticonvulsants, corticosteroids). May cause reduction in growth velocity in pediatrics. Glaucoma, increased intraocular pressure (IOP), cataracts, rare cases of systemic eosinophilic conditions, and vasculitis consistent with Churg-Strauss syndrome reported. Paradoxical bronchospasm with immediate increase in wheezing may occur; d/c immediately, treat, and institute appropriate therapy. Not indicated for relief of acute bronchospasm.

ADVERSE REACTIONS: Upper respiratory tract infection, throat irritation, headache, sinusitis/sinus infection, N/V, rhinitis, cough, muscle pain, oral candidiasis, arthralgia, articular rheumatism, fatigue, nasal congestion/blockage, malaise.

INTERACTIONS: Not recommended with strong CYP3A4 inhibitors (eg, ritonavir, atazanavir, clarithromycin, indinavir, itraconazole, nefazodone, nelfinavir, saquinavir, ketoconazole, telithromycin) as increased systemic corticosteroid adverse effects may occur. May increase levels and reduce cortisol levels with ritonavir and ketoconazole; coadministration is not recommended.

PREGNANCY: Category C, caution in nursing.

MECHANISM OF ACTION: Corticosteroid; potent anti-inflammatory activity, inhibits multiple cell types and mediator production or secretion involved in asthmatic response.

PHARMACOKINETICS: Absorption: Acts locally in lung, absolute bioavailability (7.8%). **Distribution:** (IV) V_d=4.2L/kg; plasma protein binding (99%). **Metabolism:** Liver via CYP3A4; 17 β-carboxylic acid derivative (metabolite). **Elimination:** (PO) Feces, urine (<5%); (IV) $T_{1/2}$=7.8 hrs.

NURSING CONSIDERATIONS

Assessment: Assess for hypersensitivity to milk proteins, status asthmaticus, acute bronchospasm, rapidly deteriorating asthma, risk factors for decreased bone mineral content, history of increased IOP, glaucoma, cataracts, active or quiescent pulmonary TB, ocular herpes simplex, untreated systemic infection, hepatic disease, pregnancy/nursing status, and possible drug interactions. Obtain baseline BMD, eye exam, and lung function prior to therapy.

Monitoring: Monitor for localized oral *Candida albicans* infections, upper airway symptoms, worsening of acutely deteriorating asthma, development of glaucoma, increased IOP, adrenal insufficiency, cataracts, hypercorticism, adrenal suppression, paradoxical bronchospasm, eosinophilic conditions, and hypersensitivity reactions. Monitor growth rate in pediatric patients. Monitor BMD and lung function periodically.

Patient Counseling: Advise to use at regular intervals and rinse mouth after inhalation; do not use with a spacer. Advise that localized infections with *Candida albicans* may occur in the mouth and pharynx. Advise that product is not a bronchodilator and not intended as a rescue medication for acute asthma exacerbations; contact physician immediately if deterioration of asthma occurs. Inform not to d/c unless directed by physician and on administration instructions. Instruct to avoid exposure to chickenpox or measles; consult physician if exposed, if existing TB infections, fungal/bacterial/viral/parasitic infections, ocular herpes simplex symptoms do not improve or worsen, or if hypersensitivity reactions occur. Counsel on risks of decreased BMD and reduced growth velocity in children. Instruct to get regular eye examinations. Inform not to exceed recommended dose. Instruct not to use with a spacer device. Instruct to carry a warning card indicating the need for supplementary systemic corticosteroids during periods of stress or a severe asthma attack.

Administration: Oral inhalation route. After use, rinse mouth with water without swallowing. Refer to PI for further administration instructions. **Storage:** 20-25°C (68-77°F). Keep in a dry place, away from direct heat or sunlight. Device is not reusable. Discard in 6 weeks (50mcg) or 2 months (100mcg and 250mcg) after removal from pouch or when the indicator reads "0", whichever comes first.

FLOVENT HFA
RX
fluticasone propionate (GlaxoSmithKline)

THERAPEUTIC CLASS: Corticosteroid

INDICATIONS: Maint treatment of asthma as prophylactic therapy in patients ≥4 yrs, and for patients requiring oral corticosteroid therapy for asthma.

DOSAGE: *Adults:* Previous Bronchodilator Only: Initial: 88mcg bid. Max: 440mcg bid. Previous Inhaled Corticosteroids: Initial: 88-220mcg bid. May consider starting doses >88mcg bid with poorer asthma control or previous high-dose inhaled corticosteroid requirement. Max: 440mcg bid. Previous Oral Corticosteroids: Initial: 440mcg bid. Max: 880mcg bid. Reduce PO prednisone

dose no faster than 2.5-5mg/day on a weekly basis beginning after at least 1 week of fluticasone therapy. Titrate: Reduce to lowest effective dose once asthma stability is achieved. Increase to higher strength if response to initial dose is inadequate after 2 weeks.
Pediatrics: ≥12 yrs: Previous Bronchodilator Only: Initial: 88mcg bid. Max: 440mcg bid. Previous Inhaled Corticosteroids: Initial: 88-220mcg bid. May consider starting doses >88 mcg bid with poorer asthma control or previous high-dose inhaled corticosteroid requirement. Max: 440mcg bid. Previous Oral Corticosteroids: Initial: 440mcg bid. Max: 880mcg bid. Reduce PO prednisone dose no faster than 2.5-5mg/day on a weekly basis beginning after at least 1 week of fluticasone therapy. Titrate: Reduce to lowest effective dose once asthma stability is achieved. Increase to higher strength if response to initial dose is inadequate after 2 weeks. 4-11 yrs: Initial/Max: 88mcg bid.

HOW SUPPLIED: MDI: 44mcg/inh [10.6g], 110mcg/inh [12g], 220mcg/inh [12g]

CONTRAINDICATIONS: Primary treatment of status asthmaticus or other acute episodes of asthma where intensive measures are required.

WARNINGS/PRECAUTIONS: *Candida albicans* infections of mouth and pharynx reported; treat and/or interrupt treatment if needed. Not indicated for rapid relief of bronchospasm. Increased susceptibility to infections (eg, chickenpox, measles) with immunosuppression, may lead to serious/fatal course; if exposed, consider prophylaxis/treatment. Caution with tuberculosis (TB), untreated systemic fungal, bacterial, viral, or parasitic infections, and ocular herpes simplex; potential for worsening these infections. Deaths due to adrenal insufficiency have been reported with transfer from systemic to inhaled corticosteroid (ICS); if oral corticosteroid is required, wean slowly from systemic corticosteroid use after transferring to ICS. Resume oral corticosteroids during periods of stress or a severe asthma attack if patient previously withdrawn from systemic corticosteroids. Transfer from systemic corticosteroid therapy may unmask conditions previously suppressed (eg, rhinitis, conjunctivitis, eczema, arthritis, eosinophilic conditions). Observe for systemic corticosteroid withdrawal effects. Reduce dose slowly if hypercorticism and adrenal suppression/crisis appear. Hypersensitivity reactions may occur. Decrease in bone mineral density (BMD) reported with long-term use; caution with major risk factors for decreased bone mineral content, such as prolonged immobilization, family history of osteoporosis, postmenopausal status, tobacco use, advanced age, poor nutrition, or chronic use of drugs that can reduce bone mass (eg, anticonvulsants, corticosteroids). May cause reduction in growth velocity in pediatrics. Glaucoma, increased intraocular pressure (IOP), cataracts, rare cases of systemic eosinophilic conditions, and vasculitis consistent with Churg-Strauss syndrome reported. Paradoxical bronchospasm with immediate increase in wheezing may occur; d/c immediately, treat, and institute alternative therapy.

ADVERSE REACTIONS: Upper respiratory tract infection, throat irritation, sinusitis/sinus infection, upper respiratory tract inflammation, dysphonia, candidiasis, cough, bronchitis, headache.

INTERACTIONS: Not recommended with strong CYP3A4 inhibitors (eg, ritonavir, atazanavir, clarithromycin, indinavir, itraconazole, nefazodone, nelfinavir, saquinavir, ketoconazole, telithromycin) as increased systemic corticosteroid adverse effects may occur. Ritonavir and ketoconazole may increase levels and reduce cortisol levels; coadministration is not recommended.

PREGNANCY: Category C, caution in nursing.

MECHANISM OF ACTION: Corticosteroid; possesses potent anti-inflammatory activity. Inhibits multiple cell types (eg, mast cells, eosinophils, basophils, lymphocytes, macrophages, neutrophils) and mediator production or secretion (eg, histamine, eicosanoids, leukotrienes, cytokines) involved in the asthmatic response.

PHARMACOKINETICS: Absorption: Acts locally in lung. **Distribution:** (IV) V_d=4.2L/kg; plasma protein binding (99%). **Metabolism:** Liver via CYP3A4; 17 β-carboxylic acid (metabolite). **Elimination:** (PO) Feces, urine (<5%); (IV) $T_{1/2}$=7.8 hrs.

NURSING CONSIDERATIONS

Assessment: Assess for status asthmaticus, acute asthma episode, acute bronchospasm, active or quiescent TB, ocular herpes simplex; untreated systemic infections, risk factors for decreased bone mineral content, history of increased IOP, glaucoma or cataracts, vision changes, hepatic disease, previous hypersensitivity to the drug, pregnancy/nursing status, and possible drug interactions. Obtain baseline lung function test, BMD, and eye exam. In pediatrics, obtain baseline height.

Monitoring: Monitor for signs of infection, immunosuppression, systemic corticosteroid effects, adrenal insufficiency, hypersensitivity reactions, decreased BMD, glaucoma, increased IOP, cataracts, bronchospasm, eosinophilic conditions, asthma instability, and adrenal insufficiency. Monitor growth in pediatric patients. Monitor lung function (FEV_1) or morning peak expiratory flow, β-agonist use, and asthma symptoms during oral corticosteroid withdrawal. Monitor patients with hepatic disease.

Patient Counseling: Advise that localized infections with *Candida albicans* may occur in the mouth and pharynx; advise to rinse mouth after use. Inform that product is not intended for acute asthma exacerbations; instruct to contact physician immediately if deterioration of asthma occurs. Instruct to avoid exposure to chickenpox or measles. Inform of potential worsening of existing TB, fungal, bacterial, viral, or parasitic infections, or ocular herpes simplex. Counsel on risks of systemic corticosteroid effects, decreased BMD, and reduced growth velocity in children. Inform that long-term use may increase risk of some eye problems. Instruct to d/c therapy if a hypersensitivity reaction occurs. Instruct to use at regular intervals as directed and not to stop use abruptly; advise to contact physician immediately if use is d/c.

Administration: Oral inhalation. After use, rinse mouth with water without swallowing. Shake well before use. Refer to PI for further administration instructions. **Storage:** 25°C (77°F); excursions permitted to 15-30°C (59-86°F). Store inhaler with mouthpiece down. Inhaler should be at room temperature before use. Discard when the counter reads 000.

FLUDROCORTISONE   RX   F

fludrocortisone acetate (Various)

THERAPEUTIC CLASS: Corticosteroid

INDICATIONS: Partial replacement therapy for primary & secondary adrenocortical insufficiency in Addison's disease. Treatment of salt-losing adrenogenital syndrome.

DOSAGE: *Adults:* Addison's Disease: Usual: 0.1mg/day with concomitant cortisone 10-37.5mg/day or hydrocortisone 10-30mg/day in divided doses. Dose Range: 0.1mg 3 times weekly to 0.2mg/day. If HTN develops, reduce to 0.05mg/day. Salt-Losing Adrenogenital Syndrome: 0.1-0.2mg/day.

HOW SUPPLIED: Tab: 0.1mg* *scored

CONTRAINDICATIONS: Systemic fungal infections.

WARNINGS/PRECAUTIONS: Treatment of conditions other than those indicated is not advised. May mask signs of infection, and new infections may appear; may decrease resistance and inability to localize infection. Prolonged use may produce posterior subcapsular cataracts or glaucoma with possible optic nerve damage, and may enhance the establishment of secondary ocular infection due to fungi or viruses. Can cause HTN, salt and water retention, and hypokalemia; monitor carefully for the dosage and salt intake. Serum electrolyte monitoring is advised with prolonged use; salt restriction diet and K$^+$ supplementation may be necessary. May increase calcium excretion. Reactivation of tuberculosis (TB) may occur. Caution with hypothyroidism, cirrhosis, ocular herpes simplex, HTN, ulcerative colitis, diverticulitis, intestinal anastomosis, peptic ulcer, renal insufficiency, osteoporosis and myasthenia gravis. Avoid exposure to chickenpox or measles. Psychic derangements may appear. Adverse reactions produced if large doses used or upon rapid withdrawal. May affect the nitrobluetetrazolium test for bacterial infections and produce false-negative results.

ADVERSE REACTIONS: HTN, congestive heart failure, edema, cardiac enlargement, hypokalemia, hypokalemic alkalosis.

INTERACTIONS: Decreases pharmacologic effect of aspirin; monitor salicylate levels or therapeutic effect of aspirin. Enhanced hypokalemia with amphotericin B and potassium-depleting diuretics (eg, furosemide, ethacrynic acid). Increased risk of digitalis toxicity and arrhythmias with hypokalemia when given with digitalis glycosides. Decreased effects with rifampin, barbiturates, and phenytoin. Decrease PT with oral anticoagulants; monitor for PT. Diminish effects of oral hypoglycemics and insulin. Enhanced edema with other anabolic steroids (eg, oxymethalone, norethandrolone). Adjust dose with initiation or termination of estrogen. Avoid live virus vaccines (including smallpox) and other immunizations.

PREGNANCY: Category C, caution in nursing.

MECHANISM OF ACTION: Synthetic adrenocortical steroid; acts on electrolyte balance and carbohydrate metabolism and on distal tubules of kidney to enhance reabsorption of sodium ions from tubular fluid into the plasma. Increases urinary excretion of both K$^+$ and hydrogen ions.

PHARMACOKINETICS: Distribution: Found in breast milk. **Elimination**: $T_{1/2}$=3.5 hrs (Plasma), 18-36 hr (Biological).

NURSING CONSIDERATIONS

Assessment: Assess for hypersensitivity reactions to drug, systemic fungal infections, other current infections, active TB, vaccination, HTN, heart disease, renal/hepatic impairment, unusual stress, psychotic tendencies, thyroid function, hypoprothrombinemia, osteoporosis, myasthenia gravis, peptic ulcers with/without impending perforation, fresh intestinal anastomosis, diverticulitis/ulcerative colitis, possible drug/lab test interactions (eg, nitrobluetetrazolium test for bacterial infection) and pregnancy/nursing status.

Monitoring: Monitor for occurrence of infections, edema, weight gain, psychic derangement, cataracts, and frequent measuring of serum electrolytes, TSH, LFTs, glucose, intraocular pressure, and BP.

Patient Counseling: Inform drug increases susceptibility to infections. Instruct to avoid exposure to chickenpox or measles. Counsel to carry supply of medication for emergency use. Advise on the importance of regular follow-up visits and to use medication exactly as directed. Advise to notify physician of dizziness, severe or continuing headaches, swelling of feet or lower legs, or unusual weight gain. Advise to report any medical history of heart disease, HTN, kidney or liver disease, and to report current use of any medicines. Inform patient to keep medication out of reach of children.

Administration: Oral route. **Storage:** 15-30°C (59-86°F). Avoid excessive heat. Dispense in a tightly-closed, light-resistant container.

FLUZONE   RX
influenza virus vaccine (Sanofi Pasteur)

OTHER BRAND NAMES: Fluzone High-Dose (Sanofi Pasteur) - Fluzone Intradermal (Sanofi Pasteur)

THERAPEUTIC CLASS: Vaccine

INDICATIONS: Active immunization against influenza disease caused by influenza virus subtypes A and type B contained in the vaccine in persons (Fluzone) ≥6 months, (High-Dose [HD]) ≥65 yrs, (Intradermal [ID]) 18-64 yrs.

DOSAGE: *Adults:* (Fluzone) 0.5mL IM as 1 dose. (HD) ≥65 yrs: 0.5mL IM as 1 dose. (ID) 18-64 yrs: 0.1mL ID as 1 dose.
Pediatrics: Previously Unvaccinated/Vaccinated for the First Time Last Season With 1 Dose: 36 months-8 yrs: 0.5mL IM, 2 doses at least 1 month apart. 6-35 months: 0.25mL IM, 2 doses at least 1 month apart. Vaccinated 2 Doses Last Season/Received at Least 1 Dose ≥2 Yrs Ago/ Patients ≥9 yrs: ≥36 months: 0.5mL IM as 1 dose. 6-35 months: 0.25mL IM as 1 dose.

HOW SUPPLIED: Inj: (Fluzone) 0.25mL, 0.5mL [prefilled syringe], 0.5 mL [vial], 5mL [MDV]; (HD) 0.5mL [prefilled syringe]; (ID) 0.1mL [prefilled micro-inj system]

CONTRAINDICATIONS: Hypersensitivity to egg proteins.

WARNINGS/PRECAUTIONS: Caution if Guillain-Barre syndrome has occurred within 6 weeks of previous influenza vaccination. Medical treatment and supervision must be available to manage possible anaphylactic reactions. Expected immune response may not be obtained in immunocompromised persons. Vaccination may not protect all recipients. (Fluzone/HD) Prefilled syringes may contain natural rubber latex which may cause allergic reactions in latex-sensitive individuals.

ADVERSE REACTIONS: Injection-site reactions (pain, tenderness, erythema, swelling, induration, ecchymosis, pruritus), myalgia, malaise, headache, fever, shivering.

INTERACTIONS: Patients receiving immunosuppressive therapy may not obtain expected immune response.

PREGNANCY: (Fluzone/HD) Category C, (ID) category B; caution in nursing.

MECHANISM OF ACTION: Vaccine; stimulates the immune system to produce antibodies that may protect against influenza virus subtypes A and B.

NURSING CONSIDERATIONS

Assessment: Assess immunization and health/medical status, immunosuppression, previous hypersensitivity to egg proteins or any of its components, sensitivity to rubber latex, pregnancy/nursing status, and possible drug interactions.

Monitoring: Monitor for hypersensitivity reactions, injection-site reactions, Guillain-Barre syndrome, and other adverse events.

Patient Counseling: Inform patients or guardians of benefits/risks of treatment. Advise to inform physician if adverse reactions occur. Counsel that vaccine does not prevent other respiratory infections, and that annual vaccination is recommended. Inform that vaccine contains killed viruses, and cannot cause influenza.

Administration: IM/ID route. Inspect visually for particulate matter and/or discoloration prior to administration. Shake the micro-inj system, syringe or single-dose vial before administering and the multidose vial each time before withdrawing a dose. (Fluzone) Administer in deltoid muscle in patients ≥12 months or anterolateral aspect of thigh in infants (6-11 months). (HD) Administer in deltoid muscle. (ID) Refer to PI for administration instructions. **Storage:** 2-8°C (35-46°F). Do not freeze; discard if frozen. Between uses, return the multidose vial to recommended storage conditions.

FML

fluorometholone (Allergan)

OTHER BRAND NAMES: FML Forte (Allergan)

THERAPEUTIC CLASS: Corticosteroid

INDICATIONS: Treatment of corticosteroid-responsive inflammation of the palpebral and bulbar conjunctiva, cornea, and anterior segment of the globe.

DOSAGE: *Adults:* Apply a small amount (1/2 inch ribbon) qd-tid (oint) or instill 1 drop bid-qid (sus) into conjunctival sac. May reduce dose but caution not to d/c therapy prematurely. Reevaluate if signs/symptoms do not improve after 2 days. (0.1%) May increase to 1 application q4h during the initial 24-48 hrs.
Pediatrics: ≥2 yrs: Apply a small amount (1/2 inch ribbon) qd-tid (oint) or instill 1 drop bid-qid (sus) into conjunctival sac. May reduce dose but caution not to d/c therapy prematurely. Reevaluate if signs/symptoms do not improve after 2 days. (0.1%) May increase to 1 application q4h during the initial 24-48 hrs.

HOW SUPPLIED: Oint: 0.1% [3.5g]; Sus: 0.1% [5mL, 10mL, 15mL], (Forte) 0.25% [5mL, 10mL, 15mL]

CONTRAINDICATIONS: Viral diseases of the cornea and conjunctiva (eg, epithelial herpes simplex keratitis, vaccinia, varicella), mycobacterial infection of the eye, and fungal diseases of ocular structures.

WARNINGS/PRECAUTIONS: Prolonged use may result in glaucoma with damage to the optic nerve, defects in visual acuity and fields of vision, and in posterior subcapsular cataract formation. Prolonged use may suppress host immune response and increase hazard of secondary ocular infections. Use in the presence of thin corneal or scleral tissue, which may be caused by various ocular diseases or long-term use of topical corticosteroids, may lead to perforation. May enhance activity of or mask acute purulent infections of the eye. Routinely monitor intraocular pressure (IOP) if used for ≥10 days. Caution with glaucoma. Use after cataract surgery may delay healing and increase incidence of bleb formation. May prolong course and may exacerbate severity of many viral infections of the eye; use with extreme caution with history of herpes simplex. Not effective in mustard gas keratitis and Sjogren's keratoconjunctivitis. Fungal infections of the cornea may develop coincidentally with long-term use; suspect fungal invasion in any persistent corneal ulceration. Withdraw treatment by gradually decreasing frequency of application in chronic condition. (Oint) May retard corneal healing.

ADVERSE REACTIONS: Elevation of IOP, glaucoma, optic nerve damage, posterior subcapsular cataract formation, delayed wound healing, acute anterior uveitis, globe perforation.

PREGNANCY: Category C, not for use in nursing.

MECHANISM OF ACTION: Corticosteroid; not established. Suspected to act by induction of phospholipase A_2 inhibitory proteins called lipocortins, which control the biosynthesis of potent inflammation mediators (eg, prostaglandins, leukotrienes) by inhibiting release of their precursor, arachidonic acid.

PHARMACOKINETICS: Distribution: Found in breast milk (systemic use).

NURSING CONSIDERATIONS

Assessment: Assess for viral diseases of cornea and conjunctiva, mycobacterial infection of the eye, fungal diseases of ocular structures, hypersensitivity to drug or other corticosteroids, history of herpes simplex, thin corneal or scleral tissue, glaucoma, cataract surgery, and pregnancy/nursing status.

Monitoring: Monitor for glaucoma, optic nerve damage, visual acuity and fields of vision defects, posterior subcapsular cataracts, secondary ocular infections, perforation of the cornea/sclera, exacerbation of viral infections of eye, fungal invasion, and other adverse reactions. Routinely monitor IOP if used for ≥10 days. Monitor for improvement of signs/symptoms.

Patient Counseling: Advise to d/c use and consult physician if inflammation or pain persists >48 hrs or becomes aggravated. Instruct to use caution to avoid touching the bottle tip to eyelids or to any other surface to prevent contamination. Instruct to keep bottle tightly closed when not in use and to keep it out of reach of children. (Sus) Inform that the preservative benzalkonium chloride may be absorbed by soft contact lenses; instruct those wearing soft contact lenses to wait at least 15 min after instilling sus to insert soft contact lenses.

Administration: Ocular route. (Sus) Shake well before use. **Storage:** (Oint) 15-25°C (59-77°F). Avoid exposure to temperatures >40°C (104°F). (Sus) 2-25°C (36-77°F) or (Forte) ≤25°C (77°F). Protect from freezing.

FOCALIN
dexmethylphenidate HCl (Novartis)

> Caution with history of drug dependence or alcoholism. Marked tolerance and psychological dependence with varying degrees of abnormal behavior may occur with chronic abusive use. Frank psychotic episodes may occur. Careful supervision is necessary during withdrawal from abusive use, since severe depression may occur. Withdrawal after chronic use may unmask symptoms of underlying disorder that may require follow-up.

THERAPEUTIC CLASS: Sympathomimetic amine

INDICATIONS: Treatment of attention-deficit hyperactivity disorder (ADHD).

DOSAGE: *Adults:* Take bid at least 4 hrs apart. Methylphenidate-Naive: Initial: 5mg/day (2.5mg bid). Titrate: May increase weekly by 2.5-5mg/day. Max: 20mg/day (10mg bid). Currently on Methylphenidate: Initial: Take 1/2 of methylphenidate dose. Max: 20mg/day (10mg bid). Reduce or d/c if paradoxical aggravation of symptoms occur. D/C if no improvement after appropriate dosage adjustments over 1 month.
Pediatrics: ≥6 yrs: Take bid at least 4 hrs apart. Methylphenidate-Naive: Initial: 5mg/day (2.5mg bid). Titrate: May increase weekly by 2.5-5mg/day. Max: 20mg/day (10mg bid). Currently on Methylphenidate: Initial: Take 1/2 of methylphenidate dose. Max: 20mg/day (10mg bid). Reduce or d/c if paradoxical aggravation of symptoms occur. D/C if no improvement after appropriate dosage adjustments over 1 month.

HOW SUPPLIED: Tab: 2.5mg, 5mg, 10mg

CONTRAINDICATIONS: Marked anxiety, tension, agitation; glaucoma, motor tics or family history or diagnosis of Tourette's syndrome. Treatment with or within 14 days of MAOI use.

WARNINGS/PRECAUTIONS: Avoid with known serious structural cardiac abnormalities, cardiomyopathy, serious heart rhythm abnormalities, or other serious cardiac problems; sudden death reported in children and adolescents with structural cardiac abnormalities or other serious heart problems. Sudden death, stroke, myocardial infarction (MI) reported in adults. May cause modest increase in HR and BP; caution with HTN, heart failure, recent MI or ventricular arrhythmia. Prior to treatment, perform a physical exam and medical history (including assessment for family history of sudden death or ventricular arrhythmia). Promptly evaluate if symptoms of cardiac disease develop during treatment. May exacerbate symptoms of behavior disturbance and thought disorder with preexisting psychotic disorder. Caution in patients with comorbid bipolar disorder; may cause induction of mixed/manic episodes. May cause treatment-emergent psychotic or manic symptoms (eg, hallucinations, delusional thinking, mania) in children and adolescents without prior history of psychotic illness or mania at usual doses; d/c may be appropriate. Aggressive behavior or hostility reported in children with ADHD. Suppression of growth reported with long-term use; monitor height and weight. May lower convulsive threshold; d/c in the presence of seizures. Difficulties with accommodation and blurred vision reported. Monitor CBC, differential, and platelets with prolonged therapy. Not for use in pediatrics <6 yrs.

ADVERSE REACTIONS: Abdominal pain, fever, anorexia, nausea, nervousness, insomnia. (Pediatrics) Loss of appetite, weight loss, tachycardia.

INTERACTIONS: See Contraindications. May decrease the effectiveness of drugs used to treat HTN. Caution with pressor agents. May inhibit metabolism of coumarin anticoagulants, anticonvulsants (eg, phenobarbital, phenytoin, primidone) and some antidepressants (eg, TCAs, SSRIs); adjust dose. May possibly interact with venlafaxine.

PREGNANCY: Category C, caution in nursing.

MECHANISM OF ACTION: Sympathomimetic amine; CNS stimulant. Mechanism in ADHD has not been established; suspected to block the reuptake of norepinephrine and dopamine into the presynaptic neuron and increase release of these monoamines into extraneuronal space.

PHARMACOKINETICS: Absorption: Readily absorbed; T_{max}=2.9 hrs (fed), 1.5 hrs (fasted). **Metabolism:** Via de-esterification (d-ritalinic acid; primary metabolite). **Elimination:** Urine (90%); $T_{1/2}$=2.2 hrs.

NURSING CONSIDERATIONS

Assessment: Assess for marked anxiety, agitation, tension, glaucoma, tics, family history of or diagnosis of Tourette's syndrome, preexisting psychotic disorders, seizure disorder, bipolar disorder, history of drug dependence or alcoholism, pregnancy/nursing status, and for possible drug interactions. Assess for medical conditions that might be compromised by increases in BP and HR (eg, HTN, heart failure, recent MI, ventricular arrhythmia), structural cardiac abnormalities, cardiomyopathy, serious heart rhythm abnormalities, or other serious cardiac problems. Perform physical exam and obtain a medical history prior to therapy.

Monitoring: Monitor for symptoms of cardiac disease (eg, exertional chest pain, unexplained syncope), MI, stroke, exacerbations of behavioral disturbances and thought disorders, bipolar disorder, worsening of aggressive behavior or hostility, emergent psychotic or manic symptoms (eg, hallucinations, delusional thinking, mania), seizures, and for visual disturbances. During prolonged use, perform periodic monitoring of CBC, differential, and platelet counts. In pediatric patients, monitor height and weight. Monitor BP and HR.

Patient Counseling: Inform about risks and benefits of treatment. Advise that may take with or without food. Advise to notify physician of all medications currently taking and if any adverse events develop.

Administration: Oral route. **Storage:** 25°C (77°F); excursions permitted to 15-30°C (59-86°F). Protect from light and moisture.

FOCALIN XR
dexmethylphenidate HCl (Novartis)

CII

F

> Caution with history of drug dependence or alcoholism. Marked tolerance and psychological dependence with varying degrees of abnormal behavior may occur with chronic abusive use. Frank psychotic episodes may occur. Careful supervision is required during withdrawal from abusive use, since severe depression may occur. Withdrawal after chronic use may unmask symptoms of underlying disorder that may require follow-up.

THERAPEUTIC CLASS: Sympathomimetic amine

INDICATIONS: Treatment of attention-deficit hyperactivity disorder (ADHD) in patients ≥6 yrs.

DOSAGE: *Adults:* Individualize dose. Methylphenidate-Naive: Initial: 10mg qam. Titrate: May adjust weekly in 10mg increments. Max: 40mg/day. Currently on Methylphenidate: Initial: 1/2 of methylphenidate total daily dose. Currently on Dexmethylphenidate Immediate-Release: Switch to same daily dose of the extended-release. Reduce or d/c if paradoxical aggravation of symptoms occurs. D/C if no improvement after appropriate dosage adjustments over 1 month. *Pediatrics:* ≥6 yrs: Individualize dose. Methylphenidate-Naive: Initial: 5mg qam. Titrate: May adjust weekly in 5mg increments. Max: 30mg/day. Currently on Methylphenidate: Initial: 1/2 of methylphenidate total daily dose. Currently on Dexmethylphenidate Immediate-Release: Switch to same daily dose of extended-release. Reduce or d/c if paradoxical aggravation of symptoms occurs. D/C if no improvement after appropriate dosage adjustments over 1 month.

HOW SUPPLIED: Cap, Extended-Release: 5mg, 10mg, 15mg, 20mg, 25mg, 30mg, 35mg, 40mg

CONTRAINDICATIONS: Marked anxiety, tension, agitation, glaucoma, motor tics or family history or diagnosis of Tourette's syndrome. Treatment with or within a minimum of 14 days following d/c of an MAOI.

WARNINGS/PRECAUTIONS: Avoid with known serious structural cardiac abnormalities, cardiomyopathy, serious heart rhythm abnormalities, or other serious cardiac problems; sudden death reported in children and adolescents with structural cardiac abnormalities or other serious heart problems. Sudden death, stroke, myocardial infarction (MI) reported in adults. May cause modest increase in BP and HR; caution with HTN, heart failure, recent MI, or ventricular arrhythmia. Prior to treatment, perform a physical exam and medical history (including assessment for family history of sudden death or ventricular arrhythmia). Promptly evaluate if symptoms of cardiac disease develop during treatment. May exacerbate symptoms of behavior disturbance and thought disorder in patients with preexisting psychotic disorder. Caution in patients with comorbid bipolar disorder; may cause induction of mixed/manic episodes. May cause treatment-emergent psychotic or manic symptoms (eg, hallucinations, delusional thinking, mania) in children and adolescents without prior history of psychotic illness or mania at usual doses; d/c may be appropriate. Aggressive behavior or hostility reported in children with ADHD. Suppression of growth reported with long-term use in pediatric patients; monitor height and weight. May lower convulsive threshold; d/c in the presence of seizures. Difficulties in accommodation and blurring of vision reported. Monitor CBC, differential, and platelets with prolonged therapy.

ADVERSE REACTIONS: Dyspepsia, headache, anxiety. **Adults:** Dry mouth, pharyngolaryngeal pain, feeling jittery, dizziness. **Pediatrics:** Decreased appetite, insomnia, depression, vomiting, anorexia, irritability, nasal congestion, pruritus.

INTERACTIONS: See Contraindications. May decrease the effectiveness of drugs used to treat HTN. Caution with pressor agents. May inhibit metabolism of coumarin anticoagulants, anticonvulsants (eg, phenobarbital, phenytoin, primidone), and tricyclic drugs (eg, imipramine, clomipramine, desipramine); adjust dose. Coadministration with antacids or acid suppressants could alter the release of dexmethylphenidate. May possibly interact with venlafaxine.

PREGNANCY: Category C, caution in nursing.

MECHANISM OF ACTION: Sympathomimetic amine; CNS stimulant. Mechanism in ADHD not established; suspected to block reuptake of norepinephrine and dopamine into the presynaptic neuron and increase release of these monoamines into extraneuronal space.

PHARMACOKINETICS: Absorption: Absolute bioavailability (22-25%); T_{max}=1.5 hrs (1st peak), 6.5 hrs (2nd peak). **Distribution:** Plasma protein binding (12-15%, racemic methylphenidate); V_d=2.65L/kg. **Metabolism:** De-esterification; d-ritalinic acid (metabolite). **Elimination:** Urine (90%, racemic methylphenidate); $T_{1/2}$=2-4.5 hrs (adults), 2-3 hrs (children).

F

NURSING CONSIDERATIONS

Assessment: Assess for history of drug dependence or alcoholism, presence of cardiac disease, medical conditions that might be compromised by increases in BP and HR, preexisting psychotic disorders, comorbid bipolar disorder, seizures, any conditions where treatment is contraindicated, pregnancy/nursing status, and possible drug interactions.

Monitoring: Monitor for symptoms of cardiac disease, exacerbations of behavioral disturbance and thought disorder, psychotic or manic symptoms, worsening of aggressive behavior or hostility, seizures, and visual disturbances. During prolonged use, perform periodic monitoring of CBC, differential, and platelet counts. In pediatric patients, monitor growth. Monitor BP and HR.

Patient Counseling: Inform about risks/benefits of therapy. Instruct to take drug qam, swallow whole, and never crush or chew. If unable to swallow, instruct to sprinkle cap contents over spoonful of applesauce and consume immediately in its entirety. Instruct to read Medication Guide.

Administration: Oral route. Swallow whole or sprinkle contents on applesauce. Do not crush, chew, or divide. **Storage:** 25°C (77°F), excursions permitted to 15-30°C (59-86°F).

FOLIC ACID   RX
folic acid (Various)

THERAPEUTIC CLASS: Erythropoiesis agent

INDICATIONS: Treatment of megaloblastic anemia due to folic acid deficiency and in anemias of nutritional origin, pregnancy, infancy, or childhood.

DOSAGE: *Adults:* Usual: Up to 1mg/day. Maint: 0.4mg qd. Pregnancy/Nursing: Maint: 0.8mg qd. Max: 1mg/day. Increase maintenance dose with alcoholism, hemolytic anemia, anticonvulsant therapy, chronic infection.
Pediatrics: Usual: Up to 1mg/day. Maint: Infants: 0.1mg qd. <4 yrs: 0.3mg qd. ≥4 yrs: 0.4mg qd.

HOW SUPPLIED: Inj: 5mg/mL; Tab: (OTC) 0.4mg, 0.8mg, (RX) 1mg

WARNINGS/PRECAUTIONS: Not for monotherapy in pernicious anemia and other megaloblastic anemias with B12 deficiency. May obscure pernicious anemia in dosage >0.1mg/day. Decreased B12 serum levels with prolonged therapy.

ADVERSE REACTIONS: Allergic sensitization.

INTERACTIONS: Antagonizes phenytoin effects. Methotrexate, phenytoin, primidone, barbiturates, alcohol, alcoholic cirrhosis, nitrofurantoin, and pyrimethamine increase loss of folate. Increased seizures with phenytoin, primidone, and phenobarbital reported. Tetracycline may cause false low serum and red cell folate due to suppression of *Lactobacillus casei*.

PREGNANCY: Category A, requirement increases during nursing.

MECHANISM OF ACTION: Acts as cofactor for transformylation reactions in biosynthesis of purines and thymidylates of nucleic acids; acts on megaloblastic bone marrow to produce normoblastic marrow; required for nucleoprotein synthesis and maintenance of normal erythropoiesis.

PHARMACOKINETICS: Absorption: Rapid (small intestine); T_{max}=1 hr. **Distribution:** Found in breast milk. **Metabolism:** Liver via reduced diphosphopyridine nucleotide and folate reductase. **Elimination:** Urine, feces.

NURSING CONSIDERATIONS

Assessment: Assess for alcoholism, chronic infection, and pernicious, megaloblastic, and hemolytic anemias, and for possible drug interactions.

Monitoring: Monitor for allergic/hypersensitivity reactions.

Patient Counseling: Advise to seek medical attention if symptoms of allergic/hypersensitivity reaction occurs.

Administration: Oral route. **Storage:** 20-25°C (68-77°F).

FOLOTYN   RX
pralatrexate (Allos Therapeutics, Inc.)

THERAPEUTIC CLASS: Dihydrofolic acid reductase inhibitor

INDICATIONS: Treatment of patients with relapsed or refractory peripheral T-cell lymphoma.

DOSAGE: *Adults:* Usual: 30mg/m² IV push over 3-5 min once weekly for 6 weeks in 7-week cycles until progressive disease or unacceptable toxicity. Vitamin Supplementation: Start low-dose (1.0-1.25mg) PO folic acid on a daily basis during the 10-day period preceding the 1st dose and continue during the full course of therapy and for 30 days after the last dose. Give vitamin B12 (1mg) IM inj no more than 10 weeks prior to the 1st dose and q8-10 weeks thereafter. Subsequent vitamin B12 inj may be given the same day as treatment with pralatrexate. Refer to PI for dose modifications following mucositis and hematologic/treatment-related toxicities.

HOW SUPPLIED: Inj: 20mg/mL [1mL, 2mL]

WARNINGS/PRECAUTIONS: May suppress bone marrow function, manifested by thrombocytopenia, neutropenia, and anemia. May cause mucositis; omit dose if ≥Grade 2 mucositis occurs. Dermatologic reactions reported; monitor closely; if severe, withhold or d/c therapy. Tumor lysis syndrome reported; monitor closely and treat for complications. Supplement with folic acid and vitamin B12 to potentially reduce treatment-related hematological toxicity and mucositis. May cause fetal harm if used during pregnancy. Caution with moderate to severe renal impairment; monitor renal function and for systemic toxicity. Not recommended in patients with end-stage renal disease undergoing dialysis. LFTs abnormalities reported; monitor liver function.

ADVERSE REACTIONS: Mucositis, thrombocytopenia, N/V, fatigue, pyrexia, sepsis, febrile neutropenia, dehydration, dyspnea, anemia, constipation, edema, cough, epistaxis.

INTERACTIONS: Delayed clearance with increasing doses of probenecid. Monitor closely for signs of systemic toxicity due to increased drug exposure with probenecid or other drugs that may affect relevant transporter systems (eg, NSAIDs).

PREGNANCY: Category D, not for use in nursing.

MECHANISM OF ACTION: Folate analog metabolic inhibitor; competitively inhibits dihydrofolate reductase. Also a competitive inhibitor for polyglutamylation by the enzyme folylpolyglutamyl synthetase. This inhibition results in the depletion of thymidine and other biological molecules, the synthesis of which depends on single carbon transfer.

PHARMACOKINETICS: Distribution: V_d=105L (S-diastereomer), 37L (R-diastereomer); plasma protein binding (67%). **Elimination:** Urine (31% S-diastereomer, 38% R-diastereomer); $T_{1/2}$=12-18 hrs.

NURSING CONSIDERATIONS

Assessment: Assess for renal/hepatic impairment, pregnancy/nursing status, and for possible drug interactions. Perform serum chemistry tests prior to the start of the 1st and 4th dose of a given cycle.

Monitoring: Monitor for bone marrow suppression, mucositis, dermatologic reactions, tumor lysis syndrome, systemic toxicity, and for other adverse reactions. Monitor renal function and LFTs. Monitor CBC and severity of mucositis weekly.

Patient Counseling: Instruct to take folic acid and vitamin B12 as a prophylactic measure to reduce possible side effects. Inform of the risk of low blood cell counts; instruct to contact physician if signs of infection, bleeding, or symptoms of anemia occur. Inform of signs and symptoms of mucositis, ways to reduce the risk of development, and/or ways to maintain nutrition and control discomfort from mucositis if it occurs. Counsel about signs and symptoms of dermatologic reactions and instruct to notify physician immediately if any skin reactions occur. Inform of signs and symptoms of tumor lysis syndrome and instruct to notify physician if symptoms occur. Advise to inform physician if taking any concomitant medications, including prescription and nonprescription drugs. Instruct to notify physician if pregnant, planning to become pregnant, or if nursing.

Administration: IV route. Refer to PI for further preparation and administration instructions.
Storage: 2-8°C (36-46°F) in original carton to protect from light. Unopened Vials: Stable at room temperature for 72 hrs in original carton; discard if left in room temperature for >72 hrs. Discard any unused portion remaining after inj.

FORADIL RX
formoterol fumarate (Merck)

Long-acting β_2-adrenergic agonists (LABA) may increase the risk of asthma-related death. Contraindicated in asthma without use of a long-term asthma control medication (eg, inhaled corticosteroid). Do not use for asthma adequately controlled on low- or medium-dose inhaled corticosteroids. LABA may increase risk of asthma-related hospitalization in pediatrics and adolescents; ensure adherence with both long-term asthma control medication and LABA.

THERAPEUTIC CLASS: Beta$_2$-agonist

INDICATIONS: Treatment of asthma and prevention of bronchospasm only as concomitant therapy with long-term asthma control medication (eg, inhaled corticosteroid) in adults and children ≥5 yrs with reversible obstructive airway disease, including nocturnal asthma. For acute prevention of exercise-induced bronchospasm (EIB) in adults and children ≥5 yrs, PRN basis. Long-term maintenance treatment of bronchoconstriction in chronic obstructive pulmonary disease (COPD), including chronic bronchitis and emphysema.

DOSAGE: *Adults:* Asthma/COPD: 12mcg q12h using Aerolizer Inhaler. Max: 24mcg/day. EIB: 12mcg at least 15 min before exercise PRN; additional doses should not be used for 12 hrs after administration or if already receiving bid dosing for asthma. Re-evaluate regimen if previously effective dose fails to provide usual response.

Pediatrics: ≥5 yrs: Asthma: 12mcg q12h using Aerolizer Inhaler. Max: 24mcg/day. EIB: 12mcg at least 15 min before exercise PRN; additional doses should not be used for 12 hrs after administration or if already receiving bid dosing for asthma. Re-evaluate regimen if previously effective dose fails to provide usual response.

HOW SUPPLIED: Cap, Inhalation: 12mcg [12^s, 60^s]

CONTRAINDICATIONS: Asthma without use of long-term asthma control medication (eg, inhaled corticosteroid).

WARNINGS/PRECAUTIONS: Do not use with significantly worsening/acutely deteriorating asthma, other LABA, or for acute asthma symptoms. Not a substitute for inhaled or PO corticosteroids. D/C regular use of inhaled, short-acting β_2-agonist; use only for relief of acute asthma symptoms. Deterioration of asthma may occur; monitor for signs of worsening asthma. D/C if paradoxical bronchospasm or cardiovascular (CV) effects occur. Caution with CV disorders (eg, coronary insufficiency, cardiac arrhythmias, HTN), convulsive disorders, thyrotoxicosis, and unusual response to sympathomimetic amines. ECG changes and immediate hypersensitivity reactions may occur. Changes in blood glucose and serum potassium may occur. Contains lactose; allergic reactions may occur in patients with severe milk protein allergy.

ADVERSE REACTIONS: Viral infection, upper respiratory tract infection, CV events, asthma exacerbations, bronchitis, back pain, pharyngitis, chest pain.

INTERACTIONS: Adrenergic drugs may potentiate effects; use with caution. Xanthine derivatives, steroids, or diuretics may potentiate any hypokalemic effect. ECG changes and/or hypokalemia that may result from non-K$^+$ sparing diuretics (eg, loop/thiazide diuretics) can be acutely worsened; use with caution. MAOIs, TCAs, and drugs known to prolong QTc interval may potentiate effect on CV system; use with extreme caution. Use with β-blockers may block effects and produce severe bronchospasm in asthmatic patients; if needed, consider cardioselective β-blocker with caution.

PREGNANCY: Category C, caution in nursing.

MECHANISM OF ACTION: LABA (β_2-agonist); acts as bronchodilator, stimulates intracellular adenyl cyclase, the enzyme that catalyzes the conversion of ATP to cAMP. Increased cAMP levels cause relaxation of bronchial smooth muscle and inhibition of release of mediators of immediate hypersensitivity from cells, especially from mast cells.

PHARMACOKINETICS: Absorption: Rapid; C_{max}=92pg/mL, T_{max}=5 min. **Distribution:** Plasma protein binding (61-64%). **Metabolism:** Direct glucuronidation, O-demethylation via CYP2D6, 2C19, 2C9, 2A6. **Elimination:** With Asthma: Urine (10%, unchanged; 15-18%, conjugates); COPD: Urine (7%, unchanged; 6-9%, conjugates). $T_{1/2}$=10 hrs.

NURSING CONSIDERATIONS

Assessment: Assess for asthma and use of asthma control medication, previous hypersensitivity to the drug, CV disorders, convulsive disorders, thyrotoxicosis, unusual response to sympathomimetic amines, diabetes mellitus (DM), pregnancy/nursing status, and possible drug interactions. Obtain baseline serum K$^+$ and blood glucose levels.

Monitoring: Monitor for paradoxical bronchospasm, signs of worsening asthma, CV effect, hypersensitivity reactions, aggravation of DM and ketoacidosis. Monitor pulse rate, BP, ECG changes, serum K$^+$ and blood glucose levels.

Patient Counseling: Inform of the risk and benefits of therapy. Instruct not to use to relieve acute asthma symptoms. Advise to seek medical attention if symptoms worsen, if treatment becomes less effective, or if more than usual inhalations of short-acting β_2-agonist is needed. Instruct not to swallow capsules. Instruct not to exceed prescribed dose, d/c, or reduce without medical advice. Inform that treatment may lead to palpitations, chest pain, rapid HR, tremor, or nervousness. Inform not to use with a spacer and never to exhale into the device. Advise to avoid exposing caps to moisture and to handle with dry hands. Advise to always use new Aerolizer Inhaler that comes with each refill. Advise to contact physician if pregnant/nursing or severe milk protein allergy. Inform that in rare cases, caps might break into small pieces; pierce caps only once.

Administration: Oral inhalation route. Do not ingest/swallow caps orally. Refer to PI for proper administration. **Storage:** Prior to dispensing: 2-8°C (36-46°F). After dispensing: 20-25°C (68-77°F). Protect from heat and moisture. Always store caps in blister and remove only from blister immediately before use.

FORTAMET

RX

metformin HCl (Shionogi)

Lactic acidosis reported (rare). May occur in association with other conditions such as diabetes mellitus (DM) with significant renal insufficiency, congestive heart failure (CHF), and conditions with risk of hypoperfusion and hypoxemia. Increased risk with the degree of renal dysfunction and age. Avoid in patients ≥80 yrs unless renal function is normal. Avoid with clinical/laboratory evidence of hepatic disease. Temporarily d/c prior to IV radiocontrast studies or surgical procedures. Caution against excessive alcohol intake; may potentiate effects of metformin on lactate metabolism. Withhold in the presence of any condition associated with hypoxemia, dehydration, or sepsis. Regularly monitor renal function and use minimum effective dose to decrease risk. If lactic acidosis is suspected, immediately d/c and institute general supportive measures.

THERAPEUTIC CLASS: Biguanide

INDICATIONS: Adjunct to diet and exercise to improve glycemic control in type 2 DM.

DOSAGE: *Adults:* ≥17 yrs: Take with evening meal. Initial: 500-1000mg qd. With Insulin: Initial: 500mg qd. Titrate: May increase by 500mg/week. Max: 2500mg/day. Decrease insulin dose by 10-25% if FPG <120mg/dL. Elderly/Debilitated/Malnourished: Dose conservatively; do not titrate to max.

HOW SUPPLIED: Tab, Extended-Release: 500mg, 1000mg

CONTRAINDICATIONS: Renal disease/dysfunction (eg, SrCr ≥1.5mg/dL [males], ≥1.4mg/dL [females], or abnormal CrCl), acute or chronic metabolic acidosis, including diabetic ketoacidosis with or without coma.

WARNINGS/PRECAUTIONS: Lactic acidosis may be suspected in diabetic patients with metabolic acidosis lacking evidence of ketoacidosis (ketonuria and ketonemia). Caution with concomitant medications that may affect renal function, result in significant hemodynamic change, or interfere with the disposition of metformin. Temporarily d/c prior to surgical procedures associated with restricted oral intake. Temporarily withhold drug before, during, and 48 hrs after radiologic studies with IV iodinated contrast materials; reinstitute only when renal function is normal. D/C in hypoxic states (eg, shock, CHF, acute myocardial infarction [MI]), dehydration, and sepsis. Avoid with hepatic impairment. May decrease vitamin B12 levels. Increased risk of hypoglycemia in elderly, debilitated/malnourished, adrenal or pituitary insufficiency, or alcohol intoxication. Temporarily withhold metformin and administer insulin if loss of glycemic control occurs due to stress; reinstitute metformin after acute episode is resolved.

ADVERSE REACTIONS: Lactic acidosis, infection, diarrhea, nausea, headache, dyspepsia, rhinitis, flatulence, abdominal pain.

INTERACTIONS: Furosemide, nifedipine, cimetidine, and cationic drugs (eg, amiloride, digoxin, morphine, procainamide, quinidine, quinine, ranitidine, triamterene, trimethoprim, vancomycin) may increase metformin levels. Thiazides, other diuretics, corticosteroids, phenothiazines, thyroid products, estrogens, oral contraceptives, phenytoin, nicotinic acid, sympathomimetics, calcium channel blockers, and isoniazid may cause hyperglycemia and loss of glycemic control. May decrease furosemide levels.

PREGNANCY: Category B, not for use in pregnancy or nursing.

MECHANISM OF ACTION: Biguanide; decreases hepatic production and intestinal absorption of glucose, and improves insulin sensitivity by increasing peripheral glucose uptake and utilization.

PHARMACOKINETICS: Absorption: C_{max}=2849ng/mL, T_{max}=6 hrs, AUC=26811ng•hr/mL. **Elimination:** Urine (90%); $T_{1/2}$=6.2 hrs (plasma), 17.6 hrs (blood).

NURSING CONSIDERATIONS

Assessment: Assess for hypoxic states (eg, acute CHF, acute MI, cardiovascular collapse), septicemia, acute/chronic metabolic acidosis, adrenal/pituitary insufficiency, alcoholism, pregnancy/nursing status, and possible drug interactions. Evaluate for other medical/surgical conditions and for possible drug interactions. Assess FPG, HbA1c, renal function, LFTs, and hematologic parameters (eg, Hgb/Hct, RBC indices).

Monitoring: Monitor for lactic acidosis, hypoglycemia, prerenal azotemia, hypoxic states, hypersensitivity reactions, and other adverse reactions. Monitor FPG, HbA1c, renal function (eg, SrCr), LFTs, and hematologic parameters (eg, Hgb/Hct, RBC indices).

Patient Counseling: Inform of the potential risks, benefits, and alternative modes of therapy. Inform about the importance of adherence to dietary instructions, regular exercise programs, and regular testing of blood glucose, HbA1c, renal function, and hematologic parameters. Inform of the risk of lactic acidosis with therapy and to contact physician if unexplained hyperventilation, myalgia, malaise, unusual somnolence, or other nonspecific symptoms occur. Counsel against excessive alcohol intake. Explain risks, symptoms, and conditions that predispose to the development of hypoglycemia when initiating combination therapy. Instruct that drug must be taken with food, swallowed whole with a full glass of water and should not be chewed, cut, or crushed, and that inactive ingredients may be eliminated in the feces as a soft mass.

Administration: Oral route. **Storage:** 20-25°C (68-77°F); excursions permitted to 15-30°C (59-86°F). Keep tightly closed. Protect from light and moisture. Avoid excessive heat and humidity.

FORTAZ   RX
ceftazidime (GlaxoSmithKline)

THERAPEUTIC CLASS: Cephalosporin (3rd generation)

INDICATIONS: Treatment of lower respiratory tract (eg, pneumonia), skin and skin structure (SSSI), bone/joint, gynecologic, CNS (eg, meningitis), intra-abdominal (eg, peritonitis), and urinary tract infections (UTI); and bacterial septicemia caused by susceptible strains of microorganisms. Treatment of sepsis.

DOSAGE: *Adults:* Usual: 1g IM/IV q8-12h. Uncomplicated UTI: 250mg IM/IV q12h. Complicated UTI: 500mg IM/IV q8-12h. Bone and Joint Infection: 2g IV q12h. Uncomplicated Pneumonia/Mild SSSI: 500mg-1g IM/IV q8h. Serious Gynecological and Intra-Abdominal/Meningitis/Severe Life-Threatening Infection: 2g IV q8h. Lung Infection Caused by *Pseudomonas* spp. in Cystic Fibrosis (Normal Renal Function): 30-50mg/kg IV q8h. Max: 6g/day. Renal Impairment: Refer to PI. *Pediatrics:* 1 month-12 yrs: 30-50mg/kg IV q8h. Max: 6g/day. Use higher doses for immunocompromised patients with cystic fibrosis or meningitis. Neonates (0-4 weeks): 30mg/kg IV q12h. Renal Impairment: Refer to PI.

HOW SUPPLIED: Inj: 500mg, 1g, 2g; 1g, 2g [Add-Vantage]; 1g/50mL, 2g/50mL [Galaxy]. Also available as a Pharmacy Bulk Package.

WARNINGS/PRECAUTIONS: Prolonged use may result in overgrowth of nonsusceptible organisms. Cross hypersensitivity among β-lactam antibiotics reported; caution with penicillin (PCN) sensitivity. D/C if allergic reaction occurs. *Clostridium difficile*-associated diarrhea (CDAD) reported and may range in severity from mild diarrhea to fatal colitis; d/c if suspected/confirmed. Elevated levels with renal insufficiency may lead to seizures, encephalopathy, coma, asterixis, myoclonia, and neuromuscular excitability. Associated with fall in prothrombin activity; caution with renal/hepatic impairment, poor nutritional state, and protracted course of antimicrobial therapy. Caution with colitis, history of GI disease, and elderly. Distal necrosis may occur after inadvertent intra-arterial administration. False (+) for urine glucose with Benedict's solution, Fehling's solution, and Clinitest tabs. Increased risk of development of drug-resistant bacteria if used in the absence of a proven or strongly suspected bacterial infection or prophylactic indication.

ADVERSE REACTIONS: Allergic reactions, increased ALT/AST/GGT/LDH, eosinophilia, local/GI reactions.

INTERACTIONS: Nephrotoxicity reported with aminoglycosides or potent diuretics (eg, furosemide). Avoid with chloramphenicol. Risk of fall in prothrombin activity with a protracted course of antimicrobial therapy. May reduce efficacy of combined oral estrogen/progesterone contraceptives.

PREGNANCY: Category B, caution in nursing.

MECHANISM OF ACTION: 3rd-generation cephalosporin; bactericidal, inhibits enzymes responsible for cell-wall synthesis.

PHARMACOKINETICS: Absorption: (IV/IM) Administration of variable doses resulted in different parameters. **Distribution:** Plasma protein binding (<10%); found in breast milk. **Elimination:** Urine (80-90%, unchanged); $T_{1/2}$=1.9 hrs (IV), 2 hrs (IM).

NURSING CONSIDERATIONS

Assessment: Assess for history of hypersensitivity to cephalosporins/PCNs, history of GI disease, colitis, renal/hepatic impairment, nursing status, and for possible drug interactions.

Monitoring: Monitor for signs and symptoms of hypersensitivity reactions, CDAD, LDH, LFTs, renal function, PT, hemolytic anemia, superinfection. Monitor for seizures, encephalopathy, coma, asterixis, neuromuscular excitability, and myoclonia with renal impairment. Perform periodic susceptibility testing.

Patient Counseling: Inform therapy only treats bacterial, not viral infections (eg, common cold). Instruct to take exactly as directed; skipping doses or not completing full course may decrease effectiveness and increase resistance. Advise that may experience diarrhea; notify physician if watery/bloody stools (with/without stomach cramps and fever) occur.

Administration: IM/IV route. Refer to PI for administration, preparation of solutions, use of frozen plastic container, compatibility and stability, and instructions for constitution of ADD-Vantage vials. **Storage:** 15-30°C (59-86°F), in dry state. Protect from light. Frozen as premixed solution should not be stored above -20°C.

FORTEO   RX
teriparatide (Lilly)

> Prescribe only when benefits outweigh risks; do not prescribe for patients who are at increased baseline risk for osteosarcoma (including those with Paget's disease of bone or unexplained alkaline phosphatase elevations, pediatric and young adult patients with open epiphyses, or prior external beam or implant radiation therapy involving the skeleton).

THERAPEUTIC CLASS: Recombinant human parathyroid hormone

INDICATIONS: Treatment of postmenopausal women with osteoporosis at high risk for fracture. To increase bone mass in men with primary or hypogonadal osteoporosis at high risk for fracture. Treatment of men and women with glucocorticoid-induced osteoporosis at high risk for fracture.

DOSAGE: *Adults:* 20mcg qd SQ into thigh or abdominal wall.

HOW SUPPLIED: Inj: 250mcg/mL [2.4mL]

WARNINGS/PRECAUTIONS: Use for >2 yrs is not recommended. Do not give in patients with bone metastases or history of skeletal malignancies, metabolic bone diseases other than osteoporosis, preexisting hypercalcemia, underlying hypercalcemic disorder (eg, primary hyperparathyroidism). May transiently increase serum calcium and exacerbate hypercalcemia. Consider measurement of urinary calcium excretion if active urolithiasis or preexisting hypercalciuria is suspected; caution in patients with active or recent urolithiasis. Transient episodes of symptomatic orthostatic hypotension reported within 1st several doses; administer initially under circumstances where patient can sit or lie down if symptoms of orthostatic hypotension occur.

ADVERSE REACTIONS: Pain, arthralgia, rhinitis, asthenia, N/V, dizziness, headache, HTN, increased cough, pharyngitis, constipation, dyspepsia, diarrhea, rash.

INTERACTIONS: Hypercalcemia may predispose to digitalis toxicity; use caution with digoxin.

PREGNANCY: Category C, not for use in nursing.

MECHANISM OF ACTION: Recombinant human parathyroid hormone; binds to specific high-affinity cell-surface receptors. Stimulates new bone formation on trabecular and cortical (periosteal and/or endosteal) bone surfaces by preferential stimulation of osteoblastic activity over osteoclastic activity. Produces an increase in skeletal mass, markers of bone formation and resorption, and bone strength.

PHARMACOKINETICS: Absorption: Rapid. Absolute bioavailability (95%); T_{max}=30 min. **Distribution:** (IV) V_d=0.12L/kg. **Metabolism:** Liver (nonspecific enzymatic mechanisms). **Elimination:** Kidney; $T_{1/2}$=1 hr.

NURSING CONSIDERATIONS

Assessment: Assess for increased baseline risk for osteosarcoma, bone metastases or history of skeletal malignancies, metabolic bone disease other than osteoporosis, hypercalcemia, hypercalcemic disorder, hypercalciuria, active or recent urolithiasis, previous hypersensitivity to the drug, pregnancy/nursing status, and possible drug interactions. Consider measurement of urinary calcium excretion if active urolithiasis or preexisting hypercalciuria is suspected.

Monitoring: Monitor for signs/symptoms of osteosarcoma, orthostatic hypotension, and other adverse reactions.

Patient Counseling: Inform of potential risk of osteosarcoma and encourage to enroll in the voluntary Forteo Patient Registry. Instruct to sit or lie down if lightheadedness or palpitations following inj develop; if symptoms persist or worsen, advise to contact physician before continuing treatment. Instruct to contact physician if persistent symptoms of hypercalcemia (eg, N/V, constipation, lethargy, muscle weakness) develop. Counsel on roles of supplemental calcium and/or vitamin D, weight-bearing exercise, and modification of certain behavioral factors (eg, smoking, alcohol use). Instruct on proper use of delivery device (pen) and proper disposal of needles; advise not to share pen with other patients and not to transfer contents to a syringe. Instruct to discard pen after the 28-day use period. Counsel to read Medication Guide and pen User Manual before starting therapy and each time the prescription is renewed.

Administration: SQ route. Inject into thigh or abdominal wall. Administer initially under circumstances where patient can sit or lie down if symptoms of orthostatic hypotension occur. **Storage:** 2-8°C (36-46°F). Recap pen when not in use. Minimize time out of the refrigerator during the use period; deliver dose immediately following removal from the refrigerator. Do not freeze; do not use if has been frozen.

FORTESTA GEL
testosterone (Endo)

> Virilization reported in children secondarily exposed to testosterone gel. Children should avoid contact with unwashed or unclothed application sites in men using testosterone gel. Advise patients to strictly adhere to recommended instructions for use.

THERAPEUTIC CLASS: Androgen

INDICATIONS: Replacement therapy in males for conditions associated with a deficiency or absence of endogenous testosterone (congenital or acquired primary hypogonadism or hypogonadotropic hypogonadism).

DOSAGE: *Adults:* Initial: Apply 40mg (4 pump actuations) qam to intact skin of the thighs. May adjust between 10-70mg based on serum testosterone concentration from a single blood draw 2 hrs after application, 14 days, and 35 days after starting treatment or following dose adjustment. Max: 70mg. Total Serum Testosterone Concentration: ≥2500ng/dL: Decrease daily dose by 20mg (2 pump actuations). ≥1250-<2500ng/dL: Decrease daily dose by 10mg (1 pump actuation). ≥500-<1250ng/dL: Continue on current dose. <500ng/dL: Increase daily dose by 10mg (1 pump actuation).

HOW SUPPLIED: Gel: 10mg/actuation [60g]

CONTRAINDICATIONS: Prostate or breast carcinoma in men, women who are or may become pregnant, or nursing mothers.

WARNINGS/PRECAUTIONS: Application site and dose are not interchangeable with other topical testosterone products. Patients with BPH may be at increased risk for worsening of signs/symptoms of BPH. May increase risk for prostate cancer; evaluate for prostate cancer prior to and during therapy. Risk of virilization in women and children due to secondary exposure; d/c until cause of virilization is identified. Increases in Hct and red blood cell mass may increase risk for thromboembolic events; may require reduction or d/c of drug. Suppression of spermatogenesis may occur. Prolonged use may cause serious hepatic effects (eg, peliosis hepatis, hepatic neoplasms, cholestatic hepatitis, jaundice). Risk of edema with or without congestive heart failure (CHF) with preexisting cardiac, renal, or hepatic disease. Gynecomastia may develop and persist. May potentiate sleep apnea, especially with obesity or chronic lung diseases. Changes in serum lipid profile reported. Caution in cancer patients at risk of hypercalcemia and associated hypercalciuria. May decrease concentrations of thyroxin-binding globulins, resulting in decreased total T4 serum concentrations and increased resin uptake of T3 and T4. Gel is flammable; avoid fire, flame, or smoking until dry.

ADVERSE REACTIONS: Application-site reactions, prostatic-specific antigen (PSA) increased, abnormal dreams.

INTERACTIONS: Changes in insulin sensitivity or glycemic control reported. Concurrent use with adrenocorticotropic hormone or corticosteroids may increase fluid retention. Changes in anticoagulant activity may occur; frequently monitor INR and PT in patients taking anticoagulants.

PREGNANCY: Category X, contraindicated in nursing.

MECHANISM OF ACTION: Androgen; responsible for normal growth and development of male sex organs and for maintenance of secondary sex characteristics.

PHARMACOKINETICS: Metabolism: Estradiol and DHT (active metabolites). **Elimination:** (IM) Urine (90% glucuronic and sulfuric acid conjugates), feces (6% unconjugated); $T_{1/2}$=10-100 min.

NURSING CONSIDERATIONS

Assessment: Assess for conditions where treatment is contraindicated, BPH, cardiac/renal/hepatic disease, obesity, chronic lung disease, and for possible drug interactions. Assess use in cancer patients at risk of hypercalcemia. Obtain baseline Hct.

Monitoring: Monitor for prostate carcinoma, hepatic toxicity, edema with or without CHF, gynecomastia, and sleep apnea. In patients with BPH, monitor for signs/symptoms of worsening BPH. Perform periodic monitoring of Hgb, Hct, PSA, serum lipid profile, LFTs, and serum testosterone levels. In cancer patients at risk for hypercalcemia, regularly monitor serum Ca^{2+} levels.

Patient Counseling: Inform that men with known or suspected prostate/breast cancer should not use androgen therapy. Report signs/symptoms of secondary exposure in children (eg, penis/clitoris enlargement, premature development of pubic hair, increased erections) and in women (eg, changes in hair distribution, increase in acne). Advise family members to avoid contact with unwashed or unclothed application site of men. Apply product as directed; wash hands with soap and water after application, cover application site with clothing after gel dries, and wash application site with soap and water prior to direct skin-to-skin contact with others. Inform about possible adverse reactions. Advise to read the Medication Guide prior to therapy and reread each time prescription is renewed. Inform that drug is flammable until dry. Keep out of reach of children.

Administration: Topical route. Prime the canister pump in upright position, slowly and fully depress the actuator eight times. Refer to PI for administration details. **Storage:** 20-25°C (68-77°F); excursions permitted to 15-30°C (59-86°F). Do not freeze.

FORTICAL RX
calcitonin-salmon (rdna origin) (Upsher-Smith)

THERAPEUTIC CLASS: Hormonal bone resorption inhibitor

INDICATIONS: Treatment of postmenopausal osteoporosis in women >5 yrs postmenopause with low bone mass relative to healthy postmenopausal women; recommended in conjunction with an adequate calcium and vitamin D intake.

DOSAGE: *Adults:* 200 IU qd intranasally. Alternate nostrils daily.

HOW SUPPLIED: Nasal Spray: 200 IU/activation

WARNINGS/PRECAUTIONS: Possibility of systemic allergic reactions (eg, anaphylaxis, anaphylactic shock). Allergic reactions should be differentiated from generalized flushing and hypotension. Consider skin testing if sensitivity suspected. Development of mucosal alterations or transient nasal conditions reported; perform periodic nasal exams. Rhinitis, epistaxis, sinusitis most commonly reported in postmenopausal patients. D/C if severe ulceration of nasal mucosa occurs (indicated by ulcers >1.5mm diameter or penetrating below mucosa, or associated with heavy bleeding). Incidence of rhinitis, irritation, erythema, and excoriation higher in geriatric patients.

ADVERSE REACTIONS: Rhinitis, nasal symptoms, back pain, arthralgia, epistaxis, headache, influenza-like symptoms, fatigue, erythematous rash, arthrosis, myalgia, sinusitis, bronchospasm, HTN, constipation.

INTERACTIONS: May reduce lithium levels; dose of lithium may need to be adjusted. Prior diphosphonate use appears to reduce the anti-resorptive response to calcitonin-salmon nasal spray in patients with Paget's disease.

PREGNANCY: Category C, not for use in nursing.

MECHANISM OF ACTION: Hormonal bone resorption inhibitor; actions on bone not fully established. Calcitonin receptors have been found in osteoclasts and osteoblasts. Initially causes a marked transient inhibition of the ongoing bone resorptive process. Prolonged use causes a smaller decrease in the rate of bone resorption. Associated with inhibition of osteoclast function and increased osteoblastic activity.

PHARMACOKINETICS: Absorption: T_{max}=13 min; Bioavailability (3%). **Elimination:** $T_{1/2}$=18 min.

NURSING CONSIDERATIONS

Assessment: Assess for previous allergy to calcitonin-salmon; perform skin testing if sensitivity suspected. Assess for pregnancy/nursing status and for possible drug interactions. Perform nasal and bone mineral density examination prior to treatment. Assess patient's intake of calcium and vitamin D and recommend adequate intake (at least 1000mg/day elemental calcium and 400 IU/day vitamin D) to retard progressive loss of bone mass.

Monitoring: Monitor for signs/symptoms of allergic reaction (eg, anaphylactic shock, anaphylaxis), nasal mucosal alterations, rhinitis, epistaxis, and sinusitis. Perform periodic nasal exams of nasal mucosa, turbinates, septum, and mucosal blood vessels. Perform periodic monitoring of urine sediment. Measure lumbar vertebral bone mass periodically to monitor for efficacy.

Patient Counseling: Counsel to notify physician of significant nasal irritation. Advise to seek emergency help if serious allergic reaction occurs (eg, troubled breathing, swelling of face, throat or tongue, rapid heartbeat, chest pain, feeling faint or dizzy). Advise to store new, unassembled medication in refrigerator away from light, and not to freeze. Instruct that before priming pump and using new medication, allow to reach room temperature. Inform that after opening, store at room temperature, in upright position; discard unused medication 30 days after 1st use. Recommend adequate intake of calcium and vitamin D.

Administration: Intranasal route. To prime pump, hold bottle upright and depress the 2 white side arms of pump toward the bottle at least 5X until a full spray is produced. To administer, carefully place the nozzle into the nostril with the head in upright position and pump firmly depressed toward the bottle. Do not prime pump before each daily use. **Storage:** Unopened: 2-8°C (36-46°F). Protect from freezing. Opened: 20-25°C (68-77°F); excursions permitted to 15-30°C (59-86°F). Store in upright position. Discard 30 days after 1st use.

FOSAMAX RX
alendronate sodium (Merck)

THERAPEUTIC CLASS: Bisphosphonate

INDICATIONS: Treatment and prevention of osteoporosis in postmenopausal women. Treatment to increase bone mass in men with osteoporosis. Treatment of glucocorticoid-induced osteoporosis. Treatment of Paget's disease.

DOSAGE: *Adults:* Osteoporosis: Treatment: 70mg once weekly or 10mg qd. Prevention: 35mg once weekly or 5mg qd. Glucocorticoid-Induced: 5mg qd; 10mg qd for postmenopausal women not on estrogen. Paget's Disease: 40mg qd for 6 months. Take ≥30 min before the 1st food, beverage (other than plain water), or other medication. Take tabs with 6-8 oz. of plain water. Follow oral sol with 2 oz. of plain water. Do not lie down for ≥30 min and until after 1st food of the day.

HOW SUPPLIED: Sol: 70mg [75mL]; Tab: 5mg, 10mg, 35mg, 40mg, 70mg

CONTRAINDICATIONS: Esophageal abnormalities that delay esophageal emptying (eg, stricture or achalasia); inability to stand or sit upright for ≥30 min; hypocalcemia. Patients at increased risk of aspiration (oral sol).

WARNINGS/PRECAUTIONS: Not recommended with severe renal insufficiency (CrCl <35mL/min). May cause local irritation of the upper GI mucosa; caution with active upper GI problems (eg, Barrett's esophagus, dysphagia, esophageal diseases, gastritis, duodenitis, ulcers). Esophageal adverse events and gastric and duodenal ulcers reported. D/C if dysphagia, odynophagia, retrosternal pain, new or worsening heartburn develops. Supervise therapy in those who cannot comply with dosing instructions due to mental disability. Treat hypocalcemia or other mineral metabolism disorders prior to therapy; hypocalcemia reported; ensure adequate calcium and vitamin D intake. Severe, incapacitating bone, joint, and/or muscle pain reported; d/c if severe symptoms develop. Osteonecrosis of the jaw (ONJ) reported; d/c to reduce risk of ONJ in patients requiring invasive dental procedures. Atypical, low-energy, or low-trauma fractures of the femoral shaft reported; consider interrupting therapy. In patients with glucocorticoid-induced osteoporosis, ascertain hormonal status and consider replacement therapy; measure bone mineral density (BMD) at initiation and repeat after 6-12 months after combined alendronate and glucocorticoid treatment.

ADVERSE REACTIONS: Nausea, abdominal pain, musculoskeletal pain (bone, muscle, or joint), acid regurgitation, flatulence, dyspepsia, constipation, diarrhea, dyspepsia.

INTERACTIONS: Calcium supplements and other multivalent cations, antacids, and some oral medications will interfere with absorption; take ≥1/2 hour after alendronate. Increased GI irritation with aspirin-containing products and alendronate >10mg. Caution with NSAID use due to associated GI irritation. Concomitant use with IV ranitidine may double bioavailability of oral alendronate. Concomitant use with hormone-replacement therapy (eg, estrogen ± progestin) may lead to a greater degree of suppression of bone turnover. Increased oral bioavailability with oral prednisone. May increase risk of atypical femur fractures with glucocorticoids (eg, prednisone). Caution with risk factors for ONJ (eg, chemotherapy, corticosteroids). Reduced bioavailability with concomitant coffee or orange juice.

PREGNANCY: Category C, caution in nursing.

MECHANISM OF ACTION: Bisphosphonate; binds to hydroxyapatite found in bone, specifically inhibits the osteoclast-mediated bone resorption.

PHARMACOKINETICS: Absorption: Absolute bioavailability: Women (0.64%), men (0.59%). **Distribution:** V_d=28L; plasma protein binding (78%). **Elimination:** (IV) Urine (50%), feces (little or none); $T_{1/2}$>10 yrs.

NURSING CONSIDERATIONS

Assessment: Assess for esophageal abnormalities, ability to stand or sit upright for ≥30 min, hypocalcemia, active upper GI problems, mineral metabolism disorders, risk factors (invasive dental procedures, diagnosed cancer, chemotherapy, corticosteroids, poor oral hygiene, comorbid disorders) of ONJ, renal impairment (eg, CrCl <35mL/min), hypersensitivity, pregnancy/nursing status, and possible drug interactions. Obtain BMD if taking glucocorticoids. Assess for risk of aspiration if using oral sol.

Monitoring: Monitor for signs/symptoms of ONJ, atypical fracture, esophageal reactions, musculoskeletal pain, hypocalcemia, mineral metabolism disorders. Monitor serum alkaline phosphatase especially in patients with Paget's disease and BMD q6-12 months if taking glucocorticoids.

Patient Counseling: Inform about risks and benefits of therapy and to read Medication Guide. Instruct to take supplemental calcium and vitamin D if dietary intake is inadequate. Counsel to consider weight-bearing exercise, modifying behavioral factors (eg, cigarette smoking, excessive alcohol use), to take medication with plain water in the am ≥30 min before the 1st food, beverage, or medication, and to swallow each tab with a full glass of water (6-8 oz.). If taking oral sol, advise to take ≥2 oz. of water after administration. Instruct to avoid chewing or sucking on tab, taking at hs or before arising for the day, and lying down for ≥30 min following administration and until after 1st food of the day. Advise to d/c and contact physician if symptoms of esophageal disease develop. Instruct to take the following am if dose is missed and return to taking dose on regularly scheduled day; avoid taking 2 doses at the same time.

Administration: Oral route. Refer to PI for proper administration. **Storage:** Tab: 15-30°C (59-86°F). Store in a well-closed container. Oral sol: 25°C (77°F); excursions permitted to 15-30°C (59-86°F). Do not freeze.

FOSAMAX PLUS D RX
alendronate sodium - cholecalciferol (Merck)

THERAPEUTIC CLASS: Bisphosphonate/vitamin D analog

INDICATIONS: Treatment of osteoporosis in postmenopausal women. Treatment to increase bone mass in men with osteoporosis.

DOSAGE: *Adults:* 1 tab (70mg-2800 IU or 70mg-5600 IU) once weekly. Usual: 70mg-5600 IU once weekly. Take with 6-8 oz. of plain water ≥30 min before the 1st food, beverage, or other medication of the day. Do not lie down for ≥30 min and until after 1st food of the day.

HOW SUPPLIED: Tab: (Alendronate Sodium-Cholecalciferol) 70mg-2800 IU, 70mg-5600 IU

CONTRAINDICATIONS: Esophageal abnormalities that delay esophageal emptying (eg, stricture or achalasia), inability to stand or sit upright for ≥30 min, hypocalcemia.

WARNINGS/PRECAUTIONS: Not recommended with severe renal insufficiency (CrCl <35mL/min). May cause local irritation of the upper GI mucosa; caution with active upper GI problems (eg, Barrett's esophagus, dysphagia, esophageal diseases, gastritis, duodenitis, ulcers). Esophageal adverse events and gastric and duodenal ulcers reported; d/c if dysphagia, odynophagia, retrosternal pain, or new/worsening heartburn develops. Supervise therapy in patients who cannot comply with dosing instructions due to mental disability. May decrease serum calcium and phosphate; treat hypocalcemia or other mineral metabolism disorders prior to therapy. Severe and occasionally incapacitating bone, joint, and/or muscle pain reported; d/c if severe symptoms develop. Osteonecrosis of the jaw (ONJ) reported; discontinuation may reduce risk in patients requiring invasive dental procedures. Atypical, low-energy or low trauma fractures of the femoral shaft reported; consider interrupting therapy. Do not use alone to treat vitamin D deficiency. Vitamin D3 supplementation may worsen hypercalcemia and/or hypercalciuria in patients with diseases associated with unregulated overproduction of 1,25-dihydroxyvitamin D (eg, leukemia, lymphoma, sarcoidosis); monitor urine and serum calcium.

ADVERSE REACTIONS: Decreases in serum calcium and phosphate, abdominal pain, musculoskeletal pain, acid regurgitation, flatulence, nausea, dyspepsia, constipation, diarrhea.

INTERACTIONS: NSAID associated with GI irritation; use with caution. Alendronate: Antacids, some oral medications, and products containing calcium and other multivalent cations may interfere with absorption; take ≥1/2 hour after alendronate. Increased upper GI adverse events with aspirin-containing products and alendronate >10mg. Doubled bioavailability reported with IV ranitidine. Risk factors for ONJ include concomitant chemotherapy or corticosteroids. May increase risk of atypical femur fractures with glucocorticoids (eg, prednisone). Reduced bioavailability reported with coffee or orange juice. Cholecalciferol: Impaired absorption with olestra, mineral oils, orlistat, bile acid sequestrants (eg, cholestyramine, colestipol); consider additional supplementation. Increased catabolism with anticonvulsants, cimetidine, and thiazides; consider additional supplementation.

PREGNANCY: Category C, caution in nursing.

MECHANISM OF ACTION: Alendronate: Bisphosphonate; binds to bone hydroxyapatite and specifically inhibits the activity of osteoclasts, the bone-resorbing cells. Reduces bone resorption with no direct effect on bone formation. Cholecalciferol: Vitamin D analog; increases intestinal absorption of calcium and phosphate. Regulates serum calcium, renal calcium and phosphate excretion, bone formation, and bone resorption.

PHARMACOKINETICS: Absorption: Alendronate: Absolute bioavailability: Women (0.64%), men (0.59%). Cholecalciferol: (2800 IU) C_{max}=4.0ng/mL; T_{max}=10.6 hrs; AUC=120.7ng•hr/mL. See PI. **Distribution:** Alendronate: V_d ≥28L; plasma protein binding (78%). Cholecalciferol: Found in breast milk. **Metabolism:** Cholecalciferol: Liver (rapid) via hydroxylation to 25-hydroxyvitamin D3; subsequently metabolized in kidney to 1,25-dihydroxyvitamin D3 (active metabolite). **Elimination:** Alendronate: (IV) Urine (50%), feces (little or none); (PO) $T_{1/2}$=>10 yrs. Cholecalciferol: (IV) Urine (2.4%), feces (4.9%); (PO) $T_{1/2}$=14 hrs.

NURSING CONSIDERATIONS

Assessment: Assess for esophageal abnormalities, ability to stand or sit upright for ≥30 min, hypocalcemia, active upper GI problems, mineral metabolism disorders, diseases associated with unregulated overproduction of 1,25 dihydroxyvitamin D, risk factors for ONJ (invasive dental procedures, diagnosed cancer, concomitant therapies [eg, chemotherapy, corticosteroids], poor oral hygiene, comorbid disorders), renal insufficiency, hypersensitivity, pregnancy/nursing status, and possible drug interactions.

Monitoring: Monitor for signs/symptoms of esophageal reactions, hypocalcemia, mineral metabolism disorders, musculoskeletal pain, ONJ, and atypical fractures. Monitor urine/serum calcium and renal function in patients with conditions in which treatment is cautioned. Reevaluate the need for therapy periodically.

Patient Counseling: Inform of risks and benefits and to read Medication Guide before starting therapy. Instruct to take supplemental calcium and vitamin D if dietary intake is inadequate. Counsel to consider weight-bearing exercise and modifying certain behavioral factors (eg, cigarette smoking, excessive alcohol use). Instruct to take medication with plain water the 1st thing upon arising for the day ≥30 min before the 1st food, beverage, or medication, and to swallow each tab with a full glass of water (6-8 oz.). Instruct to avoid chewing or sucking on tab, taking at hs or before arising for the day, and lying down for ≥30 min following administration and until after 1st food of the day. Advise to d/c and contact physician if symptoms of esophageal disease develop. If dose is missed, instruct to take dose the following am and return to taking dose on regularly scheduled day; advise to avoid taking 2 tabs on the same day.

Administration: Oral route. **Storage:** 20-25°C (68-77°F); excursions permitted to 15-30°C (59-86°F). Protect from moisture and light. Store in original package until use.

FOSINOPRIL   RX
fosinopril sodium (Various)

> ACE inhibitors can cause death/injury to developing fetus during 2nd and 3rd trimesters. D/C therapy if pregnancy detected.

THERAPEUTIC CLASS: ACE inhibitor

INDICATIONS: Treatment of HTN may be used alone or with thiazide diuretics. Adjunct therapy for heart failure (HF).

DOSAGE: *Adults:* HTN: If possible, d/c diuretic 2-3 days before therapy. Initial: 10mg qd, monitor carefully if cannot d/c diuretic. Maint: 20-40mg qd. Resume diuretic if BP not controlled. Max: 80mg qd. HF: Initial: 10mg qd, 5mg with moderate to severe renal failure or vigorous diuresis. Titrate: Increase over several weeks. Maint: 20-40mg qd. Max: 40mg qd. Elderly: Start at low end of dosing range.
Pediatric: >50kg: HTN: 5-10mg qd.

HOW SUPPLIED: Tab: 10mg*, 20mg, 40mg *scored

CONTRAINDICATIONS: History of ACE inhibitor associated angioedema.

WARNINGS/PRECAUTIONS: Head, neck, and intestinal angioedema reported; d/c if laryngeal stridor or angioedema of the face, lips, mucous membranes, tongue, glottis, or extremities occur. Anaphylactoid reactions during desensitization and during membrane exposure reported. Monitor for hypotension in high-risk patients (eg, HF, volume and/or salt depletion, surgery/anesthesia). May cause agranulocytosis; consider monitoring WBCs in patients with collagen vascular disease, especially if associated with renal impairment. Rarely associated with cholestatic jaundice that progresses to fulminant hepatic necrosis and sometimes death; d/c if jaundice or if marked elevations of hepatic enzymes occur. Caution in patients with impaired liver function. May cause changes in renal function; caution in patients with severe CHF, renal artery stenosis, and in patients with pre-existing renal impairment. May cause hyperkalemia; caution in patients with risk factors for hyperkalemia (eg, diabetes mellitus (DM), renal dysfunction). Persistent nonproductive cough reported. Less effective on BP and more reports of angioedema in blacks than nonblacks. Caution in elderly.

ADVERSE REACTIONS: Dizziness, cough, hypotension, musculoskeletal pain, headache, fatigue, diarrhea, N/V.

INTERACTIONS: May increase lithium levels. Hypotension risk with diuretics. Increased risk of hyperkalemia with K⁺-sparing diuretics (eg, spironolactone, amiloride, triamterene), K⁺-containing salt substitutes, or K⁺ supplements. Decreased absorption with antacids; space dosing by 2 hrs. Nitritoid reactions (eg, facial flushing, N/V, hypotension) reported rarely with injectable gold.

PREGNANCY: Category D, not for use in nursing.

MECHANISM OF ACTION: ACE inhibitor; inhibition results in decreased plasma angiotensin II, which leads to decreased vasopressor activity and decreased aldosterone secretion.

PHARMACOKINETICS: **Absorption:** Slow; T_{max}=3 hrs. **Distribution:** Plasma protein binding (99.4%); found in breast milk. **Metabolism:** Hepatic; glucuronidation; fosinoprilat (active metabolite). **Elimination:** Urine, feces; (HTN) $T_{1/2}$=11.5 hrs. (HF) $T_{1/2}$=14 hrs.

NURSING CONSIDERATIONS

Assessment: Assess for history of ACE inhibitor associated angioedema. Assess for volume and/or salt depletion, renal artery stenosis, CHF, pregnancy/nursing status, renal/hepatic function, hypersensitivity to drug, and for possible drug interactions. Assess for risk factors for developing hyperkalemia (eg, DM).

Monitoring: Monitor for signs/symptoms of head/neck and intestinal angioedema, anaphylactoid reactions, hypotension, agranulocytosis, hepatic failure, renal impairment, hyperkalemia, and for persistent non-productive cough. Monitor renal function. In patients with collagen vascular disease, consider monitoring WBC count.

Patient Counseling: Inform that angioedema including laryngeal edema can occur; instruct to immediately report to physician and d/c therapy if any signs or symptoms of angioedema (eg, swelling of face, eyes, lips, tongue, extremities; difficulty swallowing or breathing) occur. Lightheadedness may occur, instruct to d/c therapy if syncope occurs until physician has been contacted. Inadequate fluid intake or excessive perspiration, diarrhea, or vomiting can lead to an excessive fall in BP. Avoid using K$^+$ supplements or salt substitutes containing K$^+$ unless physician has been notified. Counsel to report any signs of infection (eg, sore throat, fever). Inform of potential risks of therapy if used during pregnancy.

Administration: Oral route. **Storage:** 25°C (77°F); excursions permitted to 15-30°C (59-86°F). Protect from moisture; keep bottle tightly closed.

FOSINOPRIL/HCTZ RX
fosinopril sodium - hydrochlorothiazide (Various)

ACE inhibitors can cause injury/death to developing fetus during 2nd and 3rd trimesters. D/C therapy if pregnancy detected.

THERAPEUTIC CLASS: ACE inhibitor/thiazide diuretic

INDICATIONS: Treatment of hypertension.

DOSAGE: *Adults:* Not Controlled with Fosinopril/HCTZ monotherapy: 10mg-12.5mg tab or 20mg-12.5mg tab qd.

HOW SUPPLIED: Tab: (Fosinopril-HCTZ) 10mg-12.5mg, 20mg-12.5mg

CONTRAINDICATIONS: Anuric patients and hypersensitivity to other sulfonamide-derived drugs.

WARNINGS/PRECAUTIONS: Angioedema involving the face, extremities, lips, tongue, glottis, larynx, and intestines reported; d/c if laryngeal stridor or angioedema of the face, tongue, or glottis occur. Anaphylactoid reactions during desensitization and during membrane exposure reported. Can cause symptomatic hypotension; most likely to occur in volume- and/or salt-depleted patients and patients undergoing surgery or during anesthesia with agents that produce hypotension. Correct volume and/or salt depletion prior to therapy. Enhanced effects with postsympathectomy patients. May cause changes in renal function (eg, increase SrCr, BUN, azotemia); caution in patients with severe congestive heart failure (CHF), severe renal disease, renal artery stenosis, or preexisting renal impairment. Associated with neutropenia/agranulocytosis; monitor WBC in patients with collagen-vascular disease and impaired renal function. Rarely, associated with syndrome that starts with cholestatic jaundice and progresses to fulminant necrosis and sometimes death; d/c if experience jaundice or marked elevations of hepatic enzymes. Caution in patients with impaired hepatic function or progressive liver disease. May exacerbate or activate systemic lupus erythematosus (SLE). Monitor electrolytes to detect possible electrolyte imbalance. Dilutional hyponatremia may occur in edematous patients. May cause hypercalcemia, hypophosphatemia, hypomagnesemia, reduce glucose tolerance and raise serum levels of cholesterol, TG, and uric acid. Persistent nonproductive cough reported. Avoid if CrCl ≤30mL/min/1.73m^2.

ADVERSE REACTIONS: Headache, cough, fatigue, dizziness.

INTERACTIONS: Caution with other antihypertensives. May alter insulin requirements. Nitritoid reactions (eg, facial flushing, N/V, hypotension) reported rarely with injectable gold. Increased risk of lithium toxicity. Fosinopril: Increased risk of hyperkalemia with K$^+$-sparing diuretics, K$^+$ supplements, or K$^+$-containing salt substitutes. Antacids may impair absorption; separate dose by 2 hrs. HCTZ: Potentiate effects of ganglionic or peripheral adrenergic-blocking agents. May decrease effects of methenamine. May increase responsiveness to tubocurarine. May decrease arterial responsiveness to norepinephrine. NSAIDs decrease diuretic, natriuretic, and antihypertensive effects. Potentiates orthostatic hypotension with alcohol, barbiturates, and narcotics. Reduced absorption with cholestyramine, colestipol. Increase risk of hypokalemia with corticosteroids and adrenocorticotropic hormone.

PREGNANCY: Category C (1st trimester) and D (2nd and 3rd trimesters), not for use in nursing.

MECHANISM OF ACTION: Fosinopril: ACE inhibitor; inhibition results in decreased plasma angiotensin II, which leads to decreased vasopressor activity and decreased aldosterone secretion. HCTZ: Thiazide diuretic; affects renal tubular mechanism of electrolyte reabsorption directly increasing excretion of Na$^+$ and Cl$^-$.

PHARMACOKINETICS: Absorption: Fosinoprilat: T_{max}=3 hrs; HCTZ: T_{max}=1-2.5 hrs. **Distribution:** Found in breast milk. Fosinoprilat: Plasma protein binding (95%). HCTZ: V_d =3.6-7.8L/kg; plasma protein binding (67.9%), crosses placenta. **Metabolism:** Fosinopril: Hepatic, glucuronidation; fosinoprilat (active metabolite). **Elimination:** Fosinopril: Urine, feces, $T_{1/2}$=11.5 hrs. HCTZ: Renal; $T_{1/2}$=5-15 hrs.

NURSING CONSIDERATIONS

Assessment: Assess for anuria, history of allergy to sulfonamides, salt- and/or volume-depletion due to prolonged diuretic therapy, dietary salt restriction, diarrhea, vomiting, preexisting CHF, renal disease, collagen-vascular disease, SLE, impaired hepatic function or progressive liver disease, severe renal disease, renal artery stenosis, and preexisting renal vascular disease, pregnancy/nursing status and for possible drug interactions. Obtain baseline electrolytes (eg, K^+, Ca^{2+}, Mg^{2+}), SrCr and BUN.

Monitoring: Monitor for laryngeal stridor; angioedema of the face, tongue, or glottis; abdominal pain; anaphylactoid reactions, especially during desensitization or membrane exposure; symptomatic hypotension; jaundice; infections; and marked elevation of hepatic enzymes. Monitor BP, serum electrolytes, serum uric acid, and glucose tolerance. Monitor WBC in patients with collagen-vascular disease.

Patient Counseling: Inform about fetal risks if taken during pregnancy. Caution that inadequate fluid intake, excessive perspiration, diarrhea, or vomiting can lead to excessive fall in BP, with the same consequences of lightheadedness and possible syncope. Advise not to use salt or K^+ supplements. Counsel about signs/symptoms of neutropenia (infections), angioedema, electrolyte imbalance (thirst, weakness, lethargy), and other adverse effects; advise to seek prompt medical attention.

Administration: Oral route. **Storage:** 20-25°C (68-77°F); excursions permitted to 15-30°C (59-86°F). Protect from moisture.

FRAGMIN   RX
dalteparin sodium (Eisai)

Epidural or spinal hematomas may occur in patients anticoagulated with low molecular weight heparins or heparinoids and who are receiving neuraxial anesthesia or undergoing spinal puncture; long-term or permanent paralysis may result. Increased risk of developing epidural or spinal hematomas in patients using indwelling epidural catheters, concomitant use of other drugs that affect hemostasis (eg, NSAIDs, platelet inhibitors, other anticoagulants), history of traumatic or repeated epidural or spinal puncture, or a history of spinal deformity or spinal surgery. Monitor frequently for signs/symptoms of neurologic impairment; urgent treatment is necessary if neurologic compromise occurs. Consider benefits and risks before neuraxial intervention in patients anticoagulated or to be anticoagulated for thromboprophylaxis.

THERAPEUTIC CLASS: Low molecular weight heparin

INDICATIONS: Prophylaxis of ischemic complications in unstable angina and non-Q-wave myocardial infarction (MI) in conjunction with aspirin (ASA) therapy. Prophylaxis of deep vein thrombosis (DVT), which may lead to pulmonary embolism (PE), in hip replacement surgery, abdominal surgery in patients at risk for thromboembolic complications, and for those at risk for thromboembolic complications due to severely restricted mobility during acute illness. Extended treatment of symptomatic venous thromboembolism (VTE) (proximal DVT and/or PE) to reduce the recurrence of VTE in patients with cancer.

DOSAGE: *Adults:* Administer SQ. Prophylaxis of Ischemic Complications in Unstable Angina/Non-Q-Wave MI: 120 IU/kg q12h with PO ASA (75-165mg qd) until clinically stabilized. Usual Duration: 5-8 days. Max: 10,000 IU q12h. Prophylaxis of VTE Following Hip Replacement Surgery: Preop (Starting Day of Surgery): Usual: 2500 IU within 2 hrs preop, then 2500 IU 4-8 hrs postop. Preop (Starting Evening Prior to Surgery): Usual: 5000 IU 10-14 hrs preop, then 5000 IU 4-8 hrs postop. Postop Start: Usual: 2500 IU 4-8 hrs postop. Maint (Pre/Postop): 5000 IU qd for 5-10 days postop (up to 14 days). Abdominal Surgery: Risk of Thromboembolic Complications: 2500 IU 1-2 hrs pre-op then qd for 5-10 days postop. Abdominal Surgery with High Thromboembolic Risk: 5000 IU pm preop then qd for 5-10 days postop. Abdominal Surgery with Malignancy: 2500 IU 1-2 hrs preop, followed by 2500 IU 12 hrs later, then 5000 IU qd for 5-10 days postop. Severely Restricted Mobility During Acute Illness: 5000 IU qd for 12-14 days. Treatment of Symptomatic VTE in Cancer Patients: 200 IU/kg qd for 1st 30 days, then 150 IU/kg qd for months 2-6. Max: 18,000 IU/day. Platelet Count 50,000-100,000/mm³: Reduce dose by 2500 IU until platelet count ≥100,000/mm³. Platelet Count <50,000/mm³: D/C therapy until platelet count >50,000/mm³. Severe Renal Impairment (CrCl <30mL/min): Monitor anti-Xa levels to determine appropriate dose.

HOW SUPPLIED: Inj: (Syringe) 2500 IU/0.2mL, 5000 IU/0.2mL, 7500 IU/0.3mL, 10,000 IU/0.4mL, 10,000 IU/1mL, 12,500 IU/0.5mL, 15,000 IU/0.6mL, 18,000 IU/0.72mL; (MDV) 95,000 IU/3.8mL, 95,000 IU/9.5 mL

CONTRAINDICATIONS: Active major bleeding, history of heparin-induced thrombocytopenia or heparin-induced thrombocytopenia with thrombosis, patients undergoing epidural/neuraxial anesthesia, as treatment for unstable angina/non-Q wave MI and for prolonged VTE prophylaxis, and hypersensitivity to pork products.

WARNINGS/PRECAUTIONS: Not for IM inj. Not indicated for acute treatment of VTE. Extreme caution in patients with increased risk of hemorrhage (eg, severe uncontrolled HTN, bacterial endocarditis, bleeding disorders, active ulceration, and angiodysplastic GI disease, hemorrhagic stroke, or shortly after brain, spinal or ophthalmological surgery). Increased risk of bleeding with thrombocytopenia or platelet defects, severe liver/kidney insufficiency, hypertensive or diabetic retinopathy, and recent GI bleeding. May cause heparin-induced thrombocytopenia with or without thrombosis; d/c or reduce dose if platelet count <100,000/mm³. Multi-dose vials (MDV) contain benzyl alcohol; caution in pregnant women. In premature infants, benzyl alcohol reported to be associated with fatal "gasping syndrome". Caution in elderly with low body weight (<45kg) and those predisposed to decreased renal function.

ADVERSE REACTIONS: Bleeding, injection-site pain, thrombocytopenia, elevation of serum transaminases (ALT, AST), injection-site hematoma.

INTERACTIONS: See Boxed Warning and Contraindications. Caution with oral anticoagulants, platelet inhibitors, and thrombolytic agents due to increased risk of bleeding.

PREGNANCY: Category B, caution in nursing.

MECHANISM OF ACTION: Low molecular weight heparin; enhances inhibition of factor Xa and thrombin by antithrombin, while only slightly affecting the activated partial thromboplastin time.

PHARMACOKINETICS: Absorption: Absolute bioavailability (87%); C_{max}=0.19 IU/mL (2500 IU), 0.41 IU/mL (5000 IU), 0.82 IU/mL (10,000 IU); T_{max}=4 hrs. **Distribution:** V_d=40-60mL/kg; found in breast milk. **Elimination:** $T_{1/2}$=3-5 hrs.

NURSING CONSIDERATIONS

Assessment: Assess for risk factors for bleeding or developing epidural/spinal hematoma, active major bleeding, history of heparin-induced thrombocytopenia with or without thrombosis, if undergoing epidural/neuraxial anesthesia, known hypersensitivity to heparin or pork products, severe renal impairment, pregnancy/nursing status, possible drug interactions, or any other conditions where treatment is contraindicated or cautioned.

Monitoring: Monitor for signs/symptoms of neurological impairment, bleeding, thrombocytopenia, and allergic reactions. Monitor for signs/symptoms of spinal or epidural hematomas in patients receiving neuraxial anesthesia or undergoing spinal puncture. Perform periodic CBC with platelet count, blood chemistry, and stool occult blood tests. Monitor anti-Xa levels in patients with severe renal impairment or if abnormal coagulation parameters or bleeding occurs.

Patient Counseling: Inform patients who had neuraxial anesthesia/spinal puncture, particularly if taking concomitant NSAIDs, platelet inhibitors, or other anticoagulants to watch for signs/symptoms of spinal/epidural hematoma (eg, tingling, numbness, muscular weakness) and notify physician immediately if any of these occurs. Instruct to d/c use of ASA or other NSAIDs prior to therapy. Counsel about injecting instructions if therapy is to continue after discharge from hospitals. Instruct to contact physician if any unusual bleeding, bruising, or signs of thrombocytopenia (eg, rash of dark red spots under skin) develop. Advise that it will take longer than usual to stop bleeding; may bruise and/or bleed more easily while on therapy. Advise to inform health practitioners when taking medications known to affect bleeding before any surgery is scheduled or any new drug is taken. Instruct to inform physicians and dentists of all medications they are taking, including those obtained without prescription.

Administration: SQ route. Do not mix with other inj or infusions unless compatible. Refer to PI for proper administration technique. **Storage:** 20-25°C (68-77°F). MDV: Room temperature for ≤2 weeks after first penetration of the rubber stopper. Discard any unused sol after 2 weeks.

FROVA   RX
frovatriptan succinate (Endo)

THERAPEUTIC CLASS: 5-HT$_{1B/1D}$ agonist

INDICATIONS: Acute treatment of migraine with or without aura.

DOSAGE: *Adults:* 2.5mg with fluids. If headache recurs after initial relief, may repeat after 2 hrs. Max: 7.5mg/day. Safety of treating >4 migraines/30 days not known.

HOW SUPPLIED: Tab: 2.5mg

CONTRAINDICATIONS: Ischemic heart disease (eg, angina pectoris, history of myocardial infarction (MI), or documented silent ischemia), or patients who have symptoms or findings consistent with ischemic heart disease, coronary artery vasospasm (eg, Prinzmetal's angina), significant cardiovascular disease (CVD), cerebrovascular syndromes including strokes of any type as well as transient ischemic attacks (TIA), peripheral vascular disease including ischemic bowel disease, uncontrolled HTN, hemiplegic or basilar migraine, use within 24 hrs of treatment with another 5-HT$_1$ agonist, an ergotamine containing or ergot-type medications.

WARNINGS/PRECAUTIONS: Confirm diagnosis. Potential to cause coronary artery vasospasm. Not for patients in whom unrecognized CAD is predicted by presence of risk factors (eg, HTN, hypercholesterolemia, smoker, obesity, diabetes, CAD family history, menopause, males >40 yrs) unless a cardiovascular evaluation provides evidence that the patient is free of underlying CVDs. In these patients, administer 1st dose under medical supervision and obtain ECG to assess presence of cardiac ischemia; monitor cardiovascular function with long-term intermittent use. Serious adverse cardiac events, cerebrovascular events, vasospastic reactions, and HTN reported. Serotonin syndrome symptoms (eg, mental status changes, autonomic instability, neuromuscular aberrations, and GI symptoms) reported. May bind to melanin in the eye, which may lead to toxicity with long-term use.

ADVERSE REACTIONS: Dizziness, headache, paresthesia, dry mouth, fatigue, hot or cold sensation, skeletal pain, flushing, N/V, coronary vasospasm, myocardial ischemia.

INTERACTIONS: See Contraindications. Prolonged vasospastic reactions with ergot-type agents and other 5-HT$_1$ agonists. Increased plasma levels with propranolol and oral contraceptives. Decreased levels with ergotamine tartrate. Serotonin syndrome reported when combined use with an SSRI or SNRI.

PREGNANCY: Category C, caution in nursing.

MECHANISM OF ACTION: 5-HT$_{1B/1D}$ agonist; binds with high affinity to 5-HT$_{1B/1D}$ receptors. Believed to act on extracerebral, intracranial arteries and to inhibit excessive dilation of these vessels in migraine.

PHARMACOKINETICS: Absorption: Absolute bioavailability: (20%) male, (30%) female; T$_{max}$=2-4 hrs. **Distribution:** V$_d$=4.2L/kg (male), 3L/kg (female); plasma protein binding (15%). **Metabolism:** via CYP1A2. Desmethyl frovatropin (active metabolite). **Elimination:** Feces (62%), urine (32%); T$_{1/2}$=26 hrs.

NURSING CONSIDERATIONS

Assessment: Confirm diagnosis of migraine before initiating therapy. Assess for ischemic heart disease or symptoms or findings consistent with ischemic heart disease, coronary artery vasospasm (eg, Prinzmetal's angina), CAD risk, hemiplegic or basilar migraine, hepatic/renal impairment, pregnancy/nursing status, ECG changes, any other conditions where treatment is contraindicated or cautioned and possible drug interactions.

Monitoring: In patients with risk factors predictive of CAD, administration of 1st dose should be in physician's office or medically staffed and equipped facility as cardiac ischemia may occur in absence of clinical symptoms; ECG should be obtained immediately during interval in those with risk factors. Monitor for signs/symptoms of cardiac events (eg, coronary vasospasm, acute MI, arrhythmia, ECG changes), cerebrovascular events (eg, hemorrhage, stroke, TIAs), peripheral vascular ischemia, colonic ischemia with bloody diarrhea and abdominal pain, serotonin syndrome (eg, mental status changes, autonomic instability, neuromuscular aberrations and/or GI symptoms), ophthalmic effects, and increased BP.

Patient Counseling: Instruct to read PI before use. Inform about potential risks (eg, serotonin syndrome manifestations), especially if taken with SSRIs or SNRIs. Report adverse reactions to physician. Advise to take as directed. Notify physician if pregnant/nursing or planning to become pregnant.

Administration: Oral route. **Storage:** 25°C (77°F); excursions permitted to 15-30°C (59-86°F). Protect from moisture.

FUROSEMIDE RX
furosemide (Various)

> May lead to profound diuresis with excessive amounts; medical supervision required and dose and dose schedule must be adjusted to individual patient's needs.

OTHER BRAND NAMES: Lasix (Sanofi-Aventis)

THERAPEUTIC CLASS: Loop diuretic

INDICATIONS: (Inj, PO) Treatment of edema associated with congestive heart failure, liver cirrhosis, and renal disease including nephrotic syndrome in adults and pediatrics. (PO) Treatment of hypertension alone or in combination with other antihypertensive agents in adults. (Inj) Adjunct therapy for acute pulmonary edema.

DOSAGE: *Adults:* (PO): Individualize dose. HTN: Initial: 40mg bid. Concomitant Antihypertensives: Reduce dose of other agents by 50%. Edema: Initial: 20-80mg. May repeat or increase by 20-40mg after 6-8 hrs. Give individually determined single dose qd or bid. Max: 600mg/day. Dose on 2-4 consecutive days each week. Closely monitor if on >80mg/day.

Geriatrics: Start at the low end of dosing range. (Inj) Individualize dose. Edema: Initial: 20-40mg IV/IM. May repeat or increase by 20mg after 2 hrs. Give individually determined single dose qd or bid. Acute Pulmonary Edema: Initial: 40mg IV. May increase to 80mg IV after 1 hr.
Pediatrics: Edema: (PO) Initial: 2mg/kg single dose. May increase by 1-2mg/kg after 6-8 hrs. Max: 6mg/kg. (Inj) Initial: 1mg/kg IV/IM. May increase by 1mg/kg IV/IM after 2 hrs. Max: 6mg/kg. Premature Infants: Max: 1mg/kg/day.

HOW SUPPLIED: (Generic) Inj: 10mg/mL; Sol: 10mg/mL, 40mg/5mL; (Generic, Lasix) Tab: 20mg, 40mg*, 80mg *scored

CONTRAINDICATIONS: Anuria.

WARNINGS/PRECAUTIONS: Monitor for fluid/electrolyte imbalance (eg, hypokalemia), renal or hepatic dysfunction. Initiate in hospital with hepatic cirrhosis and ascites. Tinnitus, hearing impairment, deafness reported. Ototoxicity associated with rapid injection, severe renal impairment, higher than recommended doses, or hypoproteinema; control IV infusion rate. Excessive diuresis may cause dehydration, blood volume reduction with circulatory collapse, vascular thrombosis and embolism; caution particularly in elderly. Hyperglycemia and precipitation of diabetes mellitus (DM) reported. Can cause acute urinary retention, asymptomatic hyperuricemia, and precipitation of gout. May activate/exacerbate systemic lupus erythematosus (SLE). Cross-sensitivity with sulfonamide allergy. (Inj) May increase risk of patent ductus arteriosus (PDA) in premature neonates with respiratory distress syndrome. May cause hearing loss in neonates.

ADVERSE REACTIONS: Pancreatitis, jaundice, anorexia, paresthesias, ototoxicity, blood dyscrasias, dizziness, rash, urticaria, photosensitivity, fever, thrombophlebitis, restlessness.

INTERACTIONS: Ototoxicity with aminoglycosides, ethacrynic acid, cisplatin, or other ototoxic drugs. Avoid with aminoglycosides and ethacrynic acid. Caution with high-dose salicylates; risk of salicylate toxicity. Lithium toxicity. Antagonizes tubocurarine. Potentiates antihypertensives, succinylcholine, ganglionic or peripheral adrenergic blockers. Severe hypotension and renal function deterioration with ACE inhibitors or angiotensin II receptor blockers. Decreases arterial response to norepinephrine. Reduced natriuretic and antihypertensive effect with sucralfate and indomethacin. Separate by at least 2 hrs with sucralfate. Hypokalemia with adrenocorticotropic hormone, corticosteroids, licorice in large amounts, or prolonged use of laxatives. Digitalis may exacerbate metabolic effects of hypokalemia. Renal changes with NSAIDs. Orthostatic hypotension may be aggravated by alcohol, barbiturates, or narcotics. Avoid with chloral hydrate. Intestinal absorption decreased with phenytoin. Reduced effect with methotrexate and other drugs that undergo significant renal tubular secretion; conversely may increase serum levels of these drugs and potentiate toxicity of these drugs and furosemide. May increase risk of cephalosporin-induced nephrotoxicity, gouty arthritis with cyclosporine, nephrotoxicity with other nephrotoxic drugs. Higher risk of renal deterioration with radiocontrast.

PREGNANCY: Category C, caution in nursing.

MECHANISM OF ACTION: Loop diuretic; primarily inhibits reabsorption of Na^+ and Cl^- in proximal and distal tubules and in loop of Henle.

PHARMACOKINETICS: Distribution: Plasma protein binding (91-99%), found in breast milk. **Metabolism:** Biotransformation. Furosemide glucuronide (major metabolite). **Elimination:** Urine; $T_{1/2}$=2 hrs.

NURSING CONSIDERATIONS

Assessment: Assess for anuria, sulfonamide hypersensitivity, DM, SLE, possible drug interactions, hepatic/renal impairment, and pregnancy/nursing status. Obtain baseline serum electrolytes, renal function, urine, and blood glucose.

Monitoring: Monitor serum electrolytes, CO_2, creatinine and BUN frequently in first few months, then periodically; renal and hepatic function, urine, and blood glucose periodically. Monitor for signs/symptoms of electrolyte imbalance, blood dyscrasias, hyperglycemia, hyperuricemia or precipitation of gout, hypotension, ototoxicity, persistent PDA, and hypersensitivity reactions. Monitor renal function and consider renal ultrasonography in pediatrics.

Patient Counseling: Advise to seek medical attention if symptoms of electrolyte imbalance (eg, dry mouth, thirst, weakness), hypotension, ototoxicity (tinnitus, hearing impairment), or hypersensitivity reactions occur. Advise that postural hypotension can be managed by getting up slowly. K^+ supplements/dietary measures may be needed to control or avoid hypokalemia. Advise diabetics that may increase blood glucose levels and thereby affect urine glucose tests. Inform that the skin may be more sensitive to the effects of sunlight. Inform to avoid medications that may increase blood pressure, including OTC products for appetite suppression and cold symptoms.

Administration: Oral, IV/IM route. See PI for high dose parenteral therapy. **Storage:** Tab, Sol: 25°C (77°F); excursions permitted to 15-30°C (59-86°F). Protect sol from light and moisture. IV: 20-25°C (68-77°F). Protect from light.

FUSILEV

RX

levoleucovorin (Spectrum)

THERAPEUTIC CLASS: Cytoprotective agent

INDICATIONS: Rescue therapy after high-dose methotrexate (MTX) therapy in osteosarcoma. To diminish the toxicity and counteract the effects of impaired MTX elimination and of inadvertent overdosage of folic acid antagonists. For use in combination chemotherapy with 5-fluorouracil (5-FU) in the palliative treatment of patients with advanced metastatic colorectal cancer.

DOSAGE: *Adults:* Levoleucovorin Rescue: 7.5mg (5mg/m²) IV q6h for 10 doses starting 24 hrs after the beginning of MTX infusion. Continue therapy, hydration and urinary alkalinization until MTX level is <5x10⁻⁸M (0.05 micromolar). Refer to PI for guidelines on dosage adjustment and rescue extensions. Inadvertent MTX Overdosage: 7.5mg (5mg/m²) IV q6h until serum MTX is <10⁻⁸M. Titrate: Increase to 50mg/m² IV q3h until MTX level is <10⁻⁸M if 24-hr SrCr is 50% over baseline, or if 24-hr MTX level is >5x10⁻⁶M, or 48-hr level is >9 x 10⁻⁷M. Employ concurrent hydration (3L/day) and urinary alkalinization with Na bicarbonate; adjust bicarbonate dose to maintain urine pH at ≥7. Start rescue therapy as soon as possible after overdose and within 24 hrs of MTX administration when there is delayed excretion. Colorectal Cancer: 100mg/m² slow IV over a minimum of 3 min, followed by 370mg/m² 5-FU IV, daily for 5 days, or 10mg/m² IV, followed by 425mg/m² 5-FU IV, daily for 5 days. May repeat at 4-week intervals for 2 courses, then at 4- to 5-week intervals provided that the patient has completely recovered from the toxic effects of the prior treatment course. May increase 5-FU dose by 10% if no toxicity. Reduce 5-FU daily dose by 20% with moderate GI/hematologic toxicity and by 30% with severe toxicity.

HOW SUPPLIED: Inj: 50mg, 10mg/mL [17.5mL, 25mL]

WARNINGS/PRECAUTIONS: Do not inject >16mL/min. Do not administer intrathecally. Not approved for pernicious anemia and megaloblastic anemias secondary to the lack of vitamin B12; improper use may cause a hematologic remission while neurologic manifestations continue to progress. Do not initiate or continue therapy with 5-FU in patients with symptoms of GI toxicity until symptoms have completely resolved; caution in elderly and/or debilitated. Monitor patients with diarrhea until it has resolved, as rapid clinical deterioration leading to death can occur. Seizures and/or syncope reported in cancer patients, most commonly in those with CNS metastases or other predisposing factors.

ADVERSE REACTIONS: Stomatitis, N/V, diarrhea, dyspepsia, typhlitis, dyspnea, dermatitis, confusion, neuropathy, abnormal renal function, taste perversion.

INTERACTIONS: May enhance 5-FU toxicity. Seizures and/or syncope reported with fluoropyrimidine. Increased treatment failure and morbidity rates in trimethoprim-sulfamethoxazole-treated HIV patients with *Pneumocystis carinii* pneumonia. Folic acid in large amounts may counteract antiepileptic effect of phenobarbital, phenytoin, and primidone, and increase seizure frequency in children; use with caution when taken with anticonvulsants.

PREGNANCY: Category C, not for use in nursing.

MECHANISM OF ACTION: Folate analog; counteracts the therapeutic and toxic effects of folic acid antagonists, which act by inhibiting dihydrofolate reductase. Enhances therapeutic effects of fluoropyrimidines used in cancer therapy (eg, 5-FU).

PHARMACOKINETICS: Absorption: (Total-Tetrahydrofolate [THF]) C_{max}=1722ng/mL; (5-methyl-THF) C_{max}=275ng/mL, T_{max}=0.9 hrs. **Metabolism:** 5-methyl-THF (metabolite). **Elimination:** $T_{1/2}$=5.1 hrs (total-THF), 6.8 hrs (5-methyl-THF).

NURSING CONSIDERATIONS

Assessment: Assess for previous allergic reactions to folic acid or folinic acid, pernicious anemia and megaloblastic anemias secondary to the lack of vitamin B12, GI toxicity, third-space fluid accumulation (eg, ascites, pleural effusion), renal impairment, inadequate hydration, CNS metastases, pregnancy/nursing status, and possible drug interactions.

Monitoring: Monitor for GI toxicity, seizures, syncope, and hypersensitivity reactions. Monitor patients with diarrhea until it has resolved. Monitor fluid and electrolytes in patients with abnormalities in MTX excretion. Monitor SrCr and MTX levels at least qd.

Patient Counseling: Inform about risks and benefits of therapy. Advise to notify physician if any adverse reaction occurs. Instruct to inform physician if pregnant/nursing.

Administration: IV route. Do not administer with other agents in the same admixture. Administer 5-FU and levoleucovorin separately. Refer to PI for reconstitution and infusion instructions. **Storage:** (Powder) 25°C (77°F); excursions permitted from 15-30°C (59-86°F). Protect from light. Reconstitution/Dilution with 0.9% NaCl: Room temperature for ≤12 hrs. Dilution with 5% Dextrose: Room temperature for ≤4 hrs. (Sol) 2-8°C (36-46°F). Protect from light. Dilution with 0.9% NaCl or 5% Dextrose: Room temperature for ≤4 hrs.

FUZEON

RX

enfuvirtide (Roche Labs)

THERAPEUTIC CLASS: Fusion inhibitor

INDICATIONS: In combination with other antiretroviral agents for the treatment of HIV-1 infection in treatment-experienced patients with evidence of HIV-1 replication despite ongoing antiretroviral therapy.

DOSAGE: *Adults:* Usual: 90mg bid SQ into the upper arm, anterior thigh, or abdomen.
Pediatrics: 6-16 yrs: Usual: 2mg/kg bid SQ into the upper arm, anterior thigh, or abdomen. Max: 90mg SQ bid. Refer to PI for weight-based dosing chart.

HOW SUPPLIED: Inj: 90mg/mL

WARNINGS/PRECAUTIONS: Local inj-site reactions reported; monitor for signs/symptoms of cellulitis or local infection. Administration with Biojector 2000 may result in neuralgia and/or paresthesia, bruising, and hematomas. Patients with hemophilia or other coagulation disorders may have a higher risk of post-inj bleeding. May cause bacterial pneumonia; monitor for signs/ symptoms of pneumonia, especially, those predisposed to pneumonia (eg, low initial CD4 cell count, high initial viral load, IV drug use, smoking, and prior history of lung disease). Associated with systemic hypersensitivity reactions; d/c immediately if signs/symptoms develop. May lead to anti-enfuvirtide antibody production which cross reacts with HIV gp41 and could result in false-positive HIV test with an ELISA assay. Immune reconstitution syndrome reported.

ADVERSE REACTIONS: Diarrhea, local inj-site reactions, fatigue, nausea, decreased weight, sinusitis, abdominal pain, cough, herpes simplex, decreased appetite, pancreatitis.

INTERACTIONS: May result in a higher risk of post-inj bleeding with anticoagulants.

PREGNANCY: Category B, not for use in nursing.

MECHANISM OF ACTION: Fusion inhibitor; interferes with the entry of HIV-1 into cells by inhibiting fusion of viral and cellular membranes; binds to the first heptad-repeat (HR1) in the gp41 subunit of the viral envelope glycoprotein and prevents the conformational changes required for the fusion of viral and cellular membranes.

PHARMACOKINETICS: Absorption: Absolute bioavailability (84.3%); C_{max}=4.59mcg/mL; T_{max}=8 hrs; AUC=55.8mcg•hr/mL. **Distribution:** V_d=5.5L; plasma protein binding (92%). **Metabolism:** Liver via hydrolysis; M_3 (metabolite). **Elimination:** $T_{1/2}$=3.8 hrs.

NURSING CONSIDERATIONS

Assessment: Assess for risk factors for pneumonia (eg, history of lung disease, decreased CD4 cell count, increased viral load, IV drug use, smoking), infections, hemophilia, history of coagulation disorders, pregnancy/nursing status, and possible drug interactions.

Monitoring: Monitor for signs/symptoms of cellulitis or local inj-site reactions, pneumonia, immune reconstitution syndrome, post-inj bleeding, nerve pain/paresthesia, and hypersensitivity reactions.

Patient Counseling: Inform of risk for inj-site reactions; instruct to monitor for signs of cellulitis and local infections. Advise to seek medical attention if experiencing symptoms of pneumonia (eg, cough with fever, rapid breathing, SOB) and systemic hypersensitivity (eg, rash, fever, N/V, chills, rigors, hypotension). Inform that therapy is not a cure for HIV-1 infection and patients may continue to contract illnesses associated with HIV-1. Advise that the drug must be taken as a part of a combination antiretroviral regimen. Instruct on proper drug preparation (eg, use of aseptic technique), administration (eg, preferred anatomical site), and disposal. Advise to inform physician if pregnant, planning to become pregnant, or breastfeeding. Instruct not to change dosage or schedule without consulting physician.

Administration: SQ route. Refer to PI for proper administration. Do not inject into moles, scar tissue, bruises, navel, surgical scars, tattoos, burn sites, directly over a blood vessel, or near areas where large nerves course close to the skin, into a preceding site, or a site with current inj-site reaction from an earlier dose. **Storage:** Vial: 25°C (77°F); excursions permitted to 15-30°C (59-86°F). Reconstituted Sol: 2-8°C (36-46°F). Use within 24 hrs.

GABITRIL

RX

tiagabine HCl (Cephalon)

THERAPEUTIC CLASS: Nipecotic acid derivative

INDICATIONS: Adjunctive therapy in adults and children ≥12 yrs in the treatment of partial seizures.

DOSAGE: *Adults:* Induced (Patients Already Taking Enzyme-Inducing Antiepilepsy Drugs [AEDs]): Initial: 4mg qd. Titrate: May increase total daily dose by 4-8mg at weekly intervals until clinical response is achieved, or up to 56mg/day. Give total daily dose in divided doses (bid-qid). Refer to PI for Typical Dosing Titration Regimen. Non-Induced: Requires lower dose and slower dose titration. Hepatic Impairment: May require reduced initial/maint doses and/or longer dosing intervals. *Pediatrics:* 12-18 yrs: Induced: Initial: 4mg qd. Titrate: May increase total daily dose by 4mg at the beginning of Week 2, then may increase by 4-8mg at weekly intervals until clinical response is achieved, or up to 32mg/day. Give total daily dose in divided doses (bid-qid). Refer to PI for Typical Dosing Titration Regimen. Non-Induced: Requires lower dose and slower dose titration. Hepatic Impairment: May require reduced initial/maint doses and/or longer dosing intervals.

HOW SUPPLIED: Tab: 2mg, 4mg, 12mg, 16mg

WARNINGS/PRECAUTIONS: New-onset seizures and status epilepticus in patients without epilepsy reported; d/c therapy and evaluate for an underlying seizure disorder. Increased risk of suicidal thoughts or behavior may occur; monitor for emergence or worsening of depression, suicidal thoughts/behavior, and/or any unusual changes in mood or behavior. Avoid abrupt d/c; may increase seizure frequency. May affect thought processes (eg, impaired concentration, speech or language problems, confusion) and level of consciousness (eg, somnolence, fatigue). May exacerbate EEG abnormalities; caution with history of spike and wave discharges on EEG and adjust dosage. Sudden unexpected death in epilepsy reported. Moderately severe to incapacitating generalized weakness reported; weakness resolved after dose reduction or d/c. There may be a possibility of long-term ophthalmologic effects. Serious rash (eg, maculopapular, vesiculobullous, Stevens-Johnson syndrome) may occur. Caution with liver disease.

ADVERSE REACTIONS: Dizziness, asthenia, tremor, somnolence, N/V, nervousness, abdominal pain, pain, difficulty with concentration/attention, insomnia, confusion, pharyngitis, rash, diarrhea.

INTERACTIONS: May reduce valproate concentrations. Increased free concentration with valproate. Increased clearance with carbamazepine, phenytoin, and phenobarbital (primidone). Caution with drugs that may depress the nervous system (eg, ethanol, or triazolam); may cause possible additive depressive effects. Reports of new-onset seizures and status epilepticus in patients without epilepsy with concomitant drugs that lower the seizure threshold (antidepressants, antipsychotics, stimulants, narcotics). Potential interactions with drugs that induce or inhibit hepatic metabolizing enzymes. Use with highly protein-bound drugs may lead to higher free fractions of tiagabine or competing drugs.

PREGNANCY: Category C, caution in nursing.

MECHANISM OF ACTION: Nipecotic acid derivative; not established. Enhances activity of gamma aminobutyric acid (GABA), the major inhibitory neurotransmitter in the CNS. Binds to recognition sites associated with the GABA uptake carrier, thereby blocking GABA uptake into presynaptic neurons, permitting more GABA to be available for receptor binding on the surfaces of postsynaptic cells.

PHARMACOKINETICS: Absorption: Rapid, well-absorbed; absolute bioavailability (90%); T_{max}=2.5 hrs (fed), T_{max}=45 min (fasting). **Distribution:** Plasma protein binding (96%). **Metabolism:** Liver via CYP3A; thiophene ring oxidation leading to formation of 5-oxo-tiagabine and glucuronidation. **Elimination:** Urine (25%), feces (63%); $T_{1/2}$=7-9 hrs (non-induced).

NURSING CONSIDERATIONS

Assessment: Assess for underlying seizure disorder, history of status epilepticus and spike and wave discharges on EEG, depression, suicidal thoughts/behavior, history of hypersensitivity reactions, hepatic impairment, pregnancy/nursing status, and possible drug interactions.

Monitoring: Monitor for occurrence of new-onset seizures and status epilepticus in patients without a previous history of epilepsy, withdrawal seizures, cognitive and neuropsychiatric events, EEG changes, rash, emergence or worsening of depression, suicidal thoughts/behavior, unusual changes in mood or behavior, generalized weakness, ophthalmologic changes, and other adverse reactions.

Patient Counseling: Inform patients, caregivers, and families about increased risk of suicidal thoughts and behavior and to alert for the emergence or worsening of symptoms of depression, any unusual changes in mood or behavior, or emergence of suicidal thoughts, behaviors, or thoughts of self-harm; instruct to report immediately to healthcare providers. Inform that dizziness, somnolence, and other symptoms/signs of CNS depression may occur; instruct to avoid driving/operating other complex machinery until adjusted to effects. Notify physician if pregnant, intend to become pregnant, if breastfeeding or intend to breastfeed. If multiple doses are missed, instruct to contact physician for possible retitration. Encourage pregnant patients to enroll in North American Antiepileptic Drug (NAAED) Pregnancy Registry by calling 888-233-2334 or go to aedpregnancyregistry.org.

Administration: Oral route. Take with food. **Storage:** 20-25°C (68-77°F). Protect from light and moisture.

GANCICLOVIR   RX

ganciclovir sodium (Various)

Clinical toxicity includes granulocytopenia, anemia, and thrombocytopenia. Carcinogenic, teratogenic, and aspermato-
genic in animal studies. (Cap) Use only for prevention of cytomegalovirus (CMV) disease in patients with advanced HIV
infection at risk for CMV disease and in solid organ transplant recipients, and maintenance treatment of CMV retinitis
immunocompromised patients. Risk of more rapid rate of CMV retinitis progression; use as maintenance treatment only
when this risk is balanced by the benefit of avoiding daily IV infusions. (IV) Use only for the treatment of CMV retinitis in
immunocompromised patients, and prevention of CMV disease in transplant patients at risk for CMV disease.

OTHER BRAND NAMES: Cytovene IV (Genentech)

THERAPEUTIC CLASS: Synthetic guanine derivative nucleoside analogue

INDICATIONS: (Cap) Prevention of CMV disease in solid organ-transplant recipients and in advanced HIV patients at risk for CMV disease. Alternative to IV for maintenance treatment of CMV
retinitis in immunocompromised patients (eg, with AIDS) in whom retinitis is stable following appropriate induction therapy and for whom the risk of more rapid progression is balanced by the
benefit associated with avoiding daily IV infusions. (IV) Treatment of CMV retinitis in immunocompromised patients (eg, with AIDS). Prevention of CMV disease in transplant recipients at risk
for CMV disease.

DOSAGE: *Adults:* CMV Retinitis Treatment: Initial: 5mg/kg IV q12h for 14-21 days. Maint: (IV)
5mg/kg qd, 7 days/week, or 6mg/kg qd, 5 days/week; (Cap) 1000mg tid or 500mg 6X/day q3h
during waking hrs. Progression of CMV Retinitis While on Maint: Repeat induction. CMV Disease
Prevention in Advanced HIV Patients: 1000mg PO tid. CMV Disease Prevention in Transplant
Recipients: (IV) Initial: 5mg/kg q12h for 7-14 days, followed by 5mg/kg qd, 7 days/week or
6mg/kg qd, 5 days/week. (Cap) 1000mg tid. Renal Impairment: Refer to PI for dose modifications. Consider dose reduction with neutropenia, anemia, and/or thrombocytopenia.

HOW SUPPLIED: Cap: 250mg, 500mg; (Cytovene IV) Inj: 500mg

WARNINGS/PRECAUTIONS: Do not exceed recommended dose. Avoid if absolute neutrophil count (ANC) <500 cells/μL or platelet count <25,000 cells/μL. Caution with preexisting
cytopenias or history of cytopenic reactions to other drugs, chemicals, or irradiation. May cause
inhibition of spermatogenesis in men. May cause suppression of fertility in women. Women of
childbearing potential should use effective contraception during treatment and men should
practice barrier contraception during and for at least 90 days after therapy. Caution in elderly
and with renal impairment. (IV) Larger doses and more rapid infusions increase toxicity. SQ/IM
inj may cause severe tissue irritation. Administration should be accompanied by adequate hydration. Phlebitis and/or pain may occur at infusion site. Administer only into veins with adequate
blood flow. Avoid rapid or bolus IV inj.

ADVERSE REACTIONS: Fever, diarrhea, anorexia, vomiting, leukopenia, sweating, infection,
chills, thrombocytopenia, neutropenia, anemia, neuropathy, sepsis, pruritus.

INTERACTIONS: Avoid with imipenem-cilastatin. May increase levels of didanosine. May have additive toxicity with drugs that inhibit replication of rapidly dividing cell populations (eg, nucleoside analogues), amphotericin B and trimethoprim/sulfamethoxazole. Monitor renal function
with nephrotoxic drugs. (Cap) May increase exposure of zidovudine. Probenecid may increase
exposure. Didanosine (if given 2 hrs before therapy) and zidovudine may decrease exposure.

PREGNANCY: Category C, not for use in nursing.

MECHANISM OF ACTION: Synthetic guanine derivative nucleoside analogue; believed to inhibit
viral DNA synthesis by competitively inhibiting viral DNA polymerases and incorporating into
viral DNA, resulting in eventual termination of viral DNA elongation.

PHARMACOKINETICS: Absorption: (PO) Absolute bioavailability (5%) (fasted), (6-9%) (fed);
AUC_{0-24}=15.9μg•hr/mL, C_{max}=1.02μg/mL (500mg q3h, 6 times daily, fed state), AUC_{0-24}=15.4μg•hr/
mL, C_{max}=1.18μg/mL (1000mg tid, fed state). (IV) C_{max}=8.27-9μg/mL; AUC=22.1-26.8μg•hr/mL.
Distribution: Plasma protein binding (1-2%); (IV) V_d=0.74L/kg. **Elimination:** (PO) Feces (86%),
urine (5%); $T_{1/2}$= 4.8 hrs. (IV) Urine (91.3%); $T_{1/2}$=3.5 hrs.

NURSING CONSIDERATIONS

Assessment: Assess for hypersensitivity to acyclovir, preexisting cytopenias or history of cytopenic reactions to other drugs, chemicals, or irradiation, renal impairment, pregnancy/nursing
status, and possible drug interactions. Obtain baseline ANC and platelet count.

Monitoring: Perform frequent monitoring of CBC and platelet counts. Monitor SrCr or CrCl, and
for retinitis progression.

Patient Counseling: Advise of the importance of close monitoring of blood counts, and that
drug may cause infertility. Advise women of childbearing potential that drug should not be used
during pregnancy and that effective contraception should be used. Advise men to practice barrier contraception during and for at least 90 days following treatment. Inform that therapy may
be a potential carcinogen. Advise that drug is not a cure for CMV retinitis and that progression

of retinitis may continue to occur during and after treatment; instruct to have ophthalmologic follow-up examinations at a minimum of q4-6 weeks during treatment.

Administration: IV/Oral route. (IV) Administer at constant rate over 1 hr. (PO) Take with food. Refer to PI for preparation of IV sol, handling, and disposal. **Storage:** (IV) 25°C (77°F); excursions permitted to 15-30°C (59-86°F). (Cap) 20-25° (68-77°F); excursions permitted between 15-30°C (59-86°F). Reconstituted Sol in Vial: Stable at room temperature for 12 hrs. Do not refrigerate. Diluted Infusion Sol: 0.9% NaCl: Stable at 5°C for 14 days in polyvinyl chloride bags; use within 24 hrs of dilution. Do not freeze.

GARDASIL RX
human papillomavirus recombinant vaccine, quadrivalent (Merck)

G

THERAPEUTIC CLASS: Vaccine

INDICATIONS: Vaccination of girls and women 9-26 yrs of age for the prevention of cervical, vulvar, vaginal, and anal cancer caused by human papillomavirus (HPV) types 16 and 18, genital warts (condyloma acuminata) caused by HPV types 6 and 11, cervical intraepithelial neoplasia (CIN) Grade 2/3 and cervical adenocarcinoma in situ (AIS), CIN Grade 1, vulvar intraepithelial neoplasia (VIN) Grades 2 and 3, vaginal intraepithelial neoplasia (VaIN) Grades 2 and 3, and anal intraepithelial neoplasia (AIN) Grades 1, 2, and 3 caused by HPV types 6, 11, 16, and 18. Vaccination of boys and men 9-26 yrs of age for the prevention of anal cancer caused by HPV types 16 and 18, genital warts (condyloma acuminata) caused by HPV types 6 and 11, and AIN Grades 1, 2, and 3 caused by HPV types 6, 11, 16, and 18.

DOSAGE: *Adults:* ≤26 yrs: 0.5mL IM in the deltoid region of the upper arm or in the higher anterolateral area of the thigh at the following schedule: 0, 2 months, 6 months.
Pediatrics: ≥9 yrs: 0.5mL IM in the deltoid region of the upper arm or in the higher anterolateral area of the thigh at the following schedule: 0, 2 months, 6 months.

HOW SUPPLIED: Inj: 0.5mL

CONTRAINDICATIONS: Severe hypersensitivity reaction to yeast.

WARNINGS/PRECAUTIONS: Syncope may occur; observe for 15 min after administration. Appropriate medical treatment and supervision should be readily available in case of an anaphylactic reaction. Continue to undergo cervical and/or anal cancer screening. Does not protect against disease from vaccine and non-vaccine HPV types to which a person has previously been exposed through sexual activity. Not intended for treatment of active external genital lesions; cervical, vulvar, vaginal, and anal cancers; CIN; VIN; VaIN; AIN. Does not protect against diseases due to HPV types not contained in the vaccine and genital diseases not caused by HPV. Vaccination may not result in protection in all vaccine recipients. Does not prevent HPV-related CIN 2/3 or worse in women >26 yrs. Response may be diminished in immunocompromised individuals.

ADVERSE REACTIONS: Local-site reactions (eg, pain, swelling, erythema, pruritus, bruising), fever, nausea, dizziness, diarrhea, headache.

INTERACTIONS: Immunosuppressive therapies, including irradiation, antimetabolites, alkylating agents, cytotoxic drugs, and corticosteroids (used in greater than physiologic doses), may reduce the immune responses to vaccines.

PREGNANCY: Category B, caution in nursing.

MECHANISM OF ACTION: Vaccine; exact mechanism not established. Suspected to develop humoral immune response.

NURSING CONSIDERATIONS

Assessment: Assess current health and immune status, age of patient, pregnancy/nursing status, and for possible drug interactions. Assess for hypersensitivity to drug and yeast.

Monitoring: Monitor for signs/symptoms of anaphylactic reactions, syncope, tonic-clonic movements, and for seizure-like activity.

Patient Counseling: Inform about benefits and risks associated with vaccine. Advise to continue to undergo cervical and/or anal cancer screening. Advise that vaccine does not provide protection against disease from vaccine and non-vaccine HPV types to which a person has previously been exposed through sexual activity. Inform that syncope may occur following vaccination. Inform about importance of completing immunization series unless contraindicated. Advise that vaccine is not recommended during pregnancy. Instruct to report any adverse reactions to physician.

Administration: IM route. Shake well before use. Do not dilute or mix with other vaccines. Refer to PI for instructions for use. **Storage:** 2-8°C (36-46°F). Do not freeze. Protect from light. Administer as soon as possible after being removed from refrigeration; can be out of refrigeration (≤25°C/77°F) for ≤72 hrs.

GELNIQUE

RX

oxybutynin chloride (Watson)

THERAPEUTIC CLASS: Muscarinic antagonist

INDICATIONS: Treatment of overactive bladder with symptoms of urge urinary incontinence, urgency, and frequency.

DOSAGE: *Adults:* Apply contents of 1 sachet to dry, intact skin on the abdomen, upper arms/ shoulders, or thighs qd. Rotate sites.

HOW SUPPLIED: Gel: 100mg/g (10%) [30^s]

CONTRAINDICATIONS: Urinary retention, gastric retention, and uncontrolled narrow-angle glaucoma.

WARNINGS/PRECAUTIONS: For topical application only. Gel preparation is flammable; avoid open fire or smoking until gel has dried. Caution with bladder outflow obstruction, GI obstructive disorders, gastroesophageal reflux, and myasthenia gravis. May decrease gastrointestinal motility; caution with ulcerative colitis or intestinal atony. Skin hypersensitivity may occur; d/c if hypersensitivity develops. D/C and provide appropriate treatment in the event of angioedema. Skin transference may occur; cover application site with clothing after gel has dried.

ADVERSE REACTIONS: Dry mouth, application-site reactions, urinary tract/upper respiratory tract infections.

INTERACTIONS: Caution with bisphosphonates or other drugs that may cause or exacerbate esophagitis. Concomitant use with other anticholinergic (antimuscarinic) agents may increase the frequency and/or severity of dry mouth, constipation, blurred vision, somnolence, and pharmacological effects.

PREGNANCY: Category B, caution in nursing.

MECHANISM OF ACTION: Antispasmodic, antimuscarinic agent; acts as competitive antagonist of acetylcholine at postganglionic muscarinic receptors, resulting in relaxation of bladder smooth muscle.

PHARMACOKINETICS: Absorption: Abdomen: C_{max}=6.8ng/mL; AUC_{0-24}=112.7ng•hr/mL. Upper Arm/Shoulder: C_{max}=8.3ng/mL; AUC_{0-24}=133.8ng•hr/mL. Thigh: C_{max}=7ng/mL; AUC_{0-24}=125.1ng•hr/ mL. **Distribution:** (IV) V_d=193L. **Metabolism:** CYP3A4, N-desethyloxybutynin (active metabolite). **Elimination:** Urine (<0.1% unchanged); (IV) $T_{1/2}$=2 hrs.

NURSING CONSIDERATIONS

Assessment: Assess for urinary retention, gastric retention, uncontrolled narrow-angle glaucoma, bladder outflow obstruction, GI obstructive disorders, ulcerative colitis or intestinal atony, gastroesophageal reflux, myasthenia gravis, pregnancy/nursing status, and for possible drug interactions.

Monitoring: Monitor for signs/symptoms of urinary retention, gastric retention, esophagitis, angioedema, and for skin hypersensitivity reactions.

Patient Counseling: Advise that therapy is for topical application only and not to be ingested. Instruct not to apply to recently shaved skin surfaces. Instruct to wash hands immediately after product application. Advise to avoid showering or water immersion for 1 hr after product application. Counsel to cover treated sites with clothing if close skin-to-skin contact is anticipated. Instruct to avoid open fire or smoking until gel is dried. Inform that the drug may produce significant adverse reactions related to anticholinergic pharmacological activity (eg, constipation, urinary retention, and blurred vision). Advise to exercise caution in engaging in potentially dangerous activities until effects have been determined. Inform that heat prostration may occur in hot environment. Inform that alcohol may enhance drowsiness.

Administration: Topical route. **Storage:** 25°C (77°F); excursions permitted to 15-30°C (59-86°F). Protect from moisture and humidity. Apply immediately after the sachets are opened and contents expelled. Discard used sachets in a manner that prevents accidental application or ingestion by children, pets, or others.

GEMCITABINE

RX

gemcitabine (Various)

OTHER BRAND NAMES: Gemzar (Lilly)

THERAPEUTIC CLASS: Nucleoside analogue antimetabolite

INDICATIONS: In combination with carboplatin for treatment of advanced ovarian cancer that has relapsed for at least 6 months after completion of platinum-based therapy. In combination with paclitaxel for 1st-line treatment of metastatic breast cancer after failure of prior anthracycline-containing adjuvant chemotherapy, unless anthracyclines were clinically contraindicated.

In combination with cisplatin for 1st-line treatment of inoperable, locally advanced (Stage IIIA or IIIB), or metastatic (Stage IV) non-small cell lung cancer. First-line treatment of locally advanced (nonresectable Stage II or Stage III) or metastatic (Stage IV) adenocarcinoma of the pancreas in patients previously treated with 5-fluorouracil (5-FU).

DOSAGE: *Adults:* Refer to PI for dose modifications guideline for each indication. Ovarian Cancer: 1000mg/m^2 IV over 30 min on Days 1 and 8 of each 21-day cycle. Give carboplatin area under the curve 4 IV on Day 1 after gemcitabine. Breast Cancer: 1250mg/m^2 IV over 30 min on Days 1 and 8 of each 21-day cycle. Give paclitaxel 175mg/m^2 on Day 1 as 3-hr IV infusion before gemcitabine. Non-Small Cell Lung Cancer: 4-Week Cycle: 1000mg/m^2 IV over 30 min on Days 1, 8, and 15 of each 28-day cycle. Give cisplatin 100mg/m^2 IV on Day 1 after gemcitabine infusion. 3-Week Cycle: 1250mg/m^2 IV over 30 min on Days 1 and 8 of each 21-day cycle. Give cisplatin 100mg/m^2 IV on Day 1 after gemcitabine infusion. Pancreatic Cancer: 1000mg/m^2 IV over 30 min once weekly for up to 7 weeks (or until toxicity necessitates reducing or holding a dose), then 1 week off. Give subsequent cycles as once-weekly infusions for 3 consecutive weeks out of every 4 weeks.

HOW SUPPLIED: Inj: 2g; (Gemzar) 200mg, 1g

WARNINGS/PRECAUTIONS: Patients should be monitored closely by a physician experienced in the use of cancer chemotherapeutic agents. Increased toxicity with prolonged infusion time beyond 60 min and more frequent than weekly dosing. Myelosuppression is a dose-limiting toxicity; bone marrow suppression as manifested by leukopenia, thrombocytopenia, and anemia may occur. Pulmonary toxicity reported; d/c immediately and institute appropriate supportive care measures if severe lung toxicity occurs. Hemolytic uremic syndrome (HUS), renal failure, and serious hepatotoxicity reported; caution with preexisting renal impairment and hepatic insufficiency. Use in patients with concurrent liver metastases or preexisting history of hepatitis, alcoholism, or liver cirrhosis may cause exacerbation of the underlying hepatic insufficiency. May cause fetal harm.

ADVERSE REACTIONS: Myelosuppression, N/V, anemia, leukopenia, neutropenia, thrombocytopenia, elevated serum transaminases/alkaline phosphatases, proteinuria, fever, rash, hematuria, dyspnea, peripheral edema.

INTERACTIONS: Serious hepatotoxicity reported with other potentially hepatotoxic drugs. Higher incidence of myelosuppression and SrCr toxicity with cisplatin. Radiation toxicity reported with radiotherapy.

PREGNANCY: Category D, not for use in nursing.

MECHANISM OF ACTION: Nucleoside analogue antimetabolite; exhibits cell phase specificity, primarily killing cells undergoing DNA synthesis (S-phase). Blocks progression of cells through the G1/S-phase boundary.

PHARMACOKINETICS: Distribution: V_d=50L/m^2 (infusion <70 min), 370L/m^2 (infusion 70-285 min). **Metabolism:** Intracellular by nucleoside kinases to the active diphosphate (dFdCDP) and triphosphate (dFdCTP) nucleosides. **Elimination:** Urine (92-98%); $T_{1/2}$=42-94 min (infusion <70 min), 245-638 min (infusion 70-285 min).

NURSING CONSIDERATIONS

Assessment: Assess for liver metastases, history of hepatitis, alcoholism or liver cirrhosis, previous hypersensitivity to drug, preexisting renal impairment and hepatic insufficiency, pregnancy/nursing status, and possible drug interactions. Obtain CBC, including differential and platelet count, prior to each dose, and renal/hepatic function.

Monitoring: Monitor for signs/symptoms of myelosuppression, pulmonary toxicity, HUS, renal failure, hepatotoxicity, and other adverse events/toxicities that may occur. Perform periodic monitoring of hepatic function (eg, LFTs) and renal function. Monitor SrCr, K$^+$, calcium, and magnesium when using with cisplatin.

Patient Counseling: Inform about risk of low blood cell counts and instruct to immediately contact physician if any signs/symptoms of infection (eg, fever), anemia, or bleeding occurs. Inform that drug may cause fetal harm; instruct to notify physician if pregnant or nursing.

Administration: IV route. Refer to PI for proper preparation, reconstitution, and administration instructions. **Storage:** (Unopened vials) 20-25°C (68-77°F); excursions permitted to 15-30°C (59-86°F). (Reconstituted) 20-25°C (68-77°F) for 24 hrs. Discard unused portion. Do not refrigerate.

GEODON   RX
ziprasidone HCl - ziprasidone mesylate (inj) (Pfizer)

Elderly patients with dementia-related psychosis treated with antipsychotic drugs are at an increased risk of death; most deaths appeared to be cardiovascular (eg, heart failure, sudden death) or infectious (eg, pneumonia) in nature. Not approved for the treatment of dementia-related psychosis.

OTHER BRAND NAMES: Geodon for Injection (Pfizer)

THERAPEUTIC CLASS: Benzisoxazole derivative

INDICATIONS: (PO) Treatment of schizophrenia. Monotherapy for acute treatment of manic or mixed episodes associated with bipolar I disorder. Adjunct to lithium or valproate for maintenance treatment of bipolar I disorder. (IM) Treatment of acute agitation in schizophrenic patients who need IM antipsychotic medication for rapid control of agitation.

DOSAGE: *Adults:* Schizophrenia: (PO) Initial/Maint: 20mg bid. Titrate: May increase up to 80mg bid; adjust dose at intervals of not <2 days if indicated. Max: 80mg bid. Maint: No additional benefit for dose >20mg bid. Bipolar Disorder: (PO) Initial: 40mg bid. Titrate: May increase to 60 or 80mg bid on 2nd day, then adjust dose based on tolerance and efficacy within the range 40-80mg bid. Maint (as adjunct to lithium/valproate): 40-80mg bid. Take with food. Agitation: (IM) Usual: 10mg q2h-20mg q4h. Max: 40mg/day. Administration >3 consecutive days has not been studied. Elderly: Start at lower end of dosing range.

HOW SUPPLIED: Cap: (HCl) 20mg, 40mg, 60mg, 80mg; Inj: (Mesylate) 20mg/mL

CONTRAINDICATIONS: Concomitant dofetilide, sotalol, quinidine, Class Ia/III antiarrhythmics, mesoridazine, thioridazine, chlorpromazine, droperidol, pimozide, sparfloxacin, gatifloxacin, moxifloxacin, halofantrine, mefloquine, pentamidine, arsenic trioxide, levomethadyl acetate, dolasetron mesylate, probucol, tacrolimus, and drugs that prolong QT interval. History of QT prolongation (including congenital long QT syndrome), recent acute myocardial infarction (MI) and uncompensated heart failure.

WARNINGS/PRECAUTIONS: D/C if persistent QTc measurements >500 msec. Hypokalemia and/or hypomagnesemia may increase risk of QT prolongation and arrhythmia. Initiate further evaluation if symptoms of torsades de pointes (eg, dizziness, palpitations, or syncope) occur. Neuroleptic malignant syndrome (NMS) reported; d/c therapy, institute intensive treatment and medical monitoring, and treat any concomitant illness if it occurs. Tardive dyskinesia (TD) may occur; consider d/c therapy. Hyperglycemia and diabetes mellitus (DM) reported. Rash/urticaria reported; d/c therapy upon appearance of rash. Orthostatic hypotension reported; caution with cardiovascular disease (CVD), cerebrovascular disease or conditions that predispose to hypotension. Leukopenia, neutropenia, and agranulocytosis reported; d/c with severe neutropenia (absolute neutrophil count <1000/mm^3). Caution with history of seizures or conditions that may lower seizure threshold. Esophageal dysmotility and aspiration pneumonia may occur. May elevate prolactin levels. May impair physical/mental abilities. Priapism reported. May disrupt the body's ability to reduce core body temperature. Closely supervise high-risk patients for suicide attempts. Caution in elderly. Caution with renal dysfunction when administered IM. Concomitant use of IM and oral preparations in schizophrenic patients not recommended.

ADVERSE REACTIONS: Heart failure, pneumonia, asthenia, N/V, constipation, dyspepsia, diarrhea, dry mouth, extrapyramidal symptoms, somnolence, akathisia, dizziness, respiratory tract infection, rash.

INTERACTIONS: See Contraindications. Caution with centrally acting drugs. May enhance effects of antihypertensives. May antagonize effects of levodopa and dopamine agonists. Carbamazepine may decrease levels. CYP3A4 inhibitors (eg, ketoconazole) may increase levels. Serotonin syndrome may occur with serotonergic medicinal products. Periodically monitor serum K$^+$ and magnesium (Mg^{2+}) with diuretics. Caution with medication with anticholinergic activity; may elevate core body temperature.

PREGNANCY: Category C, not for use in nursing.

MECHANISM OF ACTION: Psychotropic agent; not established. Actions are mediated through a combination of dopamine type 2 (D$_2$) and serotonin type 2 (5HT$_2$) antagonism.

PHARMACOKINETICS: Absorption: (PO) Well-absorbed; absolute bioavailability (60%); T$_{max}$=6-8 hrs. (IM) Absolute bioavailability (100%); T$_{max}$=60 min. **Distribution:** (PO) V$_d$=1.5L/kg; plasma protein binding (>99%). **Metabolism:** (PO) Liver (extensive) via aldehyde oxidase (major), CYP3A4 (minor); benzisothiazole (BITP) sulphoxide, BITP-sulphone, ziprasidone sulphoxide, and S-methyl-dihydroziprasidone (major metabolites). **Elimination:** (PO) Urine (20%, <1% unchanged) and feces (66%, <4% unchanged); T$_{1/2}$=7 hrs. (IM) T$_{1/2}$=2-5 hrs.

NURSING CONSIDERATIONS

Assessment: Assess for conditions where treatment is contraindicated or cautioned. Perform baseline CBC and serum electrolytes (K$^+$, Mg^{2+}) in patients at risk for significant electrolyte disturbances. Obtain baseline fasting blood glucose (FBG) in patients with increased risk for DM. Replete serum electrolytes prior to treatment. Assess for drug hypersensitivity, pregnancy/nursing status and possible drug interactions.

Monitoring: Monitor for QT prolongation, torsades de pointes, NMS, TD, rash, orthostatic hypotension, seizures, esophageal dysmotility, aspiration pneumonia, suicidal ideation, and weight gain. Monitor renal function, prolactin levels, serum electrolytes (K$^+$, Mg^{2+}) and CBC, especially for decline of WBC with signs/symptoms of infection. Monitor for symptoms of hyperglycemia. Monitor regularly for FBG and worsening of glucose control in DM patients. Careful monitoring during the initial dosing period for some elderly.

Patient Counseling: Inform regarding the risks and benefits of therapy. Inform that use may impair mental/physical abilities. Counsel to take with food, avoid alcohol and high temperatures or humidity; drug may interfere with body's ability to regulate temperature. Advise to inform healthcare providers of the following: history of QT prolongation, recent acute MI, uncompensated heart failure, taking other QT-prolonging drugs, risk for electrolyte abnormalities, and history of cardiac arrhythmia. Instruct to report conditions that increase risk for electrolyte disturbances (eg, hypokalemia, taking diuretics, prolonged diarrhea) and if dizziness, palpitations, or syncope occurs.

Administration: Oral, IM route. (IM) Refer to PI for preparation instructions. **Storage:** Cap: 25°C (77°F), excursions permitted to 15-30°C (59-86°F). Inj: Dry form: 25°C (77°F); excursions permitted to 15-30°C (59-86°F). Protect from light. Reconstituted: 15-30°C (59-86°F) ≥24 hrs when protected from light or refrigerated at 2-8°C (36-46°F) for ≥7 days.

G

GLEEVEC   RX
imatinib mesylate (Novartis)

THERAPEUTIC CLASS: Protein-tyrosine kinase inhibitor

INDICATIONS: Treatment of newly diagnosed patients with Philadelphia chromosome-positive (Ph+) chronic myeloid leukemia (CML) in chronic phase. **Adults:** Treatment of Ph+ CML in blast crisis, accelerated phase, or in chronic phase after failure of interferon-α therapy. Treatment of relapsed or refractory Ph+ acute lymphoblastic leukemia (ALL). Treatment of myelodysplastic/myeloproliferative diseases (MDS/MPD) associated with platelet-derived growth factor receptor (PDGFR) gene rearrangements. Treatment of aggressive systemic mastocytosis (ASM) patients without the D816V c-Kit mutation or with unknown c-Kit mutational status. Treatment of hypereosinophilic syndrome (HES) and/or chronic eosinophilic leukemia (CEL) patients who have the FIP1L1-PDGFRα fusion kinase (mutational analysis or FISH demonstration of CHIC2 allele deletion) and for patients with HES and/or CEL who are FIP1L1-PDGFRα fusion kinase-negative or unknown. Treatment of unresectable, recurrent, and/or metastatic dermatofibrosarcoma protuberans (DFSP). Treatment of patients with Kit (CD117)-positive unresectable and/or metastatic malignant GI stromal tumors (GIST). Adjuvant treatment of patients following complete gross resection of Kit (CD117)-positive GIST.

DOSAGE: *Adults:* CML: Chronic Phase: Usual: 400mg qd. Titrate: May increase to 600mg qd if conditions permit. See PI. Accelerated Phase/Blast Crisis: Usual: 600mg qd. Titrate: May increase to 400mg bid if conditions permit. See PI. Relapsed/Refractory Ph+ ALL: 600mg qd. MDS or MPD/ASM without D816V c-Kit Mutation or with Unknown c-Kit Mutational Status Not Responding Satisfactorily to Other Therapies/HES and/or CEL: 400mg qd. ASM with Eosinophilia/HES or CEL with FIP1L1-PDGFRα: Initial: 100mg qd. Titrate: May increase to 400mg qd in the absence of adverse reactions and presence of insufficient response. DFSP: 800mg/day (as 400mg bid). Unresectable and/or Metastatic Malignant GIST: Usual: 400mg qd. Titrate: May increase to 400mg bid if signs/symptoms of disease progression at a lower dose are clear and in the absence of severe adverse reactions. Adjuvant Treatment after Complete Gross Resection of GIST: 400mg qd for 3 yrs. Coadministration with Strong CYP3A4 Inducers: If necessary, increase dose by at least 50% and monitor carefully. Severe Hepatic Impairment: Reduce dose by 25%. Moderate Renal Impairment (CrCl 20-39mL/min): Reduce starting dose by 50%. Titrate: As tolerated. Max: 400mg. Mild Renal Impairment (CrCl 40-59mL/min): Max: 600mg. Hepatotoxicity/Nonhematologic Adverse Reaction: If bilirubin >3X ULN or transaminases >5X ULN, withhold therapy until bilirubin <1.5X ULN and transaminases <2.5X ULN. Continue at reduced dose. Neutropenia/Thrombocytopenia: See PI for dosage adjustments. *Pediatrics:* ≥2 yrs: Newly Diagnosed CML: 340mg/m² qd or split into 2 doses (am and pm). Max: 600mg. Coadministration with Strong CYP3A4 Inducers: If necessary, increase dose by at least 50% and monitor carefully. Severe Hepatic Impairment: Reduce dose by 25%. Moderate Renal Impairment (CrCl 20-39mL/min): Reduce starting dose by 50%. Titrate: As tolerated. Max: 400mg. Mild Renal Impairment (CrCl 40-59mL/min): Max: 600mg. Hepatotoxicity/Nonhematologic Adverse Reaction: If bilirubin >3X ULN or transaminases >5X ULN, withhold drug until bilirubin <1.5X ULN and transaminases <2.5X ULN. Reduce dose to 260mg/m²/day. Neutropenia/Thrombocytopenia: See PI for dosage adjustments.

HOW SUPPLIED: Tab: 100mg*, 400mg* *scored

WARNINGS/PRECAUTIONS: Fluid retention/edema (eg, pleural effusion, pericardial effusion, pulmonary edema, ascites) reported. Hematologic toxicity (eg, anemia/neutropenia/thrombocytopenia) reported; monitor CBC weekly during 1st month, biweekly during 2nd month, and periodically thereafter. May be hepatotoxic; monitor LFTs at baseline, then monthly or PRN; interrupt and/or reduce dose if laboratory abnormalities occur. Severe congestive heart failure (CHF) and left ventricular dysfunction reported; carefully monitor patients with cardiac disease or risk factors for cardiac or history of renal failure, and evaluate/treat any patient with cardiac or renal failure. Hemorrhages reported; monitor for GI symptoms at the start of the therapy as GI tumor sites may be the source of GI hemorrhages. May cause GI irritation; GI perforation reported rarely. In patients with HES and cardiac involvement, cardiogenic shock/left ventricular dysfunction reported; reversible with administration of systemic steroids, circulatory support measures, and temporary d/c of treatment. Perform echocardiogram and determine troponin levels in patients with HES/CEL and MDS/MPD or ASM associated with high eosinophil levels; consider prophylactic use of systemic steroids (1-2mg/kg) for 1-2 weeks concomitantly at initiation of therapy if either is abnormal. Bullous dermatological reactions (eg, erythema multiforme, Stevens-Johnson syndrome) reported. Potential toxicities from long-term use. Interrupt treatment if severe nonhematologic adverse reaction develops (eg, severe hepatotoxicity, severe fluid retention); resume if appropriate. May cause fetal harm; sexually active female patients of reproductive potential should use highly effective contraception. Caution with severe renal impairment. Growth retardation reported in children and preadolescents. Tumor lysis syndrome reported in patients with CML, GIST, ALL, and eosinophilic leukemia; caution in patients at risk of tumor lysis syndrome (those with tumors with high proliferative rate or high tumor burden prior to treatment), and correct clinically significant dehydration and treat high uric acid levels prior to treatment. May impair physical/mental abilities.

ADVERSE REACTIONS: N/V, edema, muscle cramps, musculoskeletal pain, diarrhea, rash, fatigue, asthenia, abdominal pain, hemorrhage, malaise, neutropenia, anemia, anorexia.

INTERACTIONS: Increased levels with CYP3A4 inhibitors; caution with strong CYP3A4 inhibitors (eg, ketoconazole, atazanavir, indinavir, nefazodone, nelfinavir, ritonavir, saquinavir, telithromycin, voriconazole, clarithromycin, itraconazole). Avoid with grapefruit juice. Decreased levels with rifampin, St. John's wort, and enzyme-inducing antiepileptic drugs (eg, carbamazepine, oxcarbazepine, phenytoin, fosphenytoin, phenobarbital, primidone). Avoid concomitant use or increase dose by at least 50% if necessary with strong CYP3A4 inducers (eg, dexamethasone, phenytoin, carbamazepine, rifampin, rifabutin, rifampicin, phenobarbital). Caution with CYP3A4 substrates that have narrow therapeutic windows (eg, alfentanil, cyclosporine, dihydroergotamine, ergotamine, fentanyl, quinidine, sirolimus, tacrolimus, pimozide). Increases levels of simvastatin, metoprolol, and drugs metabolized by CYP3A4 (eg, dihydropyridine calcium channel blockers, triazolo-benzodiazepines, certain HMG-CoA reductase inhibitors). Switch patients on warfarin to low molecular weight or standard heparin. Caution with CYP2D6 substrates that have narrow therapeutic windows. Inhibits acetaminophen O-glucuronidate pathway in vitro. When concomitantly used with chemotherapy, liver toxicity reported; monitor hepatic function. Hypothyroidism reported in thyroidectomy patients undergoing levothyroxine replacement.

PREGNANCY: Category D, not for use in nursing.

MECHANISM OF ACTION: Protein-tyrosine kinase inhibitor; inhibits the bcr-abl tyrosine kinase, the constitutive abnormal tyrosine kinase created by the Philadelphia chromosome abnormality in CML; inhibits proliferation and induces apoptosis in bcr-abl positive cell lines as well as fresh leukemic cells from Ph+ CML. Also an inhibitor of the receptor tyrosine kinases for PDGF and stem cell factor (SCF), c-kit, and inhibits PDGF- and SCF-mediated cellular events; in vitro, inhibits proliferation and induces apoptosis in GIST cells, which express an activating c-Kit mutation.

PHARMACOKINETICS: Absorption: Well-absorbed. Absolute bioavailability (98%); T_{max}=2-4 hrs. **Distribution:** Plasma protein binding (95%); found in breast milk. **Metabolism:** Liver via CYP3A4 (major), CYP1A2, CYP2D6, CYP2C9, CYP2C19 (minor); N-demethylated piperazine derivative (major active metabolite). **Elimination:** Urine (13%, 5% unchanged), feces (68%, 20% unchanged); $T_{1/2}$=18 hrs (imatinib), 40 hrs (active metabolite).

NURSING CONSIDERATIONS

Assessment: Assess for cardiac disease, renal impairment, advanced age, pregnancy/nursing status, and for possible drug interactions. Perform echocardiogram and determine troponin levels in patients with HES/CEL and MDS/MPD or ASM associated with high eosinophil levels. Obtain baseline CBC and LFTs.

Monitoring: Monitor for signs and symptoms of fluid retention, CHF, left ventricular dysfunction, hepatotoxicity, hemorrhage, GI disorders, tumor lysis syndrome, and bullous dermatological reactions. Perform CBC for the 1st month of therapy, biweekly for the 2nd month, and periodically thereafter. Monitor LFTs monthly or as clinically indicated. Monitor for cardiogenic shock in patients with HES and growth in children. Monitor thyroid-stimulating hormone levels in thyroidectomy patients undergoing levothyroxine replacement.

Patient Counseling: Instruct to take exactly as prescribed with a meal and large glass of water. Advise to take the dose as soon as possible if missed; advise to not take if almost time for the next dose and to never double the dose. Advise women of reproductive potential to avoid becoming pregnant; instruct sexually active females to use highly effective contraception. Instruct to notify physician if pregnant and not to breastfeed while on therapy. Advise to contact physician if experience any adverse effects while on therapy. Instruct to notify physician if have history of cardiac disease or risk factors for cardiac failure. Counsel not to take any other medications, including over-the-counter medications (eg, herbal products) without consulting a physician. Advise that growth retardation has been reported in children and preadolescents; inform that growth should be monitored. Inform that undesirable effects (eg, dizziness, blurred vision, somnolence) may occur; instruct to use caution when driving/operating machinery.

Administration: Oral route. Take with food and a large glass of water. If unable to swallow tab, disperse in a glass of water or apple juice; required number of tab should be placed in the appropriate volume of beverage (approximately 50mL for 100mg tab and 200mL for 400mg tab); stir and administer sus immediately after disintegration of tab. **Storage:** 25°C (77°F); excursions permitted to 15-30°C (59-86°F). Protect from moisture.

GLIPIZIDE/METFORMIN   RX
metformin HCl - glipizide (Teva)

> Lactic acidosis reported (rare); increased risk with diabetics with significant renal insufficiency, congestive heart failure (CHF), increased age, and conditions with risk of hypoperfusion and hypoxemia. Avoid in patients ≥80 yrs unless renal function is normal. Withhold therapy in the presence of any condition associated with hypoxemia, dehydration, or sepsis. Avoid in patients with hepatic disease. Caution against excessive alcohol intake; may potentiate effects of metformin on lactate metabolism. Temporarily d/c prior to intravascular radiocontrast study or surgical procedures. D/C use and institute appropriate therapy if lactic acidosis occurs.

THERAPEUTIC CLASS: Sulfonylurea/biguanide

INDICATIONS: Adjunct to diet and exercise to improve glycemic control in adults with type 2 diabetes mellitus (DM).

DOSAGE: *Adults:* Individualize dose. Inadequate Glycemic Control on Diet/Exercise Alone: Initial: 2.5mg-250mg qd with a meal. If FPG is 280-320mg/dL, give 2.5mg-500mg bid. Titrate: Increase by 1 tab/day every 2 weeks. Max: 10mg-1000mg/day or 10mg-2000mg/day in divided doses. Inadequate Glycemic Control on Sulfonylurea and/or Metformin: Initial: 2.5mg-500mg or 5mg-500mg bid (with am and pm meals). Starting dose should not exceed daily dose of glipizide or metformin already being taken. Titrate: Increase by no more than 5mg-500mg/day up to minimum effective dose. Max: 20mg-2000mg/day. Elderly/Debilitated/Malnourished: Dose conservatively; do not titrate to max.

HOW SUPPLIED: Tab: (Glipizide-Metformin) 2.5mg-250mg, 2.5mg-500mg, 5mg-500mg

CONTRAINDICATIONS: Renal disease/dysfunction (eg, SrCr ≥1.5mg/dL [males], ≥1.4mg/dL [females], abnormal CrCl), acute/chronic metabolic acidosis, including diabetic ketoacidosis with or without coma. Use while undergoing radiologic studies with intravascular iodinated contrast materials.

WARNINGS/PRECAUTIONS: Increased risk of cardiovascular (CV) mortality reported. No conclusive evidence of macrovascular risk reduction. Hypoglycemia may occur; increased risk with renal/hepatic insufficiency, elderly, debilitated, malnourished patients, adrenal or pituitary insufficiency, or alcohol intoxication. Hemolytic anemia reported; caution with glucose-6-phosphate dehydrogenase (G6PD) deficiency and consider non-sulfonylurea alternatives. Caution with concomitant medications that may affect renal function, result in significant hemodynamic change, or interfere with the disposition of metformin. Withhold therapy before, during, and for 48 hrs after radiologic studies with IV iodinated contrast materials; reinstitute only when renal function is normal. D/C in hypoxic states (eg, shock, acute CHF or myocardial infarction [MI]), dehydration, and sepsis. Temporarily d/c prior to surgical procedures associated with restricted food/fluids intake. May decrease serum vitamin B12 levels.

ADVERSE REACTIONS: Lactic acidosis, upper respiratory tract infection, HTN, headache, diarrhea, dizziness, musculoskeletal pain, N/V, abdominal pain, hypoglycemia.

INTERACTIONS: See Boxed Warning and Contraindications. Thiazides and other diuretics, corticosteroids, phenothiazines, thyroid products, estrogens, oral contraceptives, phenytoin, nicotinic acid, sympathomimetics, calcium channel blockers, and isoniazid may cause hyperglycemia and loss of blood glucose control. Hypoglycemic action of sulfonylureas may be potentiated by NSAIDs, some azoles, and other highly protein-bound drugs, salicylates, sulfonamides, chloramphenicol, probenecid, coumarins, MAOIs, and β-blockers. Severe hypoglycemia reported with concomitant oral miconazole. Increased levels with fluconazole. Furosemide, nifedipine, cationic drugs eliminated by renal tubular secretion (eg, amiloride, digoxin, morphine, procainamide, quinidine, quinine, ranitidine, triamterene, trimethoprim, vancomycin), and cimetidine may increase metformin levels. May decrease furosemide levels.

PREGNANCY: Category C, not for use in nursing.

MECHANISM OF ACTION: Glipizide: Sulfonylurea; lowers blood glucose acutely by stimulating the release of insulin from the pancreas. Metformin: Biguanide; decreases hepatic production and intestinal absorption of glucose, and improves insulin sensitivity by increasing peripheral glucose uptake and utilization.

PHARMACOKINETICS: Absorption: Glipizide: Rapid, complete; T_{max}=1-3 hrs. Metformin: (500mg) Absolute bioavailability (50-60%) (fasted). **Distribution:** Glipizide: Plasma protein binding (98-99%); V_d=11L (IV). Metformin: (850mg) V_d=654L (PO). **Metabolism:** Glipizide: Liver (extensive). **Elimination:** Glipizide: Urine (<10% unchanged); $T_{1/2}$=2-4 hrs. Metformin: Urine (90% [PO], unchanged [IV]); $T_{1/2}$=6.2 hrs (plasma), 17.6 hrs (blood).

NURSING CONSIDERATIONS

Assessment: Assess for previous hypersensitivity to drug, renal/hepatic disease, hypoxic states, acute/chronic metabolic acidosis, adrenal/pituitary insufficiency, alcoholism, G6PD deficiency, pregnancy/nursing status, and possible drug interactions. Assess FPG, HbA1c, and hematologic parameters (eg, Hgb/Hct, RBC indices).

Monitoring: Monitor for lactic acidosis, prerenal azotemia, hypoxic states, CV disease, hypersensitivity reactions, and other adverse reactions. Monitor FPG, renal function, LFTs, hematologic parameters (eg, Hgb/Hct, RBC indices). Monitor HbA1c at intervals of approximately 3 months.

Patient Counseling: Inform about potential risks/benefits and alternative modes of therapy. Inform about the importance of adherence to dietary instructions, regular exercise programs, and regular testing of blood glucose, glycosylated Hgb, renal function, and hematologic parameters. Explain risks, symptoms, and conditions that predispose to the development of lactic acidosis and hypoglycemia. Counsel to d/c drug and report to physician if unexplained hyperventilation, myalgia, malaise, N/V, somnolence, or other nonspecific symptoms occur. Counsel against excessive alcohol intake.

Administration: Oral route. **Storage:** 20-25°C (68-77°F).

GLUCAGON RX
glucagon (Lilly)

THERAPEUTIC CLASS: Glucagon

INDICATIONS: Treatment for severe hypoglycemia. Diagnostic aid for radiologic examination of the stomach, duodenum, small bowel, and colon when diminished intestinal motility would be advantageous.

DOSAGE: *Adults:* Severe Hypoglycemia: ≥20kg: 1mg (1 U) SQ/IM/IV. After 15 min, may give additional dose if response is delayed, however seek for an emergency aid so that parenteral glucose can be given. Give supplemental carbohydrate after the patient responds to treatment. Diagnostic Aid: Stomach/Duodenum/Small Bowel: 0.25-0.5mg (0.25-0.5 U) IV, or 1mg (1 U) IM, or 2mg (2 U) IV/IM before procedure. Colon Relaxation: 2mg (2 U) IM 10 min before procedure. Elderly: Start at lower end of dosing range.
Pediatrics: Severe Hypoglycemia: ≥20kg: 1mg (1 U) SQ/IM/IV. <20kg: 0.5mg (0.5 U) or dose equivalent to 20-30mcg/kg. After 15 min, may give additional dose if response is delayed, however seek for an emergency aid so that parenteral glucose can be given. Give supplemental carbohydrate after the patient responds to treatment.

HOW SUPPLIED: Inj: 1mg/mL (1 U/mL)

CONTRAINDICATIONS: Pheochromocytoma.

WARNINGS/PRECAUTIONS: Caution with a history suggestive of insulinoma and/or pheochromocytoma. In patients with insulinoma, IV glucagon may produce an initial increase in blood glucose and then subsequently cause hypoglycemia. In the presence of pheochromocytoma, may cause the tumor to release catecholamines, which may result in a sudden and marked increase in BP. Generalized allergic reactions (eg, urticaria, respiratory distress, and hypotension) reported. Effective in treating hypoglycemia only if sufficient liver glycogen is present. Little or no help in states of starvation, adrenal insufficiency, or chronic hypoglycemia; treat with glucose.

ADVERSE REACTIONS: N/V, allergic reactions, urticaria, respiratory distress, hypotension.

INTERACTIONS: Addition of an anticholinergic during diagnostic examination may increase side effects.

PREGNANCY: Category B, caution in nursing.

MECHANISM OF ACTION: Glucagon; polypeptide hormone that increases blood glucose levels and relaxes smooth muscle of the GI tract.

PHARMACOKINETICS: Absorption: (SQ) C_{max}=7.9ng/mL, T_{max}=20 min; (IM) C_{max}=6.9ng/mL, T_{max}=13 min. **Distribution:** V_d=0.25L/kg (1mg dose). **Metabolism:** Extensively degraded in liver, kidneys, plasma. **Elimination:** $T_{1/2}$=8-18 min (1mg dose).

NURSING CONSIDERATIONS

Assessment: Assess if patient is in state of starvation, has adrenal insufficiency or chronic hypoglycemia. Assess for history suggestive of insulinoma and/or pheochromocytoma, pregnancy/nursing status, and possible drug interactions.

Monitoring: Monitor for signs/symptoms of an allergic reaction, HTN, and hypoglycemia. Monitor blood glucose levels in patients with hypoglycemia until asymptomatic.

Patient Counseling: Instruct patient and family members, in event of emergency, how to properly prepare and administer glucagon. Inform about measures to prevent hypoglycemia; including following a uniform regimen on a regular basis, careful adjustment of the insulin program, frequent testing of blood or urine for glucose, and routinely carrying hyperglycemic agents to quickly elevate blood glucose levels (eg, sugar, candy, readily absorbed carbohydrates). Inform about symptoms of hypoglycemia and how to treat it appropriately. Inform caregivers that if patient is hypoglycemic, patient should be kept alert and hypoglycemia should be treated as quickly as possible to prevent CNS damage. Advise to inform physician when hypoglycemia occurs.

Administration: IM/IV/SQ routes. Use immediately after reconstitution; discard any unused portion. Refer to PI for further instructions and directions for use. **Storage:** Before reconstitution: 20-25°C (68-77°F); excursions allowed between 15-30°C (59-86°F).

GLUCOPHAGE XR   RX
metformin HCl (Bristol-Myers Squibb)

Lactic acidosis reported (rare); increased risk with increased age, diabetes mellitus (DM), renal dysfunction, congestive heart failure (CHF), and conditions with risk of hypoperfusion and hypoxemia. Avoid use in patients ≥80 yrs unless renal function is normal. Withhold therapy in the presence of any condition associated with hypoxemia, dehydration, or sepsis. Avoid with clinical or laboratory evidence of hepatic disease. Caution against excessive alcohol intake; may potentiate the effects of metformin on lactate metabolism. Temporarily d/c prior to any IV radiocontrast study or surgical procedures. D/C use and institute appropriate therapy if lactic acidosis occurs.

OTHER BRAND NAMES: Glucophage (Bristol-Myers Squibb)

THERAPEUTIC CLASS: Biguanide

INDICATIONS: Adjunct to diet and exercise to improve glycemic control in type 2 DM.

DOSAGE: *Adults:* Individualize dose. (Tab) Initial: 500mg bid or 850mg qd with meals. Titrate: Increase by 500mg/week or 850mg q2 weeks, up to a total of 2000mg/day given in divided doses, or may increase from 500mg bid to 850mg bid after 2 weeks. Patients Requiring Additional Glycemic Control: Max: 2550mg/day. With Insulin: Initial: 500mg qd. Titrate: Increase by 500mg/week. Max: 2500mg/day. Decrease insulin dose by 10-25% when FPG <120mg/dL. Give in 3 divided doses with meals if dose is >2g/day. (Tab, ER) Initial: ≥17 yrs: 500mg qd with pm meal. Titrate: Increase by 500mg/week. Max: 2000mg/day. With Insulin: Initial: 500mg qd. Titrate: Increase by 500mg/week. Max: 2000mg/day. Decrease insulin dose by 10-25% when FPG <120mg/dL. Elderly/Debilitated/Malnourished: Dose conservatively; do not titrate to max. *Pediatrics:* 10-16 yrs: (Tab) Individualize dose. Initial: 500mg bid with meals. Titrate: Increase by 500mg/week. Max: 2000mg/day, given in divided doses.

HOW SUPPLIED: Tab: (Glucophage) 500mg, 850mg, 1000mg; Tab, Extended-Release (ER): (Glucophage XR) 500mg, 750mg

CONTRAINDICATIONS: Renal disease/dysfunction (eg, SrCr ≥1.5mg/dL [males], ≥1.4mg/dL [females], or abnormal CrCl), acute or chronic metabolic acidosis, diabetic ketoacidosis with or without coma. D/C temporarily (48 hrs) for radiologic studies with intravascular iodinated contrast materials.

WARNINGS/PRECAUTIONS: D/C therapy if conditions associated with lactic acidosis and characterized by hypoxemia states (eg, acute CHF, cardiovascular [CV] collapse, acute myocardial infarction [MI]) or prerenal azotemia develop. D/C therapy if temporary loss of glycemic control occurs due to stress; temporarily give insulin and reinstitute after acute episode is resolved. May decrease serum vitamin B12 levels. Increased risk of hypoglycemia in elderly, debilitated/malnourished, with adrenal or pituitary insufficiency, or alcohol intoxication. Consider therapeutic alternatives, including initiation of insulin, if secondary failure occurs. Caution in elderly.

ADVERSE REACTIONS: Lactic acidosis, diarrhea, N/V, flatulence, asthenia, abdominal discomfort, hypoglycemia, dizziness, dyspnea, taste disorder, chest discomfort, flu syndrome, palpitations, indigestion.

INTERACTIONS: See Boxed Warning and Contraindications. May increase levels with furosemide, nifedipine, cimetidine, cationic drugs (eg, digoxin, amiloride, procainamide, quinidine, quinine, ranitidine, trimethoprim, vancomycin, triamterene, morphine). Observe for loss of glycemic control with thiazides, other diuretics, corticosteroids, phenothiazines, thyroid products, estrogens, oral contraceptives, phenytoin, nicotinic acid, sympathomimetics, calcium channel blockers, and isoniazid. May interact with highly protein-bound drugs (eg, salicylates, sulfonamides, chloramphenicol, probenecid). May decrease furosemide, glyburide levels. Caution with drugs that may affect renal function or result in significant hemodynamic change or may interfere with the disposition of metformin. Hypoglycemia may occur with concomitant use of other glucose-lowering agents (eg, sulfonylureas, insulin). May overlap drug effects when transferred from chlorpropamide. Hypoglycemia may be difficult to recognize with β-adrenergic blocking drugs.

PREGNANCY: Category B, not for use in nursing.

MECHANISM OF ACTION: Biguanide; decreases hepatic glucose production and intestinal absorption of glucose, and improves insulin sensitivity by increasing peripheral glucose uptake and utilization.

PHARMACOKINETICS: Absorption: (Tab) Absolute bioavailability (50-60%); (Tab, ER) T_{max}=7 hrs. Administration of different doses resulted in different parameters. **Distribution:** (Tab) V_d=654L. **Elimination:** Urine (90%); $T_{1/2}$=6.2 hrs (plasma), 17.6 hrs (blood).

NURSING CONSIDERATIONS

Assessment: Assess for renal/hepatic impairment, acute/chronic metabolic acidosis, presence of a hypoxic state (eg, acute CHF, acute MI, CV collapse), dehydration, sepsis, alcoholism, nutritional status, adrenal/pituitary insufficiency, pregnancy/nursing status, and for possible drug interactions. Assess baseline renal function, FPG, HbA1c, and hematological parameters (Hct, Hgb, RBC indices).

Monitoring: Monitor for lactic/metabolic acidosis, ketoacidosis, hypoglycemia, hypoxemia (eg, CV collapse, acute CHF, acute MI), prerenal azotemia, and for decreases in vitamin B12 levels. Monitor FPG, HbA1c, renal function (eg, SrCr, CrCl), and hematological parameters (eg, Hgb, Hct, RBC indices).

Patient Counseling: Inform of the potential risks and benefits of therapy. Inform about the importance of adherence to dietary instructions and a regular exercise program. Inform of the risk of developing lactic acidosis during therapy; advise to d/c therapy immediately and contact physician if unexplained hyperventilation, myalgia, malaise, unusual somnolence, or other nonspecific symptoms occur. Instruct to avoid excessive alcohol intake. Counsel to take tab with meals and tab ER with pm meal. Instruct that ER tab must be swallowed whole and not crushed or chewed.

Administration: Oral route. (Tab, ER) Must be swallowed whole; do not crush or chew. **Storage:** 20-25°C (68-77°F); excursions permitted to 15-30°C (59-86°F).

GLUCOTROL   RX
glipizide (Pfizer)

THERAPEUTIC CLASS: Sulfonylurea (2nd generation)

INDICATIONS: Adjunct to diet and exercise to improve glycemic control in adults with type 2 diabetes mellitus (DM).

DOSAGE: *Adults:* Take 30 min before meals. Initial: 5mg qd before breakfast; give 2.5mg if elderly or with liver disease. Titrate: Increase by 2.5-5mg; several days should elapse between titration. May divide dose if unsatisfactory response to single dose. Maint: Total daily doses >15mg/day should be divided and given with meals of adequate caloric content. May give total daily doses >30mg bid to long-term patients. Max: 15mg qd or 40mg/day. Switch From Insulin: If ≤20 U/day: D/C insulin and start at 5mg qd. If >20 U/day: Reduce insulin dose by 50% and begin at 5mg qd. Titration: Several days should elapse between titration. Switching from Other Oral Hypoglycemics: No transition period necessary. Elderly/Debilitated/Malnourished/Renal or Hepatic Impairment: Dose conservatively.

HOW SUPPLIED: Tab: 5mg*, 10mg* *scored

CONTRAINDICATIONS: Type 1 DM, diabetic ketoacidosis, with or without coma.

WARNINGS/PRECAUTIONS: Increased risk of cardiovascular (CV) mortality reported; inform patient of potential risks, advantages, and alternative therapy. May produce severe hypoglycemia; proper patient selection, dosage, and instructions are important. Increased risk of hypoglycemia with elderly, debilitated, malnourished, renal/hepatic disease, adrenal or pituitary insufficiency. Loss of blood glucose control may occur when exposed to stress (eg, fever, trauma, infection, or surgery); d/c therapy and administer insulin. Secondary failure may occur over period of time. May cause hemolytic anemia in patients with glucose 6-phosphate dehydrogenase (G6PD) deficiency; observe caution and consider a non-sulfonylurea alternative. Caution in elderly.

ADVERSE REACTIONS: Hypoglycemia, GI disturbances, allergic skin reactions, dizziness, drowsiness, headache, leukopenia, thrombocytopenia, hemolytic anemia.

INTERACTIONS: Hypoglycemic effects potentiated by NSAIDs, some azoles, other highly protein-bound drugs, salicylates, sulfonamides, chloramphenicol, probenecid, coumarins, MAOIs, and β-blockers. Severe hypoglycemia reported with oral miconazole. Increase levels with fluconazole. Hyperglycemia and possible loss of glycemic control with thiazides and other diuretics, corticosteroids, phenothiazines, thyroid products, estrogens, oral contraceptives, phenytoin, nicotinic acid, sympathomimetics, calcium channel blockers, and isoniazid. Increased likelihood of hypoglycemia with alcohol and use of >1 glucose lowering drug. Caution with salicylates or dicumarol.

PREGNANCY: Category C, not for use in nursing.

MECHANISM OF ACTION: Sulfonylurea; lowers blood glucose acutely by stimulating the insulin release from the pancreas.

PHARMACOKINETICS: Absorption: Rapid and complete; T_{max}=1-3 hrs. **Distribution:** Plasma protein binding (98-99%); (IV) V_d=11L. **Metabolism**: Extensive via liver. **Elimination**: Urine (<10% unchanged); $T_{1/2}$=2-4 hrs.

NURSING CONSIDERATIONS

Assessment: Assess previous hypersensitivity, FPG, HbA1c, renal/hepatic function, LFTs, type 1 DM, diabetic ketoacidosis, GI disease, age, debilitated or malnourished patients, adrenal or pituitary insufficiency, G6PD deficiency, pregnancy/nursing status and for possible drug interactions.

Monitoring: Monitor blood and urine glucose, HbA1c, renal and hepatic function, SGOT, LDH, alkaline phosphate, BUN, creatinine, signs/symptoms of hypoglycemia, endocrine/metabolic/hematologic reactions, and any adverse reactions.

Patient Counseling: Instruct to take 30 min before meals. Inform about importance of adhering to dietary instructions, a regular exercise program, and regular testing of urine/blood glucose. Educate on risks/benefits of therapy; signs/symptoms of hypoglycemia/hyperglycemia, predisposing conditions, and treatment of hypoglycemia; and primary and secondary failure. Emphasize that diet is the primary form of treatment for type 2 diabetic patients; caloric restriction and weight loss for obese diabetic patient. Inform that regular physical activity is important, and CV risk factors should be identified and managed.

Administration: Oral route. **Storage:** <30°C (86°F).

GLUCOTROL XL   RX
glipizide (Pfizer)

OTHER BRAND NAMES: Glipizide ER (Various)

THERAPEUTIC CLASS: Sulfonylurea (2nd generation)

INDICATIONS: Adjunct to diet and exercise, to improve glycemic control in adults with type 2 diabetes mellitus (DM).

DOSAGE: *Adults:* Initial: 5mg qd with breakfast; use lower doses if sensitive to hypoglycemics. Titrate: Based on lab measures of glycemic control. Maint: 5-10mg qd. Max: 20mg/day. Switch from Immediate-Release (IR) Glipizide: Give a qd dose at nearest equivalent total daily dose. If receiving IR formulation, may titrate to ER starting with 5mg qd. Combination Therapy: Initial: 5mg qd. Switch From Insulin: If ≤20 U/day: D/C insulin and start at 5mg qd. If >20 U/day: Reduce insulin dose by 50% and begin at 5mg qd. Titrate: Several days should elapse between titration. Switching from Other Oral Hypoglycemics: No transition period necessary. Elderly/Debilitated/Malnourished/Renal or Hepatic Impairment: Dose conservatively.

HOW SUPPLIED: Tab, Extended-Release: 2.5mg, 5mg, 10mg

CONTRAINDICATIONS: Type 1 DM, diabetic ketoacidosis, with or without coma.

WARNINGS/PRECAUTIONS: Increased risk of cardiovascular (CV) mortality reported; inform patient of potential risks, advantages, and alternative therapy. Markedly reduced GI retention times reported. May produce severe hypoglycemia; proper patient selection, dosage, and instructions are important. Increased risk of hypoglycemia with elderly, debilitated, malnourished, renal/hepatic disease, adrenal or pituitary insufficiency. Loss of blood glucose control may occur when exposed to stress (eg, fever, trauma, infection, or surgery); d/c therapy and administer insulin. Secondary failure may occur over period of time. May cause hemolytic anemia in patients with glucose 6-phosphate dehydrogenase (G6PD) deficiency; observe caution and consider a non-sulfonylurea alternative.

ADVERSE REACTIONS: Hypoglycemia, asthenia, headache, dizziness, diarrhea, nervousness, tremor, flatulence.

INTERACTIONS: Hypoglycemic effects potentiated by NSAIDs, other highly protein-bound drugs, salicylates, sulfonamides, chloramphenicol, probenecid, coumarins, MAOIs, and β-blockers. Severe hypoglycemia reported with oral miconazole. Increased levels with fluconazole. Hyperglycemia and possible loss of glycemic control with thiazides and other diuretics, corticosteroids, phenothiazines, thyroid products, estrogens, oral contraceptives, phenytoin, nicotinic acid, sympathomimetics, calcium channel blockers, and isoniazid. Increased likelihood of hypoglycemia with alcohol and use of >1 glucose lowering drug. Caution with salicylates or dicumarol.

PREGNANCY: Category C, not for use in nursing.

MECHANISM OF ACTION: Sulfonylurea; lowers blood glucose acutely by stimulating the release of insulin from the pancreas.

PHARMACOKINETICS: Absorption: Rapid and complete (IR); absolute bioavailability (100%); T_{max}=6-12 hrs. **Distribution:** V_d=10L; plasma protein binding (98-99%). **Metabolism:** Liver; aromatic hydroxylation products (major metabolites). **Elimination:** Urine (80%, <10% unchanged), feces (10%, <10% unchanged); $T_{1/2}$=2-5 hrs.

NURSING CONSIDERATIONS

Assessment: Assess previous hypersensitivity, FPG, HbA1c, renal/hepatic function, LFTs, type 1 DM, ketoacidosis, GI disease, preexisting severe GI narrowing, debilitated or malnourished patients, adrenal or pituitary insufficiency, G6PD deficiency, pregnancy/nursing status and for possible drug interactions.

Monitoring: Monitor blood and urine glucose, HbA1c q3 months, renal and hepatic function, LFTs, signs/symptoms of hypoglycemia, loss control of blood glucose, hemolytic anemia, endocrine/metabolic/hematologic reactions, and any adverse reactions.

Patient Counseling: Counsel to swallow whole with breakfast; do not chew, divide, or crush. Inform that patients may notice something that looks like a tablet in their stool and about importance of adhering to dietary instructions, a regular exercise program, and regular testing of urine/blood glucose. Educate on risks/benefits and of therapy; signs/symptoms of hypoglycemia/hyperglycemia, predisposing conditions and treatment of hypoglycemia; and primary and secondary failure.

Administration: Oral route. Swallow whole; do not chew, divide, or crush tab. **Storage:** 15-30°Ç (59°-86°F). Protect from moisture and humidity.

G

GLUCOVANCE RX
metformin HCl - glyburide (Bristol-Myers Squibb)

> Lactic acidosis reported (rare); increased risk with increased age, DM with renal insufficiency, congestive heart failure (CHF), and conditions with risk of hypoperfusion and hypoxemia. Avoid use in patients ≥80 yrs unless renal function is normal. Withhold therapy in the presence of any condition associated with hypoxemia, dehydration, or sepsis. Avoid in patients with clinical or laboratory evidence of hepatic disease. Caution against excessive alcohol intake, may potentiate the effects of metformin on lactate metabolism. Temporarily D/C prior to any IV radiocontrast study or surgical procedures. D/C use and institute appropriate therapy if lactic acidosis occur. Monitor renal function and for metabolic acidosis.

THERAPEUTIC CLASS: Sulfonylurea/biguanide

INDICATIONS: Adjunct to diet and exercise to improve glycemic control in adults with type 2 diabetes mellitus (DM).

DOSAGE: *Adults:* Individualize dose. Inadequate Glycemic Control on Diet/Exercise Alone: Initial: 1.25mg-250mg qd-bid with meals. If HbA1c >9% or fasting plasma glucose (FPG) >200mg/dL, give 1.25mg-250mg bid (with morning and evening meals). Titrate: Increase by 1.25mg-250mg/day every 2 weeks. Do not use 5mg-500mg for initial therapy. Inadequate Glycemic Control on a Sulfonylurea and/or Metformin: Initial: 2.5mg-500mg or 5mg-500mg bid with meals. Starting dose should not exceed daily doses of glyburide or metformin already being taken. Titrate: Increase by no more than 5mg-500mg/day. Max: 20mg-2000mg/day. With Concomitant Thiazolidinediones (TZDs): Initiate and titrate TZD as recommended. If hypoglycemia occurs, reduce glyburide component. Elderly/Debilitated/Malnourished: Do not titrate to maximum dose.

HOW SUPPLIED: Tab: (Glyburide-Metformin) 1.25mg-250mg, 2.5mg-500mg, 5mg-500mg

CONTRAINDICATIONS: Renal disease or dysfunction (SrCr ≥1.5mg/dL [males], ≥1.4mg/dL [females], or abnormal CrCl), metabolic acidosis, including diabetic ketoacidosis. D/C temporarily for radiologic studies involving intravascular iodinated contrast materials.

WARNINGS/PRECAUTIONS: Increased risk of cardiovascular (CV) mortality. Increased risk of hypoglycemia with deficient caloric intake, in elderly, debilitated, malnourished, adrenal/pituitary insufficiency or alcohol intoxication. Caution in patients with glucose-6-phosphate dehydrogenase (G6PD) deficiency; may lead to hemolytic anemia. D/C if CV collapse (shock), acute CHF, acute myocardial infarction (MI), or prerenal azotemia occur. Temporarily suspend therapy before any surgical procedure (except minor procedures not associated with restricted intake of foods and fluids), and do not restart until oral intake has resumed and renal function returns to normal. May decrease serum vitamin B12 levels; caution in those with inadequate vitamin B12 or calcium intake or absorption.

ADVERSE REACTIONS: Upper respiratory infection, N/V, abdominal pain, headache, dizziness, diarrhea.

INTERACTIONS: See Boxed Warning & Contraindications. Furosemide, nifedipine, and cimetidine may increase metformin levels. Hypoglycemia is potentiated by ciprofloxacin, miconazole, thiazolidinedione, salicylates, sulfonamides, chloramphenicol, probenecid, coumarins, MAOIs, NSAIDs, highly protein-bound drugs, other glucose lowering agents, phenylbutazone, warfarin and β-blockers. Thiazides and other diuretics, corticosteroids, phenothiazines, thyroid products, estrogens, oral contraceptives, phenytoin, nicotinic acid, sympathomimetics, calcium channel blockers, and isoniazid may cause hyperglycemia. Monitor LFTs and weight gain with TZD and rosiglitazone. May compete for common renal tubular transport systems with cationic drugs (eg, amiloride, digoxin, morphine, procainamide, quinidine, ranitidine, triamterene, trimethoprim, or vancomycin).

PREGNANCY: Category B, not for use in nursing.

MECHANISM OF ACTION: Glyburide: Sulfonylurea; stimulates release of insulin from the pancreas. Metformin: Biguanide; decreases hepatic glucose production and intestinal absorption of glucose, and improves insulin sensitivity by increasing peripheral glucose uptake and utilization.

PHARMACOKINETICS: Absorption: Glyburide: T_{max}=4 hrs. Metformin: absolute bioavailability (50-60%). **Distribution:** Glyburide: plasma protein binding (extensive). Metformin: V_d=654L. **Metabolism:** Glyburide: metabolites: 4-trans-hydroxy (major) and 3-cis hydroxy derivative. **Elimination:** Glyburide: bile, urine (50% each route); $T_{1/2}$=10 hrs. Metformin: urine (90%); $T_{1/2}$=6.2 hrs (plasma), 17.6 hrs (blood).

NURSING CONSIDERATIONS

Assessment: Assess for renal disease/dysfunction, metabolic acidosis, diabetic ketoacidosis, patients who have undergone radiologic studies using intravascular iodinated contrast materials or surgical procedures, CHF, conditions with risk of hypoperfusion and hypoxemia, septicemia, hydration status, patient's age, hepatic disease, alcoholism, CV disease, caloric intake, adrenal/pituitary insufficiency, G6PD deficiency, vitamin B12 or calcium deficiency, hypersensitivity, pregnancy/nursing status and for possible drug interactions. Assess FPG, HbA1c levels, renal function (eg, CrCl), LFTs, hematologic parameters (eg, Hgb, Hct and RBC indices).

Monitoring: Monitor for hypoglycemia, lactic acidosis, prerenal azotemia, CHF, CV disease, shock, acute MI, metabolic acidosis and hypersensitivity reactions. Monitor FPG, HbA1c, renal function (eg, SrCr), LFTs, hematologic parameters (eg, Hgb/Hct, CBC). Evaluate serum electrolytes and ketones, blood glucose, blood pH, lactate, pyruvate, and metformin levels in the evidence of ketoacidosis or lactic acidosis.

Patient Counseling: Inform about potential risks and benefits of drug and alternative modes of therapy. Inform that drug is adjunct to diet and exercise to control diabetes. Inform about importance of adherence to dietary instructions, regular exercise programs, and regular testing of blood glucose, glycosylated Hgb, renal function, and hematologic parameters. Report unexplained hyperventilation, myalgia, malaise, N/V, and somnolence. Explain risk of lactic acidosis, its signs/symptoms, and conditions that predispose its development. Explain risk of hypoglycemia. Counsel against excessive alcohol intake.

Administration: Oral route. **Storage:** 25°C (77°F). Dispense in light-resistant container.

GLUMETZA   RX
metformin HCl (Depomed)

> Lactic acidosis may occur due to metformin accumulation; increased risk with conditions such as sepsis, dehydration, excess alcohol intake, hepatic/renal impairment, and acute congestive heart failure (CHF). If acidosis is suspected, d/c and hospitalize patient immediately.

THERAPEUTIC CLASS: Biguanide

INDICATIONS: Adjunct to diet and exercise to improve glycemic control in adults with type 2 diabetes mellitus (DM).

DOSAGE: *Adults:* Individualize dose. Initial: 500mg qd. Titrate: May increase by 500mg no sooner than q1-2 weeks if higher dose is needed and there are no GI adverse reactions. Max: 2000mg/day. Take with pm meal. Elderly: Start at lower end of dosing range.

HOW SUPPLIED: Tab, Extended-Release: 500mg, 1000mg

CONTRAINDICATIONS: Renal impairment (SrCr ≥1.5mg/dL [males], ≥1.4mg/dL [females], or abnormal CrCl), acute or chronic metabolic acidosis, including diabetic ketoacidosis.

WARNINGS/PRECAUTIONS: Not for treatment of type 1 diabetes or diabetic ketoacidosis. Verify renal function is normal prior to starting therapy and at least annually thereafter. Avoid use in patients ≥80 yrs unless renal function is not reduced. Avoid in hepatic impairment. D/C if conditions associated with hypoxemia, cardiovascular (CV) collapse, acute myocardial infarction (MI), acute CHF, or prerenal azotemia develop. Acute alteration of renal function and lactic acidosis reported with intravascular iodinated contrast materials (eg, IV urogram, IV cholangiography, angiography, and computed tomography); temporarily d/c at time of or prior to procedure, withhold for 48 hrs subsequent to procedure, and reinstitute only after renal function is normal. D/C prior to any surgical procedure necessitating restricted food/fluid intake; restart after oral intake resumed and renal function found to be normal. May decrease serum vitamin B12 levels; measure hematologic parameters annually. Increased risk of hypoglycemia in elderly, debilitated/malnourished, adrenal/pituitary insufficiency, and alcohol intoxication. Caution in elderly.

ADVERSE REACTIONS: Lactic acidosis (signs may include malaise, myalgia, respiratory distress, increasing somnolence, abdominal distress), hypoglycemia, diarrhea, nausea.

INTERACTIONS: Hypoglycemia may occur with other glucose-lowering agents (eg, sulfonylureas and insulin) or ethanol; may require lower doses of insulin secretagogues (eg, sulfonylurea) or insulin. Alcohol may potentiate effect on lactate metabolism; caution against excessive alcohol intake. Caution with medications that may affect renal function or result in significant hemodynamic change or may interfere with the disposition of metformin, such as cationic drugs (eg, amiloride, cimetidine, digoxin, morphine, procainamide, quinidine, quinine, ranitidine, triamterene, trimethoprim, or vancomycin) that are eliminated by renal tubular secretion; dosage adjustment recommended. Caution with topiramate or other carbonic anhydrase inhibitors (eg, zonisamide, acetazolamide or dichlorphenamide); may increase risk of lactic acidosis. Risk of hyperglycemia and loss of blood glucose control with thiazides and other diuretics, corticosteroids, phenothiazines, thyroid products, estrogens, oral contraceptives, phenytoin, nicotinic acid, sympathomimetics, calcium channel blockers, and isoniazid.

PREGNANCY: Category B, not for use in nursing.

MECHANISM OF ACTION: Biguanide; decreases hepatic glucose production, decreases intestinal absorption of glucose, and improves insulin sensitivity by increasing peripheral glucose uptake and utilization.

PHARMACOKINETICS: Absorption: T_{max}=7-8 hrs (1000mg, single dose). **Distribution:** V_d=654L (850mg immediate release, single dose). **Elimination:** Urine (90%, unchanged); $T_{1/2}$=6.2 hrs (plasma), 17.6 hrs (blood).

NURSING CONSIDERATIONS

Assessment: Assess for DM type, diabetic ketoacidosis, metabolic acidosis, sepsis, dehydration, excess alcohol intake, hepatic/renal impairment, CHF, hypoperfusion, hypoxemia, adequate vitamin B12 or calcium intake/absorption, adrenal/pituitary insufficiency, caloric intake, general health status, pregnancy/nursing status, and possible drug interactions. Obtain baseline FPG, HbA1c, SrCr, CrCl, and LFTs. Evaluate for other medical/surgical conditions.

Monitoring: Monitor for hypoglycemia, lactic acidosis, malaise, myalgia, respiratory distress, somnolence, abdominal distress, hypoxemia, dehydration, sepsis, hypothermia, hypotension, resistant bradyarrhythmias, CV collapse, acute CHF, acute MI, or prerenal azotemia. Monitor renal/hepatic function, HbA1c, FPG, and hematologic parameters. Monitor serum vitamin B12 measurements at 2-3 yr intervals if inadequate B12 or calcium intake/absorption.

Patient Counseling: Inform of the potential risks and benefits of the drug and of alternative modes of therapy. Counsel about the importance of adherence to dietary instructions, regular exercise program, regular testing of blood glucose, and HbA1c. Advise to seek medical advice during periods of stress (eg, fever, trauma, infection, surgery). Counsel about the risks/symptoms of, and conditions that predispose to the development of lactic acidosis. D/C and promptly seek medical attention if symptoms of unexplained hyperventilation, myalgia, malaise, unusual somnolence, or other nonspecific symptoms occur. Inform about the importance of regular testing of renal function and hematological parameters. Counsel against excessive alcohol intake, either acute or chronic, while on therapy. Inform that hypoglycemia may occur when used in conjunction with insulin secretagogues (eg, sulfonylureas and insulin). Instruct to swallow tab whole; do not crush or chew; if a dose is missed, do not take 2 doses of 2000mg the same day. Inactive ingredients may occasionally be eliminated in the feces as soft mass resembling the tab.

Administration: Oral route. Swallow whole; do not split, crush or chew. **Storage:** 20-25°C (68-77°F); excursions permitted to 15-30°C (59-86°F).

GLYNASE PRESTAB   RX
glyburide (Pharmacia & Upjohn)

THERAPEUTIC CLASS: Sulfonylurea (2nd generation)

INDICATIONS: Adjunct to diet and exercise, to improve glycemic control in adults with type 2 diabetes mellitus (DM).

DOSAGE: *Adults:* Initial: 1.5-3mg qd with breakfast or 1st main meal; give 0.75mg if sensitive to hypoglycemic drugs. Titrate: Increase by increments of ≤1.5mg at weekly intervals based on patient's response. Maint: 0.75-12mg qd or in divided doses. Max: 12mg/day. Transfer from Other Oral Antidiabetic Agents: Initial: 1.5-3mg/day. Retitrate when transferring from other glyburide products or oral hypoglycemic agents. Exercise particular care during 1st 2 weeks when transferring patients from chlorpropamide. Switch From Insulin: If <20 U/day: 1.5-3mg qd. If 20-40 U/day: 3mg qd. If >40 U/day, decrease insulin dose by 50% and give 3mg qd. Titrate: Progressive withdrawal of insulin, and increase in increments of 0.75-1.5mg every 2-10 days. Concomitant Metformin: Add glyburide gradually to max dose of metformin monotherapy after 4 weeks if needed. Elderly/Debilitated/Malnourished/Renal or Hepatic Impairment: Conservative initial and maintenance dose.

HOW SUPPLIED: Tab: 1.5mg*, 3mg*, 6mg* *scored

CONTRAINDICATIONS: Diabetic ketoacidosis with or without coma, type 1 DM.

WARNINGS/PRECAUTIONS: Increased risk of cardiovascular mortality reported. Risk of hypoglycemia, especially with renal/hepatic and adrenal/pituitary insufficiency, elderly, debilitated, and malnourished. Loss of blood glucose control may occur when exposed to stress (eg, fever,

455

trauma, infection, surgery); d/c therapy and start insulin. Secondary failure may occur over period of time. Caution with glucose 6-phosphate dehydrogenase (G6PD) deficiency; treatment may lead to hemolytic anemia; thus, consider a non-sulfonylurea alternative.

ADVERSE REACTIONS: Hypoglycemia, liver function abnormalities, GI disturbances, leukopenia, agranulocytosis, thrombocytopenia, hemolytic anemia, aplastic anemia, pancytopenia, hyponatremia, changes in accommodation, blurred vision, allergic reactions.

INTERACTIONS: Hypoglycemic effects may be potentiated by NSAIDs, other drugs that are highly protein-bound, ciprofloxacin, salicylates, sulfonamides, chloramphenicol, probenecid, coumarins, MAOIs, alcohol, and β-adrenergic blocking agents. Severe hypoglycemia reported with oral hypoglycemics and oral miconazole. Hypoglycemia may occur with >1 glucose-lowering drug used. Certain drugs, including thiazides and other diuretics, corticosteroids, phenothiazines, thyroid products, estrogens, oral contraceptives, phenytoin, nicotinic acid, sympathomimetics, calcium channel blockers, and isoniazid, tend to cause hyperglycemia and may lead to loss of glycemic control. May overlap drug effects when transferred from chlorpropamide. May be displaced from protein binding sites by phenylbutazone, warfarin, and salicylates. Possible interaction with ciprofloxacin. Decrease levels with metformin.

PREGNANCY: Category B, not for use in nursing.

MECHANISM OF ACTION: Sulfonylurea; lowers blood glucose acutely by stimulating the release of insulin from the pancreas.

PHARMACOKINETICS: Absorption: C_{max}=106ng/mL (3mg); AUC=568ng•hr/mL (3mg); T_{max}=2-3 hrs. **Distribution:** Plasma protein binding (extensive). **Metabolism:** 4-trans-hydroxy derivative (major metabolite). **Elimination:** Bile (50%), urine (50%); $T_{1/2}$=4 hrs.

NURSING CONSIDERATIONS

Assessment: Assess for diabetic ketoacidosis, type 1 DM, renal/hepatic function, presence of debilitation or malnourishment, adrenal/pituitary insufficiency, G6PD deficiency, pregnancy/nursing status, and for possible drug interactions. Assess FPG and HbA1c levels. Assess adherence to diet before classifying secondary failure.

Monitoring: Monitor for signs/symptoms of hypoglycemia, hemolytic anemia, therapeutic response to therapy, primary/secondary failure. Periodically monitor FPG, HbA1c, and urine glucose.

Patient Counseling: Inform of the potential risks and advantages of therapy and of alternative modes of therapy. Instruct to take with breakfast or first main meal. Advise about the importance of adhering to dietary instructions, a regular exercise program, and regular testing of urine and/or blood glucose. Inform of risks of hypoglycemia, symptoms and treatment, and conditions that predispose to its development. Counsel about primary/secondary failure.

Administration: Oral route. **Storage:** 20-25°C (68-77°F).

GLYSET   RX
miglitol (Pharmacia & Upjohn)

THERAPEUTIC CLASS: Alpha-glucosidase inhibitor

INDICATIONS: Adjunct to diet and exercise to improve glycemic control in adults with type 2 diabetes mellitus.

DOSAGE: *Adults:* Initial: 25mg tid. May give 25mg qd (to minimize GI side effects) and gradually increase to tid. Titrate: After 4-8 weeks, increase to 50mg tid for 3 months. Maint: 50mg tid. May increase to 100mg tid if needed. Max: 100mg tid. One hour postprandial plasma glucose may be used to determine minimum effective dose. Take with first bite of each main meal.

HOW SUPPLIED: Tab: 25mg, 50mg, 100mg

CONTRAINDICATIONS: Diabetic ketoacidosis, inflammatory bowel disease, colonic ulceration, partial intestinal obstruction or predisposal to intestinal obstruction. Chronic intestinal diseases associated with digestion or absorption disorders or conditions that may deteriorate with increased gas formation in the intestine.

WARNINGS/PRECAUTIONS: Use oral glucose (dextrose) not sucrose (cane sugar) to treat mild-moderate hypoglycemia. Temporary insulin therapy may be necessary at times of stress such as fever, trauma, infection, or surgery. Not recommended with significant renal dysfunction (SrCr >2mg/dL).

ADVERSE REACTIONS: Flatulence, diarrhea, abdominal pain, skin rash, low serum iron.

INTERACTIONS: Intestinal absorbents (eg, charcoal) and digestive enzyme preparations containing carbohydrate-splitting enzmes (eg, amylase, pancreatin) may reduce effects. May reduce bioavailability of ranitidine and propranolol. Levels may be lowered with glyburide, metformin, or digoxin.

PREGNANCY: Category B, not for use in nursing.

MECHANISM OF ACTION: α-glucosidase inhibitor; reversibly inhibits membrane-bound intestinal α-glucosidase hydrolase enzymes.

PHARMACOKINETICS: Absorption: Complete, T_{max}=2-3 hrs. **Distribution:** V_d=0.18L/kg; plasma protein binding (<4.0%); found in breast milk. **Elimination:** Urine (95% unchanged); $T_{1/2}$=2 hrs.

NURSING CONSIDERATIONS

Assessment: Assess for diabetic ketoacidosis, inflammatory bowel disease, colonic ulceration, partial intestinal obstruction, chronic intestinal disease, renal function, pregnancy/nursing status, hypersensitivity, and possible drug interactions.

Monitoring: Monitor for hypoglycemia, FPG, HbA1c, renal function, diabetic ketoacidosis, GI symptoms, skin rash, serum iron.

Patient Counseling: Inform that drug is adjunct to diet and exercise. Counsel that during periods of stress (fever, trauma, infection, or surgery), medication requirements may change; patients should seek medical advice promptly. Counsel about dose-related gastrointestinal effects (eg, flatulence, soft stools, diarrhea, or abdominal discomfort). Inform that if side effects occur, they usually develop during the first few weeks of therapy. Advise to continue to adhere to dietary instructions, regular exercise program and regular testing of urine and/or blood glucose. Advise to take with the first bite of each meal.

Administration: Oral route. **Storage:** 25°C (77°F); excursions permitted to 15-30°C (59-86°F).

GRALISE
gabapentin (Depomed)

RX

THERAPEUTIC CLASS: GABA analog

INDICATIONS: Management of postherpetic neuralgia.

DOSAGE: *Adults:* Take with evening meal. Initial: Day 1: 300mg qd. Titrate: Day 2: 600mg qd. Days 3-6: 900mg qd. Days 7-10: 1200mg qd. Days 11-14: 1500mg qd. Day 15: 1800mg qd. Dose Reduction/Substitution/Withdrawal: Should be done gradually over ≥1 week. Renal Dysfunction: Initial: 300mg qd. Titrate: Follow the same schedule listed above; individualize daily dosing. CrCl ≥60mL/min: 1800mg qd. CrCl 30-60mL/min: 600mg-1800mg qd.

HOW SUPPLIED: Tab: 300mg, 600mg

WARNINGS/PRECAUTIONS: Not interchangeable with other gabapentin products. Increased risk of suicidal thoughts or behavior reported; monitor for the emergence or worsening of depression, suicidal thoughts or behavior, and/or any unusual changes in mood or behavior. Possible tumorigenic potential. Drug reaction with eosinophilia and systemic symptoms (DRESS)/multiorgan hypersensitivity reported; evaluate immediately and d/c if etiology be established. Avoid with CrCl <30mL/min or in patients undergoing hemodialysis.

ADVERSE REACTIONS: Dizziness, somnolence, headache, peripheral edema, diarrhea.

INTERACTIONS: Increased gabapentin absorption with naproxen. Reduced hydrocodone C_{max} and area under the curve (AUC). Increased gabapentin AUC values with hydrocodone and morphine. Decreased oral clearance when coadministered with cimetidine. Increased C_{max} of norethindrone. Reduced bioavailability with an antacid containing aluminum hydroxide and magnesium hydroxide; take ≥2 hrs following the antacid.

PREGNANCY: Category C, caution in nursing.

MECHANISM OF ACTION: Gamma-aminobutyric acid analog; not established. Suspected to prevent allodynia and hyperalgesia.

PHARMACOKINETICS: Absorption: (1800mg qd) C_{max}=9585ng/mL; T_{max}=8 hrs; AUC_{0-24}=132808ng•hr/mL. **Distribution:** (150mg IV) V_d=58L; plasma protein binding (<3%); found in breast milk. **Elimination:** Kidneys (unchanged); (gabapentin immediate release 1200-3000mg/day) $T_{1/2}$=5-7 hrs.

NURSING CONSIDERATIONS

Assessment: Assess for epilepsy, renal function, preexisting tumors, hypersensitivity to the drug, pregnancy/nursing status, and possible drug interactions.

Monitoring: Monitor for suicidal thoughts or behavior, emergence or worsening of depression, mood and behavioral changes, new or worsening preexisting tumors, dizziness, DRESS, hypersensitivity reactions, and other adverse reactions.

Patient Counseling: Inform to take as prescribed. Advise that the drug is not interchangeable with other formulations of gabapentin. Inform that the drug may cause dizziness, somnolence, and other signs and symptoms of CNS depression. Advise patients not to drive or operate machinery; may impair mental/physical abilities. Advise to notify physician if signs of CNS depression develop with concomitant treatment of morphine. If dose is missed, instruct to take drug with food as soon as it is remembered or to skip the missed dose if it is almost time for the next dose and take next dose at regular time; do not take two doses at the same time. Inform patients, caregivers, and families that the drug may increase suicidal thoughts and behavior, and to report immediately to physician if there is emergence or worsening of symptoms of depression, unusual mood or behavioral changes, or emergence of suicidal thoughts, behavior, or thoughts about self-harm. Advise patients to call their healthcare provider or poison control center, or got to the nearest emergency room right away. Advise to take with evening meal and to swallow whole; do not split, crush, or chew tablets.

Administration: Oral route. Swallow whole; do not split, crush, or chew tabs. **Storage:** 25°C (77°F); excursions permitted to 15-30°C (59-86°F).

GRANISETRON   RX
granisetron HCl (Various)

THERAPEUTIC CLASS: 5-HT$_3$ receptor antagonist

INDICATIONS: (Inj/PO) Prevention of N/V associated with initial and repeat courses of emetogenic cancer therapy (eg, high-dose cisplatin). (PO) Prevention of N/V associated with radiation (eg, total body irradiation and fractionated abdominal radiation).

DOSAGE: *Adults:* Emetogenic Chemotherapy: (PO) 2mg qd up to 1 hr before chemotherapy or 1mg tab bid up to 1 hr before chemotherapy and 12 hrs later. (IV) 10mcg/kg, undiluted over 30 sec or diluted (with 0.9% NaCl or D5W) over 5 min, within 30 min before chemotherapy. Prevention of N/V with Radiation: (PO) 2mg qd within 1 hr of radiation.
Pediatrics: 2-16 yrs: Emetogenic Chemotherapy: 10mcg/kg IV within 30 min before chemotherapy.

HOW SUPPLIED: Inj: 0.1mg/mL [1mL]; 1mg/mL [1mL, 4mL]; Tab: 1mg

WARNINGS/PRECAUTIONS: Does not stimulate gastric or intestinal peristalsis; do not use instead of nasogastric suction. May mask progressive ileus or gastric distension. QT prolongation reported; caution with preexisting arrhythmias, cardiac conduction disorders, cardiac disease, and electrolyte abnormalities. (Inj) Hypersensitivity reactions may occur in patients who exhibited hypersensitivity to other selective 5-HT$_3$ receptor antagonists.

ADVERSE REACTIONS: Headache, asthenia, somnolence, diarrhea, constipation, insomnia, fever, ALT/AST elevation.

INTERACTIONS: Hepatic CYP450 enzyme inducers or inhibitors may alter clearance and T$_{1/2}$. Caution with cardiotoxic chemotherapy, drugs known to prolong QT interval and/or arrhythmogenic drugs. May inhibit metabolism with ketoconazole. (Inj) Increased total plasma clearance with phenobarbital.

PREGNANCY: Category B, caution in nursing.

MECHANISM OF ACTION: 5-HT$_3$ receptor antagonist; blocks serotonin stimulation and subsequent vomiting after emetogenic stimuli.

PHARMACOKINETICS: Absorption: C_{max}=63.8ng/mL (IV, 40mcg/kg), 5.99ng/mL (PO). **Distribution:** Plasma protein binding (65%). V_d=3.07L/kg (IV, 40mcg/kg). **Metabolism:** CYP3A; N-demethylation, aromatic ring oxidation, conjugation. **Elimination:** (PO) Urine (11% unchanged, 48% metabolites), feces (38% metabolites). (IV) Urine (12% unchanged, 49% metabolites), feces (34% metabolites); T$_{1/2}$=8.95 hrs (IV, 40mcg/kg).

NURSING CONSIDERATIONS

Assessment: Assess for preexisting arrhythmias, cardiac conduction disorders, cardiac disease, electrolyte abnormalities, previous hypersensitivity to drug, pregnancy/nursing status, and possible drug interactions.

Monitoring: Monitor for masking of progressive ileus and gastric distention, QT prolongation and hypersensitivity reactions.

Patient Counseling: Inform about risks/benefits of therapy. Advise patients to report any adverse events to their healthcare provider.

Administration: Oral, IV route. Refer to PI for inj stability and compatibility. Undiluted IV should be administered over 30 sec. Diluted sol should be infused over 5 min. **Storage:** 20-25°C (68-77°F). Protect from light. Retain in carton until time of use. (Inj) Excursions permitted to 15-30°C (59-86°F). Diluted Sol: 0.9% NaCl or D5W: Stable at room temperature for 24 hrs under normal lighting conditions. Do not freeze. Once the multidose vial is penetrated, use within 30 days.

GRIS-PEG   RX
griseofulvin (Pedinol)

THERAPEUTIC CLASS: *Penicillium*-derived antifungal

INDICATIONS: Treatment of the following ringworm infections: tinea corporis, tinea pedis, tinea cruris, tinea barbae, tinea capitis, and tinea unguium when caused by one or more species of *Microsporum, Epidermophyton,* and *Trichophyton.*

DOSAGE: *Adults:* T. corporis/T. cruris/T. capitis: 375mg/day in single or divided doses. T. corporis: Treat for 2-4 weeks. T. capitis: Treat for 4-6 weeks. Difficult Fungal Infections to Eradicate/T. pedis/ T. unguium: 750mg/day, given in a divided dose. T. pedis: Concomitant topical agents required. Treat for 4-8 weeks. T. unguium: Treat for at least 4 months (fingernails) and at least 6 months (toenails), depending on rate of growth.
Pediatrics: >2 yrs: Usual: 3.3mg/lb/day. 35-60 lbs: 125-187.5mg/day. >60 lbs: 187.5-375mg/day. T. capitis: Treat for 4-6 weeks. T. corporis: Treat for 2-4 weeks. T. pedis: Treat for 4-8 weeks. T. unguium: Treat for at least 4 months (fingernail) and at least 6 months (toenails), depending on rate of growth.

HOW SUPPLIED: Tab: 125mg*, 250mg* *scored

CONTRAINDICATIONS: Porphyria, hepatocellular failure, pregnancy.

WARNINGS/PRECAUTIONS: Not for prophylactic use. Severe skin reactions (eg, Stevens-Johnson syndrome [SJS], toxic epidermal necrolysis) reported; d/c if these occur. Elevations in AST, ALT, bilirubin and jaundice reported; monitor for hepatic adverse events and d/c if warranted. Periodically organ system function including renal, hepatic, and hematopoietic functions if on prolonged therapy; d/c if granulocytopenia occurs. Cross-sensitivity with penicillin (PCN) may exist. Photosensitivity reported. Lupus erythematosus or lupus-like syndromes reported. Clinical relapse may occur if therapy not continued until infecting organism eradicated.

ADVERSE REACTIONS: Hypersensitivity reactions (eg, skin rashes, urticaria, erythema multiforme-like reactions), granulocytopenia, oral thrush, N/V, epigastric distress, diarrhea, headache, dizziness, insomnia, mental confusion.

INTERACTIONS: Anticoagulants (warfarin-type) may require dosage adjustment. Decreased effect with barbiturates. Possible interaction with oral contraceptives. Increased alcohol effect, producing tachycardia and flush.

PREGNANCY: Contraindicated in pregnancy, safety not known in nursing.

MECHANISM OF ACTION: *Penicillium*-derived antifungal; fungistatic with *in vitro* activity against various species of *Microsporum, Epidermophyton,* and *Trichophyton.*

PHARMACOKINETICS: Absorption: (250mg unaltered tab) C_{max}=600.61ng/mL; T_{max}=4.04 hrs; AUC=8,618.89ng•hr/mL. (250mg physically altered tab [crushed in applesauce]) C_{max}=672.61ng/mL; T_{max}=3.08 hrs; AUC=9,023.71ng•hr/mL.

NURSING CONSIDERATIONS

Assessment: Assess for identification of fungi responsible for infection (eg, cultures, microscopic exam). Assess for hepatocellular failure, porphyria, hypersensitivity to PCN, pregnancy/nursing status, and for possible drug interactions.

Monitoring: Monitor for signs/symptoms of serious skin reactions (eg, SJS, erythema multiforme), hepatotoxicity, photosensitivity reactions, and for lupus erythematosus or lupus-like syndromes. Perform periodic monitoring of organ system function including renal, hepatic, and hematopoietic functions in patients on prolonged therapy.

Patient Counseling: Inform of the importance of compliance with full course of therapy. Counsel to avoid intense natural or artificial sunlight while on medication. Instruct to take proper hygienic precautions to prevent spread of infection. Advise females to avoid pregnancy while on therapy. Instruct to notify physician if any adverse reactions occur.

Administration: Oral route. Swallow whole or crushed and sprinkled onto 1 tbsp of applesauce and swallow immediately without chewing. **Storage:** 15-30°C (59-86°F). Store in tight, light-resistant container.

HALAVEN   RX
eribulin mesylate (Eisai)

THERAPEUTIC CLASS: Antimicrotubule agent

INDICATIONS: Treatment of metastatic breast cancer in patients who have previously received at least 2 chemotherapeutic regimens for the treatment of metastatic disease. Prior therapy should have included an anthracycline and a taxane in either the adjuvant or metastatic setting.

DOSAGE: *Adults:* Administer IV over 2-5 min on Days 1 and 8 of a 21-day cycle. Usual: 1.4mg/m². Mild Hepatic (Child-Pugh A)/Moderate Renal (CrCl 30-50 mL/min) Impairment: Usual: 1.1mg/m². Moderate Hepatic Impairment (Child-Pugh B): Usual: 0.7mg/m². Refer to PI for dose modifications.

HOW SUPPLIED: Inj: 0.5mg/mL [2mL]

WARNINGS/PRECAUTIONS: Severe neutropenia (absolute neutrophil count <500/mm^3) reported; monitor CBC prior to each dose, increase frequency of monitoring if Grade 3 or 4 cytopenias develop. Peripheral neuropathy reported; monitor closely for signs of peripheral motor and sensory neuropathy. May cause fetal harm during pregnancy. QT prolongation reported; monitor ECG in patients with congestive heart failure (CHF), bradyarrhythmias, and electrolyte abnormalities. Correct hypokalemia or hypomagnesemia prior to therapy and monitor these electrolytes periodically during therapy. Avoid with congenital long QT syndrome. Not studied in patients with severe hepatic (Child-Pugh C) and severe renal (CrCl <30mL/min) impairment.

ADVERSE REACTIONS: Neutropenia, anemia, peripheral neuropathy, headache, asthenia/fatigue, pyrexia, weight decreased, constipation, diarrhea, N/V, arthralgia, dyspnea, alopecia.

INTERACTIONS: Monitor ECG with drugs known to prolong the QT interval (eg, Class Ia and III antiarrhythmics).

PREGNANCY: Category D, not for use in nursing.

MECHANISM OF ACTION: Antimicrotubule agent; inhibits the growth phase of microtubules via tubulin-based antimitotic mechanism leading to G$_2$/M cell-cycle block, disruption of mitotic spindles, and apoptotic cell death after prolonged mitotic blockage.

PHARMACOKINETICS: Distribution: V$_d$=43-114L/m^2; plasma protein binding at concentrations of 100-1000ng/mL (49-65%). **Metabolism:** Liver via CYP3A4. **Elimination:** Urine (9%, 91% unchanged), feces (82%, 88% unchanged); T$_{1/2}$=40 hrs.

NURSING CONSIDERATIONS

Assessment: Assess for renal/hepatic impairment, CHF, bradyarrhythmias, congenital long QT syndrome, electrolyte abnormalities, pregnancy/nursing status, and possible drug interactions. Assess for peripheral neuropathy and obtain CBC.

Monitoring: Monitor for signs of neuropathy and other adverse reactions. Monitor ECG in patients with CHF, bradyarrhythmias, and electrolyte abnormalities. Monitor K$^+$ and magnesium levels periodically. Monitor CBC prior to each dose and increase frequency of monitoring if Grade 3 or 4 cytopenias develop.

Patient Counseling: Advise to contact healthcare provider for a fever ≥100.5°F or other signs/symptoms of infection (eg, chills, cough, or burning or pain on urination). Advise women of childbearing potential to avoid pregnancy and use effective contraception during treatment.

Administration: IV route. Do not dilute in or administer through IV line containing sol with dextrose. Do not administer in same IV line with the other medicinal products. Refer to PI for the preparation and administration instructions. **Storage:** 25°C (77°F); excursions permitted to 15-30°C (59-86°F). Do not freeze. Undiluted/Diluted Sol: Up to 4 hrs at room temperature or for up to 24 hrs under refrigeration (40°F or/ 4°C). Discard unused portions of the vial.

HALCION   CIV
triazolam (Pharmacia & Upjohn)

THERAPEUTIC CLASS: Benzodiazepine

INDICATIONS: Short-term treatment of insomnia (generally 7-10 days).

DOSAGE: *Adults:* Individualize dose. Usual: 0.25mg at bedtime. Max: 0.5mg. Elderly/Debilitated: Initial: 0.125mg. Max: 0.25mg.

HOW SUPPLIED: Tab: 0.125mg, 0.25mg* *scored

CONTRAINDICATIONS: Pregnancy, concomitant use of ketoconazole, itraconazole, nefazodone, medications that significantly impair the oxidative metabolism mediated by CYP3A.

WARNINGS/PRECAUTIONS: Initiate only after careful evaluation; failure of insomnia to remit after 7-10 days of treatment may indicate presence of psychiatric and/or medical illness. Use lowest effective dose especially in elderly. Complex behaviors (eg, sleep-driving) reported; d/c if sleep-driving occurs. Severe anaphylactic and anaphylactoid reactions reported; do not rechallenge if angioedema develops. Increased daytime anxiety, abnormal thinking, and behavioral changes reported. Worsening of depression, including suicidal thinking, reported in primarily depressed patients. May impair mental/physical abilities. Anterograde amnesia, paradoxical reactions, and traveler's amnesia reported. Respiratory depression and apnea reported in patients with compromised respiratory function. Caution with renal/hepatic impairment, chronic pulmonary insufficiency, and sleep apnea. Tolerance to and dependence on drug may develop; caution with history of alcoholism, drug abuse, or with marked personality disorders, due to increased risk of dependence. Withdrawal symptoms reported following abrupt d/c; avoid abrupt d/c, and taper dose.

ADVERSE REACTIONS: Drowsiness, dizziness, lightheadedness, headache, nervousness, coordination disorders, ataxia, N/V.

INTERACTIONS: See Contraindications. Caution and consider dose reduction with drugs inhibiting CYP3A to a lesser but significant degree. Not recommended with azole-type antifungals. Macrolide antibiotics (eg, erythromycin, clarithromycin) and cimetidine may increase levels; caution and consider dose reduction with macrolides and cimetidine. Isoniazid, oral contraceptives, grapefruit juice, and ranitidine may increase levels. Additive CNS depression and increased risk of complex behaviors with psychotropic medications, anticonvulsants, antihistamines, alcohol, and other CNS depressants. Caution with fluvoxamine, diltiazem, verapamil, sertraline, paroxetine, ergotamine, cyclosporine, amiodarone, nicardipine, and nifedipine.

PREGNANCY: Category X, not for use in nursing.

MECHANISM OF ACTION: Triazolobenzodiazepine hypnotic agent.

PHARMACOKINETICS: Absorption: C_{max}=1-6ng/mL, T_{max}=2 hrs. **Metabolism:** Hydroxylation via CYP3A. **Elimination:** Urine (79.9% two primary metabolites); $T_{1/2}$=1.5-5.5 hrs.

NURSING CONSIDERATIONS

Assessment: Assess for primary psychiatric and/or medical illness, depression, renal/hepatic impairment, chronic pulmonary insufficiency, sleep apnea, history of seizures, alcoholism, or drug abuse, marked personality disorders, hypersensitivity, pregnancy/nursing status, and possible drug interactions.

Monitoring: Monitor for complex behaviors, anaphylactic/anaphylactoid reactions, angioedema, increased daytime anxiety, emergence of any new behavioral signs/symptoms, tolerance, withdrawal effects, and other adverse reactions.

Patient Counseling: Inform of benefits/risks of therapy and potential for physical/psychological dependence. Caution against hazardous tasks (operating machinery/driving). Instruct to immediately report to physician if any adverse reactions such as sleep-driving and other complex behaviors develop. Advise to avoid alcohol consumption. Instruct to notify physician if pregnant, planning to become pregnant, or if nursing.

Administration: Oral route. **Storage:** 20-25°C (68-77°F).

HALFLYTELY

RX

bisacodyl - polyethylene glycol 3350 - sodium bicarbonate - potassium chloride - sodium chloride (Braintree)

THERAPEUTIC CLASS: Bowel cleanser/stimulant laxative

INDICATIONS: Colon cleansing prior to colonoscopy.

DOSAGE: *Adults:* Consume only clear liquids on day of preparation. Take 1 bisacodyl tab with water. Do not crush or chew tab. After 1st bowel movement (or max of 6 hrs) drink sol, at a rate of 8 oz. q10 mins. Drink all sol. Drink each portion at longer intervals or d/c sol temporarily if abdominal distension/discomfort occurs until symptoms improve.

HOW SUPPLIED: Kit: Tab, Delayed-Release: (Bisacodyl) 5mg. Sol: (Polyethylene Glycol 3350-Potassium Chloride-Sodium Bicarbonate-Sodium Chloride) 210g-0.74g-2.86g-5.6g [2000mL].

CONTRAINDICATIONS: Ileus, GI obstruction, gastric retention, bowel perforation, toxic colitis, toxic megacolon.

WARNINGS/PRECAUTIONS: Serious arrhythmias reported rarely; caution in patients at increased risk of arrhythmias (eg, history of prolonged QT, uncontrolled arrhythmias, recent myocardial infarction [MI], unstable angina, congestive heart failure [CHF], or cardiomyopathy), and consider pre-dose and post-colonoscopy ECGs. Perform post-colonoscopy lab tests (electrolytes, creatinine, BUN) if patient develops vomiting or signs of dehydration. Hydrate patients adequately before, during, and after administration. Caution in patients with increased risk for seizure, renal impairment, and fluid and electrolyte disturbances. Correct electrolyte abnormalities prior to treatment. Caution in severe active ulcerative colitis (UC). Caution in patients with impaired gag reflex and patients prone to regurgitation/aspiration. Ischemic colitis reported; evaluate if severe abdominal pain or rectal bleeding develops. Generalized tonic-clonic seizures reported with the use of large volume (4L) polyethylene glycol-based colon preparation products; caution in patients with a history of seizures and patients at risk of seizure or with known or suspected hyponatremia. Monitor closely with impaired water handling. Do not add additional ingredients other than flavor packs provided.

ADVERSE REACTIONS: N/V, abdominal fullness, abdominal cramping, overall discomfort.

INTERACTIONS: Oral medications taken within 1 hr of start of administration may not be absorbed from GI tract. Avoid bisacodyl delayed release tablets within 1 hr of taking an antacid. Caution with drugs that lower the seizure threshold (eg, tricyclic antidepressants), in patients withdrawing from alcohol or benzodiazepines, drugs that increase the risk of electrolyte abnormalities (eg, diuretics); monitor baseline and post-colonoscopy laboratory tests (Na, K^+, calcium, creatinine, BUN). Caution with drugs that may increase the risk of adverse events of arrhythmias and prolonged QT with fluid and electrolyte abnormalities. Caution with drugs that may affect renal function (eg, diuretics, ACE inhibitors, ARBs, NSAIDs); consider baseline and post-colonoscopy labs (electrolytes, SrCr, BUN) in these patients.

PREGNANCY: Category C, caution in nursing.

MECHANISM OF ACTION: Polyethylene glycol-3350: Osmotic laxative; causes water to be retained within the GI tract. Bisacodyl: Simulant laxative; active metabolite acts directly on the colonic mucosa to produce colonic peristalsis. The stimulant laxative effect of bisacodyl, together with the osmotic effect of the unabsorbed PEG when ingested with a large volume of water, produces watery diarrhea.

PHARMACOKINETICS: Absorption: Polyethylene glycol-3350: Minimal. **Metabolism:** Bisacodyl: Hydrolysis by intestinal brush border enzymes and colonic bacteria to form bis-(p-hydroxyphenyl) pyridyl-2 methane (active metabolite).

NURSING CONSIDERATIONS

Assessment: Assess for GI obstruction, bowel perforation, electrolyte/fluid abnormalities, history of seizures, known or suspected hyponatremia, renal impairment, any other conditions where treatment is contraindicated or cautioned, hypersensitivity, pregnancy/nursing status, and possible drug interactions. Obtain baseline electrolytes, Na, K+, Ca, SrCr, and BUN in patients at risk for seizures and patients with renal impairment. Perform baseline ECGs in patients at risk for arrhythmias.

Monitoring: Perform baseline and post-colonoscopy lab tests in patients with seizure risk (eg, known/suspected hyponatremia), and consider these tests in patients with impaired renal function. Monitor for hypersensitivity reactions, aspiration, cardiac arrhythmias, abdominal pain, rectal bleeding, ischemic colitis, and seizures.

Patient Counseling: Oral medication administered within 1 hr of start of administration of sol may be flushed from GI tract—hence, not absorbed. Instruct to take exactly as directed. Advise not to take other laxatives while taking HalfLytely and Bisacodyl Tablet Bowel Prep Kit. Notify physician if they have trouble swallowing or are prone to regurgitation or aspiration. Instruct to slow or temporarily d/c administration if severe bloating, distention or abdominal pain occurs until symptoms abate and notify physician. Advise to d/c administration and contact physician if hives, rashes, allergic reaction, signs and symptoms of dehydration develops.

Administration: Oral route. **Storage:** 20-25°C (68-77°F); excursions permitted to 15-30°C (59-86°F). Refrigerate reconstituted solution and use within 48 hrs.

HALOPERIDOL   RX
haloperidol (Various)

> Elderly patients with dementia-related psychosis treated with antipsychotic drugs are at an increased risk of death; most deaths appeared to be cardiovascular (CV) (eg, heart failure, sudden death) or infectious (eg, pneumonia) in nature. Not approved for the treatment of patients with dementia-related psychosis.

OTHER BRAND NAMES: Haldol (Ortho-McNeil)

THERAPEUTIC CLASS: Butyrophenone

INDICATIONS: (Inj) Treatment of schizophrenia and control of tics and vocal utterances of Tourette's disorder in adults. (Sol/Tab) Management of manifestations of psychotic disorders. Control of tics and vocal utterances of Tourette's disorder in children and adults. Treatment of severe behavior problems in children with combative, explosive, hyperexcitability and for short-term treatment of children with hyperactivity showing excessive motor activity accompanied by conduct disorders that failed to respond to psychotherapy and medications other than antipsychotics.

DOSAGE: *Adults:* Individualize dose. (PO) Initial: Moderate Symptoms/Elderly/Debilitated: 0.5-2mg bid or tid. Severe Symptoms/Chronic/Resistant: 3-5mg bid or tid. Doses up to 100mg/day may be needed to achieve optimal response. Doses >100mg/day have been used for severe resistant patients but safety on prolonged use not demonstrated. Refer to PI for dose adjustments/maint dosing. (Inj) 2-5mg IM for prompt control of acute agitation with moderately severe or very severe symptoms. May give subsequent doses as often as every hour, although 4-8 hr intervals may be satisfactory, depending on response. Refer to PI for switchover procedure.
Pediatrics: 3-12 yrs (15-40kg): (PO) Individualize dose. Initial: Lowest possible dose of 0.5mg/day. Increase by increments of 0.5mg/day at 5-7 day intervals until desired therapeutic effect obtained. May divide total dose to be given bid or tid. Psychotic Disorders: 0.05-0.15mg/kg/day. May require higher doses in severely disturbed psychotic children. Nonpsychotic Behavior Disorders/Tourette's Disorder: 0.05-0.075mg/kg/day. Short term treatment for severely disturbed nonpsychotic/hyperactive children with behavior disorders may suffice. Refer to PI for dose adjustments/maint dosing.

HOW SUPPLIED: Inj: 5mg/mL (Haldol); Sol: 2mg/mL [15mL, 120mL]; Tab: 0.5mg*, 1mg*, 2mg*, 5mg*, 10mg*, 20mg* *scored

CONTRAINDICATIONS: Severe toxic CNS depression or comatose states, Parkinson's disease.

WARNINGS/PRECAUTIONS: Risk of tardive dyskinesia (TD), especially in the elderly; consider d/c if signs/symptoms develop. Neuroleptic malignant syndrome (NMS) reported; d/c and treat immediately. Hyperpyrexia, heat stroke, and bronchopneumonia reported. Use only during pregnancy if benefits justifies risk to fetus. Caution with severe cardiovascular disease (CVD), history of seizures, EEG abnormalities, and known/history of allergic reactions to drugs. May cause transient hypotension and/or anginal pain with severe CVD; treat hypotension with metaraminol, phenylephrine, or norepinephrine. May cause rapid mood swing to depression when used to control mania in cyclic disorders, severe neurotoxicity in patients with thyrotoxicosis, and increased prolactin levels. Caution in elderly. May impair mental/physical abilities. (Inj/Tab) Sudden death, QT prolongation, and torsades de pointes may occur. Caution with other QT-prolonging conditions (eg, electrolyte imbalance, underlying cardiac abnormalities, hypothyroidism, and familial long QT-syndrome). Leukopenia, neutropenia, and agranulocytosis reported; d/c if severe neutropenia (absolute neutrophil count <1000/mm^3) develops. Monitor CBC and d/c at 1st sign of decline in WBC if with preexisting low WBC count or history of drug-induced leukopenia/neutropenia. (Inj) Not approved for IV administration.

ADVERSE REACTIONS: Extrapyramidal symptoms, TD, dystonia, ECG changes, ventricular arrhythmias, tachycardia, hypotension, HTN, N/V, constipation, diarrhea, dry mouth, blurred vision, urinary retention.

INTERACTIONS: Encephalopathic syndrome followed by irreversible brain damage may occur with lithium. Caution with anticonvulsants and anticoagulants (eg, phenindione). Anticholinergics, including antiparkinson agents, may increase intraocular pressure. May potentiate CNS depressants (eg, alcohol, anesthetics, opiates); avoid with alcohol. Avoid with epinephrine for hypotension treatment. (Inj/Tab) Caution with drugs prolonging QT interval or cause electrolyte imbalance. Rifampin may decrease levels. (Inj) Ketoconazole (400mg/day) and paroxetine (20mg/day) may increase QTc. CYP3A4 or CYP2D6 substrates/inhibitors may increase levels. Carbamazepine may decrease levels.

PREGNANCY: Safety not known in pregnancy, not for use in nursing.

MECHANISM OF ACTION: Butyrophenone; mechanism not established.

PHARMACOKINETICS: Distribution: (Inj) Found in breast milk.

NURSING CONSIDERATIONS

Assessment: Assess for history of dementia-related psychosis or any other conditions where treatment is cautioned or contraindicated. Assess for hypersensitivity to drug, pregnancy/ nursing status, and possible drug interactions. Obtain baseline CBC, ECG, EEG, and serum electrolytes.

Monitoring: Monitor for signs/symptoms of NMS, TD, bronchopneumonia, hypersensitivity reactions, and other adverse reactions. Monitor for neurotoxicity in patients with thyrotoxicosis. Monitor vital signs, CBC, ECG, EEG, serum electrolytes, and cholesterol levels.

Patient Counseling: Inform about risks/benefits of therapy. Instruct to use caution in performing hazardous tasks (eg, operating machinery/driving). Instruct to avoid alcohol due to possible additive effects and hypotension. Advise to inform physician if nursing, pregnant, or plan to get pregnant.

Administration: Oral and IM route. (Inj) Inspect visually for particulate matter and discoloration prior to administration. Do not give IV. **Storage:** (Tab/Sol) 20-25°C (68-77°F). (Inj) 15-30°C (59-86°F). (Inj/Sol) Do not freeze. Protect from light.

Havrix   RX
hepatitis A vaccine (GlaxoSmithKline)

THERAPEUTIC CLASS: Vaccine

INDICATIONS: Active immunization against disease caused by hepatitis A virus (HAV) in persons ≥12 months of age.

DOSAGE: *Adults:* 1mL IM, then 1mL IM booster anytime between 6-12 months later. *Pediatrics:* 1-18 yrs: 0.5mL IM, then 0.5mL IM booster anytime between 6-12 months later.

HOW SUPPLIED: Inj: 720 EL U/0.5mL, 1440 EL U/mL

CONTRAINDICATIONS: Previous severe allergic reaction to neomycin.

WARNINGS/PRECAUTIONS: Prefilled syringes may contain natural rubber latex; may cause allergic reactions in latex-sensitive individuals. Syncope may occur and can be accompanied by transient neurological signs. Appropriate treatment and supervision must be available for possible anaphylactic reactions. Immunocompromised persons may have a diminished immune response.

May not prevent hepatitis A infection in patients who have an unrecognized hepatitis A infection at time of vaccination. May not protect all individuals. Lower antibody response reported in patients with chronic liver disease. Primary immunization should be administered at least 2 weeks prior to expected exposure to HAV.

ADVERSE REACTIONS: Inj-site reactions (eg, induration, soreness, redness, swelling, pain), headache, irritability, fever, fatigue, malaise, anorexia, nausea, loss of appetite, drowsiness.

INTERACTIONS: Immunosuppressive therapies, including irradiation, antimetabolites, alkylating agents, cytotoxic drugs, and corticosteroids (used in greater than physiological doses) may reduce immune response.

PREGNANCY: Category C, caution in nursing.

MECHANISM OF ACTION: Vaccine; presence of antibodies confers protection against HAV infection.

NURSING CONSIDERATIONS

Assessment: Assess for history of hypersensitivity reactions to previous dose of hepatitis A vaccine, neomycin, latex sensitivity, chronic liver disease, presence of immunosuppression, immunization status/vaccination history, pregnancy/nursing status, and possible drug interactions.

Monitoring: Monitor for allergic reactions, inj-site reactions (eg, pain, redness, swelling), syncope, and any other possible adverse events. Monitor immune response.

Patient Counseling: Inform of potential benefits/risks of immunization. Counsel about potential adverse reactions and that the vaccine contains noninfectious killed viruses and cannot cause hepatitis A infection. Instruct to report any adverse events to physician.

Administration: IM route. Do not administer in the gluteal region; administer in the anterolateral aspect of the thigh in young children or in the deltoid region in older children and adults. Shake well before use. Do not dilute to administer. Coadministration of other vaccines or immune globulin should be given at different inj site; do not mix with any other vaccine or product in the same syringe or vial. **Storage:** 2-8°C (36-46°F). Do not freeze; discard if frozen.

HELIDAC   RX
tetracycline HCl - bismuth subsalicylate - metronidazole (Prometheus)

> Metronidazole has been shown to be carcinogenic in mice and rats. Unnecessary use of the drug should be avoided. Its use should be reserved for the eradication of *Helicobacter pylori* for treatment of patients with *H. pylori* infection and duodenal ulcer disease.

THERAPEUTIC CLASS: *H. pylori* treatment combination

INDICATIONS: In combination with an H_2 antagonist for eradication of *H. pylori* for treatment of patients with *H. pylori* infection and duodenal ulcer disease (active or history of duodenal ulcer).

DOSAGE: *Adults:* (Bismuth) (2 tabs) 525mg + (Metronidazole) 250mg + (Tetracycline) 500mg, all qid for 14 days with an H_2 antagonist taken as directed. Take at mealtime and hs. Chew and swallow bismuth tabs. Take metronidazole tab and tetracycline cap with a full glass of water; swallow whole.

HOW SUPPLIED: Cap: (Tetracycline) 500mg; Tab: (Metronidazole) 250mg; Tab, Chewable: (Bismuth Subsalicylate) 262.4mg

CONTRAINDICATIONS: Pregnancy, nursing, pediatrics, renal/hepatic impairment, known allergy to aspirin (ASA) or salicylates.

WARNINGS/PRECAUTIONS: Use in the absence of a proven or strongly suspected bacterial infection or prophylactic indication is unlikely to provide benefit and increases the risk of development of drug-resistant bacteria. Caution in elderly. Bismuth subsalicylate: Rare reports of neurotoxicity with excessive doses. May cause temporary and harmless darkening of the tongue and/or black stool. May interfere with x-ray diagnostic procedures of the GI tract. Metronidazole: Encephalopathy, peripheral neuropathy, convulsive seizures, aseptic meningitis reported; d/c if abnormal neurological signs develop. Caution in patients with CNS disease. May produce teratogenic effects. Mild leukopenia reported; caution with evidence of or history of blood dyscrasias. Known or previously unrecognized candidiasis may present more prominent symptoms. May interfere with blood chemistry tests (eg, AST, ALT, lactate dehydrogenase, TG, hexokinase glucose). Tetracycline: May cause permanent discoloration of the teeth during tooth development (last half of pregnancy, infancy, and childhood up to 8 yrs). Enamel hypoplasia reported. Photosensitivity manifested by an exaggerated sunburn reaction reported; d/c at first evidence of skin erythema. May increase BUN. May result in overgrowth of nonsusceptible organisms (eg, fungi); d/c if superinfection occurs. Pseudotumor cerebri (benign intracranial hypertension) in adults reported.

ADVERSE REACTIONS: Nausea, diarrhea, abdominal pain, melena.

INTERACTIONS: Bismuth subsalicylate: Increases risk of bleeding when administered with anticoagulant therapy. May enhance hypoglycemic effect of antidiabetic agents. Caution with ASA, probenecid, and sulfinpyrazone. Tetracycline: Depressed plasma prothrombin activity with anticoagulants. Impaired absorption reported with antacids containing aluminum, calcium, or magnesium; preparations containing iron, zinc, or sodium bicarbonate; or milk or dairy products. Possible reduced absorption with bismuth or calcium carbonate. May interfere with bactericidal action of penicillin; avoid concomitant use. May render oral contraceptives less effective; breakthrough bleeding reported. Fatal renal toxicity with methoxyflurane reported. Metronidazole: Potentiates anticoagulant effect of warfarin and other oral coumarin anticoagulants, resulting in prolonged PT. Coadministration of drugs that decrease microsomal liver enzyme activity (eg, cimetidine) may prolong the half-life and decrease plasma clearance of metronidazole. Accelerated elimination leading to reduced plasma levels of metronidazole reported with drugs that induce microsomal liver enzymes (eg, phenytoin, phenobarbital). May impair phenytoin clearance. May increase lithium levels which may lead to toxicity. Avoid alcohol during and at least 1 day after therapy. Psychotic reactions reported in alcoholics with concomitant disulfiram; metronidazole should not be given to patients who have taken disulfiram within the last 2 weeks.

PREGNANCY: Category D, not for use in nursing.

MECHANISM OF ACTION: Antimicrobial; combination therapy with activity against *H. pylori*.

PHARMACOKINETICS: Absorption: (Salicylic acid, 525mg) C_{max}=13.1mcg/mL. (Metronidazole, 250mg) Well-absorbed; C_{max}=6mcg/mL; T_{max}=1-2 hrs. (Tetracycline) Readily absorbed. **Distribution**: (Bismuth) Plasma protein binding (>90%). (Salicylic acid) V_d=170mL/kg; plasma protein binding (90%). (Metronidazole) Plasma protein binding (<20%), appears in CSF, saliva, breast milk. (Tetracycline) Crosses placenta, found in fetal tissues, secreted in breast milk. **Metabolism**: (Salicyclic acid) Extensive. (Metronidazole) Side chain oxidation, glucuronide conjugation; 2-hydroxymethyl (metabolite). **Elimination**: (Bismuth) Urine, bile; $T_{1/2}$=21-72 days. (Salicylic acid, 525mg) Urine (10%, unchanged); $T_{1/2}$=2-5 hrs. (Metronidazole) Urine (60-80%), feces (6-15%); $T_{1/2}$=8 hrs. (Tetracycline) Urine, feces.

NURSING CONSIDERATIONS

Assessment: Assess for renal/hepatic impairment, hypersensitivity to ASA/salicylates or any component of drug therapy, candidiasis, CNS diseases, presence/history of blood dyscrasias, other conditions where therapy is contraindicated or cautioned, pregnancy/nursing status, and possible drug interactions.

Monitoring: Monitor for signs/symptoms of encephalopathy, peripheral/optic neuropathy, convulsive seizures, aseptic meningitis, pseudotumor cerebri, neurotoxicity, photosensitivity, candidiasis, overgrowth of nonsusceptible organisms, BUN, leukopenia, and other adverse reactions.

Patient Counseling: Instruct to take exactly as directed to maintain effectiveness of treatment and to prevent development of bacterial resistance. Inform that therapy does not treat viral infections. Instruct to chew and swallow bismuth subsalicylate tabs, and to swallow tetracycline cap and metronidazole tab whole with a full glass of water. Advise to take tetracycline, particularly the bedtime dose, with an adequate amount of fluid to prevent esophageal irritation and ulceration. Inform that if a dose is missed, continue normal dosing until medication is done and do not double the dose; advise to contact physician if >4 doses are missed. Advise to consult physician if ringing in the ears occurs while taking ASA. Inform that therapy may make oral contraceptives less effective, and to use a different or additional form of contraception. Advise to notify physician if breakthrough bleeding or pregnancy occurs while on therapy. Instruct to avoid alcohol while on medication and for 1 day after d/c. Counsel to avoid exposure to sun/sun lamps. Inform that harmless and temporary darkening of tongue and/or black stool may occur.

Administration: Oral route. **Storage**: 20-25°C (68-77°F).

HEPARIN SODIUM   RX
heparin sodium (Various)

OTHER BRAND NAMES: Heparin Sodium in Dextrose 5% (Various)

THERAPEUTIC CLASS: Glycosaminoglycan

INDICATIONS: Prophylaxis and treatment of venous/arterial thrombosis and its extension, pulmonary embolism (PE) and peripheral arterial embolism; atrial fibrillation with embolization. Diagnosis and treatment of acute and chronic consumptive coagulopathies/disseminated intravascular coagulation (DIC). Prevention of clotting in arterial and cardiac surgery. (Heparin Sodium Inj) Prevention of postoperative deep vein thrombosis and PE with major abdominothoracic surgery or at risk of developing thromboembolic disease. May be used as anticoagulant in blood transfusion, extracorporeal circulation, dialysis procedures, and in blood samples for laboratory purposes.

DOSAGE: *Adults:* Adjust dose according to coagulation test results. See PI for details in specific disease states. Based on 150 lb/68kg: (Heparin Sodium Inj) Deep SQ Inj: Initial: 5000 U IV, then

10,000-20,000 U SQ. Maint: 8000-10,000 U q8h or 15,000-20,000 U q12h. Intermittent IV Injection: Initial: 10,000 U IV. Maint: 5000-10,000 U q4-6h. Continuous IV Infusion: Initial: 5000 U IV. Maint: 20,000-40,000 U/24 hrs. (Heparin Sodium in Dextrose 5%) Initial: 5000 U IV, then 20,000-40,000 U q24hr IV.
Pediatrics: Initial: 50 U/kg IV. Maint: 100 U/kg IV q4h or 20,000 U/m^2/24 hrs continuously.

HOW SUPPLIED: Inj: (Heparin Sodium Inj) (preservative-free) 1000 U/mL, 5000 U/0.5mL; (with benzyl alcohol) 5000 U/mL; (with parabens) 1000 U/mL [1mL, 10mL, 30mL], 5000 U/mL, 10,000 U/mL [1mL, 5mL], 20,000 U/mL. (Heparin Sodium in Dextrose 5%) 20,000 U [500mL], 25,000 U [250mL, 500mL].

CONTRAINDICATIONS: Severe thrombocytopenia, if blood coagulation tests cannot be performed at appropriate intervals (with full-dose heparin), uncontrollable active bleeding state (except in DIC). (Heparin Sodium in Dextrose 5%) Allergy to corn or corn products.

WARNINGS/PRECAUTIONS: Hemorrhage can occur at any site; extreme caution in disease states with increased danger of hemorrhage (eg, severe HTN, subacute bacterial endocarditis, surgery, increased bleeding tendencies, ulcerative lesions and continuous tube drainage of the stomach or small intestine, menstruation, liver disease with impaired hemostasis). Thrombocytopenia, heparin-induced thrombocytopenia and thrombosis (HIT/HITT), and hyperaminotransferasemia reported. D/C if platelet count <100,000/mm^3, recurrent thrombosis develops, coagulation tests unduly prolonged, or hemorrhage occurs. Increased heparin resistance with fever, thrombosis, thrombophlebitis, infections with thrombosing tendencies, myocardial infarction, cancer, and postop patients. Higher bleeding incidence in women >60 yrs. Not recommended for IM use. Do not use as a catheter lock flush product. Fatal hemorrhage reported in pediatrics due to medication errors (eg, confused with "catheter lock flush" vials). (Heparin Sodium in Dextrose 5%) Without electrolytes, do not administer simultaneously with blood through same administration set; agglomeration may occur. Sulfite sensitivity may occur; caution especially in asthmatics. Caution with diabetes mellitus (DM).

ADVERSE REACTIONS: Thrombocytopenia, hemorrhage, local irritation, erythema, mild pain, hematoma, chills, fever, urticaria, asthma, lacrimation, N/V, anaphylactoid reactions, HIT/HITT.

INTERACTIONS: May prolong PT when taken with dicumarol or warfarin; wait at least 5 hrs after last IV dose or 24 hrs after last SQ dose, and if a valid PT is to be obtained. Platelet inhibitors (eg, aspirin [ASA], dextran, phenylbutazone, ibuprofen, indomethacin, dipyridamole, hydroxychloroquine, other drugs that interfere with platelet-aggregation reactions) may induce bleeding; use with caution. Digitalis, tetracyclines, nicotine, or antihistamines may partially counteract anticoagulant action. Decreased PTT with IV nitroglycerin; monitor PTT and adjust heparin dose with concurrent use.

PREGNANCY: Category C, (preservative-free) safe in nursing; (preserved with benzyl alcohol) not for use in nursing.

MECHANISM OF ACTION: Glycosaminoglycan; inhibits reactions that lead to blood clotting and the formation of fibrin clots. Acts at multiple sites in the normal coagulation system.

PHARMACOKINETICS: Absorption: (SQ) T$_{max}$=2-4 hrs. **Metabolism:** Liver and reticuloendothelial system. **Elimination:** T$_{1/2}$=10 min.

NURSING CONSIDERATIONS

Assessment: Assess for severe thrombocytopenia, pregnancy status, and possible drug interactions. Assess use in disease states at risk for hemorrhage and use in older patients (>60 yrs). Assess that suitable coagulation tests (eg, whole blood clotting time, PTT) can be performed at appropriate intervals in patients on full-dose heparin. Assess for thrombocytopenia, HIT, and HITT. Obtain baseline CBC, including platelet counts. (Heparin Sodium in Dextrose 5%) Assess for corn and sulfite hypersensitivity, and DM.

Monitoring: Monitor for signs/symptoms of hemorrhage, thrombocytopenia, heparin resistance, hypersensitivity reactions, and hyperaminotransferasemia. Perform periodic monitoring of platelet counts, Hct, and tests for occult blood in stool during entire therapy course, and frequent coagulation tests if given therapeutically. If given by continuous IV infusion, monitor coagulation time every 4 hrs in early stages of treatment. If given intermittently by IV inj, monitor coagulation tests before each inj during the initial phase of treatment and then at appropriate intervals thereafter.

Patient Counseling: Counsel about increased risk of bleeding tendencies while on medication. Instruct to notify physician if any type of unusual bleeding or hypersensitivity reaction occurs. Advise that periodic lab monitoring is required during treatment.

Administration: (Heparin Sodium Inj) IV/SQ routes. (Heparin Sodium in Dextrose 5%) IV route. **Storage:** (Heparin Sodium Inj) 20-25°C (68-77°F). (Heparin Sodium in Dextrose 5%) 25°C; brief exposure up to 40°C does not adversely affect product. Avoid excessive heat.

HEPSERA RX
adefovir dipivoxil (Gilead Sciences)

Lactic acidosis and severe hepatomegaly with steatosis, including fatal cases, reported with the use of nucleoside analogues. Severe acute exacerbations of hepatitis reported upon d/c of therapy; closely monitor hepatic function for at least several months. If appropriate, resumption of anti-hepatitis B therapy may be warranted. Chronic use may result in nephrotoxicity in patients at risk of or having underlying renal dysfunction; monitor renal function and adjust dose if required. HIV resistance may occur in patients with unrecognized or untreated HIV infection.

THERAPEUTIC CLASS: Nucleotide analogue reverse transcriptase inhibitor

INDICATIONS: Treatment of chronic hepatitis B in patients ≥12 yrs with evidence of active viral replication and either evidence of persistent elevations in serum aminotransferases (ALT/AST) or histologically active disease.

DOSAGE: *Adults:* 10mg qd. Renal Impairment: CrCl 30-49mL/min: 10mg q48h. CrCl 10-29mL/min: 10mg q72h. Hemodialysis Patients: 10mg q7 days following dialysis. *Pediatrics:* ≥12 yrs: 10mg qd.

HOW SUPPLIED: Tab: 10mg

WARNINGS/PRECAUTIONS: Caution in adolescents with underlying renal dysfunction; monitor renal function closely. In HBV-infected patients, offer HIV-1 antibody testing before initiating therapy. Obesity and prolonged nucleoside exposure may be risk factors for lactic acidosis and severe hepatomegaly with steatosis. Caution with known risk factors for liver disease; d/c if lactic acidosis or pronounced hepatotoxicity develop. Resistance to the drug can result in viral load rebound which may result in exacerbation of hepatitis B, leading to liver decompensation and possible fatal outcome. To reduce risk of resistance in patients with lamivudine-resistant hepatitis B virus (HBV), use adefovir dipivoxil in combination with lamivudine and not as monotherapy. To reduce risk of resistance in patients receiving monotherapy, consider modification of treatment if serum HBV DNA remains above >1000 copies/mL with continued treatment. Caution in elderly.

ADVERSE REACTIONS: Nephrotoxicity, lactic acidosis, severe hepatomegaly with steatosis, asthenia, headache, abdominal pain, nausea, flatulence, diarrhea, dyspepsia.

INTERACTIONS: Avoid with tenofovir disoproxil fumarate (TDF) or TDF-containing products. Drugs that reduce renal function or compete for active tubular secretion may increase levels of either adefovir and/or the coadministered drugs. Caution with nephrotoxic agents (eg, cyclosporine, tacrolimus, aminoglycosides, vancomycin, and NSAIDs).

PREGNANCY: Category C, not for use in nursing.

MECHANISM OF ACTION: Nucleotide analogue reverse transcriptase inhibitor; inhibits HBV DNA polymerase (reverse transcriptase) by competing with natural substrate deoxyadenosine triphosphate and by causing DNA chain termination after incorporation into viral DNA.

PHARMACOKINETICS: Absorption: Bioavailability (59%); C_{max}=18.4ng/mL; T_{max}=1.75 hrs; AUC=220ng•h/mL. Refer to PI for pharmacokinetic parameters in pediatrics and in patients with varying degrees of renal function. **Distribution:** V_d=392mL/kg (IV, 1mg/kg/day), 352mL/kg (IV, 3mg/kg/day); plasma protein binding (≤4%). **Elimination:** Urine (45%); $T_{1/2}$=7.48 hrs.

NURSING CONSIDERATIONS

Assessment: Assess for renal dysfunction, risk factors for lactic acidosis and liver disease, hypersensitivity, pregnancy/nursing status, and possible drug interactions. Perform HIV antibody testing and assess CrCl.

Monitoring: Monitor for signs/symptoms of lactic acidosis, hepatotoxicity, nephrotoxicity, clinical resistance, and other adverse reactions. Monitor renal function and (after d/c) hepatic function.

Patient Counseling: Inform of risks, benefits, and alternative modes of therapy. Instruct to follow a regular dosing schedule to avoid missing doses. Advise to immediately report any severe abdominal pain, muscle pain, yellowing of eyes, dark urine, pale stools, and/or loss of appetite. Instruct to notify physician if any unusual/known symptom develops, persists, or worsens. Advise not to d/c therapy without first informing physician. Advise that routine laboratory monitoring and follow-up is important during therapy. Inform of importance of obtaining HIV antibody testing prior to starting therapy. Counsel women of childbearing age about risks of drug exposure during pregnancy, and to notify physician if the patient becomes pregnant while on therapy. Inform pregnant patients about the pregnancy registry.

Administration: Oral route. **Storage:** 25°C (77°F); excursions permitted to 15-30°C (59-86°F).

HERCEPTIN   RX
trastuzumab (Genentech)

May result in cardiac failure; incidence and severity highest with anthracycline-containing chemotherapy regimens. Evaluate left ventricular function prior to and during treatment; d/c in patients receiving adjuvant therapy and withhold in patients with metastatic disease for clinically significant decrease in left ventricular function. May result in serious and fatal infusion reactions and pulmonary toxicity; interrupt infusion for dyspnea or clinically significant hypotension, and monitor until symptoms completely resolve. D/C for anaphylaxis, angioedema, interstitial pneumonitis, or acute respiratory distress syndrome. Exposure during pregnancy may result in oligohydramnios and oligohydramnios sequence manifesting as pulmonary hypoplasia, skeletal abnormalities, and neonatal death.

THERAPEUTIC CLASS: Monoclonal antibody/HER2-blocker

INDICATIONS: Adjuvant treatment of HER2-overexpressing node-positive or node-negative breast cancer as part of a treatment regimen consisting of doxorubicin, cyclophosphamide, and either paclitaxel or docetaxel, with docetaxel and carboplatin, or as single agent following multimodality anthracycline-based therapy. In combination with paclitaxel for 1st-line treatment of HER2-overexpressing metastatic breast cancer, or as single agent for treatment of HER2-overexpressing breast cancer in patients who have received ≥1 chemotherapy regimens for metastatic disease. In combination with cisplatin and capecitabine or 5-fluorouracil for treatment of patients with HER2-overexpressing metastatic gastric or gastroesophageal junction adenocarcinoma who have not received prior treatment for metastatic disease.

DOSAGE: *Adults:* Breast Cancer Adjuvant Treatment: Administer for 52 weeks. During and Following Paclitaxel, Docetaxel, or Docetaxel/Carboplatin: Initial: 4mg/kg IV infusion over 90 min, then at 2mg/kg IV infusion over 30 min weekly during chemotherapy for the first 12 weeks (paclitaxel or docetaxel) or 18 weeks (docetaxel/carboplatin). One week following the last weekly dose, give 6mg/kg IV infusion over 30-90 min q3 weeks. As Single Agent within 3 Weeks Following Completion of Multimodality Anthracycline-Based Chemotherapy Regimens: Initial: 8mg/kg IV infusion over 90 min. Maint: 6mg/kg IV infusion over 30-90 min q3 weeks. Breast Cancer Metastatic Treatment: Initial: 4mg/kg as 90-min IV infusion. Maint: 2mg/kg once weekly as 30-min IV infusion until disease progression. Metastatic Gastric Cancer: Initial: 8mg/kg as 90-min IV infusion. Maint: 6mg/kg IV infusion over 30-90 min q3 weeks until disease progression. Refer to PI for dose modifications.

HOW SUPPLIED: Inj: 440mg

WARNINGS/PRECAUTIONS: Monitor left ventricular ejection fraction (LVEF) prior to initiation, q3 months during and upon completion of therapy, and q6 months for ≥2 yrs following completion as a component of adjuvant therapy. Repeat LVEF measurement at 4 week intervals if therapy withheld for significant left ventricular cardiac dysfunction. Patients with symptomatic intrinsic lung disease or extensive tumor involvement of the lungs, resulting in dyspnea at rest, may have more severe pulmonary toxicity. Use FDA-approved tests for the specific tumor type to assess HER2 protein overexpression and HER2 gene amplification.

ADVERSE REACTIONS: Cardiac failure, infusion reactions, pulmonary toxicity, fever, N/V, headache, nasopharyngitis, diarrhea, infections, fatigue, anemia, neutropenia, rash, weight loss.

INTERACTIONS: See Boxed Warning. Higher incidence of neutropenia with myelosuppressive chemotherapy. Paclitaxel may increase trough concentrations.

PREGNANCY: Category D, not for use in nursing.

MECHANISM OF ACTION: Monoclonal antibody (IgG1 kappa)/HER2 blocker; inhibits proliferation of human tumor cells that overexpress HER2.

PHARMACOKINETICS: Absorption: C_{max}=377mcg/mL (500mg), 123mcg/mL (4mg/kg initial, then 2mg/kg weekly), 216mcg/mL (8mg/kg initial, then 6mg/kg q3 weeks). **Distribution:** V_d=44mL/kg. **Elimination:** $T_{1/2}$=2 days (10mg), 12 days (500mg), 6 days (4mg/kg initial, then 2mg/kg weekly), 16 days (8mg/kg initial, then 6mg/kg q3 weeks).

NURSING CONSIDERATIONS

Assessment: Assess cardiac function, including history, physical exam, and baseline LVEF. Assess HER2 protein overexpression and HER2 gene amplification. Assess for symptomatic intrinsic lung disease or extensive tumor involvement of lungs, pregnancy/nursing status, and for possible drug interactions.

Monitoring: Monitor for infusion reactions, pulmonary toxicity, neutropenia, and other adverse reactions. Monitor LVEF q3 months during and upon completion of therapy, and q6 months for ≥2 yrs following completion as a component of adjuvant therapy.

Patient Counseling: Advise to contact physician immediately for new onset or worsening SOB, cough, swelling of ankles/legs or face, palpitations, weight gain of >5 lbs in 24 hrs, dizziness, or loss of consciousness. Inform that drug may cause fetal harm. Advise women of childbearing potential to use effective contraceptive methods during and ≥6 months following therapy. Instruct not to breastfeed during treatment.

Administration: IV route. Do not administer as IV push or bolus. Do not mix with other drugs. Refer to PI for preparation and administration instructions. **Storage:** 2-8°C (34-46°F). Reconstituted with Bacteriostatic Water for Inj: 2-8°C (34-46°F) for 28 days. Reconstituted with Unpreserved Sterile Water for Inj: Use immediately. Diluted in Polyvinylchloride or Polyethylene Bags containing 0.9% Sodium Chloride Inj: 2-8°C (34-46°F) for ≤24 hrs prior to use. Do not freeze following reconstitution/dilution.

HIBERIX   RX
haemophilus B conjugate - tetanus toxoid (GlaxoSmithKline)

THERAPEUTIC CLASS: Vaccine

INDICATIONS: Active immunization as a booster dose for the prevention of invasive disease caused by *Haemophilus influenza* type b in children 15 months-4 yrs (prior to 5th birthday).

DOSAGE: *Pediatrics:* 15 months-4 yrs: Single dose (0.5mL) IM into the anterolateral aspect of the thigh or deltoid.

HOW SUPPLIED: Inj: 0.5mL

WARNINGS/PRECAUTIONS: Use as a booster dose in children who have received a primary series with a *Haemophilus* b Conjugate Vaccine. Evaluate potential benefits and risks if Guillain-Barre syndrome occurs within 6 weeks of receipt of a prior tetanus toxoid-containing vaccine. Tip caps of prefilled syringe may contain natural rubber latex; allergic reactions may occur in latex-sensitive individuals. Syncope may occur and can be accompanied by transient neurological signs. Review immunization history for possible vaccine hypersensitivity; appropriate treatment should be available for possible anaphylactic reactions. Expected immune response may not be obtained in immunosuppressed children. Urine antigen detection may not have a diagnostic value within 1-2 weeks after receipt of vaccine. Not a substitute for routine tetanus immunization.

ADVERSE REACTIONS: Fever, fussiness, loss of appetite, restlessness, sleepiness, diarrhea, vomiting, inj-site reactions (eg, redness, pain, swelling).

INTERACTIONS: Immunosuppressive therapies, including irradiation, antimetabolites, alkylating agents, cytotoxic drugs, and corticosteroids (used in greater than physiologic doses) may reduce immune response to vaccine.

PREGNANCY: Category C, safety not known in nursing.

MECHANISM OF ACTION: Vaccine; protects against invasive disease due to *H. influenzae* type b.

NURSING CONSIDERATIONS

Assessment: Review immunization history, current health/medical status (eg, immunosuppression), and known allergic reaction to previous dose of any *H. influenzae* type b vaccination or tetanus toxoid-containing vaccine. Assess for latex hypersensitivity and possible drug interactions.

Monitoring: Monitor for allergic reactions, signs/symptoms of Guillian-Barre syndrome, inj-site reactions (eg, pain, redness, swelling), syncope, and for any other possible adverse events. Monitor immune response.

Patient Counseling: Inform patient's parents/guardians about benefits/risks of immunization. Counsel about the potential for adverse reactions; instruct to notify physician if any adverse reactions occur.

Administration: IM route. Do not administer SQ, intradermally, or IV. Do not mix with any other vaccine in the same syringe or vial. Refer to PI for reconstitution instructions. **Storage:** 2-8°C (36-46°F). Protect from light. Diluent: 2-8°C (36-46°F) or at 20-25°C (68-77°F). Do not freeze. After Reconstitution: 2-8°C (36-46°F). Do not freeze. Discard if not used within 24 hrs or if has been frozen.

HIZENTRA   RX
immune globulin subcutaneous (human) (CSL Behring)

THERAPEUTIC CLASS: Immunoglobulin

INDICATIONS: Replacement therapy for primary humoral immunodeficiency (eg, humoral immune defect in congenital agammaglobulinemia, common variable immunodeficiency, X-linked agammaglobulinemia, Wiskott-Aldrich syndrome, and severe combined immunodeficiencies) in adults and pediatric patients ≥2 yrs of age.

DOSAGE: *Adults:* SQ: Individualize dose based on clinical response and IgG trough levels. Before receiving treatment, patients need to have received Immune Globulin Intravenous (Human) (IGIV) treatment at regular intervals for at least 3 months; start treatment 1 week after last IGIV infusion. Initial: Weekly dose may be calculated by dividing the previous IGIV dose in grams by the number of weeks between IGIV doses; then multiply this by the dose adjustment factor of 1.53. Multiply the calculated dose by 5 to convert to mL. For the 1st infusion, do not exceed volume of 15mL/site. Volume may be increased to 20mL/site after the fourth infusion to a max volume of 25mL/site as tolerated. For the first infusion, the max recommended flow rate is 15mL/hr/site. For subsequent infusions, the flow rate may be increased to a max of 25mL/hr/site as tolerated. Max Flow Rate: 50mL/hr for all sites combined at any time. Measure serum IgG trough level after 2 to 3 months of treatment. Refer to PI for dose adjustment information. Risk of Measles Exposure: Minimum: 200mg/kg/week for 2 consecutive weeks. If exposed to measles, give dose as soon as possible after exposure.

Pediatrics: ≥2 yrs: SQ: Individualize dose based on clinical response and IgG trough levels. Before receiving treatment, patients need to have received IGIV treatment at regular intervals for at least 3 months; start treatment 1 week after last IGIV infusion. Initial: Weekly dose may be calculated by dividing the previous IGIV dose in grams by the number of weeks between IGIV doses; then multiply this by the dose adjustment factor of 1.53. Multiply the calculated dose by 5 to convert to mL. For the 1st infusion, do not exceed volume of 15mL/site. Volume may be increased to 20mL/site after the fourth infusion to a max volume of 25mL/site as tolerated. For the first infusion, the max recommended flow rate is 15mL/hr/site. For subsequent infusions, the flow rate may be increased to a max of 25mL/hr/site as tolerated. Max Flow Rate: 50mL/hr for all sites combined at any time. Measure serum IgG trough level after 2 to 3 months of treatment. Refer to PI for dose adjustment information. Risk of Measles Exposure: Minimum: 200mg/kg/week for 2 consecutive weeks. If exposed to measles, give dose as soon as possible after exposure.

HOW SUPPLIED: Inj: 1g/5mL, 2g/10mL, 4g/20mL

CONTRAINDICATIONS: Hyperprolinemia; IgA-deficient patients with antibodies against IgA and a history of hypersensitivity.

WARNINGS/PRECAUTIONS: May cause severe hypersensitivity reactions; patients with known antibodies to IgA may have a greater risk. D/C immediately if hypersensitivity reaction occurs. Thrombotic events may occur; caution with those at increased risk; administer minimum rate practicable if at risk of developing thrombotic event. May cause aseptic meningitis syndrome (AMS); rule out other causes of meningitis. Renal dysfunction/failure, osmotic nephropathy and death may occur. Patient should not be volume-depleted prior to initiation. Monitor renal function and urine output in high-risk patients; administer at the minimum practicable rate; may d/c if renal function deteriorates. Can contain blood group antibodies that may cause hemolysis and a positive Coombs' test. Noncardiogenic pulmonary edema may occur; if transfusion-related acute lung injury (TRALI) is suspected, test for presence of anti-neutrophil antibodies in both product and patient's serum. May carry risk of transmitting infectious agents (eg, viruses, Creutzfeldt-Jakob disease agent). Various passively transferred antibodies in Ig preparations may lead to misinterpretation of results of serological testing.

ADVERSE REACTIONS: Local reactions (eg, swelling, redness, heat, pain, and itching at injection site), headache, diarrhea, back pain, N/V, pain in extremity, fatigue, cough, rash

INTERACTIONS: Caution with nephrotoxic drugs; may increase risk of renal dysfunction/failure. May interfere with response to live viral vaccines (eg, measles, mumps, rubella). Caution with estrogen-containing products; may increase risk of thrombosis.

PREGNANCY: Category C, safety not known in nursing.

MECHANISM OF ACTION: Immune globulin (human); not fully established. Supplies broad spectrum of opsonizing and neutralizing IgG antibodies against a wide variety of bacterial and viral agents.

PHARMACOKINETICS: Absorption: C_{max}=1616mg/dL; AUC=10560 day•mg/dL; T_{max}=2.9 days.

NURSING CONSIDERATIONS

Assessment: Assess for history of anaphylactic or severe systemic reaction to human immune globulin, hyperprolinemia, IgA deficiency with antibodies to IgA, history of atherosclerosis, multiple CV risk factors, impaired cardiac output, hypercoagulable disorder, prolonged immobilization, known or suspected hyperviscosity, renal impairment, pregnancy/nursing status, and for possible drug interactions. Assess risk for acute renal failure (eg, preexisting renal insufficiency, DM, hypovolemia, overweight, or using concomitant nephrotoxic products). Obtain baseline BUN and SrCr levels.

Monitoring: Monitor for signs and symptoms of hypersensitivity/anaphylactic reactions, thrombotic events, renal dysfunction, AMS, hemolysis, and for infections. Monitor for pulmonary adverse reactions; if TRALI suspected, test for presence of anti-neutrophil antibodies.

Patient Counseling: Instruct patients on self administration, if appropriate. Inform that therapy may contain infectious agents and interfere with the response to live viral vaccines. Advise to report immediately to physician any signs/symptoms of renal dysfunction (eg, decreased urine output, sudden weight gain, fluid retention/edema), TRALI (eg, severe breathing problems), thrombotic/embolic events (eg, SOB, mental status changes), AMS (eg, fever, drowsiness, neck stiffness, painful eye movements), hemolysis (eg, increased HR, yellowing of skin or eyes), and if local reaction lasts more than a few days.

Administration: SQ route. Do not inject into a blood vessel. Do not mix with other products. May infuse into multiple injection sites (≤4). Inj sites should be ≥2 inches apart. Refer to PI for further preparation and administration instructions. **Storage:** Up to 25°C (77°F). Do not freeze and shake. Do not use if frozen. Keep in original carton to protect from light.

HORIZANT
gabapentin enacarbil (GlaxoSmithKline)

RX

THERAPEUTIC CLASS: GABA analog

INDICATIONS: Treatment of moderate to severe primary restless legs syndrome in adults.

DOSAGE: *Adults:* 600mg qd with food at about 5 pm. Renal Impairment: CrCl ≥60mL/min: 600mg/day. CrCl 30-59mL/min: Initial: 300mg/day. Titrate: Increase to 600mg PRN. CrCl 15-29mL/min: 300mg/day. CrCl <15mL/min: 300mg qod.

HOW SUPPLIED: Tab, Extended Release: 300mg, 600mg

WARNINGS/PRECAUTIONS: Not recommended in patients with CrCl <15mL/min on hemodialysis or who are required to sleep during the day and remain awake at night. Drug causes significant driving impairment, somnolence, sedation, and dizziness. Not interchangeable with other gabapentin products. Increases the risk of suicidal thoughts or behavior; monitor for the emergence or worsening of depression, suicidal thoughts/behavior, and/or any unusual changes in mood or behavior. Drug reaction with eosinophilia and systemic symptoms (DRESS)/multiorgan hypersensitivity reported; evaluate immediately if signs/symptoms (eg, hypersensitivity, fever, lymphadenopathy) are present and d/c if alternative etiology cannot be established. If recommended daily dose is exceeded, reduce dose to 600mg daily for 1 week prior to d/c to minimize potential for withdrawal seizure. May have tumorigenic potential. Caution in elderly and with renal impairment.

ADVERSE REACTIONS: Somnolence, sedation, dizziness, headache, nausea, dry mouth, flatulence, fatigue, irritability, feeling drunk/abnormal, peripheral edema, weight increase, vertigo, depression.

INTERACTIONS: Cimetidine may increase exposure and decrease renal clearance.

PREGNANCY: Category C, not for use in nursing.

MECHANISM OF ACTION: Gamma-aminobutiric acid analog; not established. Prodrug of gabapentin; binds with high affinity to the α2delta subunit of voltage-activated calcium channels.

PHARMACOKINETICS: Absorption: Bioavailability (75% [fed], 42-65% [fasted]); T_{max}=5 hrs (fasted), 7.3 hrs (fed). **Distribution:** Plasma protein binding (<3%); V_d=76L. **Metabolism:** Extensive 1st-pass hydrolysis to gabapentin (active form). **Elimination:** Kidney (unchanged); urine (94%), feces (5%); $T_{1/2}$=5.1-6 hrs.

NURSING CONSIDERATIONS

Assessment: Assess for renal function (CrCl), preexisting tumors, depression, pregnancy/nursing status, and possible drug interactions. Assess if patient is on hemodialysis or required to sleep during the day and remain awake at night.

Monitoring: Monitor for withdrawal seizures with treatment d/c, somnolence, sedation, dizziness, emergence or worsening of depression, suicidal thoughts/behavior, and/or any unusual changes in mood/behavior, DRESS, development or worsening of tumors, renal function, and hypersensitivity reactions.

Patient Counseling: Instruct patients to read the Medication Guide before starting therapy and to reread it upon prescription renewal. Inform that the therapy can cause significant driving impairment, somnolence, and dizziness; advise not to drive or operate dangerous machinery. Counsel that treatment may increase the risk of suicidal thoughts and behavior; advise to report to physician any behaviors of concern. Advise that multiorgan hypersensitivity reactions/DRESS may occur; instruct to contact their physician if they experience any signs or symptoms of these conditions. Advise that product is not interchangeable with other gabapentin products. Instruct to take only as prescribed and to take with food at about 5 pm. If the dose is missed, instruct to take the next dose at about 5 pm the following day. Advise to swallow tab whole and not to cut, crush, or chew.

Administration: Oral route. **Storage:** 25°C (77°F); excursions permitted to 15-30°C (59-86°F). Protect from moisture.

HUMALOG
insulin lispro, rdna origin (Lilly)

RX

THERAPEUTIC CLASS: Insulin

INDICATIONS: To improve glycemic control in adults and children with diabetes mellitus.

DOSAGE: *Adults:* Individualize dose. Usual Requirement: 0.5-1 unit/kg/day. Give within 15 min ac or immediately pc. Continuous SQ Insulin Infusion (CSII) by External Pump: Initial: Based on the total daily insulin dose of the previous regimen. Usual: 50% of total dose given as meal-related boluses and the remainder as basal infusion. Renal/Hepatic Impairment: May need to reduce dose.

Pediatrics: ≥3 yrs: Individualize dose. Usual Requirement: 0.5-1 unit/kg/day. Give within 15 min ac or immediately pc. CSII by External Pump: Initial: Based on the total daily insulin dose of the previous regimen. Usual: 50% of total dose given as meal-related boluses and the remainder as basal infusion. Renal/Hepatic Impairment: May need to reduce dose.

HOW SUPPLIED: Inj: 100 U/mL [10mL, vial]; [3mL, Pen, KwikPen, Cartridge]

CONTRAINDICATIONS: Episodes of hypoglycemia.

WARNINGS/PRECAUTIONS: Any change in insulin regimen should be made cautiously and under medical supervision. Changes in strength, manufacturer, type or method of administration may result in the need for a change in dosage. Stress, major illness, changes in exercise, or meal patterns may alter insulin requirements. Hypoglycemia may occur; caution in patients with hypoglycemia unawareness and patients predisposed to hypoglycemia (eg, pediatrics, patients who fast or have erratic food intake). Hypokalemia may occur; caution in patients who may be at risk. Severe, life-threatening, generalized allergy, including anaphylaxis may occur. Do not mix with insulin preparations other than NPH insulin or with other insulins for use in an external SQ infusion pump. Malfunction of the insulin pump or infusion set or insulin degradation can rapidly lead to hyperglycemia or ketosis; prompt identification and correction of the cause is necessary. Interim SQ injections with the drug may be required if using SQ infusion pump. Train patients using continuous SQ infusion pump therapy to administer by injection; alternate insulin therapy should be available in case of pump failure.

ADVERSE REACTIONS: Hypoglycemia, flu syndrome, pharyngitis, rhinitis, headache, pain, cough increased, infection, nausea, fever, abdominal pain, asthenia, bronchitis, diarrhea, myalgia.

INTERACTIONS: May require dose adjustment and close monitoring with drugs that may increase blood glucose-lowering effect and susceptibility to hypoglycemia (oral antidiabetics, salicylates, sulfonamide antibiotics, MAOIs, fluoxetine, pramlintide, disopyramide, fibrates, propoxyphene, pentoxifylline, ACE inhibitors, angiotensin II receptor blocking agents, and somatostatin analogs [eg, octreotide]), drugs that may reduce blood glucose-lowering effect (corticosteroids, isoniazid, niacin, estrogens, oral contraceptives, phenothiazines, danazol, diuretics, sympathomimetic agents [eg, epinephrine, albuterol, terbutaline], somatropin, atypical antipsychotics, glucagon, protease inhibitors, and thyroid hormones), or drugs that may increase or reduce blood glucose-lowering effect (β-blockers, clonidine, lithium salts, and alcohol). Pentamidine may cause hypoglycemia, sometimes followed by hyperglycemia. Hypoglycemic signs may be reduced or absent with sympatholytics (eg, β-blockers, clonidine, guanethidine, and reserpine). Caution with K^+-lowering drugs or drugs sensitive to serum K^+ levels.

PREGNANCY: Category B, caution in nursing.

MECHANISM OF ACTION: Insulin lispro (rDNA origin); regulates glucose metabolism. Lowers blood glucose by stimulating peripheral glucose uptake, and by inhibiting hepatic glucose production. Inhibits lipolysis and proteolysis, and enhances protein synthesis.

PHARMACOKINETICS: Absorption: (0.1-0.2 U/kg) Absolute bioavailability (55-77%); (0.1-0.4 U/kg) T_{max}=30-90 min. **Distribution:** V_d=0.26-0.36L/kg. **Elimination:** $T_{1/2}$=1 hr.

NURSING CONSIDERATIONS

Assessment: Assess for predisposal to hypoglycemia, risk for hypokalemia, alcohol consumption, exercise routines, hypersensitivity, pregnancy/nursing status, and possible drug interactions. Obtain baseline renal function, LFTs, FPG, and HbA1c.

Monitoring: Monitor for signs and symptoms of hypoglycemia, hypokalemia, lipodystrophy, allergic reactions, and other adverse effects. Monitor FPG, HbA1c, K^+ levels, and renal/hepatic function.

Patient Counseling: Instruct on self-management procedures (eg, glucose monitoring, proper injection technique, management of hypoglycemia/hyperglycemia). Advise on handling of special situations such as intercurrent conditions (eg, illness, stress, emotional disturbance), inadequate or skipped doses, inadvertent administration of an increased dose, inadequate food intake, and skipped meals. Instruct diabetic women to inform physician if pregnant or are contemplating pregnancy. Instruct to always check label before injection to avoid medication errors such as accidental mix-ups. Instruct on how to use external infusion pump.

Administration: SQ route. Inject SQ in the abdominal wall, thigh, upper arm, or buttocks. Refer to PI for preparation, handling, and administration techniques. **Storage:** Refer to PI for storage conditions. Pump: Change the drug in the reservoir at least q7 days, and the infusion sets and the infusion set insertion site at least q3 days or after exposure to >37°C (98.6°F). Discard cartridge used in the D-Tron pumps after 7 days even if still contains the drug. Diluted Humalog: 5°C (41°F) for 28 days and 30°C (86°F) for 14 days. Do not dilute drug contained in a cartridge or drug used in an external insulin pump.

HUMALOG MIX 75/25
insulin lispro protamine - insulin lispro, rdna origin (Lilly)

RX

THERAPEUTIC CLASS: Insulin

INDICATIONS: Treatment of diabetes mellitus (DM) for the control of hyperglycemia.

DOSAGE: *Adults:* Individualize dose. Inject SQ within 15 min ac. Renal/Hepatic Impairment: May need to reduce/adjust dose.

HOW SUPPLIED: Inj: (Insulin Lispro Protamine-Insulin Lispro) 75 U-25 U/mL [10mL, vial]; [3mL, Pen, KwikPen]

CONTRAINDICATIONS: Episodes of hypoglycemia.

WARNINGS/PRECAUTIONS: Any change of insulin should be made cautiously and only under medical supervision. Changes in strength, manufacturer, type, species, or method of manufacture may result in the need for a change in dosage. Hypoglycemia and hypokalemia may occur; caution in patients who are fasting or have autonomic neuropathy. Lipodystrophy and hypersensitivity may occur. May require dose adjustments with change in physical activity or usual meal plan. Stress, illness, or emotional disturbance may alter insulin requirements. Monitor glucose levels and adjust dose with hepatic/renal impairment. Inj-site reactions (eg, redness, swelling, itching), and severe, life-threatening, generalized allergy, including anaphylaxis, may occur. Contains metacresol as excipient; localized reactions and generalized myalgia reported with cresol-containing injectable products. Antibody production reported. Not for IV use.

ADVERSE REACTIONS: Hypoglycemia, hypokalemia, allergic reactions, inj-site reactions, lipodystrophy, pruritus, rash.

INTERACTIONS: May increase insulin requirements with corticosteroids, isoniazid, certain lipid-lowering drugs (eg, niacin), estrogens, oral contraceptives, phenothiazines, thyroid replacement therapy. May decrease insulin requirements with oral antidiabetic drugs, salicylates, sulfa antibiotics, MAOIs, ACE inhibitors, angiotensin II receptor blocking agents, β-blockers, inhibitors of pancreatic function (eg, octreotide), and alcohol. β-blockers may mask symptoms of hypoglycemia. Caution with K$^+$-lowering drugs or drugs sensitive to serum K$^+$ levels.

PREGNANCY: Category B, caution in nursing.

MECHANISM OF ACTION: Insulin; regulates glucose metabolism.

PHARMACOKINETICS: Absorption: (0.3 U/kg) T$_{max}$=30-240 min. **Distribution:** V$_d$=0.26-0.36L/kg (insulin lispro).

NURSING CONSIDERATIONS

Assessment: Assess for predisposal to hypoglycemia, risk of hypokalemia, alcohol consumption, exercise routines, hypersensitivity, pregnancy/nursing status, and possible drug interactions. Obtain baseline renal function, LFTs, FPG, and HbA1c.

Monitoring: Monitor for signs and symptoms of hypoglycemia, hypokalemia, lipodystrophy, allergic reactions, antibody production, and other adverse effects. Monitor FPG, HbA1c, K$^+$ levels, and renal/hepatic function.

Patient Counseling: Inform about potential risks and benefits of drug and alternative therapies. Instruct not to mix drug with any other insulin. Inform of the importance of proper insulin storage, inj techniques, timing of dosage, adherence to meal planning, regular physical activity, regular blood glucose monitoring, periodic HbA1c testing, recognition and management of hypo/hyperglycemia, and periodic assessment for DM complications. Instruct to inform physician if pregnant or intend to become pregnant. Instruct how to use the delivery device. Instruct not to share the medication with others.

Administration: SQ route. **Storage:** Unopened: <30°C (86°F) for 28 days (vial) or 10 days (Pen, KwikPen), or at 2-8°C (36-46°F). Do not use if frozen. Opened: <30°C (86°F) for 28 days (vial) or 10 days (Pen, KwikPen). Do not refrigerate Pen/KwikPen. Protect from direct heat and light.

HUMATROPE
somatropin rdna origin (Lilly)

RX

THERAPEUTIC CLASS: Human growth hormone

INDICATIONS: Treatment of pediatrics with growth failure due to inadequate secretion of endogenous growth hormone (GH), short stature associated with Turner syndrome (TS), idiopathic short stature (ISS), short stature or growth failure with short stature homeobox-containing gene (SHOX) deficiency, and for growth failure in children born small for gestational age (SGA) who fail to demonstrate catch-up growth by 2-4 yrs. Replacement of endogenous GH in adults with adult-onset or childhood-onset growth hormone deficiency (GHD).

DOSAGE: *Adults:* GHD: Non-Weight-Based: Initial: 0.2mg/day SQ (range, 0.15-0.30mg/day). Titrate: Increase gradually q1-2 months by 0.1-0.2mg/day based on response and insulin-like growth factor-I (IGF-I) concentrations. Weight-Based: Initial: ≤0.006mg/kg/day (6mcg/kg/day) SQ. Titrate: Increase based on individual requirement. Max: 0.0125mg/kg/day (12.5mcg/kg/day). Elderly: Lower starting dose and smaller dose increments. Estrogen-replete women may need higher doses than men.
Pediatrics: Individualize dose. GHD: 0.026-0.043mg/kg/day SQ (0.18-0.30mg/kg/week). TS: ≤0.054mg/kg/day SQ (0.375mg/kg/week). ISS: ≤0.053mg/kg/day SQ (0.37mg/kg/week). SHOX Deficiency: 0.050mg/kg/day SQ (0.35mg/kg/week). SGA: ≤0.067mg/kg/day SQ (0.47mg/kg/week). Refer to PI for further details.

HOW SUPPLIED: Inj: 5mg [vial]; 6mg, 12mg, 24mg [cartridge]

CONTRAINDICATIONS: Pediatrics with closed epiphyses. Active proliferative or severe non-proliferative diabetic retinopathy. Active malignancy. Acute critical illness due to complications following open heart or abdominal surgery, multiple accidental trauma, or acute respiratory failure. Prader-Willi syndrome with severe obesity, with history of upper airway obstruction or sleep apnea, or with severe respiratory impairment.

WARNINGS/PRECAUTIONS: Avoid use of cartridge if allergic to metacresol or glycerin. Examine for progression/recurrence of underlying disease in those with preexisting tumors or GHD secondary to intracranial lesion. Monitor for malignant transformation of skin lesions. May unmask undiagnosed impaired glucose tolerance and overt diabetes mellitus (DM); monitor glucose levels. New onset type 2 DM reported. Intracranial HTN with papilledema, visual changes, headache, N/V reported; perform funduscopic exam before initiation and during therapy; d/c if papilledema occurs. Monitor other hormonal replacement treatments in patients with hypopituitarism. Undiagnosed/untreated hypothyroidism may prevent optimal response. Hypothyroidism may worsen or develop; perform periodic thyroid function tests. Slipped capital femoral epiphysis, fluid retention, or systemic allergic reactions may occur. Progression of scoliosis may occur in pediatrics with rapid growth. Increased risk of ear/hearing disorders and cardiovascular (CV) disorders in patients with TS. Pancreatitis reported (rare). Tissue atrophy may occur when administered at the same site over a long period of time. Serum levels of inorganic phosphorus, alkaline phosphatase, parathyroid hormone and IGF-I may increase after therapy. Caution in the elderly.

ADVERSE REACTIONS: Ear disorder, arthrosis, pain, edema, arthralgia, myalgia, HTN, paraesthesias, glucose intolerance, scoliosis, otitis media, hyperlipidemia, rhinitis, flu syndrome, headache.

INTERACTIONS: Use with glucocorticoid therapy may attenuate growth-promoting effects in children; carefully adjust glucocorticoid replacement dosing in children. May inhibit 11β-hydroxysteroid dehydrogenase type 1 (11βHSD-1), resulting in reduced serum cortisol concentrations; may need glucocorticoid replacement or dose adjustments in glucocorticoid therapy. May increase clearance of antipyrine. May alter clearance of compounds metabolized by CYP450 liver enzymes (eg, corticosteroids, sex steroids, anticonvulsants, cyclosporine). May require larger dose with oral estrogen replacement. May need to adjust dose of insulin and/or oral hypoglycemic agents in diabetic patients and hormone replacement therapy in patients with thyroid dysfunction.

PREGNANCY: Category C, caution in nursing.

MECHANISM OF ACTION: Human growth hormone; binds to dimeric GH receptors located within the cell membranes of target tissue cells, resulting in intracellular signal transduction and subsequent induction of transcription and translation of GH-dependent proteins, including IGF-1, IGF BP-3, and acid labile subunit.

PHARMACOKINETICS: Absorption: Absolute bioavailabilty (75%); C_{max}=63.3ng/mL; AUC=585ng•hr/mL. **Distribution:** V_d=0.957L/kg. **Metabolism:** Liver and kidney (protein catabolism). **Elimination:** Urine. $T_{1/2}$=3.81 hrs.

NURSING CONSIDERATIONS

Assessment: Assess for causes of poor growth, hypersensitivity to either metacresol or glycerin, pregnancy/nursing status, possible drug interactions, or any other conditions where treatment is contraindicated or cautioned. Perform funduscopic exam. In patients with TS, assess for otitis media, other ear disorders, and CV disorders.

Monitoring: Monitor for growth, clinical response, compliance, malignant transformation of skin lesions, symptoms of slipped capital femoral epiphysis, progression of preexisting scoliosis in pediatric patients, pancreatitis, fluid retention, and allergic reactions. Monitor patients with hypopituitarism who are on other hormone replacement therapy. Perform periodic thyroid function test and funduscopic exam. In patients with TS, monitor for signs or symptoms of ear disorders (eg, otitis media) and CV disorders. In patients with preexisting tumors or GH deficiency secondary to an intracranial lesion, monitor for progression or recurrence of underlying disease process.

Patient Counseling: Inform of the potential benefits and risks of therapy, proper administration, usage and disposal, and caution against any reuse of needles and syringes. Instruct to dispose used needles and syringes in a puncture-resistant container.

Administration: SQ route. Refer to PI for reconstitution, administration, and preparation. **Storage:** (Vial) 2-8°C (36-46°F). Reconstituted: 2-8°C (36-46°F); stable up to 14 days. Reconstituted with sterile water: 2-8°C (36-46°F); use within 24 hrs; use only one dose per vial and discard unused portion. (Cartridge) 2-8°C (36-46°F). Reconstituted: 2-8°C (36-46°F); stable for 28 days. Avoid freezing.

HUMIRA   RX
adalimumab (Abbott)

Increased risk of serious infections (eg, active tuberculosis [TB], TB reactivation, invasive fungal infections, bacterial/viral or other opportunistic infections) leading to hospitalization or death, mostly with immunosuppressants (eg, methotrexate [MTX] or corticosteroids). D/C if serious infection or sepsis develops. Active/latent reactivation TB may present with disseminated, extrapulmonary disease; test for latent TB and treat prior to initiation of therapy. Invasive fungal infection reported; consider empiric antifungal therapy in patients at risk who develop severe systemic illness. Consider risks and benefits prior to therapy with chronic or recurrent infections. Monitor for development of infection during and after treatment including development of TB in patients who tested negative for latent TB infection prior to therapy. Lymphoma and other malignancies reported in children and adolescents. Aggressive and fatal hepatosplenic T-cell lymphoma (HSTCL) reported majority in patients with Crohn's disease (CD) or ulcerative colitis in adolescent and young adult males with concomitant azathioprine or 6-mercaptopurine.

THERAPEUTIC CLASS: Monoclonal antibody/TNF-alpha receptor blocker

INDICATIONS: Reduce signs/symptoms, induce major clinical response, inhibit progression of structural damage, and improve physical function of moderate-severe active adult rheumatoid arthritis (RA) with/without MTX or nonbiologic disease-modifying antirheumatic drugs (DMARDs). Reduce signs/symptoms of active adult ankylosing spondylitis (AS) and moderate-severe active polyarticular juvenile idiopathic arthritis (JIA) in pediatric patients ≥4 yrs with/without MTX. Reduce signs/symptoms, inhibit progression of structural damage, and improve physical function in active adult psoriatic arthritis (PsA) with/without nonbiologic DMARDs. Reduce signs/symptoms and induce/maintain clinical remission in moderate-severe active adult CD with inadequate response to conventional therapy and lost response/intolerant to infliximab. Treatment of moderate-severe chronic adult plaque psoriasis (Ps) for who are candidates for systemic or phototherapy and when other systemic therapies are medically less appropriate.

DOSAGE: *Adults:* RA/PsA/AS: 40mg SQ every other week. Some patients with RA not taking concomitant MTX may derive additional benefit from increasing to 40mg every week. CD: Initial: 160mg SQ at Day 1 (given as 4 inj of 40mg in 1 day or as 2 inj of 40mg/day for 2 consecutive days); then 80mg after 2 weeks (Day 15). Maint: 40mg every other week beginning at Week 4 (Day 29). Ps: Initial: 80mg SQ followed by 40mg every other week starting 1 week after initial dose. *Pediatrics:* 4-17 yrs: Polyarticular JIA: 15kg (33 lbs)-<30kg (66 lbs): 20mg SQ every other week. ≥30kg (≥66 lbs): 40mg SQ every other week.

HOW SUPPLIED: Inj: 40mg/0.8mL [Prefilled pen]; 20mg/0.4mL, 40mg/0.8mL [Prefilled syringe]

WARNINGS/PRECAUTIONS: Treatment in CD and Ps >1 yr has not been clinically evaluated. Cases of acute and chronic leukemia, and lymphoma in adults as well as other malignancies including breast, colon, prostate, lung, melanoma and nonmelanoma skin cancer reported. Anaphylaxis and angioneurotic edema reported (rare); d/c immediately and initiate appropriate therapy. Increase risk of HBV reactivation in carriers; d/c and start antiviral therapy if occurs. New onset or exacerbation of CNS/peripheral demyelinating disease reported; caution with pre-existing or recent-onset CNS/peripheral nervous system demyelinating disorders. Rare reports of pancytopenia including aplastic anemia reported; seek medical attention if signs/symptoms of blood dyscrasias/infection develop and d/c for significant hematologic abnormalities. New onset or worsening of congestive heart failure (CHF) reported; caution with heart failure. May result in autoantibody formation; d/c if lupus-like syndrome develops. Caution in elderly.

ADVERSE REACTIONS: Lymphoma, HSCTL, upper respiratory tract infections, inj-site pain/reactions, headache, rash, sinusitis, nausea, urinary tract infections, flu syndrome, abdominal pain, hyperlipidemia, hypercholesterolemia, back pain, hematuria.

INTERACTIONS: See Boxed Warning. Reduced clearance with MTX. Concomitant use of anakinra or abatacept is not recommended in RA due to increased risk of serious infections. Avoid with live vaccines.

PREGNANCY: Category B, not for use in nursing.

MECHANISM OF ACTION: Recombinant human IgG1 TNF-α monoclonal antibody; binds specifically to TNF-α and blocks its interaction with p55 and p75 cell surface TNF receptors. Lyses surface TNF-expressing cells *in vitro* in the presence of complement. Modulates biological responses that are induced or regulated by TNF. In plaque psoriasis, therapy reduces the epidermal thickness and infiltration of inflammatory cells.

PHARMACOKINETICS: Absorption: (40mg SQ single dose) Absolute bioavailability (64%), C_{max}=4.7mcg/mL, T_{max}=131 hrs. **Distribution:** (0.25-10mg/kg IV dose) V_d=4.7-6L. **Elimination:** (0.25-10mg/kg IV dose) $T_{1/2}$=2 weeks.

NURSING CONSIDERATIONS

Assessment: Assess for active/latent infection, history of chronic/recurrent infection, infection risk, TB risk factors, HBV infection status, demyelinating disease, CHF, hypersensitivity to drug, latex allergy, pregnancy/nursing status, and possible drug interactions. Assess for history of travel to infection-endemic areas. Assess for immunization history in pediatric patients. Test for latent TB.

Monitoring: Monitor for serious infections, active/reactivation TB, malignancies (eg, lymphoma), hypersensitivity reactions, HBV reactivation, demyelinating disease, hematological reactions, worsening/new onset CHF, lupus-like syndrome, and other adverse reactions.

Patient Counseling: Inform about benefits/risks of therapy. Inform that therapy may lower the ability of immune system to fight infection; instruct to contact physician if any symptoms of infection, including TB, invasive fungal infection, and reactivation of HBV, occur. Counsel about risk of malignancies. Advise to seek immediate medical attention if any symptoms of severe allergic reactions develop. Advise latex-sensitive patients that the needle cap of prefilled syringe contains latex. Advise to report any signs of new/worsening medical conditions (eg, CHF, neurological disease, autoimmune disorder) or any symptoms suggestive of a cytopenia (eg, bleeding, bruising, or persistent fever). Instruct on proper inj technique, as well as proper syringe and needle disposal.

Administration: SQ route. Rotate inj sites; avoid in areas where skin is tender, bruised, red, or hard. Inject full amount in the syringe. Refer to PI for instructions on how to use inj. **Storage:** 2-8°C (36-46°F). Do not freeze. Protect prefilled syringe from exposure to light. Store in original carton until time of administration.

Humulin 70/30   OTC
insulin human, rdna origin - insulin, human (isophane/regular) (Lilly)

THERAPEUTIC CLASS: Insulin

INDICATIONS: To control hyperglycemia in diabetes.

DOSAGE: *Adults:* Individualize dose.
Pediatrics: Individualize dose.

HOW SUPPLIED: Inj: (Isophane-Regular) 70 U-30 U/mL [3mL, 10mL]

WARNINGS/PRECAUTIONS: Any change of insulin should be made cautiously and only under medical supervision. Changes in strength, manufacturer, type, species, or method of manufacturing may result in the need for a change in dosage. Some patients may require a change in dose from that used with other insulins; adjustment may occur with the 1st dose, or during the 1st several weeks or months if needed. Hypoglycemia may occur with too much insulin, missing or delaying meals, exercising, or working more than usual. Illness/infection (especially with N/V), pregnancy, exercise, and travel may change insulin requirements. SQ administration may result in lipoatrophy or lipohypertrophy. May cause local (redness, swelling, itching at inj site that usually clears up in a few days to a few weeks) or generalized (rash over the whole body, SOB, wheezing, BP reduction, fast pulse, sweating) allergy. Not for IM or IV use.

ADVERSE REACTIONS: Hypoglycemia.

INTERACTIONS: Increased insulin requirements with oral contraceptives, corticosteroids, or thyroid replacement therapy. Reduced insulin requirements with oral antidiabetics, salicylates (eg, aspirin), sulfa antibiotics, alcohol, certain antidepressants, and some kidney and BP medicines. Early warning symptoms of hypoglycemia may be different or less pronounced with β-blockers.

PREGNANCY: Safety not known in pregnancy/nursing.

MECHANISM OF ACTION: Insulin; regulates glucose metabolism.

NURSING CONSIDERATIONS

Assessment: Assess for risk of hypoglycemia, alcohol consumption, exercise routines, pregnancy/nursing status, and possible drug interactions. Obtain baseline FPG and HbA1c.

Monitoring: Monitor for signs and symptoms of hypoglycemia, lipodystrophy, and allergic reactions. Monitor FPG and HbA1c.

Patient Counseling: Advise to never share needles or syringes, use the proper and correct syringe type, use disposable syringes and needles only once, and discard properly. Counsel on proper dose preparation and administration techniques. Instruct to always carry a quick source of sugar (hard candy or glucose tabs). Counsel about signs/symptoms of hypoglycemia, importance of frequent monitoring of blood glucose levels, and need for a balanced diet and regular exercise. Advise to keep an extra/spare supply of syringes and needles on hand and always wear diabetic identification. Instruct to notify physician if pregnant/nursing or plan to become pregnant, and of any medications concurrently being taken. **Administration:** SQ route. Inject SQ in abdomen, thigh, or arms. Refer to PI for preparation and administration instructions. **Storage:** Unopened: Refrigerate. Do not freeze. Opened: <30°C (86°F). Protect from heat and light.

HUMULIN N   OTC
insulin, nph - insulin human, rdna origin (Lilly)

THERAPEUTIC CLASS: Insulin

INDICATIONS: To control hyperglycemia in diabetes.

DOSAGE: *Adults:* Individualize dose.
Pediatrics: Individualize dose.

HOW SUPPLIED: Inj: 100 U/mL [3mL, 10mL]

WARNINGS/PRECAUTIONS: Any change of insulin should be made cautiously and only under medical supervision. Changes in strength, manufacturer, type, species, or method of manufacturing may result in the need for a change in dosage. Some patients may require a change in dose from that used with other insulins; adjustment may occur with the 1st dose, or during the 1st several weeks or months if needed. Hypoglycemia may occur with too much insulin, missing or delaying meals, exercising, or working more than usual. Illness/infection (especially with N/V), pregnancy, exercise, and travel may change insulin requirements. SQ administration may result in lipoatrophy or lipohypertrophy. May cause local (redness, swelling, itching at inj site that usually clears up in a few days to a few weeks) or generalized (rash over the whole body, SOB, wheezing, BP reduction, fast pulse, sweating) allergy. Not for IM or IV use.

ADVERSE REACTIONS: Hypoglycemia.

INTERACTIONS: Increased insulin requirements with oral contraceptives, corticosteroids, or thyroid replacement therapy. Reduced insulin requirements with oral antidiabetics, salicylates (eg, aspirin), sulfa antibiotics, alcohol, certain antidepressants, and some kidney and BP medicines. Early warning symptoms of hypoglycemia may be different or less pronounced with β-blockers.

PREGNANCY: Safety not known in pregnancy/nursing.

MECHANISM OF ACTION: Insulin; regulates glucose metabolism.

NURSING CONSIDERATIONS

Assessment: Assess for risk of hypoglycemia, alcohol consumption, exercise routines, pregnancy/nursing status, and possible drug interactions. Obtain baseline FPG and HbA1c.

Monitoring: Monitor for signs and symptoms of hypoglycemia, lipodystrophy, and allergic reactions. Monitor FPG and HbA1c.

Patient Counseling: Advise to never share needles or syringes, use the proper and correct syringe type, use disposable syringes and needles only once, and discard properly. Counsel on proper dose preparation and administration techniques. Instruct to always carry a quick source of sugar (hard candy or glucose tabs). Counsel about signs/symptoms of hypoglycemia, importance of frequent monitoring of blood glucose levels, and need for a balanced diet and regular exercise. Advise to keep extra/spare supply of syringes and needles on hand and always wear diabetic identification. Instruct to notify physician if pregnant/nursing or plan to become pregnant, and of any medications concurrently being taken.

Administration: SQ route. Inject SQ in abdomen, thigh, or arms. Refer to PI for preparation and administration instructions. **Storage:** Unopened: Refrigerate. Do not freeze. Opened: <30°C (86°F). Protect from heat and light.

HUMULIN R   OTC
insulin human, rdna origin - insulin, human regular (Lilly)

THERAPEUTIC CLASS: Insulin

INDICATIONS: Adjunct to diet and exercise to improve glycemic control in adults and children with type 1 and 2 diabetes mellitus.

DOSAGE: *Adults:* Individualize dose. (SQ) ≥3X daily ac. Inj should be followed by a meal within 30 min. (IV) 0.1-1 U/mL in infusion systems with 0.9% NaCl. Renal/Hepatic Impairment: May need to reduce dose.
Pediatrics: Individualize dose. (SQ) ≥3X daily ac. Inj should be followed by a meal within 30 min.

(IV) 0.1-1 U/mL in infusion systems with 0.9% NaCl. Renal/Hepatic Impairment: May need to reduce dose.

HOW SUPPLIED: Inj: 100 U/mL [3mL, 10mL]

CONTRAINDICATIONS: Episodes of hypoglycemia.

WARNINGS/PRECAUTIONS: Any change in insulin should be made cautiously and only under medical supervision. Changes in strength, manufacturer, type, species, or method of administration may result in the need for a change in dosage. May require dose adjustments with change in physical activity or usual meal plan. Stress, illness, or emotional disturbance may alter insulin requirements. Hypoglycemia may occur; caution in patients with hypoglycemia unawareness and those predisposed to hypoglycemia (eg, pediatrics, those who fast or have erratic food intake). Hyperglycemia, diabetic ketoacidosis, or hyperosmolar coma may develop if taken less than needed. Hypokalemia may occur; caution in patients who may be at risk. Severe, life-threatening, generalized allergy, including anaphylaxis, may occur. Contains metacresol as excipient; localized reactions and generalized myalgia reported. May be administered IV under medical supervision; close monitoring of blood glucose and K^+ is required.

ADVERSE REACTIONS: Hypoglycemia, hypokalemia, lipodystrophy, weight gain, peripheral edema.

INTERACTIONS: May require dose adjustment and close monitoring with drugs that may increase blood glucose-lowering effect and susceptibility to hypoglycemia (eg, oral antihyperglycemics, salicylates, sulfa antibiotics, MAOIs, SSRIs, pramlintide, disopyramide, fibrates, fluoxetine, propoxyphene, pentoxifylline, ACE inhibitors, angiotensin II receptor blocking agents, inhibitors of pancreatic function [eg, octreotide]), drugs that may reduce blood-glucose-lowering effect (eg, corticosteroids, isoniazid, certain lipid-lowering drugs [eg, niacin], estrogens, oral contraceptives, phenothiazines, danazol, diuretics, sympathomimetic agents, somatropin, atypical antipsychotics, glucagon, protease inhibitors, thyroid replacement therapy), or drugs that may increase or decrease blood glucose-lowering effect (eg, β-adrenergic blockers, clonidine, lithium salts, alcohol). Pentamidine may cause hypoglycemia which may sometimes be followed by hyperglycemia. β-adrenergic blockers, clonidine, guanethidine, and reserpine may mask the signs of hypoglycemia. Caution with K^+-lowering medications or medications sensitive to serum K^+ concentrations.

PREGNANCY: Category B, caution in nursing.

MECHANISM OF ACTION: Insulin; regulates glucose metabolism. Lowers blood glucose by stimulating peripheral glucose uptake and by inhibiting hepatic glucose production. Inhibits lipolysis, proteolysis, and gluconeogenesis, and enhances protein synthesis.

NURSING CONSIDERATIONS

Assessment: Assess for predisposal to hypoglycemia, risk of hypokalemia, hypersensitivity, pregnancy/nursing status, and possible drug interactions. Obtain baseline renal function, LFTs, FPG, and HbA1c.

Monitoring: Monitor for signs and symptoms of hypoglycemia, lipodystrophy, allergic reactions, and other adverse effects. Monitor renal function, LFTs, FPG, HbA1c, and serum K^+ levels.

Patient Counseling: Advise to use the proper and correct syringe type. Counsel on proper dose preparation and administration techniques. Instruct to always carry a quick source of sugar (hard candy or glucose tabs). Counsel about signs/symptoms of hypoglycemia, importance of frequent monitoring of blood glucose levels, and need for a balanced diet and regular exercise. Instruct to exercise caution when driving or operating machinery. Instruct to notify physician if pregnant/nursing or plan to become pregnant, and of any medications concurrently being taken.

Administration: SQ/IV route. Inject SQ in abdomen, thigh, or upper arms. Rotate inj sites. Refer to PI for preparation and administration instructions. **Storage:** Unopened: 2-8°C (36-46°F). Do not freeze. Opened: <30°C (86°F). Protect from heat and light. Use within 31 days. Admixture: 2-8°C (36-46°F) for 48 hrs, then may use at room temperature for up to an additional 48 hrs.

HYALGAN   RX
sodium hyaluronate (Fidia Pharma)

THERAPEUTIC CLASS: Hyaluronan

INDICATIONS: Treatment of pain in osteoarthritis of the knee in patients who have failed to respond adequately to conservative nonpharmacologic therapy and to simple analgesics (eg, acetaminophen).

DOSAGE: *Adults:* 2mL intra-articularly into the affected knee once a week for a total of 5 inj. Some patients may experience benefit with 3 inj given at weekly intervals.

HOW SUPPLIED: Inj: 10mg/mL [2mL]

CONTRAINDICATIONS: Intra-articular inj with presence of infections or skin diseases in the area of the inj site.

WARNINGS/PRECAUTIONS: Avoid use with disinfectants for skin preparation containing quaternary ammonium salts; may result in precipitate formation. Anaphylactoid and allergic reactions reported. Transient increases in inflammation in the injected knee reported in patients with inflammatory arthritis (eg, rheumatoid arthritis, gouty arthritis). Safety and effectiveness of use with other intra-articular injectables, or into the joints other than the knee have not been established. Caution with allergy to avian proteins, feathers, and egg products. Remove joint effusion if present, and inject SQ lidocaine or similar local anesthetic prior to treatment.

ADVERSE REACTIONS: GI complaints, inj-site pain, knee swelling/effusion, local skin reactions (eg, rash, ecchymosis), pruritus, headache.

PREGNANCY: Safety not known in pregnancy/nursing.

MECHANISM OF ACTION: Hyaluronan.

NURSING CONSIDERATIONS

Assessment: Assess for previous hypersensitivity to hyaluronate preparations; allergy to avian proteins, feathers, and egg products; infections or skin diseases in the area of inj site; use of disinfectants containing quaternary ammonium salts; and signs of acute inflammation prior to administration.

Monitoring: Monitor for anaphylactic and allergic reactions, transient increase of inflammation in inj site, and other adverse reactions.

Patient Counseling: Inform that transient pain/swelling of injected joint may occur after inj. Instruct to avoid strenuous activities or prolonged (>1 hr) weight-bearing activities (eg, jogging, tennis) within 48 hrs following therapy.

Adminstration: Intra-articular route. Use strict aseptic technique. Inject using 20-gauge needle. Use separate vial for each knee if treatment is bilateral. **Storage:** <25°C (77°F). Protect from light. Do not freeze. Discard any unused portions.

HYDROCHLOROTHIAZIDE   RX
hydrochlorothiazide (Various)

THERAPEUTIC CLASS: Thiazide diuretic

INDICATIONS: Management of HTN alone or in combination with other antihypertensives, and edema in pregnancy due to pathologic causes. (Tab) Adjunct therapy in edema associated with congestive heart failure, hepatic cirrhosis, corticosteroid and estrogen therapy, and renal dysfunction (eg, nephrotic syndrome, acute glomerulonephritis, chronic renal failure).

DOSAGE: *Adults:* (Cap) Initial: 12.5mg qd. Max: 50mg/day. Elderly: Initial: 12.5mg. Titrate: Increase by 12.5mg increments if needed. (Tab) Individualize dose according to response. Use lowest effective dose. Edema: Usual: 25-100mg daily as single or divided dose. May give qod or 3-5 days/week. HTN: Initial: 25mg qd. Titrate: May increase to 50mg daily as a single or in 2 divided doses.
Pediatrics: (Tab) Diuresis/HTN: 1-2mg/kg/day given as single or 2 divided doses. Max: 2-12 yrs: 100mg/day. Infants up to 2 yrs: 37.5mg/day. <6 months: Up to 3mg/kg/day given in 2 divided doses may be required.

HOW SUPPLIED: Cap: 12.5mg; Tab: 12.5mg, 25mg*, 50mg* *scored

CONTRAINDICATIONS: Anuria, hypersensitivity to sulfonamide-derived drugs.

WARNINGS/PRECAUTIONS: Caution with severe renal disease. May precipitate azotemia and cumulative effects may develop with impaired renal function. Caution with impaired hepatic function or progressive liver disease; may precipitate hepatic coma. May cause idiosyncratic reaction, resulting in acute transient myopia and acute angle-closure glaucoma; d/c as rapidly as possible. Fluid or electrolyte imbalance (eg, hyponatremia, hypochloremic alkalosis, hypokalemia, hypomagnesemia) may develop; monitor serum electrolytes periodically. Hypokalemia may develop, especially with brisk diuresis, with severe cirrhosis, or after prolonged therapy; may use potassium-sparing diuretics, potassium supplements, or foods high in potassium to avoid or treat hypokalemia. Dilutional hyponatremia may occur in edematous patients in hot weather; appropriate therapy of water restriction rather than salt administration should be instituted except for life-threatening hyponatremia. Hyperuricemia may occur or acute gout may be precipitated. Hyperglycemia may occur. Latent diabetes mellitus (DM) may manifest. May decrease urinary calcium excretion. D/C prior to parathyroid function tests. (Cap) Pathologic changes in parathyroid glands, with hypercalcemia and hypophosphatemia, observed on prolonged therapy. (Tab) Sensitivity reactions may occur. May exacerbate/activate systemic lupus erythematosus (SLE). Enhanced antihypertensive effects in postsympathectomy patients. Consider withholding or d/c therapy if progressive renal impairment becomes evident. May cause intermittent and slight elevation of serum calcium in the absence of known disorders of calcium metabolism. May be associated with increases in cholesterol and TG levels.

ADVERSE REACTIONS: Weakness, hypotension (including orthostatic hypotension), pancreatitis, jaundice, diarrhea, vomiting, blood dyscrasias, rash, photosensitivity, electrolyte imbalance, impotence, renal dysfunction/failure, interstitial nephritis.

INTERACTIONS: Potentiation of orthostatic hypotension may occur with alcohol, barbiturates, and narcotics. Dosage adjustment of antidiabetic drugs (insulin or oral hypoglycemic agents) may be required. May potentiate or have an additive effect with other antihypertensives. Cholestyramine and colestipol resins may reduce absorption. Intensified electrolyte depletion, particularly hypokalemia, with concomitant corticosteroids and adrenocorticotropic hormone use. May decrease response to pressor amines (eg, norepinephrine). May increase responsiveness to nondepolarizing skeletal muscle relaxants (eg, tubocurarine). Increased risk of lithium toxicity; avoid concomitant use. NSAIDs may reduce diuretic, natriuretic, and antihypertensive effects. Hypokalemia and hypomagnesemia may sensitize or exaggerate the response of the heart to toxic effects of digitalis.

PREGNANCY: Category B, not for use in nursing.

MECHANISM OF ACTION: Thiazide diuretic; has not been established. Affects distal renal tubular mechanism of electrolyte reabsorption, increasing excretion of Na^+ and Cl^-.

PHARMACOKINETICS: Absorption: C_{max}=70-490ng/mL; T_{max}=1-5 hrs. **Distribution:** Plasma protein binding (40%-68%); crosses placenta; found in breast milk. **Elimination:** Urine (55%-77%, >95% unchanged [Cap]; ≥61% [Tab]); $T_{1/2}$=6-15 hrs (Cap), 5.6-14.8 hrs (Tab).

NURSING CONSIDERATIONS

Assessment: Assess for anuria, SLE, DM, sulfonamide or penicillin hypersensitivity, history of allergy or bronchial asthma, hepatic/renal impairment, pregnancy/nursing status, and possible drug interactions. Obtain baseline serum electrolytes.

Monitoring: Monitor serum electrolytes periodically. Monitor for signs/symptoms of fluid or electrolyte imbalance, exacerbation or activation of SLE, hyperglycemia, hyperuricemia or precipitation of gout, hypersensitivity reactions, myopia, angle-closure glaucoma, renal/hepatic dysfunction, and increases in cholesterol and TG.

Patient Counseling: Advise to seek medical attention if symptoms of electrolyte imbalance (eg, dry mouth, thirst, weakness) or hypersensitivity reactions occur. Counsel to take as directed.

Administration: Oral route. **Storage:** 20-25°C (68-77°F). (Cap) Protect from light, moisture, freezing, -20°C (-4°F).

HYDROXYZINE HCL   RX
hydroxyzine HCl (Various)

THERAPEUTIC CLASS: Piperazine antihistamine

INDICATIONS: (PO) Symptomatic relief of anxiety and tension associated with psychoneurosis and adjunct in organic disease states in which anxiety is manifested. Sedative when used as premedication and following general anesthesia. Management of pruritus due to allergic conditions (eg, chronic urticaria, atopic/contact dermatitis) and histamine-mediated pruritus. (Inj) Total management of anxiety, tension, and psychomotor agitation in conditions of emotional stress. Useful in alleviating the manifestations of anxiety and tension as in the preparation for dental procedures and in acute emotional problems. Management of anxiety associated with organic disturbances (eg, certain types of heart disease) and as adjunctive therapy in alcoholism and allergic conditions with strong emotional overlay (eg, asthma, chronic urticaria, pruritus). Treatment of acutely disturbed or hysterical patients and acute/chronic alcoholism with anxiety withdrawal symptoms or delirium tremens. As pre-/postoperative and pre-/postpartum adjunctive medication to permit reduction in narcotic dosage, allay anxiety, and control emesis. To control N/V, excluding that of pregnancy.

DOSAGE: *Adults:* (PO) Anxiety/Tension: 50-100mg qid. Pruritus: 25mg tid-qid. Sedation: 50-100mg. (IM) N/V, Pre-/Postoperative and Pre-/Postpartum Adjunct: 25-100mg. Psychiatric/Emotional Emergencies: 50-100mg immediately and q4-6h PRN. Adjust dose according to response to therapy. Elderly: Start at lower end of dosing range.
Pediatrics: (PO) Anxiety/Tension/Pruritus: >6 yrs: 50-100mg/day in divided doses. <6 yrs: 50mg/day in divided doses. Sedation: 0.6mg/kg. (IM) N/V, Pre-/Postoperative Adjunct: 0.5mg/lb. Adjust dose according to response to therapy.

HOW SUPPLIED: Inj: 25mg/mL [1mL], 50mg/mL [1mL, 2mL, 10mL]; Sol: 10mg/5mL [30mL, 120mL, 473mL, 3785mL]; Syrup: 10mg/5mL [118mL, 473mL]; Tab: 10mg, 25mg, 50mg

CONTRAINDICATIONS: Early pregnancy. (Inj) SQ, intra-arterial, or IV administration.

WARNINGS/PRECAUTIONS: May impair mental/physical abilities. Effectiveness in long-term use (>4 months) has not been established. Caution in elderly.

ADVERSE REACTIONS: Dry mouth, drowsiness, involuntary motor activity.

INTERACTIONS: Potentiates CNS depression with other CNS depressants (eg, narcotics, non-narcotic analgesics, barbiturates, alcohol); dose reduction of other CNS depressants recommended. Rare cases of cardiac arrest and death have been reported following the combined use of the inj and other CNS depressants. May potentiate meperidine; use with great caution and at reduced dosage. (PO) Caution with alcohol; may increase effects when used simultaneously.

PREGNANCY: Contraindicated in early pregnancy, not for use in nursing.

MECHANISM OF ACTION: Piperazine antihistamine; believed to suppress activity in key regions of subcortical area of CNS and shown to have primary skeletal muscle relaxation, bronchodilator activity, antihistaminic, antispasmodic, antiemetic, and analgesic effects.

PHARMACOKINETICS: Absorption: (PO) Rapid.

NURSING CONSIDERATIONS

Assessment: Assess hypersensitivity to drug, pregnancy/nursing status and possible drug interactions.

Monitoring: Monitor for response to treatment, drowsiness, and other adverse reactions.

Patient Counseling: Inform about risks/benefits of therapy. Caution against concomitant use with alcohol or other CNS depressants. May impair mental/physical abilities.

Administration: Oral, IM routes. (Inj) May be administered without further dilution. Must be injected well within the body of a relatively large muscle. Refer to PI for administration sites for adults/pediatrics. **Storage:** 20-25°C (68-77°F). (Syrup) Protect from freezing. (Inj) Excursions permitted to 15-30°C (59-86°F). Discard unused portion of the single dose vial. (Inj/Syrup) Protect from light.

HYZAAR   RX
losartan potassium - hydrochlorothiazide (Merck)

> **Drugs that act directly on the renin-angiotensin system can cause injury/death to developing fetus during 2nd and 3rd trimesters. D/C when pregnancy is detected.**

THERAPEUTIC CLASS: Angiotensin II receptor antagonist/thiazide diuretic

INDICATIONS: Treatment of HTN. Reduction of risk of stroke in patients with HTN and left ventricular hypertrophy (LVH) (may not apply to Black patients).

DOSAGE: *Adults:* Individualize dose. HTN: Usual: 50mg-12.5mg qd. Max: 100mg-25mg qd. Uncontrolled BP on Losartan Monotherapy or HCTZ Alone/Uncontrolled BP on 25mg qd HCTZ/Controlled BP on 25mg qd HCTZ with Hypokalemia: Switch to 50mg-12.5mg qd. Titrate: If BP remains uncontrolled after 3 weeks, increase to 100mg-25mg qd. Uncontrolled BP on 100mg Losartan Monotherapy: Switch to 100mg-12.5mg qd. Titrate: If BP remains uncontrolled after 3 weeks, increase to 100mg-25mg qd. Severe HTN: Initial: 50mg-12.5mg qd. Titrate: If inadequate response after 2-4 weeks, increase to 100mg-25mg qd. Max: 100mg-25mg qd. HTN with LVH: Initial: Losartan 50mg qd. If inadequate BP reduction, add 12.5mg HCTZ or substitute losartan-HCTZ 50mg-12.5mg. If additional BP reduction needed, substitute with losartan 100mg and HCTZ 12.5mg or losartan-HCTZ 100mg-12.5mg, followed by losartan 100mg and HCTZ 25mg or losartan-HCTZ 100mg-25mg. Replacement Therapy: Combination may be substituted for titrated components.

HOW SUPPLIED: Tab: (Losartan-HCTZ) 50mg-12.5mg, 100mg-12.5mg, 100mg-25mg

CONTRAINDICATIONS: Anuria, hypersensitivity to other sulfonamide-derived drugs.

WARNINGS/PRECAUTIONS: Not indicated for initial therapy of HTN. Symptomatic hypotension may occur in intravascular volume-depleted patients; correct volume depletion before therapy. Not recommended with hepatic impairment requiring losartan titration. Not recommended with severe renal impairment (CrCl ≤30mL/min). Angioedema reported. HCTZ: Caution with hepatic impairment or progressive liver disease; may precipitate hepatic coma. Hypersensitivity reactions may occur. May exacerbate or activate systemic lupus erythematosus (SLE). May cause idiosyncratic reaction, resulting in acute transient myopia and acute angle-closure glaucoma; d/c as rapidly as possible. Observe for signs of fluid or electrolyte imbalance (hyponatremia, hypochloremic alkalosis, and hypokalemia). Hyperuricemia may occur or frank gout may be precipitated. Hyperglycemia, hypomagnesemia, and hypercalcemia may occur. D/C before testing for parathyroid function. Enhanced effects in postsympathectomy patients. Increased cholesterol, TG levels reported. May precipitate azotemia with renal disease. Losartan: Oliguria and/or progressive azotemia and (rarely) acute renal failure and/or death may occur in patients whose renal function is dependent on the renin-angiotensin-aldosterone system (eg, severe congestive heart failure [CHF]). May increase BUN and SrCr levels with renal artery stenosis. Dual blockade of the renin-angiotensin-aldosterone system is associated with increased risk of hypotension, syncope, hyperkalemia, and changes in renal function (including acute renal failure); closely monitor BP, renal function, and electrolytes with concomitant ACE inhibitors.

ADVERSE REACTIONS: Hypokalemia, dizziness, upper respiratory infection, abdominal pain, palpitations, back pain, sinusitis, rash, cough, edema/swelling.

INTERACTIONS: May decrease effects of diuretics and angiotensin II receptor antagonists and may further deteriorate renal function with NSAIDs, including selective cyclooxygenase-2 inhibitors. Clearance of lithium may be reduced. HCTZ: Avoid with lithium. Potentiation of orthostatic hypotension may occur with alcohol, barbiturates, or narcotics. Dose adjustment of antidiabetic drugs (eg, oral agents, insulin) may be required. Additive effect or potentiation of other antihypertensives. Anionic exchange resins (eg, cholestyramine, colestipol) may impair absorption. Corticosteroids, adrenocorticotropic hormone, or glycyrrhizin (found in liquorice) may intensify electrolyte depletion, particularly hypokalemia. May decrease response to pressor amines (eg, norepinephrine). May increase response to nondepolarizing skeletal muscle relaxants (eg, tubocurarine). Losartan: Rifampin or phenobarbital may decrease levels. Fluconazole may decrease levels of the active metabolite and increase levels of losartan. Cimetidine or erythromycin may increase area under the curve. K^+-sparing diuretics (eg, spironolactone, triamterene, amiloride), K^+ supplements, or salt substitutes containing K^+ may increase serum K^+.

PREGNANCY: Category C (1st trimester) and D (2nd and 3rd trimesters), not for use in nursing.

MECHANISM OF ACTION: Losartan: Angiotensin II receptor antagonist; blocks vasoconstrictor and aldosterone-secreting effects of angiotensin II by selectively blocking binding of angiotensin II to AT_1 receptor. HCTZ: Thiazide diuretic; has not been established. Affects the renal tubular mechanisms of electrolyte reabsorption, directly increasing excretion of Na^+ and chloride in approximately equivalent amounts.

PHARMACOKINETICS: Absorption: Losartan: Well absorbed; T_{max}=1 hr, 3-4 hrs (active metabolite). **Distribution:** Losartan: V_d=34L, 12L (active metabolite); plasma protein binding (98.7%, 99.8% active metabolite). HCTZ: Crosses placenta; found in breast milk. **Metabolism:** Losartan: CYP2C9, 3A4; carboxylic acid (active metabolite). **Elimination:** Losartan: Urine (35%, 4% unchanged, 6% active metabolite), feces (60%); $T_{1/2}$=2 hrs, 6-9 hrs (active metabolite). HCTZ: Kidney (≥61% unchanged); $T_{1/2}$=5.6-14.8 hrs.

NURSING CONSIDERATIONS

Assessment: Assess for hypersensitivity to drugs and its components, anuria, sulfonamide hypersensitivity, history of penicillin allergy, volume/salt depletion, SLE, diabetes mellitus (DM), CHF, hepatic/renal function, postsympathectomy status, cirrhosis, renal artery stenosis, pregnancy/nursing status, and possible drug interactions. Obtain baseline BP.

Monitoring: Monitor for signs/symptoms of fluid/electrolyte imbalance, exacerbation/activation of SLE, idiosyncratic reaction, hypotension, latent DM, hyperglycemia, hypomagnesemia, hypercalcemia, hyperuricemia or precipitation of gout, hypersensitivity reactions, and other adverse reactions. Monitor BP, serum electrolytes, renal function, cholesterol, and TG levels periodically.

Patient Counseling: Inform of pregnancy risks and instruct to report pregnancy to their physician immediately. Counsel that lightheadedness may occur especially during the 1st days of therapy; instruct to report to physician. Instruct to d/c therapy and consult physician if syncope occurs. Advise that inadequate fluid intake, excessive perspiration, diarrhea, or vomiting may result in an excessive fall in BP, leading to lightheadedness or syncope. Instruct not to use K^+ supplements or salt substitutes containing K^+ without consulting physician.

Administration: Oral route. **Storage:** 25°C (77°F); excursions permitted to 15-30°C (59-86°F). Keep container tightly closed. Protect from light.

IMITREX RX
sumatriptan succinate - sumatriptan (GlaxoSmithKline)

THERAPEUTIC CLASS: $5-HT_1$-agonist

INDICATIONS: Acute treatment of migraine attacks with or without aura in adults. (Inj) Acute treatment of cluster headache episodes.

DOSAGE: *Adults:* ≥18 yrs: (Inj) Max Single Dose: 6mg SQ. Max Dose/24 hrs: Two 6mg inj separated by at least 1 hr. (Spray) Individualize dose. 5mg, 10mg, or 20mg single dose administered into 1 nostril; may repeat once after 2 hrs if headache returns. 10mg dose may be obtained by administering a single 5mg dose in each nostril. Max: 40mg/24 hrs. (Tab) Individualize dose. Initial: 25mg, 50mg, or 100mg single dose. May repeat after 2 hrs if headache returns or with partial response. Max: 200mg/24 hrs. If headache returns after initial treatment with inj dose, may give additional single tabs (up to 100mg/day), with an interval of at least 2 hrs between tab doses. Safety of treating >4 headaches/30 days not known. Hepatic Disease: Max: 50mg/single dose.

HOW SUPPLIED: Inj: 4mg/0.5mL, 6mg/0.5mL; Spray: 5mg, 20mg [6^s]; Tab: 25mg, 50mg, 100mg

CONTRAINDICATIONS: History, symptoms, or signs of ischemic cardiac syndromes (eg, angina pectoris, myocardial infarction [MI], silent myocardial ischemia), cerebrovascular syndromes (eg, strokes, transient ischemic attacks), and peripheral vascular syndromes (eg, ischemic bowel disease). Other significant underlying cardiovascular diseases, uncontrolled HTN, hemiplegic or basilar migraine, severe hepatic impairment, and use within 24 hrs of another 5-HT$_1$ agonist, ergotamine-containing or ergot-type medications (eg, dihydroergotamine, methysergide). (Inj) IV administration. (Spray, Tab) Concurrent administration of MAO-A inhibitors or use within 2 weeks of d/c of an MAO-A inhibitor.

WARNINGS/PRECAUTIONS: Has potential to cause coronary artery vasospasm; do not give with documented ischemic/vasospastic coronary artery disease (CAD). Avoid in patients whom unrecognized CAD is predicted by presence of risk factors (eg, HTN, hypercholesterolemia, smoker, obesity, diabetes, CAD family history, menopause, males >40 yrs) unless with a satisfactory cardiovascular evaluation; administer 1st dose under medical supervision; obtain ECG on the 1st occasion of therapy during the interval immediately following administration. Perform periodic cardiovascular evaluation in patients on long-term intermittent use with risk factors for CAD. Serious adverse cardiac events reported. Cerebral/subarachnoid hemorrhage, stroke, other cerebrovascular events, vasospastic reactions, and peripheral vascular/colonic ischemia with abdominal pain and bloody diarrhea reported. Serotonin syndrome may occur; d/c if serotonin syndrome is suspected. HTN and hypertensive crisis reported rarely. Hypersensitivity reactions may occur. Caution with controlled HTN. Chest discomfort, jaw or neck tightness reported. Evaluate for atherosclerosis or predisposition to vasospasm if signs/symptoms suggestive of decreased arterial flow occurs. Caution with diseases that may alter the absorption, metabolism, or excretion of drugs (eg, hepatic or renal impairment). Rare reports of seizures; caution with history of epilepsy or conditions associated with a lower seizure threshold. Exclude other potentially serious neurologic conditions before therapy. Reconsider the diagnosis of migraine before giving a 2nd dose. Overuse of acute migraine drugs may lead to exacerbation of headache. Not recommended in elderly. (Inj) Possible long-term ophthalmic effects. Should only be used when a clear diagnosis of migraine or cluster headache has been established. (Spray, Tab) Should only be used with a clear diagnosis of migraine headache has been established. (Spray) May cause irritation in the nose and throat.

ADVERSE REACTIONS: (Inj) Atypical sensations, flushing, chest discomfort, neck pain/stiffness. (Spray) Nasal cavity or sinuses disorder/discomfort, N/V, bad/unusual taste. (Tab) pain sensation, pressure sensation, malaise/fatigue.

INTERACTIONS: See Contraindications. Serotonin syndrome reported with SSRIs or SNRIs. (Inj) May increase levels with MAO-A inhibitor; coadministration not generally recommended; if clinically warranted, suitable dose adjustment and appropriate observation is advised.

PREGNANCY: Category C, avoid breast feeding for 12 hrs after administration.

MECHANISM OF ACTION: Selective 5-HT$_1$ receptor subtype agonist; activates vascular 5-HT$_1$ receptors on the basilar artery and in the vasculature of human dura mater and mediates vasoconstriction. Also activates 5-HT$_1$ receptors on peripheral terminals of the trigeminal nerve innervating cranial blood vessels.

PHARMACOKINETICS: Absorption: (Nasal Spray, 5mg) C_{max}=5ng/mL; (Nasal Spray, 20mg) C_{max}=16ng/mL; (PO, 25mg) C_{max}=18ng/mL; (PO, 100mg) C_{max}=51ng/mL; (SQ, 6mg) Deltoid: C_{max}=74ng/mL, T_{max}=12 min. Thigh: C_{max}=52ng/mL. **Distribution:** (PO) V_d=2.4L/kg, (SQ) V_d=2.7L/kg; plasma protein binding (14-21%); (SQ) found in breast milk. **Metabolism:** Via monoamine oxidase-A (major); indole acetic acid (metabolite). **Elimination:** (Nasal Spray) Urine (3% unchanged and 42% as metabolite), $T_{1/2}$=2 hrs; (PO) Urine (60%), feces (40%), $T_{1/2}$=2.5 hrs; (SQ) Urine (22%, unchanged; 38%, metabolite), $T_{1/2}$=115 min.

NURSING CONSIDERATIONS

Assessment: Confirm diagnosis of migraine and (Inj) cluster headache before therapy. Assess for cardiovascular diseases, HTN, hemiplegic/basilar migraine, ECG changes, and for other conditions where treatment is cautioned or contraindicated. Assess hepatic/renal function, pregnancy/nursing status, and for possible drug interactions.

Monitoring: Monitor for signs/symptoms of cardiac events (eg, coronary vasospasm, acute MI, arrhythmia, ECG changes), cerebrovascular events (eg, hemorrhage, stroke, transient ischemic attacks), peripheral vascular ischemia, colonic ischemia with bloody diarrhea and abdominal pain, serotonin syndrome, hypersensitivity reactions, hypertension, and other adverse reactions.

Patient Counseling: Inform about potential risks of therapy and instruct to report adverse reactions to physician. Advise to notify physician of all medications currently taking and if pregnant or nursing. (Inj) Counsel about proper use of autoinjector. Advise about inj sites with an adequate skin and SQ thickness to accommodate length of needle.

Administration: Oral, SQ, or nasal route. **Storage:** 2-30°C (36-86°F). Protect from light.

IMURAN   RX
azathioprine (Prometheus)

Increased risk of malignancy with chronic immunosuppression. Malignancy (eg, post-transplant lymphoma and hepatos-plenic T-cell lymphoma [HSTCL]) reported in patients with inflammatory bowel disease. Physician should be familiar with this risk as well as mutagenic potential and possible hematologic toxicities.

THERAPEUTIC CLASS: Purine antagonist antimetabolite

INDICATIONS: Adjunct therapy for prevention of rejection in renal homotransplantation. Management of active rheumatoid arthritis (RA) to reduce signs and symptoms.

DOSAGE: *Adults:* Renal Homotransplantation: Individualize dose. Initial: 3-5mg/kg/day, beginning at the time of transplant. Usually given as a single dose on the day of, and minority of cases 1-3 days before, transplantation. Maint: 1-3mg/kg daily. RA: Initial: 1mg/kg/day (50-100mg) qd-bid. Titrate: Increase by 0.5mg/kg/day after 6-8 weeks, then q4 week if no serious toxicities and initial response is unsatisfactory. Max: 2.5mg/kg/day. Maint: May decrease by 0.5mg/kg/day or 25mg/day q4 weeks to lowest effective dose. May be considered refractory if no improvement after 12 weeks. Renal Dysfunction: Give lower doses.

HOW SUPPLIED: Tab: 50mg* *scored

CONTRAINDICATIONS: (RA) Pregnancy, patients previously treated with alkylating agents (eg, cyclophosphamide, chlorambucil, melphalan).

WARNINGS/PRECAUTIONS: Renal transplant patients are known to have an increased risk of malignancy. Post-transplant lymphomas may be increased with aggressive immunosuppressive treatment. Acute myelogenous leukemia as well as solid tumors reported in patients with RA. Severe leukopenia, thrombocytopenia, macrocytic anemia, pancytopenia, and severe bone marrow suppression may occur. Increased risk of myelotoxicity with low or absent thiopurine S-methyl transferase (TPMT) activity; may increase risk of myelotoxicity with intermediate TPMT activity. Monitor CBCs, including platelet counts, weekly during the 1st month, twice monthly for the 2nd and 3rd months of therapy, then monthly or more frequently if dose/therapy changes. Reduce dose or d/c temporarily if rapid fall in, or persistently low leukocyte count, or other evidence of bone marrow depression occurs. Serious infections (eg, fungal, viral, bacterial, and protozoal) may be fatal and should be treated vigorously; reduce dose and/or consider use of other drugs. May cause fetal harm. Gastrointestinal hypersensitivity reaction characterized by severe N/V reported.

ADVERSE REACTIONS: Malignancy, HSTCL, post-transplant lymphoma, hematologic toxicities, leukopenia, infections, N/V.

INTERACTIONS: See Contraindications. Combined use with disease-modifying antirheumatic drugs is not recommended. Caution with concomitant aminosalicylates (eg, sulphasalazine, mesalazine, olsalazine); may inhibit TPMT enzyme. Allopurinol inhibits one inactivation pathway; reduce dose to approximately 1/3-1/4 of the usual dose. Drugs affecting myelopoiesis (eg, co-tri-moxazole) may exaggerate leukopenia. ACE inhibitors may induce anemia and severe leukopenia. May inhibit anticoagulant effects of warfarin. Use of ribavirin for hepatitis C has been reported to induce severe pancytopenia and may increase the risk of azathioprine-related myelotoxicity.

PREGNANCY: Category D, not for use in nursing.

MECHANISM OF ACTION: Purine antagonist antimetabolite; an imidazolyl derivative of 6-mer-captopurine (6-MP). In homograft survival, it suppresses hypersensitivities of the cell-mediated type and causes variable alterations in antibody production. Immuno-inflammatory response mechanisms not established; suppresses disease manifestation and underlying pathology in autoimmune disease.

PHARMACOKINETICS: Absorption: Well absorbed; T_{max}=1-2 hrs. **Distribution:** Plasma protein binding (30%); crosses placenta, found in breast milk. **Metabolism:** Liver and erythrocytes (extensive); 6-MP activated to 6-thioguanine nucleotides (major metabolites); inactivated via thiol methylation by TPMT and oxidation by xanthine oxidase. **Elimination:** Urine; $T_{1/2}$=5 hrs (decay rate of S-containing metabolites of azathioprine).

NURSING CONSIDERATIONS

Assessment: Assess for drug hypersensitivity, renal/hepatic dysfunction, previous treatment of RA with alkylating agents, pregnancy/nursing status, and for possible drug interactions. Assess for patient's underlying disease or concomitant therapies. Conduct TPMT genotyping/phenotyping to identify absent or reduced enzymatic activity. Obtain baseline CBC with platelet counts.

Monitoring: Monitor for signs/symptoms of bone marrow suppression, malignancies, infections, and for GI hypersensitivity reactions. Monitor CBC, serum transaminases, alkaline phosphatase, and bilirubin levels. Consider TPMT testing in patients with abnormal CBC results unresponsive to dose reduction.

Patient Counseling: Inform about necessity of periodic CBC while on therapy. Instruct to report any unusual bleeding or bruising or signs of infections. Inform about risk of malignancy. Inform of the danger of infection while on therapy; instruct to notify physician if signs and symptoms of infection occur. Educate about careful dosage instructions, especially with impaired renal function or concomitant use with allopurinol. Inform of the potential risks during pregnancy and nursing; advise to notify physician if pregnant or nursing.

Administration: Oral route. Refer to PI for parenteral administration. **Storage:** 15-25°C (59-77°F). Protect from light and store in a dry place.

INCIVEK   RX
telaprevir (Vertex)

THERAPEUTIC CLASS: Protease inhibitor

INDICATIONS: Treatment of genotype 1 chronic hepatitis C in combination with peginterferon alfa and ribavirin in adults with compensated liver disease who are treatment-naive or who have previously been treated with interferon-based treatment.

DOSAGE: *Adults:* Combination Therapy with Peginterferon Alfa/Ribavirin: 750mg tid (q7-9h) with food (not low fat) for 12 weeks. Monitor HCV-RNA levels at weeks 4 and 12 to determine treatment duration and futility. Refer to PI for recommended treatment duration, dose reduction and discontinuation.

HOW SUPPLIED: Tab: 375mg

CONTRAINDICATIONS: Women who are or may become pregnant and men whose female partners are pregnant. Concomitant CYP3A substrates with a narrow therapeutic index, or strong CYP3A inducers (eg, alfuzosin, rifampin, dihydroergotamine, ergonovine, ergotamine, methylergonovine, cisapride, St. John's wort, lovastatin, simvastatin, sildenafil or tadalafil when used for treatment of pulmonary arterial HTN, pimozide, oral midazolam, triazolam). Refer to the individual monographs for peginterferon alfa and ribavirin.

WARNINGS/PRECAUTIONS: Women of childbearing potential and men must use 2 forms of effective contraception during treatment and for 6 months after treatment d/c; perform monthly pregnancy tests during this time. Serious skin reactions, including drug rash with eosinophilia and systemic symptoms (DRESS) and Stevens-Johnson syndrome reported rarely; d/c combination therapy immediately and promptly refer patients to urgent medical care if serious reaction occurs. Mild to moderate rash may occur; monitor and d/c if rash becomes severe. Peginterferon alfa and ribavirin may be continued unless no signs of improvement or rash has not resolved. Anemia reported with peginterferon alfa and ribavirin; combination therapy may cause additional decrease in Hgb. Monitor Hgb prior to and at least every 4 weeks during combination treatment and consider dose reduction of ribavirin; do not restart after d/c from anemia. Do not reduce dose or restart after d/c from rash. Caution in elderly. Not recommended with moderate/severe hepatic impairment or with decompensated liver disease.

ADVERSE REACTIONS: Rash, pruritus, anemia, N/V, hemorrhoids, diarrhea, anorectal discomfort, dysgeusia, fatigue, anal pruritus.

INTERACTIONS: See Contraindications. Dose adjustments of concomitant drugs made during treatment should be readjusted after completion of therapy. Avoid with colchicine in patients with renal/hepatic impairment; risk of toxicity. Not recommended with voriconazole, high doses of itraconazole or ketoconazole, rifabutin, systemic corticosteroids, salmeterol, and darunavir, fosamprenavir or lopinavir (all with ritonavir). May increase levels of atorvastatin; avoid concomitant use. May increase levels of antiarrhythmics, digoxin, macrolide antibacterials, desipramine, trazodone, azole antifungals, rifabutin, alprazolam, IV midazolam, amlodipine and other calcium channel blockers, corticosteroids, bosentan, atazanavir, tenofovir, immunosuppressants, salmeterol, and PDE5 inhibitors for erectile dysfunction. May decrease levels of escitalopram, zolpidem, efavirenz, ethinyl estradiol, and methadone. Use lowest digoxin dose initially with careful titration and monitoring of serum digoxin concentrations. May alter concentrations of warfarin (monitor INR) or anticonvulsants (monitor drug levels). Macrolide antibacterials, azoles, and other CYP3A4/P-glycoprotein inhibitors may increase levels. Anticonvulsants, rifabutin, HIV protease inhibitors, and efavirenz may decrease levels.

PREGNANCY: Category B, Category X when used with peginterferon alfa and ribavirin, not for use in nursing.

MECHANISM OF ACTION: Hepatitis C virus (HCV) NS3/4A protease inhibitor; direct-acting antiviral agent against HCV.

PHARMACOKINETICS: Absorption: (750mg q8h) C_{max}=3510ng/mL; AUC_{8h}=22,300ng•h/mL. (Single dose) T_{max}=4-5 hrs. **Distribution:** V_d=252L; plasma protein binding (59-76%). **Metabolism:** Extensively metabolized by liver via CYP3A4, involving hydrolysis, oxidation, and reduction. **Elimination:** Urine (1%), feces (82%, 31.9% unchanged), exhaled air (9%); $T_{1/2}$=4-4.7 hrs.

NURSING CONSIDERATIONS

Assessment: Assess for pregnancy/nursing status, men whose female partners are of childbearing potential, hepatic function, and possible drug interactions. Obtain CBC (with WBC differential count).

Monitoring: Monitor for DRESS and other adverse reactions. Monitor HCV-RNA levels at Weeks 4, 12, and as clinically indicated. Perform hematology evaluations (including white cell differential count) at Weeks 2, 4, 8, and 12 or as clinically appropriate thereafter. Perform chemistry evaluations (electrolytes, SrCr, uric acid, hepatic enzymes, bilirubin, TSH) as frequently as the hematology evaluations or as clinically indicated and a routine monthly pregnancy test in females. Monitor Hgb at least every 4 weeks.

Patient Counseling: Inform that drug must be used in combination with peginterferon alfa and ribavirin. Instruct to notify healthcare provider immediately if pregnant. Advise women of childbearing potential and men to use 2 nonhormonal methods of effective contraception. Inform that combination treatment may cause rash; report any skin changes or itching. Advise not to stop treatment due to rash unless instructed. Inform that the effect of treatment of hepatitis C on transmission is unknown and that appropriate precautions to prevent transmission should be taken. In case a dose is missed within 4 hrs of the time it is usually taken, instruct to take the prescribed dose with food as soon as possible and if >4 hrs has passed, do not take the missed dose and resume to the usual dosing schedule. Counsel to ingest food containing around 20g of fat within 30 min prior to dose.

Administration: Oral route. **Storage:** 25°C (77°F); excursions permitted to 15-30°C (59-86°F).

INDERAL LA   RX
propranolol HCl (Akrimax)

THERAPEUTIC CLASS: Nonselective beta-blocker

INDICATIONS: Management of HTN, angina pectoris due to coronary atherosclerosis, and hypertrophic subaortic stenosis. Common migraine headache prophylaxis.

DOSAGE: *Adults:* HTN: Initial: 80mg qd. Maint: 120-160mg qd. Angina: Initial: 80mg qd. Titrate: Increase gradually at 3-7 day intervals. Maint: 160mg qd. Max: 320mg qd. Migraine: Initial: 80mg qd. Maint: 160-240mg qd. D/C gradually if unsatisfactory response within 4-6 weeks after reaching maximal dose. Hypertrophic Subaortic Stenosis: Usual: 80-160mg qd.

HOW SUPPLIED: Cap, Extended-Release: 60mg, 80mg, 120mg, 160mg

CONTRAINDICATIONS: Cardiogenic shock, sinus bradycardia and >1st-degree block, bronchial asthma.

WARNINGS/PRECAUTIONS: Exacerbation of angina and myocardial infarction (MI) following abrupt d/c reported. Caution with well-compensated cardiac failure, bronchospastic lung disease, Wolff-Parkinson-White (WPW) syndrome, tachycardia, and hepatic/renal impairment. Do not routinely withdraw chronic therapy prior to surgery. May mask acute hypoglycemia or hyperthyroidism signs/symptoms. Avoid abrupt d/c. May reduce intraocular pressure (IOP). May be more reactive to repeated challenge with history of severe anaphylactic reaction to variety of allergens; may be unresponsive to usual doses of epinephrine. Elevated serum K+, transaminases and alkaline phosphatase observed in HTN. Elevated BUN reported in severe heart failure (HF). Hypersensitivity reactions and cutaneous reactions (eg, Stevens-Johnson syndrome [SJS]) reported. Continued use in patients without history of HF may cause cardiac failure. Caution in elderly. Not for treatment of hypertensive emergencies.

ADVERSE REACTIONS: Bradycardia, congestive heart failure (CHF), hypotension, lightheadedness, mental depression, N/V, agranulocytosis.

INTERACTIONS: Administration with CYP450 (2D6, 1A2, 2C19) substrates, inducers, and inhibitors may lead to clinically relevant drug interactions. Increased levels with CYP2D6 substrates/inhibitors (eg, amiodarone, cimetidine, delavirdine, fluoxetine, paroxetine, quinidine, ritonavir), CYP1A2 substrates/inhibitors (eg, imipramine, cimetidine, ciprofloxacin, fluvoxamine, isoniazid, ritonavir, theophylline, zileuton, zolmitriptan, rizatriptan), and CYP2C19 substrates/inhibitors (eg, fluconazole, cimetidine, fluoxetine, fluvoxamine, teniposide, tolbutamide). Decreased blood levels with hepatic enzyme inducers (eg, rifampin, ethanol, phenytoin, phenobarbital, cigarette smoking). Increased levels of propafenone, lidocaine, zolmitriptan, rizatriptan, nifedipine, diazepam and its metabolites. Increased levels with nisoldipine, nicardipine, chlorpromazine. Decreased theophylline clearance. Increased thioridazine plasma and metabolite concentrations with doses ≥160mg/day. Decreased levels with aluminum hydroxide gel, cholestyramine, colestipol, lovastatin, pravastatin. Decreased levels of lovastatin and pravastatin. Increased warfarin levels and PT. Caution with drugs that slow atrioventricular (AV) nodal conduction (eg, digitalis, lidocaine, calcium channel blocker). Bradycardia, hypotension, high-degree heart block, and HF reported with diltiazem. Bradycardia, HF, and cardiovascular collapse reported with verapamil. May cause hypotension with ACE inhibitors. May antagonize effects of clonidine. May prolong 1st dose hypotension with prazosin. Postural hypotension reported with terazosin or doxazosin. May reduce resting sympathetic nervous activity with catecholamine-depleting drugs (eg, reserpine). May experience uncontrolled HTN with epinephrine. Effects can be reversed by β-agonists (eg, dobutamine or isoproterenol). May reduce efficacy with indomethacin and NSAIDs. May depress myocardial contractility with methoxyflurane and trichloroethylene. Hypotension and cardiac arrest reported with haloperidol. May lower T3 concentration with thyroxine. May exacerbate hypotensive effects of MAOIs or TCAs. May augment the risks of general anesthesia. May need to adjust dose of insulin. Increased levels with alcohol.

PREGNANCY: Category C, caution in nursing.

MECHANISM OF ACTION: Nonselective β-adrenergic receptor blocker; not established. Proposed to decrease cardiac output, inhibit renin release, and lessen tonic sympathetic nerve outflow from vasomotor centers in the brain.

PHARMACOKINETICS: Absorption: Almost complete; T_{max}=6 hrs. **Distribution:** V_d=4L/kg; plasma protein binding (90%); crosses placenta, blood-brain barrier; found in breast milk. **Metabolism:** CYP2D6 (hydroxylation), CYP1A2, 2D6 (oxidation), N-dealkylation, glucuronidation. Propranolol glucuronide, naphthyloxylactic acid, glucuronic acid, sulfate conjugates (major metabolites). **Elimination:** $T_{1/2}$=10 hrs.

NURSING CONSIDERATIONS

Assessment: Assess for bronchial asthma, sinus bradycardia, AV heart block, cardiogenic shock, CHF, bronchospastic disease, hyperthyroidism, diabetes mellitus, WPW syndrome, history of HF, hepatic/renal function, hypersensitivity to drug, pregnancy/nursing status, and possible drug interactions.

Monitoring: Monitor for signs/symptoms of cardiac failure, hypoglycemia, decreased IOP, thyrotoxicosis, withdrawal symptoms (eg, angina, MI), hypersensitivity reactions, and other adverse reactions.

Patient Counseling: Instruct not to interrupt or d/c therapy without consulting physician. Inform that drug may mask signs of thyrotoxicosis and hypoglycemia. Advise to contact physician if symptoms of HF, withdrawal, or hypersensitivity reactions occur. Inform that therapy may interfere with glucoma screening test.

Administration: Oral route. **Storage:** 20-25°C (68-77°F); excursions permitted to 15-30°C (59-86°F). Protect from light, moisture, freezing, and excessive heat.

INDOMETHACIN   RX
indomethacin (Various)

NSAIDs may cause an increased risk of serious cardiovascular (CV) thrombotic events, myocardial infarction (MI), stroke, and serious GI adverse events including bleeding, ulceration, and perforation of the stomach or intestines. Contraindicated for the treatment of perioperative pain in the setting of coronary artery bypass graft (CABG) surgery.

OTHER BRAND NAMES: Indocin (Iroko)

THERAPEUTIC CLASS: NSAID

INDICATIONS: Management of moderate to severe rheumatoid arthritis (RA), including acute flares of chronic disease, ankylosing spondylitis (AS), and osteoarthritis (OA), acute painful shoulder (bursitis and/or tendinitis) and/or acute gouty arthritis.

DOSAGE: *Adults:* RA/AS/OA: Initial: 25mg (5mL) PO bid-tid. Titrate: May increase by 25mg (5mL) or 50mg (10mL) at weekly intervals. Max: 150-200mg (30-40mL) per day. Bursitis/Tendinitis: 75-150mg (15-30mL) per day given in 3 or 4 divided doses for 7-14 days. Acute Gouty Arthritis: 50mg (10mL) PO tid until pain is tolerable, then d/c.
Pediatrics: >14 yrs: RA/AS/OA: Initial: 25mg (5mL) PO bid-tid. Titrate: May increase by 25mg (5mL) or 50mg (10mL) at weekly intervals. Max: 150-200mg (30-40mL) per day. Bursitis/Tendinitis: 75-150mg (15-30mL) per day given in 3 or 4 divided doses for 7-14 days. Acute Gouty Arthritis: 50mg (10mL) PO tid until pain is tolerable, then d/c.

HOW SUPPLIED: Cap: 25mg, 50mg; Sus: (Indocin) 25mg/5mL [237mL]

CONTRAINDICATIONS: Aspirin (ASA) or other NSAID allergy that precipitates acute asthmatic attack, urticaria, or rhinitis. Treatment of perioperative pain in the setting of CABG surgery.

WARNINGS/PRECAUTIONS: Not a substitute for corticosteroids or to treat corticosteroid insufficiency. May lead to onset of new HTN or worsening of preexisting HTN; monitor BP closely. Fluid retention and edema reported; caution with fluid retention or heart failure (HF). Renal papillary necrosis and other renal injury reported after long-term use. Not recommended for use with advanced renal disease; if therapy must be initiated, monitor renal function. Anaphylactoid reactions may occur; avoid in patient with ASA-triad. May cause serious skin adverse events (eg, exfoliative dermatitis, Stevens-Johnson syndrome [SJS], and toxic epidermal necrolysis [TEN]); d/c at the first appearance of skin rash or any other signs of hypersensitivity. Avoid in late pregnancy; may cause premature closure of ductus arteriosis. May cause elevations of LFTs; d/c if liver disease develops or systemic manifestations occur. Anemia may occur; with long-term use, monitor Hgb/Hct if signs or symptoms of anemia develop. May inhibit platelet aggregation and prolong bleeding time; monitor with coagulation disorders. Caution with preexisting asthma and avoid with ASA-sensitive asthma. Corneal deposits and retinal disturbances reported with prolonged therapy; d/c if such changes are observed. Blurred vision may be significant; perform eye exams at periodic intervals during prolonged therapy. May aggravate depression or other psychiatric disturbances, epilepsy, and parkinsonism; use with caution. D/C if severe CNS adverse reactions develop. May impair mental/physical abilities. Caution in elderly.

ADVERSE REACTIONS: Headache, dizziness, upper GI ulcers, GI bleeding, GI perforation, N/V, dyspepsia, heartburn, epigastric pain, indigestion.

INTERACTIONS: May diminish antihypertensive effect of ACE inhibitors (eg, captopril) and angiotensin II antagonists (eg, losartan). Avoid with ASA, salicylates, diflunisal, triamterene, and other NSAIDs. May reduce the diuretic, natriuretic, and antihypertensive effects of loop, K^+-sparing, and thiazide diuretics. Increase levels of digoxin reported. Reduced basal plasma renin activity (PRA), as well as those elevations of PRA induced by furosemide reported. May decrease lithium clearance; monitor for toxicity. Caution with methotrexate; may enhance methotrexate toxicity. May increase levels with probenecid. Caution with cyclosporine and anticoagulants. Blunting of the antihypertensive effects of β-blockers reported. May increase risk of serious GI bleeding when used concomitantly with oral corticosteroids or anticoagulants, alcohol, or smoking.

PREGNANCY: Category C, not for use in nursing.

MECHANISM OF ACTION: NSAID; not established; exhibits antipyretic, analgesic, and anti-inflammatory properties. Suspected to inhibit prostaglandin synthesis.

PHARMACOKINETICS: Absorption: Readily absorbed. (Cap) Bioavailability (100%); C_{max}=1-2mcg/mL; T_{max}=2 hrs. **Distribution:** Plasma protein binding (99%); crosses blood-brain barrier and placenta; found in breast milk. **Metabolism:** desmethyl, desbenzoyl, desmethyldesbenzoyl (metabolites). **Elimination:** Urine (60% as drug/metabolites), feces (33% as drug); $T_{1/2}$=4.5 hrs.

NURSING CONSIDERATIONS

Assessment: Assess for history of asthma, urticaria or allergic-type reaction after previous use of NSAIDs, perioperative pain in setting of CABG surgery, cardiovascular disease (CVD) or risk factors for CVD, HTN, fluid retention or HF, hyponatremia, history ulcer disease or GI bleeding, coagulation disorders or anticoagulant therapy, concomitant use of corticosteroids, NSAIDs therapy, smoking, alcohol use, age, health status, anemia, renal/hepatic impairment, rhinitis with or without nasal polyps, pregnancy/nursing status, depression or other psychiatric disturbances, epilepsy, parkinsonism, and possible drug interactions.

Monitoring: Monitor BP during initiation of therapy and thereafter. Monitor platelet function, CBCs, LFTs, dexamethasone suppression tests, renal function, and chemistry profile. Monitor signs/symptoms of anaphylactic/anaphylactoid reactions, adverse skin events (eg, exfoliative dermatitis, SJS, TEN), eosinophilia, rash, corneal deposits and retinal disturbances with periodic ophthalmic exam, CNS effects, aggravation of depression or other psychiatric disturbances, GI bleeding/ulceration and perforation, anemia, CV thrombotic events, MI, stroke, new or worsening HTN, renal toxicity, renal papillary necrosis, other renal injury, and hyperkalemia.

Patient Counseling: Inform about potential serious side effects (eg, CV side effects such as MI or stroke); seek medical attention if signs/symptoms of chest pain, SOB, weakness, slurred speech, skin rash, blisters or fever, GI effects, bleeding, ulceration and perforation, signs of anaphylactic/anaphylactoid reaction, or hepatic toxicity occurs. Caution while performing hazardous tasks (eg, operating machinery/driving). Advise to notify physician if weight gain/edema occurs. Inform of risks if used during pregnancy.

Administration: Oral route. Take with food. **Storage:** (Cap) 20-25°C (68-77°F). Protect from light. Dispense in a tight, light-resistant container. (Sus) Below 30°C (86°F); avoid >50°C (122°F). Protect from freezing.

INFERGEN   RX
interferon alfacon-1 (Three Rivers)

> May cause or aggravate fatal or life-threatening neuropsychiatric, autoimmune, ischemic, and infectious disorders. Monitor closely with periodic clinical and laboratory evaluations. D/C with persistently severe or worsening signs/symptoms of these conditions. When used with ribavirin, refer to the individual monograph.

THERAPEUTIC CLASS: Biological response modifier

INDICATIONS: Treatment of chronic hepatitis C (CHC) in patients ≥18 yrs with compensated liver disease.

DOSAGE: *Adults:* Monotherapy: Initial: 9mcg SQ three times per week for 24 weeks. Tolerated Previous Interferon Therapy but did not Respond/Relapsed: 15mcg SQ three times per week for up to 48 weeks. Reduce to 7.5mcg if severe adverse reactions occur. Combination Treatment with Ribavirin: 15mcg SQ qd with weight-based ribavirin 1000mg-1200mg (<75kg and ≥75kg) PO in two divided doses for up to 48 weeks. Take with food. Reduce dose from 15mcg to 9mcg and from 9mcg to 6mcg if serious adverse reactions occur. Refer to PI for dose modifications and d/c based on depression or laboratory parameters. D/C if persistent or recurrent serious adverse effects despite dose adjustment, or failure to achieve at least a 2 $\log_{10}$ drop after 12 weeks or undetectable HCV-RNA levels after 24 weeks.

HOW SUPPLIED: Inj: 9mcg/0.3mL, 15mcg/0.5mL

CONTRAINDICATIONS: Hepatic decompensation (Child-Pugh score >6 [class B and C]), autoimmune hepatitis. When used with ribavirin, refer to the individual monograph.

WARNINGS/PRECAUTIONS: May cause severe psychiatric adverse events; extreme caution with history of depression. If patients develop psychiatric problems, monitor during treatment and in the 6-month follow-up period; d/c if psychiatric symptoms persist/worsen or suicidal ideation/aggressive behavior towards others identified. Cardiovascular events (eg, arrhythmia, cardiomyopathy, myocardial infarction [MI]) reported. Caution with cardiovascular disease (CVD); monitor with history of MI and arrhythmic disorder. Dyspnea, pulmonary infiltrates, pneumonia, bronchiolitis obliterans, interstitial pneumonitis, pulmonary HTN, and sarcoidosis, resulting in fatal respiratory failure may occur; d/c if persistent or unexplained pulmonary infiltrates/pulmonary function impairment develops. Risk of hepatic decompensation in CHC patients with cirrhosis; d/c if symptoms of hepatic decompensation occur. Increases in SrCr, including renal failure reported; monitor for signs/symptoms of toxicity. Ischemic and hemorrhagic cerebrovascular events reported. May suppress bone marrow function resulting in severe cytopenias; d/c if severe decreases in neutrophil (<0.5x10⁹/L) or platelet counts (<50x10⁹/L). Caution with abnormally low peripheral blood cell counts, transplant/chronically immunosuppressed patients. Autoimmune disorders reported; caution with autoimmune disorders. Hemorrhagic/ischemic colitis, pancreatitis, serious acute hypersensitivity reactions, ophthalmologic disorders (eg, retinopathy including macular edema) reported; d/c therapy if these occur. Caution with history of endocrine disorders. Hyperthyroidism/hypothyroidism, diabetes mellitus (DM) reported; d/c if uncontrollable. Neutropenia, thrombocytopenia, hypertriglyceridemia, and thyroid disorders reported; perform laboratory tests prior to therapy, 2 weeks after initiation, and periodically thereafter. Caution in elderly. Use with ribavirin: Avoid pregnancy at least 6 months after d/c of ribavirin. Caution in patients with low baseline neutrophil counts (<1500 cells/mm³); d/c for severe neutropenia. Avoid with history of significant/unstable cardiac disease.

ADVERSE REACTIONS: Depression, insomnia, pharyngitis, headache, fatigue, fever, myalgia, rigors, body pain, arthralgia, back pain, abdominal pain, nausea, diarrhea, nervousness.

INTERACTIONS: Peripheral neuropathy reported with telbivudine. Caution with agents that cause myelosuppression. When used with ribavirin, refer to the individual monograph.

PREGNANCY: Category C (monotherapy) and X (combination with ribavirin), not for use in nursing.

MECHANISM OF ACTION: Type-I interferon; binds to the interferon cell-surface receptor, leading to the production of several interferon-stimulated gene products.

NURSING CONSIDERATIONS

Assessment: Assess for neuropsychiatric, autoimmune, ischemic, and infectious disorders. Assess for hepatic impairment (eg, cirrhosis, hepatic decompression, autoimmune hepatitis), hypersensitivity reactions, myelosuppression (including concurrent use of myelosuppressive therapy), preexisting cardiac disease (eg, MI, arrhythmias), renal impairment, preexisting ophthalmologic disorders, history of pulmonary disease, history of endocrine disorders (eg, DM, thyroid disease), pregnancy/nursing status, and possible drug interactions. Obtain baseline CBC with platelet count, SrCr/CrCl, serum albumin, bilirubin, TSH/T4, and eye exam. Obtain electrocardiogram with preexisting cardiac abnormalities before combination therapy. Assess use with transplant or chronically immunosuppressed patients.

Monitoring: Monitor for occurrence or aggravation of neuropsychiatric, autoimmune, ischemic, and infectious disorders. Monitor for neutropenia, thrombocytopenia, depression, psychiatric symptoms, CV events, persistent or unexplained pulmonary infiltrates, pulmonary function impairment, hepatic/renal function during treatment, colitis, pancreatitis, hypersensitivity reactions, ocular symptoms, occurrence or aggravation of hyper- or hypothyroidism, DM, hyperglycemia, and hypertriglyceridemia. Monitor for signs/symptoms of interferon toxicity, including increases in SrCr with impaired renal function. Perform periodic ophthalmologic exam in patients with preexisting ophthalmologic disorder (eg, diabetic retinopathy or hypertensive retinopathy). Monitor laboratory tests (eg, CBC with platelet count, SrCr/CrCl, serum albumin, bilirubin, TSH, and T4) 2 weeks after initiation and periodically thereafter.

Patient Counseling: Inform about the benefits and risks associated with therapy. Instruct to avoid pregnancy during and for 6 months post-treatment with combination therapy; recommend monthly pregnancy tests during this period. Do not initiate therapy until a report of negative pregnancy test has been obtained. Inform that there are no data regarding whether therapy will prevent transmission of HCV infection to others. Instruct about the importance of proper disposal procedures and cautioned against reuse of needles, syringes, or re-entry of vial. Advise to report signs/symptoms of depression or suicidal ideation or other adverse reactions to physician. Inform that laboratory evaluations are required before and during therapy. Instruct patients to keep well-hydrated.

Administration: SQ route. **Storage:** 2-8°C (36-46°F). Do not freeze; avoid vigorous shaking and exposure to direct sunlight. May allow to reach room temperature prior to injection. Discard unused portion.

INFUMORPH
morphine sulfate (Baxter)

> **Risk of severe adverse reactions; observe patient for 24 hrs following test dose, and for first several days after catheter implantation.**

THERAPEUTIC CLASS: Opioid analgesic

INDICATIONS: Treatment of intractable chronic pain in microinfusion devices.

DOSAGE: *Adults:* Lumbar Intrathecal: Opioid-Intolerant: 0.2-1mg/day. Opioid-Tolerant: 1-10mg/day. Max: Must be individualized. Caution with >20mg/day. Epidural: Opioid-Intolerant: 3.5-7.5mg/day. Opioid-Tolerant: 4.5-10mg/day. May increase to 20-30mg/day. Max: Must be individualized. Starting dose must be based on in-hospital evaluation of response to serial single-dose intrathecal/epidural bolus injections of regular morphine sulfate.

HOW SUPPLIED: Inj: 10mg/mL (200mg), 25mg/mL (500mg)

CONTRAINDICATIONS: For neuraxial analgesia: Infection at injection site, anticoagulants, uncontrolled bleeding diathesis, any therapy or condition that may render intrathecal or epidural administration hazardous.

WARNINGS/PRECAUTIONS: Have resuscitation equipment, oxygen, and antidote (eg, naloxone) available; severe respiratory depression may occur. Use only if less invasive means of controlling pain fail. Not for single-dose IV, IM, or SQ administration. May be habit-forming. Caution with determining refill frequency. Make sure needle is properly placed in the filling port of device. Myoclonic-like spasm of the lower extremities reported if dose >20mg/day; may need detoxification. Caution with head injury, increased ICP, decreased respiratory reserve, hepatic/renal dysfunction (epidural injection), elderly. Avoid with chronic asthma, upper airway obstruction, other chronic pulmonary disorders. Biliary colic reported. May cause micturition disturbances especially with BPH. Increased risk of orthostatic hypotension with reduced circulating blood volume and impaired myocardial function. Avoid abrupt withdrawal. Risk of withdrawal in patients maintained on parenteral/oral narcotics. Not for routine use in obstetric labor/delivery.

ADVERSE REACTIONS: Respiratory depression, myoclonus convulsions, dysphoric reactions, pruritus, urinary retention, constipation, lumbar puncture-type headache, peripheral edema, orthostatic hypotension.

INTERACTIONS: Depressant effect may be potentiated by CNS depressants (eg, alcohol, sedatives, antihistamines, psychotropics). Increased risk of respiratory depression with neuroleptics. Contraindicated with anticoagulants. Risk of withdrawal with narcotic antagonists. Increased risk of orthostatic hypotension with sympatholytic drugs.

PREGNANCY: Category C, safety in nursing not known.

MECHANISM OF ACTION: Opioid analgesic; analgesic effects are produced via at least 3 areas of the CNS: the periaqueductal-periventricular gray matter, the ventromedial medulla, and the spinal cord. Interacts predominantly with μ-receptors which are found distributed in the brain, spinal cord, and in the trigeminal nerve.

PHARMACOKINETICS: Absorption: (Epidural): Rapid absorption; C_{max}=33-40ng/mL, T_{max}=10-15 min; (Intrathecal): C_{max}≤1-7.8ng/mL, T_{max}=5-10 min. **Distribution:** Plasma protein binding (36%); Muscle tissue binding (54%). Readily passes into fetal circulation, found in breast milk. (IV): V_d=1.0-4.7L/kg. **Metabolism:** Hepatic glucuronidation. **Elimination:** Kidneys (major), urine (2-12% unchanged), feces (10%); $T_{1/2}$=1.5-4.5 hrs.

NURSING CONSIDERATIONS

Assessment: Assess for level of pain intensity, patient's general condition, age, and medical status, or any other conditions where treatment is contraindicated or cautioned. Assess for history of hypersensitivity, pregnancy/nursing status, renal/hepatic function, and possible drug interactions.

Monitoring: Monitor for signs/symptoms of respiratory depression and/or respiratory arrest, myoclonic events, seizures, dysphoric reactions, toxic psychoses, biliary colic, urinary retention, drug abuse and dependence. If administered intrathecally or via epidural, closely monitor for 24 hrs for signs/symptoms of respiratory depression.

Patient Counseling: Counsel to notify physician immediately if develop signs/symptoms of respiratory depression. Avoid using other CNS depressants and alcohol during therapy. Medication has potential for abuse and dependence. Avoid abrupt withdrawal of medication; withdrawal symptoms may occur. Instruct that if accidental skin contact occurs, wash affected area with water.

Administration: IV, epidural, or intrathecal route. Proper placement of needle or catheter should be verified before epidural injection. **Storage:** 20-25°C (68-77°F); excursions permitted to 15-30°C (59-86°F). Protect from light. Do not freeze.

INNOHEP   RX
tinzaparin sodium (Leo Pharma)

Epidural or spinal hematomas resulting in long-term or permanent paralysis may occur in patients anticoagulated with low molecular weight heparins, heparinoids, or fondaparinux sodium and who are receiving neuraxial anesthesia or undergoing spinal puncture. Increased risk with indwelling epidural catheters, concomitant use of other drugs that affect hemostasis (eg, NSAIDs, platelet inhibitors, other anticoagulants), history of traumatic or repeated epidural or spinal puncture, or a history of spinal deformity or spinal surgery. Monitor frequently for signs/symptoms of neurologic impairment; if neurologic compromise noted, urgent treatment is necessary. Consider benefit and risks before neuraxial intervention in patients anticoagulated or to be anticoagulated for thromboprophylaxis.

THERAPEUTIC CLASS: Low molecular weight heparin

INDICATIONS: Treatment of acute symptomatic deep vein thrombosis (DVT) with or without pulmonary embolism (PE) in conjunction with warfarin.

DOSAGE: *Adults:* 175 anti-Xa IU/kg SQ qd for at least 6 days and until anticoagulated with warfarin (INR ≥2 for 2 consecutive days). Begin warfarin within 1-3 days of therapy. Refer to PI for dosing chart.

HOW SUPPLIED: Inj: 20,000 anti-Xa IU/mL [2mL]

CONTRAINDICATIONS: Hypersensitivity to heparin, sulfite, benzyl alcohol, or pork. Active major bleeding, or in patients with history of heparin-induced thrombocytopenia (HIT).

WARNINGS/PRECAUTIONS: Not for IM/IV injection. Cannot use interchangeably unit for unit with heparin or other low molecular weight heparins. Increased risk for death in elderly patients with renal insufficiency; consider alternative therapy. Extreme caution in patients at increased risk of bleeding (severe uncontrolled HTN, bacterial endocarditis, congenital or acquired bleeding disorders, active or recent ulceration and angiodysplastic GI disease, hemorrhagic stroke, diabetic retinopathy, or shortly after brain, spinal or ophthalmological surgery). Bleeding and thrombocytopenia may occur during therapy. D/C if severe hemorrhage occurs or if platelets <100,000/mm³. Sulfite sensitivity, especially in asthmatic patients, reported. Priapism reported (rare). Contains benzyl alcohol; "Gasping syndrome" in premature infants reported; caution in pregnant women. Periodic CBC including platelets, Hct, Hgb and stool occult blood test recommended.

ADVERSE REACTIONS: Bleeding, injection-site hematoma, asymptomatic increase in AST and ALT, urinary tract infection.

INTERACTIONS: See Boxed Warning. Prior to initiation of therapy, d/c agents that may enhance the risk of hemorrhage (eg, anticoagulants, platelet inhibitors, thrombolytics) unless the agents are essential; if coadministration is necessary, monitor closely for hemorrhage.

PREGNANCY: Category B, caution use in nursing.

MECHANISM OF ACTION: Low molecular weight heparin; inhibits reactions that lead to blood clotting, including the formation of fibrin clots. Acts as a potent co-inhibitor of several activated coagulation factors, including factors Xa and IIa (thrombin). Primary inhibitory activity mediated through plasma protease inhibitor, antithrombin.

PHARMACOKINETICS: Absorption: (4500 IU, Single Dose) C_{max}=0.25 IU/mL, T_{max}=3.7 hrs, AUC=2.0 IU•hr/mL. (175 IU/kg, Day 1) C_{max}=0.87 IU/mL, T_{max}=4.4 hrs, AUC=9.0 IU•hr/mL. (175 IU/kg, Day 5) C_{max}=0.93 IU/mL, T_{max}=4.6 hrs, AUC=9.7 IU•hr/mL; absolute bioavailability (86.7%). **Distribution:** V_d=3.1-5.0L. **Metabolism:** Partially metabolized by desulphation and depolymerization. **Elimination:** Renal; $T_{1/2}$=3-4 hrs.

NURSING CONSIDERATIONS

Assessment: Assess for signs of active major bleeding; presence or history of HIT; severe renal impairment; hypersensitivity to heparin, sulfites, benzyl alcohol or pork products; pregnancy/nursing status, and possible drug interactions. Assess use in conditions with increased risk of hemorrhage.

Monitoring: Monitor for signs/symptoms of bleeding (eg, decreases in Hct, Hgb, BP), thrombocytopenia, hypersensitivity reactions, and priapism. If concomitant therapy with neuraxial anesthesia, monitor for epidural or spinal hematomas and for neurological impairment. Perform periodic monitoring of CBC including platelet count, Hgb, Hct, and stool test for occult blood.

Patient Counseling: Advise about increased risk of bleeding during therapy. Instruct to notify physician if unusual bleeding or hypersensitivity reaction occurs. During pregnancy, advise risk of "Gasping syndrome." Counsel on the proper way to administer: patients should be lying down or sitting when administering SQ Injection; alternate between left and right anterolateral and posterolateral abdominal wall; hold skin fold between thumb and forefinger; insert whole length of needle into skin; to minimize bruising, do not rub injection site after administration.

Administration: SQ route. Patients should be lying down or sitting when administering SQ injection. Alternate between left and right anterolateral and posterolateral abdominal wall. **Storage:** Store at 25°C (77°F); excursions permitted to 15-30°C (59-86°F).

INNOPRAN XL   RX

propranolol HCl (GlaxoSmithKline)

> Exacerbation of angina and myocardial infarction (MI) reported following abrupt d/c; reduce dose gradually over at least a few weeks prior to d/c. Caution against interruption or cessation of therapy without a physician's advice. Reinstitute if exacerbation of angina occurs; take other measures for management of angina pectoris. Coronary artery disease (CAD) may be unrecognized; follow the above advice in patients at risk of having atherosclerotic heart disease who are given propranolol for other indications.

THERAPEUTIC CLASS: Nonselective beta-blocker

INDICATIONS: Management of HTN.

DOSAGE: *Adults:* Individualize dose. Initial: 80mg qhs (approximately 10 pm) taken consistently, either on empty stomach or with food. May titrate to 120mg qhs. Elderly: Start at low end of dosing range.

HOW SUPPLIED: Cap, Extended-Release: 80mg, 120mg

CONTRAINDICATIONS: Cardiogenic shock, sinus bradycardia, sick sinus syndrome and >1st-degree heart block (unless a permanent pacemaker is in place), bronchial asthma.

WARNINGS/PRECAUTIONS: Caution with congestive heart failure (CHF); may precipitate more severe failure. Hypersensitivity reactions and cutaneous reactions (eg, Stevens-Johnson syndrome [SJS]) reported. Caution with bronchospastic lung disease, hepatic or renal impairment, prolonged physical exertion, labile insulin-dependent diabetics, underlying skeletal muscle disease, and Wolff-Parkinson-White (WPW) syndrome and tachycardia. Avoid routine withdrawal before surgery. Exacerbation of myopathy and myotonia reported. May mask acute hypoglycemia and hyperthyroidism signs/symptoms. Abrupt withdrawal may exacerbate hyperthyroidism, including thyroid storm. May reduce intraocular pressure (IOP); may interfere with glaucoma screening test. May be more reactive to repeated challenge with history of severe anaphylactic reaction to variety of allergens; may be unresponsive to usual doses of epinephrine. Elevated serum K$^+$, transaminases and alkaline phosphatase observed. Elevated BUN reported in severe heart failure. Not for treatment of hypertensive emergencies. Caution in elderly.

ADVERSE REACTIONS: Fatigue, dizziness, constipation.

INTERACTIONS: Administration with CYP450 (CYP2D6, 1A2, 2C19) substrates, inhibitors or inducers may lead to relevant drug interactions. Increased levels and/or toxicity with CYP2D6 substrates/inhibitors (eg, fluoxetine, paroxetine, quinidine, ritonavir), CYP1A2 substrates/inhibitors (eg, imipramine, ciprofloxacin, fluvoxamine, isoniazid, theophylline, zileuton, zolmitriptan, rizatriptan), CYP2C19 substrates/inhibitors (eg, fluconazole, fluoxetine, fluvoxamine, teniposide, tolbutamide). Caution with drugs that slow down atrioventricular (AV) conduction (eg, digitalis, lidocaine, calcium channel blockers [CCBs]). Increased levels with nisoldipine, nicardipine, propafenone, cimetidine, and acute alcohol use. ACE inhibitors can cause hypotension. May antagonize clonidine effects; caution when withdrawing from clonidine. Potentiated by propafenone and amiodarone. Decreased levels with hepatic metabolism inducers (eg, rifampin, cigarette smoking). Decreased clearance of lidocaine, bupivacaine, mepivacaine, and theophylline. Caution with amide anesthetics. May prolong 1st dose hypotension with prazosin. Postural hypotension reported with terazosin, doxazosin, quinidine. May experience uncontrolled HTN with epinephrine. May reduce resting sympathetic nervous activity with catecholamine-depleting drugs (eg, reserpine). Methoxyflurane and trichloroethylene may depress myocardial contractility. Effects can be reversed by β-agonists (eg, dobutamine, isoproterenol). May exacerbate hypotensive effects of MAOIs or TCAs. Hypotension and cardiac arrest reported with haloperidol. May reduce efficacy with indomethacin and NSAIDs. May lower T3 levels with thyroxine. Increased levels of nifedipine, diazepam, zolmitriptan, rizatriptan, and thioridazine. Decreased levels with aluminum hydroxide gel, cholestyramine, colestipol, chronic alcohol use. Coadministration with chlorpromazine may increase levels of both drugs. Increased warfarin levels and PT. Decreased levels of lovastatin and pravastatin. May augment risks of general anesthesia. May be more difficult to adjust insulin dosage.

PREGNANCY: Category C, caution in nursing.

MECHANISM OF ACTION: Nonselective β-adrenergic receptor blocker; not established. Proposed to decrease cardiac output, inhibit renin release by the kidneys, and diminish tonic sympathetic nerve outflow from vasomotor centers in the brain.

PHARMACOKINETICS: Absorption: Almost complete; T_{max}=12-14 hrs (fasted). **Distribution:** V_d=4L; plasma protein binding (90%); found in breast milk. **Metabolism:** Liver (extensive); CYP2D6 (aromatic hydroxylation), CYP1A2, 2D6 (oxidation), CYP2C19, P-glycoprotein, N-dealkylation, glucuronidation. Propranolol glucuronide, naphthyloxylactic acid, and glucuronic acid and sulfate conjugates of 4-hydroxy propranolol (major metabolites). **Elimination:** $T_{1/2}$=8 hrs.

NURSING CONSIDERATIONS

Assessment: Assess for atherosclerotic heart disease, cardiogenic shock, sinus bradycardia, sick sinus syndrome, AV block, presence of pacemaker, bronchial asthma, CHF, bronchospastic lung disease, hepatic or renal impairment, prolonged physical exertion, underlying skeletal muscle disease, hyperthyroidism, diabetes, WPW syndrome, history of anaphylactic reactions, possible drug interactions, and pregnancy/nursing status. Obtain baseline vital signs, serum K⁺, transaminase, alkaline phosphatase, and thyroid function tests.

Monitoring: Monitor for signs/symptoms of cardiac failure, hypoglycemia, decreased IOP, thyrotoxicosis, myopathy, myotonia, withdrawal symptoms, hypersensitivity reactions, cutaneous reactions, and other adverse reactions. Monitor vital signs, serum K⁺, transaminase, alkaline phosphatase, LFTs, and renal/thyroid function tests.

Patient Counseling: Inform about risks and benefits of therapy. Instruct not to interrupt or d/c therapy without consulting physician. Advise to contact physician if symptoms of heart failure, withdrawal (angina), or hypersensitivity reactions occur. May interfere with glaucoma screening test.

Administration: Oral route. **Storage:** 25°C (77°F); excursions permitted to 15-30°C (59-86°F). Keep tightly closed.

INSPRA   RX
eplerenone (Pfizer)

THERAPEUTIC CLASS: Aldosterone blocker

INDICATIONS: Improve survival of stable patients with left ventricular systolic dysfunction and congestive heart failure (CHF) post-myocardial infarction (MI). Treatment of hypertension, alone or with other antihypertensives.

DOSAGE: *Adults:* CHF Post-MI: Initial: 25mg qd. Titrate: Increase to 50mg qd within 4 weeks. Maint: 50mg qd. Adjust dose based on K⁺ level: See table in PI. HTN: Initial: 50mg qd. May increase to 50mg bid if effect on BP is inadequate. Max: 100mg/day. With Moderate CYP3A4 Inhibitors: Initial: 25mg qd.

HOW SUPPLIED: Tab: 25mg, 50mg

CONTRAINDICATIONS: All Indications: Serum K⁺ >5.5mgEq/L at initiation, CrCl ≤30mL/min, concomitant potent CYP3A4 inhibitors (eg, ketoconazole, itraconazole, nefazodone, troleandomycin, clarithromycin, ritonavir, nelfinavir). When treating HTN: Type 2 diabetes with microalbuminuria, SrCr >2mg/dL (males) or >1.8mg/dL (females), CrCl <50mg/min, concomitant K⁺ supplements or K⁺-sparing diuretics (eg, amiloride, spironolactone, triamterene).

WARNINGS/PRECAUTIONS: Minimize risk of hyperkalemia (>5.5mEq/L) with proper patient selection and monitoring. Patients with CHF post-MI, with SrCr >2mg/dL (males) or >1.8mg/dL (females), CrCl ≤50mL/min, or are diabetic (especially those with proteinuria) should be treated cautiously. Increased risk of hyperkalemia with decreased renal function.

ADVERSE REACTIONS: Headache, dizziness, hyperkalemia, increased SrCr/TG/GGT, angina/MI, hypokalemia, diarrhea, coughing, fatigue, flu-like symptoms.

INTERACTIONS: See Contraindications. Increased levels with other CYP3A4 inhibitors (eg, erythromycin, verapamil, saquinavir, fluconazole). In HTN, use caution with ACE inhibitors and angiotensin II receptor antagonists; increased risk of hyperkalemia, especially with diabetics with microalbuminuria. Monitor lithium levels. Monitor antihypertensive effect with NSAIDs.

PREGNANCY: Category B, not for use in nursing.

MECHANISM OF ACTION: Aldosterone blocker; binds to mineralocorticoid receptor and blocks binding of aldosterone.

PHARMACOKINETICS: Absorption: Absolute bioavailability (69%); T_{max}=1.5 hrs. **Distribution:** V_d=43-90L; plasma protein binding (50%). **Metabolism:** CYP3A4. **Elimination:** Urine (67%, <5% unchanged), feces (32%, <5% unchanged); $T_{1/2}$=4-6 hrs.

NURSING CONSIDERATIONS

Assessment: Assess serum K⁺, SrCr. Assess for type 2 DM with microalbuminuria, proteinuria, impaired renal function, pregnancy/nursing status, and possible drug interactions.

Monitoring: Monitor serum K⁺, BP, and renal function tests periodically. Monitor for signs/symptoms of hyperkalemia and hypersensitivity reactions.

Patient Counseling: Advise against use of K⁺ supplements or salt substitutes containing K⁺, and strong CYP3A4 inhibitors. Advise to seek medical attention if symptoms of hyperkalemia, dizziness, diarrhea, vomiting, rapid or irregular heartbeat, lower extremity edema, difficulty breathing, or hypersensitivity reactions occur.

Administration: Oral route. **Storage:** 25°C (77°F); excursions permitted to 15-30°C (59-86°F).

INTEGRILIN   RX
eptifibatide (Merck)

THERAPEUTIC CLASS: Glycoprotein IIb/IIIa inhibitor

INDICATIONS: Treatment of acute coronary syndrome (ACS) (unstable angina/non-ST-segment elevation myocardial infarction), including patients being medically managed and those undergoing percutaneous coronary intervention (PCI), including intracoronary stenting.

DOSAGE: *Adults:* ACS: 180mcg/kg IV bolus, then 2mcg/kg/min IV infusion until discharge or initiation of coronary artery bypass graft (CABG) surgery, up to 72 hrs. If undergoing PCI, continue until discharge or for up to 18-24 hrs post-PCI, whichever comes 1st, allowing up to 96 hrs of therapy. Non-Dialysis with CrCl <50mL/min: 180mcg/kg IV bolus as soon as possible following diagnosis, immediately followed by 1mcg/kg/min IV infusion. PCI: 180mcg/kg IV bolus immediately before PCI, then 2mcg/kg/min IV infusion. Give 2nd bolus of 180mcg/kg 10 min after 1st bolus. Continue until discharge or for up to 18-24 hrs post-PCI, whichever comes 1st. A minimum of 12 hrs of infusion is recommended. Non-Dialysis with CrCl <50mL/min: 180mcg/kg IV bolus immediately before PCI, immediately followed by 1mcg/kg/min IV infusion. Give 2nd bolus of 180mcg/kg 10 min after 1st bolus. See PI for concomitant aspirin (ASA) and heparin doses and dosing charts by weight.

HOW SUPPLIED: Inj: 20mg [10mL]; 75mg, 200mg [100mL]

CONTRAINDICATIONS: Active abnormal bleeding, history of bleeding diathesis, or stroke within past 30 days. Severe HTN not adequately controlled on antihypertensives, major surgery within preceding 6 weeks, history of hemorrhagic stroke, current or planned concomitant parenteral glycoprotein IIb/IIIa inhibitor, renal dialysis dependency.

WARNINGS/PRECAUTIONS: Bleeding reported, mostly at arterial access site for cardiac catheterization, GI tract, or genitourinary tract. Caution in patients undergoing PCI; d/c infusion and heparin immediately if bleeding not controlled with pressure. Caution with renal dysfunction (CrCl <50mL/min). D/C infusion and heparin if acute profound thrombocytopenia occurs or platelet decreases to <100,000/mm³; monitor serial platelet counts, assess the drug-dependent antibodies, and treat as appropriate. Minimize arterial/venous puncture, IM inj, and the use of urinary catheters, nasotracheal intubation, and NG tubes. Avoid noncompressible sites (eg, subclavian or jugular veins) when obtaining IV access. Monitor Hct, Hgb, platelet counts, SrCr, and PT/aPTT before therapy (and activated clotting time [ACT] before PCI). Check aPTT/ACT prior to arterial sheath removal; do not remove unless aPTT is <45 sec or ACT <150 sec. If CrCl <50mL/min, d/c before CABG surgery.

ADVERSE REACTIONS: Bleeding (eg, intracranial hemorrhage, hematuria, hematemesis), thrombocytopenia, hypotension.

INTERACTIONS: See Contraindications. Caution with other drugs that affect hemostasis (eg, thrombolytics, oral anticoagulants, NSAIDs, dipyridamole). Cerebral, pulmonary, GI hemorrhage reported with ASA and heparin. Increased incidence of bleeding and transfusions with streptokinase; use with caution.

PREGNANCY: Category B, caution in nursing.

MECHANISM OF ACTION: Glycoprotein IIb/IIIa inhibitor; reversibly inhibits platelet aggregation by preventing the binding of fibrinogen, von Willebrand factor, and other adhesive ligands to GP IIb/IIIa.

PHARMACOKINETICS: Distribution: Plasma protein binding (25%). **Elimination:** Urine; T₁/₂=2.5 hrs.

NURSING CONSIDERATIONS

Assessment: Assess for drug hypersensitivity, history of bleeding diathesis or stroke, or active abnormal bleeding within previous 30 days, severe HTN, major surgery within the preceding 6 weeks, history of hemorrhagic stroke, dependency on renal dialysis, renal insufficiency, pregnancy/nursing status, and for possible drug interactions. Obtain baseline Hgb, Hct, platelet counts, SrCr, and PT/aPTT. In patients undergoing PCI, obtain baseline ACT.

Monitoring: Monitor for signs/symptoms of bleeding, thrombocytopenia, and hypersensitivity reactions. Monitor aPTT and ACT. Monitor platelets in patients with low platelet counts.

Patient Counseling: Inform about bleeding tendency and risks and benefits of therapy. Contact physician if signs of unusual bleeding develops.

Administration: IV route. Refer to PI for instructions for administration. **Storage:** 2-8°C (36-46°F). May store at 25°C (77°F) for ≤2 months with excursions permitted to 15-30°C (59-86°F). Protect from light. Discard any unused portion in the vial.

INTELENCE   RX
etravirine (Tibotec)

THERAPEUTIC CLASS: Non-nucleoside reverse transcriptase inhibitor

INDICATIONS: Treatment of HIV-1 infection in combination with other antiretrovirals, for antiretroviral treatment-experienced adult patients who have evidence of viral replication and HIV-1 strains resistant to a non-nucleoside reverse transcriptase inhibitor (NNRTI) and other antiretrovirals.

DOSAGE: *Adults:* Usual: 200mg (one 200mg tab or two 100mg tabs) bid pc.

HOW SUPPLIED: Tab: 100mg, 200mg

WARNINGS/PRECAUTIONS: Severe, potentially life-threatening, and fatal skin reactions (eg, erythema multiforme, toxic epidermal necrolysis, Stevens-Johnson syndrome), and hypersensitivity reactions reported; d/c immediately if this occurs and initiate appropriate therapy. Immune reconstitution syndrome and redistribution/accumulation of body fat reported. Risks and benefits have not been established in treatment naive adult patients. Caution in elderly.

ADVERSE REACTIONS: Rash, peripheral neuropathy.

INTERACTIONS: May alter therapeutic effect and adverse reaction profile with drugs that induce, inhibit, or are substrates of CYP3A, CYP2C9 and CYP2C19, or are transported by P-glycoprotein. Avoid with other NNRTIs, delavirdine, atazanavir (ATV) without low-dose ritonavir (RTV), ATV/RTV, fosamprenavir (FPV) without low-dose RTV, FPV/RTV, tipranavir/RTV, indinavir without low-dose RTV, nelfinavir without low-dose RTV, RTV (600mg bid), carbamazepine, phenobarbital, phenytoin, rifampin, rifapentine, and St. John's wort. Caution with digoxin; use lowest dose initially. May increase levels of nelfinavir without RTV, digoxin, warfarin (monitor INR), anticoagulants, 14-OH-clarithromycin, diazepam, and fluvastatin. May increase maraviroc levels in the presence of a potent CYP3A inhibitor (eg, RTV boosted protease inhibitor). May decrease levels of maraviroc, antiarrhythmics, clarithromycin, rifabutin, systemic dexamethasone, atorvastatin, lovastatin, simvastatin, immunosuppressant, and clopidogrel (active) metabolite. Fluconazole, omeprazole, voriconazole, itraconazole or ketoconazole, clarithromycin may increase levels. Efavirenz, nevirapine, ranitidine, darunavir/RTV, lopinavir/RTV, saquinavir/RTV, rifabutin, tenofovir disoproxil fumarate may decrease levels. Consider alternatives to clarithromycin such as azithromycin for treatment of *Mycobacterium avium* complex. Monitor for withdrawal symptoms when coadministered with methadone, buprenorphine, buprenorphine/naloxone. May need to alter sildenafil dose.

PREGNANCY: Category B, not for use in nursing.

MECHANISM OF ACTION: Non-nucleoside reverse transcriptase inhibitor of HIV-1; binds directly to reverse transcriptase and blocks the RNA-dependent and DNA-dependent DNA polymerase activities by causing a disruption of the enzyme's catalytic site.

PHARMACOKINETICS: Absorption: T_{max}=2.5-4 hrs. **Distribution:** Plasma protein binding (99.9%). **Metabolism:** Liver via CYP3A, CYP2C9, and CYP2C19; (methyl hydroxylation). **Elimination:** Feces (93.7%); urine (1.2%); $T_{1/2}$=41 hrs.

NURSING CONSIDERATIONS

Assessment: Assess treatment history, pregnancy/nursing status, and possible drug interactions. Perform resistance testing where possible.

Monitoring: Monitor for signs/symptoms of severe skin/hypersensitivity reactions, body fat redistribution/accumulation, immune reconstitution syndrome (eg, opportunistic infections), and other adverse reactions. Monitor clinical status including liver transaminases.

Patient Counseling: Inform that product is not a cure for HIV; opportunistic infections may still occur. Inform that therapy does not reduce risk of HIV transmission to others; take precaution to avoid transmission (eg, safe sex practices). Advise to take medication following a meal bid ud. Instruct to always use with other antiretrovirals. Advise not to alter dose or d/c therapy without consultation. If a dose is missed within 6 hrs of time usually taken, take as soon as possible with a meal; if scheduled time exceeds 6 hrs, do not take missed dose; resume normal dosing schedule.

Advise to report use of other Rx, OTC, or herbal products (eg, St. John's wort). Counsel to d/c and notify physician if severe rash develops. Advise that redistribution or accumulation of body fat may occur. Instruct mothers to avoid nursing to reduce risk of HIV transmission.

Administration: Oral route. Tabs may be dispersed in glass of water if unable to swallow tab whole. Stir and drink immediately once dispersed. Rinse glass several times, with each rinse completely swallowed to ensure entire dose is consumed. **Storage:** 25°C (77°F); excursions permitted to 15-30°C (59-86°F). Store in the original bottle. Protect from moisture.

INTRON A   RX
interferon alfa-2b (Schering)

May cause or aggravate fatal or life-threatening neuropsychiatric, autoimmune, ischemic, and infectious disorders. Monitor closely with periodic clinical and laboratory evaluations. D/C with severe or worsening signs/symptoms of these conditions.

THERAPEUTIC CLASS: Biological response modifier

INDICATIONS: Treatment of hairy cell leukemia in patients ≥18 yrs. Adjuvant to surgical treatment in patients ≥18 yrs with malignant melanoma who are free of disease but at high risk for systemic recurrence, within 56 days of surgery. Initial treatment of clinically aggressive follicular non-Hodgkin's lymphoma with anthracycline-containing combination chemotherapy in patients ≥18 yrs. Treatment of AIDS-related Kaposi's sarcoma and intralesional treatment of condylomata acuminata involving external surfaces of the genital and perianal areas in selected patients ≥18 yrs. Treatment of chronic hepatitis C with compensated liver disease who have a history of blood or blood-product exposure and/or are HCV antibody positive in patients ≥18 yrs. Treatment of chronic hepatitis C with compensated liver disease in patients ≥3 yrs previously untreated with alfa-interferon therapy, and in patients ≥18 yrs who have relapsed following alfa-interferon therapy, in combination with ribavirin; refer to ribavirin PI. Treatment of chronic hepatitis B in patients ≥1 yr with compensated liver disease and those who are serum HBsAg positive for ≥6 months and have evidence of HBV replication with elevated serum ALT.

DOSAGE: *Adults:* ≥18 yrs: Hairy Cell Leukemia: 2 MIU/m² IM/SQ 3X/week up to 6 months. Malignant Melanoma: Induction: 20 MIU/m² IV, over 20 min, 5 consecutive days/week for 4 weeks. Maint: 10 MIU/m² SQ 3X/week for 48 weeks. Follicular Lymphoma: 5 MIU SQ 3X/week for up to 18 months. Condylomata Acuminata: 1 MIU/lesion 3X/week alternating days for 3 weeks. Max: 5 lesions/course. An additional course may be administered at 12-16 weeks. Kaposi's Sarcoma: 30 MIU/m²/dose IM/SQ 3X/week until disease progression or maximal response has been achieved after 16 weeks of treatment. Hepatitis C: 3 MIU IM/SQ 3X/week for 18-24 months. Hepatitis B: 5 MIU IM/SQ qd or 10 MIU IM/SQ 3X/week for 16 weeks. Refer to PI for dose adjustments, route of administration and dosage forms/strengths selection for each indication. *Pediatrics:* ≥3 yrs: Hepatitis C: 3 MIU IM/SQ 3X/week for 18-24 months. ≥1 yr: Hepatitis B: 3 MIU/m² SQ 3X/week for 1 week, then 6 MIU/m² SQ 3X/week for total therapy of 16-24 weeks. Max: 10 MIU/m² 3X/week. Refer to PI for dose adjustments, route of administration and dosage forms/strengths selection for each indication.

HOW SUPPLIED: Inj: 18 MIU, 30 MIU, 60 MIU [pen]; 10 MIU, 18 MIU, 50 MIU [powder]; 18 MIU, 25 MIU [vial]

CONTRAINDICATIONS: Autoimmune hepatitis, decompensated liver disease. When used with Rebetol, refer to PI for additional contraindications.

WARNINGS/PRECAUTIONS: Caution with coagulation disorders, severe myelosuppression, debilitating conditions (eg, pulmonary disease, diabetes mellitus [DM] prone to ketoacidosis). Caution with history of cardiovascular disease (CVD); monitor closely. Supraventricular arrhythmias, ischemic and hemorrhagic cerebrovascular events reported. Neuropsychiatric events reported; caution with history of psychiatric disorders. Monitor patients during treatment and in 6-month follow-up period if psychiatric problems develop; d/c therapy if symptoms persist or worsen. Obtundation, coma, and encephalopathy may occur in elderly treated with higher doses. May suppress bone marrow function; d/c if severe decreases in neutrophil or platelet counts occur. Ophthalmology disorders may be induced or aggravated; conduct baseline eye exam and monitor periodically with preexisting disorders. D/C if new or worsening ophthalmologic disorders occur. Thyroid abnormalities and DM reported; d/c therapy if conditions develop and cannot be normalized by medication. Hepatotoxicity, pulmonary, and autoimmune disorders reported; monitor or d/c therapy if appropriate. Avoid in patients with history of autoimmune disease or immunosuppressed transplant recipients. Pulmonary disorders may be induced or aggravated; obtain chest x-ray if respiratory symptoms develop. The powder formulation contains albumin; carries an extremely remote risk for transmission of viral diseases and Creutzfeldt-Jakob disease. Should not be used with rapidly progressive visceral disease. Peripheral neuropathy reported when used in combination with telbivudine. May cause birth defects and/or death of unborn child and hemolytic anemia when used in combination with ribavirin. Acute serious hypersensitivity reactions may occur; d/c immediately if it occurs. New onset or exacerbated psoriasis or sarcoidosis, and hypertriglyceridemia reported. D/C if persistently elevated TG associated with symptoms of potential pancreatitis occurs. Do not interchange brands. Caution in elderly.

ADVERSE REACTIONS: Flu-like symptoms, fatigue, fever, neutropenia, abnormal granulocyte count, myalgia, anorexia, decreased WBC count, N/V, asthenia, increased AST, headache, chills, GI disorders.

INTERACTIONS: May increase levels of theophylline. Caution with myelosuppressive agents (eg, zidovudine). Higher incidence of neutropenia with zidovudine.

PREGNANCY: Category C, Category X (with ribavirin), not for use in nursing.

MECHANISM OF ACTION: α-Interferon; binds to specific membrane receptors on cell surface initiating induction of enzymes, suppression of cell proliferation, immunomodulating activities, and inhibition of virus replication.

PHARMACOKINETICS: Absorption: (IM/SQ) C_{max}=18-116 IU/mL, T_{max}=3-12 hrs; (IV) C_{max}=135-273 IU/mL. **Elimination:** (IM/SQ) $T_{1/2}$=2-3 hrs; (IV) $T_{1/2}$=2 hrs.

NURSING CONSIDERATIONS

Assessment: Assess for history of psychiatric disorders, CVD, autoimmune and ophthalmologic disorders, hepatic/renal impairment, hypersensitivity reactions, pregnancy/nursing status, possible drug interactions, or any other condition where treatment is contraindicated or cautioned. Obtain baseline CBC, blood chemistry, and eye exam. Perform ECG in patients with preexisting cardiac abnormalities. Perform liver biopsy and test for presence of HCV antibody.

Monitoring: Monitor for CVD, bone marrow toxicity, neuropsychiatric, cerebrovascular, ocular, endocrine, gastrointestinal, pulmonary, or autoimmune disorders. Monitor for hypersensitivity reactions, psoriasis, sarcoidosis, renal/hepatic dysfunction. Closely monitor patients with history of MI or arrhythmic disorder, liver/pulmonary function abnormalities, WBC in myelosuppressed patients. Monitor LFTs, PT, alkaline phosphatase, albumin and bilirubin levels periodically and at approximately 2-week intervals during ALT flare. Monitor serum TSH, TG, electrolytes, ECG, chest x-ray periodically. Repeat CBC and platelet count 1-2 weeks after initiation of therapy, and monthly thereafter. Evaluate serum ALT at approximately 3-month intervals. Repeat TSH testing at 3 and 6 months during therapy. Evaluate HBeAg, HBsAg, and ALT at the end of therapy, then at 3 and 6 months post-therapy. Perform periodic ophthalmologic exams with those who develop ocular symptoms and with preexisting ophthalmologic disorders.

Patient Counseling: Inform of risks and benefits associated with treatment. Instruct on proper use of product. Advise to seek medical attention for symptoms of depression, cardiovascular, ophthalmologic toxicity, pancreatitis or colitis, and cytopenias (eg, high persistent fevers, bruising, dyspnea). Keep well-hydrated. Inform that use of antipyretic may ameliorate some of the flu-like symptoms. Instruct self-administering patients on the proper disposal of needles and syringes and caution against reuse. In combination with Ribavirin: Inform of the risks to fetus; instruct female patients and female partners of male patients to use 2 forms of birth control during treatment and for 6 months after therapy is d/c. Instruct to brush teeth bid and have regular dental examinations when used in combination with ribavirin.

Administration: IM, SQ, IV, and intralesional route. Refer to Medication Guide for proper administration. **Storage:** 2-8°C (36-46°F). (Powder) Use immediately after reconstitution; may store up to 24 hrs at 2-8°C (36-46°F). (Sol for Inj/Sol for Inj in Multidose Pens) Do not freeze. Keep away from heat.

INTUNIV   RX
guanfacine (Shire)

THERAPEUTIC CLASS: Alpha$_{2A}$-agonist

INDICATIONS: Treatment of attention-deficit hyperactivity disorder (ADHD) as monotherapy and as adjunctive therapy to stimulant medications.

DOSAGE: *Pediatrics:* 6-17 yrs: Monotherapy/Adjunctive Therapy: Initial: 1mg qd. Titrate: Adjust in increments of ≤1mg/week. Maint: 1-4mg qd for 9 weeks based on clinical response and tolerability. Range: (Monotherapy) 0.05-0.08mg/kg qd; if well tolerated, doses up to 0.12mg/kg qd may provide additional benefit. Max: 4mg/day. (Adjunctive Therapy) 0.05-0.12mg/kg/day. Switching from Immediate-Release: D/C immediate-release, and titrate with extended-release according to the recommended schedule. D/C: Taper in decrements of ≤1mg q3-7 days. Refer to PI for dosage reinitiation and adjustment.

HOW SUPPLIED: Tab, Extended-Release: 1mg, 2mg, 3mg, 4mg

WARNINGS/PRECAUTIONS: Hypotension, bradycardia, syncope, somnolence, and sedation reported. Caution with history of hypotension, heart block, bradycardia, cardiovascular disease (CVD), and syncope or condition(s) that predispose to syncope (eg, orthostatic hypotension, dehydration). Not intended for use in patients who exhibit symptoms secondary to environmental factors and/or other primary psychiatric disorders, including psychosis. May impair mental/physical abilities.

ADVERSE REACTIONS: Hypotension, decreased appetite, somnolence/sedation, headache, fatigue, abdominal pain, nausea, lethargy, dizziness, irritability, dry mouth, constipation.

INTERACTIONS: CYP3A4 inducers (eg, rifampin) may decrease exposure; consider increasing guanfacine dose. May increase valproic acid concentrations; adjust dose of valproic acid. Additive effects with antihypertensives and CNS depressants (eg, sedative/hypnotics, benzodiazepines, barbiturates, phenothiazines, antipsychotics); caution during coadministration. Use with caution with other antihypertensives or other drugs that reduce BP or HR or increase risk of syncope. Avoid with alcohol. Caution with ketoconazole or other strong CYP3A4/5 inhibitors. Avoid with other guanfacine-containing products. Increased exposure and C_{max} with lisdexamfetamine dimesylate.

PREGNANCY: Category B, caution in nursing.

MECHANISM OF ACTION: Alpha$_{2A}$-adrenergic agonist; mechanism not established in ADHD. Reduces sympathetic nerve impulses from the vasomotor center to the heart and blood vessels, resulting in decreased peripheral vascular resistance and reduction in HR.

PHARMACOKINETICS: Absorption: Children (6-12 yrs): C_{max}=10ng/mL; AUC=162ng•hr/mL. Adolescents (13-17 yrs): C_{max}=7ng/mL; AUC=116ng•hr/mL. **Pediatrics:** T_{max}=5 hrs. **Distribution:** Plasma protein binding (70%). **Metabolism:** CYP3A4. **Elimination:** $T_{1/2}$=18 hrs (adults).

NURSING CONSIDERATIONS

Assessment: Assess HR and BP. Assess for history of hypotension, bradycardia, heart block, CVD, syncope, and hypersensitivity to drug, renal/hepatic impairment, pregnancy/nursing status, and possible drug interactions.

Monitoring: Monitor HR and BP following dose increases and periodically while on therapy. Monitor for orthostatic hypotension, syncope, somnolence, and sedation.

Patient Counseling: Instruct to swallow tab whole with water, milk, or other liquid; do not crush, chew, or break before swallowing. Inform that taking drug with high-fat meal raises blood levels. Instruct caregiver to supervise the child or adolescent taking the therapy. Inform of the adverse reactions that may occur. Caution against operating heavy equipment or driving. Advise to avoid becoming dehydrated or overheated, and to avoid use with alcohol.

Administration: Oral route. Do not crush, chew, or break tabs before swallowing. Avoid with high-fat meals. **Storage:** 25°C (77°F); excursions permitted to 15-30°C (59-86°F).

INVANZ   RX
ertapenem (Merck)

THERAPEUTIC CLASS: Carbapenem

INDICATIONS: Treatment of complicated intra-abdominal infections, complicated skin and skin structure infections (cSSSI) including diabetic foot infections without osteomyelitis, complicated urinary tract infections (UTI) including pyelonephritis, community-acquired pneumonia (CAP), and acute pelvic infections including postpartum endomyometritis, septic abortion, and postsurgical gynecologic infections caused by susceptible isolates of microorganisms. Prevention of surgical-site infection in adults following elective colorectal surgery.

DOSAGE: *Adults:* 1g IM/IV qd. Infuse IV over 30min. Duration: Complicated Intra-Abdominal Infections: 5-14 days. cSSSI: 7-14 days. Diabetic Foot: ≤28 days. CAP/Complicated UTI: 10-14 days. Acute Pelvic Infections: 3-10 days. Max Duration: IV: 14 days. IM: 7 days. Prophylaxis Following Colorectal Surgery: 1g IV single dose given 1 hr prior to surgical incision. Hemodialysis/CrCl ≤30mL/min/1.73m^2: 500mg IM/IV qd; give 150mg IM/IV if 500mg IM/IV was administered within 6 hours prior to hemodialysis.
Pediatrics: ≥13 years: 1g IM/IV qd. 3 months-12 yrs: 15mg/kg IV/IM bid. Max: 1g/day. Infuse IV over 30min. Duration: Complicated Intra-Abdominal Infections: 5-14 days. cSSSI: 7-14 days. Diabetic Foot: ≤28 days. CAP/Complicated UTI: 10-14 days. Acute Pelvic Infections: 3-10 days. Max Duration: IV: 14 days. IM: 7 days.

HOW SUPPLIED: Inj: 1g

CONTRAINDICATIONS: (IM) Hypersensitivity to amide-type local anesthetics (when using lidocaine HCl diluent).

WARNINGS/PRECAUTIONS: Serious and occasionally fatal hypersensitivity (anaphylactic) reactions reported. D/C immediately if an allergic reaction occurs. Seizures and other CNS adverse experiences reported, most commonly in patients with CNS disorders and/or compromised renal function. If focal tremors, myoclonus, or seizures occur, evaluate and treat as needed; may need to reduce dose or d/c therapy. *Clostridium difficile*-associated diarrhea (CDAD) reported. Caution with IM administration; avoid inadvertent inj into a blood vessel. May result in bacterial resistance with prolonged use or use in the absence of a proven/suspected bacterial infection, or a prophylactic indication; take appropriate measures if superinfection develops. Periodically assess organ system function (eg, renal, hepatic, and hematopoietic) during prolonged therapy. Caution in elderly. Not recommended in infants <3 months and for the treatment of meningitis in pediatrics.

ADVERSE REACTIONS: Diarrhea, infused vein complication, N/V, anemia, headache, edema/swelling, fever, abdominal pain, constipation, altered mental status, insomnia, vaginitis, ALT/AST increase.

INTERACTIONS: Increased plasma levels with concomitant probenecid use; coadministration not recommended. May decrease serum levels of valproic acid or divalproex sodium; increased risk of breakthrough seizures. Concomitant use not recommended, but if necessary, consider supplemental anticonvulsant therapy.

PREGNANCY: Category B, caution in nursing.

MECHANISM OF ACTION: Carbapenem; bactericidal activity results from the inhibition of cell wall synthesis and is mediated through binding to penicillin (PCN)-binding proteins.

PHARMACOKINETICS: Absorption: (IM) Almost complete; bioavailability (90%); T_{max}=2.3 hrs. **Distribution:** V_d=0.12L/kg (adults), 0.16L/kg (13-17 yrs), 0.2L/kg (3 months-12 yrs); plasma protein binding (85%-95%); found in breast milk. **Metabolism:** Hydrolysis of the β-lactam ring; inactive ring-opened derivative (major metabolite). **Elimination:** (IV) Urine (80%, 38% unchanged, 37% metabolite), feces (10%); $T_{1/2}$=4 hrs (adults, 13-17 yrs), 2.5 hrs (3 months-12 yrs).

NURSING CONSIDERATIONS

Assessment: Assess for hypersensitivity reactions to PCNs, cephalosporins, other β-lactams, amide type local anesthetics and other allergens, CNS disorders, renal impairment, pregnancy/nursing status, and possible drug interactions.

Monitoring: Monitor for anaphylactoid or hypersensitivity reactions, CDAD, superinfections, CNS disorders, seizures, drug toxicity, and other adverse reactions. Monitor organ system function including renal, hepatic, hematopoietic function periodically during prolonged therapy.

Patient Counseling: Advise that serious allergic reactions could occur and may require immediate treatment. Advise to report any previous hypersensitivity reactions to the medication, other β-lactams, or other allergens. Counsel to inform physician if taking valproic acid or divalproex sodium. Instruct to use ud; inform that skipping doses or not completing full course may decrease effectiveness and increase resistance. Inform that diarrhea may occur, even as late as ≥2 months after last dose of therapy; notify physician as soon as possible if watery/bloody stools (with or without stomach cramps and fever) occur.

Administration: IV/IM route. Do not mix or coinfuse with other medications. Do not use diluents containing dextrose (α-D-glucose). Refer to PI for reconstitution and administration instructions.
Storage: Before Reconstitution: Do not store >25°C (77°F). Reconstituted and Infusion Sol: 25°C and used within 6 hrs, or under refrigeration (5°C) for 24 hrs and used within 4 hrs after removal from refrigeration. Do not freeze sol.

INVEGA   RX
paliperidone (Janssen)

> Elderly patients with dementia-related psychosis treated with antipsychotic drugs are at an increased risk of death; most deaths appeared to be cardiovascular (CV) (eg, heart failure, sudden death) or infectious (eg, pneumonia) in nature. Not approved for the treatment of patients with dementia-related psychosis.

THERAPEUTIC CLASS: Benzisoxazole derivative

INDICATIONS: Treatment of schizophrenia in adults and adolescents. Treatment of schizoaffective disorder as monotherapy and an adjunct to mood stabilizers and/or antidepressant therapy in adults.

DOSAGE: *Adults:* Schizophrenia: 6mg qd. Titrate: If indicated may increase by 3mg/day; dose increases >6mg/day should be made at intervals >5 days. Usual: 3-12mg/day. Max: 12mg/day. Schizoaffective Disorder: 6mg qd. Titrate: If indicated may increase by 3mg/day at intervals of >4 days. Usual: 3-12mg/day. Max: 12mg/day. Renal Impairment: Individualize dose. CrCl ≥50-<80mL/min: Initial: 3mg qd. Max: 6mg qd. CrCl ≥10-<50mL/min: Initial: 1.5mg qd. Max: 3mg qd. Elderly: Adjust dose according to renal function.
Pediatrics: 12-17 yrs: Schizophrenia: Initial: 3mg qd. Titrate: If indicated may increase by 3mg/day at intervals of >5 days. Max: <51kg: 6mg/day. ≥51kg: 12mg/day.

HOW SUPPLIED: Tab, Extended-Release: 1.5mg, 3mg, 6mg, 9mg

WARNINGS/PRECAUTIONS: Neuroleptic malignant syndrome (NMS) and tardive dyskinesia (TD) reported; d/c if these occur. May increase QTc interval; avoid with congenital long QT syndrome and history of cardiac arrhythmias. Hyperglycemia and diabetes mellitus (DM), in some cases extreme and associated with ketoacidosis or hyperosmolar coma or death reported;

monitor for hyperglycemia and perform fasting blood glucose testing at the beginning of therapy, and periodically in patients at risk for DM. Undesirable alterations in lipids and weight gain reported. May elevate prolactin levels. Avoid with preexisting severe GI narrowing. May induce orthostatic hypotension and syncope; caution with known CV disease, cerebrovascular disease, or conditions that predispose to hypotension. Leukopenia, neutropenia, and agranulocytosis reported; d/c in cases of severe neutropenia (absolute neutrophil count <1000/mm³). Somnolence reported. May impair mental/physical abilities. Seizures reported; caution with history of seizures or conditions that lower the seizure threshold. May cause esophageal dysmotility and aspiration; caution with risk of aspiration pneumonia. May induce priapism; severe cases may require surgical intervention. May disrupt body's ability to reduce core body temperature; caution with conditions that may contribute to an elevated core body temperature. May have an antiemetic effect that may mask signs/symptoms of overdosage with certain drugs or of conditions (eg, intestinal obstruction, Reye's syndrome, brain tumor). Patients with Parkinson's disease or dementia with Lewy bodies may have increased sensitivity to therapy. Caution with suicidal tendencies, renal impairment, and in elderly. Not recommended with CrCl <10mL/min.

ADVERSE REACTIONS: Extrapyramidal symptoms, tachycardia, somnolence, akathisia, dyskinesia, dyspepsia, dizziness, nasopharyngitis, headache, nausea, hyperkinesia, constipation, weight gain, parkinsonism, tremors.

INTERACTIONS: Consider additive exposure with risperidone. Avoid with other drugs known to prolong QTc interval, including Class 1A (eg, quinidine, procainamide) or Class III (eg, amiodarone, sotalol) antiarrhythmics, antipsychotics (eg, chlorpromazine, thioridazine), and antibiotics (eg, gatifloxacin, moxifloxacin). Caution with other centrally acting drugs, alcohol, and drugs with anticholinergic activity. May antagonize the effect of levodopa and other dopamine agonists. Additive effect may be observed with other agents that cause orthostatic hypotension. Carbamazepine may decrease levels. Paroxetine (a potent CYP2D6 inhibitor) may increase exposure in CYP2D6 extensive metabolizers. Divalproex sodium may increase levels; consider dose reduction with valproate.

PREGNANCY: Category C, not for use in nursing.

MECHANISM OF ACTION: Benzisoxazole derivative; not established. Proposed to be mediated through a combination of central dopamine type 2 (D_2) and serotonin type 2 ($5HT_{2A}$) receptor antagonism.

PHARMACOKINETICS: Absorption: Absolute bioavailability (28%); T_{max}=24 hrs. **Distribution**: Plasma protein binding (74%); V_d=487L; found in breast milk. **Metabolism**: CYP2D6, 3A4 (limited); (immediate-release) dealkylation, hydroxylation, dehydrogenation, and benzisoxazole scission. **Elimination**: (Immediate-release) Urine (80%; 59% unchanged), feces (11%); $T_{1/2}$=23 hrs.

NURSING CONSIDERATIONS

Assessment: Assess for dementia-related psychosis, congenital long QT syndrome, history of cardiac arrhythmias, DM, risk factors for DM, severe GI narrowing, history of clinically significant low WBCs or drug-induced leukopenia/neutropenia, Parkinson's disease, dementia with Lewy bodies, other conditions where treatment is contraindicated or cautioned, renal impairment, pregnancy/nursing status, and possible drug interactions. Obtain baseline FPG in patients at risk for DM.

Monitoring: Monitor for NMS, TD, QT prolongation, hyperprolactinemia, orthostatic hypotension, syncope, cognitive and motor impairment, seizures, esophageal dysmotility, aspiration, priapism, and disruption of body temperature. Monitor for signs of hyperglycemia; perform periodic monitoring of FPG levels in patients with DM or at risk for DM. Monitor for signs/symptoms of leukopenia/neutropenia; perform frequent monitoring of CBC in patients with history of clinically significant low WBC or drug-induced leukopenia/neutropenia. Monitor weight and renal function.

Patient Counseling: Inform of the risk of orthostatic hypotension during initiation/reinitiation or dose increases. Inform that therapy has the potential to impair judgment, thinking, or motor skills; advise to use caution when operating hazardous machinery (eg, automobiles). Advise to avoid alcohol during therapy. Instruct to notify physician of all prescription and nonprescription drugs currently taking, and if pregnant, intending to become pregnant, or breastfeeding. Counsel on appropriate care in avoiding overheating and dehydration. Inform that medication must be swallowed whole with liquids; advise not to chew, divide, or crush. Advise that tab shell, along with insoluble core components, may be found in stool.

Administration: Oral route. Swallow whole with liquids; do not crush, divide, or chew. **Storage**: Up to 25°C (77°F); excursions permitted to 15-30°C (59-86°F). Protect from moisture.

INVEGA SUSTENNA

RX

paliperidone palmitate (Janssen)

> Elderly patients with dementia-related psychosis treated with antipsychotic drugs are at an increased risk of death; most deaths appeared to be cardiovascular (CV) (eg, heart failure, sudden death) or infectious (eg, pneumonia) in nature. Not approved for the treatment of patients with dementia-related psychosis.

THERAPEUTIC CLASS: Benzisoxazole derivative

INDICATIONS: Acute and maintenance treatment of schizophrenia in adults.

DOSAGE: *Adults:* Initial: 234mg IM on Day 1, then 156mg 1 week later (in deltoid muscle). Maint: 117mg/month (in deltoid or gluteal muscle). Range: 39-234mg based on tolerability and/or efficacy. Adjust dose monthly. Reassess periodically to determine need for continued treatment. Mild Renal Impairment (CrCl ≥50-<80mL/min)/Elderly with Decreased Renal Function: Initial: 156mg IM on Day 1, then 117mg 1 week later (in deltoid muscle). Maint: 78mg/month (in deltoid or gluteal muscle). Switching from Oral Antipsychotics: D/C oral antipsychotics when initiating IM therapy. See PI for conversion. Switching from Long-Acting Injectable Antipsychotics: Initiate treatment in place of the next scheduled inj and continue at monthly intervals. Reevaluate periodically. Refer to PI for instructions on missed doses.

HOW SUPPLIED: Inj, Extended-Release: 39mg, 78mg, 117mg, 156mg, 234mg

WARNINGS/PRECAUTIONS: Neuroleptic malignant syndrome (NMS) and tardive dyskinesia (TD) reported; d/c if these occur. May increase QTc interval; avoid with congenital long QT syndrome and history of cardiac arrhythmias. Hyperglycemia and diabetes mellitus (DM), in some cases extreme and associated with ketoacidosis or hyperosmolar coma or death, reported; monitor for hyperglycemia and perform FPG testing at the beginning of therapy, and periodically in patients at risk for DM. Undesirable alterations in lipids and weight gain reported. May elevate prolactin levels. May induce orthostatic hypotension and syncope; caution with known CV disease, cerebrovascular disease, or conditions that predispose to hypotension. Leukopenia, neutropenia, and agranulocytosis reported; d/c in cases of severe neutropenia (absolute neutrophil count <1000/mm³). Somnolence, sedation, and dizziness reported. May impair mental/physical abilities. Seizures reported; caution with history of seizures or conditions that lower the seizure threshold. May cause esophageal dysmotility and aspiration; caution with risk of aspiration pneumonia. May induce priapism; severe cases may require surgical intervention. May disrupt body's ability to reduce core body temperature; caution with conditions that may contribute to an elevated core body temperature. May have an antiemetic effect that may mask signs/symptoms of overdosage with certain drugs or of conditions (eg, intestinal obstruction, Reye's syndrome, brain tumor). Patients with Parkinson's disease or dementia with Lewy bodies may have increased sensitivity to therapy. Caution with suicidal tendencies, renal impairment, and in elderly. Not recommended with CrCl <50mL/min. Intended for IM inj; avoid inadvertent inj into a blood vessel.

ADVERSE REACTIONS: Upper abdominal pain, constipation, N/V, inj-site reactions, nasopharyngitis, weight gain, dizziness, akathisia, extrapyramidal disorder, headache, somnolence/sedation, agitation, anxiety, insomnia.

INTERACTIONS: Caution with other centrally acting drugs and alcohol. May antagonize the effect of levodopa and other dopamine agonists. An additive effect may be observed with other agents that cause orthostatic hypotension. Avoid with other drugs known to prolong QTc interval, including Class 1A (eg, quinidine, procainamide) or Class III (eg, amiodarone, sotalol) antiarrhythmics, antipsychotics (eg, chlorpromazine, thioridazine), or antibiotics (eg, gatifloxacin, moxifloxacin). Carbamazepine may decrease levels. Additive exposure with oral paliperidone or oral or injectable risperidone. Caution with anticholinergics; may contribute to an elevated body temperature. Paroxetine (a potent CYP2D6 inhibitor) may increase exposure in CYP2D6 extensive metabolizers.

PREGNANCY: Category C, not for use in nursing.

MECHANISM OF ACTION: Benzisoxazole derivative; not established. Proposed to be mediated through a combination of central dopamine Type 2 (D_2) and serotonin Type 2 ($5HT_{2A}$) receptor antagonism.

PHARMACOKINETICS: Absorption: T_{max}=13 days. **Distribution:** V_d=391L; plasma protein binding (74%); found in breast milk. **Metabolism:** Dealkylation, hydroxylation, dehydrogenation, and benzisoxazole scission; CYP2D6, 3A4 (limited). **Elimination:** (39-234mg IM single-dose) $T_{1/2}$=25-49 days.

NURSING CONSIDERATIONS

Assessment: Assess for dementia-related psychosis, congenital long QT syndrome, history of cardiac arrhythmias, DM, risk factors for DM, history of clinically significant low WBCs or drug-induced leukopenia/neutropenia, Parkinson's disease, dementia with Lewy bodies, or conditions where treatment is contraindicated or cautioned, renal impairment, pregnancy/nursing status, and possible drug interactions. Obtain baseline FPG in patients at risk for DM.

Monitoring: Monitor for NMS, TD, QT prolongation, hyperprolactinemia, orthostatic hypotension, syncope, cognitive and motor impairment, seizures, aspiration, priapism, and disruption of body temperature. Monitor for signs of hyperglycemia; perform periodic monitoring of FPG levels in patients with DM or at risk for DM. Monitor for signs/symptoms of leukopenia/neutropenia; perform frequent monitoring of CBC in patients with history of clinically significant low WBC or drug-induced leukopenia/neutropenia. Monitor weight and renal function.

Patient Counseling: Advise patients on risk of orthostatic hypotension. Caution about operating machinery/driving. Avoid concomitant use of alcohol. Advise to avoid overheating and becoming dehydrated. Instruct to inform physician about any concomitant medications. Advise to notify physician if become pregnant or intend to become pregnant. Instruct not to breastfeed.

Administration: IM route. Inject slowly, deep into muscle. Avoid inadvertent inj into a blood vessel. Do not administer dose in divided inj. Refer to PI for proper instructions for use. **Storage:** 25°C (77°F); excursions permitted to 15-30°C (59-86°F).

INVIRASE   RX
saquinavir mesylate (Roche Labs)

THERAPEUTIC CLASS: Protease inhibitor

INDICATIONS: Treatment of HIV-1 infection in combination with ritonavir and other antiretroviral agents in adults >16 yrs.

DOSAGE: *Adults:* >16 yrs: Combination Therapy with Ritonavir 100mg BID: 1000mg bid within 2 hrs after a meal. Combination Therapy with Lopinavir/Ritonavir (400/100mg): 1000mg bid (with no additional ritonavir).

HOW SUPPLIED: Cap: 200mg; Tab: 500mg

CONTRAINDICATIONS: Congenital long QT syndrome, refractory hypokalemia or hypomagnesemia, complete atrioventricular (AV) block without implanted pacemakers, severe hepatic impairment, in patients at high risk of complete AV block, and with drugs that both increase saquinavir plasma concentrations and prolong the QT interval. Coadministration with CYP3A substrates for which increased plasma concentrations may result in serious and/or life-threatening reactions (eg, alfuzosin, amiodarone, bepridil, dofetilide, flecainide, lidocaine [systemic], propafenone, quinidine, trazodone, rifampin, dihydroergotamine, ergonovine, ergotamine, methylergonovine, cisapride, lovastatin, simvastatin, pimozide, sildenafil [for treatment of pulmonary arterial HTN], triazolam, orally administered midazolam).

WARNINGS/PRECAUTIONS: Refer to the individual monograph of ritonavir. Interrupt therapy if serious or severe toxicity occurs until etiology identified or toxicity resolves. May prolong PR and QT intervals in a dose-dependent fashion. 2nd-or 3rd-degree AV block and torsade de pointes reported. Monitor ECG with congestive heart failure (CHF), bradyarrhythmias, hepatic impairment, electrolyte abnormalities, in patients with increased risk for cardiac conduction abnormalities, underlying structural heart disease, pre-existing conduction system abnormalities, cardiomyopathies, and ischemic heart disease. Correct hypokalemia/hypomagnesemia prior to therapy and monitor periodically. New onset or exacerbation of diabetes mellitus (DM), hyperglycemia or diabetic ketoacidosis, immune reconstitution syndrome, redistribution/accumulation of body fat, spontaneous bleeding with hemophilia A and B reported. Worsening liver disease in patients with underlying hepatitis B or C, cirrhosis, chronic alcoholism, and/or other underlying liver abnormalities reported. Elevated cholesterol and/or TG levels observed; marked elevation in TG is a risk factor for pancreatitis. (Cap) contained amount of lactose should not induce specific symptoms of intolerance. Continued administration of therapy may increase likelihood of cross-resistance with other protease inhibitors. Caution with severe renal impairment, end-stage renal disease, and in elderly.

ADVERSE REACTIONS: Diarrhea, abdominal pain, pruritus, fever, rash, N/V, fatigue, pneumonia, lipodystrophy.

INTERACTIONS: See Contraindications. Not recommended with garlic capsules, fluticasone, salmeterol, ketoconazole or itraconazole >200mg/day, and tipranavir/ritonavir combination. Avoid with colchicine in patients with renal/hepatic impairment and with IV midazolam. Caution with drugs that prolong PR interval (eg, calcium channel blockers, β-blockers, digoxin, atazanavir), lopinavir/ritonavir, ibutilide, sotalol, erythromycin, halofantrine, pentamidine, dexamethasone, methadone, proton pump inhibitors, neuroleptics, and anticonvulsants. Drugs that affect CYP3A and/or P-gp may modify pharmacokinetics. May increase levels of bosentan, maraviroc, warfarin (monitor INR), colchicine, ketoconazole, rifabutin, tricyclic antidepressants, benzodiazepines, midazolam, CCBs, digoxin, salmeterol, fluticasone, HMG-CoA reductase inhibitors, immunosuppressants, clarithromycin, and PDE5 inhibitors for erectile dysfunction. May decrease levels of methadone and ethinyl estradiol. Delavirdine, atazanavir, indinavir, clarithromycin, and omeprazole may increase levels. Efavirenz, nevirapine, dexamethasone, St. John's wort, garlic capsules, potent CYP3A inducers (eg, phenobarbital, phenytoin, carbamazepine) may decrease levels.

PREGNANCY: Category B, not for use in nursing.

MECHANISM OF ACTION: HIV protease inhibitor; binds to the protease active site and inhibits activity of the enzyme, preventing cleavage of the viral polyproteins and resulting in formation of immature, noninfectious virus particles.

PHARMACOKINETICS: Absorption: Administration of variable doses and combinations resulted in different parameters. **Distribution:** Plasma protein binding (98%). (12mg IV) V_d=700L. **Metabolism:** Hepatic via CYP3A4. **Elimination:** (600mg PO) Urine (1%), feces (88%). (10.5mg IV); Urine (3%), feces (81%).

NURSING CONSIDERATIONS

Assessment: Assess for conditions where treatment is contraindicated or cautioned, renal/hepatic impairment, drug hypersensitivity, pregnancy/nursing status, and possible drug interactions. Obtain serum K^+ and magnesium, TG and cholesterol levels, and ECG prior to initiation of treatment.

Monitoring: Periodically monitor ECG, serum K^+ and magnesium levels, TG and cholesterol levels and hepatic/renal function. Monitor for signs/symptoms of AV block, QT prolongation, cardiac conduction abnormalities, torsades de pointes, worsening liver disease, pancreatitis, spontaneous bleeding, immune reconstitution syndrome, fat redistribution/accumulation, new onset DM, and other adverse reactions.

Patient Counseling: Inform the drug is not a cure for HIV; opportunistic infections may still occur. Inform that drug therapy has not been shown to reduce the risk of transmitting HIV to others through sexual contact or blood contamination. Advise to report use of other Rx, OTC, or herbal products (eg, St. John's wort). Inform that changes in the ECG (PR interval or QT interval prolongation) may occur; instruct to consult health care provider if experiencing dizziness, lightheadedness, or palpitations. Inform that redistribution or accumulation of body fat may occur. Advise that it should be used in combination with ritonavir. Instruct to take drug within 2 hrs after a full meal. Advise the importance of taking medication everyday; do not alter dose or d/c therapy without consulting physician. If dose is missed, instruct to take as soon as possible and not to double next dose.

Administration: Oral route. **Storage:** 25°C (77°F); excursions permitted to 15-30°C (59-86°F).

ISENTRESS

RX

raltegravir (Merck)

THERAPEUTIC CLASS: HIV-integrase strand transfer inhibitor

INDICATIONS: Treatment of HIV-1 infection in combination with other antiretroviral agents in adults and pediatrics ≥2 yrs and weighing ≥10kg.

DOSAGE: *Adults:* (Tab) 400mg bid. With Rifampin: 800mg bid.
Pediatrics: (Tab) ≥12 yrs: 400mg bid. 6-<12 yrs (≥25kg): 400mg bid. (Tab, Chewable) 2-<12 yrs: ≥40kg: 300mg bid. 28-<40kg: 200mg bid. 20-<28kg: 150mg bid. 14-<20kg: 100mg bid. 10-<14kg: 75mg bid. Max: 300mg bid.

HOW SUPPLIED: Tab: 400mg; Tab, Chewable: 25mg, 100mg* *scored

WARNINGS/PRECAUTIONS: Do not substitute chewable tabs for the 400mg film-coated tab; not bioequivalent. Severe, potentially life-threatening, and fatal skin reactions (eg, Stevens-Johnson syndrome, toxic epidermal necrolysis), and hypersensitivity reactions reported; d/c therapy and other suspect agents if signs/symptoms develop. Immune reconstitution syndrome may occur. Caution in elderly. Avoid dosing before dialysis session. (Tab, Chewable) Contains phenylalanine; caution in patients with phenylketonuria.

ADVERSE REACTIONS: Hyperglycemia, ALT/AST elevation, hyperbilirubinemia, serum lipase elevation, insomnia, low absolute neutrophil count, serum creatine kinase increase, pancreatic amylase increase, thrombocytopenia.

INTERACTIONS: UGT1A1 inhibitors (eg, atazanavir, atazanavir/ritonavir) and drugs that increase gastric pH (eg, omeprazole) may increase levels. Rifampin, efavirenz, etravirine, and tipranavir/ritonavir may decrease levels. Caution with drugs that cause myopathy or rhabdomyolysis.

PREGNANCY: Category C, not for use in nursing.

MECHANISM OF ACTION: HIV-1 integrase strand transfer inhibitor; inhibits the catalytic activity of HIV-1 integrase (an HIV-1 encoded enzyme required for viral replication) thus preventing the formation of HIV-1 provirus, resulting in the prevention of propagation of the viral infection.

PHARMACOKINETICS: Absorption: (Tab) T_{max}=3 hrs (fasting). Refer to PI for parameters in different age groups in pediatric studies. **Distribution:** Plasma protein binding (83%). **Metabolism:**

Glucuronidation via UGT1A1; raltegravir-glucuronide (metabolite). **Elimination:** Urine (9% unchanged; 23% raltegravir-glucuronide), feces (51%); T$_{1/2}$=9 hrs.

NURSING CONSIDERATIONS

Assessment: Assess for opportunistic infections, history of psychiatric illness, risk of myopathy or rhabdomyolysis, liver disease, pregnancy/nursing status, and possible drug interactions. Assess if patient is undergoing dialysis session. (Tab, Chewable) Assess for phenylketonuria.

Monitoring: Monitor for signs/symptoms of severe skin/hypersensitivity reactions, and immune reconstitution syndrome.

Patient Counseling: Instruct to d/c therapy immediately and seek medical attention if rash, fever, generally ill feeling, extreme tiredness, muscle or joint aches, blisters, oral lesions, eye inflammation, facial swelling, swelling of the eyes, lips, mouth, breathing difficulty, and/or signs and symptoms of liver problems (eg, yellowing of the skin or whites of the eyes, dark- or tea-colored urine, pale-colored stools/bowel movements, N/V, loss of appetite) develops. Advise that therapy is not a cure for HIV or AIDS and that opportunistic infections may still develop. Instruct to practice safe sex by using barrier methods (eg, condoms). Advise to never reuse or share needles, other inj equipment, or personal items that can have blood or body fluids on them. If a dose is missed, instruct to take as soon as remembered; if not remembered until next dose, instruct to skip missed dose and go back to regular dosing schedule. Advise not to double the next dose or take more than the prescribed dose. Instruct to contact physician if unusual symptom develops or if any known symptom persists or worsens.

Administration: Oral route. (Tab) Swallow whole. (Tab, Chewable) Chew or swallow whole. **Storage:** 20-25°C (68-77°F); excursions permitted to 15-30°C (59-86°F). (Tab, Chewable) Store in the original package with the bottle tightly closed. Keep the desiccant in the bottle to protect from moisture.

ISONIAZID RX
isoniazid (Various)

> Severe, fatal hepatitis may develop. Monitor LFTs monthly. D/C drug if signs and symptoms of hepatic damage occur. Patients with tuberculosis (TB) who have isoniazid-induced hepatits should have appropriate treatment with alternative drugs. Defer preventive treatment in persons with acute hepatic disease.

THERAPEUTIC CLASS: Isonicotinic acid hydrazide

INDICATIONS: Prevention and treatment of TB.

DOSAGE: *Adults:* Active TB: 5mg/kg as a single dose. Max: 300mg qd or 15mg/kg 2 to 3 times/week. Max: 900mg/day. Use with other antituberculosis agents. Prevention: 300mg qd single dose.
Pediatrics: Active TB: 10-15mg/kg as a single dose. Max: 300mg qd or 20-40mg/kg 2 to 3 times/week. Max: 900mg/day. Use with other antituberculosis agents. Prevention: 10mg/kg qd single dose. Max: 300mg qd.

HOW SUPPLIED: Inj: 100mg/mL; Syrup: 50mg/5mL; Tab: 100mg, 300mg

CONTRAINDICATIONS: Severe hypersensitivity reactions including drug-induced hepatitis, previous INH-associated hepatic injury, severe adverse effects (eg, drug fever, chills, arthritis), acute liver disease of any etiology.

WARNINGS/PRECAUTIONS: D/C if hypersensitivity occurs. Monitor closely with liver or renal disease, daily alcohol users, pregnancy, age >35, and concurrent chronic medications. Precaution with HIV seropositive patients. Take with vitamin B$_6$ in malnourished and those predisposed to neuropathy.

ADVERSE REACTIONS: Peripheral neuropathy, N/V, anorexia, epigastric distress, elevated serum transaminases, bilirubinemia, jaundice, hepatitis, skin eruptions, pyridoxine deficiency.

INTERACTIONS: Alcohol is associated with hepatitis. May increase phenytoin, theophylline, and valproate serum levels. Do not take with food. Severe acetaminophen toxicity reported. Decreases carbamazepine metabolism and AUC of ketoconazole. Avoid tyramine- and histamine-containing foods.

PREGNANCY: Category C, caution in nursing.

MECHANISM OF ACTION: Isonicotinic acid hydrazide; inhibits mycoloic acid synthesis and acts against actively growing tuberculosis bacilli.

PHARMACOKINETICS: Absorption: T$_{max}$: 1-2 hrs. **Distribution:** Crosses placenta, found in breast milk. **Metabolism:** Acetylation and dehydrazination. **Elimination:** Urine (50-70%).

NURSING CONSIDERATIONS

Assessment: Assess for previous isoniazid-associated hepatic injury, acute liver disease, HIV status, pregnancy status, age, and drug interactions. Document reasons for therapy, culture, and susceptibility.

Monitoring: Prior to therapy and periodically thereafter, measure hepatic enzymes (AST, ALT). D/C at first sign of hypersensitivity reaction. Monitor for peripheral neuropathy, convulsions, N/V, agranulocytosis, hemolytic anemia, SLE-like syndrome, metabolic and endocrine reactions (hyperglycemia, pyridoxine deficiency, pellagra).

Patient Counseling: Immediately report signs/symptoms consistent with liver damage or other adverse events (unexplained anorexia, N/V, dark urine, icterus, rash, persistent paresthesias of the hands and feet, persistent fatigue, weakness or fever of >3 days duration, and/or abdominal tenderness). Drug should not be taken with food. Take pyridoxine tablets if peripheral neuropathy develops.

Administration: Oral and IM route. **Storage:** Tab: 20-25°C (68-77°F). Syrup: 15-30°C (59-86°F). Protect from light and moisture. Dispense in tight, light-resistant container. Inj: 20-25°C (68-77°F). Protect from light. If vial contents crystallize, warm vial to room temperature to redissolve crystals before use.

ISOSORBIDE DINITRATE   RX

isosorbide dinitrate (Various)

OTHER BRAND NAMES: Isordil Titradose (Biovail)

THERAPEUTIC CLASS: Nitrate vasodilator

INDICATIONS: Prevention of angina pectoris due to coronary artery disease. (Tab, SL) Prevention and treatment of angina pectoris due to coronary artery disease.

DOSAGE: *Adults:* (Isordil Titradose/Tab) Initial: 5-20mg bid-tid. Maint: 10-40mg bid-tid. Allow a dose-free interval of ≥14 hrs. (Tab, Extended-Release) Refer to PI. (Tab, SL) Take 1 tab (2.5-5mg) 15 min before activity. Elderly: Start at lower end of dosing range.

HOW SUPPLIED: Tab, SL (Generic): 2.5mg, 5mg; Tab (Generic): 5mg*, 10mg*, 20mg*, 30mg*; Tab, Extended-Release (Generic): 40mg*; Tab (Isordil Titradose): 5mg*, 40mg* *scored.

WARNINGS/PRECAUTIONS: Severe hypotension, particularly with upright posture, may occur. Not for use with acute myocardial infarction (MI) or congestive heart failure (CHF); perform careful clinical or hemodynamic monitoring if used for these conditions. Hypotension may be accompanied by paradoxical bradycardia and increased angina pectoris. May aggravate angina caused by hypertrophic cardiomyopathy. Caution with volume depletion, hypotension, and elderly. May develop tolerance. Chest pain, acute MI and sudden death reported during temporary withdrawal. (Tab, SL) Not the 1st drug of choice for abortion of acute anginal episode.

ADVERSE REACTIONS: Headache, lightheadedness, hypotension, syncope, crescendo angina, rebound HTN.

INTERACTIONS: Severe hypotension with sildenafil. Additive vasodilation with other vasodilators (eg, alcohol).

PREGNANCY: Category C, caution in nursing.

MECHANISM OF ACTION: Nitrate vasodilator; relaxes vascular smooth muscle and dilates peripheral arteries and veins; venous dilatation reduces left ventricular end diastolic pressure and pulmonary capillary wedge pressure (preload); arteriolar relaxation reduces systemic vascular resistance, systolic arterial pressure, and mean arterial pressure (afterload); dilates the coronary artery.

PHARMACOKINETICS: Absorption: Nearly complete (Tab/Isordil Titradose). Bioavailability (10-90%) (Tab/Isordil Titradose); (40-50%) (Tab, SL). T_{max}=1 hr (Tab/Isordil Titradose); 10-15 min (Tab, SL). **Distribution:** V_d=2-4L/kg. **Metabolism:** Liver; extensive first-pass metabolism (Tab/Tab, Extended-Release/Isordil Titradose); 2-mononitrate, 5-mononitrate (active metabolites). **Elimination:** $T_{1/2}$=1 hr; 5 hrs (5-mononitrate), 2 hrs (2-mononitrate).

NURSING CONSIDERATIONS

Assessment: Assess for drug hypersensitivity, hypotension, acute MI, CHF, volume depletion, hypertrophic cardiomyopathy, alcohol intake, pregnancy/nursing status, and possible drug interactions.

Monitoring: Careful clinical or hemodynamic monitoring for hypotension and tachycardia in patients with MI or CHF. Monitor for paradoxical bradycardia, increased angina pectoris, hypotension, hemodynamic rebound, decreased exercise tolerance, chest pain, acute MI, and other adverse reactions.

Patient Counseling: Counsel to carefully follow prescribed dosing regimen. Inform that headaches accompany therapy and are markers of drug activity; instruct not to alter schedule of therapy since loss of headache may be associated with simultaneous loss of anti-anginal efficacy. Inform that lightheadedness on standing may occur which may be more frequent with alcohol consumption.

Administration: Oral/SL route. **Storage:** (Isordil Titradose) 25°C (77°F); excursions permitted to 15-30°C (59-86°F). Protect from light. (Tab) 25°C (77°F). Protect from light. (Tab, SL/Tab, Extended-Release) 20-25°C (68-77°F). (Tab, SL) Protect from light and moisture.

ISOSORBIDE MONONITRATE   RX
isosorbide mononitrate (Kremers Urban)

THERAPEUTIC CLASS: Nitrate vasodilator

INDICATIONS: Prevention of angina pectoris due to coronary artery disease.

DOSAGE: *Adults:* Initial: 30mg (single tab or as 1/2 of a 60mg tab) or 60mg (single tab) qd in am. Titrate: May increase to 120mg (single tab or as two 60mg tabs) qd in am. Rarely, 240mg/day may be required. Elderly: Start at lower end of dosing range.

HOW SUPPLIED: Tab, Extended-Release: 30mg*, 60mg*, 120mg *scored

WARNINGS/PRECAUTIONS: Not useful in aborting acute anginal episode. Not recommended for use in patients with acute myocardial infarction (MI) or congestive heart failure. Severe hypotension, particularly with upright posture, may occur. Caution in volume depleted, hypotensive, and elderly. Nitrate-induced hypotension may be accompanied by paradoxical bradycardia and increased angina pectoris. May aggravate angina caused by hypertrophic cardiomyopathy. May develop tolerance. Chest pain, acute MI, and sudden death reported during temporary withdrawal.

ADVERSE REACTIONS: Headache, dizziness, dry mouth, asthenia, cardiac failure, abdominal pain, earache, arrhythmia, hyperuricemia, arthralgia, purpura, anxiety, hypochromic anemia, atrophic vaginitis, bacterial infection.

INTERACTIONS: Sildenafil amplifies vasodilatory effects resulting in severe hypotension. Vasodilating effects may be additive with those of other vasodilators. Alcohol has been found to exhibit additive effects. Marked symptomatic orthostatic hypotension reported with calcium channel blockers; dose adjustments of either class of agents may be necessary.

PREGNANCY: Category B, caution with nursing.

MECHANISM OF ACTION: Nitrate vasodilator; relaxes vascular smooth muscle, producing dilatation of the peripheral arteries and veins, especially the latter. Dilation of veins leads to reducing the left ventricular end-diastolic pressure and pulmonary capillary wedge pressure (preload). Arteriolar relaxation reduces systemic vascular resistance, systolic arterial pressure, and mean arterial pressure (afterload). It also dilates the coronary artery.

PHARMACOKINETICS: Absorption: (Sol/Immediate-release tab) Absolute bioavailability (100%), T_{max}=30-60 min. **Distribution:** V_d=0.6-0.7L/kg (IV); plasma protein binding (5%). **Metabolism:** Liver. Cleared through denitration to isosorbide and glucuronidation as the mononitrate. **Elimination:** Urine (96%, 2% unchanged), feces (1%); $T_{1/2}$=5 hrs.

NURSING CONSIDERATIONS

Assessment: Assess for drug hypersensitivity, severe hypotension, volume depletion, angina caused by hypertrophic cardiomyopathy, any other conditions where treatment is contraindicated or cautioned, pregnancy/nursing status, and possible drug interactions.

Monitoring: Monitor for hypotension with paradoxical bradycardia, tachycardia, aggravation of angina, tolerance, chest pain, acute MI, and other adverse reactions.

Patient Counseling: Inform about the risks and benefits of therapy. Instruct to take tab in the morning upon arising. Advise that daily headaches may accompany treatment; avoid altering schedule of treatment as the headaches are a marker of the activity of the medication and loss of headache may be associated with loss of antianginal efficacy. Inform to swallow tab whole with half-glassful of fluid; do not crush or chew tabs. Advise to not be concerned if occasionally something that looks like a tab is noticed in the stool. Counsel to carefully follow dosing regimen.

Administration: Oral route. Swallow tab whole with half glass of fluid; do not crush or chew. Do not break 30mg tab. **Storage:** 20-30°C (68-86°F).

IXEMPRA   RX
ixabepilone (Bristol-Myers Squibb)

> **Contraindicated in combination with capecitabine in patients with AST/ALT >2.5X ULN or bilirubin >1X ULN due to increased risk of toxicity and neutropenia-related death.**

THERAPEUTIC CLASS: Antimicrotubule agent

INDICATIONS: In combination with capecitabine for treatment of patients with metastatic or locally advanced breast cancer resistant to treatment with an anthracycline and a taxane, or whose cancer is taxane resistant and for whom further anthracycline therapy is contraindicated. As monotherapy for treatment of metastatic or locally advanced breast cancer in patients whose tumors are resistant or refractory to anthracyclines, taxanes, and capecitabine.

DOSAGE: *Adults:* Usual: 40mg/m² IV infusion over 3 hrs every 3 weeks. Patients with BSA >2.2m² should be dosed based on 2.2m². Adjust dose based on toxicities (see PI). Patient should not begin a new cycle of treatment unless the neutrophil count is ≥1500 cells/mm³, the platelet count is ≥100,000 cell/mm³, and nonhematologic toxicities have improved to grade 1 (mild) or resolved. If toxicities recur, an additional 20% dose reduction should be made. Hepatic Impairment: Combination Therapy: AST and ALT ≤2.5X ULN and Bilirubin ≤1X ULN: 40mg/m². Monotherapy: Mild (AST and ALT ≤2.5X ULN and Bilirubin ≤1X ULN): 40mg/m². AST and ALT ≤10X ULN and Bilirubin ≤1.5X ULN: 32mg/m². Moderate (AST and ALT ≤10X ULN and Bilirubin >1.5 to ≤3X ULN): 20-30mg/m². Strong CYP3A4 Inhibitors: Avoid or reduce dose to 20mg/m². If d/c, allow a wash-out period of approximately 1 week before adjusting dose to the indicated dose. Strong CYP3A4 Inducers: Avoid or gradually increase dose to 40-60mg/m² given as a 4 hr IV infusion. If d/c, re-turn to dose used prior to initiation of strong inducer. Premedicate all patients with H₁-antagonist (eg, diphenhydramine 50mg PO) and H₂-antagonist (eg, ranitidine 150-300mg PO) approximate-ly 1 hr before infusion. Premedicate with corticosteroids (eg, dexamethasone 20mg IV, 30 min before infusion or PO 60 min before infusion) if prior hypersensitivity reaction experienced.

HOW SUPPLIED: Inj: 15mg, 45mg

CONTRAINDICATIONS: History of severe (CTC Grade 3/4) hypersensitivity reaction to Cremophor EL or derivatives (eg, polyoxyethylated castor oil). Neutrophil count <1500 cells/mm³ or platelet count <100,000 cells/mm³. In combination with capecitabine patients with AST or ALT >2.5X ULN or bilirubin >1X ULN.

WARNINGS/PRECAUTIONS: Peripheral neuropathy may occur early during treatment; monitor for symptoms and manage by dose adjustment, dose delays or d/c. Caution with diabetes mel-litus (DM) or preexisting peripheral neuropathy. Myelosuppression, primarily neutropenia, may occur and is dose-dependent; monitor with frequent peripheral blood cell counts and adjust dose PRN. Avoid monotherapy if AST or ALT >10X ULN or bilirubin >3X ULN and use caution if AST or ALT >5X ULN. Premedicate all patients with H₁- and H₂-antagonists 1 hr before treatment; d/c and institute aggressive supportive treatment if hypersensitivity occurs. May cause fetal harm; avoid during pregnancy. Caution with history of cardiac disease. D/C if cardiac ischemia or impaired cardiac function develops. Potential cognitive impairment may occur from excipients (eg, dehydrated alcohol USP).

ADVERSE REACTIONS: Peripheral neuropathy, fatigue/asthenia, myalgia/arthralgia, alopecia, N/V, stomatitis/mucositis, diarrhea, musculoskeletal pain, palmar-plantar erythrodysesthesia (hand-foot) syndrome, anorexia, abdominal pain.

INTERACTIONS: CYP3A4 inhibitors may increase levels; avoid or reduce dose with strong CYP3A4 inhibitors (eg, ketoconazole, itraconazole, clarithromycin, atazanavir, nefazodone, saqui-navir, telithromycin, ritonavir, amprenavir, indinavir, nelfinavir, delavirdine, voriconazole, grape-fruit juice); use caution with mild/moderate CYP3A4 inhibitors (eg, erythromycin, fluconazole, verapamil), and monitor all patients closely for acute toxicities. Strong CYP3A4 inducers (eg, dexamethasone, phenytoin, carbamazepine, rifampin, rifabutin, phenobarbital) may decrease levels; avoid or consider gradual dose adjustment or alternative agents. Avoid St. John's wort; may decrease levels.

PREGNANCY: Category D, not for use in nursing.

MECHANISM OF ACTION: Microtubule inhibitor; binds directly to β-tubulin subunits on microtu-bules, leading to suppression of microtubule dynamics. Blocks the mitotic phase of cell division, leading to cell death.

PHARMACOKINETICS: Absorption: C_{max}=252ng/mL; T_{max}=3 hrs; AUC=2143ng•hr/mL. **Distribution:** V_d= >1000L. Plasma protein binding (67-77%). **Metabolism:** Liver (extensive); oxida-tion via CYP3A4. **Elimination:** Urine (21%, 5.6% unchanged), feces (65%, 1.6% unchanged); $T_{1/2}$=52 hrs.

NURSING CONSIDERATIONS

Assessment: Assess for hypersensitivity to Cremophor EL or polyoxyethylated castor oil, DM, preexisting peripheral neuropathy, history of cardiac disease, renal dysfunction, hepatic impair-ment, pregnancy/nursing status, and possible drug interactions. Obtain baseline LFTs and peripheral blood cell count.

Monitoring: Monitor LFTs and peripheral blood cell counts periodically. Monitor for signs/symp-toms of neuropathy, myelosuppression, fever/neutropenia, cardiac adverse reactions, hepatic toxicity, and hypersensitivity reactions.

Patient Counseling: Advise to seek medical attention if symptoms of peripheral neuropathy (eg, numbness, tingling in hands or feet), fever/neutropenia (eg, chills, cough, burning, or pain urinat-ing), hypersensitivity reaction (eg, urticaria, pruritus, rash, flushing, swelling, chest tightness, dyspnea), or cardiac events (eg, chest pain, difficulty breathing, palpitations, unusual weight gain) occur. Instruct to avoid grapefruit juice. Inform of pregnancy/nursing risks; advise to use effective contraceptive methods to prevent pregnancy and avoid nursing during treatment.

Administration: IV infusion. Refer to PI for proper instructions of preparation and administration.
Storage: Unreconstituted: 2-8°C (36-46°F). Protect from light. Reconstituted Sol: Stable at room temperature/light for a max of 1 hr. Diluted with Infusion Fluid: Stable at room temperature/light for a max of 6 hrs at a pH of 6.0-9.0.

JALYN   RX
tamsulosin HCl - dutasteride (GlaxoSmithKline)

THERAPEUTIC CLASS: 5-alpha reductase inhibitor/alpha antagonist

INDICATIONS: Treatment of symptomatic benign prostatic hyperplasia (BPH) in men with an enlarged prostate.

DOSAGE: *Adults:* Usual: 1 cap qd, 30 min after the same meal each day.

HOW SUPPLIED: Cap: (Dutasteride-Tamsulosin) 0.5mg-0.4mg

CONTRAINDICATIONS: Pregnancy, women of childbearing potential, pediatrics.

WARNINGS/PRECAUTIONS: Not approved for the prevention of prostate cancer. Orthostatic hypotension/syncope may occur; caution to avoid situations where syncope could result in an injury. Prior to initiating treatment, consideration should be given to other urological conditions that may cause similar symptoms; BPH and prostate cancer may coexist. Risk to male fetus; cap should not be handled by pregnant women or women who may become pregnant. May reduce serum prostate specific antigen (PSA) concentration during therapy; establish a new baseline PSA at least 3 months after starting therapy and monitor PSA periodically thereafter. Any confirmed increase from the lowest PSA value during treatment may signal the presence of prostate cancer. May increase the risk of high-grade prostate cancer. Avoid blood donation until ≥6 months following the last dose. Reduced total sperm count, semen volume, and sperm motility reported. May cause priapism, which may lead to permanent impotence if not properly treated. Intraoperative floppy iris syndrome (IFIS) reported during cataract surgery. Caution with sulfa allergy; allergic reaction has been reported.

ADVERSE REACTIONS: Ejaculation disorders, impotence, decreased libido, breast disorders, dizziness.

INTERACTIONS: Avoid with strong inhibitors of CYP3A4 (eg, ketoconazole); may increase tamsulosin exposure. Caution with moderate inhibitors of CYP3A4 (eg, erythromycin), strong (eg, paroxetine) or moderate (eg, terbinafine) inhibitors of CYP2D6; potential for significant increase in tamsulosin exposure. Caution with cimetidine and warfarin. Avoid with other α-adrenergic antagonists; may increase the risk of symptomatic hypotension. Caution with phosphodiesterase type 5 inhibitors; may cause symptomatic hypotension.

PREGNANCY: Category X, not for use in nursing.

MECHANISM OF ACTION: Dutasteride: Type I, II 5α-reductase inhibitor; inhibits the conversion of testosterone to dihydrotestosterone, the androgen primarily responsible for the initial development and subsequent enlargement of the prostate gland. Tamsulosin: $α_{1A}$ antagonist; selective blockade of $α_1$ adrenoceptors in the prostate results in relaxation of the smooth muscles of the bladder neck and prostate, improving urine flow and reducing symptoms.

PHARMACOKINETICS: Absorption: Dutasteride: (Fed) C_{max}=2.14ng/mL, T_{max}=3 hrs, AUC=39.6ng•hr/mL. Tamsulosin: Complete; (Fed) C_{max}=11.3ng/mL, T_{max}=6 hrs, AUC=187.2ng•hr/mL. **Distribution:** Dutasteride: V_d=300-500L, plasma protein binding (99% albumin, 96.6% α-1 acid glycoprotein). Tamsulosin: Plasma protein binding (94-99%). **Metabolism:** Dutasteride: Extensive. CYP3A4, 3A5; 4'-hydroxydutasteride, 1,2-dihydroxydutasteride, 6-hydroxydutasteride (major metabolites). Tamsulosin: Liver (extensive); CYP3A4, CYP2D6. **Elimination:** Dutasteride: Urine (<1% unchanged), feces (5% unchanged, 40% metabolites); $T_{1/2}$=5 weeks. Tamsulosin: Urine (76%, <10% unchanged), feces (21%); $T_{1/2}$=14-15 hrs, 9-13 hrs (healthy).

NURSING CONSIDERATIONS

Assessment: Assess for BPH, drug hypersensitivity, sulfa allergy, urologic diseases, and possible drug interactions.

Monitoring: Monitor for signs/symptoms of prostate cancer, other urological diseases, orthostatic hypotension, syncope, priapism, IFIS, and allergic reactions. Obtain new baseline PSA ≥3 months after starting treatment and monitor PSA periodically thereafter.

Patient Counseling: Inform about the possible occurrence of symptoms related to orthostatic hypotension (eg, dizziness and vertigo) and the potential risk of syncope; caution to avoid situations where injury could result if syncope occurs. Inform of an increase in high-grade prostate cancer in men reported. Inform females who are pregnant or intend to become pregnant not to handle drug due to potential risk to fetus; inform that if patient comes in contact with leaking cap, wash area immediately with soap and water. Inform that cap should be swallowed whole and not chewed, crushed, or opened. Inform that may become deformed and/or discolored if kept at high temperatures; instruct to avoid use if this occurs. Advise about the possibility of priapism (rare) that may lead to permanent erectile dysfunction if not brought to immediate medical attention. Advise not to donate blood for ≥6 months following the last dose. If considering cataract surgery, advise to inform ophthalmologist of therapy.

Administration: Oral route. Swallow cap whole; do not chew or open. **Storage:** 25°C (77°F); excursions permitted to 15-30°C (59-86°F).

JANUMET   RX
metformin HCl - sitagliptin (Merck)

> Lactic acidosis may occur due to metformin accumulation; risk increases with conditions such as sepsis, dehydration, excess alcohol intake, hepatic insufficiency, renal impairment, and acute congestive heart failure (CHF). If acidosis is suspected, d/c and hospitalize patient immediately.

THERAPEUTIC CLASS: Dipeptidyl peptidase-4 inhibitor/biguanide

INDICATIONS: Adjunct to diet and exercise to improve glycemic control in adults with type 2 diabetes mellitus (DM) when treatment with both sitagliptin and metformin is appropriate.

DOSAGE: *Adults:* Individualize dose. Take bid with meals, with gradual dose escalation to reduce GI side effects of metformin. Not Currently on Metformin: Initial: 50mg sitagliptin/500mg metformin bid. On Metformin: Initial: 50mg bid (100mg/day) of sitagliptin and current metformin dose. On Metformin 850mg bid: Initial: 50mg sitagliptin/1000mg metformin bid. Max: 100mg sitagliptin/2000mg metformin. With Insulin/Insulin Secretagogue (eg, sulfonylurea): May require lower dose of insulin secretagogue or insulin.

HOW SUPPLIED: Tab: (Metformin-Sitagliptin) 500mg-50mg, 1000mg-50mg

CONTRAINDICATIONS: Renal disease or renal dysfunction (eg, SrCr ≥1.5mg/dL [male], ≥1.4mg/dL [female], or abnormal CrCl). Acute or chronic metabolic acidosis, including diabetic ketoacidosis, with or without coma. Temporarily d/c if undergoing radiologic studies involving intravascular administration of iodinated contrast materials.

WARNINGS/PRECAUTIONS: Not for use in type 1 DM or for treatment of diabetic ketoacidosis. Acute pancreatitis reported; d/c if pancreatitis is suspected. Avoid with hepatic impairment. Worsening renal function, including acute renal failure reported; d/c with evidence of renal impairment. May decrease vitamin B12 levels; monitor hematologic parameters annually. Suspend temporarily for any surgical procedures (except minor procedures not associated with restricted food and fluid intake); restart when oral intake is resumed and renal function is normal. Evaluate for evidence of ketoacidosis or lactic acidosis if laboratory abnormalities or clinical illness develops; d/c if acidosis occurs. D/C in hypoxic states (eg, acute CHF, shock, acute myocardial infarction). Temporary loss of glycemic control may occur when exposed to stress (eg, fever, trauma, infection, surgery); withhold therapy and temporarily administer insulin. Serious hypersensitivity reactions reported; d/c if hypersensitivity reaction is suspected and institute alternative treatment. No conclusive evidence of macrovascular risk reduction. Avoid in patients ≥80 yrs unless renal function is normal. Caution in elderly.

ADVERSE REACTIONS: Lactic acidosis, diarrhea, upper respiratory infection, headache, N/V, abdominal pain.

INTERACTIONS: See Contraindications. May slightly increase digoxin levels; monitor appropriately. Hypoglycemia may occur with other glucose-lowering agents (eg, sulfonylureas, insulin) and ethanol; may require lower doses of sulfonylurea or insulin. Metformin: Furosemide, nifedipine, and cationic drugs (eg, digoxin, amiloride, procainamide, quinidine, quinine, ranitidine, trimethoprim, vancomycin, triamterene, morphine, cimetidine) may increase levels. Less likely to interact with highly protein-bound drugs (eg, salicylates, sulfonamides, chloramphenicol, probenecid). Observe for loss of glycemic control with thiazides and other diuretics, corticosteroids, phenothiazines, thyroid products, estrogens, oral contraceptives, phenytoin, nicotinic acid, sympathomimetics, calcium channel blockers, and isoniazid. Alcohol may potentiate effect of metformin on lactate metabolism. Caution with drugs that may affect renal function or result in significant hemodynamic change or may interfere with the disposition of metformin (eg, cationic drugs eliminated by renal tubular secretion). May decrease furosemide and glyburide levels. May be difficult to recognize hypoglycemia with β-adrenergic blocking drugs.

PREGNANCY: Category B, caution in nursing.

MECHANISM OF ACTION: Sitagliptin: Dipeptidyl peptidase-4 inhibitor; slows the inactivation of incretin hormones thus increases insulin release and decreases glucagon levels in the circulation in a glucose-dependent manner. Metformin: Biguanide; decreases hepatic glucose production, decreases intestinal absorption of glucose, and improves insulin sensitivity by increasing peripheral glucose uptake and utilization.

PHARMACOKINETICS: Absorption: Sitagliptin: Absolute bioavailability (87%). Metformin: Absolute bioavailability (50-60%) (fasted). **Distribution:** Sitagliptin: (IV) V_d=198L; plasma protein binding (38%). Metformin: V_d=654L. **Metabolism:** Sitagliptin: Via CYP3A4 and CYP2C8. **Elimination:** Sitagliptin: Feces (13%), urine (87%, 79% unchanged); $T_{1/2}$=12.4 hrs. Metformin: Urine (90%); $T_{1/2}$=6.2 hrs (plasma), 17.6 hrs (blood).

NURSING CONSIDERATIONS

Assessment: Assess for metabolic acidosis, renal/hepatic function, previous hypersensitivity to the drug, history of pancreatitis, type 1 DM, diabetic ketoacidosis, pregnancy/nursing status, and possible drug interactions. Assess if patient is planning to undergo any surgical procedure or is under any form of stress. Obtain baseline FPG, HbA1c, and CrCl.

Monitoring: Monitor for lactic acidosis, pancreatitis, clinical illness, hypoxic states, and hypersensitivity reactions. Monitor renal function, especially in elderly, at least annually. Monitor vitamin B12 levels in patients predisposed to develop subnormal vitamin B12 levels. Monitor FPG, HbA1c, renal/hepatic function, and hematologic parameters periodically.

Patient Counseling: Inform of risks, benefits, and alternative modes of therapy. Advise on importance of adherence to diet and exercise, regular physical activity, periodic blood glucose monitoring, HbA1c testing, recognition/management of hypoglycemia/hyperglycemia, and assessment of diabetic complications. Advise of the risk of lactic acidosis. Counsel against excessive alcohol intake. Inform that GI symptoms and acute pancreatitis may occur. Instruct to seek medical advice during periods of stress (eg, fever, trauma, infection, surgery) as medication needs may change. Advise to d/c and notify physician if symptoms of allergic reactions, unexplained hyperventilation, myalgia, malaise, unusual somnolence, dizziness, slow or irregular heart beat, sensation of feeling cold (especially in the extremities), or other nonspecific symptoms occur. Inform that incidence of hypoglycemia is increased when added to sulfonylurea or insulin and a lower dose of sulfonylurea or insulin may be required. Counsel to inform physician if any unusual symptom develops, or if any known symptom persists or worsens.

Administration: Oral route. Take with meals. **Storage:** 20-25°C (68-77°F); excursions permitted to 15-30°C (59-86°F).

JANUMET XR   RX
metformin HCl - sitagliptin (Merck)

> Lactic acidosis may occur due to metformin accumulation; risk increases with conditions such as sepsis, dehydration, excess alcohol intake, hepatic impairment, renal impairment, and acute congestive heart failure (CHF). If acidosis is suspected, d/c and hospitalize patient immediately.

THERAPEUTIC CLASS: Dipeptidyl peptidase-4 inhibitor/biguanide

INDICATIONS: Adjunct to diet and exercise to improve glycemic control in adults with type 2 diabetes mellitus (DM) when treatment with both sitagliptin and metformin ER is appropriate.

DOSAGE: *Adults:* Individualize dose. Take qd with meal, preferably in pm. Not Currently on Metformin: Initial: 100mg-1000mg; if metformin dose is inadequate to achieve glycemic control, titrate gradually (to reduce GI side effects of metformin) up to max recommended daily dose. On Metformin: Initial: 100mg sitagliptin and previously prescribed metformin dose. On Metformin Immediate-Release (IR) 850mg bid or 1000mg bid: Initial: Two 50mg-1000mg tabs taken together qd. Max Daily Dose: 100mg-2000mg. Changing Between Janumet and Janumet XR: Maintain the same total daily dose of sitagliptin and metformin; if metformin dose is inadequate to achieve glycemic control, titrate gradually up to max recommended daily dose. With Insulin/Insulin Secretagogue (eg, sulfonylurea): May require lower dose of insulin secretagogue or insulin.

HOW SUPPLIED: Tab, Extended-Release: (Sitagliptin-Metformin ER) 50mg-500mg, 50mg-1000mg, 100mg-1000mg

CONTRAINDICATIONS: Renal impairment (eg, SrCr ≥1.5mg/dL [men], ≥1.4mg/dL [women], or abnormal CrCl), acute or chronic metabolic acidosis, including diabetic ketoacidosis.

WARNINGS/PRECAUTIONS: Not for use in type 1 DM or for treatment of diabetic ketoacidosis. Acute pancreatitis reported; d/c if pancreatitis is suspected. Avoid with hepatic impairment. Worsening renal function, including acute renal failure reported; d/c with evidence of renal impairment. May decrease vitamin B12 levels; monitor hematologic parameters annually. Suspend temporarily for any surgical procedures (except minor procedures not associated with restricted food and fluid intake); restart when oral intake is resumed and renal function is normal. Evaluate for evidence of ketoacidosis or lactic acidosis if laboratory abnormalities or clinical illness develops; d/c if acidosis occurs. Temporarily d/c if undergoing radiologic studies involving intravascular iodinated contrast materials. D/C in hypoxic states (eg, acute CHF, shock, acute myocardial infarction). Temporary loss of glycemic control may occur when exposed to stress (eg, fever, trauma, infection, surgery); withhold therapy and temporarily administer insulin. Serious hypersensitivity reactions reported; d/c if hypersensitivity reaction is suspected and institute alternative treatment. No conclusive evidence of macrovascular risk reduction. Caution with history of angioedema to another dipeptidyl peptidase-4 (DPP4) inhibitor and in elderly.

ADVERSE REACTIONS: Lactic acidosis, diarrhea, upper respiratory infection, headache, N/V, abdominal pain.

INTERACTIONS: Topiramate or other carbonic anhydrase inhibitors (eg, zonisamide, acetazolamide, dichlorphenamide) may induce metabolic acidosis; use with caution. Hypoglycemia may occur with other glucose-lowering agents (eg, sulfonylureas, insulin) or ethanol; may require lower doses of insulin secretagogue or insulin. Metformin: Cationic drugs that are eliminated by renal tubular secretion (eg, cimetidine, amiloride, digoxin, morphine, procainamide, quinidine, quinine, ranitidine, triamterene, trimethoprim, vancomycin) may potentially produce an interaction; monitor and adjust dose. Observe for loss of glycemic control with thiazides and other diuretics, corticosteroids, phenothiazines, thyroid products, estrogens, oral contraceptives, phenytoin, nicotinic acid, sympathomimetics, calcium channel blockers, and isoniazid. Alcohol may potentiate effect of metformin on lactate metabolism. Caution with drugs that may affect renal function or result in significant hemodynamic change or may interfere with the disposition of metformin (eg, cationic drugs eliminated by renal tubular secretion). May be difficult to recognize hypoglycemia with β-adrenergic blocking drugs.

PREGNANCY: Category B, caution in nursing.

MECHANISM OF ACTION: Sitagliptin: DPP4 inhibitor; slows the inactivation of incretin hormones thus increases insulin release and decreases glucagon levels in the circulation in a glucose-dependent manner. Metformin: Biguanide; decreases hepatic glucose production, decreases intestinal absorption of glucose, and improves insulin sensitivity by increasing peripheral glucose uptake and utilization.

PHARMACOKINETICS: Absorption: Sitagliptin: Absolute bioavailability (87%); T_{max}=3 hrs (median). Metformin: (ER) T_{max}=8 hrs (median); (IR) C_{max}=5mcg/mL. **Distribution:** Sitagliptin: (IV) V_d=198L; plasma protein binding (38%). Metformin IR: V_d=654L. **Metabolism:** Sitagliptin: Via CYP3A4 and CYP2C8. **Elimination:** Sitagliptin: Feces (13%), urine (87%, 79% unchanged); $T_{1/2}$=12.4 hrs. Metformin: Urine (90%); $T_{1/2}$=6.2 hrs (plasma), 17.6 hrs (blood).

NURSING CONSIDERATIONS

Assessment: Assess for metabolic acidosis, risk factors for lactic acidosis, renal/hepatic function, previous hypersensitivity to the drug or other drugs of same class, history of pancreatitis, type 1 DM, diabetic ketoacidosis, pregnancy/nursing status, and possible drug interactions. Assess if patient is planning to undergo any surgical procedure or is under any form of stress. Obtain baseline FPG, HbA1c, CrCl, and hematologic parameters.

Monitoring: Monitor for signs/symptoms of lactic acidosis, pancreatitis, clinical illness, hypoxic states, and hypersensitivity reactions. Monitor renal function, especially in elderly, at least annually. Monitor vitamin B12 levels in patients predisposed to develop subnormal vitamin B12 levels. Monitor FPG, HbA1c, renal/hepatic function, and hematologic parameters periodically.

Patient Counseling: Inform of risks, benefits, and alternative modes of therapy. Advise on importance of adherence to dietary instructions, regular physical activity, periodic blood glucose monitoring, HbA1c testing, regular testing of renal function and hematological parameters, recognition/management of hypoglycemia/hyperglycemia, and assessment of diabetic complications. Instruct to seek medical advice during periods of stress (eg, fever, trauma, infection, surgery) as medication needs may change. Advise of the risk of lactic acidosis. Inform that GI symptoms, acute pancreatitis, and allergic reactions may occur. Advise to d/c and notify physician if symptoms of allergic reactions, persistent severe abdominal pain, unexplained hyperventilation, myalgia, malaise, unusual somnolence, dizziness, slow or irregular heart beat, sensation of feeling cold (especially in the extremities), or other nonspecific symptoms occur. Counsel against excessive alcohol intake. Inform that incidence of hypoglycemia is increased when added to sulfonylurea or insulin and a lower dose of sulfonylurea or insulin may be required. Counsel to inform physician if any unusual symptom develops, or if any known symptom persists or worsens.

Administration: Oral route. Take qd with a meal, preferably in pm. Do not split, break, crush, or chew before swallowing. Take 100mg Sitagliptin/1000mg Metformin ER tab as single tab qd. Patients using 2 tabs should take the 2 tabs together qd. **Storage:** 20-25°C (68-77°F); excursions permitted to 15-30°C (59-86°F).

JANUVIA   RX
sitagliptin (Merck)

THERAPEUTIC CLASS: Dipeptidyl peptidase-4 inhibitor

INDICATIONS: Adjunct to diet and exercise to improve glycemic control in adults with type 2 diabetes mellitus (DM).

DOSAGE: *Adults:* Usual: 100mg qd. Renal Insufficiency: Moderate (CrCl ≥30 to <50mL/min): 50mg qd. Severe (CrCl <30mL/min)/End Stage Renal Disease Requiring Hemodialysis or Peritoneal Dialysis: 25mg qd. With Insulin/Insulin Secretagogue (eg, sulfonylurea): May require lower dose of insulin secretagogue or insulin.

HOW SUPPLIED: Tab: 25mg, 50mg, 100mg

WARNINGS/PRECAUTIONS: Do not use in type 1 DM or for treatment of diabetic ketoacidosis. Acute pancreatitis reported; d/c if pancreatitis is suspected. Use caution to ensure that correct dose is prescribed with moderate/severe renal impairment. Worsening renal function, including acute renal failure reported. Serious hypersensitivity reactions reported; d/c if hypersensitivity reaction is suspected and institute alternative treatment. No conclusive evidence of macrovascular risk reduction. Caution in elderly.

ADVERSE REACTIONS: Nasopharyngitis, upper respiratory infection, headache.

INTERACTIONS: May slightly increase digoxin levels; monitor appropriately. May require lower dose of insulin secretagogue (eg, sulfonylurea) or insulin therapy to reduce risk of hypoglycemia.

PREGNANCY: Category B, caution in nursing.

MECHANISM OF ACTION: Dipeptidyl peptidase-4 inhibitor; slows inactivation of incretin hormones thus increases insulin release and decreases glucagon levels in the circulation in a glucose-dependent manner.

PHARMACOKINETICS: Absorption: Rapid. Absolute bioavailability (87%); T_{max}=1-4 hrs; AUC=8.52μM•hr; C_{max}=950nM. **Distribution:** (IV) V_d=198L; plasma protein binding (38%). **Metabolism:** Via CYP3A4 and CYP2C8. **Elimination:** Feces (13%), urine (87%, 79% unchanged); $T_{1/2}$=12.4 hrs.

NURSING CONSIDERATIONS

Assessment: Assess renal function, for previous hypersensitivity to the drug, history of pancreatitis, type 1 DM, diabetic ketoacidosis, pregnancy/nursing status, and possible drug interactions. Obtain baseline FPG, HbA1c, and CrCl.

Monitoring: Monitor for pancreatitis and hypersensitivity reactions. Monitor FPG, HbA1c, and renal function periodically.

Patient Counseling: Inform of risks, benefits, and alternative modes of therapy. Advise on the importance of adherence to dietary instructions, regular physical activity, periodic blood glucose monitoring, HbA1c testing, recognition/management of hypoglycemia/hyperglycemia, and assessment of diabetic complications. Instruct to seek medical advice during periods of stress (eg, fever, trauma, infection, surgery) as medication needs may change. Instruct to d/c use and notify physician if signs and symptoms of pancreatitis or allergic reactions occur. Inform that incidence of hypoglycemia is increased when added to sulfonylurea or insulin and a lower dose of sulfonylurea or insulin may be required. Counsel to inform physician if any unusual symptom develops, or if any known symptom persists or worsens.

Administration: Oral route. May be taken with or without food. **Storage:** 20-25°C (68-77°F); excursions permitted to 15-30°C (59-86°F).

JENLOGA   RX
clonidine HCl (Shionogi)

THERAPEUTIC CLASS: Alpha-adrenergic agonist

INDICATIONS: Treatment of hypertension, alone or with other antihypertensives.

DOSAGE: *Adults:* Individualize dose. Initial: 0.1mg hs. Titrate: If inadequate reduction in BP, may increase in increments of 0.1mg/day at weekly intervals. Doses >0.1mg/day should be divided and taken am and hs. If am and hs doses are not equal, hs dose should be the larger of the two. Usual: 0.2-0.6mg/day. Max: 0.6mg/day. Renal Impairment: Initial: 0.1mg/day. Increase dose slowly. Carefully monitor to prevent excessive blood pressure lowering or bradycardia.

HOW SUPPLIED: Tab: 0.1mg

WARNINGS/PRECAUTIONS: Avoid abrupt d/c; reduce dose gradually over 2 to 4 days. Rare instances of hypertensive encephalopathy, cerebrovascular accidents (CVA) and death reported after withdrawal. Caution with severe coronary insufficiency, conduction disturbances, recent myocardial infarction (MI), cerebrovascular disease, or chronic renal failure; uptitrate dose slowly. In patients who have developed localized contact sensitization to a clonidine transdermal system, substitution of PO clonidine may result in the development of a generalized skin rash. In patients who develop an allergic reaction from a clonidine transdermal system, substitution of oral clonidine may elicit an allergic reaction (eg, generalized rash, urticaria, angioedema). Monitor BP during surgery; additional measures to control BP should be available. Continue to within 4 hrs of surgery and resume as soon as possible thereafter.

ADVERSE REACTIONS: Dry mouth, fatigue, dizziness, headache, nausea, somnolence, insomnia.

INTERACTIONS: May potentiate CNS depression with alcohol, barbiturates, or other sedating drugs. Hypotensive effect may be reduced by tricyclic antidepressants. Monitor HR with agents that affect sinus node function or AV nodal conduction (eg, digitalis, calcium channel blockers, β-blockers). Sinus bradycardia reported with diltiazem or verapamil. D/C β-blockers several days before the gradual withdrawal of clonidine in patients taking both.

PREGNANCY: Category C, not for use in nursing.

MECHANISM OF ACTION: Centrally acting alpha-2 adrenergic agonist; stimulates α-adrenoreceptors in the brain stem, reducing sympathetic outflow from CNS and decreasing peripheral resistance, renal vascular resistance, HR, and BP.

PHARMACOKINETICS: Absorption: T_{max}=4-7 hrs. **Distribution:** Found in breast milk. **Metabolism:** Liver. **Elimination:** Urine (40-60%, unchanged); $T_{1/2}$=13 hrs.

NURSING CONSIDERATIONS

Assessment: Assess for severe coronary insufficiency, conduction disturbances, recent MI, cerebrovascular disease, renal impairment, pregnancy/nursing status, and for possible drug interactions.

Monitoring: Monitor BP and renal function periodically. Monitor for withdrawal signs/symptoms (eg, hypertensive encephalopathy, CVA), presence of generalized skin rash, and allergic reactions.

Patient Counseling: Caution against interruption of therapy without physician's advice. Caution in engaging in hazardous activities (eg, operating machinery or driving). Inform that sedative effect may be increased by concomitant use of alcohol, barbiturates, or other sedating drugs. Inform that medication may cause dryness of the eyes; caution with contact lenses.

Administration: Oral route. **Storage:** 20-25°C (68-77°F).

JEVTANA   RX
cabazitaxel (Sanofi-Aventis)

> Neutropenic deaths reported. Perform frequent blood cell counts to monitor for neutropenia. Avoid with neutrophil counts of ≤1500 cells/mm³. Severe hypersensitivity reactions reported; d/c immediately if this occurs and administer appropriate therapy. Patients should receive premedication. Contraindicated in patients with history of severe hypersensitivity reactions to this medication or drugs formulated with polysorbate 80.

THERAPEUTIC CLASS: Antimicrotubule agent

INDICATIONS: In combination with prednisone for the treatment of hormone-refractory metastatic prostate cancer previously treated with a docetaxel-containing treatment regimen.

DOSAGE: *Adults:* Individualize dose based on BSA. Initial: 25mg/m² over 1-hr IV infusion q3 weeks with PO prednisone 10mg qd. Reduce dose to 20mg/m² if patients experience prolonged Grade ≥3 neutropenia (>1 week) despite appropriate medications (including granulocyte-colony stimulating factor [G-CSF]), febrile neutropenia, or Grade ≥3 diarrhea or persisting diarrhea despite appropriate medication, fluid, and electrolyte replacement. Delay treatment until improvement or resolution of febrile neutropenia, diarrhea, and until neutrophil count is >1500 cells/mm³. Use G-CSF for secondary prophylaxis for neutropenia and febrile neutropenia. D/C treatment if patient continues to experience any of these reactions at 20mg/m². Premedicate at least 30 min prior to each dose with antihistamine (dexchlorpheniramine 5mg, diphenhydramine 25mg, or equivalent antihistamine), corticosteroid (dexamethasone 8mg or equivalent steroid), H_2 antagonist (ranitidine 50mg or equivalent H_2 antagonist). Also give antiemetics as prophylaxis (PO or IV) PRN.

HOW SUPPLIED: Inj: 60mg/1.5mL

CONTRAINDICATIONS: Neutrophil counts ≤1500/mm³.

WARNINGS/PRECAUTIONS: May cause GI symptoms (N/V, severe diarrhea), and intensive treatment measures may be required; may need to delay treatment or reduce dose with Grade ≥3 diarrhea. Renal failure, including cases with fatal outcome, reported; identify cause and treat aggressively. Caution with severe renal impairment (CrCl <30mL/min) and in patients with end-stage renal disease. Avoid with hepatic impairment (total bilirubin ≥ULN, or AST and/or ALT ≥1.5X ULN). May cause fetal harm; avoid during pregnancy. Caution in elderly. Caution when handling or preparing sol.

ADVERSE REACTIONS: Hypersensitivity reactions, neutropenia, anemia, leukopenia, thrombocytopenia, diarrhea, fatigue, N/V, constipation, asthenia, abdominal pain, anorexia, back pain, hematuria.

INTERACTIONS: Avoid with strong CYP3A inhibitors (eg, ketoconazole, itraconazole, clarithromycin, atazanavir, indinavir, nefazodone, nelfinavir, ritonavir, saquinavir, telithromycin, voriconazole), strong CYP3A inducers (eg, phenytoin, carbamazepine, rifampin, rifabutin, rifapentin, phenobarbital), and St. John's wort. Caution with concomitant use of moderate CYP3A inhibitors.

PREGNANCY: Category D, not for use in nursing.

MECHANISM OF ACTION: Antimicrotubule agent; binds to tubulin and promotes its assembly into microtubules while simultaneously inhibiting disassembly which results in the inhibition of mitotic and interphase cellular functions.

PHARMACOKINETICS: Absorption: C_{max}=226 ng/mL; AUC=991 ng•hr/mL; T_{max}=1 hr. **Distribution**: V_{ss}=4,864L; plasma protein binding (89%-92%). **Metabolism**: Liver (extensive) via CYP3A4/5, and to a lesser extent CYP2C8. **Elimination**: Urine (3.7%) (2.3%, unchanged), feces (76%); $T_{1/2}$= 95 hrs

NURSING CONSIDERATIONS

Assessment: Assess for hypersensitivity to drugs formulated with polysorbate 80, hepatic/severe renal impairment, pregnancy/nursing status, and possible drug interactions. Obtain baseline neutrophil count. Assess for high-risk clinical features that may predispose to increased neutropenia complications.

Monitoring: Monitor CBC on weekly basis during Cycle 1 and before each treatment cycle thereafter. Monitor for signs/symptoms of severe neutropenia, febrile neutropenia, infections, severe diarrhea, dehydration, renal failure, and hypersensitivity reactions.

Patient Counseling: Counsel about the risk of potential hypersensitivity; instruct to immediately report signs of hypersensitivity reactions. Advise on the importance of routine blood cell counts. Instruct to immediately report any occurrence of fever. Inform to report if not compliant with PO corticosteroid regimen. Counsel about side effects associated with exposure such as severe and fatal infections, dehydration, and renal failure. Advise to report significant vomiting or diarrhea, decreased urinary output, and hematuria. Advise to inform physician before taking any other medications. Advise women of childbearing age not to become pregnant while taking this drug. Inform elderly that certain side effects may be more frequent or severe.

Administration: IV infusion; refer to PI for preparation and administration procedures. Use first diluted sol within 30 min. Use second diluted sol within 8 hrs at ambient temperature (including the 1-hr infusion); 24 hrs (including the 1-hr infusion) under refrigeration. Do not use PVC infusion containers or polyurethane infusions sets. **Storage**: Undiluted: 25°C (77°F); excursions permitted to 15-30°C (59-86°F). Do not refrigerate. Diluted Second Sol: 0.9% NaCl or D5W: 24 hrs under refrigerated conditions.

JUVISYNC   RX
simvastatin - sitagliptin (Merck)

THERAPEUTIC CLASS: Dipeptidyl peptidase-4 inhibitor/HMG-CoA reductase inhibitor

INDICATIONS: Adjunct to diet and exercise to improve glycemic control in adults with type 2 diabetes mellitus (DM). Adjunct to diet to reduce total mortality risk by reducing coronary heart disease (CHD) deaths, risk of nonfatal myocardial infarction and stroke, and need for coronary/noncoronary revascularization procedures in patients at high risk of coronary events because of existing CHD, DM, peripheral vessel disease, history of stroke or other cerebrovascular disease. Reduce elevated total cholesterol (total-C), LDL-C, apolipoprotein B (Apo B), and TG, and to increase HDL-C in primary hyperlipidemia (Fredrickson Type IIa, heterozygous familial and nonfamilial) or mixed dyslipidemia (Fredrickson Type IIb). Reduce elevated TG in hypertriglyceridemia (Fredrickson Type IV hyperlipidemia). Reduce elevated TG and VLDL-C in primary dysbetalipoproteinemia (Fredrickson Type III hyperlipidemia). Reduce total-C and LDL-C in homozygous familial hypercholesterolemia as adjunct to other lipid-lowering treatments or if treatments are unavailable.

DOSAGE: *Adults:* Usual: 100mg-10mg, 100mg-20mg, or 100mg-40mg qd. Take as a single dose in the pm. Initial: 100mg-40mg/day. Patients on Simvastatin with or without Sitagliptin 100mg/day: Initial: 100mg sitagliptin and dose of simvastatin already taken. Analyze lipid levels after ≥4 weeks and adjust dose PRN. With Insulin/Insulin Secretagogue (eg, sulfonylurea): May require lower dose of insulin secretagogue or insulin. Concomitant Verapamil/Diltiazem: Max: 100mg-10mg qd. Concomitant Amiodarone/Amlodipine/Ranolazine: Max: 100mg-20mg qd. Homozygous Familial Hypercholesterolemia: Usual: 100mg-40mg qd. Chinese Patients taking Lipid-Modifying Doses (≥1g/day niacin) of Niacin-Containing Products: Caution with 100mg-40mg qd.

HOW SUPPLIED: Tab: (Sitagliptin-Simvastatin) 100mg-10mg, 100mg-20mg, 100mg-40mg

CONTRAINDICATIONS: Concomitant strong CYP3A4 inhibitors (eg, itraconazole, ketoconazole, posaconazole, HIV protease inhibitors, erythromycin, clarithromycin, telithromycin, and nefazodone), gemfibrozil, cyclosporine, or danazol. Active liver disease or unexplained persistent elevations in hepatic transaminase levels, women who are or may become pregnant, nursing mothers.

WARNINGS/PRECAUTIONS: Not for use in type 1 DM or for treatment of diabetic ketoacidosis. Not recommended with moderate or severe renal impairment or end-stage renal disease. Caution in elderly. Sitagliptin: Acute pancreatitis reported; d/c if pancreatitis is suspected. Worsening renal function, including acute renal failure, reported. Serious hypersensitivity reactions reported; d/c if hypersensitivity reaction is suspected and institute alternative treatment. Angioedema reported; caution with history of angioedema. Simvastatin: Myopathy and rhabdomyolysis reported; predisposing factors include advanced age (≥65 yrs), female gender, uncontrolled hypothyroidism, and renal impairment. The risk of myopathy, including rhabdomyolysis, is dose related. D/C therapy if myopathy is suspected/diagnosed, or if markedly elevated CPK levels occur. Temporarily withhold in any patient experiencing an acute or serious condition predisposing to the development of renal failure secondary to rhabdomyolysis (eg, sepsis; hypotension; major surgery; trauma; severe metabolic, endocrine, or electrolyte disorders; uncontrolled epilepsy). Persistent increases in serum transaminases reported; monitor LFTs before and during treatment when clinically indicated. Increase in HbA1c and fasting serum glucose levels reported. Caution with heavy alcohol use and history of hepatic disease.

ADVERSE REACTIONS: Nasopharyngitis, upper respiratory infection, headache, abdominal pain, myalgia, constipation, nausea, atrial fibrillation, gastritis, DM, insomnia, vertigo, bronchitis, eczema, hypoglycemia.

INTERACTIONS: See Contraindications. May slightly elevate plasma digoxin concentrations. Sitagliptin: May require lower dose of insulin secretagogue (eg, sulfonylurea) or insulin therapy to reduce risk of hypoglycemia. Simvastatin: Avoid large quantities of grapefruit juice (>1 quart daily). Voriconazole may inhibit metabolism; may need to adjust dose. Increased risk of myopathy with fibrates and colchicine; caution when prescribed. Increased risk of myopathy, including rhabdomyolysis, with amiodarone, ranolazine, calcium channel blockers (eg, verapamil, diltiazem, or amlodipine), lipid-modifying doses of niacin-containing products (≥1g/day niacin), and CYP3A4 inhibitors. May potentiate effect of coumarin anticoagulants; monitor PT.

PREGNANCY: Category X, not for use in nursing.

MECHANISM OF ACTION: Sitagliptin: Dipeptidyl peptidase-4 inhibitor; slows inactivation of incretin hormones thus increases insulin release and decreases glucagon levels in the circulation in a glucose-dependent manner. Simvastatin: HMG-CoA reductase inhibitor; inhibits enzyme that catalyzes the conversion of HMG-CoA to mevalonate, an early and rate-limiting step in the biosynthetic pathway for cholesterol. Reduces VLDL, TG, and increases HDL-C.

PHARMACOKINETICS: Absorption: Sitagliptin: Rapid. Absolute bioavailability (87%); T_{max}=1-4 hrs; AUC=8.52μM•hr; C_{max}=950nM. Simvastatin: Bioavailability (<5%); T_{max}=1.5 hrs(simvastatin lactone), 4-6 hrs (simvastatin acid). **Distribution:** Sitagliptin: (IV) V_d=198L; plasma protein binding (38%). Simvastatin: Plasma protein binding (95%). **Metabolism:** Sitagliptin: Via CYP3A4 and CYP2C8. Simvastatin: Liver (extensive 1st pass); β-hydroxyacid, 6'-hydroxy, 6'-hydroxymethyl, and 6'-exomethylene (major active metabolites). **Elimination:** Sitagliptin: Feces (13%), urine (87%, 79% unchanged); $T_{1/2}$=12.4 hrs. Simvastatin: Feces (60%), urine (13%).

NURSING CONSIDERATIONS

Assessment: Assess renal function, for previous hypersensitivity to the drug, history of pancreatitis, type 1 DM, diabetic ketoacidosis, active liver disease or unexplained persistent elevations in serum transaminases, risk factors for developing myopathy (eg, advanced age, uncontrolled hypothyroidism, renal impairment), pregnancy/nursing status, and possible drug interactions. Assess use in patients who consume substantial quantities of alcohol and/or have a past history of liver disease. Obtain baseline lipid profile (total-C, LDL-C, HDL-C, TG), LFTs, FPG, HbA1c, and CrCl.

Monitoring: Monitor for pancreatitis, hypersensitivity reactions, signs/symptoms of myopathy (eg, muscle pain, tenderness, weakness), rhabdomyolysis, and liver dysfunction. Monitor patients receiving digoxin. Periodically monitor lipid levels (LDL-C), creatine kinase levels, LFTs, FPG, HbA1c, and renal function.

Patient Counseling: Inform of risks, benefits, and alternative modes of therapy. Advise on the importance of adherence to dietary instructions, regular physical activity, periodic blood glucose monitoring, HbA1c testing. Educate on recognition/management of hypoglycemia/hyperglycemia and assessment for diabetic complications. Instruct to seek medical advice during periods of stress (eg, fever, trauma, infection, surgery) as medication needs may change. Instruct to d/c use and notify physician if signs and symptoms of pancreatitis or allergic reactions occur. Counsel to inform physician if any unusual symptom develops, or if any known symptom persists or worsens. Advise to adhere to their National Cholesterol Education Program recommended diet, regular exercise program, and periodic testing of a fasting lipid panel. Inform of the risk of myopathy, including rhabdomyolysis; advise to contact physician immediately if unexplained muscle pain, tenderness, or weakness occurs. Inform that liver function will be checked prior to and during treatment. Advise to d/c therapy and contact physician if pregnant. Inform that drug should not be taken if breastfeeding. Advise females of childbearing potential to use effective contraception. Inform of the substances that should not be taken concomitantly with the drug. Instruct to swallow tab whole; do not split, crush, or chew.

Administration: Oral route. Swallow whole; do not split, chew, or crush. **Storage:** 20-25°C (68-77°F); excursions permitted to 15-30°C (59-86°F). Store in a dry place with cap tightly closed.

KADIAN
morphine sulfate (Actavis)

> Contains morphine sulfate, a Schedule II controlled substance, that has a high potential for abuse and is subject to misuse, addiction, and criminal diversion. 100mg and 200mg cap are for use in opioid-tolerant patients only; these strengths may cause fatal respiratory depression in non-opioid tolerant patients. Not for use as a prn analgesic. Swallow whole or sprinkle contents on applesauce. Do not chew, crush, or dissolve.

THERAPEUTIC CLASS: Opioid analgesic

INDICATIONS: Management of moderate to severe pain when continuous, around-the-clock opioid analgesic is needed for an extended period of time.

DOSAGE: *Adults:* Individualize dose. Conversion from Other Oral Morphine: Give 50% of daily oral morphine dose q12h or give 100% oral morphine dose q24h. Do not give more frequently than q12h. Conversion from Parenteral Morphine: Dose of oral morphine 3x the daily parenteral morphine dose may be sufficient in chronic-use settings. Conversion from Other Parenteral or Oral Opioids: Initial: Give 50% of estimated daily morphine demand and supplement with IR morphine. 1st dose may be taken with the last dose of any IR morphine. Conversion from Other Non-Opioids and Intermittent Use of Moderate or Strong Opioids: Give 50% of estimated total daily oral morphine dose q12h or q24h. Titrate: No more frequently than qod to stabilize before escalating the dose. Breakthrough Pain: Supplement dose with <20% of daily dose of short-acting analgesic. Switch to bid dosing after excessive sedation to qd dosing or inadequate analgesia before next dose. Opioid Non-Tolerant: 10-20mg. Titrate: Increase not >20mg qod. Refer to PI for considerations in dosing adjustments and conversion to other formulations or other opioids. Elderly: Start at low end of dosing range.

HOW SUPPLIED: Cap, Extended-Release: 10mg, 20mg, 30mg, 50mg, 60mg, 80mg, 100mg, 200mg

CONTRAINDICATIONS: Respiratory depression in the absence of resuscitative equipment or in unmonitored settings, acute or severe bronchial asthma or hypercarbia, has or suspected of having paralytic ileus.

WARNINGS/PRECAUTIONS: Not indicated for pain in the immediate postoperative period or if pain is mild or not expected to persist for an extended period of time. Do not use as 1st opioid. Increased risk of respiratory depression in elderly, debilitated patients, those suffering from conditions accompanied by hypoxia, hypercapnia, or upper airway obstruction. Caution and consider non-opioid analgesics with chronic obstructive pulmonary disease or cor pulmonale, substantially decreased respiratory reserve (eg, severe kyphoscoliosis), or preexisting respiratory depression. Respiratory depression and potential to elevate CSF pressure may be markedly exaggerated in the presence of head injury, other intracranial lesions, or preexisting increase in ICP; may obscure neurologic signs of further increases in pressure with head injuries. May cause orthostatic hypotension and syncope in ambulatory patients. May cause severe hypotension in an individual whose ability to maintain BP has been compromised by a depleted blood volume. Caution in patients with circulatory shock. Avoid with GI obstruction, especially paralytic ileus; may obscure diagnosis or clinical course with acute abdominal conditions. Rare cases of anaphylaxis reported. Caution in renal/hepatic/pulmonary impairment, hypothyroidism, myxedema, adrenocortical insufficiency (eg, Addison's disease), CNS depression or coma, toxic psychosis, prostatic hypertrophy, urethral stricture, acute alcoholism, delirium tremens, kyphoscoliosis, inability to swallow, and convulsive disorders. May aggravate convulsions with convulsive disorders. Caution with biliary tract disease and acute pancreatitis; may cause spasm of the sphincter of Oddi. Tolerance and physical dependence may occur. Avoid abrupt withdrawal. May impair mental/physical abilities. D/C 24 hrs before procedure that interrupts pain transmission pathways (eg, cordotomy); give short-acting parenteral opioid. May cause neonatal withdrawal symptoms. Caution in elderly/debilitated.

ADVERSE REACTIONS: Respiratory depression, drowsiness, dizziness, constipation, nausea, anxiety.

INTERACTIONS: Caution with CNS depressants (including sedatives, hypnotics, general anesthetics, antiemetics, phenothiazines, tranquilizers, other opioids, illicit drugs, alcohol); may increase the risk of respiratory depression, hypotension, profound sedation, or coma. May enhance neuromuscular blocking action and increases respiratory depression with skeletal relaxants. Caution with agonist/antagonist analgesics (eg, pentazocine, nalbuphine, butorphanol); may reduce analgesic effects or precipitate withdrawal symptoms. Potentiated by MAOIs; avoid during or within 14 days of use. May reduce diuretic effects. Confusion and severe respiratory depression reported with cimetidine. Risk of hypotension with phenothiazines or general anesthetics.

PREGNANCY: Category C, not for use in nursing.

MECHANISM OF ACTION: Opioid analgesic; not established. Acts as a pure agonist, binding with and activating opioid receptors at sites in the peri-aqueductal and periventricular gray matter, the ventromedial medulla, and the spinal cord to produce analgesia.

PHARMACOKINETICS: Absorption: Various doses resulted in different parameters. **Distribution:** V_d=3-4L/kg; plasma protein binding (30-35%); crosses the placenta, found in breast milk. **Metabolism:** Liver (conjugation) to glucuronide metabolites; morphine-3-glucuronide, morphine-6-glucuronide. **Elimination:** Urine (10% unchanged); bile (small amount); feces (7-10%); $T_{1/2}$=2-4 hrs.

NURSING CONSIDERATIONS

Assessment: Assess for degree of opioid tolerance, previous opioid dose, level of pain intensity, type and severity of pain, patient's general condition and medical status, or any other conditions where treatment is contraindicated or cautioned. Assess for history of hypersensitivity, pregnancy/nursing status, renal/hepatic function, and possible drug interactions.

Monitoring: Monitor for signs/symptoms of respiratory depression, hypotension, anaphylaxis, convulsions, tolerance and physical dependence (eg, withdrawal symptoms), and signs of medication misuse or abuse, and other adverse reactions.

Patient Counseling: Advise to take medication only ud and do not adjust dose without consulting physician. Instruct to swallow cap whole or sprinkle on small amount of applesauce; do not chew, crush, or dissolve. Advise that 100mg and 200mg caps are for use only in opioid-tolerant patients. Counsel to report episodes of breakthrough pain and adverse experiences during therapy. Inform that drug may impair mental/physical ability. Advise not to take alcohol or other CNS depressants (eg, sleeping medication, tranquilizers) except if directed by physician. Instruct to inform physician if pregnant, become pregnant, or plan to become pregnant prior to therapy. Counsel on the importance of safely tapering the dose and that abrupt d/c of therapy may precipitate withdrawal symptoms. Inform of the potential for drug abuse and must be protected from theft. Inform that severe constipation may occur. Instruct to keep in a secure place out of reach of children and when no longer needed destroy the unused cap by flushing down the toilet.

Administration: Oral route. Refer to PI for alternative methods of administration. **Storage:** 25°C (77°F); excursions permitted to 15-30°C (59-86°F). Protect from light and moisture.

KALETRA   RX
ritonavir - lopinavir (Abbott)

THERAPEUTIC CLASS: Protease inhibitor

INDICATIONS: Treatment of HIV-1 infection in combination with other antiretrovirals.

DOSAGE: *Adults:* 400mg-100mg bid. Less than 3 Lopinavir Resistance-Associated Substitutions: 800mg-200mg qd. Concomitant Therapy with Efavirenz, Nevirapine, Amprenavir, Nelfinavir: (Tabs) 500mg-125mg bid; (Sol) 533mg-133mg (6.5mL) bid.
Pediatrics: 6 months-18 yrs: (Sol) ≥15-40kg: 10mg-2.5mg/kg bid. <15kg: 12mg-3mg/kg bid. Max: 400mg-100mg bid. (Tab) >35kg: 400mg-100mg bid. >25-35kg: 300mg-75mg bid. 15-25kg: 200mg-50mg bid. 14 days-6 months: (Sol) 16mg-4mg/kg bid. Concomitant Therapy with Efavirenz, Nevirapine, Amprenavir, Nelfinavir: Treatment-Naive and Treatment-Experienced: 6 months-18 yrs: (Sol) ≥15-45kg: 11mg-2.75mg/kg bid. <15kg: 13mg-3.25mg/kg bid. Max: 533mg-133mg bid. (Tab) >45kg: 500mg-125mg bid. >30-45kg: 400mg-100mg bid. >20-30kg: 300mg-75mg bid. 15-20kg: 200mg-50mg bid. Refer to PI for BSA-based dosing.

HOW SUPPLIED: Tab: (Lopinavir-Ritonavir) 100mg-25mg, 200mg-50mg; Sol: 80mg-20mg/mL [160mL]

CONTRAINDICATIONS: Coadministration with CYP3A substrates for which elevated plasma concentrations are associated with serious and/or life-threatening reactions and with potent CYP3A inducers where significantly reduced lopinavir levels may be associated with the potential for loss of virologic response and possible resistance and cross-resistance (eg, alfuzosin, rifampin, dihydroergotamine, ergonovine, ergotamine, methylergonovine, St. John's wort, cisapride, lovastatin, simvastatin, sildenafil [when used to treat pulmonary arterial HTN], pimozide, triazolam, oral midazolam).

WARNINGS/PRECAUTIONS: Avoid sol in preterm neonates; may be at increased risk of propylene glycol-associated adverse events and other toxicities. Pancreatitis including marked TG elevations reported; evaluate and suspend therapy if clinically appropriate. Underlying hepatitis B or C or marked serum transaminase elevations prior to treatment may be at increased risk for developing or worsening of transaminase elevations or hepatic decompensation; conduct appropriate laboratory testing prior to therapy and monitor during treatment. New onset or exacerbation of diabetes mellitus (DM), hyperglycemia, diabetic ketoacidosis, immune reconstitute syndrome, fat redistribution, lipid elevations, and increased bleeding with hemophilia A and B reported. PR and QT interval prolongation, torsade de pointes, and cases of second/third degree atrioventricular block reported; caution with those at increased risk for conduction abnormalities, or coadministration of drugs that prolong PR interval. Avoid use with congenital long QT syndrome and hypokalemia. Once-daily regimen is not recommended for adults with ≥3 lopinavir

K

resistance associated substitutions or in pediatric patients. Caution with hepatic impairment and in elderly.

ADVERSE REACTIONS: Asthenia, diarrhea, N/V, dysgeusia, hepatotoxicity, pancreatitis, rash, abdominal pain, dyspepsia, headache, decreased weight, insomnia.

INTERACTIONS: See Contraindications. Avoid with colchicine in patients with renal/hepatic impairment, tadalafil for pulmonary arterial hypertension during initiation, oral midazolam, and tipranavir/ritonavir combination. Not recommended with voriconazole, high doses of itraconazole or ketoconazole, and salmeterol. May increase levels of fentanyl, tenofovir, amprenavir, indinavir, nelfinavir, saquinavir, maraviroc, antiarrhythmics, anticancer agents, trazodone, azole antifungals (eg, ketoconazole), rifabutin, clarithromycin in patients with renal impairment, IV midazolam, dihydropyridine calcium channel blockers, bosentan, HMG-CoA reductase inhibitors, immunosuppressants, inhaled steroids, salmeterol, and PDE5 inhibitors for erectile dysfunction. May decrease levels of methadone, phenytoin, bupropion, atovaquone, ethinyl estradiol, abacavir, zidovudine, and voriconazole. Delavirdine and CYP3A inhibitors may increase levels. May alter concentrations of warfarin; monitor INR. Efavirenz, nevirapine, amprenavir, nelfinavir, and anticonvulsants may decrease levels; not for qd dosing regimen. Rifampin, fosamprenavir/ritonavir, and dexamethasone may decrease levels. Sol contains alcohol; may produce disulfiram-like reactions with disulfiram or metronidazole.

PREGNANCY: Category C, not for use in nursing.

MECHANISM OF ACTION: Lopinavir: HIV-1 protease inhibitor; prevents cleavage of the Gag-Pol polyprotein, resulting in the production of immature, noninfectious viral particles. Ritonavir: HIV-1 protease inhibitor; CYP3A inhibitor that inhibits metabolism of lopinavir, increasing its plasma levels.

PHARMACOKINETICS: Absorption: Lopinavir: (400mg-100mg bid) C_{max}=9.8µg/mL, T_{max}=4 hrs, AUC=92.6µg•h/mL. Refer to PI for pediatric parameters. **Distribution:** Lopinavir: Plasma protein binding (98-99%). **Metabolism:** Lopinavir: Hepatic via CYP3A (extensive). Ritonavir: Induces own metabolism. **Elimination:** Unchanged lopinavir: Urine (2.2%), feces (19.8%).

NURSING CONSIDERATIONS

Assessment: Assess for history of hypersensitivity reactions, history of pancreatitis, hepatitis B or C, cirrhosis, DM or hyperglycemia, hyperlipidemia, hemophilia type A or B, structural heart disease, preexisting conduction system abnormalities, ischemic heart disease or cardiomyopathies, congenital long QT syndrome, hypokalemia, renal/hepatic impairment, pregnancy/nursing status, and for possible drug interactions. Obtain baseline TG, serum transaminase, total cholesterol levels. Assess children for the ability to swallow intact tab.

Monitoring: Monitor for signs/symptoms of pancreatitis, hyperglycemia, hepatic dysfunction, infection, fat redistribution, hypersensitivity reactions, and other adverse reactions. Monitor infants for increase in serum osmolality, SrCr, and toxicity (eg, hyperosmolality, renal toxicity, CNS depression, seizures, hypotonia, cardiac arrhythmias, ECG changes, hemolysis) if benefit of using oral sol immediately after birth outweighs the potential risks. Monitor LFTs, lipid profile, glucose, total bilirubin, ECG changes, serum lipase, and serum amylase levels.

Patient Counseling: Instruct to take prescribed dose as directed; sol should be taken with food and tabs may be taken with or without food. Instruct to inform physician if weight changes in children occurs. If a dose is missed, take dose as soon as possible and return to normal schedule; do not double next dose. Advise that product is not a cure for HIV; opportunistic infections may still occur. Advise to use additional or alternative contraceptive measures if receiving estrogen-based hormonal contraceptives. Inform that skin rashes, liver function changes, electrocardiogram changes, redistribution/accumulation of body fat, new onset or worsening of preexisting diabetes, and hyperglycemia may occur; seek medical attention if symptoms of worsening liver disease (eg, abdominal pain, jaundice), dizziness, abnormal heart rhythm, or loss of consciousness occur. Inform of greater chance of developing diarrhea with qd regimen. Instruct to notify physician if using other Rx/OTC or herbal products, particularly St. John's wort. When taking didanosine, advise to take tab at the same time without food or take 1 hr before or 2 hrs after sol. Inform that hypotension, visual changes, sustained erection may occur if receiving sildenafil, tadalafil, or vardenafil; report any symptoms to physician. Advise not to expose tabs to high humidity outside original container >2 weeks.

Administration: Oral route. Swallow tab whole; do not crush, break, or chew. Take sol with food. **Storage:** (Tab) 20-25°C (68-77°F); excursions permitted to 15-30°C (59-86°F). (Sol) 2-8°C (36-46°F). Avoid exposure to excessive heat. If stored at room temperature up to 25°C (77°F), sol should be used within 2 months.

KAPVAY ER   RX
clonidine HCl (Shionogi)

THERAPEUTIC CLASS: Alpha$_2$-agonist

INDICATIONS: Treatment of attention deficit hyperactivity disorder (ADHD) as monotherapy and as adjunctive therapy to stimulant medications.

DOSAGE: *Pediatrics:* 6-17 yrs: Initial: 0.1mg hs. Titrate: Adjust in increments of 0.1mg/day at weekly intervals until desired response is achieved. Max: 0.4mg/day. D/C in in decrements of no more than 0.1 mg every 3 to 7 days. Refer to PI for further dosing information.

HOW SUPPLIED: Tab, Extended-Release: 0.1mg, 0.2mg

WARNINGS/PRECAUTIONS: May cause dose related decreases in BP and HR; measure HR and BP prior to initiation of therapy, following dose increases, and periodically while on therapy. Somnolence and sedation reported. May impair mental/physical abilities. Avoid abrupt d/c; sudden cessation may result in headache, tachycardia, nausea, flushing, warm feeling, light-headedness, tightness in chest, and anxiety. Caution with history of hypotension, heart block, bradycardia, CV disease, syncope, severe coronary insufficiency, conduction disturbances, recent myocardial infarction (MI), cerebrovascular disease, and chronic renal failure. May elicit allergic reactions (eg, generalized rash, urticaria, angioedema).

ADVERSE REACTIONS: Somnolence, fatigue, upper respiratory infection, nasal congestion, nightmares, throat pain, increased body temperature, insomnia, emotional disorder, constipation, dry mouth, ear pain.

INTERACTIONS: May potentiate the CNS-depressive effects of alcohol, barbiturates or other sedating drugs. Decreased hypotensive effects with TCAs. Caution with agents known to affect sinus node function or AV nodal conduction (eg, digitalis, calcium channel blockers, β-blockers). Additive pharmacodynamic effects with other antihypertensives. Avoid with other products containing clonidine.

PREGNANCY: Category C, caution in nursing.

MECHANISM OF ACTION: Centrally acting alpha$_2$-adrenergic agonist; not established. Stimulates alpha$_2$-adrenergic receptors in the brain.

PHARMACOKINETICS: Absorption: (Adults) (Fed) C_{max}=235pg/mL, AUC=6505hr•pg/mL, T_{max}=6.8 hrs; (fasted) C_{max}=258pg/mL, AUC=6729hr•pg/mL, T_{max}=6.5 hrs; Absolute bioavailability (89%). **Distribution:** Found in breast milk. **Elimination:** (Adults) $T_{1/2}$=12.67 hrs (fed), 12.65 hrs (fasted).

NURSING CONSIDERATIONS

Assessment: Assess for history of hypotension, heart block, bradycardia, CVD, syncope, HTN, severe coronary insufficiency, conduction disturbances, recent MI, cerebrovascular disease, chronic renal failure, pregnancy/nursing status, and for possible drug interactions. Obtain baseline HR and BP.

Monitoring: Monitor for somnolence, sedation, hypotension, bradycardia, allergic reactions (eg, generalized rash, urticaria, angioedema), and for the presence of other side effects. Perform periodic BP and HR monitoring while on therapy.

Patient Counseling: Inform about risks and benefits of therapy and counsel appropriately. Advise not to d/c abruptly. If total daily dose does not allow equal bid dosing, instruct to take higher of two doses at bedtime. Instruct to swallow tab whole and never crush, cut or chew. Advise to consult a physician if pregnant, nursing or thinking of becoming pregnant. Caution against operating heavy equipment or driving until treatment response has been evaluated.

Administration: Oral route. **Storage:** 20-25°C (68-77°F).

K-Dur   RX
potassium chloride (Schering)

THERAPEUTIC CLASS: K⁺ supplement

INDICATIONS: (For those unable to tolerate liquid or effervescent potassium preparations). Treatment and prevention of hypokalemia with or without metabolic alkalosis. Treatment of digitalis intoxication and hypokalemic familial periodic paralysis.

DOSAGE: *Adults:* Prevention: 20mEq/day. Hypokalemia: 40-100mEq/day. Divide dose if >20mEq. Take with meals and a full glass of water or liquid. Tab can be broken in half or dissolved in water.

HOW SUPPLIED: Tab, Extended-Release: 10mEq, 20mEq* *scored

CONTRAINDICATIONS: Hyperkalemia, esophageal ulceration, delay in GI passage (from structural, pathological, pharmacologic causes [eg, anticholinergic agents]), cardiac patients with esophageal compression due to enlarged left atrium.

WARNINGS/PRECAUTIONS: Potentially fatal hyperkalemia may occur. Extreme caution with acidosis, cardiac and renal disease; monitor ECG and electrolytes. Hypokalemia with metabolic acidosis should be treated with an alkalinizing potassium salt (eg, potassium bicarbonate, potassium citrate). May produce ulcerative or stenotic GI lesions.

ADVERSE REACTIONS: Hyperkalemia, GI effects (obstruction, bleeding, ulceration), N/V, abdominal pain, flatulence, diarrhea.

INTERACTIONS: See Contraindications. Risk of hyperkalemia with ACE inhibitors (eg, captopril, enalapril), K⁺-sparing diuretics and K⁺ supplements.

PREGNANCY: Category C, safe for use in nursing.

MECHANISM OF ACTION: K⁺ supplement (electrolyte replenisher); potassium ions participate in maintenance of intracellular tonicity, transmission of nerve impulses, contraction of cardiac, skeletal, and smooth muscle, and maintenance of normal renal function.

NURSING CONSIDERATIONS

Assessment: Assess for chronic renal disease, conditions which impair K⁺ excretion, esophageal compression due to enlarged left atrium, structural/pathologic cause for arrest/delay in passing through GI (diabetic gastroparesis), and possible drug interactions. Obtain baseline serum K⁺ levels and renal function test.

Monitoring: Monitor serum K⁺ levels, renal function, ECG, and acid-base balance. Monitor for hyperkalemia, signs of acute metabolic acidosis, acute dehydration, GI ulcerations, and hypersensitivity reactions.

Patient Counseling: Instruct to report symptoms of GI bleeding (tarry stools), ulcerations/perforations (severe vomiting, abdominal pain, distention), trouble swallowing, or tablet sticking in throat. Take with meals and full glass of water; swallow whole, do not crush, chew, or suck. If difficulty swallowing whole tablet; break tablet in half. Take each half separately with glass of water or place whole tab in 1/2 glass of water and allow 2 min to disintegrate, stir for half min after disintegration, swirl suspension and drink content. Add another 1oz of water, swirl, and drink immediately and repeat once more.

Administration: Oral route. **Storage:** 25°C (77°F); excursions permitted to 15-30°C (59-86°F). Keep tightly closed.

KEPIVANCE   RX
palifermin (Biovitrum)

THERAPEUTIC CLASS: Keratinocyte growth factor

INDICATIONS: To decrease the incidence and duration of severe oral mucositis in patients with hematologic malignancies receiving myelotoxic therapy requiring hematopoietic stem cell support. As supportive care for preparative regimens predicted to result in ≥World Health Organization Grade 3 mucositis in the majority of patients.

DOSAGE: *Adults:* 60mcg/kg/day IV bolus for 3 consecutive days before myelotoxic therapy (give 3rd dose 24-48 hrs before myelotoxic therapy) and 3 consecutive days after myelotoxic therapy (give 1st of these doses on the day of stem cell infusion after the infusion is completed, and >4 days after last palifermin dose), for a total of 6 doses.

HOW SUPPLIED: Inj: 6.25mg

WARNINGS/PRECAUTIONS: Safety and efficacy not established with nonhematologic malignancies. Shown to enhance growth of human epithelial tumor cell lines in vitro and increase rate of tumor cell line growth in a human carcinoma xenograft model.

ADVERSE REACTIONS: Rash, serum amylase/lipase elevation, fever, pruritus, erythema, edema, mouth/tongue discoloration or thickening, alteration of taste, pain, dysesthesia (hyperesthesia/hypoesthesia/paresthesia), arthralgia.

INTERACTIONS: Not recommended for use with melphalan 200mg/m² as a conditioning regimen. Do not administer 24 hrs before, during infusion, or 24 hrs after administration of myelotoxic chemotherapy; may result in increased severity and duration of oral mucositis. May interact with unfractionated as well as low molecular weight heparins. Heparin may increase (5-fold) systemic exposure; avoid coadministration.

PREGNANCY: Category C, not for use in nursing.

MECHANISM OF ACTION: Keratinocyte growth factor (KGF); binds to the KGF receptor, which results in proliferation, differentiation, and migration of the epithelial cells.

PHARMACOKINETICS: Elimination: $T_{1/2}$=4.5 hrs.

NURSING CONSIDERATIONS

Assessment: Assess for pregnancy/nursing status and possible drug interactions.

Monitoring: Monitor for tumor growth.

Patient Counseling: Instruct to report to physician occurrence of rash, skin reddening, itchiness, tongue swelling, mouth and tongue sensation changes, and taste alteration. Inform of the evidence of tumor growth and stimulation in cell culture and in animal models of nonhematopoietic human tumors.

Administration: IV route. Refer to PI for proper preparation and administration. **Storage:** Powder: 2-8°C (36-46°F). Reconstituted Sol: 2-8°C (36-46°F) for up to 24 hrs. Do not freeze. Protect from light.

KEPPRA
levetiracetam (UCB)

RX

THERAPEUTIC CLASS: Pyrrolidine derivative

INDICATIONS: (PO) Adjunctive therapy in the treatment of partial onset seizures in adults and children ≥1 month with epilepsy. Adjunctive therapy in the treatment of myoclonic seizures in adults and adolescents ≥12 yrs with juvenile myoclonic epilepsy (JME). Adjunctive therapy in the treatment of primary generalized tonic-clonic (PGTC) seizures in adults and children ≥6 yrs with idiopathic generalized epilepsy (IGE). (IV) Alternative for adults ≥16 yrs when PO administration is temporarily not feasible in the adjunctive therapy of partial onset seizures with epilepsy, myoclonic seizures with JME, and PGTC with IGE.

DOSAGE: *Adults:* ≥16 yrs: (IV) Administer as a 15-min IV infusion following dilution. (IV/PO) Partial Onset Seizures/Myoclonic Seizures with JME/PGTC Seizures with IGE: Initial: 500mg bid. Titrate: Increase by 1000mg/day q2 weeks. Max: 3000mg/day. Renal Impairment: Individualize dose: CrCl 50-80mL/min: 500mg-1000mg q12h. CrCl 30-50mL/min: 250mg-750mg q12h. CrCl <30mL/min: 250mg-500mg q12h. End-Stage Renal Disease with Dialysis: 500mg-1000mg q24h. A supplemental dose of 250mg-500mg following dialysis is recommended for female patients. (IV) Replacement Therapy: Initial total daily dose should be equivalent to the total daily dose and frequency of PO formulation. (PO) Switching to PO: Switch at equivalent daily dose and frequency of IV administration at the end of IV treatment period.
Pediatrics: (PO) Myoclonic Seizures with JME: ≥12 yrs: Initial: 500mg bid. Titrate: Increase by 1000mg/day q2 weeks. Max: 3000mg/day. Partial Onset Seizures: 4-<16 yrs: Initial: 10mg/kg bid. Titrate: Increase by 20mg/kg/day q2 weeks. Max: 30mg/kg bid or 3000mg/day. (Tab) >40kg: Initial: 500mg bid. Titrate: Increase by 1000mg/day q2 weeks. Max: 1500mg bid. 20-40kg: Initial: 250mg bid. Titrate: Increase by 500mg/day q2 weeks. Max: 750mg bid. (Sol) Refer to PI for weight-based dosing calculation. 6 months-<4 yrs: Initial: 10mg/kg bid. Titrate: Increase by 20mg/kg/day in 2 weeks. Max: 25mg/kg bid. Reduce daily dose if cannot tolerate 50mg/kg/day. 1 month-<6 months: Initial: 7mg/kg bid. Titrate: Increase by 14mg/kg/day q2 weeks. Max: 21mg/kg bid. PGTC Seizures with IGE: 6-<16 yrs: Initial: 10mg/kg bid. Titrate: Increase by 20mg/kg/day q2 weeks. Max: 30mg/kg bid.

HOW SUPPLIED: Inj: 100mg/mL [5mL]; Sol: 100mg/mL [16 fl. oz.]; Tab: 250mg*, 500mg*, 750mg*, 1000mg* *scored

WARNINGS/PRECAUTIONS: May cause somnolence, fatigue, coordination difficulties, and behavioral abnormalities. May impair mental/physical abilities. Withdraw gradually to minimize the potential of increased seizure frequency. Hematologic abnormalities may occur. Caution with renal impairment and in elderly. (IV) LFT abnormalities may occur. (PO) Increased risk of suicidal thoughts or behavior reported; monitor for emergence or worsening of depression, suicidal thoughts/behavior, and/or any unusual changes in mood or behavior. Serious dermatological reactions (eg, Stevens-Johnson syndrome [SJS] and toxic epidermal necrolysis [TEN]) reported; d/c at the 1st sign of rash, do not resume and consider alternative therapy if signs/symptoms suggest SJS/TEN. Increased diastolic BP reported. Monitor patients during pregnancy and continue close monitoring through postpartum, especially if the dose was changed during pregnancy.

ADVERSE REACTIONS: Somnolence, asthenia, headache, infection, pain, anorexia, dizziness, nervousness, vertigo, ataxia, pharyngitis, rhinitis, irritability, depression, diarrhea.

INTERACTIONS: Increased metabolite concentration and decreased metabolite renal clearance with probenecid. (PO) Increased clearance with enzyme-inducing antiepileptic drugs in pediatrics.

PREGNANCY: Category C, not for use in nursing.

MECHANISM OF ACTION: Pyrrolidine derivative; not established. Proposed to inhibit burst firing without affecting normal neuronal excitability, suggesting that it may selectively prevent hypersynchronization of epileptiform burst firing and propagation of seizure activity.

PHARMACOKINETICS: Absorption: Rapid, (IV) almost complete; (PO) bioavailability (100%), T_{max}=1 hr. **Distribution:** Plasma protein binding (<10%); found in breast milk. **Metabolism:** Enzymatic hydrolysis of acetamide group; ucb L057 (metabolite). **Elimination:** Urine (66%, unchanged); $T_{1/2}$=7 hrs.

K

NURSING CONSIDERATIONS

Assessment: Assess for renal impairment, depression, suicidal thoughts/behavior, pregnancy/ nursing status, and possible drug interactions.

Monitoring: Monitor for somnolence, fatigue, coordination difficulties and behavioral abnormalities, increased seizure frequency, and other adverse reactions. Monitor renal function and hematological changes. (IV) Monitor LFTs. (PO) Monitor for dermatologic reactions, emergence or worsening of depression, suicidal thoughts/behavior, and any unusual changes in mood or behavior. Monitor patients during pregnancy and continue close monitoring through postpartum, especially if the dose was changed during pregnancy.

Patient Counseling: Counsel on the benefits and risks of therapy. Instruct to take drug exactly as directed. Advise not to drive or operate heavy machinery until accustomed to the effects of medication. Advise that the drug may cause changes in behavior and patients may experience psychotic symptoms. Instruct to report any symptoms of depression and/or suicidal ideation to the physician. Advise to notify their physician if pregnant or intend to become pregnant prior to therapy. (PO) Inform that the drug may increase the risk of suicidal thoughts and behavior; advise to be alert if signs/symptoms of depression, any unusual changes in mood/behavior, suicidal thoughts/behavior, or thoughts about self-harm emerge or worsen, and instruct to notify physician immediately. Inform that serious dermatological adverse reactions reported; advise to notify physician if rash develops.

Administration: Oral/IV route. (PO) Swallow tab whole; do not crush or chew. Give PO sol using a calibrated measuring device for patients ≤20kg. (IV) Refer to PI for preparation and administration. **Storage:** 25°C (77°F); excursions permitted to 15-30°C (59-86°F). (IV) Diluted Sol: Stable for ≥24 hrs and stored in polyvinyl chloride bags at 15-30°C (59-86°F).

KEPPRA XR   RX
levetiracetam (UCB)

THERAPEUTIC CLASS: Pyrrolidine derivative

INDICATIONS: Adjunct therapy for treatment of partial onset seizures in patients ≥16 yrs with epilepsy.

DOSAGE: *Adults:* Initial: 1000mg qd. Titrate: Adjust dose in increments of 1000mg/day q2 weeks. Max: 3000mg/day. Renal Impairment: Individualize dose. CrCl 50-80mL/min/1.73m²: 1000-2000mg q24h. CrCl 30-50mL/min/1.73m²: 500-1500mg q24h. CrCl <30mL/min/1.73m²: 500-1000mg q24h. End-Stage Renal Disease on Dialysis: Use immediate-release formulation. *Pediatrics:* ≥16 yrs: Initial: 1000mg qd. Titrate: Adjust dose in increments of 1000mg/day q2 weeks. Max: 3000mg/day.

HOW SUPPLIED: Tab, Extended-Release: 500mg, 750mg

WARNINGS/PRECAUTIONS: Increased risk of suicidal thoughts or behavior reported; monitor for emergence or worsening of depression, suicidal thoughts/behavior, and/or any unusual changes in mood or behavior. May cause somnolence, dizziness, fatigue, coordination difficulties, and behavioral abnormalities. Withdraw gradually to minimize the potential of increased seizure frequency. Hematologic abnormalities and changes in LFTs may occur. Caution with moderate to severe renal impairment, if on hemodialysis, and in elderly.

ADVERSE REACTIONS: Somnolence, influenza, nasopharyngitis, irritability, dizziness, nausea.

INTERACTIONS: Increased metabolite concentration and decreased metabolite renal clearance with probenecid.

PREGNANCY: Category C, not for use in nursing.

MECHANISM OF ACTION: Pyrrolidine derivative; not established. Proposed to inhibit burst firing without affecting normal neuronal excitability, suggesting that it may selectively prevent hypersynchronization of epileptiform burst firing and propagation of seizure activity.

PHARMACOKINETICS: Absorption: Almost complete; T_{max} =4 hrs. **Distribution:** Plasma protein binding (<10%); found in breast milk. **Metabolism:** Enzymatic hydrolysis of acetamide group; ucb L057 (metabolite). **Elimination:** Urine (66%, unchanged); $T_{1/2}$ =7 hrs.

NURSING CONSIDERATIONS

Assessment: Assess for renal impairment, depression, suicidal thoughts/behavior, unusual changes in mood/behavior, pregnancy/nursing status, and possible drug interactions.

Monitoring: Monitor for emergence or worsening of depression, suicidal thoughts/behavior, and any unusual changes in mood or behavior, CNS adverse effects, increased seizure frequency, and other adverse reactions. Monitor for hematological/hepatic changes and renal function.

Patient Counseling: Instruct to take drug exactly as directed and to swallow tab whole; do not chew, break, or crush. Inform that the drug may increase the risk of suicidal thoughts and behavior; advise to be alert if signs/symptoms of depression, any unusual changes in mood/behavior, suicidal thoughts/behavior, or thoughts about self-harm emerge or worsen; instruct to notify physician immediately. Counsel that medication may cause irritability and aggression. Advise to notify physician if they become pregnant or intend to become pregnant. Encourage pregnant patients to enroll in North American Antiepileptic Drug Pregnancy registry by calling 1-888-233-2334. Inform that dizziness and somnolence may occur; advise not to drive or operate heavy machinery or engage in other hazardous activities until adjusted to effects.

Administration: Oral route. **Storage:** 25°C (77°F); excursions permitted to 15-30°C (59-86°F).

KETEK   RX
telithromycin (Sanofi-Aventis)

> **Contraindicated with myasthenia gravis. Fatal and life-threatening respiratory failure in patients with myasthenia gravis reported.**

THERAPEUTIC CLASS: Ketolide antibiotic

INDICATIONS: Treatment of mild to moderate community-acquired pneumonia (CAP) due to susceptible strains of microorganisms for patients ≥18 yrs.

DOSAGE: *Adults:* 800mg qd for 7-10 days. Severe Renal Impairment (CrCl <30mL/min): 600mg qd. Hemodialysis: 600mg qd, given after dialysis session on dialysis days. Severe Renal Impairment (CrCl <30mL/min) with Hepatic Impairment: 400mg qd.

HOW SUPPLIED: Tab: 300mg, 400mg

CONTRAINDICATIONS: Myasthenia gravis, history of hepatitis and/or jaundice associated with use of telithromycin or any macrolide antibiotic, hypersensitivity to macrolide antibiotics, concomitant use with cisapride or pimozide, and concomitant use with colchicine in patients with renal or hepatic impairment.

WARNINGS/PRECAUTIONS: Acute hepatic failure and severe liver injury, including fulminant hepatitis and hepatic necrosis, reported; monitor closely and d/c if any signs/symptoms of hepatitis occur. Permanently d/c if hepatitis or transaminase elevations combined with systemic symptoms occur. May prolong QTc interval leading to risk for ventricular arrhythmias including torsades de pointes; avoid in patients with congenital prolongation of QTc interval, with ongoing proarrhythmic conditions (eg, uncorrected hypokalemia/hypomagnesemia), and in clinically significant bradycardia. Visual disturbances and loss of consciousness reported; minimize hazardous activities such as driving and operating heavy machinery. *Clostridium difficile*-associated diarrhea (CDAD) reported; d/c if CDAD is suspected or confirmed. Unlikely to provide benefit and increases risk of drug resistance if used in the absence of bacterial infection or for prophylactic indication.

ADVERSE REACTIONS: Diarrhea, nausea, headache, dizziness.

INTERACTIONS: See Contraindications. Avoid with simvastatin, lovastatin, atorvastatin, rifampin, ergot alkaloid derivatives (eg, ergotamine, dihydroergotamine), Class IA (eg, quinidine, procainamide) or Class III (eg, dofetilide) antiarrhythmics. May increase levels of theophylline, midazolam, digoxin, simvastatin, metoprolol, levonorgestrel, substrates of OATP1 (B1, B3) family members, drugs metabolized by the CYP450 system (eg, carbamazepine, cyclosporine, tacrolimus, sirolimus, hexobarbital, phenytoin), especially CYP3A4. May decrease levels of sotalol. Itraconazole and ketoconazole may increase levels. CYP3A4 inducers (eg, phenytoin, carbamazepine, phenobarbital, rifampin) may decrease levels. May potentiate effects of oral anticoagulants. Theophylline may worsen GI effects; take 1 hr apart from therapy. May cause hypotension, bradyarrhythmia, and loss of consciousness with calcium channel blockers metabolized by CYP3A4 (eg, verapamil, amlodipine, diltiazem). High levels of HMG-CoA reductase inhibitors increase risk of myopathy and rhabdomyolysis; monitor for signs and symptoms. Caution with benzodiazepines metabolized by CYP3A4 (eg, triazolam) and metoprolol in patients with heart failure.

PREGNANCY: Category C, caution in nursing.

MECHANISM OF ACTION: Ketolide antibiotic; blocks protein synthesis by binding to domains II and V of 23S rRNA of 50S ribosomal subunit and may also inhibit assembly of nascent ribosomal units.

PHARMACOKINETICS: Absorption: Absolute bioavailability (57%); C_{max}=1.9µg/mL (single dose), 2.27µg/mL (multiple dose); T_{max}=1 hr; $AUC_{(0-24)}$=8.25µg•hr/mL (single dose), 12.5µg•hr/mL (multiple dose). **Distribution:** V_d=2.9L/kg; plasma protein binding (60-70%). **Metabolism:** Via CYP3A4 dependent and independent pathways. **Elimination:** Urine (13% unchanged); feces (7% unchanged); $T_{1/2}$=7.16 hrs (single dose), 9.81 hrs (multiple dose).

NURSING CONSIDERATIONS

Assessment: Assess for myasthenia gravis, history of hepatitis and/or jaundice, previous hypersensitivity to telithromycin or macrolides, renal/hepatic impairment, LFTs, QTc prolongation risk (eg, congential prolongation, proarrhythmic conditions, significant bradycardia), pregnancy/nursing status, and possible drug interactions. Perform culture and susceptibility testing.

Monitoring: Monitor LFTs and ECG for QTc prolongation. Monitor for visual disturbances, hepatitis, loss of consciousness associated with vagal syndrome, renal impairment, CDAD, pancreatitis, allergic reactions (eg, angioedema, anaphylaxis), and signs/symptoms of hepatitis.

Patient Counseling: Inform that therapy treats bacterial, not viral, infections. Advise against operating machinery or driving and to seek physician's advice if visual difficulties (eg, blurred vision, difficulty focusing, and objects looking doubled), loss of consciousness, confusion, or hallucination is experienced. Advise that therapy is contraindicated with myasthenia gravis. Instruct to d/c and seek medical attention if signs and symptoms of liver injury develop (eg, nausea, fatigue, anorexia, jaundice, dark urine, light colored stools, pruritus, tender abdomen). Instruct to report any fainting during therapy and to inform physician of history of QTc prolongation, proarrhythmic conditions, or significant bradycardia. Advise to take as directed; skipping doses or not completing full course may decrease effectiveness and increase antibiotic resistance. Advise to contact physician if diarrhea (watery/bloody stools) occurs. Advise to inform physician of any other medications taken concurrently with telithromycin.

Administration: Oral route. Can be given with or without food. **Storage:** 25°C (77°F); excursions permitted to 15-30°C (59-86°F).

KETOCONAZOLE   RX

ketoconazole (Various)

K

> Associated with hepatic toxicity, including fatalities; monitor closely. Coadministration of terfenadine, astemizole, or cisapride is contraindicated due to reported cases of serious cardiovascular adverse events (eg, torsades de pointes, ventricular fibrillation, ventricular tachycardia).

THERAPEUTIC CLASS: Azole antifungal

INDICATIONS: Treatment of the following systemic fungal infections: candidiasis, chronic mucocutaneous candidiasis, oral thrush, candiduria, blastomycosis, coccidioidomycosis, histoplasmosis, chromomycosis, and paracoccidioidomycosis. Treatment of patients with severe recalcitrant cutaneous dermatophyte infections who have not responded to topical therapy or oral griseofulvin, or who are unable to take griseofulvin.

DOSAGE: *Adults:* Initial: 200mg qd. May be increased to 400mg qd in very serious infections or if responsiveness is insufficient within the expected time.
Pediatrics: >2 yrs: Single dose of 3.3-6.6mg/kg.

HOW SUPPLIED: Tab: 200mg* *scored

CONTRAINDICATIONS: Coadministration of terfenadine, astemizole, cisapride, or oral triazolam.

WARNINGS/PRECAUTIONS: Several cases of hepatitis reported in children. Monitor LFTs prior to therapy and at frequent intervals during treatment. Transient minor liver enzyme elevations reported; d/c if these persist, worsen, or if accompanied by symptoms of possible liver injury. Anaphylaxis reported (rare) after the 1st dose. Hypersensitivity reactions reported. Suppresses adrenal corticosteroid secretion at high doses. May lower serum testosterone levels. In cases of achlorhydria, dissolve each tab in 4mL aqueous sol of 0.2 N HCl; use drinking straw to avoid contact with teeth, followed with a cup of tap water. Should not be used for fungal meningitis. Minimum treatment for recalcitrant dermatophyte infections is 4 weeks in cases involving glabrous skin, minimum treatment for candidiasis is 1-2 weeks, minimum treatment for chronic mucocutaneous candidiasis requires maint therapy, minimum treatment for other indicated systemic mycoses is 6 months.

ADVERSE REACTIONS: N/V, abdominal pain, pruritus.

INTERACTIONS: See Boxed Warning and Contraindications. Reduced absorption with drug-induced achlorhydria; give antacids, anticholinergics, and H_2 blockers at least 2 hrs after administration. Caution with hepatotoxic drugs. May potentiate and prolong hypnotic and sedative effects of midazolam or triazolam. Severe hypoglycemia may occur with oral hypoglycemics. May enhance anticoagulant effect of coumarin-like drugs; carefully titrate and monitor anticoagulant effect. Reduced levels with rifampin; avoid concomitant use. Concentrations are adversely affected with isoniazid; avoid concomitant use. May increase levels of cyclosporine, tacrolimus, methylprednisolone, digoxin, loratadine, and drugs metabolized by CYP3A4. Disulfiram-like reactions may occur with alcohol.

PREGNANCY: Category C, not for use in nursing.

MECHANISM OF ACTION: Azole antifungal; impairs synthesis of ergosterol, a vital component of fungal cell membranes.

PHARMACOKINETICS: Absorption: C_{max}=3.5μg/mL; T_{max}=1-2 hrs. **Distribution:** Plasma protein binding (99%); found in breast milk. **Metabolism:** Via oxidation, degradation of imidazole and piperazine rings, oxidative dealkylation, and aromatic hydroxylation. **Elimination:** Biphasic. $T_{1/2}$=2 hrs; bile (major), urine (13%, 2-4% unchanged).

NURSING CONSIDERATIONS

Assessment: Assess for drug hypersensitivity, achlorhydria, LFTs, pregnancy/nursing status, and possible drug interactions.

Monitoring: Monitor LFTs, signs/symptoms of hepatotoxicity, and hypersensitivity reactions.

Patient Counseling: Inform patient about risk of hepatic toxicity. Advise to report any signs/symptoms of liver dysfunction (eg, fatigue, anorexia, N/V, jaundice, dark urine, or pale stools) to their physician.

Administration: Oral route. **Storage:** 20-25°C (68-77°F). Protect from moisture.

KETOROLAC   RX
ketorolac tromethamine (Various)

For short-term (up to 5 days in adults) use only. Increasing the recommended dose will increase risk of serious adverse events. May cause peptic ulcers, GI bleeding, and/or perforation. Elderly are at greater risk for serious GI events. Contraindicated with active or history of peptic ulcer disease/GI bleeding, recent GI bleeding/perforation, prophylactic analgesic before any major surgery, advanced renal impairment, risk of renal failure due to volume depletion, cerebrovascular bleeding, hemorrhagic diathesis, incomplete hemostasis, high risk of bleeding, labor and delivery, nursing, with concurrent aspirin (ASA) or NSAIDs, and for minor or chronic painful conditions. (Inj) Contraindicated in intrathecal/epidural use. (Tab) Used only as continuation therapy and the combined duration of use of IV/IM. May cause an increased risk of cardiovascular thrombotic events, myocardial infarction, and stroke. Contraindicated in perioperative pain in coronary artery bypass graft (CABG) surgery and in pediatric patients.

THERAPEUTIC CLASS: NSAID

INDICATIONS: Short-term (≤5 days) management of moderately severe acute pain that requires analgesia at the opioid level, usually in postoperative setting.

DOSAGE: *Adults:* Single-Dose: (IM) <65 yrs: 60mg. ≥65 yrs/Renal Impairment/<50kg: 30mg. (IV) <65 yrs: 30mg. ≥65 yrs/Renal Impairment/<50kg: 15mg. Multiple-Dose: (IM/IV) <65 yrs: Usual: 30mg q6h. Max: 120mg/day. ≥65 yrs/Renal Impairment/<50kg: Usual: 15mg q6h. Max: 60mg/day. Transition from IM/IV to PO: 17-64 yrs: 20mg PO single dose, then 10mg PO q4-6h PRN. Max: 40mg/day. ≥65 yrs/Renal Impairment/<50kg: 10mg single dose, then 10mg PO q4-6h. Max: 40mg/day. Refer to PI for dosing instructions. Elderly: Start at lower end of dosing range. *Pediatrics:* 2-16 yrs: Single-Dose: (IM) 1mg/kg. Max: 30mg. (IV) 0.5mg/kg. Max: 15mg.

HOW SUPPLIED: Inj: 15mg/mL, 30mg/mL [1mL, 2mL]; Tab: 10mg

CONTRAINDICATIONS: Active/history of peptic ulcer, recent/history of GI bleeding/perforation, advanced renal impairment or risk of renal failure, labor/delivery, nursing mothers, ASA or NSAID allergy, as prophylactic analgesic before major surgery, cerebrovascular bleeding, hemorrhagic diathesis, incomplete hemostasis, high risk of bleeding, and concomitant use with ASA, NSAIDs, probenecid, or pentoxifylline. (Inj) Neuraxial (epidural or intrathecal) administration. (Tab) Treatment of perioperative pain in CABG surgery.

WARNINGS/PRECAUTIONS: May develop minor upper GI adverse problems (eg, dyspepsia). Increased risk for GI ulceration/bleeding with smoking, older age, and poor general health status; use lowest effective dose for shortest possible duration. May exacerbate inflammatory bowel disease (eg, ulcerative colitis, Crohn's disease). Caution with hepatic impairment or history of liver disease, coagulation disorders, in postoperative setting when hemostasis is critical, patients on therapeutic doses of anticoagulants. Avoid perioperative use. Acute renal failure, interstitial nephritis, and nephrotic syndrome reported; caution with impaired renal function, dehydration, heart failure, liver dysfunction, and those taking diuretics. May cause anaphylactic/anaphylactoid reactions and serious skin adverse events (eg, exfoliative dermatitis, Steven-Johnson syndrome (SJS), and toxic epidermal necrolysis [TEN]); d/c at the first appearance of skin rash or any other signs of hypersensitivity. May lead to new HTN or worsening of preexisting HTN. Avoid in late pregnancy; may cause premature closure of ductus arteriosus. Edema, retention of NaCl, oliguria, elevations of BUN and creatinine have been reported; caution with cardiac decompensation, HTN or similar conditions. Not used as a substitute for corticosteroid insufficiency. May elevate LFTs. Liver disease may develop; d/c if systemic manifestations (eg, eosinophilia, rash) occur. Caution with asthma; may lead to severe bronchospasm. Caution in elderly.

ADVERSE REACTIONS: Nausea, dyspepsia, abdominal pain, diarrhea, edema, headache, drowsiness, dizziness.

INTERACTIONS: See Boxed Warning and Contraindication. Binding of warfarin to plasma proteins is slightly reduced. Binding reduced with concomitant use with salicylate/ASA. May increase risk of serious bleeding with anticoagulants (eg, warfarin/heparin), SSRIs, NSAIDs, alcohol, oral corticosteroids, and possibly with dextran. May reduce natriuretic response to furosemide and thiazide diuretics; may impair response. May elevate plasma lithium levels and reduction in renal lithium clearance; monitor for lithium toxicity. May enhance methotrexate toxicity. May increase risk of renal impairment with ACE inhibitors/angiotensin receptor antagonists; use with caution. Seizures have been reported with concomitant use of antiepileptic drugs (eg, phenytoin, carbamazepine). Hallucinations reported with psychoactive drugs (eg, fluoxetine, thiothixene, alprazolam). May cause apnea with nondepolarizing muscle relaxants.

PREGNANCY: Category C, not for use in nursing.

MECHANISM OF ACTION: NSAID; has not been established. Suspected to inhibit prostaglandin synthetase.

PHARMACOKINETICS: Absorption: (PO) Absolute oral bioavailability (100%). Refer to PI for other pharmacokinetic parameters. **Distribution:** V_d=13L; plasma protein binding (99%); found in breast milk. **Metabolism:** Liver; hydroxylation, conjugation. **Elimination:** Urine (92%; 40% metabolites, 60% unchanged), feces (6%); $T_{1/2}$=5-6 hrs.

NURSING CONSIDERATIONS

Assessment: Assess for risk factors for GI events (eg, GI bleeding/perforation, history of peptic ulcer disease, smoking), or any other conditions where therapy is cautioned/contraindicated. Assess for possible drug interactions.

Monitoring: Monitor for signs/symptoms of GI events, fluid retention, anaphylactic/anaphylactoid/skin (eg, exfoliative dermatitis, SJS, TEN) reactions, myocardial infarction, stroke, new-onset or worsening preexisting HTN, renal impairment, and other adverse reactions. Monitor BP, LFTs, renal function, CBC, and chemical profile. Carefully monitor patients with coagulation disorders.

Patient Counseling: Inform about potential risks/benefits of the medication. Instruct not to use for more than 5 days. Instruct to seek medical attention for signs and symptoms of GI ulceration/ bleeding (eg, epigastric pain, dyspepsia, melena, and hematemesis), cardiovascular events (eg, chest pain, SOB, weakness, slurring speech), hepatotoxicity (eg, nausea, fatigue, jaundice), skin reactions (eg, rash, blisters), anaphylactoid reaction (eg, difficulty breathing, swelling of face/ throat), or if unexplained weight gain or edema occurs. Caution against use in late pregnancy.

Administration: IM/IV/Oral routes. IV bolus must be given ≥15 sec. (Inj) Refer to PI for list of incompatible products. **Storage:** 20-25°C (68-77°F). (Inj) Protect from light.

KINERET   RX
anakinra (Amgen)

THERAPEUTIC CLASS: Interleukin-1 receptor antagonist

INDICATIONS: Reduce the signs/symptoms and slow the progression of structural damage in moderately to severely active rheumatoid arthritis (RA) in patients ≥18 yrs who have failed ≥1 disease modifying antirheumatic drugs (DMARDs). Can be used alone or in combination with DMARDs other than TNF-blocking agents.

DOSAGE: *Adults:* 100mg SQ qd at approximately the same time every day. CrCl <30mL/min: 100mg SQ qod.

HOW SUPPLIED: Inj: 100mg/0.67mL

CONTRAINDICATIONS: Hypersensitivity to *E. coli*-derived proteins.

WARNINGS/PRECAUTIONS: Hypersensitivity reactions and increased incidence of serious infections reported; d/c if severe hypersensitivity reaction or serious infection occurs. Avoid with active infection. May decrease neutrophil count; obtain neutrophil count before therapy, monthly for 3 months, and thereafter quarterly for ≤1 yr. Needle cover of prefilled syringe contains dry latex rubber; caution in patients who are sensitive to latex. Caution in elderly.

ADVERSE REACTIONS: Injection-site reactions, development of antibodies, infections, worsening of RA, upper respiratory infection, headache, nausea, neutropenia, diarrhea, sinusitis, arthralgia, flu-like symptoms, abdominal pain, serious infections.

INTERACTIONS: Neutropenia and higher rate of infections reported with etanercept; use with TNF-blocking agents is not recommended. Avoid concomitant use with live vaccines.

PREGNANCY: Category B, caution in nursing.

MECHANISM OF ACTION: Interleukin-1 (IL-1) receptor antagonist; blocks biologic activity of IL-1 by competitively inhibiting IL-1 binding to the IL-1 type I receptor, which is expressed in a wide variety of tissues and organs.

PHARMACOKINETICS: Absorption: Absolute bioavailability (95%); T_{max}=3-7 hrs. **Elimination:** $T_{1/2}$=4-6 hrs.

NURSING CONSIDERATIONS

Assessment: Assess for known hypersensitivity to *E. coli*-derived proteins, active and/or chronic infection, immunosuppression, severe renal insufficiency or end-stage renal disease, latex sensitivity, pregnancy/nursing status, and possible drug interactions. Obtain neutrophil count.

Monitoring: Monitor for signs/symptoms of serious infections, hypersensitivity reactions, neutropenia, and malignancies. Monitor neutrophil count monthly for 3 months, and thereafter quarterly for ≤1 yr.

Patient Counseling: Counsel about proper dosage, administration, and disposal of medication; caution against reuse of needles, syringes, and drug product. Counsel about signs/symptoms of allergic and other adverse drug reactions and appropriate actions to be taken if any signs/symptoms are experienced. Inform that the needle cover of prefilled syringe contains dry natural rubber, which should not be handled by latex-sensitive individuals.

Administration: SQ route. Administer only 1 dose/day. **Storage:** 2-8°C (36-46°F). Do not freeze or shake. Protect from light.

KLOR-CON M   RX
potassium chloride (Upsher-Smith)

OTHER BRAND NAMES: Klor-Con (Upsher-Smith)

THERAPEUTIC CLASS: K⁺ supplement

INDICATIONS: Treatment of hypokalemia with or without metabolic alkalosis, in digitalis intoxication, and in patients with hypokalemic familial periodic paralysis. Prevention of hypokalemia in patients at risk (eg, digitalized patients, cardiac arrhythmias).

DOSAGE: *Adults:* Individualize dose. Prevention: 20mEq/day. Hypokalemia: 40-100mEq/day. Divide dose if >20mEq. Elderly: Start at low end of dosing range. Take with meals and fluids. (Klor-Con M) May break Klor-Con M in half or mix with 4 oz. of water. (Klor-Con Extended-Release Tab): Swallow tab whole; do not crush, chew, or suck. (Klor-Con M) May break Klor-Con M in half or mix with 4 oz. of water.

HOW SUPPLIED: (Klor-Con M) Tab, Extended-Release: 10mEq, 15mEq, 20mEq; (Klor-Con) Pow: 20mEq, 25mEq; Tab, Extended-Release: 8mEq, 10mEq

CONTRAINDICATIONS: (Tab, ER) Hyperkalemia, cardiac patients with esophageal compression due to an enlarged left atrium. Structural, pathological (eg, diabetic gastroparesis) or pharmacological (eg, use of anticholinergic agents or other agents with anticholinergic properties) cause for arrest or delay through the GI tract with all solid dosage forms. (Powder) Hyperkalemia.

WARNINGS/PRECAUTIONS: (Tab, Extended-Release; Powder) Potentially fatal hyperkalemia and cardiac arrest may occur; monitor serum K⁺ levels and adjust dose appropriately. Extreme caution with acidosis and cardiac and renal disease; monitor ECG and electrolytes. Hypokalemia with metabolic acidosis should be treated with an alkalinizing K⁺ salt (eg, K⁺ bicarbonate, K⁺ citrate, K⁺ acetate, K⁺ gluconate). (Tab, Extended-Release) Solid oral dosage forms may produce ulcerative and/or stenotic lesions of the GI tract; d/c use if severe vomiting, abdominal pain, distention or GI bleeding occurs. Reserve use of ER preparations for those who cannot tolerate, cannot comply, or refuse to take liquid or effervescent preparations. Caution in elderly.

ADVERSE REACTIONS: Hyperkalemia, GI effects (eg, obstruction, bleeding, ulceration), N/V, abdominal pain/discomfort, flatulence, diarrhea.

INTERACTIONS: (Tab, Extended-Release) See Contraindications. Risk of hyperkalemia with ACE inhibitors (eg, captopril, enalapril). (Tab, Extended-Release; Powder) Risk of hyperkalemia with K⁺-sparing diuretics (eg, spironolactone, triamterene, amiloride).

PREGNANCY: Category C, (Tab, Extended-Release) Safe for use in nursing, (Powder) caution in nursing.

MECHANISM OF ACTION: K⁺ supplement (electrolyte replenisher); participates in a number of essential physiological processes, including the maintenance of intracellular tonicity, the transmission of nerve impulses, the contraction of cardiac, skeletal, and smooth muscle, and the maintenance of normal renal function.

PHARMACOKINETICS: Absorption: (Klor-Con Extended-Release Tab) GI tract. **Elimination:** (Klor-Con Extended-Release Tab) Urine and feces.

NURSING CONSIDERATIONS

Assessment: Assess for hyperkalemia, chronic renal failure, systemic acidosis, cardiac patients, if patient cannot tolerate, refuses to take, or cannot comply with taking liquid or effervescent K+ preparations prior to administration of an ER tab formulation. Obtain baseline ECG, serum electrolyte levels, and renal function.

Monitoring: Monitor for signs/symptoms of hyperkalemia and other adverse events that may occur. In patients taking solid oral dosage forms, monitor for signs/symptoms of GI lesions. In patients with cardiac disease, acidosis, or renal disease, monitor acid-base balance and perform appropriate monitoring of serum electrolytes, ECG, renal function, and the clinical status of the patient.

Patient Counseling: Inform about benefits and risks of therapy. Report to physician if develop any type of GI symptoms (eg, tarry stools or other evidence of GI bleeding, vomiting, abdominal pain/distention) or if other adverse events occur. Instruct to contact physician if develop difficulty swallowing or if the tablets are sticking in the throat. (Klor-Con): Swallow tablets whole and to take with meals and full glass of water or other liquid. Follow the frequency and amount prescribed by the physician, especially if also taking diuretics and/or digitalis preparations. (Klor-Con M): Take each dose with meals and with full glass of water or other liquid. Inform that may break tablets in half or make an oral aqueous suspension with tablets and 4 oz. of water (see PI for proper preparation). Inform that aqueous suspension not taken immediately should be discarded and use of other liquids for suspending is not recommended.

Administration: Oral route. (Klor-Con M) Refer to PI for preparation of aqueous suspension.
Storage: (Klor-Con): 15-30°C (59-86°F). (Klor-Con M): 20-25°C (68-77°F); excursions permitted to 15-30°C (59-86°F).

KOMBIGLYZE XR RX

metformin HCl - saxagliptin (Bristol-Myers Squibb/ AstraZeneca)

> **Lactic acidosis may occur due to metformin accumulation; risk increases with conditions such as sepsis, dehydration, excess alcohol intake, hepatic impairment, renal impairment, and acute congestive heart failure (CHF). If acidosis is suspected, d/c and hospitalize patient immediately.**

THERAPEUTIC CLASS: Dipeptidyl peptidase-4 inhibitor/biguanide

INDICATIONS: Adjunct to diet and exercise to improve glycemic control in adults with type 2 diabetes mellitus (DM) when treatment with both saxagliptin and metformin is appropriate.

DOSAGE: *Adults:* Individualize dose. Take qd with evening meal, with gradual dose titration to reduce GI side effects of metformin. On Metformin: Dose should provide metformin at the dose already being taken, or the nearest therapeutically appropriate dose. Adjust dose accordingly if switched from metformin immediate release (IR) to extended release (ER); monitor glycemic control. Need 5mg of Saxagliptin and not Currently Treated with Metformin: Initial: 5mg-500mg qd. Need 2.5mg of Saxagliptin in Combination with Metformin ER: Initial: 2.5mg-1000mg qd. Need 2.5mg Saxagliptin who are Metformin Naive/Require a Dose of Metformin >1000mg: Use individual components. Max: 5mg for saxagliptin and 2000mg for metformin ER. With Strong CYP3A4/5 Inhibitors: Max: 2.5mg-1000mg qd. With Insulin Secretagogue (eg, sulfonylurea)/Insulin: May require lower doses of insulin secretagogue or insulin.

HOW SUPPLIED: Tab, Extended-Release: (Saxagliptin-Metformin ER) 5mg-500mg, 5mg-1000mg, 2.5-1000mg

CONTRAINDICATIONS: Renal impairment (eg, SrCr ≥1.5mg/dL [men], ≥1.4mg/dL [women], or abnormal CrCl), acute or chronic metabolic acidosis, including diabetic ketoacidosis.

WARNINGS/PRECAUTIONS: Not for use for the treatment of type 1 DM. Not studied with history of pancreatitis. Acute pancreatitis reported; d/c if suspected. D/C with evidence of renal impairment. Avoid with hepatic disease/impairment. May decrease vitamin B12 levels; monitor hematological parameters annually. Suspend temporarily for any surgical procedure (except minor procedures not associated with restricted intake of foods and fluids); restart when oral intake is resumed and renal function is normal. Evaluate for evidence of ketoacidosis or lactic acidosis if laboratory abnormalities or clinical illness develops; d/c if acidosis occurs. Temporarily d/c if undergoing radiologic studies involving intravascular administration of iodinated contrast materials. D/C in hypoxic states (eg, shock, acute CHF, acute myocardial infarction [MI]). Serious hypersensitivity reactions reported; d/c if suspected. Avoid in patients ≥80 yrs unless renal function is not reduced. Caution in elderly, debilitated, patients with history of angioedema, malnourished patients and those with adrenal/pituitary insufficiency or alcohol intoxication.

ADVERSE REACTIONS: Lactic acidosis, diarrhea, N/V, upper respiratory tract infection, urinary tract infection, headache, nasopharyngitis.

INTERACTIONS: Increased risk of hypoglycemia with other glucose-lowering agents (eg, sulfonylureas, insulin) or ethanol; lower dose of sulfonylurea or insulin may be required. Metformin: Concomitant use with cationic drugs that are eliminated by renal tubular secretion (eg, cimetidine, digoxin, amiloride, procainamide, quinidine, quinine, ranitidine, trimethoprim, vancomycin, triamterene, morphine) may potentially produce an interaction; monitor and adjust dose if necessary. Observe for loss of glycemic control with thiazides and other diuretics, corticosteroids, phenothiazines, thyroid products, estrogens, oral contraceptives, phenytoin, nicotinic acid, sympathomimetics, calcium channel blockers, and isoniazid. Alcohol may potentiate the effect of metformin on lactate metabolism. Caution with drugs that may affect renal function or result in significant hemodynamic change or may interfere with the disposition of metformin (eg, cationic drugs eliminated by renal tubular secretion). May be difficult to recognize hypoglycemia with β-adrenergic blocking drugs. Saxagliptin: Increased plasma concentrations with ketoconazole and other strong CYP3A4/5 inhibitors (eg, atazanavir, clarithromycin, indinavir, itraconazole, nefazodone, nelfinavir, ritonavir, saquinavir, and telithromycin). Strong CYP3A4/5 inducers and inhibitors may alter pharmacokinetics of saxagliptin and its active metabolite.

PREGNANCY: Category B, caution in nursing.

MECHANISM OF ACTION: Metformin: Biguanide; decreases hepatic glucose production, decreases intestinal absorption of glucose, and improves insulin sensitivity by increasing peripheral glucose uptake and utilization. Saxagliptin: Dipeptidyl peptidase-4 inhibitor; slows the inactivation of the incretin hormones, thereby increasing their bloodstream concentrations and reducing fasting and postprandial glucose concentrations in a glucose-dependent manner in type 2 DM.

PHARMACOKINETICS: Absorption: Saxagliptin: C_{max}=24ng/mL; AUC=78ng•hr/mL; T_{max}=2 hrs. 5-hydroxy saxagliptin: C_{max}=47ng/mL; AUC=214ng•hr/mL; T_{max}=4 hrs. Metformin: T_{max}=7 hrs. **Distribution:** Metformin: V_d=654L. **Metabolism:** Saxagliptin: Hepatic via CYP3A4/5; 5-hydroxy saxagliptin (active metabolite). **Elimination:** Saxagliptin: Feces (22%), urine (24% unchanged, 36% active metabolite); $T_{1/2}$=2.5 hrs (saxagliptin), 3.1 hrs (5-hydroxy saxagliptin). Metformin: Urine (90%); $T_{1/2}$=6.2 hrs (plasma), 17.6 hrs (blood).

NURSING CONSIDERATIONS

Assessment: Assess for metabolic acidosis, renal/hepatic function, previous hypersensitivity to the drug, history of pancreatitis, type 1 DM, diabetic ketoacidosis, presence of a hypoxic state (eg, CHF, acute MI, cardiovascular collapse), pregnancy/nursing status, and for possible drug interactions. Assess if patient is planning to undergo any surgical procedure or is under any form of stress. Obtain baseline FPG, HbA1c, CrCl, and hematological parameters.

Monitoring: Monitor for lactic acidosis, pancreatitis, hypoglycemia, clinical illness, hypoxic states, hypersensitivity reactions, and for decreases in vitamin B12 levels. Monitor for prerenal azotemia in patients with hypoxic conditions. Monitor FPG, HbA1c, renal/hepatic function, and hematological parameters periodically.

Patient Counseling: Inform of the potential risks, benefits, and alternative modes of therapy. Advise on the importance of adherence to dietary instructions, regular physical activity, periodic blood glucose monitoring and HbA1c testing, regular testing of renal function and hematological parameters, recognition and management of hypoglycemia and hyperglycemia, and assessment of diabetes complications. Instruct to seek medical advise promptly during periods of stress (eg, fever, trauma, infection, or surgery); medication requirements may change. Inform of the risk of developing lactic acidosis during therapy; advise to d/c therapy immediately and contact physician if unexplained hyperventilation, myalgia, malaise, unusual somnolence, dizziness, slow or irregular heart beat, sensation of feeling cold (especially in the extremities) or other nonspecific symptoms occur, persist, or worsen. Counsel against excessive alcohol intake. Instruct to swallow tab whole and do not chew, cut, or crush. Inform that inactive ingredients may be eliminated in the feces as a soft mass that may resemble the original tab.

Administration: Oral route. **Storage:** 20-25°C (68-77°F); excursions permitted to 15-30°C (59-86°F).

KRISTALOSE   RX
lactulose (Cumberland)

THERAPEUTIC CLASS: Osmotic laxative

INDICATIONS: Treatment of constipation.

DOSAGE: *Adults:* 10-20g/day. Max 40g/day. Dissolve pkt contents in 4 oz. of water.

HOW SUPPLIED: Powder (crystals for suspension): 10g/pkt, 20g/pkt [1ˢ, 30ˢ]

CONTRAINDICATIONS: Patients who require a low galactose diet.

WARNINGS/PRECAUTIONS: Caution in DM due to galactose and lactose content. Monitor electrolytes periodically in elderly or debilitated if used for >6 months. Potential for explosive reaction with electrocautery procedures during proctoscopy or colonoscopy.

ADVERSE REACTIONS: Flatulence, intestinal cramps, diarrhea, N/V.

INTERACTIONS: Nonabsorbable antacids may decrease effects.

PREGNANCY: Category B, caution in nursing.

MECHANISM OF ACTION: Osmotic laxative; increases osmotic pressure and slight acidification of the colonic contents.

PHARMACOKINETICS: Absorption: Poorly absorbed from GI tract. **Elimination:** Urine (≤3%).

NURSING CONSIDERATIONS

Assessment: Assess for DM, patients requiring a low-galactose diet.

Monitoring: Monitor serum electrolytes (potassium, sodium, chloride, carbon dioxide), diarrhea, vomiting.

Patient Counseling: May be diluted with fruit juice, water, or milk. Report any potential adverse effects.

Administration: Oral route. Dissolve contents of packet in 4 oz. of water. **Storage:** Store 15-30°C (59-86°F).

KRYSTEXXA   RX
pegloticase (Savient)

> Anaphylaxis and infusion reactions reported during and after administration; generally manifests within 2 hrs of infusion. Delayed-type hypersensitivity reactions also reported. Closely monitor for an appropriate period of time for anaphylaxis after administration. Premedicate with antihistamines and corticosteroids. Monitor serum uric acid levels prior to infusions and consider d/c treatment if levels increase >6mg/dL, particularly when 2 consecutive levels >6mg/dL are observed.

THERAPEUTIC CLASS: Recombinant urate-oxidase enzyme

INDICATIONS: Treatment of chronic gout in adults refractory to conventional therapy.

DOSAGE: *Adults:* 8mg IV infusion q2 weeks. Do not administer as IV push or bolus.

HOW SUPPLIED: Inj: 8mg/mL

CONTRAINDICATIONS: Glucose-6-phosphate dehydrogenase (G6PD) deficiency.

WARNINGS/PRECAUTIONS: Not recommended for treatment of asymptomatic hyperuricemia. Gout flares may occur after initiation; gout flare prophylaxis with an NSAID or colchicine is recommended starting ≥1 week before initiation of therapy and lasting ≥6 months, unless medically contraindicated or not tolerated. Caution with congestive heart failure (CHF); monitor closely following infusion. May increase risk of anaphylaxis and infusion reactions in re-treated patients due to immunogenicity.

ADVERSE REACTIONS: Gout flare, infusion reaction, N/V, contusion/ecchymosis, nasopharyngitis, constipation, chest pain, anaphylaxis, delayed-type hypersensitivity reactions.

PREGNANCY: Category C, not for use in nursing.

MECHANISM OF ACTION: Recombinant urate-oxidase enzyme; catalyzes oxidation of uric acid to allantoin, thereby lowering serum uric acid.

NURSING CONSIDERATIONS

Assessment: Assess for G6PD deficiency, asymptomatic hyperuricemia, CHF, and pregnancy/nursing status. Obtain serum uric acid levels prior to infusion.

Monitoring: Monitor for signs/symptoms of anaphylaxis, infusion reactions, and gout flares. Monitor serum uric acid levels.

Patient Counseling: Instruct to read Medication Guide, inform that anaphylaxis and infusion reactions can occur while on therapy, and about the importance of adherence to help prevent or lessen the severity of these reactions. Instruct to seek immediate medical attention if an allergic reaction occurs. Inform that gout flares may initially increase when starting therapy and that medications to help reduce flares may need to be taken regularly for the 1st few months after therapy is started. Instruct patients with G6PD deficiency not to take the drug.

Administration: IV route. Inspect for particulate matter and discoloration prior to administration. Do not mix or dilute with other drugs. Refer to PI for further preparation and administration instructions. **Storage:** 2-8°C (36-46°F). Protect from light. Do not shake or freeze. Diluted Sol: Stable for 4 hrs at 2-8°C (36-46°F) and at 20-25°C (68-77°F).

K-TAB   RX
potassium chloride (Abbott)

THERAPEUTIC CLASS: K⁺ supplement

INDICATIONS: (For those unable to tolerate or refuse liquid or effervescent potassium preparations). Treatment of hypokalemia with or without metabolic alkalosis, in digitalis intoxication, and in hypokalemic familial periodic paralysis. Prevention of hypokalemia in patients who would be at particular risk if hypokalemia were to develop (eg, digitalized patients, significant cardiac arrhythmia).

DOSAGE: *Adults:* Individualize dose. Prevention of Hypokalemia: 20mEq/day. Hypokalemia: 40-100mEq/day. Divide dose if >20mEq/day such that no more than 20mEq is given as a single dose. Elderly: Start at low end of dosing range. Take with meals and full glass of water or liquid.

HOW SUPPLIED: Tab, Extended-Release: 10mEq

CONTRAINDICATIONS: Hyperkalemia, cardiac patients with esophageal compression due to enlarged left atrium, arrest/delay in GI passage (from structural, pathological, pharmacologic causes [eg, anticholinergic agents]).

WARNINGS/PRECAUTIONS: Potentially fatal hyperkalemia may occur. Carefully monitor serum K$^+$ with chronic renal disease or any other condition which impairs K$^+$ excretion. Extreme caution with acidosis, cardiac and renal disease; monitor ECG, acid-base balance and electrolytes. Hypokalemia with metabolic acidosis should be treated with an alkalinizing potassium salt (eg, potassium bicarbonate, potassium citrate, potassium acetate, potassium gluconate). May produce ulcerative or stenotic GI lesions. D/C if severe vomiting, abdominal pain, distention, or GI bleeding occurs. Caution in elderly.

ADVERSE REACTIONS: Hyperkalemia, GI effects (obstruction, bleeding, ulceration, perforation), N/V, abdominal pain/discomfort, flatulence, diarrhea, rash.

INTERACTIONS: See Contraindications. Risk of hyperkalemia with ACE inhibitors (eg, captopril, enalapril), K$^+$-sparing diuretics.

PREGNANCY: Category C, safe for use in nursing.

MECHANISM OF ACTION: K$^+$ supplement; helps in maintenance of intracellular tonicity, transmission of nerve impulses, contraction of cardiac, skeletal, and smooth muscle, and maintenance of normal renal function.

NURSING CONSIDERATIONS

Assessment: Assess for chronic renal disease, conditions that impair K$^+$ excretion, hyperkalemia, esophageal compression due to enlarged left atrium, structural/pathologic/pharmacologic cause for arrest/delay in passing tablet through GI tract (eg, diabetic gastroparesis), and possible drug interactions. Obtain baseline serum K$^+$ levels and renal function.

Monitoring: Monitor serum K$^+$ levels, renal function, ECG, and acid-base balance. Monitor for hyperkalemia, signs of acute metabolic acidosis, acute dehydration, GI ulcerations, and hypersensitivity reactions.

Patient Counseling: Advise to report symptoms of GI bleeding (tarry stools), ulcerations/obstructions/perforations (severe vomiting, abdominal pain, distention), trouble swallowing, or tablet sticking in throat. Instruct to take with meals and full glass of water or other liquid. Instruct to swallow whole; do not crush, chew, or suck tablets. Instruct to follow frequency and amount as directed by physician.

Administration: Oral route. **Storage:** Below 30°C (86°F).

KUVAN   RX
sapropterin dihydrochloride (Biomarin)

THERAPEUTIC CLASS: Synthetic tetrahydrobiopterin

INDICATIONS: To reduce blood phenylalanine (Phe) levels in patients with hyperphenylalaninemia (HPA) due to tetrahydrobiopterin-(BH4)-responsive phenylketonuria (PKU) in conjunction with a Phe-restricted diet.

DOSAGE: *Adults:* Initial: 10mg/kg/day qd. Titrate: Adjust dose within the range of 5-20mg/kg/day. Max: 20mg/kg/day. Take with food.

HOW SUPPLIED: Tab: 100mg

WARNINGS/PRECAUTIONS: Monitor blood Phe levels during treatment. Active management of dietary Phe intake is required to ensure Phe control and nutritional balance. Caution in patients with hepatic impairment. Monitor for allergic reactions.

ADVERSE REACTIONS: Headache, diarrhea, abdominal pain, upper respiratory tract infection, pharyngolaryngeal pain, N/V.

INTERACTIONS: Use with caution when coadministering with drugs that inhibit folate metabolism (eg, methotrexate). Use with caution when coadministered with PDE-5 inhibitors such as sildenafil and vardenafil; may induce vasorelaxation. May cause exacerbation of convulsions, overstimulation, or irritability when coadministered with levodopa.

PREGNANCY: Category C, caution in nursing.

MECHANISM OF ACTION: Synthetic tetrahydrobiopterin; activates residual phenylalanine hydroxylase (PAH) enzyme, improves the normal oxidative metabolism of phenylalanine, and decreases phenylalanine levels.

PHARMACOKINETICS: Elimination: T$_{1/2}$=6.7 hrs.

NURSING CONSIDERATIONS

Assessment: Assess for hepatic and renal impairment, pregnancy status, nursing status, and possible drug interactions. Obtain baseline blood phenylalanine levels.

Monitoring: Monitor for signs and symptoms of an allergic reaction. Monitor for response to treatment; blood phenylalanine levels should be checked one week after initiating treatment and periodically thereafter for up to one month. If no response at 20mg/kg/day after one month, d/c medication. Monitor dietary intake of phenylalanine. Monitor hepatic or renal function if impairment exists.

Patient Counseling: Inform that should be on a phenylalanine restricted diet. Instruct to take medication at the same time everyday with food. Dissolve tablet in 4-8 oz. (120-240mL) of water or apple juice; take within 15 min of dissolution. Instruct that if remnants still exist, add more water or apple juice to ensure that full dose is taken. Instruct that if miss a dose, take as soon as possible; do not take 2 doses on the same day. Notify physician of all medications currently taking or if pregnant. Contact physician if develop any signs of an allergic reaction.

Administration: Oral route. **Storage:** 20-25°C (68-77°F); excursions allowed between 15-30°(59-86°F). Keep container tightly closed. Protect from moisture.

LABETALOL   RX
labetalol HCl (Various)

THERAPEUTIC CLASS: Nonselective beta-blocker/alpha₁ blocker

INDICATIONS: (Tab) Management of hypertension. (Inj) Management of severe hypertension.

DOSAGE: *Adults:* (Tab) HTN: Initial: 100mg bid. Titrate: 100mg bid every 2-3 days. Maint: 200-400mg bid. Severe HTN: 1200-2400mg/day given bid-tid. Increments should not exceed 200mg bid for titration. (Inj) Severe HTN: Administer in supine position. Repeated IV Infusion: Initial: 20mg over 2 min. Titrate: Give additional 40mg or 80mg at 10-min intervals if needed. Max: 300mg. Slow Continuous Infusion: 200mg at rate of 2mg/min. Usual Dose Range: 50-200mg. Max: 300mg. May adjust dose according to BP. Switch to tabs when BP is stable while in hospital. Initial: 200mg, then 200-400mg 6-12 hrs later on Day 1. Titrate: May increase at 1-day interval.

HOW SUPPLIED: Inj: 5mg/mL; Tab: 100mg*, 200mg*, 300mg *scored

CONTRAINDICATIONS: Bronchial asthma, overt cardiac failure, >1st-degree heart block, cardiogenic shock, severe bradycardia, other conditions associated with severe and prolonged hypotension, history of obstructive airway disease.

WARNINGS/PRECAUTIONS: Severe hepatocellular injury reported; caution with hepatic dysfunction. Monitor LFTs periodically; d/c at 1st sign of liver injury or jaundice. Caution in well-compensated patients with a history of heart failure; CHF may occur. Avoid abrupt withdrawal; may exacerbate ischemic heart disease. Avoid with bronchospastic disease and in overt cardiac failure. Caution with pheochromocytoma; paradoxical HTN reported. Caution with DM; may mask symptoms of hypoglycemia. Withdrawal before surgery is controversial. Several deaths reported during surgery. Caution when reducing severely elevated BP; cerebral infarction, optic nerve infarction, angina and ECG ischemic changes reported. Avoid injection with low cardiac indices and elevated systemic vascular resistance.

ADVERSE REACTIONS: Fatigue, dizziness, dyspepsia, N/V, nasal stuffiness, somnolence, ejaculation failure, postural hypotension, increased sweating, paresthesia.

INTERACTIONS: Increased tremors with TCAs. Potentiated by cimetidine; may need to reduce dose. Synergistic antihypertensive effects blunt the reflex tachycardia with nitroglycerin. Caution with calcium antagonists. May need to adjust dose of antidiabetic drugs. Antagonizes effects of β-agonists (bronchodilators). May block epinephrine effects. (Inj) Synergistic effects with halothane; do not use ≥3% halothane.

PREGNANCY: Category C, caution in nursing.

MECHANISM OF ACTION: α₁ and nonselective β-adrenergic receptor blocker; produces dose-related falls in BP without reflex tachycardia and significant reduction in heart rate.

PHARMACOKINETICS: Absorption: Complete; T_{max}=1-2 hrs. **Distribution:** Plasma protein binding (50%); found in breast milk; crosses placenta. **Metabolism:** Liver (conjugation and glucuronidation). **Elimination:** Urine (IV, 55-60% unchanged), feces; (Tab) $T_{1/2}$=6-8 hrs, (IV) $T_{1/2}$=5.5 hrs.

NURSING CONSIDERATIONS

Assessment: Assess for bronchospastic disease, heart block, severe bradycardia, cardiogenic shock, overt cardiac failure, DM, pheochromocytoma, ischemic heart disease, severe or prolonged hypotension, hepatic impairment, history of heart failure, and possible drug interactions.

Monitoring: Monitor LFTs periodically. Monitor for signs/symptoms of cardiac failure, HTN, exacerbation of ischemia following abrupt withdrawal, bronchospastic disease, hypoglycemia, hypersensitivity reactions, and hepatic dysfunction.

Patient Counseling: Instruct to remain supine during and immediately following (for up to 3 hrs) injection; advise on how to proceed gradually to become ambulatory. Instruct not to interrupt or d/c therapy without consulting physician. Instruct to report signs/symptoms of cardiac failure or hepatic dysfunction (eg, pruritus, dark urine, persistent anorexia, jaundice, RUQ tenderness, or unexplained flu-like symptoms). Transient scalp itching may occur, usually when treatment with tabs is initiated.

Administration: Oral, IV route; refer to PI for administration technique. **Storage**: Tab: 15-30°C (59-86°F). IV: 20-25°C (68-77°F). Protect from light and freezing.

LACTULOSE   RX
lactulose (Various)

OTHER BRAND NAMES: Constulose (Actavis) - Enulose (Alpharma) - Generlac (Morton Grove)

THERAPEUTIC CLASS: Osmotic laxative

INDICATIONS: Treatment of constipation. Prevention and treatment of portal-systemic encephalopathy, including stages of hepatic pre-coma and coma.

DOSAGE: *Adults:* Constipation: 15-30mL qd. Max 60mL/day. May mix with fruit juice, water, or milk. Portal-Systemic Encephalopathy: 30-45mL tid-qid. Adjust dose every 1 or 2 days to produce 2-3 soft stools daily. Rectal Use: Reversal of Coma: Mix 300mL with 700mL of water or saline and retain for 30-60 min. May repeat q4-6h. Oral doses should be started before completely stopping enema.
Pediatrics: Portal-Systemic Encephalopathy: Older Children/Adolescents: 40-90mL/day divided tid-qid adjusted to produce 2-3 soft stools daily. *Infants:* 2.5-10mL in divided doses to produce 2-3 soft stools daily.

HOW SUPPLIED: Sol: 10g/15mL

CONTRAINDICATIONS: Patients who require a low galactose diet.

WARNINGS/PRECAUTIONS: Caution in DM due to galactose and lactose content. Monitor electrolytes periodically in elderly or debilitated if used >6 months. Potential for explosive reaction with electrocautery procedures during proctoscopy or colonoscopy.

ADVERSE REACTIONS: Flatulence, intestinal cramps, diarrhea, N/V.

INTERACTIONS: Decreased effect with nonabsorbable antacids.

PREGNANCY: Category B, caution in nursing.

MECHANISM OF ACTION: Synthetic disaccharide; broken down primarily to lactic acid, by the action of colonic bacteria, resulting in increased osmotic pressure and slight acidification of colonic content, causing an increase in stool water content and softens the stool. In portal-systemic encephalopathy, acidification of colonic contents results in retention of ammonia in colon as ammonium ion; ammonia then migrates from blood into colon to form ammonium ion, which traps and prevents absorption of ammonia; finally, laxative actions expels trapped ammonium ion from colon.

PHARMACOKINETICS: Absorption: Poor. **Elimination:** Urine (≤3%).

NURSING CONSIDERATIONS

Assessment: Assess for DM. Assess patients requiring a low-galactose diet and those requiring electrocautery procedures.

Monitoring: Monitor serum electrolytes (potassium, sodium, chloride, carbon dioxide) periodically, diarrhea, vomiting.

Patient Counseling: Drug may be diluted with fruit juice, water, or milk. Report potential adverse effects.

Administration: Oral route. **Storage:** 25°C (77°F); excursions permitted to 15-30°C (59-86°F). Dispense in tight, light-resistant container with child-resistant closure.

LAMICTAL   RX
lamotrigine (GlaxoSmithKline)

> Serious life-threatening rash, including Stevens-Johnson syndrome (SJS), toxic epidermal necrolysis (TEN), and/or rash-related death reported. Serious rash occurs more often in pediatrics than in adults. D/C at first sign of rash unless rash is clearly not drug related. Potential increased risk with concomitant valproate (including valproic acid and divalproex sodium) or exceeding the recommended initial dose/dose escalation.

OTHER BRAND NAMES: Lamictal ODT (GlaxoSmithKline)

THERAPEUTIC CLASS: Phenyltriazine

INDICATIONS: Adjunctive therapy in patients (≥2 yrs) with partial seizures, primary generalized tonic-clonic seizures, and for generalized seizures of Lennox-Gastaut syndrome. For conversion to monotherapy in adults (≥16 yrs) with partial seizures receiving a single antiepileptic drug (AED) (carbamazepine, phenytoin, phenobarbital, primidone, or valproate). Maint treatment of bipolar I disorder to delay the time to occurrence of mood episodes (depression, mania, hypomania, mixed episodes) in adults (≥18 yrs) treated for acute mood episodes with standard therapy.

DOSAGE: *Adults:* Epilepsy: Concomitant Valproate: Weeks 1 and 2: 25mg qod. Weeks 3 and 4: 25mg qd. Week 5 Onward: Increase q1-2 weeks by 25-50mg/day. Maint: 100-200mg/day with valproate alone or 100-400mg/day with valproate and other drugs inducing glucuronidation in 1 or 2 divided doses. Patients not Taking Carbamazepine, Phenytoin, Phenobarbital, Primidone, or Valproate: Weeks 1 and 2: 25mg qd. Weeks 3 and 4: 50mg qd. Week 5 Onward: Increase q1-2 weeks by 50mg/day. Maint: 225-375mg/day in 2 divided doses. Concomitant Carbamazepine, Phenytoin, Phenobarbital, Primidone without Valproate: Weeks 1 and 2: 50mg/day. Weeks 3 and 4: 100mg/day in 2 divided doses. Week 5 Onward: Increase q1-2 weeks by 100mg/day. Maint: 300-500mg/day in 2 divided doses. Conversion to Monotherapy: See PI. Bipolar Disorder: Patients not Taking Carbamazepine, Phenytoin, Phenobarbital, Primidone, or Valproate: Weeks 1 and 2: 25mg qd. Weeks 3 and 4: 50mg qd. Week 5: 100mg qd. Weeks 6 and 7: 200mg qd. Concomitant Valproate: Weeks 1 and 2: 25mg qod. Weeks 3 and 4: 25mg qd. Week 5: 50mg qd. Weeks 6 and 7: 100mg qd. Concomitant Taking Carbamazepine, Phenytoin, Phenobarbital, Primidone without Valproate: Weeks 1 and 2: 50mg qd. Weeks 3 and 4: 100mg qd. Week 5: 200mg qd. Week 6: 300mg qd. Week 7: Up to 400mg qd. Weeks 3-7: Take in divided doses. Following d/c of Psychotropic Drugs Excluding Carbamazepine, Phenytoin, Phenobarbital, Primidone, or Valproate: Maintain current dose. Following d/c of Valproate with Current Dose of Lamotrigine 100mg qd: Week 1: 150mg qd. Week 2 Onward: 200mg qd. Following d/c of Carbamazepine, Phenytoin, Phenobarbital, Primidone with Current Dose of Lamotrigine 400mg qd: Week 1: 400mg qd. Week 2: 300mg qd. Week 3 Onward: 200mg qd. Concomitant/Starting/Stopping Estrogen-Containing Oral Contraceptives: See PI. Hepatic Impairment: Moderate and Severe: Reduce by 25%. Severe with Ascites: Reduce by 50%. Adjust maint and escalation doses based on clinical response. Elderly: Start at lower end of dosing range.
Pediatrics: Epilepsy: ≥16 yrs: Conversion to Monotherapy: See PI. >12 yrs: Same as adults. 2-12 yrs: Give in 1-2 divided doses, rounded down to the nearest whole tab. Concomitant Valproate: Weeks 1 and 2: 0.15mg/kg/day. Weeks 3 and 4: 0.3mg/kg/day. Week 5 Onward: Increase q1-2 weeks by 0.3mg/kg/day. Maint: 1-3mg/kg/day with valproate alone or 1-5mg/kg/day. Max: 200mg/day. Initial Weight-Based Dosing Guide (Weeks 1-4): See PI. Patients not Taking Carbamazepine, Phenytoin, Phenobarbital, Primidone, or Valproate: Weeks 1 and 2: 0.3mg/kg/day. Weeks 3 and 4: 0.6mg/kg/day. Week 5 Onward: Increase q1-2 weeks by 0.6mg/kg/day. Maint: 4.5-7.5mg/kg/day. Max: 300mg/day. Concomitant Carbamazepine, Phenytoin, Phenobarbital, Primidone without Valproate: Weeks 1 and 2: 0.6mg/kg/day. Weeks 3 and 4: 1.2 mg/kg/day. Week 5 Onward: Increase q1-2 weeks by 1.2mg/kg/day. Maint: 5-15mg/kg/day. Max: 400mg/day. <30kg: May increase maint dose by up to 50% based on clinical response.

HOW SUPPLIED: Tab: 25mg*, 100mg*, 150mg*, 200mg*; Tab, Chewable: (CD) 2mg, 5mg, 25mg; Tab, Disintegrating: (ODT) 25mg, 50mg, 100mg, 200mg *scored

WARNINGS/PRECAUTIONS: Multiorgan hypersensitivity reactions (also known as Drug Reaction with Eosinophilia and Systemic Symptoms) reported. Fatalities from acute multiorgan failure and various degrees of hepatic failure reported. Isolated liver failure without rash or involvement of other organs reported. D/C if alternative etiology for signs/symptoms of early manifestations of hypersensitivity cannot be established. Blood dyscrasias (eg, neutropenia, leukopenia, anemia, thrombocytopenia, pancytopenia, aplastic anemia, pure red cell aplasia) reported. Increased risk of suicidal thoughts or behavior; balance risk of suicidal thoughts or behavior with risk of untreated illness prior to therapy. Worsening of depressive symptoms and/or emergence of suicidal ideation and behaviors (suicidality) may be experienced in bipolar disorder; consider d/c. Write prescriptions for smallest quantity of tabs to reduce risk of overdose. Increases risk of developing aseptic meningitis; evaluate for other causes of aseptic meningitis and treat appropriately. Avoid abrupt withdrawal due to risk of withdrawal seizures; taper dose over a period of at least 2 weeks. Sudden unexplained death in epilepsy reported. Status epilepticus reported. May cause toxicity of the eyes and other melanin-containing tissues due to melanin binding. Medication errors reported. Caution with renal/hepatic impairment and in elderly.

ADVERSE REACTIONS: Dizziness, diplopia, infection, headache, ataxia, blurred vision, N/V, somnolence, fever, pharyngitis, rhinitis, rash, diarrhea, abdominal pain.

INTERACTIONS: See Boxed Warning. Phenytoin, carbamazepine, phenobarbital, primidone, rifampin, and estrogen-containing oral contraceptives may decrease levels. May decrease levels of levonorgestrel. Valproate may increase levels. May increase carbamazepine epoxide levels. May inhibit dihydrofolate reductase; caution with other medications that inhibit folate metabolism. May affect clearance with drugs known to induce or inhibit glucuronidation; may require dose adjustment. Higher incidence of headache, dizziness, nausea, and somnolence may occur with oxcarbazepine. May increase topiramate levels. Ethinyl estradiol and levonorgestrel may increase clearance.

PREGNANCY: Category C, caution in nursing.

MECHANISM OF ACTION: Phenyltriazine; mechanism not established. Suspected to inhibit voltage-sensitive Na channels, thereby stabilizing neuronal membranes and consequently modulating presynaptic transmitter release of excitatory amino acids (eg, glutamate, aspartate).

PHARMACOKINETICS: Absorption: Rapid and complete. Absolute bioavailability (98%); T_{max}=1.4-4.8 hrs. **Distribution:** V_d=0.9-1.3L/kg; plasma protein binding (55%); found in breast milk.

Metabolism: Liver via glucuronic acid conjugation; 2-N-glucuronide conjugate (major metabolite, inactive). **Elimination:** Urine (94%; 10% unchanged, 76% 2-N-glucuronide), feces (2%). Refer to PI for variable parameters with concomitant AEDs.

NURSING CONSIDERATIONS

Assessment: Assess for history of allergy/rash to other AEDs, renal/hepatic impairment, depression, systemic lupus erythematosus or other autoimmune diseases, hypersensitivity, pregnancy/nursing status, and possible drug interactions. If restarting after d/c, assess for initial dosing recommendations.

Monitoring: Monitor for signs/symptoms of rash, multiorgan hypersensitivity reactions, multiorgan failure, status epilepticus, blood dyscrasias, emergence/worsening of depression, suicidal thoughts or behavior, unusual mood/behavior changes, aseptic meningitis, and ophthalmologic effects. Monitor drug levels with concomitant medications or if dosage adjustments are being made. Monitor effectiveness of long-term use (>16 weeks).

Patient Counseling: Instruct to notify physician immediately if rash, signs/symptoms of hypersensitivity (eg, fever, lymphadenopathy), blood dyscrasias, multiorgan hypersensitivity reactions, acute multiorgan failure, or aseptic meningitis occur. Inform about increased risk of suicidal thoughts and behavior; advise to be alert if signs/symptoms of depression, any unusual changes in mood/behavior, suicidal thoughts/behavior, or thoughts about self-harm emerge or worsen, and instruct to notify physician immediately. Advise to notify physician if worsening of seizure control occurs. Inform that CNS depression may occur; advise to avoid operating machinery/driving until adjusted to effects. Advise to notify physician if pregnant or intend to become pregnant, or breastfeeding. Discuss the benefits/risks of continuing breastfeeding; instruct to monitor their child for potential adverse effects. Advise females to notify physician if they plan to start or stop oral contraceptives or other hormonal preparations. Advise to report changes in menstrual patterns. Instruct not to abruptly d/c therapy; if therapy is stopped, advise to notify physician before restarting. Instruct to visually inspect tab and verify if correct, as well as formulation, each time prescription is filled.

Administration: Oral route. Refer to PI for proper administration. **Storage:** (Tab/Tab, Chewable) 25°C (77°F); excursions permitted to 15-30°C (59-86°F) in a dry place. (Tab) Protect from light. (Tab, Disintegrating) 20-25°C (68-77°F); excursions permitted between 15-30°C (59-86°F).

LAMISIL   RX
terbinafine HCl (Novartis)

THERAPEUTIC CLASS: Allylamine antifungal

INDICATIONS: (Granules) Treatment of tinea capitis in patients ≥4 yrs. (Tabs) Treatment of onychomycosis of toenail or fingernail due to dermatophytes (tinea unguium).

DOSAGE: *Adults:* (Tab) Onychomycosis: Fingernail: 250mg qd for 6 weeks. Toenail: 250mg qd for 12 weeks. (Granules) Tinea Capitis: Take qd with food for 6 weeks. <25kg: 125mg/day. 25-35kg: 187.5mg/day. >35kg: 250mg/day. Elderly: Start at lower end of dosing range.
Pediatrics: ≥4 yrs: (Granules) Tinea Capitis: Take qd with food for 6 weeks. <25kg: 125mg/day. 25-35kg: 187.5mg/day. >35kg: 250mg/day.

HOW SUPPLIED: Granules: 125mg/pkt, 187.5mg/pkt; Tab: 250mg

WARNINGS/PRECAUTIONS: Cases of liver failure, some leading to liver transplant or death, reported in individuals with and without preexisting liver disease; d/c therapy if evidence of liver injury develops. Not recommended for patients with chronic or active liver disease. Hepatotoxicity may occur. D/C if any symptoms of persistent N/V, anorexia, fatigue, right upper abdominal pain or jaundice, dark urine or pale stools occur and evaluate liver function immediately. Taste/smell disturbance reported; d/c if symptoms of taste/smell disturbance occur. Depressive symptoms may occur. Transient decreases in absolute lymphocyte counts, and cases of severe neutropenia reported; d/c and start supportive management if the neutrophil count is ≤1000 cells/mm³. Serious skin reactions (eg, Stevens-Johnson syndrome and toxic epidermal necrolysis) reported; d/c if progressive skin rash occurs. Precipitation and exacerbation of cutaneous and systemic lupus erythematosus reported. Measure serum transaminases (ALT and AST) prior to initiating therapy.

ADVERSE REACTIONS: Headache, diarrhea, liver enzyme abnormalities, rash. (Granules) Nasopharyngitis, pyrexia, cough, vomiting, upper respiratory tract infection, upper abdominal pain. (Tabs) Dyspepsia.

INTERACTIONS: Coadministration with drugs predominantly metabolized by CYP2D6 (eg, TCAs, β-blockers, SSRIs, antiarrhythmics class 1C, MAOIs type B) should be done with careful monitoring and may require dose reduction of the 2D6-metabolized drug. Increased levels of desipramine. Increased dextromethorphan/dextrorphan ratio in urine in patients who are extensive metabolizers of dextromethorphan. Increased clearance of cyclosporine. Decreased clearance of caffeine. May increase levels with fluconazole. May increase systemic exposure with other inhibitors of both CYP2C9 and CYP3A4 (eg, ketoconazole, amiodarone). Clearance increased by rifampin and decreased by cimetidine. Altered PT with warfarin.

PREGNANCY: Category B, not for use in nursing.

MECHANISM OF ACTION: Allylamine antifungal; acts by inhibiting squalene epoxidase enzyme, thus blocking biosynthesis of ergosterol, an essential component of fungal cell membrane.

PHARMACOKINETICS: Absorption: (Tab) Well-absorbed; bioavailability (40%); (250mg single dose) C_{max}=1μg/mL, T_{max}=2 hrs, AUC =4.56μg•hr/mL. **Distribution:** Plasma protein binding (>99%); found in breast milk. **Metabolism:** Extensive, (Granules) rapid; CYP2C9, CYP1A2, CYP3A4, CYP2C8, CYP2C19 (major). **Elimination:** Urine (70%); (Tab) $T_{1/2}$=200-400 hrs, (Granules) (125mg dose) $T_{1/2}$=26.7 hrs; (187.5mg dose) $T_{1/2}$=30.5 hrs.

NURSING CONSIDERATIONS

Assessment: Assess for known hypersensitivity, liver disease, immunodeficiency, lupus erythematosus, nursing status, and possible drug interactions. Prior to treatment, obtain LFTs (eg, measurement of serum transaminases), and appropriate nail specimens for lab testing (potassium hydroxide preparation, fungal culture, or nail biopsy) to confirm diagnosis of onychomycosis.

Monitoring: Monitor for signs of hepatotoxicity, taste/smell disturbances, occurrence of progressive skin rash, depressive symptoms, and signs/symptoms of lupus erythematosus. Monitor CBC with immunodeficiency if therapy continues for >6 weeks, or if signs of secondary infection occur.

Patient Counseling: Instruct to take exactly as directed. Advise to report immediately to their physician and d/c treatment if any symptoms of N/V, right upper abdominal pain, jaundice, dark urine or pale stool, taste/smell disturbance, anorexia, fatigue, depressive symptoms, hives, mouth sores, blistering and peeling skin, swelling of the face, lips, tongue or throat, or difficulty breathing or swallowing occurs. Instruct patient to report to their physician for any symptoms of new or worsening lupus erythematosus or skin rash. Inform that photosensitivity reaction may occur; instruct to minimize exposure to natural and artificial sunlight (tanning beds or UVA/B treatment) while on therapy. Advise to have serum transaminases (ALT/AST) be measured before treatment. Advise to notify physician if taken too many doses.

Administration: Oral route. (Granules) Sprinkle contents of each pkt on a spoonful of pudding or other soft, non-acidic food, such as mashed potatoes, and swallow the entire spoonful (without chewing); do not use applesauce or fruit-based foods. Refer to PI for the complete administration instruction. **Storage:** (Tab) <25°C (77°F); in a tight container. Protect from light. (Granules) 25°C (77°F); excursions permitted to 15-30°C (59-86°F).

LANOXIN   RX
digoxin (GlaxoSmithKline)

OTHER BRAND NAMES: Digoxin (Various)

THERAPEUTIC CLASS: Cardiac glycoside

INDICATIONS: Treatment of mild to moderate heart failure and control of ventricular response rate in patients with chronic atrial fibrillation (A-fib).

DOSAGE: *Adults:* Individualize dose. Heart Failure: May be accomplished rapidly or gradually. Rapid Digitalization: LD: (Inj) 0.4-0.6mg IV, (Tab) 0.5-0.75mg PO, or (Sol) 10-15mcg/kg PO. Additional Doses: (Inj) 0.1-0.3mg or (Tab) 0.125-0.375mg at 6-8 hr intervals until clinical effect noted. (Sol) Give at 4-8 hr intervals until clinical effect noted. Gradual Digitalization: (Tab) Initial: 0.25mg qd (good renal function), 0.125mg qd (>70 yrs/impaired renal function), 0.0625 qd (marked renal impairment). Titrate: May increase every 2 weeks based on response. (Tab) Maint: 0.125-0.5mg qd; refer to PI for dose requirements based on weight and renal function. (Sol) Maint: 3-4.5mcg/kg/day (good renal function); refer to PI for dose requirements based on weight and renal function. A-Fib: Titrate to minimum dose that achieves desired response. Elderly: Start at low end of dosing range.

Pediatrics: Individualize dose. Heart Failure: May be accomplished rapidly or gradually. Rapid Digitalization: LD (Inj): Give 1/2 of total digitalizing dose. Digitalizing Dose (with normal renal function): Premature Infants: 15-25mcg/kg. Full-Term Infants: 20-30mcg/kg. 1-24 months: 30-50mcg/kg. 2-5 yrs: 25-35mcg/kg. 5-10 yrs: 15-30mcg/kg. >10 yrs: 8-12mcg/kg. LD (Sol): Premature Infants: 20-30mcg/kg. Full-Term Infants: 25-35mcg/kg. 1-24 months: 35-60mcg/kg. 2-5 yrs: 30-45mcg/kg. 5-10 yrs: 20-35mcg/kg. >10 yrs: 10-15mcg/kg. Additional Doses (Inj/Sol): Give in fractions every 4-8 hr intervals until clinical response noted. Renal Disease: Start at low doses; carefully titrate based on clinical response. Gradual Digitalization: Begin with maint dose. (Inj) Maint: Premature Infants: 20-30% of IV digitalizing dose/day. Full-Term Infants to >10 yrs: 25-35% of IV digitalizing dose/day. (Sol) Maint: Premature Infants: 4.7-7.8mcg/kg/day. Full-Term Infants: 7.5-11.3mcg/kg/day. 1-24 months: 11.3-18.8mcg/kg/day. 2-5 yrs: 9.4-13.1mcg/kg/day. 5-10 yrs: 5.6-11.3mcg/kg/day. >10 yrs: 3-4.5mcg/kg/day; refer to PI for dose requirements based on weight and renal function. (Tab) Maint: 2-5 yrs: 10-15mcg/kg. 5-10 yrs: 7-10mcg/kg. >10 yrs: 3-5mcg/kg. A-Fib: (Inj/Tab) Titrate to minimum dose that achieves desired response.

HOW SUPPLIED: Sol: 50mcg/mL [60mL]; Inj: (Lanoxin) 0.25mg/mL, (Lanoxin Pediatric) 0.1mg/mL; (Lanoxin) Tab: 0.125mg*, 0.25mg* *scored

CONTRAINDICATIONS: Ventricular fibrillation.

WARNINGS/PRECAUTIONS: May cause severe sinus bradycardia or sinoatrial block with pre-existing sinus node disease and may cause advanced or complete heart block with preexisting incomplete atrioventricular (AV) block; consider insertion of a pacemaker before treatment. Increased risk of ventricular fibrillation in patients with Wolff-Parkinson-White (WPW) syndrome; do not use with accessory AV pathway unless conduction down the pathway has been blocked pharmacologically or by surgery. Avoid with preserved left ventricular ejection (eg, restrictive cardiomyopathy, constrictive pericarditis, amyloid heart disease, acute cor pulmonale); increased risk of toxicity. Avoid with idiopathic hypertrophic subaortic stenosis and myocarditis. Reduce usual maint dose with impaired renal function. Toxicity may occur in patients with hypokalemia, hypomagnesemia, or hypercalcemia; maintain electrolytes during treatment. Hypocalcemia may nullify the effects of treatment. Hypothyroidism may reduce digoxin requirements. Atrial arrhythmias associated with hypermetabolic states may be resistant to the treatment; use caution to avoid toxicity. Caution with acute myocardial infarction; may result in increased myocardial oxygen demand and ischemia. May result in potentially detrimental increases in coronary vascular resistance. Inadequate response in patients with beri beri heart disease; treat underlying thiamine deficiency. Causes prolongation of PR interval and depression of ST segment. May produce false positive ST-T changes on ECG during exercise testing. Caution with identifying etiology of toxicity; signs and symptoms of digoxin toxicity may be mistaken for worsening symptoms of congestive heart failure.

ADVERSE REACTIONS: Heart block, rhythm disturbances, anorexia, N/V, diarrhea, visual disturbances, headache, weakness, dizziness, mental disturbances.

INTERACTIONS: Increased risk of arrhythmias with calcium, sympathomimetics, and succinylcholine. Increased digoxin dose requirement with thyroid supplements. Additive effects on AV node conduction with calcium channel blockers and β-blockers. Increased serum concentrations with quinidine, verapamil, amiodarone, propafenone, indomethacin, itraconazole, alprazolam, spironolactone, propantheline, diphenoxylate, erythromycin/clarithromycin (possibly other macrolides), tetracycline, carvedilol. Decreased serum concentrations with antacids, anti-cancer drugs, cholestyramine, kaolin-pectin, meals high in bran, metoclopramide, neomycin, rifampin, sulfasalazine. (Inj/Tab) Risk of digitalis toxicity with K⁺-depleting diuretics. Caution with drugs that deteriorate renal function. Altered levels with quinine and penicillamine. (Sol) Increased serum concentrations with captopril, nitrendipine, ranolazine, ritonavir, diltiazem, nifedipine, rabeprazole, telmisartan, azithromycin, cyclosporine, diclofenac, epoprostenol, esomeprazole, ketoconazole, lansoprazole, metformin, omeprazole. Decreased concentrations with acarbose, activated charcoal, albuterol, colestipol, exenatide, miglitol, salbutamol, St. John's wort, sucralfate, sulfasalazine. Higher rate of torsades de pointes with dofetilide. Increased PR interval and QRS duration reported with moricizine. Teriparatide transiently increases serum calcium; caution with coadministration. Potential to alter pharmacokinetics with P-glycoprotein inducers/inhibitors.

PREGNANCY: Category C, caution in nursing.

MECHANISM OF ACTION: Cardiac glycoside; inhibits Na⁺-K⁺ ATPase, leading to increase in intracellular concentration of Na⁺ and thus an increase in intracellular concentration of Ca^{2+}.

PHARMACOKINETICS: Absorption: (Tab) Absolute bioavailability (60-80%), T_{max}=1-3 hrs. (Sol) Absolute bioavailability (70-85%), T_{max}=30-90 min. (Inj) Absolute bioavailability (100%). **Distribution:** Plasma protein binding (25%); crosses placenta; found in breast milk. **Metabolism:** Hydrolysis, oxidation, and conjugation; 3 β-digoxigenin, 3-ketodigoxigenin (metabolites). **Elimination:** Urine (50-70%); $T_{1/2}$= (healthy volunteer) 1.5-2 days, (anuric patients) 3.5-5 days. (Sol) $T_{1/2}$=18-36 hrs (pediatrics), 36-48 hrs (adults).

NURSING CONSIDERATIONS

Assessment: Assess for known hypersensitivity, ventricular fibrillation, myocarditis, thyroid and electrolyte disorders, hypermetabolic states, sinus node disease, incomplete AV block, renal impairment, accessory AV pathway (WPW syndrome), heart failure with preserved ventricular ejection fraction, idiopathic hypertrophic subaortic stenosis, acute myocardial infarction, beri beri heart disease, pregnancy/nursing status, and possible drug interactions.

Monitoring: Monitor serum electrolytes and renal function periodically. Monitor for signs/symptoms of sinoatrial block, severe sinus bradycardia, complete AV block, electrolyte imbalance, drug toxicity, vasoconstriction, and hypersensitivity reactions. Monitor serum digoxin levels.

Patient Counseling: Instruct to take the drug as prescribed and not to adjust dose without consulting the physician. Advise to notify physician if taking any OTC medications, including herbal medication, or are started on a new prescription. Inform that blood tests will be necessary to ensure the appropriate digoxin dose. Instruct to contact physician if N/V, persistent diarrhea, confusion, weakness, or visual disturbances occur. Advise parents or caregivers that symptoms of digoxin toxicity may be difficult to recognize in infants and pediatric patients; symptoms such as weight loss, failure to thrive in infants, abdominal pain, and behavioral disturbances may be indications of digoxin toxicity. Suggest to monitor and record heart rate and BP daily. Instruct women of childbearing potential who become or are planning to become pregnant to consult physician prior to initiation or continuing therapy with digoxin. (Sol) Instruct to use calibrated dropper to measure the dose and to avoid less precise measuring tools (eg, tsp).

Administration: Oral/IV route. Refer to PI for dilution instructions. **Storage:** 25°C (77°F); excursions permitted to 15-30°C (59-86°F). Protect from light. (Tab) Store in dry place. Diluted Sol: Use immediately.

LANTUS   RX
insulin glargine, rdna origin (Sanofi-Aventis)

THERAPEUTIC CLASS: Insulin

INDICATIONS: To improve glycemic control in adults with type 1 or type 2 diabetes mellitus (DM) and in children with type 1 DM.

DOSAGE: *Adults:* Individualize dose. Inject SQ qd at same time every day. Type 1 DM: Initial: 1/3 of total daily insulin requirement. Type 2 DM Not Currently Treated With Insulin: Initial: 10 U (or 0.2 U/kg) qd. Adjust according to patient's needs. Switching From QD NPH Insulin: Initial: Same as NPH dose being d/c. Switching From BID NPH Insulin: Initial: 80% of the total NPH dose being d/c. Renal/Hepatic Impairment: May need to reduce dose.
Pediatrics: ≥6 yrs: Individualize dose. Inject SQ qd at same time every day. Type 1 DM: Initial: 1/3 of total daily insulin requirement. Switching From QD NPH Insulin: Initial: Same as NPH dose being d/c. Switching From BID NPH Insulin: Initial: 80% of the total NPH dose being d/c. Renal/ Hepatic Impairment: May need to reduce dose.

HOW SUPPLIED: Inj: 100 U/mL [10mL, vial]; [3mL, OptiClik, SoloStar]

WARNINGS/PRECAUTIONS: Not recommended for the treatment of diabetic ketoacidosis. Use in regimens with short-acting insulin with type 1 DM. Glucose monitoring is essential for all patients receiving insulin therapy. Any change of insulin should be made cautiously and only under medical supervision. Changing from one insulin product to another or changing the strength may result in the need for a change in dosage. Not for IV use or via an insulin pump; may result in severe hypoglycemia if usual SQ dose is given IV. Do not mix or dilute with any other insulin or sol. Do not share disposable or reusable insulin devices or needles between patients; may carry a risk for transmission of blood-borne pathogens. Hypoglycemia may occur; caution in patients with hypoglycemia unawareness and patients predisposed to hypoglycemia (pediatrics, patients who fast or have erratic food intake). Hypoglycemia may impair ability of concentration and react. Severe, life-threatening, generalized allergy, including anaphylaxis, may occur. Not recommended during periods of rapidly declining renal/hepatic function. Caution in elderly.

ADVERSE REACTIONS: Hypoglycemia, allergic reactions, headache, lipodystrophy, injection-site reactions, rash, pruritus, upper respiratory tract infection, peripheral edema, HTN, influenza, cataracts, arthralgia, infection, pain in extremities.

INTERACTIONS: May require dose adjustment and close monitoring with drugs that may increase the blood glucose-lowering effect and susceptibility to hypoglycemia (eg, oral antidiabetics, pramlintide, ACE inhibitors, disopyramide, fibrates, fluoxetine, MAOIs, propoxyphene, pentoxifylline, salicylates, somatostatin analogs, sulfonamide antibiotics), decrease the blood glucose-lowering effect (eg, corticosteroids, niacin, danazol, diuretics, sympathomimetics [eg, epinephrine, albuterol, terbutaline], glucagon, isoniazid, phenothiazines derivatives, somatropin, thyroid hormones, estrogens, progestogens [eg, in oral contraceptives], protease inhibitors, atypical antipsychotics [eg, olanzapine and clozapine]), and potentiate or weaken the blood glucose-lowering effect (β-blockers, clonidine, lithium salts, alcohol). Pentamidine may cause hypoglycemia, sometimes followed by hyperglycemia. Signs of hypoglycemia may be reduced or absent with sympatholytics (eg, β-blockers, clonidine, guanethidine, reserpine).

PREGNANCY: Category C, caution in nursing.

MECHANISM OF ACTION: Insulin glargine (rDNA origin); regulates glucose metabolism. Lowers blood glucose by stimulating peripheral glucose uptake and by inhibiting hepatic glucose production. Inhibits lipolysis and proteolysis, and enhances protein synthesis.

PHARMACOKINETICS: Metabolism: M1 (21^A-Gly-insulin) and M2 (21^A-Gly-des-30^B-Thr-insulin) (active metabolites).

NURSING CONSIDERATIONS

Assessment: Assess for diabetic ketoacidosis, predisposition to hypoglycemia, hypersensitivity, renal/hepatic impairment, pregnancy/nursing status, and possible drug interactions. Obtain baseline blood glucose and HbA1c levels.

Monitoring: Monitor for signs/symptoms of hypoglycemia, concentration/reaction impairment, lipodystrophy, allergic reactions, and other adverse reactions. Monitor blood glucose and HbA1c levels.

Patient Counseling: Inform about potential side effects (eg, lipodystrophy, weight gain, allergic reactions, hypoglycemia). Inform that the ability to concentrate and react may be impaired as a result of hypoglycemia; advise to use caution when driving or operating machinery. Instruct to always check the insulin label before each inj. Instruct to inspect sol for particles and discoloration before use. Advise not to share disposable or reusable insulin devices or needles. Instruct on self-management procedures (eg, glucose monitoring, proper inj technique, management of hypoglycemia and hyperglycemia) and handling of special situations (eg, intercurrent conditions, inadequate or skipped dose, inadvertent administration of increased insulin dose, inadequate food intake, skipped meals). Advise to inform physician if pregnant or contemplating pregnancy.

Administration: SQ route. Inject in the abdomen, thigh, or upper arm. Rotate inj sites. Refer to PI for administration techniques. **Storage:** Unopened: 2-8°C (36-46°F). Open (In-Use): 30°C (86°F). Discard after 28 days. Protect from direct heat and light. Do not refrigerate opened (in-use) vial/cartridge/SoloStar.

LASTACAFT   RX
alcaftadine (Allergan)

THERAPEUTIC CLASS: H_1-antagonist

INDICATIONS: Prevention of itching associated with allergic conjunctivitis.

DOSAGE: *Adults:* 1 drop in each eye qd.
Pediatrics: ≥2 yrs: 1 drop in each eye qd.

HOW SUPPLIED: Sol: 0.25% [3mL]

WARNINGS/PRECAUTIONS: For topical ophthalmic use only. Caution not to touch the dropper tip to eyelids or surrounding areas to minimize contamination. Do not wear contact lens if the eye is red. Not for treatment of contact lens-related irritation. Do not instill while wearing contact lenses; reinsert lenses after 10 min following administration.

ADVERSE REACTIONS: Eye irritation, burning and/or stinging upon instillation, eye redness, eye pruritus.

PREGNANCY: Category B, caution in nursing.

MECHANISM OF ACTION: H_1-receptor antagonist; inhibits release of histamine from mast cells, decreases chemotaxis, and inhibits eosinophil activation.

PHARMACOKINETICS: Absorption: C_{max}=60pg/mL, 3ng/mL (active metabolite); T_{max}=15 min (median), 1 hr after dosing (active metabolite). **Distribution:** Plasma protein binding (39.2%), (62.7%, active metabolite). **Metabolism:** non-CYP450 cytosolic enzymes; carboxylic acid metabolite (active metabolite). **Excretion:** Urine (unchanged); $T_{1/2}$=2 hrs (active metabolite).

NURSING CONSIDERATIONS

Assessment: Assess for contact lens-related irritation and pregnancy/nursing status.

Monitoring: Monitor for possible adverse reactions.

Patient Counseling: Advise to avoid touching the tip of dropper to any surface to avoid contamination. Advise not to wear contact lenses if the eye is red. Advise not to use to treat contact lens-related irritation. Advise to remove contact lenses prior to instillation, then reinsert lenses after 10 min following administration. Inform that the drug is for topical ophthalmic administration only.

Administration: Ocular route. **Storage:** 15-25°C (59-77°F). Keep bottle tightly closed when not in use.

LATISSE   RX
bimatoprost (Allergan)

THERAPEUTIC CLASS: Prostaglandin analog

INDICATIONS: Treatment of hypotrichosis of the eyelashes.

DOSAGE: *Adults:* 1 drop qd in pm using the disposable sterile applicator supplied. Apply evenly along the skin of upper eyelid margin at the base of eyelashes.

HOW SUPPLIED: Sol: 0.03% [1.5mL, 3mL, 5mL]

WARNINGS/PRECAUTIONS: May lower intraocular pressure (IOP) when instilled directly to the eye. Increased iris pigmentation reported. May cause pigment changes (darkening) to periorbital pigmented tissues and eyelashes. May cause hair growth to occur in areas where sol comes in repeated contact with the skin surface. Caution with active intraocular inflammation (eg, uveitis); inflammation may be exacerbated. Macular edema, including cystoid macular edema, reported during treatment of elevated IOP; caution with aphakic patients, pseudophakic patients with torn posterior lens capsule, or patients at risk of macular edema. Avoid contact of bottle tip to any other surface. Use the accompanying sterile applicators on 1 eye, then discard; reuse of applicators increases the potential for contamination and infections. Bacterial keratitis associated with the use of multidose containers reported. Contact lenses should be removed prior to application and may be reinserted 15 min following its administration.

ADVERSE REACTIONS: Eye pruritus, conjunctival hyperemia, skin hyperpigmentation, ocular irritation, dry eye symptoms, erythema of the eyelid.

INTERACTIONS: May interfere with the desired reduction in IOP with IOP-lowering prostaglandin analogs.

PREGNANCY: Category C, caution in nursing.

MECHANISM OF ACTION: Prostaglandin analog; has not been established. Believed that growth of eyelashes occur by increasing the percent of hairs in, and the duration of the anagen or growth phase.

PHARMACOKINETICS: Absorption: C_{max}=0.08ng/mL, AUC=0.09ng•hr/mL, T_{max}=10 min. **Distribution:** V_d=0.67L/kg. **Metabolism:** Oxidation, N-deethylation, and glucuronidation. **Elimination:** (IV) Urine (67%), feces (25%); $T_{1/2}$=45 min.

NURSING CONSIDERATIONS

Assessment: Assess for active intraocular inflammation, aphakia, pseudophakia with a torn posterior lens capsule, risk for macular edema, pregnancy/nursing status, and possible drug interactions.

Monitoring: Monitor for IOP changes, increased iris pigmentation, pigment changes (darkening) to periorbital pigmented tissues and eyelashes, macular edema (eg, cystoid macular edema), bacterial keratitis, and other adverse reactions.

Patient Counseling: Instruct to apply medication every pm using only the accompanying sterile applicators, not to apply to lower eyelash line, and to blot any excess sol outside the upper eyelid margin with tissue or other absorbent material. Counsel that if any sol gets into the eye proper, it will not cause harm; eye should not be rinsed. Counsel that the effect is not permanent and can be expected to gradually return to original level upon d/c. Instruct that bottle must be maintained intact and to avoid contaminating the bottle tip or applicator. Advise to notify physician if new ocular condition (eg, trauma or infection) develops, sudden decrease in visual acuity occurs, have ocular surgery, and if any ocular reactions (eg, conjunctivitis, eyelid reactions) develop. Advise about the potential for increased brown iris pigmentation (may be permanent), eyelid skin darkening, and unexpected hair growth or eyelash changes. Advise that contact lenses should be removed prior to application, and may be reinserted 15 min following its administration.

Administration: Ocular route. Refer to PI for further application instructions. **Storage:** 2-25°C (36-77°F).

LATUDA   RX
lurasidone HCl (Sunovion)

> Elderly patients with dementia-related psychosis treated with antipsychotic drugs are at an increased risk of death; most deaths appeared to be cardiovascular (CV) (eg, heart failure, sudden death) or infectious (eg, pneumonia) in nature. Not approved for the treatment of dementia-related psychosis.

THERAPEUTIC CLASS: Benzoisothiazol derivative

INDICATIONS: Treatment of schizophrenia.

DOSAGE: *Adults:* Initial: 40mg qd. Max: 80mg/day. Moderate-Severe Renal/Hepatic Impairment or Concomitant Moderate CYP3A4 Inhibitors (eg, Diltiazem): Max: 40mg/day. Take with food (at least 350 calories).

HOW SUPPLIED: Tab: 20mg, 40mg, 80mg

CONTRAINDICATIONS: Concomitant use with strong CYP3A4 inhibitors (eg, ketoconazole) and strong CYP3A4 inducers (eg, rifampin).

WARNINGS/PRECAUTIONS: Neuroleptic malignant syndrome (NMS) reported; d/c if this occurs. Tardive dyskinesia (TD) reported; consider d/c if this occurs. May cause metabolic changes (hyperglycemia, dyslipidemia, weight gain) that may increase CV and cerebrovascular risk. Hyperglycemia, in some cases extreme and associated with ketoacidosis or hyperosmolar coma or death reported; monitor for hyperglycemia, and perform FPG testing at the beginning of therapy and periodically in patients at risk for diabetes mellitus (DM). Undesirable alterations in lipids and weight gain reported. May elevate prolactin levels. Leukopenia, neutropenia, and agranulocytosis reported; d/c at 1st sign of decline in WBC without other causative factors in patients with preexisting low WBC or history of drug-induced leukopenia/neutropenia or if severe neutropenia (absolute neutrophil count <1000/mm³) develops. May cause orthostatic hypotension and syncope; caution with CV disease, cerebrovascular disease, or conditions that predispose to hypotension (eg, dehydration, hypovolemia, and treatment with antihypertensives). Caution with history of seizures or with conditions that lower the seizure threshold. May impair mental/physical abilities. May disrupt body's ability to reduce core body temperature; caution with conditions that may contribute to an elevated core body temperature (eg, strenuous exercise, concomitant medication with anticholinergic activity). May lead to suicide attempts; supervision should accompany therapy in patients at high risk. May cause esophageal dysmotility and aspiration; avoid use in patients at risk for aspiration pneumonia.

ADVERSE REACTIONS: Somnolence, akathisia, N/V, parkinsonism, agitation, dyspepsia, fatigue, back pain, dystonia, dizziness, insomnia, anxiety, restlessness.

INTERACTIONS: See Contraindications. Caution with other centrally acting drugs and alcohol. May increase levels of digoxin and midazolam; dose adjustment not required. Diltiazem (moderate CYP3A4 inhibitor) may increase levels; do not exceed 40mg/day if coadministered. Lithium may increase levels; dose adjustment not required.

PREGNANCY: Category B, caution in nursing.

MECHANISM OF ACTION: Benzoisothiazol derivative; not established. Suggested that the efficacy is mediated through a combination of dopamine type 2 (D_2) and serotonin type 2 ($5HT_{2A}$) receptor antagonism.

PHARMACOKINETICS: Absorption: T_{max}=1-3 hrs. **Distribution:** (40mg dose) V_d= 6173L; plasma protein binding (99%). **Metabolism:** Mainly via CYP3A4; oxidative N-dealkylation, hydroxylation of norbornane ring, and S-oxidation; ID-14283, ID-14326 (active metabolites). **Elimination:** Urine (9%), feces (80%); (40mg dose) $T_{1/2}$=18 hrs.

NURSING CONSIDERATIONS

Assessment: Assess for dementia-related psychosis, preexisting low WBCs or drug-induced leukopenia/neutropenia, CV disease, cerebrovascular disease, conditions that predispose to hypotension, conditions that lower the seizure threshold, risk of aspiration pneumonia, risk factors for DM, hepatic/renal impairment, conditions where treatment is contraindicated or cautioned, pregnancy/nursing status, and possible drug interactions. Obtain baseline FPG in patients at risk for DM.

Monitoring: Monitor for signs/symptoms of NMS, TD, hyperprolactinemia, orthostatic hypotension, syncope, cognitive and motor impairment, seizures, aspiration, hyperglycemia, disruption of body temperature, dyslipidemia, suicide attempts, and other possible side effects. Monitor FPG, lipid profile, weight gain, and CBC (in patients with preexisting low WBC or drug-induced leukopenia/neutropenia). In patients with clinically significant neutropenia, monitor for fever or other symptoms or signs of infection.

Patient Counseling: Advise that elderly patients with dementia-related psychosis are at increased risk of death. Counsel about signs/symptoms of NMS (eg, hyperpyrexia, muscle rigidity, altered mental status, autonomic instability), hyperglycemia, and DM. Advise of risk of orthostatic hypotension particularly at time of initiating/reinitiating treatment, or increasing dose. Advise that some patients may need blood glucose and/or CBC monitoring during therapy. Counsel to notify physician if taking any other medications and if intending to become pregnant or if become pregnant during therapy. Advise to use caution when operating hazardous machinery/ driving. Advise to avoid alcohol while on treatment. Advise to take appropriate care in avoiding overheating and dehydration.

Administration: Oral route. Take with food (at least 350 calories). **Storage:** 25°C (77°F); excursions permitted to 15-30°C (59-86°F).

LAZANDA   CII
fentanyl (Archimedes)

> Contains fentanyl with abuse liability similar to other opioid analgesics. Do not substitute for any other fentanyl product. Contraindicated for use in opioid non-tolerant patients and management of acute or postoperative pain. Life-threatening respiratory depression could occur at any dose in opioid non-tolerant patients. Do not convert patients on a mcg-per-mcg basis from another fentanyl product to Lazanda. Use special care when dosing. Use only in opioid-tolerant patients with cancer and only by healthcare professionals who are knowledgeable/skilled in the use of Schedule II opioids to treat cancer pain. Must be kept out of reach of children. Concomitant use with CYP3A4 inhibitors may increase plasma levels, and may cause fatal respiratory depression. Available only through Lazanda REMS (Risk Evaluation and Mitigation Strategy) program.

THERAPEUTIC CLASS: Opioid analgesic

INDICATIONS: Management of breakthrough pain in cancer patients ≥18 yrs who are already receiving and are tolerant to opioid therapy for their underlying persistent cancer pain.

DOSAGE: *Adults:* ≥18 yrs: Initial (including switching from another fentanyl product): 100mcg (one 100mcg spray in one nostril). Maint: If adequate analgesia obtained within 30 min with 100mcg, treat subsequent episodes with this dose. Titrate: Individualize. If adequate analgesia not achieved with the 100mcg dose, escalate dose in a stepwise manner (200mcg [one 100mcg spray in each nostril], then 400mcg [one 400mcg spray in one nostril], then 800mcg [one 400mcg spray in each nostril]) over consecutive breakthrough episodes until adequate analgesia with tolerable side effects is achieved; allow ≥2 hrs before treating another episode. Max: 800mcg. Maint: Use the established dose for each subsequent breakthrough episodes; limit to ≤4 doses/day and allow ≥2 hrs before treating another episode. May use rescue medication if pain relief is inadequate after 30 min following dosing, or a separate breakthrough episode occurs before the next dose is permitted (within 2 hrs). Refer to PI for instructions on titration, re-adjustment, and d/c of therapy.

HOW SUPPLIED: Spray: 100mcg/spray, 400mcg/spray

CONTRAINDICATIONS: Opioid non-tolerant patients, management of acute or postoperative pain (eg, headache/migraine, dental pain, or use in emergency room).

WARNINGS/PRECAUTIONS: Serious or fatal respiratory depression may occur even at recommended doses; more likely to occur with underlying respiratory disorders and in elderly/debilitated, or when given with other drugs that depress respiration. May impair mental and/or physical abilities. Cautiously adjust dose in patients with chronic obstructive pulmonary disease or pre-existing medical conditions predisposing to respiratory depression; may further decrease respiratory drive to the point of respiratory failure. Extreme caution in patients particularly susceptible to intracranial effects of CO_2 retention (eg, evidence of increased intracranial pressure or impaired consciousness). May obscure clinical course of head injuries. Caution with bradyarrhythmias and hepatic/renal dysfunction. Potential for misuse, abuse, addiction, and overdose.

ADVERSE REACTIONS: Respiratory depression, N/V, somnolence, dizziness, headache, constipation, pyrexia.

INTERACTIONS: See Boxed Warning. May produce increased depressant effects with other CNS depressants (eg, other opioids, sedatives/hypnotics, general anesthetics, phenothiazines, tranquilizers, skeletal muscle relaxants, sedating antihistamines, alcoholic beverages); dose adjustment may be required. May decrease levels and efficacy with CYP3A4 inducers (eg, barbiturates, carbamazepine, glucocorticoids, phenytoin, pioglitazone). Lower peak plasma concentrations and delayed T_{max} with vasoconstrictive nasal decongestants (eg, oxymetazoline); may decrease efficacy. Not recommended with MAOIs, or within 14 days of d/c of MAOIs.

PREGNANCY: Category C, not for use in nursing.

MECHANISM OF ACTION: Pure opioid agonist; mechanism not established. μ-opioid receptor agonist. Specific CNS opioid receptors for endogenous compounds with opioid-like activity have been identified throughout the brain and spinal cord and play a role in analgesic effects.

PHARMACOKINETICS: Absorption: Administration of various doses led to different parameters. **Distribution:** V_d=4L/kg; plasma protein binding (80-85%); crosses placenta, found in breast milk. **Metabolism:** Liver and intestinal mucosa via CYP3A4; norfentanyl (metabolite). **Elimination:** Urine (<7%, unchanged), feces (1%, unchanged); $T_{1/2}$=21.9 hrs (100mcg), 24.9 hrs (200mcg and 800mcg), 15 hrs (400mcg).

NURSING CONSIDERATIONS

Assessment: Assess for degree of opioid tolerance, previous opioid dose, level/intensity/type of pain, general condition and medical status, and conditions where treatment is contraindicated or cautioned. Assess for pregnancy/nursing status, renal/hepatic function, and possible drug interactions.

Monitoring: Monitor for signs/symptoms of respiratory depression, impairment of mental/physical abilities, abuse/addiction, and hypersensitivity reactions.

Patient Counseling: Counsel that therapy may be fatal in children, individuals for whom it is not prescribed, and who are not opioid tolerant; keep out of reach of children. Do not take medication for acute or postoperative pain, pain from injuries, headache, migraine, or any other short-term pain. Take drug as prescribed, and avoid sharing it with anyone else, and combining it with alcohol, sleep aids, or tranquilizers except by order of prescribing physician. Must wait ≥2 hrs before treating another episode. Medication has potential for abuse. Can affect one's ability to perform activities that require high level of attention. Notify physician if breakthrough pain is not alleviated or worsens after taking the medication. Counsel female patients on the effects that drug may have on them and their unborn child if they become or plan to become pregnant. Dispose of bottle and start a new one if it has been ≥5 days since the bottle was last used and ≥14 days since the bottle was primed. Counsel on proper administration and disposal, and the meaning of opioid tolerance.

Administration: Intranasal route. Refer to PI for proper administration and disposal. **Storage:** ≤25°C. Do not freeze. Return bottle to child-resistant container after each use. Protect from light.

LESCOL XL

RX

fluvastatin sodium (Novartis)

OTHER BRAND NAMES: Lescol (Novartis)

THERAPEUTIC CLASS: HMG-CoA reductase inhibitor

INDICATIONS: Adjunct to diet, to reduce total cholesterol (total-C), LDL, TG, and apolipoprotein B (Apo B) levels, and to increase HDL in primary hypercholesterolemia and mixed dyslipidemia (Types IIa and IIb) when response to nonpharmacological measures is inadequate, and to reduce total-C, LDL, and Apo B levels in adolescent boys and girls who are ≥1 yr postmenarche, 10-16 yrs of age, with heterozygous familial hypercholesterolemia unresponsive to dietary restriction and LDL ≥190mg/dL or LDL ≥160mg/dL with a positive family history of premature CV disease or ≥2 other CV disease risk factors present. To reduce risk of undergoing coronary revascularization procedures and to slow the progression of coronary atherosclerosis in patients with coronary heart disease.

DOSAGE: *Adults:* Usual: 20-80mg/day. Do not take two 40mg cap at one time. LDL Reduction ≥25%: Initial: 40mg cap qpm or 80mg tab qd or 40mg cap bid. LDL Reduction <25%: Initial: 20mg cap qpm. Hypercholesterolemia/Mixed Dyslipidemia: Initial: 40mg cap qpm or 40mg cap bid or 80mg tab qd. Concomitant Cyclosporine/Fluconazole: Max: 20mg cap bid.
Pediatrics: 10-16 yrs: Heterozygous Familial Hypercholesterolemia: Initial: One 20mg cap. Titrate: Adjust dose at 6-week intervals. Max: 40mg cap bid or 80mg tab qd. Concomitant Cyclosporine/Fluconazole: Max: 20mg cap bid.

HOW SUPPLIED: Cap: (Lescol) 20mg, 40mg; Tab, Extended-Release: (Lescol XL) 80mg

CONTRAINDICATIONS: Active liver disease or unexplained, persistent elevations of serum transaminases, pregnancy, nursing mothers.

WARNINGS/PRECAUTIONS: Rhabdomyolysis with acute renal failure secondary to myoglobinuria reported; caution in patients with predisposing factors to myopathy (eg, age ≥65 yrs, renal impairment, and inadequately treated hypothyroidism). D/C if myopathy is suspected/diagnosed or if markedly elevated CPK levels occur. Temporarily withhold if experiencing acute or serious condition predisposing to development of renal failure secondary to rhabdomyolysis. Increases in serum transaminases reported; perform LFTs before initiation and if signs/symptoms of liver injury occur. Hepatic failure reported; promptly interrupt therapy if serious liver injury and/or hyperbilirubinemia or jaundice occurs and do not restart if no alternate etiology found. Caution with heavy alcohol use or history of liver disease and in elderly. Increase in HbA1c and fasting serum glucose levels reported. May blunt adrenal and/or gonadal steroid hormone production. Evaluate if endocrine dysfunction develops. May cause CNS toxicity. Caution with severe renal impairment at doses >40mg.

ADVERSE REACTIONS: Dyspepsia, abdominal pain, headache, sinusitis, nausea, diarrhea, myalgia, flu-like symptoms, abnormal LFTs.

INTERACTIONS: Increased risk of myopathy and/or rhabdomyolysis with cyclosporine, erythromycin, fibrates, niacin, colchicine, and gemfibrozil; avoid with gemfibrozil, caution with colchicine and fibrates, and consider dose reduction with niacin. Caution with drugs that decrease levels of endogenous steroid hormones (eg, ketoconazole, spironolactone, cimetidine). Bleeding and/or increased PT reported with coumarin anticoagulants; monitor PT of patients on warfarin-type anticoagulants when therapy is initiated or dosage is changed. Increased glyburide and phenytoin levels. (Cap) Cyclosporine and fluconazole may increase levels; limit therapy to 20mg bid. May increase levels of diclofenac and warfarin. Glyburide, phenytoin, cimetidine, ranitidine, omeprazole, diclofenac, warfarin, and digoxin may increase levels. Cholestyramine, rifampicin, and propranolol may decrease levels. (Tab, XL) Clopidogrel may alter levels.

PREGNANCY: Category X, not for use in nursing.

MECHANISM OF ACTION: HMG-CoA reductase inhibitor; inhibits conversion of HMG-CoA to mevalonate (precursor of sterols, including cholesterol). Inhibition of cholesterol biosynthesis reduces cholesterol in hepatic cells, which stimulates the synthesis of LDL receptors, thereby increasing uptake of LDL particles, resulting in reduction of plasma cholesterol concentration.

PHARMACOKINETICS: Absorption: Absolute bioavailability (24%); T_{max}=<1 hr. Tab: Relative bioavailability (relative to cap) (29%); T_{max}=3 hrs (fasting), 2.5 hrs (low-fat meal), 6 hrs (high-fat meal). **Distribution:** V_d=0.35L/kg, plasma protein binding (98%). **Metabolism:** Liver via CYP2C9, 2C8 and 3A4 through hydroxylation, N-dealkylation, and β-oxidation pathways. **Elimination:** Feces (90% metabolites, <2% unchanged), urine (5%); $T_{1/2}$=3 hrs.

NURSING CONSIDERATIONS

Assessment: Assess for active liver disease or unexplained, persistent elevations in serum transaminase, pregnancy/nursing status, predisposing factors for myopathy, heavy alcohol intake, history of liver disease, and possible drug interactions. Obtain baseline lipid profile (total-C, LDL, HDL, TG) and LFTs.

Monitoring: Monitor for signs/symptoms of myopathy (unexplained muscle pain, tenderness, weakness), rhabdomyolysis, liver/renal/endocrine dysfunction, CNS toxicity, and other adverse reactions. Perform periodic monitoring of lipid profile.

Patient Counseling: Inform of the substances that should not be taken concomitantly with the drug. Counsel to inform other healthcare professionals that they are taking the drug. Instruct to report promptly unexplained muscle pain, tenderness, or weakness, fatigue, anorexia, right upper abdominal discomfort, dark urine, or jaundice. Inform women of childbearing age to use an effective method of birth control, stop taking drug if they become pregnant, and not to breastfeed while on therapy.

Administration: Oral route. **Storage:** 25°C (77°F); excursions permitted to 15-30°C (15-86°F). Dispense in a tight container. Protect from light.

LETAIRIS   RX
ambrisentan (Gilead)

> Contraindicated in pregnancy; may cause serious birth defects. Exclude pregnancy before treatment and prevent during treatment and for 1 month after stopping treatment by using 2 acceptable methods of contraception, unless the patient has had tubal sterilization or chooses to use Copper T 380A IUD or LNg 20 IUS, in which case no additional contraception is needed. Obtain monthly pregnancy tests. Available only through a restricted program under a Risk Evaluation and Mitigation Strategy called the Letairis Education and Access Program (LEAP); prescribers, patients, and pharmacies must enroll in the program.

THERAPEUTIC CLASS: Endothelin receptor antagonist

INDICATIONS: Treatment of pulmonary arterial HTN (WHO Group 1) to improve exercise ability and delay clinical worsening.

DOSAGE: *Adults:* Initial: 5mg qd. Titrate: May increase to 10mg qd if 5mg is tolerated. Max: 10mg qd.

HOW SUPPLIED: Tab: 5mg, 10mg

CONTRAINDICATIONS: Women who are or may become pregnant.

WARNINGS/PRECAUTIONS: May cause peripheral edema; reported with greater frequency and severity in elderly patients. If clinically significant fluid retention develops, evaluate further to determine cause and possible need for treatment or d/c of therapy. If acute pulmonary edema occurs during initiation, consider the possibility of pulmonary veno-occlusive disease; d/c if confirmed. May decrease sperm count. Decreases in Hgb and Hct, that may result in anemia requiring transfusion, reported; measure Hgb prior to initiation, at 1 month, and periodically thereafter. Not recommended with clinically significant anemia. Consider d/c if clinically significant Hgb decrease is observed and other causes have been excluded. Not recommended with moderate/severe hepatic impairment. Investigate for the cause of liver injury if hepatic impairment develops; d/c with aminotransferase elevations >5X ULN or if elevations are accompanied by bilirubin >2X ULN, or by signs/symptoms of liver dysfunction, and other causes are excluded.

ADVERSE REACTIONS: Peripheral edema, nasal congestion, flushing, sinusitis.

INTERACTIONS: Cyclosporine may increase exposure; limit dose to 5mg qd when coadministered with cyclosporine. Rifampin may increase area under the curve; no dose adjustment required.

PREGNANCY: Category X, not for use in nursing.

MECHANISM OF ACTION: Endothelin receptor antagonist; selective for endothelin type-A receptor, blocks the vasoconstriction and cell proliferation effects of endothelin-1 in vascular smooth muscle and endothelium.

PHARMACOKINETICS: Absorption: T_{max}=2 hrs. **Distribution:** Plasma protein binding (99%). **Metabolism:** Liver via CYP3A, 2C19, and UGTs 1A9S, 2B7S, and 1A3S. **Elimination:** $T_{1/2}$=15 hrs.

NURSING CONSIDERATIONS

Assessment: Assess for anemia, hepatic impairment, pregnancy/nursing status, and possible drug interactions. Obtain baseline Hgb levels.

Monitoring: Monitor for fluid retention, pulmonary edema, pulmonary veno-occlusive disease, hepatic impairment, and for improvements in WHO class symptoms and exercise ability. Obtain monthly pregnancy tests. Measure Hgb at 1 month and periodically thereafter.

Patient Counseling: Advise that drug is available only through a restricted program called LEAP and from Certified Specialty Pharmacies enrolled in LEAP. Instruct to read Medication Guide each time the medication is received. Advise to complete a patient enrollment form. Inform that drug may cause serious birth defects if used by pregnant women. Educate and counsel women of childbearing potential to use highly reliable contraception during and for 1 month after stopping treatment. If IUD or tubal sterilization is used, inform that additional contraception is not needed. Instruct to contact physician if pregnancy is suspected. Instruct to report to physician if symptoms of liver injury (eg, anorexia, N/V, fever, malaise, fatigue, right upper quadrant abdominal discomfort, jaundice, dark urine, itching) occur. Advise of the importance of Hgb testing. Inform of other risks associated with therapy (eg, decreases in Hgb, Hct, and sperm count, fluid overload).

Administration: Oral route. Do not split, crush, or chew tabs. May be taken with or without food.

Storage: 25°C (77°F); excursions permitted to 15-30°C (59-86°F). Store in original packaging.

LEUKERAN   RX
chlorambucil (GlaxoSmithKline)

> Can severely suppress bone marrow function. Potentially carcinogenic, mutagenic, and teratogenic. Produces infertility.

THERAPEUTIC CLASS: Nitrogen mustard alkylating agent

INDICATIONS: Treatment of chronic lymphatic (lymphocytic) leukemia, malignant lymphomas including lymphosarcoma, giant follicular lymphoma, and Hodgkin's disease.

DOSAGE: *Adults:* Usual: 0.1-0.2mg/kg/day for 3-6 weeks as required. Adjust according to response; reduce with abrupt fall in WBC count. Hodgkin's Disease: Usual: 0.2mg/kg/day. Other Lymphomas/Chronic Lymphocytic Leukemia: Usual: 0.1mg/kg/day. Lymphocytic Infiltration of Bone Marrow/Hypoplastic Bone Marrow: Max: 0.1mg/kg/day. Maint: 2-4mg/day or less, depending on the status of blood counts. Hepatic Impairment: Reduce dose. Elderly: Start at the lower end of dosing range.

HOW SUPPLIED: Tab: 2mg

CONTRAINDICATIONS: Prior resistance to therapy.

WARNINGS/PRECAUTIONS: Should not be given for conditions other than chronic lymphatic leukemia or malignant lymphomas. Convulsions, leukemia and secondary malignancies observed. Acute leukemia reported; risk increases with chronic treatment and large cumulative doses. Weigh benefit on an individual basis against possible risk of induction of secondary malignancy. Causes chromatid or chromosome damage and sterility. Rare instances of skin rash progressing to erythema multiforme, toxic epidermal necrolysis, or Stevens-Johnson syndrome reported; d/c if skin reactions develop. May cause fetal harm; women of child bearing potential should avoid becoming pregnant. Slowly progressive lymphopenia reported; lymphocyte count usually returns to normal upon completion of therapy. Caution with history of seizures, head trauma, or who are receiving other potentially epileptogenic drugs, hepatic impairment, and in elderly. Avoid live vaccines in the immunocompromised.

ADVERSE REACTIONS: Bone marrow suppression, anemia, leukopenia, neutropenia, thrombocytopenia, pancytopenia, infertility.

INTERACTIONS: Caution within 4 weeks of full course of radiation or chemotherapy because of the vulnerability of the bone marrow to damage; do not give at full dosages.

PREGNANCY: Category D, not for use in nursing.

MECHANISM OF ACTION: Nitrogen mustard alkylating agent; interferes with DNA replication and induces cellular apoptosis via the accumulation of cytosolic p53 and subsequent activation of Bax, an apoptosis promoter.

PHARMACOKINETICS: Absorption: Rapid and complete. (0.6-1.2 mg/kg) T_{max}=1 hr; (0.2mg/kg) C_{max}=492ng/mL, T_{max}=0.83 hrs, AUC=883ng•hr/mL; (Phenylacetic acid mustard [PAAM]) C_{max}=306ng/mL, T_{max}=1.9 hrs; AUC=1204ng•hr/mL. **Distribution:** V_d=0.31L/kg, plasma protein binding (99%). **Metabolism:** Liver (extensive); oxidative degradation to monohydroxy/dihydroxy derivatives; PAAM (major metabolite). **Elimination:** Urine (20-60%, <1% chlorambucil or PAAM); $T_{1/2}$=1.5 hrs (0.6-1.2mg/kg dose), 1.3 hrs (0.2mg/kg dose), 1.8 hrs (PAAM).

NURSING CONSIDERATIONS

Assessment: Assess for prior resistance, history of seizures or head trauma, hepatic impairment, pregnancy/nursing status and possible drug interactions. Obtain baseline Hgb, WBC, and platelet count.

Monitoring: Monitor for signs/symptoms of bone marrow suppression, cross-hypersensitivity reactions, secondary malignancies, convulsions, infertility, leukemia, and skin reactions. Monitor Hgb levels, total and differential leukocyte counts, and quantitative platelet counts weekly. During 1st 3-6 weeks of therapy, blood counts should be made 3 or 4 days after each weekly CBC. Monitor for toxicity in patients with hepatic impairment.

Patient Counseling: Advise to avoid vaccinations with live vaccines. Inform that major toxicities are related to hypersensitivity, drug fever, myelosuppression, hepatotoxicity, infertility, seizures, GI toxicity, and secondary malignancies. Instruct not to take without medical supervision. Advise to consult a physician if skin rash, bleeding, fever, jaundice, persistent cough, seizures, N/V, amenorrhea, or unusual lumps/masses occur. Advise women of childbearing potential to avoid becoming pregnant.

Administration: Oral route. **Storage:** 2-8°C (36-46°F).

LEVAQUIN RX
levofloxacin (Janssen)

> Fluoroquinolones are associated with an increased risk of tendinitis and tendon rupture in all ages. Risk is further increased with patients >60 yrs, patients taking corticosteroids, and with kidney, heart, or lung transplants. May exacerbate muscle weakness with myasthenia gravis; avoid in patients with known history of myasthenia gravis.

THERAPEUTIC CLASS: Fluoroquinolone

INDICATIONS: Treatment of uncomplicated and complicated skin and skin structure infections (SSSI), uncomplicated and complicated urinary tract infections (UTI), acute bacterial sinusitis, acute bacterial exacerbation of chronic bronchitis (ABECB), community-acquired pneumonia (CAP), nosocomial pneumonia, chronic bacterial prostatitis, and acute pyelonephritis (AP), including cases with concurrent bacteremia caused by susceptible strains of microorganisms in adults ≥18 yrs. To reduce the incidence or progression of disease following anthrax exposure in adults and pediatrics.

DOSAGE: *Adults:* ≥18 yrs: PO/IV: CAP: 750mg qd for 5 days or 500mg qd for 7-14 days. Acute Bacterial Sinusitis: 750mg qd for 5 days or 500mg qd for 10-14 days. ABECB: 500mg qd for 7 days. Complicated SSSI/Nosocomial Pneumonia: 750mg qd for 7-14 days. Uncomplicated SSSI: 500mg qd for 7-10 days. Chronic Bacterial Prostatitis: 500mg qd for 28 days. Complicated UTI/AP: 750mg qd for 5 days or 250mg qd for 10 days. Uncomplicated UTI: 250mg qd for 3 days. Inhalational Anthrax: 500mg qd for 60 days. Refer to PI for dose adjustment with renal impairment (CrCl <50mL/min). IV: Infuse over 60 min q24h (250-500mg) or over 90 min q24h (750mg).
Pediatrics: ≥6 months: PO/IV: Inhalational Anthrax: >50kg: 500mg q24h for 60 days. <50kg: 8mg/kg q12h for 60 days. Max: 250mg/dose. IV: Infuse over 60 min q24h (250-500mg).

HOW SUPPLIED: Inj: 25mg/mL [vial], 5mg/mL in 5% Dextrose [pre-mixed]; Sol: 25mg/mL; Tab: 250mg, 500mg, 750mg

WARNINGS/PRECAUTIONS: D/C if experience pain, swelling, inflammation, or rupture of a tendon. Serious and sometimes fatal hypersensitivity reactions reported; d/c if skin rash, jaundice, or any other sign of hypersensitivity appears and institute appropriate therapy. Severe hepatotoxicity including acute hepatitis and fatal events reported; d/c if signs and symptoms of hepatitis occur. Convulsions, toxic psychoses, and increased intracranial pressure (including pseudotumor cerebri) reported. CNS stimulation may occur; d/c and institute appropriate measures if CNS events occur. Caution with CNS disorders (eg, severe cerebral arteriosclerosis, epilepsy) or risk factors that may predispose to seizures or lower seizure threshold. *Clostridium difficile*-associated diarrhea (CDAD) reported. Rare cases of sensory or sensorimotor axonal polyneuropathy resulting in paresthesias, hypoesthesias, dysesthesias and weakness reported; d/c if symptoms of neuropathy occur. May prolong QT interval; avoid with known QT interval prolongation or uncorrected hypokalemia. Increased incidence of musculoskeletal disorders in pediatric patients. Blood glucose disturbances reported in diabetics; d/c if hypoglycemic reactions occur. May cause photosensitivity/phototoxicity reactions; d/c if photosensitivity/phototoxicity occurs. Avoid excessive exposure to sun/UV light. Increased risk of development of drug-resistant bacteria if used in the absence of a strongly suspected bacterial infection. Crystalluria and cylindruria reported; maintain adequate hydration. Caution in elderly and in patients with renal impairment.

ADVERSE REACTIONS: Tendinitis, tendon rupture, nausea, diarrhea, constipation, headache, insomnia, dizziness.

INTERACTIONS: See Boxed Warning. Caution with drugs that may lower the seizure threshold. Avoid with class IA (eg, quinidine, procainamide) and class III (eg, amiodarone, sotalol) antiarrhythmics. NSAIDs may increase risk of CNS stimulation and convulsive seizures. May enhance effects of warfarin; monitor PT and INR. May increase theophylline levels and increase risk of theophylline-related adverse reactions; monitor theophylline levels closely. Disturbances of blood glucose in diabetic patients receiving a concomitant antidiabetic agent reported; monitor glucose levels. Reduced renal clearance with either cimetidine or probenecid. (PO) Antacids containing magnesium, aluminum, as well as sucralfate, metal cations such as iron, and multivitamins preparations with zinc, or didanosine may substantially interfere with the gastrointestinal absorption and lower systemic concentrations; take at least two hours before or two hours after PO levofloxacin.

PREGNANCY: Category C, not for use in nursing.

MECHANISM OF ACTION: Fluoroquinolone; inhibits bacterial topoisomerase IV and DNA gyrase (both of which are type II topoisomerases), which are enzymes required for DNA replication, transcription, repair, and recombination.

PHARMACOKINETICS: Absorption: (PO) Rapid and complete; (Tab) absolute bioavailability (99%); administration of variable doses resulted in different parameters. **Distribution:** V_d=74-112L;

plasma protein binding (24-38%); found in breast milk. **Metabolism:** Limited. **Elimination:** (PO) Urine (87% unchanged, <5% desmethyl and N-oxide metabolites), feces (<4%); $T_{1/2}$=6-8 hrs.

NURSING CONSIDERATIONS

Assessment: Assess for risk factors for developing tendinitis and tendon rupture, history of myasthenia gravis, drug hypersensitivity, CNS disorders or risk factors that may predispose to seizures or lower seizure threshold, QT interval prolongation, uncorrected hypokalemia, renal/hepatic function, pregnancy/nursing status, and possible drug interactions.

Monitoring: Monitor for ECG changes (eg, QT interval prolongation), anaphylactic reactions, hepatotoxicity, arrhythmias, CNS events, CDAD, peripheral neuropathy, musculoskeletal disorders (pediatrics), tendon rupture, tendinitis, and for photosensitivity/phototoxicity reactions. Monitor hydration status, blood glucose levels, and renal function. Monitor for muscle weakness in patients with myasthenia gravis. Monitor for evidence of bleeding if currently taking warfarin.

Patient Counseling: Inform that drug treats only bacterial, not viral, infections. Advise to take as prescribed; inform that skipping doses or not completing the full course of therapy may decrease effectiveness and increase drug resistance. Advise to take oral sol 1 hr before or 2 hrs after eating, to take tab without regard to meals, to take medication at same time each day, to drink fluids liberally, and that antacids, metal cations, and multivitamins should be taken at least 2 hrs before or 2 hrs after PO administration. Notify physician if symptoms of pain, swelling, or inflammation of a tendon, or weakness or inability to move joints develop. Notify physician of any history of convulsions, QT prolongation, or myasthenia gravis. D/C use and notify physician if allergic reaction, skin rash, signs/symptoms of liver injury or peripheral neuropathy occur. Caution in activities requiring mental alertness and coordination. Instruct to contact physician immediately if watery and bloody diarrhea (with or without stomach cramps and fever) develop. Inform physician if child has tendon or joint-related problems prior to, during, or after therapy. Advise to minimize or avoid exposure to natural or artificial sunlight. Instruct diabetic patients being treated with antidiabetic agents to d/c therapy and notify physician if hypoglycemia occurs. Inform physician if taking warfarin.

Administration: IV, Oral route. (PO) Administer antacids containing magnesium or aluminum, sucralfate, metal cations such as iron, multivitamin preparations with zinc, or didanosine chewable/buffered tab or pediatric powder for oral sol at least 2 hrs before or 2 hrs after PO levofloxacin administration. (Sol) Administer 1 hr before or 2 hrs after eating. (Inj) Refer to PI for more information on administration, preparation, stability, compatibility, and thawing instructions. **Storage:** (Tab) 15-30°C (59-86°F). (Sol) 25°C (77°F); excursions permitted to 15-30°C (59-86°F). (Inj) Single-use Vials: Controlled room temperature and protected from light. Diluted in Plastic IV Container (5mg/mL): Stable at ≤25°C (77°F) for 72 hrs; 5°C (41°F) for 14 days; -20°C (-4°F) for 6 months. Premixed Sol: ≤25°C (77°F); brief exposure ≤40°C (104°F). Avoid excessive heat and protect from freezing and light.

LEVBID   RX
hyoscyamine sulfate (Alaven)

THERAPEUTIC CLASS: Anticholinergic

INDICATIONS: Adjunct treatment of peptic ulcer, irritable bowel syndrome, neurogenic bladder, and neurogenic bowel disturbances. Management of functional intestinal disorders (eg, mild dysenteries, diverculitis, acute enterocolitis). To control gastric secretion, visceral spasm, and hypermotility in spastic colitis, spastic bladder, cystitis, pylorospasm, and associated abdominal cramps. Drying agent for symptomatic relief of acute rhinitis. Symptomatic relief of biliary and renal colic with concomitant morphine or other narcotics. To reduce rigidity and tremors and to control associated sialorrhea and hyperhidrosis in parkinsonism. Antidote for anticholinesterase poisoning.

DOSAGE: *Adults:* 1-2 tabs q12h. Max: 4 tabs/24 hrs. Elderly: Start at low end of dosing range. *Pediatrics:* ≥12 yrs: 1-2 tabs q12h. Max: 4 tabs/24 hrs.

HOW SUPPLIED: Tab, Extended-Release: 0.375mg

CONTRAINDICATIONS: Glaucoma; obstructive uropathy; obstructive GI tract disease; paralytic ileus, intestinal atony of elderly/debilitated; unstable cardiovascular (CV) status in acute hemorrhage; severe ulcerative colitis; toxic megacolon complicating ulcerative colitis, myasthenia gravis.

WARNINGS/PRECAUTIONS: Risk of heat prostration with high environmental temperature. May impair physical/mental abilities. Caution with diarrhea, autonomic neuropathy, hyperthyroidism, coronary heart disease, congestive heart failure, cardiac arrhythmias, HTN, renal disease, and hiatal hernia associated with reflux esophagitis. Psychosis reported in sensitive patients.

ADVERSE REACTIONS: Anticholinergic effects, drowsiness, headache, nervousness, N/V, diarrhea.

INTERACTIONS: May have additive effects with other antimuscarinics, amantadine, haloperidol, phenothiazines, MAOIs, TCAs, and some antihistamines. Antacids may interfere with absorption.

PREGNANCY: Category C, caution in nursing.

MECHANISM OF ACTION: Belladonna alkaloid; inhibits action of acetylcholine on structures innervated by postganglionic cholinergic nerves and on smooth muscles that respond to acetylcholine but lack cholinergic innervation, inhibiting GI propulsive motility, decreasing gastric acid secretion, and controlling excess pharyngeal, tracheal, and bronchial secretions.

PHARMACOKINETICS: Absorption: Complete; T_{max}=4.2 hrs. **Distribution:** Crosses placenta and blood-brain barrier; found in breast milk. **Metabolism:** Partial hydrolysis; tropic acid, tropine (metabolites). **Elimination:** Urine (unchanged); $T_{1/2}$=7.47 hrs.

NURSING CONSIDERATIONS

Assessment: Assess for glaucoma, obstructive uropathy, GI obstruction, paralytic ileus, intestinal atony, unstable CV status in acute hemorrhage, other conditions where treatment is contraindicated/cautioned, pregnancy/nursing status, and possible drug interactions.

Monitoring: Monitor for signs/symptoms of heat prostration, incomplete intestinal obstruction, blurred vision, psychosis, CNS events, diarrhea, and other adverse reactions. Monitor renal function.

Patient Counseling: Advise against engaging in activities requiring mental alertness (eg, operating a motor vehicle or other machinery) or performing hazardous work while on treatment. Inform that heat prostration may occur with drug use (fever and heat stroke due to decreased sweating); use caution if febrile, or exposed to high environmental temperatures.

Administration: Oral route. Do not crush or chew. **Storage:** 20-25°C (68-77°F); excursions permitted to 15-30°C (59-86°F). Dispense in tight, light-resistant container with child-resistant closure.

LEVEMIR   RX
insulin detemir, rdna origin (Novo Nordisk)

THERAPEUTIC CLASS: Insulin

INDICATIONS: To improve glycemic control in adults and children with diabetes mellitus (DM).

DOSAGE: *Adults:* Individualize dose. Administer SQ qd (with pm meal or at hs) or bid (give pm dose with pm meal, at hs, or 12 hrs after am dose). Initial: Type 2 DM Not Currently Treated With Insulin: 10 U (or 0.1-0.2 U/kg). Type 1 DM: 1/3 of total daily insulin requirement. Use rapid or short-acting pre-meal insulin to satisfy remaining daily insulin requirement. Titrate: Adjust based on blood glucose measurements. Conversion From Insulin Glargine/NPH Insulin: Switch on a unit-to-unit basis. More units may be required in some type 2 DM on NPH insulin. Hepatic/Renal Impairment: May need to adjust dose.
Pediatrics: ≥6 yrs: Individualize dose. Administer SQ qd (with pm meal or at hs) or bid (give pm dose with pm meal, at hs, or 12 hrs after am dose). Initial: Type 1 DM: 1/3 of total daily insulin requirement. Use rapid or short acting pre-meal insulin to satisfy remaining daily insulin requirement. Titrate: Adjust based on blood glucose measurements. Conversion From Insulin Glargine/NPH Insulin: Switch on a unit-to-unit basis. Hepatic/Renal Impairment: May need to adjust dose.

HOW SUPPLIED: Inj: 100 U/mL [10mL, vial]; [3mL, Flexpen]

WARNINGS/PRECAUTIONS: Not for the treatment of diabetic ketoacidosis. Not for use in insulin infusion pump. Any change of insulin dose should be made cautiously and under medical supervision. Changes in strength, manufacturer, type or method of administration may result in the need for a change in dosage. Not for IV or IM use. Do not dilute or mix with any other insulin or sol. Hypoglycemia may occur; caution in patients with hypoglycemia unawareness and patients predisposed to hypoglycemia (eg, pediatrics, patients who fast or have erratic food intake). Hypoglycemia may impair ability to concentrate and react. Severe, life-threatening, generalized allergy, including anaphylaxis, may occur. Careful glucose monitoring and dose adjustments with renal/hepatic impairment. Lipodystrophy may occur; rotate inj sites within the same region. Caution in elderly.

ADVERSE REACTIONS: Hypoglycemia, upper respiratory tract infection, headache, pharyngitis, influenza-like illness, abdominal pain, back pain, gastroenteritis, bronchitis, pyrexia, cough, viral infection, N/V, rhinitis.

INTERACTIONS: May require dose adjustment and close monitoring with drugs that may increase blood glucose-lowering effect and susceptibility to hypoglycemia (eg, oral antidiabetic drugs, pramlintide acetate, ACE inhibitors, disopyramide, fibrates, fluoxetine, MAOIs, propoxyphene, pentoxifylline, salicylates, somatostatin analogs, and sulfonamide antibiotics), drugs that may reduce blood-glucose-lowering effects (eg, corticosteroids, niacin, danazol, diuretics, sympathomimetic agents [eg, epinephrine, albuterol, terbutaline], glucagon, isoniazid, phenothiazine derivatives, somatropin, thyroid hormones, estrogens, progestogens [eg, in oral contraceptives), protease inhibitors, and atypical antipsychotic medications [eg, olanzapine and clozapine], or drugs that may either increase or decrease blood-glucose-lowering effects (eg, β-blockers, clonidine, lithium salts, and alcohol). Pentamidine may cause hypoglycemia, sometimes followed by hyperglycemia. Hypoglycemic signs may be reduced or absent with anti-adrenergic drugs (eg, β-blockers, clonidine, guanethidine, and reserpine).

PREGNANCY: Category B, caution in nursing.

MECHANISM OF ACTION: Insulin detemir (rDNA origin); regulates glucose metabolism and lowers blood glucose by facilitating cellular uptake of glucose into skeletal muscle and adipose tissue and by inhibiting the output of glucose from the liver. Inhibits lipolysis in the adipocyte, inhibits proteolysis, and enhances protein synthesis.

PHARMACOKINETICS: Absorption: Absolute bioavailability (60%); T_{max}=6-8 hrs. **Distribution:** Plasma protein binding (>98%); V_d=0.1L/kg. Crosses placenta. **Elimination:** $T_{1/2}$=5-7 hrs.

NURSING CONSIDERATIONS

Assessment: Assess predisposition to hypoglycemia, hypersensitivity, renal/hepatic function pregnancy/nursing status, and possible drug interactions.

Monitoring: Monitor for signs/symptoms of hypoglycemia, lipodystrophy, allergic reactions, inj-site reactions, and other adverse effects. Monitor FPG, HbA1c, and renal/hepatic function.

Patient Counseling: Inform about potential risks and benefits of taking insulin, including possible side effects. Instruct on self-management procedures including glucose monitoring, proper inj technique, and management of hypoglycemia and hyperglycemia. Advise to use caution when driving or operating machinery. Instruct to always check label before inj to avoid medication errors such as accidental mix-ups. Instruct on handling of special situations such as intercurrent conditions, inadequate or skipped insulin dose, inadvertent administration of an increased insulin dose, inadequate food intake, or skipped meals. Advise to use only if sol is clear and colorless with no visible particles. Notify physician if pregnant/plan to become pregnant.

Administration: SQ route. Inject in thigh, abdominal wall, or upper arm. Rotate inj sites. Refer to PI for instructions on preparation, handling and administration. **Storage:** 2-8°C (36-46°F) until expiration date or <30°C (86°F) for up to 42 days if refrigeration not possible. Keep in carton until time of use. Discard opened vial after 42 days after initial use. FlexPen After Initial Use: <30°C (86°F) for up to 42 days; do not refrigerate or store with needle in place. Do not freeze or use if frozen. Keep from direct heat and light.

LEVITRA   RX
vardenafil HCl (Merck)

THERAPEUTIC CLASS: Phosphodiesterase type 5 inhibitor

INDICATIONS: Treatment of erectile dysfunction (ED).

DOSAGE: *Adults:* Initial: 10mg 1 hr prior to sexual activity. Titrate: May decrease to 5mg or increase to max of 20mg based on response. Max: 1 tab/day. Elderly: ≥65 yrs: Initial: 5mg. Moderate Hepatic Impairment (Child-Pugh B): Initial: 5mg. Max: 10mg. Concomitant Ritonavir: Max: 2.5mg/72 hrs. Concomitant Indinavir/Saquinavir/Atazanavir/Clarithromycin/Ketoconazole 400mg daily/Itraconazole 400mg daily: Max: 2.5mg/24 hrs. Concomitant Ketoconazole 200mg daily/Itraconazole 200mg daily/Erythromycin: Max: 5mg/24 hrs. Concomitant Stable α-blocker: Initial: 5mg; 2.5mg when used with certain CYP3A4 inhibitors.

HOW SUPPLIED: Tab: 2.5mg, 5mg, 10mg, 20mg

CONTRAINDICATIONS: Concomitant nitrates or nitric oxide donors.

WARNINGS/PRECAUTIONS: Avoid when sexual activity is inadvisable due to underlying cardiovascular (CV) status. Increased sensitivity to vasodilation effects with left ventricular outflow obstruction. Decrease in supine BP reported. Avoid with unstable angina, hypotension (resting SBP <90 mmHg), uncontrolled HTN (>170/110 mmHg), recent history of stroke, life-threatening arrhythmia, myocardial infarction (MI) within last 6 months, severe cardiac failure, severe hepatic impairment (Child-Pugh C), end-stage renal disease (ESRD) requiring dialysis, hereditary degenerative retinal disorders including retinitis pigmentosa, congenital QT prolongation. Rare reports of prolonged erections >4 hrs and priapism. Caution with bleeding disorders, peptic ulcers, anatomical deformation of the penis or predisposition to priapism. Rare reports of non-arteritic anterior ischemic optic neuropathy (NAION) with phosphodiesterase type 5 (PDE5) inhibitors. Sudden decrease or loss of hearing accompanied by tinnitus and dizziness reported.

ADVERSE REACTIONS: Headache, flushing, rhinitis, dyspepsia, sinusitis, flu syndrome, dizziness, nausea.

INTERACTIONS: See Contraindications. Avoid use with Class IA (eg, quinidine, procainamide) or Class III (eg, amiodarone, sotalol) antiarrhythmics and other agents for ED. Caution with medications known to prolong QT interval. Increased levels with CYP3A4 inhibitors (eg, ritonavir, indinavir, saquinavir, atazanavir, ketoconazole, itraconazole, clarithromycin, erythromycin). Additive hypotensive effect, which may lead to symptomatic hypotension when used with α-blockers. Reduced clearance with CYP3A4/5 and CYP2C9 inhibitors.

PREGNANCY: Category B, not for use in nursing.

MECHANISM OF ACTION: PDE5 inhibitor; increases the amount of cGMP, which causes smooth muscle relaxation, allowing increased blood flow into the penis, resulting in erection.

PHARMACOKINETICS: Absorption: Rapid, absolute bioavailability (15%); T_{max}=30 min-2 hrs. **Distribution:** V_d=208L; plasma protein binding (95%). **Metabolism:** Via CYP3A4, CYP3A5, CYP2C. M1 (major metabolite). **Elimination:** Feces (91-95%), urine (2-6%); $T_{1/2}$=4-5 hrs.

NURSING CONSIDERATIONS

Assessment: Assess for CV disease, left ventricular outflow obstruction (eg, aortic stenosis, idiopathic hypertrophic subaortic stenosis), congenital QT prolongation, retinitis pigmentosa, bleeding disorders, active peptic ulceration, anatomical deformation of the penis or conditions that predispose to priapism (eg, sickle cell anemia, multiple myeloma, leukemia), and renal/hepatic impairment. Assess potential underlying causes of ED and for possible drug interactions.

Monitoring: Monitor potential for cardiac risk due to sexual activity, hypotension, color vision changes or other eye adverse events (eg, NAION), hypersensitivity reactions, and hearing impairment. Monitor for adverse events when used in combination with other drugs.

Patient Counseling: Discuss risks and benefits of therapy. Seek medical assistance if erection persists >4 hrs. Inform that postural hypotension may occur. Advise of potential BP-lowering effect of nitrates, α-blockers and antihypertensive medications, and cardiac risk of sexual activity. Counsel about protective measures necessary to guard against STDs, including HIV; drug does not protect against STDs. D/C and inform doctor if sudden loss of vision or hearing occur. Counsel to take as prescribed.

Administration: Oral route. **Storage:** 25°C (77°F); excursions permitted to 15-30°C (59-86°F).

LEVOPHED   RX
norepinephrine bitartrate (Hospira)

> To prevent sloughing and necrosis in area of extravasation, area should be infiltrated with 10-15mL saline sol containing 5-10mg of Regitine (brand of phentolamine), an adrenergic blocking agent. Sympathetic blockade with phentolamine causes immediate and conspicuous local hyperemic changes if infiltrated within 12 hrs. Give phentolamine as soon as possible after the extravasation is noted.

THERAPEUTIC CLASS: Alpha-adrenergic agonist

INDICATIONS: For BP control in certain acute hypotensive states (eg, pheochromocytomectomy, sympathectomy, poliomyelitis, spinal anesthesia, myocardial infarction, septicemia, blood transfusion, and drug reactions). As an adjunct in the treatment of cardiac arrest and profound hypotension.

DOSAGE: *Adults:* Average Dosage: Initial: 8-12mcg/min (2-3mL) as IV infusion until low normal BP (80-100mmHg systolic) is established and maintained by adjusting rate of flow. Maint: 2-4mcg/min (0.5-1mL). High Dosage: Individualize dose (as high as 68mg/day). Elderly: Start at lower end of dosing range.

HOW SUPPLIED: Inj: 4mg/4mL

CONTRAINDICATIONS: Hypotension from blood volume deficits except as an emergency measure to maintain coronary and cerebral artery perfusion until blood volume replacement therapy can be completed, mesenteric or peripheral vascular thrombosis (unless administration is necessary as a life-saving procedure in the opinion of the attending physician), profound hypoxia or hypercarbia, concomitant use of cyclopropane and halothane anesthetics.

WARNINGS/PRECAUTIONS: Contains sodium metabisulfite; may cause allergic-type reactions (eg, anaphylactic symptoms, life-threatening or less severe asthmatic episodes). May produce dangerously high BP with overdoses due to potency and varying response; monitor BP q2 min from initial administration until desired BP is obtained, then q5 min if administration is to be continued. Headache may be a symptom of HTN due to overdosage; monitor rate of flow constantly. Infusions should be given into a large vein, particularly an antecubital vein whenever possible. Avoid a catheter tie-in technique if possible. Occlusive vascular diseases (eg, atherosclerosis, arteriosclerosis, diabetic endarteritis, Buerger's disease) more likely to occur in the lower than in the upper extremity; avoid leg veins in elderly or in those suffering from such disorders. Gangrene in lower extremity reported when given in an ankle vein. Check infusion site frequently for free flow. Avoid extravasation into the tissues; local necrosis might ensue. Blanching may occur; consider changing the infusion site at intervals to allow effects of local vasoconstriction to subside. Caution in elderly.

ADVERSE REACTIONS: Ischemic injury, bradycardia, arrhythmias, anxiety, headache, respiratory difficulty, extravasation necrosis at inj site.

INTERACTIONS: See Contraindications. Caution with MAOI or triptyline/imipramine antidepressants; severe, prolonged HTN may result.

PREGNANCY: Category C, caution in nursing.

MECHANISM OF ACTION: Alpha-adrenergic agonist; peripheral vasoconstrictor (α-adrenergic action) and inotropic stimulator of the heart and dilator of coronary arteries (β-adrenergic action).

NURSING CONSIDERATIONS

Assessment: Assess hypotension and need for blood volume replacement. Assess use as emergency measure or life-saving procedure (eg, hypotension from blood volume deficits to maintain coronary and cerebral artery perfusion until blood volume replacement therapy can be completed, mesenteric or peripheral vascular thrombosis). Assess for profound hypoxia or hypercarbia, sulfite sensitivity, pregnancy/nursing status, and possible drug interactions. Assess use in elderly and occlusive vascular diseases. Obtain baseline BP.

Monitoring: Monitor for HTN, headache, gangrene, extravasation, blanching, and hypersensitivity/allergic reactions. Monitor infusion site, rate of flow, BP, and central venous pressure.

Patient Counseling: Inform of risks/benefits of therapy. Advise to inform physician if headache occurs.

Administration: IV route. Refer to PI for proper dilution and administration. **Storage:** 20-25°C (68-77°F); (vial) excursions permitted to 15-30° (59-86°F). Protect from light.

LEVOTHROID   RX
levothyroxine sodium (Forest)

Do not use for the treatment of obesity or weightloss; doses within range of daily hormonal requirements are ineffective for weight reduction in euthyroid patients. Serious or life-threatening manifestations of toxicity, particularly when given in association with sympathomimetic amines (those used for their anorectic effects).

THERAPEUTIC CLASS: Thyroid replacement hormone

INDICATIONS: Hypothyroidism. As a pituitary TSH suppressant for nonendemic goiter and for chronic lymphocytic thyroiditis. Diagnostic agent in suppression tests to differentiate mild hyperthyroidism or thyroid gland autonomy. Adjunct therapy with antithyroid drugs to treat thyrotoxicosis. Adjunct to surgery and radioiodine therapy for TSH-dependent thyroid cancer.

DOSAGE: *Adults:* Hypothyroidism: Usual: 100-200mcg/day. Endocrine/Cardiovascular Complications: Initial: 50mcg/day. Titrate: Increase by 50mcg/day every 2-4 weeks until euthyroid. Hypothyroid with Angina: Initial: 25mcg/day. Titrate: Increase by 25-50mcg every 2-4 weeks until euthyroid.
Pediatrics: Hypothyroidism: >12 yrs: Usual: 100-200mcg/day. 6-12 yrs: 4-5mcg/kg/day. 1-5 yrs: 5-6mcg/kg/day. 6-12 months: 6-8mcg/kg/day. 0-6 months: 10-15mcg/kg/day. May crush tab and sprinkle over food (applesauce) or mix with 5-10mL water, formula (non-soy), or breast milk.

HOW SUPPLIED: Tab: 25mcg*, 50mcg*, 75mcg*, 88mcg*, 100mcg*, 112mcg*, 125mcg*, 137mcg*, 150mcg*, 175mcg*, 200mcg*, 300mcg* *scored

CONTRAINDICATIONS: Untreated thyrotoxicosis, acute myocardial infarction (MI), and uncorrected adrenal insufficiency.

WARNINGS/PRECAUTIONS: Do not use in the treatment of obesity; larger doses in euthyroid patients can cause serious or even life-threatening toxicity. Caution with cardiovascular (CV) disease, HTN. May aggravate diabetes mellitus (DM) or insipidus and adrenal cortical insufficiency. Excessive doses in infants may produce craniosynostosis. Add glucocorticoid with myxedema coma.

ADVERSE REACTIONS: Lactose hypersensitivity, transient partial hair loss in children.

INTERACTIONS: Monitor insulin and oral hypoglycemic requirements. May potentiate anticoagulant effects of warfarin; adjust warfarin dose and monitor PT/INR. Increased adrenergic effects of catecholamines; caution with CAD. Decreased absorption with cholestyramine and colestipol; space dosing by 4-5 hrs. Estrogens increase thyroxine-binding globulin; increase in thyroid dose may be needed. Large dose may cause life-threatening toxicities with sympathomimetic amines. Avoid mixing crushed tabs with foods/formula with large amounts of iron, soybean or fiber.

PREGNANCY: Category A, caution in nursing.

MECHANISM OF ACTION: Thyroid hormone; not understood, suspected to control DNA transcription and protein synthesis. Regulates multiple metabolic processes.

PHARMACOKINETICS: Distribution: Plasma protein binding (99%). **Metabolism:** Deiodination (major pathway), conjugation (minor pathway) in liver (mainly), kidneys, and other tissues. **Elimination:** Urine; T4 (feces 20% unchanged); $T_{1/2}$=6-7 days; $T_{1/2}$=≤2 days (T3).

NURSING CONSIDERATIONS

Assessment: Assess for drug hypersensitivity, CV disease, angina pectoris, acute MI, suppressed serum TSH level with normal T3 and T4 levels, overt thyrotoxicosis, DM, clotting disorder, adrenal/pituitary gland problems, malabsorption, autoimmune polyglandular syndrome, undergoing surgery, and possible drug and test interactions. Assess infants with congenital hypothyrodism for other congenital anomalies.

Monitoring: Requires frequent lab tests and clinical evaluation of thyroid function by TSH levels, and also glucose/lipid metabolism, urinary glucose in diabetics, and clotting status. Monitor for CV signs such as arrhythmia and coronary insufficiency, growth/development, bone metabolism, cognitive function, emotional state, GI function, reproductive function, partial hair loss in children, and signs/symptoms of thyrotoxicosis.

Patient Counseling: Counsel to take 1 hr before breakfast, and not to to use as part of weight control regimen. Inform that replacement therapy is essential for life, except in cases of transient hypothyroidism. Advise to notify physician if pregnant/nursing or intend to become pregnant or if taking any other drugs. Counsel to not d/c or change dosage. Report signs/symptoms of thyroid toxicity.

Administration: Oral route. **Storage:** 25°C (77°F); excursions permitted to 15-30°C (59-86°F). Protect from light and moisture.

LEVOXYL   RX
levothyroxine sodium (King)

> Do not use for the treatment of obesity or weight loss; doses within range of daily hormonal requirements are ineffective for weight reduction in euthyroid patients. Serious or life-threatening manifestations of toxicity may occur when given in larger doses, particularly when given in association with sympathomimetic amines.

THERAPEUTIC CLASS: Thyroid replacement hormone

INDICATIONS: Replacement or supplemental therapy in congenital or acquired hypothyroidism of any etiology, except transient hypothyroidism during the recovery phase of subacute thyroiditis. Treatment or prevention of various types of euthyroid goiters, including thyroid nodules, subacute or chronic lymphocytic thyroiditis, multinodular goiter, and as an adjunct to surgery and radioiodine therapy for thyrotropin-dependent well-differentiated thyroid cancer.

DOSAGE: *Adults:* Individualize dose. Adjust dose based on periodic assessment of patient's clinical response and laboratory parameters. Take in am at least 30 minutes before food. Take with water. Take at least 4 hrs apart from drugs that are known to interfere with absorption. Hypothyroidism: Usual: 1.7mcg/kg/day. Doses >200mcg/day seldom required. >50 yrs/<50 yrs with Cardiac Disease: Initial: 25-50mcg/day. Titrate: Increase by 12.5-25mcg increments every 6-8 weeks as needed. Elderly with Cardiac Disease: Initial: 12.5-25mcg/day. Titrate: Increase by 12.5-25mcg increments every 4-6 weeks until euthyroid. Severe Hypothyroidism: Initial: 12.5-25mcg/day. Titrate: Increase by 25mcg/day every 2-4 weeks until TSH level normalized. Pregnancy: May increase dose requirements. Subclinical Hypothyroidism: Lower doses may be adequate to normalize the TSH level (eg, 1mcg/kg/day). TSH Suppression in Well-Differentiated Thyroid Cancer and Thyroid Nodules: Individualize dose based on the specific disease and the patient being treated. Refer to PI for further details.
Pediatrics: Individualize dose. Adjust dose based on periodic assessment of patient's clinical response and laboratory parameters. Take in AM at least 30 minutes before food. Take with water. Take at least 4 hrs apart from drugs that are known to interfere with absorption. Hypothyroidism: Growth/Puberty Complete: Usual: 1.7mcg/kg/day. >12 yrs (Growth/Puberty Incomplete): 2-3mcg/kg/day. 6-12 yrs: 4-5mcg/kg/day. 1-5 yrs: 5-6mcg/kg/day. 6-12 months: 6-8mcg/kg/day. 3-6 months: 8-10mcg/kg/day. 0-3 months: 10-15mcg/kg/day. Infants at Risk for Cardiac Failure: Use lower dose (eg, 25mcg/day). Titrate: Increase dose every 4-6 weeks as needed. Infants with Serum T4 <5mcg/dL: Initial: 50mcg/day. Chronic/Severe Hypothyroidism: Children: Initial: 25mcg/day. Titrate: Increase by 25mcg increments every 2-4 weeks until desired effect is achieved. Minimize Hyperactivity in Older Children: Initial: Give 1/4 of full replacement dose. Titrate: Increase on a weekly basis by an amount equal to 1/4 the full recommended replacement dose until the full recommended replacement dose is reached. May crush tab and mix with 5-10mL of water.

HOW SUPPLIED: Tab: 25mcg, 50mcg, 75mcg, 88mcg, 100mcg, 112mcg, 125mcg, 137mcg, 150mcg, 175mcg, 200mcg

CONTRAINDICATIONS: Untreated subclinical (suppressed serum TSH level with normal T3 level and T4 levels) or overt thyrotoxicosis of any etiology, acute myocardial infarction (MI), and uncorrected adrenal insufficiency.

WARNINGS/PRECAUTIONS: Should not be used in the treatment of male or female infertility unless associated with hypothyroidism. Contraindicated in patients with nontoxic diffuse goiter or nodular thyroid disease, particularly in elderly or with underlying cardiovascular (CV) disease if serum TSH level is already suppressed; use with caution if TSH level is not suppressed and carefully monitor thyroid function. Has narrow therapeutic index; carefully titrate dose to avoid over- or under-treatment. May decrease bone mineral density (BMD) with long term use; give minimum dose necessary to achieve desired clinical and biochemical response. Caution with CV disorders and the elderly. If cardiac symptoms develop or worsen, reduce or withhold dose for 1 week and then restart at lower dose. May produce CV effects (eg, increase HR, increase in cardiac wall thickness, increase in cardiac contractility, precipitation of angina or arrhythmias). Monitor patients with coronary artery disease (CAD) closely during surgical procedures; may precipitate cardiac arrhythmias. Caution in patients with diabetes mellitus (DM). Patients with concomitant adrenal insufficiency should be treated with replacement glucocorticoids prior to therapy.

ADVERSE REACTIONS: Fatigue, increased appetite, weight loss, heat intolerance, headache, hyperactivity, irritability, insomnia, palpitations, arrhythmias, dyspnea, hair loss, menstrual irregularities, pseudotumor cerebri (children), slipped capital femoral epiphysis (children).

INTERACTIONS: Concurrent sympathomimetics may increase effects of sympathomimetics or thyroid hormone and may increase risk of coronary insufficiency with CAD. Upward dose adjustments may be needed for insulin and oral hypoglycemic agents. May decrease absorption with soybean flour, cottonseed meal, walnuts, and dietary fiber. May potentiate oral anticoagulant effects; adjust dose and monitor PT. May decrease levels and effects of digitalis glycosides. Reduced TSH secretion with dopamine/dopamine agonists, glucocorticoids, octreotide. Decreased thyroid hormone secretion with aminoglutethimide, amiodarone, iodine (including iodine-containing radiographic contrast agents), lithium, methimazole, propylthiouracil (PTU), sulfonamides, tolbutamide. May increase thyroid hormone secretion with amiodarone and iodide. May decrease T4 absorption with antacids (aluminum & magnesium hydroxides), simethicone, bile acid sequestrants (cholestyramine, colestipol), calcium carbonate, cation exchange resins (kayexalate), ferrous sulfate, orlistat, and sucralfate; administer at least 4 hrs apart. May increase serum thyroxine-binding globulin (TBG) concentrations with clofibrate, estrogen-containing oral contraceptives, oral estrogens, heroin/methadone, 5-fluorouracil, mitotane, and tamoxifen. May decrease serum TBG concentrations with androgens/anabolic steroids, asparaginase, glucocorticoids, and slow-release nicotinic acid. May cause protein-binding site displacement with furosemide (>80mg IV), heparin, hydantoins, NSAIDs (fenamates, phenylbutazone), and salicylates (>2g/day). May alter T4 and T3 metabolism with carbamazepine, hydantoins, phenobarbital, and rifampin. May decrease T4 5'-deiodinase activity with amiodarone, β-adrenergic antagonists (eg, propranolol >160mg/day), glucocorticoids (eg, dexamethasone >4mg/day), and PTU. Concurrent use with tri/tetracyclic antidepressants may increase the therapeutic and toxic effects of both drugs. Coadministration with sertraline in patients stabilized on levothyroxine may result in increased levothyroxine requirements. Interferon-α may cause development of antithyroid microsomal antibodies and may cause transient hypothyroidism, hyperthyroidism, or both. Interleukin-2 has been associated with transient painless thyroiditis. Excessive use with growth hormones (eg, somatropin, somatrem) may accelerate epiphyseal closure. Ketamine may produce marked HTN and tachycardia. May reduce uptake of radiographic agents. Decreased theophylline clearance may occur in hypothyroid patients. Altered levels of thyroid hormone and/or TSH levels with choral hydrate, diazepam, ethionamide, lovastatin, metoclopramide, 6-mercaptopurine, nitroprusside, para-aminosalicylate sodium, perphenazine, resorcinol (excessive topical use), and thiazide diuretics.

PREGNANCY: Category A, caution in nursing.

MECHANISM OF ACTION: Thyroid replacement hormone; mechanism not established. Suspected that principal effects are exerted through control of DNA transcription and protein synthesis.

PHARMACOKINETICS: Absorption: Majority absorbed from jejunum and upper ileum. **Distribution:** Plasma protein binding (>99%); found in breast milk. **Metabolism:** Sequential deiodination and conjugation in liver (mainly), kidneys, and other tissues. **Elimination:** Urine, feces (20% unchanged); $T_{1/2}$=6-7days (T4), ≤2 days (T3).

NURSING CONSIDERATIONS

Assessment: Assess for untreated subclinical or overt thyrotoxicosis, acute MI, uncorrected adrenal insufficiency, age, CAD, CV disorders, nontoxic diffuse goiter, nodular thyroid disease, DM, drug hypersensitivity, pregnancy/nursing status, and for possible drug interactions. In patients with secondary or tertiary hypothyroidism, assess for additional hypothalamic/pituitary hormone deficiencies. Assess for weight, TSH levels. In infants with congenital hypothyroidism, assess for other congenital anomalies.

Monitoring: Monitor for CV effects. In patients on long-term therapy, monitor for signs/symptoms of decreased BMD. In patients with nontoxic diffuse goiter or nodular thyroid disease, monitor for precipitation of thyrotoxicosis. In adults with primary hypothyroidism, perform periodic monitoring of serum TSH levels. In pediatric patients with congenital hypothyroidism, perform periodic monitoring of serum TSH levels and total or free T4 levels. In patients with secondary and tertiary hypothyroidism, perform periodic monitoring of serum free T4 levels.

Patient Counseling: Instruct to notify physician if allergic to any food or medicine, pregnant or plan to become pregnant, breastfeeding or taking any other drugs, including prescriptions and over-the-counter preparations. Notify physician of any other medical conditions, particularly heart disease, diabetes, clotting disorders, and adrenal or pituitary gland problems. Instruct not to stop or change dose unless directed by physician. Take on empty stomach, with a full glass of water, at least 1/2 hr before eating any food. Advise that partial hair loss may occur during the first few months of therapy, but is usually temporary. Notify physician or dentist prior to surgery about levothyroxine therapy. Inform that drug should not be used for weight control. Inform patients that tablets may rapidly swell and disintegrate resulting in choking, gagging, tablet getting stuck in throat or difficulty swallowing. Instruct to notify physician if rapid or irregular heartbeat, chest pain, SOB, leg cramps, headache, or any other unusual medical event.

Administration: Oral route. Take with water. **Storage:** 20-25°C (68-77°F); excursions permitted to 15-30°C (59-86°F). Store away from heat, moisture, and light.

LEXAPRO RX
escitalopram oxalate (Forest)

Antidepressants increased the risk of suicidal thinking and behavior (suicidality) in short-term studies in children, adolescents, and young adults with major depressive disorder (MDD) and other psychiatric disorders. Monitor and observe closely for clinical worsening, suicidality, or unusual changes in behavior in patients who are started on antidepressant therapy. Not approved for use in pediatric patients <12 yrs of age.

THERAPEUTIC CLASS: Selective serotonin reuptake inhibitor

INDICATIONS: Acute and maintenance treatment of MDD in adults and adolescents 12-17 yrs. Acute treatment of generalized anxiety disorder (GAD) in adults.

DOSAGE: *Adults:* MDD: Initial: 10mg qd. Titrate: May increase to 20mg after ≥1 week. GAD: Initial: 10mg qd. Titrate: May increase to 20mg after ≥1 week. Efficacy >8 weeks not studied. Elderly/Hepatic Impairment: 10mg qd. Periodically assess need for maint. Allow ≥14 days interval between d/c of MAOI and initiation of escitalopram, or vice versa.
Pediatrics: 12-17 yrs: MDD: Initial: 10mg qd. Titrate: May increase to 20mg after ≥3 weeks. Periodically assess need for maint. Hepatic Impairment: 10mg qd. Allow ≥14 days interval between d/c of MAOI and initiation of escitalopram, or vice versa.

HOW SUPPLIED: Sol: 5mg/5mL; Tab: 5mg, 10mg*, 20mg* *scored

CONTRAINDICATIONS: Concomitant use of MAOI or pimozide.

WARNINGS/PRECAUTIONS: Serotonin syndrome or neuroleptic malignant syndrome (NMS)-like reactions may occur. Avoid abrupt d/c; gradually decrease dose. Activation of mania/hypomania reported; caution with history of mania. May increase the risk of bleeding events. Hyponatremia may occur; caution in elderly and volume-depleted patients. D/C if symptomatic hyponatremia occurs and institute appropriate intervention. Convulsions reported. Caution with history of seizures, conditions that alter metabolism or hemodynamic responses, severe renal impairment. May impair mental/physical abilities.

ADVERSE REACTIONS: N/V, insomnia, ejaculation disorder, increased sweating, somnolence, fatigue, diarrhea, dry mouth, headache, constipation, indigestion, neck/shoulder pain, anorgasmia.

INTERACTIONS: See Contraindications. Increased risk of serotonin syndrome or NMS-like reactions with serotonergic drugs (including triptans), antipsychotics, dopamine antagonists, linezolid, lithium, tramadol, St. John's wort; use with caution. Use with other SSRIs, serotonin and norepinephrine reuptake inhibitors, tryptophan, or alcohol is not recommended. Caution with other CNS drugs, and drugs metabolized by CYP2D6 (eg, desipramine). Increased risk of bleeding with NSAIDs, aspirin (ASA), warfarin, and other anticoagulants. Rare reports of weakness, hyperreflexia, and incoordination with sumatriptan. May increase levels with cimetidine. May decrease levels of ketoconazole. May increase levels of metoprolol. May increase clearance with carbamazepine. Increased risk of hyponatremia with diuretics.

PREGNANCY: Category C, caution in nursing.

MECHANISM OF ACTION: SSRI; presumed to be linked to potentiation of serotonergic activity in the CNS resulting from its inhibition of CNS neuronal reuptake of serotonin.

PHARMACOKINETICS: Absorption: T_{max}=5 hrs. **Distribution:** Plasma protein binding (56%); found in breast milk. **Metabolism:** Hepatic; N-demethylation via CYP3A4, 2C19. **Elimination:** Urine (8%); $T_{1/2}$=27-32 hrs.

NURSING CONSIDERATIONS

Assessment: Assess for history of seizures, history of mania/hypomania, volume depletion, disease/condition that alters metabolism or hemodynamic response, hepatic/renal impairment, drug hypersensitivity, pregnancy/nursing status, and possible drug interactions. Obtain detailed psychiatric history.

Monitoring: Monitor for signs/symptoms of clinical worsening, suicidality, unusual changes in behavior, serotonin syndrome, NMS-like reactions, abnormal bleeding, hyponatremia, seizures, cognitive and motor impairment, and hepatic/renal dysfunction. Regularly monitor weight and growth in pediatrics.

Patient Counseling: Advise to look for emergence of anxiety, agitation, panic attacks, insomnia, irritability, hostility, aggressiveness, impulsivity, akathisia, hypomania, mania, behavioral changes, worsening depression, or suicidal ideation; instruct to report such symptoms, especially if severe, abrupt in onset, or not part of presenting symptoms. Caution about risk of serotonin syndrome with concomitant triptans, tramadol, other serotonergic agents, and risk of bleeding with ASA, warfarin, or other drugs that affect coagulation. Notify physician if taking or plan to take any prescribed or over-the-counter drugs. May notice improvement in 1-4 weeks; continue therapy as directed. Caution against hazardous tasks (eg, operating machinery and driving). Avoid alcohol. Notify physician if become pregnant, intend to become pregnant, or are breastfeeding. Inform of the need for comprehensive treatment program.

Administration: Oral route. Administer qd, in am or pm, with or without food. **Storage:** 25°C (77°F); excursions permitted to 15-30°C (59-86°F).

LIALDA   RX
mesalamine (Shire)

THERAPEUTIC CLASS: 5-Aminosalicylic acid derivative

INDICATIONS: Induction of remission in patients with active, mild to moderate ulcerative colitis (UC), and for maintenance of remission of UC.

DOSAGE: *Adults:* Induction of Remission: 2-4 tabs qd with a meal. Maint of Remission: 2 tabs qd with a meal. Elderly: Start at lower end of dosing range.

HOW SUPPLIED: Tab, Delayed-Release: 1.2g

WARNINGS/PRECAUTIONS: Renal impairment, including minimal change nephropathy, acute and chronic interstitial nephritis, and renal failure reported; caution with renal dysfunction or history of renal disease. Evaluate renal function prior to therapy and periodically thereafter. May cause acute intolerance syndrome; d/c if such syndrome is suspected. Caution with sulfasalazine hypersensitivity. Cardiac hypersensitivity reactions (myocarditis, pericarditis) reported; caution in patients with conditions predisposing to the development of myocarditis or pericarditis. Reports of hepatic failure in patients with preexisting liver disease; caution in patients with liver disease. Patients with pyloric stenosis or other organic/functional upper GI tract obstruction may have prolonged gastric retention, which could delay drug release in the colon. Caution in elderly.

ADVERSE REACTIONS: Headache, flatulence, acute intolerance syndrome, ulcerative colitis.

INTERACTIONS: May increase risk of renal reactions with nephrotoxic agents (eg, NSAIDs). May increase risk for blood disorders with azathioprine or 6-mercaptopurine.

PREGNANCY: Category B, caution in nursing.

MECHANISM OF ACTION: 5-aminosalicylic acid derivative; not established. Suspected to diminish inflammation by blocking cyclooxygenase and inhibiting prostaglandin production in colon.

PHARMACOKINETICS: Absorption: Administration of variable doses resulted in different parameters. **Distribution:** Plasma protein binding (43%); found in breast milk; crosses placenta. **Metabolism:** Liver and intestinal mucosa (acetylation); N-acetyl-5-aminosalicylic acid (major metabolite). **Elimination:** Urine (<8% unchanged, >13% N-acetyl-5-aminosalicylic acid); $T_{1/2}$=7-9 hrs (2.4g), 8-12 hrs (4.8g).

NURSING CONSIDERATIONS

Assessment: Assess for conditions predisposing to development of myocarditis and pericarditis, pyloric stenosis or other organic/functional upper GI tract obstruction, sensitivity to sulfasalazine, renal/hepatic function, pregnancy/nursing status, and possible drug interactions.

Monitoring: Monitor for signs/symptoms of acute intolerance syndrome, hypersensitivity reactions, renal/hepatic function, and blood cell counts in geriatric patients.

Patient Counseling: Instruct not to take drug if hypersensitive to salicylates (eg, aspirin) or other mesalamines. Inform to notify physician of all medications taken, and if allergic to sulfasalazine, salicylates, or mesalamine; taking NSAIDs, other nephrotoxic agents, azathioprine, or 6-mercaptopurine; experiencing cramping, abdominal pain, bloody diarrhea, fever, headache, or rash during therapy; are pregnant, plan to become pregnant, or are breastfeeding. Instruct to swallow tab whole and not to break outer coating.

Administration: Oral route. **Storage:** 15-25°C (59-77°F); excursions permitted to 30°C (86°F).

LIBRAX

RX

chlordiazepoxide HCl - clidinium bromide (Valeant)

THERAPEUTIC CLASS: Benzodiazepine/anticholinergic

INDICATIONS: Adjunctive therapy in the treatment of irritable bowel syndrome, acute entero-colitis, and peptic ulcer.

DOSAGE: *Adults:* Individualize dose. Usual/Maint: 1-2 caps tid-qid ac and hs. Elderly/Debilitated: Initial: Not more than 2 caps/day. Titrate: Increase gradually PRN.

HOW SUPPLIED: Cap: (Chlordiazepoxide-Clidinium) 5mg-2.5mg

CONTRAINDICATIONS: Glaucoma, prostatic hypertrophy, benign bladder neck obstruction.

WARNINGS/PRECAUTIONS: May impair mental/physical abilities. Risk of congenital malforma-tions during first trimester of pregnancy; avoid use. Inhibition of lactation may occur. Paradoxical reactions (eg, excitement, stimulation, and acute rage) reported in psychiatric patients. Caution in treatment of anxiety states with evidence of impending depression; suicidal tendencies may be present. Caution in elderly and with renal or hepatic dysfunction. Use lowest effective dose in debilitated patients. Avoid abrupt withdrawal after extended therapy; withdrawal symptoms reported following d/c.

ADVERSE REACTIONS: Drowsiness, ataxia, confusion, skin eruptions, edema, extrapyramidal symptoms, dry mouth, nausea, constipation, altered libido, blood dyscrasias, jaundice, hepatic dysfunction, blurred vision, urinary hesitancy.

INTERACTIONS: Additive effects with alcohol and CNS depressants. Coadministration with other psychotropic agents not recommended; caution with MAOIs and phenothiazines. Altered coagu-lation effects reported with oral anticoagulants. Constipation may occur when coadministered with other spasmolytic agents.

PREGNANCY: Not for use in pregnancy, safety not known in nursing.

MECHANISM OF ACTION: Chlordiazepoxide: Benzodiazepine; antianxiety agent. Clidinium: Anticholinergic; shown to have a pronounced antispasmodic and antisecretory effect on the GI tract.

NURSING CONSIDERATIONS

Assessment: Assess for glaucoma, prostatic hypertrophy, benign bladder neck obstruction, re-nal/hepatic dysfunction, alcohol intake, history of drug abuse, drug hypersensitivity, pregnancy/nursing status, and possible drug interactions.

Monitoring: Monitor for ataxia, oversedation, drowsiness, confusion, and other adverse reactions. Monitor for paradoxical reactions (eg, excitement, stimulation, acute rage) in psychiatric patients. Periodic blood counts and LFTs are advisable when treatment is protracted. Monitor for signs of impending depression, or any suicidal tendencies.

Patient Counseling: Inform that psychological and physical dependence may develop, and to consult physician before increasing dose or abruptly d/c. Advise to observe caution when performing hazardous tasks (eg, operating machinery/driving). Advise to notify physician if pregnant/breastfeeding or plan to become pregnant. Inform of potential additive effects with alcohol and other CNS depressants.

Administration: Oral route. **Storage:** 25°C (77°F); excursions permitted to 15-30°C (59-86°F).

LIBRIUM

chlordiazepoxide HCl (Valeant)

THERAPEUTIC CLASS: Benzodiazepine

INDICATIONS: Management of anxiety disorders and short-term relief of anxiety symptoms, withdrawal symptoms of acute alcoholism, and preoperative apprehension and anxiety.

DOSAGE: *Adults:* Individualize dose. Mild-Moderate Anxiety: 5-10mg tid-qid. Severe Anxiety: 20-25mg tid-qid. Alcohol Withdrawal: 50-100mg; repeat until agitation controlled. Max: 300mg/day. Preoperative Anxiety: 5-10mg tid-qid on days prior to surgery. Elderly/Debilitated: 5mg bid-qid. *Pediatrics:* ≥6 yrs: Individualize dose. Usual: 5mg bid-qid. May increase to 10mg bid-tid.

HOW SUPPLIED: Cap: 5mg, 10mg, 25mg

WARNINGS/PRECAUTIONS: May impair mental/physical abilities, including mental alertness in children. Risk of congenital malformations during first trimester of pregnancy; avoid use. Paradoxical reactions (eg, excitement, stimulation, and acute rage) reported in psychiatric patients, and in hyperactive aggressive pediatric patients. Caution in treatment of anxiety states with evidence of impending depression; suicidal tendencies may be present. Caution with porphyria, renal or hepatic dysfunction. Use lowest effective dose in elderly and debilitated patients. Avoid abrupt withdrawal after extended therapy; withdrawal symptoms reported following d/c.

ADVERSE REACTIONS: Drowsiness, ataxia, confusion, skin eruptions, edema, nausea, constipation, extrapyramidal symptoms, libido changes, EEG changes.

INTERACTIONS: Additive effects with CNS depressants and alcohol. Coadministration with other psychotropic agents not recommended; caution with MAOIs and phenothiazines. Altered coagulation effects reported with oral anticoagulants.

PREGNANCY: Not for use in pregnancy, safety not known in nursing.

MECHANISM OF ACTION: Benzodiazepine; not established. Has antianxiety, sedative, appetite stimulating, and weak analgesic actions; blocks EEG arousal from stimulation of brain stem reticular formation.

PHARMACOKINETICS: Elimination: Urine (1-2% unchanged, 3-6% conjugates); $T_{1/2}$=24-48 hrs.

NURSING CONSIDERATIONS

Assessment: Assess for pregnancy status, hepatic/renal function, and possible drug interactions.

Monitoring: Monitor elderly/debilitated patients for ataxia and oversedation, drowsiness, confusion. Monitor for paradoxical reactions in psychiatric patients and in hyperactive aggressive pediatric patients. Periodic blood counts and LFTs are advisable when treatment is protracted. Monitor for signs of impending depression or any suicidal tendencies.

Patient Counseling: Inform that psychological/physical dependence may occur; consult physician before increasing dose or abruptly d/c. Advise to notify physician if become pregnant during therapy or plan to become pregnant. May impair mental/physical abilities; caution while operating machinery/driving. May impair mental alertness in children. Avoid alcohol and other CNS depressant drugs.

Administration: Oral route. **Storage:** 25°C (77°F); excursions permitted to 15-30°C (59-86°F).

L

LIDODERM PATCH   RX
lidocaine (Endo)

THERAPEUTIC CLASS: Acetamide local anesthetic

INDICATIONS: Relief of pain associated with post-herpetic neuralgia.

DOSAGE: *Adults:* Apply to intact skin to cover the most painful area. Apply up to 3 patches, once for up to 12 hrs within 24-hr period. May cut patches into smaller sizes before removal of the release liner. Debilitated/Impaired Elimination: Treat smaller areas. Remove patch if irritation or burning occurs; may reapply when irritation subsides.

HOW SUPPLIED: Patch: 5% [30^s]

WARNINGS/PRECAUTIONS: Serious adverse events may occur in children or pets if ingested; keep out of reach. Excessive dosing by applying to larger areas or for longer than the recommended wearing time may result in serious adverse effects. Increased risk of toxicity in patients with severe hepatic disease. Caution with history of drug sensitivities, smaller patients and patients with impaired elimination. Avoid broken or inflamed skin, placement of external heat (eg, heating pads, electric blankets) and eye contact.

ADVERSE REACTIONS: Application-site reactions (eg, erythema, edema, bruising, papules, vesicles, discoloration, depigmentation, burning sensation, pruritus, dermatitis, petechia, blisters, exfoliation, abnormal sensation).

INTERACTIONS: Additive toxic effects with concomitant Class I antiarrhythmics (eg, tocainide, mexiletine); use caution. Consider total amount absorbed from all formulations containing other local anesthetics.

PREGNANCY: Category B, caution in nursing.

MECHANISM OF ACTION: Local anesthetic; stabilizes neuronal membranes by inhibiting ionic fluxes required for initiation and conduction of impulses.

PHARMACOKINETICS: Absorption: C_{max}=0.13mcg/mL; T_{max}=11 hrs. **Distribution:** V_d=0.7-2.7L/kg (IV); plasma protein binding (70%). Crosses placenta; found in breast milk. **Metabolism:** Liver (rapid); monoethylglycinexylidide, glycinexylidide (active metabolites). **Elimination:** Urine (<10%, unchanged); $T_{1/2}$=81-149 min (IV).

NURSING CONSIDERATIONS

Assessment: Assess for history of drug sensitivities to local anesthetics of the amide type and para-aminobenzoic acid derivatives, hepatic disease, pregnancy/nursing status, and for possible drug interactions.

Monitoring: Monitor for local skin reactions, allergic/anaphylactoid reactions, liver function, pain intensity, and pain relief periodically and other adverse reactions.

Patient Counseling: Instruct to remove patch and not to reapply if irritation or burning sensation occurs during application until irritation subsides. If eye contact occurs, immediately wash with water or saline and protect eye until sensation returns. Counsel to avoid application to larger areas and for longer than recommended wearing time. Avoid applying to broken or inflamed skin. Instruct to wash hands after handling patch and to fold used patches so adhesive side sticks to itself. Keep out of reach of children and pets.

Administration: Transdermal route. Refer to PI for proper handling and disposal. **Storage:** Store at 25°C (77°F); excursions permitted to 15-30°C (59-86°F).

LIPITOR   RX
atorvastatin calcium (Parke-Davis/Pfizer)

THERAPEUTIC CLASS: HMG-CoA reductase inhibitor

INDICATIONS: To reduce the risk of myocardial infarction (MI), stroke, revascularization procedures, and angina in adults without clinically evident coronary heart disease (CHD) but with multiple risk factors for CHD. To reduce the risk of MI and stroke in patients with type 2 diabetes, and without clinically evident CHD, but with multiple risk factors for CHD. To reduce the risk of nonfatal MI, fatal and nonfatal stroke, revascularization procedures, hospitalization for congestive heart failure, and angina in patients with clinically evident CHD. Adjunct to diet for treatment of primary hypercholesterolemia (heterozygous familial and nonfamilial) and mixed dyslipidemia (Types IIa and IIb). Adjunct to diet for treatment of patients with elevated serum TG levels (Type IV). Treatment of primary dysbetalipoproteinemia (Type III) inadequately responding to diet. Adjunct to other lipid-lowering treatments or if treatments are unavailable, for treatment of homozygous familial hypercholesterolemia. Adjunct to diet for treatment of boys and postmenarchal girls, 10-17 yrs of age, with heterozygous familial hypercholesterolemia.

DOSAGE: *Adults:* Individualize dose. Hyperlipidemia/Mixed Dyslipidemia: Initial: 10mg or 20mg qd (or 40mg qd for LDL reduction >45%). Titrate: Adjust dose accordingly at 2- to 4-week intervals. Usual: 10-80mg qd. Homozygous Familial Hypercholesterolemia: 10-80mg qd. Concomitant Lopinavir plus Ritonavir: Use lowest dose necessary. Concomitant Clarithromycin/Itraconazole/Fosamprenavir/Ritonavir plus Saquinavir, Darunavir, or Fosamprenavir: Limit to 20mg; use lowest dose necessary. Concomitant Nelfinavir: Limit to 40mg; use lowest dose necessary.
Pediatrics: 10-17 yrs: Individualize dose. Heterozygous Familial Hypercholesterolemia: Initial: 10mg/day. Titrate: Adjust dose at intervals of ≥4 weeks. Max: 20mg/day.

HOW SUPPLIED: Tab: 10mg, 20mg, 40mg, 80mg

CONTRAINDICATIONS: Active liver disease which may include unexplained persistent elevations in hepatic transaminases, women who are pregnant or may become pregnant, and nursing mothers.

WARNINGS/PRECAUTIONS: Rare cases of rhabdomyolysis with acute renal failure secondary to myoglobinuria reported. Increased risk of rhabdomyolysis in patients with history of renal impairment; closely monitor for skeletal muscle effects. D/C if markedly elevated CPK levels occur or if myopathy is diagnosed or suspected. Temporarily withhold or d/c if acute, serious condition suggestive of myopathy occurs or if with risk factor predisposing to development of renal failure secondary to rhabdomyolysis. Persistent increases in serum transaminases reported; obtain liver enzyme tests prior to initiation and repeat as clinically indicated. Fatal and nonfatal hepatic failure (rare) reported; promptly interrupt therapy if serious liver injury with clinical symptoms and/or hyperbilirubinemia or jaundice occurs and do not restart if no alternate etiology found. Caution in patients who consume substantial quantities of alcohol and/or have history of liver disease. Increases in HbA1c and FPG levels reported. May blunt adrenal and/or gonadal steroid production. Increased risk of hemorrhagic stroke in patients with recent stroke or transient ischemic attack (TIA). Caution in elderly.

ADVERSE REACTIONS: Nasopharyngitis, arthralgia, diarrhea, diabetes, pain in extremity, urinary tract infection, dyspepsia, nausea, musculoskeletal pain, muscle spasms, myalgia, insomnia.

INTERACTIONS: Avoid with cyclosporine, telaprevir, gemfibrozil, or combination of tipranavir plus ritonavir. Caution with fibrates and drugs that decrease levels or activity of endogenous steroid hormones (eg, ketoconazole, spironolactone, cimetidine). Increased risk of myopathy with fibric acid derivatives, erythromycin, lipid-modifying doses of niacin, strong CYP3A4 inhibitors (eg, clarithromycin, HIV protease inhibitors), and azole antifungals; consider lower initial and maint doses. Strong CYP3A4 inhibitors (eg, clarithromycin, several combinations of HIV protease inhibitors, telaprevir, itraconazole) and grapefruit juice may increase levels. CYP3A4 inducers (eg, efavirenz, rifampin) may decrease levels; simultaneous coadministration with rifampin recommended. May increase digoxin levels; monitor appropriately. May increase area under the curve of norethindrone and ethinyl estradiol. Myopathy, including rhabdomyolysis, reported with colchicine; use with caution. OATP1B1 inhibitors (eg, cyclosporine) may increase bioavailability.

PREGNANCY: Category X, not for use in nursing.

MECHANISM OF ACTION: HMG-CoA reductase inhibitor; inhibits conversion of HMG-CoA to mevalonate (precursor of sterols, including cholesterol).

PHARMACOKINETICS: Absorption: Rapid; absolute bioavailability (14%); T_{max}=1-2 hrs. **Distribution:** V_d=381L; plasma protein binding (≥98%). **Metabolism:** CYP3A4 (extensive); ortho- and parahydroxylated derivatives (active metabolites). **Elimination:** Bile (major), urine (<2%); $T_{1/2}$=14 hrs.

NURSING CONSIDERATIONS

Assessment: Assess for active or history of liver disease, unexplained and persistent elevations in serum transaminase levels, pregnancy/nursing status, history of renal impairment, risk factors predisposing to the development of renal failure secondary to rhabdomyolysis, alcohol intake, recent stroke or TIA, hypersensitivity to drug, and possible drug interactions. Obtain baseline LFTs.

Monitoring: Monitor for signs/symptoms of rhabdomyolysis and myopathy (unexplained muscle pain, tenderness, weakness). Monitor lipid profile and CPK levels. Perform LFTs as clinically indicated.

Patient Counseling: Advise to adhere to the National Cholesterol Education Program-recommended diet, a regular exercise program, and periodic testing of a fasting lipid panel. Inform of the substances that should not be taken concomitantly with the drug. Advise to inform other healthcare professionals that they are taking the drug. Inform of the risk of myopathy; instruct to report promptly any unexplained muscle pain, tenderness, or weakness. Inform that liver function will be checked prior to initiation and if signs or symptoms of liver injury occurs; instruct to report promptly any symptoms that may indicate liver injury (eg, fatigue, anorexia, right upper abdominal discomfort, dark urine, or jaundice). Instruct women of childbearing age to use effective method of birth control to prevent pregnancy. Advise to d/c therapy and contact physician if pregnancy occurs. Instruct not to use the drug if breastfeeding.

Administration: Oral route. Administer as a single dose at any time of the day, with or without food. **Storage:** 20-25°C (68-77°F).

LIPOFEN   RX
fenofibrate (Kowa)

THERAPEUTIC CLASS: Fibric acid derivative

INDICATIONS: Treatment of hypertriglyceridemia (Types IV and V) as adjunct to diet. Reduction of elevated total cholesterol, LDL, apolipoprotein B (Apo B), TG, and to increase HDL in primary hypercholesterolemia or mixed dyslipidemia (Types IIa and IIb) as adjunct to diet.

DOSAGE: *Adults:* Hypercholesterolemia/Mixed Dyslipidemia: Initial: 150mg qd. Hypertriglyceridemia: Initial : 50-150mg/day. Titrate: Adjust if needed after repeat lipid determinations at 4-8 week intervals. Max: 150mg/day. Renal Dysfunction/Elderly: Initial: 50mg/day. Titrate: Adjust if needed after lipid determinations and evaluation of the effects on renal function.

HOW SUPPLIED: Cap: 50mg, 150mg

CONTRAINDICATIONS: Pre-existing gallbladder disease, unexplained persistent liver function abnormality, hepatic or severe renal dysfunction (including primary biliary cirrhosis).

WARNINGS/PRECAUTIONS: Monitor LFTs regularly; d/c if >3X ULN. May cause cholelithiasis; d/c if gallstones found. D/C if myopathy or marked creatine phosphokinase (CPK) elevation occurs. Decreased Hgb, Hct, WBCs, thrombocytopenia, and agranulocytosis reported; monitor CBC during first 12 months of therapy. Acute hypersensitivity reactions (rare) and pancreatitis reported. Minimize dose in severe renal impairment. Increased rate of pulmonary embolus (PE) and deep vein thrombosis (DVT) reported. Not indicated for patients with Type I hyperlipoproteinemia.

ADVERSE REACTIONS: Abdominal/back pain, headache, abnormal LFTs, respiratory disorder, increased CPK, ALT/AST increase.

INTERACTIONS: Potentiates coumarin anticoagulants; reduce anticoagulant dose and monitor PT/INR. Avoid HMG-CoA reductase inhibitors unless benefits outweigh risks. Bile acid sequestrants may impede absorption; take at least 1 hr before or 4-6 hrs after the resin. Evaluate benefits/risks with immunosuppressants (eg, cyclosporine) and other nephrotoxic agents. Medication known to exacerbate hypertriglyceridemia (eg, β-blockers, thiazides, estrogens) should be discontinued or changed if possible prior to initiating therapy.

PREGNANCY: Category C, not for use in nursing.

MECHANISM OF ACTION: Fibric acid derivative; activates peroxisome proliferator-activated receptor α (PPARα), increasing lipolysis and elimination of triglyceride-rich particles from plasma by activating lipoprotein lipase and reducing production of apoprotein C-III (lipoprotein lipase inhibitor). Activation of PPARα also induces an increase in synthesis of Apo A-I and A-II, and HDL-cholesterol. Reduces serum uric acid levels in hyperuricemic and healthy individuals by increasing the urinary excretion of uric acid.

PHARMACOKINETICS: Absorption: Well absorbed. **Distribution:** Plasma protein binding (99%). **Metabolism:** Hydrolysis, glucuronidation; fenofibric acid (active metabolite). **Elimination:** Urine (60%), feces (25%); $T_{1/2}$=10-35 hrs.

NURSING CONSIDERATIONS

Assessment: Assess for hepatic/renal dysfunction, preexisting gallbladder disease, pregnancy/ nursing status, and drug interactions. Obtain baseline lipid levels.

Monitoring: Monitor for signs/symptoms of liver dysfunction, cholelithiasis, pancreatitis, hypersensitivity reactions, hematological changes (eg, thrombocytopenia, agranulocytosis), myopathies, rhabdomyolysis, PE, DVT, and elevations in SrCr. Periodically monitor liver function (eg, ALT, AST), cholesterol levels, and blood counts. Evaluate CPK levels in patients suspected of having myopathies. Monitor for clinical response; if adequate response not seen after 2 months with maximum dose, d/c therapy.

Patient Counseling: Advise to immediately contact physician if unexplained muscle pain, tenderness, or weakness develop, particularly when accompanied by malaise or fever. Recommend appropriate lipid-lowering diet. Instruct to take with/without meals.

Administration: Oral route. **Storage:** 15°-30°C (59°-86°F). Keep out of reach of children. Protect from moisture.

LITHIUM ER
lithium carbonate (Various)

RX

> Lithium toxicity is closely related to serum levels, and can occur at doses close to therapeutic levels. Facilities for prompt and accurate serum lithium determinations should be available before initiating therapy.

OTHER BRAND NAMES: Lithobid (Noven)

THERAPEUTIC CLASS: Antimanic agent

INDICATIONS: Treatment of manic episodes of bipolar disorder and maintenance treatment of bipolar disorder.

DOSAGE: *Adults:* Individualize dose. Acute Mania: 900mg bid or 600mg tid to achieve effective serum levels of 1-1.5mEq/L; monitor levels twice weekly until stabilized. Maint: 900-1200mg/day, given bid-tid to maintain serum levels of 0.6-1.2mEq/L; monitor levels every 2 months. Elderly: Start at lower end of dosing range.
Pediatrics: ≥12 yrs: Individualize dose. Acute Mania: 900mg bid or 600mg tid to achieve effective serum levels of 1-1.5mEq/L; monitor levels twice weekly until stabilized. Maint: 900-1200mg/day, given bid-tid to maintain serum levels of 0.6-1.2 mEq/L; monitor levels every 2 months.

HOW SUPPLIED: Tab, Extended-Release: 300mg, 450mg*; (Lithobid) 300mg *scored

WARNINGS/PRECAUTIONS: Avoid with significant renal or cardiovascular disease (CVD), severe debilitation, dehydration, or sodium depletion. Chronic therapy may be associated with diminution of renal concentrating ability; carefully manage to avoid dehydration with resulting lithium retention and toxicity. Morphologic changes with glomerular and interstitial fibrosis and nephron-atrophy reported; assess kidney function prior to and during therapy. Decreased tolerance reported to ensue from protracted sweating or diarrhea; if occur, administer supplemental fluid and salt. Reduce dose or d/c with sweating, diarrhea, or infection with elevated temperatures. Caution with hypothyroidism; monitor thyroid function. May impair mental/physical abilities. May decrease sodium reabsorption which could lead to sodium depletion; maintain normal diet, including salt, and adequate fluid intake. Caution in elderly. May be associated with the unmasking of Brugada syndrome; avoid with or those suspected of having Brugada syndrome.

ADVERSE REACTIONS: Fine hand tremor, polyuria, mild thirst, general discomfort, diarrhea, N/V, drowsiness, muscular weakness, lack of coordination, ataxia, giddiness, tinnitus, blurred vision, large output of diluted urine.

INTERACTIONS: Risk of encephalopathic syndrome (eg, weakness, lethargy, fever, tremulousness, confusion, EPS) followed by irreversible brain damage with haloperidol and other neuroleptics; monitor for evidence of neurological toxicity and d/c therapy if such signs appear. May prolong effects of neuromuscular blockers; use with caution. May increase risk of neurotoxic effects with calcium channel blockers or carbamazepine. Increased levels with indomethacin, piroxicam, and other NSAIDs (eg, cyclooxygenase-2 inhibitors); monitor lithium levels closely when initiating or d/c NSAID use. Acetazolamide, urea, xanthine preparations, and alkalinizing agents (eg, sodium bicarbonate) may decrease levels. May produce hypothyroidism with iodide preparations. May provoke lithium toxicity with metronidazole; monitor closely. Risk of lithium toxicity with diuretics and ACE inhibitors due to reduced renal clearance; avoid concomitant use. Extreme caution when concomitant use with diuretics or ACE inhibitors is necessary; monitor lithium levels and adjust dose if necessary. Fluoxetine may increase/decrease lithium levels; monitor closely. Caution with selective serotonin reuptake inhibitors. May interact with methyldopa or phenytoin.

PREGNANCY: Category D, not for use in nursing.

MECHANISM OF ACTION: Antimanic agent; not established. Suspected to alter sodium transport in nerve and muscle cells and effects a shift toward intraneuronal metabolism of catecholamines.

PHARMACOKINETICS: Distribution: Found in breast milk. **Elimination:** Urine (primary), feces (insignificant). $T_{1/2}$=24 hrs.

NURSING CONSIDERATIONS

Assessment: Assess for CVD, severe debilitation, dehydration, sodium depletion. Assess renal function (urinalysis, SrCr), thyroid function with history of thyroid disease, pregnancy/nursing status, and possible drug interactions. Assess for Brugada syndrome or patients with risk factors.

Monitoring: Monitor for diminution of renal concentrating ability (eg, nephrogenic diabetes insipidus), glomerular and interstitial fibrosis, and nephron atrophy in patients on long-term therapy, encephalopathic syndrome, renal function, thyroid function in patients with a history of hypothyroidism, serum lithium levels, signs of lithium toxicity, and other adverse effects. Monitor for unexplained syncope or palpitations.

Patient Counseling: Counsel about clinical signs of lithium toxicity (eg, diarrhea, vomiting, tremor, mild ataxia, drowsiness, muscle weakness); advise to d/c therapy and notify physician if any of these signs occur. Inform of the risks and benefits of therapy. Advise to seek immediate emergency assistance if fainting, lightheadedness, abnormal heartbeat, SOB, or other adverse reactions develop. Inform that lithium may impair mental/physical abilities; caution in activities requiring alertness.

Administration: Oral route. **Storage:** (Lithobid) 15-30°C (59-86°F). Protect from moisture. (300mg) 20-25°C (68-77°F) or (450mg) 25°C (77°F); excursions permitted to 15-30°C (59-86°F).

LIVALO   RX L
pitavastatin (Kowa)

THERAPEUTIC CLASS: HMG-CoA reductase inhibitor

INDICATIONS: Adjunctive therapy to diet to reduce elevated total-C, LDL, apolipoprotein B (Apo B), TG, and to increase HDL in adults with primary hyperlipidemia or mixed dyslipidemia.

DOSAGE: *Adults:* Individualize dose. Initial: 2mg qd. Usual: 1-4mg qd. Max: 4mg qd. After initiation or upon titration, analyze lipid levels after 4 weeks and adjust dose accordingly. Moderate/Severe Renal Impairment (GFR 30-59mL/min/1.73m^2 and GFR 15-29mL/min/1.73m^2 not receiving hemodialysis, respectively)/End-Stage Renal Disease Receiving Hemodialysis: Initial: 1mg qd. Max: 2mg qd. Concomitant Erythromycin: Max: 1mg qd. Concomitant Rifampin: Max: 2mg qd.

HOW SUPPLIED: Tab: 1mg, 2mg, 4mg

CONTRAINDICATIONS: Active liver disease including unexplained persistent elevations of hepatic transaminase levels, women who are pregnant or may become pregnant, nursing mothers, and coadministration with cyclosporine.

WARNINGS/PRECAUTIONS: Myopathy and rhabdomyolysis with acute renal failure secondary to myoglobinuria reported. Caution with predisposing factors for myopathy (eg, advanced age [>65 yrs], renal impairment, and inadequately treated hypothyroidism). D/C if markedly elevated creatine kinase (CK) levels occur or myopathy is diagnosed/suspected. Temporarily withhold if experiencing acute, serious condition suggestive of myopathy or predisposing to the development of renal failure secondary to rhabdomyolysis (eg, sepsis, hypotension, dehydration, trauma, major surgery, severe metabolic, endocrine, and electrolyte disorders, or uncontrolled seizures). Increases in serum transaminases (eg, AST, ALT) reported; perform LFTs before the initiation of therapy and if signs or symptoms of liver injury occur. Fatal and nonfatal hepatic failure reported (rare); promptly interrupt therapy if serious liver injury with clinical symptoms and/or hyperbilirubinemia or jaundice occurs. Increases in HbA1c and fasting serum glucose levels reported. Caution in patients who consume substantial quantities of alcohol. Increased risk for severe myopathy with doses >4mg qd.

ADVERSE REACTIONS: Back pain, constipation, myalgia, diarrhea, pain in extremity, arthralgia, headache, influenza, nasopharyngitis.

INTERACTIONS: See Contraindications. Significantly increased exposure with erythromycin and rifampin. Increased risk of myopathy/rhabdomyolysis with fibrates; avoid with gemfibrozil and use caution with other fibrates. May enhance risk of skeletal muscle effects with niacin; caution with lipid-modifying doses of niacin and consider dose reduction of pitavastatin. Monitor PT and INR with warfarin.

PREGNANCY: Category X, not for use in nursing.

MECHANISM OF ACTION: HMG-CoA reductase inhibitor; inhibits the rate-determining enzyme involved with biosynthesis of cholesterol, in a manner of competition with the substrate so that it inhibits cholesterol synthesis in the liver.

PHARMACOKINETICS: Absorption: (Oral Sol) Absolute bioavailability (51%); T_{max}=1 hr. **Distribution:** Plasma protein binding (>99%); V_d=148L. **Metabolism:** CYP2C9, 2C8; lactone (major metabolite) via glucuronide conjugate by uridine 5'-diphosphate (UDP) glucuronosyltransferase (UGT1A3 and UGT2B7). **Elimination:** Urine (15%), feces (79%); $T_{1/2}$=12 hrs.

NURSING CONSIDERATIONS

Assessment: Assess for active liver disease or unexplained elevations in serum transaminase levels, renal impairment, inadequately treated hypothyroidism, substantial consumption of alcohol, pregnancy/nursing status, possible drug interactions, and other conditions where treatment is cautioned/contraindicated. Obtain baseline lipid profile and LFTs prior to therapy.

Monitoring: Monitor signs/symptoms of myopathy, rhabdomyolysis, acute renal failure, and hypersensitivity reactions. Monitor for increases in HbA1c and fasting serum glucose levels. Perform periodic monitoring of lipid profile and CK levels. Analyze lipid levels 4 weeks after initiation/titration. Perform LFTs if signs or symptoms of liver injury occurs. Monitor PT and INR when using warfarin.

Patient Counseling: Inform that the drug can be taken at any time of the day with or without food. Advise to inform physician immediately if experiencing unexplained muscle pain, tenderness, or weakness. Counsel women of childbearing age to use effective method of birth control to prevent pregnancy during therapy. Instruct pregnant or breastfeeding women to d/c therapy and consult physician. Inform that liver enzymes will be checked before therapy and if signs or symptoms of liver injury occurs (eg, fatigue, anorexia, right upper abdominal discomfort, dark urine, or jaundice).

Administration: Oral route. **Storage:** 15-30°C (59-86°F). Protect from light.

LO/OVRAL
RX

norgestrel - ethinyl estradiol (Wyeth)

> Cigarette smoking increases the risk of serious cardiovascular (CV) side effects. Risk increases with age (>35 yrs) and with heavy smoking (≥15 cigarettes/day). Women who use oral contraceptives should be strongly advised not to smoke.

OTHER BRAND NAMES: Low-Ogestrel (Watson) - Cryselle (Duramed)

THERAPEUTIC CLASS: Estrogen/progestogen combination

INDICATIONS: Prevention of pregnancy.

DOSAGE: *Adults:* Start 1st Sunday after menses begins or the 1st day of menses. First cycle use: 1 white tab qd for 21 days followed by 1 pink /peach (inert) tab qd for 7 consecutive days. After the first cycle use: Begin next and all subsequent courses after taking the last pink/peach tab. Follow same dosing schedule. (Lo/Ovral) Switching from 21-day regimen: Start 7 days after taking last dose. Switching from progestin-only pill: Start the next day after last dose. Switching from implant/injection: Start on the day of implant removal or the day the next injection would be due. Use after pregnancy/abortion/miscarriage: Start on day 28 postpartum in nonlactating mother or after a second-trimester abortion.
Pediatrics: Postpubertal adolescents: Start 1st Sunday after menses begins or the 1st day of menses. First cycle use: 1 white tab qd for 21 days followed by 1 pink/peach (inert) tab qd for 7 consecutive days. After the first cycle use: Begin next and all subsequent courses after taking the last pink/peach tab. Follow same dosing schedule. (Lo/Ovral) Switching from 21-day regimen: Start 7 days after taking last dose. Switching from progestin-only pill: Start the next day after last dose. Switching from implant/injection: Start on the day of implant removal or the day the next injection would be due. Use after pregnancy/abortion/miscarriage: Start on day 28 postpartum in nonlactating mother or after a second-trimester abortion.

HOW SUPPLIED: Tab: (Ethinyl Estradiol-Norgestrel) 0.03mg-0.3mg

CONTRAINDICATIONS: Thrombophlebitis, thromboembolic disorders, history of DVT or thromboembolic disorders, cerebrovascular or coronary artery disease (current or past history), known or suspected carcinoma of the breast or personal history of breast cancer, carcinoma of the endometrium or other known or suspected estrogen-dependent neoplasia, undiagnosed abnormal genital bleeding, cholestatic jaundice of pregnancy or jaundice with prior pill use, pregnancy, hepatic adenomas or carcinomas or benign liver tumors. (Lo/Ovral) Active liver disease, valvular heart disease with thrombogenic complications, thrombogenic rhythm disorders, hereditary or acquired thrombophilias, major surgery with prolonged immobilization, diabetes with vascular involvement, headaches with focal neurological symptoms, uncontrolled HTN.

WARNINGS/PRECAUTIONS: Increased risk of venous and arterial thrombotic and thromboembolic events (eg, MI, thromboembolism, stroke), hepatic neoplasia, gallbladder disease. Retinal thrombosis reported; d/c use if unexplained partial or complete loss of vision occurs, onset of proptosis or diplopia, papilledema, or retinal vascular lesions develop. May cause glucose intolerance; monitor prediabetic and diabetic patients. May cause fluid retention and increase BP; monitor closely with HTN and d/c if significant elevation of BP occurs. May cause onset or exacerbation of migraine or development of headaches with new pattern. Breakthrough bleeding and spotting reported; rule out malignancy or pregnancy. Ectopic and intrauterine pregnancy may occur in contraceptive failures. Monitor closely with hyperlipidemias; consider non-hormonal contraception with uncontrolled dyslipidemias. D/C if jaundice develops. Monitor closely with depression and d/c if depression recurs to significant degree. May develop visual changes or changes in lens tolerance with contact-lens wearers. Diarrhea and/or vomiting may reduce hormone absorption. Perform annual physical exam. Use before menarche is not indicated. Does not protect against HIV infection (AIDS) and other sexually transmitted diseases (STDs). May affect certain endocrine, LFTs and blood components. Should not be used to induce withdrawal bleeding as a test for pregnancy, or to treat threatened or habitual abortion during pregnancy.

ADVERSE REACTIONS: N/V, breakthrough bleeding, spotting, amenorrhea, migraine, depression, vaginal candidiasis, edema, weight changes, abdominal cramps/bloating, menstrual flow changes, cervical erosion and secretion.

INTERACTIONS: Reduced contraceptive effectiveness resulting in unintended pregnancy and breakthrough bleeding with antibiotics (eg, ampicillin, other penicillins, tetracyclines), anticonvulsants and other drugs that increase the metabolism of contraceptive steroids (eg rifampin, rifabutin, barbiturates, primidone, phenylbutazone, phenytoin, dexamethasone, carbamazepine, felbamate, oxcarbazepine, topiramate, griseofulvin, St. John's wort and modafinil). Significant changes (increase or decrease) in plasma levels with anti-HIV protease inhibitors; safety and efficacy may be affected. Increased levels with atorvastatin, ascorbic acid, acetaminophen and CYP3A4 inhibitors (eg, indinavir, itraconazole, ketoconazole, fluconazole, troleandomycin). Increased risk of intrahepatic cholestasis with troleandomycin. Increased plasma levels of cyclosporin, prednisolone and other corticosteroids, and theophylline. Decreased plasma concentrations of acetaminophen and increased clearance of temazepam, salicylic acid, morphine and clofibric acid.

PREGNANCY: Category X, not for use in nursing.

MECHANISM OF ACTION: Estrogen/progestogen combination oral contraceptive; acts by suppressing gonadotropins. Primarily acts by inhibiting ovulation. Also responsible for causing changes in cervical mucus (increases difficulty of sperm entry into uterus) and in endometrium (reduces likelihood of implantation).

PHARMACOKINETICS: Distribution: Found in breast milk.

NURSING CONSIDERATIONS

Assessment: Assess for presence or history of breast cancer, estrogen dependent neoplasia, abnormal genital bleeding, active liver disease, and known/suspected pregnancy or any other conditions where treatment is cautioned or contraindicated. Assess use in patients who are >35 yrs and heavy smokers (≥15 cigarettes/day). Assess use with HTN, hyperlipidemias, obesity, DM, or in patients at increased risk for thrombosis. Assess for possible drug interactions.

Monitoring: Monitor for bleeding irregularities, thromboembolic events, onset or exacerbation of headaches or migraines, and ectopic pregnancy. Monitor fasting blood glucose levels in DM and prediabetic patients, BP with history of HTN, lipid levels with a history of hyperlipidemia. Monitor for signs of liver dysfunction (eg, jaundice) and signs of depression with previous history. Refer patients with contact lenses to an ophthalmologist if visual changes occur. Perform annual history and physical exam.

Patient Counseling: Counsel about possible adverse effects of drug. Advise to avoid smoking while on medication. Inform that drug does not protect against HIV infection and other STDs. Instruct women to use additional method of birth control until after first 7 days of administration in initial cycle. Take medication at same time every day and at intervals not exceeding 24 hrs. If dose is missed, take next pill as soon as possible, then take next dose at regular time. If patient skips 2 or more doses, advise to use another method of contraception until patient has taken medication for 7 consecutive days. If spotting or breakthrough bleeding occurs, continue taking medication; notify physician if bleeding is persistent or prolonged.

Administration: Oral route. **Storage:** 20-25°C (68-77°F). (Low-Ogestrel) 15-25°C (59-77°F).

LOCOID RX
hydrocortisone butyrate (Ferndale)

THERAPEUTIC CLASS: Corticosteroid

INDICATIONS: (Cre, Oint) Corticosteroid-responsive dermatoses. (Sol) Seborrheic dermatitis.

DOSAGE: *Adults:* (Cre, Oint) Apply bid-tid. May use occlusive dressings for psoriasis or recalcitrant conditions. D/C dressings if infection develops. (Sol) Apply bid-tid.

Pediatrics: (Cre, Oint) Apply bid-tid. May use occlusive dressings for psoriasis or recalcitrant conditions. D/C dressings if infection develops. (Sol) Apply bid-tid. Use least amount effective for condition.

HOW SUPPLIED: Cre, Oint: 0.1% [15g, 45g]; Sol: 0.1% [20mL, 60mL]

WARNINGS/PRECAUTIONS: May produce reversible HPA axis suppression, manifestations of Cushing's syndrome, hyperglycemia, and glucosuria. D/C if irritation occurs. Use appropriate antifungal or antibacterial agent with dermatological infections. Pediatric patients may be more susceptible to systemic toxicity. Caution when applied to large surface areas. Avoid contact with eyes. Limit to smallest amount compatible with an effective therapeutic regimen. Chronic corticosteroid therapy may interfere with the growth and development of children; use least amount effective for condition.

ADVERSE REACTIONS: Burning, itching, irritation, dryness, folliculitis, hypertrichosis, acneiform eruptions, hypopigmentation, perioral dermatitis, allergic dermatitis, skin maceration, secondary infection, skin atrophy, striae, miliaria.

PREGNANCY: Category C, caution in nursing.

MECHANISM OF ACTION: Corticosteroid; possesses anti-inflammatory, anti-pruritic, and vaso-constrictive properties. Anti-inflammatory actions not established.

PHARMACOKINETICS: Absorption: Percutaneous; inflammation, other disease states, and occlusive dressings may increase absorption. **Distribution:** Bound to plasma proteins to varying degrees. Systemically administered corticosteroids found in breast milk. **Metabolism:** Liver. **Elimination:** Renal (major), bile.

NURSING CONSIDERATIONS

Assessment: Assess for severity of infection and use in pregnant/nursing patients.

Monitoring: Monitor for signs/symptoms dermatological infections (eg, fungal, bacterial). For patients on large doses or in patients using occlusive dressings, perform periodic monitoring for HPA-axis suppression using urinary free cortisol and ACTH stimulation tests. Monitor for signs/symptoms of systemic toxicity in pediatrics.

Patient Counseling: Counsel to use externally and exactly as directed; avoid contact with eyes. Report signs of adverse reactions; do not bandage, cover or wrap treated skin area. Inform care-givers of pediatric patients to avoid using tight-fitting diapers or plastic pants on treatment area.

Administration: Topical route. **Storage:** Cre: 15-25°C (59-77°F), Oint: 2-30°C (36-86°F), Sol: 5-25°C (41-77°F).

LOESTRIN 21   RX
norethindrone acetate - ethinyl estradiol (Duramed)

> Cigarette smoking increases the risk of serious cardiovascular (CV) side effects. Risk increases with age (>35 yrs) and with heavy smoking (≥15 cigarettes/day). Women who use oral contraceptives should be strongly advised not to smoke.

OTHER BRAND NAMES: Junel 1.5/30 (Barr) - Junel 1/20 (Barr) - Microgestin 1/20 (Watson) - Microgestin 1.5/30 (Watson) - Loestrin 21 1.5/30 (Duramed) - Loestrin 21 1/20 (Duramed)

THERAPEUTIC CLASS: Estrogen/progestogen combination

INDICATIONS: Prevention of pregnancy.

DOSAGE: *Adults:* 1 tab qd for 21 days, stop 7 days, then repeat. Start 1st Sunday after menses begin or the 1st day of menses.
Pediatrics: Postpubertal: 1 tab qd for 21 days, stop 7 days, then repeat. Start 1st Sunday after menses begin or the 1st day of menses.

HOW SUPPLIED: Tab: (Ethinyl Estradiol-Norethindrone) (1/20) 20mcg-1mg, (1.5/30) 30mcg-1.5mg

CONTRAINDICATIONS: Thrombophlebitis, thromboembolic disorders, past history of deep vein thrombophlebitis or thromboembolic disorders, cerebral vascular or coronary artery disease (CAD), known or suspected carcinoma of the breast, carcinoma of the endometrium or other known or suspected estrogen-dependent neoplasia, undiagnosed abnormal genital bleeding, cholestatic jaundice of pregnancy or jaundice with prior pill use, hepatic adenomas or carcinomas, and pregnancy.

WARNINGS/PRECAUTIONS: Increased risk of myocardial infarction (MI), thromboembolism, stroke, hepatic neoplasia, gallbladder disease, and vascular disease. Increased risk of morbidity and mortality with HTN, hyperlipidemia, obesity, and diabetes. Caution in women with CV disease risk factors. Start use ≤4-6 weeks postpartum if not breastfeeding. May increase risk of breast cancer and cancer of the reproductive organs. Retinal thrombosis reported; d/c if unexplained partial or complete loss of vision occurs, onset of proptosis or diplopia, papilledema, or retinal vascular lesions develop. Should not be used to induce withdrawal bleeding as a test for pregnancy, or to treat threatened or habitual abortion during pregnancy. May cause glucose intolerance; monitor prediabetic and diabetic patients. May elevate BP; monitor closely and d/c use if significant BP elevation occurs. New onset/exacerbation of migraine, or recurrent, persistent, severe headache may develop; d/c therapy if these occur. Breakthrough bleeding and spotting reported; rule out malignancy or pregnancy. May cause serum TG or other lipid changes (eg, elevated LDL). May be poorly metabolized with impaired liver function; d/c if jaundice develops. May cause fluid retention; caution with conditions that aggravate fluid retention. Caution with history of depression; d/c if depression recurs to serious degree. May develop changes in vision or lens tolerance in contact lens wearers. Does not protect against HIV infection (AIDS) and other sexually transmitted diseases (STDs). Perform annual history and physical exam. Use before menarche is not indicated. May affect certain endocrine, LFTs, and blood components in laboratory tests.

ADVERSE REACTIONS: N/V, breakthrough bleeding, spotting, amenorrhea, migraine, mental depression, vaginal candidiasis, edema, weight changes, abdominal cramps/bloating, menstrual flow changes, melasma.

INTERACTIONS: Reduced effects, increased breakthrough bleeding, and menstrual irregularities with rifampin. Reduced effects and increased incidence of breakthrough bleeding with phenylbutazone. Increased metabolism and reduced contraceptive effectiveness with anticonvulsants (phenobarbital, phenytoin, carbamazepine). Pregnancy reported with antimicrobials (ampicillin, griseofulvin, and tetracyclines). Increased levels with atorvastatin, ascorbic acid, and acetaminophen (APAP). Increased plasma levels of cyclosporine, prednisolone, and theophylline. Decreased levels of APAP. Increased clearance of temazepam, salicylic acid, morphine, and clofibric acid. Reduced plasma levels with troglitazone resulting in reduced contraceptive effectiveness.

PREGNANCY: Category X, not for use in nursing.

MECHANISM OF ACTION: Estrogen/progestogen oral contraceptive; acts by suppressing gonadotropins, primarily inhibiting ovulation, and causing other alterations, including changes in cervical mucus (increases difficulty of sperm entry into uterus) and endometrium (reduces likelihood of implantation).

PHARMACOKINETICS: Absorption: Ethinyl Estradiol: Absolute bioavailability (43%). Norethindrone: Rapid and complete. Absolute bioavailability (64%). **Distribution:** V_d=2-4L/kg; plasma protein binding (>95%); found in breast milk. **Metabolism:** Ethinyl Estradiol: Extensive via CYP3A4; oxidation, sulfate/glucuronide conjugation; 2-hydroxy ethinyl estradiol (primary oxidative metabolite). Norethindrone: Extensive; reduction, sulfate/glucuronide conjugation. **Elimination:** Urine, feces.

NURSING CONSIDERATIONS

Assessment: Assess for presence or history of breast cancer, estrogen dependent neoplasia, abnormal genital bleeding, active liver disease, and known/suspected pregnancy or any other conditions where treatment is cautioned or contraindicated. Assess use in patients who are >35 yrs and heavy smokers (≥15 cigarettes/day). Assess use with HTN, hyperlipidemias, obesity, DM, or in patients at increased risk for thrombosis. Assess for possible drug interactions.

Monitoring: Monitor for bleeding irregularities, thromboembolic events, onset or exacerbation of headaches or migraines, and ectopic pregnancy. Monitor fasting blood glucose levels in DM and prediabetic patients, BP with history of HTN, lipid levels with a history of hyperlipidemia. Monitor for signs of liver dysfunction (eg, jaundice) and signs of depression with previous history. Refer patients with contact lenses to an ophthalmologist if visual changes occur. Perform annual history and physical exam.

Patient Counseling: Counsel about potential adverse effects. Inform that drug does not protect against HIV infection and other STDs. Instruct to use additional method of protection until after the 1st week of administration in the initial cycle when utilizing the Sunday-Start Regimen. Instruct to take exactly as directed and at intervals not exceeding 24 hrs. Take drug regularly with meal or hs; if dose is missed, take as soon as remembered, then take next dose at regularly scheduled time; continue regimen if spotting or breakthrough bleeding occurs; notify physician if bleeding persists. Avoid smoking while on medication.

Administration: Oral route. Refer to PI for special notes on administration. **Storage:** 20-25°C (68-77°F).

LOFIBRA   RX
fenofibrate (Gate)

THERAPEUTIC CLASS: Fibric acid derivative

INDICATIONS: Adjunct to diet for treatment of adults with hypertriglyceridemia (Fredrickson Types IV and V hyperlipidemia) and for the reduction of LDL, total-C, TG, and apolipoprotein B in adults with primary hypercholesterolemia or mixed dyslipidemia (Fredrickson Types IIa and IIb).

(Tab) Adjunct to diet to increase HDL-C in adults with primary hypercholesterolemia or mixed dyslipidemia (Fredrickson Types IIa and IIb).

DOSAGE: *Adults:* Primary Hypercholesterolemia/Mixed Hyperlipidemia: Initial: (Cap) 200mg/day. (Tab) 160mg/day. Hypertriglyceridemia: Individualize dose. Initial: (Cap) 67-200mg/day. (Tab) 54-160mg qd. Titrate: Adjust PRN after repeat lipid levels at 4-8 week intervals. Max: (Cap) 200mg/day. (Tab) 160mg/day. Renal Dysfunction: Initial: (Cap) 67mg/day. (Tab) 54mg/day. Increase only after evaluation of the effects on renal function and lipid levels at this dose. Elderly: Initial: (Cap) Limit to 67mg/day. (Tab) Limit to 54mg/day. Consider lowering dose if lipid levels fall significantly below targeted range.

HOW SUPPLIED: Cap: 67mg, 134mg, 200mg; Tab: 54mg, 160mg

CONTRAINDICATIONS: Hepatic or severe renal dysfunction (including primary biliary cirrhosis and unexplained persistent liver function abnormality), preexisting gallbladder disease.

WARNINGS/PRECAUTIONS: Hepatocellular, chronic active and cholestatic hepatitis and cirrhosis (rare) reported. Increases in serum transaminases (AST or ALT) reported; monitor LFTs regularly and d/c if enzyme level persists to >3X ULN. May cause cholelithiasis; d/c if gallstones found. May cause myositis, myopathy, or rhabdomyolysis; determine serum creatine kinase (CK) level if muscle pain, tenderness, or weakness occur; d/c if myopathy/myositis is suspected/diagnosed or marked CPK elevation occurs. Control lipids with appropriate diet, exercise, and weight loss in obese patients and control any medical problems (eg, diabetes mellitus, hypothyroidism) that are contributing to lipid abnormalities prior to therapy. Measure lipid levels prior to therapy and during initial treatment; d/c if inadequate response after 2 months on max dose of 200mg/day (Cap) or 145 mg/day (Tab). Acute hypersensitivity reactions (rare) and pancreatitis reported. Mild to moderate decrease in Hgb, Hct, and WBCs reported; periodically monitor CBC during the first 12 months of therapy. Thrombocytopenia and agranulocytosis reported (rare). Caution in renally impaired elderly. (Tab) Pulmonary embolus, deep vein thrombosis, and elevated SrCr observed.

ADVERSE REACTIONS: Abnormal LFTs, abdominal/pain, respiratory disorder, back pain, increases in ALT or AST, headache, increased CPK.

INTERACTIONS: Caution with anticoagulants due to potentiation of coumarin/coumarin-type anticoagulants; reduce anticoagulant dose to maintain desirable PT/INR. Avoid HMG-CoA reductase inhibitors unless benefits outweigh risks; rhabdomyolysis, markedly elevated CK levels, and myoglobinuria leading to acute renal failure reported. Bile acid sequestrants may impede absorption; take at least 1 hr before or 4-6 hrs after bile acid binding resin. Evaluate benefits/risks with immunosuppressants (eg, cyclosporine) and other nephrotoxic agents; use lowest effective dose. Prior to therapy, d/c or change if possible, medications that are known to exacerbate hypertriglyceridemia (eg, beta-blockers, thiazides, estrogens). (Tab) Increased plasma concentrations with pravastatin, glimepiride, and fluvastatin. Decreased plasma concentrations with atorvastatin.

PREGNANCY: Category C, not for use in nursing.

MECHANISM OF ACTION: Fibric acid derivative; activates peroxisome proliferator activated receptor α (PPARα), increasing lipolysis and elimination of TG-rich particles from plasma by activating lipoprotein lipase and reducing production of apoprotein C-III. Activation of PPARα induces an increase in the synthesis of apoproteins A-I, A-II, and HDL.

PHARMACOKINETICS: Absorption: Well absorbed; T_{max}=6-8 hrs. **Distribution:** Plasma protein binding (99%). **Metabolism:** Rapid, via hydrolysis by esterases to fenofibric acid (active metabolite), conjugation. **Elimination:** Urine (60% metabolite), feces (25%); $T_{1/2}$=20 hrs.

NURSING CONSIDERATIONS

Assessment: Assess for hypersensitivity, hepatic/renal impairment, pre-existing gallbladder disease, severe hypertriglyceridemia, pregnancy/nursing status, and possible drug interactions. Assess for body weight and alcohol intake. Obtain CPK, lipid levels and LFTs prior to therapy.

Monitoring: Monitor for signs/symptoms of myositis, myopathy, and rhabdomyolysis; measure serum creatine kinase levels if myopathy is suspected. Monitor for signs/symptoms of increases in serum transaminases, hepatitis, and cirrhosis; perform periodic monitoring of LFTs. Monitor for signs/symptoms of cholelithiasis; perform gallbladder studies if cholelithiasis is suspected. Monitor for signs/symptoms of pancreatitis, hypersensitivity reactions, (Tab) PE and DVT. Periodically monitor blood counts (eg, Hgb, Hct, and WBC) and lipid levels.

Patient Counseling: Inform of risks/benefits of therapy. Advise to immediately notify physician if unexplained muscle pain, tenderness, or weakness, with malaise or fever occur. Recommend appropriate lipid-lowering diet.

Administration: Oral route. Place on an appropriate lipid-lowering diet before treatment, and continue diet during treatment. Take with meals. **Storage:** 20-25°C (68-77°F). Protect from moisture.

LOMOTIL
diphenoxylate HCl - atropine sulfate (Pfizer)

THERAPEUTIC CLASS: Opioid/anticholinergic

INDICATIONS: Adjunctive therapy for management of diarrhea.

DOSAGE: *Adults:* Initial: 2 tabs or 10mL qid. Titrate: Reduce dose after symptoms are controlled. Maint: 2 tabs or 10mL qd. Max: 20mg/day diphenoxylate. D/C if symptoms not controlled after 10 days at max dose of 20mg/day (diphenoxylate).
Pediatrics: 2-12 yrs: Initial: 0.3-0.4mg/kg/day of solution in four divided doses. Titrate: Reduce dose after symptoms are controlled. Maint: May be as low as 25% of initial dose. D/C if no improvement within 48 hrs.

HOW SUPPLIED: (Diphenoxylate-Atropine) Sol: 2.5mg-0.025mg/5mL [60mL]; Tab: 2.5mg-0.025mg

CONTRAINDICATIONS: Obstructive jaundice, diarrhea associated with pseudomembranous enterocolitis or enterotoxin-producing bacteria.

WARNINGS/PRECAUTIONS: Avoid in children <2 yrs. Overdosage may result in severe respiratory depression and coma, leading to brain damage or death. Avoid use with severe dehydration or electrolyte imbalance until corrective therapy is initiated. May induce toxic megacolon with acute ulcerative colitis; d/c if abdominal distention occurs or untoward symptoms develop. May cause intestinal fluid retention. Avoid with diarrhea associated with organisms that penetrate the intestinal mucosa, and with pseudomembranous enterocolitis. Extreme caution with advanced hepatorenal disease and liver dysfunction. Caution in pediatrics, especially with Down's syndrome.

ADVERSE REACTIONS: Numbness of extremities, dizziness, anaphylaxis, drowsiness, toxic megacolon, N/V, urticaria, pruritus, anorexia, pancreatitis, paralytic ileus, euphoria, malaise/lethargy.

INTERACTIONS: MAOIs may precipitate hypertensive crisis. (Diphenoxylate) May potentiate barbiturates, tranquilizers, and alcohol. Potential to prolong $T_{1/2}$ of drugs for which the rate of elimination is dependent on the microsomal drug metabolizing enzyme system.

PREGNANCY: Category C, caution in nursing.

MECHANISM OF ACTION: Diphenoxylate: Antidiarrheal. Atropine: Anticholinergic.

PHARMACOKINETICS: Absorption: (4 tabs) C_{max}=163ng/mL; T_{max}=2 hrs. **Metabolism:** Rapid and extensive metabolism through ester hydrolysis to diphenoxylic acid (major metabolite). **Elimination:** Urine (14%), feces (49%). $T_{1/2}$=12-14 hrs (diphenoxylic acid).

NURSING CONSIDERATIONS

Assessment: Assess for hypersensitivity, obstructive jaundice, diarrhea associated with pseudomembranous enterocolitis or enterotoxin-producing bacteria, severe dehydration, electrolyte imbalance, hepatic dysfunction, hepatorenal disease, ulcerative colitis, Down's syndrome, diarrhea (caused by *Escherichia coli*, *Salmonella*, *Shigella*), pregnancy/nursing status, and possible drug interactions.

Monitoring: Monitor for severe dehydration, electrolyte imbalance, renal function, toxic megacolon in ulcerative colitis, abdominal distention, signs of atropinism, and other adverse reactions.

Patient Counseling: Instruct to take as directed and not to exceed the recommended dosage. Inform of consequences of overdosage, including severe respiratory depression and coma, possibly leading to permanent brain damage or death. Instruct to exercise caution while operating machinery/driving. Advise to avoid alcohol and other CNS depressants. Advise to keep medicines out of reach of children. Inform patient that drowsiness or dizziness may occur.

Administration: Oral route. Plastic dropper should be used when measuring liquid for administration to children. **Storage:** Dispense liquids in original container.

LOPID
gemfibrozil (Parke-Davis)

THERAPEUTIC CLASS: Fibric acid derivative

INDICATIONS: Adjunctive therapy to diet for treatment of Types IV and V hyperlipidemia with risk of pancreatitis not responding to dietary management (usually TG >2000mg/dL). May consider therapy if TG 1000-2000mg/dL with history of pancreatitis or recurrent abdominal pain typical of pancreatitis. Risk reduction of coronary artery disease in Type IIb patients without history or symptoms of existing coronary heart disease inadequately responding to weight loss, dietary therapy, exercise, and other pharmacologic agents and with triad of low HDL, and elevated LDL, and TG levels.

L

DOSAGE: *Adults:* 600mg bid. Give 30 min before am and pm meals.

HOW SUPPLIED: Tab: 600mg* *scored

CONTRAINDICATIONS: Hepatic or severe renal dysfunction including primary biliary cirrhosis, pre-existing gallbladder disease, combination therapy with repaglinide.

WARNINGS/PRECAUTIONS: Cholelithiasis reported. May be associated with myositis. D/C if myositis and gallstones suspected/diagnosed, abnormal LFTs persist, and significant lipid response not obtained. Severe anemia, leukopenia, thrombocytopenia, and bone marrow hypoplasia (rare) reported; monitor blood counts periodically during 1st 12 months. May worsen renal insufficiency. Control serum lipids with appropriate diet, exercise, and weight loss in obese patients, and other medical problems that contribute to lipid abnormalities (eg, diabetes mellitus [DM], hypothyroidism) prior to therapy.

ADVERSE REACTIONS: Dyspepsia, abdominal pain, diarrhea, fatigue, bacterial and viral infections, musculoskeletal symptoms, abnormal LFTs, hematologic changes, hypesthesia, paresthesia, taste perversion.

INTERACTIONS: See Contraindications. Caution with anticoagulants; reduce anticoagulant dose and monitor PT. Increased risk of myopathy and rhabdomyolysis with HMG-CoA reductase inhibitors. Reduced exposure with resin-granule drugs (eg, colestipol); spaced dosing required.

PREGNANCY: Category C, not for use in nursing.

MECHANISM OF ACTION: Fibric acid derivative; not established. Suspected to inhibit peripheral lipolysis, decrease hepatic extraction of free fatty acids, thus reducing hepatic TG production and inhibiting synthesis and increasing clearance of VLDL carrier apolipoprotein B, leading to decreased VLDL production.

PHARMACOKINETICS: Absorption: Complete; T_{max}=1-2 hrs. **Metabolism:** Oxidation to form hydroxymethyl and carboxyl metabolites. **Elimination:** Urine (70%, <2% unchanged), feces (6%).

NURSING CONSIDERATIONS

Assessment: Assess for hepatic/renal dysfunction, primary biliary cirrhosis, gallbladder disease, consistent abnormal lipid levels, DM, hypothyroidism, coronary heart disease, previous hypersensitivity to drug, pregnancy/nursing status, and possible drug interactions.

Monitoring: Monitor for development of myositis, cholelithiasis, gallstones, and cataracts. Periodically monitor serum lipids and creatine kinase levels, CBC, LFTs, and renal function.

Patient Counseling: Inform about potential risks/benefits of therapy. Advise to report signs of myositis (eg, muscle pain, tenderness, or weakness). Notify physician if pregnant/nursing or planning to become pregnant.

Administration: Oral route. **Storage:** 20-25°C (68-77°F). Protect from light and humidity.

LOPRESSOR   RX
metoprolol tartrate (Novartis)

Exacerbation of angina and myocardial infarction (MI) reported following abrupt d/c. When d/c chronic therapy, particularly with ischemic heart disease, taper over 1-2 weeks with careful monitoring. If worsening of angina or acute coronary insufficiency develop, reinstate therapy promptly, at least temporarily, and take other appropriate measures. Avoid interruption or d/c of therapy without physician's advice.

THERAPEUTIC CLASS: Selective beta$_1$-blocker

INDICATIONS: (Tab) Treatment of HTN alone or in combination with other antihypertensives. Long-term treatment of angina pectoris. (Inj/Tab) To reduce cardiovascular mortality in hemodynamically stable patients with definite or suspected acute MI.

DOSAGE: *Adults:* HTN: Individualize dose. Initial: 100mg/day PO in single or divided doses given alone or with a diuretic. Titrate: May increase at weekly (or longer) intervals. Usual: 100-450mg/day. Max: 450mg/day. Angina: Individualize dose. Initial: 100mg/day PO in 2 divided doses. Titrate: Increase weekly until optimum clinical response is achieved or pronounced slowing of HR. Usual: 100-400mg/day. Max: 400mg/day. Upon d/c, taper gradually over 1-2 weeks. MI (Early Phase): 5mg IV bolus q2 min for 3 doses (monitor BP, HR, and ECG). If tolerated, give 50mg PO q6h for 48 hrs. Maint: 100mg bid. If not tolerated, give 25-50mg PO q6h. D/C if with severe intolerance. Initiate PO dose 15 min after last IV dose. MI (Late Phase): 100mg bid for ≥3 months. Elderly: Start at lower end of dosing range. Take tab with or immediately following meals.

HOW SUPPLIED: Inj: 1mg/mL [5mL]; Tab: 50mg*, 100mg* *scored

CONTRAINDICATIONS: (Tab) Sinus bradycardia, >1st-degree heart block, cardiogenic shock, overt cardiac failure, sick sinus syndrome, severe peripheral arterial circulatory disorders. (Inj/Tab) HR <45 beats/min, 2nd- and 3rd-degree heart block, significant 1st-degree heart block, systolic BP <100mmHg, moderate to severe cardiac failure.

WARNINGS/PRECAUTIONS: Caution in hypertensive and angina patients who have congestive heart failure (CHF) controlled by digitalis and diuretics. Continued myocardial depression may lead to cardiac failure; d/c if cardiac failure continues despite adequate digitalization and diuretic therapy. Avoid with bronchospastic diseases. Avoid withdrawal prior to major surgery. May mask tachycardia occurring with hypoglycemia; caution in diabetics. May cause paradoxical increase in BP with pheochromocytoma if administered alone; always initiate α-blocker before starting therapy. May mask clinical signs of hyperthyroidism; if suspected to develop thyrotoxicosis, avoid abrupt withdrawal. May decrease sinus HR or slow atrioventricular (AV) conduction; d/c if heart failure/block occur or atropine therapy fails. Hypotension may occur; d/c therapy, assess hemodynamic status and extent of myocardial damage. Caution with impaired hepatic function and in elderly.

ADVERSE REACTIONS: Bradycardia, tiredness, dizziness, depression, SOB, diarrhea, pruritus, rash, heart block, heart failure, hypotension.

INTERACTIONS: Additive effects with catecholamine-depleting drugs (eg, reserpine). May block epinephrine effects. Caution with digitalis; both agents slow AV conduction and decrease HR. May enhance cardiodepressant effect with some inhalational anesthetics. May increase levels with potent CYP2D6 inhibitors (eg, antidepressants, antipsychotics, antiarrhythmics, antiretrovirals, antihistamines, antimalarials, antifungals, stomach ulcer drugs); caution when coadministering. When given concomitantly with clonidine, d/c several days before clonidine is withdrawn.

PREGNANCY: Category C, caution in nursing.

MECHANISM OF ACTION: β-blocker; not established. Proposed to competitively antagonize catecholamines at peripheral adrenergic-neuronal sites; has central effect leading to reduced sympathetic outflow to periphery and suppression of renin activity.

PHARMACOKINETICS: Absorption: Rapid, complete. **Distribution:** Found in breast milk. **Metabolism:** Liver (extensive) via CYP2D6 (oxidation). **Elimination:** PO: Urine (<5%, unchanged), IV: Urine (10%, unchanged); $T_{1/2}$=2.8 hrs (extensive metabolizers); $T_{1/2}$=7.5 hrs (poor metabolizers).

NURSING CONSIDERATIONS

Assessment: Assess for sinus bradycardia, heart block, cardiogenic shock, cardiac failure, CHF, ischemic heart disease, bronchospastic diseases, hyperthyroidism, diabetes mellitus, sick sinus syndrome, severe peripheral arterial circulatory disorders, pheochromocytoma, hepatic function, hypersensitivity to the drug, pregnancy/nursing status, and possible drug interactions. Obtain baseline BP, HR, and ECG.

Monitoring: Monitor BP, HR, ECG and hemodynamic status periodically. Monitor for signs/symptoms of cardiac failure, hypoglycemia, thyrotoxicosis, withdrawal symptoms (angina, MI), hypotension, and hypersensitivity reactions. Monitor patients with ischemic heart disease.

Patient Counseling: Instruct to take regularly and continuously, as directed, with or immediately following meals. If a dose is missed, take next dose at scheduled time (without doubling). Avoid d/c without consulting physician. Caution in tasks requiring alertness (eg, operating machinery/driving). Contact physician before any surgery or if difficulty of breathing, or other adverse reactions occur.

Administration: Oral, IV route. (Inj) Inspect for particulate matter and discoloration prior to administration. **Storage:** 25°C (77°F); excursions permitted to 15-30°C (59-86°F). (Tab) Protect from moisture. (Inj) Protect from light.

LORCET CIII
hydrocodone bitartrate - acetaminophen (Forest)

> Associated with cases of acute liver failure, at times resulting in liver transplant and death. Most cases associated with acetaminophen (APAP) doses >4000 mg/day and involved more than one APAP-containing product.

OTHER BRAND NAMES: Lorcet Plus (Forest)

THERAPEUTIC CLASS: Opioid analgesic

INDICATIONS: Relief of moderate to moderately severe pain.

DOSAGE: *Adults:* Adjust dose according to severity of pain and response. Usual: 1 tab q4-6h PRN for pain. Max: 6 tabs/day. Elderly: Start at lower end of dosing range.

HOW SUPPLIED: Tab: (Hydrocodone-APAP) 10mg-650mg*, (Plus) 7.5mg-650mg* *scored

WARNINGS/PRECAUTIONS: May produce dose-related respiratory depression and irregular/periodic breathing. Respiratory depressant effects and elevation of CSF pressure may be exaggerated in the presence of head injury, other intracranial lesions, or a preexisting increase in intracranial pressure. May obscure diagnosis or clinical course of acute abdominal conditions or head injuries. Hypersensitivity/anaphylaxis reported; d/c if signs/symptoms occur. Caution in elderly, debilitated, severe hepatic/renal dysfunction, hypothyroidism, Addison's disease, prostatic hypertrophy, and urethral stricture. Increased risk of acute liver failure in patients with underlying liver disease. May be habit-forming. Suppresses cough reflex; caution with pulmonary disease and postoperative use.

ADVERSE REACTIONS: Acute liver failure, dizziness, lightheadedness, sedation, N/V.

INTERACTIONS: Additive CNS depression with other narcotics, antianxiety agents, antihistamines, antipsychotics, other CNS depressants (eg, alcohol); reduce dose. Increased effect of antidepressants or hydrocodone with MAOIs or TCAs. Increased risk of acute liver failure with alcohol ingestion.

PREGNANCY: Category C, not for use in nursing.

MECHANISM OF ACTION: Hydrocodone: Narcotic analgesic and antitussive; not established. Suspected to relate to existence of opiate receptors in the CNS. APAP: Nonopiate, nonsalicylate analgesic and antipyretic; not established. Antipyretic activity is mediated through hypothalamic heat regulating centers; inhibits prostaglandin synthetase.

PHARMACOKINETICS: Absorption: Hydrocodone: (10mg) C_{max}=23.6ng/mL; T_{max}=1.3 hrs. APAP: Rapid. **Distribution:** APAP: Found in breast milk. **Metabolism:** Hydrocodone: O-demethylation, N-demethylation, and 6-keto reduction. APAP: Liver (conjugation). **Elimination:** Hydrocodone: $T_{1/2}$=3.8 hrs. APAP: Urine (85%); $T_{1/2}$=1.25-3 hrs.

NURSING CONSIDERATIONS

Assessment: Assess for level of pain intensity, type of pain, patient's general condition and medical status, or any other conditions where treatment is contraindicated or cautioned. Assess for history of hypersensitivity, pregnancy/nursing status, renal/hepatic function, and possible drug interactions.

Monitoring: Monitor for signs/symptoms of hypersensitivity reactions, respiratory depression, elevated CSF pressure, drug dependence, and drug abuse. Monitor serial hepatic/renal function tests with severe hepatic/renal disease.

Patient Counseling: Instruct to d/c and seek medical attention if signs of allergy (eg, rash, difficulty breathing) develop. Instruct patients to not use more than one APAP-containing product. Inform to not take >4000mg/day of APAP, and to seek medical attention if take more than the recommended dose. Advise that medication may impair mental/physical abilities; avoid hazardous tasks (eg, operating machinery/driving). Instruct not to take with alcohol/other CNS depressants. Counsel that drug may be habit-forming and instruct to take ud.

Administration: Oral route. **Storage:** 20-25°C (68-77°F).

LORTAB   CIII
hydrocodone bitartrate - acetaminophen (UCB)

> Associated with cases of acute liver failure, at times resulting in liver transplant and death. Most cases associated with acetaminophen (APAP) doses >4000 mg/day and involved more than one APAP-containing product.

OTHER BRAND NAMES: Hycet (Eclat)

THERAPEUTIC CLASS: Opioid analgesic

INDICATIONS: Relief of moderate to moderately severe pain.

DOSAGE: *Adults:* Adjust dose according to severity of pain and response. (5mg-500mg) Usual: 1 or 2 tabs q4-6h PRN. Max: 8 tabs/day. (7.5mg-500mg, 10mg-500mg) Usual: 1 tab q4-6h PRN. Max: 6 tabs/day. (Sol) Usual: 1 tbsp q4-6h PRN. Max: 6 tbsp/day. Elderly: Start at lower end of dosing range.
Pediatrics: ≥2 yrs: Adjust dose according to severity of pain and response. (Sol) Usual: Give q4-6h PRN. ≥46kg: 1 tbsp. Max: 6 tbsp/day. 32-45kg: 2 tsp. Max: 12 tsp/day. 23-31kg: 1 1/2 tsp. Max: 9 tsp/day. 16-22kg: 1 tsp. Max: 6 tsp/day. 12-15kg: 3/4 tsp. Max: 4 1/2 tsp/day.

HOW SUPPLIED: (Hydrocodone-APAP) Sol: (Hycet) 7.5mg-325mg/15mL, (Lortab) 7.5mg-500mg/15mL; Tab: (Lortab) 5mg-500mg*, 7.5mg-500mg*, 10mg-500mg* *scored

WARNINGS/PRECAUTIONS: May produce dose-related respiratory depression, and irregular/periodic breathing. Respiratory depressant effects and elevation of CSF pressure may be exaggerated in the presence of head injury, other intracranial lesions, or preexisting increase in intracranial pressure. May obscure diagnosis or clinical course of acute abdominal conditions or head injuries. Hypersensitivity/anaphylaxis reported; d/c if signs/symptoms occur. Caution in elderly, debilitated, severe hepatic or renal dysfunction, hypothyroidism, Addison's disease, prostatic hypertrophy, and urethral stricture. Increased risk of acute liver failure in patients with underlying liver disease. Suppresses cough reflex; caution with pulmonary disease and postoperative use. May be habit-forming. (Sol) Infants may have increased sensitivity to respiratory depression; administer cautiously in substantially reduced initial doses by personnel experienced in administering opioids to infants, and monitor intensively.

ADVERSE REACTIONS: Acute liver failure, lightheadedness, dizziness, sedation, N/V.

INTERACTIONS: Additive CNS depression with other narcotics, antihistamines, antipsychotics, antianxiety agents, or other CNS depressants (including alcohol); reduce dose. Increased effect of antidepressants or hydrocodone with MAOIs or TCAs. Increased risk of acute liver failure with alcohol ingestion.

PREGNANCY: Category C, not for use in nursing.

MECHANISM OF ACTION: Hydrocodone: Narcotic analgesic and antitussive; not established. Suspected to relate to existence of opiate receptors in CNS. APAP: Nonopiate, nonsalicylate analgesic and antipyretic; not established. Antipyretic activity is mediated through hypothalamic heat-regulating centers; inhibits prostaglandin synthetase.

PHARMACOKINETICS: Absorption: Hydrocodone: (10mg) C_{max}=23.6ng/mL; T_{max}=1.3 hrs. APAP: Rapid. **Distribution:** Hydrocodone: Crosses placenta. APAP: Found in breast milk. **Metabolism:** Hydrocodone: O-demethylation, N-demethylation, and 6-keto reduction. APAP: Liver (conjugation). **Elimination:** Hydrocodone: $T_{1/2}$=3.8 hrs. APAP: Urine (85%); $T_{1/2}$=1.25-3 hrs.

NURSING CONSIDERATIONS

Assessment: Assess for level of pain intensity, type of pain, patient's general condition and medical status, or any other conditions where treatment is contraindicated or cautioned. Assess for history of hypersensitivity, pregnancy/nursing status, renal/hepatic function, and possible drug interactions.

Monitoring: Monitor for signs/symptoms of hypersensitivity reactions, respiratory depression, elevated CSF pressure, drug dependence, and drug abuse. Monitor serial hepatic/renal function tests with severe hepatic/renal disease.

Patient Counseling: Instruct to d/c and seek medical attention if signs of allergy (eg, rash, difficulty breathing) develop. Instruct patients to not use more than one APAP-containing product. Inform to not take >4000mg/day of APAP, and to seek medical attention if take more than the recommended dose. Advise that medication may impair mental/physical abilities; avoid hazardous tasks (eg, operating machinery/driving). Instruct not to take with alcohol/other CNS depressants. Counsel that drug may be habit-forming and instruct to take ud.

Administration: Oral route. **Storage:** 20-25°C (68-77°F).

LOSEASONIQUE   RX
ethinyl estradiol - levonorgestrel (Duramed)

Cigarette smoking increases the risk of serious CV events from combination oral contraceptive (COC) use. This risk increases with age and with number of cigarettes smoked. Women who are >35 yrs and smoke should not use COCs.

THERAPEUTIC CLASS: Estrogen/progestogen combination

INDICATIONS: Prevention of pregnancy.

DOSAGE: *Adults:* 1 tablet qd for 91 days. Begin taking on first Sunday after the onset of menstruation. If menses begin on Sunday, start on that day. Use non-hormonal back-up method of contraception (eg, condoms, spermicide) until levonorgestrel-ethinyl estradiol tablet has been taken daily for 7 consecutive days. Begin next and all subsequent 91 day cycles without interruption on same day of week (Sunday) upon which first course began, following the same schedule. Postpartum women should start COC no earlier than 4-6 weeks postpartum.
Pediatrics: Postpubertal: 1 tablet qd for 91 days. Begin taking on first Sunday after the onset of menstruation. If menses begin on Sunday, start on that day. Use non-hormonal back-up method of contraception (eg, condoms, spermicide) until levonorgestrel-ethinyl estradiol tablet has been taken daily for 7 consecutive days. Begin next and all subsequent 91 day cycles without interruption on same day of week (Sunday) upon which first course began, following the same schedule. Postpartum women should start COC no earlier than 4-6 weeks postpartum.

HOW SUPPLIED: Tab: (Ethinyl Estradiol-Levonorgestrel) 0.02mg-0.1mg; Tab: (Ethinyl Estradiol) 0.01mg.

CONTRAINDICATIONS: Patients with high risk of arterial or venous thrombotic diseases (eg, women who smoke, if over age 35; presence or history of deep vein thrombosis or pulmonary embolism; cerebrovascular or coronary artery disease; thrombogenic valvular or thrombogenic rhythm diseases of the heart; hypercoagulopathies; uncontrolled HTN; diabetes with vascular disease; headaches with focal neurological symptoms or migraine headaches with or without aura if over age 35), presence or history of breast cancer or other estrogen or progestin sensitive cancer, liver tumors (benign or malignant) or liver disease, and pregnancy.

WARNINGS/PRECAUTIONS: Increases the risk of venous thromboembolism, arterial thromboses (eg, stroke, MI); d/c if arterial or deep venous thrombotic event occurs. D/C if unexplained loss of vision, proptosis, diplopia, papilledema, or retinal vascular lesions occur; evaluate for retinal vein thrombosis. May increase risk of cervical cancer or intraepithelial neoplasia. D/C if jaundice develops. Increases risk of hepatic adenomas, hepatocellular carcinoma, and gallbladder disease.

Oral contraceptive cholestasis may occur in women with history of pregnancy related cholestasis. May cause HTN; d/c if BP rises significantly in women with history of well controlled HTN. May decrease glucose tolerance; monitor prediabetic and diabetic women. May affect lipid levels; consider alternate therapy in patients with uncontrolled dyslipidemias. Breakthrough bleeding and spotting may occur, especially during the first 3 months; if bleeding persists, check for causes. Amenorrhea may occur during use; check for pregnancy. Amenorrhea or oligomenorrhea may occur after d/c therapy. May change the results of some laboratory tests (eg, coagulation factors, lipids, glucose tolerance, binding proteins). May need to increase dose of thyroid hormone in patients on thyroid hormone replacement therapy.

ADVERSE REACTIONS: Headaches, irregular and/or heavy uterine bleeding, dysmenorrhea, N/V, back pain, breast tenderness, mood changes, acne, weight gain.

INTERACTIONS: Use with drugs or herbal products that induce enzymes, including CYP3A4, that metabolize contraceptive hormones, may decrease the plasma concentrations and the effectiveness of the hormonal contraceptive or cause breakthrough bleeding; counsel to use additional contraception or a different method of contraception. Barbiturates, bosentan, carbamazepine, felbamate, griseofulvin, oxcarbazepine, phenytoin, rifampin, St. John's wort, and topiramate may decrease contraceptive effectiveness. HIV protease inhibitors may increase or decrease levels. Reports of pregnancy with antibiotic use. Increased levels with atorvastatin, ascorbic acid, acetaminophen, and CYP3A4 inhibitors (eg, itraconazole, ketoconazole). Decreases levels of lamotrigine and may reduce seizure control; may require dosage adjustment of lamotrigine.

PREGNANCY: Safety not known in pregnancy, caution in nursing.

MECHANISM OF ACTION: Estrogen/progestogen combination oral contraceptive; primarily suppresses ovulation. Also responsible for causing changes in cervical mucus (increases difficulty in sperm entry into uterus) and endometrium (reduces likelihood of implantation).

PHARMACOKINETICS: Absorption: Rapid; Levonorgestrel: Absolute bioavailability (nearly 100%); T_{max} =1.6 hrs; C_{max} = 6.0ng/mL; AUC=76.5ng•hr/mL. Ethinyl estradiol: Absolute bioavailability (43%); T_{max}=1.8 hrs; C_{max}=122.8pg/mL; AUC=1335.8pg•hr/mL. **Distribution:** Found in breast milk; Levonorgestrel: V_d=1.8L/kg; plasma protein binding (97.5%-99%). Ethinyl estradiol: V_d=4.3L/kg; plasma protein binding (95%-97%). **Metabolism:** Levonorgestrel: Sulfate and glucuronide conjugates. Ethinyl estradiol: 1st past metabolism in gut wall, Hepatic, via CYP3A4 (hydroxylation), methylation, conjugation. **Elimination:** Levonorgestrel: Urine (45%), feces (32%); $T_{1/2}$=28.5 hrs. Ethinyl estradiol: Urine, feces; $T_{1/2}$=17.5 hrs.

NURSING CONSIDERATIONS

Assessment: Assess for presence or history of breast cancer, estrogen dependent neoplasia, abnormal genital bleeding, active liver disease, and known/suspected pregnancy or any other conditions where treatment is cautioned or contraindicated. Assess use in patients who are >35 yrs and heavy smokers (≥15 cigarettes/day). Assess use with HTN, hyperlipidemias, obesity, DM, or in patients at increased risk for thrombosis. Assess for possible drug interactions.

Monitoring: Monitor for signs/symptoms of venous thromboembolism, arterial thromboses (eg, stroke, MI), cervical cancer or intraepithelial neoplasia, retinal vein thrombosis, jaundice, hepatic adenomas, hepatocellular carcinoma, gallbladder disease, headaches, bleeding irregularities, and for interference with laboratory tests. Monitor glucose levels in DM or prediabetic patients. Monitor for HTN, cholestasis in women who have a history of pregnancy related cholestasis.

Patient Counseling: Inform that drug does not protect against HIV infection (AIDS) and other STDs. Advise not to smoke while on medication. Instruct to take medication by mouth at the same time everyday, and what to do in the event pills are missed. Counsel to use back-up or alternative method of contraception when enzyme inducers are used with COCs. Counsel COCs may reduce breast milk production. Counsel any patient who uses COCs postpartum, and have not yet had a period, to use an additional method of contraception until she has taken a levonorgestrel-ethinyl estradiol tablet for 7 consecutive days.

Administration: Oral route. **Storage:** 20-25°C (68-77°F).

LOTEMAX SUSPENSION   RX
loteprednol etabonate (Bausch & Lomb)

THERAPEUTIC CLASS: Corticosteroid

INDICATIONS: Treatment of inflammation of the palpebral and bulbar conjunctiva, cornea and anterior segment of the globe. Management of postoperative inflammation.

DOSAGE: *Adults:* Steroid-Responsive Disease: 1-2 drops qid, may increase up to 1 drop every hr within the 1st week of treatment. Re-evaluate after 2 days if no improvement. Postoperative: 1-2 drops qid starting 24 hrs postop and continue for 2 weeks.

HOW SUPPLIED: Sus: 0.5% [2.5mL, 5mL, 10mL, 15mL]

CONTRAINDICATIONS: Viral diseases of the cornea and conjunctiva including epithelial herpes simplex keratitis, vaccinia, and varicella. Mycobacterial infection and fungal diseases of the eye.

WARNINGS/PRECAUTIONS: Caution with glaucoma, history of herpes simplex, and diseases causing thinning of cornea/sclera. Prolonged use can cause glaucoma, optic nerve damage, defects in visual acuity and fields of vision, cataracts, or secondary ocular infections (eg, fungal). Monitor IOP after 10 days of therapy. Re-evaluate if no response after 2 days. May delay healing and increase incidence of bleb formation after cataract surgery. May mask or enhance existing infection in acute, purulent conditions.

ADVERSE REACTIONS: Elevated IOP, abnormal vision, chemosis, discharge, dry eyes, burning on instillation, epiphora, itching, photophobia, foreign body sensation, optic nerve damage, visual field defects.

PREGNANCY: Category C, caution in nursing.

MECHANISM OF ACTION: Glucocorticoid; anti-inflammatory agent. Not established; suspected to inhibit edema, fibrin deposition, capillary dilation and deposition of collagen and scar formation by the induction of phospholipase A_2 inhibitory proteins, lipocortins.

NURSING CONSIDERATIONS

Assessment: Assess for viral diseases of cornea and conjunctiva, dendritic keratitis, vaccinia, varicella, mycobacterial infection, fungal disease of ocular structures, glaucoma, thinning of corneal/scleral epithelium, hypersensitivity, cataract surgery.

Monitoring: Frequent measuring of IOP and slit lamp microscopy exam where appropriate, fluorescein staining for monitoring of glaucoma with damage to optic nerve with defects in visual acuity and fields of vision, posterior subscapsular cataract, delayed corneal healing, thinning of cornea and sclera, ulceration, perforation, secondary ocular infections or masking of existing infections.

Patient Counseling: Advise to d/c drug and notify physician if symptoms persist or worsen. Instruct to not wear soft contact lenses during treatment. Counsel to avoid touching bottle tip to eyelids or any other surface.

Administration: Ocular route. Shake vigorously before using. **Storage:** 15-25°C (59-77°F). Do not freeze.

L

LOTENSIN   RX
benazepril HCl (Novartis)

> D/C when pregnancy is detected. Drugs that act directly on the renin-angiotensin system can cause injury/death to the developing fetus.

THERAPEUTIC CLASS: ACE inhibitor

INDICATIONS: Treatment of HTN. May be used alone or in combination with thiazide diuretics.

DOSAGE: *Adults:* Not Receiving Diuretic: Initial: 10mg qd. Maint: 20-40mg/day as single dose or in 2 equally divided doses. Dose adjustment should be based on measurement of peak (2-6 hrs after dosing) and trough responses. If no adequate trough response when given qd, increase dose or consider divided administration. May add diuretic if BP not controlled. Max: 80mg/day. Currently Receiving Diuretic: D/C diuretic 2-3 days prior to therapy if possible. If Cannot D/C Diuretic: Initial: 5mg. CrCl <30mL/min: Initial: 5mg qd. May titrate upward until BP is controlled. Max: 40mg/day.
Pediatrics: ≥6 yrs: Initial: 0.2mg/kg qd. Max: 0.6mg/kg or 40mg/day.

HOW SUPPLIED: Tab: 5mg, 10mg, 20mg, 40mg

CONTRAINDICATIONS: History of angioedema.

WARNINGS/PRECAUTIONS: Not recommended in pediatric patients with GFR <30mL. Less effect on BP and more reports of angioedema in blacks than nonblacks. Anaphylactoid reactions reported. Angioedema reported; d/c and administer appropriate therapy if laryngeal stridor or angioedema of the face, tongue, or glottis occurs. Intestinal angioedema reported; monitor for abdominal pain. Anaphylactoid reactions reported during desensitization with hymenoptera venom, dialysis with high-flux membranes, and LDL apheresis with dextran sulfate absorption. Symptomatic hypotension may occur and is most likely with volume and/or salt depletion (eg, diuretic therapy, dietary salt restriction, dialysis, diarrhea, vomiting); correct volume and/or salt depletion prior to therapy. Excessive hypotension associated with oliguria, azotemia, acute renal failure, or death may occur with congestive heart failure (CHF); monitor patients during first 2 weeks of therapy and whenever dose is increased. May cause agranulocytosis and bone marrow depression; monitor WBC in patients with renal and collagen vascular disease. Rarely, associated with syndrome of cholestatic jaundice or hepatitis progressing to fulminant hepatic necrosis and death; d/c if jaundice or marked LFT elevation occurs. May increase BUN and SrCr in patients with renal disease; reduce dose and d/c diuretic. Hyperkalemia and persistent nonproductive cough reported. Hypotension may occur with surgery or during anesthesia. Caution in elderly.

ADVERSE REACTIONS: Headache, dizziness, fatigue, somnolence, nausea, cough.

INTERACTIONS: Hypotension risk, and increased BUN and SrCr with diuretics. Increased risk of hyperkalemia with K^+-sparing diuretics (eg, spironolactone, triamterene, amiloride), K^+-containing salt substitutes, or K^+ supplements; monitor K^+ levels. Increased lithium levels and symptoms of lithium toxicity; use caution and monitor frequently. Nitritoid reactions (eg, facial flushing, N/V, hypotension) reported when used concomitantly with injectable gold (sodium aurothiomalate). Hypoglycemia may develop with concomitant use with oral antidiabetics or insulin in diabetics. NSAIDs, including selective cyclooxygenase-2 inhibitors, may decrease effects of ACE inhibitors and may further deteriorate renal function.

PREGNANCY: Category D, safety not known in nursing.

MECHANISM OF ACTION: ACE inhibitor; catalyzes the conversion of angiotensin I to the vasoconstrictor, angiotensin II that stimulates aldosterone secretion by adrenal cortex. Inhibition results in decreased plasma angiotensin II, which leads to decreased vasopressor activity and to decreased aldosterone secretion.

PHARMACOKINETICS: Absorption: T_{max} = 0.5-1 hr, 1-2 hrs (metabolite, fasting), 2-4 hrs (metabolite, nonfasting); bioavailability ($\geq$37%). **Distribution:** Plasma protein binding (96.7%; 95.3% metabolite); crosses placenta; found in breast milk. **Metabolism:** Liver, cleavage of ester group; benazeprilat (active metabolite). **Elimination:** Urine (trace amounts, unchanged; 20% metabolite; 4% benazepril glucuronide; 8% benazeprilat glucuronide); $T_{1/2}$=10-11 hrs (metabolite, adults), 5 hrs (metabolite, pediatrics).

NURSING CONSIDERATIONS

Assessment: Assess for history of angioedema, hypersensitivity, volume/salt depletion, collagen-vascular disease (eg, systemic lupus erythematosus, scleroderma), CHF, diabetes mellitus, renal artery stenosis, renal/hepatic impairment, pregnancy/nursing status, and possible drug interactions. Obtain baseline BP, BUN, and SrCr.

Monitoring: Monitor for angioedema, anaphylactoid reactions, hyperkalemia, and cough. Monitor WBCs in patient with collagen and renal disease, BP, LFTs, and renal/hepatic function.

Patient Counseling: Inform of pregnancy risks and discuss treatment options with women planning to become pregnant; advise to report pregnancy to physician as soon as possible. Instruct to d/c therapy and to immediately report signs/symptoms of angioedema or syncope. Inform that lightheadedness may occur, especially during 1st days of therapy; instruct to report to physician. Inform that inadequate fluid intake or excessive perspiration, diarrhea, or vomiting may lead to excessive drop in BP resulting in lightheadedness or syncope. Avoid K^+ supplements or salt substitutes containing K^+ without consulting physician. Report promptly if symptoms of infection (eg, sore throat, fever) develop.

Administration: Oral route. Refer to PI for suspension preparation instructions. **Storage:** $\leq$30°C (86°F). Protect from moisture.

LOTENSIN HCT   RX
benazepril HCl - hydrochlorothiazide (Novartis)

> D/C when pregnancy is detected. Drugs that act directly on the renin-angiotensin system can cause injury/death to the developing fetus.

THERAPEUTIC CLASS: ACE inhibitor/thiazide diuretic

INDICATIONS: Treatment of HTN.

DOSAGE: *Adults:* Not Controlled with Benazepril Monotherapy: Initial: 10mg-12.5mg or 20mg-12.5mg. Titrate: Based on clinical response. May increase HCTZ dose after 2-3 weeks. Controlled with 25mg HCTZ/day with Hypokalemia: Switch to 5mg-6.25mg. Replacement Therapy: Substitute for individually titrated components.

HOW SUPPLIED: Tab: (Benazepril-HCTZ) 5mg-6.25mg*, 10mg-12.5mg*, 20mg-12.5mg*, 20mg-25mg* *scored

CONTRAINDICATIONS: Anuria, hypersensitivity to other sulfonamide-derived drugs, history of angioedema.

WARNINGS/PRECAUTIONS: Not for initial therapy. Avoid use if CrCl $\leq$30mL/min. Caution in elderly. Caution with impaired hepatic function or progressive liver disease; may precipitate hepatic coma. Symptomatic hypotension may occur and is most likely with volume and/or salt depletion (eg, diuretic therapy); correct volume and/or salt depletion prior to therapy. Interrupt for few days prior to parathyroid function test. Benazepril: Angioedema reported; d/c and administer appropriate therapy if laryngeal stridor or angioedema of the face, tongue, or glottis occur. Intestinal angioedema reported; monitor for abdominal pain. Anaphylactoid reactions reported during desensitization with hymenoptera venom, dialysis with high-flux membranes, and LDL apheresis with dextran sulfate absorption. May increase BUN and SrCr levels in patients with renal disease; reduce dose and d/c. May cause agranulocytosis and bone marrow depression; monitor WBC in patients with renal and collagen vascular disease. Excessive hypotension associated with oliguria, azotemia, acute renal failure, or death may occur with congestive heart failure (CHF); monitor patients during first 2 weeks of therapy and whenever dose is increased. Rarely, associated with syndrome of cholestatic jaundice or hepatitis progressing to fulminant hepatic necrosis and death; d/c if jaundice or marked LFT elevation occurs. Hyperkalemia and persistent, nonproductive cough reported. Hypotension may occur with surgery or during anesthesia. HCTZ: May precipitate azotemia with renal disease. May cause hypersensitivity reactions, exacerbation or activation of systemic lupus erythematosus (SLE), hyperuricemia or precipitation of frank gout, hyperglycemia, hypomagnesemia, and manifestations of latent diabetes mellitus (DM). May cause idiosyncratic reaction, resulting in acute transient myopia and acute-angle glaucoma; d/c as rapidly as possible. Observe for signs of fluid or electrolyte imbalance (eg, hyponatremia, hypochloremic alkalosis, hypokalemia). Altered parathyroid glands, with hypercalcemia and hypophosphatemia, seen with prolonged therapy. May reduce glucose tolerance and increase cholesterol, TG, and uric acid levels. Enhanced effects in postsympathectomy patients.

ADVERSE REACTIONS: Dizziness, fatigue, postural dizziness, headache, cough, nausea.

INTERACTIONS: NSAIDs, including selective cyclooxygenase-2 inhibitors, may decrease effects of diuretics and ACE inhibitors and may further deteriorate renal function. Increased lithium levels and symptoms of lithium toxicity; use caution and monitor frequently. Benazepril: Increased risk of hyperkalemia with K^+-sparing diuretics (eg, spironolactone, triamterene, amiloride), K^+-containing salt substitutes, or K^+ supplements; monitor K^+ levels. Nitritoid reactions (eg, facial flushing, N/V, hypotension) reported when used concomitantly with injectable gold (sodium aurothiomalate). HCTZ: Insulin requirements in diabetics may need adjustment. May decrease arterial responsiveness to norepinephrine. May potentiate other antihypertensives, especially ganglionic or peripheral adrenergic-blocking drugs. May increase responsiveness to tubocurarine. Anionic exchange resins (eg, cholestyramine or colestipol) may impair absorption. Increased risk of hypokalemia with concomitant corticosteroids or adrenocorticotropic hormone. Alcohol, barbiturates, and narcotics may potentiate orthostatic hypotension. May increase absorption with agents that reduce GI motility.

PREGNANCY: Category D, not for use in nursing.

MECHANISM OF ACTION: Benazepril: ACE inhibitor; effects appear to result from suppression of renin-angiotensin-aldosterone system. Inhibition results in decreased plasma angiotensin II, which leads to decreased vasopressor activity and decreased aldosterone secretion. HCTZ: Thiazide diuretic; has not been established. Affects renal tubular mechanisms of electrolyte reabsorption, directly increasing excretion of Na^+ and Cl^- in approximately equivalent amounts.

PHARMACOKINETICS: Absorption: Benazepril: T_{max}=0.5-1 hr, 1-2 hrs (metabolite, fasting), 2-4 hrs (metabolite, nonfasting); bioavailability (≥37%). HCTZ: T_{max}=1-2.5 hrs; bioavailability (50-80%). **Distribution:** Found in breast milk; crosses placenta. Benazepril: Plasma protein binding (96.7%, 95.3% metabolite). HCTZ: Plasma protein binding (67.9%); V_d= 3.6-7.8L/kg. **Metabolism:** Benazepril: Liver, cleavage of ester group; benazeprilat (active metabolite). **Elimination:** Benazepril: Urine (trace amounts, unchanged; 20% metabolite; 4% benazepril glucuronide; 8% benazeprilat glucuronide); $T_{1/2}$=10-11 hrs (metabolite). HCTZ: Kidney; $T_{1/2}$=5-15 hrs.

NURSING CONSIDERATIONS

Assessment: Assess for hypersensitivity, anuria, sulfonamide-derived drug hypersensitivity, history of angioedema, allergy or bronchial asthma, volume/salt depletion, CHF, SLE, renal/hepatic function, electrolyte levels, pregnancy/nursing status, possible drug interactions, and any other conditions where treatment is contraindicated or cautioned. Obtain baseline BP, BUN, and SrCr.

Monitoring: Monitor for angioedema, anaphylactoid reactions, hyperkalemia, cough, hypotension, jaundice, hypersensitivity reactions, SLE, idiosyncratic reaction, myopia, and angle-closure glaucoma. Periodically monitor WBCs in patients with collagen vascular disease. Monitor serum electrolytes, BP, LFTs, renal function (BUN, SrCr), and cholesterol/TG levels. Monitor patients closely for the 1st 2 weeks of therapy and during dose increases (CHF).

Patient Counseling: Inform of pregnancy risks and discuss treatment options; advise to report pregnancy to physician as soon as possible. Instruct to d/c therapy and to immediately report signs/symptoms of angioedema or syncope. Inform that lightheadedness may occur, especially during 1st days of therapy; instruct to report to physician. Inadequate fluid intake or excessive perspiration, diarrhea, or vomiting may lead to excessive drop in BP resulting in lightheadedness or syncope. Avoid K^+ supplements or salt substitutes containing K^+ without consulting physician. Report promptly if symptoms of infection (eg, sore throat, fever) develop.

Administration: Oral route. **Storage:** ≤30°C (86°F). Protect from moisture and light.

Lotrel
RX

benazepril HCl - amlodipine besylate (Novartis)

> D/C when pregnancy is detected. Drugs that act directly on the renin-angiotensin system can cause death/injury to the developing fetus.

THERAPEUTIC CLASS: Calcium channel blocker (dihydropyridine)/ACE inhibitor

INDICATIONS: Treatment of HTN not adequately controlled on monotherapy with either agent.

DOSAGE: *Adults:* Usual: Dose qd. Add-On Therapy: Use if not adequately controlled with amlodipine (or another dihydropyridine) alone or benazepril (or another ACE inhibitor) alone. If adequately controlled with amlodipine but experience unacceptable edema, combination therapy may achieve similar (or better) BP control with less edema. Replacement Therapy: May substitute for titrated components. Elderly/Hepatic Impairment: Initial: 2.5mg amlodipine. Refer to PI for dosing for individual components.

HOW SUPPLIED: Cap: (Amlodipine-Benazepril) 2.5mg-10mg, 5mg-10mg, 5mg-20mg, 5mg-40mg, 10mg-20mg, 10mg-40mg

CONTRAINDICATIONS: History of angioedema.

WARNINGS/PRECAUTIONS: Symptomatic hypotension may occur, most likely in volume- or salt-depleted patients (eg, prolonged diuretic therapy, dietary salt restriction, dialysis, diarrhea, vomiting). Avoid with severe renal disease (CrCl <30mL/min). Hyperkalemia reported; risk factors include diabetes mellitus (DM) and renal insufficiency. Caution in elderly. Benazepril: Angioedema reported; d/c and institute appropriate treatment if laryngeal stridor or angioedema of the face, tongue, or glottis occurs. More reports of angioedema in blacks than in nonblacks. Intestinal angioedema reported; monitor for abdominal pain. Anaphylactoid reactions reported during desensitization with hymenoptera venom, dialysis with high-flux membranes, and LDL apheresis with dextran sulfate absorption. Excessive hypotension associated with oliguria, azotemia, and acute renal failure or death may occur in congestive heart failure (CHF); monitor patients during first 2 weeks of therapy and whenever dose is increased or a diuretic is added/increased. Rarely associated with cholestatic jaundice that progresses to fulminant hepatic necrosis and sometimes death; d/c if jaundice or marked elevations of hepatic enzymes occur. May increase SrCr and BUN in patients with renal artery stenosis; monitor renal function during the 1st few weeks of therapy. Persistent nonproductive cough reported. Hypotension may occur with surgery or during anesthesia. Amlodipine: Increased frequency, duration, or severity of angina or acute myocardial infarction (MI) reported, particularly in those with severe obstructive coronary artery disease (CAD).

ADVERSE REACTIONS: Cough, headache, dizziness, edema, angioedema.

INTERACTIONS: Hypotension risk and increased BUN and SrCr with diuretics. Benazepril: NSAIDs, including selective cyclooxygenase-2 inhibitors, may decrease effects of ACE inhibitors and may further deteriorate renal function. Increased risk of hyperkalemia with K⁺ supplements, K⁺-sparing diuretics (eg, spironolactone, amiloride, triamterene), or K⁺-containing salt substitutes; frequently monitor serum K⁺. Increased lithium levels and symptoms of lithium toxicity reported; frequently monitor lithium levels. Nitritoid reactions (eg, facial flushing, N/V, hypotension) reported with injectable gold (sodium aurothiomalate). Amlodipine: May increase exposure to simvastatin; limit dose of simvastatin to 20mg daily.

PREGNANCY: Category D, not for use in nursing.

MECHANISM OF ACTION: Amlodipine: Calcium channel blocker (dihydropyridine); inhibits transmembrane influx of calcium ions into vascular smooth muscle and cardiac muscle. Acts directly on vascular smooth muscle to cause a reduction in peripheral vascular resistance and reduction in BP. Benazepril: ACE inhibitor; effects appear to result from suppression of renin-angiotensin-aldosterone system. Inhibition results in decreased plasma angiotensin II, which leads to decreased vasopressor activity and to decreased aldosterone secretion.

PHARMACOKINETICS: Absorption: Amlodipine: T_{max}=6-12 hrs; bioavailability (64-90%). Benazepril: T_{max}=0.5-2 hrs, 1.5-4 hrs (benazeprilat); bioavailability (≥37%). **Distribution:** Amlodipine: V_d=21L/kg; plasma protein binding (93%). Benazepril: V_d=0.7L/kg; crosses the placenta; found in breast milk. **Metabolism:** Amlodipine: Liver (extensive). Benazepril: Liver, cleavage of ester group; benazeprilat (active metabolite). **Elimination:** Amlodipine: Urine (10% unchanged, 60% metabolites); $T_{1/2}$=2 days. Benazepril: Urine (trace unchanged, 20% benazeprilat), bile (11-12% benazeprilat); $T_{1/2}$=10-11 hrs (benazeprilat).

NURSING CONSIDERATIONS

Assessment: Assess for history of angioedema, hypersensitivity to drug or ACE inhibitors, severe aortic stenosis, CHF, severe obstructive CAD, volume/salt depletion, DM, renal artery stenosis, hepatic/renal impairment, pregnancy/nursing status, and possible drug interactions.

Monitoring: Monitor for signs/symptoms of hypotension, anaphylactoid or hypersensitivity reactions, head/neck and intestinal angioedema, increased angina or MI, hepatic function, and other adverse reactions. Monitor BP, serum K⁺ levels, and renal function (for the 1st few weeks in patients with renal artery stenosis).

Patient Counseling: Inform of the consequences of exposure to the medication during pregnancy and of treatment options in women planning to become pregnant. Advise to report pregnancies to physician as soon as possible. Advise to seek medical attention if symptoms of hypotension, anaphylactoid or hypersensitivity reactions, angioedema (head/neck, intestinal), infection, trouble swallowing, breathing problems (eg, wheezing or asthma), and hepatic dysfunction (eg, itching, yellow eyes/skin, flu-like symptoms) occur.

Administration: Oral route. **Storage:** 25°C (77°F); excursions permitted to 15-30°C (59-86°F). Protect from moisture.

LOTRISONE   RX
betamethasone dipropionate - clotrimazole (Schering)

THERAPEUTIC CLASS: Corticosteroid/azole antifungal

INDICATIONS: Topical treatment of symptomatic inflammatory tinea pedis, tinea cruris, and tinea corporis caused by *Trichophyton rubrum*, *Trichophyton mentagrophytes*, and *Epidermophyton floccosum* in patients ≥17 yrs.

DOSAGE: *Adults:* ≥17 yrs: Massage sufficient amount into affected skin area(s) bid (am and pm). Do not use for >2 weeks for the treatment of tinea cruris and tinea corporis or for >4 weeks for the treatment of tinea pedis. Amounts of cream >45g/week or of lotion >45mL/week should not be used.

HOW SUPPLIED: (Betamethasone Dipropionate-Clotrimazole) Cre: 0.643mg-10mg/g [15g, 45g]; Lot: 0.643mg-10mg/g [30mL]

WARNINGS/PRECAUTIONS: Systemic absorption of corticosteroids may produce reversible HPA axis suppression, Cushing's syndrome, hyperglycemia, and glucosuria. Use over large surface areas, prolonged use, and use under occlusive dressings augment systemic absorption. Not for use with occlusive dressing. D/C if irritation develops. Pediatrics may be more susceptible to systemic toxicity. Not recommended for patients <17 yrs or patients with diaper dermatitis.

ADVERSE REACTIONS: Cre, Lot: Itching, irritation, folliculitis, hypertrichosis, acneiform eruptions, hypopigmentation. Cre: Paresthesia, rash, edema, secondary infection. Lot: Burning, dry skin, stinging.

PREGNANCY: Category C, caution in nursing.

MECHANISM OF ACTION: Corticosteroid/azole antifungal agent. Clotrimazole: Imidazole antifungal agent; inhibits 14-α-demethylation of lanosterol in fungi by binding to 1 of the CYP450 enzymes. Leads to accumulation of 14-α-methylsterols and reduced concentrations of ergosterol, a sterol essential for a normal fungal cytoplasmic membrane. The methylsterols may affect the electron transport system, thereby inhibiting growth of fungi. Betamethasone: Corticosteroid; has been shown to have topical systemic pharmacologic and metabolic effects characteristic of this class of drugs.

PHARMACOKINETICS: Metabolism: Liver. **Elimination:** Renal, biliary.

NURSING CONSIDERATIONS

Assessment: Assess for hypersensitivity to other corticosteroids or imidazoles. Assess pregnancy/nursing status.

Monitoring: Monitor for signs/symptoms of hypothalmic-pituitary-adrenal-axis suppression, skin irritation. When used on large surface areas and/or with occlusive dressings, perform periodic monitoring for HPA-axis suppression using adrenocorticotropic hormone test, morning plasma cortisol test, and urinary free-cortisol level test. Monitor for systemic toxicity, Cushing's syndrome, and delayed weight gain.

Patient Counseling: Counsel to use exactly as directed for fully prescribed treatment period. Advise to avoid contact with eyes, mouth, or intravaginally. Inform to contact physician if no improvement after 1 week of treatment for tinea cruris or tinea corporis, or 2 weeks for tinea pedis. Instruct to avoid using occlusive dressings or tight-fitting clothing on treated areas and not to use with other corticosteroids. Counsel the patient to use only for 2 weeks if the affected area is the groin and notify physician if condition persists after 2 weeks. Advise that the medication should be used only for the disorder for which it was prescribed. Counsel on adverse events.

Administration: Topical route. Shake lotion well before each use. **Storage:** 25C°(77°F), excursions permitted to 15-30°C (59-86°F). Store lotion in upright position.

LOTRONEX

RX

alosetron HCl (Prometheus)

> Serious GI adverse events (eg, ischemic colitis, serious constipation complications) reported. Only prescribers enrolled in Prometheus Prescribing Program should prescribe this medication. Patients must read and sign the Patient Acknowledge Form before receiving initial prescription. D/C immediately if constipation or symptoms of ischemic colitis develop; do not resume therapy in patients with ischemic colitis. Indicated only for women with severe diarrhea-predominant irritable bowel syndrome (IBS) who have not responded adequately to conventional therapy.

THERAPEUTIC CLASS: 5-HT$_3$ receptor antagonist

INDICATIONS: Treatment for women with severe diarrhea-predominant IBS who have chronic symptoms (≥6 months), exclusion of anatomic or biochemical abnormalities of GI tract, failure to respond to conventional therapy.

DOSAGE: *Adults:* Initial: 0.5mg bid for 4 weeks. D/C if constipation occurs, then restart at 0.5mg qd if constipation resolves. D/C if constipation recurs at lower dose. Titrate: If tolerated and IBS symptoms are not adequately controlled, may increase to up to 1mg bid. D/C after 4 weeks if symptoms are not controlled on 1mg bid.

HOW SUPPLIED: Tab: 0.5mg, 1mg

CONTRAINDICATIONS: Current constipation. History of chronic/severe constipation or sequelae from constipation, intestinal obstruction, stricture, toxic megacolon, GI perforation/adhesions, ischemic colitis, impaired intestinal circulation, thrombophlebitis or hypercoagulable state, Crohn's disease, ulcerative colitis, diverticulitis, severe hepatic impairment. Inability to understand/comply with Patient Acknowledgment Form. Concomitant administration with fluvoxamine.

WARNINGS/PRECAUTIONS: Caution in elderly and debilitated patients; may be at greater risk for complications of constipation. Caution with mild/moderate hepatic impairment.

ADVERSE REACTIONS: Constipation, ischemic colitis, abdominal discomfort/pain, nausea, GI discomfort/pain.

INTERACTIONS: See Contraindications. Increased risk of constipation with medications that decrease GI motility. Inducers and inhibitors of CYP1A2, with minor contributions from CYP3A4 and CYP2C9, drug-metabolizing enzymes may alter clearance. Avoid with quinolone antibiotics and cimetidine. Caution with strong CYP3A4 inhibitors (eg, ketoconazole, clarithromycin, telithromycin, protease inhibitors, voriconazole, itraconazole).

PREGNANCY: Category B, caution in nursing.

MECHANISM OF ACTION: 5-HT$_3$ receptor antagonist; inhibits activation of non-selective cation channels, which results in the modulation of the enteric nervous system.

PHARMACOKINETICS: Absorption: Rapidly absorbed, absolute bioavailability (50-60%), 9ng/mL (young women); T$_{max}$=1 hr. **Distribution:** V$_d$=65-95L, plasma protein binding (82%). **Metabolism:** via Liver (extensive). **Elimination:** Urine (74%, metabolites), feces (11%, <1% unchanged); T$_{1/2}$=1.5 hrs.

NURSING CONSIDERATIONS

Assessment: Assess for history of chronic or severe constipation or sequelae from constipation, intestinal obstruction or stricture, toxic megacolon, GI perforation or adhesion, ischemic colitis, impaired intestinal circulation, thrombophlebitis or hypercoagulable state, Crohn's disease or ulcerative colitis, diverticulitis, severe hepatic impairment, pregnancy/nursing status and possible drug interactions.

Monitoring: Monitor LFTs, signs/symptoms of ischemic colitis and serious complications of constipation, perforation and other adverse reactions.

Patient Counseling: Counsel on the risk and benefits of the treatment. Review side effects and advise to report if any develop. Inform that tab may be taken with or without meals. Do not start if patient is constipated. D/C and contact prescriber if become constipated, have symptoms of ischemic colitis, or if IBS symptoms are not controlled after 4 weeks of taking 1mg bid.

Administration: Oral route. **Storage:** 25°C (77°F); excursions permitted to 15-30°C (59-86°F).

LOVASTATIN

RX

lovastatin (Various)

OTHER BRAND NAMES: Mevacor (Merck)

THERAPEUTIC CLASS: HMG-CoA reductase inhibitor

INDICATIONS: To reduce risk of myocardial infarction, unstable angina, and coronary revascularization procedures in patients without symptomatic cardiovascular disease (CVD), average to moderately elevated total-C and LDL, and below average HDL. To slow progression of coronary atherosclerosis in patients with coronary heart disease by lowering total-C and LDL to target levels. Adjunct to diet for treatment of primary hypercholesterolemia (Types IIa and IIb), and for treatment of adolescents who are ≥1 yr postmenarche (10-17 yrs) with heterozygous familial hypercholesterolemia whose LDL remains >189mg/dL or LDL remains >160mg/dL and a positive family history of premature CVD or ≥2 other CVD risk factors are present after an adequate trial of diet therapy.

DOSAGE: *Adults:* Individualize dose. Initial: 20mg qd with pm meal. Usual: 10-80mg/day in single or 2 divided doses. Max: 80mg/day. Requiring LDL Reduction of ≥20%: Initial: 20mg/day. May consider starting dose of 10mg if smaller reductions required. Titrate: Adjust at ≥4-week intervals. Consider dose reduction if cholesterol levels fall significantly below the targeted range. Concomitant Danazol/Diltiazem/Verapamil: Initial: 10mg/day. Max: 20mg/day. Concomitant Amiodarone: Max: 40mg/day. Severe Renal Insufficiency (CrCl <30mL/min): Carefully consider dosage increases >20mg/day; give cautiously if deemed necessary.
Pediatrics: 10-17 yrs: Individualize dose. Heterozygous Familial Hypercholesterolemia: Usual: 10-40mg/day. Max: 40mg/day. Requiring LDL Reduction of ≥20%: Initial: 20mg/day. May consider starting dose of 10mg if smaller reductions required. Titrate: Adjust at ≥4-week intervals. Concomitant Danazol/Diltiazem/Verapamil: Initial: 10mg/day. Max: 20mg/day. Concomitant Amiodarone: Max: 40mg/day. Severe Renal Insufficiency (CrCl <30mL/min): Carefully consider dosage increases >20mg/day; give cautiously if deemed necessary.

HOW SUPPLIED: Tab: 10mg, (Mevacor) 20mg, 40mg

CONTRAINDICATIONS: Active liver disease or unexplained persistent elevations of serum transaminases, pregnancy, women of childbearing age who may become pregnant, and nursing mothers. Concomitant strong CYP3A4 inhibitors (eg, itraconazole, ketoconazole, posaconazole, HIV protease inhibitors, boceprevir, telaprevir, erythromycin, clarithromycin, telithromycin, nefazodone).

WARNINGS/PRECAUTIONS: Myopathy/rhabdomyolysis reported; d/c if markedly elevated CPK levels occur or myopathy is diagnosed/suspected, and temporarily withhold in any patient experiencing acute or serious condition predisposing to development of renal failure secondary to rhabdomyolysis. Persistent increases in serum transaminases reported; obtain liver enzyme tests prior to initiation and repeat as clinically indicated. Fatal and nonfatal hepatic failure (rare) reported; promptly interrupt therapy if serious liver injury with clinical symptoms and/or hyperbilirubinemia or jaundice occurs and do not restart if no alternate etiology found. Caution in patients who consume substantial quantities of alcohol and/or have history of liver disease. Increases in HbA1c and FPG levels reported. Evaluate patients who develop endocrine dysfunction.

ADVERSE REACTIONS: Headache, constipation, flatulence, myalgia, creatine kinase (CK) elevations.

INTERACTIONS: See Contraindications. Voriconazole may increase concentration and may increase risk of myopathy/rhabdomyolysis; consider dose adjustment. Avoid with gemfibrozil, cyclosporine, and large quantities of grapefruit juice (>1 quart/day). Caution with fibrates or lipid-lowering doses (≥1g/day) of niacin as these may cause myopathy when given alone. Do not exceed 20mg qd with danazol, diltiazem, or verapamil, and 40mg qd with amiodarone. Caution with colchicine and consider dose adjustment with ranolazine due to increased risk of myopathy/rhabdomyolysis. Determine PT before initiation and frequently during therapy with coumarin anticoagulants. Caution with drugs that may decrease the levels or activity of endogenous steroid hormones (eg, spironolactone, cimetidine).

PREGNANCY: Category X, not for use in nursing.

MECHANISM OF ACTION: HMG-CoA reductase inhibitor; involves reduction of VLDL concentration and induction of LDL receptor, leading to reduced production and/or increased catabolism of LDL.

PHARMACOKINETICS: Absorption: T_{max}=2-4 hrs (active and total inhibitors). **Distribution:** Plasma protein binding (>95%). **Metabolism:** Liver (extensive), by hydrolysis via CYP3A4; β-hydroxyacid and 6'-hydroxy derivative (major active metabolites). **Elimination:** Feces (83%), urine (10%).

NURSING CONSIDERATIONS

Assessment: Assess for active liver disease or unexplained serum transaminase elevations, history of alcohol consumption, pregnancy/nursing status, renal impairment, and possible drug interactions. Obtain baseline renal function, LFTs, and cholesterol levels.

Monitoring: Monitor for signs/symptoms of myopathy, rhabdomyolysis, endocrine dysfunction, and other adverse effects. Monitor cholesterol levels, CK, and LFTs.

Patient Counseling: Advise about substances to be avoided and to report promptly unexplained muscle pain, tenderness, or weakness, and any symptoms that may indicate liver injury (eg, fatigue, anorexia, right upper abdominal discomfort, dark urine, jaundice). Counsel adolescent females on appropriate contraceptive methods while on therapy.

Administration: Oral route. **Storage:** 20-25°C (68-77°F). Protect from light.

Lovaza RX
omega-3-acid ethyl esters (GlaxoSmithKline)

THERAPEUTIC CLASS: Lipid-regulating agent

INDICATIONS: Adjunct to diet to reduce TG levels in adults with severe (≥500mg/dL) hypertriglyceridemia.

DOSAGE: *Adults:* 4g/day (4 caps qd or 2 caps bid).

HOW SUPPLIED: Cap: 1g

WARNINGS/PRECAUTIONS: Contains ethyl esters of omega-3 fatty acids (EPA and DHA) obtained from oil of several fish sources; unknown whether patients allergic to fish and/or shellfish are at an increased risk of an allergic reaction. Caution with known hypersensitivity to fish and/or shellfish. Increase in ALT levels without concurrent increase in AST levels reported. May increase LDL-C levels.

ADVERSE REACTIONS: Eructation, taste perversion, dyspepsia.

INTERACTIONS: Possible prolongation of bleeding time with concomitant anticoagulants or other drugs affecting coagulation (aspirin [ASA], NSAIDs, warfarin, coumarin); monitor periodically. D/C or change medications known to exacerbate hypertriglyceridemia (eg, β-blockers, thiazides, estrogens) prior to consideration of therapy.

PREGNANCY: Category C, caution in nursing.

MECHANISM OF ACTION: Lipid-regulating agent; not established. Inhibits acyl CoA:1,2-diacylglycerol acyltransferase, increases mitochondrial and peroxisomal β-oxidation in the liver, decreases lipogenesis in the liver, and increases plasma lipoprotein lipase activity. May reduce the synthesis of TG in the liver because EPA and DHA are poor substrates for the enzymes responsible for TG synthesis, and EPA and DHA inhibit esterification of other fatty acids.

NURSING CONSIDERATIONS

Assessment: Assess for persistent abnormal TG levels, hypersensitivity (eg, anaphylactic reaction), pregnancy/nursing status, other conditions which may affect treatment, and possible drug interactions. Attempt to control serum TG levels with appropriate diet, exercise, and weight loss in obese patients before instituting therapy.

Monitoring: Periodically monitor ALT/AST/LDL-C levels, coagulation parameters (during concomitant use with drugs affecting coagulation) and check for possible adverse effects.

Patient Counseling: Caution patients with known sensitivity or allergy to fish and/or shellfish. Advise that the use of lipid-regulating agents does not reduce the importance of adhering to diet. Capsules should be swallowed whole and not altered in any way.

Administration: Oral route. Swallow whole. Do not break open, crush, dissolve, or chew. **Storage:** 25°C (77°F); excursions permitted to 15-30°C (59-86°F). Do not freeze.

Lovenox RX
enoxaparin sodium (Sanofi-Aventis)

Epidural or spinal hematomas resulting in long-term or permanent paralysis may occur in patients anticoagulated with low molecular weight heparins (LMWH) or heparinoids and are receiving neuraxial anesthesia or undergoing spinal puncture. Increased risk with indwelling epidural catheters, concomitant use of other drugs that affect hemostasis (eg, NSAIDs, platelet inhibitors, other anticoagulants), history of traumatic or repeated epidural or spinal puncture, or a history of spinal deformity or spinal surgery. Monitor frequently for signs/symptoms of neurologic impairment; if neurologic compromise noted, urgent treatment is necessary. Consider benefit and risks before neuraxial intervention in patients anticoagulated or to be anticoagulated for thromboprophylaxis.

THERAPEUTIC CLASS: Low molecular weight heparin

INDICATIONS: Prophylaxis of deep vein thrombosis (DVT) in patients undergoing abdominal surgery who are at risk for thromboembolic complications, or undergoing hip replacement surgery during and following hospitalization, or undergoing knee replacement surgery, or medical patients who are at risk for thromboembolic complications due to severely restricted mobility during acute illness. Inpatient treatment of acute DVT with or without pulmonary embolism (PE) in conjunction with warfarin. Outpatient treatment of acute DVT without PE in conjunction with warfarin. Prophylaxis of ischemic complications of unstable angina and non-Q-wave myocardial infarction (MI) when administered with aspirin (ASA). Treatment of acute ST-segment elevation MI (STEMI) when administered with ASA in patients receiving thrombolysis and being medically managed or with percutaneous coronary intervention (PCI).

DOSAGE: *Adults:* SQ: DVT Prophylaxis: Abdominal Surgery: 40mg qd with initial dose given 2 hrs preop for up to 12 days (usually 7-10 days). Hip/Knee Replacement Surgery: 30mg q12h with initial dose given 12-24 hrs postop for up to 14 days (usually 7-10 days). Consider 40mg qd with initial dose given 9-15 hrs pre-op for up to 3 weeks as thromboprophylaxis in hip surgery. Acute Medical Illness: 40mg qd for up to 14 days (usually 6-11 days). Acute DVT Treatment: Outpatient without PE: 1mg/kg q12h for up to 17 days (usually 7 days). Inpatient with or without PE: 1mg/kg q12h, or 1.5mg/kg qd, up to 17 days (usually 5-7 days), administered at the same time daily. Initiate concomitant warfarin therapy when appropriate usually within 72 hrs. Unstable Angina/Non-Q-Wave MI: 1mg/kg q12h in conjunction with ASA therapy (100-325mg/day) for up to 12.5 days (usually 2-8 days). Treatment of Acute STEMI: <75 yrs: 30mg single IV bolus plus a 1mg/kg SQ dose, followed by 1mg/kg q12h SQ. Max: 100mg for the first 2 doses only, followed by 1mg/kg dosing for the remaining doses for ≥8 days or until hospital discharge. ≥75 yrs: Do not use initial IV bolus. Initial: 0.75mg/kg SQ q12h. Max: 75mg for the first 2 doses only, followed by 0.75mg/kg dosing for the remaining doses for ≥8 days or until hospital discharge. All patients should receive 75-325mg/day ASA as soon as they are identified as having STEMI. In Conjunction with Thrombolytic Therapy: Give enoxaparin between 15 min before and 30 min after start of fibrinolytic therapy. Continue treatment for ≥8 days or until hospital discharge. PCI: If last dose is given <8 hrs before balloon inflation, no additional dosing is needed. If last dose is given >8 hrs before balloon inflation, give an IV bolus of 0.3mg/kg. Refer to PI for dosage regimen with severe renal impairment (CrCl <30mL/min).

HOW SUPPLIED: Inj: (Multi-dose vial) 300mg/3mL; (Syringe) 30mg/0.3mL, 40mg/0.4mL, 60mg/0.6mL, 80mg/0.8mL, 100mg/mL, 120mg/0.8mL, 150mg/mL

CONTRAINDICATIONS: Active major bleeding, thrombocytopenia associated with a positive *in vitro* test for antiplatelet antibody in the presence of enoxaparin sodium, hypersensitivity to heparin or pork products, hypersensitivity to benzyl alcohol (only with the multi-dose formulation).

WARNINGS/PRECAUTIONS: Not for IM injection. Extreme caution with increased risk of hemorrhage (eg, bacterial endocarditis, congenital or acquired bleeding disorders, active ulcerative and angiodysplastic GI disease, hemorrhagic stroke, or shortly after brain, spinal, or ophthalmological surgery) and with history of heparin-induced thrombocytopenia. Major hemorrhages including retroperitoneal and intracranial bleeding reported. To minimize the risk of bleeding following vascular instrumentation during treatment of unstable angina, non-Q-wave MI, and acute STEMI, adhere precisely to the intervals recommended between doses. Observe for signs of bleeding or hematoma formation at the site of the procedure. Caution in patients with bleeding diathesis, uncontrolled arterial HTN or history of a recent GI ulceration, diabetic retinopathy, renal dysfunction, and hemorrhage. Thrombocytopenia reported; d/c if platelet count <100,000/mm³. Cannot be used interchangeably (unit for unit) with heparin or other LMWH. Pregnant women with mechanical prosthetic heart valves may be at higher risk for thromboembolism and have a higher rate of fetal loss; monitor anti-Factor Xa levels, and adjust dosage PRN. Multi-dose vial contains benzyl alcohol which crosses the placenta and has been associated with fatal "gasping syndrome" in premature neonates; use with caution or only when clearly needed in pregnant women. Periodic CBC including platelet count and stool occult blood tests are recommended during course of treatment. Anti-Factor Xa may be used to monitor anticoagulant activity in patients with significant renal impairment or if abnormal coagulation parameters or bleeding occur. Caution with hepatic impairment.

ADVERSE REACTIONS: Hemorrhage, ecchymosis, anemia, peripheral edema, fever, hematoma, dyspnea, nausea, ALT/AST elevations.

INTERACTIONS: See Boxed Warning. D/C agents that may enhance the risk of hemorrhage prior to therapy (eg, anticoagulants, platelet inhibitors such as acetylsalicylic acid, salicylates, NSAIDs [including ketorolac tromethamine], dipyridamole, or sulfinpyrazone). If coadministration is essential, conduct close monitoring. May increase risk of hyperkalemia with K⁺-sparing drugs, and administration of K⁺.

PREGNANCY: Category B, not for use in nursing.

MECHANISM OF ACTION: LMWH; has antithrombotic properties.

PHARMACOKINETICS: Absorption: (SQ) Administration of variable doses resulted in different parameters. Absolute bioavailability (100%). T_{max}=3-5 hrs. **Distribution:** (Anti-Factor Xa activity) V_d=4.3L. **Metabolism:** Liver; via desulfation and/or depolymerization. **Elimination:** Urine; $T_{1/2}$=4.5-7 hrs.

NURSING CONSIDERATIONS

Assessment: Assess for presence of active major bleeding, thrombocytopenia, hypersensitivity to heparin or pork products, hypersensitivity to benzyl alcohol, renal dysfunction, any other conditions where treatment is cautioned, nursing/pregnancy status, and for possible drug interactions.

Monitoring: Monitor for signs/symptoms of hemorrhage and thrombocytopenia. Monitor for epidural or spinal hematomas, and for neurological impairment if used concomitantly with spinal/epidural anesthesia or spinal puncture. Monitor for signs/symptoms of hyperkalemia. Periodically monitor CBC including platelet count, stool occult blood tests. If bleeding occurs, monitor anti-factor Xa levels.

Patient Counseling: Inform of the benefits and risks of therapy. Inform to watch for signs/symptoms of spinal or epidural hematoma (tingling, numbness, muscular weakness) if patients have had neuraxial anesthesia or spinal puncture, particularly, if they are taking concomitant NSAIDs, platelet inhibitors, or other anticoagulants; contact physician if these occur. Advise to seek medical attention if unusual bleeding, bruising, signs of thrombocytopenia, and allergic reactions develop. Counsel that it will take longer than usual to stop bleeding; may bruise and/or bleed more easily when treated with enoxaparin. Inform of instructions for injecting if therapy is to continue after discharge. Instruct to notify physicians and dentists of enoxaparin therapy prior to surgery or taking a new drug.

Administration: SQ or IV (for multi-dose vial) route. Inspect visually for particulate matter and discoloration. Use tuberculin syringe or equivalent when using multi-dose vial. Refer to PI for administration techniques. **Storage:** 25°C (77°F); excursions permitted to 15-30°C (59-86°F). Do not store multi-dose vials for >28 days after first use.

LUCENTIS RX
ranibizumab (Genentech)

THERAPEUTIC CLASS: Monoclonal antibody/VEGF-A blocker

INDICATIONS: Treatment of neovascular (Wet) age-related macular degeneration (AMD) and macular edema following retinal vein occlusion (RVO).

DOSAGE: *Adults:* AMD/RVO: Administer 0.5mg (0.05mL) by intravitreal inj once a month (approximately 28 days). AMD: May reduce to 1 inj q3 months after the 1st four inj if monthly inj are not feasible.

HOW SUPPLIED: Inj: 10mg/mL

CONTRAINDICATIONS: Ocular or periocular infections.

WARNINGS/PRECAUTIONS: Intravitreal inj have been associated with endophthalmitis and retinal detachments; use proper aseptic inj technique. Increases in intraocular pressure (IOP) noted within 60 min of intravitreal inj. Risk of arterial thromboembolic events (eg, nonfatal stroke, nonfatal myocardial infarction, vascular death).

ADVERSE REACTIONS: Conjunctival hemorrhage, eye pain, vitreous floaters, increased IOP, intraocular inflammation, cataract, nasopharyngitis, foreign body sensation in the eyes, eye irritation, lacrimation increased, visual disturbances/vision blurred, ocular hyperemia, dry eye, maculopathy, headache.

INTERACTIONS: May develop serious intraocular inflammation when used adjunctively with verteporfin photodynamic therapy (PDT); incidence reported when drug was administered 7 days after verteporfin PDT.

PREGNANCY: Category C, caution in nursing.

MECHANISM OF ACTION: Monoclonal antibody/human vascular endothelial growth factor A (VEGF-A) blocker; binds to receptor binding site of VEGF-A; prevents the interaction of VEGF-A with its receptors (VEGFR1 and VEGFR2) on the surface of endothelial cells, thereby reducing endothelial cell proliferation, vascular leakage, and new blood vessel formation.

PHARMACOKINETICS: Absorption: C_{max}=1.5ng/mL; T_{max}=1 day. **Elimination:** $T_{1/2}$=9 days.

NURSING CONSIDERATIONS

Assessment: Assess for ocular or periocular infections, hypersensitivity to drug, pregnancy/nursing status, and possible drug interaction.

Monitoring: Monitor for signs/symptoms of endophthalmitis, retinal detachments, arterial thromboembolic events, and hypersensitivity reactions. Monitor IOP and perfusion of the optic nerve head. Perform tonometry within 30 min following inj. Monitor during the week following the inj to permit early treatment should an infection occur.

Patient Counseling: Inform about risks of developing endophthalmitis following administration. Instruct to seek immediate care from an ophthalmologist if the eye becomes red, sensitive to light, painful, or develops a change in vision.

Administration: Ophthalmic intravitreal inj. Refer to PI for preparation for administration. **Storage:** 2-8°C (36-46°F). Do not freeze. Protect from light and store in the original carton until time of use.

LUMIGAN RX
bimatoprost (Allergan)

THERAPEUTIC CLASS: Prostaglandin analog

INDICATIONS: Reduction of elevated intraocular pressure (IOP) in patient with open-angle glaucoma or ocular HTN.

DOSAGE: *Adults:* Usual: 1 drop in affected eye(s) qd in pm. Max: Once-daily dosing. Space dosing with other ophthalmic drugs by at least 5 min.
Pediatrics: ≥16 yrs: Usual: 1 drop in affected eye(s) qd in pm. Max: Once-daily dosing. Space dosing with other ophthalmic drugs by at least 5 min.

HOW SUPPLIED: Sol: 0.01%, 0.03% [2.5mL, 5mL, 7.5mL]

WARNINGS/PRECAUTIONS: Changes to pigmented tissues, including increased pigmentation of iris (may be permanent), eyelid, and eyelashes (may be reversible) reported. Regularly examine patients with noticeably increased iris pigmentation. May cause changes to eyelashes and vellus hair in the treated eye. Caution with active intraocular inflammation (eg, uveitis); inflammation may be exacerbated. Macular edema, including cystoid macular edema, reported; caution with aphakic patients, pseudophakic patients with torn posterior lens capsule, or patients at risk of macular edema. Bacterial keratitis reported with multi-dose container. Remove contact lenses prior to instillation; may reinsert 15 min after administration.

ADVERSE REACTIONS: Eyelash changes, conjunctival hyperemia, ocular pruritus/dryness/burning, visual disturbances, foreign body sensation, eye pain, periocular skin pigmentation, blepharitis, cataracts, periorbital erythema, eyelash darkening, superficial punctate keratitis, infections.

PREGNANCY: Category C, caution in nursing.

MECHANISM OF ACTION: Synthetic prostaglandin analog; selectively mimics the effects of naturally occurring substances, prostamides. Believed to lower IOP by increasing outflow of aqueous humor through both the trabecular meshwork and uveoscleral routes.

PHARMACOKINETICS: Absorption: (0.03%) C_{max}=0.08ng/mL, T_{max}=10 min, AUC=0.09ng•hr/mL. **Distribution:** (0.03%) V_d=0.67L/kg. **Metabolism:** Via oxidation, N-deethylation, and glucuronidation. **Elimination:** (IV) Urine (67%), feces (25%); $T_{1/2}$=45 min.

NURSING CONSIDERATIONS

Assessment: Assess for active intraocular inflammation (eg, uveitis), aphakic/pseudophakic patient with torn posterior lens capsule; angle-closure, inflammatory, or neovascular glaucoma; and pregnancy/nursing status.

Monitoring: Monitor for changes to pigmented tissue (eg, increased pigmentation of the iris, periorbital tissue [eyelid]), changes in eyelashes and vellus hair, exacerbation of intraocular inflammation, macular edema (eg, cystoid macular edema), and bacterial keratitis.

Patient Counseling: Inform about the potential for increased brown pigmentation of iris (may be permanent) and the possibility of darkening of eyelid skin (may be reversible after d/c). Inform about the possibility of eyelash and vellus hair changes in the treated eye during treatment. Advise to avoid touching tip of dispensing container to contact the eye, surrounding structures, fingers, or any other surface in order to avoid contamination of the solution. Advise to consult physician if having ocular surgery, or developed an intercurrent ocular condition (eg, trauma or infection) or ocular reaction. Instruct to remove contact lenses prior to instillation; reinsert 15 min after administration. Instruct to administer at least 5 min apart if using more than 1 topical ophthalmic drug.

Administration: Ocular route. **Storage:** 2-25°C (36-77°F).

LUNESTA   CIV
eszopiclone (Sunovion)

THERAPEUTIC CLASS: Nonbenzodiazepine hypnotic agent

INDICATIONS: Treatment of insomnia.

DOSAGE: *Adults:* Individualize dose. Initial: 2mg immediately before hs. Titrate: May be initiated at or raised to 3mg, if clinically indicated. Elderly: Use lowest possible effective dose. Difficulty Falling Asleep: Initial: 1mg immediately before hs. Titrate: May increase to 2mg, if clinically indicated. Difficulty Staying Asleep: 2mg immediately before hs. Severe Hepatic Impairment: Initial: 1mg. With Potent CYP3A4 Inhibitors: Initial: Not to exceed 1mg. Titrate: May be raised to 2mg, if needed.

HOW SUPPLIED: Tab: 1mg, 2mg, 3mg

WARNINGS/PRECAUTIONS: Abnormal thinking and behavioral changes reported. Complex behavior such as "sleep driving" has been reported; d/c if episode of "sleep driving" occur. Amnesia and other neuropsychiatric symptoms may occur. Worsening of depression, including suicidal thoughts and actions, reported in primarily depressed patients. Evaluate carefully and immediately for the emergence of new behavioral signs and symptoms. Avoid rapid dose decrease or abrupt d/c. Should only be taken immediately prior to bed or after going to bed and experiencing difficulty falling asleep. Rare cases of angioedema (involving tongue, glottis, or larynx) reported; if occurs do not rechallenge. Taking medications while still up and about may result in short-term memory impairment, hallucinations, impaired coordination, dizziness, and lightheadedness. Caution in conditions affecting metabolism or hemodynamic responses, and compromised respiratory function. Caution with signs and symptoms of depression. May impair physical/mental ability.

ADVERSE REACTIONS: Headache, unpleasant taste, somnolence, dry mouth, dizziness, infection, rash, chest pain, N/V, peripheral edema, migraine.

INTERACTIONS: May produce additive CNS-depressant effects with other psychotropic medications, anticonvulsants, antihistamines, ethanol, and other drugs that produce CNS depression. Avoid with alcohol. Decreased exposure with rifampicin. Increased levels with ketoconazole and other strong CYP3A4 inhibitors (eg, itraconazole, clarithromycin, nefazodone, troleandomycin, ritonavir, nelfinavir). Decreased levels with and of lorazepam. Coadministration with olanzapine produced a decrease in Digit Symbol Substitution Test (DSST) score.

PREGNANCY: Category C, caution in nursing.

MECHANISM OF ACTION: Nonbenzodiazepine hypnotic agent; mechanism not established. Suspected to interact with GABA-receptor complexes at binding domains located close to or allosterically coupled to benzodiazepine receptor.

PHARMACOKINETICS: Absorption: Rapidly absorbed; T_{max}=1 hr. C_{max} reduced by 21%, T_{max} delayed by 1 hr with high-fat meal. **Distribution:** Plasma protein binding (52-59%). **Metabolism:** Liver (extensive); oxidation and demethylation pathways via CYP3A4 and CYP2E1. Primary Metabolites: (S)-zopiclone-N-oxide and (S)-N-desmethyl zopiclone. **Elimination:** Urine (75% metabolite), (<10% parent drug); $T_{1/2}$=6 hrs, 9 hrs (elderly).

NURSING CONSIDERATIONS

Assessment: Assess for psychiatric or physical illness, diseases/conditions that could affect metabolism or hemodynamic response. Assess for depression, suicidal ideations, respiratory function, hepatic impairment, hypersensitivity reactions, pregnancy/nursing status, and other possible drug interactions.

Monitoring: Monitor for anaphylactic/anaphylactoid reactions, insomnia, angioedema, severe sedation, memory disorders, coordination, dizziness, lightheadedness, abnormal thinking/behavioral changes (eg, aggressiveness or extroversion that seem out of character), complex/bizarre behavior, worsening of depression, physical/psychological dependence, respiratory depression, motor or cognitive performance in elderly, withdrawal-emergent anxiety, and rebound insomnia.

Patient Counseling: Inform about potential benefits/risks of drug and possibility of physical/ psychological dependence. Instruct to take immediately before hs when patient can dedicate 8 hrs to sleep. Advise not to take with alcohol, other sedating drugs, with or immediately after a heavy/high-fat meal. Report to physician if "sleep driving" and other complex behavior occurred. Caution in performing hazardous tasks (eg, operating machinery, driving).

Administration: Oral route. **Storage:** 25°C (77°F), excursions permitted to 15-30°C (59-86°F).

LUPRON DEPOT-PED   RX
leuprolide acetate (Abbott)

THERAPEUTIC CLASS: Synthetic gonadotropin releasing hormone analog

INDICATIONS: Treatment of children with clinically diagnosed central precocious puberty (CPP) with onset of secondary sexual characteristics <8 yrs in females and <9 yrs in males associated with pubertal pituitary gonadotropin activation.

DOSAGE: *Pediatrics:* ≥2 yrs: Individualize dose. (1-Month) Administer single IM inj once a month. Starting dose: >37.5kg: 15mg. >25-37.5kg: 11.25mg. ≤25kg: 7.5mg. Titrate: May increase to next available higher dose (eg, 11.25mg or 15mg at the next monthly inj), if adequate hormonal and clinical suppression is not achieved. May also adjust dose with changes in body weight. Maint: Dose resulting in adequate hormonal suppression. (3-Month) Administer single IM inj q3 months (12 weeks). D/C therapy at appropriate age of onset of puberty.

HOW SUPPLIED: Inj: (1-Month) 7.5mg, 11.25mg, 15mg; (3-Month Kit) 11.25mg, 30mg

CONTRAINDICATIONS: Women who are or may become pregnant.

WARNINGS/PRECAUTIONS: Increase in clinical signs and symptoms of puberty may occur in early phase due to rise in gonadotropins and sex steroids. Postmarketing reports of convulsions observed; caution especially with history of seizures, epilepsy, cerebrovascular disorders, central nervous system anomalies or tumors. If noncompliant with schedule or dose is inadequate, gonadotropins and/or sex steroids may increase or rise above prepubertal levels. (3-Month) Do not use partial syringe or combination of syringes to achieve a particular dose; each formulation and strength have different release characteristics.

ADVERSE REACTIONS: Inj-site reactions/pain including abscess, general pain, headache, emotional lability, vasodilation, acne/seborrhea, rash including erythema multiforme, vaginal bleeding/discharge, vaginitis.

INTERACTIONS: Postmarketing reports of convulsions observed in patients on concomitant medications that have been associated with convulsions, such as bupropion and SSRIs.

PREGNANCY: Category X, not for use in nursing.

MECHANISM OF ACTION: Synthetic gonadotropin releasing hormone (GnRH) analog; potent inhibitor of gonadotropin secretion, resulting in suppression of testicular and ovarian steroidogenesis.

PHARMACOKINETICS: Absorption: (7.5mg in adults) C_{max}=20ng/mL, T_{max}=4 hrs; (11.5mg) C_{max}=19.1ng/mL; (30mg) C_{max}=52.5ng/mL; (11.5mg and 30mg) T_{max}=1 hr. **Distribution:** Plasma protein binding (43-49%), V_d=27L (IV). **Elimination:** (3.75mg) Urine (<5% parent and M-I), (1mg IV) $T_{1/2}$=3 hrs.

NURSING CONSIDERATIONS

Assessment: Assess for height and weight measurements, GnRH stimulation response, sex steroid levels, bone age versus chronological age, pregnancy, and hypersensitivity to drug. Rule out congenital adrenal hyperplasia, chorionic gonadotropin-secreting tumor, steroid-secreting tumor, and intracranial tumor. Confirm diagnosis of CPP (refer to PI).

Monitoring: Monitor GnRH stimulation response and sex steroid levels, hormonal and clinical parameters, measurements of bone age for advancement every 6-12 months, convulsions, and other adverse reactions. (1-Month) Monitor during treatment (eg, at month 2-3, month 6, and further as judged clinically appropriate). (3-Month) Monitor after 1-2 months of initiating therapy, with dose changes or periodically during treatment, to ensure adequate suppression.

Patient Counseling: Inform females that pregnancy is contraindicated and instruct to inform physician if patient becomes pregnant during treatment. Counsel about the importance of continuous therapy and adherence to drug administration schedule. Inform females that signs of puberty (eg, vaginal bleeding) may occur during first few weeks of therapy; notify physician if symptoms continue beyond 2nd month. Advise that some pain and irritation is expected; report if more severe or other unusual signs or symptoms occur. Advise parents/caregivers to notify physician if new or worsened symptoms develop after beginning treatment.

Administration: IM route. Must be administered under physician's supervision. Inj site should be varied periodically. Refer to PI for administration instructions. **Storage:** 25°C (77°F); excursions permitted to 15-30°C (59-86°F). Reconstituted Sus: Discard if not used within 2 hrs.

LUSEDRA `CIV`
fospropofol disodium (Eisai)

THERAPEUTIC CLASS: Anesthetic agent

INDICATIONS: For monitored anesthesia care (MAC) sedation in adult patients undergoing diagnostic or therapeutic procedures.

DOSAGE: *Adults:* Individualize dose. Standard Dosing Regimen: 18-<65 yrs who are Healthy or Patients With Mild Systemic Disease (ASA P1 or P2): Initial: 6.5mg/kg IV bolus. Supplemental: 1.6mg/kg IV as necessary. Max: 16.5mL (initial dose) and 4mL (supplemental dose). Modified Dosing Regimen: ≥65 yrs or Patients with Severe Systemic Disease (ASA P3 or P4): Initial/ Supplemental: 75% of the standard dosing regimen. Give supplemental doses only when patients can demonstrate purposeful movement in response to verbal or light tactile stimulation and no more frequently than every 4 min. Refer to PI for specific information regarding standard and modified dosing regimens. Use supplemental oxygen in all patients undergoing sedation.

HOW SUPPLIED: Inj: 35mg/mL

WARNINGS/PRECAUTIONS: Only trained persons in general anesthesia administration and not involved in the conduct of the diagnostic or therapeutic procedure should administer fospropofol. Sedated patients should be continuously monitored and facilities for maintenance of patent airway, providing artificial ventilation, administration of supplemental oxygen, and instituting of cardiovascular resuscitation must be immediately available. Respiratory depression and hypoxemia reported. Hypotension reported; caution in patients with compromised myocardial function, reduced vascular tone, or reduced intravascular volume. May cause unresponsiveness or minimal responsiveness to vigorous tactile or painful stimulation. Caution in hepatic impairment.

ADVERSE REACTIONS: Paresthesia, pruritus, N/V, hypoxemia, hypotension.

INTERACTIONS: Concomitant use with other cardiorespiratory depressants (eg, benzodiazepines, sedative-hypnotics, narcotic analgesics) may produce additive cardiorespiratory effects.

PREGNANCY: Category B, not for use in nursing.

MECHANISM OF ACTION: Sedative-hypnotic agent. Prodrug of propofol; metabolized by alkaline phosphatases following IV injection.

PHARMACOKINETICS: Absorption: (Fospropofol) AUC=19mcg•h/mL. (Propofol) AUC=1.2mcg•h/mL **Distribution:** (Fospropofol) V_d=0.33L/kg. (Propofol) V_d=5.8L/kg; plasma protein binding (98%). Crosses placenta, found in breast milk. **Metabolism:** Complete via alkaline phosphatases to propofol, formaldehyde, and phosphate; further metabolized to propofol glucuronide, quinol-4-sulfate, quinol-1-glucuronide, quinol-4-glucuronide (major metabolites). **Elimination:** (Fospropofol) $T_{1/2}$=0.88 hrs. (Propofol) $T_{1/2}$=1.13 hrs.

NURSING CONSIDERATIONS

Assessment: Assess for respiratory depression, hypotension or risk of hypotension (eg, compromised myocardial function, reduced vascular tone, reduced intravascular volume), hepatic impairment, pregnancy/nursing status, and for possible drug interactions.

Monitoring: Monitor continuously during sedation and recovery process for early signs of hypotension, apnea, airway obstruction, and/or oxygen desaturation. Monitor responsiveness to vigorous tactile or painful stimulation.

Patient Counseling: Inform that paresthesias (including burning, tingling, stinging) and/or pruritus are frequently experienced during the 1st injection and are typically mild to moderate in intensity, last a short time, and require no treatment. Counsel that a patient escort may be required after procedure. Instruct to avoid engaging in activities requiring complete alertness, coordination and/or physical dexterity (eg, operating hazardous machinery, signing legal documents, driving a motor vehicle) until physician has approved of performing such tasks.

Administration: IV route. **Storage:** 25°C (77°F); excursions permitted 15-30°C (59-86°F).

Luvox CR   RX

fluvoxamine maleate (Jazz Pharmaceuticals, Inc.)

> Antidepressants increased the risk of suicidal thinking and behavior (suicidality) in short-term studies in children, adolescents, and young adults with major depressive disorder (MDD) and other psychiatric disorders. Monitor and observe closely for clinical worsening, suicidality, or unusual changes in behavior in patients who are started on antidepressant therapy. Not approved for use in pediatric patients.

THERAPEUTIC CLASS: Selective serotonin reuptake inhibitor

INDICATIONS: Treatment of obsessive compulsive disorder (OCD) and social anxiety disorder (social phobia).

DOSAGE: *Adults:* Initial: 100mg qhs. Titrate: May increase by 50mg every week until maximum therapeutic response is achieved. Maint: 100-300mg/day. Max: 300mg/day. Maint/Continuation of Extended Treatment: Lowest effective dose. Periodically reassess need to continue. Switching to/from MAOI: Allow ≥14 days between d/c and initiation of therapy. Elderly/Hepatic Impairment: Titrate slowly. 3rd Trimester Pregnancy: Taper dose.

HOW SUPPLIED: Cap, Extended-Release: 100mg, 150mg

CONTRAINDICATIONS: Concomitant use of alosetron, tizanidine, thioridazine, or pimozide. Use during or within 14 days of MAOI therapy.

WARNINGS/PRECAUTIONS: Serotonin syndrome or neuroleptic malignant syndrome (NMS)-like reactions reported. May precipitate mixed/manic episode in patients at risk for bipolar disorder; screen for risk for bipolar disorder prior to initiating treatment. D/C should be gradual. May increase risk of bleeding events; caution with NSAIDs, aspirin (ASA), or other drugs that affect coagulation. Activation of mania/hypomania, syndrome of inappropriate antidiuretic hormone secretion, hyponatremia reported. Caution with history of mania or hepatic dysfunction, conditions that alter metabolism or hemodynamic responses. Caution with patients taking diuretics or who are volume depleted, especially the elderly; d/c if symptomatic hyponatremia occurs. Seizures reported; caution with history of convulsive disorders, avoid with unstable epilepsy and monitor patients with controlled epilepsy; d/c if seizures occur or seizure frequency increases. Consider potential risks and benefits of treatment during 3rd trimester of pregnancy. Decreased appetite and weight loss reported in children; monitor weight and growth.

ADVERSE REACTIONS: Headache, asthenia, nausea, diarrhea, anorexia, dyspepsia, insomnia, somnolence, nervousness, dizziness, anxiety, dry mouth, tremor, abnormal ejaculation.

INTERACTIONS: See Contraindications. Known potent inhibitor of CYP1A2, CYP3A4, CYP2C9, CYP2C19, and weak inhibitor of CYP2D6. Increased plasma concentrations of methadone, TCAs, propranolol, metoprolol, warfarin, alosetron, and alprazolam. Increased area under the curve (AUC), C_{max} of alprazolam, tacrine, ramelteon, and alosetron. Increased serum levels of clozapine; risk of adverse events may be higher. Increased levels of carbamazepine and symptoms of toxicity reported. Decreased clearance levels of mexiletine, theophylline, and benzodiazepines like alprazolam, midazolam, triazolam, and diazepam. Bradycardia reported; caution with diltiazem. Concomitant use of serotonergic drugs and with drugs that impair metabolism of serotonin may cause serotonin syndrome and NMS-like reactions. Caution with tryptophan; may enhance serotonergic effects and severe vomiting may occur. Weakness, hyperreflexia, incoordination with SSRIs and sumatriptan reported. Risk of seizures with lithium. Altered anticoagulation effects with warfarin. Diuretics may increase the risk of hyponatremia. A clinically significant interaction is possible with drugs having narrow therapeutic ratio such as pimozide, warfarin, theophylline, certain benzodiazepines, omeprazole, and phenytoin. Smoking increases metabolism. Avoid alcohol.

PREGNANCY: Category C, not for use in nursing.

MECHANISM OF ACTION: SSRI; inhibits neuronal uptake of serotonin.

PHARMACOKINETICS: Absorption: C_{max} (at doses 100mg, 200mg, 300mg) =47ng/mL, 161ng/mL, 319ng/mL. **Distribution:** V_d=25L/kg; plasma protein binding (80%); found in breast milk. **Metabolism:** Liver (extensive) via oxidative demethylation and deamination. **Elimination:** Urine (94%), $T_{1/2}$ =16.3 hrs.

NURSING CONSIDERATIONS

Assessment: Assess for MDD, risk for bipolar disorder, depressive symptoms, history of mania, seizures, suicide, drug abuse, disease/condition that alters metabolism or hemodynamic response, hepatic impairment, history of hypersensitivity to drug, pregnancy/nursing status and possible drug interactions. Obtain a detailed psychiatric history prior to therapy.

Monitoring: Monitor for signs/symptoms of clinical worsening (suicidality, unusual changes in behavior), serotonin syndrome, NMS-like reactions (muscle rigidity, hyperthermia, mental status changes), abnormal bleeding, hyponatremia, seizures, hepatic dysfunction, and other adverse reactions. If d/c therapy (particularly if abrupt), monitor for symptoms of dysphoric mood, irritability, agitation, dizziness, sensory disturbances, anxiety, confusion, headache, lethargy, emotional lability, insomnia, and hypomania.

Patient Counseling: Advise to avoid alcohol. Caution on risk of serotonin syndrome with concomitant use of triptans, tramadol, or other serotonergic agents. Seek medical attention for symptoms of serotonin syndrome (mental status changes, tachycardia, hyperthermia, N/V, diarrhea, incoordination), NMS, allergic reactions (rash, hives), abnormal bleeding (particularly if using NSAIDs or ASA), hyponatremia, activation of mania, seizures, clinical worsening (suicidal ideation, unusual changes in behavior), and discontinuation symptoms (eg, irritability, agitation, dizziness, anxiety, headache, insomnia). Instruct not to crush or chew; may be taken with or without food. Caution against hazardous tasks (eg, operating machinery and driving). Notify physician if pregnant, intend to become pregnant, or breastfeeding. Counsel about benefits and risks of therapy. Inform physician if taking or plan to take any over-the-counter medications.

Administration: Oral route. **Storage:** Store at 25°C (77°F); excursions permitted to 15-30°C (59-86°F). Avoid exposure to >30°C (86°F). Protect from high humidity. Keep out of reach of children.

LUXIQ   RX
betamethasone valerate (Stiefel)

THERAPEUTIC CLASS: Corticosteroid

INDICATIONS: Relief of the inflammatory/pruritic manifestations of corticosteroid-responsive dermatoses of the scalp.

DOSAGE: *Adults:* Apply to affected scalp area bid (am and pm). Repeat until entire affected scalp area is treated.

HOW SUPPLIED: Foam: 0.12% [50g, 100g]

WARNINGS/PRECAUTIONS: May produce reversible hypothalamic-pituitary-adrenal (HPA) axis suppression, manifestations of Cushing's syndrome, hyperglycemia, and glucosuria; pediatric patients are at greater risk. Caution when applied to large surface areas, for prolonged use, or under occlusive dressings; may increase systemic absorption. Evaluate periodically for HPA suppression; d/c or reduce frequency of application or substitute a less potent steroid if noted. D/C if irritation develops. Use appropriate antifungal or antibacterial agent with dermatological infections; if infection does not clear, d/c until infection is controlled. Administration to children should be limited to smallest amount compatible with an effective therapeutic regimen; may interfere with growth and development. Flammable; avoid fire, flame, or smoking during and immediately after application.

ADVERSE REACTIONS: Burning, stinging, pruritus, paresthesia, acne, alopecia, conjunctivitis.

PREGNANCY: Category C, caution in nursing.

MECHANISM OF ACTION: Corticosteroid; possesses anti-inflammatory, antipruritic, and vasoconstrictive properties. Anti-inflammatory mechanism not established. Suspected to induce phospholipase A_2 inhibitory proteins, lipocortins. Lipocortins control biosynthesis of potent mediators of inflammation (eg, prostaglandins, leukotrienes) by inhibiting release of their precursor, arachidonic acid.

PHARMACOKINETICS: Absorption: Percutaneous; occlusion, inflammation, and other diseases may increase absorption. **Distribution:** Systemically administered corticosteroids are found in breast milk. **Metabolism:** Liver. **Elimination:** Renal (major), bile.

NURSING CONSIDERATIONS

Assessment: Assess for hypersensitivity to corticosteroids and pregnancy/nursing status.

Monitoring: Monitor for signs/symptoms of HPA-axis suppression, Cushing's syndrome, hyperglycemia, glucosuria, local skin irritation, allergic contact dermatitis (eg, failure to heal), and for the development of dermatological infections (eg, fungal, bacterial). Monitor for signs of glucocorticoid insufficiency following withdrawal from treatment. In patients on high doses or using occlusive dressings, perform periodic monitoring for HPA-axis suppression using adrenocorticotropic hormone (ACTH) stimulation, am plasma cortisol, and urinary free cortisol tests. In pediatric patients, monitor for signs/symptoms of systemic toxicity and growth.

Patient Counseling: Inform to use exactly as directed; avoid contact with eyes. Counsel on proper dispensing and application. Instruct not to bandage, cover, or wrap treated scalp area unless directed by physician. Contact physician if no improvement within 2 weeks of starting therapy or if adverse reactions develop. Avoid fire, flame, or smoking during and immediately following drug application. Advise patient to wash hands immediately after application. Keep out of reach of children.

Administration: Topical route. Invert can and dispense foam onto saucer or other cool surface first, then apply in small amounts to scalp. Gently massage into affected area until foam disappear. **Storage:** 20-25°C (68-77°F). Do not expose to heat or store at temperatures above 49°C (120°F). Do not puncture or incinerate container. Contents under pressure.

LYBREL   RX
ethinyl estradiol - levonorgestrel (Wyeth)

> Cigarette smoking increases the risk of serious cardiovascular (CV) side effects from oral contraceptive use. Risk increases with age (>35yrs) and with heavy smoking (≥15 cigarettes/day). Women who use oral contraceptives should be strongly advised not to smoke.

THERAPEUTIC CLASS: Estrogen/progestogen combination

INDICATIONS: Prevention of pregnancy.

DOSAGE: *Adults:* 1 tab qd. No Current Contraceptive Therapy: Start on Day 1 of menstrual cycle. Current 21- or 28-day Contraceptive Regimen: Start on Day 1 of withdrawal bleed (at the latest 7 days after last active tablet). Current Progestin-Only Pill Regimen: Start on the day after taking progestin-only pill. Current Implant Regimen: Start on the day of implant removal. Current Inj Regimen: Start on the day the next inj is due. Use nonhormonal back-up method of birth control for 1st 7 days of therapy when initiating after progestin-only pill, implant, or inj. Start no earlier than Day 28 postpartum in the nonlactating mother or after second trimester abortion.
Pediatrics: Postpubertal adolescents: 1 tab qd. No Current Contraceptive Therapy: Start on Day 1 of menstrual cycle. 21- or 28-day Regimen: Start on Day 1 of withdrawal bleed (at the latest 7 days after last active tablet). Progestin-Only Pill: Start on the day after taking progestin-only pill. Implant: Start on the day of implant removal. Inj: Start on the day the next inj is due. Use nonhormonal back-up method of birth control for 1st 7 days of therapy when initiating after progestin-only pill, implant, or inj. Start no earlier than Day 28 postpartum in the nonlactating mother or after second trimester abortion.

HOW SUPPLIED: Tab: (Ethinyl Estradiol-Levonorgestrel) 20mcg-90mcg

CONTRAINDICATIONS: Thrombophlebitis or history of deep vein thrombophlebitis (DVT), thromboembolic disorders or history of thromboembolic disorders, current or past history of cerebrovascular or coronary artery disease (CAD), valvular heart disease with thrombogenic complications, thrombogenic rhythm disorders, uncontrolled HTN, diabetes with vascular involvement, headaches with focal neurological symptoms such as aura, major surgery with prolonged immobilization, hereditary or acquired thrombophilia, known or suspected breast carcinoma or personal history of breast carcinoma, carcinoma of the endometrium or other known or suspected estrogen-dependent neoplasia, undiagnosed abnormal genital bleeding, cholestatic jaundice of pregnancy or jaundice with prior pill use, hepatic adenomas or carcinomas or active liver disease, known or suspected pregnancy.

WARNINGS/PRECAUTIONS: Increased risk of MI, vascular disease, venous thromboembolic and thrombotic disease, cerebrovascular disease (thrombotic and hemorrhagic stroke), transient ischemic attacks (TIA), hepatic neoplasia, and gallbladder disease. Increased risk of morbidity and mortality in patients with inherited or acquired thrombophilias, HTN, hyperlipidemia, obesity, diabetes mellitus (DM) and surgery or trauma with increased risk of thrombosis. May increase risk of breast and cervical cancer. Retinal thrombosis reported; d/c if unexplained partial or complete loss of vision, onset of proptosis or diplopia, papilledema, or retinal vascular lesions develops. Should not be used to induce withdrawal bleeding as a test for pregnancy, or to treat threatened or habitual abortion during pregnancy. May cause glucose intolerance; monitor prediabetic and diabetic patients. May cause fluid retention and increase BP; monitor closely with HTN and d/c if significant elevation of BP occurs. D/C with onset or exacerbation of migraine headache. May cause unscheduled breakthrough bleeding and spotting. Ectopic and intrauterine pregnancies may occur with contraceptive failures. Caution in patients with history of depression; d/c if significant depression develops. Monitor closely with hyperlipidemias; may elevate LDL and/or plasma TG. D/C if jaundice develop. Visual changes or changes in lens tolerance may develop with contact lens use. Diarrhea and/or vomiting may reduce serum concentrations. Perform annual physical exam. May affect certain endocrine, LFTs, and blood components. Does not protect against HIV infection (AIDS) or other STDs. Use before menarche is not indicated.

ADVERSE REACTIONS: Acne, Budd-Chiari syndrome, change in cervical erosion and secretion, dizziness, edema/fluid retention, focal nodular hyperplasia, GI symptoms, hirsutism, infertility, lactation, persistent melasma/chloasma, N/V, pancreatitis, rash (allergic), loss of scalp hair.

INTERACTIONS: Reduced contraceptive effectiveness leading to unintended pregnancy or unscheduled bleeding with antibiotics, anticonvulsants, and other drugs that increase the metabolism of contraceptive steroids (eg, rifampin, rifabutin, barbiturates, phenylbutazone, primidone, dexamethasone, phenytoin, carbamazepine, felbamate, oxcarbazepine, griseofulvin, topiramate, and modafinil). Contraceptive failures and unscheduled bleeding reported with ampicillins and other penicillins and tetracyclines. Decreased enterohepatic recirculation with substances that reduce gastric transit time. Anti-HIV protease inhibitors may increase or decrease levels. Reduce effectiveness with St. John's wort (*Hypericum perforatum*). Atorvastatin, ascorbic acid, acetaminophen, CYP3A4 inhibitors (eg, itraconazole, ketoconazole) may increase hormone levels. Troleandomycin may increase risk for intrahepatic cholestasis. May increase levels of cyclosporine, theophylline, prednisolone, and other corticosteroids. May decrease levels of acetaminophen and lamotrigine. Increases clearance of temazepam, salicylic acid, morphine, clofibric acid.

PREGNANCY: Category X, not for use in nursing.

MECHANISM OF ACTION: Estrogen/progesterone combination oral contraceptive. Acts by suppression of gonadotropins. Primarily inhibits ovulation. Also responsible for changes in cervical mucus (increasing difficulty of sperm entry into uterus) and in endometrium (reducing likelihood of implantation).

PHARMACOKINETICS: Absorption: Oral administration on variable days resulted in different parameters. Levonorgestrel: Rapid and completely absorbed, absolute bioavailability (100%); Ethinyl estradiol: Rapid and completely absorbed, absolute bioavailability (between 38% and 43%). **Distribution:** Levonorgestrel: Sex hormone-binding globulin (SHBG). Ethinyl Estradiol: Plasma protein binding (97%). **Metabolism:** Levonorgestrel: Reduction, hydroxylation and conjugation. Ethinyl Estradiol: Liver; hydroxylation via CYP3A4; methylation sulfation, glucuronidation. **Elimination:** Levonorgestrel: Urine (40-68%), feces (16-48%); $T_{1/2}$=36 hrs. Ethinyl Estradiol: Urine, feces; $T_{1/2}$=21 hrs.

NURSING CONSIDERATIONS

Assessment: Assess for presence or history of breast cancer, estrogen dependent neoplasia, abnormal genital bleeding, active liver disease, and known/suspected pregnancy or any other conditions where treatment is cautioned or contraindicated. Assess use in patients who are >35 yrs and heavy smokers (≥15 cigarettes/day). Assess use with HTN, hyperlipidemias, obesity, DM, or in patients at increased risk for thrombosis. Assess for possible drug interactions.

Monitoring: Monitor bleeding irregularities, thromboembolic events, onset or exacerbation of headaches or migraines, and ectopic pregnancy. Monitor fasting blood glucose levels in DM and prediabetic patients, BP with history of HTN, lipid levels with a history of hyperlipidemia. Monitor for signs of liver dysfunction (eg, jaundice) and signs of depression with previous history. Refer patients with contact lenses to an ophthalmologist if visual changes occur. Perform annual history and physical exam.

Patient Counseling: Instruct that medication does not protect against HIV infection (AIDS) and other STDs. Counsel about potential adverse effects. May experience spotting/bleeding; continue therapy and notify physician if persists. Advise to avoid smoking. Instruct to take pill at same time every day. Inform that if 1 pill missed, take as soon as remembered; take next pill at next regular scheduled time. Advise that pregnancy can occur if patient has sexual intercourse during 7 days after restarting pills; use nonhormonal birth control method during that time.

Administration: Oral route. **Storage:** 25°C (77°F); excursions permitted to 15-30°C (59-86°F).

L

Lyrica

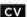

pregabalin (Pfizer)

THERAPEUTIC CLASS: GABA analog

INDICATIONS: Management of neuropathic pain associated with diabetic peripheral neuropathy, postherpetic neuralgia, and fibromyalgia. Adjunctive therapy for adult patients with partial onset seizures.

DOSAGE: *Adults:* Neuropathic Pain: Initial: 50mg tid. Titrate: May increase to 300mg/day within 1 week based on efficacy and tolerability. Max: 300mg/day (100mg tid). Postherpetic Neuralgia: Initial: 75mg bid or 50mg tid (150mg/day). Titrate: May increase to 300mg/day within 1 week based on efficacy and tolerability. If tolerated, may increase up to 600mg/day divided bid or tid if no sufficient pain relief experienced following 2-4 weeks of treatment with 300mg/day. Usual: 150-300mg/day. Partial-Onset Seizures: Initial: 150mg/day divided bid-tid. Titrate: May increase based on response and tolerability up to max dose of 600mg/day. Fibromyalgia: Initial: 75mg bid. Titrate: May increase to 300mg/day (150mg bid) within 1 week based on efficacy and tolerability, then further increase to 450mg/day (225mg bid) if sufficient benefit not experienced. Usual: 300-450mg/day. Max: 450mg/day. Refer to PI for dosage adjustment based on renal function. D/C: Taper over minimum of 1 week.

HOW SUPPLIED: Cap: 25mg, 50mg, 75mg, 100mg, 150mg, 200mg, 225mg, 300mg. Sol: 20mg/mL [16 fl. oz.]

WARNINGS/PRECAUTIONS: Angioedema reported; d/c if angioedema with respiratory compromise occurs. Caution in patients who had a previous episode of angioedema. Hypersensitivity reactions reported; d/c immediately if symptoms occur. Avoid abrupt withdrawal; gradually taper over a minimum of 1 week. Increased risk of suicidal thoughts/behavior; monitor for emergence or worsening of depression, suicidal thought/behavior, and/or unusual changes in mood/behavior. May cause weight gain and peripheral edema; caution with congestive heart failure (CHF). May cause dizziness and somnolence; may impair physical/mental abilities. New or worsening of preexisting tumors reported. Blurred vision, decreased visual acuity, visual field changes, and funduscopic changes reported. Creatine kinase (CK) elevations and rhabdomyolysis reported; d/c if myopathy is diagnosed or suspected or if markedly elevated CK levels occur. Associated with a decrease in platelet counts and PR interval prolongation. Caution in patients with renal impairment.

ADVERSE REACTIONS: Dizziness, somnolence, ataxia, peripheral edema, weight gain, blurred vision, diplopia, tremor, dry mouth, abnormal thinking, infection, headache, fatigue, constipation, euphoric mood.

INTERACTIONS: May increase risk of angioedema with other drugs associated with angioedema (eg, ACE inhibitors). Additive effects on cognitive and gross motor functioning with oxycodone, lorazepam, and ethanol. Caution with thiazolidinedione class of antidiabetic drugs; higher frequencies of weight gain and peripheral edema reported. Gabapentin reported to cause a small reduction in absorption rate.

PREGNANCY: Category C, not for use in nursing.

MECHANISM OF ACTION: Gamma-aminobutyric acid derivative; not fully established; binds with high affinity to the α_2-delta site (an auxiliary subunit of voltage-gated calcium channels) in CNS tissues.

PHARMACOKINETICS: Absorption: Well absorbed; T_{max}=1.5 hrs (fasting), 3 hrs (fed). **Distribution:** V_d=0.5L/kg. **Metabolism:** Negligible metabolism. N-methylated derivative (major metabolite). **Elimination:** Urine (90% unchanged); $T_{1/2}$=6.3 hrs.

NURSING CONSIDERATIONS

Assessment: Assess for hypersensitivity, renal impairment, preexisting tumors, history of drug abuse, history of depression, previous episode of angioedema, CHF, pregnancy/nursing status, and possible drug interactions. Obtain baseline weight.

Monitoring: Monitor for angioedema, hypersensitivity reactions, peripheral edema, weight gain, new tumors or worsening of preexisting tumors, opthalmological effects, rhabdomyolysis, dizziness, somnolence, emergence or worsening of depression, suicidal thoughts or behavior, and/or changes in behavior. Monitor CK levels and platelet counts. Monitor ECG for PR interval prolongation.

Patient Counseling: Instruct to d/c therapy and seek medical attention if hypersensitivity reactions or symptoms of angioedema occur. Inform patients and caregivers to be alert for the emergence or worsening of depression, unusual changes in mood or behavior, or the emergence of suicidal thoughts, behavior, or thoughts of self-harm; immediately report behaviors of concern to physician. Dizziness, somnolence, blurred vision, and other CNS signs and symptoms may occur; advise to use caution when operating machinery/driving. Weight gain and edema may occur. Do not d/c therapy abruptly/rapidly. Visual disturbances may occur; contact physician if any changes in vision occur. Report unexplained muscle pain, tenderness, or weakness, particularly if accompanied by malaise or fever to physician. Do not consume alcohol while on therapy. Notify physician if pregnant, intend to become pregnant, breastfeeding or intend to breastfeed. Inform men on therapy who plan to father a child, of the potential risk of male-mediated teratogenicity. Instruct diabetic patients to pay attention to skin integrity while on therapy.

Administration: Oral route. **Storage:** 25°C (77°F); excursions permitted to 15-30°C (59-86°F).

LYSTEDA   RX
tranexamic acid (Ferring)

THERAPEUTIC CLASS: Antifibrinolytic agent

INDICATIONS: Treatment of cyclic heavy menstrual bleeding.

DOSAGE: *Adults:* Usual: 2 tabs tid for max of 5 days during monthly menstruation. Renal Impairment: SrCr >1.4-≤2.8mg/dL: 2 tabs bid for max of 5 days during menstruation. SrCr >2.8-≤5.7mg/dL: 2 tabs qd for max of 5 days during menstruation. SrCr >5.7mg/dL: 1 tab qd for max of 5 days during menstruation.

HOW SUPPLIED: Tab: 650mg

CONTRAINDICATIONS: Active thromboembolic disease (eg, deep vein thrombosis [DVT], pulmonary embolism, or cerebral thrombosis); history of thrombosis or thromboembolism (including retinal vein or artery occlusion) or intrinsic risk of thrombosis or thromboembolism (eg, thrombogenic valvular disease, thrombogenic cardiac rhythm disease, or hypercoagulopathy).

WARNINGS/PRECAUTIONS: Exclude endometrial pathology prior to treatment. Retinal venous and arterial occlusion reported; d/c immediately and refer to ophthalmologist if visual and ocular symptoms occur. Severe allergic reactions reported involving dyspnea, throat tightening, and facial flushing that required medical treatment. Anaphylactic shock reported with IV bolus administration. Cerebral edema and cerebral infarction may occur in women with subarachnoid hemorrhage. Ligneous conjunctivitis reported.

ADVERSE REACTIONS: Headache, nasal and sinus symptoms, back pain, abdominal pain, musculoskeletal pain, arthralgia, muscle cramps/spasms, migraine, anemia, fatigue.

INTERACTIONS: Combination hormonal contraceptives may increase thromboembolic risk; use only if there is strong medical need and caution in obese and smokers especially >35 yrs old. Not recommended with Factor IX complex concentrates or anti-inhibitor coagulant concentrates. Caution with all-trans retinoic acid for remission induction of acute promyelocytic leukemia. Tissue plasminogen activators may decrease efficacy of both drugs.

PREGNANCY: Category B, caution in nursing.

MECHANISM OF ACTION: Antifibrinolytic; synthetic lysine amino acid derivative, which diminishes the dissolution of hemostatic fibrin by plasmin. Reversibly binds to the lysine receptor binding sites of plasmin for fibrin, preventing binding to fibrin monomers, thus preserving and stabilizing fibrin's matrix structure.

PHARMACOKINETICS: Absorption: Absolute bioavailability (45%); T_{max}=2.5 hrs, (single dose) AUC_{inf}=80.19μg•h/mL, C_{max}=13.83mcg/mL; (multiple dose) C_{max}=16.41μg/mL. **Distribution:** V_d=0.18L/kg; V_{ss}=0.39L/kg; plasma protein bound (3%); crosses placenta; found in breast milk. **Elimination:** Urine (>95%, unchanged); $T_{1/2}$=11.08 hrs.

NURSING CONSIDERATIONS

Assessment: Assess for endometrial disease, active thromboembolic disease, history of thrombosis or thromboembolism or intrinsic risk for such conditions, acute promyelocytic leukemia, subarachnoid hemorrhage, renal impairment, pregnancy/nursing status, hypersensitivity, and possible drug interactions.

Monitoring: Monitor for venous thromboembolism, arterial thromboses, severe allergic reactions and anaphylactic shock, retinal venous and arterial occlusion, visual and ocular symptoms, ligneous conjunctivitis, cerebral edema, and cerebral infarction.

Patient Counseling: Instruct to take as prescribed; inform to adhere to dosing regimen. Instruct to d/c and notify physician if eye symptoms or change in vision, severe allergic reactions (eg, SOB or throat tightening), and if menstrual bleeding persists or worsens. Inform that headache, sinus and nasal symptoms, back pain, abdominal pain, musculoskeletal pain, joint pain, muscle cramps, migraine, anemia, and fatigue may occur.

Administration: Oral route. Do not chew or break apart; swallow whole. **Storage:** 25°C (77°F); excursions permitted to 15-30°C (59-86°F).

MACROBID

RX

nitrofurantoin monohydrate - nitrofurantoin macrocrystals (Procter & Gamble)

THERAPEUTIC CLASS: Imidazolidinedione antibacterial

INDICATIONS: Treatment of acute uncomplicated urinary tract infections (acute cystitis) caused by caused by susceptible strains of *Escherichia coli* or *Staphylococcus saprophyticus*.

DOSAGE: *Adults:* 100mg q12h for 7 days.
Pediatrics: >12 yrs: 100mg q12h for 7 days.

HOW SUPPLIED: Cap: 100mg

CONTRAINDICATIONS: Anuria, oliguria, significant impairment of renal function (CrCl <60mL/min or clinically significant elevated SrCr), pregnancy at term (38-42 weeks gestation), labor and delivery or when onset of labor is imminent, and neonates <1 month of age, and previous history of nitrofurantoin-associated cholestatic jaundice/hepatic dysfunction.

WARNINGS/PRECAUTIONS: Not for treatment of pyelonephritis or perinephric abscesses. Acute, subacute, or chronic pulmonary reactions (diffuse interstitial pneumonitis, pulmonary fibrosis, or both) reported; d/c and take appropriate measures if these occur. Closely monitor pulmonary condition if on long term therapy. Hepatic reactions (eg, hepatitis, cholestatic jaundice, chronic active hepatitis, hepatic necrosis) occur rarely. Monitor for liver injury; d/c and take appropriate measures if hepatitis occurs. Peripheral neuropathy reported; risk may be increased with renal impairment, anemia, diabetes mellitus (DM), electrolyte imbalance, vitamin B deficiency, and debilitating disease. Monitor periodically for changes in renal function if on long term therapy. Optic neuritis reported rarely. May induce hemolytic anemia of the primaquine-sensitivity type. *Clostridium difficile*-associated diarrhea (CDAD) reported. False (+) reaction for glucose in urine with Benedict's and Fehling's solutions. Use in the absence of a proven or strongly suspected bacterial infection or a prophylactic indication is unlikely to provide benefit and increases risk of the development of drug-resistant bacteria.

ADVERSE REACTIONS: Nausea, headache, flatulence.

INTERACTIONS: Antacids containing magnesium trisilicate reduce both the rate and extent of absorption. Increased serum levels, decreased urinary levels, and decreased efficacy with uricosuric drugs (eg, probenecid, sulfinpyrazone).

PREGNANCY: Category B, not for use in nursing.

MECHANISM OF ACTION: Imidazolidinedione antibacterial; inhibits protein synthesis, aerobic energy metabolism, DNA, RNA, and cell-wall synthesis.

PHARMACOKINETICS: Absorption: C_{max}=<1mcg/mL. **Distribution:** Found in breast milk. **Elimination:** Urine (20-25% unchanged).

NURSING CONSIDERATIONS

Assessment: Assess for anuria, oliguria, significant renal impairment, history of nitrofurantoin-associated cholestatic jaundice/hepatic dysfunction, glucose-6-phosphate dehydrogenase deficiency, DM, anemia, electrolyte imbalance, vitamin B deficiency, debilitating disease, drug hypersensitivity, pregnancy/nursing status, and for possible drug interactions. Obtain urine specimens for culture and susceptibility testing prior to therapy.

Monitoring: Monitor for persistence or reappearance of bacteriuria, acute/subacute/chronic pulmonary reactions, hepatic reactions (eg, hepatitis, cholestatic jaundice, chronic active hepatitis, hepatic necrosis), peripheral neuropathy, optic neuritis, hematologic manifestations, and CDAD. Monitor LFTs periodically. Monitor renal and pulmonary function periodically during long-term therapy. Obtain urine specimens for culture and susceptibility testing after completion of therapy.

Patient Counseling: Advise to take with food to enhance tolerance and improve drug absorption. Instruct to complete full course of therapy and to contact physician if any unusual symptoms occur. Do not use antacids containing magnesium trisilicate. Therapy treats bacterial, not viral infections. Advise to take exactly ud; skipping doses or not completing full course may decrease effectiveness and increase drug resistance. Diarrhea is a common problem and usually ends when antibiotic is d/c. Watery and bloody stools (with/without stomach cramps and fever) may develop as late as ≥2 months after last dose; notify physician immediately if this occurs.

Administration: Oral route. Take with food. **Storage:** 15-30°C (59-86°F).

MACRODANTIN

RX

nitrofurantoin macrocrystals (Procter & Gamble)

THERAPEUTIC CLASS: Imidazolidinedione antibacterial

INDICATIONS: Treatment of urinary tract infections cause by susceptible strains of microorganisms.

DOSAGE: *Adults:* 50-100mg qid for 1 week or at least 3 days after sterility of the urine obtained. Long-term Suppressive Use: 50-100mg qhs.
Pediatrics: ≥1 month: 5-7mg/kg/day given in 4 divided doses for 1 week or at least 3 days after sterility of the urine obtained. Long-term Suppressive Use: 1mg/kg/day given in single dose or in 2 divided doses.

HOW SUPPLIED: Cap: 25mg, 50mg, 100mg

CONTRAINDICATIONS: Anuria, oliguria, significant impairment of renal function (CrCl <60mL/min or clinically significant elevated SrCr), pregnancy at term (38-42 weeks' gestation), use during labor and delivery, or when the onset of labor is imminent, neonates <1 month, and previous history of nitrofurantoin-associated cholestatic jaundice/hepatic dysfunction.

WARNINGS/PRECAUTIONS: Not for treatment of pyelonephritis or perinephric abscesses. Acute, subacute, or chronic pulmonary reactions (diffuse interstitial pneumonitis, pulmonary fibrosis, or both) reported; d/c and take appropriate measures if these occur. Closely monitor pulmonary condition if on long term therapy. Hepatic reactions (eg, hepatitis, cholestatic jaundice, chronic active hepatitis, and hepatic necrosis) occur rarely. Monitor for liver injury; d/c and take appropriate measures if hepatitis occurs. Peripheral neuropathy reported; risk may be increased with renal impairment, anemia, diabetes mellitus (DM), electrolyte imbalance, vitamin B deficiency, and debilitating disease. Monitor periodically for changes in renal function if on long-term therapy. Optic neuritis reported rarely. May cause hemolytic anemia of the primaquine-sensitivity type. *Clostridium difficile*-associated diarrhea (CDAD) reported. False (+) reaction for glucose in urine with Benedict's and Fehling's solutions. Use in the absence of a proven or strongly suspected bacterial infection or a prophylactic indication is unlikely to provide benefit and increases risk of the development of drug-resistant bacteria.

ADVERSE REACTIONS: Pulmonary hypersensitivity reactions, hepatic reactions, peripheral neuropathy, exfoliative dermatitis, erythema multiforme, lupus-like syndrome, nausea, emesis, anorexia.

INTERACTIONS: Antacids containing magnesium trisilicate reduce both the rate and extent of absorption. Increased serum levels, decreased urinary levels, and decreased efficacy with uricosuric drugs (eg, probenecid, sulfinpyrazone).

PREGNANCY: Category B, not for use in nursing.

MECHANISM OF ACTION: Imidazolidinedione antibacterial; inhibits protein synthesis, aerobic energy metabolism, DNA, RNA, and cell-wall synthesis.

PHARMACOKINETICS: Distribution: Found in breast milk. **Elimination:** Urine (100mg qid for 7 days: Day 1: 37.9%; Day 7:35%).

NURSING CONSIDERATIONS

Assessment: Assess for anuria, oliguria, significant renal impairment, history of nitrofurantoin-associated cholestatic jaundice/hepatic dysfunction, glucose-6-phosphate dehydrogenase deficiency, DM, anemia, electrolyte imbalance, vitamin B deficiency, debilitating disease, drug hypersensitivity, pregnancy/nursing status, and possible drug interactions. Obtain urine specimen for culture and susceptibility testing prior to therapy.

Monitoring: Monitor for persistence or reappearance of bacteriuria, acute/subacute/chronic pulmonary reactions, hepatic reactions (eg, hepatitis, cholestatic jaundice, chronic active hepatitis, hepatic necrosis), peripheral neuropathy, optic neuritis, hematologic manifestations, and CDAD. Monitor LFTs periodically. Monitor renal and pulmonary function periodically during long-term therapy. Obtain urine specimens for culture and susceptibility testing after completion of therapy.

Patient Counseling: Advise to take with food to enhance tolerance and improve drug absorption. Instruct to complete full course of therapy and to contact physician if any unusual symptoms occur. Do not use antacids containing magnesium trisilicate. Therapy treats bacterial, not viral infections. Instruct to take exactly ud; skipping doses or not completing full course may decrease effectiveness and increase drug resistance. Diarrhea is a common problem and ends when antibiotic is d/c. Watery and bloody stools (with/without stomach cramps and fever) may develop as late as ≥2 months after last dose; notify physician immediately if this occurs.

Administration: Oral route. Take with food.

MALARONE   RX
proguanil HCl - atovaquone (GlaxoSmithKline)

OTHER BRAND NAMES: Malarone Pediatric (GlaxoSmithKline)
THERAPEUTIC CLASS: Pyrimidine synthesis inhibitor

INDICATIONS: Prophylaxis or treatment of acute, uncomplicated malaria caused by *Plasmodium falciparum*.

DOSAGE: *Adults:* Prevention: Begin 1-2 days before entering malaria-endemic area, continue daily during stay and for 7 days after return. 250mg-100mg qd. Treatment: 1000mg-400mg qd for 3 days.
Pediatrics: Prevention: Begin 1-2 days before entering endemic area, continue during stay and for 7 days after return. >40kg: 250mg-100mg (1 adult strength tab) qd. 31-40kg: 187.5mg-75mg qd. 21-30kg: 125mg-50mg qd. 11-20kg: 62.5mg-25mg qd. Treatment: Treat for 3 consecutive days. >40kg: 1000mg-400mg qd (4 adult strength tabs). 31-40kg: 750mg-300mg (3 adult strength tabs). 21-30kg: 500mg-200mg qd (2 adult strength tabs). 11-20kg: 250mg-100mg (1 adult strength tab). 9-10kg: 187.5mg-75mg qd. 5-8kg: 125mg-50mg qd.

HOW SUPPLIED: Tab: (Atovaquone-Proguanil) 62.5mg-25mg (Pediatric), 250mg-100mg

CONTRAINDICATIONS: Prophylaxis in patients with severe renal impairment (CrCl <30mL/min).

WARNINGS/PRECAUTIONS: Rare cases of anaphylaxis reported. Not evaluated for treatment of cerebral malaria or other severe manifestations of complicated malaria, including hyperparasitemia, pulmonary edema, or renal failure. Patients with severe malaria are not candidates for PO therapy. Elevated LFTs and rare cases of hepatitis reported with prophylactic use. Diarrhea or vomiting may reduce absorption; monitor for parasitemia and consider use of an antiemetic in patients who are vomiting. Alternative therapy may be required with severe or persistent diarrhea or vomiting. Parasite relapse occurred commonly when used as monotherapy to treat *P. vivax*. Treat with a different blood schizonticide in the event of recrudescent *P. falciparum* infections or failure of chemoprophylaxis. Caution in elderly.

ADVERSE REACTIONS: Abdominal pain, headache, N/V, pruritus, diarrhea, elevated LFTs, asthenia, anorexia, dizziness, gastritis, cough.

INTERACTIONS: Not recommended with rifampin or rifabutin. Atovaquone: Concomitant use of rifampin, rifabutin, or tetracycline may decrease levels. Reduced bioavailability with metoclopramide. Caution with indinavir; may decrease trough levels of indinavir. Proguanil: May potentiate anticoagulant effect of warfarin and other coumarin-based anticoagulants; caution when initiating and withdrawing therapy.

PREGNANCY: Category C, caution in nursing.

MECHANISM OF ACTION: Pyrimidine synthesis inhibitors. Atovaquone: Acts as a selective inhibitor of parasite mitochondrial electron transport. Proguanil: Acts via its metabolite, cycloguanil, which inhibits dihydrofolate reductase in the malaria parasite, disrupting deoxythymidylate synthesis.

PHARMACOKINETICS: Absorption: Atovaquone: Absolute bioavailability (23% with food). Proguanil: Extensively absorbed. **Distribution:** Atovaquone: V_d=8.8L/kg; plasma protein binding (>99%). Proguanil: V_d=1617-2502L (patients >15 yrs with body weight 31-110kg), V_d=462-966L (patients ≤15 yrs with body weight 11-56kg). Plasma protein binding (75%); found in breast milk. **Metabolism:** Proguanil: Cycloguanil (active metabolite) via CYP2C19. **Elimination:** Atovaquone: Feces (94% unchanged), urine (<0.6%). $T_{1/2}$=2-3 days (adult). Proguanil: Urine (40-60%); $T_{1/2}$=12-21 hrs (adult and pediatric patients).

NURSING CONSIDERATIONS

Assessment: Assess for cerebral malaria, hyperparasitemia, pulmonary edema, diarrhea, vomiting, decreased hepatic/renal function, pregnancy/nursing status, and possible drug interactions.

Monitoring: Monitor for parasitemia and parasite relapse to determine if antiemetic or alternative antimalarial therapy is needed. Monitor for adverse reactions.

Patient Counseling: Instruct patients to take tab at the same time each day with food or a milky drink; repeat dose if vomiting occurs within 1 hr after dosing. Instruct patient if dose is missed, to take as soon as possible and then return to normal dosing schedule. Advise not to double the dose if a dose is skipped. Counsel about serious adverse events associated with therapy. Instruct to consult physician about alternative forms of prophylaxis if drug is prematurely d/c for any reason. Inform that protective clothing, insect repellants, and bednets are important components of malaria prophylaxis. Instruct to seek medical attention for any febrile illness that occurs during or after return from a malaria-endemic area. Discuss with pregnant/nursing women anticipating travel to malarious areas about the risks/benefits of such travel.

Administration: Oral route. Take at the same time each day with food or a milky drink. Repeat dose in the event of vomiting within 1 hr after dosing. May crush and mix with condensed milk just prior to administration for children who may have difficulty swallowing tablets. **Storage:** 25°C (77°F); excursions permitted to 15-30°C (59-86°F).

MARINOL
dronabinol (Abbott)

THERAPEUTIC CLASS: Cannabinoid

INDICATIONS: Treatment of anorexia associated with weight loss in AIDS patients and N/V associated with cancer chemotherapy in patients who have failed to respond adequately to conventional antiemetic treatments.

DOSAGE: *Adults:* Individualize dose. Appetite Stimulation: Initial: 2.5mg bid before lunch and supper. Titrate: Reduce dose to 2.5mg qpm or qhs if 5mg/day dose is intolerable. Max: 20mg/day in divided doses. Antiemetic: Initial: 5mg/m^2 1-3 hrs before chemotherapy, then q2-4h after chemotherapy, for a total of 4-6 doses/day. Titrate: May increase dose by 2.5mg/m^2 increments. Max: 15mg/m^2/dose.
Pediatrics: Antiemetic: Initial: 5mg/m^2 1-3 hrs before chemotherapy, then q2-4h after chemotherapy, for a total of 4-6 doses/day. Titrate: May increase dose by 2.5mg/m^2 increments. Max: 15mg/m^2/dose.

HOW SUPPLIED: Cap: 2.5mg, 5mg, 10mg

CONTRAINDICATIONS: Allergy to sesame oil.

WARNINGS/PRECAUTIONS: May impair mental/physical abilities. Seizure and seizure-like activity reported; d/c immediately if seizures develop. Caution with history of seizure disorders, substance abuse, and cardiac disorders due to occasional hypotension, possible HTN, syncope, or tachycardia. Caution in patients with mania, depression, or schizophrenia; exacerbation of these illnesses may occur. Caution in elderly (particularly those with dementia), pregnancy, nursing, and pediatrics.

ADVERSE REACTIONS: Abdominal pain, N/V, dizziness, euphoria, paranoid reaction, somnolence, abnormal thinking.

INTERACTIONS: May displace highly protein-bound drugs; dose requirement changes may be needed. Additive or synergistic CNS effects with sedatives, hypnotics, or other psychoactive drugs. Additive HTN, tachycardia, and possible cardiotoxicity with sympathomimetics (eg, amphetamines, cocaine). Additive or super-additive tachycardia, and drowsiness with anticholinergics (eg, atropine, scopolamine, antihistamines). Additive tachycardia, HTN, and drowsiness with TCAs (eg, amitriptyline, amoxapine, desipramine). Additive drowsiness and CNS depression with CNS depressants (eg, barbiturates, benzodiazepines, ethanol, lithium, opioids, buspirone, antihistamines, muscle relaxants). May result in hypomanic reaction with disulfiram and fluoxetine in patients who smoked marijuana. May decrease clearance of antipyrine and barbiturates. May increase theophylline metabolism in patients who smoked marijuana/tobacco.

PREGNANCY: Category C, not for use in nursing.

MECHANISM OF ACTION: Cannabinoid; has complex effects on the CNS, including central sympathomimetic activity.

PHARMACOKINETICS: Absorption: Administration of variable doses resulted in different pharmacokinetic parameters. **Distribution:** V_d=10L/kg; plasma protein binding (97%); found in breast milk. **Metabolism:** Liver via microsomal hydroxylation; 11-OH-delta-9-THC (active metabolite). **Elimination:** Urine (10-15%), bile/feces (50%, <5% unchanged); $T_{1/2}$=25-36 hrs.

NURSING CONSIDERATIONS

Assessment: Assess for history of hypersensitivity to the drug and sesame oil, history of seizure disorders, substance abuse (including alcohol abuse/dependence), cardiac disorders, mania, depression, schizophrenia, pregnancy/nursing status, hepatic/renal impairment, and possible drug interactions.

Monitoring: Monitor for psychiatric illness exacerbation, abdominal pain, N/V, dizziness, euphoria, paranoid reaction, somnolence, abnormal thinking, hypotension or HTN, syncope, tachycardia, for psychological and physiological dependence, and other adverse reactions.

Patient Counseling: Inform about additive CNS depression effect if taken concomitantly with alcohol or other CNS depressants (eg, benzodiazepines, barbiturates). Advise to use caution while performing hazardous tasks (eg, operating machinery/driving) until effect is well tolerated. Inform of mood changes and other behavioral effects that may occur during therapy. Advise that patients must be under constant supervision of a responsible adult during initial use and following dosage adjustments. Instruct to immediately report to physician any adverse effects and notify if pregnant or breastfeeding.

Administration: Oral route. **Storage:** 8-15°C (46-59°F). Protect from freezing.

MAVIK

RX

trandolapril (Abbott)

> D/C when pregnancy is detected. Drugs that act directly on the renin-angiotensin system can cause injury/death to the developing fetus.

THERAPEUTIC CLASS: ACE inhibitor

INDICATIONS: Treatment of HTN alone or in combination with other antihypertensives (eg, HCTZ). For use in stable patients with evidence of left-ventricular systolic dysfunction or who are symptomatic from congestive heart failure (CHF) within the 1st few days after sustaining acute myocardial infarction (MI).

DOSAGE: *Adults:* HTN: Not Receiving Diuretics: Initial: 1mg qd in nonblack patients; 2mg qd in black patients. Titrate: Adjust dose at intervals of at least 1 week based on BP response. Usual: 2-4mg qd. Max: 8mg qd. May give 4mg bid if inadequately treated with qd dosing. May add diuretic if not adequately controlled. Receiving Diuretics: D/C diuretic 2-3 days prior to therapy if possible, then resume diuretic if BP is not controlled. If diuretic cannot be d/c, use initial dose of 0.5mg. Titrate to the optimal response. Heart Failure/Left-Ventricular Dysfunction Post-MI: Initial: 1mg qd. Titrate: Increase to target dose of 4mg qd as tolerated; if not tolerated, continue with the greatest tolerated dose. CrCl <30mL/min or Hepatic Cirrhosis: Initial: 0.5mg qd. Titrate to optimal response.

HOW SUPPLIED: Tab: 1mg*, 2mg, 4mg *scored

CONTRAINDICATIONS: Hereditary/idiopathic angioedema, history of ACE inhibitor-associated angioedema.

WARNINGS/PRECAUTIONS: Anaphylactoid reactions reported during desensitization with hymenoptera venom, dialysis with high-flux membranes, and LDL apheresis with dextran sulfate absorption. Angioedema reported; d/c, treat appropriately, and monitor until swelling disappears if laryngeal stridor or angioedema of the face, tongue or glottis occurs. Intestinal angioedema reported; monitor for abdominal pain. Higher rate of angioedema in blacks than nonblacks. Symptomatic hypotension may occur and is most likely with volume and/or salt depletion; correct depletion prior to therapy. Excessive hypotension associated with oliguria, azotemia, acute renal failure, or death may occur in patients with CHF; monitor during first 2 weeks of therapy and whenever dose is increased. Caution with ischemic heart disease, aortic stenosis, or cerebrovascular disease; avoid hypotension. Consider lowering dose if transient hypotension occurs. May cause agranulocytosis and bone marrow depression; periodically monitor WBCs in patients with collagen vascular disease and/or renal disease. Rarely, associated with syndrome of cholestatic jaundice, fulminant hepatic necrosis, and death; d/c if jaundice develops. May cause changes in renal function. Increases in BUN and SrCr reported in patients with renal artery stenosis and without preexisting renal vascular disease; reduce dose and/or d/c. Hyperkalemia reported; risk factors include renal insufficiency and diabetes mellitus (DM). Persistent nonproductive cough reported. Hypotension may occur with major surgery or during anesthesia.

ADVERSE REACTIONS: Cough, dizziness, hypotension, elevated serum uric acid, elevated BUN, syncope, hyperkalemia, elevated creatinine, cardiogenic shock, intermittent claudication.

INTERACTIONS: Hypotension risk, increased BUN and SrCr with diuretics. K⁺-sparing diuretics (spironolactone, triamterene, or amiloride), K⁺ supplements, or K⁺-containing salt substitutes may increase risk of hyperkalemia; use with caution and monitor serum K⁺. May increase blood glucose lowering effect of antidiabetic medications (insulin or oral hypoglycemic agents). Increased lithium levels and symptoms of lithium toxicity reported; monitor lithium levels. Diuretic (with lithium) may increase risk of lithium toxicity. NSAIDs, including selective cyclooxygenase-2 inhibitors, may deteriorate renal function; monitor renal function periodically. Antihypertensive effect may be attenuated by NSAIDs; increase BP monitoring. Nitritoid reactions (eg, facial flushing, N/V, hypotension) reported with injectable gold (sodium aurothiomalate). May enhance hypotensive effect of certain inhalation anesthetics.

PREGNANCY: Category D, not for use in nursing.

MECHANISM OF ACTION: ACE inhibitor; reduces angiotensin II formation, decreases vasoconstriction and aldosterone secretion, and increases plasma renin.

PHARMACOKINETICS: Absorption: Trandolapril: Absolute bioavailability (10%); T_{max}=1 hr. Trandolaprilat: Absolute bioavailability (70%); T_{max}=4-10 hrs. **Distribution:** V_d=18L; plasma protein binding (80% trandolapril; 65-94% trandolaprilat). **Metabolism:** Liver via glucuronidation and deesterification; trandolaprilat (active metabolite). **Elimination:** Urine (33%), feces (66%); $T_{1/2}$=6 hrs (trandolapril), 22.5 hrs (trandolaprilat).

NURSING CONSIDERATIONS

Assessment: Assess for hereditary/idiopathic angioedema, history of ACE inhibitor-associated angioedema, volume/salt depletion, CHF, ischemic heart disease, aortic stenosis, cerebrovascular disease, collagen vascular disease (eg, systemic lupus erythematosus, scleroderma), DM, renal/hepatic impairment, hypersensitivity to drug, pregnancy/nursing status, and possible drug interactions.

Monitoring: Monitor for anaphylactoid reactions, angioedema, hypotension, jaundice, hyperkalemia, cough, and other adverse effects. Periodically monitor WBCs in patients with collagen vascular disease and/or renal disease. Monitor BP and renal/hepatic function.

Patient Counseling: Advise to d/c and consult physician if any signs/symptoms of angioedema (swelling of the face, extremities, eyes, lips, tongue, difficulty in swallowing or breathing) or if syncope occurs. Inform that lightheadedness may occur, especially during 1st days of therapy; report to physician. Inform that inadequate fluid intake, excessive perspiration, diarrhea, or vomiting may lead to excessive fall in BP with same consequences of lightheadedness and possible syncope. Advise to inform physician of therapy prior to surgery and/or anesthesia. Advise to avoid use of K⁺ supplements or salt substitutes containing K⁺ without consulting physician. Instruct to immediately report any signs/symptoms of infection (eg, sore throat, fever). Inform about the consequences of exposure during pregnancy in females of childbearing age. Instruct to report pregnancies to physician as soon as possible.

Administration: Oral route. **Storage:** 20-25°C (68-77°F).

MAXAIR RX
pirbuterol acetate (Graceway)

THERAPEUTIC CLASS: Beta₂-agonist

INDICATIONS: Prevention and reversal of bronchospasm in patients ≥12 yrs with reversible bronchospasm including asthma as monotherapy or with theophylline and/or corticosteroids.

DOSAGE: *Adults:* 1-2 inh q4-6h. Max: 12 inh/day.
Pediatrics: ≥12 yrs: 1-2 inh q4-6h. Max: 12 inh/day.

HOW SUPPLIED: MDI: 200mcg/actuation [2.8g, 14g]

WARNINGS/PRECAUTIONS: D/C if cardiovascular (CV) effects occurr. ECG changes reported. Caution with CV disorders (eg, coronary insufficiency, ischemic heart disease, HTN, arrhythmias), hyperthyroidism, diabetes mellitus (DM), convulsive disorders, and patients who are unusually responsive to sympathomimetic amines. Can produce paradoxical bronchospasm; d/c immediately if this develops and institute alternative therapy. Consider adding anti-inflammatory agents to therapy (eg, corticosteroids) to adequately control asthma. Reevaluate patient and treatment regimen if deterioration of asthma observed. Changes in systolic and diastolic BP and hypokalemia may occur.

ADVERSE REACTIONS: Nervousness, tremor, headache, dizziness, palpitations, tachycardia, cough, nausea.

INTERACTIONS: Avoid with other short-acting aerosol β₂ agonists. May potentiate action on the vascular system with MAOIs or TCAs. May worsen the ECG changes and/or hypokalemia caused by non-K⁺ sparing diuretics (eg, loop or thiazide diuretics); caution with use. Pulmonary effect blocked by β-blockers. Caution with cardioselective β-blockers.

PREGNANCY: Category C, caution in nursing.

MECHANISM OF ACTION: β₂-adrenergic bronchodilator; stimulates the intracellular adenyl cyclase, the enzyme that converts adenosine triphosphate to cyclic adenosine monophosphate (cAMP). Increased cAMP levels are associated with relaxation of bronchial smooth muscle and inhibition of release of mediators of immediate hypersensitivity from cells.

PHARMACOKINETICS: Elimination: Urine (51%); $T_{1/2}$=2 hrs.

NURSING CONSIDERATIONS

Assessment: Assess for previous hypersensitivity to the drug, CV disorders, HTN, unusual response to sympathomimetic amines, convulsive disorders, hyperthyroidism, DM, pregnancy/nursing status, and possible drug interactions.

Monitoring: Monitor pulse rate, BP, ECG changes, for CV effects, paradoxical bronchospasm and hypokalemia, hypersensitivity reactions, and deterioration of asthma.

Patient Counseling: Instruct patient to take as directed. Seek medical attention if treatment becomes less effective, symptoms becomes worse, and/or more frequent use is needed. Contact physician if pregnant/nursing, and/or experiencing adverse reactions. Instruct not to use with any other inhalation aerosol canister or any other actuator. Advise to keep out of reach of children and avoid spraying in eyes. Advise to prime before use for the first time and if not used in 48 hrs.

Administration: Oral inhalation route. Shake well. **Storage:** 15-30°C (59-86°F). Do not use or store near heat or open flame.

M

MAXALT
RX
rizatriptan benzoate (Merck)

OTHER BRAND NAMES: Maxalt-MLT (Merck)

THERAPEUTIC CLASS: 5-HT$_{1B/1D}$ agonist

INDICATIONS: Acute treatment of migraine attacks with or without aura in adults.

DOSAGE: *Adults:* Individualize dose. Usual: 5-10mg single dose. Separate doses by ≥2 hrs. Max: 30mg/24 hrs. Concomitant Propranolol: Use 5mg dose. Max: 3 doses/24 hrs. (MLT) Dissolve on tongue and swallow with saliva.

HOW SUPPLIED: Tab: 5mg, 10mg; (MLT) Tab, Disintegrating: 5mg, 10mg

CONTRAINDICATIONS: Ischemic heart disease (IHD) (eg, angina pectoris, history of myocardial infarction [MI], or documented silent ischemia), symptoms or findings consistent with IHD, coronary artery vasospasm (eg, Prinzmetal's variant angina), other significant underlying cardiovascular disease (CVD), uncontrolled HTN, hemiplegic/basilar migraine, concurrent use of MAOIs or use within 2 weeks of d/c of MAOI therapy, concomitant use with another 5-HT1 agonist or an ergotamine-containing or ergot-type medication (eg, dihydroergotamine, methysergide) within 24 hrs.

WARNINGS/PRECAUTIONS: Safety and effectiveness not established for cluster headache. Not intended for prophylactic therapy. Use only when diagnosis is confirmed. May cause coronary vasospasm. Avoid with unrecognized coronary artery disease (CAD) predicted by presence of risk factors (eg, HTN, hypercholesterolemia, smoker, obesity, diabetes, strong family history of CAD, female with surgical/physiological menopause, males >40 yrs) unless with a satisfactory cardiovascular (CV) evaluation; administer 1st dose under medical supervision and obtain ECG to assess presence of cardiac ischemia. Perform periodic interval CV evaluation with intermittent long-term use. Serious adverse cardiac events, including acute MI, reported within few hours following administration. Cerebrovascular events (eg, cerebral/subarachnoid hemorrhage, stroke), vasospastic reactions (eg, peripheral vascular/colonic ischemia with abdominal pain and bloody diarrhea), BP elevation, and hypertensive crisis reported. Sensations of tightness, pain, pressure, and heaviness in precordium, throat, neck, and jaw not associated with arrhythmias or ischemic ECG changes reported. Serotonin syndrome may occur; symptoms may include mental status changes, autonomic instability, neuromuscular aberrations, and GI symptoms. Caution with renal dialysis, moderate hepatic insufficiency, and diseases that may alter absorption, metabolism, or excretion of drugs. May possibly cause long-term ophthalmologic effects. (MLT) Contains phenylalanine; caution with phenylketonuria.

ADVERSE REACTIONS: Paresthesia, dry mouth, nausea, dizziness, somnolence, asthenia/fatigue, pain/pressure sensation.

INTERACTIONS: See Contraindications. Increased plasma levels with propranolol. Serotonin syndrome reported with SSRIs or serotonin norepinephrine reuptake inhibitors (SNRIs).

PREGNANCY: Category C, caution in nursing.

MECHANISM OF ACTION: 5-HT$_{1B/1D}$ receptor agonist; binds with high affinity to human cloned 5-HT$_{1B/1D}$ receptors on extracerebral, intracranial blood vessels, and on trigeminal system nerve terminals resulting in cranial vessel constriction, neuropeptide release inhibition, and reduced transmission in trigeminal pain pathways.

PHARMACOKINETICS: Absorption: Complete; (Tab) absolute bioavailability (45%), T_{max}=1-1.5 hrs; (MLT) T_{max}=1.6-2.5 hrs. **Distribution:** V_d=140L (male), 110L (female); plasma protein binding (14%). **Metabolism:** Oxidative deamination via monoamine oxidase-A (MAO-A). N-monodesmethyl-rizatriptan (active metabolite). **Elimination:** Urine (82%), (14% unchanged, 51% indole acetic acid metabolite), feces (12%); $T_{1/2}$=2-3 hrs.

NURSING CONSIDERATIONS

Assessment: Confirm diagnosis before instituting therapy. Assess for IHD, coronary artery vasospasm, CVD, HTN, hemiplegic/basilar migraine, risk factors for CAD, hepatic/renal function, diseases that may alter absorption, metabolism, or excretion of drugs, phenylketonuria, pregnancy/nursing status, drug hypersensitivity, and possible drug interactions. Perform CV evaluation prior to therapy.

Monitoring: Monitor for signs/symptoms of coronary vasospasm, CV adverse events, cerebrovascular events, peripheral vascular ischemia, colonic ischemia with bloody diarrhea and abdominal pain, serotonin syndrome, ophthalmologic effects, increased BP, and other adverse reactions. Monitor ECG during the interval immediately following therapy in patients with CAD risk factors. Perform periodic interval CV evaluation with intermittent long-term use.

Patient Counseling: Inform that the drug may cause somnolence and dizziness; evaluate ability to perform complex tasks during attacks and after administration. Caution about the risk of serotonin syndrome, especially if combined with SSRIs or SNRIs. Instruct to read patient package insert before taking the drug. (MLT) Instruct not to remove blister from outer pouch until just prior to dosing; peel open with dry hands and place disintegrating tab on tongue, where it will be dissolved and swallowed with saliva.

Administration: Oral route. **Storage:** 15-30°C (59-86°F).

MAXITROL   RX
neomycin sulfate - polymyxin B sulfate - dexamethasone (Alcon)

THERAPEUTIC CLASS: Antibacterial/corticosteroid combination

INDICATIONS: For steroid-responsive inflammatory ocular conditions for which a corticosteroid is indicated and where bacterial infection or the risk of bacterial ocular infection exist.

DOSAGE: *Adults:* (Oint) Apply 1/2 inch in conjunctival sac(s) up to 3-4 times daily. Max: 8g for initial prescription. (Sus) Instill 1-2 drops in conjunctival sac(s) up to 4-6 times daily in mild disease and qh in severe disease. Taper to d/c as inflammation subsides. Max: 20mL for initial prescription.

HOW SUPPLIED: Oint: (Dexamethasone-Neomycin sulfate-Polymyxin sulfate) 0.1%-3.5mg-10,000 U/g [3.5g]; Sus: (Dexamethasone-Neomycin sulfate-Polymyxin sulfate) 0.1%-3.5mg-10,000 U/mL [5mL]

CONTRAINDICATIONS: Epithelial herpes simplex keratitis (dendritic keratitis), vaccinia, varicella, and other viral diseases of the cornea and conjunctiva, mycobacterial infection of the eye, fungal diseases of ocular structures.

WARNINGS/PRECAUTIONS: For topical ophthalmic use only; not for injection. Glaucoma with damage to the optic nerve, defects in visual acuity and fields of vision, and posterior subcapsular cataract formation may occur after prolonged use. May cause perforations when used with diseases causing thinning of cornea or sclera. May mask infection or enhance existing infection in acute purulent conditions of the eye. Monitor intraocular pressure (IOP) if used for ≥10 days. Prolonged use may suppress host response, increase risk of secondary ocular infections, or cause persistent fungal infections of the cornea. May cause cutaneous sensitization. Caution in the treatment of herpes simplex. Perform eye exam (eg, slit lamp biomicroscopy, fluorescein staining) prior to therapy and renewal of medication. (Sus) Usage after cataract surgery may delay healing and increase incidence of bleb formation. May prolong course and exacerbate severity of ocular viral infections (eg, herpes simplex). Do not inject subconjunctivally, nor directly introduce into anterior chamber of the eye. If no improvement is seen after 2 days, re-evaluate patient. Suspect fungal invasion in any persistent corneal ulceration during/after therapy; take fungal cultures when appropriate.

ADVERSE REACTIONS: Allergic sensitizations, elevated IOP, posterior subcapsular cataract formation, delayed wound healing, secondary infections.

PREGNANCY: Category C, caution in nursing.

MECHANISM OF ACTION: Antibacterial/Corticosteroid. Dexamethasone: Corticosteroid; suppresses the inflammatory response to a variety of agents. May inhibit the body's defense mechanism against infection.

PHARMACOKINETICS: Distribution: (Systemically administered) found in breast milk.

NURSING CONSIDERATIONS

Assessment: Assess for active viral diseases of the cornea and conjunctiva, epithelial herpes simplex keratitis, vaccinia, varicella, mycobacterial infection of the eye, fungal disease of ocular structures, diseases causing thinning of sclera or cornea, acute purulent conditions, history of cataract surgery, hypersensitivity to the drug or its components, and pregnancy/nursing status. Perform eye exam (eg, slit lamp biomicroscopy, flourescein staining) prior to therapy.

Monitoring: Monitor for signs and symptoms of glaucoma, optic nerve damage, visual acuity and visual field defects, subcapsular cataract, ocular/corneal perforations, cutaneous sensitizations, bacterial, viral, fungal infections. Monitor IOP and perform eye exams (eg, slit lamp biomicroscopy, flourescein staining) prior to renewal of medication. (Sus) Monitor use after cataract surgery. Perform fungal cultures when fungal invasion is suspected.

Patient Counseling: Advise not to touch dropper tip to any surface; may contaminate drug. Keep out of reach of children. Use medication as prescribed. Medication is for topical ophthalmic use only. Inform physician if pregnant or breastfeeding. (Oint) Advise not to wear contact lenses if signs and syptoms of bacterial ocular infection are present. Instruct not to use product if the imprinted carton seals have been damaged or removed. (Sus) Advise to d/c and consult physician if inflammation or pain persists >48 hrs or becomes aggravated. Use of the same bottle by more than one person may spread infection. Shake well before use and keep bottle tightly closed when not in use.

Administration: Ocular route. (Oint) Tilt head back. Place finger on cheek just under the eye and gently pull down until a "V" pocket is formed between eyeball and lower lid. Place small amount of ointment in the "V" pocket. Look downward before closing the eye. **Storage:** Oint: 2-25°C (36-77°F). Sus: 8-27°C (46-80°F). Store upright.

Maxzide   RX
triamterene - hydrochlorothiazide (Mylan Bertek)

> Abnormal elevation of serum K⁺ levels (≥5.5mEq/L) may occur with all K⁺-sparing diuretic combinations. Hyperkalemia is more likely to occur with renal impairment and diabetes (even without evidence of renal impairment), and in elderly or severely ill; monitor serum K⁺ levels at frequent intervals.

OTHER BRAND NAMES: Maxzide-25 (Mylan Bertek)

THERAPEUTIC CLASS: K⁺-sparing diuretic/thiazide diuretic

INDICATIONS: Treatment of HTN or edema if hypokalemia occurs on HCTZ alone, or when a thiazide diuretic is required and cannot risk hypokalemia. May be used alone or as an adjunct to other antihypertensives, such as β-blockers.

DOSAGE: *Adults:* (Maxzide-25) 1-2 tabs qd, given as a single dose or (Maxzide) 1 tab qd.

HOW SUPPLIED: Tab: (Triamterene-HCTZ) (Maxzide) 75mg-50mg*, (Maxzide-25) 37.5mg-25mg* *scored

CONTRAINDICATIONS: Elevated serum K⁺ (≥5.5mEq/L), anuria, acute or chronic renal insufficiency or significant renal impairment, sulfonamide hypersensitivity, K⁺-sparing agents (eg, spironolactone, amiloride, or other formulations containing triamterene), K⁺ supplements, K⁺ salt substitutes, K⁺-enriched diets.

WARNINGS/PRECAUTIONS: Obtain ECG if hyperkalemia is suspected. Avoid in severely ill in whom respiratory or metabolic acidosis may occur; if used, frequent evaluations of acid/base balance and serum electrolytes are necessary. May cause idiosyncratic reaction, resulting in acute transient myopia and acute angle-closure glaucoma; d/c as rapidly as possible. Monitor for fluid/electrolyte imbalances. May manifest latent diabetes mellitus (DM). Caution with hepatic impairment or progressive liver disease; minor alterations in fluid and electrolyte balance may precipitate hepatic coma. May cause hypochloremia. Dilutional hyponatremia may occur in edematous patients in hot weather. Caution with history of renal lithiasis. May increase BUN and SrCr; d/c if azotemia increases. May contribute to megaloblastosis in folic acid deficiency. Hyperuricemia may occur or acute gout may be precipitated. May decrease serum PBI levels. Decreased calcium excretion reported. Changes in parathyroid glands with hypercalcemia and hypophosphatemia reported during prolonged use. Sensitivity reactions may occur. May exacerbate or activate systemic lupus erythematosus (SLE). May interfere with the fluorescent measurement of quinidine.

ADVERSE REACTIONS: Hyperkalemia, jaundice, pancreatitis, N/V, taste alteration, drowsiness, dry mouth, depression, anxiety, tachycardia, fluid/electrolyte imbalances.

INTERACTIONS: See Contraindications. Increased risk of hyperkalemia with ACE inhibitors. Hypokalemia may develop with corticosteroids, adrenocorticotropic hormone, or amphotericin B. Insulin requirements may be increased, decreased, or unchanged. May potentiate other antihypertensives (eg, β-blockers); dosage adjustments may be necessary. Avoid with lithium due to risk of lithium toxicity. Acute renal failure reported with indomethacin; caution with NSAIDs. May increase responsiveness to tubocurarine. May decrease arterial responsiveness to norepinephrine. Alcohol, barbiturates, or narcotics may aggravate orthostatic hypotension. May cause hypokalemia, which can sensitize or exaggerate the response of the heart to the toxic effects of digitalis (eg, increased ventricular irritability).

PREGNANCY: Category C, not for use in nursing.

MECHANISM OF ACTION: Triamterene: K⁺-sparing diuretic; exerts diuretic effect on distal renal tubule to inhibit the reabsorption of Na⁺ in exchange for K⁺ and H⁺. HCTZ: Thiazide diuretic; blocks renal tubular absorption of Na⁺ and Cl⁻ ions. This natriuresis and diuresis is accompanied by a secondary loss of K⁺ and bicarbonate.

PHARMACOKINETICS: Absorption: Well absorbed. HCTZ: T_{max}=2 hrs. Triamterene: Rapid, T_{max}=1 hr. **Distribution:** Crosses placenta; found in breast milk. **Metabolism:** Triamterene: Sulfate conjugation; hydroxytriamterene (metabolite). **Elimination:** HCTZ: Urine (unchanged).

NURSING CONSIDERATIONS

Assessment: Assess for conditions where treatment is contraindicated or cautioned, diabetes, risk for respiratory or metabolic acidosis, SLE, pregnancy/nursing status, and for possible drug interactions. Obtain baseline BUN, SrCr, and serum electrolytes.

Monitoring: Monitor for signs/symptoms of hyperkalemia, idiosyncratic reaction, hypokalemia, azotemia, renal stones, hepatic coma, and for fluid/electrolyte imbalances. Monitor serum K⁺ levels, BUN, SrCr, folic acid levels. Monitor serum and urine electrolytes if vomiting or receiving parenteral fluids.

Patient Counseling: Inform about risks/benefits of therapy. Advise to seek medical attention if symptoms of hyperkalemia (eg, paresthesias, muscular weakness, fatigue), hypokalemia, renal stones, electrolyte imbalance (eg, dry mouth, thirst, weakness), or hypersensitivity reactions occur. Notify physician if pregnant/nursing.

Administration: Oral route. **Storage:** 20-25°C (68-77°F). Protect from light.

MEDROL RX
methylprednisolone (Pharmacia & Upjohn)

THERAPEUTIC CLASS: Glucocorticoid

INDICATIONS: Steroid-responsive disorders.

DOSAGE: *Adults:* Individualize dose. Initial: 4-48mg/day depending on disease and response. Maint: Decrease dose by small amounts to lowest effective dose. Withdraw gradually after long-term therapy. Acute Exacerbations of Multiple Sclerosis: 200mg/day for 1 week followed by 80mg qod for 1 month. Alternate Day Therapy (ADT): Twice the usual daily dose administered every other am. Refer to PI for detailed information for ADT.
Pediatric: Individualize dose. Initial: 4-48mg/day depending on disease and response. Maint: Decrease dose by small amounts to lowest effective dose. Withdraw gradually after long-term therapy. Acute Exacerbations of Multiple Sclerosis: 200mg/day for 1 week followed by 80mg qod for 1 month. Alternate Day Therapy (ADT): Twice the usual daily dose administered every other am. Refer to PI for detailed information for ADT.

HOW SUPPLIED: Tab: 2mg*, 4mg*, 8mg*, 16mg*, 32mg*; (Dose-Pak) 4mg* [21⁵] *scored

CONTRAINDICATIONS: Systemic fungal infections.

WARNINGS/PRECAUTIONS: May need to increase dose before, during, and after stressful situations. May mask signs of infection or cause new infections. Possible benefits should be weighed against potential hazards if used during pregnancy/nursing. Prolonged use may produce glaucoma, optic nerve damage, and secondary ocular infections. May cause BP elevation, increased K⁺ excretion, and salt/water retention. More severe/fatal course of infections reported with chickenpox, measles. Caution with strongyloides, latent tuberculosis (TB), hypothyroidism, cirrhosis, ocular herpes simplex, HTN, diverticulitis, fresh intestinal anastomoses, ulcerative colitis, osteoporosis, myasthenia gravis, renal insufficiency, and peptic ulcer disease. Kaposi's sarcoma reported. Growth and development of children on prolonged therapy should be monitored. Monitor for psychic disturbances. Avoid abrupt withdrawal.

ADVERSE REACTIONS: Fluid and electrolyte disturbances, HTN, osteoporosis, muscle weakness, Cushingoid state, menstrual irregularities, impaired wound healing, convulsions, ulcerative esophagitis, excessive sweating, increased intracranial pressure, glaucoma, abdominal distention, headache, decreased carbohydrate tolerance.

INTERACTIONS: Reduced efficacy with hepatic enzyme inducers (eg, phenobarbital, phenytoin, and rifampin). Increases clearance of chronic high-dose aspirin (ASA). Caution with ASA in hypoprothrombinemia. Effects on oral anticoagulants are variable; monitor PT. Increased insulin and oral hypoglycemic requirements in diabetics. Avoid live vaccines with immunosuppressive doses. Possible decreased vaccine response with killed or inactivated vaccines with immunosuppressive doses. Mutual inhibition of metabolism with cyclosporine; convulsions reported. Potentiated by ketoconazole and troleandomycin. Concomitant administration with immunosuppressive agents may be associated with development of infections.

PREGNANCY: Safety in pregnancy and nursing not known.

MECHANISM OF ACTION: Anti-inflammatory glucocorticoid; causes profound and varied metabolic effects and modifies the body's immune responses to diverse stimuli.

PHARMACOKINETICS: Absorption: Readily absorbed from GI tract.

NURSING CONSIDERATIONS

Assessment: Assess for systemic fungal infections, current infections, active TB, vaccination history, ulcerative colitis, diverticulitis, peptic ulcer with impending perforation, renal/hepatic insufficiency, septic arthritis/unstable joint, HTN, osteoporosis, myasthenia gravis, thyroid status, psychotic tendencies, drug hypersensitivity and possible drug interactions.

Monitoring: Monitor for adrenocortical insufficiency, occurrence of infection, psychic derangement, cataracts, acute myopathy, Kaposi's sarcoma, and fluid retention. Monitor serum electrolytes, TSH, LFTs, intraocular pressure, and BP. Monitor urinalysis, blood sugar, weight, chest x-ray, and upper GI x-ray (if ulcer history) regularly during prolonged therapy. Monitor growth and development of infants and children on prolonged corticosteroids therapy.

Patient Counseling: Advise not to d/c abruptly or without medical supervision. Inform that susceptibility to infections may increase. Avoid exposure to chickenpox or measles; report immediately if exposed. Dietary salt restriction and supplementation of K⁺ is advised.

Administration: Oral route. **Storage:** 20-25°C (68-77°F).

MEFLOQUINE   RX
mefloquine HCl (Various)

THERAPEUTIC CLASS: Quinolinemethanol derivative

INDICATIONS: Treatment and prophylaxis of mild to moderate acute malaria caused by *Plasmodium falciparum* and/or *Plasmodium vivax*.

DOSAGE: *Adults:* Treatment: 5 tabs (1250mg) single dose. If no improvement within 48 to 72 hrs, use alternative therapy. Prophylaxis: 250mg once weekly. Start 1 week before arrival in endemic area and continue for additional 4 weeks after leaving. Take at same day of each week, after the main meal.
Pediatrics: ≥20kg: Treatment: ≥6 months: 20-25mg/kg in 2 divided doses (taken 6-8 hrs apart). If no improvement within 48 to 72 hours, use alternative therapy. If vomiting occurs <30 min after dose, give a 2nd full dose. If vomiting occurs 30-60 min after dose, give additional half-dose. If vomiting recurs, consider alternative treatment if no improvement within a reasonable period of time. Prophylaxis: 5mg/kg once weekly. >45kg: 1 tab/week. 30-45kg: 3/4 tab once weekly. 20-30kg: 1/2 tab once weekly.

HOW SUPPLIED: Tab: 250mg* *scored

CONTRAINDICATIONS: Use as prophylaxis in patients with active or recent history of depression, generalized anxiety disorder, psychosis, schizophrenia, or other major psychiatric disorders, or with a history of convulsions.

WARNINGS/PRECAUTIONS: Do not use for curative treatment if previous prophylaxis has failed. High risk of relapse seen with acute *P. vivax*; after initial treatment, subsequently treat with 8-aminoquinoline (eg, primaquine). Use IV antimalarials in life-threatening, serious or overwhelming malaria infection due to *P. falciparum*; may give tab after completion of IV treatment. May cause psychiatric symptoms. During prophylactic use, d/c if psychiatric symptoms of acute anxiety, depression, restlessness, or confusion occur. Increased risk of convulsions in epileptic patients; use only for curative treatment if there are compelling medical reasons for its use in such patients. May impair mental/physical abilities. In long term therapy, monitor LFTs and perform ophthalmic exams. Caution with cardiac disease, psychiatric disturbances, hepatic impairment, and elderly.

ADVERSE REACTIONS: N/V, myalgia, fever, dizziness, headache, syncope, sleep disorders, chills, diarrhea, abdominal pain, fatigue, tinnitus, loss of appetite, skin rash.

INTERACTIONS: Do not administer with halofantrine or ketoconazole within 15 weeks of the last dose of mefloquine tab; may prolong QTc interval. Concomitant administration with other related compounds (eg, quinine, quinidine, chloroquine) may cause ECG abnormalities and increase risk of convulsions; delay mefloquine dose at least 12 hrs after last dose of these drugs. Avoid propranolol; cardiopulmonary arrest reported. Coadministration of drugs known to alter cardiac conduction (eg, anti-arrhythmic or β-blockers, CCBs, antihistamines or H1-blockers, TCAs, and phenothiazines) may contribute to prolongation of QTc interval. May reduce seizure control by lowering plasma levels of anticonvulsants (eg, valproic acid, carbamazepine, phenobarbital, and phenytoin); monitor blood levels and adjust dosage accordingly. Complete vaccinations with live, attenuated vaccines (eg, typhoid vaccine) at least 3 days before mefloquine therapy. Caution with anticoagulants, antidiabetic agents, and rifampin. May increase/decrease plasma concentration with CYP450 inhibitors or inducers.

PREGNANCY: Category C, not for use in nursing.

MECHANISM OF ACTION: Quinolinemethanol derivative; suspected to act as blood schizonticide. Exact mechanism is not known.

PHARMACOKINETICS: Absorption: C_{max}=1000-2000mcg/L (250mg/week); T_{max}=6-24 hrs (single dose), 7-10 weeks (250mg/week). **Distribution:** V_d=20L/kg; plasma protein binding (98%); crosses placenta; found in breast milk. **Metabolism:** Extensive. Liver via CYP3A4; 2,8-bis-trifluoromethyl-4-quinoline carboxylic acid. **Elimination:** Bile/feces, urine (9% unchanged, 4% metabolite); $T_{1/2}$=2-4 weeks.

NURSING CONSIDERATIONS

Assessment: Assess LFTs, ECG. Assess for active/history of depression, generalized anxiety disorder, psychosis, schizophrenia, other major psychiatric disorders, or convulsions, epilepsy, central/peripheral nervous system disorders, hepatic impairment, cardiac disease, pregnancy status/nursing, drug hypersensitivity, and possible drug interactions.

Monitoring: Monitor for psychiatric symptoms, convulsions, QTc interval prolongation, and other adverse reactions. Monitor hepatic function and ECG periodically. Periodic ophthalmic exams recommended.

Patient Counseling: Inform that malaria can be a life-threatening infection and that drug is prescribed to help prevent/treat this serious infection. Inform that dizziness, vertigo, or loss of balance may occur. Instruct to start therapy one week prior to arrival in an endemic area if used as a prophylaxis. Inform that psychiatric symptoms (eg, acute anxiety, depression, restlessness, confusion) may be a prodrome to a more serious event; d/c therapy and contact physician. Advise that no chemoprophylactic regimen is 100% effective; use of protective clothing, insect repellants, and bednets are important components of malaria prophylaxis. Instruct to seek medical attention for any febrile illness that occurs after return from a malarious area and inform physician that they may have been exposed to malaria. Advise females to use effective birth control during prophylaxis and for up to 3 months thereafter.

Administration: Oral route. Do not take on empty stomach and administer with at least 8 oz. (240mL) of water. May crush and suspend tab in small amount of water, milk, or other beverages for small children/other persons unable to swallow tab whole. **Storage:** 20-25°C (68-77°F). Protect from light and moisture.

MEGACE ES
megestrol acetate (Par)

RX

OTHER BRAND NAMES: Megace (Bristol-Myers Squibb)

THERAPEUTIC CLASS: Progesterone

INDICATIONS: Treatment of anorexia, cachexia, or unexplained significant weight loss in AIDS patients.

DOSAGE: *Adults:* Initial: 800mg/day (20mL/day). Usual: 400-800mg/day. (ES) Initial/Usual: 625mg/day (5mL/day). Elderly: Start at lower end of dosing range.

HOW SUPPLIED: Sus: 40mg/mL [240mL], (ES) 125mg/mL [150mL]

CONTRAINDICATIONS: Known or suspected pregnancy.

WARNINGS/PRECAUTIONS: New onset or exacerbation of preexisting diabetes mellitus (DM) and overt Cushing's syndrome reported. Adrenal insufficiency reported in patients receiving or being withdrawn from chronic therapy; laboratory evaluation for adrenal insufficiency and consideration of replacement or stress doses of a rapidly acting glucocorticoid are strongly recommended. Caution with history of thromboembolic disease and in elderly. Institute therapy only after treatable causes of weight loss are sought and addressed.

ADVERSE REACTIONS: Diarrhea, impotence, rash, flatulence, N/V, HTN, asthenia, insomnia, anemia, fever, decreased libido, dyspepsia, headache, hyperglycemia.

INTERACTIONS: (ES) Decreased exposure of indinavir; consider higher dose of indinavir.

PREGNANCY: Category X, not for use in nursing.

MECHANISM OF ACTION: Progesterone; not established; has appetite-enhancing property.

PHARMACOKINETICS: Absorption: (800mg/day) C_{max}=753ng/mL, AUC=10476ng•hr/mL, T_{max}=5 hrs. (750mg/day) C_{max}=490ng/mL, AUC=6779ng•hr/mL, T_{max}=3 hrs. **Elimination:** Urine (66.4%), feces (19.8%); (ES) $T_{1/2}$=20-50 hrs.

NURSING CONSIDERATIONS

Assessment: Assess for preexisting DM, history of thromboembolic disease, renal dysfunction, hypersensitivity to drug, pregnancy/nursing status, and possible drug interactions.

Monitoring: Monitor for new/worsening DM, Cushing's syndrome, and adrenal insufficiency.

Patient Counseling: Instruct to use as directed by physician. Inform about product differences to avoid overdosing or underdosing. Advise to report any adverse reaction experiences, use contraception if capable of becoming pregnant, and notify physician if pregnancy occurs.

Administration: Oral route. Shake well before use. **Storage:** 15-25°C (59-77°F). Protect from heat.

MENACTRA
meningococcal polysaccharide diphtheria toxoid conjugate vaccine (Sanofi Pasteur)

RX

THERAPEUTIC CLASS: Vaccine

INDICATIONS: Active immunization to prevent invasive meningococcal disease caused by *Neisseria meningitidis* serogroups A, C, Y, and W-135 for persons 9 months-55 yrs.

DOSAGE: *Adults:* ≤55 yrs: 0.5mL IM.
Pediatrics: ≥2 yrs: 0.5mL IM. 9-23 months: 0.5mL IM and repeat after 3 months.

HOW SUPPLIED: Inj: 0.5mL

WARNINGS/PRECAUTIONS: Guillain-Barre syndrome (GBS) reported; may be at increased risk of GBS if previously diagnosed with GBS. Epinephrine and other appropriate agents must be immediately available for possible acute anaphylactic reactions. Immunocompromised persons may have diminished immune response to therapy. May not protect all recipients.

ADVERSE REACTIONS: Inj-site reactions, headache, fatigue, malaise, arthralgia, anorexia, chills, fever, diarrhea, drowsiness, irritability, rash, vomiting.

INTERACTIONS: Immunosuppressive therapies (eg, irradiation, antimetabolites, alkylating agents, cytotoxic drugs, and corticosteroids [used in greater than physiologic doses]) may reduce immune response. Tetanus and diphtheria toxoids vaccine may increase serum bactericidal assay to meningococcal serogroups A, C, Y, and W-135; higher rate of systemic adverse events with concomitant use. Pneumococcal antibody responses to some serotypes in pneumococcal conjugate vaccine 7 (PCV7) were decreased following coadministration with PCV7.

PREGNANCY: Category C, caution in nursing.

MECHANISM OF ACTION: Vaccine; leads to production of bactericidal antibodies directed against the capsular polysaccharides of serogroups A, C, Y, and W-135.

NURSING CONSIDERATIONS

Assessment: Assess current health and immune status, for history of GBS, pregnancy/nursing status, and possible drug interactions. Review immunization history for possible vaccine sensitivity and previous vaccination-related adverse reactions.

Monitoring: Monitor for GBS, allergic/anaphylactic reactions, and for other potential adverse effects.

Patient Counseling: Inform of the potential benefits/risks of immunization therapy. Instruct to report any adverse reactions to physician.

Administration: IM route. Do not administer IV or SQ. Do not administer if particulate matter and discoloration present. Do not mix with any other vaccine in the same syringe. **Storage:** 2-8°C (35-46°F). Do not freeze.

MENVEO   RX
meningococcal (groups A, C, Y and W-135) oligosaccharide diphtheria crm 197 congugate
(Novartis)

THERAPEUTIC CLASS: Vaccine

INDICATIONS: Active immunization to prevent invasive meningococcal disease caused by *Neisseria meningitidis* serogroups A, C, Y and W-135 for persons 2-55 yrs.

DOSAGE: *Adults:* ≤55 yrs: Single 0.5mL IM preferably into the deltoid muscle (upper arm). *Pediatrics:* ≥2 yrs: Single 0.5mL IM preferably into the deltoid muscle (upper arm). 2-5 yrs (Continued High Risk of Meningococcal Disease): May administer second dose 2 months after first dose.

HOW SUPPLIED: Inj: 0.5mL

WARNINGS/PRECAUTIONS: Appropriate medical treatment must be available should an acute allergic reaction, including an anaphylactic reaction occur. Syncope associated with seizure-like movements reported; observe for 15 min after administration to prevent and manage syncopal reactions. Expected immune response may not be obtained in immunocompromised persons. May increase risk of Guillain-Barre syndrome (GBS). Avoid with bleeding disorders unless potential benefit outweighs risk.

ADVERSE REACTIONS: Pain at injection site, local erythema, induration at injection site, irritability, sleepiness, change in eating, diarrhea, headache, myalgia, malaise, N/V, rash, chills, arthralgia.

INTERACTIONS: Immunosuppressive therapies (eg, irradiation, antimetabolites, alkylating agents, cytotoxic drugs, and corticosteroids [used in greater than physiologic doses]) may reduce immune response. Avoid with anticoagulants unless potential benefit outweighs risk. Lower geometric mean antibody concentrations (GMCs) for antibodies to the pertussis antigens filamentous hemagglutinin (FHA) and pertactin observed when coadministered with Boostrix and Gardasil as compared with Boostrix alone.

PREGNANCY: Category B, caution in nursing.

MECHANISM OF ACTION: Vaccine; leads to production of bactericidal antibodies directed against the capsular polysaccharides of meningococcal serogroups A, C, Y and W-135.

NURSING CONSIDERATIONS

Assessment: Assess for previous hypersensitivity to vaccine or other vaccines containing similar components, bleeding disorders, immune system status, *N. meningitidis* serogroup B infections, pregnancy/nursing status and possible drug interactions. Assess children 2-5 yrs for continued high risk of meningococcal disease. Review immunization history for possible vaccine sensitivity and previous vaccination-related adverse reactions.

Monitoring: Monitor for allergic reactions, syncope, seizure-like activity, GBS, inj-site reactions, immune response, and other adverse effects.

Patient Counseling: Inform of the potential benefits/risks of immunization therapy. Educate about the potential adverse reactions temporally associated with the vaccine. Instruct to report any side effects to the physician. Inform about the Novartis pregnancy registry as appropriate (1-877-311-8972).

Administration: IM route. Not for IV, SQ, or intradermal use. Do not mix with any other vaccine or diluent in the same syringe or vial. Refer to PI for reconstitution instructions. **Storage:** 2-8°C (36-46°F); maintain at 36-46°F during transport. Do not freeze or use frozen/previously frozen product. Protect from light. Do not use after expiration date; use reconstituted vaccine immediately, but may be held at or below 25°C (77°F) for up to 8 hrs.

MEPERIDINE   CII
meperidine HCl (Roxane)

OTHER BRAND NAMES: Demerol (Sanofi-Aventis)

THERAPEUTIC CLASS: Opioid analgesic

INDICATIONS: Relief of moderate to severe pain.

DOSAGE: *Adults:* Usual: 50-150mg q3-4h PRN. Concomitant Phenothiazines/Other Tranquilizers: Reduce dose by 25-50%.
Pediatrics: Usual: 1.1-1.8mg/kg, up to the adult dose, q3-4h PRN. Concomitant Phenothiazines/Other Tranquilizers: Reduce dose by 25-50%.

HOW SUPPLIED: Sol: 50mg/5mL; Tab: 50mg*, 100mg*; (Demerol) Tab: 50mg*, 100mg *scored

CONTRAINDICATIONS: During or within 14 days of MAOI use. (Demerol) Severe respiratory insufficiency.

WARNINGS/PRECAUTIONS: May be habit forming. Not for chronic pain; may increase risk of toxicity (eg, seizures) with prolonged use. Respiratory depressant effects and elevation of CSF pressure may be exaggerated in the presence of head injury, other intracranial lesions, or preexisting increase in intracranial pressure. May obscure diagnosis or clinical course of head injuries or acute abdominal conditions. Extreme caution with acute asthmatic attack, chronic obstructive pulmonary disease or cor pulmonale, or other respiratory conditions. May cause severe hypotension in postoperative patients or individuals whose ability to maintain BP has been compromised by depleted blood volume. May impair mental/physical abilities. May produce orthostatic hypotension in ambulatory patients. Not recommended during labor. Caution in elderly, debilitated, patients with atrial flutter or other supraventricular tachycardias, and other special risk patients; refer to PI. May aggravate preexisting convulsions. Caution with alcoholism or other drug dependencies; may develop tolerance, dependence, addiction, or abuse. Avoid abrupt d/c.

ADVERSE REACTIONS: Lightheadedness, dizziness, sedation, N/V, sweating, respiratory/circulatory depression.

INTERACTIONS: See Contraindications. Additive effects with alcohol, other opioids, or illicit drugs that cause CNS depression. Caution and consider dose reduction with other CNS depressants (eg, sedatives or hypnotics, general anesthetics, phenothiazines, other tranquilizers, alcohol); may result in respiratory depression, hypotension, profound sedation, or coma. Caution with agonist/antagonist analgesics (eg, pentazocine, nalbuphine, butorphanol, buprenorphine); may reduce the analgesic effect and/or precipitate withdrawal symptoms. Acyclovir may increase levels. Cimetidine may reduce clearance and Vd; caution with coadministration. Phenytoin may enhance hepatic metabolism; use caution. Avoid with ritonavir; may increase levels of active metabolite. May enhance neuromuscular blocking action of skeletal muscle relaxants. May result in severe hypotension with phenothiazines or certain anesthetics.

PREGNANCY: Category C, not for use in nursing.

MECHANISM OF ACTION: Narcotic analgesic; produces actions similar to morphine most prominently involving the CNS and organs composed of smooth muscle. Produces analgesic and sedative effects.

PHARMACOKINETICS: Metabolism: Liver; normeperidine (metabolite). **Distribution:** Crosses placental barrier; found in breast milk.

NURSING CONSIDERATIONS

Assessment: Assess for intensity/type of pain, patient's general condition and medical status, any other conditions where treatment is contraindicated or cautioned, renal/hepatic function, pregnancy/nursing status, and possible drug interactions.

M

Monitoring: Monitor for signs/symptoms of tolerance or dependence, misuse or abuse, increase in CSF pressure, hypotension, respiratory depression, convulsions, and toxicity.

Patient Counseling: Advise to report pain or adverse events occurring during treatment. Instruct not to adjust dose or abruptly d/c therapy without consulting physician. Counsel that drug may impair mental and/or physical ability required for driving, operating heavy machinery, or other potentially hazardous tasks. Instruct not to drink alcohol or take other CNS depressants (eg, sleep aids, tranquilizers). Advise women who become or are planning to become pregnant about the effects of the drug in pregnancy. Inform that medication has potential for drug abuse; counsel to protect from theft and use by anyone other than the prescribed patient. Instruct to keep medication in a secure place and flush unused tab if no longer needed.

Administration: Oral route. (Sol) Take each dose in 1/2 glass of water. **Storage:** 25°C (77°F); excursions permitted to 15-30°C (59-86°F).

MERREM   RX
meropenem (AstraZeneca)

THERAPEUTIC CLASS: Carbapenem

INDICATIONS: Treatment of intra-abdominal infections (complicated appendicitis and peritonitis), bacterial meningitis, and complicated skin and skin structure infections (cSSSI) caused by susceptible strains of microorganisms.

DOSAGE: *Adults:* IV: Usual: cSSSI: 500mg q8h. Intra-Abdominal Infections: 1g q8h. Renal Impairment: CrCl >25-50mL/min: Give usual dose q12h. CrCl 10-25mL/min: Give 1/2 usual dose q12h. CrCl <10mL/min: Give 1/2 usual dose q24h. Administer as infusion over 15-30 min; doses of 1g may be given as bolus inj (5-20mL) over 3-5 min.
Pediatrics: ≥3 months: IV: >50kg: Intra-Abdominal Infections: 1g q8h. Meningitis: 2g q8h. cSSSI: 500mg q8h. ≤50kg: Intra-Abdominal Infections: 20mg/kg q8h. Max: 1g q8h. Meningitis: 40mg/kg q8h. Max: 2g q8h. cSSSI: 10mg/kg q8h. Max: 500mg q8h. Administer as infusion over 15-30 min, or as bolus inj (5-20mL) over 3-5 min.

HOW SUPPLIED: Inj: 500mg, 1g

WARNINGS/PRECAUTIONS: Serious and fatal hypersensitivity reactions reported. Carefully assess previous reactions to penicillins, cephalosporins, other β-lactams, and other allergens; d/c immediately if allergic reaction occurs. Seizures and other adverse CNS effects reported, particularly with history of seizures or CNS disorders, brain lesions, bacterial meningitis, use of concomitant medications with seizure potential, and compromised renal function. Evaluate patients neurologically if focal tremors, myoclonus, or seizures occur; consider anticonvulsant therapy and examine the need to reduce dose or d/c meropenem therapy. *Clostridium difficile*-associated diarrhea (CDAD) reported; d/c if CDAD is suspected or confirmed. May result in bacterial resistance with prolonged use in the absence of proven or suspected bacterial infection, or a prophylactic indication; take appropriate measures if superinfection develops. Thrombocytopenia reported with renal impairment. Inadequate information on use in patients on peritoneal dialysis or hemodialysis.

ADVERSE REACTIONS: Diarrhea, N/V, rash, headache, constipation, anemia, pain.

INTERACTIONS: Probenecid inhibits renal excretion; avoid concomitant use. May reduce valproic acid or divalproex sodium levels, thereby increasing risk of breakthrough seizures; concomitant use generally not recommended, but if necessary, consider supplemental anticonvulsant therapy.

PREGNANCY: Category B, caution in nursing.

MECHANISM OF ACTION: Broad-spectrum carbapenem; penetrates bacterial cell walls to reach penicillin-binding-protein targets, thus inhibiting cell wall synthesis, resulting in cell death.

PHARMACOKINETICS: Absorption: 30-min infusion: C_{max}=23mcg/mL (500mg); 49mcg/mL (1g). 5-min bolus inj: C_{max}=45mcg/mL (500mg); 112mcg/mL (1g). **Distribution:** Plasma protein binding (2%). **Elimination:** Urine (70%, unchanged); $T_{1/2}$=1 hr (patients ≥2 yrs), 1.5 hrs (pediatrics 3 months-2 yrs).

NURSING CONSIDERATIONS

Assessment: Assess for previous β-lactam hypersensitivity, history of seizure or brain lesions, renal impairment, pregnancy/nursing status, and possible drug interactions.

Monitoring: Monitor for signs/symptoms of anaphylactic/hypersensitivity reactions, CDAD, superinfections, and seizures. Periodically monitor organ system functions (eg, renal, hepatic, hematopoietic) during prolonged use.

Patient Counseling: Instruct to take as directed; skipping doses or not completing full course may decrease effectiveness and increase antibiotic resistance. Inform that diarrhea may occur, even as late as ≥2 months after last dose of therapy; advise to contact physician as soon as possible if watery/bloody stools (with/without stomach cramps/fever) occur. Counsel to inform physician if taking valproic acid or divalproex sodium.

Administration: IV route. Refer to PI for preparation of solution and stability information.
Storage: Dry Powder: 20-25°C (68-77°F).

METADATE CD
methylphenidate HCl (UCB)

> Caution with history of drug dependence or alcoholism. Marked tolerance and psychological dependence may result from chronic abusive use. Frank psychotic episodes may occur, especially with parenteral abuse. Careful supervision required during withdrawal from abusive use since severe depression may occur. Withdrawal following chronic use may unmask symptoms of underlying disorder that may require follow-up.

THERAPEUTIC CLASS: Sympathomimetic amine

INDICATIONS: Treatment of attention-deficit hyperactivity disorder (ADHD).

DOSAGE: *Pediatrics:* ≥6 yrs: Individualize dose. Initial: 20mg qam before breakfast. Titrate: May adjust in weekly 10-20mg increments to a max of 60mg/day based on tolerability/efficacy. Max: 60mg/day. Maint/Extended Treatment: Periodically reevaluate long-term usefulness for individual patients with trials off medication to assess functioning without pharmacotherapy. Reduce dose or d/c if necessary, if paradoxical aggravation of symptoms or other adverse events occur. D/C if no improvement after appropriate dose adjustments over 1 month.

HOW SUPPLIED: Cap, Extended-Release: 10mg, 20mg, 30mg, 40mg, 50mg, 60mg

CONTRAINDICATIONS: Rare hereditary problems of fructose intolerance, glucose-galactose malabsorption or sucrase-isomaltase insufficiency, marked anxiety/tension/agitation, glaucoma, motor tics, family history or diagnosis of Tourette's syndrome, severe HTN, angina pectoris, cardiac arrhythmias, heart failure (HF), recent myocardial infarction (MI), hyperthyroidism or thyrotoxicosis, during or within 14 days of MAOI use, on the day of surgery.

WARNINGS/PRECAUTIONS: Sudden death, stroke, and MI reported; avoid with known structural cardiac abnormalities, cardiomyopathy, serious heart abnormalities, coronary artery disease or other serious cardiac problems. May increase BP and HR; caution with preexisting HTN, heart failure, MI, or ventricular arrhythmias. Assess patients for cardiac disease prior to initiating therapy; promptly perform cardiac evaluation if symptoms suggestive of cardiac disease develop. May exacerbate symptoms of behavior disturbance and thought disorder in patients with a preexisting psychotic disorder. May induce mixed/manic episode in patients with bipolar disorder; assess for bipolar disease before starting therapy. May cause treatment-emergent psychotic or manic symptoms in children and adolescents without prior history of psychotic illness or mania at usual doses. Aggressive behavior or hostility reported. May cause growth suppression in children. May lower seizure threshold; d/c if seizures occur. Visual disturbances reported. May produce positive results during drug testing. Not well established with long-term effects in children.

ADVERSE REACTIONS: Headache, abdominal pain, anorexia, insomnia, nervousness.

INTERACTIONS: See Contraindications. May inhibit metabolism of coumarin anticoagulants, anticonvulsants (eg, phenobarbital, phenytoin, primidone), phenylbutazone, and some antidepressants (eg, tricyclics and SSRIs); may need to adjust dose of these drugs downward; and monitor plasma drug levels (coagulation times, for coumarin) when initiating or d/c methylphenidate therapy. Caution with pressor agents. Clearance might be affected by urinary pH; either increased with acidifying agents or decreased with alkalinizing agents. Risk of sudden BP increase with halogenated anesthetics during surgery.

PREGNANCY: Category C, caution in nursing.

MECHANISM OF ACTION: CNS stimulant; not established, thought to block reuptake of norepinephrine and dopamine into presynaptic neuron and increase release of these monoamines into extraneuronal space.

PHARMACOKINETICS: Absorption: Readily absorbed. Administration of variable doses resulted in different parameters. **Metabolism:** Via deesterification. Metabolite: α-phenyl-piperidine acetic acid (ritalinic acid). **Elimination:** $T_{1/2}$=6.8 hrs.

NURSING CONSIDERATIONS

Assessment: Assess for agitation, anxiety, tension, glaucoma, tics, family history or diagnosis of Tourette's syndrome, cardiovascular conditions, structural cardiac abnormalities, hyperthyroidism or thyrotoxicosis, bipolar illness, seizure disorder or history of seizures, history of drug dependence or alcoholism, if undergoing surgery and hereditary problems of fructose intolerance, glucose-galactose malabsorption, or sucrase-isomaltase insufficiency, and possible drug interactions.

Monitoring: Monitor for cardiac abnormalities, increased BP and HR, exacerbations of behavior disturbances and thought disorders, psychotic or manic symptoms, aggression, hostility, seizures, and visual disturbances. In patients with bipolar disorder, monitor for mixed/manic episode. Perform periodic monitoring of CBC, differential and platelet count during prolonged therapy. Monitor growth in children.

M

Patient Counseling: Inform about the benefits and risks of therapy, appropriate use, and drug abuse/dependence. Instruct to take 1 dose in the morning before breakfast. Instruct that capsule may be swallowed whole or opened and sprinkled in 1 tbsp of applesauce and given immediately, and not stored for future use; advise not to crush or chew. Instruct patient, their families, and caregivers to read the Medication Guide.

Administration: Oral route. **Storage:** 25°C (77°F); excursions permitted to 15-30°C (59-86°F).

METADATE ER
methylphenidate HCl (UCB)

> Caution with history of drug dependence or alcoholism. Marked tolerance and psychological dependence with varying degrees of abnormal behavior may occur with chronic abusive use. Frank psychotic episodes may occur. Careful supervision is required during withdrawal from abusive use since severe depression may occur. Withdrawal after chronic use may unmask symptoms of underlying disorder that may require follow-up.

THERAPEUTIC CLASS: Sympathomimetic amine

INDICATIONS: Treatment of attention-deficit disorder (ADHD) and narcolepsy.

DOSAGE: *Adults:* Individualize dose. (Immediate-Release [IR] Methylphenidate) 10-60mg/day given in divided doses bid-tid 30-45 min ac. Take last dose before 6 pm if unable to sleep. (Tab, ER) May use in place of IR tabs when 8-hr dose corresponds to titrated 8-hr IR dose. *Pediatrics:* ≥6 yrs: Individualize dose. Initiate in small doses with gradual weekly increments. Max: 60mg/day. (IR Methylphenidate) Initial: 5mg bid before breakfast and lunch. Titrate: Increase gradually by 5-10mg weekly. (Tab, ER) May use in place of IR tabs when the 8-hr dose corresponds to the titrated 8-hr IR dose. Reduce dose or d/c if paradoxical aggravation of symptoms occur. D/C if no improvement after appropriate dose adjustment over a 1-month period.

HOW SUPPLIED: Tab, Extended-Release (ER): 20mg

CONTRAINDICATIONS: Marked anxiety, tension, and agitation; glaucoma; motor tics or family history or diagnosis of Tourette's syndrome; severe HTN, angina pectoris, cardiac arrhythmias, heart failure (HF), recent myocardial infarction (MI), hyperthyroidism or thyrotoxicosis; surgery; during or within 14 days of MAOI use; Lapp lactase deficiency or glucose-galactose malabsorption.

WARNINGS/PRECAUTIONS: Sudden death, stroke, and MI reported; avoid with known serious structural cardiac abnormalities, cardiomyopathy, serious heart rhythm abnormalities, coronary artery disease, or other serious cardiac problems. May cause modest increase in BP and HR; caution with HTN, HF, recent MI, or ventricular arrhythmia. Assess for presence of cardiac disease prior to initiating therapy; promptly perform cardiac evaluation if symptoms suggestive of cardiac disease develop. May exacerbate symptoms of behavior disturbance and thought disorder in patients with preexisting psychotic disorder. Caution in patients with comorbid bipolar disorder; may cause induction of mixed/manic episodes. May cause treatment-emergent psychotic or manic symptoms in children and adolescents without prior history of psychotic illness or mania at usual doses; d/c treatment if appropriate. Aggressive behavior or hostility reported in children and adolescents with ADHD. Suppression of growth reported with long-term use in pediatric patients; monitor height and weight. May lower convulsive threshold; d/c if seizures occur. Difficulties with accommodation and blurring of vision reported. Patients with an element of agitation may react adversely; d/c if necessary. Not indicated in all cases of this behavioral syndrome, and in symptoms associated with acute stress reactions. D/C drug periodically to assess child's condition; therapy should not be indefinite. Monitor CBC, differential, and platelet counts during prolonged therapy.

ADVERSE REACTIONS: Nervousness, insomnia, hypersensitivity reactions, anorexia, nausea, dizziness, palpitations, headache, dyskinesia, drowsiness, BP and pulse changes, tachycardia, angina, arrhythmia.

INTERACTIONS: See Contraindications. Caution with pressor agents. May decrease effectiveness of antihypertensives. May inhibit metabolism of coumarin anticoagulants, anticonvulsants (eg, phenobarbital, phenytoin, primidone), phenylbutazone, and tricyclic drugs (eg, imipramine, clomipramine, desipramine); may need to adjust dose. Monitor coagulation times with coumarin when initiating or d/c treatment. Clearance may be affected by agents that alter urinary pH. Possible occurrence of neuroleptic malignant syndrome (NMS) with concurrent therapies associated with NMS; single report of NMS-like event possibly related to concurrent use of venlafaxine.

PREGNANCY: Category C, caution in nursing.

MECHANISM OF ACTION: Sympathomimetic amine; not established. Mild CNS stimulant; presumably activates brainstem arousal system and cortex to produce stimulant effect.

PHARMACOKINETICS: Absorption: Slowly absorbed. T_{max}=1.3-8.2 hrs (sustained-release tab), 0.3-4.4 hrs (IR tab).

NURSING CONSIDERATIONS

Assessment: Assess for cardiac disease, psychotic disorders, bipolar disorder, seizures, history of drug dependence or alcoholism, acute stress reactions, and any other conditions where treatment is contraindicated or cautioned. Assess pregnancy/nursing status and possible drug interactions. Obtain baseline height/weight in children, and CBC, differential, and platelet counts.

Monitoring: Monitor for signs and symptoms of cardiac disease, increased BP and HR, exacerbations of behavior disturbances and thought disorders, psychotic or manic symptoms, aggression, hostility, seizures, and visual disturbances. Monitor growth in children. In patients with bipolar disorder, monitor for mixed/manic episode. Perform periodic monitoring of CBC, differential, and platelet counts during prolonged therapy.

Patient Counseling: Inform about potential risks, benefits, and appropriate use of treatment. Instruct to read the Medication Guide. Instruct to swallow whole tab; do not chew or crush. Advise to take 30-45 min ac and last dose before 6 pm to avoid insomnia. Advise that medication contains lactose.

Administration: Oral route. **Storage:** 20-25°C (77°F); excursions permitted to 15-30°C (59-86°F). Protect from moisture.

METHADOSE   CII
methadone HCl (Mallinckrodt)

> Deaths due to cardiac and respiratory effects reported during initiation and conversion from other opioid agonists. Respiratory depression and QT prolongation observed. Only certified/approved opioid treatment programs can dispense oral methadone for treatment of narcotic addiction. Use as analgesic should be initiated only if benefits outweigh risks. (Powder) For oral administration only and must be used in the preparation of a liquid by dissolving powder in an appropriate vehicle. Preparation must not be injected.

THERAPEUTIC CLASS: Opioid analgesic

INDICATIONS: Detoxification and maintenance treatment of opioid addiction (heroin or other morphine-like drugs) in conjunction with appropriate social and medical services. (Tab) Treatment of moderate to severe pain not responsive to non-narcotic analgesics.

M

DOSAGE: Adults: Detoxification: Initial/Induction: 20-30mg/day. Titrate: Give 5-10mg 2-4 hrs later if needed. Max: 40mg on first day. Adjust dose to control withdrawal symptoms over first week. Short-Term Detoxification: Titrate to 40mg/day given in divided doses to achieve adequate stabilizing level. Stabilization can continue for 2-3 days, then decrease dose every 1-2 days depending on symptoms. Maint: Titrate to a dose at which symptoms prevented for 24 hrs. Usual: 80-120mg/day. Medically Supervised Withdrawal After a Period of Maintenance Treatment: Dose reductions should be <10% of established tolerance or maintenance dose, and 10- to 14-day intervals should elapse between dose reductions. Pregnancy: May increase dose or decrease dosing interval. (Tab) Pain in Opioid Non-Tolerant: Initial: 2.5-10mg q8-12h, slowly titrated to effect. Conversion From Parenteral: Use a 1:2 dose ratio parenteral to oral. Switching From Other Chronic Opioids: Use caution; see PI for dosing details.

HOW SUPPLIED: Oral Concentrate: 10mg/mL; Powder (generic): 50g, 100g, 500g, 1kg; Tab: 5mg*, 10mg*; Tab, Dispersible: 40mg *scored

CONTRAINDICATIONS: In any situation where opioids are contraindicated such as respiratory depression (in the absence of resuscitative equipment or in unmonitored settings), acute bronchial asthma or hypercarbia, and paralytic ileus.

WARNINGS/PRECAUTIONS: Can cause respiratory depression and elevate CSF pressure; caution with decreased respiratory reserve, hypoxia, hypercapnia, head injuries, other intracranial lesions or a preexisting increase in intracranial pressure (ICP). Cases of QT interval prolongation and serious arrhythmia observed; caution in patients with risk of prolonged QT interval and evaluate for risk factors. Caution in elderly. Caution in patients with severe hepatic/renal impairment, hypothyroidism, Addison's disease, prostatic hypertrophy, or urethral stricture. Risk of tolerance, dependence, and abuse. May obscure the diagnosis or clinical course of acute abdominal conditions. May impair mental/physical abilities. Patients tolerant to other opioids may be incompletely tolerant to methadone. Infants born to opioid-dependent mothers may exhibit respiratory difficulties and withdrawal symptoms. May produce hypotension.

ADVERSE REACTIONS: Lightheadedness, dizziness, sedation, sweating, N/V.

INTERACTIONS: Inhibitors and inducers of CYP3A4, CYP2B6, CYP2C19, CYP2C9, and CYP2D6 may alter metabolism and effects. Opioid antagonists, mixed agonist/antagonists, and partial agonists may precipitate withdrawal symptoms. Concomitant use with other opioid analgesics, general anesthetics, phenothiazines, tranquilizers, sedative-hypnotics, or other CNS depressants may cause respiratory depression, hypotension, profound sedation, or coma. Deaths reported when abused in conjunction with benzodiazepines. Caution with drugs that may prolong QT interval. MAOIs may cause severe reactions. May increase levels of desipramine. Abacavir, amprenavir, efavirenz, nelfinavir, nevirapine, ritonavir, lopinavir + ritonavir (combination) may increase clearance or decrease levels. May decrease levels of didanosine and stavudine. May increase area under the curve of zidovudine.

PREGNANCY: Category C, not for use in nursing.

MECHANISM OF ACTION: Synthetic opioid analgesic; μ-agonist. Produces actions similar to morphine; acts on CNS and organs composed of smooth muscle. May also act as an N-methyl-D-aspartate (NMDA) receptor antagonist.

PHARMACOKINETICS: Absorption: Bioavailability (36-100%); C_{max}=124-1255ng/mL; T_{max}=1-7.5 hrs. **Distribution:** V_d=1-8L/kg; plasma protein binding (85-90%); found in breast milk and umbilical cord plasma. **Metabolism:** Hepatic N-demethylation; CYP3A4, 2B6, 2C19 (major); 2C9, 2D6 (minor). **Elimination:** Urine, feces; $T_{1/2}$=7-59 hrs; (Tab) $T_{1/2}$=8-59 hrs.

NURSING CONSIDERATIONS

Assessment: Assess for respiratory status, history of acute bronchial asthma or COPD, CNS depression, cardiac conduction abnormalities, increased ICP, acute abdominal conditions, volume depletion, hepatic/renal impairment, or any other conditions where treatment is contraindicated or cautioned. Assess hypersensitivity to drug, pregnancy/nursing status, and possible drug interactions.

Monitoring: Monitor for signs/symptoms of respiratory depression, QT prolongation and arrhythmias, misuse or abuse of medication, physical dependence and tolerance, withdrawal symptoms, elevations in CSF pressure, orthostatic hypotension, and hypersensitivity reactions.

Patient Counseling: Inform that medication may impair mental/physical abilities; use caution when performing hazardous tasks (eg, operating machinery/driving). Advise to avoid using alcohol and other CNS depressants. Instruct to seek immediate medical care if signs/symptoms of arrhythmia (eg, palpitations, dizziness, syncope) or difficulty in breathing develops. Orthostatic hypotension may occur. Instruct to keep out of reach of children. Avoid abrupt withdrawal; taper dosing with medical supervision. Inform patients treated for opioid dependence that d/c may lead to relapse of illicit drug use. Educate about potential for abuse and to protect from theft. Reassure that dose of methadone will "hold" for longer periods of time as treatment progresses after initiation.

Administration: Oral route. **Storage:** 20-25°C (68-77°F).

METHOTREXATE   RX
methotrexate (Various)

> Should only be used by physicians with knowledge and experience in the use of antimetabolite therapy. Use only for life-threatening neoplastic diseases, or in patients with psoriasis or rheumatoid arthritis (RA) with severe, recalcitrant, disabling disease not adequately responsive to other forms of therapy. Deaths in the treatment of malignancy, psoriasis, and RA reported. Monitor for bone marrow, liver, lung, and kidney toxicities. Patients should be informed of the risks involved and should be under physician's care throughout therapy. Fetal death and/or congenital anomalies reported. Reduced elimination with impaired renal function, ascites, or pleural effusions; monitor for toxicity, reduce dose, and d/c in some cases. Unexpectedly severe, sometimes fatal, bone marrow suppression, aplastic anemia, and GI toxicity reported with usually high dosage along with some NSAIDs. May cause hepatotoxicity, fibrosis, and cirrhosis (generally only after prolonged use). Acutely, liver enzyme elevations frequently seen. Periodic liver biopsies recommended for psoriatic patients on long-term therapy. Drug-induced lung disease (including acute/chronic interstitial pneumonitis), and potentially fatal opportunistic infections may occur. Interrupt therapy if pulmonary symptoms (especially dry, nonproductive cough), or diarrhea and ulcerative stomatitis occur. Malignant lymphomas may occur with low-dose therapy, and thus, may not require cytotoxic treatment; d/c therapy 1st, and if lymphoma does not regress, institute appropriate treatment. May induce tumor lysis syndrome in patients with rapidly growing tumors; may be prevented/alleviated with appropriate supportive and pharmacologic measures. Severe, occasionally fatal, skin reactions reported. Concomitant radiotherapy may increase risk of soft tissue necrosis and osteonecrosis. (Inj) Use of high dose regimens recommended for osteosarcoma requires meticulous care. Formulations and diluents containing preservatives must not be used for intrathecal or high dose therapy.

THERAPEUTIC CLASS: Dihydrofolic acid reductase inhibitor

INDICATIONS: Treatment of gestational choriocarcinoma, chorioadenoma destruens, and hydatidiform mole. Used in maintenance therapy with other chemotherapeutic agents. Used alone or in combination with other anticancer agents in the treatment of breast cancer, epidermoid cancer of the head and neck, advanced mycosis fungoides (cutaneous T-cell lymphoma), and lung cancer, particularly squamous cell and small cell types. Treatment of advanced stage non-Hodgkin's lymphomas in combination with other chemotherapeutic agents. Symptomatic control of severe, recalcitrant, disabling psoriasis not adequately responsive to other forms of therapy, but only when the diagnosis has been established, as by a biopsy and/or after dermatologic consultation. Management of severe, active RA (ACR criteria) in selected adults or children with active polyarticular-course juvenile RA, who had insufficient response to, or are intolerant of, adequate trial of 1st-line therapy (including NSAIDs). (Inj) Prophylaxis and treatment of meningeal leukemia, and maintenance therapy in combination with other chemotherapeutic agents in acute lymphocytic leukemia. Followed by leucovorin rescue with other chemotherapeutic agents, prolong relapse-free survival in non-metastatic osteosarcoma patients who have undergone surgical resection or amputation for the primary tumor.

DOSAGE: *Adults:* Choriocarcinoma/Trophoblastic Disease: 15-30mg/day PO/IM for 5 days. May repeat 3-5X as required with rest period of ≥1 week interposed between courses until manifesting toxic symptoms subside. Leukemia: Induction: 3.3mg/m² with prednisone 60mg/m²/day. Remission Maintenance: 30mg/m²/week PO/IM given twice weekly or 2.5mg/kg IV every 14 days. If and when relapse does occur, obtain reinduction of remission by repeating the initial induction regimen. Meningeal Leukemia: Prophylaxis/Treatment: 12mg/m² intrathecally. Treatment: Give at 2-5 day intervals. Max: 15mg. Burkitt's Tumor: Stages I-II: 10-25mg/day PO for 4-8 days. Lymphosarcoma: Stage III: 0.625-2.5mg/kg/day with other antineoplastic agents. Treatment in all stages consist of several courses with 7-10 day rest periods. Mycosis Fungoides: Early Stage: 5-50mg once weekly. If poor response, give 15-37.5mg twice weekly. Adjust dose based on response and hematologic monitoring. Combination chemotherapy regimens that includes IV therapy with higher doses with leucovorin rescue has been used for advanced stages. Osteosarcoma: Initial: 12g/m² IV, increase to 15g/m² if peak serum levels of 1000 micromolar not reached at end of infusion. Psoriasis: Initial: 10-25mg PO/IM/IV weekly until adequate response or use divided oral dose schedule, 2.5mg at 12 hr intervals for 3 doses. Titrate: Increase gradually until optimal response. Maint: Reduce to lowest effective dose. Max: 30mg/week. RA: Initial: 7.5mg PO once weekly, or 2.5mg q12h for 3 doses given as a course once weekly. Titrate: Gradual increase. Max: 20mg/week. After response, reduce dose to lowest effective amount of drug. See PI for proper leucovorin rescue therapy.
Pediatrics: Meningeal Leukemia: Prophylaxis/Treatment: ≥3yrs: 12mg. 2 yrs: 10mg. 1 yr: 8mg. <1 yr: 6mg. Give intrathecally. If dosing based on weight: 12mg/m². Max: 15mg. Treatment: Give at 2-5 day intervals. Juvenile RA: 2-16 yrs: Initial: 10mg/m² once weekly. Adjust dose gradually to achieve optimal response. Max: 30mg/m²/week.

HOW SUPPLIED: Inj: 25mg/mL [2mL, 4mL, 8mL, 10mL], 1g; Tab: 2.5mg* *scored

CONTRAINDICATIONS: Pregnant women with psoriasis or RA (should be used in treatment of pregnant women with neoplastic diseases only when potential benefit outweighs risk to the fetus), nursing mothers. Psoriasis or RA patients with alcoholism, alcoholic liver disease, chronic liver disease, immunodeficiency syndromes, and preexisting blood dyscrasias.

WARNINGS/PRECAUTIONS: Toxicity may be related in frequency and severity to dose/frequency of administration; reduce dose or d/c therapy and take corrective measures when toxicity occurs; may include use of leucovorin calcium and/or acute, intermittent hemodialysis with high-flux dialyzer if necessary. If therapy is reinstituted, carry it out with caution and with adequate consideration of further need for the drug and increased alertness as to possible recurrence of toxicity. Caution in elderly; consider low doses and monitor for early signs of toxicity. Avoid pregnancy if either partner is receiving therapy. (Inj) May affect mental/physical abilities. Fatal gasping syndrome reported in neonates; formulations containing benzyl alcohol as preservative is not recommended for use in neonates. In RA, appear at first use and duration of therapy have been reported as risk factor for hepatotoxicity; LFT and liver biopsy should be performed. Methotrexate given by intrathecal routes appear significantly in the systemic circulation and may cause systemic methotrexate toxicity; systemic antileukemic therapy with the drug should be appropriately adjusted, reduced or d/c.

ADVERSE REACTIONS: Ulcerative stomatitis, leukopenia, N/V, abdominal distress, malaise, fatigue, chills, fever, dizziness, decreased resistance to infection, elevated LFTs, thrombocytopenia, rash, pruritus.

INTERACTIONS: See Boxed Warning. Caution with NSAIDs or salicylates during low doses and nephrotoxic chemotherapeutic agents (eg, cisplatin) during high doses of therapy. Increased toxicity due to displacement by sulfonamides, phenytoin, phenylbutazone, and salicylates. Renal tubular transport diminished by probenecid. May increase levels of mercaptopurine. Oral antibiotics (eg, tetracycline, chloramphenicol, nonabsorbable broad spectrum) may decrease intestinal absorption or interfere with enterohepatic circulation. Penicillins may decrease renal clearance; hematologic and GI toxicity observed. Closely monitor with hepatotoxins (eg, azathioprine, retinoids, sulfasalazine) for increased risk of hepatotoxicity. May decrease theophylline clearance. Trimethoprim/sulfamethoxazole may increase bone marrow suppression by decreasing tubular secretion and/or additive antifolate effects. Immunization with live virus vaccines is generally not recommended. (Inj) NSAIDs with high doses of therapy may elevate and prolong serum levels; avoid NSAIDs with high doses of therapy. Folic acid or its derivatives may decrease response to drug. High doses of leucovorin may reduce the efficacy of intrathecal administration of drug.

PREGNANCY: Category X, not for use in nursing.

MECHANISM OF ACTION: Dihydrofolic acid reductase inhibitor; interferes with DNA synthesis, repair, and cellular replication. Mechanism in RA not established; may affect immune function.

PHARMACOKINETICS: Absorption: (PO, Healthy) Well-absorbed. Bioavailability (60%); T_{max}=1-2 hrs. Oral administration resulted in different parameters according to disease state and dosing; refer to PI for further information. (Inj) Complete. T_{max}=30-60 min (IM). **Distribution:** (IV) V_d=0.18L/kg (Initial), 0.4-0.8L/kg (Steady state); plasma protein binding (50%); found in breast milk. **Metabolism:** Hepatic and intracellular; 7-hydroxymethotrexate (metabolite). **Elimination:**

M

(IV) Urine (80-90% unchanged), bile (≤10%); T$_{1/2}$=0.7-5.8 hrs (pediatrics with acute lymphocytic leukemia), 0.9-2.3 hrs (juvenile RA), 3-10 hrs (psoriasis, RA, low-dose), 8-15 hrs (high dose).

NURSING CONSIDERATIONS

Assessment: Assess pregnancy/nursing status, alcoholism, chronic liver disease, immunodeficiency, blood dyscrasias, ascites, pleural effusions, and possible drug interactions. Obtain baseline CBC with differential and platelet counts, hepatic enzymes, renal function tests, liver biopsy, and chest x-ray.

Monitoring: Monitor for toxicities of bone marrow, liver, lung, kidney and GI, diarrhea, ulcerative stomatitis, tumor lysis syndrome, skin reactions, and opportunistic infections. Monitor hematology at least monthly, and renal/hepatic function every 1-2 months during therapy of RA and psoriasis. Perform more frequent monitoring of laboratory parameters during antineoplastic therapy. If drug-induced lung disease is suspected, perform pulmonary function tests.

Patient Counseling: Advise about early signs/symptoms of toxicity, the need to see their physician promptly if any are experienced, and the need for close follow-up including periodic laboratory test to monitor toxicity. Emphasize to the patient that the recommended dose is taken weekly in RA and psoriasis, and that mistaken daily use of recommended dose has led to fatal toxicity; prescriptions should not be written or refilled on a PRN basis. Counsel about risks/benefits of therapy, and effects on reproduction.

Administration: Oral, IM, IV, intra-arterial, or intrathecal route. (Inj) Refer to PI for reconstitution and dilution instructions. **Storage:** 20-25°C (68-77°F). Protect from light.

METHYLIN
methylphenidate HCl (Mallinckrodt)

> Caution with history of drug dependence or alcoholism. Marked tolerance and psychological dependence may result from chronic abusive use. Frank psychotic episodes may occur, especially with parenteral abuse. Careful supervision required during withdrawal from abusive use since severe depression may occur. Withdrawal following chronic use may unmask symptoms of underlying disorder that may require follow-up.

THERAPEUTIC CLASS: Sympathomimetic amine

INDICATIONS: Treatment of attention deficit disorder and narcolepsy.

DOSAGE: *Adults:* Individualize dose. (Sol/Tab/Tab, Chewable) 10-60mg/day given in divided doses bid or tid 30-45 min ac. Take last dose before 6 pm if insomnia occurs. (ER) May be used in place of immediate-release (IR) tab when 8-hr dose corresponds to titrated 8-hr IR dose. *Pediatrics:* ≥6 yrs: Individualize dose. Reduce dose or d/c if paradoxical aggravation of symptoms occurs. D/C if no improvement after appropriate dose adjustment over a 1-month period. (Sol/Tab/Tab, Chewable) Initial: 5mg bid before breakfast and lunch. Titrate: Increase gradually in increments of 5-10mg weekly. Max: 60mg/day. (ER) May be used in place of IR tab when 8-hr dose corresponds to titrated 8-hr IR dose.

HOW SUPPLIED: Sol: 5mg/5mL [500mL], 10mg/5mL [500mL]; Tab: 5mg, 10mg*, 20mg*; Tab, Chewable: 2.5mg, 5mg, 10mg*; Tab, Extended-Release (ER): 10mg, 20mg *scored

CONTRAINDICATIONS: Marked anxiety, tension, agitation, glaucoma, motor tics or family history or diagnosis of Tourette's syndrome. Treatment with or within a minimum of 14 days following d/c of a MAOI.

WARNINGS/PRECAUTIONS: Sudden death, stroke, and myocardial infarction (MI) reported; avoid with known structural cardiac abnormalities, cardiomyopathy, serious heart rhythm abnormalities, coronary artery disease or other serious cardiac problems. May increase BP and HR; caution with preexisting HTN, heart failure, MI, or ventricular arrhythmias. Assess patients for cardiac disease prior to initiating therapy; promptly perform cardiac evaluation if symptoms suggestive of cardiac disease develop. May exacerbate symptoms of behavior disturbance and thought disorder in patients with a preexisting psychotic disorder. May induce mixed/manic episode in patients with bipolar disorder; assess for bipolar disease before starting therapy. May cause treatment-emergent psychotic or manic symptoms in children and adolescents without prior history of psychotic illness or mania at usual doses. Aggressive behavior or hostility reported. May cause growth suppression in children. May lower convulsive threshold; d/c if seizures occur. Visual disturbances reported. Patients with an element of agitation may react adversely; d/c therapy if necessary. Not indicated in all cases of this behavioral syndrome, and in symptoms associated with acute stress reactions. D/C drug periodically to assess child's condition; therapy should not be indefinite. (Sol/Tab, Chewable) Not well established with long-term effects in children.

ADVERSE REACTIONS: Nervousness, insomnia, hypersensitivity, anorexia, nausea, dizziness, headache, dyskinesia, drowsiness, BP and pulse changes, tachycardia, weight loss, abdominal pain, decreased appetite.

INTERACTIONS: See Contraindications. Caution with pressor agents. May inhibit metabolism of coumarin anticoagulants, anticonvulsants (eg, phenobarbital, phenytoin, primidone), TCAs (eg, imipramine, clomipramine, desipramine); may need to adjust dose of these drugs downward; and monitor plasma drug levels (coagulation times, for coumarin) when initiating or d/c methylphenidate therapy for tab and ER. (Sol/Tab, Chewable) May decrease hypotensive effect of guanethidine. (Tab/ER) Serious adverse reactions reported with clonidine. May decrease the effectiveness of antihypertensives.

PREGNANCY: (Tab/ER) Category C, caution in nursing. (Tab, Chewable/Sol) Safety not known in pregnancy and nursing.

MECHANISM OF ACTION: Sympathomimetic amine; not been established. CNS stimulant, thought to block the reuptake of norepinephrine and dopamine into the presynaptic neuron and increase the release of monoamines into the extraneuronal space. Presumably activates the brain stem arousal system and cortex to produce stimulant effect.

PHARMACOKINETICS: Absorption: (ER/Tab) Extensive. (ER) T_{max}=4.7 hrs (children). (Tab) T_{max}=1.9 hrs (children). (Tab, Chewable) C_{max}=10ng/mL (20mg); T_{max}=1-2 hrs. (Sol) C_{max}=9ng/mL (20mg); T_{max}=1-2 hrs. **Metabolism:** Deesterification to α-phenyl-piperidine acetic acid; α-phenyl-2-piperidine acetic acid (major metabolite). **Elimination:** (Tab, Chewable/Sol) Urine (90%; 80% metabolite). (Sol) $T_{1/2}$=2.7 hrs (20mg). (Tab, Chewable) $T_{1/2}$=3 hrs (20mg).

NURSING CONSIDERATIONS

Assessment: Assess for cardiac disease, psychotic disorders, bipolar disorder, seizures, history of drug dependence or alcoholism, acute stress reactions, and any other conditions where treatment is contraindicated or cautioned. Assess pregnancy/nursing status, and for possible drug interactions.

Monitoring: Monitor for signs and symptoms of cardiac disease, increased BP and HR, exacerbations of behavior disturbances and thought disorders, psychotic or manic symptoms, aggression, hostility, seizures, and visual disturbances. Monitor growth in children. In patients with bipolar disorder, monitor for mixed/manic episode. Perform periodic monitoring of CBC, differential, and platelet counts during prolonged therapy.

Patient Counseling: Inform patients and families/caregivers about risks, benefits, and appropriate use of treatment. Instruct to read the Medication Guide. (Tab, Chewable) Advise not to take the drug if have difficulty swallowing. Seek medical attention if experienced chest pain, vomiting, difficulty in swallowing or breathing after taking the drug. Take with a full glass of water or other fluid. Contains phenylalanine.

Administration: Oral route. (ER) Swallow whole; do not chew or crush. (Tab, Chewable) Take with at least 8 oz. of water or other fluid. **Storage:** 20-25°C (68-77°F). (Tab) Protect from light. (ER/Tab, Chewable) Protect from moisture.

METOCLOPRAMIDE   RX
metoclopramide (Various)

May cause tardive dyskinesia (TD); d/c if signs/symptoms of TD develop; avoid use for >12 weeks of therapy unless benefit outweighs risk.

OTHER BRAND NAMES: Reglan Tablets (ANI) - Reglan Injection (Baxter)

THERAPEUTIC CLASS: Dopamine antagonist/prokinetic

INDICATIONS: (PO) Short-term therapy (4-12 weeks) for adults with symptomatic, documented gastroesophageal reflux disease (GERD) who fail to respond to conventional therapy. (Inj, PO) Relief of symptoms associated with acute and recurrent diabetic gastric stasis in adults. (Inj) Prevention of postoperative or chemotherapy-induced N/V. Facilitates small bowel intubation in adults and pediatric patients in whom the tube does not pass the pylorus with conventional maneuvers. Stimulates gastric emptying and intestinal transit of barium in cases where delayed emptying interferes with radiological examination of the stomach and/or small intestines.

DOSAGE: *Adults:* (PO) GERD: 10-15mg up to qid 30 min before each meal and hs. Sensitive to Metoclopramide/Elderly: 5 mg/dose. Intermittent Symptoms: ≤20mg as single dose prior to the provoking situation. If esophageal lesions are present, 15mg qid. Max: 12 weeks of therapy. (PO, Inj) Diabetic Gastroparesis: 10mg PO 30 min before each meal and hs for 2-8 weeks. If severe, begin with IM or IV (may give 10mg IV slowly over 1-2 min); may need inj ≤10 days before symptoms subside, at which time PO administration may be instituted. (Inj) Antiemetic: (Postop) 10-20mg IM near end of surgery. (Chemotherapy-Induced) 1-2mg/kg IV infusion over a period of ≥15 min, 30 min before chemotherapy then q2h for 2 doses, then q3h for 3 doses. Give 2mg/kg for highly emetogenic drugs for initial 2 doses. Small Bowel Intubation/Radiological Exam: 10mg by slow IV as single dose (undiluted) over 1-2 min. Renal Impairment: CrCl <40mL/min: Initial: 50% of normal dose. May adjust as appropriate. Elderly: Start at lower end of dosing range.
Pediatrics: (Inj) Small Bowel Intubation: Administer single dose (undiluted) by slow IV over 1-2

min. >14 yrs: 10mg. 6-14 yrs: 2.5-5mg. <6 yrs: 0.1mg/kg. Renal Impairment: CrCl <40mL/min: Initial: 50% of normal dose. May adjust as appropriate.

HOW SUPPLIED: Inj (Reglan): 5mg/mL [2mL, 10mL, 30mL]; Sol: 5mg/5mL; Tab (Reglan): 5mg, 10mg* *scored

CONTRAINDICATIONS: When GI motility stimulation is dangerous (eg, perforation, mechanical obstruction, GI hemorrhage), pheochromocytoma, epilepsy, and concomitant drugs that cause extrapyramidal symptoms (EPS).

WARNINGS/PRECAUTIONS: Neuroleptic malignant syndrome (NMS) reported; d/c and institute intensive symptomatic treatment and medical monitoring if NMS occurs. Extrapyramidal symptoms (EPS) (primarily as acute dystonic reactions) may occur. May cause Parkinsonian-like symptoms; more common within first 6 months after beginning treatment; generally subside within 2-3 months of d/c; caution with preexisting Parkinson's disease. Mental depression may occur; caution with prior history of depression. Not to be used for symptomatic control of TD. Caution with HTN, renal impairment, and/or in elderly. Risk of developing fluid retention and volume overload, especially with cirrhosis or congestive heart failure (CHF); d/c if these occur. May increase risk of developing methemoglobinemia and/or sulfhemoglobinemia with NADH-cytochrome b_5 reductase deficiency. May experience withdrawal symptoms after d/c.

ADVERSE REACTIONS: TD, fatigue, restlessness, lassitude, drowsiness.

INTERACTIONS: See Contraindications. May decrease gastric absorption of some drugs (eg, digoxin) and increase rate and/or extent of intestinal absorption of others (eg, acetaminophen, tetracycline, levodopa, ethanol, and cyclosporine). Additive sedation with alcohol, sedatives, hypnotics, narcotics, or tranquilizers. Caution with MAOIs; catecholamines released in patients with HTN. GI motility effect antagonized by anticholinergics and narcotic analgesics. Insulin dose or timing of dose may require adjustment. Rare cases of hepatotoxicity with drugs with hepatotoxic potential. Inhibits the central and peripheral effects of apomorphine.

PREGNANCY: Category B, caution in nursing.

MECHANISM OF ACTION: Dopamine antagonist/promotility agent; mechanism not established, appears to sensitize tissues to the action of acetylcholine; stimulates motility of upper GI tract without stimulating gastric, biliary or pancreatic secretions and accelerates gastric emptying and intestinal transit; increases resting tone of lower esophageal sphincter. Antiemetic; antagonizes central and peripheral dopamine receptors, thereby blocking stimulation of chemoreceptor trigger zone.

PHARMACOKINETICS: Absorption: Rapid and well absorbed; absolute bioavailability (80%); (PO) T_{max}=1-2 hrs; IV administration in pediatrics resulted in different parameters. **Distribution:** Plasma protein binding (30%); V_d=3.5L/kg; found in breast milk. **Elimination:** (PO) Urine (85%); $T_{1/2}$=5-6 hrs.

NURSING CONSIDERATIONS

Assessment: Assess for conditions when GI motility stimulation is dangerous, pheochromocytoma, epilepsy, sensitivity or tolerance to the drug, CHF, cirrhosis, history of depression, Parkinson's disease, HTN, NADH-cytochrome b_5 reductase and glucose-6-phosphate dehydrogenase deficiency, diabetes mellitus, renal impairment, pregnancy/nursing status, and for possible drug interactions.

Monitoring: Monitor for signs/symptoms of depression, EPS, Parkinsonian-like symptoms, TD, NMS, HTN, fluid retention/volume overload, and hypersensitivity reactions. (PO) Monitor for withdrawal symptoms.

Patient Counseling: Instruct to read the Medication Guide. Inform that drug may impair mental and physical abilities; use caution while operating machinery/driving. (PO) Inform that drug is recommended for adults only.

Administration: Oral, IV/IM route. (Inj) IV inj of undiluted drug should be made slowly, allowing 1-2 min for 10mg. Administration of diluted drug should be slow, over a period of ≥15 min. For doses >10mg, dilute in 50mL of parenteral solution. Refer to PI for IV admixture compatibilities. **Storage:** 20-25°C (68-77°F). (Inj) If diluted with NaCl, may be stored frozen for ≤4 weeks. Diluted solutions may be stored ≤48 hrs (without freezing) if protected from light. In normal light conditions, may be stored ≤24 hrs.

METOPROLOL/HCTZ   RX
metoprolol tartrate - hydrochlorothiazide (Various)

> Exacerbation of angina and, in some cases, myocardial infarction (MI) reported following abrupt d/c. When d/c therapy, avoid abrupt withdrawal even without overt angina pectoris. Caution patients against interruption of therapy without physician's advice.

OTHER BRAND NAMES: Lopressor HCT (Novartis)

THERAPEUTIC CLASS: Selective beta$_1$-blocker/thiazide diuretic

INDICATIONS: Management of HTN.

DOSAGE: *Adults:* Individualize dose. Combination Therapy: Metoprolol: 100-200mg/day given qd or in divided doses. HCTZ: 25-50mg/day given qd or in divided doses. Max: 50mg/day. May gradually add another antihypertensive when necessary, beginning with 50% of the usual recommended starting dose. Elderly: Start at lower end of dosing range.

HOW SUPPLIED: Tab: (Metoprolol-HCTZ) 50mg-25mg*, 100mg-25mg*, 100mg-50mg*; (Lopressor HCT) 50mg-25mg*, 100mg-25mg* *scored

CONTRAINDICATIONS: Sinus bradycardia, >1st-degree heart block, cardiogenic shock, overt cardiac failure, sick sinus syndrome, severe peripheral arterial circulatory disorders, anuria, hypersensitivity to sulfonamide-derived drugs.

WARNINGS/PRECAUTIONS: Not for initial therapy. Caution with hepatic dysfunction and in elderly. Metoprolol: May cause/precipitate heart failure; d/c if cardiac failure continues despite adequate treatment. Avoid with bronchospastic diseases, but may use with caution if unresponsive to/intolerant of other antihypertensives. Avoid withdrawal of chronically administered therapy prior to major surgery; however, may augment risks of general anesthesia and surgical procedures. Caution with diabetic patients; may mask tachycardia occurring with hypoglycemia. Paradoxical BP increase reported with pheochromocytoma; give in combination with and only after initiating α-blocker therapy. May mask hyperthyroidism. Avoid abrupt withdrawal in suspected thyrotoxicosis; may precipitate thyroid storm. HCTZ: Caution with severe renal disease; may precipitate azotemia. If progressive renal impairment becomes evident, d/c therapy. May precipitate hepatic coma in patients with liver dysfunction/disease. Sensitivity reactions are more likely to occur with history of allergy or bronchial asthma. May exacerbate/activate systemic lupus erythematosus (SLE). May cause idiosyncratic reaction, resulting in acute transient myopia and acute angle-closure glaucoma; d/c HCTZ as rapidly as possible. Fluid/electrolyte imbalance (eg, hyponatremia, hypochloremic alkalosis, hypokalemia) may develop. May cause hyperuricemia and precipitation of frank gout. Latent diabetes mellitus (DM) may manifest during therapy. Enhanced effects seen in postsympathectomy patients. D/C prior to parathyroid function test. Decreased calcium excretion observed. Altered parathyroid gland, with hypercalcemia and hypophosphatemia, observed with prolonged therapy. May increase urinary excretion of magnesium, resulting in hypomagnesemia.

ADVERSE REACTIONS: Fatigue, lethargy, dizziness, vertigo, flu syndrome, drowsiness, somnolence, hypokalemia, headache, bradycardia.

INTERACTIONS: Metoprolol: May exhibit additive effect with catecholamine-depleting drugs (eg, reserpine). Digitalis glycosides may increase risk of bradycardia. Some inhalation anesthetics may enhance cardiodepressant effect. May be unresponsive to usual doses of epinephrine. Potent CYP2D6 inhibitors (eg, certain antidepressants, antipsychotics, antiarrhythmics, antiretrovirals, antihistamines, antimalarials, antifungals, stomach ulcer drugs) may increase levels. Increased risk for rebound HTN following clonidine withdrawal; d/c metoprolol several days before withdrawing clonidine. Effects can be reversed by β-agonists (eg, dobutamine or isoproterenol). HCTZ: Hypokalemia can sensitize/exaggerate cardiac response to toxic effects of digitalis. Risk of hypokalemia with steroids or adrenocorticotropic hormone. Insulin requirements may change in diabetic patients. May decrease arterial responsiveness to norepinephrine. May increase responsiveness to tubocurarine. May increase risk of lithium toxicity. Rare reports of hemolytic anemia with methyldopa. NSAIDs may reduce diuretic, natriuretic, and antihypertensive effects. Impaired absorption reported with cholestyramine and colestipol. Alcohol, barbiturates, and narcotics may potentiate orthostatic hypotension. May potentiate other antihypertensive drugs (eg, ganglionic or peripheral adrenergic blocking drugs).

PREGNANCY: Category C, not for use in nursing.

MECHANISM OF ACTION: Metoprolol: β$_1$-adrenergic receptor blocker; not established. Proposed to competitively antagonize catecholamines at peripheral adrenergic-neuron sites, have central effect leading to reduced sympathetic outflow to periphery, and suppress renin activity. HCTZ: Thiazide diuretic; not established. Affects renal tubular mechanism of electrolyte reabsorption and increases excretion of Na$^+$ and Cl$^-$.

PHARMACOKINETICS: Absorption: Metoprolol: Rapid and complete. HCTZ: Rapid; T$_{max}$=1-2.5 hrs. **Distribution:** Found in breast milk. Metoprolol: Plasma protein binding (12%); found in CSF. HCTZ: V$_d$=3.6-7.8L/kg; plasma protein binding (67.9%); crosses the placenta. **Metabolism:** Metoprolol: Liver (extensive) via CYP2D6 (oxidation). **Elimination:** Metoprolol: Urine (<5%, unchanged); T$_{1/2}$=2.8 hrs (extensive metabolizers), 7.5 hrs (poor metabolizers). HCTZ: Urine (72-97%); T$_{1/2}$=10-17 hrs.

NURSING CONSIDERATIONS

Assessment: Assess for history of heart failure, sulfonamide hypersensitivity, SLE, hyperthyroidism, DM, pheochromocytoma, hepatic/renal impairment, any other conditions where treatment is contraindicated/cautioned, pregnancy/nursing status, and possible drug interactions. Obtain baseline serum electrolytes.

M

Monitoring: Monitor for signs/symptoms of cardiac failure, hypoglycemia, thyrotoxicosis, electrolyte imbalance, exacerbation/activation of SLE, hyperuricemia or precipitation of gout, hypersensitivity reactions, hepatic/renal dysfunction, myopia, angle-closure glaucoma, and other adverse reactions. Monitor serum electrolytes.

Patient Counseling: Instruct to take regularly and continuously ud with or immediately following meals. If dose is missed, advise to take next dose at scheduled time (without doubling the dose) and not to d/c without consulting physician. Instruct to avoid driving, operating machinery, or engaging in tasks requiring alertness until response to therapy is determined. Advise to contact physician if difficulty in breathing or other adverse reactions occur, and to inform physician/dentist of drug therapy before undergoing any type of surgery.

Administration: Oral route. **Storage:** (Lopressor HCT) 25°C (77°F); excursions permitted to 15-30°C (59-86°F). (Metoprolol-HCTZ) 20-25°C (68-77°F). Protect from moisture.

METROGEL RX
metronidazole (Galderma)

OTHER BRAND NAMES: MetroLotion (Galderma)

THERAPEUTIC CLASS: Imidazole antibiotic

INDICATIONS: (1% Gel) Treatment of inflammatory lesions of rosacea. (0.75% Gel, Lot) Treatment of inflammatory papules and pustules of rosacea.

DOSAGE: *Adults:* Wash affected area before application. (Gel) Apply and rub in a thin film to the entire affected area(s) bid, am and pm (0.75%) or qd (1%). (Lot) Apply a thin layer to the entire affected area(s) bid, am and pm or ud.

HOW SUPPLIED: Gel: (Generic) 0.75% [45g], 1% [60g]; Lot: 0.75% [59mL]

WARNINGS/PRECAUTIONS: Not for PO, ophthalmic, or intravaginal use. Avoid eye contact; tearing of the eyes reported. Caution with evidence or history of blood dyscrasia. (0.75% Gel, Lot) Decrease frequency of use or d/c if local irritation occurs. (1% Gel) Peripheral neuropathy reported; reevaluate therapy immediately if abnormal neurologic signs appear. Caution with CNS diseases. Irritant and allergic contact dermatitis reported; consider d/c if occurs.

ADVERSE REACTIONS: Burning/stinging, skin irritation, dryness, transient redness, metallic taste, tingling or numbness of extremities, nausea.

INTERACTIONS: PO metronidazole may potentiate the anticoagulant effect of warfarin and coumarin anticoagulants resulting in prolongation of PT.

PREGNANCY: Category B, not for use in nursing.

MECHANISM OF ACTION: Imidazole antibiotic; action in the treatment of rosacea unknown, but appear to include an anti-inflammatory effect.

PHARMACOKINETICS: Absorption: (1% Gel) C_{max}=32ng/mL; T_{max}=6-10 hrs; AUC_{0-24}=595ng•hr/mL. (0.75% Lot) C_{max}=96ng/mL; AUC_{0-24}=962ng•hr/mL. **Distribution:** Crosses placenta. (PO) Found in breast milk.

NURSING CONSIDERATIONS

Assessment: Assess for drug hypersensitivity, evidence/history of blood dyscrasia, CNS diseases, pregnancy/nursing status, and for possible drug interactions.

Monitoring: Monitor for peripheral neuropathy, irritant/allergic contact dermatitis or local irritation, and for other adverse reactions.

Patient Counseling: Advise to use medication exactly as directed. Instruct to avoid contact with eyes and cleanse affected area(s) before applying. Counsel to notify physician if any adverse reactions develop. Inform that may use cosmetics following application.

Administration: Topical route. **Storage:** 20-25°C (68-77°F). (1% Gel) Excursions permitted between 15-30°C (59-86°F). (Lot) Protect from freezing.

METROGEL-VAGINAL RX
metronidazole (Medicis)

THERAPEUTIC CLASS: Nitroimidazole

INDICATIONS: Treatment of bacterial vaginosis.

DOSAGE: *Adults:* Usual: 1 applicatorful intravaginally qd or bid for 5 days. For qd dosing, administer at hs.

HOW SUPPLIED: Gel: 0.75% [70g]

WARNINGS/PRECAUTIONS: Not for ophthalmic, dermal, or PO use. Convulsive seizures and peripheral neuropathy reported; d/c promptly if abnormal neurologic signs appear. Caution with

CNS diseases and severe hepatic disease. Known or previously unrecognized vaginal candidiasis may present more prominent symptoms during therapy. May develop symptomatic *Candida* vaginitis during or immediately after therapy. Contains ingredients that may cause burning and irritation of the eye; rinse with copious amounts of cool tap water in the event of accidental contact. May interfere with certain types of determinations of serum chemistry values (eg, AST, ALT, LDH, TG, and glucose hexokinase).

ADVERSE REACTIONS: Symptomatic *Candida* cervicitis/vaginitis, vaginal discharge, pelvic discomfort, N/V, headache, vulva/vaginal irritation, GI discomfort.

INTERACTIONS: May potentiate anticoagulant effect of warfarin and other coumarin anticoagulants resulting in prolongation of PT. Elevation of serum lithium levels and signs of lithium toxicity may occur in short-term therapy with high doses of lithium. Cimetidine may prolong $T_{1/2}$ and decrease plasma clearance. May cause disulfiram-like reaction with alcohol. May cause psychotic reactions in alcoholic patients using disulfiram concurrently; do not administer within 2 weeks of d/c of disulfiram.

PREGNANCY: Category B, not for use in nursing.

MECHANISM OF ACTION: Nitroimidazole; intracellular targets of action on anaerobes unknown. Reduced by metabolically active anaerobes and the reduced form of the drug interacts with bacterial DNA.

PHARMACOKINETICS: Absorption: C_{max}=214ng/mL (Day 1), 294ng/mL (Day 5); T_{max}=6-12 hrs; AUC=4977ng•hr/mL. **Distribution:** Found in breast milk (PO); crosses the placenta.

NURSING CONSIDERATIONS

Assessment: Assess for hypersensitivity to drug, CNS/severe hepatic diseases, vaginal candidiasis, alcohol intake, nursing status, and possible drug interactions. Assess for clinical diagnosis of bacterial vaginosis.

Monitoring: Monitor for convulsive seizures, peripheral neuropathy, *Candida* vaginitis, and other adverse reactions.

Patient Counseling: Caution about drinking alcohol while on therapy. Instruct not to engage in vaginal intercourse during treatment. Inform to avoid contact with eyes and instruct to rinse with copious amounts of cool tap water in the event of accidental contact.

Administration: Intravaginal route. Refer to PI for administration instructions. **Storage:** 15-30°C (59-86°F). Protect from freezing.

M

MIACALCIN
RX
calcitonin-salmon (Novartis)

THERAPEUTIC CLASS: Hormonal bone resorption inhibitor

INDICATIONS: Treatment of postmenopausal osteoporosis in females >5 yrs postmenopause. (Inj) Treatment of Paget's disease of bone and hypercalcemia.

DOSAGE: *Adults:* (Inj) Paget's Disease: Initial: 100 IU IM/SQ qd. 50 IU IM/SQ qd or qod may be sufficient in some patients; maintain higher dose with serious deformity and neurological involvement. Hypercalcemia: Initial: 4 IU/kg IM/SQ q12h. Titrate: May increase to 8 IU/kg q12h after 1-2 days, then to 8 IU/kg q6h after 2 days if response is unsatisfactory. Max: 8 IU/kg q6h. Postmenopausal Osteoporosis: (Inj) Usual: 100 IU IM/SQ qod. If >2mL, use multiple injection sites and IM route. Take with supplemental calcium (1.5g calcium carbonate qd) and vitamin D (400 IU qd). (Spray) Usual: 1 spray (200 IU) qd, alternating nostrils daily.

HOW SUPPLIED: Inj: 200 IU/mL; Spray: 200 IU/actuation

WARNINGS/PRECAUTIONS: Serious allergic-type reactions (eg, bronchospasm, swelling of tongue or throat, anaphylactic shock) reported. Skin testing should be considered prior to treatment with suspected sensitivity to calcitonin. Urinary casts reported; monitor urine sediment periodically. (Spray) Perform periodic nasal exams. D/C if severe ulceration (ulcers >1.5mm diameter, penetrating below mucosa or if with heavy bleeding) of the nasal mucosa occurs. (Inj) May lead to possible hypocalcemic tetany; provisions for parenteral calcium administration should be available during the first several administrations of calcitonin.

ADVERSE REACTIONS: (Inj) N/V, injection-site inflammatory reactions, flushing of face or hands. (Spray) Nasal symptoms, rhinitis, back pain, headache, arthralgia, epistaxis, abdominal pain, angina pectoris, arthrosis, conjunctivitis, constipation.

INTERACTIONS: Concomitant use with lithium may lead to reduced plasma lithium; lithium dose may need to be adjusted. (Spray) Prior use of diphosphonate reduced the anti-resorptive response with Paget's disease.

PREGNANCY: Category C, not for use in nursing.

MECHANISM OF ACTION: Hormonal bone resorption inhibitor; actions on bone has not been fully established. Calcitonin receptors have been found in osteoclasts and osteoblasts. Initially causes a marked transient inhibition of the ongoing bone resorptive process. Prolonged use causes a smaller decrease in the rate of bone resorption which is associated with a decreased number of osteoclasts as well as decrease in their resorptive activity.

PHARMACOKINETICS: Absorption: (Spray) T_{max}=13 min. (Inj): Absolute bioavailability (66% IM), (71% SQ); T_{max}=23 min (SQ). **Distribution:** V_d=0.15-0.3L/kg. **Metabolism:** Kidney, blood, peripheral tissues. **Elimination:** (Spray) $T_{1/2}$=18 min. (Inj) Urine; $T_{1/2}$=58 min (IM), $T_{1/2}$=59-64 min (SQ).

NURSING CONSIDERATIONS

Assessment: Assess for hypersensitivity to medication, and consider skin testing for patients with suspected sensitivity to calcitonin. Assess for pregnancy/nursing status and possible drug interactions. (Spray) Obtain baseline nasal exam (eg, visualization of the nasal mucosa, turbinates, septum, and mucosal blood vessel status). (Inj) For treatment of osteoporosis, obtain baseline measurement of biochemical markers of bone resorption/turnover and bone mineral density.

Monitoring: Monitor for signs/symptoms of serious allergic reactions (eg, bronchospasm, swelling of tongue or throat, anaphylactic shock). Perform periodic exams of urine sediment. (Spray) Monitor for nasal mucosal alterations, transient nasal conditions, and ulceration of nasal mucosa; perform periodic nasal exams. Perform periodic measurements of lumbar vertebral bone mass. (Inj) Monitor for hypocalcemic tetany. For treatment of Paget's disease, perform periodic measurement of serum alkaline phosphatase and 24-hr urinary hydroxyproline. For treatment of osteoporosis, monitor biochemical markers of bone resorption/turnover and bone mineral density.

Patient Counseling: (Spray) Instruct how to assemble and prime pump, and introduce medication in the nasal passages. Advise to contact physician if allergic reaction or nasal irritation occurs. Inform that new, unassembled bottles should be refrigerated and protected from freezing. Instruct to allow medication to reach room temperature before priming pump and using a new bottle. Instuct to store opened bottle upright at room temperature for ≤35 days. Inform that after 30 doses, each spray may not deliver correct amount of medication; keep track of number of doses used. (Inj) Instruct about sterile injection technique.

Administration: Intranasal/IM/SQ routes. **Storage:** (Spray) Unopened: 2-8°C (36-46°F). Protect from freezing. Used: 15-30°C (59-86°F) in upright position for ≤35 days. (Inj) 2-8°C (36-46°F).

MICARDIS

telmisartan (Boehringer Ingelheim)

RX

D/C when pregnancy is detected. Drugs that act directly on the renin-angiotensin system can cause injury/death to the developing fetus.

THERAPEUTIC CLASS: Angiotensin II receptor antagonist

INDICATIONS: Treatment of HTN alone or in combination with other antihypertensives. Reduction of risk of myocardial infarction, stroke, or death from cardiovascular causes in patients ≥55 yrs at high risk of developing major cardiovascular events who are unable to take ACE inhibitors.

DOSAGE: *Adults:* HTN: Individualize dose. Initial: 40mg qd. Usual: 20-80mg/day. If additional BP reduction is required beyond that achieved with the 80mg dose, a diuretic may be added. Cardiovascular Risk Reduction: Usual: 80mg qd. Monitor BP and adjust dose of medications that lower BP if needed. Biliary Obstructive Disorders/Hepatic Insufficiency: Start at low doses and titrate slowly.

HOW SUPPLIED: Tab: 20mg, 40mg, 80mg

WARNINGS/PRECAUTIONS: May develop orthostatic hypotension in patients on dialysis. Symptomatic hypotension may occur in patients with an activated renin-angiotensin system (eg, volume- and/or salt-depleted patients receiving high doses of diuretics); correct this condition before therapy or monitor closely. Hyperkalemia may occur, particularly in patients with advanced renal impairment, heart failure (HF), and on renal replacement therapy; monitor serum electrolytes periodically. Caution in patient with hepatic impairment (eg, biliary obstructive disorders); reduced clearance may be expected. Oliguria and/or progressive azotemia and (rarely) acute renal failure and/or death may occur in patients whose renal function is dependent on the renin-angiotensin-aldosterone system (eg, severe congestive heart failure [CHF]). Changes in renal function may occur in susceptible patients and with the dual blockade of the renin-angiotensin-aldosterone system (eg, adding an ACE inhibitor); monitor renal function. May increase SrCr/BUN in patients with renal artery stenosis.

ADVERSE REACTIONS: Upper respiratory tract infection, back pain, sinusitis, diarrhea, intermittent claudication, skin ulcer.

INTERACTIONS: Avoid with ACE inhibitor. Increased exposure to ramipril and ramiprilat; concomitant use is not recommended. Hyperkalemia may occur with K^+ supplements, K^+-sparing diuretics, K^+-containing salt substitutes or other drugs that increase K^+ levels. May increase digoxin levels; monitor digoxin levels upon initiating, adjusting, and d/c therapy. May increase serum lithium levels/toxicity; monitor lithium levels during concomitant use. NSAIDs, including selective cyclooxygenase-2 inhibitors, may deteriorate renal function; monitor renal function periodically. Antihypertensive effect may be attenuated by NSAIDs.

PREGNANCY: Category D, not for use in nursing.

MECHANISM OF ACTION: Angiotensin II receptor antagonist; blocks the vasoconstrictor and aldosterone-secreting effects of angiotensin II by selectively blocking the binding of angiotensin II to the AT_1 receptor in many tissues, such as vascular smooth muscle and adrenal gland.

PHARMACOKINETICS: Absorption: Absolute bioavailability: 40mg (42%), 160mg (58%); T_{max}=0.5-1 hr. **Distribution:** V_d=500L; plasma protein binding (>99.5%). **Metabolism:** Conjugation. **Elimination:** Feces (>97%, unchanged), urine (0.49%); $T_{1/2}$=24 hrs.

NURSING CONSIDERATIONS

Assessment: Assess for known hypersensitivity (eg, anaphylaxis or angioedema), biliary obstructive disorders, HF/CHF, unilateral/bilateral renal artery stenosis, hepatic/renal impairment, volume/salt depletion, dialysis patients, pregnancy/nursing status, and possible drug interactions.

Monitoring: Monitor for symptomatic hypotension and other adverse reactions. Monitor BP, ECG, hepatic/renal function, serum electrolytes.

Patient Counseling: Inform women of childbearing age about the consequences of exposure to the medication during pregnancy. Discuss treatment options with women planning to become pregnant. Instruct to report pregnancies to the physician as soon as possible.

Administration: Oral route. **Storage:** 25°C (77°F); excursions permitted to 15-30°C (59-86°F).

MICARDIS HCT
telmisartan - hydrochlorothiazide (Boehringer Ingelheim)

RX

M

D/C when pregnancy is detected. Drugs that act directly on the renin-angiotensin system can cause injury/death to the developing fetus.

THERAPEUTIC CLASS: Angiotensin II receptor antagonist/thiazide diuretic

INDICATIONS: Treatment of HTN.

DOSAGE: *Adults:* Uncontrolled BP on 80mg Telmisartan/Controlled BP on 25mg/day of HCTZ but with Hypokalemia: Initial: 80mg-12.5mg tab qd. Uncontrolled BP on 25mg/day of HCTZ: Initial: 80mg-12.5mg qd or 80mg-25mg tab qd. Titrate/Max: Increase to 160mg-25mg if BP uncontrolled after 2-4 weeks. Biliary Obstruction/Hepatic Insufficiency: Initial: 40mg-12.5mg tab under qd. Replacement Therapy: May substitute combination for titrated components.

HOW SUPPLIED: Tab: (Telmisartan-HCTZ) 40mg-12.5mg, 80mg-12.5mg, 80mg-25mg

CONTRAINDICATIONS: Anuria, hypersensitivity to sulfonamide-derived drugs.

WARNINGS/PRECAUTIONS: Not for initial therapy. Hypotension may occur in patients with activated renin-angiotensin system such as volume- or Na⁺-depleted (eg, vigorously treated with diuretics); correct these conditions prior to therapy and monitor closely. Not recommended with severe renal impairment (CrCl ≤30mL/min) and severe hepatic impairment. HCTZ: Caution with hepatic impairment or progressive liver disease; may precipitate hepatic coma. May cause hypersensitivity reactions, exacerbation or activation of systemic lupus erythematosus (SLE), hyperuricemia or precipitation of frank gout, hyperglycemia, hypomagnesemia, hypercalcemia, and latent diabetes mellitus (DM). May cause an idiosyncratic reaction, resulting in acute transient myopia and acute angle-closure glaucoma; d/c as rapidly as possible. Observe for clinical signs of fluid or electrolyte imbalance (hyponatremia, hypochloremic alkalosis, and hypokalemia). Hypokalemia may develop, especially with brisk diuresis, severe cirrhosis, or after prolonged therapy. Hypokalemia may cause cardiac arrhythmia and may sensitize/exaggerate the response of the heart to toxic effects of digitalis. D/C before testing for parathyroid function. Enhanced effects in postsympathectomy patients. Increased cholesterol and TG levels reported. Caution with severe renal disease; may precipitate azotemia with renal disease. Telmisartan: Oliguria and/or progressive azotemia and (rarely) acute renal failure and/or death may occur in patients whose renal function is dependent on the renin-angiotensin-aldosterone system (eg, severe congestive heart failure [CHF]). Changes in renal function may occur in susceptible patients and with the dual blockade of the renin-angiotensin-aldosterone system (eg, adding an ACE inhibitor); monitor renal function. May increase SrCr/BUN in patients with renal artery stenosis.

ADVERSE REACTIONS: Upper respiratory tract infection, dizziness, sinusitis, fatigue, diarrhea.

INTERACTIONS: NSAIDs, including selective cyclooxygenase-2 inhibitors, may decrease effects of diuretics and angiotensin II receptor antagonists and may further deteriorate renal function. May increase risk of lithium toxicity; avoid concurrent use. HCTZ: Alcohol, barbiturates, or narcotics may potentiate orthostatic hypotension. Dosage adjustment of antidiabetic drugs (eg, PO agents, insulin) may be required. Additive effect or potentiation with other antihypertensive drugs. Anionic exchange resins (eg, cholestyramine and colestipol resins) may impair absorption. Corticosteroids and adrenocorticotropic hormone may intensify electrolyte depletion, particularly hypokalemia. May decrease response to pressor amines (eg, norepinephrine). May increase responsiveness to nondepolarizing skeletal muscle relaxant (eg, tubocurarine). Telmisartan: May increase digoxin levels; monitor digoxin levels. May increase exposure to ramipril; concomitant use not recommended. May slightly decrease warfarin levels. Possible inhibition of drugs metabolized by CYP2C19.

PREGNANCY: Category D, not for use in nursing.

MECHANISM OF ACTION: Telmisartan: Angiotensin II receptor antagonist; blocks the vasoconstrictor and aldosterone-secreting effects of angiotensin II by selectively blocking the binding of angiotensin II to the AT_1 receptor in many tissues, such as vascular smooth muscle and adrenal gland. HCTZ: Thiazide diuretic; affects renal tubular mechanisms of electrolyte reabsorption, directly increasing excretion of Na^+ salt and chloride in approximately equivalent amounts.

PHARMACOKINETICS: Absorption: Telmisartan: Absolute bioavailability: 40mg (42%), 160mg (58%); T_{max}=0.5-1 hr. **Distribution:** Telmisartan: V_d=500L; plasma protein binding (>99.5%). HCTZ: Crosses placenta; found in breast milk. **Metabolism:** Telmisartan: Conjugation. **Elimination:** Telmisartan: Feces (>97%, unchanged), urine (0.49%); $T_{1/2}$=24 hrs. HCTZ: Urine (61%, unchanged); $T_{1/2}$=5.6-14.8 hrs.

NURSING CONSIDERATIONS

Assessment: Assess for hypersensitivity to drugs and its components, anuria, sulfonamide-derived hypersensitivity, history of penicillin allergy, volume/salt depletion, SLE, DM, CHF, hepatic/renal impairment, biliary obstructive disorder, renal artery stenosis, cirrhosis, postsympathectomy patients, pregnancy/nursing status, and possible drug interactions. Obtain baseline BP.

Monitoring: Monitor for exacerbation/activation of SLE, idiosyncratic reaction, latent DM manifestations, hyperglycemia, hypercalcemia, hyperuricemia or precipitation of gout, hypersensitivity reactions, and other adverse reactions. Monitor BP, serum electrolytes, and renal function periodically.

Patient Counseling: Inform women of childbearing age about the consequences of exposure to the medication during pregnancy. Discuss treatment options with women planning to become pregnant. Instruct to report pregnancies to the physician as soon as possible. Caution that lightheadedness may occur, especially during the 1st days of therapy and should be instructed to report to physician. Instruct to d/c therapy and consult physician if syncope occurs. Caution patients that inadequate fluid intake, excessive perspiration, diarrhea, or vomiting can lead to an excessive fall in BP, with the same consequences of lightheadedness and possible syncope. Advise patient not to use K^+ supplements or salt substitutes that contain K^+ without consulting the prescribing physician.

Administration: Oral route. **Storage:** 25°C (77°F); excursions permitted to 15-30°C (59-86°F).

MICRO-K   RX
potassium chloride (Ther-Rx)

THERAPEUTIC CLASS: K^+ supplement

INDICATIONS: (For those unable to tolerate liquid or effervescent potassium preparations). Treatment and prevention of hypokalemia with or without metabolic alkalosis. Treatment of digitalis intoxication and hypokalemic familial periodic paralysis.

DOSAGE: *Adults:* Prevention: 20mEq/day. Hypokalemia: 40-100mEq/day. Divide dose if >20mEq. Take with meal and full glass of water or liquid. May sprinkle on soft food; swallow without chewing.

HOW SUPPLIED: Cap, Extended-Release: 8mEq, 10mEq

CONTRAINDICATIONS: Hyperkalemia, esophageal ulceration, delay in GI passage (from structural, pathological, pharmacologic causes [eg, anticholinergic agents]), cardiac patients with esophageal compression due to enlarged left atrium.

WARNINGS/PRECAUTIONS: Potentially fatal hyperkalemia may occur. Extreme caution with acidosis, cardiac and renal disease; monitor ECG and electrolytes. Hypokalemia with metabolic acidosis should be treated with an alkalinizing potassium salt (eg, potassium bicarbonate, potassium citrate). May produce ulcerative or stenotic GI lesions.

ADVERSE REACTIONS: Hyperkalemia, GI effects (obstruction, bleeding, ulceration), N/V, abdominal pain, diarrhea.

INTERACTIONS: See Contraindications. Risk of hyperkalemia with ACE inhibitors (eg, captopril, enalapril), K^+-sparing diuretics, and K^+ supplements.

PREGNANCY: Category C, safe for use in nursing.

MECHANISM OF ACTION: K$^+$ supplement; helps in maintenance of intracellular tonicity, transmission of nerve impulses, contraction of cardiac, skeletal, and smooth muscle, and maintenance of normal renal function.

NURSING CONSIDERATIONS

Assessment: Assess for conditions that impair excretion of K$^+$, hyperkalemia, esophageal compression due to enlarged left atrium, conditions causing arrest or delay in passage through GI, renal insufficiency, DM, and possible drug interactions.

Monitoring: Monitor serum K$^+$ levels regularly; renal function, ECG, and acid-base balance. Monitor for GI ulceration/obstruction/perforation, hyperkalemia, renal dysfunction, and hypersensitivity reactions.

Patient Counseling: Instruct to take with meals; swallow with full glass of water or other suitable liquid. Do not crush, chew, or suck. Seek medical attention if symptoms of GI ulceration, obstruction, perforation (vomiting, abdominal pain, distention, GI bleeding), hyperkalemia, or hypersensitivity reactions occur.

Administration: Oral route. **Storage:** 20-25°C (68-77°F).

MICROZIDE   RX
hydrochlorothiazide (Watson)

THERAPEUTIC CLASS: Thiazide diuretic

INDICATIONS: Management of HTN either alone or in combination with other antihypertensives.

DOSAGE: *Adults:* Initial: 12.5mg qd. Max: 50mg/day.

HOW SUPPLIED: Cap: 12.5mg

CONTRAINDICATIONS: Anuria, sulfonamide hypersensitivity.

WARNINGS/PRECAUTIONS: May cause idiosyncratic reaction, resulting in acute transient myopia and acute angle-closure glaucoma; d/c as rapidly as possible. May manifest latent diabetes mellitus (DM). May precipitate azotemia with renal impairment. Hypokalemia reported; monitor serum electrolytes and for sign/symptoms of fluid/electrolyte disturbances. Dilutional hyponatremia may occur in edematous patients in hot weather. Hyperuricemia or acute gout may be precipitated. Caution with hepatic impairment; hepatic coma may occur with severe liver disease. Decreased calcium excretion and changes in parathyroid glands with hypercalcemia and hypophosphatemia reported during prolonged use. D/C prior to parathyroid test.

ADVERSE REACTIONS: Weakness, hypotension, pancreatitis, jaundice, diarrhea, vomiting, hematologic abnormalities, anaphylactic reactions, electrolyte imbalance, muscle spasm, vertigo, renal failure, erythema multiforme, transient blurred vision, impotence.

INTERACTIONS: Potentiation of orthostatic hypotension with alcohol, barbiturates, narcotics. Additive effect or potentiation with antihypertensive drugs. Dose adjustment of antidiabetic drugs (oral agents or insulin) may be required. Reduced absorption with cholestyramine or colestipol. Increased risk of electrolyte depletion (eg, hypokalemia) with corticosteroids and adrenocorticotropic hormone. May decrease response to pressor amines (eg, norepinephrine). May increase responsiveness to nondepolarizing skeletal muscle relaxants (eg, tubocurarine). Increased risk of lithium toxicity; avoid with lithium. NSAIDs may reduce diuretic, natriuretic, and antihypertensive effects. May cause hypokalemia, which can sensitize or exaggerate the response of the heart to the toxic effects of digitalis.

PREGNANCY: Category B, not for use in nursing.

MECHANISM OF ACTION: Thiazide diuretic; blocks reabsorption of Na$^+$ and Cl$^-$ ions, thereby increasing the quantity of Na$^+$ traversing the distal tubule and the volume of water excreted. Also decreases the excretion of calcium and uric acid, may increase the excretion of iodide and may reduce GFR.

PHARMACOKINETICS: Absorption: Well absorbed; C_{max}=70-490ng/mL; T_{max}=1-5 hrs. **Distribution:** Plasma protein binding (40-68%); crosses placenta; found in breast milk. **Elimination:** Urine (55-77%, >95% unchanged); $T_{1/2}$=6-15 hrs.

NURSING CONSIDERATIONS

Assessment: Assess for anuria, known hypersensitivity to sulfonamide-derived drugs, history of penicillin allergy, DM, risk for developing hypokalemia, impaired renal/hepatic function, edema, pregnancy/nursing status, and for possible drug interactions. Obtain baseline serum electrolytes.

Monitoring: Monitor for signs/symptoms of decreased visual acuity, ocular pain, azotemia, hypokalemia, fluid/electrolyte disturbances, dilutional hyponatremia, hyperuricemia or acute gout, and hepatic coma. Periodically monitor serum electrolytes in patients with risk for developing hypokalemia.

M

Patient Counseling: Counsel about signs/symptoms of fluid and electrolyte imbalance and advise to seek prompt medical attention.

Administration: Oral route. **Storage:** 20-25°C (68-77°F). Protect from light, moisture, freezing, -20°C (-4°F). Keep container tightly closed.

MINIPRESS   RX
prazosin HCl (Pfizer)

THERAPEUTIC CLASS: Alpha₁-blocker (quinazoline)

INDICATIONS: Treatment of hypertension either alone or in combination with other antihypertensive drugs.

DOSAGE: *Adults:* Initial: 1mg bid-tid. Titrate: Slowly increase to 20mg/day in divided doses. Maint: 6-15mg qd in divided doses. Max: 40mg/day. Concomitant with Diuretic/Antihypertensive Agent: Reduce to 1-2mg tid, then retitrate.

HOW SUPPLIED: Cap: 1mg, 2mg, 5mg

WARNINGS/PRECAUTIONS: Syncope with sudden loss of consciousness may occur, usually after initial dose or dose increase; Patient should be placed in the recumbent position and treated with supportive care. Due to excessive postural hypotensive effect, caution to avoid situations where injury could result should syncope occur during initiation of therapy. Always start on 1mg cap. Possible adverse effects (eg, dizziness, lightheadedness) may occur. Intraoperative floppy iris syndrome (IFIS) may occur during cataract surgery. False (+) for pheochromocytoma may occur. D/C with elevated urinary VMA levels and retest after 1 month.

ADVERSE REACTIONS: Dizziness, headache, drowsiness, lack of energy, weakness, palpitations, N/V, edema, orthostatic hypotension, dyspnea, syncope, depression, urinary frequency, diarrhea, and blurred vision.

INTERACTIONS: Additive hypotensive effects with diuretics, PDE5 inhibitors, β-blockers, or other antihypertensives. Dizziness or syncope may occur with alcohol.

PREGNANCY: Category C, caution in nursing.

MECHANISM OF ACTION: α₁ blocker, quinazoline derivative; not established. Blocks the postsynaptic α-adrenoreceptors resulting in vasodilation and reduction in total peripheral resistance.

PHARMACOKINETICS: Absorption: T_{max}=3 hrs. **Distribution:** Plasma protein binding (highly bound). Found in breast milk. **Metabolism:** Demethylation and conjugation. **Elimination:** Bile and feces; $T_{1/2}$=2-3 hrs.

NURSING CONSIDERATIONS

Assessment: Assess BP, LFTs, urinary VMA levels, hypersensitivity, pregnancy/nursing status, and for possible drug interactions.

Monitoring: Monitor BP, LFTs, HR, urinary VMA levels. Monitor for orthostatic hypotension, edema, epistaxis, lichen planus, angina pectoris and hypersensitivity reactions.

Patient Counseling: Inform that dizziness or drowsiness may occur after first dose; avoid driving or performing hazardous tasks for first 24 hrs. Dizziness, lightheadedness or fainting may occur; get up slowly when rising from a lying or sitting position. Instruct to be careful in the amount of alcohol taken. Counsel to use extra care during exercise or hot weather, or if standing for long periods.

Administration: Oral route. **Storage:** Below 30°C (86°F).

MINOCIN   RX
minocycline HCl (Triax)

THERAPEUTIC CLASS: Tetracycline derivative

INDICATIONS: Treatment of the following infections caused by susceptible microorganisms: Rocky Mountain spotted fever; typhus fever and the typhus group; Q fever; rickettsialpox; tick fevers; respiratory tract infections; lymphogranuloma venereum; psittacosis (ornithosis); trachoma; inclusion conjunctivitis; nongonococcal urethritis, endocervical, or rectal infections in adults; relapsing fever; chancroid (PO only); plague; tularemia; cholera; *Campylobacter fetus* infections; brucellosis; bartonellosis; granuloma inguinale. Treatment of infections caused by *Escherichia coli, Enterobacter aerogenes, Shigella* species, *Acinetobacter* spp. Respiratory tract infections caused by *Haemophilus influenzae,* respiratory tract and urinary tract infections caused by *Klebsiella* spp. Treatment of upper respiratory tract infections caused by *Streptococcus pneumoniae,* skin and skin structure infections caused by *Staphylococcus aureus.* When penicillin is contraindicated, treatment of the following infections caused by susceptible microorganisms: uncomplicated urethritis is men due to *Neisseria gonorrhoeae* and for the treatment of other gonococcal infections (PO only), infections in women caused by *N. gonorrhoeae* (PO only), meningitis (IV only), syphilis, yaws, listeriosis, anthrax, Vincent's infection, actinomycosis, infections caused by *Clostridium* species. Adjunct in acute intestinal amebiasis. (PO) May be used to treat asymptomatic carriers of *N. meningitidis* to eliminate meningococci from the nasopharynx. Limited clinical data show that it has been used successfully in the treatment of infections caused by *Mycobacterium marinum*.

DOSAGE: *Adults:* Usual: 200mg initially, then 100mg q12 hrs. Max: (IV) 400mg/24 hrs. (Cap) Alternative: 100-200mg initially, then 50mg qid. Uncomplicated Gonococcal Infections (Men, Other Than Urethritis and Anorectal Infections)/(Sus) Gonorrhea in Patients Sensitive to Penicillin: 200mg initially, then 100mg q12 hrs for minimum 4 days, with post-therapy cultures within 2-3 days. (Cap/Sus) Uncomplicated Gonococcal Urethritis (Men): 100mg q12 hrs for 5 days. Syphilis: Administer usual dose for 10-15 days. Meningococcal Carrier State: 100mg q12 hrs for 5 days. *Mycobacterium marinum:* 100mg q12 hrs for 6-8 weeks. Uncomplicated Urethral, Endocervical, or Rectal Infection Caused by *Chlamydia trachomatis* or *Ureaplasma urealyticum:* 100mg q12 hrs for at least 7 days. Renal Dysfunction: Max: 200mg/24 hrs. (Cap) Take with plenty of fluids.
Pediatrics: >8 yrs: 4mg/kg initially followed by 2mg/kg q12 hrs, not to exceed adult dose. Renal Impairment (CrCl < 80mL/min): Max: 200mg/24 hrs. (PO) Take with plenty of fluids.

HOW SUPPLIED: Cap: 50mg, 100mg; Inj: 100mg; Sus: 50mg/5mL [60mL]

WARNINGS/PRECAUTIONS: May cause fetal harm during pregnancy. Do not use during tooth development (last half of pregnancy, infancy, ≤8 yrs); may cause permanent discoloration of the teeth or enamel hypoplasia. Decrease in fibula growth rate has been observed when given to premature infants given PO tetracycline (25mg/kg q6h); reversible upon d/c. Drug rash with eosinophilia and systemic symptoms (DRESS) including fatal cases reported; d/c if this syndrome is recognized. Caution in renal impairment; may increase BUN and lead to azotemia, hyperphosphatemia, acidosis. Photosensitivity reported. May impair mental/physical abilities. CNS effects (light-headedness, dizziness or vertigo) reported; symptoms may disappear during therapy and upon d/c. *Clostridium difficile*-associated diarrhea (CDAD) reported; ranges from mild diarrhea to fatal colitis. Consider CDAD in all patients who present diarrhea after use (over 2 months after administration). If CDAD develops, d/c antibiotic not directed against *C. difficile* and initiate appropriate therapy. May cause superinfection; d/c and institute appropriate therapy. Pseudotumor cerebri (benign intracranial HTN) in adults associated with use. Clinical manifestations are headache and blurred vision. May cause bulging fontanels in infants. Hepatotoxicity reported; caution in hepatic dysfunction. Caution in elderly. False elevations of urinary catecholamine levels due to intolerance with fluorescence test may occur. (Sus) Safety during pregnancy not established. Contains Na+ sulfite, may cause allergic-type reactions (eg, anaphylactic symptoms and life-threatening or less severe asthmatic episodes) in certain susceptible people.

ADVERSE REACTIONS: Neutropenia, agranulocytosis, hypersensitivity syndrome, lupus-like syndrome, serum sickness-like syndrome, fever, N/V, diarrhea, increased LFTs, renal toxicity, rash, exfoliative dermatitis, Stevens-Johnson syndrome, skin and mucous membrane pigmentation, headache, tooth discoloration.

INTERACTIONS: May require downward adjustments of anticoagulant dosage. May interfere with bactericidal action of penicillin; avoid concurrent use when possible. May decrease efficacy of oral contraceptives. Fatal renal toxicity with methoxyflurane reported. Avoid isotretinoin shortly before, during and after therapy; each drug alone is associated with pseudotumor cerebri. Caution with other hepatotoxic drugs. Increased risk of ergotism with ergot alkaloids. (PO) Impaired absorption with antacids containing aluminum or calcium or magnesium and iron-containing products.

PREGNANCY: Category D, not for use in nursing.

MECHANISM OF ACTION: Tetracycline; bacteriostatic, thought to inhibit protein synthesis.

PHARMACOKINETICS: Absorption: (Cap) C_{max}=3.5µg/mL; T_{max}=2.1 hrs (fasted). **Distribution:** Crosses placenta (IV). **Elimination:** (Cap/Sus) Urine, feces; $T_{1/2}$=15.5 hrs (Cap), 11-17 hrs (Sus), 15-23 hrs (IV), 11-16 hrs (hepatic dysfunction), 18-69 hrs (renal dysfunction).

NURSING CONSIDERATIONS

Assessment: Assess for age, bacterial infection, hepatic/renal impairment, gonorrhea, syphilis, hypersensitivity, pregnancy/nursing status, possible drug interactions. (Sus) Assess for sulfite sensitivity.

Monitoring: Monitor growth rate, syphilis, organ systems, including hematopoietic, renal (BUN and creatinine) and hepatic, periodically. Monitor for signs/symptoms of thyroid cancer, DRESS, hepatotoxicity, hypersensitivity syndrome, lupus-like syndrome, serum sickness-like syndrome, photosensitivity, CNS effects, superinfection, CDAD, and pseudotumor cerebri. (Cap) When coexistent syphilis is suspected, monitor blood serology monthly for at least 4 months. (Sus, IV) Serologic test for syphilis after 3 months.

Patient Counseling: Inform that therapy treats bacterial, not viral (eg, common cold), infections. Take as directed; skipping doses or not completing full course may decrease effectiveness and

M

increase bacterial resistance. May experience diarrhea. If watery/bloody stools, with or without cramps and fever occur, notify physician as soon as possible. Inform pregnant patients about the potential hazard to the fetus. (PO) Swallow whole and take with full glass of liquid. Advise that photosensitivity manifested by an exaggerated sunburn reaction can occur; d/c treatment at the 1st evidence of skin erythema. Caution in patients who experience CNS symptoms about driving vehicles or using hazardous machinery. May decrease efficacy of oral contraceptives. Discard by expiration date.

Administration: Oral and IV route. (IV) Avoid rapid administration. Refer to PI for further information. **Storage:** 20-25°C (68-77°F). (Cap) Protect from light, moisture, and excessive heat. (Sus) Do not freeze.

MiraLax OTC
polyethylene glycol 3350 (Schering-Plough)

THERAPEUTIC CLASS: Osmotic laxative

INDICATIONS: Relief of occasional constipation.

DOSAGE: *Adults:* Stir and dissolve 17g in 4-8 oz. of beverage (cold/hot/room temperature) and drink qd. Use for ≤7 days.
Pediatrics: ≥17 yrs: Stir and dissolve 17g in 4-8 oz. of beverage (cold/hot/room temperature) and drink qd. Use for ≤7 days.

HOW SUPPLIED: Powder: 17g/dose

WARNINGS/PRECAUTIONS: Avoid in patients with allergy to the drug and in kidney disease unless directed by physician. D/C if rectal bleeding or diarrhea develop, or if nausea, bloating, cramping, or abdominal pain gets worse.

ADVERSE REACTIONS: Loose, watery, more frequent stools.

PREGNANCY: Safety not known in pregnancy and nursing.

MECHANISM OF ACTION: Osmotic laxative.

NURSING CONSIDERATIONS

Assessment: Assess for allergy to the drug, kidney disease, N/V or abdominal pain, sudden change in bowel habits that lasts >2 weeks, irritable bowel syndrome, pregnancy/nursing status, and if taking prescription drugs.

Monitoring: Monitor for rectal bleeding, diarrhea, or worsening of nausea, bloating, cramping, abdominal pain.

Patient Counseling: Inform patient not to take more than directed. Keep out of reach of children; instruct to contact Poison Control Center right away in case of overdose. Instruct to inform physician if laxative needs to be used for > 1 week.

Administration: Oral route. **Storage:** 20-25°C (68-77°F)

Mirapex RX
pramipexole dihydrochloride (Boehringer Ingelheim)

THERAPEUTIC CLASS: Non-ergot dopamine agonist

INDICATIONS: Treatment of signs/symptoms of idiopathic Parkinson's disease. Treatment of moderate to severe primary restless legs syndrome (RLS).

DOSAGE: *Adults:* Parkinson's: Initial: 0.125mg tid. Titrate: May increase every 5-7 days (eg, Week 2: 0.25mg tid; Week 3: 0.5mg tid; Week 4: 0.75mg tid; Week 5: 1mg tid; Week 6: 1.25mg tid; Week 7: 1.5mg tid). Maint: 0.5-1.5mg tid. Max: 1.5mg tid. Renal Impairment: Mild: CrCl >60mL/min: Initial: 0.125mg tid. Max: 1.5mg tid. Moderate: CrCl 35-59mL/min: Initial: 0.125mg bid. Max: 1.5mg bid. Severe: CrCl 15-34mL/min: Initial: 0.125mg qd. Max: 1.5mg qd. Recommend to d/c over a period of 1 week. RLS: Initial: 0.125mg qd, 2-3 hrs before hs. Titrate: May double dose every 4-7 days up to 0.5mg/day. Moderate/Severe Renal Impairment (CrCl 20-60mL/min): Increase duration between titration steps to 14 days.

HOW SUPPLIED: Tab: 0.125mg, 0.25mg*, 0.5mg*, 0.75mg, 1mg*, 1.5mg* *scored

WARNINGS/PRECAUTIONS: Somnolence, symptomatic hypotension, hallucinations and rhabdomyolysis reported. May impair mental/physical abilities. Caution with renal insufficiency. May potentiate dyskinesia. May cause retinal pathology, fibrotic complications, withdrawal-emergent hyperpyrexia, and confusion. Consider d/c if significant daytime sleepiness or sudden onset of sleep occurs during daily activities. Rebound and augmentation in RLS reported. Patient's with Parkinson's disease have higher risk of developing melanoma; monitor regularly.

ADVERSE REACTIONS: Nausea, dizziness, somnolence, insomnia, constipation, asthenia, hallucinations, anorexia, peripheral edema, amnesia, confusion, headache, diarrhea, dreaming abnormalities.

INTERACTIONS: May increase risk of drowsiness with concomitant sedating medications and medications that increase pramipexole plasma levels. Decreased oral clearance with drugs secreted by the cationic transport system (eg, cimetidine, ranitidine, diltiazem, triamterene, verapamil, quinidine, and quinine) and amantidine. May increase levels with cimetidine. May increase peak plasma concentration of levodopa. Decreased effects with dopamine antagonists (eg, phenothiazines, butyrophenones, thioxanthenes, metoclopramide).

PREGNANCY: Category C, not for use in nursing.

MECHANISM OF ACTION: Non-ergot dopamine agonist; not established. Suspected to stimulate dopamine receptors in the striatum.

PHARMACOKINETICS: Absorption: Rapid, absolute bioavailability (>90%), T_{max}=2 hrs. **Distribution:** V_d=500L; plasma protein binding (15%). **Elimination:** Urine (90% unchanged); $T_{1/2}$=8 hrs (healthy), 12 hrs (elderly).

NURSING CONSIDERATIONS

Assessment: Assess for symptomatic hypotension, sleep disorders, dyskinesia, retinal exam, cardiovascular disease, orthostatic hypotension, hypersensitivity to drug, pregnancy/nursing status, and possible drug interactions. Obtain baseline BP and renal function test.

Monitoring: Monitor BP, renal function test, signs/symptoms of rhabdomyolysis, orthostatic hypotension, melanomas, fibrotic complications, hallucinations, impulse control behaviors/compulsive behaviors, and hypersensitivity reactions. Continually reassess for drowsiness or sleepiness.

Patient Counseling: Instruct to take with/without food. Caution while operating machinery/driving. Counsel about impulse control disorders/compulsive behaviors and report side effects. Advise to inform physician regarding concomitant medications (eg, other sedating medications, alcohol) being taken. Advise that hallucination may occur, especially in the elderly with Parkinson's disease. Notify physician if intense urge to gamble, increased sexual urges, and other intense urges occur. Inform that postural hypotension may develop with/without symptoms. Notify physician if pregnant or intend to be pregnant during therapy, intend to breastfeed, or are breastfeeding.

Administration: Oral route. **Storage:** 25°C (77°F); excursions permitted to 15-30°C (59-86°F). Protect from light.

M

MIRCETTE RX
desogestrel - ethinyl estradiol (Duramed)

> Cigarette smoking increases risk of serious cardiovascular (CV) side effects. Risk increases with age (>35 yrs) and heavy smoking (≥15 cigarettes/day). Women who use oral contraceptives should be strongly advised not to smoke.

OTHER BRAND NAMES: Kariva (Barr)

THERAPEUTIC CLASS: Estrogen/progestogen combination

INDICATIONS: Prevention of pregnancy.

DOSAGE: *Adults:* 1 tab qd for 28 days, then repeat. Start 1st Sunday after menses begin or 1st day of menses.
Pediatrics: Postpubertal: 1 tab qd for 28 days, then repeat. Start 1st Sunday after menses begin or 1st day of menses.

HOW SUPPLIED: Tab: (Ethinyl Estradiol-Desogestrel) 0.02mg-0.15mg, (Ethinyl Estradiol) 0.01mg

CONTRAINDICATIONS: Thrombophlebitis, thromboembolic disorders, past history of deep vein thrombophlebitis or thromboembolic disorders, cerebral vascular or coronary artery disease, known or suspected carcinoma of the breast, carcinoma of the endometrium or other known or suspected estrogen-dependent neoplasia, undiagnosed abnormal genital bleeding, cholestatic jaundice of pregnancy or jaundice with prior pill use, hepatic adenomas or carcinomas, known or suspected pregnancy.

WARNINGS/PRECAUTIONS: Increased risk of myocardial infarction (MI), vascular disease, thromboembolism, stroke, hepatic neoplasia, and gallbladder disease. Increased risk of morbidity and mortality with HTN, hyperlipidemia, obesity, and diabetes mellitus (DM). D/C at least 4 wks prior to and 2 wks post-elective surgery with increased risk of thromboembolism and during or following prolonged immobilization. Caution in women with CV disease risk factors. May develop visual changes with contact lens. Retinal thrombosis reported; d/c if unexplained partial or complete loss of vision or other ophthalmic irregularities. May cause glucose intolerance, elevated LDL, other lipid abnormalities, or exacerbate migraine headaches. May cause increased BP and fluid retention; d/c if significant BP elevations occur. Breakthrough bleeding and spotting reported; rule out malignancies or pregnancy. Not indicated for use before menarche. May affect certain endocrine, LFTs, and blood components in laboratory tests. Perform annual history/ physical exam; monitor women with history of breast cancer.

ADVERSE REACTIONS: N/V, breakthrough bleeding, spotting, amenorrhea, migraine, mental depression, vaginal candidiasis, edema, weight changes, cholestatic jaundice, menstrual flow changes, pulmonary embolism, MI, HTN.

INTERACTIONS: Reduced effects resulting in increased breakthrough bleeding and menstrual irregularities seen with rifampin, barbiturates, phenylbutazone, phenytoin sodium, carbamazepine, and possibly with griseofulvin, ampicillin, and tetracyclines. May decrease lamotrigine levels; dosage adjustment of lamotrigine may be necessary.

PREGNANCY: Category X, not for use in nursing.

MECHANISM OF ACTION: Estrogen/progestogen combination; acts by suppression of gonadotropins and inhibition of ovulation. Also causes changes in cervical mucus (increasing difficulty of sperm entry into uterus) and changes in endometrium (reducing likelihood of implantation).

PHARMACOKINETICS: Absorption: Desogestrel: Rapid, complete; relative bioavailability (100%). Ethinyl estradiol: Rapid, almost complete; relative bioavailability (93-99%). **Distribution:** Desogestrel: Sex hormone-binding globulin (99%, metabolite). Ethinyl estradiol: Plasma albumin binding (98.3%); found in breast milk. **Metabolism:** Desogestrel: Liver and intestinal mucosa via hydroxylation, glucuronidation and sulfate conjugation; etonogestrel (metabolite). Ethinyl estradiol: Conjugation. **Elimination:** Urine, bile, feces. Desogestrel: $T_{1/2}$=27.8 hrs (metabolite). Ethinyl estradiol: $T_{1/2}$=23.9 hrs.

NURSING CONSIDERATIONS

Assessment: Assess for current or history of thrombophlebitis or thromboembolic disorders, history of HTN, hyperlipidemia, DM, obesity, breast cancer, and any other conditions where treatment is contraindicated or cautioned. Assess use in women >35 yrs, smokers (≥15 cigarettes/day). Assess pregnancy/nursing status and for possible drug interactions.

Monitoring: Monitor bleeding irregularities, thromboembolic events, other vascular problems, malignant neoplasms, ocular lesions, onset or exacerbation of headaches or migraines, MI, stroke, hepatic neoplasia, and ectopic pregnancy. Monitor fasting blood glucose levels in DM and prediabetic patients, BP with history of HTN, lipid levels with a history of hyperlipidemia, signs of liver dysfunction (eg, jaundice), and signs of worsening depression with previous history. Refer patients with contact lenses to an ophthalmologist if visual changes occur. Monitor LFTs, PT, thyroxine binding globulin, T3 and T4, and serum folate levels.

Patient Counseling: Counsel about potential adverse effects. Inform that drug does not protect against HIV infection and other sexually transmitted diseases. Instruct to avoid smoking. Instruct to take as directed at intervals not exceeding 24 hrs. Instruct that if dose is missed, take as soon as remembered, then take next dose at regularly scheduled time. Counsel that light bleeding is possible. Caution that some drugs decrease efficacy, consult physician before use to determine appropriate back-up contraceptive method and report any side effects experienced.

Administration: Oral route. **Storage:** 20-25°C (68-77°F).

MIRENA   RX
levonorgestrel (Bayer Healthcare)

THERAPEUTIC CLASS: Progestogen

INDICATIONS: Intrauterine contraception up to 5 yrs. Treatment of heavy menstrual bleeding in women who choose to use intrauterine contraception as their method of contraception. Recommended for women who had ≥1 child.

DOSAGE: *Adults:* Initial release rate is 20mcg/day. Rate decreases by 50% after 5 yrs. Replace every 5 yrs. Initial insertion into uterine cavity is recommended within 7 days of menstruation onset or immediately after 1st trimester abortion. May replace at any time during menstrual cycle. May insert 6 weeks postpartum or until uterine involution is complete. If involution is substantially delayed, consider waiting until 12 weeks postpartum.

HOW SUPPLIED: Intrauterine Insert: 52mg

CONTRAINDICATIONS: Pregnancy, congenital or acquired uterine anomaly, acute or history of pelvic inflammatory disease (PID) unless there has been a subsequent intrauterine pregnancy, postpartum endometritis, infected abortion in the past 3 months, uterine or cervical neoplasia or unresolved, abnormal Pap smear, genital bleeding of unknown etiology, untreated acute cervicitis or vaginitis including bacterial vaginosis or other lower genital tract infections until infection is controlled, acute liver disease, liver tumor (benign or malignant), conditions associated with increased susceptibility to pelvic infections, previously inserted intrauterine device (IUD) that is not removed, breast carcinoma.

WARNINGS/PRECAUTIONS: If pregnancy occurs while device is in place, evaluate for ectopic pregnancy and remove device; may increase the risk of septic abortion, congenital anomalies, premature labor/delivery, and miscarriage. Group A streptococcal sepsis (GAS) reported. Does not protect against sexually transmitted disease (STD). Associated with an increased risk of PID and actinomycosis; remove device and initiate antibiotic therapy. Can alter bleeding patterns and result in spotting, irregular bleeding, heavy bleeding, oligomenorrhea, and amenorrhea; if bleeding irregularities develop during prolonged treatment, rule out endometrial pathology. Perforation or penetration of the uterine wall or cervix or embedment in myometrium may occur; may result in pregnancy; remove when this occurs. May increase risk of perforation in fixed retroverted uteri, during lactation, and postpartum. Partial or complete expulsion may occur; replace within 7 days of menstrual period after pregnancy has been ruled out. May cause enlarged ovarian follicles. Breast cancer reported. May affect glucose tolerance. Caution with increased risk of infective endocarditis and/or have coagulopathies. Remove device if with: new onset menorrhagia and/or metrorrhagia producing anemia; STD; endometritis; jaundice (first time); intractable pelvic pain; severe dyspareunia; endometrial or cervical malignancy. Remove if the following occurs for the 1st time: migraine, focal migraine with asymmetrical visual loss or other symptoms indicating transient cerebral ischemia, exceptionally severe headache; marked BP increase; or severe arterial disease (eg, stroke or MI).

ADVERSE REACTIONS: Uterine/vaginal bleeding alterations, amenorrhea, intramenstrual bleeding, spotting, abdominal/pelvic pain, ovarian cysts, headache/migraine, acne, depressed/altered mood, menorrhagia, vaginal discharge, IUD expulsion, breast tenderness/pain.

INTERACTIONS: May decrease serum concentrations of progestins with drugs or herbal products that induce enzymes such as CYP3A4 (eg, barbiturates, bosentan, carbamazepine, felbamate, griseofulvin, oxcarbazepine, phenytoin, rifampin, St. John's wort, topiramate). Significant changes (increase or decrease) in serum concentrations of progestin with HIV protease inhibitors, non-nucleoside reverse transcriptase inhibitors. Caution if receiving anticoagulants.

PREGNANCY: Contraindicated in pregnancy. Not for use in nursing.

MECHANISM OF ACTION: Progestogen; not conclusively demonstrated. Thickens cervical mucus (preventing passage of sperm into uterus), inhibits sperm capacitation or survival, and alters endometrium.

PHARMACOKINETICS: Distribution: V_d=1.8L/kg, plasma protein binding (97.5-99%). Found in breast milk. **Metabolism:** Sulfate and glucuronide (lesser extent) conjugates (metabolites). **Excretion:** Urine (45%), feces (32%); $T_{1/2}$=17 hrs.

NURSING CONSIDERATIONS

Assessment: Perform complete medical and social history (including that of partner) and physical exam including a pelvic exam, Pap smear, breast exam and appropriate tests for STDs. Assess for any conditions where treatment is contraindicated or cautioned. Assess for pregnancy/nursing status. Assess for migraine, focal migraine with asymmetrical visual loss or other symptoms indicating transient cerebral ischemia, exceptionally severe headache; marked BP increase; jaundice (first time) or with severe arterial disease and possible drug interactions. Prior to insertion, determine degree of patency of the endocervical canal and internal os and the direction and depth of the uterine cavity.

Monitoring: Re-examine/evaluate 4-12 weeks after insertion and at least once a year. Monitor for pregnancy, ectopic pregnancy, intrauterine pregnancy, GAS, PID, and other adverse effects. Monitor blood glucose in diabetics and monitor for marked BP increase. During insertion, monitor for decrease pulse, perspiration, or pallor. See if thread is still visible and for length of thread.

Patient Counseling: Drug does not protect against HIV infection (AIDS) and other STDs. Inform of risks/benefits of the drug device. Immediately report any symptoms of PID (eg, unusual vaginal discharge, abdominal/pelvic pain/tenderness, chills) and if partner becomes HIV-positive or acquires an STD. Inform that some bleeding (eg, irregular or prolonged bleeding, spotting) may occur during 1st few weeks; contact healthcare provider if symptoms continue or become severe. Contact healthcare provider if experiencing stroke or heart attack, develops very severe or migraine headaches, unexplained fever, yellowing of skin or whites in the eyes, may be pregnant, pelvic pain or pain during sex, HIV positive, exposed to STDs, unusual vaginal discharge, genital sores, severe or prolonged vaginal bleeding, or cannot feel threads. Instruct how to check after menstrual period that threads still protrude from cervix and caution not to pull on threads and displace drug device. No contraceptive protection exists if device is displaced or expelled.

Administration: Intrauterine route. Refer to PI for insertion, continuing care, and removal instructions. **Storage:** 25°C (77°F); excursions permitted to 15-30°C (59-86°F).

M-M-R II   RX

rubella vaccine live - measles vaccine live - mumps vaccine live (Merck)

THERAPEUTIC CLASS: Vaccine

INDICATIONS: Vaccination against measles, mumps, and rubella in individuals ≥12 months.

DOSAGE: *Adults:* 0.5mL SQ into outer aspect of upper arm.
Pediatrics: 12-15 months: 0.5mL SQ into outer aspect of upper arm. Repeat before elementary school entry. If first vaccinated <12 months of age, repeat dose between 12-15 months and then revaccinate before elementary school entry.

HOW SUPPLIED: Inj: 0.5mL

CONTRAINDICATIONS: Pregnant females; avoid pregnancy for 3 months after vaccination. Anaphylactic/anaphylactoid reactions to neomycin, febrile respiratory illness or other active febrile infection, immunosuppressive therapy (except corticosteroids as replacement therapy), blood dyscrasias, leukemia, lymphoma of any type, malignant neoplasms affecting bone marrow or lymphatic system, primary and acquired immunodeficiency states (including immunosuppression associated with AIDS, other clinical manifestation of HIV infection, cellular immune deficiencies, hypogammaglobulinemic and dysgammaglobulinemic states), and family history of congenital or hereditary immunodeficiency.

WARNINGS/PRECAUTIONS: Caution with history of cerebral injury, individual or family history of convulsions or any other condition in which stress due to fever should be avoided. Caution with history of anaphylactic/anaphylactoid, or other immediate reactions to egg ingestion; may increase risk of hypersensitivity reactions. Have epinephrine (1:1000) available should an anaphylactic/anaphylactoid reaction occur. May develop severe thrombocytopenia in individuals with current thrombocytopenia. Evaluate serologic status to determine need for additional doses. Ensure that injection does not enter a blood vessel. Excretion of small amounts of the live attenuated rubella virus from the nose or throat 7-28 days after vaccination reported. Avoid with active untreated tuberculosis.

ADVERSE REACTIONS: Atypical measles, fever, syncope, headache, dizziness, malaise, diarrhea, local reactions, N/V, arthralgia, arthritis, pneumonitis, sore throat, Stevens-Johnson syndrome.

INTERACTIONS: See Contraindications. Do not give with immune globulin; may interfere with expected immune response. May be given 1 month before or after administration of other live viral vaccines. Defer vaccination for ≥3 months following administration of immune globulin (human), blood or plasma transfusions. Do not give concurrently with diphtheria, tetanus, pertussis (DTP) and/or oral poliovirus vaccines (OPV). May result in temporary depression of tuberculin skin sensitivity if given individually; administer test either before or simultaneously.

PREGNANCY: Category C, caution in nursing.

MECHANISM OF ACTION: Live virus vaccine; may induce antibodies that protect against measles, mumps, and rubella.

PHARMACOKINETICS: Distribution: Found in breast milk (live attenuated rubella).

NURSING CONSIDERATIONS

Assessment: Assess for immune and current health/medical status, vaccination history, thrombocytopenia, active untreated tuberculosis, conditions where treatment is contraindicated or cautioned, nursing status, and possible drug interactions.

Monitoring: Monitor for anaphylactic/anaphylactoid reactions, thrombocytopenia, vaccine-preventable diseases in HIV patients, and other adverse reactions.

Patient Counseling: Inform of benefits/risks of vaccination. Instruct to report any serious adverse reactions. Inform that pregnancy should be avoided for 3 months after vaccination.

Administration: SQ route. Refer to PI for proper reconstitution and administration procedures.
Storage: Unreconstituted: -50 to 8°C (-58 to 46°F). Protect from light. Before Reconstitution: 2-8°C (36-46°F). May refrigerate diluent or store separately at room temperature; do not freeze. Reconstituted: 2-8°C (36-46°F), store in a dark place; discard if not used within 8 hrs.

MOBIC   RX
meloxicam (Boehringer Ingelheim)

> NSAIDs may cause an increased risk of serious cardiovascular thrombotic events, myocardial infarction, stroke, and serious GI adverse events, including bleeding, ulceration, and perforation of the stomach or intestines. Elderly patients at greater risk for serious GI events. Contraindicated for the treatment of perioperative pain in the setting of coronary artery bypass graft (CABG) surgery.

THERAPEUTIC CLASS: NSAID

INDICATIONS: Relief of signs and symptoms of osteoarthritis (OA) and rheumatoid arthritis (RA). Relief of signs and symptoms of pauciarticular/polyarticular course juvenile RA in patients ≥2 yrs.

DOSAGE: *Adults:* OA/RA: Initial/Maint: 7.5mg qd. Max: 15mg/day. Hemodialysis: Max: 7.5mg/day. *Pediatrics:* ≥2 yrs: Juvenile RA: Individualize dose. Usual: 0.125mg/kg qd. Max: 7.5mg/day.

HOW SUPPLIED: Sus: 7.5mg/5mL; Tab: 7.5mg, 15mg

CONTRAINDICATIONS: Aspirin (ASA) or other NSAID allergy that precipitates asthma, urticaria, or allergic-type reactions. Treatment of perioperative pain in the setting of CABG surgery.

WARNINGS/PRECAUTIONS: Use lowest effective dose for the shortest duration possible. Extreme caution with history of ulcer disease or GI bleeding. May cause elevations of LFTs; d/c if liver disease develops, or if systemic manifestations occur. May lead to onset of new HTN, or worsening of preexisting HTN. Fluid retention and edema reported. Renal papillary necrosis, renal insufficiency, acute renal failure, and other renal injury reported after long-term use. Not recommended for use with severe renal impairment (CrCl <20mL/min). Caution in patients with considerable dehydration; rehydrate 1st, then start therapy. Caution in debilitated patients, with preexisting kidney disease, and asthma. Closely monitor patients with significant renal impairment. Avoid with ASA-triad/ASA-sensitive asthma. May cause anaphylactoid reactions and serious skin adverse events (eg, exfoliative dermatitis, Stevens-Johnson syndrome, toxic epidermal necrolysis); d/c at 1st appearance of rash or other signs of hypersensitivity. Avoid use starting at 30 weeks gestation; may cause premature closure of ductus arteriosus. Not a substitute for corticosteroids or for treatment of corticosteroid insufficiency. May mask signs of inflammation and fever. Anemia may occur; with long-term use, monitor Hgb/Hct if symptoms of anemia develop. May inhibit platelet aggregation and prolong bleeding time. May be associated with a reversible delay in ovulation; not recommended in women with difficulties conceiving, or who are undergoing investigation of infertility.

ADVERSE REACTIONS: Abdominal pain, diarrhea, dyspepsia, nausea, headache, anemia, arthralgia, insomnia, upper respiratory tract infection, urinary tract infection, dizziness, pain, pharyngitis, edema, influenza-like symptoms.

INTERACTIONS: Patients taking ACE inhibitors, thiazides, and loop diuretics (eg, furosemide) may have impaired response to these therapies. Risk of renal toxicity when coadministered with diuretics, ACE inhibitors, and angiotensin II receptor antagonists. Increased risk of GI bleeding with anticoagulants (eg, warfarin), smoking, alcohol, and oral corticosteroids. May diminish antihypertensive effect of ACE inhibitors. Not recommended with ASA; increased rate of GI ulceration or other complications with low-dose ASA. May elevate lithium plasma levels; observe for signs of lithium toxicity. May increase cyclosporine and methotrexate toxicities. (Sus) Not recommended with sodium polystyrene sulfonate (Kayexalate).

PREGNANCY: Category C (<30 weeks gestation) and D (≥30 weeks gestation), not for use in nursing.

MECHANISM OF ACTION: NSAIDs; has not been established. Suspected to inhibit prostaglandin synthetase, resulting in reduced formation of prostaglandins, thromboxanes, and prostacyclin.

PHARMACOKINETICS: Absorption: Administration of variable doses in different populations resulted in different parameters. Absolute bioavailability (89%). **Distribution:** V_d=10L, plasma protein binding (99.4%); crosses placenta. **Metabolism:** Liver (extensive); oxidation via CYP2C9 (major), CYP3A4 (minor). **Elimination:** Urine (0.2% unchanged), feces (1.6% unchanged); $T_{1/2}$=15-20 hrs.

NURSING CONSIDERATIONS

Assessment: Assess for cardiovascular disease (CVD), risk factors for CVD, ASA-triad, coagulation disorders, any other conditions where treatment is contraindicated or cautioned, renal/hepatic function, pregnancy/nursing status, and possible drug interactions. Assess use in elderly and debilitated patients.

Monitoring: Monitor for signs/symptoms of cardiovascular thrombotic events, HTN, GI events, fluid retention, edema, and anaphylactoid/skin reactions. Monitor BP, renal function, and LFTs. Perform periodic monitoring of CBC and chemistry profile with long-term use.

Patient Counseling: Advise to seek medical attention if symptoms of cardiovascular events (eg, chest pain, SOB, weakness, slurring of speech), GI ulceration and bleeding (eg, epigastric pain, dyspepsia, melena, hematemesis), hepatotoxicity (eg, nausea, fatigue, lethargy, pruritus, jaundice, right upper quadrant tenderness, flu-like symptoms), anaphylactoid reaction (eg, difficulty breathing, swelling of face/throat), skin rash, blisters, fever, hypersensitivity reaction (eg, itching), weight gain, or edema occur. Instruct to avoid use starting at 30 weeks gestation. Advise females of reproductive potential who desire pregnancy that drug may be associated with a reversible delay in ovulation.

Administration: Oral route. (Sus) Shake gently before using. **Storage:** 25°C (77°F); excursions permitted to 15-30°C (59-86°F). Keep tab in a dry place.

MONODOX RX
doxycycline monohydrate (Aqua)

THERAPEUTIC CLASS: Tetracycline derivative

INDICATIONS: Treatment of rocky mountain spotted fever, typhus fever and the typhus group, Q fever, rickettsialpox, ticks fever, respiratory tract infections, urinary tract infections, skin and skin structure infections, inclusion conjunctivitis, uncomplicated urethral/endocervical/rectal infections caused by *Chlamydia trachomatis*, nongonococcal urethritis caused by *C. trachomatis* and

U. urealyticum, relapsing fever, lymphogranuloma venereum, psittacosis, trachoma, tularemia, *Campylobacter fetus*, chancroid, plague, cholera, brucellosis, bartonellosis, granuloma inguinale, and anthrax. Treatment of infections caused by *E. coli, Enterobacter aerogenes, Shigella* species, and *Acinetobacter* species. Treatment of uncomplicated gonorrhea, syphilis, yaws, listeriosis, Vincent's infection, actinomycosis, and *Clostridium* species infections when penicillin is contraindicated. Adjunct therapy for acute intestinal amebiasis and severe acne.

DOSAGE: *Adults:* Usual: 100mg q12h or 50mg q6h on 1st day. Maint: 100mg qd or 50mg q12h. Severe Infection: 100mg q12h. Uncomplicated Gonococcal Infections (Except Anorectal Infections in Men): 100mg bid for 7 days or 300mg stat, then repeat in 1 hr. Acute Epididymo-Orchitis caused by *N. gonorrhoeae* or *C. trachomatis*: 100mg bid for ≥10 days. Primary/Secondary Syphilis: 300mg/day in divided doses for ≥10 days. Uncomplicated Urethral/Endocervical/Rectal Infection caused by *C. trachomatis*: 100mg bid for ≥7 days. Nongonococcal Urethritis caused by *C. trachomatis* and *U. urealyticum*: 100mg bid for ≥7 days. Inhalational Anthrax (Post-Exposure): 100mg bid for 60 days. Streptococcal Infections: Continue for 10 days.
Pediatrics: >8 yrs: ≤100 lbs: 2mg/lb divided in 2 doses on 1st day. Maint: 1mg/lb as qd or 2 divided doses, on subsequent days. Severe Infection: >100 lbs: Use usual adult dose. ≤100 lbs: ≤2mg/lb/day. Inhalation Anthrax (Post-Exposure): ≥100 lbs: 100mg bid for 60 days. <100 lbs: 1mg/lb bid for 60 days. Streptococcal Infections: Continue for 10 days.

HOW SUPPLIED: Cap: 50mg, 75mg, 100mg

WARNINGS/PRECAUTIONS: May cause permanent tooth discoloration during tooth development (last half of pregnancy, infancy, <8 yrs). Enamel hypoplasia reported. *Clostridium difficile*-associated diarrhea (CDAD) reported; d/c if CDAD is suspected or confirmed. May increase BUN. Photosensitivity reported; avoid direct sunlight or UV light and d/c treatment at the first evidence of skin erythema. May result in overgrowth of non-susceptible organisms including fungi; d/c if superinfection occurs. Intracranial HTN in adults reported. Use in the absence of proven or strong suspected bacterial infection is unlikely to provide benefit and increases the risk of drug resistant bacteria. May cause fetal harm.

ADVERSE REACTIONS: Esophagitis, esophageal ulceration, diarrhea, hepatotoxicity, anorexia, N/V, hypersensitivity reactions.

INTERACTIONS: Decreased $T_{1/2}$ with carbamazepine, barbiturates, phenytoin. Depresses prothrombin activity; may require downward adjustment of anticoagulant dose. May interfere with bactericidal action of penicillin; avoid use. May decrease effects of oral contraceptives. Impaired absorption with antacids containing aluminum, calcium, or magnesium and iron-containing products. Fatal renal toxicity may occur with methoxyflurane.

PREGNANCY: Category D, not for use in nursing.

MECHANISM OF ACTION: Tetracycline; bacteriostatic, thought to inhibit protein synthesis.

PHARMACOKINETICS: Absorption: C_{max}=3.61mcg/mL; T_{max}=2.6 hrs. **Distribution:** Found in breast milk. **Elimination:** Urine, feces; $T_{1/2}$=16.33 hrs.

NURSING CONSIDERATIONS

Assessment: Assess for known hypersensitivity, pregnancy/nursing status, and possible drug interactions. In venereal disease, when coexistent syphilis is suspected, perform a dark field examination before treatment.

Monitoring: Monitor for signs/symptoms of hypersensitivity reactions, photosensitivity (skin erythema), superinfection, CDAD, and benign intracranial HTN. In long-term therapy, perform periodic laboratory evaluation of organ systems, including hematopoietic, renal, and hepatic studies. In venereal disease, when coexistent syphilis is suspected, repeat blood serology monthly for ≥4 months.

Patient Counseling: Inform of pregnancy risks. Inform to avoid excessive sunlight or artificial UV light, and to d/c therapy if phototoxicity (eg, skin eruptions) occurs. Instruct to wear sunscreen or sunblock. Advise to drink fluids liberally. Inform that therapy treats bacterial, not viral, infections. Instruct patients to take as directed; skipping doses or not completing full course may decrease effectiveness and increase antibiotic resistance. Inform patient that they may experience diarrhea. Inform that absorption of drug is reduced by calcium-containing products and bismuth subsalicylate. Instruct to notify physician if photosensitivity or watery/bloody stools occur. May increase incidence of vaginal candidiasis.

Administration: Oral route. Take with full glass of water. Take with food if GI irritation occurs. **Storage**: 20-25°C (68-77°F).

MORPHINE

morphine sulfate (Various)

> Oral sol is available in 10mg/5mL, 20mg/5mL, and 100mg/5mL concentrations. The 100mg/5mL (20mg/mL) concentration is indicated for use in opioid-tolerant patients only. Use caution when prescribing and administering to avoid dosing errors due to confusion between different concentrations and between mg and mL, which could result in accidental overdose and death. Ensure the proper dose is communicated and dispensed. Keep out of reach of children. Seek emergency medical help immediately in case of accidental ingestion.

THERAPEUTIC CLASS: Opioid analgesic

INDICATIONS: Relief of moderate to severe acute and chronic pain where use of an opioid analgesic is appropriate. (Sol, 100mg/5mL) Relief of moderate to severe acute and chronic pain in opioid-tolerant patients.

DOSAGE: *Adults:* Individualize dose. Opioid-Naive Patients: Initial: 10-20mg (sol) or 15-30mg (tab) q4h PRN for pain. Titrate based upon the individual patient's response to the initial dose. Conversion from Parenteral to PO Formulation: Anywhere from 3-6mg PO dose may be required to provide pain relief equivalent to 1mg parenteral dose. Conversion from Parenteral PO Non-Morphine Opioids to PO Morphine: Close observation and dose adjustment is required. Refer to published relative potency information. Conversion from Controlled-Release PO Formulation to PO Formulation: Dose adjustment with close observation is necessary. Maint: Continue to re-evaluate with special attention to the maint of pain control and side effects. Periodically reassess the continued need for opioid analgesic use during chronic use especially for non-cancer-related pain (or pain associated with other terminal illness). Taper dose gradually. Elderly: Start at lower end of dosing range.

HOW SUPPLIED: Sol: 10mg/5mL [100mL, 500mL], 20mg/5mL [100mL, 500mL], 100mg/5mL [30mL, 120mL]; Tab: 15mg*, 30mg* *scored

CONTRAINDICATIONS: Respiratory depression in absence of resuscitative equipment, acute or severe bronchial asthma or hypercarbia, has or suspected of having paralytic ileus.

WARNINGS/PRECAUTIONS: Increased risk of respiratory depression in elderly or debilitated patients and in those with conditions accompanied by hypoxia, hypercapnia, or upper airway obstruction. Caution and consider alternative non-opioid analgesics with chronic obstructive pulmonary disease or cor pulmonale, substantially decreased respiratory reserve (eg, severe kyphoscoliosis), hypoxia, hypercapnia, or preexisting respiratory depression. Contains morphine sulfate, a Schedule II controlled substance, that has a high potential for abuse and is subject to misuse, abuse, or diversion. The possible respiratory depressant effects and the potential to elevate CSF pressure may be markedly exaggerated in the presence of head injury, intracranial lesions, or preexisting increase in intracranial pressure (ICP); may obscure neurologic signs of further increased ICP in patients with head injuries. May cause orthostatic hypotension and syncope in ambulatory patients. May cause severe hypotension when ability to maintain BP has been compromised by a depleted blood volume. Caution with circulatory shock. Avoid with GI obstruction, especially paralytic ileus; may obscure diagnosis or clinical course with acute abdominal conditions. Caution with biliary tract disease including acute pancreatitis; may cause spasm of the sphincter of Oddi and diminish biliary and pancreatic secretions. Caution with and reduce dose in patients with severe renal or hepatic impairment, Addison's disease, hypothyroidism, prostatic hypertrophy, or urethral stricture, and in elderly or debilitated. Caution with CNS depression, toxic psychosis, acute alcoholism, and delirium tremens. May aggravate convulsions in patients with convulsive disorders and may aggravate or induce seizures. May impair mental/physical abilities.

ADVERSE REACTIONS: Respiratory depression, apnea, circulatory depression, respiratory arrest, shock, cardiac arrest, lightheadedness, dizziness, constipation, somnolence, sedation, N/V, sweating.

INTERACTIONS: Caution with CNS depressants (eg, sedatives, hypnotics, general anesthetics, antiemetics, phenothiazines, tranquilizers, other opioids, illicit drugs, alcohol); may increase the risk of respiratory depression, hypotension, profound sedation, or coma. May enhance the neuromuscular blocking action of skeletal muscle relaxants and produce an increased degree of respiratory depression. Avoid with mixed agonist/antagonist analgesics (eg, pentazocine, nalbuphine, butorphanol). Precipitated apnea, confusion, and muscle twitching reported with cimetidine. Potentiated action by MAOIs; allow at least 14 days after stopping MAOIs before initiating treatment. May result in increased risk of urinary retention and/or severe constipation, which may lead to paralytic ileus with anticholinergics or other medications with anticholinergic activity. Caution with P-glycoprotein inhibitors.

PREGNANCY: Category C, not for use in nursing.

MECHANISM OF ACTION: Opioid analgesic; precise mechanism unknown. Specific CNS opiate receptors and endogenous compounds with morphine-like activity have been identified throughout the brain and spinal cord and are likely to play a role in the expression and perception of analgesic effects. Causes respiratory depression, in part by a direct effect on the brainstem

M

respiratory centers, and depresses cough reflex by direct effect on the cough center in the medulla.

PHARMACOKINETICS: Absorption: Bioavailability (<40%); C_{max}=78ng/mL (tab), 58ng/mL (sol). **Distribution:** V_d=1-6L/kg; plasma protein binding (20-35%); crosses placenta, found in breast milk. **Metabolism:** Liver via conjugation; 3- and 6-glucuronide (metabolites). **Elimination:** Urine (10% unchanged), feces (7-10%); $T_{1/2}$=2 hrs (IV).

NURSING CONSIDERATIONS

Assessment: Assess for degree of opioid tolerance, level of pain intensity, type of pain, patient's general condition and medical status, or any other conditions where treatment is contraindicated or cautioned, pregnancy/nursing status, and possible drug interactions.

Monitoring: Monitor for respiratory depression, CSF pressure elevation, orthostatic hypotension, syncope, hypotension, aggravation of convulsions/seizures, and other adverse reactions.

Patient Counseling: Advise to take only ud and not to adjust dose without consulting a physician. Inform physician if pregnant or plan to become pregnant prior to therapy. Counsel on the importance of safely tapering the dose. Inform of potential for severe constipation. Inform that therapy may produce physical or psychological dependence. Caution against performing hazardous tasks (eg, operating machinery/driving). Advise to avoid alcohol or CNS depressants except by the orders of the prescribing physician during therapy. Keep in a secure place out of reach of children and when no longer needed, instruct to destroy the unused tabs by flushing down the toilet.

Administration: Oral route. (Sol, 100mg/5mL) Used only for patients who have already been titrated to a stable analgesic regimen using lower strengths and who can benefit from use of a smaller volume of sol; always use the enclosed calibrated PO syringe. **Storage:** 15-30°C (59-86°F). Protect from moisture.

MOXATAG   RX
amoxicillin (Middlebrook)

THERAPEUTIC CLASS: Semisynthetic ampicillin derivative

INDICATIONS: Treatment of tonsillitis and/or pharyngitis secondary to *Streptococcus pyogenes* in adults and pediatric patients ≥12 yrs.

DOSAGE: *Adults:* Take 775mg qd within 1 hr of finishing a meal for 10 days. Do not chew or crush. *Pediatrics:* ≥12 yrs: Take 775mg qd within 1 hr of finishing a meal for 10 days. Do not chew or crush.

HOW SUPPLIED: Tab, Extended Release: 775mg

WARNINGS/PRECAUTIONS: Serious, fatal anaphylactic reactions and superinfections may occur; d/c and treat accordingly. *Clostridium difficile*-associated diarrhea (CDAD) ranging from mild diarrhea to fatal colitis reported; d/c and treat accordingly. May cause erythematous skin rash in these patients; avoid use in patients with mononucleosis. Increases risk of the development of drug-resistant bacteria when used prophylactically or in the absence of bacterial infection. High urine concentrations of amoxicillin may result in false-positive urinary glucose tests; glucose-tests based on enzymatic glucose oxidase reactions may be used. Not recommended for use in severe renal impairment (CrCl <30mL/min) or hemodialysis.

ADVERSE REACTIONS: Vulvovaginal mycotic infection, diarrhea, N/V, abdominal pain, headache.

INTERACTIONS: Concurrent use with probenecid may increase and prolong blood levels; decreases renal tubular secretion of amoxicillin. Chloramphenicol, macrolides, sulfonamides, and tetracyclines may interfere with bactericidal effects. Lowers estrogen reabsorption and reduces efficacy of combined oral estrogen/progesterone contraceptives.

PREGNANCY: Category B, caution in nursing.

MECHANISM OF ACTION: Ampicillin analog; bactericidal action against susceptible organisms during the stage of multiplication; acts through inhibition of biosynthesis of cell wall mucopeptide.

PHARMACOKINETICS: Absorption: C_{max} =6.6 mcg/mL. T_{max}=3.1 hrs. **Distribution:** Plasma protein binding (20%). **Elimination:** Urine (unchanged); $T_{1/2}$=1.5 hrs.

NURSING CONSIDERATIONS

Assessment: Assess for history of allergic reaction to PCNs, cephalosporins, or other allergens, infectious mononucleosis, phenylketonurics, pregnancy/nursing status, and for possible drug interactions.

Monitoring: Monitor for serious anaphylactic reactions, erythematous skin rash, development of drug resistance or superinfection with mycotic or bacterial pathogen, signs/symptoms of CDAD (may range from mild diarrhea to fatal colitis). Monitor for false (+) reactions for urinary glucose test. Caution in dose selection in elderly; monitor renal function.

Patient Counseling: Do not chew or crush. Inform drug treats bacterial, not viral, infections. Instruct to take exactly as directed; skipping doses or not completing full course may decrease effectiveness and increase resistance. Inform about potential benefits/risks; notify physician if experience watery/bloody diarrhea (with/without stomach cramps and fever) which may occur as late as 2 months after treatment. Notify physician of serious hypersensitivity reactions, pregnancy, or nursing.

Administration: Oral route. **Storage:** 25°C (77°F). Excursion permitted to 15-30°C (59-86°)

MOXEZA   RX
moxifloxacin HCl (Alcon)

THERAPEUTIC CLASS: Fluoroquinolone

INDICATIONS: Treatment of bacterial conjunctivitis caused by susceptible strains of organisms.

DOSAGE: *Adults:* 1 drop bid for 7 days in the affected eye(s).
Pediatrics: ≥4 months: 1 drop bid for 7 days in the affected eye(s).

HOW SUPPLIED: Sol: 0.5% [3mL]

WARNINGS/PRECAUTIONS: For topical ophthalmic use only; should not be introduced directly into the anterior chamber of the eye. Serious and sometimes fatal hypersensitivity reactions reported with systemic use; d/c and institute appropriate therapy if allergic reaction occurs. Prolonged use may cause overgrowth of nonsusceptible organisms, including fungi. D/C use and consider alternative therapy if superinfection occurs. Avoid wearing contact lenses when signs/symptoms of bacterial conjunctivitis are present.

ADVERSE REACTIONS: Eye irritation, pyrexia, conjunctivitis.

PREGNANCY: Category C, caution in nursing.

MECHANISM OF ACTION: Fluoroquinolone antibiotic; inhibition of topoisomerase II (DNA gyrase) and topoisomerase IV. DNA gyrase is an essential enzyme involved in replication, transcription, and repair of bacterial DNA. Topoisomerase IV is an enzyme known to play a key role in partitioning of chromosomal DNA during bacterial cell division.

PHARMACOKINETICS: Absorption: AUC=8.17ng•hr/mL. **Distribution:** Presumed to be excreted in breast milk.

NURSING CONSIDERATIONS

Assessment: Assess severity of infection, symptoms, and pregnancy/nursing status.

Monitoring: Monitor for signs/symptoms of hypersensitivity/anaphylactic reactions and other adverse reactions. Monitor for superinfection; examine with magnification (eg, slit lamp biomicroscopy) and fluorescein staining, where appropriate.

Patient Counseling: Advise on proper use to prevent bacterial contamination. D/C medication and contact physician if rash or allergic reaction occurs. Advise not to wear contact lenses if signs/symptoms of bacterial conjunctivitis are present.

Administration: Ocular route. Do not inject into eye. **Storage:** 2-25°C (36-77°F).

MS CONTIN   CII
morphine sulfate (Purdue Pharma)

> Indicated for opioid-tolerant patients only. Contains morphine sulfate, a Schedule II controlled substance that has a high potential for abuse and is subject to misuse, addiction, and criminal diversion. 100mg and 200mg tabs are for use in opioid-tolerant patients only; these strengths may cause fatal respiratory depression in non-opioid tolerant patients. Not indicated for use in the management of acute or postoperative pain and is not intended for use as a prn analgesic. Swallow whole. Do not break, chew, dissolve, crush or inject tabs.

THERAPEUTIC CLASS: Opioid analgesic

INDICATIONS: Management of moderate to severe pain when a continuous, around-the-clock opioid analgesic is needed for an extended period of time. Postoperative use if the patient is already receiving the drug prior to surgery or if postoperative pain is expected to be moderate to severe and persist for an extended period of time.

DOSAGE: *Adults:* Individualize dose. Conversion from Immediate-Release Oral Morphine: Give 1/2 of patient's 24-hr requirement q12h or give 1/3 of daily requirement q8h. Conversion from Parenteral Morphine: Initial: Estimates of oral to parenteral potency vary. A dose of oral morphine only 3 times the daily parenteral morphine requirement may be sufficient in chronic settings.

Reassess periodically for need of continued around-the-clock therapy. Swallow whole; do not crush, chew, break or dissolve. Elderly: Start at the low end of dosing range.

HOW SUPPLIED: Tab, Controlled-Release: 15mg, 30mg, 60mg, 100mg, 200mg

CONTRAINDICATIONS: Paralytic ileus, respiratory depression in the absence of resuscitative equipment, acute or severe bronchial asthma or hypercarbia.

WARNINGS/PRECAUTIONS: Do not use as a first opioid. May cause respiratory depression; caution with conditions accompanied by hypoxia, hypercapnia, or decreased respiratory reserve such as asthma, COPD or cor pulmonale, severe obesity, sleep apnea, myxedema, kyphoscoliosis, or CNS depression. Avoid with head injury, intracranial lesions, or pre-existing elevated intracranial pressure. May obscure neurologic signs if further increases in intracranial pressure in patients with head injury. May aggravate convulsions with convulsive disorders. May cause severe hypotension; caution in patients with circulatory shock. Caution with severe hepatic/renal dysfunction, adrenocortical insufficiency, coma, toxic psychosis, prostatic hypertrophy, urethral stricture, alcoholism, delirium tremens, and inability to swallow. May cause neonatal withdrawal syndrome. May increase biliary tract pressure; caution with inflammatory or obstructive bowel disorder, acute pancreatitis secondary to biliary tract disease, and in biliary surgery. May cause mental/physical impairment. Avoid abrupt withdrawal. Tolerance and physical dependence may occur. Rare cases of anaphylaxis reported. Does not release morphine continuously over the course of dosing interval. Caution with elderly/debilitated.

ADVERSE REACTIONS: Constipation, lightheadedness, dizziness, sedation, N/V, sweating, dysphoria, euphoria.

INTERACTIONS: Additive depressant effects with other CNS depressants (eg, sedatives, hypnotics, general anesthetics, phenothiazines, tranquilizers, alcohol). Enhances neuromuscular blocking effects and increases respiratory depression with skeletal muscle relaxants. Caution with agonist/antagonist analgesics (eg, pentazocine, nalbuphine, butorphanol, buprenorphine); may reduce analgesic effect or cause withdrawal symptoms. Risk of hypotension with phenothiazines or general anesthetics.

PREGNANCY: Category C, not for use in nursing.

MECHANISM OF ACTION: Opioid analgesic; principal actions are analgesia and sedation. Precise mechanism of analgesic effects not established. Binds to CNS opiate receptors, producing analgesic effects. Also produces respiratory depression by direct action on brain stem respiratory centers, and depresses cough reflex by direct action on cough center in the medulla.

PHARMACOKINETICS: Absorption: (Immediate-release) Bioavailability (50%). **Distribution:** V_d=4L/kg; crosses placental membranes; found in breast milk. **Metabolism:** Liver to glucuronide metabolites, M3G (major metabolite), M6G (active metabolite). **Elimination:** Renal (primary), bile; (IV) $T_{1/2}$=2-4 hrs.

NURSING CONSIDERATIONS

Assessment: Assess for degree of opioid tolerance, previous opioid dose, level of pain intensity, type of pain, patient's general condition and medical status, or any other conditions where treatment is contraindicated or cautioned. Assess for history of hypersensitivity, pregnancy/nursing status, renal/hepatic function, and possible drug interactions.

Monitoring: Monitor for signs/symptoms of respiratory depression, elevation in CSF pressure, hypotension, convulsions, tolerance and physical dependence, and misuse or abuse.

Patient Counseling: Advise that the drug contains morphine and should be taken only as directed. Do not change the dose without consulting physician. Drug is designed to work properly only if swallowed whole. Report episodes of breakthrough pain and adverse experiences. May impair mental and/or physical ability required to perform hazardous tasks (eg, operating machinery/driving). Avoid alcohol or other CNS depressants. Avoid abrupt withdrawal if on medication for more than a few weeks; taper dose. Special care must be taken to avoid accidental ingestion or use by individuals other than the patient for whom it was originally prescribed. Advise to flush unused medication down toilet; has drug abuse potential; protect from theft. May pass empty matrix "ghosts" (tablets) via colostomy or in the stool. Inform physician if pregnant or planning to become pregnant.

Administration: Oral route. **Storage:** 25°C (77°F); excursions permitted between 15-30°C (59-86°F). Dispense in a tight, light-resistant container.

MULTAQ   RX

dronedarone (Sanofi-Aventis)

> Doubles the risk of death in patients with symptomatic heart failure (HF) with recent decompensation requiring hospitalization or NYHA Class IV HF; contraindicated in these patients. Doubles the risk of death, stroke, and hospitalization for HF in patients with permanent atrial fibrillation (A-fib); contraindicated in patients in A-fib who will not or cannot be cardioverted into normal sinus rhythm.

THERAPEUTIC CLASS: Class III antiarrhythmic

INDICATIONS: To reduce the risk of hospitalization for A-fib in patients in sinus rhythm with a history of paroxysmal or persistent A-fib.

DOSAGE: *Adults:* 400mg bid. Take as 1 tab with am meal and 1 tab with pm meal.

HOW SUPPLIED: Tab: 400mg

CONTRAINDICATIONS: Permanent A-fib, symptomatic HF with recent decompensation requiring hospitalization or NYHA Class IV symptoms, 2nd- or 3rd-degree atrioventricular block or sick sinus syndrome (except when used with a functioning pacemaker), bradycardia <50 bpm, liver toxicity related to previous use of amiodarone, QTc Bazett interval ≥500 msec or PR interval >280 msec, severe hepatic impairment, pregnancy, nursing mothers. Concomitant use of strong CYP3A inhibitors (eg, ketoconazole, itraconazole, voriconazole, cyclosporine, telithromycin, clarithromycin, nefazodone, ritonavir), drugs or herbal products that prolong QT interval and might increase risk of torsades de pointes (eg, phenothiazine antipsychotics, TCAs, certain oral macrolide antibiotics, Class I and III antiarrhythmics).

WARNINGS/PRECAUTIONS: Monitor cardiac rhythm no less often than q3 months. New onset or worsening of HF reported; d/c if HF develops or worsens and requires hospitalization. Hepatocellular injury (including acute liver failure requiring transplant) reported; d/c if hepatic injury is suspected and test serum enzymes, AST, ALT, alkaline phosphatase, and serum bilirubin. Do not restart therapy without another explanation for observed liver injury. K⁺ levels should be within normal range prior to and during therapy. May induce moderate QTc (Bazett) prolongation. Increased SrCr and BUN levels reported; reversible upon d/c. Periodically monitor renal function. Premenopausal women who have not undergone hysterectomy/oophorectomy must use effective contraception while on therapy.

ADVERSE REACTIONS: QT prolongation, SrCr increase, diarrhea, N/V, abdominal pain, asthenic conditions, rashes, pruritus, eczema, dermatitis, allergic dermatitis.

INTERACTIONS: See Contraindications. Hypokalemia/hypomagnesemia may occur with K⁺-depleting diuretics. Increased digoxin levels and increased GI disorders observed with digoxin. Digoxin may also potentiate electrophysiologic effects; halve the dose of digoxin and closely monitor serum levels and for toxicity if digoxin treatment is continued. Calcium channel blockers (CCBs) (eg, verapamil, diltiazem) may potentiate effects on conduction and may increase exposure. Bradycardia more frequently observed with β-blockers. Give a low dose of CCB or β-blockers initially and increase only after ECG verification of good tolerability. Avoid grapefruit juice, and rifampin or other CYP3A inducers (eg, phenobarbital, carbamazepine, phenytoin, St. John's wort). May increase exposure of simvastatin/simvastatin acid, verapamil, diltiazem, nifedipine, dabigatran, P-glycoprotein substrates, and CYP2D6 substrates (eg, β-blockers, TCAs, SSRIs). Avoid doses >10mg qd of simvastatin. May increase plasma levels of tacrolimus, sirolimus, and other CYP3A substrates with a narrow therapeutic range; monitor and adjust dosage appropriately. Clinically significant INR elevations with oral anticoagulants and increased S-warfarin exposure reported; monitor INR after initiating therapy.

PREGNANCY: Category X, not for use in nursing.

MECHANISM OF ACTION: Benzofuran derivative; not established. Has antiarrhythmic properties belonging to all 4 Vaughan-Williams classes.

PHARMACOKINETICS: Absorption: Absolute bioavailability (4% without food, 15% with high fat meal); T_{max}=3-6 hrs. **Distribution:** Plasma protein binding (>98% in vitro); (IV) V_d=1400L. **Metabolism:** Extensive via CYP3A; N-debutylation, oxidative deamination, and direct oxidation; N-debutyl metabolite (active). **Elimination:** Urine (6%, metabolites), feces (84%, metabolites); $T_{1/2}$=13-19 hrs.

NURSING CONSIDERATIONS

Assessment: Assess for recent HF decompensation, permanent A-fib, any other conditions where treatment is contraindicated/cautioned, pregnancy/nursing status, and possible drug interactions. Obtain baseline serum K⁺ levels.

Monitoring: Monitor for signs/symptoms of new/worsening HF, hepatic injury, and QT interval prolongation. Monitor cardiac rhythm no less often than every 3 months, hepatic serum enzymes periodically during first 6 months, and renal function periodically.

Patient Counseling: Instruct to take with meals and not to take with grapefruit juice. If a dose is missed, advise to take next dose at the regularly scheduled time and to not double the dose. Counsel to consult physician if signs/symptoms of HF or potential hepatic injury occur. Advise to inform physician of any history of HF, rhythm disturbance other than A-fib or atrial flutter, or predisposing conditions, such as uncorrected hypokalemia. Advise to report any use of other prescription, nonprescription medication, or herbal products, particularly St. John's wort. Counsel patients of childbearing potential about appropriate contraceptive choices while on therapy.

Administration: Oral route. **Storage:** 25°C (77°F); excursions permitted to 15-30°C (59-86°F).

MYCAMINE
micafungin sodium (Astellas)

RX

THERAPEUTIC CLASS: Glucan synthesis inhibitor

INDICATIONS: Treatment of candidemia, acute disseminated candidiasis, *Candida* peritonitis and abscesses, and esophageal candidiasis. Prophylaxis of *Candida* infections in patients undergoing hematopoietic stem cell transplantation (HSCT).

DOSAGE: *Adults:* Candidemia/Acute Disseminated Candidiasis/*Candida* Peritonitis and Abscesses: 100mg IV qd (usual range 10-47 days). Esophageal Candidiasis: 150mg IV qd (usual range 10-30 days). *Candida* Infections Prophylaxis in HSCT: 50mg IV qd (usual range 6-51 days).

HOW SUPPLIED: Inj: 50mg, 100mg [vial]

WARNINGS/PRECAUTIONS: Isolated cases of serious hypersensitivity reactions (eg, anaphylaxis, anaphylactoid reactions, shock) reported; d/c infusion and administer appropriate treatment. Acute intravascular hemolysis, hemolytic anemia, and hemoglobinuria reported; monitor for worsening of hemolysis and hemolytic anemia and evaluate for risk/benefits of continuing therapy. LFT abnormalities reported; monitor for worsening hepatic function and evaluate for risk/benefits of continuing therapy. Hepatic abnormalities, hepatic impairment, hepatitis, and hepatic failure reported with multiple concomitant medications in patients with serious underlying conditions. Significant renal dysfunction, acute renal failure, and elevations in BUN and creatinine reported; monitor for worsening of renal function. Efficacy against infections caused by fungi other than *Candida* has not been established. Has not been studied in patients with endocarditis, osteomyelitis, and meningitis due to *Candida* infections. Caution in elderly.

ADVERSE REACTIONS: Diarrhea, pyrexia, neutropenia, hypomagnesemia, cough, rash, headache, insomnia, HTN, bacteremia, tachycardia, N/V, mucosal inflammation, constipation.

INTERACTIONS: Monitor for sirolimus, nifedipine, or itraconazole toxicity; reduce dose of these drugs if necessary.

PREGNANCY: Category C, caution in nursing.

MECHANISM OF ACTION: Antifungal agent; inhibits the synthesis of 1,3-β-D-glucan, a component of fungal cell walls.

PHARMACOKINETICS: Absorption: IV infusion of variable doses resulted in different parameters. **Distribution:** V_d=0.39L/kg (terminal phase); plasma protein binding (>99%). **Metabolism:** Metabolized to M-1 (catechol form) by arylsulfatase and further metabolized to M-2 (methoxy form) by catechol-O-methyltransferase. M-5 is formed (hydroxylation) catalyzed by CYP450 isoenzymes. **Elimination:** (25mg) Urine and feces (82.5%); feces (71%).

NURSING CONSIDERATIONS

Assessment: Assess drug hypersensitivity, cultures and other diagnostic tests prior to therapy, pregnancy/nursing status, and for possible drug interactions.

Monitoring: Monitor for hypersensitivity reactions, LFTs, renal dysfunction, hematological effects (hemolysis, hemolytic anemia), and other adverse reactions.

Patient Counseling: Counsel about the benefits and risk of treatment. Inform of the common adverse effects and instruct to notify physician if signs/symptoms of hypersensitivity or anaphylaxis reactions, hematological reactions, hepatic effects, or renal complications develop, persists, or worsens. Advise to inform their physician if taking any other medications including over-the-counter medications.

Administration: IV (infusion) route. Do not mix or coinfuse with other medications. Refer to PI for directions for reconstitution, dilution, and administration. **Storage:** Unopened vial: 25°C (77°F); excursions permitted to 15-30°C (59-86°F). Reconstituted/Diluted infusions: 25°C (77°F) for up to 24 hrs. Diluted infusion should be protected from light.

MYFORTIC
mycophenolic acid (Novartis)

RX

Immunosuppression may lead to increased susceptibility to infection and possible development of lymphoma and other neoplasms. Only physicians experienced in immunosuppressive therapy and management of organ transplant recipients should use mycophenolic acid. Manage patient in facilities equipped and staffed with adequate laboratory and supportive medical resources. Physician responsible for administration should have complete information requisite for patient follow-up. Female users of childbearing potential must use contraception. Use during pregnancy is associated with increased risks of pregnancy loss and congenital malformations.

THERAPEUTIC CLASS: Inosine monophosphate dehydrogenase inhibitor

INDICATIONS: Prophylaxis of organ rejection in patients receiving allogeneic renal transplants, administered in combination with cyclosporine and corticosteroids.

DOSAGE: *Adults:* 720mg bid (1440mg total daily dose). Elderly: Max: 720mg bid. *Pediatrics:* 400mg/m^2 BSA bid. Max: 720mg bid. BSA >1.58m^2: 1440mg daily dose (4 tabs 180mg or 2 tabs 360mg bid). BSA 1.19-1.58m^2: 1080mg daily dose (3 tabs 180mg or 1 tab 180mg +1 tab 360mg bid). BSA <1.19m^2: Cannot be accurately administered using currently available formulations.

HOW SUPPLIED: Tab, Delayed-Release: 180mg, 360mg

WARNINGS/PRECAUTIONS: Risk of developing lymphomas and other malignancies, particularly of the skin. Limit exposure to sunlight and UV light by wearing protective clothing and using sunscreen with high protection factor. Increased susceptibility to infections including opportunistic infections (eg, polyomavirus), fatal infections, and sepsis. Polyomavirus infections may produce serious and fatal outcomes including progressive multifocal leukoencephalopathy (PML) and Polyomavirus associated nephropathy (PVAN). Monitor for blood dyscrasias (eg, neutropenia or anemia); interrupt or reduce dose if blood dyscrasias occur (eg, neutropenia [absolute neutrophil count <1.3x10^3/μL] or anemia). Must have negative serum/urine pregnancy test sensitivity of at least 25 mIU/mL within 1 week before therapy. Two reliable forms of contraception are required four weeks before therapy, during therapy, and 6 weeks following d/c. Intestinal perforations, GI hemorrhage, gastric ulcers, and duodenal ulcers rarely observed; caution with active serious digestive system disease. Caution in patients with delayed graft function. Avoid with rare hereditary deficiency of hypoxanthine-guanine phosphoribosyl-transferase (HGPRT) (eg, Lesch-Nyhan and Kelley-Seegmiller syndrome). May have increased levels in patients with severe chronic renal impairment (GFR <25mL/min/1.73m^2 BSA). Caution in elderly.

ADVERSE REACTIONS: Constipation, diarrhea, leukopenia, N/V, anemia, dyspepsia, cytomegalovirus infection, urinary tract infection, insomnia, postoperative pain, herpes simplex, herpes zoster, candida.

INTERACTIONS: Avoid concomitant use with azathioprine and mycophenolate mofetil. Reduced efficacy with drugs that interfere with enterohepatic recirculation (eg, cholestyramine) and drugs that bind bile acids (eg, bile acid sequestrants, oral activated charcoal). Decreased effects of live attenuated vaccines; avoid concomitant use. Increased levels of both drugs with acyclovir/ganciclovir in the presence of renal impairment. Decreased levels with magnesium- and aluminum-containing antacids; do not administer simultaneously. Decreased effects of oral contraceptives. Cases of pure red cell aplasia reported with other immunosuppressive agents. May disrupt enterohepatic recirculation with drugs that alter the GI flora.

PREGNANCY: Category D, not for use in nursing.

MECHANISM OF ACTION: Inosine monophosphate dehydrogenase inhibitor; inhibits the de novo pathway of guanosine nucleotide synthesis without incorporation to deoxyribonucleic acid.

PHARMACOKINETICS: Absorption: Absolute bioavailability (72%); T_{max}=1.5-2.75 hrs. **Distribution:** V_d=54L; plasma protein binding (>98%, mycophenolic acid [MPA]), (82%, MPAG). **Metabolism:** Glucuronyl transferase (mycophenolic acid glucuronide [MPAG], major metabolite). **Elimination:** Urine (>60% MPAG, 3% unchanged MPA), bile; $T_{1/2}$=8-16 hrs (MPA), 13-17 hrs (MPAG).

NURSING CONSIDERATIONS

Assessment: Assess for hepatic/renal impairment, inherited deficiency of HGPRT (eg, Lesch-Nyhan and Kelley-Seegmiller syndromes), pregnancy/nursing status, and for possible drug interactions.

Monitoring: Monitor for signs of delayed graft rejection, lymphomas, skin cancer, GI bleeding/perforation, infections (eg, sepsis, PML), PVAN, and for blood dyscrasias (eg, neutropenia, anemia). Monitor CBC weekly during the 1st month, twice monthly for the 2nd and 3rd months, and then monthly through 1st year.

Patient Counseling: Counsel to take on an empty stomach (1 hr before or 2 hrs after food intake) and to swallow tab whole; do not crush, chew, or cut. Give complete dosage instructions and inform about increased risk of lymphoproliferative disease, and certain other malignancies. Instruct to avoid prolonged exposure to sunlight and UV light by wearing protective clothing and using sunscreen. Inform that use in pregnancy is associated with an increased risk of 1st trimester pregnancy loss and birth defects; instruct to use effective contraception (two methods) 4 weeks prior, during therapy, and for 6 weeks after d/c.

Administration: Oral route. **Storage:** 25°C (77°F); excursions permitted to 15-30°C (59-86°F). Protect from moisture.

MYLERAN   RX
busulfan (GlaxoSmithKline)

> Do not use unless CML diagnosis is established. May induce severe bone marrow hypoplasia; reduce dose or d/c if unusual depression of bone marrow function occurs.

THERAPEUTIC CLASS: Alkylating agent

INDICATIONS: Palliative treatment of chronic myelogenous leukemia (CML).

DOSAGE: *Adults:* 60mcg/kg/day or 1.8mg/m²/day. Reserve dose >4mg/day for the most compelling symptoms. Remission Induction: Range: 4-8mg/day.
Pediatrics: 60mcg/kg/day or 1.8mg/m²/day. Reserve dose >4mg/day for the most compelling symptoms.

HOW SUPPLIED: Tab: 2mg

CONTRAINDICATIONS: Lack of definitive diagnosis of CML.

WARNINGS/PRECAUTIONS: Induction of bone marrow failure resulting in severe pancytopenia reported. Bronchopulmonary dysplasia with pulmonary fibrosis, cellular dysplasia, malignant tumors, acute leukemias, hepatic veno-occlusive disease reported. Ovarian suppression and amenorrhea with menopausal symptoms have occurred. Cardiac tamponade in patients with thalassemia and seizures reported. Caution with compromised bone marrow reserve from prior irradiation/chemotherapy. Seizures reported.

ADVERSE REACTIONS: Myelosuppression, pulmonary fibrosis, cardiac tamponade, hyperpigmentation, weakness, fatigue, weight loss, N/V, melanoderma, hyperuricemia, myasthenia gravis, hepatic veno-occlusive disease.

INTERACTIONS: Additive myelosuppression with myelosuppressive drugs. Additive pulmonary toxicity with cytotoxic drugs. Increased clearance of cyclophosphamide and busulfan with phenytoin pretreatment. Decreased clearance with concomitant cyclophosphamide alone. Reduced clearance with itraconazole; monitor for signs of toxicity. Concurrent thioguanine was associated with portal HTN and esophageal varices with abnormal LFTs; caution with long-term therapy.

PREGNANCY: Category D, not for use in nursing.

MECHANISM OF ACTION: Bifunctional alkylating agent.

PHARMACOKINETICS: Absorption: (IV, PO) Absolute bioavailability (adults 80%, children 68%); C_{max}(2mg, 4mg)=30ng/mL, 68ng/mL; T_{max}=0.9 hrs; AUC (4mg) =269ng•hr/mL **Distribution**: Plasma protein binding (32%); crosses blood-brain barrier. **Metabolism**: Liver (extensive); 3-hydroxytetrahydrothiophene-1, 1-dioxide (major metabolite). **Elimination**: Urine (>2% unchanged); $T_{1/2}$=2.69 hrs.

NURSING CONSIDERATIONS

Assessment: Assess for chronic myelogenous leukemia, history of seizure disorder, head trauma, if receiving other potentially epileptogenic drugs, pregnancy/nursing status. Note other diseases/conditions and drug therapies.

Monitoring: Periodically measure serum transaminases, alkaline phosphatase, and bilirubin for early detection of hepatotoxicity, and evaluate weekly Hgb/Hct, total WBC count and differential, quantitative platelet count, and bone marrow exam for evaluation of marrow status. Monitor for signs/symptoms of busulfan toxicity and bronchopulmonary dysplasia with pulmonary fibrosis, secondary malignancies, chromosomal aberrations.

Patient Counseling: Counsel about need for periodic blood counts and to report unusual bleeding, fever, breathing difficulty, anorexia, weight loss, or melanoderma.

Administration: Oral route. **Storage**: 25°C (77°F); excursions permitted to 15-30°C (59-86°F).

NABI-HB   RX
hepatitis B immune globulin (Biotest)

THERAPEUTIC CLASS: Vaccine

INDICATIONS: Treatment for acute exposure to blood containg HBsAg, perinatal exposure of infants born to HBsAg-positive mothers, sexual exposure to HBsAg-positive persons, and household exposure to persons with acute HBV infection.

DOSAGE: *Adults:* Acute Exposure to Blood Containing HBsAg: 0.06mL/kg IM after exposure and within 24 hrs. Sexual Exposure to HBsAg-Positive Person(s): 0.06mL/kg IM (single dose) and start hepatitis B vaccine series within 14 days of the last sexual contact or if sexual contact with the infected person will continue. Refer to PI for recommendations for hepatitis B prophylaxis following percutaneous or permucosal exposure.
Pediatrics: Prophylaxis of Infant to HBsAg-Positive Mother: 0.5mL IM within 12 hrs. Prophylaxis of Infant (<12 months) Exposed to Mother or Caregiver with Acute HBV-Infection: 0.5mL IM. Refer to PI for recommended schedule of hepatitis B immunoprophylaxis to prevent perinatal transmission.

HOW SUPPLIED: Inj: >312 IU [1mL]; >1560 IU [5mL]

CONTRAINDICATIONS: Anaphylactic or severe systemic reaction to human globulin or IgA-deficiency disorder.

WARNINGS/PRECAUTIONS: Caution in patients with severe thrombocytopenia or coagulation disorders that contraindicate IM administration; give only if expected benefits outweigh the potential risks. Products made from human plasma may contain infectious agents and cause disease. Must be administered IM.

ADVERSE REACTIONS: Headache, erythema, myalgia, malaise, nausea, injection-site pain, elevated alkaline phosphatase levels.

INTERACTIONS: May interfere with live virus vaccines; defer until 3 months following the last dose of vaccine.

PREGNANCY: Category C, caution in nursing.

MECHANISM OF ACTION: Vaccine; passive immunization from HBV exposure resulting in reduction of HBV infection rate.

PHARMACOKINETICS: Absorption: T_{max}=6.5 days. **Distribution:** V_d=11.2L. **Excretion:** $T_{1/2}$=23.1 days.

NURSING CONSIDERATIONS

Assessment: Assess HBsAg/HBeAg, thrombocytopenia, coagulation disorder, IgA-deficiency, previous history of severe anaphylactic or systemic reaction to human globulin, live virus vaccination, and pregnancy/nursing status. Assess for acute exposure to blood of HBsAg-positive mothers, sexual contact with HBsAg-positive persons, and household persons with acute HBV infection.

Monitoring: Monitor for erythema, headache, myalgia, malaise, nausea, and elevated alkaline phosphatase levels.

Patient Counseling: Advise to avoid live virus vaccination for 3 months after hepatitis B immune globulin administration; revaccinate persons immediately after live virus administration.

Administration: IM administration only for post-exposure prophylaxis. Preferred sites are anterolateral aspect of the upper thigh and deltoid muscle. **Storage:** 2-8°C (36-46°F). Do not freeze. Use within 6 hrs once opened; do not reuse or save for future use and partially used vials should be discarded.

NABUMETONE   RX
nabumetone (Various)

N

> NSAIDs may cause an increased risk of serious cardiovascular (CV) thrombotic events, myocardial infarction (MI), stroke and serious GI adverse events including bleeding, ulceration, and perforation of the stomach or intestines. Contraindicated for the treatment of perioperative pain in the setting of coronary artery bypass graft (CABG) surgery.

THERAPEUTIC CLASS: NSAID

INDICATIONS: Relief of signs and symptoms of osteoarthritis and rheumatoid arthritis.

DOSAGE: *Adults:* Initial: 1000mg qd with or without food. Titrate: May give 1500-2000mg depending on clinical response to initial therapy. Max: 2000mg/day given qd-bid. Renal impairment: Moderate: Initial : ≤750mg qd. Severe: Initial: ≤500mg qd.

HOW SUPPLIED: Tab: 500mg, 750mg

CONTRAINDICATIONS: History of asthma, urticaria, or allergic-type reactions after taking aspirin (ASA) or other NSAIDs. Treatment of perioperative pain in the setting of CABG surgery.

WARNINGS/PRECAUTIONS: Use lowest effective dose for shortest duration possible to minimize risk for CV events and adverse GI events. May lead to onset of new HTN or worsening of pre-existing HTN; caution with HTN and monitor BP closely. Fluid retention and edema reported; caution with fluid retention or heart failure. Renal papillary necrosis and other renal injury reported after long-term use. Not recommended for use with advanced renal disease; if therapy must be initiated, monitor renal function closely. Anaphylactoid reactions may occur. Should not be given with ASA triad. May cause serious skin adverse events (eg, exfoliative dermatitis, Stevens-Johnson syndrome, and toxic epidermal necrolysis). Avoid in late pregnancy; may cause premature closure of ductus arteriosus. May cause elevations of LFTs; d/c if liver disease develops or systemic manifestations occur. Caution in elderly. Anemia may occur; with long-term use, monitor Hgb/Hct if signs or symptoms of anemia develop. May inhibit platelet aggregation and prolong bleeding time; monitor with coagulation disorders. Caution with asthma and avoid with ASA-sensitive asthma. May induce photosensitivity.

ADVERSE REACTIONS: Diarrhea, dyspepsia, abdominal pain, constipation, flatulence, N/V, positive stool guaiac, dizziness, headache, pruritus, rash, tinnitus, edema.

INTERACTIONS: Caution with warfarin and other protein bound drugs. May decrease natriuretic effect of furosemide and thiazides; possible renal failure risk. May elevate lithium and methotrexate levels. May diminish antihypertensive effect of ACE inhibitors. Avoid concomitant ASA. May increase risk of GI bleeding with concomitant use of oral corticosteroids, anticoagulants or alcohol.

PREGNANCY: Category C, not for use in nursing.

MECHANISM OF ACTION: NSAID (naphthylalkanone derivative); suspected to inhibit prostaglandin synthesis, exerts anti-inflammatory, analgesic, and antipyretic actions.

PHARMACOKINETICS: Absorption: Well-absorbed (GIT). PO administration of variable doses resulted in different parameters. **Distribution:** Plasma protein binding (>99%). **Metabolism:** Liver (extensive biotransformation), 6-methoxy-2-naphthylacetic acid (active metabolite). **Elimination:** Urine (approximately 80%), feces (9%); $T_{1/2}$=24 hrs.

NURSING CONSIDERATIONS

Assessment: Assess LFTs, renal function, CBC, and coagulation profile. Assess for history of CABG surgery, asthma and allergic reactions to ASA or other NSAIDs, active ulceration or chronic inflammation of GI tract, CVD, asthma, alcohol intake, pregnancy/nursing status. Note other diseases/conditions and drug therapies.

Monitoring: Monitor for hypersensitivity reactions, CV thrombotic events, MI, stroke, GI bleeding, asthma, and skin adverse effects. Monitor BP, LFTs, renal function, CBC with differential and platelet count, coagulation profile, ocular effects, and photosensitivity.

Patient Counseling: Counsel about potential side effects; seek medical attention if any develop, especially serious CV events or adverse GI events. Counsel about possible drug interactions and to take as prescribed. Advise women not to use in late pregnancy.

Administration: Oral route. **Storage:** 20-25°C (68-77°F). Dispense in tight, light-resistant container.

NAMENDA   RX
memantine HCl (Forest)

OTHER BRAND NAMES: Namenda XR (Forest)

THERAPEUTIC CLASS: NMDA receptor antagonist

INDICATIONS: Treatment of moderate to severe dementia of the Alzheimer's type.

DOSAGE: *Adults:* (Sol, Tab) Initial: 5mg qd. Titrate: Increase at intervals ≥1 week in 5mg increments to 10mg/day (5mg bid), 15mg/day (5mg and 10mg as separate doses), and 20mg/day (10mg bid). Severe Renal Impairment: (CrCl 5-29mL/min): Target Dose: 5mg bid. (Cap, ER) Initial: 7mg qd. Titrate: Increase at intervals ≥1 week in 7mg increments to 28mg qd. Max: 28mg qd. Severe Renal Impairment (CrCl 5-29mL/min): Target dose: 14mg/day. Switching from Tabs to ER, Caps: Switch from 10mg bid tabs to 28mg qd caps the day following last dose of 10 mg tab. Severe Renal Impairment: Switch from 5mg bid tabs to 14mg qd caps the day following last dose of 5mg tab.

HOW SUPPLIED: Sol: 2mg/mL [360mL]; Tab: 5mg, 10mg; Titration-Pak: 5mg [28^s], 10mg [21^s]. Cap, Extended-Release: 7mg, 14mg, 21mg, 28mg.

WARNINGS/PRECAUTIONS: Use not evaluated with seizure disorders. Conditions that raise urine pH may decrease the urinary elimination resulting in increased plasma levels. Caution in patients with severe hepatic impairment. Consider dose reduction with severe renal impairment.

ADVERSE REACTIONS: Dizziness, headache, constipation, confusion, HTN, coughing, somnolence, hallucination, vomiting, back pain, pain, diarrhea.

INTERACTIONS: Caution with other NMDA antagonists (eg, amantadine, ketamine, dextromethorphan), urinary alkalinizers (eg, carbonic anhydrase inhibitors, sodium bicarbonate). Drugs eliminated via renal (cationic system) mechanism, including HCTZ, triamterene, metformin, cimetidine, ranitidine, quinidine, nicotine, may alter levels of both agents.

PREGNANCY: Category B, caution in nursing.

MECHANISM OF ACTION: NMDA receptor antagonist; postulated to exert its therapeutic effect through its action as a low to moderate affinity uncompetitive (open-channel) NMDA receptor antagonist which binds preferentially to the NMDA receptor-operated cation channels.

PHARMACOKINETICS: Absorption: (Sol, Tab) T_{max}=3-7 hrs. (Cap, ER) T_{max}=9-12 hrs. **Distribution:** V_d=9-11L/kg. Plasma protein binding (45%). **Metabolism:** Liver (partial); N-glucuronide conjugate, 6-hydroxy memantine, 1-nitroso-deaminated memantine (metabolites). **Elimination:** Urine (48%, unchanged); $T_{1/2}$=60-80 hrs.

NURSING CONSIDERATIONS

Assessment: Assess for conditions that raise urine pH, presence of a seizure disorder, renal/hepatic impairment, pregnancy/nursing status, and for possible drug interactions.

Monitoring: Monitor renal/hepatic function and for adverse events.

Patient Counseling: (Cap, ER; Sol; Tab) Instruct to take as prescribed. Inform about possible side effects and instruct to notify physician if any develop. (Cap, ER) Instruct to swallow cap whole or inform that cap may be opened and sprinkled on applesauce and the entire contents should be consumed. Inform that caps should not be divided, chewed, or crushed and can be taken with/without food.

Administration: Oral route. Refer to PI for instructions for oral solution. **Storage:** 25°C (77°F); excursions permitted to 15-30°C (59-86°F).

NAPRELAN   RX
naproxen sodium (Shionogi)

NSAIDs may increase risk of serious cardiovascular thrombotic events, myocardial infarction (MI), and stroke; increased risk with duration of use and with cardiovascular disease (CVD) or risk factors for CVD. Increased risk of serious GI adverse events (eg, bleeding, ulceration, and stomach/intestinal perforation) that can be fatal and occur anytime during use without warning symptoms; elderly patients are at a greater risk. Contraindicated for treatment of perioperative pain in the setting of coronary artery bypass graft (CABG) surgery.

THERAPEUTIC CLASS: NSAID

INDICATIONS: Treatment of rheumatoid arthritis (RA), osteoarthritis (OA), ankylosing spondylitis (AS), tendinitis, bursitis, acute gout, and primary dysmenorrhea. Relief of mild to moderate pain.

DOSAGE: *Adults:* RA/OA/AS: Initial: 750mg or 1g qd. Titrate: Adjust dose/frequency up or down depending on clinical response; may increase to 1.5g qd for limited periods if patient can tolerate lower doses well. Pain/Primary Dysmenorrhea/Tendinitis/Bursitis: Initial: 1g qd (or 1.5g qd for a limited period). Max: 1g/day thereafter. Acute Gout: 1st Day: 1-1.5g qd. Succeeding Days: 1g qd until attack subsides. Elderly/Renal/Hepatic Impairment: Start at lower end of dosing range.

HOW SUPPLIED: Tab, Controlled-Release: 375mg, 500mg, 750mg

CONTRAINDICATIONS: History of asthma, urticaria, or allergic-type reactions with aspirin (ASA) or other NSAIDs. Treatment of perioperative pain in the setting of CABG surgery.

WARNINGS/PRECAUTIONS: Use lowest effective dose for the shortest duration possible. May cause HTN or worsen preexisting HTN; monitor BP closely. Fluid retention and edema reported; caution with fluid retention or heart failure. Caution with prior history of ulcer disease, GI bleeding, or risk factors for GI bleeding (eg, prolonged NSAID therapy, older age, poor general health status); monitor for GI ulceration/bleeding and d/c if serious GI event occurs. Renal injury reported with long-term use; increased risk with renal/hepatic impairment, heart failure, and elderly. Not recommended with advanced renal disease or moderate to severe renal impairment (CrCl <30mL/min); monitor renal function closely if therapy is initiated. Anaphylactoid reactions may occur. Caution with asthma and avoid with ASA-sensitive asthma and the ASA-triad. May cause serious skin reactions (eg, exfoliative dermatitis, Stevens-Johnson syndrome, toxic epidermal necrolysis); d/c at 1st appearance of skin rash/hypersensitivity. Avoid in late pregnancy; may cause premature closure of ductus arteriosus. Not a substitute for corticosteroids nor treatment for corticosteroid insufficiency; may mask signs of inflammation and fever. May cause elevated LFTs or severe hepatic reactions (eg, jaundice, fulminant hepatitis, liver necrosis, hepatic failure); d/c if liver disease or systemic manifestations occur, and if abnormal LFTs persist/worsen. Anemia reported; monitor Hgb/Hct if anemia develops. May inhibit platelet aggregation and prolong bleeding time; monitor patients with coagulation disorders.

ADVERSE REACTIONS: Cardiovascular thrombotic events, MI, stroke, GI events, headache, dyspepsia, flu syndrome, pain, infection, nausea, diarrhea, constipation, rhinitis, sinusitis, urinary tract infection.

INTERACTIONS: Increased risk of GI bleeding with oral corticosteroids, anticoagulants, alcohol use, and smoking. Risk of renal toxicity with diuretics and ACE inhibitors. Monitor patients receiving anticoagulants. May diminish antihypertensive effect of ACE inhibitors. Not recommended with ASA. May reduce natriuretic effect of loop (eg, furosemide) or thiazide diuretics; monitor for signs of renal failure and diuretic efficacy. May increase lithium levels; monitor for lithium toxicity. May enhance methotrexate toxicity; caution with concomitant use. Synergistic effect on GI bleeding with warfarin.

PREGNANCY: Category C, not for use in nursing.

MECHANISM OF ACTION: NSAID; not established. Inhibition of prostaglandin synthesis thought to be involved in anti-inflammatory effect.

PHARMACOKINETICS: Absorption: Rapid and complete. Bioavailability (95%); (1g qd multiple dose) C_{max}=94mcg/mL, T_{max}=5 hrs, AUC=1448mcg•hr/mL. **Distribution:** V_d=0.16L/kg; plasma protein binding (>99%); found in breast milk. **Metabolism:** Extensive; 6-0-desmethyl naproxen metabolite. **Elimination:** Urine (<1% unchanged, <1% 6-0-desmethyl naproxen, 66-92% conjugates), feces (<5%); $T_{1/2}$=15 hrs.

NURSING CONSIDERATIONS

Assessment: Assess for history of asthma, urticaria, or allergic-type reactions with ASA or other NSAIDs, ASA-triad, CVD, risk factors for CVD, HTN, fluid retention, heart failure, history of ulcer disease, history of/risk factors for GI bleeding, general health status, renal/hepatic function,

N

coagulation disorders, pregnancy/nursing status, and possible drug interactions. Obtain baseline CBC and BP.

Monitoring: Monitor BP, CBC, bleeding time, LFTs, renal function, and chemistry profile periodically. Monitor for GI bleeding/ulceration/perforation, CV thrombotic events, MI, stroke, HTN, fluid retention, edema, and skin/allergic reactions.

Patient Counseling: Inform to seek medical advice if symptoms of CV events (eg, chest pain, SOB, weakness, slurred speech), GI ulceration/bleeding (eg, epigastric pain, dyspepsia, melena, hematemesis), skin/hypersensitivity reactions (eg, rash, blisters, fever, itching), unexplained weight gain or edema, hepatotoxicity (eg, nausea, fatigue, lethargy, pruritus, jaundice, right upper quadrant tenderness, flu-like symptoms), or anaphylactoid reactions (eg, face/throat swelling, difficulty breathing) occur. Instruct to avoid in late pregnancy.

Administration: Oral route. **Storage:** 20-25°C (68-77°F).

NAPROSYN   RX
naproxen sodium (Genentech)

> NSAIDs may increase risk of serious cardiovascular thrombotic events, myocardial infarction (MI), and stroke; increased risk with duration of use and with cardiovascular disease (CVD) or risk factors for CVD. Increased risk of serious GI adverse events (eg, bleeding, ulceration, and stomach/intestinal perforation) that can be fatal and occur anytime during use without warning symptoms; elderly patients are at a greater risk. Contraindicated for treatment of perioperative pain in the setting of coronary artery bypass graft (CABG) surgery.

OTHER BRAND NAMES: Anaprox DS (Genentech) - Anaprox (Genentech) - EC-Naprosyn (Genentech)

THERAPEUTIC CLASS: NSAID

INDICATIONS: Relief of signs and symptoms of rheumatoid arthritis (RA), osteoarthritis (OA), ankylosing spondylitis (AS), and juvenile arthritis (JA). (Naprosyn/Anaprox/Anaprox DS) Relief of signs and symptoms of tendonitis, bursitis, and acute gout, and management of pain and primary dysmenorrhea.

DOSAGE: *Adults:* RA/OA/AS: (Naprosyn) 250mg, 375mg, or 500mg bid. (EC-Naprosyn) 375mg or 500mg bid. (Anaprox) 275mg bid. (Anaprox DS) 550mg bid. Titrate: Adjust dose/frequency up or down depending on clinical response; may increase to 1500mg/day for ≤6 months if patient can tolerate lower doses well. Pain/Dysmenorrhea/Tendonitis/Bursitis: (Anaprox/Anaprox DS) Initial: 550mg, then 550mg q12h or 275mg q6-8h PRN. Max: 1375mg/day initially, then 1100mg/day thereafter. Acute Gout: (Naprosyn) Initial: 750mg, then 250mg q8h until attack subsides. (Anaprox) Initial: 825mg, then 275mg q8h until attack subsides. Elderly/Renal/Hepatic Impairment: Start at lower end of dosing range.
Pediatrics: ≥2 yrs: JA: (Sus) 5mg/kg bid. Refer to PI for additional information. Renal/Hepatic Impairment: Start at lower end of dosing range.

HOW SUPPLIED: Sus: (Naprosyn) 125mg/5mL; Tab: (Naprosyn) 250mg*, 375mg, 500mg*, (Anaprox) 275mg, (Anaprox DS) 550mg*; Tab, Delayed-Release: (EC-Naprosyn) 375mg, 500mg *scored

CONTRAINDICATIONS: History of asthma, urticaria, or other allergic-type reactions with aspirin (ASA) or other NSAIDs. Treatment of perioperative pain in the setting of CABG surgery.

WARNINGS/PRECAUTIONS: Use lowest effective dose for the shortest duration possible. May cause HTN or worsen preexisting HTN; monitor BP closely. Fluid retention and edema reported; caution with fluid retention, HTN, or heart failure. Caution with prior history of ulcer disease, GI bleeding, risk factors for GI bleeding (eg, prolonged NSAID therapy, smoking, older age, poor general health status); monitor for GI ulceration/bleeding and d/c if serious GI event occurs. May exacerbate inflammatory bowel disease (IBD) (eg, ulcerative colitis, Crohn's disease). Renal injury reported with long-term use; increased risk with renal/hepatic impairment, hypovolemia, heart failure, salt depletion, and in elderly. Not recommended with advanced renal disease or CrCl <30mL/min; monitor renal function closely. D/C if renal injury occurs. Anaphylactoid reactions may occur. Caution with asthma and avoid with ASA-sensitive asthma and the ASA-triad. May cause serious skin adverse events (eg, exfoliative dermatitis, Stevens-Johnson syndrome, toxic epidermal necrolysis); d/c at 1st appearance of skin rash/hypersensitivity. Avoid in late pregnancy; may cause premature closure of ductus arteriosus. Not a substitute for corticosteroids or for the treatment for corticosteroid insufficiency; may mask signs of inflammation and fever. Periodically monitor Hgb if initial Hgb ≤10g and receiving long-term therapy. Perform ophthalmic studies if visual changes/disturbances occur. May cause elevations of LFTs or severe hepatic reactions (eg, jaundice, fulminant hepatitis, liver necrosis, and hepatic failure); d/c if liver disease or systemic manifestations occur, or if abnormal LFTs persist/worsen. Caution with chronic alcoholic liver disease and other diseases with decreased/abnormal plasma proteins if high doses are administered; dosage adjustment may be required. Anemia reported; monitor Hgb/Hct if anemia develops. May inhibit platelet aggregation and prolong bleeding time; monitor patients with coagulation disorders. Monitor CBC and chemistry profile periodically with long-term treatment. (Sus, Anaprox/Anaprox DS) Contains sodium; caution with severely restricted sodium intake. (EC-Naprosyn) Not recommended for initial treatment of acute pain.

ADVERSE REACTIONS: Cardiovascular thrombotic events, MI, stroke, GI adverse events, edema, drowsiness, dizziness, constipation, heartburn, abdominal pain, nausea, headache, tinnitus, dyspnea, pruritus.

INTERACTIONS: Avoid with other naproxen products. Not recommended with ASA. Risk of renal toxicity with diuretics and ACE inhibitors. Coadministration may decrease efficacy of thiazide or loop (eg, furosemide) diuretics; monitor for signs of renal failure and diuretic efficacy. May diminish antihypertensive effect of ACE inhibitors and β-blockers (eg, propranolol). May enhance methotrexate toxicity; caution with concomitant use. May increase lithium levels; monitor for lithium toxicity. Increased risk of GI bleeding with SSRIs, oral corticosteroids, anticoagulants, and alcohol; monitor carefully. Synergistic effect on GI bleeding with warfarin. Potential for interaction with other albumin-bound drugs (eg, coumarin-type anticoagulants, sulfonylureas, hydantoins, other NSAIDs, ASA); observe for possible dose adjustment with hydantoins, sulfonamides or sulfonylureas. Probenecid significantly increases plasma levels and $T_{1/2}$. Antacids, sucralfate, and cholestyramine can delay absorption. (EC-Naprosyn) Not recommended with H_2-blockers, sucralfate, or intensive antacid therapy.

PREGNANCY: Category C, not for use in nursing.

MECHANISM OF ACTION: NSAID; not established. May be related to prostaglandin synthetase inhibition.

PHARMACOKINETICS: Absorption: Rapid and complete. Bioavailability (95%). Naprosyn: C_{max}=97.4mcg/mL, AUC=767mcg•hr/mL, T_{max}=2-4 hrs (tab), 1-4 hrs (sus). EC-Naprosyn: C_{max}=94.9mcg/mL, AUC=845mcg•hr/mL, T_{max}=4 hrs. Anaprox: T_{max}=1-2 hrs. **Distribution:** V_d=0.16L/kg; plasma protein binding (>99%); found in breast milk. **Metabolism:** Liver (extensive); 6-0-desmethyl naproxen (metabolite). **Elimination:** Urine (95%; <1% unchanged, <1% 6-0-desmethyl naproxen, 66-92% conjugates), feces (≤3%); $T_{1/2}$=12-17 hrs.

NURSING CONSIDERATIONS

Assessment: Assess for history of asthma, urticaria, or allergic-type reactions with ASA or other NSAIDs, ASA-triad, CVD, risk factors for CVD, HTN, fluid retention, heart failure, salt restriction, history of ulcer disease, history of/risk factors for GI bleeding, general health status, history of IBD, renal/hepatic impairment, hypovolemia, decreased/abnormal plasma proteins, coagulation disorders, tobacco/alcohol use, pregnancy/nursing status, and for possible drug interactions. Obtain baseline CBC and BP.

Monitoring: Monitor BP, CBC, LFTs, renal function, and chemistry profile periodically. Monitor for GI bleeding/ulceration/perforation, cardiovascular thrombotic events, MI, stroke, HTN, fluid retention, edema, and skin/allergic reactions.

Patient Counseling: Inform to seek medical advice if symptoms of cardiovascular events (eg, chest pain, SOB, weakness, slurring of speech), GI ulceration/bleeding (eg, epigastric pain, dyspepsia, melena, hematemesis), skin/hypersensitivity reactions (eg, rash, itching, blisters, fever), unexplained weight gain or edema, hepatotoxicity (eg, nausea, fatigue, lethargy, pruritus, jaundice, right upper quadrant tenderness, flu-like symptoms), or anaphylactoid reactions (eg, difficulty breathing, face/throat swelling) occur. Instruct to avoid in late pregnancy. Instruct to use caution when performing activities that require alertness if drowsiness, dizziness, vertigo, or depression occurs.

Administration: Oral route. (EC-Naprosyn) Do not chew, crush, or break. (Sus) Shake gently before use. **Storage:** 15-30°C (59-86°F). (Sus) Avoid excessive heat, >40°C (104°F).

NARDIL RX
phenelzine sulfate (Parke-Davis)

Antidepressants increased the risk of suicidal thinking and behavior (suicidality) in children, adolescents, and young adults in short-term studies of major depressive disorder and other psychiatric disorders. Monitor and observe closely for clinical worsening, suicidality, or unusual changes in behavior in patients who are started on antidepressant therapy. Not approved for use in pediatric patients.

THERAPEUTIC CLASS: Monoamine oxidase inhibitor

INDICATIONS: Treatment of atypical, nonendogenous or neurotic depression not responsive to other antidepressants.

DOSAGE: *Adults:* Initial: 15mg tid. Titrate: Increase to 60-90mg/day at a fairly rapid pace consistent with patient tolerance until maximum benefit. Maint: Reduce slowly over several weeks to 15mg qd or qod.

HOW SUPPLIED: Tab: 15mg

CONTRAINDICATIONS: Pheochromocytoma, congestive heart failure (CHF), severe renal impairment or renal disease, history of liver disease, and abnormal LFTs. Concomitant use of meperidine, guanethidine, sympathomimetic drugs (eg, amphetamines, cocaine, methylpheni-date, dopamine, epinephrine, norepinephrine), or related compounds (eg, methyldopa, L-dopa, L-tryptophan, L-tyrosine, phenylalanine), high tyramine- or dopamine-containing food, excessive caffeine and chocolate, dextromethorphan, CNS depressants (eg, alcohol, certain narcotics), local anesthesia containing sympathomimetic vasoconstrictors, and spinal anesthesia. Elective surgery requiring general anesthesia. ≥14 days should elapse between d/c of therapy and start of another antidepressant (including other MAOIs), buspirone HCl, bupropion HCl, and serotonin reuptake inhibitor (except fluoxetine). Allow ≥5 weeks between d/c of fluoxetine and initiation of therapy.

WARNINGS/PRECAUTIONS: Hypertensive crises and intracranial bleeding reported; monitor BP frequently and d/c use if palpitation or frequent headaches occur. Postural hypotension may occur. Caution with epilepsy, diabetes mellitus (DM), and patients on insulin or hypoglycemic agents. Hypomania and agitation reported following long-term use. May cause excessive stimulation in schizophrenics.

ADVERSE REACTIONS: Dizziness, headache, drowsiness, sleep disturbances, fatigue, weakness, tremors, constipation, dry mouth, GI disturbances, elevated serum transaminases, weight gain, postural hypotension, edema, sexual disturbances.

INTERACTIONS: See Contraindications. Avoid with sauerkraut, any spoiled or improperly refrigerated, handled, or stored protein-rich foods such as meats, fish, and dairy products, and over-the-counter (OTC) cold and cough preparations, nasal decongestants (tabs, drops, or spray), hay-fever/sinus/asthma inhalant medications, antiappetite medicines, weight-reducing preparations, and "pep" pills. Reduce dose of barbiturates. Caution with rauwolfia alkaloids. Exaggerated hypotensive effects with antihypertensives (eg, thiazides, β-blockers); use with caution. May potentiate hypoglycemic agents; requirements for insulin or oral hypoglycemic agents may be decreased.

PREGNANCY: Safety not known in pregnancy/nursing.

MECHANISM OF ACTION: MAOI; inhibits MAO activity.

PHARMACOKINETICS: Absorption: (30mg) C_{max}=19.8ng/mL, T_{max}=43 mins. **Metabolism:** Extensive; oxidation via MAO; acetylation (minor). **Elimination:** Urine (73%); $T_{1/2}$=11.6 hrs (30mg).

NURSING CONSIDERATIONS

Assessment: Assess for pheochromocytoma, CHF, history of liver disease, bipolar disorder risk (detailed psychiatric history, family history of suicide, bipolar disorder, and depression), epilepsy, schizophrenia, manic-depressive state, DM, renal/hepatic impairment, drug hypersensitivity, pregnancy/nursing status, and possible drug interactions.

Monitoring: Monitor for clinical worsening, suicidality, unusual changes in behavior, hypertensive crisis, postural hypotension, hypomania, increased insulin sensitivity, increased psychosis, and activation of mania. Monitor BP frequently.

Patient Counseling: Inform patients, families, and caregivers about benefits/risks of therapy, including potential for clinical worsening and suicide risk. Instruct to notify physician if symptoms/adverse reactions occur during treatment or when adjusting the dose (eg, palpitations, tachycardia). Counsel to avoid concomitant intake of alcohol, foods with high tyramine content, certain OTC (eg, dextrometorphan) and prescription drugs, excessive quantities of caffeine and chocolate.

Administration: Oral route. **Storage:** 15-30°C (59-86°F).

NASACORT AQ   RX
triamcinolone acetonide (Sanofi-Aventis)

THERAPEUTIC CLASS: Corticosteroid

INDICATIONS: Treatment of nasal symptoms of seasonal and perennial allergic rhinitis in adults and children ≥2 yrs.

DOSAGE: *Adults:* Initial/Max: 2 sprays/nostril qd. Titrate to minimum effective dose. Reduce dose to 1 spray/nostril qd if max benefit/symptom control achieved. Elderly: Start at lower end of dosing range.
Pediatrics: ≥12 yrs: Initial/Max: 2 sprays/nostril qd. Titrate to minimum effective dose. Reduce dose to 1 spray/nostril qd if max benefit/symptom control achieved. 6-12 yrs: Initial: 1 spray/nostril qd. Max: 2 sprays/nostril qd. Reduce dose to 1 spray/nostril qd if symptoms controlled. 2-5 yrs: Initial/Max: 1 spray/nostril qd.

HOW SUPPLIED: Spray: 55mcg/spray [16.5g]

WARNINGS/PRECAUTIONS: May cause local nasal effects (eg, epistaxis, *Candida* infections of the nose and pharynx, nasal septum perforation, impaired wound healing). Avoid with recent nasal ulcers, surgery, or trauma. Glaucoma and/or cataracts may develop; monitor closely in patients with change in vision, history of increased intraocular pressure (IOP), glaucoma, and/ or cataracts. May increase susceptibility to infections; caution with active/quiescent tuberculosis (TB), ocular herpes simplex, or untreated bacterial, fungal, and systemic viral or parasitic infections. Avoid exposure to chickenpox and measles. D/C slowly if hypercorticism and adrenal suppression occur. Risk of adrenal insufficiency and withdrawal symptoms when replacing systemic corticosteroids with topical corticosteroids. Potential for reduced growth velocity in pediatrics. Caution in elderly.

ADVERSE REACTIONS: Pharyngitis, epistaxis, increased cough, flu syndrome, bronchitis, dyspepsia, tooth disorder, headache, pharyngolaryngeal pain, nasopharyngitis, upper abdominal pain, diarrhea, asthma, rash, excoriation.

PREGNANCY: Category C, caution in nursing.

MECHANISM OF ACTION: Corticosteroid; mechanism not established. Shown to have wide range of actions on multiple cell types (eg, mast cells, eosinophils, neutrophils, macrophages, lymphocytes) and mediators (eg, histamine, eicosanoids, leukotrienes, cytokines) involved in inflammation.

PHARMACOKINETICS: Absorption: Minimal; C_{max}=0.5ng/mL; T_{max}=1.5 hrs; AUC (110mcg, 400mcg)=1.4ng•hr/mL, 4.7ng•hr/mL. **Distribution:** V_d=99.5L (IV). **Elimination:** $T_{1/2}$=3.1 hrs.

NURSING CONSIDERATIONS

Assessment: Assess for history of hypersensitivity, increased IOP, glaucoma or cataracts, recent nasal ulcers/surgery/trauma, active or quiescent TB, untreated local or systemic infections, ocular herpes simplex, suppressed immune system, asthma or other conditions requiring chronic systemic corticosteroid therapy, and pregnancy/nursing status.

Monitoring: Monitor for acute adrenal insufficiency, hypercorticism, chickenpox, measles, suppression of growth velocity in children, nasal septum perforation, vision changes, glaucoma, cataracts, increased IOP, epistaxis, wound healing, worsening of infections, hypoadrenalism (in infants born to mothers who recieved corticosteroids during therapy), and other adverse reactions. Examine periodically for evidence of nasal or pharyngeal *Candida* infections.

Patient Counseling: Counsel to take as directed at regular intervals. Inform of possible local nasal effects, cataracts, glaucoma, and immunosuppression. Advise not to use with recent nasal ulcers, surgery, or trauma until healing has occurred. Instruct to avoid exposure to chickenpox and measles. Instruct to consult physician if symptoms do not improve, the condition worsens, or change in vision occurs. Advise to avoid spraying into eyes.

Administration: Intranasal route. Shake well before each use. Refer to PI for proper administration. **Storage:** 20-25°C (68-77°F).

NASONEX   RX

mometasone furoate monohydrate (Schering Corporation)

THERAPEUTIC CLASS: Corticosteroid

INDICATIONS: Treatment of nasal symptoms of seasonal and perennial allergic rhinitis and relief of nasal congestion associated with seasonal allergic rhinitis in patients ≥2 yrs. Prophylaxis of nasal symptoms of seasonal allergic rhinitis in patients ≥12 yrs. Treatment of nasal polyps in patients ≥18 yrs.

DOSAGE: *Adults:* Treatment (Seasonal/Perennial Allergic Rhinitis)/Prophylaxis and Treatment of Nasal Congestion (Seasonal Allergic Rhinitis): 2 sprays/nostril qd. Prophylaxis may start 2-4 weeks before pollen season. Nasal Polyps: 2 sprays/nostril qd-bid.
Pediatrics: ≥12 yrs: Treatment (Seasonal/Perennial Allergic Rhinitis)/Prophylaxis and Treatment of Nasal Congestion (Seasonal Allergic Rhinitis): 2 sprays/nostril qd. Prophylaxis may start 2-4 weeks before pollen season. 2-11 yrs: Treatment (Seasonal/Perennial Allergic Rhinitis)/Nasal Congestion (Seasonal Allergic Rhinitis): 1 spray/nostril qd.

HOW SUPPLIED: Spray: 50mcg/spray [17g]

WARNINGS/PRECAUTIONS: Local nasal effects (eg, epistaxis, *Candida* infections of nose and pharynx, nasal septum perforation, impaired wound healing) may occur; d/c when infection occurs. Glaucoma and/or cataracts may develop; monitor closely in patients with change in vision, history of increased intraocular pressure (IOP), glaucoma, and/or cataracts. D/C if hypersensitivity reactions, including instances of wheezing, occur. May increase susceptibility to infections; caution with active/quiescent tuberculosis (TB), ocular herpes simplex, or untreated bacterial, fungal, and systemic viral infections. Hypercorticism and adrenal suppression may appear when used at higher than recommended doses or in susceptible individuals at recommended doses; d/c slowly if such changes occur. May reduce growth velocity of pediatrics; monitor growth routinely.

ADVERSE REACTIONS: Headache, viral infection, pharyngitis, epistaxis/blood-tinged mucus, cough, upper respiratory tract infection, dysmenorrhea, musculoskeletal pain, sinusitis, N/V.

INTERACTIONS: May increase plasma concentrations with ketoconazole.

PREGNANCY: Category C, caution with nursing.

MECHANISM OF ACTION: Corticosteroid; not established. Demonstrates anti-inflammatory properties and is shown to have wide range of effects on multiple cell types (eg, mast cells, eosinophils, neutrophils, macrophages, lymphocytes) and mediators (eg, histamine, eicosanoids, leukotrienes, cytokines) involved in inflammation.

PHARMACOKINETICS: Absorption: Bioavailability (<1%). **Distribution:** Plasma protein binding (98-99%). **Metabolism:** Liver (extensive) via CYP3A4. **Elimination:** Bile (as metabolites); urine (limited extent); (IV) $T_{1/2}$=5.8 hrs.

NURSING CONSIDERATIONS

Assessment: Assess for previous hypersensitivity, active/quiescent TB, infections, ocular herpes simplex, change in vision, history of IOP, glaucoma or cataracts, recent nasal septum ulcers, nasal surgery/trauma, pregnancy/nursing status, and possible drug interactions.

Monitoring: Monitor for acute adrenal insufficiency, hypercorticism, nasal or pharyngeal *Candida* infections, suppression of growth velocity in children, hypersensitivity reactions, wheezing, nasal septum perforation, changes in vision, glaucoma, cataracts, increased IOP, epistaxis, wound healing, worsening of infections, and other adverse reactions.

Patient Counseling: Advise to take as directed at regular intervals and not to increase prescribed dosage. Inform patients that treatment may be associated with adverse reactions (eg, epistaxis, nasal septum perforation, *Candida* infection). Inform that glaucoma and/or cataracts may develop. Counsel to avoid exposure to chickenpox or measles and to immediately consult a physician if exposed. Contact physician if symptoms worsen or do not improve. Supervise young children during administration. Advise patient to take missed dose as soon as remembered. Counsel on proper priming and administration techniques.

Administration: Intranasal route. Refer to PI for proper administration. **Storage:** 25°C (77°F); excursions permitted to 15-30°C (59-86°F). Protect from light.

NATACYN   RX
natamycin (Alcon)

THERAPEUTIC CLASS: Tetraene polyene antifungal

INDICATIONS: Treatment of fungal blepharitis, conjunctivitis, and keratitis caused by susceptible organisms. Effectiveness as a single agent in fungal endophthalmitis has not been established.

DOSAGE: *Adults:* Keratitis: 1 drop q1-2h for 3-4 days, then 1 drop 6-8 times daily for 14-21 days or until the resolution of infection. Reduce dose at 4-7 day intervals. Blepharitis/Conjunctivitis: 1 drop 4-6 times daily.

HOW SUPPLIED: Sus: 5% [15mL]

WARNINGS/PRECAUTIONS: For topical ophthalmic use only, not for injection. Failure of improvement of keratitis following 7-10 days of administration suggests that the infection may be caused by a microorganism not susceptible to natamycin. Continuation of therapy should be based on clinical re-evaluation and additional laboratory studies. Adherence of suspension to areas of epithelial ulceration or retention of the suspension in the fornices occurs regularly.

ADVERSE REACTIONS: Allergic reaction, change in vision, chest pain, corneal opacity, dyspnea, eye discomfort, eye edema, eye hyperemia, eye irritation, eye pain, foreign body sensation, paresthesia, tearing.

PREGNANCY: Category C, caution in nursing.

MECHANISM OF ACTION: Tetraene polyene antifungal; binds to sterol moiety of the fungal cell membrane. Polyenesterol complex alters permeability of membrane to produce depletion of essential cellular constituents.

PHARMACOKINETICS: Absorption: GI (poor).

NURSING CONSIDERATIONS

Assessment: Assess proper diagnosis through clinical and lab evaluation (eg, smear and culture of corneal scrapings). Assess use in pregnant/nursing females.

Monitoring: Monitor for clinical response. In patients with keratitis, reassess therapy if no response within 7 to 10 days.

Patient Counseling: Advise not to touch dropper tip to any surface to avoid contamination of suspension. Instruct not to wear contact lenses if have signs/symptoms of fungal blepharitis, conjunctivitis, and keratitis.

Administration: Ocular route. Shake well before use. **Storage:** 2-24°C (36-75°F). Do not freeze. Avoid exposure to light and excessive heat.

NATAZIA
estradiol valerate - dienogest (Bayer Healthcare)

RX

Cigarette smoking increases risk of serious cardiovascular (CV) events from combination oral contraceptive (COC) use. Risk increases with age (>35 yrs) and with the number of cigarettes smoked. Should not be used by women who are >35 yrs and smoke.

THERAPEUTIC CLASS: Estrogen/progestogen combination

INDICATIONS: Prevention of pregnancy.

DOSAGE: *Adults:* 1 tab qd at the same time for 28 days, then repeat. Take in the order directed on the blister pack. Start on Day 1 of menses or not earlier than 4 weeks postpartum for postpartum women who do not breastfeed or after 2nd trimester abortion. When starting therapy, use a nonhormonal back-up contraceptive method for first 9 days of therapy. Regard as a missed tab if vomiting/diarrhea occurs within 3-4 hrs after taking a colored tab. Refer to PI when switching from combination hormonal method or progestin-only method.
Pediatrics: Postpubertal: 1 tab qd at the same time for 28 days, then repeat. Take in the order directed on the blister pack. Start on Day 1 of menses or not earlier than 4 weeks postpartum for postpartum women who do not breastfeed or after 2nd trimester abortion. When starting therapy, use a nonhormonal back-up contraceptive method for first 9 days of therapy. Regard as a missed tab if vomiting/diarrhea occurs within 3-4 hrs after taking a colored tab. Refer to PI when switching from combination hormonal method or progestin-only method.

HOW SUPPLIED: Tab: (Estradiol valerate) 1mg, 3mg; Tab: (Estradiol valerate-Dienogest) 2mg-2mg, 2mg-3mg

CONTRAINDICATIONS: High risk of arterial/venous thrombotic diseases (eg, smoking if >35 yrs, history/presence of deep vein thrombosis/pulmonary embolism, cerebrovascular disease, coronary artery disease, thrombogenic valvular or thrombogenic rhythm diseases of the heart [eg, subacute bacterial endocarditis with valvular disease, or atrial fibrillation], inherited/acquired hypercoagulopathies, uncontrolled HTN, diabetes mellitus [DM] with vascular disease, headaches with focal neurological symptoms or migraine with/without aura if >35 yrs), undiagnosed abnormal uterine bleeding, history/presence of breast or other estrogen-/progestin-sensitive cancer, benign/malignant liver tumors, liver disease, pregnancy.

WARNINGS/PRECAUTIONS: Increased risk of venous thromboembolism and arterial thrombosis (eg, stroke, MI). D/C if arterial or deep venous thrombotic event occurs. D/C at least 4 weeks before and through 2 weeks after major surgery or other surgeries known to have an elevated risk of thromboembolism. Caution with CV disease risk factors. D/C if there is unexplained loss of vision, proptosis, diplopia, papilledema, or retinal vascular lesions; evaluate for retinal vein thrombosis immediately. May increase risk of breast or cervical cancer, intraepithelial neoplasia, gallbladder disease, hepatic adenomas, and hepatocellular carcinoma; d/c if jaundice develops. Cholestasis may occur with history of pregnancy-related cholestasis. Increased BP reported; d/c if BP rises significantly. May decrease glucose tolerance; monitor prediabetic and diabetic women. Consider alternative contraception with uncontrolled dyslipidemia. Increased risk of pancreatitis with hypertriglyceridemia or family history thereof. If new headaches develop that are recurrent, persistent, or severe, evaluate cause and d/c if indicated. May increase frequency or severity of migraines. May cause bleeding irregularities (eg, breakthrough bleeding, spotting, amenorrhea); rule out pregnancy or malignancies. Not for use as a test for pregnancy. Caution with history of depression; d/c if depression recurs to serious degree. May change results of laboratory tests (eg, coagulation factors, lipids, glucose tolerance, binding proteins). May induce/exacerbate angioedema in patients with hereditary angioedema. Chloasma may occur; avoid sun exposure or UV radiation in women with a tendency to chloasma. Not indicated for use before menarche.

ADVERSE REACTIONS: N/V, headache, migraine, irregular menstruation, metrorrhagia, breast pain/discomfort/tenderness, acne, increased weight.

INTERACTIONS: Agents that induce certain enzymes, including CYP3A4 may decrease contraceptive efficacy and/or increase breakthrough bleeding; consider alternative contraceptive or a back-up method when using moderate or weak inducers and continue back-up contraception for 28 days after d/c of the inducer. Avoid with strong CYP3A4 inducers (eg, carbamazepine, phenytoin, rifampicin, St. John's wort) and for at least 28 days after d/c of these inducers. Strong CYP3A4 inhibitors (eg, ketoconazole) and moderate CYP3A4 inhibitors (eg, erythromycin) may increase dienogest and estradiol levels. Other CYP3A4 inhibitors (eg, azole antifungals, cimetidine, verapamil, macrolides) may increase dienogest levels. Significant changes (increase/decrease) in plasma estrogen and progestin levels may occur with some HIV/Hepatitis C virus protease inhibitors or with non-nucleoside reverse transcriptase inhibitors. Pregnancy reported with antibiotics. May decrease plasma concentrations of lamotrigine and reduce seizure control;

may need dosage adjustment. May need to increase dose of thyroid hormone in patients on thyroid hormone replacement therapy.

PREGNANCY: Contraindicated in pregnancy, not for use in nursing.

MECHANISM OF ACTION: Estrogen/progestin combination oral contraceptive; acts primarily by suppressing ovulation. Also causes cervical mucus changes that inhibit sperm penetration and endometrial changes that reduce the likelihood of implantation.

PHARMACOKINETICS: Absorption: Dienogest: Bioavailability (91%); C_{max}=91.7ng/mL, T_{max}=1 hrs, $AUC_{(0-24\ hr)}$=964ng/mL; Estradiol: C_{max}=73.3pg/mL, T_{max}=6 hrs, $AUC_{(0-24\ hr)}$=1301pg•hr/mL. **Distribution:** Estradiol: V_d=1.2L/kg (IV); bound to sex hormone-binding globulin (38%) and albumin (60%); found in breast milk. Dienogest: V_d=46L (IV); bound to albumin (90%); found in breast milk. **Metabolism:** Estradiol: Extensive 1st pass effect; CYP3A; estrone and its sulfate or glucuronide conjugates (main metabolites); Dienogest: extensive (hydroxylation, conjugation), CYP3A4 (main). **Elimination:** Estradiol: Urine (main), feces (10%), $T_{1/2}$=14 hrs; Dienogest: Renal (main); $T_{1/2}$=11 hrs.

NURSING CONSIDERATIONS

Assessment: Assess for risk factors of arterial or venous thrombotic diseases, current or history of DVT or pulmonary embolism, cerebrovascular disease, CAD, pregnancy/nursing status, or any other condition where treatment is contraindicated or cautioned. Assess for possible drug interactions.

Monitoring: Monitor for signs/symptoms of CV disorders (eg, MI, stroke, venous thrombosis), breast cancer, liver tumors or liver disease (eg, jaundice), gallbladder disease, retinal vascular thrombosis, elevations in BP, headache, pancreatitis, migraine aggravation, depression, bleeding irregularities and amenorrhea. Monitor thyroid function in patients on thyroid replacement therapy. Monitor liver function. Monitor glucose levels in prediabetic and diabetic women.

Patient Counseling: Counsel that cigarette smoking increases the risk of serious CV events and to avoid use in women who are >35 yrs old and smoke. Inform that therapy does not protect against HIV infection and other STDs. Advise to take 1 tab daily by mouth at the same time every day in the exact order noted on the blister. Instruct what to do in the event pills are missed. Inform of possible drug interactions. Advise to notify physician if breastfeeding or planning to breastfeed. Counsel any patient who starts medication postpartum, and who has not yet had a period, to use an additional method of contraception until have taken medication for 9 consecutive days. Inform that amenorrhea may occur. Instruct to avoid exposure to sun or UV radiation in women with tendency to chloasma.

Administration: Oral route. Do not skip a dose or delay intake by >12 hrs. **Storage:** 25°C (77°F); excursions permitted to 15-30°C (59-86°F).

NATRECOR   RX
nesiritide (Scios Inc.)

THERAPEUTIC CLASS: Human B-type natriuretic peptide

INDICATIONS: Treatment of acutely decompensated congestive heart failure with dyspnea at rest or with minimal activity.

DOSAGE: *Adults:* 2mcg/kg IV bolus over 60 sec, then 0.01mcg/kg/min continuous IV infusion. Refer to PI for Weight-Adjusted Bolus Volume and Infusion Flow Rate.

HOW SUPPLIED: Inj: 1.5mg

CONTRAINDICATIONS: As primary therapy for cardiogenic shock or systolic BP (SBP) <90mmHg.

WARNINGS/PRECAUTIONS: Avoid with low cardiac filling pressures. Use precaution for parenteral administration of protein pharmaceuticals or *Escherichia coli*-derived products; may cause allergic or untoward reaction. Avoid when vasodilators are inappropriate (eg, significant valvular stenosis, restrictive/obstructive cardiomyopathy, constrictive pericarditis, pericardial tamponade, conditions where cardiac output is dependent on venous return or for patients suspected to have low cardiac filling pressures). May affect renal function; azotemia reported in severe heart failure. May cause hypotension; reduce dose or d/c use if hypotension occurs. Increased risk of hypotension with drugs that may cause hypotension (eg, oral ACE inhibitors). Caution with BP <100mmHg at baseline.

ADVERSE REACTIONS: N/V, bradycardia, angina pectoris, abdominal pain, insomnia, hypotension, headache, nausea, back pain, ventricular tachycardia, ventricular extrasystoles, dizziness, anxiety.

PREGNANCY: Category C, caution in nursing.

MECHANISM OF ACTION: Human B-type natriuretic peptide; binds to the particulate guanylate cyclase receptor of vascular smooth muscle and endothelial cells, leading to increased intracellular concentrations of cGMP and smooth muscle relaxation.

PHARMACOKINETICS: Distribution: V_d=0.19L/kg. **Elimination:** Renal; $T_{1/2}$=18 min.

NURSING CONSIDERATIONS

Assessment: Assess for cardiogenic shock or SBP <90mmHg, low cardiac filling pressures, conditions where vasodilators are inappropriate, pregnancy/nursing status, possible drug interactions, and known hypersensitivity to drug or any of its components.

Monitoring: Monitor renal function, HR, BP, cardiac index/status, and hemodynamic parameters. Monitor for hypotension.

Patient Counseling: Counsel about potential adverse effects of drug.

Administration: IV route. Refer to PI for preparation and administration instructions. **Storage:** <25°C. Do not freeze. Protect from light. Reconstituted Sol: 2-25°C (36-77°F) for up to 24 hrs.

NATROBA   RX
spinosad (ParaPRO/Pernix Therapeutics)

THERAPEUTIC CLASS: Pediculocide

INDICATIONS: Topical treatment of head lice infestation in patients ≥4 yrs.

DOSAGE: *Adults:* Apply ≤120mL to adequately cover dry scalp and hair. Leave on for 10 min, then thoroughly rinse off with warm water. Apply 2nd treatment if live lice seen 7 days after the 1st. *Pediatrics:* ≥4 yrs: Apply ≤120mL to adequately cover dry scalp and hair. Leave on for 10 min, then thoroughly rinse off with warm water. Apply 2nd treatment if live lice seen 7 days after the 1st.

HOW SUPPLIED: Sus: 0.9% [120mL]

WARNINGS/PRECAUTIONS: Not for oral, ophthalmic, or intravaginal use. Contains benzyl alcohol; avoid in neonates and infants <6 months.

ADVERSE REACTIONS: Application site erythema, irritation, ocular erythema.

PREGNANCY: Category B, caution in nursing.

MECHANISM OF ACTION: Pediculocide; causes neuronal excitation in insects; lice become paralyzed and die after periods of hyperexcitation.

NURSING CONSIDERATIONS

Assessment: Assess pregnancy/nursing status.

Monitoring: Monitor for presence of live lice after 7 days of 1st treatment.

Patient Counseling: Advise to use only on dry scalp and hair. Instruct not to swallow. Instruct to rinse thoroughly with water if medication gets in or near the eyes. Advise to wash hands after application. Inform to use on children only under direct supervision of an adult. Consult physician if pregnant/breastfeeding.

Administration: Topical route. Shake well before use. Avoid contact with eyes. **Storage:** 25°C (77°F); excursions permitted between 15-30°C (59-86°F).

NAVANE   RX
thiothixene (Pfizer)

> Elderly patients with dementia-related psychosis treated with antipsychotic drugs are at an increased risk of death; most deaths appeared to be cardiovascular (CV) (eg, heart failure, sudden death) or infectious (eg, pneumonia) in nature. Navane is not approved for the treatment of patients with dementia-related psychosis.

THERAPEUTIC CLASS: Thioxanthene

INDICATIONS: Management of schizophrenia.

DOSAGE: *Adults:* Individualize dose. Mild Condition: Initial: 2mg tid. Titrate: May increase to 15mg/day. Severe Condition: Initial: 5mg bid. Usual: 20-30mg/day. Max: 60mg/day. *Pediatrics:* ≥12 yrs: Individualize dose. Mild Condition: Initial: 2mg tid. Titrate: May increase to 15mg/day. Severe Condition: Initial: 5mg bid. Usual: 20-30mg/day. Max: 60mg/day.

HOW SUPPLIED: Cap: 1mg, 2mg, 5mg, 10mg

CONTRAINDICATIONS: Circulatory collapse, comatose states, CNS depression, blood dyscrasias.

WARNINGS/PRECAUTIONS: May cause tardive dyskinesia (TD) and neuroleptic malignant syndrome (NMS); d/c if this develops. May impair mental/physical abilities. May mask signs of overdosage of toxic drugs and obscure conditions, such as intestinal obstruction and brain tumor. Caution with history of convulsive disorders or in a state of alcohol withdrawal; may lower convulsive threshold. Monitor for pigmentary retinopathy and lenticular pigmentation. Caution with CV disease, extreme heat exposure, activities requiring alertness. May elevate prolactin levels. May cause leukopenia, neutropenia, and agranulocytosis; consider d/c at 1st sign of significant decline in WBC in absence of other causes, and d/c when absolute neutrophil count (ANC) is <1000/mm³. False positive pregnancy tests may occur. Risk for extrapyramidal symptoms (EPS) and/or withdrawal symptoms following delivery in neonates exposed during 3rd trimester of pregnancy.

ADVERSE REACTIONS: NMS, TD, tachycardia, hypotension, lightheadedness, syncope, drowsiness, restlessness, agitation, insomnia, EPS, cerebral edema, CSF abnormalities, allergic reactions, hematologic effects.

INTERACTIONS: Possible additive effects with hypotensive agents, CNS depressants, and alcohol. Increased clearance with hepatic microsomal enzyme inducers (eg, carbamazepine). Potentiates the actions of barbiturates. Caution with atropine or related drugs. Paradoxical effects (lowering of BP) with pressor agents (eg, epinephrine).

PREGNANCY: Safety is not known in pregnancy and nursing.

MECHANISM OF ACTION: Thioxanthene derivative; antipsychotic agent.

NURSING CONSIDERATIONS

Assessment: Assess for dementia-related psychosis in elderly, history of convulsive disorders, history of CV disorders, CNS depression, circulatory collapse, comatose state, blood dyscrasias, alcohol intake, infections, intestinal obstruction, brain tumor, possibility of extreme heat exposure, previous hypersensitivity to the drug, pregnancy/nursing status, and possible drug interactions. Obtain baseline vital signs, CBC, LFTs, prolactin levels.

Monitoring: Monitor for hypersensitivity reactions, TD, NMS, CV effects, visual disturbances, and EPS. Monitor LFTs, bilirubin, CBC, prolactin, and blood glucose.

Patient Counseling: Inform about the risks of the treatment particularly about the possibility of developing TD. Advise about risk of chronic use of drug. Use caution when performing hazardous tasks (operating machinery/driving). Warn about possible additive effects (eg, hypotension) when drug is combined with hypotensive agents, CNS depressants and/or alcohol.

Administration: Oral route.

NEORAL   RX
cyclosporine (Novartis)

> Should only be prescribed by physicians experienced in management of systemic immunosuppressive therapy for indicated diseases. Increased susceptibility to infection and development of neoplasia (eg, lymphoma) may result from immunosuppression. Cyclosporine may be coadministered with other immunosuppressive agents in kidney, liver, and heart transplant patients. Not bioequivalent to Sandimmune and cannot be used interchangeably without physician supervision. Caution in switching from Sandimmune. Monitor cyclosporine blood concentrations in transplant and rheumatoid arthritis (RA) patients to avoid toxicity due to high concentrations. Dose adjustments should be made to minimize possible organ rejection due to low concentrations in transplant patients. Increased risk of developing skin malignancies in psoriasis patients previously treated with PUVA, methotrexate (MTX) or other immunosuppressive agents, UVB, coal tar, or radiation therapy. Cyclosporine may cause systemic HTN and nephrotoxicity. Monitor renal function for renal dysfunction including, structural kidney damage, during therapy.

THERAPEUTIC CLASS: Cyclic polypeptide immunosuppressant

INDICATIONS: Prophylaxis of organ rejection in kidney, liver, and heart allogeneic transplants. Treatment of severe, active RA where disease has not adequately responded to MTX. May be used in combination with MTX in RA not responding adequately to MTX alone. Treatment of nonimmunocompromised adults with severe (eg, extensive and/or disabling), recalcitrant, plaque psoriasis who failed to respond to at least one systemic therapy (eg, PUVA, retinoids, MTX) or in patients for whom other systemic therapies are contraindicated, or cannot be tolerated.

DOSAGE: *Adults:* Always give bid. Administer on a consistent schedule with regard to time of day and relation to meals. Newly Transplanted Patients: Initial: May give 4-12 hrs prior to transplant or postoperatively. Dose may vary depending on transplanted organ and other immunosuppressive agents included in protocol. Renal Transplant: 9±3mg/kg/day. Liver Transplant: 8±4mg/kg/day. Heart Transplant: 7±3mg/kg/day. Adjust subsequent dose to achieve a pre-defined blood concentration. Adjunct therapy with adrenal corticosteroid recommended initially. Conversion from Sandimmune: Start with same daily dose as was previously used with Sandimmune, (1:1 dose conversion). Adjust subsequent dose to attain a pre-conversion blood trough concentration. Monitor blood levels every 4-7 days while adjusting to trough levels. Transplant Patients with Poor Sandimmune Absorption: Caution when converting patients at doses >10mg/kg/day. Titrate dose individually based on trough concentrations, tolerability, and clinical response. Measure blood trough concentration at least 2X a week until stabilized within desired range. RA: Initial: 2.5mg/kg/day. Titrate: May be increased by 0.5-0.75mg/kg/day after 8 weeks and again after

12 weeks. Max: 4mg/kg/day. Combined with MTX (up to 15mg/week): ≤3mg/kg/day. D/C therapy if no benefit is seen by 16 weeks of treatment. Psoriasis: Initial: 2.5mg/kg/day for 4 weeks. If no significant clinical improvement occurs, may increase dosage at 2-week intervals. Titrate: May increase approximately 0.5mg/kg/day based on clinical response. Max: 4mg/kg/day. D/C if satisfactory response cannot be achieved after 6 weeks at 4mg/kg/day or the patient's maximum tolerated dose. (RA/Psoraisis) Reduce dose by 25-50% if adverse events (eg, HTN) occur. D/C if reduction is not effective. Elderly: Start at lower end of dosing range.

HOW SUPPLIED: Cap: 25mg, 100mg; Sol: 100mg/mL [50mL]

CONTRAINDICATIONS: Psoriasis/RA: Abnormal renal function, uncontrolled HTN, malignancies. Psoriasis: Concomitant PUVA or UVB therapy, MTX, other immunosuppressants, coal tar, or radiation therapy.

WARNINGS/PRECAUTIONS: May cause hepatotoxicity. Structural kidney damage and persistent renal dysfunction associated with therapy if not properly monitored and doses are not properly adjusted. Elevation of SrCr and BUN may occur and reflect a reduction in GFR; may require close monitoring of impaired renal function and frequent dose adjustment. Elevations in SrCr and BUN levels do not necessarily indicate rejection; evaluate patient before initiating dose adjustment. Increase in SrCr is generally reversible upon dose reduction and upon d/c. May develop syndrome of thrombocytopenia and microangiopathic hemolytic anemia resulting in graft failure. Significant hyperkalemia and hyperuricemia reported. Avoid excessive sun exposure. Increased risk for opportunistic infections, including activation of latent viral infections. BK virus-associated nephropathy reported; reduce immunosuppression if it develops. Encephalopathy and optic disc edema reported. Evaluate before and during treatment for development of malignancies. In RA patients, monitor BP on two occassions before treatment, obtain two baseline SrCr levels, then monitor BP and SrCr q2 weeks for the first 3 months of therapy, and then monthly if the patient is stable or more frequently during dose adjustments. In psoriasis patients, obtain baseline SrCr, BUN, CBC, Mg+, K+, uric acid, and lipids, then monitor q2 weeks for the first 3 months of therapy, and then monthly if the patient is stable or more frequently during dose adjustments. Monitor CBC and LFTs monthly with MTX. Monitor SrCr after initiation or increases in NSAID dose for RA. Caution in elderly.

ADVERSE REACTIONS: Renal dysfunction, HTN, hirsutism/hypertrichosis, tremor, headache, gingival hyperplasia, diarrhea, N/V, paresthesia, dyspepsia, stomatitis, hypomagnesemia, BK virus-associated nephropathy.

INTERACTIONS: See Boxed Warning and Contraindications. Avoid with K+-sparing diuretics, caution with K+-sparing drugs (eg, ACE inhibitors, angiotensin II receptor antagonists), K+-containing drugs, and K+-rich diet. Ciprofloxacin, gentamicin, tobramycin, vancomycin, SMZ/TMP, melphalan, amphotericin B, ketoconazole, azapropazon, colchicine, diclofenac, naproxen, sulindac, cimetidine, ranitidine, tacrolimus, fibric acid derivatives (eg, bezafibrate, fenofibrate), MTX, and NSAIDs may potentiate renal dysfunction. Monitor levels and adjust dose with CYP3A4 and/or P-glycoprotein (P-gp) inducers and inhibitors. Avoid with orlistat. Diltiazem, nicardipine, verapamil, fluconazole, itraconazole, ketoconazole, voriconazole, azithromycin, clarithromycin, erythromycin, quinupristin/dalfopristin, methylprednisolone, allopurinol, amiodarone, bromocriptine, colchicine, danazol, imatinib, metoclopramide, nefazodone, oral contraceptives may increase levels. Avoid with grapefruit and grapefruit juice. Nafcillin, rifampin, carbamazepine, oxcarbazepine, phenobarbital, phenytoin, bosentan, octreotide, orlistat, sulfinpyrazone, terbinafine, ticlopidine, St. John's wort may decrease levels. Caution with rifabutin. May double diclofenac blood levels. May increase MTX levels and decrease levels of active metabolite of MTX. Increases levels of CYP3A4 and/or P-gp substrates. May reduce clearance of digoxin, colchicine, prednisolone, HMG-CoA reductase inhibitors, and etoposide. Increased levels with sirolimus; give 4 hrs after cyclosporine administration. Vaccinations may be less effective; avoid live vaccines during therapy. Convulsions reported with high dose methylprednisolone. Frequent gingival hyperplasia with nifedipine. Caution with nephrotoxic drugs and HIV protease inhibitors (eg, indinavir, nelfinavir, ritonavir, and saquinavir). May increase levels of repaglinide and thereby increase risk of hypoglycemia.

PREGNANCY: Category C, not for use in nursing.

MECHANISM OF ACTION: Cyclic polypeptide immunosuppressant; results from specific and reversible inhibition of immunocompetent lymphocytes in the G_0- and G_1-phase of the cell cycle. T-lymphocytes are preferentially inhibited with T-helper cell as main target while also possibly suppressing T-suppressor cells. Also inhibits lymphokine production and release (eg, interleukin-2).

PHARMACOKINETICS: Absorption: Incomplete; T_{max}=1.5-2 hrs. Pharmacokinetic parameters varied with different indications (renal, liver, RA and/or psoriasis). **Distribution:** V_d=3-5L/kg (IV); plasma protein binding (90%); found in breast milk. **Metabolism:** (Extensive) Liver via CYP3A4, to a lesser extent GI tract and kidneys. M1, M9, and M4N (major metabolites); oxidation and demethylation pathways. **Elimination:** Bile (primary), urine (6%, 0.1% unchanged); $T_{1/2}$=8.4 hrs.

N

NURSING CONSIDERATIONS

Assessment: Assess for hypersensitivity to the drug, abnormal renal function, uncontrolled HTN, presence of malignancies, pregnancy/nursing status, and possible drug interactions. RA: Before initiating treatment, assess BP (on at least 2 occasions) and obtain 2 SrCr levels. Psoriasis: Prior to treatment, perform dermatological and physical examination, including measuring BP. Assess for presence of occult infections and for the presence of tumors initially. Assess for atypical skin lesions and biopsy them. Obtain baseline SrCr (at least twice), BUN, LFTs, bilirubin, CBC, Mg$^+$, K$^+$, uric acid, and lipid levels.

Monitoring: Monitor for renal/hepatic impairment. Monitor cyclosporine blood concentrations routinely in transplant patients and periodically in RA patients. RA: Monitor BP and SrCr every 2 weeks during the initial 3 months of treatment, then monthly if patient is stable. Monitor SrCr and BP after an increase of the dose of NSAIDs and after initiation of new NSAID therapy. If coadministered with MTX, monitor CBC and LFTs monthly. Psoriasis: Monitor for occult infections and tumors. Monitor SrCr, BUN, BP, CBC, uric acid, K$^+$, lipids, and Mg$^+$ levels every 2 weeks during first 3 months of treatment, then monthly if stable.

Patient Counseling: Instruct to contact physician before changing formulations of cyclosporine, which may require dose changes. Inform that repeated laboratory tests are required while on therapy. Advise of the potential risks if used during pregnancy and inform of the increased risk of neoplasia, HTN, and renal dysfunction. Inform that vaccinations may be less effective and to avoid live vaccines during therapy. Advise to take the medication on a consistent schedule with regard to time and meals, and to avoid grapefruit and grapefruit juice.

Administration: Oral route. Dilute oral sol with orange or apple juice that is at room temperature. Avoid diluting oral sol with grapefruit juice. **Storage:** Cap/Sol: 20-25°C (68-77°F). Use within 2 months upon opening. Sol: Do not refrigerate. At <20°C (68°F) may form gel; light flocculation, or formation of light sediment may occur; warm at 25°C (77°C) to reverse changes.

NEULASTA RX
pegfilgrastim (Amgen)

THERAPEUTIC CLASS: Granulocyte colony stimulating factor

INDICATIONS: To decrease the incidence of infection, as manifested by febrile neutropenia, in patients with non-myeloid malignancies receiving myelosuppressive anticancer drugs associated with a clinically significant incidence of febrile neutropenia.

DOSAGE: *Adults:* 6mg SQ once per chemotherapy cycle.

HOW SUPPLIED: Inj: 6mg/0.6mL

WARNINGS/PRECAUTIONS: Not for the mobilization of peripheral blood progenitor cells for hematopoietic stem cell transplantation. May cause splenic rupture; evaluate for an enlarged spleen or splenic rupture in patients who report left upper abdominal or shoulder pain. May cause acute respiratory distress syndrome (ARDS); evaluate patients who develop fever and lung infiltrates or respiratory distress; d/c if ARDS develops. Serious allergic reactions (eg, anaphylaxis) reported; d/c permanently if occurs. Do not administer with history of serious allergic reactions to the drug. May cause severe and sometimes fatal sickle cell crises in patients with sickle cell disorders. May act as a growth factor for any tumor type; not approved for myeloid malignancies and myelodysplasia. Needle cover on prefilled syringe contains latex; do not administer in persons with latex allergies.

ADVERSE REACTIONS: Bone pain, pain in extremity.

INTERACTIONS: Do not administer between 14 days before and 24 hrs after cytotoxic chemotherapy.

PREGNANCY: Category C, caution in nursing.

MECHANISM OF ACTION: Granulocyte colony stimulating factor; acts on hematopoietic cells by binding to specific cell surface receptors, thereby stimulating proliferation, differentiation, commitment, and end cell functional activation.

PHARMACOKINETICS: Elimination: $T_{1/2}$=15-80 hrs.

NURSING CONSIDERATIONS

Assessment: Assess for myeloid malignancies, myelodysplasia, history of hypersensitivity to the drug, latex allergy, sickle cell disorders, pregnancy/nursing status, and possible drug interactions.

Monitoring: Monitor for signs/symptoms of serious allergic reactions, splenic rupture, ARDS, sickle cell crises (in patients with sickle cell disorders), and tumor growth.

Patient Counseling: Advise of risks (eg, splenic rupture, ARDS, serious allergic reactions, sickle cell crisis). Instruct to notify physician and report if left upper quadrant or shoulder pain, SOB, signs/symptoms of sickle cell crisis or infection, flushing, dizziness, or rash occurs. Advise women to notify physician if become pregnant during treatment.

Administration: SQ route. **Storage:** Refrigerate at 2-8°C (36-46°F) in the carton to protect from light. Do not shake. Discard syringes stored at room temperature for >48 hrs. Avoid freezing; if frozen, thaw in the refrigerator before administration. Discard syringe if frozen more than once.

NEUMEGA   RX
oprelvekin (Wyeth)

| Allergic or hypersensitivity reactions, including anaphylaxis, reported; permanently d/c if this develops. |

THERAPEUTIC CLASS: Thrombopoietic agent

INDICATIONS: Prevention of severe thrombocytopenia and reduction of the need for platelet transfusions following myelosuppressive chemotherapy in adults with nonmyeloid malignancies who are at high risk of severe thrombocytopenia.

DOSAGE: *Adults:* 50mcg/kg SQ qd. Initiate 6-24 hrs after chemotherapy completion. Continue therapy until post-nadir platelet count is ≥50,000/μL. Max: 21 days/treatment course. D/C at least 2 days before starting the next chemotherapy cycle. May give for up to 6 cycles following chemotherapy. Severe Renal Impairment (CrCl <30mL/min): 25mcg/kg SQ.

HOW SUPPLIED: Inj: 5mg

WARNINGS/PRECAUTIONS: Not indicated following myeloablative chemotherapy. May cause serious fluid retention; caution in congestive heart failure (CHF) patients, patients who may be susceptible to developing CHF, patients receiving aggressive hydration, patients with history of heart failure who are well-compensated and receiving appropriate medical therapy, or patients who may develop fluid retention as a result of associated medical conditions or whose medical condition may be exacerbated by fluid retention . Monitor preexisting fluid collections; consider drainage if medically indicated. Moderate decreases in Hgb, Hct, and RBCs reported. Cardiovascular events including arrhythmias and pulmonary edema reported. Caution with history of atrial arrhythmias. Papilledema reported; caution in patients with preexisting papilledema, or with tumors involving the CNS. Changes in visual acuity and/or visual field defects may occur in patients with papilledema. Obtain CBC before chemotherapy and at regular intervals during therapy. Monitor platelet counts during expected nadir time and until adequate recovery has occurred (post-nadir counts ≥50,000/μL).

ADVERSE REACTIONS: Edema, dyspnea, tachycardia, conjunctival injection, palpitations, atrial arrhythmias, pleural effusions, syncope, pneumonia, neutropenic fever, headache, N/V, mucositis, diarrhea.

INTERACTIONS: Perform close monitoring of fluid and electrolyte status in patients receiving chronic diuretic therapy.

PREGNANCY: Category C, not for use in nursing.

MECHANISM OF ACTION: Thrombopoietic agent; stimulates megakaryocytopoiesis and thrombopoiesis.

PHARMACOKINETICS: Absorption: Absolute bioavailability (>80%); C_{max}=17.4ng/mL; T_{max}=3.2 hrs. **Elimination:** Urine; $T_{1/2}$=6.9 hrs.

NURSING CONSIDERATIONS

Assessment: Assess for conditions where treatment is contraindicated or cautioned, pregnancy/nursing status, and possible drug interactions. Obtain baseline CBC prior to chemotherapy.

Monitoring: Monitor for signs/symptoms of hypersensitivity reactions, papilledema, fluid retention, pleural/pericardial effusion, atrial arrhythmias, and other adverse reactions. Periodically monitor CBC (including platelet counts), fluid balance, fluid and electrolyte status (chronic diuretic therapy).

Patient Counseling: Inform of pregnancy risks. Instruct on the proper dose, method for reconstituting and administering, and importance of proper disposal of the product when used outside of the hospital or office setting. Inform of the serious and most common adverse reactions associated with the product. Advise to immediately seek medical attention if any of the signs or symptoms of allergic or hypersensitivity reactions (edema, difficulty breathing, swallowing or talking, SOB, wheezing, chest pain, throat tightness, lightheadedness), worsening of dyspnea, or symptoms attributable to atrial arrhythmia occur.

Administration: SQ route. Administer in either the abdomen, thigh, or hip (upper arm if not self-injecting). Refer to PI for preparation of the product. **Storage:** 2-8°C (36-46°F). Protect powder from light. Do not freeze. Reconstituted: 2-8°C (36-46°F) or up to 25°C (77°F). Do not freeze or shake.

NEUPOGEN

RX

filgrastim (Amgen)

THERAPEUTIC CLASS: Granulocyte colony stimulating factor

INDICATIONS: To decrease incidence of infection, as manifested by febrile neutropenia in patients with nonmyeloid malignancies receiving myelosuppressive anticancer drugs associated with significant incidence of severe neutropenia with fever. To reduce the time to neutrophil recovery and duration of fever, following consolidation chemotherapy treatment of adults with acute myeloid leukemia (AML). To reduce the duration of neutropenia and neutropenia-related clinical sequelae in patients with nonmyeloid malignancies undergoing myeloablative chemotherapy followed by marrow transplantation. For mobilization of hematopoietic progenitor cells into the peripheral blood for collection by leukapheresis. For chronic administration to reduce incidence and duration of sequelae of neutropenia in symptomatic patients with congenital neutropenia, cyclic neutropenia, or idiopathic neutropenia.

DOSAGE: *Adults:* Myelosuppressive Chemotherapy: Initial: 5mcg/kg qd SQ bolus, short IV infusion (15-30 min), or continuous SQ/IV infusion. Titrate: May increase in increments of 5mcg/kg for each chemotherapy cycle, according to duration and severity of ANC nadir. Should be administered no earlier than 24 hrs after the administration of cytotoxic chemotherapy. Should not be administered in the period 24 hrs before the administration of chemotherapy. Continue therapy after chemotherapy daily for up to 2 weeks, until the post nadir absolute neutrophil count (ANC) =10,000/mm³ is reached. D/C if ANC surpasses 10,000/mm³ after the expected chemotherapy-induced neutrophil nadir. Bone Marrow Transplant: 10mcg/kg/day by IV infusion of 4 or 24 hrs or by continuous 24-hr SQ infusion. First dose at least 24 hrs after cytotoxic chemotherapy and at least 24 hrs after bone marrow infusion. Dose Adjustment: Adjust according to ANC; see PI. Peripheral Blood Progenitor Cell Collection: 10mcg/kg/day SQ, either as a bolus or continuous infusion. Should be given at least four days before the 1st leukapheresis procedure and continue until the last leukapheresis. Monitor neutrophils after 4 days and consider dose modification if WBC >100,000/mm³. Chronic Neutropenia: Congenital Neutropenia: Initial: 6mcg/kg SQ bid. Idiopathic or Cyclic Neutropenia: Initial: 5mcg/kg SQ qd. Adjust dose based on clinical course and ANC.

HOW SUPPLIED: Inj: 300mcg/0.5mL, 300mcg/mL, 480mcg/0.8mL, 480mcg/1.6mL

CONTRAINDICATIONS: Hypersensitivity to *Esherichia coli*-derived proteins.

WARNINGS/PRECAUTIONS: Allergic-type reactions reported. Splenic rupture reported, some fatal. Evaluate for enlarged spleen or splenic rupture if complaints of left upper abdominal and/or shoulder tip pain. Acute respiratory distress syndrome (ARDS) reported; d/c until resolved. Alveolar hemorrhage manifesting as pulmonary infiltrates and hemoptysis requiring hospitalization reported. Severe sickle cell crises reported with sickle cell disorders. Confirm diagnosis of severe chronic neutropenia prior to therapy. Avoid simultaneous use with chemotherapy and radiation therapy. CBC monitoring is recommended twice a week during therapy to avoid potential complications of excessive leukocytosis. Potential for immunogenicity. Avoid premature d/c of therapy prior to time of recovery from expected neutrophil nadir. Cutaneous vasculitis reported; continue therapy at a reduced dose.

ADVERSE REACTIONS: N/V, skeletal pain, alopecia, diarrhea, neutropenic fever, mucositis, fatigue, anorexia, dyspnea, headache, cough, skin rash, splenomegaly, thrombocytopenia.

INTERACTIONS: Caution with drugs that may potentiate the release of neutrophils (eg, lithium). Transient positive bone imaging changes have been associated with increased hematopoietic activity of the bone marrow in response to growth factor therapy.

PREGNANCY: Category C, caution in nursing.

MECHANISM OF ACTION: Granulocyte colony-stimulating factor (G-CSF); acts on hematopoietic cells by binding to specific cell surface receptors. Stimulates proliferation, differentiation commitment, and some end-cell functional activation.

PHARMACOKINETICS: Absorption: (SQ, 3.45mcg/kg, 11.5mcg/kg): C_{max}=4ng/mL, 49ng/mL; T_{max}=2-8 hrs. **Distribution**: V_d=150mL/kg. **Elimination**: $T_{1/2}$=3.5 hrs, (IV) $T_{1/2}$=231 min (34.5mcg/kg), (SQ) $T_{1/2}$=210 min (3.45mcg/kg).

NURSING CONSIDERATIONS

Assessment: Obtain CBC with differential and platelet count. Assess for severe chronic neutropenia, history of chemotherapy/radiation therapy, history of hypersensitivity to *E. coli*-derived proteins, pregnancy/nursing status, and for possible drug interactions.

Monitoring: Monitor CBC with differential and platelet count 2-3 times a week. Perform annual bone marrow and cytogenetic evaluations throughout treatment for patients with congenital neutropenia. Monitor for hypersensitivity reactions, splenic rupture, ARDS, alveolar hemorrhage, hemoptysis, and sickle cell crises (in patients with sickle cell disease).

Patient Counseling: Counsel about potential adverse effects; seek medical attention if any develop. Report any left upper abdominal or shoulder tip pain. Refer patients to Information for Patients and Caregivers included with package insert in each dispensing pack. **Administration:** SQ/IV route. Refer to PI for dilution and administration instructions. **Storage:** 2-8°C (36-46°F). Avoid shaking. Discard vial or prefilled syringe if left at room temperature >24 hrs.

NEURONTIN   RX
gabapentin (Parke-Davis)

THERAPEUTIC CLASS: GABA analog

INDICATIONS: Adjunctive therapy for partial seizures with and without secondary generalization in patients >12 yrs with epilepsy. Adjunctive therapy for partial seizures in pediatrics 3-12 yrs. Management of postherpetic neuralgia (PHN) in adults.

DOSAGE: *Adults:* Epilepsy: Initial: 300mg tid. Titrate: If necessary, may increase up to 1800mg/day divided tid. The max time between doses in the tid schedule should not exceed 12 hrs. Max: 3600mg/day. PHN: Initial: 300mg single dose on Day 1, then 300mg bid on Day 2, and 300mg tid on Day 3. Titrate: Increase PRN for pain up to 600mg tid. Refer to PI for dosage in renal impairment. Elderly: Start at lower end of dosing range. If d/c or reducing dose, perform gradually over ≥1 week.
Pediatrics: Epilepsy: >12 yrs: Initial: 300mg tid. Titrate: If necessary, may increase up to 1800mg/day divided tid. Max: 3600mg/day. 3-12 yrs: Initial: 10-15mg/kg/day divided tid. Titrate: Increase to effective dose over a period of 3 days. Usual: ≥5 yrs: 25-35mg/kg/day divided tid. 3-4 yrs: 40mg/kg/day divided tid. Max: 50mg/kg/day. Refer to PI for dosage in renal impairment. If d/c or reducing dose, perform gradually over ≥1 week.

HOW SUPPLIED: Cap: 100mg, 300mg, 400mg; Sol: 250mg/5mL [470mL]; Tab: 600mg*, 800mg* *scored

WARNINGS/PRECAUTIONS: Increased risk of suicidal thoughts or behavior reported; monitor for emergence or worsening of depression, suicidal thoughts or behavior, and/or any unusual changes in mood and behavior. Associated with neuropsychiatric adverse events (eg, emotional lability, hostility, thought disorder, hyperkinesia) in pediatrics 3-12 yrs. Avoid abrupt withdrawal; may increase seizure frequency. May have tumorigenic potential. Sudden and unexplained deaths reported. Drug reaction with eosinophilia and systemic symptoms (DRESS)/multiorgan hypersensitivity reported; evaluate immediately if signs/symptoms are present and d/c if etiology for the signs and symptoms cannot be established. Caution in elderly.

ADVERSE REACTIONS: Somnolence, dizziness, peripheral edema, ataxia, nystagmus, fatigue, tremor, rhinitis, N/V, infection, diarrhea, asthenia, dry mouth, constipation.

INTERACTIONS: Decreased levels when taken with Maalox; take 2 hrs following antacid. Increased levels with controlled-release morphine and naproxen sodium. Hydrocodone increases gabapentin area under the curve while gabapentin decreases hydrocodone levels in a dose-dependent manner.

PREGNANCY: Category C, caution in nursing.

MECHANISM OF ACTION: GABA analog; not established. Anticonvulsant activity: Suspected to bind to different areas of the brain, including neocortex and hippocampus. Analgesic effects: Prevents allodynia and hyperalgesia.

PHARMACOKINETICS: Distribution: (150mg IV) V_d=58L. Plasma protein binding (<3%); found in breast milk. **Metabolism:** Not appreciably metabolized. **Elimination:** Renal (unchanged); $T_{1/2}$=5-7 hrs.

NURSING CONSIDERATIONS

Assessment: Assess for renal impairment, hypersensitivity, preexisting tumors, pregnancy/nursing status, and possible drug interactions.

Monitoring: Monitor for neuropsychiatric events in pediatrics, withdrawal-precipitated seizures, status epilepticus, emergence or worsening of depression, suicidal thoughts, changes in behavior, adverse reactions, development of new tumors, worsening of preexisting tumors, renal function, DRESS, and hypersensitivity reactions.

Patient Counseling: Instruct that medication may be taken with or without food and to take only as prescribed. Advise that scored tabs can be broken in half; the remaining half tab should be administered at the next dose, or discarded if unused after several days. Inform that may cause dizziness, somnolence, and other signs/symptoms of CNS depression; caution against operating machinery/driving until accustomed to effects of medication. Encourage patients to enroll in North American Antiepileptic Drug Pregnancy Registry if they become pregnant. Advise patients to be alert for and to contact physician if experience emergence/worsening of depression, unusual changes in mood/behavior, or the emergence of suicidal thoughts, behavior, or thoughts about self-harm. Advise to immediately report to physician any rash or other signs/symptoms of hypersensitivity (eg, fever, lymphadenopathy).

Administration: Oral route. **Storage:** Cap/Tab: 25°C (77°F); excursions permitted to 15-30°C (59-86°F). Sol: 2-8°C (36-46°F).

NEVANAC

RX

nepafenac (Alcon)

THERAPEUTIC CLASS: NSAID

INDICATIONS: Treatment of pain and inflammation associated with cataract surgery.

DOSAGE: *Adults:* 1 drop to affected eye tid beginning 1 day prior to cataract surgery. Continue on day of surgery and throughout first 2 weeks of postoperative period.
Pediatrics: ≥10 yrs: 1 drop to affected eye tid beginning 1 day prior to cataract surgery. Continue on day of surgery and throughout first 2 weeks of postoperative period.

HOW SUPPLIED: Sus: 0.1% [3mL]

WARNINGS/PRECAUTIONS: Potential for increased bleeding time due to interference with thrombocyte aggregation. Increased bleeding of ocular tissue (eg, hyphemas); caution with known bleeding tendencies which may prolong bleeding time. May slow or delay healing, or result in keratitis. Continued use may be sight threatening due to epithelial breakdown, corneal thinning, erosion, ulceration, or perforation; d/c if corneal epithelial breakdown occurs. Caution with complicated ocular surgeries, corneal denervation, corneal epithelial defects, diabetes mellitus (DM), ocular surface diseases (eg, dry eye syndrome), rheumatoid arthritis (RA), or repeat ocular surgeries within a short period of time. Increased risk for occurence and severity of corneal adverse events if used >1 day prior to surgery or use beyond 14 days post-surgery. Avoid use with contact lenses and during late pregnancy.

ADVERSE REACTIONS: Capsular opacity, decreased visual acuity, foreign body sensation, increased intraocular pressure, sticky sensation, conjunctival edema, corneal edema, dry eye, lid margin crusting, ocular discomfort, ocular hyperemia/pain/pruritus, photophobia, tearing.

INTERACTIONS: Increased potential for healing problems with topical steroids. Caution with agents that may prolong bleeding time.

PREGNANCY: Category C, caution in nursing.

MECHANISM OF ACTION: NSAID; inhibits prostaglandin biosynthesis.

PHARMACOKINETICS: Absorption: C_{max}=0.310ng/mL (nepafenac), 0.422ng/mL (amfenac, metabolite). **Metabolism:** Hydrolysis via ocular tissue hydrolases to amfenac.

NURSING CONSIDERATIONS

Assessment: Assess for drug hypersensitivity, bleeding tendencies, complicated or repeated ocular surgeries, corneal denervation, corneal epithelial defects, DM, ocular surface diseases, RA, if using contact lenses, pregnancy/nursing status, and possible drug interactions.

Monitoring: Monitor for hypersensitivity reactions, wound healing problems, keratitis, bleeding time, bleeding of ocular tissues in conjunction with ocular surgery, and evidence of epithelial corneal breakdown.

Patient Counseling: Inform of possibility that slow or delayed healing may occur. Advise on proper use to prevent bacterial contamination, and shake bottle well before use. Instruct if using >1 ophthalmic medication separate by 5 minutes, and not use while wearing contact lenses. Instruct to immediately notify physician if intercurrent ocular condition (eg, trauma or infection) occurs or undergoing ocular surgery to assess continuation of therapy.

Administration: Intraocular route. Administer 5 minutes apart if using >1 topical medication. **Storage:** 2-25°C (36-77°F).

NEXAVAR

RX

sorafenib (Bayer Healthcare)

THERAPEUTIC CLASS: Multikinase inhibitor

INDICATIONS: Treatment of unresectable hepatocellular carcinoma and advanced renal cell carcinoma.

DOSAGE: *Adults:* 400mg bid without food (≥1 hr ac or 2 hrs pc). Continue until no longer clinically benefiting from therapy or until unacceptable toxicity occurs. Temporarily interrupt or reduce dose to 400mg qd or qod if adverse events suspected. Refer to PI for dose modifications for skin toxicity.

HOW SUPPLIED: Tab: 200mg

CONTRAINDICATIONS: Squamous cell lung cancer when given in combination with carboplatin and paclitaxel.

WARNINGS/PRECAUTIONS: HTN, cardiac ischemia and/or infarction reported; temporary or permanent d/c should be considered. Increased risk of bleeding may occur; consider d/c if bleeding necessitates medical intervention. Hand-foot skin reaction and rash reported; may require topical treatment, temporary interruption, and/or dose modification, or permanent d/c in severe or persistent cases. D/C if GI perforation occurs. Temporarily interrupt therapy when undergoing major surgical procedures. May prolong QT/QTc interval; avoid with congenital long QT syndrome. May cause fetal harm.

ADVERSE REACTIONS: HTN, fatigue, weight loss, rash/desquamation, hand-foot skin reaction, alopecia, pruritus, diarrhea, N/V, anorexia, constipation, hemorrhage, dyspnea.

INTERACTIONS: See Contraindications. Avoid with gemcitabine/cisplatin in squamous cell lung cancer. Avoid with strong CYP3A4 inducers (eg, carbamazepine, dexamethasone, phenobarbital, phenytoin, rifabutin, rifampin, St. John's wort). May increase systemic exposure of UGT1A1 and UGT1A9 substrates. Infrequent bleeding or increased INR with warfarin; monitor for PT changes, INR, or bleeding episodes. May increase concentrations of P-glycoprotein substrates. May decrease levels with oral neomycin. Monitor use with drugs known to prolong the QT interval (eg, Class Ia and III antiarrhythmics).

PREGNANCY: Category D, not for use in nursing.

MECHANISM OF ACTION: Multikinase inhibitor; inhibits multiple intracellular (CRAF, BRAF, and mutant BRAF) and cell surface kinases (KIT, FLT-3, RET, VEGFR-1, VEGFR-2, VEGFR-3, and PDGFR-β) thought to be involved in tumor cell signaling, angiogenesis, and apoptosis.

PHARMACOKINETICS: Absorption: Relative bioavailability (38-49%); T_{max}=3 hrs. **Distribution:** Plasma protein binding (99.5%). **Metabolism:** Liver via oxidation and glucuronidation; CYP3A4, UGT1A9; pyridine N-oxide (metabolite). **Elimination:** (100mg dose sol) Feces (77%, 51% unchanged), urine (19% glucuronidated metabolites); $T_{1/2}$=25-48 hrs.

NURSING CONSIDERATIONS

Assessment: Assess for squamous cell lung cancer on carboplatin and paclitaxel therapy, bleeding problems, renal/hepatic dysfunction, major surgical procedures, congestive heart failure, bradyarrhythmias, electrolyte abnormalities, drug hypersensitivity, pregnancy/nursing status, and possible drug interactions. Note other diseases/conditions and drug therapies.

Monitoring: Monitor BP weekly during the first 6 weeks and periodically thereafter. Monitor for cardiac ischemia/infarction, hemorrhage, HTN, dermatologic toxicities, GI perforation, and QT/QTc prolongation. Monitor electrolyte abnormalities with on-treatment ECG and electrolytes (eg, magnesium, calcium, K$^+$). Monitor changes in PT, INR, or clinical bleeding episodes when given with warfarin.

Patient Counseling: Counsel about possible side effects; report any episodes of bleeding, chest pain, or other symptoms of cardiac ischemia and/or infarction. Inform patient with history of prolonged QT interval that treatment can worsen the condition. Advise of possible occurrence of hand-foot skin reaction and rash during therapy and appropriate countermeasures. Inform that HTN may develop especially during the first 6 weeks; advise that BP should be monitored regularly during therapy. Inform female patients that the drug may cause birth defects or fetal loss during pregnancy and that they should not become pregnant during therapy or for at least 2 weeks after stopping therapy; both males and females should use effective birth control during treatment to avoid conception. Consult physician if become pregnant while on therapy. Advise against breastfeeding.

Administration: Oral route. **Storage:** 25°C (77°F); excursions permitted to 15-30°C (59-86°F). Store in dry place.

NEXIUM RX
esomeprazole magnesium (AstraZeneca)

THERAPEUTIC CLASS: Proton pump inhibitor

INDICATIONS: Short-term treatment (4-8 weeks) and maintenance (up to 6 months) in the healing and symptomatic resolution of erosive esophagitis. Short-term treatment (up to 6 weeks) of erosive esophagitis due to acid-mediated gastroesophageal reflux disease (GERD) in infants 1 month to <1 yr. Short-term treatment (4-8 weeks) of heartburn and other symptoms associated with GERD in adults and children ≥1 yr. Reduction in occurrence of gastric ulcers associated with continuous NSAID therapy in patients at risk for developing gastric ulcers. Long term-treatment of pathological hypersecretory conditions (eg, Zollinger-Ellison syndrome). In combination with amoxicillin and clarithromycin for the treatment of *Helicobacter pylori* infection and duodenal ulcer disease (active or history of within the past 5 yrs) to eradicate *H. pylori*.

DOSAGE: *Adults:* Erosive Esophagitis: Healing: 20mg or 40mg qd for 4-8 weeks; may extend treatment for additional 4-8 weeks if not healed. Maint of Healing: 20mg qd for up to 6 months. Symptomatic GERD: 20mg qd for 4 weeks; may extend treatment for additional 4 weeks if symptoms not resolved completely. Risk Reduction of NSAID-Associated Gastric Ulcer: 20mg or 40mg qd for up to 6 months. *H. pylori* Eradication: Triple Therapy: 40mg qd + amoxicillin 1000mg bid + clarithromycin 500mg bid, all for 10 days. Pathological Hypersecretory Conditions: 40mg bid; adjust dose PRN. Doses up to 240mg qd have been administered. Severe Liver Impairment (Child-Pugh Class C): Max: 20mg/day. Take ≥1 hr before meals.
Pediatrics: 12-17 yrs: GERD: 20mg or 40mg qd for up to 8 weeks. 1-11 yrs: Symptomatic GERD: 10mg qd for up to 8 weeks. Max: 1mg/kg/day. Healing of Erosive Esophagitis: ≥20kg: 10mg or 20mg qd for 8 weeks. Max: 1mg/kg/day. <20kg: 10mg qd for 8 weeks. Max: 1mg/kg/day. Erosive Esophagitis due to Acid-Mediated GERD: 1 month-<1 yr: >7.5-12kg: 10mg qd for up to 6 weeks. >5-7.5kg: 5mg qd for up to 6 weeks. 3-5kg: 2.5mg qd for up to 6 weeks. Max: 1.33mg/kg/day. Severe Liver Impairment (Child-Pugh Class C): Max: 20mg/day. Take ≥1 hr before meals.

HOW SUPPLIED: Cap, Delayed-Release: 20mg, 40mg; Sus, Delayed-Release: 2.5mg, 5mg, 10mg, 20mg, 40mg (granules/pkt)

WARNINGS/PRECAUTIONS: Symptomatic response does not preclude the presence of gastric malignancy. Atrophic gastritis reported with long-term use. May increase risk for osteoporosis-related fractures of the hip, wrist, or spine especially with high-dose and long term therapy; use lowest dose and shortest duration possible. Hypomagnesemia reported and may require magnesium replacement and d/c of therapy; consider monitoring of magnesium levels prior to and periodically during therapy with prolonged treatment. Drug-induced decrease in gastric acidity results in enterochromaffin-like cell hyperplasia and increased chromogranin A levels; may interfere with investigations for neuroendocrine tumors.

ADVERSE REACTIONS: Headache, diarrhea, nausea, flatulence, abdominal pain, constipation, dry mouth.

INTERACTIONS: CYP2C19 or 3A4 inducers may decrease levels; avoid concomitant use of St. John's wort or rifampin. May reduce atazanavir and nelfinavir levels; concomitant use not recommended. May change absorption or levels of antiretrovirals. May increase saquinavir and cilostazol levels; consider dose reduction. May interfere with absorption of drugs where gastric pH is an important determinant of bioavailability (eg, ketoconazole, atazanavir, iron salts, digoxin); may increase systemic exposure of digoxin. Monitor for increases in INR and PT with warfarin. May increase levels of tacrolimus, methotrexate, and diazepam. Increased levels with combined inhibitors of CYP2C19 and 3A4 (eg, voriconazole). Increased levels of esomeprazole and 14-hydroxyclarithromycin with amoxicillin and clarithromycin. May inhibit metabolism of CYP2C19 substrates. Caution with digoxin or other drugs that may cause hypomagnesemia (eg, diuretics).

PREGNANCY: Category B, not for use in nursing.

MECHANISM OF ACTION: Proton pump inhibitor (PPI); suppresses gastric acid secretion by specific inhibition of the H^+/K^+-ATPase in the gastric parietal cell. Blocks the final step of acid production.

PHARMACOKINETICS: Absorption: C_{max}=2.1µmol/L (20mg), 4.7µmol/L (40mg); T_{max}=1.6 hrs; AUC=4.2µmol•hr/L (20mg), 12.6µmol•hr/L (40mg). Refer to PI for pharmacokinetic parameters in pediatrics. **Distribution:** V_d=16L; plasma protein binding (97%). **Metabolism:** Liver (extensive) via CYP2C19 (hydroxylation, desmethylation), CYP3A4. **Elimination:** Urine (80% metabolites, <1% unchanged), feces; $T_{1/2}$=1.2 hrs (20mg), 1.5 hrs (40mg).

NURSING CONSIDERATIONS

Assessment: Assess for hypersensitivity to PPIs, hepatic function, risk for osteoporosis-related fractures, pregnancy/nursing status, and possible drug interactions. Obtain baseline magnesium levels.

Monitoring: Monitor for signs/symptoms of atrophic gastritis, bone fractures, hypomagnesemia, hypersensitivity reactions, and other adverse reactions. Monitor magnesium levels periodically. Monitor LFTs.

Patient Counseling: Advise to notify physician if taking other medications. Inform that antacids may be used while on therapy. Advise to take medication ≥1 hr ac. Instruct not to chew or crush cap; if opening cap to mix granules with food, mix with applesauce only. Instruct proper technique for administration of opened cap or oral sus. Counsel regarding the correct amount of water to use when mixing dose of oral sus. Advise to immediately report and seek care if cardiovascular/neurological symptoms occur (eg, palpitations, dizziness, seizures, and tetany); these may be signs of hypomagnesemia.

Administration: Oral route. May be given via gastric/NG route. Take ≥1 hr ac. Refer to PI for preparation and administration instructions. **Storage:** 25°C (77°F); excursions permitted to 15-30°C (59-86°F).

NEXIUM IV
RX

esomeprazole sodium (AstraZeneca)

THERAPEUTIC CLASS: Proton pump inhibitor

INDICATIONS: Short-term treatment of gastroesophageal reflux disease with erosive esophagitis in adults and pediatrics 1 month to 17 yrs, when PO therapy is not possible or appropriate.

DOSAGE: *Adults:* 20mg or 40mg qd IV inj (≥3 min) or infusion (10-30 min) for up to 10 days. Severe Liver Impairment (Child-Pugh Class C): Max: 20mg/day. D/C and switch to PO as soon as possible/appropriate.
Pediatrics: IV infusion over (10-30 min). 1-17 yrs: ≥55kg: 20mg qd. <55kg: 10mg qd. 1 month-<1 yr: 0.5mg/kg qa. Severe Liver Impairment (Child-Pugh Class C): Max: 20mg/day. D/C and switch to PO as soon as possible/appropriate.

HOW SUPPLIED: Inj: 20mg, 40mg

WARNINGS/PRECAUTIONS: Symptomatic response does not preclude the presence of gastric malignancy. Atrophic gastritis reported with long-term use. May increase risk of osteoporosis-related fractures of the hip, wrist, or spine especially with high-dose and long-term therapy; use lowest dose and shortest duration possible. Hypomagnesemia reported and may require magnesium replacement and d/c of therapy; consider monitoring of magnesium levels prior to and periodically during therapy with prolonged treatment. Drug-induced decrease in gastric acidity results in enterochromaffin-like cell hyperplasia and increased chromogranin A levels; may interfere with investigations for neuroendocrine tumors.

ADVERSE REACTIONS: Headache, flatulence, nausea, abdominal pain, diarrhea, dry mouth.

INTERACTIONS: CYP2C19 or 3A4 inducers may decrease levels; avoid concomitant use of St. John's wort or rifampin. May reduce atazanavir and nelfinavir levels; concomitant use not recommended. May change absorption or levels of antiretrovirals. May increase saquinavir and cilostazol levels; consider dose reduction. Monitor for increases in INR and PT with warfarin. May increase levels of tacrolimus, methotrexate, and diazepam. Decreased clearance of diazepam. Increased levels with combined inhibitors of CYP2C19 and 3A4 (eg, voriconazole). Decreased absorption of ketoconazole, atazanavir, iron salts, and erlotinib. Increase absorption of and exposure to digoxin; monitor levels. May inhibit metabolism of CYP2C19 substrates. Caution with digoxin or other drugs that may cause hypomagnesemia (eg, diuretics).

PREGNANCY: Category B, not for use in nursing.

MECHANISM OF ACTION: Proton pump inhibitor; suppresses gastric acid secretion by specific inhibition of the H^+/K^+-ATPase in the gastric parietal cell. Blocks the final step of acid production.

PHARMACOKINETICS: Absorption: C_{max}=3.86µmol/L (20mg), 7.51µmol/L (40mg). AUC=5.11µmol•hr/L (20mg), 16.21µmol•hr/L (40mg). **Distribution:** V_d=16L; plasma protein binding (97%). **Metabolism:** Liver (extensive) via CYP2C19 (hydroxylation, desmethylation), 3A4. **Elimination:** Urine (primary, <1% unchanged), feces. $T_{1/2}$=1.05 hrs (20mg), 1.41 hrs (40mg).

NURSING CONSIDERATIONS

Assessment: Assess for hypersensitivity to drug or substituted benzimidazoles, hepatic function, risk for osteoporosis-related fractures, pregnancy/nursing status, and possible drug interactions. Obtain baseline magnesium levels.

Monitoring: Monitor for signs/symptoms of atrophic gastritis, bone fractures, hypomagnesemia, hypersensitivity reactions, and other adverse reactions. Monitor magnesium levels periodically. Monitor LFTs.

Patient Counseling: Advise to notify physician if taking other medications. Inform that antacids may be used while on therapy. Advise to report and seek care if cardiovascular/neurological symptoms occur (eg, palpitations, dizziness, seizures, and tetany); these may be signs of hypomagnesemia.

Administration: IV route. Refer to PI for preparation and administration instructions. Should not be administered concomitantly with any other medications through same IV site or tubing. Always flush IV line both prior to and after administration. **Storage:** 25°C (77°F); excursions permitted to 15-30°C (59-86°F). Protect from light. Store in carton until time of use. Reconstituted Sol: up to 30°C (86°F); use within 12 hrs after reconstitution.

NEXTERONE
RX

amiodarone HCl (Baxter)

THERAPEUTIC CLASS: Class III antiarrhythmic

INDICATIONS: Initiation of treatment and prophylaxis of frequently recurring ventricular fibrillation (VF) and hemodynamically unstable ventricular tachycardia (VT) refractory to other therapies. Treatment of patients with VT/VF for whom oral amiodarone is indicated, but who are unable to take oral medication.

DOSAGE: *Adults:* May individualize 1st 24-hr dose. Max Initial Infusion Rate: 30mg/min. LD: 150mg IV over 1st 10 min (15mg/min), then 360mg IV over next 6 hrs (1mg/min). Maint: 540mg IV over remaining 18 hrs (0.5mg/min). After 1st 24 hrs, continue with infusion rate of 720mg/24 hrs (0.5mg/min) for 2-3 weeks; may increase rate to achieve arrhythmia suppression. Max Concentration (Infusions >1 hr): 2mg/mL (unless a central venous catheter is used). Breakthrough Episodes of VF/Hemodynamically Unstable VT: Supplemental 150mg IV over 10 min. Switching to Oral Amiodarone (assuming a 720mg/day IV infusion): <1 week of IV Infusion: Initial: 800-1600mg/day; 1-3 weeks of IV Infusion: Initial: 600-800mg/day; >3 weeks of IV Infusion: Initial: 400mg/day. Elderly: Start at lower end of dosing range.

HOW SUPPLIED: Inj: 50mg/mL

CONTRAINDICATIONS: Cardiogenic shock, marked sinus bradycardia, 2nd- or 3rd-degree atrioventricular (AV) block unless a functioning pacemaker is available.

WARNINGS/PRECAUTIONS: Hypotension reported; treat initially by slowing the infusion. Bradycardia and AV block reported; ensure availability of temporary pacemaker in patients with known predisposition to bradycardia or AV block. Elevations of hepatic enzymes reported. Acute centrolobular confluent hepatocellular necrosis leading to hepatic coma and acute renal failure may occur at a much higher LD concentration and much faster rate of infusion than recommended. Consider d/c or reducing rate of administration with evidence of progressive hepatic injury. May worsen or precipitate a new arrhythmia; monitor for QTc prolongation. Pulmonary toxicity/fibrosis and adult respiratory distress syndrome (ARDS) reported. Optic neuropathy/neuritis may occur; perform ophthalmic examination if symptoms of visual impairment appear. Not intended for long-term maint use. Hypo- and hyperthyroidism, thyroid nodules/cancer/dysfunction reported; evaluate thyroid function prior to treatment and periodically thereafter. Hyperthyroidism may result in thyrotoxicosis and arrhythmia breakthrough or aggravation. May cause fetal harm. Corneal refractive laser surgery may be contraindicated. Correct hypokalemia or hypomagnesemia prior to initiation of therapy. Caution in elderly.

ADVERSE REACTIONS: Hypotension, asystole, cardiac arrest, pulseless electrical activity (PEA), cardiogenic shock, congestive heart failure, bradycardia, liver function test abnormalities, VT, AV block.

INTERACTIONS: Potential for drug interactions may persist after d/c due to long half-life. CYP3A inhibitors (eg, protease inhibitors, cimetidine) may increase levels. Do not take grapefruit juice during treatment. QT prolongation and torsades de pointes (TdP) with loratadine and trazodone reported. CYP2C8 inhibitors may increase levels. May increases levels of CYP1A2/CYP2C9/CYP2D6/CYP3A and P-glycoprotein substrates. May elevate plasma levels of cyclosporine, digoxin, quinidine, procainamide, phenytoin, flecainide. D/C or reduce digitalis dose by 50%. Reduce quinidine and procainamide doses by one-third. Myopathy/rhabdomyolysis reported with HMG-CoA reductase inhibitors that are CYP3A4 substrates (eg, atorvastatin, lovastatin, simvastatin). May potentiate bradycardia, sinus arrest, and AV block with β-receptor blocking agents (eg, propranolol) or calcium channel antagonists (eg, verapamil, diltiazem). May increase PT with warfarin. Concomitant use with clopidogrel may result in ineffective inhibition of platelet aggregation. CYP3A inducers (eg, rifampin, St. John's wort) may decrease levels. Concomitant use with fentanyl may cause hypotension, bradycardia, and decreased cardiac output. Cholestyramine may decrease levels and half-life. QTc prolongation with disopyramide, fluoroquinolones, macrolides, and azoles. Concomitant use with propranolol, diltiazem, verapamil may result in hemodynamic and electrophysiologic interactions. May be more sensitive to myocardial depressant and conduction defects of halogenated inhalational anesthetics. May impair metabolism of phenytoin, dextromethorphan, and methotrexate. Seizures and sinus bradycardia reported with concomitant use of lidocaine. Action of antithyroid drugs may be delayed in amiodarone-induced thyrotoxicosis. Radioactive iodine therapy is contraindicated with amiodarone-induced hyperthyroidism. Monitor electrolyte and acid-base balance with concomitant diuretics. Initiate any added antiarrhythmic drug at a lower than usual dose.

PREGNANCY: Category D, not for use in nursing.

MECHANISM OF ACTION: Class III antiarrhythmic; blocks sodium, calcium, and potassium channels; exerts noncompetitive antisympathetic action, and negative chronotropic and dromotropic effects; lengthens cardiac action potential, decreases cardiac workload and myocardial oxygen consumption.

PHARMACOKINETICS: Absorption: C_{max}=7-26mg/L (150mg IV). **Distribution:** Plasma protein binding (>96%); crosses the placenta, found in breast milk. **Metabolism:** CYP3A, 2C8; N-desethylamiodarone (major active metabolite). **Elimination:** Urine, bile; $T_{1/2}$=9-36 days (amiodarone); 9-30 days (N-desethylamiodarone).

NURSING CONSIDERATIONS

Assessment: Assess for cardiogenic shock, marked sinus bradycardia, 2nd- or 3rd-degree AV block, functioning pacemaker, thyroid dysfunction, hypersensitivity, pregnancy/nursing status, and possible drug interactions. Prior to initiation, correct hypokalemia and hypomagnesemia.

Monitoring: Monitor for hypotension, bradycardia, AV block, acute centrolobular hepatocellular necrosis, hepatic coma, acute renal failure, hepatic injury, worsening of existing or precipitation of new arrhythmia, ARDS, pulmonary toxicity, pulmonary fibrosis, optic neuropathy/neuritis, hypo/hyperthyroidism, thyroid nodules, thyroid cancer, QTc prolongation. Monitor LFTs and thyroid function. Perform perioperative monitoring for patients undergoing general anesthesia. Perform regular ophthalmic examination (eg, fundoscopy and slit-lamp exams) during administration.

Patient Counseling: Inform about benefits and risks of therapy. Instruct to d/c nursing while on therapy. Advise that corneal refractive laser surgery may be contraindicated. Counsel to not take grapefruit juice, over-the-counter cough medicine (that commonly contains dextromethorphan), and St. John's wort during therapy. Inform of the symptoms of hypo- and hyperthyroidism, particularly if transitioned to oral therapy.

Administration: IV route. May be diluted in D$_5$W or saline and administered in polyvinyl chloride (PVC), polyolefin, or glass containers. Do not use evacuated glass containers for admixing. Refer to PI for further instructions on administration and preparation. **Storage:** 20-25°C (68-77°F); excursions permitted to 15-30°C (59-86°F). Protect from light and excessive heat.

NIASPAN   RX
niacin (Abbott)

THERAPEUTIC CLASS: Nicotinic acid

INDICATIONS: To reduce elevated total cholesterol (TC), LDL-C, TG, and apolipoprotein B levels, and to increase HDL-C in primary hyperlipidemia and mixed dyslipidemia. With concomitant lovastatin or simvastatin, to treat primary hyperlipidemia and mixed dyslipidemia when treatment with monotherapy is inadequate. To reduce the risk of recurrent nonfatal myocardial infarction (MI) with history of MI and hyperlipidemia. To slow progression/promote regression of atherosclerotic disease with concomitant bile acid binding resin, in patients with history of coronary artery disease and hyperlipidemia, and to reduce elevated TC and LDL-C levels in adult patients with primary hyperlipidemia. Adjunct therapy for treatment of severe hypertriglyceridemia in adult patients with risk of pancreatitis and who do not respond adequately to diet.

DOSAGE: *Adults:>*16 yrs: Take at hs after low-fat snack. Individualize dose. Initial: 500mg. Titrate: Increase by 500mg q4 weeks. After Week 8, titrate to patient response and tolerance. If inadequate response with 1000mg qd, increase dose to 1500mg qd; may subsequently increase dose to 2000mg qd. Do not increase daily dose by more than 500mg in any 4-week period. Maint: 1000-2000mg qhs. Max: 2000mg/day. With Lovastatin/Simvastatin: Adjust dose at intervals of ≥4 weeks. Max: Niacin: 2000mg qd, Lovastatin/Simvastatin 40mg qd. May take aspirin (ASA) (up to 325mg) 30 min before administration to reduce flushing. Women may respond at lower doses than men. Do not interchange 3 of 500mg and 2 of 750mg tab. If d/c therapy for an extended period of time, reinstitution should include titration phase.

HOW SUPPLIED: Tab, Extended-Release: 500mg, 750mg, 1000mg

CONTRAINDICATIONS: Active liver disease or unexplained persistent elevations in hepatic transaminases, active peptic ulcer disease, arterial bleeding.

WARNINGS/PRECAUTIONS: Do not substitute with equivalent doses of immediate-release niacin; severe hepatic toxicity including fulminant hepatic necrosis may occur. If switching from immediate-release niacin, initiate with low doses and titrate to desired therapeutic response. Caution with heavy alcohol use and/or past history of liver disease, renal impairment, unstable angina, and acute phase of MI. Closely observe patients with history of jaundice, hepatobiliary disease, or peptic ulcer. Myopathy and rhabdomyolysis reported. Associated with abnormal LFTs; d/c if transaminase levels progress (3X ULN and are persistent), or if associated with nausea, fever, and/or malaise. May increase FPG; caution in diabetic patients. May reduce platelet count and phosphorus levels; periodically monitor phosphorus levels in patients at risk for hypophosphatemia. May increase PT; caution in patients undergoing surgery. Elevated uric acid levels reported; caution in patients predisposed to gout.

ADVERSE REACTIONS: Flushing, diarrhea, N/V, increased cough, pruritus, rash.

INTERACTIONS: Increased levels of lovastatin and simvastatin, and decreased levels of lovastatin acid. Reduced bioavailability with lovastatin and simvastatin. Increased risk of rhabdomyolysis/myopathy with HMG-CoA reductase inhibitors (eg, lovastatin, simvastatin). May potentiate effects of ganglionic blocking agents and vasoactive drugs resulting in postural hypotension. Separate dosing from bile acid binding resins (eg, colestipol, cholestyramine) by at least 4-6 hrs. May decrease metabolic clearance of nicotinic acid with ASA. May potentiate adverse effects of niacin with vitamins or other nutritional supplements containing large doses of niacin or related compounds (eg, nicotinamide). May increase flushing and pruritus with alcohol, hot drinks, or spicy foods; avoid around time of administration. Caution with anticoagulants; monitor platelet counts and PT. Caution in patients with unstable angina or acute phase MI receiving vasoactive drugs (eg, nitrates, calcium channel blockers, adrenergic blockers). Adjustment of hypoglycemic therapy may be necessary.

PREGNANCY: Category C, not for use in nursing.

MECHANISM OF ACTION: Nicotinic acid; not established. May partially inhibit release of free fatty acids from adipose tissue, and increase lipoprotein lipase activity, which may increase the rate of chylomicron TG removal from plasma. Decreases the rate of hepatic synthesis of VLDL and LDL, and does not appear to affect fecal excretion of fats, sterols, or bile acids.

PHARMACOKINETICS: Absorption: T_{max}=5 hrs. **Distribution:** Found in breast milk. **Metabolism:** Liver (rapid and extensive); nicotinamide adenine dinucleotide, and (via conjugation) nicotinuric acid (metabolites). **Elimination:** Urine (60-76%; up to 12%, unchanged).

NURSING CONSIDERATIONS

Assessment: Assess for history of jaundice, hepatobiliary disease or peptic ulcer, diabetes, uncontrolled hypothyroidism, risk for hypophosphatemia, any other conditions where treatment is contraindicated or cautioned, upcoming surgery, pregnancy/nursing status, and possible drug interactions. Assess LFTs and lipid levels.

Monitoring: Monitor for signs/symptoms of hepatotoxicity, rhabdomyolysis, decreases in platelet counts, and increases in PT and uric acid levels. Monitor phosphorus levels in patients at risk for hypophosphatemia. Monitor LFTs (eg, AST, ALT) every 6-12 weeks during 1st year and periodically thereafter. Monitor periodically serum creatine phosphokinase, K+, and lipid levels. Monitor glucose levels frequently.

Patient Counseling: Advise to adhere to recommended diet, a regular exercise program, and periodic testing of a fasting lipid panel. Counsel to take at hs, after a low-fat snack. Advise not to break, crush, or chew tab; swallow whole. Contact physician before restarting therapy if dosing is interrupted for any length of time and inform that retitration is recommended. Instruct to notify physician of any unexplained muscle pain, tenderness or weakness, dizziness, changes in blood glucose if diabetic, and all medications being taken (eg, vitamins or other nutritional supplements containing niacin or nicotinamide). Inform that flushing may occur but may subside after several weeks of consistent use; get up slowly if awakened by flushing at night. Inform that taking ASA 30 min before dosing may minimize flushing. Avoid ingestion of alcohol, spicy foods, or hot drinks with administration to prevent flushing. Advise to d/c use and contact physician if pregnancy occurs. Advise breastfeeding women not to use drug.

Administration: Oral route. **Storage:** 20-25°C (68-77°F).

NIFEDIPINE   RX
nifedipine (Various)

OTHER BRAND NAMES: Procardia (Pfizer)

THERAPEUTIC CLASS: Calcium channel blocker (dihydropyridine)

INDICATIONS: Management of vasospastic angina and chronic stable angina without evidence of vasospasm in patients who remain symptomatic despite adequate doses of β-blockers and/or organic nitrates or who cannot tolerate those agents.

DOSAGE: *Adults:* Initial: 10mg tid. Usual: 10-20mg tid or 20-30mg tid-qid with evidence of coronary artery spasm. Titrate over a 7-14 day period. If symptoms warrant (eg, activity level, attack frequency, SL nitroglycerin consumption) dose may be increased from 10mg tid to 20mg tid, then 30mg tid over a 3-day period. Ischemic hospitalized patients may increase in 10mg increments over 4- to 6-hr periods; single dose should rarely exceed 30mg. Max: 180mg/day. Elderly: Start at the low end of the dosing range.

HOW SUPPLIED: Cap: 10mg (Procardia), 20mg

WARNINGS/PRECAUTIONS: May cause hypotension; monitor BP initially and with titration. Not for acute reduction of BP or control of essential HTN. May increase frequency, duration and/or severity of angina or acute myocardial infarction (MI), particularly with severe obstructive coronary artery disease (CAD). Avoid with acute coronary syndrome and within 1 or 2 weeks after MI. May develop congestive heart failure (CHF) especially with aortic stenosis. Peripheral edema associated with vasodilation may occur; patients with angina complicated by CHF, rule out peripheral edema caused by left ventricular dysfunction. Transient elevations of enzymes (eg, alkaline phosphatase, CPK, LDH, SGOT, SGPT), cholestasis with/without jaundice, and allergic hepatitis reported. May decrease platelet aggregation and increase bleeding time. Positive direct Coombs test with/without hemolytic anemia reported. Reversible elevation in BUN and SrCr reported rarely in patients with chronic renal insufficiency. Caution in elderly. Taper dose upon d/c.

ADVERSE REACTIONS: Dizziness, lightheadedness, giddiness, flushing, heat sensation, heart-burn, muscle cramps, tremor, headache, weakness, nausea, peripheral edema, nervousness/mood changes, palpitation.

INTERACTIONS: β-blockers may increase risk of CHF, severe hypotension, or angina exacerba-tion; avoid abrupt β-blocker withdrawal. Severe hypotension and/or increased fluid volume reported together with β-blockers and fentanyl or other narcotic analgesics. May increase digoxin levels; monitor when initiating, adjusting, and d/c therapy to avoid over- or under-digita-lization. May decrease plasma levels of quinidine. May increase PT with coumarin anticoagulants. Cimetidine and grapefruit juice may increase levels. Monitor with other medications known to lower BP.

PREGNANCY: Category C, safety not known in nursing.

MECHANISM OF ACTION: Calcium channel blocker; inhibits calcium ion influx into cardiac muscle and smooth muscle. Angina: Has not been established; believed to act by relaxation and prevention of coronary artery spasm and reduction of oxygen utilization.

PHARMACOKINETICS: Absorption: Rapid and fully absorbed; T_{max}=30 min. **Distribution:** Plasma protein binding (92-98%). **Metabolism:** Liver, extensive. **Elimination:** Urine (80%); $T_{1/2}$=2 hrs.

NURSING CONSIDERATIONS

Assessment: Assess for CHF, severe obstructive CAD, aortic stenosis, hepatic/renal impairment, essential HTN, recent MI, recent β-blocker withdrawal, pregnancy/nursing status, and possible drug interactions.

Monitoring: Monitor for excessive hypotension, increased frequency, duration and/or severity of angina and/or acute MI (especially during initiation and dose titration), CHF, peripheral edema (determine cause), cholestasis with or without jaundice and allergic hepatitis. Monitor BP, LFTs, BUN, SrCr, for decreased platelet aggregation, and increased bleeding time.

Patient Counseling: Inform about potential risks/benefits of drug. Advise to swallow capsule whole.

Administration: Oral route. Swallow capsule whole. **Storage:** 15-25°C (59-77°F). Protect from light and moisture.

NILANDRON RX N
nilutamide (Sanofi-Aventis)

> Interstitial pneumonitis reported. Reports of interstitial changes including pulmonary fibrosis that led to hospitalization and death reported rarely. Symptoms included exertional dyspnea, cough, chest pain, and fever. X-rays showed interstitial or alveolo-interstitial changes, and pulmonary function tests revealed a restrictive pattern with decreased DLco. Perform routine chest x-ray prior to initiating treatment; consider baseline pulmonary function tests. Instruct patients to report any new or worsening SOB during treatment. If symptoms occur, d/c immediately until it can be determined if symptoms are drug related.

THERAPEUTIC CLASS: Nonsteroidal antiandrogen

INDICATIONS: In combination with surgical castration for the treatment of metastatic prostate cancer (Stage D_2).

DOSAGE: *Adults:* Usual: 300mg qd for 30 days, followed thereafter by 150mg qd.

HOW SUPPLIED: Tab: 150mg

CONTRAINDICATIONS: Severe hepatic impairment, severe respiratory insufficiency.

WARNINGS/PRECAUTIONS: For max benefit, begin treatment on the same day as or on the day after surgical castration. Hepatotoxicity reported; measure serum transaminase levels prior to initiation, at regular intervals for 1st 4 months of treatment, and periodically thereafter. Obtain LFTs at 1st sign/symptom suggestive of liver dysfunction; d/c immediately if jaundice develops or ALT >2X ULN and closely monitor LFTs until resolution. Not for use in women, particularly for non-serious or non-life-threatening conditions. Isolated cases of aplastic anemia reported. Patients whose disease progresses while on therapy may experience clinical improvement with d/c.

ADVERSE REACTIONS: Interstitial pneumonitis, hot flushes, impaired adaptation to dark, nausea, urinary tract infection, increased AST/ALT, dizziness, constipation, abnormal vision, dyspnea, HTN.

INTERACTIONS: May reduce metabolism of CYP450 substrates in vitro; may increase serum $T_{1/2}$ of drugs with a low therapeutic margin (eg, vitamin K antagonists, phenytoin, theophylline), leading to a toxic level; dosage of these drugs or others with similar metabolism may need to be modified. Monitor PT and reduce dose of vitamin K antagonists if necessary.

PREGNANCY: Category C, safety not known in nursing.

MECHANISM OF ACTION: Nonsteroidal antiandrogen; blocks effects of testosterone at the androgen receptor level in vitro and interacts with the androgen receptor and prevents the normal androgenic response in vivo.

PHARMACOKINETICS: Absorption: Rapid and complete. **Metabolism:** Extensive, via oxidation. **Elimination:** Urine (62%, <2% unchanged), feces (1.4%-7%); $T_{1/2}$=38-59.1 hrs (100-300mg single dose).

NURSING CONSIDERATIONS

Assessment: Assess for severe hepatic impairment, severe respiratory insufficiency, hypersensitivity to drug or any of its component, and possible drug interactions. Perform routine chest X-ray, and obtain baseline pulmonary function tests and hepatic enzymes.

Monitoring: Monitor for signs/symptoms of interstitial pneumonitis, hepatotoxicity, and disease progression. Measure serum transaminase levels at regular intervals for 1st 4 months of treatment, and periodically thereafter. Obtain LFTs at 1st sign/symptom suggestive of liver dysfunction.

Patient Counseling: Inform that therapy should be started on the day of, or on the day after, surgical castration; advise not to interrupt or d/c dosing without consulting physician. Instruct to report any new or worsening dyspnea. Advise to consult physician should N/V, abdominal pain, or jaundice occur. Instruct to avoid intake of alcoholic beverages if experiencing alcohol intolerance. Counsel to wear tinted glasses to alleviate the delayed adaptation to dark; caution about driving at night and through tunnels.

Administration: Oral route. **Storage:** 25°C (77°F); excursions permitted between 15-30°C (59-86°F). Protect from light.

NIRAVAM
alprazolam (Azur)

CIV

THERAPEUTIC CLASS: Benzodiazepine

INDICATIONS: Treatment of generalized anxiety disorder and panic disorder, with or without agoraphobia.

DOSAGE: *Adults:* Individualize dose. Anxiety: Initial: 0.25-0.5mg tid. Titrate: May increase every 3-4 days. Max: 4mg/day in divided doses. Panic Disorder: Initial: 0.5mg tid. Titrate: May increase by no more than 1mg/day every 3-4 days depending on response; slower titration to doses >4mg/day. Usual: 1-10mg/day. Daily Dose Reduction/Discontinuation: Decrease dose gradually (no more than 0.5mg/day every 3 days). Elderly/Advanced Liver Disease/Debilitating Disease: Initial: 0.25mg bid-tid. Titrate: Increase gradually PRN and as tolerated.

HOW SUPPLIED: Tab, Disintegrating: 0.25mg*, 0.5mg*, 1mg*, 2mg* *scored

CONTRAINDICATIONS: Acute narrow-angle glaucoma, coadministration with potent CYP3A4 inhibitors (eg, ketoconazole, itraconazole).

WARNINGS/PRECAUTIONS: Seizures, including status epilepticus reported with dose reduction or abrupt d/c. Use may lead to physical and psychological dependence; prescribe for short periods and periodically reassess the need for continued treatment. Increased risk of dependence with doses >4mg/day, treatment for >12 weeks, and in panic disorder patients. May cause fetal harm. Avoid use during 1st trimester of pregnancy; may increase risk of congenital anomalies. May impair mental/physical abilities. Hypomania and mania reported in patients with depression. Early morning anxiety and emergence of anxiety symptoms between doses reported; give same total daily dose divided as more frequent administrations. Withdrawal reactions may occur; reduce dose or d/c therapy gradually. Has a weak uricosuric effect. Decreased systemic elimination rate with alcoholic liver disease and obesity. Caution with severe depression, suicidal ideation/plans, impaired renal/hepatic/pulmonary function, elderly, and debilitated. Slow disintegration or dissolution, resulting in slowed or decreased absorption with diseases that cause dry mouth or raise stomach pH.

ADVERSE REACTIONS: Sedation, fatigue/tiredness, impaired coordination, irritability, memory impairment, increased/decreased appetite, cognitive disorder, weight gain/loss, constipation, dysarthria, lightheadedness, dry mouth, decreased/increased libido.

INTERACTIONS: See Contraindications. Avoid with other azole-type antifungals. Caution with alcohol, other CNS depressants, propoxyphene, diltiazem, isoniazid, macrolide antibiotics (eg, erythromycin, clarithromycin), grapefruit juice, sertraline, paroxetine, ergotamine, cyclosporine, amiodarone, nicardipine, nifedipine, and other CYP3A inhibitors. Increased plasma levels of imipramine and desipramine. Additive CNS depressant effects with psychotropics, anticonvulsants, antihistaminics, alcohol, and other drugs which themselves produce CNS depression. Slow disintegration or dissolution, resulting in slowed or decreased absorption with drugs that cause dry mouth or raise stomach pH. Increased concentration with nefazodone, fluvoxamine, and cimetidine; consider dose reduction of alprazolam. Increased concentration with fluoxetine and oral contraceptives; use with caution. Decreased levels with CYP3A inducers, propoxyphene, carbamazepine, and smoking.

PREGNANCY: Category D, not for use in nursing.

MECHANISM OF ACTION: Benzodiazepine; not established. Binds to gamma aminobutyric acid (GABA) receptors in the brain and enhances GABA-mediated synaptic inhibition; such actions may be responsible for the efficacy in anxiety disorder and panic disorder.

PHARMACOKINETICS: Absorption: Readily absorbed; C_{max}=8-37ng/mL (0.5-3mg); T_{max}=1.5-2 hrs. **Distribution:** Plasma protein binding (80%); crosses placenta; found in breast milk. **Metabolism:** Extensive. Liver via CYP3A4; 4-hydroxyalprazolam and α-hydroxyalprazolam (major metabolites). **Elimination:** Urine, $T_{1/2}$=12.5 hrs.

NURSING CONSIDERATIONS

Assessment: Assess for known sensitivity to drug, acute narrow-angle glaucoma, depression, suicidal ideation, renal/hepatic/pulmonary impairment, debilitation, obesity, diseases that cause dry mouth or raise stomach pH, history of alcohol/substance abuse, history of seizures/epilepsy, pregnancy/nursing status, and possible drug interactions. Assess for risk of dependence among panic disorder patients.

Monitoring: Monitor for dependence, rebound/withdrawal symptoms (eg, seizures), early morning anxiety and emergence of anxiety symptoms, CNS depression, hypomania, mania, suicidality, and other treatment-emergent symptoms. Reassess usefulness of therapy periodically.

Patient Counseling: Instruct not to remove tab from the bottle until just prior to dosing and inform of proper administration. Advise to inform physician about any alcohol consumption and medicine taken; alcohol should generally be avoided while taking this medication. Instruct to inform physician of pregnancy/nursing status. Advise not to drive or operate dangerous machinery until become familiar with the effects of this medication. Advise not to increase/decrease dose or abruptly d/c therapy without consulting physician; instruct to follow gradual dosage tapering schedule. Inform of risks associated with doses >4mg/day.

Administration: Oral route. Remove tab from bottle with dry hands and immediately place tab on top of the tongue. Refer to PI for additional handling/administration instructions. **Storage:** 20-25°C (68-77°F); excursions permitted to 15-30°C (59-86°F). Protect from moisture.

NITRO-DUR   RX
nitroglycerin (Schering)

OTHER BRAND NAMES: Nitrek (Mylan Bertek) - Minitran (Graceway)

THERAPEUTIC CLASS: Nitrate vasodilator

INDICATIONS: Prevention of angina pectoris. Not for acute attack.

DOSAGE: *Adults:* Initial: 0.2-0.4mg/hr for 12-14 hrs. Remove for 10-12 hrs.

HOW SUPPLIED: Patch: (Minitran) 0.1mg/hr, 0.2mg/hr, 0.4mg/hr, 0.6mg/hr [30s]; (Nitrek) 0.2mg/hr, 0.4mg/hr, 0.6mg/hr [30s]; (Nitro-Dur) 0.1mg/hr, 0.2mg/hr, 0.3mg/hr, 0.4mg/hr, 0.6mg/hr, 0.8mg/hr [30s]

CONTRAINDICATIONS: Allergy to adhesives in NTG patches.

WARNINGS/PRECAUTIONS: Severe hypotension may occur; caution with volume depletion or hypotension. May aggravate angina caused by hypertrophic cardiomyopathy. Tolerance to other nitrate forms may decrease effects. Monitor with acute MI or CHF. Do not discharge defibrillator/cardioverter through the patch.

ADVERSE REACTIONS: Headache, lightheadedness, hypotension, syncope.

INTERACTIONS: Additive vasodilating effects with other vasodilators (eg, alcohol). Marked orthostatic hypotension reported with CCBs. Vasodilatory effects with phosphodiesterase inhibitors (eg, sildenafil) can result in severe hypotension.

PREGNANCY: Category C, caution in nursing.

MECHANISM OF ACTION: Nitrate vasodilator; relaxes vascular smooth muscle, and consequent dilatation of peripheral arteries and veins, especially the latter. Dilatation of veins leads to reduced left ventricular end-diastolic pressure and pulmonary capillary wedge pressure (preload). Arteriolar relaxation reduces systemic vascular resistance, systolic arterial pressure, and mean arterial pressure (afterload). It also dilates the coronary artery.

PHARMACOKINETICS: Absorption: T_{max}=2 hrs. **Distribution:** V_d=3L/kg. **Metabolism:** Extrahepatic metabolism (RBC and vascular walls). Inorganic nitrate and the 1,2- and 1,3- dinitroglycerols. Dinitrates are metabolized to mononitrates and to glycerol and CO_2. **Elimination:** $T_{1/2}$=3 min.

NURSING CONSIDERATIONS

Assessment: Assess for severe hypotension or volume depletion, angina caused by hypertrophic cardiomyopathy, alcohol intake, pregnancy/nursing status, and possible drug interactions.

Monitoring: Monitor for hypotension and tachycardia. Monitor for paradoxical bradycardia and increased angina pectoris, decreased exercise tolerance and hemodynamic rebound, headaches and lightheadedness on standing, manifestation of true physical dependence (chest pain, acute MI), and methemoglobinemia.

Patient Counseling: Counsel to carefully follow dosing regimen. Inform about headaches (markers of drug activity) and lightheadedness on standing. Avoid alcohol consumption.

Administration: Transdermal route. **Storage:** 15-30°C (59-86°F).

NITROLINGUAL SPRAY   RX
nitroglycerin (Arbor Pharmaceuticals)

OTHER BRAND NAMES: NitroMist (Akrimax)

THERAPEUTIC CLASS: Nitrate vasodilator

INDICATIONS: Acute relief of an attack or prophylaxis of angina pectoris due to coronary artery disease.

DOSAGE: *Adults:* Acute: 1-2 sprays at onset of attack onto or under the tongue. May repeat (Nitrolingual) q3-5 min or (Nitromist) q5 min PRN. Max: 3 sprays/15 min. If chest pain persist after a total of 3 sprays, prompt medical attention is recommended. Prophylaxis: 1-2 sprays onto or under the tongue 5-10 min before activity that may cause acute attack. (NitroMist) Elderly: Start at lower end of dosing range.

HOW SUPPLIED: Spray: 400mcg/spray

CONTRAINDICATIONS: Concomitant use with selective inhibitor of cyclic guanosine monophosphate (cGMP)-specific phosphodiesterase type 5 (PDE5), as PDE5 inhibitors such as sildenafil, vardenafil, and tadalafil. (NitroMist) Severe anemia and increased intracranial pressure (ICP).

WARNINGS/PRECAUTIONS: Severe hypotension may occur; caution with volume depletion or hypotension. May aggravate angina caused by hypertrophic cardiomyopathy. (NitroMist) Dose-related headaches reported. Excessive use may lead to development of tolerance; use only the smallest number of doses required for effective response. (Nitrolingual) Tolerance and cross-tolerance to other nitrates/nitrites may occur.

ADVERSE REACTIONS: Headache, flushing, drug rash, exfoliative dermatitis.

INTERACTIONS: See Contraindications. Marked orthostatic hypotension reported with calcium channel blockers. (Nitrolingual) Alcohol may enhance sensitivity to the hypotensive effects. Decreased or increased effect with other agents that depend on vascular smooth muscle. (NitroMist) Additive hypotensive effects with antihypertensive drugs, and β-adrenergic blockers (eg, labetolol). Increased levels with aspirin. May reduce anticoagulant effect of heparin. Decreased 1st-pass metabolism of dihydroergotamine; avoid ergotamine and related drugs. Caution with tissue-type plasminogen activator; may decrease thrombolytic effect.

PREGNANCY: Category C, caution in nursing.

MECHANISM OF ACTION: Nitrate vasodilator; relaxation of vascular smooth muscle, producing a vasodilator effect on both peripheral arteries and veins with more prominent effects on the latter.

PHARMACOKINETICS: Absorption: (Nitrolingual) C_{max}=1041pg/mL•min, T_{max}=7.5 min, AUC=12,769pg/mL•min. (NitroMist) C_{max}=0.8ng/mL, T_{max}=8 min; (1,2-dinitroglycerin) C_{max}=3.7ng/mL, T_{max}=34 min; (1,3-dinitroglycerin) C_{max}=1ng/mL, T_{max}=41 min. **Metabolism:** Liver via reductase enzyme to glycerol nitrate metabolites and inorganic nitrates; hydrolysis to 1,2- and 1,3-dinitroglycerin (active metabolites). **Elimination:** (Nitrolingual) $T_{1/2}$=3 min, 10 min (1,2-dinitroglycerin), 11 min (1,3-dinitroglycerin).

NURSING CONSIDERATIONS

Assessment: Assess for hypotension, volume-depletion, angina caused by hypertrophic cardiomyopathy, pregnancy/nursing status, and possible drug interactions. (NitroMist) Assess for severe anemia and increased ICP.

Monitoring: Monitor for hypotension with paradoxical bradycardia, increased angina, and tolerance. Perform clinical or hemodynamic monitoring with acute myocardial infarction.

Patient Counseling: Inform about side effects of the drug. Instruct not to take with drugs used for erectile dysfunction. Instruct not to open the bottle forcibly or use near open flame. Instruct how to prime device prior to use and if device has not been used within 6 weeks. (Nitrolingual) Instruct to use 5-10 min prior to engaging in activities which might provoke an acute attack.

Administration: Oral transmucosal route. Do not inhale. (Nitrolingual) Do not expectorate medication or rinse mouth for 5-10 min after administration. **Storage:** 25°C (77°F); excursions permitted to 15-30°C (59-85°F).

NITROSTAT   RX
nitroglycerin (Parke-Davis)

THERAPEUTIC CLASS: Nitrate vasodilator

INDICATIONS: Acute relief of an attack or acute prophylaxis of angina pectoris due to coronary artery disease.

DOSAGE: *Adults:* Treatment: 1 tab SL or in buccal pouch at 1st sign of acute attack. May repeat every 5 min until relief is obtained. If pain persists after a total of 3 tabs in 15 min, or if pain is different than typically experienced, prompt medical attention is recommended. Prophylaxis: Take 5-10 min prior to engaging in activities that may cause acute attack. Elderly: Start at lower end of dosing range.

HOW SUPPLIED: Tab, SL: 0.3mg, 0.4mg, 0.6mg

CONTRAINDICATIONS: Early myocardial infarction (MI), severe anemia, increased intracranial pressure (ICP), patients who are using a phophodiesterase-5 inhibitor (eg, sildenafil citrate, tadalafil, vardenafil hydrochloride).

WARNINGS/PRECAUTIONS: Use smallest dose required for effective relief of acute attack; excessive use may lead to tolerance. Severe hypotension, particularly with upright posture, may occur with small doses; caution with volume-depletion or hypotension. Nitroglycerin-induced hypotension may be accompanied by paradoxical bradycardia and increased angina pectoris. May aggravate angina caused by hypertrophic cardiomyopathy. As tolerance to other forms of nitroglycerin develops, effect on exercise tolerance is blunted. Physical dependence may occur. D/C if blurred vision or dry mouth occurs. Excessive dosage may produce severe headaches. SL nitroglycerin may cause nitrate tolerance in patients who maintain high continuous nitrate levels for more than 10-12 hrs daily. Caution in elderly.

ADVERSE REACTIONS: Headache, vertigo, dizziness, weakness, palpitation, syncope, flushing, drug rash, exfoliative dermatitis.

INTERACTIONS: See Contraindications. Antihypertensive drugs, β-adrenergic blockers, or phenothiazines may cause additive hypotensive effects. Calcium channel blockers may cause marked orthostatic hypotension. Alcohol may cause hypotension. Aspirin may enhance vasodilatory and hemodynamic effects. Caution with alteplase therapy. IV nitroglycerin reduces anticoagulant effect of heparin; monitor activated PTT during concomitant use. TCAs (eg, amitriptyline, desipramine, doxepin) and anticholinergics may make SL tab dissolution difficult. Avoid ergotamine and related drugs or monitor for ergotism symptoms if unavoidable. Long-acting nitrates may decrease therapeutic effect.

PREGNANCY: Category C, caution in nursing.

MECHANISM OF ACTION: Nitrate vasodilator; forms free radical nitric oxide which activates guanylate cyclase, resulting in an increase of guanosine 3'5' monophosphate in smooth muscle and other tissues leading to dephosphorylation of myosin light chains, which regulate contractile state in smooth muscle, resulting in vasodilatation.

PHARMACOKINETICS: Absorption: (SL) Rapid. Absolute bioavailability (40%). (0.3mg x 2 doses) C_{max}=2.3ng/mL, T_{max}=6.4 min, AUC=14.9ng•mL/min; (0.6mg x 1 dose) C_{max}=2.1ng/mL, T_{max}=7.2 min, AUC=14.9ng•mL/min. **Distribution:** (IV) V_d=3.3L/kg; plasma protein binding (60%). **Metabolism:** Liver via reductase enzyme to glycerol nitrate metabolites to glycerol and organic nitrate; 1,2- and 1,3-dinitroglycerin (major metabolites). **Elimination:** $T_{1/2}$=2.8 min (0.3mg x 2 doses), 2.6 min (0.6mg x 1 dose).

NURSING CONSIDERATIONS

Assessment: Assess for early MI, severe anemia, increased ICP, hypotension, volume depletion, angina caused by hypertrophic cardiomyopathy, known hypersensitivity to the drug, pregnancy/ nursing status, and possible drug interactions.

Monitoring: Monitor for hypotension, paradoxical bradycardia, increased/aggravated angina pectoris, tolerance, physical dependence, blurring of vision, drying of mouth, headache, and other adverse reactions. In patients with an acute MI or congestive heart failure, perform careful clinical or hemodynamic monitoring for hypotension and tachycardia.

Patient Counseling: Counsel on the proper dosage and administration of the drug. Instruct to take tab sublingually; do not chew, crush, or swallow. Advise to sit down when taking the drug and to use caution when returning to standing position. Inform about side effects of the drug (eg, headaches, lightheadedness upon standing, burning or tingling sensation when administered SL). Counsel that lightheadedness may be more frequent in patients who have consumed alcohol. Instruct to keep in original glass container and to tightly cap after each use.

Administration: SL route. Do not swallow tabs; intended for SL or buccal administration. Administer in sitting position. **Storage:** 20-25°C (68-77°F).

NIZATIDINE

RX

nizatidine (Sandoz)

OTHER BRAND NAMES: Axid (Braintree)

THERAPEUTIC CLASS: H_2-blocker

INDICATIONS: Treatment of active duodenal ulcer (DU) and benign gastric ulcer (GU) for up to 8 weeks. Maintenance therapy for DU after healing of an active DU. Treatment of endoscopically diagnosed esophagitis, including erosive and ulcerative esophagitis, and heartburn due to gastroesophageal reflux disease (GERD) for up to 12 weeks. (Sol) Treatment of endoscopically diagnosed esophagitis, including erosive and ulcerative esophagitis, and heartburn due to gastroesophageal reflux disease (GERD) for up to 8 weeks in pediatrics ≥12 yrs.

DOSAGE: *Adults:* Active DU/Active Benign GU: Usual: 300mg qhs or 150mg bid up to 8 weeks. Maint of Healed Active DU: 150mg qhs up to 1 yr. GERD: 150mg bid up to 12 weeks. Renal Impairment: CrCl 20-50mL/min: 150mg/day. Maint: 150mg qod. CrCl <20mL/min: 150mg qod. Maint: 150mg every 3 days. Elderly: Caution with dose selection.
Pediatrics: ≥12 yrs: (Sol) Erosive Esophagitis/GERD: 150mg bid up to 8 weeks. Max: 300mg/day. Renal Impairment: CrCl 20-50mL/min: 150mg/day. Maint: 150mg qod. CrCl <20mL/min: 150mg qod. Maint: 150mg every 3 days.

HOW SUPPLIED: Cap: 150mg, 300mg; Sol: (Axid) 15mg/mL [480mL]

WARNINGS/PRECAUTIONS: Caution with moderate to severe renal insufficiency; reduce dose. Symptomatic response does not preclude the presence of gastric malignancy. False positive tests for urobilinogen with Multistix may occur. Caution in elderly. (Cap) Safety and effectiveness in pediatrics not established.

ADVERSE REACTIONS: Headache, abdominal pain, pain, asthenia, diarrhea, N/V, flatulence, dyspepsia, rhinitis, pharyngitis, dizziness, cough, fever, irritability.

INTERACTIONS: May elevate serum salicylate levels with high dose (3900mg/day) aspirin. Inhibits gastric acid secretion stimulated by caffeine, betazole, and pentagastrin. May decrease absorption with antacids consisting of aluminum and magnesium hydroxides with simethicone. Fatal thrombocytopenia reported with concomitant use of another H_2-receptor antagonist.

PREGNANCY: Category B, not for use in nursing.

MECHANISM OF ACTION: H_2-receptor antagonist; competitive, reversible inhibitor of histamine at the histamine H_2-receptors, particularly those in the gastric parietal cells.

PHARMACOKINETICS: Absorption: Absolute bioavailability (>70%); C_{max}=700-1,800mcg/L (150mg dose), 1400-3600mcg/L (300mg dose), T_{max}=0.5-3 hrs. **Distribution:** Plasma protein binding (35%); found in breast milk. **Metabolism:** N2-monodesmethylnizatidine (principal metabolite). **Elimination:** Urine (>90%, 60% unchanged); feces (<6%); $T_{1/2}$=1-2 hrs, 3.5-11 hrs (anepheric patients).

NURSING CONSIDERATIONS

Assessment: Assess for hypersensitivity to other H_2 receptor antagonists, renal dysfunction, presence of gastric malignancy, pregnancy/nursing status, and possible drug interactions.

Monitoring: Monitor for signs/symptoms of hypersensitivity and other adverse reactions. Monitor for signs of clinical improvement.

Patient Counseling: Inform of the risks/benefits of therapy. Advise to take medication exactly as prescribed. Instruct to contact physician if signs/symptoms of hypersensitivity or other adverse reaction develops. Counsel pregnant/nursing females about risks of use.

Administration: Oral route. **Storage:** Cap: 20-25° (68-77°F). Sol: 25° (77°F); excursions permitted to 15-30°C (59-86°F).

NORCO

CIII

hydrocodone bitartrate - acetaminophen (Watson)

> Associated with cases of acute liver failure, at times resulting in liver transplant and death, mostly associated with acetaminophen (APAP) use at doses >4000mg/day, and often involved >1 APAP-containing product.

OTHER BRAND NAMES: Maxidone (Watson)

THERAPEUTIC CLASS: Opioid analgesic

INDICATIONS: Relief of moderate to moderately severe pain.

DOSAGE: *Adults:* Adjust dose according to severity of pain and response. (5mg-325mg) Usual: 1 or 2 tabs q4-6h PRN. Max: 8 tabs/day. (7.5mg-325mg, 10mg-325mg) Usual: 1 tab q4-6h PRN. Max: 6 tabs/day. (Maxidone) Usual: 1 tab q4-6h PRN. Max: 5 tabs/day. Elderly: Start at lower end of dosing range.

HOW SUPPLIED: Tab: (Hydrocodone-APAP) (Norco) 5mg-325mg*, 7.5mg-325mg*, 10mg-325mg*; (Maxidone) 10mg-750mg* *scored

WARNINGS/PRECAUTIONS: Increased risk of acute liver failure in patients with underlying liver disease. Hypersensitivity and anaphylaxis reported; d/c if signs/symptoms occur. May produce dose-related respiratory depression at high doses or in sensitive patients, and irregular/periodic breathing. Respiratory depressant effects and CSF pressure elevation capacity may be exaggerated in the presence of head injury, intracranial lesions, or preexisting increase in intracranial pressure. May obscure diagnosis or clinical course of acute abdominal conditions or head injuries. Caution in elderly, debilitated, severe hepatic/renal impairment, hypothyroidism, Addison's disease, prostatic hypertrophy, and urethral stricture. Suppresses cough reflex; caution with pulmonary disease and in postoperative use. Dependence and tolerance may develop.

ADVERSE REACTIONS: Acute liver failure, lightheadedness, dizziness, sedation, N/V.

INTERACTIONS: Additive CNS depression with narcotics, antipsychotics, antihistamines, antianxiety agents, alcohol, or other CNS depressants; reduce dose. Use with MAOIs or TCAs may increase the effect of either the antidepressant or hydrocodone. Increased risk of acute liver failure with alcohol.

PREGNANCY: Category C, not for use in nursing.

MECHANISM OF ACTION: Hydrocodone: Opioid analgesic; not established. Believed to relate to existence of opiate receptors in the CNS. APAP: Nonopiate, nonsalicylate analgesic and antipyretic; not established. Antipyretic activity mediated through hypothalamic heat-regulating centers; inhibits prostaglandin synthetase.

PHARMACOKINETICS: Absorption: Hydrocodone: (10mg) C_{max}=23.6ng/mL, T_{max}=1.3 hrs. APAP: Rapid. **Distribution:** APAP: Found in breast milk. **Metabolism:** Hydrocodone: O-demethylation, N-demethylation, and 6-ketoreduction. APAP: Liver via conjugation. **Elimination:** Hydrocodone: (10mg) $T_{1/2}$=3.8 hrs. APAP: Urine (85%); $T_{1/2}$=1.25-3 hrs.

NURSING CONSIDERATIONS

Assessment: Assess for level of pain intensity, type of pain, patient's general condition and medical status, or any other conditions where treatment is contraindicated or cautioned. Assess for history of hypersensitivity, renal/hepatic impairment, pregnancy/nursing status, and possible drug interactions.

Monitoring: Monitor for acute liver failure, hypersensitivity reactions, respiratory depression, drug dependence or tolerance, and other adverse reactions. Monitor serial hepatic/renal function tests with severe hepatic/renal disease.

Patient Counseling: Instruct to look for APAP on package labels and not to use >1 APAP-containing product. Instruct to seek medical attention immediately upon ingestion of >4000mg/day of APAP or more than recommended dose of therapy, even if feeling well. Advise to d/c and contact physician if signs of allergy (eg, rash, difficulty breathing) develop. Inform that drug may impair mental/physical abilities; instruct to use caution if performing hazardous tasks (eg, operating machinery/driving). Instruct to avoid alcohol and other CNS depressants, and to take drug exactly as prescribed.

Administration: Oral route. **Storage:** (5mg-325mg) 15-30°C (59-86°F). (7.5mg-325mg, 10mg-325mg)/(Maxidone) 20-25°C (68-77°F).

NORDITROPIN   RX
somatropin rdna origin (Novo Nordisk)

OTHER BRAND NAMES: Norditropin FlexPro (Novo Nordisk) - Norditropin Nordiflex (Novo Nordisk)

THERAPEUTIC CLASS: Human growth hormone

INDICATIONS: (Adults) Replacement of endogenous growth hormone (GH) with adult-onset or childhood-onset growth hormone deficiency (GHD). (Pediatrics) Treatment for growth failure due to inadequate endogenous growth hormone secretion. Treatment for short stature associated with Noonan syndrome and Turner syndrome (TS). Treatment for short stature born small for gestational age (SGA) with no catch-up growth by age 2-4 yrs.

DOSAGE: *Adults:* GHD: Weight-Based: Initial: ≤0.004mg/kg/day SQ. Titrate: Increase to ≤0.016mg/kg/day after 6 weeks according to individual requirements. Non-Weight Based: Initial: 0.2mg/day SQ (range, 0.15-0.30mg/day). Titrate: Increase gradually every 1-2 months by 0.1-0.2mg/day based on response and insulin-like growth factor-I (IGF-I) concentrations. Elderly: Lower starting dose and smaller dose increments. Estrogen-replete women may need higher doses than men.

Pediatrics: Individualize dose. GHD: 0.024-0.034mg/kg/day SQ 6-7X/week. Noonan Syndrome: ≤0.066mg/kg/day SQ. TS/SGA: ≤0.067mg/kg/day SQ. Refer to PI for further details.

HOW SUPPLIED: Inj: 5mg/1.5mL, 15mg/1.5mL [cartridge]; (FlexPro) 5mg/1.5mL, 10mg/1.5mL, 15mg/1.5mL [prefilled pen]; (Nordiflex) 5mg/1.5mL, 10mg/1.5mL, 15mg/1.5mL, 30mg/3mL [prefilled pen].

CONTRAINDICATIONS: Acute critical illness due to complications following open heart surgery, abdominal surgery or multiple accidental trauma, or acute respiratory failure (ARF); Prader-Willi syndrome with severe obesity, history of upper airway obstruction or sleep apnea, or severe respiratory impairment; active malignancy; active proliferative or severe non-proliferative diabetic retinopathy; pediatrics with closed epiphyses.

WARNINGS/PRECAUTIONS: Increased mortality reported with acute critical illness; weigh benefit against the potential risk for treatment continuation if these illnesses develop during therapy. Not indicated for growth failure due to genetically confirmed Prader-Willi syndrome. In patients with pre-existing tumors or GHD secondary to an intracranial lesion, monitor for progression or recurrence of underlying disease. Interrupt therapy if signs of upper airway obstruction, onset of or increased snoring, and/or new onset sleep apnea develops. Monitor for potential malignant transformation of skin lesions. May unmask undiagnosed impaired glucose tolerance and overt diabetes mellitus (DM); monitor glucose levels. New onset type 2 DM reported. Intracranial HTN with papilledema, visual changes, headache, N/V reported; perform funduscopic exam before initiation and during therapy and d/c if papilledema occurs. Fluid retention may occur. Undiagnosed/untreated hypothyroidism may prevent optimal response. Hypothyroidism may become evident or worsen; perform periodic thyroid function tests. Slipped capital femoral epiphysis may occur; pediatric patients with onset of a limp or complaints of hip or knee pain during therapy should be evaluated. Progression of scoliosis may occur in pediatrics with rapid growth; caution with history of scoliosis. Increased risk of ear/hearing disorders and cardiovascular (CV) disorders in patients with TS. Patients with epiphyseal closure who were treated in childhood should be re-evaluated before continuation of therapy as adults. Tissue atrophy may occur when administered at the same site over a long period of time. Allergic reactions may occur. Pancreatitis reported (rare); consider pancreatitis if persistent severe abdominal pain develops. Caution in elderly. Serum levels of inorganic phosphorus, alkaline phosphatase, parathyroid hormone and IGF-I may increase after therapy. Treatment for short stature should be d/c when the epiphyses are fused.

ADVERSE REACTIONS: Edema, infection, arthralgia, headache, increased sweating, leg edema, myalgia, bronchitis, flu-like symptoms, HTN, gastroenteritis, paresthesia, skeletal pain, laryngitis, otitis media.

INTERACTIONS: Use with glucocorticoid therapy may attenuate growth-promoting effects in children; carefully adjust glucocorticoid replacement dosing. May inhibit 11β-hydroxysteroid dehydrogenase type 1 (11βHSD-1), resulting in reduced serum cortisol concentrations; may need glucocorticoid replacement or dose adjustments in glucocorticoid therapy. May alter the clearance of compounds metabolized by CYP450 liver enzymes (eg, corticosteroids, sex steroids, anticonvulsants, cyclosporine). May increase clearance of antipyrine. May require larger dose with oral estrogen replacement. May require dose adjustment of insulin or oral/injectable hypoglycemic agents in diabetic patients and thyroid hormone replacement therapy in patients with thyroid dysfunction.

PREGNANCY: Category C, caution in nursing.

MECHANISM OF ACTION: Human GH; binds to dimeric GH receptor in cell membrane of target cells, resulting in intracellular signal transduction and a host of pharmacodynamic effects.

PHARMACOKINETICS: Absorption: T_{max}=4-5 hrs; C_{max}=13.8ng/mL (4mg), 17.1ng/mL (8mg). **Elimination**: $T_{1/2}$=7-10 hrs.

NURSING CONSIDERATIONS

Assessment: Assess for any condition where treatment is contraindicated or cautioned. Assess for pregnancy/nursing status, drug hypersensitivity, and possible drug interactions. In patients with TS, assess for otitis media, other ear disorders, and CV disorders. In patients with epiphyseal closure who were treated with somatropin replacement therapy in childhood, reevaluate before continuing therapy as adults. Perform funduscopic exam. Assess for short stature in patients with Noonan syndrome.

Monitoring: Monitor for upper airway obstruction, onset of or increased snoring, sleep apnea, malignant transformation of skin lesions, intracranial HTN, fluid retention, slipped capital femoral epiphysis, progression of scoliosis, tissue atrophy at injection site, allergic reactions, and pancreatitis. Monitor growth response and IGF-I concentrations. Perform periodic thyroid function tests, funduscopic exam, and measurement of glucose levels. Monitor for progression of underlying disease process with pre-existing tumors or GHD secondary to intracranial lesion. In patients with TS, monitor for signs/symptoms of otitis media and for CV disorders.

Patient Counseling: Inform about benefits/risks of therapy. Instruct on proper usage and disposal, and caution against reuse of needles. Seek medical attention if symptoms of allergic reactions, slipped capital femoral epiphysis (onset of limp, hip or knee pain), respiratory infections (eg, otitis media or ear/CV disorders) and/or progression of scoliosis occurs.

Administration: SQ route. Always rotate inj sites. **Storage:** Unused: 2-8°C (36-46°F). Do not freeze. Avoid direct light. In-use: 5mg, 10mg: 2-8°C (36-46°F) and use within 4 weeks or store ≤25°C (77°F) for ≤3 weeks. Discard unused portion. 15mg, 30mg: 2-8°C (36-46°F) and use within 4 weeks; discard unused portion after 4 weeks.

NORINYL 1/50   RX
| mestranol - norethindrone (Watson)

Cigarette smoking increases the risk of serious CV side effects. Risk increases with age (>35 yrs) and with heavy smoking (≥15 cigarettes/day). Women who use oral contraceptives should be strongly advised not to smoke.

OTHER BRAND NAMES: Necon 1/50 (Watson)

THERAPEUTIC CLASS: Estrogen/progestogen combination

INDICATIONS: Prevention of pregnancy.

DOSAGE: *Adults:* 1 tab qd for 28 days, then repeat. Start 1st Sunday after menses begin or 1st day of menses.
Pediatrics: Postpubertal Adolescents: 1 tab qd for 28 days, then repeat. Start 1st Sunday after menses begin or 1st day of menses.

HOW SUPPLIED: Tab: (Mestranol-Norethindrone) 0.05mg-1mg

CONTRAINDICATIONS: Thrombophlebitis, thromboembolic disorders, history of deep vein thrombophlebitis (DVT), cerebral vascular or coronary artery disease (CAD), carcinoma of the endometrium or other known or suspected estrogen-dependent neoplasia, undiagnosed abnormal genital bleeding, cholestatic jaundice of pregnancy or jaundice with prior pill use, hepatic adenomas or carcinomas, known or suspected carcinoma of the breast, and pregnancy. (Norinyl 1/50) Benign liver tumors.

WARNINGS/PRECAUTIONS: Increased risk of MI, vascular disease, thromboembolism, stroke, gallbladder disease, and hepatic neoplasia. Increased risk of morbidity and mortality in patients with HTN, hyperlipidemias, obesity and diabetes. May increase risk of breast cancer and cancer of the reproductive organs. Retinal thrombosis reported; d/c if unexplained partial or complete loss of vision occurs, onset of proptosis or diplopia, papilledema, or retinal vascular lesions develop. May cause glucose intolerance; monitor prediabetic and diabetic patients. May cause fluid retention and increase BP; monitor closely and d/c if significant elevation of BP occurs. Breakthrough bleeding and spotting reported; rule out malignancy or pregnancy. May cause onset or exacerbation of a migraine or development of a headache. May develop visual changes with contact lens. May elevate LDL levels or cause other lipid effects. D/C if jaundice develops. Caution with history of depression; d/c if depression recurs to serious degree. Not indicated for use before menarche. Does not protect against HIV infection (AIDS) and other sexually transmitted diseases (STDs). May affect certain endocrine, LFTs, and blood components in laboratory tests. Ectopic and intrauterine pregnancies may occur with contraceptive failures. Should not be used to induce withdrawal bleeding as a test for pregnancy, or to treat threatened or habitual abortion during pregnancy.

ADVERSE REACTIONS: N/V, breakthrough bleeding, spotting, amenorrhea, migraine, mental depression, vaginal candidiasis, edema, weight changes, abdominal cramps/bloating, menstrual flow changes, melasma.

INTERACTIONS: Reduced effects, increased breakthrough bleeding, and menstrual irregularities with rifampin, barbiturates, phenylbutazone, phenytoin Na⁺, and possibly with griseofulvin, ampicillin, tetracyclines, and (Necon 1/50) carbamazepine.

PREGNANCY: Category X, not for use in nursing.

MECHANISM OF ACTION: Estrogen/progestogen oral contraceptive; suppresses gonadotropins. Primarily inhibits ovulation. Also causes changes in cervical mucus (increases difficulty of sperm entry into uterus) and endometrium (reduces likelihood of implantation).

PHARMACOKINETICS: Distribution: Found in breast milk.

NURSING CONSIDERATIONS

Assessment: Assess for thrombophlebitis, thromboembolic disorders, history of DVT or thromboembolic disorders, any other conditions where treatment is contraindicated or cautioned. Assess for pregnancy/nursing status, and for possible drug interactions. Assess use in patients with hyperlipidemia, HTN, obesity, diabetes, history of depression, and in patients >35 yrs who smoke ≥15 cigarettes/day. (Norinyl 1/50) Assess for benign liver tumors.

Monitoring: Monitor for MI, thromboembolism, stroke, and other adverse effects. Monitor glucose levels in diabetic or prediabetic patients, BP with history of HTN, and lipid levels with history of hyperlipidemia. Monitor for signs of liver dysfunction (eg, jaundice), and signs of worsening depression with previous history. Refer patients with contact lenses to ophthalmologist if ocular changes develop. Perform annual physical exam while on therapy.

Patient Counseling: Inform that therapy does not protect against HIV infection and other STDs. Inform of potential risks/benefits of oral contraceptives. When initiating treatment, instruct to use additional form of contraception until after 7 days on therapy. Take 1 pill at same time daily at intervals not exceeding 24 hrs. If dose is missed, take as soon as possible; take next dose at regularly scheduled time. Continue medication if spotting or breakthrough bleeding occur; notify physician if symptoms persist. Inform that missing a pill can cause spotting or light bleeding. Advise not to smoke while on therapy.

Administration: Oral route. **Storage:** 15-25°C (59-77°F) (Norinyl 1/50); 20-25°C (68-77°F) (Necon 1/50).

NOROXIN RX
norfloxacin (Merck)

> Fluoroquinolones are associated with an increased risk of tendinitis and tendon rupture in all ages. Risk further increased in patients >60 yrs, patients taking corticosteroids, and in patients with kidney, heart, or lung transplants. May exacerbate muscle weakness with myasthenia gravis; avoid in patients with known history of myasthenia gravis.

THERAPEUTIC CLASS: Fluoroquinolone

INDICATIONS: Treatment of complicated and uncomplicated urinary tract infections (UTI), including cystitis, uncomplicated urethral and cervical gonorrhea, and prostatitis caused by susceptible strains of designated microorganisms.

DOSAGE: *Adults:* Uncomplicated UTI due to *E. coli, K. pneumoniae,* or *P. mirabilis*: 400mg q12h for 3 days. Uncomplicated UTIs due to Other Organisms: 400mg q12h for 7-10 days. Complicated UTIs: 400mg q12h for 10-21 days. CrCl ≤30mL/min: 400mg qd. Uncomplicated Gonorrhea: 800mg single dose. Acute/Chronic Prostatitis: 400mg q12h for 28 days.

HOW SUPPLIED: Tab: 400mg

CONTRAINDICATIONS: History of tendinitis or tendon rupture associated with use of quinolones.

WARNINGS/PRECAUTIONS: D/C if experience pain, swelling, inflammation, or rupture of tendon. Convulsions, increased intracranial pressure (ICP) (including pseudotumor cerebri), and toxic psychoses reported. May cause CNS stimulation which may lead to tremors, restlessness, lightheadedness, confusion, and hallucinations. D/C and institute appropriate measures if a CNS reaction occurs. Caution with known or suspected CNS disorders (eg, severe cerebral arteriosclerosis, epilepsy) or other factors which predispose to seizures. Serious and sometimes fatal hypersensitivity reactions reported; d/c if skin rash, jaundice, or any other sign of hypersensitivity appears and institute appropriate therapy. *Clostridium difficile*-associated diarrhea (CDAD) reported. Rare cases of sensory or sensorimotor axonal polyneuropathy, resulting in paresthesias, hypoesthesias, dysesthesias, and weakness reported; d/c if symptoms of neuropathy or deficits in light touch, pain, temperature, position sense, vibratory sensation, and/or motor strength occur. Maintain adequate hydration. Not shown to be effective for syphilis. May mask or delay symptoms of incubating syphilis if used in high doses for short periods of time to treat gonorrhea. All patients with gonorrhea should have a serologic test for syphilis at the time of diagnosis; repeat test after 3 months of treatment. Photosensitivity/phototoxicity reactions may occur; d/c if phototoxicity occurs. Avoid excessive exposure to sun/UV light. Hemolytic reactions reported with glucose-6-phosphate dehydrogenase (G6PD) deficiency. Caution with risk factors for torsades de pointes (eg, known QT prolongation, uncorrected hypokalemia). Caution in elderly and in patients with renal impairment.

ADVERSE REACTIONS: Tendinitis, tendon rupture, muscle weakness exacerbation, dizziness, nausea, headache, abdominal cramping, asthenia, rash.

INTERACTIONS: See Boxed Warning. May increase theophylline and cyclosporine levels. May enhance effects of oral anticoagulants including warfarin or its derivatives; closely monitor PT or other suitable coagulation tests. Diminished urinary excretion with probenecid. Avoid with nitrofurantoin; may antagonize antibacterial effect in urinary tract. Multivitamins, or other products containing iron or zinc, antacids or sucralfate, and didanosine (chewable/buffered tabs, pediatric oral sol) may interfere with absorption; space dose by 2 hrs. May reduce clearance of caffeine. Coadministration with NSAIDs may increase risk of CNS stimulation and convulsive seizures. On rare occasions, may result in severe hypoglycemia if coadministered with glyburide (a sulfonylurea agent); monitor blood glucose levels. Drugs metabolized by CYP1A2 (eg, caffeine, clozapine, ropinirole, tacrine, theophylline, tizanidine) may result in increased substrate drug concentrations when given usual doses. Caution with drugs that can result in prolongation of the QTc interval (eg, class IA or class III antiarrhythmics).

PREGNANCY: Category C, not for use in nursing.

MECHANISM OF ACTION: Fluoroquinolone; inhibits bacterial DNA synthesis, inhibits ATP-dependent DNA supercoiling reaction catalyzed by DNA gyrase, inhibits relaxation of super-coiled DNA, and promotes double-stranded DNA breakage.

PHARMACOKINETICS: Absorption: C_{max}=0.8μg/mL (200mg), 1.5μg/mL (400mg), 2.4μg/mL (800mg); T_{max}=1 hr. Refer to PI for different pharmacokinetic parameters of different age groups. **Distribution:** Plasma protein binding (10-15%). **Elimination:** Urine (26-32% unchanged, 5-8% active metabolites); feces (30%); $T_{1/2}$=3-4 hrs, 4 hrs (elderly).

NURSING CONSIDERATIONS

Assessment: Assess for risk factors for developing tendinitis and tendon rupture. Assess for myasthenia gravis, drug hypersensitivity, CNS disorders or factors that may predispose to seizures, risk factors for torsades de pointes, G6PD deficiency, renal impairment, pregnancy/nursing status, and for possible drug interactions. Obtain baseline culture and susceptibility test, and serologic test for syphilis.

Monitoring: Monitor for tendinitis, tendon rupture, convulsions, increased ICP, toxic psychoses, CNS stimulation, CDAD, neuropathy, photosensitivity reactions, hypersensitivity reactions, and other adverse reactions. Repeat culture and susceptibility testing performed periodically. Perform follow-up serologic test for syphilis after 3 months.

Patient Counseling: Instruct to notify physician if symptoms of pain, swelling, or inflammation of a tendon, or weakness or inability to move joints occur; rest and refrain from exercise and d/c therapy. Advise that therapy may cause changes in the ECG (eg, QTc interval prolongation), dizziness, lightheadedness, and worsening of myasthenia gravis symptoms. Instruct to notify physician if have history of QTc prolongation or proarrhythmic conditions, or if have a history of convulsions. Advise to d/c and contact physician if symptoms of peripheral neuropathies develop or at first sign of skin rash or other allergic reaction. Instruct to take at least 1 hr ac or at least 2 hrs pc or ingestion of dairy products. Inform to drink fluids liberally and to take exactly as directed; advise that skipping doses or not completing full course may decrease effectiveness and increase resistance. Advise to contact physician if diarrhea occurs. Counsel that the drug treats bacterial, not viral infections. Instruct to avoid exposure to natural or artificial sunlight. Counsel on possible drug interactions. Inform that multivitamins or other products containing iron or zinc, antacids, or didanosine should not be taken 2 hrs before or within 2 hrs after taking the drug.

Administration: Oral route. **Storage:** 25°C (77°F); excursions permitted to 15-30°C (59-86°F). Keep container tightly closed.

NORPACE   RX
disopyramide phosphate (Pharmacia & Upjohn)

> In a long-term clinical study in patients with asymptomatic non-life-threatening ventricular arrhythmias who had a myocardial infarction, an excessive mortality or non-fatal cardiac arrest rate was seen in patients treated with encainide or flecainide compared to placebo. Considering the known proarrhythmic properties of Norpace or Norpace CR and the lack of evidence of improved survival, its use should be reserved for patients with life-threatening ventricular arrhythmias.

OTHER BRAND NAMES: Norpace CR (Pharmacia & Upjohn)

THERAPEUTIC CLASS: Class I antiarrhythmic

INDICATIONS: Treatment of documented life-threatening ventricular arrhythmias.

DOSAGE: *Adults:* Usual: 400-800mg/day in divided dose. Recommended: 150mg q6h immediate-release (IR) or 300mg q12h extended-release (CR). Adjust dose with anticholinergic effects. Weight <110 lbs/Moderate Hepatic or Renal Insufficiency (CrCl >40mL/min): 100mg q6h IR or 200mg q12h CR. Severe Renal Insufficiency (with or without initial 150mg LD): CrCl 30-40mL/min: 100mg q8h IR. CrCl 15-30mL/min: 100mg q12h IR. CrCl <15mL/min: 100mg q24h IR. Rapid Control of Ventricular Arrhythmia: LD: 300mg IR (200mg if <110 lbs). Follow with maint dose. Cardiomyopathy/Cardiac Decompensation: Initial: 100mg q6-8h IR. Adjust gradually. See PI if no response or toxicity occurs. Elderly: Start at low end of dosing range. *Pediatrics:* 12-18 yrs: 6-15mg/kg/day. 4-12 yrs: 10-15mg/kg/day. 1-4 yrs: 10-20mg/kg/day. <1 yrs: 10-30mg/kg/day. Give in equally divided doses q6h. Hospitalize patient during initial therapy. Start dose titration at lower end of range.

HOW SUPPLIED: Cap: (Norpace) 100mg, 150mg; Cap, Extended-Release: (Norpace CR) 100mg, 150mg

CONTRAINDICATIONS: Cardiogenic shock, 2nd- or 3rd-degree AV block (if no pacemaker present), congenital QT prolongation.

WARNINGS/PRECAUTIONS: May cause or worsen congestive heart failure (CHF) and produce hypotension due to negative inotropic properties. Reduce dose if 1st-degree heart block occurs. Avoid with urinary retention, glaucoma, and myasthenia gravis unless adequate over-riding measures taken. Atrial flutter/fibrillation; digitalize first. Monitor closely or withdraw

673

if QT prolongation >25% occurs and ectopy continues. D/C if QRS widening >25% occurs. Avoid LD with cardiomyopathy or cardiac decompensation. Correct K⁺ abnormalities before therapy. Reduce dose with renal/hepatic dysfunction; monitor ECG. Avoid CR formulation with CrCl ≤40mL/min. Caution with sick sinus syndrome, Wolff-Parkinson-White syndrome, bundle branch block, or elderly. May significantly lower blood glucose.

ADVERSE REACTIONS: Dry mouth, urinary retention/frequency/urgency, constipation, blurred vision, GI effects, dizziness, fatigue, headache.

INTERACTIONS: Avoid type IA and IC antiarrhythmics, and propranolol except in unresponsive, life-threatening arrhythmias. Hepatic enzyme inducers may lower levels. Avoid within 48 hrs before or 24 hrs after verapamil. Possible fatal interactions with CYP3A4 inhibitors. Monitor blood glucose with β-blockers, alcohol.

PREGNANCY: Category C, not for use in nursing.

MECHANISM OF ACTION: Type I antiarrhythmic; decreases rate of diastolic depolarization in cells with augmented automaticity, decreases upstroke velocity, and increases action potential duration of normal cardiac cells. Decreases disparity in refractoriness between infracted and adjacent normally perfused myocardium and has no effect on α- or β-adrenergic receptors.

PHARMACOKINETICS: Absorption: Rapid and complete; C_{max}=2.22mcg/mL, T_{max}=4.5 hrs. **Distribution:** Plasma protein binding (50-65%). **Metabolism:** Liver. **Elimination:** Urine (50% unchanged), (20% mono-N-dealkylated metabolite), (10% other metabolite); $T_{1/2}$=11.65 hrs.

NURSING CONSIDERATIONS

Assessment: Prior to therapy, patients with atrial flutter or AF should be digitalized and K⁺ abnormalities should be corrected. Assess for cardiogenic shock, pre-existing 2nd- or 3rd-degree heart block, presence of functioning pacemaker, sick sinus syndrome (bradycardia/tachycardia syndrome), Wolff-Parkinson-White syndrome, bundle branch block, congenital QT prolongation, MI, life-threatening arrhythmia, CHF, cardiomyopathy or myocarditis, chronic malnutrition, hepatic/renal impairment, alcohol intake, glaucoma, myasthenia gravis, urinary retention or BPH, pregnancy/nursing status, and possible drug interactions.

Monitoring: Monitor for hypotension, HF, PR interval prolongation, widening of QRS, hypoglycemia, heart block, urinary retention, and myasthenia crisis.

Patient Counseling: Inform about risks/benefits; report adverse reactions. Notify if pregnant/nursing.

Administration: Oral route. **Storage:** 25°C (77°F); excursions permitted to 15-30°C (59-86°F).

NORVASC   RX
amlodipine besylate (Pfizer)

THERAPEUTIC CLASS: Calcium channel blocker (dihydropyridine)

INDICATIONS: Treatment of HTN or coronary artery disease (CAD), including chronic stable or vasospastic (Prinzmetal's/variant) angina, alone or in combination with other antihypertensives or antianginals, respectively. To reduce risks of hospitalization due to angina and to reduce the risk of coronary revascularization procedure in patients with recently documented CAD by angiography and without heart failure or ejection fraction <40%.

DOSAGE: *Adults:* HTN: Initial: 5mg qd. Titrate over 7-14 days. Adjust dosage according to patient's need. Max: 10mg qd. Small/Fragile/Elderly/Hepatic Insufficiency/Concomitant Antihypertensive: 2.5mg qd. Chronic Stable/Vasospastic Angina: Usual: 5-10mg qd. Elderly/Hepatic Insufficiency: Give lower dose. CAD: Usual: 5-10mg qd. Elderly: Start at lower end of dosing range.
Pediatrics: 6-17 yrs: HTN: Usual: 2.5-5mg qd. Max: 5mg qd.

HOW SUPPLIED: Tab: 2.5mg, 5mg, 10mg

WARNINGS/PRECAUTIONS: May cause symptomatic hypotension, particularly in patients with severe aortic stenosis. Worsening angina and acute myocardial infarction (MI) may develop after starting or increasing the dose, particularly with severe obstructive CAD. Not a β-blocker and gives no protection against dangers of abrupt β-blocker withdrawal. Titrate slowly with severe hepatic impairment, and caution in elderly.

ADVERSE REACTIONS: Edema, palpitations, dizziness, headache, fatigue, flushing.

INTERACTIONS: Diltiazem increased systemic exposure in elderly hypertensive patients. Strong inhibitors of CYP3A4 (eg, ketoconazole, itraconazole, ritonavir) may increase plasma concentrations to a greater extent; monitor for symptoms of hypotension and edema with CYP3A4 inhibitors. Monitor BP if coadministered with CYP3A4 inducers. May increase simvastatin exposure; limit dose of simvastatin to 20mg daily.

PREGNANCY: Category C, not for use in nursing.

MECHANISM OF ACTION: Calcium channel blocker (dihydropyridine); inhibits the transmembrane influx of calcium ions into vascular smooth muscle and cardiac muscle. Acts directly on vascular smooth muscle to cause a reduction in peripheral vascular resistance and reduction in BP.

PHARMACOKINETICS: Absorption: Absolute bioavailability (64-90%); T_{max}=6-12 hrs. **Distribution:** Plasma protein binding (93%). **Metabolism:** Hepatic. **Elimination:** Urine (10% parent compound; 60% metabolites), $T_{1/2}$=30-50 hrs.

NURSING CONSIDERATIONS

Assessment: Assess for hypersensitivity to the drug, severe aortic stenosis, hepatic function, pregnancy/nursing status, and possible drug interactions. Obtain baseline BP.

Monitoring: Monitor for worsening of angina, MI, and other adverse reactions. Monitor BP.

Patient Counseling: Inform of the risks/benefits of therapy. Counsel about potential adverse effects; advise to seek medical attention if any develop. Instruct to take as prescribed.

Administration: Oral route. **Storage:** 15-30°C (59-86°F).

NORVIR   RX
ritonavir (Abbott)

> Coadministration with several classes of drugs, including sedative hypnotics, antiarrhythmics, or ergot alkaloid preparations, may result in potentially serious and/or life-threatening adverse events due to possible effects on hepatic metabolism of certain drugs. Review medications taken by patients prior to prescribing ritonavir or when prescribing other medications to patients already taking ritonavir.

THERAPEUTIC CLASS: Protease inhibitor

INDICATIONS: Treatment of HIV-1 infection in combination with other antiretrovirals.

DOSAGE: *Adults:* Initial: 300mg bid. Titrate: Increase every 2-3 days by 100mg bid. Maint/Max: 600mg bid. Reduce dose with other protease inhibitors. Elderly: Start at low end of dosing range. Take with meals.
Pediatrics: >1 month: Initial: 250mg/m² bid. Titrate: Increase every 2-3 days by 50mg/m² bid. Maint: 350-400mg/m² bid or highest tolerated dose. Max: 600mg bid. Reduce dose with other protease inhibitors. Take with meals. Refer to PI for pediatric dosage guidelines.

HOW SUPPLIED: Cap: 100mg; Sol: 80mg/mL [240mL]; Tab: 100mg

CONTRAINDICATIONS: Coadministration with CYP3A substrates, such as voriconazole, St. John's wort, or drugs for which elevated plasma concentrations are associated with serious and/or life-threatening reactions (eg, alfuzosin HCl, amiodarone, flecainide, propafenone, quinidine, dihydroergotamine, ergonovine, ergotamine, methylergonovine, cisapride, lovastatin, simvastatin, pimozide, sildenafil when used for treatment of pulmonary arterial HTN, triazolam, oral midazolam).

WARNINGS/PRECAUTIONS: Hepatic transaminase elevation >5X ULN, clinical hepatitis, and jaundice reported; increased risk for transaminase elevations with underlying hepatitis B or C. Caution with preexisting liver disease, liver enzyme abnormalities or hepatitis; consider increased AST/ALT monitoring, especially during first 3 months of therapy. Not recommended in severe hepatic impairment. Pancreatitis observed; d/c if diagnosed. Allergic reactions, anaphylaxis, Stevens-Johnson syndrome, toxic epidermal necrolysis reported; d/c if severe reactions develop. Prolonged PR interval, 2nd- or 3rd-degree atrioventricular (AV) block may occur; caution with underlying structural heart disease, preexisting conduction system abnormalities, ischemic heart disease, and cardiomyopathies. May elevate TG and total cholesterol levels. New onset or exacerbation of diabetes mellitus (DM), hyperglycemia, diabetic ketoacidosis, cross-resistance with other protease inhibitors, increased bleeding with hemophilia A and B, redistribution/accumulation of body fat, autoimmune disorders, and immune reconstitution syndrome reported. Caution in elderly.

ADVERSE REACTIONS: Diarrhea, anorexia, N/V, abdominal pain, asthenia, headache, dizziness, taste perversion, circumoral/peripheral paresthesia, dyspepsia, fever.

INTERACTIONS: See Boxed Warning and Contraindications. Not recommended with fluticasone, salmeterol, and high doses of itraconazole or ketoconazole. Avoid with colchicine in patients with renal/hepatic impairment. Fluconazole, fluoxetine, clarithromycin, and delavirdine may increase levels. Rifampin and St. John's wort may decrease levels. May increase levels of CYP3A or 2D6 substrates, atazanavir, darunavir, amprenavir, saquinavir, tipranavir, maraviroc, normeperidine, vincristine, vinblastine, antiarrhythmics, carbamazepine, clonazepam, ethosuximide, antidepressants, desipramine, trazodone, dronabinol, ketoconazole, itraconazole, salmeterol, fluticasone, colchicine, clarithromycin, rifabutin, quinine, β-blockers, PDE5 inhibitors (eg, vardenafil, sildenafil, tadalafil), calcium channel blockers, digoxin, bosentan, atorvastatin, rosuvastatin, immunosuppressants, neuroleptics, sedative/hypnotics, IV midazolam, methamphetamine, fentanyl, dasatinib, and nilotinib. May decrease levels of voriconazole, didanosine, meperidine, theophylline, divalproex, lamotrigine, phenytoin, bupropion, atovaquone, methadone, and ethinyl estradiol. Caution with drugs that prolong PR interval. Cardiac and neurologic events reported with disopyramide, mexiletine, nefazodone, fluoxetine, and β-blockers. May alter concentrations of warfarin (monitor INR) and indinavir. May require initiation or dose adjustments of insulin or oral hypoglycemics. May need dose decrease of tramadol, propoxyphene, and steroids (eg, dexamethasone, fluticasone, prednisone). (Cap/Sol) Contain alcohol; may produce disulfiram-like reactions with disulfiram or metronidazole. May increase levels of HMG-CoA reductase inhibitors, narcotic analgesics. Caution with anticoagulants, anticonvulsants, and antiarrhythmics.

PREGNANCY: Category B, not for use in nursing.

MECHANISM OF ACTION: HIV protease inhibitor; renders enzyme incapable of processing Gag-Pol polyprotein precursor, which leads to production of noninfectious immature HIV-1 particles.

PHARMACOKINETICS: Absorption: C_{max}=11.2mcg/mL; (Sol) T_{max}=2 hrs (fasting), 4 hrs (fed); (Cap) AUC=121.7mcg•hr/mL, (Sol) AUC=129mcg•hr/mL. **Distribution:** Plasma protein binding (98-99%). **Metabolism:** CYP3A, CYP2D6 (oxidation); isopropylthiazole (major metabolite). **Elimination:** (Sol) Urine (11.3%, 3.5% unchanged), feces (86.4%, 33.8% unchanged); $T_{1/2}$=3-5 hrs.

NURSING CONSIDERATIONS

Assessment: Assess for preexisting liver disease, hepatitis, DM, hemophilia, underlying cardiac problems, lipid disorders, previous hypersensitivity to drug, pregnancy/nursing status, and possible drug interactions. Obtain baseline ECG, AST, ALT, gamma-glutamyl transferase (GGT), CPK, uric acid, TG, and cholesterol levels.

Monitoring: Monitor for signs/symptoms of anaphylaxis or allergic reactions, hepatitis, jaundice, hepatic dysfunction, new onset or exacerbation of DM, hyperglycemia, diabetic ketoacidosis, pancreatitis, AV block, cardiac conduction abnormalities, immune reconstitution syndrome, fat redistribution or accumulation. Monitor for bleeding in patients with hemophilia. Monitor ECG, LFTs, GGT, CPK, uric acid, TG, and cholesterol levels.

Patient Counseling: Inform about risks and benefits of therapy. Inform that therapy does not reduce risk of HIV transmission to others and it is not a cure for HIV-1 infection; opportunistic infections may still occur. Inform to take every day as prescribed and to take with food. Instruct not to alter dose or d/c without consult. If a dose is missed, instruct to take next dose as soon as possible but if a dose is stopped, instruct not to double the dose. Inform about potential adverse effects. Notify physician if using other Rx, OTC or herbal products, particularly St. John's wort. Use with PDE5 inhibitors for erectile dysfunction may increase risk of adverse events; promptly report any symptoms. If taking oral contraceptives, an alternative contraceptive measure should be used. Instruct to report symptoms, such as dizziness, lightheadedness, abnormal heart rhythm, or loss of consciousness.

Administration: Oral route. (Tab) Swallow whole; do not crush, break, or chew. (Sol) Shake well before use. May mix with chocolate milk, Ensure, or Advera within 1 hr of dosing. **Storage:** Cap: 2-8°C (36-46°F). May not require refrigeration if used within 30 days and stored below 25°C (77°F). Protect from light. Avoid exposure to excessive heat. Sol: 20-25°C (68-77°F). Do not refrigerate. Avoid exposure to excessive heat. Tab: 20-25°C (68-77°F); excursions permitted to 15-30°C (59-86°F).

NOVACORT RX
pramoxine HCl - hydrocortisone acetate (Primus)

THERAPEUTIC CLASS: Corticosteroid/anesthetic

INDICATIONS: Relief of the inflammatory and pruritic manifestations of corticosteroid-responsive dermatoses.

DOSAGE: *Adults:* Apply to affected area(s) tid-qid. May use occlusive dressings for psoriasis or recalcitrant conditions. D/C dressings if infection develops.
Pediatrics: Apply to affected area(s) tid-qid. May use occlusive dressings for psoriasis or recalcitrant conditions. D/C dressings if infection develops. Use least amount effective for condition.

HOW SUPPLIED: Gel: (Hydrocortisone-Pramoxine) 2%-1% [29g]

WARNINGS/PRECAUTIONS: May produce reversible hypothalamic-pituitary-adrenal axis suppression, manifestations of Cushing's syndrome, hyperglycemia, and glucosuria. Caution when applied to large surface areas, under occlusive dressings, or with prolonged use. Use appropriate antifungal or antibacterial agent with dermatological infections; d/c if infection does not clear. Pediatrics may be more susceptible to systemic toxicity. D/C if irritation develops.

ADVERSE REACTIONS: Burning, itching, irritation, dryness, folliculitis, hypertrichosis, acneiform eruptions, hypopigmentation, perioral dermatitis, allergic dermatitis, skin maceration, secondary infection, skin atrophy, striae, miliaria.

PREGNANCY: Category C, caution in nursing.

MECHANISM OF ACTION: Topical corticosteroid/anesthetic. Hydrocortisone: Possesses anti-inflammatory, anti-pruritic, and vasoconstrictive properties. Anti-inflammatory mechanism not established. Pramoxine: Stabilizes neuronal membrane of nerve endings with which it comes into contact.

PHARMACOKINETICS: Absorption: Percutaneous; occlusion, inflammation, other disease states may increase absorption. **Distribution:** Bound to plasma protein in varying degrees. Systemically administered corticosteroids found in breast milk. **Metabolism:** Liver. **Elimination:** Kidney (major), bile.

NURSING CONSIDERATIONS

Assessment: Assess for severity of dermatoses and use in pregnant/nursing patients.

Monitoring: Monitor for signs/symptoms of reversible HPA-axis suppression, Cushing's syndrome, hyperglycemia, glucosuria, skin irritation, and dermatological infections (eg, fungal, bacterial). In patients on large doses of therapy and in patients using occlusive dressings, perform frequent monitoring of HPA-axis suppression using urinary free cortisol and adrenocorticotropic hormone stimulation tests. Monitor for signs of steroid withdrawal following d/c of therapy. In pediatric patients, monitor for signs/symptoms of systemic toxicity, HPA-axis suppression, Cushing's syndrome, and intracranial HTN.

Patient Counseling: Instruct to use medication exactly as directed; avoid contact with eyes. Report adverse reactions. Do not bandage, cover, or wrap treated skin unless directed by physician to do so. Advise caregivers of pediatric patients to avoid tight-fitting diapers or plastic pants on treatment diaper area.

Administration: Topical. **Storage:** Store at 15-30°C (59-86°F). Keep tightly closed.

NOVOLIN 70/30   OTC
insulin human, rdna origin - insulin, human (isophane/regular) (Novo Nordisk)

THERAPEUTIC CLASS: Insulin

INDICATIONS: To control hyperglycemia in diabetes.

DOSAGE: *Adults:* Individualize dose.
Pediatrics: Individualize dose.

HOW SUPPLIED: Inj: (Isophane-Regular) 70 U-30 U/mL [10mL]

WARNINGS/PRECAUTIONS: Avoid in patients with hypoglycemia. Any change of insulin should be made cautiously and only under medical supervision. Hyperglycemia may occur if dosage is not taken. Hyperglycemia may lead to diabetic ketoacidosis if not treated; may cause loss of consciousness, coma, or death. May need to change dosage with illness, stress, diet change, physical activity/exercise, other medicines or surgery. May impair physical and mental abililities. Hypoglycemia may occur; monitor for symptoms of hypoglycemia (eg, sweating, dizziness, hunger, blurred vision, headache). Serious allergic reaction, inj-site reaction, hand/feet swelling, vision changes, and hypokalemia may occur. May cause lipodystrophy; rotate inj site.

ADVERSE REACTIONS: Hypoglycemia, allergic reaction, inj-site reaction, lipodystrophy, hand/feet swelling, vision changes, hypokalemia.

INTERACTIONS: Avoid with alcohol (eg, beer, wine); may affect blood glucose.

PREGNANCY: Safety not known in pregnancy/nursing.

MECHANISM OF ACTION: Insulin; structurally identical to insulin produced by the human pancreas that is used to control high blood glucose in patients with diabetes mellitus.

NURSING CONSIDERATIONS

Assessment: Assess for medical conditions, hypoglycemia, alcohol consumption, hypersensitivity, pregnancy/nursing status, and for possible drug interactions. Obtain baseline blood glucose levels.

Monitoring: Monitor for signs of hypoglycemia, hypokalemia, vision changes, lipodystrophy, inj-site reaction, hand/feet swelling, and allergic reactions. Monitor blood glucose levels.

Patient Counseling: Inform about potential risks and benefits of taking insulin and possible adverse reactions. Counsel on proper administration techniques, lifestyle management, regular blood glucose monitoring, signs and symptoms of hypoglycemia/hyperglycemia, management of hypoglycemia/hyperglycemia, and proper storage of insulin. Advise to consult physician during periods of stress, if with illness, diet/physical activity changes, or surgery for possible changes in insulin dosage. Instruct to exercise caution when driving or operating machinery. Instruct to always check carefully for correct type of insulin before administering. Instruct to notify physician of all medicines that are being taken.

Administration: SQ route. Inject in abdomen, upper arms, buttocks, or upper legs. Rotate inj site. Do not mix with any insulins. Refer to labeling for administration techniques. **Storage:**

(Unopened) 2-8°C (36-46°F) or if refrigeration not possible, ≤25°C (77°F) for ≤6 weeks. Do not freeze. Protect from light. (Opened) <25°C (77°F) for ≤6 weeks; discard unused portion after 6 weeks. Keep away from direct heat/light.

Novolin R   OTC
insulin, human regular (Novo Nordisk)

THERAPEUTIC CLASS: Insulin

INDICATIONS: To improve glycemic control in adults and children with diabetes mellitus.

DOSAGE: *Adults:* Individualize dose. Usual: 0.5-1 U/kg/day. (SQ) Inject approximately 30 min prior to the start of a meal. Use with intermediate- or long-acting insulin. (IV) 0.05-1 U/mL in infusion systems with 0.9% NaCl, 5% dextrose, or 10% dextrose with 40 mmol/L of potassium chloride. Renal/Hepatic Impairment: May need to reduce dose.
Pediatrics: Individualize dose. Usual: 0.5-1 U/kg/day. (SQ) Inject approximately 30 min prior to the start of a meal. Use with intermediate- or long-acting insulin. (IV) 0.05-1 U/mL in infusion systems with 0.9% NaCl, 5% dextrose, or 10% dextrose with 40 mmol/L of potassium chloride. Renal/Hepatic Impairment: May need to reduce dose.

HOW SUPPLIED: Inj: 100 U/mL [10mL]

CONTRAINDICATIONS: Episodes of hypoglycemia.

WARNINGS/PRECAUTIONS: Any change of insulin dose should be made cautiously and only under medical supervision. Changing from one insulin product to another or changing the strength may result in the need for a change in dosage. The time course of therapy's action may vary in different individuals or at different times in the same individual and is dependent on dose, site of inj, local blood supply, temperature, and physical activity. May require dose adjustments in patients who change their level of physical activity or meal plan. Stress, illness, or emotional disturbance may alter insulin requirements. Hypoglycemia may occur; caution in patients with hypoglycemia unawareness and those predisposed to hypoglycemia (eg, those who fast or have erratic food intake, pediatrics, elderly). Hypoglycemia may impair mental/physical abilities. Hypokalemia may occur; caution in patients who may be at risk. Hyperglycemia, diabetic ketoacidosis, or hyperosmolar hyperglycemic non-ketotic syndrome may develop if taken less than needed. Redness, swelling, or itching at inj site may occur. Contains metacresol as excipient; localized reactions and generalized myalgias reported. Severe, life-threatening, generalized allergy (eg, anaphylaxis) may occur. Insulin mixtures should not be administered IV. Increases in titers of anti-insulin antibodies reported. May be administered IV under medical supervision; close monitoring of blood glucose and K⁺ is required. Use in insulin pumps not recommended. Has not been studied in patients <2 yrs or pediatric patients with type 2 diabetes.

ADVERSE REACTIONS: Hypoglycemia, inj-site reaction, lipodystrophy, weight gain, peripheral edema, transitory reversible ophthalmologic refraction disorder, diabetic retinopathy worsening, peripheral neuropathy.

INTERACTIONS: May require dose adjustment and close monitoring with drugs that may increase blood glucose-lowering effect and susceptibility to hypoglycemia (oral antidiabetic drugs, pramlintide acetate, ACE inhibitors, disopyramide, fibrates, fluoxetine, MAOIs, propoxyphene, salicylates, somatostatin analogs [eg, octreotide], sulfonamide antibiotics), drugs that may reduce blood glucose-lowering effect leading to worsening of glycemic control (corticosteroids, niacin, danazol, diuretics, sympathomimetic agents [eg, epinephrine, salbutamol, terbutaline], isoniazid, phenothiazine derivatives, somatropin, thyroid hormones, estrogens, progestogens, atypical antipsychotics), or drugs that may either potentiate or weaken blood glucose-lowering effect (β-blockers, clonidine, lithium salts). Alcohol may increase susceptibility to hypoglycemia. Pentamidine may cause hypoglycemia, sometimes followed by hyperglycemia. Hypoglycemic signs may be reduced or absent with sympatholytics (eg, β-blockers, clonidine, guanethidine, reserpine). Caution with K⁺-lowering drugs or drugs sensitive to serum K⁺ concentrations.

PREGNANCY: Category B, caution in nursing.

MECHANISM OF ACTION: Insulin; regulates glucose metabolism. Binds to insulin receptors on muscle and adipocytes and lowers blood glucose by facilitating the cellular uptake of glucose and simultaneously inhibiting the output of glucose from the liver.

PHARMACOKINETICS: Absorption: T_{max}=1.5-2.5 hrs (0.1 U/kg SQ).

NURSING CONSIDERATIONS

Assessment: Assess for predisposal to hypoglycemia, risk of hypokalemia, hypersensitivity, renal/hepatic impairment, pregnancy/nursing status, and possible drug interactions. Obtain baseline blood glucose and HbA1c levels.

Monitoring: Monitor for signs and symptoms of hypoglycemia, lipodystrophy, allergic reactions, and other adverse effects. Monitor blood glucose, HbA1c, and K⁺ concentrations (frequently during IV).

Patient Counseling: Inform about potential risks and benefits of therapy, including possible adverse reactions. Counsel on inj technique, lifestyle management, regular glucose monitoring, periodic HbA1c testing, recognition and management of hypo- and hyperglycemia, adherence to meal planning, complications of therapy, timing of dose, instruction in the use of inj devices, and proper storage. Instruct to exercise caution when driving or operating machinery. Instruct to inform physician if pregnant/breastfeeding or intend to become pregnant. Instruct to always carefully check that they are administering the correct insulin to avoid medication errors.

Administration: SQ/IV route. Inject SQ in abdomen, buttocks, thigh, or upper arm. Rotate inj sites within same region. **Storage:** Unopened: 2-8°C (36-46°F) or, if carried as a spare or if refrigeration not possible, <25°C (77°F) for 42 days. Do not freeze. Protect from light. Do not expose to heat/light. Opened: <25°C (77°F) for 42 days, away from heat/light. Do not refrigerate after 1st use.

NOVOLOG   RX
insulin aspart, rdna origin (Novo Nordisk)

THERAPEUTIC CLASS: Insulin

INDICATIONS: To improve glycemic control in adults and children with diabetes mellitus.

DOSAGE: *Adults:* Individualize dose. Usual Requirement: 0.5-1 unit/kg/day. Give immediately within 5-10 min ac; use with an intermediate or long-acting insulin. Continuous SQ Insulin Infusion (CSII) by External Pump: Infuse pre-meal boluses immediately (within 5-10 min) ac. Initial: Based on the total daily insulin dose of the previous regimen. Usual: 50% of total dose given as meal-related boluses and the remainder given as basal infusion. Renal/Hepatic Impairment: May need to reduce dose.
Pediatrics: ≥2 yrs: Individualize dose. Usual requirement: 0.5-1 unit/kg/day. Give immediately within 5-10 min ac; use with an intermediate or long-acting insulin. CSII by External Pump: Infuse pre-meal boluses immediately (within 5-10 min) ac. Initial: Based on the total daily insulin dose of the previous regimen. Usual: 50% of total dose given as meal-related boluses and the remainder given as basal infusion. Renal/Hepatic Impairment: May need to reduce dose.

HOW SUPPLIED: Inj: 100 U/mL [10mL, vial]; [3mL, Flexpen, Penfill]

CONTRAINDICATIONS: Episodes of hypoglycemia.

WARNINGS/PRECAUTIONS: Any change of insulin dose should be made cautiously and under medical supervision. Changing from one insulin product to another or changing the insulin strength may result in the need for a change in dosage. May require dose adjustments in patients who change physical activity level or meal plan. Illness, emotional disturbances, or other stresses may alter insulin requirements. Hypoglycemia may occur; caution in patients with hypoglycemia unawareness and patients predisposed to hypoglycemia (eg, patients who fast or have erratic food intake). Hypokalemia may occur; caution in patients who may be at risk. Redness, swelling, or itching at the inj site may occur. Severe, life-threatening, generalized allergic reactions including anaphylaxis may occur. Increases in anti-insulin antibodies observed. Do not mix with any other insulin or diluent for use in an external SQ infusion pump. Malfunction of the insulin pump or infusion set or insulin degradation can rapidly lead to hyperglycemia or ketosis; prompt identification and correction of the cause is necessary. Interim SQ inj with the drug may be required if using SQ infusion pump. Train patients using continuous SQ infusion pump therapy to administer by inj; alternate insulin therapy should be available in case of pump failure.

ADVERSE REACTIONS: Hypoglycemia, headache, nausea, diarrhea, hyporeflexia, onychomycosis, sensory disturbance, urinary tract infection, chest pain, lipodystrophy, abdominal pain, skin disorder, inj-site reaction, sinusitis.

INTERACTIONS: May require dose adjustment and close monitoring with drugs that may increase blood glucose-lowering effect and susceptibility to hypoglycemia (oral antidiabetic products, pramlintide, ACE inhibitors, disopyramide, fibrates, fluoxetine, MAOIs, propoxyphene, salicylates, somatostatin analog [eg, octreotide], sulfonamide antibiotics), drugs that may reduce blood-glucose-lowering effects (corticosteroids, niacin, danazol, diuretics, sympathomimetic agents [eg, epinephrine, salbutamol, terbutaline], isoniazid, phenothiazine derivatives, somatropin, thyroid hormones, estrogens, progestogens [eg, in oral contraceptives], atypical antipsychotics), or drugs that may potentiate or weaken glucose-lowering effects (β-blockers, clonidine, lithium salts, and alcohol). Pentamidine may cause hypoglycemia, sometimes followed by hyperglycemia. Hypoglycemic signs may be reduced or absent with sympatholytics (eg, β-blockers, clonidine, guanethidine, and reserpine). Caution with K+ lowering drugs or drugs sensitive to serum K+ levels.

PREGNANCY: Category B, caution in nursing.

MECHANISM OF ACTION: Insulin aspart (rDNA origin); regulates glucose metabolism. Binds to the insulin receptors on muscle and fat cells and lowers blood glucose by facilitating the cellular uptake of glucose and simultaneously inhibiting the output of glucose from the liver.

PHARMACOKINETICS: Absorption: C_{max}=82mU/L; T_{max}=40-50 min. **Distribution:** Plasma protein binding (<10%). **Elimination:** $T_{1/2}$=81 min.

NURSING CONSIDERATIONS

Assessment: Assess for predisposal to hypoglycemia, risk of hypokalemia, alcohol consumption, exercise routines, hypersensitivity, pregnancy/nursing status, and possible drug interactions. Obtain baseline renal function, LFTs, FPG, and HbA1c.

Monitoring: Monitor for signs and symptoms of hypoglycemia, hypokalemia, lipodystrophy, allergic reactions, and other adverse effects. Monitor FPG, HbA1c, K⁺ levels, and renal/hepatic function.

Patient Counseling: Inform about potential risks and benefits of taking insulin and possible adverse reactions. Counsel on proper administration techniques, lifestyle management, regular glucose monitoring, periodic HbA1c testing, recognition and management of hypo- and hyperglycemia, complications of insulin therapy, timing of dose, instruction in the use of inj or SQ infusion device, and proper storage of insulin. Advise to always check carefully when administering appropriate insulin to avoid medication errors. Instruct on how to use external infusion pump.

Administration: SQ/ IV route. Inject SQ in the abdomen, buttocks, thigh, upper arm, or give by continuous SQ infusion by an external insulin pump. Rotate inj sites. Refer to PI for preparation, handling, and administration techniques. **Storage:** Refer to PI for storage conditions for vial, cartridges, and FlexPen. Pump: Discard after at least every 6 days of use or after exposure to >37°C (98.6°F). Change infusion set and infusion set insertion site at least every 3 days. Diluted Novolog: <30°C (86°F) for 28 days. Infusion Fluids: Room temperature for 24 hrs.

NOVOLOG MIX 70/30 RX

insulin aspart protamine - insulin aspart, rdna origin (Novo Nordisk)

THERAPEUTIC CLASS: Insulin

INDICATIONS: To improve glycemic control in patients with diabetes mellitus (DM).

DOSAGE: *Adults:* Individualize dose. Type 1 DM: Inject SQ bid within 15 min ac. Type 2 DM: Inject SQ bid within 15 min ac or pc. Hepatic/Renal Impairment: May need to reduce dose. Elderly: Start at lower end of dosing range.

HOW SUPPLIED: Inj: (Insulin Aspart Protamine-Insulin Aspart) 70 U-30 U/mL [10mL, vial]; [3mL, Flexpen]

CONTRAINDICATIONS: Episodes of hypoglycemia.

WARNINGS/PRECAUTIONS: Do not mix with other insulins or use IV or in insulin pumps. Any change of insulin should be made cautiously and only under medical supervision. Changing from one insulin product to another or changing the insulin strength may result in the need for a change in dosage. Stress, illness, changes in meals or exercise may alter insulin requirements. Hypoglycemia may occur; caution in patients with hypoglycemia unawareness and patients predisposed to hypoglycemia. Hypokalemia may occur; caution in patients who may be at risk. Inj-site reactions (eg, erythema, edema, pruritus) may occur. Severe, life-threatening, generalized allergic reactions, including anaphylaxis may occur. Insulin antibodies may develop during treatment. Caution in elderly.

ADVERSE REACTIONS: Hypoglycemia, headache, influenza-like symptoms, dyspepsia, back pain, diarrhea, pharyngitis, rhinitis, skeletal pain, upper respiratory tract infection, neuropathy, abdominal pain, lipodystrophy, weight gain, peripheral edema.

INTERACTIONS: May require dose adjustment and close monitoring with drugs that may increase blood glucose-lowering effect and susceptibility to hypoglycemia (oral antidiabetic products, pramlintide, ACE inhibitors, disopyramide, fibrates, fluoxetine, MAOIs, propoxyphene, salicylates, somatostatin analog [eg, octreotide], sulfonamide antibiotics), drugs that may reduce blood glucose-lowering effect (corticosteroids, niacin, danazol, diuretics, sympathomimetic agents [eg, epinephrine, salbutamol, terbutaline], isoniazid, phenothiazine derivatives, somatropin, thyroid hormones, estrogens, progestogens [eg, in oral contraceptives], atypical antipsychotics), or drugs that may potentiate or weaken blood glucose-lowering effect (β-blockers, clonidine, lithium salts, and alcohol). Pentamidine may cause hypoglycemia, which may sometimes be followed by hyperglycemia. Hypoglycemic signs may be reduced or absent with sympatholytics (eg, β-blockers, clonidine, guanethidine, and reserpine). Caution with K⁺ lowering drugs or drugs sensitive to serum K⁺ levels.

PREGNANCY: Category B, caution in nursing.

MECHANISM OF ACTION: Insulin; regulates glucose metabolism. Binds to the insulin receptors on muscle, liver, and fat cells and lowers blood glucose by facilitating the cellular uptake of glucose and simultaneously inhibiting the output of glucose from the liver.

PHARMACOKINETICS: Absorption: Rapid; (0.2 U/kg) C_{max}=23.4mU/L, T_{max}=60 min; (0.3 U/kg) C_{max}=61.3mU/L, T_{max}=85 min. **Distribution:** Plasma protein binding (0-9%). **Elimination:** $T_{1/2}$=8-9 hrs.

NURSING CONSIDERATIONS

Assessment: Assess for predisposal to hypoglycemia, risk of hypokalemia, alcohol consumption, exercise routines, hypersensitivity, pregnancy/nursing status, and possible drug interactions. Obtain baseline renal function, LFTs, FPG, and HbA1c.

Monitoring: Monitor for signs and symptoms of hypoglycemia, hypokalemia, lipodystrophy, allergic reactions, and other adverse effects. Monitor FPG, HbA1c, K^+ levels, and renal/hepatic function.

Patient Counseling: Inform about potential risks and benefits of taking insulin. Counsel on proper administration techniques, lifestyle management, regular glucose monitoring, periodic HbA1c testing, recognition and management of hypo- and hyperglycemia, complications of insulin therapy, timing of dose, instruction in the use of device, and proper storage of insulin. Instruct to exercise caution when driving or operating machinery. Instruct to always check carefully when administering appropriate insulin to avoid medication errors.

Administration: SQ route. Inject SQ in the abdomen, buttocks, thigh, or upper arm. Rotate inj sites. Refer to PI for resuspension instruction and administration technique. **Storage:** Refer to PI for storage conditions for vial and FlexPen.

NOXAFIL   RX
posaconazole (Schering)

THERAPEUTIC CLASS: Azole antifungal

INDICATIONS: Prophylaxis of invasive *Aspergillus* and *Candida* infections in patients ≥13 yrs, who are at high risk of developing these infections due to being severely immunocompromised. Treatment of oropharyngeal candidiasis, including oropharyngeal candidiasis refractory to itraconazole and/or fluconazole.

DOSAGE: *Adults:* Prophylaxis of Invasive Fungal Infections: 200mg (5mL) tid. Base duration of therapy on recovery from neutropenia or immunosuppression. Oropharyngeal Candidiasis: LD: 100mg (2.5mL) bid on 1st day, then 100mg qd for 13 days. Oropharyngeal Candidiasis Refractory to Itraconazole and/or Fluconazole: 400mg (10mL) bid. Base duration of therapy on severity of underlying disease and clinical response.
Pediatrics: ≥13 yrs: Prophylaxis of Invasive Fungal Infections: 200mg (5mL) tid. Base duration of therapy on recovery from neutropenia or immunosuppression. Oropharyngeal Candidiasis: LD: 100mg (2.5mL) bid on 1st day, then 100mg qd for 13 days. Oropharyngeal Candidiasis Refractory to Itraconazole and/or Fluconazole: 400mg (10mL) bid. Base duration of therapy on severity of underlying disease and clinical response.

HOW SUPPLIED: Sus: 40mg/mL [105mL]

CONTRAINDICATIONS: Coadministration with sirolimus, CYP3A4 substrates that prolong the QT interval (eg, pimozide, quinidine), simvastatin, ergot alkaloids.

WARNINGS/PRECAUTIONS: Prolongation of QT interval and rare cases of torsades de pointes reported; caution with potentially proarrhythmic conditions. Hepatic reactions (eg, mild to moderate elevations in ALT, AST, alkaline phosphatase, total bilirubin, and/or clinical hepatitis) reported. Cholestasis or hepatic failure reported in patients with serious underlying medical conditions. D/C if signs/symptoms of liver disease develop that may be attributable to therapy. Monitor closely for breakthrough fungal infections with severe renal impairment.

ADVERSE REACTIONS: Fever, headache, rigors, anemia, neutropenia, diarrhea, N/V, abdominal pain, coughing, dyspnea, anorexia, fatigue, asthenia, pain.

INTERACTIONS: See Contraindications. Elevated cyclosporine and tacrolimus levels reported; frequently monitor levels and consider dose adjustment of cyclosporine or tacrolimus. Avoid with cimetidine, esomeprazole, rifabutin, phenytoin, and efavirenz unless benefits outweigh risks. If concomitant phenytoin is required, monitor closely and consider phenytoin dose reduction. If concomitant rifabutin is required, monitor CBC and adverse events. Monitor adverse events with benzodiazepines metabolized through CYP3A4 (eg, midazolam, alprazolam, triazolam). May increase levels of vinca alkaloids; consider dose adjustment of vinca alkaloid. Consider dose reduction of concomitant statins that are metabolized through CYP3A4. Monitor for adverse events and toxicity with calcium channel blockers (eg, verapamil, diltiazem, nifedipine, nicardipine, felodipine) and drugs that are metabolized through CYP3A4 (eg, atazanavir, ritonavir); dose reduction of these drugs may be needed. Decreased levels with cimetidine, esomeprazole, and metoclopramide; monitor for breakthrough fungal infections. Increased digoxin levels; monitor digoxin plasma concentrations. Inhibitors or inducers of UDP glucuronidation or P-glycoprotein (P-gp) may affect posaconazole concentrations. Monitor glucose concentration with glipizide.

PREGNANCY: Category C, not for use in nursing.

N

MECHANISM OF ACTION: Triazole antifungal agent; blocks synthesis of ergosterol, a key component of fungal cell membrane, through inhibition of the enzyme lanosterol 14α-demethylase and accumulation of methylated sterol precursors.

PHARMACOKINETICS: Administration: Administration of variable doses resulted in different parameters. **Distribution:** V_d=1774L; plasma protein binding (>98%). **Metabolism:** Via UDP glucuronidation; glucuronide conjugates (metabolites). **Elimination:** Feces (71%), urine (13%); $T_{1/2}$=35 hrs.

NURSING CONSIDERATIONS

Assessment: Assess for drug hypersensitivity, renal function, proarrhythmic conditions, LFTs, pregnancy/nursing status, and for possible drug interactions.

Monitoring: Monitor for signs/symptoms of hypersensitivity reactions, hepatic reactions, QT prolongation, torsades de pointes, and LFTs. In patients with severe renal impairment, monitor for breakthrough fungal infections.

Patient Counseling: Instruct to take medication with full meal; if cannot eat full meal, may take with liquid nutritional supplement or acidic carbonated beverage. Inform physician of all medications being taken. Inform physician if severe diarrhea or vomiting develops, have a heart or circulatory condition, are pregnant or plan to become pregnant, nursing, have liver disease, flu-like symptoms, experience itching, eyes/skin turn yellow, feel more tired than usual, or had an allergic reaction to other antifungal medications.

Administration: Oral route. **Storage:** 25°C (77°F); excursions permitted to 15-30°C (59-86°F). Do not freeze.

NPLATE   RX
romiplostim (Amgen)

THERAPEUTIC CLASS: Thrombopoietin receptor agonist

INDICATIONS: Treatment of thrombocytopenia in patients with chronic immune thrombocytopenia (ITP) who have had an insufficient response to corticosteroids, immunoglobulins, or splenectomy.

DOSAGE: *Adults:* Administer weekly. Initial: 1mcg/kg SQ based on actual body weight. Titrate: Adjust weekly dose by increments of 1mcg/kg until platelet count is ≥50 x 10⁹/L. Max: 10mcg/kg/week. Platelet Count <50 x 10⁹/L: Increase dose by 1mcg/kg. Platelet Count >200 x 10⁹/L for 2 Consecutive Weeks: Reduce dose by 1mcg/kg. Platelet Count >400 x 10⁹/L: Do not dose; continue assessing platelet count weekly. After platelet count falls to <200 x 10⁹/L, resume therapy at a dose reduced by 1mcg/kg. D/C if platelet count does not increase to a sufficient level after 4 weeks of therapy at the max weekly dose. With Other Medical ITP Therapies (eg, Corticosteroids, Danazol, Azathioprine, IV Immunoglobulin, and Anti-D Immunoglobulin): May reduce or d/c medical ITP therapies if platelet count is ≥50 x 10⁹/L.

HOW SUPPLIED: Inj: 250mcg, 500mcg

WARNINGS/PRECAUTIONS: Use only in patients with ITP whose degree of thrombocytopenia and clinical condition increases the risk for bleeding; do not use to normalize platelet counts. Use lowest dose to achieve and maintain platelet count ≥50 x 10⁹/L. Progression from myelodysplastic syndromes (MDS) to acute myelogenous leukemia has been observed; do not use for the treatment of thrombocytopenia due to MDS or any cause of thrombocytopenia other than chronic ITP. Thrombotic/thromboembolic complications may occur. Portal vein thrombosis reported in patients with chronic liver disease. May increase risk for development or progression of reticulin fiber formation within bone marrow; consider bone marrow biopsy if new or worsening blood morphological abnormalities or cytopenias occur. D/C may worsen thrombocytopenia; following d/c, obtain weekly CBCs, including platelet counts for at least 2 weeks, and consider alternative treatments for worsening thrombocytopenia. If hyporesponsiveness or failure to maintain a platelet response occurs, search for causative factors (eg, neutralizing antibodies). Caution with renal/hepatic impairment and in elderly.

ADVERSE REACTIONS: Headache, arthralgia, dizziness, insomnia, myalgia, pain in extremity, abdominal pain, shoulder pain, dyspepsia, development of antibodies, paresthesia.

PREGNANCY: Category C, not for use in nursing.

MECHANISM OF ACTION: Thrombopoietin (TPO) receptor agonist; increases platelet production through binding and activation of the TPO receptor.

PHARMACOKINETICS: Absorption: T_{max}=7-50 hrs. **Elimination:** $T_{1/2}$=1-34 days.

NURSING CONSIDERATIONS

Assessment: Assess for degree of thrombocytopenia, hepatic/renal impairment, and pregnancy/nursing status.

Monitoring: Monitor CBCs, including platelet count, weekly during dose adjustment phase, then monthly after establishment of a stable dose, and then weekly for at least 2 weeks after d/c. Monitor for thrombotic/thromboembolic complications, bone marrow reticulin fiber formation, new/worsening morphological abnormalities or cytopenias, worsening thrombocytopenia (after d/c), and hyporesponsiveness, or failure to maintain platelet response with therapy.

Patient Counseling: Inform of risks and benefits of therapy. Advise that the risks associated with long-term administration are unknown. Counsel to avoid situations or medications that may increase risk for bleeding. Inform pregnant women to enroll in pregnancy registry.

Administration: SQ route. Refer to PI for preparation/reconstitution and administration instructions. **Storage:** 2-8°C (36-46°F). Do not freeze. Reconstituted: 25°C (77°F) or at 2-8°C (36-46°F) for up to 24 hrs prior to administration. Protect from light. Discard unused portion.

NUCYNTA
tapentadol (Janssen)

`CII`

THERAPEUTIC CLASS: Central acting analgesic

INDICATIONS: Relief of moderate to severe acute pain in patients ≥18 yrs.

DOSAGE: *Adults:* Individualize dose. Usual: 50mg, 75mg, or 100mg q4-6h depending on pain intensity. Day 1: 2nd dose may be given 1 hr after 1st dose if pain relief is inadequate, then 50mg, 75mg, or 100mg q4-6h. Adjust dose to maintain adequate analgesia with acceptable tolerability. Max: 700mg on Day 1, then 600mg/day thereafter. Moderate Hepatic Impairment: Initial: 50mg q8h or longer between doses. Max: 3 doses/24 hrs. Elderly: Start at lower end of dosing range.

HOW SUPPLIED: Tab: 50mg, 75mg, 100mg

CONTRAINDICATIONS: Significant respiratory depression, acute/severe bronchial asthma, or hypercapnia (in unmonitored settings or the absence of resuscitative equipment); paralytic ileus; MAOI use during or within 14 days of treatment.

WARNINGS/PRECAUTIONS: May cause respiratory depression; occurs more frequently in elderly, debilitated, and patients with hypoxia, hypercapnia, or upper airway obstruction. Caution with asthma, chronic obstructive pulmonary disease (COPD), cor pulmonale, severe obesity, sleep apnea syndrome, myxedema, kyphoscoliosis, CNS depression, and coma. Can raise CSF pressure; avoid in those susceptible to such effects. May obscure clinical course of patients with head injury; caution with head injury, intracranial lesions, or other sources of preexisting increased intracranial pressure (ICP). May be abused in a manner similar to other opioids; carefully monitor for signs of abuse and addiction. May impair mental/physical abilities. Caution with history of seizure disorder, conditions that put patient at risk of seizures, and moderate hepatic impairment. Potentially life-threatening serotonin syndrome may occur. Withdrawal symptoms may occur upon abrupt d/c. May cause spasm of sphincter of Oddi; caution with biliary tract disease, including acute pancreatitis. Avoid use with severe renal/hepatic impairment.

ADVERSE REACTIONS: N/V, dizziness, somnolence, constipation, pruritus, dry mouth, hyperhidrosis, fatigue.

INTERACTIONS: See Contraindications. May exhibit additive CNS depression with other opioid analgesics, general anesthetics, phenothiazines, antiemetics, other tranquilizers, sedatives, hypnotics, other CNS depressants (eg, alcohol); consider dose reduction. Serotonin syndrome may occur, particularly with serotonergic drugs (eg, SSRIs, SNRIs, TCAs, MAOIs, and triptans) and drugs that may impair metabolism of serotonin.

PREGNANCY: Category C, not for use in nursing.

MECHANISM OF ACTION: Centrally-acting synthetic analgesic; not established. Suspected to be due to mu-opioid agonist activity and the inhibition of norepinephrine reuptake.

PHARMACOKINETICS: Absorption: T_{max}=1.25 hrs; absolute bioavailability (32%). **Distribution:** (IV) V_d=540L; plasma protein binding (20%). **Metabolism:** Conjugation (extensive); tapentadol-O-glucuronide (major metabolite). **Elimination:** Kidneys (99%); urine (3% unchanged, 70% conjugated); $T_{1/2}$=4 hrs.

NURSING CONSIDERATIONS

Assessment: Assess for pain intensity, pregnancy/nursing status, possible drug interactions, and conditions where treatment is contraindicated or cautioned.

Monitoring: Monitor for signs of respiratory depression especially high-risk patients (eg, asthma, COPD), increased CSF pressure in patients with head injury or preexisting increased ICP, abuse or addiction, withdrawal symptoms, mental/physical impairment, and for serotonin syndrome. Monitor hepatic/renal function.

Patient Counseling: Instruct to report episodes of breakthrough pain and adverse experiences during therapy. Counsel to take only as directed; instruct to not adjust dose without consulting the physician. Advise that it may be appropriate to taper dosing when discontinuing as withdrawal symptoms may occur. Inform of potential for drug abuse and that mental/physical abilities may be impaired. Advise to notify physician if pregnant/planning to become pregnant. Avoid breastfeeding and alcohol use. Inform of risk of seizures and serotonin syndrome. Instruct to notify physician of any prescription or OTC drugs currently taking.

Administration: Oral route. **Storage:** 25°C (77°F); excursions permitted to 15-30°C (59-86°F). Protect from moisture.

NUCYNTA ER

tapentadol (Janssen)

Contains tapentadol, a μ-opioid and Schedule II controlled substance with abuse liability similar to other opioid analgesics. Consider the risk of misuse, abuse, or diversion when prescribing, or dispensing. Not intended for use as PRN analgesic and for the management of acute or postoperative pain. Avoid with alcohol or medications containing alcohol; may result in potentially fatal overdose of tapentadol when given concomitantly. Swallow whole; do not split, break, chew, dissolve, or crush.

THERAPEUTIC CLASS: Central acting analgesic

INDICATIONS: Management of moderate to severe chronic pain in adults, when a continuous, around-the-clock opioid analgesic is needed for an extended period of time.

DOSAGE: *Adults:* Individualize dose. Take 1 tab at a time with enough water to ensure complete swallowing. Titrate to adequate analgesia with dose increases of 50mg no more than bid every 3 days. Max: 500mg/day. Opioid-Naive Patients: Initial: 50mg bid (approximately q12h). Titrate within therapeutic range of 100-250mg bid. Opioid-Experienced Patients: Initial: 50mg titrated to an effective and tolerable dose within the therapeutic range of 100-250mg bid. Conversion from Nucynta to Nucynta ER: Convert using the equivalent total daily dose of Nucynta and divide into 2 equal doses of Nucynta ER by approximately 12-hr interval. Taper the dose when d/c. Moderate Hepatic Impairment: Initial: 50mg once q24h. Max: 100mg qd. Elderly: Start at lower end of dosing range.

HOW SUPPLIED: Tab, Extended Release: 50mg, 100mg, 150mg, 200mg, 250mg

CONTRAINDICATIONS: Significant respiratory depression, severe bronchial asthma, or hypercapnia (in unmonitored settings or the absence of resuscitative equipment); paralytic ileus; MAOI use during or within 14 days of treatment.

WARNINGS/PRECAUTIONS: D/C all other tapentadol and tramadol products when beginning treatment. May cause respiratory depression; occurs more frequently in elderly, debilitated, and patients with hypoxia, hypercapnia, or upper airway obstruction. Caution with asthma, chronic obstructive pulmonary disease (COPD), cor pulmonale, severe obesity, sleep apnea syndrome, myxedema, kyphoscoliosis, CNS depression, or coma. Can raise CSF pressure; avoid in those susceptible to such effects. May obscure clinical course of patients with head injury; caution with head injury, intracranial lesions, or other sources of preexisting increased intracranial pressure (ICP). May cause severe hypotension. May impair mental/physical abilities. Caution with history of seizure disorder, conditions that put patient at risk of seizures, moderate hepatic impairment, adrenocortical insufficiency, delirium tremens, myxedema or hypothyroidism, prostatic hypertrophy, or urethral stricture, and toxic psychosis. Potentially life-threatening serotonin syndrome may occur. Withdrawal symptoms may occur upon abrupt d/c; taper dose to reduce symptoms. May cause spasm of sphincter of Oddi; caution with biliary tract disease, including acute pancreatitis. Avoid use with severe renal/hepatic impairment.

ADVERSE REACTIONS: N/V, dizziness, constipation, headache, somnolence, fatigue, dry mouth, hyperhidrosis, pruritus, insomnia, dyspepsia.

INTERACTIONS: See Contraindications. May exhibit additive CNS depression with other opioid analgesics, general anesthetics, phenothiazines, other tranquilizers, antiemetics, sedatives, hypnotics, centrally acting muscle relaxants, other CNS depressants (eg, alcohol); consider dose reduction of one or both agents. Serotonin syndrome may occur, particularly with serotonergic drugs (eg, SSRIs, serotonine norepinephrine reuptake inhibitors [SNRIs], TCAs, and triptans), drugs that affect serotonergic neurotransmitter system (eg, mirtazapine, trazodone, and tramadol) and drugs that may impair metabolism of serotonin (including MAOIs). May increase serum levels and cause a potentially fatal overdose of tapentadol with alcohol; avoid use. Not recommended with mixed agonist/antagonist (eg, butorphanol, nalbuphine, pentazocine) and partial agonists (eg, buprenorphine); may reduce analgesic effects. May increase risk of urinary retention and/or severe constipation, which may lead to paralytic ileus, with anticholinergic products.

PREGNANCY: Category C, not for use in nursing.

MECHANISM OF ACTION: Centrally-acting synthetic analgesic; not established. Suspected to be due to μ-opioid agonist activity and the inhibition of norepinephrine reuptake.

PHARMACOKINETICS: Absorption: T_{max}=3-6 hrs; absolute bioavailability (32%). **Distribution:** (IV) V_d=540L; plasma protein binding (20%). **Metabolism:** Conjugation; N-desmethyl tapentadol by CYP2C9 and CYP2C19; hydroxy tapentadol by CYP2D6. **Elimination:** Kidneys (99%); urine (3% unchanged, 70% conjugated); $T_{1/2}$=5 hrs.

NURSING CONSIDERATIONS

Assessment: Assess for history or risk factors for abuse or addiction, age, general condition and medical status, opioid exposure/tolerance, pain intensity, previous opioid daily dose, potency and type of analgesic, balance between pain management and adverse reactions, pregnancy/ nursing status, possible drug interactions, and conditions where treatment is contraindicated or cautioned.

Monitoring: Monitor for improvement in pain, medical status, dose selection, signs of respiratory depression especially in high-risk patients (eg, asthma, COPD), increased CSF pressure in patients with head injury or preexisting increased ICP, abuse or addiction, withdrawal symptoms, mental/physical impairment, hypotension, and for serotonin syndrome. Monitor hepatic/renal function.

Patient Counseling: Instruct to report episodes of breakthrough pain and adverse experiences during therapy. Take only as directed; do not adjust dose without consulting the physician. Notify physician if experience changes in pain level or if need a change in dosage. Advise that it may be appropriate to taper dosing upon d/c as withdrawal symptoms may occur. Advise to swallow whole; do not split, break, chew or crush, or dissolve. Take one tab at a time; do not pre-soak, lick, or wet the tablet prior to placing in the mouth. Take each tablet with enough water to ensure complete swallowing. Flush tablets down the toilet if no longer needed. Keep in a childproof container, protect from theft and do not give to individual if not prescribed. Respiratory depression and hypotension may occur. Inform of potential for drug abuse and that mental/physical abilities may be impaired. Notify physician if pregnant/plan to become pregnant. Avoid breastfeeding and alcohol use. Inform of risk of seizures and serotonin syndrome. Notify physician of any prescription or OTC drugs currently taking.

Administration: Oral route. **Storage:** 25°C (77°F); excursions permitted to 15-30°C (59-86°F). Protect from moisture.

NUEDEXTA   RX

quinidine sulfate - dextromethorphan hydrobromide (Avanir)

THERAPEUTIC CLASS: NMDA receptor antagonist

INDICATIONS: Treatment of pseudobulbar affect (PBA).

DOSAGE: *Adults:* Initial: 1 cap PO qd for 7 days. On 8th day of therapy and thereafter, 1 cap q12h.

HOW SUPPLIED: Cap: (Dextromethorphan HBr-Quinidine sulfate) 20mg-10mg

CONTRAINDICATIONS: Drug-induced thrombocytopenia, hepatitis, bone marrow depression or lupus-like syndrome. Prolonged QT interval, congenital long QT syndrome or history suggestive to torsades de pointes and patients with heart failure. Complete atrioventricular (AV) block without implanted pacemakers, or patients with high risk of complete AV block. During or within 14 days of MAOI therapy. Concomitant use with quinidine, quinine, or mefloquine, drugs that both prolong QT interval and metabolized by CYP2D6 (eg, thioridazine and pimozide).

WARNINGS/PRECAUTIONS: Quinidine may cause immune-mediated thrombocytopenia; d/c immediately if this occurs. Quinidine has also been associated with lupus-like syndrome involving polyarthritis, rash, bronchospasm, lymphadenopathy, hemolytic anemia, vasculitis, uveitis, angioedema, agranulocytosis, sicca syndrome, myalgia, skeletal-muscle enzymes elevation and pneumonitis. Hepatitis, including granulomatous hepatitis, reported. Fever and other signs of hypersensitivity may occur. QT prolongation reported; may cause torsades de pointes-type ventricular tachycardia. ECG evaluation should be conducted at baseline and 3-4 hrs after first dose in patients with left ventricular hypertrophy (LVH), left ventricular dysfunction (LVD), those taking drugs that prolong the QT interval, and drugs that are strong or moderate CYP3A4 inhibitors. Reevaluate ECG if risk factors of arrhythmia change during therapy. Hypokalemia and hypomagnesemia should be corrected prior to therapy and monitor during treatment. D/C if cardiac arrhythmia (eg, syncope or palpitations) occurs. May cause dizziness; caution in patients with motor impairment affecting gait or with history of falls. May cause serotonin syndrome. Monitor for worsening clinical condition in myasthenia gravis and other conditions adversely affected by anticholinergic effects.

ADVERSE REACTIONS: Diarrhea, dizziness, cough, vomiting, asthenia, peripheral edema, urinary tract infection (UTI), influenza, increased gamma-glutamyltransferase, flatulence.

INTERACTIONS: See Contraindications. Recommend ECG when taking moderate or strong CYP3A4 inhibitors. Concomitant use with SSRIs or TCAs increases risk of serotonin syndrome. Adjust doses of desipramine and paroxetine if given together. Concomitant administration with digoxin may result in increased digoxin levels; monitor plasma digoxin concentration and reduce dose if necessary. Additive effect with memantine. Caution in combination with alcohol and other centrally acting drugs.

PREGNANCY: Category C, caution in nursing.

MECHANISM OF ACTION: (Dextromethorphan) NMDA receptor antagonist; mechanism has not been established; sigma-1 receptor and uncompetitive NMDA receptor antagonist. (Quinidine) increases plasma levels of dextromethorphan by competitively inhibiting cytochrome P450 2D6, which catalyzes a major biotransformation pathway for dextromethorphan.

PHARMACOKINETICS: Absorption: Quinidine: C_{max}=2-5mcg/mL, T_{max}=1-2 hrs; Dextromethorphan: T_{max}=3-4 hrs. **Distribution:** Dextromethorphan: Plasma protein binding (60-70%). Quinidine: 3-hydroxyquinidine (major metabolite), plasma protein binding (80-89%). **Metabolism:** Liver. Dextromethorphan: CYP2D6. Quinidine: CYP3A4. **Elimination:** Dextromethorphan: $T_{1/2}$=13 hrs. Quinidine: Urine (20%, unchanged), $T_{1/2}$=7 hrs.

NURSING CONSIDERATIONS

Assessment: Assess for drug hypersensitivity, history of drug-induced thrombocytopenia, chronic HTN, known CAD, history of stroke, electrolyte abnormality (eg, hypokalemia, hypomagnesemia), bradycardia, family history of QT abnormality, or any other condition where treatment is contraindicated or cautioned. Assess renal/hepatic function, pregnancy/nursing status and possible drug interactions. Obtain baseline ECG and genotyping.

Monitoring: Monitor for development of thrombocytopenia, lightheadedness, chills, fever, N/V, fatal hemorrhage, lupus-like syndrome, polyarthritis, rash, bronchospasm, lymphadenopathy, hemolytic anemia, vasculitis, uveitis, angioedema, agranulocytosis, sicca syndrome, myalgia, skeletal-muscle enzyme elevation, pneumonitis, hepatitis including granulomatous hepatitis, fever, hypersensitivity, QTc prolongation, torsades de pointes, ventricular tachycardia, cardiac arrhythmias, dizziness, serotonin syndrome, hypokalemia, hypomagnesemia and other possible adverse reactions. Monitor ECG 3-4 hrs after the first dose in patients at risk of QT prolongation and torsades de pointes, plasma digoxin levels, worsening of myasthenia gravis and other conditions that may be affected by anticholinergic effects. Reevaluate ECG if risk factors of arrhythmia change during therapy.

Patient Counseling: Inform about the risks and benefits of the treatment. Report any adverse effects to healthcare provider. Take medication as prescribed; do not take >2 caps in 24-hr period and make sure there is an approximate 12-hr interval between doses, and do not double dose after a missed dose. Inform healthcare provider about all medications they are taking and planning to take. Advise patients to seek immediate medical attention if hypersensitivity reactions, fainting or loss of consciousness occur. Inform healthcare providers of personal or family history of QTc prolongation. Instruct not to share or give medication to others even if with the same symptoms. Contact healthcare providers if PBA persists or worsens. Advise to use precautions to reduce risk of falls as dizziness may occur.

Administration: Oral route. **Storage:** 25°C (77°F); excursions permitted to 15-30°C (59-86°F).

NULOJIX   RX
belatacept (Bristol-Myers Squibb)

> Increased risk for developing post-transplant lymphoproliferative disorder (PTLD), predominantly involving the CNS. Recipients without immunity to Epstein-Barr virus (EBV) are at a particularly increased risk; use in EBV seropositive patients only. Do not use in transplant recipients who are EBV seronegative or with unknown serostatus. Only physicians experienced in immunosuppressive therapy and management of kidney transplant patients should prescribe belatacept. Increased susceptibility to infection and the possible development of malignancies may result from immunosuppression. Use in liver transplant patients is not recommended due to an increased risk of graft loss and death.

THERAPEUTIC CLASS: Selective costimulation modulator

INDICATIONS: Prophylaxis of organ rejection in adults receiving a kidney transplant in combination with basiliximab induction, mycophenolate mofetil, and corticosteroids.

DOSAGE: *Adults:* Initial Phase: 10mg/kg on Day 1 (day of transplantation, prior to implantation), Day 5, and end of week 2, 4, 8, and 12 after transplantation. Maint Phase: 5mg/kg at end of week 16 after transplantation and every 4 weeks (±3 days) thereafter. Dose should be evenly divisible by 12.5mg.

HOW SUPPLIED: Inj: 250mg

CONTRAINDICATIONS: Transplant recipients who are EBV seronegative or with unknown EBV serostatus.

WARNINGS/PRECAUTIONS: T-cell depleting therapies to treat acute rejection should be used cautiously. Avoid prolonged exposure to UV light and sunlight. Progressive multifocal leukoencephalopathy (PML) reported; consider in the differential diagnosis if new or worsening neurological, cognitive or behavioral signs and symptoms reported; recommended doses should not be exceeded. Increased risk of developing bacterial, viral (cytomegalovirus [CMV] and herpes), fungal, protozoan, including opportunistic infections; prophylaxis for CMV (≥3 months) and *Pneumocystis jiroveci* are recommended after transplantation. Tuberculosis (TB) reported; evaluate for TB and test/treat for latent infection prior to initiation. Polyoma virus-associated nephropathy reported and associated with deteriorating renal function and kidney graft loss; consider reduction in immunosuppression. Not recommended in liver transplant patient.

ADVERSE REACTIONS: Anemia, diarrhea, urinary tract infection, peripheral edema, constipation, HTN, pyrexia, graft dysfunction, cough, N/V, headache, hypokalemia, hyperkalemia, leukopenia.

INTERACTIONS: Avoid use of live vaccines. *In vitro*, belatacept inhibits the production of certain cytokines during alloimune response; be aware of potentially altered CYP450 metabolism of drugs. Increase in C_{max} and area under the curve (AUC) of mycophenolic acid when mycophenolate mofetil is given in combination.

PREGNANCY: Category C, not for use in nursing.

MECHANISM OF ACTION: Selective T-cell costimulation blocker; binds to CD80 and CD86 on antigen-presenting cells thereby blocking CD28 mediated costimulation of T lymphocytes.

PHARMACOKINETICS: Absorption: (10mg/kg) C_{max}=247µg/mL; AUC=22252µg•hr/mL. (5mg/kg) C_{max}=139µg/mL; AUC=14090µg•hr/mL. **Distribution:** V_d=0.11L/kg (10mg/kg), 0.12L/kg (5mg/kg). **Elimination:** $T_{1/2}$=9.8 days (10mg/kg), 8.2 days (5mg/kg).

NURSING CONSIDERATIONS

Assessment: Assess for EBV serostatus, possible drug interactions, pregnancy/nursing status, and any other conditions where treatment is cautioned.

Monitoring: Monitor BP, CBC, lipid profile, glucose levels, and renal function parameters. Monitor for signs and symptoms of PTLD, PML, infections, malignancies, TB, polyoma virus nephropathy, and other adverse reactions.

Patient Counseling: Instruct patients to report neurological, cognitive, or behavioral signs and symptoms (eg, changes in mood or usual behavior, confusion, problem thinking, loss of memory, changes in walking or talking, decreased strength or weakness on one side of the body, changes in vision). Inform about increased risk of PTLD, malignancies (eg, skin cancer), PML, and infections. Instruct to limit exposure to sunlight and UV light by wearing protective clothing and using sunscreen with high protection factor. Advise to avoid live vaccines. Inform about pregnancy/nursing risks.

Administration: IV route. Refer to PI for compatibility/preparation/administration instructions. Infuse in a separate line. Infusion must be completed within 24 hrs of reconstitution. **Storage:** 2-8°C (36-46°F). Transfer reconstituted sol into infusion bag/bottle immediately. Reconstituted Sol: 2-8°C (36-46°F) and protected from light for up to 24 hrs; 4 hrs of the total 24 hrs can be at room temperature (20-25°C [68-77°F]) and room light.

NUTROPIN   RX
somatropin (Genentech)

OTHER BRAND NAMES: Nutropin AQ (Genentech)

THERAPEUTIC CLASS: Human growth hormone

INDICATIONS: (Adults) Replacement of endogenous growth hormone (GH) in GH deficiency (GHD). (Pediatrics) Long-term treatment of growth failure due to lack of adequate endogenous GH secretion, in short stature associated with Turner syndrome, and in idiopathic short stature (ISS). Treatment of growth failure associated with chronic renal insufficiency (CRI) up to the time of renal transplantation.

DOSAGE: *Adults:* GHD: Initial: Up to 0.006mg/kg/day SQ. Max: <35 yrs: 0.025mg/kg qd. ≥35 yrs: 0.0125mg/kg/day. Alternatively may use 0.2mg/day (range: 0.15-0.30mg/day). Increase every 1-2 months by increments of 0.1-0.2mg qd. Elderly: Start at low end of dosing range. *Pediatrics:* GHD: Usual: 0.3mg/kg/week divided into daily SQ doses. Pubertal Patients: Up to 0.7mg/kg/week divided into daily SQ doses. CRI: 0.35mg/kg/week divided into daily SQ doses. Continue until renal transplantation. Hemodialysis: Give qhs or 3-4 hrs post-dialysis. Chronic Cycling Peritoneal Dialysis: Give in am after dialysis. Chronic Ambulatory Peritoneal Dialysis: Give qhs during overnight exchange. Turner Syndrome: Up to 0.375mg/kg/week SQ in divided doses 3-7x/week. ISS: 0.3mg/kg/week divided into daily SQ doses.

HOW SUPPLIED: Inj: 5mg, 10mg, (AQ) 10mg/2mL, 20mg/2mL, (AQ NuSpin) 5mg/2mL, 10mg/2mL, 20mg/2mL

CONTRAINDICATIONS: Acute critical illness after serious surgeries (eg, open heart or abdominal surgery, accidental trauma, acute respiratory failure), closed epiphyses in pediatrics, active proliferative or severe nonproliferative diabetic retinopathy, active neoplasia, evidence of recurrence or progression of an intracranial tumor. Prader-Willi syndrome (unless also diagnosed with GH deficiency) with severe obesity or respiratory impairment.

WARNINGS/PRECAUTIONS: Caution with epiphyseal closure in adults treated with GH-replacement therapy in childhood. Recurrence/progression reported with intracranial lesions. Renal osteodystrophy may occur with growth failure secondary to renal impairment. Scoliosis and slipped capital femoral epiphysis may develop in rapid growth. Caution with Turner syndrome and ISS. Intracranial HTN with papilledema, visual changes, headache, N/V has been reported. Monitor for malignant transformation of skin lesions. Injecting SQ in same site over long period of time may cause tissue atrophy. May decrease insulin sensitivity. Caution in elderly.

ADVERSE REACTIONS: Antibodies to the protein, leukemia, transient peripheral edema, arthralgia, carpal tunnel syndrome, malignant transformations, gynecomastia, pancreatitis.

INTERACTIONS: Decreased effects with glucocorticoids. May reduce insulin sensitivity; may need insulin adjustment. May need to increase dose in adult women on estrogen replacement.

PREGNANCY: Category C, caution in nursing.

MECHANISM OF ACTION: Human growth hormone; increases growth rate and serum insulin-like growth factor-I levels.

PHARMACOKINETICS: Absorption: (SQ) Absolute bioavailability (81%), C_{max}=71.1mcg/L, T_{max}=3.9 hrs, AUC=677 mcg•hr/L. **Distribution:** V_d=50mL/kg. **Metabolism:** Liver and kidneys. **Elimination:** (SQ) $T_{1/2}$=2.1 hrs. (IV) $T_{1/2}$=19.5 min.

NURSING CONSIDERATIONS

Assessment: Assess for any conditions where treatment is contraindicated or cautioned, pre-existing type 1 or type 2 DM or impaired glucose tolerance, history of scoliosis, pre-existing papilledema, hypothyroidism, diagnostic imaging (rule out pituitary or intracranial tumor), hypopituitarism and possible drug interactions. Obtain baseline funduscopic exam. Chronic renal insufficiency (pediatrics): Baseline x-ray of hips. Prader-Willi syndrome: Evaluate for signs of upper airway obstruction or sleep apnea before initiation. Turner syndrome: Evaluate for otitis media or other ear disorders, and for CV disorders before initiation.

Monitoring: Monitor FPG, and thyroid function tests periodically, periodic funduscopic exam, weight control (Prader-Willi), signs/symptoms of malignant transformation of skin lesions, intracranial HTN, renal osteodystrophy, slipped capital femoral epiphysis (onset of limp, hip or knee pain), hypersensitivity/allergic reactions, respiratory infections (Prader-Willi), otitis media or ear disorders, CV disorders (Turner syndrome), and progression of scoliosis.

Patient Counseling: Instruct on proper usage and disposal, and caution against reuse of needles and syringes. Seek medical attention if symptoms of slipped capital femoral epiphysis (onset of limp, hip or knee pain), hypersensitivity/allergic reactions, respiratory infections (Prader-Willi), otitis media or ear disorders and CV disorders (Turner syndrome), and progression of scoliosis occur.

Administration: SQ route. Do not shake. Refer to PI for proper administration. **Storage:** Before and after reconstitution: 2-8°C (36-46°F). Avoid freezing. AQ: Stable for 28 days after initial use. Protect from light. Nutropin: Stable 14 days after reconstitution.

NuvaRing

RX

etonogestrel - ethinyl estradiol (Organon)

> Cigarette smoking increases risk of serious cardiovascular (CV) side effects. Risk increases with age (>35 yrs) and heavy smoking (≥15 cigarettes/day). Women who use combination hormonal contraception should be strongly advised not to smoke.

THERAPEUTIC CLASS: Estrogen/progestogen combination

INDICATIONS: Prevention of pregnancy.

DOSAGE: *Adults:* Insert ring vaginally. Ring is to remain in place continuously for 3 weeks. It should be removed for 1-week break and then a new ring should be inserted on same day of week as the last ring was removed. No Hormonal Contraceptive Use in the Preceding Cycle: Insert ring on Day 1-5 of menstrual bleeding. If inserted on Days 2-5 of cycle, use an additional barrier method of contraception (eg, condom, spermicide) for 1st 7 days. Changing from Combined Hormonal Contraceptive: May switch any day, but at the latest on the day following the usual hormone-free interval. Changing from Progestin-Only Method (minipill, implant, or injection) or from Progestogen-Releasing Intrauterine System (IUS): May switch on any day from the minipill. May switch from an implant or IUS on the day of its removal and from an injectable on the day when the next injection is due. In all cases, additional barrier method (eg, condom, spermicide) should be use for the 1st 7 days.
Pediatrics: Postpubertal: Insert ring vaginally. Ring is to remain in place continuously for 3 weeks. It should be removed for 1-week break and then a new ring should be inserted on same day of week as the last ring was removed. No Hormonal Contraceptive Use in the Preceding Cycle: Insert ring on Day 1-5 of menstrual bleeding. If inserted on Days 2-5 of cycle, use an additional barrier method of contraception (eg, condom, spermicide) for 1st 7 days. Changing from

Combined Hormonal Contraceptive: May switch any day, but at the latest on the day following the usual hormone-free interval. Changing from Progestin-Only Method (minipill, implant, or injection) or from Progestogen-Releasing Intrauterine System (IUS): May switch on any day from the minipill. May switch from an implant or IUS on the day of its removal and from an injectable on the day when the next injection is due. In all cases, additional barrier method (eg, condom, spermicide) should be use for the 1st 7 days.

HOW SUPPLIED: Vaginal ring: (Ethinyl estradiol-Etonogestrel) 0.015mg-0.120mg/day

CONTRAINDICATIONS: Thrombophlebitis, history of deep vein thrombophlebitis, active or history of thromboembolic disorders, current or history of cerebral vascular disease, current or history of coronary artery disease, valvular heart disease with thrombogenic complications, severe HTN, diabetes with vascular involvement, headaches with focal neurological symptoms, major surgery with prolonged immobilization, breast carcinoma or history of breast carcinoma, carcinoma of the endometrium or other estrogen-dependent neoplasia, undiagnosed abnormal genital bleeding, cholestatic jaundice of pregnancy or jaundice with prior hormonal contraceptive use, hepatic tumors (benign or malignant) or active liver disease, pregnancy, heavy smoking (≥15 cigarettes per day) and >35 yrs.

WARNINGS/PRECAUTIONS: Increases risk of MI, thromboembolism, stroke, hepatic neoplasia, vascular disease, gallbladder disease, and HTN. Increased risk of morbidity and mortality in certain inherited thrombophilias, HTN, hyperlipidemias, obesity, and diabetes. May increase risk of breast cancer and cancer of the reproductive organs. Retinal thrombosis reported; d/c if unexplained partial or complete loss of vision, onset of proptosis or diplopia, papilledema, or retinal vascular lesions develop. May cause decreased glucose tolerance, fluid retention, breakthrough bleeding, and spotting. May increase BP; d/c if significant elevation in BP occurs. May elevate LDL levels or cause other lipid changes. May cause or exacerbate migraine headaches; d/c if severe or recurrent headache or migraine develops. D/C if jaundice or if significant depression develops. May develop visual changes with contact lens. May be expelled while removing tampons on rare occasions. Toxic shock syndrome reported. Older women who take hormonal contraceptive should take the lowest possible dose formulation that is effective. Ectopic as well as intrauterine pregnancy may occur in contraceptive failures. Does not protect against HIV infection (AIDS) and other STDs. Vaginal/cervical erosion or ulceration rarely reported. May affect certain endocrine, LFTs, and blood components in laboratory tests.

ADVERSE REACTIONS: Vaginitis, headache, upper respiratory tract infection, vaginal secretion, sinusitis, weight gain, nausea.

INTERACTIONS: Reduced contraceptive effectiveness when co-administered with some antifungals, anticonvulsants, and other drugs that increase the metabolism of contraceptive steroids (eg, barbiturates, griseofulvin, rifampin, phenylbutazone, phenytoin, carbamazepine, felbamate, oxcarbazepine, topiramate, modafinil); use additonal form of contraception when taking such medications. HIV protease inhibitors may increase or decrease estrogen and progestin levels. St. John's wort may reduce contraceptive effectiveness and may cause breakthrough bleeding. Atorvastatin, ascorbic acid, acetaminophen, CYP3A4 inhibitors (eg, itraconazole, ketoconazole), vaginal miconazole nitrate may increase plasma hormone levels. May increase levels of cyclosporine, prednisolone, and theophylline. May decrease levels of acetaminophen and increase clearance of temazepam, salicylic acid, morphine, and clofibric acid.

PREGNANCY: Category X, not for use in nursing.

MECHANISM OF ACTION: Estrogen/progestogen combination; suppresses gonadotropins, leading to inhibition of ovulation, and increases difficulty of sperm entry into uterus and reduces likelihood of implantation by producing changes in cervical mucus and endometrium, respectively.

PHARMACOKINETICS: Absorption: Etonogestrel: Rapid; bioavailability (100%); C_{max}=1716pg/mL; T_{max}=200.3 hrs. Ethinyl estradiol: Rapid; absolute bioavailability (56%); C_{max}=34.7pg/mL; T_{max}=59.3 hrs. **Distribution:** Found in breast milk. Etonogestrel: Serum albumin binding (66%), sex hormone-binding globulin (32%). Ethinyl estradiol: Serum albumin binding (98.5%). **Metabolism:** Hepatic via CYP3A4. **Elimination:** Urine, bile, feces; Etonogestrel: $T_{1/2}$=29.3 hrs; Ethinyl estradiol: $T_{1/2}$=44.7 hrs.

NURSING CONSIDERATIONS

Assessment: Assess for conditions in which treatment is contraindicated or cautioned. Assess for pregnancy/nursing status, and for possible drug interactions. Assess if a heavy smoker and if over 35 yrs. Assess use in patients who have inherited thrombophilias, HTN, hyperlipidemias, obesity, or DM.

Monitoring: Monitor for signs and symptoms of MI, thromboembolism, stroke, and other adverse effects. Monitor lipid levels with history of hyperlipidemia; monitor BP if have history of HTN; monitor serum glucose levels in DM or prediabetic patients. Refer patients with contact lenses to an opthalmologist if visual changes or changes in lens tolerance occur. Perform annual physical exam.

Patient Counseling: Counsel that drug does not protect against HIV infection/AIDS or other STDs and to take as directed. Counsel about possibility of light spotting. Avoid smoking to prevent cardiovascular side effects. Seek immediate medical attention if develop sharp chest pain, coughing blood, shortness of breath, pain in the calf, chest pain or chest heaviness, vision or speech abnormalities, severe headache, severe vomiting, severe dizziness, severe abdominal pain, sudden fever or sunburn rash, breast lumps, irregular vaginal bleeding or spotting, urination problems, swelling of fingers or ankles, or if develop sleeping disturbances or fatigue. Caution that some medications decrease efficacy and should not be used without physician instructions. Inform that if ring is accidentally expelled and left outside of the vagina for less than three hours, contraceptive efficacy is not reduced; ring can be rinsed with cool to lukewarm water and reinserted as soon as possible or a new ring can be inserted and the regimen should continue without alteration.

Administration: Intravaginal route. Refer to PI for specific instructions. **Storage:** 2-8°C (36-46°F). After dispensing, store up to 4 months at 25°C (77°F); excursions permitted to 15-30°C (59-86°F). Avoid direct sunlight or above 30°C (86°F).

NUVIGIL
armodafinil (Cephalon)

THERAPEUTIC CLASS: Wakefulness-promoting agent

INDICATIONS: To improve wakefulness in patients with excessive sleepiness associated with narcolepsy, obstructive sleep apnea (OSA), and shift work disorder (SWD). As adjunct to standard treatment for underlying obstruction in OSA.

DOSAGE: *Adults:* ≥17 yrs: OSA/Narcolepsy: 150mg or 250mg qam. SWD: 150mg qd 1 hr prior to work shift. Elderly: Consider dose reduction.

HOW SUPPLIED: Tab: 50mg, 150mg, 250mg

WARNINGS/PRECAUTIONS: May cause severe or life-threatening rash, including Stevens-Johnson syndrome (SJS), toxic epidermal necrolysis (TEN), and drug rash with eosinophilia and systemic symptoms (DRESS); d/c treatment at first sign of rash. Angioedema, anaphylactoid reactions, multi-organ hypersensitivity and psychiatric adverse experiences reported; d/c treatment if symptoms develop. Caution with history of psychosis, depression, or mania. Caution if recent myocardial infarction (MI) or unstable angina. Avoid in patients with history of left ventricular hypertrophy or with mitral valve prolapse who have experienced mitral valve prolapse syndrome (eg, ischemic ECG changes, chest pain, arrhythmia) with CNS stimulants. May impair mental/physical abilities. Reduce dose with severe hepatic impairment. Use low dose in elderly.

ADVERSE REACTIONS: Headache, nausea, dizziness, insomnia, diarrhea, dry mouth, anxiety, depression, rash.

INTERACTIONS: Potent CYP3A4/5 inducers (eg, carbamazepine, phenobarbital, rifampin) or inhibitors (eg, ketoconazole, erythromycin) may alter plasma levels. Effectiveness of CYP3A substrates (eg, cyclosporine, ethinyl estradiol, midazolam, triazolam) may be reduced; consider dose adjustment. May cause moderate inhibition of CYP2C19 activity; dosage reduction may be required for some CYP2C19 substrates (eg, omeprazole, diazepam, phenytoin, propranolol, clomipramine). Weakly induces CYP1A2; may affect CYP1A2 substrates. Methylphenidate or dextroamphetamine may delay absorption. Caution with MAOIs. Monitor PT/INR with warfarin. Effectiveness of steroidal contraceptives may be reduced during and for 1 month after d/c of therapy; alternate or concomitant methods of contraception are recommended.

PREGNANCY: Category C, caution in nursing.

MECHANISM OF ACTION: Wakefulness-promoting agent; not established. Binds to the dopamine transporter and inhibits dopamine reuptake.

PHARMACOKINETICS: Absorption: Readily absorbed. T_{max}=2 hrs (fasted), delayed by 2-4 hrs (fed). **Distribution:** V_d=42L; plasma protein binding (60%, based on modafinil). **Metabolism:** Liver via hydrolytic deamidation, S-oxidation, aromatic ring hydroxylation, and glucuronide conjugation; CYP3A4/5. **Elimination:** Feces (1%), urine (80%, <10% parent compound); $T_{1/2}$=15 hrs.

NURSING CONSIDERATIONS

Assessment: Assess for hypersensitivity, hepatic impairment, pregnancy/nursing status, possible drug interactions, and a history of psychosis, depression, mania, left ventricular hypertrophy, or mitral valve prolapse. Assess for a recent history of MI or unstable angina. Use only in patients who have had a complete evaluation of their excessive sleepiness, and in whom a diagnosis of either narcolepsy, OSA, and/or SWD has been made.

Monitoring: Monitor for serious rash, SJS, TEN, DRESS, angioedema, hypersensitivity, multi-organ hypersensitivity reactions, psychiatric adverse symptoms, and other adverse reactions. Monitor BP. If used adjunctively with continuous positive airway pressure (CPAP), monitor for CPAP compliance. Periodically re-evaluate long-term usefulness if prescribed for an extended time.

Patient Counseling: Advise that this is not a replacement for sleep. Inform that drug may improve but does not eliminate sleepiness. Advise to avoid taking alcohol during therapy. Caution against hazardous tasks (eg, driving, operating machinery) or performing other activities that require mental alertness. Advise to notify physician if pregnant or intend to become pregnant or if nursing during therapy. Caution about increased risk of pregnancy when using steroidal contraceptives and for 1 month after d/c therapy. Inform physician if taking or planning to take any prescribed or OTC drugs. Instruct to contact physician if rash, depression, anxiety, or signs of psychosis or mania develop. Inform of importance of continuing previously prescribed treatments. Advise to d/c and notify physician if rash, hives, mouth sores, blisters, peeling skin, trouble swallowing or breathing or other allergic reactions develop.

Administration: Oral route. **Storage:** 20-25°C (68-77°F).

NYSTATIN ORAL   RX
nystatin (Various)

THERAPEUTIC CLASS: Polyene antifungal

INDICATIONS: (Sus) Treatment of oral candidiasis. (Tab) Treatment of non-esophageal mucus membrane GI candidiasis.

DOSAGE: *Adults:* (Sus) Oral Candidiasis: 4-6mL qid (1/2 of dose in each side of mouth). Retain in mouth as long as possible before swallowing. Continue treatment for at least 48 hrs after perioral symptoms disappeared and cultures demonstrate eradication of *Candida albicans.* (Tab) Non-Esophageal GI Candidiasis: 1-2 tab tid. Continue treatment for at least 48 hrs after clinical cure. *Pediatrics:* (Sus) Oral Candidiasis: 4-6mL qid (1/2 of dose in each side of mouth). Retain in mouth as long as possible before swallowing. Infants: 2mL qid. Premature/Low Birth Weight Infants: 1mL qid. Use dropper to place 1/2 of dose in each side of mouth and avoid feeding for 5-10 min. Continue treatment for at least 48 hrs after perioral symptoms disappeared and cultures demonstrate eradication of *Candida albicans.*

HOW SUPPLIED: Sus: 100,000 U/mL [60mL, 473mL, 3785mL]; Tab: 500,000 U

WARNINGS/PRECAUTIONS: Not for use in treatment of systemic mycoses. D/C if sensitization/irritation occurs. Caution with renal insufficiency.

ADVERSE REACTIONS: Oral irritation/sensitization, diarrhea, N/V, GI upset/disturbances.

PREGNANCY: Category C, caution in nursing.

MECHANISM OF ACTION: Polyene antifungal; binds to sterols in the cell membrane of susceptible *Candida* species with a resultant change in membrane permeability, allowing leakage of intracellular components.

PHARMACOKINETICS: Elimination: Feces (unchanged).

NURSING CONSIDERATIONS

Assessment: Assess for history of hypersensitivity to the drug or any of its components, renal insufficiency, and pregnancy/nursing status. Confirm diagnosis of candidiasis.

Monitoring: Monitor for oral irritation/sensitization, other adverse reactions, and renal function.

Patient Counseling: Inform about the risks and benefits of therapy. Advise to notify physician if any adverse reactions (eg, sensitization, irritation) occur. Instruct to inform physician if pregnant, planning to become pregnant, or breastfeeding.

Administration: Oral route. (Sus) Shake well before using. Protect from freezing. **Storage:** 20-25°C (68-77°F).

NYSTOP   RX
nystatin (Paddock)

THERAPEUTIC CLASS: Polyene antifungal

INDICATIONS: Treatment of cutaneous or mucocutaneous mycotic infections caused by *Candida albicans* and other susceptible *Candida* species.

DOSAGE: *Adults:* Apply to lesions bid-tid until healing is complete. *Candida* Infection of the Feet: Dust the powder on the feet and in all footwear. *Pediatrics:* Apply to lesions bid-tid until healing is complete. *Candida* Infection of the Feet: Dust the powder on the feet and in all footwear.

HOW SUPPLIED: Powder: 100,000 U/g [15g, 30g, 60g]

WARNINGS/PRECAUTIONS: Not for systemic, PO, intravaginal, or ophthalmic use. D/C if irritation or sensitization develops and institute appropriate measures. Confirm diagnosis of *Candida*

infection using potassium hydroxide smears, cultures, or other diagnostic methods; repeat test if there is a lack of therapeutic response.

ADVERSE REACTIONS: Allergic reactions, burning, itching, rash, eczema, pain on application site.

PREGNANCY: Category C, caution in nursing.

MECHANISM OF ACTION: Polyene antifungal; binds to sterols in the cell membrane of susceptible species resulting in a change in membrane permeability and subsequent leakage of intracellular components.

NURSING CONSIDERATIONS

Assessment: Assess for history of hypersensitivity to the drug or any of its components and pregnancy/nursing status. Confirm diagnosis of *Candida* infection using appropriate diagnostic methods.

Monitoring: Monitor for irritation or sensitization, other adverse reactions, and therapeutic response. Reassess diagnosis if there is a lack of therapeutic response.

Patient Counseling: Instruct to use exactly ud, including replacement of missed dose. Advise not to use the medication for any disorder other than prescribed. Instruct not to interrupt or d/c therapy until treatment is completed, even if symptomatic relief occurs within the first few days of treatment. Advise to notify physician promptly if skin irritation develops.

Administration: Topical route. **Storage:** 15-30°C (59-86°F). Avoid excessive heat (40°C [104°F]).

OFIRMEV   RX
acetaminophen (Cadence)

THERAPEUTIC CLASS: Analgesic

INDICATIONS: Management of mild to moderate pain, management of moderate to severe pain with adjunctive opioid analgesics and for reduction of fever.

DOSAGE: *Adults:* ≥50kg: Usual: 1000mg q6h or 650mg q4h. Max Daily Dose: 4000mg/day. Max Single Dose:1000mg/dose. <50kg: 15mg/kg q6h or 12.5mg/kg q4h. Max Daily Dose: 75g/kg/day. Max Single Dose: 15mg/kg/dose. Dosing interval must be a minimum of 4 hrs.
Pediatrics: ≥13 yrs: ≥50kg: Usual: 1000mg q6h or 650mg q4h. Max Daily dose: 4000mg/day. Max Single Dose: 1000mg/dose. <50kg: 15mg/kg q6h or 12.5mg/kg q4h. Max Daily Dose: 75mg/kg/day. Max Single Dose:15mg/kg q6h or 12.5mg/kg q4h. ≥2-12 yrs: 15mg/kg q6h or 12.5mg/kg q4h. Max Daily Dose: 75mg/kg/day (up to 3750mg). Max Single Dose: 15mg/kg/dose (up to 750mg). Dosing interval must be a minimum of 4 hrs.

HOW SUPPLIED: Inj: 10mg/mL

CONTRAINDICATIONS: Severe hepatic impairment or severe active liver disease.

WARNINGS/PRECAUTIONS: May result in hepatic injury (eg, severe hepatotoxicity, death) in doses higher than recommended; do not exceed maximum recommended daily dose. Caution with hepatic impairment or active hepatic disease, alcoholism, chronic malnutrition, severe hypovolemia, or severe renal impairment (CrCl ≤30mL/min). Hypersensitivity and anaphylaxis reported; d/c immediately if symptoms associated with allergy/hypersensitivity occur. Life-threatening anaphylaxis requiring emergent medical attention reported.

ADVERSE REACTIONS: N/V, headache, insomnia, constipation, pruritus, agitation, atelectasis.

INTERACTIONS: Altered metabolism and increased hepatotoxic potential with substances that induce or regulate CYP2E1. Excessive alcohol use may induce hepatic cytochromes. Ethanol may inhibit metabolism. Increased international normalized ratio (INR) in some patients stabilized on warfarin.

PREGNANCY: Category C, caution in nursing.

MECHANISM OF ACTION: Analgesic/antipyretic; not established. Thought to primarily involve central actions.

PHARMACOKINETICS: Absorption: Variable doses to different age groups resulted in different parameters; refer to PI. **Distribution:** Plasma protein binding (10-25%); widely distributed throughout body tissues except fat; (PO) found in breast milk. **Metabolism:** Liver; glucuronide and sulfate conjugation, and oxidation via CYP2E1; N-acetyl-p-benzoquinone imine (NAPQI) (metabolite). **Elimination:** Urine (<5% unconjugated, >90% within 24 hrs).

NURSING CONSIDERATIONS

Assessment: Assess for previous hypersensitivity, severe hepatic impairment or severe active liver disease, alcoholism, chronic malnutrition, severe hypovolemia, or severe renal impairment (CrCl ≤30mL/min). Assess for pregnancy/nursing status and possible drug interactions.

Monitoring: Monitor for signs and symptoms of hypersensitivity and anaphylaxis (eg, swelling of face, mouth, and throat, respiratory distress, urticaria, rash, and pruritus), and other adverse reactions.

Patient Counseling: Inform about the risks and benefits of therapy. Warn not to exceed the recommended dose. Notify physician if any adverse reactions occur or if pregnant/nursing or planning to become pregnant. Counsel about possible drug interactions.

Administration: IV route. Administer by IV infusion. Do not add other medications to the vial or infusion device. Refer to PI for administration technique. **Storage:** 20-25°C (68-77°F). Use within 6 hrs after opening. Do not refrigerate or freeze.

OFLOXACIN   RX
ofloxacin (Various)

Fluoroquinolones are associated with an increased risk of tendinitis and tendon rupture in all ages. Risk is further increased in patients >60 yrs, taking corticosteroids, and with kidney, heart or lung transplants. May exacerbate muscle weakness with myasthenia gravis; avoid with known history of myasthenia gravis.

THERAPEUTIC CLASS: Fluoroquinolone

INDICATIONS: Treatment of complicated urinary tract infections (UTI), uncomplicated skin and skin structure infections (SSSI), acute bacterial exacerbation of chronic bronchitis (ABECB), community-acquired pneumonia (CAP), acute uncomplicated urethral and cervical gonorrhea, nongonococcal urethritis and cervicitis, mixed infections of urethra and cervix, acute pelvic inflammatory disease (PID), uncomplicated cystitis, and prostatitis caused by susceptible strains of microorganisms.

DOSAGE: *Adults:* ABECB/CAP/SSSI: 400mg q12h for 10 days. Cervicitis/Urethritis: 300mg q12h for 7 days. Gonorrhea: 400mg single dose. PID: 400mg q12h for 10-14 days. Uncomplicated Cystitis: 200mg q12h for 3 days (*Escherichia coli* or *Klebsiella pneumoniae*) or 7 days (other pathogens). Complicated UTI: 200mg q12h for 10 days. Prostatitis: *(E. coli)* 300mg q12h for 6 weeks. CrCl 20-50mL/min: After regular initial dose, give q24h. CrCl <20mL/min: After regular initial dose, give 50% of normal dose q24h. Severe Hepatic Impairment: Max: 400mg/day.

HOW SUPPLIED: Tab: 200mg, 300mg, 400mg

WARNINGS/PRECAUTIONS: Convulsions, increased ICP, toxic psychosis, CNS stimulation, and serious, sometimes fatal, hypersensitivity reactions reported; d/c if any occur. Rare cases of sensory or sensorimotor axonal polyneuropathy reported; d/c if symptoms of neuropathy occur. *Clostridium difficile*-associated diarrhea (CDAD) and ruptures of shoulder, hand, and Achilles' tendon reported. Not shown to be effective for syphilis. Maintain adequate hydration. Caution with renal or hepatic dysfunction, risk for seizures, CNS disorder with predisposition to seizures. Avoid excessive sunlight. Monitor blood, renal and hepatic function with prolonged therapy. D/C immediately at the first appearance of skin rash, jaundice, or any other sign of hypersensitivity and supportive measures instituted. Drug therapy should be d/c if photosensitivity/phototoxicity occurs. Avoid in patients with known prolongation of the QT interval, and with uncorrected hypokalemia. Caution in elderly taking corticosteroids.

ADVERSE REACTIONS: N/V, insomnia, headache, dizziness, diarrhea, external genital pruritus in women, vaginitis.

INTERACTIONS: See Boxed Warning. Decreased absorption with antacids, sucralfate, multivitamins, zinc, didanosine; separate dosing by 2 hrs. Cimetidine may interfere with elimination. Cyclosporine levels may be elevated. NSAIDs may increase risk of seizures. Probenecid may affect renal tubular secretion. Avoid in patients receiving Class IA (quinidine, procainamide), or Class III (amiodarone, sotalol) antiarrhythmic agents. May potentiate theophylline, warfarin. May potentiate insulin, oral hypoglycemics; d/c if hypoglycemia occurs. May increase half-life of drugs metabolized by CYP450.

PREGNANCY: Category C, not for use in nursing.

MECHANISM OF ACTION: Fluoroquinolone; synthetic broad-spectrum antimicrobial agent; inhibits topoisomerase II (DNA gyrase) and topoisomerase IV, which are required for bacterial DNA replication, transcription, repair, and recombination.

PHARMACOKINETICS: **Absorption:** Oral administration of variable doses resulted in different parameters; T_{max}=1-2 hrs; bioavailability (98%). **Distribution:** Plasma protein binding (32%), found in breast milk. **Elimination:** Biphasic ($T_{1/2}$=4-5 hrs, 20-25 hrs), renal.

NURSING CONSIDERATIONS

Assessment: Assess for risk factors for developing tendinitis and tendon rupture, myasthenia gravis, renal function, LFTs, pregnancy/nursing status, history of seizures, QTc prolongation, and possible drug interactions. Obtain baseline culture and susceptibility test and serologic test for syphilis.

O

Monitoring: Monitor for tendinitis or tendon rupture, convulsions, increased ICP, toxic psychosis, CNS events, CDAD, peripheral neuropathy, photosensitivity reactions, and hypersensitivity reactions. Assess renal function and perform follow-up serologic test for syphilis after 3 months.

Patient Counseling: Notify physician if experience symptoms of pain, swelling, or inflammation of a tendon, or weakness or inability to move joints; rest and refrain from exercise and d/c therapy. Call physician if muscle weakness or breathing problems worsen. Inform that drug treats bacterial, not viral, infections. Take exactly as directed; skipping doses or not completing full course may decrease effectiveness and increase resistance. Inform about potential benefits/risks. D/C and notify physician if experience skin rash, other allergic reaction, watery or bloody stools, or symptoms of peripheral neuropathy develop. Use caution in activities requiring mental alertness and coordination. Advise diabetic patients to use caution; hypoglycemia may develop during therapy. Inform to take with or without meals, and to drink fluids. Avoid sun exposure.

Administration: Oral route. **Storage:** 25°C (77°F), excursions permitted to 15-30°C (59-86°F).

OFLOXACIN OTIC SOLUTION 0.3% RX

ofloxacin (Various)

OTHER BRAND NAMES: Floxin Otic Singles Solution (Daiichi Sankyo)

THERAPEUTIC CLASS: Fluoroquinolone

INDICATIONS: Treatment of otitis externa in patients ≥6 months, chronic suppurative otitis media in patients ≥12 yrs with perforated tympanic membranes, and acute otitis media in patients ≥1 yr with tympanostomy tubes, caused by susceptible isolates of designated microorganisms.

DOSAGE: *Adults:* Otitis Externa: 10 drops (0.5mL) or 2 single-dispensing containers (SDCs) into affected ear qd for 7 days. Chronic Suppurative Otitis Media with Perforated Tympanic Membrane: 10 drops (0.5mL) or 2 SDCs bid into affected ear for 14 days. Pump tragus 4 times by pushing inward to facilitate penetration into the middle ear.
Pediatrics: Otitis Externa: ≥13 yrs: 10 drops (0.5mL) or 2 SDCs into affected ear qd for 7 days. 6 months-13 yrs: 5 drops (0.25mL) or 1 single-dispensing container (SDC) into affected ear qd for 7 days. Chronic Suppurative Otitis Media with Perforated Tympanic Membrane: ≥12 yrs: 10 drops (0.5mL) or 2 SDCs bid into affected ear for 14 days. Acute Otitis Media with Tympanostomy Tubes: 1-12 yrs: 5 drops (0.25mL) or 1 SDC bid into affected ear for 10 days. Pump tragus 4 times by pushing inward to facilitate penetration into the middle ear.

HOW SUPPLIED: Sol: 0.3% [5mL, 10mL], (Singles) 0.3% [20s]

WARNINGS/PRECAUTIONS: D/C if hypersensitivity reaction occurs. Prolonged use may result in overgrowth in nonsusceptible organisms; re-evaluate if no improvement after one week. If otorrhea persists after a full course, or if two or more episodes occur within 6 months, further evaluation is recommended. Not for injection and ophthalmic use.

ADVERSE REACTIONS: Pruritus, application site reaction, taste perversion.

PREGNANCY: Category C, not for use in nursing.

MECHANISM OF ACTION: Fluoroquinolone; exerts antibacterial activity by inhibiting DNA gyrase (a bacterial topoisomerase), an essential enzyme which controls DNA topology and assists in DNA replication, repair, deactivation, and transcription.

PHARMACOKINETICS: Absorption: (Perforated tympanic membrane) C_{max}=10ng/mL.

NURSING CONSIDERATIONS

Assessment: Assess for drug hypersensitivity, preexisting cholesteatoma, foreign body or tumor, pregnancy/nursing status.

Monitoring: Monitor for anaphylactic reactions, cardiovascular collapse, loss of consciousness, angioedema, airway obstruction, dyspnea, urticaria and itching, overgrowth of nonsusceptible organisms (fungi), for improvement/persistence of otorrhea.

Patient Counseling: Counsel to avoid touching applicator tip to fingers or other surfaces to avoid contamination. D/C and instruct to contact physician if signs of allergy occur. Instruct patients to warm bottle by holding for 1-2 min, to avoid dizziness which may result from instillation of a cold solution. Instruct to lie with affected ear upward, before instilling the drops; maintain position for 5 min. Repeat if necessary, for opposite ear.

Administration: Otic route. **Storage:** 20-25°C (68-77°F). Protect from light.

OFORTA   RX
fludarabine phosphate (Sanofi-Aventis)

> **Severe neurologic effects, including blindness, coma, and death, reported with use of high doses (4X greater than recommended); similar toxicity rarely reported with use within recommended dose range. Periodic neurological assessments are recommended. Life-threatening and sometimes fatal autoimmune hemolytic anemia reported; evaluate and closely monitor for hemolysis. High incidence of fatal pulmonary toxicity reported in combination with pentostatin (deoxycoformycin); use not recommended.**

THERAPEUTIC CLASS: Antimetabolite

INDICATIONS: Treatment of adults with B-cell chronic lymphocytic leukemia whose disease is unresponsive to or has progressed during or after treatment with at least 1 standard alkylating agent-containing regimen.

DOSAGE: *Adults:* Usual: 40mg/m^2 qd for 5 consecutive days. Commence each 5-day course every 28 days. May decrease or delay dose based on evidence of hematologic or nonhematologic toxicity. Administer 3 additional cycles following achievement of maximal response, then d/c. CrCl 30-70mL/min/1.73m^2: Reduce dose by 20%. CrCl <30mL/min/1.73m^2: Reduce dose by 50%.

HOW SUPPLIED: Tab: 10mg

WARNINGS/PRECAUTIONS: Consider delaying or d/c therapy if neurotoxicity occurs. Patients with advanced age, renal impairment, and bone marrow impairment may be predisposed to increased toxicity; closely monitor and modify dose accordingly. Severe bone marrow suppression, notably anemia, thrombocytopenia and neutropenia, reported; perform careful hematologic monitoring. Fatalities due to infection reported; monitor for signs and symptoms of infection. Caution in patients with large tumor burdens; tumor lysis syndrome reported. Transfusion-associated graft-versus-host disease rarely reported after transfusion of non-irradiated blood; consider use of irradiated blood if transfusion is required. Caution with renal impairment. May cause fetal harm; women of childbearing potential and fertile males must take contraceptive measures during and at least 6 months after cessation of therapy.

ADVERSE REACTIONS: Myelosuppression, CNS toxicity, autoimmune hemolytic anemia, fever, chills, infections, N/V, malaise, fatigue, anorexia, weakness, pain, cough.

INTERACTIONS: See Boxed Warning.

PREGNANCY: Category D, not for use in nursing.

MECHANISM OF ACTION: Antimetabolite; not established. Inhibits DNA polymerase α, gamma, and delta, and inhibits ribonucleoside diphosphate reductase. Also inhibits DNA primase and DNA ligase I.

PHARMACOKINETICS: Absorption: Absolute bioavailability (50-65%); T$_{max}$=1-2 hrs. **Distribution:** Plasma protein binding (19-29%) (IV). **Metabolism:** Rapid dephosphorylation to 2F-ara-A (active metabolite). **Elimination:** T$_{1/2}$=20 hrs (IV).

NURSING CONSIDERATIONS

Assessment: Assess for age, renal and bone marrow impairment, risk of tumor lysis syndrome, pregnancy/nursing status, and possible drug interactions.

Monitoring: Monitor for bone marrow suppression, severe neurologic effects, autoimmune hemolytic anemia, hemolysis, signs of hematologic/nonhematologic toxicity, tumor lysis syndrome, infection, renal function and other adverse events. Periodically monitor peripheral blood counts/hematologic profile.

Patient Counseling: Inform of the importance of periodic blood count assessment. Instruct to notify physician if fever or other signs of infection develop. Advise women of childbearing potential and fertile males to take contraceptive measures during and for at least 6 months after cessation of therapy. Instruct to exercise caution in handling the drug; advise not to crush tab, and to avoid direct skin or mucous membrane contact or inhalation. If contact occurs, instruct to wash thoroughly with soap and water or wash the eyes immediately with gently flowing water for at least 15 min. Advise to consult healthcare provider in case of skin reaction or eye contact.

Administration: Oral route. Swallow whole with water; do not chew or break. **Storage:** 25°C (77°F) under normal lighting condition; excursions permitted to 15-30°C (59-86°F).

OLEPTRO   RX
trazodone HCl (Angelini Labopharm)

> **Antidepressants increased the risk of suicidal thinking and behavior (suicidality) in children, adolescents and young adults in short-term studies of major depressive disorder (MDD) and other psychiatric disorders. Monitor and observe closely for clinical worsening, suicidality, or unusual changes in behavior in patients who are started on antidepressant therapy. Trazodone is not approved for use in pediatric patients.**

THERAPEUTIC CLASS: Triazolopyridine derivative

INDICATIONS: Treatment of MDD.

DOSAGE: *Adults:* Initial: 150mg qd. Titrate: May increase by 75mg qd every 3 days. Max: 375mg qd. Once adequate response is achieved, reduce dose gradually, with subsequent adjustment depending on therapeutic response. Maintain on the lowest effective dose and periodically reassess to determine the continued need for maintenance treatment.

HOW SUPPLIED: Tab, Extended Release: 150mg*, 300mg* *scored

WARNINGS/PRECAUTIONS: Monitor for withdrawal symptoms when treatment is stopped; reduce dose gradually whenever possible. Serotonin syndrome (eg, mental status changes, autonomic instability, neuromuscular aberrations, GI symptoms) or neuroleptic malignant syndrome (NMS)-like reactions may occur. Screen patients (including psychiatric history, family history) for bipolar disorder; not approved in treating bipolar depression. Caution in patients with cardiac disease (eg, myocardial infarction [MI]); may cause cardiac arrhythmias. May cause QT/QTc interval prolongation and GI bleeding. Priapism rarely reported; caution in men with sickle cell anemia, multiple myeloma, leukemia or in men with penile anatomical deformation (eg, angulation, cavernosal fibrosis, Peyronie's disease). Hyponatremia may occur; d/c and institute appropriate medical intervention. Orthostatic hypotension and syncope reported. May impair mental/physical abilities. Caution in hepatic/renal impairment and elderly.

ADVERSE REACTIONS: Somnolence, sedation, headache, dry mouth, dizziness, nausea, fatigue, diarrhea, constipation, back pain, blurred vision, sexual dysfunction.

INTERACTIONS: May cause serotonin syndrome or NMS-like reactions with other serotogenic drugs (SSRIs, SNRIs and triptans), MAOIs, other antipsychotics, or dopamine antagonists. Not recommended with serotonin precursors (eg, tryptophan). May enhance response to alcohol, barbiturates and other CNS depressants. Increase risk of cardiac arrhythmia with drugs that prolong QT interval or CYP3A4 inhibitors. CYP3A4 inhibitors (eg, ritonavir, ketoconazole, indinavir, itraconazole, nefazodone) may increase levels; consider lower dose. Carbamazepine decreases levels; monitor to determine if a dose increase is required. Increased serum digoxin or phenytoin levels; monitor serum levels and adjust dose as needed. May affect PT time in patients on warfarin. Concomitant use with an antihypertensive may require reduction in the dose of the antihypertensive drug. Not for use in combination or within 14 days of d/c treatment with an MAOI. Monitor and use caution with NSAIDs, ASA, and other drugs that affect coagulation or bleeding. Increased risk of hyponatremia with diuretics.

PREGNANCY: Category C, caution in nursing.

MECHANISM OF ACTION: Triazolopyridine derivative; mechanism not established. Suspected to potentiate serotonergic activity in the CNS. Preclinical trials shows selective inhibition of neuronal reuptake of serotonin and activity as an antagonist at 5HT-2A/2 serotonin receptors.

PHARMACOKINETICS: Absorption: Well absorbed; (100mg tid dose) AUC=33058ng•h/mL, C_{max}=3118ng/mL; (300mg qd dose) AUC=29131ng•h/mL, C_{max}=1812ng/mL. **Distribution:** Plasma protein binding (89-95%). **Metabolism:** Liver (extensive); CYP3A4 via oxidative cleavage; m-chlorophenylpiperazine (active metabolite). **Elimination:** Urine (70-75%). $T_{1/2}$=10 hrs.

NURSING CONSIDERATIONS

Assessment: Assess for psychiatric history (eg, suicide, depression, bipolar disorder), family history, cardiac disease (eg, MI), serotonin syndrome, bleeding events, sickle cell anemia, multiple myeloma, leukemia, penile anatomical deformation in men, syndrome of inappropriate antidiuretic hormone secretion (SIADH), arrhythmias, hepatic/renal impairment, pregnancy/nursing status, and for possible drug interactions. Obtain baseline vital signs, serum electrolytes, ECG, hepatic/renal function.

Monitoring: Monitor for signs/symptoms of clinical worsening, suicidality, unusual behavior changes or mental status changes, neuromuscular aberrations, GI symptoms, priapism, arrhythmias, hyponatremia (eg, headache, confusion, weakness), bleeding events, hepatic/renal impairment, hypotension, and withdrawal symptoms when d/c treatment. Monitor vital signs, serum electrolytes, ECG, hepatic/renal function.

Patient Counseling: Inform about the benefits and risks of therapy. Advise patients, families and caregivers of need to observe for signs/symptoms of clinical worsening and suicidality (eg, agitation, anxiety, panic attacks, mania, changes in behavior) and sleep disturbances; instruct to contact physician if these and other symptoms occur. Counsel to avoid alcohol, sedatives and other CNS depressants. Instruct males to d/c use and contact physician if prolonged or inappropriate penile erection develops. Inform that mental and/or physical ability required for performing potentially hazardous tasks (eg, operating machinery, driving) may be impaired. Instruct to notify physician if pregnant or intend to become pregnant and if nursing.

Administration: Oral route. Do not chew or crush. Take at the same time everyday, preferably at bedtime, on empty stomach. **Storage:** 15-30°C. Keep in tight, light-resistant containers.

OLUX   RX
clobetasol propionate (Connetics)

THERAPEUTIC CLASS: Corticosteroid

INDICATIONS: Short-term topical treatment of inflammatory and pruritic manifestations of moderate to severe corticosteroid-responsive dermatoses of the scalp and mild to moderate plaque-type psoriasis of non-scalp regions, excluding the face and intertriginous areas.

DOSAGE: *Adults:* Apply to affected area bid (am and pm). Use smallest amount possible that sufficiently covers the area, no more than 1.5 capfuls/application. Max Dose: 50g/week. Max Duration: 2 consecutive weeks.
Pediatrics: ≥12 yrs: Apply to affected area bid (am and pm). Use smallest amount possible that sufficiently covers the area, no more than 1.5 capfuls/application. Max Dose: 50g/week. Max Duration: 2 consecutive weeks.

HOW SUPPLIED: Foam: 0.05% [50g, 100g]

WARNINGS/PRECAUTIONS: Shown to suppress the adrenals at a dose of 7g/day. May produce reversible hypothalamic-pituitary-adrenal axis suppression, manifestations of Cushing's syndrome, hyperglycemia, and glucosuria. Evaluate for adrenal suppression when applied to large surface areas or under occlusive dressings; withdraw, reduce frequency, or substitute for a less potent steroid if adrenal suppression noted. Use appropriate antifungal or antibacterial agent with dermatological infections; d/c until infection controlled. Pediatric patients may be more susceptible to systemic toxicity. D/C if irritation occurs. Avoid extensive or prolonged use in pregnant patients. Caution in elderly. Flammable; avoid fire, flame, or smoking during and immediately following application.

ADVERSE REACTIONS: Adrenal suppression, application site burning/reaction, pruritus, irritation, erythema, folliculitis, cracking/fissuring of skin, numbness of fingers, telangiectasia, skin atrophy.

PREGNANCY: Category C, caution in nursing.

MECHANISM OF ACTION: Corticosteroid; anti-inflammatory activity has not been established. Also has antipruritic and vasoconstrictive properties. Suspected to act by induction of phospholipase A_2 inhibitory proteins (lipocortins), which may inhibit the release of arachidonic acid.

PHARMACOKINETICS: Absorption: Percutaneous. **Metabolism:** Liver. **Elimination**: Kidney (major), bile.

NURSING CONSIDERATIONS

Assessment: Assess for previous drug hypersensitivity, dermatological infections, and pregnancy/nursing status.

Monitoring: Monitor for development of skin irritation and infection. Monitor response to treatment, adrenal suppression (using adrenocorticotropin hormone stimulation, am plasma cortisol test, urinary free cortisol test), Cushing's syndrome, and other adverse effects if used for long term treatment.

Patient Counseling: Counsel patient on the signs/symptoms of adverse reactions and to contact physician if any occur. Counsel to use exactly as directed, externally, and not longer than the prescribed time. Advise not to bandage, cover, or wrap treated skin area, unless directed by physician. Advise to avoid contact with eyes.

Administration: Topical route. Refer to PI for administration instructions. **Storage:** 20-25°C (68-77°F). Do not puncture/incinerate container, expose to heat, or store above 49°C (120°F).

OLUX-E   RX
clobetasol propionate (Stiefel)

THERAPEUTIC CLASS: Corticosteroid

INDICATIONS: Treatment of inflammatory and pruritic manifestations of corticosteroid-responsive dermatoses in patients ≥12 yrs.

DOSAGE: *Adults:* Apply a thin layer to affected area(s) bid (am and pm), for up to 2 consecutive weeks. Max: 50g/week or 21 capfuls/week.
Pediatrics: ≥12 yrs: Apply a thin layer to affected area(s) bid (am and pm), for up to 2 consecutive weeks. Max: 50g/week or 21 capfuls/week.

HOW SUPPLIED: Foam: 0.05% [50g, 100g]

WARNINGS/PRECAUTIONS: May cause reversible hypothalamic pituitary adrenal (HPA) axis suppression with the potential for glucocorticosteroid insufficiency, Cushing's syndrome, hyperglycemia, and unmasking of latent diabetes mellitus. Periodically evaluate for HPA axis suppression; withdraw, reduce frequency, or substitute a less potent steroid if HPA axis suppression occurs. Manifestations of adrenal insufficiency may require systemic corticosteroids. Pediatric patients may be more susceptible to systemic toxicity. Local adverse reactions more likely to occur with occlusive use, prolonged use, or use of higher potency corticosteroids. D/C if irritation occurs. Use appropriate antimicrobial agent with skin infections; d/c until infection is treated. Avoid application to eyes, face, groin, axillae, and area of skin atrophy. Flammable; avoid fire, flame, or smoking during and immediately following application. Do not apply on the chest if used during lactation. D/C if control is achieved.

ADVERSE REACTIONS: Application-site reaction, application-site atrophy, folliculitis, acneiform eruptions, hypopigmentation, perioral dermatitis, allergic contact dermatitis, secondary infection, irritation, striae, miliaria.

INTERACTIONS: Use of >1 corticosteroid-containing products may increase the total systemic corticosteroid exposure.

PREGNANCY: Category C, caution in nursing.

MECHANISM OF ACTION: Corticosteroid; has not been established. Plays a role in cellular signaling, immune function, inflammation, and protein regulation.

PHARMACOKINETICS: Absorption: Percutaneous. C_{max}=59pg/mL, T_{max}=5 hrs (post-dose on day 8). **Distribution:** Found in breast milk (systemically administered). **Metabolism:** Liver. **Elimination:** Kidneys, bile.

NURSING CONSIDERATIONS

Assessment: Assess for presence of concomitant skin infections, severity of dermatoses, use in pediatric patients, factors that predispose to HPA axis suppression, pregnancy/nursing status, and possible drug interaction.

Monitoring: Monitor for signs/symptoms HPA axis suppression, Cushing's syndrome, hyperglycemia, irritation, allergic contact dermatitis (eg, failure to heal), and skin infections. Monitor for systemic toxicity, HPA axis suppression, Cushing's syndrome, linear growth retardation, delayed weight gain, and intracranial HTN in pediatrics. Monitor response to therapy.

Patient Counseling: Counsel to use externally and exactly as directed; avoid use on face, skin folds (eg, underarms, groin), eyes or other mucous membranes. Advise to wash hands after use. Instruct not to use for any disorder other than for which it was prescribed. Advise not to bandage or wrap treatment area, unless directed by physician. Counsel to contact physician if any local or systemic adverse reactions occur, if no improvement is seen after 2 weeks, or if surgery is contemplated. Advise that foam is flammable; avoid fire, flame, or smoking during application. Advise to d/c when control is achieved.

Administration: Topical route. Shake can, hold upside down, and depress the actuator. Dispense small amount (about a capful) and gently massage into affected area. **Storage:** 20-25°C (68-77°F). Do not puncture or incinerate container. Do not expose to heat or store above 49°C (120°F).

OMNARIS   RX
ciclesonide (Sunovion)

THERAPEUTIC CLASS: Non-halogenated glucocorticoid

INDICATIONS: Treatment of nasal symptoms associated with seasonal allergic rhinitis in adults/children ≥6 yrs and with perennial allergic rhinitis in adults/adolescents ≥12 yrs.

DOSAGE: *Adults:* Seasonal/Perennial Allergic Rhinitis: 2 sprays/nostril qd. Max: 2 sprays/nostril/day (200mcg/day). Elderly: Start at low end of dosing range.
Pediatrics: Perennial Allergic Rhinitis: ≥12 yrs: 2 sprays/nostril qd. Max: 2 sprays/nostril/day (200mcg/day). Seasonal Allergic Rhinitis: ≥6 yrs: 2 sprays/nostril qd. Max: 2 sprays/nostril/day (200mcg/day).

HOW SUPPLIED: Spray: 50mcg/spray [12.5g]

WARNINGS/PRECAUTIONS: Epistaxis reported. *Candida albicans* infections of nose or pharynx may occur; examine periodically and treat accordingly. Caution with active or quiescent tuberculosis (TB) infections, untreated local/systemic fungal/bacterial infections, systemic viral or parasitic infections, or ocular herpes simplex. Risk for more severe/fatal course of infections (eg, chickenpox, measles); avoid exposure in patients who have not had these diseases or have not been properly immunized. Nasal septal perforation may occur; avoid spraying directly onto nasal septum. Risk of acute adrenal insufficiency and withdrawal symptoms when replacing systemic corticosteroids with topical corticosteroids; monitor closely. D/C slowly if symptoms of hypercorticism and adrenal suppression occur. May exacerbate symptoms of asthma and other conditions requiring long-term systemic corticosteroid use with rapid dose decrease. May cause reduced growth velocity in pediatrics. May impair wound healing; avoid in recent nasal septal ulcers, nasal surgery, or nasal trauma until healed. Glaucoma and/or cataracts may develop; caution with vision changes, history of increased intraocular pressure (IOP), glaucoma and/or cataracts. Caution in elderly.

ADVERSE REACTIONS: Headache, epistaxis, nasopharyngitis, back pain, pharyngolaryngeal pain, sinusitis, influenza, nasal discomfort, bronchitis, urinary tract infection, cough.

INTERACTIONS: Ketoconazole may increase levels of the active metabolite des-ciclesonide.

PREGNANCY: Category C, caution in nursing.

MECHANISM OF ACTION: Non-halogenated glucocorticoid; mechanism not established. Shown to have a wide range of effects on multiple cell types (eg, mast cells, eosinophils, neutrophils, macrophages, and lymphocytes) and mediators (eg, histamine, eicosanoids, leukotrienes, and cytokines) involved in allergic inflammation.

PHARMACOKINETICS: Absorption: Des-ciclesonide: C_{max}=<30pg/mL. **Distribution:** (IV) V_d=2.9L/kg (Ciclesonide), 12.1L/kg (des-ciclesonide); plasma protein binding (≥99%). **Metabolism:** Hydrolyzed to des-ciclesonide (active metabolite); further metabolism in liver, via CYP3A4, CYP2D6. **Elimination:** (IV) Feces (66%), urine (≤20%).

NURSING CONSIDERATIONS

Assessment: Assess patients who have not been immunized or exposed to infections such as measles or chickenpox. Assess for drug hypersensitivity, TB, any infections, ocular herpes simplex, history of increased IOP, glaucoma, cataracts, recent nasal septal ulcers, nasal surgery/ trauma, use of other inhaled or systemic corticosteroids, pregnancy/nursing status, and possible drug interactions.

Monitoring: Monitor for hypercorticism, adrenal suppression, TB, infections, ocular herpes simplex, chickenpox, and measles. Monitor for epistaxis, nasal septal perforation, growth velocity in children, wound healing, visual changes, hypoadrenalism in infants born to mothers receiving corticosteroids during pregnancy, and hypersensitivity reactions. Monitor for adrenal insufficiency and withdrawal symptoms in the event of replacing systemic with topical corticosteroids.

Patient Counseling: Counsel on appropriate priming and administration of spray. Avoid spraying in eyes or directly onto nasal septum. Take as directed at regular intervals; do not exceed prescribed dosage. Contact physician if symptoms do not improve by a reasonable time (over 1-2 weeks in seasonal allergic rhinitis and 5 weeks in perennial allergic rhinitis) or if condition worsens. Counsel about risks of epistaxis, nasal ulceration, *Candida* infections, and other adverse reactions. Instruct to avoid exposure to chickenpox or measles and to consult physician if exposed to chickenpox or measles. Inform that worsening of existing TB infections, fungal/bacterial/viral/parasitic infections, or ocular herpes simplex may occur. Glaucoma and cataracts may develop; inform physician if change in vision occurs.

Administration: Intranasal route. Shake bottle gently and prime pump by actuating 8 times before use. Reprime with 1 spray if not used for 4 consecutive days. **Storage:** 25°C (77°F); excursions permitted to 15-30°C (59-86°F). Do not freeze. Discard after 4 months after removal from pouch or after 120 actuations following initial priming, whichever comes first.

OMNITROPE   RX
somatropin rdna origin (Sandoz)

THERAPEUTIC CLASS: Recombinant human growth hormone

INDICATIONS: Treatment of pediatrics with growth failure due to inadequate secretion of endogenous growth hormone (GH), Prader-Willi syndrome (PWS), and Turner syndrome (TS). Treatment of growth failure in pediatrics born small for gestational age (SGA) who fail to manifest catch-up growth by age 2 yrs, and idiopathic short stature (ISS) in pediatrics whose epiphyses are not closed. Replacement of endogenous GH in adults with adult-onset or childhood-onset GH deficiency (GHD).

DOSAGE: *Adults:* Divide weekly dose over 6 or 7 days of SQ inj (preferably in pm). GHD: Weight-Based: Initial: Not more than 0.04mg/kg/week given as daily SQ inj. Titrate: May increase at 4- to 8-week intervals. Max: 0.08mg/kg/week. Non Weight-Based: Initial: 0.2mg/day (range, 0.15-0.30mg/day). Titrate: May increase gradually q1-2 months by increments of 0.1-0.2mg/day based on clinical response and serum insulin-like growth factor-I (IGF-I) concentrations. Maint: Individualize dose. Elderly: Start at lower end of dosing range and consider smaller dose increments.
Pediatrics: Individualize dose. Divide weekly dose over 6 or 7 days of SQ inj (preferably in pm). GHD: 0.16-0.24mg/kg/week. PWS: 0.24mg/kg/week. SGA: Up to 0.48mg/kg/week. TS: 0.33mg/kg/week. ISS: Up to 0.47mg/kg/week.

HOW SUPPLIED: Inj: 5.8mg (vial); 5mg/1.5mL, 10mg/1.5mL (cartridge)

CONTRAINDICATIONS: Acute critical illness due to complications following open heart surgery, abdominal surgery, multiple accidental trauma, or with acute respiratory failure. Patients with PWS who are severely obese, with history of upper airway obstruction or sleep apnea, or with severe respiratory impairment. Active malignancy, or progression or recurrence of underlying intracranial tumor. Active proliferative or severe non-proliferative diabetic retinopathy, pediatrics with closed epiphyses.

WARNINGS/PRECAUTIONS: Increased mortality reported in patients with acute critical illness. Fatalities reported in pediatric patients with PWS. Evaluate PWS patients for signs of upper airway obstruction and sleep apnea before treatment; d/c therapy if these signs occur (eg, new/increased snoring). Implement effective weight control in patients with PWS and treat respiratory infections aggressively. Examine for progression/recurrence of underlying disease process in those with preexisting tumors or GHD secondary to intracranial lesion. Monitor for malignant transformation of skin lesions. May decrease insulin sensitivity, as well as unmask undiagnosed impaired glucose tolerance and overt diabetes mellitus (DM). New-onset type 2 DM reported; monitor glucose levels. Intracranial HTN with papilledema, visual changes, headache, N/V reported; perform fundoscopic exam before and during therapy and d/c if papilledema occurs. Fluid retention in adults may occur. Monitor other hormonal replacement treatments in patients with hypopituitarism. Undiagnosed/untreated hypothyroidism may prevent optimal response. Hypothyroidism may become evident/worsen in patients with GHD; perform periodic thyroid function tests. Slipped capital femoral epiphysis and progression of scoliosis may occur. Increased risk of ear/hearing and cardiovascular disorders reported in TS patients. Tissue atrophy may occur when administered at the same site over prolonged periods; can be avoided by rotating the inj site. Local/systemic allergic reactions may occur. Serum levels of inorganic phosphorus, alkaline phosphatase, parathyroid hormone, and IGF-I may increase. Pancreatitis rarely reported. Caution in elderly. (5mg/1.5mL cartridge, 5.8mg/vial) Contains benzyl alcohol.

ADVERSE REACTIONS: Elevated HbA1c, eosinophilia, hematoma.

INTERACTIONS: Use with glucocorticoid therapy may attenuate growth-promoting effects in children; carefully adjust glucocorticoid replacement dosing. May inhibit 11β-hydroxysteroid dehydrogenase type 1, resulting in reduced serum cortisol concentrations; may need glucocorticoid replacement/dose adjustments of glucocorticoid therapy (eg, cortisone acetate, prednisone). May increase clearance of antipyrine. May alter clearance of compounds metabolized by CYP450 liver enzymes (eg, corticosteroids, sex steroids, anticonvulsants, cyclosporine); monitor carefully. May require larger dose with oral estrogen replacement. May need to adjust dose of insulin and/or oral hypoglycemic agents in diabetic patients and thyroid hormone replacement therapy in patients with thyroid dysfunction.

PREGNANCY: Category B, caution in nursing.

MECHANISM OF ACTION: Recombinant human GH; binds to dimeric GH receptor in cell membrane of target cells resulting in intracellular signal transduction.

PHARMACOKINETICS: Absorption: C_{max}=72-74mcg/L; T_{max}=4 hrs. **Metabolism:** Liver and kidneys (proteolytic degradation). **Elimination:** $T_{1/2}$=2.5-2.8 hrs.

NURSING CONSIDERATIONS

Assessment: Assess for PWS, preexisting DM or impaired glucose tolerance, diabetic retinopathy, active malignancy, history of scoliosis, hypothyroidism, hypopituitarism, otitis media/other ear disorders in TS, pregnancy/nursing status, possible drug interactions, or any other conditions where treatment is contraindicated or cautioned. Perform funduscopic exam.

Monitoring: Monitor for growth, clinical response, compliance, malignant transformation of skin lesions, fluid retention, allergic reactions, pancreatitis, and slipped capital femoral epiphysis and progression of scoliosis in pediatrics. Perform periodic thyroid function tests, funduscopic exam, and monitoring of glucose levels. In patients with PWS, monitor weight as well as signs of respiratory infections, sleep apnea, and upper airway obstruction. In patients with preexisting tumors or GHD secondary to intracranial lesion, monitor for progression/recurrence of underlying disease process. In patients with TS, monitor for ear/hearing/cardiovascular disorders.

Patient Counseling: Inform about potential benefits and risks of therapy, proper administration, usage and disposal, and caution against any reuse of needles and syringes.

Administration: SQ route. Refer to PI for preparation and administration instructions. **Storage:** 2-8°C (36-46°F). Keep in carton to protect from light. Do not freeze. (Cartridge) After First Use: Keep in pen at 2-8°C (36-46°F) for a max of 28 days. (Vial) Reconstituted: Use within 3 weeks. After First Use: Store in carton at 2-8°C (36-46°F).

ONGLYZA   RX

saxagliptin (Bristol-Myers Squibb/ AstraZeneca)

THERAPEUTIC CLASS: Dipeptidyl peptidase-4 inhibitor

INDICATIONS: Adjunct to diet and exercise to improve glycemic control in adults with type 2 diabetes mellitus (DM).

DOSAGE: *Adults:* 2.5mg or 5mg qd. Moderate or Severe Renal Impairment/Hemodialysis with End-Stage Renal Disease (ESRD) (CrCl ≤50mL/min): 2.5mg qd. Concomitant Strong CYP3A4/5 Inhibitors: 2.5mg qd. Concomitant Insulin Secretagogue (eg, sulfonylurea)/Insulin: May require lower dose of insulin secretagogue or insulin.

HOW SUPPLIED: Tab: 2.5mg, 5mg

WARNINGS/PRECAUTIONS: Do not use in type 1 DM or for treatment of diabetic ketoacidosis. Acute pancreatitis reported; d/c if suspected and initiate appropriate management. Serious hypersensitivity reactions reported; d/c if suspected, assess for other potential causes for the event, and institute alternative treatment for DM. No conclusive evidence of macrovascular risk reduction. Caution with history of angioedema to another dipeptidyl peptidase-4 inhibitor and in elderly.

ADVERSE REACTIONS: Upper respiratory tract infection, urinary tract infection, nasopharyngitis, headache, peripheral edema, hypoglycemia.

INTERACTIONS: Strong CYP3A4/5 inducers and inhibitors may alter pharmacokinetics. May require lower dose of insulin secretagogue (eg, sulfonylurea) or insulin to minimize risk of hypoglycemia. Ketoconazole or other strong CYP3A4/5 inhibitors (eg, atazanavir, clarithromycin, indinavir, itraconazole, nefazodone, nelfinavir, ritonavir, saquinavir, and telithromycin) may increase plasma concentrations.

PREGNANCY: Category B, caution in nursing.

MECHANISM OF ACTION: Dipeptidyl peptidase-4 inhibitor; slows the inactivation of the incretin hormones, thereby increasing their bloodstream concentrations and reducing fasting and postprandial glucose concentrations in a glucose-dependent manner.

PHARMACOKINETICS: Absorption: C_{max}=24ng/mL, 47ng/mL (5-hydroxy saxagliptin); AUC=78ng•hr/mL, 214ng•hr/mL (5-hydroxy saxagliptin); T_{max}=2 hrs, 4 hrs (5-hydroxy saxagliptin). **Metabolism:** CYP3A4/5; 5-hydroxy saxagliptin (active metabolite). **Elimination:** Feces (22%), urine (24% unchanged, 36% 5-hydroxy saxagliptin); $T_{1/2}$=2.5 hrs, 3.1 hrs (5-hydroxy saxagliptin).

NURSING CONSIDERATIONS

Assessment: Assess renal function, for previous hypersensitivity to drug or to another dipeptidyl peptidase-4 inhibitor, history of pancreatitis, type 1 DM, diabetic ketoacidosis, pregnancy/nursing status, and possible drug interactions. Obtain baseline FPG and HbA1c.

Monitoring: Monitor for pancreatitis and hypersensitivity reactions. Monitor FPG, HbA1c, and renal function periodically. Measure lymphocyte count when clinically indicated (eg, settings of unusual or prolonged infection).

Patient Counseling: Inform of potential risks, benefits, and alternative modes of therapy. Advise on the importance of adherence to dietary instructions, regular physical activity, periodic blood glucose monitoring and HbA1c testing, recognition/management of hypoglycemia/hyperglycemia, and assessment of diabetic complications. Instruct to seek medical advice promptly during periods of stress (eg, fever, trauma, infection, surgery) and if unusual symptom develops or existing symptom persists or worsens. Instruct to d/c use and notify physician if signs and symptoms of pancreatitis (eg, persistent severe abdominal pain) or allergic reactions occur. Inform that if a dose was missed, take the next dose as prescribed, unless otherwise instructed by physician; instruct not to take an extra dose the next day.

Administration: Oral route. Do not split or cut tab. Administer following hemodialysis with ESRD requiring hemodialysis. **Storage:** 20-25°C (68-77°F); excursions permitted to 15-30°C (59-86°F).

ONSOLIS
fentanyl (Meda)

CII

> Contains fentanyl with abuse liability similar to other opioid analgesics. Must be used only in opioid-tolerant patients. Contraindicated for use in opioid non-tolerant patients and management of acute or postoperative pain, including headache/migraine, dental pain, or use in the emergency room. Do not convert on a mcg-per-mcg basis to Onsolis from other transmucosal fentanyl products. Life-threatening respiratory depression in opioid non-tolerant patients reported. Do not substitute for any other fentanyl product; may result in fatal overdose. If breakthrough pain is not relieved, patients should wait at least 2 hrs for the next dose. Keep out of reach of children and dispose of unneeded films properly. Concomitant use with CYP3A4 inhibitors may cause fatal respiratory depression. Use only by knowledgeable/skilled Schedule II opioid specialists. Available only through restricted distribution program (FOCUS).

THERAPEUTIC CLASS: Opioid analgesic

INDICATIONS: Management of breakthrough pain in patients with cancer (≥18 yrs) who are already receiving and who are tolerant to opioid therapy for their underlying persistent cancer pain.

DOSAGE: *Adults:* Initial: 200mcg. Titrate: May titrate by using multiples of 200mcg (for doses of 400mcg, 600mcg, or 800mcg) if adequate pain relief is not achieved after initiation. Do not use more than four of 200mcg films simultaneously. If adequate pain relief is not achieved after

800mcg, and patient has tolerated the 800mcg dose, may treat next episode by using one 1200mcg film. Max: 1200mcg. Single doses should only be used once per episode, and should be separated by at least 2 hrs. If adequate pain relief is not achieved within 30 min, use rescue medication ud. Limit to ≤4 doses/day. If >4 breakthrough pain episodes a day, may increase around-the-clock opioid medicine used for persistent cancer pain. Switching From Another Oral Transmucosal Fentanyl: Initial: ≤200mcg. Do not switch on a mcg-per-mcg basis.

HOW SUPPLIED: Film, Buccal: 200mcg, 400mcg, 600mcg, 800mcg, 1200mcg

CONTRAINDICATIONS: Opioid non-tolerant patients and management of acute or postoperative pain including headache/migraine, dental pain, or use in the emergency room.

WARNINGS/PRECAUTIONS: Caution with COPD (chronic obstructive pulmonary disease), pre-existing medical conditions predisposing to hypoventilation, severe renal or hepatic disease and bradyarrhythmias. Extreme caution with evidence of increased intracranial pressure or impaired consciousness; may obscure the clinical course of a patient with head injury. May impair physical/mental abilities. Caution in elderly.

ADVERSE REACTIONS: Respiratory depression, circulatory depression, hypotension, shock, constipation, asthenia, fatigue, anorexia, N/V, constipation, dehydration, dizziness, dyspnea, headache.

INTERACTIONS: See Boxed Warning. Increased depressant effects with other CNS depressants (eg, other opioids, sedatives or hypnotics, general anesthetics, phenothiazines, tranquilizers, sedating antihistamines, skeletal muscle relaxants, alcoholic beverages). CYP3A4 inducers (eg, barbiturates, carbamazepine, efavirenz, glucocorticoids, modafinil, nevirapine, oxcarbazepine, phenobarbital, phenytoin, pioglitazone, rifabutin, rifampin, St. John's wort, or troglitazone) decrease plasma concentration and may reduce efficacy. Avoid use within 14 days of MAOIs. Respiratory depression reported with other drugs that depress respiration.

PREGNANCY: Category C, not for use in nursing.

MECHANISM OF ACTION: Pure opioid agonist; produces analgesia. Precise analgesic action not established; known to be μ-opioid receptor agonist. Specific CNS opioid receptors for endogenous compounds with opioid-like activity are found throughout the brain and spinal cord and are involved in producing analgesic effects.

PHARMACOKINETICS: Absorption: Rapid (buccal mucosa) and prolonged (GI tract). Absolute bioavailability (71%); various doses resulted in different parameters. **Distribution:** V_d=4L/kg; plasma protein binding (80-85%). Crosses the placenta; found in breast milk. **Metabolism:** Liver and intestinal mucosa via CYP3A4; norfentanyl (metabolite). **Elimination:** Urine (<7% unchanged), feces (1% unchanged); $T_{1/2}$=14 hrs.

NURSING CONSIDERATIONS

Assessment: Assess for degree of opioid tolerance, previous opioid dose, level of pain intensity, type of pain, patient's general condition, age and medical status, or any other conditions where treatment is contraindicated or cautioned. Assess for history of hypersensitivity, pregnancy/nursing status, renal/hepatic function, and possible drug interactions.

Monitoring: Monitor for signs/symptoms of respiratory depression, drug abuse, physical dependence, bradycardia, opioid toxicity, hypersensitivity, anaphylaxis, signs of increased drug activity.

Patient Counseling: Notify physician if signs/symptoms of respiratory depression develop. Inform that film contains medicine in an amount that can be fatal in children, in individuals for whom it is not prescribed, and in those who are not opioid tolerant. Safely dispose any unneeded films remaining from a prescription as soon as possible by removing from foil package, and flushing the film down the toilet; do not flush the foil packages or cartons. Notify physician if breakthrough pain is not alleviated or worsens. Avoid using concomitant therapy with other CNS depressants and alcohol. May cause mental/physical impairment and has potential for abuse. Encourage patients to read the Medication Guide. Patients must enroll in FOCUS program by calling 1-877-466-7654 (1-877-4Onsolis) or visit online.

Administration: Oral (buccal) route. May be placed on both sides of the mouth not on top of each other when multiple films are used. Do not cut or tear prior to use. Refer to PI for proper administration. **Storage:** 20-25°C (68-77°F); excursions permitted between 15-30°C (59-86°F) until ready to use. Protect from freezing and moisture. Do not use if the foil package has been opened.

OPANA ER   CII
oxymorphone HCl (Endo)

> (Tab, Extended-Release) Increased risk of misuse, abuse, or diversion. For continuous analgesia only; not intended for PRN use. To be swallowed whole; not to be broken, chewed, dissolved, or crushed. Avoid with alcohol or medications containing alcohol.

OTHER BRAND NAMES: Opana (Endo)

THERAPEUTIC CLASS: Opioid analgesic

INDICATIONS: (Tab) Relief of moderate to severe acute pain. (Tab, ER) Relief of moderate to severe pain in patients requiring continuous, around-the-clock opioid treatment for extended period of time.

DOSAGE: *Adults:* Individualize dose. (Tab) Initial: Opioid-Naive: 10-20mg q4-6h. May start with 5mg (eg, for renal/hepatic impairment, geriatrics) if necessary. Max: 20mg. Conversion from Parenteral Oxymorphone: Give 10x total daily parenteral oxymorphone dose in 4 or 6 equally divided doses (eg, [IV dose x 10] divided by 4 or 6). Conversion from Other Oral Opioids: Give 50% of calculated total daily dose in 4-6 equally divided doses, q4-6h. Maint: Identify source of increased pain and adjust dose. (Tab, ER) Opioid-Naive: Initial: 5mg q12h. Titrate: Increase dose individually at increments of 5-10mg q12h every 3-7 days. Conversion from Opana: Give half of total daily Opana dose as ER, q12h. Conversion from Parenteral Oxymorphone: Give 10x total daily parenteral oxymorphone dose in 2 equally divided doses (eg, [IV dose x 10] divided by 2). Conversion from Other Oral Opioids: Give 50% of calculated total daily dose (refer to PI for conversion ratios) in 2 divided doses, q12h. Gradually adjust initial dose until adequate pain relief and acceptable side effects are achieved. Maint: Titrate if necessary; follow the same method as Initial Therapy. (Tab/Tab, ER) Mild Hepatic/Renal Impairment (CrCl <50mL/min): Start with lowest dose and titrate slowly while carefully monitoring side effects. With CNS Depressants: Start at 1/3 to 1/2 of usual dose. Elderly: Start at lower end of dosing range and slowly titrate to adequate analgesia. Cessation Therapy: Taper gradually. Take on an empty stomach ≥1 hr prior to or 2 hrs after eating.

HOW SUPPLIED: Tab: 5mg, 10mg; Tab, Extended-Release (ER): 5mg, 10mg, 20mg, 30mg, 40mg

CONTRAINDICATIONS: Respiratory depression (Tab: except in monitored settings with resuscitative equipment), acute/severe bronchial asthma or hypercarbia, paralytic ileus, moderate/severe hepatic impairment.

WARNINGS/PRECAUTIONS: Schedule II controlled substance with abuse liability. Respiratory depression may occur; extreme caution in elderly or debilitated patients, with hypoxia, hypercapnia, or decreased respiratory reserve such as asthma, chronic obstructive pulmonary disease (COPD) or cor pulmonale, severe obesity, sleep apnea syndrome, myxedema, kyphoscoliosis, CNS depression, or coma. With head injury, intracranial lesions or a pre-existing increase in intracranial pressure (ICP), possible respiratory depressant effects and potential to elevate CSF pressure may be markedly exaggerated; effects on papillary response and consciousness may obscure neurologic signs of further increases in ICP with head injuries. May cause severe hypotension. Caution with increased ICP, impaired consciousness, circulatory shock, adrenocortical insufficiency (eg, Addison's disease), prostatic hypertrophy or urethral stricture, severe pulmonary impairment, moderate/severe renal dysfunction, mild hepatic impairment and toxic psychosis. May aggravate convulsions with convulsive disorders and may induce/aggravate seizures. May obscure diagnosis or clinical course in patients with acute abdominal conditions. May cause spasm of the sphincter of Oddi; caution with biliary tract disease (including acute pancreatitis). May impair physical/mental abilities. May produce tolerance and dependence. Avoid abrupt d/c; may cause abstinence syndrome in physically dependent patients. (Tab, ER) Not indicated for pre-emptive analgesia (administration pre-operatively for the management of post-operative pain). Only indicated for post-operative use if already receiving drug prior to surgery or if post-operative pain is expected to be moderate or severe and persist for an extended period of time.

ADVERSE REACTIONS: Constipation, N/V, pyrexia, somnolence, headache, dizziness, pruritus, increased sweating, xerostomia, sedation, confusion, anxiety.

INTERACTIONS: See Boxed Warning. Additive CNS depression with other CNS depressants (eg, sedatives, hypnotics, tranquilizers, general anesthetics, phenothiazines, other opioids, alcohol). Caution with MAOIs; avoid within 14 days of MAOIs use. Anticholinergics may increase risk of urinary retention and/or severe constipation, which may lead to paralytic ileus. CNS side effects (eg, confusion, disorientation, respiratory depression, apnea, seizures) reported with cimetidine. Reduced effect and/or precipitate withdrawal symptoms with mixed agonist/antagonist analgesics (eg, pentazocine, nalbuphine, butorphanol, buprenorphine). Severe hypotension with phenothiazines or other agents that compromise vasomotor tone.

PREGNANCY: Category C, caution with nursing.

MECHANISM OF ACTION: Opioid analgesic; pure opioid agonist. Has not been established. Suspected that specific CNS opiate receptors and endogenous compounds with morphine-like activity have been identified throughout the brain and spinal cord and are likely to play a role in the expression and perception of analgesic effects.

PHARMACOKINETICS: Absorption: Absolute bioavailability (10%). Administration of variable doses resulted in different pharmacokinetic parameters. Refer to PI. **Distribution:** Plasma protein binding (10-12%); crosses placenta. **Metabolism:** Liver (reduction or conjugation); oxymorphone-3-glucuronide, 6-OH-oxymorphone (major metabolites). **Elimination:** Urine (<1% unchanged, 33-38% oxymorphone-3-glucuronide, 0.25-0.62% 6-OH-oxymorphone), feces.

NURSING CONSIDERATIONS

Assessment: Assess for patient's prior analgesic treatment, degree of opioid tolerance, type and severity of pain, age, patient's general condition and medical status, history or risk factors for abuse and addiction, respiratory depression, paralytic ileus, acute/severe bronchial asthma or hypercarbia, or any other conditions where treatment is cautioned. Assess for drug hypersensitivity, pregnancy/nursing status, renal/hepatic function, and possible drug interactions.

Monitoring: Monitor for signs/symptoms of respiratory depression, presence of elevated CSF pressure, hypotension, convulsions, spasms of sphincter of Oddi, physical dependence and tolerance, and abuse or misuse of medication. Monitor patients closely to evaluate for adequate analgesia and side effects. Monitor all patients closely when converting to ER tab from methadone to other opioid agonists. Monitor for decreased bowel motility in post-operative patients. Periodically reassess continued need for around-the-clock opioid therapy.

Patient Counseling: Instruct to take as directed. ER tab should be swallowed whole; do not break, chew, dissolve, or crush. Inform that if broken or chewed, contents of tab may release all at once and cause fatal overdose. Instruct to take on empty stomach, ≥1 hr prior to or 2 hrs after eating. Caution in performing hazardous tasks (eg, operating machinery/driving). Avoid alcohol, medications containing alcohol or other CNS depressants. Report episodes of breakthrough pain or adverse events. Contact physician if inadequate pain control and avoid adjusting dose without consulting physician. Inform that drug has potential for abuse and should be protected from theft. Counsel on the importance of safely tapering dose and abrupt d/c if receiving treatment for more than a few days to weeks. Advise of the potential for severe constipation. Advise women regarding effects in pregnancy and nursing. Instruct to keep out of reach of children and dispose any unused tablet by flushing down in the toilet as soon as they are no longer needed.

Administration: Oral route. **Storage:** 25°C (77°F); excursions permitted to 15-30°C (59-86°F). Dispense in tight container with child-resistant closure.

OPTIVAR   RX
azelastine HCl (Meda)

THERAPEUTIC CLASS: H$_1$-antagonist

INDICATIONS: Treatment of itching of the eye associated with allergic conjunctivitis.

DOSAGE: *Adults:* Usual: 1 drop into each affected eye bid.
Pediatrics: ≥3 yrs: Usual: 1 drop into each affected eye bid.

HOW SUPPLIED: Sol: 0.05% [6mL]

WARNINGS/PRECAUTIONS: For ocular use only; not for inj or PO use.

ADVERSE REACTIONS: Eye burning/stinging, headaches, bitter taste, asthma, conjunctivitis, dyspnea, eye pain, fatigue, influenza-like symptoms, pharyngitis, pruritus, rhinitis, temporary blurring.

PREGNANCY: Category C, caution in nursing.

MECHANISM OF ACTION: Selective H$_1$ antagonist; inhibits release of histamine and other mediators from cells (eg, mast cells) involved in the allergic response and decreases chemotaxis and activation of eosinophils.

PHARMACOKINETICS: Absorption: Low. **Distribution:** V$_d$=14.5L/kg (IV/PO); plasma protein binding (88%). **Metabolism:** CYP450; N-desmethylazelastine (principal metabolite). **Elimination:** (PO) Feces (75%, <10% unchanged); T$_{1/2}$= 22 hrs (IV/PO).

NURSING CONSIDERATIONS

Assessment: Assess for drug hypersensitivity and pregnancy/nursing status.

Monitoring: Monitor for adverse events.

Patient Counseling: Advise not to touch dropper tip to any surface to prevent contamination. Instruct to keep bottle tightly closed when not in use. Advise not to wear contact lenses if eye is red. Inform that drug is not used to treat contact lens-related irritation. Instruct patients who wear soft contact lenses and whose eyes are not red to wait at least 10 min after instillation before inserting contact lenses.

Administration: Ocular route. **Storage:** 2-25°C (36-77°F).

ORACEA   RX
doxycycline (Galderma)

THERAPEUTIC CLASS: Tetracycline derivative

INDICATIONS: Treatment of only inflammatory lesions (papules and pustules) of rosacea in adults.

DOSAGE: *Adults:* 40mg qd in am. Take on empty stomach, preferably at least 1 hr prior or 2 hrs after meals.

HOW SUPPLIED: Cap: 40mg

WARNINGS/PRECAUTIONS: May cause fetal harm during pregnancy. Use during tooth development (eg, last half of pregnancy, infancy, ≤8 yrs) may cause permanent tooth discoloration or enamel hypoplasia. Pseudomembranous colitis reported, diarrhea may occur; initiate appropriate treatment. Photosensitivity reported. Autoimmune syndrome reported; monitor LFTs, ANA, CBC. Tissue hyperpigmentation reported. Superinfection reported; caution in patients with history of or predisposition to candidiasis overgrowth. Bacterial resistance may develop; use only as indicated. May increase BUN; caution in patients with renal impairment. Bulging fontanels in infants and pseudotumor cerebri (benign intracranial HTN) in adults reported.

ADVERSE REACTIONS: Nasopharyngitis, sinusitis, diarrhea, HTN.

INTERACTIONS: May require downward adjustment of anticoagulant dosage. May interfere with bactericidal action of penicillin; avoid concurrent use when possible. Concomitant use with methoxyflurane may result in fatal renal toxicity. Bismuth subsalicylate, proton pump inhibitors, antacids containing aluminum, calcium or magnesium and iron-containing preparations may impair absorption. May interfere with the effectiveness of oral contraceptives. Avoid concurrent use with oral retinoids (eg, isotretinoin, acitretin). Barbiturates, carbamazepine, and phenytoin decrease the half-life of doxycycline.

PREGNANCY: Category D, not for use in nursing.

MECHANISM OF ACTION: Tetracycline-derivative antibacterial agent; has not been established.

PHARMACOKINETICS: Absorption: Single dose: C_{max}=510ng/mL; T_{max}=3 hrs; AUC=9227ng•hr/ mL. Steady-state: C_{max}=600ng/mL; T_{max}=2 hrs; AUC=7543ng•hr/mL. **Distribution**: Plasma protein binding (>90%); crosses the placenta, found in breast milk. **Elimination**: Urine (unchanged), feces (unchanged); $T_{1/2}$=21.2 hrs (single dose), 23.2 hrs (steady-state).

NURSING CONSIDERATIONS

Assessment: Assess for pregnancy/nursing status, renal impairment, history of or predisposition to candidiasis overgrowth, and those with gastric insufficiencies (eg, patients with gastrectomy, gastric bypass surgery, or in patients who are achlorhydric), visual disturbances prior to therapy, and possible drug interactions.

Monitoring: Monitor for signs/symptoms of pseudomembranous colitis, infection, autoimmune syndrome, bulging fontanels in infants, and benign intracranial HTN in adults. Routinely monitor for papilledema during therapy. Monitor BUN level, LFTs, ANA, CBC. Monitor for signs/symptoms of azotemia, hyperphosphatemia, and acidosis in patients with renal insufficiencies. Perform periodic monitoring of drug serum levels in patients with renal impairment.

Patient Counseling: Take medication as directed (1 hr before or 2 hrs after meals with fluid); exceeding recommended dosage may increase incidence of side effects including the development of resistant microorganisms. Medication is not for treatment or prevention of infections. Minimize/avoid exposure to natural or artificial sunlight (eg, tanning beds). Wear loose-fitting clothing to protect skin from sun exposure; d/c at first evidence of sunburn. Medication may cause autoimmune disorders; contact physician if arthralgia, fever, rash, or malaise develop. Drug may cause discoloration of skin, scars, teeth, or gums. Inform females drug may render oral contraceptives less effective, and to avoid if pregnant or nursing. Counsel males and females who are attempting to conceive a child not to use. Inform that diarrhea, headache, blurred vision may occur; seek medical help if symptoms develop.

Administration: Oral route. **Storage**: 15-30°C (59-86°F). Dispense in tight, light-resistant containers.

ORAVIG   RX
miconazole (Strativa)

THERAPEUTIC CLASS: Azole antifungal

INDICATIONS: Local treatment of oropharyngeal candidiasis.

DOSAGE: *Adults:* ≥16 yrs: Apply 1 buccal tab to the upper gum region (canine fossa) qd for 14 consecutive days.

HOW SUPPLIED: Tab, Buccal: 50mg

CONTRAINDICATIONS: Hypersensitivity to milk protein concentrate.

WARNINGS/PRECAUTIONS: Allergic reactions, including anapylactic reactions reported; d/c at 1st sign of hypersensitivity. Caution in patients with hepatic impairment.

ADVERSE REACTIONS: Oral pain/discomfort, tongue/mouth ulceration, loss of/altered taste, N/V, diarrhea, headache, gingival pruritus/swelling.

INTERACTIONS: Caution with warfarin; may enhance anticoagulant effects. Closely monitor PT/INR and for evidence of bleeding. May interact with drugs metabolized through CYP2C9 and CYP3A4 (eg, oral hypoglycemics, phenytoin, ergot alkaloids).

PREGNANCY: Category C, caution in nursing.

MECHANISM OF ACTION: Azole antifungal; inhibits 14α-demethylase, inhibiting ergosterol synthesis (an essential part of the fungal cell membrane) and affects the synthesis of triglycerides and fatty acids and inhibits oxidative/peroxidative enzymes.

PHARMACOKINETICS: Absorption: C_{max}=15.1mcg/mL; T_{max}=7 hrs; AUC=55.23mcg•hr/mL. **Metabolism:** Hepatic (major), no active metabolites. **Elimination:** $T_{1/2}$=24 hrs, urine (<1%, unchanged).

NURSING CONSIDERATIONS

Assessment: Assess for possible drug interactions, pregnancy/nursing status, hypersensitivity to milk protein concentrate, hepatic impairment.

Monitoring: Closely monitor PT/INR and evidence of bleeding with concomitant anticoagulants. Monitor for hypersensitivity reactions, signs and symptoms of hepatic impairment, and other adverse events.

Patient Counseling: Apply buccal tab in the morning, after brushing teeth and with dry hands. Place rounded side of tab against the upper gum just above the incisor tooth and hold in place for 30 sec to ensure adhesion. Subsequent applications should be made to alternate sides of mouth. Allow tab to dissolve slowly; food/drink can be taken; avoid chewing gum and situations that could interfere with the sticking of the tab (eg, touching tab, hitting tab when brushing teeth, rinsing mouth too vigorously, wearing upper denture). If tab does not adhere or falls off within 1st 6 hrs, inform that the same tab should be repositioned immediately. If tab still does not adhere, apply a new tab. If swallowed within 1st 6 hrs, drink a glass of water and apply a new tab only once. If tab falls off or is swallowed after in place for 6 hrs or more, do not apply a new tab until the next scheduled dose. Do not crush, chew, or swallow. Report adverse events to physician.

Administration: Buccal route. **Storage:** 20-25°C (68-77°F); excursions between 15-30°C permitted at room temperature. Protect from moisture.

ORENCIA   RX
abatacept (Bristol-Myers Squibb)

THERAPEUTIC CLASS: Selective costimulation modulator

INDICATIONS: To reduce signs and symptoms, induce major clinical response, inhibit progression of structural damage, and improve physical function in adults with moderate to severe active rheumatoid arthritis (RA). May be used as monotherapy or concomitantly with disease-modifying antirheumatic drugs other than TNF-antagonists. To reduce signs and symptoms in pediatric patients ≥6 yrs with moderate to severe active polyarticular juvenile idiopathic arthritis (JIA). May be used alone or in combination with methotrexate.

DOSAGE: *Adults:* RA: IV Regimen: Give as an IV infusion over 30 min. Initial: >100kg: 1000mg. 60-100kg: 750mg. <60kg: 500mg. Maint: Give at 2 and 4 weeks after the 1st infusion and q4 weeks thereafter. SQ Regimen: Following a single IV LD, give the 1st 125mg inj within a day, followed by 125mg inj once weekly. Patients Unable to Receive IV Infusion: Initiate weekly SQ inj without an IV LD. Switching from IV to SQ: Give the 1st 125mg SQ dose instead of the next scheduled IV dose.
Pediatrics: 6-17 yrs: JIA: Give as an IV infusion over 30 min. ≥75kg: Follow adult IV dosing regimen. Max: 1000mg. <75kg: Initial: 10mg/kg IV. Maint: Give at 2 and 4 weeks after the 1st infusion and q4 weeks thereafter.

HOW SUPPLIED: Inj: 125mg/1mL [prefilled syringe], 250mg

WARNINGS/PRECAUTIONS: Anaphylaxis or anaphylactoid reactions reported. Serious infections including sepsis and pneumonia reported. Caution with a history of recurrent infections, underlying conditions that may predispose to infections, or chronic, latent, or localized infections; monitor new infection and d/c if serious infections develop. Screen for latent tuberculosis (TB) infection and viral hepatitis prior to initiation of therapy. Hepatitis B reactivation may occur with antirheumatic therapies. JIA patients should be up to date with all immunizations prior to initiation of therapy. Caution with chronic obstructive pulmonary disease (COPD); monitor for worsening of respiratory status. May affect host defenses against infections and malignancies. Caution in elderly. (IV) Contains maltose that may react with glucose dehydrogenase pyrroloquinolinequinone (GDH-PQQ) based glucose monitoring and may result in falsely elevated blood glucose readings on the day of infusion.

ADVERSE REACTIONS: Headache, nasopharyngitis, dizziness, cough, back pain, HTN, dyspepsia, urinary tract infection, rash, pain in extremities, upper respiratory tract infection, nausea, sinusitis, influenza, bronchitis.

INTERACTIONS: Concomitant use with TNF-antagonist may increase risk of serious infections, and is not recommended. Concomitant use with other biologic RA therapy, such as anakinra, is not recommended. Do not use live vaccines concurrently or within 3 months of d/c. Serious infections reported with concomitant immunosuppressive therapy.

PREGNANCY: Category C, not for use in nursing.

MECHANISM OF ACTION: Selective costimulation modulator; inhibits T cell activation by binding to CD80 and CD86, thereby blocking interaction with CD28.

PHARMACOKINETICS: Absorption: C_{max}=295mcg/mL (RA patients, IV), 48.1mcg/mL (RA patients, SQ), 217mcg/mL (JIA patients). **Distribution:** V_d=0.07L/kg (RA patients, IV), 0.11L/kg (RA patients, SQ). **Elimination:** $T_{1/2}$=13.1 days (RA patients, IV), 14.3 days (RA patients, SQ).

NURSING CONSIDERATIONS

Assessment: Assess for immunization history in pediatrics, history of recurrent infections, chronic/latent/localized infections, underlying conditions that may predispose to infection, COPD, pregnancy/nursing status, and possible drug interactions. Screen for latent TB infection and viral hepatitis.

Monitoring: Monitor for signs/symptoms of hypersensitivity, infection, immunosuppression, malignancies, hepatitis B reactivation, exacerbation of COPD, cough, rhonchi, dyspnea, and worsening of respiratory status. Monitor blood glucose in diabetic patients using methods not based on GDH-PQQ.

Patient Counseling: Instruct to immediately contact physician if allergic reaction or infection occurs. Ask about history of recurrent infection, chronic/latent/localized infections, conditions which may predispose to infection, positive skin test to TB infection. Inform that patient may be tested for TB prior to therapy. Instruct not to receive live vaccines during therapy or within 3 months following d/c. Instruct to inform doctor if pregnant/nursing or plan to become pregnant. Inform diabetic patients that the infusion contains maltose, which can give falsely elevated blood glucose readings on the day of administration; advise to consider alternative monitoring methods that do not react with maltose.

Administration: IV/SQ routes. Refer to PI for complete preparation and administration instructions. Diluted sol must be fully infused within 24 hrs of reconstitution. **Storage:** 2-8°C (36-46°F). Protect from light; store in original package until time of use. Do not allow prefilled syringe to freeze. Diluted Sol: Room temperature or 2-8°C (36-46°F); discard after 24 hrs.

ORTHO EVRA   RX
ethinyl estradiol - norelgestromin (Janssen)

Cigarette smoking increases the risk of serious cardiovascular (CV) events. Risk increases with age (>35 yrs) and with the number of cigarettes smoked. Should not be used by women who are >35 yrs of age and smoke. Has higher steady state concentrations and lower peak concentrations than oral contraceptives. May increase risk of venous thromboembolism for current users of Ortho Evra.

THERAPEUTIC CLASS: Estrogen/progestogen combination

INDICATIONS: Prevention of pregnancy.

DOSAGE: *Adults:* Start 1st Sunday after menses begins or 1st day of menses. Apply patch every week on same day for 3 weeks. Week 4 is patch-free. There should not be more than a 7-day patch-free interval between cycles. Apply to clean, dry, intact skin on upper outer arm, abdomen, buttock, or back in a place where it won't be rubbed by tight clothing. Only 1 patch should be worn at a time. Refer to PI for further dosing guidelines.
Pediatrics: Postpubertal: Start 1st Sunday after menses begins or 1st day of menses. Apply patch every week on same day for 3 weeks. Week 4 is patch-free. There should not be more than a 7-day patch-free interval between cycles. Apply to clean, dry, intact skin on upper outer arm, abdomen, buttock or back in a place where it won't be rubbed by tight clothing. Only 1 patch should be worn at a time. Refer to PI for further dosing guidelines.

HOW SUPPLIED: Patch: (Ethinyl Estradiol-Norelgestromin): 0.75mg-6mg [1ˢ, 3ˢ]

CONTRAINDICATIONS: Thrombophlebitis or past history of deep vein thrombophlebitis, thromboembolic disorders (current or past history), known thrombophilic conditions, cerebrovascular or coronary artery disease (current or history), valvular heart disease with complications, persistent BP ≥160mmHg systolic or ≥100mmHg diastolic, diabetes with vascular involvement, headaches with focal neurological symptoms, major surgery with prolonged immobilization, known or suspected carcinoma of the breast or personal history of breast cancer, carcinoma of the endometrium or other known or suspected estrogen-dependent neoplasia, undiagnosed abnormal genital bleeding, cholestatic jaundice of pregnancy or jaundice with prior hormonal contraceptive use, acute/chronic hepatocellular disease with abnormal liver function, hepatic adenomas or carcinomas, known or suspected pregnancy.

WARNINGS/PRECAUTIONS: Increased risk of myocardial infarction (MI), vascular disease, thromboembolism, thrombotic disease, stroke, hepatic neoplasia/adenoma, and gallbladder disease. May increase risk of breast cancer and cancer of the reproductive organs. Increased risk of morbidity and mortality with HTN, hyperlipidemia, obesity, and diabetes. D/C at least 4 wks prior to and 2 wks post-elective surgery with increased risk of thromboembolism and during and following prolonged immobilization. Caution in women with CV disease risk factors. May develop visual changes with contact lens. Retinal thrombosis reported; d/c if unexplained partial or complete loss of vision or other ophthalmic irregularities occur. May cause glucose intolerance, hypertriglyceridemia, elevated LDL, and other lipid abnormalities. May cause fluid retention and increase BP; d/c if persistent elevation of BP occurs (≥160mmHg systolic or ≥100mmHg diastolic). D/C with onset or exacerbation of migraine headache or headache with a new pattern that is recurrent, persistent, or severe. Breakthrough bleeding and spotting reported; rule out malignancies or pregnancy. Ectopic and intrauterine pregnancies may occur with contraceptive failures. May be less effective in women ≥198 lbs. D/C if jaundice develops. Caution in patients with history of depression; d/c if significant depression develops. May affect certain endocrine tests and LFTs and blood components. Perform annual history/physical exam; monitor women with family history of breast cancer.

ADVERSE REACTIONS: Breast symptoms (eg, breast discomfort, engorgement, pain), irregular uterine bleeding, dysmenorrhea, emotional lability, diarrhea, headache, application-site disorder, N/V, abdominal pain, dizziness.

INTERACTIONS: Reduce effects or increase incidence of breakthrough bleeding with drugs that induce enzymes (eg, CYP3A4) that metabolize contraceptive hormones (eg, barbiturates, bosentan, carbamazepine, felbamate, griseofulvin, oxcarbazepine, phenytoin, rifampin, St. John's wort, topiramate); additional or a different method of contraception is needed. Protease inhibitors and non-nucleoside reverse transcriptase inhibitors may increase or decrease levels. Pregnancy reported with antibiotics. HMG-CoA reductase inhibitors (eg, atorvastatin, rosuvastatin), ascorbic acid, acetaminophen (APAP), and CYP3A4 inhibitors (eg, itraconazole, ketoconazole, voriconazole, fluconazole, grapefruit juice) may increase ethinyl estradiol levels. May increase levels of cyclosporine, prednisolone, and theophylline. May decrease levels of APAP, clofibric acid, morphine, salicylic acid, and temazepam. May decrease lamotrigine levels; dosage adjustment of lamotrigine may be necessary.

PREGNANCY: Category X, not for use in nursing.

MECHANISM OF ACTION: Estrogen/progestogen contraceptive; acts by suppressing gonadotropins. Primarily inhibits ovulation. Also produces other alterations including changes in the cervical mucus (increases difficulty of sperm entry into uterus) and endometrium (reduces likelihood of implantation).

PHARMACOKINETICS: Absorption: Ethinyl estradiol: AUC_{0-168}=12971pg•h/mL; C_{max}=97.4pg/mL. Norelgestromin: AUC_{0-168}=145ng•h/mL; C_{max}=1.12ng/mL. Refer to PI for additional parameters. **Distribution:** Found in breast milk. Ethinyl estradiol: Serum albumin binding (extensive). Norelgestromin: Serum protein binding (>97%). **Metabolism:** Ethinyl estradiol: Hydroxylated, glucuronide, and sulfate conjugates (metabolites). Norelgestromin: Hepatic; hydroxylated and conjugated metabolites, norgestrel (metabolites). **Elimination:** Urine, feces; $T_{1/2}$=17 hrs (ethinyl estradiol), 28 hrs (norelgestromin).

NURSING CONSIDERATIONS

Assessment: Assess for current or history of thrombophlebitis or thromboembolic disorders, thrombophilic conditions, or any other conditions where treatment is contraindicated or cautioned. Assess for pregnancy/nursing status and possible drug interactions. Assess use in patients with HTN, hyperlipidemias, obesity, diabetes, and in patients >35 yrs who smoke.

Monitoring: Monitor for signs/symptoms of thromboembolism, MI, stroke, and other adverse effects. Monitor for signs of HTN; perform regular monitoring of BP throughout duration of therapy. Monitor for changes in lipid levels; measure lipid levels periodically. Monitor serum glucose levels in prediabetic and diabetic patients. Refer patients with contact lenses to an ophthalmologist if visual changes or changes in lens tolerance develop. Perform annual physical exam.

Patient Counseling: Inform that drug does not protect against HIV (AIDS) and other sexually transmitted diseases. Advise to avoid smoking and inform about possible adverse effects. Instruct to have annual physical exam and medical evaluation while on therapy. Instruct to apply patch to clean, dry, intact healthy skin (on upper outer arm, abdomen, buttock, or back) where it will not be rubbed by tight clothing. Inform not to place patch on red, irritated, or cut skin, or on the breasts. Advise that there may be spotting, light bleeding, breast tenderness, or nausea during use; instruct that if symptoms persist, notify physician. Counsel to wear only one patch at a time. Advise not to skip patches and to never have the patch off for >7 days in a row. Instruct to use nonhormonal back up method when started using on the 1st Sunday after menses begin for the first 7 days of the first cycle only.

Administration: Transdermal route. Apply immediately upon removal from protective pouch. Apply each new patch to a new spot. Refer to PI for further administration instruction. **Storage:** 25°C (77°F); excursions permitted to 15-30°C (59-86°F). Store patches in their protective pouches. Do not store in refrigerator or freezer.

ORTHO TRI-CYCLEN
ethinyl estradiol - norgestimate (Ortho-McNeil)

RX

Cigarette smoking increases risk of serious cardiovascular (CV) side effects. Risk increases with age (>35 yrs) and heavy smoking (≥15 cigarettes/day). Women who use oral contraceptives should be strongly advised not to smoke.

OTHER BRAND NAMES: Tri-Sprintec (Barr) - Trinessa (Watson) - Tri-Previfem (Qualitest)

THERAPEUTIC CLASS: Estrogen/progestogen combination

INDICATIONS: Prevention of pregnancy. Treatment of moderate acne vulgaris in females ≥15 yrs who have no known contraindication to oral contraceptive therapy, desires oral contraception, and have achieved menarche.

DOSAGE: *Adults:* Contraception/Acne: 1 tab qd for 28 days, then repeat. Start 1st Sunday after menses begin or 1st day of menses.
Pediatrics: Postpubertal: Contraception/Acne (≥15 yrs): 1 tab qd for 28 days, then repeat. Start 1st Sunday after menses begin or 1st day of menses.

HOW SUPPLIED: Tab: (Ethinyl Estradiol-Norgestimate) 0.035mg-0.18mg, 0.035mg-0.215mg, 0.035mg-0.25mg

CONTRAINDICATIONS: Thrombophlebitis or thromboembolic disorders, past history of deep vein thrombophlebitis or thromboembolic disorders, cerebral vascular or coronary artery disease (CAD) (current), known or suspected carcinoma of the breast, carcinoma of the endometrium or other known or suspected estrogen-dependent neoplasia, undiagnosed abnormal genital bleeding, cholestatic jaundice of pregnancy or jaundice with prior pill use, hepatic adenomas or carcinomas, known or suspected pregnancy. (Ortho Tri-Cyclen, TriNessa, Tri-Previfem) History of cerebral vascular/CAD or breast cancer, valvular heart disease with complications, severe HTN, diabetes with vascular involvement, headaches with focal neurological symptoms, major surgery with prolonged immobilization, acute or chronic hepatocellular disease with abnormal liver function.

WARNINGS/PRECAUTIONS: Increased risk of myocardial infarction (MI), vascular disease, thromboembolism, stroke, hepatic neoplasia, and gallbladder disease. May increase risk of breast cancer and cancer of the reproductive organs. Increased risk of morbidity and mortality with HTN, hyperlipidemia, obesity, and diabetes mellitus (DM). D/C at least 4 wks prior to and 2 wks post-elective surgery with increased risk of thromboembolism and during or following prolonged immobilization. Caution in women with CV disease risk factors. May develop visual changes with contact lens. Retinal thrombosis reported; d/c if unexplained partial or complete loss of vision or other ophthalmic irregularities. May cause glucose intolerance, elevated LDL, other lipid abnormalities, or exacerbate migraine headaches. May cause increased BP and fluid retention; d/c if significant BP elevations occur. Breakthrough bleeding and spotting reported; rule out malignancies or pregnancy. Not indicated for use before menarche. May affect certain endocrine, LFTs, and blood components in laboratory tests. Perform annual history/physical exam; monitor women with history of breast cancer.

ADVERSE REACTIONS: N/V, breakthrough bleeding, GI symptoms (eg, abdominal cramps, bloating), spotting, menstrual flow changes, amenorrhea, migraine, depression, vaginal candidiasis, edema, weight changes, cervical erosion, and secretion.

INTERACTIONS: Reduced effects resulting in breakthrough bleeding or unintended pregnancy may occur when coadministered with antibiotics, anticonvulsants, and other drugs that increase metabolism (eg, rifampin, barbiturates, phenylbutazone, phenytoin, carbamazepine, griseofulvin, and (Tri-Sprintec) possibly with ampicillin and tetracyclines. (TriNessa, Ortho-Tri Cyclen, Tri-Previfem) Reduced effects resulting in breakthrough bleeding with felbamate, oxcarbazepine, topiramate, and St. John's wort. Atorvastatin, ascorbic acid, acetaminophen (APAP), CYP3A4 inhibitors (eg, itraconazole, ketoconazole) may increase hormone levels. Increase levels of cyclosporine, prednisolone, and theophylline. Decrease levels of APAP. Increases clearance of temazepam, salicylic acid, morphine, and clofibric acid. Anti-HIV protease inhibitors may significantly change (increase/decrease) hormone levels. (Ortho Tri Cylcen, TriNessa) May significantly decrease plasma levels of lamotrigine; dosage adjustment of lamotrigine may be necessary. Decreased concentrations of contraceptive hormones with bosentan; risk of unintended pregnancy and unscheduled bleeding.

PREGNANCY: Category X, not for use in nursing.

MECHANISM OF ACTION: Estrogen/progestogen oral contraceptive; acts by suppressing gonadotropins and inhibits ovulation. Also produces other alterations including changes in the cervical mucus (increases difficulty of sperm entry into uterus) and endometrium (reduces likelihood of implantation).

PHARMACOKINETICS: Absorption: Rapidly absorbed. Oral administration on various days during dosing led to altered parameters; refer to PI. **Distribution:** Found in breast milk. Norgestimate: Serum protein binding (>97%). Ethinyl estradiol: Serum albumin binding (>97%). **Metabolism:** Norgestimate: GI tract and/or liver (1st pass mechanism). Norelgestromin (primary active metabolite): Hepatic, norgestrel (active metabolite). Ethinyl estradiol: Hydroxylated, glucuronide, and sulfate conjugates. **Elimination:** Norgestimate: Urine (47%), feces (37%).

NURSING CONSIDERATIONS

Assessment: Assess for current or history of thrombophlebitis, thromboembolic disorders, breast cancer, HTN, hyperlipidemias, DM, obesity, or any other conditions where treatment is contraindicated or cautioned. Assess use in patients >35 who smoke ≥15 cigarettes/day. Assess pregnancy/nursing status and for possible drug interactions.

Monitoring: Monitor for signs/symptoms of MI, thromboembolism/thrombotic disease, stroke, and other adverse effects. Monitor BP with history of HTN, serum glucose levels in DM or predia-betic patients, lipid levels with history of hyperlipidemia, and for signs of worsening depression with previous history. Monitor liver function and for signs of liver toxicity (eg, jaundice). Refer to an ophthalmologist if ocular changes develop. Monitor serum folate levels in patient who becomes pregnant shortly after d/c. Perform annual physical exam.

Patient Counseling: Inform that drug does not protect against HIV infection (AIDS) and other sexually transmitted diseases. Advise to avoid smoking while on medication. Counsel about potential adverse effects. Instruct to take exactly as directed at intervals not exceeding 24 hrs. Advise about risk of pregnancy if dose is missed. D/C if pregnancy confirmed/suspected. Instruct that if one dose missed, take as soon as possible; take next pill at regularly scheduled time. May experiece spotting, light bleeding, or stomach sickness during first 1-3 packs of pills; advise not to d/c medication and if symptoms persist, notify physician.

Administration: Oral route. **Storage:** (Ortho Tri-Cyclen, TriNessa) 25°C (77°F), excursions per-mitted to 15-30°C (59-86°F); (Tri-Previfem) 20-25°C (68-77°F). Protect from light. (Tri-Sprintec) 20-25°C (68-77°).

ORTHO TRI-CYCLEN LO   RX
ethinyl estradiol - norgestimate (Ortho-McNeil)

> Cigarette smoking increases risk of serious cardiovascular (CV) side effects. Risk increases with age (>35 yrs) and with heavy smoking (≥15 cigarettes/day). Women who use oral contraceptives are strongly advised not to smoke.

THERAPEUTIC CLASS: Estrogen/progestogen combination

INDICATIONS: Prevention of pregnancy.

DOSAGE: *Adults:* 1 tab qd for 28 days, then repeat. Start 1st Sunday after menses begins or 1st day of menses.
Pediatrics: Postpubertal: 1 tab qd for 28 days, then repeat. Start 1st Sunday after menses begins or 1st day of menses.

HOW SUPPLIED: Tab: (Ethinyl Estradiol-Norgestimate) 0.025mg-0.18mg, 0.025mg-0.215mg, 0.025mg-0.25mg

CONTRAINDICATIONS: Thrombophlebitis or past history of deep vein thrombophlebitis, thromboembolic disorders (current or past history), cerebral vascular or coronary artery disease (current or past history), valvular heart disease with complications, severe HTN, diabetes mellitus (DM) with vascular involvement, headaches with focal neurological symptoms, major surgery with prolonged immobilization, breast cancer (current or past history), endometrial cancer, other known or suspected estrogen dependent neoplasia, undiagnosed abnormal genital bleeding, cholestatic jaundice of pregnancy or jaundice with prior pill use, hepatic adenomas or carcino-mas, known or suspected pregnancy.

WARNINGS/PRECAUTIONS: Increased risk of myocardial infarction (MI), vascular disease, thromboembolism, stroke, hepatic neoplasia, and gallbladder disease. May increase risk of breast cancer and cancer of the reproductive organs. Increased risk of morbidity and mortality with HTN, hyperlipidemia, obesity, and DM. D/C at least 4 wks prior to and 2 wks post-elective surgery with increased risk of thromboembolism and during or following prolonged immobiliza-tion. Caution in women with CV disease risk factors. May develop visual changes with contact lens. Retinal thrombosis reported; d/c if unexplained partial or complete loss of vision or other ophthalmic irregularities. May cause glucose intolerance, elevated LDL, other lipid abnormalities, or exacerbate migraine headaches. May cause increased BP and fluid retention; d/c if signifi-cant BP elevations occur. Breakthrough bleeding and spotting reported; rule out malignancies or pregnancy. Not indicated for use before menarche. May affect certain endocrine, LFTs, and blood components in laboratory tests. Perform annual history/physical exam; monitor women with history of breast cancer.

ADVERSE REACTIONS: N/V, breakthrough bleeding, spotting, amenorrhea, migraine, depression, vaginal candidiasis, edema, weight changes, melasma, breast changes, changes in cervical erosion and secretion, allergic rash.

INTERACTIONS: Reduced effects result in pregnancy or breakthrough bleeding with antibiotics, anticonvulsants, and other drugs that increase the metabolism of contraceptive steroids (eg, rifampin, barbiturates, phenylbutazone, phenytoin, carbamazepine, felbamate, oxcarbazepine, griseofulvin, topiramate, ampicillin, tetracyclines, St. John's wort). Anti-HIV protease inhibitors may increase or decrease plasma levels. Atorvastatin, ascorbic acid, acetaminophen (APAP), CYP3A4 inhibitors (eg, itraconazole, ketoconazole) may increase plasma ethinyl estradiol levels. Increased plasma levels of cyclosporine, prednisolone, and theophylline have been reported. Decreased plasma concentration in APAP and increased the clearance of temazepam, salicylic acid, morphine, and clofibric acid. May significantly decrease plasma levels of lamotrigine; dosage adjustment of lamotrigine may be necessary.

PREGNANCY: Category X, not for use in nursing.

MECHANISM OF ACTION: Estrogen/progestogen oral contraceptive; acts by suppression of gonadotropins and inhibits ovulation. Also produces alterations/changes in the cervical mucus (increases difficulty of sperm entry into uterus) and the endometrium (reduces likelihood of implantation).

PHARMACOKINETICS: Absorption: Rapid. **Distribution:** Found in breast milk. Norgestimate/Ethinyl estradiol: Serum protein binding (>97%). **Metabolism:** Norgestimate: GI tract and/or liver, 1st pass mechanism. Norelgestromin (active major metabolite): Hepatic, norgestrel (active metabolite). Ethinyl estradiol: Hydroxylated, glucuronide, and sulfate conjugates. **Elimination:** Urine, feces; $T_{1/2}$=28.1 hrs (norelgestromin), 36.4 hrs (norgestrel), 17.7 hrs (ethinyl estradiol).

NURSING CONSIDERATIONS

Assessment: Assess for current or history of thrombophlebitis or thromboembolic disorders, history of HTN, hyperlipidemia, DM, obesity, breast cancer, and any other conditions where treatment is contraindicated or cautioned. Assess use in women >35 yrs, smokers (≥15 cigarettes/day). Assess pregnancy/nursing status and for possible drug interactions.

Monitoring: Monitor for signs/symptoms of MI, thromboembolism, stroke, hepatic neoplasia, and other adverse effects. Monitor BP with history of HTN, serum glucose levels in DM or prediabetic patients, lipid levels with history of hyperlipidemia, and for signs of worsening depression with previous history. Monitor liver function and for signs of liver toxicity (eg, jaundice). Refer to an ophthalmologist if ocular changes develop.

Patient Counseling: Inform that the drug does not protect against HIV infection (AIDS) and other sexually transmitted diseases. Counsel about potential adverse effects. Advise to avoid smoking. Instruct to take exactly as directed at intervals not exceeding 24 hrs. Advise about risks of pregnancy if dose is missed. If one dose is missed, take as soon as possible and take next pill at regular scheduled time. May experience spotting, light bleeding, or nausea during the first 1-3 packs of pills; advise not to d/c medication and if symptoms persist, notify physician. D/C if pregnancy is confirmed/suspected.

Administration: Oral route. **Storage:** 25°C (77°F); excursions permitted to 15-30°C (59-86°F). Protect from light.

ORTHO-CYCLEN   RX
ethinyl estradiol - norgestimate (Ortho-McNeil)

Cigarette smoking increases risk of serious cardiovascular (CV) side effects. Risk increases with age (>35 yrs) and heavy smoking (≥15 cigarettes/day). Women who use oral contraceptives should be strongly advised not to smoke.

OTHER BRAND NAMES: Sprintec (Barr) - MonoNessa (Watson)

THERAPEUTIC CLASS: Estrogen/progestogen combination

INDICATIONS: Prevention of pregnancy.

DOSAGE: *Adults:* 1 tab qd for 28 days, then repeat. Start 1st Sunday after menses begin or 1st day of menses.
Pediatrics: Postpubertal Adolescents: 1 tab qd for 28 days, then repeat. Start 1st Sunday after menses begin or 1st day of menses.

HOW SUPPLIED: Tab: (Ethinyl Estradiol-Norgestimate) 0.035mg-0.25mg

CONTRAINDICATIONS: Thrombophlebitis or past history of deep vein thrombophlebitis, thromboembolic disorders (current or past history of), cerebral vascular or coronary artery disease (current or past history of), carcinoma of the breast (current or past history of), carcinoma of the endometrium or other known or suspected estrogen dependent neoplasia, undiagnosed abnormal genital bleeding, cholestatic jaundice of pregnancy or jaundice with prior pill use, hepatic adenomas or carcinomas, known or suspected pregnancy. (Mononessa, Ortho-Cyclen) Valvular heart disease with complications, severe HTN, diabetes with vascular involvement, headaches with focal neurological symptoms, major surgery with prolonged immobilization, acute or chronic hepatocellular disease with abnormal liver function.

WARNINGS/PRECAUTIONS: Increased risk of myocardial infarction (MI), vascular disease, thromboembolism, stroke, gallbladder disease, and hepatic neoplasia. May increase risk of breast cancer and cancer of the reproductive organs. Retinal thrombosis reported; d/c if unexplained partial or complete loss of vision, onset of proptosis or diplopia, papilledema, or retinal vascular lesions develop. May cause glucose intolerance, fluid retention, breakthrough bleeding, and spotting. May increase BP; d/c if significant elevations in BP occur. May elevate LDL levels or cause other lipid changes. May cause or exacerbate migraine headaches. May develop visual changes with contact lens. Increased risk of morbidity and mortality with HTN, hyperlipidemia, obesity, and diabetes mellitus (DM). D/C if jaundice or if significant depression develops. Not indicated for use before menarche. Does not protect against HIV infection (AIDS) or other sexually transmitted diseases (STDs). May affect certain endocrine, LFTs, and blood components in laboratory tests.

ADVERSE REACTIONS: N/V, breakthrough bleeding, GI symptoms (such as abdominal cramps, bloating), spotting, menstrual flow changes, amenorrhea, migraine, depression, vaginal candidiasis, edema, weight changes, cervical erosion and secretion.

INTERACTIONS: Reduced effects resulting in breakthrough bleeding or unintended pregnancy may occur when coadministered with antibiotics, anticonvulsants, and other drugs that increase metabolism (eg, rifampin, barbiturates, phenylbutazone, phenytoin, carbamazepine, felbamate, oxcarbazepine, griseofulvin, ampicillin, tetracyclines, topiramate, bosentan, St. John's wort). (Mononessa, Ortho-Cyclen) Atorvastatin, ascorbic acid, acetaminophen, CYP3A4 inhibitors (eg, itraconazole, ketoconazole) may increase hormone levels. Increases levels of cyclosporine, prednisolone, and theophylline. Decreases levels of acetaminophen. Increases clearance of temazepam, salicylic acid, morphine, and clofibric acid. May significantly decrease plasma levels of lamotrigine; dosage adjustment of lamotrigine may be necessary. Anti-HIV protease inhibitors may significantly change (increase and decrease) hormone levels.

PREGNANCY: Category X, not for use in nursing.

MECHANISM OF ACTION: Estrogen/progestogen combination oral contraceptive; acts by suppression of gonadotropins. Inhibits ovulation and produces changes in cervical mucus (increases difficulty of sperm entry into uterus) and the endometrium (reduces likelihood of implantation).

PHARMACOKINETICS: Absorption: Rapid. Oral administration of various doses led to altered parameters. Refer to PI for specific parameters for norelgestromin, norgestrel, and ethinyl estradiol. **Distribution:** Found in breast milk. Norelgestromin and norgestrel: Albumin binding (>97%). Ethinyl estradiol: Albumin binding (>97%). **Metabolism:** Norgestimate: GI tract and/or liver (1st pass mechanism); norelgestromin (primary active metabolite), norgestrel (active metabolite). Ethinyl estradiol: Hydroxylated, glucuronide, sulfate conjugates. **Elimination:** Norgestimate: Urine (47%), feces (37%).

NURSING CONSIDERATIONS

Assessment: Assess for thrombophlebitis or past history of deep vein thrombophlebitis, current or history of thromboembolic disorders, or any other conditions where treatment is contraindicated or cautioned. Assess use in patients >35 yrs old who smoke ≥15 cigarettes/day. Assess use with history of HTN, hyperlipidemia, obesity, or DM. Assess pregnancy/nursing status and for possible drug interactions.

Monitoring: Monitor for signs/symptoms of MI, thromboembolism, stroke, hepatic neoplasia, and other adverse effects. Monitor serum glucose levels in DM and prediabetic patients. Monitor BP with history of HTN, lipid levels with history of hyperlipidemia, and for signs of worsening depression with previous history. Refer patients to an ophthalmologist if ocular changes develop. Perform annual physical exam while on therapy. Monitor liver function and for signs of liver toxicity (eg, jaundice).

Patient Counseling: Inform that drug does not protect against HIV infection (AIDS) and other STDs. Advise to avoid smoking while on medication. Counsel about potential adverse effects. Instruct to take exactly as directed at intervals not exceeding 24 hrs. Advise about risk of pregnancy if dose is missed. Instruct that if one dose missed, take as soon as possible; take next pill at regularly scheduled time; this means you may take 2 pills in 1 day. May experience spotting, light bleeding, or stomach sickness during first 1-3 packs of pills; advise not to d/c medication and if symptoms persist, notify physician.

Administration: Oral route. **Storage:** (Mononessa, Ortho-Cyclen) 25°C (77°F); excursions permitted to 15-30°C (59-86°F). Protect from light. (Sprintec) 20-25°C (68-77°F).

ORTHO-NOVUM 1/35 RX

ethinyl estradiol - norethindrone (Ortho-McNeil)

Cigarette smoking increases risk of serious cardiovascular (CV) side effects. Risk increases with age (>35 yrs) and with heavy smoking (≥15 cigarettes/day). Women who use oral contraceptives are strongly advised not to smoke.

OTHER BRAND NAMES: Nortrel 1/35 (Barr) - Norinyl 1/35 (Watson) - Necon 1/35 (Watson)

THERAPEUTIC CLASS: Estrogen/progestogen combination

INDICATIONS: Prevention of pregnancy.

DOSAGE: *Adults:* 28 day regimen: 1 tab qd for 28 days, then repeat. Start 1st Sunday after menses begins or 1st day of menses. (Nortrel) 21 day regimen: 1 tab qd for 21 days, then stop for 7 days, then repeat. Start 1st Sunday after menses begins or 1st day of menses.
Pediatrics: Postpubertal: 28 day regimen: 1 tab qd for 28 days, then repeat. Start 1st Sunday after menses begins or 1st day of menses. (Nortrel) 21 day regimen: 1 tab qd for 21 days, then stop for 7 days, then repeat. Start 1st Sunday after menses begins or 1st day of menses.

HOW SUPPLIED: Tab: (Ethinyl Estradiol-Norethindrone) 0.035mg-1mg

CONTRAINDICATIONS: Thrombophlebitis or past history of deep vein thrombophlebitis, thromboembolic disorders (current or past history), cerebral vascular or coronary artery disease (CAD), known or suspected carcinoma of the breast, carcinoma of the endometrium or other known or suspected estrogen-dependent neoplasia, undiagnosed abnormal genital bleeding, cholestatic jaundice of pregnancy or jaundice with prior pill use, hepatic adenomas or carcinomas, known or suspected pregnancy. (Ortho-Novum) History of cerebral vascular or CAD, valvular heart disease with complications, severe HTN, diabetes with vascular involvement, headaches with focal neurological symptoms, major surgery with prolonged immobilization, acute or chronic hepatocellular disease with abnormal liver function. (Norinyl) Benign liver tumors.

WARNINGS/PRECAUTIONS: Increased risk of myocardial infarction (MI), vascular disease, thromboembolism, stroke, hepatic neoplasia, and gallbladder disease. Increased risk of morbidity and mortality with HTN, hyperlipidemias, obesity, and diabetes mellitus (DM). D/C at least 4 wks prior to and 2 wks post-elective surgery with increased risk of thromboembolism and during or following prolonged immobilization. Caution in women with CV disease risk factors. May increase risk of breast cancer and cervical intraepithelial neoplasia. Benign hepatic adenomas and hepatocellular carcinoma reported. D/C if jaundice develops. May develop visual changes with contact lenses. Retinal thrombosis reported; d/c if unexplained partial or complete loss of vision or other ophthalmic irregularities develop. May cause glucose intolerance, lipid abnormalities, or exacerbate migraine headaches. May cause fluid retention and increase BP; monitor closely and d/c if significant elevation of BP occurs. Breakthrough bleeding and spotting reported; rule out malignancy or pregnancy. Perform annual physical exam. Monitor closely with depression and d/c if depression recurs to serious degree. Not indicated for use before menarche. May affect certain endocrine, LFTs, and blood components in laboratory tests. (Necon, Nortrel, Ortho-Novum) Ectopic and intrauterine pregnancies may occur with contraceptive failure.

ADVERSE REACTIONS: N/V, breakthrough bleeding, spotting, amenorrhea, migraine, mental depression, vaginal candidiasis, edema, weight changes, abdominal cramps/bloating, menstrual flow changes, melasma.

INTERACTIONS: Reduced effects, increased breakthrough bleeding, and menstrual irregularities with rifampin, barbiturates, phenylbutazone, phenytoin Na⁺, and possibly with griseofulvin, ampicillin, tetracyclines (Necon, Nortrel, Ortho-Novum) carbamazepine. (Ortho-Novum) Reduced effects resulting in unintended pregnancy or breakthrough bleeding may occur when coadministered with antibiotics, anticonvulsants, and other drugs that increase the metabolism of contraceptive steroids (eg, felbamate, oxcarbazepine, topiramate, bosentan), and St. John's wort. Anti-HIV protease inhibitors may increase or decrease plasma levels. Atorvastatin, ascorbic acid, acetaminophen (APAP), and CYP3A4 inhibitors (eg, itraconazole, ketoconazole) may increase plasma estradiol levels. Bosentan may decrease hormone levels. Increased levels of cyclosporine, prednisolone, and theophylline have been reported. Decreased levels of APAP and lamotrigine. Increased clearance of temazepam, salicylic acid, morphine, and clofibric acid.

PREGNANCY: Category X, not for use in nursing.

MECHANISM OF ACTION: Estrogen/progestogen oral contraceptive; acts by suppression of gonadotropins and inhibits ovulation. Also produces alterations/changes in the cervical mucus (increases difficulty of sperm entry into uterus) and the endometrium (reduces likelihood of implantation).

PHARMACOKINETICS: Distribution: Found in breast milk.

NURSING CONSIDERATIONS

Assessment: Assess for current history of thrombophlebitis or thromboembolic disorders, history of HTN, hyperlipidemia, DM, obesity, breast cancer, and any other conditions where

O

treatment is contraindicated or cautioned. Assess use in women >35 yrs, smokers (≥15 cigarettes/day). Assess pregnancy/nursing status and for possible drug interactions.

Monitoring: Monitor for signs/symptoms of MI, thromboembolism, stroke, hepatic neoplasia, and other adverse effects. Monitor BP with history of HTN, serum glucose levels in diabetic and pre-diabetic patients, lipid levels with history of hyperlipidemia, and for signs of worsening depression with previous history. Monitor LFTs and for signs of liver dysfunction (eg, jaundice). Refer to an ophthalmologist if ocular changes develop.

Patient Counseling: Inform that the drug does not protect against HIV infection (AIDS) and other sexually transmitted diseases. Counsel about potential adverse effects. Advise to avoid smoking. Instruct to take exactly as directed at intervals not exceeding 24 hrs. Advise about risks of pregnancy if dose is missed. Instruct that if one dose is missed, take as soon as possible, and then take next dose at regular scheduled time. Inform that spotting, light bleeding, or nausea may occur during the first 1-3 packs of pills; advise not to d/c medication and if symptoms persist, notify physician. D/C if pregnancy is confirmed/suspected.

Administration: Oral route. **Storage:** (Ortho-Novum) 25°C (77°F); excursions permitted to 15-30°C (59-86°F). (Norinyl) 15-25°C (59-77°F). (Necon) 20-25°C (68-77°F).

OSMOPREP   RX
monobasic sodium phosphate monohydrate - dibasic sodium phosphate (Salix)

> Rare, but serious reports of acute phosphate nephropathy. Some cases resulted in permanent renal impairment requiring long-term dialysis. Patients at increased risk may include those with increased age, hypovolemia, increased bowel transit time (eg, bowel obstruction), active colitis, baseline kidney disease, and using medicines that affect renal perfusion or function (eg, diuretics, angiotensin converting enzyme [ACE] inhibitors, angiotensin receptor blockers [ARBs], and possibly NSAIDs). Use the recommended dose and dosing regimen (pm/am split dose).

THERAPEUTIC CLASS: Bowel cleanser

INDICATIONS: For cleansing the colon in preparation for colonoscopy in adults ≥18 yrs of age.

DOSAGE: *Adults:* ≥18 yrs: Evening Before Colonoscopy Procedure: 4 tabs with 8 oz. of clear liquids q15min for a total of 20 tabs. Day of Colonoscopy Procedure: Starting 3-5 hrs before procedure, 4 tabs with 8 oz. of clear liquids q15min for a total of 12 tabs. Drink only clear liquids. Do not use within 7 days of previous administration. Do not take any additional enema or laxative, particularly one containing sodium phosphate.

HOW SUPPLIED: Tab: (Sodium Phosphate Monobasic Monohydrate-Sodium Phosphate Dibasic Anhydrous) 1.102g-0.398g

CONTRAINDICATIONS: Patients with biopsy-proven acute phosphate nephropathy.

WARNINGS/PRECAUTIONS: Fatalities reported due to significant fluid shifts, severe electrolyte abnormalities, and cardiac arrhythmias. Adequately hydrate before, during and after use. Use with caution in elderly, impaired renal function, congestive heart failure (CHF), ascites, unstable angina, acute bowel obstruction, bowel perforation, toxic megacolon, gastric retention, ileus, pseudo-obstruction of the bowel, severe chronic constipation, acute colitis, gastric bypass, stapling surgery, hypomotility syndrome, history of acute phosphate nephropathy and known or suspected electrolyte disturbances. Correct electrolyte abnormalities before treatment. Rare reports of generalized tonic-clonic seizures and/or loss of consciousness. Caution in patients with history of seizures and in patients at higher risk of seizures (eg, patients withdrawing from alcohol or benzodiazepines, patients with known or suspected hyponatremia). Rare reports of serious arrhythmias; caution in patients with high risk of arrhythmias (eg, patients with prolonged QT, history of cardiomyopathy, history of uncontrolled arrhythmias, and recent history of myocardial infarction [MI]). Prolongation of QT interval reported. May induce colonic mucosal aphthous ulcerations and exacerbate inflammatory bowel disease (IBD).

ADVERSE REACTIONS: Abdominal bloating, abdominal pain, N/V, colonic mucosal aphthous ulcers, renal impairment, acute phosphate nephropathy.

INTERACTIONS: See Boxed Warning. Medications administered in close proximity to sodium phosphate tablets may not be absorbed from the GI tract. Caution if taking medications that may affect electrolyte levels (eg, diuretics), reduce seizure threshold (eg, tricyclic antidepressants), or prolong the QT interval.

PREGNANCY: Category C, safety not known in nursing.

MECHANISM OF ACTION: Purgative: Mechanism not established, primary mode of action thought to be through the osmotic effect of Na^+, causing large amounts of water to be drawn into the colon, promoting evacuation.

NURSING CONSIDERATIONS

Assessment: Assess if at increased risk of developing acute phosphate nephropathy or biopsy-proven acute phosphate nephropathy. Assess use in patients with severe renal insufficiency or renal impairment, or in any other conditions where treatment is contraindicated or cautioned. Consider baseline labs (phosphate, calcium, K⁺, Na⁺, SrCr, BUN) in patients who may be at increased risk for serious adverse events. Consider pre-dose ECG in patients with known prolonged QT or in patients with serious risk of cardiac arrhythmias. Assess hypersensitivity, pregnancy/nursing status, and for possible drug interactions.

Monitoring: Monitor for signs and symptoms of acute phosphate nephropathy, fluid shifts, severe electrolyte abnormalities, cardiac arrhythmias, renal failure, nephrocalcinosis, generalized tonic-clonic seizures, loss of consciousness, QT prolongation and colonic mucosal aphthous ulcerations. Consider performing post-colonoscopy labs (phosphate, calcium, Na⁺, K⁺, SrCr, BUN) in patients at increased risk for adverse events or if develop vomiting or signs of dehydration. Consider post-colonoscopy ECG in patients with high risk of serious cardiac arrhythmias or in patients with known prolonged QT.

Patient Counseling: Stress importance of adequate hydration before, during and after use. Instruct to drink 8 oz. of clear liquid with each 4-tab dose. Instruct to contact physician if experience symptoms of dehydration. Instruct not to use within 7 days of previous administration and not to administer additional laxative or purgative agents. Instruct to contact physician if develop worsening of bloating, abdominal pain, N/V, or headache.

Administration: Oral route. **Storage:** 25°C (77°F); excursions permitted to 15-30°C (59-86°F). Discard any unused portion.

OVCON-35　　　RX
ethinyl estradiol - norethindrone (Warner Chilcott)

Cigarette smoking increases the risk of serious cardiovascular (CV) side effects. Risk increases with age (>35 yrs) and with heavy smoking (≥15 cigarettes/day). Women who use oral contraceptives should be strongly advised not to smoke.

OTHER BRAND NAMES: Balziva (Barr) - Ovcon-50 (Warner Chilcott)

THERAPEUTIC CLASS: Estrogen/progestogen combination

INDICATIONS: Prevention of pregnancy.

DOSAGE: *Adults:* 1 tab qd for 28 days, then repeat regimen on the next day after the last tab. Start on the 1st day of menses or 1st Sunday after menses begin. For the 1st cycle of a Sunday start regimen, use back-up method if had intercourse before having taken the seven pills. *Pediatrics:* Postpubertal Adolescents: 1 tab qd for 28 days, then repeat regimen on the next day after the last tab. Start on the 1st day of menses or 1st Sunday after menses begin. For the 1st cycle of a Sunday start regimen, use back-up method if had intercourse before having taken the seven pills.

HOW SUPPLIED: Tab: (Ethinyl Estradiol-Norethindrone) (Ovcon 35, Balziva) 0.035mg-0.4mg; (Ovcon 50) 0.05mg-1mg

CONTRAINDICATIONS: Thrombophlebitis, current or history of thromboembolic disorders, past history of deep vein thrombophlebitis, cerebrovascular or coronary artery disease (CAD), known or suspected carcinoma of the breast, endometrial carcinoma or other known or suspected estrogen-dependent neoplasia, undiagnosed abnormal genital bleeding, cholestatic jaundice of pregnancy or jaundice with prior pill use, hepatic adenomas or carcinomas, known or suspected pregnancy.

WARNINGS/PRECAUTIONS: Increased risk of myocardial infarction (MI), thromboembolism, cerebrovascular events, gallbladder disease, and hepatic neoplasia. May increase risk of breast cancer and cervical intraepithelial neoplasia. May cause benign hepatic adenomas. Retinal thrombosis reported; d/c if unexplained partial or complete loss of vision, onset of proptosis or diplopia, papilledema, or retinal vascular lesions develop. Increased risk of gallbladder surgery reported. May cause glucose intolerance; caution with prediabetic and diabetic patients. May cause fluid retention and increase BP; monitor closely with HTN and d/c if significant elevation of BP occurs. May cause migraine or development of headaches; d/c and evaluate the cause. Breakthrough bleeding and spotting reported; rule out malignancy or pregnancy. Does not protect against HIV infection (AIDS) or other sexually transmitted diseases (STD). D/C if jaundice develops. Monitor closely with depression and d/c if depression recurs to serious degree. May develop visual changes or changes in contact lense tolerance. Not indicated for use before menarche. Use back-up method of contraception with significant GI disturbance.

ADVERSE REACTIONS: N/V, breakthrough bleeding, GI symptoms (eg, abdominal cramps, bloating), spotting, menstrual flow changes, amenorrhea, migraine, depression, vaginal candidiasis, edema, weight changes, cervical ectropion and secretion changes.

INTERACTIONS: Reduced effects, increased breakthrough bleeding, and menstrual irregularities with rifampin, barbiturates, phenylbutazone, phenytoin sodium, and possibly with griseofulvin, ampicillin, and tetracyclines.

PREGNANCY: Category X, not for use in nursing.

MECHANISM OF ACTION: Estrogen/progestogen combination oral contraceptive; acts by suppressing gonadotropins. Primarily inhibits ovulation but also produces other alterations, including changes in the cervical mucus (increases difficulty of sperm entry into uterus) and endometrium (reduces likelihood of implantation).

PHARMACOKINETICS: Distribution: Found in breast milk.

NURSING CONSIDERATIONS

Assessment: Assess for pregnancy/nursing status, possible drug interactions, and conditions where treatment is contraindicated or cautioned. Assess use in patients >35 yrs who smoke ≥15 cigarettes/day, and with HTN, hyperlipidemia, obesity, and DM.

Monitoring: Monitor for signs/symptoms of thromboembolism, stroke, MI, and other adverse effects. Monitor BP in patients with a history of HTN, HTN-related disease, or renal disease. Monitor for signs of depression in patients with a history of depression. Perform annual history and physical exam. Monitor serum glucose levels in prediabetic and diabetic patients. Monitor lipid levels in patients with a history of hyperlipidemia.

Patient Counseling: Inform that medication does not protect against HIV/AIDS and other STDs. Counsel about possible serious side effects. Advise to avoid smoking while on therapy. If dose is missed, refer to PI for instructions. If spotting, light bleeding, or nausea occurs during first 1-3 packs of pills, advise not to d/c medication and if symptoms persist, notify physician. Inform if vomiting or diarrhea occurs or if taking other medications, efficacy may decrease; use backup method of contraception. Refer patients with contact lenses to an ophthalmologist if changes in vision or lens tolerance develop.

Administration: Oral route. Take 1 pill at the same time every day until the pack is empty. If on 28 day regimen, start the next pack the day after the last inactive tablet and do not wait any days between packs. **Storage:** (Ovcon 35, Balziva) 20-25°C (68-77°F). (Ovcon 50) Below 30°C (86°F).

OXYBUTYNIN   RX
oxybutynin chloride (Various)

OTHER BRAND NAMES: Ditropan (Ortho-Mcneil/Janssen)

THERAPEUTIC CLASS: Anticholinergic

INDICATIONS: Relief of symptoms of bladder instability associated with voiding in patients with uninhibited neurogenic or reflex neurogenic bladder (eg, urgency, frequency, urinary leakage, urge incontinence, dysuria).

DOSAGE: *Adults:* Usual: 5mg bid-tid. Max: 5mg qid. Frail Elderly: Initial: 2.5mg bid-tid. *Pediatrics:* ≥5 yrs: Usual: 5mg bid. Max: 5mg tid.

HOW SUPPLIED: Syrup: 5mg/5mL [473mL]; Tab: (Ditropan) 5mg* *scored

CONTRAINDICATIONS: Urinary retention, gastric retention and other severe decreased GI motility conditions, uncontrolled narrow-angle glaucoma, and in patients at risk for these conditions.

WARNINGS/PRECAUTIONS: Angioedema of the face, lips, tongue and/or larynx reported; d/c if involves the tongue, hypopharynx, or larynx. Associated with anticholinergic CNS effects; consider dose reduction or d/c if occur. May aggravate symptoms of hyperthyroidism, coronary heart disease (CHD), congestive heart failure (CHF), arrhythmias, hiatal hernia, tachycardia, HTN, myasthenia gravis, and prostatic hypertrophy. Caution with preexisting dementia treated with cholinesterase inhibitors, hepatic/renal impairment, myasthenia gravis, clinically significant bladder outflow obstruction, GI obstructive disorders, ulcerative colitis, intestinal atony, gastroesophageal reflux disorder (GERD), and in frail elderly.

ADVERSE REACTIONS: Dry mouth, constipation, somnolence, headache, nausea, blurred vision, dyspepsia, dizziness, urinary tract infection, urinary hesitation, nervousness, insomnia, urinary retention.

INTERACTIONS: May increase frequency and/or severity of adverse effects with other anticholinergics. May alter GI absorption of other drugs due to GI motility effects. Ketoconazole may increase levels. Caution with CYP3A4 inhibitors (eg, antimycotics, macrolides) and drugs (eg, bisphosphonates) that may cause or exacerbate esophagitis.

PREGNANCY: Category B, caution in nursing.

MECHANISM OF ACTION: Antispasmodic/anticholinergic agent; inhibits muscarinic action of acetylcholine on smooth muscle exerting direct antispasmodic effect; relaxes smooth muscle of bladder.

PHARMACOKINETICS: Absorption: Rapid; absolute bioavailability (6%); T_{max}=1 hr. Refer to PI for pediatric, isomer, and metabolite parameters. **Distribution:** (IV) V_d=193L. **Metabolism:** Liver via CYP3A4; desethyloxybutynin (active metabolite). **Elimination:** Urine (<0.1% unchanged); $T_{1/2}$=2-3 hrs.

NURSING CONSIDERATIONS

Assessment: Assess for bladder outflow obstruction, GI obstructive disorders, decreased GI motility conditions, GERD, GI narrowing, narrow-angle glaucoma, myasthenia gravis, hyperthyroidism, CHD, CHF, arrhythmias, hiatal hernia, tachycardia, HTN, prostatic hypertrophy, preexisting dementia, previous hypersensitivity to the drug, hepatic/renal function, pregnancy/nursing status, and possible drug interactions.

Monitoring: Monitor for aggravation of myasthenia gravis, hyperthyroidism, CHD, CHF, arrhythmias, hiatal hernia, tachycardia, HTN, prostatic hypertrophy symptoms. Monitor for signs of anticholinergic CNS effects, hypersensitivity reactions, GI narrowing, hepatic/renal impairment, and other adverse reactions.

Patient Counseling: Inform patients that angioedema may occur and could result in life-threatening airway obstruction; advise to promptly d/c therapy and seek medical attention if edema involves tongue, hypopharynx, or larynx. Inform that heat prostration (fever, heat stroke) may occur when administered in high environmental temperature. Inform that oxybutynin may produce blurred vision and drowsiness which may be enhanced by alcohol; advise to exercise caution.

Administration: Oral route. **Storage:** 15-30°C (59-86°F).

OXYCODONE IMMEDIATE-RELEASE `CII`
oxycodone HCl (Various)

THERAPEUTIC CLASS: Opioid analgesic

INDICATIONS: Moderate to moderately severe pain.

DOSAGE: *Adults:* Usual: 5mg q6h prn for pain.

HOW SUPPLIED: Cap: 5mg

CONTRAINDICATIONS: Respiratory depression, acute or severe bronchial asthma, hypercarbia, paralytic ileus, situations where opioids are contraindicated.

WARNINGS/PRECAUTIONS: Extreme caution with COPD, cor pulmonale, decreased respiratory reserve, hypoxia, hypercapnia, pre-existing respiratory depression. Caution with circulatory shock, delirium tremens, acute alcoholism, adrenocortical insufficiency, CNS depression, myxedema or hypothyroidism, BPH, severe hepatic/renal/pulmonary impairment, toxic psychosis, biliary tract disease, increased ICP, or head injury, elderly or debilitated. May cause severe hypotension. May produce drug dependence; caution in known drug abuse. May aggravate convulsive disorders and mask abdominal disorders. May impair mental/physical abilities.

ADVERSE REACTIONS: Lightheadedness, dizziness, N/V, sedation.

INTERACTIONS: Respiratory depression, hypotension and profound sedation with other CNS depressants (eg, sedatives, anesthetics, phenothiazines, alcohol). Mixed agonist/antagonist analgesics may reduce the analgesic effect and/or cause withdrawal. Risk of severe hypotension with phenothiazines, or other agents that compromise vasomotor tone. May enhance skeletal muscle relaxant effects and increase respiratory depression. May interact with CYP2D6 inhibitors (eg, amiodarone, quinidine, polycyclic antidepressants). Caution with MAOIs.

PREGNANCY: Category B, not for use in nursing.

MECHANISM OF ACTION: Opioid analgesic; pure agonist opioid whose principal therapeutic effect is analgesia. Precise action not established. However, specific CNS opioid receptors for endogenous compounds with opioid-like activity are found throughout the brain and spinal cord and play a role in analgesic effects.

PHARMACOKINETICS: Distribution: Found in breast milk. **Metabolism:** Via CYP2D6 to oxymorphone (metabolite).

NURSING CONSIDERATIONS

Assessment: Assess for adrenocortical insufficiency (eg, Addison's disease), kyphoscoliosis associated with respiratory depression, prostatic hypertrophy or urethral stricture, acute pancreatitis, or any other conditions where treatment is contraindicated or cautioned. Assess for pregnancy/nursing status and possible drug interactions.

Monitoring: Monitor for signs/symptoms of respiratory depression, hypotension, convulsions, medication dependence and tolerance, medication abuse, sphincter of Oddi spasms, elevations in CSF pressure, and elevations in serum amylase levels.

Patient Counseling: Advise not to adjust dosing without consulting physician. Inform that medication may impair mental/physical abilities required for performing hazardous tasks (eg, operating machinery/driving). Counsel to avoid alcohol and other CNS depressants. Inform medication has potential for abuse; protect from theft. Advise not to abruptly d/c medication if on therapy for a few weeks; taper dosing.

Administration: Oral route. **Storage:** 20-25°C (68-77°F); protect from moisture and dispense in tight, light-resistant container.

OxyContin

`CII`

oxycodone HCl (Purdue Pharma)

> Contains oxycodone, a schedule II controlled substance with abuse liability similar to morphine. Not intended for use as a PRN analgesic. 60mg and 80mg tabs, a single dose >40mg, or a total daily dose >80mg are only for use in opioid-tolerant patients; may cause fatal respiratory depression with intolerant patients. Abuse potential; assess for risks of opioid abuse/addiction prior to therapy. Swallow tab whole; do not cut, break, chew, crush, or dissolve. Concomitant use with CYP3A4 inhibitors (eg, macrolides, azole-antifungals, protease inhibitors) may cause fatal respiratory depression.

THERAPEUTIC CLASS: Opioid analgesic

INDICATIONS: Management of moderate to severe pain when a continuous, around-the-clock analgesic is needed for an extended period of time. For use following the immediate postoperative period (1st 12-24 hours after surgery) in patients already receiving the drug before surgery or those expected to have moderate to severe pain for an extended period of time.

DOSAGE: *Adults:* Individualize dose. Opioid-Naive: 10mg q12h. Titrate: Determine dose that provides adequate analgesia and minimizes adverse reactions while maintaining q12h dosing regimen. May increase total daily dose by 25-50% of the current dose every 1-2 days. Opioid-Tolerant Patients: Refer to PI for conversion to oxycodone from other opioid analgesics. Hepatic Impairment/With Concurrent CNS Depressants/Debilitated, Non-Opioid Tolerant: Start at 1/3 to 1/2 the usual starting dose. Reassess continued need for around-the-clock opioid therapy regularly (eg, every 6-12 months). Taper dose gradually upon d/c of therapy.

HOW SUPPLIED: Tab, Controlled-Release: 10mg, 15mg, 20mg, 30mg, 40mg, 60mg, 80mg

CONTRAINDICATIONS: Significant respiratory depression, acute or severe bronchial asthma, known or suspected paralytic ileus.

WARNINGS/PRECAUTIONS: Not to be used for pre-emptive analgesia, mild pain, pain not expected to persist for an extended period of time, or pain in immediate postoperative period. May cause CNS and respiratory depression. Extreme caution with chronic obstructive pulmonary disease (COPD), cor pulmonale, decreased respiratory reserve, hypoxia, hypercapnia, and preexisting respiratory depression. May induce or aggravate convulsions/seizures; caution with history of seizure disorders. Caution in patients who have difficulty swallowing or underlying GI disorders that may predispose to obstruction. May obscure diagnosis or clinical course of acute abdominal conditions; caution in patients who are at risk of developing ileus. Respiratory depressant effects may be exaggerated in the presence of head injury, intracranial lesions, or other sources of preexisting increased intracranial pressure (ICP). May produce miosis independent of ambient light and altered consciousness, which may obscure neurologic signs associated with ICP in persons with head injuries. May cause severe hypotension; caution in circulatory shock. May cause spasm of sphincter of Oddi and increases in serum amylase; caution with biliary tract disease, including acute pancreatitis. Gradually increase dose if tolerance develops. Caution with alcoholism, delirium tremens, adrenocortical insufficiency, CNS depression, debilitation, kyphoscoliosis associated with respiratory compromise, myxedema or hypothyroidism, prostatic hypertrophy or urethral stricture, severe hepatic/renal/pulmonary impairment, and toxic psychosis. May impair mental and physical abilities.

ADVERSE REACTIONS: Respiratory depression, constipation, N/V, somnolence, dizziness, pruritus, headache, dry mouth, asthenia, sweating, apnea, respiratory arrest, circulatory depression, hypotension.

INTERACTIONS: See Boxed Warning. Respiratory depression, hypotension, and profound sedation or coma may occur with other CNS depressants (eg, sedatives, hypnotics, anxiolytics, neuroleptics, tranquilizers, centrally acting antiemetics, general anesthetics, phenothiazines, alcohol, other opioids). Risk of severe hypotension with phenothiazines or other agents that compromise vasomotor tone. May enhance neuromuscular blocking action of skeletal muscle relaxants (eg, pancuronium) and increase respiratory depression. May increase levels with voriconazole. May decrease levels with CYP450 inducers (eg, rifampin, carbamazepine, phenytoin). Caution with MAOIs. Mixed agonist/antagonist analgesics (eg, pentazocine, nalbuphine, butorphanol) may reduce analgesic effect and/or cause withdrawal.

PREGNANCY: Category B, not for use in nursing.

MECHANISM OF ACTION: Opioid analgesic; pure μ-receptor opioid agonist. Precise analgesic action not established. However, specific CNS opioid receptors have been found throughout the brain and spinal cord and play a role in analgesic effect.

PHARMACOKINETICS: Absorption: Administration of variable doses resulted in different parameters. **Distribution:** V_d=2.6L/kg; plasma protein binding (45%); crosses placenta; found in breast milk. **Metabolism:** Extensively via CYP3A and CYP2D6 to noroxycodone, noroxymorphone (major metabolites), and oxymorphone. **Elimination:** Urine; $T_{1/2}$=4.5 hrs.

NURSING CONSIDERATIONS

Assessment: Assess for risk factors for abuse or addiction, family history of substance abuse, history of mental illness or depression, degree of opioid tolerance, previous opioid dose, level of pain intensity, type of pain, respiratory depression, COPD, hypoxia, hypercapnia, emotional status, or any other conditions where treatment is contraindicated or cautioned. Assess for pregnancy/nursing status, renal/hepatic function, and possible drug interactions.

Monitoring: Monitor for signs/symptoms of respiratory depression, CNS depression, seizures/convulsions, elevations in CSF pressure, hypotension, spasm of sphincter of Oddi, tolerance and physical dependence. Monitor BP and serum amylase levels. Routinely monitor for signs of misuse, abuse and addiction.

Patient Counseling: Instruct to swallow tab whole; do not cut, break, chew, dissolve, or crush. Instruct not to presoak, lick, or wet tab prior to placing in the mouth. Advise to report episodes of breakthrough pain or adverse events (eg, respiratory depression). Instruct not to adjust dose without consulting physician. Inform that mental/physical abilities may be impaired; instruct to avoid alcohol or other CNS depressants. Inform that the drug has potential for abuse and to protect from theft. Inform that if taking medication for more than a few weeks, to avoid abrupt withdrawal; advise that dosing will need to be tapered. Counsel to not share or permit use by other individuals. Counsel to notify physician if pregnant or plan to become pregnant. Instruct to dispose any unused medication by flushing down the toilet.

Administration: Oral route. Take 1 tab at a time with enough water. **Storage:** 25°C (77°F); excursions permitted to 15-30°C (59-86°F).

OXYTROL   RX
oxybutynin (Watson)

THERAPEUTIC CLASS: Anticholinergic

INDICATIONS: Treatment of overactive bladder with symptoms of urge urinary incontinence, urgency, and frequency.

DOSAGE: *Adults:* One 3.9mg/day system applied twice weekly (every 3-4 days) to dry, intact skin on the abdomen, hip, or buttock. Avoid reapplication to same site within 7 days.

HOW SUPPLIED: Patch: 3.9mg/day [8s]

CONTRAINDICATIONS: Urinary retention, gastric retention, uncontrolled narrow-angle glaucoma, and in patients at risk for these conditions.

WARNINGS/PRECAUTIONS: Angioedema may occur; d/c and provide appropriate therapy. Caution with hepatic/renal impairment, bladder outflow obstruction, GI obstructive disorders, ulcerative colitis, intestinal atony, myasthenia gravis, and gastroesophageal reflux. May decrease GI motility.

ADVERSE REACTIONS: Application-site reactions (pruritus, erythema, vesicles, rash), dry mouth, diarrhea, constipation.

INTERACTIONS: Other anticholinergics and other agents that produce dry mouth, constipation, somnolence, and/or other anticholinergic-like effects may increase frequency and/or severity of anticholinergic effects. Caution with bisphosphonates or other drugs that may exacerbate esophagitis. May alter GI absorption of other drugs due to GI motility effects.

PREGNANCY: Category B, caution in nursing.

MECHANISM OF ACTION: Antispasmodic, anticholinergic agent; acts as competitive antagonist of acetylcholine at postganglionic muscarinic receptors, resulting in relaxation of bladder smooth muscle.

PHARMACOKINETICS: Absorption: Administration using variable dosing studies resulted in different parameters. **Distribution:** (IV) V_d=193L. **Metabolism:** Liver (extensive); CYP3A4, N-desethyloxybutynin (active metabolite). **Elimination:** Urine (<0.1% unchanged, <0.1% N-desethyloxybutynin); (IV) $T_{1/2}$=2 hrs.

NURSING CONSIDERATIONS

Assessment: Assess for bladder outflow obstruction, urinary/gastric retention, uncontrolled narrow-angle glaucoma, gastroesophageal reflux, GI obstructive disorder, ulcerative colitis, intestinal atony, esophagitis, myasthenia gravis, renal/hepatic impairment, pregnancy/nursing status, and possible drug interactions.

Monitoring: Monitor for signs/symptoms of angioedema, gastric retention, urinary retention, decreased gastric motility, renal/hepatic dysfunction, and for exacerbation of esophagitis.

Patient Counseling: Advise that heat prostration may occur in hot environment. Counsel that dizziness, drowsiness, and blurred vision may occur and alcohol may enhance drowsiness. Inform that angioedema has been reported and instruct to d/c therapy and seek medical attention when angioedema occurs. Instruct to apply to dry, intact skin on abdomen, hip, or buttock; advise to avoid reapplication to same site within 7 days.

Administration: Transdermal route. Apply immediately after removal from protective pouch.
Storage: 25°C (77°F); excursions permitted to 15-30°C (59-86°F). Protect from moisture and humidity. Do not store outside the sealed pouch.

OZURDEX   RX
dexamethasone (Allergan)

THERAPEUTIC CLASS: Corticosteroid

INDICATIONS: Treatment of macular edema following branch retinal vein occlusion or central retinal vein occlusion and treatment of noninfectious uveitis affecting the posterior segment of the eye.

DOSAGE: *Adults:* 0.7mg intravitreal inj via Novadur drug delivery system.

HOW SUPPLIED: Intravitreal Implant: 0.7mg

CONTRAINDICATIONS: Advanced glaucoma, active or suspected ocular or periocular infections including most viral diseases of the cornea and conjunctiva, including active epithelial herpes simplex keratitis (dendritic keratitis), vaccinia, varicella, mycobacterial infections, and fungal diseases.

WARNINGS/PRECAUTIONS: Intravitreal inj has been associated with endophthalmitis, eye inflammation, increased intraocular pressure (IOP), and retinal detachments; regularly monitor patients following inj. May produce posterior subcapsular cataracts, increased IOP, glaucoma, and may enhance the establishment of secondary ocular infections due to bacteria, fungi, or viruses. Caution with history of ocular herpes simplex. Risk of implant migration into the anterior chamber in patients whom posterior capsule of the lens is absent or has a tear.

ADVERSE REACTIONS: Increased IOP, conjunctival hemorrhage, eye pain, conjunctival hyperemia, ocular HTN, cataract, headache.

PREGNANCY: Category C, caution in nursing.

MECHANISM OF ACTION: Corticosteroid; suppresses inflammation by inhibiting multiple inflammatory cytokines resulting in decreased edema, fibrin deposition, capillary leakage, and migration of inflammatory cells.

PHARMACOKINETICS: Absorption: C_{max} =94pg/mL.

NURSING CONSIDERATIONS

Assessment: Assess for glaucoma and for active or suspected ocular or periocular infections (eg, herpes simplex keratitis, vaccinia, varicella, mycobacterial infections, or fungal diseases), pregnancy/nursing status, and hypersensitivity to product components.

Monitoring: Monitor for elevated IOP and endophthalmitis by checking for perfusion of the optic nerve head immediately after inj, tonometry within 30 min of application, and biomicroscopy between 2-7 days after administration. Monitor for eye inflammation and retinal detachment, posterior subcapsular cataracts, glaucoma and secondary ocular infections, and other adverse events that may occur.

Patient Counseling: Inform of risks for potential complications including development of endophthalmitis and increased IOP. If the eye becomes red, sensitive to light, painful, or develops a change in vision, advise to immediately consult an ophthalmologist. Inform that temporary visual blurring may occur after receiving the treatment; instruct to avoid driving/using machines until this has resolved.

Administration: Intravitreal route. Procedure should be carried out under controlled aseptic conditions. Adequate anesthesia and a broad-spectrum microbicide applied to the periocular skin, eyelid and ocular surface should be given prior to inj. Refer to PI for administration instructions.
Storage: 15-30°C (59-86°F).

PACLITAXEL   RX
paclitaxel (Various)

> Should be administered under supervision of a physician experienced in the use of cancer chemotherapeutic agents. Anaphylaxis and severe hypersensitivity reactions reported; pretreat with corticosteroids, diphenhydramine, and H_2 antagonists. Fatal reactions have occured despite premedication. Do not rechallenge if severe hypersensitivity reaction occurs. Should not be given to patients with solid tumors having baseline neutrophil counts of <1500 cells/mm³ and with AIDS-related Kaposi's sarcoma having baseline neutrophil count of <1000 cells/mm³. Perform peripheral blood cell counts frequently to monitor occurrence of bone marrow suppression, primarily neutropenia.

THERAPEUTIC CLASS: Antimicrotubule agent

INDICATIONS: First-line (in combination with cisplatin) and subsequent therapy for the treatment of advanced ovarian carcinoma. Adjuvant treatment of node-positive breast cancer administered sequentially to standard doxorubicin-containing combination chemotherapy. Treatment of breast cancer after failure of combination chemotherapy for metastatic disease or relapse within 6 months of adjuvant chemotherapy. Second-line treatment of AIDS-related Kaposi's sarcoma. First-line treatment of non-small cell lung cancer (NSCLC) in combination with cisplatin in patients who are not candidates for potentially curative surgery and/or radiation therapy.

DOSAGE: *Adults:* Premedicate with dexamethasone (20mg PO 12 and 6 hrs before inj), diphehydramine or its equivalent (50mg IV 30-60 min prior to inj), and cimetidine (300mg) or ranitidine (50 mg) IV 30-60 min before inj. Ovarian Carcinoma: Previously Untreated: 175mg/m^2 IV over 3 hrs or 135mg/m^2 IV over 24 hrs every 3 weeks followed by cisplatin 75mg/m^2. Previously Treated: Usual: 135mg/m^2 IV or 175mg/m^2 IV over 3 hrs every 3 weeks. Breast Cancer: Adjuvant Therapy: Usual: 175mg/m^2 IV over 3 hrs every 3 weeks for 4 courses given sequentially to doxorubicin-containing combination chemotherapy. Failure of Initial Chemotherapy for Metastatic Disease or Relapse within 6 Months of Chemotherapy: 175mg/m^2 IV over 3 hrs every 3 weeks. NSCLC: Usual: 135mg/m^2 IV over 24 hrs every 3 weeks followed by cisplatin 75mg/m^2. Kaposi's Sarcoma: Usual: 135mg/m^2 IV over 3 hrs every 3 weeks or 100mg/m^2 IV over 3 hrs every 2 weeks. Reduce dose by 20% for subsequent courses of paclitaxel inj in patients who experience severe neutropenia (neutrophils <500 cells/mm^3 for a week or longer) or severe peripheral neuropathy. Refer to PI for dosing in patients with hepatic impairment and modifications in patients with advanced HIV disease.

HOW SUPPLIED: Inj: 30mg/5mL, 100mg/16.7mL, 150mg/25mL, 300mg/50mL

CONTRAINDICATIONS: Hypersensitivity to drugs formulated in polyoxyl 35 castor oil, NF; solid tumor patients with baseline neutrophils <1500 cells/mm^3, or AIDS-related Kaposi's sarcoma patients with baseline neutrophils <1000 cells/mm^3.

WARNINGS/PRECAUTIONS: Severe conduction abnormalities reported; administer appropriate therapy and perform continuous cardiac monitoring during subsequent therapy. May cause fetal harm during pregnancy. Hypotension, bradycardia, and HTN reported. Contains dehydrated alcohol; CNS and other alcohol effects may occur. Caution in patients with bilirubin >2X ULN and in elderly. Inj-site reactions and peripheral neuropathy reported.

ADVERSE REACTIONS: Anaphylaxis, bone marrow suppression, neutropenia, infections, bleeding, abnormal ECG, hypotension, peripheral neuropathy, myalgia/arthralgia, N/V, diarrhea, alopecia, inj-site reactions.

INTERACTIONS: Myelosuppression more profound when given after cisplatin than with the alternate sequence. Caution with CYP3A4 substrates (eg, midazolam, buspirone, felodipine, lovastatin, eletriptan, sildenafil, simvastatin, triazolam), inducers (eg, rifampicin, carbamazepine), and inhibitors (eg, atazanavir, clarithromycin, indinavir, itraconazole, ketoconazole, nefazodone, nelfinavir, ritonavir, saquinavir, telithromycin). Caution with CYP2C8 substrates (eg, repaglinide and rosiglitazone), inhibitors (eg, gemfibrozil), and inducers (eg, rifampin). May increase doxorubicin levels.

PREGNANCY: Category D, not for use in nursing.

MECHANISM OF ACTION: Antimicrotubule agent; promotes assembly of microtubules from tubulin dimers and stabilizes microtubules by preventing depolymerization and induces abnormal arrays or bundles of microtubules throughout the cell cycle and multiple asters of microtubules during mitosis.

PHARMACOKINETICS: Absorption: IV administration of multiple doses resulted in different parameters. **Distribution:** V_d=227-688L/m^2; plasma protein binding (89-98%). **Metabolism:** Liver via CYP2C8 (major), CYP3A4 (minor). 6α-hydroxypaclitaxel (major metabolite); 3'-*p*-hydroxypaclitaxel and 6α, 3'-*p*-dihydroxypaclitaxel (minor metabolites). **Elimination:** Urine (1.3-12.6% unchanged), feces (71%, 5% unchanged).

NURSING CONSIDERATIONS

Assessment: Assess for hypersensitivity (polyoxyl 35 castor oil, NF), hepatic impairment, bilirubin levels, pregnancy/nursing status, and possible drug interactions. Assess for baseline neutrophil count in patients with solid tumors or with Kaposi's sarcoma.

Monitoring: Monitor for signs/symptoms of anaphylaxis/hypersensitivity reactions, inj-site reactions, myelosuppression, toxicity, and other adverse reactions. Monitor blood count frequently and vital signs frequently during 1st hr of infusion. Monitor cardiac function in patients with serious conduction abnormalities and when used in combination with doxorubicin.

Patient Counseling: Inform about risks and benefits of therapy. Advise that drug may cause fetal harm; advise women of childbearing potential to avoid becoming pregnant. Advise to report to healthcare provider for any signs of an allergic reaction or signs of infection. Advise to inform physician if with liver/heart problems and are breastfeeding or plan to breastfeed.

Administration: IV route. Refer to PI for preparation and administration procedures. **Storage:** Undiluted: 20-25°C (68-77°F). Retain in the original package to protect from light. Diluted Sol: Ambient temperature approximately 25°C (77°F) and room lighting conditions for up to 27 hrs.

P

PAMELOR   RX
nortriptyline HCl (Mallinckrodt)

> Antidepressants increased the risk of suicidal thinking and behavior (suicidality) in short-term studies in children, adolescents, and young adults with major depressive disorder (MDD) and other psychiatric disorders. Monitor and observe closely for clinical worsening, suicidality, or unusual changes in behavior in patients who are started on antidepressant therapy. Nortriptyline is not approved for use in pediatric patients.

THERAPEUTIC CLASS: Tricyclic antidepressant

INDICATIONS: Relief of symptoms of depression.

DOSAGE: *Adults:* 25mg tid-qid. Max: 150mg/day. Total daily dose may be given once a day. Monitor serum levels if dose >100mg/day. Elderly/Adolescents: 30-50mg/day in single or divided doses.

HOW SUPPLIED: Cap: 10mg, 25mg, 50mg, 75mg; Sol: 10mg/5mL

CONTRAINDICATIONS: MAOI use within 14 days, acute recovery period following MI.

WARNINGS/PRECAUTIONS: MI, arrhythmia, strokes have occurred. Caution with cardiovascular disease (CVD), glaucoma, history of urinary retention, hyperthyroidism. May lower seizure threshold, exacerbate psychosis or activate schizophrenia, cause symptoms of mania in bipolar disease, or alter glucose levels. D/C several days prior to elective surgery.

ADVERSE REACTIONS: Arrhythmias, hypotension, HTN, tachycardia, MI, heart block, stroke, confusion, hallucination, insomnia, tremors, ataxia, dry mouth, blurred vision, skin rash.

INTERACTIONS: See Contraindications. May block guanethidine effects. Arrhythmia risk with thyroid agents. Alcohol may potentiate effects. "Stimulating" effect with reserpine. Monitor with anticholinergic and sympathomimetic drugs. Increased plasma levels with cimetidine. Hypoglycemia reported with chlorpropamide. SSRIs, antidepressants, phenothiazines, propafenone, flecainide and CYP2D6 inhibitors (eg, quinidine) may potentiate effects. Decreased clearance with quinidine.

PREGNANCY: Safety during pregnancy and nursing not known.

MECHANISM OF ACTION: Tricyclic antidepressant; inhibits activity of histamine, 5-hydroxytryptamine, and acetylcholine; increases pressor effect of NE, blocks pressor response of phenethylamine, and interferes with transport, release, and storage of catecholamine.

NURSING CONSIDERATIONS

Assessment: Assess for acute recovery period after MI, bipolar disorder risk, history of mania, unrecognized/history of schizophrenia, possible drug interactions, history of seizures, CVD, hyperthyroidism, DM, glaucoma, urinary retention, history of agitation or overactivity, and pregnancy/nursing status.

Monitoring: Periodically monitor blood glucose. Monitor for signs/symptoms of clinical worsening (suicidality, unusual changes in behavior), mania, cardiovascular events, increasing psychosis, increasing anxiety/agitation, mydriasis, hypo/hyperglycemia, seizures, cognitive/motor impairment.

Patient Counseling: Advise to avoid alcohol. Seek medical attention for symptoms of activation of mania, seizures, clinical worsening (suicidal ideation, unusual changes in behavior), cardiovascular events, increasing psychosis, increasing anxiety/agitation, mydriasis, and hypo/hyperglycemia. May impair physical/mental abilities.

Administration: Oral route. **Storage:** 20-25°C (68-77°F).

PANCREAZE   RX
pancrelipase (Janssen)

THERAPEUTIC CLASS: Pancreatic enzyme supplement

INDICATIONS: Treatment of exocrine pancreatic insufficiency due to cystic fibrosis or other conditions.

DOSAGE: *Adults:* Individualize dose based on clinical symptoms, degree of steatorrhea present, and fat content of diet. Start at the lowest recommended dose and increase gradually. Initial: 500 lipase U/kg/meal. Max: 2500 lipase U/kg/meal (or ≤10,000 lipase U/kg/day) or <4000 lipase U/g fat ingested/day. Give half of the dose used for an individualized full meal with each snack. Reduce dose in older patients. Refer to PI for the dosing limitations.
Pediatrics: Individualize dose based on clinical symptoms, degree of steatorrhea present, and fat content of diet. Start at the lowest recommended dose and increase gradually. ≥4 yrs: Initial: 500 lipase U/kg/meal. Max: 2500 lipase U/kg/meal (or ≤10,000 lipase U/kg/day) or <4000 lipase U/g fat ingested/day. Give half of the dose used for an individualized full meal with each

snack. >12 months-<4 yrs: Initial: 1000 lipase U/kg/meal. Max: 2500 lipase U/kg/meal (or ≤10,000 lipase U/kg/day) or <4000 lipase U/g fat ingested/day. ≤12 months: May give 2000-4000 lipase U/120mL of formula or per breastfeeding. Refer to PI for the dosing limitations.

HOW SUPPLIED: Cap, Delayed-Release: (Lipase-Protease-Amylase) (MT 4) 4200 U-10,000 U-17,500 U; (MT 10) 10,500 U-25,000 U-43,750 U; (MT 16) 16,800 U-40,000 U-70,000 U; (MT 20) 21,000 U-37,000 U-61,000 U

WARNINGS/PRECAUTIONS: Fibrosing colonopathy reported; monitor closely for progression to stricture formation. Caution with doses >2500 lipase U/kg/meal (or >10,000 lipase U/kg/day); use only if these doses are documented to be effective by 3-day fecal fat measures. Examine patients receiving >6000 lipase U/kg/meal; immediately decrease dose or titrate dose downward to a lower range. Should not be crushed or chewed or mixed in foods with pH >4.5; may disrupt enteric coating of cap resulting in early release of enzymes, irritation of oral mucosa, and/or loss of enzyme activity. Ensure that no drug is retained in the mouth. Caution with gout, renal impairment, or hyperuricemia; may increase blood uric acid levels. Risk for transmission of viral diseases. Caution with known allergy to proteins of porcine origin; may cause severe allergic reactions. Not interchangeable with other pancrelipase products. Should not be mixed directly into formula or breast milk.

ADVERSE REACTIONS: Abdominal pain, flatulence, diarrhea, N/V, constipation, pruritus, urticaria, rash.

PREGNANCY: Category C, caution in nursing.

MECHANISM OF ACTION: Pancreatic enzyme supplement; catalyze the hydrolysis of fats to monoglyceride, glycerol and free fatty acids, proteins into peptides and amino acids, and starches into dextrins and short chain sugars, such as maltose and maltriose in the duodenum and proximal small intestine, thereby acting like digestive enzymes physiologically secreted by the pancreas.

NURSING CONSIDERATIONS

Assessment: Assess for allergy to porcine proteins, gout, renal impairment, hyperuricemia, and pregnancy/nursing status.

Monitoring: Monitor for fibrosing colonopathy, stricture formation, oral mucosa irritation, viral diseases, and for allergic reactions. Monitor serum uric acid levels and renal function.

Patient Counseling: Instruct to take medication with food. Inform that if a dose is missed to take next dose with the next meal/snack as directed; instruct that doses should not be doubled. Counsel not to crush or chew the caps and its contents. Instruct to swallow intact caps with adequate amounts of liquid at mealtimes. Inform that contents can also be sprinkled in soft acidic foods if necessary. Instruct to notify physician if pregnant/breastfeeding or are thinking of becoming pregnant/breastfeeding during therapy. Advise to contact physician immediately if allergic reactions develop.

Administration: Oral route. Take during meals or snacks, with sufficient fluid. Swallow caps whole. Refer to PI for further administration instructions. **Storage:** Do not store >25°C (77°F). Avoid heat. Store in a dry place in the original container. Keep container tightly closed between uses; protect from moisture.

PARCOPA

RX

levodopa - carbidopa (Schwarz)

THERAPEUTIC CLASS: Dopa-decarboxylase inhibitor/dopamine precursor

INDICATIONS: Treatment of symptoms of idiopathic Parkinson's disease, postencephalitic parkinsonism, and symptomatic parkinsonism.

DOSAGE: *Adults:* 25mg-100mg tab: Initial: 1 tab tid. Titrate: Increase by 1 tab qd or qod until 8 tabs/day. 10mg-100mg tab: Initial: 1 tab tid-qid. Titrate: Increase 1 tab qd or qod until 2 tabs qid. 70-100mg/day carbidopa required. Max: 200mg/day carbidopa. Levodopa must be d/c 12 hrs before starting carbidopa-levodopa.

HOW SUPPLIED: Tab, Disintegrating: (Carbidopa-Levodopa) 10mg-100mg*, 25mg-100mg*, 25mg-250mg* *scored

CONTRAINDICATIONS: MAOIs during or within 14 days of use; narrow-angle glaucoma; suspicious, undiagnosed skin lesions; history of melanoma.

WARNINGS/PRECAUTIONS: Dyskinesias and mental disturbances may occur. Caution with severe cardiovascular(CV) or pulmonary disease, bronchial asthma, renal or hepatic disease, endocrine disease, chronic wide-angle glaucoma, peptic ulcer, and MI with residual arrhythmias. Neuroleptic malignant syndrome (NMS) reported during dose reduction or withdrawal. Dark color may appear in saliva, urine, or sweat. May cause false (+) ketonuria or false (-) glucosuria (glucose-oxidase method).

ADVERSE REACTIONS: Dyskinesias, choreiform, dystonia and other involuntary movements, nausea.

INTERACTIONS: See Contraindications. Risk of postural hypotension with antihypertensives, selegiline. HTN and dyskinesia may occur with TCAs. Reduced effects with dopamine D_2 antagonists (eg, phenothiazines, butyrophenones, risperidone), isoniazid. Antagonized by phenytoin, papaverine, metoclopramide. Reduced bioavailability with iron salts, high-protein diets.

PREGNANCY: Category C, caution in nursing

MECHANISM OF ACTION: Carbidopa: Inhibits decarboxylation of peripheral levodopa. Levodopa: Crosses blood-brain barrier, converting into dopamine and thereby increasing concentrations in the brain.

PHARMACOKINETICS: Absorption: Carbidopa: Bioavailability (99%). **Elimination:** Urine.

NURSING CONSIDERATIONS

Assessment: Assess for glaucoma, CV or pulmonary disease, melanoma, asthma, phenylketonuria, or any other conditions where treatment is contraindicated or cautioned. Assess LFTs, renal function, CBC, pregnancy/nursing status, and possible drug interactions.

Monitoring: Monitor for cardiac, hepatic/renal functions during initial dosage adjustment period, depression and suicidal ideation, worsening of dyskinesia, rhabdomyolysis, diarrhea, hallucinations, fibrotic complications, hyperpyrexia, melanomas, IOP, and hypersensitivity reactions.

Patient Counseling: Instruct to take as prescribed. Caution while operating machinery/driving. Discoloration of body fluids may occur. High-protein diet, excessive acidity, and iron salts reduce clinical effectiveness. Wearing-off effect may be seen at end of dosing interval. Report any adverse effects. Place tablet on tongue and dissolve with saliva.

Administration: Oral route. **Storage:** 20-25°C (68-77°F); excursions permitted to 15-30°C (59-86°F).

PARLODEL   RX
bromocriptine mesylate (Novartis)

THERAPEUTIC CLASS: Dopamine receptor agonist

INDICATIONS: Treatment of dysfunctions associated with hyperprolactinemia, including amenorrhea with or without galactorrhea, infertility, or hypogonadism. Treatment of prolactin-secreting adenomas, acromegaly, and signs and symptoms of idiopathic or postencephalitic Parkinson's disease.

DOSAGE: *Adults:* Take with food. Hyperprolactinemia: Initial: 1/2-1 tab qd. Titrate: Additional 1 tab (2.5mg) may be added as tolerated every 2-7 days until optimal therapeutic response. Usual: 2.5-15mg/day. Acromegaly: Initial: 1/2-1 tab on retiring for 3 days. Titrate: Additional 1/2-1 tab should be added as tolerated every 3-7 days until optimal therapeutic benefit is obtained. Reevaluate monthly and adjust dose based on reductions of growth hormone (GH) or clinical response. Usual: 20-30mg/day. Max: 100mg/day. Withdraw for 4-8 weeks on a yearly basis if being treated with pituitary irradiation. Parkinson's Disease: Maintain levodopa dose during introductory period, if possible. Initial: 1/2 tab bid. Titrate: Individualize; may increase every 14-28 days by 2.5mg/day until max therapeutic response. If levodopa dose has to be reduced because of adverse reactions, increase the daily dose of bromocriptine gradually in small (2.5mg) increments. Max: 100mg/day. Elderly: Start at lower end of dosing range.
Pediatrics: Take with food. ≥16 yrs: Hyperprolactinemia: Initial: 1/2-1 tab qd. Titrate: Additional 1 tab (2.5mg) may be added as tolerated every 2-7 days until optimal therapeutic response. Usual: 2.5-15mg/day. Acromegaly: Initial: 1/2-1 tab on retiring for 3 days. Titrate: Additional 1/2-1 tab should be added as tolerated every 3-7 days until optimal therapeutic benefit is obtained. Reevaluate monthly and adjust dose based on reductions of GH or clinical response. Usual: 20-30mg/day. Max: 100mg/day. Withdraw for 4-8 weeks on a yearly basis if being treated with pituitary irradiation. Parkinson's Disease: Maintain levodopa dose during introductory period, if possible. Initial: 1/2 tab bid. Titrate: Individualize; may increase every 14-28 days by 2.5mg/day until max therapeutic response. If levodopa dose has to be reduced because of adverse reactions, increase the daily dose of bromocriptine gradually in small (2.5mg) increments. Max: 100mg/day. 11-15 yrs: Prolactin-Secreting Pituitary Adenoma: Initial: 1/2-1 tab qd. Titrate: May increase dose as tolerated until a therapeutic response is achieved. Usual: 2.5-10mg/day.

HOW SUPPLIED: Cap: 5mg; Tab: 2.5mg* *scored

CONTRAINDICATIONS: Uncontrolled HTN, postpartum period in women with history of coronary artery disease (CAD) and other severe cardiovascular (CV) conditions unless withdrawal is medically contraindicated, pregnancy if treating hyperprolactinemia. Hypertensive disorders of pregnancy if used to treat acromegaly, prolactinoma, or Parkinson's disease, unless withdrawal is medically contraindicated.

WARNINGS/PRECAUTIONS: Perform complete evaluation of pituitary before treatment. Carefully observe if pregnancy occurs; safety during pregnancy not established. Somnolence and sudden sleep onset may occur, particularly to patients with Parkinson's disease; consider dose reduction or d/c. May impair physical/mental abilities. Symptomatic hypotension may occur. HTN, myocardial infarction (MI), seizures, and strokes reported (rare) in postpartum women; avoid in prevention of physiological lactation. D/C if HTN, severe, progressive or unremitting headache, or evidence of CNS toxicity develops. Pleural and pericardial effusions, pleural and pulmonary fibrosis, constrictive pericarditis, and retroperitoneal fibrosis reported, particularly on long-term and high-dose treatment; consider d/c if diagnosed or suspected. Caution with history of psychosis or CV disease. Avoid with hereditary problems of galactose intolerance, severe lactase deficiency, or glucose-galactose malabsorption. Visual field deterioration may develop; monitor visual fields with macroprolactinoma and consider dose reduction. Use contraceptive measures, other than PO contraceptives, during treatment. Cerebrospinal fluid rhinorrhea reported in patients with prolactin-secreting adenomas. Cold-sensitive digital vasospasm and possible tumor expansion reported in acromegalic patients; d/c if tumor expansion develops. May cause severe GI bleeding in patients with peptic ulcers. Safety during long-term use (>2 yrs) for Parkinson's disease not established. Evaluate hepatic, hematopoietic, CV, and renal function periodically. May cause confusion and mental disturbances with high-doses; caution with dementia. Reduce dose or d/c if hallucination occurs. May cause intense urges (eg, to gamble, have sex, or spend money uncontrollably); consider dose reduction or d/c. Caution with history of MI with residual atrial, nodal, or ventricular arrhythmia. Regularly monitor for melanomas. Symptom complex resembling the neuroleptic malignant syndrome (NMS) reported with rapid dose reduction, withdrawal of, or changes in antiparkinsonian therapy. Caution in elderly.

ADVERSE REACTIONS: Confusion, hallucinations, headache, drowsiness, visual disturbance, hypotension, nasal congestion, N/V, dizziness, constipation, anorexia, dry mouth, dyspepsia.

INTERACTIONS: Not recommended with other ergot alkaloids. May potentiate side effects with alcohol. May interact with dopamine antagonists, butyrophenones, and certain other agents. May decrease efficacy with phenothiazines, haloperidols, metoclopramide, and pimozide. Caution with strong CYP3A4 inhibitors (eg, azole antimycotics, HIV protease inhibitors). May increase plasma levels with macrolide antibiotics (eg, erythromycin), octreotide, and inhibitors and/or potent substrates for CYP3A4. Caution with drugs that can alter blood pressure (eg, vasoconstrictor such as sympathomimetics); concomitant use in puerperium is not recommended.

PREGNANCY: Category B, not for use in nursing.

MECHANISM OF ACTION: Dopamine receptor agonist; activates postsynaptic dopamine receptors and modulates prolactin secretion from anterior pituitary by secreting prolactin inhibitory factor.

PHARMACOKINETICS: Absorption: C_{max}=465ng/mL (fasted, 2 x 2.5mg), 628pg/mL (5mg bid); AUC=2377pg•hr/mL; T_{max}=2.5 hrs. **Distribution:** Plasma protein binding (90-96%). **Metabolism:** Liver (extensive), via CYP3A; hydroxylation. **Elimination:** Feces (82%), urine (5.6%); $T_{1/2}$=4.85 hrs.

NURSING CONSIDERATIONS

Assessment: Assess for previous hypersensitivity to ergot alkaloids, uncontrolled HTN, history of CAD or other severe CV conditions, pituitary tumors, dementia, history of psychosis, pleuropulmonary disorders, history of peptic ulcer or GI bleeding, hereditary problems of galactose intolerance, severe lactase deficiency or glucose-galactose malabsorption, macroadenomas, renal/hepatic disease, pregnancy/nursing status, and for possible drug interactions. Perform complete pituitary evaluation.

Monitoring: Monitor for GI bleeding, somnolence, sudden sleep onset, hypotension, HTN, seizures, stroke, MI, pleural and pericardial effusions, pleural and pulmonary fibrosis, constrictive pericarditis, retroperitoneal fibrosis, visual disturbances, cold sensitive digital vasospasm, peptic ulcers, enlargement of preexisiting prolactin-secreting tumor, symptom complex resembling NMS, confusion and mental disturbances. Monitor BP, CBC, prolactin levels, LFTs, and renal function. Monitor visual fields in patients with macroprolactinoma; rapidly progressive visual field loss should be evaluated by a neurosurgeon. Evaluate periodically for hepatic, hematopoietic, CV, and renal function.

Patient Counseling: Inform that dizziness, drowsiness, faintness, fainting, and syncope may occur during treatment. Advise that somnolence and episodes of sudden sleep onset may occur and instruct not to engage in activities that require alertness (eg, driving or operating machinery), when experiencing these episodes. Instruct patients with hyperprolactinemic states associated with macroadenoma or those who have had previous transsphenoidal surgery to report any persistent watery nasal discharge. Inform patients with macroadenoma that d/c of therapy may be associated with rapid regrowth of tumor and recurrence of their original symptoms. Advise of the possibility that patients may experience intense urges to gamble, have sex, or spend money uncontrollably and the inability to control these urges while on therapy. Inform that hypotensive reactions may occasionally occur and result in reduced alertness.

Administration: Oral route. **Storage:** <25°C (77°F).

P

PARNATE   RX

tranylcypromine sulfate (GlaxoSmithKline)

> Antidepressants increased the risk of suicidal thinking and behavior (suicidality) in short-term studies in children, adolescents, and young adults with major depressive disorder (MDD) and other psychiatric disorders. Monitor and observe closely for clinical worsening, suicidality, or unusual changes in behavior in patients who are started on antidepressant therapy. Tranylcypromine is not approved for use in pediatric patients.

THERAPEUTIC CLASS: Monoamine oxidase inhibitor

INDICATIONS: Treatment of major depressive episode without melancholia.

DOSAGE: *Adults:* Usual: 30mg qd in divided doses. Titrate: If no improvement after 2 weeks, may increase by 10mg/day increments every 1-3 weeks. Max: 60mg/day.

HOW SUPPLIED: Tab: 10mg

CONTRAINDICATIONS: Concomitant use with MAO inhibitors or dibenzazepine derivatives, sympathomimetics (eg, amphetamines) or OTC drugs such as cold, hay fever, weight-reducing products that contain vasoconstrictors, some CNS depressants (eg, narcotics and alcohol), antihypertensive agents, diuretics, antihistamine, sedative or anesthetic drugs, bupropion, buspirone, dextromethorphan, SSRIs (eg, fluoxetine, paroxetine, sertraline), meperidine, anesthetic agents, anti-parkinsonism drugs, cheese or other foods with a high tyramine content, or excessive quantities of caffeine. Cerebrovascular disorders, cardiovascular disease (CVD), HTN, history of headaches, pheochromocytoma, history of liver disease, abnormal LFTs. Elective surgery requiring general anesthesia.

WARNINGS/PRECAUTIONS: Anxiety, agitation, panic attacks, insomnia, irritability, hostility, aggressiveness, impulsivity, akathisia, hypomania, mania reported. D/C if hypertensive crisis (eg, occipital headache, neck stiffness or soreness, N/V, tachycardia, bradycardia), palpitations, and/or frequent headaches occur. Hypotension reported. Caution in epileptic patients; may lower seizure threshold. D/C at first sign of hepatic dysfunction or jaundice; monitor LFTs periodically. Caution in patients with renal dysfunction, hyperthyroidism, elderly and diabetics taking insulin or glycemic agents. Drug dependency possible in doses excessive of the therapeutic range. May suppress anginal pain in myocardial ischemia. May precipitate mixed/manic episode in patients at risk for bipolar disorder; adequately screen patients to determine risk prior to initiating treatment. May impair mental/physical abilities.

ADVERSE REACTIONS: Restlessness, insomnia, weakness, drowsiness, nausea, diarrhea, tachycardia, anorexia, edema, tinnitus, muscle spasm, overstimulation, dizziness, dry mouth.

INTERACTIONS: See Contraindications. Caution with disulfiram. Additive hypotensive effects with phenothiazines. Tryptophan may precipitate disorientation, memory impairment and other neurological and behavioral signs. Avoid metrizamide; d/c 48 hrs before myelography and may resume 24 hrs post-procedure. Concurrent use with guanethidine, methyldopa, reserpine, dopamine, levodopa may precipitate HTN, headache and related symptoms.

PREGNANCY: Safety in pregnancy and nursing not known.

MECHANISM OF ACTION: Non-hydrazine MAOI; inhibits monoamine oxidase, increasing concentration of epinephrine, norepinephrine, and serotonin in storage sites throughout the nervous system.

NURSING CONSIDERATIONS

Assessment: Assess for risk of bipolar disorder, history of CVD, HTN, history of headaches, cerebrovascular disease, pheochromocytoma, seizure disorder, hyperthyroidism, DM, history of hepatic impairment, severe renal impairment, suicidal thinking and behavior, pregnancy/nursing status, and possible drug interactions.

Monitoring: Monitor BP, HR, renal/hepatic function, for signs and symptoms of clinical worsening, hypertensive crisis, seizures in epileptic patients, postural hypotension, and hypoglycemia in diabetics.

Patient Counseling: Inform family and caregivers the need to monitor for emergence of agitation, irritability, unusual changes in behavior, suicidality; notify healthcare provider if symptoms occur. Report occurrences of headache or other unusual symptoms (eg, palpitations, tachycardia, severe constriction in the throat or chest, N/V). Advise to seek medical attention for symptoms of hypertensive crisis, hypoglycemia, or seizures. Inform of the possibility of hypotension, faintness, drowsiness. May impair performance of potentially hazardous tasks, such as driving a car or operating machinery. Advise to avoid concomitant intake of alcohol, foods with a high tyramine content (eg, cheese), dextromethorphan, excessive quantities of caffeine. Caution not to take concomitant prescription or OTC medications without advice of a physician.

Administration: Oral route. **Storage:** 15-30°C (59-86°F). Dispense in tight, light-resistant container.

PASER   RX
aminosalicylic acid (Jacobus)

THERAPEUTIC CLASS: Hydroxybenzoic acid derivative

INDICATIONS: Treatment of tuberculosis (TB) in combination with other active agents.

DOSAGE: *Adults:* 4g tid. Sprinkle on applesauce, yogurt, or mix with tomato or orange juice. *Pediatrics:* Use smaller doses corresponding to the adult dose (4g tid). Sprinkle on applesauce, yogurt, or mix with tomato or orange juice.

HOW SUPPLIED: Granules, Delayed-Release: 4g/pkt

CONTRAINDICATIONS: Severe renal disease.

WARNINGS/PRECAUTIONS: Monitor for rash, or signs of intolerance during first 3 months. D/C if hypersensitivity (rash), fever, or other premonitory signs of intolerance occur. Can desensitize by administering small, gradually increasing doses.

ADVERSE REACTIONS: Diarrhea, N/V, abdominal pain, fever, dermatitis, lymphoma-like syndrome, leukocytosis, eosinophilia, agranulocytosis, thrombocytopenia, Coombs' positive hemolytic anemia, jaundice, hypoglycemia.

INTERACTIONS: Reduces acetylation of isoniazid, especially in rapid acetylators. Decreases vitamin B_{12} absorption; consider vitamin B12 maintenance treatment. Decreases digoxin levels.

PREGNANCY: Category C, safety in nursing not known.

MECHANISM OF ACTION: Bacteriostatic agent; believed to inhibit folic acid synthesis and/or inhibition of synthesis of the cell-wall component, mycobactin, thus reducing iron uptake by *Mycobacterium tuberculosis.*

PHARMACOKINETICS: Absorption: C_{max}=20mcg/mL; T_{max}=6 hrs. **Distribution:** Plasma protein binding (50-60%), CSF penetration occurs only if the meninges is inflamed. **Metabolism:** Via acetylation. **Excretion:** Urine (80%); $T_{1/2}$=26.4 min.

NURSING CONSIDERATIONS

Assessment: Assess for hepatic/renal impairment, hypersensitivity reactions, pregnancy/nursing status, and possible drug interactions. Obtain baseline CBC and platelet count, FPG, urinalysis, hepatic/renal function.

Monitoring: Monitor for N/V, diarrhea, abdominal pain, hepatomegaly, lymphadenopathy, leucocytosis, eosinophilia. Monitor for rash or signs of intolerance during first 3 months. Monitor CBC and platelet count, FPG, urinalysis, hepatic/renal function.

Patient Counseling: Inform about risks and benefits of therapy. Instruct to d/c if hypersensitivity (eg, rash, fever, diarrhea) occurs. Inform that poor compliance in taking anti-TB drugs leads to treatment failure and resistance against organisms. Skeleton of the granules may be seen in stool. Sprinkle granules on acidic foods such as applesauce or yogurt or stir into a fruit drink and swirl to protect the coating from sinking. Store in refrigerator or freezer. Instruct not to use and inform pharmacist or physician if packets are swollen or the granules have lost their tan color and are dark brown or purple.

Administration: Oral route. Administer tid by suspension in an acidic drink or food (eg, applesauce, yogurt, tomato/orange juice) with pH<5. **Storage:** Store below 15°C (59°F), refrigerate or freeze. Packets may be stored at room temperature for short periods of time. Avoid excessive heat.

PATANOL   RX
olopatadine HCl (Alcon)

THERAPEUTIC CLASS: H_1-antagonist and mast cell stabilizer

INDICATIONS: Allergic conjunctivitis.

DOSAGE: *Adults:* 1 drop bid, q6-8h.
Pediatrics: ≥3 yrs: 1 drop bid, q6-8h.

HOW SUPPLIED: Sol: 0.1% [5mL]

WARNINGS/PRECAUTIONS: May re-insert contact lens 10 min after dosing if eye is not red. Not for injection or oral use.

ADVERSE REACTIONS: Headache, asthenia, blurred vision, burning, stinging, cold syndrome, dry eye, foreign body sensation, hyperemia, hypersensitivity, keratitis, lid edema, nausea, pharyngitis, pruritus, rhinitis.

PREGNANCY: Category C, caution in nursing.

MECHANISM OF ACTION: Antihistaminic drug; relatively selective histamine H_1-antagonist; inhibits the type 1 immediate hypersensitivity reaction, including inhibition of histamine induced effects on human conjunctival epithelial cells.

PHARMACOKINETICS: Absorption: C_{max}=0.5-1.3ng/mL; T_{max}=2 hrs. **Metabolism:** Metabolites: Mono-desmethyl and N-oxide. **Elimination:** Urine (60-70% parent drug).

NURSING CONSIDERATIONS

Assessment: Assess for drug hypersensitivity.

Monitoring: Monitor for headache and other adverse reactions.

Patient Counseling: Counsel not to wear contact lenses if eye is red; wait at least 10 min after instillation to wear contact lenses. Instruct to avoid touching tip of container to eye or any other surface to avoid contamination.

Administration: Ocular route. **Storage:** 4-25°C (39-77°F). Keep bottle tightly closed.

PAXIL   RX
paroxetine HCl (GlaxoSmithKline)

> Antidepressants increased the risk of suicidal thinking and behavior (suicidality) in short-term studies in children, adolescents, and young adults with major depressive disorder (MDD) and other psychiatric disorders. Monitor and observe closely for clinical worsening, suicidality, or unusual changes in behavior in patients who are started on antidepressant therapy. Not approved for use in pediatric patients.

THERAPEUTIC CLASS: Selective serotonin reuptake inhibitor

INDICATIONS: Treatment of MDD, panic disorder with or without agoraphobia, obsessive compulsive disorder (OCD), social anxiety disorder (SAD), generalized anxiety disorder (GAD), and post-traumatic stress disorder (PTSD).

DOSAGE: *Adults:* Give qd, usually in the am. To titrate, may increase in 10mg/day increments at intervals of ≥1 week. Maintain on the lowest effective dose and reassess periodically to determine the need for continued treatment. MDD: Initial: 20mg/day. Max: 50mg/day. Maint: Efficacy is maintained for periods of up to 1 year with doses that averaged about 30mg. OCD: Initial: 20mg/day. Usual: 40mg qd. Max: 60mg/day. Panic Disorder: Initial: 10mg/day. Usual: 40mg/day. Max: 60mg/day. GAD: Initial/Usual: 20mg/day. Dose range: 20-50mg/day. SAD: Initial/Usual: 20mg/day. Dose range: 20-60mg/day; no additional benefit for doses >20mg/day. PTSD: Initial: 20mg/day. Dose range: 20-50mg/day. Elderly/Debilitated/Severe Renal/Hepatic Impairment: Initial: 10mg/day. Max: 40mg/day. 3rd Trimester Pregnancy: Taper dose. Allow ≥14-day interval between d/c of MAOI and start of paroxetine HCl and vice versa. Use with Reversible MAOIs (eg, linezolid, methylene blue) and D/C of Treatment: Refer to PI.

HOW SUPPLIED: Sus: 10mg/5mL [250mL]; Tab: 10mg*, 20mg*, 30mg, 40mg *scored

CONTRAINDICATIONS: Use with MAOIs intended to treat depression with, or within 14 days of treatment. Do not start treatment in patients being treated with a reversible MAOI (eg, linezolid, methylene blue). Concomitant use with thioridazine or pimozide.

WARNINGS/PRECAUTIONS: Not approved for treatment of bipolar depression. Serotonin syndrome (eg, mental status changes, autonomic instability, neuromuscular aberrations, and/or GI symptoms) or neuroleptic malignant syndrome (NMS)-like reactions reported. Increased risk of congenital malformations reported in 1st trimester of pregnancy. Neonatal complications requiring prolonged hospitalization, respiratory support, and tube feeding may develop in neonates exposed in the late third trimester. Activation of mania/hypomania reported; caution in patients with a history of mania. Caution with history of seizures; d/c if seizures occur. Adverse reactions (eg, dysphoric mood, irritability) upon d/c reported; avoid abrupt withdrawal. Akathisia may develop. Hyponatremia reported; caution in elderly and volume-depleted patients. May increase risk of bleeding events. Bone fracture risk reported; consider pathological fracture in patients with unexplained bone pain, point tenderness, swelling, or bruising. Caution with disease/conditions that could affect metabolism or hemodynamic responses, narrow-angle glaucoma, severe renal/hepatic impairment, and in elderly and debilitated patients. May impair mental/physical abilities.

ADVERSE REACTIONS: Suicidality, somnolence, headache, insomnia, nausea, asthenia, abnormal ejaculation, dry mouth, constipation, dizziness, diarrhea, decreased libido, sweating, decreased appetite, tremor.

INTERACTIONS: See Contraindications. Serotonin syndrome or NMS-like reactions reported when used alone and in combination with serotonergic drugs (eg, triptans, fentanyl, lithium, tramadol, or St. John's wort), drugs that impair serotonin metabolism, antipsychotics, and dopamine antagonists. Use with other SSRIs, serotonin and norepinephrine reuptake inhibitors (SNRIs), or tryptophan is not recommended. Avoid alcohol. Concomitant use with aspirin (ASA), NSAIDs, warfarin, and other anticoagulants may increase risk of bleeding events. Use with diuretics may increase risk of developing hyponatremia. Metabolism and pharmacokinetics of paroxetine may be affected by induction or inhibition of drug-metabolizing enzymes. Increased levels with cimetidine. Reduced levels with phenobarbital, phenytoin, fosamprenavir/ritonavir. Increased phenytoin level after 4 weeks of coadministration reported. Caution with drugs that are metabolized by CYP2D6 (eg, antidepressants, phenothiazines, risperidone, type 1C antiarrhythmics) and with drugs that inhibit CYP2D6 (eg, quinidine). May increase levels of desipramine, risperidone, atomoxetine. May reduce efficacy of tamoxifen. May inhibit metabolism of TCAs; caution with concomitant use. May displace other highly protein-bound drugs. Decreased levels of digoxin seen; use caution. May increase procyclidine levels; reduce dose if anticholinergic effects are seen. Severe hypotension reported when added to chronic metoprolol treatment. May elevate theophylline levels. Caution with lithium.

PREGNANCY: Category D, caution in nursing.

MECHANISM OF ACTION: SSRI; inhibits CNS neuronal reuptake of serotonin.

PHARMACOKINETICS: Absorption: Complete; Tab (30mg): C_{max}=61.7ng/mL; T_{max}=5.2 hrs. **Distribution:** Plasma protein binding (93-95%); found in breast milk. **Metabolism:** Extensive; oxidation and methylation via CYP2D6. **Elimination:** Sol (30 mg): Urine (62%, metabolites; 2%, parent compound); feces (36%, metabolites; <1%, parent compound); Tab (30 mg): $T_{1/2}$=21 hrs.

NURSING CONSIDERATIONS

Assessment: Assess for history of seizures or mania, volume depletion, diseases/conditions that alter metabolism or hemodynamic responses, hepatic/renal impairment, narrow-angle glaucoma, previous hypersensitivity, pregnancy/nursing status, and for possible drug interactions. Assess use in the elderly or debilitated patients. Screen for bipolar disorder.

Monitoring: Monitor for signs/symptoms of clinical worsening, serotonin syndrome or NMS-like reactions, seizures, manic episodes, akathisia, bone fracture, hyponatremia especially in the elderly, and abnormal bleeding. Upon d/c, monitor for d/c symptoms. Periodically assess for need of therapy. Regularly monitor weight and growth of children and adolescents.

Patient Counseling: Instruct to swallow whole, not to chew or crush, and to avoid alcohol. Notify physician of all prescription, over-the-counter drugs currently taking or planning to take. Caution on risk of serotonin syndrome with concomitant use of triptans, tramadol, or other serotonergic agents. Instruct patient, families, and caregivers to report emergence of anxiety, agitation, panic attacks, insomnia, irritability, hostility, aggressiveness, impulsivity, akathisia, hypomania, mania, unusual changes in behavior, worsening of depression, and suicidal ideation, especially during drug initiation or dose adjustment. Caution against hazardous tasks (eg, operating machinery, driving). Inform that improvement may be noticed in 1-4 weeks; continue therapy as directed. Notify physician if pregnant/intend to become pregnant, or breastfeeding. Caution about concomitant use with NSAIDs, ASA, warfarin, or other drugs that affect coagulation.

Administration: Oral route. (Sus) Shake well before use. **Storage:** (Tab): 15-30°C (59-86°F). (Sus): ≤25°C (77°F).

P

PAXIL CR   RX
paroxetine HCl (GlaxoSmithKline)

> Antidepressants increased the risk of suicidal thinking and behavior (suicidality) in short-term studies in children, adolescents, and young adults with major depressive disorder (MDD) and other psychiatric disorders. Monitor and observe closely for clinical worsening, suicidality, or unusual changes in behavior in patients who are started on antidepressant therapy. Not approved for use in pediatric patients.

THERAPEUTIC CLASS: Selective serotonin reuptake inhibitor

INDICATIONS: Treatment of MDD, panic disorder with or without agoraphobia, social anxiety disorder (SAD), and premenstrual dysphoric disorder (PMDD).

DOSAGE: *Adults:* Give qd, usually in the am with/without food. MDD: Initial: 25mg/day. Titrate: May increase by 12.5mg/day at intervals of ≥1 week. Max: 62.5mg/day. Panic Disorder: Initial: 12.5mg/day. Titrate: May increase by 12.5mg/day at intervals of ≥1 week. Max: 75mg/day. Maint: Lowest effective dose. SAD: Initial: 12.5mg/day. Titrate: May increase by 12.5mg/day at intervals of ≥1 week. Max: 37.5mg/day. Maint: Lowest effective dose. PMDD: Initial: 12.5mg/day. Give either qd throughout menstrual cycle or limited to luteal phase. 25mg/day also shown to be effective. Titrate: Changes should occur at intervals of ≥1 week. Elderly/Debilitated/Severe Renal/Hepatic Impairment: Initial: 12.5mg/day. Max: 50mg/day. Third Trimester Pregnancy: Taper dose. Allow ≥14-day interval between d/c MAOI and start of paroxetine HCl and vice versa. Use with Reversible MAOIs (eg, linezolid, methylene blue) and D/C of Treatment: Refer to PI.

HOW SUPPLIED: Tab, Controlled-Release: 12.5mg, 25mg, 37.5mg

CONTRAINDICATIONS: Use with MAOIs intended to treat depression with, or within 14 days of treatment. Do not start treatment in patients being treated with a reversible MAOI (eg, linezolid, methylene blue). Concomitant use with thioridazine or pimozide.

WARNINGS/PRECAUTIONS: Not approved for treatment of bipolar depression. Serotonin syndrome (eg, mental status changes, autonomic instability, neuromuscular aberrations, and/or GI symptoms) or neuroleptic malignant syndrome (NMS)-like reactions reported. Increased risk of congenital malformations reported in first trimester of pregnancy. Neonatal complications requiring prolonged hospitalization, respiratory support, and tube feeding may develop in neonates exposed in the late third trimester. Activation of mania/hypomania reported; caution with a history of mania. Caution with history of seizures; d/c if seizures occur. Adverse reactions upon d/c (eg, dysphoric mood, irritability) reported; avoid abrupt withdrawal. Akathisia may develop. Hyponatremia reported; caution in elderly and volume-depleted patients. May increase risk of bleeding events. Bone fracture risk reported; consider pathological fracture in patients with unexplained bone pain, point tenderness, swelling, or bruising. Caution with disease/conditions that could affect metabolism or hemodynamic responses, narrow-angle glaucoma, severe renal/hepatic impairment, and in elderly and debilitated patients. May impair mental/physical abilities.

ADVERSE REACTIONS: Suicidality, somnolence, insomnia, nausea, asthenia, abnormal ejaculation, dry mouth, constipation, dizziness, diarrhea, decreased libido, sweating, abnormal vision, headache, tremor.

INTERACTIONS: See Contraindications. Serotonin syndrome or NMS-like reactions reported when used alone and in combination with serotonergic drugs (eg, triptans, fentanyl, lithium, tramadol, or St. John's wort), drugs that impair serotonin metabolism, antipsychotics, and dopamine antagonists. Use with other SSRIs, serotonin and norepinephrine reuptake inhibitors (SNRIs), or tryptophan is not recommended. Avoid alcohol. Concomitant use with aspirin (ASA), NSAIDs, warfarin, and other drugs that may affect coagulation may increase risk of bleeding events. Use with diuretics may increase risk of developing hyponatremia. Metabolism and pharmacokinetics may be affected by induction or inhibition of drug-metabolizing enzymes. Increased levels with cimetidine. Reduced levels with phenobarbital, phenytoin, fosamprenavir/ritonavir. Increased phenytoin level after 4 weeks of coadministration reported. Caution with drugs that are metabolized by CYP2D6 (eg, antidepressants, phenothiazines, risperidone, tamoxifen, type 1C antiarrhythmics) and with drugs that inhibit CYP2D6 (eg, quinidine). May increase levels of desipramine, risperidone, atomoxetine. May reduce efficacy of tamoxifen. May inhibit metabolism of TCAs; caution with concomitant use. May displace or be displaced by other highly protein-bound drugs. Decreased levels of digoxin seen; use caution. May increase procyclidine levels; reduce dose if anticholinergic effects are seen. Severe hypotension may occur when added to chronic metoprolol treatment. May elevate theophylline levels. Caution with lithium.

PREGNANCY: Category D, caution in nursing.

MECHANISM OF ACTION: SSRI; inhibits CNS neuronal reuptake of serotonin.

PHARMACOKINETICS: Absorption: Complete; administration of variable doses resulted in different parameters; T_{max}=6-10 hrs. **Distribution:** Plasma protein binding (93-95%); found in breast milk. **Metabolism:** Extensive; oxidation and methylation via CYP2D6. **Elimination:** Sol: Urine (62%, metabolites; 2%, parent); feces (36%, metabolites; <1%, parent). $T_{1/2}$=15-20 hrs.

NURSING CONSIDERATIONS

Assessment: Assess for history of seizures or mania, volume depletion, diseases/conditions that affect metabolism or hemodynamic response, hepatic/renal impairment, narrow-angle glaucoma, previous hypersensitivity, pregnancy/nursing status, and for possible drug interactions. Assess use in the elderly or debilitated patients. Screen for bipolar disorder.

Monitoring: Monitor for signs/symptoms of clinical worsening, serotonin syndrome or NMS-like reactions, seizures, mania, akathisia, bone fracture, hyponatremia especially in the elderly, and abnormal bleeding. Upon d/c, monitor for d/c symptoms. Periodically assess for need of therapy. Regularly monitor weight and growth of children and adolescents.

Patient Counseling: Inform patient to swallow whole, not to chew or crush, and to avoid alcohol use. Notify physician of all prescription, over-the-counter drugs currently taking or planning to take. Caution on risk of serotonin syndrome with concomitant use of triptans, tramadol, or other serotonergic agents. Instruct patient, families, and caregivers to report emergence of anxiety, agitation, panic attacks, insomnia, irritability, hostility, aggressiveness, impulsivity, akathisia, hypomania, mania, unusual changes in behavior, worsening of depression, and suicidal ideation, especially during drug initiation or dose adjustment. Caution against hazardous tasks (eg, operating machinery, driving). Inform that improvement may be noticed in 1-4 weeks; continue therapy as directed. Notify physician if pregnant/intend to become pregnant, or breastfeeding. Caution on concomitant use with NSAIDs, ASA, warfarin, or other drugs that affect coagulation.

Administration: Oral route. **Storage:** ≤25°C (77°F). (Generic) 20-25°C (68-77°F).

PEDIAPRED   RX
prednisolone sodium phosphate (CellTech)

THERAPEUTIC CLASS: Glucocorticoid

INDICATIONS: Steroid-responsive dermatoses.

DOSAGE: *Adults:* Initial: 5-60mg/day depending on disease and response. Maint: Decrease dose by small amounts to lowest effective dose. MS Exacerbations: 200mg qd for 1 week, then 80mg qod for 1 month.
Pediatrics: Initial: 0.14-2mg/kg/day given tid-qid. Nephrotic Syndrome: 20mg/m² tid for 4 weeks, then 40mg/m² qod for 4 weeks. Uncontrolled Asthma: 1-2mg/kg/day in single or divided doses until peak expiratory rate of 80% is achieved (usually 3-10 days).

HOW SUPPLIED: Sol: 5mg/5mL [120mL]

CONTRAINDICATIONS: Systemic fungal infections.

WARNINGS/PRECAUTIONS: May produce reversible hypothalamic-pituitary-adrenal axis suppression. Adjust dose during stress or change in thyroid status. May mask signs of infection or cause new infections. May activate latent amebiasis. Avoid with cerebral malaria. Avoid exposure to chickenpox or measles. Not for treatment of optic neuritis or active ocular herpes simplex. May cause elevation of BP or IOP, cataracts, glaucoma, optic nerve damage, Kaposi's sarcoma, psychic derangements, salt/water retention, increased excretion of K⁺ and/or calcium, osteoporosis, growth suppression in children, secondary ocular infections. Caution with strongyloides, chronic heart failure, diverticulitis, HTN, renal insufficiency, fresh intestinal anastomoses, active or latent peptic ulcer, ulcerative colitis. Enhanced effect in hypothyroidism or cirrhosis. Avoid abrupt withdrawal. Caution in elderly, increased risk of corticosteroid-induced side effects; start at low end of dosing range; monitor bone mineral density.

ADVERSE REACTIONS: Edema, fluid/electrolyte disturbances, osteoporosis, muscle weakness, pancreatitis, peptic ulcer, impaired wound healing, increased intracranial pressure, cushingoid state, hirsutism, menstrual irregularities, growth suppression in children, glaucoma, nausea, weight gain.

INTERACTIONS: Enhanced metabolism with barbiturates, phenytoin, ephedrine, and rifampin. Use with cyclosporine may increase activity of both drugs; convulsions reported with concomitant use. Decreased metabolism with estrogens or ketoconazole. May inhibit response to warfarin. Increased risk of GI side effects with aspirin or other NSAIDs. May increase clearance of salicylates. High doses or concurrent neuromuscular drugs may cause acute myopathy. Enhanced possibility of hypokalemia when given with K⁺-depleting agents. May produce severe weakness in myasthenia gravis patients on anticholinesterase agents. Avoid live vaccines with immunosuppressive doses. Possible diminished response with killed or inactivated vaccines. May increase blood glucose; adjust antidiabetic agents. May suppress reactions to skin tests.

PREGNANCY: Category C, caution in nursing.

MECHANISM OF ACTION: Synthetic adrenocorticoid steroid; promotes gluconeogenesis, increases deposition of glycogen in the liver, inhibits glucose utilization, increases catabolism of protein, lipolysis, glomerular filtration that leads to increased urinary excretion of urate and calcium.

PHARMACOKINETICS: Absorption: Rapidly absorbed from GI tract. **Distribution:** Plasma protein binding (70-90%); found in breast milk. **Metabolism:** Liver. **Elimination:** Urine (as sulfate and glucuronide congugates); $T_{1/2}$=2-4 hrs.

NURSING CONSIDERATIONS

Assessment: Assess for systemic fungal/other infections, active TB, vaccination history, HTN, CHF, renal insufficiency, ophthalmic disease, osteoporosis, thyroid status, hepatic impairment, nonspecific ulcerative colitis, ulcers, pregnancy/nursing status, and possible drug interactions.

Monitoring: Monitor for adrenocortical insufficiency, occurrence of infections, psychic derangement, cataracts, acute myopathy, Kaposi's sarcoma, fluid retention, and measurement of serum electrolytes, TSH, LFTs, glucose, IOP, and BP.

Patient Counseling: Advise not to d/c therapy abruptly or without medical supervision. Avoid exposure to chickenpox or measles; report immediately if exposed. Dietary salt restriction and K⁺ supplementation is advised.

Administration: Oral route. **Storage:** 4-25°C (39-77°F).

PEDIARIX   RX

pertussis vaccine acellular, adsorbed - hepatitis B (recombinant) - poliovirus vaccine, inactivated - diphtheria toxoid - tetanus toxoid (GlaxoSmithKline)

THERAPEUTIC CLASS: Vaccine/toxoid combination

INDICATIONS: Active immunization against diphtheria, tetanus, pertussis, all known subtypes of hepatitis B virus (HBV), and poliomyelitis in infants born of HBsAg-negative mothers, beginning as early as 6 weeks through 6 years (prior to 7th birthday).

DOSAGE: *Pediatrics:* 6 weeks to 6 yrs: 3 doses of 0.5mL IM at 2, 4, and 6 months (6-8 week intervals, preferably 8 weeks). May be used to complete the first 3 doses of DTaP series in children who have received 1 or 2 doses of Infanrix and are also scheduled to receive other vaccine components of Pediarix. May be used to complete the HBV vaccination series following 1 or 2 doses of another HBV vaccine including vaccines from other manufacturers in children born of HBsAg-negative mothers who are also scheduled to receive the other components of Pediarix. May be used to complete first 3 doses of the inactivated poliovirus vaccine (IPV) series in children who have received 1 or 2 doses of IPV from other manufacturers and are scheduled to receive other components of Pediarix. May use Infanrix and Kinrix to complete DTaP and IPV series; refer to prescribing information for further details.

HOW SUPPLIED: Inj: 0.5mL

CONTRAINDICATIONS: Encephalopathy (eg, coma, decreased level of consciousness, prolonged seizures) within 7 days of administration of a previous pertussis-containing vaccine that is not attributable to another identifiable cause, progressive neurologic disorder (including infantile spasms, uncontrolled epilepsy, or progressive encephalopathy). Hypersensitivity to yeast, neomycin, or polymyxin B.

WARNINGS/PRECAUTIONS: Use in infants is associated with higher risk of fever relative to separately administered vaccines. Evaluate potential benefits and risks if Guillain-Barre syndrome occurs within 6 weeks of receipt of a prior tetanus toxoid-containing vaccine. Tip cap and rubber plunger of prefilled syringes contain dry natural rubber latex; allergic reactions may occur in latex-sensitive individuals. Syncope may occur and can be accompanied by transient neurological signs. Caution if any of the following occur in temporal relation to receipt of a pertussis-containing vaccine: temperature ≥40.5°C (105°F) within 48 hrs not due to another identifiable cause; collapse or shock-like state occurring within 48 hrs; persistent, inconsolable crying lasting ≥3 hrs occurring within 48 hrs; or if seizures occur within 3 days. May administer an antipyretic at the time of vaccination and for the ensuing 24 hrs for children at higher risk for seizures. Apnea in premature infants following IM administration observed; decisions about when to administer vaccine should be based on consideration of potential benefits, medical status, and possible risks. Review immunization history for possible vaccine sensitivity; appropriate treatment should be available for possible allergic reactions.

ADVERSE REACTIONS: Local inj-site reactions (pain, redness, swelling), fever, irritability/fussiness, drowsiness, loss of appetite.

INTERACTIONS: Immunosuppressive therapies, including irradiation, antimetabolites, alkylating agents, cytotoxic drugs, and corticosteroids (used in greater than physiologic doses), may reduce immune response to vaccine.

PREGNANCY: Category C, safety not known in nursing.

MECHANISM OF ACTION: Vaccine/toxoid combination; stimulates immune system to elicit immune response, which produces neutralizing antibodies that may protect against diphtheria toxin, tetanus toxin, pertussis, hepatitis B, and poliovirus infections.

NURSING CONSIDERATIONS

Assessment: Review immunization history, current health/medical status (eg, immunosuppression), previous sensitivity related to yeast, neomycin, or polymyxin B. Assess for previous sensitivity/vaccination-related adverse reactions, progressive neurologic disorder, possible drug interactions, or for any other condition where treatment is cautioned or contraindicated. Assess use in premature infants.

Monitoring: Monitor for signs/symptoms of Guillain-Barre syndrome, allergic reactions, apnea in premature infants, syncope, and other adverse reactions.

Patient Counseling: Inform parents/guardians about potential benefits/risks of immunization, and of the importance of completing the immunization series. Advise parents/guardians about the potential for adverse reactions; instruct to report any adverse events to healthcare provider.

Administration: IM route. Do not administer IV, intradermally, or SQ. Refer to PI for preparation and administration instructions. Do not mix with any other vaccine in the same syringe or vial. Administer other vaccines separately, at different inj site. **Storage:** 2-8°C (36-46°F). Do not freeze. Discard if frozen.

PEGASYS RX
peginterferon alfa-2a (Roche)

> May cause or aggravate fatal or life-threatening neuropsychiatric, autoimmune, ischemic, and infectious disorders. Monitor closely with periodic clinical and laboratory evaluations. D/C with severe or worsening signs or symptoms of these conditions. Use with ribavirin may cause birth defects, fetal death, and hemolytic anemia. Refer to the individual PI for more information on ribavirin.

THERAPEUTIC CLASS: Pegylated virus proliferation inhibitor

INDICATIONS: Treatment of chronic hepatitis C (CHC) virus infection, alone or in combination with Copegus, in patients ≥5 yrs of age with compensated liver disease and not previously treated with interferon-alfa. Treatment of HBeAg-positive and HBeAg-negative chronic hepatitis B (CHB) in adults with compensated liver disease, evidence of viral replication, and liver inflammation.

DOSAGE: *Adults:* CHC: 180mcg SQ once weekly for 48 weeks. With Copegus: 180mcg SQ once weekly. Genotype 2 and 3: Treat for 24 weeks. Genotype 1 and 4: Treat for 48 weeks. CHC w/ HIV Coinfection: 180mcg SQ once weekly for 48 weeks. With Copegus: 180mcg SQ once weekly for 48 weeks, regardless of genotype. CHB: 180mcg SQ once weekly for 48 weeks. Refer to PI for dose modification and discontinuation. Renal Impairment: CrCl 30-50mL/min: 180mcg once weekly; CrCl <30mL/min, and with Hemodialysis: 135mcg once weekly. *Pediatrics:* ≥5 yrs: CHC: With Copegus: 180mcg/1.73m² x BSA SQ once weekly. Max: 180mcg SQ once weekly. Genotype 2 and 3: Treat for 24 weeks. For Other Genotypes: Treat for 48 weeks. Refer to PI for dose modification for neutropenia, increased ALT, and decreased platelets.

HOW SUPPLIED: Inj: 180mcg/0.5mL [prefilled syringe]; 180mcg/0.5mL, 135mcg/0.5mL [ProClick autoinjector]; 180mcg/mL [vial]

CONTRAINDICATIONS: Autoimmune hepatitis, hepatic decompensation (Child-Pugh score >6 [class B and C]) in cirrhotic patients before treatment, hepatic decompensation with Child-Pugh score ≥6 in cirrhotic CHC patients coinfected with HIV before treatment, neonates, and infants (contains benzyl alcohol). When used with Copegus, refer to PI for additional contraindications.

WARNINGS/PRECAUTIONS: Life-threatening neuropsychiatric reactions may occur; extreme caution with history of depression; d/c immediately in severe cases and institute psychiatric intervention. Caution with preexisting cardiac disease and autoimmune disorders. May cause bone marrow suppression and severe cytopenias; d/c if severe decrease in neutrophil or platelet count develop. May cause or aggravate hypothyroidism, hyperthyroidism, and pulmonary disorders. Hypoglycemia, hyperglycemia, diabetes mellitus (DM), ischemic and hemorrhagic cerebrovascular events, autoimmune/ophthalmologic disorders reported. CHC patients with cirrhosis may be at risk for hepatic decompensation and death. Exacerbation of hepatitis B reported; d/c immediately if hepatic decompensation with increase in ALT occurs. Serious infections, hypersensitivity reactions, ulcerative or hemorrhagic/ischemic colitis, and pancreatitis reported; d/c if any of these develop. D/C with new or worsening ophthalmologic disorders, pulmonary infiltrates or pulmonary function impairment, and pancytopenia. Peripheral neuropathy reported in combination with telbivudine. May delay growth in pediatric patients. Caution with CrCl <50mL/min and in elderly.

ADVERSE REACTIONS: Injection-site reactions, fatigue/asthenia, diarrhea, pyrexia, rigors, N/V, neutropenia, myalgia, headache, irritability/anxiety/nervousness, insomnia, depression.

INTERACTIONS: May inhibit CYP1A2 and increase area under the curve levels of theophylline; monitor theophylline serum levels and consider dose adjustments. May increase levels of methadone; monitor for toxicity. Hepatic decompensation can occur with concomitant use of nucleoside reverse transcriptase inhibitors (NRTIs) and peginterferon alfa-2a/ribavirin; refer to PI for respective NRTIs for guidance regarding toxicity management. Concomitant use of peginterferon alfa-2a/ribavirin with zidovudine may cause severe neutropenia and severe anemia; reduce dose or d/c if worsening clinical toxicities occur.

PREGNANCY: Category C, Category X (with ribavirin); not for use in nursing.

MECHANISM OF ACTION: Interferon alfa-2a; binds to human type 1 interferon receptor leading to receptor dimerization which activates multiple intracellular signal transduction pathways initially mediated by the JAK/STAT pathway. Expected to have pleiotropic biological effects in the body.

PHARMACOKINETICS: Absorption: T_{max}=72-96 hrs. **Elimination:** $T_{1/2}$=160 hrs (CHC).

NURSING CONSIDERATIONS

Assessment: Assess for neuropsychiatric, autoimmune, ischemic or infectious disorders, hepatic/renal impairment, risk of severe anemia, known hypersensitivity reactions, pregnancy/nursing status, possible drug interactions, or any other conditions where treatment is contraindicated or cautioned. Obtain baseline CBC, SrCr, TSH, LFTs, CD4⁺ (HIV), Hgb, Hct, and eye exam. Perform ECG for preexisting cardiac diseases prior to therapy. Obtain pregnancy test in women of childbearing potential.

Monitoring: Monitor for neuropsychiatric, autoimmune, ischemic, infectious disorders, bone marrow toxicities, CV disorders, cerebrovascular disorders, or other adverse effects. Monitor hematological (Weeks 2 and 4), biochemical tests (Week 4), LFTs, TSH (every 12 weeks). Perform periodic eye exams in patients with preexisting ophthalmologic disorders. Perform monthly pregnancy tests if on combination therapy with Copegus and for 6 months after d/c. Monitor CBC, clinical status, and hepatic/renal function.

Patient Counseling: Counsel on benefits and risks of therapy. Advise not to use drug in combination with Copegus for pregnant women or men whose female partners are pregnant; perform monthly pregnancy tests. Inform of the teratogenic/embryocidal risks; use two forms of effective

P

contraception during and for 6 months post therapy. Inform that drug is not known to prevent transmission of HCV/HBV infection to others; laboratory evaluation is required prior to therapy, and periodically thereafter. Counsel to avoid alcohol, and avoid driving or operating machinery if dizziness, confusion, somnolence, or fatigue occurs. Instruct to remain well hydrated, and not to switch to other brand of interferon without consulting physician. Instruct on the proper preparation, administration, and disposal techniques; do not reuse any needles and syringes.

Administration: SQ route. Administer in abdomen or thigh. **Storage:** 2-8°C (36-46°F). Do not leave out of the refrigerator for ≥24 hrs. Do not freeze or shake. Protect from light. Discard any unused portion.

PEG-INTRON RX

peginterferon alfa-2b (Schering)

> May cause or aggravate fatal or life-threatening neuropsychiatric, autoimmune, ischemic, and infectious disorders. Monitor closely with periodic clinical and laboratory evaluations. D/C with severe or worsening signs/symptoms of these conditions. Use with ribavirin may cause birth defects, fetal death, and hemolytic anemia. Refer to individual PI for more information on ribavirin.

THERAPEUTIC CLASS: Pegylated virus proliferation inhibitor

INDICATIONS: Treatment of chronic hepatitis C (CHC) in patients with compensated liver disease in combination with Rebetol (ribavirin) and an approved hepatitis C virus (HCV) NS3/4A protease inhibitor in patients ≥18 yrs with HCV genotype 1 infection. Treatment of CHC in patients with compensated liver disease in combination with Rebetol in patients with genotypes other than 1, pediatric patients (3-17 yrs), or in patients with genotype 1 infection where use of an HCV NS3/4A protease inhibitor is not warranted based on tolerability, contraindications or other clinical factors. Treatment of CHC as monotherapy in patients with compensated liver disease if there are contraindications to or significant intolerance of Rebetol and for use only in previously untreated adult patients.

DOSAGE: *Adults:* ≥18 yrs: Monotherapy: 1mcg/kg/week SQ for 1 yr. Combination Therapy: 1.5mcg/kg/week SQ with 800-1400mg Rebetol PO based on body weight; refer to PI of the specific HCV NS3/4A protease inhibitor for dosing regimen. Treatment with PegIntron/Rebetol of Interferon Alfa-Naive Patients: Genotype 1: Treat for 48 weeks. Genotype 2 and 3: Treat for 24 weeks. Retreatment with PegIntron/Rebetol of Prior Treatment Failures: Retreat for 48 weeks, regardless of HCV genotype. Refer to PI for volume of PegIntron to be injected, dose modifications, and discontinuation. CrCl 30-50mL/min: Reduce dose by 25%. Hemodialysis/CrCl 10-29mL/min: Reduce dose by 50%.
Pediatrics: 3-17 yrs: Combination with Rebetol: 60mcg/m²/week SQ with 15mg/kg/day Rebetol PO in 2 divided doses. Remain on pediatric dosing regimen if 18th birthday was reached while receiving therapy. Genotype 1: Treat for 48 weeks. Genotype 2 and 3: Treat for 24 weeks. Refer to PI for volume of PegIntron to be injected, dose modifications, and discontinuation. CrCl 30-50mL/min: Reduce dose by 25%. Hemodialysis/CrCl 10-29mL/min: Reduce dose by 50%.

HOW SUPPLIED: Inj: 50mcg/0.5mL, 80mcg/0.5mL, 120mcg/0.5mL, 150mcg/0.5mL [vial, Redipen]

CONTRAINDICATIONS: Autoimmune hepatitis, hepatic decompensation (Child-Pugh score >6 [class B and C]) in cirrhotic CHC patients before or during treatment. When used with Rebetol, refer to PI for additional contraindications.

WARNINGS/PRECAUTIONS: Life-threatening or fatal neuropsychiatric events reported; caution with history of psychiatric disorders. Monitor during treatment and in 6-month follow-up period if psychiatric problems develop; d/c therapy if symptoms persist or worsen. Cases of encephalopathy reported with higher doses. Cardiovascular (CV) events reported; caution with cardiovascular disease (CVD). Monitor patients with history of myocardial infarction (MI) and arrhythmia. May cause or aggravate hypothyroidism and hyperthyroidism. Ophthalmologic disorders may be induced or aggravated; conduct baseline eye exam and monitor periodically with preexisting conditions. D/C if new or worsening ophthalmologic disorders occur. Ischemic and hemorrhagic cerebrovascular events reported. May suppress bone marrow function; d/c if severe decreases in neutrophil or platelet count develop. May rarely be associated with aplastic anemia. Hyperglycemia, diabetes mellitus, autoimmune/pulmonary/dental/ and periodontal disorders, pancreatitis, colitis, increase in SrCr and ALT, hypersensitivity reactions, and elevated TG have been observed. Caution with autoimmune disorders and history of pulmonary disease. D/C if pancreatitis, ulcerative or hemorrhagic/ischemic colitis, or hypersensitivity reactions occur. CHC patients with cirrhosis may be at risk for hepatic decompensation and death. Monitor patients with renal impairment for toxicity; adjust dose or d/c therapy. Use caution and avoid concomitant Rebetol in CrCl <50mL/min. Peripheral neuropathy reported when used in combination with telbivudine. Inhibited growth velocity reported in pediatric use with combination therapy. Caution in elderly.

ADVERSE REACTIONS: Headache, fatigue/asthenia, rigors, N/V, abdominal pain, anorexia, emotional lability/irritability, myalgia, inj-site inflammation/erythema/reaction, fever, neutropenia.

INTERACTIONS: May increase methadone concentrations; monitor signs/symptoms of increased narcotic effect. May decrease therapeutic effects of CYP2C8/9 (eg, warfarin, phenytoin, tolbutamide) or CYP2D6 (eg, flecainide, dextromethorphan) substrates. Concomitant use of peginterferon alfa-2a/Rebetol with zidovudine may cause severe neutropenia and severe anemia.

PREGNANCY: Category C, Category X (with Rebetol); not for use in nursing.

MECHANISM OF ACTION: Pegylated virus proliferation inhibitor; binds to and activates the human type 1 interferon receptor. Upon binding, the receptor subunits dimerize and activate multiple intracellular signal transduction pathways.

PHARMACOKINETICS: Absorption: T_{max}=15-44 hrs. **Elimination:** $T_{1/2}$=40 hrs (HCV-infected).

NURSING CONSIDERATIONS

Assessment: Assess for history of psychiatric disorders, CVD, autoimmune and ophthalmologic disorders, hepatic/renal impairment, hypersensitivity reactions, pregnancy/nursing status, possible drug interactions, or any other condition where treatment is contraindicated or cautioned. Obtain baseline CBC, blood chemistry, and eye exam. Perform ECG in patients with preexisting cardiac abnormalities.

Monitoring: Monitor periodically CBC, blood chemistry, LFTs, renal function, TG levels, HCV RNA, and complete eye exam. Monitor for signs/symptoms of autoimmune, ischemic, infectious, endocrine, pulmonary, ophthalmologic, and cerebrovascular disorders, neuropsychiatric events, encephalopathy, bone marrow toxicity, hepatic decompensation, CV events, ulcerative or hemorrhagic/ischemic colitis, pancreatitis, hypersensitivity reactions, and cutaneous eruptions.

Patient Counseling: Inform about the benefits and risks associated with therapy. Advise to report any symptoms of depression or suicidal ideation to physician. Instruct to avoid pregnancy during treatment with combination therapy and for 6 months after therapy is d/c. Advise to administer drug hs or use antipyretics to minimize flu-like symptoms. Instruct to brush teeth bid and have regular dental examinations when used in combination with Rebetol. Inform that chest x-ray or other tests may be needed if fever, cough, SOB, or other symptoms of lung problems develop. Advise to keep well-hydrated. Instruct self-administering patients on the proper disposal of needles and syringes, caution against reuse, and to rotate inj sites.

Administration: SQ route. Refer to PI for preparation and instructions for use. Monotherapy: Administer on the same day of the week. Combination with Rebetol: Take with food. **Storage:** (Redipen) 2-8°C (36-46°F). Do not reuse. (Vials) 25°C (77°F); excursions permitted to 15-30°C (59-86°F). (Redipen/Vial) Reconstituted Sol: Use immediately, but may store for up to 24 hrs at 2-8°C (36-46°F). Do not freeze. Keep away from heat.

P

PENICILLIN VK   RX
penicillin V potassium (Various)

THERAPEUTIC CLASS: Penicillin

INDICATIONS: Treatment of mild to moderately severe bacterial infections, including infections of the respiratory tract, oropharynx, skin and soft tissue, and infections such as scarlet fever or mild erysipelas caused by susceptible strains of microorganisms. Prevention of recurrence following rheumatic fever and/or chorea. May be useful as prophylaxis against bacterial endocarditis in patients with congenital heart disease or rheumatic or other acquired valvular heart disease who are undergoing dental procedures and surgical procedures of the upper respiratory tract.

DOSAGE: *Adults:* Usual: Streptococcal Infections (Scarlet Fever/Erysipelas/Upper Respiratory Tract): 125-250mg q6-8h for 10 days. Pneumococcal Infections (Otitis Media/Respiratory Tract): 250-500mg q6h until afebrile for at least 2 days. Staphylococcus Infections (Skin/Soft Tissue)/Fusospirochetosis (Oropharnyx): 250-500mg q6-8h. Rheumatic Fever/Chorea Prevention: 125-250mg bid. Bacterial Endocarditis Prophylaxis: 2g one hr before procedure and then 1g after 6 hrs.
Pediatrics: ≥12 yrs: Usual: Streptococcal Infections (Scarlet Fever/Erysipelas/Upper Respiratory Tract): 125-250mg q6-8h for 10 days. Pneumococcal Infections (Otitis Media/Respiratory Tract): 250-500mg q6h until afebrile for at least 2 days. Staphylococcus Infections (Skin/Soft Tissue)/Fusospirochetosis (Oropharnyx): 250-500mg q6-8h. Rheumatic Fever/Chorea Prevention: 125-250mg bid. Bacterial Endocarditis Prophylaxis: 2g or 1g (<60 lbs) one hr before procedure and then 1g or 500mg (<60 lbs) after 6 hrs.

HOW SUPPLIED: Sus: 125mg/5mL [100mL, 200mL], 250mg/5mL [100mL, 200mL]; Tab: 250mg, 500mg

WARNINGS/PRECAUTIONS: Not for severe pneumonia, empyema, bacteremia, pericarditis, meningitis, and arthritis during the acute stage. PO (PCN) should not be used in patients at particularly high risk for endocarditis. Should not be used as adjunctive prophylaxis for genitourinary instrumentation/surgery, lower intestinal tract surgery, sigmoidoscopy, and childbirth. Serious and fatal anaphylactic reactions reported; caution with a history of hypersensitivity to PCN, cephalosporins, and/or multiple allergens. Caution with history of significant allergies and/or asthma. D/C if an allergic reaction occurs and institute appropriate therapy. *Clostridium difficile*-associated diarrhea (CDAD) reported. May result in bacterial resistance with prolonged use or use in the absence of a proven/suspected bacterial infection or a prophylactic indication; take appropriate measures if superinfection develops. May not be effective with severe illness, N/V, gastric dilatation, cardiospasm, or intestinal hypermotility. Obtain cultures following completion of treatment for streptococcal infections.

ADVERSE REACTIONS: Epigastric distress, N/V, diarrhea, hypersensitivity reactions, black hairy tongue, fever, eosinophilia.

PREGNANCY: Safety in pregnancy/nursing not known.

MECHANISM OF ACTION: PCN; exerts a bactericidal action against PCN-sensitive microorganisms during the stage of active multiplication. Acts through inhibition of biosynthesis of cell wall mucopeptide.

PHARMACOKINETICS: Distribution: Plasma protein binding (80%). **Elimination:** Urine.

NURSING CONSIDERATIONS

Assessment: Assess for previous hypersensitivity reactions to PCNs/cephalosporins or other allergens, history of asthma, N/V, gastric dilatation, severe illness, cardiospasm, intestinal hypermotility, and pregnancy/nursing status. Obtain cultures and sensitivity tests especially in suspected staphylococcal infections.

Monitoring: Monitor for signs/symptoms of hypersensitivity reactions, CDAD, overgrowth of nonsusceptible organisms, superinfections, and other adverse reactions. Obtain cultures following completion of treatment streptococcal infections.

Patient Counseling: Counsel that therapy only treats bacterial and not viral infections (eg, common cold). Instruct to take ud; inform that skipping doses or not completing the full course of therapy may decrease effectiveness of treatment and increase likelihood that bacteria may develop resistance to treatment. Inform that diarrhea may occur. Instruct to seek medical attention if watery and bloody stools occur even after two or more months of d/c therapy.

Administration: Oral route. **Storage:** 20-25°C (68-77°F). (Reconstituted Sus) Store in a refrigerator. Discard any unused portion after 14 days.

PENLAC RX
ciclopirox (Dermik)

THERAPEUTIC CLASS: Broad-spectrum antifungal

INDICATIONS: Mild to moderate onychomycosis of fingernails or toenails without lunula involvement due to *Trichophyton rubrum* (in immunocompetent patients).

DOSAGE: *Adults:* Apply qhs (or 8 hrs before washing) to nail bed, hyponychium, and under surface when it is free of nail bed. Apply daily over previous coat and remove with alcohol every 7 days. Repeat cycle up to 48 weeks.

HOW SUPPLIED: Sol: 8% [6.6mL]

WARNINGS/PRECAUTIONS: Only for use on nails and adjacent skin. Caution with removal of infected nail in insulin-dependent DM or diabetic neuropathy.

ADVERSE REACTIONS: Periungual erythema, erythema of proximal nail fold, nail shape change, nail irritation, ingrown toenail, nail discoloration.

INTERACTIONS: Avoid nail polish or other nail cosmetics on treated nails.

PREGNANCY: Category B, caution in nursing.

MECHANISM OF ACTION: Broad spectrum antifungal; acts by chelation of polyvalent cations (Fe^{+3} or Al^{+3}), resulting in the inhibition of the metal-dependent enzymes responsible for degradation of peroxides within fungal cell.

PHARMACOKINETICS: Absorption: Serum levels range from 12-80ng/mL following topical administration. **Elimination:** Urine (<5% of applied topical dose).

NURSING CONSIDERATIONS

Assessment: Assess use with insulin-dependent DM, diabetic neuropathy, and in pregnant/nursing females.

Monitoring: Monitor for signs/symptoms of sensitivity reactions and chemical irritation. Perform frequent (eg, monthly) removal of unattached infected nails, trimming of onycholic nails, and filing of any excess horny material.

Patient Counseling: Advise to avoid contact with eyes and mucous membranes. Apply medication evenly over entire nail plate and 5mm of surrounding skin. Notify physician if signs of increased irritation at the application site develop. File away (with emery board) loose nail material and trim nails as required. Do not use nail polish or other nail cosmetic products on the treated nails. Instruct not to use medication near open flame. Inform that it may take up to 48 weeks of daily application of the medication (including monthly professional removal of unattached infected nails) before a clear or almost clear nail is seen.

Administration: Topical route. **Storage:** 15-30°C (59-86°F). Flammable; keep away from heat and flame.

PENNSAID   RX
diclofenac sodium (Mallinckrodt)

NSAIDs may cause an increased risk of serious cardiovascular thrombotic events, MI, stroke and serious GI adverse events including bleeding, ulceration, and perforation of the stomach or intestines. Contraindicated for the treatment of perioperative pain in the setting of coronary artery bypass graft (CABG) surgery.

THERAPEUTIC CLASS: NSAID

INDICATIONS: Treatment of signs and symptoms of osteoarthritis of the knee(s).

DOSAGE: *Adults:* Usual: 40 drops per knee qid. Apply to clean, dry skin. Dispense 10 drops into the hand, or directly onto the knee. Spread evenly around front, back and sides of the knee. Repeat the procedure until 40 drops have been applied and the knee is completely covered. To treat the other knee, repeat the procedure.

HOW SUPPLIED: Sol: (1.5%) 150mL

CONTRAINDICATIONS: Aspirin (ASA) or other NSAID allergy that precipitates asthma, urticaria, or allergic reactions. Setting of coronary artery bypass graft (CABG) surgery.

WARNINGS/PRECAUTIONS: Not evaluated for use on spine, hip, or shoulder. May lead to onset of new HTN or worsening of preexisting HTN; monitor BP closely. Fluid retention and edema reported; caution with fluid retention or heart failure. Renal papillary necrosis and other renal injury reported after long-term use. Not recommended for use with advanced renal disease; if therapy must be initiated, monitor renal function. Anaphylactoid reactions may occur. May cause serious skin adverse events (eg, exfoliative dermatitis, Stevens-Johnson syndrome [SJS], and toxic epidermal necrolysis [TEN]). Avoid in late pregnancy; may cause premature closure of ductus arteriosus. May cause elevations of LFTs; d/c if liver disease develops or systemic manifestations occur. To minimize the potential for adverse liver-related events, use the lowest effective dose for the shortest duration possible. Caution in elderly. Anemia may occur; with long-term use, monitor Hgb/Hct if signs or symptoms of anemia develop. May inhibit platelet aggregation and prolong bleeding time; monitor with coagulation disorders. Caution with asthma and avoid with ASA-sensitive asthma. Patients should minimize or avoid exposure to natural or artificial sunlight on treated areas. Caution with history of ulcer or GI bleeding; monitor for signs or symptoms of GI bleeding. May diminish utility of diagnostic signs (eg, inflammation, fever) in detecting infectious complications of presumed noninfectious, painful conditions.

ADVERSE REACTIONS: Dyspepsia, dry skin, rash, pharyngitis, abdominal pain, infection, contact dermatitis, flatulence, pruritus, diarrhea, nausea, constipation, edema, paresthesia.

INTERACTIONS: Increased adverse effects with ASA; avoid use. Synergistic effects of anticoagulants such as warfarin on GI bleeding. May reduce natriuretic effect of furosemide and thiazides; monitor for signs of renal failure. May increase levels of lithium. Caution with methotrexate. Increased nephrotoxicity with cyclosporine. Avoid use with oral NSAID. Caution with drugs that are potentially hepatotoxic (eg, acetaminophen, certain antibiotics, antiepileptics). May impair response to therapies with ACE inhibitors, thiazide or loop diuretics.

PREGNANCY: Category C (prior to 30 weeks gestation); Category D (starting 30 weeks gestation), not for use in nursing.

MECHANISM OF ACTION: NSAID; inhibits enzyme, cyclooxygenase (COX), resulting in the reduced formation of prostaglandins, thromboxanes, and prostacylin.

PHARMACOKINETICS: Absorption: (Single Dose) C_{max}=8.1ng/mL; T_{max}=11 hrs; AUC_{0-t}=177.5ng.h/mL, AUC_{0-inf}=196.3ng.h/mL. (Multiple Dose) C_{max}=19.4ng/mL; T_{max}=4 hrs; AUC_{0-t}=695.4ng.h/mL, AUC_{0-inf}=745.2ng.h/mL. **Distribution:** Plasma protein binding (99%). **Metabolism:** 4'-hydroxy-diclofenac (major metabolite); glucuronidation or sulfation and oxidation. **Elimination:** Bile and urine; $T_{1/2}$= 36.7 hrs (single dose), 79 hrs (multiple dose).

NURSING CONSIDERATIONS

Assessment: Assess for hypersensitivity to ASA or NSAIDs, history of ulcer or GI bleeding, HTN, fluid retention, CHF, asthma, cardiovascular disease (or risk factors), renal/hepatic impairment, pregnancy/nursing status and possible drug interactions. Obtain baseline BP.

P

Monitoring: Monitor BP, LFTs, and renal function periodically. Monitor for signs/symptoms of cardiovascular events, GI events (eg, ulcerations, bleeding), hepatotoxicity, renal dysfunction, HTN, skin reactions, anemia, blood loss and hypersensitivity reactions.

Patient Counseling: Inform about the possible effects of the drug (eg, cardiovascular effects, GI effects, hepatotoxicity, weight gain/edema, anaphylactoid reactions, effects during pregnancy). Avoid contact with eyes and mucosa. Do not apply to open skin wounds, infections, inflammations or exfoliative dermatitis. Avoid exposure on treated knees to natural or artificial sunlight. Avoid showering/bathing for at least 30 min after application. Wash and dry hands after use. Do not apply external heat and/or occlusive dressings to treated area. Avoid wearing clothing or applying other topical products until treated knee is dry.

Administration: Topical route. **Storage:** 25°C (77°F); excursions permitted to 15°-30°C (50°-86°F).

PENTASA   RX
mesalamine (Shire)

THERAPEUTIC CLASS: 5-Aminosalicylic acid derivative

INDICATIONS: Induction of remission and for treatment of mild to moderate active ulcerative colitis.

DOSAGE: *Adults:* 1g qid. Can be given up to 8 weeks.

HOW SUPPLIED: Cap, Controlled-Release: 250mg, 500mg

WARNINGS/PRECAUTIONS: Caution with hepatic and renal dysfunction; monitor closely. Nephrotoxicity should be suspected in patients developing renal dysfunction during treatment. D/C if acute intolerance syndrome develops (eg, cramping, bloody diarrhea, abdominal pain, headache). If rechallenge is considered, perform under careful observation.

ADVERSE REACTIONS: Diarrhea, headache, nausea, abdominal pain.

PREGNANCY: Category B, caution in nursing.

MECHANISM OF ACTION: 5-aminosalicylic acid derivative; mechanism unknown. Suspected to diminish inflammation by blocking cyclooxygenase and inhibiting prostaglandin production in the colon.

PHARMACOKINETICS: Absorption: C_{max}=1mcg/mL, T_{max}=3 hrs. (N-acetylmesalamine) C_{max}=1.8mcg/mL, T_{max}=3 hrs. **Distribution:** Crosses the placenta; found in breast milk. **Metabolism:** N-acetylmesalamine (Metabolite). **Elimination:** Feces, urine (19-30%, N-acetylmesalamine).

NURSING CONSIDERATIONS

Assessment: Assess for preexisting renal disease, hepatic/renal function, hypersensitivity to the drug or salicylates, and pregnancy/nursing status. Obtain baseline LFTs, BUN, creatinine, and urinalysis (protein).

Monitoring: Monitor LFTs, BUN, creatinine, and urinalysis (protein) periodically. Monitor signs/symptoms of hepatotoxicity, acute intolerance syndrome (cramping, acute abdominal pain, bloody diarrhea), hypersensitivity, allergic reactions, and nephrotoxicity.

Patient Counseling: Advise to take as prescribed. Seek medical attention if symptoms of hepatotoxicity, acute intolerance syndrome (cramping, acute abdominal pain, bloody diarrhea), hypersensitivity and allergic reactions occur.

Administration: Oral route. **Storage:** 25°C (77°F); excursions permitted to 15-30°C (59-86°F).

PERCOCET   CII
oxycodone HCl - acetaminophen (Endo)

Associated with cases of acute liver failure, at times resulting in liver transplant and death. Most cases associated with acetaminophen (APAP) doses >4000 mg/day and involved more than one APAP-containing product.

OTHER BRAND NAMES: Endocet (Endo)

THERAPEUTIC CLASS: Opioid analgesic

INDICATIONS: Relief of moderate to moderately severe pain.

DOSAGE: *Adults:* Individualize dose. (325mg-2.5mg) 1 or 2 tabs q6h. Max: 12 tabs/day. (325mg-5mg) 1 tab q6h prn. Max: 12 tabs/day. (325mg-7.5mg) 1 tab q6h prn. Max: 8 tabs/day. (500mg-7.5mg) 1 tab q6h prn. Max: 8 tabs/day. (325mg-10mg) 1 tab q6h prn. Max: 6 tabs/day. (650mg-10mg) 1 tab q6h prn. Max: 6 tabs/day. Do not exceed 4g/day of APAP.

HOW SUPPLIED: Tab: (APAP-Oxycodone) 325mg-5mg*, 325mg-7.5mg, 325mg-10mg, 500mg-7.5mg, 650mg-10mg, (Percocet) 325mg-2.5mg *scored

CONTRAINDICATIONS: Oxycodone: Significant respiratory depression (in unmonitored settings or absence of resuscitative equipment), acute or severe bronchial asthma or hypercarbia, suspected or known paralytic ileus.

WARNINGS/PRECAUTIONS: Caution with CNS depression, elderly/debilitated, severe hepatic/renal/pulmonary impairment, hypothyroidism, Addison's disease, prostatic hypertrophy, urethral stricture, acute alcoholism, delirium tremens, kyphoscoliosis with respiratory depression, myxedema, and toxic psychosis. May obscure the diagnosis or clinical course of acute abdominal conditions. Oxycodone: May cause drug dependence and tolerance; has abuse potential. May cause respiratory depression; extreme caution in acute asthma, chronic obstructive pulmonary disease, cor pulmonale, or preexisting respiratory impairment; consider non-opioid alternatives or use lowest effective dose and monitor carefully. Respiratory depressant effects may be exaggerated with head injury, intracranial lesions, or pre-existing increased intracranial pressure; may obscure neurological signs of worsening in patients with head injuries. May cause severe hypotension in patients whose ability to maintain blood pressure has been compromised and orthostatic hypotension in ambulatory patients. May decrease bowel motility; monitor for ileus in postoperative patients. May cause spasm of the sphincter of Oddi and increase in serum amylase; caution with biliary tract disease including acute pancreatitis. May aggravate convulsions and seizures. Avoid abrupt d/c; may precipitate withdrawal symptoms. Anaphylaxis reported in patients with codeine hypersensitivity. APAP: Hypersensitivity/anaphylaxis reported; d/c if signs/symptoms occur. Increased risk of acute liver failure with underlying liver disease.

ADVERSE REACTIONS: Lightheadedness, dizziness, drowsiness, N/V, sedation, respiratory depression, apnea, respiratory arrest, circulatory depression, hypotension, shock.

INTERACTIONS: Oxycodone: Severe hypotension may occur when coadministered with drugs which compromise vasomotor tone (eg, phenothiazines). May enhance neuromuscular-blocking action of skeletal muscle relaxants and increase respiratory depression. Additive CNS depression with other opioid analgesics, general anesthetics, centrally acting anti-emetics, phenothiazines, tranquilizers, sedatives-hypnotics, and other CNS depressants (eg, alcohol); reduce dose of one or both agents. Caution with concurrent agonist/antagonist analgesics (eg, pentazocine, nalbuphine, naltrexone and butorphanol) use; may reduce analgesic effect of oxycodone and/or precipitate withdrawal symptoms. May produce paralytic ileus with anticholinergics. APAP: Increased risk of acute liver failure with alcohol ingestion; hepatotoxicity reported in chronic alcoholics. Increase in glucuronidation and plasma clearance as well as decreased half-life with oral contraceptives. Increased effects with propranolol and probenecid. May decrease effects of loop diuretics, lamotrigine, and zidovudine.

PREGNANCY: Category C, not for use in nursing.

MECHANISM OF ACTION: Oxycodone: Opioid analgesic; semisynthetic pure opioid agonist whose principal therapeutic action is analgesia. Effects mediated by CNS receptors (eg, μ and kappa) for endogenous opioid-like compounds (eg, endorphins, enkephalins). APAP: Nonopiate, nonsalicyclic analgesic, and antipyretic; not established. Antipyretic effect produced through inhibition of endogenous pyrogen action on the hypothalamic heat-regulating centers.

PHARMACOKINETICS: Absorption: APAP: Rapid. Oxycodone: Absolute bioavailability (87%). **Distribution:** APAP/Oxycodone: Found in breast milk. Oxycodone: Plasma protein binding (45%); (IV) V_d=211.9L; crosses the placenta. **Metabolism:** APAP: Liver via CYP450, conjugation with glucuronic acid, sulfuric acid and cysteine; NAPQI (toxic metabolite). Oxycodone: N-dealkylation, O-demethylation via CYP2D6; noroxycodone, oxymorphone (metabolites). **Elimination:** APAP: Urine (90-100%). Oxycodone: Urine (8-14% unchanged); $T_{1/2}$=3.51 hrs.

NURSING CONSIDERATIONS

Assessment: Assess for drug hypersensitivity, severity and type of pain, respiratory depression, bronchial asthma, hypercarbia, paralytic ileus, level of consciousness, alcohol consumption, pregnancy/nursing status, renal/hepatic function, drug abuse potential, possible drug interactions, or any other conditions where treatment is contraindicated or cautioned.

Monitoring: Monitor for signs/symptoms of respiratory depression, elevations in CSF pressure, altered consciousness, hypotension, hepatotoxicity, convulsions, anaphylactic reactions, decreased bowel motility in postoperative patients, spasm of sphincter of Oddi, serum amylase levels, physical dependence and tolerance, abuse or misuse of medication, hypersensitivity reactions, and withdrawal syndrome during d/c.

Patient Counseling: Advise to d/c and contact physician immediately if develop signs of allergy (eg, rash, difficulty breathing). Inform to not take >4g/day of APAP and to contact physician if exceed the recommended dose. Advise to dispose of unused drug by flushing down toilet. Inform that drug may impair mental/physical abilities required to perform hazardous tasks (eg, operating machinery/driving). Instruct to avoid alcohol or other CNS depressants. Advise to not adjust dose without consulting physician and to not abruptly d/c if on treatment for more than a few weeks. Advise that drug has a potential for abuse; protect from theft. Notify physician if pregnant, planning to become pregnant or are breastfeeding.

Administration: Oral route. **Storage:** 20-25°C (68-77°F).

PERCODAN CII
oxycodone HCl - aspirin (Endo)

OTHER BRAND NAMES: Endodan (Endo)

THERAPEUTIC CLASS: Opioid analgesic

INDICATIONS: Management of moderate to moderately severe pain.

DOSAGE: *Adults:* Usual: 1 tab q6h PRN for pain. Dose should be adjusted according to severity of pain and patient response. Max: (aspirin [ASA]) Should not exceed 4g/day or 12 tabs/day.

HOW SUPPLIED: Tab: (ASA-Oxycodone HCl) 325mg-4.8355mg* *scored

CONTRAINDICATIONS: ASA: Hemophilia, viral infection in children/teens with or w/o fever. Oxycodone: Significant respiratory depression (in unmonitored settings or absence of resuscitative equipment), acute/severe bronchial asthma or hypercarbia, known/suspected paralytic ileus.

WARNINGS/PRECAUTIONS: Oxycodone: May cause drug dependence and tolerance; potential for abuse. May cause respiratory depression; extreme caution in acute asthma, chronic obstructive pulmonary disease, cor pulmonale, or preexisting respiratory impairment; use lowest dose and carefully supervise administration, or consider non-opioid alternatives; may use reversal agent (eg, naloxone hydrochloride). Caution in elderly/debilitated. Respiratory depressant effects may be markedly exaggerated in the presence of head injury, intracranial lesions, or pre-existing increased intracranial pressure and may obscure neurological signs of worsening in patients with head injuries. May cause severe hypotension in patients whose ability to maintain blood pressure has been compromised and orthostatic hypotension in ambulatory patients. Monitor for decreased bowel motility in postoperative patients. May cause spasm of the sphincter of Oddi and increase in serum amylase; caution with biliary tract disease including acute pancreatitis. Caution with acute alcoholism, hypothyroidism, Addison's disease, prostatic hypertrophy, urethral stricture, delirium tremens, kyphoscoliosis with respiratory depression, myxedema, toxic psychosis, and biliary disease. May aggravate convulsions and seizures. Avoid abrupt d/c; may cause the precipitation of withdrawal symptoms. ASA: May inhibit platelet function and cause gastric mucosal irritation and bleeding; caution with peptic ulcer or coagulation abnormalities and alert for GI ulceration and bleeding even without previous GI symptoms. Avoid in pregnancy, especially during the third trimester and during labor and delivery, severe renal failure (GFR <10mL/min), and severe hepatic insufficiency. May cause elevated hepatic enzymes, BUN, creatinine, and amylase, hyperkalemia, proteinuria, and prolonged bleeding time.

ADVERSE REACTIONS: Respiratory depression, apnea, respiratory arrest, circulatory depression, hypotension, shock, dependence, tolerance.

INTERACTIONS: ASA: May lead to high serum concentrations of acetazolamide. May diminish hyponatremic and hypotensive effects of angiotensin converting enzyme inhibitors. May increase serum concentrations of acetazolamide, causing toxicity. Increased risk for bleeding with anticoagulants (eg, warfarin, heparin) and chronic, heavy alcohol use. May decrease the total concentration of phenytoin and increase serum valproic acid levels. May diminish hypotensive effects of β-blockers. May diminish effectiveness of diuretics. Avoid NSAIDs; may increase bleeding or lead to decreased renal function. May enhance the serious side effects and toxicity of ketorolac and methotrexate. Antagonizes the uricosuric action of probenecid or sulfinpyrazone. May increase the serum glucose-lowering action of insulin and sulfonylureas leading to hypoglycemia. Oxycodone: May enhance neuromuscular-blocking action of skeletal muscle relaxants. Additive CNS depression with other opioid analgesics, general anesthetics, centrally acting anti-emetics, phenothiazines, tranquilizers, sedatives-hypnotics, and other CNS depressants (eg, alcohol); reduce dose of one or both agents. May cause severe hypotension with drugs which compromise vasomotor tone (eg, phenothiazines). Agonist/antagonist analgesics (eg, pentazocine, nalbuphine, naltrexone, and butorphanol) may reduce analgesic effect and/or may precipitate withdrawal symptoms; administer with caution. (Percodan) Decreased clearance with CYP3A4 inhibitors and increase/prolong opioid effects. Decreased plasma concentration with CYP450 inducers, reducing opioid efficacy or causing abstinence syndrome in physical dependence. Caution when initiating therapy and consider dose adjustment until stable drug effects achieved.

PREGNANCY: Category B (Oxycodone) and D (ASA), not for use in nursing.

MECHANISM OF ACTION: ASA: Acetylsalicylic acid; inhibits prostaglandin production, including those involved in inflammation. In CNS, works on hypothalamus heat-regulating center to reduce fever. Oxycodone: Semisynthetic pure opioid agonist; principal therapeutic effect is analgesia. Other effects include anxiolysis, euphoria, and feelings of relaxation. Effects mediated by CNS receptors (eg, μ, kappa) for endogenous opioid-like compounds (eg, endorphins, enkephalins).

PHARMACOKINETICS: Absorption: ASA: Rapidly absorbed. Oxycodone: Absolute bioavailability (87%). **Distribution:** ASA: Found in most body tissues, fluids (eg, fetal tissues, breast milk, CNS, liver, kidneys); variable serum protein binding; crosses placenta. Oxycodone: Plasma protein binding (45%); found in breast milk, crosses placenta and blood brain barrier; (IV) V_d=211.9L. **Metabolism:** ASA: Liver (first pass) via microsomal enzymes and gut wall, hydrolysis to salicylate, salicyluric acid, salicyl phenolic glucuronide, salicyl acyl glucuronide, gentisic acid, gentisuric acid (major metabolites). Oxycodone: Extensive, liver (first pass); N-dealkylation, O-demethylation, glucuronidation, N-demethylation, ketoreduction; CYP3A4 (major), CYP2D6; noroxycodone (primary), oxymorphone, noroxymorphone (active metabolites). **Elimination:** ASA: Urine (80%-100%; 10% unchanged salicylates, 90% metabolites); $T_{1/2}$=15 min (ASA), 2-3 hrs (salicylates). Oxycodone: Urine (8-14% parent compound; metabolites); $T_{1/2}$=3.51 hrs.

NURSING CONSIDERATIONS

Assessment: Assess for drug hypersensitivity, bleeding disorders, viral infection, respiratory depression, bronchial asthma, hypercarbia, paralytic ileus, level of consciousness, alcohol consumption, pregnancy/nursing status, drug abuse potential, possible drug interactions, or any other conditions where treatment is contraindicated or cautioned.

Monitoring: Monitor for signs/symptoms of respiratory depression, presence of elevated CSF pressure and level of consciousness, GI ulceration and/or bleeding, platelet function/coagulation panel, anaphylactic reactions, decreased bowel motility in post-op patients, spasms of sphincter of Oddi, physical dependence and tolerance, abuse or misuse of medication, hypersensitivity reactions, and withdrawal syndrome during d/c.

Patient Counseling: Instruct if accidental ingestion occurs, seek medical attention. Advise to dispose of unused drug via toilet. Advise to consult physician before adjusting dosing. Warn patient that drug has potential for abuse and may impair mental/physical abilities. Instruct to avoid alcohol and other CNS depressants; report adverse events (eg, respiratory depression); protect drug from theft and do not give to anyone; consult physician before taking the product if pregnant, plan to become pregnant, and nursing. Advise that drug may cause or worsen constipation.

Administration: Oral route. In cessation of therapy, taper dose gradually until d/c. **Storage:** 25°C (77°F); excursions permitted to 15-30°C (59-86°F). Dispense in a tight, light-resistant container.

PERFOROMIST RX
formoterol fumarate (Dey)

Long-acting β_2-adrenergic agonists (LABA) may increase risk of asthma-related death. Contraindicated in asthma without use of a long-term asthma control medication.

THERAPEUTIC CLASS: Beta$_2$-agonist

INDICATIONS: Long-term maint treatment of bronchoconstriction in patients with chronic obstructive pulmonary disease (COPD), including chronic bronchitis and emphysema.

DOSAGE: *Adults:* 20mcg bid (am and pm) by nebulization. Max: 40mcg/day.

HOW SUPPLIED: Sol, Inhalation: 20mcg/2mL

CONTRAINDICATIONS: Asthma without use of a long-term asthma control medication.

WARNINGS/PRECAUTIONS: Not for acutely deteriorating COPD, or relief of acute symptoms (eg, as rescue therapy for treatment of acute episodes of bronchospasm). Cardiovascular (CV) effects and fatalities reported with excessive use; do not use excessively or with other LABA. D/C if paradoxical bronchospasm or CV effects occur. ECG changes reported. Caution with CV disorders (eg, coronary insufficiency, cardiac arrhythmias, HTN), convulsive disorders, thyrotoxicosis, and unusual responsiveness to sympathomimetic amines. Hypokalemia, hyperglycemia, and immediate hypersensitivity reactions may occur.

ADVERSE REACTIONS: Diarrhea, nausea, CV events, COPD exacerbation, nasopharyngitis, dry mouth.

INTERACTIONS: Adrenergic drugs may potentiate sympathetic effects; use with caution. Xanthine derivatives, steroids, or diuretics may potentiate any hypokalemic effect. ECG changes and/or hypokalemia that may result from non-K$^+$ sparing diuretics (eg, loop/thiazide diuretics) can be acutely worsened; use with caution. MAOIs, TCAs, and drugs known to prolong QTc interval may potentiate effect on CV system; use with extreme caution. β-blockers may block effects and produce severe bronchospasm in COPD patients; if needed, consider cardioselective β-blocker with caution.

PREGNANCY: Category C, caution in nursing.

MECHANISM OF ACTION: LABA (β_2-agonist); acts as bronchodilator, stimulates intracellular adenyl cyclase, the enzyme that catalyzes the conversion of ATP to cyclic-3',5'-adenosine monophosphate (cAMP). Increased cAMP levels cause relaxation of bronchial smooth muscle and inhibition of release of mediators of immediate hypersensitivity from cells, especially from mast cells.

PHARMACOKINETICS: Distribution: Plasma protein binding (61-64%). **Metabolism:** Direct glucuronidation via UGT1A1, 1A8, 1A9, 2B7, 2B15; O-demethylation via CYP2D6, 2C19, 2C9, 2A6. **Elimination:** Urine (1.1-1.7%, unchanged).

NURSING CONSIDERATIONS

Assessment: Assess for acute COPD deteriorations, asthma, use of control medication, CV disorders, convulsive disorders, thyrotoxicosis, unusual responsiveness to sympathomimetic amines, diabetes mellitus (DM), pregnancy/nursing status, and possible drug interactions.

Monitoring: Monitor for signs of COPD destabilization, serious asthma exacerbations, paradoxical bronchospasm, CV effects, hypokalemia, hyperglycemia, aggravation of DM and ketoacidosis, and immediate hypersensitivity reactions. Monitor pulse rate, BP, ECG changes, serum K⁺ and blood glucose levels.

Patient Counseling: Inform of the risks and benefits of therapy. Instruct to seek medical attention if symptoms worsen despite recommended doses, if treatment becomes less effective, or if needs more inhalations of a short-acting β_2-agonist than usual. Advise not to ingest inhalation sol, and not to exceed prescribed dose or d/c unless directed by physician. Instruct to d/c regular use of short-acting β_2-agonists (eg, albuterol) and use only for symptomatic relief of acute symptoms. Counsel not to use with other inhalers containing LABA or mix with other drugs. Inform of the common adverse reactions (eg, palpitations, chest pain, rapid heart rate).

Administration: Oral inhalation route. Administer only via standard jet nebulizer (PARI-LC Plus) connected to an air compressor (Proneb) with adequate airflow and equipped with a facemask or mouthpiece. Remove from foil pouch only immediately before use. **Storage:** Prior to Dispensing: 2-8°C (36-46°F). After Dispensing: 2-25°C (36-77°F) for ≤3 months. Protect from heat.

PEXEVA   RX
paroxetine mesylate (Noven)

Antidepressants increased the risk of suicidal thinking and behavior (suicidality) in short-term studies in children, adolescents, and young adults with major depressive disorder (MDD) and other psychiatric disorders. Monitor and observe closely for clinical worsening, suicidality or unusual changes in behavior in patients who are started on antidepressant therapy. Paroxetine is not approved for use in pediatric patients.

THERAPEUTIC CLASS: Selective serotonin reuptake inhibitor

INDICATIONS: Treatment of MDD, obsessive compulsive disorder (OCD), panic disorder with or without agoraphobia, and generalized anxiety disorder (GAD).

DOSAGE: *Adults:* Give qd, usually in the am. To titrate, may increase weekly by 10mg/day. MDD: Initial: 20mg/day. Max: 50mg/day. OCD: Initial: 20mg/day. Usual: 40mg/day. Max: 60mg/day. Panic Disorder: Initial: 10mg/day. Usual: 40mg/day. Max: 60mg/day. GAD: Initial: 20mg/day. Usual: 20-50mg/day. Elderly/Debilitated/Severe Renal or Hepatic Impairment: Initial: 10mg/day. Max: 40mg/day.

HOW SUPPLIED: Tab: 10mg, 20mg*, 30mg, 40mg *scored

CONTRAINDICATIONS: Concomitant use of MAOIs, thioridazine, and pimozide.

WARNINGS/PRECAUTIONS: Avoid use in bipolar depression. Potentially life-threatening serotonin syndrome and neuroleptic malignant syndrome (NMS)-like reactions reported. Increased risk of congenital malformations reported in infants. Activation of mania/hypomania reported; caution with history of mania. Caution with history of seizures; d/c if seizures occur. Akathisia may develop. Hyponatremia reported, caution in elderly and volume-depleted patients. May increase risk of bleeding events. Caution with conditions that affect metabolism or hemodynamic responses, narrow-angle glaucoma and hepatic/renal impairment. May impair mental/physical abilities. Dysphoric mood, irritability, agitation, dizziness, sensory disturbances, anxiety, confusion, headache, lethargy, emotional lability, insomnia, and hypomania reported upon d/c; avoid abrupt withdrawal.

ADVERSE REACTIONS: Asthenia, sweating, nausea, decreased appetite, somnolence, dizziness, insomnia, tremor, nervousness, abnormal ejaculation, dry mouth, constipation, decreased libido, impotence, headache.

INTERACTIONS: See Contraindications. Serotonin syndrome or NMS-like reactions reported when used alone and in combination with serotonergic drugs (eg, triptans, linezolid, lithium, tramadol, or St. John's wort), drugs that impair serotonin metabolism, antipsychotics, and dopamine antagonists. Use with other SSRIs, SNRIs, or tryptophan is not recommended. Caution with warfarin, phenobarbital, phenytoin, lithium, and digoxin. Avoid alcohol. Concomitant use with ASA, NSAIDs, warfarin, and other anticoagulants may increase risk of bleeding events. Use with diuretics may increase risk of developing hyponatremia. Increased levels with cimetidine. Caution with drugs that are metabolized by CYP2D6 (eg, antidepressants, phenothiazines, risperidone, Type 1C antiarrhythmics) and with drugs that inhibit CYP2D6 (eg, quinidine). May increase levels of risperidone. May increase levels of atomoxetine; may require dose adjustments. May impair metabolism of TCAs, caution with concomitant use. May shift concentrations when concomitantly used with highly protein-bound drugs. May increase procyclidine and theophylline levels. Severe hypotension reported when added to chronic metoprolol treatment. Decreased level with fosamprenavir/ritonavir.

PREGNANCY: Category D, caution in nursing.

MECHANISM OF ACTION: SSRI; inhibits CNS neuronal reuptake of serotonin.

PHARMACOKINETICS: Absorption: Complete; C_{max}=81.3ng/mL; T_{max}=8.1 hrs. **Distribution:** Plasma protein binding (95%); found in breast milk. **Metabolism:** Extensive; oxidation and methylation via CYP2D6. **Elimination:** Urine (62% metabolites; 2% parent compound); feces (36% metabolites; <1% parent compound); $T_{1/2}$=33.2 hrs.

NURSING CONSIDERATIONS

Assessment: Assess for bipolar disorder risk, history of seizures, history of mania, volume depletion, diseases/conditions that alter metabolism or hemodynamic responses, hepatic/renal impairment, narrow-angle glaucoma, pregnancy/nursing status, and for possible drug interactions. Assess use in the elderly.

Monitoring: Monitor for signs/symptoms of clinical worsening (eg, suicidality, unusual changes in behavior), serotonin syndrome or NMS-like reactions, seizures, and hyponatremia. Upon d/c, monitor for symptoms of dysphoric mood, irritability, agitation, dizziness, sensory disturbances, anxiety, confusion, headache, lethargy, emotional lability, insomnia, and hypomania.

Patient Counseling: Instruct to swallow whole, not to chew or crush. Advise to avoid alcohol. Seek medical attention for symptoms of serotonin syndrome, abnormal bleeding (particularly if using NSAIDs, ASA, warfarin), akathisia, hyponatremia, mydriasis, activation of mania, seizures, clinical worsening, or d/c symptoms (irritability, agitation, dizziness, anxiety, headache, insomnia). Caution against hazardous tasks (eg, operating machinery and driving). Inform may notice improvement in 1-4 weeks; continue therapy as directed. Notify physician if pregnant, intend to become pregnant, or are breastfeeding. Counsel about benefits and risks of therapy. Inform physician if taking, or plan to take, any prescription or OTC drugs.

Administration: Oral route. **Storage:** 25°C (77°F); excursions permitted to 15-30°C (59-86°F). Protect from humidity.

PHENERGAN INJECTION RX
promethazine HCl (Baxter)

Do not use in pediatric patients <2 yrs because of potential for fatal respiratory depression. Caution when used in pediatrics ≥2 yrs. Injection may cause severe chemical irritation and damage to tissue regardless of the route of administration. Irritation and damage may result from perivascular extravasation, unintentional intra-arterial injection, or intraneuronal/perineuronal infiltration; surgical intervention may be required. Preferred route of administration is deep IM injection.

THERAPEUTIC CLASS: Phenothiazine derivative

INDICATIONS: Amelioration of allergic reactions to blood or plasma. In anaphylaxis as an adjunct to epinephrine and other standard measures after acute symptoms have been controlled. For other uncomplicated allergic conditions of the immediate type when oral therapy is not possible or contraindicated. For sedation and relief of apprehension to produce light sleep. Active treatment of motion sickness. Prevention and control of N/V associated with certain types of anesthesia and surgery. Adjunct to analgesics for the control of postoperative pain. Preoperative, postoperative, and obstetric (during labor) sedation. IV in special surgical situations such as repeated bronchoscopy, ophthalmic surgery, and poor-risk patients, with reduced amounts of meperidine or other narcotic analgesic as adjunct to anesthesia and analgesia.

DOSAGE: *Adults:* (IM/IV) IM route is preferred. Allergy: Initial: 25mg, may repeat within 2 hrs. Adjust to the smallest adequate amount to relieve symptoms. For continued therapy, oral route preferred. Sedation: 25-50mg qhs in hospitalized patients. N/V: Usual: 12.5-25mg, not to be repeated more frequently than q4h. Preoperative/Postoperative Adjunct: 25-50mg. May be combined with appropriately reduced doses of analgesics and atropine-like drugs. Obstetrics: 50mg in early stages of labor, 25-75mg in established labor may be given with an appropriately reduced dose of any desired narcotic, may repeat once or twice q4h in normal labor. Max: 100mg/24 hrs of labor. Do not give IV administration >25mg/mL and at a rate >25mg/min. Elderly: Start at lower end of dosing range.
Pediatrics: ≥2 yrs: Dose should not exceed half of suggested adult dose. Premedication Adjunct: Usual: 1.1 mg/kg body weight in combination with an appropriately reduced dose of narcotic or barbiturate and appropriate dose of an atropine-like drug. Do not give IV administration >25mg/mL and at a rate >25mg/min.

HOW SUPPLIED: Inj: 25mg/mL, 50mg/mL

CONTRAINDICATIONS: Children <2 yrs, comatose states, intra-arterial or SQ injection.

WARNINGS/PRECAUTIONS: Not recommended for uncomplicated vomiting in pediatrics. May impair physical/mental ability. Fatal respiratory depression reported; avoid with compromised respiratory function or patients at risk of respiratory failure (eg, COPD, sleep apnea). May lower seizure threshold. Caution with bone marrow depression; leukopenia and agranulocytosis reported. Neuroleptic malignant syndrome (NMS) reported. Sulfite sensitivity may occur; caution especially in asthmatics. Avoid in pediatrics with Reye's syndrome or other hepatic diseases. Hallucinations and convulsions may occur in pediatrics. Increased susceptibility to dystonias in acutely ill pediatric patients with dehydration. May inhibit platelet aggregation in the newborn when used in pregnant women within 2 weeks of delivery. Caution with narrow-angle glaucoma, prostatic hypertrophy, stenosing peptic ulcer, bladder-neck or pyloroduodenal obstruction, cardiovascular (CV) disease, hepatic dysfunction. Cholestatic jaundice reported. May cause false interpretations of diagnostic pregnancy tests and may increase blood glucose. Caution in elderly.

ADVERSE REACTIONS: Respiratory depression, severe tissue injury, drowsiness, dizziness, tinnitus, blurred vision, dry mouth, increased or decreased BP, urticaria, N/V, blood dyscrasia, gangrene.

INTERACTIONS: Concomitant use with respiratory depressants in pediatric patients may result in death. May increase, prolong, or intensify sedation when used concomitantly with CNS depressants (eg, alcohol, sedative/hypnotics [including barbiturates], general anesthetics, narcotics, TCAs, tranquilizers); avoid concomitant use or reduce dose. Reduce dose of barbiturates by at least 50% if given concomitantly. Reduce dose of narcotics by 25-50% if given concomitantly. Caution with drugs that alter seizure threshold (eg, narcotics, local anesthetics). Leukopenia and agranulocytosis reported when used with other known marrow-toxic agents. Do not use epinephrine for promethazine injection overdose. Caution with anticholinergics. Possible adverse reactions with MAOIs. NMS reported alone and in combination with antipsychotics.

PREGNANCY: Category C, not for use in nursing.

MECHANISM OF ACTION: Phenothiazine derivative/H_1 receptor antagonist; possesses antihistamine (does not block release of histamine), sedative, anti-motion sickness, antiemetic, and anticholinergic effects.

PHARMACOKINETICS: Metabolism: Liver; sulfoxides, N-desmethylpromethazine (metabolites). **Elimination:** Urine; $T_{1/2}$=9-16 hrs (IV), 9.8 hrs (IM).

NURSING CONSIDERATIONS

Assessment: Assess for history of seizure disorder, compromised respiratory function or risk of respiratory failure (eg, COPD, sleep apnea), bone marrow depression, sulfite hypersensitivity, asthma, narrow-angle glaucoma, prostatic hypertrophy, stenosing peptic ulcer, pyloroduodenal obstruction, bladder-neck obstruction, CV disease, hepatic impairment, pregnancy/nursing status, and for possible drug interactions. Assess age of patient and presence of a comatose state. In pediatrics, assess for Reye's syndrome or presence of acute illness with dehydration.

Monitoring: Monitor for signs/symptoms of respiratory depression, seizures, leukopenia, agranulocytosis, NMS, cholestatic jaundice, injection-site reactions, and for hypersensitivity reactions. Monitor for hallucinations, convulsions, extrapyramidal symptoms and dystonia in pediatrics. In newborns, monitor platelet count, when used in pregnant women within 2 weeks of delivery.

Patient Counseling: Advise regarding risk of respiratory depression and risk of tissue injury. May impair physical/mental abilities. Seek medical attention if symptoms of respiratory depression, seizures, infections, NMS (hyperpyrexia, muscle rigidity, autonomic instability), injection site reactions (burning, pain, erythema), or hypersensitivity reactions occur. Avoid alcohol, certain other medications with possible interactions, and prolonged sun exposure.

Administration: IV, IM route. If pain occurs during IV injection, stop immediately and evaluate for possible arterial injection or perivascular extravasation. Inspect before use and discard if either color or particulate is observed. **Storage:** 20-25°C (68-77°F). Protect from light.

PHENOBARBITAL
phenobarbital (Various)

THERAPEUTIC CLASS: Barbiturate

INDICATIONS: Treatment of generalized, tonic-clonic and cortical focal seizures. For relief of anxiety, tension and apprehension. Short-term treatment of insomnia.

DOSAGE: *Adults:* Sedation: 30-120mg/day given bid-tid. Max: 400mg/24h. Hypnotic: 100-200mg. Seizures: 60-200mg/day. Elderly/Debilitated/Renal or Hepatic Dysfunction: Reduce dosage.
Pediatrics: Seizures: 3-6mg/kg/day.

HOW SUPPLIED: Elixir: 20mg/5mL; Tab: 15mg, 30mg, 32.4mg, 60mg, 64.8mg, 100mg

CONTRAINDICATIONS: Respiratory disease with dyspnea or obstruction, porphyria, severe liver dysfunction. Large doses with nephritic patients.

WARNINGS/PRECAUTIONS: May be habit-forming. Avoid abrupt withdrawal. Caution with acute or chronic pain; may mask symptoms or paradoxical excitement may occur. Cognitive deficits reported in children with febrile seizures. May cause excitement in children; excitement, depression or confusion in elderly, debilitated. Caution with hepatic dysfunction, borderline hypoadrenal function, depression.

ADVERSE REACTIONS: Drowsiness, residual sedation, lethargy, vertigo, somnolence, respiratory depression, hypersensitivity reactions, N/V, headache.

INTERACTIONS: May be potentiated by MAOIs, antihistamines, alcohol, tranquilizers, sedative/hypnotics, other CNS depressants. Decreases effects of oral anticoagulants and oral contraceptives. Increases corticosteroid metabolism. Decreases absorption of griseofulvin. Decreases half-life of doxycycline. May alter phenytoin metabolism. Increased levels with sodium valproate and valproic acid.

PREGNANCY: Category D, caution in nursing.

MECHANISM OF ACTION: Barbiturate; nonselective CNS depressant. Capable of producing all levels of CNS mood alteration. Responsible for depressing the sensory cortex, decreasing motor activity, altering cerebellar function, causing sedation and hypnosis.

PHARMACOKINETICS: Distribution: Distributed to all tissues and fluids. High concentrations found in the brain, liver, and kidneys. Found in breast milk. **Metabolism:** Hepatic. **Elimination:** Urine (primary), feces; $T_{1/2}$=79 hrs (adults), 110 hrs (children and newborns less than 48 hrs old).

NURSING CONSIDERATIONS

Assessment: Assess for history of manifest or latent porphyria, hepatic impairment, or respiratory disease with evidence of dyspnea or obstruction. Assess use in children, pregnant/nursing women, history of drug abuse, elderly or debilitated patients, acute or chronic pain, borderline hypoadrenal function, and history of depression or suicidal tendencies. Assess for possible drug interactions.

Monitoring: For patients on prolonged therapy, perform periodic evaluations of hematopoietic, renal/hepatic function. Monitor for signs of psychological/physical dependence, cognitive deficits in children, signs/symptoms of CNS depression, acute intoxication of medication (eg, unsteady gait, slurred speech), signs of chronic intoxication (eg, confusion, insomnia), and for exfoliative dermatitis (eg, Stevens-Johnson syndrome, toxic epidermal necrosis). Monitor for withdrawal symptoms (eg, anxiety, muscle twitching, weakness, convulsions, delirium) after d/c medication.

Patient Counseling: Inform psychological/physical dependence may result. Instruct not to increase dosage without consulting physician. Inform medication may impair mental/physical abilities; use caution when performing hazardous tasks. Avoid alcohol or other CNS depressants while on medication. Notify physician if any type of rash develops.

Administration: Oral route. **Storage:** 15-30°C (59-86°F).

PHENYTEK   RX   P
phenytoin sodium (Mylan)

THERAPEUTIC CLASS: Hydantoin

INDICATIONS: Control of generalized tonic-clonic (grand mal) and complex partial (psychomotor, temporal lobe) seizures. Prevention and treatment of seizures occurring during or following neurosurgery.

DOSAGE: *Adults:* Individualize dose. No Previous Treatment: Initial: 100mg tid. Titrate: May increase at 7- to 10-day intervals. Maint: 100mg tid-qid. May increase up to 200mg tid. QD Dosing: May consider 300mg qd if controlled with divided doses of three 100mg caps daily. LD (clinic/hospital): 1g in 3 divided doses (400mg, 300mg, 300mg) given 2 hrs apart. Start maint dose 24 hrs later. Avoid LD with renal and hepatic disease.
Pediatrics: Individualize dose. Initial: 5mg/kg/day given in 2 or 3 equally divided doses. Titrate: May increase at 7- to 10-day intervals. Maint: 4-8mg/kg/day. Max: 300mg/day. >6 yrs: May require minimum adult dose (300mg/day).

HOW SUPPLIED: Cap, Extended-Release: 200mg, 300mg

WARNINGS/PRECAUTIONS: Avoid abrupt withdrawal; may precipitate status epilepticus. May increase risk of suicidal thoughts/behavior; monitor for worsening of depression and any unusual changes in mood or behavior, or thoughts of self-harm. Lymphadenopathy (benign lymph node hyperplasia, pseudolymphoma, lymphoma, and Hodgkin's disease) with or without serum sickness-like reactions reported; observe for an extended period and use alternative antiepileptic drugs. May exacerbate porphyria; use with caution. Caution in pregnancy; increased seizure frequency in mothers, congenital malformations (orofacial clefts, cardiac defects, dysmorphic facial features, nail and digit hypoplasia, growth abnormalities and mental deficiency), and malignancies (eg, neuroblastoma) observed. Life-threatening bleeding disorder may occur in newborns exposed to phenytoin in utero; give vitamin K to mother before delivery and to neonate after birth. Caution with hepatic impairment, elderly or if gravely ill; may show early signs of toxicity. D/C if rash (exfoliative, purpuric, bullous, lupus erythematosus, Stevens-Johnson syndrome [SJS], toxic epidermal necrolysis [TEN]) occurs. For milder types of rash (measles-like or scarlatiniform), may resume therapy after rash has completely disappeared. If rash recurs after

745

reinstitution, further phenytoin medication is contraindicated. Hyperglycemia and osteomalacia reported. Avoid use for seizures due to hypoglycemia or other metabolic causes. Not effective for absence (petit mal) seizures. Confused states referred to as delirium, psychosis, encephalopathy, or irreversible cerebellar dysfunction reported with increased levels; reduce dose or d/c if symptoms persist. May increase serum glucose, alkaline phosphatase, gamma glutamyl transpeptidase (GGT) levels, interfere with dexamethasone and metyrapone tests, and decrease T4 concentration. Avoid with enteral feeding preparation.

ADVERSE REACTIONS: Nystagmus, ataxia, slurred speech, decreased coordination, confusion.

INTERACTIONS: Increased levels with acute alcohol intake, amiodarone, chloramphenicol, chlordiazepoxide, cimetidine, diazepam, dicumarol, disulfiram, estrogens, ethosuximide, fluoxetine, H_2-antagonists, halothane, isoniazid, methylphenidate, phenothiazines, phenylbutazone, salicylates, succinamides, sulfonamides, ticlopidine, tolbutamide, trazodone. Decreased levels with chronic alcohol use, carbamazepine, reserpine, sucralfate. Impaired efficacy of corticosteroids, coumarin anticoagulants, digitoxin, doxycycline, estrogens, furosemide, oral contraceptives, paroxetine, quinidine, rifampin, theophylline, vitamin D. May increase or decrease levels with phenobarbital, sodium valproate, valproic acid. Calcium antacids decrease absorption; space dosing. Moban (molindone) contains calcium ions that interfere with absorption. TCAs may precipitate seizures; may need to adjust dose.

PREGNANCY: Category D, not for use in nursing.

MECHANISM OF ACTION: Hydantoin; inhibits seizure activity by promoting Na efflux from neurons, stabilizing the threshold against hyperexcitability caused by excessive stimulation or environmental changes capable of reducing membrane sodium gradient. Reduces the post-tetanic potentiation at synapses, which prevents cortical seizure foci from detonating adjacent cortical areas.

PHARMACOKINETICS: Absorption: Slow and extended. T_{max}=4-12 hrs. **Distribution:** Protein binding (high). **Metabolism:** Hepatic via hydroxylation. **Elimination:** Bile (inactive metabolite) and urine; $T_{1/2}$=22 hrs.

NURSING CONSIDERATIONS

Assessment: Assess for alcohol use, impaired liver function, grave illness, porphyria, seizures due to hypoglycemic or other metabolic causes, absence (petit mal) seizures, pregnancy/nursing status, possible drug interactions, and hypersensitivity reactions. Obtain baseline serum phenytoin levels.

Monitoring: Monitor alcohol use, alkaline phosphatase, GGT, phenytoin levels and serum concentrations of T4. Monitor for signs and symptoms of status epilepticus, skin rash, hyperglycemia, osteomalacia, phenytoin toxicity (eg, delirium, psychosis, encephalopathy or irreversible cerebellar dysfunction), development of lymphadenopathy, serum sickness-like reactions, increased seizure frequency in pregnancy, and hypersensitivity reactions. Monitor for worsening of depression, suicidal thoughts/behavior, unusual change in mood/behavior, or thoughts of self-harm.

Patient Counseling: Advise of importance of strictly adhering to prescribed dosage regimen, and of informing physician of any clinical condition in which it is not possible to take the drug orally. Caution with the use of other drugs or alcohol while on medication. Notify physician if skin rash develops. Stress good dental hygiene to minimize development of gingival hyperplasia and its complications. May increase risk of suicidal thoughts and behavior; advise to report to healthcare provider immediately if emergence/worsening of depression, unusual change in mood/behavior, suicidal thoughts/behavior occurs. Notify physician if pregnant or intend to become pregnant. Encourage patients to enroll in North American Antiepileptic Drug (NAAED) Pregnancy Registry by calling 888-233-2334 or go to www.aedpregnancyregistry.org.

Administration: Oral route. **Storage:** 20-25°C (68-77°F). Protect from light and moisture.

PHOSLYRA   RX
calcium acetate (Fresenius)

THERAPEUTIC CLASS: Phosphate binder

INDICATIONS: To reduce serum phosphorus in end stage renal disease patients.

DOSAGE: *Adults:* Initial: 10mL with each meal. Titrate: Every 2-3 weeks until acceptable serum phosphorus level is reached. Increase dose gradually to lower serum phosphate levels to the target range, as long as hypercalcemia does not develop. Maint: 15-20mL with each meal.

HOW SUPPLIED: Sol: 667mg/5mL [473mL]

CONTRAINDICATIONS: Hypercalcemia.

WARNINGS/PRECAUTIONS: May develop hypercalcemia. Monitor serum calcium twice weekly during early dose adjustment period. If hypercalcemia develops, reduce dose or d/c immediately depending on severity. Chronic hypercalcemia may lead to vascular calcification and other soft-tissue calcification; radiographic evaluation of suspected anatomical region may be helpful in early detection of soft-tissue calcification. Maintain serum calcium-phosphate (CaXP) product <55mg^2/dL^2. Caution in elderly.

ADVERSE REACTIONS: Diarrhea, dizziness, edema, weakness.

INTERACTIONS: Avoid with other calcium supplements, including calcium-based nonprescription antacids. Hypercalcemia may aggravate digitalis toxicity. May induce laxative effect with other products containing maltitol. May decrease bioavailability of tetracyclines or fluoroquinolones. Administer oral medication where a reduction in the bioavailability of that medication would have a clinically significant effect on its safety/efficacy 1 hr before or 3 hrs after therapy. Monitor blood levels of concomitant drugs that have a narrow therapeutic range. Decreased bioavailability of ciprofloxacin when coadministered.

PREGNANCY: Category C, caution in nursing.

MECHANISM OF ACTION: Phosphate binder; combines with dietary phosphate to form insoluble calcium- phosphate complex resulting in decreased serum phosphorus concentrations.

PHARMACOKINETICS: Distribution: Found in breast milk.

NURSING CONSIDERATIONS

Assessment: Assess for hypercalcemia, pregnancy/nursing status, and for possible drug interactions.

Monitoring: Monitor for hypercalcemia, confusion, delirium, stupor, coma, anorexia, N/V, vascular and other soft-tissue calcification. Monitor serum calcium twice weekly early in treatment, during dose adjustment and periodically thereafter. Monitor for serum phosphorus levels periodically.

Patient Counseling: Instruct to take with meals, adhere to prescribed diets, and to avoid use of nonprescription antacids. Inform about symptoms of hypercalcemia. Advise patients who are taking oral medication to take the drug 1 hr before or 3 hrs after calcium acetate.

Administration: Oral route. **Storage:** 25°C (77°F); excursions permitted to 15-30°C (59-86°F).

PINDOLOL　　　　　　　　　　RX
pindolol (Various)

THERAPEUTIC CLASS: Nonselective beta-blocker

INDICATIONS: Management of HTN.

DOSAGE: *Adults:* Initial: 5mg bid. Titrate: May increase by 10mg/day after 3-4 weeks. Max: 60mg/day.

HOW SUPPLIED: Tab: 5mg, 10mg

CONTRAINDICATIONS: Bronchial asthma, overt cardiac failure, cardiogenic shock, second- and third-degree heart block, severe bradycardia.

WARNINGS/PRECAUTIONS: Caution with well-compensated heart failure, nonallergic bronchospasm, renal or hepatic impairment. Can cause cardiac failure. Avoid abrupt withdrawal. Withdrawal before surgery is controversial. May mask hypoglycemia or hyperthyroidism symptoms.

ADVERSE REACTIONS: Dizziness, fatigue, insomnia, nervousness, dyspnea, edema, joint pain, muscle cramps/pain.

INTERACTIONS: Additive hypotension and/or bradycardia with catecholamine-depleting drugs. Both thioridazine and pindolol levels may increase when used concomitantly.

PREGNANCY: Category B, not for use in nursing.

MECHANISM OF ACTION: Nonselective β-blocker; inhibits β-adrenergic receptor with intrinsic sympathomimetic activity.

PHARMACOKINETICS: Absorption: Rapid; T_{max}=1 hr. **Distribution:** V_d=2L/kg; plasma protein binding (40%). **Metabolism:** Metabolized to hydroxy-metabolites, which are excreted as glucoronides and ethereal sulfates. **Elimination:** Urine (35-40%), feces (6-9%); $T_{1/2}$=approximately 3-4 hrs, $T_{1/2}$=8 hrs (metabolites).

NURSING CONSIDERATIONS

Assessment: Assess for history of anaphylactic reaction, bronchial asthma, overt cardiac failure, cardiogenic shock, second- or third-degree heart block, severe bradycardia, bronchospastic disease, DM, thyrotoxicosis, LFTs, renal function, pregnancy/nursing status, and possible drug interactions. D/C drug well before any surgeries.

Monitoring: Monitor for anaphylactic reactions, LFTs, dizziness, fatigue, edema, dyspnea, muscle pain, heart block, hypotension, claudication, visual disturbances, impotence, CBC with differential and platelet count, Peyronie's disease, CHF, bronchospasm.

Patient Counseling: Instruct not to interrupt or d/c therapy without consulting physician. Counsel about signs/symptoms of CHF, bronchospasm, and other adverse effects; seek prompt medical assistance if any develop.

Administration: Oral route. **Storage:** Below 30°C (86°F); tight, light-resistant container.

PLAQUENIL RX
hydroxychloroquine sulfate (Sanofi-Aventis)

> Be familiar with complete prescribing information before prescribing hydroxychloroquine.

THERAPEUTIC CLASS: Quinine derivative

INDICATIONS: Suppression and treatment of acute attacks of malaria in adults and children. Treatment of discoid and systemic lupus erythematosus and rheumatoid arthritis (RA) in adults.

DOSAGE: *Adults:* Malaria Suppression: 400mg weekly. Begin 2 weeks before exposure and continue for 8 weeks after leaving endemic area. Give 400mg q6h for 2 doses if therapy is not begun before exposure. Acute Attack: 800mg, then 400mg 6-8 hrs later, then 400mg for 2 more days. RA: Initial: 400-600mg qd with food or milk; increase until optimum response. Maint: After 4-12 weeks, 200-400mg qd with food or milk. Lupus Erythematosus: Initial: 400mg qd-bid for several weeks depending on response. Maint: 200-400mg/day. *Pediatrics:* Malaria Suppression: 5mg/kg (base) weekly, max 400mg/dose. Begin 2 weeks before exposure and continue for 8 weeks after leaving endemic area. Acute Attack: 10mg base/kg, max 800mg/dose; then 5mg base/kg, max 400mg/dose at 6, 24 and 48 hrs after 1st dose.

HOW SUPPLIED: Tab: 200mg (200mg tab=155mg base)

CONTRAINDICATIONS: Long-term therapy in children or if retinal/visual field changes due to 4-aminoquinoline compounds.

WARNINGS/PRECAUTIONS: Caution with hepatic disease, glucose-6-phosphate-dehydrogenase deficiency, alcoholism, psoriasis, and porphyria. Perform baseline and periodic (3 months) ophthalmologic exams and blood cell counts with prolonged therapy. Test periodically for muscle weakness. D/C if blood disorders occur. Avoid if possible in pregnancy. D/C after 6 months if no improvement in RA.

ADVERSE REACTIONS: Headache, dizziness, diarrhea, loss of appetite, muscle weakness, nausea, abdominal cramps, bleaching of hair, dermatitis, ocular toxicity, visual field defects.

INTERACTIONS: Caution with hepatotoxic drugs.

PREGNANCY: Safety in pregnancy and nursing not known.

MECHANISM OF ACTION: Quinine derivative; has antimalarial action. Precise mechanism not established.

NURSING CONSIDERATIONS

Assessment: Assess for retinal or visual field defects, psoriasis, hepatic disease, alcoholism, *Plasmodium* deficiency, chloroquine-resistant strains of *P. falciparum*, auditory damage, pregnancy/nursing status. Note other diseases/conditions and drug therapies.

Monitoring: Monitor CBC with differential and platelet count, dermatologic reactions, chloroquine retinopathy, psychosis, irritability, myopathy, abnormal nerve conduction, depression of deep tendon reflexes, and allergic reactions.

Patient Counseling: Counsel about adverse effects and to d/c drug and seek medical attention if any signs/symptoms develop. Advise about need for periodic follow-up.

Administration: Oral route. **Storage:** Room temperature up to 30°C (86°F).

PLAVIX RX
clopidogrel bisulfate (Bristol-Myers Squibb/Sanofi-Aventis)

> Effectiveness is dependent on activation to an active metabolite via CYP2C19. Poor metabolizers of CYP2C19 treated with clopidogrel at recommended doses exhibit higher cardiovascular (CV) event rates following acute coronary syndrome (ACS) or undergoing percutaneous coronary intervention than patients with normal CYP2C19 function. Tests are available to indentify a patient's CYP2C19 genotype and to determine therapeutic strategy. Consider alternative treatment in poor metabolizers.

THERAPEUTIC CLASS: Platelet aggregation inhibitor

INDICATIONS: To decrease the rate of combined endpoint of CV death, myocardial infarction (MI), stroke, or refractory ischemia in patients with non-ST-segment elevation ACS (unstable angina [UA]/non-ST-elevation MI [NSTEMI]), including those who are managed medically and those with coronary revascularization. To reduce the rate of death from any cause and the rate of combined endpoint of death, reinfarction, or stroke in patients with ST-elevation MI (STEMI). To reduce the rate of combined endpoint of new ischemic stroke or MI, and other vascular deaths in patients with history of recent MI or stroke, or established peripheral arterial disease (PAD).

DOSAGE: *Adults:* Recent MI/Stroke or PAD: 75mg qd. UA/NSTEMI: Initial: LD: 300mg. Maint: 75mg qd with aspirin (ASA) (75-325mg qd). STEMI: 75mg qd with ASA (75-325mg qd), with or without thrombolytics. May initiate with or without a LD.

HOW SUPPLIED: Tab: 75mg, 300mg

CONTRAINDICATIONS: Active pathological bleeding (eg, peptic ulcer, intracranial hemorrhage).

WARNINGS/PRECAUTIONS: Increased risk of bleeding; d/c 5 days before surgery if antiplatelet effect is not desired. Avoid therapy lapses; if need to temporarily d/c, restart as soon as possible. Premature d/c increases risk of CV events. Thrombotic thrombocytopenic purpura (TTP) reported.

ADVERSE REACTIONS: TTP, bleeding, epistaxis, hematuria, bruising, hematoma, pruritus.

INTERACTIONS: Avoid with omeprazole or esomeprazole; if a proton pump inhibitor is required, use another acid reducing agent with minimal or no inhibitory effect on formation of clopidogrel active metabolite (eg, dexlansoprazole, lansoprazole, pantoprazole). Warfarin, NSAIDs, or ASA may increase risk of bleeding. Certain CYP2C19 inhibitors may reduce platelet inhibition.

PREGNANCY: Category B, not for use in nursing.

MECHANISM OF ACTION: Platelet activation and aggregation inhibitor; irreversibly and selectively inhibits the binding of adenosine diphosphate (ADP) to its platelet $P2Y_{12}$ receptor and subsequent ADP-mediated activation of the glycoprotein GPIIb/IIIa complex.

PHARMACOKINETICS: Absorption: Rapid. Bioavailability (≥50%); T_{max}=30-60 min. **Metabolism:** Liver (extensive) via CYP450 (active thiol metabolite) and hydrolysis. **Elimination:** Urine (50%), feces (46%); $T_{1/2}$=6 hrs.

NURSING CONSIDERATIONS

Assessment: Assess for presence of active pathological bleeding, previous hypersensitivity to the drug, reduced CYP2C19 function, pregnancy/nursing status, and possible drug interactions. Assess use in patients at risk for increased bleeding (eg, undergoing surgery).

Monitoring: Monitor for signs/symptoms of TTP (eg, thrombocytopenia, microangiopathic hemolytic anemia, neurological findings, renal dysfunction, fever) and bleeding.

Patient Counseling: Inform about the benefits and risks of treatment. Instruct to take exactly as prescribed and not to d/c without consulting the prescribing physician. Inform that they may bruise and/or bleed more easily and that bleeding will take longer than usual to stop. Advise to report to physician any unanticipated, prolonged, or excessive bleeding, or blood in stool or urine. Inform that TTP, a rare but serious condition, has been reported; instruct to seek prompt medical attention if unexplained fever, weakness, extreme skin paleness, purple skin patches, yellowing of the skin or eyes, or neurological changes occur. Instruct to notify physician or dentist about therapy before scheduling any invasive procedure. Inform about possible drug interaction with drugs such as omeprazole, warfarin, or NSAIDs.

Administration: Oral route. **Storage:** 25°C (77°F); excursions permitted to 15-30°C (59-86°F).

PLETAL   RX
cilostazol (Otsuka America)

Contraindicated with congestive heart failure (CHF) of any severity due to possible decrease in survival.

THERAPEUTIC CLASS: Phosphodiesterase III inhibitor

INDICATIONS: Reduction of symptoms of intermittent claudication.

DOSAGE: *Adults:* Usual: 100mg bid, at least 1/2 hr before or 2 hrs after breakfast and dinner. Concomitant CYP3A4/CYP2C19 Inhibitors: Consider 50mg bid.

HOW SUPPLIED: Tab: 50mg, 100mg

CONTRAINDICATIONS: CHF of any severity. Hemostatic disorders or active pathologic bleeding (eg, peptic ulcer, intracranial bleeding).

WARNINGS/PRECAUTIONS: Thrombocytopenia/leukopenia progressing to agranulocytosis rarely reported. Special caution with moderate/severe hepatic impairment, severe renal impairment (CrCl <25mL/min). Caution with thrombocytopenia and in patients at risk of bleeding from surgery or pathologic processes.

ADVERSE REACTIONS: Headache, palpitation, tachycardia, abnormal stools, diarrhea, peripheral edema, dizziness, infection, rhinitis, pharyngitis, nausea, back pain, dyspepsia.

INTERACTIONS: May increase levels with CYP3A4 inhibitors (eg, ketoconazole, itraconazole, fluconazole, miconazole, fluvoxamine, fluoxetine, nefazodone, sertraline, diltiazem, erythromycin, clarithromycin, other macrolide antibiotics, grapefruit juice) or CYP2C19 inhibitors (eg, omeprazole); use with caution and consider reducing dose. Caution with clopidogrel and other antiplatelet agents. Smoking may decrease levels.

PREGNANCY: Category C, not for use in nursing.

MECHANISM OF ACTION: Phosphodiesterase III inhibitor; not established. Suspected to inhibit phosphodiesterase activity and suppress cyclic AMP (cAMP) degradation resulting in an increase of cAMP in platelets and blood vessels, leading to inhibition of platelet aggregation and vasodilation.

PHARMACOKINETICS: Distribution: Plasma protein binding (95-98%). **Metabolism:** Liver (extensive) via CYP450 3A4 (primary), 2C19; 3,4-dehydro-cilostazol, 4'-trans-hydroxy-cilostazol (major active metabolites). **Elimination:** Urine (74%), feces (20%); $T_{1/2}$=11-13 hrs.

NURSING CONSIDERATIONS

Assessment: Assess for CHF, hemostatic disorders, active pathologic bleeding, renal/hepatic function, hypersensitivity to drug, pregnancy/nursing status, and possible drug interactions.

Monitoring: Monitor for signs/symptoms of thrombocytopenia, leukopenia, agranulocytosis, and other adverse reactions.

Patient Counseling: Advise to take at least 30 mins before or 2 hrs after food. Inform that benefits of medication may not be immediate; treatment may be required for up to 12 weeks before beneficial effect is experienced.

Administration: Oral route. **Storage:** 25°C (77°F); excursions permitted to 15-30°C (59-86°F).

PNEUMOVAX 23   RX
pneumococcal vaccine polyvalent (Merck)

THERAPEUTIC CLASS: Vaccine

INDICATIONS: Active immunization for the prevention of pneumococcal disease caused by the 23 serotypes contained in the vaccine in persons ≥50 yrs of age and persons aged ≥2 yrs who are at increased risk for pneumococcal disease.

DOSAGE: *Adults:* Usual/Revaccination: Single 0.5mL dose SQ/IM into the deltoid muscle or lateral mid-thigh.
Pediatrics: ≥2 yrs: Usual/Revaccination: Single 0.5mL dose SQ/IM into the deltoid muscle or lateral mid-thigh.

HOW SUPPLIED: Inj: 0.5mL

WARNINGS/PRECAUTIONS: Defer vaccination in patients with moderate or severe acute illness. Caution with severely compromised cardiovascular (CV) and/or pulmonary function in whom systemic reaction would be a significant risk. Does not replace the need for antibiotic prophylaxis against pneumococcal infection; continue use of antibiotic prophylaxis after vaccination. Response may be diminished in immunocompromised individuals. May not prevent pneumococcal meningitis in patients with chronic CSF leakage resulting from congenital lesions, skull fractures, or neurosurgical procedures. Will not prevent disease caused by capsular types of pneumococcus other than those contained in the vaccine. Avoid routine revaccination of immunocompetent patients previously vaccinated with a 23-valent vaccine.

ADVERSE REACTIONS: Local inj-site reactions (eg, pain, soreness, tenderness, swelling, induration, erythema), asthenia, fatigue, myalgia, headache.

INTERACTIONS: Immunosuppressive therapies may reduce immune response. Reduced immune response to zoster vaccine live; separate vaccination by at least 4 weeks.

PREGNANCY: Category C, caution in nursing.

MECHANISM OF ACTION: Vaccine; induce antibodies that enhance opsonization, phagocytosis, and killing of pneumococci by leukocytes and other phagocytic cells.

NURSING CONSIDERATIONS

Assessment: Assess for history of hypersensitivity to any component of the vaccine, health/immunity status, vaccination history, compromised CV and pulmonary function, chronic CSF leakage, moderate or severe acute illness, pregnancy/nursing status, and possible drug interactions.

Monitoring: Monitor patients with compromised CV and pulmonary function. Monitor for hypersensitivity reactions and for other possible adverse reactions.

Patient Counseling: Inform of potential benefits/risks of vaccination. Inform that the vaccine may not result in protection of all vaccinees. Instruct to report any adverse reactions to physician.

Administration: IM or SQ route into the deltoid muscle or lateral mid-thigh. Do not mix with other vaccines in the same syringe or vial. **Storage:** 2-8°C (36-46°F).

POTABA
potassium P-aminobenzoate (Glenwood)
RX

THERAPEUTIC CLASS: Vitamin B complex

INDICATIONS: Possibly effective for the treatment of Peyronie's disease, dermatomyositis, linear scleroderma, pemphigus.

DOSAGE: *Adults:* Usual: 12g/day, in 4 to 6 divided doses. Take with meals or snacks. Tabs should be taken with plenty of liquid. Dissolve powder in water or juice.
Pediatrics: 1g/day for each 10 lbs of body wt given in divided doses. Dissolve powder in water or juice. Take with food and plenty of liquid.

HOW SUPPLIED: Cap: 0.5g; Pow: 2g/envule [50s]; Tab: 0.5g

CONTRAINDICATIONS: Concomitant sulfonamides.

WARNINGS/PRECAUTIONS: Suspend therapy if anorexia, nausea, occurs. D/C if hypersensitivity reaction develops. Caution with renal disease.

ADVERSE REACTIONS: Anorexia, nausea, fever, rash.

PREGNANCY: Safety in pregnancy or nursing not known.

MECHANISM OF ACTION: Vitamin B complex; anti-fibrosis action due to its mediation of increased oxygen uptake at tissue level.

NURSING CONSIDERATIONS

Assessment: Assess for renal function, pregnancy/nursing status, and possible drug interaction (eg, sulfonamides).

Monitoring: Monitor for anorexia, nausea, and hypoglycemia.

Patient Counseling: Advise to take with food and adequate amount of liquid to prevent GI upset.

Administration: Oral route.

PRADAXA
dabigatran etexilate mesylate (Boehringer Ingelheim)
RX

THERAPEUTIC CLASS: Thrombin inhibitor

INDICATIONS: To reduce risk of stroke and systemic embolism in patients with non-valvular atrial fibrillation.

DOSAGE: *Adults:* CrCl >30mL/min: 150mg bid. CrCl 15-30mL/min: 75mg bid. Concomitant Dronedarone/Systemic Ketoconazole with CrCl 30-50mL/min: Reduce to 75mg bid. Conversion from Warfarin: D/C warfarin and start when INR <2.0. Conversion to Warfarin: Start warfarin 3 days (CrCl ≥50mL/min), 2 days (CrCl 30-50mL/min), or 1 day (CrCl 15-30mL/min) before d/c. Conversion from Parenteral Anticoagulants: Start 0-2 hrs before time of the next dose of parenteral drug was to have been administered, or at time of d/c of a continuously administered parenteral drug (eg, IV unfractionated heparin). Conversion to Parenteral Anticoagulant: Wait 12 hrs (CrCl ≥30mL/min), or 24 hrs (CrCl <30mL/min) after last dose before initiating parenteral drug. Surgery and Interventions: D/C 1-2 days (CrCl ≥50mL/min) or 3-5 days (CrCl <50mL/min) before invasive or surgical procedures. Consider longer times for patients undergoing major surgery, spinal puncture, or placement of a spinal or epidural catheter or port in whom complete hemostasis may be required.

HOW SUPPLIED: Cap: 75mg, 150mg

CONTRAINDICATIONS: Active pathological bleeding.

WARNINGS/PRECAUTIONS: Periodically monitor renal function as clinically indicated; adjust therapy accordingly. D/C with acute renal failure; consider alternative therapy. Increases risk of bleeding and may cause significant and, sometimes, fatal bleeding; promptly evaluate for any signs/symptoms of blood loss. Renal impairment may increase anticoagulant activity and $T_{1/2}$. Consider administration of platelet concentrates in cases where thrombocytopenia is present. Discontinuing for active bleeding, elective surgery, or invasive procedures may increase the risk of stroke. Minimize lapses in therapy.

ADVERSE REACTIONS: GI reactions.

INTERACTIONS: Risk factors for bleeding include the use of drugs that increase the risk of bleeding (eg, anti-platelet agents, heparin, fibrinolytics, chronic use of NSAIDs). Consider administration of platelet concentrates in cases where long-acting antiplatelet drugs have been used. P-glycoprotein (P-gp) inducers (eg, rifampin) may reduce exposure; avoid use. In patients with renal impairment, P-gp inhibitors (eg, dronedarone, systemic ketoconazole) may increase exposure; consider reducing dose in moderate renal impairment (CrCl 30-50mL/min). Avoid use

P

with P-gp inhibitors in patients with severe renal impairment (CrCl 15-30mL/min). Oral verapamil, amiodarone, quinidine, or clopidogrel may increase levels.

PREGNANCY: Category C, caution in nursing.

MECHANISM OF ACTION: Direct thrombin inhibitor; prevents the development of a thrombus. Both free and clot-bound thrombin, and thrombin-induced platelet aggregation are inhibited by the active moieties.

PHARMACOKINETICS: Absorption: Absolute bioavailability (3-7%); T_{max}=1 hr (fasted). **Distribution:** Plasma protein binding (35%); V_d=50-70L. **Metabolism:** Hydrolysis, conjugation; acyl glucuronides (active metabolite). **Elimination:** Urine (7%), feces (86%); $T_{1/2}$=12-17 hrs. Refer to PI for pharmacokinetic parameters of renally impaired.

NURSING CONSIDERATIONS

Assessment: Assess for active pathological bleeding, renal function, risk factors for bleeding, history of hypersensitivity reaction to the drug, pregnancy/nursing status, and possible drug interactions.

Monitoring: Monitor for bleeding, GI adverse reactions, hypersensitivity reactions, and for increased risk of stroke on temporary d/c. Periodically monitor renal function as clinically indicated. When necessary, monitor anticoagulant activity by using aPTT or ECT, and not INR.

Patient Counseling: Instruct to take exactly as prescribed and not to d/c without talking to physician. Keep caps in the original bottle to protect from moisture. When >1 bottle is dispensed, instruct to open only one bottle at a time. Counsel to remove only one cap from the opened bottle at the time of use; immediately and tightly close bottle. Do not to chew, break, or open caps and take the pellets alone. Inform that they may bleed longer and more easily. Instruct to call physician for any signs/symptoms of bleeding, dyspepsia, or gastritis. Instruct to inform physician if taking dabigatran before any invasive procedure (including dental procedures) is scheduled. Advise to list all prescription/over-the-counter medications, or dietary supplements they are taking or planning to take. Instruct that if a dose is missed, take that dose as soon as possible on the same day or skip it if cannot be taken at least 6 hrs before the next scheduled dose. Instruct not to double dose.

Administration: Oral route. **Storage:** 25°C (77°F); excursions permitted to 15-30°C (59-86°F). Store in the original package to protect from moisture. (Bottles) Once opened, must use within 4 months. Keep tightly closed.

PRANDIMET   RX
metformin HCl - repaglinide (Novo Nordisk)

> Lactic acidosis may occur due to metformin accumulation; risk increases with sepsis, dehydration, excess alcohol intake, hepatic impairment, renal impairment, and acute congestive heart failure (CHF). If acidosis suspected, d/c and hospitalize patient immediately.

THERAPEUTIC CLASS: Biguanide/Meglitinide

INDICATIONS: Adjunct to diet and exercise to improve glycemic control in adults with type 2 diabetes mellitus (DM) who are already treated with a meglitinide and metformin, or who have inadequate glycemic control on a meglitinide alone or metformin alone.

DOSAGE: *Adults:* Individualize dose. Administer bid-tid up to 4mg-1000mg/meal. Take dose within 15-30 min ac. Max: 10mg-2500mg/day. Patient Inadequately Controlled on Metformin Monotherapy: Initial: 1mg-500mg bid with meals. Titrate: Gradually escalate dose to reduce risk of hypoglycemia. Patient Inadequately Controlled w/ Meglitinide Monotherapy: Initial: 500mg of metformin component bid. Titrate: Gradually escalate dose to reduce GI side effects. Concomitant use of Repaglinide/Metformin: Initiate at dose of repaglinide and metformin similar to (but not exceeding) current doses. Titrate to maximum daily dose as necessary to achieve targeted glycemic control.

HOW SUPPLIED: Tab: (Repaglinide-Metformin) 1mg-500mg, 2mg-500mg

CONTRAINDICATIONS: Renal impairment (eg, SrCr ≥1.5mg/dL [males], ≥1.4mg/dL [females], or abnormal CrCl). Acute or chronic metabolic acidosis, including diabetic ketoacidosis. Concomitant gemfibrozil.

WARNINGS/PRECAUTIONS: Not for use for the treatment of type 1 DM or diabetic ketoacidosis. Suspend prior to any surgical procedures (except minor procedures not associated with restricted food and fluid intake); restart when oral intake is resumed and renal function is normal. D/C at the time of or prior to intravascular contrast studies with iodinated materials; withhold for 48 hrs subsequent to procedure and restart only if renal function is normal. May cause hypoglycemia; risk increased in elderly, debilitated or malnourished, and those with adrenal or pituitary insufficiency. Temporary loss of glycemic control may occur when exposed to stress (eg, fever, infection, trauma, surgery); withhold therapy and temporarily administer insulin. Evaluate for evidence of ketoacidosis or lactic acidosis if laboratory abnormalities or clinical illness develops; d/c if acidosis occurs. D/C in hypoxic states (eg, acute CHF, shock, acute myocardial infarction [MI]). May decrease vitamin B12 levels; monitor hematologic parameters annually. Avoid with hepatic/renal impariment. D/C if renal impairment occurs. Avoid in patients ≥80 yrs unless CrCl measurement demonstrates that renal function is not reduced. No conclusive evidence of macrovascular risk reduction.

ADVERSE REACTIONS: Lactic acidosis, hypoglycemia, headache, diarrhea, N/V, upper respiratory tract infection.

INTERACTIONS: See Contraindications. Metformin: Cimetidine, furosemide, nifedipine, and ibuprofen may increase levels. Propranolol may decrease levels. Cationic drugs (eg, amiloride, digoxin, morphine, procainamide, quinidine, quinine, ranitidine, triamterene, trimethoprim, vancomycin) may compete for common renal tubular transport systems. Alcohol potentiates effect on lactate metabolism. May decrease levels of furosemide. Caution with drugs that may affect renal function or result in significant hemodynamic change or may interfere with the disposition of metformin (eg, cationic drugs eliminated by renal tubular secretion). Repaglinide: CYP2C8 inhibitors (eg, gemfibrozil, trimethoprim, deferasirox), CYP3A4 inhibitors (eg, itraconazole, ketaconazole), or CYP2C8/3A4 inducers (eg, rifampin) may alter the pharmacokinetics and pharmacodynamics. Not for use in combination with NPH-insulin. Levonorgestrel/ethinyl estradiol may decrease levels and increase C_{max}. Clarithromycin, ketoconazole, itraconazole, deferasirox, gemfibrozil, simvastatin, trimethoprim, and OATP1B1 inhibitors (eg, cyclosporine) may increase levels. Nifedipine and rifampin may decrease levels. May increase levels of ethinyl estradiol.

PREGNANCY: Category C, not for use in nursing.

MECHANISM OF ACTION: Metformin: Biguanide; improves glucose tolerance by lowering both basal and postprandial plasma glucose. Decreases hepatic glucose production, decreases intestinal absorption of glucose, and improves insulin sensitivity by increasing peripheral glucose uptake and utilization. Repaglinide: Meglitinide; lowers blood glucose levels by stimulating the release of insulin from the pancreas.

PHARMACOKINETICS: Absorption: Metformin: Absolute bioavailabilty (50%-60%, fasted); C_{max}=799.4-838.8ng/mL; AUC=5871.6-6041.9ng•h/mL. Repaglinide: Absolute bioavailability (56%); C_{max}=12.9-26ng/mL; AUC=17.6-35ng•h/mL. T_{max}=1 hr. **Distribution:** Metformin: V_d=654L. Repaglinide: (IV) V_d=31L; plasma protein binding (>98%). **Metabolism:** Repaglinide: CYP2C8, 3A4; oxidation and direct conjugation with glucuronic acid; oxidized dicarboxylic acid (M2), aromatic amine (M1), acyl glucuronide (M7) (major metabolites). **Elimination:** Metformin: Urine (90%); $T_{1/2}$=6.2 hrs (plasma), 17.6 hrs (blood). Repaglinide: Feces (90%, <2% unchanged), urine (8%, 0.1% unchanged); $T_{1/2}$=1 hr.

NURSING CONSIDERATIONS

Assessment: Assess for diabetic ketoacidosis, acute or chronic metabolic acidosis, renal/hepatic impairment, type 1 DM, cardiovascular (CV) risk factors, adrenal/pituitary insufficiency, pregnancy/nursing status, possible drug interactions, or any other conditions where treatment is contraindicated or cautioned. Assess if scheduled to undergo any radiologic studies with iodinated materials, surgical procedure, or under any form of stress. Obtain FPG, HbA1c, renal/hepatic function, and hematological parameters.

Monitoring: Monitor for signs/symptoms of hypoglycemia, lactic acidosis, CV collapse (shock), acute CHF, acute MI, and renal/hepatic impairment. Monitor vitamin B12 levels in patients predisposed to developing subnormal vitamin B12 levels. Perform periodic monitoring of FPG, HbA1c, and hematologic parameters. Monitor renal function at least annually. Monitor serum electrolytes and ketones, blood glucose/blood pH, lactate levels, pyruvate, and metformin levels if clinical illness develops.

Patient Counseling: Inform about risks/benefits of therapy. Instruct to take 15-30 min ac; skip dose for skipped meal. Counsel against excessive alcohol intake. Inform of importance of adherence to dietary instructions, a regular exercise program, regular testing of blood glucose, HbA1c, renal function, and hematologic parameters. Instruct to seek medical advice during periods of stress. Inform about risks of hypoglycemia, its symptoms and treatment, and predisposing conditions. Inform of risk of lactic acidosis, and predisposing conditions; advise to d/c immediately and contact physician if unexplained hyperventilation, myalgia, malaise, unusual somnolence, GI symptoms, or other nonspecific symptoms occur. Advise to notify physician of all concomitant medications and if pregnant/nursing.

Administration: Oral route. **Storage:** Do not store above 25°C (77°F). Protect from moisture.

PRANDIN   RX
repaglinide (Novo Nordisk)

THERAPEUTIC CLASS: Meglitinide
INDICATIONS: Adjunct to diet and exercise to improve glycemic control in adults with type 2 diabetes mellitus (DM).

DOSAGE: *Adults:* Take dose within 15-30 min ac bid-qid in response to changes in meal pattern. Initial: Treatment-Naive or HbA1c <8%: 0.5mg ac. Previous Therapy with Blood Glucose-Lowering Drugs and HbA1c ≥8%: 1mg or 2mg ac. Titrate: May double preprandial dose up to 4mg at no less than 1-week intervals until response is achieved. Maint: 0.5-4mg ac. Max: 16mg/day. Occurrence of Hypoglycemia with Metformin or Thiazolidinedione Combination: Reduce repaglinide dose. Replacement Therapy of Other Oral Hypoglycemic Agents: Start repaglinide on the day after final dose is given. Combination Therapy with Metformin or Thiazolidinedione: Starting dose and dose adjustments same as for repaglinide monotherapy. Severe Renal Impairment (CrCl 20-40mL/min): Initial: 0.5mg ac; titrate carefully. Hepatic Dysfunction: Longer intervals between dose adjustments.

HOW SUPPLIED: Tab: 0.5mg, 1mg, 2mg

CONTRAINDICATIONS: Diabetic ketoacidosis with or without coma, type 1 diabetes, concomitant gemfibrozil.

WARNINGS/PRECAUTIONS: No conclusive evidence of macrovascular risk reduction. May cause hypoglycemia; risk increased in elderly, debilitated or malnourished patients, and with adrenal, pituitary, hepatic, or severe renal insufficiency. Loss of glycemic control may occur when exposed to stress (eg, fever, trauma, infection, or surgery); may need to d/c therapy and administer insulin. Secondary failure may occur; assess adequate adjustment of dose and adherence to diet before classifying a patient as a secondary failure. Caution with hepatic impairment.

ADVERSE REACTIONS: Hypoglycemia, upper respiratory infection, headache, rhinitis, sinusitis, bronchitis, arthralgia, back pain, N/V, diarrhea, dyspepsia, cardiovascular events, constipation, paresthesia, chest pain.

INTERACTIONS: See Contraindications. Not for use in combination with NPH-insulin. CYP3A4 and/or 2C8 inducers (eg, rifampin, barbiturates, carbamazepine), CYP3A4 inhibitors (eg, ketoconazole, itraconazole, erythromycin), and CYP2C8 inhibitors (eg, trimethoprim, gemfibrozil, and montelukast) may alter metabolism; use caution. OATP1B1 inhibitors (eg, cyclosporine), gemfibrozil, itraconazole, ketoconazole, clarithromycin, trimethroprim, and deferasirox may increase levels. Rifampin may decrease levels. May potentiate hypoglycemic action with NSAIDs, other highly protein-bound drugs, salicylates, sulfonamides, cyclosporine, chloramphenicol, coumarins, probenecid, MAOIs, β-adrenergic blocking agents, and alcohol; observe closely for hypoglycemia. Thiazides and other diuretics, corticosteroids, phenothiazines, thyroid products, estrogens, phenytoin, nicotinic acid, oral contraceptives, sympathomimetics, calcium channel blockers, and isoniazid tend to produce hyperglycemia and may lead to loss of glycemic control. β-adrenergic blockers may mask hypoglycemia. Levonorgestrel/ethinyl estradiol combination may increase repaglinide, levonorgestrel, and ethinyl estradiol C_{max} and ethinyl estradiol area under the curve. Simvastatin may increase repaglinide C_{max}.

PREGNANCY: Category C, not for use in nursing.

MECHANISM OF ACTION: Meglitinide; lowers blood glucose levels by stimulating the release of insulin from the pancreas.

PHARMACOKINETICS: Absorption: Rapid and complete; absolute bioavailability (56%); T_{max} =1 hr. See PI for parameters of different doses. **Distribution:** (IV) V_d=31L; plasma protein binding (>98%). **Metabolism:** CYP2C8, 3A4; oxidation, and direct conjugation with glucuronic acid; oxidized dicarboxylic acid (M2), aromatic amine (M1), acyl glucuronide (M7) (major metabolites). **Elimination:** Feces (90%, <2% unchanged), urine (8%, 0.1% unchanged); $T_{1/2}$=1-1.4 hr.

NURSING CONSIDERATIONS

Assessment: Assess for diabetic ketoacidosis, type 1 DM, adrenal/pituitary/renal/hepatic insufficiency, pregnancy/nursing status, and possible drug interactions. Obtain baseline blood glucose (FPG, postprandial glucose [PPG]) and HbA1c).

Monitoring: Monitor for hypo/hyperglycemia, headache, and other adverse events. Monitor FPG, PPG, HbA1c every 3 months, and renal/hepatic function.

Patient Counseling: Inform about risks/benefits of therapy, alternative modes of therapy, and primary/secondary failure. Inform about importance of adherence to dietary instructions, regular exercise program, regular blood glucose monitoring, and periodic HbA1c testing. Inform about risks of hypoglycemia, its symptoms and treatment, and predisposing conditions. Inform physician if rhinitis, sinusitis, headache, and other adverse events occur. Instruct to take ac (2, 3, or 4x a day preprandially); skip dose if skipping a meal and add dose if adding a meal.

Administration: Oral route. **Storage:** Do not store above 25°C (77°F). Protect from moisture.

PRAVACHOL RX
pravastatin sodium (Bristol-Myers Squibb)

THERAPEUTIC CLASS: HMG-CoA reductase inhibitor

INDICATIONS: To reduce risk of myocardial infarction (MI), revascularization procedures, and cardiovascular mortality (with no increase in death from noncardiovascular causes), in hypercholesterolemic patients without clinically evident coronary heart disease (CHD). To reduce risk of total morbidity (by reducing coronary death), MI, revascularization procedures, stroke and stroke/transient ischemic attack, and to slow progression of coronary atherosclerosis, in patients with clinically evident CHD. Adjunct to diet for treatment of primary hypercholesterolemia and mixed dyslipidemia (Types IIa and IIb). Adjunct to diet for treatment of patients with elevated serum TG levels (Type IV). Treatment of patients with primary dysbetalipoproteinemia (Type III) who do not respond adequately to diet. Adjunct to diet and lifestyle modification for treatment of heterozygous familial hypercholesterolemia in children and adolescents ≥8 yrs.

DOSAGE: *Adults:* Initial: 40mg qd. Titrate: May increase to 80mg qd if 40mg qd does not achieve desired cholesterol levels. Significant Renal Impairment: Initial: 10mg qd. Concomitant Lipid-Altering Therapy: Give either 1 hr or more before or at least 4 hrs following the resin. Concomitant Immunosuppressive: Initial: 10mg qhs. Titrate: Increase dose cautiously. Usual Max: 20mg/day. Concomitant Cyclosporine: Limit to 20mg qd. Concomitant Clarithromycin: Limit to 40mg qd.
Pediatrics: 14-18 yrs: Initial: 40mg qd. Max: 40mg. 8-13 yrs: Usual: 20mg qd. Max: 20mg. Concomitant Lipid-Altering Therapy: Give either 1 hr or more before or at least 4 hrs following the resin. Concomitant Immunosuppressive: Initial: 10mg qhs. Titrate: Increase dose cautiously. Usual Max: 20mg/day. Concomitant Cyclosporine: Limit to 20mg qd. Concomitant Clarithromycin: Limit to 40mg qd.

HOW SUPPLIED: Tab: 10mg, 20mg, 40mg, 80mg

CONTRAINDICATIONS: Active liver disease or unexplained, persistent elevations of transaminase, women who are pregnant or may become pregnant, and nursing mothers.

WARNINGS/PRECAUTIONS: Rare cases of rhabdomyolysis with acute renal failure secondary to myoglobinuria reported. Increased risk of rhabdomyolysis in patients with history of renal impairment; closely monitor for skeletal muscle effects. Uncomplicated myalgia and myopathy reported; d/c therapy if markedly elevated CPK levels occur or myopathy is diagnosed or suspected. Temporarily withhold in any patient experiencing an acute or serious condition predisposing to development of renal failure secondary to rhabdomyolysis. May cause biochemical liver function abnormalities; perform LFTs prior to initiation of therapy and PRN. Caution with recent (<6 months) history of liver disease, signs that may suggest liver disease, in heavy alcohol users, and elderly. Fatal and nonfatal hepatic failure (rare) reported; promptly interrupt therapy if serious liver injury with clinical symptoms and/or hyperbilirubinemia or jaundice occurs, and do not restart if alternate etiology is not found. May blunt adrenal or gonadal steroid hormone production. Evaluate patients who display clinical evidence of endocrine dysfunction.

ADVERSE REACTIONS: N/V, diarrhea, sinus abnormality, rash, fatigue, musculoskeletal pain and trauma, cough, muscle cramps, dizziness, headache, upper respiratory tract infection, influenza, chest pain.

INTERACTIONS: Increased risk of myopathy with cyclosporine, fibrates, niacin (nicotinic acid), erythromycin, clarithromycin, colchicine, and gemfibrozil; caution with colchicine and fibrates, and avoid with gemfibrozil. Niacin may enhance risk of skeletal muscle effects; consider dose reduction. Caution with drugs that may diminish levels or activity of steroid hormones (eg, ketoconazole, spironolactone, cimetidine).

PREGNANCY: Category X, not for use in nursing.

MECHANISM OF ACTION: HMG-CoA reductase inhibitor; inhibits the conversion of HMG-CoA to mevalonate, an early and rate limiting step in biosynthetic pathway for cholesterol. Reduces VLDL and TG and increases HDL.

PHARMACOKINETICS: Absorption: Absolute bioavailability (17%); T_{max}=1-1.5 hrs; (fasted) C_{max}=26.5ng/mL, AUC=59.8ng•hr/mL. **Distribution:** Plasma protein binding (50%); found in breast milk. **Metabolism:** Liver (extensive) via isomerization and enzymatic ring hydroxylation; 3α-hydroxyisomeric (active metabolite). **Elimination:** Feces (70%), urine (20%); $T_{1/2}$=1.8 hrs.

NURSING CONSIDERATIONS

Assessment: Assess for active liver disease or unexplained, persistent elevations of serum transaminases, hypersensitivity to drug, predisposing factors for myopathy, alcohol intake, pregnancy/nursing status, and possible drug interactions. Obtain baseline LFTs.

Monitoring: Monitor for signs/symptoms of rhabdomyolysis and myopathy, endocrine dysfunction, and other adverse reactions. Monitor lipid profile and CPK levels. Perform LFTs when clinically indicated.

Patient Counseling: Advise to report promptly unexplained muscle pain, tenderness, or weakness, particularly if accompanied by malaise or fever, or any symptoms of liver injury, including fatigue, anorexia, right upper abdominal discomfort, dark urine, or jaundice. Counsel females of childbearing potential on appropriate contraceptive methods while on therapy.

Administration: Oral route. **Storage:** 25°C (77°F); excursions permitted to 15-30°C (59-86°F). Protect from light.

P

PRECEDEX

RX

dexmedetomidine HCl (Hospira)

THERAPEUTIC CLASS: Alpha$_2$-agonist

INDICATIONS: For sedation of initially intubated and mechanically ventilated patients during treatment in an intensive care setting. For sedation of non-intubated patients prior to and/or during surgical and other procedures.

DOSAGE: *Adults:* Individualize dose. Not indicated for infusions >24 hrs. ICU Sedation: Initial: Up to 1mcg/kg IV infusion over 10 min. Conversion from Alternate Sedative Therapy: Initial: A loading dose may be required. Maint: 0.2-0.7mcg/kg/hr. Adjust to achieve desired level of sedation. Procedural Sedation: Initial: 1mcg/kg IV infusion over 10 min. Maint: 0.6mcg/kg/hr. Titrate: 0.2-1mcg/kg/hr. Adjust to achieve desired level of sedation. Elderly (>65 yrs): Initial: 0.5mcg/kg IV infusion over 10 min. Less Invasive Procedures (eg, ophthalmic surgery): Initial: 0.5mcg/kg IV infusion over 10 min. Awake Fiberoptic Intubation: Initial: 1mcg/kg IV infusion over 10 min. Maint: 0.7mcg/kg/hr until endotracheal tube is secured. Elderly (>65 yrs)/Hepatic Impairment: Dose reduction should be considered.

HOW SUPPLIED: Inj: 100mcg/mL

WARNINGS/PRECAUTIONS: Should only be administered by persons skilled in the management of patients in an intensive care setting. Monitor patients continuously. Hypotension, bradycardia and sinus arrest reported; treat appropriately. Hypotension and/or bradycardia may be more pronounced in patients with hypovolemia, diabetes mellitus (DM), or chronic HTN and in elderly patients. Caution with advanced heart block and/or severe ventricular dysfunction. Transient HTN observed primarily during the loading dose. Arousability and alertness reported in some patients upon stimulation. Withdrawal events (eg, N/V, agitation) reported within 24-48 hrs after d/c therapy. If tachycardia and/or HTN occurs after d/c, supportive therapy is indicated. Use for >24 hrs associated with tolerance, tachyphylaxis, and a dose related increase in adverse events.

ADVERSE REACTIONS: Hypotension, HTN, bradycardia, dry mouth, respiratory depression, tachycardia, N/V, atrial fibrillation, fever, hyperglycemia, anemia, hypovolemia, hypoxia, atelectasis.

INTERACTIONS: Concurrent use with anesthetics, sedatives, hypnotics, and opioids (eg, sevoflurane, isoflurane, propofol, alfentanil, midazolam) may potentiate effects; consider dose reduction. Caution with concomitant use of other vasodilators or negative chronotropic agents; may have additive effects.

PREGNANCY: Category C, caution in nursing.

MECHANISM OF ACTION: Selective α_2-adrenergic agonist; possesses sedative properties.

PHARMACOKINETICS: Distribution: V$_d$=118L, plasma protein binding (94%). **Metabolism:** Liver via direct glucuronidation and CYP2A6 (aliphatic hydroxylation). **Elimination:** Feces (4%), urine (95%); T$_{1/2}$= 2 hrs.

NURSING CONSIDERATIONS

Assessment: Assess for advanced heart block, severe ventricular dysfunction, hepatic impairment, hypovolemia, DM, chronic HTN, pregnancy/nursing status, and for possible drug interactions. Obtain baseline vital signs, ECG, and LFTs.

Monitoring: Monitor for hypotension, bradycardia, sinus arrest, transient HTN. Monitor for tolerance and tachyphylaxis if use of therapy >24 hrs.

Patient Counseling: If infused for >6 hrs, instruct to report nervousness, agitation and headaches that may occur for up to 48 hrs. Instruct to report symptoms that may occur within 48 hrs after administration (eg, weakness, confusion, excessive sweating, weight loss, abdominal pain, salt cravings, diarrhea, constipation, dizziness or lightheadedness).

Administration: IV route. Refer to PI for preparation and administration instructions. **Storage:** 25°C (77°F); excursions allowed 15-30°C (59-86°F).

PRECOSE

RX

acarbose (Bayer Healthcare)

THERAPEUTIC CLASS: Alpha-glucosidase inhibitor

INDICATIONS: Adjunct to diet and exercise to improve glycemic control in adults with type 2 diabetes mellitus.

DOSAGE: *Adults:* Individualize dose. Initial: 25mg tid with first bite of each main meal. May also initiate at 25mg qd to minimize GI side effects then increase gradually to 25mg tid. Titrate: After reaching 25mg tid, may increase to 50mg tid at 4-8 week intervals, then further to 100mg tid PRN. Maint Range: 50-100mg tid. Max: ≤60kg: 50mg tid. >60kg: 100mg tid. If no further reduction in postprandial glucose or HbA1c observed with 100mg tid, consider reducing dose.

HOW SUPPLIED: Tab: 25mg, 50mg, 100mg

CONTRAINDICATIONS: Diabetic ketoacidosis, cirrhosis, inflammatory bowel disease, colonic ulceration, partial intestinal obstruction or predisposition to it, chronic intestinal diseases with marked disorders of digestion or absorption, and conditions that may deteriorate from increased intestinal gas formation.

WARNINGS/PRECAUTIONS: Not recommended with significant renal dysfunction (SrCr >2mg/dL). Elevated serum transaminase levels, fulminant hepatitis, and hyperbilirubinemia reported; monitor serum transaminase levels every 3 months for first year, then periodically. Reduce dose or d/c if elevated serum transaminases persist. Loss of control of blood glucose may occur when exposed to stress (eg, fever, trauma, infection, surgery); temporary insulin therapy may be necessary. Pneumatosis cystoides intestinalis reported; d/c and perform appropriate diagnostic imaging if this is suspected. Reduce dose temporarily or permanently if strongly distressing symptoms develop in spite of adherence to the diabetic diet. Inhibits hydrolysis of sucrose to glucose and fructose; use oral glucose (dextrose) instead of sucrose (cane sugar) in treatment of mild to moderate hypoglycemia.

ADVERSE REACTIONS: Flatulence, diarrhea, abdominal pain.

INTERACTIONS: Closely observe for loss of blood glucose control with thiazides and other diuretics, corticosteroids, phenothiazines, thyroid products, estrogens, oral contraceptives, phenytoin, nicotinic acid, sympathomimetics, calcium channel blockers, and isoniazid. Intestinal adsorbents (eg, charcoal) and digestive enzyme preparations containing carbohydrate-splitting enzymes (eg, amylase, pancreatin) may reduce effect; avoid concomitant use. May affect digoxin bioavailability; may require dose adjustment of digoxin. May reduce peak plasma level of metformin. Increased potential for hypoglycemia with insulin or sulfonylureas; adjust dose if hypoglycemia occurs.

PREGNANCY: Category B, not for use in nursing.

MECHANISM OF ACTION: α-glucosidase inhibitor; competitively and reversibly inhibits pancreatic α-amylase and membrane-bound intestinal α-glucoside hydrolase enzymes.

PHARMACOKINETICS: Absorption: Active Drug: Bioavailability (<2%); T_{max}=1 hr. **Metabolism:** GI tract by intestinal bacteria and digestive enzymes; 4-methylpyrogallol derivatives (major metabolites). **Elimination:** Urine (<2%), feces (51%, unabsorbed); $T_{1/2}$=2 hrs.

NURSING CONSIDERATIONS

Assessment: Assess for renal dysfunction, diabetic ketoacidosis, cirrhosis, inflammatory bowel disease, colonic ulceration, partial intestinal obstruction or predisposition to it, chronic intestinal diseases with marked disorders of digestion or absorption, conditions that may deteriorate from increased intestinal gas formation, previous hypersensitivity to the drug, pregnancy/nursing status, and possible drug interactions.

Monitoring: Monitor FPG, HbA1c, LFTs, and renal function. Monitor serum transaminases every 3 months for 1st year, then periodically. Monitor for signs/symptoms of hypoglycemia and pneumatosis cystoides intestinalis.

Patient Counseling: Instruct to take tid at the start of each main meal. Inform about importance of adhering to dietary instructions, a regular exercise program, and regular testing of urine and blood glucose. Counsel about risks, signs/symptoms, treatment of hypoglycemia, and conditions that predispose to its development. Instruct to have readily available source of glucose (dextrose, D-glucose) to treat symptoms of low blood sugar. Inform that side effects (GI effects such as flatulence, diarrhea, abdominal discomfort) usually develop during the 1st few weeks of therapy and generally diminish in frequency and intensity with time.

Administration: Oral route. **Storage:** ≤25°C (≤77°F). Protect from moisture.

PRED FORTE   RX
prednisolone acetate (Allergan)

THERAPEUTIC CLASS: Corticosteroid

INDICATIONS: Treatment of inflammation of the palpebral and bulbar conjunctiva, cornea and anterior segment of the globe.

DOSAGE: *Adults:* 1-2 drops bid-qid. May dose more frequently during initial 24-48 hrs. Re-evaluate after 2 days if no improvement.

HOW SUPPLIED: Sus: 1% [1mL, 5mL, 10mL, 15mL]

CONTRAINDICATIONS: Viral diseases of the cornea and conjunctiva including epithelial herpes simplex keratitis, vaccinia, and varicella. Mycobacterial infection and fungal diseases of the eye.

WARNINGS/PRECAUTIONS: Caution with glaucoma, herpes simplex, diseases causing thinning of cornea/sclera and other ocular viral infections. Prolonged use can cause glaucoma or secondary ocular infections (eg, fungal). Monitor IOP after 10 days of therapy. Re-evaluate if no response after 2 days. May delay healing and increase incidence of bleb formation after cataract surgery. Avoid abrupt withdrawal with chronic use. Contains sodium bisulfite.

ADVERSE REACTIONS: Elevation of IOP, glaucoma, infrequent optic nerve damage, posterior subcapsular cataract formation, delayed wound healing, burning/stinging upon instillation, ocular irritation, secondary infection, visual disturbance.

PREGNANCY: Category C, not for use in nursing.

MECHANISM OF ACTION: Glucocorticoid; anti-inflammatory agent; inhibits edema, fibrin deposition, capillary dilation, deposition of collagen, and scar formation.

NURSING CONSIDERATIONS

Assessment: Assess for viral disease of cornea and conjunctiva, dendritic keratitis, vaccinia and varicella, mycobacterial infection and/or fungal disease of ocular structures, glaucoma, mustard gas keratitis, Sjogren's keratoconjunctivitis, thinning of corneal/scleral epithelium, hypersensitivity to sulfite, asthma, cataract surgery, and pregnancy/nursing status.

Monitoring: Monitor for anaphylactic symptoms and asthma attacks. Frequent measuring of IOP and slit lamp microscopy exam where appropriate, fluorescein staining for monitoring of glaucoma with damage to the optic nerve with defects in visual acuity and fields of vision, posterior subcapsular cataract, delayed corneal healing, thinning of cornea and sclera, ulceration, perforation, and secondary ocular infections (or masking of existing infections).

Patient Counseling: Advise to d/c drug and consult physician if symptoms persist or worsen. Instruct to wait 15 min after instillation to wear soft contact lenses. Counsel to avoid touching bottle tip to eyelids or any other surface.

Administration: Ocular route. **Storage:** 25°C (77°F). Protect from freezing. Keep tightly closed.

PREDNISONE   RX
prednisone (Roxane)

THERAPEUTIC CLASS: Glucocorticoid

INDICATIONS: Steroid-responsive disorders.

DOSAGE: *Adults:* Initial: 5-60mg/day depending on disease and response. Maint: Decrease dose by small amounts to lowest effective dose.
Pediatrics: Initial: 5-60mg/day depending on disease and response. Maint: Decrease dose by small amounts to lowest effective dose.

HOW SUPPLIED: Sol: 5mg/mL, 5mg/5mL; Tab: 1mg, 2.5mg, 5mg, 10mg, 20mg, 50mg

CONTRAINDICATIONS: Systemic fungal infections.

WARNINGS/PRECAUTIONS: May need to increase dose before, during, and after stressful situations. May mask signs of infection or cause new infections. Prolonged use may produce glaucoma, optic nerve damage, secondary ocular infections. Increases BP, salt/water retention, K⁺ excretion. More severe/fatal course of infections reported with chickenpox, measles. Caution with latent TB, hypothyroidism, cirrhosis, ocular herpes simplex, HTN, diverticulitis, fresh intestinal anastomosis, ulcerative colitis, osteoporosis, myasthenia gravis, renal insufficiency, peptic ulcer disease. Growth and development of children on prolonged therapy should be monitored. Monitor for psychic disturbances. Avoid abrupt withdrawal.

ADVERSE REACTIONS: Fluid and electrolyte disturbances, HTN, osteoporosis, muscle weakness, cushingoid state, menstrual irregularities, nervousness, insomnia, impaired wound healing, DM, ulcerative esophagitis, excessive sweating, increased ICP, carbohydrate intolerance, glaucoma, cataracts, weight gain, nausea, malaise.

INTERACTIONS: Increases clearance of high dose aspirin (ASA); caution in hypoprothrombinemia. Increased insulin and oral hypoglycemic requirements in diabetes mellitus. Avoid smallpox vaccine, and live vaccines with immunosuppressive doses. Possible decreased vaccine response with killed or inactivated vaccines with immunosuppressive doses. Increased clearance with hepatic enzyme inducers. Decreased metabolism with troleandomycin, ketoconazole. Variable effect on oral anticoagulants.

PREGNANCY: Safety in pregnancy and nursing not known.

MECHANISM OF ACTION: Anti-inflammatory glucocorticoid; causes profound and varied metabolic effects and modifies the body's immune responses to diverse stimuli.

PHARMACOKINETICS: Absorption: Readily absorbed (GI tract).

NURSING CONSIDERATIONS

Assessment: Assess unusual stress, fungal/other current infections, active TB, thyroid status, vaccination status, hepatic/liver impairment, hypoprothrombinemia, psychiatric tendencies, ulcerative colitis, diverticulitis, peptic ulcer with/without impending perforation, intestinal anastamoses, HTN, osteoporosis, myasthenia gravis, pregnancy/nursing status, and possible drug interactions.

Monitoring: In pediatrics, monitor for hypoadrenalism, growth and development. Monitor for psychiatric derangements, infection, cataracts, fluid retention, adrenocortical insufficiency, intestinal perforation/peritoneal irritation, serum electrolytes, TSH, glucose, LFTs, BP, IOP.

Patient Counseling: Avoid exposure to chickenpox or measles; report immediately if exposed. Advise regarding dietary salt restriction and K⁺ supplementaion.

Administration: Oral route. **Storage:** 25°C (77°F); excursions permitted to 15-30°C.

PREMARIN TABLETS   RX
conjugated estrogens (Wyeth)

> Estrogens increase the risk of endometrial cancer. Perform adequate diagnostic measures (eg, endometrial sampling), to rule out malignancy with undiagnosed persistent or recurring abnormal genital bleeding. Should not be used for the prevention of cardiovascular (CV) disease or dementia. Increased risks of myocardial infarction (MI), stroke, invasive breast cancer, pulmonary embolism (PE), and deep vein thrombosis (DVT) in postmenopausal women (50-79 yrs of age) reported. Increased risk of developing probable dementia in postmenopausal women ≥65 yrs of age reported. Should be prescribed at the lowest effective dose for the shortest duration consistent with treatment goals and risks.

THERAPEUTIC CLASS: Estrogen

INDICATIONS: Treatment of moderate to severe vasomotor symptoms and/or vulvar/vaginal atrophy due to menopause. Treatment of hypoestrogenism due to hypogonadism, castration, or primary ovarian failure. Palliative treatment of breast cancer in patients with metastatic disease. Palliative treatment of advanced androgen-dependent carcinoma of the prostate. Prevention of postmenopausal osteoporosis.

DOSAGE: *Adults:* Vasomotor Symptoms/Vulvar and Vaginal Atrophy/Prevention of Osteoporosis: Initial: 0.3mg qd continuously or cyclically (eg, 25 days on, 5 days off). Adjust subsequent dose based on response (including bone mineral density [BMD] response for osteoporosis). Female Hypogonadism: 0.3 or 0.625mg qd cyclically (eg, 3 weeks on and 1 week off). Adjust dose based on severity of symptoms and response of the endometrium. Female Castration/Primary Ovarian Failure: 1.25mg qd cyclically. Adjust dose based on severity of symptoms and response. Breast Cancer (palliation): 10mg tid for minimum 3 months. Prostate Cancer (palliation): 1.25-2.5mg (two 1.25mg) tid. Use lowest effective dose for the shortest duration consistent with treatment goals and risk. Re-evaluate at 3- to 6-month intervals.

HOW SUPPLIED: Tab: 0.3mg, 0.45mg, 0.625mg, 0.9mg, 1.25mg

CONTRAINDICATIONS: Undiagnosed abnormal genital bleeding, known/suspected/history of breast cancer unless being treated for metastatic disease, known/suspected estrogen-dependent neoplasia, active or history of DVT/PE, active or recent arterial thromboembolic disease (eg, stroke, MI), liver dysfunction or disease, thrombophilic disorders (eg, protein C, protein S, or antithrombin deficiency), known/suspected pregnancy.

WARNINGS/PRECAUTIONS: Increased risk of stroke, DVT, PE, and MI reported; d/c immediately if any of these events occur or are suspected. Caution in patients with risk factors for arterial vascular disease (eg, HTN, diabetes mellitus [DM], tobacco use, hypercholesterolemia, obesity) and/or venous thromboembolism (eg, personal history or family history of venous thromboembolism, obesity, systemic lupus erythematosus [SLE]). If feasible, d/c at least 4 to 6 weeks before surgery of the type associated with an increased risk of thromboembolism, or during periods of prolonged immobilization. May increase risk of breast/endometrial/ovarian cancer, and gallbladder disease. May lead to severe hypercalcemia with breast cancer and bone metastases; d/c and take appropriate measures if hypercalcemia occurs. Retinal vascular thrombosis reported; if visual abnormalities or migraine occurs, d/c pending examination. If examination reveals papilledema or retinal vascular lesions, d/c permanently. Cases of anaphylaxis reported. Angioedema involving tongue, larynx, face, hands, and feet requiring medical intervention occurred. Patients who develop an anaphylactic reaction with or without angioedema after treatment should not receive treatment again. May induce or exacerbate symptoms of angioedema, particularly in women with hereditary angioedema. Consider addition of a progestin if no hysterectomy. May elevate BP and thyroid-binding globulin levels. May elevate plasma TG; consider d/c if pancreatitis or other complications develop. Caution with history of cholestatic jaundice associated with past estrogen use or with pregnancy; d/c in case of recurrence. May cause fluid retention; caution with cardiac/renal dysfunction. Caution with hypoparathyroidism; hypocalcemia may occur. May exacerbate endometriosis, asthma, DM, epilepsy, migraine, porphyria, SLE, and hepatic hemangiomas; use with caution. May affect certain endocrine and blood components in laboratory tests.

P

ADVERSE REACTIONS: Abdominal pain, asthenia, back pain, headache, infection, pain, arthralgia, leg cramps, breast pain, vaginal hemorrhage, vaginitis, flatulence, flu syndrome, diarrhea, nausea.

INTERACTIONS: CYP3A4 inducers (eg, St. John's wort, phenobarbital, carbamazepine, rifampin) may decrease levels, which may decrease therapeutic effects and/or change uterine bleeding profile. CYP3A4 inhibitors (eg, erythromycin, clarithromycin, ketoconazole, itraconazole, ritonavir, grapefruit juice) may increase levels, which may result in side effects. Patients concomitantly receiving thyroid hormone replacement therapy and estrogens may require increased doses of their thyroid replacement therapy.

PREGNANCY: Contraindicated in pregnancy, not for use in nursing.

MECHANISM OF ACTION: Estrogen; binds to nuclear receptors in estrogen-responsive tissues. Circulating estrogens modulate pituitary secretion of the gonadotropins, luteinizing hormone, and follicle-stimulating hormone, through negative-feedback mechanism. Reduces elevated levels of these hormones in postmenopausal women.

PHARMACOKINETICS: Absorption: Well absorbed; oral administration of variable doses resulted in different parameters. **Distribution:** Largely bound to sex hormone-binding globulin and albumin; found in breast milk. **Metabolism:** Liver, to estrone (metabolite) and estriol (major urinary metabolite); sulfate and glucuronide conjugation (liver); gut hydrolysis; CYP3A4 (partial metabolism). **Elimination:** Urine (parent drug and metabolites).

NURSING CONSIDERATIONS

Assessment: Assess for undiagnosed abnormal genital bleeding, presence or history of breast cancer, estrogen-dependent neoplasia, DVT or PE, or any other conditions where treatment is contraindicated or cautioned. Assess for pregnancy/nursing status and possible drug interactions. Assess need for progestin therapy in women who have not had a hysterectomy. Assess for cardiac or renal dysfunction.

Monitoring: Monitor for signs/symptoms of CV disorders, malignant neoplasms, dementia, gallbladder disease, hypercalcemia, visual abnormalities, increased BP, elevations in plasma triglycerides, pancreatitis, hypertriglyceridemia, cholestatic jaundice, hypothyroidism, fluid retention, exacerbation of endometriosis and other conditions (eg, asthma, DM, epilepsy, migraines, SLE). Perform annual mammography, regular monitoring of BP, and periodic evaluation (every 3-6 months), including BMD to determine need of therapy. Monitor thyroid function in patients on thyroid replacement therapy. Monitor if undiagnosed persistent or recurring genital bleeding occurs; perform adequate diagnostic measures (eg, endometrial sampling) to rule out malignancies.

Patient Counseling: Inform that drug increases risk for uterine cancer, heart attack, stroke, breast cancer, blood clots, and dementia. Instruct to report any breast lumps, unusual vaginal bleeding, dizziness and faintness, changes in speech, severe headaches, chest pain, SOB, leg pains, changes in vision, or vomiting. Advise to notify physician if planning surgery or bedrest. Instruct to take medication at same time daily and to perform monthly self-breast exams. Counsel that if dose is missed, take as soon as possible; if almost time for next dose, skip dose, and go back to normal dosing schedule.

Administration: Oral route. **Storage:** 20-25°C (68-77°F); excursions permitted to 15-30°C (59-86°F).

PREMARIN VAGINAL   RX
conjugated estrogens (Wyeth)

> Estrogens increase the risk of endometrial cancer. Perform adequate diagnostic measures, including endometrial sampling, to rule out malignancy with undiagnosed persistent or recurring abnormal genital bleeding. Should not be used for the prevention of cardiovascular disease (CVD) or dementia. Increased risks of myocardial infarction (MI), stroke, invasive breast cancer, pulmonary embolism (PE), and deep vein thrombosis (DVT) in postmenopausal women (50-79 yrs of age) reported. Increased risk of developing probable dementia in postmenopausal women ≥65 yrs of age reported. Should be prescribed at the lowest effective dose for the shortest duration consistent with treatment goals and risks.

THERAPEUTIC CLASS: Estrogen

INDICATIONS: Treatment of atrophic vaginitis and kraurosis vulvae, and moderate to severe dyspareunia, a symptom of vulvar and vaginal atrophy due to menopause.

DOSAGE: *Adults:* Atrophic Vaginitis/Kraurosis Vulvae: Initial: 0.5g intravaginally cyclically (21 days on, then 7 days off). Titrate: May increase to 0.5-2g based on individual response. Moderate To Severe Dyspareunia: 0.5g intravaginally 2X/week (eg, Monday and Thursday) continuously or cyclically (21 days on, then 7 days off).

HOW SUPPLIED: Cre: 0.625mg/g [42.5g]

CONTRAINDICATIONS: Undiagnosed abnormal genital bleeding, known/suspected/history of breast cancer, known/suspected estrogen-dependent neoplasia, active/history of DVT/PE, active/history of arterial thromboembolic disease (eg, stroke, MI), liver dysfunction/disease, thrombophilic disorders (eg, protein C, protein S, or antithrombin deficiency), or known/suspected pregnancy.

WARNINGS/PRECAUTIONS: D/C therapy immediately if stroke, DVT, PE, or MI occurs or are suspected. Caution in patients with risk factors for arterial vascular disease (eg, HTN, diabetes mellitus [DM], tobacco use, hypercholesterolemia, obesity) and/ or venous thromboembolism (VTE) (eg, personal history or family history of VTE, obesity, systemic lupus erythematosus [SLE]). If feasible, d/c at least 4 to 6 weeks before surgery of the type associated with an increased risk of thromboembolism, or during periods of prolonged immobilization. May increase risk of gallbladder disease requiring surgery and ovarian cancer. May lead to severe hypercalcemia in patients with breast cancer and bone metastases; d/c and take appropriate measures if hypercalcemia occurs. Retinal vascular thrombosis reported; if visual abnormalities or migraine occurs, d/c pending examination. If examination reveals papilledema or retinal vascular lesions, d/c permanently. Increased risk of endometrial cancer with unopposed estrogens in women with intact uteri; consider addition of progestin to in postmenopausal women with a uterus or in posthysterectomy for endometriosis. May elevate BP, thyroid-binding globulin levels, and plasma TG. Consider d/c if pancreatitis occurs. Caution with history of cholestatic jaundice associated with past estrogen use or pregnancy; d/c in case of recurrence. May cause fluid retention; caution with cardiac/renal dysfunction. Caution with hypoparathyroidism; hypocalcemia may occur. Anaphylaxis and angioedema reported with PO treatment. May induce or exacerbate symptoms of angioedema in women with hereditary angioedema. May exacerbate endometriosis, asthma, DM, epilepsy, migraine, porphyria, SLE, and hepatic hemangiomas; use with caution. May weaken and contribute to the failure of condoms, diaphragms, or cervical caps made of latex or rubber. May affect certain endocrine and blood components in laboratory tests.

ADVERSE REACTIONS: Breast pain, headache.

INTERACTIONS: CYP3A4 inducers (eg, St. John's wort, phenobarbital, carbamazepine, rifampin) may decrease levels which may decrease therapeutic effects and/or change uterine bleeding profile. CYP3A4 inhibitors (eg, erythromycin, clarithromycin, ketoconazole, itraconazole, ritonavir, grapefruit juice) may increase levels which may result in side effects. Patients concomitantly receiving thyroid hormone replacement therapy and estrogens may require increased doses of thyroid replacement therapy.

PREGNANCY: Contraindicated in pregnancy, not for use in nursing.

MECHANISM OF ACTION: Estrogen; binds to nuclear receptors in estrogen-responsive tissues. Circulating estrogens modulate pituitary secretion of gonadotropins, luteinizing hormone and follicle stimulating hormone, through negative feedback mechanism. Reduces elevated levels of these hormones in postmenopausal women.

PHARMACOKINETICS: Absorption: Well absorbed through the skin and mucus membranes. **Distribution:** Largely bound to sex hormone-binding globulin and albumin; found in breast milk. **Metabolism:** Liver to estrone (metabolite), estriol (major urinary metabolite); sulfate and glucuronide conjugation (liver); gut hydrolysis; CYP3A4 (partial metabolism). **Elimination:** Urine (parent compound and metabolites).

NURSING CONSIDERATIONS

Assessment: Assess for abnormal genital bleeding, estrogen-dependent neoplasia, presence or history of breast cancer, arterial thromboembolic disease, DVT or PE, hereditary angioedema, thrombophilic disorders, or any other conditions where treatment is contraindicated or cautioned. Assess use in women ≥65 yrs, nursing patients, and those with DM, asthma, epilepsy, migraines or porphyria, SLE, and hepatic hemangiomas. Assess for pregnancy/nursing status and possible drug interactions.

Monitoring: Monitor for signs/symptoms of CV events, malignant neoplasms, dementia, gallbladder disease, hypercalcemia, visual abnormalities, pancreatitis, hypertriglyceridemia, cholestatic jaundice, hypothyroidism, fluid retention, exacerbation of endometriosis and other conditions. Perform annual breast exam and regular monitoring of BP. Monitor thyroid function in patients on thyroid replacement therapy. Perform periodic evaluation to determine need for treatment. Monitor if undiagnosed persistent or recurring genital bleeding occurs, perform adequate diagnostic measures (eg, endometrial sampling) to rule out malignancies.

Patient Counseling: Advise to notify physician if signs/symptoms of unusual vaginal bleeding occur. Inform about possible serious adverse reactions (eg, CVD, malignant neoplasms, and probable dementia) and possible less serious but common adverse reactions (eg, headache, breast pain/tenderness, N/V). Instruct on how to use the applicator. Instruct to perform monthly breast self-examination. Inform that medication may weaken barrier contraceptives (eg, latex or rubber condoms, diaphragms, cervical caps).

Administration: Intravaginal route. Refer to PI for instructions on use of applicator. **Storage:** 20-25°C (68-77°F); excursions permitted to 15-30°C (59-86°F).

PREMPHASE   RX
medroxyprogesterone acetate - conjugated estrogens (Wyeth)

Estrogens increase the risk of endometrial cancer. Perform adequate diagnostic measures, including endometrial sampling, to rule out malignancy in postmenopausal women with undiagnosed persistent or recurring abnormal genital bleeding. Should not be used for the prevention of cardiovascular disease (CVD) or dementia. Increased risk of myocardial infarction (MI), stroke, invasive breast cancer, pulmonary embolism (PE), and deep vein thrombosis (DVT) in postmenopausal women (50-79 yrs) reported. Increased risk of developing probable dementia in postmenopausal women ≥65 yrs reported. Should be prescribed at the lowest effective dose and for the shortest duration consistent with treatment goals and risks.

OTHER BRAND NAMES: Prempro (Wyeth)

THERAPEUTIC CLASS: Estrogen/progestogen combination

INDICATIONS: Treatment of moderate to severe vasomotor symptoms and/or vulvar and vaginal atrophy due to menopause and prevention of postmenopausal osteoporosis.

DOSAGE: *Adults:* (Premphase) 0.625mg tab qd on Days 1-14 and 0.625mg-5mg tab qd on Days 15-28. (Prempro) 1 tab qd. Reevaluate treatment need periodically.

HOW SUPPLIED: Tab: (Premphase) (Conjugated Estrogens) 0.625mg, (Conjugated Estrogens-Medroxyprogesterone) 0.625mg-5mg; (Prempro) (Conjugated Estrogens-Medroxyprogesterone) 0.3mg-1.5mg, 0.45mg-1.5mg, 0.625mg-2.5mg, 0.625mg-5mg

CONTRAINDICATIONS: Undiagnosed abnormal genital bleeding, known/suspected/history of breast cancer, known/suspected estrogen-dependent neoplasia, active or history of DVT/PE/arterial thromboembolic disease (eg, stroke, MI), known liver dysfunction/disease or thrombophilic disorders (eg, protein C, protein S, or antithrombin deficiency), known/suspected pregnancy.

WARNINGS/PRECAUTIONS: Increased risk of CVD; d/c immediately if this occurs or is suspected. Caution in patients with risk factors for arterial vascular disease (eg, HTN, diabetes mellitus [DM], tobacco use, hypercholesterolemia, obesity) and/or venous thromboembolism (eg, personal history of venous thromboembolism, obesity, systemic lupus erythematosus [SLE]). If feasible, d/c at least 4 to 6 weeks before surgery of the type associated with an increased risk of thromboembolism, or during periods of prolonged immobilization. May increase risk of gallbladder disease requiring surgery and ovarian cancer. May lead to severe hypercalcemia in patients with breast cancer and bone metastases; d/c and take appropriate measures if hypercalcemia occurs. Retinal vascular thrombosis reported; if visual abnormalities or migraine occurs, d/c pending examination. If examination reveals papilledema or retinal vascular lesions, d/c permanently. May elevate BP, plasma TG (with preexisting hypertriglyceridemia), and thyroid-binding globulin levels; d/c if pancreatitis occurs. Caution with history of cholestatic jaundice associated with past estrogen use or with pregnancy; d/c in case of recurrence. May cause fluid retention; caution with cardiac/renal dysfunction. Caution with hypoparathyroidism; hypocalcemia may result. May induce or exacerbate symptoms of angioedema, particularly in women with hereditary angioedema. May exacerbate endometriosis, asthma, DM, epilepsy, migraine, porphyria, SLE, and hepatic hemangiomas; use with caution. Consider addition of a progestin to estrogen monotherapy with residual endometriosis post-hysterectomy. May affect certain endocrine and blood components in laboratory tests.

ADVERSE REACTIONS: Breast pain, headache, abdominal pain, infection, back pain, flu syndrome, pharyngitis, dysmenorrhea, nausea, depression, asthenia, arthralgia, leukorrhea, rhinitis, flatulence.

INTERACTIONS: CYP3A4 inducers (eg, St. John's wort, phenobarbital, carbamazepine, rifampin) may decrease levels, which may decrease therapeutic effects and/or change uterine bleeding profile. CYP3A4 inhibitors (eg, erythromycin, clarithromycin, ketoconazole, itraconazole, ritonavir, grapefruit juice) may increase levels, which may result in side effects. Aminoglutethimide may significantly depress bioavailability of medroxyprogesterone acetate (MPA). Patients receiving concomitant thyroid hormone replacement therapy may require increased doses of thyroid replacement therapy.

PREGNANCY: Contraindicated in pregnancy, not for use in nursing.

MECHANISM OF ACTION: Conjugated Estrogens: Estrogen; binds to nuclear receptors in estrogen-responsive tissues. Circulating estrogens modulate pituitary secretion of gonadotropins, luteinizing hormone, and follicle-stimulating hormone, through negative-feedback mechanism. Reduces elevated levels of these hormones in postmenopausal women. MPA: Progesterone derivative; parenterally administered MPA inhibits gonadotropin production, which prevents follicular maturation and ovulation. Decreases nuclear estrogen receptors and suppresses epithelial DNA synthesis in endometrial tissue.

PHARMACOKINETICS: Absorption: Well-absorbed. Oral administration of various doses resulted in different parameters. **Distribution:** Found in breast milk. Estrogen: Largely bound to sex hormone-binding globulin and albumin. MPA: Plasma protein binding (90%). **Metabolism:** Estrogen: Liver, to estrone (metabolite); estriol (major urinary metabolite); enterohepatic recirculation via sulfate and glucuronide conjugation in the liver; biliary secretion of conjugates into the intestine; hydrolysis in the intestine; reabsorption. MPA: Liver via hydroxylation, with subsequent conjugation. **Elimination:** Estrogen: Urine (parent compound and metabolites). MPA: Urine (metabolites).

NURSING CONSIDERATIONS

Assessment: Assess for abnormal genital bleeding, presence or history of breast cancer, estrogen-dependent neoplasia, active or history of DVT/PE/arterial thromboembolic disease, liver dysfunction/disorder, thrombophilic disorders, known/suspected pregnancy, and any other conditions where treatment is cautioned. Assess for possible drug interactions.

Monitoring: Monitor for signs/symptoms of CVD, malignant neoplasms, dementia, gallbladder disease, hypercalcemia, visual abnormalities, BP elevations, elevations in plasma TG, pancreatitis, cholestatic jaundice, hypothyroidism, fluid retention, and exacerbation of endometriosis and other conditions. Perform annual breast examinations; schedule mammography based on patient age, risk factors, and prior mammogram results. Monitor thyroid function in patients on thyroid hormone replacement therapy. Perform adequate diagnostic measures (eg, endometrial sampling) in patients with undiagnosed persistent or recurring genital bleeding. Perform periodic evaluation to determine treatment need.

Patient Counseling: Inform postmenopausal women of the importance of reporting abnormal vaginal bleeding as soon as possible. Inform of possible serious adverse reactions of therapy (eg, CVD, malignant neoplasms, probable dementia) and possible less serious but common adverse reactions (eg, headache, breast pain and tenderness, N/V). Advise to have yearly breast examinations by a healthcare provider and perform monthly breast self-examinations.

Administration: Oral route. **Storage**: 20-25°C (68-77°F); excursions permitted to 15-30°C (59-86°F).

PREVACID   RX
lansoprazole (Takeda)

OTHER BRAND NAMES: Prevacid Solutab (Takeda)

THERAPEUTIC CLASS: Proton pump inhibitor

INDICATIONS: Short-term treatment of active duodenal ulcer (DU), active benign gastric ulcer (GU), and erosive esophagitis (EE). Maintenance of healing of DU and EE. Treatment and risk reduction of NSAID-associated GU. Treatment of heartburn and other symptoms associated with gastroesophageal reflux disease (GERD). Long-term treatment of pathological hypersecretory conditions (eg, Zollinger-Ellison syndrome). Combination therapy with amoxicillin +/- clarithromycin for *Helicobacter pylori* eradication to reduce the risk of DU recurrence.

DOSAGE: *Adults:* DU: Short-Term Treatment: 15mg qd for 4 weeks. Maintenance of Healing: 15mg qd. Short-term Treatment of Benign GU: 30mg qd for up to 8 weeks. NSAID-associated GU: Healing: 30mg qd for 8 weeks. Risk Reduction: 15mg qd for up to 12 weeks. GERD: Short-term Treatment of Symptomatic GERD: 15mg qd for up to 8 weeks. Short-Treatment of EE: 30mg qd for up to 8 weeks. May give for 8 more weeks if healing does not occur. If there is recurrence of EE, an additional 8-week course may be considered. Maintenance of Healing of EE: 15mg qd. Pathological Hypersecretory Conditions (eg, Zollinger-Ellison Syndrome): Initial: 60mg qd. Titrate: Adjust to individual patient needs. Max: 90mg bid. Divide dose if >120mg/day. *H. pylori* Eradication to Reduce Risk of DU Recurrence: Triple Therapy: 30mg + amoxicillin 1000mg + clarithromycin 500mg, all bid (q12h) for 10 or 14 days. Dual Therapy: 30mg + amoxicillin 1000mg, both tid (q8h) for 14 days. Severe Hepatic Impairment: Consider dose adjustment. Take before eating.
Pediatrics: 12-17 yrs: Short-Term Treatment of Symptomatic GERD: Nonerosive GERD: 15mg qd for up to 8 weeks. EE: 30mg qd for up to 8 weeks. 1-11 yrs: Short-Term Treatment of Symptomatic GERD/EE: ≤30kg: 15mg qd for up to 12 weeks. Titrate: May increase after ≥2 weeks of treatment if remain symptomatic. Max: 30mg bid. >30kg: 30mg qd for up to 12 weeks. Titrate: May increase after ≥2 weeks of treatment if remain symptomatic. Max: 30mg bid. Severe Hepatic Impairment: Consider dose adjustment. Take before eating.

HOW SUPPLIED: Cap, Delayed-Release: 15mg, 30mg; Tab, Disintegrating (SoluTab): 15mg, 30mg

WARNINGS/PRECAUTIONS: Symptomatic response does not preclude the presence of gastric malignancy. May increase risk for osteoporosis-related fractures of the hip, wrist, or spine especially with high-dose and long-term therapy; use lowest dose and shortest duration appropriate to the condition being treated. Hypomagnesemia reported; magnesium replacement and d/c of therapy may be required. (Tab, Disintegrating) Contains phenylalanine.

ADVERSE REACTIONS: Abdominal pain, constipation, diarrhea, nausea, dizziness, headache.

INTERACTIONS: Substantially decreases atazanavir concentrations; avoid concomitant use. May alter absorption of other drugs where gastric pH is an important determinant of oral bioavailability (eg, ketoconazole, ampicillin esters, digoxin, iron salts). Delayed absorption and reduced

P

bioavailability with sucralfate; give ≥30 mins prior to sucralfate. May increase theophylline clearance; may require dose adjustment. Monitor for increases in INR and PT with warfarin. May increase tacrolimus levels. May decrease mean area under the curve of active metabolite of clopidogrel. Caution with digoxin or other drugs that may cause hypomagnesemia (eg, diuretics).

PREGNANCY: Category B, not for use in nursing.

MECHANISM OF ACTION: Proton pump inhibitor; suppresses gastric acid secretion by specific inhibition of the (H^+, K^+)-ATPase enzyme system at the secretory surface of the gastric parietal cell.

PHARMACOKINETICS: Absorption: Rapid; absolute bioavailability (>80%); T_{max}=1.7 hrs. **Distribution:** Plasma protein binding (97%). **Metabolism:** Liver (extensive). **Elimination:** Urine (1/3), feces (2/3); $T_{1/2}$=<2 hrs.

NURSING CONSIDERATIONS

Assessment: Assess for hepatic insufficiency, osteoporosis, phenylketonuria, previous hypersensitivity to drug, pregnancy/nursing status, and possible drug interactions. Obtain baseline magnesium levels.

Monitoring: Monitor for signs/symptoms of bone fractures, hypersensitivity reactions, and other adverse reactions. Monitor magnesium levels periodically.

Patient Counseling: Advise to contact physician if any adverse events develop while on therapy; seek immediate medical attention if develop cardiovascular/neurological symptoms of hypomagnesemia (eg, palpitations, dizziness, seizures, tetany). Instruct to take missed dose as soon as possible; do not take missed dose if next scheduled dose is due. Advise to not take two doses at the same time to make up for a missed dose. Instruct to take before eating. Inform of alternative methods of administration if have swallowing difficulties.

Administration: Oral route. May also be administered via NG tube. Do not crush, break, cut, or chew. Swallow caps whole. Allow tab to disintegrate on the tongue until particles can be swallowed. Refer to PI for additional administration instructions. **Storage:** 25°C (77°F); excursions permitted to 15-30°C (59-86°F).

PREVPAC   RX
amoxicillin - clarithromycin - lansoprazole (TAP)

THERAPEUTIC CLASS: H. pylori treatment combination

INDICATIONS: Treatment of H. pylori infection associated with active duodenal ulcer and to reduce the risk of duodenal ulcer recurrence.

DOSAGE: *Adults:* 1g amoxicillin, 500mg clarithromycin and 30mg lansoprazole, all bid (am and pm) before meals for 10 or 14 days. Swallow each pill whole. Renal Impairment (with or without hepatic impairment): Decrease clarithromycin dose or prolong intervals.

HOW SUPPLIED: Cap: (Amoxicillin) 500mg, Tab: (Clarithromycin) 500mg, Cap, Delayed-Release: (Lansoprazole) 30mg

CONTRAINDICATIONS: Concomitant use with cisapride, pimozide, astemizole, terfenadine, ergotamine or dihydroergotamine.

WARNINGS/PRECAUTIONS: Serious and occasional fatal hypersensitivity reactions reported in patients on penicillin therapy. Avoid if CrCl <30mL/min. Caution with cephalosporin/PCN allergy; anaphylactic reactions have been reported. Pseudomembranous colitis reported. D/C if superinfections occur. Caution in elderly. Do not use clarithromycin during pregnancy. Symptomatic response to lansoprazole does not preclude the presence of gastric malignancy. *Clostridium difficile*-associated diarrhea (CDAD) reported. D/C if confirmed. Exacerbation of symptoms with myasthenia gravis and new onset of myasthenic syndrome reported with clarithromycin.

ADVERSE REACTIONS: Diarrhea, taste perversion, headache, abdominal pain, dark stools, myalgia, confusion, respiratory disorders, skin reactions, vaginitis.

INTERACTIONS: See Contraindications. Lansoprazole: May interfere with absorption of drugs dependent on gastric pH for bioavailability (eg, atazanavir, ketoconazole, ampicillin esters, iron salts, digoxin). Monitor increase in INR and prothrombin time with concomitant use of warfarin. Amoxicillin: May decrease renal tubular secretion when coadministered with probenecid. May interfere with bactericidal effects of penicillin with chloramphenicol, macrolides, sulfonamides and tetracycline. Clarithromycin: May increase theophylline and carbamazepine levels. Simultaneous administration with zidovudine resulted in decreased steady-state zidovudine levels in HIV-infected patients. Elevated digoxin levels in patients receiving concomitant digoxin. May lead to increased exposure to colchicine when coadministered; monitor for toxicity. May increase or prolong both therapeutic and adverse effects with erythromycin. Torsades de pointes may occur with quinidine or disopyramide. May increase systemic exposure of sildenafil; consider dose reduction.

PREGNANCY: Category C, not for use in nursing.

MECHANISM OF ACTION: Lansoprazole: Substituted benzimidazole; inhibits gastric acid secretion. Amoxicillin: Semi-synthetic antibiotic; has broad spectrum of bactericidal activity against many gram-positive and gram-negative microorganisms. Clarithromycin: Semi-synthetic macrolide antibiotic.

PHARMACOKINETICS: Absorption: Lansoprazole: Rapidly absorbed; absolute bioavailability (80%); T_{max}=1.7 hrs. Amoxicillin: Rapidly absorbed. Clarithromycin: Rapidly absorbed; absolute bioavailability (50%); T_{max}=2-2.5 hrs. **Distribution:** Lansoprazole: Plasma protein binding (97%); found in breast milk. Amoxicillin: Plasma protein binding (approximately 20%). Clarithromycin: Found in breast milk. **Metabolism:** Lansoprazole: Liver (extensive). Clarithromycin: 14-OH clarithromycin (active metabolite). **Elimination:** Lansoprazole: Urine, feces; $T_{1/2}$=<2 hrs. Amoxicillin: Urine (60%); $T_{1/2}$=61.3 mins. Clarithromycin: Urine (30%); $T_{1/2}$=5-7 hrs; (metabolite) $T_{1/2}$=7-9 hrs.

NURSING CONSIDERATIONS

Assessment: Assess for hypersensitivity to other macrolides, PCNs, or cephalosporins. Assess for proper diagnosis of susceptible bacteria (eg, cultures), pregnancy/nursing status, renal impairment, gastric malignancy, presence of bacterial infection, and possible drug interactions.

Monitoring: Monitor for signs/symptoms of drug interactions (eg, cardiac arrhythmias), hypersensitivity reactions (eg, anaphylaxis), pseudomembranous colitis and CDAD, and development of superinfections.

Patient Counseling: Instruct to take each dose twice per day before eating; swallow pill whole. Notify physician of all medications currently being taken. Inform that drug treats bacterial, not viral, infections. Take exactly as directed; skipping doses may decrease effectiveness and increase antibiotic resistance. Instruct to avoid pregnancy/nursing during therapy and contact physician if diarrhea occurs.

Administration: Oral route. **Storage:** 20-25°C (68-77°F). Protect from light and moisture.

PREZISTA
darunavir (Janssen)

RX

THERAPEUTIC CLASS: Protease inhibitor

INDICATIONS: Treatment of HIV-1 infection in adult and pediatric (≥3 yrs) patients in combination with ritonavir (RTV) and other antiretroviral agents.

DOSAGE: *Adults:* Treatment-Naive/Treatment-Experienced with No Darunavir Resistance Associated Substitutions: 800mg (two 400mg tabs or two 4mL sus administrations) with RTV 100mg qd. Treatment-Experienced with ≥1 Darunavir Resistance Associated Substitution Or with No Feasible Genotypic Testing: 600mg (one 600mg tab or 6mL sus) with RTV 100mg bid. *Pediatrics:* 3-<18 yrs: Give bid. ≥40 kg: 600mg tab or 6mL sus with RTV 100mg. ≥30-<40kg: 450mg tab or 4.6mL sus with RTV 100mg. ≥15-<30kg: 375mg tab or 3.8mL sus with RTV 50mg. Sus should be used with RTV sol if unable to swallow. ≥14-<15kg: 2.8mL sus with RTV sol 0.6mL. ≥13-<14kg: 2.6mL sus with RTV sol 0.5mL. ≥12-<13kg: 2.4mL sus with RTV sol 0.5mL. ≥11-<12kg: 2.2mL sus with RTV sol 0.4mL. ≥10-<11kg: 2mL sus with RTV sol 0.4mL. Do not exceed recommended dose for treatment-experienced adults.

HOW SUPPLIED: Sus: 100mg/mL [200mL]; Tab: 75mg, 150mg, 400mg, 600mg

CONTRAINDICATIONS: Coadministration with CYP3A substrates for which elevated plasma concentrations are associated with serious and/or life-threatening reactions (eg, alfuzosin, dihydroergotamine, ergonovine, ergotamine, methylergonovine, cisapride, pimozide, oral midazolam, triazolam, St. John's wort, lovastatin, simvastatin, rifampin, sildenafil [when used to treat pulmonary arterial HTN]).

WARNINGS/PRECAUTIONS: Must be coadministered with RTV and food to achieve desired effect. Drug-induced hepatitis (eg, acute hepatitis, cytolytic hepatitis) and liver injury reported; consider interruption or d/c therapy if evidence of new/worsening liver dysfunction occurs. Avoid in patients with severe hepatic impairment. Severe skin reactions including Stevens-Johnson syndrome (SJS) and toxic epidermal necrolysis (TEN) reported; d/c if severe skin reaction develops. Caution with sulfonamide allergy. Increased bleeding in hemophilia type A and B, new onset/exacerbation of diabetes mellitus (DM), diabetic ketoacidosis, hyperglycemia, and redistribution/accumulation of body fat reported. Immune reconstitution syndrome may occur. Caution in elderly.

ADVERSE REACTIONS: Diarrhea, N/V, headache, abdominal pain, rash.

INTERACTIONS: See Contraindications. Avoid with colchicine in renal/hepatic impairment and voriconazole. Not recommended with lopinavir, saquinavir, telaprevir, salmeterol, and other protease inhibitors (except atazanavir and indinavir). May increase levels of CYP3A substrates, CYP2D6 substrates, indinavir, maraviroc, antiarrhythmics, digoxin, carbamazepine, trazodone, desipramine, clarithromycin, ketoconazole, itraconazole, rifabutin, β-blockers, parenteral mid-azolam, calcium channel blockers, inhaled fluticasone, bosentan, pravastatin, atorvastatin, rosuvastatin, immunosuppressants, norbuprenorphine, neuroleptics, sildenafil for erectile dysfunction, vardenafil, and tadalafil. May decrease levels of phenytoin, phenobarbital, methadone, ethinyl estradiol, norethindrone, sertraline, and paroxetine. May decrease levels of warfarin; monitor INR. CYP3A inhibitors, ketoconazole, itraconazole, indinavir, and rifabutin may increase levels. CYP3A inducers and systemic dexamethasone may decrease levels. Administer didanosine 1 hr before/2 hrs after.

PREGNANCY: Category C, not for use in nursing.

MECHANISM OF ACTION: Protease inhibitor; selectively inhibits the cleavage of HIV-1 encoded Gag-Pol polyproteins in infected cells, thereby preventing the formation of mature virus particles.

PHARMACOKINETICS: Absorption: Absolute oral bioavailability (37%) darunavir, (82%) darunavir/RTV; T_{max}=2.5-4 hrs. **Distribution:** Plasma protein binding (95%). **Metabolism:** Hepatic (extensive); oxidation via CYP3A. **Elimination:** Darunavir/RTV: Feces (79.5%), urine (13.9%); $T_{1/2}$=15 hrs.

NURSING CONSIDERATIONS

Assessment: Assess for sulfonamide allergy, liver dysfunction, hemophilia, preexisting DM, pregnancy/nursing status, and for possible drug interactions. Assess ability to swallow tablets. In treatment experienced patients, assess treatment history and perform phenotypic and genotypic testing.

Monitoring: Monitor for signs/symptoms of severe skin reactions (eg, SJS, TEN), new onset/exacerbation of DM, diabetic ketoacidosis, hyperglycemia, bleeding episodes, fat redistribution, immune reconstitution syndrome, and for hepatic impairment. Perform therapeutic drug monitoring for drug interactions as recommended.

Patient Counseling: Inform that drug does not cure HIV infection. Advise to stay on continuous HIV therapy to control infection and decrease related illnesses. Instruct to practice safer sex using latex or polyurethane condoms. Counsel not to share personal items that can have blood or body fluids on them. Inform to never to reuse or share needles. Advise to take with food and to swallow tab whole with a drink; instruct not to alter dose or d/c without consulting physician. Counsel to take drug immediately for missed dose <6 hrs and <12 hrs for bid and qd dosing respectively, and take the next dose at regular scheduled time. Instruct that if a dose is missed by >6 hrs or >12 hrs for bid and qd dosing respectively, take the next dose as scheduled; instruct not to double the dose. Counsel to report use of any other Rx, OTC, or herbal medication (eg, St. John's wort). Instruct to use alternative contraceptive measures if on estrogen-based contraceptive during therapy. Advise about the signs/symptoms of liver problems (eg, jaundice, dark urine, pale colored stools, N/V, loss of appetite, or pain/aching/sensitivity in the right upper quadrant of the abdomen) and severe skin reactions (eg, fever, general malaise, fatigue, muscle/joint aches, blisters, oral lesions, conjunctivitis, hepatitis, eosinophilia). Inform that redistribution and accumulation of fat may occur.

Administration: Oral route. Take with food. (Sus) Shake well before use. **Storage:** 25°C (77°F); excursions permitted to 15-30°C (59-86°F). (Sus) Do not refrigerate or freeze. Avoid exposure to excessive heat. Store in the original container.

PRILOSEC   RX
omeprazole magnesium - omeprazole (AstraZeneca)

THERAPEUTIC CLASS: Proton pump inhibitor

INDICATIONS: Short-term treatment of active duodenal ulcer (DU) and active benign gastric ulcer (GU) in adults. Treatment of heartburn and other symptoms associated with gastroesophageal reflux disease (GERD) in adults and pediatrics. Short-term treatment and maintenance of healing of erosive esophagitis in adults and pediatrics. Long-term treatment of pathological hypersecretory conditions (eg, Zollinger-Ellison syndrome, multiple endocrine adenomas, systemic mastocytosis) in adults. Combination therapy with clarithromycin +/- amoxicillin in *Helicobacter pylori* infection and duodenal ulcer disease for *H. pylori* eradication.

DOSAGE: *Adults:* Active DU: 20mg qd for 4 weeks; some may require additional 4 weeks. GERD: Without Esophageal Lesions: 20mg qd for up to 4 weeks. With Erosive Esophagitis and Accompanying Symptoms: 20mg qd for 4-8 weeks. May continue for an additional 4 weeks if do not respond after 8 weeks. Consider additional 4-8 week courses if recurrence of symptoms/erosive esophagitis. GU: 40mg qd for 4-8 weeks. Maint of Healing of Erosive Esophagitis: 20mg qd for up to 12 months. Hypersecretory Conditions: Initial: 60mg qd; adjust if needed and continue for as long as clinically indicated. Divide dose if >80mg/day. Max: 120mg tid. *H. pylori* Eradication: Triple Therapy: omeprazole 20mg + clarithromycin 500mg + amoxicillin 1000mg, all bid for 10 days. Give additional 18 days of omeprazole 20mg qd if ulcer present at initiation of therapy. Dual Therapy: omeprazole 40mg qd + clarithromycin 500mg tid for 14 days. Give additional 14 days of omeprazole 20mg qd if ulcer present at initiation of therapy. (Cap) Take before eating and swallow whole.

Pediatrics: 1-16 yrs: GERD/Maint of Healing of Erosive Esophagitis: ≥20kg: 20mg/day. 10-<20kg: 10mg/day. 5-<10kg: 5mg/day. (Cap) Take before eating and swallow whole.

HOW SUPPLIED: Cap, Delayed-Release (Omeprazole): 10mg, 20mg, 40mg; Sus, Delayed-Release (Omeprazole magnesium): 2.5mg, 10mg (granules/pkt)

WARNINGS/PRECAUTIONS: Symptomatic response does not preclude the presence of gastric malignancy. Atrophic gastritis reported with long-term use. May increase risk for osteoporosis-related fractures of the hip, wrist, or spine especially with high-dose and long term therapy; use lowest dose and shortest duration appropriate to the condition being treated. Hypomagnesemia reported rarely; consider monitoring magnesium levels prior to and periodically during therapy with prolonged treatment.

ADVERSE REACTIONS: Headache, diarrhea, abdominal pain, N/V, flatulence; (pediatrics) fever, respiratory disorders.

INTERACTIONS: May reduce atazanavir and nelfinavir levels; use is not recommended. May change levels of antiretrovirals. May increase saquinavir levels; monitor for possible toxicity and consider dose reduction. May interfere with absorption of drugs where gastric pH is an important determinant of bioavailability (eg, ketoconazole, ampicillin esters, iron salts). May prolong elimination of drugs metabolized by oxidation in the liver (eg, diazepam, warfarin, and phenytoin); omeprazole is an inhibitor of CYP2C19. Monitor patients taking drugs metabolized by CYP450 (eg, cyclosporine, disulfiram, benzodiazepines). Monitor for increases in INR and PT with warfarin. Concomitant administration with voriconazole (a combined inhibitor of CYP2C19 and 3A4) resulted in more than doubling of omeprazole exposure. Decreased levels with drugs known to induce CYP2C19 or CYP3A4 (eg, St. John's wort, rifampin); avoid concomitant use. Avoid use with clopidogrel; coadministration reduces platelet inhibition. When used with clarithromycin, the levels of both drugs may be increased. Increased levels of tacrolimus and cilostazol; consider cilostazol dose reduction. Digoxin absorption may be increased with concomitant use. Caution with digoxin or other drugs that may cause hypomagnesemia (eg, diuretics).

PREGNANCY: Category C, not for use in nursing.

MECHANISM OF ACTION: Proton pump inhibitor; suppresses gastric acid secretion by specific inhibition of the H^+/K^+ ATPase enzyme system at the secretory surface of the gastric parietal cell.

PHARMACOKINETICS: Absorption: (Cap) Rapid; absolute bioavailability (30-40%); T_{max}=0.5-3.5 hrs. **Distribution:** Plasma protein binding (95%); found in breast milk. **Metabolism:** Extensive via CYP450. **Elimination:** Urine (77%), feces; (Cap) $T_{1/2}$=0.5-1 hr.

NURSING CONSIDERATIONS

Assessment: Assess for hypersensitivity to the drug or its components, gastric malignancy, hepatic impairment, risk for osteoporosis-related fractures, pregnancy/nursing status, and possible drug interactions. Obtain baseline LFTs and magnesium levels.

Monitoring: Monitor for signs/symptoms of atrophic gastritis, bone fractures, hypomagnesemia, hypersensitivity reactions, and other adverse reactions. Monitor LFTs. Monitor INR and PT when given with warfarin. Monitor magnesium levels periodically.

Patient Counseling: Advise to contact physician if any adverse events develop while on therapy; seek immediate medical attention if cardiovascular/neurological symptoms of hypomagnesemia (eg, palpitations, dizziness, seizures, tetany) develop. Instruct to take before eating. Inform of alternative methods of administration if have swallowing difficulties.

Administration: Oral route. (Sus) May also be given via gastric/nasogastric route. Refer to PI for administration instructions. **Storage:** (Cap) 15-30°C (59-86°F). Protect from light and moisture. (Sus) 25°C (77°F); excursions permitted to 15-30°C (59-86°F).

PRIMAXIN I.M.   RX
cilastatin sodium - imipenem (Merck)

THERAPEUTIC CLASS: Thienamycin/dehydropeptidase I inhibitor

INDICATIONS: Treatment of lower respiratory tract (LRTI), skin and skin structure (SSSI), intra-abdominal, and gynecologic infections caused by susceptible strains of microorganisms.

DOSAGE: *Adults:* Mild to Moderate LRTI/SSSI/Gynecologic Infection: 500mg or 750mg IM q12h depending on severity. Mild to Moderate Intra-Abdominal Infection: 750mg IM q12h. Continue for at least 2 days after signs and symptoms resolve; do not treat >14 days. Max: 1500mg/day. Elderly: Start at lower end of dosing range.

Pediatrics: ≥12 yrs: Mild to Moderate LRTI/SSSI/Gynecologic Infections: 500mg or 750mg IM q12h depending on severity. Mild to Moderate Intra-Abdominal Infection: 750mg IM q12h. Continue for at least 2 days after signs and symptoms resolve; do not treat >14 days. Max: 1500mg/day.

HOW SUPPLIED: Inj: (Imipenem-Cilastatin) 500mg-500mg, 750mg-750mg

Primaxin I.V.

CONTRAINDICATIONS: Severe shock, heart block, hypersensitivity to local anesthetics of amide type (due to lidocaine diluent).

WARNINGS/PRECAUTIONS: Not intended for severe or life-threatening infections. Serious and occasionally fatal hypersensitivity (anaphylactic) reactions reported. Carefully assess previous reactions to penicillin (PCN), cephalosporins, other β-lactams, and other allergens. Seizures and other CNS adverse experiences such as myoclonic activity reported, particularly in patients with CNS disorders (eg, brain lesions or history of seizures) who also have compromised renal function. *Clostridium difficile*-associated diarrhea (CDAD) reported. May result in bacterial resistance with prolonged use or use in the absence of a proven/suspected bacterial infection or a prophylactic indication; take appropriate measures if superinfection develops. Avoid inadvertent injection into a blood vessel. Caution in elderly. Safety and efficacy not established in patients with CrCl <20 mL/min/1.73m².

ADVERSE REACTIONS: Injection-site pain, N/V, diarrhea, rash.

INTERACTIONS: Minimal increases in plasma levels and $T_{1/2}$ with probenecid; concomitant use not recommended. May decrease levels of valproic acid or divalproex sodium, thereby increasing risk of breakthrough seizures; concomitant use is generally not recommended, but if necessary, consider supplemental anticonvulsant therapy.

PREGNANCY: Category C, caution in nursing.

MECHANISM OF ACTION: (Imipenem) Thienamycin; inhibits cell-wall synthesis. (Cilastatin) Dehydropeptidase I inhibitor; prevents renal metabolism of imipenem.

PHARMACOKINETICS: Absorption: Imipenem: Bioavailability (75%), C_{max}=10mcg/mL (500mg), 12mcg/mL (750mg); T_{max}=2 hrs. Cilastatin: Bioavailability (95%), C_{max}=24mcg/mL (500mg), 33mcg/mL (750mg); T_{max}=1 hr. **Distribution:** Imipenem: Plasma protein binding (20%). Cilastatin: Plasma protein binding (40%). **Metabolism:** Imipenem: Kidneys by dehydropropeptidase I. **Elimination:** Imipinem: Urine (50%); $T_{1/2}$=2-3 hrs. Cilastatin: Urine (75%).

NURSING CONSIDERATIONS

Assessment: Assess for severity and type of infection. Assess for hypersensitivity to local anesthetics (amide type), PCN, cephalosporins, β-lactams, and other allergens. Assess for severe shock, heart block, CNS disorders (eg, brain lesions, history of seizures), renal function, pregnancy/nursing status, and possible drug interactions.

Monitoring: Monitor for CNS adverse events (eg, seizures or myoclonic activity), hypersensitivity reactions, CDAD, superinfection, and other possible adverse events.

Patient Counseling: Counsel to inform physician if taking valproic acid or divalproex sodium. Instruct to take as directed; skipping doses or not completing full course may decrease effectiveness and increase resistance. Inform that diarrhea may occur, even as late as ≥2 months after last dose of therapy; notify physician as soon as possible if watery/bloody stools (with/without stomach cramps and fever) occur.

Administration: IM route. Administer by deep IM injection into large muscle mass (eg, gluteal muscles or lateral part of the thigh). Do not mix or physically add with other antibiotics; may be administered concomitantly but at separate sites with antibiotics such as aminoglycosides. Refer to PI for preparation instructions. **Storage:** Before reconstitution: Below 25°C (77°F). Reconstituted with lidocaine: Use within 1 hr after reconstitution.

PRIMAXIN I.V.   RX

cilastatin sodium - imipenem (Merck)

THERAPEUTIC CLASS: Thienamycin/dehydropeptidase I inhibitor

INDICATIONS: Treatment of lower respiratory tract, complicated and uncomplicated urinary tract (UTI), intra-abdominal, gynecologic, skin and skin structure, bone and joint, and polymicrobic infections, septicemia, and endocarditis caused by susceptible strains of microorganisms.

DOSAGE: *Adults:* Dose based on severity or type of infection. ≥70kg and CrCl ≥71mL/min: Uncomplicated UTI: 250mg q6h. Complicated UTI: 500mg q6h. Fully susceptible organisms (eg, gram-positive and gram-negative aerobes and anaerobes): Mild: 250mg q6h. Moderate: 500mg q8h or 500mg q6h. Severe: 500mg q6h. Moderately susceptible organisms (eg, *Pseudomona aeruginosa*): Mild: 500mg q6h. Moderate: 500mg q6h or 1g q8h. Severe: 1g q8h or 1g q6h. Max: 50mg/kg/day or 4g/day, whichever is lower. May use up to 90mg/kg/day, not exceeding 4g/day with cystic fibrosis. Renal Impairment (CrCl ≤70mL/min) and/or <70kg: Refer to PI. CrCl 6-20mL/min or CrCl ≤5mL/min with Hemodialysis: 125 or 250mg q12h.
Pediatrics: ≥3 months: Dose based on severity or type of infection. Non-CNS Infections: 15-25mg/kg q6h. Max: 2g/day if fully susceptible or 4g/day if moderately susceptible. May use up to 90mg/kg/day (not exceeding 4g/day) in older children (>12 yrs) with cystic fibrosis. 4 weeks-3 months and ≥1500g: 25mg/kg q6h. 1-4 weeks and ≥1500g: 25mg/kg q8h. <1 week and ≥1500g: 25mg/kg q12h.

HOW SUPPLIED: Inj: (Imipenem-Cilastatin) 250mg-250mg, 500mg-500mg

WARNINGS/PRECAUTIONS: Serious and occasionally fatal hypersensitivity (anaphylactic) reactions reported. Carefully assess previous reactions to penicillins (PCNs), cephalosporins, β-lactams, and other allergens. Seizures and other CNS adverse experiences such as confusional states and myoclonic activity reported, particularly when recommended dosages were exceeded or when given to patients with CNS disorders (eg, brain lesions or history of seizures) and/or compromised renal function. *Clostridium difficile*-associated diarrhea (CDAD) reported. May result in bacterial resistance with prolonged use or use in the absence of a proven/suspected bacterial infection or a prophylactic indication; take appropriate measures if superinfection develops. If focal tremors, myoclonus, or seizures occur, perform neurological evaluation, institute anticonvulsant therapy, and examine whether to decrease dose or d/c therapy. Avoid with CrCl ≤5mL/min unless hemodialysis is instituted within 48 hrs. Caution with CrCl <20mL/min; potential increased risk of seizures. Use in patients on hemodialysis is recommended only when benefits outweigh seizure risk. Not recommended in pediatric patients with CNS infections and <30kg with impaired renal function. Caution in elderly.

ADVERSE REACTIONS: Phlebitis/thrombophlebitis, convulsions, diarrhea, rash, fever, hypotension, seizures, dizziness, pruritus, urticaria, somnolence, N/V.

INTERACTIONS: Seizures reported with ganciclovir; avoid concomitant use. Minimal increases in plasma levels and $T_{1/2}$ with probenecid; concomitant use not recommended. May decrease levels of valproic acid or divalproex sodium, thereby increasing risk of breakthrough seizures; concomitant use is generally not recommended, but if necessary, consider supplemental anticonvulsant therapy.

PREGNANCY: Category C, caution in nursing.

MECHANISM OF ACTION: Imipenem: Thienamycin; inhibits cell-wall synthesis. Cilastatin: Dehydropeptidase I inhibitor; prevents renal metabolism of imipenem.

PHARMACOKINETICS: Absorption: Imipenem: 14-24mcg/mL (250mg), 21-58mcg/mL (500mg), 41-83mcg/mL (1000mg). Cilastatin: 15-25mcg/mL (250mg), 31-49mcg/mL (500mg), 56-88mcg/mL (1000mg). **Distribution:** Imipenem: Plasma protein binding (20%). Cilastatin: Plasma protein binding (40%). **Metabolism:** Imipenem: Kidneys by dehydropeptidase I. **Elimination:** Imipenem: Urine (70%); $T_{1/2}$=1 hr. Cilastatin: Urine (70%); $T_{1/2}$=1 hr.

NURSING CONSIDERATIONS

Assessment: Assess for severity and type of infection. Assess for renal impairment, weight, history of hypersensitivity to PCNs, cephalosporins, β-lactams, and other allergens, use of hemodialysis, CNS disorders (eg, brain lesions, history of seizures), pregnancy/nursing status, and possible drug interactions. Obtain CrCl.

Monitoring: Periodically monitor organ system function (eg, renal, hepatic, and hematopoietic) with prolonged therapy. Monitor for CNS adverse events (eg, seizures, myoclonic activity and confusional states), hypersensitivity reactions, CDAD, and superinfections. Monitor CrCl.

Patient Counseling: Counsel to inform physician if taking valproic acid or divalproex sodium. Instruct to take as directed; skipping doses or not completing full course may decrease effectiveness and increase resistance. Inform that diarrhea may occur, even as late as ≥2 months after last dose of therapy; notify physician as soon as possible if watery/bloody stools (with/without stomach cramps and fever) occur.

Administration: IV route. Each 125mg, 250mg, or 500mg dose should be infused over 20-30 min. Each 750mg or 1000mg dose should be infused over 40-60 min. Do not mix or physically add to other antibiotics; may be administered concomitantly with other antibiotics, such as aminoglycosides. Refer to PI for preparation instructions. **Storage:** Dry powder: Below 25°C (77°F). Reconstituted: Stable for 4 hrs at room temperature or for 24 hrs under refrigeration (5°C). Do not freeze.

P

PRINIVIL   RX
lisinopril (Merck)

ACE inhibitors can cause death/injury to the developing fetus during 2nd and 3rd trimesters. D/C if pregnancy is detected.

THERAPEUTIC CLASS: ACE inhibitor

INDICATIONS: Treatment of HTN used alone as initial therapy or concomitantly with other classes of antihypertensive agents. Adjunct therapy in heart failure (HF) inadequately responding to diuretics and digitalis. Adjunct therapy in hemodynamically stable patients within 24 hrs of acute myocardial infarction (AMI) to improve survival.

DOSAGE: *Adults:* HTN: Initial: 10mg qd. Adjust dose according to BP response. Usual: 20-40mg qd. Max: 80mg/day. May add a low-dose diuretic if BP not controlled. Diuretic-Treated Patients: D/C diuretic 2-3 days prior to therapy. Adjust dose according to BP response. If diuretic cannot be d/c, give initial lisinopril dose of 5mg under medical supervision for ≥2 hrs and until BP has stabilized for additional 1 hr. CrCl 10-30mL/min: Initial: 5mg qd. CrCl <10mL/min: Initial: 2.5mg qd. Titrate: May increase until BP is controlled. Max: 40mg/day. HF: Initial: 5mg qd. Usual: 5-20mg qd. HF with Hyponatremia or CrCl ≤30mL/min or SrCr >3mg/dL: Initial: 2.5mg qd under close medical supervision. AMI: Initial: 5mg within 24 hrs, then 5mg after 24 hrs, then 10mg after 48 hrs, then 10mg qd. Maint: 10mg qd for 6 weeks. Patients with Systolic BP (SBP) ≤120mmHg when Treatment is Started or During First 3 Days After the Infarct: 2.5mg. Maint: 5mg/day with temporary reductions to 2.5mg PRN if SBP ≤100mmHg; d/c if SBP <90mmHg for >1 hr. Elderly: Start at lower end of dosing range.

Pediatrics: ≥6 yrs: HTN: Initial: 0.07mg/kg qd (up to 5mg total). Adjust dose according to BP response. Max: 0.61mg/kg qd (40mg).

HOW SUPPLIED: Tab: 5mg*, 10mg*, 20mg* *scored

CONTRAINDICATIONS: History of ACE inhibitor-associated angioedema, hereditary or idiopathic angioedema.

WARNINGS/PRECAUTIONS: Anaphylactoid reactions reported during desensitization with hymenoptera venom, dialysis with high-flux membranes, and LDL apheresis with dextran sulfate absorption. Angioedema reported; d/c and administer appropriate therapy. Intestinal angioedema reported; monitor for abdominal pain. More reports of angioedema in blacks than nonblacks. Excessive hypotension rarely seen with uncomplicated HTN. Some BP reduction common with HF; caution when initiating therapy. Patients with AMI in a study had a higher incidence of persistent hypotension; do not initiate if at risk of further serious hemodynamic deterioration or cardiogenic shock. Reduce dose or d/c if symptomatic hypotension develops. Rare cases of leukopenia/neutropenia and bone marrow depression reported; monitor WBCs in patients with renal disease and collagen vascular disease. Agranulocytosis may occur. Rarely, associated with syndrome of cholestatic jaundice or hepatitis progressing to fulminant hepatic necrosis and death. May cause changes in renal function. D/C if jaundice or marked hepatic enzyme elevation and renal dysfunction occur. Oliguria and/or progressive azotemia and rarely acute renal failure and/or death may occur with severe congestive HF patients whose renal function is dependent on the renin-angiotensin-aldosterone system. May increase BUN/SrCr with renal artery stenosis or with no preexisting renal vascular disease. Hyperkalemia and persistent nonproductive cough reported. Caution with left ventricular outflow obstruction, renal dysfunction, and in elderly. Not recommended in pediatrics with GFR <30mL/min/1.73m². Dual blockade of the renin-angiotensin-aldosterone system is associated with increased risk of hypotension, syncope, hyperkalemia, and changes in renal function (including acute renal failure); closely monitor BP, renal function, and electrolytes with concomitant angiotensin II receptor antagonists. Hypotension may occur with major surgery or during anesthesia.

ADVERSE REACTIONS: Hypotension, dizziness, headache, diarrhea, cough, chest pain, hyperkalemia.

INTERACTIONS: Hypotension risk, and increased BUN and SrCr with diuretics. Increased hypoglycemic risk with insulin or oral hypoglycemics. NSAIDs, including selective cyclooxygenase-2 (COX-2) inhibitors and indomethacin, may diminish antihypertensive effect and may cause further deterioration of renal function in patients with compromised renal function. Increased risk of hyperkalemia with K⁺-sparing diuretics, K⁺-containing salt substitutes, or K⁺ supplements; monitor K⁺ levels. Concomitant K⁺-sparing agents should generally not be used with HF. Lithium toxicity with lithium; monitor lithium levels. Nitritoid reactions with injectable gold.

PREGNANCY: Category C (1st trimester) and D (2nd and 3rd trimesters), not for use in nursing.

MECHANISM OF ACTION: ACE inhibitor; decreases plasma angiotensin II, which leads to decreased vasopressor activity and decreased aldosterone secretion.

PHARMACOKINETICS: Absorption: Adults: T_{max}=7 hrs. **Pediatrics:** T_{max}=6 hrs. **Distribution:** Crosses placenta. **Elimination:** Urine (unchanged); $T_{1/2}$=12 hrs.

NURSING CONSIDERATIONS

Assessment: Assess for history of ACE inhibitor-associated angioedema, hereditary or idiopathic angioedema, risk of excessive hypotension, left ventricular outflow obstruction, renal artery stenosis, risk of hyperkalemia, renal function, hypersensitivity to drug, pregnancy/nursing status, and possible drug interactions.

Monitoring: Monitor for angioedema, anaphylactoid reactions, hyperkalemia, and cough. Monitor WBCs in patients with collagen vascular and renal disease, BP, LFTs, and renal function.

Patient Counseling: Inform about fetal risks if taken during pregnancy; report pregnancy to physician as soon as possible. Inform that excessive perspiration, dehydration, and other causes of volume depletion (eg, diarrhea, vomiting) may lead to fall in BP. Instruct to report lightheadedness, to d/c therapy and consult physician if actual syncope occurs, not to use salt substitutes containing K⁺ without consulting physician, to immediately report any signs/symptoms of infection (eg, fever, sore throat), and to d/c and immediately report angioedema (swelling of face, extremities, eyes, lips, tongue, difficulty swallowing or breathing). Instruct diabetics treated with antidiabetic agents to monitor for hypoglycemia.

Administration: Oral route. Refer to PI for instruction for preparation of sus. Shake sus before use. **Storage:** (Tab) 15-30°C (59-86°F). Protect from moisture. (Sus) ≤25°C (77°F) for ≤4 weeks.

PRINZIDE   RX
lisinopril - hydrochlorothiazide (Merck)

> ACE inhibitors can cause death/injury to developing fetus during 2nd and 3rd trimesters. D/C if pregnancy is detected.

THERAPEUTIC CLASS: ACE inhibitor/thiazide diuretic

INDICATIONS: Treatment of HTN.

DOSAGE: *Adults:* Not Controlled with Lisinopril/HCTZ Monotherapy: Initial: 10mg-12.5mg or 20mg-12.5mg qd. Titrate: May increase HCTZ dose after 2-3 weeks. Controlled on 25mg HCTZ qd with Hypokalemia: Switch to 10mg-12.5mg qd. Max: 80mg-50mg. Replacement Therapy: Substitute combination for titrated individual components. Elderly: Start at lower end of dosing range.

HOW SUPPLIED: Tab: (Lisinopril-HCTZ) 10mg-12.5mg, 20mg-12.5mg* *scored

CONTRAINDICATIONS: History of ACE inhibitor-associated angioedema, hereditary or idiopathic angioedema, anuria, hypersensitivity to other sulfonamide-derived drugs.

WARNINGS/PRECAUTIONS: Not for initial therapy of HTN. Avoid with CrCl ≤30mL/min. Caution in elderly. Lisinopril: Angioedema (face, extremities, lips, tongue, glottis, and/or larynx) reported rarely; d/c promptly and administer appropriate therapy. Intestinal angioedema reported; monitor for abdominal pain. More reports of angioedema in blacks than non-blacks. Anaphylactoid reactions reported during desensitization with hymenoptera venom, dialysis with high-flux membranes, and LDL apheresis with dextran sulfate absorption. Excessive hypotension associated with oliguria and/or progressive azotemia, and rarely with acute renal failure and/or death may occur with congestive heart failure (CHF); monitor closely. Neutropenia, agranulocytosis, and bone marrow depression may occur; monitor WBCs with collagen vascular disease and renal disease. Rarely, syndrome that starts with cholestatic jaundice or hepatitis progressing to fulminant hepatic necrosis and (sometimes) death reported; d/c if jaundice or marked elevations of hepatic enzymes occur. Caution with left ventricular outflow obstruction. May cause changes in renal function. Increased BUN/SrCr reported with renal artery stenosis. Hyperkalemia, persistent nonproductive cough reported. Dual blockade of the renin-angiotensin-aldosterone system is associated with increased risk of hypotension, syncope, hyperkalemia, and changes in renal function (including acute renal failure); closely monitor BP, renal function, and electrolytes with concomitant angiotensin II receptor antagonists. Hypotension may occur with major surgery or during anesthesia. HCTZ: May precipitate azotemia with renal disease. Caution with hepatic impairment or progressive liver disease; may precipitate hepatic coma. Sensitivity reactions may occur. May exacerbate/activate systemic lupus erythematosus (SLE). May cause idiosyncratic reaction, resulting in acute transient myopia and acute angle-closure glaucoma; d/c as rapidly as possible. Observe for signs of fluid or electrolyte imbalance (hyponatremia, hypochloremic alkalosis, hypokalemia). Hyperuricemia, gout precipitation, hypercalcemia, hyperglycemia, and hypomagnesemia may occur. D/C before testing for parathyroid function. Enhanced effects with postsympathectomy patients. Increased cholesterol, TG levels reported.

ADVERSE REACTIONS: Dizziness, headache, cough, fatigue, orthostatic effects, muscle cramps, angioedema, hypotension.

INTERACTIONS: NSAIDs, including selective cyclooxygenase-2 inhibitors, may diminish effects of diuretic and ACE inhibitors, and may cause further deterioration of renal function. Increased risk of lithium toxicity; avoid with lithium. Lisinopril: Hypotension risk, and increased BUN and SrCr with diuretics. Increased serum K$^+$ with K$^+$-sparing diuretics (eg, spironolactone, triamterene, amiloride), K$^+$ supplements, K$^+$-containing salt substitutes. Nitritoid reactions reported rarely with injectable gold. HCTZ: Potentiates orthostatic hypotension with alcohol, barbiturates, and narcotics. Dose adjustment of antidiabetic drugs (eg, oral agents and insulin) may be needed. Cholestyramine and colestipol resins impair absorption. Corticosteroids and adrenocorticotropic hormone may intensify electrolyte depletion, particularly, hypokalemia. May decrease response to pressor amines (eg, norepinephrine). May have additive effect or potentiation of other antihypertensives. Increased responsiveness to nondepolarizing skeletal muscle relaxants (eg, tubocurarine).

PREGNANCY: Category C (1st trimester) and D (2nd and 3rd trimesters), not for use in nursing.

MECHANISM OF ACTION: Lisinopril: ACE inhibitor; decreases plasma angiotensin II, which leads to decreased vasopressor activity and decreased aldosterone secretion. HCTZ: Thiazide diuretic; not established. Affects distal renal tubular mechanism of electrolyte reabsorption. Increases excretion of Na$^+$ and Cl$^-$.

PHARMACOKINETICS: Absorption: Lisinopril: T$_{max}$=7 hrs. **Distribution:** Crosses placenta. HCTZ: Found in breast milk. **Elimination:** Lisinopril: Urine (unchanged); T$_{1/2}$=12 hrs. HCTZ: Renal (≥61% unchanged); T$_{1/2}$=5.6-14.8 hrs.

NURSING CONSIDERATIONS

Assessment: Assess for renal/hepatic impairment, collagen vascular disease (eg, SLE), history of ACE inhibitor-associated and hereditary/idiopathic angioedema, anuria, hypersensitivity to other sulfonamide/penicillin-derived drugs, CHF, left ventricle outflow obstruction, DM, severe cirrhosis, postsympathectomy, renal artery stenosis, risk factors for hyperkalemia, allergy or bronchial asthma, pregnancy/nursing status, and possible drug interactions. Obtain baseline BP, electrolytes (eg, K^+), blood glucose, cholesterol, TG, and uric acid.

Monitoring: Monitor for signs/symptoms of angioedema, fluid/electrolyte imbalance, exacerbation/activation of SLE, idiosyncratic reaction, hypotension, latent DM, hyperglycemia, hypomagnesemia, hypercalcemia, hyperuricemia or precipitation of gout, hypersensitivity reactions, and other adverse reactions. Monitor BP, serum electrolytes, renal function, cholesterol, and TG levels periodically. Monitor WBCs in patients with collagen vascular and renal disease.

Patient Counseling: Inform about fetal risks if taken during pregnancy; report pregnancy to physician as soon as possible. Inform that excessive perspiration, dehydration, and other causes of volume depletion (eg, diarrhea, vomiting) may lead to fall in BP. Instruct to report lightheadedness, to d/c therapy and consult physician if actual syncope occurs, not to use salt substitutes containing K^+ without consulting physician, to immediately report any signs/symptoms of infection (eg, fever, sore throat), and to d/c and immediately report angioedema (swelling of face, extremities, eyes, lips, tongue, difficulty swallowing or breathing).

Administration: Oral route. **Storage:** 15-30°C (59-86°F). Protect from excessive light and humidity.

PRISTIQ   RX
desvenlafaxine (Wyeth)

> Antidepressants increased the risk of suicidal thinking and behavior (suicidality) in children, adolescents, and young adults in short-term studies of major depressive disorder (MDD) and other psychiatric disorders. Monitor and observe closely for clinical worsening, suicidality, or unusual changes in behavior. Not approved for use in pediatric patients.

THERAPEUTIC CLASS: Serotonin and norepinephrine reuptake inhibitor

INDICATIONS: Treatment of MDD.

DOSAGE: *Adults:* 50mg qd. Moderate Renal Impairment (CrCl 30-50mL/min): 50mg/day. Severe Renal Impairment (CrCl <30mL/min) or End-Stage Renal Disease (ESRD): 50mg qod. Do not give supplemental doses after dialysis. Do not escalate doses with moderate or severe renal impairment or ESRD. Hepatic Impairment: 50mg/day. Max: 100mg/day.

HOW SUPPLIED: Tab, Extended-Release: 50mg, 100mg

CONTRAINDICATIONS: Concomitant use of MAOIs or use within 14 days of taking MAOIs; allow ≥7 days after stopping drug before starting an MAOI.

WARNINGS/PRECAUTIONS: Not approved for treatment of bipolar depression. Serotonin syndrome or neuroleptic malignant syndrome (NMS)-like reactions reported; d/c immediately and initiate supportive symptomatic treatment. May cause sustained increases in BP; consider dose reduction or d/c. May increase risk of bleeding events. Mydriasis reported; monitor patients with raised intraocular pressure (IOP) or those at risk of acute narrow-angle glaucoma. Activation of mania/hypomania reported; caution with history or family history of mania/hypomania. Caution with cardiovascular (CV), cerebrovascular, or lipid metabolism disorders. Dose-related elevations of fasting serum total cholesterol, LDL, and TG reported. D/C symptoms may occur; gradually taper dose. Avoid abrupt withdrawal or dose reduction. Caution with renal or hepatic impairment. Seizures reported; caution with seizure disorders. May cause hyponatremia; consider d/c if symptomatic and institute appropriate medical intervention. Consider d/c of therapy if interstitial lung disease and eosinophilic pneumonia occur. Caution in elderly.

ADVERSE REACTIONS: Headache, N/V, dry mouth, diarrhea, dizziness, insomnia, somnolence, hyperhidrosis, constipation, anxiety, decreased appetite, male sexual function disorders, fatigue.

INTERACTIONS: See Contraindications. May cause serotonin syndrome or NMS-like reactions with serotonergic drugs (eg, triptans), drugs which impair serotonin metabolism, antipsychotics, or other dopamine antagonists; d/c immediately if these occur. Not recommended with serotonin precursors (eg, tryptophan). Aspirin, NSAIDs, warfarin, and other anticoagulants may add to risk of bleeding. Diuretics may increase risk of hyponatremia. Avoid with products containing venlafaxine or alcohol. Caution with CNS-active drugs. Potent CYP3A4 inhibitors (eg, ketoconazole) may increase levels. May increase levels of CYP2D6 substrates (eg, desipramine). May decrease levels of CYP3A4 substrates (eg, midazolam).

PREGNANCY: Category C, not for use in nursing.

MECHANISM OF ACTION: Selective serotonin and norepinephrine reuptake inhibitors (SNRI); potentiates neurotransmitter activity in CNS by inhibiting neuronal serotonin and norepinephrine reuptake.

PHARMACOKINETICS: Absorption: Absolute bioavailability (80%); T_{max}=7.5 hrs. **Distribution:** Plasma protein binding (30%); V_d=3.4L/kg (IV); found in breast milk. **Metabolism:** Conjugation via UGT isoforms, and (minor) N-demethylation via CYP3A4. **Elimination:** Urine (45% unchanged, 19% glucuronide metabolite, <5% oxidative metabolite); $T_{1/2}$=11 hrs.

NURSING CONSIDERATIONS

Assessment: Assess for HTN, increased IOP, risk factors for acute narrow-angle glaucoma, history or family history of mania/hypomania, CV/cerebrovascular/lipid metabolism disorders, hepatic/renal impairment, seizures, volume depletion, hypersensitivity to drug, pregnancy/nursing status, and possible drug interactions.

Monitoring: Monitor for signs/symptoms of clinical worsening, suicidality, unusual changes in behavior, serotonin syndrome or NMS-like reactions, abnormal bleeding, mydriasis, activation of mania/hypomania, seizures, hyponatremia, interstitial lung disease, and eosinophilic pneumonia. Monitor HR, BP, LFTs, renal function, and serum lipid levels. Monitor for d/c symptoms when d/c therapy. Periodically reevaluate the need for continued treatment.

Patient Counseling: Advise about the benefits and risks of therapy and its appropriate use. Instruct patients and caregivers to notify physician if signs of clinical worsening, changes in behavior, or suicidality occur. Caution about the risk of serotonin syndrome or NMS-like reactions. Advise to have BP monitored regularly, to observe for signs and symptoms of activation of mania/hypomania, to avoid alcohol, and not to d/c therapy without notifying physician. Inform that drug may impair physical/mental ability and that remains of tab passing in the stool may be noticed. Instruct to notify physician if nursing, become pregnant, or intend to become pregnant.

Administration: Oral route. Swallow tab whole with fluid; do not divide, crush, chew, or dissolve. Take at same time each day. **Storage:** 20-25°C (68-77°F); excursions permitted to 15-30°C (59-86°F).

PROAIR HFA   RX
albuterol sulfate (Teva)

THERAPEUTIC CLASS: Beta$_2$-agonist

INDICATIONS: Treatment or prevention of bronchospasm in patients ≥4 yrs with reversible obstructive airway disease. Prevention of exercise-induced bronchospasm (EIB) in patients ≥4 yrs.

DOSAGE: *Adults*: Treatment/Prevention of Bronchospasm: 2 inh q4-6h or 1 inh q4h. EIB Prevention: 2 inh 15-30 min before exercise. Elderly: Start at lower end of dosing range. *Pediatrics:* ≥4 yrs: Treatment/Prevention of Bronchospasm: 2 inh q4-6h or 1 inh q4h. EIB Prevention: 2 inh 15-30 min before exercise.

HOW SUPPLIED: MDI: 90mcg/inh [8.5g]

WARNINGS/PRECAUTIONS: Deterioration of asthma may occur; monitor for signs of worsening asthma and consider adding anti-inflammatory agents (eg, corticosteroids) to therapeutic regimen. D/C if paradoxical bronchospasm or cardiovascular (CV) effects occur. Caution with CV disorders (eg, coronary insufficiency, cardiac arrhythmias, HTN), convulsive disorders, hyperthyroidism, diabetes mellitus (DM), and unusual response to sympathomimetic amines. ECG changes and immediate hypersensitivity reactions may occur. Fatalities reported with excessive use. May produce significant hypokalemia. Caution in elderly and when administering higher doses with renal impairment.

ADVERSE REACTIONS: Pharyngitis, headache, rhinitis, dizziness, pain, tachycardia.

INTERACTIONS: Avoid other short-acting sympathomimetic aerosol bronchodilators; caution with additional adrenergic drugs administered by any route. Avoid β-blockers; if not possible, use cardioselective β-blockers with caution. Extreme caution with MAOIs, TCAs during or within 2 weeks of d/c. Monitor digoxin levels. ECG changes and/or hypokalemia caused by non-K$^+$-sparing diuretics (eg, loop or thiazide diuretics) may be worsened.

PREGNANCY: Category C, not for use in nursing.

MECHANISM OF ACTION: β$_2$-agonist; activates β$_2$-adrenergic receptors on airway smooth muscle leading to activation of adenylcyclase and to an increase in intracellular cyclic-3',5'-adenosine monophosphate (cAMP). This increased cAMP leads to activation of protein kinase A, which inhibits the phosphorylation of myosin and lowers intracellular ionic calcium concentrations, resulting in relaxation of smooth muscle of all airways, from the trachea to terminal bronchioles.

PHARMACOKINETICS: Absorption: C$_{max}$=4100pg/mL; AUC=28,426pg•hr/mL. (Pediatrics) C$_{max}$=1100pg/mL; AUC=5120pg•hr/mL. **Metabolism:** GI tract by SULTIA3 (sulfotransferase). **Elimination:** Urine (80-100%), feces (<20%); $T_{1/2}$=6 hrs. (Pediatrics) $T_{1/2}$=166 min.

NURSING CONSIDERATIONS

Assessment: Assess for convulsive disorders, hyperthyroidism, DM, CV disorders, renal impairment, hypersensitivity, pregnancy/nursing status, and possible drug interactions. Assess use in patients unusually responsive to sympathomimetic amines.

Monitoring: Monitor for possible paradoxical bronchospasm, deterioration of asthma, CV effects, hypokalemia, immediate hypersensitivity reactions, and other adverse effects. Monitor BP, HR, ECG changes, and blood glucose.

Patient Counseling: Instruct to use as prescribed and not to increase dose or frequency of doses without consulting physician. Instruct on how to properly prime, clean, and use inhaler. Inform to take other concomitant drugs/asthma medications as directed. Counsel to report lack of response or the occurrence of any adverse side effect. Instruct to inform physician if pregnant or nursing. Counsel to keep out of reach of children.

Administration: Oral inhalation route. Shake well before use. **Storage:** 15-25°C (59-77°F). Protect from freezing and prolonged exposure to direct sunlight.

PROAMATINE   RX
midodrine HCl (Shire)

> Can cause marked elevation of supine BP. Clinical benefits of improving ability to carry out activities of daily living have not been verified.

THERAPEUTIC CLASS: Alpha$_1$-agonist

INDICATIONS: Treatment of symptomatic orthostatic hypotension.

DOSAGE: *Adults:* Initial: 10mg tid; at 3-4 hr intervals, while awake. Max: 30mg/day. To avoid supine HTN during sleep, do not give <4 hrs before bedtime or after evening meal. Renal Dysfunction: Initial: 2.5mg tid.

HOW SUPPLIED: Tab: 2.5mg*, 5mg*, 10mg* *scored

CONTRAINDICATIONS: Severe organic heart disease, acute renal disease, urinary retention, pheochromocytoma, thyrotoxicosis, persistent and excessive supine HTN.

WARNINGS/PRECAUTIONS: Risk of supine HTN; monitor for symptoms of supine HTN (eg, pounding in ears, headache, blurred vision) and supine and standing BP; d/c if supine HTN persists. Caution with urinary retention, diabetes, renal or hepatic dysfunction. May decrease HR due to vagal reflex.

ADVERSE REACTIONS: Supine and sitting HTN, paresthesia, scalp pruritus, goosebumps, chills, urinary urge/retention/frequency.

INTERACTIONS: Caution with concomitant use of drugs that cause vasoconstriction (eg, phenylephrine, ephedrine, phenylpropanolamine, dihydroergotamine, pseudoephedrine); monitor BP. Fludrocortisone may potentiate supine HTN due to salt-retaining properties. OTC cold and diet products may potentiate pressor effects. Antagonized by alpha-blockers (eg, prazosin, terazosin, doxazosin). Metformin, cimetidine, ranitidine, procainamide, triamterene, flecainide, and quinidine may increase clearance. Caution with cardiac glycosides (eg, digitalis), psychopharmacologics, β-blockers, or other drugs that directly or indirectly reduce HR.

PREGNANCY: Category C, caution in nursing.

MECHANISM OF ACTION: Desglymidodrine (major metabolite); a$_1$-agonist; exerts its actions via activation of the α-adrenergic receptors of the arteriolar and venous vasculature, producing an increase in vascular tone and elevation of BP.

PHARMACOKINETICS: Absorption: Midodrine (prodrug): Rapid; absolute bioavailability (93%); T$_{max}$=1/2 hr. Desglymidodrine: T$_{max}$=1-2 hrs. **Distribution:** Poor; across blood-brain barrier. **Metabolism:** Liver via deglycination to desglymidodrine (major metabolite). **Elimination:** Urine (80%, metabolite); T$_{1/2}$=3-4 hrs (metabolite).

NURSING CONSIDERATIONS

Assessment: Assess for severe organic heart disease, acute renal impairment, urinary retention, hepatic impairment, pheochromocytoma or thyrotoxicosis, orthostatic hypotension with DM, history of visual problems, pregnancy/nursing status, and for possible drug interactions. Evaluate baseline renal and LFTs.

Monitoring: Monitor for signs/symptoms of supine HTN (eg, cardiac awareness, pounding in the ears, headache, blurred vision) and for bradycardia (eg, pulse slowing, increased dizziness, syncope, cardiac awareness). Monitor supine and sitting BP, HR, and renal/hepatic function.

Patient Counseling: Inform that certain OTC products (eg, cold remedies, diet aids) can elevate BP and may potentiate the pressor effect of the drug. Inform about the signs/symptoms of supine HTN; instruct to not take dose if supine for any length of time.

Administration: Oral route. Take during daytime, not to be taken after evening meals or <4 hrs before bedtime. **Storage:** 25°C (77°F); excursions permitted to 15-30°C (59-86°F).

PROBENECID/COLCHICINE RX
colchicine - probenecid (Various)

THERAPEUTIC CLASS: Uricosuric

INDICATIONS: Chronic gouty arthritis complicated by frequent, recurrent acute gout attacks.

DOSAGE: *Adults:* Initial: 1 tab qd for 1 week, then 1 tab bid. Maint: Continue dosage that will maintain normal serum urate levels. May reduce dose by 1 tab q6 months if acute attacks absent ≥6 months and normal serum urate levels. Renal Impairment: 2 tabs/day. Titrate: May increase dose by 1 tab q4 weeks if symptoms not controlled. Max: 4 tabs/day. Decrease dose if gastric intolerance occurs.

HOW SUPPLIED: Tab: (Probenecid-Colchicine) 500mg-0.5mg

CONTRAINDICATIONS: Blood dyscrasias, uric acid kidney stones, children <2 yrs, pregnancy, initiating therapy before acute gout attack subsides, coadministration with salicylates.

WARNINGS/PRECAUTIONS: Exacerbation of gout may occur. Severe allergic reactions and anaphylaxis reported rarely; d/c if hypersensitivity occurs. Caution with history of peptic ulcer. Hematuria, renal colic, costovertebral pain, and formation of uric acid stones reported; maintain liberal fluid intake and alkalization of urine. May not be effective in chronic renal insufficiency (GFR ≤30mL/min). Reversible azoospermia reported. Colchicine is an established mutagen; may be carcinogenic.

ADVERSE REACTIONS: Headache, dizziness, fever, pruritus, acute gouty arthritis, purpura, leukopenia, peripheral neuritis, muscular weakness, N/V, urticaria, anemia, dermatitis, alopecia.

INTERACTIONS: See Contraindications. Salicylates and pyrazinamide antagonize uricosuric effects; use acetaminophen (APAP) if mild analgesic is needed. Probenecid increases plasma levels of penicillin and other β-lactams; psychic disturbances reported. Methotrexate levels increased with coadministration; reduce dose and monitor levels. May prolong/enhance effects of sulfonylureas; increased risk of hypoglycemia. Increased $T_{1/2}$ and levels of indomethacin, naproxen, ketoprofen, meclofenamate, lorazepam, APAP, rifampin. Increased levels of sulindac and sulfonamides; monitor sulfonamide levels with prolonged use. Inhibits renal transport of amino hippuric acid, aminosalicylic acid, indomethacin, sodium iodomethamate and related iodinated organic acids, 17-ketosteroids, pantothenic acid, phenolsulfonphthalein, sulfonamides and sulfonylureas. Possible falsely high plasma levels of theophylline. Decreases hepatic/renal excretion of sulfobromophthalein. May require significantly less thiopental for induction of anesthesia.

PREGNANCY: Contraindicated in pregnancy; safety not known in nursing.

MECHANISM OF ACTION: Probenecid: Uricosuric/renal tubular blocking agent; inhibits tubular reabsorption of urate, increasing urinary excretion of uric acid and decreasing serum urate levels. Colchicine: Colchicum alkaloid; not been established. Has prophylactic, suppressive effect helping to reduce incidence of acute attacks and to relieve residual pain and mild discomfort.

NURSING CONSIDERATIONS

Assessment: Assess for known blood dyscrasias, uric acid kidney stones, acute/chronic gout attack, history of peptic ulcer, patient's age, renal function, hypersensitivity to drug, pregnancy/nursing status, and possible drug interactions.

Monitoring: Monitor for signs/symptoms of gout exacerbation, allergic reactions, hematuria, renal colic, costovertebral pain, and uric acid stone formation. Monitor serum uric acid levels.

Patient Counseling: Inform about the risks and benefits of therapy and importance of liberal fluid intake. Advise to seek medical attention if symptoms of allergic reaction, hematuria, renal colic, or costovertebral pain occur.

Administration: Oral route. **Storage:** 20-25°C (68-77°F). Protect from light.

PROCARDIA XL RX
nifedipine (Pfizer)

OTHER BRAND NAMES: Nifedical XL (Teva)

THERAPEUTIC CLASS: Calcium channel blocker (dihydropyridine)

INDICATIONS: Management of vasospastic angina and chronic stable angina without evidence of vasospasm in patients who remain symptomatic despite adequate doses of β-blockers and/or organic nitrates or who cannot tolerate those agents. Treatment of HTN alone or with other antihypertensive agents.

DOSAGE: *Adults:* Angina/HTN: Initial: 30 or 60mg qd. Titrate over a 7-14 day period (usual) but may proceed more rapidly if symptoms warrant. Max: 120mg/day. Caution with doses >90mg for angina. Switching from Nifedipine Capsules Alone or with Other Antianginal Agents: Use nearest equivalent daily dose. Titrate as clinically warranted.

HOW SUPPLIED: Tab, Extended-Release: (Nifedical XL) 30mg, 60mg; (Procardia XL) 30mg, 60mg, 90mg

WARNINGS/PRECAUTIONS: May cause hypotension; monitor BP initially and with titration. May increase frequency, duration, and/or severity of angina or acute myocardial infarction (MI), particularly with severe obstructive coronary artery disease (CAD). May develop congestive heart failure (CHF), especially with tight aortic stenosis. GI obstruction and bezoars reported; caution with altered GI anatomy and hypomotility disorders. Peripheral edema associated with vasodilation may occur; rule out peripheral edema caused by left ventricular dysfunction in patients with angina or HTN complicated by CHF. Transient elevations of enzymes (eg, alkaline phosphatase, CPK, LDH, SGOT, SGPT), cholestasis with/without jaundice, and allergic hepatitis reported rarely. May decrease platelet aggregation and increase bleeding time. Positive direct Coombs test with or without hemolytic anemia reported. Reversible elevation in BUN and SrCr reported rarely in patients with chronic renal insufficiency. (Procardia XL) Tablet adherence to GI wall with ulceration reported.

ADVERSE REACTIONS: Dizziness, headache, nausea, fatigue, constipation, edema.

INTERACTIONS: β-Blockers may increase risk of CHF, severe hypotension, or angina exacerbation; avoid abrupt β-blocker withdrawal. Severe hypotension and/or increased fluid volume reported together with β-blockers and fentanyl or other narcotic analgesics. May increase digoxin levels; monitor digoxin levels when initiating, adjusting, and d/c therapy to avoid over- or under-digitalization. May increase PT with coumarin anticoagulants. Cimetidine may increase levels. Decreased serum K^+ levels with diuretics. Monitor with other medications known to lower BP. Increased risk of GI obstruction with H_2-histamine blockers, NSAIDs, laxatives, anticholinergic agents, levothyroxine, (Procardia XL) opiates, and neuromuscular blocking agents.

PREGNANCY: Category C, safety not known in nursing.

MECHANISM OF ACTION: Calcium channel blocker; inhibits calcium ion influx into cardiac muscle and smooth muscle. Angina: Has not been established; believed to act by relaxation and prevention of coronary artery spasm and reduction of oxygen utilization. HTN: Peripheral arterial vasodilation resulting in reduction in peripheral vascular resistance.

PHARMACOKINETICS: Absorption: Complete. Bioavailability (86%). **Distribution:** Plasma protein binding (92-98%, [Procardia XL]) (90-98%, [Nifedical XL]). **Metabolism:** Liver, extensive. **Elimination:** Urine (60-80%, metabolites; <0.1%, unchanged), feces (metabolites); $T_{1/2}$=2 hrs.

NURSING CONSIDERATIONS

Assessment: Assess for CHF, severe obstructive CAD, aortic stenosis, hepatic/renal impairment, altered GI anatomy (eg, severe GI narrowing, colon cancer, small bowel obstruction, bowel resection, gastric bypass, vertical banded gastroplasty, colostomy, diverticulitis, diverticulosis, and inflammatory bowel disease), hypomotility disorders (eg, constipation, gastroesophageal reflux disease, ileus, obesity, hypothyroidism, diabetes), recent β-blocker withdrawal, pregnancy/nursing status, and possible drug interactions.

Monitoring: Monitor for excessive hypotension, increased frequency, duration and/or severity of angina and/or acute MI (especially during initiation and dose titration), CHF, signs/symptoms of GI obstruction, peripheral edema (determine cause), cholestasis with/without jaundice and allergic hepatitis. Monitor BP, LFTs, BUN, SrCr, for decreased platelet aggregation, and increased bleeding time.

Patient Counseling: Advise to take exactly as prescribed. Instruct to swallow tablet whole; not to chew, divide, or crush. Counsel about adverse effects; advise to report any. (Procardia XL) Inform that it is normal to occasionally observe a tablet-like material in the stool.

Administration: Oral route. **Storage:** Protect from moisture and humidity. (Procardia XL) <30°C (86°F). (Nifedical XL) 25°C (77°F); excursions permitted to 15-30°C (59-86°F).

PROCHLORPERAZINE   RX

prochlorperazine (Various)

> Elderly patients with dementia-related psychosis treated with antipsychotic drugs are at an increased risk of death; most deaths appeared to be cardiovascular (CV) (eg, heart failure, sudden death) or infectious (eg, pneumonia) in nature. Treatment with conventional antipsychotic drugs may similarly increase mortality. Not approved for the treatment of patients with dementia-related psychosis.

THERAPEUTIC CLASS: Phenothiazine derivative

INDICATIONS: Control of severe N/V. Treatment of schizophrenia. Maleate: Short-term treatment of generalized nonpsychotic anxiety.

DOSAGE: *Adults:* Adjust dose according to individual response. Begin with the lowest recommended dosage. N/V: (Tab) Usual: 5mg or 10mg PO tid-qid. Daily dose >40mg should only be used in resistant cases. (IM) Initial: 5-10mg IM q3-4h PRN. Max: 40mg/day. (IV) 2.5-10mg slow IV or infusion at rate ≤5mg/min. Max: 10mg single dose and 40mg/day. N/V with Surgery: (IM) 5-10mg IM 1-2 hrs before induction of anesthesia (repeat once in 30 min PRN). (IV) 5-10mg as slow IV injection or infusion 15-30 min before induction of anesthesia. To control acute symptoms during or after surgery, repeat once PRN. Max: 40mg/day. Nonpsychotic Anxiety: (Tab) Usual: 5mg tid-qid. Max: 20mg/day, not longer than 12 weeks. Psychotic Disorders (Schizophrenia): (Tab) Mild/Outpatient: 5-10mg tid-qid. Moderate-Severe/Hospitalized: Initial: 10mg tid-qid. May increase dose gradually in small increments every 2-3 days. Severe: (Tab) 100-150mg/day. (IM) Initial: 10-20mg, may repeat q2-4h PRN (or, in resistant cases, every hr). Switch to PO after obtaining control at the same dosage level or higher. Prolonged Parenteral Therapy: 10-20mg IM q4-6h. Debilitated or Emaciated *Adults:* Increase more gradually. Elderly: Start at lower end of dosing range and increase more gradually.
Pediatrics: N/V: ≥2 yrs, ≥20 lbs: Adjust dosage and frequency according to the severity of symptoms and response. (Tab) 20-29 lbs: Usual: 2.5mg qd-bid. Max: 7.5mg/day. 30-39 lbs: 2.5mg bid-tid. Max: 10mg/day. 40-85 lbs: 2.5mg tid or 5mg bid. Max: 15mg/day. Severe N/V: (IM) Calculate each dose on the basis of 0.06mg/lb of body weight. Control is usually obtained with 1 dose. Psychotic Disorders (Schizophrenia): (Tab) 2-12 yrs: Initial: 2.5mg bid-tid. Do not give >10mg on the 1st day. Increase dose based on patient's response. 6-12 yrs: Max: 25mg/day. 2-5 yrs: Max: 20mg/day. (IM) <12 yrs: Calculate each dose on the basis of 0.06mg/lb of body weight. Control is usually obtained with 1 dose. Switch to PO after obtaining control at the same dosage level or higher.

HOW SUPPLIED: Inj: (Edisylate) 5mg/mL [2mL, 10mL]; Tab: (Maleate) 5mg, 10mg

CONTRAINDICATIONS: Comatose states, concomitant large doses of CNS depressants (eg, alcohol, barbiturates, narcotics), pediatric surgery, pediatrics <2 yrs or <20 lbs.

WARNINGS/PRECAUTIONS: Secondary extrapyramidal symptoms can occur. Tardive dyskinesia (TD) may develop, especially in elderly and during long term use. Neuroleptic malignant syndrome (NMS) reported; d/c if it occurs and institute appropriate treatment; caution during reintroduction of therapy as NMS recurrence reported. Avoid in patients with bone marrow depression, previous hypersensitivity reaction, and in pregnant women. May impair mental and/ or physical abilities especially during the first few days of therapy; caution if operating vehicle or machinery. May mask symptoms of overdose of other drugs, and obscure diagnosis of intestinal obstruction, brain tumor, and Reye's syndrome; avoid in children/adolescents whose signs and symptoms suggest Reye's syndrome. May cause hypotension; caution with large doses and parenteral administration in patients with impaired CV system. May interfere with thermoregulation; caution in patients exposed to extreme heat. Evaluate therapy periodically with prolonged use. Leukopenia/neutropenia/agranulocytosis reported; monitor during first few months of therapy, and d/c at first sign of leukopenia or if severe neutropenia (absolute neutrophil count <1000/mm³) occur. Caution with glaucoma, in children with dehydration or acute illness, and in elderly. May produce α-adrenergic blockade, lower seizure threshold, or elevate prolactin levels. D/C 48 hrs before myelography; may resume after 24 hrs postprocedure.

ADVERSE REACTIONS: NMS, cholestatic jaundice, leukopenia, agranulocytosis, drowsiness, dizziness, amenorrhea, blurred vision, skin reactions, hypotension, motor restlessness, extrapyramidal symptoms, TD, dystonia, pseudoparkinsonism.

INTERACTIONS: See Contraindications. May intensify and prolong action of CNS depressants (opiates, alcohol, anesthetics, barbiturates, narcotics, analgesics, antihistamines), atropine, and organophosphorus insecticides. May decrease oral anticoagulant effects. Thiazide diuretics accentuate orthostatic hypotension. Increased levels of both drugs with propranolol. Anticonvulsants may need dosage adjustment. May lower convulsive threshold. May interfere with metabolism of phenytoin and precipitate toxicity. Risk of encephalopathic syndrome occurs with lithium. May antagonize antihypertensive effects of guanethidine and related compounds. Avoid use prior to myelography with metrizamide; vomiting as a sign of toxicity of cancer chemotherapeutic drugs may be obscured by the antiemetic effect. May reverse effect of epinephrine. May cause paradoxical further lowering of BP with epinephrine and other pressor agents (excluding norepinephrine bitartrate and phenylephrine HCl).

PREGNANCY: Safety is not known in pregnancy; caution in nursing.

MECHANISM OF ACTION: Phenothiazine derivative; antiemetic and antipsychotic.

PHARMACOKINETICS: Distribution: Excreted in breat milk.

NURSING CONSIDERATIONS

Assessment: Assess for Reye's syndrome, TD, pregnancy/nursing status, possible drug interactions, impaired CV system, breast cancer, glaucoma, bone marrow depression, preexisting low WBC count, history of drug induced leukopenia/neutropenia, history of psychosis, and seizure disorder. Assess use in children with acute illness or dehydration, elderly, debilitated, or emaciated patients.

Monitoring: Monitor for extrapyramidal symptoms, signs/symptoms of TD, NMS, hypotension, fever, sore throat, infection, jaundice, motor restlessness, dystonia, pseudoparkinsonism, and hypersensitivity reactions. Monitor CBC, WBC, and prolactin levels. Conduct liver studies if fever with grippe-like symptoms occur.

Patient Counseling: Inform about the risks and benefits of therapy. Avoid engaging in hazardous activities (eg, operating vehicles or machinery) and exposure to extreme heat. Seek medical attention if symptoms of TD, NMS (hyperpyrexia, muscle rigidity, altered mental status), hypotension, mydriasis, encephalopathic syndrome (weakness, lethargy, fever), sore throat, infection, deep sleep, or hypersensitivity reactions occur.

Administration: IV, IM, Oral route. (Inj) Inspect visually for particulate matter and discoloration. Discard if marked discoloration noted. Inject deeply into upper, outer quadrant of the buttock. SQ is not advisable because of local irritation. May be administered either undiluted or diluted in isotonic solution. When given IV, do not use bolus injection. Do not mix with other agents in the syringe. Avoid getting injection solution on hands or clothing because of potential contact dermatitis. **Storage:** Tab, Inj: 20-25°C (68-77°F). Protect from light. (Inj) Do not freeze.

PROCRIT   RX
epoetin alfa (Centocor)

> Increased risk of death, myocardial infarction, stroke, venous thromboembolism, thrombosis of vascular access, and tumor progression or recurrence. Use the lowest dose sufficient to reduce/avoid the need for RBC transfusions. Chronic Kidney Disease (CKD): Greater risks for death, serious adverse cardiovascular (CV) reactions, and stroke when administered to target Hgb level >11g/dL. Cancer: Shortened overall survival and/or increased risk of tumor progression or recurrence in patients with breast, non-small cell lung, head and neck, lymphoid, and cervical cancers. Must enroll in and comply with the ESA APPRISE Oncology Program to prescribe and/or dispense to patients. Use only for anemia from myelosuppressive chemotherapy. Not indicated for patients receiving myelosuppressive chemotherapy when anticipated outcome is cure. D/C following completion of chemotherapy course. Perisurgery: Due to increased risk of deep venous thrombosis (DVT), consider DVT prophylaxis.

THERAPEUTIC CLASS: Erythropoiesis stimulator

INDICATIONS: Treatment of anemia due to CKD, including patients on/not on dialysis; anemia due to zidovudine administered at ≤4200mg/week in HIV-infected patients with endogenous serum erythropoietin levels of ≤500 mU/mL; anemic patients with nonmyeloid malignancies where anemia is due to the effect of concomitant myelosuppressive chemotherapy, and upon initiation, there is a minimum of 2 additional months of planned chemotherapy. To reduce the need for allogeneic RBC transfusions in patients with perioperative Hgb >10 to ≤13g/dL who are at high risk for perioperative blood loss from elective, noncardiac, nonvascular surgery.

DOSAGE: *Adults:* Initiate when Hgb is <10g/dL (see PI for additional parameters). CKD on Dialysis/Not on Dialysis: Initial: 50-100 U/kg IV/SQ TIW. IV route recommended for patients on dialysis. Titrate: Adjust dose based on Hgb levels; see PI. Zidovudine-Treated HIV Patients: Initial: 100 U/kg IV/SQ TIW. Titrate: Adjust dose based on Hgb levels; see PI. Malignancy: Initial: 150 U/kg SQ TIW or 40,000 U SQ weekly until completion of a chemotherapy course. Titrate: Adjust dose based on Hgb levels; see PI. Surgery Patients: Usual: 300 U/kg/day SQ for 10 days before, on day of, and for 4 days after surgery; or 600 U/kg SQ in 4 doses administered 21, 14, and 7 days before surgery and on the day of surgery. DVT prophylaxis recommended. Individualize dose selection and adjustment for the elderly to achieve/maintain target Hgb.
Pediatrics: Initiate when Hgb is <10g/dL (see PI for additional parameters). 5-18 yrs: Malignancy: Initial: 600 U/kg IV weekly until completion of a chemotherapy course. Titrate: Adjust dose based on Hgb levels; see PI. Max: 60,000 U weekly. 1 month-16 yrs: CKD on Dialysis: Initial: 50 U/kg IV/SQ TIW. IV route is recommended for patients on dialysis. Titrate: Adjust dose based on Hgb levels; see PI.

HOW SUPPLIED: Inj: Single-dose: 2000 U/mL, 3000 U/mL, 4000 U/mL, 10,000 U/mL, 40,000 U/mL; Multidose: 10,000 U/mL, 20,000 U/mL

CONTRAINDICATIONS: Uncontrolled HTN, pure red cell aplasia (PRCA) that begins after treatment with epoetin alfa or other erythropoietin drugs. Multidose: Neonates, infants, pregnant women, and nursing mothers.

WARNINGS/PRECAUTIONS: Not indicated in patients with cancer receiving hormonal agents, biologic products, or radiotherapy, unless also receiving concomitant myelosuppressive chemotherapy, in patients scheduled for surgery who are willing to donate autologous blood, in patients undergoing cardiac/vascular surgery, and as substitute for RBC transfusions in patients requiring immediate correction of anemia. Correct/exclude other causes of anemia (eg, vitamin deficiency, metabolic/chronic inflammatory conditions, bleeding) prior to therapy. Increased risk of congestive heart failure, deep venous thrombosis undergoing orthopedic procedures, other thromboembolic events, and death in patients undergoing coronary artery bypass surgery. Hypertensive encephalopathy and seizures reported with CKD. Reduce/withhold therapy if BP becomes difficult to control. PRCA and severe anemia (with or without other cytopenias), with neutralizing antibodies to erythropoietin reported. Withhold and evaluate for neutralizing antibodies to erythropoietin if severe anemia and low reticulocyte count occur; d/c permanently if PRCA develops. Immediately and permanently d/c if serious allergic/anaphylactic reactions occur. Contains albumin; may carry an extremely remote risk for transmission of viral diseases or Creutzfeldt-Jakob disease. May require adjustment in dialysis prescriptions and increased anticoagulation with heparin to prevent clotting of extracorporeal circuit during hemodialysis. Multidose vial contains benzyl alcohol; benzyl alcohol associated with serious adverse events and death, particularly in pediatrics.

ADVERSE REACTIONS: CV/thromboembolic reactions, pyrexia, N/V, HTN, cough, arthralgia, myalgia, pruritus, rash, headache, injection-site pain, stomatitis, dizziness.

PREGNANCY: Category C, caution in nursing.

MECHANISM OF ACTION: Erythropoiesis stimulating protein; stimulates erythropoiesis by the same mechanism as endogenous erythropoietin.

PHARMACOKINETICS: Absorption: Adults and Pediatrics with CKD: (SQ) T_{max}=5-24 hrs. Anemic Cancer Patients: (SQ) T_{max}=5-24 hrs. **Elimination:** Adults and Pediatrics with CKD: (IV) $T_{1/2}$=4-13 hrs. Anemic Cancer Patients: (SQ) $T_{1/2}$=16-67 hrs.

NURSING CONSIDERATIONS

Assessment: Assess for uncontrolled HTN, previous hypersensitivity to the drug, causes of anemia, pregnancy/nursing status, and other conditions where treatment is cautioned/contraindicated. Obtain baseline iron status, Hgb levels, transferrin saturation, and serum ferritin.

Monitoring: Monitor for signs/symptoms of an allergic reaction, CV/thromboembolic events, stroke, premonitory neurologic symptoms, PRCA, severe anemia. Monitor Hgb (weekly until stable and then monthly for CKD), BP, iron status, transferrin saturation, and progression or recurrence of tumor in cancer patients. Monitor serum ferritin; supplemental iron is recommended if ferritin is <100mcg/L or serum transferrin saturation is <20%.

Patient Counseling: Inform about risks/benefits of therapy, increased risks of mortality, serious CV events, thromboembolic events, stroke, tumor progression/recurrence, need to have regular lab tests for Hgb, and for cancer patients to sign the patient-physician acknowledgment form prior to therapy. Instruct to undergo regular BP monitoring, adhere to prescribed antihypertensive regimen, and follow recommended dietary restrictions. Advise to contact physician for new onset neurologic symptoms or change in seizure frequency, and other possible side effects of therapy. Inform that risks are associated with benzyl alcohol in neonates, infants, pregnant women, and nursing mothers. Instruct of proper disposal, and caution against the reuse of needles, syringes, or drug product.

Administration: IV/SQ route. IV route recommended in hemodialysis patients. Do not dilute and do not mix with other solutions; refer to PI for admixing exceptions. **Storage:** 2-8°C (36-46°F). Do not freeze or shake. Protect from light. Discard unused portions of multidose vials 21 days after initial entry.

PROGRAF RX
tacrolimus (Astellas)

> Increased risk of lymphoma and other malignancies, particularly of the skin, due to immunosuppression. Increased susceptibility to infections (bacterial, viral, fungal, protozoal, opportunistic). Should only be prescribed by physicians experienced in immunosuppressive therapy and management of organ transplant patients. Patients should be managed in facilities equipped and staffed with adequate laboratory and supportive medical resources. Physician responsible for maint therapy should have complete information requisite for the follow-up of the patient.

THERAPEUTIC CLASS: Macrolide immunosuppressant

INDICATIONS: Prophylaxis of organ rejection in allogeneic kidney, liver, and heart transplants with concomitant adrenal corticosteroids. In heart and kidney transplant patients, azathioprine or mycophenolate mofetil (MMF) coadministration is recommended.

DOSAGE: *Adults:* Initial: Administer no sooner than 6 hrs after liver/heart transplant. May administer within 24 hrs of kidney transplant, but should be delayed until renal function has recovered. Adjunct therapy with adrenal corticosteroids is recommended early post-transplant. (Inj) Give as continuous IV infusion if cannot tolerate PO. D/C as soon as patient can tolerate PO, usually within 2-3 days. Initial: Kidney/Liver Transplant: 0.03-0.05mg/kg/day. Heart Transplant: 0.01mg/kg/day. (PO) Initial: Administer daily dose as 2 divided doses, q12h. Titrate based on clinical assessments of rejection and tolerability. Maint: Lower dosage may be sufficient. If receiving IV infusion, the first dose of PO therapy should be given 8-12 hrs after d/c of IV infusion. Liver Transplant: Initial: 0.10-0.15mg/kg/day. Kidney Transplant: Initial: 0.2mg/kg/day in combination with azathioprine or 0.1mg/kg/day in combination with MMF/IL-2 receptor antagonist. Black patients may require higher doses. Heart Transplant: Initial: 0.075mg/kg/day. Refer to PI for dose adjustments in renal/hepatic impairment. Elderly: Start at lower end of dosing range.

P

Pediatrics: Liver Transplant: Initial: (PO) 0.15-0.2mg/kg/day as 2 divided doses, q12h. (Inj) 0.03-0.05mg/kg/day IV if necessary. Refer to PI for dose adjustments in renal/hepatic impairment.

HOW SUPPLIED: Cap: 0.5mg, 1mg, 5mg; Inj: 5mg/mL

CONTRAINDICATIONS: (Inj) Hypersensitivity to polyoxyl 60 hydrogenated castor oil (HCO-60).

WARNINGS/PRECAUTIONS: Increased risk for polyoma virus infections, cytomegalovirus (CMV) viremia and CMV disease. Progressive multifocal leukoencephalopathy (PML) reported; consider PML in differential diagnosis in patients reporting neurological symptoms and consider consultation with a neurologist. May cause new onset diabetes mellitus; closely monitor blood glucose concentrations. May cause acute/chronic nephrotoxicity; closely monitor patients with renal dysfunction. Consider changing to another immunosuppressive therapy in patients with persistent SrCr elevations unresponsive to dose adjustments. May cause neurotoxicity (eg, posterior reversible encephalopathy syndrome [PRES], delirium, coma); if PRES is suspected or diagnosed, maintain BP control and immediately reduce immunosuppression. Hyperkalemia and HTN reported. Myocardial hypertrophy reported; consider dose reduction or d/c therapy if diagnosed. Pure red cell aplasia (PRCA) reported; d/c therapy if diagnosed. Caution in elderly. (Inj) Anaphylactic reactions may occur; should be reserved for patients unable to take cap orally. Patients should be under continuous observation for at least the first 30 min following the start of infusion and at frequent intervals thereafter; stop infusion if signs/symptoms of anaphylaxis occur.

ADVERSE REACTIONS: Lymphoma, malignancies, infection, tremor, HTN, abnormal renal function, headache, insomnia, hyperglycemia, hyperkalemia, hypomagnesemia, diarrhea, N/V, paresthesia.

INTERACTIONS: Do not use simultaneously with cyclosporine; d/c at least 24 hrs before initiating the other. Use with sirolimus is not recommended in liver and heart transplants. Increased blood concentrations with drugs/substances known to inhibit CYP3A enzymes (eg, lansoprazole, omeprazole, cimetidine). Decreased blood concentrations with drugs known to induce CYP3A enzymes. May increase mycophenolic acid (MPA) exposure after crossover from cyclosporine to tacrolimus in patients concomitantly receiving MPA-containing products. Avoid grapefruit or grapefruit juice and (unless the benefits outweigh the risks) nelfinavir. Monitor whole blood concentrations and adjust dose with concomitant protease inhibitors (eg, ritonavir), verapamil, diltiazem, nifedipine, nicardipine, erythromycin, clarithromycin, troleandomycin, chloramphenicol, rifampin, rifabutin, phenytoin, carbamazepine, phenobarbital, St. John's wort, magnesium and aluminum hydroxide antacids, bromocriptine, nefazodone, metoclopramide, danazol, ethinyl estradiol, or methylprednisolone, or when concomitant use of antifungal drugs (eg, azoles, caspofungin) with tacrolimus is initiated or d/c. Monitor phenytoin plasma concentrations and adjust phenytoin dose PRN when tacrolimus and phenytoin are administered concomitantly. Caution with CYP3A4 inhibitors (eg, antifungals, calcium channel blockers, macrolide antibiotics). Additive/synergistic impairment of renal function with drugs that may be associated with renal dysfunction (eg, aminoglycosides, ganciclovir, amphotericin B, cisplatin, nucleotide reverse transcriptase inhibitors, protease inhibitors). Caution prior to use of other agents or antihypertensive agents associated with hyperkalemia (eg, K⁺-sparing diuretics, ACE inhibitors, angiotensin receptor blockers). Strong CYP3A4-inhibitors and strong inducers not recommended without close monitoring of tacrolimus whole blood trough concentrations. Avoid live vaccines (eg, intranasal influenza, measles, mumps, rubella, oral polio, BCG, yellow fever, varicella, TY21a typhoid).

PREGNANCY: Category C, not for use in nursing.

MECHANISM OF ACTION: Macrolide immunosuppressant; not established. Suspected to inhibit T-lymphocyte activation. Binds to intracellular protein, FKBP-12. Complex of tacrolimus-FKBP-12, calcium, calmodulin, and calcineurin is then formed and phosphatase activity of calcineurin inhibited. Effect may prevent dephosphorylation and translocation of nuclear factor of activated T-cells (NF-AT), a nuclear component thought to initiate gene transcription for the formation of lymphokines. Results in inhibition of T-lymphocyte activation.

PHARMACOKINETICS: Absorption: (PO) Incomplete and variable. Refer to PI for parameters in different populations. **Distribution:** Plasma protein binding (99%), crosses placenta, found in breast milk. **Metabolism:** Hepatic, via CYP3A (demethylation and hydroxylation); 13-demethyl tacrolimus (major metabolite); 31-demethyl (active metabolite). **Elimination:** (PO) Feces (92.6%), urine (2.3%). (IV) Feces (92.4%); urine (<1% unchanged). Refer to PI for $T_{1/2}$ values in different populations.

NURSING CONSIDERATIONS

Assessment: Assess for hypersensitivity to drug, Epstein Barr Virus/CMV seronegativity, pregnancy/nursing status, and possible drug interactions. Assess hepatic/renal function. (Inj) Assess for hypersensitivity to HCO-60 (polyoxyl 60 hydrogenated castor oil).

Monitoring: Monitor tacrolimus blood concentrations in conjunction with other laboratory and clinical parameters (hepatic/renal dysfunction, addition or d/c of potential interacting drugs, post-transplant time). Monitor for signs/symptoms of neurotoxicity, lymphomas and other malignancies (skin), anaphylactic reactions, HTN, myocardial hypertrophy, PRCA, and various infections. Monitor serum K+ and glucose concentrations.

Patient Counseling: Advise to take medicine at the same 12-hr interval everyday. Instruct to take consistently either with or without food. Advise to limit exposure to sunlight and UV light by wearing protective clothing and to use sunscreen with high protection factor. Advise to contact physician if frequent urination, increased thirst, hunger, vision changes, deliriums, or tremors develop. Instruct to attend all visits and complete all blood tests ordered by medical team. Instruct to inform physician when start or stop taking any medication (prescription and nonprescription, natural/herbal, nutritional supplements, vitamins). Instruct to inform physician if planning to become pregnant or to breastfeed.

Administration: Oral/IV routes. Refer to PI for preparation and administration instructions.
Storage: Cap: 25°C (77°F); excursions permitted to 15-30°C (59-86°F). Inj: 5-25°C (41-77°F). Store diluted infusion in glass or polyethylene containers and discard after 24 hrs.

PROLIA RX
denosumab (Amgen)

THERAPEUTIC CLASS: IgG_2 monoclonal antibody

INDICATIONS: Treatment of postmenopausal women with osteoporosis at high risk for fracture (eg, history of osteoporotic fracture, multiple risk factors for fracture) or patients who have failed or are intolerant to other available osteoporosis therapy. As treatment to increase bone mass in women at high risk for fracture receiving adjuvant aromatase inhibitor therapy for breast cancer. As treatment to increase bone mass in men at high risk for fracture receiving androgen deprivation therapy for nonmetastatic prostate cancer.

DOSAGE: *Adults*: 60mg as single SQ injection once q6 months. Administer in the upper arm, upper thigh, or abdomen. If a dose is missed, administer as soon as patient is available and schedule inj q6 months from date of last inj. All patients should receive calcium 1000mg daily and at least 400 IU vitamin D daily.

HOW SUPPLIED: Inj: 60mg/mL

CONTRAINDICATIONS: Hypocalcemia.

WARNINGS/PRECAUTIONS: Should be administered by a healthcare professional. Should not be given with other drugs having the same active ingredient (eg, Xgeva). Hypocalcemia may be exacerbated; correct preexisting hypocalcemia prior to initiating therapy. Monitor calcium and mineral levels (phosphorus and magnesium) in patients predisposed to hypocalcemia and disturbances of mineral metabolism (eg, history of hypoparathyroidism, thyroid/parathyroid surgery, malabsorption syndromes, excision of small intestine, severe renal impairment or receiving dialysis). Endocarditis and serious skin, abdomen, urinary tract, and ear infections leading to hospitalization reported. Caution in patients with impaired immune system; may be at increased risk for serious infections. Epidermal and dermal adverse events (eg, dermatitis, eczema, rashes) may occur; d/c if severe symptoms develop. Osteonecrosis of the jaw (ONJ) may occur; routine oral exam should be performed prior to initiation of treatment. Significant suppression of bone remodeling as evidenced by markers of bone turnover and bone histomorphometry reported.

ADVERSE REACTIONS: Back pain, anemia, vertigo, upper abdominal pain, peripheral edema, cystitis, upper respiratory tract infection, pneumonia, hypercholesterolemia, pain in extremity, musculoskeletal pain, bone pain, sciatica, insomnia.

INTERACTIONS: Immunosuppressant agents may increase the risk of serious infections. Concomitant use with chemotherapy and corticosteroids may increase risk of ONJ.

PREGNANCY: Category C, not for use in nursing.

MECHANISM OF ACTION: IgG2 monoclonal antibody; binds to receptor activator of nuclear factor kappa-B ligand (RANKL) and prevents RANKL from activating its receptor, RANK, on the surface of osteoclasts and their precursors, thereby decreasing bone resorption and increasing bone mass and strength in both cortical and trabecular bone.

PHARMACOKINETICS: Absorption: (60mg SQ, after fasting) C_{max}=6.75mcg/mL; T_{max}=10 days; $AUC_{0-16\ weeks}$=316mcg•day/mL. **Elimination:** $T_{1/2}$=25.4 days.

NURSING CONSIDERATIONS

Assessment: Assess for preexisting hypocalcemia, history of hypoparathyroidism, thyroid/parathyroid surgery, malabsorption syndromes, excision of small intestine, renal impairment, risk factors for ONJ, pregnancy/nursing status, and possible drug interactions.

Monitoring: Monitor calcium and mineral levels (phosphorus and magnesium). Monitor for signs and symptoms of hypocalcemia, infections including cellulitis, and dermatological reactions (dermatitis, rashes, and eczema). Monitor for long-term consequences of the degree of suppression of bone remodeling (eg, ONJ, atypical fractures, delayed fracture healing).

P

Patient Counseling: Counsel not to take with other drugs with the same active ingredient. Inform about the symptoms of hypocalcemia and the importance of maintaining calcium levels with adequate calcium and vitamin D supplementation. Advise to seek prompt medical attention if develop signs and symptoms of hypocalcemia, infections including cellulitis, and dermatological reactions (dermatitis, rashes, and eczema). Advise to maintain good oral hygiene during treatment and to inform dentist prior to dental procedures of current treatment. Instruct to inform physician or dentist if experience persistent pain and/or slow healing of the mouth or jaw after dental surgery. Counsel to adhere to doctor appointments every 6 months.

Administration: SQ route. Refer to PI for preparation and administration instructions. **Storage:** 2-8°C (36-46°F). Do not freeze. Prior to Administration: ≤25°C (77°F). Use within 14 days. Protect from direct light and heat. Avoid vigorous shaking.

PROMACTA   RX
eltrombopag (GlaxoSmithKline)

May cause hepatotoxicity. Measure serum ALT, AST, and bilirubin prior to initiation, every 2 weeks during the dose adjustment phase, and monthly following establishment of a stable dose. If bilirubin is elevated, perform fractionation. Evaluate abnormal serum liver tests with repeat testing within 3-5 days. If the abnormalities are confirmed, monitor liver tests weekly until the abnormality(ies) resolve, stabilize, or return to baseline levels. D/C if ALT levels increase to ≥3X ULN and are progressive, or persistent for ≥4 weeks, or accompanied by increased direct bilirubin, or accompanied by clinical symptoms of liver injury or evidence for hepatic decompensation.

THERAPEUTIC CLASS: Thrombopoietin receptor agonist

INDICATIONS: Treatment of thrombocytopenia in patients with chronic immune (idiopathic) thrombocytopenia purpura (ITP) who have had an insufficient response to corticosteroids, immunoglobulins, or splenectomy.

DOSAGE: *Adults:* Initial: 50mg qd. East Asian Ancestry/Mild-to-Severe Hepatic Impairment (Child-Pugh Class A, B, C): Initial: 25mg qd. East Asian Ancestry with Hepatic Impairment (Child-Pugh Class A, B, C): Consider initiating at a reduced dose of 12.5mg qd. Titrate: Adjust the dose to achieve and maintain platelet count ≥50 x 10⁹/L. Max: 75mg/day. Platelet Count <50 x 10⁹/L following at least 2 Weeks of Therapy: Increase daily dose by 25mg to a max of 75mg/day. For patients taking 12.5mg qd, increase dose to 25mg/day before increasing the dose amount by 25mg. Platelet Count ≥200 x 10⁹/L to ≤400 x 10⁹/L at any Time: Decrease daily dose by 25mg. Wait 2 weeks to assess effects of this and any subsequent dose adjustments. Platelet count >400 x 10⁹/L: D/C therapy; increase the frequency of platelet monitoring to 2x weekly. Once platelet count is <150 x 10⁹/L, reinitiate therapy at a daily dose reduced by 25mg. For patients taking 25mg qd, reinitiate therapy at a daily dose of 12.5mg. Platelet Count >400 x 10⁹/L after 2 Weeks of Therapy at Lowest Dose: D/C therapy. Hepatic Impairment (Child-Pugh A, B, C): After initiating therapy or after any subsequent dosing increase, wait 3 weeks before increasing the dose. D/C if no increase in platelet counts to a sufficient level after 4 weeks of therapy at max daily dose of 75mg.

HOW SUPPLIED: Tab: 12.5mg, 25mg, 50mg, 75mg

WARNINGS/PRECAUTIONS: Use only in patients with ITP whose degree of thrombocytopenia and clinical condition increase the risk for bleeding; not to be used to normalize platelet counts. If d/c due to ≥3X ULN ALT, reinitiation is not recommended; may cautiously reintroduce if potential benefit outweighs risk for hepatotoxicity. May increase risk for development or progression of reticulin fiber deposition within the bone marrow; consider bone marrow biopsy if new or worsening blood morphological abnormalities or cytopenias occur. Thrombotic/thromboembolic complications may result from increase in platelet counts; caution in patients with known risk factors for thromboembolism (eg, factor V Leiden, ATIII deficiency, antiphospholipid syndrome, chronic liver disease). May increase the risk for hematological malignancies. Development or worsening of cataracts reported. Caution with hepatic impairment (Child-Pugh Class A, B, C) and in elderly.

ADVERSE REACTIONS: Headache, N/V, diarrhea, upper respiratory tract infection, hyperbilirubinemia, increased ALT/AST, myalgia, cataract, urinary tract infection, oropharyngeal pain, fatigue, pharyngitis, back pain.

INTERACTIONS: Monitor for signs/symptoms of excessive exposure with moderate/strong inhibitors of CYP1A2 (eg, ciprofloxacin, fluvoxamine) or CYP2C8 (eg, gemfibrozil, trimethoprim), moderate/strong inhibitors of breast cancer resistance protein (BCRP), and moderate/strong inhibitors of UGT1A1 or UGT1A3. Polyvalent cations (eg, iron, calcium, aluminum, magnesium, selenium, zinc) may reduce absorption due to chelation; do not take within 4 hrs of any medications or products containing polyvalent cations (eg, antacids, dairy products, and mineral supplements). Monitor closely for signs/symptoms of excessive exposure to substrates of UGT1A1, UGT1A3, UGT1A4, UGT1A6, UGT1A9, UGT2B7, and UGT2B15 (eg, acetaminophen, narcotics, NSAIDs). Caution with substrates of organic anion transporting polypeptide OATP1B1 or BCRP (eg, benzylpenicillin, atorvastatin, fluvastatin, pravastatin, rosuvastatin, methotrexate, nateglinide, repaglinide, rifampin, doxorubicin); monitor for signs/symptoms of excessive exposure and consider dose reduction of these drugs.

PREGNANCY: Category C, not for use in nursing.

MECHANISM OF ACTION: Thrombopoietin (TPO)-receptor agonist; interacts with the transmembrane domain of the human TPO-receptor and initiates signaling cascades that induce proliferation and differentiation of megakaryocytes from bone marrow progenitor cells.

PHARMACOKINETICS: Absorption: AUC=108mcg•hr/mL (50mg), 168mcg•hr/mL (75mg); C_{max}=8.01mcg/mL (50mg), 12.7mcg/mL (75mg); T_{max}=2-6 hrs. **Distribution:** Plasma protein binding (>99%). **Metabolism:** Extensive; cleavage, oxidation (via CYP1A2, CYP2C8), and conjugation with glucuronic acid (via UGT1A1, UGT1A3), glutathione, or cysteine. **Elimination:** Urine (31%), feces (59%, 20% unchanged); $T_{1/2}$=26-35 hrs (ITP).

NURSING CONSIDERATIONS

Assessment: Assess for degree of thrombocytopenia, risk factors for thromboembolism, hepatic impairment, pregnancy/nursing status, and for possible drug interactions. Obtain baseline CBC with differentials including platelet counts. Obtain baseline LFTs and ocular exam.

Monitoring: Monitor for bone marrow reticulin deposition, thrombotic/thromboembolic complications, cataracts, hematologic malignancies, and other adverse reactions. Monitor LFTs. Perform regular ocular exam. Monitor CBCs with differentials including platelet counts weekly during the dose adjustment phase and then monthly after establishment of a stable dose and then weekly for at least 4 weeks after d/c.

Patient Counseling: Inform about the risks and benefits of therapy. Therapy may be associated with hepatobiliary lab abnormalities and that laboratory monitoring will be required prior to, during, and after therapy. Avoid situations or medications that may increase risk for bleeding and to report to physician any signs/symptoms of liver problems (eg, yellowing of the skin or the whites of the eyes, unusual darkening of the urine, unusual tiredness, right upper stomach area pain). Thrombocytopenia and risk of bleeding may recur following d/c, particularly when d/c while on anticoagulants/antiplatelet agents. Inform about the risk of reticulin fiber formation within bone marrow and risk for thrombotic/thromboembolic complications with excessive dose. Counsel that platelet counts and CBCs must be performed regularly and that patients should be monitored weekly until stable dose is achieved, then monthly while on therapy, and for ≥4 weeks after d/c. Take on an empty stomach and to space ≥4 hrs between therapy and foods, mineral supplements, and antacids containing polyvalent cations. Notify physician if pregnant, planning to become pregnant, or if nursing.

Administration: Oral route. Take on empty stomach (1 hr before or 2 hrs after a meal). Do not take >1 dose within 24 hrs. **Storage:** 25°C (77°F); excursions permitted to 15-30°C (59-86°F).

P

PROMETHAZINE   RX
promethazine HCl (Various)

> Promethazine HCl should not be used in patients <2 yrs; potential for fatal respiratory depression. Caution when administering to patients ≥2 yrs; use lowest effective dose and avoid concomitant administration of respiratory depressants.

OTHER BRAND NAMES: Phenadoz (Paddock) - Promethegan (G & W Labs)

THERAPEUTIC CLASS: Phenothiazine derivative

INDICATIONS: Allergic and vasomotor rhinitis, allergic conjunctivitis, allergic reactions to blood or plasma, dermographism, mild allergic skin manifestation of urticaria and angioedema. Preoperative, postoperative, or obstetric sedation. Adjunct in anaphylactic reactions. Prevention and control of N/V with certain types of anesthesia and surgery. Active and prophylactic treatment of motion sickness. Sedation, relief of apprehension, production of light sleep. Adjunct with meperidine or other analgesics for postoperative pain. Antiemetic in postoperative patients.

DOSAGE: *Adults:* Allergy: Usual: 25mg qhs or 12.5mg ac and hs; may give 6.25-12.5mg tid. Adjust to lowest effective dose after initiation. Motion Sickness: Initial: 25mg 30-60 min before travel, repeat after 8-12 hrs prn. Maint: 25mg bid, on arising and before pm meal. Prevention/Control of N/V: Prevention: Usual: 25mg, may repeat q4-6h PRN. Control: Usual: 25mg, then 12.5-25mg q4-6h prn. Sedation: 25-50mg qhs. Preoperative: 50mg night before surgery, then 50mg preoperatively. Postoperative/Adjunctive with analgesics: 25-50mg.
Pediatrics: ≥2 yrs: Allergy: Usual: 25mg qhs or 12.5mg ac and hs; may give 6.25-12.5mg tid. Adjust to lowest effective dose after initiation. Motion Sickness: 12.5-25mg bid. Prevention/Control of N/V: Prevention: Usual: 25mg, may repeat q4-6h PRN. Control: Usual: 25mg or 0.5mg/lb, then 12.5-25mg q4-6h prn. Adjust dose based on patient age/weight and severity of condition. Sedation: 12.5-25mg hs. Preoperative: 12.5-25mg night before surgery, then 0.5mg/lb preoperatively. Postoperative/Adjunctive with analgesics: 12.5-25mg.

HOW SUPPLIED: Sup: (Phenadoz, Promethazine) 12.5mg, 25mg, (Promethegan) 50mg; Syrup: (Promethazine): 6.25mg/5mL [118mL, 237mL, 473mL] Tab: (Promethazine) 12.5mg*, 25mg*, 50mg *scored

CONTRAINDICATIONS: Treatment of lower respiratory tract symptoms, including asthma. Comatose states, pediatric patients <2 yrs.

WARNINGS/PRECAUTIONS: Avoid in pediatrics whose signs and symptoms may suggest Reye's syndrome or other hepatic diseases. May impair mental/physical abilities. May lower seizure threshold; caution with seizure disorders. May lead to potentially fatal respiratory depression; avoid with compromised respiratory function (eg, chronic obstructive pulmonary disease, sleep apnea). Caution with bone marrow depression; leukopenia and agranulocytosis reported. Neuroleptic malignant syndrome (NMS) reported; d/c immediately. Hallucinations and convulsions may occur in pediatrics. Acutely ill pediatrics who are dehydrated may have increased susceptibility to dystonias. Not recommended for uncomplicated vomiting in pediatrics; should be limited to prolonged vomiting of known etiology. Caution with narrow-angle glaucoma, prostatic hypertrophy, stenosing peptic ulcer, bladder-neck or pyloroduodenal obstruction, cardiovascular (CV) disease, hepatic impairment. Cholestatic jaundice reported. Caution in elderly.

ADVERSE REACTIONS: Drowsiness, sedation, blurred vision, dizziness, increased or decreased BP, urticaria, dry mouth, N/V, respiratory depression, hallucination, leukopenia, apnea, NMS.

INTERACTIONS: See Boxed Warning. May increase rates of extrapyramidal effects with concomitant MAOI use. May increase, prolong, or intensify the sedative action of other CNS depressants, such as alcohol, sedatives/hypnotics (including barbiturates), narcotics, narcotic analgesics, general anesthetics, TCAs, tranquilizers; avoid such agents or reduce dosages. Reduce barbiturate dose by at least one-half and narcotic analgesics by one-quarter to one-half. May reverse vasopressor effect of epinephrine. Caution with medications that may affect seizure threshold (eg, narcotics, local anesthetics). Caution with anticholinergics. Leukopenia and agranulocytosis reported, usually with marrow-toxic agents. NMS reported in combination with antipsychotics.

PREGNANCY: Category C, not for use in nursing.

MECHANISM OF ACTION: Phenothiazine derivative; H_1 receptor-blocking agent (antihistaminic action) and provides sedative and antiemetic effects.

PHARMACOKINETICS: Absorption: Well absorbed from GI tract. **Metabolism:** Liver; sulfoxides, N-demethylpromethazine (metabolites). **Elimination:** Urine.

NURSING CONSIDERATIONS

Assessment: Assess for drug hypersensitive or idiosyncratic reaction, or any other conditions where treatment is contraindicated or cautioned. Assess for pregnancy/nursing status and for possible drug interaction. Assess for signs/symptoms of Reye's syndrome, hepatic diseases, or encephalopathy in pediatrics.

Monitoring: Monitor for signs/symptoms of CNS/respiratory depression, NMS, seizures, cholestatic jaundice, leukopenia, agranulocytosis. Monitor for hallucinations, convulsions, extrapyramidal symptoms, respiratory depression, dystonias in pediatrics. Monitor for false positive and false negative pregnancy tests, blood glucose levels, and BP. Monitor platelet count in newborns when used in pregnant women within 2 weeks of delivery.

Patient Counseling: Inform that drowsiness or impairment of mental and/or physical abilities may occur. Counsel to report involuntary muscle movements. Instruct to avoid alcohol use, prolonged sun exposure, and concomitant use of other CNS depressants.

Administration: Oral and rectal route. **Storage:** (Tab) 20-25°C (68-77°F). Protect from light. (Sup) 2-8°C (36-46°F).

PROMETHAZINE VC/CODEINE
phenylephrine HCl - promethazine HCl - codeine phosphate (Qualitest)

> Contraindicated in pediatrics <6 yrs of age. Concomitant administration of promethazine products with other respiratory depressants is associated with respiratory depression, and sometimes death, in pediatrics. Respiratory depression, including fatalities, have been reported with use of promethazine HCl in patients <2 yrs.

THERAPEUTIC CLASS: Phenothiazine derivative/antitussive/sympathomimetic

INDICATIONS: Temporary relief of coughs and upper respiratory symptoms (eg, nasal congestion) associated with allergy or the common cold.

DOSAGE: *Adults:* 5mL q4-6h. Max: 30mL/24hr. Elderly: Start at lower end of dosing range. *Pediatrics:* ≥12 yrs: 5mL q4-6h. Max: 30mL/24hr. 6-<12 yrs: 2.5-5mL q4-6h. Max: 30mL/24hr.

HOW SUPPLIED: Syrup: (Codeine Phosphate-Promethazine Hydrochloride-Phenylephrine Hydrochloride) 10mg-6.25mg-5mg/5mL [118mL, 237mL, 473mL]

CONTRAINDICATIONS: Concomitant use with MAOIs, comatose states, treatment of lower respiratory tract symptoms (eg, asthma), HTN, peripheral vascular insufficiency, pediatric patients <6 yrs.

WARNINGS/PRECAUTIONS: Should only be given to a pregnant woman if clearly needed. Caution in elderly. Codeine: Do not increase dose if cough fails to respond to treatment. May cause/aggravate constipation. Caution in atopic children. Capacity to elevate CSF pressure and respiratory depressant effects may be markedly exaggerated in head injury, intracranial lesions, or with preexisting increase in intracranial pressure. May obscure clinical course in patients with head injuries. Avoid with acute febrile illness with productive cough or in chronic respiratory disease. May produce orthostatic hypotension in ambulatory patients. Give with caution and reduce initial dose with acute abdominal conditions, convulsive disorders, significant hepatic/renal impairment, fever, hypothyroidism, Addison's disease, ulcerative colitis, prostatic hypertrophy, recent GI or urinary tract surgery, and in the very young, elderly, or debilitated. Use lowest effective dose for the shortest period of time. Potential for abuse and dependence. Promethazine: May impair mental/physical abilities. May lead to potentially fatal respiratory depression; avoid with compromised respiratory function (eg, chronic obstructive pulmonary disease, sleep apnea). May lower seizure threshold; caution with seizure disorders. Leukopenia and agranulocytosis reported, especially when given with other marrow toxic agents; caution with bone marrow depression. Neuroleptic malignant syndrome (NMS) reported; d/c immediately if NMS occurs. Hallucinations and convulsions may occur in pediatrics. Acutely ill pediatric patients who are dehydrated may have increased susceptibility to dystonias. Cholestatic jaundice reported. Caution with narrow-angle glaucoma, prostatic hypertrophy, stenosing peptic ulcer, pyloroduodenal/bladder-neck obstruction, cardiovascular disease, or with impaired liver function. May increase blood glucose. Phenylephrine: Caution with diabetes mellitus, thyroid, and heart diseases. May cause urinary retention in men with symptomatic benign prostatic hypertrophy. May decrease cardiac output; use extreme caution with arteriosclerosis, elderly, and/or patients with initially poor cerebral or coronary circulation.

ADVERSE REACTIONS: Drowsiness, dizziness, anxiety, sedation, tremor, blurred vision, dry mouth, increased or decreased BP, N/V, respiratory depression, urinary retention, NMS, constipation.

INTERACTIONS: See Boxed Warning and Contraindications. Promethazine: May increase, prolong, or intensify the sedative action of other CNS depressants, such as alcohol, sedatives/hypnotics (eg, barbiturates), narcotics, narcotic analgesics, general anesthetics, TCAs, and tranquilizers; avoid such agents or administer in reduced doses. Reduce dose of barbiturate by at least 1/2 and narcotic analgesics by 1/4-1/2. May reverse vasopressor effect of epinephrine. Caution with other agents with anticholinergic properties and drugs that also affect seizure threshold (eg, narcotics, local anesthetics). Phenylephrine: Pressor response increased with TCAs and decreased with prior administration of phentolamine or other α-adrenergic blockers. Ergot alkaloids may cause excessive rise in BP. Tachycardia or other arrhythmias may occur with bronchodilator sympathomimetics, epinephrine, or other sympathomimetics. Reflex bradycardia blocked and pressor response enhanced with atropine sulfate. Cardiostimulating effects blocked with prior administration of propranolol or other β-adrenergic blockers. Synergistic adrenergic response with diet preparations (eg, amphetamines, phenylpropanolamine).

PREGNANCY: Category C, caution in nursing.

MECHANISM OF ACTION: Codeine: Narcotic analgesic/antitussive; primary effects are on CNS and GI tract. Promethazine: Phenothiazine derivative; blocks H_1 receptor and provides sedative and antiemetic effects. Phenylephrine: Sympathomimetic amine; potent postsynaptic-α-receptor agonist with little effect on β-receptors of heart. Causes vasoconstriction and has a mild central stimulant effect.

PHARMACOKINETICS: Absorption: Codeine/Promethazine: Well-absorbed. Phenylephrine: Irregularly absorbed. **Distribution:** Codeine: Crosses placenta; found in breast milk. **Metabolism:** Codeine: Liver via O-demethylation, N-demethylation, and partial conjugation with glucuronic acid. Promethazine: Liver; sulfoxides and N-demethylpromethazine (metabolites). Phenylephrine: Liver and intestine via monoamine oxidase. **Elimination:** Codeine: Urine (primary); inactive metabolites and free/conjugated morphine), feces (negligible amount; parent compound and metabolites). Promethazine: Urine (metabolites).

NURSING CONSIDERATIONS

Assessment: Assess for drug hypersensitivity or idiosyncracy, history of drug abuse/dependence, or any other conditions where treatment is contraindicated or cautioned. Assess BP, pregnancy/nursing status, and for possible drug interactions.

Monitoring: Monitor for signs/symptoms of CNS and respiratory depression, constipation, leukopenia, agranulocytosis, cholestatic jaundice, seizures, NMS, and orthostatic hypotension. Monitor for urinary retention in men with BPH. Monitor pediatric patients for hallucinations, convulsions, and dystonias. Monitor glucose levels. Reevaluate 5 days or sooner if cough is unresponsive to treatment.

P

Patient Counseling: Instruct to measure medication with an accurate measuring device. Inform that therapy may cause marked drowsiness and may impair mental and/or physical abilities required for performing hazardous tasks (eg, driving, operating machinery); advise to avoid such activities until it is known that they do not become drowsy or dizzy with the therapy. Counsel to avoid the use of alcohol and other CNS depressants while on therapy. Report any involuntary muscle movements. Avoid prolonged sun exposure. Inform that therapy may produce orthostatic hypotension. Inform about risks and the signs of morphine overdose (extreme sleepiness, confusion, shallow breathing). Instruct nursing mothers to watch for signs of morphine toxicity in their infants (eg, increased sleepiness more than usual, difficulty breastfeeding, breathing difficulties, or limpness). Notify pediatrician immediately if these signs are noticed or get emergency medical attention.

Administration: Oral route. **Storage:** 20-25°C (68-77°F).

PROMETHAZINE W/CODEINE
promethazine HCl - codeine phosphate (Various)

> Contraindicated in pediatrics <6 yrs of age. Concomitant administration of promethazine products with other respiratory depressants is associated with respiratory depression, and sometimes death, in pediatrics. Respiratory depression, including fatalities, have been reported with use of promethazine in pediatrics <2 yrs.

OTHER BRAND NAMES: Prometh w/ Codeine (Actavis)

THERAPEUTIC CLASS: Phenothiazine derivative/antitussive

INDICATIONS: Temporary relief of cough and upper respiratory symptoms associated with allergy or the common cold.

DOSAGE: *Adults:* 5mL q4-6h. Max: 30mL/24hr. Elderly: Start at lower end of dosing range. *Pediatrics:* ≥12 yrs: 5mL q4-6h. Max: 30mL/24hr. 6-<12 yrs: 2.5-5mL q4-6h. Max: 30mL/24hr.

HOW SUPPLIED: Syrup: (Codeine Phosphate-Promethazine Hydrochloride) 10mg-6.25mg/5mL [118mL, 273mL, 473mL]

CONTRAINDICATIONS: Comatose states, treatment of lower respiratory tract symptoms (eg, asthma), pediatric patients <6 yrs.

WARNINGS/PRECAUTIONS: Should only be given to a pregnant woman if clearly needed. Caution in elderly. Codeine: Do not increase dose if cough fails to respond to treatment. May cause/aggravate constipation. Caution in atopic children. Capacity to elevate CSF pressure and respiratory depressant effects may be markedly exaggerated in head injury, intracranial lesions, or with preexisting increase in intracranial pressure. May obscure clinical course in patients with head injuries. Avoid with acute febrile illness with productive cough or in chronic respiratory disease. May produce orthostatic hypotension in ambulatory patients. Give with caution and reduce initial dose with acute abdominal conditions, convulsive disorders, significant hepatic/renal impairment, fever, hypothyroidism, Addison's disease, ulcerative colitis, prostatic hypertrophy, recent GI or urinary tract surgery, and in the very young, elderly, or debilitated. Use lowest effective dose for the shortest period of time. Potential for abuse and dependence. Promethazine: May impair mental/physical abilities. May lead to potentially fatal respiratory depression; caution with compromised respiratory function (eg, chronic obstructive pulmonary disease, sleep apnea). May lower seizure threshold; caution with seizure disorders. Leukopenia and agranulocytosis reported, especially when given with other marrow toxic agents; caution with bone marrow depression. Neuroleptic malignant syndrome (NMS) reported; d/c immediately if NMS occurs. Hallucinations and convulsions may occur in pediatrics. Acutely ill pediatric patients who are dehydrated may have increased susceptibility to dystonias. Cholestatic jaundice reported. Caution with narrow-angle glaucoma, prostatic hypertrophy, stenosing peptic ulcer, pyloroduodenal/bladder-neck obstruction, cardiovascular disease, or with impaired liver function. May increase blood glucose.

ADVERSE REACTIONS: Drowsiness, dizziness, sedation, blurred vision, dry mouth, increased or decreased BP, N/V, constipation, urinary retention, leukopenia, agranulocytosis, respiratory depression, NMS.

INTERACTIONS: See Boxed Warning. Possible interaction with MAOIs (eg, increased incidence of extrapyramidal effects); consider initial small test dose. Promethazine: May increase, prolong, or intensify the sedative action of other CNS depressants, such as alcohol, sedative/hypnotics (including barbiturates), narcotics, narcotic analgesics, general anesthetics, TCAs, and tranquilizers; avoid such agents or administer in reduced doses. Reduce dose of barbiturate by at least 1/2 and narcotic analgesic by 1/4-1/2. May reverse vasopressor effect of epinephrine. Caution with other agents with anticholinergic properties and drugs that also affect seizure threshold (eg, narcotics, local anesthetics).

PREGNANCY: Category C, caution in nursing.

MECHANISM OF ACTION: Codeine: Narcotic analgesic/antitussive; primary effects are on CNS and GI tract. Promethazine: Phenothiazine derivative; blocks H_1 receptor and provides sedative and antiemetic effects.

PHARMACOKINETICS: Absorption: Well-absorbed. **Distribution:** Codeine: Crosses placenta; found in breast milk. **Metabolism:** Codeine: Liver via O-demethylation, N-demethylation, and partial conjugation with glucuronic acid. Promethazine: Liver; sulfoxides and N-demethylpromethazine (metabolites). **Elimination:** Codeine: Urine (primary; inactive metabolites and free/conjugated morphine), feces (negligible amount; parent compound and metabolites). Promethazine: Urine (metabolites).

NURSING CONSIDERATIONS

Assessment: Assess for drug hypersensitivity or idiosyncracy, history of drug abuse/dependence, or any other conditions where treatment is contraindicated or cautioned. Assess BP, pregnancy/nursing status, and for possible drug interactions.

Monitoring: Monitor for signs/symptoms of CNS and respiratory depression, constipation, leukopenia, agranulocytosis, cholestatic jaundice, seizures, NMS, orthostatic hypotension, and abuse and dependence. Monitor pediatric patients for hallucinations, convulsions, and dystonias. Monitor glucose levels. Reevaluate 5 days or sooner if cough is unresponsive to treatment.

Patient Counseling: Instruct to measure medication with an accurate measuring device. Inform that therapy may cause drowsiness and may impair mental and/or physical abilities required for performing potentially hazardous tasks (eg, driving, operating machinery); advise to avoid such activities until it is known that they do not become drowsy or dizzy with the therapy. Avoid the use of alcohol and other CNS depressants while on therapy. Report any involuntary muscle movements. Avoid prolonged sun exposure. Inform that therapy may produce orthostatic hypotension. Inform about risks and the signs of morphine overdose (extreme sleepiness, confusion, shallow breathing). Instruct nursing mothers to watch for signs of morphine toxicity in their infants (eg, increased sleepiness more than usual, difficulty breastfeeding, breathing difficulties, or limpness); notify pediatrician immediately if these signs are noticed or get emergency medical attention.

Administration: Oral route. **Storage:** 20-25°C (68-77°F).

PROPECIA   RX
finasteride (Merck)

THERAPEUTIC CLASS: Type II 5 alpha-reductase inhibitor

INDICATIONS: Treatment of male pattern hair loss (androgenetic alopecia) in men only.

DOSAGE: *Adults:* Usual: 1mg qd for ≥3 months. Continued use is recommended to sustain benefit; re-evaluate periodically. Withdrawal of treatment may lead to reversal of effect within 12 months.

HOW SUPPLIED: Tab: 1mg

CONTRAINDICATIONS: Pregnancy.

WARNINGS/PRECAUTIONS: Not for use in pediatrics or women. Efficacy not established in bitemporal recession. Caution with liver function abnormalities. Pregnant women or women who may potentially be pregnant should not handle crushed or broken tabs because of potential risk to a male fetus. May increase risk of development of high-grade prostate cancer.

ADVERSE REACTIONS: Decreased libido, erectile dysfunction, decreased volume of ejaculate, ejaculation disorder.

PREGNANCY: Category X, not for use in nursing.

MECHANISM OF ACTION: Type II 5α-reductase inhibitor; blocks peripheral conversion of testosterone to 5α-dihydrotestosterone (DHT), resulting in significant decreases in serum and tissue DHT concentrations.

PHARMACOKINETICS: Absorption: Mean bioavailability (65%); C_{max}=9.2ng/mL; T_{max}=1-2 hrs; $AUC_{(0-24 hr)}$=53ng•hr/mL. **Distribution:** V_d=76L; plasma protein binding (90%); crosses blood brain barrier. **Metabolism:** Liver (extensive); via CYP3A4. **Elimination:** (Oral) Urine (39% metabolites), feces (57%); $T_{1/2}$=4.5 hrs (IV), 5-6 hrs (18-60 yrs), 8 hrs (>70 yrs).

NURSING CONSIDERATIONS

Assessment: Assess liver function and for hypersensitivity to drug and its components. Obtain baseline prostate-specific antigen levels (PSA).

Monitoring: Monitor for hypersensitivity reactions or other adverse reactions. Monitor PSA levels.

Patient Counseling: Instruct pregnant or potentially pregnant females not to handle broken or crushed tabs due to potential risk to male fetus. Notify physician if changes in breast (eg, lumps, pain, nipple discharge) occur. Inform of possible adverse reactions (eg, decreased volume of ejaculate, impotence, decreased libido).

Administration: Oral route. **Storage:** 15-30°C (59-86°F).

PROPRANOLOL
RX

propranolol HCl (Various)

THERAPEUTIC CLASS: Nonselective beta-blocker

INDICATIONS: (Tab) Management of HTN, angina pectoris, hypertrophic subaortic stenosis, atrial fibrillation (A-fib), reduction of cardiovascular mortality post-myocardial infarction (MI), and familial or hereditary essential tremor. Adjunct to control BP and reduce symptoms of pheochromocytoma. Common migraine headache prophylaxis. (Inj) For cardiac arrhythmias (supraventricular/ventricular tachycardia, tachyarrhythmia of digitalis intoxication, resistant tachyarrhythmia due to excessive catecholamine action during anesthesia).

DOSAGE: *Adults:* (Tab) Individualize dose. HTN: Initial: 40mg bid. Titrate: Increase gradually until adequate BP control. Maint: 120-240mg/day. Angina: 80-320mg/day bid-qid. To d/c, reduce gradually over several weeks. A-Fib: 10-30mg tid-qid before meals and hs. MI: Initial: 40mg tid. Titrate: 60-80mg tid after 1 month as tolerated. Usual: 180-240mg/day in divided doses. Max: 240mg/day. Migraine: Initial: 80mg/day in divided doses. Usual: 160-240mg/day. May increase gradually for optimum prophylaxis. D/C if unsatisfactory within 4-6 weeks after max dose; withdraw gradually over several weeks. Tremor: Initial: 40mg bid. Usual/Maint: 120mg/day. Hypertrophic Subaortic Stenosis: Usual: 20-40mg tid-qid, before meals and hs. Pheochromocytoma: Usual: 60mg/day in divided doses for 3 days before surgery with α-adrenergic blocker. Inoperable Tumor: Usual: 30mg/day in divided doses with α-adrenergic blocker. (Inj) Arrhythmia: Usual: 1-3mg IV at ≤1mg/min. May give second dose if necessary after 2 min then avoid additional drugs <4 hrs. Hepatic Impairment: Consider lower dose. (Inj/Tab) Elderly: Start at lower end of dosing range.

HOW SUPPLIED: Inj: 1mg/mL; Tab: 10mg*, 20mg*, 40mg*, 60mg*, 80mg* *scored

CONTRAINDICATIONS: Cardiogenic shock, sinus bradycardia and >1st-degree block, bronchial asthma.

WARNINGS/PRECAUTIONS: Exacerbation of angina and MI following abrupt d/c reported. Caution with well-compensated cardiac failure, bronchospastic lung disease, Wolff-Parkinson-White (WPW) syndrome, tachycardia, and hepatic/renal impairment. Withdrawal before surgery is controversial. May mask acute hypoglycemia or hyperthyroidism signs/symptoms. Avoid abrupt d/c. May reduce intraocular pressure (IOP). May be more reactive to repeated challenge with history of severe anaphylactic reaction to variety of allergens; may be unresponsive to usual doses of epinephrine. Elevated serum K⁺, transaminases and alkaline phosphatase observed. Elevated BUN reported in severe heart failure. Not for treatment of hypertensive emergencies. Caution in elderly. (Inj) Risk of anaphylactic reaction. (Tab) Hypersensitivity reactions and cutaneous reactions (eg, Stevens-Johnson syndrome [SJS]) reported. Continued use in patients without history of heart failure may cause cardiac failure.

ADVERSE REACTIONS: Bradycardia, CHF, hypotension, lightheadedness, mental depression, N/V, agranulocytosis.

INTERACTIONS: Administration with CYP450 (2D6, 1A2, 2C19) substrates, inducers, and inhibitors may lead to clinically relevant drug interactions. Increased levels with CYP2D6 substrates/inhibitors (eg, amiodarone, cimetidine, delavirdine, fluoxetine, paroxetine, quinidine, ritonavir), CYP1A2 substrates/inhibitors (eg, imipramine, cimetidine, ciprofloxacin, fluvoxamine, isoniazid, ritonavir, theophylline, zileuton, zolmitriptan, rizatriptan), and CYP2C19 substrates/inhibitors (eg, fluconazole, cimetidine, fluoxetine, fluvoxamine, teniposide, tolbutamide). Decreased blood levels with hepatic enzyme inducers (eg, rifampin, ethanol, phenytoin, phenobarbital, cigarette smoking). Increased levels of propafenone, lidocaine, zolmitriptan, rizatriptan, diazepam and its metabolites. Increased levels with nisoldipine, nicardipine, chlorpromazine. Decreased theophylline clearance. Increased thioridazine plasma and metabolite concentrations with doses ≥160mg/day. Decreased levels with aluminum hydroxide gel, cholestyramine, colestipol, lovastatin, pravastatin. Decreased levels of lovastatin, pravastatin. Increased warfarin levels and PT. Caution with drugs that slow atrioventricular nodal conduction (eg, digitalis, lidocaine, calcium channel blocker). Bradycardia, hypotension, high degree heart block, and heart failure reported with diltiazem. May cause hypotension with ACE inhibitors. May antagonize effects of clonidine. May prolong first dose hypotension with prazosin. Postural hypotension reported with terazosin or doxazosin. May reduce resting sympathetic nervous activity with catecholamine-depleting drugs (eg, reserpine). May experience uncontrolled HTN with epinephrine. Effects can be reversed by β-agonists (eg, dobutamine or isoproterenol). May reduce efficacy with indomethacin and NSAIDs. May depress myocardial contractility with methoxyflurane and trichloroethylene. Hypotension and cardiac arrest reported with haloperidol. May lower T3 concentration with thyroxine. May exacerbate hypotensive effects of MAOIs or TCAs. May augment the risks of general anesthesia. May need to adjust dose of insulin. (Inj) Severe bradycardia, asystole, and heart failure reported with disopyramide. (Tab) Increased levels with alcohol.

PREGNANCY: Category C, caution in nursing.

MECHANISM OF ACTION: Nonselective β-adrenergic receptor blocker; not established. (Tab) Proposed to decrease cardiac output, inhibit renin release and lessen tonic sympathetic nerve outflow from vasomotor centers in the brain. (Inj) Decreases normal and ectopic pacemaker cells and AV nodal conduction velocity.

PHARMACOKINETICS: Absorption: (Tab) Almost complete; T_{max}=1-4 hrs. **Distribution:** V_d=4-5L/kg; plasma protein binding (90%). (Tab) Crosses placenta; (Inj/Tab) found in breast milk. **Metabolism:** CYP2D6 (hydroxylation), CYP1A2, 2D6 (oxidation), N-dealkylation, glucuronidation. Propranolol glucuronide, naphthyloxylactic acid, glucuronic acid, sulfate conjugates (major metabolites). **Elimination:** $T_{1/2}$=3-6 hrs (PO), 2-5.5 hrs (Inj).

NURSING CONSIDERATIONS

Assessment: Assess for bronchial asthma, sinus bradycardia, AV heart block, cardiogenic shock, CHF, bronchospastic disease, hyperthyroidism, diabetes mellitus, WPW syndrome, history of heart failure, hepatic/renal function, hypersensitivity to drug, pregnancy/nursing status, and possible drug interactions.

Monitoring: Monitor for signs/symptoms of cardiac failure, hypoglycemia, decreased IOP, thyrotoxicosis, withdrawal symptoms, hypersensitivity reactions, and other adverse reactions. (Inj) Monitor ECG and central venous pressure during anesthesia. (Tab) For HTN, measure BP near end of dosing interval to determine satisfactory BP control.

Patient Counseling: Instruct not to interrupt or d/c therapy without consulting physician. Contact physician if symptoms of heart failure, withdrawal, or hypersensitivity reactions occur. May interfere with glaucoma screening test.

Administration: Oral and IV route. (Inj) Inspect visually for particulate matter/discoloration. **Storage:** 20-25°C (68-77°F). (Inj) Protect from freezing/excessive heat. (Tab) Dispense in tight, light-resistant container.

PROPYLTHIOURACIL   RX
propylthiouracil (Various)

> Severe liver injury and acute liver failure reported; some cases have been fatal or required liver transplantation. Reserve use only for those who cannot tolerate methimazole and in whom radioactive iodine therapy or surgery are not appropriate for the management of hyperthyroidism. Treatment of choice during or just prior to the 1st trimester of pregnancy due to risk of fetal abnormalities associated with methimazole.

THERAPEUTIC CLASS: Thiourea-derivative antithyroid agent

INDICATIONS: Patients with Grave's disease with hyperthyroidism or toxic multinodular goiter who are intolerant of methimazole and for whom surgery or radioactive iodine therapy is not an appropriate treatment option. To ameliorate symptoms of hyperthyroidism in preparation for thyroidectomy or radioactive iodine therapy in patients who are intolerant of methimazole.

DOSAGE: *Adults:* Initial: 300mg/day. Severe Hyperthyroidism/Very Large Goiters: Initial: 400mg/day; occassionally may require 600-900mg/day. Maint: 100-150mg/day. Give daily dose in 3 equal doses, q8h. Elderly: Start at lower end of dosing range.
Pediatrics: ≥6 yrs: Initial: 50mg/day in 3 equal doses, q8h. Titrate: Carefully increase based on clinical response and evaluation of TSH and free T4 levels.

HOW SUPPLIED: Tab: 50mg* *scored

WARNINGS/PRECAUTIONS: Not recommended for pediatric patients except when methimazole is not well-tolerated and surgery or radioactive iodine therapy are not appropriate. D/C if hepatic dysfunction, agranulocytosis, aplastic anemia, pancytopenia, anti-neutrophilic cytoplasmic antibodies (ANCA)-positive vasculitis, hepatitis, interstitial pneumonitis, fever or exfoliative dermatitis develops. May cause hypothyroidism; adjust dose to maintain euthyroid state. Fetal goiter and cretinism may occur when given during pregnancy. May cause hypoprothrombinemia and bleeding; monitor PT especially before surgery. Monitor thyroid function tests periodically.

ADVERSE REACTIONS: Agranulocytosis, liver injury, liver failure, thrombocytopenia, aplastic anemia, hepatitis, periarteritis, hypoprothrombinemia, skin rash, urticaria, N/V, epigastric distress, arthralgia, paresthesias.

INTERACTIONS: May increase activity of oral anticoagulants (eg, warfarin); consider additional monitoring of PT/INR. Hyperthyroidism may increase clearance of β-blockers; may need reduced β-blocker dose when patient becomes euthyroid. Digitalis glycoside levels may be increased when patient becomes euthyroid; may need to reduce digitalis dose. Theophylline clearance may decrease when patient becomes euthyroid; may need reduced theophylline dose. Caution with other drugs that cause agranulocytosis.

PREGNANCY: Category D, safety not known in nursing.

MECHANISM OF ACTION: Antithyroid agent; inhibits the synthesis of thyroid hormones and the conversion of thyroxine to triiodothyronine in peripheral tissues.

P

PHARMACOKINETICS: Absorption: Readily absorbed. **Distribution:** Found in breast milk, crosses placenta. **Metabolism:** Extensive. **Elimination:** Urine (35%).

NURSING CONSIDERATIONS

Assessment: Assess for previous hypersensitivity to the drug, hepatic impairment, pregnancy/nursing status, and possible drug interactions.

Monitoring: Monitor for signs/symptoms of hepatic dysfunction, agranulocytosis, leukopenia, thrombocytopenia, aplastic anemia, pancytopenia, ANCA-positive vasculitis, interstitial pneumonitis, fever, exfoliative dermatitis, and hypothyroidism. Monitor CBC with differential, PT, TSH, free T4 levels, AST, ALT, bilirubin, and alkaline phosphatase.

Patient Counseling: Instruct to inform physician if pregnant/nursing or planning to become pregnant. Advise to report signs/symptoms of illness (eg, fever, sore throat, skin eruptions, headache, general malaise) and hepatic dysfunction (anorexia, pruritus, upper quadrant pain, jaundice, light colored stools, dark urine). Inform about the risk of liver failure.

Administration: Oral route. **Storage:** 15-30°C (59-86°F).

PROQUAD   RX

varicella virus vaccine live - rubella vaccine live - measles vaccine live - mumps vaccine live
(Merck)

THERAPEUTIC CLASS: Vaccine

INDICATIONS: Active immunization for the prevention of measles, mumps, rubella, and varicella in children 12 months through 12 yrs of age.

DOSAGE: *Pediatrics:* 12 months-12 yrs: 0.5mL SQ (first dose usually at 12-15 months). If a second dose is needed, administer at 4-6 yrs of age.

HOW SUPPLIED: Inj: 0.5mL

CONTRAINDICATIONS: Concomitant administration with immunosuppressive therapy (including high-dose corticosteroids) or immunosuppressant drugs. History of hypersensitivity to gelatin, history of anaphylactoid reaction to neomycin, blood dyscrasias, leukemia, lymphomas of any type, or other malignant neoplasms affecting the bone marrow or lymphatic systems, primary and acquired immunodeficiency states, including AIDS or other clinical manifestations of infection with human immunodeficiency virus (HIV); cellular immune deficiencies; hypogammaglobulinemic and dysgammaglobulinemic states, family history of congenital or hereditary immunodeficiency, active untreated tuberculosis (TB) or active febrile illness with fever >101.3°F; pregnancy.

WARNINGS/PRECAUTIONS: Higher rates of fever and febrile seizures at 5-12 days after vaccination in children 12-23 months old who have not been previously vaccinated against measles, mumps, rubella, or varicella. Caution with history of cerebral injury, individual or family history of convulsions or any other condition in which stress due to fever should be avoided. Caution with history of anaphylactic/anaphylactoid reactions to egg ingestion; may increase risk of immediate-type hypersensitivity reactions. Neomycin allergy manifested as a contact dermatitis is not a contraindication. Caution in children with thrombocytopenia or in those who experienced thrombocytopenia after vaccination with previous dose of measles, mumps, rubella, and/or varicella vaccine. Contains albumin; remote risk for transmission of viral diseases. Vaccine recipients should attempt to avoid close association with high-risk individuals susceptible to varicella for ≤6 weeks following vaccination; refer to PI for information on high-risk individuals. Defer vaccination for ≥3 months following blood or plasma transfusions, or administration of immune globulins. Avoid pregnancy for 3 months following vaccination. May result in temporary depression of tuberculin skin sensitivity if given individually; administer test either any time before, simultaneously with, or ≥4-6 weeks after administration.

ADVERSE REACTIONS: Injection-site reactions (pain/tenderness/soreness, erythema, swelling), fever, irritability, measles-like rash, rubella-like rash, arthralgia, arthritis.

INTERACTIONS: See Contraindications. Avoid use of salicylates for 6 weeks after vaccination; Reye's syndrome reported. ≥1 month should elapse between a dose of measles-containing vaccine (eg, M-M-R II), and ≥3 months between a dose of varicella-containing vaccine.

PREGNANCY: Category C, not for use in nursing.

MECHANISM OF ACTION: Vaccine; stimulates immune system to elicit immune response to produce antibodies that may protect against measles, mumps, rubella, and varicella.

NURSING CONSIDERATIONS

Assessment: Assess for health status, immunization history, conditions where treatment is contraindicated or cautioned, and possible drug interactions. Assess for high-risk individuals susceptible to varicella.

Monitoring: Monitor for signs/symptoms of allergic reactions, fever, thrombocytopenia, Reye's syndrome, and injection-site reactions (eg, pain, tenderness, soreness, erythema, swelling, ecchymosis, rash).

Patient Counseling: Inform of potential benefits/risk associated with vaccination. Advise to avoid use of salicylates for 6 weeks after vaccination. Instruct post-pubertal females to postpone pregnancy for 3 months after vaccination. Inform that vaccination may not offer 100% protection. Instruct to report any adverse reactions to physician.

Administration: SQ route. Inspect for particulate matter and discoloration before administration. Inject SQ into the outer aspect of the deltoid region of the upper arm or into the higher anterolateral area of the thigh. Refer to PI for preparation/administration. **Storage:** Frozen between -50 to -15°C (-58 to +5°F) or refrigerate at 2-8°C (36-46°F) for up to 72 hrs prior to reconstitution. Discard if stored at 2-8°C and not used within 72 hrs of removal from 5°F (-15°C). Protect from light. Discard if reconstituted vaccine not used within 30 min and was stored at room temperature. Do not freeze reconstituted vaccine. Store diluent separately at 20-25°C (68-77°F), or at 2-8°C (36-46°F). Refer to PI for more storage information.

PROQUIN XR   RX

ciprofloxacin (Depomed)

Fluoroquinolones are associated with an increased risk of tendinitis and tendon rupture in all ages. Risk is further increased in patients >60 yrs, patients taking corticosteroids, and patients with kidney, heart, or lung transplants. May exacerbate muscle weakness with myasthenia gravis; avoid in patients with known history of myasthenia gravis.

THERAPEUTIC CLASS: Fluoroquinolone

INDICATIONS: Treatment of uncomplicated urinary tract infections (UTI) (acute cystitis) caused by *Escherichia coli* and *Klebsiella pneumoniae*.

DOSAGE: *Adults:* 500mg qd, preferably with pm meal, for 3 days.

HOW SUPPLIED: Tab, Extended-Release: 500mg

WARNINGS/PRECAUTIONS: D/C if experience pain, swelling, inflammation, or rupture of tendon. Convulsions, increased intracranial pressure (ICP), and toxic psychosis reported; d/c if CNS events (eg, dizziness, confusion, tremors, hallucinations, depression, or suicidal thoughts/acts) occur. Caution with CNS disorders or other risk factors that may predispose them to seizures or lower the seizure threshold. Severe and occasionally fatal hypersensitivity reactions reported; d/c immediately if signs of hypersensitivity appear. *Clostridium difficile*-associated diarrhea (CDAD) reported. May result in bacterial resistance with prolonged use or use in the absence of a proven/suspected bacterial infection or a prophylactic indication; take appropriate measures if superinfection develops. Rare cases of sensory or sensorimotor axonal polyneuropathy reported; d/c if symptoms of neuropathy occur. Crystalluria and cylindruria reported; maintain adequate hydration. Photosensitivity/phototoxicity reactions may occur; d/c if phototoxicity occurs. Not interchangeable with other ciprofloxacin extended-release or immediate-release formulations. Caution with risk factors for torsades de pointes (eg, known QT prolongation, uncorrected hypokalemia). Caution in elderly and with renal impairment.

ADVERSE REACTIONS: Fungal infection, nasopharyngitis, headache, micturition urgency.

INTERACTIONS: See Boxed Warning. Increased levels of and serious and fatal reactions reported with theophylline; monitor levels and adjust dose. Magnesium- or aluminum-containing antacids, sucralfate, didanosine chewable/buffered tablets or pediatric powder, and products containing calcium, iron, or zinc decrease absorption; administer ≥4 hrs before or 2 hrs after these drugs. May alter serum levels of phenytoin. Severe hypoglycemia with glyburide (rare). Increased levels with probenecid. Reduced clearance of caffeine. Transient SrCr elevations with cyclosporine. Enhances oral anticoagulant effects of warfarin or its derivatives; monitor PT or other coagulation tests. May increase risk of methotrexate toxic reactions due to inhibition of renal tubular transport. High-dose quinolones shown to provoke convulsions with NSAIDs (not aspirin). Caution with drugs that can result in prolongation of the QT interval (eg, class IA or III antiarrhythmics). Caution with concomitant use of drugs that may lower the seizure threshold. Avoid taking with milk products or calcium-fortified juices alone.

PREGNANCY: Category C, not for use in nursing.

MECHANISM OF ACTION: Fluoroquinolone; inhibits topoisomerase II (DNA gyrase) and topoisomerase IV (both type II topoisomerases), which are required for bacterial DNA replication, transcription, repair, and recombination.

PHARMACOKINETICS: Absorption: C_{max}=0.82mcg/mL; T_{max}=6.1 hrs; AUC=7.67mcg•hr/mL. **Distribution:** Plasma protein binding (9.9-36.6%). Found in breast milk. **Metabolism:** Desethylenecipfrofloxacin, sulfocipfrofloxacin, oxocipfrofloxacin, and formylcipfrofloxacin (metabolites). **Elimination:** Urine (26.9%, unchanged) (over 24 hrs), (41%) (over 96 hrs), feces (43%); $T_{1/2}$=4.5 hrs.

NURSING CONSIDERATIONS

Assessment: Assess for risk factors for developing tendinitis and tendon rupture, myasthenia gravis, drug hypersensitivity, renal function, risk factors for torsades de pointes, CNS disorders or factors that may predispose to seizures or lower seizure threshold, pregnancy/nursing status, and possible drug interactions.

Monitoring: Monitor for tendinitis or tendon rupture, convulsions, increased ICP, toxic psychosis, CNS events, CDAD, superinfections, peripheral neuropathy, photosensitivity reactions, and hypersensitivity reactions. Assess renal function.

Patient Counseling: Instruct to take exactly as directed; skipping doses or not completing full course may decrease effectiveness and increase bacterial resistance. Inform to notify physician if experience pain, swelling, or inflammation of a tendon, or weakness or inability to move joints; rest and refrain from exercise and d/c therapy. Instruct to d/c and notify physician if an allergic reaction, skin rash, watery and bloody stools, or symptoms of peripheral neuropathy. Notify physician if worsening muscle weakness or breathing problems, or sunburn-like reaction occurs, if pregnant/nursing, and of all current medications and supplements. Instruct to take with main meal of day, preferably with evening meal. Avoid concomitant use with dairy products or calcium-fortified juices alone and to avoid breastfeeding. Avoid exposure to natural or artificial sunlight. Instruct to see how they react to therapy before engaging in activities that require mental alertness or coordination.

Administration: Oral route. Swallow whole; do not split, crush, or chew. Administer ≥4 hrs before or 2 hrs after magnesium- or aluminum-containing antacids, sucralfate, didanosine chewable/buffered tab or pediatric powder, metal cations (eg, iron), multivitamins with zinc. **Storage:** 25°C (77°F); excursions permitted to 15-30°C (59-86°F).

PROSCAR   RX
finasteride (Merck)

THERAPEUTIC CLASS: Type II 5 alpha-reductase inhibitor

INDICATIONS: Treatment of symptomatic benign prostatic hyperplasia (BPH) in men with an enlarged prostate to improve symptoms, reduce risk of acute urinary retention, and reduce risk of the need for surgery, including transurethral resection of the prostate (TURP) and prostatectomy. To reduce risk of symptomatic progression of BPH (a confirmed ≥4 point increase in American Urological Association symptom score) in combination with doxazosin.

DOSAGE: *Adults:* 5mg qd, monotherapy or in combination with doxazosin.

HOW SUPPLIED: Tab: 5mg

CONTRAINDICATIONS: Pregnancy.

WARNINGS/PRECAUTIONS: Not approved for the prevention of prostate cancer. Not for use in pediatrics or women. Pregnant women or women who may potentially be pregnant should not handle crushed or broken tabs because of potential risk to a male fetus. Perform appropriate evaluation to identify other conditions that might mimic BPH (eg, infection, prostate cancer, stricture disease, hypotonic bladder, or other neurogenic disorders). Patients with large residual urinary volume and/or severely diminished urinary flow may not be candidates for therapy; monitor for obstructive uropathy. Caution with liver dysfunction. May decrease serum prostate specific antigen (PSA) levels in patients with BPH or prostate cancer; any confirmed increase should be carefully evaluated. May increase the risk of development of high-grade prostate cancer.

ADVERSE REACTIONS: Impotence, decreased libido, decreased ejaculate volume, asthenia, postural hypotension, dizziness, abnormal ejaculation.

PREGNANCY: Category X, not for use in nursing.

MECHANISM OF ACTION: Type II 5α-reductase inhibitor; competitively inhibits type II 5α-reductase with which it forms a stable enzyme complex inhibiting metabolism of testosterone to 5α-dihydrotestosterone.

PHARMACOKINETICS: Absorption: Mean bioavailability (63%); C_{max}=37ng/mL; T_{max}=1-2 hrs. Refer to PI for different pharmacokinetic parameters of different age groups. **Distribution:** V_d=76L; plasma protein binding (90%). **Metabolism:** Liver (extensive) via CYP3A4. **Elimination:** (Oral) Urine (39% metabolites), feces (57%); $T_{1/2}$=6 hrs (45-60 yrs), 8 hrs (≥70 yrs).

NURSING CONSIDERATIONS

Assessment: Assess for hypersensitivity to drug and its components, conditions which may mimic BPH and for liver function abnormalities. Assess for patients with large residual urinary volume and/or severely diminished urinary flow. Obtain baseline PSA levels.

Monitoring: Monitor for obstructive uropathy in patients with large residual urinary volume and/or severely diminished urinary flow. Monitor for hypersensitivity reactions and other adverse reactions. Monitor PSA levels.

Patient Counseling: Inform that there was an increase in high-grade prostate cancer in men treated with 5α-reductase inhibitors indicated for BPH treatment. Instruct pregnant or potentially pregnant females not to handle crushed or broken tabs due to potential risk to male fetus. Inform males that the volume of ejaculate may decrease and impotence/decreased libido may occur. Advise to notify physician if changes in breast (eg, lumps, pain, nipple discharge) occurs.

Administration: Oral route. **Storage:** <30°C (86°F).

PROTAMINE SULFATE   RX
protamine sulfate (Various)

> May cause severe hypotension, cardiovascular (CV) collapse, noncardiogenic pulmonary edema, catastrophic pulmonary vasoconstriction, and pulmonary HTN; risk factors include high dose/overdose, rapid/previous administration, repeated doses, and current/previous use of protamine-containing drugs. Risk to benefit of administration should be carefully considered with presence of any risk factors. Should not be given when bleeding occurs without prior heparin use.

THERAPEUTIC CLASS: Heparin antagonist

INDICATIONS: Management of heparin overdose.

DOSAGE: *Adults:* Administer as very slow IV infusion over 10 min in doses not to exceed 50mg. Determine dose by blood coagulation studies. Each mg neutralizes not less than 100 USP heparin units.

HOW SUPPLIED: Inj: 10mg/mL [5mL, 25mL]

WARNINGS/PRECAUTIONS: May cause allergic reactions with fish hypersensitivity. Rapid administration may cause severe hypotensive and anaphylactoid-like reactions. Caution in cardiac surgeries; hyperheparinemia or bleeding reported. Previous exposure to protamine/protamine-containing insulin may induce humoral immune response; severe hypersensitivity reaction, including life-threatening anaphylaxis reported. Increased risk of antiprotamine antibodies in infertile or vasectomized men.

ADVERSE REACTIONS: Hypotension, bradycardia, transitory flushing/feeling of warmth, lassitude, dyspnea, N/V, back pain, anaphylaxis that causes severe respiratory distress, circulatory collapse, noncardiogenic pulmonary edema, acute pulmonary HTN.

INTERACTIONS: Incompatible with certain antibiotics, such as cephalosporins and penicillins. Concomitant or previous use of protamine-containing drugs (eg, NPH insulin, protamine zinc insulin, certain beta-blockers) is risk factor for severe adverse events; see Boxed Warning.

PREGNANCY: Category C, caution in nursing.

MECHANISM OF ACTION: Heparin antagonist; has anticoagulant effects when administered alone, however, when given in presence of heparin, a stable salt is formed and anticoagulant activity of both drugs is lost.

NURSING CONSIDERATIONS

Assessment: Assess for fish allergy, previous vasectomy, previous exposure, severe left ventricular dysfunction, abnormal preoperative pulmonary hemodynamics, and possible drug interactions. Assess blood coagulation studies for appropriate dosage.

Monitoring: Monitor for hypersensitivity/allergic reactions, hypotension, CV collapse, pulmonary edema, and pulmonary HTN. Monitor blood coagulation studies.

Administration: Slow IV infusion. Large-size 25mL vials are designed for antiheparin treatment only when large doses of heparin have been given during surgery. **Storage:** 20-25°C (68-77°F). Do not freeze.

PROTONIX   RX
pantoprazole sodium (Wyeth)

OTHER BRAND NAMES: Protonix IV (Wyeth)

THERAPEUTIC CLASS: Proton pump inhibitor

INDICATIONS: (Tab/Sus) Short-term treatment (≤8 weeks) in the healing and symptomatic relief of erosive esophagitis (EE) associated with gastroesophageal reflux disease (GERD) in adults and pediatrics ≥5 yrs. Maintenance of healing of EE and reduction in relapse rates of daytime and nighttime heartburn symptoms in adults with GERD. Long-term treatment of pathological hypersecretory conditions, including Zollinger-Ellison syndrome. (IV) Short-term treatment (7-10 days) of adults with GERD and history of EE. Treatment of pathological hypersecretory conditions, including Zollinger-Ellison syndrome in adults.

DOSAGE: *Adults:* (Tab/Sus) Short-Term Treatment of EE Associated with GERD: 40mg qd for ≤8 weeks. May consider additional 8-week course if no healing after 8 weeks of treatment.

P

Maintenance of Healing of EE: 40mg qd. Pathological Hypersecretory Conditions Including Zollinger-Ellison Syndrome: Initial: 40mg bid. Adjust to patient's needs and continue for as long as clinically indicated. Max: 240mg/day. If unable to swallow 40mg tab, give two 20mg tabs. (IV) GERD Associated with History of EE: 40mg qd IV infusion for 7-10 days. D/C as soon as the patient is able to receive treatment with tab/sus. Pathological Hypersecretion Including Zollinger-Ellison Syndrome: Individualize dose. Usual: 80mg q12h IV infusion. May adjust frequency based on acid output; may increase to 80mg q8h if higher dosage is needed. Max: 240mg/day. Duration >6 days not studied.

Pediatrics: ≥5 yrs: (Tab/Sus) Short-Term Treatment of EE Associated with GERD: ≥15kg-<40kg: 20mg qd for ≤8 weeks. ≥40kg: 40mg qd for ≤8 weeks. If unable to swallow 40mg tab, give two 20mg tabs. Do not divide 40mg pkt to create 20mg dosage for pediatrics unable to take tab.

HOW SUPPLIED: Inj: 40mg; Sus, Delayed-Release: 40mg (granules/pkt); Tab, Delayed-Release: 20mg, 40mg

WARNINGS/PRECAUTIONS: Symptomatic response does not preclude the presence of gastric malignancy. May increase risk of osteoporosis-related fractures of hip, wrist, or spine with high-dose (multiple daily doses) and long-term therapy (a year or longer); use lowest dose and shortest duration appropriate to the condition being treated. Hypomagnesemia reported; magnesium replacement and d/c of therapy may be required. Consider monitoring magnesium levels prior to and periodically during therapy for patients expected to be on prolonged treatment. Anaphylaxis and other serious reactions (eg, erythema multiforme, Stevens-Johnson syndrome, toxic epidermal necrolysis) reported. (Tab/Sus) Atrophic gastritis noted with long-term therapy particularly in patients who were *Helicobacter pylori* positive. Vitamin B12 deficiency caused by hypo- or achlorhydria possible with long-term use (>3 yrs). (IV) Thrombophlebitis reported. Consider zinc supplementation in patients prone to zinc deficiency. Mild, transient transaminase elevations observed in clinical studies.

ADVERSE REACTIONS: Headache, diarrhea, N/V, abdominal pain, flatulence, dizziness, arthralgia, rash. (Tab/Sus) Fever, upper respiratory infection.

INTERACTIONS: May substantially decrease plasma levels of atazanavir or nelfinavir; concomitant use not recommended. Monitor for increases in INR and PT with warfarin. May interfere with the absorption of drugs where gastric pH is an important determinant of bioavailability (eg, ketoconazole, ampicillin esters, iron salts, digoxin). Caution with digoxin or other drugs that may cause hypomagnesemia (eg, diuretics). May decrease mean area under the curve (AUC) of active metabolite of clopidogrel. (IV) Caution with other EDTA-containing products.

PREGNANCY: Category B, not for use in nursing.

MECHANISM OF ACTION: Proton pump inhibitor; suppresses final step in gastric acid production by covalently binding to the (H^+, K^+)-ATPase enzyme system at the secretory surface of gastric parietal cell.

PHARMACOKINETICS: Absorption: (Tab) Absolute bioavailability (77%). (40mg) C_{max}=2.5µg/mL; T_{max}=2.5 hrs; AUC=4.8µg•hr/mL. (40mg IV) C_{max}=5.52µg/mL; AUC=5.4µg•hr/mL. **Distribution:** V_d=11.0-23.6L; plasma protein binding (98%); (PO) found in breast milk. **Metabolism:** Liver (extensive) via demethylation, by CYP2C19, with subsequent sulfation; oxidation by CYP3A4. **Elimination:** Urine (71%), feces (18%); $T_{1/2}$=1 hr.

NURSING CONSIDERATIONS

Assessment: Assess for gastric malignancy, osteoporosis, hypersensitivity, pregnancy/nursing status, and possible drug interactions. Assess magnesium levels in patients expected to be on prolonged treatment. (IV) Assess for zinc deficiency.

Monitoring: Monitor for signs/symptoms of bone fractures, hypomagnesemia, hypersensitivity reactions, and other adverse reactions. Monitor magnesium levels periodically in patients expected to be on prolonged treatment. (Tab/Sus) Monitor for signs/symptoms of atrophic gastritis, vitamin B12 deficiency, and GI tumors. (IV) Monitor for acid output measurements, anaphylaxis and other serious reactions, thrombophlebitis, zinc deficiency, transaminase elevations, and other adverse reactions.

Patient Counseling: (IV) Inform of the most frequently occurring adverse reactions. Instruct to inform physician if any unusual symptom develops, or if any known symptom persists or worsens. Instruct to inform healthcare provider of any other medications currently taking, including over-the-counter medications, as well as allergies to any medications. (Tab/Sus) Advise not to split, crush, or chew. Advise to immediately report and seek care for any cardiovascular or neurological symptoms, including palpitation, dizziness, seizures, and tetany as these may be signs of hypomagnesemia. (Tab) Instruct to swallow whole, with or without food in stomach. Counsel that concomitant administration of antacids does not affect absorption. (Sus) Instruct to administer in apple juice or applesauce approximately 30 min ac; do not place in water, other liquids, or foods. Advise not to divide PO sus pkt to make smaller dose.

Administration: Oral and IV route. (Tab) Swallow whole, with or without food. (Sus) May also be administered via NG/gastrostomy tube. Do not administer in liquids other than apple juice or foods other than applesauce. Refer to PI for administration instructions. (IV) Flush IV lines prior to and after administration with 5% Dextrose Inj, USP, 0.9% NaCl Inj, USP, or Lactated Ringer's Inj, USP. May be administered over a period of ≥2 min or 15 min (7mL/min) infusion. Refer to PI for reconstitution and administration instructions. **Storage:** 20-25°C (68-77°F); excursions permitted to 15-30°C (59-86°F). (IV) Protect from light. Refer to PI for reconstituted and admixed sol storage information.

PROTOPIC RX
tacrolimus (Astellas)

> Rare cases of malignancy (eg, skin and lymphoma) reported with topical calcineurin inhibitors, including tacrolimus oint, although causal relationship has not been established. Avoid long-term use, and application should be limited to areas of involvement with atopic dermatitis. Not indicated for children <2 yrs; only 0.03% oint is indicated for children 2-15 yrs.

THERAPEUTIC CLASS: Macrolide immunosuppressant

INDICATIONS: Second-line therapy for short-term and noncontinuous chronic treatment of moderate to severe atopic dermatitis in non-immunocompromised adults and children who have failed to respond adequately to other topical prescription treatments for atopic dermatitis, or when those treatments are not advisable.

DOSAGE: *Adults:* (0.03% or 0.1%) Apply thin layer to the affected skin bid until signs and symptoms resolve. Reexamine patient if signs and symptoms do not improve within 6 weeks. *Pediatrics:* 2-15 yrs: (0.03%) Apply thin layer to the affected skin bid until signs and symptoms resolve. Reexamine patient if signs and symptoms do not improve within 6 weeks.

HOW SUPPLIED: Oint: 0.03%, 0.1% [30g, 60g, 100g]

WARNINGS/PRECAUTIONS: Long-term safety, beyond 1 yr of noncontinuous use, has not been established. Avoid with premalignant and malignant skin conditions. Not recommended for oral application, or in patients having skin conditions with a skin barrier defect where there is potential for increased systemic absorption (eg, Netherton's syndrome, lamellar ichthyosis, generalized erythroderma, cutaneous graft versus host disease). May cause local symptoms, such as skin burning (burning sensation, stinging, soreness) or pruritus and may improve as the lesions of atopic dermatitis resolve. Resolve bacterial or viral infections at treatment sites before starting treatment. Increased risk of varicella zoster (chickenpox or shingles) and herpes simplex virus (HSV) infection, or eczema herpeticum. Lymphadenopathy reported; d/c if etiology of lymphadenopathy is unknown, or in the presence of acute infectious mononucleosis. Minimize or avoid natural or artificial sunlight exposure during treatment. Rare cases of acute renal failure reported; caution in patients predisposed to renal impairment. Not for ophthalmic use. Do not use with occlusive dressings.

ADVERSE REACTIONS: Skin burning, pruritus, flu-like symptoms, allergic reaction, skin erythema, headache, skin infection, fever, herpes simplex, rhinitis, increased cough, asthma, pharyngitis, pustular rash, folliculitis.

INTERACTIONS: Caution with CYP3A4 inhibitors (eg, erythromycin, itraconazole, ketoconazole, fluconazole, calcium channel blockers, cimetidine) in patients with widespread and/or erythrodermic disease.

PREGNANCY: Category C, not for use in nursing.

MECHANISM OF ACTION: Macrolide immunosuppressant; not established in atopic dermatitis. Inhibits T-lymphocyte activation by 1st binding to an intracellular protein, FKBP-12. A complex of tacrolimus-FKBP-12, calcium, calmodulin, and calcineurin is then formed and the phosphatase activity of calcineurin is inhibited. This has been shown to prevent the dephosphorylation and translocation of nuclear factor of activated T-cells (NF-AT), a nuclear component thought to initiate gene transcription for the formation of lymphokines.

PHARMACOKINETICS: Absorption: Absolute bioavailability (0.5%), C_{max}=<2ng/mL. **Distribution:** Plasma protein binding (99%); crosses placenta; found in breast milk. **Metabolism:** Extensive via CYP3A; demethylation and hydroxylation; 13-demethyl tacrolimus (major metabolite).

NURSING CONSIDERATIONS

Assessment: Assess for history of hypersensitivity to drug, premalignant/malignant skin conditions, conditions where there is potential for increased systemic absorption, bacterial or viral infections at treatment sites, renal impairment, pregnancy/nursing status, and possible drug interactions.

Monitoring: Monitor for skin malignancy, lymphoma, infections (eg, varicella zoster virus, HSV, eczema herpeticum), local symptoms, lymphadenopathy, and acute renal failure. Monitor improvement of signs/symptoms of atopic dermatitis within 6 weeks.

Patient Counseling: Instruct to use drug exactly as prescribed, only on areas of skin that have eczema, and not to use continuously for prolonged period. Advise to d/c medication when signs/symptoms of eczema (eg, itching, rash, redness) subside. Instruct to consult physician if symptoms get worse, a skin infection develops, or if symptoms do not improve after 6 weeks. Advise caregivers applying the oint or patients not treating their hands, to wash hands with soap and water after application. Counsel not to bathe, shower, or swim right after application. Advise to avoid getting oint in the eyes or mouth. Instruct to avoid artificial sunlight exposure during treatment, limit sun exposure, wear loose-fitting clothing that protects treated area from the sun, and not to cover treated skin with bandages, dressings, or wraps.

Administration: Topical route. Rub in the minimum amount of oint gently and completely.
Storage: 25°C (77°F); excursions permitted to 15-30°C (59-86°F).

PROVENGE   RX
sipuleucel-T (Dendreon)

THERAPEUTIC CLASS: Immunomodulatory agent

INDICATIONS: Treatment of asymptomatic or minimally symptomatic metastatic castrate resistant (hormone refractory) prostate cancer.

DOSAGE: *Adults:* Usual: 3 complete doses (250mL each) given at approximately 2-week intervals via IV infusion over 60 min. If unable to give scheduled infusion, additional leukapheresis is needed. Premedication: PO acetaminophen and antihistamine (eg, diphenhydramine) 30 min prior to administration.

HOW SUPPLIED: Sus: 250mL

WARNINGS/PRECAUTIONS: For autologous use only. Acute infusion reactions reported; infusion rate may be decreased or stopped depending on severity of reaction and administer appropriate medical therapy PRN. Monitor closely with cardiac or pulmonary conditions. May transmit infectious diseases to health care professionals handling the product; employ universal precautions. Do not infuse until confirmation of product release has been received.

ADVERSE REACTIONS: Chills, fatigue, fever, back pain, N/V, joint ache, headache, paresthesia, anemia, constipation, infusion reactions, citrate toxicity, pain, dizziness.

INTERACTIONS: Immunosuppressive agents may alter efficacy and/or safety; evaluate patients whether it is appropriate to reduce or d/c immunosuppressive agents prior to treatment.

PREGNANCY: Safety in pregnancy and nursing not known.

MECHANISM OF ACTION: Immunomodulatory agent (autologous cellular immunotherapy); not established. Induces an immune response targeted against prostatic acid phosphatase, an antigen expressed in most prostate cancer.

NURSING CONSIDERATIONS

Assessment: Assess for history of cardiac or pulmonary conditions, and possible drug interactions.

Monitoring: Monitor for signs and symptoms of infusion reactions especially with cardiac or pulmonary conditions. Monitor for infectious sequelae in patients with central venous catheters.

Patient Counseling: Counsel on adhering to preparation instructions for leukapheresis procedure, possible side effects, and post-procedure care. Advise to report signs and symptoms of acute infusion reactions (eg, fever, chills, fatigue, breathing problems, dizziness, high blood pressure, N/V, headache or muscle aches) and symptoms suggestive of cardiac arrhythmia. Notify physician if taking immunosuppressive agents. Inform of the need for a central venous catheter placement if peripheral venous access is not adequate and counsel on the importance of catheter care; advise to inform physician if fever or any swelling or redness around the catheter site occurs. Inform of the need to undergo an additional leukapheresis if a scheduled dose is missed.

Administration: IV route. Begin infusion prior to expiration date and time; do not infuse expired product. Do not use a cell filter. Infuse IV over 60 min; observe patient for at least 30 min after each infusion. Refer to PI for modification for infusion reactions and preparation instructions.
Storage: Infusion bag must remain within the insulated polyurethane container until the time of administration; stable for ≤3 hrs at room temperature once removed. Do not remove from the outer cardboard shipping box. Refer to PI for complete handling instructions.

PROVERA   RX
medroxyprogesterone acetate (Pharmacia & Upjohn)

> Should not be used for the prevention of cardiovascular disease (CVD) or dementia. Increased risks of myocardial infarction (MI), stroke, invasive breast cancer, pulmonary embolism (PE), and deep vein thrombosis (DVT) in postmenopausal women (50-79 yrs) reported. Increased risk of developing probable dementia in postmenopausal women ≥65 yrs of age reported. Should be prescribed at the lowest effective dose and for the shortest duration consistent with treatment goals and risks.

THERAPEUTIC CLASS: Progestogen

INDICATIONS: Treatment of secondary amenorrhea and abnormal uterine bleeding due to hormonal imbalance in the absence of organic pathology, such as fibroids or uterine cancer. Reduce incidence of endometrial hyperplasia in non-hysterectomized postmenopausal women receiving daily oral 0.625mg conjugated estrogen.

DOSAGE: *Adults:* Secondary Amenorrhea: 5 or 10mg/day for 5-10 days; 10mg/day for 10 days, beginning at anytime, is used to induce optimum secretory transformation of primed endometrium. Abnormal Uterine Bleeding: 5 or 10mg/day for 5-10 days beginning on Day 16 or 21 of cycle; 10mg/day for 10 days, beginning on Day 16 of the cycle is recommended to produce an optimum secretory transformation of primed endometrium. Endometrial Hyperplasia: 5 or 10mg/day for 12-14 consecutive days per month beginning on Day 1 or 16 of cycle.

HOW SUPPLIED: Tab: 2.5mg*, 5mg*, 10mg* *scored

CONTRAINDICATIONS: Undiagnosed abnormal genital bleeding, known/suspected/history of breast cancer, known/suspected estrogen- or progesterone-dependent neoplasia, active or history of DVT/PE, active or recent arterial thromboembolic disease (eg, stroke, MI), known liver dysfunction or disease, missed abortion, known/suspected pregnancy, as a diagnostic test for pregnancy.

WARNINGS/PRECAUTIONS: Increased risk of cardiovascular events. Caution in patients with risk factors for arterial vascular disease (eg, HTN, diabetes mellitus, tobacco use, hypercholesterolemia, obesity) and/or venous thromboembolism (eg, personal history or family history of venous thromboembolism, obesity, systemic lupus erythematosus [SLE]). Unopposed estrogen in women with a uterus has been associated with increased risk of endometrial cancer. May increase risk of ovarian cancer. If visual abnormalities or migraine occurs, d/c pending examination. If examination reveals papilledema or retinal vascular lesions, d/c permanently. Consider addition of a progestin if no hysterectomy. In cases of undiagnosed abnormal vaginal bleeding, perform adequate diagnostic measures. Withdrawal bleeding may occur within 3-7 days after d/c therapy. May elevate BP. May increase plasma TG leading to pancreatitis and other complications with pre-existing hypertriglyceridemia. Caution with history of cholestatic jaundice; d/c in case of recurrence. May cause fluid retention; caution with cardiac/renal dysfunction. Caution with severe hypocalcemia. May exacerbate asthma, DM, epilepsy, migraine, porphyria, SLE, and hepatic hemangiomas; use with caution. May affect certain endocrine, LFTs, and blood components in laboratory tests.

ADVERSE REACTIONS: Abnormal uterine bleeding, breast tenderness, galactorrhea, urticaria, pruritus, edema, rash, menstrual changes, change in weight, mental depression, insomnia, somnolence, dizziness, headache, nausea.

INTERACTIONS: Patients on thyroid replacement therapy may require higher doses of thyroid hormone.

PREGNANCY: Category X, not for use in nursing.

MECHANISM OF ACTION: Progestogen; transforms proliferative endometrium into secretory endometrium.

PHARMACOKINETICS: Absorption: Rapid. Administration of different doses resulted in different pharmacokinetic parameters; refer to PI. **Distribution:** Plasma protein binding (90%); found in breast milk. **Metabolism:** Extensive (hepatic) via hydroxylation with subsequent conjugation. **Elimination:** Urine.

NURSING CONSIDERATIONS

Assessment: Assess for abnormal genital bleeding, presence or history of breast cancer, estrogen/progesterone-dependent neoplasias, DVT, PE, active or recent (within past yr) arterial thromboembolic disease, and any other conditions where treatment may be contraindicated or cautioned, and for possible drug interactions.

Monitoring: Monitor for signs/symptoms of CVD, malignant neoplasms, visual abnormalities, hypertriglyceridemia, fluid retention, exacerbation of asthma, hypersensitivity reactions, and other conditions. Perform annual mammography, regular monitoring of BP, and periodic evaluation (q3-6 months) to determine need of therapy. Monitor thyroid function in patients on thyroid replacement therapy. In cases of undiagnosed, persistent, or recurrent vaginal bleeding in women with uterus, perform adequate diagnostic measures (eg, endometrial sampling) to rule out malignancies.

Patient Counseling: Counsel about risk of birth defects if exposed to drug. Inform that drug may increase risk for breast cancer, uterine cancer, stroke, heart attack, blood clots, and dementia. Instruct to report breast lumps, unusual vaginal bleeding, dizziness/faintness, changes in speech, severe headaches, chest pain, SOB, leg pain, visual changes, or vomiting. Instruct to have an annual pelvic exam, breast exam, and mammogram. Advise to perform monthly self breast exams.

Administration: Oral route. **Storage:** 20-25°C (68-77°F).

P

PROVIGIL
modafinil (Cephalon)

THERAPEUTIC CLASS: Wakefulness-promoting agent

INDICATIONS: To improve wakefulness in patients with excessive sleepiness associated with narcolepsy, obstructive sleep apnea (OSA), shift work disorder (SWD). As adjunct to standard treatment for underlying obstruction in OSA.

DOSAGE: *Adults:* ≥17 yrs: 200mg qd. Max: 400mg/day as single dose. Narcolepsy/OSA: Take as single dose in am. SWD: Take 1 hr prior to start of work shift. Severe Hepatic Impairment: 100mg qd. Elderly: Consider dose reduction.

HOW SUPPLIED: Tab: 100mg, 200mg* *scored

WARNINGS/PRECAUTIONS: Rare cases of severe or life-threatening rash, including Stevens-Johnson syndrome (SJS), toxic epidermal necrolysis (TEN), and drug rash with eosinophilia and systemic symptoms (DRESS) reported; d/c treatment at first sign of rash. Angioedema, anaphylactoid reactions, multi-organ hypersensitivity and psychiatric adverse experiences reported; d/c treatment if symptoms develop. Caution with a history of psychosis, depression or mania. Caution with recent myocardial infarction (MI) or unstable angina. Avoid in patients with history of left ventricular hypertrophy or with mitral valve prolapse who have experienced mitral valve prolapse syndrome (eg, ischemic ECG changes, chest pain, arrhythmia) with CNS stimulants. May impair mental/physical abilities. Reduce dose with severe hepatic impairment. Use low dose in elderly. Doses up to 400mg/day have been well tolerated but there is no evidence that this dose confers additional benefit.

ADVERSE REACTIONS: Headache, nausea, nervousness, anxiety, insomnia, rhinitis, diarrhea, back pain, dizziness, dyspepsia, flu syndrome, dry mouth, anorexia, pharyngitis.

INTERACTIONS: Methylphenidate and dextroamphetamine may delay absorption. May reduce efficacy of steroidal contraceptives up to 1 month after d/c. Caution with MAOIs. CYP3A4 inducers (eg, carbamazepine, phenobarbital, rifampin) may decrease levels. CYP3A4 inhibitors (eg, ketoconazole, itraconazole) may increase levels. May increase levels of drugs metabolized by CYP2C19 (eg, diazepam, propranolol, phenytoin) or CYP2C9 (eg, warfarin). Monitor for toxicity with CYP2C19 substrates and PT/INR with warfarin. May increase levels of certain TCAs (eg, clomipramine, desipramine) and SSRIs in CYP2D6 deficient patients. May decrease levels of drugs metabolized by CYP3A4 (eg, cyclosporine, ethinyl estradiol, triazolam). May induce CYP1A2 and CYP2B6; caution with CYP1A2 and CYP2B6 substrates.

PREGNANCY: Category C, caution in nursing.

MECHANISM OF ACTION: Wakefulness promoting agent; not established. Binds to dopamine transporter, inhibits dopamine reuptake, and results in increased extracellular dopamine levels in some brain regions.

PHARMACOKINETICS: Absorption: Rapid. T_{max}=2-4 hrs, delayed by 1 hr (fed). **Distribution:** V_d=0.9L/kg; plasma protein binding (60%). **Metabolism:** Liver via hydrolytic deamination, S-oxidation, aromatic ring hydroxylation, and glucuronide conjugation; CYP3A4. **Elimination:** Feces (1%), urine (80%, <10% parent compound); $T_{1/2}$=15 hrs.

NURSING CONSIDERATIONS

Assessment: Assess for hypersensitivity, hepatic impairment, pregnancy/nursing status, possible drug interactions, and a history of psychosis, depression, mania, left ventricular hypertrophy, or mitral valve prolapse. Assess for a recent history of MI or unstable angina. Use only in patients who have had complete evaluation of their excessive sleepiness, and in whom a diagnosis of either narcolepsy, OSA, and/or SWD has been made.

Monitoring: Monitor for serious rash, SJS, TEN, DRESS, angioedema, hypersensitivity, multi-organ hypersensitivity reactions, psychiatric adverse symptoms, and other adverse reactions. Monitor BP. If used adjunctively with continuous positive airway pressure (CPAP), monitor for CPAP compliance. Periodically re-evaluate long-term usefulness if prescribed for an extended time.

Patient Counseling: Advise that this is not a replacement for sleep. Inform that drug may improve but does not eliminate sleepiness. Avoid taking alcohol during therapy. Caution against hazardous tasks (eg, driving, operating machinery) or performing other activities that require mental alertness. Notify physician if pregnant or intend to become pregnant or if nursing during therapy. Caution about increased risk of pregnancy when using steroidal contraceptives and for 1 month after d/c therapy. Inform physician if taking or planning to take any prescribed or OTC drugs. Contact physician if chest pain, rash, depression, anxiety, or signs of psychosis or mania develop. Inform of importance of continuing previously prescribed treatments. D/C and notify physician if rash, hives, mouth sores, blisters, peeling skin, trouble swallowing or breathing or other allergic reactions develop.

Administration: Oral route. **Storage:** 20-25°C (68-77°F).

PROZAC
fluoxetine HCl (Lilly)

RX

Antidepressants increased the risk of suicidal thinking and behavior (suicidality) in short-term studies in children, adolescents, and young adults with major depressive disorder (MDD) and other psychiatric disorders. Monitor and observe closely for clinical worsening, suicidality, or unusual changes in behavior in patients who started on antidepressant therapy. Approved for use in pediatric patients with MDD and obsessive compulsive disorder (OCD).

THERAPEUTIC CLASS: Selective serotonin reuptake inhibitor

INDICATIONS: Acute and maintenance treatment of MDD in patients ≥8 yrs. Acute and maintenance treatment of OCD in patients ≥7 yrs, binge-eating and vomiting behaviors in adults with moderate to severe bulimia nervosa, and acute treatment of panic disorder with or without agoraphobia in adults. Acute treatment of depressive episodes associated with bipolar I disorder, and treatment-resistant depression (MDD patients who failed to respond to 2 separate trials of different antidepressants) in adults in combination with olanzapine.

DOSAGE: *Adults:* MDD: Initial: 20mg/day qam. Titrate: May increase after several weeks if improvement is insufficient. Doses >20mg/day may be given qd (am) or bid (am and noon). Max: 80mg/day. (Cap, Delayed-Release) 1 cap/week starting 7 days after the last daily dose of 20mg cap. Consider reestablishing a daily dosing regimen if satisfactory response is not maintained. OCD: Initial: 20mg/day qam. Titrate: May increase after several weeks if improvement is insufficient. Doses >20mg/day may be given qd (am) or bid (am and noon). Usual: 20-60mg/day. Max: 80mg/day. Bulimia Nervosa: 60mg/day qam. May titrate up to this target dose over several days. Max: 60mg/day. Panic Disorder: Initial: 10mg/day. Titrate: Increase to 20mg/day after 1 week. May consider additional dose increase after several weeks if no clinical improvement. Max: 60mg/day. Depressive Episodes Associated with Bipolar I Disorder/Treatment-Resistant Depression: Initial: 20mg + 5mg olanzapine qpm. Titrate: Adjust dose based on efficacy and tolerability. Usual: 20-50mg + 5-12.5mg olanzapine (depressive episodes associated with bipolar I disorder) or 5-20mg olanzapine (treatment-resistant depression). Max: 75mg + 18mg olanzapine. Predisposed to Hypotensive Reactions/Hepatic Impairment/With Factors That Slow Metabolism of Olanzapine or Fluoxetine in Combination/Sensitive to Olanzapine: Initial: 20mg + 2.5-5mg olanzapine. Titrate: If indicated, increase dose cautiously. Hepatic Impairment (Cirrhosis)/Elderly: Use lower or less frequent dosage. Third Trimester Pregnancy: Taper dose. Periodically reassess need for continued treatment.
Pediatrics: MDD: ≥8 yrs: Initial: 10 or 20mg/day. Titrate: Increase to 20mg/day after 1 week at 10mg/day. Lower Weight Children: Initial/Target: 10mg/day. Titrate: May increase to 20mg/day after several weeks if improvement is insufficient. OCD: ≥7 yrs: Adolescents and Higher Weight Children: Initial: 10mg/day. Titrate: Increase to 20mg/day after 2 weeks. May consider additional dose increases after several more weeks if improvement is insufficient. Usual: 20-60mg/day. Lower Weight Children: Initial: 10mg/day. Titrate: May consider additional dose increases after several more weeks if improvement is insufficient. Usual: 20-30mg/day. Max: 60mg/day. Periodically reassess need for continued treatment.

HOW SUPPLIED: Cap: 10mg, 20mg, 40mg; Cap, Delayed-Release (Prozac Weekly): 90mg

CONTRAINDICATIONS: During or within 14 days of d/c MAOI therapy, use of thioridazine during or within 5 weeks of d/c fluoxetine, concomitant pimozide use.

WARNINGS/PRECAUTIONS: Avoid abrupt withdrawal; taper dose to minimize the risk of d/c symptoms (eg, dysphoric mood, irritability, agitation, dizziness, sensory disturbances). Serotonin syndrome or neuroleptic malignant syndrome (NMS)-like reactions reported; d/c therapy and initiate supportive symptomatic treatment. Convulsions, rash and/or urticaria, anorexia and weight loss, mania/hypomania, anxiety, insomnia, nervousness, mydriasis reported. Hyponatremia reported; elderly, patients taking diuretics or who are volume-depleted are at greater risk. May increase risk of bleeding reactions. D/C if unexplained allergic reaction (eg, rash), or symptomatic hyponatremia occurs. May alter glycemic control in patients with diabetes. Caution with diseases/conditions that could affect hemodynamic responses or metabolism, increased intraocular pressure (IOP) or risk for acute narrow-angle glaucoma, history of seizures, hepatic impairment, and in elderly. May impair mental/physical abilities. May precipitate mixed/manic episode in patients at risk for bipolar disorder. Not indicated for the treatment of depressive episodes associated with bipolar I disorder, and treatment-resistant depression as monotherapy.

ADVERSE REACTIONS: Somnolence, anorexia, anxiety, asthenia, diarrhea, dry mouth, dyspepsia, headache, insomnia, abnormal dreams, impotence, flu syndrome, constipation, nausea, nervousness.

INTERACTIONS: See Contraindications. Caution with CNS active drugs, drugs that may affect serotonergic neurotransmitter systems (eg, triptans, linezolid, tramadol, lithium, St. John's wort), and drugs metabolized by CYP2D6, including certain antidepressants (eg, TCA), antipsychotics (eg, phenothiazines and most atypicals), and antiarrhythmics (eg, propafenone, flecainide). Consider decreasing dose of CYP2D6 substrates with narrow therapeutic index (eg, flecainide, propafenone, vinblastine, and TCAs). May increase levels of phenytoin, carbamazepine, haloperidol, clozapine, alprazolam, imipramine, desipramine, and olanzapine. May prolong $T_{1/2}$ of diazepam. May increase/decrease lithium levels; lithium toxicity and increased serotonergic effects reported. May cause a shift in plasma concentration with drugs that are tightly bound to protein (eg, warfarin, digitoxin), resulting in an adverse effect. Increased risk of bleeding with aspirin (ASA), NSAIDs, warfarin, and other drugs affecting coagulation. Serotonin syndrome/NMS-like reactions reported with serotonergic drugs (eg, triptans), drugs that impair metabolism of serotonin, antipsychotics, and dopamine antagonists. Not recommended with serotonin precursors (eg, tryptophan), SNRIs, or other SSRIs. Antidiabetic drugs (eg, insulin, oral hypoglycemics) may require dose adjustment. Rare reports of prolonged seizures with electroconvulsive therapy.

PREGNANCY: Category C, not for use in nursing.

MECHANISM OF ACTION: SSRI; not established. Suspected to inhibit CNS neuronal reuptake of serotonin.

PHARMACOKINETICS: Absorption: C_{max}=15-55ng/mL, T_{max}=6-8 hrs. (Cap, Delayed-Release) Delayed onset by 1-2 hrs. **Distribution:** Plasma protein binding (94.5%); crosses the placenta; found in breast milk. **Metabolism:** Liver (extensive) via CYP2D6; demethylation to norfluoxetine (active metabolite). **Elimination:** Kidney; $T_{1/2}$=1-3 days (acute administration), 4-6 days (chronic administration), 4-16 days (norfluoxetine).

NURSING CONSIDERATIONS

Assessment: Assess for risk of bipolar disorder, volume depletion, history of mania/seizures, disease/condition that affects metabolism or hemodynamic response, diabetes, increased IOP or risk of acute narrow-angle glaucoma, hepatic function, pregnancy/nursing status, and possible drug interactions.

Monitoring: Monitor for signs/symptoms of clinical worsening, suicidality and unusual changes in behavior (especially during initial few months, and dosage changes), hypersensitivity reactions, serotonin syndrome, bleeding reactions, altered appetite and weight, hyponatremia, seizures, hypo/hyperglycemia, and other adverse reactions. Monitor height and weight periodically in children. Periodically reassess need for continued treatment.

Patient Counseling: Inform of the risks, benefits, and appropriate use of therapy. Advise to monitor for unusual changes in behavior, worsening of depression, and suicidal ideation on a day-to-day basis, and to report such symptoms to physician. Instruct to seek medical attention if symptoms associated with serotonin syndrome or NMS-like reactions, severe allergic reaction, increased/unusual bruising/bleeding (particularly if using NSAIDs or ASA), or hyponatremia occur. Advise to avoid operating hazardous machinery or driving a car until effects of drug are known and will not affect performance. Advise to inform physician if taking or planning to take any other medications or alcohol, and if pregnant/intend to become pregnant, or breastfeeding. Instruct to take drug exactly as prescribed, not to stop without consulting physician, and to consult physician if symptoms do not improve.

Administration: Oral route. **Storage:** 15-30°C (59-86°F). Protect from light.

PULMICORT   RX
budesonide (AstraZeneca)

OTHER BRAND NAMES: Pulmicort Respules (AstraZeneca) - Pulmicort Flexhaler (AstraZeneca)

THERAPEUTIC CLASS: Corticosteroid

INDICATIONS: (Flexhaler) Maintenance treatment of asthma as prophylactic therapy in patients ≥6 yrs. (Respules) Maintenance treatment of asthma and as prophylactic therapy in children 12 months to 8 yrs.

DOSAGE: *Adults:* (Flexhaler) ≥18 yrs: Individualize dose. Initial: 180-360mcg bid. Max: 720mcg bid. Titrate to the lowest effective dose once asthma stability is achieved. Elderly: Start at lower end of dosing range.
Pediatrics: ≥6 yrs: (Flexhaler) Individualize dose. Initial: 180-360mcg bid. Max: 360mcg bid. 1-8 yrs: (Respules) Previous Bronchodilators Alone: Initial: 0.5mg qd or 0.25mg bid. Max: 0.5mg/day. Previous Inhaled Corticosteroids: Initial: 0.5mg qd or 0.25mg bid up to 0.5mg bid. Max: 1mg/day. Previous Oral Corticosteroids: Initial: 1mg qd or 0.5mg bid. Max: 1mg/day. Not Responding to Non-Steroidal Therapy: Initial: 0.25mg qd. Titrate to the lowest effective dose once asthma stability is achieved. After 1 week of budesonide, gradually reduce PO corticosteroid dose. If once-daily treatment does not provide adequate control, increase total daily dose and/or administer as a divided dose.

HOW SUPPLIED: Powder, Inhalation: (Flexhaler) 90mcg/dose, 180mcg/dose. Sus, Inhalation: (Respules) 0.25mg/2mL, 0.5mg/2mL, 1mg/2mL [2mL]

CONTRAINDICATIONS: Primary treatment of status asthmaticus or other acute episodes of asthma where intensive measures are required. (Flexhaler) Severe hypersensitivity to milk proteins.

WARNINGS/PRECAUTIONS: *Candida albicans* infections of mouth and pharynx reported; treat and/or d/c if needed. Not indicated for the rapid relief of bronchospasm or other acute episodes of asthma; may require oral corticosteroids. Increased susceptibility to infections (eg, chickenpox, measles), may lead to serious/fatal course; if exposed consider prophylaxis/treatment. Caution with tuberculosis (TB), untreated systemic fungal, bacterial, viral or parasitic infections, and ocular herpes simplex. Deaths due to adrenal insufficiency reported with transfer from systemic to inhaled corticosteroids (ICS); if oral corticosteroids required weane slowly from systemic steroid use after transferring to ICS. Transfer from systemic to inhalation therapy may unmask allergic conditions (eg, rhinitis, conjunctivitis). Observe for systemic corticosteroid withdrawal effects. Appearance of hypercorticism and adrenal suppression; reduce dose slowly. Decreases in bone mineral density (BMD) reported; caution with major risk factors for decreased bone mineral content including chronic use of drugs that can reduce bone mass (eg, anticonvulsants, corticosteroids). May cause reduction in growth velocity in pediatrics. Glaucoma, increased intraocular pressure, and cataracts reported. Bronchospasm, with immediate increase in wheezing, may occur; d/c immediately. Rare cases of systemic eosinophilic conditions and vasculitis consistent with Churg-Strauss syndrome reported. Hypersensitivity reactions reported; d/c if signs and symptoms occur. (Flexhaler) Caution in elderly and patients with severe milk protein allergy.

ADVERSE REACTIONS: Respiratory infection. (Flexhaler) Nasopharyngitis, headache, fever, sinusitis, pain, N/V, insomnia, dry mouth, weight gain. (Respules) Rhinitis, otitis media, coughing, viral infection, ear infection, gastroenteritis.

INTERACTIONS: Oral ketoconazole increases plasma levels of oral budesonide. Inhibition of metabolism and increased exposure with CYP3A4 inhibitor. Caution with ketoconazole and other known strong CYP3A4 inhibitors (eg, ritonavir, clarithromycin, itraconazole, nefazodone).

PREGNANCY: Category B, caution in nursing

MECHANISM OF ACTION: Corticosteroid; not established. Shown to have inhibitory activities against multiple cell types (eg, mast cells, eosinophils, neutrophils, macrophages, lymphocytes) and mediators (eg, histamine, eicosanoids, leukotrienes, cytokines) involved in inflammatory and asthmatic response.

PHARMACOKINETICS: Absorption: Respules: (4-6 yrs) Absolute bioavailability (6%); C_{max}=2.6nmol/L; T_{max}=20 min. Flexhaler: (Adults) T_{max}=10 min; C_{max}=0.6nmol/L (180mcg qd), 1.6nmol/L (360mcg bid). (Peds) T_{max}=15-30 min; C_{max}=0.4nmol/L (180mcg qd), 1.5nmol/L (360mcg bid). **Distribution:** V_d=3L/kg; plasma protein binding (85-90%); found in breast milk. **Metabolism:** Liver (extensive) via CYP450 and CYP3A4; 16α-hydroxyprednisolone and 6β-hydroxybudesonide (major metabolites). **Elimination:** Urine and feces (metabolites); (IV) Urine (60%). Respules: $T_{1/2}$=2.3 hrs. Flexhaler: $T_{1/2}$=2-3 hrs.

NURSING CONSIDERATIONS

Assessment: Assess for concomitant diseases (eg, status asthmaticus, acute bronchospasm, other acute episodes of asthma), infections, major risk factors for decreased bone mineral content, history of eye disorders, hypersensitivity, pregnancy/nursing status, and possible drug interactions. Obtain baseline cortisol production. Assess lung function in oral corticosteroids withdrawal. (Flexhaler) Assess for severe milk protein hypersensitivity and hepatic disease.

Monitoring: Monitor for localized oral infections with *C. albicans*, worsening or acutely deteriorating asthma, systemic corticosteroid effects, decreased BMD, height in children, vision change, bronchospasm, and hypersensitivity reactions. (Flexhaler) Monitor for hepatic disease.

Patient Counseling: Advise to use at regular intervals and rinse mouth after inhalation; effectiveness depends on regular use. Instruct to d/c if oral candidiasis or hypersensitivity reactions occur. Inform that medication is not meant to relieve acute asthma symptoms and extra doses should not be used for that purpose. Instruct not to d/c without physician's guidance; symptoms may recur after d/c. Warn to avoid exposure to chickenpox or measles; if exposed, consult physician. Counsel that maximum benefit may not be achieved for ≥1-2 weeks (Flexhaler) or ≥4-6 weeks (Respules); instruct to notify physician if symptoms worsen or do not improve in that time frame. (Flexhaler) Instruct not to repeat inhalation even if they did not feel medication when inhaling; discard whole device after labeled number of inhalations have been used. Advise to carry a warning card indicating need for supplement systemic corticosteroid during periods of stress or severe asthma attack if chronic systemic corticosteroids have been reduced or withdrawn. Consult physician if pregnant/breastfeeding or intend to become pregnant.

Administration: Oral inhalation route. After use, rinse mouth with water without swallowing. (Flexhaler) Prime prior to initial use and inhale deeply and forcefully each time the device is used. (Respules) Administer via jet nebulizer connected to air compressor with adequate air flow, equipped with mouthpiece or suitable face mask. Refer to PI for proper administration. **Storage:** (Flexhaler, Turbuhaler): 20-25°C (68-77°F). Cover tightly. Store in a dry place. (Respules): 20-25°C (68-77°F). Protect from light. Do not freeze. After aluminum foil opened, unused ampules stable for 2 weeks. Once opened, use promptly.

P

PURINETHOL   RX
mercaptopurine (Gate)

THERAPEUTIC CLASS: Purine analog

INDICATIONS: Maintenance therapy of acute lymphatic (lymphocytic, lymphoblastic) leukemia as part of a combination regimen.

DOSAGE: *Adults:* Maint: Once complete hematologic remission is obtained. Usual: 1.5-2.5mg/kg/day as single dose. Concomitant Allopurinol: Reduce mercaptopurine dose to 1/3-1/4 of usual dose. Hepatic Impairment/Thiopurine-S-methyltransferase (TPMT) Deficiency: Reduce dose. Elderly/Renal impairment: Start at the low end of the dosing range.
Pediatrics: Maint: Once complete hematologic remission is obtained. Usual: 1.5-2.5mg/kg/day as single dose. Concomitant Allopurinol: Reduce mercaptopurine dose to 1/3-1/4 of usual dose. Hepatic Impairment/TPMT Deficiency: Reduce dose. Renal Impairment: Start at lower dose.

HOW SUPPLIED: Tab: 50mg* *scored

CONTRAINDICATIONS: Prior resistance to mercaptopurine or thioguanine.

WARNINGS/PRECAUTIONS: Should not be used unless a diagnosis of acute lymphatic leukemia is established. Not effective for prophylaxis or treatment of CNS leukemia. Not effective in acute myelogenous/chronic lymphatic leukemia, the lymphomas (including Hodgkins disease), or solid tumors. May increase risk of neoplasia; hepatosplenic T-cell lymphoma reported in patients treated for inflammatory bowel disease. Risk of dose-related bone marrow suppression. Life-threatening infections and bleeding reported; d/c at first sign of unexpectedly abnormal large fall in any formed elements of the blood not attributable to other drug or disease process. Increased sensitivity to myelosuppressive effects with TPMT gene deficiency; consider TPMT testing with evidence of severe toxicity. Hepatotoxicity (especially with >2.5mg/kg dose) and hepatic encephalopathy reported; allow early detection of hepatotoxicity. D/C with deterioration of liver function, toxic hepatitis and biliary stasis. Risk of immunosuppression which may manifest decreased cellular hypersensitivities and decreased allograft rejection; induction of immunity to infectious agents or vaccines. May cause fetal harm. Monitor patient clinical status and modify therapy depending on response and manifestations of toxicity. Caution in elderly, renal, and hepatic impairment.

ADVERSE REACTIONS: Bone marrow toxicity, hepatotoxicity, anemia, thrombocytopenia, leukopenia, myelosuppression, jaundice.

INTERACTIONS: Severe toxicity with allopurinol; reduce mercaptopurine dose to 1/3 to 1/4 of the usual dose. Reduce dose with other myelosuppressants. Enhanced marrow suppression reported with trimethoprim-sulfamethoxazole. Exacerbation of bone marrow toxicity with drugs that inhibit TPMT (eg, olsalazine, mesalazine, sulphasalazine). Inhibition of the anticoagulant effect of warfarin reported. Hepatotoxicity reported with doxorubicin. Subnormal induction of immunity to vaccines may occur with concomitant use.

PREGNANCY: Category D, not for use in nursing.

MECHANISM OF ACTION: Purine analog; competes with hypoxanthine and guanine for hypoxanthine-guanine phosphoribosyltransferase (HGPRTase) and is converted to thioinosinic acid, which then inhibits glutamine-5-phosphoribosylpyrophosphate amidotransferase of the de novo pathway for purine ribonucleotide synthesis.

PHARMACOKINETICS: Absorption: Incomplete. **Distribution:** Plasma protein binding (19%). **Metabolism:** Via HGPRTase. **Elimination:** (PO) Urine (46%). (IV) $T_{1/2}$=21 min (pediatric); 47 min (adult).

NURSING CONSIDERATIONS

Assessment: Assess for CNS leukemia, acute myelogenous/chronic lymphatic leukemia, the lymphomas (including Hodgkins disease), solid tumors, prior drug resistance, pre-existing liver/renal disease, TPMT gene defect, pregnancy/nursing status, and for possible drug interactions. Obtain baseline WBC with differential, Hgb/Hct, platelet count, serum transaminase levels, alkaline phosphatase levels, bilirubin levels, and renal function.

Monitoring: Monitor for signs/symptoms of bone marrow toxicity, hypersensitivity reactions, hepatoxicity, and immunosuppression. Monitor WBC with differential, Hgb/Hct, and platelet count weekly; increase monitoring frequency during induction phase. Monitor serum transaminase levels, alkaline phosphatase, and bilirubin levels weekly at beginning of therapy and then at monthly intervals thereafter; monitor more frequently with preexisting liver disease. Perform bone marrow exam for evaluation of marrow status. Consider performing TPMT testing if evidence of severe bone marrow toxicity develops. Monitor patient clinical status and need to modify therapy based on response and manifestations of toxicity.

Patient Counseling: Inform of major toxicities related to therapy (eg, myelosuppression, hepatotoxicity, GI toxicity). Advise women of childbearing potential to avoid becoming pregnant while on therapy. Advise to take under medical supervision. Advise to seek medical attention if symptoms of fever, sore throat, jaundice, N/V, signs of local infection, bleeding from any site, or if symptoms suggestive of anemia develop.

Administration: Oral route. **Storage:** 15-25°C (59-77°F) in a dry place.

PYLERA RX

tetracycline HCl - bismuth subcitrate potassium - metronidazole (Axcan Scandipharm)

THERAPEUTIC CLASS: *H. pylori* treatment combination

INDICATIONS: Treatment of *Helicobacter pylori* infection and duodenal ulcer disease (active or history of within the past 5 years) to eradicate *H. pylori*, in combination with omeprazole.

DOSAGE: *Adults:* Usual: 3 caps qid for 10 days, pc and at hs. Take with omeprazole 20mg bid after am and pm meals.

HOW SUPPLIED: Cap: (Bismuth Subcitrate Potassium-Metronidazole-Tetracycline HCl) 140mg-125mg-125mg

CONTRAINDICATIONS: Severe renal impairment, concomitant use with methoxyflurane, disulfiram taken within last 2 weeks, and alcoholic beverages or other products containing propylene glycol during therapy and for at least 3 days after therapy.

WARNINGS/PRECAUTIONS: Use in the absence of a proven or strongly suspected bacterial infection or a prophylactic indication is unlikely to provide benefit and increases the risk of the development of drug-resistant bacteria. Caution with hepatic impairment and in elderly. (Bismuth) Neurotoxicity associated with excessive doses reported. May cause temporary and harmless darkening of the tongue and/or black stool. May interfere with x-ray diagnostic procedures of the GI tract. (Metronidazole) Encephalopathy, optic and peripheral neuropathy, convulsive seizures, and aseptic meningitis reported. Known or previously unrecognized candidiasis may present more prominent symptoms; treat with an antifungal agent. Caution with evidence or history of blood dyscrasia. Mild leukopenia reported; obtain total and differential leukocyte counts prior to and after therapy. May interfere with certain serum chemistry values (eg, AST, ALT, LDH, TG, and hexokinase glucose). (Tetracycline) May cause fetal harm. May cause permanent teeth discoloration during tooth development (last half of pregnancy, infancy, and childhood to the age of 8 yrs) and enamel hypoplasia; avoid use in this age group. Maternal hepatotoxicity may occur if given during pregnancy at high doses (>2g IV). Pseudotumor cerebri reported. May cause overgrowth of non-susceptible organisms; d/c if superinfection occurs. Photosensitivity reported; avoid sun or sun lamps exposure and d/c if skin erythema occurs. May increase BUN. Higher serum tetracycline levels may lead to azotemia, hyperphosphatemia, and acidosis in patients with renal impairment.

ADVERSE REACTIONS: Abnormal feces, nausea, diarrhea, abdominal pain, asthenia, headache, dysgeusia.

INTERACTIONS: See Contraindications. May alter anticoagulant effects of warfarin and other oral coumarin anticoagulants; monitor PT, INR, or other suitable anticoagulation tests and for evidence of bleeding. (Metronidazole) Short term use may increase serum lithium concentrations and signs of lithium toxicity with high doses of lithium. Decreased plasma clearance and prolonged $T_{1/2}$ with drugs that inhibit microsomal liver enzymes (eg, cimetidine). Accelerated elimination and reduced plasma concentrations with drugs that induce liver enzymes (eg, phenytoin, phenobarbital). Impaired phenytoin clearance; monitor phenytoin concentrations. (Tetracycline) Oral contraceptives may become less effective and may cause breakthrough bleeding if given concomitantly. Antacids containing aluminum, calcium, or magnesium; preparations containing iron, zinc, or sodium bicarbonate; or milk and dairy products may reduce absorption; do not consume concomitantly. May interfere with bactericidal effects of penicillin; avoid coadministration.

PREGNANCY: Category D, not for use in nursing.

MECHANISM OF ACTION: *H. pylori* treatment combination; antimicrobial agent. (Bismuth) Antibacterial action not well understood. (Metronidazole) Metabolized through reductive pathways into reactive intermediates that have cytotoxic action. (Tetracycline HCl) Interacts with 30S subunit of the bacterial ribosome and inhibits protein synthesis.

PHARMACOKINETICS: Absorption: Metronidazole: Well-absorbed. Tetracycline: 60-90% (stomach and upper small intestine). Administration of the individual drugs as separate cap formulations or as Pylera resulted in variable pharmacokinetic parameters. **Distribution:** Bismuth: Plasma protein binding (>90%). Metronidazole: Plasma protein binding (<20%); found in breast milk. Tetracycline: Plasma protein binding (varying degrees); crosses placenta, found in breast milk. **Metabolism:** Metronidazole: Side-chain oxidation and glucuronide conjugation. **Elimination:** Bismuth: $T_{1/2}$=5 days (blood and urine); urinary, biliary. Metronidazole: $T_{1/2}$=8 hrs, urine (60-80%), feces (6-15%). Tetracycline: Urine, feces.

NURSING CONSIDERATIONS

Assessment: Assess for age, history of blood dyscrasia, known or previously unrecognized candidiasis, hepatic/renal function, drug hypersensitivity, pregnancy/nursing status, and possible drug interactions. Obtain total and differential leukocyte counts prior to therapy.

Monitoring: Monitor for renal/hepatic impairment, encephalopathy, neuropathy, convulsive seizures, aseptic meningitis, leukopenia, enamel hypoplasia pseudomotor cerebri, superinfection, photosensitivity reactions, skin erythema, and other adverse reactions. Monitor total and differential leukocyte counts and BUN levels.

Patient Counseling: Advise pregnant women that therapy may cause fetal harm. Advise to avoid breastfeeding while on therapy or discard breast milk during and for 24 hrs after the last dose. Inform that allergic reactions may occur; d/c therapy if urticaria, erythematosus rash, flushing, or fever occur. Inform of the risks of central/peripheral nervous system effects; d/c and notify physician immediately if any neurologic symptoms develop. Instruct to avoid exposure to sun or sun lamps. Instruct to notify physician of all medications currently taking. Inform that temporary and harmless darkening of tongue and/or black stool may occur. Inform of proper dosing information. Advise not to take double doses; if a dose is missed, continue normal dosing schedule until medication is gone. Instruct to inform physician if >4 doses are missed. Instruct to swallow cap whole with full glass of water. Counsel that therapy should only be used to treat bacterial, not viral infections.

Administration: Oral route. Swallow cap whole with a full glass of water (8 oz). **Storage:** 20-25°C (68-77°F).

QUINIDINE GLUCONATE INJECTION RX
quinidine gluconate (Various)

THERAPEUTIC CLASS: Class IA antiarrhythmic/schizonticide antimalarial

INDICATIONS: Treatment of life-threatening *Plasmodium falciparum* malaria. Conversion of atrial fibrillation/flutter (A-Fib/Flutter) to normal sinus rhythm. Treatment of ventricular arrhythmias.

DOSAGE: *Adults:* Malaria: LD: 15mg/kg base (24mg/kg gluconate) over 4 hrs. Maint: After 8 hrs, 7.5mg/kg (12mg/kg gluconate) IV q8h for 7 days. Alternate: Initial: 6.25mg/kg base (10mg/kg gluconate) IV over 1-2 hrs. Maint: 12.5mcg/kg/min base (20mcg/kg/min gluconate) for 72hr. A-Fib/Flutter: 0.25mg/kg/min. Max: 5-10mg/kg. Consider alternate therapy if conversion to sinus rhythm not achieved. Ventricular Arrhythmia: Dosing regimens not adequately studied. Generally similar to A-Fib/Flutter. Renal/Hepatic Impairment or CHF: Reduce dose. Elderly: Start at low end of dosing range.
Pediatrics: Malaria: LD: 15mg/kg base (24mg/kg gluconate) over 4 hrs. Maint: After 8 hrs, 7.5mg/kg (12mg/kg gluconate) IV q8h for 7 days. Alternate: Initial: 6.25mg/kg base (10mg/kg gluconate) IV over 1-2 hrs. Maint: 12.5mcg/kg/min base (20mcg/kg/min gluconate) for 72hr.

HOW SUPPLIED: Inj: 80mg/mL [10mL]

CONTRAINDICATIONS: In the absence of a functional artificial pacemaker any cardiac rhythm dependent upon a junctional or idioventricular pacemaker (including with complete atrioventricular [AV] block), thrombocytopenic purpura with previous treatment, patients adversely affected by anticholinergics (eg, myasthenia gravis).

WARNINGS/PRECAUTIONS: Rapid infusion can cause peripheral vascular collapse and severe hypotension. May prolong QTc interval and may lead to torsades de pointes. Paradoxical increase in ventricular rate in A-Fib/Flutter. Caution in those at risk of complete AV block without implanted pacemakers, renal/hepatic dysfunction, elderly, and congestive heart failure (CHF). Physical/pharmacologic maneuvers to terminate paroxysmal supraventricular tachycardia may be ineffective. Exacerbated bradycardia in sick sinus syndrome.

ADVERSE REACTIONS: Upper GI distress, lightheadedness, fatigue, palpitations, weakness, visual problems, N/V, diarrhea, changes in sleeping habits, rash, headache, diarrhea, angina-like pain.

INTERACTIONS: Urine alkalinizers (eg, carbonic anhydrase inhibitors, sodium bicarbonate, thiazide diuretics) reduce renal elimination. CYP3A4 inducers (eg, phenobarbital, phenytoin, rifampin) may accelerate elimination. Verapamil, diltiazem decrease clearance. Caution with drugs metabolized by CYP2D6 (eg, mexiletine, phenothiazines, polycyclic antidepressants, codeine, hydrocodone) or by CYP3A4 (eg, nifedipine, felodipine, nicardipine, nimodipine). β-blockers may decrease clearance. May slow metabolism of nifedipine. Increases levels of digoxin, digitoxin, procainamide and haloperidol. Increased levels with ketoconazole, amiodarone, cimetidine. Potentiates warfarin, depolarizing and nondepolarizing neuromuscular blockers. Additive effects with anticholinergics, vasodilators, and negative inotropes. Antagonistic effects with cholinergics, vasoconstrictors, and positive inotropes.

PREGNANCY: Category C, not for use in nursing.

MECHANISM OF ACTION: Antimalarial schizonticide and antiarrhythmic agent with class 1a activity. Slows phase-0 depolarization by depressing the inward depolarizing Na⁺ current, which slows conduction, prolongs effective refractory period, and reduces automaticity in the heart. Also has anticholinergic activity, negative ionotropic activity, and acts peripherally as an α-adrenergic antagonist.

PHARMACOKINETICS: Absorption: T_{max}=<2 hrs. **Distribution:** V_d=2-3L/kg; plasma protein binding (80-88%) in adults and older children, (50-70%) in pregnant women, infants and neonates; found in breast milk. **Metabolism:** Liver, via CYP3A4 pathway. 3-hydroxy-quinidine (3HQ); major metabolite. **Elimination:** Urine (20% unchanged); $T_{1/2}$=6-8 hrs (adults), 3-4 hrs (pediatrics), and 12 hrs (3HQ).

NURSING CONSIDERATIONS

Assessment: Assess for structural heart disease, pre-existing long-QT syndrome, implanted pacemaker, history of torsades de pointes, other conduction defects, thrombocytopenic purpura, CHF, renal/hepatic dysfunction, myasthenia gravis, pregnancy/nursing status, and possible drug/diet interactions.

Monitoring: Monitor for exacerbated bradycardia, paradoxical increase in ventricular rate in atrial flutter/fibrillation, torsades de pointes, life-threatening ventricular arrhythmia, hypotension, ventricular extrasystoles/tachycardia/flutter and ventricular fibrillation. Continuously/carefully monitor ECG and BP.

Patient Counseling: Inform about risks/benefits of drug and report any adverse reactions. Notify physician if pregnant/nursing. Avoid grapefruit juice.

Administration: IV route. **Storage:** 25°C (77°F); excursions permitted to 15-30°C (59-86°F).

QUIXIN   RX
levofloxacin (Vistakon)

THERAPEUTIC CLASS: Fluoroquinolone

INDICATIONS: Treatment of bacterial conjunctivitis caused by susceptible strains of organisms.

DOSAGE: *Adults:* Days 1-2: 1-2 drops in affected eye(s) q2h while awake, up to 8x/day. Days 3-7: 1-2 drops in affected eye(s) q4h while awake, up to qid.
Pediatrics: ≥1 yr: Days 1-2: 1-2 drops in affected eye(s) q2h while awake, up to 8x/day. Days 3-7: 1-2 drops in affected eye(s) q4h while awake, up to qid.

HOW SUPPLIED: Sol: 0.5% [5mL]

WARNINGS/PRECAUTIONS: Should not be injected subconjunctivally nor introduced directly to anterior chamber of the eye. D/C if allergic reaction or superinfection occurs; prolonged use may cause overgrowth of non-susceptible organisms. Avoid wearing contact lenses if signs/symptoms of conjunctivitis present.

ADVERSE REACTIONS: Transient ocular burning, transient decreased vision, fever, foreign body sensation, headache, ocular pain/discomfort, pharyngitis, photophobia.

INTERACTIONS: Systemic quinolone therapy may increase theophylline levels, interfere with caffeine metabolism, enhance warfarin effects, and elevate SrCr with cyclosporine.

PREGNANCY: Category C, caution in nursing.

MECHANISM OF ACTION: Fluoroquinolone; inhibits bacterial topoisomerase IV and DNA gyrase, which are enzymes required for DNA replication, transcription, repair, and recombination.

PHARMACOKINETICS: Absorption: C_{max}=0.94ng/mL (single dose), 2.15ng/mL (multiple doses). **Distribution:** Presumed to be excreted in breast milk.

NURSING CONSIDERATIONS

Assessment: Assess for hypersensitivity to the drug or to other quinolones, use of contact lenses, pregnancy/nursing status, possible drug interactions, or any other conditions where treatment is contraindicated or cautioned.

Monitoring: Monitor for signs/symptoms of hypersensitivity or anaphylactic reaction, and overgrowth of nonsusceptible organisms. Perform eye exam using magnification (eg, slit-lamp biomicroscopy, fluorescein staining) if necessary.

Patient Counseling: Instruct to avoid contaminating applicator tip with material from eye, fingers, or other sources. Advise not to wear contact lenses if there are signs/symptoms of bacterial conjunctivitis. Instruct to d/c medication and contact physician if signs of hypersensitivity reaction (eg, rash) develop.

Administration: Ocular route. Do not inject subconjunctivally or introduce directly into anterior chamber of eye. **Storage:** 15-25°C (59-77°F).

QUTENZA   RX
capsaicin (NeurogesX)

THERAPEUTIC CLASS: Analgesic

INDICATIONS: Management of neuropathic pain associated with postherpetic neuralgia.

DOSAGE: *Adults:* Apply single patch for 60 min; up to 4 patches may be applied. May repeat q3 months or as warranted by the return of pain (not more frequently than q3 months). Apply to dry, intact skin.

HOW SUPPLIED: Patch: 179mg [8%]

WARNINGS/PRECAUTIONS: Do not apply to the face, scalp, or broken skin. Do not use near eyes or mucous membranes. Aerosolization may occur upon rapid removal; remove gently and slowly by rolling the adhesive side inward. If irritation of eyes or airways occur, flush with cool water. Inhalation can result in coughing or sneezing; provide supportive medical care if SOB develops. If skin not intended to be treated comes into contact with patch, apply cleansing gel for 1 min, then wipe off with dry gauze and wash with soap and water. May experience substantial procedural pain; treat with local cooling (eg, ice pack) and/or analgesic medication, such as opioids; use of opioids may impair mental/physical abilities. HTN reported; monitor periodically. Increased risk of cardiovascular (CV) effects with unstable/poorly controlled HTN and history of CV/cerebrovascular events.

ADVERSE REACTIONS: Application-site erythema, pain, pruritus, papules, edema, nasopharyngitis, N/V.

PREGNANCY: Category B, safety not known in nursing.

MECHANISM OF ACTION: TRPV1 channel agonist; causes an initial enhanced stimulation of the TRPV1-expressing cutaneous nociceptors that may be associated with painful sensations followed by pain relief thought to be mediated by a reduction in TRPV1-expressing nociceptive nerve endings.

PHARMACOKINETICS: Absorption: C_{max}=4.6ng/mL.

NURSING CONSIDERATIONS

Assessment: Assess application site, unstable/poorly controlled HTN, history of CV/cerebrovascular events, and pregnancy/nursing status.

Monitoring: Monitor for any hypersensitivity reactions and monitor BP periodically during treatment. Monitor for occurrence of possible side effects.

Patient Counseling: Inform that exposure of the skin to the patch may result in transient erythema and burning sensation. Instruct not to touch patch; may produce burning and/or stinging sensation. Inform physician if pregnant/breastfeeding, side effects becomes severe or if eye/airway irritation occurs. Inform that treated area may be heat sensitive (eg, hot showers/bath, direct sunlight, vigorous exercise) for a few days after treatment. Inform patients that they may be given medications such as opioids that may impair mental/physical abilities. Inform that a small transient increase in BP may occur during and shortly after treatment. Instruct to inform physician if have experienced any recent CV event.

Administration: Topical route. May cut patch to match size/shape of treatment. Refer to PI for instructions for use. **Storage:** 20-25°C (68-77°F); excursions permitted between 15-30°C (59-86°F). Keep in sealed pouch immediately before use.

QVAR   RX
beclomethasone dipropionate (Teva)

THERAPEUTIC CLASS: Corticosteroid

INDICATIONS: Maintenance treatment of asthma as prophylactic therapy in patients ≥5 yrs. To reduce or eliminate the need for systemic corticosteroids in asthma patients requiring systemic corticosteroids.

DOSAGE: *Adults:* Previously on Bronchodilators Alone: 40-80mcg bid. Max: 320mcg bid. Previously on Inhaled Corticosteroids: 40-160mcg bid. Max: 320mcg bid. Taper to the lowest effective dose once desired effect is achieved. Maintained on Systemic Corticosteroids: Initial: Should be used concurrently with the usual maint dose of systemic corticosteroids. May attempt gradual reduction of systemic corticosteroid dose after 1 week on inhaled therapy by reducing the daily or alternate daily dose. Elderly: Start at lower end of dosing range.
Pediatrics: ≥12 yrs: Previously on Bronchodilators Alone: 40-80mcg bid. Max: 320mcg bid. Previously on Inhaled Corticosteroids: 40-160mcg bid. Max: 320mcg bid. 5-11 yrs: Previously on Bronchodilators Alone/Inhaled Corticosteroids: 40mcg bid. Max: 80mcg bid. Taper to the lowest effective dose once desired effect is achieved. Maintained on Systemic Corticosteroids: Initial:

Should be used concurrently with the usual maint dose of systemic corticosteroids. May attempt gradual reduction of systemic corticosteroid dose after 1 week on inhaled therapy by reducing the daily or alternate daily dose.

HOW SUPPLIED: MDI: 40 mcg/inh, 80 mcg/inh [7.3g, 8.7g]

CONTRAINDICATIONS: Primary treatment of status asthmaticus or other acute episodes of asthma where intensive measures are required.

WARNINGS/PRECAUTIONS: Not indicated for the relief of acute bronchospasm. Deaths due to adrenal insufficiency have occurred with transfer from systemic corticosteroids to inhaled corticosteroids. Resume oral corticosteroids (in large doses) immediately during stress or severe asthma attack. Transfer from systemic to inhalation therapy may unmask allergic conditions (eg, rhinitis, conjunctivitis, eczema). Increased susceptibility to infections (eg, chickenpox, measles); if exposed, consider prophylaxis/treatment. Not a bronchodilator and is not indicated for rapid relief of bronchospasm. D/C, treat, and institute alternative therapy if bronchospasm occurs after dosing. Observe for systemic corticosteroid effects (eg, hypercorticism and adrenal suppression); if changes appear, reduce dose slowly. May cause reduction in growth velocity in pediatrics. Caution with active or quiescent tuberculosis (TB) infection, untreated systemic fungal, bacterial, parasitic, or viral infections, or ocular herpes simplex. Rare cases of glaucoma, increased intraocular pressure (IOP), and cataracts reported. Caution in elderly.

ADVERSE REACTIONS: Headache, pharyngitis, upper respiratory tract infection, rhinitis, increased asthma symptoms, sinusitis, dysphonia, dysmenorrhea, coughing.

PREGNANCY: Category C, not for use in nursing.

MECHANISM OF ACTION: Corticosteroid; have multiple anti-inflammatory effects, inhibiting both inflammatory cells (eg, mast cells, eosinophils, basophils, lymphocytes, macrophages, and neutrophils) and release of inflammatory mediators (eg, histamine, eicosanoids, leukotrienes, and cytokines). These anti-inflammatory actions contribute to the efficacy in asthma.

PHARMACOKINETICS: Absorption: (Beclomethasone) C_{max}=88pg/mL, T_{max}= 0.5 hr; (Beclomethasone-17-monopropionate [17-BMP]) C_{max}=1419pg/mL, T_{max}=0.7hr. **Distribution:** Found in breast milk; plasma protein binding (94-96%, 17-BMP) (*in vitro*). **Metabolism:** Liver (biotransformation) via CYP3A4; 17-BMP, beclomethasone-21-monopropionate, beclomethasone (major metabolites). **Elimination:** Feces, urine (<10%); $T_{1/2}$= 2.8 hrs (17-BMP).

NURSING CONSIDERATIONS

Assessment: Assess for status asthmaticus, active or quiescent pulmonary TB, untreated systemic fungal, bacterial, parasitic or viral infections, ocular herpes simplex, exposure to chickenpox or measles, pregnancy/nursing status, and possible drug interactions.

Monitoring: Monitor for bronchospasm, growth suppression in children, glaucoma, increased IOP, cataracts, adrenal insufficiency, hypersensitivity reactions, and other adverse effects. Monitor for relief or worsening of symptoms.

Patient Counseling: Inform about the risks and benefits of therapy. Advise to avoid exposure to chickenpox or measles or to seek medical advice if exposed to these diseases. Instruct to use drug as directed and should not be stopped abruptly. Inform that drug is not intended for treatment of acute asthma. Counsel about the proper use of inhaler and advise to rinse mouth after use. Advise to seek medical attention if worsening of existing TB, infections, or ocular herpes simplex occur, if symptoms do not improve or worsen, or during periods of stress or severe asthmatic attack.

Administration: Oral inhalation. Prime prior to intial use or if not used for over 10 days. Refer to PI for directions for use. Should only be used with product's actuator and should not be used with any other inhalation drug product. **Storage:** 25°C (77°F); excursions permitted to 15-30° (59-86°F). For optimal results, canister should be at room temperature when used.

RANEXA

RX

ranolazine (Gilead Sciences)

THERAPEUTIC CLASS: Miscellaneous antianginal

INDICATIONS: Treatment of chronic angina; may be used with β-blockers, nitrates, calcium channel blockers, antiplatelet therapy, lipid-lowering therapy, angiotensin-converting enzyme inhibitors, and angiotensin receptor blockers.

DOSAGE: *Adults:* Initial: 500mg bid. Titrate: May increase to 1000mg bid, PRN, based on clinical symptoms. Max: 1000mg bid. Concurrent Use with Moderate CYP3A Inhibitors (eg, diltiazem, verapamil, erythromycin): Max: 500mg bid. Concurrent Use with P-glycoprotein (P-gp) Inhibitors (eg, cyclosporine): Titrate dose based on clinical response. Elderly: Start at lower end of dosing range.

HOW SUPPLIED: Tab, Extended-Release: 500mg, 1000mg

CONTRAINDICATIONS: Liver cirrhosis, concomitant use with CYP3A inducers (eg, rifampin, rifabutin, rifapentine, phenobarbital, phenytoin, carbamazepine, St. John's wort) or strong CYP3A inhibitors (eg, ketoconazole, itraconazole, clarithromycin, nefazodone, nelfinavir, ritonavir, indinavir, saquinavir).

WARNINGS/PRECAUTIONS: May prolong QTc interval in a dose-related manner. Caution with renal impairment and in elderly. Produces small reductions in HbA1c in patients with diabetes; should not be considered a treatment for diabetes.

ADVERSE REACTIONS: Dizziness, headache, constipation, N/V, abdominal pain, anorexia, asthenia, bradycardia, confusion, dyspepsia, dyspnea, peripheral edema, hematuria, hyperhidrosis.

INTERACTIONS: See Contraindications. Diltiazem and verapamil may increase levels; limit dose to 500mg bid with moderate CYP3A inhibitors (eg, fluconazole, diltiazem, verapamil, erythromycin, grapefruit juice or grapefruit-containing products). P-gp inhibitors (eg, cyclosporine) may increase concentrations; titrate dose based on clinical response. May increase levels of simvastatin; limit simvastatin dose to 20mg qd. May increase concentrations of sensitive CYP3A substrates (eg, lovastatin) and CYP3A substrates with a narrow therapeutic range (eg, cyclosporine, tacrolimus, sirolimus); may require dose adjustment of these drugs. Increased exposure to digoxin and CYP2D6 substrates (eg, TCAs, antipsychotics); may adjust digoxin dose and lower doses of CYP2D6 substrates. Rifampin may decrease concentrations. Paroxetine may increase concentrations. May increase concentrations of immediate-release metoprolol. Partially inhibits formation of the main metabolite of dextromethorphan (dextrorphan).

PREGNANCY: Category C, not for use in nursing.

MECHANISM OF ACTION: Antianginal; not established. Can inhibit the cardiac late Na current.

PHARMACOKINETICS: Absorption: Highly variable. C_{max}=2600ng/mL (1000mg bid), T_{max}=2-5 hrs. **Distribution:** Plasma protein binding (62%). **Metabolism:** Intestine and liver (rapid and extensive) by CYP3A (major) and CYP2D6 (minor). **Elimination:** Urine (75%), feces (25%) (sol); (<5% unchanged in urine and feces); $T_{1/2}$=7 hrs, 6-22 hrs (metabolites).

NURSING CONSIDERATIONS

Assessment: Assess for liver cirrhosis, QT interval prolongation, renal impairment, pregnancy/nursing status, and possible drug interactions.

Monitoring: Monitor for ECG changes (eg, QT interval prolongation). Monitor HbA1c and SrCr levels.

Patient Counseling: Inform that drug will not abate an acute angina episode. Advise to inform physician of any other concurrent medications, including over-the-counter drugs, and of any history of QTc prolongation or congenital long QT syndrome. Instruct to limit grapefruit juice/products. Advise that if a dose is missed, take the prescribed dose at the next scheduled time; instruct not to double the next dose. Instruct to swallow tab whole; do not crush, break, or chew. Advise that drug may be taken with or without meals. Instruct to contact physician if fainting spells occur. Advise that therapy may cause dizziness and lightheadedness; instruct to know how to react to drug before engaging in activities requiring mental alertness or coordination (eg, operating machinery, driving).

Administration: Oral route. Swallow tab whole; do not crush, break, or chew. **Storage:** 25°C (77°F); excursions permitted to 15-30°C (59-86°F).

RAPAFLO   RX
silodosin (Watson)

THERAPEUTIC CLASS: Alpha$_1$-antagonist

INDICATIONS: Treatment of the signs and symptoms of benign prostatic hyperplasia (BPH).

DOSAGE: *Adults:* 8mg qd with a meal. Moderate Renal Impairment (CrCl 30-50mL/min): 4mg qd with a meal.

HOW SUPPLIED: Cap: 4mg, 8mg

CONTRAINDICATIONS: Severe renal impairment (CrCl <30mL/min), severe hepatic impairment (Child-Pugh score ≥10), and concomitant administration with strong CYP3A4 inhibitors (eg, ketoconazole, clarithromycin, itraconazole, ritonavir).

WARNINGS/PRECAUTIONS: Postural hypotension and syncope may occur. May impair mental/physical abilities. Caution in patients with moderate renal impairment. Patients thought to have BPH should be examined prior to therapy to rule out prostate cancer. Intraoperative floppy iris syndrome observed during cataract surgery in some patients on α$_1$-blockers or previously treated with α$_1$-blockers.

ADVERSE REACTIONS: Retrograde ejaculation, dizziness, diarrhea, orthostatic hypotension, headache, nasopharyngitis, nasal congestion.

INTERACTIONS: See Contraindications. Concomitant administration with moderate CYP3A4 inhibitors (eg, diltiazem, erythromycin, verapamil) may increase plasma concentrations. Caution with antihypertensives; monitor for possible adverse events. Avoid with strong P-gp inhibitors (eg, cyclosporine) and other α-blockers. Concomitant use with PDE5 inhibitors can potentially cause symptomatic hypotension.

PREGNANCY: Category B, safety not known in nursing.

MECHANISM OF ACTION: $α_1$-antagonist; blocks $α_1$-adrenoreceptors, causing relaxation of smooth muscles in the bladder neck and prostate, resulting in improved urine flow and reduction in BPH symptoms.

PHARMACOKINETICS: Absorption: Absolute bioavailability (32%), C_{max}=61.6ng/mL, T_{max}=2.6 hrs, AUC_{ss}=373.4ng•hr/mL. **Distribution:** V_d=49.5L; plasma protein binding (97%). **Metabolism:** Via glucuronidation, alcohol and aldehyde dehydrogenase, CYP3A4; KMD-3213G (main metabolite), KMD-3293 (second major metabolite). **Elimination:** Urine (33.5%), feces (54.9%); $T_{1/2}$=13.3 hrs.

NURSING CONSIDERATIONS

Assessment: Assess for severe renal/hepatic impairment, prostate cancer, and possible drug interactions.

Monitoring: Monitor for signs/symptoms of postural hypotension and adverse reactions. Monitor for degree of renal impairment.

Patient Counseling: Instruct to take medication with a meal. Counsel about possible symptoms of postural hypotension (eg, dizziness); caution about driving, operating machinery, or performing hazardous tasks. Inform that orgasm with reduced or no semen does not pose a safety concern and is reversible when drug is d/c. Notify ophthalmologist about the use of silodosin before cataract surgery or other eye procedures, even if no longer taking silodosin.

Administration: Oral route. **Storage:** Store at 25°C (77°F); excursions permitted to 15°-30°C (59°-86°F). Protect from light and moisture.

RAPAMUNE   RX
sirolimus (Wyeth)

Increased susceptibility to infection and possible development of lymphoma and other malignancies may result from immunosuppression. Only physicians experienced in immunosuppressive therapy and management of renal transplant patients should use sirolimus. Use not recommended in liver or lung transplant patients. Excess mortality and graft loss in combination with tacrolimus reported in liver transplant patients. Increased hepatic artery thrombosis with cyclosporine or tacrolimus in liver transplant patients. Cases of bronchial anastomotic dehiscence, most fatal, reported in lung transplant patients.

THERAPEUTIC CLASS: Macrocyclic lactone immunosuppressant

INDICATIONS: Prophylaxis of organ rejection in patients ≥13 yrs receiving renal transplants.

DOSAGE: *Adults:* Take initial dose as soon as possible after transplantation. Take 4 hrs after cyclosporine. Maintain on a dose for at least 7-14 days before further dose adjustment. Refer to full PI for maintenance dose adjustments. Max: 40mg/day. If estimated dose is >40mg/day due to addition of LD, LD should be administered over 2 days. Monitor trough concentration at least 3-4 days after LD(s). Low-Moderate Immunologic Risk: Initial: Take with cyclosporine and corticosteroids. Give LD equivalent to 3x the maintenance dose. Progressively d/c cyclosporine over 4-8 weeks at 2-4 months following transplantation. Adjust dose to maintain blood trough concentration within target range. High-Immunologic Risk: Take with cyclosporine and corticosteroids for the first 12 months. LD: Up to 15mg on Day 1 post-transplantation. Maint: 5mg/day beginning on Day 2. Obtain trough level between Days 5 and 7 and adjust daily dose thereafter. Mild or Moderate Hepatic Impairment: Reduce maintenance dose by 1/3. Severe Hepatic Impairment: Reduce maintenance by 1/2. Low Body Weight (<40kg): Adjust initial dose based on BSA to 1mg/m²/day with a LD of 3mg/m². Elderly: Start at lower end of dosing range.
Pediatrics: ≥13 yrs: Take initial dose as soon as possible after transplantation. Take 4 hrs after cyclosporine. Maintain on a dose for at least 7-14 days before further dose adjustment. Refer to full PI for maintenance dose adjustments. Max: 40mg/day. If estimated dose is >40mg/day due to addition of LD, LD should be administered over 2 days. Monitor trough concentration at least 3-4 days after LD(s). Low-Moderate Immunologic Risk: Initial: Take with cyclosporine and corticosteroids. Give LD equivalent to 3x the maintenance dose. Progressively d/c cyclosporine over 4-8 weeks at 2-4 months following transplantation. Adjust dose to maintain blood trough concentration within target range. Mild or Moderate Hepatic Impairment: Reduce maintenance dose by 1/3. Severe Hepatic Impairment: Reduce maintenance by 1/2. Low Body Weight (<40kg): Adjust initial dose based on BSA to 1mg/m²/day with a LD of 3mg/m².

HOW SUPPLIED: Sol: 1mg/mL [60mL]; Tab: 0.5mg, 1mg, 2mg

WARNINGS/PRECAUTIONS: Hypersensitivity reactions reported. Associated with the development of angioedema. Impaired wound healing, lymphocele, wound dehiscence, and fluid accumulation (eg, peripheral edema, lymphedema, pleural effusion, ascites, pericardial effusions) reported. May increase serum cholesterol and TG that may require treatment. May delay recovery of renal function in patients with delayed graft function. Proteinuria commonly observed. Increased risk for opportunistic infections, including activation of latent viral infections (eg, BK virus-associated nephropathy). Progressive multifocal leukoencephalopathy (PML) reported. Reduce immunosuppression if BK virus nephropathy is suspected or PML develops. Interstitial lung disease (eg, pneumonitis, bronchiolitis obliterans organizing pneumonia, pulmonary fibrosis) reported. Safety and efficacy of de novo use without cyclosporine is not established in renal transplant patients. Provide 1 year prophylaxis for *Pneumocystis carinii* pneumonia and 3 months for cytomegalovirus after transplant. Patient sample concentration values from different assays may not be interchangeable. Increased risk of skin cancer; limit exposure to sunlight and UV light. Caution in elderly.

ADVERSE REACTIONS: Infection, lymphoma, malignancy, graft loss, peripheral edema, hypertriglyceridemia, HTN, constipation, hypercholesterolemia, increased creatinine, abdominal pain, diarrhea, headache.

INTERACTIONS: See Boxed Warning. CYP3A4 and P-gp inducers may decrease sirolimus concentrations. CYP3A4 and P-gp inhibitors may increase sirolimus concentrations. Avoid with strong inhibitors (eg, ketoconazole, voriconazole, itraconazole, erythromycin, telithromycin, clarithromycin) and strong inducers (eg, rifampin, rifabutin) of CYP3A4 and P-gp. May increase levels with cyclosporine, bromocriptine, cimetidine, cisapride, clotrimazole, danazol, diltiazem, fluconazole, HIV-protease inhibitors (eg, ritonavir, indinavir), metoclopramide, nicardipine, troleandomycin, and verapamil. May decrease levels with carbamazepine, phenobarbital, phenytoin, rifapentine, St. John's wort. May increase verapamil concentration. Vaccines may be less effective; avoid live vaccines. Increased risk of angioedema with angiotensin converting anzyme inhibitors. Increase risk of calcineurin inhibitor-induced hemolytic uremic syndrome/thrombotic thrombocytopenic purpura/thrombotic microangiography. Do not dilute or take with grapefruit juice. Caution with other nephrotoxic drugs (eg, aminoglycosides, amphotericin B). Monitor for possible development of rhabdomyolysis with HMG-CoA inhibitor and/or fibrate.

PREGNANCY: Category C, not for use in nursing.

MECHANISM OF ACTION: Immunosuppressant; inhibits T-lymphocyte activation and proliferation that occurs in response to antigenic and cytokine (interleukin [IL]-2, IL-4, and IL-15) stimulation by a mechanism distinct from that of other immunosuppressants. Also inhibits antibody production.

PHARMACOKINETICS: Absorption: (Sol) AUC=194ng•hr/mL, C_{max}=14.4ng/mL, T_{max}=2.1 hrs. (Tab) AUC=230ng•hr/mL, C_{max}=15ng/mL, T_{max}=3.5 hrs. Different pharmacokinetic data resulted from concentration-controlled trials of pediatric renal transplants. **Distribution:** V_d=12L/kg; plasma protein binding (92%). **Metabolism:** Intestinal wall and liver (extensive) via O-demethylation and hydroxylation; hydroxy, demethyl, and hydroxymethyl (major metabolites). **Elimination:** Feces (91%), urine (2.2%); $T_{1/2}$=62 hrs.

NURSING CONSIDERATIONS

Assessment: Assess for drug hypersensitivity, immunologic risk, hepatic impairment, body weight/body mass index, hyperlipidemia, infections, pregnancy/nursing status, and possible drug interactions.

Monitoring: Monitor for infections including opportunistic infections and activation of latent infections, development of PML, lymphoma/lymphoproliferative disease, other malignancies particularly of the skin, signs and symptoms of graft loss, hypersensitivity reactions, interstitial lung disease, and hyperlipidemia. Monitor trough concentrations especially in patients with altered drug metabolism, who weigh <40kg, and with hepatic impairment, and when a change is made during concurrent administration of strong CYP3A4 inducers or inhibitors. Monitor urinary protein excretion, renal/hepatic functions, cholesterol, TG, and BP.

Patient Counseling: Instruct to avoid prolonged exposure to sunlight and UV light. Instruct not to take when nursing and inform of the potential risks with pregnancy; instruct to use effective contraception prior to, during therapy and 12 weeks after therapy has been stopped. Inform to take with/without food, but do not crush, chew, or split.

Administration: Oral route. Give consistently with or without food. (Tab) Do not crush, chew, or split. (Sol) Refer to PI for proper dilution and administration. **Storage:** (Sol) 2-8°C (36-46°F), should be used within 1 month once opened. May store up to 25°C (77°F) for a short period of time (eg, not >15 days). (Tab) 20-25°C (68-77°F). Protect from light.

RAZADYNE ER

RX

galantamine hbr (Ortho-McNeil)

OTHER BRAND NAMES: Razadyne (Ortho-McNeil)
THERAPEUTIC CLASS: Acetylcholinesterase inhibitor

INDICATIONS: Treatment of mild to moderate dementia of the Alzheimer's type.

DOSAGE: *Adults:* (Sol, Tab) Initial: 4mg bid with am and pm meals. Titrate: Increase to 8mg bid after 4 weeks if tolerated, then increase to 12mg bid after 4 weeks if tolerated. Usual: 16-24mg/day. Max: 24mg/day. (Cap, ER) Initial: 8mg qd with am meal. Titrate: Increase to 16mg qd after 4 weeks, then increase to 24mg qd after 4 weeks if tolerated. Usual: 16-24mg/day. Max: 24mg/day. If therapy is interrupted, restart at lowest dose and increase to current dose. Moderate Renal/Hepatic Impairment (Child-Pugh: 7-9): Caution during dose titration. Max: 16mg/day. Avoid use with severe renal (CrCl <9mL/min) and severe hepatic impairment (Child-Pugh: 10-15).

HOW SUPPLIED: Sol: (Razadyne) 4mg/mL [100mL]; Tab: (Razadyne) 4mg, 8mg, 12mg. Cap, Extended-Release: (Razadyne ER) 8mg, 16mg, 24mg.

WARNINGS/PRECAUTIONS: Vagotonic effects; caution with supraventricular conduction disorder. May cause bradycardia and/or heart block. Caution with asthma or obstructive pulmonary disease. Monitor for active or occult GI bleeding and ulcers due to increased gastric acid secretion. Risk of generalized convulsions or bladder outflow obstruction. Ensure adequate fluid intake during treatment. Deaths reported with mild cognitive impairment.

ADVERSE REACTIONS: N/V, diarrhea, anorexia, weight loss, fatigue, dizziness, headache, depression, insomnia, abdominal pain, dyspepsia, UTI.

INTERACTIONS: Potential to interfere with anticholinergics. Synergistic effect with succinylcholine, other cholinesterase inhibitors, similar neuromuscular blockers, or cholinergic agonists (eg, bethanechol). Increased levels with cimetidine, ketoconazole, and paroxetine. Caution with drugs that slow HR due to vagotonic effects. Monitor for GI bleeding with NSAIDs.

PREGNANCY: Category B, not for use in nursing.

MECHANISM OF ACTION: Unknown; suspected to inhibit acetylcholinesterase-enhancing cholinergic function by increasing concentration of acetylcholine through reversible inhibition of its hydrolysis.

PHARMACOKINETICS: Absorption: Rapid and complete, bioavailability (90%), T_{max}=1 hr. **Distribution:** V_d=175L; plasma protein binding (18%). **Metabolism:** Liver (glucuronidation). CYP450 enzymes: 2D6, 3A4. **Elimination:** Urine (unchanged); $T_{1/2}$=7 hrs.

NURSING CONSIDERATIONS

Assessment: Assess for drug hypersensitivity, cardiovascular conduction defects, GI bleeding, ulcer disease, severe asthma or COPD, renal/hepatic function, and possible drug interactions.

Monitoring: Monitor closely for symptoms of active or occult GI bleeding, and cardiac conduction defects. Monitor for common adverse events (eg, N/V, anorexia, dizziness, syncope).

Patient Counseling: Take drug preferably with morning and evening meals. Ensure adequate fluid intake during treatment. If therapy has been interrupted for several days or longer, physician must restart patient at lowest dose and gradually increase to current dose. Report any adverse effects.

Administration: Oral route. **Storage:** 25°C (77°F); excursions permitted to 15-30°C (59-86°F). Do not freeze.

R

REBETOL   RX
ribavirin (Schering)

> Not for monotherapy treatment of chronic hepatitis C (CHC) virus infection. Primary toxicity is hemolytic anemia. Anemia associated with therapy may result in worsening of cardiac disease and lead to fatal and nonfatal myocardial infarctions (MI). Avoid with significant or unstable cardiac disease. Contraindicated in women who are pregnant and male partners of pregnant women. Extreme care must be taken to avoid pregnancy during therapy and for 6 months after completion of therapy. Use at least 2 reliable forms of effective contraception during therapy and 6 months after d/c.

THERAPEUTIC CLASS: Nucleoside analogue

INDICATIONS: In combination with interferon alfa-2b (pegylated and nonpegylated) for treatment of CHC in patients ≥3 yrs with compensated liver disease.

DOSAGE: *Adults:* Combination Therapy with Peg-Intron: 800-1400mg/day PO based on body weight (Refer to PI). With Peg-Intron 1.5mcg/kg/week SQ. Interferon Alfa-Naive: Genotype 1: Treat for 48 weeks. Genotype 2 and 3: Treat for 24 weeks. Retreatment: Treat for 48 weeks, regardless of HCV genotype. Combination Therapy with Intron A: ≤75kg: 400mg qam and 600mg qpm. >75kg: 600mg qam and 600mg qpm. With Intron A 3 million IU three times weekly SQ. Interferon Alfa-Naive: Treat for 24-48 weeks. Retreatment: Treat for 24 weeks. Individualize duration of treatment depending on baseline disease characteristics, response to therapy, and tolerability of regimen. Elderly: Start at lower end of dosing range. Refer to PI for dose modifications and d/c.
Pediatrics: ≥3 yrs: Combination Therapy with Peg-Intron/Intron A: <47kg: (Sol) 15mg/kg/day

divided into two doses. 47-59kg: 400mg qam and 400mg qpm. 60-73kg: 400mg qam and 600mg qpm. >73kg: 600mg qam and 600mg qpm. With Intron A 3 million IU/m² three times weekly SQ for 25-61kg (refer to adult dosing for >61kg) or Peg-Intron 60mcg/m²/week SQ. May use sol regardless of body weight. Genotype 1: Treat for 48 weeks. Genotype 2 or 3: Treat for 24 weeks. Remain on pediatric dosing if reached 18th birthday while receiving therapy in combination with Peg-Intron. Refer to PI for dose modifications and d/c.

HOW SUPPLIED: Cap: 200mg; Sol: 40mg/mL [100mL]

CONTRAINDICATIONS: Women who are or may become pregnant and men whose female partners are pregnant, autoimmune hepatitis, hemoglobinopathies (eg, thalassemia major, sickle cell anemia), CrCl <50mL/min, and combination with didanosine.

WARNINGS/PRECAUTIONS: Suspend therapy in patients with signs and symptoms of pancreatitis and d/c therapy in patients with confirmed pancreatitis. Pulmonary symptoms (eg, dyspnea, pulmonary infiltrates, pneumonitis, pulmonary HTN, pneumonia, sarcoidosis, or exacerbation of sarcoidosis) reported; closely monitor or d/c therapy if appropriate. Alpha interferons may induce or aggravate ophthalmologic disorders (eg, decrease or loss of vision, retinopathy). Perform eye examination in all patients prior to therapy, periodically with preexisting ophthalmologic disorders (eg, diabetic or hypertensive retinopathy), and if symptoms develop during therapy. D/C if new or worsening ophthalmologic disorders develop. Severe decreases in neutrophil and platelet counts, and hematologic, endocrine (eg, TSH), and hepatic abnormalities may occur in combination with Peg-Intron; perform hematology and blood chemistry testing prior to therapy and periodically thereafter. Dental/periodontal disorders reported with combination therapy. Weight changes and growth inhibition reported with combination therapy in pediatric patients. Combination therapy associated with significant adverse reactions (eg, severe depression, suicidal ideation, suppression of bone marrow function, autoimmune and infectious disorders, diabetes). Caution with preexisting cardiac disease; d/c if cardiovascular status deteriorates. Caution in elderly. (Cap) Not for treatment of HIV infection, adenovirus, respiratory syncytial virus, parainfluenza, or influenza infections.

ADVERSE REACTIONS: Hemolytic anemia, headache, fatigue/asthenia, rigors, fever, N/V, anorexia, myalgia, arthralgia, insomnia, irritability, depression, neutropenia.

INTERACTIONS: See Contraindications. Closely monitor for toxicities (eg, hepatic decompensation, anemia) with nucleoside reverse transcriptase inhibitors (NRTIs); consider d/c or reduce dose. May inhibit phosphorylation of lamivudine, stavudine, and zidovudine. Severe pancytopenia, bone marrow suppression, and myelotoxicity reported with azathioprine.

PREGNANCY: Category X, not for use in nursing.

MECHANISM OF ACTION: Nucleoside analogue; not established. Has direct antiviral activity in tissue culture against many RNA viruses; increases mutation frequency in the genomes of several viruses and ribavirin triphosphate inhibits HCV polymerase in a biochemical reaction.

PHARMACOKINETICS: Absorption: Rapid and extensive; (Cap) C_{max}=782ng/mL, T_{max}=1.7 hrs, AUC=13400ng•h/mL, absolute bioavailability (64%). (Sol) C_{max}=872ng/mL, T_{max}=1 hr, AUC=14098ng•h/mL. **Distribution:** (Cap) V_d=2825L. **Metabolism:** Nucleated cells (phosphorylation); deribosylation and amide hydrolysis. **Elimination:** Urine (61%), feces (12%). (Cap) $T_{1/2}$=43.6 hrs.

NURSING CONSIDERATIONS

Assessment: Assess for history of hemoglobinopathies (eg, thalassemia major, sickle-cell anemia), depression, hepatic/renal/pulmonary function, autoimmune hepatitis, pregnancy status (including female partners of male patients), nursing status, preexisting ophthalmologic disorders, cardiac disease, and possible drug interactions. Prior to initiation, conduct pregnancy test, hematologic tests (CBC with differential, Hct, Hgb, neutrophil and platelet count), blood chemistries (LFTs, TSH), ECG in patients with preexisting cardiac disease, and eye examination. Confirm use of ≥2 reliable forms of effective contraception.

Monitoring: Monitor CBC, LFTs, TSH, platelet and neutrophil count, ECG and HCV-RNA periodically. Monitor height and weight in pediatrics. Obtain Hct and Hgb (Week 2 and 4, more if needed). Perform pregnancy test monthly and 6 months after d/c of therapy (including female partners of male patients). Monitor the use of effective contraception during therapy and for 6 months after therapy. Schedule regular dental exams. Perform periodic ophthalmologic exams in patients with preexisting ophthalmologic disorders. Monitor for anemia, worsening of cardiac disease, MI, pancreatitis, renal/hepatic dysfunction, cardiovascular deterioration, pulmonary impairment, new/worsening ophthalmologic disorders, dental/periodontal disorders, suicidal ideation, depression, bone marrow suppression, autoimmune and infectious disorders, diabetes, and other adverse reactions. Monitor patients >50 yrs and those with impaired renal function with respect to development of anemia.

Patient Counseling: Inform that anemia may develop. Advise that laboratory evaluations are required prior to starting therapy and periodically thereafter. Instruct to take with food and keep well hydrated; do not open, break, or crush capsules before swallowing. Inform of pregnancy risks; instruct to use ≥2 forms of contraception during therapy and 6 months after d/c of therapy (including female partners of male patients). Advise to notify physician in the event of pregnancy. Counsel on risk/benefits associated with treatment. Inform that appropriate precautions to prevent hepatitis C virus transmission should be taken. Inform to take missed doses as soon as possible during the same day; do not double next dose. Advise to have a regular dental examinations.

Administration: Oral route. **Storage:** Cap: 25°C (77°F); excursions permitted to 15-30°C (59-86°F). Sol: 2-8°C (36-46°F) or 25°C (77°F); excursions permitted to 15-30°C (59-86°F).

REBIF
interferon beta-1a (EMD Serono)

RX

THERAPEUTIC CLASS: Biological response modifier

INDICATIONS: Treatment of patients with relapsing forms of multiple sclerosis (MS) to decrease the frequency of clinical exacerbations and delay the accumulation of physical disability.

DOSAGE: *Adults:* Initial: 20% of prescribed dose SQ TIW. Titrate: Increase over a 4-week period to either 22mcg or 44mcg SQ TIW. Administer at the same time (preferably late afternoon or pm) on the same 3 days at least 48 hrs apart each week. Refer to PI for full schedule for patient titration. If With Leukopenia/Elevated LFTs: Reduce dose or d/c until toxicity resolves. Elderly: Start at lower end of dosing range.

HOW SUPPLIED: Inj, prefilled syringe: 22mcg, 44mcg; (Titration Pack) 8.8mcg and 22mcg

CONTRAINDICATIONS: Hypersensitivity to human albumin.

WARNINGS/PRECAUTIONS: Caution with depression. Increased frequency of depression and suicidal ideation/attempts reported; d/c if depression develops. Liver injury reported; reduce dose if SGPT >5X ULN, or d/c if jaundice or other symptoms of liver dysfunction appear. Caution with active liver disease, alcohol abuse, increased serum SGPT (>2.5X ULN) or history of significant liver disease. Mild to severe allergic reactions, including anaphylaxis reported (some occurred after prolonged use). Contains albumin; may carry extremely remote risk of viral disease and Creutzfeldt-Jakob disease (CJD) transmission. Seizures, leukopenia, and new or worsening thyroid abnormalities reported; monitor regularly for these conditions. Caution with preexisting seizure disorders and in elderly.

ADVERSE REACTIONS: Injection-site reactions, influenza-like symptoms, headache, fatigue, fever, rigors, chest pain, back pain, myalgia, abdominal pain, depression, elevation of liver enzymes, hematologic abnormalities.

INTERACTIONS: May cause neutropenia and lymphopenia with myelosuppressive agents. Consider potential for hepatic injury with hepatotoxic agents or new agents added to the regimen.

PREGNANCY: Category C, caution in nursing.

MECHANISM OF ACTION: Biological response modifier; mechanism in MS not established. Binding of interferon β to its receptors initiates a complex cascade of intracellular events that leads to the expression of numerous interferon-induced gene products and markers, including 2', 5'-oligoadenylate synthetase, β_2-microglobulin and neopterin, which may mediate some of the biological activities.

PHARMACOKINETICS: Absorption: C_{max}=5.1 IU/mL, T_{max}=16 hrs, AUC_{0-96}=294 IU•hr/mL. **Elimination:** $T_{1/2}$=69 hrs.

NURSING CONSIDERATIONS

Assessment: Assess for history of drug hypersensitivity, depression, liver disease, alcohol abuse, thyroid dysfunction, preexisting seizure disorder, myelosuppression, pregnancy/nursing status, and possible drug interactions.

Monitoring: Monitor for signs/symptoms of depression, suicidal ideation, suicide attempts, allergic reaction, and seizures. Monitor CBC and LFTs at 1, 3, and 6 month after initiation, then periodically thereafter. Monitor thyroid function tests q6 months or as clinically indicated.

Patient Counseling: Inform about risks/benefits of drug; report any adverse reactions. Instruct not to change dosage or schedule without consulting physician. Advise to notify physician if symptoms of depression and/or suicidal ideation occur. Inform about the abortifacient potential of the drug; advise to notify physician if pregnant/nursing or plan to become pregnant. Instruct on aseptic technique when administering drug and on importance of proper syringe disposal. Inform of the importance of rotating injection sites.

Administration: SQ route. Refer to PI for instruction on preparation and self-injection. **Storage:** 2-8°C (36-46°F). Do not freeze. If refrigerator is not available, store at or below 25°C (77°F) for up to 30 days, away from heat and light.

RECLAST   RX
zoledronic acid (Novartis)

THERAPEUTIC CLASS: Bisphosphonate

INDICATIONS: Treatment and prevention of osteoporosis in postmenopausal women, glucocorticoid-induced osteoporosis in men and women who are either initiating or continuing systemic glucocorticoids in a daily dosage equivalent to 7.5mg or greater of prednisone, and who are expected to remain on glucocorticoids for at least 12 months. Treatment to increase bone mass in men with osteoporosis and of Paget's disease of bone in men and women.

DOSAGE: *Adults:* Infuse IV over no less than 15 min at a constant rate. Treatment of Osteoporosis (Men/Postmenopausal Women) and Treatment/Prevention of Glucocorticoid-Induced Osteoporosis: 5mg once a yr. Paget's disease: 5mg. Refer to PI for retreatment. Prevention of Osteoporosis (Postmenopausal Women): 5mg once q2 yrs. Recommended Intake of Calcium in Osteoporosis: At least 1200mg/day. Recommended Intake of Vitamin D in Osteoporosis: 800-1000 IU/day. Recommended Intake of Calcium in Paget's Disease: 1500mg/day in 2-3 divided doses, especially during the 2 weeks following administration. Refer to PI for information on retreatment. Recommended Intake of Vitamin D in Paget's Disease: 800 IU/day, especially during the 2 weeks following administration. May give acetaminophen to reduce acute phase reaction symptoms.

HOW SUPPLIED: Inj: 5mg/100mL

CONTRAINDICATIONS: Hypocalcemia, CrCl <35mL/min, and with evidence of acute renal impairment.

WARNINGS/PRECAUTIONS: Contains same active ingredient as Zometa; do not treat concomitantly. Treat preexisting hypocalcemia and disturbances of mineral metabolism prior to treatment; clinical monitoring of calcium and mineral levels highly recommended. Risk of hypocalcemia in Paget's disease. Withhold therapy until normovolemic status has been achieved if history or physical signs suggest dehydration. Caution with chronic renal impairment. Acute renal impairment, including renal failure, may occur, especially in patients with preexisting renal compromise, advanced age, or severe dehydration; calculate CrCl based on actual body weight before each dose, and assess fluid status in patients at increased risk of acute renal failure. Osteonecrosis of the jaw (ONJ) reported; perform routine oral exam prior to treatment, and avoid invasive dental procedures while on treatment in patients with concomitant risk factors if possible. Atypical, low-energy, or low trauma fractures of the femoral shaft reported; evaluate patients with thigh/groin pain to rule out incomplete femur fracture and consider interruption of therapy. Avoid pregnancy; may cause fetal harm. Musculoskeletal (bone, joint, muscle) pain reported; withhold future treatment if severe symptoms develop. Caution with aspirin (ASA) sensitivity; may cause bronchoconstriction. Reevaluate the need for continued therapy on a periodic basis.

ADVERSE REACTIONS: Pain, chills, dizziness, osteoarthritis, fatigue, hypocalcemia, headache, HTN, influenza-like illness, myalgia, arthralgia, pyrexia, N/V, acute phase reaction.

INTERACTIONS: Caution with aminoglycosides; may have an additive effect to lower serum calcium levels for prolonged periods. Caution with loop diuretics; may increase risk of hypocalcemia. Caution with other nephrotoxic drugs (eg, NSAIDs) and diuretics; may cause acute renal impairment. Exposure to concomitant medications that are primarily renally excreted (eg, digoxin) may increase in patients with renal impairment.

PREGNANCY: Category D, not for use in nursing.

MECHANISM OF ACTION: Bisphosphonate; acts primarily on bone. Inhibits osteoclast-mediated bone resorption.

PHARMACOKINETICS: Distribution: Plasma protein binding (28% at 200ng/mL), (53% at 50ng/mL). **Elimination:** Urine (39% within 24 hrs); $T_{1/2}$=146 hrs.

NURSING CONSIDERATIONS

Assessment: Assess for hypocalcemia and disturbances of mineral metabolism, renal function, risk factors for developing renal impairment and ONJ, hypersensitivity, ASA sensitivity, pregnancy/nursing status, and possible drug interactions. Calculate CrCl based on actual body weight before each dose. Assess fluid status in patients at increased risk of acute renal failure. Perform oral exam and consider appropriate preventive dentistry in patients with history of concomitant risk factors.

Monitoring: Monitor for signs and symptoms of hypocalcemia, acute phase reactions, ONJ, atypical femur fracture, musculoskeletal pain, bronchoconstriction, and other adverse events that may develop. Monitor renal function, serum calcium/mineral levels, and alkaline phosphatase.

Patient Counseling: Inform about benefits and risks of therapy, and the importance of calcium and vitamin D supplementation. Notify physician if kidney problems exist, taking any other medications, unable to take calcium supplements, had surgery to remove some or all of parathyroid glands, had sections of intestine removed, and sensitive to ASA. Inform that drug may cause fetal harm; avoid becoming pregnant and breastfeeding. Advise on day of treatment to eat and drink normally (at least 2 glasses of fluid [eg, water] within a few hrs prior to infusion). Instruct to contact physician or dentist if persistent pain and/or non-healing sore of the mouth or jaw, fever, flu-like symptoms, myalgia, arthralgia, headache, bone/joint/muscle pain, and other adverse events develop.

Administration: IV route. Hydrate prior to administration. IV infusion should be followed by a 10mL normal saline flush of the IV line. Do not allow to come in contact with any calcium or other divalent cation-containing sol. Administer as a single IV sol through a separate vented infusion line. Inspect visually for particulate matter and discoloration prior to administration. **Storage:** 25°C (77°F); excursions permitted to 15-30°C (59-86°F). Stable for 24 hrs at 2-8°C (36-46°F) after opening. If refrigerated, allow to reach room temperature before administration.

RECOMBIVAX HB
hepatitis B (recombinant) (Merck)

RX

OTHER BRAND NAMES: Recombivax HB Adult (Merck) - Recombivax HB Dialysis (Merck) - Recombivax HB Pediatric/Adolescent (Merck)

THERAPEUTIC CLASS: Vaccine

INDICATIONS: Vaccination against infection caused by all known subtypes of hepatitis B virus.

DOSAGE: *Adults:* ≥20 yrs: 3-Dose Regimen: 10mcg IM into the deltoid muscle at 0, 1, 6 months. May be given SQ if at risk of hemorrhage. Predialysis/Dialysis (Dialysis Formulation): 40mcg at 0, 1, 6 months; consider booster/revaccination if anti-hepatitis B surface (HBs) level <10 mIU/mL 1-2 months after third dose. Known/Presumed Exposure to Hepatitis B Surface Antigen (HBsAg): Follow 3-Dose Regimen giving first dose within 7 days of exposure. Give 0.06mL/kg hepatitis B immune globulin (HBIG) immediately after exposure or within 24 hrs IM at a separate site. *Pediatrics:* Give IM into anterolateral thigh in infants/young children. May be given SQ if at risk of hemorrhage. 0-19 yrs: 3-Dose Regimen (Pediatric/Adolescent Formulation) 5mcg at 0, 1, 6 months. 11-15 yrs: 2-Dose Regimen (Adult Formulation): 10mcg at 0 and 4-6 months. Infants Born to HBsAg Positive/Unknown Status Mothers: Follow 3-Dose Regimen above. Give 0.5mL HBIG immediately in the opposite anterolateral thigh if the mother is determined to be HBsAg positive within 7 days of delivery. Known/Presumed Exposure to Hepatitis B Surface Antigen (HBsAg): Follow 3-Dose Regimen giving first dose within 7 days of exposure. Give 0.06mL/kg hepatitis B immune globulin (HBIG) immediately after exposure or within 24 hrs IM at a separate site.

HOW SUPPLIED: Inj: (Pediatric/Adolescent) 5mcg/0.5mL, (Adult) 10mcg/mL, (Dialysis) 40mcg/mL

CONTRAINDICATIONS: Hypersensitivity to yeast.

WARNINGS/PRECAUTIONS: Do not continue therapy if hypersensitivity occurs after inj. May not prevent hepatitis B with unrecognized infection at time of vaccination. Anaphylactoid reactions may occur; have epinephrine (1:1000) immediately available. Tip cap, vial stopper, and syringe plunger stopper may contain natural latex rubber, which may cause allergic reactions in latex-sensitive individuals; use with caution. Delay use with serious active infection (eg, febrile illness). Caution with severely compromised cardiopulmonary status and in those where a febrile or systemic reaction could pose a significant risk. Do not give intradermally or IV. Avoid injection of a blood vessel.

ADVERSE REACTIONS: Irritability, fever, diarrhea, fatigue/weakness, diminished appetite, rhinitis, inj-site reactions.

PREGNANCY: Category C, caution in nursing.

MECHANISM OF ACTION: Vaccine; may produce immune response for protection against infection caused by all known subtypes of hepatitis B virus.

NURSING CONSIDERATIONS

Assessment: Assess current health status, hypersensitivity to yeast or any component of the vaccine, and pregnancy/nursing status. Review immunization history for possible vaccine sensitivity and previous vaccination-related adverse reactions.

Monitoring: Monitor for signs/symptoms of hypersensitivity reactions, inj-site reactions, immune response, and for systemic reactions. Perform annual antibody testing in hemodialysis patients to assess the need for booster doses.

Patient Counseling: Inform of potential benefits/risks of vaccination and the importance of completing the immunization series. Instruct to report inj-site reactions or any severe adverse reactions to physician.

Administration: IM route. May be given SQ if at risk of hemorrhage. Shake well before use. Inspect for particulate matter and discoloration prior to administration. **Storage:** 2-8°C (36-46°F). Do not freeze.

REFLUDAN   RX
lepirudin (Bayer Healthcare)

THERAPEUTIC CLASS: Thrombin inhibitor

INDICATIONS: Anticoagulant for heparin-induced thrombocytopenia (HIT) and associated thromboembolic disease.

DOSAGE: *Adults:* LD: 0.4mg/kg (max 44mg) IV over 15-20 seconds. Initial: 0.15mg/kg/hr (max 16.5mg/hr) continuous infusion for 2-10 days. Adjust dose based on aPTT. If aPTT is above target range, stop infusion for 2 hrs and restart at 50% of previous rate. Check aPTT 4 hrs later. If aPTT is below target range, increase rate in steps of 20% and check aPTT 4 hrs later. Do not exceed 0.21mg/kg/hr. Renal Impairment: LD: 0.2mg/kg. Initial: CrCl 45-60mL/min: 0.075mg/kg/hr. CrCl 30-44mL/min: 0.045mg/kg/hr. CrCl 15-29 mL/min: 0.0225mg/kg/hr. CrCl <15mL/min/ Hemodialysis: Avoid or stop infusion. Concomitant Thrombolytic Therapy: LD: 0.2mg/kg. Initial: 0.1mg/kg/hr.

HOW SUPPLIED: Inj: 50mg

WARNINGS/PRECAUTIONS: Risk of bleeding. Weigh risks/benefits with recent puncture of large vessels or organ biopsy, anomaly of vessels or organs, recent cerebrovascular accident (CVA), stroke, intracerebral surgery or other neuraxial procedures, severe uncontrolled HTN, bacterial endocarditis, advanced renal impairment, hemorrhagic diathesis, recent major surgery or bleeding. Avoid with baseline aPTT ≥2.5. Monitor aPTT 4 hrs after initiating infusion and at least once daily. Liver injury may enhance anticoagulant effects. Antihirudin antibodies reported; may increase anticoagulant effects.

ADVERSE REACTIONS: Hemorrhagic events (eg, bleeding, anemia, hematoma, hematuria, epistaxis, hemothorax), fever, liver dysfunction, pneumonia, sepsis, allergic skin reactions, multiorgan failure.

INTERACTIONS: Thrombolytics increase risk of life-threatening intracranial bleeding or other bleeding complications and may enhance the effect on aPTT prolongation. Increased risk of bleeding with coumarin derivatives and other drugs that affect platelet function.

PREGNANCY: Category B, not for use in nursing.

MECHANISM OF ACTION: Thrombin inhibitor; binds to thrombin and thereby blocks its thrombogenic activity.

PHARMACOKINETICS: Absorption: C_{max}=1500ng/mL. **Distribution:** V_d=12.2L. **Metabolism:** Catabolic hydrolysis. **Elimination:** Urine (48%); $T_{1/2}$=1.3 hrs.

NURSING CONSIDERATIONS

Assessment: Assess for bleeding risk (eg, recent puncture of large vessels, recent cerebrovascular accident, severe uncontrolled HTN, bacterial endocarditis, hemorrhagic diasthesis), presence of hepatic/renal dysfunction, nursing status, and drug interactions. Obtain baseline aPTT ratio.

Monitoring: Monitor for signs/symptoms of bleeding complications (eg, intracranial bleeding) and allergic reactions (eg, anaphylactic reactions). Monitor aPTT ratio 4 hrs after start of infusion and perform once daily thereafter during treatment.

Patient Counseling: Instruct to notify physician immediately if develop any type of allergic reaction (eg, anaphylaxis). Advise about increased risk of bleeding during therapy. Laboratory monitoring is needed during therapy.

Administration: IV route. Do not mix with other drugs. Reconstitute: 1) Use Sterile Water for Inj, USP; or 0.9% for NaCl Inj, USP. 2) For rapid, complete reconstitution, inject 1mL of diluent into the vial and shake it gently. 3) Further dilute to final concentration of 5mg/mL. Dilute using 0.9% NaCl Inj USP, or 5% Dextrose Inj USP. 4) Warm to room temperature prior to administration. **Storage:** Unopened vials: 2-25°C (35.6-77°F). Reconstituted: Use immediately; will remain stable for 24 hrs at room temperature.

RELENZA   RX
zanamivir (GlaxoSmithKline)

THERAPEUTIC CLASS: Neuraminidase inhibitor

INDICATIONS: Treatment of uncomplicated acute illness due to influenza A and B virus in patients ≥7 yrs who have been symptomatic for no more than 2 days. Prophylaxis of influenza in patients ≥5 yrs.

DOSAGE: *Adults:* Treatment: 2 inh (10mg) q12h for 5 days. Take 2 doses on 1st day at least 2 hrs apart, then 12 hrs apart on subsequent days. Prophylaxis: Administer at same time each day. Community Outbreaks: 2 inh (10mg) qd for 28 days. Household Setting: 2 inh (10mg) qd for 10 days.
Pediatrics: Treatment: ≥7 yrs: 2 inh (10mg) q12h for 5 days. Take 2 doses on 1st day at least 2 hrs apart, then 12 hrs apart on subsequent days. Prophylaxis: ≥5 yrs: Administer at same time each day. Community Outbreaks: 2 inh (10mg) qd for 28 days. Household Setting: 2 inh (10mg) qd for 10 days.

HOW SUPPLIED: Powder, Inhalation: 5mg/inh [4 blisters/disk]

CONTRAINDICATIONS: History of allergic reaction to milk proteins.

WARNINGS/PRECAUTIONS: Not a substitute for early vaccination on an annual basis. No evidence for efficacy in any illness caused by agents other than influenza viruses types A and B. Consider available information on influenza drug susceptibility patterns and treatment effects when deciding whether to use therapy. Not shown to reduce risk of transmission of influenza to others nor shown to be effective for prophylaxis in the nursing home setting. Not recommended for use with underlying airway disease (eg, asthma, chronic obstructive pulmonary disease). Serious cases of bronchospasm reported; d/c if bronchospasm or decline in respiratory function develops. Allergic-like reactions (eg, oropharyngeal edema, serious skin rashes, anaphylaxis) reported; d/c and institute appropriate treatment if an allergic reaction occurs or is suspected. Delirium and abnormal behavior reported; monitor for abnormal behavior and evaluate risks and benefits of continuing treatment if neuropsychiatric symptoms occur. Not studied with high-risk underlying medical conditions. Has not been shown to prevent serious bacterial infections initially presenting with influenza-like symptoms or that may coexist with/occur as complications during course of influenza. Must not be made into an extemporaneous sol for administration by nebulization or mechanical ventilation. Administer only using provided device.

ADVERSE REACTIONS: Bronchospasm, headache, diarrhea, nausea, sinusitis, cough, ear/nose/throat infections, nasal symptoms, throat/tonsil discomfort and pain, muscle pain, malaise, fatigue, viral respiratory infection, temperature regulation disturbances.

INTERACTIONS: Avoid administration of live attenuated influenza vaccines within 2 weeks before or 48 hrs after zanamivir unless medically indicated.

PREGNANCY: Category C, caution in nursing.

MECHANISM OF ACTION: Neuraminidase inhibitor; inhibits influenza virus neuraminidase, affecting release of viral particles.

PHARMACOKINETICS: Absorption: C_{max}=17-142ng/mL, T_{max}=1-2 hrs, AUC_{inf}=111-1364ng•hr/mL. **Distribution:** Plasma protein binding (<10%). **Elimination:** Urine (unchanged), feces (unabsorbed); $T_{1/2}$=2.5-5.1 hrs.

NURSING CONSIDERATIONS

Assessment: Assess for history of allergic reaction to milk proteins, airway disease and other underlying medical conditions, pregnancy/nursing status, and for possible drug interactions.

Monitoring: Monitor for signs/symptoms of bronchospasm, allergic reactions, neuropsychiatric events (eg, delirium, abnormal behavior), and other adverse reactions.

Patient Counseling: Advise to seek medical attention if symptoms of bronchospasm, an allergic reaction, or neuropsychiatric events (eg, seizures, confusion, unusual behavior) occur. If taking inhaled bronchodilators, counsel to use bronchodilators before drug. Inform that the use of the drug does not reduce the risk of transmission of influenza to others. Instruct on proper use of Diskhaler. If prescribed for children, instruct parents or caregivers on proper administration and supervision.

Administration: Oral inhalational route. Refer to PI for instructions for use. **Storage:** 25°C (77°F); excursions permitted to 15-30°C (59-86°F). Do not puncture any blister until taking a dose using the Diskhaler.

RELISTOR   RX
methylnaltrexone bromide (Salix)

THERAPEUTIC CLASS: Opioid antagonist

INDICATIONS: Treatment of opioid-induced constipation in patients with advanced illness who are receiving palliative care, when response to laxative therapy has not been sufficient.

DOSAGE: *Adults:* Usual: 1 dose qod PRN. Max: 1 dose/24 hrs. 38-<62kg (84-<136 lbs): 8mg. 62-114kg (136-251 lbs): 12mg. <38kg (<84 lbs) or >114kg (>251 lbs) 0.15mg/kg; calculate inj volume by multiplying weight in lbs by 0.0034 or weight in kg by 0.0075 and round up volume to nearest 0.1mL. Severe Renal Impairment (CrCl <30mL/min): Reduce dose by one-half. Do not prescribe pre-filled syringes to patients requiring dosing calculated on a mg/kg basis; prescribe only in patients requiring an 8mg or 12mg dose.

HOW SUPPLIED: Inj: 12mg/0.6mL [vial, pre-filled syringe], 8mg/0.4mL [pre-filled syringe]

CONTRAINDICATIONS: Known/suspected mechanical GI obstruction.

WARNINGS/PRECAUTIONS: D/C therapy if severe/persistent diarrhea occurs and/or worsening abdominal symptoms develop during treatment. GI perforations (eg, stomach, duodenum, colon) reported in advanced illness associated with localized/diffused reduction of structural integrity in the wall of GI tract (eg, cancer, peptic ulcer, Ogilvie's syndrome). Caution with known/suspected lesions of the GI tract. Use beyond 4 months or in patients with peritoneal catheters has not been studied.

ADVERSE REACTIONS: Abdominal pain, flatulence, nausea, dizziness, hyperhidrosis, diarrhea.

PREGNANCY: Category B, caution in nursing.

MECHANISM OF ACTION: Opioid antagonist; peripherally acting mu-opioid receptor antagonist in tissues such as GI tract, thereby decreasing constipating effects of opioids without impacting opioid-mediated analgesic effects on the CNS.

PHARMACOKINETICS: Absorption: Rapid; T_{max}=0.5 hrs. Administration of variable doses resulted in different pharmacokinetic parameters. **Distribution:** V_d=1.1L/kg; plasma protein binding (11-15.3%). **Metabolism:** Methyl-6-naltrexol isomers, methylnaltrexone sulfate (metabolites). **Elimination:** 85% unchanged; urine (approximately 50%), feces (<50%); $T_{1/2}$=8 hrs.

NURSING CONSIDERATIONS

Assessment: Assess for mechanical GI obstruction, presence of peritoneal catheters, severe renal impairment (CrCl <30mL/min), presence of advanced illness associated with localized/diffused reduction of structural integrity of the GI tract wall (eg, cancer, peptic ulcer, Ogilvie's syndrome), patients with GI tract lesions, and pregnancy/nursing status.

Monitoring: Monitor for signs/symptoms of severe/persistent diarrhea and abdominal symptoms, GI perforations (eg, stomach, duodenum, colon), and other adverse reactions. Monitor CrCl.

Patient Counseling: Instruct that usual schedule is 1 dose qod, PRN but no more frequently than 1 dose in a 24-hr period. Advise to be within close proximity to toilet facilities once drug is administered. Inform to d/c therapy if experiencing severe/persistent diarrhea and/or worsening abdominal symptoms; contact physician. Counsel that common side effects include transient abdominal pain and N/V. Inform to d/c if opioid pain medication is stopped.

Administration: SQ route. Inject in the upper arm, abdomen, or thigh. Refer to PI for preparation and administration instructions. **Storage:** 20-25°C (68-77°F); excursions permitted to 15-30°C (59-86°F). Do not freeze. Protect from light. Once drawn into the syringe, store at ambient room temperature and administer within 24 hrs if immediate administration is not possible.

RELPAX   RX
eletriptan hydrobromide (Pfizer)

THERAPEUTIC CLASS: $5-HT_{1B/1D}$ agonist

INDICATIONS: Acute treatment of migraine with or without aura.

DOSAGE: *Adults:* Individualize dose. Initial: 20 or 40mg at onset of headache. May repeat after 2 hrs if headache recurs after initial relief. Max: 40mg/dose or 80mg/day.

HOW SUPPLIED: Tab: 20mg, 40mg

CONTRAINDICATIONS: Ischemic heart disease (eg, angina pectoris, history of myocardial infarction [MI], or documented silent ischemia) or symptoms/findings consistent with ischemic heart disease, coronary artery vasospasm (eg, Prinzmetal's variant angina), or other significant underlying cardiovascular disease, cerebrovascular syndromes (eg, stroke, transient ischemic attacks), peripheral vascular disease (eg, ischemic bowel disease), uncontrolled HTN, hemiplegic/basilar migraine, use of other $5-HT_1$ agonists or ergotamine-containing/ergot-type agents (eg, dihydroergotamine, methysergide) within 24 hrs, severe hepatic impairment.

WARNINGS/PRECAUTIONS: Has potential to cause coronary artery vasospasm; do not give with documented ischemic/vasospastic coronary artery disease (CAD). Not for patients in whom unrecognized CAD is predicted by presence of risk factors (eg, HTN, hypercholesterolemia, smoker, obesity, diabetes, CAD family history, menopause, males >40 yrs) unless with a satisfactory cardiovascular evaluation; administer 1st dose under medical supervision and obtain ECG during interval immediately after administration to assess for cardiac ischemia. Monitor cardiovascular function with long-term intermittent use. Serious adverse cardiac events (eg, acute MI, life-threatening arrhythmias), cerebrovascular events, and vasospastic reactions (eg, coronary artery vasospasm, peripheral vascular ischemia, colonic ischemia) reported. Serotonin syndrome may occur; symptoms may include mental status changes, autonomic instability, neuromuscular aberrations, and GI symptoms. HTN and hypertensive crisis reported rarely. Caution with hepatic dysfunction. Possible long-term ophthalmologic effects. Avoid in elderly.

ADVERSE REACTIONS: Asthenia, dizziness, drowsiness, nausea, headache, paresthesia, dry mouth, flushing/feeling of warmth, chest tightness/pain/pressure, abdominal pain/cramps, dyspepsia, dysphagia.

INTERACTIONS: See Contraindications. Avoid use within 72 hrs of potent CYP3A4 inhibitors (eg, ketoconazole, itraconazole, nefazodone, troleandomycin, clarithromycin, ritonavir, nelfinavir). May cause additive prolonged vasospastic reaction with ergot-containing drugs. Serotonin syndrome reported with SSRIs or SNRIs. Propranolol, erythromycin, verapamil, and fluconazole may increase levels.

PREGNANCY: Category C, caution in nursing.

MECHANISM OF ACTION: Selective $5HT_{1D/1B}$ agonist; binds with high affinity to $5HT_{1D/1B/1F}$ receptors. Suspected to perform its action by (1) activation of $5\text{-}HT_{1D/1B}$ receptors located on intracranial blood vessels, including those on arteriovenous anastomoses, which leads to vasoconstriction and is correlated with relief of migraine headache, or (2) activation of $5\text{-}HT_{1D/1B}$ receptors in trigeminal system, which results in inhibition of pro-inflammatory neuropeptide release.

PHARMACOKINETICS: Absorption: Well-absorbed; absolute bioavailability (50%); T_{max}=1.5 hrs. **Distribution:** V_d=138L; plasma protein binding (85%). **Metabolism:** via CYP3A4; N-demethylated metabolite (active). **Elimination:** Urine. $T_{1/2}$= 4 hrs (parent drug), 13 hrs (metabolite).

NURSING CONSIDERATIONS

Assessment: Confirm diagnosis of migraine before therapy. Assess for ischemic heart disease (eg, angina pectoris, Prinzmetal's variant angina, MI or documented silent MI), ECG changes, or any other conditions where treatment is contraindicated or cautioned. Assess for hepatic/renal impairment, pregnancy/nursing status, and possible drug interactions.

Monitoring: Monitor for signs/symptoms of cardiac events (eg, coronary vasospasm, acute MI, arrhythmia), cerebrovascular events (eg, stroke), peripheral vascular ischemia, colonic ischemia, serotonin syndrome (eg, mental status changes), hypersensitivity reactions, ophthalmologic changes, and other adverse reactions. For patients with CAD risk factors, administration of first dose should be done in physician's office or medically staffed and equipped facility; obtain ECG during interval immediately after administration to assess for cardiac ischemia. For patients on long-term intermittent therapy or with CAD risk factors, periodically monitor cardiovascular function. Monitor BP, weight, and LFTs.

Patient Counseling: Inform about potential risks of therapy (eg, serotonin syndrome) and possible drug interactions. Advise to take exactly as prescribed. Instruct to notify physician if any adverse reactions occur, or if pregnant/nursing or plan to become pregnant.

Administration: Oral route. **Storage:** 25°C (77°F); excursions permitted to 15-30°C (59-86°F).

REMERON   RX
mirtazapine (Schering)

R

Antidepressants increased the risk of suicidal thinking and behavior (suicidality) in short-term studies in children, adolescents, and young adults with major depressive disorder (MDD) and other psychiatric disorders. Monitor and observe closely for clinical worsening, suicidality, or unusual changes in behavior in patients who are started on antidepressant therapy. Not approved for use in pediatric patients.

OTHER BRAND NAMES: RemeronSolTab (Schering)

THERAPEUTIC CLASS: Piperazino-azepine

INDICATIONS: Treatment of MDD.

DOSAGE: *Adults:* Initial: 15mg qhs. Titrate: May increase at intervals of at least 1-2 weeks. Max: 45mg/day. Reassess periodically to determine the need for maint treatment.

HOW SUPPLIED: Tab: 15mg*, 30mg*, 45mg; Tab, Disintegrating: 15mg, 30mg, 45mg *scored

CONTRAINDICATIONS: Use during or within 14 days of initiating or d/c of therapy with MAOI.

WARNINGS/PRECAUTIONS: Not approved for treatment of bipolar depression. Agranulocytosis and severe neutropenia reported; d/c if sore throat, fever, stomatitis, or other signs of infection develop, along with low WBC count. Serotonin syndrome or neuroleptic malignant syndrome (NMS)-like reactions reported, particularly with serotonergic drugs (eg, triptans), drugs that impair metabolism of serotonin, antipsychotics, and dopamine antagonists. D/C therapy and initiate supportive symptomatic treatment if mental status changes (eg, agitation, hallucinations), autonomic instability (eg, tachycardia, labile blood pressure), neuromuscular aberrations (eg, hyperreflexia, incoordination), and/or GI symptoms occur. Avoid abrupt d/c. Akathisia/psychomotor restlessness reported; increasing the dose may be detrimental in patients with these symptoms. May impair mental/physical abilities. Hyponatremia, dizziness, increased appetite, weight gain, seizures, mania/hypomania, and elevation in cholesterol, TG, and ALT reported. Caution with hepatic/renal impairment, diseases/conditions affecting metabolism or hemodynamic responses, history of seizures and mania/hypomania, and elderly. May cause orthostatic hypotension;

caution with cardiovascular (CV) or cerebrovascular disease that could be exacerbated by hypotension and conditions that predispose to hypotension (eg, dehydration, hypovolemia).

ADVERSE REACTIONS: Somnolence, increased appetite, weight gain, dizziness, dry mouth, constipation, asthenia, flu syndrome, abnormal dreams, abnormal thinking, increased cholesterol/TG levels.

INTERACTIONS: See Contraindications. Caution with drugs that may affect serotonergic neurotransmitter systems (eg, tryptophan, triptans, linezolid, serotonin reuptake inhibitors, venlafaxine, lithium, tramadol, St. John's wort). Caution with antihypertensives and drugs known to cause hyponatremia. Alcohol and diazepam increase cognitive and motor skill impairment; avoid concomitant use. Decreased levels with phenytoin, carbamazepine, and other hepatic metabolism inducers (eg, rifampicin). Cimetidine and ketoconazole may increase levels. Caution with potent CYP3A4 inhibitors, HIV protease inhibitors, azole antifungals, erythromycin, or nefazodone. Increased INR with warfarin. Not recommended with serotonin precursors (eg, tryptophan).

PREGNANCY: Category C, caution in nursing.

MECHANISM OF ACTION: Piperazino-azepine group; not established. Acts as an antagonist at central presynaptic α_2 adrenergic inhibitory autoreceptors and heteroreceptors, an action that is postulated to result in an increase in central noradrenergic and serotonergic activity.

PHARMACOKINETICS: Absorption: Rapid and complete; absolute bioavailability (50%); T_{max}=2 hrs. **Distribution:** Plasma protein binding (85%). **Metabolism:** Extensive; demethylation and hydroxylation via CYP2D6, CYP1A2, and CYP3A followed by glucuronide conjugation. **Elimination:** Urine (75%), feces (15%); $T_{1/2}$=20-40 hrs.

NURSING CONSIDERATIONS

Assessment: Assess for psychiatric history (including history of suicide, mania/hypomania, bipolar disorder, depression), CV or cerebrovascular diseases (including history of myocardial infarction, angina, or ischemic stroke), predisposition for hypotension, renal/hepatic impairment, diseases/conditions affecting metabolism or hemodynamic response, pregnancy/nursing status, and possible drug interactions.

Monitoring: Monitor for signs/symptoms of clinical worsening, suicidality, and unusual changes in behavior (especially during initial few months, and dosage changes), signs of infection (eg, sore throat, fever, stomatitis), serotonin syndrome/NMS-like reactions, altered appetite and weight, hyponatremia, and seizures. Monitor LFTs, renal function tests, absolute neutrophil count, and cholesterol and TG levels.

Patient Counseling: Inform about benefits/risks associated with therapy. Advise families and caregivers of the need for close observation for signs of clinical worsening and suicidal risks and to report such signs to physician. Warn about risk of developing agranulocytosis and instruct to contact physician if signs of infection (eg, fever, chills, sore throat, mucous membrane ulceration) develop. Caution against operating machinery/driving. Advise to continue therapy as directed, to inform physician on concomitant medications, and to avoid alcohol. Inform physician if pregnant/nursing or planning to become pregnant. (Tab, Disintegrating) Inform phenylketonurics that the tab contains phenylalanine.

Administration: Oral route. (Tab, Disintegrating) Use immediately after removal from blister. Do not split the tab. Place tab on the tongue and can be swallowed by saliva. **Storage:** 25°C (77°F); excursions permitted to 15-30°C (59-86°F). Protect from light and moisture.

R

REMICADE   RX
infliximab (Janssen)

Increased risk for developing serious infections (eg, active tuberculosis [TB], latent TB reactivation, invasive fungal infections, bacterial/viral infections, and opportunistic infections) leading to hospitalization or death, mostly with immunosuppressants (eg, methotrexate [MTX] or corticosteroids). D/C if serious infection or sepsis develops. Active/latent reactivation TB may present with disseminated, extrapulmonary disease; test for latent TB and treat prior to initiation of therapy. Invasive fungal infection reported; consider empiric antifungal therapy in patients at risk who develop severe systemic illness. Consider risks and benefits prior to therapy with chronic or recurrent infections. Monitor for development of infection during and after treatment, including development of TB in patients who tested negative for latent TB infection prior to therapy. Lymphoma and other malignancies reported in children and adolescents. Aggressive and fatal hepatosplenic T-cell lymphoma (HSTCL) reported in patients with Crohn's disease (CD) or ulcerative colitis (UC) and the majority were adolescent and young adult males; all of these patients were treated concomitantly with azathioprine or 6-mercaptopurine.

THERAPEUTIC CLASS: Monoclonal antibody/TNF-alpha receptor blocker

INDICATIONS: Reduce signs/symptoms, induce and maintain clinical remission in adults and pediatrics ≥6 yrs with moderately to severely active Crohn's disease (CD) when response to conventional therapy is inadequate. Reduce the number of draining enterocutaneous and rectovaginal fistulas and maintain fistula closure in adults with fistulizing CD. Reduce signs/symptoms, induce and maintain clinical remission in adults and pediatrics ≥6 yrs, induce and maintain mucosal healing, and eliminate corticosteroid use in adults with moderately to severely active ulcerative colitis (UC) when response to conventional therapy is inadequate. Reduce signs/symptoms, inhibit progression of structural damage, and improve physical function with moderately to severely active rheumatoid arthritis (RA) (in combination with MTX) and psoriatic arthritis. Reduce signs/symptoms with active ankylosing spondylitis (AS). Treatment of adults with chronic, severe (eg, extensive and/or disabling) plaque psoriasis who are candidates for systemic therapy and when other systemic therapies are medically less appropriate.

DOSAGE: *Adults:* CD/Fistulizing CD: Induction Regimen: 5mg/kg IV at 0, 2, and 6 weeks. Maint: 5mg/kg q8 weeks. Patients Who Respond and Lose Their Response: May increase to 10mg/kg. Consider d/c if no response by Week 14. UC/Psoriatic Arthritis (with or without MTX)/Plaque Psoriasis: Induction Regimen: 5mg/kg IV at 0, 2, and 6 weeks. Maint: 5mg/kg q8 weeks. RA (with MTX): Induction Regimen: 3mg/kg IV at 0, 2, and 6 weeks. Maint: 3mg/kg q8 weeks. Incomplete Response: May increase up to 10mg/kg or give q4 weeks. AS: Induction Regimen: 5mg/kg IV at 0, 2, and 6 weeks. Maint: 5mg/kg q6 weeks. Refer to PI for premedication regimens.
Pediatrics: ≥6 yrs: CD/UC: Induction Regimen: 5mg/kg IV at 0, 2, and 6 weeks. Maint: 5mg/kg q8 weeks. Refer to PI for premedication regimens.

HOW SUPPLIED: Inj: 100mg [20mL]

CONTRAINDICATIONS: Hypersensitivity to murine proteins. Moderate to severe heart failure (New York Heart Association Class III/IV) with doses >5mg/kg.

WARNINGS/PRECAUTIONS: Do not initiate with an active infection. Increased risk of infection with elderly or patients with comorbid conditions; consider the risks prior to therapy for those who have resided or travelled in areas of endemic TB or mycoses, and with any underlying conditions predisposing to infection. Cases of acute/chronic leukemia and non-melanoma skin cancers (NMSCs) reported. Caution in patients with moderate to severe chronic obstructive pulmonary disease (COPD), history of malignancy or in continuing treatment in patients who develop malignancy during therapy. Hepatitis B virus (HBV) reactivation reported; if reactivation occurs, d/c and initiate antiviral therapy with appropriate supportive treatment. Severe hepatic reactions (eg, acute liver failure, jaundice, hepatitis, cholestasis) reported; d/c if jaundice or marked elevations of liver enzymes (eg, ≥5X ULN) develop. New onset (rare) or worsening of heart failure reported; d/c if new or worsening symptoms of heart failure occur. Leukopenia, neutropenia, thrombocytopenia, and pancytopenia reported; seek medical attention if signs/symptoms of blood dyscrasias/infection develop and d/c if significant hematologic abnormalities. Hypersensitivity reactions reported; d/c if occur. Systemic vasculitis, seizures, and new onset/exacerbation of CNS demyelinating disorders reported (rare); consider d/c if these disorders develop. Caution when switching from one biologic disease-modifying antirheumatic drug to another; overlapping biological activity may further increase risk of infection. May cause autoantibody formation; d/c if lupus-like syndrome develops. Caution in administration of live vaccines to infants born to female patients treated with infliximab during pregnancy. All pediatric patients should be up to date with vaccinations prior to therapy. Caution in elderly.

ADVERSE REACTIONS: Infections, infusion reactions, nausea, rash, headache, sinusitis, pharyngitis, coughing, abdominal pain, diarrhea, bronchitis, dyspepsia, fatigue, HTN, arthralgia.

INTERACTIONS: See Boxed Warning. Avoid with live vaccines. Avoid use with tocilizumab; possible increased immunosuppression and increased risk of infection. Not recommended with anakinra or abatacept; may increase risk of serious infections. May decrease the incidence of anti-infliximab antibody production and increase infliximab concentrations with MTX. Monitoring of the effects (eg, warfarin) or drug concentrations (eg, cyclosporine, theophylline) and dose adjustments may be needed with CYP450 substrates with narrow therapeutic index.

PREGNANCY: Category B, not for use in nursing.

MECHANISM OF ACTION: Monoclonal antibody/TNF-α receptor blocker; neutralizes biological activity of TNF-α by binding with high affinity to the soluble and transmembrane forms of TNF-α and inhibits binding of TNF-α with its receptors.

PHARMACOKINETICS: Distribution: Crosses placenta. **Elimination:** $T_{1/2}$=7.7-9.5 days.

NURSING CONSIDERATIONS

Assessment: Assess for active/chronic/recurrent infection (eg, TB, HBV), history of an opportunistic infection, recent travel in areas of endemic TB or endemic mycoses, underlying conditions that may predispose to infection, heart failure, history of heavy smoking, history of malignancy, moderate to severe COPD, inflammatory bowel disease, presence or history of significant hematologic abnormalities, neurologic disorders, pregnancy/nursing status, known hypersensitivity to murine proteins, and for possible drug interactions. Assess for vaccination history in pediatric patients. Perform test for latent TB infection.

Monitoring: Monitor for sepsis, TB (active, reactivation, or latent), invasive fungal infections, or bacterial, viral, and other infections caused by opportunistic pathogens during and after therapy. Monitor for development of lymphoma, HSTCL, or other malignancies. Monitor for NMSCs in psoriasis patients, new or worsening symptoms of heart failure, active HBV infection, hepatotoxicity, hematological events, hypersensitivity reactions, CNS demyelinating disorders, and lupus-like syndrome. Monitor LFTs.

Patient Counseling: Advise of potential risks and benefits of therapy. Inform that therapy may lower the ability of immune system to fight infections; instruct to immediately contact physician if experience signs/symptoms of infection, including TB and HBV reactivation. Counsel about risks of lymphoma and other malignancies while on therapy. Advise to report signs of new or worsening medical conditions (eg, heart disease, neurological diseases, or autoimmune disorders) and symptoms of cytopenia (eg, bruising, bleeding, persistent fever).

Administration: IV route. Refer to PI for administration and preparation instructions. **Storage:** 2-8°C (36-46°F).

RENAGEL   RX
sevelamer HCl (Genzyme)

THERAPEUTIC CLASS: Phosphate binder

INDICATIONS: Control of serum phosphorus in patients with chronic kidney disease on dialysis.

DOSAGE: *Adults:* Take with meals. Not Taking Phosphate Binder: Initial: Serum Phosphorus >5.5 and <7.5mg/dL: 800mg tid. Serum Phosphorus ≥7.5 and <9mg/dL: 1200-1600mg tid. Serum Phosphorus ≥9mg/dL: 1600mg tid. Switching from Calcium Acetate (667mg tab): Initial: Calcium acetate 1 tab/meal: 800mg/meal. Calcium acetate 2 tabs/meal: 1200-1600mg/meal. Calcium acetate 3 tabs/meal: 2000mg-2400mg/meal. Titrate: All Patients: Adjust based on serum phosphorus concentrations. Serum Phosphorus >5.5mg/dL: Increase by 1 tab/meal at 2-week interval PRN. Serum Phosphorus 3.5-5.5mg/dL: Maintain current dose. Serum Phosphorus <3.5mg.dL: Decrease by 1 tab/meal at 2-week interval PRN. Elderly: Start at lower end of dosing range.

HOW SUPPLIED: Tab: 400mg, 800mg

CONTRAINDICATIONS: Bowel obstruction.

WARNINGS/PRECAUTIONS: Dysphagia and esophageal tablet retention reported with use of tab formulations; consider use of sus formulations in patients with history of swallowing disorder. Bowel obstruction and perforation reported. Monitor bicarbonate and chloride levels, and for reduced vitamin D, E and K (clotting factors), and folic acid levels. Caution in elderly.

ADVERSE REACTIONS: N/V, abdominal pain, constipation, diarrhea, flatulence, dyspepsia, peritonitis.

INTERACTIONS: May decrease ciprofloxacin bioavailability by 50%. Very rare cases of increased TSH levels reported with levothyroxine; monitor TSH levels. When giving oral medication where reduction in bioavailability would have a clinically significant effect on its safety or efficacy, administer the drug ≥1 hr before or 3 hrs after sevelamer hydrochloride and monitor blood levels of the drug. Caution with antiarrhythmic or anti-seizure medications.

PREGNANCY: Category C, safety not known in nursing.

MECHANISM OF ACTION: Phosphate binder; contains multiple amines which exist in a protonated form in the intestine, and bind phosphate molecules through ionic and hydrogen bonding and decrease absorption, hence lowering phosphate concentration in the serum.

NURSING CONSIDERATIONS

Assessment: Assess for presence of bowel obstruction and other GI disorders (eg, dysphagia, swallowing disorders, GI motility disorders, GI tract surgery), pregnancy/nursing status, and possible drug interactions.

Monitoring: Monitor for bowel obstruction and perforation, dysphagia, esophageal tablet retention, and other adverse reactions. Monitor for bicarbonate, chloride, and folic acid levels, and for reduced vitamins D, E, and K (clotting factors).

Patient Counseling: Inform to take with meals and adhere to prescribed diets. Instruct to take other concomitant medications dose apart from sevelamer hydrochloride. Advise to report new onset or worsening of existing constipation to physician.

Administration: Oral route. **Storage:** 25°C (77°F); excursions permitted to 15-30°C (59-86°F). Protect from moisture.

RENVELA   RX
sevelamer carbonate (Genzyme)

THERAPEUTIC CLASS: Phosphate binder

INDICATIONS: Control of serum phosphorus in patients with chronic kidney disease on dialysis.

DOSAGE: *Adults:* Take with meals. Not Taking Phosphate Binder: Initial: Serum Phosphorus >5.5 and <7.5mg/dL: 0.8g tid. Serum Phosphorus ≥7.5mg/dL: 1.6g tid. Switching from Sevelamer HCl/ Switching Between Sevelamer Carbonate Tab and Powder: Use same dose in grams. Further titration may be necessary to achieve desired phosphorus levels. Switching from Calcium Acetate (667mg tab): Initial: 0.8g/meal if previously taking 1 tab calcium acetate/meal. 1.6g/meal if previously taking 2 tabs calcium acetate/meal. 2.4g/meal if previously taking 3 tabs calcium acetate/meal. Titrate: All Patients: May increase dose by 0.8g tid with meals at 2-week intervals PRN. Elderly: Start at low end of dosing range.

HOW SUPPLIED: Tab: 800mg; Powder: 0.8g/pkt, 2.4g/pkt

CONTRAINDICATIONS: Bowel obstruction.

WARNINGS/PRECAUTIONS: Dysphagia and esophageal tablet retention reported with use of tab formulation; consider use of sus in patient with history of swallowing disorder. Bowel obstruction and perforation reported. Safety not established in patients with dysphagia, swallowing disorders, severe GI motility disorders including severe constipation, or major GI tract surgery. Monitor bicarbonate and chloride levels, and for reduced vitamins D, E, and K (clotting factors), and folic acid levels. Caution in elderly.

ADVERSE REACTIONS: N/V, diarrhea, dyspepsia, abdominal pain, flatulence, constipation.

INTERACTIONS: May decrease ciprofloxacin bioavailability by 50%; consider dosing ≥1 hr before or 3 hrs after and monitor. Rare cases of increased TSH levels reported with levothyroxine; monitor TSH levels and for signs of hypothyroidism when used concomitantly.

PREGNANCY: Category C, safety not known in nursing.

MECHANISM OF ACTION: Phosphate binder; contains multiple amines which exist in a protonated form in the intestine, and bind phosphate molecules through ionic and hydrogen bonding and decrease absorption, hence lowering phosphate concentration in the serum.

NURSING CONSIDERATIONS

Assessment: Assess for presence of bowel obstruction and other GI disorders (eg, dysphagia, swallowing disorders, GI motility disorders, GI tract surgery), pregnancy/nursing status, and possible drug interactions.

Monitoring: Monitor for bowel obstruction and perforation, dysphagia, esophageal tablet retention, bicarbonate and chloride levels, and for reduced vitamins D, E, and K (clotting factors), and folic acid levels.

Patient Counseling: Inform to take with meals and adhere to prescribed diets. If taking an oral medication where reduced bioavailability would produce a clinically significant effect on safety or efficacy, advise to take medication ≥1 hr before or 3 hrs after dosing. Advise to report new onset or worsening of existing constipation to physician.

Administration: Oral route. Powder Preparation: Empty contents of packet in cup and mix thoroughly with appropriate amount of water. Minimum Amount of Water: 0.8g: 1 oz./30mL/6 tsp/2 tbsp. 2.4g: 2 oz./60mL/4 tbsp. Vigorously stir just before drinking. Drink within 30min. **Storage:** 25°C (77°C); excursions permitted to 15-30°C (59-86°F). Protect from moisture.

R

REOPRO
abciximab (Lilly)

RX

THERAPEUTIC CLASS: Glycoprotein IIb/IIIa inhibitor

INDICATIONS: Adjunct to percutaneous coronary intervention (PCI) for prevention of cardiac ischemic complications in patients undergoing PCI or with unstable angina unresponsive to conventional therapy when PCI is planned within 24 hrs. Intended for use with aspirin and heparin.

DOSAGE: *Adults:* PCI: 0.25mg/kg IV bolus given 10-60 min before start PCI, followed by 0.125mcg/kg/min IV infusion (Max: 10mcg/min) for 12 hrs. Unstable Angina: 0.25mg/kg IV bolus followed by 10mcg/min infusion for 18-24 hrs, concluding 1 hr after PCI.

HOW SUPPLIED: Inj: 2mg/mL

CONTRAINDICATIONS: Active internal bleeding, recent (within 6 weeks) significant GI or genitourinary (GU) bleeding, cerebrovascular accident (CVA) within 2 yrs, CVA with significant residual neurological deficit, bleeding diathesis, oral anticoagulants within 7 days (unless PT ≤1.2X control), thrombocytopenia, recent (within 6 weeks) major surgery or trauma, intracranial neoplasm, arteriovenous malformation, aneurysm, severe uncontrolled HTN, history of vasculitis, IV dextran use before PCI or during an intervention. Hypersensitivity to murine proteins.

WARNINGS/PRECAUTIONS: Increased risk of bleeding. Monitor all potential bleeding sites (eg, catheter insertion sites, arterial and venous puncture sites, cutdown sites). Arterial/venous punctures, intramuscular injections, and use of urinary catheters, nasotracheal intubation, nasogastric tubes, and automatic blood pressure cuffs should be minimized. When obtaining intravenous access, non-compressible sites (eg, subclavian or jugular veins) should be avoided. Minimize vascular and other trauma. D/C if serious, uncontrollable bleeding, thrombocytopenia, or emergency surgery occurs. Anaphylaxis may occur. Antibody (HACA) formation may occur; risk of hypersensitivity, thrombocytopenia, decreased benefit with readministration. Monitor platelets, PT, APTT, ACT before infusion.

ADVERSE REACTIONS: Bleeding, thrombocytopenia, hypotension, bradycardia, N/V, back/chest pain, headache.

INTERACTIONS: Caution with other drugs that affect hemostasis (eg, thrombolytics, heparin, oral anticoagulants, NSAIDs, dipyridamole, ticlopidine). Increased risk of bleeding with anticoagulants, thrombolytics, and antiplatelets. If have HACA titers, possible allergic reactions with monoclonal antibody agents.

PREGNANCY: Category C, caution in nursing.

MECHANISM OF ACTION: Glycoprotein IIb/IIIa inhibitor; binds to the GPIIb/IIIa receptor and inhibits platelet aggregation by preventing the binding of fibrinogen, von Willebrand factor, and other adhesive molecules to GPIIb/IIIa receptor sites on activated platelets. Also binds to vitronectin receptor, which mediates the procoagulant properties of platelets and the proliferative properties of vascular endothelial and smooth muscle cells.

PHARMACOKINETICS: Elimination: $T_{1/2}$=30 min.

NURSING CONSIDERATIONS

Assessment: Assess for active internal bleeding, recent GI or GU bleeding, history of CVA, bleeding diathesis, thrombocytopenia, recent major surgery or trauma, intracranial neoplasm, arteriovenous malformation, aneurysm, severe uncontrolled HTN, presence or history of vasculitis, pregnancy/nursing status, and drug interactions. Obtain baseline prothrombin time, ACT, aPTT, and platelet counts.

Monitoring: Monitor for signs/symptoms of bleeding; document and monitor vascular puncture sites. If hematoma develops, monitor for enlargement. Monitor for allergic reactions (eg, anaphylaxis) and thrombocytopenia. Check aPTT or ACT prior to arterial sheath removal; should not be removed unless aPTT ≤50 seconds or ACT ≤175 seconds. Monitor platelet counts 2-4 hrs following bolus dose and 24 hrs prior to discharge.

Patient Counseling: Counsel to contact physician if develop hypersensitivity reactions (eg, anaphylaxis). Inform patients that they will bleed and bruise more easily and take longer to stop bleeding. Instruct to report any unusual bleeding to physician.

Administration: IV infusion. In case of hypersensitivity reaction, epinephrine, dopamine, theophylline, antihistamines, and corticosteroids should be available for immediate use. Refer to PI for administration and preparation instructions. **Storage:** Store at 2-8°C (36-46°F). Do not freeze. Do not shake. Discard any unused portion left in vial.

REQUIP   RX
ropinirole HCl (GlaxoSmithKline)

OTHER BRAND NAMES: Requip XL (GlaxoSmithKline)

THERAPEUTIC CLASS: Non-ergoline dopamine agonist

INDICATIONS: (Tab/Tab, Extended-Release) Treatment of signs and symptoms of idiopathic Parkinson's disease. (Tab) Treatment of moderate-to-severe primary Restless Legs Syndrome (RLS).

DOSAGE: *Adults:* Parkinson's: Tab: Initial: 0.25mg tid. Titrate: May increase weekly by 0.25mg tid (0.75mg/day) for 4 weeks. After Week 4, may increase weekly by 1.5mg/day up to 9mg/day, then by 3mg/day weekly to 24mg/day. Max: 24mg/day. Withdrawal: Decrease dose to bid for 4 days, then qd for 3 days. Tab, XL: Initial: 2mg qd for 1-2 weeks. Titrate: May increase by 2mg/day at ≥1 week intervals, depending on therapeutic response and tolerability. Max: 24mg/day. Swallow whole; do not chew, crush, or divide. Switching from Immediate-Release (IR) to XL: Initial dose should match total daily dose of IR formulation. Refer to PI for conversion from IR to XL. RLS: Tab: Initial: 0.25mg qd, 1-3 hrs before bedtime. Titrate: 0.5mg qd Days 3-7, 1mg qd Week 2, then increase by 0.5mg weekly. Max: 4mg.

HOW SUPPLIED: Tab: 0.25mg, 0.5mg, 1mg, 2mg, 3mg, 4mg, 5mg; Tab, Extended-Release: (XL) 2mg, 4mg, 6mg, 8mg, 12mg

WARNINGS/PRECAUTIONS: (Tab/Tab, XL) Falling asleep during activities of daily living reported; if significant, d/c or warn patient to refrain from dangerous activities. Syncope, bradycardia, postural hypotension, and hallucinations reported. Caution with hepatic dysfunction. Symptom complex similar to neuroleptic malignant syndrome (NMS), fibrotic complications, and melanoma reported. (Tab, XL) May cause elevation of BP and changes in HR. May exacerbate psychosis.

ADVERSE REACTIONS: (Tab) Neuralgia, hallucinations, somnolence, vomiting, headache, edema, fatigue, syncope, orthostatic symptoms. (Tab, XL) Dyskinesia, nausea, dizziness, constipation, abdominal pain/discomfort, back pain.

INTERACTIONS: Adjust dose if CYP1A2 inhibitor or estrogen is stopped or started during treatment. Potentiated by ciprofloxacin. Decreased effects with dopamine antagonists (eg, phenothiazines, butyrophenones, thioxanthenes, metoclopramide). Caution with alcohol, CNS depressants, and sedatives which may increase drowsiness. May increase clearance with smoking. May potentiate dopaminergic side effects of L-dopa and cause or exacerbate preexisting dyskinesia.

PREGNANCY: Category C, not for use in nursing.

MECHANISM OF ACTION: Non-ergoline dopamine agonist; believed to stimulate postsynaptic D_2-type receptors within the caudate-putamen in the brain.

PHARMACOKINETICS: Absorption: Rapid; absolute bioavailability (45-55%), T_{max}=1-2 hrs (IR), 6-10 hrs (XL). **Distribution:** V_d=7.5L/kg, plasma protein binding (40%). **Metabolism:** Liver via CYP1A2 (extensive); N-despropylation and hydroxylation. **Elimination:** Urine (<10%, unchanged), $T_{1/2}$=6 hrs.

NURSING CONSIDERATIONS

Assessment: Assess for presence of sleep disorder, history of cardiovascular disease, dyskinesia, major psychotic disorder, pregnancy/nursing status and possible drug interactions. Assess LFTs, renal function tests, and CBC.

Monitoring: Perform dermatological screening periodically. Monitor eye exams and for symptoms of NMS, impulse control symptoms (eg, compulsive behaviors such as pathological gambling and hypersexuality), fibrotic complications, melanomas, signs/symptoms of postural hypotension, hallucinations.

Patient Counseling: Caution while operating machinery/driving. Counsel on potential for drowsiness, daytime sleepiness, falling asleep during activity; d/c if these events occurs. Risk of symptomatic hypotension. Take as prescribed; avoid alcohol or concurrent CNS depressants. Report lack of response or severe adverse effects. Notify physician if new or increased gambling urges, increased sexual urges, or other intense urges occur.

Administration: Oral route. **Storage:** (Tab) 20-25°C (68-77°F). Protect from light and moisture. (Tab, Extended-Release) 25°C (77°F); excursions permitted to 15-30°C (59-86°F).

RESCRIPTOR   RX
delavirdine mesylate (ViiV Healthcare)

THERAPEUTIC CLASS: Non-nucleoside reverse transcriptase inhibitor

INDICATIONS: Treatment of HIV-1 infection in combination with at least 2 other active antiretrovirals.

DOSAGE: *Adults:* Usual: 400mg (four 100mg or two 200mg tab) tid. Take with acidic beverage (eg, orange/cranberry juice) if achlorhydric.
Pediatrics: ≥16 yrs: Usual: 400mg (four 100mg or two 200mg tab) tid. Take with acidic beverage (eg, orange/cranberry juice) if achlorhydric.

HOW SUPPLIED: Tab: 100mg, 200mg

CONTRAINDICATIONS: Concomitant CYP3A substrates that are associated with serious and/or life-threatening events at elevated plasma concentrations (eg, astemizole, terfenadine, dihydroergotamine, ergonovine, ergotamine, methylergonovine, cisapride, pimozide, alprazolam, midazolam, triazolam).

WARNINGS/PRECAUTIONS: Immune reconstitution syndrome and redistribution/accumulation of body fat reported. May confer cross-resistance to the other non-nucleoside reverse transcriptase inhibitors (NNRTIs). Severe rash (eg, erythema multiforme, Stevens-Johnson syndrome) reported; d/c use if this occurs. Caution with hepatic impairment and in elderly.

ADVERSE REACTIONS: Headache, fatigue, N/V, diarrhea, increased ALT/AST, rash, maculopapular rash, pruritus, erythema, insomnia, upper respiratory infection.

INTERACTIONS: See Contraindications. Not recommended with lovastatin, simvastatin, St. John's wort, phenytoin, phenobarbital, carbamazepine, rifabutin, rifampin, or chronic use of H_2-receptor antagonists and proton pump inhibitors (PPI). Caution with HMG-CoA reductase inhibitors metabolized by CYP3A4 (eg, atorvastatin, cerivastatin); increased risk of myopathy and rhabdomyolysis. May increase levels of nelfinavir, saquinavir, clarithromycin, sildenafil, amprenavir, indinavir, lopinavir, ritonavir, amphetamines, trazodone, antiarrhythmics, warfarin (monitor INR), calcium channel blockers, atorvastatin, cerivastatin, fluvastatin, immunosuppressants, fluticasone propionate, methadone, and ethinyl estradiol. May decrease levels of didanosine. Ketoconazole, fluoxetine, and CYP3A inhibitors may increase levels. Nelfinavir, didanosine, antacids, CYP3A inducers, H$_2$-receptor antagonists, PPI, and dexamethasone may decrease levels. Concomitant use of didanosine and antacids should be separated by at least 1 hr.

PREGNANCY: Category C, not for use in nursing.

MECHANISM OF ACTION: NNRTI; binds directly to reverse transcriptase and blocks RNA-dependent and DNA-dependent DNA polymerase activities.

PHARMACOKINETICS: Absorption: Rapid; (400mg tid) C$_{max}$=35µM, AUC=180µM•hr; T$_{max}$=1 hr. Bioavailability (relative to oral sol) (85%). **Distribution:** Plasma protein binding (98%). **Metabolism:** Hepatic (N-desalkylation, pyridine hydroxylation) via CYP3A (major), 2D6. **Elimination:** (300mg tid multiple dose) Urine (51%, <5% unchanged), feces (44%); (400mg tid) T$_{1/2}$=5.8 hrs.

NURSING CONSIDERATIONS

Assessment: Assess for hepatic dysfunction, hypersensitivity, achlorhydria, pregnancy/nursing status, and possible drug interactions.

Monitoring: Monitor for severe rash or rash accompanied by symptoms (eg, fever, blistering, oral lesions, conjunctivitis, swelling, muscle joint aches), immune reconstitution syndrome (eg, opportunistic infections), cross-resistance to other NNRTIs, fat redistribution, and other adverse events.

Patient Counseling: Instruct to read patient package insert before therapy. Inform that drug is not a cure for HIV-1 infection and that they may continue to acquire illnesses associated with HIV-1 infection and it has not been shown to reduce the risk of HIV-1 transmission. Inform to take as prescribed, not to alter dose without consulting doctor. Advise patients with achlorhydria to take with acidic beverage (orange/cranberry juice). Inform to take at least 1 hr apart if taking antacids, and to take with/without food. Advise to d/c and seek medical attention if severe rash or rash with symptoms of fever, blistering, oral lesions, conjunctivitis, swelling, muscle and joint aches occur. Counsel that fat redistribution may occur. Advise to report use of any prescription or nonprescription medication or herbal products, particularly St. John's wort. Inform patients receiving sildenafil about increased risk of sildenafil-associated adverse events (eg, hypotension, visual changes, priapism). Counsel to notify physician if pregnant or breastfeeding and encourage exposed pregnant women to enroll in an Antiretroviral Pregnancy Registry.

Administration: Oral route. May disperse 100-mg tab in at least 3 oz. of water (200-mg tab is not dispersible). Refer to PI on how to prepare dispersion. **Storage:** 20-25°C (68-77°F). Protect from high humidity.

RESTASIS   RX
cyclosporine (Allergan)

THERAPEUTIC CLASS: Topical immunomodulator

INDICATIONS: To increase tear production in patients whose tear production is presumed to be suppressed due to ocular inflammation associated with keratoconjunctivitis sicca.

DOSAGE: *Adults:* Instill 1 drop bid ou, q12h. With Artificial Tears: Allow 15 min interval between products.
Pediatrics: ≥16 yrs: Instill 1 drop bid ou, q12h. With Artificial Tears: Allow 15 min interval between products.

HOW SUPPLIED: Emulsion: 0.05% [0.4mL]

CONTRAINDICATIONS: Active ocular infections.

WARNINGS/PRECAUTIONS: For ophthalmic use only. Not studied in patients with a history of herpes keratitis.

ADVERSE REACTIONS: Ocular burning, conjunctival hyperemia, discharge, epiphora, eye pain, foreign body sensation, pruritus, stinging, visual disturbance (eg, blurring).

PREGNANCY: Category C, caution in nursing.

MECHANISM OF ACTION: Topical immunomodulator; not established. Thought to act as a partial immunomodulator.

PHARMACOKINETICS: Distribution: Found in breast milk (systemic administration).

NURSING CONSIDERATIONS

Assessment: Assess for presence of active ocular infection, history of herpes keratitis, and pregnancy/nursing status.

Monitoring: Monitor for signs/symptoms of ocular burning and other adverse reactions.

Patient Counseling: Inform to use single-use vial immediately after opening and discard remaining contents following use. Instruct that the tip of the vial should not touch the eye or any surface to avoid contamination. Advise to remove contact lenses before administration; inform that lenses may be reinserted 15 min following administration.

Administration: Ocular route. Invert unit dose vial a few times to obtain uniform, white, opaque emulsion before using. **Storage:** 15-25°C (59-77°F).

RESTORIL
temazepam (Mallinckrodt)

CIV

THERAPEUTIC CLASS: Benzodiazepine

INDICATIONS: Short-term treatment of insomnia (7-10 days).

DOSAGE: *Adults:* Administer at bedtime. Usual: 15mg. Range: 7.5-30mg. Transient Insomnia: 7.5mg may be sufficient. Elderly/Debilitated: Initiate with 7.5mg until individual response is determined.

HOW SUPPLIED: Cap: 7.5mg, 15mg, 22.5mg, 30mg

CONTRAINDICATIONS: Women who are or may become pregnant.

WARNINGS/PRECAUTIONS: Initiate only after careful evaluation; failure of insomnia to remit after 7-10 days of treatment may indicate primary psychiatric and/or medical illness. Worsening of insomnia and emergence of thinking or behavior abnormalities may occur especially in elderly; use lowest possible effective dose. Behavioral changes (eg, decreased inhibition, bizarre behavior, agitation, hallucinations, depersonalization) and complex behavior (eg, sleep-driving) reported; strongly consider d/c if sleep-driving episode occurs. Amnesia and other neuropsychiatric symptoms may occur unpredictably. Worsening of depression, including suicidal thinking, reported. Withdrawal symptoms may occur after abrupt d/c. Rare cases of angioedema (eg, tongue, glottis, larynx) and anaphylaxis reported; do not rechallenge if angioedema develops. Oversedation, confusion, and/or ataxia may develop with large doses in elderly and debilitated patients. Caution with hepatic/renal impairment, chronic pulmonary insufficiency, debilitated, severe or latent depression, and elderly. Abnormal LFTs, renal function tests, and blood dyscrasias reported.

ADVERSE REACTIONS: Drowsiness, headache, fatigue, nervousness, lethargy, dizziness, nausea.

INTERACTIONS: Increased risk of complex behaviors with alcohol and CNS depressants. Potential additive effects with hypnotics and CNS depressants. Possible synergistic effect with diphenhydramine.

PREGNANCY: Category X, caution in nursing.

MECHANISM OF ACTION: Benzodiazepine hypnotic agent.

PHARMACOKINETICS: Absorption: Well absorbed; C_{max}=865ng/mL; T_{max}=1.5 hrs. **Distribution:** Plasma protein binding (96% unchanged); crosses placenta. **Metabolism:** Complete; conjugation. **Elimination:** Urine (80-90%); $T_{1/2}$=3.5-18.4 hrs.

NURSING CONSIDERATIONS

R

Assessment: Assess for physical and/or psychiatric disorder, medical illness, severe or latent depression, renal/hepatic dysfunction, chronic pulmonary insufficiency, pregnancy/nursing status, alcohol use, and possible drug interactions.

Monitoring: Monitor for signs/symptoms of withdrawal, tolerance, abuse, dependence, abnormal thinking, behavioral changes, agitation, depersonalization, hallucinations, complex behaviors (including "sleep-driving"), amnesia, anxiety, neuropsychiatric symptoms, worsening of depression, suicidal thoughts and actions, angioedema (tongue, glottis, or larynx), driving/psychomotor impairment, worsening of insomnia, thinking or behavioral abnormalities, possible abuse/dependence.

Patient Counseling: Inform about the benefits and risks of treatment. Instruct patient to take as prescribed. Inform about the risks and possibility of physical/psychological dependence, memory problems, and complex behaviors (eg, sleep-driving). Caution against hazardous tasks (eg, operating machinery/driving). Advise not to drink alcohol. Instruct to notify physician if pregnant/planning to become pregnant.

Administration: Oral route. **Storage:** 20-25°C (68-77°F).

RETAVASE
reteplase (EKR)

RX

THERAPEUTIC CLASS: Thrombolytic agent

INDICATIONS: Management of acute myocardial infarction (AMI) in adults for the improvement of ventricular function following AMI, reduction of the incidence of congestive heart failure (CHF), and the reduction of mortality associated with AMI.

DOSAGE: *Adults:* Administer two 10 U bolus injections. Administer each bolus as IV inj over 2 mins. Give 2nd bolus 30 mins after 1st bolus inj. Do not administer other medications simultaneously via the same IV line.

HOW SUPPLIED: Inj: 10.4 U (18.1mg)

CONTRAINDICATIONS: Active internal bleeding; history of cerebrovascular accident (CVA); recent intracranial or intraspinal surgery or trauma; intracranial neoplasm; arteriovenous malformation, or aneurysm; known bleeding diathesis; severe uncontrolled HTN.

WARNINGS/PRECAUTIONS: Bleeding is the most common complication during therapy; careful attention to all potential bleeding sites is required. If arterial puncture is necessary during administration, use an upper extremity vessel that is accessible to manual compression. Avoid IM inj and nonessential handling of patients. Perform venipuncture carefully and only if required. Weigh benefits/risks of therapy with recent major surgery, previous puncture of noncompressible vessels, cerebrovascular disease, recent GI or genitourinary (GU) bleeding, recent trauma, HTN, high likelihood of left heart thrombus, acute pericarditis, subacute bacterial endocarditis, hemostatic defects, severe hepatic or renal dysfunction, pregnancy, diabetic hemorrhagic retinopathy or other hemorrhagic ophthalmic conditions, septic thrombophlebitis or occluded AV cannula at a seriously infected site, advanced age, any other condition in which bleeding would constitute a significant hazard or be difficult to manage. Cholesterol embolism reported. Coronary thrombolysis may result in arrhythmias associated with reperfusion. Do not administer second bolus if an anaphylactoid reaction occurs. May affect results of coagulation tests and/or measurements of fibrinolytic activity.

ADVERSE REACTIONS: Bleeding, allergic reactions.

INTERACTIONS: Increased risk of bleeding with heparin, vitamin K antagonists, and drugs that alter platelet function (eg, ASA, dipyridamole, abciximab) if administered before, during, or after therapy. Concomitant use of anticoagulant therapy should be terminated if serious bleeding occurs.

PREGNANCY: Category C, caution in nursing.

MECHANISM OF ACTION: Thrombolytic agent; recombinant plasminogen activator which catalyzes the cleavage of endogenous plasminogen to generate plasmin. Plasmin in turn degrades the fibrin matrix of the thrombus, thereby exerting its thrombolytic action.

PHARMACOKINETICS: Metabolism: Hepatic. **Elimination:** Renal; $T_{1/2}$=13-16 min.

NURSING CONSIDERATIONS

Assessment: Assess for active internal bleeding, history of CVA, or any other conditions where treatment is contraindicated or cautioned. Assess for age, renal/hepatic function, pregnancy/nursing status, and possible drug interactions.

Monitoring: Monitor for signs/symptoms of bleeding, internal and superficial bleeding sites, bleeding at recent puncture sites, cholesterol embolism (eg, livedo reticularis, "purple toe" syndrome, MI, cerebral infarction, HTN, gangrenous digits), and arrhythmias. Monitor renal/hepatic function.

Patient Counseling: Inform the patient about the risks and benefits of the therapy. Instruct to contact physician if any unusual bleeding occurs or if any other adverse reaction develops. Advise to avoid IM injections while on therapy.

Administration: IV route. Refer to the PI for administration and reconstitution instructions.
Storage: Unused vial: 2-25°C (36-77°F). Box should remain sealed until use to protect the lyophilisate from exposure to light. Reconstituted: 2-30°C (36-86°F); use within 4 hrs.

RETIN-A   RX
tretinoin (Ortho Neutrogena)

OTHER BRAND NAMES: Retin-A Micro (Ortho Neutrogena)

THERAPEUTIC CLASS: Retinoid

INDICATIONS: Topical treatment of acne vulgaris.

DOSAGE: *Adults:* Cleanse area thoroughly, then apply qhs. May temporarily d/c or reduce dosing frequency if irritation occurs.
Pediatrics: ≥12 yrs: (Gel: 0.04%, 0.1%) Cleanse area thoroughly, then apply qhs. May temporarily d/c or reduce dosing frequency if irritation occurs.

HOW SUPPLIED: (Retin-A) Cre: 0.025%, 0.05%, 0.1% [20g, 45g]; Gel: 0.01%, 0.025% [15g, 45g]; Sol: 0.05% [28mL]; (Retin-A Micro) Gel: 0.04%, 0.1% [20g, 45g]

WARNINGS/PRECAUTIONS: Avoid eyes, lips, paranasal creases, mucous membranes, and sunburned skin. Acne exacerbation during early weeks of therapy may occur. D/C if sensitivity or irritation occurs. Severe irritation with eczematous skin. Causes photosensitivity. Extreme weather (eg, cold, wind) may irritate skin.

ADVERSE REACTIONS: Local skin reactions (red, edematous, blistered, crusted), photosensitivity, temporary skin pigmentation changes.

INTERACTIONS: Caution with topical agents with strong drying effects, high concentration of alcohol, astringents, spices, or lime. Caution with sulfur, resorcinol, or salicylic acid; allow effects of these agents to subside before application of tretinoin.

PREGNANCY: Category C, caution in nursing.

MECHANISM OF ACTION: Retinoic acid derivative; not established. Responsible for decreasing cohesiveness of follicular epithelial cells with decreased microcomedo formation. Also stimulates mitotic activity and increases turnover of follicular epithelial cells, causing extrusion of comedones.

NURSING CONSIDERATIONS

Assessment: Assess for presence of sunburn and eczematous skin, pregnancy/nursing status, and possible drug interactions.

Monitoring: Monitor for signs/symptoms of a skin sensitivity reaction (eg, red, edematous, blistered, or crusted skin) or chemical irritation.

Patient Counseling: Avoid exposure to sunlight/sunlamps during therapy. Advise using effective sunscreen when outdoors and protective clothing during extended sun exposure. If sunburn occurs, instruct to d/c until skin is recovered. Avoid excessive exposure to wind or cold. Medication is flammable; avoid fire, flame, or smoking during use. Keep away from eyes, mouth, angles of the nose, and mucous membranes. Notify physician if severe skin irritation occurs.

Administration: Topical administration. **Storage:** Liq, Gel: Below 86°F; Cre: Below 80°F.

RETROVIR   RX
zidovudine (ViiV Healthcare)

> Associated with hematologic toxicity (eg, neutropenia, severe anemia), particularly with advanced HIV-1 disease. Symptomatic myopathy associated with prolonged use. Lactic acidosis and severe hepatomegaly with steatosis, including fatal cases, reported with nucleoside analogues; suspend treatment if lactic acidosis or pronounced hepatotoxicity occur.

THERAPEUTIC CLASS: Nucleoside reverse transcriptase inhibitor

INDICATIONS: Treatment of HIV-1 infection in combination with other antiretrovirals. Prevention of maternal-fetal HIV-1 transmission.

DOSAGE: *Adults:* HIV-1 Infection: (PO) 600mg/day in divided doses in combination with other antiretroviral agents. (Inj) 1mg/kg IV over 1 hr 5-6 times/day. Use only until oral therapy can be administered. Maternal-Fetal HIV Transmission: >14 weeks pregnancy: Maternal Dosing: 100mg PO 5 times/day until start of labor. During Labor and Delivery: 2mg/kg IV over 1 hr followed by continuous 1mg/kg/hr IV infusion until clamping of umbilical cord. End-Stage Renal Disease On Dialysis: 100mg PO q6-8h or 1mg/kg IV q6-8h. Significant Anemia/Neutropenia: May require dose interruption and may resume therapy with adjunctive epoetin alfa therapy if marrow recovery occurs. Elderly: Start at low end of dosing range.
Pediatrics: HIV-1 Infection: 4 weeks-<18 yrs: (PO) BSA Based: 480mg/m²/day PO in divided doses (240mg/m² bid or 160mg/m² tid). Weight Based: ≥30kg: 300mg bid or 200mg tid. ≥9-<30kg: 9mg/kg bid or 6mg/kg tid. 4-<9kg: 12mg/kg bid or 8mg/kg tid. Maternal-Fetal HIV Transmission: Neonates: 2mg/kg PO q6h or 1.5mg/kg IV over 30 min q6h, starting within 12 hrs after birth and continuing through 6 weeks of age. End-Stage Renal Disease On Dialysis: 100mg PO q6-8h or 1mg/kg IV q6-8h. Significant Anemia/Neutropenia: May require dose interruption and may resume therapy with adjunctive epoetin alfa therapy if marrow recovery occurs.

HOW SUPPLIED: Cap: 100mg; Inj: 10mg/mL [20mL]; Syrup: 50mg/5mL [240mL]; Tab: 300mg

WARNINGS/PRECAUTIONS: Adverse reactions increase with disease progression. Caution with granulocyte count <1000 cells/mm³ or Hgb <9.5g/dL; monitor blood counts frequently with advanced symptomatic HIV disease, and with poor bone marrow reserve. Pancytopenia reported. D/C if neutropenia or anemia develops. Obesity and prolonged nucleoside exposure may be risk factors for lactic acidosis and severe hepatomegaly with steatosis. Caution with known risk factors for liver disease and in elderly. Immune reconstitution syndrome reported. Autoimmune disorders (eg, Grave's disease, polymyositis, Guillain-Barre syndrome) reported and can occur many months after initiation of treatment. Redistribution/accumulation of body fat observed (PO). Dose reduction in severe renal impairment (CrCl <15mL/min).

ADVERSE REACTIONS: Hematologic toxicity (eg, anemia, neutropenia), lactic acidosis, hepatomegaly with steatosis, hepatotoxicity, headache, N/V, malaise, anorexia, asthenia, constipation, abdominal pain/cramps, arthralgia, chills.

INTERACTIONS: Avoid with stavudine, nucleoside analogues affecting DNA replication (eg, ribavirin), doxorubicin, and other combination products containing zidovudine. Hepatic decompensation may occur in HIV/hepatitis C virus coinfected patients receiving interferon-alfa with

R

or without ribavirin. May increase risk of hematologic toxicities with ganciclovir, interferon-alfa, ribavirin, bone marrow suppressives, and cytotoxic agents. May decrease levels of phenytoin. Lamivudine, atovaquone, fluconazole, methadone, probenecid, and valproic acid may increase levels. Nelfinavir, ritonavir, rifampin, and clarithromycin may decrease levels.

PREGNANCY: Category C, not for use in nursing.

MECHANISM OF ACTION: Nucleoside analogue; inhibits reverse transcriptase via DNA chain termination after incorporation of the nucleotide analogue.

PHARMACOKINETICS: Absorption: (PO): Rapid. Bioavailability (64%). T_{max}=0.5-1.5 hrs. (IV) C_{max}=1.06mcg/mL. **Distribution:** V_d=1.6L/kg; plasma protein binding (<38%); crosses the placenta; found in breast milk. **Metabolism:** Hepatic. 3'-azido-3'-deoxy-5'-O-β-D-glucopyranuronosylthymidine (major metabolite). **Elimination:** (PO): Urine (14% unchanged, 74% metabolite). $T_{1/2}$=0.5-3 hrs. (IV): Urine (18% unchanged, 60% metabolite). $T_{1/2}$=1.1 hrs. Refer to PI for pediatric and renal impairment pharmacokinetic parameters.

NURSING CONSIDERATIONS

Assessment: Assess for advanced symptomatic HIV disease, risk of liver disease, obesity, prolonged use of antiretroviral nucleoside analogues, signs/symptoms of bone marrow compromise, renal/hepatic function, drug hypersensitivity, ability to swallow cap or tab in children, pregnancy/nursing status, and possible drug interactions.

Monitoring: Monitor for signs/symptoms of lactic acidosis, severe hepatomegaly with steatosis, hypersensitivity reaction, myopathy, anemia, liver/renal dysfunction, bone marrow suppression, immune reconstitution syndrome (eg, opportunistic infections), and other treatment-associated toxicities. Monitor for blood counts/hematologic indices periodically and need for dosage adjustment.

Patient Counseling: Inform that therapy is not cure for HIV, does not reduce risk of transmission of HIV and that opportunistic infections may develop. Advise to avoid doing things that can spread HIV-1 infection to others (eg, sharing of needles/inj equipment/personal items that can have blood or body fluids on them, having sex without protection, breastfeeding). Inform that major toxicities are neutropenia and/or anemia; may require transfusions or d/c drug if toxicity develops. Inform of importance of frequent blood counts while on therapy. Inform that drug may cause myopathy, myositis, lactic acidosis with liver enlargement, redistribution/accumulation of body fat (PO), headache, malaise, N/V, anorexia in adults, fever, cough, and digestive disorder in pediatrics. Advise to consult a physician if muscle weakness, SOB, symptoms of hepatitis or pancreatitis, and any other adverse events occur. Inform pregnant women that HIV transmission may still occur to their infants despite therapy; do not breastfeed to prevent postnatal transmission. Counsel that use of other medications may exacerbate toxicity. Instruct not to share medication or exceed recommended dose; take as prescribed.

Administration: IV or oral route. (IV) Avoid rapid infusion and bolus injection. Should not be given IM. **Storage:** (IV): 15-25°C (59-77°F); protect from light. (Diluted): Stable for 24 hrs at room temperature, and for 48 hrs if refrigerated at 2-8°C (36-46°F). Administer within 8 hrs if stored at 25°C (77°F) or 24 hrs if refrigerated at 2-8°C to minimize contamination. (PO): 15-25°C (59-77°F); protect caps from moisture.

REVATIO   RX
sildenafil (Pfizer)

THERAPEUTIC CLASS: Phosphodiesterase type 5 inhibitor

INDICATIONS: Treatment of pulmonary arterial HTN (PAH) (WHO Group I) to improve exercise ability and delay clinical worsening.

DOSAGE: *Adults:* PO: 20mg tid, 4-6 hrs apart. Max: 20mg tid. IV: 10mg IV bolus tid.

HOW SUPPLIED: Inj: 10mg [12.5mL]; Tab: 20mg

CONTRAINDICATIONS: Coadministration with organic nitrates in any form, either regularly or intermittently.

WARNINGS/PRECAUTIONS: Caution with myocardial infarction (MI), stroke or life-threatening arrhythmia within last 6 months, coronary artery disease (CAD) causing unstable angina, and HTN (BP >170/110). Vasodilatory effects may adversely affect patients with resting hypotension (BP <90/50), fluid depletion, severe left ventricular outflow obstruction, or autonomic dysfunction. Not recommended with pulmonary veno-occlusive disease (PVOD); consider possibility of associated PVOD if signs of pulmonary edema occur. Caution in patients with bleeding disorders or active peptic ulceration. Non-arteritic anterior ischemic optic neuropathy (NAION) reported; seek immediate medical attention if sudden loss of vision in one or both eyes occurs. Caution with previous NAION in one eye and with retinitis pigmentosa. Sudden decrease or loss of hearing reported. Caution in patients with anatomical penile deformation or with predisposition to priapism. Penile tissue damage and permanent loss of potency may result if priapism is not immediately treated. Vaso-occlusive crises requiring hospitalization reported in patients with pulmonary HTN secondary to sickle cell disease. Caution in elderly. (Inj) May be used as continued treatment in patients currently taking tab and who are temporarily unable to take PO medication.

ADVERSE REACTIONS: Epistaxis, headache, flushing, dyspepsia, insomnia, erythema, dyspnea exacerbated, rhinitis, diarrhea, myalgia, pyrexia, gastritis, sinusitis, paresthesia.

INTERACTIONS: See Contraindications. Reports of epistaxis with oral vitamin K antagonists. Retinal and eye hemorrhage reported with anticoagulants. May potentiate anti-aggregatory effect of sodium nitroprusside. Avoid with ritonavir or other potent CYP3A inhibitors, and other PDE5 inhibitors (eg, Viagra). Increased clearance with CYP3A and CYP2C9 inducers. Increased plasma concentrations with cimetidine. Increased area under the curve (AUC) with erythromycin. Increased C_{max} and AUC with saquinavir. Decreased clearance with CYP3A and CYP2C9 inhibitors. Greater decrease in plasma levels with potent CYP3A inducers. Slight decrease of sildenafil exposure with epoprostenol. Reduced clearance or increased oral bioavailability with CYP3A substrates and the combination of CYP3A substrates and β-blockers. Caution with α-blockers (eg, doxazosin) due to its additive BP-lowering effects. Additional reduction of supine BP with oral amlodipine reported. Decreased AUC and C_{max} with bosentan and increased AUC of bosentan; caution with coadministration.

PREGNANCY: Category B, caution in nursing.

MECHANISM OF ACTION: Phosphodiesterase type-5 (PDE5) inhibitor; increases cGMP within pulmonary vascular smooth muscle cells resulting in relaxation. This can lead to vasodilation of pulmonary vascular bed and, to a lesser degree, vasodilation in the systemic circulation.

PHARMACOKINETICS: Absorption: (PO) Rapid; absolute bioavailability (41%); T_{max}=60 min (fasted state). **Distribution:** V_d=105L; plasma protein binding (96%). **Metabolism:** CYP3A (major route) and CYP2C9 (minor route); N-desmethyl metabolite (active metabolite). **Elimination:** (PO) Feces (80%), urine (13%); $T_{1/2}$=4 hrs.

NURSING CONSIDERATIONS

Assessment: Assess for hypotension, fluid depletion, left ventricular outflow obstruction, autonomic dysfunction, PVOD, CAD causing unstable angina, HTN, active peptic ulceration or bleeding problems, previous NAION in one eye, retinitis pigmentosa, anatomical deformities of the penis, conditions predisposing to priapism, pulmonary HTN secondary to sickle cell disease, drug hypersensitivity, nursing/pregnancy status, and possible drug interactions. Assess for MI, stroke or life-threatening arrhythmia within last 6 months. Obtain baseline BP.

Monitoring: Monitor for signs of pulmonary edema, decreased/sudden loss of vision or hearing, tinnitus, dizziness, epistaxis, priapism, and hypersensitivity reactions. Monitor BP.

Patient Counseling: Counsel about risks and benefits of the drug. Inform that drug is also marketed as Viagra for male erectile dysfunction. Advise not to take Viagra or other PDE5 inhibitors and organic nitrates during therapy. Advise to notify physician if sudden decrease/loss of vision or hearing occur. Instruct to seek immediate medical attention if an erection persists >4 hrs.

Administration: Oral, IV route. **Storage:** 25°C (77°F); excursions permitted to 15-30°C (59-86°F).

R

ReVia   RX
naltrexone HCl (Duramed)

THERAPEUTIC CLASS: Opioid antagonist

INDICATIONS: Treatment of alcohol dependence and to block effects of exogenously administered opioids.

DOSAGE: *Adults:* Alcoholism: 50mg qd up to 12 weeks. Opioid Dependence: Begin 7-10 days after opioid-free period and no signs of withdrawal. Initial: 25mg qd. Maint: 50mg qd. Naloxone Challenge Test: 0.2mg IV, observe for 30 sec, then 0.6mg IV, observe for 20 min; or 0.8mg SQ, observe for 20 min.

HOW SUPPLIED: Tab: 50mg* *scored

CONTRAINDICATIONS: Acute hepatitis or liver failure, failed naloxone challenge test or positive urine screen for opioids, opioid-dependent, concomitant opioid analgesics, acute opioid withdrawal.

WARNINGS/PRECAUTIONS: Hepatotoxicity with excessive doses; does not appear to be a hepatotoxin at recommended doses. Only treat patients opioid-free for 7-10 days. Attempting to overcome opiate blockade is very dangerous. More sensitive to lower doses of opioids after naltrexone is d/c. Safety in ultra-rapid opiate detoxification is not known. Increased risk of suicide in substance abuse patients. Severe opioid withdrawal syndromes reported with accidental ingestion in opioid-dependent patients. Monitor closely during blockade reversal. Caution in renal or hepatic impairment. Perform naloxone challenge test if question of opioid dependence.

ADVERSE REACTIONS: N/V, headache, dizziness, nervousness, fatigue, restlessness, insomnia, anxiety, somnolence.

INTERACTIONS: See Contraindications. Do not use with disulfiram unless benefits outweigh risk of hepatotoxicity. Lethargy and somnolence reported with thioridazine. Antagonizes opioid-containing cough and cold, antidiarrheal, and analgesic agents.

PREGNANCY: Category C, caution in nursing.

MECHANISM OF ACTION: Opioid antagonist; markedly attenuates or completely blocks (reversibly) the subjective effects of IV-administered opioids.

PHARMACOKINETICS: Absorption: Rapid and complete. Bioavailability (5-40%); T_{max}=1 hr. **Distribution:** V_d=1350L; plasma protein binding (21%). **Metabolism:** Liver , 6β-naltrexol (major metabolite). **Elimination:** Urine (2% unchanged), (43% conjugated); (naltrexone, β-naltrexol) $T_{1/2}$=4 hrs, 13 hrs.

NURSING CONSIDERATIONS

Assessment: Start treatment only under medical judgment of prescribing physician. Assess potential of opioid use within past 7-10 days. If question of occult opioid dependence, perform naloxone challenge test. Assess for acute hepatitis or liver failure and possible drug interactions.

Monitoring: Monitor LFTs, symptoms/signs of respiratory depression, hepatotoxicity, idiopathic thrombocytopenic purpura, suicide attempts, withdrawal symptoms in opioid-dependent patients.

Patient Counseling: Instruct to take as prescribed. Drug treats alcoholism or drug dependence. Carry identification card to alert medical personnel of naltrexone use and to ensure adequate treatment in a medical emergency. Caution against taking heroin or any other opioid drug with therapy; may lead to serious injury, including coma. Notify physician if pregnant/nursing.

Administration: Oral route. **Storage:** 20-25°C (68-77°F).

REVLIMID   RX
lenalidomide (Celgene)

A known human teratogen that causes severe life-threatening human birth defects. Avoid during pregnancy; may cause birth defects or death to a developing baby. Women of childbearing potential should have 2 negative pregnancy tests prior to treatment and must use 2 forms of contraception or continuously abstain from heterosexual sex during and for 4 weeks after treatment. Available only under a restricted distribution program called "RevAssist". May cause neutropenia and thrombocytopenia. Patients on therapy for del 5q myelodysplastic syndromes (MDS) should have their CBC monitored weekly for the 1st 8 weeks of therapy and monthly thereafter; patients may require dose interruption and/or reduction and use of blood product support and/or growth factors. Increased risk of deep vein thrombosis (DVT) and pulmonary embolism (PE) in patients with multiple myeloma. Observe for signs and symptoms of thromboembolism.

THERAPEUTIC CLASS: Thalidomide Analog

INDICATIONS: Treatment for transfusion-dependent anemia due to low- or intermediate-1-risk myelodysplastic syndromes (MDS) associated with a deletion 5q cytogenetic abnormality with or without additional cytogenetic abnormalities. In combination with dexamethasone for the treatment of multiple myeloma (MM) in patients who have received at least 1 prior therapy.

DOSAGE: *Adults:* MDS: Initial: 10mg qd with water. Renal Impairment: Moderate (CrCl 30-60mL/min): 5mg q24h. Severe without Dialysis (CrCl <30mL/min): 5mg q48h. End Stage Renal Disease (ESRD) with Dialysis (CrCl <30mL/min): 5mg 3x a week following each dialysis. MM: Initial: 25mg qd with water on Days 1-21 of repeated 28-day cycles. Give with dexamethasone 40mg qd on Days 1-4, 9-12, and 17-20 of each 28-day cycle for the 1st 4 cycles then on Days 1-4 every 28 days. Renal Impairment: Moderate (CrCl 30-60mL/min): 10mg q24h. Severe without Dialysis (CrCl <30mL/min): 15mg q48h. ESRD with Dialysis (CrCl <30mL/min): 5mg qd; on dialysis days, administer dose following dialysis. For Grade 3/4 toxicities, hold treatment and restart at next lower dose when toxicity resolved to ≤Grade 2. Refer to PI for dose adjustments for hematologic toxicities based on platelet and/or absolute neutrophil counts. Do not break, chew or open caps.

HOW SUPPLIED: Cap: 5mg, 10mg, 15mg, 25mg

CONTRAINDICATIONS: Pregnancy and childbearing potential.

WARNINGS/PRECAUTIONS: Angioedema and serious dermatologic reactions including Stevens-Johnson syndrome (SJS) and toxic epidermal necrolysis (TEN) reported. D/C if angioedema, SJS, TEN, Grade 4 rash, exfoliative or bullous rash develops. Consider treatment interruption or d/c for Grade 2-3 skin rash. Avoid with a prior history of Grade 4 rash associated with thalidomide treatment. Tumor lysis syndrome reported; caution in patients with high tumor burden prior to treatment and monitor closely. Tumor flare reaction (characterized by tender lymph node swelling, low grade fever, pain, rash) occurred during investigational use for chronic lymphocytic leukemia (CLL) and lymphoma; treatment of CLL or lymphoma outside a well-monitored clinical trial is discouraged. Caution with renal impairment.

ADVERSE REACTIONS: Thrombocytopenia, neutropenia, pruritus, rash, diarrhea, constipation, nausea, nasopharyngitis, fatigue, arthralgia, cough, pyrexia, peripheral edema, anemia, asthenia.

INTERACTIONS: May increase digoxin levels; monitor periodically. Caution in multiple myeloma with erythropoietic agents or other agents that may increase risk of thrombosis such as estrogen containing therapies.

PREGNANCY: Category X, not for use in nursing.

MECHANISM OF ACTION: Thalidomide analogue; not established, possesses antineoplastic, immunomodulatory and antiangiogenic properties. Inhibits secretion of pro-inflammatory cytokines such as tumor necrosis factor (TNF-α) from peripheral blood mononuclear cells and also inhibits expression of cyclooxygenase-2 (COX-2) in vitro.

PHARMACOKINETICS: Absorption: Rapid, T_{max}=0.625-1.5 hrs (healthy); T_{max}=0.5-4.0 hrs (multiple myeloma). **Distribution:** Plasma protein binding (30%). **Elimination:** Urine (2/3, unchanged); $T_{1/2}$=3 hrs.

NURSING CONSIDERATIONS

Assessment: Assess for pregnancy/nursing status, renal impairment, history of Grade 4 rash, patients with high tumor burden, hypersensitivity to the drug and possible drug interactions. Obtain pregnancy test (sensitivity of ≥50 mIU/mL) 10-14 days before and 24 hrs before initiating therapy. Confirm use of 2 forms of effective contraception beginning 4 weeks prior to therapy.

Monitoring: Monitor the use of effective contraception during therapy, therapy interruptions, and for 4 weeks after therapy. Perform pregnancy test weekly during the 1st month, then monthly thereafter in women with regular menstrual cycles and every 2 weeks with irregular menstrual cycles. Monitor CBC weekly for 1st 8 weeks of therapy and monthly thereafter (MDS); every 2 weeks for 1st 12 weeks and monthly thereafter (MM). Monitor for signs/symptoms of hypersensitivity reactions, DVT, PE, thromboembolism, neutropenia, thrombocytopenia, angioedema, Grade 2-3 rash, exfoliative/bullous rash, SJS, TEN, tumor lysis syndrome, and tumor flare reaction. Monitor renal function, especially in elderly.

Patient Counseling: Instruct not to break, chew, or open caps. Counsel on potential risk of teratogenicity. Inform that treatment should only be initiated following a negative pregnancy test. Explain the importance of performing monthly pregnancy tests. Instruct to use 2 effective contraceptive methods during therapy, during therapy interruptions, and for at least 4 weeks after completing therapy. Instruct males receiving therapy to always use a latex condom during any sexual contact, even if with successful vasectomy; inform physician if he has had unprotected sexual contact with a woman who can become pregnant. Instruct to immediately d/c therapy if the patient becomes pregnant, misses her menstrual period, experiences unusual bleeding, stops taking birth control, or thinks that she may be pregnant. Inform that therapy is associated with significant neutropenia and thrombocytopenia. Seek medical attention if symptoms of thromboembolism, hypersensitivity reactions, or infection occur. Inform that the therapy in combination with dexamethasone has demonstrated significant increased risk of DVT and PE in MM.

Administration: Oral route. Do not break, chew, or open the caps; wash thoroughly if powder gets in contact with the skin or mucous membranes. **Storage:** 25°C (77°F); excursions permitted to 15-30°C (59-86°F). Dispense no more than a 28-day supply.

R

REYATAZ   RX
atazanavir sulfate (Bristol-Myers Squibb)

THERAPEUTIC CLASS: Protease inhibitor

INDICATIONS: Treatment of HIV-1 infection in combination with other antiretrovirals.

DOSAGE: *Adults:* Therapy-Naive: 300mg with ritonavir (RTV) 100mg qd. If intolerant to RTV, give atazanavir (ATV) 400mg qd. End Stage Renal Disease (ESRD) with Hemodialysis: 300mg with RTV 100mg. Therapy-Experienced: 300mg with RTV 100mg qd. 2nd/3rd Trimester Pregnancy with H_2-Receptor Antagonist or Tenofovir: 400mg with RTV 100mg qd. Concomitant Therapy: Refer to PI for proper administration and dose adjustments. Moderate Hepatic Impairment (Child-Pugh Class B) Without Prior Virologic Failure: 300mg qd. Take with food. *Pediatrics:* 6-<18 yrs: ≥40kg: 300mg with RTV 100mg qd. 20-<40kg: 200mg with RTV 100mg qd. 15-<20kg: 150mg with RTV 100mg qd. Therapy-Naive: ≥13 yrs and ≥40kg: If intolerant to RTV, give ATV 400mg qd. Concomitant Tenofovir/H_2-receptor Antagonists/Proton-Pump Inhibitors (PPIs): Do not administer without RTV. Do not exceed recommended adult dose. Take with food.

HOW SUPPLIED: Cap: 100mg, 150mg, 200mg, 300mg

CONTRAINDICATIONS: Coadministration with CYP3A or UGT1A1 substrates for which elevated plasma concentrations are associated with serious and/or life-threatening events (eg, alfuzosin, rifampin, irinotecan, triazolam, oral midazolam, dihydroergotamine, ergotamine, ergonovine, methylergonovine, cisapride, St. John's wort, lovastatin, simvastatin, pimozide, sildenafil when used for pulmonary arterial HTN, indinavir).

WARNINGS/PRECAUTIONS: Not recommended without RTV for treatment-experienced adults/pediatrics with prior virologic failure and during pregnancy or postpartum period. Should not be administered to HIV treatment-experienced patients with ESRD managed with hemodialysis. Caution with mild to moderate hepatic impairment. Avoid with severe hepatic impairment. ATV/RTV is not recommended with hepatic impairment. May prolong PR-interval; caution with preexisting conduction system diseases or with drugs that prolong PR interval. May cause rash, including Stevens-Johnson syndrome, erythema multiforme, and toxic skin eruptions; d/c if severe rash develops. May cause hyperbilirubinemia; dose reduction is not recommended and alternative antiretroviral therapy may be considered with jaundice or scleral icterus. Increased risk for further transaminase elevations or hepatic decompensation in patients with underlying hepatitis B or C infections or marked transaminase elevations; monitor prior to and during treatment. Nephrolithiasis reported; may temporarily interrupt or d/c therapy if symptoms occur. New onset or exacerbation of diabetes mellitus (DM), hyperglycemia, and diabetic ketoacidosis, immune reconstitution syndrome, redistribution/accumulation of body fat, increased risk of bleeding with hemophilia A and B reported. Various degrees of cross-resistance observed. Caution in elderly.

ADVERSE REACTIONS: N/V, jaundice/scleral icterus, rash, myalgia, headache, abdominal pain, insomnia, peripheral neurologic symptoms, diarrhea, fever, AST/ALT elevations, neutropenia.

INTERACTIONS: See Contraindications. Not recommended with nevirapine, salmeterol, or (without RTV) tenofovir, bosentan, and buprenorphine. ATV/RTV is not recommended with other protease inhibitors, voriconazole, or fluticasone. Avoid with efavirenz or PPIs in treatment-experienced patients. Avoid with colchicine in renally/hepatically impaired. Caution with CYP2C8 substrates with narrow therapeutic indices (eg, paclitaxel, repaglinide). CYP3A4 inducers, tenofovir, nevirapine, bosentan, efavirenz, PPIs (eg, omeprazole), antacids, buffered medications, H_2-receptor antagonists may decrease levels. Administer at least 2 hrs before or 1 hr after buffered formulations (eg, didanosine buffered formulations) and antacids, and 12 hrs after PPIs. RTV, clarithromycin, voriconazole may increase levels. May increase levels of tenofovir, saquinavir, antiarrhythmics (eg, amiodarone, bepridil, lidocaine [systemic], quinidine), TCAs, trazodone, nevirapine, azole antifungals (eg, itraconazole, ketoconazole), colchicine, rifabutin, IV midazolam, warfarin (monitor INR), diltiazem and other calcium channel blockers, bosentan, atorvastatin, rosuvastatin, norgestimate, norethindrone, fluticasone, clarithromycin, buprenorphine, immunosuppressants, phosphodiesterase-5 inhibitors. May decrease levels of didanosine, 14-OH clarithromycin (clarithromycin active metabolite). May alter levels of ethinyl estradiol.

PREGNANCY: Category B, not for use in nursing.

MECHANISM OF ACTION: HIV-1 protease inhibitor; selectively inhibits virus-specific processing of viral Gag and Gag-Pol polyproteins in HIV-1 infected cells, preventing formation of mature virions.

PHARMACOKINETICS: Absorption: Rapid. C_{max}=3152ng/mL, T_{max}=2.5 hrs, AUC=22262ng•h/mL. **Distribution:** Plasma protein binding (86%). **Metabolism:** Liver (extensive); mono- and dioxygenation via CYP3A. **Elimination:** Urine (13%, 7% unchanged), feces (79%, 20% unchanged); $T_{1/2}$=7 hrs.

R | NURSING CONSIDERATIONS

Assessment: Assess renal/liver function, treatment history, hepatitis B or C infection, transaminase elevations, known hypersensitivity, DM, hemophilia, conduction system disease, pregnancy/nursing status, and possible drug interactions. Obtain baseline ECG.

Monitoring: Monitor for cardiac conduction abnormalities, PR interval prolongation, rash, hyperbilirubinemia, nephrolithiasis, new onset or exacerbation of DM, hyperglycemia, diabetic ketoacidosis, immune reconstitution syndrome, fat redistribution/accumulation, and cross-resistance among protease inhibitors. Monitor LFTs in patients with underlying hepatitis B or C infection and serum transaminase elevations. Monitor for bleeding in patients with hemophilia. Monitor closely for adverse events during the 1st 2 months postpartum.

Patient Counseling: Inform that therapy is not cure for HIV, has not shown to reduce risk of HIV transmission, that opportunistic infections may develop, and to take with food as prescribed. Instruct not to open cap. Advise that if dose is missed, take as soon as possible and return to normal schedule; however, if dose is skipped, advise not to double the next dose. Instruct to report use of any other medications or herbal products. Inform that mild rashes, redistribution, and accumulation of body fat, or yellowing of the skin or eyes may occur. Advise to consult physician if dizziness or lightheadedness occurs. Advise to d/c and seek medical evaluation immediately if signs or symptoms of severe skin reactions or hypersensitivity reactions develop.

Administration: Oral route. Take with food. **Storage:** 25°C (77°F); excursions permitted to 15-30°C (59-86°F).

RHINOCORT AQUA
budesonide (AstraZeneca)

RX

THERAPEUTIC CLASS: Corticosteroid

INDICATIONS: Treatment of nasal symptoms of seasonal or perennial allergic rhinitis in adults and children ≥6 yrs.

DOSAGE: *Adults*: Initial: 1 spray/nostril qd. Max: 4 sprays/nostril qd.
Pediatrics: ≥12 yrs: Initial: 1 spray/nostril qd. Max: 4 sprays/nostril qd. 6-<12 yrs: Initial: 1 spray/nostril qd. Max: 2 sprays/nostril qd.

HOW SUPPLIED: Spray: 32mcg/spray [8.6g]

WARNINGS/PRECAUTIONS: Local nasal effects (eg, epistaxis, *Candida* infections of the nose and pharynx, nasal septal perforation, impaired wound healing) may occur. May need to d/c treatment when *Candida* infection develops. Avoid in patients with recent nasal surgery, trauma, or septal ulcers until healing has occurred. Hypersensitivity reactions may occur. May cause immunosuppresion; caution with active or quiescent tuberculosis (TB), untreated fungal, bacterial, systemic viral or parasitic infections; or ocular herpes simplex. Hypercorticism and adrenal suppression may appear with higher than recommended dose or in susceptible individuals at recommended dose; d/c slowly. Adrenal insufficiency and withdrawal symptoms may occur when replacing a systemic with a topical corticosteroid. May reduce growth velocity in pediatrics. Glaucoma, increased intraocular pressure (IOP) and cataracts reported; monitor closely in patients with change in vision, history of IOP, glaucoma, and/or cataracts. Caution with hepatic dysfunction.

ADVERSE REACTIONS: Pharyngitis, epistaxis, cough, bronchospasm, nasal irritation.

INTERACTIONS: Oral ketoconazole and other known strong CYP3A4 inhibitors (eg, ritonavir, atazanavir, clarithromycin, indinavir, itraconazole, nefazodone, nelfinavir, saquinavir, telithromycin) may increase plasma levels; use with caution.

PREGNANCY: Category B, caution in nursing.

MECHANISM OF ACTION: Corticosteroid; not established. Possesses a wide range of inhibitory activities against multiple cell types (eg, mast cells, eosinophils, neutrophils, macrophages, lymphocytes) and mediators (eg, histamine, leukotrienes, eicosanoids, cytokines) involved in allergic-mediated inflammation.

PHARMACOKINETICS: Absorption: Absolute bioavailability (34%); C_{max}=0.3nmol/L; T_{max}=0.5 hr. **Distribution:** V_d=2-3L/kg, plasma protein binding (85-90%), found in breast milk. **Metabolism:** Liver (rapid, extensive) via CYP3A4; 16a-hydroxyprednisolone and 6β-hydroxybudesonide (major metabolites). **Elimination:** Urine (2/3 metabolites), feces; $T_{1/2}$=2-3 hrs.

NURSING CONSIDERATIONS

Assessment: Assess for history of hypersensitivity, increased IOP, glaucoma and/or cataracts. Assess for recent nasal ulcers, surgery/trauma, active or quiescent TB, untreated local or systemic fungal or bacterial infections, systemic viral or parasitic infections, ocular herpes simplex, suppressed immune system, asthma or other conditions requiring chronic systemic corticosteroid therapy, pregnancy/nursing status, and possible drug interactions.

Monitoring: Monitor for acute adrenal insufficiency and withdrawal symptoms when replacing systemic corticosteroid with topical corticosteroid. Monitor for hypercorticism and/or HPA-axis suppression, disseminated infections (eg, chickenpox and measles), nasal or pharyngeal *Candida* infections, suppression of growth velocity in children, nasal septal perforation, epistaxis, glaucoma, increased IOP, and cataracts.

Patient Counseling: Inform about the benefits and risks of the treatment. Take as directed at regular intervals. Avoid exposure to chickenpox or measles. Instruct to consult physician immediately if exposed to chickenpox or measles, if existing infection worsens, or if episodes of epistaxis or nasal discomfort occur. Inform physician if a change in vision occurs.

Administration: Intranasal route. Shake gently before use. Refer to PI for further administration instructions. **Storage:** 20-25°C (68-77°F) with the valve up. Do not freeze. Protect from light.

R

RIASTAP
fibrinogen concentrate (human) (CSL Behring)

RX

THERAPEUTIC CLASS: Plasma glycoprotein

INDICATIONS: Treatment of acute bleeding episodes in patients with congenital fibrinogen deficiency, including afibrinogenemia and hypofibrinogenemia.

DOSAGE: *Adults:* Individualize dose. Known Baseline Fibrinogen Level: Target plasma fibrinogen level based on bleeding type, actual measured plasma fibrinogen level, and body weight.

Dose calculated as [target level (mg/dL)-measured level (mg/dL)]/1.7 (mg/dL per mg/kg body weight). Unknown Baseline Fibrinogen Level: Usual: 70mg/kg IV. Monitor fibrinogen level during treatment. A target fibrinogen level of 100mg/dL should be maintained until hemostasis is obtained.

HOW SUPPLIED: Inj: 900mg-1300mg

WARNINGS/PRECAUTIONS: For IV use only. Administer under medical supervision. Not indicated for dysfibrinogenemia. Allergic reactions may occur; d/c if symptoms of allergic or early signs of hypersensitivity reactions occur. Thromboembolic events reported; monitor for signs and symptoms of thrombosis. Made from human plasma; may contain infectious agents (eg, viruses) and theoretically, the Creutzfeldt-Jakob (CJD) agent that can cause disease. All infections thought to have been transmitted by product should be reported to manufacturer.

ADVERSE REACTIONS: Allergic reactions, chills, fever, headache, N/V, thromboembolic episodes.

PREGNANCY: Category C, safety not known in nursing.

MECHANISM OF ACTION: Plasma glycoprotein; physiological substrate of thrombin, factor XIIIa, and plasmin. Replaces the missing or low coagulation factor.

PHARMACOKINETICS: Absorption: C_{max}=140mg/dL, AUC=124.3mg•hr/mL (70mg/kg dose). **Distribution:** V_d=52.7mL/kg. **Elimination:** $T_{1/2}$=78.7 hrs.

NURSING CONSIDERATIONS

Assessment: Assess for drug hypersensitivity, dysfibrinogenemia, and pregnancy/nursing status. Assess fibrinogen levels.

Monitoring: Monitor for signs/symptoms of allergic/hypersensitivity reactions, thrombosis, and infection (eg, viruses). Monitor fibrinogen levels.

Patient Counseling: Inform of the signs of allergic/hypersensitivity reactions (eg, hives, chest tightness, wheezing, hypotension, anaphylaxis) and thrombotic events (eg, unexplained pleuritic, chest and/or leg pain or edema, hemoptysis, dyspnea, tachypnea, neurologic symptoms) and advise to report to physician if any of these occur. Inform of risks/benefits of therapy.

Administration: IV route. Refer to PI for preparation, reconstitution, and administration instructions. **Storage:** 2-25°C (36-77°F) up to 30 months. Protect from light. Do not freeze. Reconstituted: 20-25°C for 8 hrs. Do not freeze.

RIFAMATE   RX
rifampin - isoniazid (Sanofi-Aventis)

Isoniazid associated with severe and sometimes fatal hepatitis. Monitor LFTs on a monthly basis.

THERAPEUTIC CLASS: Isonicotinic acid hydrazide/rifamycin derivative

INDICATIONS: For pulmonary tuberculosis (TB). Not for initial therapy or prevention.

DOSAGE: *Adults:* 2 caps qd. Take 1 hr before or 2 hrs after meals. Give with pyridoxine in the malnourished, those predisposed to neuropathy (eg, alcoholics, diabetics), and adolescents.

HOW SUPPLIED: Cap: (Isoniazid-Rifampin) 150mg-300mg

CONTRAINDICATIONS: Previous isoniazid-associated hepatic injury, severe adverse reactions to isoniazid (eg, drug fever, chills, and arthritis), acute liver disease.

WARNINGS/PRECAUTIONS: Monitor LFTs before therapy, periodically thereafter. Not for intermittent therapy. Urine, feces, saliva, sputum, sweat, and tears may be colored red-orange; may stain soft contact lenses permanently. Caution with chronic liver disease or severe renal dysfunction. Perform periodic ophthalmoscopic exams.

ADVERSE REACTIONS: Headache, drowsiness, fatigue, ataxia, dizziness, confusion, visual disturbances, weakness, GI effects, peripheral neuropathy, pyridoxine deficiency, anorexia, nausea, renal or hepatic insufficiency, blood dyscrasias.

INTERACTIONS: Anticoagulants may need dose increase. May decrease activity of methadone, oral hypoglycemics, digitoxin, quinidine, disopyramide, dapsone, and corticosteroids. Higher incidence of isoniazid hepatitis with daily alcohol ingestion. Risk of phenytoin toxicity. Caution with other hepatotoxic agents and phenytoin. May decrease effects of oral contraceptives; use alternative measures.

PREGNANCY: Safety in pregnancy not known, caution in nursing.

MECHANISM OF ACTION: Isonicotinic acid hydrazide/rifamycin derivative. Isoniazid/Rifampin: Exhibits bacterial activity against intracellular and extracellular *Mycobacterium tuberculosis*. Inhibits DNA-dependent RNA polymerase activity in susceptible cells; interacts with bacterial RNA polymerase but does not inhibit the mammalian enzyme. Inhibits mycoloic acid synthesis and acts against actively growing tubercle bacilli.

PHARMACOKINETICS: Absorption: Rifampin: C_{max}=10mcg/mL, T_{max}=1.5-3 hrs. Isoniazid: T_{max}=1-2 hrs. **Distribution:** Isoniazid: Diffuses into body fluids; crosses placental barrier and into milk. **Metabolism:** Isoniazid: Acetylation and dehydrazination. **Elimination:** Rifampin: Bile, urine; $T_{1/2}$=3 hrs.

NURSING CONSIDERATIONS

Assessment: Assess for previous isoniazid-associated hepatic injury, acute liver disease, HIV status, pregnancy/nursing status, and drug interactions. Document reasons for therapy, culture and susceptibility.

Monitoring: Prior to therapy and periodically thereafter, measure hepatic enzymes (AST, ALT). D/C at first sign of hypersensitivity reactions. Monitor for peripheral neuropathy, convulsions, N/V, agranulocytosis, hemolytic anemia, systemic lupus erythematosus like syndrome, metabolic and endocrine reactions (hyperglycemia, pyridoxine deficiency, pellagra), visual disturbances, serum uric acid levels. Perform periodic ophthalmoscopic exams.

Patient Counseling: Advise to immediately report signs/symptoms consistent with liver damage or other adverse events (eg, unexplained anorexia, N/V, dark urine, icterus, rash, persistent paresthesias of the hands and feet, persistent fatigue, weakness or fever of >3 days duration and/or abdominal tenderness). Counsel not to administer with food, take as prescribed, take pyridoxine tablets if peripheral neuropathy develops. Inform that drug may produce reddish urine, sweat, sputum, and tears. Periodic eye exams are recommended when visual symptoms occur.

Administration: Oral route. **Storage:** Keep tightly closed. Store in a dry place. Avoid excessive heat.

RIFATER   RX
rifampin - isoniazid - pyrazinamide (Sanofi-Aventis)

Isoniazid associated with severe and sometimes fatal hepatitis. Monitor LFTs on a monthly basis. D/C promptly if symptoms of hepatitis occur. Defer treatment in persons with acute hepatic diseases.

THERAPEUTIC CLASS: Isonicotinic acid hydrazide/rifamycin derivative/nicotinamide analogue

INDICATIONS: For initial phase of pulmonary tuberculosis (TB) treatment.

DOSAGE: *Adults:* ≤44kg: 4 tabs single dose qd. 45-54kg: 5 tabs single dose qd. ≥55kg: 6 tabs single dose qd. Give pyridoxine in malnourished, if predisposed to neuropathy (eg, alcoholics, diabetics), and adolescents. Take 1 hr before or 2 hrs after meals with full glass of water. Treatment usually lasts 2 months.
Pediatrics: ≥15 yrs: ≤44kg: 4 tabs single dose qd. 45-54kg: 5 tabs single dose qd. ≥55kg: 6 tabs single dose qd. Give pyridoxine in malnourished, if predisposed to neuropathy (eg, alcoholics, diabetics), and adolescents. Take 1 hr before or 2 hrs after meals with full glass of water. Treatment usually lasts 2 months.

HOW SUPPLIED: Tab: (Isoniazid-Pyrazinamide-Rifampin) 50mg-300mg-120mg

CONTRAINDICATIONS: Severe hepatic damage, adverse reactions to isoniazid (eg, drug fever, chills, arthritis), acute liver disease, acute gout. Concomitant administration of atazanavir, darunavir, fosamprenavir, saquinavir, tipranavir, and ritonavir-boosted saquinavir.

WARNINGS/PRECAUTIONS: Liver dysfunction, hyperbilirubinemia, and hyperuricemia with acute gouty arthritis reported. Caution in patients with impaired liver function; monitor LFTs (every 2-4 weeks) and serum uric acid. Perform regular ophthalmologic exams. Caution with diabetes mellitus (DM), and severe renal dysfunction. Doses of rifampin >600mg given once daily or twice weekly resulted in higher incidence of adverse reactions ("flu syndrome", hematopoietic, cutaneous, GI, and hepatic reactions, SOB, shock, anaphylaxis, and renal failure). Rifampin is not recommended for intermittent therapy. May produce reddish coloration of urine, sweat, sputum, and tears. May permanently stain soft contact lenses. Caution in elderly.

ADVERSE REACTIONS: Cutaneous reactions, N/V, digestive pain, diarrhea, arthralgia, sweating, headache, insomnia, anxiety, tightness in chest, coughing, angina, palpitation, anxiety, phlebitis.

INTERACTIONS: See Contraindications. Rifampin may accelerate metabolism of anticonvulsants, digitoxin, antiarrhythmics, oral anticoagulants, antifungals, barbiturates, β-blockers, calcium channel blockers, chloramphenicol, clarithromycin, fluoroquinolones, corticosteroids, cyclosporine, cardiac glycosides, clofibrate, oral or systemic hormonal contraceptives, dapsone, diazepam, doxycycline, haloperidol, oral hypoglycemics, levothyroxine, methadone, narcotic analgesics, TCAs, progestins, quinine, tacrolimus, theophylline and zidovudine. Decreased concentration of atovaquone, ketoconazole, enalaprilat and sulfapyridine. Increased rifampin concentrations with probenecid and cotrimoxazole. Antacids may reduce rifampin absorption. Avoid foods containing tyramine and histamine (eg, cheese, red wine, tuna). Anticoagulants may need dose increase. Higher incidence of isoniazid (INH) hepatitis with daily alcohol ingestion. Avoid halothane. Monitor renal function with enflurane. INH inhibits certain CYP450 enzymes. Decreased

R

levels with corticosteroids. Increased levels with para-aminosalicylic acid. Exaggerates CNS effects of meperidine, cycloserine, disulfiram. Excess catecholamine stimulation with L-dopa. **PREGNANCY:** Category C, not for use in nursing.

MECHANISM OF ACTION: Rifampin: Rifamycin derivative; inhibits DNA-dependent RNA polymerase activity in susceptible *Mycobacterium tuberculosis* organism. Interacts with bacterial RNA polymerase, but does not inhibit the mammalian enzyme. Isoniazid: Isonicotinic acid hydrazide; inhibits the biosynthesis of mycolic acids, which are major component of the cell wall of *Mycobacterium tuberculosis*. Pyrazinamide: Nicotinamide analog; has not been established.

PHARMACOKINETICS: Absorption: Isoniazid: Bioavailability (100.6%), C_{max}=3.09mcg/mL, T_{max}=1-2 hrs. Rifampin: Bioavailability (88.8%), C_{max}=11.04mcg/mL. Pyrazinamide: Bioavailability (96.8%), C_{max}=28.02mcg/mL. **Distribution:** Isoniazid: Passes through placental barrier and into milk. Pyrazinamide: Plasma protein binding (10%), distributed in liver, lungs, and CSF; found in breast milk. Rifampin: Protein binding (80%). **Metabolism:** Isoniazid: Acetylation and dehydrazination. Pyrazinamide: Liver, via hydroxylation; pyrazinoic acid (major active metabolite). Rifampin: Via deacetylation. **Elimination:** Rifampin: Urine (30%), bile; $T_{1/2}$=3.35 hrs. Pyrazinamide: Urine (70%), (4-14% unchanged); $T_{1/2}$=9-10 hrs. Isoniazid: Urine (50-70%); $T_{1/2}$=1-4 hrs.

NURSING CONSIDERATIONS

Assessment: Assess for previous isoniazid-associated hepatic injury, acute gout, HIV status, pregnancy/nursing status, DM, and drug interactions. Document reasons for therapy, culture, and susceptibility.

Monitoring: Prior to therapy and periodically thereafter, measure hepatic enzymes (AST, ALT) every 2-4 weeks with impaired liver function. D/C at first sign of hypersensitivity reactions. Monitor for peripheral neuropathy, convulsions, N/V, agranulocytosis, hemolytic anemia, systemic lupus erythematosus-like syndrome, metabolic and endocrine reactions (hyperglycemia, pyridoxine deficiency, pellagra), visual disturbances, serum uric acid levels. Perform regular ophthalmologic exams.

Patient Counseling: Immediately report signs/symptoms consistent with liver damage or other adverse events (unexplained anorexia, N/V, dark urine, icterus, rash, persistent paresthesias of hands and feet, persistent fatigue, weakness or fever of >3 days' duration and/or abdominal tenderness). Do not administer with food; take as prescribed. Take pyridoxine tablets if peripheral neuropathy develops. Drug may produce reddish urine, sweat, sputum, and tears. Periodic ophthalmologic examination is recommended. Avoid tyramine- and histamine-containing foods. Effectiveness of oral contraceptives may be decreased; consider alternative contraceptive methods.

Administration: Oral route. **Storage:** 15-30°C (59-86°F). Protect from excessive humidity.

RILUTEK   RX
riluzole (Sanofi-Aventis)

THERAPEUTIC CLASS: Benzothiazole

INDICATIONS: Treatment of amyotrophic lateral sclerosis (ALS). Extends survival and/or time to tracheostomy.

DOSAGE: *Adults:* 50mg q12h. Take 1 hr before or 2 hrs after meals.

HOW SUPPLIED: Tab: 50mg

WARNINGS/PRECAUTIONS: Caution with hepatic impairment; monitor LFTs. D/C if ALT levels ≥5 x ULN or clinical jaundice develops. Clinical hepatitis reported. Neutropenia may occur; monitor WBC count with febrile illness. Interstitial lung disease reported; perform chest radiography if respiratory symptoms develop such as dry cough and/or dyspnea. May impair mental/physical abilities. Caution in elderly.

ADVERSE REACTIONS: Asthenia, N/V, dizziness, decreased lung function, diarrhea, abdominal pain, vertigo, circumonal paresthesia, anorexia, somnolence, headache, anorexia, rhinitis, HTN.

INTERACTIONS: Caution with concomitant use with potentially hepatotoxic drugs (eg, allopurinol, methyldopa, sulfasalazine). CYP1A2 inhibitors may decrease elimination. CYP1A2 inducers may increase elimination.

PREGNANCY: Category C, not for use in nursing.

MECHANISM OF ACTION: Benzothiazole; mechanism not established. May inhibit the effect on glutamate release, inactivates voltage-dependent sodium channels, and interferes with intracellular events that follow transmitter binding at excitatory amino acid receptors.

PHARMACOKINETICS: Absorption: Well absorbed; absolute bioavailability (60%). **Distribution:** Plasma protein binding (96%). **Metabolism:** Extensive; liver via CYP450 by hydroxylation and glucuronidation; N-hydroxyriluzole (major metabolite). **Elimination:** Urine (90% metabolites, 2% unchanged), feces (5%); $T_{1/2}$=12 hrs.

NURSING CONSIDERATIONS

Assessment: Assess for hepatic impairment, pregnancy/nursing status, alcohol intake, hypersensitivity and possible drug interactions. Perform baseline LFTs.

Monitoring: Perform baseline LFTs before therapy, every month during first 3 months, every 3 months for the remainder of the first year, then periodically thereafter. Take WBC count and chest radiography if necessary. Monitor for signs/symptoms of febrile illness, liver toxicity, and hypersensitivity reactions.

Patient Counseling: Notify healthcare professional of any signs of febrile illness. Caution about hazardous tasks (eg, operating machinery/driving). Notify healthcare professional if cough or SOB occur. Avoid use with excessive intake of alcohol. Instruct patient if a dose is missed, take next tablet as originally planned.

Administration: Oral route. **Storage:** 20-25°C (68-77°F); protect from bright light.

RIOMET   RX
metformin HCl (Ranbaxy)

Lactic acidosis reported (rare); increased risk with increased age, DM, renal dysfunction, congestive heart failure (CHF), and conditions with risk of hypoperfusion and hypoxemia. Avoid use in patients ≥80 yrs unless renal function is normal. Withhold therapy in the presence of any condition associated with hypoxemia, dehydration, or sepsis. Avoid in patients with clinical or laboratory evidence of hepatic disease. Caution against excessive alcohol intake;may potentiate the effects of metformin on lactate metabolism. Temporarily D/C prior to any IV radiocontrast study or surgical procedures. D/C use and institute appropriate therapy if lactic acidosis occur.

THERAPEUTIC CLASS: Biguanide

INDICATIONS: Adjunct to diet and exercise, to improve glycemic control in type 2 diabetes mellitus (DM).

DOSAGE: *Adults:* Individualize dose. Initial: 500mg bid or 850mg qd with meals. Titrate: Increase by 500mg/week or 850mg every 2 weeks, or may increase from 500mg bid to 850mg bid after 2 weeks. Max: 2550mg/day. Give in 3 divided doses with meals if dose is >2g/day. With Insulin: Initial: 500mg qd. Titrate: Increase by 500mg/week. Max: 2500mg/day. Decrease insulin dose by 10-25% when FPG <120mg/dL. Elderly/Debilitated/Malnourished: Conservative dosing; do not titrate to max.
Pediatrics: 10-16 yrs: Individualize dose. Initial: 500mg bid with meals. Titrate: Increase by 500mg/week. Max: 2000mg/day, given in divided doses.

HOW SUPPLIED: Sol: 500mg/5mL

CONTRAINDICATIONS: Renal disease/dysfunction (eg, SrCr ≥1.5mg/dL [males], ≥1.4mg/dL [females], or abnormal CrCl), metabolic acidosis, diabetic ketoacidosis with or without coma. D/C temporarily (48 hrs) for radiologic studies with intravascular iodinated contrast materials.

WARNINGS/PRECAUTIONS: Avoid in renal/hepatic impairment. D/C therapy in the presence of hypoxemia (eg, acute CHF, acute MI, cardiovascular collapse), dehydration, sepsis, or if loss of blood glucose occurs due to stress (give insulin). Temporarily d/c therapy prior to any surgical procedure (except minor procedures not associated with restricted intake of food and fluids). May decrease serum vitamin B12 levels. Increased risk of hypoglycemia in elderly, debilitated/ malnourished, adrenal or pituitary insufficiency, or alcohol intoxication.

ADVERSE REACTIONS: Lactic acidosis, diarrhea, N/V, flatulence, asthenia, abdominal discomfort, hypoglycemia, dizziness, dyspnea, taste disorder, chest discomfort, flu syndrome, palpitations, indigestion, headache.

INTERACTIONS: See Boxed Warning and Contraindications. Furosemide, nifedipine, cimetidine, cationic drugs (eg, digoxin, amiloride, procainamide, quinidine, quinine, ranitidine, trimethoprim, vancomycin, triamterene, morphine) may increase levels. Thiazides, other diuretics, corticosteroids, phenothiazines, thyroid products, estrogens, oral contraceptives, phenytoin, nicotinic acid, sympathomimetics, CCBs, and isoniazid may cause hyperglycemia. May interact with highly protein-bound drugs (eg, salicylates, sulfonamides, chloramphenicol, probenecid). May decrease furosemide levels. Caution with drugs that may affect renal function or result in significant hemodynamic change or may interfere with the disposition of metformin. Hypoglycemia may occur with concomitant use of other glucose-lowering agents.

PREGNANCY: Category B, not for use in nursing.

MECHANISM OF ACTION: Biguanide; decreases hepatic glucose production, decreases intestinal absorption of glucose, and improves insulin selectivity by increasing peripheral glucose uptake and utilization.

PHARMACOKINETICS: Absorption: Absolute bioavailability (50-60%); T_{max}=2.5 hrs. **Distribution:** V_d=654L. **Elimination:** Urine (90%); $T_{1/2}$=6.2 hrs (plasma), 17.6 hrs (blood).

NURSING CONSIDERATIONS

Assessment: Assess for renal/hepatic impairment, acute or chronic metabolic acidosis, presence of a hypoxic state (eg, CHF, acute MI, cardiovascular collapse), dehydration, sepsis, alcoholism, nutritional status, adrenal or pituitary insufficiency, pregnancy/nursing status, and for possible drug interactions. Assess baseline renal function, FPG, HbA1c, and hematological parameters (Hct, Hgb, red blood cell indices).

Monitoring: Monitor for lactic acidosis, ketoacidosis, hypoglycemia, hypoxemia, prerenal azotemia, and for decreases in Vitamin B12 levels. Monitor FPG, HbA1c, renal function (eg, SrCr), and hematological parameters.

Patient Counseling: Inform about the importance of adherence to dietary instructions and a regular exercise program. Inform of the risk of developing lactic acidosis during therapy; advise to d/c therapy immediately and contact physician if unexplained hyperventilation, myalgia, malaise, unusual somnolence, or other nonspecific symptoms occur. Instruct to avoid excessive alcohol intake. Inform that regular follow-up is needed. Counsel to take with meals.

Administration: Oral route. **Storage:** 15-30°C (59-86°F).

RISPERDAL   RX
risperidone (Ortho-McNeil/Janssen)

> Elderly patients with dementia-related psychosis treated with antipsychotic drugs are at an increased risk of death; most deaths appeared to be cardiovascular (CV) (eg, heart failure, sudden death) or infectious (eg, pneumonia) in nature. Not approved for treatment of patients with dementia-related psychosis.

OTHER BRAND NAMES: Risperdal M-Tab (Ortho-Mcneil/Janssen)

THERAPEUTIC CLASS: Benzisoxazole derivative

INDICATIONS: Acute and maintenance treatment of schizophrenia in adults. Treatment of schizophrenia in adolescents 13-17 yrs. Short-term treatment of acute manic or mixed episodes associated with bipolar I disorder as monotherapy (adults and pediatrics 10-17 yrs) or in combination with lithium or valproate (adults). Treatment of irritability associated with autistic disorder in children and adolescents 5-16 yrs, including symptoms of aggression toward others, deliberate self-injuriousness, temper tantrums, and quickly changing moods.

DOSAGE: *Adults:* Schizophrenia: Initial: 2mg/day qd or bid. Titrate: May increase to 4-8mg/day, by 1-2mg/day at intervals ≥24 hrs, as tolerated. Range: 4-16mg/day. Max: 16mg/day. Maint: 2-8mg/day. Periodically reassess need for maint treatment. Refer to PI if reinitiating treatment or switching from other antipsychotics. Bipolar Mania: Initial: 2-3mg qd. Titrate: Adjust at intervals ≥24 hrs in increments/decrements of 1mg/day. Range: 1-6mg/day. Max: 6mg/day. Elderly/Debilitated/Predisposed to Hypotension/Severe Renal or Hepatic Impairment: Initial: 0.5mg bid. Titrate: May increase by ≤0.5mg bid. Increases to doses >1.5mg bid should occur at intervals of ≥1 week. If qd dosing regimen in elderly/debilitated is being considered, titrate on bid regimen for 2-3 days at the target dose. Subsequent switches to a qd dosing regimen can be done thereafter. *Pediatrics:* Schizophrenia: 13-17 yrs: Initial: 0.5mg qd in am or pm. Titrate: May increase to 3mg/day, by 0.5 or 1mg/day at intervals ≥24 hrs, as tolerated. Max: 6mg/day. If with persistent somnolence, give half the daily dose bid. Refer to PI if reinitiating treatment or switching from other antipsychotics. Bipolar Mania: 10-17 yrs: Initial: 0.5mg qd in am or pm. Titrate: May increase to 2.5mg/day, by 0.5 or 1mg/day at intervals ≥24 hrs, as tolerated. Range: 0.5-6mg/day. Max: 6mg/day. If with persistent somnolence, give half the daily dose bid. Irritability Associated With Autistic Disorder: 5-16 yrs: Individualize dose. Initial: <20kg: 0.25mg/day qd or bid; ≥20kg: 0.5mg/day qd or bid. Titrate: May increase to 0.5mg/day (<20kg) or 1mg/day (≥20kg) after ≥4 days from initiation. Maint: ≥14 days. Inadequate Response: Increase by 0.25mg/day (<20kg) or 0.5mg/day (≥20kg) at ≥2-week intervals. Caution in patients <15kg. Max: <20kg: 1mg/day; ≥20kg: 2.5mg/day; >45kg: 3mg/day. If with persistent somnolence, give qd dose at hs or half the daily dose bid, or reduce dose.

HOW SUPPLIED: Sol: 1mg/mL [30mL]; Tab: 0.25mg, 0.5mg, 1mg, 2mg, 3mg, 4mg; Tab, Disintegrating: (M-Tab) 0.5mg, 1mg, 2mg, 3mg, 4mg

WARNINGS/PRECAUTIONS: Neuroleptic malignant syndrome (NMS), tardive dyskinesia (TD), and hyperprolactinemia reported. Associated with metabolic changes (eg, hyperglycemia and diabetes mellitus [DM], dyslipidemia, weight gain) that may increase CV/cerebrovascular risk. May induce orthostatic hypotension; caution with CV disease, cerebrovascular disease, and conditions that predispose to hypotension. Leukopenia, neutropenia, and agranulocytosis reported; d/c in cases of severe neutropenia (absolute neutrophil count <1000/mm³). May impair mental/physical abilities. Seizures reported; caution with history of seizures. Esophageal dysmotility and aspiration reported; caution in patients at risk for aspiration pneumonia. Priapism and thrombotic thrombocytopenic purpura (TTP) reported. May disrupt body temperature regulation; caution when exposed to extreme temperatures. May produce antiemetic effect that may mask signs/symptoms of overdosage with certain drugs or certain conditions (eg, intestinal obstruction,

Reye's syndrome, brain tumor). Closely supervise patients at high risk of suicide. Increased sensitivity reported in patients with Parkinson's disease or dementia with Lewy bodies. Caution with diseases/conditions affecting metabolism or hemodynamic responses, renal/hepatic impairment, and in elderly. Evaluate for history of drug abuse; observe for drug misuse/abuse in these patients.

ADVERSE REACTIONS: Somnolence, increased appetite, fatigue, N/V, cough, constipation, parkinsonism, upper abdominal pain, anxiety, dizziness, tremor, insomnia, sedation, akathisia.

INTERACTIONS: Caution with other centrally acting drugs and alcohol. May enhance hypotensive effects of antihypertensive drugs. May antagonize effects of levodopa and dopamine agonists. Increased bioavailability with cimetidine and ranitidine. Increased exposure with ranitidine. Decreased clearance with chronic use of clozapine. Increased valproate peak plasma concentration. Increased concentrations with fluoxetine, paroxetine, and CYP2D6 inhibitors; titrate dose accordingly when fluoxetine/paroxetine is coadministered. Decreased concentrations with carbamazepine and other known enzyme inducers (eg, phenytoin, rifampin, phenobarbital); titrate dose accordingly.

PREGNANCY: Category C, not for use in nursing.

MECHANISM OF ACTION: Benzisoxazole derivative; not established. In schizophrenia, proposed to be mediated through a combination of dopamine type 2 (D_2) and serotonin type 2 ($5HT_2$) receptor antagonism.

PHARMACOKINETICS: Absorption: Well absorbed. Absolute bioavailability (70%). Risperidone: T_{max}=1 hr. 9-hydroxyrisperidone: T_{max}=3 hrs (extensive metabolizers), 17 hrs (poor metabolizers). **Distribution:** V_d=1-2L/kg; plasma protein binding (risperidone, 90%) (9-hydroxyrisperidone, 77%); found in breast milk. **Metabolism:** Liver (extensive); hydroxylation via CYP2D6 to 9-hydroxyrisperidone (major metabolite); N-dealkylation (minor pathway). **Elimination:** Urine (70%), feces (14%). Risperidone: $T_{1/2}$=3 hrs (extensive metabolizers), 20 hrs (poor metabolizers). 9-hydroxyrisperidone: $T_{1/2}$=21 hrs (extensive metabolizers), 30 hrs (poor metabolizers).

NURSING CONSIDERATIONS

Assessment: Assess for dementia-related psychosis, DM, or any other conditions where treatment is contraindicated or cautioned. Assess for hepatic/renal impairment, pregnancy/nursing status, and possible drug interactions. Obtain baseline FPG in patients at risk for DM.

Monitoring: Monitor for NMS, TD, hyperprolactinemia, orthostatic hypotension, cognitive and motor impairment, seizures, esophageal dysmotility, aspiration, priapism, TTP, metabolic changes, and disruption of body temperature. Monitor for signs of hyperglycemia; perform periodic monitoring of FPG levels in patients with DM or at risk for DM. Monitor for signs/symptoms of leukopenia, neutropenia (eg, fever, infection), and agranulocytosis; perform frequent monitoring of CBC in patients with history of clinically significant low WBC or drug-induced leukopenia/neutropenia. Monitor liver/renal function and weight.

Patient Counseling: Advise of risk of orthostatic hypotension. Inform that therapy has the potential to impair judgment, thinking, or motor skills; advise to use caution when operating hazardous machinery (eg, automobiles). Instruct to notify physician if pregnant or plan to become pregnant, and of all medications currently being taken. Instruct not to breastfeed while on therapy. Advise to avoid alcohol during treatment. Inform that disintegrating tab contains phenylalanine.

Administration: Oral route. Refer to PI for administration/directions for use of sol and orally disintegrating tab. **Storage:** 15-25°C (59-77°F). (Sol) Protect from light and freezing. (Tab) Protect from light and moisture.

R

RISPERDAL CONSTA   RX
risperidone (Ortho-McNeil/Janssen)

> Elderly patients with dementia-related psychosis treated with antipsychotic drugs are at an increased risk of death; most deaths appeared to be cardiovascular (CV) (eg, heart failure, sudden death) or infectious (eg, pneumonia) in nature. Not approved for the treatment of patients with dementia-related psychosis.

THERAPEUTIC CLASS: Benzisoxazole derivative

INDICATIONS: Treatment of schizophrenia. As monotherapy or adjunctive therapy to lithium or valproate for maintenance treatment of bipolar I disorder.

DOSAGE: *Adults:* In PO risperidone-naive patients, establish tolerability with PO risperidone prior to treatment with risperidone inj. Give 1st inj with PO risperidone or other antipsychotic; continue for 3 weeks, then d/c PO therapy. Upward dose adjustment should not be made more frequently than q4 weeks. Schizophrenia/Bipolar I Disorder: Usual: 25mg IM q2 weeks. Titrate: May increase to 37.5mg or 50mg based on response. Max: 50mg q2 weeks. Hepatic/Renal Impairment: Prior to initiating IM therapy, administer PO dosage, 0.5mg bid during the 1st week. Titrate: May increase PO dosage to 1mg bid or 2mg qd during the 2nd week. If total daily PO dose of ≥2mg is tolerated, start at 12.5mg or 25mg IM q2 weeks. Elderly: 25mg IM q2 weeks. Reinitiation: Supplement with PO risperidone or other antipsychotic. Switching from Other Antipsychotics: Continue previous antipsychotic for 3 weeks after 1st risperidone inj. Poor Tolerability: Initial: 12.5mg IM. Coadministration with Enzyme Inducers/Fluoxetine/Paroxetine: Titrate accordingly.

HOW SUPPLIED: Inj: 12.5mg, 25mg, 37.5mg, 50mg

WARNINGS/PRECAUTIONS: Neuroleptic malignant syndrome (NMS), tardive dyskinesia (TD), hyperprolactinemia reported. Associated with metabolic changes (eg, hyperglycemia and diabetes mellitus [DM], dyslipidemia, weight gain) that may increase CV/cerebrovascular risk. May induce orthostatic hypotension; caution with CV disease, cerebrovascular disease, or conditions that predispose to hypotension. Leukopenia, neutropenia, and agranulocytosis reported; d/c in cases of severe neutropenia (absolute neutrophil count <1000/mm³). May impair mental/physical abilities. Seizures reported; caution with history of seizures. Esophageal dysmotility and aspiration reported; caution in patients at risk for aspiration pneumonia. Priapism and thrombotic thrombocytopenic purpura (TTP) reported. May disrupt body temperature regulation; caution when exposed to extreme temperatures. May produce an antiemetic effect that may mask signs/symptoms of overdosage with certain drugs or conditions (eg, intestinal obstruction, Reye's syndrome, brain tumor). Closely supervise patients at high-risk of suicide. Increased sensitivity reported in patients with Parkinson's disease or dementia with Lewy bodies. Caution with diseases/conditions affecting metabolism or hemodynamic responses, renal/hepatic impairment, and in elderly. Intended for IM inj; avoid inadvertent inj into a blood vessel.

ADVERSE REACTIONS: Headache, dizziness, constipation, dyspepsia, akathisia, parkinsonism, weight increased, dry mouth, fatigue, pain in extremity, tremor, nausea, sedation, cough, pain.

INTERACTIONS: Caution with other centrally-acting drugs and alcohol. May enhance hypotensive effects of antihypertensive drugs. May antagonize effects of levodopa and dopamine agonists. Increases bioavailability of PO risperidone with cimetidine or ranitidine. Increased exposure with ranitidine. Decreased clearance with chronic use of clozapine. Increased valproate peak plasma concentrations with PO risperidone. Increased concentrations with fluoxetine, paroxetine, and other CYP2D6 inhibitors. Decreased concentrations with carbamazepine and other CYP3A4 enzyme inducers.

PREGNANCY: Category C, not for use in nursing.

MECHANISM OF ACTION: Benzisoxazole derivative; not established. In schizophrenia, proposed to be mediated through a combination of dopamine type 2 (D_2) and serotonin type 2 ($5HT_2$) receptor antagonism.

PHARMACOKINETICS: Distribution: Rapid; V_d=1-2L/kg; plasma protein binding (risperidone, 90%), (9-hydroxyrisperidone, 77%); found in breast milk. **Metabolism**: Liver (extensive) via CYP2D6; hydroxylation, N-dealkylation; 9-hydroxyrisperidone (major metabolite). **Elimination**: Urine (70%), feces (14%); $T_{1/2}$=3-6 days.

NURSING CONSIDERATIONS

Assessment: Assess for dementia-related psychosis, DM, or any other conditions where treatment is contraindicated or cautioned. Assess for hepatic/renal impairment, pregnancy/nursing status, and for possible drug interactions. Obtain baseline FPG in patients at risk for DM.

Monitoring: Monitor for NMS, TD, hyperprolactinemia, orthostatic hypotension, cognitive and motor impairment, seizures, esophageal dysmotility, aspiration, priapism, TTP, metabolic changes, and disruption of body temperature. Monitor for signs of hyperglycemia; perform periodic monitoring of FPG levels in patients with DM or at risk for DM. Monitor for signs/symptoms of leukopenia, neutropenia (eg, fever, infection), and agranulocytosis; perform frequent monitoring of CBC in patients with history of clinically significant low WBC or drug-induced leukopenia/neutropenia. Monitor liver/renal function and weight.

Patient Counseling: Advise of risk of orthostatic hypotension and of nonpharmacologic interventions that will help reduce its occurrence. Inform that therapy has the potential to impair judgment, thinking, or motor skills; advise to use caution when operating hazardous machinery (eg, automobiles). Instruct to notify physician if pregnant or plan to become pregnant, and of all medications currently being taken. Instruct not to breastfeed while on therapy and for ≥12 weeks after last inj. Advise to avoid alcohol during treatment.

Administration: IM route. Deep IM into the gluteal or deltoid muscle q2 weeks. Not for IV use. Refer to PI for complete instructions for use. **Storage**: 2-8°C (36-46°F). Protect from light. If refrigeration is unavailable, store at ≤25°C (77°F) for ≤7 days prior to administration.

RITALIN
methylphenidate HCl (Novartis)

> Caution with history of drug dependence or alcoholism. Marked tolerance and psychological dependence may result from chronic abusive use. Frank psychotic episodes may occur, especially with parenteral abuse. Careful supervision required for withdrawal from abusive use to avoid severe depression. Withdrawal following chronic use may unmask symptoms of underlying disorder that may require follow-up.

OTHER BRAND NAMES: Ritalin LA (Novartis) - Ritalin SR (Novartis)

THERAPEUTIC CLASS: Sympathomimetic amine

INDICATIONS: (Cap, Extended-Release) Treatment of attention deficit hyperactivity disorder. (Tab; Tab, Sustained-Release) Treatment of attention deficit disorders and narcolepsy.

DOSAGE: *Adults:* Individualize dose. Reduce dose or d/c if paradoxical aggravation of symptoms occurs. D/C if no improvement after appropriate dose adjustment over a 1-month period. (Tab) 10-60mg/day divided bid-tid 30-45 min ac. Take last dose before 6 pm if insomnia occurs. (Tab, SR) May be used in place of immediate-release (IR) tab when the 8-hr dose corresponds to the titrated 8-hr IR dose. Swallow whole; do not crush or chew. (Cap, ER) Initial: 10-20mg qam. Titrate: May adjust weekly by 10mg. Max: 60mg/day. Currently on Methylphenidate: May be used in place of IR or SR tabs with a qd equivalent dose; refer to PI for recommended dosing. Swallow whole; do not crush, chew, or divide.
Pediatrics: ≥6 yrs: Individualize dose. Reduce dose or d/c if paradoxical aggravation of symptoms occurs. D/C if no improvement after appropriate dose adjustment over a 1-month period. (Tab) Initial: 5mg bid before breakfast and lunch. Titrate: Increase gradually by 5-10mg weekly. Max: 60mg/day. (Tab, SR) May be used in place of IR tab when the 8-hr dose corresponds to the titrated 8-hr IR dose. Swallow whole; do not crush or chew. (Cap, ER) Initial: 10-20mg qam. Titrate: May adjust weekly by 10mg. Max: 60mg/day. Currently on Methylphenidate: May be used in place of IR or SR tabs with a qd equivalent dose; refer to PI for recommended dosing. Swallow whole; do not crush, chew, or divide.

HOW SUPPLIED: Cap, Extended-Release (Ritalin LA): 10mg, 20mg, 30mg, 40mg; Tab (Ritalin): 5mg, 10mg*, 20mg*; Tab, Sustained-Release (Ritalin SR): 20mg *scored

CONTRAINDICATIONS: Marked anxiety, tension, agitation, glaucoma, motor tics or family history or diagnosis of Tourette's syndrome. Treatment with or within a minimum of 14 days following d/c of a MAOI.

WARNINGS/PRECAUTIONS: Sudden death, stroke, and myocardial infarction (MI) reported; avoid with known structural cardiac abnormalities, cardiomyopathy, serious heart rhythm abnormalities, coronary artery disease or other serious cardiac problems. May increase BP and HR; caution with pre-existing HTN, heart failure, MI, or ventricular arrhythmias. Assess patients for cardiac disease prior to initiating therapy; promptly perform cardiac evaluation if symptoms suggestive of cardiac disease develop. May exacerbate symptoms of behavior disturbance and thought disorder in patients with a pre-existing psychotic disorder. May induce mixed/manic episode in patients with bipolar disorder; assess for bipolar disease before starting therapy. May cause treatment-emergent psychotic or manic symptoms in children and adolescents without prior history of psychotic illness or mania at usual doses. Aggressive behavior or hostility reported. May cause growth suppression in children. May lower convulsive threshold; d/c if seizures occur. Visual disturbances reported. Not for use in children <6 yrs. (Tab; Tab, SR) Patients with an element of agitation may react adversely; d/c therapy if necessary. Not indicated in all cases of this behavioral syndrome, and in symptoms associated with acute stress reactions. D/C drug periodically to assess child's condition; therapy should not be indefinite. (Cap, ER) Periodically re-evaluate the usefulness of therapy.

ADVERSE REACTIONS: Nervousness, insomnia, hypersensitivity, anorexia, nausea, dizziness, headache, dyskinesia, drowsiness, BP and pulse changes, tachycardia, weight loss, abdominal pain, decreased appetite.

INTERACTIONS: See Contraindications. Caution with pressor agents. May decrease effectiveness of antihypertensives. May inhibit metabolism of coumarin anticoagulants, anticonvulsants, TCAs; may need to adjust dose of these drugs downward and monitor plasma drug levels/coagulation times when starting/stopping methylphenidate therapy. Possible occurrence of neuroleptic malignant syndrome (NMS) with concurrent therapies associated with NMS; single report of NMS-like event possibly related with concurrent use of venlafaxine. (Cap, ER) Release may be altered by antacids or acid suppressants. May be associated with pharmacodynamic interaction when coadministered with direct and indirect dopamine agonists (eg, DOPA and TCAs) as well as dopamine antagonists (antipsychotics, eg, haloperidol).

PREGNANCY: Category C, caution in nursing.

MECHANISM OF ACTION: Sympathomimetic amine; not established. CNS stimulant, thought to block the reuptake of norepinephrine and dopamine into the presynaptic neuron and increase

R

the release of monoamines into the extraneuronal space. Presumably activates the brain stem arousal system and cortex to produce stimulant effect.

PHARMACOKINETICS: Absorption: (Cap, ER 20mg) **Adults:** T_{max1}=2 hrs, C_{max1}=5.3ng/mL, T_{max2}=5.5 hrs, C_{max2}=6.2ng/mL, AUC=45.8ng•hr/mL. **Pediatrics:** T_{max1}=2 hrs, C_{max1}=10.3ng/mL, T_{max2}=6.6 hrs, C_{max2}=10.2ng/mL, AUC=86.6ng•hr/mL. **Distribution:** (Cap, ER) Plasma protein binding (10%-33%); V_d=2.65L/kg (d-methylphenidate), 1.8L/kg (l-methylphenidate). **Metabolism:** Rapid and extensive by carboxylesterase CES1A1; α-phenyl-2-piperidine acetic acid (major metabolite). **Elimination:** (Tab) Urine (78-97% metabolites, <1% unchanged), feces (1-3% metabolites). (Tab, SR) Urine (86% adults; 67% pediatrics). (Tab; Cap, ER) $T_{1/2}$=3.5 hrs (adults), 2.5 hrs (pediatrics).

NURSING CONSIDERATIONS

Assessment: Assess for cardiac disease, psychotic disorders, bipolar disorder, seizures, history of drug dependence or alcoholism, acute stress reactions, and any other conditions where treatment is contraindicated or cautioned. Assess pregnancy/nursing status, and for possible drug interactions. Obtain baseline height/weight in children, and CBC, differential and platelet counts.

Monitoring: Monitor for signs and symptoms of cardiac disease, increased BP and HR, exacerbations of behavior disturbances and thought disorders, psychotic or manic symptoms, aggression, hostility, seizures, and visual disturbances. Monitor growth in children. In patients with bipolar disorder, monitor for mixed/manic episode. Perform periodic monitoring of CBC, differential, and platelet counts during prolonged therapy.

Patient Counseling: Inform about risks, benefits, and appropriate use of treatment. Instruct to read the Medication Guide.

Administration: Oral route. (Cap, ER) May sprinkle contents over spoonful of applesauce if desired. **Storage:** 25°C (77°F); excursions permitted to 15-30°C (59-86°F). (Tab) Protect from light. (Tab, SR) Protect from moisture.

RITUXAN   RX
rituximab (Genentech/Biogen Idec)

Serious, including fatal, infusion reactions reported; deaths ≤24 hrs of infusion have occurred. D/C and treat for Grade 3/4 reactions. Acute renal failure, sometimes fatal, reported in the setting of tumor lysis syndrome (TLS) following treatment of non-Hodgkin's lymphoma (NHL). Severe, including fatal, mucocutaneous reactions may occur. JC virus infection resulting in progressive multifocal leukoencephalopathy (PML) and death may occur.

THERAPEUTIC CLASS: Monoclonal antibody/CD20-blocker

INDICATIONS: Treatment of NHL in patients with: relapsed or refractory, low-grade or follicular, CD20-positive, B-cell NHL as a single agent; previously untreated follicular, CD20-positive, B-cell NHL in combination with 1st-line chemotherapy, and in patients achieving a complete or partial response in combination with chemotherapy, as single agent maintenance therapy; non-progressing (including stable disease), low-grade, CD20-positive, B-cell NHL, as a single agent, after 1st-line cyclophosphamide, vincristine, and prednisone (CVP) chemotherapy; previously untreated diffuse large B-cell, CD20-positive NHL in combination with cyclophosphamide, doxorubicin, vincristine, and prednisone (CHOP) or other anthracycline-based chemotherapy regimens. Treatment of previously untreated and previously treated CD20-positive chronic lymphocytic leukemia (CLL) in combination with fludarabine and cyclophosphamide (FC). Treatment of moderately to severely active rheumatoid arthritis (RA) (who had inadequate response to ≥1 TNF-antagonist therapies) in combination with methotrexate. Treatment of Wegener's Granulomatosis (WG) and Microscopic Polyangiitis (MPA) with glucocorticoids.

DOSAGE: *Adults:* Premedicate before each infusion with acetaminophen and antihistamine. Administer as IV infusion only. Relapsed/Refractory, Low-Grade/Follicular, CD20-Positive, B-Cell NHL: 375mg/m² once weekly for 4 or 8 doses. Retreatment: 375mg/m² once weekly for 4 doses. Previously Untreated, Follicular, CD20-Positive, B-Cell NHL: 375mg/m² on Day 1 of each chemotherapy cycle for up to 8 doses. Maint: Initiate 8 weeks after completion of rituximab/chemotherapy. Give 375mg/m² as single agent q8 weeks for 12 doses. Non-progressing, Low-Grade, CD20-Positive, B-Cell NHL: After completion of 6-8 CVP chemotherapy cycles, give 375mg/m² once weekly for 4 doses at 6-month intervals to max of 16 doses. Diffuse Large B-Cell NHL: 375mg/m² on Day 1 of each chemotherapy cycle for up to 8 infusions. CLL: 375mg/m² the day prior to initiation of FC chemotherapy, then 500mg/m² on Day 1 of cycles 2-6 (q28 days). Refer to PI for dosing as a component of Zevalin. RA (with methotrexate): Two-1000mg separated by 2 weeks. Give methylprednisolone 100mg IV (or equivalent) 30 min prior to each infusion. Give subsequent courses q24 weeks or based on evaluation, but not sooner than q16 weeks. WG/MPA: 375mg/m² once weekly for 4 weeks. Give methylprednisolone 1000mg/day IV for 1-3 days followed by oral prednisone 1mg/kg/day (≤80mg/day and taper clinical need) to treat severe vasculitis symptoms. Begin regimen within 14 days prior to or with rituximab therapy; continue during and after 4 weeks course of treatment.

HOW SUPPLIED: Inj: 100mg/10mL, 500mg/50mL

WARNINGS/PRECAUTIONS: Not recommended for use with severe, active infections. Hepatitis B virus (HBV) reactivation with fulminant hepatitis, hepatic failure, and death may occur; monitor closely for HBV carriers; d/c and institute appropriate treatment if viral hepatitis develops. Serious, including fatal, bacterial, fungal, and new/reactivated viral infections may occur during and ≤1 yr after complete therapy; d/c for serious infections and institute anti-infective therapy. D/C if serious/life-threatening cardiac arrhythmias occur. Perform cardiac monitoring during and after all infusions if arrhythmias develop or with history of arrhythmias/angina. Severe renal toxicity may occur in NHL; d/c if SrCr rises or oliguria occurs. *Pneumocystis jiroveci pneumonia* (PCP) and anti-herpetic viral prophylaxis is recommended for patients with CLL during treatment and for ≤12 months following treatment as appropriate. Potential for immunogenicity. Follow current immunization guidelines and administer non-live vaccines ≥4 weeks prior to therapy for RA patients. Not recommended in patients with RA who have not had prior inadequate response to one or more TNF-antagonists and with severe active infections. Obtain CBC and platelet count prior to therapy, at weekly to monthly intervals (more frequently if cytopenia develops), and at 2- to 4-month intervals during therapy in RA, WG, or MPA patients. Abdominal pain, bowel obstruction and perforation may occur.

ADVERSE REACTIONS: Infusion reactions, mucocutaneous reactions, renal failure, JC virus infection, PML, fever, chills, rash, asthenia, lymphopenia, infection, leukopenia, neutropenia, headache, night sweats.

INTERACTIONS: Renal toxicity reported with cisplatin. Vaccination with live viral vaccines not recommended. Observe closely for signs of infection if biologic agents and/or disease modifying anti-rheumatic drugs are used concomitantly.

PREGNANCY: Category C, caution in nursing.

MECHANISM OF ACTION: Chimeric murine/human monoclonal IgG$_1$ kappa antibody/CD20 antigen blocker; binds to CD20 antigen on B-lymphocytes and Fc domain, recruits immune effector functions to mediate B-cell lysis, possibly by complement-dependent cytotoxicity and antibody-dependent cell-mediated cytotoxicity.

PHARMACOKINETICS: Absorption: RA: C_{max}=157mcg/mL (1st infusion), 183mcg/mL (2nd infusion), 318mcg/mL (2x500mg dose), 381mcg/mL (2x1000mg dose). **Distribution:** RA: V_d=3.1L. WG/MPA: V_d=4.5L. **Elimination:** NHL: $T_{1/2}$=22 days, RA: $T_{1/2}$=18 days, CLL: $T_{1/2}$=32 days. WG/MPA: $T_{1/2}$=23 days.

NURSING CONSIDERATIONS

Assessment: Assess for severe active infections, preexisting cardiac/pulmonary conditions, high number of circulating malignant cells (>25,000/mm³), history of arrhythmias or angina, high tumor burden, electrolyte abnormalities, hematologic malignancies or autoimmune diseases, risk/pre-existing HBV infection, possible drug interactions, pregnancy/nursing status. Assess history of immunization, renal function, fluid and electrolyte balance, CBC, and platelet count.

Monitoring: Monitor fluid and electrolyte balance, cardiac/renal function, CBC and platelet count periodically. Monitor for signs/symptoms of HBV reactivation, viral hepatitis, infusion reactions, TLS, arrhythmias, bacterial, fungal, and new/reactivated viral infections, mucocutaneous reactions, PML, cytopenias, bowel obstruction/perforation, new-onset neurologic manifestations, and hypersensitivity reactions. Monitor closely for infusion reactions in patients with preexisting cardiac/pulmonary conditions, and those with high numbers of circulating malignant cells. Monitor HBV infection in hepatitis B carriers.

Patient Counseling: Inform of risks of therapy and importance to assess overall health status at each visit. Drug is detectable in serum for up to 6 months following complete therapy. Use effective contraception during and for 12 months after therapy.

Administration: IV route. Do not administer as IV push/bolus; for IV infusion only. Refer to PI for infusion instructions and preparation for administration. **Storage:** 2-8°C (36-46°F). Protect from direct sunlight. Do not freeze or shake. Sol for infusion: 2-8°C (36-46°F) for 24 hrs. Stable for additional 24 hrs at room temperature.

R

ROBAXIN   RX
methocarbamol (Schwarz)

OTHER BRAND NAMES: Robaxin Injection (Baxter) - Robaxin-750 (Schwarz)

THERAPEUTIC CLASS: Muscular analgesic (central-acting)

INDICATIONS: Adjunct for relief of acute, painful musculoskeletal conditions.

DOSAGE: *Adults:* (PO) Initial: (500mg tab) 1500mg qid for 2-3 days. Maint: 1000mg qid. Initial: (750mg tab) 1500mg qid for 2-3 days. Maint: 750mg q4h or 1500mg tid. Max: 6g/d for 2-3 days; 8g/d if severe. (Inj) Moderate Symptoms: 10mL IV/IM. IV Max Rate: 3mL undiluted drug/min. IM Max: 5mL into each gluteal region. Severe/Post-Op Condition: Max: 20-30mL/day up to 3 consecutive days. If feasible, continue with PO. Tetanus: 10-20mL up to 30mL. May repeat q6h until

NG tube can be inserted. Continue with crushed tabs. Max: 24g/day PO.
Pediatrics: Tetanus: Initial: 15mg/kg or 500mg/m². Repeat q6h prn. Max: 1.8g/m² for 3 consecutive days. Administer by injection into tubing or IV infusion.

HOW SUPPLIED: Inj: 100mg/mL [10mL]; Tab: 500mg, 750mg

CONTRAINDICATIONS: (Inj) Renal pathology with injection due to propylene glycol content.

WARNINGS/PRECAUTIONS: May impair mental/physical abilities. May cause color interference in certain screening tests for 5-hydroxy-indoleacetic acid (5-HIAA) and vanillylmandelic acid (VMA). Caution in epilepsy with the injection. Injection rate should not exceed 3mL/min. Avoid extravasation with injection. Avoid use of injection particularly during early pregnancy.

ADVERSE REACTIONS: Lightheadedness, dizziness, drowsiness, nausea, urticaria, pruritus, rash, conjunctivitis, nasal congestion, blurred vision, headache, fever, seizures, syncope, flushing.

INTERACTIONS: Additive adverse effects with alcohol and other CNS depressants. May inhibit effect of pyridostigmine; caution in patients with myasthenia gravis receiving anticholinergics.

PREGNANCY: Category C, caution in nursing.

MECHANISM OF ACTION: Carbamate derivative of guaifenesin; not established, suspected to have CNS depressant with sedative and musculoskeletal relaxant properties.

PHARMACOKINETICS: Distribution: Plasma protein binding (46-50%). Found in breast milk. **Metabolism:** Via dealkylation, hydroxylation, and conjugation pathways. **Elimination:** Urine; $T_{1/2}$=1-2 hrs.

NURSING CONSIDERATIONS

Assessment: Assess for renal/hepatic impairment, myasthenia gravis, seizures, pregnancy/nursing status, alcohol intake, and drug interactions.

Monitoring: Monitor for congenital and fetal abnormalities if taken during pregnancy, for color interference in certain screening tests for 5-HIAA using nitrosonaphthol reagent and in screening tests for urinary VMA using Gitlow method.

Patient Counseling: Caution while performing hazardous tasks (operating machinery/driving). Avoid alcohol or other CNS depressants. Notify if pregnant/nursing or if planning to become pregnant.

Administration: Oral route, IV infusion, and IM; careful supervision of dose and rate of injection. **Storage:** 20-25°C (68-77°F), in tight container; excursions permitted to 15-30°C (59-86°F).

ROCALTROL   RX
calcitriol (Validus)

THERAPEUTIC CLASS: Vitamin D analog

INDICATIONS: Management of secondary hyperparathyroidism and resultant metabolic bone disease with moderate to severe chronic renal failure (CrCl 15-55mL/min) in patients not yet on dialysis. Management of hypocalcemia and resultant metabolic bone disease in patients undergoing chronic renal dialysis. Management of hypocalcemia and its clinical manifestations in patients with postsurgical hypoparathyroidism, idiopathic hypoparathyroidism, and pseudohypoparathyroidism.

DOSAGE: *Adults:* Hypoparathyroidism: Initial: 0.25mcg/day qam. Titrate: May increase at 2- to 4-week intervals if no satisfactory response observed. Usual: 0.5-2mcg/day qam. Predialysis: Initial: 0.25mcg/day. Titrate: May increase to 0.5mcg/day if necessary. Dialysis: Initial: 0.25mcg/day. Titrate: May increase by 0.25mcg/day at 4- to 8-week intervals. Patients with normal or slightly reduced calcium levels may respond to 0.25mcg qod. Usual: 0.5-1mcg/day. D/C with hypercalcemia; when calcium levels return to normal, continue therapy at a daily dose 0.25mcg lower than that previously used. Elderly: Start at lower end of dosing range. *Pediatrics:* Hypoparathyroidism: ≥6 yrs: Usual: 0.5-2mcg/day qam. 1-5yrs: Usual: 0.25-0.75mcg/day qam. Predialysis: ≥3 yrs: Initial: 0.25mcg/day. Titrate: May increase to 0.5mcg/day if necessary. <3 yrs: Initial: 10-15ng/kg/day. D/C with hypercalcemia; when calcium levels return to normal, continue therapy at a daily dose 0.25mcg lower than that previously used.

HOW SUPPLIED: Cap: 0.25mcg, 0.5mcg; Sol: 1mcg/mL [15mL]

CONTRAINDICATIONS: Hypercalcemia or evidence of vitamin D toxicity.

WARNINGS/PRECAUTIONS: Administration in excess of daily requirements may cause hypercalcemia, hypercalciuria, and hyperphosphatemia. Chronic hypercalcemia may lead to generalized vascular calcification, nephrocalcinosis, and other soft tissue calcification. Serum calcium times phosphate (Ca x P) product should not exceed 70 mg²/dL². May increase inorganic phosphate levels in serum leading to ectopic calcification in patients with renal failure; use non-aluminum phosphate binders and low phosphate diet to control serum phosphate in dialysis patients. Caution in elderly and immobilized patients. If treatment switched from ergocalciferol, may take several months for ergocalciferol level in blood to return to baseline. In patients with normal renal function, chronic hypercalcemia may be associated with an increase in SrCr. Avoid dehydration in patients with normal renal function. When indicated, an estimate of daily dietary calcium intake should be made and the intake be adjusted.

ADVERSE REACTIONS: Hypercalcemia, hypercalciuria, SrCr elevation, weakness, N/V, dry mouth, constipation, muscle and bone pain, metallic taste, polyuria, polydipsia, weight loss, hypersensitivity reactions.

INTERACTIONS: Avoid pharmacological doses of vitamin D products and derivatives during therapy. Avoid uncontrolled intake of additional calcium-containing preparations. Avoid with magnesium-containing preparations (eg, antacids) in patients on chronic renal dialysis; use may lead to hypermagnesemia. May impair intestinal absorption with cholestyramine. Reduced blood levels with phenytoin or phenobarbital. Caution with thiazides; may cause hypercalcemia. Reduced serum endogenous concentrations with ketoconazole reported. Hypercalcemia may precipitate cardiac arrhythmias in patients on digitalis; use with caution. Functional antagonism with corticosteroids. Adjust dose of concomitant phosphate-binding agent.

PREGNANCY: Category C, not for use in nursing.

MECHANISM OF ACTION: Synthetic vitamin D analog; regulates absorption of calcium from the GI tract and its utilization in the body.

PHARMACOKINETICS: Absorption: Rapid (intestine). T_{max}=3-6 hrs, 8-12 hrs (hemodialysis); C_{max}=116pmol/L (pediatrics). **Distribution:** Found in breast milk. **Metabolism:** Hydroxylation to 1α, 25R(OH)$_2$-26, 23S-lactone D$_3$ (major metabolite). **Elimination:** Feces (primary), urine (10%, 1mcg dose); $T_{1/2}$=5-8 hrs (normal subjects), 16.2 hrs and 21.9 hrs (hemodialysis).

NURSING CONSIDERATIONS

Assessment: Assess for hypercalcemia, evidence of vitamin D toxicity, renal function, presence of immobilization, pregnancy/nursing status, and possible drug interactions. Obtain baseline levels of serum calcium, phosphorus, alkaline phosphatase, creatinine, and intact parathyroid hormone (iPTH).

Monitoring: Monitor for hypercalcemia, hypercalciuria, and hyperphosphatemia. For dialysis patients, perform periodic monitoring of serum calcium, phosphorus, magnesium, and alkaline phosphatase. For hypoparathyroid patients, perform periodic monitoring of serum calcium, phosphorus, and 24-hr urinary calcium. For predialysis patients, perform monthly monitoring of serum calcium, phosphorus, alkaline phosphatase, and creatinine for 6 months; then periodically, and periodic monitoring of iPTH every 3- to 4-months. Monitor serum calcium levels ≥2X weekly after all dosage changes and during titration periods.

Patient Counseling: Inform about compliance with dosage instructions, adherence to instructions about diet and calcium supplementation, and avoidance of the use of unapproved nonprescription drugs. Carefully inform about symptoms of hypercalcemia. Advise to maintain adequate calcium intake at a minimum of 600mg/day.

Administration: Oral route. **Storage:** 15-30°C (59-86°F). Protect from light.

ROMAZICON   RX

flumazenil (Roche Labs)

THERAPEUTIC CLASS: Benzodiazepine antagonist

INDICATIONS: Complete or partial reversal of sedative effects of benzodiazepines (BZDs) given with general anesthesia, or diagnostic and therapeutic procedures, and for the management of BZD overdose in adults. For reversal of BZD-induced conscious sedation in pediatrics (1-17 yrs old).

DOSAGE: *Adults:* Reversal of Conscious Sedation/General Anesthesia: Give IV over 15 seconds. Initial: 0.2mg. May repeat dose after 45 sec and again at 60 sec intervals up to a max of 4 additional times until reach desired level of consciousness. Max Total Dose: 1mg. In event of resedation, repeated doses may be given at 20-min intervals. Max: 1mg/dose (0.2mg/min) and 3mg/hr. BZD Overdose: Give IV over 30 sec. Initial: 0.2mg. May repeat with 0.3mg after 30 sec and then 0.5mg at 1-min intervals until reach desired level of consciousness. Max Total Dose: 3mg. In event of resedation, repeated doses may be given at 20-min intervals. Max: 1mg/dose (0.5mg/min); 3mg/hr.
Pediatrics: >1 yr: Give IV over 15 sec. Initial: 0.01mg/kg (up to 0.2mg). May repeat dose after 45 sec and again at 60-sec intervals up to a max of 4 additional times until reach desired level of consciousness. Max Total Dose: 0.05mg/kg or 1mg, whichever is lower.

HOW SUPPLIED: Inj: 0.1mg/mL

CONTRAINDICATIONS: Patients given BZDs for life-threatening conditions (eg, control of ICP or status epilepticus), signs of serious cyclic antidepressant overdose.

WARNINGS/PRECAUTIONS: Caution in overdoses involving multiple drug combinations. Risk of seizures, especially with long-term BZD-induced sedation, cyclic antidepressant overdose, concurrent major sedative-hypnotic drug withdrawal, recent therapy with repeated doses of parenteral BZDs, myoclonic jerking or seizure prior to administration. Monitor for resedation, respiratory depression, or other residual BZD effects (up to 2 hrs). Avoid use in the ICU; increased risk of unrecognized BZD dependence. Caution with head injury, alcoholism, and other drug dependencies. Does not reverse respiratory depression/hypoventilation or cardiac depression. May provoke panic attacks with history of panic disorder. Adjust subsequent doses in hepatic dysfunction. Not for use as treatment for BZD dependence or for management of protracted abstinence syndromes. May trigger dose-dependent withdrawal syndromes. Extravasation may occur; administer IV into a large vein.

ADVERSE REACTIONS: N/V, dizziness, injection-site pain, increased sweating, headache, abnormal or blurred vision, agitation.

INTERACTIONS: Avoid use until neuromuscular blockade effects are reversed. Toxic effects (eg, convulsions, cardiac dysrhythmias) may occur with mixed drug overdose (eg, cyclic antidepressants).

PREGNANCY: Category C, caution in nursing.

MECHANISM OF ACTION: Benzodiazepine receptor antagonist; inhibits activity at the benzodiazepine recognition site on the GABA/benzodiazepine receptor complex.

PHARMACOKINETICS: Absorption: C_{max}=24ng/mL; AUC=15ng•hr/mL. **Distribution:** V_d=1L/kg (steady state); plasma protein binding (50%). **Metabolism:** Complete (99%). **Elimination**: Urine (90-95%), feces (5-10%); $T_{1/2}$=54 min.

NURSING CONSIDERATIONS

Assessment: Assess patients using BZD for control of potentially life-threatening condition, and those showing signs of serious cyclic antidepressant overdose. Assess for head injury, history of convulsions, panic disorders, lung disease, hepatic impairment, and possible drug interactions.

Monitoring: Monitor for occurrence of seizure, re-sedation, respiratory depression, or other residual BZD effects, dizziness, injection-site pain, increased sweating, headache, and abnormal or blurred vision.

Patient Counseling: Advise not to engage in activities requiring complete alertness (eg, operating machinery/driving) during first 24 hrs after discharge. Advise not to take alcohol or non-prescription drugs during first 24 hrs after administration, or if effects of the benzodiazepine persist.

Administration: IV route. **Storage:** Undiluted: 25°C (77°F); excursions permitted to 15-30°C (59-86°F). If drawn into syringe or diluted (0.9% NaCl, D5W, or LR) discard after 24 hrs. Store in vial until just before use.

RotaTeq
RX
rotavirus vaccine, live (Merck)

R

THERAPEUTIC CLASS: Vaccine

INDICATIONS: Prevention of rotavirus gastroenteritis in infants and children caused by the serotypes G1, G2, G3, and G4 when administered as a 3-dose series to infants between the ages of 6-32 weeks.

DOSAGE: *Pediatrics:* 6-32 weeks: Administer series of 3 doses. Initial: 2mL PO starting at 6-12 weeks of age, with subsequent doses at 4- to 10-week intervals. Third dose should not be given after 32 weeks of age.

HOW SUPPLIED: Sol: 2mL

CONTRAINDICATIONS: Severe combined immunodeficiency disease (SCID), history of intussusception.

WARNINGS/PRECAUTIONS: Caution with administration to potentially immunocompromised infants or to infants with a history of GI disorders and abdominal surgery. May increase risk of intussusception. Shedding and transmission of vaccine virus observed; caution when administering to individuals with immunodeficient close contacts. Consider delaying use with febrile illness. May not protect all vaccine recipients against rotavirus. No clinical data available for postexposure prophylaxis and administration with incomplete regimen.

ADVERSE REACTIONS: Irritability, fever, diarrhea, vomiting, bronchospasm, nasopharyngitis, otitis media, bronchiolitis, gastroenteritis, pneumonia, urinary tract infection, intussusception, hematochezia, seizures, Kawasaki disease.

INTERACTIONS: Immunosuppressive therapies including irradiation, antimetabolites, alkylating agents, cytotoxic drugs, and corticosteroids (used in greater than physiologic doses) may reduce the immune response to vaccines.

PREGNANCY: Category C, safety not known in nursing.

MECHANISM OF ACTION: Vaccine; exact immunologic mechanism is unknown. Replicates in small intestine and induces immunity.

NURSING CONSIDERATIONS

Assessment: Assess for previous hypersensitivity to the vaccine, SCID, immunization history, immunocompromised conditions, history of GI disorders, febrile illness, and possible drug interactions.

Monitoring: Monitor for hypersensitivity reactions and possible adverse events.

Patient Counseling: Inform parent/guardian of potential benefits and risks. Instruct parent/guardian to inform physician of the current health status of patient and to report if patient has close contact with a family/household member who has a weak immune system. Advise to contact physician immediately if patient develops vomiting, diarrhea, severe stomach pain, blood in stool, or change in bowel movements. Instruct parents/guardians to report other adverse reaction to their healthcare provider.

Administration: Oral route. Administer as soon as possible after being removed from refrigeration. Do not mix with any other vaccines or solutions. Do not reconstitute or dilute. Refer to PI for instructions for use. **Storage:** 2-8°C (36-46°F). Protect from light.

ROXICET CII
oxycodone HCl - acetaminophen (Roxane)

THERAPEUTIC CLASS: Analgesic combination

INDICATIONS: Relief of moderate to moderately severe pain.

DOSAGE: *Adults:* Usual: (5mg-325mg): 1 tab or 5mL sol q6h prn. (5mg-500mg): 1 tab q6h prn. Titrate: May need to exceed usual dose based on individual response, pain severity and tolerance. Max: 12 tabs/day or 60mL/day. Do not exceed acetaminophen (APAP) 4g/day.

HOW SUPPLIED: (Oxycodone-Acetaminophen) Sol: 5mg-325mg/5mL [5mL, 500mL]; Tab: 5mg-325mg*, 5mg-500mg* *scored

CONTRAINDICATIONS: Oxycodone: Significant respiratory depression (in unmonitored settings or absence of resuscitative equipment), acute or severe bronchial asthma or hypercarbia, known/suspected paralytic ileus.

WARNINGS/PRECAUTIONS: May cause physical dependence and tolerance; d/c gradually to avoid withdrawal symptoms. Potential for misuse, abuse or diversion. May cause respiratory depression, induce or aggravate convulsions/seizures, produce severe hypotension in compromised patients and orthostatic hypotension in ambulatory patients. May decrease bowel motility. May obscure the diagnosis or clinical course with head injuries or acute abdominal conditions. Caution with circulatory shock, head injury, other intracranial lesions, pre-existing increase in intracranial pressure (ICP), elderly, debilitated, CNS depression, nontolerant patients, hepatic, pulmonary or renal impairment, liver disease, hypothyroidism, Addison's disease, prostatic hypertrophy, urethral stricture, acute alcoholism, delirium tremens, kyphoscoliosis with respiratory depression, myxedema, toxic psychosis, biliary tract disease (eg, acute pancreatitis). Caution with acute asthma, chronic obstructive pulmonary disease, cor pulmonale, preexisting respiratory impairment; may decrease respiratory drive leading to apnea even at therapeutic doses. May increase serum amylase levels. Anaphylactic reactions reported.

ADVERSE REACTIONS: Respiratory depression, apnea, respiratory arrest, circulatory depression, hypotension, shock, lightheadedness, dizziness, sedation, N/V, euphoria, dysphoria, constipation, pruritus.

INTERACTIONS: Oxycodone: May enhance neuromuscular-blocking action of skeletal muscle relaxants and increase respiratory depression. Additive CNS depression with other opioid analgesics, general anesthetics, centrally acting anti-emetics, phenothiazines, tranquilizers, sedative-hypnotics, alcohol and other CNS depressants; reduce dose of one or both agents. Agonist/antagonist analgesics (eg, pentazocine, nalbuphine and butorphanol) may reduce analgesic effect of oxycodone and/or may precipitate withdrawal symptoms; administer with caution. May produce paralytic ileus with anticholinergics. APAP: Hepatotoxicity occured in chronic alcoholics. Increase in glucuronidation, plasma clearance and decreased half-life with oral contraceptives. Increased effect with propranolol. Decreases loop diuretic effects. Reduces serum lamotrigine concentrations producing decreased therapeutic effects. Increases therapeutic effectiveness with probenecid. Decreased zidovudine pharmacologic effects.

PREGNANCY: Category C, not for use in nursing.

MECHANISM OF ACTION: Oxycodone: Pure opioid agonist; principal therapeutic effect is analgesia. Effects mediated by CNS receptors (eg, µ and kappa) for endogenous opioid-like compounds (eg, endorphins, enkephalins). APAP: Non-opiate, non-salicylate; site and mechanism for analgesic effect not established. Antipyretic effect occurs through inhibition of endogenous pyrogen action on the hypothalamic heat-regulating centers.

PHARMACOKINETICS: Absorption: Oxycodone: Absolute bioavailability (87%). APAP: Rapid and almost complete. **Distribution:** Oxycodone: Plasma protein binding (45%); (IV) V_d=211.9L; found in breast milk. APAP: Plasma protein binding (20-50%) (variable); found in most body fluids, breast milk. **Metabolism:** Oxycodone: N-dealkylation to noroxycodone (metabolite); CYP2D6, O-demethylation to oxymorphone (metabolite). APAP: Liver via CYP450 (conjugation), N acetyl-p-benzoquinoneimine, N-acetylimidoquinone (NAPQI, toxic metabolite). **Excretion:** Oxycodone: Urine (parent compound and metabolites); $T_{1/2}$=3.51 hrs. APAP: Urine (90-100%).

NURSING CONSIDERATIONS

Assessment: Assess for level of pain intensity, type of pain, patient's general condition and medical status, or any other conditions where treatment is contraindicated or cautioned. Assess for history of hypersensitivity, pregnancy/nursing status, renal/hepatic function, and possible drug interactions.

Monitoring: Monitor for signs/symptoms of respiratory depression, anaphylactic reactions, elevations of CSF pressure, ileus, decreased bowel motility in postoperative patients, hypotension, hepatotoxicity, convulsions, anaphylactic reactions, sphincter of Oddi spasms, abuse, tolerance and physical dependence. Monitor serum amylase.

Patient Counseling: Instruct to keep out of reach of children. Dispose of unused drug down toilet. Do not adjust dosing without consulting physician. Drug may impair mental/physical abilities required to perform hazardous tasks (eg, operating machinery/driving). Avoid alcohol and other CNS depressants. If on medication for more than a few weeks, consult physician for gradual d/c dose schedule. Medication has potential for abuse; protect from theft. May interfere with home blood glucose measurement system and cross react with assays for detection of cocaine or cannabinoids (eg, marijuana) in human urine.

Administration: Oral route. **Storage:** (Sol/Tab) 20-25°C (68-77°F). Protect from moisture.

ROXICODONE CII
oxycodone HCl (Xanodyne)

THERAPEUTIC CLASS: Opioid analgesic

INDICATIONS: Management of moderate to severe pain.

DOSAGE: *Adults:* Individualize dose. Initial: Opioid-Naive: 5-15mg q4-6h PRN. Titrate: Based on individual response. For chronic pain, give around-the-clock. For severe chronic pain, give q4-6h at lowest effective dose. Conversion from Fixed Ratio Opioid/Non-Opioid Analgesic: D/C non-opioid analgesic; titrate dose in response to level of analgesia and adverse effects. Continuing Concomitant Non-Opioid Analgesic: Initial dose based upon most recent dose of opioid as a baseline for further titration. Conversion from Different Opioid: Consider potency of prior opioid in selection of total daily dose and adjust dosage based on patient's response. May administer supplemental analgesia for breakthrough or incident pain and titrate as needed. Reassess the need for continued use. D/C gradually by decrements of 25-50% daily. If withdrawal symptoms occur, raise dose to previous level and titrate down more slowly.

HOW SUPPLIED: Sol: 5mg/5mL [500mL], 20mg/mL [30mL]; Tab: 5mg*, 15mg*, 30mg* *scored

CONTRAINDICATIONS: Significant respiratory depression (in unmonitored settings or the absence of resuscitative equipment), acute or severe bronchial asthma, hypercarbia, paralytic ileus.

WARNINGS/PRECAUTIONS: Potential for tolerance and physical dependence. May cause respiratory depression; caution in elderly/debilitated patients, significant chronic obstructive pulmonary disease, cor pulmonale, decreased respiratory drive, hypoxia, hypercapnia or preexisting respiratory depression. May markedly exaggerate respiratory depressant effects in head injuries, other intracranial lesions or increased ICP. May obscure the clinical course of patients with head injuries and acute abdominal conditions. May cause severe hypotension in patients with compromised ability to maintain BP due to depleted volume and orthostatic hypotension. May aggravate convulsions and seizures. Caution with acute alcoholism, adrenocortical insufficiency (eg, Addison's disease), convulsive disorders, CNS depression or coma, delirium tremens, kyphoscoliosis associated with respiratory depression, myxedema or hypothyroidism, prostatic hypertrophy or urethral stricture, severe hepatic or renal impairment, toxic psychosis and biliary tract disease (eg, acute pancreatitis). May increase serum amylase. Avoid giving to women during and prior to labor. Withdrawal symptoms reported. May impair mental/physical abilities.

ADVERSE REACTIONS: Respiratory depression/arrest, circulatory depression, cardiac arrest, hypotension, shock, N/V, constipation, headache, pruritus, insomnia, dizziness, asthenia, somnolence.

INTERACTIONS: Additive CNS depression with narcotic analgesics, general anesthetics, phenothiazines, tranquilizers, sedative-hypnotics, alcohol, and other CNS depressants; reduce dose. Mixed agonist/antagonist analgesics may reduce analgesic effect and/or cause withdrawal symptoms. May enhance effect of neuromuscular blockers. May intensify effects with MAOIs; avoid within 14 days of stopping MAOIs. Severe hypotension may occur with phenothiazines or other agents that compromise vasomotor tone. Possible interaction with CYP2D6 inhibitors.

PREGNANCY: Category B, not for use in nursing.

R

MECHANISM OF ACTION: Opioid analgesic; pure opioid agonist whose principal therapeutic effect is analgesia. Precise mechanism of analgesic effect has not been established. Specific CNS opioid receptors for endogenous compounds with opioid-like activity are found in the brain and spinal cord and play a role in analgesic effects.

PHARMACOKINETICS: Absorption: Various doses resulted in different parameters; refer to PI. **Distribution:** Plasma protein binding (45%), (IV) V_d=2.6L/kg; found in breast milk. **Metabolism:** Hepatic (extensively); noroxycodone (major metabolite); CYP2D6 to oxymorphone (metabolite) and glucuronides. **Elimination:** Urine; $T_{1/2}$=3.5-4 hrs.

NURSING CONSIDERATIONS

Assessment: Assess for level of pain intensity, type of pain, patient's general condition and medical status or any other conditions where treatment is contraindicated or cautioned. Assess for history of hypersensitivity, pregnancy/nursing status, renal/hepatic function, and possible drug interactions.

Monitoring: Monitor for signs/symptoms of respiratory depression, hypotension, elevations in CSF pressure, convulsions/seizures, tolerance and physical dependence. Monitor serum amylase.

Patient Counseling: Report episodes of breakthrough pain and adverse events. Avoid adjusting dose without consulting physician. May impair mental/physical abilities required to perform hazardous tasks (eg, operating machinery/driving). Avoid alcohol consumption and other CNS depressants. Advise drug has potential for abuse; protect from theft. Counsel that if on medication for more than a few weeks and need to d/c therapy, taper dosing to avoid abrupt withdrawal. Women of childbearing potential should consult physician regarding analgesic effects and other drug use during pregnancy.

Administration: Oral route. **Storage:** 25°C (77°F); excursions permitted to 15-30°C (59-86°F). (Tab) Protect from moisture.

ROZEREM   RX
ramelteon (Takeda)

THERAPEUTIC CLASS: Melatonin receptor agonist

INDICATIONS: Treatment of insomnia characterized by difficulty with sleep onset.

DOSAGE: *Adults:* Usual: 8mg within 30 min of hs. Max: 8mg/day.

HOW SUPPLIED: Tab: 8mg

CONTRAINDICATIONS: Coadministration with fluvoxamine.

WARNINGS/PRECAUTIONS: Angioedema (of the tongue, glottis, larynx) reported; do not rechallenge if angioedema develops. Sleep disturbances may manifest as a physical and/or psychiatric disorder; symptomatic treatment of insomnia should be initiated only after careful evaluation. Failure of insomnia to remit after 7-10 days of therapy may indicate presence of psychiatric and/or medical illness; evaluate. Cognitive and behavior changes, hallucinations, amnesia, anxiety, other neuro-psychiatric symptoms, and complex behaviors reported; d/c if complex sleep behavior occurs. Worsening of depression (eg, suicidal ideation, and completed suicides) reported in primarily depressed patients. May impair physical/mental abilities. May affect reproductive hormones (eg, decreased testosterone levels, increased prolactin levels). Not recommended with severe sleep apnea. Do not use with severe hepatic impairment. Caution with moderate hepatic impairment.

ADVERSE REACTIONS: Dizziness, somnolence, fatigue, nausea, exacerbated insomnia.

INTERACTIONS: See Contraindications. Decreased efficacy with strong CYP inducers (eg, rifampin). Caution with less strong CYP1A2 inhibitors, strong CYP3A4 inhibitors (eg, ketoconazole), strong CYP2C9 inhibitors (eg, fluconazole). Increased levels with donepezil and doxepin; monitor patients closely. Increased T_{max} of zolpidem; avoid use. Increased risk of complex behaviors with alcohol and other CNS depressants. Additive effect with alcohol; avoid alcohol use.

PREGNANCY: Category C, caution in nursing.

MECHANISM OF ACTION: Melatonin receptor agonist; activity at MT_1 and MT_2 receptors believed to contribute to sleep-promoting properties. These receptors, acted upon by endogenous melatonin, are thought to be involved in the maintenance of the circadian rhythm underlying the normal sleep-wake cycle.

PHARMACOKINETICS: Absorption: Rapid. Absolute bioavailability (1.8%); T_{max}=0.75 hr (fasted). **Distribution:** Plasma protein binding (82%). **Metabolism:** Oxidation via CYP1A2 (major), CYP2C, CYP3A4 (minor). M-II, M-IV, M-I, M-III (principal metabolites). **Elimination:** Urine and feces (<0.1% parent compound); $T_{1/2}$=1-2.6 hrs, 2-5 hrs (M-II). Refer to PI for PK parameters in elderly.

R

NURSING CONSIDERATIONS

Assessment: Assess for hepatic impairment, manifestations of physical and/or psychiatric disorder, depression, sleep apnea, other comorbid diagnoses, hypersensitivity, pregnancy/nursing status, and possible drug interactions.

Monitoring: Monitor for signs/symptoms of angioedema, exacerbations of insomnia, emergence of cognitive or behavioral abnormalities, worsening of depression, complex sleep behaviors, and anaphylactic/anaphylactoid reactions.

Patient Counseling: Inform patients, families and caregivers about benefits and risks associated with treatment. Counsel for appropriate use and instruct to read Medication Guide. Inform that severe anaphylactic and anaphylactoid reactions may occur; advise to seek immediate medical attention. Instruct to report sleep-driving to doctor immediately. Instruct to consult healthcare provider if cessation of menses, galactorrhea in females, decreased libido, or fertility problems occur. Take within 30 min prior to hs and confine activities to those necessary to prepare for bed. Instruct to swallow tab whole; do not break.

Administration: Oral route. Do not take with or immediately after high-fat meal. **Storage:** 25°C (77°F); excursions permitted to 15-30°C (59-86°F). Protect from moisture and humidity.

RYTHMOL   RX
propafenone HCl (GlaxoSmithKline)

> Increased rate of death or reversed cardiac arrest rate was seen in patients treated with encainide or flecainide (Class 1C antiarrhythmics) in a long-term, multi-center, randomized, double-blind study of patients with asymptomatic non-life-threatening ventricular arrhythmias who had a myocardial infarction (MI) >6 days but <2 yrs previously. Consider any 1C antiarrhythmics to have significant proarrhythmic risk in patients with structural heart disease. Avoid in patients with non-life-threatening ventricular arrhythmias, even if the patients are experiencing unpleasant, but not life-threatening signs or symptoms.

THERAPEUTIC CLASS: Class IC antiarrhythmic

INDICATIONS: To prolong the time to recurrence of paroxysmal atrial fibrillation/flutter (PAF) and paroxysmal supraventricular tachycardia (PSVT) associated with disabling symptoms in patients without structural heart disease. Treatment of life-threatening documented ventricular arrhythmias (eg, sustained ventricular tachycardia).

DOSAGE: *Adults:* Initial: 150mg q8h. Titrate: Individualize based on response and tolerance. May increase at a minimum of 3-4 day intervals to 225mg q8h, then to 300mg q8h PRN. Max: 900mg/day. Elderly/Ventricular Arrhythmia with Marked Previous Myocardial Damage: Increase more gradually during initial phase. QRS Widening/2nd- or 3rd-degree AV Block: Reduce dose. Hepatic Dysfunction: Give 20%-30% of normal dose. Elderly: Start at the low end of dosing range.

HOW SUPPLIED: Tab: 150mg*, 225mg* *scored

CONTRAINDICATIONS: Uncontrolled congestive heart failure (CHF); cardiogenic shock; bradycardia; marked hypotension; bronchospastic disorders; electrolyte imbalance; and sinoatrial, atrioventricular (AV), and intraventricular disorders of impulse generation and/or conduction (eg, sick sinus node syndrome, AV block) in the absence of an artificial pacemaker.

WARNINGS/PRECAUTIONS: Do not use to control ventricular rate during atrial fibrillation (A-fib) or in bronchospastic disease. Use of concomitant drugs that increase the functional AV refractory period is recommended. May cause new or worsened arrhythmias and CHF. Patients with CHF should be fully compensated before receiving therapy; d/c if CHF worsens (unless CHF is due to cardiac arrhythmia) and, if indicated, restart at lower dose. Caution with hepatic or renal dysfunction. Conduction disturbances (eg, 1st-degree heart block), agranulocytosis, positive antinuclear antibody (ANA) titers, and exacerbation of myasthenia gravis reported. D/C if persistent or worsening elevation of ANA titers detected. May alter pacing and sensing thresholds of artificial pacemakers. Reversible short-term drop (within normal range) in sperm count may occur. Caution in elderly.

ADVERSE REACTIONS: Unusual taste, N/V, dizziness, constipation, headache, fatigue, blurred vision, 1st-degree AV block, intraventricular conduction delay, weakness, dry mouth, dyspnea, diarrhea, proarrhythmia, angina.

INTERACTIONS: Avoid with quinidine. Amiodarone can affect conduction and repolarization; coadministration not recommended. Increased levels with inhibitors of CYP2D6 (eg, desipramine, paroxetine, ritonavir, sertraline), CYP1A2 (eg, amiodarone), CYP3A4 (eg, ketoconazole, ritonavir, saquinavir, erythromycin, grapefruit juice); monitor closely. May increase levels of drugs metabolized by CYP2D6 (eg, desipramine, imipramine, haloperidol, venlafaxine). May increase CNS side effects of lidocaine. May increase levels of digoxin, propranolol, metoprolol, warfarin. Increased levels with cimetidine. May increase levels with fluoxetine in extensive metabolizers. Rifampin may decrease levels and may increase norpropafenone (an active metabolite) levels. May result in severe adverse events (eg, convulsion, AV block, and acute circulatory failure) with abrupt cessation of orlistat.

PREGNANCY: Category C, not for use in nursing.

MECHANISM OF ACTION: Class 1C antiarrhythmic; has local anesthetic effects and direct stabilizing action on myocardial membranes. Reduces upstroke velocity (phase 0) of the monophasic action potential. In Purkinje fibers, and to a lesser extent myocardial fibers, reduces the fast inward current carried by Na$^+$ ions. Diastolic excitability threshold is increased and effective refractory period prolonged. Reduces spontaneous automaticity and depresses triggered activity.

PHARMACOKINETICS: **Absorption:** Complete; absolute bioavailability (3.4%, 150mg dose), (10.6%, 300mg dose); T_{max}=3.5 hrs. **Metabolism:** Liver (rapid, extensive) via CYP3A4, CYP1A2 and CYP2D6. 5-hydroxypropafenone, N-depropylpropafenone (active metabolites). **Elimination:** $T_{1/2}$=2-10 hrs.

NURSING CONSIDERATIONS

Assessment: Assess for HF; cardiogenic shock; sinoatrial, AV and intraventricular disorders of impulse generation or conduction (eg, sick sinus node syndrome, AV block); implanted functioning pacemaker; bradycardia; marked hypotension; bronchospastic disorders; marked electrolyte imbalance; MI; renal/hepatic dysfunction; pregnancy/nursing status; and possible drug interactions. Evaluate ECG prior to therapy.

Monitoring: Monitor for proarrhythmic effects, signs/symptoms of conduction disturbances, agranulocytosis, HF, and exacerbation of myasthenia gravis. Monitor implanted pacemakers during therapy and re-program accordingly. Evaluate ECG during therapy. Monitor ANA titers, LFTs, and renal function.

Patient Counseling: Inform about risks/benefits of therapy. Advise to report signs of electrolyte imbalance or any adverse reactions to physician. Instruct to report the development of signs of infection such as fever, sore throat, or chills.

Administration: Oral route. **Storage:** 25°C (77°F); excursions permitted to 15-30°C (59-86°F).

RYTHMOL SR   RX
propafenone HCl (GlaxoSmithKline)

> Increased rate of death or reversed cardiac arrest rate was seen in patients treated with encainide or flecainide (Class 1C antiarrhythmics) in a long-term, multi-center, randomized, double-blind study of patients with asymptomatic non-life-threatening ventricular arrhythmias who had a myocardial infarction (MI) >6 days but <2 yrs previously. Consider any 1C antiarrhythmics to have significant proarrhythmic risk in patients with structural heart disease. Avoid in patients with non-life-threatening ventricular arrhythmias, even if the patients are experiencing unpleasant, but not life-threatening signs or symptoms.

THERAPEUTIC CLASS: Class IC antiarrhythmic

INDICATIONS: To prolong the time to recurrence of symptomatic atrial fibrillation (A-fib) in patients with episodic (most likely paroxysmal or persistent) A-fib who do not have structural heart disease.

DOSAGE: *Adults:* Initial: 225mg q12h. Titrate: Individualize based on response and tolerance. May increase at a minimum of 5-day interval to 325mg q12h. If additional therapeutic effect needed, increase to 425mg q12h. Hepatic Impairment/Significant QRS Widening/2nd- or 3rd-degree AV Block: Reduce dose.

HOW SUPPLIED: Cap, Extended-Release: 225mg, 325mg, 425mg

CONTRAINDICATIONS: Heart failure (HF), cardiogenic shock, bradycardia, marked hypotension, bronchospastic disorders or severe obstructive pulmonary disease, marked electrolyte imbalance, or sinoatrial, atrioventricular (AV) and intraventricular disorders of impulse generation or conduction (eg, sick sinus node syndrome, AV block) in the absence of an artificial pacemaker.

WARNINGS/PRECAUTIONS: Do not use to control ventricular rate during A-fib. Concomitant treatment with drugs that increase the functional AV nodal refractory period is recommended. May cause new or worsened arrhythmias; evaluate ECG prior to and during therapy to determine if response supports continued treatment. May provoke overt HF. Caution with hepatic or renal dysfunction. Conduction disturbances (eg, 1st-degree AV block), agranulocytosis, positive antinuclear antibody (ANA) titers, and exacerbation of myasthenia gravis reported. D/C if persistent or worsening elevation of ANA titers detected. May alter pacing and sensing thresholds of implanted pacemakers and defibrillators. Reversible, short-term drop (within normal range) in sperm count may occur.

ADVERSE REACTIONS: Dizziness, chest pain, palpitations, taste disturbance, dyspnea, nausea, constipation, anxiety, fatigue, upper respiratory tract infection, influenza, edema.

INTERACTIONS: Withhold Class Ia and III antiarrhythmics for ≥5 half-lives prior to dosing with propafenone. Avoid with Class Ia and III antiarrhythmics (eg, quinidine, amiodarone). Inhibitors of CYP2D6 (eg, desipramine, paroxetine, ritonavir, sertraline) and CYP3A4 (eg, ketoconazole, ritonavir, saquinavir, erythromycin, grapefruit juice) may increase levels; avoid concomitant use. Amiodarone can affect conduction and repolarization and is not recommended. May increase

CNS side effects of lidocaine. May increase levels of digoxin, propranolol, metoprolol, and warfarin; monitor closely. Fluoxetine may increase levels in extensive metabolizers. Rifampin may decrease levels and may increase norpropafenone (an active metabolite) levels. May result in severe adverse events (eg, convulsion, AV block, and acute circulatory failure) with abrupt cessation of orlistat. Increased plasma levels with CYP1A2 inhibitors (eg, amiodarone, tobacco smoke) and cimetidine.

PREGNANCY: Category C, not for use in nursing.

MECHANISM OF ACTION: Class 1C antiarrhythmic; has local anesthetic effects and direct stabilizing action on myocardial membranes. Reduces upstroke velocity (Phase 0) of the monophasic action potential. In Purkinje fibers, and to a lesser extent myocardial fibers, propafenone reduces the fast inward current carried by Na^+ ions. Diastolic excitability is increased and effective refractory period is prolonged. Reduces spontaneous automaticity and depresses triggered activity.

PHARMACOKINETICS: Absorption: T_{max}=3-8 hrs. **Distribution:** V_d=252L (IV); plasma protein binding (>95%); found in breast milk. **Metabolism:** Rapid and extensive (>90% of patients), via CYP2D6, 3A4 and 1A2. 5-hydroxypropafenone and N-depropylpropafenone (active metabolites). **Elimination:** $T_{1/2}$=2-10 hrs (>90% of patients), $T_{1/2}$=10-32 hrs (<10% of patients).

NURSING CONSIDERATIONS

Assessment: Assess for HF; cardiogenic shock; sinoatrial, AV, and intraventricular disorders of impulse generation or conduction (eg, sick sinus node syndrome, AV block); implanted functioning pacemaker; bradycardia; marked hypotension; bronchospastic disorders or severe obstructive pulmonary disease; marked electrolyte imbalance; MI; renal/hepatic dysfunction; pregnancy/nursing status; and possible drug interactions. Evaluate ECG prior to therapy.

Monitoring: Monitor for proarrhythmic effects, signs/symptoms of conduction disturbances, agranulocytosis, HF, impaired spermatogenesis, and exacerbation of myasthenia gravis. Monitor implanted pacemakers and defibrillators during and after therapy and reprogram accordingly. Evaluate ECG during therapy. Monitor ANA titers, LFTs, and renal function.

Patient Counseling: Inform about risks/benefits of therapy. Advise to report signs of electrolyte imbalance. Advise to notify physician of all prescription, herbal/natural preparations, and over-the-counter medications currently being taken or of any changes with these products. Instruct not to double the next dose if a dose is missed; take next dose at the usual time. Instruct not to crush or further divide capsule contents.

Administration: Oral route. Do not crush or further divide capsule contents. May take with or without food. **Storage:** 25°C (77°F); excursions permitted to 15-30°C (59-86°F).

RYZOLT   RX
tramadol HCl (Purdue Pharma)

THERAPEUTIC CLASS: Central acting analgesic

INDICATIONS: Management of moderate to moderately severe chronic pain in adults who require around-the-clock treatment for an extended period of time.

DOSAGE: *Adults:* Take qd. Individualize dose. Not Currently on Tramadol Immediate Release (IR): Initial: 100mg/day. Titrate: Adjust by 100mg/day increments q2-3 days to achieve a balance between adequate pain control and tolerability. If 300mg/day required, titration should take at least 4 days. Usual: 200 or 300mg/day. Maint: Use lowest effective dose. Max: 300mg/day. Currently on Tramadol IR: Initial: Calculate 24-hr IR dose and round down to next lowest 100mg increment. Max: 300mg/day. Elderly: Start at lower end of dosing range. Do not repeat dose within 24 hrs.

HOW SUPPLIED: Tab, Extended-Release: 100mg, 200mg, 300mg

CONTRAINDICATIONS: Significant respiratory depression, acute or severe bronchial asthma, or hypercapnia in unmonitored settings or the absence of resuscitative equipment.

WARNINGS/PRECAUTIONS: Seizures reported; risk increases with epilepsy, history of seizures, risk for seizures (eg, head trauma, certain metabolic disorders, alcohol/drug withdrawal, CNS infections), and doses above recommended range. Anaphylactoid reactions and serotonin syndrome reported. Avoid in suicidal or addiction-prone patients. Reports of tramadol-related deaths in history of emotional disturbances, suicidal ideation/attempts, misuse of tranquilizers/alcohol/CNS active drugs. Caution if at risk for respiratory depression; treat with naloxone (for overdose) with caution. Caution with increased intracranial pressure (ICP) or head injury; miosis may obscure existence, extent, or course of intracranial pathology. May impair mental or physical abilities. Do not d/c abruptly; withdrawal symptoms may occur. Potential for abuse, misuse, or diversion. May complicate clinical assessment of acute abdominal conditions. Avoid in hepatic or severe renal impairment (CrCl <30mL/min). Caution in elderly.

ADVERSE REACTIONS: Dizziness, N/V, constipation, pruritus, headache, somnolence, increased sweating, dry mouth, fatigue.

R

INTERACTIONS: Increased seizure risk with SSRIs, TCAs, other tricyclic compounds (eg, cyclobenzaprine, promethazine, etc), opioids, MAOIs, neuroleptics, or other drugs that reduce seizure threshold. CYP2D6 inhibitors (eg, quinidine, fluoxetine, paroxetine, amitriptyline) and CYP3A4 inhibitors (eg, ketoconazole, erythromycin) may reduce clearance of tramadol and increase risk for serious adverse events. Caution with other drugs that may affect the serotonergic neurotransmitter systems (eg, SSRIs, anorectics, SNRIs, MAOIs, triptans, a_2-adrenergic blockers, linezolid, lithium, St. John's wort); may increase risk of seizures and/or serotonin syndrome. Not recommended with carbamazepine; reduced analgesic effect. Possible digoxin toxicity and altered warfarin effects. Caution and reduce dose with CNS depressants (eg, alcohol, opioids, anesthetics, narcotics, phenothiazines, tranquilizers, sedative hypnotics). Additive effects with alcohol and CNS depressants may occur. Large dose with anesthetics or alcohol may cause respiratory depression. Altered exposure with CYP3A4 inducers (eg, rifampin, St. John's wort). In drug overdose, naloxone administration may increase risk of seizures.

PREGNANCY: Category C, not for use in nursing.

MECHANISM OF ACTION: Centrally acting synthetic opioid analgesic; not established. Suspected to be due to binding of parent and M1 metabolite to μ-opioid receptors and weak inhibition of norepinephrine and serotonin reuptake.

PHARMACOKINETICS: Absorption: T_{max}=4 hrs, 5 hrs (M1 metabolite); C_{max}=345ng/mL, 71ng/mL (M1); AUC_{0-24}=5991ng•h/mL, 1361ng•h/mL (M1). **Distribution:** (IV) V_d=2.6L/kg (male), 2.9L/kg (female); plasma protein binding (20%). Crosses placenta; found in breast milk. **Metabolism:** Liver (extensive); N-and O-demethylation and glucuronidation or sulfation via CYP3A4, 2D6. O-desmethyltramadol (M1 active metabolite). **Elimination:** Urine (30% unchanged, 60% metabolite); $T_{1/2}$=6.5 hrs, 7.5 hrs (M1).

NURSING CONSIDERATIONS

Assessment: Assess for hypersensitivity to drug and other opioids, risk of respiratory depression or seizure, bronchial asthma, hypercapnia, increased ICP, acute abdominal conditions, renal/hepatic impairment, pregnancy/nursing status, other conditions where treatment is cautioned or contraindicated, and possible drug interactions.

Monitoring: Monitor for anaphylactoid reactions, respiratory/CNS symptoms, physical dependence/abuse, seizures, serotonin syndrome, and other adverse reactions.

Patient Counseling: Inform that drug may cause seizures and/or serotonin syndrome with concomitant use of serotonergic agents or drugs that reduce tramadol clearance. Take qd, at the same time and not to exceed the recommended maximum daily dose. Inform that drug may impair mental/physical abilities; use caution when performing hazardous tasks (eg, operating machinery, driving). Advise not to take with alcoholic beverages. Advise to use caution with medications such as tranquilizers, hypnotics, or other opiate-containing analgesics. Inform physician if pregnant or plan to become pregnant.

Administration: Oral route. Swallow whole with liquid; do not split, chew, dissolve, or crush tab.
Storage: 25°C (77°F); excursions permitted between 15-30°C (59-86°F).

SABRIL   RX
vigabatrin (Lundbeck)

> Causes permanent vision loss in infants, children, and adults; timing of onset is unpredictable. Causes permanent bilateral concentric visual field constriction in a high percentage of adult patients; in some cases may damage central retina and may decrease visual acuity. Risk increases with dose and cumulative exposure; use lowest effective dose and shortest exposure. Risk may persist after d/c therapy. D/C in patients who fail to show clinical benefit within 2-4 weeks (peds) or 3 months (adults) of initiation, or as soon as treatment failure is obvious. Vision testing is required at baseline, while on therapy, and after d/c. Unless benefit clearly outweighs the risk, avoid use with other drugs associated with serious adverse ophthalmic effects (eg, retinopathy, glaucoma) and in patients with, or at high risk of, other types of irreversible vision loss. Available only through restricted distribution program (SHARE).

THERAPEUTIC CLASS: GABA analog

INDICATIONS: (Powder) Monotherapy for pediatrics (1 month-2 yrs) with infantile spasms (IS) for whom the potential benefits outweigh the potential risk of vision loss. (Tab) Adjunctive therapy for adults with refractory complex partial seizures (CPS) who have inadequately responded to several alternative treatments and for whom the potential benefits outweigh the risk of vision loss.

DOSAGE: *Adults:* Refractory CPS: (Tab) Initial: 500mg bid (1g/day). Titrate: May increase in 500mg increments at weekly intervals depending on response. Maint: 1.5g bid (3g/day). Renal Impairment: CrCl >50-80mL/min: Decrease dose by 25%. CrCl >30-50mL/min: Decrease dose by 50%. CrCl >10-<30mL/min: Decrease dose by 75%. Withdraw gradually to d/c therapy. *Pediatrics:* 1 month-2 yrs: IS: (Powder) Initial: 50mg/kg/day in 2 divided doses. Titrate: May increase by 25-50mg/kg/day increments every 3 days. Max: 150mg/kg/day. Refer to PI for volume of individual doses. Withdraw gradually to d/c therapy.

HOW SUPPLIED: Powder: 500mg/pkt [50ˢ]; Tab: 500mg* *scored

WARNINGS/PRECAUTIONS: Vision testing required no later than 4 weeks after starting therapy, at least every 3 months during therapy, and 3-6 months after d/c of therapy. Abnormal MRI signal changes involving the thalamus, basal ganglia, brain stem, and cerebellum observed in some infants. May increase risk of suicidal thoughts/behavior; monitor for worsening/emergence of depression, suicidal thoughts or behavior, and/or any unusual changes in mood or behavior. May cause anemia, somnolence, fatigue, peripheral neuropathy, weight gain, and edema. Should be withdrawn gradually when necessary. Caution in elderly.

ADVERSE REACTIONS: Vision loss/visual field defects, tremor, headache, fatigue, drowsiness, dizziness, irritability, nystagmus, upper respiratory tract infection, weight gain, diarrhea, abnormal coordination, fever, otitis media.

INTERACTIONS: See Boxed Warning. May decrease phenytoin plasma levels. May increase C_{max} and decrease T_{max} of clonazepam.

PREGNANCY: Category C, not for use in nursing.

MECHANISM OF ACTION: Gamma-aminobutyric acid (GABA) analog; not established; may be due to irreversible inhibition of GABA transaminase, which results in increased levels of GABA in the CNS.

PHARMACOKINETICS: Absorption: Complete; T_{max}=1 hr (Adults/Children), 2.5 hrs (Infants). **Distribution:** V_d=1.1L/kg. Found in breast milk. **Elimination:** Urine (95%); $T_{1/2}$=7.5 hrs (Adults), 5.7 hrs (Infants).

NURSING CONSIDERATIONS

Assessment: Assess for renal impairment, pregnancy/nursing status, underlying suicidal behavior/ideation, pregnancy/nursing status, and for drug interactions. Perform baseline vision test.

Monitoring: Monitor for worsening vision/visual field changes; perform vision testing every 3 months during therapy and 3-6 months after d/c therapy. Monitor for abnormal MRI signal changes, suicidal thoughts/behavior, worsening/emergence of depression, unusual changes in thoughts or behavior, anemia, somnolence, fatigue, peripheral neuropathy, weight gain, and for edema. Monitor CBC, Hgb, Hct, and renal function. Monitor response to therapy and continued need for treatment periodically.

Patient Counseling: Inform patients of the risk of permanent vision loss and the need for vision monitoring; if changes in vision occur, instruct to notify physician. Advise that therapy may increase the risk of suicidal thoughts and behavior; instruct to notify physician if any abnormal behaviors develop. Inform of the possibility of developing abnormal MRI signal changes. Advise to notify physician if pregnant, planning on becoming pregnant, or if breastfeeding. Instruct not to abruptly withdraw from therapy.

Administration: Oral route. (Powder) Empty contents of pkt into empty cup and dissolve with 10mL of cold/room temperature water using oral syringe. Final sol concentration should be 50mg/mL. Prepare each dose immediately prior to administration. Refer to PI for administration instructions. **Storage:** 20-25°C (68-77°F).

S

SAMSCA
RX

tolvaptan (Otsuka America)

> Initiate and reinitiate therapy in hospitalized patients only; monitor serum Na closely. Osmotic demyelination resulting in dysarthria, mutism, dysphagia, lethargy, affective changes, spastic quadriparesis, seizures, coma, or death may occur due to rapid correction of hyponatremia (eg, >12mEq/L/24 hrs). Slower rates of correction may be advisable in susceptible patients (eg, with severe malnutrition, alcoholism, or advanced liver disease).

THERAPEUTIC CLASS: Arginine vasopressin antagonist

INDICATIONS: Treatment of clinically significant hypervolemic and euvolemic hyponatremia (eg, serum Na <125mEq/L or less marked hyponatremia that is symptomatic and has resisted correction with fluid restriction), including patients with heart failure, cirrhosis, and syndrome of inappropriate antidiuretic hormone.

DOSAGE: *Adults:* Initial: 15mg qd. Titrate: Increase to 30mg qd, after at least 24 hrs. Max: 60mg qd, PRN to achieve desired levels.

HOW SUPPLIED: Tab: 15mg, 30mg

CONTRAINDICATIONS: Urgent need to raise serum Na acutely, inability to auto-regulate fluid balance, hypovolemic hyponatremia, anuria, and concomitant use of ketoconazole or other strong CYP3A inhibitors (eg, clarithromycin, itraconazole, ritonavir, indinavir, nelfinavir, saquinavir, nefazodone, telithromycin).

WARNINGS/PRECAUTIONS: Frequently monitor for changes in serum electrolytes and volume status during initiation and titration. Avoid fluid restriction during the 1st 24 hrs of therapy. Allow to continue fluid ingestion in response to thirst. Resume fluid restriction and monitor for serum Na and volume status changes following d/c of therapy. D/C or interrupt therapy if patient develops too rapid elevation in serum Na; consider hypotonic fluid administration. GI bleeding reported in cirrhotic patients; use only when the need to treat outweighs the risk. May induce copious aquaresis. Dehydration and hypovolemia may occur, especially in potentially volume-depleted patients receiving diuretics or those who are fluid restricted; interrupt or d/c therapy and provide supportive care with careful management of vital signs, fluid balance, and electrolytes. Concomitant use with hypertonic saline is not recommended. Increased serum K⁺ levels may occur; monitor serum K⁺ levels after initiation of therapy in patients with a serum K⁺ >5mEq/L and those receiving drugs known to increase serum K⁺ levels.

ADVERSE REACTIONS: Thirst, dry mouth, asthenia, constipation, pollakiuria/polyuria, hyperglycemia, pyrexia, anorexia, nausea.

INTERACTIONS: See Contraindications. Marked increased exposure with ketoconazole and strong CYP3A inhibitors. Avoid with moderate CYP3A inhibitors (eg, erythromycin, fluconazole, aprepitant, diltiazem, verapamil). Coadministration with CYP3A inducers may reduce exposure of tolvaptan; doses may have to be increased as expected clinical effects may not be observed at usual doses. Dose reduction may be required with P-gp inhibitors (eg, cyclosporine). Increased exposure with grapefruit juice. Increase exposure of digoxin and lovastatin. Higher adverse reactions of hyperkalemia with angiotensin receptor blockers, ACE inhibitors, and K⁺-sparing diuretics.

PREGNANCY: Category C, not for use in nursing.

MECHANISM OF ACTION: Arginine vasopressin antagonist; antagonizes the effect of vasopressin and causes an increase in urine water excretion resulting in an increase in free water clearance (aquaresis), a decrease in urine osmolality, and an increase serum Na concentrations.

PHARMACOKINETICS: Absorption: T_{max}=2-4 hrs. **Distribution:** V_d=3L/kg; plasma protein binding (99%). **Metabolism:** Via CYP3A. **Elimination:** $T_{1/2}$=12 hrs.

NURSING CONSIDERATIONS

Assessment: Assess serum Na levels, neurologic status, ability to respond to thirst, for any other conditions where treatment is cautioned or contraindicated, pregnancy/nursing status, and possible drug interactions.

Monitoring: Monitor for osmotic demyelination, changes in serum Na/electrolytes/volume, neurologic status, signs/symptoms of hypovolemia, and serum K⁺ levels.

Patient Counseling: Advise to continue ingestion of fluid in response to thirst. Advise to avoid fluid restriction during the first 24 hrs of therapy. Instruct to inform physician of any prescription or over-the-counter drugs being taken, including use of strong or moderate CYP3A inhibitors, or P-glycoprotein inhibitors. Advise not to breastfeed during therapy.

Administration: Oral route. **Storage:** 25°C (77°F); excursions permitted between 15-30°C (59-86°F).

SANCTURA XR   RX
trospium chloride (Allergan)

OTHER BRAND NAMES: Sanctura (Allergan)

THERAPEUTIC CLASS: Muscarinic antagonist

INDICATIONS: Treatment of overactive bladder with symptoms of urge urinary incontinence, urgency, and urinary frequency.

DOSAGE: *Adults:* (Tab) 20mg bid. Give at least 1 hr ac or on an empty stomach. CrCl <30mL/min: 20mg qd at hs. Elderly (≥75 yrs): May be titrated down to 20mg qd based upon tolerability. (Cap) 60mg qd. Give in am with water on an empty stomach, at least 1 hr ac.

HOW SUPPLIED: Cap, Extended-Release: 60mg; Tab: 20mg

CONTRAINDICATIONS: Active or risk of urinary/gastric retention and uncontrolled narrow-angle glaucoma.

WARNINGS/PRECAUTIONS: Angioedema of the face, lips, tongue, and/or larynx reported. Angioedema with upper airway swelling may be life-threatening; d/c and institute appropriate therapy if involvement of the tongue, hypopharynx, or larynx occurs. Caution with significant bladder outflow obstruction, GI obstructive disorders, moderate or severe hepatic dysfunction, and patients treated for controlled narrow-angle glaucoma. May decrease GI motility; caution with ulcerative colitis, intestinal atony, and myasthenia gravis. (Cap) Not recommended with severe renal impairment (CrCl <30mL/min). Alcohol should not be consumed within 2 hrs of administration.

ADVERSE REACTIONS: Dry mouth, constipation. (Cap) Urinary tract infection. (Tab) Headache.

INTERACTIONS: Other antimuscarinic agents may increase the frequency and/or severity of dry mouth, constipation, and other anticholinergic pharmacologic effects. May alter the absorption of some concomitantly administered drugs due to anticholinergic effects on GI motility. May interact with some drugs that are actively secreted by the kidney by competing for renal tubular secretion (eg, procainamide, pancuronium, morphine, vancomycin, tenofovir). May enhance drowsiness with alcohol. (Cap) Antacids containing aluminum hydroxide and magnesium carbonate may alter exposure. Metformin may reduce levels.

PREGNANCY: Category C, caution in nursing.

MECHANISM OF ACTION: Antispasmodic, antimuscarinic agent; reduces the tonus of smooth muscle in the bladder by antagonizing the effect of acetylcholine on muscarinic receptors.

PHARMACOKINETICS: Absorption: (Tab) Absolute bioavailability (9.6%); C_{max}=3.5ng/mL; T_{max}=5.3 hrs; AUC=36.4ng/mL•hr. (Cap) C_{max}=2ng/mL; T_{max}=5 hrs; AUC=18ng•hr/mL. **Distribution:** (Tab/Cap) Plasma protein binding (50-85%); V_d=395L (Tab), >600L (Cap). **Metabolism:** Ester hydrolysis with subsequent conjugation. **Elimination:** (Tab) Feces (85.2%), urine (5.8%, 60% unchanged); $T_{1/2}$=18.3 hrs (Tab), 35 hrs (Cap).

NURSING CONSIDERATIONS

Assessment: Assess for drug hypersensitivity, other conditions where treatment is contraindicated or cautioned, hepatic/renal impairment, pregnancy/nursing status, and for possible drug interactions.

Monitoring: Monitor for signs/symptoms of urinary/gastric retention, decreased gastric motility, angioedema, and for other adverse reactions. Monitor hepatic/renal function.

Patient Counseling: Inform that therapy may produce angioedema that could result in life-threatening airway obstruction; instruct to d/c and seek medical attention if edema of the tongue or laryngopharynx, or difficulty breathing occurs. Inform that heat prostration may occur when used in a hot environment. Advise that alcohol may enhance drowsiness. (Cap) Advise to take cap in the am with water on an empty stomach, at least 1 hr ac. (Tab) Instruct to take tab 1 hr ac or on empty stomach.

Administration: Oral route. **Storage:** 20-25°C (68-77°F); (Cap) excursions permitted at 15-30°C (59-86°F).

SANCUSO   RX
granisetron (Prostrakan)

THERAPEUTIC CLASS: 5-HT$_3$ receptor antagonist

INDICATIONS: Prevention of N/V in patients receiving moderately and/or highly emetogenic chemotherapy regimens of up to 5 consecutive days.

DOSAGE: *Adults:* Apply single patch to upper outer arm a minimum of 24 hrs before chemotherapy. May be applied up to a max of 48 hrs before chemotherapy as appropriate. Remove patch a minimum of 24 hrs after completion of chemotherapy. Can be worn for up to 7 days depending on duration of chemotherapy regimen.

HOW SUPPLIED: Patch: 3.1mg/24 hrs

WARNINGS/PRECAUTIONS: Avoid placing on red, irritated, or damaged skin. May mask progressive ileus and/or gastric distention caused by the underlying condition. Application-site reactions reported; remove patch if a generalized skin reaction or serious skin reactions occur. Avoid direct natural or artificial sunlight. Cover application site in case of risk of exposure to sunlight throughout the period of wear and for 10 days following removal. Caution in elderly.

ADVERSE REACTIONS: Constipation.

INTERACTIONS: Hepatic CYP450 enzyme (CYP1A1 and CYP3A4) inducers or inhibitors may alter clearance and $T_{1/2}$. In vitro inhibition of metabolism reported with ketoconazole. (IV) Increased total plasma clearance with phenobarbital.

PREGNANCY: Category B, caution in nursing.

MECHANISM OF ACTION: 5-HT$_3$ receptor antagonist; blocks serotonin stimulation and subsequent vomiting after emetogenic stimuli.

PHARMACOKINETICS: Absorption: T_{max}=48 hrs; C_{max}=5ng/mL; $AUC_{0-168hr}$=527ng•hr/mL. **Distribution:** Plasma protein binding (65%). **Metabolism:** N-demethylation and aromatic ring oxidation mediated by CYP450 3A. **Elimination:** (IV) Urine (12% unchanged, 49% metabolites), feces (34%).

NURSING CONSIDERATIONS

Assessment: Assess for drug hypersensitivity, GI history, pregnancy/nursing status, and possible drug interactions.

Monitoring: Monitor for hypersensitivity reactions, application-site or generalized skin reactions, and other adverse events.

Patient Counseling: Instruct to apply to clean, dry, intact healthy skin on upper outer arm and not to place on skin that is red, irritated, or damaged. Advise to inform physician if abdominal pain or swelling occurs. Advise to remove patch if severe or generalized skin reactions occur. Instruct to peel off gently. Advise to cover patch application site (eg, with clothing) if there is a risk of exposure to sunlight or sunlamps during the period of wear and for 10 days after removal. **Administration:** Topical route. Refer to PI for proper application techniques. **Storage:** 20-25°C (68-77°F); excursions permitted between 15-30°C (59-86°F).

SANDOSTATIN LAR RX
octreotide acetate (Novartis)

THERAPEUTIC CLASS: Somatostatin analog

INDICATIONS: Long-term maintenance therapy in acromegalic patients with inadequate response to surgery and/or radiotherapy or for whom surgery and/or radiotherapy is not an option. Long-term treatment of severe diarrhea and flushing episodes associated with metastatic carcinoid tumors, and profuse watery diarrhea associated with vasoactive intestinal peptide-secreting tumors (VIPomas).

DOSAGE: *Adults:* Administer IM in the gluteal region. Patients not currently receiving octreotide should begin therapy with Sandostatin injection; see PI for dosing. Acromegaly: Initial: 20mg at 4-week intervals for 3 months. Titrate: See PI for dose adjustment based on growth hormone (GH), insulin-like growth factor-1 (IGF-1) and/or clinical symptoms. Max: 40mg every 4 weeks. Withdraw yearly for 8 weeks to assess disease activity after pituitary irradiation. Resume therapy if GH or IGF-1 levels increase, and signs and symptoms recur. Carcinoid Tumors/VIPomas: Initial: 20mg at 4-week intervals for 2 months. Continue with Sandostatin injection SQ for at least 2 weeks before the switch. Titrate: If symptoms not controlled, increase to 30mg every 4 weeks. If symptoms controlled at 20mg, consider dose reduction to 10mg for a trial period. If symptoms recur increase dose to 20mg every 4 weeks. Max: 30mg every 4 weeks. For exacerbation of symptoms, give Sandostatin Inj SQ for a few days at the dosage received prior to switching to depot. When symptoms are again controlled, the Sandostatin Inj SQ can be d/c. Patients must be considered responders and tolerate the injection before switching to the depot. Renal Failure Requiring Dialysis/Cirrhotic Patients: Initial: 10mg every 4 weeks. Elderly: Start at lower end of dosing range.

HOW SUPPLIED: Inj, Depot: 10mg, 20mg, 30mg

WARNINGS/PRECAUTIONS: May inhibit gallbladder contractility and decrease bile secretion which may lead to gallbladder abnormalities or sludge. May alter balance between the counter-regulatory hormones, insulin, glucagon, and GH and lead to hypo- or hyperglycemia; monitor blood glucose levels when treatment is initiated or dose is altered and adjust antidiabetic treatment periodically. May result in hypothyroidism; monitor thyroid levels periodically. Cardiac conduction and other cardiovascular (CV) abnormalities may occur; caution in patients at risk. Depressed vitamin B12 levels and abnormal Schilling's test reported. Therapy may alter dietary fats absorption. Serum zinc may rise excessively when fluid loss is reversed for patients on TPN; monitor zinc levels. Caution in the elderly.

ADVERSE REACTIONS: Diarrhea, N/V, abdominal pain, flatulence, constipation, injection-site pain, upper respiratory infection, influenza-like symptoms, fatigue, dizziness, headache, cholelithiasis, back pain.

INTERACTIONS: May alter absorption of orally administered drugs. May decrease cyclosporine levels. May need dose adjustments of insulin, oral hypoglycemics, and bradycardia-inducing drugs (eg, β-blockers). Increased availability of bromocriptine. May decrease the metabolic clearance of drugs metabolized by CYP450; caution with other drugs metabolized by CYP3A4 with a low therapeutic index (eg, quinidine, terfenadine).

PREGNANCY: Category B, caution in nursing.

MECHANISM OF ACTION: Somatostatin analog; long acting. Exerts similiar actions to natural hormone somatostatin, but is more potent in inhibiting GH, glucagon, and insulin. Like somatostatin, it also suppresses luteinizing hormone response to gonadotropin releasing hormone, decreases splanchnic blood flow and inhibits release of serotonin, gastrin, vasoactive intestinal peptide, secretin, motilin, and pancreatic polypeptide.

PHARMACOKINETICS: Absorption: (SQ) Rapid, complete. C_{max}=5.2ng/mL; T_{max}=0.4 hrs; acromegaly: C_{max}=2.8ng/mL, T_{max}=0.7 hr. **Distribution:** V_d=13.6L; plasma protein binding (65%); acromegaly: V_d=21.6L, plasma protein binding (41.2%). **Elimination:** Urine (32%, unchanged); $T_{1/2}$=1.7-1.9 hrs.

NURSING CONSIDERATIONS

Assessment: Assess for renal/hepatic impairment, cardiac dysfunction, pregnancy/nursing status, and for possible drug interactions. Assess GH and IGF-1 levels and obtain baseline thyroid function tests (TSH, total and/or free T4).

S

Monitoring: Monitor for signs/symptoms of biliary tract abnormalities (eg, gallstones, biliary duct dilatation), hypo- and hyperglycemia, hypothyroidism, cardiac conduction abnormalities, and pancreatitis. Monitor zinc levels if receiving TPN. With acromegaly: Monitor GH and IGF-1 levels. With carcinoids: Monitor urinary 5-hydroxyindoleacetic acid, plasma serotonin levels, and plasma Substance P levels. With VIPoma: Monitor VIP levels. Monitor total and/or free T4 and vitamin B12 levels during chronic therapy.

Patient Counseling: Inform of risks and benefits of treatment. Advise patients with carcinoid tumors and VIPomas to adhere closely to scheduled return visits for reinjection to minimize exacerbation of symptoms. Advise patients with acromegaly to adhere to return visit schedule to help ensure steady control of GH and IGF-1 levels. Instruct to notify physician if any adverse reactions develop.

Administration: IM route. Avoid deltoid inj. Not for IV/SQ routes. Refer to PI for preparation and administration instructions. **Storage:** Refrigerate between 2-8°C (36-46°F). Protect from light until time of use.

SAPHRIS   RX
asenapine (Merck)

Elderly patients with dementia-related psychosis treated with antipsychotic drugs are at an increased risk of death; most deaths appeared to be cardiovascular (CV) (eg, heart failure, sudden death) or infectious (eg, pneumonia) in nature. Not approved for treatment of dementia-related psychosis.

THERAPEUTIC CLASS: Dibenzapine derivative

INDICATIONS: Treatment of schizophrenia. As monotherapy or adjunctive therapy with either lithium or valproate for the acute treatment of manic or mixed episodes associated with bipolar I disorder.

DOSAGE: *Adults:* Schizophrenia: Initial/Usual: 5mg bid. Titrate: May increase to 10mg bid after 1 week based on tolerability. Max: 10mg bid. Reassess periodically to determine need for maint treatment. Bipolar Disorder: Monotherapy: Initial/Usual: Max: 10mg bid. Titrate: May decrease to 5mg bid if warranted by adverse effects or based on tolerability. Adjunctive Therapy (with lithium/valproate): Initial/Usual: 5mg bid. Titrate: May increase to 10mg bid based on response and tolerability. Max: 10mg bid. Continue treatment beyond acute response in responding patients. Reevaluate periodically the long-term risks/benefits for individual patients.

HOW SUPPLIED: Tab, SL: 5mg, 10mg

WARNINGS/PRECAUTIONS: Neuroleptic malignant syndrome (NMS) and tardive dyskinesia (TD) reported; d/c if these occur. Hyperglycemia, in some cases extreme and associated with ketoacidosis or hyperosmolar coma or death, reported; monitor for hyperglycemia and perform FPG at the beginning of therapy, and periodically in patients at risk for diabetes mellitus (DM). May cause weight gain. Hypersensitivity reactions reported usually after the 1st dose. May induce orthostatic hypotension and syncope; monitor orthostatic vital signs and consider dose reduction if hypotension occurs. Caution with CV disease, cerebrovascular disease, or conditions that predispose to hypotension. Leukopenia, neutropenia, agranulocytosis reported; d/c with absolute neutrophil count <1000/mm³ or at 1st sign of decline in WBC. May prolong QTc interval; avoid use with history of cardiac arrhythmias or in circumstances that may increase risk of torsades de pointes. May elevate prolactin levels. Seizures reported; caution with history of seizures or conditions that lower seizure threshold. Somnolence reported. May impair physical/ mental abilities. May disrupt body's ability to reduce core body temperature. Caution with those at risk for suicide and in elderly. May cause esophageal dysmotility and aspiration; avoid with risk of aspiration pneumonia. Not recommended with severe hepatic impairment (Child-Pugh C). Minimize period of overlapping antipsychotic administration.

ADVERSE REACTIONS: Somnolence, insomnia, headache, dizziness, extrapyramidal symptoms, akathisia, vomiting, oral hypoesthesia, constipation, weight increase, fatigue, increased appetite, anxiety, arthralgia, dyspepsia.

INTERACTIONS: Avoid use with other drugs known to prolong QTc including Class 1A antiarrhythmics (eg, quinidine, procainamide), Class 3 antiarrhythmics (eg, amiodarone, sotalol), antipsychotics (eg, ziprasidone, chlorpromazine, thioridazine), and antibiotics (gatifloxacin, moxifloxacin). Caution with other centrally acting drugs, alcohol, CYP2D6 substrates and inhibitors, drugs that can induce hypotension, bradycardia, respiratory or central nervous system depression, and drugs with anticholinergic activity. May enhance effects of antihypertensive agents; use with caution. Fluvoxamine may increase levels; use with caution. Imipramine may increase levels. Paroxetine, cimetidine, and carbamazepine may decrease levels.

PREGNANCY: Category C, not for use in nursing.

MECHANISM OF ACTION: Dibenzapine derivative; not established. Suggested that efficacy may be mediated through a combination of antagonist activity at dopamine type 2 (D_2) and serotonin type 2A ($5\text{-}HT_{2A}$) receptors.

PHARMACOKINETICS: Absorption: Rapid; (5mg) absolute bioavailability (35%); C_{max}=4ng/mL; T_{max}=1 hr. **Distribution:** V_d=20-25L/kg; plasma protein binding (95%). **Metabolism:** Glucuronidation via UGT1A4 and oxidation via CYP1A2. **Elimination:** Urine (50%), feces (40%); $T_{1/2}$=24 hrs.

NURSING CONSIDERATIONS

Assessment: Assess for dementia-related psychosis, history of cardiac arrhythmias, factors that may increase risk of torsades de pointes, patients at risk for aspiration pneumonia, and conditions where treatment is cautioned. Assess for hepatic function, pregnancy/nursing status, known hypersensitivity to the drug, and possible drug interactions. Obtain baseline FBG in patients with DM or at risk for DM. Perform baseline CBC if at risk for leukopenia/neutropenia.

Monitoring: Monitor for QT prolongation, NMS, TD, hyperglycemia, orthostatic hypotension, seizures, esophageal dysmotility, aspiration, suicidal ideation, hypersensitivity reactions, and other adverse effects. Monitor renal function, prolactin levels, serum transaminases, creatine kinase, total cholesterol, TG, and CBC, especially for decline of WBC with signs/symptoms of infection. Monitor for fever or other signs/symptoms of infections with neutropenia. Monitor CBC frequently in patients with preexisting low WBC or a history of drug-induced leukopenia/ neutropenia. Monitor regularly for FBG and worsening of glucose control in DM patients. Monitor orthostatic vital signs and weight regularly. Periodically reassess to determine the need for maintenance treatment.

Patient Counseling: Inform that tab should not be chewed, crushed, or swallowed; place under tongue and allow to dissolve. Instruct to avoid eating or drinking for 10 min after administration. Advise of the risks/benefits of therapy. Inform of the signs and symptoms of serious allergic reactions; instruct to seek immediate consult if serious allergic reaction develops. Inform about risk of developing NMS and counsel about its signs and symptoms. Inform of the need to monitor blood glucose in patients with DM or risk factors of diabetes. Advise that weight gain may be experienced. Inform about risk of developing orthostatic hypotension. Advise that patients with preexisting low WBC or history of drug-induced leukopenia/neutropenia should have their CBC monitored. Caution about performing activities requiring mental alertness (eg, driving/operating machinery). Instruct to avoid overheating or dehydration. Advise to notify physician if taking or plan to take any prescription or OTC medications, or if pregnant or intend to become pregnant. Advise not to breastfeed and avoid alcohol use while on therapy.

Administration: SL route. Place under tongue and allow to dissolve completely. Do not crush, chew, or swallow. Do not eat or drink for 10 min after administration. **Storage:** 15-30°C (59-86°F).

SAVELLA   RX
milnacipran HCl (Forest)

> Antidepressants increased the risk of suicidal thinking and behavior (suicidality) in children, adolescents, and young adults in short-term studies of major depressive disorder (MDD) and other psychiatric disorders. Monitor appropriately and observe closely for clinical worsening, suicidality, or unusual behavioral changes in patients who are started on milnacipran. Not approved for use in treatment of MDD and in pediatric patients.

THERAPEUTIC CLASS: Serotonin and norepinephrine reuptake inhibitor

INDICATIONS: Management of fibromyalgia.

DOSAGE: *Adults:* Usual: 50mg bid. Titrate: Day 1: 12.5mg once. Days 2-3: 12.5mg bid. Days 4-7: 25mg bid. After Day 7: 50mg bid. May increase to 100mg bid based on individual response. Max: 200mg/day. Severe Renal Impairment (CrCl 5-29mL/min): Reduce maint dose by 50% to 25mg bid. Titrate: May increase to 50mg bid based on individual response. Switching to or from MAOI: Start MAOI after ≥5 days of milnacipran d/c or start milnacipran after ≥14 days of MAOI d/c.

HOW SUPPLIED: Tab: 12.5mg, 25mg, 50mg, 100mg

CONTRAINDICATIONS: Uncontrolled narrow-angle glaucoma, concomitant use with MAOIs or within 14 days of stopping an MAOI.

WARNINGS/PRECAUTIONS: Serotonin syndrome, neuroleptic malignant syndrome (NMS)-like reactions, seizures, increased BP, HR, and liver enzymes, and severe liver injury reported. Caution with HTN, cardiac disease, and history of seizure disorder. If sustained increase in BP or HR occurs, reduce dose or d/c therapy. D/C if jaundice or liver dysfunction develops. Withdrawal symptoms and physical dependence reported; taper and avoid abrupt d/c. Hyponatremia may occur; consider d/c in patients with symptomatic hyponatremia. May increase risk of bleeding events. Caution with history of mania; dysuria, notably in males with prostatic hypertrophy; prostatitis; and other lower urinary tract obstructive disorders. Males may experience testicular pain or ejaculation disorders. Mydriasis reported; caution with controlled narrow-angle glaucoma. Avoid with substantial alcohol use or chronic liver disease; may aggravate preexisting liver disease. Caution with moderate renal and severe hepatic impairment. Not recommended with end-stage renal disease.

ADVERSE REACTIONS: N/V, headache, constipation, hot flushes, insomnia, hyperhidrosis, palpitations, upper respiratory infection, increased HR, dry mouth, HTN, anxiety, dizziness.

INTERACTIONS: See Contraindications. Risk of serotonin syndrome and NMS-like reactions with drugs that may affect serotonergic neurotransmitter systems (eg, triptans, lithium, antipsychotics, and dopamine antagonists). Not recommended with other SSRI, SNRI, or serotonin precursors (eg, tryptophan). May cause paroxysmal HTN and possible arrhythmia with epinephrine and norepinephrine. Switch from clomipramine may increase risk of euphoria and postural hypotension; caution with other centrally acting drugs. Digoxin may potentiate adverse hemodynamic effects. Risks of postural hypotension and tachycardia with IV digoxin; avoid with IV digoxin. May inhibit antihypertensive effect of clonidine. May increase risk of bleeding events with aspirin (ASA), NSAIDs, warfarin, and other anticoagulants. Increased risk of hyponatremia with diuretics.

PREGNANCY: Category C, not for use in nursing.

MECHANISM OF ACTION: Selective SNRI; not established. Potent inhibition of neuronal norepinephrine and serotonin reuptake without directly affecting uptake of dopamine or other neurotransmitters.

PHARMACOKINETICS: Absorption: Well absorbed. Absolute bioavailability (85%-90%); T_{max}=2-4 hrs. **Distribution:** (IV) V_d=400L; plasma protein binding (13%). **Metabolism:** l-milnacipran carbamoyl-O-glucuronide (major metabolite). **Elimination:** Urine (55%, unchanged). $T_{1/2}$=6-8 hrs.

NURSING CONSIDERATIONS

Assessment: Assess for uncontrolled narrow-angle glaucoma, concomitant use of MAOIs, pre-existing tachyarrhythmias and liver disease, cardiac diseases, history of seizure disorder, mania, psychiatric disorders, renal impairment, dysuria, prostatic hypertrophy, prostatitis, lower urinary tract obstructive disorders, hypersensitivity, pregnancy/nursing status, and possible drug interactions. Obtain baseline BP, HR, and LFTs.

Monitoring: Monitor BP, HR, LFTs, sodium levels. Monitor for suicidality, worsening of depression, emergence of agitation, irritability, unusual changes in behavior, serotonin syndrome (eg, mental status changes, autonomic instability, neuromuscular aberrations, GI symptoms), NMS-like signs and symptoms (eg, hyperthermia, muscle rigidity, autonomic instability with possible rapid fluctuation of vital signs), withdrawal symptoms, physical dependence, hyponatremia, and abnormal bleeding.

Patient Counseling: Counsel patients, families, and caregivers about the risks and benefits of therapy. Instruct families and caregivers to notify physician if patient experiences agitation, irritability, suicidality, or unusual changes in behavior. Inform about the risk of serotonin syndrome with concomitant use of triptans, tramadol, or other serotonergic agents. Advise that BP and pulse should be monitored regularly. Caution about the increased risk of abnormal bleeding with concomitant use of NSAIDs, ASA, and other anticoagulants. Caution against operating machinery or driving motor vehicles until effects of drug are known. Counsel to avoid consumption of alcohol. Advise that withdrawal symptoms may occur with abrupt d/c. Instruct to notify physician if pregnant or intend to become pregnant, or if breastfeeding.

Administration: Oral route. **Storage:** 25°C (77°F); excursions permitted to 15-30°C (59-86°F).

SEASONALE   RX
ethinyl estradiol - levonorgestrel (Duramed)

> Cigarette smoking increases the risk of serious cardiovascular (CV) side effects. Risk increases with age (>35 yrs) and with heavy smoking (≥15 cigarettes/day). Women who use oral contraceptives should be strongly advised not to smoke.

OTHER BRAND NAMES: Jolessa (Barr) - Quasense (Watson)

THERAPEUTIC CLASS: Estrogen/progestogen combination

INDICATIONS: Prevention of pregnancy.

DOSAGE: *Adults*: 1 tab qd for 91 days, then repeat. Start on 1st Sunday after the onset of menses. If menses begins on Sunday, start on that day. Intervals between doses should not exceed 24 hrs. *Pediatrics*: Postpubertal: 1 tab qd for 91 days, then repeat. Start on 1st Sunday after the onset of menses. If menses begins on Sunday, start on that day. Intervals between doses should not exceed 24 hrs.

HOW SUPPLIED: Tab: (Ethinyl Estradiol-Levonorgestrel) 0.03mg/0.15mg

CONTRAINDICATIONS: Thrombophlebitis or past history of deep vein thrombophlebitis, thromboembolic disorders (current or past history), cerebral vascular or coronary artery disease (current or past history), valvular heart disease with thrombogenic complications, uncontrolled HTN, diabetes mellitus (DM) with vascular involvement, headaches with focal neurological symptoms, major surgery with prolonged immobilization, breast cancer (current or past history), endometrial cancer, other known or suspected estrogen dependent neoplasia, undiagnosed abnormal genital bleeding, cholestatic jaundice of pregnancy or jaundice with prior pill use, hepatic adenomas/carcinomas or active liver disease, known or suspected pregnancy.

WARNINGS/PRECAUTIONS: Increased risk of myocardial infarction (MI), vascular disease, thromboembolism, stroke, hepatic neoplasia, and gallbladder disease. Increased risk of morbidity and mortality with HTN, hyperlipidemia, obesity, and DM. D/C at least 4 wks prior to and 2 wks postelective surgery with increased risk of thromboembolism and during or following prolonged immobilization. Caution in women with CV disease risk factors. May develop visual changes with contact lenses. Retinal thrombosis reported; d/c if unexplained partial or complete loss of vision or other ophthalmic irregularities. May cause glucose intolerance, elevated LDL, or other lipid abnormalities, or exacerbate migraine headaches. May cause increased BP and fluid retention; d/c if significant BP elevations occur. Breakthrough bleeding and spotting reported; rule out malignancies or pregnancy. Not indicated for use before menarche. May affect certain endocrine tests, LFTs, and blood components in laboratory tests. Perform annual history/physical exam; monitor women with history of breast cancer.

ADVERSE REACTIONS: N/V, breakthrough bleeding, GI symptoms (eg, abdominal cramps, bloating), spotting, amenorrhea, migraine, depression, vaginal candidiasis, edema, weight changes, changes in cervical erosion and secretion.

INTERACTIONS: Reduced effects result in pregnancy or breakthrough bleeding with antibiotics, anticonvulsants, and other drugs that increase the metabolism of contraceptive steroids (eg, rifampin, barbiturates, phenylbutazone, phenytoin, carbamazepine, felbamate, oxcarbazepine, griseofulvin, topiramate, ampicillin, tetracyclines, St. John's wort). Anti-HIV protease inhibitors may increase or decrease plasma levels. Atorvastatin, ascorbic acid, acetaminophen (APAP), CYP3A4 inhibitors (eg, itraconazole, ketoconazole) may increase plasma ethinyl estradiol levels. Increased plasma levels of cyclosporine, prednisolone, and theophylline have been reported. Decreased plasma concentration in APAP. Increased the clearance of temazepam, salicylic acid, morphine, and clofibric acid. May significantly decrease plasma levels of lamotrigine; dosage adjustment of lamotrigine may be necessary.

PREGNANCY: Category X, not for use in nursing.

MECHANISM OF ACTION: Estrogen/progestogen combination oral contraceptive; acts by suppression of gonadotropins. Inhibits ovulation and causes changes in the cervical mucus (increasing difficulty of sperm entry into uterus) and endometrium (reducing likelihood of implantation).

PHARMACOKINETICS: Absorption: Levonorgestrel: Rapid and complete. Absolute bioavailability (100%), C_{max}=5.6ng/mL, T_{max}=1.4 hrs, AUC=60.8ng•hr/mL. Ethinyl estradiol: Rapid. Absolute bioavailability (43%), C_{max}=145pg/mL, T_{max}=1.6 hrs, AUC=1307pg•hr/mL. **Distribution:** Found in breast milk. Levonorgestrel: V_d=1.8L/kg, plasma protein binding (97.5-99%) and principally to sex hormone binding globulin (SHBG). Ethinyl estradiol: V_d=4.3L/kg, plasma protein binding (95-97%). **Metabolism:** Levonorgestrel: Sulfate and glucuronide conjugates. Ethinyl estradiol: First-pass metabolism, hepatic via CYP3A4 (hydroxylation), methylation, conjugation. **Elimination:** Levonorgestrel: Urine (45%), feces (32%); $T_{1/2}$=30 hrs. Ethinyl estradiol: Urine, feces; $T_{1/2}$=15 hrs.

NURSING CONSIDERATIONS

Assessment: Assess for current or history of thrombophlebitis or thromboembolic disorders, history of HTN, hyperlipidemia, DM, obesity, breast cancer, and any other conditions where treatment is contraindicated or cautioned. Assess use in women >35 yrs, smokers (≥15 cigarettes/day). Assess pregnancy/nursing status and for possible drug interactions.

Monitoring: Monitor for signs/symptoms of MI, thromboembolism, stroke, hepatic neoplasia and other adverse effects. Monitor BP with history of HTN, serum glucose levels in DM or prediabetic patients, lipid levels with history of hyperlipidemia, and for signs of worsening depression with previous history. Monitor liver function and for signs of liver toxicity (eg, jaundice). Refer to an ophthalmologist if ocular changes develop.

Patient Counseling: Inform that the drug does not protect against HIV infection (AIDS) and other sexually transmitted diseases. Counsel about potential adverse effects. Avoid smoking. Take exactly as directed at intervals not exceeding 24 hrs. Advise about risks of pregnancy if dose is missed. If one dose is missed, take as soon as possible and take next pill at regular, scheduled time. May experience spotting, light bleeding, or nausea during the first few weeks to months; advise not to d/c medication and if symptoms persist, notify physician. D/C if pregnancy is confirmed/suspected.

Administration: Oral route. Refer to PI for proper administration procedure. **Storage:** 20-25°C (68-77°F).

S

SEASONIQUE

RX

ethinyl estradiol - levonorgestrel (Duramed)

> Cigarette smoking increases the risk of serious cardiovascular (CV) events from combination oral contraceptive (COC) use. Risk increases with age (>35 yrs) and with heavy smoking (≥15 cigarettes/day). Women who are >35 yrs and smoke should not use COCs.

THERAPEUTIC CLASS: Estrogen/progestogen combination

INDICATIONS: Prevention of pregnancy.

DOSAGE: *Adults:* Take 1 blue-green tab qd for 84 consecutive days, followed by 1 yellow tab qd for 7 days. Begin taking on first Sunday after the onset of menstruation. If menses begin on Sunday, start on that day. Postpartum women who choose not to breastfeed should start COC no earlier than 4-6 weeks postpartum.
Pediatrics: Postpubertal adolescents: Take 1 blue-green tab qd for 84 consecutive days, followed by 1 yellow tab qd for 7 days. Begin taking on first Sunday after the onset of menstruation. If menses begin on Sunday, start on that day.

HOW SUPPLIED: Tab: (Ethinyl Estradiol-Levonorgestrel) 0.03mg-0.15mg (blue-green); Tab: (Ethinyl Estradiol) 0.01mg (yellow)

CONTRAINDICATIONS: Patients with high risk of arterial or venous thrombotic diseases (eg, women who smoke, if over age 35; presence or history of deep vein thrombosis or pulmonary embolism; cerebrovascular or coronary artery disease; thrombogenic valvular or thrombogenic rhythm diseases of the heart such as subacute bacterial endocarditis with valvular disease, or atrial fibrillation; inherited or acquired hypercoagulopathies; uncontrolled HTN; diabetes with vascular disease; headaches with focal neurological symptoms or migraines with or without aura if over age 35), undiagnosed abnormal genital bleeding, presence or history of breast cancer or other estrogen- or progestin-sensitive cancer, liver tumors or liver disease, and pregnancy.

WARNINGS/PRECAUTIONS: Increased risk of venous and arterial thromboembolism and cerebrovascular events. D/C if arterial or deep venous thrombotic events, unexplained loss of vision, proptosis, diplopia, papilledema, or retinal vascular lesions occur. D/C at least 4 weeks before and through 2 weeks after major surgery or other surgeries with an elevated risk of thromboembolism. May increase risk of cervical cancer or intraepithelial neoplasia and gall-bladder disease. Hepatic adenoma and increased risk of hepatocellular carcinoma reported; d/c if jaundice develops. Cholestasis may occur with history of pregnancy-related cholestasis. Increased BP reported; for well-controlled HTN, monitor BP and d/c if BP rises significantly. May decrease glucose tolerance (dose-related). Consider alternative contraception with uncontrolled dyslipidemias. Increased risk of pancreatitis with hypertriglyceridemia or history thereof. May increase frequency or severity of migraine; d/c if new headaches are recurrent, persistent, or severe. Unscheduled (breakthrough) bleeding and spotting may occur; if bleeding persists, check for causes (eg, pregnancy or malignancy). Should not be used to test for pregnancy. Caution in history of depression; d/c if depression recurs or worsens. May change results of laboratory tests (eg, coagulation factors, lipids, glucose tolerance and binding proteins). Caution with hereditary angioedema; exogenous estrogens may induce or exacerbate symptoms of angioedema. Chloasma may occur especially with history of chloasma; avoid sun exposure or ultraviolet radiation. Not indicated for use before menarche.

ADVERSE REACTIONS: Irregular and/or heavy uterine bleeding, weight gain, acne, migraine, cholecystitis, cholelithiasis, pancreatitis, abdominal pain, major depressive disorder.

INTERACTIONS: Reduced effectiveness, decreased plasma concentrations of contraceptive hormones, or increased incidence of breakthrough bleeding with drugs or herbal products that induce enzymes (eg, CYP3A4) that metabolize contraceptive hormones (eg, barbiturates, bosentan, carbamazepine, felbamate, griseofulvin, oxcarbazepine, phenytoin, rifampin, St. John's wort, topiramate). Significant changes (increase or decrease) in plasma levels with protease inhibitors or non-nucleoside reverse transcriptase inhibitors. Pregnancy reported with use of hormonal contraceptives and antibiotics. Increased levels with atorvastatin, ascorbic acid, acetaminophen, and CYP3A4 inhibitors (eg, itraconazole, ketoconazole). Decreases levels of lamotrigine and may reduce seizure control; may require dosage adjustment of lamotrigine. May need to increase dose of thyroid hormone in patients on thyroid hormone replacement therapy due to increased thyroid binding globulin.

PREGNANCY: Contraindicated in pregnancy; not for use in nursing.

MECHANISM OF ACTION: Estrogen/progestogen combination oral contraceptive; primarily suppresses ovulation. May change cervical mucus (inhibiting sperm penetration) and endometrium (reducing likelihood of implantation).

PHARMACOKINETICS: Absorption: T_{max}=2 hrs; Levonorgestrel: Complete; absolute bioavailability (100%). Ethinyl estradiol: Absolute bioavailability (43%). Oral administration of variable doses resulted in different parameters. **Distribution:** Levonorgestrel: V_d=1.8L/kg; plasma protein binding (97.5-99%). Ethinyl estradiol: V_d=4.3L/kg; plasma protein binding (95-97%).

S

Metabolism: Levonorgestrel: Sulfate and glucuronide conjugates. Ethinyl estradiol: 1st pass metabolism in gut wall, Hepatic, via CYP3A4 (hydroxylation), methylation, conjugation. **Elimination:** Levonorgestrel: Urine (45%), feces (32%); T$_{1/2}$=34 hrs. Ethinyl estradiol: Urine, feces; T$_{1/2}$=18 hrs.

NURSING CONSIDERATIONS

Assessment: Assess for risk of arterial or venous thrombotic diseases, uncontrolled dyslipidemias, hypertriglyceridemia, or any other conditions where treatment is contraindicated or cautioned. Assess for pregnancy/nursing status and for possible drug interactions.

Monitoring: Monitor for venous or arterial thrombotic and thromboembolic events, cervical cancer or intraepithelial neoplasia, retinal vein thrombosis (eg, loss of vision, proptosis, diplopia, papilledema, retinal vascular lesions), increasing BP, jaundice, acute or chronic disturbances in liver function, worsening headaches or migraines, and unscheduled bleeding or spotting. Monitor for cholestasis with history of pregnancy-related cholestasis, glucose levels in DM or prediabetes, and recurrence of depression with previous history.

Patient Counseling: Inform that drug does not protect against HIV infection and other STDs. Cigarette smoking increases the risk of serious cardiovascular events from COC use, and women who are >35 yrs and smoke should not use COCs. Counsel on Warnings and Precautions associated with COCs. Take at the same time everyday, what to do in the event pills are missed, and to use a back-up or alternative method of contraception when enzyme inducers are used with COCs. COCs may reduce breast milk production if breastfeeding. Counsel any patient who starts COCs postpartum, and who has not yet had a period, to use an additional method of contraception until she has taken a light blue-green tablet for 7 consecutive days. Pregnancy should be considered if amenorrhea occurs and should be ruled out if amenorrhea is associated with symptoms of pregnancy (eg, morning sickness or unusual breast tenderness).

Administration: Oral route. **Storage:** 20-25°C (68-77°F).

SECTRAL   RX
acebutolol HCl (Promius Pharma)

THERAPEUTIC CLASS: Selective beta$_1$-blocker

INDICATIONS: Management of HTN alone or in combination with other antihypertensive agents (eg, thiazide-type diuretics) in adults. Management of ventricular premature beats.

DOSAGE: *Adults:* Mild-Moderate HTN: Initial: 400mg/day, given qd-bid. Usual: 200-800mg/day. Severe/Inadequate Control HTN: 1200mg/day, given bid. Ventricular Arrhythmia: Initial: 200mg bid. Maint: Increase gradually to 600-1200mg/day. Gradually reduce dose over a period of about 2 weeks to d/c. CrCl <50mL/min: Reduce daily dose by 50%. CrCl <25mL/min: Reduce daily dose by 75%. Elderly: Start at lower end of dosing range. Max: 800mg/day.

HOW SUPPLIED: Cap: 200mg, 400mg

CONTRAINDICATIONS: Persistently severe bradycardia, 2nd- and 3rd-degree heart block, overt cardiac failure, cardiogenic shock.

WARNINGS/PRECAUTIONS: Caution in patients with history of heart failure who are controlled with digitalis and/or diuretics. Cardiac failure may occur in patients with aortic or mitral valve disease or compromised left ventricular function; digitalize and/or give diuretic, and d/c acebutolol if cardiac failure continues. Exacerbation of ischemic heart disease (eg, angina pectoris, myocardial infarction [MI]) and death reported with coronary artery disease (CAD); avoid abrupt withdrawal. Caution in patients with bronchospastic disease who do not respond to or cannot tolerate alternative treatment; use low doses. Do not routinely withdraw prior to major surgery. Caution with peripheral vascular disease (PVD); can precipitate/aggravate arterial insufficiency. Caution with hepatic or renal dysfunction. May mask hypoglycemia in diabetics or hyperthyroidism symptoms (eg, tachycardia). Abrupt withdrawal may precipitate thyroid storm; thyrotoxicosis may occur; monitor closely. May be more reactive to repeated challenge with history of severe anaphylactic reaction to variety of allergens; may be unresponsive to usual doses of epinephrine. May develop antinuclear antibodies (ANA).

ADVERSE REACTIONS: Fatigue, dizziness, headache, constipation, diarrhea, dyspepsia, nausea, dyspnea, flatulence, micturition, insomnia.

INTERACTIONS: Possible additive effects with catecholamine-depleting drugs (eg, reserpine); monitor closely for hypotension and bradycardia. NSAIDs may reduce antihypertensive effects. Exaggerated hypertensive responses with α-adrenergic stimulants reported. May potentiate insulin-induced hypoglycemia. Digitalis glycosides may increase risk of bradycardia. May augment the risks of general anesthesia.

PREGNANCY: Category B, not for use in nursing.

MECHANISM OF ACTION: Cardioselective β-adrenoreceptor blocking agent; reduction in resting HR and decrease in exercise-induced tachycardia, reduction in cardiac output at rest and

S

after exercise, reduction of systolic and diastolic BP at rest and post-exercise, and inhibition of isoproterenol-induced tachycardia.

PHARMACOKINETICS: Absorption: Well-absorbed; absolute bioavailability (40%); T_{max}=2.5 hrs; 3.5 hrs (diacetolol). **Distribution:** Plasma protein binding (26%); crosses placental barrier; found in breast milk. **Metabolism:** Diacetolol (major active metabolite). **Elimination:** Renal (30-40%), nonrenal (50-60%); $T_{1/2}$=3-4 hrs (acebutolol), 8-13 hrs (diacetolol).

NURSING CONSIDERATIONS

Assessment: Assess for bradycardia, cardiogenic shock, 2nd- and 3rd-degree heart block, overt cardiac failure, thyroid problems, hepatic/renal function, history of severe anaphylactic reaction, HF, CAD, bronchospastic disease, PVD, diabetes mellitus, pregnancy/nursing status, and possible drug interactions.

Monitoring: Monitor for cardiac failure, renal dysfunction, exacerbation of angina pectoris, and MI following abrupt withdrawal, thyrotoxicosis, ANA, and other adverse reactions.

Patient Counseling: Instruct not to interrupt or d/c therapy without consulting physician. Advise to consult physician if signs/symptoms of impending congestive heart failure or unexplained respiratory symptoms develop. Warn about possible hypertensive reactions from concomitant use of α-adrenergic stimulants, such as nasal decongestants used in OTC cold preparations.

Administration: Oral route. **Storage:** 20-25°C (68-77°F). Protect from light.

SELZENTRY   RX
maraviroc (Pfizer)

> Hepatotoxicity reported; may be preceded by severe rash or evidence of systemic allergic reaction (eg, fever, eosinophilia, elevated IgE). Immediately evaluate patients with signs or symptoms of hepatitis or allergic reaction.

THERAPEUTIC CLASS: CCR5 co-receptor antagonist

INDICATIONS: In combination with other antiretroviral agents for adults infected with only CCR5-tropic HIV-1.

DOSAGE: *Adults:* ≥16 yrs: Concomitant Potent CYP3A Inhibitors (With/Without Potent CYP3A Inducer): 150mg bid. Other Concomitant Medications (Tipranavir/Ritonavir, Nevirapine, Raltegravir, NRTIs, and Enfuvirtide): 300mg bid. Concomitant Potent CYP3A Inducers (Without a Potent CYP3A Inhibitor): 600mg bid. Dose adjustment may be required with CYP3A inhibitors/inducers and P-glycoprotein (P-gp) inhibitors/inducers. Refer to PI for concomitant medications and dosing regimen based on renal function.

HOW SUPPLIED: Tab: 150mg, 300mg

CONTRAINDICATIONS: Severe renal impairment or end-stage renal disease (ESRD) (CrCl <30mL/min) in patients who are taking potent CYP3A inhibitors or inducers.

WARNINGS/PRECAUTIONS: Caution with preexisting liver dysfunction or who are coinfected with viral hepatitis B or C. Consider d/c if signs or symptoms of hepatitis or increased liver transaminases occur along with rash or other systemic symptoms. Myocardial ischemia and/or infarction, and postural hypotension reported; caution in patients at increased risk for cardiovascular (CV) events and history of postural hypotension. Increased risk of postural hypotension in patients with severe renal insufficiency or ESRD. Immune reconstitution syndrome reported. May increase risk of developing infections. May affect immune surveillance and may lead to increased risk of malignancy. Caution In elderly.

ADVERSE REACTIONS: Upper respiratory tract infections, cough, pyrexia, rash, dizziness.

INTERACTIONS: See Contraindications. Not recommended with St. John's wort; may substantially decrease levels and may lead to loss of virologic response and possible resistance. May increase metabolic ratio of debrisoquine; potential CYP2D6 inhibition at high dose. CYP3A/P-gp inhibitors may increase levels. CYP3A inducers (eg, rifampin, etravirine, and efavirenz) may decrease levels. Caution with medications known to lower blood pressure.

PREGNANCY: Category B, not for use in nursing.

MECHANISM OF ACTION: CCR5 co-receptor antagonist; selectively binds to human chemokine receptor CCR5 present on cell membrane, preventing interaction of HIV-1 gp120 and CCR5 necessary for CCR5-tropic HIV-1 to enter cells.

PHARMACOKINETICS: Absorption: T_{max}=0.5-4 hrs (1-1200mg in uninfected volunteers); absolute bioavailability (23%, 100mg), (33%, 300mg). Refer to PI for other pharmacokinetic parameters. **Distribution:** V_d=194L; plasma protein binding (76%). **Metabolism:** CYP3A (major); secondary amine (metabolite) via N-dealkylation. **Elimination:** Urine (20%, 8% unchanged), feces (76%, 25% unchanged); $T_{1/2}$=14-18 hrs.

NURSING CONSIDERATIONS

Assessment: Assess for renal and liver dysfunction or coinfection with HBV or HCV, history of postural hypotension, LFTs, risk of CV events, pregnancy/nursing status, and possible drug interactions. Conduct tropism testing to identify appropriate patients.

Monitoring: Monitor for signs/symptoms of hepatotoxicity, allergic reactions, immune reconstitution syndrome, CV events, symptoms of postural hypotension, evidence of infections, and development of malignancy.

Patient Counseling: Inform that liver problems have been reported and advise to seek medical attention if signs/symptoms of hepatitis or allergic reactions develop. Inform that therapy is not a cure for HIV, does not reduce risk of transmission of HIV, and that opportunistic infections may develop. Instruct to avoid driving/operating machinery if dizziness occurs. Advise patients to remain under the care of a physician, to take as prescribed and in combination with other antiretroviral drugs, to not change dose or dosing schedule without consulting a physician, and to take next dose as soon as possible and not double the dose if dose is missed. Counsel to notify physician if taking other medications or herbal products, are pregnant, planning to become pregnant, or become pregnant while taking therapy.

Administration: Oral route. **Storage:** 25°C (77°F); excursions permitted 15-30°C (59-86°F).

SENSIPAR   RX
cinacalcet (Amgen)

THERAPEUTIC CLASS: Calcimimetic agent

INDICATIONS: Treatment of secondary hyperparathyroidism (HPT) in patients with chronic kidney disease (CKD) on dialysis, of hypercalcemia in patients with parathyroid carcinoma, and of severe hypercalcemia in patients with primary HPT who are unable to undergo parathyroidectomy.

DOSAGE: *Adults:* Individualize dose. Secondary HPT with CKD on Dialysis: Initial: 30mg qd. Titrate: Increase no more frequently than q2-4 weeks through sequential doses of 30mg, 60mg, 90mg, 120mg, and 180mg qd to target intact parathyroid hormone (iPTH) of 150-300pg/mL. Measure serum calcium (Ca) and phosphorus within 1 week and iPTH between 1-4 weeks after initiation or dose adjustment. May be used alone or in combination with vitamin D sterols and/or phosphate binders. Hypercalcemia with Parathyroid Carcinoma/Primary HPT: Initial: 30mg bid. Titrate: Increase every 2-4 weeks through sequential doses of 30mg bid, 60mg bid, 90mg bid, and 90mg tid-qid PRN to normalize serum Ca levels.

HOW SUPPLIED: Tab: 30mg, 60mg, 90mg

CONTRAINDICATIONS: Hypocalcemia.

WARNINGS/PRECAUTIONS: Lowers serum Ca; monitor for hypocalcemia. If serum Ca <8.4mg/dL but remains >7.5mg/dL, or if symptoms of hypocalcemia occur, Ca-containing phosphate binders and/or vitamin D sterols can be used to raise serum Ca. If serum Ca <7.5mg/dL, or if symptoms of hypocalcemia persist and dose of vitamin D cannot be increased, d/c therapy until Ca levels reach 8mg/dL or symptoms of hypocalcemia are resolved. Restart treatment using the next lowest dose. Avoid use in patients with CKD not on dialysis. Seizures reported; monitor serum Ca particularly in patients with history of seizure disorder. Hypotension, worsening heart failure (HF), and/or arrhythmia reported in patients with impaired cardiac function. Adynamic bone disease may develop with iPTH levels <100pg/mL; reduce dose or d/c therapy if iPTH levels <150pg/mL. Monitor patients with moderate and severe hepatic impairment throughout treatment.

ADVERSE REACTIONS: N/V, diarrhea, myalgia, dizziness, asthenia, anorexia, paresthesia, fatigue, fracture, hypercalcemia, dehydration, anemia, arthralgia, depression.

INTERACTIONS: May require dose adjustment with CYP2D6 substrates (eg, desipramine, metoprolol, carvedilol) and particularly those with narrow therapeutic index (eg, flecainide and most TCAs). May require dose adjustment if a patient initiates or d/c therapy with strong CYP3A4 inhibitors (eg, ketoconazole, itraconazole); closely monitor iPTH and serum Ca levels. Increased area under the curve (AUC) and C_{max} with ketoconazole. Decreased AUC with Ca carbonate and sevelamer HCl. Increased AUC and decreased C_{max} with pantoprazole. May increase AUC and C_{max} of desipramine, amitriptyline, and nortriptyline. May decrease C_{max} of warfarin. May increase AUC and decrease C_{max} of midazolam.

PREGNANCY: Category C, not for use in nursing.

MECHANISM OF ACTION: Calcimimetic agent; lowers PTH levels by increasing the sensitivity of the Ca-sensing receptor to extracellular Ca.

PHARMACOKINETICS: Absorption: T_{max}=2-6 hrs. **Distribution:** V_d=1000L; plasma protein binding (93-97%). **Metabolism:** Via CYP3A4, 2D6, and 1A2; hydrocinnamic acid and glucuronidated dihydrodiols (major metabolites). **Elimination:** Urine (80%), feces (15%); $T_{1/2}$=30-40 hrs.

NURSING CONSIDERATIONS

Assessment: Assess for hypocalcemia, a history of seizure disorder, hepatic impairment, cardiac function, pregnancy/nursing status, and possible drug interactions. Assess serum Ca levels prior to administration.

Monitoring: Monitor for seizures, signs/symptoms of hypocalcemia and adynamic bone disease. In patients with impaired cardiac function, monitor for hypotension, worsening HF, and/or arrhythmias. For patients with CKD on dialysis, monitor serum Ca and phosphorus levels within 1 week and iPTH levels 1-4 weeks after initiation or dose adjustment. After maintenance dose is reached, measure serum Ca and phosphorus levels monthly, and iPTH levels every 1-3 months. For patients with parathyroid carcinoma/primary HPT, measure serum Ca levels within 1 week after drug initiation or dose adjustment; measure serum Ca levels every 2 months after maintenance dose levels have been established. Monitor iPTH/Ca/phosphorus levels with moderate and severe hepatic impairment.

Patient Counseling: Advise to take with food or shortly after a meal; instruct to take whole and not to divide. Inform of the importance of regular blood tests. Advise to report to physician if N/V and potential symptoms of hypocalcemia (eg, tingling/numbness of the skin, muscle pain/cramping) occur. Advise to report to their physician if taking medication to prevent seizures, have had seizures in the past, and experience any seizure episodes while on therapy.

Administration: Oral route. **Storage:** 25°C (77°F); excursions permitted to 15-30°C (59-86°F).

SEPTRA   RX
sulfamethoxazole - trimethoprim (King)

OTHER BRAND NAMES: Septra DS (King) - Sulfatrim Pediatric (Alpharma)

THERAPEUTIC CLASS: Sulfonamide/tetrahydrofolic acid inhibitor

INDICATIONS: Treatment of urinary tract infections (UTI), acute otitis media, acute exacerbations of chronic bronchitis (AECB), *Pneumocystis carinii* pneumonia (PCP), traveler's diarrhea, and shigellosis caused by susceptible strains of microorganisms.

DOSAGE: *Adults:* UTI/Shigellosis: 800mg-160mg PO q12h for 10-14 days (UTI) or 5 days (shigellosis). AECB: 800mg-160mg PO q12h for 14 days. Traveler's Diarrhea: 800mg-160mg PO q12h for 5 days. PCP Treatment: 15-20mg/kg TMP and 75-100mg/kg SMX per 24 hrs given PO q6h for 14-21 days. PCP Prophylaxis: 800mg-160mg PO qd. Renal Impairment: CrCl 15-30mL/min: 50% usual dose. CrCl <15mL/min: Not recommended.
Pediatrics: ≥2 months: UTI/Otitis Media/Shigellosis: 4mg/kg TMP and 20mg/kg SMX q12h for 10 days (UTI/otitis media) or 5 days (shigellosis). PCP Treatment: 15-20mg/kg TMP and 75-100mg/kg SMX per 24 hrs given q6h for 14-21 days. PCP Prophylaxis: 150mg/m²/day TMP and 750mg/m²/day SMX PO given bid, on 3 consecutive days per week. Max: 320mg TMP and 1600mg SMX per day. Renal Impairment: CrCl 15-30mL/min: 50% usual dose. CrCl <15mL/min: Not recommended.

HOW SUPPLIED: (Sulfamethoxazole [SMX]-Trimethoprim [TMP]) Sus: (Sulfatrim Pediatric, Septra) 200mg-40mg/5mL [100mL, 473mL]; Tab: (Septra) 400mg-80mg*; Tab, DS: (Septra DS) 800mg-160mg* *scored

CONTRAINDICATIONS: Megaloblastic anemia due to folate deficiency, pregnancy at term, nursing, infants <2 months old.

WARNINGS/PRECAUTIONS: Fatal hypersensitivity reactions (eg, Stevens-Johnson syndrome, toxic epidermal necrolysis, fulminant hepatic necrosis) may occur. Cough, SOB, and pulmonary infiltrates reported. Avoid with group A β-hemolytic streptococcal infections. *Clostridium difficile*-associated diarrhea (CDAD) reported. May result in bacterial resistance with prolonged use or use in the absence of a proven/suspected bacterial infection or a prophylactic indication; take appropriate measures if superinfection develops. Caution with hepatic/renal impairment, elderly, folate deficiency (eg, chronic alcoholics, anticonvulsants, malabsorption, malnutrition), bronchial asthma, and other allergies. In glucose-6-phosphate-dehydrogenase deficiency, hemolysis may occur. Increased incidence of adverse events in AIDS patients. Maintain adequate fluid intake.

ADVERSE REACTIONS: Anorexia, N/V, rash, urticaria, cough, SOB, cholestatic jaundice, agranulocytosis, anemia, hyperkalemia, renal failure, interstitial nephritis, hyponatremia, convulsions.

INTERACTIONS: Increased risk of thrombocytopenia with purpura with diuretics (especially thiazides) in the elderly. Caution with warfarin; may prolong PT. Increased effects of phenytoin, methotrexate. Concomitant ACE inhibitor therapy may cause hyperkalemia.

PREGNANCY: Category C, not for use in nursing.

MECHANISM OF ACTION: Sulfamethoxazole: Inhibits bacterial synthesis of dihydrofolic acid by competing with para-aminobenzoic acid (PABA). Trimethoprim: Blocks production of tetrahydrofolic acid from dihydrofolic acid by binding to and reversibly inhibiting required enzyme, dihydrofolate reductase; thus drug blocks 2 consecutive steps in biosynthesis of nucleic acids and proteins essential to many bacteria.

PHARMACOKINETICS: Absorption: Rapid; T_{max}=1-4 hrs. **Distribution:** Trimethoprim: Plasma protein binding (44%); Sulfamethoxazole: Plasma protein binding (70%). Crosses placenta, found in breast milk. **Metabolism:** Sulfamethoxazole: N_4 acetylation. Trimethoprim: 1- and 3-oxide, 3'-and 4'-hydroxy derivative (principal metabolites). **Elimination:** Urine, trimethoprim (66.8%), sulfamethoxazole (84.5%; 30% as free and remaining as N_4 acetylated metabolite); $T_{1/2}$=10 hrs (sulfamethoxazole), 8-10 hrs (trimethoprim).

NURSING CONSIDERATIONS

Assessment: Assess for previous drug hypersensitivity, megaloblastic anemia, renal/hepatic impairment, folate deficiency, G6PD deficiency, severe allergy or bronchial asthma, pregnancy/nursing status, and possible drug interactions.

Monitoring: Monitor for severe hypersensitivity reactions, CDAD, development of drug resistance, superinfection, signs of bone marrow depression or specific decrease in platelets with or without pupura, hyperkalemia, hyponatremia, kernicterus, and clinical signs (eg, skin rash, sore throat, fever, arthralgia, pallor, jaundice) that may be early indications of serious reactions. Monitor CBC; d/c if significant reduction is noted. Perform urinalysis with careful microscopic exam and renal function tests.

Patient Counseling: Inform that drug only treats bacterial, not viral, infections. Take exactly as directed; skipping doses or not completing full course may decrease effectiveness and increase resistance. Maintain adequate fluid intake to prevent crystalluria and stone formation. Inform about potential benefits/risks of therapy. D/C and notify physician if skin rash, watery/bloody diarrhea (with/without muscle cramps), or fever occurs (may occur up to 2 months after therapy). Notify if pregnant/nursing.

Administration: Oral route. **Storage:** 15-25°C (59-77°F); protect from light.

SEREVENT   RX
salmeterol xinafoate (GlaxoSmithKline)

Long-acting β_2-adrenergic agonists (LABA) may increase the risk of asthma-related death. Contraindicated in asthma without use of a long-term asthma control medication (eg, inhaled corticosteroid). Do not use for asthma adequately controlled on low or medium dose inhaled corticosteroids. LABA may increase risk of asthma-related hospitalization in pediatrics and adolescents; ensure adherence with both long-term asthma control medication and LABA.

THERAPEUTIC CLASS: Beta$_2$-agonist

INDICATIONS: Treatment of asthma and prevention of bronchospasm only as concomitant therapy with a long-term asthma control medication (eg, inhaled corticosteroid) in patients ≥4 yrs with reversible obstructive airway disease, including patients with symptoms of nocturnal asthma. Prevention of exercise-induced bronchospasm (EIB) in patients ≥4 yrs. For the long-term, bid (am and pm) administration in the maintenance treatment of bronchospasm associated with chronic obstructive pulmonary disease (COPD) (eg, emphysema and chronic bronchitis).

DOSAGE: *Adults:* Asthma/COPD: 1 inh bid, am and pm (12 hrs apart). EIB: 1 inh ≥30 min before exercise (additional doses should not be used for 12 hrs after administration or if already on bid dose).
Pediatrics: ≥4 yrs: Asthma: 1 inh bid, am and pm (12 hrs apart). EIB: 1 inh ≥30 min before exercise (additional doses should not be used for 12 hrs after administration or if already on bid dose).

HOW SUPPLIED: Disk, Inhalation: 50mcg/inh [28^s, 60^s]

CONTRAINDICATIONS: Treatment of asthma without concomitant use of long-term asthma control medication (eg, inhaled corticosteroid). Primary treatment of status asthmaticus or other acute episodes of asthma or COPD where intensive measures are required. Severe hypersensitivity to milk proteins.

WARNINGS/PRECAUTIONS: Should not be initiated during rapidly deteriorating or potentially life-threatening episodes of asthma or COPD. Increased use of inhaled, short-acting β_2-agonists (SABA) is a marker of deteriorating asthma; reevaluate and reassess treatment regimen. Should not be used for relief of acute symptoms; use SABA to relieve acute symptoms. At treatment initiation, regular use of an inhaled SABA should be d/c. Not a substitute for oral/inhaled corticosteroids. Should not be used more often or at higher doses than recommended; cardiovascular (CV) effects and fatalities reported with excessive use. May produce paradoxical bronchospasm; d/c immediately, treat, and institute alternative therapy. Caution with cardiovascular disorders (CVDs) (eg, coronary insufficiency, cardiac arrhythmias, HTN), convulsive disorders, thyrotoxicosis, hepatic disease, diabetes mellitus (DM), those who are unusually responsive to sympathomimetic amines, and in elderly. ECG changes (eg, flattening of T wave, QTc interval prolongation, and ST segment depression) reported. Immediate hypersensitivity reactions, hypokalemia, and dose-related changes in blood glucose and/or serum K^+ may occur.

ADVERSE REACTIONS: Nasal/sinus congestion, pharyngitis, cough, viral respiratory infection, musculoskeletal pain, rhinitis, headache, tracheitis/bronchitis, influenza, throat irritation.

INTERACTIONS: Not recommended with strong CYP3A4 inhibitors (eg, ketoconazole, ritonavir, atazanavir, clarithromycin, indinavir, itraconazole, nefazodone, nelfinavir, saquinavir, telithromycin). Avoid with other medications containing LABA. Increased exposure with ketoconazole. Caution with non-K⁺-sparing diuretics (eg, loop or thiazide diuretics). Use with β-blockers may produce severe bronchospasm; if needed, consider cardioselective β-blocker with caution. Extreme caution with MAOIs or TCAs or within 2 weeks of d/c with these agents. Increased C_{max} with erythromycin.

PREGNANCY: Category C, not for use in nursing.

MECHANISM OF ACTION: Selective LABA (β_2-agonist); stimulates intracellular adenyl cyclase, the enzyme that catalyzes the conversion of adenosine triphosphate to cyclic-3',5'-adenosine monophosphate, producing relaxation of bronchial smooth muscles and inhibits the release of mediators of immediate hypersensitivity from mast cells.

PHARMACOKINETICS: Absorption: C_{max}=167pg/mL; T_{max}=20 min. **Distribution:** Plasma protein binding (96%). **Metabolism:** Liver (aliphatic oxidation) via CYP3A4; α-hydroxysalmeterol (metabolite). **Elimination:** Urine (25%), feces (60%); $T_{1/2}$=5.5 hrs.

NURSING CONSIDERATIONS

Assessment: Assess for asthma control, hypersensitivity to milk proteins, acute bronchospasm, rapidly deteriorating asthma or COPD, CVD, convulsive disorder, thyrotoxicosis, DM, hepatic disease, pregnancy/nursing status, and possible drug interactions. Obtain baseline lung function before therapy, serum K⁺, and blood glucose levels.

Monitoring: Monitor lung function periodically. Monitor patients with hepatic disease. Monitor for paradoxical bronchospasm, CV effects, and hypersensitivity. Monitor asthma control, pulse rate, BP, ECG changes, serum K⁺, and blood glucose levels.

Patient Counseling: Inform that drug may increase risk of asthma-related death. Inform that the medication should only be used as additional therapy when long-term asthma control medications do not adequately control asthma symptoms. Counsel that the medication is not meant to relieve acute asthma or exacerbations of COPD symptoms and extra doses should not be used for that purpose. Advise that therapy is not a substitute for oral or inhaled corticosteroids. Instruct to notify physician immediately if signs of seriously worsening asthma or COPD occur. Instruct not to change dosage or stop therapy unless directed by physician. Advise that additional LABA should not be used while on therapy. Inform of adverse effects (eg, palpitations, chest pain, rapid HR, tremor, or nervousness). Inform patients treated for EIB that additional doses should not be used for 12 hrs and not to use additional doses.

Administration: Oral inhalation route. Refer to PI for proper administration and use. **Storage:** 20-25°C (68-77°F). Keep in dry place, away from direct heat or sunlight. Discard 6 weeks after removal from pouch or after all blisters have been used (when the dose indicator reads "0"), whichever comes first.

SEROQUEL RX
quetiapine fumarate (AstraZeneca)

> Elderly patients with dementia-related psychosis treated with antipsychotic drugs are at an increased risk of death; most deaths appeared to be cardiovascular (CV) (eg, heart failure, sudden death) or infectious (eg, pneumonia) in nature. Not approved for the treatment of patients with dementia-related psychosis. Antidepressants increased the risk of suicidal thinking and behavior (suicidality) in children, adolescents, and young adults in short-term studies of major depressive disorder (MDD) and other psychiatric disorders. Monitor and observe closely for clinical worsening, suicidality, or unusual changes in behavior in patients who are started on antidepressant therapy. Not approved for use in pediatric patients <10 yrs.

THERAPEUTIC CLASS: Dibenzapine derivative

INDICATIONS: Treatment of schizophrenia in adults and adolescents (13-17 yrs). Acute treatment of manic episodes associated with bipolar I disorder, both as monotherapy and as an adjunct therapy to lithium or divalproex in adults and pediatrics (10-17 yrs). Monotherapy for acute treatment of depressive episodes associated with bipolar I/II disorder in adults. Maintenance treatment of bipolar I disorder as adjunct therapy to lithium or divalproex in adults.

DOSAGE: *Adults:* Schizophrenia: Initial: 25mg bid. Titrate: Increase total daily dose by 25-50mg divided bid-tid on the 2nd and 3rd day, as tolerated, to a total dose range of 300-400mg/day by the 4th day. Adjust doses by 25-50mg divided bid at intervals of ≥2 days if indicated. Max: 800mg/day. Maint: Responding patients should continue beyond acute response at lowest dose needed to maintain remission. Reassess periodically to determine the need for maintenance treatment. Bipolar I Disorder: Manic Episodes: Monotherapy/Adjunct: Initial: 100mg/day bid on Day 1. Titrate: Increase to 400mg/day on Day 4 in increments of up to 100mg/day divided bid. May further adjust to up to 800mg/day by Day 6 in increments of ≤200mg/day. Max: 800mg/day. Maint: 400-800mg/day given bid as adjunct therapy to lithium or divalproex. Depressive Episodes: Day 1: 50mg qhs. Day 2: 100mg qhs. Day 3: 200mg qhs. Day 4: 300mg qhs.

Patients receiving 600 mg: Day 5: 400mg qhs. Day 8: 600mg qhs. Max: 600mg/day. Elderly/ Debilitated/Predisposition to Hypotension: Consider slower rate of titration and lower target dose. Hepatic Impairment: Initial: 25mg/day. Titrate: May increase by 25-50mg/day to an effective dose, depending on response and tolerability. Refer to PI for dosing when reinitiating treatment or switching from other antipsychotics.

Pediatrics: Schizophrenia: 13-17 yrs: Administer bid or tid. Day 1: 50mg/day. Day 2: 100mg/day. Day 3: 200mg/day. Day 4: 300mg/day. Day 5: 400mg/day. After Day 5, adjust dose based on response and tolerability within recommended range of 400-800mg/day in increments of ≤100mg/day. Max: 800mg/day. Maint: Responding patients should continue beyond acute response at lowest dose needed to maintain remission. Reassess periodically to determine the need for maintenance treatment. Bipolar I Disorder: Manic Episodes: 10-17 yrs: Administer bid or tid. Day 1: 50mg/day. Day 2: 100mg/day. Day 3: 200mg/day. Day 4: 300mg/day. Day 5: 400mg/day. After Day 5, adjust dose based on response and tolerability within recommended range of 400-600mg/day in increments of ≤100mg/day. Max: 600mg/day. Maint: Responding patients should continue beyond acute response at lowest dose to maintain remission. Reassess periodically to determine the need for maintenance treatment. Debilitated/Predisposition to Hypotension: Consider slower rate of titration and lower target dose. Hepatic Impairment: Initial: 25mg/day. Titrate: May increase by 25-50mg/day to an effective dose, depending on response and tolerability. Refer to PI for dosing when reinitiating treatment or switching from other antipsychotics.

HOW SUPPLIED: Tab: 25mg, 50mg, 100mg, 200mg, 300mg, 400mg

WARNINGS/PRECAUTIONS: Neuroleptic malignant syndrome (NMS) reported; d/c and treat immediately. Worsening of metabolic parameters of weight, blood glucose, and lipids reported. Hyperglycemia reported; if symptoms develop, monitor FPG. Monitor glucose control regularly in diabetes mellitus (DM) patients and FPG in patients with risk factors for DM. Undesirable alterations in lipids and weight gain reported; monitor lipids and weight regularly. May cause tardive dyskinesia (TD); consider d/c if it occurs. May induce orthostatic hypotension; caution with CV disease, cerebrovascular disease, or conditions that predispose to hypotension (eg, dehydration, hypovolemia). HTN and hypertensive crisis in children and adolescents reported; monitor BP periodically. Leukopenia, neutropenia, and agranulocytosis reported; d/c if severe neutropenia (absolute neutrophil count [ANC] <1000/mm³). Monitor CBC and d/c at first sign of decline in WBC if preexisting low WBC count or history of drug-induced leukopenia/neutropenia. Lenticular changes reported; monitor for cataracts at initiation and every 6 months. QT prolongation reported; caution with increased risk of QT prolongation. Avoid in circumstances that may increase the risk of torsades de pointes and/or sudden death. Seizures reported; caution with history of seizures or with conditions that potentially lower the seizure threshold (eg, Alzheimer's dementia). Decrease in thyroid hormone and increase in TSH levels reported. Elevations in prolactin and serum transaminases may occur. May impair mental/physical abilities. May disrupt body's ability to reduce core body temperature; caution in conditions that may elevate core temperature (eg, exercising strenuously, exposure to extreme heat, dehydration). Priapism, esophageal dysmotility, and aspiration reported; caution in patients at risk of aspiration pneumonia. Acute withdrawal symptoms (eg, N/V, insomnia) may occur after abrupt cessation; d/c gradually.

ADVERSE REACTIONS: Headache, somnolence, dizziness, dry mouth, constipation, dyspepsia, tachycardia, asthenia, agitation, pain, weight gain, ALT increased, abdominal pain, back pain, N/V.

INTERACTIONS: Caution with other centrally acting drugs; avoid alcohol. May enhance the effects of certain antihypertensives. May antagonize the effects of levodopa and dopamine agonists. Caution with drugs known to cause electrolyte imbalance. Avoid in combination with Class IA/III antiarrhythmics, antipsychotics (eg, ziprasidone, chlorpromazine, thioridazine), antibiotics (eg, gatifloxacin, moxifloxacin), or any other class of medications known to prolong QTc interval (eg, pentamidine, levomethadyl acetate, methadone). Increased clearance with phenytoin and thioridazine. Increased doses may be required when coadministered with phenytoin or other hepatic enzyme inducers (eg, carbamazepine, barbiturates, rifampin, glucocorticoids). Decreased clearance with cimetidine and ketoconazole; reduce dosage with ketoconazole and other CYP3A inhibitors (eg, itraconazole, fluconazole, erythromycin, protease inhibitors). Decreased clearance of lorazepam. Increased levels with divalproex; insignificant increase in clearance, decrease in concentration, and absorption of divalproex reported. Caution with anticholinergic medications.

PREGNANCY: Category C, not for use in nursing.

MECHANISM OF ACTION: Dibenzothiazepine derivative; not established. Suspected to be mediated through a combination of dopamine type 2 (D_2) and serotonin type 2 ($5HT_2$) antagonism.

PHARMACOKINETICS: Absorption: Rapid, T_{max}=1.5 hrs. **Distribution:** V_d=10L/kg; plasma protein binding (83%); found in breast milk. **Metabolism:** Liver (extensive) via sulfoxidation and oxidation; CYP3A4; N-desalkyl quetiapine (active metabolite). **Elimination:** Urine (73%), feces (20%); $T_{1/2}$=6 hrs.

S

NURSING CONSIDERATIONS

Assessment: Assess for history of dementia-related psychosis, DM, or any other conditions where treatment is cautioned. Assess for pregnancy/nursing status and possible drug interactions. Evaluate baseline vital signs and weight, CBC, FBG, lipid profile, LFTs, ECG, thyroid function tests, prolactin levels, and ophthalmologic examination.

Monitoring: Monitor for signs/symptoms of NMS, hyperglycemia, TD, clinical worsening, suicidality, unusual changes in behavior, worsening of glucose control in DM, orthostatic hypotension, priapism, esophageal dysmotility, and aspiration. Monitor for acute withdrawal symptoms (eg, N/V, insomnia) with abrupt withdrawal. Monitor vital signs and weight, CBC, FPG in patients with risk factors for DM, lipid profile, ANC, LFTs, ECG, thyroid function tests, prolactin levels, and ophthalmologic examination.

Patient Counseling: Inform about risks and benefits of therapy. Advise patient, family, and caregivers to be alert for signs of behavior changes, suicidal ideation, worsening of depression, signs/symptoms of NMS, symptoms of hyperglycemia and DM, weight gain, risk of orthostatic hypotension, overheating, and dehydration; notify physician if these and other adverse reactions occur. Counsel to avoid activities requiring mental alertness (eg, operating machinery/driving). Instruct to notify physician if taking other drugs, pregnant, or plan to become pregnant. Instruct to avoid breastfeeding and alcohol intake.

Administration: Oral route. May be taken with or without food. **Storage:** 25°C (77°F); excursions permitted to 15-30°C (59-86°F).

SEROQUEL XR   RX
quetiapine fumarate (AstraZeneca)

> Elderly patients with dementia-related psychosis treated with antipsychotic drugs are at an increased risk of death; most deaths appeared to be cardiovascular (CV) (eg, heart failure, sudden death) or infectious (eg, pneumonia) in nature. Not approved for the treatment of patients with dementia-related psychosis. Antidepressants increased the risk of suicidal thinking and behavior (suicidality) in children, adolescents, and young adults in short-term studies of major depressive disorder (MDD) and other psychiatric disorders. Monitor and observe closely for clinical worsening, suicidality, or unusual changes in behavior in patients who are started on antidepressant therapy. Not approved for use in pediatric patients.

THERAPEUTIC CLASS: Dibenzapine derivative

INDICATIONS: Treatment of schizophrenia. Acute treatment of manic or mixed episodes associated with bipolar I disorder, both as monotherapy and as an adjunct to lithium or divalproex. Acute treatment of depressive episodes associated with bipolar disorder. Maintenance treatment of bipolar I disorder as adjunct therapy to lithium or divalproex. Adjunctive therapy to antidepressants for treatment of MDD.

DOSAGE: *Adults:* Schizophrenia: Give qd in pm. Initial: 300mg/day. Titrate: Within dose range of 400-800mg/day depending on response and tolerance. Dose increases may be made at intervals as short as 1 day and in increments up to 300mg/day. Max: 800mg/day. Maint: 400-800mg/day for 16 weeks. Reassess periodically the need for maintenance treatment and the appropriate dose. Bipolar Disorder: Bipolar Mania: Monotherapy/Adjunct: Give qd in pm. Day 1: 300mg/day. Day 2: 600mg/day. Titrate: May adjust dose between 400-800mg beginning on Day 3 depending on response and tolerance. Maint: 400-800mg/day as adjunct therapy to lithium or divalproex. Periodically reassess the need for maintenance treatment and the appropriate dose. Depressive Episodes: Give qd in pm. Day 1: 50mg/day. Day 2: 100mg/day. Day 3: 200mg/day. Day 4: 300mg/day. MDD Adjunctive Therapy: Initial: 50mg qd in pm. Day 3: Increase dose to 150mg qd in pm. Max: 300mg/day. Elderly/Debilitated/Predisposition to Hypotension: Consider slower rate of dose titration and lower target dose. Elderly/Hepatic Impairment: Initial: 50mg/day. Titrate: May increase in increments of 50mg/day depending on response and tolerance. Refer to PI for dosing when reinitiating treatment, switching from immediate release tab, or other antipsychotics. Swallow whole and take without food or with a light meal.

HOW SUPPLIED: Tab, Extended-Release: 50mg, 150mg, 200mg, 300mg, 400mg

WARNINGS/PRECAUTIONS: Neuroleptic malignant syndrome (NMS) reported; d/c and treat immediately. Worsening of metabolic parameters of weight, blood glucose, and lipids reported. Hyperglycemia reported; if symptoms develop, monitor FPG. Monitor glucose control regularly in diabetes mellitus (DM) patients and FPG in patients with risk factors for DM. Undesirable alterations in lipids and weight gain reported; monitor lipids and weight regularly. May cause tardive dyskinesia (TD); consider d/c if it occurs. May induce orthostatic hypotension; caution with CV disease, cerebrovascular disease, or conditions that predispose to hypotension (eg, dehydration, hypovolemia). Leukopenia, neutropenia, and agranulocytosis reported; d/c if severe neutropenia (absolute neutrophil count [ANC] <1000/mm³). Monitor CBC and d/c at first sign of decline in WBC if preexisting low WBC count or history of drug-induced leukopenia/neutropenia. Lenticular changes reported; monitor for cataracts at initiation and every 6 months. QT prolongation reported; caution with increased risk of QT prolongation. Avoid in circumstances that may increase the risk of torsade de pointes and/or sudden death. Seizures reported;

caution with history of seizures or with conditions that potentially lower the seizure threshold (eg, Alzheimer's dementia). Decrease in thyroid hormone and increase in TSH levels reported. Elevations in prolactin and serum transaminases may occur. May impair mental/physical abilities. May disrupt body's ability to reduce core body temperature; caution in conditions that may elevate core temperature (eg, exercising strenuously, exposure to extreme heat, dehydration). Priapism, esophageal dysmotility, and aspiration reported; caution in patients at risk of aspiration pneumonia. Acute withdrawal symptoms (eg, N/V, insomnia) may occur after abrupt cessation; d/c gradually.

ADVERSE REACTIONS: Dry mouth, constipation, dyspepsia, somnolence, dizziness, orthostatic hypotension, weight gain, fatigue, dysarthria, nasal congestion, extrapyramidal symptoms, increased appetite, back pain, abnormal dreams.

INTERACTIONS: Caution with other centrally acting drugs; avoid alcohol. May enhance the effects of certain antihypertensives. May antagonize the effects of levodopa and dopamine agonists. Caution with drugs known to cause electrolyte imbalance. Avoid in combination with Class IA/III antiarrythmics, antipsychotics (eg, ziprasidone, chlorpromazine, thioridazine), antibiotics (eg, gatifloxacin, moxifloxacin), or any other class of medications known to prolong QTc interval (eg, pentamidine, levomethadyl acetate, methadone). Increased clearance with phenytoin and thioridazine. Increased doses may be required when coadministered with phenytoin or other hepatic enzyme inducers (eg, carbamazepine, barbiturates, rifampin, glucocorticoids). Decreased clearance with cimetidine and ketoconazole; reduce dosage with ketoconazole and other CYP3A inhibitors (eg, itraconazole, fluconazole, erythromycin, protease inhibitors). Decreased clearance of lorazepam. Increased levels with divalproex; insignificant increase in clearance, decrease in concentration, and absorption of divalproex reported. Caution with anticholinergic medications.

PREGNANCY: Category C, not for use in nursing.

MECHANISM OF ACTION: Dibenzothiazepine derivative; not established. Suspected to be mediated through a combination of dopamine type 2 (D_2) and serotonin type 2A ($5\text{-}HT_{2A}$) antagonism.

PHARMACOKINETICS: Absorption: T_{max}=6 hrs. **Distribution:** V_d=10L/kg; plasma protein binding (83%); found in breast milk. **Metabolism:** Liver (extensive) via sulfoxidation and oxidation; CYP3A4; norquetiapine (active metabolite). **Elimination:** Urine (73%), feces (20%); $T_{1/2}$=7 hrs (quetiapine), 12 hrs (norquetiapine).

NURSING CONSIDERATIONS

Assessment: Assess for history of dementia-related psychosis, DM, or any other conditions where treatment is cautioned. Assess pregnancy/nursing status and possible drug interactions. Evaluate baseline weight, CBC, FPG, lipid profile, LFTs, ECG, thyroid function tests, prolactin levels, and ophthalmologic examination.

Monitoring: Monitor for signs/symptoms of NMS, hyperglycemia, TD, clinical worsening, suicidality, unusual changes in behavior, worsening of glucose control in DM, orthostatic hypotension, priapism, esophageal dysmotility, and aspiration. Monitor for acute withdrawal symptoms (eg, N/V, insomnia) with abrupt withdrawal. Monitor weight, CBC, FPG in patients with risk factors for DM, lipid profile, ANC, LFTs, ECG, thyroid function tests, prolactin levels, and ophthalmologic examination.

Patient Counseling: Inform about risks and benefits of therapy. Advise patient, family, and caregivers to be alert for the emergence of behavior changes, suicidal ideation, worsening of depression, signs/symptoms of NMS, symptoms of hyperglycemia and DM, weight gain, risk of orthostatic hypotension, overheating, and dehydration; notify physician if these and other adverse reactions occur. Counsel to avoid activities requiring mental alertness (eg, operating machinery/driving). Instruct to notify physician if taking other drugs, pregnant or plan to become pregnant. Instruct to avoid breastfeeding and alcohol intake.

Administration: Oral route. Swallow tab whole; do not split, crush, or chew. Take without food or with a light meal (approximately 300cal). **Storage:** Store at 25°C (77°F); excursions permitted to 15-30°C (59-86°F).

SF ROWASA   RX
mesalamine (Alaven)

OTHER BRAND NAMES: Rowasa (Alaven)

THERAPEUTIC CLASS: 5-Aminosalicylic acid derivative

INDICATIONS: Treatment of active mild to moderate distal ulcerative colitis, proctosigmoiditis, or proctitis.

DOSAGE: *Adults:* Usual: 60mL units in one rectal instillation qhs for 3-6 weeks. Retain for 8 hrs.

HOW SUPPLIED: Sus: 4g/60mL

WARNINGS/PRECAUTIONS: Acute intolerance syndrome (eg, cramping, bloody diarrhea, abdominal pain, headache) may develop; d/c if signs and symptoms occur. Re-evaluate history of sulfasalazine intolerance; if rechallenge is considered, perform under close supervision. Caution with sulfasalazine hypersensitivity; d/c if rash or fever occurs. Carefully monitor with preexisting renal disease; obtain baseline/periodic urinalysis, BUN, and creatinine. Worsening of colitis or symptoms of inflammatory bowel disease, including melena and hematochezia, may occur. Pancolitis, pericarditis (rare) reported. (Rowasa) Contains potassium metabisulfite; caution with sulfite sensitivity especially in asthmatics.

ADVERSE REACTIONS: Abdominal pain/cramps/discomfort, headache, flatulence, flu, fever, nausea, malaise/fatigue.

PREGNANCY: Category B, not for use in nursing.

MECHANISM OF ACTION: 5-aminosalicylic acid; has not been established. Suspected to diminish inflammation by blocking cyclooxygenase and inhibiting prostaglandin production in the colon.

PHARMACOKINETICS: Absorption: Colon: Poor. Extent dependent on retention time. **Metabolism:** Acetylation, N-acetyl-5-ASA (Metabolite). **Elimination:** Urine (10-30%), feces, $T_{1/2}$=0.5-1.5 hrs.

NURSING CONSIDERATIONS

Assessment: Assess for history of sulfasalazine intolerance, pre-existing renal disease, hypersensitivity, pregnancy/nursing status, and possible drug interactions. Obtain baseline urinalysis, BUN, and creatinine. (Rowasa) Assess for history of asthma or atopic allergies.

Monitoring: Monitor urinalysis, BUN, and creatinine periodically. Monitor for signs/symptoms of acute intolerance syndrome (cramping, acute abdominal pain, bloody diarrhea), hypersensitivity, or allergic reaction (rash, fever).

Patient Counseling: Instruct on how to use. Advise that best results achieved if bowel emptied immediately before administration. Advise to seek medical attention if symptoms of acute intolerance syndrome (cramping, acute abdominal pain, bloody diarrhea), hypersensitivity, or allergic reactions occur. If signs of rash or fever develop, d/c therapy. Advise to choose a suitable location for administration.

Administration: Rectal route. Refer to PI for administration instructions. **Storage:** 20-25°C (68-77°F). Excursions permitted. Discard unwrapped bottles after 14 days and products with dark brown contents.

SILENOR   RX
doxepin (Somaxon)

THERAPEUTIC CLASS: H_1-antagonist

INDICATIONS: Treatment of insomnia characterized by difficulties with sleep maintenance.

DOSAGE: *Adults:* Individualized. Do not take within 3 hrs of a meal. Initial: 6mg qd within 30 min of bedtime. May decrease to 3mg. Max: 6mg/day. Elderly: ≥65 yrs: Initial: 3mg qd. May increase to 6mg. Hepatic Impairment: Initial 3mg. Concomitant use with Cimetidine: Max: 3mg.

HOW SUPPLIED: Tab: 3mg, 6mg

CONTRAINDICATIONS: Avoid with or within 2 weeks of MAOIs. Untreated narrow angle glaucoma, severe urinary retention.

WARNINGS/PRECAUTIONS: Evaluate comorbid diagnoses prior to initiation of treatment. Failure of remission after 7 to 10 days may indicate the presence of primary psychiatric and/or medical illness that should be evaluated. Complex behaviors (eg, sleep-driving), amnesia, anxiety and other neuro-psychiatric symptoms reported; consider d/c if sleep-driving episode occurs. Worsening of depression, including suicidal thoughts and actions reported. May impair physical/mental abilities. Caution in patients with compromised respiratory function. Avoid in patient with severe sleep apnea.

ADVERSE REACTIONS: Somnolence, sedation, upper respiratory tract infection, nasopharyngitis, HTN, gastroenteritis, dizziness, N/V.

INTERACTIONS: See Contraindications. Alcohol, CNS depressants, sedating antihistamines may potentiate sedative effects. Increased exposure with inhibitors of CYP2C19, CYP2D6, CYP1A2, and CYP2C9. Doubled exposure with cimetidine. Hypoglycemia reported when oral doxepin was added to tolazamide therapy. Increased blood concentration and decreased psychomotor function with sertraline.

PREGNANCY: Category C, caution in nursing.

MECHANISM OF ACTION: H_1-antagonist; mechanism unknown but is believed to exert its sleep maintenance effect by antagonizing the H_1 receptor.

PHARMACOKINETICS: Absorption: T_{max} = 3.5 hrs; **Distribution:** V_d = 11,930L; plasma protein binding (80%); found in breast milk. **Metabolism:** Extensive by oxidation and demethylation via CYP2C19, CYP2D6, CYP1A2, CYP2C9; N-desmethyldoxepin (nordoxepin)(primary metabolite). **Elimination:** Urine (<3%); $T_{1/2}$ = 15.3 hrs (doxepin), 31 hrs (nordoxepin).

NURSING CONSIDERATIONS

Assessment: Assess for untreated narrow angle glaucoma, urinary retention, presence of a primary psychiatric and/or medical illness that may cause insomnia, depression, hepatic impairment, sleep apnea, pregnancy/nursing status, and possible drug interactions.

Monitoring: Monitor treatment response, sleep-driving, and worsening of depression such as suicidal ideation and actions.

Patient Counseling: Inform of benefits and risks associated with therapy. Counsel on appropriate use of medication. Instruct to contact physician if "sleep driving" occurs or if patient performs other complex behaviors while not fully awake. Seek medical attention if worsening of insomnia, symptoms of cognitive or behavioral abnormalities. Medication may cause sedation; caution against operating machinery (eg, automobiles) during therapy. Inform that use of alcohol, sedating antihistamines, or other CNS depressants may potentiate sedative effects of drug.

Administration: Oral route. Storage: 20°-25°C (68°-77°F). Protect from light.

SILVADENE   RX
silver sulfadiazine (Monarch Pharmaceuticals Inc.)

OTHER BRAND NAMES: SSD (Par)

THERAPEUTIC CLASS: Sulfonamide

INDICATIONS: Adjunct for prevention and treatment of wound sepsis in patients with 2nd- and 3rd-degree burns.

DOSAGE: *Adults:* Apply under sterile conditions qd-bid to thickness of approximately 1/16 inch. Re-apply if removed by patient activity. Continue until wound is healed.

HOW SUPPLIED: Cre: 1% [20g, 50g, 85g, 400g, 1000g]

CONTRAINDICATIONS: Late pregnancy, premature infants, newborns during first 2 months of life.

WARNINGS/PRECAUTIONS: Potential cross-sensitivity with other sulfonamides. Hemolysis may occur in G6PD deficient patients. Drug accumulation with hepatic and renal dysfunction. Monitor renal function and serum sulfa levels with extensive burns. Fungal proliferation, including super-infection, has been reported.

ADVERSE REACTIONS: Transient leukopenia, skin necrosis, erythema multiforme, skin discoloration, burning sensation, rash, interstitial nephritis, systemic sulfonamide reactions.

INTERACTIONS: May inactivate topical proteolytic enzymes. Leukopenia increased with cimetidine.

PREGNANCY: Category B, not for use in nursing.

MECHANISM OF ACTION: Topical antimicrobial of sulfonamide class; acts on cell membrane and cell wall of many gram-negative and gram-positive bacteria and yeast to produce bactericidal effect.

NURSING CONSIDERATIONS

Assessment: Assess pregnancy/nursing status, renal/hepatic dysfunction, glucose-6-phosphate dehydrogenase deficiency, and for possible drug interactions.

Monitoring: Monitor fungal proliferation, renal/hepatic function, urine to identify sulfa crystals, serum sulfa concentrations with wounds involving extensive body surface areas, and signs/symptoms of sulfonamide reaction (eg, agranulocytosis, aplastic anemia, thrombocytopenia, leukopenia, Stevens-Johnson syndrome, exfoliative dermatitis, hepatitis and hepatocellular necrosis, CNS reactions, and toxic nephrosis).

Patient Counseling: Instruct to clean wound with soap and water and dry thoroughly prior to application. Instruct patient to reapply to any areas from which the cream has been removed by patient's activity. Inform patients that dressings can be used if needed. Instruct patient to continue therapy until satisfactory healing has occurred, burn site is ready for graft, or serious adverse events occur.

Administration: Topical. **Storage:** At room temperature.

SIMCOR   RX
niacin - simvastatin (Abbott)

THERAPEUTIC CLASS: HMG-CoA reductase inhibitor/Nicotinic acid

INDICATIONS: Adjunct to diet to reduce total-C, LDL, apolipoprotein B, non-HDL, TG, or to increase HDL with primary hypercholesterolemia and mixed dyslipidemia, and to reduce TG with hypertriglyceridemia when treatment with simvastatin monotherapy or niacin extended-release monotherapy is considered inadequate.

DOSAGE: *Adults:* Not Currently on Niacin Extended-Release or Switching from Non-Extended-Release Niacin: Initial: 500mg-20mg qhs. Additional Lipid Level Management Needed despite Simvastatin 20-40mg: Initial: 500mg-40mg qhs. Titrate: Niacin Extended-Release: Increase by ≤500mg qd q4 weeks. After Week 8, titrate to patient response and tolerance. Maint: 1000mg-20mg to 2000mg-40mg qd depending on tolerability and lipid levels. Max: 2000mg-40mg qd. D/C for >7 Days: Retitrate as tolerated. May take aspirin (ASA) (up to 325mg) 30 min before administration to reduce flushing. Concomitant Amiodarone/Amlodipine/Ranolazine: Max: 1000mg-20mg/day. Chinese Patients: Caution with >1000mg-20mg/day. Severe Renal Dysfunction: Do not start unless already tolerating ≥10mg simvastatin.

HOW SUPPLIED: Tab: (Niacin Extended-Release-Simvastatin) 500mg-20mg, 500mg-40mg, 750mg-20mg, 1000mg-20mg, 1000mg-40mg

CONTRAINDICATIONS: Active liver disease, active peptic ulcer disease, arterial bleeding, women who are pregnant or may become pregnant, and nursing mothers. Concomitant strong CYP3A4 inhibitors (eg, itraconazole, ketoconazole, posaconazole, HIV protease inhibitors, boceprevir, telaprevir, erythromycin, clarithromycin, telithromycin, nefazodone), gemfibrozil, cyclosporine, danazol, verapamil, or diltiazem.

WARNINGS/PRECAUTIONS: Myopathy and rhabdomyolysis reported; predisposing factors include age ≥65 yrs, female gender, uncontrolled hypothyroidism, and renal impairment. The risk of myopathy/rhabdomyolysis is dose-related and is disproportionately greater with simvastatin 80mg. D/C immediately if myopathy is suspected/diagnosed or if markedly elevated CPK levels occur. Monitor for any signs/symptoms of muscle pain, tenderness, or weakness; consider periodic monitoring of serum creatine kinase (CK). Caution with dose escalation with complicated medical histories predisposing to rhabdomyolysis (eg, renal insufficiency). Temporarily d/c a few days prior to elective major surgery and when any major medical/surgical condition supervenes (eg, sepsis, hypotension, dehydration, major surgery, trauma, severe metabolic/endocrine/electrolyte disorders, uncontrolled seizures). Severe hepatic toxicity, including fulminant hepatic necrosis, has occurred when substituting sustained-release niacin for immediate-release niacin at equivalent doses. Do not substitute for equivalent dose of immediate-release (crystalline) niacin or other modified-release (sustained-release or time-release) niacin preparations. Caution with renal impairment, heavy alcohol use, history of liver disease, those predisposed to gout, and in elderly. Increases in serum transaminases reported; perform LFTs before initiation and as clinically indicated. Hepatic failure reported; promptly interrupt therapy if serious liver injury and/or hyperbilirubinemia or jaundice occurs and do not restart if no alternate etiology found. May increase HbA1C and FPG levels; closely monitor diabetic/potentially diabetic patients. May need to adjust diet and/or hypoglycemic therapy or d/c medication. May reduce platelet counts. (Niacin) May reduce phosphorus levels and increase PT or uric acid levels.

ADVERSE REACTIONS: Flushing, headache, back pain, diarrhea, nausea, pruritus.

INTERACTIONS: See Contraindications. Avoid ingestion of alcohol, hot drinks, or spicy foods around time of administration; may increase flushing and pruritus. (Simvastatin) Avoid large quantities of grapefruit juice (>1 quart/day). Voriconazole may inhibit metabolism; may need to adjust dose. Increased risk of myopathy/rhabdomyolysis with fibrates; avoid combination. Increased risk of myopathy/rhabdomyolysis with concomitant amlodipine, ranolazine, and colchicine; use caution. Decreased C_{max} with propranolol. May increase digoxin levels; monitor. May potentiate the effect of coumarin anticoagulants; monitor PT. Nelfinavir may affect simvastatin exposure. (Niacin) ASA may decrease metabolic clearance. May potentiate the effects of ganglionic blocking agents and vasoactive drugs resulting in postural hypotension. Binding to bile acid sequestrants (eg, cholestyramine and colestipol) reported; separate administration by 4-6 hrs. Nutritional supplements containing large doses of niacin or related compounds may potentiate adverse effects.

PREGNANCY: Category X, not for use in nursing.

MECHANISM OF ACTION: Niacin: Nicotinic acid; not well established. Suspected to partially inhibit release of free fatty acids from adipose tissue and increase lipoprotein lipase activity, which may increase rate of chylomicron TG removal from plasma. Decreases rate of hepatic synthesis of VLDL and LDL. Simvastatin: HMG-CoA reductase inhibitor. Inhibits conversion of HMG-CoA to mevalonate. Also reduces VLDL, TG, and increases HDL.

PHARMACOKINETICS: Absorption: Niacin: T_{max}=4.6-4.9 hrs. Simvastatin: T_{max}=1.9-2 hrs. Simvastatin Acid: C_{max}=3.29ng/mL, T_{max}=6.56 hrs, $AUC_{(0-t)}$=30.81ng•hr/mL. **Distribution:** Niacin: Found in breast milk. **Metabolism:** Liver (1st pass). Niacin: Nicotinamide adenine dinucleotide and other metabolites; conjugation to nicotinuric acid (metabolite). Simvastatin: CYP3A4; β-hydroxyacid, 6'-hydroxy, 6'-hydroxymethyl, and 6'-exomethylene derivatives (major active metabolites). **Elimination:** $T_{1/2}$=4.2-4.9 hrs (simvastatin), 4.6-5 hrs (simvastatin acid). Niacin: Urine (53-77%; 3.6-7.7% unchanged). Simvastatin: Feces (60%), urine (13%).

NURSING CONSIDERATIONS

Assessment: Assess for active liver disease, hepatic transaminase elevations, active peptic ulcer disease, arterial bleeding, pregnancy/nursing status, gout, predisposing factors for myopathy, renal impairment, and possible drug interactions. Assess use in patients who consume substantial quantities of alcohol and/or have a past history of liver disease. Obtain baseline lipid profile (total-C, LDL, HDL, TG) and LFTs.

Monitoring: Monitor for signs/symptoms of myopathy, rhabdomyolysis, liver/renal/endocrine dysfunction and other adverse reactions. Monitor for decreases in platelet counts and phosphorus levels, and increases in PT and uric acid levels. Periodically monitor lipid profile, CK, and blood glucose levels.

Patient Counseling: Instruct patients to discuss all prescription and OTC medications, including vitamins or nutritional supplements containing niacin or nicotinamide, with their physician; report promptly any unexplained muscle pain, tenderness, or weakness, and any symptoms that may indicate liver injury (eg, fatigue, anorexia, right upper abdominal discomfort, dark urine, jaundice); take at hs after a low-fat snack; swallow tab whole, do not break, crush, or chew. Contact physician prior to restarting therapy if dosing is interrupted. Inform that flushing may occur but should subside after several weeks of therapy; instruct to take ASA 30 min prior to dose, and avoid alcohol, hot drinks, and spicy foods during administration time to minimize flushing. If awakened at night due to flushing, rise slowly, especially if dizzy or faint, or taking BP medications. Contact physician promptly if dizziness occurs. If diabetic, notify physician of changes in blood glucose. Use an effective method of birth control to prevent pregnancy while on therapy; if pregnant d/c therapy and notify physician. Do not breastfeed while on therapy.

Administration: Oral route. **Storage:** 20-25°C (68-77°F).

SIMPONI   RX
golimumab (Janssen)

> Increased risk for developing serious infections (eg, active tuberculosis [TB], latent TB reactivation, invasive fungal infections, bacterial/viral infections, and opportunistic infections) leading to hospitalization or death, mostly with immunosuppressants (eg, methotrexate [MTX] or corticosteroids). D/C if serious infection develops. Active/latent reactivation TB may present with disseminated, extrapulmonary disease; test for latent TB and treat prior to initiation of therapy. Invasive fungal infection reported; consider empiric antifungal therapy in patients at risk who develop severe systemic illness. Consider risks and benefits prior to therapy with chronic or recurrent infections. Monitor for development of infection during and after treatment, including development of TB in patients who tested negative for latent TB infection prior to therapy. Lymphoma and other malignancies reported in children and adolescents.

THERAPEUTIC CLASS: Monoclonal antibody/TNF-alpha receptor blocker

INDICATIONS: Treatment of adults with moderately to severely active rheumatoid arthritis (RA) in combination with MTX, active psoriatic arthritis (PsA) alone or in combination with MTX, and active ankylosing spondylitis (AS).

DOSAGE: *Adults:* May continue corticosteroids, nonbiologic disease-modifying antirheumatic drugs (DMARDs), and/or NSAIDs during treatment. RA: 50mg SQ once a month in combination with MTX. PsA/AS: 50mg SQ once a month with or without MTX or other non-biologic DMARDs.

HOW SUPPLIED: Inj: 50mg/0.5mL

WARNINGS/PRECAUTIONS: Do not initiate with an active infection. Increased risk of infection in elderly or patients with comorbid conditions; consider the risks and benefits prior to therapy for those who have resided or travelled in areas of endemic TB or mycoses, and with any underlying conditions predisposing to infection. Hepatitis B virus (HBV) reactivation reported; if reactivation occurs, d/c and initiate antiviral therapy with appropriate supportive treatment. Worsening congestive heart failure (CHF) and new onset CHF reported; monitor closely and d/c if new/worsening symptoms appear. Rare cases of new onset or exacerbation of CNS demyelinating disorders, including multiple sclerosis and peripheral demyelinating disorders (eg, Guillain-Barre syndrome) reported; caution with central or peripheral nervous system demyelinating disorders and consider d/c if these develop. Pancytopenia, leukopenia, neutropenia, aplastic anemia, and thrombocytopenia reported; caution with significant cytopenias. Serious systemic hypersensitivity reactions reported; d/c immediately and institute appropriate therapy if anaphylactic or other serious allergic reaction occurs. Caution when switching from one biologic to another. Needle cover on the prefilled syringe and prefilled syringe in autoinjector contains dry natural rubber, a derivative of latex; avoid handling by latex-sensitive persons. Caution in elderly.

ADVERSE REACTIONS: Serious infection, lymphoma, upper respiratory tract infection, nasopharyngitis, inj-site reactions.

INTERACTIONS: See Boxed Warning. Avoid with live vaccines. Increased risk of serious infections with abatacept, anakinra, and rituximab; avoid with abatacept or anakinra. Caution with CYP450 substrates with a narrow therapeutic index; monitor effect (eg, warfarin) or drug

S

concentration (eg, cyclosporine, theophylline) upon initiation or d/c of therapy; may need dose adjustments.

PREGNANCY: Category B, not for use in nursing.

MECHANISM OF ACTION: Monoclonal antibody/TNF-α receptor blocker; binds to both the soluble and transmembrane bioactive forms of human TNF-α, preventing the binding of TNF-α to its receptors, thereby inhibiting the biological activity of TNF-α.

PHARMACOKINETICS: Absorption: Absolute bioavailability (53%); C_{max}=2.5µg/mL, T_{max}=2-6 days. **Distribution:** (IV) V_d=58-126mL/kg; crosses the placenta. **Elimination:** $T_{1/2}$=2 weeks.

NURSING CONSIDERATIONS

Assessment: Assess for active/chronic/recurrent infection, TB exposure, recent travel in areas of endemic TB or mycoses, history of opportunistic infections, underlying conditions that may predispose to infection, carrier of HBV, malignancies, CHF, demyelinating disorder, significant cytopenia, latex sensitivity, pregnancy/nursing status, and possible drug interactions. Evaluate for active TB and test for latent TB infection, and HBV infection.

Monitoring: Monitor for signs/symptoms of infection, HBV reactivation, malignancies, new or worsening CHF, new onset/exacerbation of CNS demyelinating disorders, hematological events, hypersensitivity reactions, and other adverse reactions. Periodically evaluate for active TB and test for latent TB infection.

Patient Counseling: Advise of the potential risks and benefits of therapy. Instruct to read Medication Guide before initiation of therapy and each time the prescription is renewed. Inform that therapy may lower ability of the immune system to fight infections. Instruct to contact physician if any symptoms of infection develop. Counsel about the risk of lymphoma and other malignancies. Inform latex-sensitive patients that the needle cover contains dry natural rubber, a derivative of latex. Advise to report signs of new/worsening medical conditions (eg, CHF, demyelinating disorders, autoimmune diseases, liver disease, cytopenias, or psoriasis).

Administration: SQ route. Refer to PI for administration instructions. **Storage:** 2-8°C (36-46°F). Do not freeze or shake. Protect from light.

SINEMET CR   RX
levodopa - carbidopa (Merck)

OTHER BRAND NAMES: Sinemet (Merck)

THERAPEUTIC CLASS: Dopa-decarboxylase inhibitor/dopamine precursor

INDICATIONS: Treatment of symptoms of idiopathic Parkinson's disease (paralysis agitans), post-encephalitic parkinsonism, and symptomatic parkinsonism.

DOSAGE: *Adults:* Individualize dose. (Tab) 25mg-100mg: Initial: 1 tab tid. Titrate: Increase by 1 tab qd or qod until 8 tabs/day. 10mg-100mg: Initial: 1 tab tid-qid. Titrate: Increase by 1 tab qd or qod until 2 tabs qid. Maint: 70-100mg/day carbidopa required. Max: 200mg/day carbidopa. Conversion from levodopa (d/c ≥12 hr before starting): <1500mg: 1 tab (25mg-100mg) tid or qid. >1500mg: 1 tab (25mg-250mg) tid or qid. (Tab, Extended-Release) No Prior Levodopa Use: Initial: 1 tab (50mg-200mg) bid at intervals ≥6 hrs. Titrate: Increase or decrease dose or interval accordingly. Adjust dose at interval ≥3 days. Usual: 400-1600mg/day levodopa, given in 4-8 hr intervals while awake. Refer to PI for Conversion to Extended-Release Tabs, Addition of Other Antiparkinson Medication and Interruption of Therapy.

HOW SUPPLIED: Tab: (Carbidopa-Levodopa) 10mg-100mg, 25mg-100mg, 25mg-250mg; Tab, Extended-Release: (Carbidopa-Levodopa) 25mg-100mg, 50mg-200mg

CONTRAINDICATIONS: Nonselective MAOIs during or within 14 days of use; narrow-angle glaucoma; suspicious, undiagnosed skin lesions; history of melanoma.

WARNINGS/PRECAUTIONS: Dyskinesias may occur; consider dose reduction. May cause mental disturbances; carefully observe for development of depression with suicidal tendencies. Caution with past or current psychoses, severe cardiovascular (CV) or pulmonary disease, bronchial asthma, renal, hepatic or endocrine disease. Caution with history of myocardial infarction (MI) with residual arrhythmias; monitor cardiac function carefully during initial dose adjustment. May increase possibility of upper GI hemorrhage in patients with history of peptic ulcer. Neuroleptic malignant syndrome (NMS)-like symptoms reported during dose reduction or d/c. Caution with chronic wide-angle glaucoma; monitor intraocular pressure (IOP) changes during therapy. May cause somnolence and sudden onset of sleep; caution while driving or operating machines. Monitor for development of melanoma. May cause false (+) ketonuria or false (-) glucosuria (glucose-oxidase method).

ADVERSE REACTIONS: Dyskinesia, nausea, hallucination, confusion.

INTERACTIONS: See Contraindications. Caution with neuroleptics. Risk of postural hypotension with antihypertensives and selegiline. HTN and dyskinesia reported with TCAs. Reduced effects with dopamine D_2 antagonists (eg, phenothiazines, butyrophenones, risperidone) and isoniazid. Antagonized by phenytoin, papaverine, and metoclopramide. Reduced bioavailability with iron salts.

PREGNANCY: Category C, caution in nursing.

MECHANISM OF ACTION: Dopa-decarboxylase inhibitor/dopamine precursor. Carbidopa: Inhibits decarboxylation of peripheral levodopa. Levodopa: Crosses blood-brain barrier and presumably converted to dopamine in brain.

PHARMACOKINETICS: Absorption: Administration of variable doses resulted in different parameters. **Distribution:** Levodopa: Crosses the placenta; found in breast milk. **Elimination:** Levodopa: $T_{1/2}$=50 min, 1.5 hrs (in the presence of carbidopa).

NURSING CONSIDERATIONS

Assessment: Assess for glaucoma; suspicious or undiagnosed skin lesions; history of melanoma, MI, and peptic ulcer; arrhythmia; CV, pulmonary and endocrine diseases; bronchial asthma; hepatic/renal function; psychosis; previous hypersensitivity to drug; pregnancy/nursing status; and possible drug interaction.

Monitoring: Monitor for cardiac function during initial dosage adjustment period, depression and suicidal ideations, dyskinesia, upper GI hemorrhage, NMS, IOP changes, and hypersensitivity. Periodically monitor LFTs, CBC, CV and renal function during extended therapy. Monitor for melanomas frequently and on a regular basis; periodic skin examinations should be performed by a dermatologist.

Patient Counseling: Instruct to take as prescribed. Caution while operating machinery/driving. Instruct to notify physician if wearing-off effect poses a problem to lifestyle; appearance or worsening of involuntary movements occur; and gambling, sexual or other urges intensify. Advise that discoloration of body fluids may occur. Inform that high-protein diet, excessive acidity, and iron salts reduce clinical effectiveness. Instruct to swallow extended-release tab without chewing or crushing.

Administration: Oral route. **Storage:** 25°C (77°F); excursions permitted to 15-30°C (59-86°F). Store in tightly closed container. Protect from light and moisture.

SINGULAIR   RX
montelukast sodium (Merck)

THERAPEUTIC CLASS: Leukotriene receptor antagonist

INDICATIONS: Prophylaxis and chronic treatment of asthma in adults and pediatric patients ≥12 months. Relief of symptoms of seasonal allergic rhinitis in patients ≥2 yrs and perennial allergic rhinitis in patients ≥6 months. Prevention of exercise-induced bronchoconstriction (EIB) in patients ≥6 yrs.

DOSAGE: *Adults:* Asthma: 10mg qd pm. Seasonal/Perennial Allergic Rhinitis: 10mg qd. Both Asthma and Allergic Rhinitis: 1 dose qd pm. EIB: 10mg ≥2 hrs before exercise. Do not take additional dose within 24 hrs of previous dose.
Pediatrics: Asthma: ≥15 yrs: 10mg qd pm. 6-14 yrs: 5mg chewable tab qd pm. 2-5 yrs: 4mg chewable tab or 4mg PO granules pkt qd pm. 12-23 months: 4mg PO granules pkt qd pm. Seasonal/Perennial Allergic Rhinitis: ≥15 yrs: 10mg qd. 6-14 yrs: 5mg chewable tab qd. 2-5 yrs: 4mg chewable tab or 4mg PO granules pkt qd. Perennial Allergic Rhinitis: 6-23 months: 4mg PO granules pkt qd. Both Asthma and Allergic Rhinitis: 1 dose qd pm. EIB: ≥15 yrs: 10mg ≥2 hrs before exercise. 6-14 yrs: 5mg chewable tab ≥2 hrs before exercise. Do not take additional dose within 24 hrs of previous dose.

HOW SUPPLIED: Granules: 4mg/pkt; Tab, Chewable: 4mg, 5mg; Tab: 10mg

WARNINGS/PRECAUTIONS: Not for use in the reversal of bronchospasm in acute asthma attacks, including status asthmaticus. May gradually reduce dose of inhaled corticosteroid under supervision, but avoid abrupt substitution for inhaled or oral corticosteroids. Can continue therapy during acute exacerbations of asthma; have a short-acting inhaled β-agonist available. Systemic eosinophilic conditions reported. Neuropsychiatric events (eg, agitation, aggressive behavior or hostility, anxiousness, depression) reported; evaluate risks and benefits of continuing treatment if such events occur. Chewable tabs contains phenylalanine; caution with phenylketonuria. Avoid aspirin (ASA) and NSAIDs with known ASA sensitivity. Cases of cholestatic hepatitis, hepatocellular liver injury, and mixed-pattern liver injury reported with underlying potential for liver disease (eg, alcohol use).

ADVERSE REACTIONS: Headache, pharyngitis, influenza, fever, sinusitis, diarrhea, upper respiratory tract infection, cough, abdominal pain, otitis media, rhinorrhea, otitis.

INTERACTIONS: Monitor with potent CYP450 inducers (eg, phenobarbital, rifampin).

PREGNANCY: Category B, caution in nursing.

S

MECHANISM OF ACTION: Leukotriene receptor antagonist; binds to cysteinyl leukotriene receptors found on airway smooth muscle cells and macrophages and other proinflammatory cells (eg, eosinophils and certain myeloid stem cells). Inhibits physiologic actions of leukotrienes.

PHARMACOKINETICS: Absorption: Rapid. (10mg) Bioavailability (64%); T_{max}=3-4 hrs. (5mg) T_{max}=2-2.5 hrs; bioavailability (73%, fasted), (63%, fed). (4mg Chewable) Fasted 2-5 yrs: T_{max}=2 hrs. (4mg Granules) T_{max}=2.3 hrs (fasted), 6.4 hrs (fed). **Distribution:** V_d=8-11L; plasma protein binding (>99%). **Metabolism:** Liver (extensive); CYP3A4, 2C9. **Elimination:** Biliary (major), feces (86%), urine (<0.2%); $T_{1/2}$=2.7-5.5 hrs.

NURSING CONSIDERATIONS

Assessment: Assess for history of phenylketonuria, history of ASA sensitivity, drug hypersensitivity, pregnancy/nursing status, and possible drug interactions.

Monitoring: Monitor for signs/symptoms of eosinophilia, vasculitic rash, worsening pulmonary symptoms, cardiac complications, neuropathy, neuropsychiatric events, and hypersensitivity reactions.

Patient Counseling: Inform not to use for treatment of acute asthma attacks; appropriate rescue drug (eg, short-acting β_2-agonist) should be available. Seek medical attention if short-acting bronchodilators are needed more than usual while on therapy. Advise to take daily as prescribed, even if asymptomatic, as well as during periods of worsening asthma, and to contact physician if asthma is not well controlled. Instruct not to decrease dose or d/c other anti-asthma medications unless instructed by physician. Advise to notify physician if symptoms of neuropsychiatric events occur. Advise patients with ASA sensitivity to continue avoiding ASA and NSAIDs. Inform phenylketonurics that the 4mg and 5mg chewable tab contains phenylalanine.

Administration: Oral route. Refer to PI for instructions for administration of PO granules.
Storage: 25°C (77°F); excursions permitted to 15-30°C (59-86°F). Protect from light and moisture.

SKELAXIN   RX
metaxalone (King)

THERAPEUTIC CLASS: Muscular analgesic (central-acting)

INDICATIONS: Adjunct to rest, physical therapy, and other measures for the relief of discomforts associated with acute, painful musculoskeletal conditions.

DOSAGE: *Adults:* 800mg tid-qid.
Pediatrics: >12 yrs: 800mg tid-qid.

HOW SUPPLIED: Tab: 800mg* *scored

CONTRAINDICATIONS: Known tendency to drug-induced, hemolytic, and other anemias. Significantly impaired renal/hepatic function.

WARNINGS/PRECAUTIONS: Caution with preexisting liver damage; perform serial LFTs. False-positive Benedict's tests reported; glucose-specific test will differentiate findings. Taking with food may enhance general CNS depression, especially in elderly.

ADVERSE REACTIONS: Drowsiness, dizziness, headache, nervousness, irritability, N/V, GI upset.

INTERACTIONS: Additive sedative effects with other CNS depressants (eg, alcohol, benzodiazepines, opioids, TCAs); use with caution if taking >1 CNS depressant simultaneously.

PREGNANCY: Not for use in pregnancy/nursing.

MECHANISM OF ACTION: Muscular analgesic (central-acting); has not been established. Activity may be due to general depression of CNS.

PHARMACOKINETICS: Absorption: (400mg) C_{max}=983ng/mL, T_{max}= 3.3 hrs; AUC=7479ng•hr/mL. (800mg) C_{max}=1816ng/mL, T_{max}=3 hrs; AUC=15044ng•hr/mL. **Distribution:** V_d=800L. **Metabolism:** Liver; via CYP1A2, 2D6, 2E1, 3A4 and to a lesser extent, CYP2C8, 2C9, C19. **Elimination:** Urine (metabolites); $T_{1/2}$=9 hrs (400mg), 8 hrs (800mg).

NURSING CONSIDERATIONS

Assessment: Assess for known tendency to drug-induced, hemolytic, or other anemias, significant renal/hepatic impairment, hypersensitivity to the drug, pregnancy/nursing status, and possible drug interactions.

Monitoring: Perform serial LFTs with preexisting liver damage. Monitor for signs/symptoms of CNS depression.

Patient Counseling: Inform that drug may impair mental and/or physical abilities required for performance of hazardous tasks (eg, operating machinery, driving), especially when used with alcohol or other CNS depressants.

Administration: Oral route. Taking with food may enhance general CNS depression. **Storage:** 15-30°C (59-86°F).

SOLIRIS
eculizumab (Alexion)

RX

> Life-threatening and fatal meningococcal infections reported; may become rapidly life-threatening or fatal if not recognized and treated early. Comply with the most current Advisory Committee on Immunization Practices (ACIP) recommendations for meningococcal vaccination. Immunize patients with meningococcal vaccine at least 2 weeks prior to administering the 1st dose, unless risks of delaying therapy outweigh risk of meningococcal infection development. Monitor for early signs of meningococcal infections and evaluate immediately if infection suspected. Available only through a restricted program under a Risk Evaluation and Mitigation Strategy; prescribers must enroll in this program.

THERAPEUTIC CLASS: Monoclonal antibody/Protein C5 blocker

INDICATIONS: Treatment of paroxysmal nocturnal hemoglobinuria (PNH) to reduce hemolysis, and atypical hemolytic uremic syndrome (aHUS) to inhibit complement-mediated thrombotic microangiopathy (TMA).

DOSAGE: *Adults:* PNH: Initial: 600mg/week for the 1st 4 weeks. Maint: 900mg for the 5th dose 1 week later, then 900mg every 2 weeks. aHUS: 900mg/week for the 1st 4 weeks. Maint: 1200mg for the 5th dose 1 week later, then 1200mg every 2 weeks. Refer to PI for supplemental dose after plasmapheresis/plasma exchange or fresh frozen plasma infusion.
Pediatrics: aHUS: ≥40kg: Induction: 900mg/week x 4 doses. Maint: 1200mg at week 5, then 1200mg every 2 weeks. 30-<40kg: Induction: 600mg/week x 2 doses. Maint: 900mg at week 3, then 900mg every 2 weeks. 20-<30kg: Induction: 600mg/week x 2 doses. Maint: 600mg at week 3, then 600mg every 2 weeks. 10-<20kg: Induction: 600mg/week x 1 dose. Maint: 300mg at week 2, then 300mg every 2 weeks. 5-<10kg: Induction: 300mg/week x 1 dose. Maint: 300mg at week 2, then 300mg every 3 weeks. Refer to PI for supplemental dose after plasmapheresis/plasma exchange or fresh frozen plasma infusion.

HOW SUPPLIED: Inj: 10mg/mL [30mL]

CONTRAINDICATIONS: Patients with unresolved serious *Neisseria meningitidis* infection and patients not currently vaccinated against it.

WARNINGS/PRECAUTIONS: May increase susceptibility to infections, especially with encapsulated bacteria; caution with any systemic infection, and administer vaccinations for the prevention of *Streptococcus pneumoniae* and *Haemophilus influenza* type b (Hib) infections according to ACIP guidelines in pediatric patients. Monitor PNH patients after d/c for at least 8 weeks to detect hemolysis. Monitor aHUS patients for signs and symptoms of TMA complications during treatment and for at least 12 weeks after d/c; consider reinstitution of treatment, plasma therapy, or appropriate organ-specific supportive measures if TMA complications occur. May result in infusion reactions, including anaphylaxis or other hypersensitivity reactions; interrupt infusion and institute appropriate supportive measures if signs of cardiovascular instability or respiratory compromise occur.

ADVERSE REACTIONS: Meningococcal infections, headache, nasopharyngitis, back pain, N/V, urinary tract infection, HTN, upper respiratory tract infection, diarrhea, anemia, fever, cough, nasal congestion, tachycardia.

PREGNANCY: Category C, caution in nursing.

MECHANISM OF ACTION: Monoclonal antibody/protein C5 blocker; specifically binds to the complement protein C5 with high affinity, thereby inhibiting its cleavage to C5a and C5b and preventing the generation of the terminal complement complex C5b-9. Inhibits terminal complement-mediated intravascular hemolysis in PNH patients and complement-mediated TMA in patients with aHUS.

PHARMACOKINETICS: Absorption: C_{max} =194mcg/mL (PNH). **Distribution:** V_d=7.7L (PNH), 6.14L (aHUS); crosses the placenta; found in breast milk. **Elimination:** $T_{1/2}$=272 hrs (PNH), 291 hrs (aHUS).

NURSING CONSIDERATIONS

Assessment: Assess for unresolved serious *Neisseria meningitidis* infection, meningococcal vaccination status, systemic infection, and pregnancy/nursing status. Obtain baseline serum LDH, platelet count, and SrCr.

Monitoring: Monitor for signs and symptoms of meningococcal infections, other serious infections, and infusion/hypersensitivity reactions. Monitor PNH patients after d/c for at least 8 weeks to detect hemolysis. Monitor aHUS patients for TMA complications for at least 12 weeks after d/c; monitor for signs of TMA by monitoring serial platelet counts, serum lactate dehydrogenase, and SrCr during and following d/c.

Patient Counseling: Counsel about risks and benefits of therapy, in particular the risk of meningococcal infection, and the need to be monitored by a physician following d/c. Instruct to carry

S

Soliris Patient Safety Information Card at all times; keep for 3 months after last dose. Instruct to receive meningococcal vaccination at least 2 weeks prior to receiving the 1st dose of treatment if not previously vaccinated, and to receive revaccination while on therapy. Inform of the signs and symptoms of meningococcal infection, and strongly advise to seek immediate medical attention if these occur. Inform parents/caregivers that their child being treated for aHUS should be vaccinated against *Streptococcus pneumoniae* and Hib infections.

Administration: IV route. Administer by IV infusion over 35 min. Refer to PI for preparation and administration instructions. **Storage:** 2-8°C (36-46°F). Protect from light. Do not freeze or shake. (Admixed Sol) Stable for 24 hrs at 2-8°C (36-46°F) and at room temperature.

SOLODYN RX
minocycline HCl (Medicis)

THERAPEUTIC CLASS: Tetracycline derivative

INDICATIONS: Treatment of inflammatory lesions of non-nodular moderate to severe acne vulgaris in patients ≥12 yrs.

DOSAGE: *Adults:* 1mg/kg qd for 12 weeks. Refer to PI for dose equivalents based on body weight. Renal Impairment: Reduce dose and/or extend time intervals between doses. Elderly: Start at lower end of dosing range.
Pediatrics: ≥12 yrs: 1mg/kg qd for 12 weeks. Refer to PI for dose equivalents based on body weight. Renal Impairment: Reduce dose and/or extend time intervals between doses.

HOW SUPPLIED: Tab, Extended-Release: 45mg, 55mg, 65mg, 80mg, 90mg, 105mg, 115mg, 135mg

WARNINGS/PRECAUTIONS: Safety beyond 12 weeks of use has not been established. May cause fetal harm during pregnancy; avoid use during pregnancy or by individuals of either gender who are attempting to conceive a child. Avoid use during tooth development (last half of pregnancy, infancy, pediatrics ≤8 yrs); may cause permanent discoloration of the teeth and enamel hypoplasia. Reversible decrease in fibula growth rate in premature infants reported. Pseudomembranous colitis reported; initiate appropriate therapeutic measures if it occurs. Serious liver injury (eg, irreversible drug-induced hepatitis, fulminant hepatic failure), CNS side effects, and photosensitivity reported. May increase BUN; caution in patients with renal impairment. Pseudotumor cerebri (benign intracranial HTN) reported; assess for visual disturbance prior to therapy. Check for papilledema if visual disturbance occurs during treatment. Long-term use has been associated with development of autoimmune syndromes, including drug-induced lupus-like syndrome, autoimmune hepatitis and vasculitis; d/c immediately if any of these occur. Sporadic cases of serum sickness reported shortly after use. Cases of anaphylaxis, serious skin reactions (eg, Stevens-Johnson syndrome), erythema multiforme, and drug rash with eosinophilia and systemic symptoms (DRESS) syndrome reported; d/c immediately if this syndrome occurs. May induce tissue hyperpigmentation. Drug-resistant bacteria may develop; use only as indicated. May result in overgrowth of nonsusceptible organisms; d/c and initiate appropriate therapy if superinfection develops. May impair mental/physical abilities. Caution in elderly.

ADVERSE REACTIONS: Headache, fatigue, dizziness, pruritus, malaise, mood alteration.

INTERACTIONS: Avoid with isotretinoin. May require downward adjustments of anticoagulant dosage. May interfere with bactericidal action of penicillin; avoid use. Fatal renal toxicity reported with methoxyflurane. Antacids containing aluminum, calcium or magnesium, and iron-containing preparations may impair absorption. May interfere with the effectiveness of low dose oral contraceptives; female patients should use 2nd form of contraception during treatment.

PREGNANCY: Category D, not for use in nursing.

MECHANISM OF ACTION: Tetracycline derivative; not established.

PHARMACOKINETICS: Absorption: C_{max}=2.63µg/mL; T_{max}=3.5-4 hrs; AUC_{0-24}=33.32µg•hr/mL. **Distribution:** Crosses placenta, found in breast milk.

NURSING CONSIDERATIONS

Assessment: Assess for renal impairment, visual disturbances, hypersensitivity, pregnancy/nursing status, and possible drug interactions.

Monitoring: Monitor for signs/symptoms of pseudomembranous colitis (eg, diarrhea), hepatotoxicity, superinfection, pseudotumor cerebri, visual disturbance, papilledema, DRESS syndrome, CNS side effects, and autoimmune syndromes. Perform periodic laboratory evaluations of organ systems including hematopoietic, renal, and hepatic studies. In patients showing symptoms of an autoimmune syndrome, perform appropriate tests (eg, LFTs, antinuclear antibodies, CBC). Perform serum level determinations of the drug with prolonged therapy in renally impaired patients.

Patient Counseling: Instruct to avoid use if pregnant or in patients of either gender who are planning to conceive a child. Inform that pseudomembranous colitis may occur; advise to seek medical attention if watery/bloody stools develop. Instruct to seek medical advice if loss of appetite, tiredness, diarrhea, skin turning yellow, bleeding easily, confusion, and sleepiness occur. Counsel about CNS symptoms; instruct to use caution in driving or operating machinery and advise to seek medical help if persistent headache/blurred vision is experienced. Inform that drug may render oral contraceptives less effective. Inform that autoimmune syndromes may occur; instruct to d/c immediately and seek medical help if symptoms (eg, arthralgia, fever, rash, malaise) are experienced. Counsel that discoloration of skin, scars, teeth, or gums may arise during therapy. Inform that photosensitivity reactions may occur; advise to minimize/avoid exposure to sunlight, to wear loose-fitting clothes when outdoors, and to d/c at 1st evidence of skin erythema. Instruct to take exactly ud; skipping doses or not completing full course of therapy may decrease effectiveness and create bacterial resistance. Advise to swallow tab whole; do not chew, crush, or split.

Administration: Oral route. **Storage:** 25°C (77°F); excursions permitted to 15-30°C (59-86°F). Protect from light, moisture, and excessive heat.

SOLU-CORTEF   RX
hydrocortisone sodium succinate (Pharmacia & Upjohn)

THERAPEUTIC CLASS: Glucocorticoid

INDICATIONS: Steroid-responsive disorders.

DOSAGE: *Adults:* Individualize dose. Initial: 100-500mg IV/IM, depending on disease. May repeat dose at 2, 4, or 6 hrs based on clinical response and condition. High-dose therapy should continue only until patient is stabilized, usually not beyond 48-72 hrs. Maint: Decrease initial dosage in small decrements at appropriate time intervals until the lowest dosage that maintains an adequate clinical response is reached. Withdraw gradually after long-term therapy. Acute Exacerbations of Multiple Sclerosis: Usual: 800mg/day for 1 week followed by 320mg qod for 1 month.
Pediatrics: Individualize dose. Initial: 0.56-8mg/kg/day IV/IM in 3-4 divided doses (20-240mg/m²bsa/day).

HOW SUPPLIED: Inj: 100mg, 250mg, 500mg, 1000mg

CONTRAINDICATIONS: Systemic fungal infections, idiopathic thrombocytopenic purpura (IM corticosteroid preparations), intrathecal administration.

WARNINGS/PRECAUTIONS: May result in dermal and/or subdermal changes forming depressions in the skin at the injection site. Exercise caution not to exceed recommended doses. Anaphylactoid reactions (rare) may occur. May need to increase dose before, during, and after stressful situations. High doses should not be used for the treatment of traumatic brain injury. Increases BP, salt/water retention, and K⁺ and calcium excretion. Caution in patients with left ventricular free wall rupture after a recent myocardial infarction (MI). Monitor for hypothalamic-pituitary adrenal (HPA) axis suppression, Cushing's syndrome, and hyperglycemia with chronic use. May produce reversible HPA axis suppression with the potential for glucocorticosteroid insufficiency after withdrawal of treatment. Drug-induced secondary adrenocortical insufficiency may be minimized by gradual reduction of dosage. May decrease resistance and inability to localize infection. May mask signs of current infection or cause new infections; avoid use intra-articularly, intrabursally, or for intratendinous administration for local effect in the presence of acute local infection. May exacerbate systemic fungal infections. Rule out latent or active amebiasis before initiating therapy. Caution with *Strongyloides* infestation, active or latent tuberculosis (TB), HTN, congestive heart failure (CHF), renal insufficiency, osteoporosis, and ocular herpes simplex. Caution with active or latent peptic ulcers, diverticulitis, fresh intestinal anastomoses and nonspecific ulcerative colitis; may increase risk of perforation. Acute myopathy with high doses reported most often in patients with disorders of neuromuscular transmission (eg, myasthenia gravis). Enhanced effect in patients with cirrhosis. May decrease bone formation and increase bone resorption. Psychic derangements may appear and existing emotional instability or psychotic tendencies may be aggravated. May elevate intraocular pressure (IOP); monitor IOP if steroid therapy >6 weeks. More serious/fatal course of chickenpox and measles reported. Not for use in cerebral malaria, active ocular herpes simplex. Use of oral corticosteroids not recommended in the treatment of optic neuritis. Severe medical events associated with intrathecal route of administration. May produce posterior subcapsular cataracts or glaucoma with possible damage to the optic nerves, and may enhance the establishment of secondary ocular infections due to bacteria, fungi, or viruses. Kaposi's sarcoma reported. Change in thyroid status may necessitate dose adjustment. Elevation of creatinine kinase may occur. May suppress reactions to skin tests.

ADVERSE REACTIONS: Fluid/electrolyte disturbances, HTN, osteoporosis, muscle weakness, menstrual irregularities, insomnia, impaired wound healing, diabetes mellitus, ulcerative esophagitis, excessive sweating, increased intracranial pressure, carbohydrate intolerance, glaucoma, cataracts.

INTERACTIONS: May lead to a loss of corticosteroid-induced adrenal suppression with amino-glutethimide. May develop hypokalemia with K⁺-depleting agents (eg, amphotericin-B, diuretics). Case reports of cardiac enlargement and CHF with amphotericin-B. May cause a significant decrease in clearance with macrolide antibiotics. Concomitant use with anticholinesterase agents may produce severe weakness in patients with myasthenia gravis. May inhibit response to warfarin; frequently monitor coagulation indices. May increase blood glucose concentrations; dosage adjustments of antidiabetic agents may be required. May decrease serum concentrations of isoniazid. Cholestyramine may increase clearance. Convulsions reported with cyclosporine use. May increase risk of arrhythmias with digitalis glycosides. Estrogens, including oral contraceptives, may decrease hepatic metabolism and enhance effect. May enhance metabolism and require dosage increase with drugs which induce CYP3A4 (eg, barbiturates, phenytoin, carbamazepine, rifampin). May increase plasma concentrations with drugs which inhibit CYP3A4 (eg, ketoconazole, macrolide antibiotics such as erythromycin and troleandomycin). May increase risk of corticosteroid side effects with ketoconazole. May increase risk of GI side effects with aspirin or other NSAIDs. Administration of live or live, attenuated vaccines is contraindicated in patients receiving immunosuppressive doses. Killed or inactivated vaccines may be administered, although response is unpredictable.

PREGNANCY: Category C, not for use in nursing.

MECHANISM OF ACTION: Anti-inflammatory glucocorticoid; causes profound and varied metabolic effects and modifies the body's immune responses to diverse stimuli.

PHARMACOKINETICS: Distribution: Found in breast milk (systemically administered).

NURSING CONSIDERATIONS

Assessment: Assess for systemic fungal infections, other current infections, active TB, vaccination status, hypersensitivity to drug, unusual stress, ulcerative colitis, diverticulitis, HTN, recent MI, intestinal anastomoses, active or latent peptic ulcer, osteoporosis, myasthenia gravis, psychotic tendencies, pregnancy/nursing status, and possible drug interactions.

Monitoring: Monitor for HPA axis suppression, Cushing's syndrome, and hyperglycemia with chronic use. Monitor for anaphylactoid reactions, growth/development (in pediatrics), intestinal perforation and hemorrhage, infections, cataracts, osteoporosis, psychic derangements, Kaposi's sarcoma, acute myopathy. Monitor BP, HR, ECG, glucose, TSH, LFTs, creatinine kinase, serum electrolytes, IOP.

Patient Counseling: Warn not to d/c abruptly or without medical supervision. Instruct to seek medical advise at once if fever or other signs of infection develops. Warn to avoid exposure to chickenpox or measles; advise to report immediately if exposed.

Administration: IM/IV routes. Avoid injection into deltoid muscle. Refer to PI for preparation and administration. **Storage:** 20-25°C (68-77°F). Protect from light. Discard unused solution after 3 days.

SOLU-MEDROL   RX
methylprednisolone sodium succinate (Pharmacia & Upjohn)

THERAPEUTIC CLASS: Glucocorticoid

INDICATIONS: Steroid-responsive disorders when oral therapy is not feasible.

DOSAGE: *Adults:* Individualize dose. Initial: 10-40mg IV/IM inj or IV infusion, depending on disease. High-Dose Therapy: 30mg/kg IV over at least 30 min. May be repeated q4-6h for 48 hrs. High-dose therapy should continue only until patient is stabilized, usually not beyond 48-72 hrs. Maint: Decrease initial dosage in small decrements at appropriate time intervals until the lowest dosage that maintains an adequate clinical response is reached. Withdraw gradually after long-term therapy. Acute Exacerbations of Multiple Sclerosis: 160mg qd for 1 week followed by 64mg qod for 1 month.
Pediatrics: Initial: 0.11-1.6mg/kg/day in 3-4 divided doses (3.2-48mg/m²bsa/day); Uncontrolled Asthma: 1-2mg/kg/day in single or divided doses. Continue short-course ("burst") therapy until patient achieves a peak expiratory flow rate of 80% of his/her personal best or symptoms resolve (usually 3-10 d).

HOW SUPPLIED: Inj: 40mg, 125mg, 500mg, 1g, 2g

CONTRAINDICATIONS: Systemic fungal infections, idiopathic thrombocytopenic purpura (IM corticosteroid preparations), intrathecal administration. Premature infants (formulations preserved with benzyl alcohol).

WARNINGS/PRECAUTIONS: Do not dilute or mix with other solution. Formulation that contains benzyl alcohol, is associated with toxicity especially in neonates. May result in dermal and/or subdermal changes forming depressions in the skin at the injection site. Exercise caution not to exceed recommended doses. Avoid injection into deltoid muscle. Anaphylactoid reactions (rare) may occur. May need to increase dose before, during, and after stressful situations. High doses should not be used for the treatment of traumatic brain injury. May increase BP, salt/water retention, and K⁺ and calcium excretion. Caution in patients with left ventricular free wall rupture after a recent myocardial infarction (MI). Monitor for hypothalamic-pituitary-adrenal (HPA) axis suppression, Cushing's syndrome, and hyperglycemia with chronic use. May produce reversible HPA axis suppression with the potential for glucocorticosteroid insufficiency after withdrawal of treatment. Drug-induced secondary adrenocortical insufficiency may be minimized by gradual reduction of dosage. May mask signs of current infection or cause new infections; avoid use intra-articularly, intrabursally, or for intratendinous administration for local effect in the presence of acute local infection. May exacerbate systemic fungal infections; avoid use unless needed to control drug reactions. Rule out latent or active amebiasis in unexplained diarrhea or history of travel to the tropics before initiating therapy. Caution with *Strongyloides* infestation, active or latent tuberculosis (TB), HTN, congestive heart failure (CHF), renal insufficiency, osteoporosis, ocular herpes simplex. Caution with active or latent peptic ulcers, diverticulitis, fresh intestinal anastomoses and nonspecific ulcerative colitis; may increase risk of perforation. Acute myopathy with high doses reported most often in patients with disorders of neuromuscular transmission (eg, myasthenia gravis). Enhanced effect with cirrhosis. More serious/fatal course of chickenpox and measles reported. Not for use in cerebral malaria, active ocular herpes simplex. Use of oral corticosteroids not recommended in the treatment of optic neuritis. May decrease bone formation and increase bone resorption. Psychic derangements may appear and existing emotional instability or psychotic tendencies may be aggravated. May elevate intraocular pressure (IOP); monitor IOP if steroid therapy >6 weeks. Severe medical events associated with intrathecal route of administration. May produce posterior subcapsular cataracts, glaucoma with possible damage to the optic nerves, and may enhance the establishment of secondary ocular infections due to bacteria, fungi, or viruses. Kaposi's sarcoma reported. Changes in thyroid status may necessitate dose adjustment. Elevation of creatinine kinase may occur. May suppress reactions to skin tests. Avoid abrupt withdrawal.

ADVERSE REACTIONS: Fluid/electrolyte disturbances, HTN, osteoporosis, muscle weakness, menstrual irregularities, insomnia, impaired wound healing, diabetes mellitus, ulcerative esophagitis, excessive sweating, increased intracranial pressure, carbohydrate intolerance, glaucoma, cataracts.

INTERACTIONS: May lead to a loss of corticosteroid-induced adrenal suppression with aminoglutethimide. May develop hypokalemia with K⁺-depleting agents (eg, amphotericin B, diuretics). Case reports of cardiac enlargement and CHF with amphotericin B. May cause a significant decrease in clearance with macrolide antibiotics. Concomitant use with anticholinesterase agents may produce severe weakness in patients with myasthenia gravis. May inhibit response to warfarin; frequently monitor coagulation indices. May increase blood glucose concentrations; dosage adjustments of antidiabetic agents may be required. May decrease serum concentrations of isoniazid. Cholestyramine may increase clearance. Convulsions reported with cyclosporine use. May increase risk of arrhythmias with digitalis glycosides. Estrogens, including oral contraceptives, may decrease hepatic metabolism and enhance effect. May enhance metabolism and require dosage increase with drugs that induce CYP3A4 (eg, barbiturates, phenytoin, carbamazepine, rifampin). May increase plasma concentrations with drugs that inhibit CYP3A4 (eg, ketoconazole, macrolide antibiotics such as erythromycin and troleandomycin). May increase risk of corticosteroid side effects with ketoconazole. May increase risk of GI side effects with aspirin or other NSAIDs. Administration of live or live, attenuated vaccines is contraindicated in patients receiving immunosuppressive doses. Killed or inactivated vaccines may be administered, although response is unpredictable.

PREGNANCY: Category C, not for use in nursing.

MECHANISM OF ACTION: Anti-inflammatory glucocorticoid; causes profound and varied metabolic effects and modifies the body's immune responses to diverse stimuli.

PHARMACOKINETICS: Absorption: (IM) Rapid. **Distribution:** Found in breast milk (systemically administered).

NURSING CONSIDERATIONS

Assessment: Assess for systemic fungal infections, other current infections, active TB, vaccination status, hypersensitivity to drug, unusual stress, ulcerative colitis, diverticulitis, HTN, recent MI, intestinal anastomoses, active or latent peptic ulcer, osteoporosis, myasthenia gravis, psychotic tendencies, pregnancy/nursing status, and possible drug interactions.

Monitoring: Monitor for HPA axis suppression, Cushing's syndrome, and hyperglycemia with chronic use. Monitor for anaphylactoid reactions, growth/development (in pediatrics), intestinal perforation and hemorrhage, infections, cataracts, osteoporosis, psychic derangements, Kaposi's sarcoma, acute myopathy. Monitor BP, HR, ECG, glucose, TSH, LFTs, creatine kinase, serum electrolytes, IOP.

Patient Counseling: Warn not to d/c abruptly or use without medical supervision. Instruct to seek medical advice immediately if fever or other signs of infection develop. Warn to avoid exposure to chickenpox or measles; advise to report immediately if exposed.

S

Administration: IM/IV route. Avoid injection into deltoid muscle. Refer to PI for preparation and administration. **Storage:** 20-25°C (68-77°F). Protect from light. Use within 48 hrs after mixing.

SOMA RX
carisoprodol (Meda)

THERAPEUTIC CLASS: Skeletal muscle relaxant (central-acting)

INDICATIONS: Relief of discomfort associated with acute, painful musculoskeletal conditions.

DOSAGE: *Adults:* ≥16 yrs: 250-350mg tid and hs for up to 2-3 weeks.

HOW SUPPLIED: Tab: 250mg, 350mg

CONTRAINDICATIONS: History of acute intermittent porphyria.

WARNINGS/PRECAUTIONS: May impair mental/physicial abilities. Drug abuse, dependence, and withdrawal reported with prolonged use. Withdrawal symptoms reported following abrupt cessation after prolonged use. Seizures reported in postmarketing surveillance. Caution with hepatic or renal dysfunction and in addiction-prone patients. Not studied in patients >65 yrs.

ADVERSE REACTIONS: Drowsiness, dizziness, headache.

INTERACTIONS: Additive sedative effects with other CNS depressants (eg, alcohol, benzodiazepines, opioids, TCAs); caution when coadministering. Concomitant use with meprobamate is not recommended. Increased exposure of carisoprodol and decreased exposure of meprobamate with CYP2C19 inhibitors (eg, omeprazole, fluvoxamine). Decreased exposure of carisoprodol and increased exposure of meprobamate with CYP2C19 inducers (eg, rifampin, St. John's wort). Induction effect on CYP2C19 seen with low- dose aspirin.

PREGNANCY: Category C, caution in nursing.

MECHANISM OF ACTION: Centrally acting muscle relaxant; not established. Suspected to be associated with altered interneuronal activity in the spinal cord and the descending reticular formation of the brain. Meprobamate, a metabolite, has anxiolytic and sedative properties.

PHARMACOKINETICS: Absorption: Carisoprodol: (250mg) C_{max}=1.2mcg/mL, T_{max}=1.5 hrs, AUC=4.5mcg•hr/mL; (350mg) C_{max}=1.8mcg/mL, T_{max}=1.7 hrs, AUC=7.0mcg•hr/mL. Meprobamate: (250mg) C_{max}=1.8mcg/mL, T_{max}= 3.6 hrs, AUC=32mcg•hr/mL; (350mg) C_{max}=2.5mcg/mL, T_{max}=4.5 hrs, AUC=46mcg•hr/mL. **Distribution:** Found in breast milk. **Metabolism:** Liver via CYP2C19. Meprobamate (metabolite). **Elimination:** Renal/Nonrenal route. Carisoprodol: $T_{1/2}$=1.7 hrs (250mg), 2.0 hrs (350mg). Meprobamate: $T_{1/2}$=9.7 hrs (250mg), 9.6 hrs (350mg).

NURSING CONSIDERATIONS

Assessment: Assess for acute intermittent porphyria, renal/hepatic impairment, seizures, history of addiction, use of alcohol/illegal drugs/drugs of abuse, pregnancy/nursing status, and possible drug interactions.

Monitoring: Monitor for signs/symptoms of CNS depression, drug abuse/dependence, and seizures.

Patient Counseling: Advise that drug may cause drowsiness and/or dizziness; avoid taking carisoprodol before engaging in hazardous tasks (operating machinery/driving). Avoid alcohol, illegal drugs, drugs of abuse, or other CNS depressants. Drug is limited to acute use. Notify physician if musculoskeletal symptoms persist. Inform of drug dependence/abuse potential.

Administration: Oral route. **Storage:** 20-25°C (68-77°F).

SOMAVERT RX
pegvisomant (Pharmacia & Upjohn)

THERAPEUTIC CLASS: Growth hormone receptor antagonist

INDICATIONS: Treatment of acromegaly in patients who have had an inadequate response to surgery and/or radiation therapy, and/or other medical therapies, or for whom these therapies are not appropriate.

DOSAGE: *Adults:* LD: 40mg SQ. Maint: 10mg/day SQ. Titrate: Adjust dose in 5-mg increments/decrements based on insulin-like growth factor-I (IGF-I) levels measured q4-6 weeks. Max Maint: 30mg/day. Elderly: Start at lower end of dosing range. Refer to PI for dose recommendations based on LFTs.

HOW SUPPLIED: Inj: 10mg, 15mg, 20mg

WARNINGS/PRECAUTIONS: Tumors that secrete growth hormone (GH) may expand and cause complications; monitor with periodic imaging scans of the sella turcica. May increase glucose tolerance; monitor diabetic patients. May result in functional GH deficiency. AST/ALT elevations reported; avoid with >3X ULN baseline LFTs until cause is determined. D/C if ≥5X ULN LFTs or

≥3X ULN transaminases with increase in serum total bilirubin levels, or if liver injury confirmed. Lipohypertrophy reported. Caution in elderly.

ADVERSE REACTIONS: Infection, abnormal LFTs, pain, injection-site reactions, back pain, diarrhea, nausea, flu syndrome, chest pain, dizziness, paresthesia, HTN, sinusitis, peripheral edema.

INTERACTIONS: May need to reduce dosage of insulin and/or oral hypoglycemic agents. May need higher serum concentrations with concomitant use of opioids.

PREGNANCY: Category B, caution in nursing.

MECHANISM OF ACTION: GH receptor antagonist; selectively binds to GH receptors on cell surfaces, where it blocks binding of endogenous GH and interferes with GH signal transduction. This decreases serum concentrations of IGF-I, as well as other GH-responsive proteins, including IGF binding protein-3, and acid labile subunit.

PHARMACOKINETICS: Absorption: Absolute bioavailability (57%); T_{max}=33-77 hrs. **Distribution:** V_d=7L. **Elimination:** Urine (<1%); $T_{1/2}$=6 days.

NURSING CONSIDERATIONS

Assessment: Assess for previous hypersensitivity to the drug, pregnancy/nursing status, and possible drug interactions. Assess use with tumors that secrete GH, and diabetes mellitus. Obtain baseline ALT, AST, total bilirubin, and alkaline phosphatase levels.

Monitoring: Monitor for tumor growth in patients who have GH-secreting tumors; perform periodic image scans of the sella turcica. Monitor for signs/symptoms of GH deficiency and liver dysfunction. Monitor serum IGF-I concentrations for 4-6 weeks after initiation or when dose adjustments are made, and at least q6 months after levels have normalized. Refer to PI for schedule of serial LFTs monitoring in patients with normal LFTs and elevated values.

Patient Counseling: Advise to immediately contact physician and d/c therapy if jaundice develops. Instruct on how to properly reconstitute and administer drug. Inform about the need for serial monitoring of LFTs and IGF-I levels.

Administration: SQ route. Refer to PI for reconstitution and administration instructions. Administer within 6 hrs after reconstitution. **Storage:** 2-8°C (36-46°F). Protect from freezing.

Sonata
zaleplon (King)

CIV

THERAPEUTIC CLASS: Pyrazolopyrimidine (non-benzodiazepine)

INDICATIONS: Short-term treatment of insomnia.

DOSAGE: *Adults:* Individualize dose. Insomnia: 10mg qhs. Low Weight Patients: 5mg qhs. Max: 20mg/day. Elderly/Debilitated: 5mg qhs. Max: 10mg/day. Mild to Moderate Hepatic Dysfunction/ Concomitant Cimetidine: 5mg qhs. Take immediately prior to bedtime.

HOW SUPPLIED: Cap: 5mg, 10mg

WARNINGS/PRECAUTIONS: Failure to remit after 7-10 days of treatment may indicate the presence of a primary psychiatric and/or medical illness that should be evaluated. Use the lowest effective dose. Abnormal thinking and behavior changes including bizarre behavior, agitation, hallucinations, and depersonalization reported. Complex behaviors such as sleep-driving reported; d/c if sleep-driving occurs. Amnesia and other neuropsychiatric symptoms may occur unpredictably. Caution with depressed patients; worsening of depression, suicidal thoughts and actions reported. Anaphylaxis (eg, dyspnea, throat closing, N/V) and angioedema of the tongue, glottis and larynx leading to airway obstruction may occur. Patients who develop angioedema after treatment should not be rechallenged with the drug. May result in short-term memory impairment, hallucinations, impaired coordination, dizziness and lightheadedness when taken while still up. Caution in elderly. Abuse potential exists; avoid abrupt withdrawal. Caution with diseases or conditions affecting metabolism or hemodynamic responses, compromised respiratory function, and mild-to-moderate hepatic insufficiency. Not for use in severe hepatic impairment. May impair mental/physical abilities. Contains tartrazine, which may cause allergic reactions including bronchial asthma.

ADVERSE REACTIONS: Headache, dizziness, nausea, asthenia, abdominal pain, somnolence, amnesia, eye pain, dysmenorrhea, paresthesia.

INTERACTIONS: Coadministration with other psychotropic medications, anticonvulsants, antihistamines, narcotic analgesics, anesthetics, ethanol, and other CNS depressants may produce additive CNS-depressant effects. Avoid with alcohol. CYP3A4 inducers (eg, rifampin, phenytoin, carbamazepine and phenobarbital) increase clearance. CYP3A4 inhibitors (eg, erythromycin and ketoconazole) decrease clearance. Caution when coadministered with promethazine, imipramine, or thioridazine. Cimetidine reduces clearance.

PREGNANCY: Category C, not for use in nursing.

S

MECHANISM OF ACTION: Pyrazolopyrimidine class. Hypnotic agent; interacts with GABA-benzodiazepine receptor complex.

PHARMACOKINETICS: Absorption: Rapid and complete. Absolute bioavailability (30%); T_{max}=1 hr. **Distribution:** (IV) V_d=1.4L/kg; plasma protein binding (60%); found in breastmilk. **Metabolism:** Liver (extensive) via aldehyde oxidation. **Elimination:** Urine (<1% unchanged, 70% within 48 hrs, 71% within 6 days), feces (17% within 6 days); (IV, oral) $T_{1/2}$=1 hr.

NURSING CONSIDERATIONS

Assessment: Assess for primary psychiatric and/or medical illness, diseases/conditions affecting metabolism or hemodynamic responses, compromised respiratory function (COPD, sleep apnea), depression, suicidal tendencies, hepatic/renal impairment, drug abuse/addiction, alcohol intake, pregnancy/nursing status, hypersensitivity and possible drug interactions.

Monitoring: Monitor for anaphylaxis (eg, dyspnea, throat closing, N/V); angioedema of the tongue, glottis and larynx; worsening of insomnia; abnormal thinking and behavior changes (eg, bizarre behavior, agitation, hallucinations, depersonalization); complex behaviors (eg, sleep-driving); amnesia; neuropsychiatric symptoms; worsening of depression; suicidal thoughts/actions; memory impairment; impaired coordination; dizziness; lightheadedness; physical/psychological dependence; withdrawal symptoms; hepatic and pulmonary functions and possible drug interactions. Monitor elderly and debilitated patients closely.

Patient Counseling: Take drug immediately prior to bedtime. Caution against hazardous tasks (eg, operating machinery/driving). Instruct to notify physician if sleep-driving or other complex behaviors occur. Inform about the benefits/risks, possibility of physical/psychological dependence and memory disturbances. Notify if pregnant/nursing or planning to become pregnant. Do not increase dose or d/c drug before consulting physician. Avoid alcohol.

Administration: Oral route. Take immediately prior to bedtime. **Storage:** 20-25°C (68-77°F). Dispense in a light-resistant container.

SORIATANE   RX
acitretin (Stiefel)

Avoid in pregnancy or becoming pregnant ≤3 yrs after d/c of therapy; use two reliable forms of contraception simultaneously. Only use in females of reproductive potential with severe psoriasis unresponsive to or contraindicated with other therapies. Patient must have two negative urine/serum pregnancy tests with a sensitivity of at least 25 mIU/mL before receiving initial prescription. Contraception counseling should be done on a regular basis. It is not known whether residual acitretin in seminal fluid poses risk to fetus with male patients during or after therapy. Females should avoid ethanol during and 2 months after therapy because it may increase the duration of teratogenic potential; severe birth defects reported. Interferes with contraceptive effect of microdosed progestin "minipill" oral contraceptives. Caution not to self-medicate with herbal St. John's wort because a possible interaction has been suggested with hormonal contraceptives based on reports of breakthrough bleeding. Potential to induce hepatotoxicity; elevations of AST (SGOT), ALT (SGPT), GGT (GGTP) or LDH reported. D/C if hepatotoxicity is suspected.

THERAPEUTIC CLASS: Retinoid

INDICATIONS: Treatment of severe psoriasis in adults.

DOSAGE: *Adults:* Intersubject variation in pharmacokinetics, clinical efficacy, and incidence of side effects exists. Individualize dose. Initial: 25-50mg single dose qd with main meal. Maint: 25-50mg qd may be given dependent upon response to initial treatment. May treat relapses as outlined for initial therapy. Decrease concomitant phototherapy dose dependent on patient's individual response.

HOW SUPPLIED: Cap: 10mg, 17.5mg, 25mg

CONTRAINDICATIONS: See Boxed Warning. Pregnancy, severely impaired liver or kidney function, and chronic abnormally elevated blood lipid values. Combined use with methotrexate; increased risk of hepatitis. Combined use with tetracyclines; can cause increased intracranial pressure.

WARNINGS/PRECAUTIONS: Risk of hyperostosis, pancreatitis, and pseudotumor cerebri. D/C if visual difficulties occur; decreased night vision and reduced tolerance to contact lenses reported. Bone abnormalities of the vertebral column, knees, and ankles reported. Increases TG and cholesterol and decreases HDL; perform lipid tests before therapy every 1-2 weeks until lipid response established. Caution with severe hepatic/renal impairment. Transient worsening of psoriasis may occur initially. Do not donate blood during and for 3 yrs after therapy. Avoid sun lamps and excessive sun exposure. Depression and/or psychiatric symptoms (eg, aggressive feelings, thoughts of self-harm) reported. Thinning of the skin observed. Lower dose of phototherapy is required. Caution in elderly.

ADVERSE REACTIONS: Cheilitis, rhinitis, dry mouth, epistaxis, alopecia, dry skin, skin peeling, nail disorder, pruritus, paresthesia, paronychia, skin atrophy, sticky skin, xerophthalmia, arthralgia.

INTERACTIONS: See Boxed Warning and Contraindications. Potentiates the blood glucose-lowering effect of glibenclamide; careful supervision of diabetic patients is recommended. Reduced protein binding effect of phenytoin. Avoid use with vitamin A or other oral retinoids; may increase risk of hypervitaminosis A.

PREGNANCY: Category X, not for use in nursing.

MECHANISM OF ACTION: Retinoid; antipsoriatic action not established.

PHARMACOKINETICS: Absorption: C_{max}=416ng/mL; T_{max}=2-5 hrs. **Distribution:** Plasma protein binding (99.9%); found in breast milk. **Metabolism:** Extensive; via isomerization to cis-acitretin; metabolized with the parent drug into chain-shortened breakdown products and conjugates. **Elimination:** Metabolites and conjugates: feces (34-54%), urine (16-53%). Acitretin: $T_{1/2}$=49 hrs. Cis-acitretin: $T_{1/2}$=63 hrs.

NURSING CONSIDERATIONS

Assessment: Assess for pregnancy/reproductive status, renal/liver impairment, elevated blood lipid values, diabetes, obesity, alcohol intake, or a familial history of these conditions. Assess cardiovascular status, preexisting abnormalities of the spine or extremities, and possible drug interactions (eg, tetracyclines). Blood lipids and LFT levels should be evaluated prior to therapy and again at intervals of 1-2 weeks.

Monitoring: Monitor for hepatotoxicity, hyperostosis, hypertriglyceridemia, radiological changes of pre-existing abnormalities of the spine (eg, degenerative spurs, anterior bridging of spinal vertebrae, diffuse idiopathic skeletal hyperostosis, ligament calcification, and narrowing/destruction of the cervical disc space), MI or other thromboembolic events, pancreatitis, psychiatric problems, and signs/symptoms of pseudotumor cerebri (eg, headache, N/V, visual disturbances, papilledema). Monitor eyes for dryness, lash loss, irritation, Bell's palsy, blepharitis, blurred vision and cataracts. Perform LFTs, lipids and blood sugar levels. Pregnancy test must be repeated every month during therapy and for at least 3 yrs after d/c.

Patient Counseling: Inform about the Pregnancy Prevention Actively Required During and After Treatment (*Do Your P.A.R.T*) program and about the risks of therapy. Advise to use two effective forms of contraception simultaneously at least 1 month prior to initiation of therapy. Advise against donating blood during or at least 3 yrs following completion of therapy. Inform that it is required by law that medication guide be given to patient each time therapy is dispensed. Instruct not to ingest beverages or products containing ethanol while taking therapy and for 2 months after d/c of therapy. Notify physician if nursing. Caution when driving or operating a vehicle at night. Caution against taking vitamin A supplements to avoid additive toxic effects. Avoid excessive exposure to sunlight. Keep medication away from children.

Administration: Oral route. Take with food. **Storage:** 15-25°C (59-77°F). Protect from light. Avoid exposure to high temperatures and humidity after the bottle is opened.

SORILUX   RX
calcipotriene (Stiefel)

THERAPEUTIC CLASS: Vitamin D3 derivative

INDICATIONS: Treatment of plaque psoriasis in adults ≥18 yrs.

DOSAGE: *Adults:* ≥18 yrs: Apply thin layer bid to the affected areas and rub in gently and completely.

HOW SUPPLIED: Foam: 0.005% [60g, 120g]

CONTRAINDICATIONS: Hypercalcemia.

WARNINGS/PRECAUTIONS: Propellant in drug is flammable; avoid fire, flame, and/or smoking during and immediately following application. Hypercalcemia may occur; d/c treatment until normal calcium levels are restored if elevation outside normal range occurs. Avoid exposure of treated areas to natural or artificial sunlight (eg, tanning booths, sun lamps). Limit or avoid use of phototherapy. Use not evaluated with erythrodermic, exfoliative, or pustular psoriasis. Avoid contact with eyes.

ADVERSE REACTIONS: Erythema, hypercalcemia.

PREGNANCY: Category C; caution in nursing.

MECHANISM OF ACTION: Vitamin D3 analog; not established.

NURSING CONSIDERATIONS

Assessment: Assess for hypercalcemia and pregnancy/nursing status.

Monitoring: Monitor serum calcium levels.

Patient Counseling: Advise not to refrigerate or freeze the product. Instruct to avoid fire, flame, or smoking during and immediately following application and excessive exposure of the treated areas to natural or artificial sunlight (eg, tanning booths, sun lamps). If the foam gets in or near the eyes, advise to rinse eyes thoroughly with water. Instruct to consult physician if there are no improvements after 8 weeks of treatment. Counsel to wash hands after application, unless treating the hands. **Administration:** Topical route. Not for oral, ophthalmic, or intravaginal use. **Storage:** 25°C (77°F); excursions permitted to 15-30°C (59-86°F). Do not puncture or incinerate. Do not expose to heat or at >49°C (120°F).

SPIRIVA   RX
tiotropium bromide (Boehringer Ingelheim/Pfizer)

THERAPEUTIC CLASS: Anticholinergic bronchodilator

INDICATIONS: Long-term, once-daily, maintenance treatment of bronchospasm associated with chronic obstructive pulmonary disease (COPD), including chronic bronchitis and emphysema. Reduction of exacerbations in COPD patients.

DOSAGE: *Adults:* 2 inhalations of the contents of 1 cap (18mcg) qd with HandiHaler device. Do not swallow caps.

HOW SUPPLIED: Cap, Inhalation: 18mcg

WARNINGS/PRECAUTIONS: Not for initial treatment of acute episodes of bronchospasm. D/C if hypersensitivity (eg, angioedema, itching, rash) or paradoxical bronchospasm occurs. Caution with hypersensitivity to milk proteins. Caution with narrow-angle glaucoma; be alert for signs and symptoms of narrow-angle glaucoma. Caution with urinary retention; alert patients for prostatic hyperplasia or bladder-neck obstruction (eg, difficulty passing urine, painful urination). Monitor for anticholinergic effects with moderate to severe renal impairment (CrCl ≤50mL/min).

ADVERSE REACTIONS: Dry mouth, sinusitis, constipation, abdominal pain, urinary tract infection, upper respiratory tract infection, chest pain, edema, vomiting, myalgia, moniliasis, rash, dyspepsia, pharyngitis, rhinitis.

INTERACTIONS: Avoid with other anticholinergic-containing drugs; may lead to an increase in anticholinergic adverse effects. Cimetidine may increase area under the curve and decrease clearance.

PREGNANCY: Category C, caution in nursing.

MECHANISM OF ACTION: Anticholinergic bronchodilator; inhibits M_3-receptors on smooth muscle leading to bronchodilation.

PHARMACOKINETICS: Absorption: Absolute bioavailability (19.5%); T_{max}=5 min. **Distribution:** V_d=32L/kg; plasma protein binding (72%). **Metabolism:** Liver (oxidation, conjugation) via CYP2D6, 3A4. **Elimination:** Urine (14%, inhalation), feces. $T_{1/2}$=5-6 days.

NURSING CONSIDERATIONS

Assessment: Assess for hypersensitivity to atropine or its derivatives, narrow-angle glaucoma, prostatic hyperplasia, bladder-neck obstruction, renal impairment, pregnancy/nursing status, and possible drug interactions.

Monitoring: Monitor for urinary retention, acute narrow-angle glaucoma, paradoxical bronchospasm, and hypersensitivity reactions.

Patient Counseling: Inform that contents of cap are for oral inhalation only and must not be swallowed. Advise to administer only via the HandiHaler device; should not be used for other medications. Advise not to increase dose or frequency, or use as a rescue medication for immediate relief of breathing problems. Advise to seek medical attention if acute eye pain/discomfort, blurring of vision, visual halos or colored images, difficulty in passing urine, or dysuria develop. Advise to use caution when engaging in activities (eg, driving vehicle, operating appliances/machineries). Inform that paradoxical bronchospasm may occur; d/c if this develops. Instruct not to allow the powder to enter into the eyes.

Administration: Oral inhalation route. Use with HandiHaler device only. Refer to PI for illustrative and detailed administration procedures. **Storage:** 25°C (77°F); excursions permitted to 15-30°C (59-86°F). Do not expose to extreme temperatures or moisture. Do not store in HandiHaler device.

SPORANOX

itraconazole (Centocor Ortho Biotech)

Contraindicated with cisapride, pimozide, quinidine, dofetilide, or levacetylmethadol (levomethadyl). May increase plasma concentrations of drugs metabolized by potent CYP3A4 inhibitor pathway. Serious cardiovascular events (eg, QT prolongation, torsades de pointes, ventricular tachycardia, cardiac arrest, and/or sudden death) reported with cisapride, pimozide, quinidine, levacetylmethadol. (Cap) Do not use cap for onychomycosis with ventricular dysfunction such as congestive heart failure (CHF) or history of CHF. D/C use if signs/symptoms of CHF occur. (Sol) Reassess use if signs/symptoms of CHF occur.

THERAPEUTIC CLASS: Azole antifungal

INDICATIONS: (Cap) Onychomycosis of the toenail and fingernail in immunocompetent patients. Treatment of blastomycosis (pulmonary/extrapulmonary) and histoplasmosis (eg, chronic cavitary pulmonary disease, disseminated non-meningeal), and aspergillosis (pulmonary/extrapulmonary) if refractory to or intolerant of amphotericin B therapy. (Sol) Treatment of oropharyngeal and esophageal candidiasis.

DOSAGE: *Adults:* Cap: Take with full meal. If patient has achlorhydria or taking gastric acid suppressors, give with cola beverage. Aspergillosis: 200-400mg/day. Blastomycosis/Histoplasmosis: 200mg qd. May increase in 100-mg increments if no improvement. Max: 400mg/day. Give bid if dose >200mg/day. Life-Threatening Situations: LD: 200mg tid for 1st 3 days. Continue for at least 3 months and until infection subsides. Onychomycosis: Toenail: 200mg qd for 12 consecutive weeks. Fingernail: 200mg bid for 1 week, skip 3 weeks, then repeat. Sol: Take on empty stomach. Swish 10mL at a time for several seconds, then swallow. Candidiasis: Oropharyngeal: 200mg/day (20mL) for 1-2 weeks. If unresponsive/refractory to fluconazole, give 100mg (10mL) bid. Esophageal: 100mg/day for at least 3 weeks. Continue for 2 weeks following resolution of symptoms. Max: 200mg/day (20mL) based on patient's response to therapy.

HOW SUPPLIED: Cap: 100mg [Pulsepak, 7 x 4 caps]; Sol: 10mg/mL [150mL]

CONTRAINDICATIONS: Cisapride, oral midazolam, nisoldipine, pimozide, quinidine, dofetilide, triazolam and levacetylmethadol (levomethadyl), HMG CoA-reductase inhibitors (eg, lovastatin, simvastatin), ergot alkaloids (eg, dihydroergotamine, ergometrine, ergotamine, and methylergometrine). Evidence of ventricular dysfunction (eg, CHF/history of CHF). (Cap) Treatment of onychomycosis in pregnant patients or those contemplating pregnancy.

WARNINGS/PRECAUTIONS: Sol and caps not interchangeable. Rare cases of hepatotoxicity reported. Perform LFTs; d/c if hepatic dysfunction develops. Avoid with liver disease. CHF, peripheral edema, and pulmonary edema reported in patients treated for onychomycosis and/or systemic fungal infections. Caution with ischemic/valvular disease, pulmonary disease, renal failure, hepatic impairment, and other edematous disorders. Avoid with ventricular dysfunction. D/C if neuropathy or CHF occurs. Transient or permanent hearing loss reported; d/c if hearing loss symptoms occur. Caution in elderly. (Sol) Consider alternative therapy if unresponsive in patients with cystic fibrosis. Not recommended for initiation of treatment in patients at immediate risk of systemic candidiasis.

ADVERSE REACTIONS: N/V, diarrhea, abdominal pain, fever, cough, rash, increased sweating, headache, hypokalemia, myalgia, pruritus, rhinitis, sinusitis, dyspepsia.

INTERACTIONS: See Boxed Warning and Contraindications. Increased levels of antiarrhythmics (eg, digoxin, quinidine, dofetilide, disopyramide), warfarin, carbamazepine, rifabutin, antineoplastics (eg, busulfan, docetaxel, vinca alkaloids), benzodiazepines (eg, alprazolam, diazepam, midazolam), calcium channel blockers (eg, dihydropyridines, verapamil), cisapride, immunosuppressants (eg, cyclosporine, tacrolimus, sirolimus), oral hypoglycemics, protease inhibitors (eg, indinavir, ritonavir, saquinavir), HMG CoA-reductase inhibitors (eg, atorvastatin, cerivastatin, lovastatin, simvastatin), halofantrine, alfentanil, buspirone, methylprednisolone, budesonide, dexamethasone, fluticasone, trimetrexate, cilostazol, eletriptan and fentanyl. Anticonvulsants (eg, carbamazepine, phenobarbital, phenytoin), antimycobacterials (eg, isoniazid, rifabutin, rifampin), gastric acid suppressors/neutralizers (eg, antacids, H_2-receptor antagonists, proton pump inhibitors) and nevirapine decrease levels of itraconazole. Macrolide antibiotics (eg, clarithromycin, erythromycin) and protease inhibitors (eg, indinavir, ritonavir) increase levels of itraconazole. Severe hypoglycemia with oral hypoglycemics. Additive negative inotropic effects with calcium channel blockers (CCBs). Edema reported with dihydropyridine CCBs; adjust dose. Decreased absorption of caps with antacids or gastric secretion suppressors. Prolonged QT interval may occur with halofantrine, pimozide, levacetylmethadol (levomethadyl). Fatal respiratory depression reported with fentanyl. May inhibit metabolism of glucocorticoids (eg, budesonide, dexamethasone, fluticasone), CCBs (eg, nifedipine, felodipine), trimetrexate. May increase concentration of ergot alkaloids, causing ergotism. Enhanced anticoagulant effect of coumarin-like drugs (eg, warfarin). Prior treatment with itraconazole may reduce activity of polyenes (eg, amphotericin B).

PREGNANCY: Category C, not for use in nursing.

MECHANISM OF ACTION: Azole antifungal agent; inhibits the CYP450-dependent synthesis of ergosterol, which is a vital component of fungal cell membranes.

S

PHARMACOKINETICS: Absorption: (Cap/Sol) Absolute bioavailabilty (55%). Oral administration of variable doses resulted in different parameters; refer to respective PIs for further details. **Metabolism:** Liver via CYP3A4; hydroxyitraconazole (major metabolite). **Distribution:** Plasma protein binding (99.8%) itraconazole, (99.5%) hydroxyitraconazole; found in breast milk. (IV) V_d=796L. **Elimination:** (Cap/Sol) Urine (40%, inactive metabolites), feces (3-18%).

NURSING CONSIDERATIONS

Assessment: Assess for proper diagnosis of fungal infection (eg, cultures, microscopic studies), ventricular dysfunction, ischemic/valvular disease, pulmonary disease, renal failure, hepatic impairment, edematous disorders or any other conditions where treatment is contraindicated. Assess pregnancy/nursing status prior to use. Assess for possible drug interactions.

Monitoring: Monitor for signs/symptoms of CHF, QT prolongation, torsades de pointes, ventricular tachycardia, cardiac arrest, liver dysfunction, and LFTs. Blood glucose concentrations should also be monitored when coadminstered with hypoglycemic agents. Monitor for SrCr levels and prolongation of sedative effect of midazolam.

Patient Counseling: Instruct to take cap with a full meal and oral solution in fasted state and not to interchange caps and oral solution. Counsel on signs/symptoms of CHF and liver dysfunction (eg, unusual fatigue, anorexia, N/V, jaundice, dark urine or pale stools). Instruct to contact physician before taking concomitant meds with drug. Inform to d/c therapy if hearing loss occurs. Advise to avoid pregnancy while on medication and remain on contraceptives for 2 months following completion of therapy.

Administration: Oral route. **Storage:** (Cap): 15-25°C (59-77°F). Protect from light and moisture. (Sol): 25°C (77°F). Do not freeze.

SPRYCEL

RX

dasatinib (Bristol-Myers Squibb)

THERAPEUTIC CLASS: Kinase inhibitor

INDICATIONS: Treatment of adults with newly diagnosed Philadelphia chromosome-positive (Ph+) chronic myeloid leukemia (CML) in chronic phase. Treatment of adults with chronic, accelerated, or myeloid/lymphoid blast phase Ph+ CML with resistance or intolerance to prior therapy including imatinib. Treatment of adults with Ph+ acute lymphoblastic leukemia (ALL) with resistance or intolerance to prior therapy.

DOSAGE: *Adults:* Chronic Phase CML: Initial: 100mg qd. Titrate: If no response, increase to 140mg qd. Accelerated Phase CML/Myeloid or Lymphoid Blast Phase CML/Ph+ ALL: Initial: 140mg qd. Titrate: If no response, increase to 180mg qd. Concomitant Strong CYP3A4 Inducers: Avoid use. If use is necessary, consider dose increase with careful monitoring. Concomitant Strong CYP3A4 Inhibitors: Consider dose decrease to 20mg if taking 100mg qd, and to 40mg if taking 140mg qd. If therapy not tolerated after dose reduction, either d/c concomitant inhibitor and allow 1-week washout period before increasing dose, or d/c therapy until end of treatment with inhibitor. Refer to PI for dose adjustments for neutropenia and thrombocytopenia.

HOW SUPPLIED: Tab: 20mg, 50mg, 70mg, 80mg, 100mg, 140mg

WARNINGS/PRECAUTIONS: Severe thrombocytopenia, neutropenia, and anemia reported; monitor CBC weekly for 1st 2 months and monthly thereafter, or as clinically indicated. Manage myelosuppression by temporarily withholding therapy or by dose reduction. Severe CNS and GI hemorrhage, including fatalities, and other cases of severe hemorrhage reported. Severe fluid retention including ascites, generalized edema, and severe pulmonary edema reported; perform chest x-ray if symptoms suggestive of pleural effusion develop (eg, dyspnea, dry cough). May prolong QT interval; caution in patients at risk (eg, hypokalemia or hypomagnesemia, congenital long QT syndrome). Correct hypokalemia or hypomagnesemia prior to therapy. Cardiac adverse reactions reported; monitor for signs/symptoms consistent with cardiac dysfunction and treat appropriately. Elderly patients (≥65 yrs) are more likely to experience toxicity. May increase risk of developing pulmonary arterial HTN (PAH); d/c if PAH is confirmed. May cause fetal harm. Caution with hepatic impairment.

ADVERSE REACTIONS: Myelosuppression, fluid retention, diarrhea, N/V, headache, abdominal pain, hemorrhage, pyrexia, pleural effusion, dyspnea, skin rash, fatigue.

INTERACTIONS: CYP3A4 inhibitors (eg, ketoconazole, clarithromycin, ritonavir, nefazodone) or grapefruit juice may increase levels; avoid concomitant use or consider dose decrease if use is necessary. CYP3A4 inducers (eg, dexamethasone, phenytoin, carbamazepine, rifampin, rifabutin, phenobarbital) or St. John's wort may decrease levels; avoid concomitant use or consider dose increase if use is necessary. Avoid antacids (eg, aluminum hydroxide/magnesium hydroxide); separate dose by 2 hrs if necessary. H_2 blockers (eg, famotidine) or proton pump inhibitors (eg, omeprazole) may reduce exposure; concomitant use is not recommended. May increase simvastatin levels. Caution with CYP3A4 substrates with narrow therapeutic index (eg, alfentanil, astemizole, terfenadine, cisapride, cyclosporine, fentanyl, pimozide, quinidine, sirolimus, tacrolimus,

S

ergot alkaloids [eg, ergotamine, dihydroergotamine]). Caution with anticoagulants or medications that inhibit platelet function. Antiarrhythmics or other QT-prolonging agents and cumulative high-dose anthracycline therapy may increase risk of QT prolongation.

PREGNANCY: Category D, not for use in nursing.

MECHANISM OF ACTION: Kinase inhibitor; inhibits BCR-ABL, SRC family, c-KIT, EPHA2, and PDGFRβ kinases.

PHARMACOKINETICS: Absorption: T_{max}=0.5-6 hrs. **Distribution:** V_d=2505L; plasma protein binding (96% [parent], 93% [active metabolite]). **Metabolism:** Extensive, primarily via CYP3A4. **Elimination:** Feces (85%, 19% unchanged), urine (4%, 0.1% unchanged); $T_{1/2}$=3-5 hrs.

NURSING CONSIDERATIONS

Assessment: Assess for signs/symptoms of underlying cardiopulmonary disease, hepatic impairment, prolonged QTc, hypokalemia, hypomagnesemia, pregnancy/nursing status, and possible drug interactions.

Monitoring: Monitor for signs/symptoms of hemorrhage, cardiac dysfunction, myelosuppression, pleural/pericardial effusion, fluid retention, QT prolongation, PAH, and other adverse reactions. Perform chest x-ray if symptoms of pleural effusion develop. Monitor CBC weekly for 1st 2 months and monthly thereafter.

Patient Counseling: Inform of pregnancy risks and advise to avoid becoming pregnant during therapy. Instruct to seek medical attention if symptoms of hemorrhage (eg, unusual bleeding, easy bruising), myelosuppression (eg, fever, infection), fluid retention (eg, swelling, weight gain, SOB), significant N/V, diarrhea, headache, musculoskeletal pain, fatigue, or rash develop. Inform that product contains lactose. In case of missed dose, advise not to take 2 doses at the same time, and to take next scheduled dose at its regular time. Inform that drug may be taken with or without food in am/pm.

Administration: Oral route. Swallow tab whole; do not crush or cut. **Storage:** 20-25°C (68-77°F); excursions permitted between 15-30°C (59-86°F).

STALEVO   RX
entacapone - levodopa - carbidopa (Novartis)

THERAPEUTIC CLASS: Dopa-decarboxylase inhibitor/dopamine precursor/COMT inhibitor

INDICATIONS: Treatment of idiopathic Parkinson's disease; to substitute for equivalent doses of carbidopa/levodopa and entacapone previously administered as individual products, or to replace carbidopa/levodopa (without entacapone) for those experiencing signs and symptoms of end-of-dose "wearing off" (only for those taking ≤600mg/day levodopa without dyskinesias).

DOSAGE: *Adults:* ≤75 yrs: Individualize dose. Titrate: Adjust according to desired therapeutic response. Currently Taking Carbidopa/Levodopa and Entacapone: May switch directly to corresponding strength of Stalevo with same amounts of carbidopa/levodopa. Currently Taking Carbidopa/Levodopa without Entacapone: Titrate individually with carbidopa/levodopa and entacapone, then transfer to corresponding dose once stabilized. Maint: Less Levodopa Required: Decrease strength of Stalevo at each administration or decrease frequency by extending time between doses. More Levodopa Required: Take next higher strength of Stalevo and/or increase frequency of doses. Max: 8 tabs/day (Stalevo 50, 75, 100, 125, 150); 6 tabs/day (Stalevo 200). Refer to PI for further dosing information when used concomitantly with other antiparkinsonian medications or general anesthesia.

HOW SUPPLIED: Tab: (Carbidopa-Levodopa-Entacapone): Stalevo 50: 12.5mg-50mg-200mg; Stalevo 75: 18.75mg-75mg-200mg; Stalevo 100: 25mg-100mg-200mg; Stalevo 125: 31.25mg-125mg-200mg; Stalevo 150: 37.5mg-150mg-200mg; Stalevo 200: 50mg-200mg-200mg

CONTRAINDICATIONS: Narrow-angle glaucoma; suspicious, undiagnosed skin lesions; history of melanoma. Nonselective MAOIs (eg, phenelzine, tranylcypromine); d/c nonselective MAOIs at least 2 weeks prior to therapy.

WARNINGS/PRECAUTIONS: CNS adverse effects may occur; may require dose reduction if dyskinesia or exacerbation of preexisting dyskinesia develop. Mental disturbances may occur; monitor for depression and suicidal tendencies. Caution with biliary obstruction, severe cardiovascular (CV)/pulmonary disease, bronchial asthma, renal/hepatic/endocrine disease, past or current psychoses, history of myocardial infarction with residual arrhythmias, chronic wide-angle glaucoma. Caution with history of peptic ulcer; may increase the risk of upper GI hemorrhage. Symptom complex resembling neuroleptic malignant syndrome (NMS) reported in association with dose reduction or withdrawal; observe carefully if dose is reduced abruptly or d/c, especially if receiving neuroleptics. Syncope, hypotension, hallucinations, rhabdomyolysis, hyperpyrexia, confusion, and fibrotic complications reported. Diarrhea and colitis reported with entacapone use; d/c if prolonged diarrhea develops and institute appropriate therapy. Melanomas may develop; perform periodic skin examination. Abnormalities in laboratory tests, including elevated

LFTs, decreased BUN, creatinine and uric acid levels, positive Coomb's test, false-positive reaction for urinary ketone bodies, or false-negative glucose oxidase test may occur. Caution when interpreting plasma and urine levels of catecholamines and metabolites; falsely diagnosed pheochromocytoma reported. May decrease serum iron concentrations. May depress prolactin secretion and increase growth hormone levels.

ADVERSE REACTIONS: Dyskinesia, N/V, hyperkinesia, diarrhea, urine discoloration, hypokinesia, dizziness, abdominal pain, constipation, fatigue, back pain, dry mouth, dyspnea.

INTERACTIONS: See Contraindications. May result in increased HR, arrhythmias, and BP changes with drugs metabolized by catechol-O-methyltransferase (COMT) (eg, isoproterenol, epineph-rine, norepinephrine, dopamine, dobutamine, α-methyldopa, apomorphine, isoetherine, bitolterol); use with caution. Caution with drugs known to interfere with biliary excretion, glucuronidation, and intestinal β-glucuronidase which includes probenecid, cholestyramine, and some antibiotics (eg, erythromycin, rifampicin, ampicillin, chloramphenicol). Symptomatic postural hypotension reported when added with antihypertensives. Concomitant therapy with selegiline may be associated with severe orthostatic hypotension. HTN and dyskinesia may occur with tricyclic antidepressants. Reduced bioavailability with iron salts. Levodopa: Therapeutic response may be reversed by phenytoin and papaverine. Isoniazid and dopamine D2 antagonists (eg, phenothiazines, butyrophenones, risperidone) may reduce therapeutic effects. Metoclopramide may increase the bioavailability and may also adversely affect disease control by its dopamine receptor antagonistic properties.

PREGNANCY: Category C, caution in nursing.

MECHANISM OF ACTION: Dopa-decarboxylase inhibitor/dopamine precursor/COMT inhibitor. Carbidopa: Inhibits the decarboxylation of peripheral levodopa, making more levodopa available for transport to the brain. Levodopa: Crosses blood-brain barrier and presumably converts to dopamine in brain. Entacapone: Sustains plasma levels of levodopa, resulting in more constant dopaminergic stimulation in brain.

PHARMACOKINETICS: Absorption: Levodopa: Rapid. (PO) Administration of variable doses resulted in different parameters. Entacapone: Rapid. C_{max}=1200-1500ng/mL; T_{max}=0.8-1.2 hrs; AUC=1250-1750ng•hr/mL. Carbidopa: Slower; C_{max}=40-225ng/mL; T_{max}=2.5-3.4 hrs; AUC=170-1200ng•hr/mL. **Distribution:** Plasma protein binding: Levodopa: (10-30%); Entacapone: (98%); Carbidopa: (36%). Levodopa: Crosses the placenta. **Metabolism:** Levodopa: Extensive decarboxylation by dopa decarboxylase and O-methylation by COMT. Entacapone: Isomerization; cis-isomer (active metabolite). Carbidopa: α-methyl-3-methoxy-4-hydroxyphenylpropionic acid, α-methyl-3,4-dihydroxyphenylpropionic acid (metabolites). **Elimination:** Levodopa: $T_{1/2}$=1.7 hrs. Entacapone: Feces (90%), urine (10%, 0.2% unchanged); $T_{1/2}$=0.8-1 hr. Carbidopa: Urine (30%, unchanged); $T_{1/2}$=1.6-2 hrs.

NURSING CONSIDERATIONS

Assessment: Assess for narrow-angle or chronic wide-angle glaucoma, preexisting dyskinesia, or any other conditions where treatment is contraindicated or cautioned. Assess for pregnancy/nursing status and possible drug interactions. Obtain intraocular pressure (IOP) in patients with chronic wide-angle glaucoma. Assess renal/hepatic function.

Monitoring: Monitor hematopoietic, CV/renal/hepatic function, and uric acid levels. Perform skin examination periodically. Monitor for signs/symptoms of mental disturbances, depression, suicidal tendencies, new/exacerbation of dyskinesia, NMS, rhabdomyolysis, diarrhea, colitis, upper GI hemorrhage, syncope, hypotension, melanomas, hallucinations, fibrotic complications, confusion, and hyperpyrexia. Monitor IOP in chronic wide-angle glaucoma.

Patient Counseling: Advise to take as prescribed. Inform that drug begins release of ingredients within 30 min after ingestion. Take at regular intervals, not to change dose regimen, and not to add any additional antiparkinsonian medications, including other carbidopa-levodopa preparations. Advise that "wearing-off" effect may occur at end of dosing interval; notify physician for possible treatment adjustments. Inform that discoloration of saliva, urine or sweat may occur after ingestion. Counsel that high-protein diet, excessive acidity, and iron salts may reduce clinical effectiveness. Inform that hallucinations, postural (orthostatic) hypotension, dizziness, nausea, syncope, sweating, diarrhea, and increase in dyskinesia may occur. Take caution against rising rapidly after sitting or lying down, especially if in such position for prolonged periods. Instruct to avoid operating machinery/driving until sufficient experience is gained on therapy. Advise to take caution when taking other CNS depressants due to its additive sedative effects. Instruct to notify physician if pregnant, intend to become pregnant or breastfeeding. Inform physician if new or increased gambling, sexual, or other intense urges develop.

Administration: Oral route. Do not fractionate tab. Administer only 1 tab at each dosing interval.
Storage: 25°C (77°F); excursions permitted to 15-30°C (59-86°F).

STARLIX

RX

nateglinide (Novartis)

THERAPEUTIC CLASS: Meglitinide

INDICATIONS: Adjunct to diet and exercise to improve glycemic control in adults with type 2 diabetes mellitus (DM).

DOSAGE: *Adults:* Monotherapy/Combination with Metformin or a Thiazolidinedione: Initial/Maint: 120mg tid, 1-30 min ac. May use 60mg dose tid in patients near goal HbA1c when treatment is initiated.

HOW SUPPLIED: Tab: 60mg, 120mg

CONTRAINDICATIONS: Type 1 DM, diabetic ketoacidosis.

WARNINGS/PRECAUTIONS: Risk of hypoglycemia increased with strenuous exercise, adrenal/ pituitary insufficiency, severe renal impairment, and in elderly/malnourished patients. Autonomic neuropathy may mask hypoglycemia. Caution in moderate to severe hepatic impairment. Transient loss of glucose control may occur with fever, infection, trauma, or surgery; may need insulin therapy instead of nateglinide. Secondary failure (reduced effectiveness over a period of time) may occur.

ADVERSE REACTIONS: Upper respiratory infection (URI), flu symptoms, dizziness, arthropathy, diarrhea, hypoglycemia, back pain, jaundice, cholestatic hepatitis, elevated liver enzymes.

INTERACTIONS: Alcohol, NSAIDs, salicylates, MAOIs, nonselective β-blockers, guanethidine, and CYP2C9 inhibitors (eg, fluconazole, amiodarone, miconazole, oxandrolone) may potentiate hypo-glycemia. Thiazides, corticosteroids, thyroid products, sympathomimetics, somatropin, rifampin, phenytoin, and dietary supplements (St. John's wort) may reduce hypoglycemic action of drug. Somatostatin analogues may potentiate/attenuate hypoglycemia. Reduced levels reported with liquid meals. β-blockers may mask hypoglycemic effects. Caution with highly protein bound drugs.

PREGNANCY: Category C, not for use in nursing.

MECHANISM OF ACTION: Meglitinide; lowers blood glucose levels by stimulating insulin secre-tion from the pancreas.

PHARMACOKINETICS: Absorption: Rapidly absorbed. Absolute bioavailability (73%); T_{max}=1 hr. **Distribution:** V_d=10L (IV); plasma protein binding (98%). **Metabolism:** CYP2C9, 3A4; hydroxyla-tion, glucuronide conjugation. **Elimination:** Urine (75%), feces; $T_{1/2}$=1.5 hrs.

NURSING CONSIDERATIONS

Assessment: Assess for diabetic ketoacidosis, type 1 DM, renal/hepatic impairment, adrenal/ pituitary insufficiency, pregnancy/nursing status, other conditions where treatment is cautioned, and possible drug interactions. Assess FPG and HbA1c.

Monitoring: Monitor for hypo/hyperglycemia, diabetic ketoacidosis, secondary failure, URI, and other adverse reactions. Monitor FPG, HbA1c, renal function, and LFTs.

Patient Counseling: Inform of potential risks, benefits, alternate modes of therapy, and drug interactions. Instruct to take 1-30 min ac, but to skip scheduled dose if meal is skipped. Inform about importance of adherence to meal planning, regular physical activity, regular blood glucose monitoring, periodic HbA1c testing, recognition and management of hypo/hyperglycemia, and periodic assessment for diabetes complications. Advise to notify physician if any adverse events occur.

Administration: Oral route. **Storage:** 25°C (77°F); excursions permitted to 15-30°C (59-86°F).

STAVZOR

RX

valproic acid (Noven)

Hepatotoxicity, including fatalities, has occurred usually during first 6 months of treatment. Children <2 yrs are at considerably higher risk of fatal hepatotoxicity. Monitor patients closely and perform LFTs prior to therapy and at frequent intervals thereafter. Teratogenicity reported, including neural tube defects. Pancreatitis reported, including fatal hemor-rhagic cases.

THERAPEUTIC CLASS: Carboxylic acid derivative

INDICATIONS: Monotherapy and adjunctive therapy of complex partial seizures that occur in isolation or in association with other types of seizures in patients ≥10 yrs. Treatment of simple and complex absence seizures as sole and adjunctive therapy and adjunctively in patients with multiple seizure types that include absence seizures. Treatment of manic episodes associated with bipolar disorder. Prophylaxis of migraine headaches.

DOSAGE: *Adults*: Mania: Initial: 750mg/day in divided doses. Titrate: Increase dose rapidly to achieve clinical effect. Max: 60mg/kg/day. Complex Partial Seizures: Monotherapy/Conversion to Monotherapy/Adjunctive Therapy: Initial: 10-15mg/kg/day. Titrate: Increase weekly by 5-10mg/kg/day until optimal response. Max: 60mg/kg/day. When converting to monotherapy, reduce concomitant antiepilepsy drug by 25% every 2 weeks at the start of therapy or 1-2 weeks after. Simple and Complex Absence Seizures: Initial: 15mg/kg/day. Titrate: Increase weekly by 5-10mg/kg/day until optimal response. Max: 60mg/kg/day. If dose >250mg/day, give in 2-3 doses. Migraine: Initial: 250mg bid. Max: 1000mg/day. Elderly: Reduce initial dose and titrate slowly. Consider dose reduction or d/c in patients with decreased food or fluid intake or if excessive somnolence occurs.

Pediatrics: ≥10 yrs: Complex Partial Seizures: Monotherapy/Conversion to Monotherapy/Adjunctive Therapy: Initial: 10-15mg/kg/day. Titrate: Increase weekly by 5-10mg/kg/day until optimal response. Max: 60mg/kg/day. When converting to monotherapy, reduce concomitant antiepilepsy drug by 25% every 2 weeks at the start of therapy or 1-2 weeks after.

HOW SUPPLIED: Cap, Delayed-Release: 125mg, 250mg, 500mg

CONTRAINDICATIONS: Hepatic disease, significant hepatic dysfunction, and known urea cycle disorders (UCD).

WARNINGS/PRECAUTIONS: Increased risk of suicidal thoughts or behavior; monitor for the emergence of worsening and/or any unusual changes in mood or behavior. Hyperammonemic encephalopathy in UCD patients; d/c if this occurs. If unexplained lethargy, hypothermia, vomiting, or mental status changes occur, measure ammonia levels. Caution with hepatic disease; d/c if hepatic failure suspected or apparent. Caution in the elderly; monitor fluid/nutritional intake and for dehydration/somnolence. Dose-related thrombocytopenia and elevated liver enzymes reported. Monitor platelet and coagulation tests prior to therapy, then periodically. Altered thyroid function tests and urine ketone tests. May stimulate replication of HIV and cytomegalovirus. Avoid abrupt d/c. Multiorgan hypersensitivity reactions and hypothermia reported.

ADVERSE REACTIONS: Headache, asthenia, rash, N/V, abdominal pain, dyspepsia, diarrhea, anorexia, somnolence, tremor, dizziness, diplopia, flu syndrome.

INTERACTIONS: Drugs that affect level of expression of hepatic enzymes (eg, phenytoin, carbamazepine, phenobarbital, primidone) may increase valproate clearance. Concomitant use with aspirin (ASA) decreases protein binding and metabolism. Carbapenem antibiotics (eg, ertapenem, imipenem, meropenem) may reduce serum concentration to subtherapeutic levels, resulting in loss of seizure control. Rifampin increases oral clearance and may require valproate dosage adjustment. Concomitant use with felbamate leads to an increase in valproate C_{max}. Reduces the clearance of amitriptylline, nortriptyline, and lorazepam. Induces metabolism of carbamazepine. Inhibits metabolism of diazepam, ethosuximide, phenobarbital and phenytoin; monitor drug serum concentrations and adjust dose appropriately. Breakthrough seizures reported with concomitant valproate and phenytoin use. Administration with clonazepam may induce absence status in patients with absence seizures. Increases $T_{1/2}$ of lamotrigine; serious skin reactions reported. Concomitant use with topiramate associated with hyperammonemia, with or without encephalopathy, and hypothermia. May displace protein-bound warfarin; monitor coagulation tests. Additive CNS depression with other CNS depressants (eg, alcohol). May decrease clearance of zidovudine in HIV-seropositive patients.

PREGNANCY: Category D, not for use in nursing.

MECHANISM OF ACTION: Carboxylic acid derivative; proposed to increase brain concentrations of GABA.

PHARMACOKINETICS: Absorption: T_{max}=2 hrs (fasting), 4.8 hrs (fed). **Distribution:** V_d=11L/1.73m², plasma protein binding (10% at 40mcg/mL and 18.5% at 130mcg/mL), CSF distribution (10%). Found in breast milk. **Metabolism:** Liver via glucuronidation, mitochondrial β-oxidation. **Elimination:** Urine (30-50% glucuronide conjugate, <3% unchanged); $T_{1/2}$=9-16 hrs.

NURSING CONSIDERATIONS

Assessment: Assess LFTs prior to therapy, CBC with platelets, pancreatitis, plasma ammonia levels, hepatic dysfunction/disease, and pregnancy/nursing status. Note other diseases/conditions and drug therapies. Prior to therapy, evaluate for UCD in high-risk patients (eg, history of unexplained encephalopathy, coma, etc.).

Monitoring: Monitor LFTs (at frequent intervals during first 6 months), CBC with platelets, coagulation parameters, pancreatitis, ketone and thyroid function tests, plasma drug levels, hyperammonemia, and hypersensitivity reactions. Monitor for emergence/worsening of depression, suicidality, unusual changes in behavior.

Patient Counseling: Inform to take exactly as prescribed to get the most benefit and to reduce side effects. Instruct to swallow whole; do not chew. Counsel about signs/symptoms of hepatotoxicity, pancreatitis, and hyperammonemic encephalopathy. Avoid CNS depressants (eg, alcohol). Instruct that a fever associated with other organ system involvement (rash, lymphadenopathy, etc.) may be drug-related and should be reported to physician immediately. Advise not to engage in hazardous activities (driving or operating machinery). Notify physician if suicidal thoughts, behavior, or thoughts about self-harm emerge. Advise to enroll in North American Antiepileptic Drug (NAAED) Pregnancy Registry. **Administration:** Oral route. **Storage:** 25°C (77°F); excursions permitted to 15-30°C (59-86°F).

STAXYN   RX
vardenafil HCl (GlaxoSmithKline)

THERAPEUTIC CLASS: Phosphodiesterase type 5 inhibitor

INDICATIONS: Treatment of erectile dysfunction (ED).

DOSAGE: *Adults:* 10mg PO prn 60 min before sexual activity. Max: 1 tab/day. Place on tongue to disintegrate. Take without liquid.

HOW SUPPLIED: Tab, Disintegrating: 10mg

CONTRAINDICATIONS: Concomitant nitrates or nitric oxide donors.

WARNINGS/PRECAUTIONS: Avoid when sexual activity is inadvisable due to underlying cardiovascular (CV) status. Increased sensitivity to vasodilatation effects with left ventricular outflow obstruction. Decrease in supine BP reported. Avoid with unstable angina, hypotension (SBP<90 mmHg), uncontrolled HTN (>170/100 mmHg), recent history of stroke, life-threatening arrhythmia, myocardial infarction (MI) within last 6 months, severe cardiac failure, moderate or severe hepatic impairment (Child-Pugh B or C), renal dialysis, hereditary degenerative retinal disorders including retinitis pigmentosa, congenital QT prolongation, phenylketonuria, fructose intolerance. Caution with bleeding disorders, active peptic ulcers, anatomical deformation of the penis (eg, angulation, cavernosal fibrosis, Peyronie's disease) or predisposition to priapism (eg, sickle cell anemia, multiple myeloma, leukemia). Rarely, non-arteritic anterior ischemic optic neuropathy (NAION) has been reported. Sudden decrease or loss of hearing accompanied by tinnitus and dizziness reported. Contains aspartame and sorbitol.

ADVERSE REACTIONS: Headache, flushing, nasal congestion, dyspepsia, dizziness.

INTERACTIONS: See Contraindications. Avoid use with Class IA (eg, quinidine, procainamide) or Class III (eg, amiodarone, sotalol) antiarrhythmics and other treatments for ED. Increased levels with moderate or potent CYP3A4 inhibitors (eg, ritonavir, indinavir, saquinavir, atazanavir, ketoconazole, itraconazole, clarithromycin, erythromycin). Additive hypotensive effect, which may lead to symptomatic hypotension when used with α-blockers or other antihypertensive agents. Reduced clearance with CYP3A4 and CYP2C9 inhibitors. Caution with medications known to prolong QT interval.

PREGNANCY: Category B, not for use in nursing.

MECHANISM OF ACTION: Phosphodiesterase Type 5 inhibitor; enhances erectile function by increasing the amount of cyclic guanosine monophosphate (cGMP), which triggers smooth muscle relaxations, allowing increased blood flow into the penis, resulting in erection.

PHARMACOKINETICS: Absorption: T_{max}=1.5 hrs. **Distribution:** V_{ss}=208L; plasma protein binding (95%). **Metabolism:** Via CYP3A4, CYP3A5, CYP2C. M1 (major metabolite). **Excretion:** Feces (91%-95%), urine (2%-6%); $T_{1/2}$=4-6 hrs (vardenafil), 3-5 hrs (M1).

NURSING CONSIDERATIONS

Assessment: Assess for CV disease, long QT syndrome, retinitis pigmentosa, bleeding disorders, active peptic ulceration, anatomical deformation of the penis, renal/hepatic impairment. Assess potential underlying causes of erectile dysfunction, and for possible drug interactions.

Monitoring: Monitor for potential cardiac risk due to sexual activity, postural hypotension, vision changes or other eye adverse events (eg, NAION), hypersensitivity reactions and hearing impairment. Monitor therapeutic effect when used in combination with other drugs.

Patient Counseling: Discuss the risk and benefits of the therapy. Counsel patient that use of nitrates and α-blockers could cause hypotension resulting in dizziness, syncope, or even heart attack or stroke. Contact the physician or healthcare provider if not satisfied with the quality of sexual performance or in case of unwanted effect. Priapism may occur; if not treated immediately penile tissue damage and permanent loss of potency may result. Stop the medication if experiencing sudden hearing loss, NAION, loss of vision in one or both eye. Therapy does not protect against sexually transmitted diseases.

Administration: Oral route. Place on tongue to distinegrate. Take without liquid. **Storage:** 25°C (77°F); excursions permitted to 15-30°C (59-86°F).

STELARA   RX
ustekinumab (Janssen)

THERAPEUTIC CLASS: Monoclonal antibody

S

INDICATIONS: Treatment of adult patients (≥18 yrs) with moderate to severe plaque psoriasis who are candidates for phototherapy or systemic therapy.

DOSAGE: *Adults:* ≤100kg: Initial: 45mg SQ and 4 weeks later, followed by 45mg every 12 weeks. >100kg: Initial: 90mg SQ and 4 weeks later, followed by 90mg every 12 weeks.

HOW SUPPLIED: Inj: 45mg/0.5mL, 90mg/mL

WARNINGS/PRECAUTIONS: May increase risk of infections and reactivation of latent infections. Serious bacterial, fungal, and viral infections reported. Do not give with active infection or until infection resolves or is adequately treated. Caution in patients with chronic infection or history of recurrent infection. Caution with interleukin (IL)-12/IL-23-deficiency; vulnerable to disseminated infections from mycobacteria (including nontuberculous, environmental mycobacteria), salmonella (including nontyphi strains), and Bacillus Calmette-Guerin (BCG) vaccinations. Evaluate for tuberculosis (TB) infection prior to, during, and after treatment; avoid with active TB. Consider anti-TB therapy prior to initiation in patients with history of latent or active TB when adequate treatment cannot be confirmed. May increase risk of malignancy. Serious allergic reactions reported; d/c and treat appropriately. Reversible posterior leukoencephalopathy syndrome (RPLS) reported; d/c and treat appropriately if suspected. Prior to therapy, patients should receive all immunizations appropriate for age as recommended by current immunization guidelines. Needle cover on prefilled syringe contains dry natural rubber; caution in latex-sensitive individuals. Safety and efficacy not evaluated beyond 2 yrs.

ADVERSE REACTIONS: Infection, nasopharyngitis, upper respiratory tract infection, headache, fatigue.

INTERACTIONS: Avoid with live vaccines; BCG vaccines should not be given during treatment, for 1 yr prior to initiating treatment, or 1 yr following d/c of treatment. Non-live vaccinations received during course of therapy may not elicit an immune response sufficient to prevent disease. Caution in patients receiving or who have received allergy immunotherapy; may decrease protective effect of allergy immunotherapy and may increase the risk of allergic reaction to a dose of allergen immunotherapy. Monitor therapeutic effect (eg, warfarin) or drug concentrations (eg, cyclosporine) of coadministered CYP450 substrates; adjust individual dose PRN.

PREGNANCY: Category B, caution in nursing.

MECHANISM OF ACTION: Monoclonal antibody; binds with high affinity and specificity to the p40 protein subunit used by both the IL-12 and IL-23 cytokines. *In vitro* models, ustekinumab showed to disrupt IL-12 and IL-23 mediated signaling and cytokine cascades by disrupting the interaction of these cytokines with a shared cell-surface receptor chain, IL-12 β1.

PHARMACOKINETICS: Absorption: T_{max}=13.5 days (45mg), 7 days (90mg). **Distribution:** V_d=161mL/kg (45mg), 179mL/kg (90mg); found in breast milk. **Elimination:** $T_{1/2}$=14.9-45.6 days.

NURSING CONSIDERATIONS

Assessment: Assess for active/chronic infections, history of recurrent infections, IL-12/IL-23 genetical deficiency, TB, immunization history, pregnancy/nursing status, and possible drug interactions.

Monitoring: Monitor for signs/symptoms of infection, TB during and after treatment, malignancies, serious allergic reactions, and RPLS. Monitor all patients closely after administration.

Patient Counseling: Instruct patient to read the medication guide before intiation of therapy and before each prescription renewal. Inform that therapy may lower the ability of the immune system to fight infections. Instruct of the importance of communicating any history of infections to the physician, and contacting physician if any symptoms of infection develop. Counsel about the risk of malignancies while on therapy. Advise patients to seek immediate medical attention if they experience any symptoms of serious allergic reactions.

Administration: SQ route. Refer to PI for general considerations and instructions for administration. **Storage:** 2-8°C (36-46°F). Protect from light. Do not freeze or shake. Discard any unused portion. Store vials upright.

S

STRATTERA RX
atomoxetine HCl (Lilly)

Increased risk of suicidal ideation in short-term studies in children or adolescents with attention-deficit hyperactivity disorder (ADHD); balance this risk with the clinical need. Closely monitor for suicidality (suicidal thinking and behavior), clinical worsening, or unusual changes in behavior. Close observation and communication with the prescriber by families and caregivers is advised. Not approved for major depressive disorder.

THERAPEUTIC CLASS: Selective norepinephrine reuptake inhibitor

INDICATIONS: Treatment of ADHD.

DOSAGE: *Adults:* Initial: 40mg/day. Titrate: Increase after a minimum of 3 days to target dose of about 80mg/day given qam or as evenly divided doses in the am and late afternoon/early

pm. May increase to 100mg/day after 2-4 weeks if optimum response is not achieved. Max: 100mg/day. Refer to PI for dose modifications for hepatic impairment and concomitant use of CYP2D6 inhibitors.
Pediatrics: ≥6 yrs: ≤70kg: Initial: 0.5mg/kg/day. Titrate: Increase after a minimum of 3 days to target dose of about 1.2mg/kg/day given qam or as evenly divided doses in the am and late afternoon/early pm. Max: 1.4mg/kg/day or 100mg, whichever is less. >70kg: Initial: 40mg/day. Titrate: Increase after a minimum of 3 days to target dose of about 80mg/day given qam or as evenly divided doses in the am and late afternoon/early pm. Max: 100mg/day. May increase to 100mg/day after 2-4 weeks if optimal response is not achieved. Refer to PI for dose modifications for hepatic impairment and concomitant use of CYP2D6 inhibitors.

HOW SUPPLIED: Cap: 10mg, 18mg, 25mg, 40mg, 60mg, 80mg, 100mg

CONTRAINDICATIONS: Concomitant use with MAOI during or within 2 weeks after d/c of therapy, narrow-angle glaucoma, and with known/history of pheochromocytoma.

WARNINGS/PRECAUTIONS: Not intended for use with symptoms secondary to environmental factors and/or other primary psychiatric disorders, including psychoses. May cause severe liver injury in rare cases; monitor liver enzymes. D/C with jaundice or laboratory evidence of liver injury, and do not restart therapy. Reports of myocardial infarction (MI), stroke, and sudden death in adults. Avoid use with known structural cardiac abnormalities, cardiomyopathy, serious heart rhythm abnormalities, coronary artery disease (CAD), or other serious cardiac problems; physical exam and evaluation of patient history are necessary. May increase BP and HR; caution with HTN, tachycardia, cardiovascular (CV), or cerebrovascular disease. Orthostatic hypotension and syncope reported; caution in any condition that may predispose to hypotension or with abrupt HR or BP changes. Raynaud's phenomenon reported. May cause treatment-emergent psychotic or manic symptoms (eg, hallucinations, delusional thinking, mania) in children and adolescents without prior history of psychotic illness at usual doses. Screen for risk for bipolar disorder (including psychiatric history, family history of suicide, bipolar disorder, and depression). Monitor for appearance/worsening of aggressive behavior or hostility. Allergic reactions (eg, anaphylactic reactions, angioneurotic edema, urticaria, and rash) reported (uncommon). May increase risk of urinary retention and hesitation. Rare cases of priapism reported. Monitor growth in children. Caution with hepatic impairment.

ADVERSE REACTIONS: Abdominal pain, N/V, fatigue, decreased appetite, somnolence, dizziness, headache, dry mouth, insomnia, constipation, hot flushes, urinary hesitation/retention, dysmenorrhea, dyspepsia, erectile dysfunction.

INTERACTIONS: See Contraindications. May potentiate the CV effects of systemically administered albuterol or other β_2 agonists. Caution with pressor agents (eg, dopamine, dobutamine). Increased levels with CYP2D6 inhibitors (eg, paroxetine, fluoxetine, quinidine); may need dose adjustment.

PREGNANCY: Category C, caution in nursing.

MECHANISM OF ACTION: Selective norepinephrine reuptake inhibitor; mechanism not established. May selectively inhibit the presynaptic norepinephrine transporter.

PHARMACOKINETICS: Absorption: Rapid; well absorbed; absolute bioavailability (extensive metabolizers [63%], poor metabolizers [94%]); T_{max}=1-2 hrs. **Distribution:** V_d=0.85L/kg; plasma protein binding (98%). **Metabolism:** Via CYP2D6; 4-hydroxyatomoxetine (major metabolite). **Elimination:** Urine (>80% [4-hydroxyatomoxetine-O-glucuronide] and <3% [unchanged]), feces (<17%); $T_{1/2}$=5 hrs.

NURSING CONSIDERATIONS

Assessment: Assess for major depressive disorder, psychosis, other primary psychiatric disorders, and other conditions where treatment is contraindicated or cautioned. Assess for pregnancy/nursing status and possible drug interactions. Assess BP, HR, hepatic/renal function.

Monitoring: Monitor for cardiac abnormalities or symptoms of cardiac disease, mixed/manic episode, in patients at risk for bipolar disorder, suicidality, clinical worsening or unusual changes in behavior, and other adverse effects. Monitor growth in children. Monitor HR and BP at dose increases, and periodically during therapy. Perform LFTs at the 1st sign of liver dysfunction. Periodically re-evaluate long-term usefulness of therapy.

Patient Counseling: Inform about risks of treatment and appropriate use. Encourage patients, their families and caregivers to be alert for the emergence of depression, suicidal ideation and other unusual changes in behavior. Advise to contact physician if symptoms of liver injury or priapism occur. Drug is an ocular irritant; avoid contact with eyes. Caution while operating machinery/driving. Instruct to contact physician if increase in aggression or hostility, and priapism occurs. Instruct to consult physician if taking or planning to take any prescription or OTC medicines, dietary supplements, and herbal medicines or if nursing, pregnant, or planning to become pregnant. If patients miss a dose, advise to take it as soon as possible, but should not take more than the total daily dose in any 24-hr period.

Administration: Oral route. Take whole with or without food; do not open cap. **Storage:** 25°C (77°F); excursions permitted to 15-30°C (59-86°F).

STRIANT
testosterone (Columbia Labs)

THERAPEUTIC CLASS: Androgen

INDICATIONS: Testosterone replacement therapy in males with primary or hypogonadotropic hypogonadism, congenital or acquired.

DOSAGE: *Adults:* 30mg q12h to gum region, just above the incisor tooth on either side of mouth. Rotate sites with each application. Hold system in place for 30 seconds. If buccal system falls off within the 12-hr dosing interval or falls out of position within 4 hrs prior to next dose, remove and apply new system. Do not chew or swallow.

HOW SUPPLIED: Tab, Buccal: 30mg [6 blister packs, 10 buccal systems/blister]

CONTRAINDICATIONS: Women. Carcinoma of the breast or known or suspected carcinoma of the prostate. Hypersensitivity to soy products.

WARNINGS/PRECAUTIONS: Caution in elderly; increased risk of prostatic hyperplasia/carcinoma. Risk of edema with pre-existing cardiac, renal, or hepatic disease; d/c if edema occurs. May potentiate sleep apnea, especially with obesity or chronic lung diseases. Monitor Hgb, Hct, LFTs, prostate specific antigen (PSA), cholesterol, lipids, serum testosterone. Gynecomastia frequently develops and occasionally persists.

ADVERSE REACTIONS: Gum/mouth irritation, bitter taste, gum pain/tenderness, headache, gynecomastia.

INTERACTIONS: May elevate oxyphenbutazone levels. May decrease blood glucose and, therefore, insulin requirements. Adrenocorticotropic hormone/corticosteroids may enhance edema formation; caution with cardiac or hepatic disease.

PREGNANCY: Category X, not for use in nursing.

MECHANISM OF ACTION: Androgen; responsible for normal growth and development of male sex organs and maintenance of secondary sex characteristics.

PHARMACOKINETICS: Absorption: T_{max}=10-12 hrs. **Distribution:** Sex hormone-binding globulin (40%), plasma protein binding. **Metabolism:** Estradiol, dihydrotestosterone (metabolites). **Elimination:** Urine, feces; $T_{1/2}$=10-100 min.

NURSING CONSIDERATIONS

Assessment: Assess for hypersensitivity to soy products, breast or prostate carcinoma, cardiac or renal/hepatic disease, obesity, chronic lung disease, diabetes mellitus, and possible drug interactions.

Monitoring: Periodically monitor Hgb, Hct, LFTs, PSA, cholesterol and HDL. Obtain serum testosterone levels 4-12 weeks after initiation of therapy. Monitor for signs/symptoms of hypersensitivity reactions, edema with/without CHF, gynecomastia, prostatic hyperplasia/carcinoma in geriatrics, and potentiation of sleep apnea.

Patient Counseling: Instruct to apply against gums above incisors; if it fails to adhere, replace with new system. If system falls out 4 hrs prior to next dose, replace with a new one until next scheduled dose. Advise to regularly inspect gums where applying system. Contact physician if abnormal findings on gums, too frequent or persistent erections, N/V, changes in skin color, ankle swelling, breathing disturbances, or hypersensitivity reactions occur.

Administration: Buccal route. Place rounded side surface of system against gum above incisor tooth and hold firmly in place with finger over lip and against product for 30 seconds. To remove, slide gently downwards towards tooth to avoid scratching gums. **Storage:** 20-25°C (68-77°F). Protect from heat and moisture.

SUBOXONE
naloxone - buprenorphine (Reckitt Benckiser)

THERAPEUTIC CLASS: Partial opioid agonist/opioid antagonist

INDICATIONS: Maintenance treatment of opioid dependence; should be used as part of a complete treatment plan to include counseling and psychosocial support.

DOSAGE: *Adults:* Administer SL as a single daily dose in patients initially inducted using Subutex (buprenorphine) SL tab. Maint: Target Dose: 16mg-4mg/day. Titrate: Adjust dose progressively in increments/decrements of 2mg-0.5mg or 4mg-1mg to maintain treatment and suppress opioid withdrawal signs and symptoms. Range: 4mg-1mg to 24mg-6mg/day depending on the patient. D/C of Therapy: Should be made as part of a comprehensive treatment plan. Switching Between SL Film and SL Tab: Start on the same dose as the previously administered formulation, then adjust dose PRN. Hepatic Impairment: Adjust dose and observe for precipitated opioid withdrawal. Elderly: Start at low end of dosing range.

HOW SUPPLIED: Tab, SL: (Buprenorphine-Naloxone) 2mg-0.5mg, 8mg-2mg
WARNINGS/PRECAUTIONS: Not appropriate as an analgesic. Hypersensitivity reactions and anaphylaxis reported. May precipitate opioid withdrawal signs and symptoms if administered before the agonist effects of the opioid have subsided. May impair mental/physical abilities. May produce orthostatic hypotension in ambulatory patients. Caution with debilitated patients, myxedema, hypothyroidism, acute alcoholism, adrenal cortical insufficiency (eg, Addison's disease), CNS depression or coma, toxic psychoses, prostatic hypertrophy, urethral stricture, delirium tremens, kyphoscoliosis, hepatic impairment, and in elderly. Buprenorphine: Potential for abuse. Significant respiratory depression reported; caution with compromised respiratory function. May use higher doses and repeated administration of naloxone PRN to manage overdose. Accidental pediatric exposure can cause fatal respiratory depression. Chronic use produces physical dependence. Cytolytic hepatitis and hepatitis with jaundice reported; obtain LFTs prior to initiation and periodically thereafter. Neonatal withdrawal reported when used during pregnancy. May elevate CSF pressure; caution with head injury, intracranial lesions, and other circumstances when cerebrospinal pressure may be increased. Caution with biliary tract dysfunction. May produce miosis. May obscure diagnosis or clinical course of patients with acute abdominal conditions.

ADVERSE REACTIONS: Headache, infection, pain, back pain, withdrawal syndrome, diarrhea, nausea, nervousness, runny eyes, insomnia, sweating, asthenia, anxiety, depression, rhinitis.

INTERACTIONS: May cause respiratory/CNS depression, coma and death with benzodiazepines, other CNS depressants (eg, alcohol), general anesthetics, opioid analgesics, phenothiazines, tranquilizers, or sedative/hypnotics; consider dose reduction of one or both agents. Concomitant use of other potentially hepatotoxic drugs and ongoing injecting drug use may contribute to hepatic abnormalities. CYP3A4 inhibitors (eg, azole antifungals, macrolides, and HIV protease inhibitors) may require dose reduction of 1 or both agents and monitoring. Monitor for signs and symptoms of opioid withdrawal with CYP3A4 inducers (eg, efavirenz, phenobarbital, carbamazepine, phenytoin, rifampicin). Monitor dose if non-nucleoside reverse transcriptase inhibitors are added to treatment regimen. Some antiretroviral protease inhibitors with CYP3A4 inhibitory activity (nelfinavir, lopinavir/ritonavir, ritonavir) have little effect on pharmacokinetics. Atazanavir and atazanavir/ritonavir may increase levels; monitor and reduce dose of buprenorphine.

PREGNANCY: Category C, not for use in nursing.

MECHANISM OF ACTION: Buprenorphine: Partial agonist at the μ-opioid receptor and antagonist at the kappa-opioid receptor. Naloxone: Potent antagonist at the μ-opioid receptor.

PHARMACOKINETICS: Absorption: Administration of variable doses resulted in different parameters. **Distribution:** Plasma protein binding (96%, buprenorphine; 45%, naloxone); found in breast milk (buprenorphine). **Metabolism:** Buprenorphine: N-dealkylation (by CYP3A4) and glucuronidation; norbuprenorphine (active metabolite). Naloxone: Glucuronidation, N-dealkylation, and reduction; naloxone-3-glucoronide (metabolite). **Elimination:** Buprenorphine: Urine (30%), feces (69%); $T_{1/2}$=24-42 hrs. Naloxone: $T_{1/2}$=2-12 hrs.

NURSING CONSIDERATIONS

Assessment: Assess for history of hypersensivitiy reactions, elderly status, debilitation, myxedema, hypothyroidism, acute alcoholism, adrenal cortical insufficiency (eg, Addison's disease), CNS depression or coma, toxic psychoses, prostatic hypertrophy, urethral stricture, delirium tremens, kyphoscoliosis, biliary tract dysfunction or moderate and severe hepatic impairment, compromised respiratory function, head injury, intracranial lesions and other circumstances in which cerebrospinal pressure may be increased, acute abdominal conditions, pregnancy/nursing status, and possible drug interactions. Perform LFTs prior to therapy.

Monitoring: Monitor for hypersensitivity reactions, signs/symptoms of opioid withdrawal, impaired mental/physical ability, orthostatic hypotension, respiratory depression, drug abuse/dependence, cytolitic hepatitis, hepatitis with jaundice, elevation of CSF, miosis, changes in consciousness levels and other adverse reactions. Monitor LFTs periodically.

Patient Counseling: Warn patient on danger of self-administration of benzodiazepines and other CNS depressants, including alcohol, while on therapy. Advise that the drug contains opioid that can be a target for abuse; keep tabs in safe place protected from theft and children. Seek medical attention immediately upon pediatric exposure to the drug. Caution that the drug may impair mental/physical abilities and cause orthostatic hypotension. Advise to take tab qd and do not change dose without consulting physician. Inform that treatment can cause dependence and withdrawal syndrome may occur upon d/c. Advise to report to physician all medications prescribed or currently being used. Advise women regarding possible effects during pregnancy and not to breastfeed. Advise to instruct family members that, in event of emergency, the treating physician or staff should be informed that patient is physically dependent on an opioid. Advise to dispose of unopened drugs as soon as they are no longer needed by flushing the unused tabs down the toilet.

Administration: SL route. Refer to PI for further information on method of administration, clinical supervision, and unstable patients. **Storage:** 25°C (77°F); excursions permitted to 15-30°C (59-86°F).

SUBOXONE SUBLINGUAL FILM

naloxone - buprenorphine (Reckitt Benckiser)

THERAPEUTIC CLASS: Partial opioid agonist/opioid antagonist

INDICATIONS: Maintenance treatment of opioid dependence.

DOSAGE: *Adults:* Target Maint Dose: 16mg-4mg, as a single daily dose SL in patients initially inducted using Subutex (buprenorphine) SL tab. Titrate: Adjust in increments/decrements of 2mg-0.5mg or 4mg-1mg to maintain treatment and suppress opioid withdrawal effects. Range: 4mg-1mg to 24mg-6mg/day. Switching Between SL Tab and SL Film: Start on the same dosage as the previously administered product, then adjust dose PRN. Hepatic Impairment: Adjust dose. Elderly: Start at low end of dosing range.

HOW SUPPLIED: Film, SL: (Buprenorphine-Naloxone) 2mg-0.5mg, 8mg-2mg

WARNINGS/PRECAUTIONS: Potential for abuse. Re-establish adequate ventilation in case of overdose. May use higher doses and repeated administration of naloxone PRN to manage buprenorphine overdose. Caution with compromised respiratory function. Accidental pediatric exposure can cause fatal respiratory depression. Chronic use produces physical dependence. Cytolytic hepatitis and hepatitis with jaundice reported; obtain LFTs prior to therapy and monitor during treatment. Hypersensitivity reactions reported. May cause opioid withdrawal symptoms. Neonatal withdrawal reported when used during pregnancy. Not appropriate as an analgesic. May impair mental/physical abilities. May cause orthostatic hypotension in ambulatory patients. May elevate CSF pressure; caution with head injuries, intracranial lesions, and other circumstances when CSF pressure may be increased. May produce miosis and changes in the level of consciousness. May increase intracholedochal pressure; caution with biliary tract dysfunction. May obscure the diagnosis or clinical course of acute abdominal conditions. Caution in elderly or debilitated patients, myxedema/hypothyroidism, adrenal cortical insufficiency (eg, Addison's disease), CNS depression/coma, toxic psychoses, prostatic hypertrophy/urethral stricture, acute alcoholism, delirium tremens, or kyphoscoliosis.

ADVERSE REACTIONS: Oral hypoesthesia, constipation, glossodynia, oral mucosal erythema, vomiting, intoxication, disturbance in attention, palpitations, insomnia, withdrawal syndrome, hyperhidrosis, blurred vision.

INTERACTIONS: May need dose reduction with CYP3A4 inhibitors (eg, azoles such as ketoconazole, macrolides such as erythromycin, HIV protease inhibitors). Concomitant use with other potentially hepatotoxic drugs may increase risk of hepatitis or other hepatic events. Opioid analgesics, general anesthetics, benzodiazepines, phenothiazines, other tranquilizers, sedative/hypnotics or other CNS depressants (including alcohol) may increase CNS depression; consider dose reduction of one or both agents. Monitor closely for signs and symptoms of opioid withdrawal with CYP3A4 inducers (eg, efavirenz, phenobarbital, carbamazepine, phenytoin, rifampicin). Monitor dose with non-nucleoside reverse transcriptase inhibitors (NNRTIs). Some antiretroviral protease inhibitors with CYP3A4 inhibitory activity (nelfinavir, lopinavir/ritonavir, ritonavir) have little effect on pharmacokinetics. Increased levels and sedation with atazanavir, atazanavir/ritonavir. Caution with drugs that act on the CNS.

PREGNANCY: Category C, not for use in nursing.

MECHANISM OF ACTION: Buprenorphine: Partial agonist at the μ-opioid receptor and antagonist at the kappa-opioid receptor. Naloxone: Potent antagonist at the μ-opioid receptor.

PHARMACOKINETICS: Absorption: Administration of variable doses resulted in different pharmacokinetic parameters. **Distribution:** Plasma protein binding (96% buprenorphine; 45% naloxone); found in breast milk (buprenorphine). **Metabolism:** Buprenorphine: N-dealkylation via CYP3A4 and glucuronidation; norbuprenorphine (major metabolite). Naloxone: Glucuronidation, N-dealkylation, and reduction; naloxone-3-glucoronide (metabolite). **Elimination:** Buprenorphine: Urine (30%), feces (69%); $T_{1/2}$=24-42 hrs. Naloxone: $T_{1/2}$=2-12 hrs.

NURSING CONSIDERATIONS

Assessment: Assess for previous hypersensitivity, pregnancy/nursing status, possible drug interactions, and conditions where treatment is cautioned. Obtain baseline LFTs.

Monitoring: Monitor for signs/symptoms of respiratory/CNS depression, drug dependence, illicit drug use, hepatitis, hypersensitivity reactions, orthostatic hypotension, and elevation of CSF and intracholedochal pressure. Periodically monitor LFTs. Observe for signs and symptoms of precipitated opioid withdrawal in patients with hepatic impairment. Monitor for over-medication when switching from SL tab to SL film and withdrawal and under-dosing when switching from SL film to SL tab.

Patient Counseling: Warn patient on danger of self-administration of benzodiazepines and other CNS depressants, including alcohol, while taking Suboxone. Advise that the drug contains opioid that can be a target for abuse; keep films in safe place protected from theft and children. Seek medical attention immediately upon pediatric exposure to the drug. Never give the film to anyone else; selling or giving away of Suboxone is against the law. Drug may impair mental/physical abilities; use caution when performing hazardous tasks (eg, operating machinery/driving). Take film qd and do not change dose without consulting physician. Treatment can cause dependence and withdrawal syndrome may occur upon d/c. Caution about possibility of orthostatic hypotension in ambulatory individuals. Report to physician all medications prescribed or currently being used. Advise women regarding possible effects during pregnancy and not to breastfeed. Instruct family members that, in event of emergency, the treating physician or staff should be informed that patient is physically dependent on an opioid. Advise to dispose of unopened drugs as soon as they are no longer needed by removing the film from its foil pouch and flushing them in the toilet.

Administration: Sublingual route. If additional SL film is necessary, place it on the opposite side from the first film in a manner to minimize overlapping. Keep under tongue until completely dissolved. Do not chew, swallow, or move film after placement. **Storage:** 25°C (77°F); excursions permitted to 15-30°C (59-86°F).

SULAR RX
nisoldipine (Shionogi)

THERAPEUTIC CLASS: Calcium channel blocker (dihydropyridine)

INDICATIONS: Treatment of HTN alone or in combination with other antihypertensive agents.

DOSAGE: *Adults:* Initial: 17mg qd. Titrate: May increase by 8.5mg/week or longer intervals. Maint: 17-34mg qd. Max: 34mg qd. Elderly/Hepatic Dysfunction: Initial: ≤8.5mg/day.

HOW SUPPLIED: Tab, Extended-Release: 8.5mg, 17mg, 25.5mg, 34mg

WARNINGS/PRECAUTIONS: May increase angina or acute myocardial infarction (MI) in patients with severe obstructive coronary artery disease (CAD). May cause hypotension; monitor BP initially or during titration. Caution with heart failure or compromised ventricular function, especially with concomitant β-blockers. Caution with severe hepatic dysfunction and in elderly.

ADVERSE REACTIONS: Peripheral edema, headache, dizziness, pharyngitis, vasodilation, sinusitis, palpitations.

INTERACTIONS: Increased levels with cimetidine. Avoid with phenytoin, CYP3A4 inducers or inhibitors, and grapefruit juice. Decreased bioavailability with quinidine.

PREGNANCY: Category C, not for use in nursing.

MECHANISM OF ACTION: Calcium channel antagonist (dihydropyridine); inhibits transmembrane influx of calcium into vascular smooth muscle and cardiac muscle, resulting in dilation of arterioles and decreased peripheral vascular resistance.

PHARMACOKINETICS: Absorption: Well absorbed. Absolute bioavailability (5%); T_{max}=9.2 hrs. C_{max} increases up to 245% with high fat meals. **Metabolism:** CYP3A4 via hydroxylation. **Distribution:** Plasma protein binding (>99%). **Elimination:** Urine (60-80%), feces; $T_{1/2}$=13.7 hrs.

NURSING CONSIDERATIONS

Assessment: Assess for CAD, heart failure, compromised ventricular function, pregnancy/nursing status, and possible drug interactions. Obtain baseline BP and LFTs.

Monitoring: Monitor for increased angina or MI in patients with severe obstructive CAD, and other adverse effects. Monitor BP and LFTs.

Patient Counseling: Instruct to swallow whole on an empty stomach; do not bite, divide, or crush. Instruct to avoid grapefruit juice pre/post dosing. Inform that drug contains tartrazine which may cause allergic-type reactions, especially in those with aspirin hypersensitivity.

Administration: Oral route. Take on an empty stomach (1 hr ac or 2 hrs pc). Swallow whole; do not bite, divide, or crush. **Storage:** 20-25°C (68-77°F); excursions permitted to 15-30°C (59-86°F). Protect from light and moisture.

SUMAVEL DOSEPRO RX
sumatriptan (Zogenix, Inc)

THERAPEUTIC CLASS: 5-HT$_{1B/1D}$ agonist

INDICATIONS: Acute treatment of migraine attacks, with or without aura, and acute treatment of cluster headache episodes.

DOSAGE: *Adults:* Initial: 6mg SQ. May repeat after 1 hr. Max: 12mg/day. Administer to the abdomen or thigh.

HOW SUPPLIED: Inj: 6mg/0.5mL

CONTRAINDICATIONS: IV route, ischemic heart disease (eg, angina pectoris, history of myocardial infarction [MI], or documented silent ischemia) or symptoms/findings consistent with ischemic heart disease, coronary artery vasospasm (eg, Prinzmetal's variant angina), or other significant underlying cardiovascular (CV) disease, cerebrovascular syndromes (eg, stroke, transient ischemic attacks), peripheral vascular disease (eg, ischemic bowel disease), uncontrolled HTN, or hemiplegic or basilar migraine, administration of any ergot-type agents (eg, dihydroergotamine or methysergide) or other 5-HT$_1$ agonists (eg, triptan) within 24 hrs.

WARNINGS/PRECAUTIONS: Serious adverse cardiac events (eg, acute MI, life-threatening arrhythmias), cerebrovascular events, and vasospastic reactions (eg, coronary artery vasospasm, peripheral vascular ischemia, colonic ischemia) reported. Signs or symptoms suggestive of decreased arterial flow should be evaluated for atherosclerosis or predisposition to vasospasm. Sensations of tightness, pain, pressure, and heaviness in the precordium, throat, neck, and jaw are common after therapy. Serotonin syndrome may occur; symptoms may include mental status changes, autonomic instability, neuromuscular aberrations, and GI symptoms. Caution with controlled HTN. Elevation in BP including hypertensive crisis reported. May cause hypersensitivity reactions (eg, anaphylaxis/anaphylactoid). Seizures reported; caution with history of epilepsy or lowered seizure threshold. Corneal opacities may occur. Not recommended for elderly; higher risk for CAD, HTN, and decreased hepatic function.

ADVERSE REACTIONS: Injection-site reactions, tingling, warm/hot sensation, burning sensation, feeling of heaviness, pressure sensation, feeling of tightness, numbness, flushing, chest discomfort/tightness, weakness, dizziness/vertigo, drowsiness/sedation, paresthesia, N/V.

INTERACTIONS: See Contraindications. Avoid use with MAOIs; reduced sumatriptan clearance. May cause additive prolonged vasospastic reactions with ergot-containing drugs. Serotonin syndrome reported when used in combination with SSRIs or SNRIs.

PREGNANCY: Category C, caution in nursing.

MECHANISM OF ACTION: Selective 5-HT$_{1B/1D}$ agonist; binds to vascular 5-HT$_1$-type receptors in cranial arteries, basilar artery, and vasculature of isolated dura mater, which causes vasoconstriction.

PHARMACOKINETICS: Absorption: Absolute Bioavailability (97%); C$_{max}$=71.9ng/mL (thigh), 78.6ng/mL (abdomen); T$_{max}$=12 min. **Distribution:** Plasma protein binding (14-21%); found in breast milk. **Elimination:** T$_{1/2}$=103 min (thigh), 102 min (abdomen).

NURSING CONSIDERATIONS

Assessment: Assess for presence/history of ischemic heart disease, CAD, cerebrovascular or peripheral vascular disease, uncontrolled HTN, hemiplegic or basilar migraines, history of epilepsy, pregnancy/nursing status, and possible drug interactions. Establish proper diagnosis of migraine; exclude other potentially serious neurological condition. Obtain baseline vital signs, weight, CV function, ECG, LFTs.

Monitoring: Monitor for cardiac ischemia; perform ECG monitoring after administration for those with CAD risk factors. Monitor for signs/symptoms of cardiac events, colonic ischemia, bloody diarrhea, serotonin syndrome (eg, mental status changes), hypersensitivity reactions, chest/throat/jaw/neck tightness, seizures, exacerbation of headache, and ophthalmic changes. For patients on long-term therapy or with CAD risk factors, perform periodic monitoring of CV function. If patients with no risk factors develop signs/symptoms of angina after administration, stop and reevaluate for CAD or other cardiac disease. If clinical response does not occur following administration of first dose, reassess diagnosis. Monitor vital signs, weight, and LFTs.

Patient Counseling: Inform about risks and benefits of therapy, proper use, importance of follow up, and possible drug interactions. Inform to notify physician if any symptoms such as chest pain, shortness of breath, weakness, or slurring of speech occur, or if pregnant or nursing. Advise on the proper administration techniques and sites of injection (eg, abdomen, thigh); not to administer via IM/IV.

Administration: SQ route. Refer to PI for administration. **Storage:** 20-25°C (68-77°F), with excursions permitted between 15-30°C (59-86°F). Do not freeze.

SUPRAX   RX
cefixime (Lupin)

THERAPEUTIC CLASS: Cephalosporin (3rd generation)

INDICATIONS: Otitis media, pharyngitis, tonsillitis, acute bronchitis, acute exacerbation of chronic bronchitis, uncomplicated urinary tract infections (UTIs), and cervical/urethral gonorrhea caused by susceptible strains.

DOSAGE: *Adults:* Usual: 400mg qd. Gonorrhea: 400mg single dose. CrCl 21-60mL/min/Hemodialysis: Give 75% of standard dose. CrCl <20mL/min/Continuous Ambulatory Peritoneal Dialysis (CAPD): Give 50% of standard dose.

Pediatrics: >12 yrs or >50kg: (Tab/Sus) Usual: 400mg qd. ≥6 months: (Sus) 8mg/kg qd or 4mg/kg bid. Treat for at least 10 days for *Streptococcus pyogenes.* CrCl 21-60mL/min/Hemodialysis: Give 75% of standard dose. CrCl <20mL/min/CAPD: Give 50% of standard dose.

HOW SUPPLIED: Tab: 400mg; Sus: 100mg/5mL [50mL, 75mL, 100mL]

WARNINGS/PRECAUTIONS: Caution with penicillin (PCN) or other allergy, GI disease (eg, colitis). Anaphylactic/anaphylactoid reactions, pseudomembranous colitis/*Clostridium difficile*-associated diarrhea (CDAD) reported. May result in bacterial resistance with prolonged use or use in the absence of a proven/suspected bacterial infection or a prophylactic indication; take appropriate measures if superinfection develops. Lab test interactions may occur.

ADVERSE REACTIONS: Diarrhea, abdominal pain, nausea, dyspepsia, flatulence, superinfection.

INTERACTIONS: May increase carbamazepine levels. Increased PT with anticoagulants (eg, warfarin).

PREGNANCY: Category B, not for use in nursing.

MECHANISM OF ACTION: 3rd generation cephalosporin; inhibits cell-wall synthesis.

PHARMACOKINETICS: Absorption: 40-50%. C_{max}=2mcg/mL (200mg tab), 3.7mcg/mL (400mg tab), 3mcg/mL (200mg sus), 4.6mcg/mL (400mg sus); T_{max}=2-6 hrs (200mg tab, 400mg tab/sus), 2-5 hrs (200mg sus). **Distribution:** Serum protein binding (65%). **Elimination:** Urine (50% unchanged); $T_{1/2}$=3-4 up to 9 hrs.

NURSING CONSIDERATIONS

Assessment: Assess for previous hypersensitivity to cephalosporins/PCNs or other drugs, renal/hepatic impairment, GI tract disease (eg, colitis), nutritional status, protracted course of antibiotics or anticoagulants, pregnancy/nursing status, possible drug interactions.

Monitoring: Monitor for PT with vitamin K administration as indicated. Monitor for signs/symptoms of anaphylatic/anaphylactoid reactions, pseudomembranous colitis or CDAD, superinfection, pancytopenia, agranulocytosis, and lab test interferences.

Patient Counseling: Inform that therapy only treats bacterial, not viral, infections. Take exactly as directed; skipping doses or not completing full course may decrease effectiveness and increase resistance. Inform about benefits/risks. D/C and notify physician if diarrhea or allergic reactions occur. Notify if pregnant/nursing.

Administration: Oral route. **Storage:** Sus/Tab, 20-25°C (68-77°F). After mixing, store sus at room temperature or under refrigeration for 14 days; keep tightly closed and shake well before use.

SUPREP   RX
potassium sulfate - magnesium sulfate - sodium sulfate (Braintree)

THERAPEUTIC CLASS: Bowel cleanser

INDICATIONS: Cleansing of colon as a preparation of colonoscopy in adults.

DOSAGE: *Adults:* Day Prior to Colonoscopy: May consume light breakfast or have only clear liquids. Early in evening prior to colonoscopy, dilute one bottle with 16 oz. of water and drink entire amount. Drink additional 32 oz. of water over the next hour. Day of Colonoscopy: Have only clear liquids until after colonoscopy. Morning of Colonoscopy (10-12 hrs after pm dose): Repeat steps taken on day prior with second bottle. Complete all Suprep Bowel Prep Kit and required water at least 1 hr prior to colonoscopy.

HOW SUPPLIED: Sol: (Sodium Sulfate-Potassium Sulfate-Magnesium Sulfate) 17.5g-3.13g-1.6g

CONTRAINDICATIONS: GI obstruction, bowel perforation, gastric retention, ileus, toxic colitis or toxic megacolon.

WARNINGS/PRECAUTIONS: Hydrate adequately before, during, and after use. If significant vomiting or signs of dehydration occur, consider performing post-colonoscopy tests (electrolytes, creatinine, BUN). Correct electrolyte abnormalities prior to use. Caution with conditions that may increase the risk of fluid/electrolyte disturbances and renal impairment. May increase uric acid levels; caution in patients with gout or uric acid metabolism disorders. Serious arrhythmias reported rarely; caution in patients at increased risk of arrhythmias (eg, history of prolonged QT, uncontrolled arrhythmias, recent myocardial infarction, unstable angina, congestive heart failure, cardiomyopathy). Generalized tonic-clonic seizures and/or loss of consciousness reported; caution in patients with a history of seizures and in patients at increased risk of seizures (eg, hyponatremia, alcohol or benzodiazepine withdrawal). May produce colonic mucosal aphthous ulcerations and ischemic colitis. If suspected, rule out GI obstruction or perforation prior to administration. Caution in patients with impaired gag reflex and patients prone to regurgitation or aspiration; observe during administration. Not for direct ingestion.

ADVERSE REACTIONS: Overall discomfort, abdominal distention, abdominal pain, N/V.

INTERACTIONS: Caution with concomitant use of medications that increase the risk for fluid and electrolyte disturbances or increase the risk of seizures (eg, tricyclic antidepressants),

S

arrhythmias and prolonged QT. Caution with medications that may affect renal function (eg, diuretics, ACE inhibitors, angiotensin receptor blockers, NSAIDs). Concurrent use with stimulant laxatives may increase risk of colonic mucosal ulcerations and ischemic colitis. Absorption of oral medications may not occur if administered within an hour of the start of a Suprep dose.

PREGNANCY: Category C, caution in nursing.

MECHANISM OF ACTION: Bowel cleanser: sulfate salts provide sulfate anions that are poorly absorbed. The osmotic effect of the unabsorbed sulfate anions and the associated cations causes water to be retained within the GI tract.

PHARMACOKINETICS: Absorption: T_{max} = 17 hrs (1st dose), 5 hrs (2nd dose). **Elimination:** Feces (primary), $T_{1/2}$= 8.5 hrs.

NURSING CONSIDERATIONS

Assessment: Assess for GI obstruction, bowel perforation, or any other conditions where treatment is contraindicated or cautioned. Assess for pregnancy/nursing status, and for possible drug interactions. Obtain baseline electrolytes, creatinine, and BUN in patients with renal impairment. Perform baseline ECGs in patients at risk for arrhythmias.

Monitoring: Monitor for electrolyte abnormalities, cardiac arrhythmias, seizures, loss of consciousness, colonic mucosal ulcerations, ischemic colitis, and aspiration. Perform ECG in patients at increased risk of serious cardiac arrhythmias. Monitor electrolytes, creatinine, and BUN in patients with renal impairment.

Patient Counseling: Instruct to notify physician if have difficulty swallowing or prone to regurgitation or aspiration. Inform to dilute each bottle with water prior to ingestion and drink additional water as directed by instructions. Advise that ingestion of undiluted solution may increase risk of N/V and dehydration. Inform that oral medications may not be absorbed properly if they are taken within 1 hr of starting each dose of Suprep Bowel Kit. Instruct not to take additional laxatives.

Administration: Oral Route. **Storage:** 20-25°C (68-77°F); excursions permitted between 15-30°C (59-86°F).

SUSTIVA

RX

efavirenz (Bristol-Myers Squibb)

THERAPEUTIC CLASS: Non-nucleoside reverse transcriptase inhibitor

INDICATIONS: Treatment of HIV-1 infection in combination with other antiretrovirals.

DOSAGE: *Adults:* Take on an empty stomach hs. Usual: 600mg qd with a protease inhibitor and/or nucleoside analogue reverse transcriptase inhibitors. Concomitant Voriconazole: Reduce dose to 300mg qd using cap formulation; increase voriconazole maint dose to 400mg q12h. Concomitant Rifampin in Patients ≥50kg: Increase dose to 800mg qd.
Pediatrics: ≥3 yrs: Take on an empty stomach hs. Usual: ≥40kg: 600mg qd. 32.5-<40kg: 400mg qd. 25-<32.5kg: 350mg qd. 20-<25kg: 300mg qd. 15-<20kg: 250mg qd. 10-<15kg: 200mg qd.

HOW SUPPLIED: Cap: 50mg, 200mg; Tab: 600mg

CONTRAINDICATIONS: Concomitant use with drugs for which metabolism could be inhibited by the competition for CYP3A by efavirenz, which may create potential for serious and/or life-threatening reactions (eg, bepridil, cisapride, midazolam, triazolam, pimozide, ergot derivatives [dihydroergotamine, ergonovine, ergotamine, methylergonovine], and St. John's wort).

WARNINGS/PRECAUTIONS: Not for use as monotherapy or added on as a sole agent to a failing regimen to avoid virus resistance. Not recommended with other efavirenz-containing products. Serious psychiatric events reported; immediate medical evaluation is recommended if symptoms occur. CNS symptoms reported; may dose at bedtime to improve tolerability. Skin rash reported; d/c and give appropriate treatment if severe rash develops. Avoid with moderate or severe hepatic impairment and use with caution with mild hepatic impairment or in elderly. Hepatotoxicity reported; monitor liver enzymes before and during treatment with underlying hepatic disease, marked transaminase elevations, and with other medications associated with liver toxicity, and consider monitoring without preexisting hepatic dysfunction/risk factors. Convulsions reported; caution with history of seizures. Lipid elevations, Immune reconstitution syndrome, and fat redistribution/accumulation reported. Fetal harm can occur when administered during 1st trimester of pregnancy; avoid pregnancy during use.

ADVERSE REACTIONS: Dizziness, headache, insomnia, anxiety, desquamation, depression, rash, N/V, increased ALT/AST levels, hypercholesterolemia, fatigue, erythema, CNS symptoms.

INTERACTIONS: See Contraindications. CYP3A substrates, inhibitors, or inducers may alter plasma concentrations. May alter or decrease plasma concentrations of CYP3A or 2B6 substrates. May alter plasma concentrations of CYP2C9, 2C19, and 3A4 substrates. Decreased levels with CYP3A inducers (eg, phenobarbital, rifampin, rifabutin) and anticonvulsants. May decrease levels of amprenavir, atazanavir (avoid combination in treatment-experienced patients), indinavir, lopinavir, saquinavir, maraviroc, anticonvulsants (monitor levels), buproprion, sertraline, azole antifungals (eg, voriconazole, itraconazole, ketoconazole), rifabutin, clarithromycin, calcium channel blockers, atorvastatin, pravastatin, simvastatin, hormonal contraceptives (eg, norgestimate, etonogestrel), immunosuppressants, and methadone. May alter warfarin concentrations. May increase ritonavir levels. May decrease posaconazole levels; avoid concomitant use unless benefit outweighs risks. Increased levels with ritonavir and voriconazole. Additive CNS effects with alcohol or psychoactive drugs.

PREGNANCY: Category D, not for use in nursing.

MECHANISM OF ACTION: Non-nucleoside reverse transcriptase inhibitor; mediated predominantly by noncompetitive inhibition of HIV-1 reverse transcriptase.

PHARMACOKINETICS: Absorption: T_{max}= 3-5 hrs; (600mg qd) C_{max}=12.9 µM, AUC=184 µM•h. **Distribution:** Plasma protein binding (99.5-99.75%). **Metabolism:** CYP450 3A and 2B6 (major) to hydroxylated metabolites with subsequent glucuronidation. **Elimination:** Urine (14-34%, <1% unchanged), feces (16-61%); $T_{1/2}$=40-55 hrs (multiple dose), 52-76 hrs (single dose).

NURSING CONSIDERATIONS

Assessment: Assess for underlying hepatic disease, history of injection drug use, history of seizures, psychiatric history, previous hypersensitivity to the drug, pregnancy/nursing status, and possible drug interactions. Perform pregnancy test prior to therapy. Obtain baseline liver enzymes (eg, ALT, AST), gamma-glutamyltransferase, amylase, glucose levels, lipid profile (eg, cholesterol, TG), and neutrophil count.

Monitoring: Monitor for psychiatric events, CNS symptoms, skin rash, pregnancy, convulsions, immune reconstitution syndrome (eg, opportunistic infections), hypersensitivity reactions, and other adverse reactions. Monitor liver enzymes before and during treatment with underlying hepatic disease, marked transaminase elevations, and with other medications associated with liver toxicity, and consider monitoring without preexisting hepatic dysfunction/risk factors. Monitor lipid profile.

Patient Counseling: Advise to report to physician use of any other prescription/nonprescription medication or herbal products, particularly St. John's wort. Inform that therapy is not cure for HIV, has not been shown to reduce risk of transmission of HIV, and that illnesses associated with HIV (eg, opportunistic infections) may develop. Advise to take every day as prescribed. Inform that CNS symptoms (eg, dizziness, insomnia, impaired concentration, abnormal dreams) during 1st weeks of therapy, rash, psychiatric symptoms, and redistribution/accumulation of body fat may occur. Advise to avoid potentially hazardous tasks such as driving or operating machinery if experiencing CNS symptoms and to seek medical attention if symptoms of seizures, rash, serious psychiatric events, or hypersensitivity reactions occur. Advise to notify physician of any history of mental illness or substance abuse. Inform of pregnancy risks and instruct to avoid pregnancy; use of reliable barrier contraception in combination with other methods of contraception (eg, oral contraception) during therapy and 12 weeks after d/c of therapy is recommended.

Administration: Oral route. Do not break tab. **Storage:** 25°C (77°F); excursions permitted to 15-30°C (59-86°F).

SUTENT   RX
sunitinib malate (Pfizer)

S

| Hepatotoxicity has been observed; may be severe, and deaths have been reported. |

THERAPEUTIC CLASS: Multikinase inhibitor

INDICATIONS: Treatment of GI stromal tumor (GIST) after disease progression on or intolerance to imatinib mesylate, advanced renal cell carcinoma (RCC), and progressive, well-differentiated pancreatic neuroendocrine tumors (pNET) with unresectable locally advanced or metastatic disease.

DOSAGE: *Adults:* GIST/RCC: Usual: 50mg qd; 4 weeks on, 2 weeks off. pNET: Usual: 37.5mg qd continuously without a scheduled-off treatment period. Max: 50mg/day. Interrupt or increase/decrease dose by 12.5mg based on individual safety and tolerability. Concomitant Strong CYP3A4 Inhibitors: Consider dose reduction to a minimum of 37.5mg (GIST/RCC) or 25mg (pNET) daily. Concomitant CYP3A4 Inducer: Consider dose increase. Max: 87.5mg (GIST/RCC) or 62.5mg (pNET) daily.

HOW SUPPLIED: Cap: 12.5mg, 25mg, 50mg

WARNINGS/PRECAUTIONS: Interrupt therapy for Grade 3/4 hepatic adverse events; d/c if no resolution. May cause fetal harm; avoid pregnancy. Cardiovascular (CV) events, including decline in left ventricular ejection fraction (LVEF) to below lower limit of normal, reported; d/c in the presence of clinical manifestations of congestive heart failure, and interrupt and/or reduce dose with ejection fraction <50% and >20% below baseline. QT interval prolongation and torsades de pointes observed; caution with history of QT interval prolongation, or preexisting cardiac disease, bradycardia, or electrolyte disturbances. Monitor for HTN and treat PRN; suspend temporarily in cases of severe HTN. Hemorrhagic events, including tumor-related hemorrhage, reported. Observe closely for thyroid dysfunction; monitor thyroid function and treat if signs/symptoms occur. Cases of impaired wound healing reported; interrupt temporarily if patient will undergo major surgical procedures. Monitor for adrenal insufficiency in patients with stress, trauma, or severe infection.

ADVERSE REACTIONS: Fatigue, diarrhea, N/V, mucositis/stomatitis, abdominal pain, HTN, rash, hand-foot syndrome, skin discoloration, altered taste, anorexia, bleeding, hepatotoxicity.

INTERACTIONS: Caution with antiarrhythmics. Strong CYP3A4 inhibitors (eg, ketoconazole, itraconazole, clarithromycin, atazanavir, indinavir, nefazodone, nelfinavir, ritonavir, saquinavir, telithromycin, voriconazole) and grapefruit may increase plasma concentrations; consider dose reduction. CYP3A4 inducers (eg, dexamethasone, phenytoin, carbamazepine, rifampin, rifabutin, rifapentine, phenobarbital, St. John's wort) may decrease plasma concentrations; consider dose increase while monitoring for toxicity. Avoid with St. John's wort.

PREGNANCY: Category D, not for use in nursing.

MECHANISM OF ACTION: Multikinase inhibitor; inhibits multiple receptor tyrosine kinases, some of which are implicated in tumor growth, pathologic angiogenesis, and metastatic cancer progression.

PHARMACOKINETICS: Absorption: T_{max}=6-12 hrs. **Distribution:** V_d=2230L; plasma protein binding (95%). **Metabolism:** CYP3A4. **Elimination:** Feces (61%), renal (16%); $T_{1/2}$=40-60 hrs, 80-110 hrs (active metabolite).

NURSING CONSIDERATIONS

Assessment: Assess for cardiac events, electrolyte disturbances, pregnancy/nursing status, and possible drug interactions. Obtain baseline LFTs, LVEF, thyroid function, CBC with platelet count, serum chemistries (eg, phosphate), and renal function.

Monitoring: Monitor for signs/symptoms of CV events, HTN, hemorrhagic events, adrenal insufficiency, seizures, reversible posterior leukoencephalopathy syndrome, pancreatitis, hepatotoxicity, muscle toxicity, thrombotic microangiopathy, and proteinuria. Monitor LFTs, LVEF, ECG, electrolytes (magnesium, K⁺), thyroid function, CBC with platelet count, and serum chemistries (eg, phosphate).

Patient Counseling: Instruct to seek medical attention if GI disorders (eg, diarrhea, N/V, stomatitis, dyspepsia), skin discoloration, hair depigmentation, dermatological effects (eg, dryness, thickness/cracking of skin, blister/rash on palms of hands and soles of the feet), fatigue, HTN, bleeding, swelling, mouth pain/irritation, and taste disturbance occur. Advise to inform physician of all concomitant medications, including over-the-counter medications and dietary supplements. Inform of pregnancy risks; advise women of childbearing potential to avoid becoming pregnant.

Administration: Oral route. **Storage:** 25°C (77°F); excursions permitted to 15-30°C (59-86°F).

SYMBICORT RX
formoterol fumarate dihydrate - budesonide (AstraZeneca)

> Long-acting β₂-adrenergic agonists (LABA), such as formoterol, may increase the risk of asthma-related death. LABA may increase the risk of asthma-related hospitalization in pediatric and adolescent patients. Symbicort should only be used for patients not adequately controlled on a long-term asthma-control medications or whose disease severity clearly warrants initiation of treatment with both inhaled coticosteroids and LABA. Do not use Symbicort in patients whose asthma is adequately controlled on low- or medium-dose inhaled corticosteroids.

THERAPEUTIC CLASS: Corticosteroid/beta₂ agonist

INDICATIONS: Treatment of asthma in patients ≥12 yrs. Symbicort 160/4.5: Maintenance treatment of airflow obstruction in patients with chronic obstructive pulmonary disease (COPD), including chronic bronchitis and emphysema.

DOSAGE: *Adults:* Asthma: Initial: 2 inh bid (am/pm q12h). Individualize dose based on asthma severity. Max: 160/4.5mcg bid. Patients not responding to the starting dose after 1-2 weeks of therapy with 80/4.5, replace with 160/4.5 for better asthma control. COPD (160/4.5 only): 2 inh bid. If asthma symptoms or SOB occur in the period between doses, use short-acting β₂-agonist for immediate relief. Rinse mouth with water after use.
Pediatrics: ≥12 yrs: Asthma: Initial: 2 inh bid (am/pm q12h). Individualize dose based on asthma severity. Max: 160/4.5mcg bid. Patients not responding to the starting dose after 1-2 weeks of therapy with 80/4.5, replace with 160/4.5 for better asthma control. If asthma symptoms occur in the period between doses, use short-acting β₂-agonist for immediate relief. Rinse mouth with water after use.

HOW SUPPLIED: MDI: (Budesonide-Formoterol Fumarate Dihydrate)(80/4.5) 80mcg-4.5mcg/inh, (160/4.5) 160mcg-4.5mcg/inh [60 inhalations, 120 inhalations]

CONTRAINDICATIONS: Primary treatment of status asthmaticus or other acute asthma attacks or COPD requiring intensive measures.

WARNINGS/PRECAUTIONS: Should not be initiated during acutely/rapidly deteriorating or potentially life-threatening episodes of asthma or COPD. Increased use of inhaled, short-acting β_2-agonists is a marker of deteriorating asthma; reevaluate and reassess treatment regimen. Should not be used for relief of acute symptoms; inhaled short-acting β_2-agonists should be used. At treatment initiation, regular use of oral/inhaled short-acting β_2-agonists should be d/c. Should not be used more than recommended or at higher doses than recommended; cardiovascular (CV) effects & fatalities reported. Localized infection of the mouth and pharynx with *Candida albicans* reported; if develops, treat accordingly. Lower respiratory tract infections (eg, pneumonia) reported in patients with COPD. Increased susceptibility to infections; avoid exposure to chickenpox and measles. Caution in patients with active/quiescent tuberculosis; untreated systemic fungal, bacterial, viral, or parasitic infections; or ocular herpes simplex. Deaths due to adrenal insufficiency have occurred with transfer from systemic to inhaled corticosteroids. If withdrawn from systemic corticosteroids, resume oral corticosteroids during stress or severe asthma attack. Wean slowly from systemic corticosteroid use after transferring. Transferring from oral to inhalation therapy may unmask conditions (eg, rhinitis, conjunctivitis, eczema) previously suppressed by corticosteroids. Monitor for systemic corticosteroid effects such as hypercorticism and adrenal suppression (including adrenal crisis); if effects occur reduce dose slowly. May cause paradoxical bronchospasm; d/c immediately and institute alternative therapy. Immediate hypersensitivity reactions (eg, urticaria, angioedema, rash, bronchospasm) reported. CV effects may occur; caution with CV disorder (eg, coronary insufficiency, arrhythmia, HTN). Prolonged use may result in decreased bone mineral density, glaucoma, increased IOP and cataracts. May cause reduction in growth velocity in pediatric patients. Rare cases of eosinophilic conditions (eg, Churg-Strauss syndrome) reported. Caution with convulsive disorders, thyrotoxicosis, and hepatic impairment. May aggravate pre-existing diabetes mellitus and ketoacidosis. Hypokalemia and hyperglycemia may occur.

ADVERSE REACTIONS: Asthma: Nasopharyngitis, headache, upper respiratory tract infections, sinusitis, influenza, back pain, nasal congestion, stomach discomfort. COPD: nasopharyngitis, oral candidiasis, bronchitis, sinusitis, upper respiratory tract infection.

INTERACTIONS: Caution with concomitant use of strong CYP3A4 inhibitors (eg, ketoconazole, ritonavir, atazanavir, indinavir, nefazodone, nelfinavir, saquinavir, telithromycion, itraconazole, clarithromycin); may inhibit the metabolism and increase systemic exposure of budesonide. Caution with monoamine oxidase inhibitors or tricyclic antidepressants, or within 2 weeks of discontinuation of such agents. Concomitant use with β-blockers may block the pulmonary effect of formoterol and may produce severe bronchospasm in patients with asthma. Caution with non-K$^+$-sparing diuretics (eg, loop or thiazide); ECG changes and/or hypokalemia may develop. Do not use any additional inhaled LABAs for any reason, including prevention of exercise-induced bronchospasm or treatment of asthma or COPD. Caution with chronic use of drugs that can reduce bone mass (eg, anticonvulsants, oral corticosteroids).

PREGNANCY: Category C, not for use in nursing.

MECHANISM OF ACTION: Budesonide: Corticosteroid with anti-inflammatory activity; shown to have inhibitory effects on multiple cell types (eg, mast cells, eosinophils, neutrophils, macrophages, lymphocytes) and mediators (eg, histamine, eicosanoids, leukotrienes, cytokines) involved in allergic and non-allergic mediated inflammation. Formoterol: Long-acting selective β_2-adrenergic agonist; stimulates intracellular adenyl cyclase which catalyzes conversion of ATP to cAMP to produce relaxation of bronchial smooth muscle and inhibition of release of mediators of immediate hypersensitivity from cells, especially mast cells.

PHARMACOKINETICS: Absorption: (Asthma) Budesonide: Rapidly absorbed. C_{max}=4.5nmol/L; T_{max}=20 min. Formoterol: Rapidly absorbed. C_{max}=136pmol; T_{max}=10 min. (COPD) Budesonide: Rapid (lungs). C_{max}=3.3nmol/L; T_{max}=30 min. Formoterol: Rapid (GI). C_{max}=167pmol/L; T_{max}=15 min. **Distribution:** Budesonide: V_d=3L/kg; plasma protein binding (85-90%). Formoterol: Plasma protein binding (RR enantiomer, 46%), (SS enantiomer, 58%). **Metabolism:** Budesonide: Liver (rapid; extensive) via CYP3A4. Formoterol: Liver (direct glucuronidation and O-demethylation) via CYP2D6, CYP2C. **Elimination:** Budesonide: Urine (60%); feces. $T_{1/2}$=2-3 hrs. Formoterol: Urine (62%); feces (24%).

NURSING CONSIDERATIONS

Assessment: Assess if asthma is controlled by inhaled corticosteroids and occasional use of short-acting β_2-agonists. Assess for risk factors for decreased bone mineral content (eg, tobacco use, advanced age, sedentary lifestyle, family history of osteoporosis, drugs that decrease bone mass), or any other conditions where treatment is contraindicated or cautioned. Assess for pregnancy/nursing status and for possible drug interactions. Obtain baseline bone mineral density and lung function prior to therapy.

Monitoring: Monitor bone mineral density and lung function periodically. Perform periodic eye exams. Monitor for localized oral infections with *C. albicans*, decreased bone mass, upper airway symptoms, worsening or acutely deteriorating asthma, asthma instability (serial objective measures of airflow), body height in children, development of glaucoma, increased IOP, posterior subcapsular cataracts, adrenal insufficiency, paradoxical bronchospasm, eosinophilic conditions, pneumonia, and hypersensitivity reactions.

Patient Counseling: Inform about increased risk of asthma-related death and asthma-related hospitalization in pediatric and adolescent patients. Symbicort is not meant to relieve acute asthma symptoms or exacerbations of COPD and extra doses should not be used for that purpose. Notify physician immediately if experiencing decreased effectiveness of therapy, need more inhalations than usual, or significant decrease in lung function. Do not d/c without physician's guidance. Do not use with other long-acting β$_2$-agonists for asthma and COPD. Rinse the mouth after inhalation. Contact physician if develop symptoms of pneumonia. Avoid exposure to chickenpox or measles and, if exposed, consult physician without delay. Inform of potential worsening of existing tuberculosis, fungal, bacterial, viral, or parasitic infections, or ocular herpes simplex. Inform about risks of hypercorticism and adrenal suppression, decreased bone mineral density, cataracts or glaucoma and reduced growth velocity. Taper slowly from systemic corticosteroids if transferring to Symbicort. Inform of adverse effects associated with β$_2$-agonists, such as palpitations, chest pain, rapid HR, tremor, or nervousness. Keep out of reach of children.

Administration: Oral inhalation. Prime before use for the first time by releasing 2 test sprays into the air away from face; shake well for 5 sec before each spray. Prime again if inhaler has not been used for >7 days or when it has been dropped. Shake well for 5 sec before using. **Storage:** 20-25°C (68-77°F). Canister should be at room temperature before use. Store with mouthpiece down.

SYMBYAX   RX
fluoxetine HCl - olanzapine (Lilly)

> Antidepressants increased the risk of suicidal thinking and behavior (suicidality) in short-term studies in children, adolescents, and young adults with Major Depressive Disorder (MDD) and other psychiatric disorders. Monitor and observe closely for clinical worsening, suicidality or unusual changes in behavior in patients who are started on antidepressant therapy. Elderly patients with dementia-related psychosis treated with antipsychotic drugs are at an increased risk of death; most deaths appeared to be cardiovascular (eg, heart failure, sudden death) or infectious (eg, pneumonia) in nature. Symbyax is not approved for pediatric use or for the treatment of patients with dementia-related psychosis.

THERAPEUTIC CLASS: Thienobenzodiazepine/selective serotonin reuptake inhibitor

INDICATIONS: Acute treatment of depressive episodes associated with bipolar I disorder and treatment-resistant depression (MDD patients who do not respond to 2 separate trials of different antidepressants of adequate dose and duration in the current episode) in adults.

DOSAGE: *Adults:* Depressive Episodes Associated with Bipolar I Disorder/Treatment-Resistant Depression: Initial: 6mg-25mg qpm. Adjust dose based on efficacy and tolerability. Dosing Range: Depressive Episodes Associated with Bipolar I Disorder: 6mg-12mg (olanzapine) to 25mg-50mg (fluoxetine). Treatment-Resistant Depression: 6mg-18mg (olanzapine) to 25mg-50mg (fluoxetine). Max: 18mg-75mg/day. Periodically re-examine the need for continued pharmacotherapy. Hypotension Risk/Hepatic Impairment/Slow Metabolizers/Olanzapine-Sensitive: Initial: 3mg-25mg to 6mg-25mg qd. Take in the evening. Titrate: Increase cautiously. Pregnant: Taper dose of fluoxetine during 3rd trimester. Elderly: Start at the low end of dosing range.

HOW SUPPLIED: Cap: (Olanzapine-Fluoxetine HCl): 3mg-25mg, 6mg-25mg, 6mg-50mg, 12mg-25mg, 12mg-50mg

CONTRAINDICATIONS: During or within 14 days of d/c therapy with an MAOI, concomitant use with thioridazine or use of thioridazine within 5 weeks of d/c of Symbyax, and concomitant pimozide use.

WARNINGS/PRECAUTIONS: Neuroleptic malignant syndrome (NMS) reported; d/c and instill intensive symptomatic treatment and monitoring. May cause hyperglycemia; caution in patients with diabetes mellitus (DM) or having borderline increased blood glucose levels. Obtain FPG at the beginning of treatment and periodically during treatment. Hyperlipidemia reported; obtain lipid levels at baseline and periodically thereafter. May cause weight gain; regularly monitor weight. Serotonin syndrome or NMS-like reactions reported; d/c treatment and initiate supportive therapy. Anaphylactoid and pulmonary reactions reported; d/c if unexplained allergic reaction occurs. Tardive dyskinesia (TD) may develop; consider d/c if signs and symptoms of TD appear. May cause orthostatic hypotension; caution with cardiovascular disease, cerebrovascular disease, or conditions that predispose to hypotension. Leukopenia, neutropenia, and agranulocytosis reported; d/c at 1st sign of clinically significant decline in WBC without causative factors or if severe neutropenia (absolute neutrophil count <1000/mm³) develops. May cause esophageal dysmotility and aspiration. Not approved for treatment in patients with Alzheimer's disease. Caution in patients with history of seizures or with conditions that potentially lower the seizure threshold. May increase risk of bleeding events. Hyponatremia, hyperprolactinemia, and activation of mania/hypomania reported. May impair physical/mental abilities. May disrupt body's ability to reduce core body temperature. Caution with clinically significant prostatic hypertrophy, narrow-angle glaucoma, history of paralytic ileus or related conditions, cardiac patients, diseases or conditions affecting hemodynamic responses, hepatic impairment, and in elderly. Avoid abrupt withdrawal.

ADVERSE REACTIONS: Asthenia, somnolence, weight gain, increased appetite, disturbance in attention, peripheral edema, tremor, dry mouth, arthralgia, blurred vision, sedation, fatigue, flatulence, restlessness, hypersomnia.

INTERACTIONS: See Contraindications. Caution with CNS-active drugs, hepatotoxic drugs, and anticholinergic drugs. May enhance effects of certain antihypertensive agents. May potentiate orthostatic hypotension with diazepam and alcohol. Caution with other drugs that may affect the serotonergic neurotransmitter systems (eg, triptans, linezolid, lithium, tramadol, St. John's wort), and antipsychotics or other dopamine antagonists; risk for serotonin syndrome. Avoid with SSRIs, SNRIs, and tryptophan. Increased risk of bleeding events with aspirin, NSAIDs, warfarin, and other anticoagulants. Olanzapine: May antagonize levodopa and dopamine agonists. Inducers of CYP1A2 or glucuronyl transferase (eg, carbamazepine, omeprazole, rifampin) may increase clearance. CYP1A2 inhibitors (eg, fluvoxamine, some fluoroquinolone antibiotics) may decrease clearance. Fluoxetine: Monitor TCA (eg, imipramine, desipramine) and lithium levels. Increased risk of hyponatremia with diuretics. Caution with CYP2D6 substrates, including antidepressants (eg, TCAs), antipsychotics (eg, phenothiazines and most atypicals), vinblastine, and antiarrhythmics (eg, propafenone, flecainide). May increase levels of phenytoin, carbamazepine, haloperidol, clozapine, alprazolam. May cause a shift in plasma concentration with drugs that are tightly bound to protein (eg, coumadin, digitoxin) resulting in an adverse effect. May prolong half-life of diazepam. Rare reports of prolonged seizures with combined use of electroconvulsive therapy.

PREGNANCY: Category C, not for use in nursing.

MECHANISM OF ACTION: SSRI/Thienobenzodiazepine; unknown. Proposed that activation of 3 monoaminergic neural systems (serotonin, norepinephrine, and dopamine) is responsible for its enhanced antidepressant effect. Fluoxetine: SSRI; inhibits serotonin transport; weak inhibitor of norepinephrine and dopamine transporters. Olanzapine: Thienobenzodiazepine; psychotropic agent with high affinity binding to $5HT_{2a/2c}$, $5HT_6$, D_{1-4}, H_1, and adrenergic $(\alpha)_1$-receptors.

PHARMACOKINETICS: Absorption: Fluoxetine: C_{max}=15-55ng/mL, T_{max}=6-8 hrs. Olanzapine: Well absorbed; T_{max}=6 hrs. **Distribution:** Found in breast milk. Fluoxetine: Crosses placenta; plasma protein binding (94.5%). Olanzapine: V_d=1000L; plasma protein binding (93%). **Metabolism:** Fluoxetine: Liver (extensive) via CYP2D6; norfluoxetine (active metabolite). Olanzapine: Via direct glucuronidation and CYP450-mediated oxidation; 10-N-glucuronide and 4'-N-desmethyl olanzapine (major metabolites). **Elimination:** Fluoxetine: Kidneys; $T_{1/2}$=1-3 days (acute administration), 4-6 days (chronic administration). Olanzapine: Urine (57%), feces (30%); $T_{1/2}$=21-54 hrs.

NURSING CONSIDERATIONS

Assessment: Assess for MDD, bipolar mania, DM, renal/hepatic impairment, or any other conditions where treatment is contraindicated or cautioned. Assess for dementia-related psychosis, Alzheimer's disease in the elderly, pregnancy/nursing status, and possible drug interactions. Obtain baseline lipid panel, CBC, and FBG levels.

Monitoring: Monitor for signs/symptoms of NMS, serotonin syndrome, hyperglycemia, hyperlipidemia, weight gain, TD, orthostatic hypotension, and other adverse effects. Perform periodic monitoring of FPG, lipid levels, and weight of patient. Perform frequent monitoring of CBC in patients with a history of clinically significant low WBC or drug-induced leukopenia/neutropenia. In patients with clinically significant neutropenia, monitor for fever or other symptoms or signs of infection. In high-risk patients, monitor closely for a suicide attempt.

Patient Counseling: Inform about the benefits and risks of therapy. Counsel that treatment may induce clinical worsening and suicide risks. Inform that treatment is not approved for elderly patients with dementia-related psychosis. Instruct to avoid hazardous tasks (eg, operating machinery/driving), alcohol use, overheating, and dehydration. Instruct to notify physician if pregnant or intend to become pregnant, if rash or hives develop, and if taking, planning to take, or have stopped taking any prescription or over-the-counter drugs, including herbal supplements. Instruct not to breastfeed while on therapy. Inform that orthostatic hypotension, hyperglycemia, hyperlipidemia, weight gain, and hyponatremia may occur. Counsel to take exactly as prescribed; instruct to continue even if symptoms improve. Inform of the signs and symptoms associated with serotonin syndrome or NMS-like reactions and instruct to seek medical care if they develop. Counsel to report to physician any increased or unusual bruising or bleeding.

Administration: Oral route. **Storage:** 25°C (77°F); excursions permitted to 15-30°C (59-86°F). Keep tightly closed; protect from moisture.

S

SYMLIN RX
pramlintide acetate (Amylin)

> Use with insulin. Risk of insulin-induced severe hypoglycemia, particularly with type 1 diabetes mellitus (DM). Severe hypoglycemia usually occurs within 3 hrs of injection. Serious injuries may occur if severe hypoglycemia occurs while operating a motor vehicle, or heavy machinery, or other high-risk activities. Appropriate patient selection, careful patient instruction, and insulin dose adjustments are necessary to reduce this risk.

OTHER BRAND NAMES: SymlinPen (Amylin)

THERAPEUTIC CLASS: Synthetic amylin analog

INDICATIONS: Adjunct treatment in patients with type 1 or type 2 DM who use mealtime insulin therapy and who have failed to achieve desired glucose control despite optimal insulin therapy. May be used with or without sulfonylurea and/or metformin in type 2 DM.

DOSAGE: *Adults:* Before initiating therapy, reduce insulin dose by 50%. Monitor blood glucose frequently. Adjust insulin dose once target dose of pramlintide is maintained. Type 2 DM: Initial: 60mcg SQ immediately prior to meals. Titrate: 120mcg as tolerated. Type 1 DM: Initial: 15mcg SQ immediately prior to meals. Titrate: Increase by 15mcg increments to 30mcg or 60mcg as tolerated.

HOW SUPPLIED: Inj: 600mcg/mL [5mL]; Pen injector: 1000mcg/mL [1.5mL, 2.7mL]

CONTRAINDICATIONS: Confirmed diagnosis of gastroparesis; hypoglycemia unawareness.

WARNINGS/PRECAUTIONS: Do not mix with insulin; administer as separate injections.

ADVERSE REACTIONS: N/V, headache, anorexia, abdominal pain, fatigue, dizziness, coughing, pharyngitis.

INTERACTIONS: Do not administer with agents that alter GI motility (eg, anticholinergic agents such as atropine), and agents that slow intestinal absorption of nutrients (eg, α-glucosidase inhibitors). Administer analgesics and other oral agents that require rapid onset 1 hr before or 2 hrs after injection.

PREGNANCY: Category C, caution in nursing.

MECHANISM OF ACTION: Amylinomimetic agent that modulates gastric emptying, prevents postprandial rise in plasma glucagon, and produces satiety, which leads to a decreased caloric intake.

PHARMACOKINETICS: Absorption: Absolute bioavailability (30-40%); SQ administration of variable doses resulted in different parameters. **Distribution:** Not extensively bound to blood cells or albumin (40% unbound). **Metabolism:** Kidneys (primarily). Des-lys pramlintide (primary active metabolite). **Elimination:** $T_{1/2}$=48 min.

NURSING CONSIDERATIONS

Assessment: Assess whether patient does or does not have confirmed diagnosis of gastroparesis or hypoglycemia unawareness. Evaluate patient's HbA1c, recent blood glucose monitoring data, history of insulin-induced hypoglycemia, current insulin regimen, and body weight. Assess if patient has failed to achieve proper glycemic control despite individualized insulin management. Assess use in patients with visual or dexterity impairment. Assess for possible drug interactions and pregnancy/nursing status.

Monitoring: Monitor for signs/symptoms of hypoglycemia (eg, hunger, headache, sweating, tremor) when using in combination with insulin. Monitor proper glucose control through serum blood glucose levels and HbA1c test.

Patient Counseling: Instruct to never mix with insulin and not to transfer from pen injector to syringe. If dose missed, wait until next scheduled dose and administer usual amount. Administer immediately prior to each major meal (≥250 calories or ≥30g of carbohydrates). Insulin dose adjustments should be made only by healthcare professional. Patients should have fast-acting sugar (eg, hard candy, glucose tablet, juice) at all times. Self-glucose monitoring should be done on a daily basis. Counsel about signs/symptoms of hypoglycemia (eg, hunger, headache, sweating, tremor, irritability). Instruct regarding the critical importance of maintaining proper glucose control, especially when operating heavy machinery (eg, motor vehicles).

Administration: SQ injection to abdomen or thigh; administration to the arm is not recommended because of variable absorption. Rotate injection sites; injection site should be distinct from site for any concomitant insulin injection. Allow to come to room temperature before injecting. **Storage:** Pen injectors and vials not in use: 2-8°C (36-40°F). Do not freeze. Do not use if frozen. Pen injectors and vials in use: After 1st use, refrigerate or keep at a temperature <30°C (86°F). Use within 30 days.

SYNERA   RX
lidocaine - tetracaine (Endo)

THERAPEUTIC CLASS: Acetamide local anesthetic

INDICATIONS: For use on intact skin to provide local dermal analgesia for superficial venous access and superficial dermatological procedures such as excision, electrodessication, and shave biopsy of skin lesions.

DOSAGE: *Adults:* Venipuncture or IV Cannulation: Apply to intact skin for 20-30 min prior to procedure. Superficial Dermatological Procedures: Apply to intact skin for 30 min prior to procedure.
Pediatrics: ≥3 yrs: Venipuncture or IV Cannulation: Apply to intact skin for 20-30 min prior to procedure. Superficial Dermatological Procedure: Apply to intact skin for 30 min prior to procedure.

HOW SUPPLIED: Patch: (Lidocaine-Tetracaine) 70mg-70mg

CONTRAINDICATIONS: PABA hypersensitivity.

WARNINGS/PRECAUTIONS: Serious adverse events may occur in children or pets if ingested. Caution in acutely ill or debilitated patients. Risk of allergic/anaphylactoid reactions (eg, urticaria, angioedema, bronchospasm, shock). Increased risk of toxicity in severe hepatic disease. Avoid broken or inflamed skin, eye contact, use on a larger area or for longer duration than recommended.

ADVERSE REACTIONS: Erythema, blanching, edema, urticaria, angioedema, bronchospasm, shock.

INTERACTIONS: Additive toxic effect with concomitant Class I antiarrhythmics (eg, tocainide, mexiletine). Consider total amount absorbed from all formulations with other local anesthetics.

PREGNANCY: Category B, caution in nursing.

MECHANISM OF ACTION: Lidocaine: Amide-type local anesthetic; blocks Na^+ channels required for initiation and conduction of neuronal impulses. Tetracaine: Ester-type local anesthetic; blocks Na^+ channels required for initiation and conduction of neuronal impulses.

PHARMACOKINETICS: Absorption: C_{max}=1.7ng/mL (lidocaine), <0.9ng/mL (tetracaine); T_{max}=1.7 hrs. (lidocaine). **Distribution:** Lidocaine: V_d=0.8-1.3 L/kg; plasma protein binding (75%); crosses placenta. **Metabolism:** Lidocaine: CYP1A2, CYP3A4 (N-deethylation). Monoethylglycinexylidide, glycinexylidide (active metabolites). Tetracaine: Plasma esterases (hydrolysis). **Elimination:** Lidocaine: Urine; $T_{1/2}$=1.8 hrs.

NURSING CONSIDERATIONS

Assessment: Assess for pseudocholinesterase deficiency, possible drug interactions, cardiac and hepatic impairment.

Monitoring: Monitor for allergic or anaphylactoid reactions (eg, erythema, blanching, edema), cardiac and hepatic dysfunction.

Patient Counseling: Inform that use may lead to diminished or blocked sensation in treated skin. Instruct to wash hands after application; avoid contact with eyes; remove patch before MRI.

Administration: Transdermal route. **Storage:** 25°C (77°F) excursions permitted to 15-30°C (59-86°F).

SYNERCID   RX
dalfopristin - quinupristin (Monarch Pharmaceuticals Inc.)

THERAPEUTIC CLASS: Streptogramin

INDICATIONS: Treatment of complicated skin and skin structure infections (cSSSI) caused by *Staphylococcus aureus* (methicillin-susceptible) or *Streptococcus pyogenes*.

DOSAGE: *Adults:* Usual: 7.5mg/kg IV q12h for at least 7 days. Hepatic Cirrhosis (Child Pugh A or B): May need dose reduction. Infuse over 60 min.
Pediatrics: ≥12 yrs: Usual: 7.5mg/kg IV q12h for at least 7 days. Hepatic Cirrhosis (Child Pugh A or B): May need dose reduction. Infuse over 60 min.

HOW SUPPLIED: Inj: (Dalfopristin-Quinupristin) 350mg-150mg

WARNINGS/PRECAUTIONS: *Clostridium difficile*-associated diarrhea (CDAD) reported. Flush vein with D5W following infusion to minimize venous irritation; do not flush with saline or heparin. Arthralgia, myalgia, and total bilirubin elevation reported. May result in bacterial resistance with prolonged use or use in the absence of a proven/suspected bacterial infection or a prophylactic indication; take appropriate measures if superinfection develops.

ADVERSE REACTIONS: Infusion-site reactions (eg, inflammation, pain, edema), N/V, pain, rash, hyperbilirubinemia, arthralgia, myalgia.

INTERACTIONS: Caution with drugs metabolized by CYP3A4; may increase plasma levels (eg, cyclosporine A, tacrolimus, midazolam, dihydropyridine calcium channel blockers [eg, nifedipine], verapamil, diltiazem, astemizole, terfenadine, delaviridine, nevirapine, indinavir, ritonavir, vinca alkaloids [eg, vinblastine], docetaxel, paclitaxel, diazepam, cisapride, HMG-CoA reductase inhibitors [eg, lovastatin], methylprednisolone, carbamazepine, quinidine, lidocaine, disopyramide). Monitor cyclosporine levels. Avoid drugs metabolized by CYP3A4 that prolong QTc interval. May inhibit gut metabolism of digoxin.

PREGNANCY: Category B, caution in nursing.

MECHANISM OF ACTION: Streptogramin antibiotic; components act synergistically on bacterial ribosome. Dalfopristin: Inhibits the early phase of protein synthesis. Quinupristin: Inhibits the late phase of protein synthesis.

PHARMACOKINETICS: Absorption: Quinupristin: C_{max}=3.2μg/mL, AUC=7.2μg•hr/mL; Dalfopristin: C_{max}=7.96μg/mL, AUC=10.57μg•hr/mL. **Distribution:** Quinupristin: V_d=0.45L/kg; Dalfopristin: V_d=0.24L/kg. **Metabolism:** Quinupristin: 2 conjugated active metabolites (1 with glutathione; 1 with cysteine); Dalfopristin: 1 nonconjugated active metabolite, via hydrolysis. **Elimination:** Urine: 15% (quinupristin), 19% (dalfopristin), feces (75-77%); $T_{1/2}$=0.85 hrs (quinupristin), 0.70 hrs (dalfopristin).

NURSING CONSIDERATIONS

Assessment: Assess for hepatic impairment, pregnancy/nursing status, and for possible drug interactions (eg, concurrent administration with cyclosporine).

Monitoring: Monitor for CDAD, venous irritation, arthralgia, myalgia, superinfection, and for hyperbilirubinemia. Monitor liver and renal function.

Patient Counseling: Inform about risks/benefits of therapy. Instruct to notify physician if any adverse reactions occur such as watery and bloody stools (with or without stomach cramps and fever), if pregnant/nursing, and of all prescription/nonprescription drugs being taken.

Administration: IV route. Infuse over 60 min; flush only with D5W to minimize venous irritation. Inspect for particulate matter prior to administration. Do not dilute with saline solution. Refer to PI for detailed preparation and information on compatibility. **Storage:** Before reconstitution, store in refrigerator at 2-8°C (36-46°F); diluted solution stable for 5 hrs at room temperature or for 54 hrs if refrigerated at 2-8°C (36-46°F). Do not freeze.

SYNTHROID RX
levothyroxine sodium (Abbott)

> Do not use for the treatment of obesity or weight loss; doses within range of daily hormonal requirements are ineffective for weight reduction in euthyroid patients. Serious or life-threatening manifestations of toxicity may occur when given in larger doses, particularly when given in association with sympathomimetic amines.

THERAPEUTIC CLASS: Thyroid replacement hormone

INDICATIONS: Replacement or supplemental therapy in congenital or acquired hypothyroidism of any etiology, except transient hypothyroidism during the recovery phase of subacute thyroiditis. Treatment or prevention of various types of euthyroid goiters, including thyroid nodules, subacute or chronic lymphocytic thyroiditis, multinodular goiter and as an adjunct to surgery and radioiodine therapy for thyrotropin-dependent well-differentiated thyroid cancer.

DOSAGE: *Adults:* Individualize dose. Adjust dose based on periodic assessment of patient's clinical response and laboratory parameters. Give qd, preferably 30 min to 1 hr before breakfast. Take at least 4 hrs apart from drugs that are known to interfere with its absorption. Hypothyroidism: Usual: 1.7mcg/kg/day. >200mcg/day seldom required. >50 yrs/<50 yrs with Cardiac Disease: Initial: 25-50mcg/day. Titrate: Increase by 12.5-25mcg increments every 6-8 weeks as needed. Elderly with Cardiac Disease: Initial: 12.5-25mcg/day. Titrate: Increase by 12.5-25mcg increments every 4-6 weeks until euthyroid. Severe Hypothyroidism: Initial: 12.5-25mcg/day. Titrate: Increase by 25mcg/day every 2-4 weeks until TSH level normalized. Secondary (Pituitary) or Tertiary (Hypothalamic) Hypothyroidism: Titrate: Increase until clinically euthyroid and the serum free-T4 level is restored to the upper half of the normal range. Pregnancy: May increase dose requirements. Subclinical Hypothyroidism: Lower doses may be adequate to normalize the serum TSH level (eg, 1mcg/kg/day). TSH Suppression in Well-Differentiated Thyroid Cancer and Thyroid Nodules: Individualize dose based on the specific disease and the patient being treated. Refer to PI for further details.

Pediatrics: Individualize dose. Adjust dose based on periodic assessment of patient's clinical response and laboratory parameters. Give qd, preferably 30 min to 1 hr before breakfast. Take at least 4 hrs apart from drugs that are known to interfere with its absorption. Hypothyroidism: Growth/Puberty Complete: Usual: 1.7mcg/kg/day. >12 yrs (Growth/Puberty Incomplete):

2-3mcg/kg/day. 6-12 yrs: 4-5mcg/kg/day. 1-5 yrs: 5-6mcg/kg/day. 6-12 months: 6-8mcg/kg/day. 3-6 months: 8-10mcg/kg/day. 0-3 months: 10-15mcg/kg/day. Infants at Risk for Cardiac Failure: Use lower dose (eg, 25mcg/day). Titrate: Increase dose every 4-6 weeks as needed. Infants with Serum T4 <5mcg/dL: Initial: 50mcg/day. Chronic/Severe Hypothyroidism: Children: Initial: 25mcg/day. Titrate: Increase by 25mcg increments every 2-4 weeks until desired effect is achieved. Minimize Hyperactivity in Older Children: Initial: Give 1/4 of full replacement dose. Titrate: Increase on a weekly basis by an amount equal to 1/4 the full recommended replacement dose until the full recommended replacement dose is reached. May crush tab and mix with 5-10mL of water.

HOW SUPPLIED: Tab: 25mcg*, 50mcg*, 75mcg*, 88mcg*, 100mcg*, 112mcg*, 125mcg*, 137mcg*, 150mcg*, 175mcg*, 200mcg*, 300mcg* *scored

CONTRAINDICATIONS: Untreated subclinical (suppressed serum TSH level with normal T3 level and T4 levels) or overt thyrotoxicosis of any etiology, acute myocardial infarction (MI), and uncorrected adrenal insufficiency.

WARNINGS/PRECAUTIONS: Should not be used in the treatment of male or female infertility unless associated with hypothyroidism. Contraindicated in patients with nontoxic diffuse goiter or nodular thyroid disease, particularly in elderly or with underlying cardiovascular (CV) disease if serum TSH level is already suppressed; use with caution if TSH level is not suppressed and carefully monitor thyroid function. Has narrow therapeutic index; carefully titrate dose to avoid over- or under-treatment. May decrease bone mineral density (BMD) with long-term use; give minimum dose necessary to achieve desired clinical and biochemical response. Caution with CV disorders and the elderly. If cardiac symptoms develop or worsen, reduce or withhold dose for 1 week and then restart at lower dose. Overtreatment may produce CV effects (eg, increase HR, increase in cardiac wall thickness, increase in cardiac contractility, precipitation of angina or arrhythmias). Monitor patients with coronary artery disease (CAD) closely during surgical procedures; may precipitate cardiac arrhythmias. Caution in patients with diabetes mellitus (DM). Patients with concomitant adrenal insufficiency should be treated with replacement glucocorticoids prior to therapy.

ADVERSE REACTIONS: Fatigue, increased appetite, weight loss, heat intolerance, headache, hyperactivity, irritability, insomnia, palpitations, arrhythmias, dyspnea, hair loss, menstrual irregularities, pseudotumor cerebri (children), slipped capital femoral epiphysis (children).

INTERACTIONS: Concurrent sympathomimetics may increase effects of sympathomimetics or thyroid hormone and may increase risk of coronary insufficiency with CAD. Upward dose adjustments may be needed for insulin and oral hypoglycemic agents. May decrease absorption with soybean flour, cottonseed meal, walnuts, and dietary fiber. May potentiate oral anticoagulant effects; adjust dose and monitor PT. May decrease levels and effects of digitalis glycosides. Reduced TSH secretion with dopamine/dopamine agonists, glucocorticoids, octreotide. Decreased thyroid hormone secretion with aminoglutethimide, amiodarone, iodine (including iodine-containing radiographic contrast agents), lithium, methimazole, propylthiouracil (PTU), sulfonamides, tolbutamide. May increase thyroid hormone secretion with amiodarone and iodide. May decrease T4 absorption with antacids (aluminum & magnesium hydroxides), simethicone, bile acid sequestrants (cholestyramine, colestipol), calcium carbonate, cation exchange resins (kayexalate), ferrous sulfate, orlistat, and sucralfate; administer at least 4 hrs apart. May increase serum thyroxine-binding globulin (TBG) concentrations with clofibrate, estrogen-containing oral contraceptives, oral estrogens, heroin/methadone, 5-fluorouracil, mitotane, and tamoxifen. May decrease serum TBG concentrations with androgens/anabolic steroids, asparaginase, glucocorticoids, and slow-release nicotinic acid. May cause protein-binding site displacement with furosemide (>80mg IV), heparin, hydantoins, NSAIDs (fenamates, phenylbutazone), and salicylates (>2g/day). May alter T4 and T3 metabolism with carbamazepine, hydantoins, phenobarbital, and rifampin. May decrease T4 5'-deiodinase activity with amiodarone, β-adrenergic antagonists (eg, propranolol >160mg/day), glucocorticoids (eg, dexamethasone ≥4mg/day), and PTU. Concurrent use with tri/tetracyclic antidepressants may increase the therapeutic and toxic effects of both drugs. Coadministration with sertraline in patients stabilized on levothyroxine may result in increased levothyroxine requirements. Interferon-α may cause development of antithyroid microsomal antibodies and transient hypothyroidism, hyperthyroidism, or both. Interleukin-2 has been associated with transient painless thyroiditis. Excessive use with growth hormones (eg, somatropin, somatrem) may accelerate epiphyseal closure. Ketamine may produce marked HTN and tachycardia. May reduce uptake of radiographic agents. Decreased theophylline clearance may occur in hypothyroid patients. Altered levels of thyroid hormone and/or TSH levels with choral hydrate, diazepam, ethionamide, lovastatin, metoclopramide, 6-mercaptopurine, nitroprusside, para-aminosalicylate sodium, perphenazine, resorcinol (excessive topical use), and thiazide diuretics.

PREGNANCY: Category A, caution in nursing.

MECHANISM OF ACTION: Thyroid replacement hormone; mechanism not established. Suspected that principal effects are exterted through control of DNA transcription and protein synthesis.

PHARMACOKINETICS: Absorption: Majority absorbed from jejunum and upper ileum. **Distribution:** Plasma protein binding (>99%); found in breast milk. **Metabolism:** Sequential

S

deiodination and conjugation in the liver (mainly), kidneys, and other tissues. **Elimination:** Urine; feces (approximately 20% unchanged). $T_{1/2}$=6-7 days (T4), ≤2 days (T3).

NURSING CONSIDERATIONS

Assessment: Assess for untreated subclinical or overt thyrotoxicosis, acute MI, uncorrected adrenal insufficiency, age, CAD, CV disorders, nontoxic diffuse goiter, nodular thyroid disease, DM, hypersensitivity, pregnancy/nursing status, and for possible drug interactions. In patients with secondary or tertiary hypothyroidism, assess for additional hypothalamic/pituitary hormone deficiencies. Assess for weight and TSH levels. In infants with congenital hypothyroidism, assess for other congenital anomalies.

Monitoring: Monitor for CV effects. In patients on long-term therapy, monitor for signs/symptoms of decreased BMD. In patients with nontoxic diffuse goiter or nodular thyroid disease, monitor for precipitation of thyrotoxicosis. In adults with primary hypothyroidism, perform periodic monitoring of serum TSH levels. In pediatric patients with congenital hypothyroidism, perform periodic monitoring of serum TSH levels and total or free T4 levels. In patients with secondary and tertiary hypothyroidism, perform periodic monitoring of serum free T4 levels.

Patient Counseling: Instruct to notify physician if allergic to any foods or medicines, pregnant or plan to become pregnant, breastfeeding or taking any other drugs, including prescriptions and over-the-counter preparations. Notify physician of any other medical conditions particularly heart disease, diabetes, clotting disorders, and adrenal or pituitary gland problems. Instruct not to stop or change dose unless directed by physician. Take on empty stomach, at least 1/2 to 1 hr before eating breakfast. Advise that partial hair loss may occur during the first few months of therapy, but is usually temporary. Notify physician or dentist prior to surgery about levothyroxine therapy. Inform that drug should not be used for weight control. Instruct to notify physician if rapid or irregular heartbeat, chest pain, SOB, leg cramps, headache, or any other unusual medical event occurs. Inform that dose may be increased during pregnancy. Inform that drug should not be administered within 4 hrs of agents such as iron/calcium supplements and antacids.

Administration: Oral route. **Storage:** 25°C (77°F); excursions permitted to 15-30°C (59-86°F). Protect from light and moisture.

TACHOSIL RX
absorbable fibrin sealant (Baxter)

THERAPEUTIC CLASS: Topical thrombin/fibrinogen

INDICATIONS: Adjunct to hemostasis for use in cardiovascular surgery when control of bleeding by standard surgical techniques (eg, suture, ligature; or cautery) is ineffective or impractical.

DOSAGE: *Adults:* Apply the yellow, active side of the patch to the bleeding area and hold in place with gentle pressure for at least 3 min. Number of patches to be applied should be determined by the size of the bleeding area. Max: 7 patches sized 9.5 x 4.8cm, 14 patches sized 4.8 x 4.8cm, or 42 patches sized 3.0 x 2.5cm.

HOW SUPPLIED: Patch: (Human fibrinogen-Human thrombin) 5.5mg-2.0 U/cm² [9.5cm x 4.8cm, 1 patch; 4.8cm x 4.8cm, 2 patches; 3.0cm x 2.5cm, 1 patch, 5 patches]

CONTRAINDICATIONS: Intravascular application, known anaphylactic or severe systemic reaction to horse proteins.

WARNINGS/PRECAUTIONS: Do not use in renal pelvis or ureter procedures, closure of skin incisions, or neurological procedures. Do not use for the treatment of severe or brisk arterial bleeding and as a primary mode of control. Not intended as a substitute for meticulous surgical technique and proper application of suture, ligature, or conventional procedures for hemostasis. Hypersensitivity or allergic/anaphylactoid reactions may occur with 1st-time or repetitive application; d/c if this hypersensitivity reaction occurs. Do not leave patch in an infected or contaminated space; may potentiate existing infection. Avoid over-packing when placing into cavities or closed spaces; may cause tissue compression. Use only minimum amount of patches necessary to achieve hemostasis. Carefully remove or reposition unattached pieces of patch if necessary. Made from human plasma; may carry risk of transmitting infectious agents, eg, viruses and theoretically, the Creutzfeldt-Jakob disease (CJD) agent.

ADVERSE REACTIONS: Atrial fibrillation, pleural effusion, hemorrhagic anemia, tachyarrhythmia, pyrexia, pericardial effusion, post-procedural hemorrhage.

PREGNANCY: Category C, caution in nursing.

MECHANISM OF ACTION: Topical thrombin/fibrinogen; soluble fibrinogen is transformed into fibrin by enzymatic action of thrombin, which polymerizes into a fibrin clot that adheres the collagen patch to the wound surface and achieves hemostasis.

NURSING CONSIDERATIONS

Assessment: Assess for hypersensitivity reactions to human blood products or horse proteins, size of the bleeding area, and pregnancy/nursing status.

Monitoring: Monitor for signs/symptoms of hypersensitivity or allergic/anaphylactoid reactions and for the transmission of infectious agents (eg, viruses, CJD).

Patient Counseling: Advise that drug is made from human blood, and it may carry a risk of transmitting infectious agents, (eg, viruses, CJD agent). Instruct to consult physician if symptoms of B19 virus infection appear (fever, drowsiness, chills, and runny nose, followed about 2 weeks later by a rash and joint pain).

Administration: Topical route. Refer to PI for preparation and application of patch. **Storage:** 2-25°C (36-77°F). Does not require refrigeration. Do not freeze.

TAMBOCOR   RX
flecainide acetate (Graceway)

> Excessive mortality and higher rate of nonfatal cardiac arrest reported in patients with asymptomatic non-life-threatening ventricular arrhythmias and myocardial infarction (MI) >6 days but <2 yrs prior. Class 1C antiarrhythmic use is unacceptable without life-threatening ventricular arrhythmias. Not recommended for chronic atrial fibrillation. Case reports of ventricular proarrhythmic effects with atrial fibrillation/flutter (A-fib/A-flutter).

THERAPEUTIC CLASS: Class IC antiarrhythmic

INDICATIONS: Prevention of paroxysmal supraventricular tachycardias (PSVT) associated with disabling symptoms, paroxysmal A-fib/A-flutter (PAF) associated with disabling symptoms, and documented ventricular arrhythmias, such as sustained ventricular tachycardia (VT).

DOSAGE: *Adults:* PSVT/PAF: Initial: 50mg q12h. Titrate: May increase by 50mg bid q4 days. Max: 300mg/day. Sustained VT: Initial: 100mg q12h. Titrate: May increase by 50mg bid q4 days. Max: 400mg/day. Severe Renal Impairment (CrCl ≤35mL/min): Initial: 100mg qd or 50mg bid. Less Severe Renal Disease: Initial: 100mg q12h. Reduce dose by 50% with amiodarone.
Pediatrics: >6 months: Initial: 100mg/m^2/day given bid-tid. <6 months: Initial: 50mg/m^2/day given bid-tid. Max: 200mg/m^2/day. Reduce dose by 50% with amiodarone.

HOW SUPPLIED: Tab: 50mg, 100mg*, 150mg* *scored

CONTRAINDICATIONS: Right bundle branch block associated with left hemiblock (without a pacemaker), preexisting 2nd- or 3rd-degree atrioventricular (AV) block, cardiogenic shock.

WARNINGS/PRECAUTIONS: May cause or worsen congestive heart failure (CHF) and arrhythmias; caution if history of CHF or myocardial dysfunction. Slows cardiac conduction; dose-related increases in PR, QRS, and QT intervals reported. Conduction changes may cause sinus pause, sinus arrest, bradycardia, 2nd- or 3rd-degree AV block. D/C if 2nd- or 3rd-degree AV block or right bundle branch block associated with a left hemiblock occurs, unless a ventricular pacemaker is in place. Extreme caution with sick sinus syndrome. May increase endocardial pacing thresholds and suppress ventricular escape rhythms; caution in patients with permanent pacemakers or temporary pacing electrodes. Correct hypokalemia or hyperkalemia before therapy. Trough level monitoring recommended, especially with significant hepatic impairment, CHF and moderate to severe renal impairment. Start treatment of adults with sustained VT and pediatric patients in the hospital with rhythm monitoring.

ADVERSE REACTIONS: Arrhythmias, cardiac arrest, CHF, dizziness, visual disturbances, headache, fatigue, nausea, palpitations, dyspnea, chest/abdominal pain, asthenia, edema, tremor, constipation.

INTERACTIONS: Additive negative inotropic effects with β-blockers (eg, propranolol). Levels increased by cimetidine, amiodarone, CYP2D6 inhibitors (eg, quinidine); monitor trough flecainide levels when coadministered with amioradone. Coadministration may increase digoxin levels. Increased elimination with known enzyme inducers (phenytoin, phenobarbital, carbamazepine). Avoid with diltiazem, nifedipine, verapamil, disopyramide. Milk may inhibit absorption in infants; monitor flecainide levels during major changes in milk intake.

PREGNANCY: Category C, safety not known in nursing.

MECHANISM OF ACTION: Class 1C antiarrhythmic agent with local anesthetic activity; decreases intracardiac conduction in all parts of the heart with greatest effect on His-Purkinje system (H-V conduction).

PHARMACOKINETICS: Absorption: Complete; T_{max}=3 hrs. **Distribution:** Plasma protein binding (40%); found in breast milk. **Metabolism:** Extensive, via CYP2D6; meta-O-dealkylated flecainide (active metabolite). **Elimination:** Urine (30% unchanged), feces (5%); $T_{1/2}$=20 hrs, 29 hrs (at birth), 11-12 hrs (3 months), 6 hrs (1 yr), 8 hrs (1-12 yrs), and 11-12 hrs (12-15 yrs).

T

NURSING CONSIDERATIONS

Assessment: Assess for preexisting 2nd- or 3rd-degree AV block, right bundle branch block associated with a left hemiblock, asymptomatic non-life-threatening ventricular arrhythmia, A-fib/A-flutter, supraventricular tachycardia, implanted pacemaker, cardiogenic shock, MI, cardiomyopathy, preexisting CHF or low ejection fraction, sick sinus syndrome, hypersensitivity, pregnancy/nursing status, renal/hepatic impairment and possible drug interactions. Correct hypokalemia or hyperkalemia prior to therapy.

Monitoring: Determine pacing threshold in patients with pacemaker prior to therapy, after 1 week, and at regular intervals thereafter. Periodically monitor plasma levels with renal/hepatic impairment, CHF, and/or those on concurrent amiodarone therapy. Monitor HR, ECG changes, paradoxical increase in ventricular rate, proarrhythmic effects (new or worsened supraventricular/ventricular arrhythmias), worsening of CHF, effects on cardiac conduction, bradycardia, and hypersensitivity reactions.

Patient Counseling: Inform about risks/benefits of therapy and to report any adverse reactions to physician.

Administration: Oral route. Initiate treatment of sustained VT in the hospital with rhythm monitoring. **Storage:** 15-30°C (59-86°F); tight, light-resistant container.

TAMIFLU   RX
oseltamivir phosphate (Genentech)

THERAPEUTIC CLASS: Neuraminidase inhibitor

INDICATIONS: Treatment of uncomplicated acute illness due to influenza in patients ≥1 yr who have been symptomatic for no more than 2 days. Prophylaxis of influenza in patients ≥1 yr.

DOSAGE: *Adults:* Treatment: Begin within 2 days of onset of symptoms. Usual: 75mg bid for 5 days. CrCl 10-30mL/min: Usual: 75mg qd for 5 days. Prophylaxis: Begin within 2 days of exposure. Usual: 75mg qd for at least 10 days. CrCl 10-30mL/min: Usual: 75mg qod or 30mg qd. Community Outbreak: Usual: 75mg qd. May use up to 6 weeks in immunocompetent and up to 12 weeks in immunocompromised patients. Refer to PI for treatment and prophylaxis dosing using PO sus in patients who cannot swallow cap.
Pediatrics: Treatment: ≥13 yrs: Begin within 2 days of onset of symptoms. Usual: 75mg bid for 5 days. ≥1 yr: 5-Day Regimen: ≤15kg: 30mg bid. 16-23kg: 45mg bid. 24-40kg: 60mg bid. ≥41kg: 75mg bid. Prophylaxis: Begin within 2 days of exposure. ≥13 yrs: Usual: 75mg qd for at least 10 days. ≥1 yr: 10-Day Regimen: ≤15kg: 30mg qd. 16-23kg: 45mg qd. 24-40kg: 60mg qd. ≥41kg: 75mg qd. Community Outbreak: ≥13 yrs: Usual: 75mg qd. May use up to 6 weeks in immunocompetent and up to 12 weeks in immunocompromised patients. ≥1 yr: May continue dosing for up to 6 weeks. Refer to PI for treatment and prophylaxis dosing using PO sus in patients who cannot swallow cap.

HOW SUPPLIED: Cap: 30mg, 45mg, 75mg; Sus: 6mg/mL [60mL]

WARNINGS/PRECAUTIONS: Anaphylaxis and serious skin reactions (eg, toxic epidermal necrolysis, Stevens-Johnson syndrome, erythema multiforme) reported; d/c and initiate appropriate treatment if an allergic-like reaction occurs or is suspected. Neuropsychiatric events (eg, hallucinations, delirium, abnormal behavior) leading to injury and in some cases resulting in fatal outcomes reported; monitor for abnormal behavior and evaluate risks and benefits of continuing treatment if neuropsychiatric symptoms occur. Has not been shown to prevent serious bacterial infections initially presenting with influenza-like symptoms or that may coexist with/occur as complications during course of influenza. Efficacy in treatment of influenza in patients with chronic cardiac disease and/or respiratory disease not established. Efficacy in treatment or prophylaxis of influenza in immunocompromised patients and in patients who begin treatment after 48 hrs of symptoms not established. Not a substitute for early vaccination on an annual basis. No evidence for efficacy in any illness caused by agents other than influenza viruses types A and B. Consider available information on influenza drug susceptibility patterns and treatment effects when deciding whether to use therapy.

ADVERSE REACTIONS: N/V, diarrhea, cough, headache, fatigue, abdominal pain, otitis media, asthma, epistaxis.

INTERACTIONS: Avoid administration of live attenuated influenza vaccine within 2 weeks before or 48 hrs after oseltamivir unless medically indicated. Probenecid may increase exposure.

PREGNANCY: Category C, caution in nursing.

MECHANISM OF ACTION: Neuraminidase inhibitor; inhibits influenza virus neuraminidase, affecting release of viral particles.

PHARMACOKINETICS: Absorption: Readily absorbed. Oseltamivir: C_{max}=65ng/mL; AUC_{0-12h}=112ng•h/mL. Oseltamivir carboxylate: C_{max}=348ng/mL; AUC_{0-12h}=2719ng•h/mL. **Distribution:** Oseltamivir: Plasma protein binding (42%). Oseltamivir carboxylate: Plasma protein binding (3%). (IV) V_d=23-26L. **Metabolism:** Extensive via hepatic esterases; oseltamivir carboxylate (active metabolite). **Elimination:** Oseltamivir carboxylate: Renal (>99%); $T_{1/2}$=6-10 hrs. Oseltamivir: $T_{1/2}$=1-3 hrs.

NURSING CONSIDERATIONS

Assessment: Assess for drug hypersensitivity, renal impairment, pregnancy/nursing status, and possible drug interactions.

Monitoring: Monitor for signs/symptoms of neuropsychiatric events (eg, hallucinations, delirium, abnormal behavior), anaphylaxis/serious skin reactions, and other adverse reactions.

Patient Counseling: Advise of the risk of severe allergic reactions or serious skin reactions and instruct to d/c and seek immediate medical attention if an allergic-like reaction occurs or is suspected. Advise of the risk of neuropsychiatric events and instruct to contact physician if experience signs of abnormal behavior while on therapy. Instruct to begin treatment as soon as possible from the 1st appearance of flu symptoms, and as soon as possible after exposure for prevention, at the recommendation of a physician. Instruct to take missed doses as soon as remembered, unless next scheduled dose is within 2 hrs, and then continue at the usual times. Inform that the medication is not a substitute for flu vaccination. Inform that PO sus delivers 2g sorbitol/75mg dose; this is above the daily maximum limit of sorbitol for patients with hereditary fructose intolerance and may cause dyspepsia and diarrhea.

Administration: Oral route. If oral sus is not available, may open caps and mix with sweetened liquids (eg, chocolate/corn syrup, caramel topping, light brown sugar). Refer to PI for preparation of PO sus and emergency compounding of a PO sus from caps. **Storage:** Cap/Dry Powder: 25°C (77°F); excursions permitted to 15-30°C (59-86°F). Constituted Sus: 2-8°C (36-46°F) up to 17 days, or 25°C (77°F) for up to 10 days with excursions permitted to 15-30°C (59-86°F). Do not freeze.

TAMOXIFEN
tamoxifen citrate (Various)

RX

> For women with ductal carcinoma in situ (DCIS) and women at high risk for breast cancer; serious and life-threatening events including uterine malignancies (eg, endometrial adenocarcinoma, uterine sarcoma), stroke, and pulmonary embolism (PE) reported. Some of these events were fatal. Discuss the potential benefits vs. the potential risks of these serious events with women at high risk of breast cancer and women with DCIS. The benefits of tamoxifen outweigh risks in women already diagnosed with breast cancer.

THERAPEUTIC CLASS: Antiestrogen

INDICATIONS: Treatment of metastatic breast cancer in women and men. Use as an alternative to oophorectomy or ovarian irradiation in premenopausal women with metastatic breast cancer. Treatment of node-positive and axillary node-negative breast cancer in women following mastectomy, axillary dissection, and breast irradiation. To reduce risk of invasive breast cancer in women with DCIS following breast surgery and radiation. Reduction of breast cancer incidence in high risk women. ("High risk," defined as ≥35 yrs of age with 5 yrs predicted risk of breast cancer ≥1.67%, as calculated by the Gail Model). Use for up to 5 yrs.

DOSAGE: *Adults:* Breast Cancer Treatment: 20-40mg qd. Divide daily dosages >20mg into AM and PM doses. Breast Cancer Risk Reduction/DCIS: 20mg qd for 5 yrs.

HOW SUPPLIED: Tab: 10mg, 20mg

CONTRAINDICATIONS: Women who require coumarin-type anticoagulant therapy or who have a history of deep vein thrombosis (DVT), PE.

WARNINGS/PRECAUTIONS: Hypercalcemia reported in patients with bone metastases. Increased incidence of uterine malignancies (eg, endometrial carcinoma, uterine sarcoma) and endometrial changes including hyperplasia and polyps with use. Endometriosis, fibroids, ovarian cysts, and menstrual irregularities also reported. Increased incidence of thromboembolic events (eg, DVT, PE). Malignant and nonmalignant (eg, changes in liver enzyme levels) effects on the liver reported. Ocular disturbances reported. Leukopenia, anemia, thrombocytopenia, neutropenia, pancytopenia reported. Promptly evaluate abnormal vaginal bleeding if receiving or previously received tamoxifen. Patients receiving or who have previously received tamoxifen should have annual gynecological examinations and should promptly notify physician if experience any abnormal gynecological symptoms (eg, menstrual irregularities, abnormal vaginal bleeding, changes in vaginal discharge, pelvic pain or pressure). May cause fetal harm during pregnancy; avoid pregnancy within 2 months of d/c therapy. May cause hyperlipidemia; periodic monitoring of plasma TG and cholesterol may be indicated in patients with pre-existing hyperlipidemia. Does not cause infertility even with menstrual irregularity. Perform periodic CBC, including platelet counts and periodic LFTs. Second primary tumors reported.

ADVERSE REACTIONS: Hot flashes, vaginal discharge, fatigue/asthenia, mood disturbances, insomnia, pharyngitis, N/V, irregular menses, fluid retention, pain, infection, flu syndrome, HTN, (men) loss of libido, impotence.

INTERACTIONS: Increases effects of coumarin-type anticoagulants. Increased risk of thromboembolic events with cytotoxic agents. Decreases letrozole and anastrozole levels; avoid coadministration with anastrozole. Increased levels with bromocriptine. Decreased levels with rifampin, aminoglutethimide, medroxyprogesterone, and phenobarbital. Erythromycin, cyclosporine, nifedipine and diltiazem may inhibit metabolism.

PREGNANCY: Category D, not for use in nursing.

MECHANISM OF ACTION: Non-steroidal antiestrogen; competes with estrogen for binding sites in target tissues.

PHARMACOKINETICS: Absorption: C_{max}=40ng/mL; T_{max}=5 hrs. N-desmethyl tamoxifen: C_{max}=15ng/mL. **Metabolism:** N-desmethyl tamoxifen (major metabolite). **Elimination:** Feces (primary); $T_{1/2}$=5-7 days.

NURSING CONSIDERATIONS

Assessment: Assess for history of DVT and PE, hepatic impairment, hyperlipidemia, pregnancy/nursing status, risk factors (eg, age, family history of breast cancer, breast biopsy results), and possible drug interactions. Perform baseline breast exam, mammogram, and gynecologic exam.

Monitoring: Monitor for signs/symptoms of hypercalcemia, uterine malignancies, endometrial changes, thromboembolic events (eg, PE, DVT), ocular disturbances, and for hypersensitivity reactions. Monitor CBC with platelets and LFTs periodically. Monitor PT when used with coumarin-type anticoagulants. Perform breast exam, mammogram, and gynecologic exam routinely. Perform periodic monitoring of plasma TG and cholesterol levels in patients with pre-existing hyperlipidemia.

Patient Counseling: Inform of pregnancy risks; advise to use nonhormonal contraception during therapy and for 2 months after d/c. Instruct women to seek medical attention if they experience symptoms of new breast lumps, abnormal vaginal bleeding, gynecological symptoms (eg, menstrual irregularities, changes in vaginal discharge, pelvic pain or pressure), leg swelling/tenderness, unexplained SOB, or changes in vision.

Administration: Oral route. **Storage:** 20-25°C (68-77°F). Dispense in a well-closed, light-resistant container with a child-resistant closure.

TAPAZOLE   RX
methimazole (King)

THERAPEUTIC CLASS: Thyroid hormone synthesis inhibitor

INDICATIONS: Treatment of hyperthyroidism. To ameliorate hyperthyroidism prior to subtotal thyroidectomy or radioactive iodine therapy. Also indicated when thyroidectomy is contraindicated or not advisable.

DOSAGE: *Adults:* PO: Given in 3 equal doses at 8-hr intervals. Initial: Mild: 15mg/day. Moderately Severe: 30-40mg/day. Severe: 60mg/day. Maint: 5-15mg/day.
Pediatrics: PO: Given in 3 equal doses at 8-hr intervals. Initial: 0.4mg/kg/day. Maint: 1/2 of initial dose.

HOW SUPPLIED: Tab: 5mg*, 10mg* *scored

CONTRAINDICATIONS: Nursing mothers.

WARNINGS/PRECAUTIONS: Can cause fetal harm. Agranulocytosis, leukopenia, thrombocytopenia, aplastic anemia (pancytopenia) may occur; monitor bone marrow function. D/C with agranulocytosis, aplastic anemia (pancytopenia), hepatitis or exfoliative dermatitis. Fulminant hepatitis, hepatic necrosis, and encephalopathy reported; d/c with liver abnormality, including transaminases >3X ULN. Monitor thyroid function periodically. May cause hypoprothrombinemia and bleeding; monitor PT.

ADVERSE REACTIONS: Agranulocytosis, granulocytopenia, thrombocytopenia, aplastic anemia, drug fever, lupus-like syndrome, insulin autoimmune syndrome, hepatitis, periarteritis, hypoprothrombinemia, skin rash, urticaria, N/V, epigastric distress.

INTERACTIONS: May potentiate oral anticoagulants. β-blockers, digitalis, theophylline may need dose reduction when patient becomes euthyroid. Caution with other drugs that cause agranulocytosis.

PREGNANCY: Category D, contraindicated in nursing.

MECHANISM OF ACTION: Inhibits synthesis of thyroid hormones.

PHARMACOKINETICS: Absorption: Readily absorbed (GI tract). **Distribution:** Crosses placenta and found in breast milk. **Elimination:** Urine.

NURSING CONSIDERATIONS

Assessment: Assess for drug hypersensitivity, pregnancy/nursing status, and possible drug interactions.

Monitoring: Monitor for signs of illness (eg, fever, sore throat, malaise, skin eruptions, headache), and hepatic dysfunction (eg, anorexia, upper quadrant pain). Monitor CBC, LFTs, PT, and bone marrow function. Monitor thyroid function periodically.

Patient Counseling: Instruct to inform physician if pregnant/nursing or planning to become pregnant. Instruct to report signs/symptoms of illness (eg, fever, general malaise, sore throat) to physician.

Administration: Oral route. **Storage:** 15-30°C (59-86°F).

TARCEVA   RX
erlotinib (Genentech/OSI)

THERAPEUTIC CLASS: Epidermal growth factor receptor tyrosine kinase inhibitor

INDICATIONS: Treatment of locally advanced or metastatic non-small cell lung cancer (NSCLC) after failure of at least one prior chemotherapy regimen. Maintenance treatment of locally advanced or metastatic NSCLC that has not progressed after four cycles of platinum-based first-line chemotherapy. First-line treatment of locally advanced, unresectable, or metastatic pancreatic cancer in combination with gemcitabine.

DOSAGE: *Adults:* NSCLC: 150mg qd. Pancreatic Cancer: 100mg qd in combination with gemcitabine. Continue until disease progression or unacceptable toxicity. Take at least 1 hr before or 2 hrs after ingestion of food. Severe Diarrhea/Severe Skin Reactions: May require dose reduction or temporary interruption of therapy. When dose reduction is necessary, reduce dose in 50-mg decrements. Concomitant Use With Strong CYP3A4 Inhibitors or Inhibitors of Both CYP3A4 and CYP1A2: Reduce dose if severe adverse events occur. Concomitant Use With CYP3A4 Inducers (Rifampicin): Consider alternative treatment or increase the dose at 2-week intervals. Max: 450mg. Cigarette Smoker: Increase the dose. Max: 300mg.

HOW SUPPLIED: Tab: 25mg, 100mg, 150mg

WARNINGS/PRECAUTIONS: Serious interstitial lung disease (ILD)-like events, including fatalities, reported; d/c if ILD diagnosed. Hepatotoxicity, hepatorenal syndrome, renal failure/insufficiency reported. Perform periodic LFTs; interrupt or d/c if total bilirubin >3X ULN and/or transaminases >5X ULN if pretreatment values normal and if with severe LFT changes. If dehydration occurs, interrupt therapy and intensively rehydrate; periodically monitor renal function and serum electrolytes. Caution with history of peptic ulceration or diverticular disease; d/c if GI perforation develops. Bullous, blistering, and exfoliative skin conditions, corneal perforation/ulceration reported; interrupt or d/c if symptoms develop or worsen. May cause myocardial infarction (MI)/ischemia, cerebrovascular accident (CVA), microangiopathic hemolytic anemia with thrombocytopenia, and fetal harm. INR elevations and infrequent bleeding events reported.

ADVERSE REACTIONS: Rash, diarrhea, anorexia, fatigue, dyspnea, cough, N/V, infection, stomatitis, pruritus, dry skin, conjunctivitis, keratoconjunctivitis sicca, abdominal pain, decreased weight.

INTERACTIONS: Increased concentrations with ketoconazole and other strong CYP3A4 inhibitors including ciprofloxacin, atazanavir, clarithromycin, indinavir, itraconazole, nefazodone, nelfinavir, ritonavir, saquinavir, telithromycin, troleandomycin, voriconazole, and grapefruit or grapefruit juice. CYP3A4 inducers may decrease plasma concentrations; use of CYP3A4 inducers (eg, rifampin, rifabutin, rifapentine, phenytoin, carbamazepine, phenobarbital, St. John's wort) is not recommended unless alternative therapy is unavailable. Cigarette smoking may reduce area under the curve (AUC). May decrease the AUC of CYP3A4 substrate midazolam. Drugs that alter pH of upper GI tract may alter solubility and bioavailability; concomitant use of proton pump inhibitors should be avoided. PT or INR changes with warfarin or other coumarin-derivative anticoagulants. Use with anti-angiogenic agents, corticosteroids, NSAIDs, and/or taxane-based chemotherapy may increase risk of GI perforation.

PREGNANCY: Category D, not for use in nursing.

MECHANISM OF ACTION: Kinase inhibitor; inhibits the intracellular phosphorylation of tyrosine kinase associated with epidermal growth factor receptor (EGFR).

PHARMACOKINETICS: Absorption: T_{max}=4 hrs. **Distribution:** V_d=232L; plasma protein binding (93%). **Metabolism:** CYP3A4 (major); CYP1A2, 1A1 (minor). **Elimination:** Feces (83%), urine (8%); $T_{1/2}$=36.2hrs.

NURSING CONSIDERATIONS

Assessment: Assess for lung disease/infection, hepatic/renal impairment, dehydration, history of peptic ulceration or diverticular disease, pregnancy/nursing status, and possible drug interactions. Obtain baseline LFTs and renal function. If taking warfarin or other coumarin anticoagulants, obtain baseline PT/INR.

Monitoring: Monitor for signs and symptoms of ILD (eg, dyspnea, cough, fever), hepatotoxicity, hepatorenal syndrome, renal failure/insufficiency, and dehydration. Monitor LFTs (transaminases, bilirubin, alkaline phosphatase), renal function, and serum electrolytes if there is risk of dehydration. Monitor for signs/symptoms of GI perforation, bullous and exfoliative skin disorders, MI/ischemia, CVA, microangiopathic hemolytic anemia with thrombocytopenia, and ocular disorders (eg, corneal perforation/ulceration). If taking concomitant warfarin or coumarin anticoagulants, monitor PT/INR.

Patient Counseling: Inform of risks of therapy. Instruct to notify physician if notice onset or worsening of skin rash, severe or persistent diarrhea, N/V, anorexia, SOB, cough, or if eye irritation occurs. Avoid sun exposure; recommend use of sunscreen. Advise to stop smoking and to avoid becoming pregnant while on therapy.

Administration: Oral route. **Storage:** 25°C (77°F); excursions permitted to 15-30° (59-86°F).

TARKA
RX
verapamil HCl - trandolapril (Abbott)

> D/C when pregnancy is detected. Drugs that act directly on the renin-angiotensin system can cause injury/death to the developing fetus.

THERAPEUTIC CLASS: ACE inhibitor/calcium channel blocker (nondihydropyridine)

INDICATIONS: Treatment of HTN.

DOSAGE: *Adults:* Replacement Therapy: Dose qd with food. Combination may be substituted for titrated components. Severe Liver Dysfunction: Give 30% of the normal verapamil dose. Begin therapy only after patient has either (a) failed to achieve desired antihypertensive effect with monotherapy at max recommended dose and shortest dosing interval, or (b) monotherapy dose cannot be increased further because of dose-limiting side effects.

HOW SUPPLIED: Tab, Extended-Release: (Trandolapril-Verapamil ER) 2mg-180mg, 1mg-240mg, 2mg-240mg, 4mg-240mg

CONTRAINDICATIONS: Severe left ventricular dysfunction, hypotension (SBP <90mmHg), cardiogenic shock, sick sinus syndrome, 2nd- or 3rd-degree atrioventricular (AV) block (except with functioning artificial ventricular pacemaker), atrial fibrillation/atrial flutter (A-fib/A-flutter) with an accessory bypass tract (eg, Wolff-Parkinson-White, Lown-Ganong-Levine syndromes), history of ACE inhibitor-associated angioedema.

WARNINGS/PRECAUTIONS: Not for initial therapy of HTN. Caution with impaired hepatic/renal function; monitor for abnormal PR interval prolongation. Trandolapril: Symptomatic hypotension may occur and is most likely in patients who are salt- or volume-depleted; correct depletion prior to therapy. May cause excessive hypotension, which may be associated with oliguria or azotemia, and rarely, with acute renal failure and death in patients with congestive heart failure (CHF). May cause cholestatic jaundice, fulminant hepatic necrosis, and death; d/c if jaundice develops. Angioedema reported; d/c if laryngeal stridor or angioedema of the face, tongue, or glottis occurs and administer appropriate therapy. Anaphylactoid reactions reported during desensitization with hymenoptera venom, dialysis with high-flux membranes, and LDL apheresis with dextran sulfate absorption. Potential for agranulocytosis and neutropenia; monitor WBC in patients with collagen-vascular disease and/or renal disease. May increase BUN and SrCr with renal artery stenosis and without preexisting renal vascular disease; consider dose reduction or d/c. Hyperkalemia and persistent, nonproductive cough reported. Hypotension may occur with major surgery or during anesthesia. Verapamil: Has a negative inotropic effect; avoid with severe left ventricular dysfunction. Elevated transaminases with or without alkaline phosphate elevation and hepatocellular injury reported. May lead to asymptomatic 1st-degree AV block and transient bradycardia. Sinus bradycardia, 2nd-degree AV block, sinus arrest, and pulmonary edema reported in patients with hypertrophic cardiomyopathy. May decrease neuromuscular transmission in patients with Duchenne's muscular dystrophy; reduce dose with attenuated neuromuscular transmission.

ADVERSE REACTIONS: AV block, constipation, cough, dizziness, fatigue, headache, increased hepatic enzymes, chest pain, upper respiratory tract infection.

INTERACTIONS: Increased risk of lithium toxicity. Hypotension, bradyarrhythmias, and lactic acidosis seen with clarithromycin and erythromycin. May cause additive hypotensive effects with diuretics, vasodilators, β-adrenergic blockers, α-antagonists. Trandolapril: Excessive BP reduction reported with diuretics. May increase risk of hyperkalemia with K⁺-sparing diuretics, K⁺ supplements, K⁺-containing salt substitutes. May result in deterioration of renal function with NSAIDs, including selective cyclooxygenase-2 inhibitors. NSAIDs may also attenuate antihypertensive effect. Nitritoid reactions reported with injectable gold (sodium aurothiomalate). May increase blood glucose-lowering effect of antidiabetic medications (insulin or oral antidiabetic agents). Verapamil: Not recommended with colchicine. Avoid disopyramide within 48 hrs before or 24 hrs after administration. Significant hypotension with quinidine; avoid with hypertrophic cardiomyopathy. Additive negative inotropic effect and prolongation of AV conduction with flecainide. Additive negative effects on HR, AV conduction, and/or cardiac contractility with β-adrenergic blockers. Inhalational anesthetics may depress cardiovascular activity. May potentiate activity of neuromuscular blocking agents (curare-like and depolarizing); reduce dose of either or both drugs. May increase levels of digoxin, prazosin, terazosin, simvastatin, lovastatin, atorvastatin, carbamazepine, cyclosporine, sirolimus, tacrolimus, theophylline, buspirone, midazolam, almotriptan, imipramine, doxorubicin, quinidine, metoprolol, propranolol, colchicine, and glyburide. CYP3A4 inhibitors (eg, erythromycin, telithromycin, protease inhibitors [eg, ritonavir]) may increase levels. CYP3A4 inducers (eg, rifampin, phenobarbital, sulfinpyrazone, St. John's wort) may decrease levels. Myopathy/rhabdomyolysis reported with HMG-CoA reductase inhibitors that are CYP3A4 substrates; limit simvastatin dose to 10mg daily, lovastatin dose to 40mg daily, and consider lower starting and maint doses for others (eg, atorvastatin).

PREGNANCY: Category D, not for use in nursing.

MECHANISM OF ACTION: Verapamil: Calcium channel blocker; modulates influx of ionic calcium across the cell membrane of the arterial smooth muscle as well as in conductile and contractile myocardial cells. Decreases systemic vascular resistance, usually without orthostatic decreases in BP or reflex tachycardia. Trandolapril: ACE inhibitor; inhibition results in decreased plasma angiotensin II, which leads to decreased vasopressor activity and decreased aldosterone secretion.

PHARMACOKINETICS: Absorption: Verapamil: Absolute bioavailability (20-35%), T_{max}=4-15 hrs, 5-15 hrs (norverapamil). Trandolapril: Absolute bioavailability (10%), T_{max}=0.5-2 hrs, 2-12 hrs (trandolaprilat). **Distribution:** Verapamil: Plasma protein binding (90%); found in breast milk. Trandolapril: Plasma protein binding (80%). **Metabolism:** Verapamil: Liver (extensive); norverapamil (active metabolite). Trandolapril: Trandolaprilat (active metabolite). **Elimination:** Verapamil: Urine (70% metabolite, 3-4% unchanged), feces (≥16% metabolite); $T_{1/2}$=6-11 hrs. Trandolapril: Urine (33%, <1% unchanged), feces (66%); $T_{1/2}$=6 hrs.

NURSING CONSIDERATIONS

Assessment: Assess for ventricular dysfunction, cardiogenic shock, sick sinus syndrome, AV block, A-fib/A-flutter and an accessory bypass tract, history of angioedema, LFTs, renal function, CHF, hypertrophic cardiomyopathy, neuromuscular disorders, volume/salt depletion, collagen vascular disease, pregnancy/nursing status, and possible drug interactions.

Monitoring: Monitor for angioedema, cough, anaphylactoid reactions, hypotension, hepatic/renal impairment, cholestatic jaundice, fulminant hepatic necrosis, headaches, heart block, chest pains, and agranulocytosis. Monitor BP and serum K⁺. Monitor WBC in patients with collagen vascular disease.

Patient Counseling: Counsel regarding adverse effects (eg, angioedema, neutropenia, jaundice) and instruct to report any signs/symptoms. Inform of risks when taken during pregnancy; instruct to notify physician if pregnant or become pregnant. Educate about need for periodic follow-ups and blood tests to rule out adverse effects and to monitor therapeutic effects. Instruct to take with food.

Administration: Oral route. **Storage:** 15-25°C (59-77°F).

TASIGNA   RX
nilotinib (Novartis)

> Prolongs QT interval. Monitor for hypokalemia or hypomagnesemia and correct deficiencies prior to administration and periodically. Monitor QTc at baseline, 7 days after initiation, and periodically thereafter, and follow any dose adjustments. Sudden deaths reported. Do not administer to patients with hypokalemia, hypomagnesemia, or long QT syndrome. Avoid drugs known to prolong the QT interval and strong CYP3A4 inhibitors. Avoid food 2 hrs before and 1 hr after taking dose.

THERAPEUTIC CLASS: Kinase inhibitor

INDICATIONS: Treatment of adult patients with newly diagnosed Philadelphia chromosome-positive chronic myeloid leukemia (Ph+ CML) in chronic phase (CP). Treatment of CP and accelerated phase (AP) Ph+ CML in adult patients resistant or intolerant to prior therapy that included imatinib.

DOSAGE: *Adults:* Newly Diagnosed Ph+ CML-CP: 300mg bid. Resistant or Intolerant Ph+ CML-CP/CML-AP: 400mg bid. Take at approximately 12-hr intervals. Refer to PI for dose adjustments based on hematologic and nonhematologic toxicities, QT prolongation, hepatic impairment.

HOW SUPPLIED: Cap: 150mg, 200mg

CONTRAINDICATIONS: Hypokalemia, hypomagnesemia, or long QT syndrome.

WARNINGS/PRECAUTIONS: Myelosuppression (eg, neutropenia, thrombocytopenia, anemia) may occur; perform CBC every 2 weeks for the first 2 months, then monthly thereafter. Temporarily withhold therapy or reduce dose if myelosuppression occurs. Ventricular repolarization abnormalities may have contributed to sudden deaths. May increase serum lipase; caution with history of pancreatitis. Interrupt dosing and consider appropriate diagnostics if lipase elevations are accompanied by abdominal symptoms. May elevate bilirubin, AST/ALT, and alkaline phosphatase; monitor LFTs monthly or as clinically indicated. May cause hypophosphatemia,

T

hypokalemia, hyperkalemia, hypocalcemia, and hyponatremia; correct electrolyte abnormalities prior to initiation and monitor periodically during therapy. Cases of tumor lysis syndrome reported; maintain adequate hydration and correct uric acid level prior to initiation. Reduced exposure with total gastrectomy; consider frequent follow-up and dose increase or alternative therapy. Contains lactose; avoid with galactose intolerance, severe lactase deficiency with a severe degree of intolerance to lactose-containing products, or glucose-galactose malabsorption. May cause fetal harm. Caution with relevant cardiac disorders (eg, recent myocardial infarction [MI], congestive heart failure [CHF], unstable angina, clinically significant bradycardia).

ADVERSE REACTIONS: Rash, headache, nasopharyngitis, fatigue, N/V, pruritus, arthralgia, abdominal pain, constipation, fever, upper urinary tract infection, asthenia, back pain, cough, diarrhea, myalgia.

INTERACTIONS: See Boxed Warning. Avoid with strong CYP3A4 inducers (eg, dexamethasone, phenytoin, carbamazepine, rifampin, rifabutin, rifapentine, phenobarbital), strong CYP3A4 inhibitors (eg, ketoconazole, itraconazole, clarithromycin, atazanavir, indinavir, nefazodone, nelfinavir, ritonavir, saquinavir, telithromycin, voriconazole), grapefruit products and other foods that inhibit CYP3A4, St. John's wort, or antiarrhythmic drugs. May increase levels of drugs eliminated by CYP3A4 (midazolam), CYP2C8, CYP2C9, CYP2D6, and UGT1A1 enzymes and may decrease levels of drugs eliminated by CYP2B6, CYP2C8, and CYP2C9 enzymes; caution with substrates with narrow therapeutic index. Strong CYP3A4 inhibitors or inducers may increase or decrease levels significantly. May increase levels of P-glycoprotein (P-gp) substrates. Increased concentration with P-gp inhibitors. Coadministration with imatinib may increase area under the curve of both drugs. Reduced bioavailability with proton pump inhibitors (eg, esomeprazole). Caution with H$_2$ blockers and antacids; separate dose from drug by at least several hrs.

PREGNANCY: Category D, not for use in nursing.

MECHANISM OF ACTION: Kinase inhibitor; binds to and stabilizes the inactive conformation of the kinase domain of Abl protein.

PHARMACOKINETICS: Absorption: T_{max}=3 hrs. **Distribution:** Plasma protein binding (98%). **Metabolism:** Via oxidation, hydroxylation. **Elimination:** Feces (93%, 69% unchanged), $T_{1/2}$= 17 hrs.

NURSING CONSIDERATIONS

Assessment: Assess for electrolyte abnormalities, long QT syndrome, history of pancreatitis, total gastrectomy, hepatic impairment, galactose intolerance, severe lactase deficiency, glucose-galactose malabsorption, relevant cardiac disorders, pregnancy/nursing status, and possible drug interactions. Obtain baseline ECG and uric acid levels.

Monitoring: Monitor for myelosuppression; perform CBC q2 weeks for the 1st 2 months of therapy and monthly thereafter. Check chemistry panels, including lipid profile, periodically. Monitor for signs/symptoms of QT prolongation; obtain ECG 7 days after initiation, periodically thereafter, and after dose adjustments. Monitor for electrolyte abnormalities, tumor lysis syndrome, and adequate hydration. Monitor serum lipase levels and hepatic function tests monthly or as clinically indicated.

Patient Counseling: Instruct to take dose on empty stomach, at least 2 hrs after a meal; inform that may swallow caps whole with water or disperse contents on 1 tsp of applesauce and swallow immediately (within 15 min) if unable to swallow capsules. Advise to take twice daily approximately 12 hrs apart. Instruct not to consume grapefruit products and other foods known to inhibit CYP3A4 at all times during treatment. Counsel about possible drug interactions. Advise women of childbearing potential to use effective contraceptive methods while on therapy. Instruct to take as prescribed and do not d/c therapy or change dose without consulting physician. Instruct not to take a make-up dose if a dose is missed, and to take the next dose as scheduled.

Administration: Oral route. Avoid food for at least 2 hrs before and 1 hr after taking dose. Swallow cap whole with water. May disperse contents in 1 tsp applesauce if unable to swallow cap; take immediately (within 15 minutes) and do not store for future use. **Storage:** 25°C (77°F); excursions permitted between 15-30°C (59-86°F).

TASMAR   RX
tolcapone (Valeant)

Risk of fatal, acute fulminant liver failure; should be used in patients with Parkinson's disease (PD) on levodopa/carbidopa who are experiencing symptom fluctuations and are not responding satisfactorily to or are not appropriate candidates for other adjunctive therapies. Withdraw treatment if patients fail to show benefit within 3 weeks of initiation. Do not initiate therapy if liver disease is clinically evident or if ALT/AST values >ULN. D/C if hepatocellular injury develops, and do not consider retreatment. Determine baseline ALT/AST and monitor q2-4 weeks for the 1st 6 months, then periodically thereafter. Perform LFTs before increasing dose to 200mg tid. Caution with severe dyskinesia or dystonia. D/C if ALT/AST >2X ULN or if clinical signs/symptoms suggest the onset of hepatic dysfunction (eg, persistent nausea, fatigue, lethargy, anorexia, jaundice, dark urine, pruritus, and right upper quadrant tenderness).

THERAPEUTIC CLASS: COMT inhibitor

INDICATIONS: Adjunct to levodopa/carbidopa for the treatment of signs and symptoms of idiopathic PD.

DOSAGE: *Adults:* Adjunct to Levodopa/Carbidopa: Initial: 100mg tid. Use 200mg tid only if clinical benefit is justified. May need to reduce daily levodopa dose.

HOW SUPPLIED: Tab: 100mg, 200mg

CONTRAINDICATIONS: Liver disease, patients withdrawn from therapy due to drug-induced hepatocellular injury, history of nontraumatic rhabdomyolysis, hyperpyrexia, confusion related to medication.

WARNINGS/PRECAUTIONS: Dyskinesia, orthostatic hypotension/syncope, rhabdomyolysis, hallucinations, diarrhea, fibrotic complications, and hematuria. Avoid with liver disease. Caution with severe renal impairment and severe dyskinesia or dystonia. Neuroleptic malignant syndrome (NMS) reported with rapid dose reduction or withdrawal. Increased risk of melanoma with PD; monitor periodically. D/C therapy after a total of 3 weeks if expected clinical benefit is not achieved.

ADVERSE REACTIONS: Dyskinesia, dystonia, anorexia, muscle cramps, diarrhea, orthostatic symptoms, hallucination, N/V, sleep disorders, drowsiness, increased sweating, xerostomia, urine discoloration, hepatocellular injury.

INTERACTIONS: Drugs metabolized by catechol-O-methyltransferase (COMT) (eg, α-methyldopa, dobutamine, apomorphine and isoproterenol) may need dose reduction. Avoid with nonselective MAOIs (eg, phenelzine, tranylcypromine). Caution with desipramine, tolbutamide, and warfarin.

PREGNANCY: Category C, caution in nursing.

MECHANISM OF ACTION: COMT inhibitor; suspected to alter the plasma pharmacokinetics of levodopa, leading to more sustained plasma levels of drug.

PHARMACOKINETICS: Absorption: Rapidly; absolute bioavailability (65%); C_{max}=3µg/mL (100mg), 6µg/mL (200mg); T_{max}=2 hrs. **Distribution:** V_d=9L; plasma protein binding (>99.9%). **Metabolism:** Liver; glucuronidation (main), oxidation via CYP450 enzymes 3A4, 2A6. **Elimination:** Urine (60%, 0.5% unchanged), feces (40%); $T_{1/2}$=2-3 hrs.

NURSING CONSIDERATIONS

Assessment: Assess for drug hypersensitivity, liver disease, drug-induced hepatocellular injury/ confusion, history of nontraumatic rhabdomyolysis, renal function, dyskinesia, dystonia, history of cardiac disease/pulmonary pathology (nonmalignant lung lesion), pregnancy/nursing status, and for possible drug interactions. Obtain baseline LFTs.

Monitoring: Monitor for hypersensitivity reactions, LFTs (ALT/AST), renal function test, hypotension/syncope, diarrhea, dyskinesia, rhabdomyolysis, hematuria, fibrotic complications, melanomas, hallucinations, and NMS symptoms. Perform periodic skin examination.

Patient Counseling: Instruct to take as prescribed. Inform that hallucination, nausea, and possible increase in dyskinesia/dystonia may occur. Inform of the need for regular blood tests to monitor liver enzymes. Advise that orthostatic hypotension with/without symptoms (eg, dizziness, nausea, syncope, sweating) may develop; caution to rise slowly after sitting or lying down. Instruct to neither drive nor operate complex machinery until sufficient experience of effect of therapy on mental/motor performance is gained. Instruct to use caution with CNS depressants because of possible additive sedative effect. Inform of signs/symptoms of onset of hepatic injury (persistent nausea, fatigue, lethargy, anorexia, jaundice, dark urine, pruritus, and right upper quadrant tenderness); advise to contact physician if these symptoms occur. Advise to notify physician if new or increased gambling urges, sexual urges or other intense urges occur. Advise to notify physician if become pregnant, intend to become pregnant, breastfeeding, or intend to breastfeed during therapy.

Administration: Oral route. **Storage:** 20-25°C (68-77°F). Store in tight container.

TAZICEF   RX
ceftazidime (Hospira)

THERAPEUTIC CLASS: Cephalosporin (3rd generation)

INDICATIONS: Treatment of lower respiratory tract (eg, pneumonia), skin and skin structure (SSSI), bone and joint, gynecologic, intra-abdominal, CNS (eg, meningitis), and urinary tract infections (UTI), bacterial septicemia, and sepsis caused by susceptible strains of microorganisms.

DOSAGE: *Adults:* Usual: 1g IV q8-12h. Uncomplicated UTI: 250mg IM/IV q12h. Complicated UTI: 500mg IM/IV q8-12h. Bone and Joint Infections: 2g IV q12h. Uncomplicated Pneumonia/SSSI: 500mg-1g IM/IV q8h. Gynecological/Intra-Abdominal/Meningitis/Severe Life-Threatening Infection: 2g IV q8h. Lung Infection caused by *Pseudomonas* in Cystic Fibrosis (normal renal function): 30-50mg/kg IV q8h. Max: 6g/day. Renal Impairment: CrCl 31-50mL/min: 1g q12h.

T

CrCl 16-30mL/min: 1g q24h. CrCl 6-15mL/min: 500mg q24h. CrCl <5mL/min: 500mg q48h. For severe infections (6g/day), increase renal impairment dose by 50% or increase dosing interval. Apply reduced dosage recommendations after initial 1g LD is given. Hemodialysis: Give 1g LD before and 1g after each hemodialysis period. Intra-Peritoneal Dialysis/Continuous Ambulatory Peritoneal Dialysis: Give 1g LD followed by 500mg q24h, or add to fluid at 250mg/2L. *Pediatrics:* Neonates (0-4 weeks): 30mg/kg IV q12h. 1 month-12 yrs: 30-50mg/kg IV q8h. Max: 6g/day. Higher doses for patients with cystic fibrosis or when treating meningitis.

HOW SUPPLIED: Inj: 1g, 2g. Also available as a Pharmacy Bulk Package. Refer to individual package insert for more information

WARNINGS/PRECAUTIONS: Monitor renal function; potential for nephrotoxicity. Possible cross-sensitivity between penicillins (PCNs), cephalosporins, and other β-lactams. Pseudomembranous colitis reported. Elevated levels with renal insufficiency can lead to seizures, encephalopathy, asterixis, and neuromuscular excitability. Possible decrease in PT; caution with renal or hepatic impairment, poor nutritional state; monitor PT and give vitamin K if needed. Caution with colitis and other GI diseases. Distal necrosis may occur after inadvertent intra-arterial administration. Continue for 2 days after signs/symptoms of infection resolve; may require longer therapy with complicated infections. May result in bacterial resistance with prolonged use or use in the absence of a proven/suspected bacterial infection or a prophylactic indication; take appropriate measures if superinfection develops. Lab test interactions may occur. Caution in elderly.

ADVERSE REACTIONS: Phlebitis and inflammation at injection site, pruritus, rash, fever, diarrhea, N/V.

INTERACTIONS: Nephrotoxicity reported with aminoglycosides or potent diuretics (eg, furosemide). Avoid with chloramphenicol; may decrease effect of β-lactam antibiotics.

PREGNANCY: Category B, caution in nursing.

MECHANISM OF ACTION: 3rd-generation cephalosporin; inhibits enzymes responsible for cell-wall synthesis.

PHARMACOKINETICS: Absorption: C_{max}=90mcg/mL (1g IV), 39mcg/mL (1g IM); see PI for detailed info. **Distribution:** Plasma protein binding (<10%); found in breast milk. **Elimination:** Urine (80-90% unchanged); $T_{1/2}$=1.9 hrs (IV).

NURSING CONSIDERATIONS

Assessment: Assess for previous hypersensitivity reaction to cephalosporins/PCNs or other drugs, renal/hepatic impairment, poor nutritional status, patients receiving protracted course of antibiotics, GI disease (particularly colitis), pregnancy/nursing status, and possible drug interactions.

Monitoring: Monitor PT; vitamin K administration as indicated. Monitor for signs/symptoms of allergic reactions (eg, Stevens-Johnson syndrome, toxic epidermal necrolysis), pseudomembranous colitis or *Clostridium difficile*-associated diarrhea, development of drug resistance, overgrowth of nonsusceptible organisms, seizures, encephalopathy, asterixis, neuromuscular excitability, distal necrosis in inadvertent intra-atrial injection, lab test interactions, LFTs, renal function tests, and CBCs.

Patient Counseling: Only treats bacterial, not viral, infections. Take exactly as directed; skipping doses or not completing full course may decrease effectiveness and increase resistance. Inform about risks/benefits. D/C and notify physician if experience allergic reaction or diarrhea. Notify if pregnant/nursing.

Administration: IV and IM route. Do not use flexible container in series connections. **Storage:** Dry state 20-25°C (68-77°F), reconstituted solution for 24 hrs at room temperature, or for 7 days at 5°C; stable for 3 months if frozen at -20°C; thawed solution, store for up to 8 hrs at room temperature or for 4 days at 5°C; do not refreeze thawed solution.

TAZORAC   RX
tazarotene (Allergan)

THERAPEUTIC CLASS: Retinoid

INDICATIONS: (Gel 0.05%, 0.1%) Treatment of stable plaque psoriasis of up to 20% BSA involvement. (Gel 0.1%) Treatment of mild to moderate facial acne vulgaris. (Cre 0.05%, 0.1%) Treatment of plaque psoriasis. (Cre 0.1%) Treatment of acne vulgaris.

DOSAGE: *Adults:* ≥18 yrs: (Gel/Cre) Psoriasis: Start with 0.05% gel/cre, increase to 0.1% if tolerated and medically indicated. Apply thin film (enough to cover lesion) to psoriatic lesions qpm. Use gel only to ≤20% BSA. Acne: Cleanse and dry skin. Apply thin film (enough to cover affected area) of 0.1% gel/cre to acne lesions qpm.
Pediatrics: ≥12 yrs: (Gel) Psoriasis: Start with 0.05% gel, increase to 0.1% if tolerated and medically indicated. Apply thin film (enough to cover lesion and ≤20% BSA) to psoriatic lesions qpm.

(Gel/Cre) Acne: Cleanse and dry skin. Apply thin film (enough to cover affected area) of 0.1% gel/cre to acne lesions qpm.

HOW SUPPLIED: Gel: 0.05%, 0.1% [30g, 100g]; Cre: 0.05%, 0.1% [30g, 60g]

CONTRAINDICATIONS: Women who are or may become pregnant.

WARNINGS/PRECAUTIONS: Not for ophthalmic, oral, or intravaginal use. Use adequate birth-control measures in women of childbearing potential. Obtain negative pregnancy test result (sensitivity down to ≥50 mIU/mL for human chorionic gonadotropin [hCG]) within 2 weeks prior to therapy; initiate therapy during normal menstrual period. Apply only to affected area; for external use only. May cause severe irritation; do not use on eczematous skin. Avoid exposure to sunlight (including sunlamps); if exposure is necessary, use sunscreens (SPF ≥15) and protective clothing. Avoid with sunburn. May cause excessive pruritus, burning, skin redness, or peeling; d/c or reduce dosing interval if these occur, and patients with psoriasis being treated with 0.1% concentration can be switched to lower concentration. Weather extremes (eg, wind, cold) may cause irritation. (Gel) Not for use in >20% of BSA.

ADVERSE REACTIONS: Pruritus, burning/stinging, erythema, worsening of psoriasis, irritation, skin pain, desquamation, dry skin, rash, contact dermatitis, skin inflammation; (Cre) eczema, hypertriglyceridemia; (Gel) fissuring, bleeding.

INTERACTIONS: Avoid dermatologic medications and cosmetics that have a strong drying effect. Caution with photosensitizers (eg, thiazides, tetracyclines, fluoroquinolones, phenothiazines, sulfonamides). Apply emollients ≥1 hr before gel/cream application.

PREGNANCY: Category X, caution in nursing.

MECHANISM OF ACTION: Retinoid. Psoriasis: not established; suppresses expression of MRP8, a marker of inflammation; inhibits cornified envelope formation; induces expression of a gene which may be a growth suppressor in keratinocytes and may inhibit epidermal hyperproliferation in treated plaques. Acne: Not established; may be due to anti-hyperproliferative, normalizing-of-differentiation and anti-inflammatory actions.

PHARMACOKINETICS: Absorption: (Gel): After 7 days; C_{max}=0.72ng/mL; T_{max}=9 hrs after last dose; AUC=10.1ng•hr/mL. (Cre): After 14 Days: C_{max}=2.31ng/mL; T_{max}=8 hrs after last dose; AUC=31.2ng•hr/mL. **Distribution:** Tazarotenic Acid: Plasma protein binding (>99%). **Metabolism:** Esterase hydrolysis to form tazarotenic acid (active metabolite). **Excretion:** Urine, feces; Tazarotenic Acid: $T_{1/2}$=18 hrs.

NURSING CONSIDERATIONS

Assessment: Assess for eczematous skin, sunburn, considerable sun exposure due to occupation, sunlight sensitivity, hypersensitivity, pregnancy/nursing status, and possible drug interactions. Obtain negative pregnancy test result (sensitivity down to ≥50 mIU/mL for hCG) within 2 weeks prior to therapy.

Monitoring: Monitor for excessive pruritus, burning, skin redness, or peeling. Monitor application frequency, clinical therapeutic response, and skin tolerance.

Patient Counseling: Instruct to avoid contact with eyes, eyelids, and mouth; if contact occurs, rinse with water. Do not cover treated areas with dressings or bandages. Instruct to wash hands following administration. Advise not to take if pregnant, planning to become, or suspected to be pregnant. Instruct females to use effective form of contraception while on medication; advise to begin therapy during menstrual period. Instruct to avoid exposure to sunlight/sunlamps while on therapy; wear protective clothing and use sunscreen (SPF ≥15) when exposed to sunlight. Instruct not to use with sunburn. Inform that exposure to weather extremes (eg, wind, cold) may cause skin irritation. Contact physician if excessive skin irritation develops. Counsel that if dose is missed, do not make it up; return to normal dosing schedule.

Administration: Topical route. Refer to PI for proper administration. **Storage:** 25°C (77°F); excursions permitted to (Gel) 15-30°C (59-86°F), (Cre) -5 to 30°C (23-86°F).

TEFLARO   RX
ceftaroline fosamil (Forest)

THERAPEUTIC CLASS: Cephalosporin

INDICATIONS: Treatment of acute bacterial skin and skin structure infections (ABSSSI) and community-acquired bacterial pneumonia (CABP) caused by susceptible isolates of microorganisms.

DOSAGE: *Adults:* ≥18 yrs: ABSSSI: 600mg q12h IV infusion over 1 hr for 5-14 days. CABP: 600mg q12h IV infusion over 1 hr for 5-7 days. Renal Impairment: CrCl>30-≤50mL/min: 400mg IV (over 1 hr) q12h. CrCl ≥15-≤30mL/min: 300mg IV (over 1 hr) q12h. End-Stage Renal Disease (CrCl<15mL/min)/Hemodialysis: 200mg IV (over 1 hr) q12h. Elderly: Adjust dosage based on renal function.

HOW SUPPLIED: Inj: 400mg, 600mg

WARNINGS/PRECAUTIONS: Serious fatal hypersensitivity and skin reactions reported; d/c therapy if allergic reaction occurs. Caution with penicillin (PCN) or other β-lactam allergy; cross-sensitivity may occur. *Clostridium difficile*-associated diarrhea (CDAD) reported. May result in bacterial resistance with prolonged use or use in the absence of a proven/suspected bacterial infection or a prophylactic indication; take appropriate measures if superinfection develops. Seroconversion from negative to positive direct Coombs' test reported. If anemia develops, consider drug-induced hemolytic anemia. Caution in elderly and renally impaired.

ADVERSE REACTIONS: Diarrhea, nausea, rash.

PREGNANCY: Category B, caution in nursing.

MECHANISM OF ACTION: Cephalosporin; bactericidal action is mediated through binding to essential PCN-binding proteins.

PHARMACOKINETICS: Absorption: C_{max}=19mcg/mL (single 600mg dose), 21.3mcg/mL (multiple 600mg doses); T_{max}=1 hr (single 600mg dose); 0.92 hrs (multiple 600mg doses); AUC=56.8mcg•hr/mL (single 600mg dose); 56.3mcg•hr/mL (multiple 600mg doses). **Distribution:** V_d=20.3 L (single 600mg dose); plasma protein binding (20%). **Metabolism:** Via phosphatase enzyme; via hydrolysis to ceftaroline M-1 (inactive metabolite). **Elimination:** Urine (88%), (64% unchanged, 2% metabolite); feces (6%). $T_{1/2}$=1.6 hrs (single 600mg dose), 2.66 hrs (multiple 600mg doses).

NURSING CONSIDERATIONS

Assessment: Assess for PCN or other β-lactam allergy, renal impairment, pregnancy/nursing status, and for possible drug interactions. Obtain appropriate specimens for microbiological examination to identify pathogen and determine susceptibility.

Monitoring: Monitor for signs and symptoms of hypersensitivity reactions, superinfections, skin reactions, CDAD, and anemia. Monitor renal function, especially in elderly.

Patient Counseling: Advise that allergic reactions could occur and that serious reactions require immediate treatment; report any previous hypersensitivity reactions to other β-lactams (including cephalosporins) or other allergens. Advise that antibacterial drugs should be used to treat only bacterial infections; they do not treat viral infections (eg, common cold). Advise that although it is common to feel better early in the course of therapy, the medication should be taken as directed; skipping doses or not completing the full course of therapy may decrease the effectiveness and increase the likelihood that bacteria will develop resistance. Advise that diarrhea is common and is usually resolved when drug is d/c. Advise that frequent watery or bloody diarrhea may occur and may be a sign of a more serious intestinal infection; notify physician if this develops.

Administration: IV route. Refer to PI for further information on preparation and administration. **Storage:** 2-8°C (36-46°F). Use constituted sol within 6 hrs when stored at room temperature or within 24 hrs when stored under 2-8°C (36-46°F). Unrefrigerated/Unreconstituted: ≤25°C (77°F) for ≤7 days.

TEGRETOL   RX
carbamazepine (Novartis)

> Serious and fatal dermatologic reactions, including toxic epidermal necrolysis (TEN), Stevens-Johnson syndrome (SJS) reported; increased risk with presence of HLA-B*1502 allele; screen prior to initiation of therapy. Aplastic anemia and agranulocytosis reported. Obtain complete pretreatment hematological testing as a baseline. D/C if evidence of bone marrow depression develops.

OTHER BRAND NAMES: Epitol (Teva) - Tegretol-XR (Novartis)

THERAPEUTIC CLASS: Carboxamide

INDICATIONS: Treatment of partial seizures with complex symptomatology (psychomotor, temporal lobe), generalized tonic-clonic seizures (grand mal), and mixed seizure patterns of these, or other partial or generalized seizures. Treatment of pain associated with true trigeminal or glossopharyngeal neuralgia.

DOSAGE: *Adults:* Epilepsy: Initial: (Tab/Tab, ER) 200mg bid or (Sus) 100mg qid. Titrate: Increase weekly by adding up to 200mg/day given bid (Tab, ER) or tid-qid (Tab/Sus/Tab, Chewable) until optimal response. Maint: 800-1200mg/day. Max: 1200mg/day but doses up to 1600mg/day have been used in rare instances. With Other Anticonvulsants: Add gradually while other anticonvulsants are maintained or gradually decreased (except phenytoin, which may have to be increased). Trigeminal Neuralgia: Initial (Day 1): (Tab/Tab, ER) 100mg bid or (Sus) 50mg qid. Titrate: May increase by up to 200mg/day using increments of 100mg q12h (Tab/Tab, ER) or 50mg qid (Sus) PRN. Maint: 400-800mg/day. Max: 1200mg/day. Reevaluate every 3 months. Conversion from Tab to Sus: Give same mg/day in smaller, more frequent doses. *Pediatrics:* Epilepsy: >12 yrs: Initial: (Tab/Tab, ER) 200mg bid or (Sus) 100mg qid. Titrate: Increase weekly by adding up to 200mg/day given bid (Tab, ER) or tid-qid (Tab/Sus/Tab,

Chewable) until optimal response. Maint: 800-1200mg/day. Max: >15 yrs: 1200mg/day; 12-15 yrs: 1000mg/day. 6-12 yrs: Initial: (Tab/Tab, ER) 100mg bid or (Sus) 50mg qid. Titrate: Increase weekly by adding up to 100mg/day given bid (Tab, ER) or tid-qid (Tab/Sus/Tab, Chewable) until optimal response. Maint: 400-800mg/day. Max: 1000mg/day. <6 yrs: Initial: 10-20mg/kg/day given bid-tid (Tab) or qid (Sus). Titrate: (Tab/Sus) Increase weekly tid-qid. Max: 35mg/kg/day. With Other Anticonvulsants: Add gradually while other anticonvulsants are maintained or gradually decreased (except phenytoin, which may have to be increased). Conversion from Tab to Sus: Give same mg/day in smaller, more frequent doses.

HOW SUPPLIED: Sus: (Tegretol) 100mg/5mL [450mL]; Tab, Extended-Release: (Tegretol-XR) 100mg, 200mg, 400mg; (Tegretol) Tab, Chewable: 100mg*; (Tegretol, Epitol) Tab: 200mg* *scored

CONTRAINDICATIONS: History of bone marrow depression, MAOI use within 14 days, hypersensitivity to tricyclic compounds (eg, amitriptyline, desipramine, imipramine, protriptyline, nortriptyline, etc). Coadministration with nefazodone.

WARNINGS/PRECAUTIONS: Increased risk of suicidal thoughts or behavior. Caution in patients with history of cardiac conduction disturbance; cardiac, hepatic, or renal damage; adverse hematologic or hypersensitivity reactions to other drugs; increased intraocular pressure (IOP); mixed seizure disorder; previously interrupted course of carbamazepine. Atrioventricular heart block, slight elevations in LFTs, rare cases of liver failure. Multiorgan hypersensitivity reactions reported; consider d/c if hypersensitivity develops. May cause activation of latent psychosis and, in the elderly, confusion or agitation. Avoid with history of hepatic porphyria (eg, acute intermittent porphyria, variegate porphyria, porphyria cutanea tarda); acute attacks reported. Withdraw gradually to minimize potential increase in seizure frequency. May cause fetal harm with pregnancy. May impair physical/mental abilities. Avoid suspension in patients with fructose intolerance; start on lower doses and increase slowly. Not for relief of trivial aches or pains.

ADVERSE REACTIONS: Dizziness, drowsiness, unsteadiness, N/V, bone marrow depression, multiorgan hypersensitivity, aplastic anemia, agranulocytosis, leukopenia, eosinophilia, SJS, TEN, liver dysfunction, cardiovascular complications.

INTERACTIONS: See Contraindications. Do not give suspension with other medicinal liquids or diluents. CYP3A4 inhibitors (eg, cimetidine, macrolides, azoles) may increase plasma concentration. CYP3A4 inducers (eg, cisplatin, rifampin, theophylline) may decrease plasma concentration. Increases plasma levels of clomipramine, phenytoin, and primidone. Decreases levels of CYP3A4 substrates (eg, acetaminophen, alprazolam, warfarin). May render hormonal contraceptives (eg, oral, levonorgestrel subdermal implant) less effective. Increased risk of neurotoxic side effects with lithium. Alteration of thyroid function with other anticonvulsants. Increased isoniazid-induced hepatotoxicity with isoniazid. Symptomatic hyponatremia with some diuretics (eg, HCTZ, furosemide). Antagonizes effects of nondepolarizing muscle relaxants (eg, pancuronium).

PREGNANCY: Category D, not for use in nursing.

MECHANISM OF ACTION: Carboxamide; anticonvulsant: reduce polysynaptic response and block post-tetanic potentiation. Neuralgia: Depresses thalamic potential and bulbar and polysynaptic reflexes.

PHARMACOKINETICS: Absorption: T_{max}=1.5 hrs (Sus), 4-5 hrs (Tab), 3-12 hrs (Tab, ER). **Distribution:** Plasma protein binding (76%). Crosses placenta; found in breast milk. **Metabolism:** Liver via CYP3A4 to carbamazepine-10,11-epoxide (active metabolite). **Elimination:** Urine (72%; 3% unchanged), feces (28%); $T_{1/2}$=25-65 hrs (single dose); $T_{1/2}$=12-17 hrs (multiple doses).

NURSING CONSIDERATIONS

T

Assessment: Assess for history of bone marrow depression, hepatic porphyria, hypersensitivity to any tricyclic compound, increased IOP, previous adverse hematological and dermatological reactions with other medications, history of mixed seizure disorders, cardiac damage or cardiac conduction disturbances, depression, suicidal behavior and ideation, pregnancy/nursing status, and possible drug interactions. Assess renal function (eg, complete urinalysis, BUN), CBC (eg, platelets, reticulocytes), serum iron, presence of HLA-B*1502, LFTs; perform eye exam (eg, slit-lamp, funduscopy, tonometry) prior to therapy. (Cre) eczema, pertriglyceridemia; (Gel) fissuring, bleeding.

Monitoring: Monitor for hepatic failure, multiorgan hypersensitivity reactions, bone marrow depression, aplastic anemia, agranulocytosis, dermatological reactions (eg, SJS, TEN), latent psychosis, and confusion or agitation in elderly patients. Monitor for emergence of suicidal behavior and ideation, signs and symptoms of depression. Monitor LFTs, SrCr, BUN, IOP.

Patient Counseling: Counsel about signs/symptoms of hematological, dermatological, and hepatic complications (eg, fever, sore throat, easy bruising, jaundice); instruct to report any occurrence to physician. May cause drowsiness or dizziness; caution against using heavy machinery/driving. Avoid with alcohol or abrupt d/c. Notify physician if worsening of depression, unusual changes in mood or behavior, or suicidal thoughts/behavior occurs. Notify physician if pregnant or intend to become pregnant. Encourage pregnant patients to enroll in North American

Antiepileptic Drug (NAAED) Pregnancy Registry by calling 1-888-233-2334 or go to www.aed-pregnancyregistry.org/. **Administration:** Oral route. (Sus) Shake well before using. (Tab, ER) Swallow whole; do not chew or crush. **Storage:** (Sus): ≤30°C (86°F); dispense in tight, light-resistant container. (Tab & Tab, Chewable): ≤30°C (86°F); Protect from light and moisture; dispense in tight, light-resistant container. (Tab, ER): 15-30°C (59-86°F). Protect from moisture. Dispense in tight container.

TEKAMLO   RX

amlodipine - aliskiren (Novartis)

D/C when pregnancy is detected. Drugs that act directly on the renin-angiotensin system can cause injury/death to the developing fetus.

THERAPEUTIC CLASS: Renin inhibitor/calcium channel blocker (dihydropyridine)

INDICATIONS: Treatment of HTN, alone or with other antihypertensive agents. May be used as an add-on therapy in patients whose BP is not adequately controlled with aliskiren alone or amlodipine (or another dihydropyridine calcium channel blocker) alone, substituted for titrated components, or used as initial therapy in patients who are likely to need multiple drugs to achieve BP goals.

DOSAGE: *Adults:* Initial Therapy: 150mg-5mg qd. Titrate: May increase up to max of 300mg-10mg qd if BP remains uncontrolled after 2-4 weeks. Max: 300mg-10mg qd. Add-On Therapy: May use if not adequately controlled with aliskiren alone or amlodipine (or another dihydropyridine calcium channel blocker) alone. With dose-limiting adverse reactions to either component alone, switch to aliskiren-amlodipine containing a lower dose of that component. Replacement Therapy: May substitute for individually titrated components. Hepatic Impairment: Titrate slowly.

HOW SUPPLIED: Tab: (Aliskiren-Amlodipine) 150mg-5mg, 150mg-10mg, 300mg-5mg, 300mg-10mg

CONTRAINDICATIONS: Concomitant use with angiotensin receptor blockers (ARBs) or ACE inhibitors in patients with diabetes.

WARNINGS/PRECAUTIONS: Not recommended for initial therapy in patients with intravascular volume depletion. In patients with an activated renin-angiotensin-aldosterone system (eg, volume- and/or salt-depleted patients receiving high doses of diuretics), symptomatic hypotension may occur; correct these conditions prior to therapy or monitor closely. Renal function changes may occur; consider withholding or d/c therapy if clinically significant decrease in renal function develops. Caution in patients whose renal function may depend in part on the activity of the renin-angiotensin system (eg, renal artery stenosis, severe heart failure, post-myocardial infarction [MI], or volume depletion). Aliskiren: Angioedema of the face, extremities, lips, tongue, glottis, and/or larynx reported; d/c immediately and do not readminister if angioedema develops. Hyperkalemia may occur; monitor serum K⁺ periodically. Caution in patients with risk factors for development of hyperkalemia (eg, renal insufficiency, diabetes). Amlodipine: May increase frequency, duration, or severity of angina or acute MI, particularly in severe obstructive coronary artery disease (CAD). Caution with severe hepatic impairment and in elderly.

ADVERSE REACTIONS: Head/neck angioedema, hypotension, peripheral edema, hyperkalemia.

INTERACTIONS: See Contraindications. Avoid use with ARBs or ACE inhibitors in patients with moderate renal impairment (GFR <60ml/min). Increased risk for developing acute renal failure with ARBs, ACE inhibitors, or NSAIDs. Aliskiren: Cyclosporine or itraconazole may significantly increase levels; avoid concomitant use. Increased risk for developing hyperkalemia in combination with ARBs or ACE inhibitors, NSAIDs, or K⁺ supplements/K⁺-sparing diuretics. Potential for interaction with P-glycoprotein inhibitors. NSAIDs, including selective cyclooxygenase-2 inhibitors, may result in deterioration of renal function and attenuation of antihypertensive effect. Amlodipine: May increase simvastatin exposure; limit dose of simvastatin to 20mg/day.

PREGNANCY: Category D, not for use in nursing.

MECHANISM OF ACTION: Aliskiren: Direct renin inhibitor; decreases plasma renin activity and inhibits the conversion of angiotensinogen to angiotensin I. Amlodipine: Dihydropyridine calcium channel blocker; inhibits the transmembrane influx of calcium ions into vascular smooth muscle and cardiac muscle.

PHARMACOKINETICS: Absorption: Aliskiren: Poor; bioavailability (2.5%); T_{max}=1-3 hrs; AUC and C_{max} decreased by 79% and 90%, respectively, with food. Amlodipine: Absolute bioavailability (64-90%); T_{max}=6-12 hrs. **Distribution:** Amlodipine: Plasma protein binding (93%). **Metabolism:** Aliskiren: Via CYP3A4. Amlodipine: Hepatic (extensive). **Elimination:** Aliskiren: Urine (25% unchanged). Amlodipine: Urine (10% unchanged, 60% metabolites), $T_{1/2}$=30-50 hrs.

NURSING CONSIDERATIONS

Assessment: Assess for diabetes, history of angioedema, CAD, activated renin-angiotensin-aldosterone system (volume and/or salt depletion), renal artery stenosis, severe heart failure, post-MI, renal/hepatic impairment, pregnancy/nursing status, and possible drug interactions.

Monitoring: Monitor for signs/symptoms of hypotension, symptoms of angina or MI after dosage initiation or increase, hyperkalemia, angioedema of the head/neck, and airway obstruction. Monitor BP, serum K⁺ levels, and hepatic/renal function, including BUN and SrCr.

Patient Counseling: Inform of consequences of exposure during pregnancy; notify physician if pregnant/plan to become pregnant as soon as possible. Caution about lightheadedness, especially during the 1st days of therapy and advise to report physician. Instruct to d/c and consult physician if syncope occurs. Caution that inadequate fluid intake, excessive perspiration, diarrhea, or vomiting may lead to an excessive fall in BP, which may result in lightheadedness or syncope. Instruct to d/c and immediately report any signs/symptoms of angioedema (eg, swelling of the face, extremities, eyes, lips, tongue, difficulty swallowing or breathing). Instruct to avoid K⁺ supplements or salt substitutes containing K⁺ without consulting physician. Instruct to establish a routine pattern for taking medication with regard to meals; inform that high-fat meals decrease absorption substantially.

Administration: Oral route. **Storage:** 25°C (77°F); excursions permitted to 15-30°C (59-86°F). Protect from heat and moisture.

TEKTURNA

aliskiren (Novartis)

RX

> D/C when pregnancy is detected. Drugs that act directly on the renin-angiotensin system can cause injury/death to the developing fetus.

THERAPEUTIC CLASS: Renin inhibitor

INDICATIONS: Treatment of HTN.

DOSAGE: *Adults:* Initial: 150mg qd. Titrate: May increase to 300mg qd if BP is not adequately controlled. Max: 300mg/day.

HOW SUPPLIED: Tab: 150mg, 300mg

CONTRAINDICATIONS: Concomitant use with angiotensin receptor blockers (ARBs) or ACE inhibitors in patients with diabetes.

WARNINGS/PRECAUTIONS: Angioedema of the face, extremities, lips, tongue, glottis, and/or larynx reported; d/c therapy and do not readminister if angioedema occurs. In patients with an activated renin-angiotensin system (eg, volume- and/or salt-depleted patients such as those receiving high doses of diuretics), symptomatic hypotension may occur; correct these conditions prior to therapy or monitor closely. Renal function changes may occur; consider withholding or d/c therapy if clinically significant decrease in renal function develops. Caution in patients whose renal function may depend in part on renin-angiotensin system activity (eg, renal artery stenosis, severe heart failure, post-myocardial infarction [MI], or volume depletion). Hyperkalemia may occur; monitor serum K⁺ periodically. Caution in patients with risk factors for development of hyperkalemia (eg, renal insufficiency, diabetes).

ADVERSE REACTIONS: Angioedema, diarrhea, cough, hypotension, hyperkalemia, increased SrCr.

INTERACTIONS: See Contraindications. Concomitant use with ARBs or ACE inhibitor is not recommended in patients with GFR <60ml/min. Increased risk of renal impairment and hyperkalemia with ARBs or ACE inhibitors. Cyclosporine or itraconazole increase levels; avoid concomitant use. May cause hyperkalemia with K⁺-sparing diuretics, K⁺ supplements, or NSAIDs. Additive hyperuricemia with HCTZ. Possible interaction with P-glycoprotein inhibitors. NSAIDs, including selective cyclooxygenase-2 inhibitors, may result in deterioration of renal function and attenuation of antihypertensive effect.

PREGNANCY: Category D; not for use in nursing.

MECHANISM OF ACTION: Direct renin inhibitor; decreases plasma renin activity and inhibits conversion of angiotensinogen to angiotensin I.

PHARMACOKINETICS: Absorption: Poor; T_{max}=1-3 hrs; bioavailability (2.5%). **Metabolism:** Via CYP3A4. **Elimination:** Urine.

NURSING CONSIDERATIONS

Assessment: Assess for diabetes, renal impairment, renal artery stenosis, heart failure, post-MI, history of angioedema, volume-/salt-depletion, pregnancy/nursing status, and possible drug interactions. Obtain baseline BP.

Monitoring: Monitor BP, serum K⁺, renal function, and BUN levels. Monitor for angioedema of the head/neck and airway obstruction.

Patient Counseling: Counsel females of childbearing age about consequences of exposure during pregnancy; instruct to report pregnancy as soon as possible. Inform that angioedema may occur anytime during therapy; advise to d/c and report any signs/symptoms of angioedema immediately (eg, swelling of the face, extremities, eyes, lips, tongue, difficulty swallowing/breathing). Inform that lightheadedness can occur; instruct to report to physician. Advise to d/c treatment and to consult physician if syncope occurs. Inform that inadequate fluid intake, excessive perspiration, diarrhea, or vomiting can lead to an excessive fall in BP. Instruct patients not to use K⁺ supplements or salt substitutes containing K⁺ without consulting physician. Instruct to establish a routine pattern for taking medication with regard to meals and inform that high-fat meals decrease absorption substantially.

Administration: Oral route. **Storage:** 25°C (77°F); excursions permitted to 15-30°C (59-86°F). Protect from moisture.

TEKTURNA HCT

aliskiren - hydrochlorothiazide (Novartis)

RX

D/C when pregnancy is detected. Drugs that act directly on the renin-angiotensin system can cause injury/death to the developing fetus.

THERAPEUTIC CLASS: Renin inhibitor/thiazide diuretic

INDICATIONS: Treatment of HTN in patients whose BP is not adequately controlled with aliskiren or HCTZ monotherapy, is controlled with HCTZ alone but who experience hypokalemia, and in patients who experience dose-limiting adverse reactions on either component alone. Replacement therapy for the titrated components, and as initial therapy in patients likely to need multiple drugs to achieve BP goals.

DOSAGE: *Adults:* Add-On/Initial Therapy: Initial: 150mg-12.5mg qd. Titrate: May increase up to max of 300mg-25mg qd if BP remains uncontrolled after 2-4 weeks. Max: 300mg-25mg qd. Replacement Therapy: May substitute for individually titrated components.

HOW SUPPLIED: Tab: (Aliskiren-HCTZ) 150mg-12.5mg, 150mg-25mg, 300mg-12.5mg, 300mg-25mg

CONTRAINDICATIONS: Anuria, sulfonamide-derived drug hypersensitivity, and concomitant use with angiotensin receptor blockers (ARBs) or ACE inhibitors in patients with diabetes.

WARNINGS/PRECAUTIONS: Not indicated for initial therapy in patients with intravascular volume depletion. Symptomatic hypotension may occur in patients with activated renin-angiotensin system (eg, volume- and/or salt-depleted patients receiving high doses of diuretics); correct these conditions prior to therapy or monitor closely. Renal function changes may occur; caution in patients with renal artery stenosis, severe heart failure, post-myocardial infarction (MI), or volume depletion. Monitor renal function periodically and consider withholding or d/c if clinically significant decrease in renal function develops. May cause serum electrolyte abnormalities (eg, hyperkalemia, hypokalemia, hyponatremia, hypomagnesemia); correct hypokalemia and any coexisting hypomagnesemia prior to initiation of therapy and monitor periodically. D/C if hypokalemia is accompanied by clinical signs (eg, muscular weakness, paresis, or ECG alterations). Aliskiren: Angioedema of the face, extremities, lips, tongue, glottis and/or larynx reported; d/c therapy and do not readminister if angioedema occurs. Caution in patients with risk factors for development of hyperkalemia (eg, renal insufficiency, diabetes). HCTZ: May precipitate hepatic coma with hepatic impairment. May cause hypersensitivity reactions and exacerbation or activation of systemic lupus erythematosus (SLE). May cause an idiosyncratic reaction, resulting in transient myopia and acute angle-closure glaucoma; d/c as rapidly as possible. May alter glucose tolerance and increase serum cholesterol and TG levels. May cause or exacerbate hyperuricemia and precipitate gout in susceptible patients. May decrease urinary calcium excretion and cause elevations of serum calcium; monitor levels.

ADVERSE REACTIONS: Head and neck angioedema, dizziness, influenza, diarrhea, cough, vertigo, asthenia, arthralgia.

INTERACTIONS: See Contraindications. Avoid use with ARBs or ACE inhibitor in patients with GFR <60ml/min. Increased risk of renal impairment with ARBs or ACE inhibitors. Aliskiren: Cyclosporine or itraconazole increases levels; avoid concomitant use. Possible interaction with P-glycoprotein inhibitors. Increased risk of hyperkalemia with ARBs, ACE inhibitors, K⁺ supplements, K⁺ sparing diuretics, and NSAIDs. NSAIDs, including selective cyclooxygenase-2 inhibitors, may result in deterioration of renal function and attenuation of antihypertensive effect. HCTZ: Potentiation of orthostatic hypotension may occur with alcohol, barbiturates, and narcotics. Dosage adjustment of antidiabetic drugs (insulin or hypoglycemic agents) may be required. Ion exchange resins (eg, cholestyramine, colestipol) may reduce exposure; space dosing at least 4 hrs before or 4-6 hrs after the administration of ion exchange resins. May increase responsiveness to skeletal muscle relaxants (eg, curare derivatives). Thiazide-induced hypokalemia or hypomagnesemia may predispose patient to digoxin toxicity. Anticholinergic agents (eg, atropine, biperiden) may increase bioavailability. Prokinetic drugs may decrease bioavailability. May reduce renal excretion and enhance myelosuppressive effects of cytotoxic agents. Increased risk of lithium toxicity; avoid concurrent use.

PREGNANCY: Category D, not for use in nursing.

MECHANISM OF ACTION: Aliskiren: Direct renin inhibitor; decreases plasma renin activity and inhibits conversion of angiotensinogen to angiotensin I. HCTZ: Thiazide diuretic; has not been established. Affects renal tubular mechanisms of electrolyte reabsorption, directly increasing excretion of Na^+ and chloride in approximately equivalent amounts.

PHARMACOKINETICS: Absorption: Aliskiren: Poor. Bioavailability (2.5%); T_{max}=1 hr. HCTZ: Absolute bioavailability (70%); T_{max}=2.5 hrs. **Distribution:** HCTZ: Albumin binding (40-70%); crosses placenta; found in breast milk. **Metabolism:** Aliskiren: Via CYP3A4. **Elimination:** Aliskiren: Urine (25%, unchanged). HCTZ: Urine (70%, unchanged), $T_{1/2}$=10 hrs.

NURSING CONSIDERATIONS

Assessment: Assess for hepatic/renal impairment, anuria, sulfonamide-derived drug hypersensitivity, history of penicillin allergy, volume/salt depletion, history of allergy or bronchial asthma, SLE, risk for acute renal failure, history of angioedema, hypokalemia, hypomagnesemia, metabolic disturbances, heart failure, renal artery stenosis, post-MI, diabetes, pregnancy/nursing status, and possible drug interactions. Obtain baseline BP.

Monitoring: Monitor for idiosyncratic/hypersensitivity reactions, hypotension, metabolic disturbances, decreased visual acuity, ocular pain, and head/neck angioedema. Monitor BP, serum electrolytes, and renal function periodically.

Patient Counseling: Notify physician if any unusual symptoms develop or if any known symptoms persist or worsen. Counsel females of childbearing age about consequences of exposure during pregnancy; instruct to report pregnancies as soon as possible. Caution that lightheadedness may occur, especially during 1st few days of therapy; d/c and consult physician if syncope occurs. Caution that inadequate fluid intake, excessive perspiration, diarrhea, or vomiting can lead to excessive fall in BP, leading to lightheadedness and possible syncope. Instruct not to use K^+ supplements or salt substitutes containing K^+ without consulting a physician. Instruct to establish a routine pattern for taking medication with regard to meals and inform that high-fat meals decrease absorption substantially.

Administration: Oral route. **Storage:** 25°C (77°F); excursions permitted to 15-30°C (59-86°F). Protect from moisture.

TEMODAR

RX

temozolomide (Merck)

THERAPEUTIC CLASS: Alkylating agent (imidazotetrazine derivative)

INDICATIONS: Treatment of newly diagnosed glioblastoma multiforme (GBM) concomitantly with radiotherapy and as maintenance treatment. Treatment of refractory anaplastic astrocytoma (eg, patients experiencing disease progression on a drug regimen containing nitrosourea and procarbazine).

DOSAGE: *Adults:* (IV/PO) Adjust according to nadir neutrophil and platelet counts of previous cycle and at time of initiating next cycle. Newly Diagnosed High Grade GBM: 75mg/m² qd for 42 days with focal radiotherapy. Maint: Cycle 1 (28 days): 150mg/m² qd for 1st 5 days of each 28-day cycle. Cycle 2-6 (28 days): Refer to PI for specific dosing. Refractory Anaplastic Astrocytoma: Initial: 150mg/m² qd for 5 consecutive days per 28-day cycle. May continue therapy until disease progression. Refer to PI for dose modifications for hematologic and nonhematologic toxicities.

HOW SUPPLIED: Cap: 5mg, 20mg, 100mg, 140mg, 180mg, 250mg; Inj: 100mg [vial]

CONTRAINDICATIONS: Hypersensitivity to DTIC (dacarbazine).

WARNINGS/PRECAUTIONS: Myelosuppression may occur, including prolonged pancytopenia, which may result in aplastic anemia. Greater risk of myelosuppression in women and elderly. Cases of myelodysplastic syndrome and secondary malignancies, including myeloid leukemia, reported. *Pneumocystis carinii* pneumonia (PCP) prophylaxis required in all patients with newly diagnosed GBM receiving concomitant radiotherapy for 42-day regimen; higher occurrence of PCP when administered during a longer dosing regimen. Perform weekly blood counts until recovery if absolute neutrophil count <1.5 x 10⁹/L and platelet count <100 x 10⁹/L. May cause fetal harm in pregnancy. Caution in elderly and severe renal/hepatic impairment. (IV) Increased risk of infusion-related adverse reactions and suboptimal dosing with shorter or longer infusion time.

ADVERSE REACTIONS: Fatigue, alopecia, myelosuppression (eg, thrombocytopenia, neutropenia), N/V, anorexia, headache, constipation, fever, rash, convulsions, hemiparesis.

T

INTERACTIONS: May decrease clearance with valproic acid. Monitor all patients for the development of PCP, especially those receiving steroids. Concomitant use of medications associated with aplastic anemia, including carbamazepine, phenytoin, sulfamethoxazole/trimethoprim, complicate assessment.

PREGNANCY: Category D, not for use in nursing.

MECHANISM OF ACTION: Alkylating agent (imidazotetrazine derivative); exerts action by alkylation of DNA. Alkylation (methylation) occurs mainly at the O^6 and N^7 positions of guanine.

PHARMACOKINETICS: Absorption: (PO) Rapid and complete, T_{max}=1 hr; C_{max}= 7.5mcg/mL, 282ng/mL (MTIC); AUC=23.4mcg•hr/mL, 864ng•hr/mL (MTIC). (IV) C_{max}=7.3mcg/mL, 276ng/mL (MTIC); AUC=24.6mcg•hr/mL, 891ng•hr/mL (MTIC). **Distribution:** V_d=0.4L/kg; plasma protein binding (15%). **Metabolism:** Via spontaneous hydroxylation; 5-(3-methyltriazen-1-yl)-imidazole-4-carboxamide (MTIC) (major metabolite) to 5-amino-imidazole-4-carboxamide (AIC). **Elimination:** Urine (37.7%, 5.6% unchanged), feces (0.8%); $T_{1/2}$=1.8 hrs.

NURSING CONSIDERATIONS

Assessment: Assess for previous hypersensitivity, hypersensitivity to DTIC, myelosuppression, hepatic/renal functions, pregnancy/nursing status, and possible drug interactions. Obtain baseline CBC, platelet count, and ANC.

Monitoring: Monitor for CBC on Day 22 (21 days after 1st dose) or within 48 hrs of that day; repeat weekly until ANC >1.5 x 10⁹/L and platelet count >100 x 10⁹/L. Monitor for myelosuppression, pancytopenia, aplastic anemia, PCP, myelodysplastic syndrome, secondary malignancies, myeloid leukemia, infusion-related reactions, and other adverse reactions.

Patient Counseling: Take as prescribed; swallow cap whole and do not open or chew. Instruct not to open capsule; if accidentally opened or damaged, take rigorous precautions to avoid inhalation or contact with skin or mucous membranes. Counsel about adverse effects (eg, N/V); seek medical attention if any develop.

Administration: Oral and IV route. See PI for preparation and administration techniques. Swallow cap whole with water. **Storage:** (Cap) 25°C (77°F); excursions permitted to 15-30°C (59-96°F). (IV) 2-8°C (36-46°F). After reconstitution, store at 25°C (77°F); use reconstituted product within 14 hrs including infusion time.

TENORETIC   RX

atenolol - chlorthalidone (AstraZeneca)

THERAPEUTIC CLASS: Selective beta₁-blocker/monosulfamyl diuretic

INDICATIONS: Treatment of HTN.

DOSAGE: *Adults:* Individualize dose. Initial: 50mg-25mg tab qd. May increase to 100mg-25mg tab qd. CrCl 15-35mL/min: Max: 50mg atenolol/day. CrCl <15mL/min: Max: 50mg atenolol qod. Elderly: Start at low end of dosing range.

HOW SUPPLIED: Tab: (Atenolol-Chlorthalidone) 50mg-25mg, 100mg-25mg

CONTRAINDICATIONS: Sinus bradycardia, >1st-degree heart block, cardiogenic shock, overt cardiac failure, anuria, hypersensitivity to sulfonamide-derived drugs.

WARNINGS/PRECAUTIONS: Not for initial therapy. Avoid with untreated pheochromocytoma. May aggravate peripheral arterial circulatory disorders. Caution in elderly. Atenolol: May cause/precipitate heart failure; d/c if cardiac failure continues despite adequate treatment. Caution in patients with impaired renal function. Avoid abrupt d/c; exacerbation of angina and myocardial infarction reported. Avoid with bronchospastic disease, but may use with caution if unresponsive/intolerant of other antihypertensive treatment. Chronically administered therapy should not be routinely withdrawn prior to major surgery; however, may augment risks of general anesthesia and surgical procedures. Caution in diabetic patients; may mask tachycardia occurring with hypoglycemia. May mask clinical signs of hyperthyroidism and precipitate thyroid storm with abrupt d/c. Chlorthalidone: May precipitate azotemia with renal disease. If progressive renal impairment becomes evident, d/c therapy. Caution with impaired hepatic function or progressive liver disease; may precipitate hepatic coma. D/C prior to parathyroid function test. Decreased calcium excretion observed. Altered parathyroid glands, with hypercalcemia and hypophosphatemia, seen with prolonged therapy. Hyperuricemia may occur, or acute gout may be precipitated. Fluid/electrolyte imbalance (eg, hyponatremia, hypochloremic alkalosis, hypokalemia) may develop. Sensitivity reactions may occur. Exacerbation/activation of systemic lupus erythematous (SLE) reported. May enhance effects in postsympathectomy patient.

ADVERSE REACTIONS: Bradycardia, dizziness, fatigue, nausea.

INTERACTIONS: May potentiate other antihypertensive agents. Observe for hypotension and/or marked bradycardia with catecholamine-depleting drugs (eg, reserpine). Additive effects with calcium channel blockers. Atenolol: Bradycardia, heart block, and rise of left ventricular end diastolic pressure may occur with verapamil or diltiazem. May cause severe bradycardia, asystole, and heart failure with disopyramide. Additive effects with amiodarone. Prostaglandin synthase inhibitors (eg, indomethacin) may decrease hypotensive effects. Exacerbates rebound HTN with clonidine withdrawal. May be unresponsive to usual doses of epinephrine. Digitalis glycosides may slow atrioventricular conduction and increase risk of bradycardia. Chlorthalidone: May alter insulin requirements in diabetic patients; latent diabetes mellitus (DM) may become manifest. May develop hypokalemia with concomitant corticosteroids or adrenocorticotropic hormone. May decrease arterial response to norepinephrine. May increase responsiveness to tubocurarine. Avoid with lithium; risk of lithium toxicity.

PREGNANCY: Category D, caution in nursing.

MECHANISM OF ACTION: Atenolol: Cardioselective β-adrenoreceptor blocking agent; has not been established. Suspected to competitively antagonize catecholamines at peripheral adrenergic neuron sites, leading to decreased cardiac output; a central effect leading to reduced sympathetic outflow to the periphery and suppression of renin activity. Chlorthalidone: Monosulfamyl diuretic; acts on cortical diluting segment of ascending limb of Henle's loop and produces diuresis with increased excretion of Na^+ and Cl^-.

PHARMACOKINETICS: Absorption: Atenolol: Rapid, incomplete; T_{max}=2-4 hrs. **Distribution:** Crosses placenta. Atenolol: Plasma protein binding (6-16%); found in breast milk. **Elimination:** Atenolol: Renal excretion; feces (unchanged); $T_{1/2}$=6-7 hrs.

NURSING CONSIDERATIONS

Assessment: Assess for bradycardia, cardiogenic shock, >1st-degree heart block, overt cardiac failure, impaired renal/hepatic function, bronchospastic disease, peripheral vascular disease, DM, hyperthyroidism, pheochromocytoma, anuria, hypersensitivity to sulfonamide-derived drugs, serum electrolytes, parathyroid disease, pregnancy/nursing status, SLE, coronary artery disease, and possible drug interactions.

Monitoring: Monitor for cardiac failure, hepatic/renal function, withdrawal symptoms, hypersensitivity reactions, hyperuricemia or acute gout, and signs/symptoms of electrolyte imbalance. Monitor serum glucose, serum electrolytes (eg, K^+), and BP.

Patient Counseling: Instruct not to interrupt or d/c therapy without consulting physician. Notify physician if signs/symptoms of impending congestive heart failure or unexplained respiratory symptoms develop. Counsel about signs/symptoms of electrolyte imbalance (eg, dry mouth, thirst, weakness, lethargy), and advise to seek prompt medical attention. Inform that drug may cause potential harm to fetus; inform physician if pregnant/plans to become pregnant.

Administration: Oral route. **Storage:** 20-25°C (68-77°F).

TENORMIN RX
atenolol (AstraZeneca)

Avoid abrupt d/c of therapy in coronary artery disease (CAD). Severe exacerbation of angina and occurrence of myocardial infarction (MI) and ventricular arrhythmias reported in angina patients following abrupt d/c of β-blockers. If plan to d/c therapy, carefully observe and advise to limit physical activity. Promptly reinstitute therapy, at least temporarily, if angina worsens or acute coronary insufficiency develops. CAD may be unrecognized; may be prudent to avoid abrupt d/c in patients only treated for HTN.

THERAPEUTIC CLASS: Selective beta$_1$-blocker

INDICATIONS: Management of HTN alone or concomitantly with other antihypertensive agents. Long-term management of angina pectoris. Management of hemodynamically stable patients with definite or suspected acute myocardial infarction (AMI) to reduce cardiovascular mortality.

DOSAGE: *Adults:* HTN: Initial: 50mg qd, either alone or with diuretic therapy. Titrate: May increase to 100mg qd after 1-2 weeks. Max: 100mg qd. Angina: Initial: 50mg qd. Titrate: May increase to 100mg qd after 1 week. Max: 200mg qd. AMI: Initial: 5mg IV over 5 min, repeat 10 min later. If tolerated, give 50mg PO 10 min after the last IV dose, followed by another 50mg PO 12 hrs later. Maint: 100mg qd or 50mg bid for 6-9 days or until discharge from the hospital. Renal Impairment/Elderly: HTN: Initial: 25mg qd. HTN/Angina/AMI: Max: CrCl 15-35mL/min: 50mg/day. CrCl <15mL/min: 25mg/day. Hemodialysis: 25-50mg after each dialysis.

HOW SUPPLIED: Tab: 25mg, 50mg, 100mg

CONTRAINDICATIONS: Sinus bradycardia, >1st-degree heart block, cardiogenic shock, overt cardiac failure.

WARNINGS/PRECAUTIONS: May precipitate severe heart failure in patients with congestive heart failure (CHF) and cause cardiac failure in patients without history of heart failure; d/c if cardiac failure continues despite adequate treatment. Avoid with bronchospastic disease; if unresponsive to/intolerant of other antihypertensive treatment, use caution with bronchospastic disease. Chronically administered therapy should not be routinely withdrawn prior to major surgery; however, may augment risks of general anesthesia and surgical procedures. Caution in diabetic patients; may mask tachycardia occurring with hypoglycemia. May mask clinical signs of hyperthyroidism and precipitate thyroid storm with abrupt d/c. Avoid with untreated pheochromocytoma. May cause fetal harm. May aggravate peripheral arterial circulatory disorders. Caution in elderly and in patients with renal impairment.

ADVERSE REACTIONS: Tiredness, dizziness, cold extremities, depression, fatigue, dyspnea, postural hypotension, bradycardia, leg pain, lightheadedness, lethargy, diarrhea, nausea, wheeziness.

INTERACTIONS: Additive effects with thiazide-type diuretics, catecholamine-depleting drugs (eg, reserpine), calcium channel blockers, and amiodarone. Severe bradycardia, asystole, and heart failure is associated with disopyramide. Bradycardia and heart block can occur and left ventricular end diastolic pressure can rise with verapamil or diltiazem. Exacerbates rebound HTN with clonidine withdrawal. Prostaglandin synthase inhibitors (eg, indomethacin) may decrease hypotensive effects. May be unresponsive to usual doses of epinephrine. Concomitant use with digitalis glycosides may increase risk of bradycardia.

PREGNANCY: Category D, caution in nursing.

MECHANISM OF ACTION: Cardioselective β-adrenoreceptor-blocking agent; not established. Suspected to competitively antagonize catecholamines at peripheral (especially cardiac) adrenergic neuron sites, leading to decreased cardiac output; a central effect leading to reduced sympathetic outflow to the periphery and suppression of renin activity.

PHARMACOKINETICS: Absorption: Rapid, incomplete; T_{max}=2-4 hrs. **Distribution:** Plasma protein binding (6-16%); found in breast milk; crosses the placenta. **Metabolism:** Liver. **Elimination:** Urine (50%), feces (unchanged); $T_{1/2}$=6-7 hrs.

NURSING CONSIDERATIONS

Assessment: Assess for history of hypersensitivity, bradycardia, cardiogenic shock, >1st-degree heart block, overt cardiac failure, acute MI, renal dysfunction, bronchospastic disease, conduction abnormalities, left ventricular dysfunction, peripheral arterial circulatory disorders, diabetes mellitus, hyperthyroidism, pheochromocytoma, pregnancy/nursing status, and for possible drug interactions.

Monitoring: Monitor for signs/symptoms of cardiac failure, and for masking of hyperthyroidism. Monitor renal function, pulse, and BP. Following abrupt d/c monitor for thyroid storm and in patients with angina, monitor for severe exacerbation of angina, MI, and ventricular arrhythmias.

Patient Counseling: Instruct to take as prescribed. Advise not to interrupt or d/c therapy without first consulting physician. Counsel to notify physician if signs/symptoms of congestive heart failure or unexplained respiratory symptoms develop. Inform that drug may cause fetal harm; instruct to notify physician if pregnant or if considering becoming pregnant.

Administration: Oral route. **Storage:** 20-25°C (68-77°F).

TERAZOSIN RX
terazosin HCl (Various)

THERAPEUTIC CLASS: Alpha$_1$-blocker (quinazoline)

INDICATIONS: Treatment of HTN and symptomatic BPH.

DOSAGE: *Adults:* If d/c for several days or longer, restart using the initial dosing regimen. HTN: Initial: 1mg hs. Usual: 1-5mg qd. If response is substantially diminished at 24 hrs, may slowly increase dose or use bid regimen. Max: 40mg/day. BPH: Initial: 1mg qhs. Titrate: Increase stepwise to 2mg, 5mg, or 10mg qd to achieve the desired improvement of symptoms and/or flow rates. Usual: 10mg/day. Assess clinical response after 4-6 weeks. Max: 20mg/day.

HOW SUPPLIED: Cap: 1mg, 2mg, 5mg, 10mg

WARNINGS/PRECAUTIONS: May cause marked lowering of BP especially postural hypotension and syncope with the 1st dose or 1st few days of therapy; similar effect may be anticipated if therapy is d/c for several days and then restarted. May impair physical/mental abilities. Examine patients with BPH to rule out prostate cancer prior to initiation of therapy. Priapism (rare) reported. Intraoperative floppy iris syndrome observed during cataract surgery. Decreases in Hct, Hgb, WBC, total protein and albumin reported, possibly due to hemodilution.

ADVERSE REACTIONS: Asthenia, postural hypotension, headache, dizziness, dyspnea, nasal congestion, somnolence, palpitations, nausea, peripheral edema, pain in extremities.

INTERACTIONS: Caution with other antihypertensive agents (eg, verapamil); may need dose reduction or retitration of either agent with other antihypertensive agents. Increased levels with captopril. Hypotension reported with PDE-5 inhibitors.

PREGNANCY: Category C, caution in nursing.

MECHANISM OF ACTION: Alpha$_1$-blocker; (BPH) antagonizes α$_1$-receptors in bladder neck and prostate, relaxing smooth muscle; (HTN) antagonizes α$_1$-receptors decreasing total peripheral vascular resistance, causing decreased BP.

T

PHARMACOKINETICS: Absorption: Complete; T_{max}=1 hr. **Distribution:** Plasma protein binding (90-94%). **Elimination:** Feces (60%), urine (40%); $T_{1/2}$=12 hrs, 14 hrs (≥70 yrs), 11.4 hrs (20-39 yrs).

NURSING CONSIDERATIONS

Assessment: Assess BP, pregnancy/nursing status, and possible drug interactions. Rule out prostate cancer with BPH.

Monitoring: Monitor Hct, Hgb, WBC, total protein/albumin, and BP periodically. Monitor for signs/symptoms of hypotension, priapism, and hypersensitivity reactions.

Patient Counseling: Inform of possibility of syncope and orthostatic symptoms, especially at initiation of therapy. Caution against driving or hazardous tasks for 12 hrs after 1st dose, dosage increase, or when resuming therapy after interruption. Avoid situations where injury could result should syncope occur. Advise to sit or lie down when symptoms of low BP occur. Inform of possibility of priapism; advise to seek medical attention if it occurs and inform that it can lead to permanent erectile dysfunction if not brought to immediate medical attention.

Administration: Oral route. **Storage:** 20-25°C (68-77°F).

TESSALON
benzonatate (Pfizer)

RX

THERAPEUTIC CLASS: Non-narcotic antitussive

INDICATIONS: Symptomatic relief of cough.

DOSAGE: *Adults:* Usual: 100mg or 200mg tid PRN. Max: 600mg/day in 3 divided doses. *Pediatrics:* >10 yrs: Usual: 100mg or 200mg tid PRN. Max: 600mg/day in 3 divided doses.

HOW SUPPLIED: Cap: 200mg, (Perle) 100mg

WARNINGS/PRECAUTIONS: Severe hypersensitivity reactions (eg, bronchospasm, laryngospasm, cardiovascular collapse) reported, possibly related to local anesthesia. Swallow capsules without sucking/chewing to avoid local anesthesia adverse effects. Accidental ingestion resulting in death reported in children <10 yrs; keep out of reach of children. May cause adverse CNS effects; caution with prior sensitivity to related agents, such as para-amino-benzoic acid (PABA) based anesthetics (eg, procaine, tetracaine).

ADVERSE REACTIONS: Hypersensitivity, sedation, headache, constipation, nausea, GI upset, pruritus, skin eruptions, nasal congestion, numbness of the chest.

INTERACTIONS: Bizarre behavior (eg, mental confusion, visual hallucinations) reported with other prescribed drugs. May cause adverse CNS effects with concomitant medications.

PREGNANCY: Category C, caution in nursing.

MECHANISM OF ACTION: Non-narcotic antitussive agent; acts peripherally by anesthetizing the stretch receptors located in the respiratory passages, lungs, and pleura by dampening their activity, thereby reducing cough reflex at its source.

NURSING CONSIDERATIONS

Assessment: Assess for previous sensitivity to related compounds, such as PABA-based anesthetics (eg, procaine, tetracaine), pregnancy/nursing status, and for possible drug interactions.

Monitoring: Monitor for hypersensitivity reactions (eg, bronchospasm, laryngospasm, cardiovascular collapse), mental confusion, visual hallucinations, overdose signs/symptoms (eg, restlessness, tremors, clonic convulsions followed by profound CNS depression).

Patient Counseling: Advise not to break, chew, dissolve, cut, or crush the drug and to swallow whole. Instruct to avoid food or liquid ingestion if numbness or tingling of the tongue, mouth, throat, or face occurs; if symptoms worsen, advise to seek medical attention. Instruct to keep out of reach of children. Inform that overdosage may occur in adults; advise not to exceed single dose of 200mg and total daily dose of 600mg, and not to take two doses at a time.

Administration: Oral route. Swallow whole; do not break, chew, dissolve, cut, or crush. **Storage:** 25°C (77°F); excursions permitted to 15-30°C (59-86°F).

TESTIM
testosterone (Auxilium)

CIII

Virilization reported in children secondarily exposed to testosterone gel. Children should avoid contact with unwashed or unclothed application sites in men using testosterone gel. Advise patients to strictly adhere to recommended instructions for use.

THERAPEUTIC CLASS: Androgen

INDICATIONS: Replacement therapy in adult males for conditions associated with a deficiency or absence of endogenous testosterone (eg, congenital/acquired primary hypogonadism or hypogonadotropic hypogonadism).

DOSAGE: *Adults:* ≥18 yrs: Initial: Apply 5g qd, preferably in am, to clean, dry, intact skin of shoulders and/or upper arms. Allow to dry prior to dressing. Titrate: May increase to 10g qd if response not achieved or serum concentration is below normal range. Do not apply to genitals or abdomen; wash hands after application. To maintain serum testosterone levels, do not wash application site for ≥2 hrs.

HOW SUPPLIED: Gel: 1% [5g/tube, 30ˢ]

CONTRAINDICATIONS: Known/suspected prostate carcinoma or breast carcinoma in men. Use in women. Pregnant and nursing women should avoid skin contact with application sites on men. Hypersensitivity to soy products.

WARNINGS/PRECAUTIONS: Increases risk for worsening of BPH. Increases risk for prostate cancer; evaluate for prostate cancer prior to therapy, especially in elderly patients. Risk of virilization in women (eg, changes in body hair distribution, significant increase in acne) due to secondary skin exposure from contact with men using testosterone-containing gel products; d/c until cause of virilization has been identified. Risk of edema with or without congestive heart failure (CHF) with preexisting cardiac, renal, or hepatic disease; d/c if edema occurs, diuretic therapy may be required. Gynecomastia may develop and occasionally persists in patients being treated for hypogonadism. May potentiate sleep apnea, especially with risk factors such as obesity or chronic lung diseases. Advise patients to report persistent penis erections, changes in skin color, ankle swelling, unexplained N/V, or breathing disturbances.

ADVERSE REACTIONS: Application-site reactions, virilization from secondary exposure.

INTERACTIONS: May elevate oxyphenbutazone levels. May decrease blood glucose and insulin requirements in diabetics. Adrenocorticotropic hormone or corticosteroids may enhance edema; caution with cardiac or hepatic disease.

PREGNANCY: Category X, not for use in nursing.

MECHANISM OF ACTION: Androgen; responsible for normal growth and development of male sex organs and for maintenance of secondary sex characteristics.

PHARMACOKINETICS: Absorption: 10% absorbed systemically. **Distribution:** Sex hormone-binding globulin (SHBG) binding (40%), albumin- and plasma protein-binding (58%), unbound (2%). **Metabolism:** Skin, liver, male urogenital tract via 5α-reductase; estradiol and dihydrotestosterone (metabolites). **Elimination:** Urine (90%), feces (6%); $T_{1/2}$=10-100 min.

NURSING CONSIDERATIONS

Assessment: Assess for conditions where treatment is contraindicated, breast or prostate carcinoma, BPH, cardiac or renal/hepatic disease, obesity, chronic lung disease, polycythemia, pregnancy/nursing status of female partner, and possible drug interactions. Assess for hypersensitivity to soy products.

Monitoring: Monitor for signs/symptoms of hypersensitivity reactions, edema with/without CHF, gynecomastia, BPH, virilization, and worsening of BPH, prostate carcinoma in geriatrics, and potentiation of sleep apnea. Perform periodic monitoring of Hgb, Hct, LFTs, prostatic-specific antigen, HDL, and serum testosterone levels. Obtain serum testosterone levels 14 days after initiation of therapy.

Patient Counseling: Inform of pregnancy risks; avoid contact with application sites in children and women or if pregnant/nursing. If contact occurs, wash area immediately with soap and water. Instruct not to apply to the scrotum, penis, or abdomen. Cover application site with clothing after gel dries; wash application site with soap and water prior to direct skin-to-skin contact. Advise not to wash or swim until ≥2 hrs after application. Contact physician if experience changes in body hair distribution, increase in acne, virilization of female partner or child, too-frequent or persistent erections, changes in skin color, ankle swelling, unexplained N/V, breathing disturbances, or hypersensitivity reactions. Advise to carefully read Medication Guide. Apply qd at approximately the same time each day. Avoid if have known/suspected prostate or breast cancer. Keep out of reach of children. Inform that drug is flammable.

Administration: Topical route. Apply every day at same time to clean, dry skin of shoulder or upper arms. Wash hands thoroughly after application. **Storage:** 25°C (77°F); excursions permitted to 15-30°C (59-86°F).

TESTRED

CIII

methyltestosterone (Valeant)

THERAPEUTIC CLASS: Androgen

INDICATIONS: Testosterone-replacement therapy in males with primary hypogonadism or hypogonadotropic hypogonadism. To stimulate puberty in males with delayed puberty. May be used secondarily in females with advancing inoperable metastatic (skeletal) mammary cancer who are 1-5 yrs postmenopausal. Treatment in premenopausal females with breast cancer who have benefitted from oophorectomy and have a hormone-responsive tumor.

DOSAGE: *Adults:* Individualize dose (based on age, sex, and diagnosis). Adjust according to response and appearance of adverse reactions. Replacement Therapy in Androgen-Deficient Males: 10-50mg/day. Breast Carcinoma in Females: 50-200mg/day.

Pediatrics: Individualize dose (based on age, sex, and diagnosis). Adjust according to response and appearance of adverse reactions. Replacement Therapy in Androgen-Deficient Males: 10-50mg/day. Delayed Puberty in Males: Use lower range of 10-50mg/day for limited duration (eg, 4-6 months). May start on lower dose, then gradually increase as puberty progresses with/ without a decrease to maint levels, or may start on higher dose, then use a lower maint dose after puberty.

HOW SUPPLIED: Cap: 10mg

CONTRAINDICATIONS: Males with carcinomas of the breast or with known/suspected carcinomas of the prostate. Females who are or may become pregnant.

WARNINGS/PRECAUTIONS: May cause hypercalcemia in patients with breast cancer; d/c if this occurs. Peliosis hepatis and hepatic neoplasms, including hepatocellular carcinoma, reported with prolonged use of high doses. D/C if cholestatic hepatitis, jaundice, or abnormal LFTs occur. May increase risk of prostatic hypertrophy and prostatic carcinoma in elderly. Edema with or without congestive heart failure (CHF) may develop with preexisting cardiac, renal, or hepatic disease; d/c and consider diuretic therapy. Gynecomastia may develop. Caution in healthy males with delayed puberty; monitor bone maturation by assessing bone age of wrist and hand every 6 months. May accelerate bone maturation without producing compensatory gain in linear growth in children; may result in compromised adult stature. Should not be used for enhancement of athletic performance. Monitor for signs of virilization in females; d/c therapy at evidence of mild virilism.

ADVERSE REACTIONS: Amenorrhea, menstrual irregularities, inhibition of gonadotropin secretion, virilization in females, gynecomastia, excessive frequency and duration of penile erections, hirsutism, male pattern baldness, acne, fluid and electrolyte disturbances, nausea, cholestatic jaundice, alterations in LFTs, headache, anxiety.

INTERACTIONS: May decrease oral anticoagulant requirement. May increase oxyphenbutazone levels. May decrease blood glucose and insulin requirements in diabetics.

PREGNANCY: Category X, not for use in nursing.

MECHANISM OF ACTION: Androgen; responsible for normal growth and development of male sex organs and for maintenance of secondary sex characteristics.

PHARMACOKINETICS: Metabolism: Liver (less extensive compared to testosterone). **Elimination:** Urine, feces; $T_{1/2}$=Longer compared to testosterone.

NURSING CONSIDERATIONS

Assessment: Assess for breast/prostate carcinoma in males, cardiac/renal/hepatic disease, pregnancy/nursing status, other conditions where treatment is contraindicated/cautioned, and possible drug interactions.

Monitoring: Monitor for signs/symptoms of hypercalcemia, liver dysfunction, edema with/without CHF, prostatic hypertrophy/carcinoma in elderly, virilization in females, and other adverse reactions. Periodically monitor urine and serum calcium in breast cancer patients, Hgb, Hct, and LFTs. Assess bone age of the wrist and hand every 6 months in males with delayed puberty.

Patient Counseling: Instruct to report to physician any of the following: too-frequent or persistent erections of the penis (adult/adolescent males); hoarseness, acne, changes in menstrual period, more hair on the face (females); and N/V, changes in skin color or ankle swelling (all patients).

Administration: Oral route. **Storage:** 25°C (77°F); excursions permitted to 15-30°C (59-86°F).

TETANUS & DIPHTHERIA TOXOIDS ADSORBED   RX
diphtheria toxoid - tetanus toxoid (Various)

THERAPEUTIC CLASS: Toxoid combination

INDICATIONS: Active immunization for the prevention of tetanus and diphtheria (Td) in persons ≥7 yrs.

DOSAGE: *Adults:* Primary immunization: 0.5mL IM (deltoid) in a series of three doses. The first 2 doses are administered 4-8 weeks apart. Administer 3rd dose 6-12 months after 2nd dose. Routine booster immunization in persons who have completed primary immunization every 10 yrs thereafter. Tetanus prophylaxis in wound management: Preparation containing Td toxoids is preferred. Refer to PI for proper guide to tetanus prophylaxis in routine wound management.

May be used for postexposure diphtheria prophylaxis in persons who have not completed primary vaccination, whose vaccination status is unknown, or have not been vaccinated with diphtheria toxoid within the previous 5 yrs.

Pediatrics: ≥7 yrs: Primary immunization: 0.5mL IM (deltoid) in a series of three doses. The first 2 doses are administered 4-8 weeks apart. Administer 3rd dose 6-12 months after 2nd dose. Routine booster immunization in children 7 yrs and older who have completed primary immunization. Routine booster is recommended in children 11-12 yrs and every 10 yrs thereafter. Tetanus prophylaxis in wound management: Preparation containing Td toxoids is preferred. Refer to PI for proper guide to tetanus prophylaxis in routine wound management. May be used for postexposure diphtheria prophylaxis in children 7 yrs and older who have not completed primary vaccination, whose vaccination status is unknown, or have not been vaccinated with diphtheria toxoid within the previous 5 yrs.

HOW SUPPLIED: Inj: (Diphtheria toxoid - Tetanus toxoid) 2Lf-2Lf/0.5mL

WARNINGS/PRECAUTIONS: Immune response may not be obtained in immunocompromised patients. Increased incidence and severity of adverse reactions with more frequent administration. Do not give more frequently than every 10 yrs in persons who experienced an Arthus-type hypersensitivity reaction following a prior dose of a tetanus toxoid-containing vaccine. Have epinephrine (1:1000) and other appropriate agents and equipment available for anaphylactic reactions. Caution with tetanus toxoid-related Guillain-Barre syndrome. Not for pediatrics <7 yrs.

ADVERSE REACTIONS: Injection-site reactions, malaise, nausea, arthralgia, pyrexia, peripheral edema, dizziness, headache, convulsion, myalgia, musculoskeletal stiffness or pain, rash, cellulitis.

INTERACTIONS: May have reduced immune response with immunosuppressive therapy, including alkylating agents, antimetabolite, cytotoxic drugs, irradiation, or corticosteroids (used in greater than physiologic doses).

PREGNANCY: Category C, caution in nursing.

MECHANISM OF ACTION: Toxoid combination; activates neutralizing antibodies to diphtheria and tetanus toxins for protection against diphtheria and tetanus.

NURSING CONSIDERATIONS

Assessment: Assess history of vaccination to determine necessity of boosters. In cases of wound care, determine the necessity of tetanus prophylaxis. Assess for history of hypersensitivity reactions following previous dose of vaccine, current health status and health history, pregnancy/nursing status, and possible drug interaction. Assess for history of Arthus-type hypersensitivity reaction and Guillain-Barre syndrome following prior dose of a tetanus toxoid-containing vaccine.

Monitoring: Monitor for increased incidence and severity of adverse reactions and hypersensitivity reactions.

Patient Counseling: Inform of the benefits and risks of immunization and of importance of completing the primary immunization series or receiving recommended booster doses. Instruct to report any adverse reactions to healthcare provider.

Administration: IM route (deltoid). Inspect for particulate matter and/or discoloration prior to administration. Shake well before withdrawing each dose. Avoid into gluteal areas. Do not administer IV, SQ, or ID. **Storage:** 2-8°C (36-46°F). Do not freeze. Do not use after expiration date.

T

TEVETEN RX
eprosartan mesylate (Abbott)

> D/C when pregnancy is detected. Drugs that act directly on the renin-angiotensin system can cause injury/death to the developing fetus.

THERAPEUTIC CLASS: Angiotensin II receptor antagonist

INDICATIONS: Treatment of HTN, alone or with other antihypertensives (eg, diuretics, calcium channel blockers).

DOSAGE: *Adults:* Initial (Monotherapy and Not Volume-Depleted): 600mg qd. Usual: 400-800mg/day, given qd-bid. If antihypertensive effect is inadequate with qd regimen, give bid using same total daily dose or consider dose increase. Max: 800mg/day. Moderate and Severe Renal Impairment: Max: 600mg/day. Max BP reduction in most patients may take 2-3 weeks.

HOW SUPPLIED: Tab: 400mg, 600mg

WARNINGS/PRECAUTIONS: In patients with an activated renin-angiotensin system (eg, volume- and/or salt-depleted patients receiving diuretics), symptomatic hypotension may occur; correct volume or salt depletion prior to therapy or monitor closely. Renal function changes reported. Oliguria and/or progressive azotemia and acute renal failure and/or death (rare), may occur in patients whose renal function may depend on the renin-angiotensin-aldosterone system (eg, severe congestive heart failure [CHF]). Increases in SrCr or BUN reported with renal artery stenosis.

ADVERSE REACTIONS: Upper respiratory tract infection, rhinitis, pharyngitis, cough.

INTERACTIONS: NSAIDs, including selective cyclooxygenase-2 inhibitors, may deteriorate renal function; monitor renal function periodically. Antihypertensive effect may be attenuated by NSAIDs.

PREGNANCY: Category D, not for use in nursing.

MECHANISM OF ACTION: Angiotensin II receptor antagonist; blocks vasoconstrictor and aldosterone-secreting effects of angiotensin II by selectively blocking binding of angiotensin II to AT_1 receptor found in many tissues.

PHARMACOKINETICS: Absorption: (300mg) Absolute bioavailability (13%); T_{max}=1-2 hrs (fasted). **Distribution:** V_d=308L; plasma protein binding (98%). **Elimination:** Feces (90%), urine (7%; 80%, unchanged); (multiple doses of 600mg) $T_{1/2}$=20 hrs.

NURSING CONSIDERATIONS

Assessment: Assess for volume or salt depletion, renal impairment, CHF, renal artery stenosis, previous hypersensitivity to drug, pregnancy/nursing status, and for possible drug interactions.

Monitoring: Monitor for signs/symptoms of hypotension, renal function changes, and other adverse reactions. Monitor BP.

Patient Counseling: Inform of pregnancy risks and instruct to contact physician immediately if patient becomes pregnant. Instruct to notify physician if any adverse reactions develop.

Administration: Oral route. **Storage:** 20-25°C (68-77°F).

TEVETEN HCT
eprosartan mesylate - hydrochlorothiazide (Abbott)

RX

D/C when pregnancy is detected. Drugs that act directly on the renin-angiotensin system can cause injury/death to the developing fetus.

THERAPEUTIC CLASS: Angiotensin II receptor antagonist/thiazide diuretic

INDICATIONS: Treatment of HTN, alone or with other antihypertensives (eg, calcium channel blockers).

DOSAGE: *Adults:* Begin combination therapy only after failure to achieve desired effect with monotherapy. Refer to PI for monotherapy dosing. Replacement Therapy: May substitute for individual components. Usual (Not Volume-Depleted): 600mg-12.5mg qd. Titrate: May increase to 600mg-25mg qd. Max: 600mg-25mg qd. If additional BP control required, or to maintain bid dosing of monotherapy, 300mg eprosartan may be added qpm. Moderate and Severe Renal Impairment: Max: Eprosartan: 600mg qd. Max BP reduction in most patients may take 2-3 weeks.

HOW SUPPLIED: Tab: (Eprosartan-HCTZ) 600mg-12.5mg, 600mg-25mg

CONTRAINDICATIONS: Anuria, sulfonamide-derived drug hypersensitivity.

WARNINGS/PRECAUTIONS: Not for initial therapy of HTN. In patients with an activated renin-angiotensin system (eg, volume- and/or salt-depleted patients receiving diuretics), symptomatic hypotension may occur; correct volume or salt depletion prior to therapy or monitor closely. HCTZ: Caution with hepatic impairment or progressive liver disease; may precipitate hepatic coma. Hypersensitivity reactions may occur. May cause idiosyncratic reaction, resulting in acute transient myopia and acute angle-closure glaucoma; d/c as rapidly as possible. May exacerbate or activate systemic lupus erythematosus (SLE). Hyperuricemia may occur or frank gout may be precipitated. Hyperglycemia, hypomagnesemia, and hypercalcemia may occur. D/C prior to parathyroid test. May enhance effects in postsympathectomy patients. Observe for signs of fluid or electrolyte imbalance (hyponatremia, hypochloremic alkalosis, and hypokalemia). May precipitate azotemia; caution with severe renal disease. Withhold or d/c with evident progressive renal impairment. Eprosartan: Renal function changes reported. Oliguria and/or progressive azotemia and acute renal failure and/or death (rare), may occur in patients whose renal function may depend on the renin-angiotensin-aldosterone system (eg, severe congestive heart failure [CHF]). Increases in SrCr or BUN reported in patients with renal artery stenosis.

ADVERSE REACTIONS: Dizziness, headache, back pain, fatigue, myalgia, upper respiratory tract infection.

INTERACTIONS: NSAIDs, including selective cyclooxygenase-2 inhibitors, may decrease effects of diuretics and angiotensin II receptor antagonists and may further deteriorate renal function. Eprosartan: K⁺-sparing diuretics (eg, spironolactone, triamterene, amiloride), K⁺ supplements, or K⁺-containing salt substitutes may increase serum K⁺. HCTZ: Increased risk of lithium toxicity; avoid concurrent use. Alcohol, barbiturates, and narcotics may potentiate orthostatic hypotension. Dose adjustment of antidiabetic drugs (eg, oral agents, insulin) may be required. Additive effect or potentiation with other antihypertensives. Anionic exchange resins (eg, cholestyramine and colestipol resins) may impair absorption. Corticosteroids and adrenocorticotropic hormone may intensify electrolyte depletion, particularly hypokalemia. May decrease response to pressor amines (eg, norepinephrine). May increase responsiveness to nondepolarizing skeletal muscle relaxants (eg, tubocurarine).

PREGNANCY: Category D, not for use in nursing.

MECHANISM OF ACTION: Eprosartan: Angiotensin II receptor antagonist; blocks vasoconstrictor and aldosterone-secreting effects of angiotensin II by selectively blocking binding of angiotensin II to AT_1 receptor found in many tissues. HCTZ: Thiazide diuretic; has not been established. Affects the renal tubular mechanisms of electrolyte reabsorption, directly increasing excretion of Na^+ and Cl^- in approximately equivalent amounts.

PHARMACOKINETICS: Absorption: Eprosartan: (300mg) Absolute bioavailability (13%); T_{max}=1-2 hrs (fasted). **Distribution:** Eprosartan: V_d=308L; plasma protein binding (98%). HCTZ: Crosses placenta; found in breast milk. **Elimination:** Eprosartan: Feces (90%), urine (7%; 80%, unchanged); (multiple doses of 600mg) $T_{1/2}$=20 hrs. HCTZ: Urine (≥61%, unchanged); $T_{1/2}$=5.6-14.8 hrs.

NURSING CONSIDERATIONS

Assessment: Assess for anuria, sulfonamide-derived drug hypersensitivity, history of penicillin allergy, volume or salt depletion, renal/hepatic impairment, history of allergy or bronchial asthma, SLE, electrolyte imbalance, diabetes mellitus (DM), postsympathectomy status, CHF, renal artery stenosis, previous hypersensitivity to drug, pregnancy/nursing status, and possible drug interactions.

Monitoring: Monitor for signs/symptoms of hypotension, hypersensitivity reactions, renal/hepatic impairment, idiosyncratic reaction, exacerbation/activation of SLE, hyperuricemia or precipitation of gout, latent DM, and other adverse effects. Monitor BP and serum electrolytes periodically.

Patient Counseling: Inform of pregnancy risks and instruct to contact physician immediately if patient becomes pregnant. Counsel that lightheadedness may occur, especially during 1st days of therapy; instruct to d/c therapy and consult physician if syncope occurs. Advise that inadequate fluid intake, excessive perspiration, diarrhea, or vomiting may result in drop of BP, leading to lightheadedness or syncope. Instruct not to use K^+ supplements or salt substitutes containing K^+ without consulting physician.

Administration: Oral route. **Storage:** 20-25°C (68-77°F).

THALOMID
thalidomide (Celgene)

RX

> Severe birth defects or death to unborn baby may occur if taken during pregnancy. Should never be used by pregnant women or women who could become pregnant. Approved for marketing only under a special restricted distribution program called "System for Thalidomide Education and Prescribing Safety (S.T.E.P.S®)." May increase risk of venous thromboembolic events in patients with multiple myeloma, especially with standard chemotherapeutic agents including dexamethasone; observe for signs/symptoms of thromboembolism. Instruct patients to seek medical care if symptoms such as SOB, chest pain, arm or leg swelling develop. Consider thromboprophylaxis based on assessment of individual's underlying risk factors.

THERAPEUTIC CLASS: Immunomodulatory agent

INDICATIONS: Treatment of newly diagnosed multiple myeloma in combination with dexamethasone. Acute treatment of the cutaneous manifestations of moderate to severe erythema nodosum leprosum (ENL). Maintenance therapy for prevention and suppression of the cutaneous manifestations of ENL recurrence.

DOSAGE: *Adults:* Take with water, preferably at hs, and ≥1hr after evening meal. Multiple Myeloma: 200mg qd. Give with dexamethasone 40mg PO on days 1-4, 9-12, and 17-20 q28 days. ENL: Acute: Initial: 100-300mg qd. <50kg: Start at lower end of dosing range. Severe/Patients Who Previously Required Higher Doses to Control Reaction: Initial: Higher doses up to 400mg/day qd in divided doses. May use corticosteroids in moderate to severe neuritis with severe ENL; taper and d/c steroid when neuritis is ameliorated. Usual Duration: ≥2 weeks until signs/symptoms have subsided. Taper dose in 50mg decrements q2-4 weeks. Maint Therapy for Prevention/Suppression of ENL Recurrence: Use minimum dose to control reaction. Attempt tapering off therapy q3-6 months, in decrements of 50mg q2-4 weeks.
Pediatrics: ≥12 yrs: Take with water, preferably at hs, and ≥1hr after evening meal. Multiple Myeloma: 200mg qd. Give with dexamethasone 40mg PO on days 1-4, 9-12, and 17-20 q28 days. ENL: Acute: Initial: 100-300mg qd. <50kg: Start at lower end of dosing range. Severe/Patients Who Previously Required Higher Doses to Control Reaction: Initial: Higher doses up to 400mg/day qd in divided doses. May use corticosteroids in moderate to severe neuritis with severe ENL; taper and d/c steroid when neuritis is ameliorated. Usual Duration: ≥2 weeks until

signs/symptoms have subsided. Taper dose in 50mg decrements q2-4 weeks. Maintenance Therapy for Prevention/Suppression of ENL Recurrence: Use minimum dose to control reaction. Attempt tapering off therapy q3-6 months, in decrements of 50mg q2-4 weeks.

HOW SUPPLIED: Cap: 50mg, 100mg, 150mg, 200mg

CONTRAINDICATIONS: Pregnancy and women of childbearing potential.

WARNINGS/PRECAUTIONS: Male patients (including those with vasectomy) with female partners of childbearing potential must either completely abstain from sexual contact or must always use a latex/synthetic condom during any sexual contact. Women of reproductive potential should avoid contact with caps; wash exposed area with soap and water if contact with non-intact caps or powder contents occur. Healthcare providers or other caregivers should utilize appropriate precautions to prevent potential cutaneous exposure. Avoid blood or semen donation during therapy or for 4 weeks after d/c of therapy. May impair physical/mental ability. May cause irreversible peripheral neuropathy; monitor for symptoms and d/c therapy if drug-induced neuropathy develops. May cause dizziness and orthostatic hypotension; sit upright for a few minutes prior to standing. Decreased WBC, including neutropenia reported; do not initiate if absolute neutrophil count is <750/mm^3. May increase plasma HIV RNA levels in HIV-seropositive patients. Bradycardia reported; dose reduction or d/c may be required. May cause serious dermatologic reactions (eg, Stevens-Johnson syndrome [SJS], toxic epidermal necrolysis [TEN]); d/c if skin rash occurs and do not resume therapy if the rash is exfoliative, purpuric, or bullous or if SJS or TEN is suspected. Seizures, including grand mal convulsions, reported. Monitor and use caution in patients at risk of tumor lysis syndrome. Consider risks of adverse effects in choosing contraceptive methods. Hypersensitivity reported; d/c if severe reactions develop. Not indicated as monotherapy for cutaneous manifestations of moderate/severe ENL in the presence of moderate/severe neuritis.

ADVERSE REACTIONS: Drowsiness/somnolence, peripheral neuropathy, dizziness, neutropenia, rash, constipation, hypocalcemia, thrombosis/embolism, dyspnea, edema, anorexia, depression, agitation.

INTERACTIONS: See Boxed Warning. Avoid with medications that may cause drowsiness. Avoid with opioids, antihistamines, antipsychotics, antianxiety agents, or CNS depressants; may cause an additive sedative effect. Caution with drugs that may cause additive bradycardic effect (eg, calcium channel blockers, β-blockers, α/β-adrenergic blockers, digoxin, H$_2$ blockers, lithium, TCAs, neuromuscular blockers). Caution with drugs associated with peripheral neuropathy (eg, bortezomib, amiodarone, cisplatin, docetaxel, paclitaxel, vincristine, disulfiram, phenytoin, metronidazole, alcohol). Use two other effective or highly effective methods of contraception when HIV-protease inhibitors, griseofulvin, modafinil, penicillins, rifampin, rifabutin, phenytoin, carbamazepine, or certain herbal supplements such as St. John's wort are given concomitantly with hormonal contraceptive agents.

PREGNANCY: Category X, not for use in nursing.

MECHANISM OF ACTION: Immunomodulatory agent; not established. Possesses immunomodulatory, anti-inflammatory, and antiangiogenic properties. Immunologic effects may be caused by suppression of excessive TNF-α production and down-modulation of selected cell surface adhesion molecules involved in leukocyte migration. Also causes suppression of macrophage involvement in prostaglandin synthesis and modulation of interleukin-10 and -12 production by peripheral blood mononuclear cells. In multiple myeloma, increased numbers of circulating natural killer cells and plasma levels of interleukin-2 and INF-gamma are also seen.

PHARMACOKINETICS: Absorption: Administration of variable doses resulted in different parameters. **Distribution:** Plasma protein binding (55%, [+]-[R]-thalidomide and 66%, [-]-[S]-thalidomide). **Metabolism:** Hydrolysis. **Elimination:** Feces (<2%); urine (91.9%); T$_{1/2}$=5.5-7.3 hrs.

NURSING CONSIDERATIONS

Assessment: Assess use in those capable of reproduction. Assess that patients are committed to either abstaining from heterosexual contact or willing to use a latex or synthetic condom for males or two forms of reliable contraception, including one highly effective method and one additional effective method for females, beginning 4 weeks prior to treatment, during treatment, and continuing 4 weeks after treatment. Assess pregnancy status 24 hrs prior to therapy. Assess for moderate to severe neuritis, history/risk factors for seizures, drug hypersensitivity, nursing status, and possible drug interactions. Obtain baseline electrophysiological testing and neutrophil count prior to therapy.

Monitoring: Monitor for venous thromboembolic events, drowsiness, somnolence, peripheral neuropathy, dizziness, orthostatic hypotension, neutropenia, hypersensitivity reactions, bradycardia, syncope, seizures, serious dermatological reactions, missed periods, or abnormal menstrual bleeding. Perform pregnancy test weekly during first 4 weeks, then repeat at 4 weeks (regular menstrual cycle) or every 2 weeks (irregular menstrual cycle). Monitor for use of two reliable forms of contraception during and for 4 weeks after d/c therapy. Perform electrophysiologic testing every 6 months, and WBC with differential count periodically. In HIV patients, monitor viral load after 1st and 3rd months of therapy and every 3 months thereafter.

T

Patient Counseling: Inform about the potential teratogenicity of the drug; women of childbearing potential must have monthly pregnancy tests and must use two different forms of contraception including at least a highly effective form simultaneously during therapy and for at least 4 weeks after completing the therapy. Instruct to immediately d/c and contact physician if she becomes pregnant, misses her menstrual period, experiences unusual menstrual bleeding, or if she stops taking birth control. Instruct males to abstain from sexual contact or to use latex condoms during any sexual contact. Take medication as prescribed. Counsel of increased risk of deep vein thrombosis and pulmonary embolism in patients with multiple myeloma; drowsiness and somnolence may occur and impair mental/physical abilities.

Administration: Oral route. **Storage:** 25°C (77°F); excursions permitted to 15-30°C (59-86°F). Protect from light.

THEOPHYLLINE ER RX
theophylline (Various)

THERAPEUTIC CLASS: Methylxanthine

INDICATIONS: Treatment of the symptoms and reversible airflow obstruction associated with chronic asthma and other chronic lung disease (eg, emphysema, chronic bronchitis).

DOSAGE: *Adults:* 16-60 yrs: Individualize dose. Initial: 300-400mg qd (am or pm) for 3 days. Titrate: After 3 days, if tolerated, increase to 400-600mg qd. After 3 more days, if tolerated and needed, may increase dose >600mg according to blood levels. With Risk Factors for Impaired Clearance/Elderly (>60 yrs)/Not Feasible Serum Theophylline Concentrations: Max: 400mg/day. Conversion from Immediate-Release Theophylline: Give same daily dose as once daily. Refer to PI for other dosage instructions and dosage adjustment based on peak serum concentrations. *Pediatrics:* 12-15 yrs: Individualize dose. >45kg: Initial: 300-400mg qd (am or pm) for 3 days. Titrate: Increase to 400-600mg qd. After 3 more days, if tolerated and needed, may increase dose >600mg according to blood levels. <45kg: Initial: 12-14mg/kg/day up to a maximum of 300mg qd for 3 days. Titrate: After 3 days, if tolerated, increase to 16mg/kg/day up to a maximum of 400mg qd. After 3 more days, if tolerated and needed, increase to 20mg/kg/day up to a maximum of 600mg qd. With Risk Factors for Impaired Clearance/Not Feasible Serum Theophylline Concentrations: Max: 16mg/kg/day up to a maximum of 400mg/day. Conversion from Immediate-Release Theophylline: Give same daily dose as once daily. Refer to PI for other dosage instructions and dosage adjustment based on peak serum concentrations.

HOW SUPPLIED: Tab, Extended-Release: 400mg*, 600mg* *scored

WARNINGS/PRECAUTIONS: Extreme caution with active peptic ulcer disease, seizure disorders, and cardiac arrhythmias (not including bradyarrhythmias); increased risk of exacerbation. Caution with risk factor for reduced clearance, such as in neonates, children <1 yr, and elderly (>60 yrs), acute pulmonary edema, congestive heart failure, fever (≥102°F for 24 hrs or lesser temperature for longer periods), cor pulmonale, hypothyroidism, liver disease (eg, cirrhosis, acute hepatitis), reduced renal function in infants <3 months of age, sepsis with multiorgan failure, and shock; risk for fatal toxicity if total daily dose is not appropriately reduced. Hyperthyroidism and cystic fibrosis are associated with increased clearance. Withhold therapy and monitor serum levels if signs and symptoms of toxicity (eg, N/V, repetitive vomiting) occur, until they resolve. Avoid dose increase in response to acute exacerbation of symptoms of chronic lung disease. Measure peak steady-state serum theophylline concentration before increasing doses and limit dose increase to about 25% of the previous total daily dose to reduce risk of unintended excessive increase in serum levels.

ADVERSE REACTIONS: N/V, headache, insomnia, diarrhea, restlessness, tremors, hematemesis, hypokalemia, hyperglycemia, sinus tachycardia, hypotension/shock, nervousness, disorientation, arrhythmias, seizures.

INTERACTIONS: Blocks adenosine receptors. Alcohol, allopurinol, cimetidine, ciprofloxacin, clarithromycin, erythromycin, disulfiram, enoxacin, estrogen, fluvoxamine, interferon human recombinant α-A, methotrexate, mexiletine, pentoxifylline, propafenone, propranolol, tacrine, thiabendazole, ticlopidine, troleandomycin, and verapamil decreased theophylline clearance and increase its concentration. Aminoglutethimide, carbamazepine, isoproterenol (IV), moricizine, phenobarbital (after 2 weeks of phenobarbital use), phenytoin, rifampin, sulfinpyrazone increased theophylline clearance. May increase risk of ventricular arrhythmias with halothane. May lower theophylline seizure threshold with ketamine. Renal lithium clearance may increase. Concomitant use with pancuronium may antagonize its nondepolarizing neuromuscular blocking effects; larger doses may be required. Diazepam, flurazepam, midazolam, and lorazepam may require larger doses to produce desired level of sedation. Increased frequency of nausea, nervousness, and insomnia with ephedrine. Decreased concentrations with St. John's wort. Phenytoin concentrations may be decreased.

PREGNANCY: Category C, caution in nursing.

MECHANISM OF ACTION: Methylxanthine; acts via smooth muscle relaxation and suppression of airway response to stimuli. Bronchodilatation suggested to be mediated by inhibiting two isozymes of phosphodiesterase. Also increases the force of contraction of diaphragmatic muscles due to enhancement of calcium uptake through adenosine-mediated channel.

PHARMACOKINETICS: Absorption: Complete; bioavailability (59%, fasting). Administration of different doses resulted in different parameters. **Distribution:** V_d = 0.45L/kg; plasma protein binding (40%); crosses the placenta; found in breast milk. Metabolism: Liver (extensive); demethylation and hydroxylation via CYP1A2, 2E1, 3A3; caffeine and 3-methylxanthine (active metabolites). **Elimination:** Urine (10% unchanged), (50% unchanged in neonates). Elimination half-life varied based on age and physiological states; refer to PI for details.

NURSING CONSIDERATIONS

Assessment: Assess use with any conditions where treatment is contraindicated or cautioned. Assess known hypersensitivity, renal/hepatic functions, pregnancy/nursing status, and possible drug interactions.

Monitoring: Carefully monitor serum drug levels (target unbound concentration: 6-12mcg/mL) for dose adjustments, drug toxicity, worsening of chronic illness, hepatic dysfunction. Monitor plasma glucose, uric acid, free fatty acids, cholesterol, HDL, LDL, LFTs, and urine-free cortisol excretion. Monitoring for signs and symptoms of toxicity (eg, nausea, repetitive vomiting), adjust dosage based on serum levels.

Patient Counseling: Instruct to seek medical attention if N/V, persistent headache, insomnia, or rapid heartbeat occur. Counsel not to take St. John's wort concurrently; consult physician before stopping St. John's wort. Instruct to take once daily in morning or evening, consistently take with/without food, tablet may be split in half, and do not chew or crush. Inform physician if new illness (especially if accompanied with persistent fever) or worsening of chronic illness occurs, and if patient starts/stops smoking cigarettes or marijuana. Inform all physicians of theophylline use, especially if medication is being added or removed from treatment. Instruct not to alter the dose, timing of dose, or frequency of administration without consulting physician; instruct that if dose is missed, take next dose at the usual scheduled time and not to attempt to make up for the missed dose.

Administration: Oral route. **Storage:** 25°C (77°F); excursions permitted to 15-30°C (59-86°F).

Tiazac
diltiazem HCl (Forest)

RX

OTHER BRAND NAMES: Taztia XT (Andrx)

THERAPEUTIC CLASS: Calcium channel blocker (nondihydropyridine)

INDICATIONS: Treatment of HTN alone or in combination with other antihypertensives. Treatment of chronic stable angina.

DOSAGE: *Adults:* HTN: Usual: 120-240mg qd. Titrate: Adjust at 2-week intervals. Max: 540mg qd. Angina: Initial: 120-180mg qd. Titrate: Increase over 7-14 days. Max: 540mg qd. Elderly: Start at low end of dosing range.

HOW SUPPLIED: Cap, Extended-Release: 120mg, 180mg, 240mg, 300mg, 360mg; (Tiazac) 420mg

CONTRAINDICATIONS: Sick sinus syndrome and 2nd- or 3rd-degree atrioventricular (AV) block (except with a functioning pacemaker), severe hypotension (<90mmHg systolic), acute myocardial infarction (AMI), pulmonary congestion documented by x-ray.

WARNINGS/PRECAUTIONS: Prolongs AV node refractory periods. May develop asystole with Prinzmetal's angina. Caution in patients with preexisting ventricular dysfunction; worsening of congestive heart failure (CHF) reported. Symptomatic hypotension may occur. Mild elevations of transaminases (eg, alkaline phosphatase, bilirubin, LDH, SGOT, SGPT) reported. Acute hepatic injury reported. Caution in patients with impaired renal or hepatic function. Monitor LFTs and renal function with prolonged use. D/C if persistent dermatologic reactions (eg, skin eruptions progressing to erythema multiforme and/or exfoliative dermatitis) occur. Caution in elderly.

ADVERSE REACTIONS: Peripheral edema, dizziness, headache, infection, pain, pharyngitis, dyspepsia, dyspnea, bronchitis, AV block, asthenia, vasodilation.

INTERACTIONS: Potential additive effects with agents known to affect cardiac contractility and/or conduction. Increased levels of carbamazepine, midazolam, triazolam, lovastatin, and propranolol; monitor closely. Increased levels of diltiazem with cimetidine. Monitor digoxin and cyclosporine levels if used concomitantly. Potentiates cardiac contractility, conductivity, and automaticity, and vascular dilation with anesthetics. Additive cardiac conduction effects with digitalis or β-blockers. Avoid rifampin and other CYP3A4 inducers. Additive antihypertensive effect when used concomitantly with other antihypertensive agents. Other drugs that are specific substrates, inhibitors, or inducers of CYP3A4 may have a significant impact on the efficacy and side effect profile of diltiazem. (Tiazac) Increased levels of buspirone and quinidine. Increased risk of myopathy and rhabdomyolysis with statins (eg, lovastatin, simvastatin). Sinus bradycardia reported with the use of clonidine concurrently; monitor HR.

PREGNANCY: Category C, not for use in nursing.

MECHANISM OF ACTION: Calcium channel blocker; inhibits cellular influx of calcium ions during membrane depolarization of cardiac and vascular smooth muscle. HTN: Primarily by relaxation of vascular smooth muscle and the resultant decrease in peripheral vascular resistance. Angina: Reduces myocardial oxygen demand and inhibits coronary artery spasms.

PHARMACOKINETICS: Absorption: Well-absorbed; absolute bioavailability (40%). **Distribution:** Plasma protein binding (70-80%); found in breast milk. **Metabolism:** Hepatic; desacetyldiltiazem, desmethyldiltiazem (major metabolites). **Elimination:** Urine (2%-4%, unchanged); bile; $T_{1/2}$=4-9.5 hrs.

NURSING CONSIDERATIONS

Assessment: Assess for sick sinus syndrome and 2nd- or 3rd-degree AV block without a functional ventricular pacemaker, severe hypotension, acute MI, pulmonary congestion (documented by x-ray), CHF, ventricular dysfunction, renal/hepatic function, drug hypersensitivity, pregnancy/nursing status and possible drug interactions.

Monitoring: Monitor LFTs (eg, alkaline phosphatase, bilirubin, LDH, SGOT, SGPT), BP, HR, renal/hepatic/cardiac function, ECG abnormalities. Monitor for signs/symptoms of angina and dermatological reactions (eg, skin eruptions progressing to erythema multiforme and/or exfoliative dermatitis).

Patient Counseling: Counsel about signs/symptoms of adverse effects. Instruct to take as prescribed. Educate about need for routine check-up and lab exams. When administering with applesauce, it should not be hot and should be soft enough to swallow without chewing.

Administration: Oral route. May be administered by opening the capsule and sprinkling contents on a spoonful of applesauce. The applesauce should be swallowed immediately without chewing and followed with a glass of water. Do not divide contents. **Storage:** (Taztia XT) 20-25°C (68-77°F). (Tiazac) 25°C (77°F); excursions permitted to 15-30°C (59-86°F). Avoid excessive humidity.

Tıgan   RX
trimethobenzamide HCl (Various)

THERAPEUTIC CLASS: Emetic response modifier

INDICATIONS: Treatment of postoperative nausea and vomiting, and nausea associated with gastroenteritis.

DOSAGE: *Adults:* Usual: (Cap) 300mg tid-qid. (Inj) 200mg IM tid-qid. Adjust according to indication, severity of symptoms, and response. Renal Impairment (CrCl ≤70mL/min/1.73m²): Reduce dose or increase dosing interval. Elderly: Start at lower end of dosing range.

HOW SUPPLIED: Cap: 300mg; Inj: 100mg/mL

CONTRAINDICATIONS: (Inj) Pediatric patients.

WARNINGS/PRECAUTIONS: May impair physical/mental abilities. Caution with acute febrile illness, encephalitides, gastroenteritis, dehydration, electrolyte imbalance, especially in children/elderly/debilitated; CNS reactions reported. Caution in the elderly and with renal impairment. May obscure diagnosis of appendicitis and signs of toxicity due to overdosage of other drugs. (Cap) Caution in children; may cause extrapyramidal symptoms (EPS), which may be confused with CNS signs of undiagnosed primary disease (eg, Reye's syndrome, other encephalopathy) and may unfavorably alter the course of Reye's syndrome due to hepatotoxic potential. Not recommended for uncomplicated vomiting in children.

ADVERSE REACTIONS: Parkinson-like symptoms, blood dyscrasias, blurred vision, coma, convulsions, mood depression, diarrhea, disorientation, dizziness, drowsiness, headache, jaundice, muscle cramps, opisthotonos.

INTERACTIONS: Caution with CNS-acting agents (phenothiazines, barbiturates, belladonna derivatives) in acute febrile illness, encephalitides, gastroenteritis, dehydration, and electrolyte imbalance due to potential CNS reactions. Adverse drug interaction reported with alcohol.

PREGNANCY: Safety in pregnancy and nursing not known.

MECHANISM OF ACTION: Not established; thought to involve chemoreceptor trigger zone, through which emetic impulses are conveyed to vomiting center (direct impulses to vomiting center apparently not similarly inhibited).

PHARMACOKINETICS: Absorption: T_{max}=30 min (IM 200mg), 45 min (cap 300mg). **Metabolism:** Oxidation, trimethobenzamide N-oxide (major metabolite). **Elimination:** Urine (30-50%, unchanged); $T_{1/2}$=7-9 hrs.

NURSING CONSIDERATIONS

Assessment: Assess for renal/hepatic impairment, Reye's syndrome in children, alcohol intake, acute febrile illness, encephalitides, gastroenteritis, dehydration, electrolyte imbalance, appendicitis, previous hypersensitivity to the drug, possible drug interactions, and any other conditions where treatment is contraindicated or cautioned.

Monitoring: Monitor renal function, for signs of hepatotoxicity, CNS reactions (eg, opisthotonos, convulsions, coma), EPS, hydration status, and electrolytes.

Patient Counseling: May cause drowsiness; caution against performing hazardous tasks (operating machinery/driving). Advise patients to not consume alcohol due to a potential drug interaction.

Administration: Oral and IM route. **Storage:** 25°C (77°F); excursions permitted to 15-30°C (59-86°F).

TIKOSYN

RX

dofetilide (Pfizer)

> To minimize risk of arrhythmia, for a minimum of 3 days, place patients initiated or reinitiated on therapy in a facility that can provide CrCl calculation, ECG monitoring, and cardiac resuscitation. Drug is available only to hospitals and prescribers who have received appropriate dofetilide dosing and treatment initiation education.

THERAPEUTIC CLASS: Class III antiarrhythmic

INDICATIONS: Conversion of atrial fibrillation (A-fib)/atrial flutter (A-flutter) to normal sinus rhythm and maintenance of normal sinus rhythm in patients with highly symptomatic A-fib/A-flutter of >1 week duration who were converted to normal sinus rhythm.

DOSAGE: *Adults:* Individualize dose based on CrCl and QT interval (if HR <60bpm). Initial: CrCl >60mL/min: 500mcg bid. CrCl 40-60mL/min: 250mcg bid. CrCl 20-<40mL/min: 125mcg bid. Titrate: Check QTc 2-3 hrs after 1st dose and adjust dose if QTc >500msec (550msec in patients with ventricular conduction abnormalities) or increases by >15% from baseline. If initial dose is 500mcg bid, reduce dose to 250mcg bid. If initial dose is 250mcg bid, reduce dose to 125mcg bid. If initial dose is 125mcg bid, reduce dose to 125mcg qd. D/C therapy if at any time after the 2nd dose QTc >500msec (550msec in patients with ventricular conduction abnormalities). If renal function deteriorates, adjust dose following initial dosing. Max: CrCl >60mL/min: 500mcg bid. Refer to PI for complete dosing instructions.

HOW SUPPLIED: Cap: 125mcg, 250mcg, 500mcg

CONTRAINDICATIONS: Long QT syndromes, baseline QT interval or QTc >440msec (500msec with ventricular conduction abnormalities), severe renal impairment (CrCl <20mL/min). Concomitant verapamil, HCTZ, and inhibitors of renal cation transport system (eg, cimetidine, trimethoprim, ketoconazole, prochlorperazine, megestrol).

WARNINGS/PRECAUTIONS: May cause serious ventricular arrhythmias, primarily torsades de pointes (TdP). Calculate CrCl before 1st dose; adjust dose based on CrCl. Caution in severe hepatic impairment. Do not discharge patients within 12 hrs of conversion to normal sinus rhythm. Maintain normal K+ levels prior to and during administration. Patients with atrial fibrillation should be anticoagulated prior to cardioversion and may continue to use after cardioversion. Rehospitalize patient for 3 days anytime dose is increased. Consider electrical cardioversion if patient does not convert to normal sinus rhythm within 24 hrs of initiation of therapy. Allow 2 days washout period before start of potentially interacting drugs. Caution with elderly.

ADVERSE REACTIONS: Headache, chest pain, dizziness, ventricular arrhythmia, dyspnea, nausea, insomnia, ventricular tachycardia, TdP, respiratory tract infection, flu syndrome, back pain, diarrhea, rash, abdominal pain.

INTERACTIONS: See Contraindications. Hypokalemia or hypomagnesemia may occur with K+-depleting diuretics. CYP3A4 inhibitors (eg, macrolides, azole antifungals, protease inhibitors, serotonin reuptake inhibitors, amiodarone, cannabinoids, diltiazem, grapefruit juice, nefazadone, norfloxacin, quinine, zafirlukast) and drugs actively secreted by cationic secretion (eg, triamterene, metformin, and amiloride) may increase levels; caution when coadministered. Not recommended with drugs that prolong the QT interval (eg, phenothiazines, cisapride, bepridil, TCAs, certain oral macrolides, and certain fluoroquinolones). Withhold Class I and III antiarrhythmics for at least three half-lives before initiating dofetilide. Do not initiate therapy until amiodarone levels are <0.3mcg/mL or until amiodarone has been withdrawn for at least 3 months. Higher occurrence of TdP with digoxin.

PREGNANCY: Category C, not for use in nursing.

MECHANISM OF ACTION: Class III antiarrhythmic; blocks cardiac ion channel carrying rapid component of delayed rectifier K+ current, I_{Kr}.

PHARMACOKINETICS: Absorption: T_{max}=2-3 hrs (fasted). **Distribution:** V_d=3L/kg; plasma protein binding (60-70%). **Metabolism:** Liver via CYP3A4 through N-dealkylation and N-oxidation pathways. **Elimination:** Urine (80% unchanged, 20% metabolites); $T_{1/2}$=10 hrs.

NURSING CONSIDERATIONS

Assessment: Assess for previous hypersensitivity to the drug, congenital or acquired long QT syndrome, renal/hepatic impairment, pregnancy/nursing status, and possible drug interactions. Correct K⁺ levels prior to therapy. Obtain baseline ECG and CrCl prior to therapy.

Monitoring: Monitor serum K⁺ levels and for development of ventricular arrhythmias (eg, TdP). After initiation or cardioversion, continuously monitor by ECG for a minimum of 3 days, or for a minimum of 12 hrs after pharmacological conversion to normal sinus rhythm, whichever is greater. Evaluate renal function and QTc every 3 months or PRN.

Patient Counseling: Inform about risks/benefits, need for compliance with prescribed dosing, potential drug interactions, and the need for periodic monitoring of QTc and renal function. Instruct to notify physician of any changes in medications and supplements. Counsel to report immediately any symptoms associated with electrolyte imbalance (eg, excessive/prolonged diarrhea, sweating, vomiting, loss of appetite, thirst). Instruct not to double the next dose if a dose is missed.

Administration: Oral route. **Storage:** 15-30°C (59-86°F). Protect from humidity and moisture.

TIMENTIN
ticarcillin disodium - clavulanate potassium (GlaxoSmithKline)

RX

THERAPEUTIC CLASS: Broad-spectrum penicillin/beta-lactamase inhibitor

INDICATIONS: Treatment of septicemia (including bacteremia), lower respiratory tract, bone and joint, skin and skin structure, urinary tract (UTI), gynecologic, and intra-abdominal infections, caused by susceptible strains of microorganisms.

DOSAGE: *Adults:* ≥60kg: UTI/Systemic Infection: 3.1g (3g ticarcillin, 100mg clavulanate) q4-6h. Gynecologic Infections: (Based on ticarcillin content) Moderate: 200mg/kg/day in divided doses q6h. Severe: 300mg/kg/day in divided doses q4h. <60kg: (Based on ticarcillin content) 200-300mg/kg/day in divided doses q4-6h. Administer by IV over 30 min for 10-14 days but may prolong duration for difficult/complicated infections; continue for ≥2 days after signs/symptoms of infection disappear. Persistent Infections: May require treatment for several weeks; do not use doses smaller than indicated above. Renal Impairment: Refer to PI. *Pediatrics:* ≥3 months: ≥60kg: Mild to Moderate Infections: 3.1g (3g ticarcillin, 100mg clavulanate) q6h. Severe Infections: 3.1g q4h. <60kg: (Based on ticarcillin content): Usual: 50mg/kg/dose. Mild to Moderate Infections: 200mg/kg/day in divided doses q6h. Severe: 300mg/kg/day in divided doses q4h. Administer by IV over 30 min for 10-14 days but may prolong duration for difficult/complicated infections; continue for ≥2 days after signs/symptoms of infection disappear. Persistent Infections: May require treatment for several weeks; do not use doses smaller than indicated above. Renal Impairment: Refer to PI.

HOW SUPPLIED: Inj: (Ticarcillin-Clavulanate) 3g-100mg (3.1g) [Vial, Add-Vantage]; 3g-100mg/100mL [Galaxy]. Also available as a Pharmacy Bulk Package. Refer to individual package insert for more information.

WARNINGS/PRECAUTIONS: Serious, fatal hypersensitivity reactions reported; d/c and institute appropriate therapy if an allergic reaction occurs. *Clostridium difficile*-associated diarrhea (CDAD) reported. Periodically assess organ system functions (including renal, hepatic, hematopoietic function) during prolonged therapy. Risk of convulsions with high doses, especially with renal impairment. Bleeding manifestations associated with coagulation tests abnormalities (eg, clotting time, platelet aggregation, PT) may occur, especially with renal impairment; d/c therapy if occurs. Hypokalemia reported; caution with fluid and electrolyte imbalance. Periodically monitor serum K⁺ with prolonged therapy. Consider the salt content of the drug (4.51mEq/g) in patients requiring restricted salt intake. May result in bacterial resistance with prolonged use or use in the absence of a proven/suspected bacterial infection or a prophylactic indication; take appropriate measures if superinfection develops. Caution in elderly.

ADVERSE REACTIONS: Hypersensitivity reactions, headache, giddiness, taste/smell disturbances, stomatitis, N/V, diarrhea, thrombocytopenia, leukopenia, elevated AST/ALT, elevated SrCr/BUN, hemorrhagic cystitis.

INTERACTIONS: Increased serum levels and prolonged $T_{1/2}$ with probenecid. May reduce efficacy of combined oral estrogen/progesterone contraceptives. Inactivates aminoglycoside when mixed together in solutions for parenteral administration.

PREGNANCY: Category B, caution in nursing.

MECHANISM OF ACTION: Ticarcillin: Semisynthetic broad-spectrum penicillin (PCN) with bactericidal activity against many gram-positive and -negative aerobic and anaerobic bacteria.

Clavulanic acid: β-lactamase inhibitor; possesses ability to inactivate wide range of β-lactamase enzymes.

PHARMACOKINETICS: Absorption: Ticarcillin: C_{max}=330mcg/mL, 324mcg/mL (Galaxy), AUC=485mcg•hr/mL (adults), 339mcg•hr/mL (infants/children). Clavulanic acid: C_{max}=8mcg/mL, AUC=8.2mcg•hr/mL (adults), 7mcg•hr/mL (infants/children). **Distribution:** Plasma protein binding (45%, ticarcillin), (25%, clavulanic acid). **Elimination:** Ticarcillin: Urine (60-70%, unchanged); $T_{1/2}$=1.1 hrs (adults), 4.4 hrs (neonates), 1 hr (infants/children). Clavulanic acid: Urine (35-45%, unchanged); $T_{1/2}$=1.1 hrs (adults), 1.9 hrs (neonates), 0.9 hr (infants/children).

NURSING CONSIDERATIONS

Assessment: Assess for organisms causing the infection and their susceptibility to drug, previous hypersensitivity reactions to PCNs, cephalosporins, or other allergens, renal/hepatic impairment, presence of fluid/electrolyte imbalance, restricted salt intake, pregnancy/nursing status, and possible drug interactions.

Monitoring: Periodically monitor organ system functions (including renal, hepatic, hematopoietic function) and serum K^+ levels with prolonged use. Monitor for signs/symptoms of anaphylactic/allergic reactions, CDAD, drug resistance or superinfection, and bleeding manifestations.

Patient Counseling: Counsel that drug only treats bacterial, not viral (eg, common cold), infections. Instruct to take ud; inform that skipping doses or not completing the full course may decrease effectiveness and increase resistance. Inform that diarrhea is a common problem and usually ends when antibiotic is d/c. Advise that watery and bloody stools (with or without stomach cramps and fever) may develop even as late as ≥2 months after last dose; instruct to notify physician immediately if this occurs.

Administration: IV route; infuse over 30 min. Refer to individual PI for compatibility, stability, and directions for use. **Storage:** Vial: ≤24°C (75°F). Galaxy: -20°C (-4°F); Thawed Sol: 22°C (72°F) for 24 hrs or 4°C (39°F) for 7 days. Do not refreeze.

TIMOLOL   RX
timolol maleate (Various)

THERAPEUTIC CLASS: Nonselective beta-blocker

INDICATIONS: Treatment of HTN. To reduce cardiovascular mortality and risk of reinfarction with previous myocardial infarction (MI). Migraine prophylaxis.

DOSAGE: *Adults:* HTN: Initial: 10mg bid. Maint: 20-40mg/day. Wait at least 7 days between dose increases. Max: 60mg/day given bid. MI: 10mg bid. Migraine: Initial: 10mg bid. Maint: 20mg qd. Max: 30mg/day in divided doses. May decrease to 10mg qd. D/C if inadequate response after 6-8 weeks with max dose.

HOW SUPPLIED: Tab: 5mg, 10mg*, 20mg* *scored

CONTRAINDICATIONS: Active or history of bronchial asthma, severe chronic obstructive pulmonary disease (COPD), sinus bradycardia, 2nd- and 3rd-degree atrioventricular (AV) block, overt cardiac failure, cardiogenic shock.

WARNINGS/PRECAUTIONS: Caution with well-compensated cardiac failure, diabetes mellitus (DM), mild to moderate COPD, bronchospastic disease, dialysis, hepatic/renal impairment, or cerebrovascular insufficiency. Exacerbation of ischemic heart disease with abrupt cessation. May mask hyperthyroidism or hypoglycemia symptoms. Withdrawal before surgery is controversial. May potentiate weakness with myasthenia gravis. Can cause cardiac failure. Caution and consider monitoring renal function in elderly.

ADVERSE REACTIONS: Fatigue, headache, nausea, arrhythmia, pruritus, dizziness, dyspnea, asthenia, bradycardia.

INTERACTIONS: Possible additive effects and hypotension and/or marked bradycardia with catecholamine-depleting drugs. NSAIDs may reduce antihypertensive effects. Quinidine may potentiate β-blockade. AV conduction time prolonged with digitalis and either diltiazem or verapamil. Hypotension, AV conduction disturbances, left ventricular failure reported with oral calcium antagonists. Caution with IV calcium antagonists, insulin, oral hypoglycemics. Avoid calcium antagonists with cardiac dysfunction. May exacerbate rebound HTN following clonidine withdrawal. May block effects of epinephrine.

PREGNANCY: Category C, not for use in nursing.

MECHANISM OF ACTION: β_1- and β_2-adrenergic receptor blocking agent; reduces cardiac output and plasma renin activity.

PHARMACOKINETICS: Absorption: (PO) Completely absorbed (90%); T_{max}=2 hrs. **Metabolism:** Partially, by liver. **Excretion:** Kidneys; $T_{1/2}$=4 hrs.

T

NURSING CONSIDERATIONS

Assessment: Assess for bradycardia, cardiogenic shock, 2nd- and 3rd-degree heart block, overt cardiac failure, impaired hepatic/renal function, bronchospastic disease, peripheral vascular disease, DM, thyrotoxicosis, valvular heart disease, pregnancy/nursing status, and possible drug interactions.

Monitoring: Monitor for cardiac failure, HTN, renal function, exacerbation of ischemia following abrupt withdrawal, bronchospastic disease, anaphylactoid reactions, hypersensitivity reactions.

Patient Counseling: Counsel if signs suggest reduced cerebral blood flow; may need to d/c therapy. Instruct not to interrupt or d/c therapy without consulting physician. Counsel about signs/symptoms of congestive heart failure (CHF); notify physician if signs/symptoms of impending CHF or unexplained respiratory symptoms occur.

Administration: Oral route. **Storage:** 20-25°C (68-77°F); tight, light-resistant container.

TIMOPTIC   RX
timolol maleate (Aton)

OTHER BRAND NAMES: Timoptic-XE (Aton) - Timoptic in Ocudose (Aton)

THERAPEUTIC CLASS: Nonselective beta-blocker

INDICATIONS: Treatment of elevated intraocular pressure (IOP) in patients with ocular HTN or open-angle glaucoma. (Ocudose) May be used when a patient is sensitive to the preservative in timolol maleate ophthalmic sol, benzalkonium chloride, or when use with a preservative free topical medication is advisable.

DOSAGE: *Adults:* (Sol/Ocudose) Initial: 1 drop (0.25%) in affected eye(s) bid. If clinical response is not adequate, may change to 1 drop (0.5%) in affected eye(s) bid. Maint: 1 drop (0.25-0.5%) in affected eye(s) qd. Max: 1 drop (0.5%) bid. (XE) Initial: 1 drop (0.25 or 0.5%) in the affected eye(s) qd. Max: 1 drop (0.5%) qd. Dose of other topically applied ophthalmic drugs should be administered at least 10 mins prior to gel forming drops. (Sol/Ocudose/XE) Concomitant therapy can be instituted if IOP is still not at a satisfactory level. Evaluate IOP after 4 weeks.

HOW SUPPLIED: Sol: (Timoptic) 0.25% [5mL], 0.5% [5mL, 10mL]; Sol: (Timoptic Ocudose) 0.25%, 0.5% [0.2mL, 60ˢ]; Sol, Gel Forming: (Timoptic-XE) 0.25%, 0.5% [5mL]

CONTRAINDICATIONS: Bronchial asthma, history of bronchial asthma, severe chronic obstructive pulmonary disease (COPD), sinus bradycardia, 2nd- or 3rd-degree atrioventricular (AV) block, overt cardiac failure, cardiogenic shock.

WARNINGS/PRECAUTIONS: Severe cardiac and respiratory reactions, including death, due to bronchospasm in patients with asthma and, rarely, death associated with cardiac failure reported. Caution with cardiac failure; d/c at 1st sign/symptom of cardiac failure. May mask the signs and symptoms of acute hypoglycemia; caution in patients subject to spontaneous hypoglycemia or diabetes mellitus (DM). May mask certain clinical signs (eg, tachycardia) of hyperthyroidism; carefully manage patients suspected of developing thyrotoxicosis. Avoid with COPD (eg, chronic bronchitis, emphysema), history/known bronchospastic disease. Not for use alone in angle-closure glaucoma. May potentiate muscle weakness consistent with myasthenic symptoms (eg, diplopia, ptosis, generalized weakness); caution with myasthenia gravis or patients with myasthenic symptoms. Caution with cerebrovascular insufficiency; consider alternative therapy if signs/symptoms of reduced cerebral blood flow develop. Choroidal detachment after filtration reported. Caution in patients with history of atopy or history of severe anaphylactic reactions to a variety of allergens. (Sol/XE) Bacterial keratitis with the use of multiple-dose containers reported.

ADVERSE REACTIONS: Burning/stinging upon instillation. (XE) Ocular: blurred vision, pain, conjunctivitis, discharge, foreign-body sensation, itching, tearing. Systemic: headache, dizziness, upper respiratory infections.

INTERACTIONS: May potentiatially produce additive effects if used concomitantly with systemic β-blockers. Concomitant use of two topical β-adrenergic blocking agents is not recommended. Caution with oral/IV calcium antagonists because of possible AV conduction disturbances, left ventricular failure, or hypotension. Avoid oral/IV calcium antagonists with impaired cardiac function. Possible additive effects, production of hypotension and/or marked bradycardia may occur when used concomitantly with catecholamine-depleting drugs (eg, reserpine). Concomitant use with calcium antagonists and digitalis may cause additive effects in prolonging AV conduction time. Potentiated systemic β-blockade reported with concomitant use of CYP2D6 inhibitors (eg, quinidine, SSRIs). Mydriasis reported occasionally with epinephrine. May augment risks of general anesthesia in surgical procedures; protracted severe hypotension and difficulty in restarting and maintaining heartbeat reported; gradual withdrawal recommended. Caution with insulin or oral hypoglycemic agents.

PREGNANCY: Category C, not for use in nursing.

MECHANISM OF ACTION: Nonselective β-blocker; reduces elevated and normal IOP, whether or not accompanied by glaucoma. Ocular hypotensive action not clearly established; may be related to reduced aqueous formation and a slight increase in outflow capacity.

PHARMACOKINETICS: Absorption: (Sol/Ocudose) C_{max}=0.46ng/mL (morning dose), 0.35ng/mL (afternoon dose); (XE) C_{max}=0.28ng/mL (morning dose). **Distribution:** Found in breast milk.

NURSING CONSIDERATIONS

Assessment: Assess for presence or history of bronchial asthma, COPD (eg, bronchitis, emphysema), or any other conditions where treatment is contraindicated or cautioned. Assess for pregnancy/nursing status and possible drug interactions. Assess if planning to undergo major surgery. (Sol/XE) Assess for corneal disease or disruption of the ocular epithelial surface.

Monitoring: Monitor for signs/symptoms of cardiac failure, masking of signs/symptoms of hypoglycemia, masking of hyperthyroidism, thyrotoxicosis, reduced cerebral blood flow, choroidal detachment, and for anaphylaxis. Monitor BP, HR, IOP. Evaluate IOP after 4 weeks of treatment. (Sol/XE) Monitor for bacterial keratitis.

Patient Counseling: Advise not to use product if have presence or history of bronchial asthma, severe chronic obstructive pulmonary disease, sinus bradycardia, second- or third-degree AV block, or if have cardiac failure. (Sol/XE) Instruct to avoid touching tip of container to eye or surrounding structures. Counsel to seek physician's advice on continued use of product if underwent ocular surgery or develop intercurrent ocular condition (eg, trauma or infection). Handle ocular solutions properly to avoid contamination; using contaminated solution may result in serious eye damage. (Sol) Contains benzalkonium chloride which may be absorbed by soft contact lenses. Remove contact lenses prior to administration and reinsert 15 min following administration. (Ocudose) Instruct about proper administration. Advise to use immediately after opening, and discard the individual unit and any remaining contents immediately after use. (XE) Invert the closed container and shake once before each use. Administer at least 10 mins apart with other topical ophthalmic medications. May impair ability to perform hazardous tasks (eg, operating machinery, driving motor vehicle).

Administration: Ocular route. **Storage:** 15-30°C (59-86°F). Avoid freezing. Protect from light. (Ocudose) Keep unit dose container in protective foil overwrap and use within 1 month after opening.

TINDAMAX   RX
tinidazole (Mission)

Carcinogenicity has been seen in mice and rats treated chronically with metronidazole. Although not reported for tinidazole, the two drugs are structurally related and have similar biologic effects. Use only for approved indications.

THERAPEUTIC CLASS: Antiprotozoal agent

INDICATIONS: Treatment of trichomoniasis caused by *Trichomonas vaginalis*, giardiasis caused by *Giardia duodenalis*, intestinal amebiasis and amebic liver abscess caused by *Entamoeba histolytica*, and bacterial vaginosis in nonpregnant women.

DOSAGE: *Adults:* Take with food. Trichomoniasis/Giardiasis: 2g single dose. For trichomoniasis, treat sexual partner with same dose and at same time. Amebiasis: Intestinal: 2g qd for 3 days. Amebic Liver Abscess: 2g qd for 3-5 days. Bacterial Vaginosis: 2g qd for 2 days or 1g qd for 5 days. Hemodialysis: If given on same day and prior to hemodialysis, give additional dose equivalent to one-half of recommended dose at the end of dialysis.
Pediatrics: >3 yrs: Take with food. Giardiasis: 50mg/kg single dose. Amebiasis: Intestinal: 50mg/kg qd for 3 days. Amebic Liver Abscess: 50mg/kg qd for 3-5 days. Max (for all): 2g/day. May crush tabs in cherry syrup.

HOW SUPPLIED: Tab: 250mg*, 500mg* *scored

CONTRAINDICATIONS: Treatment during 1st trimester of pregnancy, nursing mothers during therapy and 3 days following last dose.

WARNINGS/PRECAUTIONS: Seizures, peripheral neuropathy reported. D/C if abnormal neurologic signs occur. Caution with hepatic impairment or blood dyscrasias. May develop vaginal candidiasis. May develop drug resistance if prescribed in absence of proven or strongly suspected bacterial infection. Caution in elderly.

ADVERSE REACTIONS: Metallic/bitter taste, N/V, vaginal fungal infection, anorexia, headache, dizziness, constipation, dyspepsia, cramps/epigastric discomfort, weakness, fatigue, malaise, convulsions, peripheral neuropathy.

INTERACTIONS: Avoid alcohol during therapy and for 3 days after use. Do not give if taken disulfiram within the last 2 weeks. May potentiate oral anticoagulants. May prolong $T_{1/2}$ and reduce clearance of phenytoin (IV). May decrease clearance of fluorouracil, causing increased side effects; if concomitant use needed, monitor for toxicities. May increase levels of lithium, cyclosporine, tacrolimus. Separate dosing with cholestyramine. Phenobarbital, rifampin, pheny-toin, fosphenytoin and other CYP3A4 inducers may decrease levels. Cimetidine, ketoconazole, other CYP3A4 inhibitors may increase levels. Therapeutic effect antagonized by oxytetracycline.

PREGNANCY: Category C, not for use in nursing.

MECHANISM OF ACTION: Antiprotozoal, antibacterial agent; nitro group of tinidazole is reduced by cell extracts of *Trichomonas*. Free nitro radical generated as a result of this reduction may be responsible for antiprotozoal activity.

PHARMACOKINETICS: Absorption: Rapid, complete. (Fasted) C_{max}=47.7mcg/mL, T_{max}=1.6 hrs, AUC=901.6mcg.hr/mL at 72 hours. **Distribution:** V_d= 50L; plasma protein binding (12%); crosses blood-brain and placental barrier; found in breast milk. **Metabolism:** Mainly via oxidation, hydroxylation, conjugation; CYP3A4 mainly involved. **Elimination:** Urine (20-25% unchanged), feces (12%); $T_{1/2}$=12-14 hrs.

NURSING CONSIDERATIONS

Assessment: Assess for blood dyscrasias, seizures, pregnancy/nursing status, hypersensitivity and possible drug interactions. Assess for proven or strongly suspected bacterial infection to avoid drug resistance.

Monitoring: Monitor for convulsive seizures, peripheral neuropathy, vaginal candidiasis, drug resistance, hypersensitivity reactions (urticaria, pruritis, angioedema, erythema multiforme, Stevens-Johnson syndrome).

Patient Counseling: Advise to take with food to minimize epigastric discomfort and other GI side effects. Avoid alcohol and preparations containing ethanol and propylene glycol during therapy and for 3 days afterward to prevent abdominal cramps, N/V, headache, and flushing. Therapy only treats bacterial, not viral, infections (eg, common cold). Instruct to take as directed; skipping doses or not completing full course may decrease effectiveness and increase resistance.

Administration: Oral route. **Storage:** 20-25°C (68-77°F); excursions permitted to 15-30°C (59-86°F). Protect contents from light.

TNKASE   RX
tenecteplase (Genentech)

THERAPEUTIC CLASS: Thrombolytic agent

INDICATIONS: To reduce mortality with acute myocardial infarction (AMI).

DOSAGE: *Adults:* Administer as single IV bolus over 5 sec. <60kg: 30mg. ≥60 to <70kg: 35mg. ≥70 to <80kg: 40mg. ≥80 to <90kg: 45mg. ≥90kg: 50mg. Max: 50mg/dose.

HOW SUPPLIED: Inj: 50mg

CONTRAINDICATIONS: Active internal bleeding, history of cerebrovascular accident (CVA), in-tracranial or intraspinal surgery or trauma within 2 months, intracranial neoplasm, arteriovenous malformation, aneurysm, bleeding diathesis, severe uncontrolled HTN.

WARNINGS/PRECAUTIONS: Weigh benefits/risks with recent major surgery, cerebrovascular disease, recent GI or genitourinary (GU) bleeding, recent trauma, HTN (systolic BP ≥180mmHg and/or diastolic BP ≥110mmHg), left heart thrombus, acute pericarditis, subacute bacterial endocarditis, hemostatic defects, severe hepatic dysfunction, pregnancy, diabetic hemorrhagic retinopathy or other hemorrhagic ophthalmic conditions, septic thrombophlebitis or occluded atriventricular (AV) cannula at a seriously infected site, elderly, any other bleeding condition that is difficult to manage. Cholesterol embolism and internal/superficial bleeding reported. Arrhythmias may occur with reperfusion. Avoid IM injection, noncompressible arterial puncture, and internal jugular or subclavian venous puncture. Caution with readministration.

ADVERSE REACTIONS: Bleeding.

INTERACTIONS: Increased risk of bleeding with heparin, vitamin K antagonists, and drugs that alter platelet function (eg, aspirin, dipyridamole, GP IIb/IIIa inhibitors) before or after therapy. Weigh benefits/risks with oral anticoagulants, GP IIb/IIIa inhibitors.

PREGNANCY: Category C, caution in nursing.

MECHANISM OF ACTION: Thrombolytic agent; modified form of human tissue plasminogen activator (tPA) that binds to fibrin and converts plasminogen to plasmin.

PHARMACOKINETICS: Metabolism: Liver. **Elimination:** $T_{1/2}$=90-130 min.

NURSING CONSIDERATIONS

Assessment: Assess for active internal bleeding, history of CVA, or any other condition in which treatment is contraindicated or cautioned. Assess for hepatic function, pregnancy/nursing status, advanced age, and drug interactions.

Monitoring: Check for signs/symptoms of bleeding; if serious bleeding occurs, concomitant heparin or antiplatelet agents should be discontinued immediately. Monitor for cholesterol embolization (eg, livedo reticularis, "purple toe" syndrome, acute renal failure), arrhythmia, and hypersensitivity reactions (eg, anaphylaxis).

Patient Counseling: Counsel about increased risk of bleeding while on therapy. Contact physician if any type of unusual bleeding or hypersensitivity reactions develop.

Administration: IV route. Reconstitute just prior to use. 1) Inject 10mL of SWFI into vial. 2) Do not shake; gently swirl until contents completely dissolved. 3) May be administered as reconstituted solution (5mg/mL). **Storage:** Lyophilized vial: Store at controlled room temperature not exceeding 30°C (86°F), or under refrigeration 2-8°C (36-46°F). Reconstituted: 2-8°C (36-46°F); use within 8 hrs.

TOBRADEX
tobramycin - dexamethasone (Alcon)

RX

OTHER BRAND NAMES: TobraDex ST (Alcon)

THERAPEUTIC CLASS: Aminoglycoside/corticosteroid

INDICATIONS: Steroid-responsive inflammatory ocular condition and risk of/with superficial bacterial ocular infection caused by susceptible strains of microorganisms.

DOSAGE: *Adults:* (Sus) 1-2 drops into the conjunctival sac(s) q4-6h. Titrate: May increase to 1-2 drops q2h during the initial 24-48 hrs. (ST) 1 drop into conjunctival sac(s) q4-6h. Titrate: May increase to 1 drop q2h during the initial 24-48 hrs. (Sus/ST) Not more than 20mL should be initially prescribed. (Oint) Apply 1/2 inch ribbon in conjunctival sac(s) up to tid-qid. Not more than 8g should be initially prescribed.
Pediatrics: ≥2 yrs: (Sus) 1-2 drops into the conjunctival sac(s) q4-6h. Titrate: May increase to 1-2 drops q2h during the initial 24-48 hrs. (ST) 1 drop into conjunctival sac(s) q4-6h. Titrate: May increase to 1 drop q2h during the initial 24-48 hrs. (Sus/ST) Not more than 20mL should be initially prescribed. (Oint) Apply 1/2 inch ribbon in conjunctival sac(s) up to tid-qid. Not more than 8g should be initially prescribed.

HOW SUPPLIED: Oint: (Tobramycin-Dexamethasone) 0.3%-0.1% [3.5g]; Sus: 0.3%-0.1% [2.5mL, 5mL, 10mL]; Sus (ST): 0.3%-0.05% [2.5mL, 5mL, 10mL]

CONTRAINDICATIONS: Viral diseases of the cornea and conjunctiva, epithelial herpes simplex keratitis (dendritic keratitis), vaccinia, varicella, mycobacterial infection, and fungal diseases of the eye.

WARNINGS/PRECAUTIONS: Prolonged use may result in glaucoma with optic nerve damage, visual acuity and field of vision defects, and posterior subcapsular cataract formation. Prolonged use may suppress host response and increase risk of secondary ocular infections. Caution with diseases causing thinning of the cornea or sclera; perforations may occur. May mask/enhance existing infection in acute purulent conditions. Fungal infections of the cornea may occur; consider fungal invasion in any persistent corneal ulceration. (Oint/Sus) Not for injection into the eye. Routinely monitor intraocular pressure (IOP). D/C if sensitivity occurs. Cross-sensitivity to other aminoglycoside antibiotics may occur; d/c and institute appropriate therapy if hypersensitivity develops. May result in overgrowth of nonsusceptible organisms, including fungi; initiate appropriate therapy if superinfection occurs. (ST) Monitor IOP if to be used for ≥10 days. Reevaluate after 2 days if patient fails to improve. Caution with history of herpes simplex; use may prolong the course and may exacerbate the severity of many viral infections of the eye (including herpes simplex). May delay healing and increase the incidence of bleb formation after cataract surgery. (Oint) May retard corneal wound healing.

ADVERSE REACTIONS: Hypersensitivity, localized ocular toxicity, secondary infection, increased IOP, posterior subcapsular cataract formation, impaired wound healing.

INTERACTIONS: Monitor total serum concentrations if used concominantly with systemic aminoglycoside antibiotics.

PREGNANCY: Category C, caution in nursing.

MECHANISM OF ACTION: Tobramycin: Aminoglycoside antibiotic; provides action against susceptible organisms. Dexamethasone: Corticoid; suppresses inflammatory response and probably delays or slows healing.

NURSING CONSIDERATIONS

Assessment: Assess for epithelial herpes simplex keratitis (dendritic keratitis), vaccinia, varicella, other viral diseases of cornea or conjunctiva, mycobacterial infection and fungal diseases of eye, diseases that may cause thinning of cornea or sclera, other existing infections, pregnancy/nursing status, and for drug interactions. (ST) Assess for history of herpes simplex.

Monitoring: Monitor for signs/symptoms of hypersensitivity reactions, glaucoma, defects in visual acuity and fields of vision, posterior subcapsular cataracts, perforations, secondary infections, delayed wound healing. (ST) Monitor for IOP if used for ≥10 days, exacerbation of ocular viral infections, and bleb formation. (Oint/Sus) Routinely monitor IOP, and for development of superinfections.

Patient Counseling: Instruct not to touch dropper tip to any surface to avoid contaminating contents and not to wear contact lenses during therapy. (Sus/ST) Inform to shake well before use.

Administration: Ocular route. (Sus/ST) Shake well before use. (Oint) Tilt head back; place finger on cheek just under the eye and gently pull down until a "V" pocket is formed between eyeball and lower lid; apply recommended dose; avoid touching tip of tube to eye; look downward before closing eye. **Storage:** (Sus) 8-27°C (46-80°F); store upright. (Oint/ST): 2-25°C (36-77°F); protect ST from light.

TOBREX   RX
tobramycin (Alcon)

THERAPEUTIC CLASS: Aminoglycoside

INDICATIONS: External infections of the eye and its adnexa.

DOSAGE: *Adults:* Mild to Moderate Infection: Apply half-inch oint bid-tid or 1-2 drops q4h. Severe Infection: Apply half-inch oint q3-4h or 2 drops hourly until improvement, reduce frequency prior to discontinuation.

HOW SUPPLIED: Oint: 0.3% [3.5g]; Sol: 0.3% [5mL]

WARNINGS/PRECAUTIONS: Oint may retard corneal wound healing. Cross-sensitivity to other aminoglycoside antibiotics may occur.

ADVERSE REACTIONS: Hypersensitivity, lid itching, swelling, conjunctival erythema, superinfection.

PREGNANCY: Category B, not for use in nursing.

MECHANISM OF ACTION: Aminoglycoside antibiotic; inhibits synthesis of proteins in bacterial cells.

NURSING CONSIDERATIONS

Assessment: Assess for proper diagnosis of causative organisms. Assess use in pregnancy/nursing.

Monitoring: Monitor for sensitivity reactions while on therapy. With prolonged therapy, monitor for overgrowth of nonsusceptible organisms (eg, fungi) and for development of superinfection. Monitor total serum drug concentrations with concomitant systemic aminoglycoside antibiotics.

Patient Counseling: Advise not to wear contact lenses if signs/symptoms of ocular infections develop. Instruct to notify physician if any sensitivity reactions occur. To avoid contamination, avoid touching tube or dropper tip to any surface.

Administration: Ocular route. Do not inject into eye. **Storage:** 8-27°C (46-80°F).

TOFRANIL   RX
imipramine HCl (Mallinckrodt)

> Antidepressants increased the risk of suicidal thinking and behavior (suicidality) in short-term studies in children, adolescents, and young adults with major depressive disorder and other psychiatric disorders. Monitor and observe closely for clinical worsening, suicidality, or unusual changes in behavior in patients who are started on antidepressant therapy. Imipramine is not approved for use in pediatric patients except for use in patients with nocturnal enuresis.

THERAPEUTIC CLASS: Tricyclic antidepressant

INDICATIONS: Relief of symptoms of depression. Temporary adjunct in enuresis in children ≥6 yrs.

DOSAGE: *Adults:* Depression: Hospitalized Patients: Initial: 100mg/day in divided doses. Titrate: Increase gradually to 200mg/day; may increase to 250-300mg/day after 2 weeks if needed. Outpatients: Initial: 75mg/day. Titrate: Increase to 150mg/day. Maint: 50-150mg/day. Max: 200mg/day. Elderly: Initial: 30-40mg/day. Max: 100mg/day.
Pediatrics: Depression: ≥12 yrs: Initial: 30-40mg/day. Max: 100mg/day. Enuresis: ≥6 yrs: Initial: 25mg/day 1 hr before hs. Titrate: 6-12 yrs: If inadequate response in 1 week, increase to 50mg before hs. ≥12 yrs: Increase to 75mg before hs after 1 week if needed. Max: 2.5mg/kg/day. Taper dose gradually when d/c.

HOW SUPPLIED: Tab: 10mg, 25mg, 50mg

CONTRAINDICATIONS: Acute recovery period following myocardial infarction, MAOI coadministration or use within 14 days after stopping MAOI therapy.

WARNINGS/PRECAUTIONS: Not approved for use in treating bipolar depression. Extreme caution with cardiovascular (CV) disease, hyperthyroidism, urinary retention, narrow-angle glaucoma, increased intraocular pressure (IOP), seizure disorders; cardiac surveillance required with CV disease. Caution with elderly, serious depression, renal and hepatic impairment. May alter glucose levels. May activate psychosis in schizophrenia. Manic or hypomanic episodes may occur; consider d/c until episode is relieved. May increase hazards with electroshock therapy. Photosensitivity reported; avoid excessive exposure to sunlight. D/C prior to elective surgery. Monitor CBC with differential if fever and sore throat develops; d/c if neutropenia occurs. May impair mental/physical abilities.

ADVERSE REACTIONS: Suicidality, unusual changes in behavior, clinical worsening, sleep disorders, tiredness, mild GI disturbances, orthostatic hypotension, HTN, confusion, hallucinations, numbness, tremors, dry mouth, urticaria, N/V

INTERACTIONS: See Contraindications. Metabolism may be inhibited by methylphenidate, CYP2D6 inhibitors (eg, quinidine, cimetidine, phenothiazines, SSRIs, other antidepressants, propafenone, flecainide); downward dosage adjustment may be required. Consider monitoring TCA plasma levels when coadministered with CYP2D6 inhibitors. Caution with SSRI coadministration and when switching between TCAs and SSRIs; wait sufficient time before starting therapy when switching from fluoxetine (eg, ≥5 weeks). Decreased levels with hepatic enzyme inducers (eg, barbiturates, phenytoin) and increased levels with hepatic enzyme inhibitors (eg, cimetidine, fluoxetine); dose adjustment of imipramine may be necessary. May block effects of clonidine, guanethidine, and similar agents. Additive effects with CNS depressants and alcohol. Extreme caution with drugs that lower BP and thyroid drugs. Additive effects (eg, paralytic ileus) with anticholinergics (including antiparkinsonism agents); monitor and adjust dosage carefully. Avoid use of preparations that contain a sympathomimetic amine (eg, epinephrine, norepinephrine); may potentiate catecholamine effects.

PREGNANCY: Not safe in pregnancy; not for use in nursing.

MECHANISM OF ACTION: Tricyclic antidepressant; mechanism unknown. Suspected to potentiate adrenergic synapses by blocking uptake of norepinephrine at nerve endings.

NURSING CONSIDERATIONS

Assessment: Assess for known hypersensitivity, renal/hepatic function, history of suicide, bipolar disorder, depression, urinary retention, narrow-angle glaucoma, hyperthyroidism, CV disease, seizures, pregnancy/nursing status, and possible drug interactions. Obtain baseline LFTs, ECG, IOP.

Monitoring: Monitor for clinical worsening, suicidality, or unusual changes in behavior (eg, anxiety, agitation, panic attacks, insomnia, irritability, hostility, aggressiveness, impulsivity, akathisia, psychomotor restlessness, hypomanic/manic episodes), psychosis, seizures, CV disease, ECG, and blood sugar levels. Monitor CBC with differential if fever and sore throat develop.

Patient Counseling: Inform patients, families and caregivers about benefits/risks of therapy. Instruct to read and understand Medication Guide, and assist in understanding the contents. Instruct to notify the physician if clinical worsening, suicidality or unusual changes in behavior occur during treatment or when adjusting the dose. Inform that drug may impair mental/physical abilities required for performance of hazardous tasks.

Administration: Oral route. **Storage:** 20-25°C (68-77°F).

TOPAMAX
topiramate (Janssen)　　　　　　　　　　　　　RX　T

OTHER BRAND NAMES: Topamax Sprinkle (Janssen)
THERAPEUTIC CLASS: Sulfamate-substituted monosaccharide antiepileptic
INDICATIONS: Initial monotherapy in patients ≥2 yrs with partial onset or primary generalized tonic-clonic seizures. Adjunct therapy in patients ≥2 yrs with partial onset seizures or primary generalized tonic-clonic seizures and with seizures associated with Lennox-Gastaut syndrome. Migraine headache prophylaxis in adults.

DOSAGE: *Adults:* Monotherapy: Epilepsy: Initial: Week 1: 25mg bid. Titrate: Week 2: 50mg bid. Week 3: 75mg bid. Week 4: 100mg bid. Week 5: 150mg bid. Week 6: 200mg bid. Adjunct Therapy: Epilepsy/Lennox-Gastaut Syndrome: ≥17 yrs: Initial: 25-50mg/day. Titrate: Increments of 25-50mg/day qweek. Partial Onset: Usual: 200-400mg/day in 2 divided doses. Tonic-Clonic: Usual: 400mg/day in 2 divided doses. Max: 1600mg/day. Migraine Prophylaxis: Initial: Week 1: 25mg qpm. Titrate: Week 2: 25mg bid. Week 3: 25mg qam and 50mg qpm. Week 4: 50mg bid. Usual: 100mg in 2 divided doses. CrCl <70mL/min/1.73m²: 50% of usual dose. Hemodialysis: May need supplemental dose. *Pediatrics:* Monotherapy: Epilepsy: ≥10 yrs: Initial: Week 1: 25mg bid. Titrate: Week 2: 50mg bid. Week 3: 75mg bid. Week 4: 100mg bid. Week 5: 150mg bid. Week 6: 200mg bid. 2-<10 yrs:

Based on weight. Initial: Week 1: 25mg/day qpm. Titrate: Week 2: Increase to 50mg/day (25mg bid) based on tolerability. May increase by 25-50mg/day each subsequent week as tolerated. Titration to min maint dose should be attempted over 5-7 weeks of the total titration period. Max Maint Dose: 25-50mg/day weekly increments. Refer to PI for maint dosing based on body weight. **Adjunct Therapy:** Epilepsy/Lennox-Gastaut Syndrome: 2-16 yrs: Initial: Week 1: 25mg/day qpm (or <25mg/day, based on range of 1-3mg/kg/day). Titrate: Increments of 1-3mg/kg/day q1-2 weeks (in 2 divided doses) to achieve clinical response. Usual: 5-9mg/kg/day in 2 divided doses. CrCl <70mL/min/1.73m²: 50% of usual dose. Hemodialysis: May need supplemental dose.

HOW SUPPLIED: Cap, Sprinkle: 15mg, 25mg; Tab: 25mg, 50mg, 100mg, 200mg

WARNINGS/PRECAUTIONS: Acute myopia and secondary angle-closure glaucoma reported; d/c immediately if occurs. Oligohidrosis and hyperthermia reported, mostly in pediatrics; monitor decreased sweating and increased body temperature. Caution in use with other agents predisposing patients to heat-related disorders (eg, carbonic anhydrase inhibitors, drugs with anticholinergic activity). May increase the risk of suicidal thoughts or behavior; monitor for the emergence or worsening of depression, suicidal thoughts or behavior, and/or any unusual changes in mood or behavior. Hyperchloremic, non-anion gap, metabolic acidosis (a condition which the use of metformin is contraindicated) reported; avoid concomitant use with carbonic anhydrase inhibitors. Cognitive-related dysfunction, psychiatric/behavioral disturbances, somnolence, or fatigue reported. May cause cleft lip and/or palate in infants if used during pregnancy. Avoid abrupt d/c to minimize the potential and frequency of seizures. Sudden unexplained death in epilepsy and hyperammonemia/encephalopathy reported without and with concomitant valproic acid. Kidney stones reported; increased risk with carbonic anhydrase inhibitors. Hydration is recommended to reduce new stone formation. Hypothermia with or without hyperammonemia reported with concomitant valproic acid use; consider d/c topiramate or valproate if hypothermia develops. Paresthesia may occur. May cause metabolic acidosis, a condition which the use of metformin is contraindicated. Caution with renal/hepatic impairment.

ADVERSE REACTIONS: Anorexia, anxiety, diarrhea, fatigue, fever, infection, weight decrease, cognitive problems, paresthesia, somnolence, taste perversion, mood problems, nausea, nervousness, confusion.

INTERACTIONS: Decreased levels with phenytoin, carbamazepine, lamotrigine, and valproic acid. Increased levels with HCTZ, diltiazem, and risperidone. Increased levels with lithium when coadministered with high dose of topiramate (monitor levels), amitriptyline, and phenytoin. Decreases levels of pioglitazone, risperidone, digoxin, diltiazem, glyburide. May cause CNS depression and cognitive/neuropsychiatric adverse events with alcohol and other CNS depressants; use with extreme caution. May decrease contraceptive efficacy and exposure with combination oral contraceptives.

PREGNANCY: Category D, caution in nursing.

MECHANISM OF ACTION: Sulfamate-substituted monosaccharide; unknown mechanism. Suspected to block voltage-dependent sodium channels, augment activity of the neurotransmitter gamma-aminobutyrate at some subtypes of the GABA-A receptor, antagonizes the AMPA/kainate subtype of the glutamate receptor, and inhibits the carbonic anhydrase enzyme, particularly isoenzymes II and IV.

PHARMACOKINETICS: Absorption: Rapid; T_{max}=2 hrs (400mg). **Distribution:** Plasma protein binding (15-41%). **Metabolism:** Hydroxylation, hydrolysis, glucuronidation. **Elimination:** Urine: (70% unchanged); $T_{1/2}$=21 hrs.

NURSING CONSIDERATIONS

Assessment: Assess for renal/hepatic function, predisposing factors for metabolic acidosis, inborn errors of metabolism, reduced hepatic mitochondrial activity, pregnancy/nursing status, and possible drug interactions. Obtain baseline serum bicarbonate and blood ammonia levels.

Monitoring: Monitor for signs/symptoms of acute myopia, secondary-angle glaucoma, oligohidrosis, hyperthermia, cognitive or neuropsychiatric adverse reactions, kidney stones, renal dysfunction, metabolic acidosis, paresthesias, and hyperammonemia. Monitor serum bicarbonate and blood ammonia levels.

Patient Counseling: Seek immediate medical attention if blurred vision, visual disturbances, periorbital pain, or suicidal thoughts or behavior occurs and to closely monitor for decreased sweating and increased body temperature. Warn about risk for metabolic acidosis. Use caution when engaging in activities (eg, driving or operating machinery). Inform about risk for hyperammonemia with or without encephalopathy; contact physician if unexplained lethargy, vomiting, or mental status changes develops. Maintain adequate fluid intake to minimize risk of kidney stones. Medication may decrease efficacy of oral contraceptives. Inform of pregnancy risks/benefits. Encourage to enroll in the North American Antiepileptic Drug (NAAED) Pregnancy Registry if patient becomes pregnant by calling 1-888-233-2334. Can be taken with or without food. May swallow sprinkle caps whole or open cap and sprinkle contents on small amount (tsp) of soft food; do not chew.

Administration: Oral route. (Cap) Swallow whole or sprinkle over food. **Storage:** Protect from moisture. Tab: 15-30°C (59-86°F). Cap, Sprinkle: ≤25°C (77°F).

TOPROL-XL   RX
metoprolol succinate (AstraZeneca)

> Exacerbation of angina and myocardial infarction (MI) reported following abrupt d/c. When d/c chronic therapy, particularly with ischemic heart disease, taper over 1-2 weeks with careful monitoring. If worsening of angina or acute coronary insufficiency develops, reinstate therapy promptly, at least temporarily, and take other appropriate measures. Avoid interruption or d/c of therapy without physician's advice.

THERAPEUTIC CLASS: Selective beta₁-blocker

INDICATIONS: Treatment of HTN alone or in combination with other antihypertensives. Long-term treatment of angina pectoris. Treatment of stable symptomatic (NYHA Class II or III) heart failure (HF) of ischemic, hypertensive, or cardiomyopathic origin.

DOSAGE: *Adults:* Individualize dose. HTN: Initial: 25-100mg qd. Titrate: May increase at weekly (or longer) intervals until optimum BP reduction is achieved. Max: 400mg/day. Angina: Initial: 100mg qd. Titrate: May gradually increase weekly until optimum clinical response has been obtained or there is pronounced slowing of HR. Max: 400mg/day. Reduce dose gradually over a period of 1-2 weeks if to be d/c. HF: Initial: (NYHA Class II HF) 25mg qd or (Severe HF) 12.5mg qd for 2 weeks. Titrate: Double dose every 2 weeks to the highest dose level tolerated. Max: 200mg. Reduce dose if experiencing symptomatic bradycardia. Dose should not be increased until symptoms of worsening HF have been stabilized. Hepatic Impairment: May require lower initial dose; gradually increase dose to optimize therapy. Elderly: Start at low initial dose.
Pediatrics: ≥6 yrs: Individualize dose. HTN: Initial: 1mg/kg qd up to 50mg qd. Adjust dose according to BP response. Max: 2mg/kg (or up to 200mg) qd.

HOW SUPPLIED: Tab, Extended-Release: 25mg*, 50mg*, 100mg*, 200mg* *scored

CONTRAINDICATIONS: Severe bradycardia, 2nd- or 3rd-degree heart block, cardiogenic shock, decompensated cardiac failure, sick sinus syndrome (unless with a permanent pacemaker).

WARNINGS/PRECAUTIONS: Worsening cardiac failure may occur during up-titration; lower dose or temporarily d/c. Avoid with bronchospastic disease; may be used only with those who do not respond to or cannot tolerate other antihypertensive treatment. Used in the setting of pheochromocytoma in combination with an α-blocker, and only after α-blocker has been initiated; may cause paradoxical increase in BP if administered alone. Avoid initiation of a high-dose regimen in patients undergoing non-cardiac surgery. Chronically administered therapy should not be routinely withdrawn prior to major surgery; however, the impaired ability of the heart to respond to reflex adrenergic stimuli may augment the risks of general anesthesia and surgical procedures. May mask tachycardia occurring with hypoglycemia. May mask symptoms of hyperthyroidism, such as tachycardia; abrupt withdrawal may precipitate thyroid storm. Patients with a history of severe anaphylactic reaction to variety of allergens may be more reactive to repeated challenge and may be unresponsive to usual doses of epinephrine. May precipitate or aggravate symptoms of arterial insufficiency with peripheral vascular disease (PVD). Caution with hepatic impairment and in elderly.

ADVERSE REACTIONS: Tiredness, dizziness, depression, diarrhea, SOB, bradycardia, rash.

INTERACTIONS: Additive effects with catecholamine-depleting drugs (eg, reserpine, MAOIs). May increase levels with CYP2D6 inhibitors (eg, quinidine, fluoxetine, paroxetine, propafenone). Caution when used with calcium channel blockers of the verapamil and diltiazem type. May increase the risk of bradycardia with digitalis glycosides, clonidine, diltiazem, and verapamil. When given concomitantly with clonidine, d/c several days before clonidine is gradually withdrawn; may exacerbate rebound HTN.

PREGNANCY: Category C, caution in nursing.

MECHANISM OF ACTION: β₁-selective adrenergic receptor blocker; not established. Proposed to competitively antagonize catecholamines at peripheral adrenergic-neuron sites leading to decreased cardiac output, has central effect leading to reduced symptomatic outflow to the periphery, and suppression of renin activity.

PHARMACOKINETICS: Absorption: Rapid, complete. **Distribution:** Plasma protein binding (12%); found in breast milk. **Metabolism:** Liver via CYP2D6. **Elimination:** Urine (<5% unchanged); $T_{1/2}$=3-7 hrs.

NURSING CONSIDERATIONS

Assessment: Assess for severe bradycardia, 2nd- or 3rd-degree heart block, cardiogenic shock, decompensated cardiac failure, sick sinus syndrome, presence of pacemaker, ischemic heart disease, bronchospastic disease, diabetes, hyperthyroidism, PVD, arterial insufficiency, hepatic impairment, pheochromocytoma, history of anaphylactic reactions, pregnancy/nursing status, and possible drug interactions. Obtain baseline BP, HR, and ECG.

Monitoring: Monitor for signs/symptoms of worsening cardiac failure during up-titration, hypoglycemia, precipitation of thyroid storm, arterial insufficiency in patients with PVD, anaphylactic reactions, and other adverse reactions. Monitor patients with ischemic heart disease. Monitor BP and HR.

Patient Counseling: Advise to take drug regularly and continuously, as directed, preferably with or immediately following meals. Counsel that if dose is missed, take only the next scheduled dose (without doubling). Instruct not to interrupt or d/c therapy without consulting physician. Advise to avoid operating automobiles and machinery or engaging in other tasks requiring mental alertness. Instruct to contact physician if any difficulty in breathing occurs. Instruct to inform physician or dentist of medication use before any type of surgery. Advise HF patients to consult physician if experience signs/symptoms of worsening HF (eg, weight gain, increasing SOB).

Administration: Oral route. Do not crush or chew; tablet may be divided. **Storage:** 25°C (77°F); excursions permitted to 15-30°C (59-86°F).

TORISEL   RX
temsirolimus (Wyeth)

THERAPEUTIC CLASS: mTOR inhibitor

INDICATIONS: Treatment of advanced renal cell carcinoma.

DOSAGE: *Adults:* 25mg IV over 30-60 min once a week. Premedication: Diphenhydramine IV (or similar antihistamine) 25-50mg 30 min before the start of each dose. Hold if absolute neutrophil count <1000/mm³, platelet count <75,000/mm³, or NCI CTCAE ≥Grade 3 adverse reactions. Once toxicities resolve to ≤Grade 2, restart with dose reduced by 5mg/week to a dose ≥15mg/week. Mild Hepatic Impairment: Reduce dose to 15mg/week. Concomitant Strong CYP3A4 Inhibitors: Consider dose reduction to 12.5mg/week. If strong inhibitor is d/c, allow washout period of about 1 week before dose readjustment. Concomitant Strong CYP3A4 Inducers: Consider dose increase up to 50mg/week.

HOW SUPPLIED: Inj: 25mg/mL

CONTRAINDICATIONS: Patients with bilirubin >1.5X ULN.

WARNINGS/PRECAUTIONS: Hypersensitivity/infusion reactions observed; may occur very early in the 1st infusion. D/C infusion and observe for 30-60 min if hypersensitivity reaction develops. Caution with hypersensitivity to an antihistamine (or patients who cannot receive an antihistamine for other medical reasons), polysorbate 80 or any other component. Give H_1 and/or H_2 receptor antagonist before restarting infusion. Caution with mild hepatic impairment; may need dose reduction. Hyperglycemia reported; monitor serum glucose before and during treatment. May cause immunosuppression; observe for infections (including opportunistic infections). Interstitial lung disease (ILD) reported; withhold and treat empirically with corticosteroids and antibiotics if clinically significant respiratory symptoms develop. Increases in serum TG and cholesterol reported; may require initiation, or increase in the dose, of lipid-lowering agents. Test serum TG and cholesterol before and during treatment. Bowel perforation may occur. Rapidly progressive and sometimes fatal acute renal failure not clearly related to disease progression reported. May cause abnormal wound healing; caution during perioperative period. Increased risk of intracerebral bleeding in patients with CNS tumors. Avoid use of live vaccines and close contact with those who have received live vaccines. May cause fetal harm; avoid pregnancy throughout treatment and for 3 months after d/c. Elderly may be more likely to experience certain adverse reactions (eg, diarrhea, edema, pneumonia). Monitor CBC weekly and chemistry panels q2 weeks.

ADVERSE REACTIONS: Rash, asthenia, mucositis, N/V, edema, anorexia, dyspnea, cough, pain, pyrexia, diarrhea, abdominal pain, constipation, laboratory abnormalities.

INTERACTIONS: Avoid strong CYP3A4 inhibitors or strong CYP3A4/5 inducers; if unavoidable, adjust dose of temsirolimus accordingly. Do not take St. John's wort concomitantly. Dose increases of insulin and/or oral hypoglycemic agent or lipid-lowering agents may be needed. P-glycoprotein (P-gp) inhibitors may increase concentrations; exercise caution. May increase concentrations of P-gp substrates; exercise caution. Sunitinib may cause dose-limiting toxicity. ACE inhibitors may cause angioneurotic edema-type reactions. Anticoagulants increase risk of intracerebral bleeding. Interferon-α may increase incidence of multiple adverse reactions.

PREGNANCY: Category D, not for use in nursing.

MECHANISM OF ACTION: mTOR inhibitor; inhibits activity of mTOR that controls cell division, resulting in G1 growth arrest in treated tumor cells, inability to phosphorylate p70S6k and S6 ribosomal protein, and reduced levels of hypoxia-inducible factors HIF-1 and HIF-2 α and the vascular endothelial growth factor.

PHARMACOKINETICS: Absorption: C_{max}=585ng/mL, AUC=1627ng•h/mL. **Distribution:** V_d=172L. **Metabolism:** Liver, via CYP3A4; sirolimus (active metabolite). **Elimination:** Urine (4.6%), feces (78%); $T_{1/2}$=17.3 hrs (temsirolimus), 54.6 hrs (sirolimus).

NURSING CONSIDERATIONS

Assessment: Assess for renal/hepatic impairment, CNS tumors, surgery within a few weeks prior to therapy, hypersensitivity, pregnancy/nursing status, and possible drug interactions. Obtain baseline bilirubin levels, lung radiograph, serum glucose, cholesterol, TG.

Monitoring: Monitor for hypersensitivity reactions, infections, ILD, clinical respiratory symptoms, bowel perforation, renal/hepatic impairment, intracerebral bleeding, wound healing complications, and other adverse events that may occur. Monitor CBC, chemistry panels, serum glucose, cholesterol, TG levels.

Patient Counseling: Inform of possible serious allergic reactions despite premedication with antihistamines. Instruct women of childbearing potential as well as male patients to use reliable contraception throughout treatment and continue for 3 months after last dose. Advise that blood glucose, TG, and/or cholesterol levels may increase. Counsel on the risk of developing infections, ILD, bowel perforation, renal failure, abnormal wound healing, and intracerebral bleeding. Instruct to report to physician if any facial swelling, difficulty of breathing, excessive thirst or frequency of urination, new/worsening respiratory symptoms, new/worsening abdominal pain, or blood in their stools occurs. Instruct to avoid people who recently received live vaccine.

Administration: IV route. Refer to PI for proper preparation and administration. **Storage:** 2-8°C (36-46°F). Concentrate-diluent mixture stable below 25°C up to 24 hrs. Protect from light.

TORSEMIDE   RX
torsemide (Various)

OTHER BRAND NAMES: Demadex (Meda)

THERAPEUTIC CLASS: Loop diuretic

INDICATIONS: Treatment of edema associated with congestive heart failure (CHF), renal disease, chronic renal failure (CRF), or hepatic disease. Treatment of HTN, alone or with other antihypertensive agents. (Inj) Indicated when a rapid onset of diuresis is desired or when oral administration is impractical.

DOSAGE: *Adults:* PO/IV (bolus over 2 min or continuous infusion): CHF: Initial: 10-20mg qd. Titrate: Double dose until desired response. Max: 200mg single dose. Chronic Renal Failure: Initial: 20mg qd. Titrate: Double dose until desired response. Max: 200mg single dose. Hepatic Cirrhosis: Initial: 5-10mg qd with aldosterone antagonist or K+-sparing diuretic. Titrate: Double dose until desired response. Max: 40mg single dose. HTN: Initial: 5mg qd. Titrate: May increase to 10mg qd in 4-6 weeks, then may add additional antihypertensive agent if needed.

HOW SUPPLIED: Inj: 10mg/mL [2mL, 5mL]; Tab: (Demadex) 5mg*, 10mg*, 20mg*, 100mg* *scored

CONTRAINDICATIONS: Anuria.

WARNINGS/PRECAUTIONS: Caution with cirrhosis and ascites in hepatic disease. Tinnitus and hearing loss (usually reversible) reported. Excessive diuresis may cause dehydration, blood-volume reduction, and possible thrombosis and embolism especially in elderly. Monitor for electrolyte imbalance, hypovolemia, or prerenal azotemia; if symptoms occur, d/c until corrected and restart at lower dose. Increased risk of hypokalemia with liver cirrhosis, brisk diuresis, and inadequate oral intake of electrolytes. May develop arrhythmias in patients with cardiovascular disease (CVD). Hyperglycemia, hypokalemia, hypomagnesemia, hypercalcemia, and symptomatic gout reported. May increase BUN, SrCr, serum uric acid, cholesterol, and TG.

ADVERSE REACTIONS: Headache, excessive urination, dizziness, hypomagnesemia.

INTERACTIONS: Caution with high-dose salicylates, aminoglycosides, ethacrynic acid, lithium, and digitalis glycoside. Indomethacin partially inhibits natriuretic effect. Avoid simultaneous cholestyramine administration; may decrease oral drug absorption. Probenecid decreases effects. Reduces spironolactone clearance. Risk of hypokalemia with adrenocorticotropic hormone and corticosteroids. Possible renal dysfunction with NSAIDs (including aspirin). Increased levels with digoxin.

PREGNANCY: Category B, caution in nursing.

MECHANISM OF ACTION: Loop diuretic; acts within lumen of thick ascending part of loop of Henle, inhibiting $Na^+/K^+/Cl^-$-carrier system.

PHARMACOKINETICS: Absorption: (Tab) Absolute bioavailability (80%); (Tab) T_{max}=1 hr. **Distribution:** V_d=12-15L; plasma protein binding (>99%). **Metabolism:** Liver; Carboxylic acid (major metabolite). **Elimination:** Urine (20%); $T_{1/2}$=3.5 hrs.

NURSING CONSIDERATIONS

Assessment: Assess for history of hypersensitivity to the drug or to sulfonylureas, anuria, CVD, renal/hepatic impairment, pregnancy/nursing status, and possible drug interactions.

Monitoring: Monitor serum electrolytes (serum K⁺ magnesium, calcium), BUN, creatinine, uric acid, blood glucose, TG, cholesterol, alkaline phosphatase, CBC. Monitor for signs/symptoms of hypokalemia, electrolyte imbalance, hypovolemia, prerenal azotemia, arrhythmias, tinnitus, hearing loss, hypersensitivity reactions, and renal/hepatic dysfunction.

Patient Counseling: Discuss risks and benefits of therapy. Advise to seek medical attention if symptoms of hypokalemia, electrolyte imbalance, hypersensitivity reactions, hearing loss or tinnitus occur.

Administration: IV and Oral route. (Inj) Visually inspect for particulate matter and discoloration prior to administration. Flush IV line with normal saline before and after administration. **Storage:** (Inj) 20-25°C (68-77°F); do not freeze. (Tab) 15-30°C (59-86°F).

TOVIAZ   RX
fesoterodine fumarate (Pfizer)

THERAPEUTIC CLASS: Muscarinic antagonist

INDICATIONS: Treatment of overactive bladder with symptoms of urge urinary incontinence, urgency, and frequency.

DOSAGE: *Adults:* Initial: 4mg qd. Titrate: May increase to 8mg qd based on individual response and tolerability. Severe Renal Impairment (CrCl <30mL/min)/With Potent CYP3A4 Inhibitors (eg, ketoconazole, itraconazole, clarithromycin): Max: 4mg/day.

HOW SUPPLIED: Tab, Extended Release: 4mg, 8mg

CONTRAINDICATIONS: Urinary retention, gastric retention, uncontrolled narrow-angle glaucoma, hypersensitivity to tolterodine tartrate tab/extended-release cap.

WARNINGS/PRECAUTIONS: Angioedema of the face, lips, tongue, and/or larynx reported; d/c and institute appropriate therapy if involvement of tongue, hypopharynx, or larynx occurs. Risk of urinary retention; caution with clinically significant bladder outlet obstruction. Caution with decreased GI motility (eg, with severe constipation), controlled narrow-angle glaucoma, and myasthenia gravis. Not recommended with severe hepatic impairment (Child-Pugh C).

ADVERSE REACTIONS: Dry mouth, constipation, urinary tract infection, dry eyes.

INTERACTIONS: May increase the frequency and/or severity of dry mouth, constipation, urinary retention, and other anticholinergic pharmacologic effects with other antimuscarinic agents that produce such effects. May alter the absorption of some concomitantly administered drugs due to anticholinergic effects on GI motility. CYP3A4 inhibitors may increase levels; doses >4mg not recommended in patients taking potent CYP3A4 inhibitors (eg, ketoconazole, itraconazole, clarithromycin). CYP2D6 inhibitors may increase levels. Rifampin or rifampicin may decrease levels.

PREGNANCY: Category C, caution in nursing.

MECHANISM OF ACTION: Competitive muscarinic receptor antagonist; inhibits muscarinic receptors in the bladder, which affects contractions of urinary bladder smooth muscle and stimulation of salivary secretion.

PHARMACOKINETICS: Absorption: Well absorbed. Bioavailability (52%, 5-hydroxymethyl tolterodine [5-HMT]); T_{max}=5 hrs (5-HMT). Variable doses resulted in different pharmacokinetic parameters in extensive and poor CYP2D6 metabolizers. **Distribution:** Plasma protein binding (50%, 5-HMT); V_d=169L (IV, 5-HMT). **Metabolism:** Rapid and extensive via hydrolysis; 5-HMT (active metabolite). 5-HMT further metabolized in liver via CYP2D6 and CYP3A4. **Elimination:** Urine (70%; 16%, 5-HMT), feces (7%); $T_{1/2}$=7 hrs (5-HMT).

NURSING CONSIDERATIONS

Assessment: Assess for hypersensitivity to drug or tolterodine tartrate, other conditions where treatment is contraindicated or cautioned, hepatic/renal function, pregnancy/nursing status, and possible drug interactions.

Monitoring: Monitor for angioedema, upper airway swelling, and other adverse reactions.

Patient Counseling: Inform that therapy may produce angioedema; instruct to d/c therapy and seek immediate medical attention if edema of the tongue/laryngopharynx or difficulty in breathing occurs. Counsel about clinically significant adverse effects (eg, constipation and urinary retention). Inform that blurred vision may occur; advise to exercise caution until effects have been determined. Inform that heat prostration may occur when used in a hot environment. Inform that alcohol may enhance drowsiness caused by therapy. Instruct to take drug with liquid and swallow whole; do not chew, divide, or crush.

Administration: Oral route. Take with liquid and swallow whole; do not crush, chew, or divide. **Storage:** 20-25°C (68-77°F); excursions permitted between 15-30°C (59-86°F). Protect from moisture.

TRADJENTA

linagliptin (Boehringer Ingelheim)

RX

THERAPEUTIC CLASS: Dipeptidyl peptidase-4 inhibitor

INDICATIONS: Adjunct to diet and exercise to improve glycemic control in adults with type 2 diabetes mellitus (DM).

DOSAGE: *Adults:* Usual: 5mg qd. With Insulin Secretagogue (eg, sulfonylurea): May require lower dose of insulin secretagogue.

HOW SUPPLIED: Tab: 5mg

WARNINGS/PRECAUTIONS: Do not use in type 1 DM or for the treatment of diabetic ketoacidosis. Has not been studied in combination with insulin. No clinical studies reported establishing conclusive evidence of macrovascular risk reduction.

ADVERSE REACTIONS: Nasopharyngitis, hypoglycemia, arthralgia, back pain, headache.

INTERACTIONS: Strong inducers of P-glycoprotein or CYP3A4 (eg, rifampin) may reduce efficacy; use of alternative treatments is strongly recommended. May require lower dose of insulin secretagogue (eg, sulfonylurea) to reduce risk of hypoglycemia.

PREGNANCY: Category B, caution in nursing.

MECHANISM OF ACTION: Dipeptidyl peptidase-4 inhibitor; degrades the incretin hormones glucagon-like peptide-1 and glucose-dependent insulinotropic polypeptide, thus increasing the concentrations of active incretin hormones, stimulating the release of insulin in a glucose-dependent manner and decreasing glucagon levels in the circulation.

PHARMACOKINETICS: Absorption: Absolute bioavailability (30%); T_{max}=1.5 hrs; AUC=139nmol•h/L; C_{max}=8.9nmol/L. **Distribution:** (IV) V_d=1100L; plasma protein binding (concentration-dependent). **Elimination:** Enterohepatic (80%), urine (5%); $T_{1/2}$=12 hrs.

NURSING CONSIDERATIONS

Assessment: Assess for history of hypersensitivity, type 1 DM, diabetic ketoacidosis, pregnancy/nursing status, and possible drug interactions.

Monitoring: Monitor for adverse reactions. Monitor for blood glucose and HbA1c levels periodically.

Patient Counseling: Inform of the potential risks and benefits of therapy, alternative modes of therapy, importance of adhering to dietary instructions, regular physical activity, periodic blood glucose monitoring and HbA1c testing, recognition/management of hypoglycemia/hyperglycemia, and assessment for diabetes complications. Instruct to promptly seek medical advice during periods of stress (eg, fever, trauma, infection, surgery) as medication requirements may change. Instruct patients to take as prescribed; advise not to double the next dose if missed. Instruct to read patient information leaflet before starting therapy and when renewing prescription. Notify doctor or pharmacist if unusual symptom develops or known symptom persists/worsens.

Administration: Oral route. **Storage:** 25°C (77°F); excursions permitted to 15-30°C (59-86°F).

TRANDATE

labetalol HCl (Prometheus)

RX

THERAPEUTIC CLASS: Nonselective beta-blocker/alpha$_1$ blocker

INDICATIONS: Management of HTN alone or in combination with other antihypertensives especially thiazide and loop diuretics.

DOSAGE: *Adults:* Individualize dose. Initial: 100mg bid. Titrate: May increase by 100mg bid every 2-3 days. Maint: 200-400mg bid. Severe HTN: 1200-2400mg/day given bid-tid. Titrate: Do not increase by >200mg bid. Elderly: Initial: 100mg bid. Titrate: May increase by 100mg bid. Maint: 100-200mg bid.

HOW SUPPLIED: Tab: 100mg*, 200mg*, 300mg* *scored

CONTRAINDICATIONS: Bronchial asthma, overt cardiac failure, greater than first-degree heart block, cardiogenic shock, severe bradycardia, other conditions associated with severe and prolonged hypotension.

WARNINGS/PRECAUTIONS: Hepatic injury, hepatic necrosis and death reported. Caution with hepatic dysfunction. Avoid abrupt withdrawal; may exacerbate ischemic heart disease. Intraoperative floppy iris syndrome (IFIS) reported during cataract surgery. Caution with latent cardiac insufficiency. Avoid in overt congestive heart failure. Avoid with bronchospastic disease; use caution if patient does not respond to or cannot tolerate other antihypertensives. Paradoxical HTN in pheochromocytoma reported. May prevent the appearance of premonitory signs and symptoms of acute hypoglycemia. Do not withdraw routinely prior to surgery.

T

ADVERSE REACTIONS: Dizziness, fatigue, N/V, dyspepsia, paresthesia, nasal stuffiness, ejaculation failure, impotence, edema, dyspnea, headache, vertigo, postural hypotension, increased sweating.

INTERACTIONS: Increased tremor with TCAs. Antagonizes effects of β-agonists (bronchodilators). Potentiated by cimetidine; may need to reduce dose. Synergistic effects with halothane anesthesia. Synergistic antihypertensive effects blunts the reflex tachycardia with nitroglycerin. Caution with calcium antagonists. May need to adjust dose of antidiabetic drugs (eg, insulin). Increase risk of bradycardia with digitalis glycosides.

PREGNANCY: Category C, caution in nursing.

MECHANISM OF ACTION: Selective $α_1$-adrenergic and nonselective β-adrenergic receptor blocking agent.

PHARMACOKINETICS: Absorption: Complete; T_{max}=1-2 hrs; absolute bioavailability (25%). **Distribution:** Plasma protein binding (50%); crosses placenta. **Metabolism:** Liver (conjugation, glucuronidation). **Elimination:** Feces, urine (55-60%); $T_{1/2}$=6-8 hrs.

NURSING CONSIDERATIONS

Assessment: Assess for bradycardia, heart block, cardiogenic shock, cardiac failure, ischemic heart disease, severe hypotension, bronchospastic disease, DM, pheochromocytoma, anaphylactic reactions, pregnancy/nursing status, and possible drug interactions.

Monitoring: Monitor for cardiac failure, HTN, renal function, exacerbation of ischemia following abrupt withdrawal, bronchospastic disease, arrhythmias, hypersensitivity reactions, CBC with platelets and differential, anaphylactic reactions.

Patient Counseling: Instruct not to interrupt or d/c without consulting physician. Report signs/symptoms of cardiac failure or hepatic dysfunction (eg, pruritus, dark urine, persistent anorexia, jaundice, right upper quadrant [RUQ] tenderness, or unexplained flu-like symptoms). Transient scalp itching may occur, usually when treatment initiated.

Administration: Oral route. **Storage:** 2-30°C (36-86°F); protect from excessive moisture.

TRANSDERM SCOP   RX
scopolamine (Novartis Consumer)

THERAPEUTIC CLASS: Anticholinergic

INDICATIONS: Prevention of N/V associated with motion sickness or recovery from anesthesia and surgery in adults.

DOSAGE: *Adults:* Motion Sickness N/V: 1 patch at least 4 hrs before the antiemetic effect is required. Replace patch after 3 days if therapy is required for >3 days. Postoperative N/V: 1 patch on the evening before surgery or 1 hr prior to cesarean section. Remove patch 24 hrs following surgery.

HOW SUPPLIED: Patch: 1.5mg [4*]

CONTRAINDICATIONS: Angle-closure (narrow angle) glaucoma.

WARNINGS/PRECAUTIONS: Apply only to skin in the postauricular area. May increase intraocular pressure (IOP) with chronic open-angle (wide-angle) glaucoma; monitor use and adjust therapy PRN. Not for use in children. May impair physical/mental abilities. Rare idiosyncratic reactions (eg, acute toxic psychosis) reported. Caution with pyloric obstruction, urinary bladder neck obstruction, and intestinal obstruction. Caution in elderly and with hepatic/renal dysfunction; increased CNS effects may occur. May aggravate seizures or psychosis; caution in patients with history of such disorders. Remove patch before undergoing a magnetic resonance imaging scan; skin burns at the patch site may occur.

ADVERSE REACTIONS: Dry mouth, drowsiness, blurred vision, dilation of pupils, dizziness, disorientation, confusion.

INTERACTIONS: May decrease absorption of PO medications due to decreased gastric motility and delayed gastric emptying. Caution with other drugs with CNS effects (eg, sedatives, tranquilizers, alcohol) and anticholinergic properties (eg, other belladonna alkaloids, antihistamines including meclizine, TCAs, and muscle relaxants).

PREGNANCY: Category C, caution in nursing.

MECHANISM OF ACTION: Anticholinergic agent; acts as competitive inhibitor at postganglionic muscarinic receptor sites of parasympathetic nervous system and on smooth muscle that responds to acetylcholine but lacks cholinergic innervation. Acts in the CNS by blocking cholinergic transmission from vestibular nuclei to higher centers in the CNS and from reticular formation to the vomiting center.

PHARMACOKINETICS: Absorption: Well-absorbed; T_{max}=24 hrs. **Distribution:** Crosses placenta; found in breast milk. **Metabolism:** Extensive; conjugation. **Elimination:** Urine (<10%; 5% unchanged); $T_{1/2}$=9.5 hrs.

NURSING CONSIDERATIONS

Assessment: Assess for known hypersensitivity to the drug, angle-closure (narrow-angle)/chronic open-angle (wide-angle) glaucoma, pyloric obstruction, urinary bladder neck obstruction, intestinal obstruction, history of seizures or psychosis, hepatic/renal dysfunction, pregnancy/nursing status, and for possible drug interactions.

Monitoring: Monitor for drowsiness, disorientation, confusion, idiosyncratic reactions (eg, confusion, agitation, rambling speech, hallucinations, paranoid behaviors, delusions), CNS effects, and aggravation of seizures or psychosis. Monitor IOP in patients with chronic open-angle (wide-angle) glaucoma.

Patient Counseling: Inform to wash hands thoroughly with soap and water immediately after handling patch so that any drug that might get on the hands will not come into contact with the eyes. Instruct to dispose the patch properly to avoid contact with children or pets. Advise to remove the patch and notify physician if symptoms of acute narrow-angle glaucoma (pain and reddening of eyes and dilation of pupils) or difficulty in urinating is experienced. Inform of the disorienting effects of the drug and advise to use caution when engaging in underwater sports, driving, or operating dangerous machineries.

Administration: Transdermal route. Apply to the hairless area behind one ear. Thoroughly wash hands after application. Wear only 1 patch at anytime. Do not cut patch. Discard patch if displaced and replace with a fresh patch. **Storage:** 20-25°C (68-77°F).

TRANXENE T-TAB
clorazepate dipotassium (Lundbeck)

`CIV`

THERAPEUTIC CLASS: Benzodiazepine

INDICATIONS: Management of anxiety disorders or for the short-term relief of the symptoms of anxiety. Adjunctive therapy in the management of partial seizures. Symptomatic relief of acute alcohol withdrawal.

DOSAGE: *Adults:* Anxiety: Initial: 15mg qhs. Usual: 30mg/day in divided doses. Max: 60mg/day. Elderly/Debilitated: Initial: 7.5-15mg/day. Alcohol Withdrawal: Day 1: 30mg, then 30-60mg/day. Day 2: 45-90mg/day. Day 3: 22.5-45mg/day. Day 4: 15-30mg. Give in divided doses. Reduce dose and continue with 7.5-15mg/day; d/c when stable. Max: 90mg/day. Antiepileptic Adjunct: Max Initial: 7.5mg tid. Titrate: Increase by no more than 7.5mg/week. Max: 90mg/day. *Pediatrics:* ≥9 yrs: Anxiety: Initial: 15mg qhs. Usual: 30mg/day in divided doses. Max: 60mg/day. Antiepileptic Adjunct: >12 yrs: Max Initial: 7.5mg tid. Titrate: Increase by no more than 7.5mg/week. Max: 90mg/day. 9-12 yrs: Max Initial: 7.5mg bid. Titrate: Increase by no more than 7.5mg/week. Max: 60mg/day.

HOW SUPPLIED: Tab: 3.75mg*, 7.5mg*, 15mg* *scored

CONTRAINDICATIONS: Acute narrow-angle glaucoma.

WARNINGS/PRECAUTIONS: Avoid with depressive neuroses or psychotic reactions. May impair mental/physical abilities. Withdrawal symptoms (eg, delirium, tremors, abdominal and muscle cramps, insomnia, irritability, memory impairment) may occur following abrupt withdrawal; taper gradually following extended therapy. Caution with known drug dependency, renal/hepatic impairment. May increase the risk of suicidal thoughts and behavior; monitor for emergence or worsening of depression, suicidal thoughts or behavior and/or any unusual changes in mood or behavior. Suicidal tendencies may be present in patients who have depression along with anxiety; least amount of drug that is feasible should be available to such patients. Monitor LFTs and blood counts periodically with long-term therapy. Caution in elderly/debilitated; use lowest effective dose and dose adjustments should be made slowly to preclude ataxia or excessive sedation.

ADVERSE REACTIONS: Drowsiness, dizziness, GI complaints, nervousness, blurred vision, dry mouth, headache, mental confusion.

INTERACTIONS: Additive CNS depression with CNS depressants, alcohol. Potentiated by barbiturates, narcotics, phenothiazines, MAOIs, other antidepressants. Increased sedation with hypnotics.

PREGNANCY: Safety in pregnancy not known, not for use in nursing.

MECHANISM OF ACTION: Benzodiazepine; antianxiety/hypnotic agent which has CNS depressant effect.

PHARMACOKINETICS: Distribution: (Nordiazepam) Found in breast milk; plasma protein binding (97-98%). **Metabolism:** Liver; rapidly decarboxylated to nordiazepam (primary metabolite); hydroxylation. **Elimination:** Urine (62-67%), feces (15-19%); (Nordiazepam) $T_{1/2}$=40-50 hrs.

T

NURSING CONSIDERATIONS

Assessment: Assess for acute narrow-angle glaucoma, renal/hepatic impairment, depressive neurosis, psychotic reactions, pregnancy/nursing status, and for possible drug interactions. Assess psychological potential for drug dependence.

Monitoring: Monitor for signs/symptoms of depression, suicidal thoughts or behavior, unusual changes in mood or behavior, and for drug dependence. Monitor for withdrawl symptoms (eg, delirium, tremors, abdominal and muscle cramps, insomnia, irritability, memory impairment) following abrupt withdrawl. In patients on prolonged therapy, monitor blood counts and LFTs periodically.

Patient Counseling: Inform about benefits/risks and appropriate use of therapy. Advise to read Medication Guide. Counsel patients, caregivers, and family members that therapy may increase the risk of suicidal thoughts and behavior and advise of the need to be alert for the emergence or worsening of the signs and symptoms of depression, any unusual changes in mood/behavior, suicidal thoughts/behavior, or thoughts about self-harm; instruct to immediately report behaviors of concern to healthcare provider. Caution against engaging in hazardous tasks requiring mental alertness (eg, operating machinery/driving). Inform that therapy may produce psychological and physical dependence; instruct to contact physician before either increasing the dose or discontinuing therapy. Advise patients to enroll in North American Antiepileptic Drug (NAAED) Pregnancy Registry if they become pregnant.

Administration: Oral route. **Storage:** 20-25°C (68-77°F). Protect from moisture; keep bottle tightly closed.

TRAVATAN Z   RX
travoprost (Alcon)

THERAPEUTIC CLASS: Prostaglandin analog

INDICATIONS: Reduction of elevated intraocular pressure (IOP) in patients with open-angle glaucoma or ocular HTN.

DOSAGE: *Adults:* 1 drop in affected eye(s) qd in pm. Space by at least 5 min if using >1 topical ophthalmic drug.
Pediatrics: ≥16 yrs: 1 drop in affected eye(s) qd in pm. Space by at least 5 min if using >1 topical ophthalmic drug.

HOW SUPPLIED: Sol: 0.004% [2.5mL, 5mL]

WARNINGS/PRECAUTIONS: Changes to pigmented tissues, including increased pigmentation of iris (may be permanent), eyelid, and eyelashes (may be reversible) reported. Regularly examine patients with noticeably increased iris pigmentation. May cause changes to eyelashes and vellus hair in the treated eye. Caution with active intraocular inflammation (eg, uveitis); inflammation may be exacerbated. Macular edema, including cystoid macular edema, reported; caution with aphakic patients, pseudophakic patients with torn posterior lens capsule, or patients at risk of macular edema. Treatment of angle-closure, inflammatory, or neovascular glaucoma has not been evaluated. Bacterial keratitis reported with multidose container. Remove contact lenses prior to instillation; may reinsert 15 min after administration.

ADVERSE REACTIONS: Ocular hyperemia, foreign body sensation, decreased visual acuity, eye discomfort/pruritus/pain.

PREGNANCY: Category C, caution in nursing.

MECHANISM OF ACTION: Prostaglandin analog; not established. Selective FP prostanoid receptor agonist believed to reduce IOP by increasing uveoscleral outflow.

PHARMACOKINETICS: Absorption: C_{max}=0.018ng/mL; T_{max}=30 min. **Metabolism:** Cornea, via esterases to active free acid and systemically to inactive metabolites via β-oxidation and reduction. **Elimination:** Urine (<2%); $T_{1/2}$=45 min.

NURSING CONSIDERATIONS

Assessment: Assess for active intraocular inflammation (uveitis), active macular edema, aphakic/pseudophakic patients with torn posterior lens capsule, angle-closure, inflammatory, or neovascular glaucoma, and pregnancy/nursing status.

Monitoring: Monitor for increased pigmentation of the iris, periorbital tissue (eyelid); changes in eyelashes (eg, increased length, thickness, and number of lashes); macular edema (including cystoid macular edema); and bacterial keratitis.

Patient Counseling: Inform about risk of brown pigmentation of iris (may be permanent) and darkening of eyelid skin (may be reversible after d/c). Inform about the possibility of eyelash and vellus hair changes. Advise to avoid touching tip of dispensing container to contact eye, surrounding structures, fingers, or any other surface in order to avoid contamination of the sol by common bacteria to cause ocular infections. Advise to consult physician if having ocular surgery or developed intercurrent ocular conditions (eg, trauma or infection) or ocular reactions. Instruct to remove contact lenses prior to instillation; reinsert 15 min after administration. Instruct to administer at least 5 min apart if using >1 topical ophthalmic drugs. **Administration:** Ocular route. **Storage:** 2-25°C (36-77°F).

TRAZODONE   RX
trazodone HCl (Various)

Antidepressants increased the risk of suicidal thinking and behavior (suicidality) in short-term studies in children and adolescents with major depressive disorder (MDD) and other psychiatric disorders. Monitor and observe closely for clinical worsening, suicidality, and unusual changes in behavior in patients who are started on antidepressant therapy. Trazodone is not approved for use in pediatric patients.

THERAPEUTIC CLASS: Triazolopyridine derivative

INDICATIONS: Treatment of depression.

DOSAGE: *Adults:* Initial: 150mg/day in divided doses pc. Titrate: May increase by 50mg/day every 3-4 days. Max: (Outpatient) 400mg/day in divided doses, (Inpatient) 600mg/day in divided doses. Maint: Lowest effective level, and may gradually reduce if adequate response is achieved.

HOW SUPPLIED: Tab: 50mg*, 100mg*, 150mg*, 300mg*, *scored

WARNINGS/PRECAUTIONS: Monitor for clinical worsening and/or suicidal ideation and behavior (suicidality), especially at initiation of therapy or dose changes. Consideration should be given to changing the therapeutic regimen, including possibly d/c medication if depression is persistently worse or if emergent suicidality or symptoms that may be precursors to worsening depression or suicidality occur. Prior to treatment, adequately screen for bipolar disorder; not approved for use in treating bipolar depression. May cause priapism; d/c use if prolonged or inappropriate erections occur. Not recommended for use during the initial recovery phase of myocardial infarction (MI). Cardiac arrhythmias may occur; caution in patients with preexisting cardiac disease, and monitor closely. Hypotension, including orthostatic hypotension, and syncope reported. D/C therapy prior to elective surgery. Occasional low WBC and low neutrophil count reported. May impair physical/mental abilities.

ADVERSE REACTIONS: Dry mouth, edema, constipation, blurred vision, fatigue, nervousness, drowsiness, dizziness, headache, insomnia, N/V, musculoskeletal pain, hypotension, confusion, priapism.

INTERACTIONS: CYP3A4 inhibitors (eg, ritonavir, ketoconazole, indinavir, itraconazole, nefazodone) may increase levels; a lower dose of trazodone may be required when used with potent CYP3A4 inhibitors. Carbamazepine decreases levels; monitor to determine if dosage increase of trazodone is required. Increases digoxin and phenytoin serum levels. Caution with MAOIs. May enhance response to alcohol, barbiturates, and other CNS depressants. May affect PT in patients on warfarin. Concomitant use with antihypertensive therapy, may require a dose reduction of the antihypertensive drug. Avoid electroshock therapy. May interact with general anesthetics.

PREGNANCY: Category C, caution in nursing.

MECHANISM OF ACTION: Triazolopyridine derivative; suspected to selectively inhibit serotonin uptake by brain synaptosomes and potentiate behavioral changes induced by the serotonin precursor, 5-hydroxytryptophan.

PHARMACOKINETICS: Absorption: Well absorbed; T_{max}=1 hr (taken on an empty stomach), 2 hrs (taken with food). **Metabolism:** Liver via CYP3A4 to m-chlorophenylpiperazine (active metabolite).

NURSING CONSIDERATIONS

Assessment: Assess for bipolar disorder, cardiac disease or recent MI, pregnancy/nursing status, and for possible drug interactions. Prior to initiating treatment, assess if patient is planning to undergo surgery.

Monitoring: Monitor for signs/symptoms of clinical worsening, suicidality, unusual changes in behavior, priapism, cardiac arrhythmias, and for hypotension.

Patient Counseling: Inform about the benefits and risks of therapy. Advise patients, families, and caregivers of need to observe for signs/symptoms of clinical worsening and suicidal risks (eg, anxiety, agitation, panic attacks, mania, changes in behavior, suicidal ideation); contact physician if such symptoms occur. Avoid alcohol, sedatives, and other CNS depressants. Instruct males to d/c use and contact physician if develop a prolonged or inappropriate penile erection. Inform that may impair the mental and/or physical ability required for performing potentially hazardous tasks (eg, driving). Take shortly after a meal or light snack.

Administration: Oral route. **Storage:** 20-25°C (68-77°F). Protect from temperatures above 40°C (104°F). Dispense in tight, light-resistant container.

TREANDA RX
bendamustine HCl (Cephalon)

THERAPEUTIC CLASS: Alkylating agent

INDICATIONS: Treatment of chronic lymphocytic leukemia (CLL) and indolent B-cell non-Hodgkin's lymphoma (NHL) that has progressed during or within six months of treatment with rituximab or a rituximab-containing regimen.

DOSAGE: *Adults:* CLL: 100mg/m² IV over 30 min on Days 1 and 2, of a 28-day cycle. Max: 6 cycles. Delay treatment for Grade 4 hematologic toxicity or clinically significant ≥Grade 2 non-hematologic toxicity. ≥Grade 3 Hematologic Toxicity: Reduce dose to 50mg/m² on Days 1 and 2 of each cycle; if ≥Grade 3 toxicity recurs, reduce dose to 25mg/m² on Days 1 and 2 of each cycle. ≥Grade 3 Non-hematologic Toxicity: Reduce dose to 50mg/m² on Days 1 and 2 of each cycle. Consider dose re-escalation in subsequent cycles. NHL: 120mg/m² IV over 60 min on Days 1 and 2 of a 21-day cycle. Max: 8 cycles. Delay treatment for Grade 4 hematologic toxicity or clinically significant ≥Grade 2 non-hematologic toxicity. Grade 4 Hematologic Toxicity: Reduce dose to 90mg/m² on Days 1 and 2 of each cycle; if Grade 4 toxicity recurs, reduce dose to 60mg/m² on Days 1 and 2 of each cycle. ≥Grade 3 Non-hematologic Toxicity: Reduce dose to 90mg/m² on Days 1 and 2 of each cycle; if ≥Grade 3 toxicity recurs, reduce dose to 60mg/m² on Days 1 and 2 of each cycle.

HOW SUPPLIED: Inj: 25mg, 100mg

CONTRAINDICATIONS: Hypersensitivity to mannitol.

WARNINGS/PRECAUTIONS: Myelosuppression may occur; monitor blood counts including leukocytes, platelets, Hgb and neutrophils closely. Infection, including pneumonia and sepsis, reported. Increased susceptibility to infection with myelosuppression. May cause infusion reactions; monitor clinically and consider d/c with Grade 3 or 4 infusion reactions. May cause tumor lysis syndrome; maintain adequate volume status and monitor blood chemistry, particularly K⁺ and uric acid levels. Skin reactions, including rash, toxic skin reactions, and bullous exanthema, reported; if severe or progressive, withhold or d/c treatment. Pre-malignant and malignant diseases (eg, myelodysplastic syndrome, myeloproliferative disorders, acute myeloid leukemia, bronchial carcinoma) reported. Do not use with moderate or severe hepatic impairment; caution with mild hepatic impairment. Do not use if CrCl <40mL/min; caution with lesser degrees of renal impairment. Extravasation reported resulting in hospitalizations from erythema, marked swelling, and pain; take precautions to avoid extravasation and monitor infusion site for redness, swelling, pain, infection and necrosis. Can cause fetal harm.

ADVERSE REACTIONS: Lymphopenia, leukopenia, neutropenia, anemia, thrombocytopenia, N/V, fatigue, diarrhea, fever, constipation, anorexia, cough, headache, weight loss, rash.

INTERACTIONS: CYP1A2 inducers (eg, omeprazole, smoking) may decrease plasma concentrations and increase plasma concentrations of active metabolites. CYP1A2 inhibitors (eg, fluvoxamine, ciprofloxacin) may increase plasma concentrations and decrease plasma concentrations of active metabolites. Cases of Stevens-Johnson syndrome (SJS) and toxic epidermal necrolysis (TEN) reported with allopurinol and other medications known to cause these syndromes. Skin reactions including rash, toxic skin reactions and bullous exanthema may occur when used concomitantly with other anticancer agents.

PREGNANCY: Category D, not for use in nursing.

MECHANISM OF ACTION: Bifunctional mechlorethamine derivative. Mechanism not established; forms electrophilic alkyl groups which form covalent bonds with electron-rich nucleophilic moieties, resulting in interstrand DNA crosslinks. Bifunctional covalent linkage can lead to cell death via several pathways. Active against both quiescent and dividing cells.

PHARMACOKINETICS: Distribution: Plasma protein binding (94-96%); V_d=25L. **Metabolism:** Hydrolysis; M3, M4 (minor metabolites) via CYP1A2. **Elimination:** Feces (90%); $T_{1/2}$=40 min (bendamustine 120mg/m²); $T_{1/2}$=3 hrs, 30 min (M3, M4).

NURSING CONSIDERATIONS

Assessment: Assess for hypersensitivity to mannitol, myelosuppression, premalignant or malignant disease, renal and hepatic impairment, pregnancy/nursing status and possible drug interactions. Obtain baseline blood counts including WBC, neutrophil, platelet count, Hgb/Hct, LFTs, CrCl.

Monitoring: Monitor CBCs, blood chemistry particularly K⁺ and uric acid levels, LFTs, SrCr levels, and renal/hepatic function periodically. Monitor for development of premalignant or malignant disease. Monitor for signs/symptoms of severe anaphylactic and anaphylactoid reactions, skin reactions, infusion reactions (eg, fever, chills, pruritus and rash) and IV infusion-site reactions (eg, redness, swelling, pain, infection, necrosis), severe myelosuppression (eg, neutropenic sepsis, alveolar hemorrhage with Grade 3 thrombocytopenia, and cytomegalovirus [CMV]), tumor lysis syndrome, infections, impaired hepatic/renal function, pregnancy/nursing status and possible drug interactions.

Patient Counseling: Contact physician if an allergic reaction (eg, rash, facial swelling, difficulty breathing during or soon after infusion) develops. Therapy may cause decrease in WBCs, platelets, and RBCs; advise to contact physician if SOB, significant fatigue, bleeding, fever, or other signs of infection develop. Advise women to avoid becoming pregnant throughout the treatment and for 3 months after the therapy; immediately report pregnancy. Avoid nursing while on therapy. Men should use reliable contraception while on therapy. May cause tiredness; avoid driving any vehicle or operating any dangerous tools or machinery. May cause N/V, diarrhea, and rash. Report any adverse reactions immediately to physician. Mild rash or itching may occur; report immediately for severity or worsening.

Administration: IV route. Administer as IV infusion only. Refer to PI for further instructions on preparation of reconstituted solution, dilution, and administration. **Storage:** 25°C (77°F); excursions permitted up to 30°C (86°F). Retain in original carton until time of use to protect from light. Sol for infusion: Stable for 24 hrs when refrigerated (2-8°C or 36°-47°F) or for 3 hrs when stored at room temperature (15-30°C or 59-86°F) and room light. Refer to PI for procedures for safe handling and disposal.

TRECATOR RX
ethionamide (Wyeth)

THERAPEUTIC CLASS: Peptide synthesis inhibitor

INDICATIONS: Treatment of active tuberculosis (TB) in patients with *Mycobacterium tuberculosis* resistant to isoniazid or rifampin, or where there is intolerance to other drugs.

DOSAGE: *Adults:* 15-20mg/kg qd with food. May give in divided doses with poor GI tolerance. Max: 1g/day. Alternate Regimen: Initial: 250mg qd then titrate gradually to optimal doses as tolerated, or 250mg qd for 1-2 days, then 250mg bid for 1-2 days, then 1g/day in 3-4 divided doses. Continue therapy until bacteriological conversion has become permanent and maximal clinical improvement occurs.
Pediatrics: ≥12 yrs: 10-20mg/kg/day in divided doses given bid or tid with food, or 15mg/kg/day as single dose. Continue therapy until bacteriological conversion has become permanent and maximal clinical improvement occurs.

HOW SUPPLIED: Tab: 250mg

CONTRAINDICATIONS: Severe hepatic impairment.

WARNINGS/PRECAUTIONS: Give with pyridoxine. Rapid development of resistance if used alone; should be used with at least 1 or 2 other drugs. Perform ophthalmologic exams before and periodically during therapy. Measure serum transaminases prior to initiation and monthly thereafter. Risk of hypoglycemia in diabetics; monitor blood glucose prior to initiation then periodically. Hypothyroidism reported; monitor TFTs.

ADVERSE REACTIONS: N/V, diarrhea, abdominal pain, excessive salivation, metallic taste, stomatitis, anorexia, psychotic disturbances, drowsiness, dizziness, hypersensitivity reactions, increase in serum bilirubin, SGOT or SGPT.

INTERACTIONS: D/C all antituberculous medication with elevated serum transaminases until resolved; reintroduce sequentially to determine which drug is responsible. May raise isoniazid levels. May potentiate adverse effects of other antituberculous drugs. Convulsions reported with cycloserine. Risk of psychotic reactions with excessive ethanol ingestion.

PREGNANCY: Category C, not for use in nursing.

MECHANISM OF ACTION: Peptide synthesis inhibitor; may be bacteriostatic or bactericidal in action.

PHARMACOKINETICS: Absorption: Completely absorbed; C_{max}=2.16mcg/mL, T_{max}=1.02 hrs, AUC=7.67mcg•hr/mL. **Distribution:** V_d=93.5L; plasma protein binding (30%); widely distributed into body tissues. **Metabolism:** Liver (extensive). **Elimination:** Urine ≤1%; $T_{1/2}$=1.92 hrs.

NURSING CONSIDERATIONS

Assessment: Assess for severe hepatic impairment, diabetes mellitus, susceptibility test, pregnancy/nursing status, and possible drug interactions.

Monitoring: Monitor for hypersensitivity reactions (eg, rash, photosensitivity), GI (eg, N/V, diarrhea) and psychotic disturbances (eg, mental depression). Determination of serum transaminases (SGOT, SGPT), blood glucose, thyroid function, and eye exams should be done periodically.

Patient Counseling: Advise to report vision loss or blurriness, with/without eye pain. Instruct to avoid excessive ethanol ingestion to avoid psychotic reaction. Take as directed; skipping doses or not completing full course may decrease effectiveness and increase resistance.

Administration: Oral route. **Storage:** 20-25°C (68-77°F). Dispense in tight container.

TRELSTAR
triptorelin pamoate (Watson)

RX

THERAPEUTIC CLASS: Synthetic gonadotropin-releasing hormone analog

INDICATIONS: Palliative treatment of advanced prostate cancer.

DOSAGE: *Adults:* 3.75mg IM q4 weeks, 11.25mg IM q12 weeks, or 22.5mg IM q24 weeks as single dose in either buttock. Alternate injection site periodically.

HOW SUPPLIED: Inj: 3.75mg, 11.25mg, 22.5mg

CONTRAINDICATIONS: Women who are or may become pregnant.

WARNINGS/PRECAUTIONS: Anaphylactic shock, hypersensitivity, angioedema reported; d/c immediately and administer appropriate supportive and symptomatic care if these occur. May cause transient increase in serum testosterone levels. Worsening/onset of new signs/symptoms (eg, bone pain, neuropathy, hematuria, urethral/bladder outlet obstruction) may occur during 1st weeks of treatment. Spinal cord compression reported. Institute standard treatment or immediate orchiectomy in extreme cases if spinal cord compression or renal impairment develops. Closely monitor patients with metastatic vertebral lesions and/or urinary tract obstruction during 1st few weeks of therapy. Hyperglycemia, increased risk of developing diabetes/myocardial infarction (MI), sudden cardiac death, and stroke reported in men receiving gonadotropin-releasing hormone (GnRH) agonists. Monitor response by measuring serum levels of testosterone periodically or as indicated. May suppress pituitary-gonadal system in therapeutic dose and mislead diagnostic tests of pituitary-gonadotropic and gonadal functions during treatment.

ADVERSE REACTIONS: Hot flushes, HTN, headache, skeletal pain, dysuria, leg edema, back pain, impotence, erectile dysfunction, testicular atrophy.

INTERACTIONS: Avoid hyperprolactinemic drugs.

PREGNANCY: Category X, not for use in nursing.

MECHANISM OF ACTION: Synthetic decapeptide agonist analog of GnRH; initially increases circulating levels of luteinizing hormone (LH), follicle-stimulating hormone (FSH), testosterone, and estradiol; chronic and continuous administration causes a sustained decrease in LH and FSH secretion and marked reduction of testicular steroidogenesis.

PHARMACOKINETICS: Absorption: (IM) C_{max} (3.75mg, 11.25mg, 22.5mg)=28.4ng/mL, 38.5ng/mL, 44.1ng/mL; T_{max}=1-3 hrs. **Distribution:** V_d (0.5mg IV)=30-33L. **Elimination:** Liver and kidneys; Urine (41.7%, unchanged); $T_{1/2}$=3 hrs.

NURSING CONSIDERATIONS

Assessment: Assess pregnancy/nursing status, metastatic vertebral lesions, urinary tract obstruction, hypersensitivity to drug, cardiovascular disease (CVD), diabetes mellitus (DM), renal/hepatic impairment, and for possible drug interactions. Obtain baseline serum testosterone, prostate specific antigen (PSA) levels, blood glucose levels, LFTs.

Monitoring: Monitor response to drug and for signs/symptoms of worsening prostate cancer, spinal cord compression, renal impairment, hypersensitivity reactions (eg, anaphylactic shock, angioedema), signs/symptoms suggestive of development of CVD, and other adverse reactions. Periodically monitor serum testosterone, PSA levels, blood glucose and/or glycosylated Hgb (HbA1c), LFTs.

Patient Counseling: Inform that patients may experience worsening of symptoms of prostate cancer during 1st weeks of treatment. Advise that the symptoms should decline 3-4 weeks following administration of therapy. Inform of the increased risk of developing DM, MI, sudden cardiac death, and stroke. Allergic reactions could occur and serious reactions require immediate treatment. Report any previous hypersensitivity to drug and its components and contact physician if any side effects develop.

Administration: IM route. Inspect visually for particulate matter/discoloration prior to administration. Refer to PI for reconstitution instructions. **Storage:** 20-25°C (68-77°F). Do not freeze with Mixject.

TRENTAL
pentoxifylline (Sanofi-Aventis)

RX

THERAPEUTIC CLASS: Blood viscosity reducer

INDICATIONS: Treatment of intermittent claudication due to chronic occlusive arterial disease of the limbs.

DOSAGE: *Adults:* 400mg tid with meals for at least 8 weeks. Reduce to 400mg bid if digestive and CNS side effects occur; d/c if side effects persist.

HOW SUPPLIED: Tab, Extended-Release: 400mg

CONTRAINDICATIONS: Recent cerebral and/or retinal hemorrhage, intolerance to methylxanthines (eg, caffeine, theophylline, theobromine).

WARNINGS/PRECAUTIONS: Monitor Hgb and Hct with risk factors complicated by hemorrhage (eg, recent surgery, peptic ulceration, cerebral/retinal bleeding). Occasional reports of angina, hypotension, and arrhythmia in patients with concurrent coronary artery and cerebrovascular diseases.

ADVERSE REACTIONS: Bloating, dyspepsia, N/V, dizziness, headache.

INTERACTIONS: Increase risk of bleeding with warfarin; monitor PT/INR more frequently. May increase theophylline levels; risk of theophylline toxicity. May increase effect of antihypertensives.

PREGNANCY: Category C, not for use in nursing.

MECHANISM OF ACTION: Blood viscosity reducer; not established. Increases blood flow to affected microcirculation and enhances tissue oxygenation. Improves erythrocyte flexibility, increases leukocyte deformability, and inhibits neutrophil adhesion and activation.

PHARMACOKINETICS: Absorption: T_{max}=1 hr. **Distribution:** Found in breast milk. **Metabolism:** 1st pass; metabolites (major): Metabolite 1 (1-[5-hydroxyhexyl]-3,7-dimethylxanthine); metabolite V (1-[3-carboxypropyl]-3,7-dimethylxanthine). **Elimination:** Urine (major), feces (<4%); $T_{1/2}$=0.4-0.8 hrs; $T_{1/2}$=0.4-0.8 hrs (metabolites).

NURSING CONSIDERATIONS

Assessment: Assess for recent cerebral and/or retinal hemorrhage, hypersensitivity to methylxanthines (eg, caffeine, theophylline, theobromine), nursing/pregnancy status, renal function, and drug interactions.

Monitoring: In presence of concurrent coronary artery disease and cerebrovascular disease, monitor for signs/symptoms of angina, arrhythmia, and hypotension. If on concomitant warfarin therapy, perform more frequent monitoring of PT time. If risk for bleeding (eg, recent surgery, peptic ulceration, recent cerebral and/or retinal bleeding), periodically monitor Hgb and/or Hct. Perform periodic monitoring of renal function in the elderly (≥65 yrs).

Patient Counseling: Inform to take with meals. Instruct to report if any digestive (eg, dyspepsia, nausea) or CNS (eg, headaches) side effects develop; dose adjustment may be needed. Report any signs/symptoms of angina or hypotension.

Administration: Oral administration. **Storage:** 15-30°C (59-86°F). Dispense in well-closed, light-resistant container. Protect blisters from light.

TREXIMET   RX
naproxen sodium - sumatriptan (GlaxoSmithKline)

> May increase risk of serious cardiovascular (CV) thrombotic events, myocardial infarction (MI), and stroke; increased risk with duration of use and with cardiovascular disease (CVD) or risk factors for CVD. Increased risk of serious GI adverse events (eg, bleeding, ulceration, and stomach/intestinal perforation) that can be fatal and occur anytime during use without warning symptoms; elderly patients are at greater risk.

THERAPEUTIC CLASS: 5-HT$_1$-agonist/NSAID

INDICATIONS: Acute treatment of migraine attacks with or without aura in adults.

DOSAGE: *Adults:* Individualize dose. Usual: 1 tab. Max: 2 tabs/24 hrs. Dosing should be at least 2 hrs apart.

HOW SUPPLIED: Tab: (Naproxen-Sumatriptan): 500mg-85mg

CONTRAINDICATIONS: History, symptoms, or signs of ischemic cardiac syndromes, cerebrovascular syndromes, or peripheral vascular syndromes (eg, ischemic bowel disease), other significant CVD, coronary artery bypass graft (CABG) surgery, hepatic impairment, uncontrolled HTN, hemiplegic or basilar migraine; concurrent administration or use within 2 weeks of MAO-A inhibitor d/c; use within 24 hrs of ergotamine-containing agents, ergot-type drugs, or other 5-HT$_1$ agonists, allergic-type reaction with NSAID/aspirin (ASA).

WARNINGS/PRECAUTIONS: May cause coronary artery vasospasm; avoid with risk factors (eg, HTN, hypercholesterolemia, smoker, obesity, diabetes, coronary artery disease (CAD) family history, menopause, males >40 yrs). Evaluate for atherosclerosis or predisposition to vasospasm if signs/symptoms suggestive of decreased arterial flow occur. Chest discomfort, jaw or neck tightness, peripheral vascular ischemia, and colonic ischemia reported. Caution with controlled HTN, fluid retention, and heart failure. Serotonin syndrome may occur; symptoms may include mental status changes, autonomic instability, neuromuscular aberrations, and GI symptoms. Anaphylactic/anaphylactoid reactions may occur; avoid in patients with ASA-triad. May cause serious skin reactions (eg, exfoliative dermatitis, Stevens-Johnson syndrome, toxic epidermal necrolysis); d/c at 1st appearance of skin rash/hypersensitivity. Avoid in late pregnancy; may cause premature closure of ductus arteriosus. Caution with diseases that may alter absorption/

metabolism/excretion, preexisting asthma, history of epilepsy or conditions associated with a lowered seizure threshold. Renal injury reported with long-term use and increased risk with renal/hepatic impairment, heart failure, and elderly; not recommended in patients with CrCl <30mL/min. Exclude potentially serious neurologic conditions before treatment in patients not previously diagnosed with migraine headache or who experience headache that is atypical for them. Anemia may occur; monitor Hgb/Hct if signs/symptoms of anemia develop. May inhibit platelet aggregation and prolong bleeding time; monitor carefully. D/C if signs and symptoms of liver/renal disease develop, systemic manifestations (eg, eosinophilia) occur, or abnormal LFTs persist or worsen. Use lowest effective dose for the shortest duration possible. Caution with prior history of ulcer disease, GI bleeding, risk factors for GI bleeding, history of inflammatory bowel disease. Overuse may lead to exacerbation of headache.

ADVERSE REACTIONS: CV thrombotic events, MI, stroke, GI events (eg, bleeding, ulceration, and perforation of the stomach or intestines), dizziness, somnolence, nausea, chest discomfort/pain; neck/throat/jaw pain, tightness, pressure.

INTERACTIONS: See Contraindications. Avoid with other naproxen-containing products. Caution with methotrexate; may prolong serum methotrexate levels. Not recommended with ASA. Increased plasma lithium levels; monitor for lithium toxicity. May reduce natriuretic effect of furosemide and thiazides. Probenecid may increase levels. May reduce the antihypertensive effect of ACE inhibitors, propranolol and other β-blockers. Increased risk of renal toxicity with diuretics and ACE inhibitors. Increased risk of GI bleeding with oral corticosteroids, warfarin, alcohol use, and smoking. Life-threatening serotonin syndrome reported with SSRIs and SNRIs.

PREGNANCY: Category C, not for use in nursing.

MECHANISM OF ACTION: Naproxen: NSAID; not established. Related to prostaglandin synthetase inhibition. Sumatriptan: $5-HT_1$ receptor agonist; mediates vasoconstriction of human basilar artery and vasculature of human dura mater, which correlates with the relief of migraine headache.

PHARMACOKINETICS: Absorption: Naproxen: Rapid and complete; bioavailability (95%); T_{max}=5 hrs. Sumatriptan: Bioavailability (15%), T_{max}=1 hr. **Distribution:** Naproxen: V_d=0.16L/kg; plasma protein binding (>99%); found in breast milk. Sumatriptan: V_d=2.4L/kg; plasma protein binding (14-21%); found in breast milk. **Metabolism:** Naproxen: Extensive; 6-0-desmethyl naproxen metabolite. Sumatriptan: Indole acetic acid (metabolite). **Elimination:** Naproxen: Urine (<1% unchanged, <1% 6-0-desmethyl naproxen, 66-92% conjugates), $T_{1/2}$=19 hrs. Sumatriptan: Urine (60%), feces (40%); $T_{1/2}$=2 hrs.

NURSING CONSIDERATIONS

Assessment: Assess for conditions where treatment is contraindicated or cautioned, pregnancy/nursing status, and possible drug interactions. Obtain ECG after 1st administration for those with CAD risk factors.

Monitoring: Monitor for signs/symptoms of cardiac events, colonic ischemia, bloody diarrhea, serotonin syndrome, hypersensitivity reactions, jaw/neck tightness, seizures, headache, signs and symptoms of GI adverse events, and clinical response. For long-term therapy or with CAD risk factors, perform periodic monitoring of CV function. Monitor vital signs, CBC, LFTs, bleeding time, renal function, and ECG periodically.

Patient Counseling: Inform to seek medical advice if symptoms of CV events (eg, chest pain, SOB, weakness, slurring of speech), GI ulcerations/bleeding (eg, epigastric pain, dyspepsia, melena, hematemesis), skin/hypersensitivity reactions (eg, rash, blisters, fever, itching), unexplained weight gain or edema, hepatotoxicity (eg, nausea, fatigue, lethargy, pruritus, jaundice, right upper quadrant tenderness, flu-like symptoms), anaphylactoid reactions (eg, difficulty breathing, swelling of the face or throat) occur. Instruct to avoid in late pregnancy. Inform about the risk of serotonin syndrome during combined use with SSRIs and SNRIs. Advise to use caution with activities that require alertness if they experience drowsiness, dizziness, vertigo, or depression during therapy.

Administration: Oral route. Give 1st dose in physician's office or similar medically staffed and equipped facility unless patient has previously received sumatriptan. Do not split, crush, or chew tab. **Storage:** 25°C (77°F); excursions permitted to 15-30°C (59-86°F).

TRIBENZOR   RX
olmesartan medoxomil - amlodipine - hydrochlorothiazide (Daiichi Sankyo)

> **D/C when pregnancy is detected. Drugs that act directly on the renin-angiotensin system can cause injury/death to the developing fetus.**

THERAPEUTIC CLASS: ARB/Calcium channel blocker (dihydropyridine)/Thiazide diuretic

INDICATIONS: Treatment of HTN.

T

DOSAGE: *Adults:* Usual: Dose qd. May increase after 2 weeks. Max: 40mg-10mg-25mg. Replacement Therapy: May substitute for individually titrated components. Add-On/Switch Therapy: Use if not adequately controlled on any 2 of the following antihypertensive classes: angiotensin receptor blockers, calcium channel blockers, and diuretics. With dose-limiting adverse reactions to any component on dual therapy, switch to triple therapy containing a lower dose of that component. Severe Hepatic Impairment/Elderly ≥75 yrs: Initial: 2.5mg amlodipine.

HOW SUPPLIED: Tab: (Olmesartan-Amlodipine-HCTZ) 20mg-5mg-12.5mg, 40mg-5mg-12.5mg, 40mg-5mg-25mg, 40mg-10mg-12.5mg, 40mg-10mg-25mg

CONTRAINDICATIONS: Anuria, hypersensitivity to sulfonamide-derived drugs.

WARNINGS/PRECAUTIONS: Not for initial therapy of HTN. Has not been studied in patients with heart failure (HF). Avoid use with severe renal impairment (CrCl ≤30mL/min). Renal impairment reported; consider withholding or d/c if progressive renal impairment becomes evident. Amlodipine: May develop increased frequency, duration, or severity of angina or acute myocardial infarction (MI), particularly with severe obstructive coronary artery disease (CAD). Rare reports of acute hypotension; caution with severe aortic stenosis. Hepatic enzyme elevations reported. HCTZ: May precipitate azotemia with renal disease, and hepatic coma due to fluid and electrolyte imbalance. Observe for clinical signs of fluid or electrolyte imbalance (eg, hyponatremia, hypochloremic alkalosis, hypokalemia). May cause metabolic acidosis, hyperuricemia or precipitation of frank gout, hyperglycemia, manifestation of latent diabetes mellitus (DM), hypomagnesemia, hypersensitivity reactions, exacerbation/activation of systemic lupus erythematosus (SLE), and increased cholesterol and TG levels. Enhanced effects in postsympathectomy patients. D/C before testing for parathyroid function. May cause idiosyncratic reaction, resulting in acute transient myopia and acute angle-closure glaucoma; d/c as rapidly as possible. Olmesartan: Symptomatic hypotension may occur in patients with an activated renin-angiotensin system (eg, volume- and/or salt-depleted patients); initiate treatment under close medical supervision. Oliguria or progressive azotemia and (rarely) acute renal failure and/or death may occur in patients whose renal function may depend on renin-angiotensin-aldosterone system activity (eg, severe congestive heart failure). May increase SrCr and BUN levels with renal artery stenosis. Hyperkalemia reported.

ADVERSE REACTIONS: Dizziness, peripheral edema, headache, fatigue, nasopharyngitis, muscle spasms, nausea.

INTERACTIONS: Amlodipine: May increase exposure to simvastatin; limit dose of simvastatin to 20mg daily. HCTZ: Potentiation of orthostatic hypotension may occur with alcohol, barbiturates, or narcotics. Dose adjustment of antidiabetic drugs (eg, oral agents, insulin) may be required. Additive effect or potentiation with other antihypertensives. Anionic exchange resins (eg, cholestyramine, colestipol) may impair absorption. Corticosteroids and adrenocorticotropic hormone may intensify electrolyte depletion, particularly hypokalemia. May decrease response to pressor amines (eg, norepinephrine). May increase response to nondepolarizing skeletal muscle relaxants (eg, tubocurarine). Increased risk of lithium toxicity; avoid concurrent use. NSAIDs may reduce diuretic, natriuretic, and antihypertensive effects. Olmesartan: May deteriorate renal function and attenuate antihypertensive effect with NSAIDs, including cyclooxygenase-2 inhibitors.

PREGNANCY: Category D, not for use in nursing.

MECHANISM OF ACTION: Amlodipine: Calcium channel blocker (dihydropyridine); inhibits transmembrane influx of calcium ions into vascular smooth muscle and cardiac muscle. Olmesartan: Angiotensin II receptor antagonist; blocks vasoconstrictor effects of angiotensin II by selectively blocking binding of angiotensin II to AT_1 receptor in vascular smooth muscle. HCTZ: Thiazide diuretic; has not been established. Affects renal tubular mechanisms of electrolyte reabsorption, directly increasing excretion of Na^+ and Cl^- and indirectly reducing plasma volume.

PHARMACOKINETICS: Absorption: Olmesartan: Rapid; absolute bioavailability (26%); T_{max}=1-2 hrs. Amlodipine: Absolute bioavailability (64-90%); T_{max}=6-12 hrs. HCTZ: T_{max}=1.5-2 hrs. **Distribution:** Olmesartan: V_d=17L; plasma protein binding (99%). Amlodipine: Plasma protein binding (93%). HCTZ: Crosses placenta; found in breast milk. **Metabolism:** Olmesartan: Ester hydrolysis. Amlodipine: Hepatic (extensive). **Excretion:** Olmesartan: Urine (35-50%), feces; $T_{1/2}$=13 hrs. Amlodipine: Urine (60% metabolites, 10% parent), $T_{1/2}$=30-50 hrs. HCTZ: Urine (≥61% unchanged); $T_{1/2}$=5.6-14.8 hrs.

NURSING CONSIDERATIONS

Assessment: Assess for anuria, sulfonamide-derived drug hypersensitivity, history of penicillin allergy, renal/hepatic function, HF, recent MI, aortic stenosis, renal artery stenosis, SLE, volume/salt depletion, electrolyte imbalances, postsympathectomy status, DM, CAD, cirrhosis, history of allergy or bronchial asthma, pregnancy/nursing status, and possible drug interactions.

Monitoring: Monitor for signs/symptoms of hypotension, hypersensitivity reactions, idiosyncratic reaction, latent DM, hepatic/renal function. Monitor BP, visual acuity, serum electrolytes, cholesterol levels, TG levels, SrCr, and BUN.

Patient Counseling: Counsel about risks/benefits of therapy and possible adverse effects. Inform of consequences of exposure during pregnancy; notify physician if pregnant/plan to become pregnant as soon as possible. Caution about lightheadedness, especially during the 1st days of therapy, and advise to report to physician. Instruct to d/c and consult physician if syncope occurs. Caution that inadequate fluid intake, excessive perspiration, diarrhea, or vomiting may lead to an excessive fall in BP, which may result in lightheadedness or syncope.

Administration: Oral route. **Storage:** 25°C (77°F); excursions permitted to 15-30°C (59-86°F).

TRICOR   RX
fenofibrate (Abbott)

THERAPEUTIC CLASS: Fibric acid derivative

INDICATIONS: Adjunct to diet for treatment of adults with severe hypertriglyceridemia. Adjunct to diet to reduce elevated LDL, total cholesterol, TG, and apolipoprotein B, and to increase HDL in patients with primary hypercholesterolemia or mixed dyslipidemia.

DOSAGE: *Adults:* Primary Hypercholesterolemia/Mixed Dyslipidemia: Initial: 145mg qd. Max: 145mg qd. Severe Hypertriglyceridemia: Individualize dose. Initial: 48-145mg/day. Titrate: Adjust dose if necessary following repeat lipid determinations at 4- to 8-week intervals. Max: 145mg qd. Mild to Moderate Renal Impairment: Initial: 48mg/day. Titrate: Increase only after evaluation of effects on renal function and lipid levels. Elderly: Dose based on renal function. Reduce dose if lipid levels significantly fall below target range. D/C if no adequate response after 2 months of treatment with max dose.

HOW SUPPLIED: Tab: 48mg, 145mg

CONTRAINDICATIONS: Severe renal impairment (including dialysis), active liver disease (including primary biliary cirrhosis and unexplained persistent liver function abnormalities), preexisting gallbladder disease, and nursing mothers.

WARNINGS/PRECAUTIONS: Increased risk of myopathy and rhabdomyolysis; d/c therapy if markedly elevated CPK levels occur or myopathy/myositis suspected or diagnosed. Increases in serum transaminases, hepatocellular, chronic active and cholestatic hepatitis, and cirrhosis (rare) reported; periodically monitor LFTs, and d/c therapy if enzyme levels persist >3X the normal limit. Elevations in SrCr reported; monitor renal function in patients with renal impairment or at risk for renal insufficiency. May cause cholelithiasis; d/c if gallstones are found. Acute hypersensitivity reactions and pancreatitis reported. Mild to moderate decreases in Hgb, Hct and WBCs, thrombocytopenia, and agranulocytosis reported; periodically monitor RBC/WBC counts during the first 12 months of therapy. May cause venothromboembolic disease (eg, pulmonary embolism [PE], deep vein thrombosis [DVT]). Estrogen therapy, thiazide diuretics, and β-blockers may be associated with massive rises in plasma TG; d/c of these drugs may obviate the need for specific drug therapy of hypertriglyceridemia.

ADVERSE REACTIONS: Abdominal pain, back pain, headache, abnormal liver function tests, increased ALT/AST and CPK, respiratory disorder.

INTERACTIONS: Increased risk of rhabdomyolysis with HMG-CoA reductase inhibitors (statins); avoid combination unless benefit outweighs risk. May potentiate coumarin anticoagulant effects; caution with use, monitor PT/INR frequently, and reduce dose of the anticoagulant. Immunosuppressants (eg, cyclosporine, tacrolimus) may produce nephrotoxicity; consider benefits and risks, use lowest effective dose, and monitor renal function with immunosuppressants and other potentially nephrotoxic agents. Bile acid resins may bind other drugs given concurrently; take at least 1 hr before or 4-6 hrs after the bile acid binding resin. Changes in exposure/levels with atorvastatin, pravastatin, fluvastatin, glimepiride, metformin, and rosiglitazone.

PREGNANCY: Category C, not for use in nursing.

MECHANISM OF ACTION: Fibric acid derivative; activates peroxisome proliferator-activated receptor α. Increases lipolysis and elimination of TG-rich particles from plasma by activating lipoprotein lipase and reducing production of apoprotein C-III (lipoprotein lipase activity inhibitor). Also induces an increase in the synthesis of apoproteins A-I, A-II, and HDL.

PHARMACOKINETICS: Absorption: Well absorbed. T_{max}=6-8 hrs. **Distribution:** Plasma protein binding (99%). **Metabolism:** Rapid by ester hydrolysis to fenofibric acid (active metabolite). **Elimination:** Urine (60%, fenofibric acid and glucuronate conjugate), feces (25%); $T_{1/2}$=20 hrs.

NURSING CONSIDERATIONS

Assessment: Assess for renal impairment, active liver disease, preexisting gallbladder disease, other medical conditions (eg, diabetes, hypothyroidism), hypersensitivity to drug, pregnancy/nursing status, and possible drug interactions.

Monitoring: Monitor for signs/symptoms of myositis, myopathy, or rhabdomyolysis; measure CPK levels in patients reporting such symptoms. Monitor for cholelithiasis, pancreatitis, hypersensitivity reactions, PE, and DVT. Monitor renal function, LFTs, CBC, and lipid levels.

Patient Counseling: Advise of potential benefits and risks of therapy, and medications to be avoided during treatment. Instruct to follow appropriate lipid-modifying diet during therapy and to take drug qd without regard to food at prescribed dose. Instruct to inform physician of all medications, supplements, and herbal preparations being taken, any changes in medical conditions, development of muscle pain, tenderness, weakness, and onset of abdominal pain or any other new symptoms.

Administration: Oral route. **Storage:** 25°C (77°F); excursions permitted to 15-30°C (59-86°F). Protect from moisture.

TRIGLIDE   RX
fenofibrate (Sciele)

THERAPEUTIC CLASS: Fibric acid derivative

INDICATIONS: Adjunct to diet for treatment of hypertriglyceridemia (Types IV and V). Reduction of LDL, total cholesterol, TG, and apolipoprotein B in primary hypercholesterolemia or mixed dyslipidemia (Types IIa and IIb).

DOSAGE: *Adults:* Hypercholesterolemia/Mixed Hyperlipidemia: 160mg qd. Hypertriglyceridemia: Initial: 50-160mg/day. Titrate: Adjust if needed after repeat lipid levels at 4-8 week intervals. Max: 160mg/day. Renal Dysfunction/Elderly: Initial: 50mg/day. Take without regard to meals.

HOW SUPPLIED: Tab: 50mg, 160mg

CONTRAINDICATIONS: Severe renal dysfunction, hepatic dysfunction (including primary biliary cirrhosis and unexplained persistent liver function abnormality), preexisting gallbladder disease.

WARNINGS/PRECAUTIONS: Increased serum transaminases (AST/ALT) reported; d/c if >3X ULN. Hepatocellular, chronic active and cholestatic hepatitis and cirrhosis reported. Monitor LFTs regularly; d/c if >3X ULN. May cause cholelithiasis; d/c if gallstones found. May cause myositis, myopathy, or rhabdomyolysis; d/c if myopathy/myositis or marked CPK elevation occurs. Decreased Hgb, Hct, WBCs, thrombocytopenia, and agranulocytosis reported; monitor CBC during first 12 months of therapy. Acute hypersensitivity reactions (eg, Stevens-Johnson syndrome [SJS], toxic epidermal necrolysis [TEN]), elevated SrCr, and pancreatitis reported. Higher rates of pulmonary embolus (PE) and deep vein thrombosis (DVT) reported. Caution in the elderly. Monitor lipids periodically initially; d/c if inadequate response after 2 months on 160mg/day. Caution in elderly.

ADVERSE REACTIONS: Abdominal pain, back pain, headache, abnormal LFTs, respiratory disorder, increased CPK/SGPT/SGOT.

INTERACTIONS: May potentiate coumarin anticoagulants; reduce anticoagulant dose and monitor PT/INR. Avoid HMG-CoA reductase inhibitors unless benefits outweigh risks. Bile acid sequestrants may impede absorption; take at least 1 hr before or 4-6 hrs after the resin. Evaluate benefits/risks with immunosuppressants (eg, cyclosporine) and other nephrotoxic agents; use lowest effective dose.

PREGNANCY: Category C, not for use in nursing.

MECHANISM OF ACTION: Fibric acid derivative; activates peroxisome proliferator-activated receptor alpha (PPARα). Causes an increase in lipolysis and elimination of triglyceride-rich particles from plasma by activating lipoprotein lipase and reducing production of apoprotein C-III. Induces an increase in apoprotein A-I, A-II, and HDL cholesterol synthesis. Reduces serum uric acid levels by increasing urinary excretion of uric acid.

PHARMACOKINETICS: Absorption: Well absorbed; T_{max}=3 hrs. **Distribution:** Plasma protein binding (99%). **Metabolism:** Hydrolysis, conjugation; fenofibric acid (active metabolite). **Elimination:** Urine (60%), feces (25%); $T_{1/2}$=16 hrs.

NURSING CONSIDERATIONS

Assessment: Assess for hepatic/renal dysfunction, primary biliary cirrhosis, unexplained persistent liver function abnormality, persistent elevation of lipid levels, hypothyroidism, preexisting gallbladder disease, and DM. Assess pregnancy/nursing status and possible drug interactions. Check baseline liver function and lipid levels.

Monitoring: Periodically monitor lipid levels, LFTs, CPK, PT, INR, CBC. Monitor for signs of myopathy (eg, unexplained muscle pain, tenderness, or weakness, with fever or malaise), cholelithiasis/cholecystitis, pancreatitis, hepatocellular, chronic active and cholestatic hepatitis, liver cirrhosis, malignancy, and hypersensitivity reaction or severe skin rash.

Patient Counseling: Advise to immediately contact physician if unexplained muscle pain, tenderness, or weakness with malaise or fever. Recommend appropriate lipid-lowering diet. May be taken with/without food.

Administration: Oral route. **Storage:** 20-25°C (68-77°F); excursions permitted between 15-30°C (59-86°F). Protect from light and moisture.

T

TRILEPTAL　　　　　　　　　　　　　　　　　　　　　RX

oxcarbazepine (Novartis)

THERAPEUTIC CLASS: Dibenzazepine

INDICATIONS: Monotherapy or adjunctive therapy in the treatment of partial seizures in adults; monotherapy in children aged ≥4 yrs with epilepsy, and adjunctive therapy in children aged ≥2 yrs with partial seizures.

DOSAGE: *Adults:* Monotherapy: Initial: 300mg bid. Titrate: Increase by 300mg/day every 3rd day. Maint: 1200mg/day. Adjunct Therapy: Initial: 300mg bid. Titrate: Increase weekly by a max of 600mg/day. Maint: 1200mg/day. Conversion to Monotherapy: Initial: 300mg bid while reducing other antiepileptic drugs (AEDs). Titrate: Increase weekly by a max of 600mg/day increment. Max dose must be reached in about 2-4 weeks. Withdraw other AEDs over 3-6 weeks. Maint: 2400mg/day. Renal Impairment: CrCl <30mL/min: Initial: 300mg/day. Titrate: Increase gradually. *Pediatrics:* 4-16 yrs: Monotherapy: Initial: 4-5mg/kg bid. Titrate: Increase by 5mg/kg/day every 3rd day. Maint (mg/day): Refer to PI for Dosing Chart. Adjunct Therapy: Initial: 4-5mg/kg bid. Max: 600mg/day. Titrate: Increase over 2 weeks. Maint: 20-29kg: 900mg/day. 29.1-39kg: 1200mg/day. >39kg: 1800mg/day. Conversion to Monotherapy: Initial: 4-5mg/kg bid while reducing other AEDs. Titrate: Increase weekly by max of 10mg/kg/day to target dose. Withdraw other AEDs over 3-6 weeks. 2-<4 yrs: Adjunct Therapy: Initial: 4-5mg/kg bid. Max: 600mg/day. <20kg: Initial: 8-10mg/kg bid. Max maint dose must be achieved over 2-4 weeks. Max: 60mg/kg/day. Renal Impairment: CrCl <30mL/min: Initial: 300mg/day. Titrate: Increase gradually.

HOW SUPPLIED: Sus: 300mg/5mL [250mL]; Tab: 150mg*, 300mg*, 600mg* *scored.

WARNINGS/PRECAUTIONS: May develop hyponatremia. D/C if anaphylaxis and angioedema involving the larynx, glottis, lips, and eyelids develop. Caution with history of hypersensitivity reactions to carbamazepine. Serious dermatologic reactions (eg, Stevens-Johnson syndrome [SJS], toxic epidermal necrolysis [TEN]) and multi-organ hypersensitivity reported. Increased risk of suicidal thoughts or behavior; monitor unusual changes in mood and behavior. Withdraw gradually to minimize the potential of increased seizure frequency. Associated with CNS adverse effects (cognitive symptoms, somnolence or fatigue, coordination abnormalities). Rare reports of agranulocytosis, leukopenia, and pancytopenia; d/c if any evidence of hematologic events develops. Monitor patients during pregnancy and continue close monitoring through postpartum. Caution with severe hepatic impairment.

ADVERSE REACTIONS: Dizziness, somnolence, diplopia, fatigue, N/V, ataxia, abnormal vision, tremor, abnormal gait, dyspepsia, abdominal pain, constipation, diarrhea, headache.

INTERACTIONS: Monitor serum Na⁺ levels during maintenance treatment, particularly with other medications also known to decrease Na⁺ levels (eg, drugs associated with inappropriate antidiuretic hormone secretion). Verapamil, valproic acid, and strong CYP450 inducers (eg, carbamazepine, phenytoin, phenobarbital) may decrease levels. Decreased plasma levels of cyclosporine, felodipine, oral contraceptives, and dihydropyridine calcium antagonists. May induce metabolism of CYP3A4/5 substrates. Increased plasma levels of phenytoin, phenobarbital, and CYP2C19 substrates. Decreased plasma levels with AEDs that are CYP450 inducers.

PREGNANCY: Category C, not for use in nursing.

MECHANISM OF ACTION: Dibenzazepine; not established. Oxcarbazepine and 10-monohydroxy metabolite (MHD) suspected to exert antiseizure effects through blockade of voltage-sensitive Na⁺ channels, resulting in stabilization of hyperexcited neural membranes, inhibition of repetitive neuronal firing, and diminution of propagation of synaptic impulses. Also, increased K⁺ conductance and modulation of high-voltage activated calcium channels may contribute to anticonvulsant activity.

PHARMACOKINETICS: Absorption: Complete; T_{max}=4.5 hrs (Tab), 6 hrs (Sus). **Distribution:** V_d=49L (MHD); plasma protein binding (40%) (MHD); found in breast milk. **Metabolism:** Liver (extensive); 10-monohydroxy derivative (MHD) (active metabolite). **Elimination:** Urine (>95%, <1% unchanged), feces (<4%); $T_{1/2}$=2 hrs (parent drug), 9 hrs (MHD). Refer to PI for pediatric parameters.

NURSING CONSIDERATIONS

Assessment: Assess hepatic and renal function. Assess for history of hypersensitivity reaction to carbamazepine, depression, pregnancy/nursing status, and possible drug interactions.

Monitoring: Monitor T4 levels. Monitor for signs/symptoms of hyponatremia, anaphylaxis and angioedema, severe dermatological reactions, cognitive or neuropsychiatric events, multiorgan hypersensitivity, hematological effects, emergence or worsening of depression, suicidal thoughts or behavior, and/or any unusual changes in mood or behavior, and other adverse reactions.

Patient Counseling: Advise to patients, their caregivers and families to be alert for the emergence or worsening of signs/symptoms of depression, any unusual changes in mood or behavior, or the emergence of suicidal thoughts, behavior, or thoughts about self-harm, and to read

Medication Guide. Immediately report signs/symptoms suggesting angioedema and blood disorders. Notify physician if fever with other organ system involvement or serious skin reaction develops. Counsel females that efficacy of oral contraceptives may decrease; use another form of contraception. Avoid alcohol and operating heavy machinery until effects of drug are gauged. May take with or without food. If pregnant, encourage to enroll in the North American Antiepileptic Drug (NAAED) Pregnancy Registry at 1-888-233-2334 or www.aedpregnancyregistry.org.

Administration: Oral route. May interchange tab and oral sus at equal doses. Sus: May mix in a small glass of water prior to administration or, swallow directly from syringe. Shake well before use. **Storage:** 25°C (77°F); excursions permitted to 15-30°C (59-86°F). Tab: Dispense in tight container. Sus: Use within 7 weeks after opening.

TRILIPIX   RX
fenofibric acid (Abbott)

THERAPEUTIC CLASS: Fibric acid derivative

INDICATIONS: Adjunct to diet in combination with a statin for treatment of mixed dyslipidemia. Adjunct to diet for treatment of severe hypertriglyceridemia, primary hyperlipidemia, or mixed dyslipidemia.

DOSAGE: *Adults:* Max: 135mg qd. Severe Hypertriglyceridemia: Individualize dose. Initial: 45-135mg qd. Titrate: May adjust dose if necessary following repeat lipid determinations at 4-8 week intervals. Primary Hyperlipidemia/Mixed Dyslipidemia: 135mg qd. Mixed Dyslipidemia With Statins: 135mg qd. Mild-to-Moderate Renal Impairment: Initial: 45mg qd. Titrate: May increase after evaluation of effects on renal function and lipid levels. Elderly: Base dose selection on renal function.

HOW SUPPLIED: Cap, Delayed-Release: 45mg, 135mg

CONTRAINDICATIONS: Severe renal impairment (including dialysis), active liver disease (including primary biliary cirrhosis and unexplained persistent liver function abnormalities), nursing mothers, and pre-existing gallbladder disease.

WARNINGS/PRECAUTIONS: Increased risk of myositis/myopathy and rhabdomyolysis; d/c therapy if myositis/myopathy or marked creatine phosphokinase (CPK) elevation occurs. Reversible elevations in SrCr reported; monitor renal function in patients with renal impairment or at risk for renal insufficiency. Increase in serum transaminases, hepatocellular, chronic active and cholestatic hepatitis, and cirrhosis (rare) reported; monitor LFTs, and d/c therapy if enzyme levels persist >3X ULN. May cause cholelithiasis; d/c if gallstones are found. Acute hypersensitivity reactions (rare) and pancreatitis reported. Mild to moderate decreases in Hgb, Hct and WBCs, rare thrombocytopenia and agranulocytosis reported. May cause venothromboembolic disease (eg, pulmonary embolism [PE], deep vein thrombosis [DVT]). Not indicated for patients with elevated chylomicrons and plasma TG, but with normal levels of VLDL. D/C medications known to exacerbate hypertriglyceridemia (β-blockers, estrogens, thiazides) prior to therapy.

ADVERSE REACTIONS: Headache, back pain, nasopharyngitis, nausea, myalgia, diarrhea, upper respiratory tract infection, abnormal liver function test, abdominal pain, arthralgia, dizziness, dyspepsia, sinusitis, constipation.

INTERACTIONS: May potentiate anticoagulant effects of oral coumarin anticoagulants; caution with use, monitor PT/INR frequently, and adjust dose of the oral anticoagulant. Bile acid resins may impede absorption; take ≥1 hr before or 4-6 hrs after the bile acid resin. Evaluate benefits/risks with immunosuppressants (eg, cyclosporine) and other potentially nephrotoxic agents; use lowest effective dose. Changes in exposure/levels with atorvastatin, ezetimibe, fluvastatin, glimepiride, metformin, omeprazole, pravastatin, rosiglitazone, rosuvastatin, and simvastatin. Increased risk of rhabdomyolysis with statins.

PREGNANCY: Category C, not for use in nursing.

MECHANISM OF ACTION: Fibric acid derivative; activates peroxisome proliferator-activated receptor α. Increases lipolysis and elimination of TG-rich particles from plasma by activating lipoprotein lipase and reducing production of APO C-III. Also induces an increase in the synthesis of HDL-C and Apo AI and AII.

PHARMACOKINETICS: Absorption: Well-absorbed. Absolute bioavailability (81%); T_{max}=4-5 hrs. **Distribution:** Plasma protein binding (99%). **Metabolism:** Conjugation with glucuronic acid. **Elimination:** Urine; $T_{1/2}$=20 hrs.

NURSING CONSIDERATIONS

Assessment: Assess for renal impairment, active liver disease, pre-existing gallbladder disease, excessive alcohol intake, pregnancy/nursing status, other medical conditions (eg, diabetes mellitus, hypothyroidism), and possible drug interactions. Obtain baseline LFTs and lipid levels.

Monitoring: Monitor for signs/symptoms of myositis, myopathy, rhabdomyolysis; measure CPK levels if myopathy is suspected. Monitor for cholelithiasis, pancreatitis, hypersensitivity reactions, DVT, and PE. Monitor renal function, LFTs, CBC, and lipid levels.

Patient Counseling: Advise of potential benefits and risks of therapy, and medications to be avoided during treatment. Instruct to read Medication Guide, follow appropriate lipid-modifying diet during therapy, return for routine monitoring, take drug qd without regard to food at prescribed dose, and swallow cap whole. Inform that if on statin therapy, both drugs may be taken at the same time. Notify physician of all medications, supplements, and herbal preparations being taken, any changes in medical conditions, development of muscle pain, tenderness, or weakness, and onset of abdominal pain or any other new symptoms.

Administration: Oral route. **Storage:** 25°C (77°F); excursions permitted to 15-30°C (59-86°F). Protect from moisture.

TRIPEDIA   RX

pertussis vaccine, acellular - diphtheria toxoid - tetanus toxoid (Sanofi Pasteur)

THERAPEUTIC CLASS: Vaccine/toxoid combination

INDICATIONS: Active immunization against diphtheria, tetanus, and pertussis in pediatrics 6 weeks-7 yrs (prior to 7th birthday). Combined with ActHIB for active immunization in pediatrics 15-18 months previously immunized against diphtheria, tetanus, and pertussis with 3 doses of whole-cell pertussis DTP or acellular pertussis vaccine and 3 or fewer doses of ActHIB within 1st year of life for prevention of *Haemophilus influenzae* type b, diphtheria, tetanus, and pertussis.

DOSAGE: *Pediatrics:* ≥6 weeks up to 7 yrs: Primary Series: 3 doses of 0.5mL IM at 4-8 week intervals. 1st dose usually at 2 months, but can give at 6 weeks up to 7th birthday. Booster: 4th dose (0.5mL IM) at 15-20 months, at least 6 months after 3rd dose, 5th dose at 4-6 yrs; prior to school entry. May give to complete 4th or 5th dose of primary series of 3 doses of whole-cell pertussis DTP (4th dose at 15-20 months and 5th dose before school if 4th dose not given on or before 4th birthday). May combine with ActHIB for 4th dose at 15-18 months.

HOW SUPPLIED: Inj: 0.5mL

CONTRAINDICATIONS: Hypersensitivity to thimerosal and gelatin, immediate anaphylactic reaction associated with previous dose, encephalopathy not due to an identifiable cause within 7 days of prior pertussis immunization. Defer during poliomyelitis outbreak or acute febrile illness.

WARNINGS/PRECAUTIONS: Caution if within 48 hrs of previous whole-cell DTP or acellular DTP vaccine, fever ≥105°F not due to another identifiable cause, collapse or shock-like state, or inconsolable crying lasting ≥3 hrs occurs, or if convulsions occur within 3 days. For high seizure risk, give acetaminophen at time of vaccination and q4-6h for 24 hrs. Caution with neurologic or CNS disorders. Avoid with coagulation disorders. Have epinephrine available. Suboptimal response may occur in immunocompromised patients.

ADVERSE REACTIONS: Local erythema and swelling, irritability, drowsiness, anorexia, fever.

INTERACTIONS: Avoid with anticoagulants. Immunosuppressive therapy (eg, irradiation, antimetabolites, alkylating agents, cytotoxic drugs, corticosteroids) may decrease response. Do not combine through reconstitution with any vaccine for infants <15 months.

PREGNANCY: Category C, safety in nursing not known.

MECHANISM OF ACTION: Active immunization against diphtheria, tetanus, and pertussis (whooping cough).

NURSING CONSIDERATIONS

Assessment: Review current health status, previous sensitivity/immunization events (eg, fever, shock, persistent crying, convulsions, Guillain-Barre syndrome), and possible drug interactions.

Monitoring: Monitor for Arthus-type hypersensitivity reactions, injection-site for erythema, swelling, and tenderness, fever, irritability, drowsiness, anorexia, N/V, high-pitched/persistent crying, and neurological complications.

Patient Counseling: Inform of potential benefits/risks; report any adverse reactions to physician. May not offer 100% protection.

Administration: IM route. Inject into anterolateral aspect of thigh or deltoid region. **Storage:** 2-8°C (36-46°F). Do not freeze.

TRIZIVIR RX

abacavir sulfate - zidovudine - lamivudine (ViiV Healthcare)

Lactic acidosis and severe hepatomegaly with steatosis, including fatal cases, reported with nucleoside analogues. Abacavir: Serious and sometimes fatal hypersensitivity reactions (multi-organ clinical syndrome) reported; d/c as soon as suspected and never restart therapy or any other abacavir-containing product. Patients with HLA-B*5701 allele are at high risk for hypersensitivity; screen for HLA-B*5701 allele prior to therapy. Zidovudine: Associated with hematologic toxicity (eg, neutropenia, severe anemia), particularly with advanced HIV-1 disease. Symptomatic myopathy associated with prolonged use. Lamivudine: Severe acute exacerbations of hepatitis B reported in patients coinfected with hepatitis B virus (HBV) upon d/c of therapy; closely monitor hepatic function for at least several months. If appropriate, initiation of anti-hepatitis B therapy may be warranted.

THERAPEUTIC CLASS: Nucleoside reverse transcriptase inhibitor

INDICATIONS: Treatment of HIV-1 infection alone or in combination with other antiretrovirals.

DOSAGE: *Adults:* ≥40kg and CrCl ≥50mL/min: Usual: 1 tab bid. Elderly: Caution with dose selection.
Pediatrics: Adolescents: ≥40kg and CrCl ≥50mL/min: Usual: 1 tab bid.

HOW SUPPLIED: Tab: (Abacavir Sulfate-Lamivudine-Zidovudine) 300mg-150mg-300mg

CONTRAINDICATIONS: Hepatic impairment.

WARNINGS/PRECAUTIONS: Obesity and prolonged nucleoside exposure may be risk factors for lactic acidosis and severe hepatomegaly with steatosis; suspend therapy if clinical or laboratory findings suggestive of lactic acidosis or pronounced hepatotoxicity develop. Immune reconstitution syndrome reported. Autoimmune disorders (eg, Graves' disease, polymyositis, and Guillain-Barre syndrome) reported to occur in the setting of immune reconstitution and can occur many months after initiation of treatment. Redistribution/accumulation of body fat may occur. Cross-resistance potential with nucleoside reverse transcriptase inhibitors reported. Caution with any known risk factors for liver disease and in elderly. Avoid use in adolescents weighing <40kg, and in patients requiring dose adjustments (eg, renal impairment [CrCl <50mL/min]). Abacavir: Increased risk of myocardial infarction (MI) reported; consider the underlying risk of coronary heart disease when prescribing therapy. Lamivudine: Emergence of lamivudine-resistant HBV reported. Zidovudine: Caution with compromised bone marrow evidenced by granulocyte count <1000 cells/mm³ or Hgb <9.5g/dL; monitor blood counts frequently with advanced HIV-1 disease and periodically with other HIV-1 infected patients. Interrupt therapy if anemia or neutropenia develops.

ADVERSE REACTIONS: Lactic acidosis, severe hepatomegaly with steatosis, hematologic toxicity, myopathy, N/V, headache, malaise, fatigue, hypersensitivity reaction, diarrhea, fever, chills, depressive disorders, skin rashes, ear/nose/throat infections.

INTERACTIONS: Avoid with other abacavir-, lamivudine-, zidovudine-, and/or emtricitabine-containing products. Hepatic decompensation may occur in HIV-1/hepatitis C virus (HCV) coinfected patients with interferon-alfa with or without ribavirin; closely monitor for treatment-associated toxicities. Abacavir: Ethanol may decrease elimination causing an increase in overall exposure. May increase PO methadone clearance. Zidovudine: Avoid with stavudine, doxorubicin, and some nucleoside analogues affecting DNA replication (eg, ribavirin). Atovaquone, fluconazole, methadone, probenecid, and valproic acid may increase area under the curve (AUC). Clarithromycin, nelfinavir, rifampin, and ritonavir may decrease AUC. May increase hematologic toxicity with ganciclovir, interferon-alfa, ribavirin, and other bone marrow suppressive or cytotoxic agents. Lamivudine: Nelfinavir and trimethoprim/sulfamethoxazole may increase levels.

PREGNANCY: Category C, not for use in nursing.

MECHANISM OF ACTION: Abacavir: Carbocyclic synthetic nucleoside analogue; inhibits HIV-1 reverse transcriptase (RT) by competing with natural substrate deoxyguanosine-5'-triphosphate and by incorporating into viral DNA. Lamivudine/Zidovudine: Synthetic nucleoside analogue; inhibits RT via DNA chain termination after incorporation of the nucleotide analogue.

PHARMACOKINETICS: Absorption: Rapid. Bioavailability: Abacavir/Lamivudine (86%), zidovudine (64%). **Distribution:** Abacavir: V_d=0.86L/kg; plasma protein binding (50%). Lamivudine: V_d=1.3L/kg; plasma protein binding (low); found in breast milk. Zidovudine: V_d=1.6L/kg; plasma protein binding (low); crosses the placenta; found in breast milk. **Metabolism:** Abacavir: Via alcohol dehydrogenase and glucuronyl transferase. Lamivudine: Trans-sulfoxide (metabolite). Zidovudine: Hepatic via glucuronyl transferase; 3'-azido-3'-deoxy-5'-O-β-D-glucopyranuronosylthymidine (GZDV) (major metabolite). **Elimination:** Abacavir: $T_{1/2}$=1.45 hrs. Lamivudine: (IV) Urine (70%, unchanged); $T_{1/2}$=5-7 hrs. Zidovudine: Urine (14% unchanged, 74% GZDV); $T_{1/2}$=0.5-3 hrs.

NURSING CONSIDERATIONS

Assessment: Assess for history of hypersensitivity, hepatic/renal impairment, risk factors for lactic acidosis, risk factors for liver and coronary heart disease, bone marrow compromise, HBV infection, pregnancy/nursing status, and possible drug interactions. Assess for HLA-B*5701 allele type. Assess for prior exposure to any abacavir-containing product.

Monitoring: Monitor for signs and symptoms of hypersensitivity reactions, hematologic toxicity, lactic acidosis, hepatomegaly with steatosis, myopathy, immune reconstitution syndrome (eg, opportunistic infections), autoimmune disorders, fat redistribution, and MI. Monitor hepatic/renal function and blood counts. Monitor hepatic function for several months after d/c therapy.

Patient Counseling: Inform patients regarding hypersensitivity reactions with abacavir; instruct to contact physician immediately if symptoms develop and not to restart or replace with any drug containing abacavir without medical consultation. Inform patients that myopathy and myositis with pathological changes may occur with prolonged use of zidovudine. Inform that the drug may cause a rare but serious condition called lactic acidosis with liver enlargement (hepatomegaly). Inform that toxicities include neutropenia and anemia; inform of the importance of having blood work done regularly. Inform patients coinfected with HBV that deterioration of liver disease has occurred in some cases when treatment with lamivudine was d/c; instruct to discuss any changes of regimen with the physician. Inform that hepatic decompensation has occurred in HIV-1-/HCV-coinfected patients with interferon alfa with or without ribavirin. Inform that redistribution/accumulation of body fat may occur. Advise that drug is not a cure for HIV-1 infection and that illness associated with HIV-1 may still be experienced. Advise to avoid doing things that can spread HIV-1 infection to others (eg, sharing of needles/inj equipment/personal items that can have blood or body fluids on them, having sex without protection, breastfeeding). Inform patients to take all HIV medications exactly as prescribed.

Administration: Oral route. **Storage:** 25°C (77°F); excursions permitted to 15-30°C (59-86°F).

TRUSOPT   RX
dorzolamide HCl (Merck)

THERAPEUTIC CLASS: Carbonic anhydrase inhibitor

INDICATIONS: Treatment of elevated intraocular pressure (IOP) in patients with ocular HTN or open-angle glaucoma.

DOSAGE: *Adults:* 1 drop in the affected eye(s) tid.
Pediatrics: 1 drop in the affected eye(s) tid.

HOW SUPPLIED: Sol: 2% [10mL]

WARNINGS/PRECAUTIONS: Systemically absorbed. Rare fatalities have occurred due to severe sulfonamide reactions; d/c if signs of hypersensitivity or other serious reactions occur. Sensitizations may recur if readministered irrespective of the route of administration. Not recommended with severe renal impairment (CrCl <30mL/min). Caution with hepatic impairment. Local ocular adverse effects (eg, conjunctivitis, lid reactions) reported with chronic use; d/c use and evaluate patient before considering restarting therapy. Bacterial keratitis with contaminated containers, and choroidal detachment following filtration procedures reported. Caution in patients with low endothelial cell counts; increased potential for corneal edema.

ADVERSE REACTIONS: Ocular burning, stinging, discomfort, bitter taste, superficial punctate keratitis, ocular allergic reactions, conjunctivitis, lid reactions, blurred vision, eye redness, tearing, dryness, photophobia.

INTERACTIONS: Acid-base disturbances reported with oral carbonic anhydrase inhibitors; caution with high-dose salicylates. Concomitant administration of oral carbonic anhydrase inhibitors not recommended due to potential additive effects.

PREGNANCY: Category C, not for use in nursing.

MECHANISM OF ACTION: Carbonic anhydrase inhibitor; decreases aqueous humor secretion, presumably by slowing the formation of bicarbonate ions with subsequent reduction in Na$^+$ and fluid transport.

PHARMACOKINETICS: Absorption: Systemic. **Distribution:** Plasma protein binding (33%). **Metabolism:** N-desethyl (metabolite). **Elimination:** Urine (unchanged, metabolite).

NURSING CONSIDERATIONS

Assessment: Assess for hypersensitivity reaction, history of sulfonamide hypersensitivity, acute angle-closure glaucoma, renal/hepatic impairment, pregnancy/nursing status, and possible drug interactions.

Monitoring: Monitor for improvement in IOP, serious reactions, sulfonamide hypersensitivity reactions (eg, Stevens-Johnson syndrome, toxic epidermal necrolysis, fulminant hepatic necrosis, agranulocytosis, aplastic anemia, blood dyscrasias), ocular reactions, bacterial keratitis, choroidal detachment, and other adverse reactions. Monitor serum electrolyte and blood pH levels.

Patient Counseling: Advise to d/c and notify physician if signs of hypersensitivity or ocular reactions (eg, conjunctivitis, lid reactions) occur. Avoid allowing tip of dispensing container to contact eye or surrounding structures. If container becomes contaminated, serious damage to the eye and loss of vision may result. Advise to immediately contact physician concerning use of present multidose container if undergoing ocular surgery or a concomitant ocular condition (eg, trauma, infection) develops. Advise to administer at least 10 min apart if using >1 ophthalmic medication. Advise to remove contact lenses prior to administration; may be reinserted 15 min after.

Administration: Ocular route. Administer at least 10 min apart if using >1 topical ophthalmic drug. **Storage:** 15-30°C (59-86°F). Protect from light.

TRUVADA
tenofovir disoproxil fumarate - emtricitabine (Gilead)

RX

> Lactic acidosis and severe hepatomegaly with steatosis, including fatal cases, reported with the use of nucleoside analogues. Not approved for chronic hepatitis B virus (HBV) infection. Severe acute exacerbations of hepatitis B reported in patients coinfected with HBV upon d/c of therapy; closely monitor hepatic function for at least several months. If appropriate, initiation of anti-hepatitis B therapy may be warranted.

THERAPEUTIC CLASS: Nucleoside analogue combination

INDICATIONS: Treatment of HIV-1 infection in combination with other antiretrovirals in adults and pediatrics ≥12 yrs.

DOSAGE: *Adults:* ≥35kg: CrCl ≥50mL/min: 1 tab qd. CrCl 30-49mL/min: 1 tab q48 hrs. *Pediatrics:* ≥12 yrs: ≥35kg: CrCl ≥50mL/min: 1 tab qd. CrCl 30-49mL/min: 1 tab q48 hrs.

HOW SUPPLIED: Tab: (Emtricitabine-Tenofovir Disoproxil Fumarate [TDF]) 200mg-300mg

WARNINGS/PRECAUTIONS: Obesity and prolonged nucleoside exposure may be risk factors for lactic acidosis and severe hepatomegaly with steatosis. Caution with known risk factors for liver disease. D/C if findings suggestive of lactic acidosis or pronounced hepatotoxicity (hepatomegaly and steatosis even without marked transaminase elevations) develop. Prior to treatment, all patients with HIV-1 should be tested for the presence of chronic HBV. Renal impairment reported; calculate CrCl prior to and during therapy. Avoid in patients with CrCl <30mL/min or patients requiring hemodialysis. Decreased bone mineral density (BMD), fractures, and osteomalacia reported; assess BMD with history of pathologic bone fracture or other risk factors for osteoporosis or bone loss. Immune reconstitution syndrome reported. Fat redistribution/accumulation may occur. Regimens that only contain three nucleoside reverse transcriptase inhibitors (NRTI) have been shown to be less effective than triple drug regimens containing two NRTIs in combination with either a non-nucleoside reverse transcriptase inhibitor or a HIV-1 protease inhibitor; early virological failure and high rates of resistance substitutions reported. Triple nucleoside regimens should be used with caution and treatment modifications should be considered. Caution in elderly.

ADVERSE REACTIONS: Diarrhea, nausea, fatigue, headache, dizziness, depression, abnormal dreams, insomnia, rash.

INTERACTIONS: Avoid with nephrotoxic agents, adefovir dipivoxil, and other drugs containing emtricitabine, TDF, or lamivudine. Drugs that are renally eliminated (eg, acyclovir, cidofovir, ganciclovir, valacyclovir, valganciclovir) may increase levels of emtricitabine, tenofovir, and/or the coadministered drug. Increases levels of didanosine (ddI) when coadministered; monitor for ddI-associated adverse effects and d/c ddI if any develop. TDF: Atazanavir, lopinavir/ritonavir may increase levels. May decrease atazanavir levels; monitor for TDF-associated adverse reactions and d/c if any develop. Atazanavir without ritonavir should not be coadministered with TDF.

PREGNANCY: Category B, not for use in nursing.

MECHANISM OF ACTION: Emtricitabine: Synthetic nucleoside analogue of cytidine; inhibits activity of HIV-1 reverse transcriptase (RT) by competing with natural substrate deoxycytidine 5'-triphosphate and by being incorporated into nascent viral DNA, resulting in chain termination. TDF: Acyclic nucleoside phosphonate diester analogue of adenosine monophosphate; inhibits activity of HIV-1 RT by competing with the natural substrate deoxyadenosine 5'-triphosphate and after incorporation into DNA, by DNA chain termination.

PHARMACOKINETICS: Absorption: Emtricitabine: Rapid. Bioavailability (92%), C_{max}=1.8mcg/mL, T_{max}=1-2 hrs, AUC=10mcg•h/mL. TDF: Bioavailability (25%), C_{max}=0.3mcg/mL, T_{max}=1 hr, AUC=2.29mcg•h/mL. **Distribution:** Emtricitabine: Plasma protein binding (<4%). TDF: Plasma protein binding (<0.7%). **Metabolism:** Emtricitabine: 3'-sulfoxide diastereomers, glucoronic acid conjugate (metabolites). **Elimination:** Emtricitabine: Urine (86%) (13%, metabolites); $T_{1/2}$=10 hrs. TDF: (IV) Urine (70-80%, unchanged); $T_{1/2}$=17 hrs.

NURSING CONSIDERATIONS

Assessment: Assess for risk factors for lactic acidosis, liver disease, HBV status, renal impairment, pregnancy/nursing status, and for possible drug interactions. Assess BMD in patient with a history of pathologic bone fracture or other risk factors for osteoporosis or bone loss. Calculate

CrCl in all patients prior to initiating therapy. In HBV-infected patients, perform HIV-1 antibody testing. In HIV-1 patients, perform testing for presence of chronic HBV.

Monitoring: Monitor for signs/symptoms of lactic acidosis, hepatomegaly with steatosis, new onset or worsening renal impairment, decreases in bone mineral density, redistribution/accumulation of body fat, and for immune reconstitution syndrome (eg, opportunistic infections). Upon d/c of therapy in HBV patients, monitor hepatic function closely and for signs/symptoms of acute exacerbation of hepatitis B. Monitor CrCl and monitor serum phosphorus levels, especially in patients at risk for renal impairment.

Patient Counseling: Inform that medication is not cure for HIV-1 and may continue to experience illness associated with HIV-1 infection, including opportunistic infections. Advise to continue to practice safe sex and to use latex or polyurethane condoms and to never reuse or share needles. Inform that tablets are for oral ingestion only. Counsel about the importance of adherence to regimen on a regular dosing schedule to avoid missing doses. Inform about the benefits/risks of therapy.

Administration: Oral route. **Storage:** 25°C (77°F), excursions permitted to 15-30°C (59-86°F).

TussiCaps

CIII

hydrocodone polistirex - chlorpheniramine polistirex (Mallinckrodt)

THERAPEUTIC CLASS: Opioid antitussive/antihistamine

INDICATIONS: Relief of cough and upper respiratory symptoms associated with allergy or a cold in adults and children ≥6 yrs.

DOSAGE: *Adults:* 1 full-strength cap q12h. Max: 2 caps/24 hrs. Elderly: Start at lower end of dosing range.
Pediatrics: ≥12 yrs: 1 full-strength cap q12h. Max: 2 caps/24 hrs. 6-11 yrs: 1 half-strength cap q12h. Max: 2 caps/24 hrs.

HOW SUPPLIED: Cap, Extended-Release: (Chlorpheniramine-Hydrocodone) 8mg-10mg (Full-Strength), 4mg-5mg (Half-Strength)

CONTRAINDICATIONS: Children <6 yrs of age.

WARNINGS/PRECAUTIONS: May produce dose-related respiratory depression and irregular/periodic breathing; may be antagonized by the use of naloxone HCl and other supportive measures when indicated. Caution with postoperative use, pulmonary disease, depressed ventilatory function, narrow-angle glaucoma, asthma, prostatic hypertrophy, severe hepatic/renal impairment, hypothyroidism, Addison's disease, or urethral stricture, and in pediatrics ≥6 yrs, elderly, or debilitated. May have exaggerated respiratory depressant effects and elevation of CSF pressure in patients with head injury, other intracranial lesions, or preexisting increase in intracranial pressure. May obscure clinical course of head injuries and acute abdominal conditions. Chronic use may result in obstructive bowel disease, especially in patients with underlying intestinal motility disorder. Carefully consider benefit to risk ratio, especially in pediatrics with respiratory embarrassment (eg, croup).

ADVERSE REACTIONS: Sedation, drowsiness, lethargy, anxiety, dysphoria, euphoria, dizziness, rash, pruritus, N/V, ureteral spasm, urinary retention, psychic dependence, mood changes.

INTERACTIONS: Additive CNS depression with narcotics, antihistamines, antipsychotics, antianxiety agents, or other CNS depressants (including alcohol); reduce dose of 1 or both agents when combined therapy is contemplated. Increased effect of either antidepressant or hydrocodone with MAOIs or TCAs. May produce paralytic ileus with other anticholinergics. Increased risk of respiratory depression in pediatrics with other respiratory depressants.

PREGNANCY: Category C, not for use in nursing.

MECHANISM OF ACTION: Hydrocodone: Semisynthetic narcotic antitussive/analgesic; not established. Believed to act directly on cough center. Chlorpheniramine: H_1-receptor antagonist; possesses anticholinergic and sedative activity. Prevents released histamine from dilating capillaries and causing edema of the respiratory mucosa.

PHARMACOKINETICS: Absorption: (Extended-Release Sus) Hydrocodone: C_{max}=22.8ng/mL, T_{max}=3.4 hrs. Chlorpheniramine: C_{max}=58.4ng/mL, T_{max}=6.3 hrs. **Elimination:** Hydrocodone: $T_{1/2}$=4 hrs. Chlorpheniramine: $T_{1/2}$=16 hrs.

NURSING CONSIDERATIONS

Assessment: Assess patient's age, use in postoperative patients, elderly/debilitated, renal/hepatic function, other conditions where treatment is cautioned or contraindicated, drug hypersensitivity, pregnancy/nursing status, and possible drug interactions.

Monitoring: Monitor for signs/symptoms of respiratory depression, hypersensitivity reactions, hepatic/renal function, and development of obstructive bowel disease.

Patient Counseling: Inform that medication may produce marked drowsiness and impair mental and/or physical abilities required for the performance of potentially hazardous tasks (eg, driving, operating machinery). Instruct not to dilute with fluids or mix with other drugs.

Administration: Oral route. **Storage:** 20-25°C (68-77°F).

TUSSIONEX PENNKINETIC
hydrocodone polistirex - chlorpheniramine polistirex (UCB)

THERAPEUTIC CLASS: Opioid antitussive/antihistamine

INDICATIONS: Relief of cough and upper respiratory symptoms associated with allergy or a cold in adults and children ≥6 yrs.

DOSAGE: *Adults:* 5mL q12h. Max: 10mL/24 hrs. Elderly: Start at lower end of dosing range. *Pediatrics:* ≥12 yrs: 5mL q12h. Max: 10mL/24 hrs. 6-11 yrs: 2.5mL q12h. Max: 5mL/24 hrs.

HOW SUPPLIED: Sus, Extended-Release: (Chlorpheniramine-Hydrocodone) 8mg-10mg/5mL [115mL, 473mL]

CONTRAINDICATIONS: Children <6 yrs of age.

WARNINGS/PRECAUTIONS: May produce dose-related respiratory depression and irregular/periodic breathing; may be antagonized by the use of naloxone HCl and other supportive measures when indicated. Caution with postoperative use, pulmonary disease, depressed ventilatory function, narrow-angle glaucoma, asthma, prostatic hypertrophy, severe hepatic/renal impairment, hypothyroidism, Addison's disease, or urethral stricture, and in pediatrics ≥6 yrs, elderly, or debilitated. May have exaggerated respiratory depressant effects and elevation of CSF pressure in patients with head injury, other intracranial lesions, or preexisting increase in intracranial pressure. May obscure clinical course of head injuries and acute abdominal conditions. Chronic use may result in obstructive bowel disease, especially in patients with underlying intestinal motility disorder. Carefully consider benefit to risk ratio, especially in pediatrics with respiratory embarrassment (eg, croup).

ADVERSE REACTIONS: Sedation, drowsiness, lethargy, anxiety, dysphoria, euphoria, dizziness, rash, pruritus, N/V, ureteral spasm, urinary retention, psychic dependence, mood changes.

INTERACTIONS: Additive CNS depression with narcotics, antihistaminics, antipsychotics, antianxiety agents, and other CNS depressants (including alcohol); reduce dose of one or both agents when combined therapy is contemplated. Increased effect of either the antidepressant or hydrocodone with MAOIs or TCAs. May produce paralytic ileus with other anticholinergics. Increased risk of respiratory depression in pediatrics with other respiratory depressants.

PREGNANCY: Category C, not for use in nursing.

MECHANISM OF ACTION: Hydrocodone: Semisynthetic narcotic antitussive/analgesic; not established. Believed to act directly on cough center. Chlorpheniramine: H$_1$-receptor antagonist; possesses anticholinergic and sedative activity. Prevents released histamine from dilating capillaries and causing edema of the respiratory mucosa.

PHARMACOKINETICS: Absorption: (Extended-Release Sus) Hydrocodone: C$_{max}$=22.8ng/mL, T$_{max}$=3.4 hrs. Chlorpheniramine: C$_{max}$=58.4ng/mL, T$_{max}$=6.3 hrs. **Elimination:** Hydrocodone: T$_{1/2}$=4 hrs. Chlorpheniramine: T$_{1/2}$=16 hrs.

NURSING CONSIDERATIONS

Assessment: Assess patient's age, use in postoperative patients, elderly/debilitated, hepatic/renal function, other conditions where treatment is cautioned or contraindicated, drug hypersensitivity, pregnancy/nursing status, and possible drug interactions.

Monitoring: Monitor for signs/symptoms of respiratory depression, hypersensitivity reactions, hepatic/renal function, and development of obstructive bowel disease.

Patient Counseling: Instruct to shake well before use. Inform that medication may produce marked drowsiness and impair mental/physical abilities required for the performance of potentially hazardous tasks (eg, operating machinery, driving). Instruct not to dilute with fluids or mix with other drugs. Advise to measure sus with accurate measuring device. Advise that a household tsp is not accurate and could lead to overdosage; a pharmacist can recommend an appropriate measuring device and provide instructions.

Administration: Oral route. Shake well before use. Measure with an accurate measuring device; rinse with water after each use. **Storage:** 20-25°C (68-77°F); excursions permitted to 15-30°C (59-86°F).

TWINJECT
epinephrine (Verus)

RX

THERAPEUTIC CLASS: Sympathomimetic catecholamine

INDICATIONS: Emergency treatment of severe allergic reactions (type 1), including anaphylaxis to insect stings or bites, allergens, foods, drugs, diagnostic testing substances, as well as idiopathic or exercise-induced anaphylaxis.

DOSAGE: *Adults:* Administer SQ or IM into thigh. 15-30kg: (Twinject 0.15mg) 0.15mg. May repeat if needed. ≥30kg: (Twinject 0.3mg) 0.3mg. May repeat if needed.
Pediatrics: Administer SQ or IM into thigh. 15-30kg: (Twinject 0.15mg) 0.15mg. May repeat if needed. ≥30kg: (Twinject 0.3mg) 0.3mg. May repeat if needed.

HOW SUPPLIED: Inj: (Twinject 0.15mg, Twinject 0.3mg) 1mg/mL

WARNINGS/PRECAUTIONS: Inject into anterolateral aspect of thigh; avoid injecting into hands, feet, or buttock. Avoid IV use. Contains sodium bisulfite. Caution with cardiac arrhythmias, coronary artery or organic heart disease, or HTN. May precipitate/aggravate angina pectoris or produce ventricular arrhythmias with coronary insufficiency or ischemic heart disease. Light-sensitive; store in tube provided.

ADVERSE REACTIONS: Anxiety, apprehensiveness, restlessness, tremor, weakness, dizziness, sweating, palpitations, pallor, N/V, headache, respiratory difficulties, HTN.

INTERACTIONS: Monitor for cardiac arrhythmias with cardiac glycosides or diuretics. Effects may be potentiated by TCAs, MAOIs, levothyroxine, and certain antihistamines (notably chlorpheniramine, tripelennamine, diphenhydramine). Cardiostimulating and bronchodilating effects antagonized by β-adrenergic blockers (eg, propranolol). Vasoconstricting and hypertensive effects antagonized by α-adrenergic blockers (eg, phentolamine). Ergot alkaloids and phenothiazines may reverse pressor effects.

PREGNANCY: Category C, safety in nursing not known.

MECHANISM OF ACTION: Acts on α- and β-adrenergic receptors.

NURSING CONSIDERATIONS

Assessment: Assess for arrhythmias, ischemic/organic heart disease, HTN, DM, hyperthyroidism, pregnancy/nursing status, Parkinson's disease, and drug interactions (eg, medications that may sensitize heart to arrhythmia such as digitalis).

Monitoring: Monitor BP, HR, blood glucose, signs of cerebral hemorrhage, ventricular arrhythmia, HTN, and anginal pain.

Patient Counseling: Inform about side effects of therapy (eg, increased pulse rate, sense of forceful heartbeat, palpitations, throbbing headache, pallor, anxiety, shakiness). Side effects may subside rapidly, especially with rest, quiet, and recumbency but may be severe or persistent with HTN or hyperthyroidism. Never inject into buttocks or by IV route.

Administration: IM or SQ route. Inject into anterolateral administration. **Storage:** 20-25°C (68-77°F); excursions permitted to 15-30°C (59-86°F). Protect from light. Avoid freezing or refrigeration. Discard if discolored.

TWINRIX
hepatitis A vaccine - hepatitis B (recombinant) (GlaxoSmithKline)

RX

THERAPEUTIC CLASS: Vaccine

INDICATIONS: Active immunization against disease caused by hepatitis A virus and infection by all known subtypes of hepatitis B virus in patients ≥18 yrs of age.

DOSAGE: *Adults:* 3-Dose Schedule: 1mL IM in deltoid region at 0, 1, and 6 months. Alternative 4-Dose Schedule: 1mL IM in deltoid region on days 0, 7, and 21-30, followed by booster dose at month 12.

HOW SUPPLIED: Inj: 1mL [vial, prefilled syringe]

CONTRAINDICATIONS: History of severe allergic reaction to yeast or neomycin.

WARNINGS/PRECAUTIONS: Tip cap and rubber plunger of prefilled syringes may contain natural latex rubber; allergic reactions may occur in latex-sensitive individuals. Review immunization history for possible vaccine sensitivity and previous vaccination-related adverse reactions to allow an assessment of benefits and risks. Appropriate treatment and supervision must be available for possible anaphylactic reactions. Delay administration with moderate or severe acute febrile illness unless at immediate risk of hepatitis A or hepatitis B infection. Immunocompromised persons may have a diminished immune response. May not prevent hepatitis A or B infection in individuals who have unrecognized hepatitis A or B infection at the time of vaccination. May not protect all individuals.

ADVERSE REACTIONS: Inj-site reactions (eg, soreness, redness, swelling), headache, fatigue, diarrhea, nausea, fever.

INTERACTIONS: Immunosuppressive therapies (eg, irradiation, antimetabolites, alkylating agents, cytotoxic drugs and corticosteroids [used in greater than physiological doses]) may reduce immune response.

PREGNANCY: Category C, caution in nursing.

MECHANISM OF ACTION: Bivalent vaccine; produces immune response against hepatitis A and all known subtypes of hepatitis B virus.

NURSING CONSIDERATIONS

Assessment: Assess for hypersensitivity to yeast, neomycin, and to latex rubber. Assess for moderate or severe acute febrile illness, immunosuppression, unrecognized hepatitis A or B infection, pregnancy/nursing status, and for possible drug interactions. Review immunization history for possible vaccine sensitivity and previous vaccination-related adverse reactions.

Monitoring: Monitor for allergic reactions, inj-site reactions, and for immune response.

Patient Counseling: Inform of potential benefits/risks of vaccination. Educate about potential side effects. Inform that components of the vaccine cannot cause hepatitis A or B infection. Instruct to report any adverse events to the healthcare provider.

Administration: IM route. Shake well before use. Do not mix with any other vaccine or product in the same syringe or vial. **Storage:** 2-8°C (36-46°F). Do not freeze; discard if has been frozen.

TWYNSTA
amlodipine - telmisartan (Boehringer Ingelheim)

RX

> D/C when pregnancy is detected. Drugs that act directly on the renin-angiotensin system can cause injury/death to the developing fetus.

THERAPEUTIC CLASS: ARB/Calcium channel blocker (dihydropyridine)

INDICATIONS: Treatment of HTN alone or with other antihypertensive agents. May also be used as initial therapy in patients likely to need multiple drugs to achieve their BP goals.

DOSAGE: *Adults:* Individualize dose. Initial: 40mg-5mg qd. Patients Requiring Large BP Reduction: Initial: 80mg-5mg qd. Titrate: May be increased after at least 2 weeks. Max: 80mg-10mg qd. Hepatic Impairment/Patients ≥75 yrs: Not recommended for initial therapy. Hepatic Impairment/Severe Renal Impairment/Patients ≥75 yrs: Titrate slowly. Add-On Therapy: May be used if not adequately controlled on amlodipine (or another dihydropyridine calcium channel blocker) alone or telmisartan (or another angiotensin receptor blocker) alone. Patients treated with amlodipine 10mg who experience dose-limiting adverse reactions may switch to 40mg-5mg qd. Replacement Therapy: May substitute for individual components; dose may be increased if inadequate BP control.

HOW SUPPLIED: Tab: (Telmisartan-Amlodipine) 40mg-5mg, 40mg-10mg, 80mg-5mg, 80mg-10mg

WARNINGS/PRECAUTIONS: Caution with renal/hepatic dysfunction and elderly. Amlodipine: May increase frequency, duration or severity of angina or acute myocardial infarction (MI), particularly with severe obstructive coronary artery disease (CAD). Caution with severe aortic stenosis. Closely monitor patients with heart failure. Telmisartan: Symptomatic hypotension may occur in patients with an activated renin-angiotensin system (eg, volume- or salt-depleted patients); correct volume/salt depletion prior to therapy or start therapy under medical supervision with a reduced dose. Risk of hyperkalemia, particularly with advanced renal impairment or heart failure; periodically monitor serum electrolytes. Caution with biliary obstructive disorders. Oliguria and/or progressive azotemia and (rarely) acute renal failure and/or death reported in patients with renal function dependent on renin-angiotensin-aldosterone system (eg, severe congestive heart failure [CHF] or renal dysfunction). May increase SrCr/BUN with renal artery stenosis. Dual blockade of the renin-angiotensin-aldosterone system (eg, by adding an ACE inhibitor to an angiotensin II receptor antagonist) should include close monitoring of renal function.

ADVERSE REACTIONS: Peripheral edema, dizziness, back pain.

INTERACTIONS: Amlodipine: May increase exposure to simvastatin; limit dose of simvastatin to 20mg daily. Telmisartan: May increase digoxin levels; monitor digoxin levels upon initiating, adjusting, and d/c therapy. May increase lithium levels/toxicity; monitor lithium levels during concurrent use. Coadministration with NSAIDs, including selective cyclooxygenase-2 inhibitors, may attenuate antihypertensive effect of angiotensin II receptor antagonists and may further deteriorate renal function. Increased levels of ramipril/ramiprilat noted during concomitant use, whereas telmisartan levels are decreased; concomitant use not recommended. Increased risk of hyperkalemia with renal replacement therapy, K+-sparing diuretics, K+ supplements, K+-containing salt substitutes, or other drugs that increase K+ levels. Possible inhibition of the metabolism of drugs metabolized by CYP2C19.

PREGNANCY: Category C (1st trimester) and D (2nd and 3rd trimester), not for use in nursing.

MECHANISM OF ACTION: Amlodipine: Dihydropyridine calcium channel blocker; inhibits transmembrane influx of calcium ions into vascular smooth muscle and cardiac muscle. Telmisartan: Angiotensin II receptor antagonist; blocks vasoconstrictor and aldosterone-secreting effects of angiotensin II by selectively blocking the binding of angiotensin II to the AT_1 receptor in many tissues, such as vascular smooth muscle and adrenal gland.

PHARMACOKINETICS: Absorption: Amlodipine: Absolute bioavailability (64-90%); T_{max}=6-12 hrs. Telmisartan: Absolute bioavailability (42%, 40mg), (58%, 160mg); T_{max}=0.5-1 hr. **Distribution:** Amlodipine: V_d=21L/kg; plasma protein binding (93%). Telmisartan: V_d=500L; plasma protein binding (>99.5%). **Metabolism:** Amlodipine: Liver (extensive). Telmisartan: Conjugation. **Elimination:** Amlodipine: Urine (10%, parent compound), (60%, metabolites); $T_{1/2}$=30-50 hrs. Telmisartan: Feces (>97%, unchanged), urine (0.49%); $T_{1/2}$=24 hrs.

NURSING CONSIDERATIONS

Assessment: Assess for angina, MI, severe obstructive CAD, severe aortic stenosis, renal artery stenosis, CHF, volume/salt depletion, hepatic/renal function, biliary obstructive disorders, hypersensitivity to drug, pregnancy/nursing status, and possible drug interactions. Obtain baseline BP.

Monitoring: Monitor hepatic/renal function and for other adverse reactions. Monitor BP and serum electrolytes especially K+ levels.

Patient Counseling: Inform of pregnancy risks. Advise to notify physician as soon as possible if pregnant. Inform patients of side effects (eg, syncope, somnolence, dizziness, vertigo) and to seek medical attention if any occur.

Administration: Oral route. **Storage:** 25°C (77°F); excursions permitted to 15-30°C (59-86°F). Do not remove from blisters until immediately before administration. Protect from light and moisture.

TYGACIL   RX
tigecycline (Wyeth)

THERAPEUTIC CLASS: Glycylcycline

INDICATIONS: Treatment of complicated skin and skin structure infections (cSSSI), complicated intra-abdominal infections (cIAI), and community-acquired bacterial pneumonia (CABP) caused by susceptible strains of indicated pathogens in patients ≥18 yrs.

DOSAGE: *Adults:* Initial: 100mg IV over 30-60 min. Maint: 50mg q12h over 30-60 min for 5-14 days (cSSSI/cIAI) or for 7-14 days (CABP). Severe Hepatic Impairment (Child-Pugh C): Initial: 100mg IV over 30-60 min. Maint: 25mg q12h over 30-60 min.

HOW SUPPLIED: Inj: 50mg/5mL, 50mg/10mL [vial]

WARNINGS/PRECAUTIONS: Anaphylaxis/anaphylactoid reactions reported. Structurally similar to tetracyclines; may have similar adverse effects: photosensitivity, pseudotumor cerebri, pancreatitis, and anti-anabolic action (may lead to increased BUN, azotemia, acidosis, and hyperphosphatemia). Caution with known hypersensitivity to tetracyclines. Isolated cases of significant hepatic dysfunction and failure reported; evaluate risk/benefit of continued therapy if hepatic function worsens. Efficacy in hospital-acquired pneumonia not demonstrated; greater mortality seen in ventilator-associated pneumonia. Acute pancreatitis reported; consider stopping therapy if suspected. May cause fetal harm in pregnant women and permanent tooth discoloration (yellow-gray-brown) when administered during tooth development (last half of pregnancy to 8 yrs). Caution when used for cIAI secondary to clinically apparent intestinal perforations. *Clostridium difficile*-associated diarrhea (CDAD) reported. May result in bacterial resistance with prolonged use or use in the absence of a proven/suspected bacterial infection or a prophylactic indication; take appropriate measures if superinfection develops.

ADVERSE REACTIONS: N/V, diarrhea, abdominal pain, infection, headache, anemia, hypoproteinemia, increased liver enzymes, anaphylaxis/anaphylactoid reactions, acute pancreatitis, asthenia, elevated BUN, dizziness, phlebitis.

INTERACTIONS: Decreased effectiveness of oral contraceptives. Monitor PT with warfarin.

PREGNANCY: Category D, caution in nursing.

MECHANISM OF ACTION: Glycylcycline; inhibits protein translation in bacteria by binding to the 30S ribosomal subunit and blocking entry of amino-acyl tRNA molecules into the A site of the ribosome.

PHARMACOKINETICS: Absorption: IV infusion of variable doses resulted in different parameters. **Distribution:** V_d=7-9L/kg; plasma protein binding (71-89%). **Metabolism:** Liver. **Elimination:** Bile (primary), urine (22%, unchanged); $T_{1/2}$=27.1 hrs (single dose), 42.4 hrs (multiple dose).

NURSING CONSIDERATIONS

Assessment: Assess for known hypersensitivity to tetracycline antibiotics, hepatic impairment, cIAI secondary to clinically apparent intestinal perforation, culture and susceptibility testing, pregnancy/nursing status, and possible drug interactions.

Monitoring: Monitor for signs/symptoms of hypersensitivity reactions, hepatic impairment, pancreatitis, photosensitivity, superinfection, and CDAD. Monitor PT with warfarin.

Patient Counseling: Inform of fetal harm during pregnancy and that therapy treats bacterial, not viral, infections. Take as directed; skipping doses or not completing full course of therapy may decrease effectiveness and increase resistance. May experience diarrhea; notify physician if with watery/bloody stools even as late as >2 months after last dose.

Administration: IV route. Refer to PI for reconstitution. Reconstituted solution should be yellow to orange in color; if not, discard solution. **Storage:** Powder: 20-25°C (68-77°F); excursions permitted to 15-30°C (59-86°F). Solution: Room temperature up to 24 hrs (up to 6 hrs in vial and remaining time in IV bag); refrigerated 2-8°C (36-46°F) up to 48 hrs following immediate transfer of reconstituted solution into IV bag.

TYKERB   RX
lapatinib (GlaxoSmithKline)

Hepatotoxicity may occur; may be severe and deaths have been reported.

THERAPEUTIC CLASS: Kinase inhibitor

INDICATIONS: In combination with capecitabine for treatment of patients with advanced/metastatic breast cancer whose tumors overexpress HER2 and who had prior therapy including an anthracycline, a taxane, and trastuzumab. In combination with letrozole for the treatment of postmenopausal women with hormone receptor-positive metastatic breast cancer that overexpresses the HER2 receptor for whom hormonal therapy is indicated.

DOSAGE: *Adults:* HER2-Positive Metastatic Breast Cancer: Usual: 1250mg qd on Days 1-21 continuously with capecitabine 2000mg/m²/day (2 doses 12 hrs apart) on Days 1-14 in a repeating 21-day cycle. Continue treatment until disease progresses or unacceptable toxicity occurs. Hormone Receptor-Positive, HER2-Positive Metastatic Breast Cancer: Usual: 1500mg qd continuously with letrozole 2.5mg qd. Refer to PI for dose modification guidelines.

HOW SUPPLIED: Tab: 250mg

WARNINGS/PRECAUTIONS: Decreased left ventricular ejection fraction (LVEF) reported; confirm normal LVEF prior to therapy and monitor during treatment. Caution with conditions that may impair left ventricular function. Monitor LFTs before treatment, every 4-6 weeks during therapy, and as clinically indicated; d/c if severe LFT changes occur. Consider reducing dose with severe preexisting hepatic impairment. Diarrhea reported; manage with antidiarrheals, replace electrolytes/fluids, and interrupt or d/c if severe diarrhea occurs. Associated with interstitial lung disease and pneumonitis; d/c if pulmonary symptoms indicative of interstitial lung disease/pneumonitis ≥Grade 3. QT prolongation observed. Caution with hypokalemia, hypomagnesemia, and congenital long QT syndrome; correct hypokalemia and hypomagnesemia before administration. May cause fetal harm.

ADVERSE REACTIONS: Hepatotoxicity, diarrhea, N/V, stomatitis, dyspepsia, palmar-plantar erythrodysesthesia, rash, dry skin, mucosal inflammation, pain in extremity, back pain, dyspnea, fatigue.

INTERACTIONS: Caution with CYP3A4 substrates, CYP2C8 substrates, P-glycoprotein (P-gp) substrates; consider dose reduction. Avoid with strong CYP3A4 inhibitors (eg, ketoconazole, itraconazole, clarithromycin, atazanavir, indinavir, nefazodone, nelfinavir, ritonavir, saquinavir, telithromycin, voriconazole) and inducers (eg, dexamethasone, phenytoin, carbamazepine, rifampin, rifabutin, rifapentin, phenobarbital, St. John's wort); if unavoidable, consider dose modification. Avoid concomitant use with grapefruit. Caution with concomitant use of antiarrhythmics or other drugs that prolong the QT interval, and with cumulative high-dose anthracycline therapy. P-gp inhibitors may increase levels. May increase concentrations of paclitaxel, midazolam, and digoxin.

PREGNANCY: Category D, not for use in nursing.

MECHANISM OF ACTION: Kinase inhibitor; inhibits both epidermal growth factor receptor (EGFR [ErbB1]) and human epidermal receptor type 2 (HER2 [ErbB2]) receptors resulting in tumor cell growth inhibition.

T

PHARMACOKINETICS: Absorption: Incomplete and variable. C_{max}=2.43mcg/mL, T_{max}=4 hrs, AUC=36.2mcg•hr/mL. **Distribution**: Plasma protein binding (>99%). **Metabolism**: Liver (extensive); (major) CYP3A4, CYP3A5; (minor) CYP2C19, CYP2C8. **Elimination**: Feces (27% parent, 14% metabolites), urine (<2%); $T_{1/2}$=14.2 hrs (single dose).

NURSING CONSIDERATIONS

Assessment: Assess for severe hepatic impairment, decreased LVEF or conditions that may impair left ventricular function, QT prolongation, hypokalemia, hypomagnesemia, pregnancy/ nursing status, and for possible drug interactions. Obtain baseline ECG, LFTs, serum K+, and magnesium levels.

Monitoring: Monitor for signs/symptoms of hepatotoxicity, diarrhea, interstitial lung disease, hypokalemia, hypomagnesemia, decreased LVEF, and for QT prolongation. Monitor ECG and electrolytes. Monitor LFTs every 4-6 weeks during therapy and as clinically indicated.

Patient Counseling: Instruct to notify physician if SOB, palpitations, or fatigue occurs. Advise that diarrhea is a common side effect and instruct on how it should be managed; instruct to contact physician is severe diarrhea occurs. Counsel to report use of any Rx/OTC drugs or herbal products. Advise to avoid grapefruit products and take ≥1 hr ac/pc. Counsel to take capecitabine with food or within 30 min after food. Instruct to take therapy once daily and inform that dividing daily dose is not recommended. Advise against doubling dose the next day for a missed dose.

Administration: Oral route. Take ≥1 hr pc/ac. **Storage:** 25°C (77°F); excursions permitted to 15-30°C (59-86°F).

TYSABRI RX
natalizumab (Elan)

> Increases risk of progressive multifocal leukoencephalopathy (PML). Cases of PML reported with recent/concomitant use of immunomodulators or immunosuppressants. Available only through a special restricted distribution program called the TOUCH® Prescribing Program. Only prescribers, infusion centers, and pharmacies associated with infusion centers registered with the program are able to prescribe, distribute, or infuse the product. Administer only to patients who are enrolled in and meet all conditions of the program. Monitor for any new signs/symptoms of PML; withhold therapy at the 1st sign/symptom suggestive of PML.

THERAPEUTIC CLASS: Monoclonal antibody/VCAM-1 blocker

INDICATIONS: Treatment of relapsing forms of multiple sclerosis (MS) to delay the accumulation of physical disability and reduce the frequency of clinical exacerbations. To induce and maintain clinical response and remission in adults with moderately to severely active Crohn's disease (CD) with evidence of inflammation who have had an inadequate response to, or are unable to tolerate, conventional CD therapies and TNF-α inhibitors.

DOSAGE: *Adults:* 300mg IV infusion over 1 hr every 4 weeks. (CD) In patients starting therapy while on chronic PO corticosteroids, commence steroid tapering as soon as therapeutic benefit has occurred. D/C therapy if no therapeutic benefit by 12 weeks, if patient cannot be tapered off corticosteroids within 6 months, or in patients who require additional steroid use that exceeds 3 months within a calendar year to control their CD.

HOW SUPPLIED: Inj: 300mg/15mL

CONTRAINDICATIONS: Progressive multifocal leukoencephalopathy (PML).

WARNINGS/PRECAUTIONS: Efficacy of therapy beyond 2 years is unknown. Safety and efficacy with chronic progressive MS have not been studied. Immune reconstitution inflammatory syndrome (IRIS) reported with PML and subsequent d/c of natalizumab; monitor for development of IRIS and treat appropriately. Hypersensitivity reactions, including anaphylaxis reported; d/c, institute appropriate therapy, and do not retreat. May increase risk for infections. Liver injury reported; d/c with jaundice or evidence of liver injury. Induces increases in circulating lymphocytes, monocytes, eosinophils, basophils, and nucleated RBCs or transient decreases in Hgb levels. Avoid in patients with serious medical conditions resulting in significantly compromised immune system function.

ADVERSE REACTIONS: Headache, fatigue, urinary tract infection, depression, lower/upper respiratory tract infection, arthralgia, abdominal discomfort, rash, gastroenteritis, vaginitis, urinary urgency/frequency, dermatitis, abnormal LFTs.

INTERACTIONS: See Boxed Warning. Avoid with immunomodulatory therapy, immunosuppressants (eg, 6-mercaptopurine, azathioprine, cyclosporine, or methotrexate) or TNF-α inhibitors. Taper corticosteroids in CD patients when starting natalizumab therapy. Antineoplastic, immunosuppressive, or immunomodulating agents may further increase risk of infections, including PML and other opportunistic infections.

PREGNANCY: Category C, safety not known in nursing.

MECHANISM OF ACTION: Monoclonal antibody/VCAM-1 blocker; recombinant humanized IgG4k monoclonal antibody that binds to α4-subunit of α4β1 and α4β7 integrins expressed on surface of all leukocytes, except neutrophils. Inhibits α4-mediated adhesion of leukocytes to their counter-receptor(s).

PHARMACOKINETICS: Absorption: (MS) C_{max}=110mcg/mL; (CD) C_{max}=101mcg/mL. **Distribution:** Found in breast milk; (MS) V_d=5.7L; (CD) V_d=5.2L. **Elimination:** (MS) $T_{1/2}$=11 days; (CD) $T_{1/2}$=10 days.

NURSING CONSIDERATIONS

Assessment: Assess for risk of PML, history of chronic immunosuppressant or immunomodulatory therapy, immunosuppression, drug hypersensitivity, pregnancy/nursing status, and possible drug interactions. Perform magnetic resonance imaging (MRI) and CSF analysis.

Monitoring: Monitor for PML, anaphylactic/hypersensitivity reactions, infections, hepatotoxicity, or development of IRIS. Antibody testing recommended if presence of persistent antibodies suspected. Monitor CBC, LFTs, and bilirubin.

Patient Counseling: Inform about TOUCH Prescribing Program. Educate on risks/benefits of therapy. Instruct to report signs of infections, hypersensitivity reactions, and liver toxicity. Counsel about the follow-up schedule (3 and 6 months after 1st infusion, then every 6 months). Instruct to seek medical attention if symptoms suggestive of PML develop, including progressive weakness on one side of the body or clumsiness of the limbs, disturbance of vision, and changes in thinking, memory, and orientation leading to confusion and personality changes.

Administration: IV route. Refer to PI for dilution/administration instructions. **Storage:** 2-8°C (36-46°F). Administer within 8 hrs of preparation. Do not shake or freeze. Protect from light.

TYVASO   RX
treprostinil (United Therapeutics)

THERAPEUTIC CLASS: Pulmonary and systemic vasodilator

INDICATIONS: Treatment of pulmonary arterial hypertension (PAH) (World Health Organization Group 1) in patients with NYHA Class III symptoms and etiologies of idiopathic or heritable PAH or PAH associated with connective tissue diseases to improve exercise ability.

DOSAGE: *Adults:* Initial: 3 breaths (18mcg) per treatment session qid. Reduce to 1-2 breaths if not tolerated and subsequently increase to 3 breaths, as tolerated. Maint: Increase by an additional 3 breaths at approx 1-2 week intervals, if tolerated, to a target dose of 9 breaths (54mcg) per treatment session qid. Max: 9 breaths per treatment session qid. Hepatic/Renal Insufficiency: Titrate slowly.

HOW SUPPLIED: Sol: 0.6mg/mL [2.9mL]

WARNINGS/PRECAUTIONS: Safety and efficacy not established with significant underlying lung disease (eg, asthma or chronic obstructive pulmonary disease [COPD]). Caution with acute pulmonary infections; monitor carefully to detect worsening of lung disease and loss of drug effect. May produce symptomatic hypotension in patients with low systemic arterial pressure. Caution with hepatic or renal impairment. May increase risk of bleeding. Caution in elderly.

ADVERSE REACTIONS: Headache, cough, throat irritation/pharyngolaryngeal pain, nausea, flushing, syncope.

INTERACTIONS: Increased risk of bleeding with anticoagulants. Increased risk of symptomatic hypotension with diuretics, antihypertensive agents, or other vasodilators. Increased exposure with CYP2C8 inhibitors (eg, gemfibrozil); decreased exposure with CYP2C8 inducers (eg, rifampin).

PREGNANCY: Category B, caution in nursing.

MECHANISM OF ACTION: Pulmonary and systemic vasodilator; causes direct vasodilation of pulmonary and systemic arterial vascular beds. Inhibits platelet aggregation.

PHARMACOKINETICS: Absorption: Absolute bioavailability (64%) (18mcg), (72%) (36mcg); (54mcg)C_{max}=0.91-1.32ng/mL, T_{max}=0.12-0.25 hr, AUC=0.81-0.97ng•hr/mL. **Distribution:** (parenteral infusion) V_d=14L/70kg; plasma protein binding (91%). **Metabolism:** Liver via CYP2C8. **Elimination:** (SQ) Urine (79%, 4% unchanged), feces (13%); $T_{1/2}$=4 hrs.

NURSING CONSIDERATIONS

Assessment: Assess for lung disease (eg, asthma, COPD), acute pulmonary infections, low systemic arterial pressure, hepatic/renal insufficiency, pregnancy/nursing status, and possible drug interactions. Obtain baseline LFTs, renal and lung functions.

Monitoring: Monitor for worsening of lung disease, loss of drug effect, hepatic/renal insufficiency, and symptomatic hypotension. Monitor LFTs, renal and lung functions.

Patient Counseling: Counsel for proper administration process, including dosing, set-up, operation, cleaning, and maintenance, according to the instructions for use. Advise to have back-up Optineb-ir device to avoid potential interruptions in drug delivery. Inform that therapy should be resumed as soon as possible if treatment session is missed or interrupted. Advise to immediately rinse with water if in contact with skin or eyes.

Administration: Oral inhalation route. Refer to PI for proper administration. **Storage:** 25°C (77°F); excursions permitted to 15-30°C (59-86°F). If opened or transferred in a device, solution should remain for no more than 1 day. Use within 7 days if foil pack is opened. Protect from light; store unopened ampules in foil pouch.

TYZEKA   RX
telbivudine (Novartis)

Lactic acidosis and severe hepatomegaly with steatosis, including fatal cases, reported with nucleoside analogues alone or in combination with other antiretrovirals. Severe acute exacerbations of hepatitis B reported in patients who d/c therapy; monitor hepatic function closely for at least several months after d/c and resume anti-hepatitis B therapy if needed.

THERAPEUTIC CLASS: Nucleoside reverse transcriptase inhibitor

INDICATIONS: Treatment of chronic hepatitis B in adults with evidence of viral replication and either evidence of persistent elevations in serum aminotransferases (ALT or AST) or histologically active disease.

DOSAGE: *Adults;* ≥16 yrs: Usual: 600mg or 30mL qd. Dose Adjustment: CrCl 30-49mL/min: 600mg q48h or 20mL qd. CrCl <30mL/min (not requiring dialysis): 600mg q72h or 10mL qd. End-Stage Renal Disease: 600mg q96h or 6mL qd. Elderly: Adjust dose accordingly.

HOW SUPPLIED: Sol: 100mg/5mL [300mL]; Tab: 600mg

CONTRAINDICATIONS: Combination with pegylated interferon alfa-2a.

WARNINGS/PRECAUTIONS: Initiate only if pretreatment HBV DNA and ALT levels are known. HBV DNA should be <9 $\log_{10}$ copies/mL and ALT ≥2X ULN in HBeAg-positive patients prior to therapy. HBV DNA should be <7 $\log_{10}$ copies/mL in HBeAg-negative patients prior to therapy. Female gender, obesity, and prolonged nucleoside exposure may be risk factors for developing lactic acidosis and hepatomegaly with steatosis; d/c therapy if lactic acidosis or hepatotoxicity develops. Caution with known risk factors for liver disease. Myopathy/myositis and peripheral neuropathy reported; interrupt therapy if suspected and d/c if confirmed. Rhabdomyolysis and uncomplicated myalgia reported. Caution in elderly.

ADVERSE REACTIONS: Fatigue, creatinine kinase increase, headache, cough, diarrhea, abdominal pain, nausea, pharyngolaryngeal pain, arthralgia, pyrexia, rash, lactic acidosis, hepatomegaly, exacerbation of hepatitis.

INTERACTIONS: See Contraindication. Drugs that alter renal function may alter plasma concentrations. Combination with pegylated interferon alfa-2a and other interferons may be associated with risk of peripheral neuropathy.

PREGNANCY: Category B, not for use in nursing.

MECHANISM OF ACTION: Thymidine nucleoside analogue; inhibits HBV DNA polymerase by competing with thymidine 5'-triphosphate and causes DNA chain termination.

PHARMACOKINETICS: Absorption: C_{max}=3.69mcg/mL, T_{max}= 2 hrs, AUC=26.1mcg•h/mL; administration with varying degrees of renal function resulted in different pharmacokinetic parameters. **Distribution:** Plasma protein binding (3.3%). **Elimination:** Urine (42%) (600mg); $T_{1/2}$=40-49 hrs.

NURSING CONSIDERATIONS

Assessment: Assess for renal/hepatic impairment, use in women, obesity, nucleoside exposure duration, risk factors for liver disease, pregnancy/nursing status, and possible drug interactions. Obtain HBV DNA and ALT prior to therapy.

Monitoring: Monitor hepatic function periodically and for several months after d/c. Monitor for exacerbation of HBV after d/c, lactic acidosis, hepatomegaly, hepatotoxicity, myopathy, and peripheral neuropathy. Monitor HBV DNA levels at 24 weeks of therapy and every 6 months thereafter. Monitor renal function in elderly patients.

Patient Counseling: Advise patients to remain under care of a physician during therapy and to discuss any new symptoms or concurrent medication. Advise to report promptly unexplained muscle weakness, tenderness or pain, numbness, tingling, and/or burning sensations in the arms and/or legs with or without difficulty walking. Inform that medication is not a cure for hepatitis B and long-term treatment benefits are unknown. Inform that deterioration of liver disease may occur in some cases if treatment is d/c; discuss any changes in regimen to the physician. Inform that therapy has not been shown to reduce risk of transmission of HBV to others through sexual contact or blood contamination and counsel on HBV prevention strategies. Advise patients on a low-sodium diet that the sol contains 47mg sodium/600mg. Advise to dispose of unused or expired drug properly, and to remove all identifying information from the original container prior to disposal.

Administration: Oral route. Administer after hemodialysis when administered on hemodialysis days. **Storage:** 25°C (77°F); excursions permitted to 15-30°C (59-86°F). (Sol) Use within 2 months after opening. Do not freeze.

ULORIC
febuxostat (Takeda)

RX

THERAPEUTIC CLASS: Xanthine oxidase inhibitor

INDICATIONS: Chronic management of hyperuricemia in patients with gout.

DOSAGE: *Adults:* Initial: 40mg qd. Titrate: If serum uric acid (sUA) is not <6mg/dL after 2 weeks, increase dose to 80mg qd. Range: 40-80mg qd.

HOW SUPPLIED: Tab: 40mg, 80mg

CONTRAINDICATIONS: Patients being treated with azathioprine or mercaptopurine.

WARNINGS/PRECAUTIONS: Not recommended for treatment of asymptomatic hyperuricemia. Increase in gout flares observed; concurrent prophylactic treatment with NSAIDs or colchicine is recommended. Increased rate of cardiovascular (CV) thromboembolic events (eg, CV deaths, myocardial infarctions [MI], strokes) reported; monitor for signs and symptoms of MI and stroke. Elevated serum transaminase levels (ALT, AST) reported; monitor LFTs periodically. Caution with severe hepatic impairment (Child-Pugh Class C) and severe renal impairment (CrCl <30mL/min). Avoid use in patients whom the rate of urate formation is greatly increased (eg, malignant disease and its treatment, Lesch-Nyhan syndrome).

ADVERSE REACTIONS: Liver function abnormalities, nausea, arthralgia, rash, dizziness.

INTERACTIONS: See Contraindications. Caution with theophylline.

PREGNANCY: Category C, caution in nursing.

MECHANISM OF ACTION: Xanthine oxidase inhibitor; achieves therapeutic effect by decreasing sUA.

PHARMACOKINETICS: Absorption: C_{max}=1.6mcg/mL (40mg), 2.6mcg/mL (80mg); T_{max}=1-1.5 hrs. **Distribution:** V_d=50L; plasma protein binding (99.2%). **Metabolism:** Conjugation via uridine diphosphate glucuronosyltransferase enzymes and oxidation via CYP450 enzymes. **Elimination:** Urine (49%), feces (45%); $T_{1/2}$=5-8 hrs.

NURSING CONSIDERATIONS

Assessment: Assess for secondary hyperuricemia, asymptomatic hyperuricemia, hepatic/renal impairment, malignant disease, Lesch-Nyhan syndrome, pregnancy/nursing status, and possible drug interactions. Obtain baseline sUA and LFTs.

Monitoring: Monitor sUA levels as early as 2 weeks after initiation and LFTs 2 and 4 months following initiation, and periodically thereafter. Monitor for signs/symptoms of MI and stroke.

Patient Counseling: Inform that medication may be taken without regard to food or antacid use. Advise of the potential benefits and risks of therapy. Inform that gout flares, elevated liver enzymes, and adverse CV events may occur. Instruct to notify physician if rash, chest pain, SOB, or neurologic symptoms suggesting a stroke occur. Inform physician of any other medications, including over-the-counter drugs currently being taken.

Administration: Oral route. **Storage:** 25°C (77°F); excursions permitted to 15-30°C (59-86°F). Protect from light.

ULTIVA
remifentanil HCl (Abbott)

CII

THERAPEUTIC CLASS: Opioid analgesic

INDICATIONS: As an analgesic agent for use during the induction and maintenance of general anesthesia. For continuation as an analgesic into the immediate postoperative period in adults under the direct supervision of an anesthesia practitioner in a postoperative anesthesia care unit or intensive care setting. As an analgesic component of monitored anesthesia care in adults.

DOSAGE: *Adults:* Continuous IV Infusion: Induction: 0.5-1mcg/kg/min. Maint: 0.4mcg/kg/min with nitrous oxide 66%; 0.25mcg/kg/min with isoflurane (0.4-1.25 MAC); 0.25mcg/kg/min with propofol (100-200mcg/kg/min). Postop Continuation: 0.1mcg/kg/min. Coronary Artery Bypass Graft: Induction/Maint/Continuation: 1mcg/kg/min. Elderly (>65 yrs): Use 50% of adult dose. Titrate carefully.
Pediatrics: Anesthesia Maint: Continuous IV Infusion: 1-12 yrs: 0.25mcg/kg/min with halothane (0.3-1.5 MAC), sevoflurane (0.3-1.5 MAC), or isoflurane (0.4-1.5 MAC). Range: 0.05-1.3mcg/kg/min. Birth-2 months: 0.4mcg/kg/min. Range: 0.4-1mcg/kg/min.

HOW SUPPLIED: Inj: 1mg, 2mg, 5mg

CONTRAINDICATIONS: Epidural or intrathecal administration, hypersensitivity to fentanyl analogs.

WARNINGS/PRECAUTIONS: Administer only with infusion device. IV bolus administration should be used only during the maintenance of general anesthesia. Interruption of infusion will result in rapid offset of effect. Use associated with apnea and respiratory depression. Not for use in diagnostic or therapeutic procedures outside the monitored anesthesia care setting. Resuscitative and intubation equipment, oxygen, and opioid antagonist must be readily available. May cause skeletal muscle rigidity, related to the dose and speed of administration. Do not administer into the same IV tubing with blood due to potential inactivation by nonspecific esterases in blood products. Continuously monitor vital signs and oxygenation. Bradycardia, hypotension, intraoperative awareness reported. Not recommended as sole agent for induction of anesthesia.

ADVERSE REACTIONS: N/V, hypotension, muscle rigidity, bradycardia, shivering, fever, dizziness, visual disturbances, respiratory depression, apnea.

INTERACTIONS: Synergism with thiopental, propofol, isoflurane, midazolam; reduce doses of these drugs by up to 75%.

PREGNANCY: Category C, caution in nursing.

MECHANISM OF ACTION: Opioid analgesic.

PHARMACOKINETICS: Distribution: V_d=100mL/kg, 350mL/kg (initial, steady-state), plasma protein binding (70%). **Metabolism**: Hydrolysis via nonspecific blood and tissue esterases to carboxylic acid metabolite. **Elimination**: $T_{1/2}$=10-20 min.

NURSING CONSIDERATIONS

Assessment: Assess for pulmonary disease, decreased respiratory reserve, pregnancy/nursing status, and possible drug interactions.

Monitoring: Monitor for cardiovascular depression (eg, bradycardia, hypotension), respiratory depression, muscle rigidity of neck and extremities, N/V, chills, arrhythmias, chest wall rigidity. Monitor vital signs routinely. Appropriate postop monitoring should ensure adequate spontaneous breathing is established and maintained prior to discharge.

Patient Counseling: Advise to use caution while performing potentially hazardous tasks (eg, operating machinery/driving). Counsel about side effects of drug and abuse potential.

Administration: IV infusion. Refer to PI for compatibility in IV fluids. Continuous infusions should only be administered using an infusion device. **Storage**: 2-25°C (36-77°F). Diluted Sol: Stable at room temperature for 24 hrs.

ULTRACET   RX
tramadol HCl - acetaminophen (Ortho-McNeil)

> Associated with cases of acute liver failure, at times resulting in liver transplant and death. Most cases associated with acetaminophen (APAP) doses >4000 mg/day and involved more than one APAP-containing product.

THERAPEUTIC CLASS: Central acting analgesic

INDICATIONS: Short-term (≤5 days) management of acute pain.

DOSAGE: *Adults:* Initial: 2 tabs q4-6h PRN for ≤5 days. Max: 8 tabs/day. CrCl <30mL/min: Max: 2 tabs q12h. Elderly: Start at lower end of dosing range.

HOW SUPPLIED: Tab: (Tramadol-APAP) 37.5mg-325mg

CONTRAINDICATIONS: Any situation where opioids are contraindicated, including acute intoxication with alcohol, hypnotics, narcotics, centrally acting analgesics, opioids, or psychotropic drugs.

WARNINGS/PRECAUTIONS: Do not exceed recommended dose. Hypersensitivity and anaphylactic reactions reported; do not prescribe for patients with a history of anaphylactoid reactions to codeine or other opioids. May complicate clinical assessment of acute abdominal conditions. Not recommended in hepatic impairment; risk of acute liver failure increased in patients with underlying liver disease. Tramadol: Seizures reported; risk increased in patients with epilepsy, history of seizures, risk of seizures (eg, head trauma, metabolic disorders, alcohol/drug withdrawal, CNS infections). Do not prescribe for suicidal or addiction-prone patients; caution with emotional disturbances or depression. Reports of tramadol-related deaths in history of emotional disturbances, suicidal ideation/attempts, misuse of tranquilizers/alcohol/CNS active drugs. Development of serotonin syndrome including mental status changes, autonomic instability, neuromuscular aberrations, and GI symptoms reported. Caution if at risk for respiratory depression, CNS depression, head injury, increased intracranial pressure, and elderly. May impair mental/physical abilities. May cause withdrawal symptoms; do not d/c abruptly.

ADVERSE REACTIONS: Constipation, somnolence, increased sweating, diarrhea, nausea, anorexia, dizziness, acute liver failure.

INTERACTIONS: See Contraindications. Do not use concomitantly with alcohol, other acetaminophen- or tramadol-containing products; increased risk of acute liver failure with alcohol ingestion. May alter effects of warfarin; periodically monitor PT with warfarin-like compounds. Tramadol: Increased seizure risk with SSRIs, TCAs, other tricyclic compounds (eg, cyclobenzaprine, promethazine, etc), MAOIs, other opioids, neuroleptics, and drugs that reduce seizure threshold. Serotonin syndrome may occur when coadministered with SSRIs, serotonin norepinephrine reuptake inhibitors (SNRIs), TCAs, MAOIs, triptans, a_2-adrenergic blockers, linezolid, lithium, St. John's wort, or drugs that impair tramadol metabolism (CYP2D6 and CYP3A4 inhibitors); observe carefully especially during initiation and dose increases. Caution and reduce dose with CNS depressants (eg, alcohol, opioids, anesthetics, narcotics, phenothiazines, tranquilizers, sedative hypnotics); increased risk of CNS/respiratory depression. Caution with antidepressants and muscle relaxants; additive CNS depressant effects. Reduced metabolic clearance and increased risk of serious adverse effects with CYP2D6 inhibitors (eg, quinidine, fluoxetine, paroxetine, amtriptyline) and/or CYP3A4 inhibitors (eg, ketoconazole, erythromycin). Drug exposure may be altered with CYP3A4 inhibitors or inducers (eg, rifampin, St. John's wort). Digoxin toxicity may occur with concomitant use. Reduced analgesic effect with carbamazepine; coadministration not recommended. In drug overdose, naloxone administration may increase the risk of seizure.

PREGNANCY: Category C, not for use in nursing.

MECHANISM OF ACTION: Tramadol: Centrally acting synthetic opioid analgesic; not established. Thought to bind to μ-opioid receptors and weakly inhibit reuptake of norepinephrine and serotonin. APAP: Nonopiate, nonsalicylate analgesic, and antipyretic.

PHARMACOKINETICS: Absorption: Tramadol: Absolute bioavailability (75%); T_{max}=2 hrs. APAP: T_{max}=1 hr. **Distribution:** Tramadol: (100mg IV) V_d=2.6L/kg (male), 2.9L/kg (female); plasma protein binding (20%); found in breast milk; crosses the placenta. APAP: V_d=0.9L/kg; plasma protein binding (20%). **Metabolism:** Tramadol: Liver (extensive); N- and O-demethylation, glucuronidation, sulfation; CYP2D6, 3A4; M1 (active metabolite). APAP: Liver; glucuronidation, sulfation, oxidation; CYP2E1, 1A2, 3A4. **Elimination:** Tramadol: Urine (30% unchanged, 60% metabolites); $T_{1/2}$=5-6 hrs. APAP: Urine (<9% unchanged); $T_{1/2}$= 2-3 hrs.

NURSING CONSIDERATIONS

Assessment: Assess for known hypersensitivity, acute intoxication with alcohol, hypnotics, narcotics, centrally acting analgesics, opioids, or psychotropic drugs. Assess for epilepsy, risk of seizure (eg, head trauma, metabolic disorders, alcohol and drug withdrawal, CNS infections), suicidal ideation, emotional disturbance or depression, risk of respiratory depression, increased intracranial pressure, drug abuse potential, renal/hepatic impairment, pregnancy/nursing status, and possible drug interactions.

Monitoring: Monitor for hepatotoxicity, anaphylactoid reactions (eg, pruritus, hives, bronchospasm, angioedema, toxic epidermal necrolysis, and Stevens-Johnson syndrome), respiratory/ CNS depression, physical dependence/abuse, misuse, seizures, development of serotonin syndrome, withdrawal symptoms with abrupt d/c.

Patient Counseling: Instruct patient to d/c therapy and notify physician if signs of allergy (eg, rash, difficulty breathing) occur. Advise patients of dose limits and to not take >4000mg of APAP per day; notify physician if exceed the recommended dose. Inform patients not to use with other tramadol or APAP-containing products, including over-the-counter preparations. Advise that seizures and serotonin syndrome may occur when use with serotonergic agents (eg, SSRIs, SNRIs, and triptans) or drugs that significantly reduce the metabolic clearance of tramadol. Inform that therapy may impair physical/mental abilities. Notify physician if are pregnant or plan to become pregnant. Inform patients to avoid alcohol-containing beverages while on therapy.

Administration: Oral route. **Storage:** 25°C (77°F); excursions permitted to 15-30°C (59-86°F).

U

ULTRAM
tramadol HCl (PRICARA)

RX

OTHER BRAND NAMES: Ultram ER (PRICARA)

THERAPEUTIC CLASS: Central acting analgesic

INDICATIONS: (Tab) Management of moderate to moderately severe pain in adults. (Tab, ER) Management of moderate to moderately severe chronic pain in adults who require around-the-clock treatment for an extended period of time.

DOSAGE: *Adults:* (Tab) ≥17 yrs: Individualize dose. Initial: 25mg/day qam. Titrate: Increase by 25mg every 3 days to 25mg qid, then increase by 50mg every 3 days to 200mg/day (50mg qid). Usual: 50-100mg q4-6h PRN. Max: 400mg/day. CrCl <30mL/min: Dose q12h. Max: 200mg/day.

Cirrhosis: 50mg q12h. Elderly: Start at lower end of dosing range. >75 yrs: Max: 300mg/day. (Tab, ER) ≥18 yrs: Not Currently on TramadolImmediate-Release: Initial: 100mg qd. Titrate: Increase by 100mg every 5 days. Max: 300mg/day. Currently on Tramadol Immediate Release: Initial: Calculate 24-hr tramadol dose and initiate total daily dose rounded down to the next lowest 100mg increment. Maint: Individualize dose. Max: 300mg/day. Elderly: Start at lower end of dosing range.

HOW SUPPLIED: Tab: 50mg*; Tab, Extended-Release: 100mg, 200mg, 300mg *scored

CONTRAINDICATIONS: Any situation where opioids are contraindicated, including acute intoxication with any of the following: alcohol, hypnotics, narcotics, centrally acting analgesics, opioids, or psychotropic drugs.

WARNINGS/PRECAUTIONS: Seizures and anaphylactoid reactions reported; seizure risk increases in patients with epilepsy, history of seizures, risk of seizures (eg, head trauma, metabolic disorders, alcohol/drug withdrawal, CNS infections). Avoid in patients with a history of anaphylactoid reactions to codeine and other opioids. Do not prescribe for suicidal or addiction-prone patients. Caution if at risk for respiratory depression, increased intracranial pressure (ICP), head injury, and in elderly. May complicate clinical assessment of acute abdominal conditions. Do not d/c abruptly; withdrawal symptoms may occur. Development of serotonin syndrome including mental status changes, autonomic instability, neuromuscular aberrations, and GI symptoms reported. Reports of drug-related deaths in patients with history of emotional disturbances, suicidal ideation/attempts, misuse of tranquilizers/alcohol/CNS active drugs. May impair mental/physical abilities. (Tab) Adjust dose with renal/hepatic impairment and in patients older than 75 yrs of age. Caution in patients with emotional disturbances or depression. (Tab, ER) Avoid in severe renal impairment (CrCl <30mL/min) and severe hepatic impairment (Child-Pugh Class C).

ADVERSE REACTIONS: Dizziness, N/V, constipation, headache, somnolence, sweating, asthenia, dyspepsia, dry mouth, diarrhea, CNS stimulation, pruritus, flushing.

INTERACTIONS: See Contraindications. Caution and reduce dose with CNS depressants (eg, alcohol, opioids, anesthetics, narcotics, phenothiazines, tranquilizers, sedative hypnotics); increased risk of CNS/respiratory depression. Caution with antidepressants and muscle relaxants; additive CNS depressant effects. Not recommended with carbamazepine; decreased analgesic efficacy. Possible digoxin toxicity and altered warfarin effects. Potential increased risk of adverse events and reduced metabolic clearance with CYP2D6 inhibitors (eg, quinidine, fluoxetine, paroxetine, amtriptyline) and CYP3A4 inhibitors (eg, ketoconazole, erythromycin). Altered exposure with CYP3A4 inducers (eg, rifampin, St. John's wort). Increased seizure risk with SSRIs, TCAs, other tricyclic compounds (eg, cyclobenzaprine, promethazine, etc), MAOIs, other opioids, neuroleptics, and drugs that reduce seizure threshold. Caution with SSRIs, SNRIs, TCAs, MAOIs, α2-adrenergic blockers, triptans, linezolid, lithium, St. John's wort, or drugs that impair tramadol metabolism; increased risk of serotonin syndrome. In drug overdose, naloxone administration may increase the risk of seizure.

PREGNANCY: Category C, not for use in nursing.

MECHANISM OF ACTION: Centrally acting synthetic opioid analgesic; not established. Suspected to be due to binding of parent and M1 metabolite to μ-opioid receptors and weak inhibition of norepinephrine and serotonin reuptake.

PHARMACOKINETICS: Absorption: (100mg Tab) Absolute bioavailability (75%), C_{max}=592ng/mL, T_{max}=2.3 hrs. (200mg Tab, ER) C_{max}=335ng/mL, T_{max}=12 hrs, AUC=5975ng•hr/mL. **Distribution:** (IV) V_d=2.6L/kg (male), 2.9L/kg (female); plasma protein binding (20%). **Metabolism:** Extensive via CYP2D6, 3A4; N- and O-demethylation and glucuronidation or sulfation (major pathway). M1 (active metabolite). **Elimination:** Urine: (30% unchanged), (60% as metabolite). (Tab) $T_{1/2}$=6.3 hrs (drug), 7.4 hrs (M1). (Tab, ER) $T_{1/2}$=7.9 hrs (drug), 8.8 hrs (M1).

NURSING CONSIDERATIONS

Assessment: Assess for known hypersensitivity, acute intoxication with alcohol, hypnotics, narcotics, centrally acting analgesics, opioids, or psychotropic drugs. Assess for epilepsy, risk of seizure (eg, head trauma, metabolic disorders, alcohol and drug withdrawal, CNS infections), suicidal ideation, emotional disturbance or depression, risk for respiratory depression, increased ICP, drug abuse potential, renal/hepatic impairment, pregnancy/nursing status, and possible drug interactions.

Monitoring: Monitor for anaphylactoid reactions (eg, pruritus, hives, bronchospasm, angioedema, toxic epidermal necrolysis, and Stevens-Johnson syndrome), respiratory/CNS depression, physical dependence/abuse, misuse, seizures, development of serotonin syndrome, withdrawal symptoms with abrupt d/c (eg, anxiety, sweating, insomnia, rigors, pain, nausea, tremors, upper respiratory symptoms, diarrhea, piloerection and rarely, hallucinations).

Patient Counseling: Advise to use caution while performing hazardous tasks (eg, operating machinery/driving). Instruct not to consume alcohol containing beverages. Inform patients to use caution when taking tranquilizers, hypnotics or opiate containing analgesics. Notify physician if pregnant/nursing or planning to become pregnant. Educate about single-dose and 24-hr dosing limits and time interval between doses.

Administration: Oral route. (Tab, ER) Swallow whole; do not chew, crush, or split. **Storage:** 25°C (77°F); excursions permitted to 15-30°C (59-86°F).

ULTRAVATE RX
halobetasol propionate (Ranbaxy)

THERAPEUTIC CLASS: Corticosteroid

INDICATIONS: Relief of the inflammatory and pruritic manifestations of corticosteroid-responsive dermatoses.

DOSAGE: *Adults:* Apply a thin layer to affected skin qd-bid ud. Rub in gently and completely. Do not use >2 weeks. Max: 50g/week. Reassess if no improvement within 2 weeks.
Pediatrics: ≥12 yrs: Apply a thin layer to affected skin qd-bid ud. Rub in gently and completely. Do not use >2 weeks. Max: 50g/week. Reassess if no improvement within 2 weeks.

HOW SUPPLIED: Cre, Oint: 0.05% [15g, 50g]

WARNINGS/PRECAUTIONS: Systemic absorption may produce reversible hypothalamic-pituitary-adrenal (HPA) axis suppression, manifestations of Cushing's syndrome, hyperglycemia, and glucosuria. Pediatric patients may be more susceptible to systemic toxicity and drug may interfere with their growth and development. Caution when applied to large surface areas or under occlusive dressings; evaluate periodically for HPA suppression. Do not use for >2 weeks at a time and treat only small areas at any one time. If HPA axis suppression occurs, reduce application frequency, substitute less potent corticosteroid, or attempt to withdraw drug. Use appropriate antifungal or antibacterial agent with concomitant dermatological infections; d/c if no prompt favorable response until infection is controlled. HPA axis suppression (eg, low plasma cortisol, no response to ACTH stimulation), linear growth retardation, delayed weight gain, Cushing's syndrome and intracranial HTN (eg, bulging fontanelles, headache, bilateral papilledema) reported in pediatrics. Not recommended for treatment of rosacea or perioral dermatitis. Do not use on face, groin, or axillae. D/C if irritation occurs and institute appropriate therapy. Failure to heal may indicate allergic contact dermatitis; corroborate with appropriate patch testing. Signs and symptoms of glucocorticosteroid insufficiency may occur after treatment withdrawal; may require supplemental systemic corticosteroids. Reassess if no improvement after 2 weeks. D/C when control is achieved. Not for ophthalmic use.

ADVERSE REACTIONS: Stinging, burning, itching, acneiform eruptions, secondary infection, miliaria, striae, folliculitis, allergic contract dermatitis, perioral dermatitis, hypertrichosis, hypopigmentation.

PREGNANCY: Category C, caution in nursing.

MECHANISM OF ACTION: Corticosteroid; possesses anti-inflammatory, antipruritic, and vasoconstrictive properties. Anti-inflammatory activity not established; suspected to act by induction of phospholipase A_2 inhibitory proteins called lipocortins. Lipocortins control biosynthesis of potent inflammation mediators (eg, prostaglandins, leukotrienes) by inhibiting release of their common precursor, arachidonic acid.

PHARMACOKINETICS: Absorption: Percutaneous; extent of absorption determined by vehicle, integrity of skin, occlusion, inflammation, and other disease states. **Distribution:** Systemically administered corticosteroids are found in breast milk.

NURSING CONSIDERATIONS

Assessment: Assess for age in pediatric patients, rosacea or perioral dermatitis, presence of concomitant skin infections, hypersensitivity and pregnancy/nursing status. Assess skin integrity at application site.

Monitoring: Monitor for signs/symptoms of HPA axis suppression, Cushing's syndrome, hyperglycemia, glucosuria, treatment-site irritation, allergic contact dermatitis (eg, failure to heal), dermatological infections, and for hypersensitivity reactions. Following withdrawal of therapy, monitor for glucocorticosteroid insufficiency. If applying to large area or to areas under occlusion, perform periodic monitoring for HPA axis suppression using ACTH stimulation, A.M. plasma cortisol and urinary free cortisol tests. In pediatric patients, monitor for signs/symptoms of systemic toxicity, HPA axis suppression, linear growth retardation, delayed weight gain, Cushing's syndrome and intracranial HTN. Monitor for signs of clinical improvement; if no improvement within 2 weeks, reassess diagnosis.

Patient Counseling: Instruct to use externally and as directed; avoid contact with eyes and avoid use on face, groin or axillae. Do not bandage or wrap treatment area so as to be occlusive unless directed by physician. Report signs of local adverse reactions (eg, irritation). Do not use for any disorder other than for which it was used/prescribed.

Administration: Topical route. **Storage:** 15-30°C (59-86°F).

U

UNASYN

RX

ampicillin sodium - sulbactam sodium (Pfizer)

THERAPEUTIC CLASS: Semisynthetic penicillin/beta-lactamase inhibitor

INDICATIONS: Treatment of skin and skin structure (SSSI), intra-abdominal, and gynecological infections caused by susceptible strains of microorganisms.

DOSAGE: *Adults:* Usual: 1.5-3g (ampicillin+sulbactam) IM/IV q6h. Max: 4g sulbactam/day. Renal Impairment: CrCl ≥30mL/min: 1.5-3g q6-8h. CrCl 15-29mL/min: 1.5-3g q12h. CrCl 5-14mL/min: 1.5-3g q24h.

Pediatrics: ≥1 yr: SSSI: Usual: 300mg/kg/day (200mg ampicillin+100mg sulbactam) IV in equally divided doses q6h. Max: 4g sulbactam/day. Therapy should not routinely exceed 14 days. ≥40kg: Dose according to adult recommendations.

HOW SUPPLIED: Inj: (Ampicillin-Sulbactam) 1g-0.5g, 2g-1g. Also available as a Pharmacy Bulk Package. Refer to individual package insert for more information

WARNINGS/PRECAUTIONS: Serious and occasional fatal hypersensitivity reactions reported with penicillin (PCN) therapy; d/c use and initiate appropriate therapy if allergic reaction occurs. *Clostridium difficile*-associated diarrhea (CDAD) reported. Increased risk of skin rash in patients with mononucleosis; avoid administering ampicillin class antibiotics. May result in bacterial resistance with prolonged use or use in the absence of a proven/suspected bacterial infection or a prophylactic indication; take appropriate measures if superinfection develops. Decrease in total conjugated estriol, estriol-glucuronide, conjugated estrone, and estradiol reported in pregnant women. Lab test interactions may occur.

ADVERSE REACTIONS: Inj-site pain, thrombophlebitis, diarrhea.

INTERACTIONS: Probenecid decreases renal tubular secretions and may increase and prolong blood levels. Increased incidence of rash with allopurinol.

PREGNANCY: Category B, caution in nursing.

MECHANISM OF ACTION: Ampicillin: Semi-synthetic PCN; acts through inhibition of cell wall mucopeptide biosynthesis. Has a broad spectrum of bactericidal activity against many gram-positive and gram-negative aerobic and anaerobic bacteria. Sulbactam: beta-lactamase inhibitor: provides good inhibitory activity against clinically important plasmid mediated β-lactamases most frequently responsible for transferred drug resistance.

PHARMACOKINETICS: Absorption: IV/IM administration of variable doses resulted in different parameters. **Distribution:** Plasma protein binding (28% ampicillin), (38% sulbactam); found in breast milk. **Elimination:** Urine (75-85% unchanged); $T_{1/2}$=1 hr.

NURSING CONSIDERATIONS

Assessment: Assess for history of hypersensitivity to cephalosporins/PCNs or other allergens, mononucleosis, renal impairment, pregnancy/nursing status, and for possible drug interactions. Document indications for therapy, culture, and susceptibility testing.

Monitoring: Monitor for signs/symptoms of hypersensitivity reactions (eg, anaphylaxis), CDAD, superinfection, and renal function. Monitor for changes in estrogen levels in pregnant women.

Patient Counseling: Inform that drug only treats bacterial, not viral infections (eg, common cold). Inform to use as directed; inform that skipping doses or not completing full course may decrease effectiveness and increase resistance. Advise that watery and bloody stools (with or without stomach cramps and fever) may develop even as late as ≥2 months after having the last dose; instruct to contact physician if occurs.

Administration: IV/IM route. Pharmacy bulk package not for direct infusion; for preparation of IV infusion sol only. Refer to PI for preparation and reconstitution instructions. (IV) Administer slowly over at least 10-15 min or 15-30 min in greater dilutions. **Storage:** Prior to reconstitution: ≤30°C (86°F). Reconstituted Sol: Refer to PI for storage requirements.

UNIRETIC

RX

moexipril HCl - hydrochlorothiazide (UCB)

> D/C when pregnancy is detected. Drugs that act directly on the renin-angiotensin system can cause death/injury to developing fetus.

THERAPEUTIC CLASS: ACE inhibitor/thiazide diuretic

INDICATIONS: Treatment of HTN.

DOSAGE: *Adults:* Uncontrolled BP on Moexipril/HCTZ Monotherapy: Initial: 7.5mg-12.5mg, 15mg-12.5mg, or 15mg-25mg qd. Titrate: Based on clinical response. May increase HCTZ dose after 2-3 weeks. Max: 30mg-50mg qd. Controlled BP on 25mg qd HCTZ with Hypokalemia: Switch to

3.75mg-6.25mg (1/2 of 7.5mg-12.5mg tab). Excessive BP Reduction with 7.5mg-12.5mg: Switch to 3.75mg-6.25mg. Replacement Therapy: May substitute for titrated components.

HOW SUPPLIED: Tab: (Moexipril-HCTZ) 7.5mg-12.5mg*, 15mg-12.5mg*, 15mg-25mg* *scored

CONTRAINDICATIONS: History of ACE inhibitor-associated angioedema, anuria, hypersensitivity to sulfonamide-derived drugs.

WARNINGS/PRECAUTIONS: Not for initial therapy. Not recommended with severe renal impairment (CrCl ≤40mL/min/1.73m²). Symptomatic hypotension may occur, most likely in patients with salt and/or volume depletion; correct such conditions before therapy. May precipitate hepatic coma with hepatic impairment or progressive liver disease. Caution in elderly. HCTZ: Enhanced antihypertensive effects in postsympathectomy patients. May precipitate azotemia with severe renal disease. May cause idiosyncratic reaction, resulting in acute transient myopia and acute angle-closure glaucoma; d/c as rapidly as possible. May cause exacerbation or activation of systemic lupus erythematosus (SLE), hyperuricemia, precipitation of frank gout, hypercalcemia, hypophosphatemia, overt gout, reduced glucose tolerance, and increased cholesterol and TG. Hypokalemia may sensitize or exaggerate the response of the heart to toxic effects of digitalis. Observe for signs of fluid and electrolyte imbalance (eg, hypokalemia, hyponatremia, hypochloremic alkalosis); monitor serum electrolytes periodically. Moexipril: Angioedema of the face, extremities, lips, tongue, glottis, and/or larynx reported; d/c and administer appropriate therapy if symptoms develop. Intestinal angioedema reported; monitor for abdominal pain. More reports of angioedema in blacks than nonblacks. Anaphylactoid reactions reported during desensitization with hymenoptera venom, dialysis with high-flux membranes, and LDL apheresis with dextran sulfate absorption. Excessive hypotension, which may be associated with oliguria or progressive azotemia, and rarely, with acute renal failure and/or death, may occur in congestive heart failure (CHF) patients; monitor closely upon initiation and during first 2 weeks of therapy and whenever dose is increased. May cause changes in renal function. May increase BUN/SrCr in patients with no preexisting renal vascular disease or with renal artery stenosis; monitor renal function during the 1st few weeks of therapy in patients with renal artery stenosis. May cause agranulocytosis and bone marrow depression; monitor WBCs with collagen vascular disease. Rarely, associated with syndrome of cholestatic jaundice, hepatic necrosis, and death; d/c if jaundice or marked hepatic enzyme elevation occurs. Hyperkalemia and persistent nonproductive cough reported. Hypotension may occur with major surgery or during anesthesia.

ADVERSE REACTIONS: Cough, dizziness, angioedema, hypotension, fatigue.

INTERACTIONS: NSAIDs, including selective cyclooxygenase-2 inhibitors, may reduce diuretic, natriuretic, and antihypertensive effects. HCTZ: Potentiation of orthostatic hypotension may occur with alcohol, barbiturates, or narcotics. Dosage adjustment of antidiabetic drugs (oral agents and insulin) may be required. Cholestyramine and colestipol resins may reduce absorption. Corticosteroids and adrenocorticotropic hormone may intensify electrolyte depletion, particularly hypokalemia. May decrease response to pressor amines (eg, norepinephrine). May increase responsiveness to nondepolarizing skeletal muscle relaxants (eg, tubocurarine). Increased absorption with guanabenz or propantheline. May potentiate action of other antihypertensives, especially ganglionic or peripheral adrenergic-blocking drugs. Moexipril: NSAIDs may deteriorate renal function. Increase lithium levels and symptoms of toxicity; use with caution and monitor lithium levels. Increased risk of hyperkalemia with K⁺-sparing diuretics (spironolactone, amiloride, triamterene), K⁺ supplements, or K⁺-containing salt substitutes; use with caution and monitor serum K⁺. Nitritoid reactions reported with injectable gold (sodium aurothiomalate).

PREGNANCY: Category D, not for use in nursing.

MECHANISM OF ACTION: Moexipril: ACE inhibitor; decreases angiotensin II formation, leading to decreased vasoconstriction, increased plasma renin activity, and decreased aldosterone secretion. HCTZ: Thiazide diuretic; not established. Affects distal renal tubular mechanisms of electrolyte reabsorption, directly increasing excretion of Na⁺ and chloride in approximately equivalent amounts.

PHARMACOKINETICS: Absorption: Moexipril: Incomplete. Bioavailability (13%, moexiprilat); T_{max}=0.8 hr, 1.5-1.6 hrs (moexiprilat); C_{max} and AUC reduced by 70% and 40%, respectively, with low-fat breakfast, or 80% and 50%, respectively, with high-fat breakfast. **Distribution:** Moexipril: V_d=2.8L/kg (moexiprilat); plasma protein binding (50%, moexiprilat). HCTZ: V_d=1.5-4.2L/kg; plasma protein binding (21-24%); crosses placenta; found in breast milk. **Metabolism:** Rapid via de-esterification; moexiprilat (active metabolite). **Elimination:** Moexipril: Urine (1% unchanged, 7% moexiprilat, 5% other metabolites), feces (1% unchanged, 52% moexiprilat); $T_{1/2}$=1.3 hrs, 2-9 hrs (moexiprilat). HCTZ: Kidney (>60% unchanged); $T_{1/2}$=5.6-14.8 hrs.

NURSING CONSIDERATIONS

Assessment: Assess for history of ACE inhibitor-associated angioedema, anuria, hypersensitivity to drug or sulfonamide-derived drugs, history of allergy or bronchial asthma, volume/salt depletion, CHF, collagen vascular disease, renal artery stenosis, SLE, risk factors for hyperkalemia, hepatic/renal function, pregnancy/nursing status, and possible drug interactions. Obtain baseline serum electrolytes.

Monitoring: Monitor for signs of angioedema, hypotension, exacerbation/activation of SLE, idiosyncratic reaction, and other adverse reactions. Monitor hepatic/renal function, BP, WBC counts (collagen vascular disease), serum electrolytes, blood glucose, cholesterol, TG, and uric acid.

Patient Counseling: Advise to take drug 1 hr ac. Instruct to d/c use and report immediately to physician if signs/symptoms of angioedema (swelling of the face, extremities, eyes, lips, tongue, difficulty in breathing) occur. Inform that lightheadedness may occur, especially during the 1st few days of therapy; instruct to d/c use and consult physician if fainting occurs. Inform that excessive perspiration, dehydration, and other causes of volume depletion (eg, diarrhea, vomiting) may lead to excessive fall in BP; advise to consult physician if these conditions develop. Instruct not to use K⁺ supplements or salt substitutes containing K⁺ without consulting physician, and to report promptly any indication of infection (eg, sore throat, fever). Inform of the consequences of exposure during pregnancy and discuss treatment options in women planning to become pregnant. Instruct to report pregnancies to physician as soon as possible.

Administration: Oral route. Take 1 hr ac. **Storage:** 20-25°C (68-77°F). Protect from excessive moisture.

UNITHROID   RX
levothyroxine sodium (Lannett)

THERAPEUTIC CLASS: Thyroid replacement hormone

INDICATIONS: Hypothyroidism. As a pituitary TSH suppressant in the treatment and prevention of euthyroid goiters, including thyroid nodules, lymphocytic thyroiditis, and multinodular goiter. Adjunct to surgery and radioiodine therapy for thyrotropin-dependent well-differentiated thyroid cancer.

DOSAGE: *Adults:* Take in am at least 1/2-1 hr before food. Hypothyroidism: Usual: 1.7mcg/kg/day. >200mcg/day (seldom). >50 yrs/<50 yrs with Cardiac Disease: Initial: 25-50mcg/day. Titrate: Increase by 12.5-25mcg/day every 6-8 weeks until euthyroid. Elderly with Cardiac Disease: Initial: 12.5-25mcg/day. Titrate: Increase by 12.5-25mcg/day every 4-6 weeks until euthyroid. Severe Hypothyroidism: Initial: 12.5-25mcg/day. Titrate: Increase by 25mcg/day every 2-4 weeks until euthyroid. Pregnancy: May increase dose requirements. Subclinical Hypothyroidism: Lower doses required.
Pediatrics: Take in am at least 1/2-1 hr before food. Hypothyroidism: 0-3 months: 10-15mcg/kg/day. 3-6 months: 8-10mcg/kg/day. 6-12 months: 6-8mcg/kg/day. 1-5 yrs: 5-6mcg/kg/day. 6-12 yrs: 4-5mcg/kg/day. >12 yrs: 2-3mcg/kg/day. Growth/Puberty Complete: 1.7mcg/kg/day. Cardiac Risk: Initial: Use lower dose. Titrate: Increase dose every 4-6 weeks until euthyroid. Infants with Serum T4 <5mcg/dL: Initial: 50mcg/day. Chronic/Severe Hypothyroidism: Children: Initial: 25mcg/day. Titrate: Increase by 25mcg/day every 2-4 weeks until desired effect. Minimize Hyperactivity in Older Children: Initial: Give 1/4 of full replacement dose. Titrate: Increase by same amount weekly until full dose achieved. May crush tab and mix with 5-10mL water.

HOW SUPPLIED: Tab: 25mcg*, 50mcg*, 75mcg*, 88mcg*, 100mcg*, 112mcg*, 125mcg*, 150mcg*, 175mcg*, 200mcg*, 300mcg* *scored

CONTRAINDICATIONS: Untreated thyrotoxicosis, acute myocardial infarction (MI), uncorrected adrenal insufficiency.

WARNINGS/PRECAUTIONS: Do not use in the treatment of obesity; larger doses in euthyroid patients can cause serious or even life threatening toxicity. Caution with cardiovascular disease, CAD, adrenal insufficiency, autonomous thyroid tissue, hypothalamic/pituitary hormone deficiencies, and the elderly with risk of occult cardiac disease. Carefully titrate dose to avoid over or under treatment. Decreased bone mineral density with long term use. With adrenal insufficiency supplement with glucocorticoids before therapy.

INTERACTIONS: Sympathomimetics may increase risk of coronary insufficiency with CAD. Upward dose adjustments needed for insulin and oral hypoglycemic agents. Decreased absorption with soybean flour (infant formula), cotton seed meal, walnuts, and fiber. May potentiate oral anticoagulant effects; adjust dose and monitor PT/INR. May decrease levels and effects of digitalis glycosides. Cholestyramine, colestipol, ferrous sulfate, aluminum hydroxide, sodium polystyrene, sucralfate may decrease absorption. Reduced TSH secretion with dopamine/ dopamine agonists, glucocorticoids, octreotide. Decreased thyroid hormone secretion with aminoglutethimide, amiodarone, iodine (including iodine-containing radiographic contrast agents), lithium, methimazole, propylthiouracil (PTU), sulfonamides, tolbutamide. Increased thyroid hormone secretion with amiodarone, iodide (including iodine-containing radiographic contrast agents). Decreased T4 absorption with antacids (aluminum & magnesium hydroxides), simethicone, bile acid sequestrants (cholestyramine, colestipol), calcium carbonate, cation exchange resins (eg, Kayexalate), ferrous sulfate, sucralfate. Increased serum thyroxine-binding globulin (TBG) concentration with clofibrate, estrogens, heroin/methadone, 5-fluorouracil, mitotane, tamoxifen. Decreased serum TBG concentration with androgens/anabolic steroids,

U

asparaginase, glucocorticoids, nicotinic acid (slow-release). Protein-binding site displacement with furosemide, heparin, hydantoins, NSAIDs, salicylates. Increased hepatic metabolism with carbamazepine, hydantoins, phenobarbital, rifampin. Decreased conversion of T4 to T3 levels with amiodarone, β-adrenergic antagonists (propranolol >160mg/day), glucocorticoids (dexamethasone >4mg/day), PTU. Additive effects of both agents with antidepressants. Interferon-(alfa) may cause development of antithyroid microsomal antibodies causing transient hypothyroidism, hyperthyroidism, or both. Interleukin-2 has been associated with transient painless thyroiditis. Excessive use with growth hormones may accelerate epiphyseal closure. Ketamine use may produce marked HTN and tachycardia. May reduce uptake of iodine-containing radiographic contrast agents. Altered levels of thyroid hormone and/or TSH level with choral hydrate, diazepam, ethionamide, lovastatin, metoclopramide, 6-mercaptopurine, nitroprusside, para-aminosalicylate sodium, perphenazine, resorcinol (excessive topical use), thiazide diuretics.

PREGNANCY: Category A, caution in nursing.

MECHANISM OF ACTION: Thyroid hormone; not understood, suspected to control DNA transcription and protein synthesis.

PHARMACOKINETICS: Distribution: Plasma protein binding (99%), found in breast milk. **Metabolism:** Liver via sequential deiodination (major pathway), conjugation in liver (mainly), kidneys, other tissues. **Elimination:** Urine, feces (20% unchanged); (T4) $T_{1/2}$=6-7 days, (T3) $T_{1/2}$≤2 days.

NURSING CONSIDERATIONS

Assessment: Assess for suppressed serum TSH with normal T3 and T4 levels, overt thyrotoxicosis, thyroid diseases (eg, nontoxic diffuse or nodular goiter), endocrine disorders (eg, hypothalmic/pituitary hormone deficiencies, autoimmune polyglandular disorders), infants for congenital anomalies, cardiovascular diseases (eg, angina pectoris, acute MI), diabetes mellitus (DM), hypersensitivity history, clotting status, upcoming surgery, and for possible drug and test interactions.

Monitoring: Perform frequent lab tests and clinical evaluations of thyroid functions (TSH and free T4 levels, lipid metabolism, blood/urinary glucose in DM, clotting parameters). Monitor cardiovascular signs (eg, arrhythmias, coronary insufficiency), growth/development, bone metabolism, cognitive function, emotional status, GI functions, reproductive functions, partial hair loss in infants, and signs/symptoms of thyroid toxicity.

Patient Counseling: Inform that drug is to be taken for life and not for treatment of obesity or weight loss. Take on empty stomach, 1 hr before breakfast with full glass of water. Notify physician if pregnant/nursing or planning to become pregnant. Notify if taking any other drugs. Do not d/c or change dosage unless directed by physician. Report any signs/symptoms of thyroid toxicity to physician.

Administration: Oral route. **Storage**: 20-25°C (68-77°F); excursions permitted to 15-30°C (59-86°F).

UNIVASC
moexipril HCl (UCB)

RX

D/C when pregnancy is detected. Drugs that act directly on the renin-angiotensin system can cause death/injury to developing fetus.

THERAPEUTIC CLASS: ACE inhibitor

INDICATIONS: Treatment of HTN alone or in combination with thiazide diuretics.

DOSAGE: *Adults:* Not Receiving Diuretics: Initial: 7.5mg qd. Titrate: Adjust dose according to BP response. If not adequately controlled, may increase or divide dose. Usual: 7.5-30mg/day given in 1 or 2 divided doses. Max: 60mg/day. Receiving Diuretics: D/C diuretic 2-3 days prior to therapy. Resume diuretic if BP is not controlled. If diuretic cannot be d/c, give initial dose of 3.75mg. CrCl ≤40mL/min/1.73m²: Initial: 3.75mg qd given cautiously. Max: 15mg/day. Elderly: Start at lower end of dosing range.

HOW SUPPLIED: Tab: 7.5mg*, 15mg* *scored

CONTRAINDICATIONS: History of ACE inhibitor-associated angioedema.

WARNINGS/PRECAUTIONS: Angioedema of the face, extremities, lips, tongue, glottis, and/or larynx reported; d/c and administer appropriate therapy if symptoms develop. Intestinal angioedema reported; monitor for abdominal pain. More reports of angioedema in blacks than non-blacks. Anaphylactoid reactions reported during desensitization with hymenoptera venom, dialysis with high-flux membranes, and LDL apheresis with dextran sulfate absorption. Symptomatic hypotension may occur, most likely with salt and volume depletion; correct depletion prior to therapy. Excessive hypotension associated with oliguria, azotemia, acute renal failure, or death may occur in congestive heart failure (CHF) patients; monitor closely upon initiation and during first 2 weeks of therapy and whenever dose is increased. May cause agranulocytosis and bone marrow depression; monitor WBCs with collagen vascular disease. Rarely, associated with syndrome of cholestatic jaundice, fulminant hepatic necrosis, and death; d/c if jaundice or marked hepatic enzyme elevation occurs. May cause changes in renal function. Increase BUN and SrCr reported in patients with renal artery stenosis and without preexisting renal vascular disease; reduce dose and/or d/c. Hyperkalemia reported; risk factors include diabetes mellitus (DM) and renal insufficiency. Hypotension may occur with major surgery or during anesthesia. Persistent nonproductive cough reported. Caution in elderly.

ADVERSE REACTIONS: Cough increased, dizziness, diarrhea, flu syndrome.

INTERACTIONS: Hypotension risk and increased BUN and SrCr with diuretics. Increased risk of hyperkalemia with K^+-sparing diuretics (spironolactone, amiloride, triamterene), K^+ supplements, or K^+-containing salt substitutes; use with caution and monitor serum K^+. Increased lithium levels and lithium toxicity symptoms reported; use with caution and monitor lithium levels. Nitritoid reactions (eg, facial flushing, N/V, hypotension) reported with injectable gold (sodium aurothiomalate). NSAIDs, including selective cyclooxygenase-2 inhibitors, may deteriorate renal function. Antihypertensive effect may be attenuated by NSAIDs.

PREGNANCY: Category D, caution in nursing.

MECHANISM OF ACTION: ACE inhibitor; reduces angiotensin II formation, decreases vasoconstriction and aldosterone secretion, and increases plasma renin.

PHARMACOKINETICS: Absorption: Incomplete. Bioavailability (13%, moexiprilat); T_{max}=1.5 hrs (moexiprilat); C_{max} and AUC reduced by 70% and 40%, respectively, with low-fat breakfast, or 80% and 50%, respectively, with high-fat breakfast. **Distribution:** V_d=183L (moexiprilat); plasma protein binding (50%, moexiprilat). **Metabolism:** Rapid via deesterification; moexiprilat (active metabolite). **Elimination:** Urine (1% unchanged, 7% moexiprilat, 5% other metabolites), feces (1% unchanged, 52% moexiprilat); $T_{1/2}$=2-9 hrs (moexiprilat).

NURSING CONSIDERATIONS

Assessment: Assess for history of ACE inhibitor-associated angioedema, hypersensitivity to drug, volume/salt depletion, CHF, collagen vascular disease, renal artery stenosis, DM, cerebrovascular disease, hepatic/renal function, pregnancy/nursing status, and possible drug interactions.

Monitoring: Monitor BP, hepatic/renal function, WBCs (collagen vascular disease), and serum K^+ levels. Monitor for head/neck and intestinal angioedema, anaphylactoid reaction, hypersensitivity reactions.

Patient Counseling: Advise to take 1 hr ac. Instruct to d/c use and report immediately to physician if signs/symptoms of angioedema (swelling of the face, extremities, eyes, lips, tongue, difficulty in breathing) occur. Inform that lightheadedness may occur, especially during the 1st few days of therapy; instruct to d/c use and consult physician if fainting occurs. Inform that excessive perspiration, dehydration, and other causes of volume depletion (eg, diarrhea, vomiting) may lead to excessive fall in BP; advise to consult physician if these conditions develop. Instruct not to use K^+ supplements or salt substitutes containing K^+ without consulting physician, and to report any signs/symptoms of infection (eg, sore throat, fever). Inform of the consequences of exposure during pregnancy and instruct to report pregnancies to physician as soon as possible.

Administration: Oral route. Take 1 hr ac. **Storage:** Room temperature. Protect from excessive moisture.

Uroxatral   RX
alfuzosin HCl (Sanofi-Aventis)

THERAPEUTIC CLASS: Alpha₁-antagonist

INDICATIONS: Treatment of signs and symptoms of benign prostatic hyperplasia (BPH).

DOSAGE: *Adults:* 10mg qd, with food and with the same meal each day.

HOW SUPPLIED: Tab, Extended-Release: 10mg

CONTRAINDICATIONS: Moderate or severe hepatic impairment (Child-Pugh categories B and C), concomitant use of potent CYP3A4 inhibitors (eg, ketoconazole, itraconazole, ritonavir).

WARNINGS/PRECAUTIONS: Postural hypotension with or without symptoms (eg, dizziness) may develop within few hours after administration; caution with symptomatic hypotension or who had a hypotensive response to other medications. Syncope may occur; caution to avoid situations in which injury could result should syncope occur. Prostate carcinoma and BPH frequently coexist and many of their symptoms are similar; rule out the presence of prostatic cancer prior to therapy. D/C if symptoms of angina pectoris occur or worsen. Caution with severe renal impairment, mild hepatic impairment, and congenital or acquired QT prolongation. Intraoperative floppy iris syndrome (IFIS) observed in some patients during cataract surgery. Priapism rarely reported; this condition can lead to permanent impotence if not properly treated. May impair mental/physical abilities. Not for treatment of HTN. Not indicated for use in women or children.

ADVERSE REACTIONS: Dizziness, upper respiratory tract infection, headache, fatigue.
INTERACTIONS: See Contraindications. Avoid use with other α-blockers. Cimetidine, atenolol, and moderate CYP3A4 inhibitors (eg, diltiazem) may increase levels. May increase risk of hypotension/postural hypotension and syncope with nitrates and other antihypertensives. Caution with medications that prolong the QT interval. Caution with PDE5 inhibitors; may potentially cause symptomatic hypotension.
PREGNANCY: Category B, safety not known in nursing.
MECHANISM OF ACTION: α₁-antagonist; selectively inhibits $α_1$-adrenergic receptors in lower urinary tract causing smooth muscle in bladder neck and prostate to relax, which results in improved urine flow and decreased symptoms of BPH.
PHARMACOKINETICS: Absorption: Absolute bioavailability (49%), C_{max}=13.6ng/mL, T_{max}=8 hrs, AUC_{0-24}=194ng•hr/mL. **Distribution:** V_d=3.2L/kg (IV); plasma protein binding (82-90%).
Metabolism: Liver (extensive) via CYP3A4 (oxidation, O-demethylation, N-dealkylation).
Elimination: Feces (69%), urine (24%, 11% unchanged); $T_{1/2}$=10 hrs.

NURSING CONSIDERATIONS

Assessment: Assess for BPH, prostatic cancer, symptomatic hypotension, history of QT prolongation, hepatic/renal impairment, cataract surgery, hypersensitivity, and possible drug interactions. Rule out the presence of prostatic cancer prior to therapy.

Monitoring: Monitor for postural hypotension, syncope, hypersensitivity reactions, IFIS, QT prolongation, hepatic/renal dysfunction, urine flow, and allergic/hypersensitivity reactions.

Patient Counseling: Inform about possible occurrence of symptoms related to postural hypotension (eg, dizziness) when beginning therapy; caution about driving, operating machinery, or performing hazardous tasks during this period. Advise to inform ophthalmologist about using the product before cataract surgery or other procedures involving the eyes, even if the patient is no longer taking the medication. Advise about the possibility of priapism resulting from treatment and to seek immediate medical attention if it occurs. Instruct to take with food and with the same meal each day. Instruct not to crush or chew tab.

Administration: Oral route. Take with food. Swallow tab whole; do not chew or crush. **Storage:** 25°C (77°F); excursions permitted to 15-30°C (59-86°F). Protect from light and moisture.

VAGIFEM   RX
estradiol (Novo Nordisk)

Estrogens increase the risk of endometrial cancer. Perform adequate diagnostic measures, including endometrial sampling, to rule out malignancy with undiagnosed persistent or recurring abnormal genital bleeding. Should not be used for prevention of cardiovascular disease (CVD) or dementia. Increased risk of myocardial infarction (MI), pulmonary embolism (PE), stroke, invasive breast cancer, and deep vein thrombosis (DVT) in postmenopausal women (50-79 yrs of age) reported. Increased risk of developing probable dementia in postmenopausal women ≥65 yrs of age reported. Should be prescribed at the lowest effective dose and for the shortest duration consistent with treatment goals and risks.

THERAPEUTIC CLASS: Estrogen

INDICATIONS: Treatment of atrophic vaginitis due to menopause.

DOSAGE: *Adults:* Usual: Insert 1 tab intravaginally qd for 2 weeks, followed by 1 tab twice weekly.

HOW SUPPLIED: Tab: 10mcg

CONTRAINDICATIONS: Undiagnosed abnormal genital bleeding, known/suspected/history of breast cancer, known or suspected estrogen-dependent neoplasia, active or history of DVT/PE/arterial thromboembolic disease (eg, stroke, MI), liver dysfunction/disease, known/suspected pregnancy.

WARNINGS/PRECAUTIONS: Caution in patients with risk factors for arterial vascular disease (eg, HTN, diabetes mellitus [DM], tobacco use, hypercholesterolemia, obesity) and/or venous thromboembolism (VTE) (eg, personal/family history of VTE, obesity, systemic lupus erythematosus [SLE]). If feasible, d/c at least 4-6 weeks before surgery of the type associated with increased risk of thromboembolism, or during prolonged immobilization. May increase risk of gallbladder disease requiring surgery and ovarian cancer. May lead to severe hypercalcemia in women with breast cancer and bone metastases; d/c and take appropriate measures if hypercalcemia occurs. Retinal vascular thrombosis reported; if visual abnormalities or migraine occurs, d/c pending examination. If examination reveals papilledema or retinal vascular lesions, d/c permanently. Consider addition of a progestin to estrogen monotherapy in postmenopausal women with a uterus or when a woman has not had a hysterectomy, or in posthysterectomy for endometriosis. May elevate BP, plasma TG with preexisting hypertriglyceridemia; d/c if pancreatitis occurs. Caution with history of cholestatic jaundice; d/c in case of recurrence. May lead to increased thyroid-binding globulin levels; monitor thyroid function. May cause fluid retention; caution with cardiac/renal dysfunction. Caution with hypoparathyroidism; hypocalcemia may result. May exacerbate endometriosis, asthma, DM, epilepsy, migraine, porphyria, SLE, and hepatic

V

hemangiomas; use with caution. Caution in women with severely atrophic vaginal mucosa; local abrasion induced by applicator reported. May affect certain endocrine and blood components in laboratory tests.

ADVERSE REACTIONS: Back pain, diarrhea, vulvovaginal mycotic infection, vulvovaginal pruritus, headache, abdominal pain, upper respiratory tract infection, moniliasis genital.

INTERACTIONS: CYP3A4 inducers (eg, St. John's wort, phenobarbital, carbamazepine, rifampin) may decrease levels, which may decrease therapeutic effects and/or change uterine bleeding profile. CYP3A4 inhibitors (eg, erythromycin, clarithromycin, ketoconazole, itraconazole, ritonavir, grapefruit juice) may increase levels, which may result in side effects. Patients concomitantly receiving thyroid replacement therapy and estrogens may require increased doses of thyroid replacement therapy.

PREGNANCY: Contraindicated in pregnancy, caution in nursing.

MECHANISM OF ACTION: Estrogen; binds to nuclear receptors in estrogen-responsive tissues. Circulating estrogens modulate the pituitary secretion of the gonadotropins, luteinizing hormone and follicle-stimulating hormone, through a negative feedback mechanism. Reduces elevated levels of these hormones in postmenopausal women.

PHARMACOKINETICS: Absorption: Well absorbed; administration of multiple doses resulted in different parameters. **Distribution:** Largely bound to sex hormone-binding globulin and albumin; found in breast milk. **Metabolism:** Liver, to estrone (metabolite) and estriol (major urinary metabolite); enterohepatic circulation via sulfate and glucuronide conjugation in the liver; biliary secretion of conjugates in the intestine; hydrolysis in the gut; reabsorption. **Elimination:** Urine (parent compound and metabolites).

NURSING CONSIDERATIONS

Assessment: Asses for presence/history of breast cancer, estrogen-dependent neoplasia, undiagnosed abnormal vaginal bleeding, active or history of DVT/PE/arterial thromboembolic disease, liver dysfunction, pregnancy, or any other conditions where treatment is contraindicated or cautioned. Assess use in women ≥65 yrs and those with asthma, DM, epilepsy, migraines or porphyria, SLE, and hepatic hemangiomas. Assess for possible drug interactions.

Monitoring: Monitor for signs/symptoms of CVD, malignant neoplasms, dementia, gallbladder disease, cholestatic jaundice, hypercalcemia, visual abnormalities, BP elevations, fluid retention, elevations in plasma TG, pancreatitis, hypothyroidism, exacerbation of endometriosis, and other conditions (eg, asthma, DM, epilepsy, migraines, epilepsy, hemangiomas). Perform annual breast exam and regular BP monitoring. Monitor thyroid function in patients on thyroid replacement therapy. In cases of undiagnosed, persistent, or recurring abnormal vaginal bleeding in patients with a uterus, perform adequate diagnostic measures (eg, endometrial sampling) to rule out malignancy. Perform periodic evaluation (3-6 month intervals) to determine need of therapy.

Patient Counseling: Inform that drug is contraindicated in pregnancy. Advise to notify physician if signs/symptoms of unusual vaginal bleeding occur. Inform about possible serious adverse reactions (eg, CVD, malignant neoplasms, and probable dementia) and possible less serious but common adverse reactions (eg, headache, breast pain/tenderness, N/V). Instruct on how to use the applicator.

Administration: Intravaginal route. **Storage:** 25°C (77°F); excursions permitted to 15-30°C (59-86°F). Do not refrigerate.

VALCYTE   RX
valganciclovir HCl (Genentech)

> Clinical toxicity includes granulocytopenia, anemia, and thrombocytopenia. Carcinogenic, teratogenic, and caused aspermatogenesis in animal studies.

THERAPEUTIC CLASS: Synthetic guanine derivative nucleoside analogue

INDICATIONS: (Tab) Treatment of cytomegalovirus (CMV) retinitis in adult patients with AIDS and prevention of CMV disease in kidney, heart, or kidney-pancreas transplant adult patients at high risk (donor CMV seropositive/recipient CMV seronegative [D+/R-]). (Tab/Sol) Prevention of CMV disease in kidney or heart transplant patients (4 months-16 yrs) at high risk.

DOSAGE: *Adults:* Treatment of CMV Retinitis: Induction: 900mg bid for 21 days. Maint: 900mg qd. Prevention of CMV Disease: Heart/Kidney-Pancreas Transplant: 900mg qd starting within 10 days of transplantation until 100 days post-transplantation. Kidney Transplant: 900mg qd starting within 10 days of transplantation until 200 days post-transplantation. Renal Impairment: CrCl 40-59mL/min: Induction: 450mg bid. Maint: 450mg qd. CrCl 25-39mL/min: Induction: 450mg qd. Maint: 450mg q2 days. CrCl 10-24mL/min: Induction: 450mg q2 days. Maint: 450mg 2X weekly. Elderly: Start at lower end of dosing range. Take with food.
Pediatrics: 4 months-16 yrs: Prevention of CMV Disease: Recommended qd dose starting within

V

10 days of transplantation until 100 days post-transplantation is based on BSA and CrCl derived from modified Schwartz formula. Refer to PI for dose calculations. Take with food.

HOW SUPPLIED: Tab: 450mg; Sol: 50mg/mL

WARNINGS/PRECAUTIONS: Severe leukopenia, neutropenia, pancytopenia, bone marrow aplasia, and aplastic anemia reported. Avoid if absolute neutrophil count (ANC) <500 cells/μL, platelet count <25,000/μL, or Hgb <8g/dL. Cytopenia may occur and may worsen with continued dosing; caution with preexisting cytopenias. May cause inhibition of spermatogenesis in men. May cause suppression of fertility in women. Women of childbearing potential should use effective contraception during and for at least 30 days following treatment. Men should practice barrier contraception during and for at least 90 days following treatment. Acute renal failure may occur. Maintain adequate hydration. Caution in elderly and with renal impairment. Not for use in liver transplant patients. Not recommended for adult patients on hemodialysis (CrCl <10mL/min). Do not substitute tab for ganciclovir caps on a 1-to-1 basis.

ADVERSE REACTIONS: Diarrhea, N/V, pyrexia, neutropenia, anemia, cough, HTN, constipation, upper respiratory tract infection, tremor, graft rejection, thrombocytopenia, granulocytopenia.

INTERACTIONS: May increase levels of zidovudine, didanosine (monitor for toxicity), and mycophenolate mofetil (with renal impairment). Probenecid (monitor for toxicity) and mycophenolate mofetil (with renal impairment) may increase levels. Zidovudine, didanosine may decrease levels. Caution with nephrotoxic drugs, myelosuppressive drugs, or irradiation.

PREGNANCY: Category C, not for use in nursing.

MECHANISM OF ACTION: Synthetic guanine derivative nucleoside analogue; inhibits viral DNA polymerase synthesis, resulting in inhibition of human CMV replication.

PHARMACOKINETICS: Absorption: Ganciclovir: Absolute bioavailability (59.4%); C_{max}=5.61μg/mL; T_{max}=1-3 hrs; AUC=29.1μg•h/mL. **Distribution:** Ganciclovir: V_d=0.703L/kg (IV); plasma protein binding (1-2%). **Metabolism:** Intestinal wall, liver; valganciclovir (prodrug) hydrolyzed to ganciclovir. **Elimination:** Ganciclovir: Renal; $T_{1/2}$=4.08 hrs. Refer to PI for different parameters.

NURSING CONSIDERATIONS

Assessment: Assess for renal impairment, preexisting cytopenia, pregnancy/nursing status, prior/current irradiation, and possible drug interactions. Obtain baseline ANC, platelet count, and Hgb.

Monitoring: Monitor for signs/symptoms of hematologic effects (eg, granulocytopenia, anemia, thrombocytopenia, cytopenia), infertility, renal dysfunction, and other adverse reactions. Monitor CBC with differential and platelet counts frequently. Perform ophthalmologic exams q4-6 weeks during therapy.

Patient Counseling: Advise not to substitute tab for ganciclovir caps on a 1-to-1 basis. Instruct adults to use tabs, not the oral sol. Inform patients of major toxicities (eg, granulocytopenia, anemia, thrombocytopenia) and of possible need to adjust dose or d/c. Inform of possible laboratory abnormalities and the importance of close monitoring of blood counts during therapy. Instruct to take with food. Advise of possible decreased fertility. Instruct women not to use during pregnancy/breastfeeding. Advise women of childbearing potential to use effective contraception during and for at least 30 days following treatment, and men to practice barrier contraception during and at least 90 days following treatment. Advise to consider the drug a potential carcinogen. Inform that therapy may impair physical/mental ability. Inform that the drug is not a cure for CMV retinitis and may continue to experience progression during or following treatment; advise to have ophthalmologic exams q4-6 weeks while being treated.

Administration: Oral route. Take with food; do not break or crush tabs. Refer to PI for preparation of oral sol. **Storage:** Tab/Dry Powder: 25°C (77°F); excursions permitted to 15-30°C (59-86°F). Reconstituted Sol: 2-8°C (36-46°F) for no longer than 49 days. Do not freeze.

V

VALIUM
diazepam (Roche Labs)

THERAPEUTIC CLASS: Benzodiazepine

INDICATIONS: Management of anxiety disorders and short-term relief of anxiety symptoms. Symptomatic relief of acute alcohol withdrawal. Adjunct therapy for convulsive disorders and relief of skeletal muscle spasms.

DOSAGE: *Adults:* Individualize dose. Anxiety Disorders/Anxiety Symptoms: 2-10mg bid-qid. Acute Alcohol Withdrawal: 10mg tid-qid for 24 hrs. Reduce to 5mg tid-qid prn. Skeletal Muscle Spasm: 2-10mg tid-qid. Convulsive Disorders: 2-10mg bid-qid. Elderly/Debilitated: 2-2.5mg qd-bid initially. May increase gradually prn if tolerated.
Pediatrics: ≥6 months: 1-2.5mg tid-qid initially. May increase gradually prn if tolerated.

HOW SUPPLIED: Tab: 2mg*, 5mg*, 10mg* *scored

CONTRAINDICATIONS: Acute narrow-angle glaucoma, patients <6 months, myasthenia gravis, severe respiratory insufficiency, severe hepatic insufficiency, sleep apnea syndrome.

WARNINGS/PRECAUTIONS: Not recommended for the treatment of psychotic patients. Increase in frequency and/or severity of grand mal seizures may occur during adjunctive therapy and may require an increase in the dose of the standard anticonvulsant medication. May temporarily increase frequency and/or severity of seizures during abrupt withdrawal. Psychiatric and paradoxical reactions may occur; d/c if these occur. Lower dose with chronic respiratory insufficiency. Caution with history of alcohol and drug abuse. Prolonged use may result in loss of response to the effects of benzodiazepines.

ADVERSE REACTIONS: Drowsiness, fatigue, muscle weakness, ataxia, confusion, vertigo, constipation, blurred vision, dizziness, hypotension, stimulation, agitation, incontinence, skin reactions, hypersalivation.

INTERACTIONS: Mutually potentiates effects with phenothiazines, antipsychotics, anxiolytics/sedatives, hypnotics, anticonvulsants, narcotic analgesics, anesthetics, sedative antihistamines, narcotics, barbiturates, MAOIs, and other antidepressants. Alcohol enhances sedative effects; avoid concomitant use. Increased and prolonged sedation with cimetidine, ketoconazole, fluvoxamine, fluoxetine, and omeprazole. Diazepam decreases metabolic elimination of phenytoin.

PREGNANCY: Category D, not for use in nursing.

MECHANISM OF ACTION: Benzodiazepine; exerts anxiolytic, sedative, muscle-relaxant, anticonvulsant, and amnestic effects. Facilitates GABA, an inhibitory neurotransmitter in the CNS.

PHARMACOKINETICS: Absorption: T_{max}=1-1.5 hrs. **Distribution:** V_d=0.8-1.0L/kg; plasma protein binding (98%); crosses blood-brain/placental barrier, and appears in breast milk. **Metabolism:** Via N-demethylation and hydroxylation by CYP3A4 and CYP2C19 enzymes, glucuronidation; N-desmethyldiazepam, temazepam, oxazepam (active metabolites). **Elimination:** Urine; $T_{1/2}$=48 hrs, 100 hrs (N-desmethyldiazepam).

NURSING CONSIDERATIONS

Assessment: Assess for anxiety disorders/symptoms, acute alcohol withdrawal, skeletal muscle spasm, convulsive disorders, depression, and other conditions where treatment is contraindicated or cautioned. Assess for pregnancy/nursing status and possible drug interactions.

Monitoring: Monitor for hypersensitivity reactions, rebound or withdrawal symptoms, seizures, psychiatric and paradoxical reactions, and respiratory depression.

Patient Counseling: Advise to consult physician before increasing dose or abruptly d/c the drug. Advise against simultaneous ingestion of alcohol and other CNS depressants during therapy. Caution against engaging in hazardous occupations requiring complete mental alertness, such as operating machinery or driving a motor vehicle.

Administration: Oral route. **Storage:** 15-30°C (59-86°F).

VALTREX   RX
valacyclovir HCl (GlaxoSmithKline)

THERAPEUTIC CLASS: Nucleoside analogue

INDICATIONS: Treatment of herpes labialis (cold sores) in patients ≥12 yrs. Treatment of herpes zoster (shingles) in immunocompetent adults. Treatment of initial and recurrent episodes of genital herpes in immunocompetent adults, chronic suppressive therapy of recurrent episodes of genital herpes in immunocompetent and in HIV-1 infected adults, and reduction of transmission of genital herpes in immunocompetent adults. Treatment of chickenpox in immunocompetent patients 2 to <18 yrs.

DOSAGE: *Adults:* Herpes Labialis: 2g q12h for 1 day. Start at earliest symptom of cold sore. Genital Herpes: Initial Episode: 1g bid for 10 days. Start within 48 hrs after onset of symptoms. Recurrent Episodes: 500mg bid for 3 days. Start at 1st sign/symptom of episode. Chronic Suppressive Therapy with Normal Immune Function: 1g qd. Alternative: History of ≤9 Episodes/Yr: 500mg qd. Chronic Suppressive Therapy with HIV-1 and CD4 ≥100 cells/mm³: 500mg bid. Reduction of Transmission of Genital Herpes: History of ≤9 Episodes/Yr: 500mg qd for the source partner. Herpes Zoster: 1g tid for 7 days. Start within 48 hrs after onset of rash. Elderly: Reduce dose. Renal Impairment: Refer to PI for dose modifications.
Pediatrics: Herpes Labialis: ≥12 yrs: 2g q12h for 1 day. Start at earliest symptom of cold sore. Chickenpox: 2 to <18 yrs: 20mg/kg tid for 5 days. Max: 1g tid. Initiate at earliest sign/symptom.

HOW SUPPLIED: Tab: 500mg, 1g* *scored

WARNINGS/PRECAUTIONS: Thrombotic thrombocytopenic purpura/hemolytic uremic syndrome (TTP/HUS) in immunocompromised patients reported at doses of 8g qd; immediately d/c if signs/symptoms occur. Acute renal failure reported. Maintain adequate hydration. CNS adverse reactions (eg, agitation, hallucinations, confusion, delirium, seizures, encephalopathy) reported when used at higher than recommended dose in patients with or without reduced renal function and in those with underlying renal disease for their level of renal function; d/c if these occur. Caution in elderly and with renal impairment.

ADVERSE REACTIONS: Headache, N/V, abdominal pain, dysmenorrhea, arthralgia, nasopharyngitis, fatigue, rash, upper respiratory tract infections, pyrexia, decreased neutrophil counts, diarrhea, elevated ALT/AST.

INTERACTIONS: Caution with potentially nephrotoxic drugs.

PREGNANCY: Category B, caution in nursing.

MECHANISM OF ACTION: Nucleoside analogue DNA polymerase inhibitor; rapidly converted to acyclovir, which stops replication of herpes viral DNA by competitive inhibition of viral DNA polymerase, incorporation into and termination of growing viral DNA chain, and inactivation of viral DNA polymerase.

PHARMACOKINETICS: Absorption: Rapid. Absolute bioavailability (54.5% acyclovir). Oral administration of variable doses resulted in different parameters. **Distribution:** Plasma protein binding (13.5-17.9%, 9-33% acyclovir); found in breast milk. **Metabolism:** Hepatic/Intestinal (1st pass) to acyclovir and L-valine. **Elimination:** Urine (46%), feces (47%); $T_{1/2}$=2.5-3.3 hrs.

NURSING CONSIDERATIONS

Assessment: Assess for immunocompromised state, renal impairment, hydration status, pregnancy/nursing status, and possible drug interactions.

Monitoring: Monitor for signs/symptoms of renal toxicity, TTP/HUS, CNS effects, and other adverse reactions.

Patient Counseling: Advise to maintain adequate hydration. Inform that drug is not a cure for cold sores or genital herpes. For patients with cold sores, instruct to initiate treatment at earliest symptom of a cold sore (eg, tingling, itching, burning); inform that treatment should not exceed 1 day (2 doses) and that doses should be taken 12 hrs apart. For patients with genital herpes, instruct to avoid contact with lesions or sexual intercourse when lesions and/or symptoms are present to avoid infecting partner(s), and to use safe sex practice in combination with suppressive therapy. For patients with herpes zoster, advise to initiate treatment as soon as possible after diagnosis. For patients with chickenpox, advise to initiate treatment at the earliest sign/symptom.

Administration: Oral route. Refer to PI for extemporaneous preparation of oral suspension. **Storage:** 15-25°C (59-77°F).

VALTROPIN   RX
somatropin (LG Life)

THERAPEUTIC CLASS: Human growth hormone

INDICATIONS: Treatment of pediatric patients who have growth failure due to inadequate secretion of endogenous growth hormone. Treatment of growth failure associated with Turner syndrome in pediatric patients who have open epiphyses. Long-term replacement therapy in adults with growth hormone deficiency (GHD) of either adult or childhood onset etiology.

DOSAGE: *Adults:* Individualize dose. Initial: 0.33mg/day SQ 6 days a week. Dosage may be increased to individual patient requirement to maximum of 0.66mg/day after 4 weeks. Alternative Dosing: 0.2mg/day (Range: 0.15-0.3mg/day). May increase gradually every 1-2 months by 0.1-0.2mg/day based on individual patient requirements.
Pediatrics: Individualize dose. Divide weekly dose into equal amounts given either daily or 6 days a week by SQ injection. GHD: 0.17-0.3mg/kg of body weight/week. Turner Syndrome: Up to 0.375mg/kg of body weight/week.

HOW SUPPLIED: Inj: 5mg

CONTRAINDICATIONS: Pediatrics with closed epiphyses. Active proliferative and severe nonproliferative diabetic retinopathy. Presence of active malignancy. Acute critical illness due to complications following open heart surgery, abdominal surgery, or multiple accidental trauma, or those with acute respiratory failure. Patients with Prader-Willi syndrome who are severely obese or have severe respiratory impairment.

WARNINGS/PRECAUTIONS: Known sensitivity to supplied diluent (metacresol). Caution in pediatric pateints with Prader-Willi syndrome and who have 1 or more risk factor (severe obesity, history of upper airway destruction or sleep apnea, or unidentified respiratory infection). May decrease insulin sensitivity. Patients with GHD secondary to intracranial lesion should be monitored closely for progression or recurrence of underlying disease process. Intracranial HTN reported. Monitor closely with DM, glucose intolerance, hypopituitarism. Funduscopic exam recommended at initiation and periodically during course of therapy. Monitor carefully for any malignant transformation of skin lesions.

V

ADVERSE REACTIONS: Headache, pyrexia, cough, respiratory tract infection, diarrhea, vomiting, pharyngitis.

INTERACTIONS: Growth-promoting effects may be inhibited by glucocorticoids. May alter clearance of compounds metabolized by CYP450 liver enzymes (eg, corticosteroids, sex steroids, anticonvulsants, cyclosporine); monitor closely. May need insulin adjustment.

PREGNANCY: Category B, caution in nursing.

MECHANISM OF ACTION: Human growth hormone; stimulates linear growth synthesis, metabolizes lipids, reduces body fat stores by increasing cellular protein, and increases plasma fatty acids.

PHARMACOKINETICS: Absorption: C_{max}=43.97ng/mL, T_{max}=4 hrs, AUC=369.9ng•hr/mL. **Metabolism:** Liver, kidneys (protein catabolism). **Elimination:** $T_{1/2}$=3.03 hrs.

NURSING CONSIDERATIONS

Assessment: Assess for hypersensitivity to benzyl alcohol, history of scoliosis, pre-existing papilledema, hypothyroidism, diagnostic imaging (pituitary or intracranial tumor), hypopituitarism, possible drug interactions, and any other condition where treatment is contraindicated or cautioned. Obtain baseline funduscopic exam. Prader-Willi syndrome: Evaluate for signs of upper airway obstruction or sleep apnea before initiation. Turner syndrome: Evaluate for otitis media or other ear disorders, and CV disorders before initiation.

Monitoring: Monitor fasting blood glucose and thyroid function tests periodically, conduct fundoscopic exam periodically, and monitor weight control (Prader-Willi syndrome), signs/symptoms of malignant transformation of skin lesions, intracranial HTN, slipped capital femoral epiphysis (eg, onset of limp, hip or knee pain), hypersensitivity/allergic reactions, respiratory infections (Prader-Willi syndrome), otitis media or ear disorders, CV disorders and progression of scoliosis.

Patient Counseling: Instruct thoroughly as to proper usage and disposal. Caution against any reuse of needles and syringes. Seek medical attention if signs/symptoms of slipped capital femoral epiphysis (eg, onset of limp, hip or knee pain), hypersensitivity/allergic reactions, respiratory infections (Prader-Willi syndrome), otitis media or CV disorders or progression of scoliosis occur.

Administration: SQ route (thighs). **Storage:** Before reconstitution: 2-8°C (36-46°F). Do not freeze. After reconstitution: 2-8°C (36-46°F) for up to 21 days. Do not freeze.

VALTURNA   RX
valsartan - aliskiren (Novartis)

> **D/C when pregnancy is detected. Drugs that act directly on the renin-angiotensin system can cause injury/death to the developing fetus.**

THERAPEUTIC CLASS: Renin inhibitor/angiotensin II receptor antagonist

INDICATIONS: Treatment of HTN. May be used as an add-on therapy in patients whose BP is not adequately controlled with aliskiren alone or valsartan (or another angiotensin receptor blocker) alone, substituted for titrated components, or used as initial therapy in patients who are likely to need multiple drugs to achieve BP goals.

DOSAGE: *Adults:* Add-On/Initial Therapy: Initial: 150mg-160mg qd. Titrate: May increase up to 300mg-320mg qd if BP remains uncontrolled after 2-4 weeks. Max: 300mg-320mg qd. Replacement Therapy: May substitute for individually titrated components.

HOW SUPPLIED: Tab: (Aliskiren-Valsartan) 150mg-160mg, 300mg-320mg

WARNINGS/PRECAUTIONS: Not recommended for use as initial therapy in patients with intravascular volume depletion. In patients with an activated renin-angiotensin-aldosterone system (eg, volume- or salt-depleted patients), symptomatic hypotension may occur; correct these conditions prior to therapy or monitor closely. Caution in use as initial therapy with heart failure (HF) or recent myocardial infarction (MI) and in those undergoing surgery/dialysis. Hyperkalemia reported; periodic determinations of serum electrolytes are recommended. Aliskiren: Angioedema of the face, extremities, lips, tongue, glottis and/or larynx reported; d/c immediately and do not readminister if angioedema develops. Valsartan: May increase SrCr and BUN with renal artery stenosis. Changes in renal function may occur in volume-depleted patients. Oliguria and/or progressive azotemia, and (rarely) acute renal failure and/or death, may occur with severe HF patients whose renal function may depend on renin-angiotensin-aldosterone system. Clearance is lowered in patients with mild to moderate hepatic impairment, including biliary obstructive disorders. Increases in BUN, SrCr, and K+ may occur in some patients with HF and preexisting renal impairment; dose reduction and/or d/c may be required.

ADVERSE REACTIONS: Hyperkalemia, fatigue, nasopharyngitis, diarrhea, upper respiratory tract infection, urinary tract infection, influenza, vertigo.

INTERACTIONS: May cause deterioration of renal function with NSAIDs (eg, cyclooxygenase-2 inhibitors); periodically monitor renal function. NSAIDs may attenuate antihypertensive effect. Aliskiren: Cyclosporine or itraconazole increases levels; avoid concomitant use. Potential drug interaction with P-glycoprotein inhibitors. Valsartan: Greater antihypertensive effect with atenolol. Inhibitors of the hepatic uptake transporter OATP1B1 (rifampin, cyclosporine) or the hepatic efflux transporter MRP2 (ritonavir) may increase systemic exposure. K^+-sparing diuretics (eg, spironolactone, triamterene, amiloride), K^+ supplements, or salt substitutes containing K^+ may increase SrCr in HF patients and serum K^+.

PREGNANCY: Category D, not for use in nursing.

MECHANISM OF ACTION: Aliskiren: Direct renin inhibitor; decreases plasma renin activity and inhibits conversion of angiotensinogen to angiotensin I. Valsartan: Angiotensin II receptor antagonist; blocks vasoconstrictor and aldosterone-secreting effects of angiotensin II by selectively blocking the binding of angiotensin II to the AT_1 receptor.

PHARMACOKINETICS: Absorption: Aliskiren: T_{max}=1 hr; AUC and C_{max} decreased by 76% and 88%, respectively, with food. Valsartan: T_{max}=3 hrs. **Distribution:** Valsartan: (IV) V_d=17L; plasma protein binding (95%). **Metabolism:** Aliskiren: Via CYP3A4. Valsartan: Via CYP2C9; valeryl-4-hydroxy valsartan (primary metabolite). **Elimination:** Aliskiren: Urine (25%, unchanged); $T_{1/2}$=34 hrs. Valsartan: (Sol) Feces (83%), urine (13%); $T_{1/2}$=12 hrs.

NURSING CONSIDERATIONS

Assessment: Assess for history of angioedema, volume/salt depletion, renal artery stenosis, renal/hepatic impairment, surgery/dialysis, HF, recent/post-MI, pregnancy/nursing status, and possible drug interactions.

Monitoring: Monitor for head/neck angioedema or airway obstruction. Monitor BP, serum electrolytes, and renal function, including BUN and SrCr.

Patient Counseling: Instruct to inform physician or pharmacist if any unusual symptoms develop, or if any known symptoms persist or worsen. Inform of consequences of exposure during pregnancy; advise to notify physician if pregnant/plan to become pregnant as soon as possible. Inform that lightheadedness may occur, especially during the 1st days of therapy; advise to report to physician. Instruct to d/c and consult a physician if syncope occurs. Inform that inadequate fluid intake, excessive perspiration, diarrhea, or vomiting may lead to an excessive fall in BP, with the same consequences of lightheadedness and possible syncope. Instruct to avoid taking K^+ supplements or salt substitutes containing K^+ without consulting a physician. Instruct to establish a routine pattern for taking medication with regard to meals; inform that high-fat meals decrease absorption substantially.

Administration: Oral route. **Storage:** 25°C (77°F); excursions permitted to 15-30°C (59-86°F). Protect from moisture.

VANCOCIN ORAL   RX
vancomycin HCl (Viro Pharma)

THERAPEUTIC CLASS: Tricyclic glycopeptide antibiotic

INDICATIONS: Treatment of *Clostridium difficile*-associated diarrhea, and enterocolitis caused by *Staphylococcus aureus* (including methicillin-resistant strains).

DOSAGE: *Adults:* Diarrhea: 125mg qid for 10 days. Enterocolitis: 500mg-2g/day in 3 or 4 divided doses for 7-10 days.
Pediatrics: 40mg/kg/day in 3 or 4 divided doses for 7-10 days. Max: 2g/day.

HOW SUPPLIED: Cap: 125mg, 250mg

WARNINGS/PRECAUTIONS: For PO use only; not systemically absorbed. Potential for systemic absorption with multiple PO doses or in some patients with inflammatory disorders of the intestinal mucosa; monitoring of serum concentrations may be appropriate in some instances (eg, renal insufficiency and/or colitis). Nephrotoxicity (eg, renal failure, renal impairment, blood creatinine increased) reported; increased risk in patients >65 yrs. Ototoxicity reported; caution in patients with underlying hearing loss; consider performing serial tests of auditory function during use to minimize ototoxicity risk. May result in bacterial resistance with prolonged use or use in the absence of a proven/suspected bacterial infection or a prophylactic indication; take appropriate measures if superinfection develops. Caution in elderly.

ADVERSE REACTIONS: N/V, abdominal pain, hypokalemia, diarrhea, pyrexia, flatulence, urinary tract infection, headache, peripheral edema, back pain, fatigue, nephrotoxicity.

INTERACTIONS: Monitor serum concentrations with concomitant use of an aminoglycoside antibiotic. Increased risk of ototoxicity when used concurrently with other ototoxic agents (eg, aminoglycosides).

PREGNANCY: Category B, not for use in nursing.

V

MECHANISM OF ACTION: Tricyclic glycopeptide antibiotic; inhibits cell-wall biosynthesis. Also alters bacterial cell-membrane permeability and RNA synthesis.

PHARMACOKINETICS: Absorption: Poor. **Distribution:** Found in breast milk (IV). **Elimination:** Urine, feces.

NURSING CONSIDERATIONS

Assessment: Assess for inflammatory disorders of the intestinal mucosa, renal insufficiency, colitis, hearing disturbances, hypersensitivity to the drug, pregnancy/nursing status, and possible drug interactions. Obtain cultures and perform susceptibility tests.

Monitoring: Monitor for signs/symptoms of nephrotoxicity, ototoxicity, superinfection, and other adverse reactions. Monitor serum concentrations when appropriate. Monitor renal function in patients >65 yrs.

Patient Counseling: Inform that drug treats only bacterial, not viral, infections. Instruct to take exactly ud; advise that skipping doses or not completing full course may decrease effectiveness and increase bacterial resistance.

Administration: Oral route. **Storage:** 59-86°F (15-30°C).

VANCOMYCIN HCL   RX
vancomycin HCl (Various)

THERAPEUTIC CLASS: Tricyclic glycopeptide antibiotic

INDICATIONS: Treatment of serious or severe infections caused by susceptible strains of methicillin-resistant (β-lactam-resistant) staphylococci. Indicated for penicillin-allergic patients who cannot receive or have failed to respond to other drugs, and for infections caused by vancomycin-susceptible organisms that are resistant to other antimicrobials. Initial therapy when methicillin-resistant staphylococci are suspected. Effective in the treatment of staphylococcal endocarditis, other infections due to staphylococci, including septicemia, bone infections, lower respiratory tract infections, and skin and skin-structure infections. Effective alone or in combination with an aminoglycoside for endocarditis caused by S. viridans or S. bovis. Effective only in combination with an aminoglycoside for endocarditis caused by enterococci (eg, E. faecalis). Effective for treatment of diphtheroid endocarditis. Successfully used in combination with either rifampin, an aminoglycoside, or both in early-onset prosthetic valve endocarditis caused by S. epidermidis or diphtheroids. Parenteral form may be administered orally for treatment of antibiotic-associated pseudomembranous colitis produced by C. difficile and for staphylococcal enterocolitis.

DOSAGE: *Adults:* Usual: 500mg IV q6h or 1g IV q12h. Administer at no more than 10mg/min or over at least 60 min, whichever is longer. Renal Impairment: Initial: Not <15mg/kg. Dosage per day in mg is about 15X the GFR in mL/min (refer to dosage table in PI). Elderly: Require greater dose reductions than expected. Functionally Anephric Patients: Initial: 15mg/kg, then 1.9mg/kg/24 hrs. Marked Renal Impairment: 250-1000mg once every several days. Anuria: 1000mg every 7-10 days. For PO Administration: 500-2000mg/day in 3-4 divided doses for 7-10 days. Max: 2000mg/day. May dilute in 1 oz. of water. May also be administered via NG tube.
Pediatrics: Usual: 10mg/kg IV q6h. Infants/Neonates: Initial: 15mg/kg, then 10mg/kg q12h for neonates in 1st week of life and q8h thereafter until 1 month of age. Administer over at least 60 min. Renal Impairment: Initial: Not <15mg/kg. Dosage per day in mg is about 15X the GFR in mL/min (refer to table in PI). Premature Infants: Requires longer dosing intervals. ADD-Vantage vials should not be used in neonates, infants, and pediatrics who require doses <500mg. For PO Administration: 40mg/kg/day in 3-4 divided doses for 7-10 days. Max: 2000mg/day. May dilute in 1 oz. of water. May also be administered via NG tube.

HOW SUPPLIED: Inj: 500mg, 1g

WARNINGS/PRECAUTIONS: Not effective by the oral route for other types of infections. Rapid bolus administration may cause hypotension and cardiac arrest (rare); administer in diluted solution over a period not <60 min. Ototoxicity reported; caution with underlying hearing loss. Caution with renal insufficiency and adjust dose with renal dysfunction. Pseudomembranous colitis reported. May result in bacterial resistance with prolonged use or use in the absence of a proven/suspected bacterial infection or a prophylactic indication; take appropriate measures if superinfection develops. Reversible neutropenia reported; monitor leukocyte count periodically. Administer via IV route. Thrombophlebitis may occur; infuse slowly and rotate injection sites. Safety and efficacy of administration via the intraperitoneal and intrathecal (intralumbar and intraventricular) routes have not been established. Administration via intraperitoneal route during continuous ambulatory peritoneal dialysis (CAPD) has resulted in a syndrome of chemical peritonitis. Caution in elderly.

ADVERSE REACTIONS: Infusion-related events, hypotension, wheezing, pruritus, chest and back muscle spasm or pain, dyspnea, urticaria, nephrotoxicity, pseudomembranous colitis, ototoxicity, neutropenia, phlebitis.

INTERACTIONS: Concomitant use of anesthetic agents associated with erythema, histamine-like flushing, and anaphylactoid reactions. Concurrent and/or sequential systemic or topical use of other potentially neurotoxic and/or nephrotoxic drugs (eg, amphotericin B, aminoglycosides, bacitracin, polymyxin B, colistin, viomycin, cisplatin) requires careful monitoring. Increased risk of ototoxicity with concomitant ototoxic agents (eg, aminoglycoside). Periodic leukocyte count monitoring with drugs that may cause neutropenia. Serial monitoring of renal function and particular care following appropriate dosing to minimize risk of nephrotoxicity with concomitant aminoglycoside.

PREGNANCY: Category C, not for use in nursing.

MECHANISM OF ACTION: Tricyclic glycopeptide antibiotic; inhibits cell-wall biosynthesis, alters bacterial cell membrane permeability and RNA synthesis.

PHARMACOKINETICS: Absorption: (1g at 2 hrs) C_{max} =23mcg/mL; (500mg at 2 hrs) C_{max}=19mcg/mL. **Distribution:** Serum protein binding (55%). **Elimination:** Urine (75%); $T_{1/2}$=4-6 hrs.

NURSING CONSIDERATIONS

Assessment: Assess for renal function, underlying hearing loss, pregnancy/nursing status and possible drug interactions. Perform culture and susceptibility testing.

Monitoring: Monitor for hypersensitivity reactions (eg, Stevens-Johnson syndrome, vasculitis), infusion reactions (eg, hypotension, arrhythmias, "red neck"), thrombophlebitis, ototoxicity, renal function, diarrhea, pseudomembranous colitis, neutropenia, superinfection, and chemical peritonitis (intraperitoneal route). Monitor leukocyte count periodically.

Patient Counseling: Inform that drug treats bacterial, not viral, infections. Take as directed; skipping doses or not completing full course may decrease effectiveness and increase bacterial resistance. May experience diarrhea; notify physician if watery/bloody stools, hypersensitivity reactions, or superinfection develops.

Administration: IV, Oral route. Refer to PI for preparation for IV use. Intermittent infusion recommended. Physically incompatible with β-lactam antibiotics. Diluted sol may be given via NGT. (PO) Common flavoring syrup may be added to improve taste. **Storage:** 20-25°C (68-77°F). After reconstitution: may refrigerate for 14 days. After further dilution: may refrigerate for 14 days or 96 hrs depending on diluent used (refer to PI).

VANOS   RX
fluocinonide (Medicis)

THERAPEUTIC CLASS: Corticosteroid

INDICATIONS: To relieve inflammatory and pruritic manifestations of corticosteroid-responsive dermatoses in patients ≥12 yrs.

DOSAGE: *Adults:* Psoriasis/Corticosteroid-Responsive Dermatoses: Apply thin layer to affected areas qd or bid ud. Atopic Dermatitis: Apply thin layer to affected areas qd ud. Max: 60g/week. Do not use >2 weeks.
Pediatrics: ≥12 yrs: Psoriasis/Corticosteroid-Responsive Dermatoses: Apply thin layer to affected areas qd or bid ud. Atopic Dermatitis: Apply thin layer to affected areas qd ud. Max: 60g/week. Do not use >2 weeks.

HOW SUPPLIED: Cre: 0.1% [30g, 60g, 120g]

WARNINGS/PRECAUTIONS: May produce reversible hypothalamic pituitary adrenal (HPA) axis suppression, Cushing's syndrome, hyperglycemia, and unmasking of latent diabetes mellitus (DM). May suppress immune system if used for >2 weeks. Caution when used over large surface areas, over prolonged periods, under occlusion, on an altered skin barrier, and with liver failure; withdraw drug, reduce application frequency, or substitute a less potent steroid if HPA axis suppression occurs. Pediatric patients may be more susceptible to systemic toxicity. Local adverse reactions may occur. D/C if favorable response does not occur. Allergic contact dermatitis reported; d/c if irritation occurs. Avoid with rosacea, perioral dermatitis; do not apply on the face, groin, or axillae. Not for ophthalmic, PO, or intravaginal use. D/C when control is achieved; reassess if no improvement seen within 2 weeks.

ADVERSE REACTIONS: Headache, application-site burning, nasopharyngitis, nasal congestion.

INTERACTIONS: Use of >1 corticosteroid-containing product at the same time may increase total systemic absorption; use with caution.

PREGNANCY: Category C, not for use in nursing.

MECHANISM OF ACTION: Corticosteroid; has not been established. Possesses anti-inflammatory and antipruritic actions; plays a role in cellular signaling, immune function, inflammation, and protein regulation.

V

PHARMACOKINETICS: Absorption: Percutaneous; extent is determined by vehicle, integrity of skin, and use of occlusive dressings. **Distribution:** Found in breast milk (systemically administered).

NURSING CONSIDERATIONS

Assessment: Assess for rosacea, perioral dermatitis, skin infections, inflammation or other skin diseases, liver function, concomitant corticosteroid use, and pregnancy/nursing status.

Monitoring: Monitor for signs/symptoms of HPA axis suppression, Cushing's syndrome, hyperglycemia, unmasking of latent DM, skin irritation, allergic contact dermatitis, and for development of skin infections. In pediatric patients, also monitor for linear growth retardation, delayed weight gain, and intracranial HTN. Monitor for signs of glucocorticosteroid insufficiency after withdrawal. Monitor clinical improvement; if no improvement seen within 2 weeks, reassess diagnosis.

Patient Counseling: Advise to use ud by physician and not to use for disorder other than for which it was prescribed. Instruct to avoid contact with eyes and not to use on face, groin, and underarms. Inform not to use >60g/week or cover, wrap, or bandage treatment areas unless directed by physician. Counsel to wash hands following application. Inform to contact physician if local adverse reactions occur or no clinical improvement seen in 2 weeks. Instruct to notify physician if surgery is contemplated or planning to use other corticosteroids.

Administration: Topical route. **Storage:** 15-30°C (59-86°F).

VANTAS   RX
histrelin acetate (Endo)

THERAPEUTIC CLASS: Synthetic gonadotropin releasing hormone analog

INDICATIONS: Palliative treatment of advanced prostate cancer.

DOSAGE: *Adults:* Usual: 1 implant SQ (into the inner aspect of the upper arm) for 12 months. Remove after 12 months and replace with new implant.

HOW SUPPLIED: Implant: 50mg

CONTRAINDICATIONS: Women who are or may become pregnant.

WARNINGS/PRECAUTIONS: May cause transient increase in serum testosterone during 1st week of treatment; patient may experience worsening or new onset of symptoms (eg, bone pain, neuropathy, hematuria, or ureteral or bladder outlet obstruction). Spinal cord compression and ureteral obstruction reported; observe closely during 1st few weeks in patients with metastatic vertebral lesions and/or urinary tract obstruction. Difficulty in locating or removing implant may be experienced. Hyperglycemia and increased risk of developing diabetes reported; monitor blood glucose periodically. Increased risk of developing MI, sudden cardiac death, and stroke reported.

ADVERSE REACTIONS: Hot flashes, fatigue, implant-site reaction (bruising/pain/soreness/tenderness), testicular atrophy, renal impairment, gynecomastia, constipation, erectile dysfunction.

PREGNANCY: Category X, not for use in nursing.

MECHANISM OF ACTION: Synthetic gonadotropin-releasing hormone analog; acts as potent inhibitor of gonadotropin secretion when given continuously in therapeutic doses. Desensitizes responsiveness of pituitary gonadotropin, causing reduction in testicular steroidogenesis.

PHARMACOKINETICS: Absorption: C_{max}=1.1ng/mL; T_{max}=12 hrs. **Distribution:** V_d=58.4L. **Metabolism:** C-terminal dealkylation and hydrolysis. **Elimination:** $T_{1/2}$=3.92 hrs.

NURSING CONSIDERATIONS

Assessment: Assess for previous hypersensitivity, pregnancy/nursing status, metastatic vertebral lesions, urinary tract obstruction, diabetes mellitus (DM), and cardiovascular (CV) risk factors. Obtain baseline serum testosterone and prostate-specific antigen (PSA) levels.

Monitoring: Monitor for anaphylactic reactions, transient worsening or onset of new symptoms, implant-site reactions, signs/symptoms suggestive of development of CV disease, and other adverse reactions. Periodically monitor serum testosterone and PSA levels, and blood glucose and HbA1c in patients with DM.

Patient Counseling: Instruct to refrain from wetting arm for 24 hrs and from heavy lifting or strenuous exertion of arm for 7 days after implant insertion. Inform that anaphylactic reactions, transient worsening of symptoms and implant-site reactions may occur. Instruct to report to physician if the implant was expelled from the body and if the patient is experiencing unusual bleeding, redness, or pain at insertion site.

Administration: SQ implant. Refer to PI for full instructions on implant insertion/removal. **Storage:** Implant: 2-8°C (36-46°F); excursions permitted to 25°C (77°F) for 7 days. Keep in the original packaging until day of insertion. Protect from light. Do not freeze. Implantation Kit: Room temperature.

VAQTA
hepatitis A vaccine (inactivated) (Merck)

RX

THERAPEUTIC CLASS: Vaccine

INDICATIONS: Prevention of disease caused by hepatitis A virus (HAV) in persons ≥12 months. For postexposure prophylaxis when given with immune globulin (IG).

DOSAGE: *Adults:* ≥19 yrs: 1mL IM followed by a booster of 1mL 6-18 months later. May be given as a booster dose at 6-12 months following the primary dose of another inactivated hepatitis A vaccine.
Pediatrics: 1-18 yrs: 0.5mL IM followed by a booster of 0.5mL 6-18 months later.

HOW SUPPLIED: Inj: 25 U/0.5mL, 50 U/mL

CONTRAINDICATIONS: Previous allergic reaction to neomycin.

WARNINGS/PRECAUTIONS: May not prevent hepatitis A in patients who have unrecognized hepatitis A infection at time of vaccination. Medical treatment and supervision must be available to manage possible hypersensitivity reactions. Caution when vaccinating latex-sensitive individuals; may cause allergic reactions. Immunocompromised persons may have diminished response and may not be protected against HAV infection after vaccination.

ADVERSE REACTIONS: Injection-site pain, tenderness, soreness, warmth, or redness; asthenia, myalgia, fever, headache, cough, diarrhea, upper respiratory infection, irritability, nausea, fatigue.

INTERACTIONS: Immunosuppressive therapy may reduce immune response.

PREGNANCY: Category C, caution in nursing.

MECHANISM OF ACTION: Vaccine; presence of antibodies confers protection against HAV infection.

NURSING CONSIDERATIONS

Assessment: Assess for hypersensitivity reactions after previous dose of hepatitis A vaccine, hypersensitivity to neomycin, immunization status/vaccination history, latex sensitivity, presence of immunosuppression, pregnancy/nursing status, and possible drug interaction.

Monitoring: Monitor for signs/symptoms of hypersensitivity reactions (eg, anaphylaxis), injection-site reactions, immune response, fever, or other possible adverse effects.

Patient Counseling: Inform of potential risks and benefits of immunization. Inform about the potential for adverse events that have been temporally associated with the vaccination. Report severe or unusual adverse events to physician or clinic where the vaccine was administered.

Administration: IM route. Shake well before use. Refer to PI for proper administration procedures. For adults, adolescents, and children >2 yrs, inject preferably into deltoid muscle. For children 12-23 months, inject at the anterolateral area of the thigh. Do not mix with any other vaccine in the same syringe or vial. **Storage:** 2-8°C (36-46°F). Do not freeze.

VARIVAX
varicella virus vaccine live (Merck)

RX

THERAPEUTIC CLASS: Vaccine

INDICATIONS: Vaccination against varicella in individuals ≥12 months of age.

DOSAGE: *Adults:* 0.5mL SQ at elected date; repeat 4-8 weeks later.
Pediatrics: ≥13 yrs: 0.5mL SQ at elected date; repeat 4-8 weeks later. 12 months-12 yrs: 0.5mL SQ. If a 2nd dose is given, administer a minimum of 3 months later.

HOW SUPPLIED: Inj: 0.5mL

CONTRAINDICATIONS: Individuals receiving immunosuppressive therapy or immunosuppressant doses of corticosteroids, history of hypersensitivity to gelatin, anaphylactoid reaction to neomycin, blood dyscrasias, leukemia, lymphomas of any type, other malignant neoplasms affecting the bone marrow or lymphatic systems, primary and acquired immunodeficiency states, including association with AIDS or other clinical manifestations of infection with HIV, cellular immune deficiencies, hypogammaglobulinemic and dysgammaglobulinemic states, family history of congenital or hereditary immunodeficiency, active untreated tuberculosis, febrile respiratory illness or other active febrile infection, and pregnancy.

WARNINGS/PRECAUTIONS: Anaphylactoid reaction may occur; have epinephrine (1:1000) available. Defer vaccine for ≥5 months after blood or plasma transfusions, or administration of immune globulin or varicella zoster immune globulin (VZIG). Defer vaccine with family history of congenital, hereditary immunodeficiency until immune system evaluated. Vaccine virus transmission may occur; avoid close association with susceptible high-risk individuals for ≤6 weeks (eg, immunocompromised patients, pregnant women without history of chickenpox). Do not inject into a blood vessel. Use separate needle and syringe for administration of each dose to prevent transfer of infectious disease. May not result in protection of all vaccinees. Pregnancy should be avoided for 3 months following vaccination.

ADVERSE REACTIONS: Fever, inj-site complaints (eg, pain/soreness, swelling and/or erythema, rash, pruritus, hematoma, induration, stiffness), varicella-like rashes.

INTERACTIONS: See Contraindications. Avoid immune globulins including VZIG for 2 months after vaccination; defer vaccination for ≥5 months following administration of immune globulin including VZIG. Avoid salicylates for 6 weeks after vaccination.

PREGNANCY: Category C, caution in nursing.

MECHANISM OF ACTION: Vaccine; induces cell-mediated immune response against varicella zoster virus infection.

NURSING CONSIDERATIONS

Assessment: Assess for allergies and any other conditions where treatment is contraindicated or cautioned, pregnancy/nursing status, and possible drug interactions. Obtain previous immunization history and previous reaction to vaccine or similar products.

Monitoring: Monitor for signs/symptoms of allergic reactions, inj-site reactions (eg, pain, swelling, rash, hematoma, pruritus), fever, and thrombocytopenia.

Patient Counseling: Inform of potential benefits and risks of vaccination. Advise to report any adverse reactions to physician. Inform that the vaccine may not result in protection of all vaccinees. Avoid use of salicylates for 6 weeks after vaccination and avoid pregnancy 3 months after vaccination.

Administration: SQ route. Inject preferably into outer aspect of deltoid or anterolateral thigh. Refer to PI for reconstitution. Administer immediately after reconstitution; discard if not used within 30 min. **Storage:** -50°C to -15°C (-58°F to 5°F). Use of dry ice may subject to temperatures colder than -50°C (-58°F). Prior to Reconstitution: 2-8°C (36-46°F) for up to 72 continuous hrs; discard if not used. Before reconstitution, protect from light. Diluent: 20-25°C (68-77°F), or in the refrigerator.

VASOTEC   RX
enalapril maleate (Valeant)

> ACE inhibitors can cause death/injury to developing fetus during 2nd and 3rd trimesters. D/C therapy if pregnancy is detected.

THERAPEUTIC CLASS: ACE inhibitor

INDICATIONS: Treatment of HTN, alone or with other antihypertensive agents (eg, thiazide diuretics). Treatment of symptomatic congestive heart failure (CHF) usually in combination with diuretics and digitalis. To decrease the rate of development of overt heart failure and decrease incidence of hospitalization for heart failure in clinically stable asymptomatic patients with left ventricular dysfunction (ejection fraction ≤35%).

DOSAGE: *Adults:* HTN: If possible, d/c diuretic 2-3 days prior to therapy. Initial: 5mg qd; 2.5mg with concomitant diuretic. Usual: 10-40mg/day given in single dose or 2 divided doses. Resume diuretic if BP not controlled. CrCl ≤30mL/min: Initial: 2.5mg qd. Dialysis: Initial: 2.5mg qd on dialysis days. Adjust according to BP response on nondialysis days. Max: 40mg/day. Heart Failure: Initial: 2.5mg qd. Usual: 2.5-20mg bid. Titrate upward, as tolerated, over a few days/weeks. Max: 40mg/day in divided doses. Asymptomatic Left Ventricular Dysfunction: Initial: 2.5mg bid. Titrate: Increase as tolerated to 20mg/day (in divided doses). Hyponatremia or SrCr >1.6mg/dL with Heart Failure: Initial: 2.5mg/day. Titrate: Increase to 2.5mg bid, then 5mg bid and higher PRN, usually at intervals of 4 days or more. Max: 40mg/day.
Pediatrics: 1 month-16 yrs: HTN: Initial: 0.08mg/kg (up to 5mg) qd. Titrate: Adjust according to BP response. Max: 0.58mg/kg/dose (or 40mg/dose).

HOW SUPPLIED: Tab: 2.5mg*, 5mg*, 10mg,* 20mg* *scored

CONTRAINDICATIONS: History of ACE inhibitor-associated angioedema and hereditary or idiopathic angioedema.

WARNINGS/PRECAUTIONS: May increase risk of angioedema in patients with history of angioedema unrelated to ACE inhibitor therapy. Angioedema of the face, extremities, lips, tongue, glottis, and larynx reported; d/c and administer appropriate therapy if this occurs. Higher incidence of angioedema reported in blacks than nonblacks. Intestinal angioedema reported; monitor for abdominal pain (with or without N/V). Anaphylactoid reactions reported during desensitization with hymenoptera venom, dialysis with high-flux membranes, and LDL apheresis with dextran sulfate absorption. Excessive hypotension sometimes associated with oliguria or azotemia, and (rarely) acute renal failure or death may occur; monitor during first 2 weeks of therapy and whenever dose is increased. Neutropenia or agranulocytosis and bone marrow depression may occur;

V

monitor WBCs in patients with renal disease and collagen vascular disease. Rarely, a syndrome that starts with cholestatic jaundice and progresses to fulminant hepatic necrosis, and sometimes death reported; d/c if jaundice or marked elevations of hepatic enzymes develop. Caution with left ventricular outflow obstruction. May cause changes in renal function. Increases in BUN and SrCr reported with renal artery stenosis; monitor renal function during the 1st few weeks of therapy. Increases in BUN and SrCr reported with no preexisting renal vascular disease. Risk of hyperkalemia with diabetes mellitus (DM) and renal dysfunction. Persistent nonproductive cough reported. Hypotension may occur with major surgery or during anesthesia. Avoid in neonates and pediatrics with GFR <30mL/min/1.73m².

ADVERSE REACTIONS: Fatigue, headache, dizziness, hypotension.

INTERACTIONS: Hypotension risk with diuretics; monitor closely. May increase BUN and SrCr with diuretics; may require dose reduction and/or d/c of diuretic and/or therapy. May deteriorate renal function with NSAIDs. NSAIDs may diminish antihypertensive effect. Increased risk of hyperkalemia with K⁺-sparing diuretics, K⁺-containing salt substitutes, or K⁺ supplements; monitor serum K⁺ frequently. Antihypertensives that cause renin release (eg, thiazides) may augment antihypertensive effect. Lithium toxicity reported with lithium; monitor serum lithium levels frequently. Nitritoid reactions (eg, facial flushing, N/V, hypotension) reported rarely with injectable gold.

PREGNANCY: Category C (1st trimester) and D (2nd and 3rd trimesters), not for use in nursing.

MECHANISM OF ACTION: ACE inhibitor; inhibition of ACE results in decreased plasma angiotensin II, which leads to decreased vasopressor activity and decreased aldosterone secretion.

PHARMACOKINETICS: Absorption: T_{max}=1 hr, 3-4 hrs (enalaprilat). **Distribution:** Crosses placenta, found in breast milk. **Metabolism:** Hydrolysis, enalaprilat (metabolite). **Elimination:** Urine and feces (94% enalapril or enalaprilat); $T_{1/2}$=11 hrs (enalaprilat).

NURSING CONSIDERATIONS

Assessment: Assess for history of angioedema, volume/salt depletion, renal dysfunction/disease, collagen vascular disease, renal artery stenosis, left ventricular outflow obstruction, DM, pregnancy/nursing status, and possible drug interactions. Obtain baseline BP, LFTs, and renal function.

Monitoring: Monitor for anaphylactoid reaction, angioedema, hypotension, hypersensitivity, and other adverse reactions. Monitor BP, LFTs, renal function, CBC with platelet count and differential, serum K⁺ levels.

Patient Counseling: Counsel about fetal risks during pregnancy. Counsel about signs/symptoms of angioedema (eg, swelling of face, extremities, eyes, lips, tongue, difficulty in swallowing or breathing); advise to d/c and seek prompt medical attention if symptoms develop. Inform about adverse effects (eg, anaphylaxis, cough, hypotension, hyperkalemia). Instruct to report lightheadedness. Caution that dehydration, excessive perspiration, diarrhea, vomiting may lead to excessive fall in BP, which can result in lightheadedness or possible syncope. Advise to d/c and consult physician if syncope occurs. Advise not to use K⁺ supplements or salt substitutes containing K⁺ without consulting physician. Advise patient to report any signs of infection.

Administration: Oral route. Refer to PI for preparation of suspension. **Storage:** 25°C (77°F); excursions permitted to 15-30°C (59-86°F). Keep container tightly closed. Protect from moisture.

VECTIBIX   RX
panitumumab (Amgen)

Dermatologic toxicities and severe infusion reactions reported. Fatal infusion reactions occurred in postmarketing experience.

THERAPEUTIC CLASS: Monoclonal antibody/EGFR-blocker

INDICATIONS: Treatment as a single agent of epidermal growth factor receptor (EGFR)-expressing, metastatic colorectal carcinoma with disease progression on or following fluoropyrimidine-, oxaliplatin-, and irinotecan-containing chemotherapy regimens.

DOSAGE: *Adults:* Usual: 6mg/kg IV infusion over 60 min q14 days. Infuse doses >1000mg over 90 min. Reduce infusion rate by 50% with mild or moderate (Grade 1 or 2) infusion reaction for duration of that infusion. Withhold for ≥Grade 3/intolerable dermatologic toxicities. Permanently d/c if toxicity does not improve to ≤Grade 2 within 1 month. Resume with 50% of original dose if toxicity improves to ≤Grade 2 and symptoms improve after withholding ≤2 doses. Permanently d/c if toxicities recur. If toxicities do not recur, may increase subsequent doses by increments of 25% of original dose until 6mg/kg is reached.

HOW SUPPLIED: Inj: 20mg/mL [5mL, 10mL, 20mL]

WARNINGS/PRECAUTIONS: D/C if severe dermatologic toxicities or infusion reactions occur. Pulmonary fibrosis reported; permanently d/c in patients developing interstitial lung disease, pneumonitis, or lung infiltrates. Hypomagnesemia and hypocalcemia may occur; monitor electrolytes periodically during and for 8 weeks after completion of therapy. May exacerbate dermatologic toxicity upon sun exposure. Interrupt or d/c therapy if acute or worsening keratitis occurs. Perform EGFR protein expression assessment to identify patients eligible for treatment. Not recommended for treatment of colorectal cancer with KRAS mutations in codon 12 or 13.

ADVERSE REACTIONS: Skin toxicities (eg, erythema, dermatitis acneiform, pruritus, exfoliation, rash, fissures), infusion reactions, hypomagnesemia, paronychia, fatigue, abdominal pain, nausea, diarrhea, constipation.

INTERACTIONS: Avoid use with chemotherapy; decreased overall survival and increased incidence of grade 3-5 adverse reactions reported.

PREGNANCY: Category C, not for use in nursing.

MECHANISM OF ACTION: IgG2 kappa monoclonal antibody; binds specifically to EGFR on both normal and tumor cells, and competitively inhibits binding of ligands for EGFR.

PHARMACOKINETICS: Absorption: C_{max}=213mcg/mL, AUC=1306mcg•day/mL. **Elimination:** $T_{1/2}$=7.5 days.

NURSING CONSIDERATIONS

Assessment: Assess electrolyte baseline levels, EGFR protein expression, pulmonary disease, pregnancy/nursing status and potential for drug interactions.

Monitoring: Monitor for signs/symptoms of dermatologic toxicities, severe infusion reactions, angioedema, pulmonary fibrosis, and keratitis. Monitor electrolytes periodically during and for 8 weeks after completion of therapy.

Patient Counseling: Advise to report skin/ocular changes, signs and symptoms of infusion reactions (eg, fever, chills, or breathing problems), persistent/recurrent coughing, wheezing, dyspnea, or new onset facial swelling, diarrhea and dehydration, and if pregnant or nursing. Advise of need for adequate contraception in both males and females during and for 6 months after therapy and periodic monitoring of electrolytes. Limit sun exposure during and for 2 months after the last dose of therapy.

Administration: IV infusion; do not administer as bolus or push. Refer to PI for preparation and administration instructions. **Storage:** (Vial) 2-8°C (36-46°F). Protect from direct sunlight. Do not freeze. (Diluted) Room temperature; use within 6 hrs, or at 2-8°C (36-46°F); stable for 24 hrs. Do not freeze.

VECTICAL   RX
calcitriol (Galderma)

THERAPEUTIC CLASS: Vitamin D analog

INDICATIONS: Treatment of mild to moderate plaque psoriasis in adults ≥18 yrs.

DOSAGE: *Adults:* Apply to affected area(s) bid (am and pm). Max: 200g/week.

HOW SUPPLIED: Oint: 3mcg/g [5g, 100g]

WARNINGS/PRECAUTIONS: Not for PO, ophthalmic, or intravaginal use. Hypercalcemia reported; if aberrations in parameters of calcium metabolism occur, d/c therapy until these parameters norrmalize. Increased absorption with occlusive use. Avoid excessive exposure of treated areas to natural or artificial sunlight (eg, tanning booths, sun lamps); avoid or limit phototherapy.

ADVERSE REACTIONS: Laboratory test abnormality, urine abnormality, psoriasis, hypercalciuria, pruritus, hypercalcemia, skin discomfort.

INTERACTIONS: Caution with medications known to increase serum calcium level (eg, thiazide diuretics), calcium supplements, or high doses of vitamin D.

PREGNANCY: Category C, caution in nursing.

MECHANISM OF ACTION: Vitamin D analog; mechanism of action in the treatment of psoriasis not established.

NURSING CONSIDERATIONS

Assessment: Assess for known/suspected calcium metabolism disorder, pregnancy/nursing status, and possible drug interactions.

Monitoring: Monitor for hypercalcemia, aberrations in parameters of calcium metabolism, and other adverse reactions.

Patient Counseling: Instruct to use as directed. Instruct to apply only to areas of the skin affected by psoriasis; advise not to apply to the eyes, lips, or facial skin. Instruct to rub gently into the skin. Advise to notify their physician if adverse reactions occur. Advise to avoid excessive exposure of treated areas to sunlight, tanning booths, sun lamps, or other artificial sunlight and to inform physician about treatment if undergoing phototherapy.

V

Administration: Topical route. **Storage:** 25°C (77°F); excursions permitted to 15°-30°C (59°-86°F). Do not freeze or refrigerate.

VELTIN GEL

RX

clindamycin phosphate - tretinoin (Stiefel)

THERAPEUTIC CLASS: Lincosamide derivative/retinoid

INDICATIONS: Topical treatment of acne vulgaris in patients ≥12 yrs.

DOSAGE: *Adults:* Apply pea-sized amount qd in pm. Gently rub the medication to lightly cover the entire affected area. Avoid the eyes, lips and mucous membranes.
Pediatrics: ≥12 yrs: Apply pea-sized amount qd in pm. Gently rub the medication to lightly cover the entire affected area. Avoid the eyes, lips and mucous membranes.

HOW SUPPLIED: Gel: (Clindamycin phosphate-Tretinoin) 1.2%-0.025% [30g, 60g]

CONTRAINDICATIONS: Regional enteritis, ulcerative colitis, or history of antibiotic-associated colitis.

WARNINGS/PRECAUTIONS: Systemic absorption of clindamycin has been demonstrated following topical use. Diarrhea, bloody diarrhea, and colitis reported with clindamycin; d/c if significant diarrhea occurs. Severe colitis reported up to several weeks following cessation of therapy. Avoid exposure to sunlight, including sunlamps. Avoid use if sunburn present. Daily use of sunscreen products and protective apparel is recommended. Weather extremes (eg, wind, cold) may be irritating while under treatment.

ADVERSE REACTIONS: Local site reactions (eg, dryness, irritation, exfoliation, erythema).

INTERACTIONS: Avoid with erythromycin-containing products due to possible antagonism to clindamycin. Caution with neuromuscular-blocking agents. Antiperistaltic agents (eg, opiates, diphenoxylate with atropine) may prolong and/or worsen severe colitis. Skin irritation may increase when used concomitantly with other topical products with strong drying effects (eg, soaps, cleansers).

PREGNANCY: Category C, caution in nursing.

MECHANISM OF ACTION: Clindamycin: Lincosamide antibiotic; binds to the 50S ribosomal subunit of susceptible bacteria and prevents elongation of peptide chains by interfering with peptidyl transfer, thereby suppressing protein synthesis. Found to have activity against *P. acnes.* Tretinoin: Retinoid; not established; suspected to decrease the cohesiveness of follicular epithelial cells with decreased microcomedone formation. Also, stimulates mitotic activity and increased turnover of follicular epithelial cells causing extrusion of the comedones.

PHARMACOKINETICS: Absorption: Clindamycin: C_{max} = 8.73ng/mL; T_{max} = 4 hrs.

NURSING CONSIDERATIONS

Assessment: Assess for regional enteritis, ulcerative colitis or history of antibiotic-associated colitis, pre-existing sunburns, pregnancy/nursing status, and for possible drug interactions. Assess use in patients whose occupations require considerable sun exposure.

Monitoring: Monitor for signs/symptoms of diarrhea, bloody diarrhea and colitis (including pseudomembranous colitis). If diarrhea, abdominal cramps, or passage of blood or mucus, perform stool culture for *Clostridium difficile* and stool assay for *C. difficile* toxin. Monitor for local skin reactions (eg, erythema, scaling, burning, dryness, itching).

Patient Counseling: Instruct to gently wash face with a mild soap and water prior to application. Do not use more than a pea-sized amount to lightly cover the face and not to apply more than once daily, only at bedtime. Avoid exposure to sunlight, sunlamps, and ultraviolet light; daily use of sunscreen products and protective apparel are recommended. Avoid other topical medications that may increase sensitivity to sunlight. Do not use other topical products that may cause an increase in skin irritation. Therapy may cause irritation such as erythema, scaling, itching, burning, or stinging. Contact physician if experience diarrhea or GI discomfort. Advise to keep out of the reach of children.

Administration: Topical route. Not for oral, ophthalmic or intravaginal use. **Storage:** 25°C (77°F); excursions permitted to 15-30°C (59-86°F). Protect from light, heat and freezing. Keep tube tightly closed.

VENLAFAXINE

RX

venlafaxine HCl (Various)

> Antidepressants increased the risk of suicidal thinking and behavior (suicidality) in children, adolescents, and young adults in short-term studies of major depressive disorder (MDD) and other psychiatric disorders. Monitor and observe closely for clinical worsening, suicidality, or unusual changes in behavior. Not approved for use in pediatric patients.

THERAPEUTIC CLASS: Serotonin and norepinephrine reuptake inhibitor

INDICATIONS: Treatment of MDD.

DOSAGE: *Adults:* Initial: 75mg/day in 2-3 divided doses with food. Titrate: May increase to 150mg/day. If needed, increase up to 225mg/day. Dose increments of ≤75mg/day at intervals of no less than 4 days. Max: 375mg/day in 3 divided doses. Hepatic Impairment (mild to moderate)/Hemodialysis: Individualize. Reduce total daily dose by 50%. Renal Impairment (mild to moderate): Individualize. Reduce total daily dose by 25%.

HOW SUPPLIED: Tab: 25mg*, 37.5mg*, 50mg*, 75mg*, 100mg* *scored

CONTRAINDICATIONS: Concomitant use of MAOI or use within 14 days of taking an MAOI; allow ≥7 days after stopping drug before starting an MAOI.

WARNINGS/PRECAUTIONS: Avoid abrupt withdrawal; gradually reduce dose and monitor for d/c symptoms. Not approved for use in treating bipolar depression. Serotonin syndrome or neuroleptic malignant syndrome (NMS)-like reactions reported; d/c immediately and initiate supportive symptomatic treatment. May cause sustained increases in BP; consider dose reduction or d/c. Mydriasis reported; monitor patients with increased intraocular pressure (IOP) or risk of acute narrow-angle glaucoma. Treatment-emergent anxiety, nervousness, insomnia, weight loss, anorexia, and activation of mania/hypomania reported. May cause hyponatremia; d/c if symptomatic hyponatremia occurs and institute appropriate intervention. Caution with history of mania or seizures and conditions affecting hemodynamic responses or metabolism; d/c if seizures occur. May increase risk of bleeding events. Elevation of cholesterol levels reported; monitor periodically. Caution with conditions that may be compromised by HR increases (eg, hyperthyroidism, heart failure [HF], recent myocardial infarction [MI]), renal/hepatic impairment. Interstitial lung disease and eosinophilic pneumonia reported rarely. Caution in elderly.

ADVERSE REACTIONS: Asthenia, sweating, N/V, headache, diarrhea, constipation, anorexia, insomnia, somnolence, dry mouth, dizziness, nervousness, anxiety, abnormal ejaculation/orgasm, impotence in men.

INTERACTIONS: See Contraindications. Serotonin syndrome or NMS-like reactions reported when used alone and in combination with serotonergic drugs (eg, triptans), drugs that impair serotonin metabolism, antipsychotics, and dopamine antagonists. Avoid alcohol, tryptophan. Increased risk of bleeding with aspirin (ASA), NSAIDs, warfarin, and other anticoagulants. Caution with cimetidine in elderly, with HTN, hepatic dysfunction. Decreases clearance of haloperidol. May inhibit metabolism of CYP2D6 substrates. Increases risperidone and desipramine plasma levels. Increased levels with ketoconazole. Decreased indinavir levels. Caution with metoprolol, CYP3A4 inhibitors, potent inhibitors of CYP3A4 and CYP2D6, CNS-active drugs, and serotonergic drugs (eg, triptans, SSRIs, other serotonin and norepinephrine reuptake inhibitors [SNRIs], linezolid, lithium, tramadol, or St. John's wort). Coadministration with weight-loss agents not recommended. Use with diuretics may increase risk of developing hyponatremia.

PREGNANCY: Category C, not for use in nursing.

MECHANISM OF ACTION: SNRI; potentiates neurotransmitter activity in CNS by inhibiting neuronal serotonin and norepinephrine reuptake.

PHARMACOKINETICS: Absorption: Well absorbed. **Distribution:** V_d=7.5L/kg, V_d=5.7L/kg (ODV); plasma protein binding (27%, 30% [ODV]); found in breast milk. **Metabolism:** Extensive. Hepatic; O-desmethylvenlafaxine (ODV) (major active metabolite). **Elimination:** Urine (87%, 5% unchanged, 29% unconjugated ODV, 26% conjugated ODV, 27% minor inactive metabolites); $T_{1/2}$=5 hrs; $T_{1/2}$=11 hrs (ODV).

NURSING CONSIDERATIONS

Assessment: Assess for bipolar disorder, history of mania and drug abuse, hyperthyroidism, HF, recent MI, history of glaucoma, increased IOP, risk factors for acute narrow-angle glaucoma, pre-existing HTN, history of seizures, disease/condition that alters metabolism or hemodynamic response, cholesterol levels, hepatic/renal impairment, drug hypersensitivity, pregnancy/nursing status, and possible drug interactions. Obtain a detailed psychiatric history.

Monitoring: Monitor HR, BP, LFTs, renal function, cholesterol, ECG changes, height and weight. Monitor for signs/symptoms of clinical worsening, suicidality, unusual changes in behavior, serotonin syndrome or NMS-like reactions, mydriasis, severe HTN, lung disease, abnormal bleeding, allergic reactions, hyponatremia, seizures, cognitive/motor impairment, and hepatic/renal dysfunction. If abruptly d/c, monitor for d/c symptoms (eg, dysphoric mood, irritability, agitation). Periodically re-evaluate long-term usefulness of therapy.

Patient Counseling: Advise to avoid alcohol. Inform about the risks and benefits associated with treatment. Instruct to read the Medication Guide. Advise to inform physician if taking, or plan to take, any prescription or OTC drugs, including herbal preparations and nutritional supplements, since there is a potential for interactions. Seek medical attention for symptoms of serotonin syndrome (eg, mental status changes, tachycardia, hyperthermia, N/V, diarrhea, incoordination), abnormal bleeding (particularly if using NSAIDs or ASA), hyponatremia (eg, headache, weakness, unsteadiness), mydriasis, severe HTN, lung disease (eg, progressive dyspnea, cough, chest discomfort), activation of mania, seizures, clinical worsening (eg, suicidal ideation, unusual changes in behavior), or d/c symptoms (eg, irritability, agitation, dizziness, anxiety, headache, insomnia). Notify physician if pregnant or breastfeeding or if rash, hives, or related allergic phenomenon develops.

Administration: Oral route. **Storage:** 20-25°C (68-77°F) in a dry place.

VENTAVIS RX
iloprost (Actelion)

THERAPEUTIC CLASS: Prostaglandin analog

INDICATIONS: Treatment of pulmonary arterial hypertension (PAH) (WHO Group I) to improve a composite endpoint consisting of exercise tolerance, symptoms (NYHA Class), and lack of deterioration in patients with NYHA Functional Class III-IV symptoms and etiologies of idiopathic or heritable PAH or PAH associated with connective tissue diseases.

DOSAGE: *Adults:* Administer via I-neb or Prodose AAD Systems. Initial: 2.5mcg. Titrate: May increase to 5mcg and maintain if well tolerated; otherwise maintain at 2.5mcg. Should be taken 6-9 times/day (no more than once q2h). Max: 45mcg/day. Child Pugh Class B or C Hepatic Impairment: Increase dosing interval (eg, 3-4 hrs between doses). Elderly: Start at lower end of dosing range.

HOW SUPPLIED: Sol, Inhalation: 10mcg/mL [1mL], 20mcg/mL [1mL]

WARNINGS/PRECAUTIONS: Avoid contact with skin or eyes. Avoid oral ingestion. Do not initiate in patients with systolic BP <85mmHg; monitor for vital signs. Exertional syncope may reflect therapeutic gap or insufficient efficacy; consider adjusting dose or changing therapy if it occurs. D/C if signs of pulmonary edema occur. May induce bronchospasm. Bronchospasm may be more severe or frequent in patients with history of hyperreactive airways. Caution in patients with COPD, severe asthma, or pulmonary infections, hepatic/renal impairment, and in the elderly.

ADVERSE REACTIONS: Increased cough, headache, vasodilation/flushing, flu syndrome, N/V, trismus, hypotension, syncope, insomnia, palpitations, increased alkaline phosphatase/GGT, back pain.

INTERACTIONS: May increase hypotensive effect of vasodilators and antihypertensive agents. Increased risk of bleeding with anticoagulants or platelet inhibitors.

PREGNANCY: Category C, not for use in nursing.

MECHANISM OF ACTION: Synthetic analogue of prostacyclin PGI_2; dilates systemic and pulmonary arterial vascular beds. Affects platelet aggregation; relevance of this effect is unknown.

PHARMACOKINETICS: Absorption: C_{max}=150pg/mL. **Distribution:** (IV) V_d=0.7-0.8L/kg; plasma protein binding (60%). **Metabolism:** Via β-oxidation. Tetranor-iloprost (main metabolite). **Elimination:** Urine (68%), feces (12%); $T_{1/2}$=20-30 min.

NURSING CONSIDERATIONS

Assessment: Assess for history of hyperreactive airways, COPD, severe asthma, acute pulmonary infection, renal/hepatic impairment, pregnancy/nursing status, and possible drug interactions. Obtain baseline BP and vitals prior to initiation of therapy.

Monitoring: Monitor for vital signs, signs and symptoms pulmonary edema, exertional syncope, bleeding, and bronchospasm.

Patient Counseling: Counsel to use as prescribed with either I-neb or Prodose AAD Systems. Instruct on proper administration techniques. Advise that a drop in BP during therapy is possible and may cause dizziness or fainting; advise to stand up slowly when getting out of a chair or bed. Consult a physician if fainting gets worse. Inform that medication should be inhaled at intervals of not <2 hrs and that acute benefits of therapy may not last 2 hrs. Inform that patients may adjust times of administration to cover planned activities. Counsel to avoid mixing with other medications.

Administration: Inhalation route. Refer to PI for preparation instructions. **Storage:** 20-25°C (68-77°F); excursions permitted to 15-30°C (59-86°F).

V

VENTOLIN HFA RX
albuterol sulfate (GlaxoSmithKline)

THERAPEUTIC CLASS: Beta$_2$-agonist

INDICATIONS: Treatment or prevention of bronchospasm in patients with reversible obstructive airway disease. Prevention of exercise-induced bronchospasm (EIB).

DOSAGE: *Adults:* Bronchospasm: 2 inh q4-6h or 1 inh q4h. EIB: 2 inh 15-30 min before exercise. Elderly: Start at lower end of dosing range.
Pediatrics: ≥4 yrs: Bronchospasm: 2 inh q4-6h or 1 inh q4h. EIB: 2 inh 15-30 min before exercise.

HOW SUPPLIED: MDI: 90mcg/inh [8g, 18g]

WARNINGS/PRECAUTIONS: D/C if paradoxical bronchospasm or CV events occur. Avoid excessive use; may be marker of destabilization of asthma and require reevaluation of the patient. Caution with convulsive disorders, coronary insufficiency, arrhythmias, HTN, diabetes mellitus (DM), hyperthyroidism, sensitivity to sympathomimetics. Hypersensitivity reactions may occur. Fatalities reported with excessive use. May need concomitant corticosteroids. May produce significant hypokalemia. Caution in elderly.

ADVERSE REACTIONS: Throat irritation, viral respiratory infections, upper respiratory inflammation, cough, musculoskeletal pain, parodoxical bronchospasm, hoarseness, arrhythmias, hypersensitivity reactions, hypokalemia, HTN, peripheral vasodilation, angina, tremor.

INTERACTIONS: Avoid other short-acting sympathomimetic bronchodilators; caution with oral sympathomimetics. Extreme caution with MAOIs, TCAs during or within 2 weeks of d/c. β-blockers may block pulmonary effects and cause severe bronchospasm. Decreases digoxin levels. ECG changes and/or hypokalemia caused by non-K⁺-sparing diuretics (eg, loop or thiazide diuretics) may be worsened.

PREGNANCY: Category C, not for use in nursing.

MECHANISM OF ACTION: β_2-adrenergic agonist; activates β_2-adrenergic receptors on airway smooth muscle leading to the activation of adenylcyclase and to an increase in the intracellular concentration of cAMP. This increase of cAMP leads to the activation of protein kinase A, which inhibits the phosphorylation of myosin and lowers intracellular ionic calcium concentrations, resulting in relaxation of the smooth muscles of all airways, from the trachea to the terminal bronchioles.

PHARMACOKINETICS: Absorption: C_{max}=3ng/mL; T_{max}=0.42 hrs. **Elimination:** $T_{1/2}$=4.6 hrs.

NURSING CONSIDERATIONS

Assessment: Assess renal/hepatic function, history of hypersensitivity to drug, CVD (eg, coronary insufficiency, HTN, cardiac arrhythmias), convulsive disorders, hyperthyroidism, DM and ketoacidosis, pregnancy/nursing status, and possible drug interactions. Assess use in patients unusually responsive to sympathomimetic amines.

Monitoring: Monitor for possible paradoxical bronchospasm, deterioration of asthma, CV effects, hypokalemia, immediate hypersensitivity reactions and common adverse effects (eg, palpitation, rapid HR, tremor and nervousness. Monitor BP, HR, ECG changes and blood glucose.

Patient Counseling: Advise to seek medical attention if treatment becomes less effective for symptomatic relief, symptoms become worse, or usage becomes more frequent than usual. Take as directed and report lack of response or adverse side effects. Instruct how to properly prime, clean and use inhaler. Prime inhaler before using for first time or if inhaler has not been used for 2 weeks, or if it has dropped by releasing 4 test sprays into air, away from face. Clean inhaler at least once a week, wash the actuator with warm water and let it air-dry completely. Use only with actuator supplied with product. Refill prescription when the counter reads 020 or discard when the counter reads 000 or if it is 12 months after removal from the moisture-protective foil pouch, whichever comes first. Advise to never immerse the canister in water to determine the amount of drug remaining in the canister. Avoid spraying in eyes and shake well before each spray.

Administration: Oral inhalation route. **Storage:** 15-25°C (59-77°F). Keep out of the reach of children. Do not puncture. Do not use or store near heat or open flame. Exposure to temperatures above 120°F may cause bursting. Store inhaler with mouthpiece down.

VERAMYST RX
fluticasone furoate (GlaxoSmithKline)

V

THERAPEUTIC CLASS: Corticosteroid

INDICATIONS: Treatment of the symptoms of seasonal and perennial allergic rhinitis in patients ≥2 yrs.

DOSAGE: *Adults:* Initial: 2 sprays/nostril qd. Titrate to minimum effective dose. Maint: 1 spray/nostril qd. Elderly: Start at low end of dosing range.
Pediatrics: ≥12 yrs: Initial: 2 sprays/nostril qd. Titrate to minimum effective dose. Maint: 1 spray/nostril qd. 2-11 yrs: Initial: 1 spray/nostril qd. Titrate: May increase to 2 sprays/nostril qd if inadequate, then return to initial dose when symptoms are controlled.

HOW SUPPLIED: Spray: 27.5mcg/spray [10g]

WARNINGS/PRECAUTIONS: May cause local nasal effects (eg, epistaxis, nasal ulceration, *Candida* infections, nasal septum perforation, and impaired wound healing). Avoid with recent nasal ulcers, surgery, or trauma. May result in glaucoma, cataracts, and increased intraocular pressure (IOP). D/C if hypersensitivity reactions (eg, anaphylaxis, angioedema, rash, urticaria) occur. May increase susceptibility to infections; caution with active or quiescent tuberculosis

(TB), untreated fungal or bacterial infections, systemic viral or parasitic infections, or ocular herpes simplex. Avoid exposure to chickenpox and measles. D/C slowly if hypercorticism and adrenal suppression occur. Risk of adrenal insufficiency and withdrawal symptoms when replacing systemic corticosteroids with topical corticosteroids. Potential for reduced growth velocity in pediatrics. Caution with severe hepatic impairment and elderly.

ADVERSE REACTIONS: Headache, epistaxis, pharyngolaryngeal pain, nasal ulceration, back pain, pyrexia, cough.

INTERACTIONS: Increased exposure with ritonavir; avoid coadministration. Reduced cortisol levels with ketoconazole; caution with ketoconazole or other potent CYP3A4 inhibitors.

PREGNANCY: Category C, caution in nursing.

MECHANISM OF ACTION: Corticosteroid; not established. Shown to have a wide range of actions on multiple cell types (eg, mast cells, eosinophils, neutrophils, macrophages, lymphocytes) and mediators (eg, histamine, eicosanoids, leukotrienes, cytokines) involved in inflammation.

PHARMACOKINETICS: Absorption: Incomplete; absolute bioavailability (0.5%). **Distribution:** (IV) V_d=608L; plasma protein binding (>99%). **Metabolism:** Hepatic via CYP3A4; hydrolysis. **Elimination:** Feces, urine; (IV) $T_{1/2}$=15.1 hrs.

NURSING CONSIDERATIONS

Assessment: Assess for previous hypersensitivity to the drug, active or quiescent TB, untreated fungal/bacterial infection, systemic viral infection, ocular herpes simplex, history of IOP, glaucoma or cataracts, recent nasal ulcers/surgery/trauma, hepatic impairment, pregnancy/nursing status, and possible drug interactions.

Monitoring: Monitor for hypercorticism, chickenpox, measles, epistaxis, nasal ulceration, nasal septal perforation, hypoadrenalism (in infants born to a mother who received corticosteroids during pregnancy), suppression of growth velocity in children, vision changes, glaucoma, cataracts, increased IOP, and hypersensitivity reactions. Examine periodically for evidence of nasal *Candida* infections.

Patient Counseling: Counsel to take as directed and to shake well before each use. Inform of possible local nasal effects, cataracts, glaucoma, immunosuppression, and hypersensitivity reactions. Advise not to use with recent nasal ulcers, surgery, or trauma until healing has occurred. Instruct to d/c if hypersensitivity reaction occurs. Instruct to avoid exposure to chickenpox and measles. Instruct to consult physician if symptoms do not improve, the condition worsens, or change in vision occurs. Advise to avoid spraying into eyes. Inform of potential drug interactions.

Administration: Intranasal route. Prime pump before 1st time use, if not used >30 days, or cap left off >5 days. **Storage:** 15-30°C (59-86°F). Store device in upright position with cap in place. Do not freeze or refrigerate.

VERDESO   RX
desonide (Stiefel)

THERAPEUTIC CLASS: Corticosteroid

INDICATIONS: Treatment of mild to moderate atopic dermatitis in patients ≥3 months.

DOSAGE: *Adults:* Apply thin layer to affected area(s) bid. D/C when control is achieved. Max Duration: 4 consecutive weeks. Dispense smallest amount necessary to adequately cover affected area(s) with thin layer. Elderly: Start at lower end of dosing range.
Pediatrics: ≥3 months: Apply thin layer to affected area(s) bid. D/C when control is achieved. Max Duration: 4 consecutive weeks. Dispense smallest amount necessary to adequately cover affected area(s) with thin layer.

HOW SUPPLIED: Foam: 0.05% [50g, 100g]

WARNINGS/PRECAUTIONS: Not for oral, ophthalmic, or intravaginal use. May suppress immune system if use of drug is prolonged. May result in systemic absorption and effects including hypothalamic pituitary adrenal (HPA) axis suppression, manifestations of Cushing's syndrome, hyperglycemia, facial swelling, glycosuria, withdrawal syndrome, and growth retardation in children. Periodic evaluation of HPA suppression is required; withdraw, reduce frequency, or substitute a less potent steroid if adrenal suppression is noted. Caution when applied to large surface areas, upon prolonged use, or with addition of occlusive dressing. Pediatric patients may be more susceptible to systemic toxicity. May cause local skin adverse reactions. D/C and institute appropriate therapy if irritation develops. D/C and institute an appropriate antifungal, antibacterial, or antiviral agent if concomitant skin infections are present or develop. Flammable; avoid fire, flame and/or smoking during and immediately following application. Cosyntropin (adrenocorticotropic hormone [ACTH]$_{1-24}$) stimulation test may be helpful in evaluating for HPA axis suppression. Caution in elderly.

ADVERSE REACTIONS: Upper respiratory tract infection, cough, application site burning.

V

INTERACTIONS: Concomitant therapy with topical corticosteroids may produce cumulative effect; use with caution.

PREGNANCY: Category C, caution in nursing.

MECHANISM OF ACTION: Corticosteroid; plays role in cellular signaling, immune function, inflammation, and protein regulation. Precise action of treatment of atopic dermatitis is unknown.

PHARMACOKINETICS: Absorption: Extent of percutaneous absorption is determined by product formulation, integrity of the epidermal barrier, and age. **Distribution:** Systemically administered corticosteroids found in breast milk. **Metabolism:** Liver. **Elimination:** Kidneys, bile (metabolites).

NURSING CONSIDERATIONS

Assessment: Assess use in pregnant/nursing females and for possible drug interactions with concomitant topical corticosteroids.

Monitoring: Monitor for signs/symptoms of reversible HPA-axis suppression, Cushing's syndrome, hyperglycemia, facial swelling, glycosuria, withdrawal syndrome, growth retardation, delayed weight gain, and intracranial HTN in children. Perform periodic monitoring of HPA axis suppression using cosyntropin (ACTH$_{1-24}$) stimulation test if medication is used on large body surface area, used with occlusive dressing, or prolonged use with the drug. Monitor for irritation, concomitant skin infections.

Patient Counseling: Instruct to use as directed; avoid contact with eyes or other mucous membranes. Instruct not to bandage, cover, or wrap so as to be occlusive unless directed. Report any signs of local or systemic adverse reactions. Inform physician about the treatment if surgery is contemplated. Advise to d/c therapy when control is achieved; contact physician if no improvement seen within 4 weeks. Instruct to avoid use of other corticosteroid-containing product without consulting the physician. Inform that medication is flammable; avoid with fire, flame, or smoking during and immediately after application.

Administration: Topical route. Refer to PI for proper administration. **Storage:** 20-25°C (68-77°F). Do not puncture or incinerate. Do not expose containers to heat, and/or store at temperatures above 49°C (120°F).

VERELAN RX
verapamil HCl (UCB)

THERAPEUTIC CLASS: Calcium channel blocker (nondihydropyridine)

INDICATIONS: Management of essential HTN.

DOSAGE: *Adults:* Individualize dose. Usual: 240mg qam. Elderly/Small People: Initial: 120mg qam. Titrate: If inadequate response with 120mg, increase to 180mg qam, then 240mg qam, then 360mg qam, then 480mg qam based on therapeutic efficacy and safety evaluated approximately 24 hrs after dosing. Switching from Immediate-Release Verapamil: Use same total daily dose. May sprinkle on applesauce. Swallow whole; do not crush or chew.

HOW SUPPLIED: Cap, Sustained-Release: 120mg, 180mg, 240mg, 360mg

CONTRAINDICATIONS: Severe left ventricular dysfunction, hypotension (systolic blood pressure [SBP] <90mmHg), cardiogenic shock, sick sinus syndrome, 2nd/3rd-degree atrioventricular (AV) block (except in patients with a functioning ventricular pacemaker), atrial fibrillation (A-fib)/atrial flutter (A-flutter), and an accessory bypass tract (eg, Wolff-Parkinson-White, Lown-Ganong-Levine syndromes).

WARNINGS/PRECAUTIONS: May cause congestive heart failure (CHF), pulmonary edema, hypotension, asymptomatic 1st-degree AV block, transient bradycardia, and PR interval prolongation. Marked 1st-degree block or progressive development to 2nd/3rd-degree AV block requires dose reduction, or d/c and institution of appropriate therapy. Elevated transaminases with and without concomitant elevation in alkaline phosphatase and bilirubin reported; monitor LFTs periodically. Hepatocellular injury reported. Ventricular response/fibrillation has occurred in patients with paroxysmal and/or chronic A-fib/flutter and a coexisting accessory AV pathway. Sinus bradycardia, pulmonary edema, severe hypotension, 2nd-degree AV block, and sinus arrest reported in patients with hypertrophic cardiomyopathy. Caution with hepatic/renal impairment; monitor for abnormal PR interval prolongation. May decrease neuromuscular transmission in patients with Duchenne's muscular dystrophy and may cause worsening of myasthenia gravis; decrease dose with attenuated neuromuscular transmission.

ADVERSE REACTIONS: Constipation, dizziness, headache, lethargy.

INTERACTIONS: May increase levels with CYP3A4 inhibitors (eg, erythromycin, ritonavir) and grapefruit juice. May decrease levels with CYP3A4 inducers (eg, rifampin). Hypotension and bradyarrhythmias reported with telithromycin. May cause myopathy/rhabdomyolysis with HMG-CoA reductase inhibitors that are CYP3A4 substrates; limit dose of simvastatin to 10mg/day or lovastatin to 40mg/day, and may need to lower doses of other CYP3A4 substrates (eg, atorvastatin). Additive negative effects on HR, AV conduction, and contractility with β-blockers;

V

avoid with ventricular dysfunction. Asymptomatic bradycardia with atrial pacemaker has been observed with concomitant use of timolol eye drops. Decreased metoprolol clearance reported. Sinus bradycardia resulting in hospitalization and pacemaker insertion has been reported with the use of clonidine; monitor HR. Chronic treatment may increase digoxin levels, which may result in digitalis toxicity. Additive effects with other antihypertensives (eg, vasodilators, ACE inhibitors, diuretics). Excessive reduction in BP with agents that attenuate α-adrenergic function (eg, prazosin). Avoid disopyramide within 48 hrs before or 24 hrs after verapamil. Additive negative inotropic effects and AV conduction prolongation with flecainide. Avoid quinidine with hypertrophic cardiomyopathy. May increase carbamazepine, cyclosporine, and alcohol effects. Increased bleeding time with aspirin. Cimetidine may either reduce or not change clearance. May increase sensitivity to neurotoxic effects of lithium; monitor lithium levels. Rifampin may reduce oral bioavailability. May increase clearance with phenobarbital. Caution with inhalation anesthetics. May potentiate neuromuscular blockers; both agents may need dose reduction.

PREGNANCY: Category C, not for use in nursing.

MECHANISM OF ACTION: Calcium ion influx inhibitor (nondihydropyridine); inhibits transmembrane influx of ionic calcium into arterial smooth muscle as well as in conductile and contractile myocardial cells.

PHARMACOKINETICS: Absorption: Administration of variable doses resulted in different pharmacokinetic parameters. T_{max}=7-9 hrs. (Immediate-release) Absolute bioavailability (20-35%) **Distribution:** Plasma protein binding (90%); crosses placenta; found in breast milk. **Metabolism:** Liver (extensive), norverapamil (metabolite). **Elimination:** Urine (70%, metabolites; 3-4%, unchanged), feces (≥16%, metabolite); $T_{1/2}$=12 hrs.

NURSING CONSIDERATIONS

Assessment: Assess for ventricular dysfunction, cardiac failure symptoms, cardiogenic shock, sick sinus syndrome, hypertrophic cardiomyopathy, Duchenne's muscular dystrophy, attenuated neuromuscular transmission, and/or any conditions where treatment is contraindicated or cautioned. Assess for pregnancy/nursing status and possible drug interactions.

Monitoring: Monitor signs/symptoms of hypotension, CHF, heart block, ventricular fibrillation, renal/hepatic dysfunction, abnormal prolongation of PR interval and hypersensitivity reactions, and other adverse reactions. Periodically monitor LFTs, BP, ECG changes, and HR.

Patient Counseling: Instruct to swallow cap whole; do not crush or chew. Advise that the entire contents of the capsule can be sprinkled onto a spoonful of applesauce; instruct to swallow the applesauce immediately without chewing and follow with a glass of cool water. Caution that the applesauce should not be hot and should be soft enough to be swallowed without chewing. Instruct to consume the mixture immediately and not store for future use; contents should not be subdivided. Advise to seek medical attention if any adverse reactions occur. Counsel not to breastfeed and to report immediately if pregnant.

Administration: Oral route. **Storage:** 20-25°C (68-77°F). Avoid excessive heat. Brief digressions above 25°C, while not detrimental, should be avoided. Protect from moisture.

VERELAN PM   RX
verapamil HCl (UCB)

THERAPEUTIC CLASS: Calcium channel blocker (nondihydropyridine)

INDICATIONS: Management of essential HTN.

DOSAGE: *Adults:* Individualize dose. Usual: 200mg qhs. Renal or Hepatic Dysfunction/Elderly/Low-Weight Patients: Initial: 100mg qhs. If Inadequate Response with 200mg: May titrate upward to 300mg qhs, then 400mg qhs. Upward titration should be based on the therapeutic efficacy and safety evaluated approximately 24 hrs after dosing. May sprinkle on applesauce. Swallow whole; do not crush or chew.

HOW SUPPLIED: Cap, Extended-Release: 100mg, 200mg, 300mg

CONTRAINDICATIONS: Severe left ventricular dysfunction, hypotension (systolic blood pressure [SBP] <90mmHg), cardiogenic shock, sick sinus syndrome or 2nd/3rd-degree atrioventricular (AV) block (except in patients with a functioning ventricular artificial pacemaker), atrial fibrillation (A-fib)/atrial flutter (A-flutter), and an accessory bypass tract (eg, Wolff-Parkinson-White, Lown-Ganong-Levine syndromes).

WARNINGS/PRECAUTIONS: May cause congestive heart failure (CHF), pulmonary edema, hypotension, asymptomatic 1st-degree AV block, transient bradycardia, and PR interval prolongation. Marked 1st-degree block or progressive development to 2nd/3rd-degree AV block requires dose reduction, or d/c and institution of appropriate therapy. Elevated transaminases with and without concomitant elevations in alkaline phosphatase and bilirubin reported; monitor LFTs periodically. Hepatocellular injury reported. Ventricular response/fibrillation has occurred in patients with paroxysmal and/or chronic A-flutter or A-fib and a coexisting accessory AV pathway.

Sinus bradycardia, pulmonary edema, severe hypotension, 2nd-degree AV block, and sinus arrest reported in patients with hypertrophic cardiomyopathy. Caution with hepatic/renal impairment; monitor for abnormal PR interval prolongation. May decrease neuromuscular transmission in patients with Duchenne's muscular dystrophy and cause worsening of myasthenia gravis; decrease dose with attenuated neuromuscular transmission.

ADVERSE REACTIONS: Headache, infection, constipation, flu syndrome, peripheral edema, dizziness, pharyngitis, sinusitis.

INTERACTIONS: May increase levels with CYP3A4 inhibitors (eg, erythromycin, ritonavir) and grapefruit juice. May decrease levels with CYP3A4 inducers (eg, rifampin). May cause myopathy/rhabdomyolysis with HMG-CoA reductase inhibitors that are CYP3A4 substrates; limit dose of simvastatin to 10mg/day or lovastatin to 40mg/day, and may need to lower doses of other CYP3A4 substrates (eg, atorvastatin). Additive negative effects on HR, AV conduction, and/or cardiac contractility with β-blockers; avoid with ventricular dysfunction. Asymptomatic bradycardia with a wandering atrial pacemaker has been observed with concomitant use of timolol eye drops. Decreased metoprolol and propranolol clearance and variable effect with atenolol reported. Chronic treatment may increase digoxin levels, which may result in digitalis toxicity. Sinus bradycardia resulting in hospitalization and pacemaker insertion reported with the use of clonidine; monitor HR. Hypotension, bradyarrhythmias, and lactic acidocis may occur with concurrent telithromycin use. Reduced absorption with cyclophosphamide, oncovin, procarbazine, prednisone (COPP) and vindesine, adriamycin, cisplatin (VAC) cytotoxic drug regimens. May decrease clearance of paclitaxel. May increase levels of doxorubicin, carbamazepine, cyclosporine, theophylline, and alcohol effects. May increase bleeding time with aspirin. Additive effects with other antihypertensives (eg, vasodilators, ACE inhibitors, diuretics). Excessive reduction in BP with agents that attenuate α-adrenergic function (eg, prazosin). Avoid quinidine with hypertrophic cardiomyopathy. Avoid disopyramide within 48 hrs before or 24 hrs after administration. Additive negative inotropic effects and AV conduction prolongation with flecainide. May increase sensitivity to neurotoxic effects of lithium with or without an increase in serum lithium levels; monitor carefully. Caution with inhalation anesthetics. May potentiate neuromuscular blockers (eg, curare-like and depolarizing); both agents may need dose reduction. Increased clearance with phenobarbital. Reduced oral bioavailability with rifampin. Reduced or unchanged clearance with cimetidine.

PREGNANCY: Category C, not for use in nursing.

MECHANISM OF ACTION: Calcium channel blocker (nondihydropyridine); inhibits transmembrane influx of ionic calcium into arterial smooth muscle as well as in conductile and contractile myocardial cells without altering serum calcium concentrations.

PHARMACOKINETICS: Absorption: Administration of variable doses resulted in different pharmacokinetic parameters. T_{max}=11 hrs. (Immediate-release) Bioavailability (33-65% [R-enantiomer], 13-34% [S-enantiomer]). **Distribution:** Plasma protein binding (94% to albumin and 92% to α-1 acid glycoprotein [R-enantiomer], 88% to albumin and 86% to α-1 acid glycoprotein [S-enantiomer]); crosses placenta, found in breast milk. **Metabolism:** Liver (extensive); O-demethylation, N-dealkylation via CYP450; norverapamil (active metabolite). **Elimination:** Urine (70%, metabolites, 3-4%, unchanged), feces (≥16%, metabolites).

NURSING CONSIDERATIONS

Assessment: Assess for ventricular dysfunction, cardiac failure symptoms, cardiogenic shock, sick sinus syndrome, hypertrophic cardiomyopathy, Duchenne's muscular dystrophy, attenuated neuromuscular transmission, and/or any conditions where treatment is contraindicated or cautioned. Assess for pregnancy/nursing status and possible drug interactions.

Monitoring: Monitor signs/symptoms of hypotension, CHF, heart block, ventricular fibrillation, renal/hepatic dysfunction, abnormal prolongation of PR interval, hypersensitivity, and other adverse reactions. Periodically monitor LFTs, BP, ECG changes, and HR.

Patient Counseling: Instruct to swallow tab whole; do not chew, break, or crush. Advise that the entire contents of the capsule can be sprinkled onto a tbsp of applesauce; instruct to swallow the applesauce immediately without chewing and follow with a glass of cool water. Caution that the applesauce should not be hot and should be soft enough to be swallowed without chewing. Instruct to consume the mixture immediately and not store for future use; contents should not be subdivided. Advise to seek medical attention if any adverse reactions occur. Counsel not to breastfeed and to report immediately if pregnant.

Administration: Oral route. May sprinkle on applesauce. Swallow whole; do not crush or chew.
Storage: 25°C (77°F); excursions permitted to 15-30°C (59-86°F). Protect from moisture.

VESICARE   RX
solifenacin succinate (Astellas)

THERAPEUTIC CLASS: Muscarinic antagonist

INDICATIONS: Treatment of overactive bladder with symptoms of urge urinary incontinence, urgency, and urinary frequency.

DOSAGE: *Adults:* Usual: 5mg qd. Titrate: May increase to 10mg qd if 5mg dose is well tolerated. Severe Renal Impairment (CrCl <30mL/min)/Moderate Hepatic Impairment (Child-Pugh B)/With Potent CYP3A4 Inhibitors: Max: 5mg qd.

HOW SUPPLIED: Tab: 5mg, 10mg

CONTRAINDICATIONS: Urinary/gastric retention, uncontrolled narrow-angle glaucoma.

WARNINGS/PRECAUTIONS: Angioedema of the face, lips, tongue, and/or larynx, and (rare) anaphylactic reactions reported; d/c and provide appropriate therapy if involvement of tongue, hypopharynx, or larynx occurs, or anaphylactic reactions develop. Risk of urinary retention; caution with clinically significant bladder outflow obstruction. Caution with decreased GI motility, controlled narrow-angle glaucoma, renal/hepatic impairment, and history of QT prolongation. Not recommended with severe hepatic impairment (Child-Pugh C).

ADVERSE REACTIONS: Dry mouth, constipation, nausea, dyspepsia, urinary tract infection, blurred vision.

INTERACTIONS: Ketoconazole may increase levels; doses >5mg not recommended in patients taking potent CYP3A4 inhibitors (eg, ketoconazole). CYP3A4 inducers may decrease concentration. Caution with medications known to prolong the QT interval.

PREGNANCY: Category C, not for use in nursing.

MECHANISM OF ACTION: Competitive muscarinic receptor antagonist; inhibits muscarinic receptors in the bladder, which affects contractions of urinary bladder smooth muscle and stimulation of salivary secretion.

PHARMACOKINETICS: Absorption: Absolute bioavailability (90%); T_{max}=3-8 hrs. **Distribution:** V_d=600L; plasma protein binding (98%). **Metabolism:** Liver (extensive) via CYP3A4 (N-oxidation, 4R-hydroxylation); 4R-hydroxy solifenacin (active metabolite). **Elimination:** Urine (69.2%, <15% unchanged), feces (22.5%); $T_{1/2}$=45-68 hrs.

NURSING CONSIDERATIONS

Assessment: Assess for hypersensitivity to drug, other conditions where treatment is contraindicated or cautioned, renal/hepatic function, pregnancy/nursing status, and possible drug interactions.

Monitoring: Monitor for angioedema, upper airway swelling, anaphylactic reactions, and other adverse reactions.

Patient Counseling: Inform that constipation may occur; advise to contact physician if severe abdominal pain or constipation ≥3 days occurs. Inform that blurred vision may occur; advise to exercise caution when engaging in potentially dangerous activities until effects have been determined. Inform that heat prostration (due to decreased sweating) may occur when used in a hot environment. Inform that angioedema may occur, which could result in fatal airway obstruction; advise to promptly d/c and seek immediate attention if tongue/laryngopharyngeal edema or difficulty breathing occurs. Instruct to take drug with water and swallow whole; may be taken with or without food.

Administration: Oral route. Take with water and swallow whole. **Storage:** 25°C (77°F); excursions permitted to 15-30°C (59-86°F).

VFEND
voriconazole (Pfizer)

RX

THERAPEUTIC CLASS: Azole antifungal

INDICATIONS: Used in patients ≥12 yrs for the treatment of invasive aspergillosis; esophageal candidiasis; candidemia in non-neutropenic patients and the following *Candida* infections: disseminated infections in skin and infections in abdomen, kidney, bladder wall, and wounds; serious fungal infections caused by *Scedosporium apiospermum* and *Fusarium* spp. including *Fusarium solani* in patients intolerant of, or refractory to, other therapy.

DOSAGE: *Adults:* Aspergillosis/Scedosporiosis/Fusariosis: LD: 6mg/kg IV q12h for 1st 24 hrs. Maint: IV: 4mg/kg q12h; continue for ≥7 days. Switch to PO form when appropriate. PO: ≥40kg: 200mg q12h; increase to 300mg q12h if inadequate response. <40kg: 100mg q12h; increase to 150mg q12h if inadequate response. Candidemia (Non-Neutropenic Patients) and other Deep Tissue *Candida* Infections: LD: 6mg/kg IV q12h for 1st 24 hrs. Maint: IV: 3-4mg/kg q12h. PO: Follow maint dose for aspergillosis. Treat for ≥14 days after resolution of symptoms or last positive culture, whichever is longer. Esophageal Candidiasis: Maint: PO: Follow maint dose for Aspergillosis. Treat for ≥14 days and for ≥7 days after resolution of symptoms. Intolerant to Dose Increase: IV: Reduce 4mg/kg q12h to 3mg/kg q12h. PO: Reduce by 50mg steps to minimum of 200mg q12h for ≥40kg or 100mg q12h for <40kg. With Phenytoin: Maint: IV: 5mg/kg q12h. PO:

≥40kg: 400mg q12h. <40kg: 200mg q12h. With Efavirenz: Maint: PO: 400mg q12h and decrease efavirenz to 300mg q24h. Mild to Moderate Hepatic Cirrhosis (Child-Pugh Class A and B): Maint: 1/2 of usual maint dose. CrCl <50mL/min: Use PO. Therapy Duration: Consider severity of disease, recovery from immunosuppression, and clinical response.

HOW SUPPLIED: Inj: 200mg; Sus: 40mg/mL; Tab: 50mg, 200mg

CONTRAINDICATIONS: Concomitant terfenadine, astemizole, cisapride, pimozide, quinidine, sirolimus, rifampin, carbamazepine, long-acting barbiturates, high-dose ritonavir (400mg q12h), rifabutin, ergot alkaloids (ergotamine and dihydroergotamine), St. John's wort. Low-dose ritonavir (100mg q12h) should be avoided unless an assessment of benefit/risk justifies the use.

WARNINGS/PRECAUTIONS: Serious hepatic reactions (eg, clinical hepatitis, cholestasis, fulminant hepatic failure) reported (uncommon); monitor LFTs at initiation and during therapy and consider d/c if liver disease develops. Optic neuritis and papilledema reported with prolonged use; monitor visual function with treatment >28 days. May cause fetal harm. Tabs contain lactose; avoid with hereditary galactose intolerance, Lapp lactase deficiency, or glucose-galactose malabsorption. May prolong QT interval, and arrhythmias may occur; caution with proarrhythmic conditions. Anaphylactoid-type reactions reported with infusion; consider d/c of infusion if reactions occur. Correct electrolyte imbalance (eg, hypokalemia, hypomagnesemia, hypocalcemia) before starting therapy. Associated with elevations in LFTs and liver damage (eg, jaundice); caution with hepatic insufficiency. Acute renal failure may occur; monitor for development of abnormal renal function. Monitor for pancreatitis in patients with risk factors for acute pancreatitis (eg, recent chemotherapy, hematopoietic stem cell transplantation) during treatment. May cause serious exfoliative cutaneous reactions (eg, Stevens-Johnson syndrome) and photosensitivity skin reaction; d/c if exfoliative cutaneous reaction or skin lesion consistent with squamous cell carcinoma or melanoma develops. Fluorosis and periostitis reported with long-term therapy; d/c if skeletal pain and radiologic findings compatible with fluorosis and periostitis develops.

ADVERSE REACTIONS: Visual disturbances, fever, chills, rash, headache, N/V, increased alkaline phosphatase.

INTERACTIONS: See Contraindications. Avoid with fluconazole. Efavirenz, phenytoin decreased levels. Non-nucleoside reverse transcriptase inhibitors (NNRTIs) may decrease levels. Cimetidine, omeprazole, oral contraceptives (containing ethinyl estradiol and norethindrone), fluconazole increased levels. HIV protease inhibitors (eg, saquinavir, amprenavir, nelfinavir), NNRTIs (eg, delavirdine) may increase levels. Increased levels of efavirenz, oral contraceptives (containing ethinyl estradiol and norethindrone), cyclosporine, fentanyl, alfentanil, oxycodone, NSAIDs (eg, ibuprofen, diclofenac, celecoxib, naproxen, lornoxicam, meloxicam), tacrolimus, phenytoin, prednisolone, omeprazole, methadone. May increase levels of HIV protease inhibitors, NNRTIs, proton pump inhibitors, statins (eg, lovastatin), benzodiazepines (eg, midazolam, triazolam, alprazolam), calcium channel blockers (eg, felodipine), sulfonylureas (eg, tolbutamide, glipizide, glyburide), vinca alkaloids (eg, vincristine, vinblastine). Increased PT with warfarin. May increase levels of oral coumarin anticoagulants and increase PT. Inhibitors or inducers of CYP2C19, CYP2C9, and CYP3A4 may increase or decrease voriconazole systemic exposure, respectively. May increase systemic exposure of other drugs metabolized by CYP2C9, CYP2C19, and CYP3A4.

PREGNANCY: Category D, not for use in nursing.

MECHANISM OF ACTION: Triazole antifungal agent; inhibits fungal CYP450-mediated 14 α-lanosterol demethylation, an essential step in fungal ergosterol biosynthesis. Accumulation of 14 α-methyl-sterols correlates with subsequent loss of ergosterol in fungal cell wall and may be responsible for antifungal activity of voriconazole.

PHARMACOKINETICS: Absorption: Administration of different doses led to varying parameters. T_{max}=1-2 hrs. **Distribution:** V_d=4.6L/kg; plasma protein binding (58%). **Metabolism:** Hepatic via CYP2C19, 2C9, and 3A4; N-oxide (major metabolite). **Elimination:** Urine (80-83%, <2% unchanged).

NURSING CONSIDERATIONS

Assessment: Obtain fungal cultures prior to therapy to properly identify causative organisms. Assess for proarrhythmic conditions, hematological malignancy, known hypersensitivity to drug or excipient, hereditary problems of galactose intolerance, Lapp lactase deficiency or glucose-galactose malabsorption, history of cardiotoxic chemotherapy, cardiomyopathy, hypokalemia, arrhythmias, hepatic/renal insufficiency, electrolyte disturbances, pregnancy/nursing status, and for possible drug interactions. Obtain baseline LFTs.

Monitoring: Monitor visual acuity, visual field, and color perception with treatment >28 days. Monitor for infusion-related reactions, hepatotoxicity, arrhythmias, QT prolongation, acute renal failure, pancreatitis, fluorosis, periostitis, and dermatological reactions (eg, Stevens-Johnson syndrome, exfoliative cutaneous reactions, skin lesions). Monitor for drug toxicity with hepatic insufficiencies. Monitor renal function (SrCr) and hepatic function (LFTs, bilirubin) during therapy.

Patient Counseling: Counsel to take tabs or oral suspension at least 1 hr ac or 1 hr pc. Advise to avoid driving at night; drug may affect vision. Counsel to avoid hazardous tasks such as driving or operating machinery while taking the drug until it is known how the drug affects the patient.

Advise to avoid intense or prolonged exposure to direct sunlight. Counsel females to use proper contraception during therapy. Inform of the signs and symptoms of liver problems, allergic reactions, vision changes, and serious skin reactions and advise to call the physician if any of the conditions above develop.

Administration: Oral and IV route. Oral Sus/Tab: Take at least 1 hr ac or 1 hr pc. Reconstitute suspension by adding 46mL of water to bottle and shake vigorously for about 1 min. Refer to PI for IV preparation instructions. Refer to PI for use with other parenteral drug products. **Storage:** Inj: Unreconstituted: 15-30°C (59-86°F). Reconstituted: 2-8°C (36-46°F) for 24 hrs. Tab: 15-30°C (59-86°F). Oral Sus: Unreconstituted: 2-8°C (36-46°F) for 18 months. Reconstituted: 15-30°C (59-86°F) for 14 days. Do not refrigerate or freeze. Keep container tightly closed.

VIAGRA   RX
sildenafil citrate (Pfizer)

THERAPEUTIC CLASS: Phosphodiesterase type 5 inhibitor

INDICATIONS: Treatment of erectile dysfunction (ED).

DOSAGE: *Adults:* Usual: 50mg qd PRN 1 hr (recommended) or 0.5 to 4 hrs prior to sexual activity. Titrate: May decrease to 25mg or increase to 100mg qd based on effectiveness and tolerance. Max: 100mg qd. Elderly/Hepatic Impairment/CrCl <30mL/min/Concomitant Potent CYP3A4 Inhibitors (eg, ketoconazole, itraconazole, erythromycin, saquinavir): Initial: 25mg qd. Concomitant Ritonavir: Max: 25mg q48h. Concomitant α-blocker: Patient should be stable on α-blocker therapy. Initiate sildenafil at lowest dose.

HOW SUPPLIED: Tab: 25mg, 50mg, 100mg

CONTRAINDICATIONS: Organic nitrates, either taken regularly and/or intermittently, in any form.

WARNINGS/PRECAUTIONS: Potential for cardiac risk of sexual activity in patients with cardiovascular disease (CVD); avoid in men where sexual activity is inadvisable due to underlying cardiovascular status. Decrease in supine BP reported; caution in patients with left ventricular outflow obstruction (eg, aortic stenosis, idiopathic hypertrophic subaortic stenosis) and severely impaired autonomic control of BP. Prolonged erection (>4 hrs) and priapism reported. Caution with myocardial infarction (MI), stroke, or life-threatening arrhythmia within last 6 months; resting hypotension (BP<90/50) or HTN (BP>170/110), unstable angina due to cardiac failure or coronary artery disease (CAD), retinitis pigmentosa, sickle cell or related anemias, anatomical penile deformation (eg, angulation, cavernosal fibrosis, Peyronie's disease), and predisposition to priapism (eg, multiple myeloma, leukemia). Not indicated for use in newborns, children, or women. Safety not known in patients with bleeding disorders and active peptic ulceration. Rare reports of non-arteritic anterior ischemic optic neuropathy (NAION) with PDE5 inhibitors. Cases of sudden decrease or loss of hearing reported.

ADVERSE REACTIONS: Headache, flushing, dyspepsia, nasal congestion, urinary tract infection, abnormal vision (eg, color tinge, increased light sensitivity, blurred vision), diarrhea.

INTERACTIONS: See Contraindications. Contraindicated with nitric oxide donors. Increased levels with CYP3A4 inhibitors (eg, ketoconazole, itraconazole, erythromycin), protease inhibitors (eg, ritonavir, saquinavir) and cimetidine. Reduced clearance with CYP2C9 inhibitors. Increased clearance with CYP3A4 inducers (eg, rifampin, bosentan) and CYP2C9 inducers. Increased levels of bosentan. Additional supine BP reduction with amlodipine reported. Additive hypotensive effect with α-blockers (eg, doxazosin) and vasodilators (eg, minoxidil). May augment BP-lowering effect of other antihypertensives. Avoid with other treatments for ED. Loop and K⁺-sparing diuretics and nonselective β-blockers increase area under the curve of N-desmethyl sildenafil. May potentiate antiaggregatory effect of sodium nitroprusside.

PREGNANCY: Category B, not for use in nursing.

MECHANISM OF ACTION: Phosphodiesterase type 5 (PDE5) inhibitor; enhances effect of nitric oxide by inhibiting PDE5, which then increase the levels of cGMP in corpus cavernosum, resulting in smooth muscle relaxation and inflow of blood to corpus cavernosum.

PHARMACOKINETICS: Absorption: Rapid; absolute bioavailability (41%). Fasted state: T_{max}=30-120 min. High fat meal: T_{max}=delayed 60 min; C_{max}=reduction of 29%. **Distribution:** V_d=105L; plasma protein binding (96%). **Metabolism:** Liver, via CYP450 3A4 (major), 2C9 (minor); N-desmethyl sildenafil (major metabolite). **Elimination:** Feces (80% metabolites), urine (13%); $T_{1/2}$=4 hrs.

NURSING CONSIDERATIONS

Assessment: Assess for previous hypersensitivity to drug, CVD, left ventricular outflow obstruction, impaired autonomic control of BP; history of MI, stroke, or arrhythmia; resting hypotension or HTN, cardiac failure, CAD, sickle cell anemia, predisposing conditions to priapism, retinitis pigmentosa, bleeding disorders, active peptic ulceration, anatomical deformation of penis, renal/hepatic impairment, potential underlying causes of ED, and possible drug interactions.

Monitoring: Monitor potential for hypersensitivity reactions, abnormalities in vision, decrease/loss of hearing, prolonged erection, priapism, and other adverse reactions.

Patient Counseling: Instruct to seek medical assistance if erection persists >4 hrs. Inform of potential BP-lowering effect with α-blockers and antihypertensive drugs, and potential cardiac risk of sexual activity in patients with preexisting CV risk factors. Instruct not to take with other PDE5 inhibitors and organic nitrates. Counsel about protective measures necessary to guard against sexually transmitted diseases, including HIV; to d/c and seek medical attention if sudden decrease/loss of vision or hearing occur; and to take a tab 1 hr before sexual activity.

Administration: Oral route. **Storage:** 25°C (77°F); excursions permitted to 15-30°C (59-86°F).

VIBATIV   RX
telavancin (Astellas)

> Women of childbearing potential should have a serum pregnancy test prior to administration. Avoid use during pregnancy unless potential benefit to the patient outweighs the potential risk to the fetus. Potential adverse developmental outcomes in humans may occur.

THERAPEUTIC CLASS: Antibacterial agent

INDICATIONS: Treatment of adult patients with complicated skin and skin structure infections (cSSSI) caused by susceptible Gram-positive microorganisms.

DOSAGE: *Adults:* cSSSI: Initial: 10mg/kg IV q24h for 7-14 days. Administer over a 60-minute period by IV infusion. Duration of therapy depend on the severity, site of infection, and patient's clinical and bacteriologial process. Renal Impairment: CrCl 30-50mL/min: 7.5 mg/kg q24h. CrCl 10-<30mL/min: 10mg/kg q48h.

HOW SUPPLIED: Inj: 250mg, 750mg

WARNINGS/PRECAUTIONS: New onset or worsening of renal impairment may occur; monitor renal function. Decreased efficacy with moderate/severe baseline renal impairment (CrCl ≤50mL/min). Infusion-related reactions (eg, "red man syndrome"-like reactions) may occur with rapid infusion. *Clostridium difficile*-associated diarrhea (CDAD) reported. May result in bacterial resistance with prolonged use or use in the absence of a proven/suspected bacterial infection or a prophylactic indication; take appropriate measures if superinfection develops. QTc interval prolongation reported; avoid in patients with congenital long QT syndrome, known prolongation of the QTc interval, uncompensated heart failure, or severe left ventricular hypertrophy. May interfere with coagulation tests such as PT, INR, activated partial thromboplastin time (aPTT), activated clotting time, and coagulation-based factor Xa; collect sample as close as possible prior to next dose.

ADVERSE REACTIONS: Taste disturbance, N/V, foamy urine, rigors, pruritus (generalized), diarrhea, dizziness, decreased appetite, rash, infusion-site pain, infusion-site erythema.

INTERACTIONS: Caution with drugs known to prolong QT interval. Higher renal adverse events rate with concomitant medications known to affect kidney function (eg, NSAIDs, ACE inhibitors, loop diuretics).

PREGNANCY: Category C, caution in nursing.

MECHANISM OF ACTION: Antibacterial agent: Lipoglycopeptide; inhibits bacterial cell wall synthesis by interfering with the polymerization and cross-linking of peptidoglycan. Binds to the bacterial membrane and disrupts membrane barrier function.

PHARMACOKINETICS: Absorption: (Single dose) C_{max}=93.6mcg/mL; AUC=747mcg•hr/mL, (Multiple Dose) C_{max}=108mcg/mL. **Distribution:** Plasma protein binding (90%). (Single dose) V_d=145mL/kg. (Multiple dose) V_d=133mL/kg. **Excretion:** Urine (76%), feces (<1%); (Single dose) $T_{1/2}$=8 hr. (Multiple dose) $T_{1/2}$=8.1 hr.

NURSING CONSIDERATIONS

Assessment: Assess for renal impairment, renal impairment risk (eg, pre-existing renal disease, DM, CHF, HTN), congenital long QT syndrome, known prolongation of the QTc interval, uncompensated heart failure, severe left ventricular hypertrophy, concomitant drugs that prolong QTc interval, nursing status, and possible drug interactions. Perform pregnancy test prior to initiation. Obtain baseline SrCr, CrCl and ECG.

Monitoring: Monitor renal function (eg, SrCr). Monitor for CDAD, superinfection, and infusion-related reactions (eg, "red man syndrome"-like reactions).

Patient Counseling: Inform patients of risk of fetal harm when used during pregnancy; perform pregnancy test prior to administration. Encourage women capable of child-bearing to use contraceptives while on therapy. Notify healthcare provider if pregnancy occurs and encourage patients to enroll themselves in pregnancy registry. Inform physicians if watery and bloody stools (with or without stomach cramps or fever) occur as late as 2 months after the last dose of antibiotics. Antibacterial drugs should only be used to treat bacterial infections and not to treat

V

viral infection. Take as directed. Skipping doses or failure to complete the full course of therapy may decrease effectiveness of immediate treatment and may increase the development of drug-resistant bacteria. Counsel about the common adverse effects; notify physician if any unusual or known symptoms persist or worsens.
Administration: IV route. Infuse over 60 min. Refer to PI for preparation and reconstitution. Additives or other medications should not be added to single-use vials or infused simultaneously through the same IV line. If same IV line is used for sequential infusion of additional medications, the line should be flushed before and after infusion. **Storage:** 2-8°C (36-46°F); excursions permitted to ambient temperature (up to 25°C [77°F]). Avoid excessive heat. (Diluted/Reconstituted) Use within 4 hrs when stored at room temperature or within 72 hrs when stored under refrigeration at 2-8°C (36-46°F).

VIBRAMYCIN   RX
doxycycline (Pfizer)

OTHER BRAND NAMES: Vibra-Tabs (Pfizer)
THERAPEUTIC CLASS: Tetracycline derivative
INDICATIONS: Treatment of the following infections caused by susceptible microorganisms: Rocky Mountain spotted fever, typhus fever and the typhus group, Q fever, rickettsialpox, tick fevers, respiratory tract infections, lymphogranuloma venereum, psittacosis (ornithosis), trachoma, inclusion conjunctivitis, uncomplicated urethral, endocervical, or rectal infections, nongonococcal urethritis, relapsing fever, chancroid, plague, tularemia, cholera, *Campylobacter fetus* infections, brucellosis, bartonellosis, granuloma inguinale, urinary tract infections (UTI), anthrax. Treatment of infections caused by susceptible strains of: *Escherichia coli, Enterobacter aerogenes, Shigella* species, *Acinetobacter* species. When penicillin is contraindicated, treatment of the following infections caused by susceptible microorganisms: uncomplicated gonorrhea, syphilis, yaws, listeriosis, Vincent's infection, actinomycosis, infections caused by *Clostridium* species. Adjunct in acute intestinal amebiasis and severe acne. Prophylaxis of malaria due to *Plasmodium falciparum.*
DOSAGE: *Adults:* Usual: 100mg q12h on Day 1. Maint: 100mg/day. Severe Infections (eg, Chronic UTI): 100mg q12h. Streptococcal Infections: Continue for 10 days. Uncomplicated Gonococcal Infections (Except Anorectal in Men): 100mg bid for 7 days or as an alternate single visit dose, 300mg stat followed in 1 hr by a 2nd 300mg dose; may take with food, including milk or carbonated beverage PRN. Uncomplicated Urethral/Endocervical/Rectal Infections and Nongonococcal Urethritis: 100mg bid for 7 days. Early Syphilis: 100mg bid for 2 weeks. Syphilis (>1 yr duration): 100mg bid for 4 weeks. Acute Epididymo-Orchitis: 100mg bid for ≥10 days. Malaria Prophylaxis: 100mg qd. Begin 1-2 days before travel and continue daily during and for 4 weeks after leaving malarious area. Inhalational Anthrax (Post-Exposure): 100mg bid for 60 days. *Pediatrics:* >8 yrs: ≤100 lbs: 1mg/lb bid on Day 1 then 1mg/lb qd or divided into 2 doses, on subsequent days. Severe Infections: up to 2mg/lb. >100 lbs: Usual: 100mg q12h on Day 1. Maint: 100mg/day. Severe Infections (eg, Chronic UTI): 100mg q12h. Streptococcal Infections: Continue for 10 days. Malaria Prophylaxis: >8 yrs: 2mg/kg qd. Max: 100mg/day. Begin 1-2 days before travel and continue daily during and for 4 weeks after leaving malarious area. Inhalation Anthrax (Post-Exposure): <100 lbs (45kg): 1mg/lb (2.2mg/kg) bid for 60 days. ≥100 lbs: 100mg bid for 60 days.
HOW SUPPLIED: Cap: (Vibramycin Hyclate) 100mg; Sus: (Vibramycin Monohydrate) 25mg/5mL [60mL]; Syrup: (Vibramycin Calcium) 50mg/5mL [473mL]; Tab: (Vibra-Tabs) 100mg
WARNINGS/PRECAUTIONS: May cause permanent tooth discoloration if administered during tooth development (last half of pregnancy, infancy, and children <8 yrs); avoid use in these age groups for indications other than anthrax. Enamel hypoplasia and *Clostridium difficile*-associated diarrhea (CDAD) reported. May result in bacterial resistance with prolonged use or use in the absence of a proven/suspected bacterial infection or a prophylactic indication; take appropriate measures if superinfection develops. May decrease fibula growth rate in premature infants or cause fetal harm during pregnancy. Photosensitivity, increased BUN, and false elevations of urinary catecholamines may occur; d/c at 1st evidence of skin erythema. Syrup contains sodium metabisulfite that may cause allergic-type reactions. Bulging fontanels in infants and benign intracranial HTN in adults reported. When used for malaria prophylaxis, patients may still transmit the infection to mosquitoes outside endemic areas.
ADVERSE REACTIONS: Anorexia, N/V, diarrhea, maculopapular/erythematous rash, Stevens-Johnson syndrome, toxic epidermal necrolysis, photosensitivity, increased BUN, hypersensitivity reactions, hemolytic anemia, thrombocytopenia, neutropenia, eosinophilia.
INTERACTIONS: May interfere with bactericidal action of penicillin; avoid concurrent use. May depress plasma prothrombin activity, may require downward adjustment of anticoagulant dose. Impaired absorption with bismuth subsalicylate; antacid containing aluminum, calcium, and magnesium; and iron-containing preparations. Decreased $T_{1/2}$ with barbiturates, carbamazepine,

V

and phenytoin. Fatal renal toxicity reported with methoxyflurane. May render oral contraceptives less effective.

PREGNANCY: Category D, not for use in nursing.

MECHANISM OF ACTION: Tetracycline derivative; thought to exert bacteriostatic effect by inhibition of protein synthesis.

PHARMACOKINETICS: Absorption: Complete; (200mg) C_{max}=2.6mcg/mL, T_{max}=2 hrs. **Distribution:** Found in breast milk. **Elimination:** Urine (40%), feces; $T_{1/2}$=18-22 hrs.

NURSING CONSIDERATIONS

Assessment: Assess for previous hypersensitivity to the drug, pregnancy/nursing status, and possible drug interactions. Perform incision and drainage in conjunction with antibiotic therapy when indicated. Document indications for therapy as well as culture and susceptibility testing results. Perform dark-field examinations and blood serology when coexistent syphilis is suspected.

Monitoring: Monitor for signs/symptoms of hypersensitivity reactions, photosensitivity, superinfection, CDAD, vaginal candidiasis, bulging fontanels in infants, and benign intracranial HTN in adults. In venereal disease with coexistent syphilis, conduct blood serology monthly for ≥4 months. Perform periodic laboratory evaluation of organ systems including hematopoietic, renal, and hepatic studies in long-term therapy.

Patient Counseling: Apprise pregnant women of the potential hazard to fetus. Inform that the therapy does not guarantee protection against malaria; use measures that help avoid contact with mosquitoes. Avoid excessive sunlight/UV light and d/c therapy if phototoxicity occurs. Avoid foods with calcium; antacids containing aluminum, calcium, or magnesium; and bismuth subsalicylate. Drink fluids liberally. Drug may increase the incidence of vaginal candidiasis. Take exactly as directed; skipping doses or not completing full course may decrease effectiveness and increase resistance. Inform that diarrhea may be experienced and advise to notify physician as soon as possible if watery/bloody stools (with or without stomach cramps and fever) even as late as ≥2 months after last dose occur. Counsel to begin malaria prophylaxis therapy 1-2 days before travel, continue while in the malarious area and for 4 weeks after return; do not exceed 4 months.

Administration: Oral route. Take caps/tabs with adequate fluids. Take with food or milk if gastric irritation occurs. **Storage:** <30°C (86°F); tight, light-resistant container.

VICODIN

CIII

hydrocodone bitartrate - acetaminophen (Abbott)

Associated with cases of acute liver failure, at times resulting in liver transplant and death. Most cases associated with acetaminophen (APAP) doses >4000 mg/day and involved more than one APAP-containing product.

OTHER BRAND NAMES: Vicodin HP (Abbott) - Vicodin ES (Abbott)

THERAPEUTIC CLASS: Opioid analgesic

INDICATIONS: Relief of moderate to moderately severe pain.

DOSAGE: *Adults:* Adjust dose according to severity of pain and response. Usual: Vicodin: 1 or 2 tab q4-6h PRN. Max: 8 tab/day. Vicodin HP: 1 tab q4-6h PRN. Max: 6 tab/day. Vicodin ES: 1 tab q4-6h PRN. Max: 5 tab/day. Elderly: Start at lower end of dosing range.

HOW SUPPLIED: Tab: (Hydrocodone-APAP) 5mg-500mg*; (Vicodin HP) 10mg-660mg*; (Vicodin ES) 7.5mg-750mg* *scored

WARNINGS/PRECAUTIONS: Hypersensitivity/anaphylaxis reported; d/c if signs/symptoms occur. May produce dose-related respiratory depression, and irregular and periodic breathing. Respiratory depressant effects and CSF pressure elevation may be markedly exaggerated in the presence of head injury, other intracranial lesions or a preexisting increased intracranial pressure. May obscure diagnosis or clinical course of head injuries or acute abdominal conditions. Potential for abuse. Caution in elderly or debilitated, severe hepatic/renal dysfunction, hypothyroidism, Addison's disease, prostatic hypertrophy, or urethral stricture. Increased risk of acute liver failure in patients with underlying liver disease. Suppresses the cough reflex; caution with pulmonary disease and in postoperative use.

ADVERSE REACTIONS: Acute liver failure, lightheadedness, dizziness, sedation, N/V.

INTERACTIONS: Additive CNS depression with other narcotic analgesics, antihistamines, antipsychotics, antianxiety agents, or other CNS depressants (eg, alcohol); reduce dose. Concomitant use with MAOIs or TCAs may increase the effect of either the antidepressant or hydrocodone. Increased risk of acute liver failure with alcohol ingestion.

PREGNANCY: Category C, not for use in nursing.

MECHANISM OF ACTION: Hydrocodone: Opioid analgesic; not established. Suspected to relate to the existence of opiate receptors in CNS. APAP: Nonopiate, nonsalicylate analgesic and antipyretic; not established. Antipyretic activity mediated through hypothalamic heat-regulating centers; inhibits prostaglandin synthetase.

PHARMACOKINETICS: Absorption: Hydrocodone: (10mg) C_{max}=23.6ng/mL; T_{max}=1.3 hrs. APAP: Rapid. **Distribution:** APAP: Found in breast milk. **Metabolism:** Hydrocodone: O-demethylation, N-demethylation, and 6-keto reduction. APAP: Liver (conjugation). **Elimination:** Hydrocodone: $T_{1/2}$=3.8 hrs. APAP: Urine (85%); $T_{1/2}$=1.25-3 hrs.

NURSING CONSIDERATIONS

Assessment: Assess for hypersensitivity to other opioids and APAP, head injury, intracranial lesions, preexisting increased intracranial pressure, acute abdominal conditions, hepatic/renal impairment, pregnancy/nursing status, possible drug interactions, or any other conditions where treatment is contraindicated or cautioned.

Monitoring: Monitor for signs/symptoms of hypersensitivity or anaphylaxis, respiratory depression, elevations in CSF pressure, drug abuse, tolerance, and dependence. Perform serial liver and/or renal function tests in patients with severe hepatic/renal disease.

Patient Counseling: Instruct to not use >1 product that contains APAP; immediately seek medical attention upon ingestion of >4000mg/day APAP. Instruct to d/c therapy and contact physician if signs of allergy (eg, rash, difficulty breathing) develop. Caution that drug may impair mental/ physical abilities required for performance of potentially hazardous tasks (eg, driving, operating machinery). Avoid alcohol and other CNS depressants. Inform that drug may be habit forming; only take ud.

Administration: Oral route. **Storage:** 25°C (77°F); excursions permitted to 15-30°C (59-86°F).

VICOPROFEN   CIII
hydrocodone bitartrate - ibuprofen (Abbott)

OTHER BRAND NAMES: Reprexain (Hawthorn Pharmaceuticals)
THERAPEUTIC CLASS: Opioid analgesic
INDICATIONS: Short-term (generally <10 days) management of acute pain.
DOSAGE: *Adults:* Usual: 1 tab q4-6h PRN. Max: 5 tabs/day. Use lowest effective dose or longest dosing interval consistent with individual treatment goals. Elderly: Reduce dose. *Pediatrics:* ≥16 yrs: Usual: 1 tab q4-6h PRN. Max: 5 tabs/day. Use lowest effective dose or longest dosing interval consistent with individual treatment goals.
HOW SUPPLIED: (Hydrocodone-Ibuprofen) Tab: (Vicoprofen) 7.5mg-200mg; (Reprexain) 2.5mg-200mg, 5mg-200mg, 10mg-200mg
CONTRAINDICATIONS: Aspirin (ASA) or other NSAID allergy that precipitates asthma, urticaria, or other allergic reactions. Perioperative pain in the setting of coronary artery bypass graft (CABG) surgery.
WARNINGS/PRECAUTIONS: Not for treatment of corticosteroid insufficiency or substitute for corticosteroids. May diminish utility of fever and inflammation as diagnostic signs in detecting complications of presumed noninfectious, painful conditions. Caution in elderly. Ibuprofen: May increase risk of serious cardiovascular (CV) thrombotic events, myocardial infarction (MI), and stroke. May cause or worsen HTN. May cause renal toxicity; not recommended with advanced renal disease. Caution with renal disease, coagulation disorders, asthma, fluid retention, heart failure, HTN, history of ulcer disease or GI bleeding. Anaphylactoid reactions may occur. Avoid with ASA-triad and ASA-sensitive asthma, and late pregnancy. May cause serious skin adverse events (eg, exfoliative dermatitis, Stevens-Johnson syndrome, toxic epidermal necrolysis). May increase risk of GI ulceration, bleeding, perforation. Anemia, fluid retention, edema, severe hepatic reactions reported. D/C if liver disease develops or if systemic manifestations occur. May inhibit platelet aggregation and prolong bleeding time. Possible risk of aseptic meningitis, especially in systemic lupus erythematosus patients. Hydrocodone: May increase risk of misuse, abuse, or diversion. May produce dose-related respiratory depression. Respiratory depressant effects and CSF pressure elevation may be markedly exaggerated in the presence of head injury, intracranial lesions, or preexisting increased intracranial pressure. May obscure diagnosis/clinical course of acute abdominal conditions or the clinical course of head injuries. Caution in debilitated, severe impairment of hepatic/renal function, hypothyroidism, Addison's disease, prostatic hypertrophy, and urethral stricture. Suppresses cough reflex; use caution postoperatively and in pulmonary disease.
ADVERSE REACTIONS: Headache, somnolence, dizziness, constipation, dyspepsia, N/V, infection, edema, nervousness, anxiety, pruritus, diarrhea, asthenia, abdominal pain.
INTERACTIONS: Additive CNS depression with other opioid analgesics, antihistamines, antipsychotics, antianxiety agents, and other CNS depressants (eg, alcohol); reduce dose of one or both agents. Ibuprofen: Increase risk of GI bleeding with oral corticosteroids or anticoagulants. May diminish antihypertensive effect of ACE inhibitors. May increase adverse effects with ASA;

concomitant administration is not recommended. Synergistic effects on GI bleeding with warfarin. May decrease natriuretic effects of furosemide and loop or thiazide diuretics; monitor for renal failure. May increase lithium levels; monitor for lithium toxicity. May enhance methotrexate toxicity; caution when coadministered. Hydrocodone: Use with MAOIs or TCAs may increase the effect of either the antidepressant or hydrocodone. Not recommended for patients taking MAOIs or within 14 days of stopping such treatment. May produce paralytic ileus with anticholinergics. Caution with concurrent agonist/antagonist analgesics (eg, pentazocine, nalbuphine, naltrexone, and butorphanol) use; may reduce analgesic effect of hydrocodone and/or precipitate withdrawal symptoms. May enhance neuromuscular-blocking action of skeletal muscle relaxants and increase respiratory depression.

PREGNANCY: Category C, not for use in nursing.

MECHANISM OF ACTION: (Hydrocodone): Semisynthetic opioid analgesic; not established. Suspected to relate to existence of opiate receptors in CNS. (Ibuprofen): Nonsteroidal anti-inflammatory agent; not established. Suspected to inhibit cyclooxygenase activity and prostaglandin synthesis. Possesses analgesic and antipyretic activity.

PHARMACOKINETICS: Absorption: Hydrocodone: C_{max}=27ng/mL; T_{max}=1.7 hrs. Ibuprofen: C_{max}=30mcg/mL; T_{max}=1.8 hrs. **Distribution:** Hydrocodone: Plasma protein binding (19-45%). Ibuprofen: Plasma protein binding (99%). **Metabolism:** Hydrocodone: CYP2D6, via O-demethylation to hydromorphone (active metabolite); CYP3A4 via N-demethylation; 6-keto reduction. Ibuprofen: Interconversion from R-isomer to S-isomer; (+)-2-4'-(2-hydroxy-2-methylpropyl) phenyl propionic acid and (+)-2-4'-(2-carboxypropyl) phenyl propionic acid (primary metabolites). **Elimination:** Hydrocodone: Urine (primary); $T_{1/2}$=4.5 hrs. Ibuprofen: Urine (50-60% metabolites, 15% unchanged, conjugate), $T_{1/2}$=2.2 hrs.

NURSING CONSIDERATIONS

Assessment: Assess for hypersensitivity to other opioids, previous reaction to ASA or NSAIDs (eg, asthma, urticaria), type of pain (eg, CABG surgery), renal/hepatic function, pregnancy/nursing status, possible drug interactions, or any other conditions where treatment is contraindicated or cautioned. Obtain baseline BP.

Monitoring: Monitor for signs/symptoms of CV thrombotic events, MI, stroke, HTN, fluid retention and edema, drug abuse and dependence, respiratory depression, elevations in cerebrospinal fluid pressure, GI effects, renal effects (eg, renal papillary necrosis), anaphylactoid reactions, skin reactions, hepatic effects (eg, elevations in hepatic enzymes, jaundice, liver necrosis), hematological effects (eg, anemia), bronchospasm, aseptic meningitis, physical dependence and tolerance, abuse or misuse of medication, hypersensitivity reactions, and withdrawal syndrome during d/c. If signs/symptoms of anemia develop, evaluate Hgb/Hct. Monitor BP while on therapy. If on long-term therapy, perform periodic monitoring of CBC and chemistry profile.

Patient Counseling: Inform that drug cannot be substituted for corticosteroids or treat corticosteroid insufficiency. Caution that drug may impair mental and/or physical abilities required to perform potentially hazardous tasks (eg, operating machinery/driving). Avoid alcohol and other CNS depressants while on therapy. Caution that drug may be habit-forming; take only for as long as prescribed, and not more frequently than prescribed. Instruct to contact physician if CV events (eg, chest pain, SOB, slurring of speech), GI effects (eg, ulcers, bleeding), edema, or weight gain occur. Immediately stop therapy and contact physician if signs/symptoms of skin reactions or hepatotoxicity (eg, nausea, fatigue, jaundice) develop. Seek immediate medical attention if any anaphylactoid reactions (eg, difficulty breathing, facial swelling) develop. Report any signs of blurred vision or other eye symptoms.

Administration: Oral route. **Storage:** 25°C (77°F); excursions permitted to 15-30°C (59-86°F).

VICTOZA   RX
liraglutide (rdna origin) (Novo Nordisk)

> Causes dose-dependent and treatment-duration-dependent thyroid C-cell tumors at clinically relevant exposures in animal studies. It is unknown whether drug causes thyroid C-cell tumors (eg, medullary thyroid carcinoma [MTC]) in humans. Contraindicated in patients with a personal or family history of MTC and with multiple endocrine neoplasia syndrome type 2 (MEN 2). It is unknown whether monitoring with serum calcitonin or thyroid ultrasound will mitigate human risk of thyroid C-cell tumors. Counsel patients on risks and symptoms of thyroid tumors.

THERAPEUTIC CLASS: Incretin mimetic

INDICATIONS: Adjunct to diet and exercise to improve glycemic control in adults with type 2 diabetes mellitus (DM).

DOSAGE: *Adults:* Initial: 0.6mg SQ qd for 1 week. Titrate: Increase to 1.2mg/day after 1 week, then to 1.8mg/day if acceptable glycemic control is not achieved. Reinitiate at 0.6mg if >3 days have elapsed since the last dose and titrate ud. With Insulin Secretagogues (eg, sulfonylureas): Consider reducing the dose of insulin secretagogues. With Insulin: Consider reducing the dose of insulin. Administer as separate inj. May inject in the same body region but the inj should not be adjacent to each other.

HOW SUPPLIED: Inj: 0.6mg, 1.2mg, 1.8mg (6mg/mL, 3mL)

CONTRAINDICATIONS: MEN 2, personal or family history of MTC.

WARNINGS/PRECAUTIONS: Not recommended as 1st-line therapy with inadequate glycemic control on diet and exercise. Not a substitute for insulin; do not use in type 1 DM or for the treatment of diabetic ketoacidosis. Refer patients with thyroid nodules and/or elevated calcitonin levels to an endocrinologist for further evaluation. Pancreatitis reported; observe for signs/symptoms after initiation/dose increases and d/c promptly if suspected and do not restart therapy if confirmed. Acute renal failure and worsening of chronic renal failure reported; caution when initiating/escalating doses in patients with renal impairment. Serious hypersensitivity reactions (eg, anaphylactic reactions, angioedema) reported; d/c if a hypersensitivity reaction occurs. Caution with history of angioedema, history of pancreatitis, and hepatic impairment.

ADVERSE REACTIONS: N/V, diarrhea, constipation, dyspepsia, headache, antibody formation, inj-site reaction.

INTERACTIONS: Consider dose reduction of insulin secretagogues (eg, sulfonylureas) or insulin; may increase the risk of hypoglycemia. May affect the absorption of PO medications; use with caution. May alter levels of digoxin, lisinopril, atorvastatin, acetaminophen, griseofulvin, and oral contraceptives containing ethinyl estradiol and levonorgestrel.

PREGNANCY: Category C, not for use in nursing.

MECHANISM OF ACTION: Human glucagon-like peptide-1 receptor agonist; increases intracellular cyclic AMP, leading to insulin release in the presence of elevated glucose concentrations. Also decreases glucagon secretion in a glucose-dependent manner and delays gastric emptying.

PHARMACOKINETICS: Absorption: Absolute bioavailability (55%), T_{max}=8-12 hrs; (0.6mg) C_{max}=35ng/mL, AUC=960ng•hr/mL. **Distribution:** Plasma protein binding (>98%); (0.6mg) V_d=13L. **Elimination:** Urine (6%), feces (5%); $T_{1/2}$=13 hrs.

NURSING CONSIDERATIONS

Assessment: Assess for previous hypersensitivity reactions, MEN 2, personal or family history of MTC, history of angioedema, history of pancreatitis, type 1 DM, diabetic ketoacidosis, renal/hepatic impairment, pregnancy/nursing status, and for possible drug interactions.

Monitoring: Monitor for signs and symptoms of thyroid tumor, pancreatitis, elevated serum calcitonin levels, and for other adverse reactions. Monitor renal function, blood glucose levels, and HbA1c levels.

Patient Counseling: Advise to report symptoms of thyroid tumors (eg, lump in the neck, hoarseness, dysphagia, dyspnea). Inform of the potential risk of dehydration due to GI adverse reactions and instruct to take precautions to avoid fluid depletion. Inform of the potential risk for worsening renal function. Instruct to d/c therapy promptly and contact physician if persistent severe abdominal pain and/or symptoms of a hypersensitivity reaction occurs. Advise not to share pen to prevent transmission of infection. Counsel on alternative modes of therapy, importance of adhering to dietary instructions, regular physical activity, periodic blood glucose monitoring and HbA1c testing, recognition/management of hypoglycemia/hyperglycemia, and assessment for diabetes complications. Advise to seek medical advice if any unusual symptoms develop or during periods of stress (eg, fever, trauma, infection, or surgery). Instruct not to take an extra dose to make up for a missed dose and to resume as prescribed with the next scheduled dose. Advise to reinitiate treatment at 0.6mg if >3 days have elapsed since the last dose and to then titrate the dose as prescribed.

Administration: SQ route. Inject into abdomen, thigh, or upper arm; may be administered qd at any time of the day, independently of meals. Inj site and timing can be changed without dose adjustment. Refer to PI for further administration instructions. **Storage:** Prior to 1st use: 2-8°C (36-46°F). Do not freeze and do not use if has been frozen. After initial use: 15-30°C (59-86°F) or 2-8°C (36-46°F) for 30 days. Keep the pen cap on when not in use. Always remove and safely discard the needle after each inj; store pen without an inj needle attached. Protect from excessive heat and sunlight.

V

VICTRELIS
boceprevir (Merck)

RX

THERAPEUTIC CLASS: Protease inhibitor

INDICATIONS: Treatment of genotype 1 chronic hepatitis C, in combination with peginterferon alfa and ribavirin, in patients ≥18 yrs with compensated liver disease, including cirrhosis, who are previously untreated or who have failed previous interferon and ribavirin therapy.

DOSAGE: *Adults:* Combination Therapy with Peginterferon Alfa/Ribavirin: 800mg tid (q7-9h) with food. Give after 4 weeks of treatment of peginterferon alfa and ribavirin regimen.

Patients without Cirrhosis and Previously Untreated or Previous Partial Responders/Relapsers to Interferon and Ribavirin Therapy: Refer to PI for duration of therapy using Response-Guided Therapy Guidelines. Patients with Cirrhosis: Treat with boceprevir in combination with peginterferon alfa and ribavirin for 44 weeks. Refer to PI for dose modification or d/c therapy.

HOW SUPPLIED: Cap: 200mg

CONTRAINDICATIONS: Pregnant women and men whose female partners are pregnant. Concomitant CYP3A4/5 substrates for which elevated plasma concentrations are associated with serious and/or life-threatening events, or potent CYP3A4/5 inducers (eg, alfuzosin, carbamazepine, phenobarbital, phenytoin, rifampin, dihydroergotamine, ergonovine, ergotamine, methylergonovine, cisapride, St. John's wort, lovastatin, simvastatin, drospirenone, sildenafil or tadalafil when used for treatment of pulmonary arterial HTN, pimozide, triazolam, oral midazolam). Refer to the individual monographs for peginterferon alfa and ribavirin.

WARNINGS/PRECAUTIONS: Women of childbearing potential and men must use ≥2 forms of effective contraception during treatment and for ≥6 months after treatment d/c; perform routine monthly pregnancy tests during this time. Anemia reported; combination therapy may cause additional decrease in Hgb. Neutropenia reported. Obtain CBC prior to treatment and monitor periodically thereafter and consider dose reduction of peginterferon alfa and/or ribavirin. Thromboembolic events reported. Caution in elderly.

ADVERSE REACTIONS: Anemia, neutropenia, N/V, dysgeusia, diarrhea, fatigue, insomnia, chills, decreased appetite, alopecia, irritability, arthralgia, dizziness, headache.

INTERACTIONS: See Contraindications. Avoid with colchicine in patients with renal/hepatic impairment; risk of toxicity. Avoid with dexamethasone or use with caution if necessary. Avoid with budesonide, fluticasone, and efavirenz. Not recommended with salmeterol and rifabutin. May increase levels of antiarrhythmics, digoxin, trazodone, desipramine, azole antifungals, clarithromycin, dihydropyridine calcium channel blockers, bosentan, atorvastatin, immunosuppressants, drospirenone, PDE5 inhibitors for erectile dysfunction, and alprazolam or IV midazolam. May decrease levels of ethinyl estradiol. Use lowest digoxin dose initially, with careful titration and monitoring of serum digoxin concentrations. May alter levels of warfarin (monitor INR), HIV protease inhibitors, methadone, or buprenorphine. Azoles and other CYP3A4/5 inhibitors may increase levels. Ritonavir, rifabutin, dexamethasone, efavirenz, and other CYP3A4/5 inducers may decrease levels.

PREGNANCY: Category B, Category X when used with peginterferon alfa and ribavirin, not for use in nursing.

MECHANISM OF ACTION: Hepatitis C virus (HCV) NS3/4A protease inhibitor; direct acting antiviral drug against HCV.

PHARMACOKINETICS: Absorption: (800mg tid) AUC=5408ng•hr/mL; C_{max}=1723ng/mL. T_{max}=2 hrs. **Distribution:** V_d=772L; Plasma protein binding (75%). **Metabolism:** Aldo-ketoreductase-mediated pathway (primary) and oxidative metabolism via CYP3A4/5. **Elimination:** Urine (9%, 3% unchanged), feces (79%, 8% unchanged); $T_{1/2}$=3.4 hrs.

NURSING CONSIDERATIONS

Assessment: Assess for pregnancy/nursing status, men whose female partners are of childbearing potential, and for possible drug interactions. Obtain baseline CBC (with WBC differential count).

Monitoring: Monitor for the development of adverse reactions. Monitor HCV-RNA levels at Treatment Weeks 4, 8, 12, 24, at end of treatment, during treatment follow-up, and as clinically indicated. Monitor CBC at Treatment Weeks 4, 8, 12, and as clinically appropriate. Perform routine monthly pregnancy tests in females.

Patient Counseling: Inform that drug must be used in combination with peginterferon alfa and ribavirin and must not be used alone. Instruct to notify healthcare provider immediately if pregnant. Advise women of childbearing potential and men to use ≥2 forms of effective contraception during therapy and for ≥6 months after treatment d/c. Advise that anemia and neutropenia may be increased and laboratory evaluations are required prior to therapy and periodically thereafter. Inform of the potential for serious drug interactions, and that some drugs should not be taken concomitantly. Instruct to take with food. Instruct to skip missed dose if a dose is missed and it is <2 hrs before next dose, but to take missed dose and resume normal dosing schedule if a dose is missed and it is ≥2 hrs before next dose. Inform that the effect of treatment of hepatitis C on transmission is unknown and that appropriate precautions to prevent transmission should be taken.

Administration: Oral route. **Storage:** 2-8°C (36-46°F) or ≤25°C (77°F) for 3 months. Avoid exposure to excessive heat.

VIDAZA   RX
azacitidine (Celgene)

THERAPEUTIC CLASS: Pyrimidine nucleoside analog

INDICATIONS: Treatment of the following French-American-British myelodysplastic syndrome subtypes: refractory anemia or refractory anemia with ringed sideroblasts (if accompanied by neutropenia or thrombocytopenia or requiring transfusions), refractory anemia with excess blasts, refractory anemia with excess blasts in transformation, and chronic myelomonocytic leukemia.

DOSAGE: *Adults:* Initial: 75mg/m^2/day SQ or IV for 7 days. Repeat cycle q4 weeks. Titrate: May increase to 100mg/m^2 if no benefit seen after 2 cycles and if no toxicity other than N/V. Treat for a minimum of 4-6 cycles; complete or partial response may require additional cycles. Refer to PI for dose adjustment based on hematology laboratory values and renal function/serum electrolytes.

HOW SUPPLIED: Inj: 100mg

CONTRAINDICATIONS: Advanced malignant hepatic tumors.

WARNINGS/PRECAUTIONS: Anemia, neutropenia, and thrombocytopenia may occur; perform CBC PRN to monitor response and toxicity (at a minimum, before each cycle). Potentially hepatotoxic in patients with severe preexisting hepatic impairment; caution with liver disease. Monitor patients with renal impairment for toxicity. Obtain liver chemistries and SrCr prior to initiation of therapy. May cause fetal harm; women of childbearing potential should avoid pregnancy, while men should not father a child during treatment. Caution in elderly.

ADVERSE REACTIONS: N/V, anemia, thrombocytopenia, pyrexia, leukopenia, diarrhea, inj-site erythema, constipation, neutropenia, ecchymosis.

INTERACTIONS: Renal abnormalities reported with IV azacitidine in combination with other chemotherapeutic agents (eg, etoposide).

PREGNANCY: Category D, not for use in nursing.

MECHANISM OF ACTION: Pyrimidine nucleoside analogue; believed to cause hypomethylation of DNA and direct cytotoxicity on abnormal hematopoietic cells in the bone marrow.

PHARMACOKINETICS: Absorption: (SQ) Rapid. Absolute bioavailability (89%); C_{max}=750ng/mL, T_{max}=0.5 hr. **Distribution:** (IV) V_d=76L. **Elimination:** (IV) Urine (85%), feces (<1%). (SQ) Urine (50%); $T_{1/2}$=41 min.

NURSING CONSIDERATIONS

Assessment: Assess for advanced malignant hepatic tumors, hypersensitivity to drug or to mannitol, renal/hepatic impairment, pregnancy/nursing status, and possible drug interactions. Obtain baseline CBC, LFTs, and SrCr.

Monitoring: Perform CBC PRN to monitor response and toxicity (at a minimum, before each cycle). Monitor LFTs, renal function, and serum electrolytes.

Patient Counseling: Instruct to inform physician of any underlying liver or renal disease, or if pregnant/breastfeeding. Advise women of childbearing potential to avoid becoming pregnant, and men not to father a child while on therapy.

Administration: IV/SQ route. Premedicate for N/V. Refer to PI for preparation and administration instructions, and for IV sol incompatibility. **Storage:** 25°C (77°F); excursions permitted to 15-30°C (59-86°F). (Reconstituted) 25°C (77°F) for up to 1 hr for immediate SQ/IV administration, or 2-8°C (36-46°F) for up to 8 hrs for delayed SQ administration.

VIDEX   RX   V
didanosine (Bristol-Myers Squibb)

Fatal and nonfatal pancreatitis reported when used alone or as part of a combination regimen. Suspend therapy in patients with suspected pancreatitis and d/c with confirmed pancreatitis. Lactic acidosis and severe hepatomegaly with steatosis, including fatal cases, reported with nucleoside analogues. Fatal lactic acidosis reported in pregnant women who received the combination of didanosine and stavudine with other antiretroviral agents; use with caution.

OTHER BRAND NAMES: Videx EC (Bristol-Myers Squibb)

THERAPEUTIC CLASS: Nucleoside reverse transcriptase inhibitor

INDICATIONS: Treatment of HIV-1 infection in combination with other antiretroviral agents.

DOSAGE: *Adults:* >18yrs: ≥60kg: (Cap) 400mg qd; (Sol) 200mg bid or 400mg qd. 25-<60kg: (Cap) 250mg qd. <60kg: (Sol) 125mg bid or 250mg qd. 20-<25kg: (Cap) 200mg qd. Renal Impairment: CrCl ≥60mL/min: ≥60kg: (Cap) 400mg qd; (Sol) 400mg qd or 200mg bid. <60kg: (Cap) 250mg qd; (Sol) 250mg qd or 125mg bid. CrCl 30-59mL/min: ≥60kg: (Cap) 200mg qd;

(Sol) 200mg qd or 100mg bid. <60kg: (Cap) 125mg qd; (Sol) 150mg qd or 75mg bid. CrCl 10-29mL/min: ≥60kg: (Cap) 125mg qd; (Sol) 150mg qd. <60kg: (Cap) 125mg qd; (Sol) 100mg qd. CrCl <10mL/min or Continuous Ambulatory Peritoneal Dialysis/Hemodialysis: ≥60kg: (Cap) 125mg qd; (Sol) 100mg qd. <60kg: (Sol) 75mg qd. Concomitant Tenofovir Disoproxil Fumarate: CrCl ≥60mL/min: ≥60kg: 250mg qd; <60kg: 200mg qd.
Pediatrics: (Cap) ≥60kg: 400mg qd. 25-<60kg: 250mg qd. 20-<25kg: 200mg qd. (Sol) >8 months-18 yrs: 120mg/m² bid. Do not exceed adult dosing recommendations. 2 weeks-8 months: 100mg/m² bid. Renal Impairment: Dose reduction recommended. Refer to PI for more information.

HOW SUPPLIED: Cap, Delayed-Release: (Videx EC) 125mg, 200mg, 250mg, 400mg; Sol: (Videx) 2g, 4g

CONTRAINDICATIONS: Concomitant use with allopurinol or ribavirin.

WARNINGS/PRECAUTIONS: Increased frequency of liver function abnormalities in patients with preexisting liver dysfunction; consider interrupting or d/c therapy with evidence of worsening liver disease. Non-cirrhotic portal HTN and peripheral neuropathy reported; d/c if they develop. Retinal changes and optic neuritis reported; perform periodic retinal exam. Immune reconstitution syndrome reported. Autoimmune disorders (eg, Graves' disease, polymyositis, Guillain-Barre syndrome) reported in the setting of immune reconstitution and can occur many months after initiation of treatment. May cause body fat redistribution/accumulation. Caution in elderly.

ADVERSE REACTIONS: Pancreatitis, lactic acidosis, hepatomegaly with steatosis, diarrhea, neuropathy, headache, N/V, rash.

INTERACTIONS: See Boxed Warning and Contraindications. Avoid with hydroxyurea with or without stavudine. Caution with drugs that may cause pancreatic toxicity or neurotoxicity (eg, stavudine). May increase levels of nelfinavir. May decrease levels of ganciclovir, ranitidine, sulfamethoxazole, zidovudine. May increase the area under the curve and decrease the C_{max} of trimethoprim. Ganciclovir, metoclopramide, ranitidine, rifabutin, trimethoprim, and tenofovir may increase levels. Methadone, ciprofloxacin, indinavir, ketoconazole, loperamide, and ritonavir may decrease levels. (Sol) Caution with aluminum- and magnesium-containing antacids. May decrease levels of delavirdine, indinavir, azole antifungals, and quinolone and tetracycline antibiotics.

PREGNANCY: Category B, not for use in nursing.

MECHANISM OF ACTION: Synthetic purine nucleoside analogue; inhibits activity of HIV-1 reverse transcriptase both by competing with natural substrate deoxyadenosine 5'-triphosphate and by its incorporation into viral DNA, causing termination of viral DNA chain elongation.

PHARMACOKINETICS: Absorption: Rapid. T_{max}=0.25-1.5 hrs. **Distribution:** Plasma protein binding (<5%). (Sol): V_d=43.70L/m² (adults), 28L/m² (pediatrics 8 months-19 yrs). (Cap): Different parameters based on body weight, refer to PI. **Elimination:** (Sol): $T_{1/2}$=1.5 hrs (adults), 0.8 hrs (pediatrics 8 months-19 yrs), 1.2 hrs (pediatrics 2 weeks-4 months). (Cap): Different parameters based on body weight; refer to PI.

NURSING CONSIDERATIONS

Assessment: Assess for risk factors for pancreatitis, lactic acidosis, or liver disease, preexisting liver dysfunction, history of neuropathy, pregnancy/nursing status, and possible drug interactions.

Monitoring: Monitor for signs/symptoms of pancreatitis, lactic acidosis, hepatotoxicity, peripheral neuropathy, portal HTN, immune reconstitution syndrome, autoimmune disorders, and fat redistribution/accumulation. Closely monitor renal and hepatic function. Perform periodic retinal exams; if portal HTN is suspected, perform appropriate laboratory testing, including liver enzymes, serum bilirubin, albumin, CBC, INR, and ultrasonography.

Patient Counseling: Inform about possible serious toxicity of pancreatitis and advise on the signs and symptoms of lactic acidosis, hepatotoxicity including fatal hepatic events, and peripheral neuropathy. Inform about reports on retinal changes, optic neuritis, fat redistribution/accumulation, and non-cirrhotic portal HTN, including cases leading to liver transplant or death. Caution about the use of medications or other substances, including alcohol, which may exacerbate drug toxicity. Inform that treatment is not a cure for HIV and patients may continue to experience illnesses associated with HIV. Avoid doing things that can spread HIV to others (eg, sharing needles, other inj equipment, or personal items that can have blood fluids on them; sex without protection; breastfeeding). Do not skip a dose. If a dose is missed, take it immediately; however, if it is almost time for the next dose, skip the missed dose and continue with the regular dosing schedule.

Administration: Oral route. Cap: Take on empty stomach; swallow intact. Pediatric Powder for Oral Sol: Refer to PI for reconstitution. Take on empty stomach, at least 30 min ac or 2 hrs pc. Shake admixture well before use. **Storage:** Cap: 25°C (77°F); excursions permitted 15-30°C (59-86°F). Store in tightly closed container. Powder: 15-30°C (59-86°F). Admixture: 2-8°C (36-46°F) for up to 30 days.

VIGAMOX RX
moxifloxacin HCl (Alcon)

THERAPEUTIC CLASS: Fluoroquinolone
INDICATIONS: Treatment of bacterial conjunctivitis.
DOSAGE: *Adults:* 1 drop tid for 7 days.
Pediatrics: ≥1 yr: 1 drop tid for 7 days.
HOW SUPPLIED: Sol: 0.5% [3mL]
WARNINGS/PRECAUTIONS: Not for injection. Do not inject subconjunctivally or into the anterior chamber of the eye. Superinfection may result with prolonged use. Fatal hypersensitivity reactions reported after first dose of systemic quinolone therapy. Avoid contact lenses when symptoms are present.
ADVERSE REACTIONS: Conjunctivitis, decreased visual acuity, dry eye, keratitis, ocular discomfort/hyperemia, ocular pain/pruritus, subconjunctival hemorrhage, tearing.
PREGNANCY: Category C, caution in nursing.
MECHANISM OF ACTION: Fluoroquinolone antibiotic; inhibits topoisomerase II (DNA gyrase) and topoisomerase IV. DNA gyrase is an essential enzyme involved in replication, transcription, and repair of bacterial DNA. Topoisomerase IV is an enzyme known to play key role in partitioning of chromosomal DNA during bacterial cell division.
PHARMACOKINETICS: Absorption: C_{max}=2.7ng/mL; AUC=45ng•hr/mL. **Distribution:** Presumed to be excreted in breast milk.

NURSING CONSIDERATIONS

Assessment: Assess for proper diagnosis of causative organisms (eg, slit lamp biomicroscopy, fluorescein staining). Assess for allergies to other quinolones. Assess use in pregnant/nursing females.
Monitoring: Monitor for signs/symptoms of hypersensitivity or anaphylactic reactions (eg, cardiovascular collapse, angioedema, airway obstruction, dyspnea, urticaria). With prolonged therapy, monitor for overgrowth of nonsusceptible organisms (eg, fungi) and for development of superinfection.
Patient Counseling: Instruct to avoid contaminating applicator tip with material from eye, fingers, or other sources. D/C medication and contact physician if rash or allergic reaction occurs. Do not wear contact lenses while experiencing bacterial conjunctivitis.
Administration: Ocular route. Do not inject into eye. **Storage:** Store at 2-25°C (36-77°F).

VIIBRYD RX
vilazodone HCl (Forest)

Antidepressants increased the risk of suicidal thinking and behavior (suicidality) in children, adolescents, and young adults in short-term studies of major depressive disorder (MDD) and other psychiatric disorders. Monitor and observe closely for clinical worsening, suicidality, or unusual changes in behavior. Not approved for use in pediatric patients.

THERAPEUTIC CLASS: Selective serotonin reuptake inhibitor/5-HT$_{1A}$-receptor partial agonist
INDICATIONS: Treatment of major depressive disorder.
DOSAGE: *Adults:* Initial: 10mg qd for 7 days. Titrate: Increase to 20mg qd for an additional 7 days, and then an increase to 40mg qd. Usual: 40mg qd. Reassess periodically to determine the need for maintenance treatment and the appropriate dose for treatment. D/C of Therapy: Gradual dose reduction is recommended. If intolerable symptoms occur following a dose decrease or upon d/c, consider resuming previously prescribed dose and decreasing the dose at a more gradual rate. Take with food.
HOW SUPPLIED: Tab: 10mg, 20mg, 40mg
CONTRAINDICATIONS: During or within 14 days of MAOI therapy.
WARNINGS/PRECAUTIONS: Serotonin syndrome or Neuroleptic Malignant Syndrome (NMS)-like reactions may occur; d/c and initiate supportive treatment. Caution with seizure disorder. May increase the risk of bleeding events. Mania/hypomania reported; caution with a history or family history of bipolar disorder, mania, or hypomania. May increase the likelihood of mixed/manic episode in patients at risk for bipolar disorder; screen for bipolar disorder prior to initiating treatment. Reports of adverse events with abrupt d/c; reduce dose gradually whenever possible. Hyponatremia may occur in association with the syndrome of inappropriate antidiuretic hormone secretion (SIADH); greater risk in elderly.

V

ADVERSE REACTIONS: Diarrhea, N/V, dizziness, dry mouth, insomnia, abnormal dreams, decreased libido, fatigue, arthralgia, dyspepsia, flatulence, gastroenteritis, somnolence, paresthesia, restlessness.

INTERACTIONS: See Contraindications. May increase risk of serotonin syndrome and NMS-like reactions with serotonergic drugs (eg, triptans, SSRIs, SNRIs, buspirone, tramadol), drugs that impair metabolism of serotonin (including MAOIs), antipsychotics or other dopamine antagonists. Caution with CNS-active drugs. Not recommended with serotonin precursors (eg, tryptophan). Risk of bleeding may be increased with psychotropic drugs, aspirin (ASA), NSAIDs, warfarin, and other anticoagulants. Increased levels with strong CYP3A4 inhibitors (eg, ketoconazole). Reduce dose for patients with intolerable adverse events if coadministered with moderate inhibitors of CYP3A4 (eg, erythromycin). Decreased levels with CYP3A4 inducers. May increase the biotransformation of mephenytoin. May inhibit the biotransformation of substrates of CYP2C8. Diuretics may increase risk of hyponatremia. Increased free concentrations with other highly protein bound drugs.

PREGNANCY: Category C, not for use in nursing.

MECHANISM OF ACTION: SSRI and 5-HT$_{1A}$ receptor partial agonist; mechanism not established; thought to enhance serotonergic activity in the CNS through selective inhibition of serotonin reuptake.

PHARMACOKINETICS: Absorption: Absolute bioavailability (72%, with food); C_{max}=156ng/mL (fed), AUC=1645ng•h/mL (fed), T_{max}=4-5 hrs. **Distribution:** Plasma protein binding (96-99%). **Metabolism:** CYP and non-CYP pathways (possibly by carboxylesterase). **Elimination:** Urine (1%, unchanged), feces (2%, unchanged); $T_{1/2}$=25 hrs.

NURSING CONSIDERATIONS

Assessment: Assess for history or family history of mania/hypomania, seizures, volume depletion, pregnancy/nursing status, and possible drug interactions. Screen for bipolar disorder. Evaluate for history of drug abuse.

Monitoring: Monitor for clinical worsening, suicidality, unusual changes in behavior, serotonin syndrome or NMS-like reactions, abnormal bleeding, activation of mania/hypomania, hyponatremia. If d/c therapy (particularly if abrupt), monitor for d/c symptoms. Monitor for signs of drug misuse or abuse (eg, development of tolerance, drug-seeking behavior, increases in dose).

Patient Counseling: Counsel about benefits and risks of therapy. Look for the emergence of suicidality, especially early during treatment and when the dose is adjusted up or down. Take with food. Do not take with an MAOI or within 14 days of stopping an MAOI and allow 14 days after stopping vilazodone HCl before starting an MAOI. Caution about risk of serotonin syndrome or NMS-like reactions, and increased risk of bleeding. Caution about use if with history of seizures. Observe for signs and symptoms of activation of mania/hypomania. Patients treated with diuretics, or who are volume-depleted or elderly, may be at greater risk of developing hyponatremia. Avoid alcohol. Notify physician if allergic reactions (eg, rash, hives, swelling, or difficulty breathing) occur. Do not d/c without notifying physician. Therapy may impair physical/mental ability. Notify physician if pregnant/nursing, become pregnant or intend to become pregnant during therapy.

Administration: Oral route. **Storage:** 25°C (77°F); excursions permitted to 15-30°C (59-86°F).

VIMOVO   RX
esomeprazole magnesium - naproxen (AstraZeneca)

> NSAIDs may increase risk of serious cardiovascular (CV) thrombotic events, myocardial infarction (MI), and stroke; increased risk with duration of use and with cardiovascular disease (CVD) or risk factors for CVD. Increased risk of serious GI adverse events (eg, bleeding, ulceration, and stomach/intestinal perforation) that can be fatal and occur anytime during use without warning symptoms; elderly patients are at greater risk. Contraindicated for the treatment of perioperative pain in the setting of coronary artery bypass graft (CABG) surgery.

THERAPEUTIC CLASS: NSAID/Proton Pump Inhibitor

INDICATIONS: Relief of signs and symptoms of osteoarthritis, rheumatoid arthritis, and ankylosing spondylitis. Decrease the risk of developing gastric ulcers in patients at risk of developing NSAID-associated gastric ulcers.

DOSAGE: *Adults:* 375mg-20mg or 500mg-20mg bid ≥30 min ac. Elderly: Use the lowest effective dose.

HOW SUPPLIED: Tab, Delayed-Release: (Naproxen-Esomeprazole): 375mg-20mg, 500mg-20mg

CONTRAINDICATIONS: Patients who have experienced asthma, urticaria, or allergic-type reactions after taking aspirin (ASA) or other NSAIDs. Patients in the late stages of pregnancy. Treatment of perioperative pain in the setting of CABG surgery.

V

WARNINGS/PRECAUTIONS: Use lowest effective dose for the shortest duration possible. Not recommended for initial treatment of acute pain. GI-symptomatic response does not preclude the presence of gastric malignancy. D/C with active and clinically significant bleeding. (Naproxen) May cause HTN or worsen preexisting HTN; monitor BP closely. Fluid retention and edema reported; caution with HTN, fluid retention, or heart failure. Caution with history of ulcer disease, GI bleeding, or risk factors for GI bleeding (eg, prolonged NSAID therapy, older age, poor general health status); monitor for GI ulceration/bleeding and d/c if serious GI event occurs. May exacerbate inflammatory bowel disease (IBD). Renal injury reported with long-term use; increased risk with renal/hepatic impairment, hypovolemia, heart failure, salt depletion, and in elderly. Not recommended with advanced renal disease or CrCl <30mL/min; closely monitor renal function if therapy is initiated. Anaphylactic reactions may occur; avoid with ASA-triad. May cause serious skin adverse events (eg, exfoliative dermatitis, Stevens-Johnson syndrome, toxic epidermal necrolysis); d/c at 1st appearance of rash or any sign of hypersensitivity. May cause elevated LFTs or severe hepatic reactions; d/c if liver disease or systemic manifestations occur, and if abnormal LFTs persist/worsen. Caution with chronic alcoholic liver disease and other diseases with decreased/abnormal plasma proteins if high doses are administered; dosage adjustment may be required. Avoid with severe hepatic impairment; monitor and consider dose reduction with mild to moderate hepatic impairment. Anemia may occur; monitor Hgb/Hct if anemia develops with long-term use. Periodically monitor Hgb if initial Hgb ≤10g and receiving long-term therapy. May inhibit platelet aggregation and prolong bleeding time; monitor patients with coagulation disorders. Caution with asthma and avoid with ASA-sensitive asthma. Not a substitute for corticosteroids nor treatment for corticosteroid insufficiency; may mask signs of inflammation and fever. Caution in elderly and debilitated. (Esomeprazole) Atrophic gastritis reported with long-term use. Increased risk for osteoporosis-related fractures of the hip, wrist, or spine, especially with high-dose (multiple daily doses) and long-term therapy (≥1 yr). Hypomagnesemia reported rarely; consider monitoring magnesium levels prior to and periodically during therapy with prolonged treatment.

ADVERSE REACTIONS: CV thrombotic events, MI, stroke, GI adverse events, flatulence, diarrhea, nausea, abdominal distension, constipation, dyspepsia, upper respiratory tract infection, upper abdominal pain, dizziness, headache.

INTERACTIONS: May enhance methotrexate (MTX) toxicity; use with caution or consider temporary d/c during high-dose MTX administration. (Naproxen) Avoid with other naproxen-containing products and NSAIDs; coadministration with ASA not recommended. Risk of renal toxicity when coadministered with diuretics and ACE inhibitors. Diminished antihypertensive effect of ACE inhibitors and β-blockers (eg, propranolol). Delayed absorption with cholestyramine. Caution with cyclosporine; increased risk of nephrotoxicity. Coadministration may decrease efficacy of thiazides and loop (eg, furosemide) diuretics; monitor for signs of renal failure and diuretic efficacy. May increase lithium levels; monitor for toxicity. Increased risk of GI bleeding with oral corticosteroids, anticoagulants (eg, warfarin, dicumarol, heparin), antiplatelets (including low-dose ASA), smoking, alcohol, and drugs that interfere with serotonin reuptake (eg, SSRIs); monitor carefully. Potential interaction with albumin-bound drugs (eg, sulfonylureas, sulfonamides, hydantoins, other NSAIDs). Increased plasma levels with probenecid. (Esomeprazole) Caution with digoxin or other drugs that may cause hypomagnesemia (eg, diuretics). Increased levels of tacrolimus. Drug-induced decrease in gastric acidity results in enterochromaffin-like cell hyperplasia and increased chromogranin A levels; may interfere with investigations for neuroendocrine tumors. May interfere with absorption of drugs where gastric pH is an important determinant of bioavailability (eg, absorption of ketoconazole, iron salts, and erlotinib may decrease, while absorption of digoxin may increase); monitor for digoxin toxicity. Decreases levels of atazanavir and nelfinavir; coadministration not recommended. Monitor for saquinavir toxicity; consider saquinavir dose reduction. May change levels of other antiretrovirals. Monitor for increases in INR and PT with warfarin. May inhibit metabolism of CYP2C19 substrates; decreased clearance of diazepam. Levels may be increased with combined CYP2C19 and 3A4 inhibitor (eg, voriconazole). Increased concentrations of cilostazol; consider dose reduction of cilostazol. Decreased levels with CYP2C19 or 3A4 inducers; avoid with St. John's wort or rifampin.

PREGNANCY: Category C (<30 weeks gestation) and D (≥30 weeks gestation), not for use in nursing.

MECHANISM OF ACTION: Naproxen: NSAID; not established. Analgesic and antipyretic activity may be related to prostaglandin synthetase inhibition. Esomeprazole: Proton pump inhibitor; suppresses gastric acid secretion by specific inhibition of the H^+/K^+ ATPase in the gastric parietal cell.

PHARMACOKINETICS: Absorption: Naproxen: Bioavailability (95%); T_{max}=3 hrs. Esomeprazole: Rapid; T_{max}=0.43-1.2 hrs. **Distribution:** Naproxen: V_d=0.16L/kg; plasma protein binding (>99%); found in breast milk. Esomeprazole: V_d=16L; plasma protein binding (97%). **Metabolism:** Naproxen: Liver (extensive) via CYP2C9 and CYP1A2 into 6-0-desmethyl naproxen (metabolite). Esomeprazole: Liver (extensive) via CYP2C19 (major) into hydroxyl and desmethyl metabolites, and via CYP3A4 into sulfone (main metabolite). **Elimination:** Naproxen: Urine (<1% unchanged, <1% 6-0-desmethyl naproxen, 66-92% conjugates), feces (≤3%); $T_{1/2}$=15 hrs. Esomeprazole: Urine (80% metabolites, <1% unchanged), feces; $T_{1/2}$=1.2-1.5 hrs.

V

NURSING CONSIDERATIONS

Assessment: Assess for history of asthma, urticaria, or allergic-type reactions with ASA or other NSAIDs, ASA-triad, CVD, risk factors for CVD, HTN, fluid retention, heart failure, history of ulcer disease, history of/risk factors for GI bleeding, history of IBD, renal/hepatic impairment, coagulation disorders, preexisting asthma, decreased/abnormal plasma proteins, tobacco/alcohol use, pregnancy/nursing status, possible drug interactions, or any other conditions where treatment is contraindicated or cautioned. Obtain baseline BP, CBC with platelet count, coagulation and chemistry profiles.

Monitoring: Monitor for CV and GI events, active bleeding, anaphylactic/hypersensitivity/skin reactions, anemia, bone fractures, and hypomagnesemia. Monitor BP, LFTs, renal function, CBC with platelet count, coagulation and chemistry profiles.

Patient Counseling: Inform to seek medical advice if symptoms of CV events (eg, chest pain, SOB, weakness, slurred speech), GI ulceration/bleeding (eg, epigastric pain, dyspepsia, melena, hematemesis), skin/hypersensitivity reactions (eg, rash, blisters, fever, itching), unexplained weight gain or edema, hepatotoxicity (eg, nausea, fatigue, lethargy, pruritus, jaundice, right upper quadrant tenderness, flu-like symptoms), anaphylactic reactions (eg, face/throat swelling, difficulty breathing), and hypomagnesemia (eg, palpitations, dizziness, seizures, tetany) occur. Inform that medication should be avoided in late pregnancy. Caution against activities requiring alertness if drowsiness, dizziness, vertigo, or depression occurs. Inform to notify physician of history of asthma or ASA-sensitive asthma.

Administration: Oral route. Swallow whole with liquid. Do not split, chew, crush, or dissolve.
Storage: 25°C (77°F); excursions permitted to 15-30°C (59-86°F). Protect from moisture.

VIMPAT
lacosamide (UCB)

`CV`

THERAPEUTIC CLASS: Sodium channel inactivator

INDICATIONS: (Tab/Sol) Adjunctive therapy for the treatment of partial-onset seizures in patients ≥17 yrs with epilepsy. (Inj) Adjunctive therapy for the treatment of partial-onset seizures in patients ≥17 yrs with epilepsy when oral administration is temporarily not feasible.

DOSAGE: *Adults:* Partial-Onset Seizures: Initial: 50mg bid (100mg/day). Titrate: May increase at weekly intervals by 100mg/day given as two divided doses. Maint: 200-400mg/day based on response and tolerability. Mild/Moderate Hepatic Impairment/Severe Renal Impairment (CrCl ≤30mL/min)/End-Stage Renal Disease (ESRD): Max: 300mg/day. Consider dosage supplementation of up to 50% after 4-hr hemodialysis treatment. Switching from Oral to IV Dosing: Initial total daily IV dosage should be equivalent to total daily dosage and frequency of PO dosing and infused over 30-60 min. Switching from IV to Oral Dosing: Give at equivalent daily dosage and frequency of IV treatment.
Pediatrics: ≥17 yrs: Partial-Onset Seizures: Initial: 50mg bid (100mg/day). Titrate: May increase, at weekly intervals by 100mg/day given as two divided doses. Maint: 200-400mg/day based on response and tolerability. Mild/Moderate Hepatic Impairment/Severe Renal Impairment (CrCl ≤30mL/min)/ESRD: Max: 300mg/day. Consider dosage supplementation of up to 50% after 4-hr hemodialysis treatment. Switching from Oral to IV Dosing: Initial total daily IV dosage should be equivalent to total daily dosage and frequency of PO dosing and infused over 30-60 min. Switching from IV to Oral Dosing: Give at equivalent daily dosage and frequency of IV treatment.

HOW SUPPLIED: Inj: 200mg/20mL [20mL]; Sol: 10mg/mL [465mL]; Tab: 50mg, 100mg, 150mg, 200mg

WARNINGS/PRECAUTIONS: May increase risk of suicidal thoughts or behavior; monitor for the emergence or worsening of depression, suicidal thoughts/behavior, and/or unusual changes in mood/behavior. May cause dizziness and ataxia; may impair physical/mental abilities. Dose-dependent prolongations in PR interval reported. Caution with known conduction abnormalities (eg, AV block, sick sinus syndrome without pacemaker) or with severe cardiac disease (eg, myocardial ischemia, heart failure). May predispose to atrial arrhythmias especially in patients with diabetic neuropathy and/or cardiovascular disease (CVD). Syncope or loss of consciousness reported in patients with diabetic neuropathy. Withdraw gradually over minimum of 1 week to minimize potential of increased seizure frequency in patients with seizure disorders. Multi-organ hypersensitivity reactions (Drug Reaction with Eosinophilia and Systemic Symptoms [DRESS]) may occur; d/c and start alternative treatment if suspected. Avoid use with severe hepatic impairment. Monitor closely during dose titration with coexisting hepatic or renal impairment. Caution in elderly. (Sol) Contains aspartame, a source of phenylalanine.

ADVERSE REACTIONS: Dizziness, headache, N/V, fatigue, diplopia, vertigo, somnolence, ataxia, tremor, skin laceration, nystagmus, balance disorder, diarrhea, blurred vision.

INTERACTIONS: Possible further PR prolongation with concomitant use with other drugs that prolong the PR interval. Small reductions in plasma concentrations with carbamazepine, pheno-

V

barbital, or phenytoin. Possibility of pharmacodynamic interactions with drugs that affect the heart conduction system. Abnormality in LFTs with concomitant anti-epileptic drugs.

PREGNANCY: Category C, not for use in nursing.

MECHANISM OF ACTION: Sodium channel inactivator; has not been established. Selectively enhances slow inactivation of voltage-gated sodium channels, resulting in stabilization of hyperexcitable neuronal membranes and inhibition of repetitive neuronal firing. Binds to collapsin response mediator protein-2 (CRMP-2), which is mainly expressed in the nervous system and is involved in neuronal differentiation and control of axonal outgrowth.

PHARMACOKINETICS: Absorption: (PO) Complete; absolute bioavailability (100%); T_{max}=1-4 hrs. **Distribution:** V_d=0.6L/kg; plasma protein binding (<15%). **Metabolism:** CYP2C19; O-desmethyl-lacosamide (major metabolite). **Elimination:** Urine (95%), feces (<0.5%); $T_{1/2}$=13 hrs.

NURSING CONSIDERATIONS

Assessment: Assess for hepatic/renal impairment, history of depression, cardiac conduction problems and/or CVD, diabetic neuropathy, phenylketonuria, pregnancy/nursing status, and possible drug interactions. Obtain baseline LFTs and ECG.

Monitoring: Monitor for ECG abnormalities, emergence or worsening of depression, suicidal thoughts or behavior and/or any unusual changes in mood or behavior, dizziness, ataxia, prolongation in PR interval, syncope or loss of consciousness, and DRESS. Monitor renal/hepatic function.

Patient Counseling: Instruct to take only as prescribed. Counsel patients/caregivers/families about high risk of suicidal thoughts and behavior and the need to be alert for the emergence or worsening symptoms of depression, any unusual changes in behavior or mood, or the emergence of suicidal thoughts. Instruct to report to physician immediately if any behaviors of concern develop. Inform about the possible adverse reactions associated with therapy. Advise not to engage in hazardous activities (eg, driving/operating complex machinery) until effects of drug are known. Instruct to notify physician if pregnant, intend to become pregnant, or are breastfeeding.

Administration: Oral/IV route. Inj: May be administered without further dilution or may be mixed with diluents. Refer to PI for compatibility and stability information. Sol: Obtain/use calibrated measuring device. **Storage:** 20-25°C (68-77°F); excursions permitted between 15-30°C (59-86°F). Inj/Sol: Do not freeze. Inj: Discard any unused portion. Sol: Discard any unused portion after 7 weeks of first opening the bottle.

VIRACEPT   RX
nelfinavir mesylate (Agouron)

THERAPEUTIC CLASS: Protease inhibitor

INDICATIONS: Treatment of HIV infection in combination with other antiretroviral agents.

DOSAGE: *Adults:* 1250mg bid (five 250mg or two 625mg tabs) or 750mg tid (three 250mg tabs). Max: 2500 mg/day. Take with meal. May dissolve whole tab in small amount of water. Once dissolved, mix cloudy liquid well and consume immediately. Rinse glass with water and swallow rinse to ensure that entire dose is consumed.
Pediatrics: 2-13 yrs: 45-55mg/kg bid or 25-35mg/kg tid (powder or 250mg tab). Take with meal. May mix powder with small amount of water, milk, formula, soy formula/milk, or dietary supplements; once mixed, entire contents must be consumed in order to obtain the full dose. If mixture is not consumed immediately, refrigerate ≤6 hrs. Acidic food or juice is not recommended to be used in combination (eg, orange juice, apple juice, applesauce). Do not reconstitute powder with water in its original container. Refer to PI for further dosing guidelines based on age and body weight.

HOW SUPPLIED: Powder: 50mg/g [144g]; Tab: 250mg, 625mg

CONTRAINDICATIONS: Concomitant use with CYP3A substrates for which elevated plasma concentrations are associated with serious and/or life threatening events (eg, alfuzosin, amiodarone, quinidine, dihydroergotamine, ergonovine, ergotamine, methylergonovine, pimozide, sildenafil when used for treatment of pulmonary arterial HTN, midazolam, triazolam).

WARNINGS/PRECAUTIONS: Powder contains phenylalanine; caution in patients with phenylketonuria. New-onset diabetes mellitus (DM), exacerbation of DM, hyperglycemia, diabetic ketoacidosis reported. Do not use in patients with moderate or severe hepatic impairment. HIV cross-resistance between protease inhibitors, increased bleeding in patients with hemophilia A and B, fat redistribution/accumulation, and immune reconstitution syndrome reported.

ADVERSE REACTIONS: Diarrhea, N/V, flatulence, rash, redistribution of body fat, jaundice, allergic reactions, bilirubinemia, hyperglycemia, metabolic acidosis, anemia, anxiety, rhinitis, pruritus.

INTERACTIONS: See Contraindications. Avoid colchicine in patients with renal/hepatic impairment. Not recommended with lovastatin, simvastatin, salmeterol, rifampin, St. John's wort, and proton pump inhibitors (PPI). May increase levels of dihydropyridine calcium channel blockers,

V

indinavir, saquinavir, trazadone, rifabutin, bosentan, HMG-CoA reductase inhibitors (eg, atorvastatin, rosuvastatin), immunosuppresants, fluticasone, azithromycin, PDE5 inhibitors. May decrease levels of delavirdine, phenytoin, methadone, ethinyl estradiol, norethindrone area under the curve (AUC). CYP3A or CYP2C19 inhibitors, delavirdine, indinavir, ritonavir may increase levels. CYP3A or CYP2C19 inducers (eg, rifampin), omeprazole, nevirapine (C_{min}), carbamazepine, phenobarbital, rifabutin may decrease levels. May affect warfarin concentrations; monitor INR. Give didanosine 1 hr before or 2 hrs after administration. May require either initiation or dose adjustments of insulin or oral hypoglycemics for treatment of DM.

PREGNANCY: Category B, not for use in nursing.

MECHANISM OF ACTION: HIV-1 protease inhibitor; prevents cleavage of *gag* and *gag-pol* polyprotein resulting in production of immature, noninfectious virus.

PHARMACOKINETICS: Absorption: 28 days: (1250mg bid) C_{max}=4mg/L; AUC=52.8mg•h/L. (750mg tid) C_{max}=3mg/L; AUC=43.6mg•h/L. 14 days: (1250mg bid) C_{max}=4.7mg/L; AUC=35.3mg•h/L. **Distribution:** V_d=2-7L/kg; plasma protein binding (>98%). **Metabolism:** Liver via CYP3A, 2C19 (oxidation). **Elimination:** Feces (78%, metabolites), (22%, unchanged), urine (1-2%); $T_{1/2}$=3.5-5 hrs.

NURSING CONSIDERATIONS

Assessment: Assess for previous hypersensitivity, hepatic impairment, DM, hemophilia, pregnancy/nursing status, and for possible drug interactions. Assess for phenylketonuria if planning to use oral powder formulation. Obtain baseline ECG and liver enzymes.

Monitoring: Monitor for signs/symptoms of hypersensitivity reactions, new onset or exacerbation of DM and hyperglycemia, immune reconstitution syndrome, fat redistribution/accumulation, and hepatic dysfunction. In patients with hemophilia, monitor for signs/symptoms of increased bleeding (eg, hematomas, hemarthrosis). Monitor ECG changes. May enroll patients in the Antiretroviral Pregnancy Registry if they become pregnant while on treatment.

Patient Counseling: Inform that therapy is not cure for HIV, does not reduce risk of transmission of HIV, and that opportunistic infections may develop. Instruct to take with food; do not alter dose or d/c without consulting physician. Instruct to notify physician if using other Rx, OTC or herbal products, particularly St. John's wort. Advise to use alternative or additional contraceptive measures if taking oral contraceptives. Inform that use with sildenafil or other PDE5 inhibitors may increase risk of hypotension, visual changes, and prolonged penile erection; instruct to contact physician if any of these symptoms occur. Inform that most frequent adverse effect is diarrhea; may use nonprescription drugs (eg, loperamide) if occurs. Inform that fat redistribution/accumulation may occur.

Administration: Oral route. Take with meal. **Storage:** Tab/Oral Powder: 15-30°C (59-86°F). Keep container tightly closed.

VIRAMUNE   RX
nevirapine (Boehringer Ingelheim)

> Severe, life-threatening, sometimes fatal, hepatotoxicity and skin reactions (eg, Stevens-Johnson syndrome, toxic epidermal necrolysis, hypersensitivity) reported. Increased risk of hepatotoxicity reported in women and patients with higher CD4+ counts, including pregnant women. Hepatic failure reported in patients without HIV taking nevirapine for postexposure prophylaxis (PEP). Use for occupational and non-occupational PEP is contraindicated. Seek medical evaluation and d/c therapy if hepatitis, increased transaminases combined with rash or other systemic symptoms, severe skin rash or hypersensitivity reactions develop; do not restart therapy. The 14-day lead-in period with 200mg qd dosing must be followed; may decrease incidence of rash. Monitor during the 1st 18 wks of therapy, especially the first 6 wks.

OTHER BRAND NAMES: Viramune XR (Boehringer Ingelheim)

THERAPEUTIC CLASS: Non-nucleoside reverse transcriptase inhibitor

INDICATIONS: Treatment of HIV-1 infection in combination with other antiretrovirals.

DOSAGE: *Adults:* (IR) 1 tab (200mg) qd for 1st 14 days (lead-in period), then 1 tab bid. Do not increase dose if mild to moderate rash without constitutional symptoms develops during the 14-day lead-in period until rash resolves. Max Duration of Lead-in Period: 28 days. Dose Interruption (>7 days): Restart with lead-in period dose for 1st 14 days, then 1 tab bid. Dialysis Patients: Add 200mg after each dialysis treatment. (ER) Not Currently Taking IR: 1 IR tab (200mg) qd for 1st 14 days, then 1 ER tab (400mg) qd. Switching from IR to ER: May switch to ER (400mg) qd without 14-day lead-in period if already taking IR (200mg) bid. Do not begin dosing with ER if mild to moderate rash without constitutional symptoms develops during 14-day lead-in period with IR until rash resolves. Dose Interruption (>7 days): Restart 14-day lead-in period dose with IR (200mg) qd.

Pediatrics: ≥15 days: 150mg/m² qd for 14 days (lead-in period), then 150mg/m² bid. Max: 400mg/day. Do not increase dose if mild to moderate rash without constitutional symptoms develops during the 14-day lead-in period until rash resolves. Max Duration of Lead-in Period: 28

days. Dose Interruption (>7 days): Restart with lead-in period dose for 1st 14 days, then 150mg/m² bid. Dialysis Patients: Add 200mg after each dialysis treatment. Refer to PI for dose calculation based on BSA.

HOW SUPPLIED: Sus: 50mg/5mL [240mL]; Tab, Immediate-Release (IR): 200mg; Tab, Extended-Release (ER): 400mg

CONTRAINDICATIONS: Moderate or severe (Child-Pugh Class B or C) hepatic impairment. Use as part of occupational and non-occupational PEP regimens.

WARNINGS/PRECAUTIONS: Not recommended for adult females with CD4⁺ cell counts >250 cells/mm³ or in adult males with CD4⁺ cell counts >400 cells/mm³. Coinfection with hepatitis B or C and/or increased transaminase elevations at the start of therapy may increase risk of later symptomatic events and asymptomatic increases in AST/ALT. Caution with hepatic fibrosis/cirrhosis; monitor for drug-induced toxicity. Rhabdomyolysis reported in some patients with skin and/or liver reactions. Monitor closely if isolated rash of any severity occurs; delay in stopping treatment after onset of rash may result in a more serious reaction. Do not use as single agent to treat HIV or add on as a sole agent to a failing regimen; resistant virus emerges rapidly when administered as monotherapy. Consider potential for cross-resistance in the choice of new antiretroviral agent for combination therapy. Immune reconstitution syndrome and redistribution/accumulation of body fat reported. Avoid use of more than one form of nevirapine at the same time. Hepatic injury may progress despite d/c. Caution in elderly.

ADVERSE REACTIONS: Hepatotoxicity, hepatitis, transaminase elevations, liver enzyme abnormalities, rash, nausea, headache, fatigue, neutropenia, anemia.

INTERACTIONS: Avoid with atazanavir, ketoconazole, itraconazole, and rifampin. Not recommended with fosamprenavir (without ritonavir), efavirenz, and St. John's wort. May increase incidence and severity of rash with prednisone during the 1st 6 weeks of therapy. May increase levels of 14-OH clarithromycin, rifabutin, darunavir/ritonavir, maraviroc, and antithrombotics (eg, warfarin) (monitor anticoagulation levels). May decrease levels of CYP3A/2B6 substrates, clarithromycin, ethinyl estradiol, norethindrone, amprenavir, indinavir, lopinavir, methadone, nelfinavir, zidovudine, antiarrhythmics, anticonvulsants, some azole antifungals, calcium channel blockers, cancer chemotherapy, ergot alkaloids, immunosuppressants, motility agents, and opiate agonists. Fluconazole may increase levels.

PREGNANCY: Category B, not for use in nursing.

MECHANISM OF ACTION: Non-nucleoside reverse transcriptase inhibitor; binds directly to reverse transcriptase and blocks RNA-dependent and DNA-dependent DNA polymerase activities by causing disruption of the enzyme's catalytic site.

PHARMACOKINETICS: Absorption: Readily absorbed. Absolute bioavailability (93%, IR), (91%, Sus); AUC=161,000ng•hr/mL (ER single dose); C_{max}=2mcg/mL (IR/Sus), 2060ng/mL (ER single dose); T_{max}=4 hrs (IR/Sus), 24 hrs (ER). Distribution: V_d=1.21L/kg (IV); plasma protein binding (60%). Crosses placenta; found in breast milk. Metabolism: Liver (extensive); glucuronide conjugation, oxidative metabolism via CYP3A/2B6. Elimination: (IR) Urine (81.3%; <3%, parent drug), feces (10.1%); $T_{1/2}$=45 hrs (single dose), 25-30 hrs (multiple dosing).

NURSING CONSIDERATIONS

Assessment: Assess for hepatic impairment, hepatitis B or C coinfection, hepatic fibrosis/cirrhosis, pregnancy/nursing status, and possible drug interactions. Obtain baseline liver enzyme tests, and CD4⁺ cell counts.

Monitoring: Monitor for hepatotoxicity, hepatitis, skin or hypersensitivity reactions, immune reconstitution syndrome (eg, opportunistic infections) and rhabdomyolysis. Monitor LFTs during the 1st 18 wks of therapy and periodically thereafter. Measure serum transaminases immediately if signs and symptoms of hepatitis, hypersensitivity reaction, rash develop. May enroll patients in the Antiretroviral Pregnancy Registry if they become pregnant while on medication. (IR) Monitor LFTs prior to dose escalation and 2 wks post-dose escalation. (ER) Monitor LFTs prior to initiation and at 2 wks after therapy, then periodically thereafter.

Patient Counseling: Inform patients that severe liver disease/skin reactions may occur. Counsel about signs/symptoms of hepatotoxicity, rash or skin reactions, and other adverse reactions, and advise to d/c and seek medical evaluation immediately if any occur. Counsel to take drug as prescribed. Instruct not to alter the dose without consulting the physician. Instruct to take next dose as soon as possible if dose is missed; however, if dose is skipped, instruct not to double the next dose. Advise that treatment combined with safe sex practices may reduce risk of transmission. Inform that drug is not a cure for HIV-1 infection. Advise to notify physician if taking any medications or herbal products. Inform females that oral contraceptives and other hormonal methods of birth control should not be used as sole method of birth control. Instruct that medication may be taken with or without food. (ER) Inform that soft remnants of the drug may be seen in their stool.

Administration: Oral route. (ER) Swallow whole; do not chew, crush, or divide. (Sus) Shake prior to administration. Use an oral dosing syringe, particularly for dose ≤5mL. If dosing cup is used, rinse thoroughly with water and the rinse should also be administered. Storage: 25°C (77°F); excursions permitted to 15-30°C (59-86°F).

VIREAD RX
tenofovir disoproxil fumarate (Gilead)

> Lactic acidosis and severe hepatomegaly with steatosis, including fatal cases, reported with the use of nucleoside analogues. Severe acute exacerbations of hepatitis reported in patients infected with hepatitis B virus (HBV) upon d/c of therapy; closely monitor hepatic function for at least several months. If appropriate, resumption of anti-hepatitis B therapy may be warranted.

THERAPEUTIC CLASS: Nucleotide analogue reverse transcriptase inhibitor

INDICATIONS: Treatment of HIV-1 infection in combination with other antiretroviral agents in adults and pediatrics ≥2 yrs. Treatment of chronic hepatitis B in adults.

DOSAGE: *Adults:* 300mg tab qd. If unable to swallow tabs, may use 7.5 scoops of oral powder. Renal Impairment: CrCl 30-49mL/min: 300mg tab q48h. CrCl 10-29mL/min: 300mg tab q72-96h. Hemodialysis: 300mg tab every 7 days or after a total of approximately 12 hrs of dialysis. *Pediatrics:* ≥2 yrs: HIV-1 Infection: 8mg/kg qd oral powder mixed in soft food not requiring chewing. Max: 300mg/day. ≥17kg and Able to Swallow Intact Tab: 1 tab qd. Refer to PI for dosing recommendation based on body weight using tab and oral powder.

HOW SUPPLIED: Powder: 40mg/g [60g]; Tab: 150mg, 200mg, 250mg, 300mg

WARNINGS/PRECAUTIONS: Obesity and prolonged nucleoside exposure may be risk factors for lactic acidosis and severe hepatomegaly with steatosis. Caution with known risk factors for liver disease; d/c if lactic acidosis or pronounced hepatotoxicity develops. Renal impairment reported; calculate CrCl prior to therapy. Monitor CrCl and serum phosphorus in patients at risk for renal impairment. Use only in HIV-1 and HBV coinfected patients as part of an appropriate antiretroviral combination regimen. In HBV-infected patients, offer HIV-1 antibody testing before initiating therapy. In HIV-1 patients, perform testing for presence of chronic hepatitis B before initiating therapy. Decreased bone mineral density (BMD), fractures, and osteomalacia reported; assess BMD with history of pathologic bone fracture or other risk factors for osteoporosis or bone loss. Body fat redistribution/accumulation may occur. Immune reconstitution syndrome reported. Autoimmune disorders (eg, Graves' disease, polymyositis, Guillain-Barre syndrome) reported in the setting of immune reconstitution and can occur many months after initiation of treatment. Early virological failure and high rates of resistance substitutions reported with certain regimens that only contain three nucleoside reverse transcriptase inhibitors; use with caution and consider treatment modifications. Caution in elderly.

ADVERSE REACTIONS: Lactic acidosis, hepatomegaly with steatosis, N/V, diarrhea, depression, asthenia, headache, pain, rash, abdominal pain, insomnia, pruritus, dizziness, pyrexia.

INTERACTIONS: Avoid with adefovir dipivoxil, atazanavir (without ritonavir), concurrent or recent use of nephrotoxic agents, and other products containing tenofovir. May increase levels of didanosine. May decrease levels of atazanavir. Coadministration with drugs that reduce renal function or compete for active tubular secretion may increase levels of tenofovir and/or other renally eliminated drugs (eg, acyclovir, cidofovir, ganciclovir, valacyclovir, valganciclovir). Atazanavir and lopinavir/ritonavir may increase levels.

PREGNANCY: Category B, not for use in nursing.

MECHANISM OF ACTION: Nucleotide analogue reverse transcriptase inhibitor; inhibits activity of HIV-1 reverse transcriptase and HBV reverse transcriptase by competing with natural substrate deoxyadenosine 5'-triphosphate and, after incorporation into DNA, by DNA chain termination.

PHARMACOKINETICS: Absorption: Adults: (Fasted) Bioavailability (25%); (Fasted, 300mg single dose) C_{max}=0.30mcg/mL, T_{max}=1 hr, AUC=2.29mcg•hr/mL. **Pediatrics:** (300mg tab) C_{max}=0.38mcg/mL, AUC=3.39mcg•hr/mL; (8mg/kg oral powder) C_{max}=0.24mcg/mL, AUC=2.59mcg•hr/mL. **Distribution:** Plasma protein binding (<0.7%); V_d=1.3L/kg (1mg/kg IV dose), 1.2L/kg (3mg/kg IV dose); found in breast milk. **Elimination:** (Fed, 300mg qd multiple doses) Urine (32%); (Single dose) $T_{1/2}$=17 hrs.

NURSING CONSIDERATIONS

Assessment: Assess for renal impairment, risk factors for lactic acidosis and liver disease, pregnancy/nursing status, and possible drug interactions. Assess BMD in patient with a history of pathologic bone fracture or other risk factors for osteoporosis or bone loss. Calculate CrCl in all patients prior to initiating therapy. In HBV-infected patients, perform HIV-1 antibody testing. In HIV-1 patients, perform testing for presence of chronic hepatitis B.

Monitoring: Monitor for signs/symptoms of lactic acidosis, severe hepatomegaly with steatosis, fat redistribution/accumulation, immune reconstitution syndrome (eg, opportunistic infections), and autoimmune disorders. Upon d/c of therapy in HBV patients, monitor with both clinical and laboratory follow-up for acute exacerbations of hepatitis. Monitor BMD with history of pathologic bone fracture or other risk factors for osteoporosis or bone loss; renal function in all patients with CrCl <50mL/min; serum phosphorus levels (in patients at risk for renal impairment) and CrCl; therapy utilizing a triple nucleoside-only regimen; and weight of pediatric patients periodically.

Patient Counseling: Inform about risks and benefits of therapy. Inform that therapy is not a cure for HIV-1 and that opportunistic infections may develop. Avoid doing things that can spread HIV or HBV to others (eg, sharing of needles/inj equipment or personal items that can have blood/body fluids on them). Advise to always practice safe sex by using latex or polyurethane condoms. Instruct to avoid breastfeeding. Inform that tablets and oral powder are for PO ingestion only. Instruct not to d/c without first informing physician. Counsel about the importance of adherence to regimen and to avoid missing doses. Instruct to contact physician if symptoms of lactic acidosis and severe hepatomegaly with steatosis (eg, N/V, stomach discomfort, weakness) occur. Inform to remain under physician's care during therapy.

Administration: Oral route. (Powder) Measure only with the supplied dosing scoop. Mix with 2-4 oz. of soft food (eg, applesauce, baby food, yogurt) that does not require chewing; ingest immediately. Do not mix with liquid. (Tab) Take without regard to food. **Storage:** 25°C (77°F); excursions permitted to 15-30°C (59-86°F).

VIROPTIC   RX
trifluridine (Monarch Pharmaceuticals Inc.)

THERAPEUTIC CLASS: Fluorinated pyrimidine nucleoside antiviral

INDICATIONS: Treatment of primary keratoconjunctivitis and recurrent epithelial keratitis due to herpes simplex virus, types 1 and 2.

DOSAGE: *Adults:* 1 drop into cornea of the affected eye q2h while awake until corneal ulcer has completely re-epithelialized. Max: 9 drops/day. Following Re-epithelialization: 1 drop q4h while awake for 7 days; minimum of 5 drops/day. If no improvement after 7 days or if complete re-epithelialization has not occurred after 14 days, consider other forms of therapy. Avoid using >21 days.
Pediatrics: ≥6 yrs: 1 drop into cornea of the affected eye q2h while awake until corneal ulcer has completely re-epithelialized. Max: 9 drops/day. Following Re-epithelialization: 1 drop q4h while awake for 7 days; minimum of 5 drops/day. If no improvement after 7 days or if complete re-epithelialization has not occurred after 14 days, consider other forms of therapy. Avoid using >21 days.

HOW SUPPLIED: Sol: 1% [7.5mL]

WARNINGS/PRECAUTIONS: Only use with a clinical diagnosis of herpetic keratitis. May cause transient, mild local irritation of the conjunctiva and cornea when instilled. Possibility of development of viral resistance.

ADVERSE REACTIONS: Burning, stinging, palpebral edema, superficial punctate keratopathy, epithelial keratopathy, hypersensitivity reaction, stromal edema, irritation, keratitis sicca, hyperemia, increased IOP.

PREGNANCY: Category C, not for use in nursing.

MECHANISM OF ACTION: Fluorinated pyrimidine nucleoside antiviral; unknown, suspected to interfere with DNA synthesis.

PHARMACOKINETICS: Absorption: Intraocular penetration; decreased corneal integrity or stromal/uveal inflammation may enhance penetration into the aqueous humor.

NURSING CONSIDERATIONS

Assessment: Assess for clinical diagnosis of herpetic keratitis and for pregnancy/nursing status.

Monitoring: Monitor for clinical signs of improvement after 7 days of therapy and complete re-epithelialization after 14 days of therapy. Monitor for signs/symptoms of mild local irritation of conjunctiva and cornea. Monitor for possible viral resistance and hypersensitivity reactions.

Patient Counseling: Advise that recommended dosage and frequency of administration should not be exceeded. Inform that continuous administration for periods exceeding 21 days should be avoided because of potential for ocular toxicity. Instruct to report any adverse reactions that develop.

Administration: Ocular route. **Storage:** Store under refrigeration 2-8°C (36-46°F).

V

VISICOL

RX

monobasic sodium phosphate - dibasic sodium phosphate (Salix)

Rare, but serious, acute phosphate nephropathy reported. Some cases resulted in permanent renal impairment requiring long-term dialysis. Increased risk of acute phosphate nephropathy with increased age, hypovolemia, increased bowel transit time (eg, bowel obstruction), active colitis or baseline kidney disease and use of medicines that affect renal perfusion or function (eg, diuretics, ACE inhibitors, angiotensin receptor blockers, and possibly NSAIDs). Use the recommended dose and dosing regimen (pm/am split dose).

THERAPEUTIC CLASS: Bowel cleanser

INDICATIONS: For cleansing the colon in preparation for colonoscopy in adults ≥18 yrs.

DOSAGE: *Adults:* Evening Before Colonoscopy Procedure: 3 tabs (last dose is 2 tabs) with 8 oz. clear liquids q15min for a total of 20 tabs. Day of Colonoscopy Procedure: Starting 3-5 hrs before procedure, 3 tabs (last dose is 2 tabs) with 8 oz. of clear liquids q15min for a total of 20 tabs.

HOW SUPPLIED: Tab: (Sodium Phosphate Monobasic Monohydrate-Sodium Phosphate Dibasic Anhydrous) 1.102g-0.398g.

CONTRAINDICATIONS: Biopsy-proven acute phosphate nephropathy.

WARNINGS/PRECAUTIONS: Fatalities reported due to significant fluid shifts, severe electrolyte abnormalities, and cardiac arrhythmias. Adequately hydrate before, during, and after use. Inadequate fluid intake may lead to excessive fluid loss, hypovolemia, and dehydration. Caution in patients with predisposing conditions; consider baseline and post-colonoscopy labs and correct electrolyte abnormalities before treatment. Rare reports of generalized tonic-clonic seizures and/or loss of conciousness; caution in patients with history of seizures or at higher risk of seizures (eg, concomitant medication that lower seizure threshold, withdrawing from alcohol or benzodiazepines, known or suspected hyponatremia). Prolongation of QT interval reported. Swallowing difficulties may occur with a history of difficulty swallowing or anatomic narrowing of the esophagus (eg, stricture). May induce colonic mucosal aphthous ulcerations; caution with inflammatory bowel disease.

ADVERSE REACTIONS: Phosphate nephropathy, renal impairment, hyperphosphatemia, hypocalcemia, abdominal bloating, N/V, hypophosphatemia, abdominal pain, hypokalemia.

INTERACTIONS: See Boxed Warning. Caution with medications that may affect electrolyte levels (eg, diuretics), lower seizure threshold (eg, tricyclic antidepressants), or prolong QT interval. Dehydration from purgation may be exacerbated by diuretics. Avoid additional laxatives/purgatives, particularly sodium phosphate-based products. Medications administered in close proximity to the drug may not be absorbed from the GI tract.

PREGNANCY: Category C, safety not known in nursing.

MECHANISM OF ACTION: Purgative; primary mode of action thought to be through osmotic action of Na^+, causing large amounts of water to be drawn into colon, promoting colon evacuation.

NURSING CONSIDERATIONS

Assessment: Assess for biopsy-proven acute phosphate nephropathy, increased risk of developing acute phosphate nephropathy, renal impairment, other conditions where treatment is contraindicated or cautioned, hypersensitivity, pregnancy/nursing status, and possible drug interactions. Consider baseline labs (phosphate, calcium, K^+, Na^+, SrCr, BUN) in patients who may be at increased risk for serious adverse events. Consider pre-dose and post-colonoscopy ECG in patients with high risk of serious cardiac arrhythmias or with known prolonged QT.

Monitoring: Monitor for signs and symptoms of acute phosphate nephropathy, fluid shifts, severe electrolyte abnormalities, cardiac arrhythmias, renal failure, nephrocalcinosis, generalized tonic-clonic seizures, loss of consciousness, QT prolongation, and colonic mucosal aphthous ulcerations. Consider performing post-colonoscopy labs (phosphate, calcium, Na^+, K^+, SrCr, BUN) in patients at increased risk for adverse events or if they develop vomiting and/or signs of dehydration.

Patient Counseling: Inform of risks/benefits of therapy. Instruct to inform healthcare provider of any concomitant medical condition or medication being taken. Instruct to follow the dose and dosing regimen. Advise to adequately hydrate before, during, and after use. Instruct to drink 8 oz. clear liquids with each 3-tab (or each 2-tab) dose; ingest total of 3.6 quarts clear liquids. Instruct not to use within 7 days of previous administration and not to take additional laxatives or purgatives, particularly additional sodium phosphate-based products.

Administration: Oral route. **Storage:** 25°C (77°F); excursions permitted to 15-30°C (59-86°F). Discard any unused portion.

V

VISTIDE

RX

cidofovir (Gilead)

> Renal impairment is the major toxicity. Cases of acute renal failure resulting in dialysis and/or contributing to death reported with as few as 1 or 2 doses; prehydrate with IV normal saline (NS) and administer probenecid with each dose. Monitor renal function (SrCr and urine protein) within 48 hrs prior to each dose. Modify dose with renal function changes. Contraindicated with nephrotoxic agents. Neutropenia reported; monitor neutrophil counts. Carcinogenic, teratogenic, and hypospermatic in animal studies.

THERAPEUTIC CLASS: Viral DNA synthesis inhibitor

INDICATIONS: Treatment of cytomegalovirus (CMV) retinitis in AIDS patients.

DOSAGE: *Adults:* IV: Induction: 5mg/kg once weekly for 2 weeks. Maint: 5mg/kg once every 2 weeks. SrCr 0.3-0.4mg/dL Above Baseline: Reduce maint from 5mg/kg to 3mg/kg D/C with increase in SrCr ≥0.5mg/dL above baseline or ≥3+ proteinuria. Administer probenecid 2g PO 3 hrs before cidofovir, then 1g at 2 hrs and 8 hrs after completion of the 1 hr cidofovir infusion (for a total of 4g). Administer at least 1L 0.9% NS IV over a 1-2 hr period immediately before infusion. If tolerated, give 2nd L over a 1-3 hr period at start of or immediately after infusion.

HOW SUPPLIED: Inj: 75mg/mL

CONTRAINDICATIONS: Initiation of therapy in patients with SrCr >1.5mg/dL, CrCl ≤55mL/min, or urine protein ≥100mg/dL (≥2+ proteinuria). Nephrotoxic agents (d/c at least 7 days before therapy), history of clinically severe hypersensitivity to probenecid or other sulfa-containing agents, direct intraocular use.

WARNINGS/PRECAUTIONS: Decreased intraocular pressure (IOP) and visual acuity reported; monitor IOP. Decreased serum bicarbonate associated with proximal tubule injury and renal wasting syndrome (including Fanconi's syndrome) reported. Cases of metabolic acidosis in association with liver dysfunction and pancreatitis resulting in death reported. Do not administer doses greater than recommended and exceed frequency or rate of administration. Uveitis or iritis reported; consider treatment with topical corticosteroids with or without topical cycloplegic agents. Monitor for signs and symptoms of uveitis/iritis.

ADVERSE REACTIONS: Renal toxicity, N/V, neutropenia, proteinuria, decreased IOP, uveitis/iritis, pneumonia, dyspnea, infection, fever, creatinine elevation ≥2mg/dL, decreased serum bicarbonate.

INTERACTIONS: See Contraindications.

PREGNANCY: Category C, not for use in nursing.

MECHANISM OF ACTION: Viral DNA synthesis inhibitor; suppresses CMV replication by selective inhibition of viral DNA synthesis.

PHARMACOKINETICS: Absorption: Administration of variable doses (with or without probenecid) resulted in different parameters. **Distribution:** V_d=537mL/kg (without probenecid), 410mL/kg (with probenecid); plasma protein binding (<6%). **Elimination:** Urine (80-100% unchanged).

NURSING CONSIDERATIONS

Assessment: Assess renal function (SrCR and urine protein) within 48 hrs prior to each dose, history of clinically severe hypersensitivity to probenecid or other sulfa-containing agents, pregnancy/nursing status, and possible drug interactions.

Monitoring: Monitor renal function and adjust dose as required. Give IV hydration to patients with proteinuria and repeat test as necessary. Monitor WBC counts with differential (prior to each dose), and neutrophil count. IOP, visual acuity, and ocular symptoms should be monitored periodically.

Patient Counseling: Inform that drug does not cure CMV retinitis; may continue to experience progression of retinitis during and following treatment. Advise to have regular follow-up ophthalmologic examinations. Advise to temporarily d/c zidovudine administration, or decrease zidovudine dose by half, on days of cidofovir administration only. Inform of the major toxicity of the drug. Counsel on importance of completing a full course of probenecid with each cidofovir dose. Warn of potential adverse events caused by probenecid. Inform that drug may cause tumors in humans. Advise women of limited enrollment of women in clinical trials. Advise men that testes weight reduction and hypospermia may occur in humans and may cause infertility. Inform of embryotoxicity in animal studies; advise women of childbearing potential to use effective contraception during and for 1 month following therapy and for men to practice barrier contraceptive methods during and for 3 months after therapy.

Administration: IV route. Infuse at constant rate over 1 hr. Refer to PI for method of preparation and administration. **Storage:** Vial: 20-25°C (68-77°F). Admixture: Under refrigeration, 2-8°C (36-46°F), for no more than 24 hrs. If refrigerated, allow admixture to equilibrate to room temperature prior to use.

V

VITRASERT

RX

ganciclovir (Bausch & Lomb)

THERAPEUTIC CLASS: Synthetic guanine derivative nucleoside analogue

INDICATIONS: Treatment of cytomegalovirus (CMV) retinitis in patients with AIDS.

DOSAGE: *Adults:* Each implant releases 4.5mg over 5-8 months. Remove and replace when evidence of retinitis progression is seen.
Pediatrics: ≥9 yrs: Each implant releases 4.5mg over 5-8 months. Remove and replace when evidence of retinitis progression is seen.

HOW SUPPLIED: Implant: 4.5mg

CONTRAINDICATIONS: Hypersensitivity to acyclovir, patients with any contraindications for intraocular surgery (eg, external infection, severe thrombocytopenia).

WARNINGS/PRECAUTIONS: For intravitreal implantation only. Does not provide treatment for systemic CMV disease; monitor for extraocular CMV disease. Potential complications from surgery include vitreous loss or hemorrhage, cataract formation, retinal detachment, uveitis, endophthalmitis, and decrease in visual acuity. May experience immediate and temporary decrease in visual acuity in the implanted eye which lasts for 2-4 weeks postoperatively. Maintain sterility of the surgical field and implant rigorously. Handle implant by the suture tab only to avoid damaging the polymer coatings. Do not resterilize implant by any method. A high level of surgical skill is required for implantation procedure; a surgeon should have observed or assisted in surgical implantation prior to attempting the procedure.

ADVERSE REACTIONS: Visual acuity loss, vitreous hemorrhage, retinal detachments, cataract formation/lens opacities, macular abnormalities, intraocular pressure spikes, optic disk/nerve changes, uveitis, hyphemas.

PREGNANCY: Category C, not for use in nursing.

MECHANISM OF ACTION: Synthetic guanine derivative nucleoside analogue; inhibits replication of herpes viruses.

NURSING CONSIDERATIONS

Assessment: Assess for proper diagnosis of CMV retinitis, any contraindications for intraocular surgery, hypersensitivity to the drug or acyclovir, and pregnancy/nursing status.

Monitoring: Monitor for extraocular CMV disease, vitreous loss or hemorrhage, cataract formation, retinal detachment, uveitis, endophthalmitis, decrease in visual acuity, and other adverse reactions.

Patient Counseling: Advise that implant is not a cure for CMV retinitis; inform that some immunocompromised patients may continue to experience progression of retinitis. Instruct to have ophthalmologic follow-up examinations of both eyes at appropriate intervals after implantation. Counsel about the potential complications following intraocular surgery. Inform that will experience immediate and temporary decrease in visual acuity for 2-4 weeks after surgery. Advise that the implant only treats eyes in which it has been implanted. Instruct women of childbearing potential to avoid pregnancy during therapy. Inform that the medication may cause infertility and may be carcinogenic.

Administration: Intravitreal implantation. Refer to PI for handling and disposal procedure.
Storage: 15-30°C (59-86°F). Protect from freezing, excessive heat, and light.

VIVELLE-DOT

RX

estradiol (Novartis)

> Estrogens increase the risk of endometrial cancer. Perform adequate diagnostic measures, including endometrial sampling, to rule out malignancy with undiagnosed persistent or recurrent abnormal vaginal bleeding. Should not be used for the prevention of cardiovascular disease (CVD). Increased risks of myocardial infarction (MI), stroke, invasive breast cancer, pulmonary emboli (PE), and deep vein thrombosis (DVT) in postmenopausal women (50-79 yrs of age) reported. Increased risk of developing probable dementia in postmenopausal women ≥65 yrs of age reported. Should be prescribed at the lowest effective dose and for the shortest duration consistent with treatment goals and risks.

THERAPEUTIC CLASS: Estrogen

INDICATIONS: Treatment of moderate to severe vasomotor symptoms and/or vulvar/vaginal atrophy associated with menopause. Treatment of hypoestrogenism due to hypogonadism, castration, or primary ovarian failure. Prevention of postmenopausal osteoporosis.

DOSAGE: *Adults:* Apply patch 2X/week to clean, dry area of the abdomen (not to breasts or waist). Rotate application sites with an interval of at least 1 week allowed between applications to a particular site. Vasomotor Symptoms/Vulvar/Vaginal Atrophy: Initial: 0.0375mg/day 2X/week. Osteoporosis Prevention: Initial: 0.025mg/day 2X/week. Not Currently on Oral Estrogens

V

or Switching from Another Estradiol Transdermal Therapy: May be initiated at once. Currently taking Oral Estrogens: Initiate 1 week after withdrawal of oral hormone therapy, or sooner if menopausal symptoms reappear in <1 week. Adjust dose PRN. May give continuously in patients with no intact uterus, or cyclically (eg, 3 weeks on, 1 week off drug) with intact uterus. Reevaluate treatment need periodically (eg, 3-6 month intervals).

HOW SUPPLIED: Patch: 0.025mg/day, 0.0375mg/day, 0.05mg/day, 0.075mg/day, 0.1mg/day [8^s]

CONTRAINDICATIONS: Undiagnosed abnormal genital bleeding, known/suspected/history of breast cancer, known/suspected estrogen-dependent neoplasia, active or history of DVT/PE, active or recent arterial thromboembolic disease (eg, stroke, MI), liver dysfunction or disease, known/suspected pregnancy.

WARNINGS/PRECAUTIONS: Increased risk of stroke, DVT, PE, and MI reported; d/c immediately if any of these events occur or are suspected. Caution in patients with risk factors for arterial vascular disease (eg, HTN, diabetes mellitus [DM], tobacco use, hypercholesterolemia, obesity) and/or venous thromboembolism (VTE) (eg, personal history or family history of venous VTE, obesity, systemic lupus erythematosus [SLE]). If feasible, d/c at least 4 to 6 weeks before surgery of the type associated with an increased risk of thromboembolism, or during periods of prolonged immobilization. May increase risk of gallbladder disease, ovarian cancer, and breast cancer. Unopposed estrogens in women with intact uteri has been associated with increased risk of endometrial cancer. May lead to severe hypercalcemia in patients with breast cancer and bone metastases; d/c and take appropriate measures if hypercalcemia occurs. Retinal vascular thrombosis reported; if visual abnormalities or migraine occurs, d/c pending examination. If examination reveals papilledema or retinal vascular lesions, d/c permanently. Consider addition of a progestin if no hysterectomy. May elevate BP, thyroid-binding globulin levels, and plasma TG leading to pancreatitis and other complications. Caution with history of cholestatic jaundice; d/c in case of recurrence. May cause fluid retention; caution with cardiac/renal dysfunction. Caution with severe hypocalcemia. May exacerbate endometriosis, asthma, DM, epilepsy, migraine, porphyria, SLE, and hepatic hemangiomas; use with caution. May affect certain endocrine, LFTs, and blood components in laboratory tests.

ADVERSE REACTIONS: Constipation, dyspepsia, pain, influenza-like illness, nausea, nasopharyngitis, sinusitis, upper respiratory tract infection, arthralgia, breast tenderness, intermenstrual bleeding, sinus congestion, depression, insomnia, headache.

INTERACTIONS: CYP3A4 inducers (eg, St. John's wort, phenobarbital, carbamazepine, rifampin) may decrease levels/therapeutic effects and/or change uterine bleeding profile. CYP3A4 inhibitors (eg, erythromycin, clarithromycin, ketoconazole, itraconazole, ritonavir, grapefruit juice) may increase levels, which may result in side effects. Patients concomitantly receiving thyroid hormone replacement therapy and estrogens may require increased doses of thyroid hormone.

PREGNANCY: Contraindicated in pregnancy, caution in nursing.

MECHANISM OF ACTION: Estrogen; binds to nuclear receptors in estrogen-responsive tissues. Circulating estrogens modulate pituitary secretion of gonadotropins, luteinizing hormone and follicle stimulating hormone, through a negative feedback mechanism. Reduces elevated levels of these hormones in postmenopausal women.

PHARMACOKINETICS: Absorption: Transdermal administration of variable doses resulted in different parameters. **Distribution:** Largely bound to sex hormone-binding globulin and albumin; found in breast milk. **Metabolism:** Liver; estrone (metabolite); estriol (major urinary metabolite); sulfate and glucuronide conjugation (liver); gut hydrolysis; CYP 3A4 (partial metabolism). **Elimination:** Urine; $T_{1/2}$=5.9-7.7 hrs.

NURSING CONSIDERATIONS

Assessment: Assess for presence or history of breast cancer, estrogen-dependent neoplasia, abnormal genital bleeding, active or history of DVT/PE, active or recent arterial thromboembolic disease, liver dysfunction/disease, known/suspected pregnancy, and any other conditions where treatment may be contraindicated or cautioned. Assess use in women ≥65 yrs, nursing patients, and those with DM, asthma, epilepsy, migraines or porphyria, SLE, and hepatic hemangiomas. Assess for possible drug interactions. Assess need for progestin therapy in women who have not had a hysterectomy.

Monitoring: Monitor for signs/symptoms of CVD, malignant neoplasms, dementia, gallbladder disease, cholestatic jaundice, hypercalcemia, visual abnormalities, BP elevations, fluid retention, elevations in plasma TG, hypothyroidism, pancreatitis, exacerbation of endometriosis and other conditions (eg, asthma, DM, epilepsy, migraines, SLE, hepatic hemangiomas). Periodically monitor BP levels at regular intervals and thyroid function in patients on thyroid replacement therapy. Perform proper diagnostic testing (eg, endometrial sampling) in patients with undiagnosed, persistent, or recurring vaginal bleeding. Perform annual breast exam. Perform periodic evaluation to determine treatment need.

Patient Counseling: Inform that therapy may increase the risk for uterine cancer and may increase chance of heart attack, stroke, breast cancer, blood clots, and dementia. Instruct to

V

report to physician any breast lumps, unusual vaginal bleeding, dizziness and faintness, changes in speech, severe headaches, chest pain, SOB, leg pains, changes in vision, or vomiting. Advise to notify physician if pregnant or nursing. Instruct to have annual breast examination by a physician and perform monthly breast self examination. Instruct to place patch on a clean, dry area of the abdomen, to avoid oily, damaged, or irritated area and should not be applied in breasts or waistline. Counsel to rotate application sites with an interval of 1 week, and to apply immediately after opening pouch. Inform that if medication system falls off, reapply same system or apply new system PRN and continue with original treatment schedule.

Administration: Topical route. Apply immediately upon removal from the protective pouch. Refer to PI for application instructions. **Storage:** 25°C (77°F); do not store unpouched.

VIVITROL   RX
naltrexone (Alkermes)

> May cause hepatocellular injury with excessive doses. Contraindicated in acute hepatitis or liver failure; caution with active liver disease. Does not appear to be a heptatotoxin at recommended doses. Warn patient of the risk of hepatic injury and advise to seek medical attention if symptoms of acute hepatitis occur. D/C in the event of symptoms and/or signs of acute hepatitis.

THERAPEUTIC CLASS: Opioid antagonist

INDICATIONS: Treatment of alcohol dependence in patients who are able to abstain from alcohol in an outpatient setting prior to initiation of therapy. Prevention of relapse to opioid dependence, following opioid detoxification.

DOSAGE: *Adults:* 380mg IM gluteal inj q4 weeks or once a month, alternating buttocks.

HOW SUPPLIED: Inj, Extended-Release: 380mg

CONTRAINDICATIONS: Acute hepatitis or liver failure, concomitant opioid analgesics, physiologic opioid dependence, acute opioid withdrawal, positive urine screen for opioids or failed naloxone challenge test.

WARNINGS/PRECAUTIONS: Cases of eosinophilic pneumonia and hypersensitivity reactions including anaphylaxis reported. May precipitate opioid withdrawal in alcohol-dependent patients using or dependent on opioids. Must be opioid-free for ≥7-10 days prior to initiation of therapy. Perform naloxone challenge test if there is a risk of precipitating withdrawal. May respond to lower doses of opioids than previously used. Opioid overdose with fatal outcomes reported in patients who use opioids at the end of a dosing interval or when missing a dose. Attempts to overcome opioid blockade could lead to fatal overdose. Monitor for development of depression or suicidal thinking. In emergency situations, suggested plan for pain management is regional analgesia or use of non-opioid analgesics. If opioid therapy is required, monitor continuously in an anesthesia care setting. Caution in renal/hepatic impairment. Does not eliminate or diminish alcohol withdrawal symptoms. Injection-site reactions reported; inadvertent SQ injection may increase likelihood of severe injection-site reactions. As with any IM inj, caution with thrombocytopenia or any coagulation disorder (eg, hemophilia and severe hepatic failure). May cross-react with certain immunoassay methods for the detection of drugs of abuse in urine.

ADVERSE REACTIONS: N/V, diarrhea, insomnia, depression, injection-site reactions, somnolence, anorexia, muscle cramps, dizziness, syncope, appetite disorder, hepatic enzyme abnormalities, nasopharyngitis, toothache.

INTERACTIONS: See Contraindications. Antagonizes effects of opioid-containing medicines (eg, cough and cold remedies, antidiarrheals, opioid analgesics).

PREGNANCY: Category C, not for use in nursing.

MECHANISM OF ACTION: Opioid antagonist; blocks the effects of opioids by competitive binding at opioid receptors.

PHARMACOKINETICS: Absorption: T_{max}=2-3 days. **Distribution:** Plasma protein binding (21%); (PO) found in breast milk. **Metabolism:** Extensive, via dihydrodiol dehydrogenase, 6β-naltrexol (primary metabolite). **Elimination:** Urine; $T_{1/2}$=5-10 days.

NURSING CONSIDERATIONS

Assessment: Assess for hepatic failure, hepatitis or active liver disease, opioid use or dependence, thrombocytopenia, coagulation disorder (eg, hemophilia, severe hepatic failure), renal impairment, pre-existing subclinical abstinence syndrome, hypersensitivity, pregnancy/nursing status, alcohol intake, and for possible drug interactions. Assess patient's body habitus to assure the needle length is adequate.

Monitoring: Monitor for severe injection-site reactions, signs/symptoms of acute hepatitis, unintended opioid withdrawal, opioid intoxication (respiratory compromise/arrest, circulatory collapse), eosinophilic pneumonia, depression, suicidal thinking, and hypersensitivity reactions. Monitor LFTs and CPK.

Patient Counseling: Alert families and caregivers to monitor for emergence of symptoms of depression and to call a doctor immediately if observed. Carry documentation to alert medical personnel to therapy. Concomitant large doses of opioids may lead to serious injury, coma, or death. If patient previously used opioids, may be more sensitive to lower doses of opioids after naltrexone is d/c. Notify if pregnant/nursing or planning to become pregnant, experience respiratory symptoms (eg, dyspnea, coughing, or wheezing), allergic reactions. Inform that injection-site reactions may occur and instruct to seek medical attention for worsening skin reactions. Avoid opioids for ≥7-10 days before therapy and inform doctor of any prior opioid use. May cause liver injury if liver disease develops from other cause. Notify physician if signs/symptoms of liver disease and pneumonia develop. Therapy treats alcohol dependence only when used as part of treatment program. May impair mental/physical abilities. May cause nausea, which tends to subside. Instruct to receive the next dose as soon as possible if a dose is missed.

Administration: IM route; gluteal region. Must be administrated by a healthcare professional. Not for IV/SQ use. Inspect for particulate matter and discoloration prior to use. Refer to PI for preparation and administration instructions. **Storage:** 2-8°C (36-46°F). Do not freeze. Can be stored at <25°C (77°F) for <7 days prior administration.

VOLTAREN GEL

RX

diclofenac sodium (Novartis Consumer)

NSAIDs may cause an increased risk of serious cardiovascular thrombotic events, myocardial infarction, stroke and serious GI adverse events including bleeding, ulceration, and perforation of the stomach or intestines, which can be fatal. Patients with cardiovascular disease (CVD) or risk factors for CVD may be at greater risk. Elderly patients are at a greater risk for GI events. Contraindicated for the treatment of perioperative pain in the setting of coronary artery bypass graft (CABG) surgery.

THERAPEUTIC CLASS: NSAID

INDICATIONS: Relief of the pain of osteoarthritis of joints amenable to topical treatment, such as knees and hands.

DOSAGE: *Adults:* Lower Extremities: Apply 4g to affected foot, knee, or ankle qid. Max: 16g/day to any single joint. Upper Extremities: Apply 2g to affected hand, elbow, or wrist qid. Max: 8g/day to any single joint. Total dose should not exceed 32g/day over all affected joints.

HOW SUPPLIED: Gel: 1% [100g]

CONTRAINDICATIONS: Asthma, urticaria, or allergic-type reactions after taking aspirin (ASA) or other NSAID, setting of CABG surgery.

WARNINGS/PRECAUTIONS: Not evaluated for use on spine, hip, or shoulder. Avoid open wounds, eyes, mucous membranes, external heat, natural or artificial sunlight and/or occlusive dressings. May lead to onset of new HTN or worsening of pre-existing HTN; monitor BP closely. Fluid retention and edema reported; caution with fluid retention or heart failure. Renal papillary necrosis and other renal injury reported after long-term use. Not recommended for use with advanced renal disease; if therapy must be initiated, monitor renal function. Anaphylactoid reactions may occur. May cause serious skin adverse events (eg, exfoliative dermatitis, Stevens-Johnson syndrome [SJS], and toxic epidermal necrolysis [TEN]). Avoid in late pregnancy; may cause premature closure of ductus arteriosus. Not a substitute for corticosteroids or to treat corticosteroid insufficiency. May cause elevations of LFTs; d/c if liver disease develops or systemic manifestations occur. To minimize the potential for adverse liver-related events, use the lowest effective dose for the shortest duration possible. Caution in elderly. Anemia may occur; with long-term use, monitor Hgb/Hct if signs or symptoms of anemia develop. May inhibit platelet aggregation and prolong bleeding time; monitor with coagulation disorders. Caution with asthma and avoid with ASA-sensitive asthma. Caution in patients with prior history of ulcer or GI bleeding; monitor for signs or symptoms of GI bleeding. May diminish utility of diagnostic signs (eg, inflammation, fever) in detecting infectious complications of presumed noninfectious, painful conditions.

ADVERSE REACTIONS: Application-site reactions, dermatitis, ALT/AST increase, gastrointestinal effects.

INTERACTIONS: May enhance methotrexate toxicity and cyclosporine nephrotoxicity; caution when coadministering. May diminish antihypertensive effect of ACE-inhibitors and impair response of loop diuretics. May reduce natriuretic effect of furosemide and thiazides; monitor for renal failure. May increase lithium levels; monitor for toxicity. Synergistic effects on GI bleeding with anticoagulants (eg, warfarin) reported. Avoid concomitant use with other topical products, including topical medications, sunscreens, lotions, moisturizers, and cosmetics, on the same skin site; may alter tolerability and absorption. Coadministration with oral NSAIDs or ASA may result in increased adverse effects; concomitant administration with ASA not recommended. Caution with concomitant hepatotoxic drugs (eg, antibiotics, anti-epileptics). May increase risk of GI bleeding with oral corticosteroids/anticoagulants, tobacco or alcohol use.

PREGNANCY: Category C, not for use in nursing.

V

MECHANISM OF ACTION: NSAID; inhibits cyclooxygenase, resulting in reduced formation of prostaglandins, thromboxanes, and prostacylin.

PHARMACOKINETICS: Absorption: (4g) C_{max}=15ng/mL; T_{max}=14 hrs; AUC_{0-24}=233ng•h/mL. (12g) C_{max}=53.8ng/mL; T_{max}=10 hrs; AUC_{0-24}=807ng•h/mL.

NURSING CONSIDERATIONS

Assessment: Assess for hypersensitivity to ASA or NSAIDs, history of ulcer or GI bleeding, HTN, fluid retention, congestive heart failure, asthma, CVD (or risk factors), renal/hepatic impairment, pregnancy/nursing status, and for possible drug interactions. Obtain baseline BP.

Monitoring: Monitor for signs/symptoms of CV events, GI events (eg, ulcerations, bleeding), hepatotoxicity, renal dysfunction, HTN, skin reactions, anemia, blood loss and hypersensitivity reactions. Monitor BP, LFTs, and renal function periodically.

Patient Counseling: Instruct to avoid contact with eyes and mucous membranes; if contact occurs, wash with water or saline and if irritation persists for >1 hr, call physician. Advise to minimize or avoid exposure of treated areas to natural or artificial sunlight. Inform to avoid late in pregnancy. Seek medical attention for symptoms of CV events (eg, chest pain, SOB, weakness, slurring of speech), GI events (eg, epigastric pain, dyspepsia, melena, hematemesis), hepatotoxicity (eg, nausea, lethargy, flu-like symptoms, right upper quadrant pain, pruritus, fatigue), unexplained weight gain or edema, skin reactions (eg, skin rash, blisters, fever, SJS, TEN, exfoliative dermatitis) or hypersensitivity reactions (eg, difficulty breathing, swelling of face/throat); d/c at first appearance of rash/hypersensitivity reactions. Stress the importance of follow-up. Instruct not to apply to open skin wounds, infections, inflammations, or exfoliative dermatitis. Instruct to avoid concomitant use with other topical products.

Administration: Topical route. Measure onto enclosed dosing card to appropriate 2g or 4g line. Avoid showering or bathing for ≥1 hr after application. Avoid wearing clothing or gloves for ≥10 min after application. **Storage:** 25°C (77°F), excursions permitted to 15-30°C (59-86°F). Keep from freezing.

VOLTAREN OPHTHALMIC   RX
diclofenac sodium (Novartis Ophthalmics)

THERAPEUTIC CLASS: NSAID

INDICATIONS: Treatment of postoperative inflammation in patients who have undergone cataract extraction. Temporary relief of pain and photophobia in patients undergoing corneal refractive surgery.

DOSAGE: *Adults:* Cataract Surgery: 1 drop to the affected eye qid beginning 24 hrs after surgery and continue throughout the 1st 2 weeks of postoperative period. Corneal Refractive Surgery: 1-2 drops to the operative eye within the hr prior to, and within 15 min after surgery. Continue qid for ≤3 days.

HOW SUPPLIED: Sol: 0.1% [2.5mL, 5mL]

WARNINGS/PRECAUTIONS: Refractive stability in patients undergoing corneal refractive procedures and treated with diclofenac sodium ophthalmic not established; monitor for 1 yr following use. May cause increased bleeding of ocular tissues. Potential for cross-sensitivity to acetylsalicylic acid, phenylacetic acid derivatives, and other NSAIDs. May slow or delay healing. May result in keratitis. Continued use may lead to sight-threatening epithelial breakdown, corneal thinning, corneal erosion, corneal ulceration, corneal perforation; d/c if evidence of corneal epithelial breakdown occurs and monitor for corneal health. Caution in patients experiencing complicated ocular surgeries, corneal denervation, corneal epithelial defects, diabetes mellitus (DM), ocular surface disease (eg, dry eye syndrome), rheumatoid arthritis (RA), repeat ocular surgeries within a short period of time or with known bleeding tendencies. Use >24 hrs prior to surgery or beyond 14 days post-surgery may increase risk for occurrence and severity of corneal adverse events. Avoid in late pregnancy.

ADVERSE REACTIONS: Transient burning/stinging, elevated intraocular pressure (IOP), lacrimation disorder, ocular allergy, abnormal vision, conjunctivitis, eyelid swelling, ocular discharge, iritis, eye itching, corneal deposits, corneal edema, corneal opacity, corneal lesions.

INTERACTIONS: Caution with other medications which may prolong bleeding time. May increase the potential for healing problems with topical steroids.

PREGNANCY: Category C, not for use in nursing.

MECHANISM OF ACTION: NSAID; demonstrated anti-inflammatory and analgesic properties. Thought to inhibit the enzyme cyclooxygenase, which is essential for biosynthesis of prostaglandins.

NURSING CONSIDERATIONS

Assessment: Assess for hypersensitivity or cross-sensitivity, history of complicated or repeated ocular surgeries, corneal denervation, corneal epithelial defects, DM, ocular surface diseases (eg, dry eye syndrome), RA, bleeding tendencies, pregnancy/nursing status, concomitant use of medications that may prolong bleeding time or delay healing and possible drug interactions.

Monitoring: Monitor for corneal thinning, erosion, ulceration, or perforation, healing problems, keratitis, increased bleeding time, bleeding of ocular tissues (hyphemas) in conjunction with ocular surgery and other adverse reactions. Monitor patients who have undergone corneal refractive procedures for a year.

Patient Counseling: Instruct not to use while currently wearing soft contact lenses except for the use of a bandage hydrogel soft contact lens during the 1st 3 days following refractive surgery.

Administration: Ocular route. **Storage:** 15-25°C (59-77°F).

VOLTAREN-XR   RX
diclofenac sodium (Novartis)

> NSAIDs may cause an increased risk of serious cardiovascular thrombotic events, myocardial infarction (MI), stroke, and serious GI adverse events including inflammation, bleeding, ulceration, and perforation of the stomach or intestines, which may be fatal. Contraindicated for the treatment of perioperative pain in the setting of coronary artery bypass graft (CABG) surgery.

THERAPEUTIC CLASS: NSAID

INDICATIONS: Relief of signs and symptoms of osteoarthritis (OA), and rheumatoid arthritis (RA).

DOSAGE: *Adults:* OA: Usual: 100mg qd. RA: Usual: 100mg qd-bid.

HOW SUPPLIED: Tab, Extended-Release: 100mg

CONTRAINDICATIONS: Aspirin (ASA) or other NSAID allergy that precipitates asthma, urticaria, or allergic-type reactions. Treatment of perioperative pain in the setting of CABG surgery.

WARNINGS/PRECAUTIONS: Use lowest effective dose for the shortest duration possible. Not a substitute for corticosteroids or to treat corticosteroid insufficiency. May lead to onset of new HTN or worsening of pre-existing HTN; monitor BP closely. Fluid retention and edema reported; caution with fluid retention or heart failure. Extreme caution with a prior history of ulcer disease, and/or GI bleeding. Caution when initiating treatment in patients with considerable dehydration. Renal papillary necrosis and other renal injury reported after long-term use. Not recommended for use with advanced renal disease; if therapy must be initiated, monitor renal function. Anaphylactoid reactions may occur; avoid in patients with ASA-triad. May cause serious skin adverse events (eg, exfoliative dermatitis, Stevens-Johnson syndrome [SJS], toxic epidermal necrolysis). Avoid in late pregnancy; may cause premature closure of ductus arteriosus. May cause elevations of LFTs; d/c if liver disease develops or systemic manifestations occur. Caution in elderly and debilitated patients. Anemia may occur; with long-term use, monitor Hgb/Hct if signs or symptoms of anemia develop. May inhibit platelet aggregation and prolong bleeding time; monitor with coagulation disorders. Caution with asthma and avoid with ASA-sensitive asthma.

ADVERSE REACTIONS: Abdominal pain, constipation, diarrhea, dyspepsia, flatulence, gross bleeding/perforation, heartburn, N/V, GI ulcers, renal function abnormalities, anemia, dizziness, edema, elevated liver enzymes.

INTERACTIONS: Increased adverse effects with ASA; avoid use. May enhance methotrexate toxicity and increase nephrotoxicity of cyclosporine; caution with coadministration. May diminish antihypertensive effect of ACE inhibitors. Patients taking thiazides and loop diuretics may have impaired response to these therapies. ACE inhibitors and diuretics may precipitate overt renal decompensation. May reduce natriuretic effect of furosemide and thiazides. May increase lithium levels; monitor for toxicity. Synergistic effects with warfarin on GI bleeding. May increase risk of GI bleeding with oral corticosteroids or anticoagulants, tobacco or alcohol use. Caution with hepatotoxic drugs (eg, antibiotics, anti-epileptics). Caution with CYP2C9 inhibitors or inducers (eg, voriconazole, rifampin); dosage adjustment may be warranted.

PREGNANCY: Category C, not for use in nursing.

MECHANISM OF ACTION: NSAID; not known, suspected to inhibit prostaglandin synthetase.

PHARMACOKINETICS: Absorption: Absolute bioavailability (55%); T_{max}=5.3 hrs. **Distribution:** V_d=1.4L/kg; plasma protein binding (>99%). **Metabolism:** Liver (glucuronidation and sulfation). **Elimination:** Urine (65%), bile (35%); $T_{1/2}$=2.3 hrs.

NURSING CONSIDERATIONS

Assessment: Assess for cardiovascular disease or risk factors, fluid retention, edema, conditions affected by platelet function alterations, GI events or risk factors, renal/hepatic function, any other conditions where treatment is contraindicated or cautioned, pregnancy/nursing status, and possible drug interactions. Assess baseline BP, CBC, and chemistry profile.

Monitoring: Monitor for signs/symptoms of GI events, cardiovascular thrombotic events, CHF, HTN, allergic or skin reactions, hematological effects (eg, anemia, prolongation of bleeding time), renal papillary necrosis or other renal injury/toxicity, hepatotoxicity. Monitor BP, CBC, and chemistry profile periodically.

Patient Counseling: Advise to seek medical attention if signs and symptoms of hepatotoxicity (eg, nausea, fatigue, pruritus), anaphylactic/anaphylactoid reactions (eg, difficulty breathing, swelling of face/throat), skin reactions (eg, skin rash, blisters, fever, itching), cardiovascular events (eg, chest pain, SOB, weakness, slurring of speech), GI ulceration or bleeding (eg, epigastric pain, dyspepsia, melena, hematemesis), weight gain, or edema occur. Inform of pregnancy risks and instruct to avoid use during late pregnancy.

Administration: Oral route. **Storage:** Protect from moisture. Do not store above 30°C (86°F).

VoSpire ER   RX
albuterol sulfate (Dava)

THERAPEUTIC CLASS: Beta$_2$-agonist

INDICATIONS: Treatment of bronchospasm in reversible obstructive airway disease.

DOSAGE: *Adults:* Usual: 4-8mg q12h. Low Body Weight: Initial: 4mg q12h. Titrate: May increase to 8mg q12h. Max: 32mg/day in divided doses. Swallow whole with liquids; do not chew or crush. *Pediatrics:* >12 yrs: Usual: 4-8mg q12h. Low Body Weight: Initial: 4mg q12h. Titrate: May increase to 8mg q12h. Max: 32mg/day in divided doses. 6-12 yrs: Usual: 4mg q12h. Max: 24mg/day in divided doses. Swallow whole with liquids; do not chew or crush.

HOW SUPPLIED: Tab, Extended-Release: 4mg, 8mg

WARNINGS/PRECAUTIONS: Hypersensitivity reactions reported. Caution with cardiovascular disorders, especially coronary insufficiency, arrhythmias and HTN. Increased doses may signify need for concomitant corticosteroids. Can produce paradoxical bronchospasm. Caution with DM, hyperthyroidism, seizures. May produce transient hypokalemia. Erythema multiforme and Stevens-Johnson syndrome (rare) reported in children.

ADVERSE REACTIONS: Tremor, headache, nervousness, tachycardia, palpitations, N/V, muscle cramps.

INTERACTIONS: Avoid oral sympathomimetic agents. Extreme caution within 14 days of MAOI or TCA therapy. Monitor digoxin. May worsen ECG changes and/or hypokalemia with non-K$^+$-sparing diuretics. Antagonized by β-blockers.

PREGNANCY: Category C, not for use in nursing.

MECHANISM OF ACTION: β$_2$-adrenergic bronchodilator; stimulates adenyl cylase, enzyme that catalyzes formation of cAMP from ATP. Increased cAMP levels associated with relaxation of bronchial smooth muscle and inhibition of release of mediators of immediate hypersensitivity.

PHARMACOKINETICS: Absorption: C_{max}=13.7ng/mL; T_{max}=6 hrs; AUC=134ng•hr/mL. **Elimination:** $T_{1/2}$=9.3 hrs.

NURSING CONSIDERATIONS

Assessment: Assess for renal/hepatic functions, history of hypersensitivity to drug, cardiovascular disorder (coronary insufficiency, HTN, cardiac arrhythmias), convulsive disorders, hyperthyroidism, DM and ketoacidosis, pregnancy/nursing status, and possible drug interactions.

Monitoring: Monitor for possible paradoxical bronchospasm, asthma deterioration, cardiovascular effects, immediate hypersensitivity reactions, CBC with differential count, ketoacidosis, hypokalemia, serum glucose concentrations, tremors.

Patient Counseling: Instruct to swallow tablet; do not chew or crush. Report lack of response or adverse effects.

Administration: Oral route. **Storage:** Store at 20-25°C (68-77°F). Dispense in well-closed, light-resistant container.

Votrient   RX
pazopanib (GlaxoSmithKline)

Severe and fatal hepatotoxicity reported; monitor hepatic function and interrupt, reduce, or d/c dosing as recommended.

THERAPEUTIC CLASS: Tyrosine kinase inhibitor

INDICATIONS: Treatment of advanced renal cell carcinoma (RCC) and for advanced soft tissue sarcoma (STS) that has been treated with prior chemotherapy.

DOSAGE: *Adults:* Usual: 800mg PO qd without food (at least 1 hr ac or 2 hrs pc). Max: 800mg. Dose Modification: RCC: Initial Dose Reduction: 400mg, and additional decrease or increase in dose should be in 200mg steps based on tolerability. STS: Decrease or increase should be in 200mg steps based on tolerability. Moderate Hepatic Impairment: Consider alternative therapy or reduce to 200mg/day. Concomitant Strong CYP3A4 Inhibitors (eg, Ketoconazole, Ritonavir, Clarithromycin): Reduce to 400mg. Further dose reductions may be needed if adverse effects occur during therapy.

HOW SUPPLIED: Tab: 200mg

WARNINGS/PRECAUTIONS: Avoid with preexisting severe hepatic impairment. Caution with history of QT interval prolongation, and relevant preexisting cardiac disease. Cardiac dysfunction (eg, decreased left ventricular ejection fraction [LVEF], congestive heart failure [CHF]) reported; perform baseline and periodic evaluation of LVEF in patients at risk for cardiac dysfunction (eg, previous anthracycline exposure). Monitor BP and manage promptly using combination antihypertensives and dose modification of therapy. Hemorrhagic events reported; avoid with history of hemoptysis, cerebral, or clinically significant GI hemorrhage in the past 6 months. Arterial thrombotic events (eg, myocardial infarction [MI], ischemia, cerebrovascular accident (CVA), transient ischemic attacks [TIA]) reported; caution in patients at risk or who have history of these events and avoid use if occurred within the past 6 months. Venous thromboembolic events (VTE), including venous thrombosis and pulmonary embolus (PE), and GI perforation/fistula reported. Reversible posterior leukoencephalopathy syndrome (RPLS) reported; d/c if develops. HTN and hypertensive crisis reported; d/c if evidence of hypertensive crisis or if HTN is severe and persistent despite antihypertensive therapy and dose reduction. May impair wound healing; d/c therapy with wound dehiscence and at least 7 days prior to scheduled surgery. Hypothyroidism reported. Proteinuria reported. Interrupt therapy and reduce dose for 24-hr urine protein ≥3g; d/c for repeat episodes despite dose reductions. Serious infections reported; institute appropriate anti-infective therapy and consider interruption or d/c if develop. May cause fetal harm during pregnancy.

ADVERSE REACTIONS: Diarrhea, HTN, hair color changes, N/V, anorexia, fatigue, asthenia, headache, weight/appetite decreased, tumor pain, dysgeusia, musculoskeletal pain, hepatotoxicity.

INTERACTIONS: Do not use in combination with other cancer therapy; increased toxicity and mortality reported with pemetrexed and lapatinib. Strong inhibitors of CYP3A4 (eg, ketoconazole, ritonavir, clarithromycin) may increase concentrations; avoid use or reduce dose of pazopanib when it must be coadministered. Avoid grapefruit juice. CYP3A4 inducers (eg, rifampin) may decrease plasma concentrations; avoid pazopanib if chronic use of strong CYP3A4 inducers cannot be avoided. Not recommended with agents with narrow therapeutic windows that are metabolized by CYP3A4, CYP2D6, or CYP2C8. Simvastatin may increase incidence of ALT elevations; follow dosing guidelines or consider alternatives to pazopanib or d/c simvastatin. Caution in patients taking antiarrhythmics or other medications that may prolong QT interval. May increase concentrations of drugs eliminated by UGT1A1 and OATP1B1.

PREGNANCY: Category D, not for use in nursing.

MECHANISM OF ACTION: Tyrosine kinase inhibitor; inhibits vascular endothelial growth factor receptor (VEGFR)-1, VEGFR-2, VEGFR-3, platelet-derived growth factor receptor-α and -β, fibroblast growth factor receptor-1 and -3, cytokine receptor, interleukin-2 receptor inducible T-cell kinase, leukocyte-specific protein tyrosine kinase, and transmembrane glycoprotein receptor tyrosine kinase.

PHARMACOKINETICS: **Absorption:** T_{max}=2-4 hrs; (800mg dose) AUC=1037μg•h/mL, C_{max}=58.1μg/mL. **Distribution:** Plasma protein binding (>99%). **Metabolism:** CYP3A4 (major), CYP1A2/CYP2C8 (minor). **Elimination:** Feces (primary), urine (<4% administered dose); (800 mg dose) $T_{1/2}$=30.9 hrs.

NURSING CONSIDERATIONS

Assessment: Assess for history of QT interval prolongation, preexisting cardiac disease/severe hepatic impairment, HTN, impaired wound healing, history of hemoptysis/cerebral or clinically significant GI hemorrhage/MI/ischemia/CVA/TIA in the past 6 months, pregnancy/nursing status, and for possible drug interactions. Obtain baseline BP, LFTs, ECG, LVEF, and urinalysis.

Monitoring: Monitor for signs/symptoms of hepatotoxicity, QT prolongation, torsades de pointes, cardiac dysfunction, hemorrhagic events, arterial thrombotic events, VTE, PE, RPLS, GI perforation or fistula, HTN/hypertensive crisis, impaired wound healing, hypothyroidism, proteinuria, serious infection, and other adverse reactions. Monitor for LFTs at least once every 4 weeks for at least 1st 4 months of therapy or as clinically indicated, and then periodically. Monitor BP early after starting treatment and then frequently to ensure BP control. Monitor ECG, LVEF, urinalysis, and thyroid function tests. Perform maint of electrolytes within the normal range.

Patient Counseling: Advise that laboratory monitoring will be required prior to and while on therapy. Instruct to report any signs/symptoms of liver dysfunction, HTN, CHF, unusual bleeding, arterial thrombosis, new onset of dyspnea, chest pain, or localized limb edema, GI perforation/fistula, infection, and worsening of neurologic function consistent with RPLS (eg, headache, seizure, lethargy, confusion, blindness). Advise to d/c treatment at least 7 days prior to a scheduled surgery. Inform that thyroid function testing and urinalysis will be performed during treatment. Advise on how to manage diarrhea and to notify healthcare provider if moderate to severe diarrhea occurs. Advise women of childbearing potential to avoid becoming pregnant during therapy. Advise to inform healthcare providers of all concomitant medications, vitamins, or dietary and herbal supplements. Advise that depigmentation of the hair or skin may occur during treatment. Instruct to take medication without food (at least 1 hr ac or 2 hrs pc). Instruct that if a dose is missed, do not take if it is <12 hrs until the next dose.

Administration: Oral route. Do not crush tabs. **Storage:** 20-25°C (68-77°F); excursions permitted to 15-30°C (59-86°F).

VPRIV   RX
velaglucerase alfa (Shire)

THERAPEUTIC CLASS: Enzyme

INDICATIONS: Long-term enzyme replacement-therapy in pediatric and adult patients with type 1 Gaucher disease.

DOSAGE: *Adults:* 60 U/kg administered every other week as a 60-min IV infusion. Switching from Imiglucerase Therapy: Begin at the same dose when switching from a stable dose of imiglucerase to velaglucerase alfa. Titrate: Adjust dose based on therapeutic goals. 15 U/kg-60 U/kg every other week have been evaluated in clinical studies.
Pediatrics: ≥4 yrs: 60 U/kg administered every other week as a 60-min IV infusion. Switching from Imiglucerase Therapy: Begin at the same dose when switching from a stable dose of imiglucerase to velaglucerase alfa. Titrate: Adjust dose based on therapeutic goals. 15 U/kg-60 U/kg every other week have been evaluated in clinical studies.

HOW SUPPLIED: Inj: 200 U, 400 U

WARNINGS/PRECAUTIONS: Hypersensitivity reactions reported; appropriate medical support should be readily available during administration. Caution in patients who have exhibited symptoms of hypersensitivity to active ingredient/excipients or to other enzyme-replacement therapy. Infusion-related reactions reported; management should be based on the severity of the reaction (eg, slowing the infusion rate, treatment with antihistamines, antipyretics, and/or corticosteroids, and/or d/c and resume treatment with increased infusion time). Pretreatment with antihistamines and/or corticosteroids may prevent subsequent reactions. Administer under the supervision of a healthcare professional. Caution in elderly.

ADVERSE REACTIONS: Headache, dizziness, abdominal pain, nausea, back pain, joint pain, upper respiratory tract infection, activated PTT prolonged, infusion-related reaction, pyrexia, asthenia/fatigue.

PREGNANCY: Category B, caution in nursing.

MECHANISM OF ACTION: Hydrolytic lysosomal glucocerebroside-specific enzyme; catalyzes the hydrolysis of glucocerebroside, reducing the amount of accumulated glucocerebroside.

PHARMACOKINETICS: Distribution: V_d=82-108mL/kg. **Elimination:** $T_{1/2}$=11-12 min.

NURSING CONSIDERATIONS

Assessment: Assess for previous hypersensitivity to the drug and for pregnancy/nursing status.

Monitoring: Monitor for symptoms of infusion-related reactions (eg, headache, dizziness, hypotension, HTN, nausea, fatigue/asthenia, pyrexia), hypersensitivity, and other adverse reactions.

Patient Counseling: Inform that therapy should be administered under the supervision of a healthcare professional. Advise that treatment may cause hypersensitivity or infusion-related reactions.

Administration: IV route. Refer to PI for preparation and administration instructions for IV infusion. **Storage:** 2-8°C (36-46°F). Do not freeze. Protect from light.

VYTORIN   RX
ezetimibe - simvastatin (Merck/Schering-Plough)

THERAPEUTIC CLASS: Cholesterol absorption inhibitor/HMG-CoA reductase inhibitor

INDICATIONS: Adjunct to diet to: Reduce elevated total-C, LDL, Apo B, TG, non-HDL, and to increase HDL in primary (heterozygous familial and non-familial) hyperlipidemia or mixed hyperlipidemia. Reduce elevated total-C and LDL in homozygous familial hypercholesterolemia, as an adjunct to other lipid-lowering treatments (eg, LDL apheresis), or if such treatments are unavailable.

DOSAGE: *Adults:* Initial: 10mg-10mg or 10mg-20mg qpm. Usual: 10mg-10mg to 10mg-40mg qpm. LDL Reduction (>55%): Initial: 10mg-40mg qpm. After initiation or titration, analyze lipid levels after ≥2 weeks and adjust dose, PRN. Restricted Dosing: Use 10mg-80mg in patients who have been taking 10mg-80mg chronically (eg, ≥12 months) without evidence of muscle toxicity. If tolerating 10mg-80mg and needs to be initiated on drug that is contraindicated or have a dose cap for simvastatin, switch to an alternative statin or statin-based regimen with less potential for drug-drug interaction. Avoid titration to 10mg-80mg and place on alternative LDL lowering treatment if unable to achieve LDL goal with 10mg-40mg. Concomitant Verapamil/Diltiazem: Max: 10mg-10mg qd. Concomitant Amiodarone/Amlodipine/Ranolazine: Max: 10mg-20mg qd. Concomitant Bile Acid Sequestrants: Take either ≥2 hrs before or ≥4 hrs after bile acid sequestrant. Homozygous Familial Hypercholesterolemia: 10mg-40mg qpm. Chronic Kidney Disease (GFR <60mL/min/1.73m^2): 10mg-20mg qpm. Chinese Patients Taking Lipid-Modifying Doses (≥1g/day) of Niacin: Caution with >10mg-20mg qd; avoid 10mg-80mg.

HOW SUPPLIED: Tab: (Ezetimibe-Simvastatin) 10mg-10mg, 10mg-20mg, 10mg-40mg, 10mg-80mg

CONTRAINDICATIONS: Concomitant administration with strong CYP3A4 inhibitors (eg, itraconazole, ketoconazole, posaconazole, HIV protease inhibitors, boceprevir, telaprevir, erythromycin, clarithromycin, telithromycin, nefazodone), gemfibrozil, cyclosporine, or danazol. Active liver disease or unexplained persistent elevations in hepatic transaminase levels, women who are or may become pregnant, nursing mothers.

WARNINGS/PRECAUTIONS: Myopathy and rhabdomyolysis reported; predisposing factors include advanced age (≥65 yrs), female gender, uncontrolled hypothyroidism, and renal impairment. The risk of myopathy, including rhabdomyolysis, is dose related and is greater with simvastatin 80mg. D/C if myopathy is suspected/diagnosed or if markedly elevated CPK levels occur. Temporarily withhold if experiencing acute or serious condition predisposing to development of renal failure secondary to rhabdomyolysis (eg, sepsis, hypotension, major surgery, trauma, severe metabolic, endocrine, electrolyte disorders, or uncontrolled epilepsy). Persistent increases in serum transaminases reported; perform LFTs before initiation and as indicated thereafter. Fatal and nonfatal hepatic failure reported; d/c therapy if serious liver injury and/or hyperbilirubinemia or jaundice occurs and do not restart if no alternate etiology found. Caution in elderly, with heavy alcohol use, or with history of hepatic disease. Avoid with moderate/severe hepatic impairment. Increases in HbA1c and fasting serum glucose levels reported. Use doses >10mg-20mg with caution and close monitoring in patients with moderate to severe renal impairment. Has not been studied in Fredrickson Type I, III, IV, and V dyslipidemias.

ADVERSE REACTIONS: Myopathy/rhabdomyolysis, liver enzyme abnormalities (eg, transaminase elevations), headache, upper respiratory tract infection, myalgia.

INTERACTIONS: See Contraindications. Avoid large quantities of grapefruit juice (>1 quart daily). Voriconazole may inhibit metabolism; may need to adjust dose. Increased risk of myopathy, including rhabdomyolysis, with amiodarone, ranolazine, calcium channel blockers (eg, verapamil, diltiazem, or amlodipine), fibrates, lipid-modifying doses of niacin (≥1 g/day of niacin), or CYP3A4 inhibitors. Reduced ezetimibe levels with cholestyramine; incremental LDL reduction may be reduced. May slightly elevate plasma digoxin concentrations. Simvastatin may potentiate effect of coumarin anticoagulants; monitor PT. Increased INR reported when ezetimibe was added to warfarin. Caution with colchicine. Increased ezetimibe levels with cimetidine. Increased total ezetimibe area under the curve and decreased ezetimibe C_{max} with glipizide. Decreased ezetimibe levels with aluminum and magnesium hydroxide antacids. Ezetimibe decreased levels of glipizide. Ezetimibe decreased ethinyl estradiol and levonorgestrel C_{max}.

PREGNANCY: Category X, not for use in nursing.

MECHANISM OF ACTION: Ezetimibe: Cholesterol absorption inhibitor. Reduces blood cholesterol by inhibiting absorption of cholesterol by small intestine. Targets the sterol transporter, Niemann-Pick C1-Like 1, which is involved in intestinal uptake of cholesterol and phytosterols. Simvastatin: HMG-CoA reductase inhibitor. Inhibits conversion of HMG-CoA to mevalonate. Also reduces VLDL, TG, and increases HDL-C.

PHARMACOKINETICS: Absorption: Simvastatin: Bioavailability (<5% as β-hydroxyacid); T_{max}=4 hrs. **Distribution:** Plasma protein binding: Ezetimibe: (>90%, ezetimibe/ezetimibe-glucuronide). Simvastatin: (95%, simvastatin/B-hydroxyacid). **Metabolism:** Ezetimibe: Small intestine, liver via glucuronide conjugation; ezetimibe-glucuronide (active metabolite). Simvastatin: Liver (1st pass); β-hydroxyacid, 6'-hydroxy, 6'-hydroxymethyl, and 6'-exomethylene (major active metabolites). **Elimination:** Ezetimibe: Feces (78%, 69% unchanged), urine (11%, 9% ezetimibe-glucuronide); $T_{1/2}$=22 hrs. Simvastatin: Feces (60%), urine (13%).

NURSING CONSIDERATIONS

Assessment: Assess for active liver disease or unexplained persistent elevations in hepatic transaminases, pregnancy/nursing status, risk factors for developing myopathy (eg, advanced age, uncontrolled hypothyroidism), renal impairment, and possible drug interactions. Assess use in patients who consume substantial quantities of alcohol and/or have a past history of liver disease. Obtain baseline lipid profile (total-C, LDL, HDL, TG) and liver function (eg, AST, ALT) parameters.

Monitoring: Monitor for signs/symptoms of myopathy (eg, unexplained muscle pain, tenderness, weakness), rhabdomyolysis, and for liver dysfunction. Perform periodic monitoring of creatine kinase levels and lipid profile. Perform LFTs as clinically indicated.

Patient Counseling: Advise to adhere to the National Cholesterol Education Program recommended diet, a regular exercise program, and periodic testing of a fasting lipid panel. Inform of the risk of myopathy; advise to contact physician immediately if unexplained muscle pain, tenderness, or weakness develops. Advise patients who use 10mg-80mg dose that the risk of myopathy, including rhabdomyolysis, is increased. Inform that liver function will be checked prior to and during treatment; instruct to report promptly any symptoms that may indicate liver injury (eg, fatigue, anorexia, right upper abdominal discomfort, dark urine, or jaundice). Advise to d/c therapy if pregnant or planning to become pregnant, and if breastfeeding. Instruct females of childbearing potential to use effective contraception. Inform of the substances that should not be taken concomitantly with the drug. Advise to inform other healthcare professionals that they are taking the drug.

Administration: Oral route. Take at pm with or without food. **Storage:** 20-25°C (68-77°F).

VYVANSE CII
lisdexamfetamine dimesylate (Shire)

Stimulants are subject to misuse, abuse, addiction, and criminal diversion. Misuse of amphetamines may cause sudden death and serious cardiovascular (CV) adverse events.

THERAPEUTIC CLASS: Sympathomimetic amine

INDICATIONS: Treatment of attention-deficit hyperactivity disorder (ADHD) in patients ≥6 yrs.

DOSAGE: *Adults:* Individualize dose. Initial: 30mg qam. Titrate: May adjust in increments of 10-20mg/week. Max: 70mg/day.
Pediatrics: ≥6 yrs: Individualize dose. Initial: 30mg qam. Titrate: May adjust in increments of 10-20mg/week. Max: 70mg/day.

HOW SUPPLIED: Cap: 20mg, 30mg, 40mg, 50mg, 60mg, 70mg

CONTRAINDICATIONS: Use with or within a minimum of 14 days following d/c of MAOI.

WARNINGS/PRECAUTIONS: Sudden death, stroke, myocardial infarction (MI) reported; avoid with known serious structural cardiac and heart rhythm abnormalities, cardiomyopathy, coronary artery disease (CAD), or other serious cardiac problems. Promptly evaluate cardiac condition if symptoms of cardiac disease develop (eg, exertional chest pain, unexplained syncope). May cause modest increase in BP and HR; caution with conditions that could be compromised by BP or HR elevation (eg, preexisting HTN, heart failure, recent MI, or ventricular arrhythmia). May exacerbate symptoms of behavior disturbance and thought disorder in patients with preexisting psychotic disorder. Caution in patients with comorbid bipolar disorder; may cause induction of mixed/manic episode. May cause treatment-emergent psychotic/manic symptoms in children and adolescents without a prior history of psychotic illness or mania; may consider d/c if symptoms occur. Aggressive behavior or hostility reported; monitor for appearance or worsening. Monitor growth (weight and height) in pediatrics; may need to d/c if patient is not growing or gaining weight as expected. May lower convulsive threshold; d/c if seizure develops. Difficulties with accommodation and blurring of vision reported. Exacerbation of motor and phonic tics, and Tourette's syndrome reported. Prescribe or dispense the least amount feasible at one time to minimize possibility of overdosage.

ADVERSE REACTIONS: N/V, insomnia, rash, upper abdominal pain, decreased appetite, dizziness, dry mouth, irritability, weight decreased, affect lability, anxiety, anorexia, diarrhea, jittery feeling.

INTERACTIONS: See Contraindications. Urinary acidifying agents (eg, ammonium chloride, sodium acid phosphate) and methenamine may increase urinary excretion. Urinary alkalinizing agents (eg, acetazolamide and some thiazides) may decrease urinary excretion. May inhibit adrenergic blockers. May counteract sedative effect of antihistamines. May antagonize the hypotensive effects of antihypertensives. May inhibit hypotensive effects of veratrum alkaloids. May delay intestinal absorption of ethosuximide, phenobarbital, and phenytoin. May produce a synergistic anticonvulsant action with phenobarbital and phenytoin. May enhance activity of TCAs or sympathomimetic agents. May potentiate analgesic effects of meperidine. Chlorpromazine and haloperidol may inhibit central stimulant effects. Lithium carbonate may inhibit anorectic and stimulatory effects. May enhance the adrenergic effect of norepinephrine. Propoxyphene overdose may potentiate CNS stimulation and cause fatal convulsions.

PREGNANCY: Category C, not for use in nursing.

MECHANISM OF ACTION: Sympathomimetic amine; prodrug of dextroamphetamine. Therapeutic action in ADHD not known; suspected to block reuptake of norepinephrine and dopamine into presynaptic neuron and increase the monoamine release into extraneuronal space.

PHARMACOKINETICS: Absorption: Rapid; T_{max}=1 hr (lisdexamfetamine), 3.5 hrs (dextroamphetamine). **Distribution:** Found in breast milk. **Metabolism:** Hydrolysis by RBC; dextroamphetamine, L-lysine (metabolites). **Elimination:** Urine (96%; 42% amphetamine, 2% unchanged), feces (0.3%); $T_{1/2}$=<1 hr.

NURSING CONSIDERATIONS

Assessment: Assess for psychiatric history (eg, family history of suicide, bipolar disorder, depression, drug abuse, or alcoholism), CV disease, tics or Tourette's syndrome, seizure, hypersensitivity or idiosyncratic reactions to other sympathomimetic amines, pregnancy/nursing status, and possible drug interactions.

Monitoring: Monitor for CV abnormalities, exacerbations of behavior disturbances and thought disorder, psychotic or manic symptoms, aggressive behavior, hostility, seizures, visual disturbances, and exacerbation of motor and phonic tics and Tourette's syndrome. Monitor BP and HR. Monitor height and weight in children.

Patient Counseling: Inform about benefits and risks of treatment, appropriate use, and drug abuse/dependence risk. Advise about serious CV risks (eg, sudden death, MI, stroke, and HTN); instruct to contact physician immediately if patient develop symptoms of cardiac disease (eg, exertional chest pain, unexplained syncope). Inform that treatment-emergent psychotic or manic symptoms may occur. Instruct parents or guardians of pediatric patients to monitor growth and weight during treatment. Advise to notify physician if pregnant or planning to become pregnant and to avoid breastfeeding. Inform that therapy may impair ability of engaging in dangerous activities (eg, operating machinery or vehicles); instruct patient to assess how the medication affects them before performing dangerous tasks.

Administration: Oral route. Take in am; avoid afternoon doses. Swallow cap whole or dissolve entire contents in glass of water; do not store once dissolved. **Storage:** 25°C (77°F); excursions permitted to 15-30°C (59-86°F).

WelChol   RX
colesevelam HCl (Daiichi Sankyo)

THERAPEUTIC CLASS: Bile acid sequestrant

INDICATIONS: As monotherapy or in combination with a statin to reduce LDL-C levels in boys and postmenarchal girls 10-17 yrs old with heterozygous familial hypercholesterolemia if after an adequate trial of diet therapy, LDL-C remains ≥190mg/dL or ≥160mg/dL and there is a positive family history of premature cardiovascular disease (CVD), or ≥2 other CVD risk factors are present. (Adults) Adjunct to diet and exercise to reduce elevated LDL-C with primary hyperlipidemia (Fredrickson Type IIa) as monotherapy or with an HMG-CoA reductase inhibitor. Adjunct to diet and exercise to improve glycemic control with type 2 diabetes mellitus (DM).

DOSAGE: *Adults:* Hyperlipidemia/Type 2 DM: (Tab) 3 tabs bid or 6 tabs qd. Take with meal and liquid. (Sus) 3.75g qd or 1.875g bid in 4-8 oz. of water, fruit juice, or diet-soft drinks. Stir well and drink. Take with meals. May be dosed at the same time as a statin or the 2 drugs can be dosed apart.
Pediatrics: 10-17 yrs: Hyperlipidemia: (Sus) 3.75g qd or 1.875g bid in 4-8 oz. of water, fruit juice, or diet-soft drinks. Stir well and drink. Take with meals. May be dosed at the same time as a statin or the 2 drugs can be dosed apart.

HOW SUPPLIED: Sus: 1.875g, 3.75g [pkt]; Tab: 625mg

CONTRAINDICATIONS: Serum TG concentrations >500mg/dL, history of hypertriglyceridemia-induced pancreatitis or bowel obstruction.

WARNINGS/PRECAUTIONS: May increase serum TG concentrations; d/c if TG levels >500mg/dL or if hypertriglyceridemia-induced pancreatitis develops. Caution in patients with TG levels >300mg/dL or with susceptibility to deficiencies of vitamin K (eg, malabsorption syndromes) or other fat-soluble vitamins. May cause constipation; avoid with gastroparesis, GI motility disorders, those who have had major GI tract surgery, or at risk for bowel obstruction. Has not been studied in type 2 DM as monotherapy or in combination with dipeptidyl peptidase 4 inhibitors and thiazolidinediones, and in Fredrickson Type I, III, IV, or V dyslipidemias. Not for treatment of type 1 DM or diabetic ketoacidosis. (Sus) Contains phenylalanine, caution with phenylketonurics. Always mix with water, fruit juice, or soft drinks to avoid esophageal distress; do not take in its dry form. (Tab) Caution in patients with dysphagia or swallowing disorders.

W

ADVERSE REACTIONS: Asthenia, cardiovascular events, constipation, dyspepsia, nausea, rhinitis, fatigue, flu syndrome, nasopharyngitis, hypoglycemia, hypertriglyceridemia, headache, influenza, pharyngitis, upper respiratory tract infection.

INTERACTIONS: May increase TG levels with insulin or sulfonylureas. May decrease absorption of vitamins A, D, E, and K; caution when treating patients susceptible to vitamin K deficiency (eg, patients on warfarin). Give drugs with reduced GI absorption when given concomitantly and those that have not been tested for interaction, especially those with narrow therapeutic index ≥4 hours prior to taking colesevelam. May increase seizure activity or decrease phenytoin levels. May elevate TSH in patients receiving thyroid hormone replacement therapy. May decrease levels of cyclosporine, glyburide, levothyroxine, repaglinide, verapamil sustained-release, and oral contraceptives containing ethinyl estradiol and norethindrone. Concomitant use with warfarin decreases INR; monitor INR.

PREGNANCY: Category B, safety not known in nursing.

MECHANISM OF ACTION: Bile acid sequestrant; non-absorbed, lipid-lowering polymer that binds bile acids in intestine, impeding their reabsorption. Consequently, compensatory effects lead to increased LDL-C clearance from blood, resulting in decreased serum LDL-C levels. Mechanism unknown in the treatment of DM.

PHARMACOKINETICS: Absorption: Not hydrolyzed by digestive enzymes and not absorbed. **Distribution:** Limited to GI tract. **Excretion:** Urine (0.05%).

NURSING CONSIDERATIONS

Assessment: Assess for history/risk of bowel obstruction, gastroparesis or other GI motility disorders, history of major GI tract surgery or hypertriglyceridemia-induced pancreatitis, susceptibility to deficiencies of vitamin K or other fat soluble vitamins, dysphagia or swallowing disorders, pregnancy/nursing status, and possible drug interactions. Obtain baseline lipid parameters (eg, TG, non-HDL-C).

Monitoring: Monitor for hypertriglyceridemia-induced pancreatitis, hypoglycemia, dysphagia, and for esophageal obstruction. Periodically monitor lipid profile (eg, TG, non-HDL-C), blood glucose, and coadministered drug levels.

Patient Counseling: Instruct to take with meal and liquid. Inform to take drugs that may interact (eg, cyclosporine, glyburide, levothyroxine, oral contraceptives) ≥4 hrs prior. Advise to consume diet that promotes bowel regularity. Instruct to promptly d/c and seek medical attention if severe abdominal pain/constipation, or symptoms of acute pancreatitis (eg, severe abdominal pain with or without N/V) occur. Counsel to adhere to the recommended diet of the National Cholesterol Education Program (NCEP), to dietary instructions, regular exercise program, and regular FPG test. Advise to notify physician if have swallowing disorders. (Sus) Instruct to empty entire contents of one packet into a glass or cup, then add 4-8 oz. of water, fruit juice, or diet-soft drinks before ingesting.

Administration: Oral route. **Storage:** 25°C (77°F); excursions permitted to 15-30°C (59-86°F). Protect from moisture. (Tab) Brief exposure to 40°C (104°F) does not affect the product.

WELLBUTRIN SR

bupropion HCl (GlaxoSmithKline)

RX

Antidepressants increased the risk of suicidal thinking and behavior (suicidality) in short-term studies in children, adolescents, and young adults with major depressive disorder (MDD) and other psychiatric disorders. Bupropion is not approved for use in pediatric patients. Wellbutrin, Wellbutrin SR, and Wellbutrin XL are not approved for smoking cessation treatment but bupropion under the name Zyban is approved for this use. Serious neuropsychiatric events including depression, suicidal ideation, suicide attempt, and completed suicide reported in patients taking bupropion for smoking cessation. Monitor and observe closely for clinical worsening, suicidality, or unusual changes in behavior, and for neuropsychiatric symptoms (eg, behavioral changes, hostility, agitation, depressed mood, and suicide-related events) or worsening of preexisting psychiatric illness. D/C if psychiatric symptoms observed.

OTHER BRAND NAMES: Budeprion SR (Teva) - Wellbutrin (GlaxoSmithKline)

THERAPEUTIC CLASS: Aminoketone

INDICATIONS: Treatment of MDD.

DOSAGE: *Adults:* (Tab) Initial: 100mg bid. May increase to 100mg tid, no sooner than 3 days after beginning therapy. Increases should not exceed 100mg/day in a 3-day period. Usual: 100mg tid, preferably with ≥6 hrs between successive doses. Max: 450mg/day, given in divided doses of not more than 150mg each (eg, 100mg qid with ≥4 hrs between successive doses). Severe Hepatic Cirrhosis: Max: 75mg qd. Mild-Moderate Hepatic Cirrhosis/Renal Impairment: Consider reduced frequency and/or dose. (Tab, SR) Initial: 150mg qam. May increase to 150mg bid on Day 4. There should be an interval of ≥8 hrs between successive doses. Usual: 150mg bid. Max: 200mg bid. Maint: Reassess periodically to determine the need for maintenance treatment and the appropriate dose. Severe Hepatic Cirrhosis: Max: 100mg/day or 150mg qod. Mild-Moderate Hepatic Cirrhosis/Renal Impairment: Consider reduced frequency and/or dose.

HOW SUPPLIED: Tab: 75mg, 100mg; Tab, Sustained-Release (SR): 100mg, 150mg, 200mg (Wellbutrin SR). 100mg, 150mg (Budeprion SR)

CONTRAINDICATIONS: Seizure disorder, bulimia or anorexia nervosa, patients treated with other medications that contain bupropion, use of MAOIs or within 14 days of use, and patients undergoing abrupt d/c of alcohol or sedatives (including benzodiazepines).

WARNINGS/PRECAUTIONS: Screen for bipolar disorder; not approved for use in treating bipolar depression. May precipitate mixed/manic episodes in bipolar disorder patients. Dose-related risk of seizures; d/c and do not restart if seizure occurs. Extreme caution with history of seizure, cranial trauma, CNS tumor, or other predisposition(s) toward seizure, and severe hepatic cirrhosis. Potential for hepatotoxicity. Neuropsychiatric signs and symptoms (eg, delusions, hallucinations, psychosis, concentration disturbance, paranoia, confusion) reported. Altered appetite/weight and HTN reported. D/C if anaphylactoid/anaphylactic reactions occur. Caution with recent myocardial infarction, unstable heart disease, renal impairment, and hepatic impairment. False-positive urine immunoassay screening tests for amphetamines reported. (Tab) Increased restlessness, agitation, anxiety, and insomnia reported after initiation of treatment. (Tab, SR) Agitation, anxiety and insomnia reported. (Budeprion SR 100mg) Contains tartrazine which may cause allergic type reactions (including bronchial asthma) in certain susceptible persons.

ADVERSE REACTIONS: Dry mouth, excessive sweating, headache/migraine, insomnia, tremor, agitation, weight loss, N/V, constipation, dizziness, sedation, blurred vision, decreased libido.

INTERACTIONS: See Contraindications. Extreme caution with drugs that lower seizure threshold (eg, antidepressants, antipsychotics, theophylline, systemic steroids); use low initial doses and gradually titrate. Increased seizure risk with excessive alcohol or sedative use; opiate, cocaine, or stimulant addiction; use of OTC stimulants or anorectics, oral hypoglycemics, insulin. Caution with levodopa and amantadine; use low initial doses and gradually titrate. Inhibits CYP2D6; caution with drugs that are metabolized by CYP2D6 (eg, SSRIs, TCAs, antipsychotics, β-blockers, type 1C antiarrhythmics); use low initial dose. May reduce efficacy of drugs that require metabolic activation by CYP2D6 (eg, tamoxifen). Monitor for HTN with nicotine replacement therapy. Caution with CYP2B6 substrates or inhibitors/inducers (eg, orphenadrine, cyclophosphamide, thiotepa, ticlopidine, clopidogrel, ritonavir, efavirenz). Carbamazepine, phenytoin, and phenobarbital may induce metabolism. Altered PT and/or INR with warfarin. Minimize or avoid alcohol. Decreased levels with ritonavir or ritonavir/lopinavir and efavirenz; may need to increase bupropion dose but do not exceed max dose. Cimetidine increased levels of some active metabolites. Increased citalopram level. Paroxetine, sertraline, norfluoxetine, nelfinavir, and fluvoxamine may inhibit metabolism.

PREGNANCY: Category C, not for use in nursing.

MECHANISM OF ACTION: Aminoketone antidepressant; not established. Weak inhibitor of the neuronal uptake of norepinephrine and dopamine.

PHARMACOKINETICS: Absorption: T_{max}=2 hrs, 3 hrs (hydroxybupropion); (Tab, SR) T_{max}=6 hrs (hydroxybupropion). **Distribution:** Plasma protein binding (84%); found in breast milk. **Metabolism:** Extensive. Hydroxylation, hydroxybupropion (active metabolite) (CYP2B6); reduction of carbonyl group, threohydrobupropion, and erythrohydrobupropion (active metabolites). **Elimination:** Urine (87%), feces (10%), (0.5% unchanged); $T_{1/2}$=21 hrs, 20 hrs, 33 hrs, 37 hrs (bupropion, hydroxybupropion, erythrohydrobupropion, threohydrobupropion, respectively).

NURSING CONSIDERATIONS

Assessment: Assess for bipolar disorder, hepatic/renal function, pregnancy/nursing status, and possible drug interactions, or any other conditions where treatment is contraindicated or cautioned. Note other diseases/conditions.

Monitoring: Monitor for clinical worsening, suicidality, or unusual changes in behavior, seizures, increased restlessness, agitation, anxiety, insomnia, neuropsychiatric signs/symptoms, changes in weight or appetite, anaphylactoid/anaphylactic reactions, delayed hypersensitivity reactions, and HTN.

Patient Counseling: Advise patients and caregivers of need for close observation for clinical worsening and/or suicidal risks. Instruct to d/c and do not restart if experience a seizure while on therapy. Inform that the drug may impair the ability to perform tasks requiring judgment or motor and cognitive skills; use caution while operating hazardous machinery/driving. Inform that excessive use or abrupt d/c of alcohol or sedatives may alter seizure threshold; advise to minimize or avoid alcohol use. Report to physician all prescription or OTC medications being taken. Contact physician if become pregnant or plan to become pregnant during therapy.

Administration: Oral route. Avoid hs dosing. (Tab, SR) Swallow whole; do not crush, divide or chew. **Storage:** (Tab) 15-25°C (59-77°F). Protect from light and moisture. (Tab, SR) 20-25°C (68-77°F).

W

WELLBUTRIN XL RX
bupropion HCl (BTA)

Antidepressants increased the risk of suicidal thinking and behavior (suicidality) in short-term studies in children, adolescents, and young adults with major depressive disorder (MDD) and other psychiatric disorders. Bupropion is not approved for use in pediatric patients. Wellbutrin, Wellbutrin SR, and Wellbutrin XL are not approved for smoking cessation treatment, but bupropion under the name Zyban is approved for this use. Serious neuropsychiatric events including depression, suicidal ideation, suicide attempt, and completed suicide reported in patients taking bupropion for smoking cessation. Monitor and observe closely for clinical worsening, suicidality, or unusual changes in behavior and for neuropsychiatric symptoms (eg, behavioral changes, hostility, agitation, depressed mood, and suicide-related events) or worsening of pre-existing psychiatric illness. D/C if psychiatric symptoms observed.

OTHER BRAND NAMES: Budeprion XL (Teva)

THERAPEUTIC CLASS: Aminoketone

INDICATIONS: Treatment of MDD and prevention of seasonal major depressive episodes in patients diagnosed with seasonal affective disorder (SAD).

DOSAGE: Adults: Give in AM. MDD: Initial: 150mg qd. May increase to 300mg qd on Day 4. There should be an interval of ≥24 hrs between successive doses. Usual: 300mg qd. Max: 450mg qd. Maint: Reassess periodically to determine the need for maintenance treatment and the appropriate dose. SAD: Individualize timing of initiation and duration of treatment. Start in autumn; stop in early spring. Initial: 150mg qd. May increase to 300mg qd after 1 week. If the 300mg dose is not adequately tolerated, the dose can be reduced to 150mg/day. Usual/Max: 300mg qd. Patients taking 300mg/day during Autumn-Winter Season: Taper dose to 150mg/day for 2 weeks prior to d/c. Mild-Moderate Hepatic Cirrhosis/Renal Impairment: Consider reduced frequency and/or dose. Severe Hepatic Cirrhosis: Max: 150mg qod. Switching from Bupropion Tab/ Sustained-Release Tab: Give the same total daily dose when possible.

HOW SUPPLIED: Tab, Extended-Release: 150mg (Budeprion XL); 150mg, 300mg (Wellbutrin XL)

CONTRAINDICATIONS: Seizure disorder, bulimia or anorexia nervosa, patients treated with other medications that contain bupropion, use of MAOIs or within 14 days of use, and patients undergoing abrupt d/c of alcohol or sedatives (including benzodiazepines).

WARNINGS/PRECAUTIONS: Dose-related risk of seizures. D/C and do not restart if seizure occurs. Extreme caution with history of seizures, cranial trauma, CNS tumor, or other predisposition(s) toward seizure, and severe hepatic cirrhosis. Screen for bipolar disorder; not approved for use in treating bipolar depression. Neuropsychiatric signs and symptoms (eg, delusions, hallucinations, psychosis, concentration disturbance, paranoia, confusion) reported. May precipitate manic episodes in bipolar disorder patients. Caution with recent myocardial infarction, unstable heart disease, and renal/hepatic impairment. D/C if anaphylactoid/anaphylactic reactions occur. Altered appetite/weight and HTN reported. Increased restlessness, agitation, anxiety, and insomnia reported after initiation of treatment. Potential for hepatotoxicity.

ADVERSE REACTIONS: Headache, dry mouth, nausea, insomnia, dizziness, nasopharyngitis, flatulence, tremor, infection, tinnitus, sweating, myalgia, anxiety, constipation, neuropsychiatric events.

INTERACTIONS: See Contraindications. Extreme caution with drugs that lower seizure threshold (eg, antidepressants, antipsychotics, theophylline, systemic steroids); use low initial doses and gradually titrate. Increased seizure risk with excessive alcohol or sedative use; opiate, cocaine, or stimulant addiction; use of OTC stimulants or anorectics, oral hypoglycemics, insulin. Caution with levodopa and amantadine; use low initial doses and gradually titrate. Inhibits CYP2D6; caution with drugs that are metabolized by CYP2D6 (eg, SSRIs, TCAs, antipsychotics, β-blockers, type 1C antiarrhythmics); use low initial dose. Monitor for HTN with nicotine replacement therapy. Caution with CYP2B6 substrates or inhibitors/inducers (eg, orphenadrine, cyclophosphamide, thiotepa, ticlopidine, and clopidogrel). Carbamazepine, phenytoin, and phenobarbital may induce metabolism. Altered PT and/or INR with warfarin. Minimize or avoid alcohol. Decreased levels with ritonavir or ritonavir/lopinavir; may need to increase bupropion dose but do not exceed max dose. Cimetidine increased levels of some active metabolites. Increased citalopram levels. Paroxetine, sertraline, norfluoxetine, nelfinavir, efavirenz, and fluvoxamine may inhibit metabolism.

PREGNANCY: Category C, not for use in nursing.

MECHANISM OF ACTION: Aminoketone antidepressant; has not been established. Weak inhibitor of the neuronal uptake of norepinephrine and dopamine.

PHARMACOKINETICS: Absorption: T_{max}=5 hrs. **Distribution**: Plasma protein binding (84%); found in breast milk. **Metabolism**: Extensive. Hydroxylation, hydroxybupropion (active metabolite) (CYP2B6); Reduction of carbonyl group, threohydrobupropion and erythrohydrobupropion (active metabolites). **Elimination**: Urine (87%), feces (10%), (0.5% unchanged); $T_{1/2}$=21 hrs, 20 hrs, 33 hrs, 37 hrs (bupropion, hydroxybupropion, erythrohydrobupropion, threohydrobupropion, respectively).

W

NURSING CONSIDERATIONS

Assessment: Assess for bipolar disorder, hepatic/renal function, and conditions where treatment is contraindicated or cautioned, pregnancy/nursing status, and possible drug interactions. Note other diseases/conditions.

Monitoring: Monitor for clinical worsening, suicidality, or unusual changes in behavior, seizures, increased restlessness, agitation, anxiety, insomnia, neuropsychiatric signs/symptoms, changes in weight or appetite, anaphylactoid/anaphylactic reactions, delayed hypersensitivity reactions, and HTN.

Patient Counseling: Advise patients and caregivers of need for close observation for clinical worsening and/or suicidal risks. Instruct to d/c and do not restart if experience seizures while on therapy. Inform that excessive use or abrupt d/c of alcohol or sedatives may alter seizure threshold; advise to minimize or avoid alcohol use. Inform that the drug may impair the ability to perform tasks requiring judgment or motor or cognitive skills; use caution while operating hazardous machinery/driving. Report to physician all prescription or OTC medications being taken. Contact physician if become pregnant or plan to become pregnant during therapy.

Administration: Oral route. Avoid hs dosing. Swallow whole; do not crush, divide, or chew.
Storage: (Budeprion XL) 20-25°C (68-77°F). (Wellbutrin XL) 25°C (77°F); excursions permitted to 15-30°C (59-86°F).

XALATAN   RX
latanoprost (Pharmacia & Upjohn)

THERAPEUTIC CLASS: Prostaglandin analog

INDICATIONS: Reduction of elevated intraocular pressure (IOP) in patients with open-angle glaucoma or ocular HTN.

DOSAGE: *Adults:* Usual: 1 drop in affected eye(s) qd in pm. Max: Once-daily dosing. Space dosing with other ophthalmic drugs by at least 5 min.

HOW SUPPLIED: Sol: 0.005% [2.5mL]

WARNINGS/PRECAUTIONS: Changes to pigmented tissues, increased pigmentation of iris (may be permanent), eyelids and eyelashes (may be reversible), growth of eyelashes reported. Regularly exam patients with noticeably increased iris pigmentation. Macular edema, including cystoid macular edema, reported; mainly occurred in aphakic patients, pseudophakic patients with a torn posterior lens capsule, and patients at risk for macular edema. Caution with history of intraocular inflammation (iritis/uveitis), patients without an intact posterior capsule, and at risk of macular edema. Avoid with active intraocular inflammation. Limited experience in treating angle-closure, inflammatory, or neovascular glaucoma. Bacterial keratitis reported with multi-dose container. Contains benzalkonium chloride; remove contact lenses prior to use and reinsert 15 min after administration.

ADVERSE REACTIONS: Eyelash changes, eyelid skin darkening, intraocular inflammation, iris pigmentation changes, macular edema, blurred vision, ocular burning/stinging, conjunctival hyperemia, foreign body sensation, ocular itching, punctuate epithelial keratopathy.

INTERACTIONS: Avoid with other prostaglandins or prostaglandin analogs; may decrease the IOP lowering effect or cause paradoxical IOP elevations.

PREGNANCY: Category C, caution in nursing.

MECHANISM OF ACTION: Selective FP prostanoid receptor agonist; believed to reduce IOP by increasing outflow of aqueous humor.

PHARMACOKINETICS: Absorption: T_{max}=2 hrs. **Distribution:** V_d=0.16L/kg. **Metabolism:** Cornea, via esterases to active acid; liver, via fatty acid β-oxidation to 1,2-dinor and 1,2,3,4-tetranor (metabolites). **Elimination:** Urine (88-98%); $T_{1/2}$=17 min.

NURSING CONSIDERATIONS

Assessment: Assess for hypersensitivity, intraocular inflammation (iritis/uveitis), active or high risk for macular edema, aphakic or pseudophakic patients with torn posterior lens capsule, patients without an intact posterior capsule, active intraocular inflammation, angle-closure, inflammatory or neovascular glaucoma, pregnancy/nursing status, and possible drug interactions.

Monitoring: Monitor for increased brown pigmentation of iris, periorbital tissue (eyelid); changes in eyelashes (eg, increased length, thickness, or growth; brown pigmentation; change in number of lashes; misdirected growth of lashes); macular edema (eg, cystoid macular edema); active intraocular inflammation, bacterial keratitis, and hypersensitivity reactions.

Patient Counseling: Inform about risk of brown pigmentation of iris, (may be permanent); darkening of eyelid skin; eyelashes and vellus hair changes. Avoid touching tip of applicator to eye or surrounding areas. Contains benzalkonium chloride; remove contact lenses prior to administration; reinsert 15 min after administration. Administer at least 5 min apart if using >1 topical

X

ophthalmic drug. Consult physician if having ocular surgery, if intercurrent ocular condition (eg, trauma or infection) develops, or if ocular reaction (conjunctivitis, lid reactions) occurs.

Administration: Ocular route. Continue with the next dose as normal if one dose is missed.

Storage: 2-8°C (36-46°F); may store opened bottle for 6 weeks at room temperature up to 25°C (77°F). During shipment to the patient, may maintain up to 40°C (104°F) for a period not exceeding 8 days. Protect from light.

XANAX
alprazolam (Pharmacia & Upjohn)

THERAPEUTIC CLASS: Benzodiazepine

INDICATIONS: Management of anxiety disorders or short-term relief of anxiety symptoms. Treatment of panic disorder, with or without agoraphobia.

DOSAGE: *Adults:* Individualize dose. Anxiety: Initial: 0.25-0.5mg tid. Titrate: May increase at intervals of 3-4 days. Max: 4mg/day in divided doses. Panic Disorder: Initial: 0.5mg tid. Titrate: May increase by ≤1mg/day at intervals of 3-4 days depending on response; slower titration for >4mg/day. Usual: 1-10mg/day. Elderly/Advanced Liver Disease/Debilitating Disease: Initial: 0.25mg bid-tid. Titrate: Increase gradually PRN and as tolerated. Daily Dose Reduction/ Discontinuation: Decrease dose gradually (≤0.5mg q3 days).

HOW SUPPLIED: Tab: 0.25mg*, 0.5mg*, 1mg*, 2mg* *scored

CONTRAINDICATIONS: Acute narrow-angle glaucoma, untreated open-angle glaucoma, concomitant ketoconazole or itraconazole.

WARNINGS/PRECAUTIONS: Risk of dependence. Seizures reported with dose reduction or abrupt d/c. Multiple seizures, status epilepticus, early morning/emergence of anxiety reported. Withdrawal reactions may occur; reduce dose or d/c therapy gradually. May impair mental/physical ability. Caution with impaired renal/hepatic/pulmonary function, severe depression, suicidal ideation/plans, debilitation, obesity, and in elderly. May cause fetal harm. Hypomania/mania reported with depression. Has a weak uricosuric effect.

ADVERSE REACTIONS: Drowsiness, lightheadedness, depression, headache, confusion, insomnia, dry mouth, constipation, diarrhea, N/V, tachycardia/palpitations, blurred vision, nasal congestion.

INTERACTIONS: See Contraindications. Not recommended with azole antifungals. Avoid with very potent CYP3A inhibitors. Additive CNS depressant effects with psychotropics, anticonvulsants, antihistaminics, and ethanol. Fluoxetine, fluvoxamine, nefazodone, cimetidine, and oral contraceptives may increase levels. CYP3A inducers (eg, carbamazepine), propoxyphene, and smoking may decrease levels. Caution with alcohol, other CNS depressants, diltiazem, isoniazid, macrolides (eg, erythromycin, clarithromycin), grapefruit juice, sertraline, paroxetine, ergotamine, cyclosporine, amiodarone, nicardipine, nifedipine, and other CYP3A inhibitors.

PREGNANCY: Category D, not for use in nursing.

MECHANISM OF ACTION: Benzodiazepine; mechanism unknown, presumed to bind at stereo specific receptors at several sites within the CNS.

PHARMACOKINETICS: Absorption: Readily absorbed; T_{max}=1-2 hrs; C_{max}=8-37ng/mL (0.5-3mg). **Distribution:** Plasma protein binding (80%); found in breast milk; crosses the placenta. **Metabolism:** Extensive. Liver via CYP3A4; 4-hydroxyalprazolam and α-hydroxyalprazolam (major metabolites). **Elimination:** Urine; $T_{1/2}$=11.2 hrs.

NURSING CONSIDERATIONS

Assessment: Assess for drug hypersensitivity, acute narrow-angle glaucoma, untreated open-angle glaucoma, depression, suicidal ideation, renal/hepatic/pulmonary function, debilitation, obesity, pregnancy/nursing status, and possible drug interactions.

Monitoring: Monitor for rebound/withdrawal symptoms (eg, seizures), episodes of hypomania/ mania, renal/hepatic/pulmonary function. Monitor CBC, urinalysis, and blood chemistry periodically. Periodically reassess usefulness of therapy.

Patient Counseling: Advise to inform their physician about any alcohol consumption and medicines taken; alcohol should generally be avoided. Instruct to inform physician if pregnant, nursing, planning to be pregnant, or become pregnant while on therapy. Advise not to drive or operate dangerous machinery. Advise not to increase/decrease dose or abruptly d/c therapy without consulting a physician.

Administration: Oral route. **Storage:** 20-25°C (68-77°F).

XANAX XR
alprazolam (Pharmacia & Upjohn)

THERAPEUTIC CLASS: Benzodiazepine

INDICATIONS: Panic disorder with or without agoraphobia.

DOSAGE: *Adults:* Individualize dose. Initial: 0.5-1mg qd, preferably in the am. Titrate: Increase by no more than 1mg/day every 3-4 days. Maint: 1-10mg/day. Usual: 3-6mg/day. Daily Dose Reduction/Discontinuation: Decrease dose slowly (≤0.5mg q3 days). Elderly/Advanced Liver Disease/Debilitated: Initial: 0.5mg qd. Switching from IR to XR: See PI.

HOW SUPPLIED: Tab, Extended-Release: 0.5mg, 1mg, 2mg, 3mg

CONTRAINDICATIONS: Acute narrow-angle glaucoma, untreated open-angle glaucoma, concomitant ketoconazole or itraconazole.

WARNINGS/PRECAUTIONS: Risk of dependence. Seizures reported with dose reduction or abrupt d/c. Withdrawal reactions may occur; reduce dose or d/c therapy gradually. Multiple seizures, status epilepticus, early morning anxiety/emergence of anxiety symptoms between doses have been reported. May impair mental/physical ability. Caution with impaired renal/hepatic/pulmonary function, severe depression, suicidal ideation/plans, obesity, debilitation, and in elderly. May cause fetal harm. Hypomania/mania reported with depression. Has a weak uricosuric effect.

ADVERSE REACTIONS: Sedation, somnolence, memory impairment, dysarthria, abnormal coordination, fatigue, depression, constipation, mental impairment, ataxia, dry mouth, nausea, decreased libido, increased/decreased appetite/weight.

INTERACTIONS: See Contraindications. Not recommended with azole antifungals. Avoid with very potent CYP3A inhibitors. Additive CNS depressant effects with psychotropics, anticonvulsants, antihistaminics, and ethanol. Fluoxetine, fluvoxamine, nefazodone, cimetidine, and oral contraceptives may increase levels. CYP3A inducers (eg, carbamazepine), propoxyphene, and smoking may decrease levels. Caution with alcohol, other CNS depressants, diltiazem, isoniazid, macrolides (eg, erythromycin, clarithromycin), grapefruit juice, sertraline, paroxetine, ergotamine, cyclosporine, amiodarone, nicardipine, nifedipine, and other CYP3A inhibitors.

PREGNANCY: Category D, not for use in nursing.

MECHANISM OF ACTION: Benzodiazepine; mechanism unknown, presumed to bind at stereo specific receptors at several sites within the CNS.

PHARMACOKINETICS: Absorption: Readily absorbed (immediate-release); mean absolute bioavailability (90%); refer to PI for additional parameters. **Distribution:** Plasma protein binding (80%); crosses the placenta; found in breast milk. **Metabolism:** Liver (extensive), via CYP3A4; 4-hydroxyalprazolam and α-hydroxyalprazolam (major metabolites). **Elimination:** Urine (unchanged and metabolites); $T_{1/2}$=10.7-15.8 hrs.

NURSING CONSIDERATIONS

Assessment: Assess for drug hypersensitivity, acute narrow-angle glaucoma, untreated open-angle glaucoma, depression, suicidal ideation, renal/hepatic/pulmonary function, pregnancy/nursing status, and possible drug interactions. Note other diseases/conditions and drug therapies.

Monitoring: Monitor for relapse, rebound or withdrawal symptoms (seizures), hepatic/renal/pulmonary function, and other adverse reactions. Monitor CBC, urinalysis, and blood chemistry periodically. Periodically reassess usefulness of therapy.

Patient Counseling: Advise to inform physician about any alcohol consumption and medicines taken; alcohol should generally be avoided. Instruct to inform physician if pregnant, nursing, planning to be pregnant, or become pregnant while on therapy. Advise not to drive or operate dangerous machinery. Advise not to increase/decrease dose or abruptly d/c therapy without consulting a physician. Advise to take in the am; do not crush or chew tabs.

Administration: Oral route. Do not chew, crush, or break tab. **Storage:** 25°C (77°F); excursions permitted to 15-30°C (59-86°F).

XARELTO   RX
rivaroxaban (Janssen)

May increase the risk of thrombotic events and stroke after d/c of therapy in atrial fibrillation patients. If anticoagulation must be d/c for a reason other than pathological bleeding, consider administering another anticoagulant. Epidural or spinal hematomas have occurred in patients treated with rivaroxaban who are receiving neuraxial anesthesia or undergoing spinal puncture; long-term or permanent paralysis may result. Increased risk of developing epidural or spinal hematomas in patients using indwelling epidural catheters, concomitant use of other drugs that affect hemostasis (eg, NSAIDs, platelet inhibitors, other anticoagulants), history of traumatic or repeated epidural or spinal puncture, and a history of spinal deformity or spinal surgery. Monitor frequently for signs/symptoms of neurologic impairment; urgent treatment is necessary if neurologic compromise occurs. Consider benefits and risks before neuraxial intervention in patients anticoagulated or to be anticoagulated for thromboprophylaxis.

THERAPEUTIC CLASS: Specific factor Xa inhibitor

INDICATIONS: Reduce the risk of stroke and systemic embolism in patients with nonvalvular atrial fibrillation. Prophylaxis of deep vein thrombosis (DVT), which may lead to pulmonary embolism (PE) in patients undergoing knee or hip replacement surgery.

DOSAGE: *Adults:* Nonvalvular Atrial Fibrillation: CrCl >50mL/min: 20mg qd with pm meal. CrCl 15-50mL/min: 15mg qd with pm meal. Refer to PI for information when switching from or to warfarin and switching from or to anticoagulants other than warfarin. Prophylaxis of DVT: 10mg qd. Give initial dose at least 6-10 hrs after surgery once hemostasis is established. Treatment Duration: Hip Replacement Surgery: 35 days. Knee Replacement Surgery: 12 days. Surgery/Intervention: If anticoagulation must be d/c with surgery or other procedures, d/c therapy at least 24 hrs before procedure. Weigh risk of bleeding against urgency of intervention, to decide whether procedure should be delayed until 24 hrs after last dose. Restart therapy after surgery or other procedures as soon as adequate hemostasis has been established.

HOW SUPPLIED: Tab: 10mg, 15mg, 20mg

CONTRAINDICATIONS: Active pathological bleeding.

WARNINGS/PRECAUTIONS: May increase risk of bleeding and cause serious or fatal bleeding; risk of thrombotic events should be weighed against the risk of bleeding before initiation of treatment. Promptly evaluate any signs/symptoms of blood loss; d/c in patients with active pathological hemorrhage. A epidural catheter should not be removed earlier than 18 hrs after last administration of therapy. The next dose should not be administered earlier than 6 hrs after catheter removal. If traumatic puncture occurs, delay administration for 24 hrs. May increase risk of pregnancy related hemorrhage; use with caution in pregnancy. Anaphylaxis reported; avoid in patients with history of severe hypersensitivity reaction to the drug. Avoid use with CrCl <15mL/min in nonvalvular atrial fibrillation, severe renal impairment (CrCl <30mL/min) in prophylaxis of DVT, moderate (Child-Pugh B) or severe (Child-Pugh C) hepatic impairment, or any hepatic disease associated with coagulopathy. Monitor for signs/symptoms of blood loss in patients with moderate renal impairment (CrCl 30-50mL/min) in prophylaxis of DVT. D/C therapy if acute renal failure develops.

ADVERSE REACTIONS: Spinal/epidural hematomas, neurological impairment, bleeding events, wound secretion, pain in extremity.

INTERACTIONS: See Boxed Warning. May have changes in exposure with inhibitors/inducers of CYP3A4/5, CYP2J2, and P-glycoprotein (P-gp) and ATP-binding cassette G2 transporters. Avoid with combined P-gp and strong CYP3A4 inhibitors (eg, ketoconazole, itraconazole, lopinavir/ritonavir, ritonavir, indinavir/ritonavir, and conivaptan) or with combined P-gp and strong CYP3A4 inducers (eg, carbamazepine, phenytoin, rifampin, St. John's wort). May have increase in exposure with fluconazole (moderate CYP3A4 inhibitor), clarithromycin. May have significant increases in exposure with combined P-gp and weak or moderate CYP3A4 inhibitors (eg, erythromycin, azithromycin, diltiazem, verapamil, quinidine, ranolazine, dronedarone, amiodarone, and felodipine) with renal impairment. Coadministration with combined P-gp and strong CYP3A4 inducer (eg, rifampicin) may decrease area under the curve and C_{max}; may decrease efficacy. Single dose of enoxaparin resulted in additive effect on anti-factor Xa activity. Concomitant use of drugs affecting hemostasis (eg, platelet aggregation inhibitors, other antithrombotic agents, fibrinolytic therapy, NSAIDs/aspirin) increases the risk of bleeding. Single dose of warfarin resulted in additive effect on factor Xa inhibition and PT. Avoid concurrent anticoagulants with prophylaxis of DVT. May increase bleeding time with clopidogrel.

PREGNANCY: Category C, not for use in nursing.

MECHANISM OF ACTION: Specific factor Xa inhibitor; selectively blocks the active site of factor Xa and does not require a cofactor for activity. Activation of factor X to factor Xa via the intrinsic and extrinsic pathways plays a central role in the cascade of blood coagulation.

PHARMACOKINETICS: Absorption: Absolute bioavailability (80-100% [10mg], 66% [20mg, fasted]); T_{max}=2-4 hrs. **Distribution:** V_d=50L; plasma protein binding (92-95%). **Metabolism:** Oxidative degradation via CYP3A4/5 and CYP2J2; hydrolysis. **Elimination:** Urine (66%, 36% unchanged), feces (28%, 7% unchanged); $T_{1/2}$=5-9 hrs (20-45 yrs), 11-13 hrs (elderly).

X

NURSING CONSIDERATIONS

Assessment: Assess for known hypersensitivity, active pathological bleeding, risk factors of developing epidural or spinal hematomas, conditions that may increase risk of bleeding, renal/hepatic function, hepatic disease, pregnancy/nursing status, and possible drug interactions.

Monitoring: Monitor for signs/symptoms of bleeding and other adverse reactions. In patients undergoing neuraxial anesthesia or spinal puncture, monitor for epidural or spinal hematomas and neurologic impairment. Monitor renal function (eg, CrCl) periodically.

Patient Counseling: Instruct to take as directed. Advise not to d/c without consulting physician. Advise to take as soon as possible on same day and continue on the following day with recommended daily dose regimen if dose is missed. Advise patients who had neuraxial anesthesia or spinal puncture to watch for signs and symptoms of spinal/epidural hematoma (eg, tingling, numbness, and muscular weakness) especially if concomitantly taking NSAIDs or platelet inhibitors; contact physician if symptoms occur. Inform that it may take longer than normal to stop bleeding, and that they may bruise and/or bleed more easily. Instruct to report any unusual bleeding or bruising. Instruct to inform their physicians and dentists if they are taking, or plan to take, any prescription or over-the-counter drugs or herbals. Inform physician immediately if nursing/pregnant or intend to nurse or become pregnant. Inform healthcare professional about therapy before any invasive procedure.

Administration: Oral route. **Storage:** 25°C (77°F); excursions permitted to 15-30°C (59-86°F).

XELODA   RX
capecitabine (Genentech)

> Altered coagulation parameters and/or bleeding, including death, reported with concomitant coumarin-derivative anticoagulants (eg, warfarin, phenprocoumon). Monitor PT and INR frequently to adjust anticoagulant dose. Postmarketing reports showed clinically significant increases in PT and INR in patients who were stabilized on anticoagulants at start of therapy. Age >60 and diagnosis of cancer independently predispose to increased risk of coagulopathy.

THERAPEUTIC CLASS: Fluoropyrimidine carbamate

INDICATIONS: First-line treatment of metastatic colorectal carcinoma and adjuvant treatment in patients with Dukes' C colon cancer who have undergone complete resection of the primary tumor when treatment with fluoropyrimidine therapy alone is preferred. Treatment of metastatic breast cancer in combination with docetaxel after failure of prior anthracycline-containing chemotherapy. Treatment of metastatic breast cancer in patients resistant to paclitaxel and anthracycline-containing chemotherapy or resistant to paclitaxel and for whom further anthracycline therapy is not indicated.

DOSAGE: *Adults:* Individualize dose. Monotherapy: Metastatic Colorectal Cancer/Metastatic Breast Cancer: Usual: 1250mg/m² bid for 2 weeks followed by 1-week rest period given as 3-week cycles. Combination with Docetaxel: Usual: 1250mg/m² bid for 2 weeks followed by 1-week rest period, combined with docetaxel 75mg/m² as 1 hr IV q3 weeks. Adjuvant Dukes' C Colon Cancer Treatment: 1250mg/m² bid for 2 weeks followed by 1-week rest period, given as 3-week cycles for total of 8 cycles (24 weeks). CrCl 30-50mL/min: Reduce to 75% of starting dose. Interrupt and/or reduce dose if toxicity occurs. Readjust according to adverse effects. Refer to PI for dose calculation according to body surface area, dose modification recommendations, and docetaxel dose reduction schedule. Swallow whole. Take with water within 30 min after am and pm meals.

HOW SUPPLIED: Tab: 150mg, 500mg

CONTRAINDICATIONS: Hypersensitivity to 5-fluorouracil (5-FU), dihydropyrimidine dehydrogenase (DPD) deficiency, severe renal impairment (CrCl <30mL/min).

WARNINGS/PRECAUTIONS: May induce diarrhea; give fluid and electrolyte replacement with severe diarrhea. Interrupt therapy if grade 2/3/4 diarrhea occurs until diarrhea resolves or decreases intensity to grade 1. Necrotizing enterocolitis reported. Caution with elderly; ≥80 yrs may experience greater incidence of grade 3/4 adverse events. Hand-and-foot syndrome may occur; interrupt therapy if grade 2/3 symptoms occur until event resolves or decreases intensity to grade 1. Cardiotoxicity (eg, myocardial infarction [MI]/ischemia, angina, dysrhythmias, cardiac arrest/failure, cardiomyopathy) observed. Hyperbilirubinemia reported; interrupt therapy if grade 3/4 elevations in bilirubin occur until hyperbilirubinemia decreases to ≤3X ULN. Neutropenia, thrombocytopenia, and decrease in hemoglobin reported. Avoid with baseline neutrophil counts of <1.5x10⁹/L and/or thrombocyte counts of <100x10⁹/L; interrupt therapy with grade 3/4 hematologic toxicity. Rarely, severe toxicity (eg, stomatitis, diarrhea, neutropenia, neurotoxicity) associated with 5-FU has been attributed to DPD deficiency. May cause fetal harm. Caution with mild to moderate hepatic dysfunction due to liver metastases. Caution with renal insufficiency.

ADVERSE REACTIONS: Diarrhea, hand-and-foot syndrome, pyrexia, anemia, N/V, fatigue/weakness, dermatitis, thrombocytopenia, constipation, taste disturbance, stomatitis, alopecia, abdominal pain, decreased appetite.

INTERACTIONS: See Boxed Warning. May increase phenytoin levels; reduce phenytoin dose and monitor carefully. Leucovorin may increase levels and toxicity of 5-FU. May increase the mean area under the curve of S-warfarin. Use in combination with irinotecan has not been adequately studied. Caution with CYP2C9 substrates. May increase levels with aluminum/magnesium hydroxide antacids.

PREGNANCY: Category D, not for use in nursing.

MECHANISM OF ACTION: Fluoropyrimidine carbamate; binds to thymidylate synthetase forming covalently bound ternary complex that inhibits formation of thymidylate from 2'-deoxyuridylate, inhibits DNA synthesis/cell division and interferes with RNA processing and protein synthesis.

PHARMACOKINETICS: Absorption: T_{max}=1.5 hrs. **Distribution:** Plasma protein binding (<60%); primarily bound to human albumin (approximately 35%). **Metabolism:** Extensive enzymatic conversion to 5-FU; hydrogenated to less toxic metabolite (FUH_2) by dihydropyrimidine dehydrogenase; cleavage of pyrimidine ring to 5-fluoro-ureido-propionic acid (FUPA); cleavage to α-fluoro-β-alanine (major metabolite). **Elimination:** Urine (95.5%) (3% unchanged) (57% major metabolite), feces (2.6%); $T_{1/2}$=0.75 hr.

NURSING CONSIDERATIONS

Assessment: Assess for hypersensitivity to 5-FU, DPD deficiency, severe renal impairment (CrCl <30mL/min), hepatic function, history of coronary artery disease, pregnancy/nursing status, and possible drug interactions. Obtain baseline neutrophil/thrombocyte counts.

Monitoring: Monitor for cardiotoxicity, severe diarrhea, hand-and-foot syndrome, hypersensitivity reactions, renal/hepatic impairment, necrotizing enterocolitis, neutropenia, thrombocytopenia, and decreases in Hgb. Perform periodic monitoring of LFTs, CBC, and renal function.

Patient Counseling: Instruct to d/c therapy if moderate/severe toxicity occurs. Inform that toxicities may include diarrhea, N/V, hand-and-foot syndrome, and stomatitis. Instruct to seek medical attention if fever (≥100.5°F) or infection occurs. Counsel about pregnancy risks; instruct to avoid pregnancy during therapy. Advise of possible drug and food interactions. Instruct to take with water within 30 min after a meal.

Administration: Oral route. Swallow whole. Do not cut or crush. **Storage:** 25°C (77°F); excursions permitted to 15-30°C (59-86°F). Keep tightly closed.

XENICAL   RX
orlistat (Genentech)

THERAPEUTIC CLASS: Lipase inhibitor

INDICATIONS: For obesity management, including weight loss and weight maint when used in conjunction with a reduced-calorie diet. To reduce the risk for weight regain after prior weight loss. For obese patients with an initial BMI ≥30kg/m² or ≥27kg/m² in the presence of other risk factors (eg, HTN, diabetes [DM], dyslipidemia).

DOSAGE: *Adults:* Usual: 120mg tid with each main meal containing fat (during or up to 1 hr after meal). Max: 120mg tid. Use with nutritionally balanced, reduced-calorie diet that contains 30% calories from fat; distribute daily intake of fat, carbohydrate, and protein over 3 main meals. Omit dose if a meal is occasionally missed or contains no fat.
Pediatrics: ≥12 yrs: Usual: 120mg tid with each main meal containing fat (during or up to 1 hr after meal). Max: 120mg tid. Use with nutritionally balanced, reduced-calorie diet that contains 30% calories from fat; distribute daily intake of fat, carbohydrate, and protein over 3 main meals. Omit dose if a meal is occasionally missed or contains no fat.

HOW SUPPLIED: Cap: 120mg

CONTRAINDICATIONS: Pregnancy, chronic malabsorption syndrome, cholestasis.

WARNINGS/PRECAUTIONS: Weight loss may affect glycemic control in patients with DM. Severe liver injury with hepatocellular necrosis or acute hepatic failure reported, with some cases resulting in liver transplant or death; d/c therapy and other suspect medications immediately and obtain LFTs (eg, ALT, AST). May increase levels of urinary oxalate; caution with a history of hyperoxaluria or calcium oxalate nephrolithiasis. Cases of oxalate nephrolithiasis and oxalate nephropathy with renal failure reported; monitor renal function. May increase risk of cholelithiasis due to substantial weight loss. Exclude organic causes of obesity (eg, hypothyroidism). GI events may increase with a high-fat diet (>30% total daily calories from fat).

ADVERSE REACTIONS: Oily spotting, flatus with discharge, fecal urgency, fatty/oily stool, oily evacuation, increased defecation, fecal incontinence.

INTERACTIONS: Vitamin K absorption may be decreased; monitor closely for changes in coagulation parameters with chronic stable doses of warfarin. Decreased prothrombin, increased INR and unbalanced anticoagulant treatment resulting in change of hemostatic parameters with anticoagulants. Reduced cyclosporine plasma levels reported; take cyclosporine at least 3 hrs before or after administration. Reduced absorption of some fat-soluble vitamins and β-carotene supplement and inhibited absorption of vitamin E acetate supplement reported. Hypothyroidism reported with levothyroxine; administer at least 4 hrs apart and monitor for thyroid function changes. May require reduction in dosage of oral hypoglycemic agents (eg, sulfonylureas) or insulin in diabetics.

PREGNANCY: Category X, caution in nursing.

MECHANISM OF ACTION: Lipase inhibitor; exerts therapeutic acitivity in the lumen of the stomach and small intestine by forming a covalent bond with the active serine residue site of gastric and pancreatic lipases. The inactivated enzymes are thus unavailable to hydrolyze dietary fats in the form of TGs into absorbable free fatty acids and monoglycerides.

PHARMACOKINETICS: Absorption: Minimal. T_{max}=8 hrs. **Distribution:** Plasma protein binding (>99%). **Metabolism:** M1 and M3 (primary and secondary metabolites). **Elimination:** Feces (97%, 83% unchanged), urine (<2%); $T_{1/2}$=1-2 hrs, 3 hrs (M1), 13.5 hrs (M3).

NURSING CONSIDERATIONS

Assessment: Assess for chronic malabsorption, cholestasis, known hypersensitivity to the drug, history of hyperoxaluria or calcium oxalate nephrolithiasis, organic causes of obesity (eg, hypothyroidism), pregnancy/nursing status, and possible drug interactions. Obtain baseline weight, FPG, and lipid profile.

Monitoring: Monitor for hepatic dysfunction, cholelithiasis, signs/symptoms of hypersensitivity reactions, GI events, and other adverse events. Monitor renal function in patients at risk for renal insufficiency.

Patient Counseling: Instruct to avoid medication if pregnant, have chronic malabsorption syndrome, cholestasis, or hypersensitivity to the drug. Ask patients if taking cyclosporine, β-carotene or vitamin E supplements, levothyroxine, or warfarin due to potential interactions. Inform of the adverse events (eg, oily spotting, flatus with discharge, fecal urgency, fatty/oily stool, oily evacuation, increased defecation, fecal incontinence) associated with the use of the drug. Inform of the potential risks that include lowered absorption of fat-soluble vitamins and potential liver injury, increased urinary oxalate, and cholelithiasis. Instruct to report any symptoms of hepatic dysfunction while on therapy. Counsel patient to take drug as directed with meals or up to 1 hr after a meal. Advise to take a multivitamin qd at least 2 hrs before or after administration, or at hs. Advise patients to adhere to dietary guidelines.

Administration: Oral route. **Storage:** 25°C (77°F); excursions permitted to 15-30°C (59-86°F).

XERESE   RX
acyclovir - hydrocortisone (Meda)

THERAPEUTIC CLASS: Corticosteroid/Anti-infective

INDICATIONS: Early treatment of recurrent herpes labialis (cold sores) to reduce the likelihood of ulcerative cold sores and to shorten the lesion healing time in adults and adolescents ≥12 yrs.

DOSAGE: *Adults:* Apply topically 5 times per day for 5 days. Start with earliest signs and symptoms (eg, during prodrome or when lesions appear).
Pediatrics: ≥12 yrs: Apply topically 5 times per day for 5 days. Start with earliest signs and symptoms (eg, during prodrome or when lesions appear).

HOW SUPPLIED: Cre: (Acyclovir-Hydrocortisone) 5%-1% [2g, 5g]

WARNINGS/PRECAUTIONS: For cutaneous use only. Do not use in the eye, inside the mouth or nose, or on the genitals. Other orofacial lesions (eg, bacterial and fungal infections) may be difficult to distinguish from cold sores. Encourage patient to seek medical advice when cold sore fails to heal within 2 weeks. Potential for irritation and contact sensitization.

ADVERSE REACTIONS: Local skin reactions, drying or flaking of skin, burning or tingling of application site, erythema, pigmentation changes, application site reactions, inflammation.

PREGNANCY: Category B, caution in nursing.

MECHANISM OF ACTION: (Acyclovir) Synthetic purine nucleoside analogue; stops herpes viral DNA replication by competitive inhibition of viral DNA polymerase, incorporation into and termination of the growing viral DNA chain, and inactivation of viral DNA polymerase. (Hydrocortisone) Corticosteroid; possesses anti-inflammatory effects which suppress the clinical manifestations of disease in a wide range of disorders where inflammation is prominent feature.

PHARMACOKINETICS: Absorption: (Hydrocortisone) Percutaneous; extent of absorption determined by many factors, including vehicle, integrity of epidermal barrier, and use of occlusive dressings; inflammation and/or other disease processes in the skin increase absorption. **Metabolism:** (Hydrocortisone) Liver. **Excretion:** (Hydrocortisone) Kidneys, bile.

X

NURSING CONSIDERATIONS

Assessment: Assess for type of lesions (eg, bacterial and fungal infections), age, hypersensitivity, inflammation and/or other disease processes of the skin, immune status, and pregnancy/nursing status.

Monitoring: Monitor lesions for clinical response, local skin reactions, irritation, contact sensitization, and other possible adverse reactions.

Patient Counseling: Inform patients that medication is not a cure for cold sores and that medication is for cutaneous use only for herpes labialis of the lips and around the mouth. Advise not to use in the eye, inside the mouth or nose, or on the genitals. Encourage patient to seek medical advice when cold sore fails to heal within 2 weeks. Counsel to use as prescribed. Advise to avoid unnecessary rubbing of the affected area to avoid aggravating or transferring the infection.

Administration: Topical route. For each dose, apply a quantity sufficient to cover the affected area, including the outer margin. **Storage:** 20-25°C (68-77°F); excursions permitted to 15-30°C (59-86°F). Do not freeze.

XGEVA   RX
denosumab (Amgen)

THERAPEUTIC CLASS: IgG$_2$ monoclonal antibody

INDICATIONS: Prevention of skeletal-related events in patients with bone metastases from solid tumors.

DOSAGE: *Adults:* 120mg SQ every 4 weeks in the upper arm, upper thigh, or abdomen.

HOW SUPPLIED: Inj: 120mg/1.7mL

WARNINGS/PRECAUTIONS: May cause severe hypocalcemia; greater risk in patients with CrCl <30mL/min or receiving dialysis. Correct pre-existing hypocalcemia prior to treatment, monitor calcium levels and administer calcium, magnesium, and vitamin D PRN. Osteonecrosis of the jaw (ONJ) may occur; avoid invasive dental procedures during therapy. Perform oral exam. May cause fetal harm.

ADVERSE REACTIONS: Fatigue/asthenia, hypophosphatemia, nausea, dyspnea, diarrhea, hypocalcemia, cough, headache.

INTERACTIONS: Monitor calcium levels more frequently with other drugs that can lower calcium levels.

PREGNANCY: Category D, not for use in nursing.

MECHANISM OF ACTION: IgG2 monoclonal antibody; binds to RANKL and prevents it from activating its receptor, RANK, on the surface of osteoclasts and their precursors. Increased osteoclast activity, stimulated by RANKL, is a mediator of bone pathology in solid tumors with osseous metastases.

PHARMACOKINETICS: Absorption: Bioavailability (62%). **Distribution:** Crosses placenta. **Elimination:** T$_{1/2}$=28 days.

NURSING CONSIDERATIONS

Assessment: Assess for hypocalcemia, renal function, pregnancy/nursing status, and possible drug interactions. Perform oral exam and appropriate preventive dentistry.

Monitoring: Monitor calcium levels. Perform oral exam and appropriate preventive dentistry periodically.

Patient Counseling: Advise to contact a healthcare professional if experiencing symptoms of hypocalcemia (eg, paresthesias or muscle stiffness, twitching, spasms, cramps), symptoms of ONJ (eg, pain, numbness, swelling of or drainage from the jaw, mouth, or teeth), persistent pain or slow healing of the mouth or jaw after dental surgery, or pregnancy/nursing. Advise of the need for proper oral hygiene and routine dental care, informing their dentist that they are receiving the drug, and avoiding invasive dental procedures during treatment. Advise that denosumab is also marketed as Prolia; instruct to inform healthcare provider if taking Prolia

Administration: SQ route. Refer to PI for preparation and administration. **Storage:** 2-8°C (36-46°F). Do not freeze. Once removed from the refrigerator, do not expose to >25°C (77°F) or direct light and discard if not used within 14 days. Protect from heat. Avoid vigorous shaking.

XIAFLEX   RX
collagenase clostridium histolyticum (Auxilium)

THERAPEUTIC CLASS: Debriding/Healing Agent

INDICATIONS: Treatment of adult patients with Dupuytren's contracture with a palpable cord.

DOSAGE: *Adults:* Initial: Inject 0.58mg (0.25mL) into a palpable cord with a contracture of a metacarpophalangeal (MP) joint or 0.58mg (0.20mL) for proximal interphalangeal (PIP) joint. After 24 hrs, perform finger extension procedure if contracture persists. After 4 weeks, if MP or PIP contracture remains, re-inject 0.58mg (0.25mL or 0.20mL) single dose; may repeat finger extension procedure after 24 hrs. Injection and finger extension procedures may be administered up to 3x/cord at approx. 4-week intervals. Please refer to PI for reconstitution/preparation, injection, and finger extension procedures.

HOW SUPPLIED: Inj: 0.9mg/vial

WARNINGS/PRECAUTIONS: Tendon rupture, ligament damage, and serious local reactions (eg, pulley rupture, complex regional pain syndrome, sensory abnormality of the hand) reported. Avoid injecting into tendons, nerves, blood vessels, or other collagen-containing structures of the hand. Severe allergic reactions may occur.

ADVERSE REACTIONS: Tendon rupture, ligament damage, peripheral edema, contusion, injection-site hemorrhage, extremity pain, lymphadenopathy, tenderness, pruritus, skin laceration, injection-site reaction, lymph node pain, tenderness, axillary pain.

INTERACTIONS: Caution in patients receiving concomitant anticoagulants (except low-dose aspirin).

PREGNANCY: Category B, caution in nursing.

MECHANISM OF ACTION: Debriding/healing agent; enzymatically disrupts collagen.

NURSING CONSIDERATIONS

Assessment: Assess for coagulation disorders, anticoagulant medication, pregnancy/nursing status, hypersensitivity, possible drug interactions.

Monitoring: Monitor for signs/symptoms of hypersensitivity reactions, tendon/ligament injury and bleeding.

Patient Counseling: Advise that serious complications may occur. After injection, instruct to limit motion of treated finger and keep injected hand elevated until bedtime. Instruct not to disrupt injected cord by self-manipulation and to return for follow-up the next day. After finger extension and split fitting procedure, instruct to avoid strenuous activity with injected hand, wear splint at bedtime up to 4 months, and perform finger flexion and extension exercises each day. Notify of pregnancy/nursing status.

Administration: IV, or intralesional route. Must be reconstituted with the provided diluent prior to use. Refer to PI for preparation of reconstituted solution, dilution and administration. Inject only one cord at a time; inject other cords with contractures in sequential order. **Storage:** Lyophilized Powder: Refrigerate at 2-8°C (36-46°F) Do not freeze. Reconstituted solution: May keep at room temperature of 20-25°C (68-77°F) up to 1 hr or refrigerate at 2-8°C (36-46°F) up to 4 hrs prior to administration.

XIFAXAN   RX
rifaximin (Salix)

THERAPEUTIC CLASS: Semisynthetic rifampin analog

INDICATIONS: (200mg) Treatment of travelers' diarrhea caused by noninvasive strains of *Escherichia coli* in patients ≥12 yrs. (550mg) For reduction in risk of overt hepatic encephalopathy (HE) recurrence in patients ≥18 yrs.

DOSAGE: *Adults:* Travelers' Diarrhea: 200mg tid for 3 days. HE: 550mg bid.
Pediatrics: Travelers' Diarrhea: ≥12 yrs: 200mg tid for 3 days.

HOW SUPPLIED: Tab: 200mg, 550mg

WARNINGS/PRECAUTIONS: Should not be used for diarrhea complicated by fever and/or blood in the stool or diarrhea due to pathogens other than *E. coli*. D/C if diarrhea symptoms worsen or persist >24-48 hrs; consider alternative antibiotic therapy. *Clostridium difficile*-associated diarrhea (CDAD) reported and may range in severity from mild diarrhea to fatal colitis; d/c if suspected or confirmed and institute appropriate management/therapy. Use in the absence of a proven or strongly suspected bacterial infection or a prophylactic indication is unlikely to provide benefit and may increase the risk of the development of drug-resistant bacteria. Caution with severe hepatic impairment (Child-Pugh Class C); may increase systemic exposure.

ADVERSE REACTIONS: Flatulence, headache, abdominal pain, rectal tenesmus, nausea, peripheral edema, dizziness, fatigue, ascites, muscle spasms, pruritus, abdominal distention, anemia, cough, depression.

PREGNANCY: Category C, not for use in nursing.

MECHANISM OF ACTION: Semisynthetic rifampin analog; binds to β-subunit of bacterial DNA-dependent RNA polymerase, resulting in inhibition of bacterial RNA synthesis.

PHARMACOKINETICS: Absorption: Administration with consecutive dosing, fasting/fed conditions, and Child-Pugh Class (A, B, C) resulted in different pharmacokinetic parameters; refer to PI. **Distribution:** Plasma protein binding; 550mg: (67.5%, healthy), (62%, hepatic impairment). **Elimination:** Feces (96.62%, unchanged), urine (0.32% mostly metabolites), (0.03%, unchanged).

NURSING CONSIDERATIONS

Assessment: If diarrhea present, assess for causative organisms and assess if diarrhea is complicated by fever or blood in stool. Assess for hepatic impairment (Child-Pugh Class C) and pregnancy/nursing status.

Monitoring: Monitor for signs/symptoms of a hypersensitivity reaction (eg, exfoliative dermatitis, angioneurotic edema, anaphylaxis), CDAD, development of drug resistant bacteria, and for worsening of symptoms.

Patient Counseling: If being treated for traveler's diarrhea, instruct to d/c therapy and contact physician if diarrhea persists for more than 24-48 hrs or worsens. Advise to contact physician if fever develops, blood in the stool develops, or if diarrhea occurs after therapy. Inform that medication may be taken with or without food. Counsel that drug only treats bacterial infections, not viral infections (eg, common cold). Advise to take as directed and to avoid skipping doses or not completing the full course of therapy.

Administration: Oral route. **Storage:** 20-25°C (68-77°F); excursions permitted to 15-30°C (59-86°F).

XOLAIR   RX
omalizumab (Genentech/Novartis)

> Anaphylaxis, presenting as bronchospasm, hypotension, syncope, urticaria, and/or angioedema of the throat or tongue has been reported as early as after the first dose or beyond 1 yr. Monitor closely for an appropriate time period after administration.

THERAPEUTIC CLASS: Monoclonal antibody/IgE-blocker

INDICATIONS: To decrease the incidence of asthma exacerbations in adults and adolescents ≥12 yrs with moderate to severe persistent asthma with a positive skin test or in vitro reactivity to a perennial aeroallergen and whose symptoms are inadequately controlled with inhaled corticosteroids.

DOSAGE: *Adults:* 150-375mg SQ q2 or 4 weeks based on body weight (kg) and pretreatment serum total IgE level (IU/mL). Max: 150mg/site. 30-90kg and IgE ≥30-100 IU/mL: 150mg q4 weeks. >90-150kg and IgE ≥30-100 IU/mL or 30-90kg and IgE >100-200 IU/mL or 30-60kg and IgE >200-300 IU/mL: 300mg q4 weeks. >90-150kg and IgE >100-200 IU/mL or 60-90kg and IgE >200-300 IU/mL or 30-70kg and IgE >300-400 IU/mL: 225mg q2 weeks. >90-150kg and IgE >200-300 IU/mL or >70-90kg and IgE >300-400 IU/mL or 30-70kg and IgE >400-500 IU/mL or 30-60kg and IgE >500-600 IU/mL: 300mg q2 weeks. >70-90kg and IgE >400-500 IU/mL or >60-70kg and IgE >500-600 IU/mL or 30-60kg and IgE >600-700 IU/mL: 375mg q2 weeks. Refer to PI for dosing adjustments.
Pediatrics: ≥12 yrs: 150-375mg SQ q2 or 4 weeks based on body weight (kg) and pretreatment serum total IgE level (IU/mL). Max: 150mg/site. 30-90kg and IgE ≥30-100 IU/mL: 150mg q4 weeks. >90-150kg and IgE ≥30-100 IU/mL or 30-90kg and IgE >100-200 IU/mL or 30-60kg and IgE >200-300 IU/mL: 300mg q4 weeks. >90-150kg and IgE >100-200 IU/mL or 60-90kg and IgE >200-300 IU/mL or 30-70kg and IgE >300-400 IU/mL: 225mg q2 weeks. >90-150kg and IgE >200-300 IU/mL or >70-90kg and IgE >300-400 IU/mL or 30-70kg and IgE >400-500 IU/mL or 30-60kg and IgE >500-600 IU/mL: 300mg q2 weeks. >70-90kg and IgE >400-500 IU/mL or >60-70kg and IgE >500-600 IU/mL or 30-60kg and IgE >600-700 IU/mL: 375mg q2 weeks. Refer to PI for dosing adjustments.

HOW SUPPLIED: Inj: 150mg/5mL [vial]

WARNINGS/PRECAUTIONS: Malignant neoplasms reported. Not for use in treatment of other allergic conditions, acute bronchospasm, or status asthmaticus. Do not abruptly d/c systemic or inhaled corticosteroids when initiating therapy. Rarely, serious systemic eosinophilia reported with clinical features of vasculitis consistent with Churg-Strauss syndrome; caution with worsening pulmonary symptoms, cardiac complications, and/or neuropathy, especially upon reduction of oral corticosteroids. Geohelminth (eg, roundworm, hookworm, whipworm, threadworm) infections reported in patients at high risk. D/C if constellation of signs/symptoms (arthritis/arthralgia, rash, fever, lymphadenopathy) with an onset 1-5 days after the first or subsequent injections develop. Serum total IgE levels may increase due to formation of Xolair: IgE complexes.

ADVERSE REACTIONS: Anaphylaxis, malignancies, injection-site reactions, viral infections, upper respiratory tract infection, sinusitis, headache, pharyngitis, pain, fatigue, arthralgia, leg pain, dizziness.

PREGNANCY: Category B, caution in nursing.

MECHANISM OF ACTION: Monoclonal antibody/IgE blocker; inhibits binding of IgE to the high-affinity IgE receptor on the surface of mast cells and basophils and limits degree of mediator release of allergic response.

PHARMACOKINETICS: Absorption: Absolute bioavailability (62%); T_{max}=7-8 days. **Distribution:** V_d=78mL/kg. **Elimination:** $T_{1/2}$=26 days.

NURSING CONSIDERATIONS

Assessment: Assess for acute bronchospasm or status asthmaticus, malignancies, hypersensitivity, risk of geohelminth infections, and pregnancy/nursing status. Obtain baseline body weight and serum IgE levels.

Monitoring: Monitor for anaphylaxis, hypersensitivity reactions, injection-site reactions, headaches, malignancies, viral/geohelminth/upper respiratory tract infections, serum sickness-like reactions, and eosinophilic conditions especially upon reduction of oral corticosteroids. Periodically reassess need for continued therapy based upon disease severity and level of asthma control. Monitor body weight, CBC (eg, eosinophils), stool exam, and IgE levels as needed.

Patient Counseling: Inform about risk of life-threatening anaphylaxis, and that injection-site reactions (eg, bruising, redness, warmth, burning, stinging) may occur; advise to immediately notify physician if these adverse reactions develop. Instruct not to decrease dose of or stop taking any other asthma medications unless otherwise instructed. Inform that immediate improvement may not be seen after beginning of therapy. Encourage pregnant women to enroll in the Pregnancy Exposure Registry.

Administration: SQ route. Refer to PI for proper preparation and administration procedures.
Storage: 2-8°C (36-46°F). Reconstituted: May be stored at 2-8°C (36-46°F) for up to 8 hrs or 4 hrs at room temperature. Protect from direct sunlight.

XOLEGEL   RX
ketoconazole (Stiefel)

THERAPEUTIC CLASS: Azole antifungal

INDICATIONS: Topical treatment of seborrheic dermatitis in immunocompetent adults and pediatrics ≥12 yrs.

DOSAGE: *Adults:* Apply qd to affected area for 2 weeks.
Pediatrics: ≥12 yrs: Apply qd to affected area for 2 weeks.

HOW SUPPLIED: Gel: 2% [45g]

WARNINGS/PRECAUTIONS: Not for oral, ophthalmic or intravaginal use. Avoid fire, flame or smoking during and immediately following application. D/C therapy if irritation occurs or disease worsens. Use caution when applying to the chest during lactation to avoid accidental ingestion by the infant.

ADVERSE REACTIONS: Application-site burning.

PREGNANCY: Category C, caution in nursing.

MECHANISM OF ACTION: Azole antifungal; not established.

PHARMACOKINETICS: Absorption: Day 7: C_{max}=1.35ng/mL; T_{max}=8 hrs; AUC_{0-24}=20.8ng•h/mL. Day 14: C_{max}=0.80ng/mL; T_{max}=7 hrs; AUC_{0-24}=15.6ng•h/mL.

NURSING CONSIDERATIONS

Assessment: Assess for immunocompetence and pregnancy/nursing status.

Monitoring: Monitor for irritation, worsening of seborrheic dermatitis and application-site burning/reactions.

Patient Counseling: Instruct to use only as directed; for external use only. Avoid contact with eyes, nostrils and mouth. Advise to wash hands after application. Notify healthcare provider of any signs of adverse reactions.

Administration: Topical route. **Storage:** 25°C (77°F); excursions permitted to 15-30°C (59-86°F). Contents are flammable.

XOPENEX   RX
levalbuterol HCl (Sunovion)

THERAPEUTIC CLASS: Beta$_2$-agonist

INDICATIONS: Treatment or prevention of bronchospasm in patients ≥6 yrs with reversible obstructive airway disease.

DOSAGE: *Adults:* Initial: 0.63mg tid q6-8h. Inadequate Response/Severe Asthma: 1.25mg tid. Administer by nebulizer.
Pediatrics: ≥12 yrs: Initial: 0.63mg tid q6-8h. Inadequate Response/Severe Asthma: 1.25mg tid. 6-11 yrs: 0.31mg tid. Max: 0.63mg tid. Administer by nebulizer.

HOW SUPPLIED: Sol, Inhalation: 0.31mg/3mL, 0.63mg/3mL, 1.25mg/3mL [24^s]

WARNINGS/PRECAUTIONS: May produce paradoxical bronchospasm; d/c immediately and institute alternative therapy. May produce cardiovascular effects and BP changes; caution with cardiovascular diseases (CVD), especially coronary insufficiency, arrhythmias, and HTN. ECG changes reported. Fatalities reported with excessive use. Immediate hypersensitivity reactions may occur. Caution with convulsive disorders, hyperthyroidism, and diabetes mellitus (DM), and in patients unusually responsive to sympathomimetic amines. May produce significant hypokalemia. Caution when administering higher doses with renal impairment.

ADVERSE REACTIONS: Nervousness, tremor, rhinitis, increased cough, diarrhea, flu syndrome, viral infection, sinusitis, fever, headache, lymphadenopathy, pharyngitis, rash, asthenia, pain.

INTERACTIONS: Caution with other short-acting sympathomimetic aerosol bronchodilators or epinephrine. Caution with additional adrenergic drugs to avoid deleterious cardiovascular effects. Antagonized by β-blockers. Extreme caution with or within 2 weeks of d/c of MAOIs and TCAs due to potentiation. Decreased digoxin levels reported. May worsen ECG changes and/or hypokalemia with non-K$^+$-sparing diuretics (eg, loop and thiazide diuretics).

PREGNANCY: Category C, not for use in nursing.

MECHANISM OF ACTION: β$_2$-adrenergic agonist; stimulates adenylcyclase, the enzyme that catalyzes formation of cAMP from ATP. Increased cAMP levels are associated with relaxation of smooth muscles of the airway and inhibition of release of mediators from mast cells.

PHARMACOKINETICS: Absorption: Administration of variable doses in different age groups resulted in different pharmacokinetic parameters. **Metabolism:** GI tract via SULT1A3 (sulfotransferase). **Elimination:** Urine (25-46%), feces (<20%); ≥12 yrs: T$_{1/2}$=3.3 hrs (1.25mg), 4 hrs (5mg).

NURSING CONSIDERATIONS

Assessment: Assess for history of hypersensitivity to drug, CVD, convulsive disorders, hyperthyroidism, DM, renal impairment, pregnancy/nursing status and possible drug interactions. Assess use in patients unusually responsive to sympathomimetic amines.

Monitoring: Monitor for paradoxical bronchospasm, deterioration of asthma, CV effects, hypokalemia, and immediate hypersensitivity reactions. Monitor BP, HR, and ECG changes.

Patient Counseling: Instruct not to increase dose/frequency of doses without consulting physician. Seek immediate medical attention if treatment becomes less effective for symptomatic relief, symptoms worsen, or need to use the product more frequently than usual. Counsel on common side effects (eg, chest pain, palpitations, rapid HR, tremor, nervousness). Notify physician if pregnant/nursing. Take concurrent inhaled/asthma medications only as directed. Vials should be used within 2 weeks once foil pouch is opened and within 1 week if not used immediately after removal from pouch. Discard vial if solution is not colorless.

Administration: Inhalation route. Refer to PI for proper administration. **Storage:** 20-25°C (68-77°F). Protect from light and excessive heat.

XOPENEX HFA   RX
levalbuterol tartrate (Sunovion)

THERAPEUTIC CLASS: Beta$_2$-agonist

INDICATIONS: Treatment or prevention of bronchospasm in patients ≥4 yrs with reversible obstructive airway disease.

DOSAGE: *Adults:* 2 inh (90mcg) q4-6h or 1 inh (45mcg) q4h. Elderly: Start at low end of dosing range.
Pediatrics: ≥4 yrs: 2 inh (90mcg) q4-6h or 1 inh (45mcg) q4h.

HOW SUPPLIED: MDI: 45mcg/inh [8.4g, 15g]

WARNINGS/PRECAUTIONS: May produce paradoxical bronchospasm; d/c immediately and institute alternative therapy. May produce clinically significant cardiovascular effects and BP changes; caution with cardiovascular diseases (CVD), especially coronary insufficiency, arrhythmias, and HTN. ECG changes reported. Fatalities reported with excessive use. Immediate hypersensitivity reactions may occur. Caution with convulsive disorders, hyperthyroidism, and diabetes mellitus (DM), and in patients unusually responsive to sympathomimetic amines. May produce significant hypokalemia. Caution when administering higher doses with renal impairment. Caution in elderly.

ADVERSE REACTIONS: Pharyngitis, rhinitis, pain, vomiting.

INTERACTIONS: Caution with other short-acting sympathomimetic aerosol bronchodilators or epinephrine. Caution with additional adrenergic drugs to avoid deleterious cardiovascular effects. Antagonized by β-blockers. Extreme caution with or within 2 weeks of d/c of MAOIs and TCAs due to potentiation. Decreased digoxin levels reported. May worsen ECG changes and/or hypokalemia with non-K⁺-sparing diuretics (eg, loop and thiazide diuretics).

PREGNANCY: Category C, not for use in nursing.

MECHANISM OF ACTION: β_2-adrenergic agonist; stimulates adenylate cyclase, the enzyme that catalyzes formation of cAMP from ATP. Increased cAMP levels are associated with relaxation of smooth muscles of the airway and inhibition of release of mediators from mast cells.

PHARMACOKINETICS: Absorption: C_{max}=0.199ng/mL (≥12 yrs), 0.163ng/mL (4-11 yrs); T_{max}=0.54 hrs (≥12 yrs), 0.76 hrs (4-11 yrs); AUC=0.695ng•hr/mL (≥12 yrs), 0.579ng•hr/mL (4-11 yrs). **Metabolism:** GI tract via SULT1A3 (sulfotransferase). **Elimination:** Urine (25-46%), feces (<20%).

NURSING CONSIDERATIONS

Assessment: Assess for history of hypersensitivity to drug, CVD, convulsive disorders, hyperthyroidism, DM, renal impairment, pregnancy/nursing status and possible drug interactions. Assess use in patients unusually responsive to sympathomimetic amines.

Monitoring: Monitor for paradoxical bronchospasm, deterioration of asthma, CV effects, hypokalemia, and immediate hypersensitivity reactions. Monitor BP, HR, and ECG changes.

Patient Counseling: Instruct not to increase dose/frequency of doses without consulting physician. Seek immediate medical attention if treatment becomes less effective for symptomatic relief, symptoms worsen, or need to use the product more frequently than usual. Keep plastic mouthpiece clean to prevent medication build-up and blockage; wash, shake to remove excess water, and air dry thoroughly at least once a week. Counsel on common side effects (eg, chest pain, palpitations, rapid HR, tremor, nervousness). Notify physician if pregnant/nursing. Keep out of reach of children. Avoid spraying in eyes and shake well before each spray. Prime inhaler before using if using for the 1st time or inhaler has not been used for >3 days.

Administration: Oral inhalation. Refer to PI for proper administration. Shake well before use. Prime inhaler by releasing 4 test sprays into the air, away from face. **Storage:** 20-25°C (68-77°F). Store with mouthpiece down. Protect from freezing and direct sunlight. Contents under pressure. Do not puncture or incinerate. Exposure to >49°C (120°F) may cause bursting.

XYLOCAINE INJECTION   RX

lidocaine HCl (APP Pharmaceuticals)

OTHER BRAND NAMES: Xylocaine-MPF (Abraxis)

THERAPEUTIC CLASS: Local anesthetic

INDICATIONS: For production of local or regional anesthesia by infiltration techniques such as percutaneous injection and IV regional anesthesia by peripheral nerve block techniques such as brachial plexus and intercostal and by central neural techniques such as lumbar and caudal epidural blocks.

DOSAGE: *Adults:* Individualize dose. Dosage varies depending on procedure, depth of anesthesia, degree of muscular relaxation, duration of anesthesia required, and the physical condition of the patient. Max: 4.5mg/kg or total daily dose of 300mg (without epinephrine), 7mg/kg or total daily dose of 500mg (with epinephrine). Continuous Epidural/Caudal Anesthesia: Max: Intervals not less than 90 min. Paracervical Block: Max: 200mg/90 min. Administer 1/2 of the dose slowly to each side, 5 minutes between sides. Regional Anesthesia: IV: Max: 4mg/kg. Elderly/Debilitated/Cardiac or Liver Disease: Reduce dose. Refer to PI for recommended dosing for various types of anesthetic procedures.
Pediatrics: Dosage varies with age and weight. Regional Anesthesia: IV: Max: 3mg/kg. Use lowest effective concentration and lowest effective dose at all times.

HOW SUPPLIED: Inj: 0.5%, 1%, 2%; (MPF) 0.5%, 1%, 1.5%, 2%

WARNINGS/PRECAUTIONS: Should only be employed by clinicians well versed in diagnosis and management of dose related toxicity and other acute emergencies which might arise; oxygen, other resuscitative drugs, and cardiopulmonary equipment should be available for immediate use. Acidosis, cardiac arrest, and death may occur if there is a delay in toxicity management. Intra-articular infusion following arthroscopic and other surgical procedures is an unapproved use and chondrolysis reported in patients who received such infusions. Local anesthetic solutions containing antimicrobial preservatives (eg, methylparaben) should not be used for epidural or spinal anesthesia. Syringe aspiration should be performed to avoid intravascular injection. Use lowest effective dose. During epidural anesthesia, administer initial test dose and monitor for CNS and cardiovascular toxicity as well as for signs of unintended intrathecal administration. Repeated doses may cause significant increases in blood levels with each repeated dose. Reduce dose with debilitated, elderly, acutely ill, and children. Extreme caution when using lumbar and

X

caudal epidural anesthesia with existing neurological disease, spinal deformities, septicemia, and severe HTN. May trigger malignant hyperthermia. Monitor cardiovascular and respiratory vital signs and state of consciousness after each injection. Caution with hepatic disease, cardiovascular disorders, and in patients with known drug sensitivities. Small doses injected into the head and neck area including retrobulbar, dental and stellate ganglion blocks, may produce adverse reactions similiar to systemic toxicity seen with unintentional intravascular injection of larger doses; circulation and respiration should be constantly monitored and observed.

ADVERSE REACTIONS: Lightheadedness, nervousness, euphoria, confusion, dizziness, drowsiness, blurred vision, vomiting, heat/cold/numbness sensations, tremors, convulsions, respiratory depression, bradycardia, hypotension, urticaria.

INTERACTIONS: Use of CNS stimulants and depressants affects the CNS levels of lidocaine required to produce overt systemic effects. Concurrent administration of vasopressor drugs (for the treatment of hypotension related to obstetric blocks) and ergot-type oxytocic drugs may cause severe, persistent HTN or CVA.

PREGNANCY: Category B, caution in nursing.

MECHANISM OF ACTION: Anesthetic; stabilizes neuronal membrane by inhibiting ionic fluxes required for initiation and conduction of impulses, thereby effecting local anesthetic action.

PHARMACOKINETICS: Absorption: Complete. **Distribution:** Crosses blood-brain and placental barriers. **Metabolism:** Liver (rapid), oxidative N-alkylation (major pathway), yields monoethylglycinexylidide and glycinexylidide (metabolites). **Elimination:** Urine, (90% metabolites), (<10% unchanged); $T_{1/2}$=1.5-2.0 hrs.

NURSING CONSIDERATIONS

Assessment: Assess for drug sensitivities, presence of debilitation, hepatic/renal disease, pregnancy/nursing status, and for possible drug interactions. If planning to use for lumbar or caudal epidural anesthesia, assess for neurological disease, spinal deformities, septicemia, and severe HTN.

Monitoring: Monitor for allergic-type reactions, CNS toxicity, and cardiotoxiciy. Monitor for increased creatine phosphokinase levels following IM injection. Perform careful and constant monitoring of cardiovascular and respiratory vital signs and the patient's state of consciousness following each injection.

Patient Counseling: Inform about possible adverse reactions. Counsel about possibilty of temporary loss of sensation and motor activity, usually in the lower half of the body, following proper administration of epidural anesthesia.

Administration: Infiltration, peripheral nerve block, central neural block. **Storage:** 25°C (77°F). Protect from light.

XYREM [CIII]
sodium oxybate (Jazz Pharmaceuticals, Inc.)

Sodium oxybate is GHB (gamma hydroxybutyrate), a known drug of abuse. Abuse has been associated with important CNS adverse events, including death. Do not use with alcohol or other CNS depressants. Use has been associated with confusion, depression, and other neuropsychiatric events. Available only through the Xyrem Success Program, call 1-866-XYREM88.

THERAPEUTIC CLASS: CNS Depressant

INDICATIONS: Treatment of excessive daytime sleepiness and cataplexy in patients with narcolepsy.

DOSAGE: *Adults:* Initial: 2.25g qhs at least 2 hrs pc, then take 2.25g 2.5-4 hrs later. Titrate: Increase by 1.5g/night (0.75g/dose) every 1-2 weeks. Range: 6-9g/night. Max: 9g/night. Hepatic Insufficiency: Initial: Decrease by 50%. Titrate dose increments to effect.
Pediatrics: ≥16 yrs: Initial: 2.25g qhs at least 2 hrs pc, then take 2.25g 2.5-4 hrs later. Titrate: Increase by 1.5g/night (0.75g/dose) every 1-2 weeks. Range: 6-9g/night. Max: 9g/night. Hepatic Insufficiency: Initial: Decrease by 50%. Titrate dose increments to effect.

HOW SUPPLIED: Sol: 500mg/mL [180mL]

CONTRAINDICATIONS: Concomitant use with sedative hypnotic agents and patients with succinic semialdehyde dehydrogenase deficiency.

WARNINGS/PRECAUTIONS: Rapid onset of CNS depressant effects; ingest only at bedtime and while in bed. May impair physical/mental abilities. May impair respiratory drive and cause sleep apnea; caution with compromised respiratory function. Confusion, sleepwalking, and other neuropsychiatric events (eg, psychosis, paranoia, hallucinations, agitation, thought disorders and/or behavior abnormalities) may occur; evaluate patients and consider appropriate intervention. Depressive symptoms reported; monitor patients with previous history of depressive illness and/or suicide attempt. Rule out underlying etiologies, including worsening sleep apnea or nocturnal seizures if urinary/fecal incontinence develops. Daily Na^+ intake ranges from 0.5g (with 3g dose) to 1.6g (with 9g dose); caution with heart failure (HF), HTN, or renal impairment. Caution with hepatic insufficiency and in elderly.

ADVERSE REACTIONS: Headache, N/V, dizziness, pain, somnolence, nasopharyngitis, diarrhea, urinary incontinence, sleepwalking, depression.

INTERACTIONS: See Contraindications. Avoid with alcohol and other CNS depressants.

PREGNANCY: Category B, caution in nursing.

MECHANISM OF ACTION: CNS depressant; effect on cataplexy not established.

PHARMACOKINETICS: Absorption: Rapid, incomplete; absolute bioavailabiltiy (25%). C_{max}=78mcg/mL (1st peak), 142mcg/mL (2nd peak); T_{max}=0.5-1.25 hr. **Distribution:** V_d=190-384mL/kg; plasma protein binding (<1%). **Metabolism:** Kreb's cycle, β-oxidation. **Elimination:** By transformation to CO_2 eliminated by expiration. Urine (<5%), feces; $T_{1/2}$=0.5-1 hr.

NURSING CONSIDERATIONS

Assessment: Assess for compromised respiratory function, history of depressive illness or suicide attempt, sleep apnea, seizures, HF, HTN, hepatic/renal impairment, pregnancy/nursing status, alcohol intake, and possible drug interactions.

Monitoring: Monitor for signs/symptoms of CNS depression, confusion, sleep apnea, psychosis, suicide attempt, urinary/fecal incontinence, sleepwalking, dosage monitoring in hepatic/renal dysfunction. Perform antinuclear antibody (ANA) test.

Patient Counseling: Inform about the Xyrem Patient Success Program, which includes detailed information about safe/proper use of therapy as well as information to help prevent accidental use or abuse of therapy by others. See a prescriber frequently during treatment to review dose titration, symptom response, and adverse reaction. Food significantly decreases the bioavailability of the drug and may affect both the efficacy and safety of therapy; first dose should be taken several hrs after meal. Urinary/fecal incontinence may occur. Lie down and sleep after each dose and do not take the drug at any time other than at night, immediately before bedtime and then 2.5-4 hrs later. Do not take with alcohol or other sedative hypnotics while on therapy. Notify if pregnant/nursing or planning to become pregnant. Keep out of reach of children.

Administration: Oral route. Prepare both doses prior to bedtime, and place 2nd dose in close proximity to the patient's bed. Dilute each dose with 2 oz. of water prior to ingestion. Take 1st dose at least 2 hrs pc. Take both doses while seated in bed. After ingestion, patient should lie down and remain in bed. **Storage:** 25°C (77°F); excursions permitted at 15-30°C (59-86°F); consume diluted solution within 24 hrs; provided with a child-resistant cap.

XYZAL
RX

levocetirizine dihydrochloride (Sanofi-Aventis/UCB)

THERAPEUTIC CLASS: H_1-antagonist

INDICATIONS: Relief of symptoms associated with allergic rhinitis: seasonal (for adults and children ≥2 yrs) and perennial (for adults and children ≥6 months of age). Treatment of uncomplicated skin manifestations of chronic idiopathic urticaria in adults and children ≥6 months of age.

DOSAGE: *Adults:* 5mg (1 tab or 2 tsp [10mL] oral sol) qd in the evening. Mild Renal Impairment (CrCl 50-80mL/min): 2.5mg qd. Moderate Renal Impairment (CrCl 30-50mL/min): 2.5mg qod. Severe Renal Impairment (CrCl 10-30mL/min): 2.5mg twice weekly (administered q3-4 days). Elderly: Start at lower end of dosing range.
Pediatrics: ≥12 yrs: 5mg (1 tab or 2 tsp [10mL] oral sol) qd in the evening. Mild Renal Impairment (CrCl 50-80mL/min): 2.5mg qd. Moderate Renal Impairment (CrCl 30-50mL/min): 2.5mg qod. Severe Renal Impairment (CrCl 10-30mL/min): 2.5mg twice weekly (administered q3-4 days). 6-11 yrs: Usual/Max: 2.5mg (1/2 tab or 1 tsp [5mL] oral sol) qd in the evening. 6 months-5 yrs: Usual/Max: 1.25mg (1/2 tsp [2.5mL] oral sol) qd in the evening.

HOW SUPPLIED: Sol: 0.5mg/mL; Tab: 5mg* *scored

CONTRAINDICATIONS: End-stage renal disease (ESRD) (CrCl <10mL/min) and patients undergoing hemodialysis, pediatrics 6-11 yrs with renal impairment.

WARNINGS/PRECAUTIONS: Somnolence, fatigue, and asthenia reported. May impair mental/physical abilities. Adjust dose in patients with both renal/hepatic impairment. Adjust dose and dosing intervals based on CrCl in patients with renal impairment. Caution in the elderly; start at low end of dosing range.

ADVERSE REACTIONS: Somnolence, fatigue, nasopharyngitis, dry mouth, constipation, diarrhea, cough, drowsiness, pyrexia, vomiting, pharyngitis, otitis media.

INTERACTIONS: Avoid alcohol and CNS depressants. Decreased clearance with theophylline and ritonavir. Increased plasma concentration with ritonavir.

PREGNANCY: Category B, not for use in nursing.

MECHANISM OF ACTION: H_1-antagonist; antihistamine that selectively inhibits H_1-receptors.

PHARMACOKINETICS: Absorption: Rapid, extensive; C_{max}=270ng/mL (single dose), 308ng/mL (multiple doses); T_{max}=0.9 hr (tab), 0.5 hr (oral sol). **Distribution:** V_d=0.4L/kg; plasma protein binding (91-92%); found in breast milk. **Metabolism:** <14% metabolized through aromatic oxidation (via CYP 450 system), N- and O-dealkylation (via CYP3A4) and taurine conjugation pathways. **Elimination:** Urine (85.4%), feces (12.9%); $T_{1/2}$=8-9 hrs. Refer to PI for pharmacokinetic parameters of different populations.

NURSING CONSIDERATIONS

Assessment: Assess for ESRD or patients on hemodialysis, hypersensitivity to the drug, renal function, pregnancy/nursing status, and possible drug interactions.

Monitoring: Monitor for adverse reactions. Monitor renal function in elderly.

Patient Counseling: Instruct to use caution against performing hazardous tasks requiring mental alertness and motor coordination (eg, operating machinery, driving). Instruct to avoid use of alcohol or other CNS depressants since additional reduction in mental alertness may occur. Advise not to ingest more than the recommended dose.

Administration: Oral route. **Storage:** 20-25°C (68-77°F), excursions permitted to 15-30°C (59-86°F).

YASMIN   RX
drospirenone - ethinyl estradiol (Bayer Healthcare)

> Cigarette smoking increases risk of serious cardiovascular effects from combination oral contraceptive (COC) use. Risk increases with age (>35 yrs) and with the number of cigarettes smoked. Should not be used by women who are >35 yrs and smoke.

OTHER BRAND NAMES: Ocella (Barr) - Syeda (Sandoz)

THERAPEUTIC CLASS: Estrogen/progestogen combination

INDICATIONS: Prevention of pregnancy.

DOSAGE: *Adults:* 1 tab qd for 28 days, then repeat. Start 1st Sunday after menses begins or on 1st day of menses. Take at the same time each day, preferably pm, pc, or hs.
Pediatrics: Postpubertal: 1 tab qd for 28 days, then repeat. Start 1st Sunday after menses begins or on 1st day of menses. Take at the same time each day, preferably pm, pc, or hs.

HOW SUPPLIED: Tab: (Drospirenone [DRSP]-Ethinyl Estradiol [EE]) 3mg-0.03mg

CONTRAINDICATIONS: Renal impairment, adrenal insufficiency, high risk of arterial/venous thrombotic disease (eg, smoking if >35 yrs, presence/history of deep vein thrombosis/pulmonary embolism, cerebrovascular disease, coronary artery disease, thrombogenic valvular or thrombogenic rhythm diseases of the heart [eg, subacute bacterial endocarditis with valvular disease, or atrial fibrillation], inherited/acquired hypercoagulopathies, uncontrolled HTN, diabetes mellitus [DM] with vascular disease, headache with focal neurological symptoms or migraine with/without aura if >35 yrs), undiagnosed abnormal uterine bleeding, presence/history of breast or other estrogen/progestin-sensitive cancer, benign/malignant liver tumors, liver disease, pregnancy.

WARNINGS/PRECAUTIONS: Increased risk of venous thromboembolism; greatest risk during the first 6 months of COC use and is present after initially starting COC or restarting the same or different COC. Increased risk of cerebrovascular events (eg, stroke) and myocardial infarction (MI). D/C if arterial or deep venous thrombotic events, unexplained loss of vision, proptosis, diplopia, papilledema, or retinal vascular lesions occur. D/C at least 4 weeks before and through 2 weeks after major surgery or other surgeries with elevated risk of thromboembolism. Start therapy no earlier than 4 weeks postpartum in women who do not breastfeed. Caution with cardiovascular disease (CVD) risk factors. May cause hyperkalemia; avoid use in patients predisposed to hyperkalemia. May increase risk of breast cancer, cervical cancer, or intraepithelial neoplasia, and gallbladder disease. Hepatic adenoma and increased risk of hepatocellular carcinoma reported; d/c if jaundice or acute/chronic disturbances of liver function occur. Cholestasis may occur with history of pregnancy-related cholestasis. Increased BP reported; d/c if BP rises significantly. May decrease glucose tolerance; monitor prediabetic and diabetic women. Consider alternative contraception with uncontrolled dyslipidemias. May increase risk of pancreatitis with hypertriglyceridemia or family history thereof. May increase frequency/severity of migraine; d/c if new headaches that are recurrent, persistent, or severe develop. Unscheduled (breakthrough) bleeding and spotting may occur; rule out pregnancy or malignancy. Caution with history of depression; d/c if depression recurs to a serious degree. May change results of laboratory tests (eg, coagulation factors, lipids, glucose tolerance, binding proteins). May induce or exacerbate angioedema in women with hereditary angioedema. Chloasma may occur; avoid sun or UV radiation exposure. Absorption may not be complete in case of severe vomiting or diarrhea; if vomiting occurs within 3-4 hrs after tablet-taking, regard this as a missed tablet.

ADVERSE REACTIONS: Premenstrual syndrome, headache, migraine, breast pain/tenderness/discomfort, N/V, abdominal pain/discomfort/tenderness, mood changes.

INTERACTIONS: Potential for an increase in serum K^+ with ACE inhibitors, angiotensin II receptor antagonists, K^+-sparing diuretics, K^+ supplementation, heparin, aldosterone antagonists, and NSAIDs. Drugs or herbal products that induce certain enzymes, including CYP3A4 (eg, phenytoin, barbiturates, carbamazepine, bosentan, felbamate, griseofulvin, oxcarbazepine, rifampicin, topiramate, and products containing St. John's wort), may reduce drug effectiveness or increase incidence of breakthrough bleeding. Significant changes (increase/decrease) in plasma estrogen and progestin levels reported with HIV/hepatitis C virus protease inhibitors or non-nucleoside reverse transcriptase inhibitors. Pregnancy reported with antibiotics. Atorvastatin, ascorbic acid, acetaminophen, CYP3A4 inhibitors (eg, itraconazole, ketoconazole) may increase hormone levels. May decrease levels of lamotrigine and reduce seizure control. May need to increase dose of thyroid hormone in patients on thyroid hormone replacement therapy due to increased thyroid-binding globulin.

PREGNANCY: Contraindicated in pregnancy, not for use in nursing.

MECHANISM OF ACTION: Estrogen/progestogen oral contraceptive; acts primarily by suppressing ovulation. Also causes changes in cervical mucus that inhibit sperm penetration and endometrial changes that reduce the likelihood of implantation.

PHARMACOKINETICS: Absorption: DRSP: Absolute bioavailability (76%); (Cycle 13/day 21) C_{max}=78.7ng/mL; T_{max}=1.6 hrs; AUC=968ng•mL. EE: Absolute bioavailability (40%); (Cycle 13/day 21) C_{max}=90.5pg/mL; T_{max}=1.6 hrs; AUC=469.5pg•h/mL. Please refer to PI for other pharmacokinetic parameters. **Distribution:** Found in breast milk; DRSP: V_d=4L/kg, plasma protein binding (97%). (EE) V_d=4-5L/kg; plasma protein binding (98.5%). **Metabolism:** DRSP: Liver, via CYP3A4 (minor). EE: Hydroxylation (via CYP3A4), conjugation (glucuronidation and sulfation). **Elimination:** DRSP: urine, feces; $T_{1/2}$=30 hrs. EE: Urine, feces; $T_{1/2}$=24 hrs.

NURSING CONSIDERATIONS

Assessment: Assess for renal impairment, abnormal uterine bleeding, adrenal insufficiency, and known/suspected pregnancy or any other conditions where treatment is cautioned or contraindicated. Assess use in patients who are >35 yrs and heavy smokers (≥15 cigarettes/day), patients with CVD risk factors, predisposition to hyperkalemia, pregnancy-related cholestasis, HTN, DM, uncontrolled dyslipidemia, history/present hypertriglyceridemia, history of depression, hereditary angioedema, and history of chloasma. Assess for possible drug interactions.

Monitoring: Monitor for bleeding irregularities, venous/arterial thrombotic and thromboembolic events (eg, MI, stroke), cervical cancer or intraepithelial neoplasia, retinal vein thrombosis or any other ophthalmic changes, jaundice, acute/chronic disturbances in liver function, new/worsening headaches or migraines, cholestasis with history of pregnancy related cholestasis, and pancreatitis in hypertriglyceridemia. Monitor K^+ levels, glucose levels in DM or prediabetes, and BP with history of HTN. Perform annual history and physical exam.

Patient Counseling: Inform that drug does not protect against HIV infection (AIDS) and other sexually transmitted diseases. Counsel to avoid smoking while on treatment. Inform that COCs may reduce breast milk. Counsel about potential adverse effects. Instruct to take drug at the same time everyday. Counsel on what to do when pills are missed or if vomiting occurs within 3-4 hrs after tablet-taking, when enzyme inducers are used with COCs, and in other cases where use of a backup or alternative method of contraception is recommended. Inform that amenorrhea may occur and pregnancy should be ruled out if amenorrhea occurs in ≥2 consecutive cycles. Advise to inform physician of preexisting medical conditions and/or drugs currently being taken. Counsel patient who starts COCs postpartum and has not yet had a period, to use additional method of contraception until drug taken for 7 consecutive days. D/C if pregnancy occurs during treatment.

Administration: Oral route. **Storage:** (Syeda) 20-25°C (68-77°F). (Yasmin, Ocella) 25°C (77°F); excursions permitted to 15-30°C (59-86°F).

YAZ   RX
drospirenone - ethinyl estradiol (Bayer Healthcare)

Cigarette smoking increases the risk of serious cardiovascular events from combination oral contraceptive (COC) use. Risk increases with age (>35 yrs) and with the number of cigarettes smoked. Should not be used by women who are >35 yrs and smoke.

Y

OTHER BRAND NAMES: Loryna (Sandoz)

THERAPEUTIC CLASS: Estrogen/progestogen combination

INDICATIONS: Prevention of pregnancy. Treatment of moderate acne vulgaris in women ≥14 yrs who have achieved menarche and who desire an oral contraceptive for birth control. YAZ: Treatment of symptoms of premenstrual dysphoric disorder (PMDD).

YAZ

DOSAGE: *Adults:* Contraception/Acne/PMDD: 1 tab qd for 28 days, then repeat. Start 1st Sunday after menses begin or 1st day of menses. Take at the same time each day, preferably pm, pc, or qhs.
Pediatrics: Postpubertal: Contraception/Acne (≥ 14yrs)/PMDD: 1 tab qd for 28 days, then repeat. Start 1st Sunday after menses begin or 1st day of menses. Take at the same time each day, preferably pm, pc, or qhs.

HOW SUPPLIED: Tab: (Ethinyl Estradiol [EE]-Drospirenone [DRSP]) 0.02mg-3mg

CONTRAINDICATIONS: Renal impairment, adrenal insufficiency, high risk of arterial/venous thrombotic disease (eg, smoking if >35 yrs, active or history of deep vein thrombosis/pulmonary embolism, cerebrovascular disease, coronary artery disease, thrombogenic valvular or thrombogenic rhythm diseases of the heart, inherited/acquired hypercoagulopathies, uncontrolled HTN, diabetes mellitus [DM] with vascular disease, headache with focal neurological symptoms or migraine with/without aura if >35 yrs), undiagnosed abnormal uterine bleeding, presence/history of breast or other estrogen/progestin-sensitive cancer, benign/malignant liver tumors, liver disease, pregnancy.

WARNINGS/PRECAUTIONS: Increased risk of venous thromboembolism and arterial thromboses (eg, stroke, myocardial infarction). D/C if arterial or deep venous thrombotic events, unexplained loss of vision, proptosis, diplopia, papilledema, or retinal vascular lesions occur. D/C at least 4 weeks before and through 2 weeks after major surgery or other surgeries with elevated risk of thromboembolism. May cause hyperkalemia; avoid use in patients predisposed to hyperkalemia (eg, renal insufficiency, hepatic dysfunction, adrenal insufficiency). May increase risk of cervical cancer or intraepithelial neoplasia and gallbladder disease. Hepatic adenoma reported; d/c if jaundice develops. Cholestasis may occur with history of pregnancy-related cholestasis. Increased BP reported; d/c if BP rises significantly. May decrease glucose intolerance; monitor prediabetic and diabetic women. Consider alternative contraception with uncontrolled dyslipidemias. Increased risk of pancreatitis with hypertriglyceridemia or family history thereof. May develop new headaches; d/c in increased frequency or severity of migraine. Unscheduled (breakthrough) bleeding and spotting may occur; rule out pregnancy or malignancy. Caution with history of depression; d/c if depression recurs to serious degree. May change results of laboratory tests (eg, coagulation factors, lipids, glucose tolerance, binding proteins). May induce or exacerbate angioedema. Chloasma may occur especially with history of chloasma gravidarum; avoid sun or UV radiation exposure. Women who do not breastfeed may start therapy no earlier than 4 weeks postpartum. Not indicated for use before menarche and in postmenopausal women. YAZ: Not for treatment of premenstrual syndrome.

ADVERSE REACTIONS: Menstrual irregularities, N/V, headache/migraine, breast pain/tenderness, mood changes, migraine, cervical dysplasia.

INTERACTIONS: Reduced effectiveness or increased breakthrough bleeding with enzyme inducers, including CYP3A4, (eg, phenytoin, barbiturates, carbamazepine, bosentan, felbamate, griseofulvin, oxcarbazepine, rifampicin, topiramate, St. John's wort). Significant increase/decrease in plasma levels with HIV protease inhibitors or non-nucleoside reverse transcriptase inhibitors. Pregnancy reported with use of hormonal contraceptives and antibiotics. Increased levels with atorvastatin, ascorbic acid, acetaminophen, and CYP3A4 inhibitors (eg, itraconazole, ketoconazole). Decreases levels of lamotrigine and may reduce seizure control; adjust dose of lamotrigine. May need to increase dose of thyroid hormone in patients on thyroid hormone replacement therapy. Risk of hyperkalemia with angiotensin converting enzyme inhibitors, angiotensin-II receptor antagonists, K⁺-sparing diuretics, K⁺ supplementation, heparin, aldosterone antagonists, and NSAIDs.

PREGNANCY: Contraindicated in pregnancy, not for use in nursing.

MECHANISM OF ACTION: Estrogen/progestogen oral contraceptive; acts by primarily suppressing ovulation. Also causes cervical mucus changes that inhibit sperm penetration and endometrial changes that reduce the likelihood of implantation.

PHARMACOKINETICS: Absorption: DRSP: Absolute bioavailability (76%); (Cycle 1/Day 21) C_{max}=70.3ng/mL; T_{max}=1.5 hrs; AUC=763ng•h/mL. EE: Absolute bioavailability (40%); (Cycle 1/Day 21) C_{max}=45.1pg/mL; T_{max}=1.5 hrs; AUC=220pg•h/mL. **Distribution:** Found in breast milk; DRSP: V_d=4L/kg; serum protein binding (97%). EE: V_d=4-5L/kg; serum albumin binding (98.5%). **Metabolism:** DRSP: Liver, via CYP3A4 (minor). EE: Hydroxylation (via CYP3A4), conjugation with glucuronide and sulfate. **Elimination:** DRSP: Urine, feces; $T_{1/2}$=30 hrs. EE: Urine, feces; $T_{1/2}$=24 hrs.

NURSING CONSIDERATIONS

Assessment: Assess for presence/history of breast cancer, estrogen-dependent neoplasia, abnormal genital bleeding, renal/hepatic/adrenal disease, pregnancy/nursing status, or any other conditions where treatment is cautioned or contraindicated. Assess use in patients who are >35 yrs and smokers. Assess use with HTN, hyperlipidemias, DM, or in patients at increased risk for thrombosis. Assess for possible drug interactions.

Monitoring: Monitor for bleeding irregularities, thromboembolic events, onset or exacerbation of headaches or migraines, signs of liver dysfunction (eg, jaundice), signs of depression if with history thereof, retinal vein thrombosis, and visual problems. Monitor fasting blood glucose levels in DM and prediabetic patients, BP with history of HTN, lipid levels with history of hyperlipidemia, and K⁺ levels during 1st treatment cycle for patients at risk of hyperkalemia. Perform annual history/physical exam.

Patient Counseling: Inform that drug does not protect against HIV infection (AIDS) and other sexually transmitted diseases. Counsel that cigarette smoking increases the risk of serious cardiovascular events from COC use, and that women who are >35 years old and smoke should not use COCs. Counsel on warnings and precautions associated with COCs. Inform that COCs may reduce breast milk. Counsel about potential adverse effects. Instruct to take drug at the same time everyday. Counsel on what to do when pills are missed, when enzyme inducers are used with COCs, and in other cases where use of a backup or alternative method of contraception is recommended. Inform that amenorrhea may occur and pregnancy should be ruled out if amenorrhea occurs in ≥2 consecutive cycles. Advise to inform physician of preexisting medical conditions and/or drugs currently being taken. D/C if pregnancy is confirmed/suspected.

Administration: Oral route. **Storage:** (YAZ) 25°C (77°F); excursions permitted to 15-30°C (59-86°F). (Loryna) 20-25°C (68-77°F).

YERVOY

RX

ipilimumab (Bristol-Myers Squibb)

> May result in severe and fatal immune-mediated adverse reactions due to T-cell activation and proliferation, which may involve any organ system; most common are enterocolitis, hepatitis, dermatitis (eg, toxic epidermal necrolysis), neuropathy, and endocrinopathy. Majority of these reactions initially manifested during treatment; however, a minority occurred weeks to months after d/c of therapy. Permanently d/c therapy and initiate systemic high-dose corticosteroid for severe immune-mediated reactions. Assess for signs and symptoms of enterocolitis, dermatitis, neuropathy, and endocrinopathy and evaluate clinical chemistries (eg, LFTs, thyroid function tests) at baseline and before each dose.

THERAPEUTIC CLASS: Monoclonal antibody

INDICATIONS: Treatment of unresectable or metastatic melanoma.

DOSAGE: *Adults:* 3mg/kg IV over 90 min q3 weeks for a total of 4 doses. Refer to PI for recommended dose modifications.

HOW SUPPLIED: Inj: 5mg/mL [10mL, 40mL]

WARNINGS/PRECAUTIONS: Withhold scheduled dose for any moderate immune-mediated adverse reactions or for symptomatic endocrinopathy. Permanently d/c therapy for any persistent moderate adverse reactions or inability to reduce corticosteroid dose to 7.5mg prednisone or equivalent/day, failure to complete full treatment course within 16 weeks from administration of 1st dose, and severe or life-threatening adverse reactions (eg, colitis with abdominal pain, fever, ileus, peritoneal signs, increase in stool frequency [≥7 over baseline], stool incontinence, need for >24 hrs IV hydration, GI hemorrhage/perforation, AST or ALT >5X ULN, total bilirubin >3X ULN, Stevens-Johnson syndrome, rash complicated by full thickness dermal ulceration, necrotic, bullous, or hemorrhagic manifestations, Guillain-Barre syndrome, myasthenia gravis, and immune-mediated ocular disease that is unresponsive to topical immunosuppressive therapy).

ADVERSE REACTIONS: Immune-mediated reactions (enterocolitis, hepatitis, dermatitis, neuropathy, and endocrinopathy), diarrhea, colitis, pruritus, rash, fatigue.

PREGNANCY: Category C, not for use in nursing.

MECHANISM OF ACTION: IgG₁ kappa human monoclonal antibody; binds to and blocks the interaction of cytotoxic T-lymphocyte-associated antigen-4 with its ligands, CD80/CD86. Mechanism of action with melanoma is indirect; possibly through T-cell mediated anti-tumor immune responses.

PHARMACOKINETICS: Distribution: V_d=7.21L; crosses the placenta. **Elimination:** $T_{1/2}$=14.7 days.

NURSING CONSIDERATIONS

Assessment: Assess for signs and symptoms of enterocolitis, dermatitis, neuropathy, and endocrinopathy. Evaluate clinical chemistries such as LFTs and thyroid function tests at baseline.

Monitoring: Monitor for signs and symptoms of enterocolitis (diarrhea, abdominal pain, mucus or blood in stool), hepatotoxicity, dermatitis (rash, pruritus), motor or sensory neuropathy, hypophysitis, adrenal insufficiency, hyper- or hypothyroidism, and other severe immune-mediated adverse reactions. Monitor LFTs (hepatic transaminase, bilirubin levels), thyroid function tests, and clinical chemistries before each dose.

Patient Counseling: Inform of the potential risk of immune-mediated adverse reactions. Advise women that drug may cause fetal harm. Advise nursing mothers not to breastfeed while on therapy.

Administration: IV route. Refer to PI for preparation and administration instructions. **Storage:** 2-8°C (36-46°F). Do not freeze. Protect from light. Diluted Sol: Store for ≤24 hrs at 2-8°C (36-46°F) or 20-25°C (68-77°F).

ZANAFLEX   RX
tizanidine HCl (Acorda)

THERAPEUTIC CLASS: Alpha$_2$-agonist

INDICATIONS: Short-term treatment of spasticity.

DOSAGE: *Adults:* Initial: 4mg single dose q6-8h. Titrate: Increase by 2-4mg. Usual: 8mg single dose q6-8h. Max: 3 doses/24h or 36mg/day.

HOW SUPPLIED: Cap: 2mg, 4mg, 6mg; Tab: 2mg*, 4mg* *scored

CONTRAINDICATIONS: Concomitant use with fluvoxamine, ciprofloxacin or potent inhibitors of CYP1A2.

WARNINGS/PRECAUTIONS: May prolong QT interval. May cause liver damage; monitor baseline LFTs at and at 1, 3, and 6 months. Retinal degeneration and corneal opacities reported. Caution with renal impairment or elderly. May cause hypotension; caution with antihypertensives. Use with extreme caution in patients with hepatic impairment. May cause sedation and hallucinations. When discontinuing, taper dose to avoid withdrawal and rebound HTN, tachycardia, and hypertonia.

ADVERSE REACTIONS: Dry mouth, somnolence, asthenia, dizziness, UTI, urinary frequency, flu-like syndrome, rhinitis.

INTERACTIONS: See Contraindications. Potentiated depressant effect with alcohol. Potentiated by oral contraceptives; avoid concomitant use. Avoid α-adrenergic agonists. Avoid with CYP1A2 inhibitors.

PREGNANCY: Category C, caution in nursing.

MECHANISM OF ACTION: Centrally acting α$_2$-adrenergic agonist: reduces spasticity by increasing presynaptic inhibition of motor neurons.

PHARMACOKINETICS: Absorption: Complete; (Fasting) T_{max}=1 hr. (Fed) Absolute bioavailability (40%); C_{max} increased by 30%; T_{max}=1.25 hrs. **Distribution:** V_d=2.4L/kg; plasma protein binding (30%); excreted in breast milk. **Metabolism:** CYP1A2. **Elimination:** Urine (60%), feces (20%); $T_{1/2}$=2.5 hrs.

NURSING CONSIDERATIONS

Assessment: Assess for hypersensitivity, hypotension, hepatic/renal dysfunction, corneal opacities, retinal degeneration, CVD, QT prolongation, pregnancy/nursing status, and possible drug interactions. Obtain baseline LFTs.

Monitoring: Monitor for hypotension, bradycardia, lightheadedness/dizziness, syncope, hepatic impairment, sedation, hallucinosis/psychotic-like symptoms, corneal opacities, retinal degeneration, dry mouth, somnolence, asthenia, and withdrawal symptoms (eg, rebound HTN, tachycardia, hypertonia). Evaluate LFTs at 1, 3, and 6 months, BP, HR, ECG.

Patient Counseling: Counsel to take exactly as directed, not to increase dose unless directed by physician, and about possibility of orthostatic hypotension. Caution against performing hazardous tasks (eg, operating machinery/driving). To avoid withdrawal symptoms, do not suddenly d/c therapy. Avoid alcohol and CNS depressants. Advise that food changes absorption; may lead to potentiation in efficacy and adverse effects. Instruct to inform physician if taking oral contraceptives, fluvoxamine, ciprofloxacin, or if pregnant/nursing.

Administration: Oral route. **Storage:** 25°C (77°F); excursions permitted to 15-30°C (59-86°F). Dispense in tight, child-resistant container.

ZANTAC   RX
ranitidine HCl (GlaxoSmithKline)

THERAPEUTIC CLASS: H$_2$-blocker

INDICATIONS: (PO) Short-term treatment of active duodenal ulcer (DU) and benign gastric ulcer (GU). Maintenance therapy for DU and GU. Treatment of pathological hypersecretory conditions (eg, Zollinger-Ellison syndrome and systemic mastocytosis) and gastroesophageal reflux disease (GERD). Treatment and maintenance of erosive esophagitis. (Inj) Hospitalized patients with pathological hypersecretory conditions or intractable DU. Short-term alternative to oral therapy in patients who are unable to take oral medication.

DOSAGE: *Adults:* (PO) DU/GU/GERD: 150mg bid or (DU) 300mg after pm meal or qhs. Maint: 150mg qhs. Erosive Esophagitis (EE): 150mg qid. Maint: 150mg bid. Intractable DU/Hypersecretory Conditions: 150mg bid. May give ≤6g/day with severe disease. (Inj) Usual:

50mg IV/IM q6-8h or 6.25mg/hr continuous IV. IV Bolus: Inject at a rate ≤4mL/min. Intermittent Infusion: Infuse at a rate ≤5-7mL/min (15-20 min). Max: 400mg/day. Zollinger Ellison: Initial: 1mg/kg/hr. Titrate: May increase after 4 hrs by 0.5mg/kg/hr increments if >10 mEq/hr gastric output or patient becomes symptomatic. Max: 2.5mg/kg/hr and 220mg/hr infusion rate. CrCl <50mL/min: 50mg IV q18-24h or 150mg PO q24h. May increase dosing frequency to q12h if necessary. Hemodialysis: Give dose at the end of treatment.
Pediatrics: 1 month-16 yrs: (PO) DU/GU: 2-4mg/kg bid. Max: 300mg/day. Maint: 2-4mg/kg qd. Max: 150mg/day. GERD/EE: 5-10mg/kg/day given as 2 divided doses. (Inj) DU: 2-4mg/kg/day IV given q6-8h. Max: 50mg q6-8h. CrCl <50mL/min: 50mg IV q18-24h or 150mg PO q24h. May increase dosing frequency to q12h if necessary. <1 month: Patients on Extracorporeal Membrane Oxygenation (ECMO): 2mg/kg IV q12-24h or as continuous infusion.

HOW SUPPLIED: Inj: 25mg/mL, 50mg/50mL; Syrup: 15mg/mL; Tab: 150mg, 300mg; Tab, Effervescent: 25mg. Also available as a Pharmacy Bulk Package. Refer to individual package insert for more information

WARNINGS/PRECAUTIONS: Symptomatic response does not preclude the presence of gastric malignancy. Caution with hepatic/renal dysfunction. Avoid with history of acute porphyria. Caution in elderly. (IV) Do not exceed recommended infusion rates; bradycardia reported with rapid infusion. SGPT elevations reported; monitor SGPT if on IV therapy for ≥5 days at dose >100mg qid.

ADVERSE REACTIONS: Headache, constipation, diarrhea, N/V, abdominal discomfort, hepatitis, blood dyscrasias, rash, injection-site reactions (IV/IM).

INTERACTIONS: Increased absorption of triazolam, midazolam, and glipizide. Decreased absorption of ketoconazole, atazanavir, delaviridine, and gefitinib. Procainamide plasma levels increased with high doses. Altered anticoagulant effects with warfarin; monitor PT closely. Avoid chronic use with delavirdine. Monitor for prolonged sedation with midazolam and triazolam. Caution with gefitinib and atazanavir. (PO) Delayed and increased peak blood levels with propantheline. Decreased absorption in fasting subjects with high potency antacids.

PREGNANCY: Category B, caution with nursing.

MECHANISM OF ACTION: H_2-blocker; competitive, reversible inhibitor of histamine at histamine H_2-receptors, including those found on gastric cells.

PHARMACOKINETICS: Absorption: (PO, 150mg) C_{max}=440-545ng/mL, T_{max}=2-3 hrs; bioavailability (50%). (IM) Rapid; C_{max}=576ng/mL, T_{max}=15 min; bioavailability (90-100%). **Distribution:** V_d=1.4L/kg; plasma protein binding (15%); found in breast milk. **Metabolism:** Liver, N-oxide (principal metabolite). **Elimination:** Feces, Urine: (PO) (30% unchanged), (IV) (70% unchanged); (PO) $T_{1/2}$=2.5-3 hrs, (IV) $T_{1/2}$=2-2.5 hrs. Refer to PI for pediatric parameters.

NURSING CONSIDERATIONS

Assessment: Assess for hypersensitivity to drug, renal/hepatic function, gastric malignancy, history of acute porphyria, pregnancy/nursing status, and possible drug interactions.

Monitoring: Monitor for signs/symptoms of hepatic effects (eg, elevations in SGPT values), cardiovascular (CV) effects, headache, GI effects (eg, constipation, diarrhea), hypersensitivity reactions, and other adverse reactions. In patients receiving IV formulation at dosages ≥100mg qid for ≥5 days, monitor SGPT daily from Day 5 to the conclusion of IV therapy.

Patient Counseling: Inform that antacids can be given as pain relief for GI symptoms. Inform that efferdose tab contains phenylalanine. If taking efferdose tab formulation, instruct not to chew tab, swallow whole, or dissolve on tongue; should be completely dissolved in ≥5mL of water before administration; may be given by medicine dropper or oral syringe. Notify physician if any adverse events develop.

Administration: Oral/IM/IV routes. Do not chew, swallow whole, or dissolve efferdose tab in tongue. Dissolve 1 tablet in ≥5mL of water in an appropriate measuring cup. Wait until the tablet is completely dissolved before administering the solution to the infant/child. (IV) Inspect visually for particulate matter and discoloration prior to administration. Refer to PI for stability instructions and premixed inj preparation. **Storage:** Tab: 15-30°C (59-86°F). Efferdose Tab: 2-30°C (36-86°F). Syrup: 4-25°C (39-77°F). Inj: 4-25°C (39-77°F); excursions permitted to 30°C (86°F). Protect from light. Premixed Inj: 2-25°C (36-77°F). Protect from light. Protect from freezing.

ZARAH   RX
drospirenone - ethinyl estradiol (Watson)

THERAPEUTIC CLASS: Estrogen/progestogen combination
INDICATIONS: Prevention of pregnancy.

DOSAGE: *Adults:* 1 blue tab (active) qd for 21 consecutive days, followed by 1 peach tab (inert) on Days 22-28. Start 1st Sunday after menses begins or 1st day of menses. Should be taken at the same time each day, preferably pm, pc, or qhs. Begin next and all subsequent regimens on the same day of the week on which the first regimen began.

Pediatrics: Postpubertal: 1 blue tab (active) qd for 21 consecutive days, followed by 1 peach tab (inert) on Days 22-28. Start 1st Sunday after menses begins or 1st day of menses. Should be taken at the same time each day, preferably pm, pc, or qhs. Begin next and all subsequent regimens on the same day of the week on which first regimen began.

HOW SUPPLIED: Tab: (Ethinyl Estradiol-Drospirenone) 0.03mg-3mg

CONTRAINDICATIONS: Renal or adrenal insufficiency, hepatic dysfunction, thrombophlebitis, thromboembolic disorders, history of deep vein thrombophlebitis or thromboembolic disorders, cerebral-vascular or coronary artery disease (CAD), valvular heart disease with thrombogenic complications, severe HTN, diabetes with vascular involvement, headaches with focal neurological symptoms, known or suspected breast carcinoma, endometrial carcinoma or other known or suspected estrogen-dependent neoplasia, undiagnosed abnormal genital bleeding, cholestatic jaundice of pregnancy or jaundice with prior pill use, liver tumor (benign or malignant) or active liver disease, pregnancy, heavy smoking (>15 cigarettes daily) and >35 yrs.

WARNINGS/PRECAUTIONS: May cause hyperkalemia in high-risk patients; avoid use in patients predisposed to hyperkalemia (eg, renal insufficiency, hepatic dysfunction, adrenal insufficiency). Monitor K^+ levels during first treatment cycle with conditions predisposed to hyperkalemia. Increased risk of myocardial infarction (MI), thromboembolism, stroke, gallbladder disease, vascular disease, and hepatic neoplasia. Increased risk of morbidity and mortality in patients with HTN, hyperlipidemia, obesity, and diabetes mellitus (DM). May increase risk of breast cancer and cervical intraepithelial neoplasia. Retinal thrombosis reported; d/c use if unexplained partial or complete loss of vision, onset of proptosis or diplopia, papilledema, or retinal vascular lesions develop. May cause glucose intolerance; monitor prediabetic and diabetic patients. May cause fluid retention. May increase BP; monitor closely with HTN and d/c if significant elevation of BP occurs. D/C with onset or exacerbation of migraine or development of headache with new pattern which is persistent, recurrent and severe. Breakthrough bleeding and spotting reported; rule out malignancy or pregnancy. Monitor closely with hyperlipidemias. D/C if jaundice develops. Monitor closely with depression and d/c if depression recurs to serious degree. Contact lens wearers may develop visual changes. Perform annual physical exam. Should not be used to induce withdrawal bleeding as a test for pregnancy or to treat threatened or habitual abortion during pregnancy. Not indicated for use before menarche. May affect certain endocrine, LFTs, and blood components in laboratory tests. Does not protect against HIV infection (AIDS) and other STDs.

ADVERSE REACTIONS: N/V, breakthrough bleeding, spotting, amenorrhea, migraine, depression, vaginal candidiasis, edema, weight changes, breast changes, GI symptoms (abdominal cramps and bloating), menstrual flow changes.

INTERACTIONS: Concomitant use with rifampin, anticonvulsants (eg, phenobarbital, phenytoin, carbamazepine), or phenylbutazone may reduce contraceptive effectiveness and increase menstrual irregularities. Pregnancy reported with antimicrobials (eg, ampicillin, tetracycline, griseofulvin). St. John's wort may reduce contraceptive effectiveness and cause breakthrough bleeding. Increased levels with atorvastatin, ascorbic acid and acetaminophen (APAP). Risk of hyperkalemia with ACE inhibitors, angiotensin-II receptor antagonists, K^+-sparing diuretics, heparin, aldosterone antagonists, and NSAIDs; monitor K^+ levels during 1st cycle. May increase levels of cyclosporine, prednisolone, and theophylline. May decrease APAP levels and increase clearance of temazepam, salicylic acid, morphine, and clofibric acid.

PREGNANCY: Category X, not for use in nursing.

MECHANISM OF ACTION: Estrogen/progestogen oral contraceptive; suppresses gonadotropins. Inhibits ovulation and produces changes in cervical mucus (increasing difficulty of sperm entry into uterus) and endometrium (reducing likelihood of implantation).

PHARMACOKINETICS: Absorption: Drospirenone (DRSP): Absolute bioavailability (76%); (Cycle 13/Day 21) C_{max}=78.7ng/mL; T_{max}=1.6 hrs; AUC=968ng•h/mL. Ethinyl estradiol (EE): Absolute bioavailability (40%); (Cycle 13/Day 21) C_{max}=90.5pg/mL; T_{max}=1.6 hrs; AUC=469.5pg•h/mL. **Distribution:** Found in breast milk; DRSP: V_d=4L/kg; serum protein binding (97%). EE: V_d=4-5L/kg; serum albumin binding (98.5%). **Metabolism:** DRSP: Liver, via CYP3A4 (minor). EE: Hydroxylation (via CYP3A4), conjugation (glucuronidation and sulfation). **Elimination:** DRSP: Urine, feces; $T_{1/2}$=30 hrs. EE: Urine, feces; $T_{1/2}$=24 hrs.

NURSING CONSIDERATIONS

Assessment: Assess for current or history of thrombophlebitis or thromboembolic disorders, cerebrovascular disorders, or any other conditions where treatment is contraindicated or cautioned. Assess for pregnancy/nursing status and for possible drug interactions. Assess use in patients with contact lenses, HTN, DM, hyperlipidemia, and obesity.

Z

Monitoring: Monitor for signs/symptoms of MI, thromboembolism, cerebrovascular disease, carcinoma of the breast, cervical intraepithelial neoplasia, hepatic neoplasia, onset or exacerbation of a migraine headache, gallbladder disease, ocular lesions, hypertriglyceridemia, HTN, bleeding irregularities, jaundice, and for fluid retention. Monitor for signs of worsening depression in patients with a history of depression. Monitor lipid levels in patients with a history of hyperlipidemia. Monitor blood glucose levels in patients with DM. Monitor BP in patients with HTN. Perform annual history and physical exam. Monitor K+ levels in patients at risk for hyperkalemia. Refer patients with contact lenses to an ophthalmologist if visual changes or changes in contact lens tolerance occur.

Patient Counseling: Inform that drug does not protect against HIV infection (AIDS) and other STDs. Inform of potential risks/benefits of oral contraceptives. Counsel not to smoke while on treatment. Instruct to take medication at the same time daily. Inform that there may be spotting, light bleeding, or nausea during first 1-3 packs; advise not to d/c medication and if symptoms persist, notify physician. If started later than the first day of the menstrual cycle, it should not be considered effective as a contraceptive until after first 7 consecutive days of administration. Instruct what to do in the event pills are missed.

Administration: Oral route. **Storage:** 20-25°C (68-77°F).

ZARONTIN
ethosuximide (Parke-Davis)

RX

OTHER BRAND NAMES: Zarontin Oral Solution (Parke-Davis)

THERAPEUTIC CLASS: Succinimide

INDICATIONS: Control of absence (petit mal) epilepsy.

DOSAGE: *Adults:* Initial: 500mg qd. Titrate: Individualize dose according to response. May increase daily dose by 250mg q4-7 days until control is achieved with minimal side effects. Caution with doses >1.5g/day, in divided doses.
Pediatrics: Initial: ≥6 yrs: 500mg qd. 3-6 yrs: 250mg qd. Titrate: Individualize dose according to response. May increase daily dose by 250mg q4-7 days until control is achieved with minimal side effects. Optimal Dose: 20mg/kg/day. Caution with doses >1.5g/day, in divided doses.

HOW SUPPLIED: Cap: 250mg; Syrup: 250mg/5mL

WARNINGS/PRECAUTIONS: Blood dyscrasias and abnormal renal and liver function studies reported; extreme caution with known liver or renal disease. Perform periodic blood counts, urinalysis, and LFTs. Systemic lupus erythematosus (SLE) reported. May increase risk of suicidal thoughts or behavior; monitor for emergence or worsening of depression and any unusual changes in mood or behavior. Cases of birth defects reported. May increase frequency of grand mal seizures when used alone in mixed types of epilepsy. May precipitate absence (petit mal) status with abrupt withdrawal; adjust dose slowly.

ADVERSE REACTIONS: Anorexia, N/V, abdominal pain, leukopenia, drowsiness, headache, urticaria, SLE, myopia, vaginal bleeding, diarrhea, euphoria, hirsutism, microscopic hematuria.

INTERACTIONS: May interact with other antiepileptic drugs (eg, may increase levels of phenytoin; increased or decreased levels reported with valproic acid); periodically determine serum level of these drugs.

PREGNANCY: Safety not known in pregnancy, caution in nursing.

MECHANISM OF ACTION: Succinimide; suppresses paroxysmal 3 cycle/sec spike and wave activity associated with lapses of consciousness which is common in absence (petit mal) seizures. Frequency of attacks is reduced by depression of motor cortex and elevation of the CNS threshold to convulsive stimuli.

PHARMACOKINETICS: Distribution: Crosses placenta, found in breast milk.

NURSING CONSIDERATIONS

Assessment: Assess for history of hypersensitivity to succinimides, depression, renal/hepatic impairment, pregnancy/nursing status, and possible drug interactions. Obtain baseline CBC, urinalysis, renal/hepatic function prior to therapy.

Monitoring: Monitor for blood dyscrasias, signs/symptoms of SLE, and infection (eg, sore throat, fever). Monitor for occurrence of grand mal seizures in patients with mixed types of epilepsy who are on monotherapy. Monitor CBC, urinalysis, renal/hepatic function. Monitor for worsening of depression, suicidal thoughts or behavior and/or any unusual changes in mood or behavior.

Patient Counseling: Inform of the importance of strictly adhering to prescribed dosage regimen. Inform that the therapy may impair mental/physical abilities. Instruct to contact physician if any signs/symptoms of infection (eg, sore throat, fever) develop. Advise to be alert for the emergence or worsening of depression, any unusual changes in mood or behavior, suicidal thoughts/

behavior, and to report to physician any behaviors of concern. If pregnant, encourage to enroll in North American Antiepileptic Drug (NAAED) Pregnancy Registry.

Administration: Oral route. **Storage:** (Cap) 25°C (77°F); excursions permitted to 15-30°C (59-86°F). (Oral Sol) 20-25°C (68-77°F). Preserve in tight containers. Protect from freezing and light.

ZAROXOLYN
metolazone (CellTech)

RX

> Do not interchange rapid and complete bioavailability metolazone formulations for other slow and incomplete bioavailability metolazone formulations; they are not therapeutically equivalent.

THERAPEUTIC CLASS: Quinazoline diuretic

INDICATIONS: Treatment of HTN and of salt and water retention in edema accompanying CHF or renal disease.

DOSAGE: *Adults:* Edema: 5-20mg qd. HTN: 2.5-5mg qd. Elderly: Start at low end of dosing range.

HOW SUPPLIED: Tab: 2.5mg, 5mg, 10mg

CONTRAINDICATIONS: Anuria, hepatic coma or precoma.

WARNINGS/PRECAUTIONS: Risk of hypokalemia, orthostatic hypotension, hypercalcemia, hyperuricemia, azotemia, and rapid-onset hyponatremia. Cross-allergy with sulfonamide-derived drugs, thiazides, or quinethazone. Sensitivity reactions may occur with 1st dose. Monitor electrolytes. May cause hyperglycemia and glycosuria in diabetics. Caution in elderly or severe renal impairment. May exacerbate or activate SLE.

ADVERSE REACTIONS: Chest pain/discomfort, orthostatic hypotension, syncope, neuropathy, necrotizing angiitis, hepatitis, jaundice, pancreatitis, blood dyscrasias, joint pain.

INTERACTIONS: Furosemide and other loop diuretics prolong fluid and electrolyte loss. Adjust dose of other antihypertensives. Potentiates hypotensive effects of alcohol, barbiturates, and narcotics. Lithium, digitalis toxicity. Corticosteroids and adrenocorticotropic hormone increase hypokalemia and salt and water retention. Enhanced neuromuscular blocking effects of curariform drugs. Salicylates and NSAIDs decrease effects. Decreased arterial response to norepinephrine. Decrease in methenamine efficacy. Adjust anticoagulants, antidiabetics.

PREGNANCY: Category B, not for use in nursing.

MECHANISM OF ACTION: Quinazoline diuretic; acts primarily to inhibit Na^+ reabsorption at cortical diluting site, and to a lesser extent, in proximal convoluted tubule.

PHARMACOKINETICS: Absorption: T_{max}=8 hrs. **Elimination:** Urine (unchanged).

NURSING CONSIDERATIONS

Assessment: Assess for anuria, SLE, DM, sulfonamide hypersensitivity, history of allergy or bronchial asthma, hepatic/renal impairment, possible drug interactions.

Monitoring: Monitor serum electrolytes periodically. Monitor for signs/symptoms of electrolyte imbalance, exacerbation or activation of SLE, hyperglycemia, hyperuricemia or precipitation of gout, hypersensitivity reactions (eg, angioedema, bronchospasm, toxic epidermal necrolysis, Stevens-Johnson syndrome), orthostatic hypotension, renal/hepatic dysfunction.

Patient Counseling: Counsel to take medication as directed and promptly report adverse reactions. Advise not to interchange formulations. Instruct to seek medical attention if symptoms of electrolyte imbalance (eg, dry mouth, thirst, weakness) or hypersensitivity reactions occur.

Administration: Oral route. **Storage:** 25°C (77°F); excursions permitted to 15-30°C (59-86°F). Protect from light.

ZEBETA
bisoprolol fumarate (Duramed)

RX

THERAPEUTIC CLASS: Selective beta$_1$-blocker

INDICATIONS: Management of HTN alone or in combination with other antihypertensive agents.

DOSAGE: *Adults:* Individualize dose. Initial: 5mg qd. Titrate: May increase to 10mg and then, if necessary, to 20mg qd. Bronchospastic Disease: Initial: 2.5mg qd. Hepatic/Renal Dysfunction (CrCl <40mL/min): Initial: 2.5mg qd; caution with dose titration.

HOW SUPPLIED: Tab: 5mg*, 10mg *scored

CONTRAINDICATIONS: Cardiogenic shock, overt cardiac failure, 2nd- or 3rd-degree atrioventricular (AV) block, marked sinus bradycardia.

WARNINGS/PRECAUTIONS: Avoid abrupt withdrawal; exacerbation of angina pectoris, myocardial infarction (MI) and ventricular arrhythmia in patients with coronary artery disease (CAD), and exacerbation of symptoms of hyperthyroidism or precipitation of thyroid storm reported. Reinstitute temporary therapy if withdrawal symptoms occur. May mask manifestations of hypoglycemia or clinical signs of hyperthyroidism (eg, tachycardia). Caution with compensated cardiac failure, diabetes mellitus (DM), bronchospastic disease, and hepatic/renal impairment. May precipitate cardiac failure; d/c at the 1st signs/symptoms of heart failure (HF) or continue therapy while HF is treated with other drugs. Caution with peripheral vascular disease (PVD); may precipitate or aggravate symptoms of arterial insufficiency. Caution with history of severe anaphylactic reaction to a variety of allergens; reactivity may increase with repeated challenge.

ADVERSE REACTIONS: Headache, upper respiratory infection (URI), peripheral edema, fatigue, ALT/AST elevation.

INTERACTIONS: Patients with a history of severe anaphylactic reaction to a variety of allergens taking β-blockers may be unresponsive to usual doses of epinephrine. D/C several days before withdrawal of clonidine. Excessive reduction of sympathetic activity with catecholamine-depleting drugs (eg, reserpine, guanethidine); monitor closely. Avoid with other β-blockers. Caution with myocardial depressants or inhibitors of AV conduction such as calcium antagonists (eg, verapamil, diltiazem) or antiarrhythmics (eg, disopyramide). Increased risk of bradycardia with digitalis glycosides. Increased clearance with rifampin. Caution with insulin or oral hypoglycemic agents. Reversed effects with bronchodilator therapy. Additive BP lowering effects in mild to moderate HTN with HCTZ.

PREGNANCY: Category C, caution in nursing.

MECHANISM OF ACTION: β_1-selective adrenoreceptor blocking agent; not established. May decrease cardiac output, inhibit renin release by the kidneys, and diminution of tonic sympathetic outflow from the vasomotor centers in the brain.

PHARMACOKINETICS: Absorption: (10mg) Absolute bioavailability (80%); C_{max}= (5mg) 16ng/mL, (20mg) 70ng/mL; (5-20mg) T_{max}=2-4 hrs. **Distribution:** Plasma protein binding (30%). **Elimination:** Urine (50%, unchanged), feces (<2%); $T_{1/2}$=9-12 hrs.

NURSING CONSIDERATIONS

Assessment: Assess for conditions where treatment is contraindicated or cautioned, pregnancy/nursing status, and possible drug interactions.

Monitoring: Monitor for hypoglycemia, hyperthyroidism, hepatic/renal function, signs/symptoms of HF, withdrawal and arterial insufficiency. Monitor HR, ECG, CBC with platelet and differential count.

Patient Counseling: Instruct not to interrupt or d/c therapy without consulting physician. Notify physician if difficulty in breathing, signs/symptoms of CHF or excessive bradycardia develop. Educate about signs/symptoms of drug's potential adverse effects. Advise to exercise caution while driving, operating machinery or other tasks requiring alertness.

Administration: Oral route. **Storage**: 20-25°C (68-77°F). Protect from moisture. Dispense in tight container.

ZEGERID   RX
sodium bicarbonate - omeprazole (Santarus)

THERAPEUTIC CLASS: Proton pump inhibitor/Antacid

INDICATIONS: Short-term treatment of erosive esophagitis (EE) diagnosed by endoscopy, active duodenal ulcer, and active benign gastric ulcer. Treatment of heartburn and other symptoms associated with gastroesophageal reflux disease (GERD). Maintain healing of EE. (Sus 40mg-1680mg) Reduction of risk of upper GI bleeding in critically ill patients.

DOSAGE: *Adults:* ≥18 yrs: Duodenal Ulcer: 20mg qd for 4-8 weeks. Gastric Ulcer: 40mg qd for 4-8 weeks. GERD with No Esophageal Erosions: 20mg qd for ≤4 weeks. GERD with EE: 20mg qd for 4-8 weeks. May give up to an additional 4 weeks if no response to 8 weeks of therapy or may consider additional 4-8 week courses if there is recurrence of EE or GERD symptoms. Maint of Healing EE: 20mg qd. Hepatic Insufficiency/Asian Population: Consider dose reduction. (Sus 40mg-1680mg): Risk Reduction of Upper GI Bleeding in Critically III Patients: Initial: 40mg, followed by 40mg after 6-8 hrs. Maint: 40mg qd for 14 days.

HOW SUPPLIED: (Omeprazole-Sodium Bicarbonate) Cap: 20mg-1100mg, 40mg-1100mg; Sus: (powder) 20mg-1680mg/pkt, 40mg-1680mg/pkt

WARNINGS/PRECAUTIONS: (Omeprazole) Symptomatic response does not preclude the presence of gastric malignancy. Atrophic gastritis reported with long-term use. May increase risk of osteoporosis-related fractures of the hip, wrist, or spine with high doses and long-term proton pump inhibitor (PPI) therapy; use lowest dose and shortest duration of PPI therapy. Hypomagnesemia reported; may require d/c of therapy and magnesium replacement. Consider monitoring magnesium levels prior to and periodically during therapy for patients expected to be on prolonged treatment. (Sodium Bicarbonate) Consider sodium content when administering to

Z

patients on a sodium-restricted diet. Caution with Bartter's syndrome, hypokalemia, hypocalce-mia, and acid-base balance problems. Chronic use may lead to systemic alkalosis, and increased sodium intake may produce edema and weight increase.

ADVERSE REACTIONS: Agitation, anemia, bradycardia, constipation, rash, tachycardia, diarrhea, fever, thrombocytopenia, hypokalemia, hypomagnesemia, hyperglycemia, nosocomial pneumo-nia, HTN, hypotension.

INTERACTIONS: Monitor with drugs metabolized by CYP450 (eg, cyclosporine, disulfiram, benzodiazepines). Long-term use of bicarbonate with calcium or milk can cause milk-alkali syndrome. May increase saquinavir levels; consider dose reduction of saquinavir. (Omeprazole) Avoid with clopidogrel, atazanivir, and nelfinavir. Caution with digoxin or other drugs that may cause hypomagnesemia (eg, diuretics). May interfere with the absorption of drugs where gastric pH is an important determinant of bioavailability (eg, ketoconazole, ampicillin esters, iron salts, digoxin). May prolong elimination of diazepam, warfarin, phenytoin, and drugs metabolized by hepatic oxidation. May increase PT and INR with warfarin. Concomitant administration with voriconazole resulted in more than doubling of the omeprazole exposure. May increase levels of clarithromycin, 14-hydroxyclarithromycin, and tacrolimus. Reported interaction with some antiretroviral drugs.

PREGNANCY: Category C, not for use in nursing.

MECHANISM OF ACTION: Omeprazole: PPI; suppresses gastric acid secretion by specific inhibition of the (H^+/K^+)-ATPase enzyme system at secretory surface of the gastric parietal cell. Sodium Bicarbonate: Antacid; raises gastric pH and thus protects omeprazole from acid degradation.

PHARMACOKINETICS: Absorption: Omeprazole: Rapid; T_{max}=30 min; (Sus) Absolute bioavail-ability (30-40%), C_{max}=1,954ng/mL, $AUC_{(0-inf)}$=1,665ng•hr/mL (after dose 1), 3,356ng•hr/mL (after dose 2). (Cap) C_{max}=1,526ng/mL. **Distribution:** Omeprazole: Plasma protein binding (95%); found in breast milk. **Metabolism:** Omeprazole: Hydroxyomeprazole and corresponding carboxylic acid (metabolites). **Elimination:** Omeprazole: Urine (77% as metabolites), feces; $T_{1/2}$=1 hr (healthy).

NURSING CONSIDERATIONS

Assessment: Assess for gastric malignancy, sodium-restricted diet, acid-base balance problems, hypocalcemia, Bartter's syndrome, hypokalemia, risk for osteoporosis-related fractures of the hip, wrist, and spine, hypersensitivity to the drug or its components, pregnancy/nursing status, and possible drug interactions. Assess dosing in Asian/hepatic-insufficient patients, particularly in maintenance of healing of erosive esophagitis. Assess magnesium levels in patients expected to be on prolonged treatment.

Monitoring: Monitor for hypersensitivity reactions, signs/symptoms of atrophic gastritis, osteo-porosis-related fractures of the hip, wrist, and spine. Monitor for milk-alkali syndrome with long-term use of bicarbonate with calcium or milk. Monitor for systemic alkalosis, edema, or weight increase due to increased sodium intake with chronic use. Monitor magnesium levels periodically in patients expected to be on prolonged therapy.

Patient Counseling: Instruct to take on empty stomach at least 1 hr before meals. Instruct about proper dosing and directions for use. Inform that different formulations are not bioequivalent and should not be used as substitute of one for the other. Advise patients on a sodium-restricted diet or patients at risk of developing congestive heart failure that drug contains sodium. Inform that chronic use may increase sodium intake, causing swelling and weight gain. Counsel pregnant women of the harmful effects of therapy on the fetus. Advise to use with caution if regularly tak-ing calcium supplements. Counsel about the most frequent adverse events. Advise to immediate-ly report and seek care for any cardiovascular/neurological symptoms (eg, palpitation, dizziness, tetany) experienced.

Administration: Oral route. Take on an empty stomach ≥1 hr before a meal. (Caps) Swallow intact with water; do not open caps and sprinkle contents into food; do not use other liquids. (Powder) Empty pkt contents to 1-2 tbsp of water, stir well, and drink immediately; refill cup with water and drink; do not use other liquids or foods. Refer to PI for administration in patients receiving continuous nasogastric/orogastric tube feeding. **Storage:** 25°C (77°F); excursions permitted to 15-30°C (59-86°F). Protect from light and moisture.

ZEGERID OTC

OTC

sodium bicarbonate - omeprazole (Schering-Plough)

THERAPEUTIC CLASS: Proton pump inhibitor/Antacid

INDICATIONS: Treatment of frequent heartburn (≥2 days per week).

DOSAGE: *Adults:* ≥18 yrs: 1 cap qd (q24h) for 14 days. Take with glass of water in am 1 hr before food. May repeat every 4 months. Do not crush, chew, open cap and sprinkle on food. Do not take >1 cap a day.

HOW SUPPLIED: Cap: (Omeprazole-Sodium Bicarbonate) 20mg-1100mg

WARNINGS/PRECAUTIONS: Each capsule contains sodium 303mg. Do not use if patient has hypersensitivity to omeprazole. Not for immediate relief of heartburn. D/C if heartburn continues or worsens, if need to take for >14 days or if need to take >1 course of treatment every 4 months. Avoid use if having trouble/pain in swallowing food, vomiting with blood or have bloody/black stools; these may be signs of a serious condition.

INTERACTIONS: Caution with warfarin, diazepam, digoxin, antifungals/anti-yeast, tacrolimus and antiretroviral agents. Sodium bicarbonate may interact with certain prescription drugs.

PREGNANCY: Safety in pregnancy and nursing not known.

MECHANISM OF ACTION: Omeprazole: Proton pump inhibitor; stops stomach acid production at the acid pump. Sodium Bicarbonate: Antacid; allows absorption of omeprazole.

NURSING CONSIDERATIONS

Assessment: Assess for proper diagnosis, hypersensitivity to omeprazole, difficulty/pain in swallowing, vomiting with blood, bloody/black stools, pregnancy/nursing status and possible drug interactions. Assess for heartburn that lasts >3 months, lightheadedness, sweating, dizziness, chest/shoulder pain with SOB, pain radiating to the arms, neck or shoulders, frequent chest pain/wheezing, unexplained weight loss, N/V, stomach pain and if on sodium-restricted diet.

Monitoring: Monitor for continuing/worsening of heartburn, treatment that lasts >14 days, >1 treatment course every 4 months, allergic/hypersensitivity reactions and relief of symptoms.

Patient Counseling: Instruct to take 1 hr before breakfast; do not chew, crush, or open and sprinkle on food. Notify that drug may take 1 to 4 days for full effect. Advise not to take >14 days or more often than every 4 months unless directed by a doctor. Consult a physician if heartburn continues/worsens. Inform of any other medications being taken. Seek medical help or contact a poison control center if overdosage occurs. Notify physician if pregnant/breastfeeding. Keep out of reach of children.

Administration: Oral route. Swallow cap with a glass of water in am 1 hr before food. Do not chew, crush or open cap and sprinkle on food. Do not use if blue band around cap is missing/broken or if foil inner seal is missing/open/broken. **Storage:** 20-25°C (68-77°F). Keep out of high heat and humidity. Protect from moisture.

ZELAPAR   RX
selegiline HCl (Valeant)

THERAPEUTIC CLASS: Monoamine oxidase inhibitor (Type B)

INDICATIONS: Adjunct in the management of Parkinson's disease in patients exhibiting a deteriorated response to levodopa/carbidopa therapy.

DOSAGE: *Adults:* 1.25mg qd for 6 weeks. Titrate: After 6 weeks, may increase to 2.5mg if desired benefit not achieved. Max: 2.5mg/day.

HOW SUPPLIED: Tab, Orally Disintegrating: 1.25mg

CONTRAINDICATIONS: Concomitant meperidine, tramadol, methadone, propoxyphene, dextromethorphan, and other MAOIs.

WARNINGS/PRECAUTIONS: Do not exceed 2.5mg/day; risk of non-selective MAO inhibition. Greater risk of orthostatic hypotension and dizziness in geriatric patients. Decrease levodopa/carbidopa to prevent exacerbation of levodopa side effects (eg, preexisting dyskinesias). Melanoma reported; perform periodic dermatologic screening. May increase frequency of mild oropharyngeal abnormality. Caution with renal or hepatic impairment. Neuroleptic malignant syndrome reported in association with rapid dose reduction, withdrawal of, or changes in antiparkinsonian therapy. Compulsive behaviors (eg, intense urges to gamble, increased sexual urges) reported.

ADVERSE REACTIONS: Nausea, dizziness, pain, headache, insomnia, rhinitis, skin disorders, dyskinesia, backache, dyspepsia, stomatitis, constipation, hallucinations, pharyngitis, rash.

INTERACTIONS: See Contraindications. Serious, sometimes fatal, reactions have been precipitated with meperidine, tramadol, methadone, and propoxyphene; avoid concomitant use. Episodes of psychosis or bizarre behavior reported with dextromethorphan; avoid concomitant use. Severe toxicity reported with SSRIs or TCAs; avoid concurrent use and allow 2 weeks between d/c of selegiline and initiation of TCAs or SSRIs. Allow 5 weeks for fluoxetine due to a longer half-life. Caution with sympathomimetics and CYP3A4 inducers (eg, phenytoin, carbamazepine, nafcillin, phenobarbital, and rifampin).

PREGNANCY: Category C, not for use in nursing.

MECHANISM OF ACTION: Irreversible MAO inhibitor; blocks catabolism of dopamine and increases net amount of dopamine available.

Z

PHARMACOKINETICS: Absorption: C_{max}(1.25mg, 2.5mg, 5mg)=3.34, 4.47, 1.12ng/mL. T_{max}(1.25mg, 2.5mg, 5mg)=10-15 min, 10-15 min, 40-90 min. **Distribution:** Plasma protein binding (85%). **Metabolism:** Liver (1st-pass metabolism). **Elimination:** Urine; $T_{1/2}$=10 hrs (steady state).

NURSING CONSIDERATIONS

Assessment: Assess renal function, LFTs, dyskinesia, phenylalanine levels, BP, melanomas, pregnancy/nursing status, and possible drug interactions.

Monitoring: Monitor LFTs, renal function, BP, exacerbation of pre-existing dyskinesia, melanomas, hyperpyrexia, hallucinations, compulsive behaviors (eg, pathological gambling, hypersexuality).

Patient Counseling: Should be taken every morning before breakfast without liquid. Do not remove blister from outer pouch until just prior to dosing. Report any side effects. Notify physician if new or increased gambling urges, sexual urges, or other urges occur.

Administration: Oral route; dissolve on tongue. **Storage:** 25°C (77°F); excursions permitted to 15-30°C (59-86°F). Use within 3 months after opening.

ZELBORAF RX
vemurafenib (Genentech)

THERAPEUTIC CLASS: Kinase inhibitor

INDICATIONS: Treatment of unresectable or metastatic melanoma with BRAF^{V600E} mutation as detected by an FDA approved test.

DOSAGE: *Adults:* Usual: 960mg (four 240mg tabs) bid; 1st dose should be taken in am and 2nd dose 12 hrs later. Treat until disease progression or unacceptable toxicity occurs. Refer to PI for dose modifications.

HOW SUPPLIED: Tab: 240mg

WARNINGS/PRECAUTIONS: Beneficial only for BRAF^{V600E} mutation positive melanoma; confirmation prior to treatment required. Not recommended for wild-type BRAF melanoma. Cutaneous squamous cell carcinoma (cuSCC), keratoacanthoma, and new primary malignant melanoma reported; perform dermatologic evaluation prior to, every 2 months during, and for 6 months after d/c of treatment. Increased risk of cuSCC in patients ≥65 yrs, with prior skin cancer, and chronic sun exposure. D/C permanently if serious dermatologic and hypersensitivity reactions occur. QT prolongation leading to an increased risk of ventricular arrhythmias, including torsade de pointes may occur; monitor ECG and electrolytes before treatment and after dose modification. Avoid in patients with uncorrectable electrolyte abnormalities or long QT syndrome. Initiation of treatment not recommended with QTc >500 msec. Interrupt temporarily if QTc >500 msec while on therapy. Give at a lower dose once QT decreases <500 msec or d/c permanently if after correction of risk factors, the QTc increase meets values of both >500 msec and >60 msec change from pretreatment values. Liver laboratory abnormalities may occur; monitor liver enzymes and bilirubin prior to and monthly during treatment or as clinically indicated. Photosensitivity reported; avoid exposure to sunlight and modify dose for ≥Grade 2 photosensitivity. Uveitis, blurred vision, iritis, retinal vein occlusion, and photophobia reported; monitor routinely for uveitis.

ADVERSE REACTIONS: Photosensitivity reaction, alopecia, rash, pruritus, arthralgia, fatigue, peripheral edema, nausea, diarrhea, headache, skin papilloma.

INTERACTIONS: Increased area under the curve (AUC) of caffeine and dextromethorphan. Decreased AUC of midazolam. Not recommended with CYP1A2, 2D6, and 3A4 substrates with narrow therapeutic index due to alteration in concentrations; if coadministration cannot be avoided, exercise caution and consider dose reduction of CYP1A2 or 2D6 substrate. S-warfarin AUC increased; use caution and consider INR monitoring. Caution with strong CYP3A4 inhibitors and inducers. Not recommended with drugs that prolong QT interval.

PREGNANCY: Category D, not for use in nursing.

MECHANISM OF ACTION: Kinase inhibitor; inhibition of some mutated forms of BRAF serine threonine kinase including BRAF^{V600E}, resulting in prevention of cell proliferation in the absence of growth factors that would normally be required for proliferation.

PHARMACOKINETICS: Absorption: T_{max}=3 hrs; C_{max}=62mcg/mL; AUC=601mcg•h/mL. **Distribution:** Plasma protein binding (>99%); V_d=106L. **Elimination:** Feces (94%), urine (1%); $T_{1/2}$=57 hrs.

NURSING CONSIDERATIONS

Assessment: Assess for BRAF^{V600E} mutation, prior skin cancer, chronic sun exposure, uncorrectable electrolyte abnormality, long QT syndrome, pregnancy/nursing status, and possible drug interactions. Perform dermatologic evaluation and obtain baseline ECG, electrolyte levels, and LFTs.

Monitoring: Monitor for development of new skin lesions, severe dermatologic and hypersensitivity reactions, photosensitivity, uveitis, and other adverse reactions. Perform dermatologic evaluation every 2 months during, and for 6 months after d/c of treatment. Monitor ECG and electrolytes after dose modifications and ECGs 15 days after initiation, monthly for the 1st 3 months, then every 3 months thereafter, or as clinically indicated. Monitor LFTs monthly or as clinically needed.

Patient Counseling: Advise of the potential benefits and risks of treatment. Inform that BRAF^{V600E} mutation assessment is required for patient selection. Advise to expect regular dermatologic examination during treatment and up to 6 months after d/c. Stress the importance of immediately reporting any skin changes. Advise to avoid sun exposure and to wear protective clothing, sunscreen, and lip balm with SPF ≥30 when outdoors. Counsel female patients on the risks if used during prenancy/nursing. Inform of commonly reported adverse events. Instruct to swallow tab whole with a glass of water and not to chew or crush. Advise that missed dose can be taken up to 4 hrs prior to next dose and not to take both doses at the same time.

Administration: Oral route. Swallow tab whole with glass of water; do not chew or crush.
Storage: 20-25°C (68-77°F); excursions permitted between 15-30°C (59-86°F).

ZEMPLAR ORAL
paricalcitol (Abbott)

RX

THERAPEUTIC CLASS: Vitamin D analog

INDICATIONS: Prevention and treatment of secondary hyperparathyroidism associated with Stage 3 and 4 chronic kidney disease (CKD), and CKD Stage 5 on hemodialysis or peritoneal dialysis.

DOSAGE: *Adults:* CKD Stages 3 and 4: Initial: Baseline Intact Parathyroid Hormone (iPTH) Level ≤500pg/mL: 1mcg qd or 2mcg 3X/week. Baseline iPTH Level >500pg/mL: 2mcg qd or 4mcg 3X/week. Administer the 3X/week dose not more often than qod. Titrate: Individualize dose and base on serum/plasma iPTH levels. Refer to PI for further dose titration recommendations. CKD Stage 5: Initial: Based on baseline iPTH level (pg/mL)/80. Treat patients only after baseline serum calcium has been adjusted to ≤9.5mg/dL. Titrate: Individualize dose and base on iPTH and serum calcium/phosphorus. Refer to PI for further dose titration recommendations. If On a Calcium-Based Phosphate Binder: Decrease dose, withhold, or switch to non-calcium-based phosphate binder.

HOW SUPPLIED: Cap: 1mcg, 2mcg, 4mcg

CONTRAINDICATIONS: Vitamin D toxicity, hypercalcemia.

WARNINGS/PRECAUTIONS: Excessive administration may cause over suppression of PTH, hypercalcemia, hypercalciuria, hyperphosphatemia, and adynamic bone disease. Overdose may cause progressive hypercalcemia. Acute hypercalcemia may exacerbate cardiac arrhythmias and seizures. Chronic hypercalcemia may cause generalized vascular calcification and other soft-tissue calcifications. If hypercalcemia or elevated Ca x P is observed, reduce or withhold dose until these parameters are normalized.

ADVERSE REACTIONS: Pain, headache, hypotension, HTN, diarrhea, N/V, constipation, edema, arthritis, dizziness, rash, diarrhea, nasopharyngitis, viral infection, hypersensitivity.

INTERACTIONS: May increase risk of hypercalcemia with high doses of calcium-containing preparations and thiazides. High intake of calcium and phosphate may lead to serum abnormalities; frequent patient monitoring and individualized dose titration required. Prescription-based doses of vitamin D and its derivatives should be withheld during treatment to avoid hypercalcemia. Aluminum-containing preparations (eg, antacids, phosphate binders) should not be administered chronically, as increased blood levels of aluminum and aluminum bone toxicity may occur. Digitalis toxicity potentiated by hypercalcemia; caution with digitalis compounds. Increased exposure with strong CYP3A inhibitors (eg, ketoconazole, atazanavir, clarithromycin, indinavir, itraconazole, nefazodone, nelfinavir, ritonavir, saquinavir, telithromycin, voriconazole); dose adjustment may be required, and iPTH and serum calcium concentrations closely monitored if therapy is initiated or d/c with strong CYP3A4 inhibitors. Drugs that may impair intestinal absorption of fat-soluble vitamins (eg, cholestyramine) may interfere with absorption. Mineral oil or other substances that may affect absorption of fat may influence absorption.

PREGNANCY: Category C, not for use in nursing.

MECHANISM OF ACTION: Vitamin D2 analog; binds to vitamin D receptor, which results in selective activation of vitamin D responsive pathways. Shown to reduce PTH levels by inhibiting PTH synthesis and secretion.

PHARMACOKINETICS: Absorption: Absolute bioavailability (72%-86%). Refer to PI for different pharmacokinetic parameters of CKD Stages. **Distribution:** V_d=34L (healthy); 44-46L (CKD Stages 3 and 4); plasma protein binding (≥99.8%). **Metabolism:** Liver (extensive), via hydroxylation and glucuronidation; metabolized by CYP24, CYP3A4, UGT1A4. 24(R)-hydroxy paricalcitol

Z

(minor metabolite). **Elimination:** Feces (70%, 2% unchanged), urine (18%); $T_{1/2}$=4-6 hrs (healthy), 14-20 hrs (CKD Stages 3, 4, 5).

NURSING CONSIDERATIONS

Assessment: Assess for vitamin D toxicity, hypercalcemia, pregnancy/nursing status, and possible drug interactions.

Monitoring: Monitor for hypercalcemia and elevated Ca x P. Monitor serum calcium, phosphorus, and serum/plasma iPTH at least every 2 weeks for 3 months, then monthly for 3 months, and every 3 months thereafter during initiation or following dose adjustment.

Patient Counseling: Inform of the most common adverse reactions (eg, diarrhea, HTN, dizziness, vomiting). Advise to adhere to instructions regarding diet and phosphorus restriction, and to return for routine monitoring. Advise to contact physician if symptoms of elevated calcium (eg, feeling tired, difficulty thinking clearly, loss of appetite, N/V, constipation, increased thirst and urination, weight loss) develop. Advise to inform physician of all medications, supplements and herbal preparations being taken, and any change in medical condition.

Administration: Oral route. **Storage:** 25°C (77°F); excursions permitted to 15-30°C (59-86°F).

ZENPEP   RX
pancrelipase (Eurand Pharmaceuticals, Inc.)

THERAPEUTIC CLASS: Pancreatic enzyme supplement

INDICATIONS: Treatment of exocrine pancreatic insufficiency due to cystic fibrosis or other conditions.

DOSAGE: *Adults:* Individualize dose based on clinical symptoms, degree of steatorrhea present, and fat content of diet. Initial: 500 lipase U/kg/meal. Max: 2500 lipase U/kg/meal (or ≤10,000 lipase U/kg/day) or <4000 lipase U/g fat ingested/day. Half of the dose used for meals should be given with each snack.
Pediatrics: Individualize dose based on clinical symptoms, degree of steatorrhea present, and fat content of diet. ≥4 yrs: Initial: 500 lipase U/kg/meal. Max: 2500 lipase U/kg/meal (or ≤10,000 lipase U/kg/day) or <4000 lipase U/g fat ingested/day. Half of the dose used for meals should be given with each snack. >12 months-<4 yrs: Initial: 1000 lipase U/kg/meal. Max: 2500 lipase U/kg/meal (or ≤10,000 lipase U/kg/day) or <4000 lipase U/g fat ingested/day. ≤12 months: 3000 lipase U/ 120mL of formula or breastfeeding.

HOW SUPPLIED: Cap, Delayed-Release: (Amylase-Lipase-Protease) (Zenpep 3) 16,000 U-3000 U-10,000 U, (Zenpep 5) 27,000 U-5000 U-17,000 U, (Zenpep 10) 55,000 U-10,000 U-34,000 U, (Zenpep 15) 82,000 U-15,000 U-51,000 U, (Zenpep 20) 109,000 U-20,000 U-68,000 U

WARNINGS/PRECAUTIONS: Fibrosing colonopathy reported; monitor closely for progression to stricture formation. Caution with doses >2500 lipase U/kg/meal (or >10,000 lipase U/kg/day); use only if these doses are documented to be effective by 3-day fecal fat measures indicating improvement. Examine patients receiving >6000 lipase U/kg/meal; immediately decrease dose or titrate dose downward to a lower range. Caution with gout, renal impairment, or hyperuricemia; may increase blood uric acid levels. Should not be crushed or chewed, or mixed in foods with pH >4.5; may disrupt enteric coating of cap and cause early release of enzymes, irritation of oral mucosa, and/or loss of enzyme activity. Ensure that no drug is retained in the mouth. Risk for transmission of viral disease. Caution with a known allergy to proteins of porcine origin; severe allergic reactions reported. Not interchangeable with other pancrelipase products. Should not be mixed directly into formula or breast milk.

ADVERSE REACTIONS: GI disorders (eg, abdominal pain and flatulence), headache, cough, weight loss, early satiety, contusion, skin disorders.

PREGNANCY: Category C, caution in nursing.

MECHANISM OF ACTION: Pancreatic enzyme supplement; catalyzes the hydrolysis of fats to monoglycerol, glycerol and fatty acids, protein into peptides and amino acids, and starch into dextrins and short chain sugars.

NURSING CONSIDERATIONS

Assessment: Assess for gout, renal impairment, hyperuricemia, known allergy to porcine proteins, and pregnancy/nursing status.

Monitoring: Monitor for fibrosing colonopathy, stricture formation, oral mucosa irritation, viral diseases, gout, and allergic reactions. Monitor serum uric acid levels and renal function.

Patient Counseling: Instruct to take as prescribed and with food. Advise that total daily dose should not exceed 10,000 lipase U/kg/day unless clinically indicated, especially for those eating multiple snacks and meals per day. Inform to take next dose with next meal/snack ud if a dose is missed; doses should not be doubled. Instruct to swallow intact cap with adequate amounts of liquid at mealtimes. Advise to contact physician immediately if an allergic reaction develops.

Inform that doses >6000 U/kg/meal have been associated with colonic strictures in children <12 yrs. Instruct to notify physician if pregnant or plan to become pregnant during treatment. **Administration:** Oral route. Refer to PI for proper administration. **Storage:** 20-25°C (68-77°F); excursion permitted to 15-40°C (59-104°F). Avoid excessive heat. Protect from moisture; keep bottle tightly closed and out of reach of children.

ZENTRIP OTC
meclizine HCl (Sato)

THERAPEUTIC CLASS: Antihistamine

INDICATIONS: Prevention and treatment of N/V, or dizziness associated with motion sickness.

DOSAGE: *Adults:* Dissolve 1-2 strips on tongue qd or ud. Prevention: ≥1 hr prior to travel. *Pediatrics:* ≥12 yrs: Dissolve 1-2 strips on tongue qd or ud. Prevention: ≥1 hr prior to travel.

HOW SUPPLIED: Strip, Oral: 25mg

WARNINGS/PRECAUTIONS: Avoid use in children <12 yrs of age. Caution with glaucoma, breathing problems (eg, emphysema, chronic bronchitis), and difficulty in urination due to an enlarged prostate gland. D/C use and consult physician if rash, redness, itching, or difficulty in urination occurs, or if symptoms of dry mouth continue or increase. Drowsiness may occur and may impair mental/physical abilities.

ADVERSE REACTIONS: Drowsiness.

INTERACTIONS: Alcohol, sedatives, and tranquilizers may increase drowsiness. Avoid alcohol use.

PREGNANCY: Safety not known in pregnancy and nursing.

MECHANISM OF ACTION: Antihistamine.

NURSING CONSIDERATIONS

Assessment: Assess for breathing problems (eg, emphysema, chronic bronchitis), glaucoma, difficulty in urination due to an enlarged prostate gland, pregnancy/nursing status, and possible drug interactions.

Monitoring: Monitor for drowsiness, rash, redness, itching, difficulty in urination and increased/continued symptoms of dry mouth.

Patient Counseling: Inform that drowsiness may occur; caution when driving a vehicle or operating machinery. Avoid alcohol use. D/C and consult physician if rash, redness, itching, or difficulty in urination occurs, or if symptoms of dry mouth continue or increase. Consult physician before use if taking sedatives or tranquilizers and if pregnant/nursing. Keep out of reach of children; in case of overdose, get medical help or contact a Poison Control Center right away.

Administration: Oral route. **Storage:** 20-30°C (68-86°F). Protect from light. Use only if safety seal intact.

ZERIT RX
stavudine (Bristol-Myers Squibb)

Lactic acidosis and severe hepatomegaly with steatosis, including fatal cases, reported with nucleoside analogues. Fatal lactic acidosis reported in pregnant women who received the combination of stavudine and didanosine with other antiretroviral agents; use with caution. Fatal and nonfatal pancreatitis reported when used as part of a combination regimen that included didanosine.

THERAPEUTIC CLASS: Nucleoside reverse transcriptase inhibitor

INDICATIONS: Treatment of HIV-1 infection in combination with other antiretroviral agents.

DOSAGE: *Adults:* ≥60kg: 40mg q12h. <60kg: 30mg q12h. Renal Impairment: CrCl >50mL/min: ≥60kg: 40mg q12h. <60kg: 30mg q12h. CrCl 26-50mL/min: ≥60kg: 20mg q12h. <60kg: 15mg q12h. CrCl 10-25mL/min/Hemodialysis: ≥60kg: 20mg q24h. <60kg: 15mg q24h. Hemodialysis: Give after the completion of hemodialysis on dialysis days and at the same time of day on non-dialysis days.
Pediatrics: ≥60kg: 40mg q12h. 30-<60kg: 30mg q12h. ≥14 days and <30kg: 1mg/kg q12h. Birth-13 days: 0.5mg/kg q12h.

HOW SUPPLIED: Cap: 15mg, 20mg, 30mg, 40mg; Sol: 1mg/mL [200mL]

WARNINGS/PRECAUTIONS: Female gender, obesity, and prolonged nucleoside exposure may be risk factors for lactic acidosis and severe hepatomegaly with steatosis. Caution with known risk factors for liver disease; suspend if findings suggestive of symptomatic hyperlactatemia, lactic acidosis, or pronounced hepatotoxicity develop, and consider permanent d/c with confirmed lactic acidosis. Increased frequency of liver function abnormalities, including severe and

Z

potentially fatal hepatic adverse events, in patients with pre-existing liver dysfunction; monitor accordingly and interrupt or d/c if worsening of liver disease is evident. Motor weakness reported rarely; d/c if this develops. Peripheral sensory neuropathy reported; consider permanent d/c if this develops. Redistribution/accumulation of body fat reported; monitor for signs/symptoms of lipoatrophy or lipodystrophy. Immune reconstitution syndrome reported. Autoimmune disorders (eg, Graves' disease, polymyositis, Guillain-Barre syndrome) reported in the setting of immune reconstitution and can occur many months after initiation of treatment. Caution with renal impairment and in elderly.

ADVERSE REACTIONS: Lactic acidosis, severe hepatomegaly with steatosis, peripheral neurologic symptoms/neuropathy, headache, diarrhea, rash, N/V, increased AST/ALT, increased GGT/amylase/lipase/bilirubin.

INTERACTIONS: See Boxed Warning. Avoid with zidovudine and hydroxyurea with or without didanosine. D/C use of agents that are toxic to the pancreas in patients with suspected pancreatitis. Hepatic decompensation may occur with interferon/ribavirin in HIV-1/HCV coinfected patients; monitor for clinical toxicities. Caution with doxorubicin or ribavirin. Increased frequency of peripheral neuropathy with other drugs associated with neuropathy.

PREGNANCY: Category C, not for use in nursing.

MECHANISM OF ACTION: Synthetic thymidine nucleoside analogue; inhibits activity of HIV-1 reverse transcriptase by competing with natural substrate thymidine triphosphate and by causing DNA chain termination following incorporation into viral DNA. Inhibits cellular DNA polymerases β and gamma and markedly reduces synthesis of mitochondrial DNA.

PHARMACOKINETICS: Absorption: Rapid. C_{max}=536ng/mL, T_{max}=1 hr; AUC_{0-24}=2,568ng•hr/mL. **Distribution:** (IV) V_d=46L (adults), 0.73L/kg (peds). **Metabolism:** Oxidized stavudine, glucuronide conjugates, and N-acetylcysteine conjugate (minor metabolites). **Elimination:** Urine (34%) (peds); $T_{1/2}$=1.6 hrs (adults), 0.96 hr (peds).

NURSING CONSIDERATIONS

Assessment: Assess for drug hypersensitivity, risk factors for lactic acidosis or liver disease, preexisting liver dysfunction, renal impairment, history of peripheral neuropathy, pancreatitis, pregnancy/nursing status, and possible drug interactions.

Monitoring: Monitor for signs/symptoms of lactic acidosis, hepatotoxicity, worsening of liver disease, motor weakness, peripheral neuropathy, pancreatitis, fat redistribution/accumulation, lipoatrophy/lipodystrophy, immune reconstitution syndrome (eg, opportunistic infections), and autoimmune disorders.

Patient Counseling: Inform that therapy is not cure for HIV and patients may continue to experience illnesses associated with HIV. Advise to avoid doing things that can spread HIV to others (eg, sharing needles, other inj equipment, or personal items that can have blood or body fluids on them, sex without protection, breastfeeding). Instruct that if a dose is missed, take as soon as possible; if it is almost time for the next dose, skip missed dose and continue the regular dosing schedule. Advise diabetic patients that oral sol contains 50mg of sucrose/mL. Advise to seek medical attention if symptoms of hyperlactatemia or lactic acidosis syndrome (eg, unexplained weight loss, abdominal discomfort, N/V, fatigue, dyspnea, motor weakness), or peripheral neuropathy (eg, numbness, tingling or pain in the hands or feet) occur. Advise to avoid alcohol while on therapy. Inform that fat redistribution/accumulation may occur.

Administration: Oral route. Refer to PI for preparation of oral sol. **Storage:** 25°C (77°F); excursions permitted between 15-30°C (59-86°F). Sol: Protect from excessive moisture. After Reconstitution: 2-8°C (36-46°F) for 30 days.

ZESTORETIC   RX
lisinopril - hydrochlorothiazide (AstraZeneca)

> D/C when pregnancy is detected. Drugs that act directly on the renin-angiotensin system can cause death/injury to developing fetus.

THERAPEUTIC CLASS: ACE inhibitor/thiazide diuretic

INDICATIONS: Treatment of HTN.

DOSAGE: *Adults:* Not Controlled with Lisinopril/HCTZ Monotherapy: Initial: 10mg-12.5mg or 20mg-12.5mg qd depending on current monotherapy dose. Titrate: May increase HCTZ dose after 2-3 weeks. May reduce dose of lisinopril after addition of diuretic. Controlled on 25mg HCTZ qd with Hypokalemia: Switch to 10mg-12.5mg qd. Replacement Therapy: Substitute combination for titrated individual components. Elderly: Start at lower end of dosing range.

HOW SUPPLIED: Tab: (Lisinopril-HCTZ) 10mg-12.5mg, 20mg-12.5mg, 20mg-25mg

CONTRAINDICATIONS: History of ACE inhibitor-associated angioedema, anuria, hypersensitivity to other sulfonamide-derived drugs.

Z

WARNINGS/PRECAUTIONS: Not for initial therapy of HTN. Avoid with CrCl ≤30mL/min. Caution in elderly. Lisinopril: Head/neck angioedema reported; d/c and administer appropriate therapy. Intestinal angioedema reported; monitor for abdominal pain. More reports of angioedema in blacks than non-blacks. Anaphylactoid reactions reported during desensitization with hymenoptera venom, dialysis with high-flux membranes, and LDL apheresis with dextran sulfate absorption. Excessive hypotension associated with oliguria and/or progressive azotemia, and rarely with acute renal failure and/or death may occur with congestive heart failure (CHF); monitor closely. Leukopenia/neutropenia and bone marrow depression reported; monitor WBCs in patients with collagen vascular disease and renal disease. Rarely, syndrome that starts with cholestatic jaundice or hepatitis progressing to fulminant hepatic necrosis and (sometimes) death reported; d/c if jaundice or marked elevations of hepatic enzymes occur. Caution with left ventricular outflow obstruction. May cause changes in renal function. May increase BUN and SrCr levels with renal artery stenosis. Hyperkalemia, persistent nonproductive cough reported. Hypotension may occur with major surgery or during anesthesia. HCTZ: May cause idiosyncratic reaction, resulting in acute transient myopia and acute angle-closure glaucoma; d/c as rapidly as possible. May precipitate azotemia with renal disease. Caution with hepatic dysfunction or progressive liver disease; may precipitate hepatic coma. Sensitivity reactions may occur. May exacerbate/activate systemic lupus erythematosus (SLE). Observe for signs of fluid or electrolyte imbalance (hyponatremia, hypochloremic alkalosis, hypokalemia). Hyperuricemia, gout precipitation, hyperglycemia, hypomagnesemia, and hypercalcemia may occur. D/C before testing for parathyroid function. Enhanced effects in postsympathectomy patients. Increased cholesterol, TG levels reported.

ADVERSE REACTIONS: Dizziness, headache, cough, fatigue, orthostatic effects, angioedema, hypotension.

INTERACTIONS: NSAIDs, including selective cyclooxygenase-2 inhibitors, may diminish effects of diuretic and ACE inhibitors, and may cause further deterioration of renal function. Increased risk of lithium toxicity; avoid with lithium. Lisinopril: Hypotension risk, and increased BUN and SrCr with diuretics. Increased risk of hyperkalemia with K+-sparing diuretics, K+ supplements, or K+-containing salt substitutes. Nitritoid reactions with injectable gold reported. HCTZ: Potentiates orthostatic hypotension with alcohol, barbiturates, and narcotics. Dose adjustment of antidiabetic drugs (eg, oral agents and insulin) may be needed. Cholestyramine and colestipol resins impair absorption. Corticosteroids and adrenocorticotropic hormone may intensify electrolyte depletion, particularly hypokalemia. May decrease response to pressor amines (eg, norepinephrine). Potentiates other antihypertensives. Increased responsiveness to nondepolarizing skeletal muscle relaxants (eg, tubocurarine).

PREGNANCY: Category D, not for use in nursing.

MECHANISM OF ACTION: Lisinopril: ACE inhibitor; decreases plasma angiotensin II, which leads to decreased vasopressor activity and decreased aldosterone secretion. HCTZ: Thiazide diuretic; not established. Affects distal renal tubular mechanism of electrolyte reabsorption. Increases excretion of Na+ and Cl-.

PHARMACOKINETICS: Absorption: Lisinopril: T_{max}=7 hrs. **Distribution:** Crosses placenta. HCTZ: Found in breast milk. **Elimination:** Lisinopril: Urine (unchanged); $T_{1/2}$=12 hrs. HCTZ: Kidneys (≥61% unchanged); $T_{1/2}$=5.6-14.8 hrs.

NURSING CONSIDERATIONS

Assessment: Assess for renal/hepatic impairment, collagen vascular disease (eg, SLE), history of ACE inhibitor-associated and hereditary/idiopathic angioedema, anuria, hypersensitivity to other sulfonamide/penicillin-derived drugs, CHF, left ventricle outflow obstruction, diabetes mellitus (DM), postsympathectomy, risk factors for hyperkalemia, allergy or bronchial asthma, pregnancy/nursing status, and possible drug interactions.

Monitoring: Monitor for signs/symptoms of angioedema, fluid/electrolyte imbalance, exacerbation/activation of SLE, idiosyncratic reaction, latent DM, hyperglycemia, hypercalcemia, hyperuricemia or precipitation of gout, hypersensitivity reactions, and other adverse reactions. Monitor BP, serum electrolytes, renal function, cholesterol, and TG levels periodically. Monitor WBCs in patients with collagen vascular and renal diseases.

Patient Counseling: Inform about fetal risks if taken during pregnancy and discuss treatment options in women planning to become pregnant; report pregnancy to physician as soon as possible. Inform that excessive perspiration, dehydration, and other causes of volume depletion (eg, diarrhea, vomiting) may lead to fall in BP. Instruct to report lightheadedness, to d/c therapy if actual syncope occurs, not to use salt substitutes containing K+ without consulting physician, and to report immediately any signs/symptoms of leukopenia/neutropenia (eg, infections, fever, sore throat) and angioedema (swelling of the face, extremities, eyes, lips, tongue, difficulty swallowing or breathing).

Administration: Oral route. **Storage:** 20-25°C (68-77°F). Protect from excessive light and humidity.

ZESTRIL   RX
lisinopril (AstraZeneca)

> ACE inhibitors can cause death/injury to developing fetus during 2nd and 3rd trimesters. D/C if pregnancy detected.

THERAPEUTIC CLASS: ACE inhibitor

INDICATIONS: Treatment of HTN alone as initial therapy or concomitantly with other antihypertensive agents. Adjunct therapy in heart failure if inadequately responding to diuretics and digitalis. Treatment of hemodynamically stable patients within 24 hrs of acute myocardial infarction (AMI) to improve survival.

DOSAGE: *Adults:* HTN: Initial: 10mg qd. Adjust dose according to BP response. Usual: 20-40mg qd. Max: 80mg/day. May add a low-dose diuretic if BP not controlled. Diuretic-Treated Patients: D/C diuretic 2-3 days before therapy. If cannot d/c diuretic; give initial dose of 5mg under medical supervision for at least 2 hrs and until BP stabilized for additional 1 hr. Renal Impairment: Initial: CrCl >30mL/min: 10mg/day. CrCl 10-30mL/min: 5mg/day. CrCl <10mL/min: 2.5mg/day. Titrate up until BP is controlled. Max: 40mg/day. Heart Failure: Initial: 5mg qd. Usual: 5-40mg qd. Titrate: May increase by 10mg every 2 weeks. Max: 40mg/day. Hyponatremia or CrCl ≤30mL/min or SrCr >3mg/dL: Initial: 2.5mg qd under close medical supervision. AMI: Initial: 5mg within 24 hrs, then 5mg after 24 hrs, 10mg after 48 hrs, and 10mg qd for 6 weeks. Low Systolic BP (≤120mmHg) When Treatment Started or During the 1st 3 Days After the Infarct: 2.5mg. Maint: 5mg qd with temporary reductions to 2.5mg PRN if systolic BP ≤100mmHg. D/C if systolic BP <90mmHg for >1 hr. Caution with SrCr >2mg/dL. Elderly: Start at lower end of dosing range. *Pediatrics:* ≥6 yrs: HTN: Initial: 0.07mg/kg qd up to 5mg total. Adjust dose according to BP response. Max: 0.61mg/kg or 40mg.

HOW SUPPLIED: Tab: 2.5mg, 5mg*, 10mg, 20mg, 30mg, 40mg *scored

CONTRAINDICATIONS: History of angioedema, hereditary or idiopathic angioedema.

WARNINGS/PRECAUTIONS: Not recommended in pediatric patients with GFR <30mL. Less effect on BP and more reports of angioedema in blacks than nonblacks. Anaphylactoid reactions reported. Angioedema of face, extremities, lips, tongue, glottis, and larynx reported; d/c promptly and administer appropriate therapy if occurs. Intestinal angioedema reported; monitor for abdominal pain. Anaphylactoid reactions reported during desensitization with hymenoptera venom, dialysis with high-flux membranes, and LDL apheresis with dextran sulfate absorption. Excessive hypotension associated with oliguria, azotemia, and rarely with acute renal failure and/or death may occur with congestive heart failure (CHF); monitor during first 2 weeks of therapy and whenever dose is increased. May cause agranulocytosis, bone marrow depression, leukopenia/neutropenia; monitor WBC in patients with renal and collagen vascular disease. Syndrome that starts with cholestatic jaundice progressing to fulminant necrotic hepatitis and death reported; d/c if jaundice or LFT elevation occurs. Caution with left ventricular outflow tract obstruction. May increase BUN and SrCr levels with renal artery stenosis and without preexisting renal vascular disease. Risk of hyperkalemia with diabetes mellitus (DM), renal dysfunction. Persistent nonproductive cough reported. Hypotension may occur with surgery or during anesthesia. Caution in elderly.

ADVERSE REACTIONS: Chest pain, cough, diarrhea, dizziness, headache, fatigue, hypotension, asthenia, N/V, upper respiratory infection, rash.

INTERACTIONS: Hypotension risk, increased BUN and SrCr with diuretics. May increase risk of hypoglycemia with insulin or oral anti-diabetics. NSAIDs, including selective cyclooxygenase-2 inhibitors, may attenuate antihypertensive effect and may cause further deterioration of renal function. Increased risk of hyperkalemia with K+-sparing diuretics (eg, spironolactone, eplerenone, triamterene, or amiloride), K+-containing salt substitutes, or K+ supplements. Lithium toxicity reported; monitor serum lithium levels if administered concomitantly with lithium. Nitritoid reactions (eg, facial flushing, N/V, hypotension) reported rarely with injectable gold (sodium aurothiomalate).

PREGNANCY: Category C (1st trimester) and D (2nd and 3rd trimesters), not for use in nursing.

MECHANISM OF ACTION: ACE inhibitor; inhibition results in decreased plasma angiotensin II, which leads to decreased vasopressor activity and aldosterone secretion.

PHARMACOKINETICS: Absorption: T_{max}=7 hrs. **Distribution:** Crosses placenta. **Elimination:** Urine (unchanged); $T_{1/2}$=12 hrs.

NURSING CONSIDERATIONS

Assessment: Assess for history and hereditary/idiopathic angioedema, collagen vascular disease (systemic lupus erythematosus, scleroderma), CHF, DM, renal artery stenosis, renal/hepatic impairment, pregnancy/nursing status, and possible drug interactions. Obtain baseline BP, BUN, and SrCr.

Monitoring: Monitor renal function periodically. Monitor for angioedema, anaphylactoid reactions, hepatic function, hypotension, hypersensitivity, hypoglycemia, and other adverse reactions. Monitor BP, LFTs, CBC with platelet count and differential, BUN, SrCr, and serum K⁺ levels. Monitor WBCs in patients with collagen vascular and renal diseases.

Patient Counseling: Instruct to d/c therapy and to immediately report signs/symptoms of angioedema. Inform that lightheadedness may occur, especially during 1st days of therapy; advise to consult with a physician. Inform that inadequate fluid intake or excessive perspiration, diarrhea, or vomiting may lead to excessive drop in BP resulting in lightheadedness or syncope. Inform to avoid K⁺ supplements or salt substitutes containing K⁺ without consulting physician. Advise to report if any indication of infection (eg, sore throat, fever) which may be a sign of leukopenia/neutropenia. Inform of pregnancy risks; advise to report pregnancy to physician as soon as possible.

Administration: Oral route. Refer to PI suspension preparation instructions. **Storage:** 20-25°C (68-77°F). Protect from moisture, freezing, and excessive heat.

ZETIA   RX
ezetimibe (Merck/Schering-Plough)

THERAPEUTIC CLASS: Cholesterol absorption inhibitor

INDICATIONS: Adjunct to diet: As monotherapy or with concomitant HMG-CoA reductase inhibitors (statins), to reduce total-C, LDL, apolipoprotein B, and non-HDL in patients with primary (heterozygous familial and non-familial) hyperlipidemia. With concomitant fenofibrate, to reduce elevated total-C, LDL, Apo B, and non-HDL in adults with mixed hyperlipidemia. Adjunct to other lipid-lowering treatments (eg, LDL apheresis) or if such treatments are unavailable, with concomitant atorvastatin or simvastatin, to reduce elevated total-C and LDL in homozygous familial hypercholesterolemia. Reduce elevated sitosterol and campesterol levels in homozygous familial sitosterolemia.

DOSAGE: *Adults:* Usual: 10mg qd. May give with a statin (with primary hyperlipidemia) or with fenofibrate (with mixed hyperlipidemia) for incremental effect. Concomitant Bile Acid Sequestrant: Give either ≥2 hrs before or ≥4 hrs after taking bile acid sequestrant.

HOW SUPPLIED: Tab: 10mg

CONTRAINDICATIONS: Active liver disease or unexplained persistent elevations in hepatic transaminase levels when used with statins, women who are or may become pregnant, nursing mothers.

WARNINGS/PRECAUTIONS: Should be in accordance with the product labeling for the concurrently administered drug (eg, specific statin or fenofibrate). Liver enzyme elevations reported. Consider withdrawal of therapy and/or statin if an increase in ALT or AST ≥3X ULN persist. Myopathy and rhabdomyolysis reported; immediately d/c therapy and any concomitant statin or fibrate if myopathy is diagnosed/suspected. Not recommended with moderate or severe hepatic impairment.

ADVERSE REACTIONS: Upper respiratory tract infection, diarrhea, arthralgia.

INTERACTIONS: See Contraindications. May increase risk of transaminase elevations with a statin; perform LFTs before initiation and as recommended thereafter. Increased risk for skeletal muscle toxicity with higher doses of statin, depending on the statin used, and concomitant use of other drugs. Caution with cyclosporine; monitor cyclosporine levels. May increase cholesterol excretion into the bile leading to cholelithiasis with fibrates; avoid with fibrates (except fenofibrate). Consider alternative lipid-lowering therapy if cholelithiasis occurs with fenofibrate. Decreased levels with cholestyramine; incremental LDL reduction may be reduced. Monitor INR levels when used with warfarin. Increased levels with gemfibrozil, cimetidine, lovastatin, pravastatin, and rosuvastatin. Decreased levels with aluminum and magnesium hydroxide combination antacid. May increase levels of lovastatin and rosuvastatin. May decrease levels of gemfibrozil, glipizide, pravastatin, and fluvastatin. Glipizide may increase area under the curve (AUC) and decrease C_{max}. May increase AUC and decrease C_{max} of digoxin. May decrease C_{max} of ethinyl estradiol and levonorgestrel. May decrease AUC and increase C_{max} of both atorvastatin and ezetimibe. Fluvastatin may decrease AUC and increase C_{max}. Caution and close monitoring when used with simvastatin >20mg in patients with moderate to severe renal impairment.

PREGNANCY: Category C, caution in nursing.

MECHANISM OF ACTION: Cholesterol absorption inhibitor; reduces blood cholesterol by inhibiting absorption of cholesterol by the small intestine. Targets the sterol transporter, Neimann-Pick C1-like 1, which is involved in intestinal uptake of cholesterol and phytosterols.

PHARMACOKINETICS: Absorption: (Fasted) C_{max}=3.4-5.5ng/mL, 45-71ng/mL (metabolite); T_{max}=4-12 hrs, 1-2 hrs (metabolite). **Distribution:** Plasma protein binding (>90%). **Metabolism:** Small intestine and liver via glucuronide conjugation; ezetimibe-glucuronide (active metabolite). **Elimination:** Feces (78%, 69% unchanged drug), urine (11%, 9% metabolite); $T_{1/2}$=22 hrs.

Z

NURSING CONSIDERATIONS

Assessment: Assess for conditions where treatment is contraindicated or cautioned, renal/hepatic impairment, pregnancy/nursing status, and possible drug interactions. If using in combination with statin therapy, assess for risk factors for skeletal muscle toxicity (eg, use with higher doses of statins, advanced age, hypothyroidism, renal impairment, concomitant drug use). Obtain baseline lipid profile (total-C, LDL, HDL, TG). If using in combination with statin therapy, obtain baseline LFTs (eg, ALT, AST).

Monitoring: Monitor for signs/symptoms of elevated liver enzymes, myopathy, rhabdomyolysis, and other adverse reactions. Periodically monitor LFTs during concomitant therapy with statin therapy. Perform periodic monitoring of lipid profile.

Patient Counseling: Instruct to adhere to recommended diet, a regular exercise program, and periodic testing of fasting lipid panel. Counsel about risk of myopathy; instruct to promptly report to the physician if any unexplained muscle pain, tenderness, or weakness occurs. Counsel women of childbearing age to use an effective method of birth control while using added statin therapy. Instruct to d/c therapy and contact physician if they become pregnant. Advise not to breastfeed if concomitantly using statins.

Administration: Oral route. **Storage:** 25°C (77°F); excursions permitted to 15-30°C (59-86°F). Protect from moisture.

ZEVALIN   RX
ibritumomab tiuxetan (Spectrum)

> Serious infusion reactions (within 24 hrs of rituximab) and severe cutaneous/mucocutaneous reactions, some fatal, may occur. D/C rituximab, In-111 ibritumomab, and Y-90 ibritumomab if this occurs. May cause severe and prolonged cytopenias; avoid if ≥25% lymphoma marrow involvement and/or impaired bone marrow reserve. Y-90 ibritumomab dose should not exceed 32mCi (1184MBq) and do not administer to patients with altered biodistribution.

THERAPEUTIC CLASS: Monoclonal antibody/CD20-blocker

INDICATIONS: Treatment of relapsed or refractory, low-grade or follicular B-cell non-Hodgkin's lymphoma (NHL) and for previously untreated follicular NHL in patients who achieve partial or complete response to first-line chemotherapy.

DOSAGE: *Adults:* Premedicate with acetaminophen 650mg PO and diphenhydramine 50mg PO prior to rituximab infusion. Day 1: Administer rituximab 250mg/m^2 IV initially at 50mg/hr. Escalate in 50mg/hr increments q30 min to max of 400mg/hr in absence of infusion reactions. Give 5mCi In-111 ibritumomab IV over 10 min within 4 hrs following completion of rituximab infusion. Day 7, 8, or 9: Verify that expected biodistribution is present at 48-72 hrs after In-111. Refer to PI for instructions for image acquisition and biodistribution determination. If acceptable, administer rituximab 250mg/m^2 IV initially at 100mg/hr and increase rate by 100mg/hr increments q30 min to max of 400mg/hr. If infusion reactions occurred on Day 1, administer only at 50mg/hr, and escalate in 50mg/hr increments q30 min to max of 400mg/hr. Give Y-90 ibritumomab 0.4mCi/kg if platelets ≥150,000/mm^3 (or 0.3mCi/kg if platelets 100,000-149,000/mm^3) over 10 min IV within 4 hrs of rituximab.

HOW SUPPLIED: Inj: 3.2mg/2mL

WARNINGS/PRECAUTIONS: Myelodysplastic syndrome (MDS) and/or acute myelogenous leukemia (AML) reported. Monitor closely for extravasation; d/c infusion if signs or symptoms occur and restart in another limb. Minimize radiation exposure to patients during and after treatment. Contains albumin; carries remote risk for transmission of viral disease and Creutzfeldt-Jakob disease (CJD). Potential for immunogenicity. May cause fetal harm. Caution in elderly.

ADVERSE REACTIONS: Infusion reactions, cytopenias (neutropenia, leukopenia, thrombocytopenia, anemia, lymphopenia), severe cutaneous and mucocutaneous reactions, fatigue, abdominal pain, nausea, nasopharyngitis, asthenia, diarrhea, cough, pyrexia, myalgia, anorexia, night sweats, influenza-like illness.

INTERACTIONS: Avoid with live vaccines. Caution with medications that interfere with platelet function or coagulation; monitor for thrombocytopenia more frequently.

PREGNANCY: Category D, not for use in nursing.

MECHANISM OF ACTION: Human monoclonal IgG1 kappa antibody/CD20 antigen blocker; binds specifically to CD20 antigen, which is expressed on pre-B and mature B lymphocytes, and on B-cell non-Hodgkin's lymphomas. The β emission from Y-90 induces cellular damage by the formation of free cell radicals in the target and neighboring cells.

PHARMACOKINETICS: Distribution: Found in breast milk. **Elimination:** Urine (7.2% over 7 days); T$_{1/2}$=30 hrs.

NURSING CONSIDERATIONS

Assessment: Assess for lymphoma marrow involvement, impaired bone marrow reserve, cytopenia, hemorrhage, severe infections, altered biodistribution, pregnancy/nursing status, and for possible drug interactions.

Monitoring: Monitor for infusion reactions within 24 hrs of rituximab infusion. Monitor for severe cutaneous/mucocutaneous reactions, extravasation, and complications (eg, febrile neutropenia, hemorrhage). Monitor CBC and platelet counts following regimen weekly until levels recover or as clinically indicated.

Patient Counseling: Advise to contact physician if signs/symptoms of infusion reactions, cytopenias (eg, bleeding, easy bruising, petechiae or purpura, pallor, weakness or fatigue), infection (eg, pyrexia), diffuse rash, bullae, or desquamation of skin or oral mucosa occur. Advise to take premedications as prescribed and avoid medications that interfere with platelet function. Counsel patients of childbearing potential to use effective contraceptive methods during treatment and for a minimum of 12 months following therapy, and to d/c nursing during and after treatment. Advise against immunization with live vaccines for 12 months after treatment.

Administration: IV route. Refer to PI for directions for medication preparation, radiochemical purity determination, and radiation dosimetry. **Storage:** 2-8°C (36-46°F). Do not freeze.

ZIAC   RX
bisoprolol fumarate - hydrochlorothiazide (Duramed)

THERAPEUTIC CLASS: Selective beta$_1$-blocker/thiazide diuretic

INDICATIONS: Management of HTN.

DOSAGE: *Adults:* Uncontrolled BP on 2.5-20mg/day Bisoprolol or Controlled BP on 50mg/day HCTZ with Hypokalemia: Initial: 2.5mg-6.25mg qd. Titrate: May increase at 14-day intervals. Max: 20mg-12.5mg (two 10mg-6.25mg tab) qd, as appropriate. Replacement therapy: May substitute for titrated individual components. Renal/Hepatic Impairment: Caution in dosing/titrating. Cessation of therapy: Withdrawal should be achieved gradually over a period of 2 weeks.

HOW SUPPLIED: Tab: (Bisoprolol fumarate-HCTZ) 2.5mg-6.25mg, 5mg-6.25mg, 10mg-6.25mg

CONTRAINDICATIONS: Cardiogenic shock, overt cardiac failure, 2nd- or 3rd-degree atrioventricular (AV) block, marked sinus bradycardia, anuria, hypersensitivity to sulfonamide-derived drugs.

WARNINGS/PRECAUTIONS: Caution with impaired hepatic function/progressive liver disease. Bisoprolol: Caution with compensated cardiac failure. May precipitate cardiac failure; consider d/c at first signs/symptoms of heart failure (HF). Exacerbations of angina pectoris, myocardial infarction, and ventricular arrhythmia with coronary artery disease (CAD) reported upon abrupt d/c; caution against interruption or d/c without physician's advice. May precipitate or aggravate symptoms of arterial insufficiency with peripheral vascular disease (PVD); exercise caution. Avoid with bronchospastic disease, but may use with caution if unresponsive/intolerant of other antihypertensives. Chronically administered therapy should not be routinely withdrawn prior to major surgery; however, may augment risks of general anesthesia and surgical procedures. Caution with diabetes mellitus (DM); may mask tachycardia occurring with hypoglycemia. May mask hyperthyroidism and precipitate thyroid storm with abrupt d/c. HCTZ: May precipitate azotemia with impaired renal function. D/C if progressive renal impairment becomes apparent. May precipitate hepatic coma with hepatic impairment. May cause idiosyncratic reaction, resulting in acute transient myopia and acute angle-closure glaucoma; d/c HCTZ as rapidly as possible. Monitor for fluid/electrolyte disturbances (eg, hyponatremia, hypochloremic alkalosis, hypokalemia, hypomagnesemia). Decreased calcium excretion and altered parathyroid glands, with hypercalcemia and hypophosphatemia, observed on prolonged therapy. Precipitation of hyperuricemia/gout and sensitivity reactions may occur. Photosensitivity reactions and exacerbation/activation of systemic lupus erythematosus (SLE) reported. Enhanced effects in postsympathectomy patient. D/C prior to parathyroid function test.

ADVERSE REACTIONS: Hyperuricemia, dizziness, fatigue, headache, diarrhea.

INTERACTIONS: May potentiate other antihypertensive agents. Avoid with other β-blockers. Excessive reduction of sympathetic activity with catecholamine-depleting drugs (eg, reserpine, guanethidine); monitor closely. D/C for several days prior to clonidine withdrawal. Caution with myocardial depressants or inhibitors of AV conduction (eg, certain calcium antagonists [particularly phenylalkylamine and benzothiazepine classes], antiarrhythmic agents [eg, disopyramide]). Bisoprolol: Digitalis glycosides may increase risk of bradycardia. Rifampin may increase clearance. May be unresponsive to usual doses of epinephrine. HCTZ: Alcohol, barbiturates, or narcotics may potentiate orthostatic hypotension. Antidiabetic drugs (eg, oral agents, insulin) may require dosage adjustments. Impaired absorption with cholestyramine and colestipol resins. Corticosteroids and adrenocorticotropic hormone may intensify electrolyte depletion, particularly hypokalemia. May decrease response to pressor amines (eg, norepinephrine). May increase

Z

response to nondepolarizing skeletal muscle relaxants (eg, tubocurarine). Do not give with lithium; increased risk of lithium toxicity. NSAIDs may reduce diuretic, natriuretic, and antihypertensive effects.

PREGNANCY: Category C, not for use in nursing.

MECHANISM OF ACTION: Bisoprolol: β_1-selective adrenoreceptor blocking agent; not established. May decrease cardiac output, inhibit renin release by the kidneys, and decrease tonic sympathetic outflow from vasomotor centers in the brain. HCTZ: Thiazide diuretic; not established. Affects renal tubular mechanisms of electrolyte reabsorption and increases excretion of Na^+ and Cl^-.

PHARMACOKINETICS: Absorption: Well absorbed. Bisoprolol: Absolute bioavailability (80%); C_{max}=9ng/mL (2.5mg-6.25mg), 19ng/mL (5mg-6.25mg), 36ng/mL (10mg-6.25mg); T_{max}=3 hrs. HCTZ: C_{max}=30ng/mL; T_{max}=2.5 hrs. **Distribution:** Bisoprolol: Plasma protein binding (30%). HCTZ: Plasma protein binding (40-68%); crosses placenta; found in breast milk. **Elimination:** Bisoprolol: Urine (55% unchanged); feces (<2%); $T_{1/2}$=7-15 hrs. HCTZ: Urine (60% unchanged); $T_{1/2}$=4-10 hrs.

NURSING CONSIDERATIONS

Assessment: Assess for cardiogenic shock, overt/compensated cardiac failure, 2nd- or 3rd-degree AV block, marked sinus bradycardia, anuria, sulfonamide hypersensitivity, CAD, PVD, bronchospastic disease, DM, hyperthyroidism, renal/hepatic impairment, history of sulfonamide/penicillin allergy, parathyroid disease, SLE, pregnancy/nursing status, and possible drug interactions. Obtain baseline serum electrolytes.

Monitoring: Monitor for signs/symptoms of HF, withdrawal, hypoglycemia, hyperthyroidism, renal/hepatic impairment, idiosyncratic reaction, fluid or electrolyte disturbances, precipitation of hyperuricemia or gout, and hypersensitivity reactions. Perform periodic monitoring of serum electrolytes.

Patient Counseling: Instruct not to d/c therapy without physician's supervision especially in patients with CAD. Advise to consult physician if any difficulty in breathing occurs, or other signs/symptoms of congestive HF or excessive bradycardia develop. Inform that hypoglycemia may be masked in patients subject to spontaneous hypoglycemia, or diabetic patients receiving insulin or oral hypoglycemic agents; instruct to use with caution. Advise to avoid driving, operating machinery, or engaging in other tasks requiring alertness until reaction to drug is known. Advise that photosensitivity reactions may occur.

Administration: Oral route. **Storage:** 20-25°C (68-77°F).

ZIAGEN   RX
abacavir sulfate (ViiV Healthcare)

Serious and sometimes fatal hypersensitivity reactions (multi-organ clinical syndrome) reported; d/c as soon as suspected and never restart therapy with any abacavir-containing product. Patients with HLA-B*5701 allele are at high risk for hypersensitivity; screen for HLA-B*5701 allele prior to therapy. Lactic acidosis and severe hepatomegaly with steatosis, including fatal cases, reported with nucleoside analogues.

THERAPEUTIC CLASS: Nucleoside reverse transcriptase inhibitor

INDICATIONS: Treatment of HIV-1 infection in combination with other antiretroviral agents.

DOSAGE: *Adults:* 300mg bid or 600mg qd. Mild Hepatic Impairment (Child-Pugh Score 5-6): 200mg (10mL) bid.
Pediatrics: Sol: ≥3 months: 8mg/kg bid. Max: 300mg bid. Tab: ≥30kg: 300mg (1 tab) bid (am and pm). >21-<30kg: 150mg (1/2 tab) am, 300mg (1 tab) pm. 14-21kg: 150mg (1/2 tab) bid (am and pm). Mild Hepatic Impairment (Child-Pugh Score 5-6): 200mg (10mL) bid.

HOW SUPPLIED: Sol: 20mg/mL [240mL]; Tab: 300mg* *scored

CONTRAINDICATIONS: Moderate or severe hepatic impairment.

WARNINGS/PRECAUTIONS: Obesity and prolonged nucleoside exposure may be risk factors for lactic acidosis and severe hepatomegaly with steatosis. Caution with known risk factors for liver disease; d/c if findings suggestive of lactic acidosis or pronounced hepatotoxicity develop. Immune reconstitution syndrome reported. Autoimmune disorders (eg, Graves' disease, polymyositis, Guillain-Barre syndrome) reported in the setting of immune reconstitution and can occur many months after initiation of treatment. Redistribution/accumulation of body fat reported. Increased risk of myocardial infarction (MI) reported; consider the underlying risk of coronary heart disease when prescribing therapy. Caution in elderly.

ADVERSE REACTIONS: Hypersensitivity reaction, lactic acidosis, severe hepatomegaly with steatosis, N/V, headache, malaise, fatigue, diarrhea, dream/sleep disorders, fever, chills, skin rashes, ear/nose/throat infection.

INTERACTIONS: Ethanol may increase exposure. May decrease levels of methadone.

PREGNANCY: Category C, not for use in nursing.

MECHANISM OF ACTION: Nucleoside analogue; inhibits HIV-1 reverse transcriptase by competing with natural substrate dGTP and by its incorporation into viral DNA.

PHARMACOKINETICS: Absorption: Rapid and extensive; absolute bioavailability (83%). (300mg bid) C_{max}= 3mcg/mL, AUC_{0-12h}=6.02mcg•hr/mL. (600mg qd) C_{max}= 4.26mcg/mL, AUC=11.95mcg•hr/mL. **Distribution:** (IV) V_d=0.86L/kg; plasma protein binding (50%). **Metabolism:** Via alcohol dehydrogenase and glucuronyl transferase. **Elimination:** Urine (1.2% abacavir, 30% 5'-carboxylic acid metabolite, 36% 5'-glucuronide metabolite, 15% unidentified minor metabolites); feces (16%); $T_{1/2}$=1.54 hrs (single dose).

NURSING CONSIDERATIONS

Assessment: Assess for previous hypersensitivity to the drug, hepatic impairment, risk factors for lactic acidosis, risk factors for coronary heart disease, pregnancy/nursing status, and possible drug interactions. Screen for HLA-B*5701 allele prior to initiation of therapy and prior to reinitiation of therapy.

Monitoring: Monitor for hypersensitivity reactions, lactic acidosis, hepatotoxicity, immune reconstitution syndrome (eg, opportunistic infections), autoimmune disorders, fat redistribution/accumulation, and MI.

Patient Counseling: Inform that therapy is not a cure for HIV and patients may continue to experience illnesses associated with HIV. Inform about the risk of hypersensitivity reactions; instruct to contact physician immediately if symptoms develop and not to restart or replace with any drug containing abacavir without medical consultation. Counsel that lactic acidosis (with liver enlargement) and fat redistribution or accumulation may occur. Advise to avoid doing things that can spread HIV to others (eg, sharing needles, other inj equipment, or personal items that can have blood fluids on them, sex without protection, breastfeeding). Instruct to take exactly as prescribed.

Administration: Oral route. **Storage:** 20-25°C (68-77°F). Sol: Do not freeze. May be refrigerated.

ZIANA   RX
clindamycin phosphate - tretinoin (Medicis)

THERAPEUTIC CLASS: Lincosamide derivative/retinoid

INDICATIONS: Topical treatment of acne vulgaris in patients ≥12 yrs.

DOSAGE: *Adults:* Apply at hs, a pea-sized amount onto 1 fingertip, dot onto the chin, cheeks, nose, and forehead, then gently rub over entire face.
Pediatrics: ≥12 yrs: Apply at hs, a pea-sized amount onto 1 fingertip, dot onto the chin, cheeks, nose, and forehead, then gently rub over entire face.

HOW SUPPLIED: Gel: (Clindamycin-Tretinoin) 1.2%-0.025% [2g, 30g, 60g]

CONTRAINDICATIONS: Regional enteritis, ulcerative colitis, or history of antibiotic-associated colitis.

WARNINGS/PRECAUTIONS: Not for oral, ophthalmic, or intravaginal use. Keep away from eyes, mouth, angles of the nose, and mucous membranes. Avoid exposure to sunlight, including sunlamps. Avoid use if sunburn is present. Daily use of sunscreen products and protective apparel are recommended. Weather extremes (eg, wind, cold) may be irritating while under treatment. Clindamycin: Systemic absorption has been demonstrated following topical use. Diarrhea, bloody diarrhea, and colitis (including pseudomembranous colitis) reported; d/c if significant diarrhea occurs. Severe colitis reported following PO or parenteral administration with an onset of up to several weeks following cessation of therapy.

ADVERSE REACTIONS: Nasopharyngitis, local skin reactions (erythema, scaling, itching, burning), GI symptoms.

INTERACTIONS: Caution with topical medications, medicated/abrasive soaps and cleansers, soaps/cosmetics with strong drying effect, products with high concentrations of alcohol, astringents, spices, or lime because skin irritation may be increased. Avoid with erythromycin-containing products. May enhance action of neuromuscular blocking agents; use with caution. Antiperistaltic agents (eg, opiates, diphenoxylate with atropine) may prolong and/or worsen severe colitis.

PREGNANCY: Category C, caution in nursing.

MECHANISM OF ACTION: Clindamycin: Lincosamide antibiotic; binds to 50S ribosomal subunits of susceptible bacteria and prevents elongation of peptide chains by interfering with peptidyl transfer, thereby suppressing bacterial protein synthesis. Found to have (in vitro) activity against *Propionibacterium acnes*. Tretinoin: Retinoid; not established. Suspected to decrease cohesiveness of follicular epithelial cells with decreased microcomedo formation. Also, stimulates mitotic activity and increased turnover of follicular epithelial cells, causing extrusion of comedones.

Z

PHARMACOKINETICS: Absorption: Tretinoin: Percutaneous (minimal). **Distribution:** Orally and parenterally administered clindamycin found in breast milk. **Metabolism:** Tretinoin: 13-cis-retinoic acid and 4-oxo-13-cis-retinoic acid (metabolites).

NURSING CONSIDERATIONS

Assessment: Assess for regional enteritis, ulcerative colitis, or history of antibiotic-associated colitis, pregnancy/nursing status, and possible drug interactions. Assess use in patients whose occupations require considerable sun exposure.

Monitoring: Monitor for signs/symptoms of diarrhea, bloody diarrhea, colitis, local skin reactions, and other adverse reactions.

Patient Counseling: Instruct to wash face gently with mild soap and warm water at hs and apply a thin layer over the entire face (excluding the eyes and lips) after patting the skin dry. Advise not to use more than recommended amount and not to apply more than qd (at hs). Instruct to apply sunscreen qam and reapply over the course of the day PRN. Advise to avoid exposure to sunlight, sunlamp, UV light, and other medicines that may increase sensitivity to sunlight. Inform that medication may cause irritation (eg, erythema, scaling, itching, burning, stinging). Instruct to d/c therapy and contact physician if severe diarrhea or GI discomfort occurs.

Administration: Topical route. **Storage:** 25°C (77°F); excursions permitted to 15-30°C (59-86°F). Protect from light and freezing. Keep away from heat. Keep tube tightly closed.

ZINACEF   RX
cefuroxime sodium (GlaxoSmithKline)

THERAPEUTIC CLASS: Cephalosporin (2nd generation)

INDICATIONS: Treatment of septicemia, meningitis, uncomplicated and disseminated gonorrhea, lower respiratory tract (including pneumonia), urinary tract (UTI), skin and skin structure (SSSI), and bone and joint infections caused by susceptible strains of microorganisms. Preoperative and perioperative prophylaxis in patients undergoing clean-contaminated or potentially contaminated surgical procedures.

DOSAGE: *Adults:* Usual: 750mg-1.5g q8h for 5-10 days. Uncomplicated Pneumonia/UTI/SSSI/ Disseminated Gonococcal Infections: 750mg q8h. Severe/Complicated Infections: 1.5g q8h. Bone and Joint Infections: 1.5g q8h. Life-Threatening Infections/Infections due to Less Susceptible Organisms: 1.5g q6h. Meningitis: Max: 3g q8h. Uncomplicated Gonococcal Infection: 1.5g IM single dose at 2 different sites with 1g PO probenecid. Surgical Prophylaxis: 1.5g IV 0.5-1 hr before initial incision, then 750mg IM/IV q8h with prolonged procedure. Open Heart Surgery (Perioperative): 1.5g IV at induction of anesthesia and q12h thereafter, for total of 6g. Renal Impairment: CrCl 10-20mL/min: 750mg q12h. CrCl <10mL/min: 750mg q24h. Hemodialysis: Give a further dose at end of dialysis. Continue therapy for a minimum of 48-72 hrs after the patient becomes asymptomatic or evidence of bacterial eradication has been obtained. *Streptococcus pyogenes* Infections: Treat for ≥10 days. Elderly: Start at the lower end of dosing range. *Pediatrics:* ≥3 months: Usual: 50-100mg/kg/day in divided doses q6-8h. Severe/Serious Infections: 100mg/kg/day (not to exceed max adult dose). Bone and Joint Infections: 150mg/kg/day in divided doses q8h (not to exceed max adult dose). Meningitis: 200-240mg/kg/day IV in divided doses q6-8h. Renal Impairment: Modify dosing frequency consistent with adult recommendations. Continue therapy for a minimum of 48-72 hrs after the patient becomes asymptomatic or evidence of bacterial eradication has been obtained. *Streptococcus pyogenes* Infections: Treat for ≥10 days.

HOW SUPPLIED: Inj: 750mg, 1.5g, 7.5g, 750mg/50mL, 1.5g/50mL

WARNINGS/PRECAUTIONS: Caution in penicillin (PCN) sensitive patients; d/c use if allergic reaction occurs. *Clostridium difficile*-associated diarrhea (CDAD) reported. May result in bacterial resistance with prolonged use or use in the absence of a proven/suspected bacterial infection or a prophylactic indication; take appropriate measures if superinfection develops. Monitor renal function. Caution with history of GI disease, particularly colitis. Hearing loss reported in pediatric patients treated for meningitis. Risk of decreased prothrombin activity with renal/hepatic impairment, poor nutritional state, or protracted course of therapy. Lab test interactions may occur. Caution in elderly.

ADVERSE REACTIONS: Local reactions, decreased Hgb and Hct, eosinophilia, ALT/AST elevation.

INTERACTIONS: Nephrotoxicity reported with concomitant aminoglycosides. Caution with potent diuretics; may adversely affect renal function. May decrease prothrombin activity; caution with anticoagulants. May affect the gut flora, leading to lower estrogen reabsorption and reduced efficacy of combined estrogen/progesterone oral contraceptives. Increased peak serum levels and serum $T_{1/2}$ with oral administration of probenecid.

PREGNANCY: Category B, caution in nursing.

MECHANISM OF ACTION: 2nd-generation cephalosporin; inhibits cell-wall synthesis.

PHARMACOKINETICS: Absorption: C_{max}=(750mg) 27mcg/mL (IM), 50mcg/mL (IV). (1.5g) 100mcg/mL (IV); T_{max}(750mg)=45 min (IM), 15 min (IV). **Distribution:** Plasma protein binding (50%); found in breast milk. **Elimination:** Urine (89%); $T_{1/2}$=80 min.

NURSING CONSIDERATIONS

Assessment: Assess for known allergy to cephalosporins, PCN, or other drugs, renal/hepatic impairment, nutritional status, history of GI disease (eg, colitis), pregnancy/nursing status, and possible drug interactions.

Monitoring: Monitor for signs/symptoms of an allergic reaction, CDAD, and for overgrowth of nonsusceptible organisms. In pediatric patients with meningitis, monitor for hearing loss. Monitor renal function and PT.

Patient Counseling: Inform that therapy only treats bacterial, not viral, infections. Instruct to take as directed. Advise that skipping doses or not completing full course may decrease effectiveness and increase resistance. Inform that diarrhea may occur and will usually end if therapy is d/c. Instruct to notify physician if watery/bloody stools (with or without stomach cramps and fever) and other adverse reactions occur.

Administration: IV/IM routes. Refer to PI for administration procedures, directions for preparation of sol and sus, use of frozen plastic container, compatibility and stability, and instructions for constitution of ADD-Vantage vials. **Storage:** (Dry State) 15-30°C (59-86°F). Protect from light. (Frozen Premixed Sol) Do not store above -20°C.

ZINECARD   RX
dexrazoxane (Pharmacia & Upjohn)

THERAPEUTIC CLASS: EDTA derivative

INDICATIONS: Reduce incidence and severity of cardiomyopathy associated with doxorubicin in women with metastatic breast cancer who received a cumulative doxorubicin dose of 300mg/m² and who will continue doxorubicin therapy to maintain tumor control.

DOSAGE: *Adults:* IV: 10:1 ratio of dexrazoxane:doxorubicin (eg, 500mg/m²:50mg/m²). Moderate to Severe Renal Dysfunction (CrCl <40mL/min): 5:1 ratio of dexrazoxane:doxorubicin (eg, 250mg/m²:50mg/m²). Hepatic Impairment: Reduce dose proportionally (maintaining the 10:1 ratio). Administer via rapid IV drip infusion. Give doxorubicin within 30 min of start of dexrazoxane infusion (administer doxorubicin after dexrazoxane infusion completed).

HOW SUPPLIED: Inj: 250mg, 500mg

CONTRAINDICATIONS: Chemotherapy regimens not containing an anthracycline.

WARNINGS/PRECAUTIONS: Not for use with initiation of doxorubicin therapy. Monitor cardiac function; potential for anthracycline induced cardiac toxicity still exists. Secondary malignancies (eg, primarily acute myeloid leukemia) reported. Obtain frequent CBCs. Caution with moderate or severe renal insufficiency; reduce dose. Caution in elderly.

ADVERSE REACTIONS: Alopecia, N/V, fatigue, malaise, anorexia, stomatitis, fever, infection, diarrhea, pain on injection, sepsis, neurotoxicity, streaking/erythema.

INTERACTIONS: See Contraindications. Avoid during initiation of FAC (fluorouracil, doxorubicin, cyclophosphamide) therapy; may reduce antitumor efficacy. Additive myelosuppression with other chemotherapeutic agents.

PREGNANCY: Category C, not for use in nursing.

MECHANISM OF ACTION: EDTA derivative; not established. Suspected to interfere with iron-mediated free radical generation thought to be responsible, in part, for anthracycline induced cardiomyopathy.

PHARMACOKINETICS: Absorption: (500mg/m²) C_{max} = 36.5µg/mL. **Distribution:** (500mg/m²) V_d=22.4L/m². (600mg/m²) V_d=22L/m². **Elimination:** Urine (42% [500mg/m²]). $T_{1/2}$=2.5 hrs (500mg/m²), 2.1 hrs (600mg/m²).

NURSING CONSIDERATIONS

Assessment: Assess cardiac/renal/hepatic function, pregnancy/nursing status, and possible drug interactions. Obtain baseline CBC, LFTs, and renal function test (eg, CrCl).

Monitoring: Monitor for myelosuppression, secondary malignancies, and other adverse reactions. Monitor CBC with differential and platelet count, and cardiac/renal/hepatic function.

Patient Counseling: Instruct to avoid nursing during therapy. Discuss signs/symptoms of adverse effects and advise to report any if they develop.

Administration: IV route. Do not administer via IV push. Refer to PI for handling and disposal instructions, and preparation of reconstituted sol. Do not mix with other drugs. **Storage:** 25°C

Z

(77°F); excursions permitted to 15-30°C (59-86°F). Reconstituted Sol: Stable for 30 min at room temperature or 2-8°C (36-46°F) for ≤3 hrs. Infusion Sol: Stable for 1 hr at room temperature or 2-8°C (36-46°F) for ≤4 hrs.

ZIPSOR   RX
diclofenac potassium (Xanodyne)

> NSAIDs may cause an increased risk of serious cardiovascular thrombotic events, MI, stroke, and serious GI adverse events including bleeding, ulceration, and perforation of the stomach or intestines. Contraindicated for the treatment of perioperative pain in the setting of coronary artery bypass graft (CABG) surgery.

THERAPEUTIC CLASS: NSAID

INDICATIONS: Relief of mild to moderate acute pain in adults ≥18 yrs.

DOSAGE: *Adults:* ≥18 yrs: 25mg qid. Elderly: Start at low end of dosing range.

HOW SUPPLIED: Cap: 25mg

CONTRAINDICATIONS: Asthma, urticaria, or allergic reactions after taking aspirin (ASA) or other NSAIDs. Hypersensitivity to bovine protein. Treatment of perioperative pain in the setting of CABG surgery.

WARNINGS/PRECAUTIONS: May lead to onset of new HTN or worsening of pre-existing HTN; monitor BP closely. Fluid retention and edema reported; caution with fluid retention or heart failure. Caution in patients with considerable dehydration. Renal papillary necrosis and other renal injury reported after long-term use. Not recommended for use with advanced renal disease. If therapy must be initiated, monitor renal function. Anaphylactoid reactions may occur. Contraindicated in ASA-triad patients. May cause serious skin adverse events (eg, exfoliative dermatitis, Stevens-Johnson syndrome, and toxic epidermal necrolysis). Avoid in late pregnancy; may cause premature closure of ductus arteriosus. May cause elevations of LFTs; d/c if liver disease develops or systemic manifestations occur. Caution in elderly and debilitated. Anemia may occur; with long-term use, monitor Hgb/Hct if signs or symptoms of anemia develop. May inhibit platelet aggregation and prolong bleeding time; monitor with coagulation disorders. Caution with asthma and avoid with ASA-sensitive asthma. May mask symptoms of infection (eg, fever, inflammation). Caution in patients with history of ulcer disease or GI bleeding, or with risk factors (eg, concomitant oral corticosteroids or anticoagulants, smoking, alcohol). Not a substitute for corticosteroids or to treat corticosteroid insufficiency.

ADVERSE REACTIONS: Abdominal pain, constipation, diarrhea, dyspepsia, N/V, dizziness, headache, somnolence, pruritus, increased sweating.

INTERACTIONS: Avoid use with other diclofenac products. Increased adverse effects with ASA. May impair therapeutic response to ACE inhibitors, thiazides or loop diuretics; monitor for renal failure. Avoid acetaminophen unless prescribed. Synergistic effects on GI bleeding with warfarin. May increase lithium levels; monitor for toxicity. May enhance methotrexate toxicity; caution when coadministering. May increase nephrotoxicity of cyclosporine; caution when coadministering. Caution with coadministration of other drugs that are substrates or inhibitors of CYP2C9.

PREGNANCY: Category C <30 weeks gestation, Category D after 30 weeks. Not for use in nursing.

MECHANISM OF ACTION: NSAID (benzeneacetic acid derivative); suspected to inhibit prostaglandin synthetase, exerts anti-inflammatory, analgesic, and antipyretic actions.

PHARMACOKINETICS: Absorption: Mean absolute bioavailability (50%), C_{max}=1087ng/mL, AUC=597ng•h/mL, T_{max}=0.5 hr. **Distribution:** V_d=1.3L/kg; serum protein binding (>99%). **Metabolism:** Metabolites: 4'-hydroxy-, 5-hydroxy-, 3'-hydroxy-, 4',5-dihydroxy- and 3'-hydroxy-4'-methoxy diclofenac. **Elimination:** Urine (65%), bile (35%); $T_{1/2}$= approximately 1 hr.

NURSING CONSIDERATIONS

Assessment: Assess LFTs, renal function, CBC and coagulation profile. Assess for history of CABG surgery, asthma and allergic reactions to ASA or other NSAIDS, active ulceration, bleeding or chronic inflammation of GI tract, cardiovascular disease (CVD), pregnancy/nursing status, and possible drug interactions. Note other diseases/conditions and drug therapies.

Monitoring: Monitor for hypersensitivity reactions, cardiac complications, stroke, GI bleeding, asthma, skin side effects. Monitor BP, LFTs, renal function, CBC with differential and platelet count, coagulation profile (especially if on anticoagulation therapy), hyperglycemia.

Patient Counseling: Counsel about potential CV, GI, hepatotoxic and dermatological events, as well as possible weight gain/edema. Take as prescribed. Caution women against using late in pregnancy.

Administration: Oral route. **Storage:** 25°C (77°F); excursions permitted to 15-30°C (59-86°F). Protect from moisture. Dispense in tight container.

ZIRGAN

ganciclovir (Bausch & Lomb)

RX

THERAPEUTIC CLASS: Synthetic guanine derivative

INDICATIONS: Treatment of acute herpetic keratitis (dendritic ulcers).

DOSAGE: *Adults:* 1 drop in affected eye 5X per day (q3h while awake) until corneal ulcer heals, then 1 drop tid for 7 days.
Pediatrics: ≥2 yrs: 1 drop in affected eye 5X per day (q3h while awake) until corneal ulcer heals, then 1 drop tid for 7 days.

HOW SUPPLIED: Gel: 0.15% [5g]

WARNINGS/PRECAUTIONS: For topical ophthalmic use only. Avoid wearing contact lenses during the course of treatment or if signs and symptoms of herpetic keratitis are present.

ADVERSE REACTIONS: Blurred vision, eye irritation, punctate keratitis, conjunctival hyperemia.

PREGNANCY: Category C, caution in nursing.

MECHANISM OF ACTION: Guanosine derivative; competitive inhibition of viral DNA-polymerase and direct incorporation into viral primer strand DNA, resulting in DNA chain termination and prevention of replication.

NURSING CONSIDERATIONS

Assessment: Assess for signs and symptoms of herpetic keratitis, and pregnancy/nursing status.

Monitoring: Monitor for eye pain, redness, itching or inflammation, and possible adverse reactions.

Patient Counseling: Counsel regarding proper use; for topical use only. Advise that dropper tip should not touch any surface, as this may contaminate gel. Advise to consult physician if pain develops, or if redness, itching, or inflammation becomes aggravated. Instruct not to wear contact lenses during treatment.

Administration: Ocular route. **Storage:** 15-25°C (59-77°F). Do not freeze.

ZITHROMAX

azithromycin (Pfizer)

RX

THERAPEUTIC CLASS: Macrolide

INDICATIONS: Treatment of the following infections caused by susceptible microorganisms: (Sus, Tab [250mg, 500mg]) Acute bacterial exacerbations of chronic obstructive pulmonary disease (COPD), acute bacterial sinusitis (ABS), community-acquired pneumonia (CAP), pharyngitis/tonsillitis, uncomplicated skin and skin structure infections (SSSIs), urethritis/cervicitis, genital ulcer disease (men), acute otitis media. (600mg Tab/Single-Dose Pkt) Treatment of nongonococcal urethritis/cervicitis. Prevention of disseminated *Mycobacterium avium* complex (MAC) disease, alone or in combination with rifabutin, in persons with advanced HIV infection. Treatment of disseminated MAC disease in combination with ethambutol in persons with advanced HIV infection. (Inj) CAP and pelvic inflammatory disease (PID).

DOSAGE: *Adults:* (Inj) CAP: 500mg IV qd for ≥2 days, then 500mg PO (two 250mg tab) qd to complete 7-10-day course. PID: 500mg IV qd for 1-2 days, then 250mg PO qd to complete 7-day course. (PO) CAP (mild severity)/Pharyngitis/Tonsillitis (2nd-line therapy)/SSSI (uncomplicated): 500mg single dose on Day 1, then 250mg qd on Days 2-5. Acute Bacterial Exacerbation of COPD (mild-moderate): 500mg qd for 3 days or 500mg single dose on Day 1, then 250mg qd on Days 2-5. ABS: 500mg qd for 3 days. Genital Ulcer Disease (Chancroid)/Nongonococcal Urethritis/Cervicitis: 1g single dose. Gonococcal Urethritis/Cervicitis: 2g single dose. Prevention of Disseminated MAC Infections: 1200mg once weekly. May be combined with rifabutin. Treatment of Disseminated MAC Infections: 600mg qd in combination with ethambutol at 15mg/kg/day. *Pediatrics:* (Inj) ≥16 yrs: CAP: 500mg IV qd for ≥2 days, then 500mg PO (two 250mg tab) qd to complete 7-10-day course. PID: 500mg IV qd for 1-2 days, then 250mg PO qd to complete 7-day course. (Sus) ≥2 yrs: Pharyngitis/Tonsillitis: 12mg/kg qd for 5 days. ≥6 months: Acute Otitis Media: 30mg/kg single dose, or 10mg/kg qd for 3 days, or 10mg/kg single dose on Day 1, then 5mg/kg/day on Days 2-5. CAP: 10 mg/kg single dose on Day 1, then 5mg/kg on Days 2-5. ABS: 10mg/kg qd for 3 days. Refer to PI for Dosing Charts.

HOW SUPPLIED: Inj: 500mg; Sus: 100mg/5mL [15mL], 200mg/5mL [15mL, 22.5mL, 30mL], 1g [pkt]; Tab: 250mg, 500mg, 600mg

CONTRAINDICATIONS: History of cholestatic jaundice/hepatic dysfunction with prior use of azithromycin.

WARNINGS/PRECAUTIONS: Serious allergic and dermatologic reactions (eg, Stevens-Johnson syndrome [SJS] and toxic epidermal necrolysis [TEN]) rarely reported; d/c if occurs and institute

Z

appropriate therapy. Abnormal liver function, hepatitis, cholestatic jaundice, hepatic necrosis, and hepatic failure reported; d/c immediately if signs/symptoms of hepatitis occur. *Clostridium difficile*-associated diarrhea (CDAD) reported. Caution with GFR <10mL/min. May increase risk of developing cardiac arrhythmia and torsades de pointes; caution in patients at increased risk for prolonged cardiac repolarization. Myasthenia gravis exacerbation and new onset of myasthenic syndrome reported. May result in bacterial resistance with prolonged use or use in the absence of a proven/suspected bacterial infection or a prophylactic indication; take appropriate measures if superinfection develops. (Sus/Tab) Should not be relied on to treat gonorrhea or syphilis. Avoid in patients with pneumonia who are judged to be inappropriate for PO therapy because of moderate to severe illness or risk factors. (Single-Dose Pkt) Do not use single-dose packet to administer doses other than 1000mg; not for pediatrics. (Inj) Local IV site reactions reported.

ADVERSE REACTIONS: Diarrhea/loose stools, N/V, abdominal pain. (IV) Pain at injection site, local inflammation.

INTERACTIONS: Monitor terfenadine, cyclosporine, hexobarbital, phenytoin levels. May increase digoxin levels. May potentiate effects of oral anticoagulants; monitor for prothrombin time. Increased serum concentrations with nelfinavir. May produce modest effect on pharmacokinetics of atorvastatin, carbamazepine, cetirizine, didanosine, efavirenz, fluconazole, indinavir, midazolam, rifabutin, sildenafil, theophylline (PO and IV), triazolam, trimethoprim/sulfamethoxazole, and zidovudine. Efavirenz or fluconazole may have a modest effect on pharmacokinetics of azithromycin. Aluminum- and magnesium-containing antacids may reduce PO levels. Acute ergot toxicity may occur with ergotamine or dihydroergotamine. (IV) Increased side effects reported (N/V, abdominal pain, etc) with metronidazole.

PREGNANCY: Category B, caution in nursing.

MECHANISM OF ACTION: Macrolide; inhibits protein synthesis by binding to the 50S ribosomal subunits of susceptible organisms, thus interfering with microbial protein synthesis.

PHARMACOKINETICS: Absorption: Administration of variable doses resulted in different parameters. **Distribution:** (PO) V_d=31.1L/kg. **Elimination:** Biliary (major), urine; $T_{1/2}$=68 hrs.

NURSING CONSIDERATIONS

Assessment: Assess for hypersensitivity to drug, history of cholestatic jaundice, liver/renal dysfunction, myasthenia gravis, GFR, pregnancy/nursing status, and possible drug interactions. Assess use in patients at risk for prolonged cardiac repolarization. In patients with sexually transmitted urethritis or cervicitis, perform serologic test for syphilis and perform appropriate cultures for gonorrhea at the time of diagnosis. In all patients, perform appropriate culture and susceptibility tests prior to treatment. (Sus/Tab) Assess for pneumonia, cystic fibrosis, nosocomial infections, known or suspected bacteremia, patients requiring hospitalization, age, debilitated condition, and underlying health problems.

Monitoring: Monitor for signs/symptoms of allergic reactions, CDAD, superinfections, arrhythmias, torsades de pointes, hepatic dysfunction, hepatitis, cholestatic jaundice, hepatic necrosis, hepatic failure, and for new onset of myasthenic syndrome or exacerbation of myasthenia gravis. Monitor PT with oral anticoagulants. (Inj) Monitor for IV-site reactions.

Patient Counseling: Inform patient to d/c immediately and contact physician if allergic reaction occurs. Inform that therapy treats bacterial, not viral, infections. Instruct to take as directed; skipping doses or not completing full course may decrease effectiveness and increase resistance. May experience diarrhea; notify physician if watery and bloody stools occur. (PO) Advise patient to not take aluminum- or magnesium-containing antacids simultaneously.

Administration: Oral/IV routes. (Inj) Refer to PI for reconstitution and dilution instructions. Infuse concentration and rate of infusion should either be 1mg/mL over 3 hrs or 2mg/mL over 1 hr. Do not give as a bolus or as an IM injection. Do not give with other IV substances, additives, or medications or infuse simultaneously through the same IV line. (Sus) Shake well before use. (Single-Dose Pkt) Mix entire content of packet with 2 oz. of water. Drink completely. **Storage:** (Tab) 15-30°C (59-86°F); (600mg Tab) ≤30°C (86°F). (Sus) Dry Powder: <30°C (86°F). Constituted: 5-30°C (41-86°F); use within 10 days. (Single-dose packet) 5-30°C (41-86°F). Reconstituted Inj: <30°C (86°F) for 24 hrs or under refrigeration 5°C (41°F) for 7 days.

ZMAX

RX

azithromycin (Pfizer)

THERAPEUTIC CLASS: Macrolide

INDICATIONS: Treatment of mild to moderate community-acquired pneumonia (CAP) in adults and children ≥6 months and acute bacterial sinusitis in adults caused by susceptible bacteria.

DOSAGE: *Adults:* 2g single dose on an empty stomach (at least 1 hr ac or 2 hrs pc).
Pediatrics: ≥6 months: 60mg/kg single dose on an empty stomach (at least 1 hr ac or 2 hrs pc).

Patients weighing ≥34kg should receive adult dose. Refer to PI for specific pediatric dosage guidelines.

HOW SUPPLIED: Sus, Extended-Release: 2g (27mg/mL)

CONTRAINDICATIONS: History of cholestatic jaundice/hepatic dysfunction associated with prior use of azithromycin.

WARNINGS/PRECAUTIONS: Serious allergic reactions (eg, angioedema, anaphylaxis, Stevens-Johnson syndrome [SJS], and toxic epidermal necrolysis) reported; institute appropriate therapy if allergic reaction occurs. Allergic symptoms may recur after initial successful symptomatic treatment. Abnormal liver function, hepatitis, cholestatic jaundice, hepatic necrosis and hepatic failure reported; d/c therapy if signs and symptoms of hepatitis occur. *Clostridium difficile*-associated diarrhea (CDAD) reported; d/c if CDAD is suspected or confirmed. Exacerbation of symptoms of myasthenia gravis and new onset of myasthenic syndrome reported. GI disturbances and prolonged cardiac repolarization and QT interval reported. Increased risk of developing drug-resistant bacteria in the absence of a proven or strongly suspected bacterial infection. Caution with GFR <10mL/min. May consider additional antibiotic if patient vomits within 5 min of administration. Consider alternative therapy if patient vomits between 5 and 60 min after administration. Neither a second dose nor alternative therapy is warranted if patient vomits ≥60 min after administration with normal gastric emptying. Consider alternative therapy in patients with delayed gastric emptying.

ADVERSE REACTIONS: Diarrhea/loose stools, N/V, abdominal pain, headache, rash.

INTERACTIONS: May potentiate the effects of oral anticoagulants (eg, warfarin); monitor PT. Nelfinavir may increase area under the curve and C_{max}. Monitor carefully with digoxin, ergotamine or dihydroergotamine, cyclosporine, hexobarbital, and phenytoin.

PREGNANCY: Category B, caution in nursing.

MECHANISM OF ACTION: Macrolide antibiotic; inhibits microbial protein synthesis by binding to the 50S ribosomal subunits of susceptible organisms.

PHARMACOKINETICS: Absorption: Oral administration of variable doses resulted in different parameters. **Distribution:** V_d=31.1L/kg; plasma protein binding (7-51%). **Elimination:** Bile (major route), urine (6%, unchanged); $T_{1/2}$=59 hrs.

NURSING CONSIDERATIONS

Assessment: Assess for hypersensitivity to the drug, renal/hepatic function, myasthenia gravis, risk for prolonged cardiac repolarization, history of cholestatic jaundice/hepatic dysfunction associated with prior use of azithromycin, pregnancy/nursing status, and possible drug interactions. Perform appropriate culture and susceptibility tests prior to treatment.

Monitoring: Monitor for signs/symptoms of hypersensitivity reactions (eg, angioedema, SJS), CDAD, GI adverse effects, cardiac repolarization or QT prolongation, arrhythmia, myasthenia gravis, hepatic dysfunction, hepatitis, cholestatic jaundice, hepatic necrosis, and hepatic failure.

Patient Counseling: Inform to take on empty stomach. Advise to immediately report to physician any signs of allergic reaction. Instruct to contact physician if vomiting occurs within 1st hr. Inform that therapy treats bacterial, not viral, infections. Instruct to take as directed; skipping doses or not completing full course may decrease effectiveness and increase resistance. Inform that diarrhea may be experienced; instruct to notify physician if watery/bloody stools occur. Advise patient to take without regard to antacids containing magnesium and/or aluminum. Instruct to shake bottle well before use.

Administration: Oral route. Reconstitute with 60mL water. Shake well. Consume reconstituted sus within 12 hrs. Discard any remaining sus after dosing in pediatrics. **Storage:** Dry Powder: ≤30°C (86°F). Reconstituted Sus: 25°C (77°F); excursions permitted to 15-30°C (59-86°F). Do not refrigerate or freeze.

ZOCOR   RX
simvastatin (Merck)

THERAPEUTIC CLASS: HMG-CoA reductase inhibitor

INDICATIONS: Adjunct to diet to reduce risk of total mortality by reducing coronary heart disease (CHD) deaths, risk of nonfatal myocardial infarction and stroke, and need for coronary/noncoronary revascularization procedures in patients at high risk of coronary events because of existing CHD, diabetes, peripheral vessel disease, history of stroke or other cerebrovascular disease. To reduce elevated total-C, LDL, Apo B, and TG, and to increase HDL in primary hyperlipidemia (Fredrickson Type IIa, heterozygous familial and nonfamilial) or mixed dyslipidemia (Fredrickson Type IIb). To reduce elevated TG in hypertriglyceridemia (Fredrickson Type IV hyperlipidemia). To reduce elevated TG and VLDL in primary dysbetalipoproteinemia (Fredrickson Type III hyperlipidemia). To reduce total-C and LDL in homozygous familial hypercholesterolemia as adjunct to other lipid-lowering agents, or if treatments are unavailable. Adjunct to diet to

Z

reduce total-C, LDL, Apo B levels in adolescent boys and girls who are at least 1 yr postmenarche, 10-17 yrs, with heterozygous familial hypercholesterolemia (HeFH), if after an adequate trial of diet therapy, LDL remains ≥190mg/dL or ≥160mg/dL and there is positive family history of premature cardiovascular disease (CVD) or ≥2 other CVD risk factors.

DOSAGE: *Adults:* Initial: 10-20mg qpm. Usual: 5-40mg qd. High Risk for CHD Events: Initial: 40mg qd. Perform lipid determinations after 4 weeks and periodically thereafter. Restricted Dosing: Use 80mg only in patients receiving 80mg chronically (eg, ≥12 months) without evidence of muscle toxicity. If tolerating 80mg and needs to be initiated on drug that is contraindicated or has a dose cap for simvastatin, switch to an alternative statin with less potential for drug-drug interaction. Avoid titration to 80mg, and place on alternative LDL lowering treatment if unable to achieve LDL goal with 40mg. Concomitant Verapamil/Diltiazem: Max: 10mg qd. Concomitant Amiodarone/Amlodipine/Ranolazine: Max: 20mg qd. Homozygous Familial Hypercholesterolemia: Usual: 40mg qpm. Chinese Patients Taking Lipid-Modifying Doses (≥1g/day niacin) of Niacin-Containing Products: Caution with >20mg qd; avoid 80mg. Severe Renal Impairment: Initial: 5mg qd; monitor closely. *Pediatrics:* HeFH: 10-17 yrs: Initial: 10mg qpm. Usual: 10-40mg qd. Individualize dose according to recommended goal of therapy. Adjust at ≥4 week intervals. Max: 40mg qd. Concomitant Verapamil/Diltiazem: Max: 10mg qd. Concomitant Amiodarone/Amlodipine/Ranolazine: Max: 20mg qd. Chinese Patients Taking Lipid-Modifying Doses (≥1g/day niacin) of Niacin-Containing Products: Caution with >20mg qd; avoid 80mg. Severe Renal Impairment: Initial: 5mg qd; monitor closely.

HOW SUPPLIED: Tab: 5mg, 10mg, 20mg, 40mg, 80mg

CONTRAINDICATIONS: Concomitant administration of strong CYP3A4 inhibitors (eg, itraconazole, ketoconazole, posaconazole, HIV protease inhibitors, boceprevir, telaprevir, erythromycin, clarithromycin, telithromycin, nefazodone), gemfibrozil, cyclosporine, or danazol. Active liver disease, which may include unexplained persistent elevations of hepatic transaminases, women who are pregnant or may become pregnant, and nursing mothers.

WARNINGS/PRECAUTIONS: Myopathy and rhabdomyolysis reported; predisposing factors include advanced age (≥65 yrs), female gender, uncontrolled hypothyroidism, and renal impairment. Risk of myopathy, including rhabdomyolysis, is dose related and greater with 80mg doses. D/C if myopathy is suspected/diagnosed or if markedly elevated CPK levels occur. Temporarily withhold if experiencing acute or serious condition predisposing to development of renal failure secondary to rhabdomyolysis (eg, sepsis, hypotension, major surgery, trauma, severe metabolic/endocrine/electrolyte disorders, uncontrolled epilepsy). Persistent increases in serum transaminases reported; monitor LFTs before initiation and as indicated thereafter. Fatal and nonfatal hepatic failure reported; d/c therapy if serious liver injury with clinical symptoms and/or hyperbilirubinemia or jaundice occurs and do not restart if no alternate etiology found. Caution in elderly, with severe renal impairment, heavy alcohol use, or history of hepatic disease. Increase in HbA1c and FPG levels reported. Not studied in conditions where the major abnormality is elevation of chylomicrons (eg, hyperlipidemia Fredrickson Types I and V).

ADVERSE REACTIONS: Abdominal pain, headache, myalgia, constipation, nausea, atrial fibrillation, gastritis, diabetes mellitus, insomnia, vertigo, bronchitis, eczema, upper respiratory infections, urinary tract infections.

INTERACTIONS: See Contraindications. Avoid large quantities of grapefruit juice (>1 quart/day). Voriconazole may inhibit metabolism; may need to adjust dose. Increased risk of myopathy with fibrates; use with caution. Increased risk of myopathy, including rhabdomyolysis, with amiodarone, ranolazine, calcium channel blockers (eg, verapamil, diltiazem, amlodipine), lipid-modifying doses of niacin (≥1g/day niacin), colchicine, and CYP3A4 inhibitors; use caution. May slightly elevate plasma digoxin concentrations. May potentiate effect of coumarin anticoagulants; monitor PT.

PREGNANCY: Category X, not for use in nursing.

MECHANISM OF ACTION: HMG-CoA reductase inhibitor; specific inhibitor of HMG-CoA reductase, the enzyme that catalyzes the conversion of HMG-CoA to mevalonate, an early and rate limiting step in the biosynthetic pathway for cholesterol. Reduces VLDL and TG and increases HDL.

PHARMACOKINETICS: Absorption: T_{max}=4 hrs. **Distribution:** Plasma protein binding (95%). **Metabolism:** Liver (extensive 1st pass); β-hydroxyacid, 6'-hydroxy, 6'-hydroxymethyl, 6'-exomethylene derivatives (active metabolites). **Elimination:** Feces (60%), urine (13%).

NURSING CONSIDERATIONS

Assessment: Assess for active liver disease or unexplained persistent elevations in serum transaminases, risk factors for developing myopathy (eg, advanced age, uncontrolled hypothyroidism, renal impairment), severe renal impairment, pregnancy/nursing status, and possible drug interactions. Assess use in patients who consume substantial quantities of alcohol and/or have a past history of liver disease. Obtain baseline lipid profile (total-C, LDL, HDL, TG) and LFTs.

Z

Monitoring: Monitor for signs/symptoms of myopathy (eg, unexplained muscle pain, tenderness, weakness), rhabdomyolysis, and for liver dysfunction. Perform periodic monitoring of creatine kinase levels, LFTs, and lipid profile.

Patient Counseling: Advise to adhere to their National Cholesterol Education Program (NCEP) recommended diet, regular exercise program, and periodic testing of a fasting lipid panel. Inform of the risk of myopathy, including rhabdomyolysis; advise to contact physician immediately if unexplained muscle pain, tenderness, or weakness occurs. Inform patients who use the 80-mg dose that the risk of myopathy, including rhabdomyolysis, is increased. Inform that liver function will be checked prior to and during treatment; instruct to report promptly any symptoms that may indicate liver injury (eg, fatigue, anorexia, right upper abdominal discomfort, dark urine, jaundice). Inform women of childbearing age to use an effective method of birth control, stop taking drug if they become pregnant, and not to breastfeed while on therapy. Inform of the substances that should not be taken concomitantly with the drug.

Administration: Oral route. **Storage:** 5-30°C (41-86°F).

ZOFRAN   RX
ondansetron HCl (GlaxoSmithKline)

OTHER BRAND NAMES: Zofran Injection (GlaxoSmithKline)

THERAPEUTIC CLASS: 5-HT$_3$ receptor antagonist

INDICATIONS: Prevention of postoperative nausea and/or vomiting (PONV). Prevention of N/V associated with initial and repeat courses of emetogenic cancer chemotherapy, including high-dose cisplatin. (PO) Prevention of N/V associated with radiotherapy (total body irradiation, single high-dose fraction, or daily fractions to the abdomen).

DOSAGE: *Adults:* Prevention of Chemotherapy-Induced N/V: (Inj) 32mg single IV dose or three 0.15mg/kg IV doses; give 1st dose (over 15 min) 30 min before chemotherapy. For the 3-dose regimen, give subsequent doses 4 and 8 hrs after 1st dose. Prevention of N/V Associated with Highly Emetogenic Chemotherapy: (Tab) 24mg (given as three 8mg tabs) 30 min before chemotherapy. Prevention of N/V Associated with Moderately Emetogenic Chemotherapy: (PO) 8mg bid; give 1st dose 30 min before chemotherapy, then 8 hrs later, then q12h for 1-2 days after completion of chemotherapy. Prevention of PONV: (Inj) 4mg IM/IV undiluted immediately before induction of anesthesia or postoperatively if prophylactic antiemetic was not received and N/V occurs within 2 hrs after surgery. As IV, infuse over 2-5 min. (PO) 16mg 1 hr before induction of anesthesia. Prevention of N/V Associated with Radiation Therapy: (PO) Usual: 8mg tid. Total Body Irradiation: (PO) 8mg 1-2 hrs before each therapy. Single High-Dose Therapy Fraction Radiotherapy to Abdomen: (PO) 8mg 1-2 hrs before therapy then q8h after 1st dose for 1-2 days after completion of therapy. Daily Fractionated Radiotherapy to Abdomen: (PO) 8mg 1-2 hrs before therapy then q8h after 1st dose for each day radiotherapy is given. (Inj/PO) Severe Hepatic Dysfunction (Child-Pugh ≥10): Max: 8mg/day. (Inj) Give (over 15 min) 30 min prior to emetogenic chemotherapy. *Pediatrics:* Prevention of Chemotherapy-Induced N/V: (Inj) 6 months-18 yrs: Three 0.15mg/kg doses; infuse over 15 min. Give 1st dose 30 min before chemotherapy, then 4 and 8 hrs after the 1st dose. Prevention of N/V Associated with Moderately Emetogenic Cancer Chemotherapy: (PO) ≥12 yrs: 8mg bid; give 1st dose 30 min before chemotherapy, then 8 hrs later, then q12h for 1-2 days after completion of chemotherapy. 4-11 yrs: 4mg tid; give 1st dose 30 min before chemotherapy, then 4 and 8 hrs after 1st dose, then q8h for 1-2 days after completion of chemotherapy. Prevention of PONV: (Inj) 1 month-12 yrs: >40kg: 4mg IV single dose. ≤40kg: 0.1mg/kg IV single dose. Infuse over 2-5 min immediately before or after induction of anesthesia or postoperatively if prophylactic antiemetic was not received and N/V occurs shortly after surgery. (Inj/PO) Severe Hepatic Dysfunction (Child Pugh ≥10): Max: 8mg/day. (Inj) Give (over 15 min) 30 min prior to emetogenic chemotherapy.

HOW SUPPLIED: Inj: 2mg/mL [2mL, 20mL]; Sol: 4mg/5mL [50mL]; Tab/Tab, Disintegrating (ODT): 4mg, 8mg

CONTRAINDICATIONS: Concomitant use with apomorphine.

WARNINGS/PRECAUTIONS: Hypersensitivity reactions reported in patients hypersensitive to other 5-HT$_3$ receptor antagonists. ECG changes, including QT interval prolongation and torsade de pointes, reported. Avoid with congenital QT syndrome. Monitor ECG for patients with electrolyte abnormalities (eg, hypokalemia or hypomagnesemia), congestive heart failure, bradyarrhythmias, or patients taking other medications that lead to QT prolongation. May mask progressive ileus and/or gastric distension following abdominal surgery, or with chemotherapy induced N/V. Does not stimulate gastric/intestinal peristalsis; do not use instead of NG suction. (ODT) Contains phenylalanine; caution in phenylketonurics.

ADVERSE REACTIONS: Headache, diarrhea, constipation, (Inj) drowsiness/sedation, injection-site reaction, fever, (PO) malaise/fatigue, dizziness.

INTERACTIONS: See Contraindications. Inducers or inhibitors of CYP3A4, CYP2D6, CYP1A2 may change the clearance and half-life of ondansetron. Potent CYP3A4 inducers (eg, phenytoin, carbamazepine, rifampicin) may significantly increase clearance and decrease blood concentration of ondansetron. May reduce analgesic activity of tramadol.

PREGNANCY: Category B, caution in nursing.

MECHANISM OF ACTION: Selective 5-HT$_3$ receptor antagonist; not established. Blocks 5-HT$_3$ receptors from serotonin, which may stimulate vagal afferents through the 5-HT$_3$ receptors and initiate the vomiting reflex.

PHARMACOKINETICS: Absorption: Various age groups resulted in different parameters. (PO) Well-absorbed from GI tract; bioavailability (56%). **Distribution:** Plasma protein binding (70-76%). **Metabolism:** Extensive; via CYP3A4, 1A2, 2D6; hydroxylation (primary), glucuronide/sulfate conjugation. **Elimination:** Urine (5%).

NURSING CONSIDERATIONS

Assessment: Assess for hepatic impairment, pregnancy/nursing status, hypersensitivity, and possible drug interactions. If planning to use ODT, assess for phenylketonuria.

Monitoring: Monitor signs/symptoms of ECG changes, hypersensitivity reactions, and LFT abnormalities. In patients who recently underwent abdominal surgery or in patients with chemotherapy-induced N/V, monitor for masking of signs of a progressive ileus and/or gastric distension.

Patient Counseling: (ODT) Do not remove from blister until just prior to dosing; do not push through foil. Use dry hands to peel blister backing completely off blister. Remove gently and immediately place on tongue to dissolve and swallow with saliva. Inform that ODT contains phenylalanine. (Inj) Inform patients that hypersensitivity reactions may occur; advise to report any signs and symptoms (eg, fever, chills, rash, or breathing problems). Advise to report the use of all medications, especially apomorphine; may cause significant drop in blood pressure and loss of consciousness. Inform patient that headache, drowsiness/sedation, constipation, fever, and diarrhea may occur.

Administration: IM/IV/Oral routes. Refer to PI for reconstitution procedures. **Storage:** (Inj/Sol/Tab) Protect from light. (Inj/ODT/Tab) 2-30°C (36-86°F). (Sol) 15-30°C (59-86°F); store upright. (Inj) Diluted Sol: 0.9% NaCl, D5W, 0.9% NaCl & D5W, 0.45% NaCl & D5W, or 3% NaCl: Stable at room temperature for 48 hrs under normal lighting. Do not use beyond 24 hrs after dilution.

ZOLADEX 1-MONTH   RX
goserelin acetate (AstraZeneca)

THERAPEUTIC CLASS: Synthetic gonadotropin releasing hormone analog

INDICATIONS: Palliative treatment of advanced prostatic carcinoma and advanced breast cancer in pre- and perimenopausal women. In combination with flutamide for management of locally confined Stage T2b-T4 (Stage B2-C) prostatic carcinoma. Management of endometriosis, including pain relief and reduction of endometriotic lesions. Use as an endometrial-thinning agent prior to endometrial ablation for dysfunctional uterine bleeding.

DOSAGE: *Adults:* Inject SQ every 28 days into anterior abdominal wall below navel line. Advanced Prostatic Carcinoma/Breast Cancer: 3.6mg every 28 days. Stage B2-C Prostatic Carcinoma: 3.6mg starting 8 weeks before radiotherapy, then 10.8mg formulation 28 days after 1st injection, or 3.6mg at 28-day intervals for 4 doses (2 before and 2 during radiotherapy). Endometriosis: 3.6mg every 28 days for 6 months. Endometrial Thinning: 3.6mg then surgery 4 weeks later, or 2 doses of 3.6mg (given 4 weeks apart) followed by surgery 2-4 weeks after 2nd dose.

HOW SUPPLIED: Implant: 3.6mg

CONTRAINDICATIONS: Pregnancy (unless used for palliative treatment of advanced breast cancer).

WARNINGS/PRECAUTIONS: Premenopausal women should use nonhormonal contraception during therapy and for 12 weeks post-therapy. Transient worsening of symptoms or occurrence of additional signs/symptoms of prostate/breast cancer may occur during initial therapy. Temporary increase in bone pain may occur. Ureteral obstruction and spinal cord compression reported with prostate cancer. Hyperglycemia, increased risk of developing diabetes/myocardial infarction (MI), sudden cardiac death, and stroke reported in men. Hypercalcemia reported in prostate/breast cancer patients with bone metastases; initiate appropriate treatment measures if it occurs. Hypersensitivity, antibody formation, and acute anaphylactic reactions may occur. Caution when dilating the cervix for endometrial ablation; may increase cervical resistance. Retreatment cannot be recommended for management of endometriosis; consider monitoring bone mineral density (BMD) if further treatment is contemplated. May suppress pituitary-gonadal system in therapeutic doses; normal function is usually restored 12 weeks after d/c treatment.

Z

ADVERSE REACTIONS: Hot flushes, sexual dysfunction, decreased erections, seborrhea, peripheral edema, breast enlargement/atrophy, pain, vaginitis, emotional lability, decreased libido, sweating, depression, headache, acne.

INTERACTIONS: Ovarian hyperstimulation syndrome reported with other gonadotropins.

PREGNANCY: Category X (endometriosis and endometrial thinning), Category D (advanced breast cancer), not for use in nursing.

MECHANISM OF ACTION: Synthetic decapeptide analog of GnRH; acts as an inhibitor of pituitary gonadotropin secretion. In males, causes initial increase in serum LH and FSH levels, causing subsequent increases in serum testosterone levels; chronic administration suppresses pituitary gonadotropins, causing fall in testosterone levels to post-castration levels. In females, chronic exposure causes decrease in serum estradiol to levels consistent with postmenopausal state, leading to reduction of ovarian size and function, reduction in size of uterus and mammary gland, and regression of sex hormone-responsive tumors.

PHARMACOKINETICS: Absorption: (Males) C_{max}=2.84ng/mL, T_{max}=12-15 days, AUC=27.8ng•day/mL; (Females) C_{max}=1.46ng/mL, T_{max}=8-22 days, AUC=18.5ng•day/mL. **Distribution:** V_d=44.1L (Males), 20.3L (Females); plasma protein binding (27.3%). **Metabolism:** Hydrolysis of C-terminal amino acids. **Elimination:** Urine (>90%, 20% unchanged); $T_{1/2}$=4.2 hrs (Sol).

NURSING CONSIDERATIONS

Assessment: Assess for hypersensitivity, cardiovascular disease (CVD), diabetes mellitus (DM), bone metastases, ureteral obstruction, spinal cord compression, pregnancy/nursing status, and possible drug interactions. Obtain baseline vital signs and weight, serum testosterone/cholesterol/blood glucose levels, PSA, LFTs.

Monitoring: Monitor for tumor flare, ureteral obstruction, spinal cord compression, renal impairment, hypersensitivity reactions, pituitary apoplexy, sexual dysfunction, occurrence/worsening of signs/symptoms of prostate/breast cancer, bone pain, signs/symptoms suggestive of development of CVD, and hypercalcemia. Monitor BMD, serum testosterone/cholesterol/blood glucose levels, glycosylated Hgb (HbA1c), PSA, LFTs.

Patient Counseling: Inform men that risk of developing ureteral obstruction, spinal cord compression, reduction in BMD, DM or loss of glycemic control with DM, MI, sudden cardiac death, and stroke may occur. Inform women that menstruation should stop with effective doses. Counsel women about potential side effects (regular menstrual bleeding, allergic reactions, hypoestrogenism, reduction in BMD, and amenorrhea); seek medical attention if any occur. Advise against pregnancy and/or breastfeeding except for palliative treatment of advanced breast cancer. Instruct to d/c use if pregnancy occurs during treatment for endometriosis/endometrial thinning. Advise premenopausal women to use nonhormonal contraception during and 12 weeks after treatment ends. Counsel to avoid initiating treatment with abnormal vaginal bleeding or known allergy. Advise to avoid use for periods >6 months in treatment of benign gynecological conditions.

Administration: SQ route. Inject into anterior abdominal wall below navel line. See PI for extensive details of administration. **Storage:** <25°C (77°F).

ZOLADEX 3-MONTH   RX
goserelin acetate (AstraZeneca)

THERAPEUTIC CLASS: Synthetic gonadotropin releasing hormone analog

INDICATIONS: Palliative treatment of advanced prostatic carcinoma. In combination with flutamide for management of locally confined Stage T2b-T4 (Stage B2-C) prostatic carcinoma.

DOSAGE: *Adults:* Inject SQ q12 weeks into anterior abdominal wall below navel line. Stage B2-C Prostatic Carcinoma: Use 3.6mg formulation starting 8 weeks before radiotherapy, then 10.8mg formulation 28 days after 1st injection. Advanced Prostatic Carcinoma: 10.8mg q12 weeks.

HOW SUPPLIED: Implant: 10.8mg

CONTRAINDICATIONS: Pregnancy.

WARNINGS/PRECAUTIONS: Goserelin 10.8mg is not indicated in women. Tumor flare phenomenon observed; transient worsening of symptoms (or occurrence of additional signs/symptoms) of prostate cancer with initial therapy. Ureteral obstruction and spinal cord compression reported. Temporary increase in bone pain may occur. Hypersensitivity, antibody formation, and acute anaphylactic reactions may occur. Hyperglycemia, increased risk of developing diabetes/myocardial infarction (MI), sudden cardiac death, and stroke reported. May suppress pituitary-gonadal system in therapeutic doses and mislead diagnostic tests of pituitary-gonadotropic and gonadal functions during treatment.

ADVERSE REACTIONS: Hot flashes, diarrhea, pain, asthenia, gynecomastia, pelvic/bone pain, erectile/sexual dysfunction and lower urinary tract symptoms.

Z

PREGNANCY: Category X, not for use in nursing.

MECHANISM OF ACTION: Synthetic decapeptide analog of GnRH; acts as an inhibitor of pituitary gonadotropin secretion. In males, causes initial increase in serum LH and FSH levels, causing subsequent increases in serum testosterone levels; chronic administration suppresses pituitary gonadotropins, causing fall in testosterone levels to postcastration levels.

PHARMACOKINETICS: Absorption: C_{max}=8.85ng/mL; T_{max}=1.8 hrs. **Distribution:** V_d=44.1L; plasma protein binding (27%). **Metabolism:** Hydrolysis of C-terminal amino acids. **Elimination:** Urine (>90%, 20% unchanged); $T_{1/2}$=4.2 hrs.

NURSING CONSIDERATIONS

Assessment: Assess for hypersensitivity, history of cardiovascular disease (CVD), diabetes mellitus (DM), bone metastases, ureteral obstruction, spinal cord compression, and possible drug interactions. Obtain baseline serum testosterone/cholesterol/blood glucose levels, prostate-specific antigen (PSA), LFTs.

Monitoring: Monitor for signs/symptoms of worsening prostate cancer, tumor flare, ureteral obstruction, spinal cord compression, renal impairment, hypersensitivity reactions, pituitary apoplexy, signs/symptoms of CVD, and hypercalcemia, bone mineral density, serum testosterone/cholesterol/blood glucose levels, glycosylated Hgb (HbA1c), PSA, and LFTs.

Patient Counseling: Inform men of the risk of developing ureteral obstruction, spinal cord compression, reduction in BMD, DM or loss of glycemic control with DM, MI, sudden cardiac death, and stroke. Advise to inform physician if other adverse events occur.

Administration: SQ route. Inject into anterior abdominal wall below navel line. Refer to PI for proper administration. **Storage:** <25°C (77°F).

ZOLINZA   RX
vorinostat (Merck)

THERAPEUTIC CLASS: Histone deacetylase inhibitor

INDICATIONS: Treatment of cutaneous manifestations in patients with cutaneous T-cell lymphoma who have progressive, persistent, or recurrent disease on or following 2 systemic therapies.

DOSAGE: *Adults:* 400mg PO qd. Intolerant to Therapy: May reduce to 300mg PO qd. May further reduce to 300mg PO qd for 5 consecutive days each week. Take with food.

HOW SUPPLIED: Cap: 100mg

WARNINGS/PRECAUTIONS: Pulmonary embolism and deep vein thrombosis (DVT) reported. Dose-related thrombocytopenia and anemia may occur; modify dose or d/c therapy if platelet counts and/or Hgb are reduced. GI disturbances (eg, N/V, diarrhea) reported; replace fluid and electrolytes to prevent dehydration. Adequately control pre-existing N/V and diarrhea before beginning therapy. Hyperglycemia observed; monitor serum glucose, especially in diabetics or potentially diabetics. Monitor blood cell counts and chemistry tests, including electrolytes (eg, K^+, magnesium, calcium), glucose, and SrCr every 2 weeks during 1st 2 months of therapy and monthly thereafter. May cause fetal harm. Caution with renal/hepatic impairment.

ADVERSE REACTIONS: Diarrhea, fatigue, N/V, thrombocytopenia, anorexia, dysgeusia, decreased weight, muscle spasms, alopecia, dry mouth, increased SrCr, chills, constipation, hyperglycemia, proteinuria.

INTERACTIONS: Prolongation of PT and INR observed with coumarin-derivative anticoagulants. Severe thrombocytopenia and GI bleeding reported with other histone deacetylase inhibitors (eg, valproic acid).

PREGNANCY: Category D, not for use in nursing.

MECHANISM OF ACTION: Histone deacetylase inhibitor; inhibits activity of histone deacetylases (HDACs) allowing for accumulation of acetyl groups on the histone lysine residues, resulting in open chromatin structure and transcriptional activation.

PHARMACOKINETICS: Absorption: (Fasted) C_{max}=1.2μM, T_{max}=1.5 hrs, AUC=4.2μM•hr. (Fed) C_{max}=1.2μM, T_{max}=4 hrs, AUC=6.0μM•hr. **Distribution:** Plasma protein binding (71%). **Metabolism:** Liver, via glucuronidation, hydrolysis, and β-oxidation. **Elimination:** Urine (<1% unchanged); $T_{1/2}$=2 hrs.

NURSING CONSIDERATIONS

Assessment: Assess for renal/hepatic impairment, history of thromboembolism, GI disturbances, diabetes, fluid imbalance, cardiac symptoms, pregnancy/nursing status, and possible drug interactions. Assess for hypokalemia and hypomagnesemia; correct prior to therapy.

Monitoring: Monitor for signs/symptoms of pulmonary embolism; monitor for signs and symptoms particularly in patients with prior history of thromboembolic events. Monitor for DVT, thrombocytopenia, anemia, GI disturbances, dehydration, and hyperglycemia. Monitor blood cell counts, chemistry tests, electrolytes, serum glucose, and SrCr every 2 weeks for 1st 2 months and monthly thereafter.

Patient Counseling: Inform about risks and benefits of therapy. Counsel to take with food, not to open or crush, and to drink ≥2L/day of fluid to prevent dehydration. Instruct to contact physician if excessive vomiting, diarrhea, unusual bleeding, signs of DVT, and if other adverse events develop. Instruct to read patient insert carefully.

Administration: Oral route. Do not open or crush. Avoid direct contact of powder in caps with skin or mucous membranes. Avoid exposure to crushed and/or broken caps. **Storage:** 20-25°C (68-77°F); excursions permitted between 15-30°C (59-86°F).

ZOLOFT   RX
sertraline HCl (Pfizer)

> Antidepressants increased the risk of suicidal thinking and behavior (suicidality) in short-term studies in children, adolescents, and young adults with major depressive disorder (MDD) and other psychiatric disorders. Monitor and observe closely for clinical worsening, suicidality, or unusual changes in behavior in patients who are started on antidepressant therapy. Not approved for use in pediatric patients except for patients with obsessive compulsive disorder (OCD).

THERAPEUTIC CLASS: Selective serotonin reuptake inhibitor

INDICATIONS: Treatment of MDD, social anxiety disorder (SAD), panic disorder with/without agoraphobia, premenstrual dysphoric disorder, and posttraumatic stress disorder (PTSD) in adults. Treatment of OCD in patients ≥6 yrs.

DOSAGE: *Adults:* MDD/OCD: 50mg qd. Max: 200mg/day. Panic Disorder/PTSD/SAD: Initial: 25mg qd. Titrate: Increase to 50mg qd after 1 week. Adjust dose at intervals of no less than 1 week. Max: 200mg/day. Premenstrual Dysphoric Disorder: Initial: 50mg qd continuous or limited to luteal phase of cycle. Titrate: Increase to 50mg/cycle up to 150mg/day for continuous or 100mg/day for luteal phase dosing if needed. If 100mg/day is established for luteal phase dosing, use a 50mg/day titration step for 3 days at the beginning of each luteal phase dosing period. Reassess to determine need for maintenance treatment. Hepatic Impairment: Use lower or less frequent doses. *Pediatrics:* OCD: Initial: 6-12 yrs: 25mg qd. 13-17 yrs: 50mg qd. Titrate: Adjust dose at intervals of no less than 1 week. Max: 200mg/day. Reassess to determine need for maintenance treatment. Hepatic Impairment: Use lower or less frequent doses.

HOW SUPPLIED: Sol: 20mg/mL [60mL]; Tab: 25mg*, 50mg*, 100mg* *scored

CONTRAINDICATIONS: MAOI use during or within 14 days after d/c or concomitant pimozide use. Concomitant disulfiram with concentrate solution.

WARNINGS/PRECAUTIONS: Not approved for treatment of bipolar depression; screen for risk factors for bipolar disorder prior to initiation of therapy. Serotonin syndrome (eg, mental status changes, autonomic instability, neuromuscular aberrations, GI symptoms) and neuroleptic malignant syndrome (NMS)-like reactions reported. Activation of mania/hypomania and altered platelet function reported. Changes in appetite and weight loss reported. Dysphoric mood, irritability, agitation, dizziness, sensory disturbances, anxiety, confusion, headache, lethargy, emotional lability, insomnia, hypomania reported upon d/c; avoid abrupt withdrawal. May increase risk of bleeding events. Caution with seizure disorder, diseases/conditions that could affect hemodynamic responses or metabolism, and hepatic impairment. Hyponatremia reported; caution in elderly and volume-depleted patients. Diabetes mellitus reported; carefully monitor glycemic control. Caution in 3rd trimester of pregnancy due to risk of serious neonatal complications. May impair mental/physical abilities.

ADVERSE REACTIONS: Ejaculation failure, dry mouth, increased sweating, somnolence, tremor, anorexia, dizziness, headache, diarrhea, dyspepsia, N/V, agitation, insomnia, nervousness, abnormal vision.

INTERACTIONS: See Contraindications. Not recommended with tryptophan, serotonin and norepinephrine reuptake inhibitors (SNRIs), and other SSRIs. May shift concentrations with other tightly plasma-bound drugs (eg, warfarin, digitoxin). Caution with other CNS active drugs; monitor lithium, phenytoin, valproate levels with appropriate dose adjustments. May potentiate drugs metabolized by CYP2D6 with a narrow therapeutic index (eg, TCAs for treatment of MDD, type 1C antiarrhythmics). Rare cases of weakness, hyperreflexia and incoordination reported with SSRIs and sumatriptan. May induce metabolism of cisapride. Increased risk of bleeding reported with NSAIDs and aspirin (ASA). Altered anticoagulant effects reported with warfarin. Serotonin syndrome/NMS-like reactions reported with serotonergic drugs (eg, triptans, fentanyl, linezolid, tramadol, or St. John's wort), drugs that impair metabolism of serotonin, antipsychotics, and dopamine antagonists. Avoid alcohol.

PREGNANCY: Category C, caution in nursing.

MECHANISM OF ACTION: SSRI; inhibits CNS neuronal uptake of serotonin.

Z

PHARMACOKINETICS: Absorption: T_{max}=4.5-8.4 hrs. **Distribution:** Plasma protein binding (98%). **Metabolism:** Liver (extensive); N-demethylation, oxidative deamination, reduction, hydroxylation, glucuronide conjugation. **Elimination:** Feces (12-14% unchanged), urine (minor); $T_{1/2}$=26 hrs.

NURSING CONSIDERATIONS

Assessment: Assess for risk of bipolar disorder, history of seizures, diseases/conditions that alter metabolism or hemodynamic response, volume depletion, hepatic/renal impairment, MAOI or pimozide therapy, pregnancy/nursing status, and possible drug interactions. Obtain baseline vital signs and weight.

Monitoring: Monitor for worsening of depression, emergence of suicidal ideation, or unusual changes in behavior. Monitor for signs/symptoms of serotonin syndrome, NMS-like reactions, hyponatremia, and other adverse events. Monitor vital signs, platelets, PT, serum Na+, and glycemic control. Periodically monitor height and weight of pediatric patients.

Patient Counseling: Counsel about benefits, risks, and appropriate use of therapy. Advise to seek medical attention if symptoms of suicidality, activation of mania, seizures, clinical worsening, hyponatremia, and other adverse events occur, including those occurring upon d/c. Inform about risk of serotonin syndrome with concomitant triptans, tramadol, or other serotonergic agents. Advise to use caution when performing hazardous tasks (eg, operating machinery, driving). Inform that concomitant use with NSAIDs, ASA, warfarin, and other drugs that affect coagulation may increase the risk of bleeding. Counsel to avoid alcohol and to use caution when using over-the-counter products. Advise to notify physician if pregnant, intend to become pregnant or breastfeeding. Instruct to mix sol with 4 oz. water, ginger ale, lemon/lime soda, lemonade, or orange juice only and not mix with any other liquids, and to take dose immediately after mixing. Inform that dropper contains dry natural rubber and to use caution if with latex sensitivity.

Administration: Oral route. **Storage:** 25°C (77°F); excursions permitted to 15-30°C (59-86°F).

ZOLPIMIST

zolpidem tartrate (ECR)

`CIV`

THERAPEUTIC CLASS: Imidazopyridine hypnotic

INDICATIONS: Short-term treatment of insomnia characterized by difficulties with sleep initiation.

DOSAGE: *Adults:* Individualize dose. 10mg qhs. Max: 10mg/day. Elderly/Debilitated/Hepatic Insufficiency: 5mg qhs.

HOW SUPPLIED: Spray: 5mg/spray [8.2g]

WARNINGS/PRECAUTIONS: Initiate only after careful evaluation; failure of insomnia to remit after 7-10 days of treatment may indicate presence of primary psychiatric and/or medical illness. Severe anaphylactic and anaphylactoid reactions reported; do not rechallenge if angioedema develops. Abnormal thinking, behavioral changes, visual/auditory hallucinations, and complex behavior (eg, sleep-driving) reported. Worsening of depression, including suicidal thoughts and actions, reported in primarily depressed patients. Withdrawal symptoms may occur with rapid dose reduction or abrupt d/c. Should only be administered immediately prior to going to bed. May impair mental/physical abilities. Closely monitor elderly and debilitated patients for impaired motor and/or cognitive performance and unusual sensitivity. Respiratory insufficiency reported mostly in patients with preexisting respiratory impairment. Caution with diseases/conditions that could affect metabolism or hemodynamic responses, compromised respiratory function, sleep apnea syndrome, myasthenia gravis, and depression. Closely monitor patients with renal/hepatic impairment and history of drug/alcohol addiction or abuse.

ADVERSE REACTIONS: Drowsiness, headache, dizziness, allergy, sinusitis, lethargy, drugged feelings, pharyngitis, dry mouth, back pain, diarrhea, N/V.

INTERACTIONS: Caution with CNS-active drugs. CNS depressants may potentially enhance effects; consider dose adjustment. Avoid with alcohol. Additive effect of decreased alertness reported with imipramine or chlorpromazine. Additive effect on psychomotor performance with chlorpromazine or alcohol. May decrease levels of imipramine. Fluoxetine may increase $T_{1/2}$. Increased C_{max} and decreased T_{max} reported with sertraline in females. CYP3A inhibitors (eg, itraconazole, ketoconazole) may increase exposure; use caution and reduce dose with ketoconazole. Rifampin may decrease levels.

PREGNANCY: Category C, safety not known in nursing.

MECHANISM OF ACTION: Imidazopyridine, non-benzodiazepine hypnotic; interacts with a gamma-aminobutyric acid-BZ receptor complex and preferentially binds to the BZ_1 receptor with a high affinity ratio of the α_1/α_5 subunits.

PHARMACOKINETICS: Absorption: Rapid, from oral mucosa and GI tract. C_{max}=114ng/mL (5mg), 210ng/mL (10mg); T_{max}=0.9 hrs. **Distribution:** Plasma protein binding (92.5%); found in breast milk. **Elimination:** Renal; $T_{1/2}$=2.7 hrs (5mg), 3 hrs (10mg).

Z

NURSING CONSIDERATIONS

Assessment: Assess for primary psychiatric and/or medical illness, diseases/conditions that could affect metabolism or hemodynamic responses, compromised respiratory function, sleep apnea syndrome, myasthenia gravis, renal/hepatic impairment, depression, history of drug/ alcohol addiction or abuse, previous hypersensitivity to the drug, pregnancy/nursing status, and possible drug interactions.

Monitoring: Monitor for anaphylactic/anaphylactoid reactions, angioedema, abnormal thinking, behavioral changes, withdrawal effects, motor/cognitive impairment, and other adverse reactions. Monitor patients with renal/hepatic impairment, or with history of drug/alcohol addiction or abuse.

Patient Counseling: Inform of the benefits, risks, and appropriate use of therapy. Advise to immediately seek medical attention if any anaphylactic/anaphylactoid reactions occur. Advise to notify physician of all concomitant medications. Instruct to immediately report events such as sleep-driving and other complex behaviors. Counsel to take drug just before hs and only when able to stay in bed a full night (7-8 hrs) before being active again. Advise not to take drug with or immediately after a meal, and when drinking alcohol.

Administration: Oral route. Hold upright with the spray opening pointed directly into the mouth and then fully press down on the pump over the tongue. Prime pump before 1st time use (5 sprays) or if not used for at least 14 days (1 spray); refer to PI. **Storage:** 25°C (77°F); excursions permitted to 15-30°C (59-86°F). Store upright. Do not freeze. Avoid prolonged exposure to temperatures >30°C (>86°F).

ZOMETA

RX

zoledronic acid (Novartis)

THERAPEUTIC CLASS: Bisphosphonate

INDICATIONS: Treatment of hypercalcemia of malignancy. Treatment of multiple myeloma and bone metastases from solid tumors, in conjunction with antineoplastic therapy.

DOSAGE: *Adults:* Hypercalcemia of Malignancy: Max: 4mg IV infused over no less than 15 min. Retreatment (if necessary): Wait ≥7 days from initial dose. Multiple Myeloma/Bone Metastases: CrCl >60mL/min: 4mg IV infused over no less than 15 min q3-4 weeks. CrCl 50-60mL/min: 3.5mg. CrCl 40-49mL/min: 3.3mg. CrCl 30-39mL/min: 3mg. Measure SrCr prior to each dose. Withhold treatment with renal deterioration; resume when SrCr returns to within 10% of baseline. Administer with PO calcium 500mg qd and multiple vitamin containing 400 IU of vitamin D qd.

HOW SUPPLIED: Inj: 4mg/5mL, 4mg/100mL

WARNINGS/PRECAUTIONS: Contains same active ingredient as Reclast; do not treat concomitantly. Adequately rehydrate before use with hypercalcemia of malignancy. Monitor hypercalcemia-related metabolic parameters (eg, serum calcium, phosphate, and magnesium). Use with caution in patients with hypercalcemia of malignancy with severe renal impairment. Not recommended with bone metastases with severe renal impairment. Osteonecrosis of the jaw (ONJ) reported; perform dental exam prior to therapy and maintain good oral hygiene. Avoid invasive dental procedures during therapy. Severe and occasionally incapacitating bone, joint, and/or muscle pain reported; d/c if severe symptoms develop. Atypical subtrochanteric and diaphyseal femoral fractures reported; examine contralateral femur in patients who have sustained femoral shaft fracture. D/C therapy pending evaluation if atypical femur fracture is suspected. Caution with aspirin (ASA) sensitivity; bronchoconstriction reported. May cause fetal harm.

ADVERSE REACTIONS: Bone pain, N/V, fever, abnormal SrCr, fatigue, anemia, constipation, dyspnea, diarrhea, weakness, myalgia, cough, arthralgia, edema lower limb.

INTERACTIONS: Caution with aminoglycosides; may have an additive effect to lower serum calcium level for prolonged periods. Loop diuretics may increase risk of hypocalcemia; do not use until patient is rehydrated and use with caution. Caution with other nephrotoxic drugs. May increase risk of atypical femur fractures with glucocorticoids (eg, prednisone, dexamethasone).

PREGNANCY: Category D, not for use in nursing.

MECHANISM OF ACTION: Bisphosphonate; inhibits bone resorption by inhibiting osteoclastic activity and inducing osteoclast apoptosis. Also blocks osteoclastic resorption of mineralized bone and cartilage through binding to bone.

PHARMACOKINETICS: Distribution: Plasma protein binding (28% at 200ng/mL), (53% at 50ng/mL). **Elimination:** Urine (39%); $T_{1/2}$=146 hrs.

NURSING CONSIDERATIONS

Assessment: Assess for hypersensitivity, ASA hypersensitivity, pregnancy/nursing status, possible drug interactions, and risk factors for ONJ. Assess renal function and hydration status. Perform dental exam with preventive dentistry prior to treatment.

Z

Monitoring: Monitor renal function, standard hypercalcemia-related parameters, and hydration status. Monitor for ONJ, local infection, osteomyelitis, musculoskeletal pain, atypical fracture, bronchoconstriction, hypersensitivity reactions, and other adverse events that may develop.

Patient Counseling: Instruct to notify physician of kidney problems. Inform that drug may cause fetal harm; avoid becoming pregnant and breastfeeding. Advise to maintain good oral hygiene, have dental exam prior to therapy, and avoid invasive dental procedures. Advise to take PO calcium supplement of 500mg and multiple vitamins containing 400 IU of vitamin D daily if with multiple myeloma or bone metastasis of solid tumors. Advise to report any thigh, hip, or groin pain. Inform about the most common adverse events that may develop. Instruct to notify physician if ASA sensitive.

Administration: IV route. Refer to PI for proper preparation of sol and method of administration. **Storage:** 25°C (77°F); excursions permitted to 15-30°C (59-86°F). Reconstituted Sol: 2-8°C (36-46°F). Equilibrate to room temperature before administration. Total time between dilution, storage in the refrigerator, and end of administration must not exceed 24 hrs.

ZOMIG   RX
zolmitriptan (AstraZeneca)

OTHER BRAND NAMES: Zomig Nasal Spray (AstraZeneca) - Zomig-ZMT (AstraZeneca)

THERAPEUTIC CLASS: 5-HT$_{1B/1D}$ agonist

INDICATIONS: Acute treatment of migraine attacks with or without aura.

DOSAGE: *Adults:* (Spray) 5mg single dose; may repeat once after 2 hrs. Max: 10mg/24 hrs. Safety of treating >4 headaches/30 days unknown. (Tab) Initial: 2.5mg or lower (2.5mg tab may be broken in 1/2); may repeat after 2 hrs. Max: 10mg/24 hrs. Safety of treating >3 headaches/30 days unknown. (ZMT) 2.5mg single dose; may repeat after 2 hrs. Max: 10mg/24 hrs. Dissolve on tongue without water. Safety of treating >3 headaches/30 days unknown. Hepatic Impairment: Use low dose and monitor blood pressure.

HOW SUPPLIED: Nasal Spray: 5mg [0.1mL, 6°]; Tab: 2.5mg*, 5mg; Tab, Disintegrating: (ZMT) 2.5mg, 5mg *scored

CONTRAINDICATIONS: Ischemic heart disease, coronary artery vasospasm (eg, Prinzmetal's angina), uncontrolled HTN, cerebrovascular syndromes, other significant cardiovascular disease, hemiplegic or basilar migraine, MAOI use during or within 14 days, other 5-HT$_1$ agonist or ergot containing medications/ergot-type agent (eg, dihydroergotamine, methysergide) use within 24 hrs.

WARNINGS/PRECAUTIONS: Confirm migraine diagnosis. Supervise 1st dose and monitor cardiac function in those at risk of CAD (eg, HTN, hypercholesterolemia, smoker, obesity, diabetes, CAD family history, postmenopausal women, males >40 yrs). Serious adverse cardiac events, cerebrovascular events, vasospastic reactions reported with 5-HT$_1$ agonists. Disintegrating tabs contain phenylalanine. Caution with hepatic dysfunction. Reconsider diagnosis before 2nd dose, if no response seen after 1st dose. Serotonin syndrome symptoms (eg, mental status changes, autonomic instability, neuromuscular aberrations, and GI symptoms) reported. Avoid in patients with symptomatic Wolff-Parkinson-White syndrome or arrhythmias associated with other cardiac accessory conduction pathway disorders.

ADVERSE REACTIONS: Paresthesia, hyperesthesia, asthenia, warm/cold sensation, neck/throat/jaw pain, dry mouth, nausea, dizziness, somnolence, unusual taste (nasal spray).

INTERACTIONS: See Contraindications. Ergot-containing agents may prolong vasospastic reactions. Serotonin syndrome reported with combined use of an SSRI or SNRI. Half-life and AUC doubled with cimetidine.

PREGNANCY: Category C, caution in nursing.

MECHANISM OF ACTION: 5-HT$_{1D/1B}$ agonist; binds with high affinity to 5-HT$_{1D/1B}$ receptors on intracranial vessels (including arteriovenous anastomoses) and sensory nerves of trigeminal system, which results in cranial vessel constriction and inhibition of pro-inflammatory neuropeptide release.

PHARMACOKINETICS: Absorption: Well-absorbed; absolute bioavailability (40%); T$_{max}$=3 hrs (ODT/Nasal Spray), 1.5 hrs (Tab). **Distribution:** (Oral) V$_d$=7L/kg, (Nasal Spray) V$_d$=8.4L/kg. Plasma protein binding (25%). **Metabolism:** N-desmethyl (active metabolite). **Elimination:** Urine (65%, 8% unchanged), feces (30% Oral); T$_{1/2}$=3 hrs (Nasal Spray).

NURSING CONSIDERATIONS

Assessment: Confirm diagnosis of migraine before therapy. Assess for ischemic heart disease (eg, angina pectoris, Prinzmetal's variant angina, MI or documented silent MI), HTN, hemiplegic or basilar migraine, presence of risk factors for CAD (eg, hypercholesterolemia, smoking, obesity, DM, strong family history of CAD, female with surgical or physiological menopause, or male

Z

>40 yrs), ECG changes, hepatic/renal impairment, pregnancy/nursing status, and possible drug interactions.

Monitoring: Administration of 1st dose should be in physician's office or medically staffed and equipped facility as cardiac ischemia may occur in absence of clinical symptoms. ECG should be obtained immediately after administration in those with risk factors. Monitor for signs/symptoms of cardiac events (eg, coronary vasospasm, acute MI, arrhythmia, ECG changes, follow-up coronary angiography), cerebrovascular events (eg, hemorrhage, stroke, TIAs), peripheral vascular ischemia, colonic ischemia with bloody diarrhea and abdominal pain, serotonin syndrome (eg, mental status changes, autonomic instability, neuromuscular aberrations and/or GI symptoms), ophthalmic effects, and increased BP.

Patient Counseling: Inform about risk of serotonin syndrome, especially if taken with SSRIs or SNRIs. Advise to notify physician if pregnant/nursing or planning to become pregnant. Counsel on proper administration technique for nasal spray.

Administration: Oral/Nasal routes. ODT: Immediately prior to dosing, remove blister from outer pouch with dry hands. Dissolve on tongue and swallow. **Storage:** 20-25°C (68-77°F).

ZONEGRAN   RX
zonisamide (Eisai)

THERAPEUTIC CLASS: Sulfonamide anticonvulsant

INDICATIONS: Adjunctive therapy in the treatment of partial seizures in adults with epilepsy.

DOSAGE: *Adults:* ≥16 yrs: Initial: 100mg/day for 2 weeks. Titrate: May increase to 200mg/day for ≥2 weeks. May then increase to 300mg/day, then to 400mg/day in ≥2-week intervals. Renal/Hepatic Disease: May require slower titration. Elderly: Start at low end of dosing range.

HOW SUPPLIED: Cap: 25mg, 100mg

WARNINGS/PRECAUTIONS: Fatal sulfonamide reactions (eg, Stevens-Johnson syndrome, toxic epidermal necrolysis, fulminant hepatic necrosis, blood dyscrasias) rarely reported; d/c immediately if signs of hypersensitivity (eg, unexplained rash) occurs. Increased risk of oligohidrosis and hyperthermia in pediatrics; safety and effectiveness not established and use not approved for pediatrics. May increase risk of suicidal thoughts or behavior; monitor for emergence/worsening of depression, suicidal thoughts or behavior, and/or any unusual changes in mood or behavior. May cause dose-dependent metabolic acidosis; d/c or reduce dose if metabolic acidosis develops/persists. If decided to continue therapy, consider alkali treatment. Conditions or therapies that predispose to acidosis (eg, renal disease, severe respiratory disorders, status epilepticus, diarrhea, ketogenic diet, or specific drugs) may be additive to the bicarbonate lowering effects. Abrupt withdrawal may precipitate increased seizure frequency or status epilepticus; reduce dose or d/c gradually. Has a significant risk to the fetus. May cause CNS-related adverse events (eg, psychiatric symptoms, psychomotor slowing, somnolence, fatigue). May impair mental/physical abilities. Kidney stone formation, increased SrCr and BUN reported; d/c if acute renal failure or if a clinically significant sustained increase in SrCr/BUN develops. Avoid with renal failure (estimated GFR <50mL/min). Sudden unexplained deaths and status epilepticus reported. May increase serum chloride and alkaline phosphatase and decrease serum bicarbonate, phosphorus, calcium, and albumin. Caution with renal/hepatic impairment and in elderly.

ADVERSE REACTIONS: Somnolence, anorexia, dizziness, ataxia, agitation/irritability, difficulty with memory and/or concentration, headache, nausea, fatigue, abdominal pain, confusion, insomnia, diplopia.

INTERACTIONS: Liver enzyme inducers may increase metabolism and clearance and may decrease half-life. CYP3A4 inducers or inhibitors may alter serum concentrations. May cause CNS depression and other cognitive/neuropsychiatric adverse events; caution with alcohol or other CNS depressants. Other carbonic anhydrase inhibitors (eg, topiramate, acetazolamide, or dichlorphenamide) may increase the severity of metabolic acidosis and may also increase the risk of kidney stone formation; monitor for the appearance or worsening of metabolic acidosis. Phenytoin and carbamazepine may increase plasma clearance. Phenytoin, valproate, or phenobarbital and carbamazepine may decrease $T_{1/2}$. Caution with drugs that predispose patients to heat-related disorders (eg, carbonic anhydrase inhibitors, anticholinergics).

PREGNANCY: Category C, not for use in nursing.

MECHANISM OF ACTION: Sulfonamide anticonvulsant; has not been established. Found to block Na^+ channels and reduce voltage-dependent, transient inward currents (T-type Ca^{2+} currents), consequently stabilizing neuronal membranes and suppressing neuronal hypersynchronization. Facilitates both dopaminergic and serotonergic neurotransmission.

PHARMACOKINETICS: Absorption: (200-400mg) C_{max}=2-5µg/mL, T_{max}=2-6 hrs (fasted), 4-6 hrs (fed). **Distribution:** V_d=1.45L/kg (400mg); plasma protein binding (40%); found in breast milk. **Metabolism:** Liver via reduction by CYP3A4 and acetylation; N-acetyl zonisamide, 2-sulfamoy-

Z

lacetyl phenol (metabolites). **Elimination:** Urine (62%, parent drug and metabolite), feces (3%); $T_{1/2}$=63 hrs.

NURSING CONSIDERATIONS

Assessment: Assess for previous hypersensitivity to sulfonamides or the drug, depression, suicidal thoughts or behavior, conditions or therapies that predispose to acidosis, risk for kidney stones formation, renal/hepatic impairment, pregnancy/nursing status, and possible drug interactions. Obtain baseline serum bicarbonate.

Monitoring: Monitor for signs/symptoms of sulfonamide reactions, hypersensitivity, oligohidrosis, hyperthermia, emergence/worsening of depression, suicidal thoughts or behavior, unusual changes in mood or behavior, metabolic acidosis, seizures (upon withdrawal), CNS-related adverse events, kidney stones, and status epilepticus. Monitor renal function (SrCr, BUN) and serum bicarbonate periodically.

Patient Counseling: Instruct to take only as prescribed. Advise not to drive a car or operate complex machinery until accustomed to effects of medication. Instruct to contact physician if skin rash develops, seizures worsen, develop signs or symptoms of kidney stone (eg, sudden back pain, abdominal pain, blood in urine) or hematological complications (eg, fever, sore throat, oral ulcers, easy bruising), and if child is not sweating as usual with or without fever. Inform to increase fluid intake to decrease risk of kidney stone formation. Counsel patients, caregivers, and families that therapy may increase risk of suicidal thoughts and behavior. Advise to contact physician if develop symptoms of depression, unusual changes in mood or behavior, or the emergence of suicidal thoughts, behavior, or thoughts about self-harm. Instruct to contact physician if fast breathing, fatigue/tiredness, loss of appetite, irregular heart beat or palpitations develop. Advise women of childbearing potential to use effective contraception while on therapy. Instruct to notify physician if pregnant, plan to become pregnant, or breastfeeding during therapy. Encourage to enroll in North American Antiepileptic Drug Pregnancy Registry if become pregnant.

Administration: Oral route. Swallow caps whole. **Storage:** 25°C (77°F); excursions permitted to 15-30°C (59-86°F), in a dry place. Protect from light.

ZORBTIVE   RX
somatropin (EMD Serono)

THERAPEUTIC CLASS: Human growth hormone

INDICATIONS: Treatment of short bowel syndrome in patients receiving specialized nutritional support.

DOSAGE: *Adults:* 0.1mg/kg qd SQ for 4 weeks. Max: 8mg/day. Rotate injection site.

HOW SUPPLIED: Inj: 8.8mg [10mL]

CONTRAINDICATIONS: Acute critical illness due to complications following open heart or abdominal surgery, multiple accidental trauma, or acute respiratory failure; active neoplasia; benzyl alcohol sensitivity.

WARNINGS/PRECAUTIONS: Benzyl alcohol associated with toxicity in newborns; if sensitivity occurs, may reconstitute with sterile water for injection. Allergic reactions may occur. May be associated with acute pancreatitis. Cases of new-onset impaired glucose intolerance, new-onset type 2 diabetes mellitus (DM), exacerbation of preexisting DM, diabetic ketoacidosis, and diabetic coma reported. Syndrome of intracranial HTN with papilledema, visual changes, headache, and N/V reported in small number of children with growth failure with growth hormone products; perform funduscopic evaluation at the initiation and during therapy. Increased tissue turgor and musculoskeletal discomfort may occur during therapy but may resolve spontaneously with analgesic therapy, or after reducing the frequency of dosing. Carpal tunnel syndrome may occur; d/c if symptoms do not resolve after reducing the dose or frequency.

ADVERSE REACTIONS: Edema, melena, rectal hemorrhage, arthritis, fungal infection, inflammation at the inj site, paresthesia, phantom pain, bronchospasm, dyspnea, purpura, skin disorder, insomnia, hypomagnesemia, dysuria.

INTERACTIONS: May impact cortisol and cortisone metabolism. May unmask previously undiagnosed primary (and secondary) hypoadrenalism requiring glucocorticoid therapy. Use of glucocorticoid replacement therapy for previously diagnosed hypoadrenalism, especially cortisone acetate or prednisone, may require an increase in maintenance or stress doses. Dose adjustment of antidiabetics may be required.

PREGNANCY: Category B, caution in nursing.

MECHANISM OF ACTION: Human growth hormone; anabolic and anticatabolic agent that exerts influence by interacting with specific receptors on a variety of cell types. On gut, actions may be direct or mediated via local or systemic production of insulin-like growth factor-1; also enhances transmucosal transport of water, electrolytes, and nutrients.

Z

PHARMACOKINETICS: Absorption: Absolute bioavailability (70-90%). **Distribution:** (IV) V_d=12L. **Metabolism:** Liver, kidneys. **Elimination:** Urine; $T_{1/2}$=3.94 hrs. (IV) $T_{1/2}$=0.58 hrs.

NURSING CONSIDERATIONS

Assessment: Assess for acute critical illness, active malignancy, hypersensitivity to benzyl alcohol, pregnancy/nursing status, and possible drug interactions. Perform baseline funduscopic exam.

Monitoring: Monitor for hypersensitivity/allergic reactions, acute pancreatitis, impaired glucose intolerance, new-onset type 2 DM, exacerbation of preexisting DM, diabetic ketoacidosis, diabetic coma, carpal tunnel syndrome, increased tissue turgor, musculoskeletal discomfort, and other adverse reactions. Perform funduscopic exam periodically.

Patient Counseling: Inform about the risks and benefits associated with the treatment. Instruct to notify physician if they experience any side effects or discomfort during treatment. Advise to properly dispose the needles and syringes; container should be used for disposing of needles and syringes. Instruct to rotate inj sites to avoid localized tissue atrophy.

Administration: SQ route. Refer to PI for proper reconstitution. **Storage:** Before reconstitution: 15-30°C (59-86°F). After Reconstitution with Bacteriostatic Water for Injection: 2-8°C (36-46°F) for up to 14 days. Avoid freezing.

ZORTRESS   RX
everolimus (Novartis)

> Immunosuppression may lead to increased susceptibility to infection and possible development of malignancies (eg, lymphoma, skin cancer). Should only be prescribed by physicians experienced in immunosuppressive therapy and management of organ transplant patients. Increased nephrotoxicity may occur with use of standard doses of cyclosporine; reduce dose of cyclosporine to reduce renal dysfunction and monitor levels. Increased risk of kidney arterial and venous thrombosis leading to graft loss, mostly within the first 30 days post-transplantation.

THERAPEUTIC CLASS: Macrolide immunosuppressant

INDICATIONS: Prophylaxis of organ rejection in adult patients at low-moderate immunologic risk receiving a kidney transplant in combination with basiliximab induction and concurrently with reduced doses of cyclosporine and corticosteroids.

DOSAGE: *Adults:* Initial: 0.75mg bid. Administer immediately after transplantation. Titrate: May adjust dose at 4-5 day intervals based on blood concentrations achieved, tolerability, individual response, change in concomitant medications and clinical situation. Recommended Trough Concentration: 3-8ng/mL. Moderate Hepatic Impairment (Child-Pugh Class B): Reduce daily dose by 50%; monitor blood concentrations for further adjustments.

HOW SUPPLIED: Tab: 0.25mg, 0.5mg, 0.75mg

WARNINGS/PRECAUTIONS: Increased risk of developing bacterial, viral, fungal, and protozoal infections, including opportunistic infections (eg, polyoma virus infections); caution with combination immunosuppressant therapy. Angioedema reported; increased risk with concomitant use of drugs known to cause angioedema (eg, angiotensin converting enzyme [ACE] inhibitors). Delayed wound healing, increased wound-related complications, and fluid accumulation including peripheral edema reported. Hyperlipidemia following initiation and proteinuria reported; increased risk with higher whole blood trough concentrations. Use of anti-lipid therapy may not normalize lipid levels. Monitor for development of rhabdomyolysis with HMG-CoA reductase inhibitors and fibrates. Caution with concomitant use of drugs known to impair renal function. BK virus associated nephropathy (BKVAN) may lead to renal dysfunction and graft loss. Non-infectious pneumonitis and male infertility reported. May increase risk of new-onset diabetes mellitus (DM) after transplant; monitor blood glucose concentrations. Avoid with rare hereditary problems of galactose intolerance (Lapp lactase deficiency, glucose-galactose malabsorption); diarrhea and malabsorption may occur. Monitor for proteinuria. May increase the risk of thrombotic microangiopathy/thrombotic thrombocytopenic purpura/hemolytic uremic syndrome with cyclosporine; monitor hematologic parameters. Limit sunlight and ultraviolet light exposure in patients at increased risk for skin cancer.

ADVERSE REACTIONS: Peripheral edema, constipation, HTN, nausea, anemia, urinary tract infection, hyperlipidemia, diarrhea, pyrexia, increased blood creatinine, hyperkalemia, headache, hypercholesterolemia, insomnia, upper respiratory tract infections.

INTERACTIONS: See Boxed Warning. Avoid with strong inhibitors (eg, ketoconazole, itraconazole, voriconazole, clarithromycin, telithromycin, ritonavir), inducers (eg, rifampin, rifabutin) of CYP3A4, simvastatin, lovastatin, live vaccines, grapefruit, and grapefruit juice. Inhibitors of P-glycoprotein (P-gp) (eg, digoxin, cyclosporine), moderate inhibitors of CYP3A4 and P-gp (eg, fluconazole, macrolide antibiotics, nicardipine, diltiazem, nelfinavir, indinavir, amprenavir), ketoconazole, erythromycin, and verapamil may increase levels. Caution with CYP3A4 and CYP2D6 substrates with a narrow therapeutic index. Increased levels with cyclosporine; dose adjustment

Z

may be needed if cyclosporine dose is altered. CYP3A4 inducers (eg, St. John's wort, carbam-azepine, phenobarbital, phenytoin, efavirenz, nevirapine), atorvastatin, pravastatin, and rifampin may decrease levels.

PREGNANCY: Category C, not for use in nursing.

MECHANISM OF ACTION: Macrolide immunosuppressant; inhibits antigenic and interleukin (IL-2 and IL-15) stimulated activation and proliferation of T and B lymphocytes. Binds to a cytoplas-mic protein, the FK506 binding protein-12 (FKBP-12), to form an immunosuppressive complex (everolimus: FKBP-12) that binds to and inhibits the mammalian target of rapamycin (mTOR), a key regulatory kinase in cells.

PHARMACOKINETICS: Absorption: (0.75mg bid) AUC=75ng•h/mL, C_{max} =11.1ng/mL, T_{max}=1-2 hrs. **Distribution:** Plasma protein binding (74%). **Metabolism:** via CYP3A4 and P-gp (monohydroxyla-tions and O-dealkylations). **Elimination:** Feces (80%), urine (5%). (0.75mg bid) $T_{1/2}$=30 hrs.

NURSING CONSIDERATIONS

Assessment: Assess for hereditary problems of galactose intolerance, hepatic impairment, hypersensitivity to the drug or to sirolimus, pregnancy/nursing status, and for possible drug interactions. Obtain lipid profile, fasting serum glucose, and CBC.

Monitoring: Monitor for clinical signs and symptoms, serious infections, angioedema, throm-bosis, wound-related complications, fluid accumulations, lymphomas and other malignan-cies, hyperlipidemia, hepatic impairment, renal function including SrCr, proteinuria, BKVAN, pneumonitis, and blood glucose concentrations. Monitor whole blood trough concentrations and hematologic parameters.

Patient Counseling: Advise to take bid approximately 12 hrs apart consistently either with or without food. Avoid grapefruit and grapefruit juice. Counsel of risk of developing lymphomas/other malignancies; limit exposure to sunlight and UV light by wearing protective clothing and using sunscreen with high protection factor. Notify physician if have hereditary disorders of ga-lactose intolerance (Lapp lactase deficiency or glucose-galactose malabsorption). Inform of risks of impaired kidney function with cyclosporine and the importance of serum creatinine monitor-ing. Avoid pregnancy throughout treatment and for 8 weeks after d/c. Notify physician of all medications and herbal/dietary supplements being taken. Advise that drug may increase the risk of kidney arterial and venous thrombosis, resulting in graft loss, usually within first 30 days post-transplantation. Inform patients that drug has been associated with impaired or delayed wound healing, and fluid accumulation; carefully observe incision site. Inform of risk of hyperlipidemia; treatment and monitoring of blood lipid concentrations may be required. Inform of increased risk of proteinuria, DM, infections, and angioedema; inform physician if symptoms develop. Avoid live vaccines.

Administration: Oral route. Do not crush; swallow whole with water. Administer consistently approximately 12 hrs apart with or without food and at the same time as cyclosporine. **Storage:** 25°C (77°F); excursions permitted to 15-30°C (59-86°F). Protect from light and moisture.

ZOSTAVAX   RX
zoster vaccine live (Merck)

THERAPEUTIC CLASS: Vaccine

INDICATIONS: Prevention of herpes zoster (shingles) in individuals ≥50 yrs.

DOSAGE: *Adults:* ≥50 yrs: Single 0.65mL SQ in the deltoid region of upper arm.

HOW SUPPLIED: Inj: 0.65mL

CONTRAINDICATIONS: History of anaphylactic/anaphylactoid reaction to gelatin or neomycin. Immunosuppression or immunodeficiency, including history of primary or acquired immunodefi-ciency states, leukemia, lymphoma or other malignant neoplasms affecting the bone marrow or lymphatic system, AIDS or other clinical manifestations of infection with HIV, those on immuno-suppressive therapy, and pregnancy.

WARNINGS/PRECAUTIONS: Avoid pregnancy for 3 months following administration. Not indicated for treatment of zoster or postherpetic neuralgia or prevention of primary varicella infection (chickenpox). Serious adverse reactions, including anaphylaxis, reported; adequate treatment provisions, including epinephrine inj (1:1000), should be available for immediate use should an anaphylactic/anaphylactoid reaction occur. Transmission of vaccine virus may occur between vaccinees and susceptible contacts. Consider deferral in acute illness (eg, fever) or with active untreated tuberculosis (TB). Duration of protection >4 yrs after vaccination is unknown. May not result in protection of all vaccine recipients.

ADVERSE REACTIONS: Inj-site reactions (erythema, pain, tenderness, swelling, pruritus, warmth), headache.

INTERACTIONS: See Contraindications. Reduced immune response with pneumococcal vaccine polyvalent; consider administration of the 2 vaccines separated by ≥4 weeks.

Z

PREGNANCY: Contraindicated in pregnancy, caution in nursing.

MECHANISM OF ACTION: Live attenuated vaccine; boosts varicella-zoster virus specific immunity; hence protects against zoster and its complications.

NURSING CONSIDERATIONS

Assessment: Assess age and for acute illness, active untreated TB, history of anaphylactic/anaphylactoid reaction to gelatin or neomycin, or any other component of the vaccine, immunosuppression/immunodeficiency, pregnancy/nursing status, and possible drug interactions.

Monitoring: Monitor for anaphylactic/anaphylactoid reactions, inj-site reactions, headache, and other adverse events that may occur.

Patient Counseling: Ask about reactions to previous vaccines. Inform about benefits/risks of vaccine, including potential risk of transmitting vaccine virus to susceptible individuals (eg, immunosuppressed/immunodeficient individuals, pregnant women who have not had chickenpox). Instruct to report any adverse reactions or any symptoms of concern to their healthcare professional.

Administration: SQ route. Administer immediately after reconstitution; discard if not used within 30 mins. Refer to PI for proper preparation, reconstitution, and administration. **Storage:** -50°C to -15°C (-58°F to 5°F) until reconstituted. May store and/or transport at 2-8°C (36-46°F) up to 72 hrs; discard if not used within 72 hrs of removal from -15°C (5°F). Diluent: 20-25°C (68-77°F) or 2-8°C (36-46°F). Do not freeze reconstituted vaccine. Protect from light.

ZOSYN   RX
tazobactam sodium - piperacillin sodium (Wyeth)

THERAPEUTIC CLASS: Broad-spectrum penicillin/beta-lactamase inhibitor

INDICATIONS: Treatment of appendicitis, peritonitis, uncomplicated/complicated skin and skin structure infections, postpartum endometritis, pelvic inflammatory disease (PID), moderate community-acquired pneumonia (CAP), and moderate to severe nosocomial pneumonia caused by susceptible strains of microorganisms.

DOSAGE: *Adults:* Infuse over 30 min. Usual: 3.375g q6h IV for 7-10 days. CrCl 20-40mL/min: 2.25g q6h. CrCl<20mL/min: 2.25g q8h. Hemodialysis/*Clostridium difficile*-associated diarrhea (CDAD): 2.25g q12h. Give one additional dose of 0.75g following each hemodialysis session. Nosocomial Pneumonia: 4.5g q6h for 7-14 days plus an aminoglycoside. CrCl 20-40mL/min: 3.375g q6h. CrCl <20mL/min: 2.25g q6h. Hemodialysis/CAPD: 2.25g q8h. Give one additional dose of 0.75g following each hemodialysis session.
Pediatrics: Infuse over 30 min. Appendicitis/Peritonitis: ≤40kg: ≥9 months: 100mg piperacillin-12.5mg tazobactam/kg q8h. 2-9 months: 80mg piperacillin-10mg tazobactam/kg q8h. >40kg: Use adult dose.

HOW SUPPLIED: Inj: (Piperacillin-Tazobactam) 2g-0.25g, 3g-0.375g, 4g-0.5g; 2g-0.25g/50mL, 3g-0.375g/50mL, 4g-0.5g/100mL. Also available as a Pharmacy Bulk Package. Refer to individual package insert for more information.

CONTRAINDICATIONS: History of allergic reactions to cephalosporins.

WARNINGS/PRECAUTIONS: Serious, fatal hypersensitivity (anaphylactic/anaphylactoid) reactions including shock reported; if these occur d/c and institute appropriate therapy. Hypersensitivity reactions more likely to occur with history of penicillin hypersensitivity or history of sensitivity to multiple allergens. CDAD reported. D/C if bleeding manifestations occur. Superinfection may develop; take appropriate measures if this occurs. May experience neuromuscular excitability or convulsions with higher than recommended dose. Caution with restricted salt intake. Increased incidence of rash and fever in cystic fibrosis reported. Monitor electrolytes periodically with low K+ reserves. Caution with renal impairment (CrCl ≤40mL/min). Caution in elderly.

ADVERSE REACTIONS: Diarrhea, headache, constipation, N/V, insomnia, rash, fever, dyspepsia, local reactions, pruritus, fever, stool changes, agitation, pain.

INTERACTIONS: May inactivate aminoglycosides. May decrease serum concentrations of tobramycin; monitor aminoglycoside serum concentrations in patients with end stage renal disease. Probenecid prolongs half-life. Test coagulation parameters more frequently with high doses of heparin, oral anticoagulants, or other drugs which may affect blood coagulation system or thrombocyte function. Piperacillin: May prolong neuromuscular blockade of vecuronium or any nondepolarizing muscle relaxant. May increase risk of hypokalemia with cytotoxic therapy or diuretics. May reduce methotrexate clearance; monitor methotrexate concentrations and for methotrexate toxicity.

PREGNANCY: Category B, caution in nursing.

Z

MECHANISM OF ACTION: Piperacillin: Broad-spectrum penicillin; exerts bactericidal activity by inhibiting septum formation and cell wall synthesis of susceptible bacteria. Tazobactam: β-lactamase enzyme inhibitor.
PHARMACOKINETICS: Absorption: Piperacillin (2.25g, 3.375g, 4.5g): C_{max}= 134µg/mL, 242µg/mL, 298µg/mL. Tazobactam (2.25g, 3.375g, 4.5g): C_{max}= 15µg/mL, 24µg/mL, 34µg/mL. T_{max}= 30 min. **Distribution:** Plasma protein binding (30%); crosses placental barrier. Piperacillin: V_d=0.243L/kg, found in breast milk. **Elimination:** Kidneys; $T_{1/2}$=0.7-1.2 hrs. Piperacillin: Urine (68% unchanged). Tazobactam: Urine (80% unchanged, 20% as single metabolite).

NURSING CONSIDERATIONS

Assessment: Assess for previous hypersensitivity reaction to penicillins, cephalosporins, or other allergens. Assess for history of a bleeding disorder, conditions with restricted salt intake, cystic fibrosis, renal impairment, hypokalemia, pregnancy/nursing status, and possible drug interactions.

Monitoring: Monitor hematopoietic function, renal function, and serum electrolytes periodically. Monitor for signs/symptoms of electrolyte imbalance (eg, hypokalemia), hypersensitivity reactions, CDAD, superinfections, leukopenia/neutropenia, bleeding manifestations, and for neuromuscular excitability or convulsions. Monitor for rash and fever in cystic fibrosis patients.

Patient Counseling: Inform about risks/benefits of therapy. Counsel that drug only treats bacterial, not viral, infections. Instruct to take as directed; inform that skipping doses or not completing full course may decrease effectiveness and increase resistance. Advise to d/c and notify physician if an allergic reaction or watery/bloody diarrhea (with or without stomach cramps and fever) occur. Instruct to notify physician if pregnant/nursing.

Administration: IV route. Refer to PI for instructions for reconstitution and dilution. **Storage:** Vial: Prior to Reconstitution: 20-25°C (68-77°F). Reconstituted: Use immediately after reconstitution. Discard any unused portion after 24 hours if stored at 20-25°C (68-77°F) or after 48 hours if stored at 2-8°C (36-46°F). Do not freeze vials after reconstitution. Galaxy Container: -20°C (-4°F). Thawed Sol: 2-8°C (36-46°F) for 14 days, or 20-25°C (68-77°F) for 24 hrs. Do not refreeze thawed antibiotics.

ZOVIRAX ORAL   RX
acyclovir (GlaxoSmithKline)

THERAPEUTIC CLASS: Nucleoside analogue
INDICATIONS: Acute treatment of herpes zoster (shingles). Treatment of initial and recurrent episodes of genital herpes. Treatment of chickenpox (varicella).
DOSAGE: *Adults:* Herpes Zoster: 800mg q4h, 5X/day for 7-10 days. Genital Herpes: Initial Therapy: 200mg q4h, 5X/day for 10 days. Chronic Therapy: 400mg bid or 200mg 3-5X/day up to 12 months, then reevaluate. Intermittent Therapy: 200mg q4h, 5X/day for 5 days; start at 1st sign/symptom of recurrence. Chickenpox: 800mg qid for 5 days; start at earliest sign/symptom. Renal Impairment: Refer to PI for dose modifications.
Pediatrics: ≥2 yrs: Chickenpox: ≤40kg: 20mg/kg qid for 5 days. >40kg: 800mg qid for 5 days. Start at earliest sign/symptom. Renal Impairment: Refer to PI for dose modifications.
HOW SUPPLIED: Cap: 200mg; Sus: 200mg/5mL [473mL]; Tab: 400mg, 800mg
CONTRAINDICATIONS: Hypersensitivity to valacyclovir.
WARNINGS/PRECAUTIONS: Renal failure sometimes resulting in death reported. Thrombotic thrombocytopenic purpura/hemolytic uremic syndrome (TTP/HUS) in immunocompromised patients reported. Maintain adequate hydration. Caution in elderly.
ADVERSE REACTIONS: N/V, diarrhea, malaise.
INTERACTIONS: Probenecid may increase levels and $T_{1/2}$ of IV formulation. May increase risk of renal impairment and/or CNS symptoms with nephrotoxic agents; use caution.
PREGNANCY: Category B, caution in nursing.
MECHANISM OF ACTION: Synthetic purine nucleoside analogue; stops replication of herpes viral DNA by competitive inhibition of viral DNA polymerase, incorporation into and termination of growing viral DNA chain, and inactivation of viral DNA polymerase.
PHARMACOKINETICS: Absorption: Oral administration of variable doses resulted in different parameters. **Distribution:** Plasma protein binding (9-33%); found in breast milk. **Elimination:** $T_{1/2}$=2.5-3.3 hrs.

NURSING CONSIDERATIONS

Assessment: Assess for immunocompromised state, hypersensitivity to valacyclovir, renal impairment, nursing status, and possible drug interactions.
Monitoring: Monitor for signs/symptoms of TTP/HUS. Monitor BUN and SrCr.

Z

Patient Counseling: Instruct to consult physician if experiencing severe or troublesome adverse reactions, if pregnant/intending to become pregnant, or intending to breastfeed. Advise to maintain adequate hydration. Inform that therapy is not a cure for genital herpes; advise to avoid contact with lesions or intercourse when lesions/symptoms are present.

Administration: Oral route. **Storage:** 15-25°C (59-77°F); protect from moisture.

ZUPLENZ RX
ondansetron (Par)

THERAPEUTIC CLASS: 5-HT$_3$ receptor antagonist

INDICATIONS: Prevention of N/V associated with highly emetogenic cancer chemotherapy, including cisplatin ≥50mg/m^2 or with initial and repeat courses of moderately emetogenic cancer chemotherapy. Prevention of N/V associated with radiotherapy (total body irradiation, single high-dose fraction, or daily fractions to the abdomen). Prevention of postoperative nausea and/or vomiting (PONV).

DOSAGE: *Adults:* Prevention of N/V Associated with Highly Emetogenic Chemotherapy: 24mg (given successively as three 8mg films) 30 min before chemotherapy. Prevention of N/V Associated with Moderately Emetogenic Chemotherapy: 8mg bid; give 1st dose 30 min before chemotherapy, then 8 hrs later, then q12h for 1-2 days after completion of chemotherapy. Prevention of N/V Associated with Radiotherapy: Usual: 8mg tid. Total Body Irradiation: 8mg 1-2 hrs before each fraction of therapy. Single High-Dose Fraction Radiotherapy to Abdomen: 8mg 1-2 hrs before therapy, then q8h after 1st dose for 1-2 days after completion of therapy. Daily Fractionated Radiotherapy to Abdomen: 8mg 1-2 hrs before therapy, then q8h after 1st dose for each day radiotherapy is given. Prevention of PONV: 16mg (given successively as two 8mg films) 1 hr before induction of anesthesia. Severe Hepatic Dysfunction (Child-Pugh ≥10): Max: 8mg/day. *Pediatrics:* ≥12 yrs: Prevention of N/V Associated with Moderately Emetogenic Chemotherapy: 8mg bid; give 1st dose 30 min before chemotherapy, then 8 hrs later, then q12h for 1-2 days after completion of chemotherapy. 4-11 yrs: 4mg tid; give 1st dose 30 min before chemotherapy, then 4 and 8 hrs later, then q8h for 1-2 days after completion of chemotherapy. Severe Hepatic Dysfunction (Child-Pugh ≥10): Max: 8mg/day.

HOW SUPPLIED: Film, Oral: 4mg, 8mg

CONTRAINDICATIONS: Concomitant use with apomorphine.

WARNINGS/PRECAUTIONS: Hypersensitivity reactions reported in patients hypersensitive to other 5-HT$_3$ receptor antagonists. ECG changes, including QT interval prolongation, reported. May mask progressive ileus and/or gastric distension following abdominal surgery, or with chemotherapy-induced N/V. Does not stimulate gastric/intestinal peristalsis; do not use instead of NG suction.

ADVERSE REACTIONS: Headache, diarrhea, malaise/fatigue, constipation, hypoxia, pyrexia, dizziness, gynecological disorder, anxiety/agitation, urinary retention, pruritus.

INTERACTIONS: See Contraindications. Inducers or inhibitors of CYP3A4, CYP2D6, and CYP1A2 may change the clearance and T$_{1/2}$ of ondansetron. Potent CYP3A4 inducers (eg, phenytoin, carbamazepine, rifampicin) may significantly increase the clearance and decrease blood concentrations of ondansetron. May reduce analgesic activity of tramadol.

PREGNANCY: Category B, caution in nursing.

MECHANISM OF ACTION: Selective 5-HT$_3$ receptor antagonist; not established. Blocks 5-HT$_3$ receptors from serotonin. Released serotonin may stimulate the vagal afferents through 5-HT$_3$ receptors and initiate the vomiting reflex.

PHARMACOKINETICS: Absorption: Well-absorbed. T$_{max}$=1.3 hrs; AUC=225ng•hr/mL, C$_{max}$=37.28ng/mL. **Distribution:** Plasma protein binding (70-76%). **Metabolism:** Extensive via CYP3A4, 1A2, 2D6; hydroxylation (primary), glucuronide/sulfate conjugation. **Elimination:** Urine (5% parent); T$_{1/2}$=4.6 hrs.

NURSING CONSIDERATIONS

Assessment: Assess for known hypersensitivity to the drug, hepatic impairment, pregnancy/nursing status, and possible drug interactions.

Monitoring: Monitor for signs/symptoms of ECG changes, hypersensitivity reactions, and hepatic impairment. In patients who recently underwent abdominal surgery or in patients with chemotherapy-induced N/V, monitor for masking of signs of a progressive ileus and/or gastric distension.

Patient Counseling: Inform that headache, malaise/fatigue, constipation, and diarrhea may occur. Advise to report the use of all medications, especially apomorphine; may cause significant drop in blood pressure and loss of consciousness. Instruct to report any signs/symptoms of hypersensitivity reaction. Instruct on proper administration techniques and advise not to chew or swallow the film. Advise patients to wash hands after taking the medicine.

Z

Administration: Oral route. Place the film on top of the tongue until dissolves then swallow with or without liquid. Allow each film to dissolve completely before giving the next film. **Storage:** 20-25°C (68-77°F).

ZYBAN   RX
bupropion HCl (GlaxoSmithKline)

Serious neuropsychiatric events, including depression, suicidal ideation, suicide attempt, and completed suicide, reported. Some cases may be complicated by nicotine withdrawal symptoms in patients who stopped smoking. Advise patients and caregivers that the patient should stop taking bupropion and contact healthcare provider immediately if agitation, hostility, depressed mood, changes in thinking or behavior, suicidal ideation, or suicidal behavior occur. Although not indicated for the treatment of depression, it contains the same active ingredient found in antidepressant medications. Antidepressants increased the risk of suicidal thinking and behavior (suicidality) in short-term studies in children, adolescents, and young adults with major depressive disorder (MDD) and other psychiatric disorders. Bupropion is not approved for use in pediatric patients.

THERAPEUTIC CLASS: Aminoketone

INDICATIONS: Aid to smoking cessation treatment.

DOSAGE: *Adults:* Initial: 150mg qd for 1st 3 days. Usual: 150mg bid. Max: 300mg/day. Separate doses by ≥8 hrs. Initiate treatment while patient is still smoking. Patients should set a "target quit date" within the first 2 weeks of treatment. Treat for 7 to 12 weeks; d/c at 7 weeks if no progress seen. Consider ongoing therapy if patient quits smoking after 7-12 weeks. Severe Hepatic Cirrhosis: Max: 150mg qod. Mild-Moderate Hepatic Cirrhosis/Renal Impairment: Consider reduced frequency.

HOW SUPPLIED: Tab, Sustained-Release: 150mg

CONTRAINDICATIONS: Seizure disorder, bulimia or anorexia nervosa, patients treated with other medications that contain bupropion, use of MAOIs or within 14 days of use, and patients undergoing abrupt d/c of alcohol or sedatives (including benzodiazepines).

WARNINGS/PRECAUTIONS: Patients with MDD may experience worsening of depression and/or emergence of suicidal ideation and behavior or unusual changes in behavior; monitor appropriately, especially during the initial few months of a course of drug therapy, or during dosing changes. Screen for bipolar disorder; not approved for use in treating bipolar depression. May precipitate mixed/manic episode in patients at risk for bipolar disorder. Dose-dependent risk of seizures; do not prescribe >300mg/day for smoking cessation. D/C and do not restart if seizure occurs. Extreme caution with history of seizure, cranial trauma, CNS tumor, or other predisposition toward seizures, and with severe hepatic cirrhosis. Potential for hepatotoxicity. Allergic reactions (eg, anaphylactoid/anaphylactic and delayed hypersensitivity), insomnia, and HTN reported. Caution with recent history of myocardial infarction, unstable heart disease, hepatic/renal impairment, and in elderly. False-(+) urine immunoassay screening tests for amphetamines reported.

ADVERSE REACTIONS: Insomnia, dry mouth, dizziness, disturbed concentration, dream abnormality, rhinitis, rash, nervousness, nausea, diarrhea, anorexia, constipation, arthralgia, anxiety, myalgia.

INTERACTIONS: See Contraindications. Extreme caution with drugs that lower seizure threshold (eg, antidepressants, antipsychotics, theophylline, systemic steroids). Increased seizure risk with excessive alcohol or sedative use; opiate, cocaine, or stimulant addiction; use of OTC stimulants or anorectics, oral hypoglycemics, insulin. Caution with levodopa and amantadine; use low initial doses and gradually titrate. Inhibits CYP2D6; caution with drugs that are metabolized by CYP2D6 (eg, SSRIs, TCAs, antipsychotics, β-blockers, type 1C antiarrhythmics); use low initial dose. May reduce efficacy of drugs that require metabolic activation by CYP2D6 to be effective (eg, tamoxifen). Monitor for HTN with nicotine replacement therapy. Caution with CYP2B6 substrates or inhibitors/inducers (eg, orphenadrine, cyclophosphamide, thiotepa, ticlopidine, clopidogrel, ritonavir, efavirenz). Carbamazepine, phenytoin, and phenobarbital may induce metabolism. Altered PT and/or INR with warfarin. Minimize or avoid alcohol. Decreased levels with ritonavir or ritonavir/lopinavir and efavirenz; may need to increase bupropion dose but do not exceed max dose. Cimetidine increased levels of some active metabolites. Increased citalopram level. Paroxetine, sertraline, norfluoxetine, nelfinavir, and fluvoxamine may inhibit metabolism.

PREGNANCY: Category C, not for use in nursing.

MECHANISM OF ACTION: Aminoketone; not established. Weak inhibitor of the neuronal uptake of norepinephrine and dopamine.

PHARMACOKINETICS: Absorption: C_{max}=136ng/mL; T_{max}=3 hrs. **Distribution:** V_d=1950L; plasma protein binding (84%); found in breast milk. **Metabolism:** Liver (extensive), kidneys. Hydroxylation, hydroxybupropion (active metabolite) (CYP2B6); reduction of carbonyl group, threohydrobupropion, and erythrohydrobupropion (active metabolites); oxidation. **Elimination:** Urine (87%), feces (10%), (0.5% unchanged); $T_{1/2}$=21 hrs, 20 hrs, 33 hrs, 37 hrs (bupropion, hydroxybupropion, erythrohydrobupropion, threohydrobupropion, respectively).

NURSING CONSIDERATIONS

Assessment: Assess for hepatic/renal impairment, seizure disorder, seizure risk, presence/history of bulimia or anorexia nervosa, MDD, bipolar disorder, recent myocardial infarction, presence of unstable heart disease, pregnancy/nursing status, and possible drug interactions. Detailed psychiatric history, including family history of suicide, bipolar disorder, and depression should be taken.

Monitoring: Monitor signs and symptoms of neuropsychiatric events, clinical worsening, suicidality, unusual changes in behavior, hepatotoxicity, allergic reactions, insomnia, activation of psychosis and/or mania, HTN, and seizures.

Patient Counseling: Inform about the benefits and risks of therapy. Advise patients and caregivers to d/c therapy and notify physician immediately if agitation, hostility, depressed mood, changes in thinking or behavior, or if suicidal ideation or suicidal behavior occurs. Inform patients that nicotine withdrawal symptoms or exacerbation of preexisting psychiatric illness may occur. Inform patient to notify physician if pregnant/nursing. Advise to continue receiving smoking cessation counseling and support even after d/c.

Administration: Oral route. Swallow whole; do not crush, divide, or chew. **Storage:** 20-25°C (68-77°F).

ZYCLARA   RX
imiquimod (Medicis)

THERAPEUTIC CLASS: Immune response modifier

INDICATIONS: Topical treatment of clinically typical visible or palpable actinic keratoses of the full face or balding scalp in immunocompetent adults. (3.75%) Treatment of external genital and perianal warts/condyloma acuminata in patients ≥12 yrs.

DOSAGE: *Adults:* Apply as a thin film qd before hs. May suspend use for several days to manage local skin reactions. Actinic Keratoses: Apply to affected area for two 2-week treatment cycles separated by a 2-week no treatment period. Rub in until no longer visible. May use up to 0.5g (2 pkts or 2 full pump actuations) at each application. Max: 56 pkts or 15g pump per treatment course. External Genital/Perianal Warts: Apply to warts until total clearance or for up to 8 weeks. May use up to 0.25g (1 pkt or 1 full pump actuation) at each application. Max: 56 pkts or 15g pump per treatment course.
Pediatrics: ≥12 yrs: External Genital/Perianal Warts: Apply as a thin layer to warts qd before hs until total clearance or for up to 8 weeks. May use up to 0.25g (1 pkt or 1 full pump actuation) at each application. Max: 56 pkts or 15g pump per treatment course. May suspend use for several days to manage local skin reactions.

HOW SUPPLIED: Cre: 2.5%, 3.75% [0.25g pkts] [7.5g, 15g pump]

WARNINGS/PRECAUTIONS: Not for oral, ophthalmic, intra-anal, or intravaginal use. Intense local skin reactions (eg, skin weeping, erosion) may occur; may require dosing interruption. May exacerbate inflammatory skin conditions, including chronic graft versus host disease. Severe local inflammatory reactions of the female external genitalia may lead to severe vulvar swelling, which may lead to urinary retention; interrupt or d/c if severe vulvar swelling occurs. Administration not recommended until the skin is healed from any previous drug or surgical treatment. Flu-like signs and symptoms may occur; consider dosing interruption and assessment of the patient. Lymphadenopathy reported. Avoid or minimize natural or artificial sunlight exposure (including sunlamps). Avoid with sunburn until fully recovered. Caution in patients who may have considerable sun exposure (eg, due to their occupation) or with inherent sensitivity to sunlight. Avoid any other imiquimod products in the same treatment area; may increase risk and severity of local skin/systemic reactions. Caution with preexisting autoimmune conditions.

ADVERSE REACTIONS: Local skin reactions (erythema, pruritus, pain, irritation, scabbing/crusting, flaking/scaling/dryness, edema, erosion/ulceration, weeping/exudate), headache, fatigue, influenza-like illness, nausea.

PREGNANCY: Category C, caution in nursing.

MECHANISM OF ACTION: Immune response modifier; has not been established. Activates immune cells; associated with increases in markers for cytokines and immune cells.

PHARMACOKINETICS: Absorption: (Actinic Keratoses) C_{max}=0.323ng/mL, T_{max}=9 hrs. (External Genital/Perianal Warts) C_{max}=0.488ng/mL, T_{max}=12 hrs. **Elimination:** (Actinic Keratoses) $T_{1/2}$=29.3 hrs. (External Genital/Perianal Warts) $T_{1/2}$=24.1 hrs.

NURSING CONSIDERATIONS

Assessment: Assess for inflammatory skin conditions, sunburn, inherent sensitivity to sunlight, preexisting autoimmune conditions, sunlight exposure, and pregnancy/nursing status.

Monitoring: Monitor for local skin reactions, severe vulvar swelling, flu-like signs/symptoms, other adverse reactions, and response to treatment.

Z

Patient Counseling: Instruct to use ud by physician, wash hands before and after application, and avoid contact with eyes, lips, nostrils, anus, and vagina. Advise not to bandage or otherwise occlude treatment area, not to reuse partially-used pkts, and to discard pumps after full treatment course completion. Inform that local skin and systemic reactions may occur; instruct to contact physician if these occur. Instruct not to extend treatment >2 weeks (actinic keratoses) or >8 weeks (external genital/perianal warts) due to missed doses or rest periods. Counsel to continue treatment for the full treatment course even if all actinic keratoses appear to be gone. Instruct to wash treatment area with mild soap and water before and 8 hrs after application. Advise to allow treatment area to dry thoroughly before application. Instruct to avoid or minimize exposure to natural or artificial sunlight (tanning beds or UVA/B treatment); encourage to use sunscreen and protective clothing (eg, hat). Inform that additional lesions may become apparent in the treatment area during treatment. (External Genital/Perianal Warts) Instruct to avoid sexual (genital, anal, oral) contact while cre is on the skin. Advise female patients to take special care during application at the vaginal opening. Instruct uncircumcised males treating warts under the foreskin to retract the foreskin and clean the area daily. Inform that new warts may develop during therapy. Inform that drug may weaken condoms and vaginal diaphragms; concurrent use not recommended. Instruct to remove cre by washing treatment area with mild soap and water if severe local skin reaction occurs.

Administration: Topical route. Leave cre on skin for approximately 8 hrs, then remove by washing the area with mild soap and water. Prime pumps before using for the 1st time by repeatedly depressing the actuator until cre is dispensed. **Storage:** 25°C (77°F); excursions permitted to 15-30°C (59-86°F). Avoid freezing.

ZYFLO CR   RX
zileuton (Cornerstone)

OTHER BRAND NAMES: Zyflo (Cornerstone)

THERAPEUTIC CLASS: Leukotriene inhibitor

INDICATIONS: Prophylaxis and chronic treatment of asthma in adults and children ≥12 yrs.

DOSAGE: *Adults:* (Tab) 600mg qid. May take with meals and at hs. (Tab, ER) 1200mg bid within 1 hr after am and pm meals. Do not chew, cut, or crush.
Pediatrics: ≥12 yrs: (Tab) 600mg qid. May take with meals and at hs. (Tab, ER) 1200mg bid within 1 hr after am and pm meals. Do not chew, cut, or crush.

HOW SUPPLIED: Tab: 600mg; Tab, Extended-Release (ER): 600mg

CONTRAINDICATIONS: Active liver disease or transaminase elevations (≥3X ULN).

WARNINGS/PRECAUTIONS: Not for use in reversal of bronchospasm in acute attacks and status asthmaticus. Elevations of one or more LFTs and bilirubin may occur; monitor serum ALT prior to therapy, once a month for first 3 months, every 2-3 months for remainder of first year, and periodically thereafter. Symptomatic hepatitis with jaundice may develop. Increased risk for ALT elevation in females >65 yrs and those with preexisting transaminase elevations. D/C and follow transaminase levels until normal if signs of liver dysfunction (eg, right upper quadrant [RUQ] pain, nausea, fatigue, lethargy, pruritus, jaundice, or flu-like symptoms) or serum transaminase ≥5X ULN occur. Caution in patients who consume substantial quantities of alcohol and/or have a past history of liver disease. Neuropsychiatric events, including sleep disorders and behavior changes, reported; evaluate risks and benefits of continuing treatment.

ADVERSE REACTIONS: Headache, elevation of hepatic function enzyme (ALT) and bilirubin, nausea, myalgia, upper respiratory tract infection, sinusitis, pharyngolaryngeal pain, diarrhea.

INTERACTIONS: May increase theophylline and propranolol concentrations; monitor levels and reduce dose as necessary. Monitor use with other β-blockers. May increase warfarin levels; monitor PT or other coagulation parameters and adjust dose appropriately. (Tab) Not recommended for use with terfenadine. Monitor use with certain drugs metabolized by CYP3A4 (eg, dihydropyridine, calcium channel blockers, cyclosporine, cisapride, and astemizole). (Tab, ER) Monitor use with CYP3A4 inhibitors such as ketoconazole.

PREGNANCY: Category C, not for use in nursing.

MECHANISM OF ACTION: Leukotriene inhibitor; antiasthmatic agent, inhibits leukotriene (LTB$_4$, LTC$_4$, LTD$_4$, and LTE$_4$) formation by inhibiting the enzyme 5-lipoxygenase.

PHARMACOKINETICS: Absorption: (Tab) Rapid; T_{max}=1.7 hrs, C_{max}=4.98µg/ml, AUC=19.2mcg•hr/ml; (Tab, ER) T_{max}=2.1 hrs (fasting), T_{max}=4.3 hrs (fed). **Distribution:** (IR) V_d=1.2L/kg; plasma protein binding (93%). **Metabolism:** Liver, via oxidation by CYP1A2, CYP2C9, CYP3A4. **Elimination:** Urine (94.5%; <0.5% unchanged, <0.5% metabolites), feces (2.2%); (Tab) $T_{1/2}$=2.5 hrs; (Tab, ER) $T_{1/2}$=3.2 hrs.

Z

NURSING CONSIDERATIONS

Assessment: Assess LFTs and for active/history of liver disease prior to initiation and periodically thereafter. Assess for acute asthma attacks, status asthmaticus, age (female >65 yrs), pre-existing transaminase elevation, neuropsychiatric conditions/events, alcohol use, hypersensitivity, pregnancy/nursing status, and possible drug interactions.

Monitoring: Monitor for LFTs and bilirubin levels. Monitor serum ALT prior to therapy, once a month for first 3 months, every 2-3 months for remainder of first year, and periodically thereafter. Monitor for signs/symptoms of hepatitis, jaundice, liver dysfunction (eg, RUQ pain, nausea, fatigue, lethargy, pruritus or flu-like symptoms), neuropsychiatric events (eg, sleep disorders, behavior changes). Monitor alcohol consumption and worsening asthma.

Patient Counseling: Inform that drug is indicated for chronic treatment, not for acute episodes, of asthma. Advise not to reduce dose or d/c other anti-asthma medications unless instructed. Instruct that if a dose is missed, take the next dose at the scheduled time and do not double the dose. Instruct to notify healthcare provider if signs/symptoms of liver dysfunction (eg, RUQ pain, nausea, fatigue, lethargy, pruritus, jaundice, flu-like symptoms) or neuropsychiatric events (eg, sleep disorders, behavior changes) occur. Advise to consult physician before starting or stopping any prescription or OTC medications. Counsel about potential for liver damage and need for liver enzyme monitoring on regular basis. (Tab, ER) Instruct to take regularly as prescribed; within 1 hr after am and pm meals. Do not cut, crush, or chew.

Administration: Oral route. **Storage:** 20-25°C (68-77°F); (Tab, ER) excursions permitted to 15-30°C (59-86°F). Protect from light.

ZYLET   RX
loteprednol etabonate - tobramycin (Bausch & Lomb)

THERAPEUTIC CLASS: Aminoglycoside/corticosteroid

INDICATIONS: Treatment of steroid-responsive inflammatory ocular conditions for which a corticosteroid is indicated and where superficial bacterial ocular infection or a risk of bacterial ocular infection exists.

DOSAGE: *Adults:* Initial: 1-2 drops q4-6h into conjunctival sac of affected eye(s). Titrate: First 24-48 hrs; may increase dosing frequency to q1-2h. Max: 20mL for initial prescription.

HOW SUPPLIED: Sus: (Loteprednol etabonate-Tobramycin) 0.5%-0.3% [2.5mL, 5mL, 10mL]

CONTRAINDICATIONS: Viral diseases of the cornea and conjunctiva including epithelial herpes simplex keratitis (dendritic keratitis), vaccinia, and varicella, and also in mycobacterial infection of the eye and fungal diseases of ocular structures.

WARNINGS/PRECAUTIONS: Not for injection into the eye. Prolonged use may result in glaucoma with optic nerve damage, visual acuity and fields of vision defects, posterior subcapsular cataract formation, host response suppression and thus increase the hazard of secondary ocular infections, overgrowth of nonsusceptible organisms, including fungi. Fungal cultures should be taken when appropriate. Caution with glaucoma. D/C if sensitivity reactions occur. Perforations may occur in those diseases causing thinning of the cornea or sclera. May mask infection or enhance existing infection in acute purulent conditions of the eye. May prolong the course and exacerbate the severity of many viral infections of the eye (including herpes simplex); caution with history of herpes simplex. May delay healing and increase incidence of bleb formation after cataract surgery. Reevaluate if signs and symptoms fail to improve after 2 days. Monitor for intraocular pressure (IOP) if to be used for ≥10 days. Cross-sensitivity to other aminoglycosides may occur; d/c if hypersensitivity occurs and institute appropriate therapy.

ADVERSE REACTIONS: Superficial punctate keratitis, increased IOP, burning, stinging, headache, secondary infection, vision disorders, discharge, itching, lacrimation disorder, photophobia, corneal deposits, ocular discomfort, eyelid disorder.

PREGNANCY: Category C, caution in nursing.

MECHANISM OF ACTION: Loteprednol etabonate: Corticosteroid; has not been established. Suspected to act by induction of phospholipase A_2 inhibitory proteins (lipocortins), which control the biosynthesis of potent inflammatory mediators by inhibiting the release of arachidonic acid. Tobramycin: Aminoglycoside antibiotic; provides action against susceptible organisms.

NURSING CONSIDERATIONS

Assessment: Assess for viral disease of cornea and conjunctiva (eg, dendritic keratitis, vaccinia, varicella), mycobacterial infection or fungal disease of eye, glaucoma, history of herpes simplex, and pregnancy/nursing status.

Monitoring: Routinely monitor IOP if use ≥10 days. Monitor for signs/symptoms of hypersensitivity reactions, glaucoma, defects in visual acuity and fields of vision, posterior subcapsular cataracts, perforations, exacerbation of many viral infections of the eye, secondary infection, delayed wound healing, incidence of bleb formation, and superinfections.

Z

Patient Counseling: Instruct not to allow dropper tip to touch any surface to avoid contamination and not to wear contact lenses during therapy. Advise to consult physician if pain develops, redness or if itching/inflammation become aggravated, or if hypersensitivity reactions, defects in vision occur. Advise to seek medical attention if signs and symptoms fail to improve after 2 days. Counsel not to d/c therapy prematurely.

Administration: Ocular route. Shake vigorously before using. **Storage:** 15-25°C (59-77°F). Protect from freezing; store upright.

ZYMAR   RX
gatifloxacin (Allergan)

THERAPEUTIC CLASS: Fluoroquinolone

INDICATIONS: Treatment of bacterial conjunctivitis.

DOSAGE: *Adults:* 1 drop q2h while awake, up to 8x/day for 2 days; then 1 drop up to qid while awake for 5 days.
Pediatrics: ≥1 yr: 1 drop q2h while awake, up to 8x/day for 2 days; then 1 drop up to qid while awake for 5 days.

HOW SUPPLIED: Sol: 0.3% [5mL]

WARNINGS/PRECAUTIONS: Not for injection. Do not inject subconjunctivally or into the anterior chamber of the eye. Superinfection may result with prolonged use. Fatal hypersensitivity reactions reported after 1st dose of systemic quinolone therapy. Avoid contact lenses when symptoms are present.

ADVERSE REACTIONS: Conjunctival irritation, increased lacrimation, keratitis, papillary conjunctivitis, chemosis, conjunctival hemorrhage, dry eye, eye discharge/irritation/pain, red eye, eyelid edema, headache, reduced visual acuity, taste disturbance.

INTERACTIONS: Systemic quinolone therapy may increase theophylline levels, interfere with caffeine metabolism, enhance warfarin effects, and elevate SrCr with cyclosporine.

PREGNANCY: Category C, caution in nursing.

MECHANISM OF ACTION: Fluoroquinolone antibiotic; inhibits topoisomerase II (DNA gyrase) and topoisomerase IV. DNA gyrase is an essential enzyme involved in replication, transcription, and repair of bacterial DNA. Topoisomerase IV is an enzyme known to play a key role in partitioning of chromosomal DNA during bacterial cell division.

NURSING CONSIDERATIONS

Assessment: Assess for proper diagnosis of causative organisms (eg, slit lamp biomicroscopy, fluorescein staining). Assess for hypersensitivity to other quinolones, possible drug interactions, and use in pregnancy/nursing.

Monitoring: Monitor for signs/symptoms of hypersensitivity or anaphylactic reactions (eg, cardiovascular collapse, loss of consciousness, angioedema). Monitor for overgrowth of nonsusceptible organisms (eg, fungi) with prolonged therapy.

Patient Counseling: Advise to avoid contaminating applicator tip with material from eye, fingers, or other sources. Instruct to d/c therapy and contact physician at first sign of rash or allergic reaction. Advise not to wear contact lenses if there are signs/symptoms of bacterial conjunctivitis.

Administration: Ocular route. Do not inject into eye. **Storage:** Store at 15-25°C (59-77°F). Protect from freezing.

ZYMAXID   RX
gatifloxacin (Allergan)

THERAPEUTIC CLASS: Fluoroquinolone

INDICATIONS: Treatment of bacterial conjunctivitis caused by susceptible strains of organisms.

DOSAGE: *Adults:* 1 drop q2h while awake, up to 8X on Day 1, then 1 drop bid-qid while awake on Days 2-7.
Pediatrics: ≥1 yr: 1 drop q2h while awake, up to 8X on Day 1, then 1 drop bid-qid while awake on Days 2-7.

HOW SUPPLIED: Sol: 0.5% [2.5mL]

WARNINGS/PRECAUTIONS: For ophthalmic use only; should not be introduced directly into the anterior chamber of the eye. Overgrowth of nonsusceptible organisms, including fungi, may result with prolonged use. D/C use and institute alternative therapy if superinfection occurs. Avoid wearing contact lenses if there are signs and symptoms of bacterial conjunctivitis or during the course of therapy.

ADVERSE REACTIONS: Worsening of the conjunctivitis, eye irritation, dysgeusia, eye pain.

PREGNANCY: Category C, caution in nursing.

MECHANISM OF ACTION: Fluoroquinolone antibiotic; inhibition of DNA gyrase and topoisomerase IV. DNA gyrase is an essential enzyme involved in replication, transcription, and repair of bacterial DNA. Topoisomerase IV is an enzyme known to play a key role in partitioning of chromosomal DNA during bacterial cell division.

NURSING CONSIDERATIONS

Assessment: Assess for conjunctivitis, proper diagnosis of causative organisms (eg, slit lamp biomicroscopy, fluorescein staining), and pregnancy/nursing status.

Monitoring: Monitor for adverse events and overgrowth of nonsusceptible organisms (eg, fungi) with prolonged therapy.

Patient Counseling: Inform that solution is for ophthalmic use only and should not be introduced directly into the anterior chamber of the eye. Advise not to wear contact lenses if there are signs and symptoms of bacterial conjunctivitis and during course of therapy. Instruct to avoid contaminating the applicator tip with material from the eyes, fingers or other sources.

Administration: Ocular route. **Storage:** 15-25°C (59-77°F). Protect from freezing.

ZYPREXA   RX
olanzapine (Lilly)

> Elderly patients with dementia-related psychosis treated with antipsychotic drugs are at an increased risk of death; most deaths appeared to be cardiovascular (eg, heart failure, sudden death) or infectious (eg, pneumonia) in nature. Not approved for the treatment of patients with dementia-related psychosis. When used with fluoxetine, refer to the Boxed Warning section of the PI for Symbyax.

OTHER BRAND NAMES: Zyprexa Zydis (Lilly)

THERAPEUTIC CLASS: Thienobenzodiazepine

INDICATIONS: (PO) Treatment of schizophrenia, acute treatment of manic or mixed episodes associated with bipolar I disorder and maintenance treatment of bipolar I disorder in adults and adolescents 13-17 yrs. Adjunct to lithium or valproate for the treatment of manic or mixed episodes associated with bipolar I disorder in adults. In combination with fluoxetine for the treatment of depressive episodes associated with bipolar I disorder and of treatment-resistant depression in adults. (IM) Treatment of acute agitation associated with schizophrenia and bipolar I mania in adults.

DOSAGE: *Adults:* (PO) Schizophrenia: Initial/Usual: 5-10mg qd. Target dose: 10mg/day. Adjust dose by increments/decrements of 5mg qd at intervals of not <1 week. Max: 20mg/day. Maint: 10-20mg/day. Bipolar I Disorder (Manic or Mixed Episodes): Initial: 10mg or 15mg qd. Adjust dose by increments/decrements of 5mg qd at intervals of not <24 hrs. Maint: 5-20mg/day. Max: 20mg/day. With Lithium or Valproate: Initial/Usual: 10mg qd. Max: 20mg/day. Depressive Episodes Associated with Bipolar I Disorder/Resistant Depression in Combination with Fluoxetine: Initial: 5mg with 20mg fluoxetine qpm. Adjust dose based on efficacy and tolerability. Usual: 5-12.5mg with 20-50mg fluoxetine (depressive episodes associated with Bipolar I disorder) or 5-20mg with 20-50mg fluoxetine (resistant depression). Max: 18mg with 75mg fluoxetine. (IM) Agitation: Usual: 10mg. Range: 2.5-10mg. Assess for orthostatic hypotension prior to subsequent dosing. Max: 3 doses of 10mg q2-4h. May initiate PO therapy in a range of 5-20mg/day when clinically appropriate. Elderly: 5mg/inj. See PI for dosing in special populations. *Pediatrics:* 13-17 yrs: (PO) Schizophrenia/Bipolar I Disorder (Manic or Mixed Episodes): Initial: 2.5mg or 5mg qd. Target dose: 10mg/day. Adjust dose by increments/decrements of 2.5mg or 5mg. Max: 20mg/day. Maint: use lowest dose to maintain remission.

HOW SUPPLIED: Inj: 10mg [vial]; Tab: 2.5mg, 5mg, 7.5mg, 10mg, 15mg, 20mg; Tab, Disintegrating: (Zydis) 5mg, 10mg, 15mg, 20mg

WARNINGS/PRECAUTIONS: May cause hyperglycemia; caution in patients with diabetes mellitus or borderline increased blood glucose levels, and monitor for worsening of glucose control. Supervision should accompany therapy in patients at high risk of attempted suicide. Neuroleptic malignant syndrome (NMS) reported; d/c if symptoms occur and instill intensive symptomatic treatment and monitoring. Tardive dyskinesia (TD) reported; d/c if signs/symptoms develop unless treatment is required despite the presence of syndrome. Hyperlipidemia, weight gain, and hyperprolactinemia reported. May cause orthostatic hypotension; caution with cardiovascular disease (CVD), cerebrovascular disease and conditions that would predispose to hypotension. May cause esophageal dysmotility and aspiration, and disruption of body temperature regulation. Not approved for use in patients with Alzheimer's disease. Seizures reported; caution in patients with history of seizures or with conditions that lower the seizure threshold (eg, Alzheimer's dementia). Leukopenia, neutropenia, and agranulocytosis reported; d/c at 1st sign of clinically significant decline in WBC without causative factors or if severe neutropenia (absolute neutrophil

Z

count <1000/mm³) develops. May cause cognitive and motor impairment. Caution in patients with clinically significant prostatic hypertrophy, narrow-angle glaucoma, history of paralytic ileus or related conditions, hepatic impairment, and in elderly.

ADVERSE REACTIONS: Postural hypotension, constipation, dry mouth, weight gain, somnolence, dizziness, personality disorder, akathisia, asthenia, dyspepsia, tremor, increased appetite, abdominal pain, headache, insomnia.

INTERACTIONS: May potentiate orthostatic hypotension with diazepam and alcohol. May enhance effects of certain antihypertensives. Increased clearance with carbamazepine, omeprazole, and rifampin (CYP1A2 inducers). Caution with other CNS-acting drugs, drugs whose effects can induce hypotension, bradycardia, or respiratory/CNS depression, and in patients being treated with potentially hepatotoxic drugs. May antagonize effects of levodopa and dopamine agonists. Decreased clearance with fluoxetine (CYP2D6) and fluvoxamine (CYP1A2 inhibitor); consider lower dose with fluvoxamine. Caution when prescribing with anticholinergic drugs; may contribute to elevation in core body temperature. (IM) Not recommended with parenteral benzodiazepines. Increased somnolence with IM lorazepam. (PO) Decreased levels with activated charcoal.

PREGNANCY: Category C, not for use in nursing.

MECHANISM OF ACTION: Thienobenzodiazepine; not established. Proposed that efficacy in schizophrenia is mediated through a combination of dopamine and serotonin type 2 (5HT2) antagonism.

PHARMACOKINETICS: Absorption: (PO) Well-absorbed, T_{max}=6 hrs; (IM) Rapid, T_{max}=15-45 min. **Distribution:** Found in breast milk. (PO) V_d=1000L; plasma protein binding (93%). **Metabolism:** Via CYP450 mediated oxidation and direct glucuronidation; 10-N-glucuronide and 4'-N-desmethyl olanzapine (major metabolites). **Elimination:** (PO) Urine (57%, 7% unchanged), feces (30%); $T_{1/2}$=21-54 hrs.

NURSING CONSIDERATIONS

Assessment: Assess for CVD, cerebrovascular disease, risk of hypotension, history of seizures or conditions that could lower the seizure threshold, prostatic hypertrophy, narrow-angle glaucoma, history of paralytic ileus, hepatic impairment, history of drug abuse, risk factors/history of drug induced leukopenia/neutropenia, clinically significant low WBC, pregnancy/nursing status, and possible drug interactions. Assess for dementia-related psychosis and Alzheimer's disease in the elderly. Obtain baseline lipid panel, CBC, and FBG levels.

Monitoring: Monitor for signs/symptoms of NMS, TD, and other adverse effects. Monitor FBG, lipid levels, CBC, and weight of patient periodically. In patients with clinically significant neutropenia, monitor for fever or other symptoms/signs of infection. Periodically reassess to determine the need for maintenance treatment.

Patient Counseling: Advise of benefits/risks of therapy. Counsel about signs and symptoms of NMS. Inform of potential risk of hyperglycemia-related adverse events. Medication may cause hyperlipidemia and weight gain. Inform that medication may cause orthostatic hypotension; instruct to contact physician if dizziness, fast or slow heart beat, or fainting occurs. Inform that medication may impair judgment, thinking, or motor skills; instruct to use caution when operating hazardous machinery. Instruct to avoid overheating and dehydration. Instruct to avoid alcohol. Inform that orally disintegrating tab contains phenylalanine. Notify physician if taking, planning to take, or have stopped taking any prescription or over-the-counter products, including herbal supplements. Notify physician if pregnant or plan to become pregnant during treatment. Advise to avoid breastfeeding during therapy.

Administration: Oral/IM routes. (Inj) Do not administer IV or SQ. Inj slowly, deep into the muscle mass. See PI for proper reconstitution procedures. (Zydis) After opening sachet, peel back foil on blister. Do not push tab through foil. Upon opening the blister, remove tab and place entire tab in the mouth using dry hands. **Storage:** Tab, Zydis, and Inj (Before Reconstitution): 20-25°C (68-77°F); excursions permitted between 15-30°C (59-86°F). Reconstituted Inj: 20-25°C (68-77°F) for up to 1 hr; excursions permitted between 15-30°C (59-86°F). Tab/Zydis: Protect from light and moisture. Inj: Protect from light. Do not freeze.

ZYPREXA RELPREVV   RX
olanzapine (Lilly)

Elderly patients with dementia-related psychosis treated with antipsychotic drugs are at an increased risk of death. Most deaths reported appeared to be cardiovascular (eg, heart failure, sudden death) or infectious (eg, pneumonia) in nature. Not approved for the treatment of patients with dementia-related psychosis. Post-inj delirium and sedation (including coma) reported. Must be administered in a registered healthcare facility with ready access to emergency response services. Observe patient for ≥3 hrs after each inj. Available only through a restricted distribution program called Zyprexa Relprevv Patient Care Program and requires prescriber, healthcare facility, patient, and pharmacy enrollment.

THERAPEUTIC CLASS: Thienobenzodiazepine

INDICATIONS: Treatment of schizophrenia.

DOSAGE: *Adults:* Usual: 150-300mg IM every 2 weeks or 405mg IM every 4 weeks. Max: 405mg IM every 4 weeks or 300mg IM every 2 weeks. Debilitated/Hypotension Risk/Slow Metabolizers/ Sensitive to Effects: Initial: 150mg IM every 4 weeks. Titrate: Increase cautiously. Establish tolerability with oral olanzapine prior to initiating treatment. Refer to PI for recommended dosing based on corresponding oral olanzapine doses.

HOW SUPPLIED: Inj, Extended-Release: 210mg, 300mg, 405mg

WARNINGS/PRECAUTIONS: May cause hyperglycemia; caution in patients with diabetes mellitus (DM) or borderline increased blood glucose levels; monitor for worsening of glucose control. Obtain fasting blood glucose (FBG) levels at beginning of treatment and periodically during treatment. Supervision should accompany therapy if patients are at high risk of attempted suicide. Neuroleptic malignant syndrome (NMS) reported; d/c if symptoms occur and instill intensive symptomatic treatment and monitoring. Tardive dyskinesia reported; d/c if signs/symptoms develop. Hyperlipidemia reported; obtain lipid levels at baseline and periodically thereafter. May cause weight gain; perform regular monitoring of weight. May induce orthostatic hypotension; caution with known cardiovascular (CV) disease, cerebrovascular disease, and conditions that would predispose to hypotension. May cause esophageal dysmotility and aspiration. Not approved for use in patients with Alzheimer's disease. Seizures reported; caution with history of seizures or with conditions that potentially lower the seizure threshold. Leukopenia, neutropenia, and agranulocytosis reported; d/c in first sign of clinically significant decline in WBC without causative factor or if severe neutropenia (ANC <1000/mm³) develops. May cause cognitive and motor impairment. Hyperprolactinemia reported. May cause disruption of body temperature regulation. Caution in patients with clinically significant prostatic hypertrophy, narrow-angle glaucoma, history of paralytic ileus or related conditions, hepatic impairment, and elderly. Not for IV or SQ use.

ADVERSE REACTIONS: Headache, sedation, dizziness, diarrhea, back pain, N/V, nasal congestion, dry mouth, nasopharyngitis, weight increased, abdominal pain, fatigue, somnolence, increased appetite.

INTERACTIONS: May potentiate orthostatic hypotension with diazepam and alcohol. May enhance effects of certain antihypertensive agents. Increased clearance with carbamazepine, a CYP1A2 inducer. Caution with other CNS-acting drugs. May antagonize effects of levodopa and dopamine agonists. Omeprazole and rifampin, inducers of CYP1A2 or glucuronyl transferase may increase clearance. Fluvoxamine, a CYP1A2 inhibitor and fluoxetine, a CYP2D6 inhibitor may decrease clearance. Caution with concomitant use of drugs whose effects can induce hypotension, bradycardia, respiratory or CNS depression. Caution with parenteral benzodiazepines. Coadministration with IM lorazepam may potentiate somnolence. Caution in patients receiving concomitant therapy with potentially hepatotoxic drugs. Caution when prescribing with anticholinergic drugs; may contribute to elevation in core body temperature.

PREGNANCY: Category C, not for use in nursing.

MECHANISM OF ACTION: Thienobenzodiazepine; not established. Proposed that efficacy in schizophrenia is mediated through a combination of dopamine and serotonin type 2 (5HT$_2$) antagonism.

PHARMACOKINETICS: Absorption: (IM) Rapid, T_{max}=15-45 min. **Distribution:** (PO) Found in breast milk; V_d=1000L; plasma protein binding (93%). **Metabolism**: (PO) Via CYP450 mediated oxidation and direct glucuronidation; 10-N-glucuronide, 4'-N-desmethyl olanzapine (major metabolites). **Elimination:** (PO) Urine (57%, 7% unchanged), feces (30%); $T_{1/2}$ =30 days (IM).

NURSING CONSIDERATIONS

Assessment: Assess for tolerability with oral olanzapine, DM, hyperlipidemia, CV or cerebrovascular disease, risk of hypotension, history of seizures or conditions that could lower the seizure threshold, prostatic hypertrophy, narrow-angle glaucoma, history of paralytic ileus, hepatic impairment, pregnancy/nursing status, and possible drug interactions. Assess for dementia-related psychosis and Alzheimer's disease in elderly. Assess for debilitated, slow metabolizers and those pharmacodynamically sensitive to olanzapine. Obtain baseline lipid panel, CBC and FBG levels.

Monitoring: Monitor for sedation and/or delirium for ≥3 hrs post-inj. Monitor for signs/symptoms of NMS, hyperglycemia, hyperlipidemia, weight gain, tardive dyskinesia, and other adverse effects. Perform periodic monitoring of FBG, lipid levels, and weight of patient. Perform frequent monitoring of CBC in patients with a history of clinically significant low WBC or drug-induced leukopenia/neutropenia. In patients with clinically significant neutropenia, monitor for fever or other symptoms or signs of infection. In high-risk patients, monitor closely for a suicide attempt.

Patient Counseling: Advise of benefits/risks of therapy. Advise of the risk of post-inj delirium/ sedation syndrome following administration. Inform that drug is not approved for elderly with dementia-related psychosis. Counsel about the signs/symptoms of NMS. Inform of potential risk of hyperglycemia-related adverse events. Medication may cause hyperlipidemia and weight gain. Medication may cause orthostatic hypotension; instruct to contact physician if dizziness, fast or slow heart beat, or fainting occurs. Medication may impair judgment, thinking, or motor

Z

skills; instruct to use caution when operating hazardous machinery. Avoid alcohol. Notify physician if taking, planning to take, or have stopped taking any prescription or over-the-counter (OTC) drugs, including herbal supplements. Notify physician if pregnant or planning to become pregnant during treatment. Avoid breastfeeding during therapy. Advise regarding appropriate care in avoiding overheating and dehydration. Reassess periodically to determine the need for continued treatment.

Administration: IM route. See PI for proper reconstitution and administration technique. **Storage:** Room temperature ≤30°C (86°F). Reconstituted Sol: May store at room temperature for 24 hrs.

ZYTIGA

abiraterone acetate (Janssen)

RX

THERAPEUTIC CLASS: Nonsteroidal antiandrogen

INDICATIONS: In combination with prednisone for the treatment of patients with metastatic castration-resistant prostate cancer who have received prior chemotherapy containing docetaxel.

DOSAGE: *Adults:* 1000mg qd with prednisone 5mg PO bid. Take on empty stomach. Baseline Moderate Hepatic Impairment (Child-Pugh Class B): Initial: 250mg qd. If ALT/AST >5X ULN or total bilirubin >3X ULN occur, d/c and do not retreat. Hepatotoxicity (ALT/AST >5X ULN or total bilirubin >3X ULN) During Treatment: Interrupt treatment. Restart at 750mg qd following return of LFTs to patient's baseline or to AST/ALT ≤2.5X ULN and total bilirubin ≤1.5X ULN. If hepatotoxicity recurs at 750mg qd, restart retreatment at 500mg qd following return of LFTs to patient's baseline or to AST/ALT ≤2.5X ULN and total bilirubin ≤1.5X ULN. If hepatotoxicity recurs at 500mg qd, d/c use.

HOW SUPPLIED: Tab: 250mg

CONTRAINDICATIONS: Women who are or may become pregnant.

WARNINGS/PRECAUTIONS: May cause HTN, hypokalemia, and fluid retention; caution with history of cardiovascular disease (CVD) or with underlying medical conditions that might be compromised by increases in BP, hypokalemia or fluid retention, and monitor for such effects at least monthly. Control HTN and correct hypokalemia before and during treatment. Adrenocortical insufficiency reported following interruption of daily steroids and/or with concurrent infection or stress; use caution and monitor for signs/symptoms, particularly if patients withdrawn from prednisone, have prednisone dose reductions, or experience unusual stresses. Increased dosage of corticosteroids may be indicated before, during, and after stressful situations. Marked increases in liver enzymes reported; measure ALT/AST and bilirubin levels at baseline, q2 weeks for the 1st 3 months (or weekly for the 1st month, then q2 weeks for the following 2 months in patients with baseline moderate hepatic impairment), and monthly thereafter. Promptly measure serum total bilirubin, AST, and ALT if signs/symptoms of hepatotoxicity develop. Avoid with baseline severe hepatic impairment (Child-Pugh Class C).

ADVERSE REACTIONS: Joint swelling or discomfort, hypokalemia, edema, muscle discomfort, hot flush, diarrhea, urinary tract infection (UTI), cough, HTN, arrhythmia, urinary frequency, nocturia, dyspepsia, fractures, upper respiratory tract infection.

INTERACTIONS: Increased levels of dextromethorphan (CYP2D6 substrate). Avoid with CYP2D6 substrates with narrow therapeutic index (eg, thioridazine). Exercise caution and consider dose reduction of concomitant CYP2D6 substrate if alternative treatments cannot be used. Avoid or use caution with strong inhibitors or inducers of CYP3A4.

PREGNANCY: Category X, not for use in nursing.

MECHANISM OF ACTION: Androgen biosynthesis inhibitor; inhibits 17 α-hydroxylase/C17,20-lyase (CYP17).

PHARMACOKINETICS: Absorption: T_{max}=2 hrs (median); C_{max}=226ng/mL; AUC=1173ng•hr/mL. **Distribution:** V_d=19,669L; plasma protein binding (>99%). **Metabolism:** Hydrolysis via esterase to abiraterone (active metabolite). **Elimination:** Feces (88%, 55% unchanged), urine (5%); $T_{1/2}$=12 hrs.

NURSING CONSIDERATIONS

Assessment: Assess for history of CVD, underlying medical conditions that might be compromised by increases in BP, hypokalemia, or fluid retention, HTN, hypokalemia, and possible drug interactions. Obtain baseline AST, ALT, and bilirubin levels.

Monitoring: Monitor for HTN, hypokalemia, and fluid retention at least monthly, and signs/symptoms of adrenocortical insufficiency and hepatotoxicity. Monitor ALT, AST, and bilirubin levels q2 weeks for the 1st 3 months (or weekly for the 1st month, then q2 weeks for the following 2 months in patients with baseline moderate hepatic impairment), and monthly thereafter. For patients who resume treatment after development of hepatotoxicity, monitor serum transaminases and bilirubin at a minimum of q2 weeks for 3 months, and monthly thereafter.

Z

Patient Counseling: Inform that drug is used together with prednisone and instruct not to interrupt or stop either of these medications without consulting physician. Inform those receiving gonadotropin-releasing hormone agonists to maintain such treatment during therapy. Advise that no food should be consumed for at least two hours before and for at least one hour after administration. Advise to swallow tablets whole with water. Inform that if a daily dose is missed, take the normal dose the following day, but if >1 daily dose is skipped, consult physician. Counsel about the common side effects (eg, peripheral edema, hypokalemia, HTN, UTI). Advise that liver function will be monitored using blood tests. Advise to use a condom if having sex with a pregnant woman, or condom and another effective method of birth control if having sex with a woman of childbearing potential; advise that these measures are required during and for 1 week after treatment. Advise to take medication ud.

Administration: Oral route. Swallow whole with water. Take on an empty stomach; do not eat for at least 2 hrs before and for at least 1 hr after the dose is taken. **Storage:** 20-25°C (68-77°F); excursions permitted to 15-30°C (59-86°F).

Z

Appendix: Reference Tables

ABBREVIATIONS, ACRONYMS, AND SYMBOLS

ABBREVIATIONS	DESCRIPTIONS
- (eg, 6-8)	to (eg, 6 to 8)
/	per
<	less than
>	greater than
≤	less than or equal to
≥	greater than or equal to
α	alpha
β	beta
5-FU	5-fluorouracil
5-HT	5-hydroxytryptamine (serotonin)
ABECB	acute bacterial exacerbation of chronic bronchitis
aa	of each
ACTH	adrenocorticotropic hormone
ad	right ear
ADHD	attention-deficit/hyperactivity disorder
A-fib	atrial fibrillation
A-flutter	atrial flutter
AIDS	acquired immunodeficiency syndrome
ALT	alanine transaminase (SGPT)
am or AM	morning
AMI	acute myocardial infarction
ANA	antinuclear antibodies
ANC	absolute neutrophil count
APAP	acetaminophen
as	left ear
ASA	aspirin
AST	aspartate transaminase (SGOT)
au	each ear
AUC	area under the curve
AV	atrioventricular
bid	twice daily
BMI	body mass index
BP	blood pressure
BPH	benign prostatic hypertrophy
BSA	body surface area
BUN	blood urea nitrogen
CABG	coronary artery bypass graft
CAD	coronary artery disease

(Continued)

Cap	capsule or gelcap
CAP	community-acquired pneumonia
CBC	complete blood count
CF	cystic fibrosis
CHF	congestive heart failure
cm	centimeter
CMV	cytomegalovirus
C_{max}	peak plasma concentration
CNS	central nervous system
COPD	chronic obstructive pulmonary disease
CrCl	creatinine clearance
Cre	cream
CRF	chronic renal failure
CSF	cerebrospinal fluid
CVA	cerebrovascular accident
CVD	cardiovascular disease
CYP450	cytochrome P450
d/c or D/C	discontinue
DHEA	dehydroepiandrosterone
DM	diabetes mellitus
DVT	deep vein thrombosis
ECG	electrocardiogram
EEG	electroencephalogram
eg	for example
EPS	extrapyramidal symptom
ESRD	end-stage renal disease
FPG	fasting plasma glucose
FSH	follicle-stimulating hormone
g	gram
GABA	gamma-aminobutyric acid
GAD	general anxiety disorder
GERD	gastroesophageal reflux disease
GFR	glomerular filtration rate
GI	gastrointestinal
GnRH	gonadotropin-releasing hormone
GVHD	graft versus host disease
HCG	human chorionic gonadotropin
Hct	hematocrit
HCTZ	hydrochlorothiazide
HDL	high-density lipoprotein
Hgb	hemoglobin

HIV	human immunodeficiency virus
HMG-CoA	3-hydroxy-3-methylglutaryl-coenzyme A
HR	heart rate
hr or hrs	hour or hours
hs	bedtime
HSV	herpes simplex virus
HTN	hypertension
IBD	inflammatory bowel disease
IBS	irritable bowel syndrome
ICH	intracranial hemorrhage
ICP	intracranial pressure
IM	intramuscular
INH	isoniazid
Inj	injection
INR	international normalized ratio
IOP	intraocular pressure
IU*	international units
IV	intravenous/intravenously
K⁺	potassium
kg	kilogram
KIU	kallikrein inhibitor unit
L	liter
lbs	pounds
LD	loading dose
LDL	low-density lipoprotein
LFT	liver function test
LH	luteinizing hormone
LHRH	luteinizing-hormone releasing hormone
Lot	lotion
Loz	lozenge
LVH	left ventricular hypertrophy
M	molar
MAC	*Mycobacterium avium* complex
Maint	maintenance
MAOI	monoamine oxidase inhibitor
Max	maximum
mcg	microgram
mEq	milli-equivalent
mg	milligram
MI	myocardial infarction
min	minute (usually as mL/min)

(Continued)

mL	milliliter
mm	millimeter
mM	millimolar
MRI	magnetic resonance imaging
MS	multiple sclerosis
msec	millisecond
MTX	methotrexate
Na	sodium
NaCl	sodium chloride
NG	nasogastric
NKA	no known allergies
NMS	neuroleptic malignant syndrome
NPO	nothing by mouth
NSAID	nonsteroidal anti-inflammatory drug
NV or N/V	nausea and vomiting
OA	osteoarthritis
OCD	obsessive-compulsive disorder
od	right eye
Oint	ointment
os	left eye
ou	each eye
PAT	paroxysmal atrial tachycardia
pc	after meals
PCN	penicillin
PCP	*Pneumocystis carinii* pneumonia
PD	Parkinson's disease
PID	pelvic inflammatory disease
pkt, pkts	packet, packets
pm	evening
po or PO	orally
PONV	postoperative nausea and vomiting
pr	rectally
prn	as needed
PSA	prostate-specific antigen
PSVT	paroxysmal supraventricular tachycardia
PT	prothrombin time
PTSD	post-traumatic stress disorder
PTT	partial thromboplastin time
PTU	propylthiouracil
PUD	peptic ulcer disease
PVD	peripheral vascular disease

q4h, q6h, q8h, etc.	every four hours, every six hours, every eight hours, etc.
qd*	once daily
qh	every hour
qid	four times daily
qod*	every other day
qs	a sufficient quantity
qs ad	a sufficient quantity up to
RA	rheumatoid arthritis
RBC	red blood cells
RDS	respiratory distress syndrome
REM	rapid eye movement
SAH	subarachnoid hemorrhage
SBP	systolic blood pressure
sec	second(s)
SGOT	serum glutamic-oxaloacetic transaminase (AST)
SGPT	serum glutamic-pyruvic transaminase (ALT)
SIADH	syndrome of inappropriate antidiuretic hormone secretion
SLE	systemic lupus erythematosus
SOB	shortness of breath
Sol	solution
SQ, SC	subcutaneous
SrCr	serum creatinine
SSRI	selective serotonin reuptake inhibitor
SSSI	skin and skin structure infection
STD	sexually transmitted disease
Sup or supp	suppository
Sus	suspension
SVT	supraventricular tachycardia
$T_{1/2}$	half-life
Tab	tablet or caplet
Taq, SL	sublingual tablet
TB	tuberculosis
TBG	thyroxine binding globulin
tbl or tbsp	tablespoonful
TCA	tricyclic antidepressant
TD	tardive dyskinesia
TFT	thyroid function test
TG	triglyceride

(Continued)

tid	three times daily
T_{max}	time to maximum concentration
TNF	tumor necrosis factor
TPN	total parenteral nutrition
TSH	thyroid stimulating hormone
tsp	teaspoonful
TTP	thrombotic thrombocytopenic purpura
U*	unit
ud	as directed
ULN	upper limit of normal
URTI/URI	upper respiratory tract infection
UTI	urinary tract infection
UV	ultraviolet
WBC	white blood cell count
V_d	volume of distribution
VTE	venous thromboembolism
X	times (eg, >2X ULN)
yr or yrs	year or years

*According to JCAHO, these abbreviations are not recommended for use and should be written out to reduce errors.

CALCULATIONS AND FORMULAS

METRIC MEASURES

1 kilogram (kg)	1000 g
1 gram (g)	1000 mg
1 milligram (mg)	0.001 g
1 microgram (mcg or µg)	0.001 mg; 1×10^{-6} g
1 liter (L)	1000 mL
1 milliliter (mL)	0.001 L; 1 cc (cubic centimeter)

APOTHECARY MEASURES (AP)

1 scruple	20 grains (gr)
1 drachm	3 scruples; 60 gr
1 ounce (oz)	8 drachms; 24 scruples; 480 gr
1 pound (lb)	12 oz; 96 drachms; 288 scruples; 5760 gr

U.S. FLUID MEASURES

1 fluidrachm	60 minim
1 fluid ounce	8 fluidrachm; 480 minim
1 pint (pt)	16 fl oz; 7680 minim
1 quart (qt)	2 pt; 32 fl oz
1 gallon (gal)	4 qt; 128 fl oz

AVOIRDUPOIS WEIGHT (AV)

1 ounce	437.5 gr
1 pound	16 oz

CONVERSION FACTORS

1 gram	15.4 gr
1 grain	64.8 mg
1 ounce (Av)	28.35 g; 437.5 gr
1 ounce (Ap)	31.1 g; 480 gr
1 pound (Av)	453.6 g; 2.68 lb (Ap); 2.20 lb (Av)
1 fluid ounce	29.57 mL
1 fluidrachm	3.697 mL
1 minim	0.06 mL

COMMON MEASURES

1 teaspoonful	5 mL; ⅙ fl oz
1 tablespoonful	15 mL; ½ fl oz
1 wineglassful	60 mL; 2 fl oz
1 teacupful	120 mL; 4 fl oz
1 gallon	3800 mL; 128 fl oz
1 quart	960 mL; 32 fl oz
1 pint	480 mL; 16 fl oz (exactly 473.2 mL)
8 fluid ounces	240 mL
4 fluid ounces	120 mL
2.2 lb	1 kg

DOSE EQUIVALENTS

WEIGHT (METRIC)	WEIGHT (APOTHECARY)
30 g	1 ounce
15 g	4 drams
10 g	2½ drams
7.5 g	2 drams
6 g	90 grains
5 g	75 grains
4 g	60 grains; 1 dram
3 g	45 grains

(Continued)

DOSE EQUIVALENTS *(Continued)*	
WEIGHT (METRIC)	**WEIGHT (APOTHECARY)**
2 g	30 grains; ½ dram
1.5 g	22 grains
1 g	15 grains
750 mg	12 grains
600 mg	10 grains
500 mg	7½ grains
400 mg	6 grains
300 mg	5 grains
250 mg	4 grains
200 mg	3 grains
150 mg	2½ grains
125 mg	2 grains
100 mg	1½ grains
75 mg	1¼ grains
60 mg	1 grain
50 mg	¾ grain
40 mg	⅔ grain
30 mg	½ grain
25 mg	⅜ grain
20 mg	⅓ grain
15 mg	¼ grain
12 mg	⅕ grain
10 mg	⅙ grain
8 mg	⅛ grain
6 mg	1/10 grain
5 mg	1/12 grain
4 mg	1/15 grain
3 mg	1/20 grain
2 mg	1/30 grain
1.5 mg	1/40 grain
1.2 mg	1/50 grain
1 mg	1/60 grain
LIQUID MEASURES (METRIC)	**LIQUID MEASURES (APOTHECARY)**
1000 mL	1 quart
750 mL	1½ pints
500 mL	1 pint
230 mL	8 fluid ounces
200 mL	7 fluid ounces
100 mL	3½ fluid ounces
50 mL	1¾ fluid ounces
30 mL	1 fluid ounce
15 mL	4 fluid drams
10 mL	2½ fluid drams
8 mL	2 fluid drams
5 mL	1½ fluid drams
4 mL	1 fluid dram
3 mL	45 minims
2 mL	30 minims
1 mL	15 minims
0.75 mL	12 minims
0.6 mL	10 minims
0.5 mL	8 minims
0.3 mL	5 minims
0.25 mL	4 minims
0.2 mL	3 minims

DOSE EQUIVALENTS *(Continued)*	
WEIGHT (METRIC)	**WEIGHT (APOTHECARY)**
0.1 mL	1½ minims
0.06 mL	1 minim
0.05 mL	¾ minim
0.03 mL	½ minim

MILLIEQUIVALENT (mEq) AND MILLIMOLE (mmol)

CALCULATIONS

moles = $\dfrac{\text{weight of a substance (grams)}}{\text{molecular weight of that substance (grams)}}$ **OR** $= \dfrac{\text{equivalent}}{\text{valence of ion}}$

millimoles = $\dfrac{\text{weight of a substance (milligrams)}}{\text{molecular weight of that substance (milligrams)}}$ **OR** $= \dfrac{\text{milliequivalents}}{\text{valence of ion}}$ **OR** $= \text{moles} \times 1000$

equivalents = moles × valence of ion

milliequivalents = millimoles × valence of ion **OR** = equivalents × 1000

CONVERSIONS

mg/100mL to mEq/L	mEq/L = $\dfrac{\text{(mg/100mL)} \times 10 \times \text{valence}}{\text{atomic weight}}$
mEq/L to mg/100mL	mg/100mL = $\dfrac{\text{(mEq/L)} \times \text{atomic weight}}{10 \times \text{valence}}$
mEq/L to volume percent of a gas	volume % = $\dfrac{\text{(mEq/L)} \times 22.4}{10}$

ACID-BASE ASSESSMENT

DEFINITIONS

PIO_2	Oxygen partial pressure of inspired gas (mmHg); 150 mmHg in room air at sea level
FiO_2	Fractional pressure of oxygen in inspired gas (0.21 in room air)
PAO_2	Alveolar oxygen partial pressure
$PACO_2$	Alveolar carbon dioxide partial pressure
PaO_2	Arterial oxygen partial pressure
$PaCO_2$	Arterial carbon dioxide partial pressure
R	Respiratory exchange quotient (typically 0.8, increases with high-carbohydrate diet, decreases with high-fat diet)

HENDERSON-HASSELBALCH EQUATION

$pH = 6.1 + \log\,[HCO_3^- / (0.03)\,(pCO_2)]$

ALVEOLAR GAS EQUATION

$PIO_2 = FiO_2 \times$ (total atmospheric pressure - vapor pressure of H_2O at 37°C)
  $= FiO_2 \times$ (760 mmHg - 47 mmHg)

$PaO_2 = PIO_2 - PaCO_2/R$

ALVEOLAR/ARTERIAL OXYGEN GRADIENT

$PAO_2 - PaO_2$

ACID-BASE DISORDERS

DISORDER	pH	HCO$_3^-$	PCO$_2$	COMPENSATION
Metabolic acidosis	<7.35	Primary decrease	Compensatory decrease	1.2-mmHg decrease in PCO$_2$ for every 1-mmol/L decrease in HCO$_3^-$ or PCO$_2$ = (1.5 × HCO$_3^-$) + 8 (±2) or PCO$_2$ = HCO$_3^-$ + 15 or PCO$_2$ = last 2 digits of pH × 100

(Continued)

ACID-BASE DISORDERS *(Continued)*

DISORDER	PH	HCO$_3^-$	PCO$_2$	COMPENSATION
Metabolic alkalosis	>7.45	Primary increase	Compensatory increase	0.6-0.75 mmHg increase in PCO$_2$ for every 1-mmol/L increase in HCO$_3^-$. PCO$_2$ should not rise above 60 mmHg in compensation.
Respiratory acidosis	<7.35	Compensatory increase	Primary increase	*Acute:* 1-2 mmol decrease in HCO$_3^-$ for every 10-mmHg decrease in PCO$_2$. *Chronic:* 3-4 mmol increase in HCO$_3^-$ for every 10-mmHg increase in PCO$_2$.
Respiratory alkalosis	>7.45	Compensatory decrease	Primary decrease	*Acute:* 1-2 mmol increase in HCO$_3^-$ for every 10-mmHg increase in PCO$_2$. *Chronic:* 4-5 mmol decrease in HCO$_3^-$ for every 10-mmHg decrease in PCO$_2$.

ACID-BASE EQUATION

H$^+$ (in mEq/L) = (24 × PaCO$_2$) divided by HCO$_3^-$

OTHER CALCULATIONS

ANION GAP

Anion gap = Na$^+$ - (Cl$^-$ + HCO$_3^-$ measured)

ALVEOLAR-ARTERIAL GRADIENT

Aa gradient [(713) (FiO$_2$ - (PaCO$_2$ divided by 0.8))] - PaO$_2$

OSMOLALITY

Definition:
Osmolality is a measure of the total number of particles in a solution.

U.S. units (sodium as mEq/L, BUN [blood urea nitrogen] and glucose as mg/dL)
Plasma osmolality (mOsm/kg) = 2([Na$^+$] + [K$^+$]) + ([BUN]/2.8) + ([glucose]/18)

SI units (all variables in mmol/L):
Plasma osmolality (mOsm/kg) = 2[Na$^+$] + [urea] + [glucose]
Normal range plasma osmolality: 280 - 303 mOsm/kg

Corrected Sodium
Corrected Na$^+$ = measured Na$^+$ + [1.5 × (glucose -150 divided by 100)]*
*Do not correct for glucose <150.

Total Serum Calcium Corrected for Albumin Level
[(Normal albumin - patient's albumin) × 0.8] + patient's measured total calcium

Water Deficit
Water deficit = 0.6 × body weight [1 - (140 divided by Na$^+$)]*
*Body weight is estimated weight in kg; Na$^+$ is serum or plasma sodium.

Bicarbonate Deficit
HCO$_3^-$ deficit = [0.4 × weight (kg)] × (HCO$_3^-$ desired - HCO$_3^-$ measured)

CHILD-PUGH SCORE

The Child-Pugh classification is used to assess the prognosis of chronic liver disease, mainly cirrhosis. Child-Pugh is also used to determine the required strength of treatment and the necessity of liver transplantation.

Score:
The score employs five clinical measures of liver disease. Each measure is scored 1-3, with 3 indicating the most severe derangement.

Measure	1 point	2 points	3 points	Units
Bilirubin (total)*	<34 (<2)	34-50 (2-3)	>50 (>3)	mol/L (mg/dL)
Serum albumin	>35	28-35	<28	mg/L
INR†	<1.7	1.71-2.20	>2.20	no unit
Ascites	None	Suppressed with medication	Refractory	no unit
Hepatic encephalopathy	None	Grade I-II (or supressed with medication)	Grade III-IV (or refractory)	no unit

*In primary sclerosing cholangitis and primary biliary cirrhosis, the bilirubin references are changed to reflect the fact that these diseases feature high conjugated bilirubin values. The upper limit for 1 point is 68 mol/L (4 mg/dL) and the upper limit for 2 points is 170 mol/L (10 mg/dL).
†Some older reference works substitute PT prolongation for INR.

Interpretation:
Chronic liver disease is classified into Child-Pugh class A to C, employing the added score from above.

Points	Class	One-year survival	Two-year survival
5-6	A	100%	85%
7-9	B	81%	57%
10-15	C	45%	35%

CREATININE CLEARANCE

Clinically, creatinine clearance is a useful measure for estimating the glomerular filtration rate (GFR) of the kidneys.

Factors	Abbreviations
Creatinine clearance	Cl_{Cr}
Plasma creatinine concentration	P_{Cr}
Serum creatinine concentration	S_{Cr}
Urine creatinine concentration	U_{Cr}
Urine flow rate	V

Calculations:
$$Cl_{Cr} = \frac{U_{Cr} \times V}{P_{Cr}}$$

Example:
Patient with P_{Cr} 1 mg/dL, U_{Cr} 60 mg/dL, and V of 0.5 dL/hr.
$$Cl_{Cr} = \frac{60 \text{ mg/dL} \times 0.5 \text{ dL/hr}}{1 \text{ mg/dL}} = 30 \text{ dl/hr}$$

Cockroft-Gault formula: Estimates creatinine clearance (mL/min).

Male:
$$Cl_{Cr} = \frac{(140 - age) \times mass (kg)}{72 \times S_{Cr} (mg/dL)}$$

Example:
Male patient, 67 years of age, weight 75 kg, and S_{Cr} 1 mg/dL.
$$Cl_{Cr} = \frac{(140 - 67) \times 75}{72 \times 1} = 76 \text{ mL/min}$$

Female:
$$Cl_{Cr} = \frac{(140 - age) \times mass (kg) \times 0.85}{72 \times S_{Cr} (mg/dL)}$$

Example:
Female patient, 67 years of age, weight 75 kg, and S_{Cr} 1 mg/dL.
$$Cl_{Cr} = \frac{(140 - 67) \times 75 \times 0.85}{72 \times 1} = 64.6 \text{ mL/min}$$

Note: Using actual body weight (ABW) in obese patients can significantly overestimate creatinine clearance. Adjusted ideal body weight (IBW) can provide a more approximate estimate. Adjusted IBW = IBW + 0.4 (ABW - IBW).

BASAL ENERGY EXPENDITURE (BEE)

Basal energy expenditure: the amount of energy required to maintain the body's normal metabolic activity (eg, respiration, maintenance of body temperature, etc).
H = height (cm), W = weight (kg), A = age (years)
Male:
BEE = 66.67 + 13.75W + 5H - 6.76A
Female:
BEE = 66.51 + 9.56W + 1.85H - 4.68A

BODY MASS INDEX (BMI)

$$BMI = \frac{weight (kg)}{[height (m)]^2}$$

BODY SURFACE AREA (BSA)

$$BSA (m^2) = \sqrt{\frac{height (in) \times weight (lb)}{3131}}$$ **OR** $$BSA (m^2) = \sqrt{\frac{height (cm) \times weight (kg)}{3600}}$$

IDEAL BODY WEIGHT (IBW)

Adults (18 years and older; IBW is in kg):
 IBW (male) = 50 + (2.3 × height [inches] over 5 feet)
 IBW (female) = 45.5 + (2.3 × height [inches] over 5 feet)

Children (IBW is in kg; height is in cm):
 For children 1-18 years old and with a height <5 feet:
 $$IBW = \frac{(height^2 \times 1.65)}{100}$$

For children 1-18 years old and with a height >5 feet:
 IBW (male) = 39 + (2.27 × height [inches] over 5 feet)
 IBW (female) = 42.2 + (2.27 × height [inches] over 5 feet)

POUNDS/KILOGRAM CONVERSION

1 POUND = 0.45359 KILOGRAM				1 KILOGRAM = 2.2 POUNDS			
lb	kg	lb	kg	lb	kg	lb	kg
1	0.45	105	47.63	210	95.25	315	142.88
5	2.27	110	49.89	215	97.52	320	145.15
10	4.54	115	52.16	220	99.79	325	147.42
15	6.80	120	54.43	225	102.06	330	149.68
20	9.07	125	56.70	230	104.33	335	151.95
25	11.34	130	58.97	235	106.59	340	154.22
30	13.61	135	61.23	240	108.86	345	156.49
35	15.88	140	63.50	245	111.13	350	158.76
40	18.14	145	65.77	250	113.40	355	161.02
45	20.41	150	68.04	255	115.67	360	163.29
50	22.68	155	70.31	260	117.93	365	165.56
55	24.95	160	72.57	265	120.20	370	167.83
60	27.22	165	74.84	270	122.47	375	170.10
65	29.48	170	77.11	275	124.74	380	172.36
70	31.75	175	79.38	280	127.01	385	174.63
75	34.02	180	81.65	285	129.27	390	176.90
80	36.29	185	83.91	290	131.54	395	179.17
85	38.56	190	86.18	295	133.81	400	181.44
90	40.82	195	88.45	300	136.08	405	183.70
95	43.09	200	90.72	305	138.34	410	185.97
100	45.36	205	92.99	310	140.61	415	188.24

TEMPERATURE CONVERSION

FAHRENHEIT TO CELSIUS = (°F - 32) × 5/9 = °C				CELSIUS TO FAHRENHEIT = (°C × 9/5) + 32 = °F			
°F	°C	°F	°C	°C	°F	°C	°F
0.0	-17.8	50.0	10.0	0.0	32.0	38.0	100.4
5.0	-15.0	55.0	12.8	5.0	41.0	39.0	102.2
10.0	-12.2	60.0	15.6	10.0	50.0	40.0	104.0
15.0	-9.4	65.0	18.3	15.0	59.0	41.0	105.8
20.0	-6.7	70.0	21.1	20.0	68.0	42.0	107.6
25.0	-3.9	75.0	23.9	25.0	77.0	43.0	109.4
30.0	-1.1	80.0	26.7	30.0	86.0	44.0	111.2
35.0	1.7	85.0	29.4	35.0	95.0	45.0	113.0
40.0	4.4	90.0	32.2	36.0	96.8	46.0	114.8
45.0	7.2	91.0	32.8	37.0	98.6	47.0	116.6

TEMPERATURE CONVERSION (Continued)

FARENHEIT TO CELSIUS = (°F - 32) × 5/9 = °C				CELSIUS TO FARENHEIT = (°C × 9/5) + 32 = °F			
°F	°C	°F	°C	°C	°F	°C	°F
92.0	33.3	101.0	38.3	48.0	118.4	59.0	138.2
93.0	33.9	102.0	38.9	49.0	120.2	60.0	140.0
94.0	34.4	103.0	39.4	50.0	122.0	65.0	149.0
95.0	35.0	104.0	40.0	51.0	123.8	70.0	158.0
96.0	35.6	105.0	40.6	52.0	125.6	75.0	167.0
97.0	36.1	106.0	41.1	53.0	127.4	80.0	176.0
98.0	36.7	107.0	41.7	54.0	129.2	85.0	185.0
98.6	37.0	108.0	42.2	55.0	131.0	90.0	194.0
99.0	37.2	109.0	42.8	56.0	132.8	95.0	203.0
100.0	37.8	110.0	43.3	57.0	134.6	100.0	212.0
				58.0	136.4	105.0	221.0

PEDIATRIC DOSAGE ESTIMATION FORMULAS

The following formulas can be used to estimate the approximate pediatric dosage of a medication. These formulas are based on the adult dose and either the child's age or weight. These formulas should be used with caution as the response to any drug is not always directly proportional to the age or weight of the child relative to the usual adult dose. Dosage will also vary based on the formula used. Care should be taken when using any of these methods to calculate the child's dosage. Some products have FDA-approved pediatric indications and dosages; always refer to the full prescribing information first before calculating a pediatric dosage.

BASED ON WEIGHT

Augsberger's Rule:
$$\frac{[(1.5 \times \text{weight [kg]}) + 10]}{100} \times \text{adult dose} = \text{approximate child's dose}$$
Example: If the child's weight is 15 kg (33 lb) and the adult dose is 50 mg then the child's dose is 16.25 mg.
$$\frac{[(1.5 \times 15 \text{ kg}) + 10]}{100} \times 50 \text{ mg} = 16.25 \text{ mg}$$

Clark's Rule:
(weight [lb]/150) × adult dose = approximate child's dose
Example: If the child's weight is 15 kg (33 lb) and the adult dose is 50 mg then the child's dose is 11 mg.
(33/150) x 50 mg = 11 mg

BASED ON AGE

Augsberger's Rule:
$$\frac{[(4 \times \text{age [years]}) + 20]}{100} \times \text{adult dose} = \text{approximate child's dose}$$
Example: If the child's age is 8 years and the adult dose is 50 mg then the child's dose is 26 mg.
[(4 × 8) + 20)/100] x 50 mg = 26 mg

Dilling's Rule:
(age [years]/20) × adult dose = approximate child's dose
Example: If the child's age is 8 years and the adult dose is 50 mg then the child's dose is 20 mg.
(8/20) x 50 mg = 20 mg

Cowling's Rule:
$$\frac{[\text{age at next birthday (years)}]}{24} \times \text{adult dose} = \text{approximate child's dose}$$
Example: If the child is going to turn 8 years old in a few months and the adult dose is 50 mg then the child's dose is 16.7 mg.
(8/24) × 50 mg = 16.7 mg

Young's Rule:
$$\frac{[\text{age (years)}]}{\text{age} + 12} \times \text{adult dose} = \text{approximate child's dose}$$
Example: If the child's age is 8 years and the adult dose is 50 mg then the child's dose is 20 mg.
[8/(8 + 12)] x 50 mg = 20 mg

Fried's Rule (younger than 1 year):
$$\frac{[\text{age (months)}]}{150} \times \text{adult dose} = \text{approximate infant's dose}$$
Example: If the child's age is 10 months and the adult dose is 50 mg then the child's dose is 3.3 mg.
(10/150) x 50 mg = 3.33 mg

COMMON LABORATORY TEST VALUES

Listed below are generally accepted normal values for a selection of common laboratory assays conducted on serum, plasma, and blood. Remember that norms may vary from laboratory to laboratory in accordance with the methodology and quality control measures employed by the facility. When in doubt, check with the laboratory that performed the analysis.

"SI range" refers to Système International d'Unités, a uniform system of reporting numerical values that permits interchangeability of information among nations and disciplines.

TEST	CONVENTIONAL UNITS	SI UNITS
Acid phosphatase	≤2.5 ng/mL	≤2.5 µg/L
Prostatic Total	≤5.8 U/L	<97 nkat/L
Alanine aminotransferase (ALT) (SGPT)	7-41 U/L	0.12-0.70 µkat/L
Albumin, serum	4.0-5.0 mg/dL	40-50 g/L
Alkaline phosphatase	33-96 U/L	0.56-1.63 µkat/L
Ammonia [NH_3^+]	19-60 µg/dL	6-47 µmol/L
Amylase, serum	20-96 U/L	0.8-3.2 µkat/L
Antinuclear antibodies (ANA)	Negative at 1:40 dilution	
Aspartate aminotransferase (AST) (SGOT)	12-38 U/L	0.20-0.65 µkat/L
Bilirubin		
Total	0.3-1.3 mg/dL	5.1-22 µmol/L
Direct	0.1-0.4 mg/dL	1.7-6.8 µmol/L
Indirect	0.2-0.9 mg/dL	3.4-15.2 µmol/L
Blood urea nitrogen	8-20 mg/dL	2.9-7.1 mmol/L
Calcium, plasma	8.5-10.5 mg/dL	2.1-2.6 mmol/L
Calcium, ionized	4.6-5.3 mg/dL	1.15-1.32 mmol/L
Calcium, urine	100-300 mg/24h	2.5-7.5 mmol/L
Chloride, serum	102-109 mEq/L	102-109 mmol/L
Cholesterol (total plasma)		
Desirable level	<200 mg/dL	<6.0 mmol/L
Moderate risk	200-240 mg/dL	6.0-7.2 mmol/L
High risk	≥240 mg/dL	>7.2 mmol/L
Copper	<60 g/d	<0.95 µmol/L
Cortisol, serum		
Fasting, 8 AM-12 noon	5-25 µg/dL	138-690 nmol/L
12 noon-8 PM	5-15 µg/dL	138-414 nmol/L
8 PM-8 AM	0-10 µg/dL	0-276 nmol/L
Creatinine kinase (CK)		
CK-MM:	97-100% of total	0.97-1.00 of total
CK-MB:	<4% of total CK	<0.27 mckat/L
CK-BB:	0% of total	0% of total
Total	Male: 51-294 U/L	Male: 0.87-5.0 µkat/L
	Female: 39-238 U/L	Female: 0.66-4.0 µkat/L
Creatinine, serum Male	0.6-1.2 mg/dL	53-106 µmol/L
Female	0.5-0.9 mg/dL	44-80 µmol/L
Creatinine clearance	90-140 mL/mi/1.73 m^2 BSA	1.5-2.3 mL/sec/1.73^2 BSA

(Continued)

TEST	CONVENTIONAL UNITS	SI UNITS
Digoxin		
Therapeutic	0.5-2.0 ng/mL	0.64-2.6 nmol/L
Toxic	>3.9 ng/mL	>5.0 nmol/L
Erythrocyte count (RBC)		
Adult males	$4.30\text{-}5.60 \times 10^6/mm^3$	$4.30\text{-}5.60 \times 10^{12}/L$
Adult females	$4.00\text{-}5.20 \times 10^6/mm^3$	$4.00\text{-}5.20 \times 10^{12}/L$
Erythrocyte sedimentation rate (ESR)		
Male	0-15 mm/hr	0-15 mm/hr
Female	0-20 mm/hr	0-20 mm/hr
Ferritin		
Male	29-248 ng/mL	28-248 µg/L
Female	10-150 ng/mL	10-150 µg/L
Folic acid	5.4-18.0 ng/mL	12.2-40.8 nmol/L
Follicle-stimulating hormone (FSH)		
Female	3.0-20 mIU/mL	3.0-20 IU/L
Ovulation	9-26 mIU/mL	9-26 IU/L
Postmenopausal	18-153 mIU/mL	18-153 IU/L
Male	1.0-12 mIU/mL	1.0-12 IU/L
Gamma-glutamyl transferase (GGT)	9-58 U/L	0.15-0.99 µkat/L
Gases, arterial blood		
pO_2	72-104 mmHg	9.6-13.8 kPa
pCO_2	32-45 mmHg	4.3-6.2 kPa
Glucose, plasma		
Fasting	75-100 mg/dL	4.2-5.6 mmol/L
Normal	100-125 mg/dL	5.6-6.9 mmol/L
Postprandial (2 h)	<140 mg/dL	<7.8 mmol/L
Immunoglobulins (Ig)		
IgG	700-1700 mg/dL	7.0-17.0 g/L
IgA	70-350 mg/dL	0.70-3.50 g/L
IgM	50-300 mg/dL	0.50-3.0 g/L
IgD	0-14 mg/dL	0-140 mg/L
IgE	1-87 IU/L	1-87 KIU/L
Iron, serum	41-141 µg/dL	7-25 µmol/L
Iron binding capacity	251-406 µg/dL	45-73 µmol/L
Iron saturation	16-35%	0.16-0.35
Lactic acid (plasma, venous)	0.5-2.0 mEq/L	0.5-2.0 mmol/L
Lactic dehydrogenase (LDH)	88-230 U/L (laboratory-specific)	1.46-3.82 mckat/L (laboratory-specific)
Lead	<10 µg/dL	<0.5 µmol/L
Leukocyte count (WBC)	$3.54\text{-}9.06 \times 10^3/mm^3$	$3.54\text{-}9.06 \times 10^9/L$
Lipase	3-43 U/L	0.51-0.73 µkat/L
Lipoproteins (desirable levels)		
Low density (LDL)	<130 mg/dL	<3.37 mmol/L
High density (HDL)	>60 mg/dL	>1.55 mmol/L
Lithium ion (therapeutic)	0.5-1.3 mEq/L	0.5-1.3 mmol/L

TEST	CONVENTIONAL UNITS	SI UNITS
Luteinizing hormone		
Female	0.6-19 mIU/mL	0.6-19 IU/L
Ovulation	22-105 mIU/mL	22-105 IU/L
Postmenopausal	16-64 mIU/mL	16-64 IU/L
Male	1-10 mU/mL	1-10 IU/L
Osmolality, plasma	275-295 mOsm/kg	285-295 mmol/kg
Phenytoin		
Therapeutic	10-20 mg/L	40-80 µmol/L
Toxic	>40 mg/L	>158 µmol/L
Phosphorus, serum	2.5-4.5 mg/dL	0.81-1.4 mmol/L
Potassium, serum	3.5-5 mEq/L	3.5-5 mmol/L
Prolactin	2-15 ng/mL	53-360 mIU/L
Prostate-specific antigen (PSA)	<4 ng/mL	<4 µg/L
Protein		
Total	6.7-8.6 g/dL	67-86 g/L
Albumin	3.5-5.5 g/dL	35-55 g/L
Globulin	2.0-3.5 g/dL	20-35 g/L
Reticulocyte count		
Adult males	0.8-2.3% red cells	0.008-0.023 red cells
Adult females	0.8-2.0% red cells	0.008-0.023 red cells
Rheumatoid factor	<15 IU/mL	<15 kIU/L
Sodium, serum	136-145 mEq/L	136-145 mmol/L
Theophylline (therapeutic)	10-20 mg/L	55-110 µmol/L
Thyroxine-binding globulin (TBG)	1.3-3.0 mg/L	13-30 mg/L
Thyroid-stimulating hormone (TSH)	0.34-4.25 µIU/mL	0.34-4.25 mIU/L
Thyroxine (T_4)		
Free	0.7-1.24 ng/dL	9.0-16 pmol/L
Total	5.4-11.7 µg/dL	70-151 nmol/L
Transferrin	200-400 µg/dL	2.0-4.0 g/L
Triglycerides	<165 µg/dL	<1.8 mmol/L
Triiodothyronine, free (fT_3)	2.4-4.2 pg/dL	3.7-6.5 pmol/L
Triiodothyronine, total (T_3)	77-135 ng/dL	1.2-2.1 nmol/L
T_3 uptake	25-35%	0.25-0.35 (proportion of 1.0)
Urea nitrogen, blood (BUN)	7-20 mg/dL	2.5-7.1 mmol/L
Uric acid		
Male	3.1-7.0 mg/dL	0.18-0.41 mmol/L
Female	2.5-5.6 mg/dL	0.15-0.33 mmol/L
Vitamin B_{12}	279-996 pg/mL	206-735 pmol/L

Sources
Longo DL, Fauci AS, Kasper DL, et al. *Harrison's Principles of Internal Medicine*, ed 18. New York, NY: McGraw Hill; 2011.
McPhee S, Papadakis M, Rabow MW. *Current Medical Diagnosis and Treatment*. New York, NY: McGraw Hill; 2011.

TABLES FOR PHARMACY CALCULATIONS

WEIGHTS AND MEASURES

Metric Measure

Weight

1 kilogram (1 kg)	=	1000 g
1 gram (g)	=	1000 mg
1 milligram (mg)	=	0.001 g
1 microgram (mcg)	=	0.001 mg
1 gamma	=	1 mcg

Liquid

1 liter (L)	=	1000 mL
1 milliliter (mL)	=	1 cc (cubic centimeter)

Apothecary (Ap)

Weight

1 scruple	=	20 grains (gr)
1 drachm	=	3 scruples
	=	60 gr
1 ounce (oz)	=	8 drachms
	=	24 scruples
	=	480 gr
1 pound (lb)	=	16 oz
	=	96 drachms
	=	288 scruples
	=	5760 gr

U.S. Fluid Measure

1 fluidrachm	=	60 minim (min)
1 fluid ounce (fl oz)	=	8 fld drachm
	=	480 min
1 pint (pt)	=	16 fl oz
	=	7680 min
1 quart (qt)	=	2 pt
	=	32 fl oz
1 gallon (gal)	=	4 qts
	=	128 fl oz

Avoirdupois (Av)

Weight

1 ounce	=	437.5 gr
1 pound	=	16 oz

Conversion Factors

1 gram	=	15.4 gr
1 grain	=	64.8 mg
1 ounce (Av)	=	28.35 g
	=	437.5 gr
1 ounce (Ap)	=	31.1 g
	=	480 gr
1 pound (Av)	=	453.6 g
1 kilogram	=	2.68 pounds Ap
	=	2.20 lbs Av

1 fluid ounce	=	29.57 mL
1 fluidrachm	=	3.697 mL
1 minim	=	0.06 mL

Converting °F to °C

For °F to °C, the formula is:
$$°C = \tfrac{5}{9}(°F-32)$$

For °C to °F, the formula is:
$$°F = (\tfrac{9}{5} \times °C) + 32$$

Common Measures

1 teaspoonful	=	5 mL
	=	⅙ fl oz
1 tablespoonful	=	15 mL
	=	½ fl oz
1 wineglassful	=	60 mL
	=	2 fl oz
1 teacupful	=	120 mL
	=	4 fl oz

TABLE OF SATURATED SOLUTIONS

This table shows the quantity of the substance and milliliters (mL) of water for 100 mL of a saturated solution at about 25°C.

Substance	Gram	mL Water
Alum	13.00	92.0
Ammonium carbonate	22.00	88.0
Ammonium chloride	28.30	79.3
Ammonium nitrate	90.20	41.8
Ammonium sulfate	53.10	71.7
Borax	5.90	98.0
Boric acid	5.10	97.0
Calcium lactate	5.00	96.0
Chloral hydrate	120.00	31.0
Citric acid	88.60	42.7
Copper sulfate	22.30	98.7
Dextrose	59.00	60.0
Ferric chloride	125.00	29.0
Ferrous sulfate	52.80	72.7
Lactose	17.00	90.0
Lead acetate	55.00	79.0
Lithium chloride	59.50	70.2
Lithium sulfate	33.00	88.5
Magnesium sulfate	72.00	58.5
Manganese chloride	90.00	54.0
Mercuric chloride	6.96	98.5
Methylene blue	4.30	97.0
Oxalic acid	10.30	94.2
Potassium bromide	56.00	82.0
Potassium carbonate	82.20	73.5
Potassium chloride	8.41	96.6
Potassium citrate	92.00	56.5
Potassium iodide	103.20	69.1
Potassium nitrate	33.40	86.0
Potassium permanganate	7.43	97.3
Resorcinol	67.20	47.2
Rochelle salt	51.90	78.8
Silver nitrate	164.00	65.5
Sodium acetate	65.00	53.0
Sodium benzoate	41.50	73.9
Sodium bicarbonate	8.80	97.6
Sodium bromide	73.00	78.0
Sodium carbonate	27.50	96.0
Sodium chloride	31.50	88.1
Codium citrate	55.50	72.5
Sodium iodide	124.30	67.7
Sodium nitrate	62.30	73.8
Sodium salicylate	67.00	58.0
Sodium sulfate	33.30	87.0
Sodium thiocyanate	87.00	51.0
Sodium thiosulfate	93.00	46.0
Tartaric acid	76.90	54.7
Urea	62.00	53.5
Zinc sulfate	93.00	56.0

DOSE EQUIVALENTS

These approximate dose equivalents have been adopted by U.S.P. XXII, N.F. XVII. They are approved by the Food and Drug Administration.

When converting specific quantities of a prescription that requires compounding, or when converting a pharmaceutical formula from one system of weights or measures to the other, the following must be used.

Weight

Metric	Apothecary
030 g	1 ounce
015 g	4 drachms

010 g	2½ drachms	30 mg	½ grain	0100 mL	3½ fluid ounces
07.5 g	2 drachms	25 mg	⅜ grain	0050 mL	1¾ fluid ounces
006 g	90 grains	20 mg	⅓ grain	0030 mL	1 fluid ounce
005 g	75 grains	15 mg	¼ grain	0015 mL	4 fluidrachms
004 g	60 grains (1 drachm)	12 mg	⅕ grain	0010 mL	2½ fluidrachms
003 g	45 grains	10 mg	⅙ grain	0008 mL	2 fluidrachms
002 g	30 grains (½ drachm)	08 mg	⅛ grain	0005 mL	1¼ fluidrachms
01.5 g	22 grains	06 mg	$\frac{1}{10}$ grain	0004 mL	1 fluidrachm
001 g	15 grains	05 mg	$\frac{1}{12}$ grain	0003 mL	45 minims
750 mg	12 grains	04 mg	$\frac{1}{15}$ grain	0002 mL	30 minims
600 mg	10 grains	03 mg	$\frac{1}{20}$ grain	0001 mL	15 minims
500 mg	7½ grains	02 mg	$\frac{1}{30}$ grain	0.75 mL	12 minims
400 mg	6 grains	1.5 mg	$\frac{1}{40}$ grain	00.6 mL	10 minims
300 mg	5 grains	1.2 mg	$\frac{1}{50}$ grain	00.5 mL	8 minims
250 mg	4 grains	01 mg	$\frac{1}{60}$ grain	00.3 mL	5 minims
200 mg	3 grains			0.25 mL	4 minims
150 mg	2½ grains	**Liquid Measure**		00.2 mL	3 minims
125 mg	2 grains	Metric	Apothecary	00.1 mL	1½ minims
100 mg	1½ grains	1000 mL	1 quart	0.06 mL	1 minim
75 mg	1¼ grains	0750 mL	1½ pints	0.05 mL	¾ minim
60 mg	1 grain	0500 mL	1 pint	0.03 mL	½ minim
50 mg	¾ grain	0250 mL	8 fluid ounces		
40 mg	⅔ grain	0200 mL	7 fluid ounces		

POISON CONTROL CENTERS

The American Association of Poison Control Centers (AAPCC) uses a single, nationwide emergency number to automatically link callers with their regional poison center. This toll-free number, **800-222-1222**, also works for **teletype lines (TTY)** for the hearing-impaired and **telecommunication devices (TDD)** for individuals who are deaf. However, a few local poison centers and the ASPCA/Animal Poison Control Center are not part of this nationwide system and continue to use separate numbers.

Most of the centers listed below are accredited by the AAPCC. **Certified centers are marked by an asterisk after the name.** Each has to meet certain criteria. It must, for example, serve a large geographic area; it must be open 24 hours a day and provide direct-dial or toll-free access; it must be supervised by a medical director; and it must have registered pharmacists or nurses available to answer questions from the public.

Within each state, centers are listed alphabetically by city. Some state poison centers also list their original emergency numbers (including TDD/TTY) that only work within that state. For these listings, callers may use either the state number or the nationwide 800 number.

ALABAMA

BIRMINGHAM

Regional Poison Control Center (*)
Children's Hospital of Alabama

1600 7th Ave South
Birmingham AL 35233-1711
Business: 205-939-9201
Emergency: 800-222-1222
www.chsys.org

TUSCALOOSA

Alabama Poison Center (*)

2503 Phoenix Dr
Tuscaloosa AL 35405
Business: 205-345-0600
Emergency: 800-222-1222
            800-462-0800 (AL)
www.alapoisoncenter.org

ALASKA

JUNEAU

Alaska Poison Control System
Section of Injury Prevention and EMS

410 Willoughby Ave – Room 109
Box 110616
Juneau AK 99811-0616
Business: 907-465-3027
Emergency: 800-222-1222
www.chems.alaska.gov

(PORTLAND, OR)

Oregon Poison Center (*)
Oregon Health and Science University

3181 SW Sam Jackson Park Rd –
Suite CB550
Portland OR 97239
Business: 503-494-8600
Emergency: 800-222-1222
www.ohsu.edu/poison

ARIZONA

PHOENIX

Banner Poison Control Center (*)
Banner Good Samaritan Medical Center

901 E Willetta St
Phoenix AZ 85006
Business: 602-495-6360
Emergency: 800-222-1222
            800-362-0101 (AZ)
            800-253-3334 (AZ)
www.bannerpoisoncontrol.com

TUCSON

Arizona Poison and Drug Information Center (*)
Arizona Health Sciences Center

1501 N Campbell Ave – Room 1156
Tucson AZ 85724
Business: 520-626-7899
Emergency: 800-222-1222
www.pharmacy.arizona.edu/outreach/poison

ARKANSAS

LITTLE ROCK

Arkansas Poison and Drug Information Center (*)
College of Pharmacy – UAMS

4301 W Markham St – MS 522-2
Little Rock AR 72205
Business: 501-686-5540
Emergency: 800-222-1222
            800-376-4766 (AR)
TDD/TTY: 800-641-3805
www.uams.edu/cop/

ASPCA/Animal Poison Control Center

1717 S Philo Rd – Suite 36
Urbana IL 61802
Business: 217-337-5030
Emergency: 888-426-4435
            800-548-2423
http://www.aspcapro.org/
animal-poison-control.php

CALIFORNIA

FRESNO/MADERA

California Poison Control System
Fresno/Madera Division (*)
Children's Hospital Central California

9300 Valley Children's Place – MB 15
Madera CA 93636
Business: 559-622-2300
Emergency: 800-222-1222
            800-876-4766 (CA)
TDD/TTY: 800-972-3323
www.calpoison.org

SACRAMENTO

California Poison Control System
Sacramento Division (*)
UC Davis Medical Center

2315 Stockton Blvd –
Room HSF 1024
Sacramento CA 95817
Business: 916-227-1400
Emergency: 800-222-1222
            800-876-4766 (CA)
TDD/TTY: 800-972-3323
www.calpoison.org

SAN DIEGO

**California Poison Control System
San Diego Division (*)
UC San Diego Medical Center**

200 W Arbor Dr
San Diego CA 92103-8925
Business: 858-715-6300
Emergency: 800-222-1222
          800-876-4766 (CA)
TDD/TTY: 800-972-3323
www.calpoison.org

SAN FRANCISCO

**California Poison Control System
San Francisco Division (*)**

UCSF Box 1369
San Francisco CA 94143
Business: 415-502-6000
Emergency: 800-222-1222
          800-876-4766 (CA)
TDD/TTY: 800-972-3323
www.calpoison.org

COLORADO

DENVER

**Rocky Mountain Poison and Drug
Center (*)**

777 Bannock St – MC 0180
Denver CO 80204-4507
Business: 303-389-1100
Emergency: 800-222-1222
TDD/TTY: 303-739-1127 (CO)
www.rmpdc.org

CONNECTICUT

FARMINGTON

**Connecticut Poison Control Center (*)
University of Connecticut Health
Center**

263 Farmington Ave
Farmington CT 06030-5365
Business: 860-679-4540
Emergency: 800-222-1222
TDD/TTY: 866-218-5372
http://poisoncontrol.uchc.edu

DELAWARE

(PHILADELPHIA, PA)

**The Poison Control Center (*)
Children's Hospital of Philadelphia**

34th St & Civic Center Blvd
Philadelphia PA 19104-4399
Business: 215-590-2003
Emergency: 800-222-1222
          800-722-7112 (DE)
TDD/TTY: 215-590-8789
http://www.chop.edu/service/
poison-control-center/home.html

DISTRICT OF COLUMBIA

WASHINGTON, DC

National Capital Poison Center (*)

3201 New Mexico Ave NW
Suite 310
Washington DC 20016
Business: 202-362-3867
Emergency: 800-222-1222
www.poison.org

FLORIDA

JACKSONVILLE

**Florida Poison Information Center-
Jacksonville (*)
SHANDS Hospital**

655 W 8th St
Jacksonville FL 32209
Business: 904-244-4465
Emergency: 800-222-1222
http://fpicjax.org

MIAMI

**Florida/USVI Poison Information
Center-Miami (*)
University of Miami, Department of
Pediatrics**

PO Box 016960 (R-131)
Miami FL 33101
Business: 305-585-5250
Emergency: 800-222-1222
www.med.miami.edu/poisoncontrol

TAMPA

**Florida Poison Information Center-
Tampa (*)
Tampa Division**

PO Box 1289
Tampa FL 33601-1289
Business: 813-844-7044
Emergency: 800-222-1222
www.poisoncentertampa.org

GEORGIA

ATLANTA

**Georgia Poison Center (*)
Hughes Spalding Children's Hospital
Grady Health System**

80 Jesse Hill Jr. Dr SE
PO Box 26066
Atlanta GA 30303
Business: 404-616-9237
Emergency: 800-222-1222
          404-616-9000 (Atlanta)
TDD: 404-616-9287
www.georgiapoisoncenter.org

HAWAII

(DENVER, CO)

**Rocky Mountain Poison and Drug
Center (*)**

777 Bannock St – MC 0180
Denver CO 80204-4507
Business: 303-389-1100
Emergency: 800-222-1222
www.rmpdc.org

IDAHO

(DENVER, CO)

**Rocky Mountain Poison and Drug
Center (*)**

777 Bannock St – MC 0180
Denver CO 80204-4507
Business: 303-739-1100
Emergency: 800-222-1222
www.rmpdc.org

ILLINOIS

CHICAGO

Illinois Poison Center (*)

222 S Riverside Plaza – Suite 1900
Chicago IL 60606
Business: 312-906-6136
Emergency: 800-222-1222
TDD/TTY: 312-906-6185
www.illinoispoisoncenter.org/

INDIANA

INDIANAPOLIS

**Indiana Poison Center (*)
Clarian Health Partners Methodist
Hospital**

I-65 at 21st Street
Indianapolis, IN 46206-1367
Business: 317-962-2335
Emergency: 800-222-1222
          800-382-9097 (IN)
317-962-2323 (Indianapolis)
www.clarian.org/poisoncontrol

IOWA

SIOUX CITY

**Iowa Statewide Poison Control
Center (*)
Iowa Health System and the
University of Iowa Hospitals and
Clinics**

2910 Hamilton Blvd – Suite 101
Sioux City IA 51101
Business: 712-279-3710
Emergency: 800-222-1222
          712-277-2222 (IA)
www.iowapoison.org

KANSAS

KANSAS CITY

Mid-America Poison Control
University of Kansas Medical Center

3901 Rainbow Blvd
Room B-400
Kansas City KS 66160-7231
Business: 913-588-6638
Emergency: 800-222-1222
                800-332-6633 (KS)
TDD: 913-588-6639
www.kumed.com/poison

KENTUCKY

LOUISVILLE

Kentucky Regional Poison Center (*)

PO Box 35070
Louisville KY 40232-5070
Business: 502-629-7264
Emergency: 800-222-1222
                502-589-8222
                (Louisville)
www.krpc.com

LOUISIANA

MONROE

Louisiana Drug and Poison
Information Center (*)
University of Louisiana at Monroe

700 University Ave
Monroe LA 71209-6430
Business: 318-342-3648
Emergency: 800-222-1222
www.lapcc.org

MAINE

PORTLAND

Northern New England Poison
Center (*)

Maine Medical Center
22 Bramhall St
Portland ME 04102
Business: 207-662-7220
Emergency: 800-222-1222
TDD/TTY   877-299-4447 (ME)
www.nnepc.org

MARYLAND

BALTIMORE

Maryland Poison Center (*)
University of Maryland at Baltimore
School of Pharmacy

20 North Pine St, PH 772
Baltimore MD 21201
Business: 410-706-7604
Emergency: 800-222-1222
TDD: 410-706-1858
www.mdpoison.com

(WASHINGTON, DC)

National Capital Poison Center (*)

3201 New Mexico Ave NW
Suite 310
Washington DC 20016
Business: 202-362-3867
Emergency: 800-222-1222
www.poison.org

MASSACHUSETTS

BOSTON

Regional Center for Poison Control
and Prevention (*)
(Serving Massachusetts and Rhode
Island)

300 Longwood Ave
Boston MA 02115
Business: 617-355-6609
Emergency: 800-222-1222
TDD/TTY   888-244-5313
www.maripoisoncenter.com

MICHIGAN

DETROIT

Regional Poison Control Center (*)
Children's Hospital of Michigan

4160 John R Harper Professional
Office Bldg – Suite 616
Detroit MI 48201
Business: 313-745-5335
Emergency: 800-222-1222
                313-745-5711 [Detroit]
www.mitoxic.org/pcc

MINNESOTA

MINNEAPOLIS

Minnesota Poison Control System (*)
Hennepin County Medical Center

701 Park Avenue, Mail Code RL
Minneapolis, MN 55415
Business: 612-873-3144
Emergency: 800-222-1222
www.mnpoison.org

MISSISSIPPI

JACKSON

Mississippi Regional Poison Control
Center
University of Mississippi Medical
Center

2500 N State St
Jackson MS 39216
Business: 601-984-1680
Emergency: 800-222-1222
http://poisoncontrol.umc.edu

MISSOURI

ST LOUIS

Missouri Regional Poison Center (*)
Cardinal Glennon Children's Medical
Center

1465 S Grand Blvd
St Louis MO 63104-1095
Business: 314-577-5610
Emergency: 800-222-1222
www.cardinalglennon.com

MONTANA

(DENVER, CO)

Rocky Mountain Poison and Drug
Center (*)

777 Bannock St – MC 0180
Denver CO 80204-4507
Business: 303-389-1100
Emergency: 800-222-1222
www.rmpdc.org

NEBRASKA

OMAHA

The Poison Center (*)
Children's Hospital

8200 Dodge St
Omaha NE 68114
Business: 402-390-5555
Emergency: 800-222-1222
www.nebraskapoison.com

NEVADA

(DENVER, CO)

Rocky Mountain Poison and Drug
Center (*)

777 Bannock St – MC 0180
Denver CO 80204-4507
Business: 303-389-1100
Emergency: 800-222-1222
www.rmpdc.org

(PORTLAND, OR)

Oregon Poison Center (*)
Oregon Health Sciences University

33181 SW Sam Jackson Park Rd
Portland OR 97201
Business: 503-494-8600
Emergency: 800-222-1222
www.ohsu.edu/poison

NEW HAMPSHIRE

(PORTLAND, ME)

Northern New England Poison Center (*)

22 Bramhall St
Portland ME 04102
Business: 207-662-7220
Emergency: 800-222-1222
www.nnepc.org

NEW JERSEY

NEWARK

New Jersey Poison Information and Education System (*)
UMDNJ

65 Bergen St
Newark NJ 07101
Business: 973-972-9280
Emergency: 800-222-1222
TDD/TTY: 973-926-8008
www.njpies.org

NEW MEXICO

ALBUQUERQUE

New Mexico Poison and Drug Information Center (*)

1 University of New Mexico
Albuquerque NM 87131-0001
Business: 505-272-4261
Emergency: 800-222-1222
http://hsc.unm.edu/pharmacy/poison

NEW YORK

MINEOLA

Long Island Regional Poison and Drug Information Center (*)
Winthrop University Hospital

259 First St
Mineola NY 11501
Business: 516-663-2650
Emergency: 800-222-1222
TDD: 516-747-3323 (Nassau)
516-924-8811 (Suffolk)
www.winthrop.org

NEW YORK CITY

New York City Poison Control Center (*)
NYC Bureau of Public Health

455 1st Ave – Room 123
New York NY 10016
Business: 212-447-8152
English
Emergency: 800-222-1222
212-340-4494
212-POISONS
(212-764-7667)
Spanish
Emergency: 212-venenos
(212-836-3667)
www.nyc.gov/html/doh/htmls/poison/
poison.shtml

ROCHESTER

Fingerlakes Regional Poison and Drug Information Center (*)
University of Rochester Medical Center

601 Elmwood Ave
Box 321
Rochester NY 14642
Business: 585-273-4155
Emergency: 800-222-1222
TTY: 585-273-3854
www.fingerlakespoison.org

SYRACUSE

Upstate New York Poison Center (*)
SUNY Upstate Medical University

750 E Adams St
Syracuse NY 13210
Business: 315-464-7078
Emergency: 800-222-1222
TTY: 315-464-5424
www.upstate.edu/poison/contactus

NORTH CAROLINA

CHARLOTTE

Carolinas Poison Center (*)
Carolinas Medical Center

PO Box 32861
Charlotte NC 28232
Business: 704-395-3795
Emergency: 800-222-1222
TDD: 800-735-8262
TYY: 800-735-2962
www.ncpoisoncenter.org

NORTH DAKOTA

(MINNEAPOLIS, MN)

Minnesota Poison Control System (*)
Hennepin County Medical Center

701 Park Avenue, Mail Code RL
Minneapolis, MN 55415
Business: 612-873-3144
Emergency: 800-222-1222
www.mnpoison.org

OHIO

CINCINNATI

Cincinnati Drug and Poison Information Center (*)
Regional Poison Control System

3333 Burnett Ave
Vermon Place, 3rd Floor
Cincinnati OH 45229
Business: 513-636-5111
Emergency: 800-222-1222
TTY: 800-253-7955
www.cincinnatichildrens.org/dpic

CLEVELAND

Greater Cleveland Poison Control Center
University Hospitals

11100 Euclid Ave – B261 MP6007
Cleveland OH 44106
Business: 216-844-1573
Emergency: 800-222-1222
216-231-4455 (OH)
www.uhhospitals.org/rainbow
children/tabid/195/default.aspx

COLUMBUS

Central Ohio Poison Center (*)
Nationwide Children's Hospital

700 Children's Dr
Room L032
Columbus OH 43205
Business: 614-722-2635
Emergency: 800-222-1222
614-228-1323
937-222-2227
(Dayton region)
www.bepoisonsmart.com

OKLAHOMA

OKLAHOMA CITY

Oklahoma Poison Control Center (*)
Children's Hospital at OU Health Science Center

940 NE 13th St – Room 3510
Oklahoma City OK 73104
Business: 405-271-5062
Emergency: 800-222-1222
www.oklahomapoison.org

OREGON

PORTLAND

Oregon Poison Center (*)
Oregon Health and Science University

3181 SW Sam Jackson Park Rd –
Suite CB550
Portland OR 97239
Business: 503-494-8600
Emergency: 800-222-1222
www.ohsu.edu/poison

PENNSYLVANIA

PHILADELPHIA

The Poison Control Center (*)
Children's Hospital of Philadelphia

34th St & Civic Center Blvd
Philadelphia PA 19104-4399
Business: 215-590-2003
Emergency: 800-222-1222
TDD/TTY: 215-590-8789
http://www.chop.edu/service/poison-control-center/home.html

PITTSBURGH

Pittsburgh Poison Center (*)
University of Pittsburgh Medical Center

200 Lothrop Street
Pittsburgh PA 15213
Business: 412-390-3300
Emergency: 800-222-1222
           412-681-6669
           (Pittsburgh)
www.upmc.com/services/poisoncenter

RHODE ISLAND

(BOSTON, MA)

Regional Center for Poison Control and Prevention (*)

300 Longwood Ave
Boston MA 02115
Business: 617-355-6609
Emergency: 800-222-1222
TDD/TTY   888-244-5313
www.maripoisoncenter.com

SOUTH CAROLINA

COLUMBIA

Palmetto Poison Center (*)
University of South Carolina College of Pharmacy

USC Columbia SC 29208
Business: 803-777-7909
Emergency: 800-222-1222
http://poison.sc.edu

SOUTH DAKOTA

(MINNEAPOLIS, MN)

Minnesota Poison Control System (*)
Hennepin County Medical Center

701 Park Ave, Mail Code RL
Minneapolis MN 55415
Business: 612-873-3144
Emergency: 800-222-1222
www.mnpoison.org

(SIOUX FALLS)

Sanford Poison Center
Sanford Health USD Medical Center

1305 W 18th St - PO box 5039
Sioux Falls SD 57117
Business: 605-333-6638
Emergency: 800-222-1222
www.sdpoison.org

TENNESSEE

NASHVILLE

Tennessee Poison Center (*)

1161 21st Ave South
501 Oxford House
Nashville TN 37232-4632
Business: 615-936-0760
Emergency: 800-222-1222
www.tnpoisoncenter.org

TEXAS

AMARILLO

Texas Panhandle Poison Center (*)
Texas Poison Center Network

1501 S Coulter Dr
Amarillo TX 79106
Business: 806-354-1630
Emergency: 800-222-1222
www.poisoncontrol.org

DALLAS

North Texas Poison Center (*)
Texas Poison Center Network
Parkland Health & Hospital System

5201 Harry Hines Blvd
Dallas TX 75235
Business: 214-589-0911
Emergency: 800-222-1222
www.poisoncontrol.org

EL PASO

West Texas Regional Poison Center (*)
Thomason Hospital

4815 Alameda Ave
El Paso TX 79905
Business: 915-534-3802
Emergency: 800-222-1222
www.poisoncontrol.org

GALVESTON

Southeast Texas Poison Center (*)
The University of Texas Medical Branch

201 University Blvd
3.112 Trauma Bldg
Galveston TX 77555-1175
Business: 409-766-4403
Emergency: 800-222-1222
www.utmb.edu/setpc

SAN ANTONIO

South Texas Poison Center (*)
The University of Texas Health Science Center-San Antonio

7703 Floyd Curl Dr-MSC 7849
Trauma Bldg
San Antonio TX 78229-3900
Business: 210-567-5762
Emergency: 800-222-1222
www.texaspoison.com

TEMPLE

Central Texas Poison Center (*)
Scott & White Memorial Hospital

2401 S 31st St
Temple TX 76508-0001
Business: 254-724-2111
Emergency: 800-222-1222
http://www.sw.org/poison-center/poison-landing

UTAH

SALT LAKE CITY

Utah Poison Control Center (*)
University of Utah

585 Komas Dr – Suite 200
Salt Lake City UT 84108-1234
Business: 801-581-7504
Emergency: 800-222-1222
http://uuhsc.utah.edu/poison

VERMONT

(PORTLAND, ME)

Northern New England Poison Center (*)
Maine Medical Center

22 Bramhall St
Portland ME 04102
Business:　207-662-7220
Emergency: 800-222-1222
www.nnepc.org

VIRGINIA

CHARLOTTESVILLE

Blue Ridge Poison Center (*)
University of Virginia School of Medicine

PO Box 800774
Charlottesville VA 22908
Business:　434-924-5118
Emergency: 800-222-1222
　　　　　800-451-1418 (VA)
www.healthsystem.virginia.edu/brpc

RICHMOND

Virginia Poison Center (*)
Virginia Commonwealth University Medical Center

PO Box 980522
Richmond VA 23298-0522
Business:　804-828-4780
Emergency: 800-222-1222
　　　　　804-828-9123
TDD/TYY:　804-828-9123
www.poison.vcu.edu

WASHINGTON

SEATTLE

Washington Poison Control Center (*)

155 NE 100th St, Suite 400
Seattle WA 98125-8007
Business:　206-517-2351
Emergency: 800-222-1222
　　　　　206-517-2394 (WA)
TDD:　　　800-572-0638 (WA)
　　　　　206-517-2394 (Seattle)
www.wapc.org

WEST VIRGINIA

CHARLESTON

West Virginia Poison Center (*)
WVU Robert C. Byrd Health Sciences Center

3110 MacCorkle Ave SE
Charleston WV 25304
Business:　304-347-1212
Emergency: 800-222-1222
www.wvpoisoncenter.org

WISCONSIN

MILWAUKEE

Wisconsin Poison Center
Children's Hospital of Wisconsin

9000 W Wisconsin Ave
PO Box 1997, Mail Station 677A
Milwaukee WI 53201
Business:　414-266-2000
Emergency: 800-222-1222
TDD/TYY:　414-964-3497
www.wisconsinpoison.org

WYOMING

(OMAHA, NE)

Nebraska Regional Poison Center (*)

8401 W Dodge Rd, Suite 115
Omaha NE 68114
Business:　402-955-5555
Emergency: 800-222-1222
www.nebraskapoison.com

CERTIFICATION PROGRAMS FOR NURSES

Organization	Website
American Nurses Credentialing Center (ANCC)	www.nursecredentialing.org

- Acute Care Nurse Practitioner
- Adult Health Clinical Nurse Specialist (formerly Med-Surg)
- Adult Nurse Practitioner
- Adult Psychiatric & Mental Health Clinical Nurse Specialist
- Adult Psychiatric & Mental Health Nurse Practitioner
- Ambulatory Care Nurse
- Cardiac Rehabilitation Nurse
- Cardiac Vascular Nurse
- Case Management Nurse
- Child/Adolescent Psychiatric & Mental Health Clinical Nurse Specialist
- Clinical Nurse Specialist (CNS) Core Exam
- College Health Nurse
- Community Health Nurse
- Diabetes Management, Advanced
- Family Nurse Practitioner
- Family Psychiatric & Mental Health Nurse Practitioner
- General Nursing Practice
- Gerontological Clinical Nurse Specialist
- Gerontological Nurse
- Gerontological Nurse Practitioner
- High-Risk Perinatal Nurse
- Home Health Clinical Nurse Specialist
- Home Health Nurse
- Informatics Nurse
- Medical-Surgical Nurse
- Nurse Executive (formerly Nursing Administration)
- Nurse Executive, Advanced (formerly Nursing Administration, Advanced)
- Nursing Professional Development
- Pain Management
- Pediatric Clinical Nurse Specialist
- Pediatric Nurse
- Pediatric Nurse Practitioner
- Perinatal Nurse
- Psychiatric and Mental Health Nurse
- Public/Community Health Clinical Nurse Specialist
- Public Health Nurse, Advanced
- School Nurse

American Academy of Medical Esthetic Professionals (AAMEP)	www.amen-usa.org

- Medical Esthetics-Certified (ME-C)

Association for the Advancement of Medical Instrumentation (AAMI)	www.aami.org

- Biomedical Equipment Technicians (CBET)
- Clinical Laboratory Equipment Specialists (CLES)
- Radiology Equipment Specialists (CRES)

American Society of Ophthalmic Registered Nurses (ASORN)	http://webeye.ophth.uiowa.edu/asorn

- Ophthalmic Registered Nurses (CORN)

American Board of Certification for Gastroenterology Nurses (ABCGN)	www.abcgn.org

- Certified Gastroenterology Registered Nurses (CGRN)

National Council of State Boards of Nursing (NCSBN)	www.ncsbn.org

- Nurse Practitioner Certification
- Nurse Licensure Compact (NLC)

National Certification Board for Diabetes Educators (NCBDE)	www.ncbde.org

- Certified Diabetes Educator

Board of Certification for Emergency Nursing (BCEN)	www.ena.org

- Certified Emergency Nursing (CEN)
- Certified Flight Registered Nurse (CFRN)

HIV/AIDS Nursing Certification Board (HANCB)	www.hancb.org

- HIV/AIDS Nursing

Organization	Website
Certification Board of Infection Control & Epidemiology (CBIC) • Infectious Disease Nursing	**www.cbic.org**
Infusion Nurses Society (INS) • Infusion Nursing	**www.ins1.org**
National Certification Corporation (NCC) • Inpatient Obstetric (INPT) • Maternal Newborn (MN) • Low-Risk Neonatal (LRN) • Neonatal Intensive Care (NIC) • Neonatal Nurse Practitioner • Women's Health Care Nurse Practitioner • Electronic Fetal Monitoring • Neonatal Pediatric Transport	**www.nccwebsite.org**
Oncology Nursing Certification Corporation • Oncology Certified Nurse (OCN®) • Certified Pediatric Hematology Oncology Nurse (CPHON®) • Advanced Oncology Certified Nurse Practitioner (AOCNP®) • Advanced Oncology Certified Clinical Nurse Specialist (AOCNS®) • Certified Breast Care Nurse (CBCN®) • Certified Pediatric Oncology Nurse (CPON®) • Advanced Oncology Certified Nurse (AOCN®)	**www.oncc.org**
American Academy of Pain Management (AAPM) • Credentialed Pain Practitioner (CPP)	**www.aapainmanage.org**
Competency & Credentialing Institute (CCI) • Perioperative Nursing (CNOR & CRNFA)	**www.cc-institute.org**
American Society of Plastic Surgical Nurses (ASPSN) • Certified Plastic Surgical Nurse (CPSN)	**www.aspsn.org**
American Board of Perianesthesia Nursing Certification (ABPANC) • Certified Post Anesthesia Nurse (CPAN®) • Certified Ambulatory Perianesthesia Nurse (CAPA®)	**www.cpancapa.org**
National Board for Certification of School Nurses (NBCSN) • School Nursing (NBCSN)	**www.nbcsn.com**
Genetic Nursing Credentialing Commission (GNCC) • Advanced Practice Nurse in Genetics (APNG) • Genetics Clinical Nurse (GCN)	**www.geneticnurse.org**
Center for Nursing Education and Testing (C-NET®) • Dermatology Nurses Certification Board (DNCB) • Certified Dermatology Nurse (DNC) • Certified Dermatology Nurse Practitioner (DCNP) • Certified Medical-Surgical Nurse (CMSRN) • Certified Hemodialysis Technician (CCHT) • Certified Dialysis Nurse (CDN) • Certified Nephrology Nurse (CNN) • Certified Nephrology Nurse Practitioner (CNN-NP) • Plastic Surgical Nursing Certification Board (PSNCB) • Radiological Nurse (RNC) • Certified Board for Urology Nurses & Associates (CBUNA) • Certified Board Urology Associate (CUA) • Certified Urology Registered Nurse (CURN) • Certified Urology Nurse Practitioner (CUNP)	**www.cnetnurse.com**
Prepared Childbirth Educators, Inc. • Certified Breastfeeding Counselor (CBC) • Certified Childbirth Educator (CCE) • Certified Labor Support Specialist (CLSS) • Certified Prenatal/Postnatal Fitness Instructor • Certified Infant Massage Instructor/Educator	**www.childbirtheducation.org**
American Association of Nurse Anesthetists • Certified Registered Nurse Anesthetist (CRNA)	**www.aana.com**

PROFESSIONAL ASSOCIATIONS FOR NURSES

COMMUNITY HEALTH

American Academy of Ambulatory Care Nursing
East Holly Ave – Box 56
Pitman NJ 08071-0056
800-262-6877
www.aaacn.org

American Public Health Association
800 I St NW
Washington DC 20001-3710
202-777-APHA (2742)
www.apha.org

CRITICAL CARE

American Association of Critical-Care Nurses
101 Columbia
Aliso Viejo CA 92656-4109
800-899-2226
www.aacn.org

Northeast Pediatric Cardiology Nurses Association
PO Box 261
Brookline MA 02446
www.npcna.org

Society of Critical Care Medicine
500 Midway Dr
Mount Prospect IL 60056
847-827-6869
www.sccm.org

EMERGENCY NURSING

Air & Surface Transport Nurses
7995 E Prentice Ave – Suite 100
Greenwood Village CO 80111
800-897-6362
www.astna.org

Emergency Nurses Association
915 Lee St
Des Plaines IL 60016-6569
800-900-9659
www.ena.org

GERIATRICS

The American Geriatrics Society
40 Fulton St, 18th Floor
New York NY 10038
212-308-1414
www.americangeriatrics.org

Gerontological Advanced Practice Nurses Association
East Holly Ave – Box 56
Pitman NJ 08071-0056
866-355-1392
www.gapna.org

The Gerontological Society of America
1220 L St NW – Suite 901
Washington DC 20005
202-842-1275
www.geron.org

MIDWIFERY

American College of Nurse-Midwives
8403 Colesville Rd – Suite 1550
Silver Spring MD 20910
240-485-1800
www.midwife.org

NEONATAL

Association of Women's Health, Obstetric and Neonatal Nurses
2000 L St NW – Suite 740
Washington DC 20036
800-673-8499
www.awhonn.org

National Association of Neonatal Nurses
4700 W Lake Ave
Glenview IL 60025
800-451-3795
www.nann.org

NEPHROLOGY

American Nephrology Nurses' Association
East Holly Ave - Box 56
Pitman NJ 08071-0056
888-600-2622
www.annanurse.org

National Kidney Foundation
30 E 33rd St
New York NY 10016
800-622-9010
www.kidney.org

NEUROSCIENCE

American Association of Neuroscience Nurses
4700 W Lake Ave
Glenview IL 60025
800-557-2266
www.aann.org

ONCOLOGY

Association of Pediatric Hematology/Oncology Nurses
4700 W Lake Ave
Glenview IL 60025-1485
847-375-4724
www.aphon.org

Oncology Nursing Society
125 Enterprise Dr
Pittsburgh PA 15275
866-257-4ONS (4667)
www.ons.org

PALLIATIVE CARE

Hospice and Palliative Nurses Association
One Penn Center West – Suite 229
Pittsburgh PA 15276
412-787-9301
www.hpna.org

PEDIATRICS

Pediatric Nursing Certification Board
800 S Frederick Ave – Suite 204
Gaithersburg MD 20877-4152
888-641-2767
www.pncb.org

PREOPERATIVE & PERIOPERATIVE

American Association of Nurse Anesthetists
222 S Prospect Ave
Park Ridge IL 60068
847-692-7050
www.aana.com

American Society of PeriAnesthesia Nurses
90 Frontage Rd
Cherry Hill NJ 08034-1424
877-737-9696
www.aspan.org

American Society of Plastic Surgical Nurses
500 Cummings Center
Suite 4550
Beverly MA 01915
877-337-9315
www.aspsn.org

Association of PeriOperative Registered Nurses (AORN)
2170 S Parker Rd – Suite 400
Denver CO 80231
800-755-2676
www.aorn.org

PSYCHIATRIC

American Psychiatric Nurses Association
1555 Wilson Blvd – Suite 530
Arlington VA 22209
866-243-2443
www.apna.org

REHABILITATION

Association of Rehabilitation Nurses
4700 W Lake Ave
Glenview IL 60025
800-229-7530
www.rehabnurse.org

SCHOOL NURSING

American School Health Association
4340 East West Hwy – Suite 403
Bethesda MD 20814
301-652-8072
www.ashaweb.org

National Association of School Nurses
8484 Georgia Ave #420
Silver Spring MD 20910
240-821-1130
www.nasn.org

STATE ASSOCIATIONS/ ANESTHETISTS

California Association of Nurse Anesthetists
MKD Associates
PO Box 1412
Sonoma CA 95476
707-480-0096
www.canainc.org

Connecticut Association of Nurse Anesthetists
377 Research Pkwy – Suite 2D
Meriden CT 06450
203-238-1207
www.ctana.net

New York State Association of Nurse Anesthetists
1450 Western Ave – Suite 101
Albany NY 12203
518-861-8876
www.nysana.com

Pennsylvania Association of Nurse Anesthetists
PO Box 1076
Camp Hill PA 17001
800-495-PANA (7262)
www.pana.org

Texas Association of Nurse Anesthetists
PO Box 40775
Austin TX 78704
512-495-9004
www.txana.org

STUDENT NURSING

National Student Nurses' Association
45 Main St – Suite 606
Brooklyn NY 11201
718-210-0705
www.nsna.org

WOUND CARE

Wound, Ostomy and Continence Nurses Society
15000 Commerce Pkwy - Suite C
Mt Laurel NJ 08054
888-224-9626
www.wocn.org

NURSE PRACTITIONER PROGRAMS BY STATE

ALABAMA

University of Alabama-Huntsville
College of Nursing
Nursing Building – Room 207
301 Sparkman Dr NW
Huntsville AL 35899
256-824-6345
http://onlinenurse.nb.uah.edu

ARIZONA

Arizona State University
College of Nursing & Health
Innovation
500 N 3rd St
Phoenix AZ 85004
602-496-2264
http://nursingandhealth.asu.edu

University of Arizona
College of Nursing
1305 N Martin St
PO Box 210203
Tucson AZ 85721
520-626-6154
www.nursing.arizona.edu

CALIFORNIA

Azusa Pacific University
School of Nursing
PO Box 7000
Azusa CA 91702
626-815-5386
www.apu.edu/nursing

California State University-Bakersfield
Department of Nursing
9001 Stockdale Hwy
Bakersfield CA 93311
661-654-2505
www.csub.edu/nursing

California State University-Fresno
Department of Nursing
College of Health & Human Services
2345 E San Ramon – M/S MH26
Fresno CA 93740
559-278-4004
www.csufresno.edu/chhs

California State University-Long Beach
Department of Nursing
College of Health & Human Services
1250 Bellflower Blvd
Long Beach CA 90840
562-985-4194
www.csulb.edu/colleges/chhs

Loma Linda University
School of Nursing
West Hall
Loma Linda CA 92350
909-558-4923
www.llu.edu/llu/nursing

UCLA School of Nursing
700 Tiverton Ave
Los Angeles CA 90095
310-825-3109
www.nursing.ucla.edu

University of California – San
Francisco
School of Nursing
2 Koret Way – N319X
UCSF Box 0602
San Francisco CA 94113
415-476-1435
www.nurseweb.ucsf.edu

University of San Diego
Hahn School of Nursing & Health
Science
5998 Alcala Park
San Diego CA 92110
619-260-4600
www.sandiego.edu/nursing

University of San Francisco
School of Nursing
2130 Fulton St
San Francisco CA 94117
415-422-5555
www.usfca.edu/nursing

COLORADO

Regis University Loretto Heights
School of Nursing
Rueckert-Hartman College for Health
Professions
3333 Regis Blvd – Mail Code G9
Denver CO 80221
800-388-2366
www.regis.edu

University of Colorado Denver
College of Nursing
Campus Box C288 – Education 2
North
13120 E 19th Ave
Aurora CO 80045
303-556-2400
www.nursing.ucdenver.edu

CONNECTICUT

Quinnipiac University
Department of Nursing
275 Mount Carmel Ave
Hamden CT 06518
203-582-5397
www.quinnipiac.edu

Saint Joseph College
Division of Nursing
1678 Asylum Ave
West Hartford CT 06117
860-232-4571
http://www.sjc.edu/academics/schools/
school-of-health-and-natural-sciences/
nursing/

Yale University
School of Nursing
100 Church St S
PO Box 9740
New Haven CT 06536
203-785-2393
www.nursing.yale.edu

DELAWARE

University of Delaware
College of Health Sciences
School of Nursing
25 N College
Newark DE 19716
302-831-1253
www.udel.edu/nursing

DISTRICT OF COLUMBIA

Catholic University of America
School of Nursing
125 Gowan Hall
620 Michigan Ave NE
Washington DC 20064
202-319-5400
http://nursing.cua.edu

Georgetown University
School of Nursing & Health Studies
St Mary's Hall
3700 Reservoir Rd NW
Washington DC 20057
202-687-4647
http://snhs.georgetown.edu

FLORIDA

Barry University
School of Nursing
11300 NE 2nd Ave
Miami Shores FL 33161
305-899-3800
http://www.barry.edu/nursing

Florida State University
College of Nursing
Vivian M Duxbury Hall
98 Varsity Way MC 4310
Tallahassee FL 32306
850-644-3296
www.nursing.fsu.edu

University of Miami
School of Nursing & Health Studies
PO Box 248153
Coral Gables FL 33124
305-284-3666
www.miami.edu/sonhs

GEORGIA

Emory University
Nell Hodgson Woodruff School of
Nursing
1520 Clifton Rd NE
Atlanta GA 30322
404-727-7980
www.nursing.emory.edu

Georgia State University
Byrdine F Lewis School of Nursing
PO Box 4019
Atlanta GA 30302
404-413-1200
http://chhs.gsu.edu/nursing

HAWAII

Hawaii Pacific University
School of Nursing
1164 Bishop St
Honolulu HI 96813
808-544-0200
www.hpu.edu/nursing

IDAHO

Boise State University
Department of Nursing
1910 University Drive
Boise ID 83725
208-426-4143
http://nursing.boisestate.edu

Idaho State University
School of Nursing
921 S 8th Ave
Pocatello ID 83209
208-282-2132
www.isu.edu/nursing

ILLINOIS

De Paul University
Lincoln Park Campus
Department of Nursing
990 W Fullerton Pkwy
Chicago IL 60604
773-325-7280
http://csh.depaul.edu/departments/
nursing/Pages/default.aspx

North Park University
School of Nursing
3225 W Foster Ave
Chicago IL 60625
773-244-4587
http://www.northpark.edu/Academics/
School-of-Nursing.aspx

Southern Illinois University – Edwardsville
School of Nursing
Alumni Hall
PO Box 1066 – Room 2117
Edwardsville IL 62026
618-650-3956
www.siue.edu/nursing

University of Illinois – Chicago
College of Nursing
845 S Damen Ave – MC 802
Chicago IL 60612
312-996-7800
www.uic.edu/nursing

INDIANA

Indiana Wesleyan University – Marion
School of Nursing
4201 S Washington St
Marion IN 46953
888-876-6498
www.indwes.edu/nursing

Purdue University
College of Health and Human
Sciences
School of Nursing
502 N University St
West Lafayette IN 47907
765-494-4004
www.nursing.purdue.edu

KENTUCKY

University of Kentucky
College of Nursing
315 College of Nursing Building
Lexington KY 40536
859-323-5108
http://academics.uky.edu/ukcon/pub/
Pages/Default.aspx

LOUISIANA

Louisiana State University
School of Nursing
1900 Gravier St – 4th Floor
New Orleans LA 70112
504-568-4106
http://nursing.lsuhsc.edu

MARYLAND

Johns Hopkins University
School of Nursing
525 N Wolfe St
Baltimore MD 21205
410-955-7548
www.son.jhmi.edu

MASSACHUSETTS

Northeastern University
College of Health Sciences
School of Nursing
102 Robinson Hall
Boston MA 02115
617-373-3649
http://www.northeastern.edu/bouve/
nursing/index.html

University of Massachusetts –
Dartmouth
College of Nursing
285 Old Westport Rd
North Dartmouth MA 02747
508-999-8586
http://umassd.edu/nursing

University of Massachusetts –
Worcester
Graduate School of Nursing, S1-853
55 Lake Ave N
Worcester MA 01655
508-856-5801
http://www.umassmed.edu/gsn/
index.aspx

MICHIGAN

Michigan State University
College of Nursing
Life Sciences Building A117
East Lansing MI 48824
800-605-6424
www.nursing.msu.edu

University of Michigan
School of Nursing Building
400 N Ingalls
Ann Arbor MI 48109
734-763-5985
www.nursing.umich.edu

University of Michigan – Flint
School of Health Professions &
Studies
2180 William S White Building
303 East Kearsley St
Flint MI 48502
810-762-3420
www.umflint.edu/nursing

MINNESOTA

University of Minnesota
School of Nursing
5-160 Weaver-Densford Hall
308 Harvard St SE
Minneapolis MN 55455
612-624-7980
www.nursing.umn.edu

MISSOURI

Missouri State University
Department of Nursing
901 S National Ave
Springfield MO 65897
417-836-5310
www.missouristate.edu/nursing

Saint Louis University
School of Nursing
3525 Caroline St
St Louis MO 63104
314-977-8900
http://www.slu.edu/nursing.xml

University of Missouri – Kansas City
School of Nursing
Health Sciences Building
2464 Charlotte
Kansas City MO 64108
816-235-1700
http://nursing.umkc.edu

NEBRASKA

Creighton University
School of Nursing
2500 California Plaza
Omaha NE 68178
800-544-5071
www.creighton.edu/nursing

NEW JERSEY

The College of New Jersey
Department of Nursing
Paul Loser Hall 206
PO Box 7718
Ewing NJ 08628
609-771-2591
http://www.tcnj.edu/~nursing/
nursing.html

Felician College
Division of Health Sciences
Nursing & Health Management
262 S Main St
Lodi NJ 07644
201-559-6000
www.felician.edu

Monmouth University
School of Nursing & Health Studies
400 Cedar Ave
West Long Branch NJ 07764
732-571-3443
http://www.monmouth.edu/
academics/departments/nursing.asp

Ramapo College of New Jersey
Nursing Programs at Ramapo
School of Theoretical & Applied
Science
505 Ramapo Valley Rd
Mahwah NJ 07430
201-684-7749
www.ramapo.edu/nursing

Rutgers College of Nursing
Ackerson Hall – Room 102
180 University Ave
Newark NJ 07102
973-353-5293
http://nursing.rutgers.edu

NEW MEXICO

New Mexico State University
School of Nursing
MSC 3185
PO Box 30001
Las Cruces NM 88003
575-646-3812
http://www.nmsu.edu/~nursing/

University of New Mexico
College of Nursing
1 University of New Mexico
MSCO9 5350
Albuquerque NM 87131
505-272-4223
http://nursing.unm.edu/

NEW YORK

Adelphi University
School of Nursing
1 South Ave
PO Box 701
Garden City NY 11530
516-877-4510
http://nursing.adelphi.edu

SUNY Binghamton University
Decker School of Nursing
4400 Vestal Pkwy E
Binghamton NY 13903
607-777-2406
http://www.binghamton.edu/dson

College of Mount Saint Vincent
Department of Nursing
6301 Riverdale Ave
Riverdale NY 10471
718-405-3351
http://www.mountsaintvincent.edu/
nursing

Columbia University
School of Nursing
630 W 168th St
PO Box 6
New York NY 10032
212-305-5756
http://cumc.columbia.edu/dept/
nursing

D'Youville College
Nursing Department
320 Porter Ave
Buffalo NY 14201
716-829-7701
http://www.dyc.edu/academics/
nursing/index.asp

Long Island University – Brooklyn
School of Nursing
1 University Plaza
Brooklyn NY 11201
718-488-1512
http://www.liu.edu/Brooklyn/
Academics/Schools/SON.aspx

Long Island University – Brookville
C W Post Campus Department of
Nursing
720 Northern Blvd
Brookville NY 11548
516-299-2485
http://www.liu.edu/CWPost/
Academics.aspx

New York University
College of Nursing
726 Broadway – 10th Floor
New York NY 10003
212-998-5300
http://www.nyu.edu/nursing

Pace University
Lienhard School of Nursing
41 Park Row – Room 300
New York NY 10038
212-346-1716
http://www.pace.edu/lienhard

SUNY Institute of Technology at Utica/
Rome
School of Nursing & Health Systems
100 Seymour Rd
PO Box 3050
Utica NY 13502
315-792-7500
http://www.sunyit.edu/nursing

University of Buffalo
School of Nursing
103 Wende Hall
3435 Main St
Buffalo NY 14214
716-829-2533
www.nursing.buffalo.edu

University of Rochester
School of Nursing
601 Elmwood Ave
Rochester NY 14642
585-273-2375
www.son.rochester.edu

NORTH CAROLINA

University of North Carolina –
Chapel Hill
School of Nursing
301 Carrington Hall – CB7460
Chapel Hill NC 27599
919-966-3638
http://nursing.ce.unc.edu

University of North Carolina –
Charlotte
School of Nursing
9201 University City Blvd
Charlotte NC 28223
704-687-7952
www.nursing.uncc.edu

OHIO

Case Western Reserve University
Frances Payne Bolton School of
Nursing
10900 Euclid Ave
Cleveland OH 44106
216-368-2529
http://fpb.case.edu

Kent State University
College of Nursing
Henderson Hall
Box 5190
Kent OH 44242
330-672-7930
www.kent.edu/nursing

Ohio State University
College of Nursing
Newton Hall
1585 Neil Ave
Columbus OH 43210
614-292-4041
www.con.ohio-state.edu

University of Akron
College of Nursing
Mary Gladwin Hall
209 Carroll St
Akron OH 44325
330-972-7111
www.uakron.edu/nursing

University of Toledo
College of Nursing
2801 W Bancroft
Toledo OH 43606
800-586-5336
www.utoledo.edu/nursing

OKLAHOMA

University of Oklahoma
College of Nursing
PO Box 26901
1100 N Stonewall Ave
Oklahoma City OK 73117
877-367-6876
http://nursing.ouhsc.edu

OREGON

Oregon Health & Sciences University
School of Nursing
3455 SW US Veterans Hospital Rd
Portland OR 97239
866-223-1811
http://www.ohsu.edu/xd/education/
schools/school-of-nursing/about

University of Portland
School of Nursing
5000 N Willamette Blvd
Portland OR 97203
503-943-7211
www.nursing.up.edu

PENNSYLVANIA

Bloomsburg University
Department of Nursing
3121 McCormick Center for Human
Services
400 E Second St
Bloomsburg PA 17815
570-389-4423
http://bloomu.edu/nursing

Drexel University
College of Nursing & Health
Professions
245 N 15th St
Philadelpha PA 19102
215-762-8347
http://www.drexel.edu/cnhp

Millersville University
Department of Nursing
1 S George St
Millersville PA 17551
717-872-3410
www.millersville.edu/nursing

Pennsylvania State University
School of Nursing Graduate Programs
201 Health & Human Development
East
University Park PA 16802
814-863-0245
http://www.nursing.psu.edu/grad/

Temple University
College of Health Professions and
Social Work
Nursing Department
3307 N Broad St
Philadephia PA 19140
215-707-4688
www.temple.edu/nursing

University of Pennsylvania
School of Nursing
Claire M Fagin Hall
418 Curie Blvd
Philadelphia PA 19104
215-898-8281
www.nursing.upenn.edu

University of Pittsburgh
School of Nursing
Victoria Building
3500 Victoria St
Pittsburgh PA 15261
412-624-4586
www.nursing.pitt.edu

Villanova University
College of Nursing
800 E Lancaster Ave
Villanova PA 19085
610-519-4500
www.villanova.edu/nursing

TENNESSEE

Belmont University
Gordon E Inman College of Health
Sciences and Nursing
School of Nursing
1900 Belmont Blvd
Nashville TN 37212
615-460-6134
www.belmont.edu/nursing

East Tennessee State University
College of Nursing
310 Roy S Nicks Hall
PO Box 70617
Johnson City TN 37614
423-439-7199
www.etsu.edu/nursing

Union University
School of Nursing
Nursing Admissions Coordinator
1050 Union University Dr
Jackson TN 38305
731-661-6545
http://www.uu.edu/academics/son/

University of Tennessee – Memphis
College of Nursing
877 Madison Ave
Memphis TN 38163
901-448-6128
www.uthsc.edu/nursing

Vanderbilt University
School of Nursing
Godchaux Hall 207
461 21st Ave S
Nashville TN 37240
615-322-4400
www.nursing.vanderbilt.edu

TEXAS

Texas A&M University – Corpus
Christi
College of Nursing & Health Sciences
6300 Ocean Dr
Corpus Christi TX 78412
361-825-5700
www.tamucc.edu

University of Texas – Austin
School of Nursing
1700 Red River St
Austin TX 78701
512-471-7311
www.utexas.edu/nursing

VIRGINIA

Marymount University
School of Health Professions
Department of Nursing
2807 N Glebe Rd
Arlington VA 22207
703-284-1500
http://www.marymount.edu/
academics/programs/nursingBSN

Shenandoah University
Division of Nursing
1775 N Sector Ct
Winchester VA 22601
540-678-4374
http://www.su.edu/0B875B3A348444
769D87E900A02AF363.asp

University of Virginia
School of Nursing
McLeod Hall
PO Box 800782
Charlottesville VA 22908
434-924-0141
www.nursing.virginia.edu

Virginia Commonwealth University
School of Nursing
PO Box 980567
Richmond VA 23298
800-828-0724
www.nursing.vcu.edu

WASHINGTON

Gonzaga University
Department of Nursing
502 E Boone Ave
Spokane WA 99528
509-313-3569
www.gonzaga.edu/nursing

Pacific Lutheran University
School of Nursing
Ramstad Building 214
Tacoma WA 98447
253-535-7672
http://www.plu.edu/nursing

Seattle University
College of Nursing
901 12th Ave
PO Box 222000
Seattle WA 98122
206-296-5660
www.seattleu.edu/nursing

University of Washington
School of Nursing
PO Box 357260
Seattle WA 98195
206-543-8736
http://nursing.uw.edu

Washington State University
Intercollegiate College of Nursing
PO Box 1495
Spokane WA 99210
509-324-7360
www.nursing.wsu.edu

WISCONSIN

University of Wisconsin – Milwaukee
College of Nursing
PO Box 413
1921 E Hartford Ave
Milwaukee WI 53201
414-229-4801
www.uwm.edu/nursing

WYOMING

University of Wyoming
College of Health Sciences
Fay W Whitney School of Nursing
Department 3065
1000 E University Ave
Laramie WY 82071
307-766-4312
www.uwyo.edu/nursing

PROFESSIONAL ASSOCIATIONS FOR NPs

NATIONAL ASSOCIATIONS

American Academy of Nurse Practitioners
PO Box 12846
Austin TX 78711-2846
512-442-4262
www.aanp.org

Gerontological Advanced Practice Nurses Association
East Holly Ave – Box 56
Pitman NJ 08071
866-355-1392
www.gapna.org

National Association of Pediatric Nurse Practitioners
20 Brace Rd – Suite 200
Cherry Hill NJ 08034-2634
856-857-9700
www.napnap.org

Nurse Practitioners in Women's Health
505 C St NE
Washington DC 20002
202-543-9693
www.npwh.org

STATE ASSOCIATIONS

ALABAMA
North Alabama Nurse Practitioner Association
PO Box 14055
Huntsville AL 35815
www.northalabamanpa.com

ALASKA
Alaska Nurse Practitioner Association
3701 E Tudor Rd – Suite 208
Anchorage AK 99507
907-222-6847
www.alaskanp.org

ARIZONA
Arizona Nurse Practitioner Council
1850 E Southern Ave – Suite 1
Tempe AZ 85282
480-831-0404
www.arizonanp.com

ARKANSAS
Arkansas Nurses Association
1123 S University – Suite 1015
Little Rock AR 72204
501-244-2363
www.arna.org

CALIFORNIA
California Association for Nurse Practitioners
1415 L Street – Suite 200
Sacramento CA 95814
916-441-1361
www.canpweb.org

COLORADO
Colorado Society of Advance Practice Nurses
PO Box 100158
Denver CO 80250-0158
303-757-7483
www.csapn.org

CONNECTICUT
Connecticut Advanced Practice Registered Nurse Society
2842 Main St - # 323
Glastonbury CT 06033
www.ctaprns.org

DELAWARE
Delaware Nurses Association
726 Loveville Rd, Suite 3000
Hockessin DE 19707
302-239-3141
www.denurses.org

DISTRICT OF COLUMBIA
Nurse Practitioner Association of DC
PO Box 77424
Washington DC 20013-7424
www.npadc.org

FLORIDA
Florida Nurses Association
PO Box 536985
Orlando FL 32803-6985
407-896-3261
www.floridanurses.org

Florida Nurse Practitioner Network
PO Box 25422
Tampa FL 33622
866-535-3676
www.fnpn.org

GEORGIA
Nurse Practitioner Council of Coastal Georgia
PO Box 14046
Savannah GA 31416
912-351-7800
www.npcouncilofcoastalga.
enpnetwork.com

IDAHO
Nurse Practitioners of Idaho
5120 W Overland Rd – PMB 218
Boise ID 83705
208-914-0138
www.npidaho.org

ILLINOIS
Illinois Nurses Association
105 W Adams St – Ste 2101
Chicago IL 60603
312-419-2900
www.illinoisnurses.com

INDIANA
Coalition of Advanced Practice Nurses of Indiana
PO Box 87925
Canton MI 48187
www.capni.org

IOWA
Iowa Nurse Practitioner Society
www.iowanpsociety.org

KENTUCKY
Kentucky Coalition of Nurse Practitioners and Nurse Midwives
1017 Ash St
Louisville KY 40217
502-333-0076
www.kcnpnm.org

LOUISIANA
Louisiana Association of Nurse Practitioners
5713 Superior Dr – Suite A5
Baton Route LA 70816
225-293-7950
www.lanp.org

MAINE
Maine Nurse Practitioner Association
11 Columbia St
Augusta ME 04330
207-621-0313
www.mnpa.us

MARYLAND
Nurse Practitioner Association of Maryland
PO Box 540
Ellicott City MD 21041-0540
888-405-NPAM (6726)
www.npamonline.org

MASSACHUSETTS
Massachusetts Coalition of Nurse Practitioners
PO Box 1153
Littleton MA 01460
781-575-1565
www.mcnpweb.org

MICHIGAN
Michigan Council of Nurse Practitioners
PO Box 87934
Canton MI 48187
734-432-9881
www.micnp.org

MINNESOTA
Association of Southeast Minnesota Nurse Practitioners
PO Box 7371
Rochester MN 55903
www.asmnp.org

MISSISSIPPI
Mississippi Nurses Association
31 Woodgreen Pl
Madison MS 39110
601-898-0670
www.msnurses.org

MISSOURI
Missouri Nurses Association
1904 Bubba Ln
PO Box 105228
Jefferson City MO 65110
573-636-4623
www.missourinurses.org

MONTANA
Montana Nurses Association
406-442-6710
www.mtnurses.org

NEVADA
Nevada Nurses Association
PO Box 34660
Reno NV 89533
757-747-2333
www.nvnurses.org

NEW HAMPSHIRE
New Hampshire Nurse Practitioner
Association
180 Mutton Road
Webster NH 03303
603-648-2233
www.npweb.org

NEW JERSEY
New Jersey State Nurses Association
1479 Pennington Rd
Trenton NJ 08618
888-UR-NJSNA (876-5762)
www.njsna.org

NEW MEXICO
New Mexico Nurse Practitioner
Council
PO Box 40682
Albuquerque NM 87196-0682
505-366-3763
www.nmnpc.org

NEW YORK
The Nurse Practitioner Association
New York State
12 Corporate Dr
Clifton Park NY 12065
518-348-0719

www.thenpa.org

NORTH CAROLINA
North Carolina Nurses Association
PO Box 12025
Raleigh NC 27605
800-626-2153
www.ncnurses.org

OHIO
Ohio Association of Advanced Practice
Nurses
5818 Wilmington Pike – # 300
Dayton OH 45459
866-668-3839
www.oaapn.org

OKLAHOMA
Oklahoma Nurse Practitioners
Association
29850 South 567 Rd
Monkey Island OK 74331
405-445-4874
www.npofoklahoma.com

OREGON
Nurse Practitioners of Oregon
18765 SW Boones Ferry Rd –
Suite 200
Tualatin OR 97062
503-293-0011
www.nursepractitionersoforegon.org

PENNSYLVANIA
Pennsylvania Coalition of Nurse
Practitioners
PO Box 1071
Jenkintown PA 19046
866-800-6206
www.pacnp.org

SOUTH DAKOTA
Nurse Practitioner Association of
South Dakota
PO Box 2822
Rapid City SD 57709
www.npasd.org

TENNESSEE
Tennessee Nurses Association
545 Mainstream Dr – Suite 405
Nashville TN 37228
615-254-0350
www.tnaonline.org

TEXAS
Texas Nurse Practitioners
4425 S Mopac Expswy – Bldg III –
Suite 405
Austin TX 78735
512-291-6224
www.texasnp.org

UTAH
Utah Nurse Practitioners
PO Box 581084
Salt Lake City UT 84108
http://utahnp.enpnetwork.com

VERMONT
Vermont Nurse Practitioners
PO Box 64773
Burlington VT 05406
www.vtnpa.org

VIRGINIA
Virginia Council of Nurse Practitioners
250 West Main St, Suite 100
Charlottesville VA 22902
434-977-3716
www.vcnp.net

WASHINGTON
ARNPs United of Washington State
10024 SE 240th St – Suite 230
Kent WA 98031
253-480-1035
www.auws.org

WEST VIRGINIA
West Virginia Nurses Association
1007 Bigley Ave – Suite 308
Charleston WV 25302
800-400-1226
304-342-1169
www.wvnurses.org

WISCONSIN
Wisconsin Nurses Association
6117 Monona Dr – Suite 1
Monona WI 53716
608-221-0383
www.wisconsinnurses.org

ANTIPYRETIC PRODUCTS

BRAND	INGREDIENT/STRENGTH	DOSAGE
ACETAMINOPHEN		
Anacin Extra Strength Aspirin Free Tablets	Acetaminophen 500mg	**Adults & Peds ≥12 yrs:** 2 tabs q6h. **Max:** 8 tabs q24h.
FeverAll Children's Suppositories	Acetaminophen 120mg	**Peds 3-6 yrs:** 1 supp q4-6h. **Max:** 6 supp q24h.
FeverAll Infants' Suppositories	Acetaminophen 80mg	**Peds 6-11 months:** 1 supp q6h. **12-36 months:** 1 supp q4h. **Max:** 6 supp q24h.
FeverAll Jr. Strength Suppositories	Acetaminophen 325mg	**Peds 6-12 yrs:** 1 supp q4-6h. **Max:** 6 supp q24h.
PediaCare Children's Fever Reducer/ Pain Reliever Acetaminophen Oral Suspension	Acetaminophen 160mg/5mL	**Peds 2-3 yrs (24-35 lbs):** 1 tsp (5mL). **4-5 yrs (36-47 lbs):** 1½ tsp (7.5mL). **6-8 yrs (48-59 lbs):** 2 tsp (10mL). **9-10 yrs (60-71 lbs):** 2½ tsp (12.5mL). **11 yrs (72-95 lbs):** 3 tsp (15mL). May repeat q4h. **Max:** 5 doses q24h.
PediaCare Infants Fever Reducer/ Pain Reliever Acetaminophen Oral Suspension	Acetaminophen 160mg/5mL	**Peds 2-3 yrs (24-35 lbs):** 5mL. May repeat q4h. **Max:** 5 doses q24h.
Triaminic Fever Reducer Pain Reliever Syrup	Acetaminophen 160mg/5mL	**Peds 2-3 yrs (24-35 lbs):** 1 tsp (5mL). **4-5 yrs (36-47 lbs):** 1½ tsp (7.5mL). **6-8 yrs (48-59 lbs):** 2 tsp (10mL). **9-10 yrs (60-71 lbs)** 2½ tsp (12.5mL). **11 yrs (72-95 lbs):** 3 tsp (15mL). May repeat q4h. **Max:** 5 doses q24h.
Triaminic Infant's Fever Reducer Pain Reliever Syrup	Acetaminophen 160mg/5mL	**Peds 2-3 yrs (24-35 lbs):** 1 tsp (5mL). May repeat q4h. **Max:** 5 doses q24h.
Tylenol 8 Hour Caplets	Acetaminophen 650mg	**Adults & Peds ≥12 yrs:** 2 tabs q8h prn. **Max:** 6 tabs q24h.
Tylenol Arthritis Caplets	Acetaminophen 650mg	**Adults:** 2 tabs q8h prn. **Max:** 6 tabs q24h.
Tylenol Arthritis Gelcaps	Acetaminophen 650mg	**Adults:** 2 caps q8h prn. **Max:** 6 caps q24h.
Tylenol Arthritis Geltabs	Acetaminophen 650mg	**Adults:** 2 tabs q8h prn. **Max:** 6 tabs q24h.
Tylenol Children's Meltaways Tablets*	Acetaminophen 80mg	**Peds 2-3 yrs (24-35 lbs):** 2 tabs. **4-5 yrs (36-47 lbs):** 3 tabs. **6-8 yrs (48-59 lbs):** 4 tabs. **9-10 yrs (60-71 lbs):** 5 tabs. **11 yrs (72-95 lbs):** 6 tabs. May repeat q4h. **Max:** 5 doses q24h.
Tylenol Children's Suspension*	Acetaminophen 160mg/5mL	**Peds 2-3 yrs (24-35 lbs):** 1 tsp (5mL). **4-5 yrs (36-47 lbs):** 1.5 tsp (7.5mL). **6-8 yrs (48-59 lbs):** 2 tsp (10mL). **9-10 yrs (60-71 lbs):** 2.5 tsp (12.5mL). **11 yrs (72-95 lbs):** 3 tsp (15mL). May repeat q4h. **Max:** 5 doses q24h.
Tylenol Extra Strength Caplets	Acetaminophen 500mg	**Adults & Peds ≥12 yrs:** 2 tabs q6h prn. **Max:** 6 tabs q24h.
Tylenol Extra Strength EZ Tablets	Acetaminophen 500mg	**Adults & Peds ≥12 yrs:** 2 tabs q6h prn. **Max:** 6 tabs q24h.
Tylenol Extra Strength Rapid Blast Liquid	Acetaminophen 500mg/15mL	**Adults & Peds ≥12 yrs:** 2 tbsp (30mL) q6h prn. **Max:** 6 tbsp (90mL) q24h.
Tylenol Extra Strength Rapid Release Gelcaps	Acetaminophen 500mg	**Adults & Peds ≥12 yrs:** 2 caps q6h prn. **Max:** 6 caps q24h.

(Continued)

BRAND	INGREDIENT/STRENGTH	DOSAGE
ACETAMINOPHEN *(Continued)*		
Tylenol Junior Meltaways Tablets*	Acetaminophen 160mg	**Peds 6-8 yrs (48-59 lbs):** 2 tabs. **9-10 yrs (60-71 lbs):** 2.5 tabs. **11 yrs (72-95 lbs):** 3 tabs. May repeat q4h. **Max:** 5 doses q24h.
Tylenol Regular Strength Tablets	Acetaminophen 325mg	**Adults & Peds ≥12 yrs:** 2 tabs q4-6h prn. **Max:** 12 tabs q24h. **Peds 6-11 yrs:** 1 tab q4-6h. **Max:** 5 tabs q24h.
NONSTEROIDAL ANTI-INFLAMMATORY DRUGS (NSAIDs)		
Advil Caplets	Ibuprofen 200mg	**Adults & Peds ≥12 yrs:** 1-2 tabs q4-6h prn. **Max:** 6 tabs q24h.
Advil Children's Suspension	Ibuprofen 100mg/5mL	**Peds 2-3 yrs (24-35 lbs):** 1 tsp (5mL). **4-5 yrs (36-47 lbs):** 1.5 tsp (7.5mL). **6-8 yrs (48-59 lbs):** 2 tsp (10mL). **9-10 yrs (60-71 lbs):** 2.5 tsp (12.5mL). **11 yrs (72-95 lbs):** 3 tsp (15mL). May repeat q6-8h. **Max:** 4 doses q24h.
Advil Gel Caplets	Ibuprofen 200mg	**Adults & Peds ≥12 yrs:** 1-2 caps q4-6h. **Max:** 6 caps q24h.
Advil Infants' Concentrated Drops*	Ibuprofen 50mg/1.25mL	**Peds 6-11 months (12-17 lbs):** 1.25mL. **12-23 months (18-23 lbs):** 1.875mL. May repeat q6-8h. **Max:** 4 doses q24h.
Advil Junior Strength Chewables	Ibuprofen 100mg	**Peds 6-8 yrs (48-59 lbs):** 2 tabs. **9-10 yrs (60-71 lbs):** 2.5 tabs. **11 yrs (72-95 lbs):** 3 tabs. May repeat q6-8h. **Max:** 4 doses q24h.
Advil Junior Strength Tablets	Ibuprofen 100mg	**Peds 6-10 yrs (60-71 lbs):** 2 tabs. **11 yrs (72-95 lbs):** 3 tabs. May repeat q6-8h. **Max:** 4 doses q24h.
Advil Liqui-Gels	Ibuprofen 200mg	**Adults & Peds ≥12 yrs:** 1-2 caps q4-6h. **Max:** 6 caps q24h.
Advil Tablets	Ibuprofen 200mg	**Adults & Peds ≥12 yrs:** 1-2 tabs q4-6h. **Max:** 6 tabs q24h.
Aleve Caplets	Naproxen sodium 220mg	**Adults & Peds ≥12 yrs:** 1 tab q8-12h. May take 1 additional tab within 1 hour of first dose. **Max:** 2 tabs q8-12h or 3 tabs q24h.
Aleve Gelcaps	Naproxen sodium 220mg	**Adults & Peds ≥12 yrs:** 1 cap q8-12h. May take 1 additional tab within 1 hour of first dose. **Max:** 2 tabs q8-12h or 3 tabs q24h.
Aleve Liquid Gels	Naproxen sodium 220mg	**Adults & Peds ≥12 yrs:** 1 cap q8-12h. May take 1 additional cap within 1 hour of first dose. **Max:** 2 caps q8-12h or 3 caps q24h.
Aleve Tablets	Naproxen sodium 220mg	**Adults & Peds ≥12 yrs:** 1 tab q8-12h. May take 1 additional tab within 1 hour of first dose. **Max:** 2 tabs q8-12h or 3 tabs q24h.
Motrin Children's Suspension*†	Ibuprofen 100mg/5mL	**Peds 2-3 yrs (24-35 lbs):** 1 tsp (5mL). **4-5 yrs (36-47 lbs):** 1.5 tsp (7.5mL). **6-8 yrs (48-59 lbs):** 2 tsp (10mL). **9-10 yrs (60-71 lbs):** 2.5 tsp (12.5mL). **11 yrs (72-95 lbs):** 3 tsp (15mL). May repeat q6-8h. **Max:** 4 doses q24h.
Motrin IB Caplets	Ibuprofen 200mg	**Adults & Peds ≥12 yrs:** 1-2 tabs q4-6h. **Max:** 6 tabs q24h.

BRAND	INGREDIENT/STRENGTH	DOSAGE
NONSTEROIDAL ANTI-INFLAMMATORY DRUGS (NSAIDs) *(Continued)*		
Motrin IB Tablets	Ibuprofen 200mg	**Adults & Peds ≥12 yrs:** 1-2 tabs q4-6h. **Max:** 6 tabs q24h.
Motrin Infants' Drops*†	Ibuprofen 50mg/1.25mL	**Peds 6-11 months (12-17 lbs):** 1.25mL. **12-23 months (18-23 lbs):** 1.875mL. May repeat q6-8h. **Max:** 4 doses q24h.
Motrin Junior Strength Caplets*†	Ibuprofen 100mg	**Peds 6-8 yrs (24-35 lbs):** 2 tabs. **9-10 yrs (60-71 lbs):** 2.5 tabs. **11 yrs (72-95 lbs):** 3 tabs. May repeat q6-8h. **Max:** 4 doses q24h.
Motrin Junior Strength Chewable Tablets*†	Ibuprofen 100mg	**Peds 2-3 yrs (24-35 lbs):** 1 tab. **4-5 yrs (36-47 lbs):** 1.5 tabs. **6-8 yrs (48-59 lbs):** 2 tabs. **9-10 yrs (60-71 lbs):** 2.5 tabs. **11 yrs (72-95 lbs):** 3 tabs. May repeat q6-8h. **Max:** 4 doses q24h.
PediaCare Children's Pain Reliever/ Fever Reducer IB Ibuprofen	Ibuprofen 100mg/5mL	**Peds 2-3 yrs (24-35 lbs):** 1 tsp (5mL). **4-5 yrs (36-47 lbs):** 1½ tsp (7.5mL). **6-8 yrs (48-59 lbs):** 2 tsp (10mL). **9-10 yrs (60-71 lbs):** 2½ tsp (12.5mL). **11 yrs (72-95 lbs):** 3 tsp (15mL). May repeat q6-8h. **Max:** 4 doses q24h.
PediaCare Infants' Pain Reliever/Fever Reducer IB Ibuprofen Concentrated Oral Suspension	Ibuprofen 50mg/1.25mL	**Peds: 6-11 months (12-17 lbs):** 1.25mL. **12-23 months (18-23 lbs):** 1.865mL. May repeat q6-8h. **Max:** 4 doses q24h.
SALICYLATES		
Bayer Aspirin Extra Strength Caplets	Aspirin 500mg	**Adults & Peds ≥12 yrs:** 1-2 tabs q4-6h. **Max:** 8 tabs q24h.
Bayer Aspirin Safety Coated Caplets	Aspirin 325mg	**Adults & Peds ≥12 yrs:** 1-2 tabs q4h. **Max:** 12 tabs q24h.
Bayer Genuine Aspirin Tablets	Aspirin 325mg	**Adults & Peds ≥12 yrs:** 1-2 tabs q4h or 3 tabs q6h. **Max:** 12 tabs q24h.
Bayer Low-Dose Aspirin Chewable Tablets*	Aspirin 81mg	**Adults & Peds ≥12 yrs:** 4-8 tabs q4h. **Max:** 48 tabs q24h.
Bayer Low-Dose Aspirin Safety Coated Tablets	Aspirin 81mg	**Adults & Peds ≥12 yrs:** 4-8 tabs q4h. **Max:** 48 tabs q24h.
Ecotrin Low Strength Tablets	Aspirin 81mg	**Adults:** 4-8 tabs q4h. **Max:** 48 tabs q24h.
Ecotrin Regular Strength Tablets	Aspirin 325mg	**Adults & Peds ≥12 yrs:** 1-2 tabs q4h. **Max:** 12 tabs q24h.
Halfprin 162mg Tablets	Aspirin 162mg	**Adults & Peds ≥12 yrs:** 2-4 tabs q4h. **Max:** 24 tabs q24h.
Halfprin 81mg Tablets	Aspirin 81mg	**Adults & Peds ≥12 yrs:** 4-8 tabs q4h. **Max:** 48 tabs q24h.
St. Joseph Aspirin Chewable Tablets	Aspirin 81mg	**Adults & Peds ≥12 yrs:** 4-8 tabs q4h. **Max:** 48 tabs q24h.
St. Joseph Enteric Safety-Coated Tablets	Aspirin 81mg	**Adults & Peds ≥12 yrs:** 4-8 tabs q4h. **Max:** 48 tabs q24h.
SALICYLATES, BUFFERED		
Bayer Extra Strength Plus Caplets	Aspirin 500mg Buffered with Calcium carbonate	**Adults & Peds ≥12 yrs:** 1-2 tabs q4-6h. **Max:** 8 tabs q24h.
Bayer Women's Low Dose Aspirin Caplets	Aspirin 81mg Buffered with Calcium carbonate 777mg	**Adults & Peds ≥12 yrs:** 4-8 tabs q4h. **Max:** 10 tabs q24h.
Bufferin Extra Strength Tablets	Aspirin 500mg Buffered with Calcium carbonate/Magnesium oxide/ Magnesium carbonate	**Adults & Peds ≥12 yrs:** 2 tabs q6h. **Max:** 8 tabs q24h.

(Continued)

BRAND	INGREDIENT/STRENGTH	DOSAGE
SALICYLATES, BUFFERED *(Continued)*		
Bufferin Tablets	Aspirin 325mg Buffered with Calcium carbonate/Magnesium oxide/Magnesium carbonate	**Adults & Peds ≥12 yrs:** 2 tabs q4h. **Max:** 12 tabs q24h.
Bufferin Low Dose Tablets	Aspirin 81mg Buffered with Calcium carbonate/Magnesium oxide/ Magnesium carbonate	**Adults & Peds ≥12 yrs:** 4-8 tabs q4h. **Max:** 48 tabs q24h.
*Multiple flavors available. †Product currently on recall, available in generic form.		

INSOMNIA PRODUCTS

BRAND	INGREDIENT/STRENGTH	DOSE
DIPHENHYDRAMINE		
Compoz Maximum Strength Caplets	Diphenhydramine 50mg	**Adults & Peds ≥12 yrs:** 1 tab hs prn.
Compoz Maximum Strength Soft Gel Liquid Capsules	Diphenhydramine 50mg	**Adults & Peds ≥12 yrs:** 1 cap hs prn.
Nytol QuickCaps Caplets	Diphenhydramine 25mg	**Adults & Peds ≥12 yrs:** 2 tabs hs prn.
Simply Sleep Nighttime Sleep Aid Caplets	Diphenhydramine 25mg	**Adults & Peds ≥12 yrs:** 2 tabs hs prn.
Sleepinal Capsule	Diphenhydramine 50mg	**Adults & Peds ≥12 yrs:** 1 cap hs prn.
Sominex Original Formula	Diphenhydramine 25mg	**Adults & Peds ≥12 yrs:** 2 tabs hs prn.
Sominex Maximum Strength Formula	Diphenhydramine 50mg	**Adults & Peds ≥12 yrs:** 1 tab hs prn.
Unisom SleepGels	Diphenhydramine 50mg	**Adults & Peds ≥12 yrs:** 1 cap hs prn.
Unisom SleepMelts	Diphenhydramine 25mg	**Adults & Peds ≥12 yrs:** 2 tabs on tongue hs prn.
DIPHENHYDRAMINE COMBINATION		
Advil PM Caplets*	Ibuprofen/Diphenhydramine Citrate 200mg-38mg	**Adults & Peds ≥12 yrs:** 2 tabs hs.
Advil PM Liqui-Gels*	Ibuprofen/Diphenhydramine HCl 200mg-25mg	**Adults & Peds ≥12 yrs:** 2 tabs hs.
Bayer PM Caplets	Aspirin/Diphenhydramine Citrate 500mg-38.3mg	**Adults & Peds ≥12 yrs:** 2 tabs hs prn.
Excedrin PM Caplets*	Acetaminophen/Diphenhydramine Citrate 500mg-38mg	**Adults & Peds ≥12 yrs:** 2 tabs hs prn.
Excedrin PM Express Gels*	Acetaminophen/Diphenhydramine Citrate 500mg-38mg	**Adults & Peds ≥12 yrs:** 2 caps hs prn.
Goody's PM Powder	Acetaminophen/Diphenhydramine Citrate 500mg-38mg per powder	**Adults & Peds ≥12 yrs:** 2 powders hs prn with a full glass of water or may stir powder into water or other liquid.
Motrin PM Caplets*	Ibuprofen/Diphenhydramine Citrate 200mg-38mg	**Adults & Peds ≥12 yrs:** 2 tabs hs.
Tylenol PM Caplets*	Acetaminophen/Diphenhydramine HCl 500mg-25mg	**Adults & Peds ≥12 yrs:** 2 tabs hs.
Tylenol PM Rapid Release Gelcaps*	Acetaminophen/Diphenhydramine HCl 500mg-25mg	**Adults & Peds ≥12 yrs:** 2 caps hs.
Tylenol PM Geltabs*	Acetaminophen/Diphenhydramine HCl 500mg-25mg	**Adults & Peds ≥12 yrs:** 2 tabs hs.
Unisom PM Pain SleepCaps	Acetaminophen/Diphenhydramine HCl 325mg-50mg	**Adults & Peds ≥12 yrs:** 1 cap hs.
DOXYLAMINE		
Unisom SleepTabs	Doxylamine Succinate 25mg	**Adults & Peds ≥12 yrs:** 1 tab 30 minutes before hs.

* Max: 2 tabs/24 hrs

SMOKING CESSATION PRODUCTS

BRAND	INGREDIENT/STRENGTH	DOSE
NicoDerm CQ Step 1 Clear Patch	Nicotine 21mg	**Adults:** Smoking >10 cigarettes/day: **Weeks 1 to 6:** Apply one 21mg patch/day. **Weeks 7 to 8:** Apply one 14mg patch/day. **Weeks 9 to 10:** Apply one 7mg patch/day. If smoking <10 cigarettes/day: **Weeks 1 to 6:** Apply one 14mg patch/day. **Weeks 7 to 8:** Apply one 7mg patch/day.
NicoDerm CQ Step 2 Clear Patch	Nicotine 14mg	Refer to NicoDerm CQ Step 1 Clear Patch Dosing.
NicoDerm CQ Step 3 Clear Patch	Nicotine 7mg	Refer to NicoDerm CQ Step 1 Clear Patch Dosing.
Nicorette 2mg Gum	Nicotine Polacrilex 2mg	**Adults:** If you smoke your first cigarette >30 min after waking up, use 2mg gum. **Weeks 1 to 6:** 1 piece q1-2h. **Weeks 7 to 9:** 1 piece q2-4h. **Weeks 10 to 12:** 1 piece q4-8h. **Max:** 24 pieces/day.
Nicorette 4mg Gum	Nicotine Polacrilex 4mg	**Adults:** If you smoke your first cigarette <30 min after waking up, use 4mg gum. **Weeks 1 to 6:** 1 piece q1-2h. **Weeks 7 to 9:** 1 piece q2-4h. **Weeks 10 to 12:** 1 piece q4-8h. **Max:** 24 pieces/day.
Nicorette 2mg mini Lozenges	Nicotine Polacrilex 2mg	**Adults:** If smoking first cigarette >30 minutes after waking up use 2mg lozenge. **Weeks 1 to 6:** 1 lozenge q1-2h. **Weeks 7 to 9:** 1 lozenge q2-4h. **Weeks 10 to 12:** 1 lozenge q4-8h. **Max:** 5 lozenges/6 hours or 20 lozenges/day.
Nicorette 4mg mini Lozenges	Nicotine Polacrilex 4mg	**Adults:** If smoking first cigarette <30 minutes after waking up use 4mg lozenge. **Weeks 1 to 6:** 1 lozenge q1-2h. **Weeks 7 to 9:** 1 lozenge q2-4h. **Weeks 10 to 12:** 1 lozenge q4-8h. **Max:** 5 lozenges/6 hours or 20 lozenges/day.
Nicorette 2mg Lozenges	Nicotine Polacrilex 2mg	**Adults:** If smoking first cigarette >30 minutes after waking up use 2mg lozenge. **Weeks 1 to 6:** 1 lozenge q1-2h. **Weeks 7 to 9:** 1 lozenge q2-4h. **Weeks 10 to 12:** 1 lozenge q4-8h. **Max:** 5 lozenges/6 hours or 20 lozenges/day.
Nicorette 4mg Lozenges	Nicotine Polacrilex 4mg	**Adults:** If smoking first cigarette <30 minutes after waking up use 4mg lozenge. **Weeks 1 to 6:** 1 lozenge q1-2h. **Weeks 7 to 9:** 1 lozenge q2-4h. **Weeks 10 to 12:** 1 lozenge q4-8h. **Max:** 5 lozenges/6 hours or 20 lozenges/day.
Habitrol Nicotine Transdermal System Patch Step 1	Nicotine 21mg	**Adults:** Smoking >10 cigarettes/day: **Weeks 1 to 4:** Apply one 21mg patch/day. **Weeks 5 to 6:** Apply one 14mg patch/day. **Weeks 7 to 8:** Apply one 7mg patch/day. If smoking ≤10 cigarettes/day: **Weeks 1 to 6:** Apply one 14mg patch/day. **Weeks 7 to 8:** Apply one 7mg patch/day.
Habitrol Nicotine Transdermal System Patch Step 2	Nicotine 14mg	Refer to Habitrol Nicotine Transdermal System Patch Step 1 Dosing.
Habitrol Nicotine Transdermal System Patch Step 3	Nicotine 7mg	Refer to Habitrol Nicotine Transdermal System Patch Step 1 Dosing.

ACNE PRODUCTS

BRAND	INGREDIENT/STRENGTH	DOSAGE
BENZOYL PEROXIDES		
Clean & Clear Advantage 3-in-1 Exfoliating Cleanser	Benzoyl peroxide 5%	Use qd to start, then gradually increase to bid prn or ud.
Clean & Clear Continuous Control Acne Cleanser	Benzoyl peroxide 10%	Use bid, AM and PM.
Clean & Clear Persa-Gel 10, Maximum Strength	Benzoyl peroxide 10%	Apply a thin layer to affected area qd up to tid.
Clearasil Daily Clear Vanishing Acne Treatment Cream	Benzoyl peroxide 10%	Apply a thin layer to affected area qd to start. May increase up to tid prn or ud.
Clearasil Daily Clear Acne Treatment Cream, Tinted	Benzoyl peroxide 10%	Apply a thin layer to affected area qd to start. May increase up to tid prn or ud.
Clearasil Ultra Rapid Action Vanishing Treatment Cream	Benzoyl peroxide 10%	Apply a thin layer to affected area qd to start. May increase up to tid prn or ud.
Neutrogena Clear Pore Cleanser/Mask	Benzoyl peroxide 3.5%	**Cleanser:** Use qd or every other day. **Mask:** Apply even layer over skin and allow to dry up to 5 min. Do not exceed 2-3 times per wk.
Neutrogena On-the-Spot Acne Treatment Vanishing Formula	Benzoyl peroxide 2.5%	Apply to affected area qd initially, then bid-tid.
Oxy Clinical Clearing Treatment	Benzoyl peroxide 5%	Apply a thin layer to affected area qd to start. May increase up to tid prn or ud.
Oxy Maximum Face Wash	Benzoyl peroxide 10%	Use bid-tid or ud.
Oxy Maximum Spot Treatment	Benzoyl peroxide 10%	Apply a thin layer to affected area qd to start. May increase up to tid-prn or ud.
PanOxyl 4% Acne Creamy Wash	Benzoyl peroxide 4%	Gently wash affected area for 1-2 minutes. Use qd to start then increase to bid-tid prn or ud.
PanOxyl 8% Acne Creamy Wash	Benzoyl peroxide 8%	Gently wash affected area for 1-2 minutes. Use qd to start then increase to bid-tid prn or ud.
PanOxyl 10% Acne Cleansing Bar	Benzoyl peroxide 10%	Gently wash affected area for 1-2 minutes. Use qd to start then increase to bid-tid prn or ud.
PanOxyl 10% Acne Foaming Wash	Benzoyl peroxide 10%	Gently wash affected area for 1-2 minutes. Use qd to start then increase to bid-tid prn or ud.
ZAPZYT Acne Treatment Gel	Benzoyl peroxide 10%	Use qd up to tid.
SALICYLIC ACIDS		
Aveeno Clear Complexion Cleansing Bar	Salicylic acid 0.5%	Use daily ud.
Aveeno Clear Complexion Daily Moisturizer	Salicylic acid 0.5%	Apply a thin layer to affected area qd to start. May increase up to tid-prn or ud.
Aveeno Active Naturals Clear Complexion Cleanser	Salicylic acid 2%	Massage product gently for 20-30 seconds ud.
Aveeno Clear Complexion Daily Cleansing Pads	Salicylic acid 0.5%	Use qd ud.
Aveeno Clear Complexion Foaming Cleanser	Salicylic acid 0.5%	Use qd ud.
Biore Warming Anti-Blackhead Cleanser	Salicylic acid 2%	Use qd ud.
Biore Blemish Treating Astringent	Salicylic acid 2%	Apply qd to start; gradually increase up to tid-prn or ud.
Biore Blemish Fighting Ice Cleanser	Salicylic acid 2%	Use qd ud.
Bye Bye Blemish Anti-Acne Serum	Salicylic acid 1%	Apply several drops daily ud.

(Continued)

BRAND	INGREDIENT/STRENGTH	DOSAGE
SALICYLIC ACIDS (Continued)		
Bye Bye Blemish Drying Lotion	Salicylic acid 2%	Apply to affected area and leave on overnight prn or ud.
Clean & Clear Advantage 3-in-1 Foaming Acne Wash	Salicylic acid 2%	Use qd ud.
Clean & Clear Advantage Acne Cleanser	Salicylic acid 2%	Use qd ud.
Clean & Clear Advantage Acne Spot Treatment	Salicylic acid 2%	Apply a thin layer qd up to tid.
Clean & Clear Advantage Blackhead Eraser	Salicylic acid 1%	Use up to 4 times a week ud.
Clean & Clear Advantage Daily Cleansing Pads	Salicylic acid 2%	Use qd ud.
Clean & Clear Advantage Mark Treatment	Salicylic acid 2%	Apply a thin layer qd up to tid.
Clean & Clear Blackhead Clearing Scrub	Salicylic acid 2%	Use qd ud.
Clean & Clear Blackhead Eraser Cleansing Mask	Salicylic acid 0.5%	Apply a thin layer and let dry for 5 minutes 1-2 times a week.
Clean & Clear Blackhead Eraser Scrub	Salicylic acid 2%	Massage product gently for 20-30 seconds qd ud.
Clean & Clear Advantage Oil-Free Acne Control Moisturizer	Salicylic acid 0.5%	Apply a thin layer qd up to tid.
Clean & Clear Deep Cleaning Astringent	Salicylic acid 2%	Apply qd to start; gradually increase up to bid-tid prn or ud.
Clean & Clear Deep Cleaning Sensitive Skin Astringent	Salicylic acid 0.5%	Apply qd to start; gradually increase up to bid-tid prn or ud.
Clean & Clear Dual Action Moisturizer	Salicylic acid 0.5%	Apply a thin layer over affected area qd to start; gradually increase to bid-tid prn or ud.
Clearasil Daily Clear Oil-Free Face Wash	Salicylic acid 2%	Use qd ud.
Clearasil Daily Clear Oil-Free Face Wash, Sensitive Skin	Salicylic acid 2%	Use qd ud.
Clearasil Daily Clear Facial Scrub	Salicylic acid 2%	Use qd ud.
Clearasil Daily Clear Pore Cleansing Pads	Salicylic acid 2%	Apply qd to start; gradually increase up to bid-tid prn or ud.
Clearasil PerfectaWash Automatic Face Wash Dispenser & Refill	Salicylic acid 2%	Use bid ud.
Clearasil PerfectaWash Automatic Face Wash Refill Soothing Plant Extracts	Salicylic acid 2%	Use bid ud.
Clearasil PerfectaWash Automatic Face Wash Refill Superfruit Splash	Salicylic acid 2%	Use bid ud.
Clearasil Ultra Acne + Marks Spot Lotion	Salicylic acid 2%	Apply a thin layer over affected area qd to start; gradually increase to bid-tid prn or ud.
Clearasil Ultra Acne + Marks Wash and Mask	Salicylic acid 2%	**Wash:** Use bid ud. **Mask:** Apply to damp skin and leave on for up to 5 minutes 1-2 times a wk ud.
Clearasil Ultra Overnight Lotion	Salicylic acid 2%	Apply a thin layer over affected area qd to start; gradually increase to bid-tid prn or ud.
Clearasil Ultra Overnight Scrub	Salicylic acid 2%	Use at night time ud.
Clearasil Ultra Overnight Wash	Salicylic acid 2%	Use at night time ud.
Clearasil Ultra Rapid Action Daily Facial Wash	Salicylic acid 2%	Use bid ud.

BRAND	INGREDIENT/STRENGTH	DOSAGE
SALICYLIC ACIDS *(Continued)*		
Clearasil Ultra Rapid Action Face Scrub	Salicylic acid 2%	Use bid ud.
Clearasil Ultra Rapid Action Pads	Salicylic acid 2%	Apply qd to start; gradually increase up to bid-tid prn or ud.
Clearasil Ultra Rapid Action Seal-to-Clear Gel	Salicylic acid 2%	Apply a thin layer over affected area qd to start; gradually increase to bid-tid prn or ud.
Clearasil Ultra Rapid Action Treatment Gel	Salicylic acid 2%	Apply a thin layer over affected area qd to start; gradually increase to bid-tid prn or ud.
L'Oreal Go 360 Clean Anti-Breakout Facial Cleanser	Salicylic acid 2%	Use bid ud.
Neutrogena All-in-1 Acne Control Daily Scrub	Salicylic acid 2%	Use bid ud.
Neutrogena All-in-1 Acne Control Facial Treatment	Salicylic acid 1%	Apply a thin layer over affected area qd to start; gradually increase to bid-tid prn or ud.
Neutrogena Blackhead Eliminating Cleanser Mask	Salicylic acid 2%	**Cleanser:** Use qd ud. **Mask:** Apply an even layer on skin and allow to dry up to 5 minutes not more than 2-3 times a wk ud.
Neutrogena Blackhead Eliminating Daily Scrub	Salicylic acid 2%	Use qd ud.
Neutrogena Men Skin Clearing Acne Wash	Salicylic acid 2%	Use bid ud.
Neutrogena Body Clear Body Scrub	Salicylic acid 2%	Use ud.
Neutrogena Oil-Free Acne Wash	Salicylic acid 2%	Use bid ud.
Neutrogena Clear Pore Oil-Eliminating Astringent	Salicylic acid 2%	Use qd-tid ud.
Neutrogena Oil-Free Acne Stress Control Power Clear Scrub	Salicylic acid 2%	Use qd ud.
Neutrogena Oil-Free Acne Stress Control Power Foam Wash	Salicylic acid 0.5%	Use qd ud.
Neutrogena Oil-Free Acne Stress Control 3-in-1 Hydrating Acne Treatment	Salicylic acid 2%	Apply a thin layer over affected area qd to start; gradually increase to bid-tid prn or ud.
Neutrogena Oil-Free Acne Wash Cleansing Cloths	Salicylic acid 2%	Use qd ud.
Neutrogena Oil-Free Acne Wash Cream Cleanser	Salicylic acid 2%	Use bid ud.
Neutrogena Rapid Clear Acne Defense Face Lotion	Salicylic acid 2%	Apply a thin layer over affected area qd to start; gradually increase to bid-tid prn or ud.
Neutrogena Rapid Clear Foaming Scrub	Salicylic acid 2%	Use bid ud.
Neutrogena Rapid Clear 2-in-1 Fight & Fade Gel	Salicylic acid 2%	Apply a thin layer over affected area qd to start; gradually increase to bid-tid prn or ud.
Neutrogena Rapid Clear Acne Eliminating Spot Gel	Salicylic acid 2%	Apply a thin layer over affected area qd to start; gradually increase to bid-tid prn or ud.
Neutrogena Oil-Free Anti-Acne Moisturizer	Salicylic acid 2%	Apply a thin layer over affected area qd to start; gradually increase to bid-tid prn or ud.
Noxzema Clean Blemish Control Daily Scrub	Salicylic acid 1%	Use qd ud.
Noxzema Clean Blemish Control Foaming Wash	Salicylic acid 1%	Use qd ud.
Noxzema Triple Clean Anti-Blemish Pads	Salicylic acid 2%	Use qd-tid.

(Continued)

BRAND	INGREDIENT/STRENGTH	DOSAGE
SALICYLIC ACIDS (Continued)		
Olay Acne Control Face Wash	Salicylic acid 2%	Use 1 to 2 pumps bid ud.
Olay Blackhead Clearing Scrub	Salicylic acid 2%	Use qd ud.
Olay Pro-X Clear Acne Protocol	**Cleanser:** Salicylic acid 1.8% **Treatment:** Salicylic acid 1.5%	Use bid ud.
Olay Total Effects Cream Cleanser Plus Blemish Control Moisturizer	Salicylic acid 2%	Apply qd-tid ud.
Oxy Clinical Advanced Face Wash	Salicylic acid 2%	Use bid ud.
Oxy Clinical Advanced Treatment Pads	Salicylic acid 2%	Apply a thin layer to affected area qd-tid ud.
Oxy Clinical Foaming Face Wash	Salicylic acid 2%	Use bid ud.
Oxy Clinical Hydrating Therapy	Salicylic acid 0.5%	Use bid, AM and PM ud.
Oxy Maximum Cleansing Pads	Salicylic acid 2%	Apply a thin layer over affected area qd to start; gradually increase to bid-tid prn or ud.
Oxy Maximum Exfoliating Body Scrub	Salicylic acid 1%	Use ud.
Oxy Maximum Face Scrub	Salicylic acid 2%	Use qd ud.
Oxy Maximum Hydrating Body Wash	Salicylic acid 2%	Use ud.
Phisoderm Anti-Blemish Body Wash	Salicylic acid 2%	Use ud.
St. Ives Naturally Clear Apricot Scrub Blemish & Blackhead Control	Salicylic acid 2%	Use qd ud up to 3-4 times a week.
Stridex Maximum Strength Pads	Salicylic acid 2%	Apply qd to start; gradually increase up to bid-tid prn or ud.
Stridex Essential Care Pads	Salicylic acid 1%	Apply qd to start; gradually increase up to bid-tid prn or ud.
Stridex Natural Control Pads	Salicylic acid 1%	Apply qd to start; gradually increase up to bid-tid prn or ud.
Stridex Sensitive Skin Pads	Salicylic acid 0.5%	Apply qd to start; gradually increase up to bid-tid prn or ud.
ZAPZYT Acne Wash	Salicylic acid 2%	Use bid ud.
ZAPZYT Pore Clearing Scrub	Salicylic acid 2%	Use bid ud.
TRICLOSANS		
Clean & Clear Foaming Facial Cleanser	Triclosan 0.25%	Use qd ud.
Noxzema Triple Clean Anti-Bacterial Cleanser	Triclosan 0.3%	Use qd ud.
COMBINATION PRODUCTS		
Clearasil Daily Clear Adult Tinted Treatment Cream	Resorcinol, Sulfur 2-8%	Apply a thin layer over affected area qd to start; gradually increase to bid-tid prn or ud.
Stridex Dual Solutions Intensive Acne Repair	**Pads:** Salicylic acid 2% **Gel:** Benzoyl peroxide 2.5%	**Pads:** Apply qd to start; gradually increase to bid-tid prn or ud. **Gel:** Apply a thin layer over affected area qd to start; gradually increase to bid-tid prn or ud.
ZAPZYT Acne Pack	**Cleanser:** Salicylic acid 2% **Day Gel:** Salicylic acid 2% **Night Gel:** Benzoyl peroxide 5%	Use ud.

ANTIFUNGAL PRODUCTS

BRAND	INGREDIENT/STRENGTH	DOSAGE
BUTENAFINE		
Lotrimin Ultra Athlete's Foot Cream	Butenafine HCl 1%	**Adults & Peds ≥12 yrs: Athlete's Foot:** Apply bid for 1 week or qd for 4 weeks. **Jock Itch/Ringworm:** Apply qd for 2 weeks.
Lotrimin Ultra Jock Itch Cream	Butenafine HCl 1%	**Adults & Peds ≥12 yrs:** Apply qd for 2 weeks.
CLOTRIMAZOLE		
Desenex Antifungal Cream	Clotrimazole 1%	**Adults & Peds ≥2 yrs: Athlete's Foot/Ringworm:** Apply bid for 4 weeks. **Jock Itch:** Apply bid for 2 weeks.
FungiCure Intensive Anti-Fungal Liquid	Clotrimazole 1%	**Adults & Peds ≥2 yrs: Athlete's Foot/Ringworm:** Apply bid for 4 weeks. **Jock Itch:** Apply bid for 2 weeks.
FungiCure Anti-Fungal Manicure & Pedicure	Clotrimazole 1%	**Adults & Peds ≥2 yrs: Athlete's Foot/Ringworm:** Apply bid for 4 weeks.
Lotrimin AF Athlete's Foot Cream	Clotrimazole 1%	**Adults & Peds ≥2 yrs: Athlete's Foot/Ringworm:** Apply bid for 4 weeks. **Jock Itch:** Apply bid for 2 weeks.
Lotrimin AF Jock Itch Cream	Clotrimazole 1%	**Adults & Peds ≥2 yrs:** Apply bid for 2 weeks.
Lotrimin AF Ringworm Cream	Clotrimazole 1%	**Adults & Peds ≥2 yrs:** Apply bid for 4 weeks.
MICONAZOLE		
Clearly Confident Antifungal Cream	Miconazole nitrate 2%	**Adults & Peds ≥2 yrs:** Apply bid for 4 weeks.
Desenex Antifungal Liquid Spray	Miconazole nitrate 2%	**Adults & Peds ≥2 yrs:** Apply bid for 4 weeks.
Desenex Antifungal Powder	Miconazole nitrate 2%	**Adults & Peds ≥2 yrs: Athlete's Foot/Ringworm:** Apply bid for 4 weeks. **Jock Itch:** Apply bid for 2 weeks.
Desenex Antifungal Spray Powder	Miconazole nitrate 2%	**Adults & Peds ≥2 yrs:** Apply bid for 4 weeks.
Lotrimin AF Athlete's Foot Deodorant Powder Spray	Miconazole nitrate 2%	**Adults & Peds ≥2 yrs: Athlete's Foot/Ringworm:** Apply bid for 4 weeks. **Jock Itch:** Apply bid for 2 weeks.
Lotrimin AF Athlete's Foot Liquid Spray	Miconazole nitrate 2%	**Adults & Peds ≥2 yrs: Athlete's Foot/Ringworm:** Apply bid for 4 weeks. **Jock Itch:** Apply bid for 2 weeks.
Lotrimin AF Athlete's Foot Powder	Miconazole nitrate 2%	**Adults & Peds ≥2 yrs: Athlete's Foot/Ringworm:** Apply bid for 4 weeks. **Jock Itch:** Apply bid for 2 weeks.
Lotrimin AF Athlete's Foot Powder Spray	Miconazole nitrate 2%	**Adults & Peds ≥2 yrs: Athlete's Foot/Ringworm:** Apply bid for 4 weeks. **Jock Itch:** Apply bid for 2 weeks.
Lotrimin AF Jock Itch Powder Spray	Miconazole nitrate 2%	**Adults & Peds ≥2 yrs:** Apply bid for 2 weeks.
Micatin Cream	Miconazole nitrate 2%	**Adults & Peds ≥2 yrs: Athlete's Foot/Ringworm:** Apply bid for 4 weeks. **Jock Itch:** Apply bid for 2 weeks.
Miranel AF Antifungal Treatment	Miconazole nitrate 2%	**Adults & Peds ≥12 yrs: Athlete's Foot:** Apply bid for 4 weeks.
Ting Spray Powder	Miconazole nitrate 2%	**Adults & Peds ≥2 yrs: Athlete's Foot/Ringworm:** Apply bid for 4 weeks. **Jock Itch:** Apply bid for 2 weeks.
Zeasorb-AF Super Absorbent Antifungal Powder	Miconazole nitrate 2%	**Adults & Peds ≥2 yrs: Athlete's Foot/Ringworm:** Apply bid for 4 weeks. **Jock Itch:** Apply bid for 2 weeks.
TERBINAFINE		
Lamisil AT Cream for Jock Itch	Terbinafine HCl 1%	**Adults & Peds ≥12 yrs:** Apply qd for 1 week.
Lamisil AT Spray for Jock Itch	Terbinafine HCl 1%	**Adults & Peds ≥12 yrs:** Apply qd for 1 week.
Lamisil AT Spray, Athlete's Foot	Terbinafine HCl 1%	**Adults & Peds ≥12 yrs: Athlete's Foot (between toes):** Apply bid for 1 week. **Jock Itch/Ringworm:** Apply qd for 1 week.

(Continued)

BRAND	INGREDIENT/STRENGTH	DOSAGE
TERBINAFINE (Continued)		
Lamisil AT Cream, Athlete's Foot	Terbinafine HCl 1%	**Adults & Peds ≥12 yrs: Athlete's Foot (between toes):** Apply bid for 1 week. **Athlete's Foot (on side or bottom of foot):** Apply bid for 2 weeks. **Jock Itch/Ringworm:** Apply qd for 1 week.
Lamisil AT Gel, Athlete's Foot	Terbinafine HCl 1%	**Adults & Peds ≥12 yrs: Athlete's Foot (between toes):** Apply qhs for 1 week. **Jock Itch/Ringworm:** Apply qd for 1 week.
TOLNAFTATE		
Flexitol Medicated Foot Cream	Tolnaftate 1%	**Adults & Peds ≥2 yrs:** Apply bid for 4 weeks.
Lamisil AF Defense Shake Powder	Tolnaftate 1%	**Adults & Peds ≥2 yrs:** Apply bid for 4 weeks. **Prevention:** Apply qd or bid.
Tinactin Athlete's Foot Cream	Tolnaftate 1%	**Adults & Peds ≥2 yrs:** Apply bid for 4 weeks.
Tinactin Deodorant Powder Spray	Tolnaftate 1%	**Adults & Peds ≥2 yrs: Athlete's Foot:** Apply bid for 4 weeks. **Prevention:** Apply qd-bid.
Tinactin Jock Itch Cream	Tolnaftate 1%	**Adults & Peds ≥2 yrs:** Apply bid for 2 weeks.
Tinactin Jock Itch Powder Spray	Tolnaftate 1%	**Adults & Peds ≥2 yrs:** Apply bid for 2 weeks.
Tinactin Liquid Spray	Tolnaftate 1%	**Adults & Peds ≥2 yrs: Athlete's Foot:** Apply bid for 4 weeks. **Prevention:** Apply qd-bid.
Tinactin Powder Spray	Tolnaftate 1%	**Adults & Peds ≥2 yrs: Athlete's Foot:** Apply bid for 4 weeks. **Prevention:** Apply qd-bid.
Tinactin Pump Spray	Tolnaftate 1%	**Adults & Peds ≥2 yrs: Athlete's Foot:** Apply bid for 4 weeks. **Prevention:** Apply qd-bid.
Tinactin Super Absorbent Powder	Tolnaftate 1%	**Adults & Peds ≥2 yrs: Athlete's Foot:** Apply bid for 4 weeks. **Prevention:** Apply qd-bid.
Ting Antifungal Cream	Tolnaftate 1%	**Adults & Peds ≥2 yrs: Athlete's Foot/Ringworm:** Apply bid for 4 weeks. **Jock Itch:** Apply bid for 2 weeks.
Ting Spray Liquid, Athlete's Foot	Tolnaftate 1%	**Adults & Peds ≥2 yrs:** Apply bid for 4 weeks.
UNDECYLENIC ACID		
DiabetiDerm Toenail & Foot Fungus Antifungal Cream	Undecylenic acid 10%	**Adults & Peds ≥2 yrs: Athlete's Foot/Ringworm:** Apply bid for 4 weeks. **Jock Itch:** Apply bid for 2 weeks.
Flexitol Anti-Fungal Liquid	Undecylenic acid 25%	**Adults & Peds ≥2 yrs: Athlete's Foot/Ringworm:** Apply bid.
Fungi Nail Anti-Fungal Solution	Undecylenic acid 25%	**Adults & Peds ≥2 yrs: Athlete's Foot/Ringworm:** Apply bid for 4 weeks.
Fungi Nail Anti-Fungal Pen	Undecylenic acid 25%	**Adults & Peds ≥2 yrs: Athlete's Foot/Ringworm:** Apply bid for 4 weeks.
FungiCure Maximum Strength Anti-Fungal Liquid	Undecylenic acid 25%	**Adults & Peds ≥2 yrs: Athlete's Foot/Ringworm:** Apply bid for 4 weeks.
Tineacide Antifungal Cream	Undecylenic acid 13%	**Adults & Peds ≥2 yrs: Athlete's Foot (between toes):** Apply bid for 4 weeks. **Jock Itch/Ringworm:** Apply bid for 2 weeks.

CONTACT DERMATITIS PRODUCTS

BRAND	INGREDIENTS/STRENGTH	DOSE
ANTIHISTAMINE		
Benadryl Itch Stopping Extra Strength Gel	Diphenhydramine HCl 2%	**Adults & Peds ≥2 yrs:** Apply to affected area ≤ tid-qid.
ANTIHISTAMINE COMBINATION		
Benadryl Extra Strength Itch Stopping Cream	Diphenhydramine HCl/Zinc acetate 2%-0.1%	**Adults & Peds ≥2 yrs:** Apply to affected area ≤ tid-qid.
Benadryl Extra Strength Spray	Diphenhydramine HCl/Zinc acetate 2%-0.1%	**Adults & Peds ≥2 yrs:** Apply to affected area ≤ tid-qid.
Benadryl Extra Strength Itch Relief Stick	Diphenhydramine HCl/Zinc acetate 2%-0.1%	**Adults & Peds ≥2 yrs:** Apply to affected area ≤ tid-qid.
Benadryl Original Strength Itch Stopping Cream	Diphenhydramine HCl/Zinc acetate 1%-0.1%	**Adults & Peds ≥2 yrs:** Apply to affected area ≤ tid-qid.
Benadryl Readymist Itch Stopping Spray	Diphenhydramine/Zinc acetate 2%-0.1%	**Adults & Peds ≥2 yrs:** Apply to affected area ≤ tid-qid.
CalaGel Anti-Itch Gel	Diphenhydramine HCl/Zinc acetate/ Benzethonium chloride 2%-0.215%-0.15%	**Adults & Peds ≥2 yrs:** Apply to affected area ≤ tid.
Ivarest Double Relief Formula	Diphenhydramine HCl/Benzyl alcohol/ Calamine 2%-10.5%-14%	**Adults & Peds ≥2 yrs:** Apply to affected area ≤ tid-qid.
ASTRINGENT		
Domeboro Astringent Solution Powder Packets	Aluminum acetate (combination of Calcium acetate 952mg and Aluminum sulfate 1347mg)	**Adults & Peds:** Dissolve 1-3 pkts in 16 oz of water and soak affected area for 15-30 min tid or apply as compress/wet dressing to affected area for 15-30 minutes as needed or as directed.
ASTRINGENT COMBINATION		
Aveeno Calamine and Pramoxine HCl Anti-Itch Cream	Calamine/Pramoxine HCl 3%-1%	**Adults & Peds ≥2 yrs:** Apply to affected area ≤ qid.
Aveeno Anti-Itch Concentrated Lotion	Calamine/Pramoxine HCl 3%-1%	**Adults & Peds ≥2 yrs:** Apply to affected area ≤ qid.
Caladryl Clear Anti-Itch Lotion	Zinc acetate/Pramoxine HCl 0.1%-1%	**Adults & Peds ≥2 yrs:** Apply to affected area ≤ tid-qid.
Calamine Lotion (generic)	Calamine/Zinc oxide 8%-8%	**Adults & Peds:** Apply to affected area prn.
Ivy-Dry Cream	Zinc acetate/Benzyl alcohol/Camphor/ Menthol 2%-10%-0.5%-0.4%	**Adults & Peds ≥2 yrs:** Apply to affected area ≤ tid.
Ivy-Dry Super	Zinc Acetate/Benzyl alcohol/Camphor/ Menthol 2%-10%-0.5%-0.25%	**Adults & Peds ≥6 yrs:** Apply to affected area ≤ tid.
CLEANSER		
Ivarest Poison Ivy Cleansing Foam	Menthol 1%	**Adults & Peds ≥2 yrs:** Gently rub into affected area and rinse under running water ≤ tid-qid.
CORTICOSTEROID		
Aveeno 1% Hydrocortisone Anti-Itch Cream	Hydrocortisone 1%	**Adults & Peds ≥2 yrs:** Apply to affected area ≤ tid-qid.
Cortaid Advanced 12-Hour Anti-Itch Cream	Hydrocortisone 1%	**Adults & Peds ≥2 yrs:** Apply to affected area ≤ tid-qid.
Cortaid Intensive Therapy Cooling Spray	Hydrocortisone 1%	**Adults & Peds ≥2 yrs:** Apply to affected area ≤ tid-qid.
Cortaid Maximum Strength Cream	Hydrocortisone 1%	**Adults & Peds ≥2 yrs:** Apply to affected area ≤ tid-qid.

(Continued)

BRAND	INGREDIENTS/STRENGTH	DOSE
CORTICOSTEROID (Continued)		
Cortizone-10 Easy Relief Applicator	Hydrocortisone 1%	**Adults & Peds ≥2 yrs:** Apply to affected area ≤ tid-qid.
Cortizone-10 Cooling Relief Gel	Hydrocortisone 1%	**Adults & Peds ≥2 yrs:** Apply to affected area ≤ tid-qid.
Cortizone-10 Creme	Hydrocortisone 1%	**Adults & Peds ≥2 yrs:** Apply to affected area ≤ tid-qid.
Cortizone-10 Ointment	Hydrocortisone 1%	**Adults & Peds ≥2 yrs:** Apply to affected area ≤ tid-qid.
Cortizone-10 Creme Plus	Hydrocortisone 1%	**Adults & Peds ≥2 yrs:** Apply to affected area ≤ tid-qid.
Cortizone-10 Intensive Healing Formula Cream	Hydrocortisone 1%	**Adults & Peds ≥2 yrs:** Apply to affected area ≤ tid-qid.
Cortizone-10 Intensive Healing Eczema Lotion	Hydrocortisone 1%	**Adults & Peds ≥2 yrs:** Apply to affected area ≤ tid-qid.
Cortizone-10 Hydraintensive Anti-Itch Soothing Lotion	Hydrocortisone 1%	**Adults & Peds ≥2 yrs:** Apply to affected area ≤ tid-qid.
Cortizone-10 Hydraintensive Anti-Itch Healing Lotion	Hydrocortisone 1%	**Adults & Peds ≥2 yrs:** Apply to affected area ≤ tid-qid.
Cortizone-10 Quick Shot Continuous Spray	Hydrocortisone 1%	**Adults & Peds ≥2 yrs:** Spray affected area ≤ tid-qid
Corticool 1% Hydrocortisone Anti-Itch Gel	Hydrocortisone 1%	**Adults & Peds ≥2 yrs:** Apply to affected area ≤ tid-qid.
LOCAL ANESTHETIC		
Aveeno Active Naturals Skin Relief Medicated Anti-Itch Treatment	Pramoxine HCl 0.5%	**Adults & Peds ≥2 yrs:** Apply to affected area tid-qid.
Solarcaine Aloe Extra Burn Relief Gel	Lidocaine HCl 0.5%	**Adults & Peds ≥2 yrs:** Apply to affected area ≤ tid-qid.
Solarcaine Aloe Extra Burn Relief Spray	Lidocaine HCl 0.5%	**Adults & Peds ≥2 yrs:** Apply to affected area ≤ tid-qid.
LOCAL ANESTHETIC COMBINATION		
Bactine Pain Relieving Cleansing Spray	Lidocaine HCl/Benzalkonium chloride 2.5%-0.13%	**Adults & Peds ≥2 yrs:** Apply to affected area qd-tid.
Gold Bond Medicated Maximum Relief Anti-Itch Cream	Pramoxine/Menthol HCl 1%-1%	**Adults & Peds ≥2 yrs:** Apply to affected area up to tid-qid.
Lanacane Anti-Itch Cream	Benzocaine/Benzethonium chloride 20%-0.1%	**Adults & Peds ≥2 yrs:** Apply to affected area ≤ qd-tid.
Lanacane Antibacterial First Aid Spray	Benzocaine/Benzethonium chloride 20%-0.2%	**Adults & Peds ≥2 yrs:** Apply to affected area qd-tid.
Solarcaine First Aid Medicated Spray	Benzocaine/Triclosan 20%-0.13%	**Adults & Peds ≥2 yrs:** Apply to affected area ≤ qd-tid.
SKIN PROTECTANT		
Aveeno Active Naturals Skin Relief 24 Hour Moisturizing Lotion	Dimethicone 1.3%	**Adults & Peds ≥2 yrs:** Apply prn.
Aveeno Active Naturals Skin Relief Moisturizing Lotion	Dimethicone 1.3%	**Adults & Peds ≥2 yrs:** Apply prn.
Aveeno Active Naturals Intense Skin Relief Overnight Cream	Dimethicone 1.3%	**Adults & Peds ≥2 yrs:** Apply prn.
Ivy Block Lotion	Bentoquatam 5%	**Adults & Peds ≥6 yrs:** Apply 15 minutes before exposure risk and q4h or sooner if needed for continued protection.

BRAND	INGREDIENTS/STRENGTH	DOSE
SKIN PROTECTANT COMBINATION		
Gold Bond Intensive Healing Anti-Itch Skin Protectant	Dimethicone/Pramoxine 6%-1%	**Adults & Peds ≥2 yrs:** Apply to affected area tid-qid.
Gold Bond Intensive Relief Medicated Anti-Itch Lotion	Dimethicone/Menthol/Pramoxine 5%-0.5%-1%	**Adults & Peds ≥2 yrs:** Apply to affected area tid-qid.
Gold Bond Extra Strength Medicated Body Lotion	Dimethicone/Menthol 5%-0.5%	**Adults & Peds ≥2 yrs:** Apply to affected area tid-qid.
Gold Bond Medicated Body Lotion	Dimethicone/Menthol 5%-0.15%	**Adults & Peds ≥2 yrs:** Apply to affected area tid-qid.
Gold Bond Medicated Body Powder	Zinc oxide/Menthol 1%-0.15%	**Adults & Peds ≥2 yrs:** Apply to affected area tid-qid.
Gold Bond Extra Strength Medicated Body Powder	Zinc oxide/Menthol 5%-0.8%	**Adults & Peds ≥2 yrs:** Apply to affected area tid-qid.
Gold Bond Medicated Baby Powder	Cornstarch/Kaolin/Zinc oxide 79%-4%-15%	**Adults & Peds ≥2 yrs:** Apply to affected area tid-qid.

DIAPER RASH PRODUCTS

BRAND	INGREDIENTS/STRENGTH	DOSE
WHITE PETROLATUM		
Aquaphor Healing Ointment	White Petrolatum 41%	**Peds:** Apply prn.
Balmex Multi-Purpose Healing Ointment	White Petrolatum 51.1%	**Peds:** Apply prn.
Desitin Multi-Purpose Ointment	White Petrolatum 60.4%	**Peds:** Apply prn.
Vaseline Petroleum Jelly	White Petrolatum 100%	**Peds:** Apply prn.
ZINC OXIDE		
Aveeno Baby Organic Harvest Diaper Rash Cream	Zinc Oxide 13%	**Peds:** Apply prn.
Aveeno Baby Soothing Relief Diaper Rash Cream	Zinc Oxide 13%	**Peds:** Apply prn.
Balmex Diaper Rash Cream Stick	Zinc Oxide 11.3%	**Peds:** Apply prn.
Boudreaux's Butt Paste, Diaper Rash Ointment	Zinc Oxide 16%	**Peds:** Apply prn.
Boudreaux's Butt Paste, Diaper Rash Ointment – All Natural	Zinc Oxide 16%	**Peds:** Apply prn.
Boudreaux's Butt Paste, Diaper Rash Ointment – Maximum Strength	Zinc Oxide 40%	**Peds:** Apply prn.
California Baby Calming Diaper Rash Cream	Zinc Oxide 12%	**Peds:** Apply prn.
Canus Li'l Goat's Milk Ointment	Zinc Oxide 40%	**Peds:** Apply prn.
Desitin Maximum Strength Original Paste	Zinc Oxide 40%	**Peds:** Apply prn.
Desitin Rapid Relief Cream	Zinc Oxide 13%	**Peds:** Apply prn.
Johnson's Baby Powder Medicated with Aloe & Vitamin E	Zinc Oxide 10%	**Peds:** Apply prn.
Johnson's Baby Powder Medicated Zinc Oxide Skin Protectant	Zinc Oxide 10%	**Peds:** Apply prn.
Mustela Bebe Vitamin Barrier Cream	Zinc Oxide 10%	**Peds:** Apply prn.
Triple Paste Medicated Ointment	Zinc Oxide 12.8%	**Peds:** Apply prn.
COMBINATION PRODUCTS		
A+D Original Ointment	Petrolatum/Lanolin 53.4%-15.5%	**Peds:** Apply prn.
A+D Zinc Oxide Cream	Dimethicone/Zinc Oxide 1%-10%	**Peds:** Apply prn.
Anti Monkey Butt Diaper Rash Cream with Calamine	Zinc-Calamine 12%-2%	**Peds:** Apply prn.
Balmex Diaper Rash Cream with ActivGuard	Cornstarch/Zinc Oxide 83.6%-11.3%	**Peds:** Apply prn.
Lansinoh Diaper Rash Ointment	Dimethicone/USP Modified Lanolin/ Zinc Oxide 5.0%-15.5%-5.5%	**Peds:** Apply prn.
Palmer's Cocoa Butter Formula Bottom Butter Diaper Rash Cream	Zinc Oxide/Dimethicone 10%-1%	**Peds:** Apply prn.

PSORIASIS PRODUCTS

BRAND	INGREDIENT/STRENGTH	DOSAGE
COAL TAR		
DHS Tar Gel Shampoo	Coal tar 0.5%	Use at least two times per week.
DHS Tar Shampoo	Coal tar 0.5%	Use at least two times per week.
Ionil-T Shampoo	Coal tar 1%	Use at least two times per week.
MG217 Medicated Tar Lotion	Coal tar 1%	Apply to affected area qd-qid.
MG217 Medicated Tar Ointment	Coal tar 2%	Apply to affected area qd-qid.
MG217 Medicated Tar Shampoo	Coal tar 3%	Use at least two times per week.
Neutrogena T/Gel Shampoo Extra Strength	Coal tar 1%	Use every other day.
Neutrogena T/Gel Shampoo Original Formula	Coal tar 0.5%	Use at least two times per week.
Neutrogena T/Gel Shampoo Stubborn Itch Control	Coal tar 0.5%	Use at least two times per week.
Psoriasin Gel	Coal tar 1.25%	**Adults:** Apply to affected area qd-qid.
Psoriasin Ointment	Coal tar 2%	**Adults:** Apply to affected area qd-qid.
CORTICOSTEROID		
Aveeno 1% Hydrocortisone Anti-Itch Cream	Hydrocortisone 1%	**Adults & Peds ≥12 yrs:** Apply to affected area tid-qid.
Cortaid Advanced 12-Hour Anti-Itch Cream	Hydrocortisone 1%	**Adults & Peds ≥12 yrs:** Apply to affected area tid-qid.
Cortaid Intensive Therapy Cooling Spray	Hydrocortisone 1%	**Adults & Peds ≥12 yrs:** Apply to affected area tid-qid.
Cortaid Intensive Therapy Moisturizing Cream	Hydrocortisone 1%	**Adults & Peds ≥12 yrs:** Apply to affected area tid-qid.
Cortaid Maximum Strength Cream	Hydrocortisone 1%	**Adults & Peds ≥12 yrs:** Apply to affected area tid-qid.
Corticool 1% Hydrocortisone Anti-Itch Gel	Hydrocortisone 1%	**Adults & Peds ≥12 yrs:** Apply to affected area tid-qid.
Cortizone-10 Cooling Relief Gel	Hydrocortisone 1%	**Adults & Peds ≥12 yrs:** Apply to affected area tid-qid.
Cortizone-10 Creme	Hydrocortisone 1%	**Adults & Peds ≥12 yrs:** Apply to affected area tid-qid.
Cortizone-10 Creme Plus	Hydrocortisone 1%	**Adults & Peds ≥12 yrs:** Apply to affected area tid-qid.
Cortizone-10 Ointment	Hydrocortisone 1%	**Adults & Peds ≥12 yrs:** Apply to affected area tid-qid.
Cortizone-10 Easy Relief Applicator	Hydrocortisone 1%	**Adults & Peds ≥12 yrs:** Apply to affected area tid-qid.
Cortizone-10 Intensive Healing Formula	Hydrocortisone 1%	**Adults & Peds ≥12 yrs:** Apply to affected area tid-qid.
SALICYLIC ACID		
Dermarest Psoriasis Medicated Moisturizer	Salicylic acid 2%	**Adults & Peds:** Apply to affected area qd-qid.
Dermarest Psoriasis Medicated Shampoo Plus Conditioner	Salicylic acid 3%	**Adults & Peds:** Use at least two times per week.
Dermarest Psoriasis Medicated Skin Treatment	Salicylic acid 3%	**Adults & Peds:** Apply to affected area qd-qid.
DHS Sal Shampoo	Salicylic acid 3%	**Adults & Peds:** Use at least two times per week.
MG217 Sal-Acid Ointment	Salicylic acid 3%	**Adults & Peds:** Apply to affected area qd-qid.
Neutrogena T/Gel Therapeutic Conditioner	Salicylic acid 2%	**Adults & Peds:** Use at least two times per week.
Neutrogena T/Sal Therapeutic Shampoo	Salicylic acid 3%	**Adults & Peds:** Use at least three times per week.
Psoriasin Therapeutic Shampoo and Body Wash	Salicylic acid 3%	**Adults & Peds:** Use at least two times per week.

WOUND CARE PRODUCTS

BRAND	INGREDIENTS/STRENGTH	DOSAGE
NEOMYCIN/POLYMYXIN B/BACITRACIN COMBINATIONS		
Bacitracin Ointment	Bacitracin 500 U	**Adults & Peds:** Apply a small amount to affected area qd-tid.
Neosporin First Aid Antibiotic Ointment	Neomycin/Polymyxin B sulfate/ Bacitracin zinc 3.5mg-5000 U-400 U/gram	**Adults & Peds:** Apply a small amount to affected area qd-tid.
Neosporin NEO TO GO! Single Use Packets	Neomycin/Polymyxin B sulfate/ Bacitracin zinc 3.5mg-5000 U-400 U/gram	**Adults & Peds:** Apply a small amount to affected area qd-tid.
Neosporin Plus Pain Relief Cream	Neomycin/Polymyxin B sulfate/ Pramoxine HCl 3.5mg-10,000 U-10mg/gram	**Adults & Peds ≥2 yrs:** Apply a small amount to affected area qd-tid.
Neosporin Plus Pain Relief Ointment	Neomycin/Polymyxin B sulfate/ Bacitracin zinc/Pramoxine HCl 3.5mg-10,000 U-400 U-10mg/gram	**Adults & Peds ≥2 yrs:** Apply a small amount to affected area qd-tid.
Polysporin First Aid Antibiotic Ointment	Polymyxin B/Bacitracin 10,000 U-500 U/gram	**Adults & Peds:** Apply a small amount to affected area qd-tid.
Polysporin First Aid Antibiotic Powder	Polymyxin B/Bacitracin 10,000 U-500 U/gram	**Adults & Peds:** Apply a light dusting of powder on affected area qd-tid.
BENZALKONIUM CHLORIDE COMBINATIONS		
Bactine Original First Aid Liquid	Benzalkonium chloride/Lidocaine HCl 0.13%-2.5%	**Adults & Peds ≥2 yrs:** Apply a small amount to affected area qd-tid.
Bactine Pain Relieving Cleansing Spray	Benzalkonium chloride/Lidocaine HCl 0.13%-2.5%	**Adults & Peds ≥2 yrs:** Apply a small amount to affected area qd-tid.
Band-Aid Hurt Free Antiseptic Wash	Benzalkonium chloride/Lidocaine HCl 0.13%-2%	**Adults & Peds ≥2 yrs:** Flush affected area no more than tid.
Neosporin NEO TO GO! First Aid Antiseptic/Pain Relieving Spray	Benzalkonium chloride/Pramoxine HCl 0.13%-1%	**Adults & Peds ≥2 yrs:** Spray a small amount on affected area qd-tid.
BENZETHONIUM CHLORIDE COMBINATIONS		
Gold Bond Quick Spray	Benzethonium chloride/Menthol 0.13%-1%	**Adults & Peds ≥2 yrs:** Apply to affected area tid-qid.
Lanacane Anti-Bacterial First Aid Spray	Benzethonium chloride/Benzocaine 0.2%-20%	**Adults & Peds ≥2 yrs:** Spray a small amount on the affected area qd-tid.
Lanacane Anti-Itch Cream	Benzethonium chloride/Benzocaine 0.1%-20%	**Adults & Peds ≥2 yrs:** Apply a small amount to affected area not more than qd-tid.
CHLORHEXIDINE GLUCONATE		
Hibiclens	Chlorhexidine gluconate 4%	**Adults:** Apply the minimum amount necessary to cover area and wash gently. Rinse again thoroughly.
Hibistat Wipes	Chlorhexidine gluconate/Isopropyl alcohol 0.5%-70%	**Adults:** Use as needed.
IODINE		
Betadine Skin Cleanser	Povidone-iodine 7.5%	**Adults & Peds:** Wet skin and apply a sufficient amount for lather to cover all surfaces. Wash vigorously for at least 15 seconds, rinse and dry throughly.
Betadine Solution	Povidone-iodine 10%	**Adults & Peds:** Apply a small amount to affected area qd-tid.
MISCELLANEOUS		
Wound Wash Saline	Sterile 0.9% sodium chloride solution	**Adults & Peds:** Flush affected area prn.

ANTACID AND HEARTBURN PRODUCTS

BRAND	INGREDIENTS/STRENGTH	DOSAGE
ANTACIDS		
Alka-Seltzer Gold Tablets	Citric acid/Potassium bicarbonate/ Sodium bicarbonate 1000mg-344mg-1050mg	**Adults ≥60 yrs:** 2 tabs q4h prn. **Max:** 6 tabs q24h. **Adults & Peds ≥12 yrs:** 2 tabs q4h prn. **Max:** 8 tabs q24h. **Peds ≤12yrs:** 1 tab q4h prn. **Max:** 4 tabs q24h.
Alka-Seltzer Heartburn Relief Tablets	Citric acid/Sodium bicarbonate 1000mg-1940mg	**Adults ≥60 yrs:** 2 tabs q4h prn. **Max:** 4 tabs q24h. **Adults & Peds ≥12 yrs:** 2 tabs q4h prn. **Max:** 8 tabs q24h.
Alka-Seltzer Lemon Lime Tablets	Aspirin/Citric acid/Sodium bicarbonate 325mg-1000mg-1700mg	**Adults ≥60 yrs:** 2 tabs q4h prn. **Max:** 4 tabs q24h. **Adults & Peds ≥12 yrs:** 2 tabs q4h prn. **Max:** 8 tabs q24h.
Alka-Seltzer Tablets, Extra-Strength	Aspirin/Citric acid/Sodium bicarbonate 500mg-1000mg-1985mg	**Adults ≥60 yrs:** 2 tabs q6h prn. **Max:** 3 tabs q24h. **Adults & Peds ≥12 yrs:** 2 tabs q6h prn. **Max:** 7 tabs q24h.
Alka-Seltzer Tablets, Original	Aspirin/Citric acid/Sodium bicarbonate 325mg-1000mg-1916mg	**Adults ≥60 yrs:** 2 tabs q4h prn. **Max:** 4 tabs q24h. **Adults & Peds ≥12 yrs:** 2 tabs q4h prn. **Max:** 8 tabs q24h.
Brioschi Powder	Sodium bicarbonate/Tartaric acid 1.80g-1.62g/dose	**Adults & Peds ≥12 yrs:** 1 capful (6g) dissolved in 4-6 oz water q1h. **Max:** 6 doses q24h. **Adults ≥60 yrs:** 1 capful (6g) dissolved in 4-6 oz water q1h. **Max:** 3 doses q24h.
Gaviscon Extra Strength Liquid	Aluminum hydroxide/Magnesium carbonate 254mg-237.5mg/5ml	**Adults:** 2-4 tsp (10-20mL) qid. **Max:** 16 tsp (80mL) q24h.
Gaviscon Extra Strength Tablets	Aluminum hydroxide/Magnesium carbonate 160mg-105mg	**Adults:** 2-4 tabs qid. **Max:** 16 doses q24h.
Gaviscon Regular Strength Liquid	Aluminum hydroxide/Magnesium carbonate 95mg-358mg/15mL	**Adults:** 1-2 tbl (15-30mL) qid. **Max:** 8 tbl (120mL) q24h.
Gaviscon Regular Strength Tablets	Aluminum hydroxide/Magnesium trisilicate 80mg-14.2mg	**Adults:** 2-4 tabs qid. **Max:** 16 tabs q24h.
Maalox Children's Relief Chewables	Calcium carbonate 400mg	**Peds 6-11 yrs (48-95 lbs):** 2 tabs prn. **Max:** 6 tabs q24h. **Peds 2-5 yrs (24-47 lbs):** 1 tab prn. **Max:** 3 tabs q24h.
Maalox Regular Strength Chewable Tablets	Calcium carbonate 600mg	**Adults:** 1-2 tabs prn. **Max:** 12 tabs q24h.
Mylanta Supreme Antacid Liquid	Calcium carbonate/Magnesium hydroxide 400mg-135mg/5mL	**Adults:** 2-4 tsp (10-20mL) qid (between meals & hs). **Max:** 18 tsp (90mL) q24h.
Mylanta Ultimate Strength Liquid	Aluminum hydroxide/Magnesium hydroxide 500mg-500mg/5mL	**Adults & Peds ≥12 yrs:** 2-4 tsp (10-20mL) prn (between meals & hs). **Max:** 9 tsp (45mL) q24h.
Pepto Bismol Children's Pepto Antacid Chewable Tablets	Calcium carbonate 400mg	**Peds 6-11 yrs (48-95 lbs):** Take 2 tabs prn. **Max:** 6 tabs q24h. **Peds 2-5 yrs (24-47 lbs):** Take 1 tab prn. **Max:** 3 tabs q24h.
Rolaids Extra Strength Softchews	Calcium carbonate 1177mg	**Adults:** 2-3 chews q1h prn. **Max:** 6 chews q24h.
Rolaids Extra Strength Tablets	Calcium carbonate/Magnesium hydroxide 675mg-135mg	**Adults:** 2-4 tabs q1h prn. **Max:** 12 tabs q24h.
Rolaids Regular Strength Tablets	Calcium carbonate/Magnesium hydroxide 550mg-110mg	**Adults:** 2-4 tabs q1h prn. **Max:** 12 tabs q24h.
Titralac Instant Relief Tablets	Calcium carbonate 420mg	**Adults:** 2 tabs q2-3h prn. **Max:** 19 tabs q24h.
Tums Regular Strength Tablets	Calcium carbonate 500mg	**Adults:** 2-4 tabs prn. **Max:** 15 tabs q24h.
Tums Extra 750 Chewable Tablets	Calcium carbonate 750mg	**Adults:** 2-4 tabs prn. **Max:** 10 tabs q24h.

(Continued)

BRAND	INGREDIENTS/STRENGTH	DOSAGE
ANTACIDS (Continued)		
Tums Extra 750 Sugar Free Chewable Tablets	Calcium carbonate 750mg	**Adults:** 2-4 tabs prn. **Max:** 10 tabs q24h.
Tums Kids Chewable Tablets	Calcium carbonate 750mg	**Peds ≥4 yrs (≥48 lbs):** 1 tab tid prn with meals. **Max:** 4 tabs q24h. **Peds 2-4 yrs (24-47 lbs):** 1/2 tab bid prn with meals. **Max:** 2 tabs q24h.
Tums Smoothies Tablets	Calcium carbonate 750mg	**Adults:** 2-4 tabs prn. **Max:** 10 tabs q24h.
Tums Ultra 1000 Chewable Tablets	Calcium carbonate 1000mg	**Adults:** 2-3 tabs prn. **Max:** 7 tabs q24h.
ANTACIDS/ANTIFLATULENTS		
Gelusil Chewable Tablets	Aluminum hydroxide/Magnesium hydroxide/Simethicone 200mg-200mg-25mg	**Adults:** 2-4 tabs q1h prn. **Max:** 12 tabs q24h.
Maalox Advanced Maximum Strength Chewable Tablets	Calcium Carbonate/Simethicone 1000mg-60mg	**Adults & Peds ≥12 yrs:** 1-2 tabs prn. **Max:** 8 tabs q24h.
Maalox Advanced Maximum Strength Liquid	Aluminum hydroxide/Magnesium hydroxide/Simethicone 400mg-400mg-40mg/5mL	**Adults & Peds ≥12 yrs:** 2-4 tsp (10-20mL) bid. **Max:** 8 tsp (40mL) q24h.
Maalox Advanced Regular Strength Liquid	Aluminum hydroxide/Magnesium hydroxide/Simethicone 200mg-200mg-20mg/5mL	**Adults & Peds ≥12 yrs:** 2-4 tsp (10-20mL) qid. **Max:** 16 tsp (80mL) q24h.
Maalox Junior Relief Chewables	Calcium carbonate/Simethicone 400mg-24mg	**Peds 6-11 yrs:** 2 tabs prn. **Max:** 6 tabs q24h.
Mylanta Maximum Strength Liquid	Aluminum hydroxide/Magnesium hydroxide/Simethicone 400mg-400mg-40mg/5mL	**Adults & Peds ≥12 yrs:** 2-4 tsp (between meals and hs) (10-20mL) qid. **Max:** 12 tsp (60mL) q24h.
Mylanta Regular Strength Liquid	Aluminum hydroxide/Magnesium hydroxide/Simethicone 200mg-200mg-20mg/5mL	**Adults & Peds ≥12 yrs:** 2-4 tsp (between meals and hs) (10-20mL) qid. **Max:** 24 tsp (120mL) q24h.
Rolaids Extra Strength Plus Gas Soft Chews	Calcium carbonate/Simethicone 1177mg-80mg	**Adults:** 2-3 chews q1h prn. **Max:** 6 chews q24h.
Rolaids Multi-Symptom Chewable Tablets	Calcium carbonate/Magnesium hydroxide/Simethicone 675mg-135mg-60mg	**Adults:** 2-4 tabs q1h prn. **Max:** 8 tabs q24h.
Titralac Plus Chewable Tablets	Calcium carbonate/Simethicone 420mg-21mg	**Adults:** 2 tabs q2-3h prn. **Max:** 19 tabs q24h.
BISMUTH SUBSALICYLATES		
Maalox Total Relief Maximum Strength Liquid	Bismuth subsalicylate 525mg/15mL	**Adults & Peds ≥12 yrs:** 2 tbl (30mL) q1h prn. **Max:** 8 tbl (120mL) q24h.
Pepto Bismol Caplets	Bismuth subsalicylate 262mg	**Adults & Peds ≥12 yrs:** 2 tabs q½-1h prn. **Max:** 8 doses (16 tabs) q24h.
Pepto Bismol Chewable Tablets	Bismuth subsalicylate 262mg	**Adults & Peds ≥12 yrs:** 2 tabs q½-1h prn. **Max:** 8 doses (16 tabs) q24h.
Pepto Bismol Liquid	Bismuth subsalicylate 262mg/15mL	**Adults & Peds ≥12 yrs:** 2 tbl (30mL) q½-1h prn. **Max:** 8 doses (16 tbl or 240mL) q24h.
Pepto Bismol Liquid Max	Bismuth subsalicylate 525mg/15mL	**Adults & Peds ≥12 yrs:** 2 tbl (30mL) q1h prn. **Max:** 8 doses (16 tbl or 240mL) q24h.
H₂-RECEPTOR ANTAGONISTS		
Axid AR	Nizatidine 75mg	**Adults & Peds ≥12 yrs:** 1 tab qd. **Max:** 2 tabs q24h.
Pepcid AC Maximum Strength EZ Chews	Famotidine 20mg	**Adults & Peds ≥12 yrs:** 1 tab qd. **Max:** 2 tabs q24h.
Pepcid AC Maximum Strength Tablets	Famotidine 20mg	**Adults & Peds ≥12 yrs:** 1 tab qd. **Max:** 2 tabs q24h.

BRAND	INGREDIENTS/STRENGTH	DOSAGE
H₂-RECEPTOR ANTAGONISTS *(Continued)*		
Pepcid AC Tablets	Famotidine 10mg	**Adults & Peds ≥12 yrs:** 1 tab qd. **Max:** 2 tabs q24h.
Tagamet HB Tablets	Cimetidine 200mg	**Adults & Peds ≥12 yrs:** 1 tab qd. **Max:** 2 tabs q24h.
Zantac 75 Tablets	Ranitidine 75mg	**Adults & Peds ≥12 yrs:** 1 tab qd. **Max:** 2 tabs q24h.
Zantac 150 Tablets	Ranitidine 150mg	**Adults & Peds ≥12 yrs:** 1 tab qd. **Max:** 2 tabs q24h.
H₂-RECEPTOR ANTAGONISTS/ANTACIDS		
Pepcid Complete Chewable Tablets	Famotidine/Calcium carbonate/ Magnesium hydroxide 10mg-800mg-165mg	**Adults & Peds ≥12 yrs:** 1 tab qd. **Max:** 2 tabs q24h.
Tums Dual Action	Famotidine/Calcium carbonate/ Magnesium hydroxide 10mg-800mg-165mg	**Adults & Peds ≥12 yrs:** 1 tab qd. **Max:** 2 tabs q24h.
PROTON PUMP INHIBITORS		
Prevacid 24 HR	Lansoprazole 15mg	**Adults:** 1 cap qd x 14 days. May repeat 14-day course q4 months.
Prilosec OTC Tablets	Omeprazole 20mg	**Adults:** 1 tab qd x 14 days. May repeat 14-day course q4 months.
Zegerid OTC	Omeprazole/Sodium bicarbonate 20mg-1100mg	**Adults:** 1 cap qd x 14 days. May repeat 14-day course q4 months.

ANTIDIARRHEAL PRODUCTS

BRAND	INGREDIENT/STRENGTH	DOSE
ABSORBENT		
Equalactin Chewable Tablets	Calcium Polycarbophil 625mg	**Adults & Peds ≥12 yrs:** 2 tabs/dose. **Max:** 8 tabs q24h. **Peds 6-12 yrs:** 1 tab/dose. **Max:** 4 tabs q24h. **Peds 2 to ≤6yrs:** 1 tab/dose. **Max:** 2 tabs q24h.
Fibercon Caplets	Calcium Polycarbophil 625mg	**Adults & Peds ≥12 yrs:** 2 tabs qd. **Max:** 8 tabs q24h.
Konsyl Fiber Caplets	Calcium Polycarbophil 625mg	**Adults & Peds ≥12 yrs:** 2 tabs qd-qid. **Peds 6-12 yrs:** 1 tab qd-tid. **Max:** 3 Tabs q24h.
ANTIPERISTALTIC		
Imodium A-D Caplets	Loperamide HCl 2mg	**Adults & Peds ≥12 yrs:** 2 tabs after first loose stool; 1 tab after each subsequent loose stool. **Max:** 4 tabs q24h. **Peds 9-11 yrs (60-95 lbs):** 1 tab after first loose stool; ½ tab after each subsequent loose stool. **Max:** 3 tabs q24h. **Peds 6-8 yrs (48-59 lbs):** 1 tab after first loose stool; ½ tab after each subsequent loose stool. **Max:** 2 tabs q24h.
Imodium A-D EZ Chews	Loperamide HCl 2mg	**Adults & Peds ≥12 yrs:** 2 tabs after first loose stool; 1 tab after each subsequent loose stool. **Max:** 4 tabs q24h. **Peds 9-11 yrs (60-95 lbs):** 1 tab after first loose stool; ½ tab after each subsequent loose stool. **Max:** 3 tabs q24h. **Peds 6-8 yrs (48-59 lbs):** 1 tab after first loose stool; ½ tab after each subsequent loose stool. **Max:** 2 tabs q24h.
Imodium A-D Liquid	Loperamide HCl 1mg/7.5mL	**Adults & Peds ≥12 yrs:** 4 tsp (20mL) after first loose stool; 2 tsp (10mL) after each subsequent loose stool. **Max:** 8 tsp (40mL) q24h. **Peds 9-11 yrs (60-95 lbs):** 2 tsp (10mL) after first loose stool; 1 tsp (5mL) after each subsequent loose stool. **Max:** 6 tsp (30mL) q24h. **Peds 6-8 yrs (48-59 lbs):** 2 tsp (10mL) after first loose stool; 1 tsp (5mL) after each subsequent loose stool. **Max:** 4 tsp (20mL) q24h.
Imodium A-D Liquid for Use In Children (Mint Flavor)	Loperamide HCl 1mg/7.5mL	**Adults & Peds ≥12 yrs:** 6 tsp (30mL) after first loose stool; 3 tsp (15mL) after each subsequent loose stool. **Max:** 12 tsp (60mL) q24h. **Peds 9-11 yrs (60-95 lbs):** 3 tsp (15mL) after first loose stool; 1½ tsp (7.5mL) after each subsequent loose stool. **Max:** 9 tsp (45mL) q24h. **Peds 6-8 yrs (48-59 lbs):** 3 tsp (15mL) after first loose stool; 1½ tsp (7.5mL) after each subsequent loose stool. **Max:** 6 tsp (30mL) q24h.
ANTIPERISTALTIC/ANTIFLATULENT		
Imodium Multi-Symptom Relief Caplets	Loperamide HCl/Simethicone 2mg-125mg	**Adults & Peds ≥12 yrs:** 2 tabs after first loose stool; 1 tab after each subsequent loose stool. **Max:** 4 tabs q24h. **Peds 9-11 yrs (60-95 lbs):** 1 tab after first loose stool; ½ tab after each subsequent loose stool. **Max:** 3 tabs q24h. **Peds 6-8 yrs (48-59 lbs):** 1 tab after first loose stool; ½ tab after each subsequent loose stool. **Max:** 2 tabs q24h.
Imodium Multi-Symptom Relief Chewable Tablets	Loperamide HCl/Simethicone 2mg-125mg	**Adults & Peds ≥12 yrs:** 2 tabs with 4-8 oz water after first loose stool; 1 tab with 4-8 oz water after each subsequent loose stool. **Max:** 4 tabs q24h. **Peds 9-11 yrs (60-95 lbs):** 1 tab with 4-8 oz water after first loose stool; ½ tab after each subsequent loose stool. **Max:** 3 tabs q24h. **Peds 6-8 yrs (48-59 lbs):** 1 tab with 4-8 oz water after first loose stool; ½ tab after each subsequent loose stool. **Max:** 2 tabs q24h.
BISMUTH SUBSALICYLATE		
Kaopectate Extra Strength Liquid	Bismuth Subsalicylate 525mg/15mL	**Adults & Peds ≥12 yrs:** 2 tbl (30mL) q1h prn. **Max:** 4 doses (8 tbl) q24h.

(Continued)

BRAND	INGREDIENT/STRENGTH	DOSE
BISMUTH SUBSALICYLATE *(Continued)*		
Kaopectate Liquid	Bismuth Subsalicylate 262mg/15mL	**Adults & Peds ≥12 yrs:** 2 tbl (30mL) q½-1h prn. **Max:** 8 doses (16 tbl) q24h.
Maalox Total Relief Liquid	Bismuth Subsalicylate 525mg/15mL	**Adults & Peds ≥12 yrs:** 2 tbl (30mL) q1h prn. **Max:** 4 doses (8 tbl) q24h.
Pepto Bismol Caplets	Bismuth Subsalicylate 262mg	**Adults & Peds ≥12 yrs:** 2 tabs q½-1h. **Max:** 8 doses (16 tabs) q24h.
Pepto Bismol Chewable Tablets	Bismuth Subsalicylate 262mg	**Adults & Peds ≥12 yrs:** 2 tabs q½-1h. **Max:** 8 doses (16 tabs) q24h.
Pepto Bismol Instacool Chewable Tablets	Bismuth Subsalicylate 262mg	**Adults & Peds ≥12 yrs:** 2 tabs q½-1h. **Max:** 8 doses (16 tabs) q24h.
Pepto Bismol Liquid	Bismuth Subsalicylate 262mg/15mL	**Adults & Peds ≥12 yrs:** 2 tbl (30mL) q½-1h prn. **Max:** 8 doses (16 tbl) q24h.
Pepto Bismol Liquid Max	Bismuth Subsalicylate 525mg/15mL	**Adults & Peds ≥12 yrs:** 2 tbl (30mL) q1h prn. **Max:** 8 doses (16 tbl) q24h.

ANTIFLATULENT PRODUCTS

BRAND	INGREDIENT/STRENGTH	DOSE
ALPHA-GALACTOSIDASE		
Beano Food Enzyme Dietary Supplement Tablets	Alpha-Galactosidase Enzyme 150 GalU	**Adults:** Take 3 tabs before meals.
Beano Meltaways Tablets	Alpha-Galactosidase Enzyme 300 GalU	**Adults:** Take 1 tab before meals.
ANTACID/ANTIFLATULENT		
PLEASE REFER TO ANTACID AND HEARTBURN PRODUCTS CHART		
SIMETHICONE		
GasAid Maximum Strength Anti-Gas Softgelsp;	Simethicone 125mg	**Adults:** Take 1-2 caps prn and qhs. **Max:** 4 caps q24h.
Baby Gas-X Infant Drops	Simethicone 20mg/0.3mL	**Peds ≥2 yrs (≥24 lbs):** 0.6mL prn. **Peds <2 yrs (<24 lbs):** 0.3mL prn. **Max:** 6 doses q24h.
Gas-X Thin Strips	Simethicone 62.5mg	**Adults:** Allow 2-4 strips to dissolve prn after meals and hs. **Max:** 8 strips q24h.
Gas-X Chewable Tablets	Simethicone 80mg	**Adults:** Take 1-2 tabs prn and qhs. **Max:** 6 tabs q24h.
Gas-X Extra Strength Chewable Tablets	Simethicone 125mg	**Adults:** Take 1-2 tabs prn and qhs. **Max:** 4 tabs q24h.
Gas-X Extra Strength Softgels	Simethicone 125mg	**Adults:** Take 1-2 caps prn and qhs. **Max:** 4 caps q24h.
Gas-X Ultra Strength Softgels	Simethicone 180mg	**Adults:** Take 1-2 caps prn after meals and qhs. **Max:** 2 caps q24h.
Little Tummys Gas Relief Drops	Simethicone 20mg/0.3mL	**Peds ≥2 yrs (≥24 lbs):** 0.6mL prn (after meals & hs). **Peds <2 yrs (<24 lbs):** 0.3mL prn (after meals & hs). **Max:** 12 doses q24h.
Mylanta Gas Maximum Strength Chewable Tablets	Simethicone 125mg	**Adults:** Chew 1-2 tabs (after meals & hs). **Max:** 4 tabs q24h.
Mylicon Infant's Gas Relief Drops	Simethicone 20mg/0.3mL	**Peds ≥2 yrs (≥24 lbs):** 0.6mL (after meals & hs). **Peds <2 yrs (<24 lbs):** 0.3mL (after meals & hs). **Max:** 12 doses q24h.
PediaCare Infants Gas Relief Drops	Simethicone 20mg/0.3mL	**Peds ≥2 yrs (≥24 lbs):** 0.6mL (after meals & hs). **Peds <2 yrs (<24 lbs):** 0.3mL (after meals & hs). **Max:** 12 doses q24h.

HEMORRHOIDAL PRODUCTS

BRAND	INGREDIENTS/STRENGTH	DOSE
ANESTHETICS/ANESTHETIC COMBINATIONS		
Hemaway Cream	Lidocaine/Phenylephrine 0.5%-0.5%	**Adults & Peds ≥12 yrs:** Apply externally to the affected area up to 4 times a day.
Nupercainal Ointment	Dibucaine 1%	**Adults & Peds ≥12 yrs:** Apply to affected area tid-qid.
Preparation H Hemorrhoidal Cream, Maximum Strength Pain Relief	Glycerin/Phenylephrine HCl/ Pramoxine HCl/White petrolatum 14.4%-0.25%-1%-15%	**Adults & Peds ≥12 yrs:** Apply to affected area prn. **Max:** 4 times q24h.
Tronolane Anesthetic Hemorrhoid Cream	Pramoxine HCl/Zinc oxide 1%-5%	**Adults & Peds ≥12 yrs:** Apply to affected area prn. **Max:** 5 times q24h.
Tucks Hemorrhoidal Ointment	Pramoxine HCl/Zinc oxide/ Mineral oil 1%-12.5%-46.6%	**Adults & Peds ≥12 yrs:** Apply to affected area prn. **Max:** 5 times q24h.
HYDROCORTISONE		
Preparation H Anti-Itch Cream	Hydrocortisone 1.0%	**Adults & Peds ≥12 yrs:** Apply to affected area tid-qid.
WITCH HAZEL/WITCH HAZEL COMBINATIONS		
Preparation H Hemorrhoidal Cooling Gel	Phenylephrine HCl/ Witch hazel 0.25%-50.0%	**Adults & Peds ≥12 yrs:** Apply to affected area prn. **Max:** 4 times q24h.
Preparation H Medicated Wipes	Witch hazel 50%	**Adults & Peds ≥12 yrs:** Apply to affected area prn. **Max:** 6 times q24h.
T.N. Dickinson's Witch Hazel Hemorrhoidal Pads	Witch hazel 50%	**Adults & Peds ≥12 yrs:** Apply to affected area prn. **Max:** 6 times q24h.
Tucks Medicated Pads	Witch hazel 50%	**Adults & Peds ≥12 yrs:** Apply to affected area prn. **Max:** 6 times q24h.
Tucks Take Alongs Medicated Towelettes	Witch hazel 50%	**Adults & Peds ≥12 yrs:** Apply to affected area prn. **Max:** 6 times q24h.
MISCELLANEOUS		
Calmol 4 Hemorrhoidal Suppositories	Cocoa butter/Zinc oxide 76%-10%	**Adults & Peds ≥12 yrs:** Insert 1 supp prn. **Max:** 6 times q24h.
Preparation H Hemorrhoidal Ointment	Mineral oil/Petrolatum/ Phenylephrine HCl/ 14%-71.9%-0.25%	**Adults & Peds ≥12 yrs:** Apply to affected area prn. **Max:** 4 times q24h.
Preparation H Hemorrhoidal Suppositories	Cocoa butter/Phenylephrine HCl/ 85.5%-0.25%	**Adults & Peds ≥12 yrs:** Insert 1 supp prn. **Max:** 4 times q24h.
Rectal Medicone Suppositories	Hard fat/Phenylephrine 88.7%-0.25%	**Adults & Peds ≥12 yrs:** Insert 1 supp prn. **Max:** 4 times q24h.
Tronolane Suppositories	Hard fat/Phenylephrine HCl 88.7%-0.25%	**Adults & Peds ≥12 yrs:** Insert 1 supp prn. **Max:** 4 times q24h.
Tucks Internal Soothers	Topical starch 51%	**Adults & Peds ≥12 yrs:** Insert 1 supp prn. **Max:** 6 times q24h.

*Please refer to the *Laxative Products* chart for stool softeners or bulk-forming laxatives adjunct therapies.

LAXATIVE PRODUCTS

BRAND	INGREDIENTS/STRENGTH	DOSE
BULK-FORMING		
Citrucel Caplets	Methylcellulose 500mg	**Adults & Peds ≥12 yrs:** 2 tabs qd prn. **Max:** 12 tabs q24h. **Peds 6-11 yrs:** 1 tab qd prn. **Max:** 6 tabs q24h.
Citrucel Orange Powder	Methylcellulose 2g/tbl	**Adults & Peds ≥12 yrs:** 1 tbl qd-tid. **Peds 6-11 yrs:** 2.5 tsp qd-tid.
Citrucel Orange Sugar Free Powder	Methylcellulose 2g/tbl	**Adults & Peds ≥12 yrs:** 1 tbl qd-tid. **Peds 6-11 yrs:** 2 tsp qd-tid.
Equalactin Chewable Tablets	Calcium polycarbophil 625mg	**Adults & Peds ≥12 yrs:** 2 tabs qd. **Max:** 8 tabs q24h. **Peds 6-11 yrs:** 1 tab qd. **Max:** 4 tabs q24h. **Peds 2-5 yrs:** 1 tab qd. **Max:** 2 tabs q24h.
Fibercon Caplets	Calcium polycarbophil 625mg	**Adults & Peds ≥12 yrs:** 2 tabs qd. **Max:** 4 tabs qd.
Konsyl Balance Orange	Inulin/Refined psyllium	**Adults & Peds ≥12 yrs:** 1 tsp qd-tid. **Peds 7-11 yrs:** ½ tsp qd-tid.
Konsyl Easy Mix Powder	Psyllium 4.3g/tsp	**Adults & Peds ≥12 yrs:** 1 tsp qd-tid. **Peds 6-11 yrs:** ½ tsp qd-tid.
Konsyl Fiber Caplets	Calcium polycarbophil 625mg	**Adults:** 2 tabs qd-qid. **Max:** 8 tabs q24h. **Peds 6-12 yrs:** 1 tab qd-tid. **Max:** 3 tabs q24h.
Konsyl Orange Powder	Psyllium 3.4g/tbl	**Adults & Peds ≥12 yrs:** 1 tbl qd-tid. **Peds 6-11 yrs:** ½ tbl qd-tid.
Konsyl Orange Sugar Free Powder	Psyllium 3.5g/tsp	**Adults & Peds ≥12 yrs:** 1 tsp qd-tid. **Peds 6-11 yrs:** ½ tsp qd-tid.
Konsyl Original Powder	Psyllium 6g/tsp	**Adults & Peds ≥12 yrs:** 1 tsp qd-tid. **Peds 6-11 yrs:** ½ tsp qd-tid.
Konsyl-D Powder	Psyllium 3.4g/tsp	**Adults & Peds ≥12 yrs:** 1 tsp qd-tid. **Peds 6-11 yrs:** ½ tsp qd-tid.
Metamucil Capsules	Psyllium 525mg	**Adults & Peds ≥12 yrs:** 2-6 caps qd-tid.
Metamucil Capsules Plus Calcium	Psyllium/Calcium 600mg-60mg	**Adults & Peds ≥12 yrs:** 2-5 caps qd-qid.
Metamucil Orange Fiber Singles	Psyllium 3.4g/packet	**Adults & Peds ≥12 yrs:** 1 packet qd-tid. **Peds 6-11 yrs:** ½ packet qd-tid.
Metamucil Orange Fiber Singles Sugar Free	Psyllium 3.4g/packet	**Adults & Peds ≥12 yrs:** 1 packet qd-tid. **Peds 6-11 yrs:** ½ packet qd-tid.
Metamucil Orange Coarse Powder	Psyllium 3.4g/tbl	**Adults & Peds ≥12 yrs:** 1 tbl qd-tid. **Peds 6-11 yrs:** ½ tbl qd-tid.
Metamucil Orange Smooth Powder	Psyllium 3.4g/tbl	**Adults & Peds ≥12 yrs:** 1 tbl qd-tid. **Peds 6-11 yrs:** ½ tbl qd-tid.
Metamucil Original Coarse Powder	Psyllium 3.4g/tsp	**Adults & Peds ≥12 yrs:** 1 tsp qd-tid. **Peds 6-11 yrs:** ½ tsp qd-tid.
Metamucil Sugar Free Powder (multi-flavor)	Psyllium 3.4g/tsp	**Adults & Peds ≥12 yrs:** 1 tsp qd-tid. **Peds 6-11 yrs:** ½ tsp qd-tid.
Metamucil Wafers	Psyllium 3.4g/dose	**Adults & Peds ≥12 yrs:** 2 wafers qd-tid.
HYPEROSMOTICS		
Dulcolax Balance	Polyethylene glycol 3350, 17g	**Adults & Peds ≥17 yrs:** 1 capful (17g) qd. **Max:** 7 days.
Fleet Glycerin Suppositories	Glycerin 2g	**Adults & Peds ≥6 yrs:** 1 supp ud.
Fleet Liquid Glycerin Suppositories	Glycerin 5.4g	**Adults & Peds ≥6 yrs:** 1 supp ud.
Fleet Mineral Oil Enema	Mineral oil 100%/118mL	**Adults & Peds ≥12 yrs:** 1 bottle (118mL). **Peds 2-11 yrs:** ½ bottle (59mL).
Fleet Pedia-Lax Glycerin Suppositories	Glycerin 1g	**Peds 2-5 yrs:** 1 supp ud.

(Continued)

BRAND	INGREDIENTS/STRENGTH	DOSE
Fleet Pedia-Lax Liquid Glycerin Suppositories	Glycerin 2.8g	**Peds 2-5 yrs:** 1 supp ud.
Miralax	Polyethylene glycol 3350, 17g	**Adults & Peds ≥17 yrs:** 1 capful (17g) qd. **Max:** 7 days.

SALINES

BRAND	INGREDIENTS/STRENGTH	DOSE
Fleet Enema	Monobasic sodium phosphate/ Dibasic sodium phosphate 19g-7g/118mL	**Adults & Peds ≥12 yrs:** 1 bottle (118mL).
Fleet Enema Extra	Monobasic sodium phosphate/ Dibasic sodium phosphate 19g-7g/197mL	**Adults & Peds ≥12 yrs:** 1 bottle (197mL).
Fleet Pedia-Lax Chewable Tablets	Magnesium hydroxide 400mg	**Peds 6-<12 yrs:** 3-6 tabs qd. **Max:** 6 tabs q24h. **Peds 2-<6 yrs:** 1-3 tabs qd. **Max:** 3 tabs q24h.
Fleet Pedia-Lax Enema	Monobasic sodium phosphate/ Dibasic sodium phosphate 9.5g-3.5g/59mL	**Peds 5-11 yrs:** 1 bottle (59mL). **Peds 2-<5 yrs:** ½ bottle (29.5mL).
Magnesium Citrate Solution	Magnesium citrate 1.75g/30mL	**Adults & Peds ≥12 yrs:** 300mL. **Peds 6-<12 yrs:** 90-210mL. **Peds 2-<6 yrs:** 60mL.
Phillips' Antacid/Laxative Chewable Tablets	Magnesium hydroxide 311mg	**Adults & Peds ≥12 yrs:** 8 tabs qd. **Peds 6-11 yrs:** 4 tabs qd. **Peds 3-5 yrs:** 2 tabs qd.
Phillips' Laxative Caplets	Magnesium 500mg	**Adults & Peds ≥12 yrs:** 2-4 tabs qd. **Max:** 4 tabs q24h.
Phillips' Concentrated Milk of Magnesia Liquid	Magnesium hydroxide 2400mg/15mL	**Adults & Peds ≥12 yrs:** 1-2 tbl qd. **Peds 6-11 yrs:** ½-1 tbl qd.
Phillips' Milk of Magnesia Liquid	Magnesium hydroxide 1200mg/15mL	**Adults & Peds ≥12 yrs:** 2-4 tbl qd. **Peds 6-11 yrs:** 1-2 tbl qd.

SALINE COMBINATION

BRAND	INGREDIENTS/STRENGTH	DOSE
Phillips' M-O Liquid	Magnesium hydroxide/Mineral oil 300mg-1.25mL/5mL	**Adults & Peds ≥12 yrs:** 3-4 tbl qd. **Peds 6-11 yrs:** 4-6 tsp qd.

STIMULANTS

BRAND	INGREDIENTS/STRENGTH	DOSE
Alophen Tablets	Bisacodyl 5mg	**Adults & Peds ≥12 yrs:** 1-3 tabs qd. **Peds 6-11 yrs:** Take 1 tab qd.
Carter's Laxative Tablets	Bisacodyl 5mg	**Adults & Peds ≥12 yrs:** 1-3 tabs (usually 2 tabs) qd. **Peds 6-<12 yrs:** 1 tab qd.
Castor Oil	Castor oil	**Adults & Peds ≥12 yrs:** 15-60mL. **Peds 2-<12 yrs:** 5-15mL.
Dulcolax Suppository	Bisacodyl 10mg	**Adults & Peds ≥12 yrs:** 1 supp qd. **Peds 6-<12 yrs:** ½ supp qd.
Dulcolax Tablets	Bisacodyl 5mg	**Adults & Peds ≥12 yrs:** 1-3 tabs qd. **Peds 6-<12 yrs:** 1 tab qd.
Ex-Lax Chocolate	Sennosides 15mg	**Adults & Peds ≥12 yrs:** 2 pieces qd-bid. **Peds 6-<12 yrs:** 1 piece qd-bid.
Ex-Lax Maximum Strength Tablets	Sennosides 25mg	**Adults & Peds ≥12 yrs:** 2 tabs qd-bid. **Peds 6-<12 yrs:** 1 tab qd-bid.
Ex-Lax Tablets	Sennosides 15mg	**Adults & Peds ≥12 yrs:** 2 tabs qd-bid. **Peds 6-<12 yrs:** 1 tab qd-bid.
Ex-Lax Ultra Stimulant Laxative Tablets	Bisacodyl 5mg	**Adults & Peds ≥12 yrs:** 1-3 tabs qd. **Max:** 3 tabs qd. **Peds 6-<12 yrs:** 1 tab qd-bid.
Fleet Bisacodyl Enema	Bisacodyl 10mg/30mL	**Adults & Peds ≥12 yrs:** 1 bottle (30mL).
Fleet Stimulant Laxative Tablets	Bisacodyl 5mg	**Adults & Peds ≥12 yrs:** 1-3 tabs qd. **Peds 6-<12 yrs:** 1 tab qd.
Perdiem Overnight Relief Tablets	Sennosides 15mg	**Adults & Peds ≥12 yrs:** 2 tabs qd-bid. **Peds 6-<12 yrs:** 1 tab qd-bid.

BRAND	INGREDIENTS/STRENGTH	DOSE
Senokot Tablets	Sennosides 8.6mg	**Adults & Peds ≥12 yrs:** 2 tabs qd. **Max:** 4 tabs bid. **Peds 6-<12 yrs:** 1 tab qd. **Max:** 2 tabs bid. **Peds 2-<6 yrs:** ½ tab qd. **Max:** 1 tab bid.
SenokotXTRA Tablets	Sennosides 17.2mg	**Adults & Peds ≥12 yrs:** 1 tab qd. **Max:** 2 tabs bid. **Peds 6-<12 yrs:** ½ tab qd. **Max:** 1 tab bid.
STIMULANT COMBINATIONS		
Peri-Colace Tablets	Sennosides/Docusate 8.6mg-50mg	**Adults & Peds ≥12 yrs:** 2-4 tabs qd. **Peds 6-<12 yrs:** 1-2 tabs qd. **Peds 2-5 yrs:** 1 tab qd.
Senna Prompt	Psyllium/Sennosides 500mg-9mg	**Adults & Peds ≥12 yrs:** 1-5 caps qd-bid.
Senokot S Tablets	Sennosides/Docusate 8.6mg-50mg	**Adults & Peds ≥12 yrs:** 2 tabs qd. **Max:** 4 tabs bid. **Peds 6-<12 yrs:** 1 tab qd. **Max:** 2 tabs bid. **Peds 2-<6 yrs:** ½ tab qd. **Max:** 1 tab bid.
SURFACTANTS (STOOL SOFTENERS)		
Colace Capsules	Docusate sodium 100mg	**Adults & Peds ≥12 yrs:** 1-3 caps qd. **Peds 2-<12 yrs:** 1 cap qd.
Colace Capsules	Docusate sodium 50mg	**Adults & Peds ≥12 yrs:** 1-6 caps qd. **Peds 2-<12 yrs:** 1-3 caps qd.
Colace Syrup	Docusate sodium 60mg/15mL	**Adults & Peds ≥12 yrs:** 1-6 tbl qd. **Peds 2-<12 yrs:** 1-2½ tbl qd.
Docusol Constipation Relief, Mini Enemas	Docusate sodium 283mg	**Adults & Peds ≥12 yrs:** 1-3 units qd. **Peds 6-12 yrs:** 1 unit qd.
Dulcolax Stool Softener Capsules	Docusate sodium 100mg	**Adults & Peds ≥12 yrs:** 1-3 caps qd. **Peds 2-<12 yrs:** 1 cap qd.
Fleet Pedia-Lax Liquid Stool Softener	Docusate 50mg/15mL	**Peds 2-<12 yrs:** 1-3 tbl qd. **Max:** 3 tbl q24h.
Fleet Sof-Lax Capsules	Docusate sodium 100mg	**Adults & Peds ≥12 yrs:** 1-3 caps qd. **Peds 2-<12 yrs:** 1 cap qd.
Surfak Stool Softener	Docusate calcium 240mg	**Adults & Peds ≥12 yrs:** 1 cap qd.
Phillips' Stool Softener Capsules	Docusate sodium 100mg	**Adults & Peds ≥12 yrs:** 1-3 caps qd. **Peds 6-<12 yrs:** 1 cap qd.

NASAL ALLERGIC RHINITIS PRODUCTS

BRAND	INGREDIENTS/STRENGTH	DOSAGE
TOPICAL NASAL DECONGESTANTS		
4-Way Fast Acting Nasal Decongestant Spray	Phenylephrine HCl 1%	**Adults & Peds ≥12 yrs:** Instill 2-3 sprays per nostril q4h.
4-Way Mentholated Nasal Decongestant Spray	Phenylephrine HCl 1%	**Adults & Peds ≥12 yrs:** Instill 2-3 sprays per nostril q4h.
Afrin Original 12 Hour Pump Mist/No Drip/Nasal Spray	Oxymetazoline HCl 0.05%	**Adults & Peds ≥6 yrs:** Instill 2-3 sprays per nostril q10-12h. **Max:** 2 doses q24h.
Afrin Extra Moisturizing No Drip 12 Hour Pump Mist	Oxymetazoline HCl 0.05%	**Adults & Peds ≥6 yrs:** Instill 2-3 sprays per nostril q10-12h. **Max:** 2 doses q24h.
Afrin Sinus 12 Hour Pump Mist/ No Drip Nasal Spray	Oxymetazoline HCl 0.05%	**Adults & Peds ≥6 yrs:** Instill 2-3 sprays per nostril q10-12h. **Max:** 2 doses q24h.
Afrin Severe Congestion 12 Hour Pump Mist/No Drip Nasal Spray	Oxymetazoline HCl 0.05%	**Adults & Peds ≥6 yrs:** Instill 2-3 sprays per nostril q10-12h. **Max:** 2 doses q24h.
Benzedrex Inhaler	Propylhexedrine 250mg	**Adults & Peds ≥6 yrs:** Inhale 2 sprays per nostril q2h. **Max:** Do not use >3 days.
Dristan 12-Hr Nasal Spray	Oxymetazoline HCl 0.05%	**Adults & Peds ≥12 yrs:** Instill 2-3 sprays per nostril q10-12h. **Max:** 2 doses q24h.
Little Noses Decongestant Nose Drops	Phenylephrine HCl 0.125%	**Peds 2-<6 yrs:** Instill 2-3 sprays per nostril q4h.
Mucinex Moisture Smart Nasal Spray	Oxymetazoline HCl 0.05%	**Adults & Peds ≥6 yrs:** Instill 2-3 sprays per nostril q10-12h. **Max:** 2 doses q24h.
Mucinex Full Force Nasal Spray	Oxymetazoline HCl 0.05%	**Adults & Peds ≥6 yrs:** Instill 2-3 sprays per nostril q10-12h. **Max:** 2 doses q24h.
Neo-Synephrine Regular Strength Nasal Spray	Phenylephrine HCl 0.5%	**Adults & Peds ≥12 yrs:** Instill 2-3 sprays per nostril q4h.
Neo-Synephrine Extra Strength Nasal Spray	Phenylephrine HCl 1%	**Adults & Peds ≥12 yrs:** Instill 2-3 sprays per nostril q4h.
Neo-Synephrine Nighttime Nasal Spray	Oxymetazoline HCl 0.05%	**Adults & Peds ≥6 yrs:** Instill 2-3 sprays per nostril q10-12h. **Max:** 2 doses q24h.
Nostrilla Fast Relief	Oxymetazoline HCl 0.05%	**Adults & Peds ≥6 yrs:** Instill 2-3 sprays per nostril q10-12h. **Max:** 2 doses q24h.
Nostrilla Complete Congestion Relief	Oxymetazoline HCl 0.05%	**Adults & Peds ≥6 yrs:** Instill 2-3 sprays per nostril q10-12h. **Max:** 2 doses q24h.
Privine Nasal Drops	Naphazoline HCl 0.05%	**Adults & Peds ≥12 yrs:** Instill 1-2 sprays per nostril q6h.
Privine Nasal Spray	Naphazoline HCl 0.05%	**Adults & Peds ≥12 yrs:** Instill 1-2 sprays per nostril q6h.
Vicks Sinex 12-Hour Decongestant UltraFine Mist Moisturizing Nasal Spray	Oxymetazoline HCl 0.05%	**Adults & Peds ≥6 yrs:** Instill 2-3 sprays per nostril q10-12h. **Max:** 2 doses q24h.
Vicks Sinex 12-Hour Decongestant UltraFine Mist Nasal Spray	Oxymetazoline HCl 0.05%	**Adults & Peds ≥6 yrs:** Instill 2-3 sprays per nostril q10-12h. **Max:** 2 doses q24h.
Vicks Sinex 12-Hour Decongestant Nasal Spray	Oxymetazoline HCl 0.05%	**Adults & Peds ≥6 yrs:** Instill 2-3 sprays per nostril q10-12h. **Max:** 2 doses q24h.
Vicks VapoInhaler	Levmetamfetamine 50mg	**Adults & Peds ≥12 yrs:** Inhale 2 sprays per nostril q2h. **Peds 6-<12 yrs:** Inhale 1 spray per nostril q2h.
Zicam Extreme Congestion Relief Nasal Gel	Oxymetazoline HCl 0.05%	**Adults & Peds ≥6 yrs:** Instill 2-3 sprays per nostril q10-12h. **Max:** 2 doses q24h.
Zicam Intense Sinus Relief Nasal Gel	Oxymetazoline HCl 0.05%	**Adults & Peds ≥6 yrs:** Instill 2-3 sprays per nostril q10-12h. **Max:** 2 doses q24h.

(Continued)

BRAND	INGREDIENTS/STRENGTH	DOSAGE
TOPICAL NASAL MOISTURIZERS		
Ayr Saline Nasal Mist	Sodium chloride 0.65%	**Adults & Peds:** Instill 1 spray per nostril prn.
Ayr Saline Nasal Drops	Sodium chloride 0.65%	**Adults & Peds:** Instill 2-6 drops per nostril prn.
Ayr Allergy & Sinus Hypertonic Saline Nasal Mist	Sodium chloride 2.65%	**Adults & Peds:** Instill 2 sprays per nostril bid-tid.
Baby Ayr Saline Nose Spray/ Drops	Sodium chloride 0.65%	**Peds:** Instill 2-6 drops per nostril.
Ayr Saline Nasal Gel No-Drip Sinus Spray	Sodium chloride*	**Adults & Peds:** Instill 1 spray per nostril.
Ayr Saline Nasal Gel	Sodium chloride*	**Adults & Peds:** Apply around nostrils and under nose prn.
Ayr Saline Nasal Gel Moisturizing Swabs	Sodium chloride 0.65%	**Adults & Peds:** Apply in nostrils prn.
Little Noses Saline Spray/Drops	Sodium chloride 0.65%	**Adults & Peds:** Instill 2-6 drops/sprays per nostril prn.
Little Noses Sterile Saline Nasal Mist	Sodium chloride 0.9%	**Adults & Peds:** Instill 1-3 short sprays per nostril prn.
Nostrilla Conditioning Double-Moisture	Sodium chloride 1.9%*	**Adults & Peds:** Instill 1 spray per nostril prn.
Ocean Gel Ultra Moisturizing Gel	Purified water, Glycerin, Carbomer 940, Trolamine, Hyaluronan, Methylparaben, Propylparaben	**Adults & Peds:** Apply around nostrils and under nose prn.
Ocean Complete Sinus Irrigation	Sodium chloride*	**Adults & Peds:** Attach white actuator and spray into each nostril prn.
Ocean Ultra Sterile Saline Mist	Sodium chloride*	**Adults & Peds:** Spray into each nostril prn.
Ocean for Kids Premium Saline Nasal Spray	Sodium chloride 0.65%	**Peds:** Instill 2 sprays per nostril prn.
Ocean Premium Saline Nasal Spray	Sodium chloride 0.65%	**Adults & Peds:** Instill 2 sprays per nostril prn.
Simply Saline Nasal Allergy and Sinus Relief	Sodium chloride 3%	**Adults & Peds:** Spray into each nostril prn.
Simply Saline Baby Nasal Relief	Sodium chloride 0.9%	**Peds:** Spray into each nostril prn.
Simply Saline Baby Nasal Moisturizer plus Aloe Vera	Sodium chloride*	**Peds:** Apply around nostrils and under nose prn.
Simply Saline Nasal Relief	Sodium chloride 0.9%	**Adults & Peds:** Spray into each nostril prn.
Simply Saline Baby Swabs	Sodium chloride*	**Peds:** Apply in nostrils prn.
MISCELLANEOUS		
NasalCrom Nasal Spray	Cromolyn sodium 5.2mg	**Adults & Peds ≥2 yrs:** Instill 1 spray per nostril q4-6h. **Max:** 6 doses q24h.
Similasan Relief Nasal Spray	*Cardiospermum* 6X, *Galphimia glauca* 6X, *Luffa operculata* 6X, *Sabadilla* 6X	**Adults & Peds:** Instill 1-3 sprays per nostril prn.
Simply Saline Children's Cold Formula plus Moisturizers	*Luffa operculata* 6X, *Sabadilla* 6X	**Adults & Peds ≥2 yrs:** Instill 1 spray per nostril prn.
Simply Saline Cold Formula plus Menthol	*Luffa operculata* 6X, *Sabadilla* 6X	**Adults & Peds ≥2 yrs:** Instill 1 spray per nostril prn.
SinoFresh Nasal & Sinus Care	*Eucalyptus globulus* 20X, Kalium bichromicum 30X	**Adults:** Instill 1-2 sprays per nostril every morning and evening. Gently sniff to distribute solution. Blow nose to clear it of loosened debris and mucus. Re-apply 1 spray to each nostril.

BRAND	INGREDIENTS/STRENGTH	DOSAGE
MISCELLANEOUS *(Continued)*		
Zicam Allergy Relief Nasal Gel	*Luffa operculata* (4X, 12X, 30X), *Galphimia glauca* (12X, 30X), Histaminum hydrochloricum (12X, 30X, 200X), Sulphur (12X, 30X, 200X)	**Adults & Peds ≥12 yrs:** Instill 1 spray per nostril q4h.
Zicam Allergy Relief Gel Swabs	*Galphimia glauca* (12X, 30X), Histaminum hydrochloricum (12X, 30X, 200X), *Luffa operculata* (4X, 12X, 30X), Sulphur (12X, 30X, 200X)	**Adults & Peds ≥12 yrs:** Apply medication just inside first nostril. Remove swab and press lightly on the outside of first nostril for 5 sec. Re-dip swab in tube and repeat with 2nd nostril q4h.

*These products may contain multiple moisturizing agents. Please check product label for a complete list of ingredients.

IS IT A COLD, THE FLU, OR AN ALLERGY?

	COLD	FLU	AIRBORNE ALLERGY
SYMPTOMS			
Chest discomfort	Mild to moderate	Common; can become severe	Sometimes
Cough	Common (hacking cough)	Sometimes	Sometimes
Diarrhea	Never	Sometimes (more common in children)	Never
Duration	3-14 days	Days to weeks	Weeks (eg, 6 weeks for ragweed or grass pollen seasons)
Extreme exhaustion	Never	Early and prominent	Never
Fatigue, weakness	Sometimes	Usual; can last up to 2-3 weeks	Sometimes
Fever	Rare	Characteristic; high (100-102°F; occasionally higher, especially in young children); lasts 3-4 days	Never
General aches, pains	Slight	Usual; often severe	Never
Headache	Rare	Common	Sometimes
Itchy eyes	Rare or never	Rare or never	Common
Runny nose	Common	Common	Common
Sneezing	Usual	Sometimes	Usual
Sore throat	Common	Sometimes	Sometimes
Stuffy nose	Common	Sometimes	Common
Vomiting	Never	Sometimes (more common in children)	Never
TREATMENT			
	Antihistamines*	Amantadine	Antihistamines*
	Decongestants*	Rimantadine	Nasal steroids*
	Nonsteroidal anti-inflammatories*	Oseltamivir	Decongestants*
		Zanamivir	
PREVENTION			
	Wash your hands often; avoid close contact with anyone with a cold	Annual vaccination Amantadine Rimantadine Oseltamivir	Avoid allergens such as pollen, house flies, dust mites, mold, pet dander, cockroaches
COMPLICATIONS			
	Sinus infection	Bronchitis	Sinus infections
	Middle ear infection	Pneumonia	Asthma
	Asthma	Can be life-threatening	
		Can worsen chronic conditions	
		Complications more likely in the elderly, those with chronic conditions, young children, and pregnant women	

Adapted from the National Institute of Allergy and Infectious Diseases, November 2008 and CDC.gov.
*Used only for temporary relief of cold symptoms.

Cough-Cold-Flu-Allergy Products

BRAND NAME	ANALGESIC	ANTIHISTAMINE	DECONGESTANT	COUGH SUPPRESSANT	EXPECTORANT	DOSAGE
ANTIHISTAMINE						
Alavert Quick Dissolving Tablets		Loratadine 10mg				**Adults & Peds ≥6 yrs:** 1 tab qd. **Max:** 1 tab q24h.
Alavert For Kids 6+		Loratadine 10mg				**Adults & Peds ≥6 yrs:** 1 tab qd. **Max:** 1 tab q24h.
Benadryl Allergy Ultratab Tablets		Diphenhydramine HCl 25mg				**Adults & Peds ≥12 yrs:** 1-2 tabs q4-6h. **Peds 6-<12 yrs:** 1 tab q4-6h. **Max:** 6 doses q24h.
Benadryl Allergy Dye-Free Liqui-Gels		Diphenhydramine HCl 25mg				**Adults & Peds ≥12 yrs:** 1-2 caps q4-6h. **Peds 6-<12 yrs:** 1 cap q4-6h. **Max:** 6 doses q24h.
Children's Benadryl Allergy Fastmelt Tablets		Diphenhydramine HCl 12.5mg				**Adults & Peds ≥12 yrs:** 2-4 tabs q4-6h. **Peds 6-<12 yrs:** 1-2 tabs q4-6h. **Max:** 6 doses q24h.
Children's Benadryl Perfect Measure Pre-Filled Single Use Spoons		Diphenhydramine HCl 12.5mg/5mL				**Adults & Peds ≥12 yrs:** 2-4 prefilled spoons (10-20mL) q4-6h. **Peds 6-<12 yrs:** 1-2 prefilled spoons (5-10mL) q4-6h. **Max:** 6 doses q24h.
Children's Benadryl Allergy Liquid		Diphenhydramine HCl 12.5mg/5mL				**Peds 6-<12 yrs:** 1-2 tsp (5-10mL) q4-6h. **Max:** 6 doses q24h.
Children's Benadryl Dye-Free Allergy Liquid		Diphenhydramine HCl 12.5mg/5mL				**Peds 6-<12 yrs:** 1-2 tsp (5-10mL) q4-6h. **Max:** 6 doses q24h.
Claritin Tablets		Loratadine 10mg				**Adults & Peds ≥6 yrs:** 1 tab qd. **Max:** 1 tab q24h.
Claritin Liqui-Gels		Loratadine 10mg				**Adults & Peds ≥6 yrs:** 1 cap qd. **Max:** 1 cap q24h.
Claritin RediTabs 24-Hour		Loratadine 10mg				**Adults & Peds ≥6 yrs:** 1 tab qd. **Max:** 1 tab q24h.
Claritin 12-Hour RediTabs		Loratadine 5mg				**Adults & Peds ≥6 yrs:** 1 tab q12h. **Max:** 2 tabs q24h.

(Continued)

BRAND NAME	ANALGESIC	ANTIHISTAMINE	DECONGESTANT	COUGH SUPPRESSANT	EXPECTORANT	DOSAGE
ANTIHISTAMINE *(Continued)*						
Claritin 24-Hour RediTabs For Kids		Loratadine 10mg				**Adults & Peds ≥6 yrs:** 1 tab qd. **Max:** 1 tab q24h.
Claritin 12-Hour RediTabs For Kids		Loratadine 5mg				**Adults & Peds ≥6 yrs:** 1 tab q12h. **Max:** 2 tabs q24h.
Children's Claritin Chewables		Loratadine 5mg				**Adults & Peds ≥6 yrs:** 2 tabs qd. **Max:** 2 tabs q24h. **Peds 2-<6 yrs:** 1 tab qd. **Max:** 1 tab q24h.
Children's Claritin Syrup		Loratadine 5mg/5mL				**Adults & Peds ≥6 yrs:** 2 tsp (10mL) qd. **Max:** 2 tsp (10mL) q24h. **Peds 2-<6 yrs:** 1 tsp (5mL) qd. **Max:** 1 tsp (5mL) q24h.
Zyrtec Liquid Gels		Cetirizine HCl 10mg				**Adults & Peds 6-<65 yrs:** 1 cap qd. **Max:** 1 cap q24h.
Zyrtec Tablets		Cetirizine HCl 10mg				**Adults & Peds 6-<65 yrs:** 1 tab qd. **Max:** 1 tab q24h.
Children's Zyrtec Perfect Measure		Cetirizine HCl 5mg/5mL				**Adults & Peds 6-<65 yrs:** 1-2 prefilled spoons (5-10mL) qd. **Max:** 2 prefilled spoons (10mL) q24h. **Adults ≥65 yrs:** 1 prefilled spoon (5mL) qd. **Max:** 1 prefilled spoon (5mL) q24h.
Children's Zyrtec Allergy Syrup		Cetirizine HCl 5mg/5mL				**Adults & Peds 6-<65 yrs:** 1-2 tsp (5-10mL) qd. **Max:** 2 tsp (10mL) q24h. **Adults ≥65 yrs:** 1 tsp qd. **Max:** 1 tsp (5mL) q24h. **Peds 2-<6 yrs:** ½-1 tsp (2.5-5mL) qd or ½ tsp q12h. **Max:** 1 tsp (5mL) q24h.
PediaCare Children's Allergy		Diphenhydramine 12.5mg/5mL				**Peds 6-<11 yrs:** 1 tsp (5mL) q4h. **Max:** 6 doses q24h.

BRAND NAME	ANALGESIC	ANTIHISTAMINE	DECONGESTANT	COUGH SUPPRESSANT	EXPECTORANT	DOSAGE
ANTIHISTAMINE (Continued)						
PediaCare Children's 24-Hr Allergy		Cetirizine HCl 5mg/5mL				**Adults & Peds 6-<65 yrs:** 1-2 tsp (5-10mL) qd. **Max:** 2 tsp (10mL) q24h. **Adults ≥65 yrs:** 1 tsp qd. **Max:** 1 tsp (5mL) q24h. **Peds 2-<6 yrs:** ½-1 tsp (2.5-5mL) qd or ½ tsp q12h. **Max:** 1 tsp (5mL) q24h.
ANTIHISTAMINE + DECONGESTANT						
Alavert Allergy & Sinus D-12		Loratadine 5mg	Pseudoephedrine sulfate 120mg			**Adults & Peds ≥12 yrs:** 1 tab q12h. **Max:** 2 tabs q24h.
Allerest PE		Chlorpheniramine maleate 4mg	Phenylephrine HCl 10mg			**Adults & Peds ≥12 yrs:** 1 tab q4h. **Peds 6-<12 yrs:** ½ tab q4h. **Max:** 6 doses q24h.
Benadryl-D Allergy Plus Sinus		Diphenhydramine HCl 25mg	Phenylephrine HCl 10mg			**Adults & Peds ≥12 yrs:** 1 tab q4h. **Max:** 6 tabs q24h.
Children's Benadryl-D Allergy & Sinus Liquid		Diphenhydramine HCl 12.5mg/5mL	Phenylephrine HCl 5mg/5mL			**Adults ≥12 yrs:** 2 tsp (10mL) q4h. **Peds 6-<12 yrs:** 1 tsp (5mL) q4h. **Max:** 6 doses q24h.
Delsym Night Time Cough & Cold Liquid		Diphenhydramine HCl 6.25mg/5mL	Phenylephrine HCl 2.5mg/5mL			**Adults ≥12 yrs:** 2 tbl (30mL) q6h. **Max:** 4 doses q24h
Children's Delsym Night Time Cough & Cold		Diphenhydramine HCl 12.5mg/5mL	Phenylephrine HCl 5mg/5mL			**Adults ≥12 yrs:** 2 tsp (10mL) q4h. **Peds 6-<12 yrs:** 1 tsp (5mL) q4h. **Max:** 6 doses q24h.
Children's Dimetapp Cold & Allergy Chewable Tablets		Brompheniramine maleate 1mg	Phenylephrine HCl 2.5mg			**Peds 6-<12 yrs:** 2 tabs q4h. **Max:** 6 doses q24h.
Children's Dimetapp Cold & Allergy Syrup		Brompheniramine maleate 1mg/5mL	Phenylephrine HCl 2.5mg/5mL			**Adults & Peds ≥12 yrs:** 4 tsp (20mL) q4h. **Peds 6-<12 yrs:** 2 tsp (10mL) q4h. **Max:** 6 doses q24h.
Children's Dimetapp Nighttime Cold & Congestion Liquid		Diphenhydramine HCl 6.25mg/5mL	Phenylephrine HCl 2.5mg/5mL			**Adults & Peds ≥12 yrs:** 4 tsp (20mL) q4h. **Peds 6-<12 yrs:** 2 tsp (10mL) q4h. **Max:** 6 doses q24h.
Claritin-D 12 Hour		Loratadine 5mg	Pseudoephedrine sulfate 120mg			**Adults & Peds ≥12 yrs:** 1 tab q12h. **Max:** 2 tabs q24h.

(Continued)

BRAND NAME	ANALGESIC	ANTIHISTAMINE	DECONGESTANT	COUGH SUPPRESSANT	EXPECTORANT	DOSAGE
ANTIHISTAMINE + DECONGESTANT *(Continued)*						
Claritin-D 24 Hour		Loratadine 10mg	Pseudoephedrine sulfate 240mg			**Adults & Peds ≥12 yrs:** 1 tab qd. **Max:** 1 tab q24h.
Sudafed PE Sinus & Allergy Tablets*		Chlorpheniramine maleate 4mg	Phenylephrine HCl 10mg			**Adults & Peds ≥12 yrs:** 1 tab q4h. **Max:** 6 tabs q24h.
Triaminic Children's Thin Strips Night Time Cold & Cough		Diphenhydramine HCl 12.5mg/strip	Phenylephrine HCl 5mg/strip			**Peds 6-12 yrs:** 1 strip q4h. **Max:** 6 strips q24h.
Triaminic Children's Syrup Night Time Cold & Cough		Diphenhydramine HCl 6.25mg/5mL	Phenylephrine HCl 2.5mg/5mL			**Peds 6–<12 yrs:** 2 tsp (10 mL) q4h. **Max:** 6 doses q24h.
Triaminic Children's Syrup Cold & Allergy		Chlorpheniramine maleate 1mg/5mL	Phenylephrine HCl 2.5mg/5mL			**Peds 6–<12 yrs:** 2 tsp (10 mL) q4h. **Max:** 6 doses q24h.
Zyrtec-D Tablets		Cetirizine HCl 5mg	Pseudoephedrine HCl 120mg			**Adults & Peds 12–<65 yrs:** 1 tab q12h. **Max:** 2 tabs q24h.
ANTIHISTAMINE + DECONGESTANT + ANALGESIC						
Advil Allergy Sinus Caplets	Ibuprofen 200mg	Chlorpheniramine maleate 2mg	Pseudoephedrine HCl 30mg			**Adults & Peds ≥12 yrs:** 1 tab q4-6h. **Max:** 6 tabs q24h.
Alka-Seltzer Plus Cold Formula Effervescent Tablets	Aspirin 325mg	Chlorpheniramine maleate 2mg	Phenylephrine bitartrate 7.8mg			**Adults & Peds ≥12 yrs:** 2 tabs q4h. **Max:** 8 tabs q24h.
Alka-Seltzer Plus Fast Crystal Packs	Acetaminophen 650mg/packet	Chlorpheniramine maleate 4mg/packet	Phenylephrine HCl 10mg/packet			**Adults & Peds ≥12 yrs:** 1 pkt q4h. **Max:** 5 pkts q24h.
Benadryl Allergy Plus Cold Kapgels*	Acetaminophen 325mg	Diphenhydramine HCl 12.5mg	Phenylephrine HCl 5mg			**Adults & Peds ≥12 yrs:** 2 caps q4h. **Max:** 12 caps q24h.
Benadryl Severe Allergy Plus Sinus Headache Caplets*	Acetaminophen 325mg	Diphenhydramine HCl 25mg	Phenylephrine HCl 5mg			**Adults & Peds ≥12 yrs:** 2 tabs q4h. **Max:** 12 tabs q24h.
Benadryl Allergy Plus Sinus Headache Kapgels*	Acetaminophen 325mg	Diphenhydramine HCl 12.5mg	Phenylephrine HCl 5mg			**Adults & Peds ≥12 yrs:** 2 caps q4h. **Max:** 12 caps q24h.
Comtrex Severe Cold & Sinus Caplets Day and Night	Acetaminophen 325mg	Chlorpheniramine maleate 2mg	Phenylephrine HCl 5mg (nighttime dose only)			**Adults & Peds ≥12 yrs:** 2 daytime tabs q4h. 2 nighttime tabs hs. **Max:** 8 daytime tabs, 4 nighttime tabs q24h.
Dristan Cold Multi-Symptom Formula Tablets	Acetaminophen 325mg	Chlorpheniramine maleate 2mg	Phenylephrine HCl 5mg			**Adults & Peds ≥12 yrs:** 2 tabs q4h. **Max:** 12 tabs q24h.
Robitussin Peak Cold Nighttime Nasal Relief	Acetaminophen 325mg	Chlorpheniramine maleate 2mg	Phenylephrine HCl 5mg			**Adults & Peds ≥12 yrs:** 2 tabs q4h. **Max:** 12 tabs q24h.

BRAND NAME	ANALGESIC	ANTIHISTAMINE	DECONGESTANT	COUGH SUPPRESSANT	EXPECTORANT	DOSAGE
ANTIHISTAMINE + DECONGESTANT + ANALGESIC *(Continued)*						
Sudafed PE Severe Cold Formula Caplets*	Acetaminophen 325mg	Diphenhydramine HCl 12.5mg	Phenylephrine HCl 5mg			**Adults & Peds ≥12 yrs:** 2 tabs q4h. **Max:** 12 tabs q24h.
Theraflu Cold & Sore Throat Powder Packets	Acetaminophen 325mg/packet	Pheniramine maleate 20mg/packet	Phenylephrine HCl 10mg/packet			**Adults & Peds ≥12 yrs:** 1 pkt q4h. **Max:** 6 pkts q24h.
Theraflu Nighttime Severe Cold & Cough Powder Packets	Acetaminophen 650mg/packet	Diphenhydramine HCl 25mg/packet	Phenylephrine HCl 10mg/packet			**Adults & Peds ≥12 yrs:** 1 pkt q4h. **Max:** 6 pkts q24h.
Theraflu Sinus & Cold	Acetaminophen 325mg/packet	Pheniramine maleate 20mg/packet	Phenylephrine HCl 10mg/packet			**Adults & Peds ≥12 yrs:** 1 pkt q4h. **Max:** 6 pkts q24h.
Theraflu Sugar-Free Nighttime Severe Cold & Cough Powder Packets	Acetaminophen 650mg/packet	Diphenhydramine HCl 25mg/packet	Phenylephrine HCl 10mg/packet			**Adults & Peds ≥12 yrs:** 1 pkt q4h. **Max:** 6 pkts q24h.
Theraflu Flu & Sore Throat Powder Packets	Acetaminophen 650mg/packets	Pheniramine maleate 20mg/packet	Phenylephrine HCl 10mg/packet			**Adults & Peds ≥12 yrs:** 1 pkt q4h. **Max:** 6 pkts q24h.
Theraflu Warming Relief Nighttime Severe Cough & Cold	Acetaminophen 325mg/15mL	Diphenhydramine HCl 12.5mg/15mL	Phenylephrine HCl 5mg/15mL			**Adults & Peds ≥12 yrs:** 2 tbl (30mL) q4h. **Max:** 6 doses (12 tbl or 180mL) q24h.
Theraflu Warming Relief Flu & Sore Throat	Acetaminophen 325mg/15mL	Diphenhydramine HCl 12.5mg/15mL	Phenylephrine HCl 5mg/15mL			**Adults & Peds ≥12 yrs:** 2 tbl (30mL) q4h. **Max:** 6 doses (12 tbl or 180mL) q24h.
Theraflu Warming Relief Sinus & Cold	Acetaminophen 325mg/15mL	Diphenhydramine HCl 12.5mg/15mL	Phenylephrine HCl 5mg/15mL			**Adults & Peds ≥12 yrs:** 2 tbl (30mL) q4h. **Max:** 6 doses (12 tbl or 180mL) q24h.
Children's Tylenol Plus Cold	Acetaminophen 160mg/5mL	Chlorpheniramine maleate 1mg/5mL	Phenylephrine HCl 2.5mg/5mL			**Peds 6-11 yrs (48-95 lbs):** 2 tsp (10mL) q4h. **Max:** 5 doses q24h.
Children's Tylenol Plus Cold and Allergy	Acetaminophen 160mg/5mL	Diphenhydramine HCl 12.5mg/5mL	Phenylephrine HCl 2.5mg/5mL			**Peds 6-11 yrs (48-95 lbs):** 2 tsp (10mL) q4h. **Max:** 5 doses q24h.
Robitussin Peak Cold Nighttime Multi-Symptom Cold	Acetaminophen 160mg/5mL	Diphenhydramine HCl 6.25mg/5mL	Phenylephrine HCl 2.5mg/5mL			**Adults & Peds ≥12 yrs:** 4 tsp (20mL) q4h. **Max:** 6 doses q24h.
Tylenol Allergy Multi-Symptom*	Acetaminophen 325mg	Chlorpheniramine maleate 2mg	Phenylephrine HCl 5mg			**Adults & Peds ≥12 yrs:** 2 tabs q4h. **Max:** 12 tabs q24h.
Tylenol Allergy Multi-Symptom Nighttime*	Acetaminophen 325mg	Diphenhydramine HCl 25mg	Phenylephrine HCl 5mg			**Adults & Peds ≥12 yrs:** 2 tabs q4h. **Max:** 12 tabs q24h.

(Continued)

BRAND NAME	ANALGESIC	ANTIHISTAMINE	DECONGESTANT	COUGH SUPPRESSANT	EXPECTORANT	DOSAGE
ANTIHISTAMINE + DECONGESTANT + ANALGESIC *(Continued)*						
Vicks NyQuil Sinex LiquiCaps	Acetaminophen 325mg	Doxylamine succinate 6.25mg	Phenylephrine HCl 5mg			**Adults & Peds ≥12 yrs:** 2 caps q4h. **Max:** 4 doses q24h.
COUGH SUPPRESSANT						
Children's Delsym Cough Medicine				Dextromethorphan HBr 30mg/5mL		**Adults & Peds ≥12 yrs:** 2 tsp (10mL) q12h. **Max:** 4 tsp (20mL) q24h. **Peds 6-<12 yrs:** 1 tsp (5mL) q12h. **Max:** 2 tsp (10mL) q24h. **Peds 4-<6 yrs:** ½ tsp (2.5mL) q12h. **Max:** 1 tsp (5mL) q24h.
Delsym Cough Medicine				Dextromethorphan HBr 30mg/5mL		**Adults & Peds ≥12 yrs:** 2 tsp (10mL) q12h. **Max:** 4 tsp (20mL) q24h. **Peds 6-<12 yrs:** 1 tsp (5mL) q12h. **Max:** 2 tsp (10mL) q24h. **Peds 4-<6 yrs:** ½ tsp (2.5mL) q12h. **Max:** 1 tsp (5mL) q24h.
Children's Robitussin Cough Long-Acting				Dextromethorphan HBr 7.5mg/5mL		**Adults & Peds ≥12 yrs:** 4 tsp (20mL) q6-8h. **Peds 6-<12 yrs:** 2 tsp (10mL) q6-8h. **Peds 4-<6 yrs:** 1 tsp (5mL) q6-8h. **Max:** 4 doses q24h.
Robitussin Cough Long-Acting				Dextromethorphan HBr 15mg/5mL		**Adults & Peds ≥12 yrs:** 2 tsp (10mL) q6-8h. **Max:** 4 doses q24h.
Robitussin Lingering Cold Long-Acting CoughGels				Dextromethorphan HBr 15mg		**Adults & Peds ≥12 yrs:** 2 caps q6-8h. **Max:** 8 caps q24h.
Triaminic Long-Acting Cough				Dextromethorphan HBr 7.5mg/5mL		**Peds 6-<12 yrs:** 2 tsp (10mL) q6-8h. **Peds 4-<6 yrs:** 1 tsp (5mL) q6-8h. **Max:** 4 doses q24h.
Vicks DayQuil Cough				Dextromethorphan HBr 15mg/5mL		**Adults & Peds ≥12 yrs:** 2 tbl (30mL) q6-8h. **Peds 6-12 yrs:** 1 tbl (15mL) q6-8h. **Max:** 4 doses q24h.
Vicks Formula 44 Custom Care Dry Cough Suppressant				Dextromethorphan HBr 30mg/15mL		**Adults & Peds ≥12 yrs:** 1 tbl (15mL) q6-8h. **Peds 6-12 yrs:** 1½ tsp (7.5mL) q6-8h. **Max:** 4 doses q24h.

BRAND NAME	ANALGESIC	ANTIHISTAMINE	DECONGESTANT	COUGH SUPPRESSANT	EXPECTORANT	DOSAGE
COUGH SUPPRESSANT *(Continued)*						
Vicks Baby Rub Soothing Vapor Ointment				Petrolatum, fragrance, aloe extract, eucalyptus oil, lavender oil, rosemary oil		**Peds ≥3 months:** Gently massage on the chest, neck, and back to help soothe and comfort
Vicks VapoRub Topical Cream				Camphor 5.2%, Menthol 2.8%, Eucalyptus 1.2%		**Adults & Peds ≥2 yrs:** Apply to chest and throat. **Max:** tid per 24h.
Vicks VapoRub Topical Ointment				Camphor 4.8%, Menthol 2.6%, Eucalyptus 1.2%		**Adults & Peds ≥2 yrs:** Apply to chest and throat. **Max:** tid per 24h.
Vicks VapoSteam				Camphor 6.2%		**Adults & Peds ≥2 yrs:** 1 tbl/quart q8h or 1½ tsp/pint q8h (for use in a hot steam vaporizer). **Max:** tid per 24h.
Vicks Vapodrops				Menthol 1.7mg (cherry); Menthol 3.3mg (menthol)		**Peds ≥5 yrs:** 3 drops (cherry), **Peds >5 yrs:** 2 drops (menthol)
COUGH SUPPRESSANT + ANTIHISTAMINE						
Coricidin HBP Cough & Cold		Chlorpheniramine maleate 4mg		Dextromethorphan HBr 30mg		**Adults & Peds ≥12 yrs:** 1 tab q6h. **Max:** 4 tabs q24h.
Children's Dimetapp Long-Acting Cough Plus Cold		Chlorpheniramine maleate 1mg/5mL		Dextromethorphan HBr 7.5mg/5mL		**Adults & Peds ≥12 yrs:** 4 tsp (20mL) q6h. **Peds 6-<12 yrs:** 2 tsp (10mL) q6h. **Max:** 4 doses q24h.
Children's Robitussin Cough & Cold Long-Acting		Chlorpheniramine maleate 1mg/5mL		Dextromethorphan HBr 7.5mg/5mL		**Adults & Peds ≥12 yrs:** 4 tsp (20mL) q6h. **Peds 6-<12 yrs:** 2 tsp (10mL) q6h. **Max:** 4 doses q24h.
Vicks Children's NyQuil Cold & Cough		Chlorpheniramine maleate 2mg/15mL		Dextromethorphan HBr 15mg/15mL		**Adults & Peds ≥12 yrs:** 2 tbl (30mL) q6h. **Peds 6-11 yrs:** 1 tbl (15mL) q6h. **Max:** 4 doses q24h.
Vicks NyQuil Cough		Doxylamine succinate 6.25mg/15mL		Dextromethorphan HBr 15mg/15mL		**Adults & Peds ≥12 yrs:** 2 tbl (30mL) q6h. **Max:** 4 doses q24h.
COUGH SUPPRESSANT + ANALGESIC						
PediaCare Children's Fever Reducer Plus Cough and Sore Throat with APAP	Acetaminophen 160mg/5mL			Dextromethorphan 5mg/5mL		**Peds 6-11 yrs (48-95 lbs):** 2 tsp (10mL) q4h. **Max:** 5 times in 24 hrs.

(Continued)

BRAND NAME	ANALGESIC	ANTIHISTAMINE	DECONGESTANT	COUGH SUPPRESSANT	EXPECTORANT	DOSAGE
COUGH SUPPRESSANT + ANALGESIC (Continued)						
Triaminic Cough & Sore Throat	Acetaminophen 160mg/5mL			Dextromethorphan HBr 5mg/5mL		**Peds 6-<12 yrs:** 2 tsp (10mL) q4h. **Peds 4-<6 yrs:** 1 tsp (5mL) q4h. **Max:** 5 doses q24h.
Tylenol Cold & Cough Daytime*	Acetaminophen 500mg/15mL			Dextromethorphan HBr 15mg/15mL		**Adults & Peds ≥12 yrs:** 2 tbl (30mL) q6h. **Max:** 8 tbl q24h.
COUGH SUPPRESSANT + ANTIHISTAMINE + ANALGESIC						
Coricidin HBP Day & Night Multi-Symptom Cold	Acetaminophen 500mg (nighttime dose only)	Chlorpheniramine maleate 2mg (nighttime dose only)		Dextromethorphan HBr 10mg (daytime dose), 15mg (nighttime dose)	Guaifenesin 200mg (daytime dose only)	(Day) **Adults & Peds ≥12 yrs:** 1-2 softgels q4h. **Max:** 6 tabs q12h. (Night) **Adults & Peds ≥12 yrs:** 2 tabs ths and q6h. **Max:** 4 tabs q12h.
Coricidin HBP Maximum Strength Flu	Acetaminophen 500mg	Chlorpheniramine maleate 2mg		Dextromethorphan HBr 15mg		**Adults & Peds ≥12 yrs:** 2 tabs q6h. **Max:** 8 tabs q24h.
Coricidin HBP Nighttime Multi-Symptom Cold Liquid	Acetaminophen 500mg/15mL	Doxylamine succinate 6.25mg/15mL		Dextromethorphan HBr 15mg/15mL		**Adults & Peds ≥12 yrs:** 2 tbl (30mL) q6h. **Max:** 4 doses q24h.
Delsym Night Time Multi-Symptom	Acetaminophen 325mg/15mL	Doxylamine succinate 6.25mg/15mL		Dextromethorphan HBr 15mg/15mL		**Adults & Peds ≥12 yrs:** 2 tbl (30mL) q6h. **Max:** 4 doses q24h.
PediaCare Children's Fever Reducer Plus Cough and Runny Nose with Acetaminophen	Acetaminophen 160mg/5mL	Chlorpheniramine maleate 1mg/5mL		Dextromethorphan HBr 5mg/5mL		**Peds 6-11 yrs (48-95 lbs):** 2 tsp (10mL) q4h. **Max:** 5 times in 24 hrs.
Triaminic Multi-Symptom Fever	Acetaminophen 160mg/5mL	Chlorpheniramine maleate 1mg/5mL		Dextromethorphan HBr 7.5mg/5mL		**Peds 6-<12 yrs:** 2 tsp (10mL) q6h. **Max:** 4 doses q24h.
Children's Tylenol Plus Cough & Runny Nose	Acetaminophen 160mg/5mL	Chlorpheniramine maleate 1mg/5mL		Dextromethorphan HBr 5mg/5mL		**Peds 6-11 yrs (48-95 lbs):** 2 tsp (10mL) q4h. **Max:** 5 doses in 24 hrs.
Tylenol Cold and Cough Nighttime Liquid*	Acetaminophen 500mg/15mL	Doxylamine 6.25mg/15mL		Dextromethorphan HBr 15mg/15mL		**Adults & Peds ≥12 yrs:** 2 tbl (30mL) q6h. **Max:** 8 tbl q24h.
Vicks Formula 44 Custom Care Cough & Cold PM	Acetaminophen 650mg/15mL	Chlorpheniramine maleate 4mg/15mL		Dextromethorphan 30mg/15mL		**Adults & Peds ≥12 yrs:** 1 tbl (15mL) q6h. **Max:** 4 doses q24h.
Vicks NyQuil Cold & Flu Relief Liquid	Acetaminophen 325mg/15mL	Doxylamine succinate 6.25mg/15mL		Dextromethorphan HBr 15mg/15mL		**Adults & Peds ≥12 yrs:** 2 tbl (30mL) q6h. **Max:** 4 doses q24h.
Vicks NyQuil Cold & Flu Relief LiquiCaps	Acetaminophen 325mg	Doxylamine succinate 6.25mg		Dextromethorphan HBr 15mg		**Adults & Peds ≥12 yrs:** 2 caps q6h. **Max:** 4 doses q24h.
Vicks Alcohol Free NyQuil, Cold and Flu Relief Liquid	Acetaminophen 325mg/15mL	Chlorpheniramine maleate 2mg/15mL		Dextromethorphan 15mg/15mL		**Adults & Peds ≥12 yrs:** 2 tbl (30mL) q6h. **Max:** 4 doses q24h.

BRAND NAME	ANALGESIC	ANTIHISTAMINE	DECONGESTANT	COUGH SUPPRESSANT	EXPECTORANT	DOSAGE
COUGH SUPPRESSANT + ANTIHISTAMINE + ANALGESIC + DECONGESTANT						
Alka-Seltzer Plus Cold & Cough Formula Effervescent Tablets	Aspirin 325mg	Chlorpheniramine maleate 2mg	Phenylephrine bitartrate 7.8mg	Dextromethorphan HBr 10mg		**Adults & Peds ≥12 yrs:** 2 tabs q4h. **Max:** 8 tabs q24h.
Alka-Seltzer Plus Cold & Cough Formula Liquid Gels	Acetaminophen 325mg	Chlorpheniramine maleate 2mg	Phenylephrine HCl 5mg	Dextromethorphan HBr 10mg		**Adults & Peds ≥12 yrs:** 2 caps q4h. **Max:** 12 caps q24h.
Alka-Seltzer Plus Flu Formula Effervescent Tablets	Acetaminophen 250mg	Chlorpheniramine maleate 2mg	Phenylephrine HCl 5mg	Dextromethorphan HBr 10mg		**Adults & Peds ≥12 yrs:** 2 tabs q4h. **Max:** 8 tabs q24h.
Alka-Seltzer Plus Night Cold Formula Effervescent Tablets	Aspirin 500mg	Doxylamine succinate 6.25mg	Phenylephrine bitartrate 7.8mg	Dextromethorphan HBr 10mg		**Adults & Peds ≥12 yrs:** 2 tabs q4-6h. **Max:** 8 tabs q24h.
Alka-Seltzer Plus Night Cold Formula Liquid Gels	Acetaminophen 325mg	Doxylamine succinate 6.25mg	Phenylephrine HCl 5mg	Dextromethorphan HBr 10mg		**Adults & Peds ≥12 yrs:** 2 caps q4h. **Max:** 12 caps q24h.
Comtrex Nighttime Cough & Cold Caplets	Acetaminophen 325mg	Chlorpheniramine maleate 2mg	Phenylephrine HCl 5mg	Dextromethorphan HBr 10mg		**Adults & Peds ≥12 yrs:** 2 tabs q4h. **Max:** 12 tabs q24h.
Children's Dimetapp Multisymptom Cold & Flu	Acetaminophen 160mg/5mL	Chlorpheniramine maleate 1mg/5mL	Phenylephrine HCl 2.5mg/5mL	Dextromethorphan HBr 5mg/5mL		**Adults & Peds ≥12 yrs:** 4 tsp (20mL) q4h. **Peds 6-<12 yrs:** 2 tsp (10mL) q4h. **Max:** 5 doses q24h.
Theraflu Warming Relief Nighttime Multi-Symptom Cold Caplets	Acetaminophen 325mg	Chlorpheniramine maleate 2mg	Phenylephrine HCl 5mg	Dextromethorphan HBr 10mg		**Adults & Peds ≥12 yrs:** 2 tabs q4h. **Max:** 12 tabs q24h.
Children's Tylenol Plus Multi-Symptom Cold	Acetaminophen 160mg/5mL	Chlorpheniramine maleate 1mg/5mL	Phenylephrine HCl 2.5mg/5mL	Dextromethorphan HBr 5mg/5mL		**Peds 6-11 yrs (48-95 lbs):** 2 tsp (10mL) q4h. **Max:** 5 doses q24h.
PediaCare Children's Fever Reducer Plus Flu Plus Acetaminophen	Acetaminophen 160mg/5mL	Chlorpheniramine maleate 1mg/5mL	Phenylephrine HCl 2.5mg/5mL	Dextromethorphan HBr 5mg/5mL		**Peds 6-11 yrs (48-95 lbs):** 2 tsp (10mL) q4h. **Max:** 5 times in 24 hrs.
PediaCare Children's Fever Reducer Plus Multi-Symptom Cold Plus Acetaminophen	Acetaminophen 160mg/5mL	Chlorpheniramine maleate 1mg/5mL	Phenylephrine HCl 2.5mg/5mL	Dextromethorphan HBr 5mg/5mL		**Peds 6-11 yrs (48-95 lbs):** 2 tsp (10mL) q4h. **Max:** 5 times in 24 hrs.
Theraflu Warming Relief Caplets Nighttime Multi-Symptom Cold	Acetaminophen 325mg	Chlorpheniramine maleate 2mg	Phenylephrine HCl 5mg	Dextromethorphan HBr 10mg		**Adults & Peds ≥12 yrs:** 2 tabs q4h. **Max:** 12 tabs q24h.
Tylenol Cold Head Congestion Nighttime	Acetaminophen 325mg	Chlorpheniramine maleate 2mg	Phenylephrine HCl 5mg	Dextromethorphan HBr 10mg		**Adults & Peds ≥12 yrs:** 2 tabs q4h. **Max:** 12 tabs q24h.
Tylenol Cold Multi-Symptom Nighttime Gelcaps	Acetaminophen 325mg	Chlorpheniramine maleate 2mg	Phenylephrine HCl 5mg	Dextromethorphan HBr 10mg		**Adults & Peds ≥12 yrs:** 2 tabs q4h. **Max:** 12 tabs q24h.

(Continued)

BRAND NAME	ANALGESIC	ANTIHISTAMINE	DECONGESTANT	COUGH SUPPRESSANT	EXPECTORANT	DOSAGE
COUGH SUPPRESSANT + ANTIHISTAMINE + ANALGESIC + DECONGESTANT (Continued)						
Tylenol Cold Multi-Symptom Nighttime Liquid	Acetaminophen 325mg/15mL	Doxylamine succinate 6.25mg/30mL	Phenylephrine HCl 5mg/15mL	Dextromethorphan HBr 10mg/15mL		**Adults & Peds ≥12 yrs:** 2 tbl (30mL) q4h. **Max:** 12 tbl (180mL) q24h.
Children's Tylenol Plus Flu	Acetaminophen 160mg/5mL	Chlorpheniramine maleate 1mg/5mL	Phenylephrine HCl 2.5mg/5mL	Dextromethorphan HBr 5mg/5mL		**Peds 6-11 yrs (48-95 lbs):** 2 tsp (10mL) q4h. **Max:** 5 times in 24 hrs.
COUGH SUPPRESSANT + ANTIHISTAMINE + DECONGESTANT						
Children's Dimetapp Cold & Cough Syrup		Brompheniramine maleate 1mg/5mL	Phenylephrine HCl 2.5mg/5mL	Dextromethorphan HBr 5mg/5mL		**Adults & Peds ≥12 yrs:** 4 tsp (20mL) q4h. **Peds 6-<12 yrs:** 2 tsp (10mL) q4h. **Max:** 6 doses q24h.
COUGH SUPPRESSANT + DECONGESTANT						
PediaCare Children's Multi-Symptom Cold			Phenylephrine HCl 2.5mg/5mL	Dextromethorphan HBr 5mg/5mL		**Peds 6-11 yrs:** 2 tsp (10mL) q4h. **Peds 4-5 yrs:** 1 tsp (5mL) q4h. **Max:** 6 doses q24h.
Children's Sudafed PE Cold & Cough Liquid			Phenylephrine HCl 2.5mg/5mL	Dextromethorphan HBr 5mg/5mL		**Peds 6-11 yrs:** 2 tsp (10mL) q4h. **Peds 4-5 yrs:** 1 tsp (5mL) q4h. **Max:** 6 doses q24h.
Day Time Triaminic Thin Strips Cold & Cough			Phenylephrine HCl 2.5mg/strip	Dextromethorphan HBr 5mg/strip		**Peds 6-<12 yrs:** 2 strips q4h. **Peds 4-<6 yrs:** 1 strip q4h. **Max:** 6 doses q24h.
Triaminic Day Time Cold & Cough			Phenylephrine HCl 2.5mg/5mL	Dextromethorphan HBr 5mg/5mL		**Peds 6-<12 yrs:** 2 tsp (10mL) q4h. **Peds 4-<6 yrs:** 1 tsp (5mL) q4h. **Max:** 6 doses q24h.
COUGH SUPPRESSANT + DECONGESTANT + ANALGESIC						
Alka-Seltzer Plus Day Non-Drowsy Cold Formula Liquid Gels	Acetaminophen 325mg		Phenylephrine HCl 5mg	Dextromethorphan HBr 10mg		**Adults & Peds ≥12 yrs:** 2 caps q4h. **Max:** 12 caps q24h.
Alka-Seltzer Plus Day & Night Cold Formula Liquid Gels	Acetaminophen 325mg	Doxylamine 6.25mg (nighttime dose only)	Phenylephrine HCl 5mg	Dextromethorphan HBr 10mg		**Adults & Peds ≥12 yrs:** 2 caps q4h. **Max:** 12 caps q24h.
Alka-Seltzer Plus Day & Night Cold Formula Effervescent Tablets	Aspirin 325mg (day); Aspirin 500mg (night)	Doxylamine 6.25mg (nighttime dose only)	Phenylephrine bitartrate 7.8mg	Dextromethorphan HBr 10mg		**Adults & Peds ≥12 yrs:** 2 tabs q4h. **Max:** 8 tabs q24h.
Theraflu Warming Relief Caplets Daytime Multi-Symptom Cold	Acetaminophen 325mg		Phenylephrine HCl 5mg	Dextromethorphan HBr 10mg		**Adults & Peds ≥12 yrs:** 2 tabs q4h. **Max:** 12 tabs q24h.

BRAND NAME	ANALGESIC	ANTIHISTAMINE	DECONGESTANT	COUGH SUPPRESSANT	EXPECTORANT	DOSAGE
COUGH SUPPRESSANT + DECONGESTANT + ANALGESIC *(Continued)*						
Theraflu Daytime Severe Cold & Cough Powder Packets	Acetaminophen 650mg/packet		Phenylephrine HCl 10mg/packet	Dextromethorphan HBr 20mg/packet		**Adults & Peds ≥12 yrs:** 1 pkt q4h. **Max:** 6 pkts q24h.
Theraflu Multi-Symptom Severe Cold with Lipton Green Tea & Honey Lemon Flavors Powder Packets	Acetaminophen 500mg/packet		Phenylephrine HCl 10mg/packet	Dextromethorphan HBr 20mg/packet		**Adults & Peds ≥12 yrs:** 1 pkt q4h. **Max:** 6 pkts q24h.
Theraflu Warming Relief Daytime Severe Cold & Cough Liquid	Acetaminophen 325mg/15mL		Phenylephrine HCl 5mg/15mL	Dextromethorphan HBr 10mg/15mL		**Adults & Peds ≥12 yrs:** 2 tbl (30mL) q4h. **Max:** 6 doses q24h.
Children's Tylenol Plus Cold & Cough	Acetaminophen 160mg/5mL		Phenylephrine HCl 2.5mg/5mL	Dextromethorphan HBr 5mg/5mL		**Peds 6-11 yrs (48-95 lbs):** 2 tsp (10mL) q4h. **Peds 4-5 yrs (36-47 lbs):** 1 tsp (5mL) q4h. **Max:** 5 doses q24h.
Tylenol Cold Head Congestion Daytime	Acetaminophen 325mg		Phenylephrine HCl 5mg	Dextromethorphan HBr 10mg		**Adults & Peds ≥12 yrs:** 2 caps q4h. **Max:** 12 caps q24h.
Tylenol Cold Multi-Symptom Daytime Gelcaps/Caplets	Acetaminophen 325mg		Phenylephrine HCl 5mg	Dextromethorphan HBr 10mg		**Adults & Peds ≥12 yrs:** 2 caps q4h. **Max:** 12 caps q24h.
Tylenol Cold Multi-Symptom Daytime Liquid	Acetaminophen 325mg/15mL		Phenylephrine HCl 5mg/15mL	Dextromethorphan HBr 10mg/15mL		**Adults & Peds ≥12 yrs:** 2 tbl (30mL) q4h. **Max:** 12 tbl (180 mL) q24h.
Vicks DayQuil Cold & Flu Relief LiquiCaps	Acetaminophen 325mg		Phenylephrine HCl 5mg	Dextromethorphan HBr 10mg		**Adults & Peds ≥12 yrs:** 2 doses q4h. **Max:** 4 doses q24h.
Vicks DayQuil Cold & Flu Relief Liquid	Acetaminophen 325mg/15mL		Phenylephrine HCl 5mg/15mL	Dextromethorphan HBr 10mg/15mL		**Adults & Peds ≥12 yrs:** 2 tbl (30mL) q4h. **Peds 6-<12 yrs:** 1 tbl (15mL) q4h. **Max:** 4 doses q24h.
COUGH SUPPRESSANT + DECONGESTANT + EXPECTORANT						
Entex PAC (Entex-T tabs + Entex-S liquid)			Pseudoephedrine HCl 60mg	Dextromethorphan HBr 20mg/5mL	Guaifenesin 375mg	**Adults & Peds ≥12 yrs:** 1 tab q4-6h. **Peds 6-<12 yrs:** ½ tab q4-6h. **Max:** 4 doses q24h. **Liquid: Adults & Peds ≥12 yrs:** 1 tsp (5mL) q4h. **Peds 6-<12 yrs:** ½ tsp (2.5mL) q4h. **Max:** 4 doses q24h.
Maximum Strength Mucinex Fast-Max Severe Congestion & Cough Liquid			Phenylephrine HCl 5mg/10mL	Dextromethorphan HBr 10mg/10mL	Guaifenesin 200mg/10mL	**Adults & Peds ≥12 yrs:** 4 tsp (20mL) q4h.

(Continued)

BRAND NAME	ANALGESIC	ANTIHISTAMINE	DECONGESTANT	COUGH SUPPRESSANT	EXPECTORANT	DOSAGE
COUGH SUPPRESSANT + DECONGESTANT + EXPECTORANT *(Continued)*						
Children's Robitussin Cough & Cold CF			Phenylephrine HCl 2.5mg/5mL	Dextromethorphan HBr 5mg/5mL	Guaifenesin 50mg/5mL	**Adults & Peds ≥12 yrs:** 4 tsp (20mL) q4h. **Peds 6–<12 yrs:** 2 tsp (10mL) q4h. **Peds 4–<6 yrs:** 1 tsp (5mL) q4h. **Max:** 6 doses q24h.
Robitussin Peak Cold Multi-Symptom Cold			Phenylephrine HCl 5mg/5mL	Dextromethorphan HBr 10mg/5mL	Guaifenesin 100mg/5mL	**Adults & Peds ≥12 yrs:** 2 tsp (10mL) q4h. **Max:** 6 doses q24h.
Children's Mucinex Multi-Symptom Cold Liquid (Very Berry Flavor)			Phenylephrine 2.5mg	Dextromethorphan HBr 5mg	Guaifenesin 100mg	**Peds 6–12 yrs:** 10mL q4h. **Peds 4–<6 yrs:** 5mL q4h. **Max:** 6 doses q24h.
COUGH SUPPRESSANT + DECONGESTANT + EXPECTORANT + ANALGESIC						
Children's Mucinex Cold, Cough & Sore Throat Liquid	Acetaminophen 325mg/10mL		Phenylephrine HCl 5mg/10mL	Dextromethorphan HBr 10mg/10mL	Guaifenesin 200mg/10mL	**Peds 6–<12 yrs:** 2 tsp (10mL) q4h. **Peds 4–<6 yrs:** 1 tsp (5mL) q4h.
Maximum Strength Mucinex Fast-Max Cold, Flu & Sore Throat Liquid	Acetaminophen 325mg/10mL		Phenylephrine HCl 5mg/10mL	Dextromethorphan HBr 10mg/10mL	Guaifenesin 200mg/10mL	**Adults & Peds ≥12 yrs:** 4 tsp (20mL) q4h.
Children's Mucinex Multi-Symptom Cold & Fever Liquid	Acetaminophen 325mg/10mL		Phenylephrine HCl 5mg/10mL	Dextromethorphan HBr 10mg/10mL	Guaifenesin 200mg/10mL	**Peds 6–<12 yrs:** 2 tsp (10mL) q4h. **Peds 4–<6 yrs:** 1 tsp (5mL) q4h.
Sudafed PE Cold & Cough Caplets*	Acetaminophen 325mg		Phenylephrine HCl 5mg	Dextromethorphan HBr 10mg	Guaifenesin 100mg	**Adults & Peds ≥12 yrs:** 2 tabs q4h. **Max:** 12 tabs q24h.
Theraflu Max-D Severe Cold & Flu Powder Packets	Acetaminophen 1000mg/packet		Pseudoephedrine HCl 60mg/packet	Dextromethorphan HBr 30mg/packet	Guaifenesin 400mg/packet	**Adults & Peds ≥12 yrs:** 1 pkt q6h. **Max:** 4 pkts q24h.
Tylenol Cold & Flu Caplets	Acetaminophen 325mg		Phenylephrine HCl 5mg	Dextromethorphan HBr 10mg	Guaifenesin 200mg	**Adults & Peds ≥12 yrs:** 2 tabs q4h. **Max:** 12 tabs q24h.
Tylenol Cold & Flu Liquid	Acetaminophen 325mg/15mL		Phenylephrine HCl 5mg/15mL	Dextromethorphan HBr 10mg/15mL	Guaifenesin 200mg/15mL	**Adults & Peds ≥12 yrs:** 2 tbl (30mL) q4h. **Max:** 12 tbl (180mL) q24h.
Tylenol Cold Multi-Symptom Severe Liquid	Acetaminophen 325mg/15mL		Phenylephrine HCl 5mg/15mL	Dextromethorphan HBr 10mg/15mL	Guaifenesin 200mg/15mL	**Adults & Peds ≥12 yrs:** 2 tbl (30mL) q4h. **Max:** 12 tbl (180mL) q24h.
Tylenol Cold Head Congestion Severe	Acetaminophen 325mg		Phenylephrine HCl 5mg	Dextromethorphan HBr 10mg	Guaifenesin 200mg	**Adults & Peds ≥12 yrs:** 2 tabs q4h. **Max:** 12 tabs q24h.
COUGH SUPPRESSANT + EXPECTORANT						
Alka-Seltzer Plus Mucus & Congestion Liquid Gels				Dextromethorphan HBr 10mg	Guaifenesin 200mg	**Adults & Peds ≥12 yrs:** 2 caps q4h. **Max:** 12 caps q24h.

BRAND NAME	ANALGESIC	ANTIHISTAMINE	DECONGESTANT	COUGH SUPPRESSANT	EXPECTORANT	DOSAGE
COUGH SUPPRESSANT + EXPECTORANT *(Continued)*						
Coricidin HBP Chest Congestion & Cough				Dextromethorphan HBr 10mg	Guaifenesin 200mg	**Adults & Peds ≥12 yrs:** 1-2 caps q4h. **Max:** 12 caps q24h.
Maximum Strength Mucinex DM				Dextromethorphan HBr 60mg	Guaifenesin 1200mg	**Adults & Peds ≥12 yrs:** 1 tab q12h. **Max:** 2 tabs q24h.
Maximum Strength Mucinex Fast-Max DM Max Liquid				Dextromethorphan HBr 10mg/10mL	Guaifenesin 200mg/10mL	**Adults & Peds ≥12 yrs:** 4 tsp (20mL) q4h.
Mucinex Cough Liquid (Cherry Flavor)				Dextromethorphan HBr 5mg/5mL	Guaifenesin 100mg/5mL	**Peds 6-<12 yrs:** 1-2 tsp (5-10mL) q4h. **Peds 4-<6 yrs:** ½-1 tsp (2.5-5mL) q4h. **Max:** 6 doses q24h.
Mucinex Cough Mini-Melts (Orange Crème Flavor)				Dextromethorphan HBr 5mg	Guaifenesin 100mg	**Adults & Peds ≥12 yrs:** 2-4 pkts q4h. **Peds 6-<12 yrs:** 1-2 pkts q4h. **Peds 4-<6 yrs:** 1 pkt q4h. **Max:** 6 doses q24h.
Mucinex DM				Dextromethorphan HBr 30mg	Guaifenesin 600mg	**Adults & Peds ≥12 yrs:** 1-2 tabs q12h. **Max:** 4 tabs q24h.
PediaCare Children's Cough & Congestion				Dextromethorphan HBr 5mg/5mL	Guaifenesin 100mg/5mL	**Peds 6-11 yrs (48-95 lbs):** 1-2 tsp (5-10mL) q4h. **Peds 4-5 yrs (36-47 lbs):** ½-1 tsp (2.5-5mL) q4h. **Max:** 6 doses q24h.
Robitussin Peak Cold Maximum Strength Cough + Chest Congestion DM				Dextromethorphan HBr 10mg/5mL	Guaifenesin 200mg/5mL	**Adults & Peds ≥12 yrs:** 2 tsp (10mL) q4h. **Max:** 6 doses q24h.
Robitussin Peak Cold Cough & Chest Congestion DM				Dextromethorphan HBr 10mg/5mL	Guaifenesin 100mg/5mL	**Adults & Peds ≥12 yrs:** 2 tsp (10mL) q4h. **Max:** 6 doses q24h.
Robitussin Peak Cold Cough & Chest Congestion Sugar-Free DM				Dextromethorphan HBr 10mg/5mL	Guaifenesin 100mg/5mL	**Adults & Peds ≥12 yrs:** 2 tsp (10mL) q4h. **Max:** 6 doses q24h.
Vicks DayQuil Mucus Control DM				Dextromethorphan HBr 10mg/15mL	Guaifenesin 200mg/15mL	**Adults & Peds ≥12 yrs:** 2 tbl (30mL) q4h. **Peds 6-12 yrs:** 1 tbl (15mL) q4h. **Max:** 6 doses q24h.
Vicks Formula 44 Custom Care Chesty Cough				Dextromethorphan HBr 20mg/15mL	Guaifenesin 200mg/15mL	**Adults & Peds ≥12 yrs:** 1 tbl (15mL) q4h. **Peds 6-<12 yrs:** 1½ tsp (7.5mL) q4h. **Max:** 6 doses q24h.

(Continued)

BRAND NAME	ANALGESIC	ANTIHISTAMINE	DECONGESTANT	COUGH SUPPRESSANT	EXPECTORANT	DOSAGE
DECONGESTANT						
Mucinex Moisture Smart Nasal Spray			Oxymetazoline HCl 0.05%			**Adults & Peds ≥6 yrs:** 2-3 sprays in each nostril q10-12h. **Max:** 2 doses q24h.
Mucinex Full Force Nasal Spray			Oxymetazoline HCl 0.05%			**Adults & Peds ≥6 yrs:** 2-3 sprays in each nostril q10-12h. **Max:** 2 doses q24h.
PediaCare Children's Decongestant			Phenylephrine HCl 2.5mg/5mL			**Peds 6-11 yrs:** 2 tsp (10mL) q4h. **Peds 4-5 yrs:** 1 tsp (5mL) q4h. **Max:** 6 doses q24h.
Children's Sudafed Nasal Decongestant Liquid			Pseudoephedrine HCl 15mg/5mL			**Peds 6-11 yrs:** 2 tsp (10mL) q4-6h. **Peds 4-5 yrs:** 1 tsp (5mL) q4-6h. **Max:** 4 doses q24h.
Children's Sudafed PE Nasal Decongestant Liquid			Phenylephrine HCl 2.5mg/5mL			**Peds 6-11 yrs:** 2 tsp (10mL) q4h. **Peds 4-5 yrs:** 1 tsp (5mL) q4h. **Max:** 6 doses q24h.
Sudafed 12-Hour Tablets			Pseudoephedrine HCl 120mg			**Adults & Peds ≥12 yrs:** 1 tab q12h. **Max:** 2 tabs q24h.
Sudafed 24-Hour Tablets			Pseudoephedrine HCl 240mg			**Adults & Peds ≥12 yrs:** 1 tab q24h. **Max:** 1 tab q24h.
Sudafed Congestion			Pseudoephedrine HCl 30mg			**Adults & Peds ≥12 yrs:** 2 tabs q4-6h **Max:** 8 tabs q24h.
Sudafed OM Sinus Congestion Spray			Oxymetazoline HCl 0.05%			**Adults & Peds ≥6 yrs:** 2-3 sprays in each nostril q10-12h. **Max:** 2 doses q24h.
Sudafed PE Congestion*			Phenylephrine HCl 10mg			**Adults & Peds ≥12 yrs:** 1 tab q4h. **Max:** 6 tabs q24h.
Vicks Sinex 12-Hour Decongestant Nasal Spray			Oxymetazoline HCl 0.05%			**Adults & Peds ≥6 yrs:** Instill 2-3 sprays per nostril q10-12h. **Max:** 2 doses q24h.
Vicks Sinex 12-Hour Decongestant UltraFine Mist			Oxymetazoline HCl 0.05%			**Adults & Peds ≥6 yrs:** Instill 2-3 sprays per nostril q10-12h. **Max:** 2 doses q24h.

BRAND NAME	ANALGESIC	ANTIHISTAMINE	DECONGESTANT	COUGH SUPPRESSANT	EXPECTORANT	DOSAGE
DECONGESTANT *(Continued)*						
Vicks VapoInhaler			Levmetamfetamine 50mg			**Adults & Peds ≥12 yrs:** 2 inhalations per nostril q2h. **Peds 6–<12 yrs:** 1 inhalation per nostril q2h.
DECONGESTANT + ANALGESIC						
Advil Cold & Sinus Caplets/ Liqui-Gels	Ibuprofen 200mg		Pseudoephedrine HCl 30mg			**Adults & Peds ≥12 yrs:** 1-2 caps q4-6h. **Max:** 6 caps q24h.
Advil Congestion Relief	Ibuprofen 200mg		Phenylephrine HCl 10mg			**Adults & Peds ≥12 yrs:** 1 tabs q4h. **Max:** 6 tabs q24h.
Alka-Seltzer Plus Sinus Formula Effervescent Tablets	Aspirin 325mg		Phenylephrine bitartrate 7.8mg			**Adults & Peds ≥12 yrs:** 2 tabs q4h. **Max:** 8 tabs q24h.
Contac Cold + Flu Maximum Strength (Non-Drowsy)	Acetaminophen 500mg		Phenylephrine HCl 5mg			**Adults & Peds ≥12 yrs:** 2 tabs q4-6h. **Max:** 8 tabs q24h.
Robitussin Peak Cold Nasal Relief	Acetaminophen 325mg		Phenylephrine HCl 5mg			**Adults & Peds ≥12 yrs:** 2 tabs q4h. **Max:** 12 tabs q24h.
Sudafed PE Pressure and Pain Caplets*	Acetaminophen 325mg		Phenylephrine HCl 5mg			**Adults & Peds ≥12 yrs:** 2 tabs q4h. **Max:** 12 tabs q24h.
Sudafed 12-Hour Pressure and Pain Caplets	Naproxen Sodium 220mg		Pseudoephedrine HCl 120mg			**Adults & Peds ≥12 yrs:** 1 tab q12h. **Max:** 2 tabs q24h.
Children's Tylenol Plus Cold & Stuffy Nose	Acetaminophen 160mg/5mL		Phenylephrine HCl 2.5mg/5mL			**Peds 6-11 yrs (48-95 lbs):** 2 tsp (10mL) q4h. **Peds 4-5 yrs (36-47 lbs):** 1 tsp (5mL) q4h. **Max:** 5 doses q24h.
Tylenol Sinus Congestion & Pain Daytime*	Acetaminophen 325mg		Phenylephrine HCl 5mg			**Adults & Peds ≥12 yrs:** 2 caps q4h. **Max:** 12 caps q24h.
DECONGESTANT + EXPECTORANT						
Entex LQ			Phenylephrine HCl 10mg/5mL		Guaifenesin 100mg/5mL	**Adults & Peds ≥12 yrs:** 1 tsp (5mL) q4h. **Peds 6-<12 yrs:** ½ tsp 2.5mL) q4h. **Peds 2-<6 yrs:** ¼ tsp (1.25mL) q4h. **Max:** 6 doses q24h.
Entex T			Pseudoephedrine HCl 60mg		Guaifenesin 375mg	**Adults & Peds ≥12 yrs:** 1 tab q4-6h. **Peds 6-<12 yrs:** ½ tab q4-6h. **Max:** 4 doses q24h.

(Continued)

BRAND NAME	ANALGESIC	ANTIHISTAMINE	DECONGESTANT	COUGH SUPPRESSANT	EXPECTORANT	DOSAGE
DECONGESTANT + EXPECTORANT (Continued)						
Maximum Strength Mucinex D			Pseudoephedrine HCl 120mg		Guaifenesin 1200mg	**Adults & Peds ≥12 yrs:** 1 tab q12h. **Max:** 2 tabs q24h.
Mucinex Cold Liquid (Mixed Berry Flavor)			Phenylephrine HCl 2.5mg/5mL		Guaifenesin 100mg/5mL	**Peds 6–12 yrs:** 2 tsp (10mL) q4h. **Peds 4–<6 yrs:** 1 tsp (5mL) q4h. **Max:** 6 doses q24h.
Mucinex D			Pseudoephedrine HCl 60mg		Guaifenesin 600mg	**Adults & Peds ≥12 yrs:** 2 tabs q12h. **Max:** 4 tabs q24h.
Sudafed PE Non-Drying Sinus Caplets*			Phenylephrine HCl 5mg		Guaifenesin 200mg	**Adults & Peds ≥12 yrs:** 2 tabs q4h. **Max:** 12 tabs q24h.
Triaminic Chest & Nasal Congestion			Phenylephrine HCl 2.5mg/5mL		Guaifenesin 50mg/5mL	**Peds 6–<12 yrs:** 2 tsp (10mL) q4h. **Peds 4–<6 yrs:** 1 tsp (5mL) q4h. **Max:** 6 doses q24h.
DECONGESTANT + EXPECTORANT + ANALGESIC						
Maximum Strength Mucinex Fast-Max Cold & Sinus Liquid	Acetaminophen 325mg/10mL		Phenylephrine HCl 5mg/10mL		Guaifenesin 200mg/10mL	**Adults & Peds ≥12 yrs:** 4 tsp (20mL) q4h.
Sudafed Triple Action Caplets*	Acetaminophen 325mg		Pseudoephedrine HCl 30mg		Guaifenesin 200mg	**Adults & Peds ≥12 yrs:** 2 tabs q4-6h. **Max:** 8 tabs q24h.
Theraflu Warming Relief Cold & Chest Congestion Liquid	Acetaminophen 325mg/15mL		Phenylephrine HCl 5mg/15mL		Guaifenesin 200mg/15mL	**Adults & Peds ≥12 yrs:** 2 tbl (30mL) q4h. **Max:** 6 doses q24h.
Tylenol Sinus Congestion & Pain Severe*	Acetaminophen 325mg		Phenylephrine HCl 5mg		Guaifenesin 200mg	**Adults & Peds ≥12 yrs:** 2 tabs q4h. **Max:** 12 tabs q24h.
Tylenol Sinus Severe Congestion Daytime*	Acetaminophen 325mg		Pseudoephedrine HCl 30mg		Guaifenesin 200mg	**Adults & Peds ≥12 yrs:** 2 tabs q4-6h. **Max:** 8 tabs q24h.
EXPECTORANT						
Maximum Strength Mucinex					Guaifenesin 1200mg	**Adults & Peds ≥12 yrs:** 1 tab q12h. **Max:** 2 tabs q24h.
Mucinex					Guaifenesin 600mg	**Adults & Peds ≥12 yrs:** 1-2 tabs q12h. **Max:** 4 tabs q24h.
Mucinex Chest Congestion Liquid (Grape Flavor)					Guaifenesin 100mg/5mL	**Peds 6–<12 yrs:** 1-2 tsp (5-10mL) q4h. **Peds 4–<6 yrs:** ½-1 tsp (2.5-5mL) q4h. **Max:** 6 doses q24h.

BRAND NAME	ANALGESIC	ANTIHISTAMINE	DECONGESTANT	COUGH SUPPRESSANT	EXPECTORANT	DOSAGE
EXPECTORANT *(Continued)*						
Mucinex Mini-Melts (Bubble Gum Flavor)					Guaifenesin 100mg/pkt	**Adults & Peds ≥12 yrs:** 2-4 pkts q4h. **Peds 6-<12 yrs:** 1-2 pkts q4h. **Peds 4-<6 yrs:** 1 pkt q4h. **Max:** 6 doses q24h.
Mucinex Mini-Melts (Grape Flavor)					Guaifenesin 50mg/pkt	**Peds 6-<12 yrs:** 2-4 pkts q4h. **Peds 4-<6 yrs:** 1-2 pkts q4h. **Max:** 6 doses q24h.
EXPECTORANT + ANALGESIC						
Theraflu Flu & Chest Congestion Powder Packets	Acetaminophen 1000mg/packet				Guaifenesin 400mg/packet	**Adults & Peds ≥12 yrs:** 1 pkt q6h. **Max:** 4 pkts q24h.
ANTIHISTAMINE + ANALGESIC						
Advil PM Caplets/Liqui-Gels	Ibuprofen 200mg	Diphenhydramine citrate 38mg				**Adults & Peds ≥12 yrs:** 2 caps hs. **Max:** 2 caps q24h.
Coricidin HBP Cold & Flu	Acetaminophen 325mg	Chlorpheniramine maleate 2mg				**Adults & Peds ≥12 yrs:** 2 tabs q4-6h **Max:** 12 tabs q24h. **Peds 6-<12 yrs:** 1 tab q4-6h. **Max:** 5 tabs q24h.
Motrin PM	Ibuprofen 200mg	Diphenhydramine citrate 38mg				**Adults & Peds ≥12 yrs:** 2 tabs hs. **Max:** 2 tabs q24h.
Tylenol Severe Allergy*	Acetaminophen 500mg	Diphenhydramine HCl 12.5mg				**Adults & Peds ≥12 yrs:** 2 tabs q4-6h. **Max:** 8 tabs q24h.

*Product currently on recall or temporarily unavailable from manufacturer but generic forms may be available.

ANALGESIC PRODUCTS

BRAND	INGREDIENTS/STRENGTH	DOSE
ACETAMINOPHEN		
Anacin Extra Strength Aspirin Free Caplets	Acetaminophen 500mg	**Adults & Peds ≥12 yrs:** 2 tabs q6h. **Max:** 8 tabs q24h.
FeverAll Children's Suppositories	Acetaminophen 120mg	**Peds 3-6 yrs:** 1 supp q4-6h. **Max:** 6 supp q24h.
FeverAll Infants' Suppositories	Acetaminophen 80mg	**Peds 6-11 months:** 1 supp q6h. **12-36 months:** 1 supp q4h. **Max:** 6 supp q24h.
FeverAll Jr. Strength Suppositories	Acetaminophen 325mg	**Peds 6-12 yrs:** 1 supp q4-6h. **Max:** 6 supp q24h.
Tylenol 8 Hour Caplets*	Acetaminophen 650mg	**Adults & Peds ≥12 yrs:** 2 tabs q8h prn. **Max:** 6 tabs q24h.
Tylenol Arthritis Caplets	Acetaminophen 650mg	**Adults:** 2 tabs q8h prn. **Max:** 6 tabs q24h.
Tylenol Arthritis Gelcaps	Acetaminophen 650mg	**Adults:** 2 gelcaps q8h prn. **Max:** 6 caps q24h.
Tylenol Children's Meltaways Tablets†	Acetaminophen 80mg	**Peds 2-3 yrs (24-35 lbs):** 2 tabs. **4-5 yrs (36-47 lbs):** 3 tabs. **6-8 yrs (48-59 lbs):** 4 tabs. **9-10 yrs (60-71 lbs):** 5 tabs. **11 yrs (72-95 lbs):** 6 tabs. May repeat q4h. **Max:** 5 doses q24h.
Tylenol Children's Suspension	Acetaminophen 160mg/5mL	**Peds 2-3 yrs (24-35 lbs):** 1 tsp (5mL). **4-5 yrs (36-47 lbs):** 1.5 tsp (7.5mL). **6-8 yrs (48-59 lbs):** 2 tsp (10mL). **9-10 yrs (60-71 lbs):** 2.5 tsp (12.5mL). **11 yrs (72-95 lbs):** 3 tsp (15mL). May repeat q4h. **Max:** 5 doses q24h.
Tylenol Extra Strength Caplets	Acetaminophen 500mg	**Adults & Peds ≥12 yrs:** 2 caps q6h prn. **Max:** 6 caps q24h.
Tylenol Extra Strength Rapid Release Gelcaps	Acetaminophen 500mg	**Adults & Peds ≥12 yrs:** 2 caps q6h prn. **Max:** 6 caps q24h.
Tylenol Extra Strength Rapid Blast Liquid	Acetaminophen 500mg/15mL	**Adults & Peds ≥12 yrs:** 2 tbl (30mL) q6h prn. **Max:** 6 tbl (90mL) q24h.
Tylenol Extra Strength EZ Tablets	Acetaminophen 500mg	**Adults & Peds ≥12 years:** 2 tabs q6h prn. **Max:** 6 tabs q24h.
Tylenol Infants' Oral Suspension Liquid*	Acetaminophen 160mg/5mL	**Peds 2-3 yrs (24-35 lbs):** 5mL q4h prn. **Max:** 5 doses q24h.
Tylenol Junior Meltaways Tablets†	Acetaminophen 160mg	**Peds 6-8 yrs (48-59 lbs):** 2 tabs. **9-10 yrs (60-71 lbs):** 2.5 tabs. **11 yrs (72-95 lbs):** 3 tabs. May repeat q4h. **Max:** 5 doses q24h.
Tylenol Regular Strength Tablets	Acetaminophen 325mg	**Adults & Peds ≥12 yrs:** 2 tabs q4-6h prn. **Max:** 12 tabs q24h. **Peds 6-11 yrs:** 1 tab q4-6h. **Max:** 5 tabs q24h.
ACETAMINOPHEN COMBINATIONS		
Excedrin Back & Body Caplets*	Acetaminophen/Aspirin buffered 250mg-250mg	**Adults & Peds ≥12 yrs:** 2 tabs q6h prn. **Max:** 8 tabs q24h.
Excedrin Extra Strength Caplets*	Acetaminophen/Aspirin/Caffeine 250mg-250mg-65mg	**Adults & Peds ≥12 yrs:** 2 tabs q6h prn. **Max:** 8 tabs q24h.
Excedrin Extra Strength Geltabs*	Acetaminophen/Aspirin/Caffeine 250mg-250mg-65mg	**Adults & Peds ≥12 yrs:** 2 tabs q6h prn. **Max:** 8 tabs q24h.

(Continued)

BRAND	INGREDIENTS/STRENGTH	DOSE
ACETAMINOPHEN COMBINATIONS *(Continued)*		
Excedrin Extra Strength Express Gels*	Acetaminophen/Aspirin/Caffeine 250mg-250mg-65mg	**Adults & Peds ≥12 yrs:** 2 tabs q6h prn. **Max:** 8 tabs q24h.
Excedrin Extra Strength Tablets*	Acetaminophen/Aspirin/Caffeine 250mg-250mg-65mg	**Adults & Peds ≥12 yrs:** 2 tabs q6h prn. **Max:** 8 tabs q24h.
Excedrin Menstrual Complete Express Gels*	Acetaminophen/Aspirin/Caffeine 250mg-250mg-65mg	**Adults & Peds ≥12 yrs:** 2 caps q4-6h prn. **Max:** 8 tabs q24h.
Excedrin Migraine Caplets*	Acetaminophen/Aspirin/Caffeine 250mg-250mg-65mg	**Adults:** 2 tabs prn. **Max:** 2 tabs q24h.
Excedrin Migraine Geltabs*	Acetaminophen/Aspirin/Caffeine 250mg-250mg-65mg	**Adults:** 2 tabs prn. **Max:** 2 tabs q24h.
Excedrin Migraine Tablets*	Acetaminophen/Aspirin/Caffeine 250mg-250mg-65mg	**Adults:** 2 tabs prn. **Max:** 2 tabs q24h.
Excedrin Sinus Headache Caplets*	Acetaminophen/Phenylephrine HCl 325mg-5mg	**Adults & Peds ≥12 yrs:** 2 tabs q4h. **Max:** 12 tabs q24h.
Excedrin Tension Headache Caplets*	Acetaminophen/Caffeine 500mg-65mg	**Adults & Peds ≥12 yrs:** 2 tabs q6h. **Max:** 8 tabs q24h.
Excedrin Tension Headache Express Gels*	Acetaminophen/Caffeine 500mg-65mg	**Adults & Peds ≥12 yrs:** 2 caps q6h. **Max:** 8 caps q24h.
Excedrin Tension Headache Geltabs*	Acetaminophen/Caffeine 500mg-65mg	**Adults & Peds ≥12 yrs:** 2 tabs q6h. **Max:** 8 tabs q24h.
Goody's Body Pain Powder	Acetaminophen/Aspirin 325mg-500mg	**Adults & Peds ≥12 yrs:** Place 1 powder on tongue q6h. **Max:** 4 powders q24h.
Goody's Cool Orange	Acetaminophen/Aspirin/Caffeine 325mg-500mg-65mg	**Adults & Peds ≥12 yrs:** Place 1 powder on tongue q6h. **Max:** 4 powders q24h.
Goody's Extra Strength Headache Powder	Acetaminophen/Aspirin/Caffeine 260mg-500mg-32.5mg	**Adults & Peds ≥12 yrs:** 1 powder q6h. **Max:** 4 powders q24h.
Midol Menstrual Complete Caplets	Acetaminophen/Caffeine/Pyrilamine maleate 500mg-60mg-15mg	**Adults & Peds ≥12 yrs:** 2 tabs q6h. **Max:** 8 tabs q24h.
Midol Complete Gelcaps	Acetaminophen/Caffeine/Pyrilamine maleate 500mg-60mg-15mg	**Adults & Peds ≥12 yrs:** 2 caps q6h. **Max:** 8 caps q24h.
Midol Teen Formula Caplets	Acetaminophen/Pamabrom 500mg-25mg	**Adults & Peds ≥12 yrs:** 2 tabs q6h. **Max:** 8 tabs q24h.
Pamprin Cramp Caplets	Acetaminophen/Magnesium salicylate/Pamabrom 250mg-250mg-25mg	**Adults & Peds ≥12 yrs:** 2 tabs q4-6h. **Max:** 8 tabs q24h.
Pamprin Max Caplets	Acetaminophen/Aspirin/Caffeine 250mg-250mg-65mg	**Adults & Peds ≥12 yrs:** 2 tabs q4-6h. **Max:** 8 tabs q24h.
Pamprin Multi-Symptom Caplets	Acetaminophen/Pamabrom/Pyrilamine 500mg-25mg-15mg	**Adults & Peds ≥12 yrs:** 2 tabs q4-6h. **Max:** 8 tabs q24h.
Premsyn PMS Caplets	Acetaminophen/Pamabrom/Pyrilamine 500mg-25mg-15mg	**Adults & Peds ≥12 yrs:** 2 tabs q4-6h. **Max:** 8 tabs q24h.
Vanquish Caplets	Acetaminophen/Aspirin/Caffeine 194mg-227mg-33mg	**Adults & Peds ≥12 yrs:** 2 tabs q6h. **Max:** 8 tabs q24h.
ACETAMINOPHEN/SLEEP AIDS		
Excedrin PM Caplets*	Acetaminophen/Diphenhydramine Citrate 500mg-38mg	**Adults & Peds ≥12 yrs:** 2 tabs qhs. **Max:** 2 tabs q24h.
Excedrin PM Express Gels*	Acetaminophen/Diphenhydramine Citrate 500mg-38mg	**Adults & Peds ≥12 yrs:** 2 tabs qhs. **Max:** 2 tabs q24h.
Goody's PM Powder	Acetaminophen/Diphenhydramine 500mg-38mg	**Adults & Peds ≥12 yrs:** 2 powders hs prn.
Midol PM Caplets	Acetaminophen/Diphenhydramine Citrate 500mg-38mg	**Adults & Peds ≥12 yrs:** 2 tabs hs prn.

BRAND	INGREDIENTS/STRENGTH	DOSE
ACETAMINOPHEN/SLEEP AIDS *(Continued)*		
Tylenol PM Caplets	Acetaminophen/Diphenhydramine 500mg-25mg	**Adults & Peds ≥12 yrs:** 2 tabs hs prn. **Max:** 2 tabs q24h.
Tylenol PM Rapid Release Gels*	Acetaminophen/Diphenhydramine 500mg-25mg	**Adults & Peds ≥12 yrs:** 2 caps hs prn. **Max:** 2 caps q24h.
Tylenol PM Geltabs	Acetaminophen/Diphenhydramine 500mg-25mg	**Adults & Peds ≥12 yrs:** 2 tabs hs prn. **Max:** 2 tabs q24h.
NSAIDs		
Advil Caplets	Ibuprofen 200mg	**Adults & Peds ≥12 yrs:** 1-2 tabs q4-6h. **Max:** 6 tabs q24h.
Advil Children's Suspension	Ibuprofen 100mg/5mL	**Peds 2-3 yrs (24-35 lbs):** 1 tsp (5mL). **4-5 yrs (36-47 lbs):** 1.5 tsp (7.5mL). **6-8 yrs (48-59 lbs):** 2 tsp (10mL). **9-10 yrs (60-71 lbs):** 2.5 tsp (12.5mL). **11 yrs (72-95 lbs):** 3 tsp (15mL). May repeat q6-8h. **Max:** 4 doses q24h.
Advil Gel Caplets	Ibuprofen 200mg	**Adults & Peds ≥12 yrs:** 1-2 tabs q4-6h. **Max:** 6 tabs q24h.
Advil Infants' Concentrated Drops	Ibuprofen 50mg/1.25mL	**Peds 6-11 months (12-17 lbs):** 1.25mL. **12-23 months (18-23 lbs):** 1.875mL. May repeat q6-8h. **Max:** 4 doses q24h.
Advil Junior Strength Chewable Tablets	Ibuprofen 100mg	**Peds 6-8 yrs (48-59 lbs):** 2 tabs. **9-10 yrs (60-71 lbs):** 2.5 tabs. **11 yrs (72-95 lbs):** 3 tabs. May repeat q6-8h. **Max:** 4 doses q24h.
Advil Junior Strength Tablets	Ibuprofen 100mg	**Peds 6-10 yrs (48-71 lbs):** 2 tabs. **11 yrs (72-95 lbs):** 3 tabs. May repeat q6-8h. **Max:** 4 doses q24h.
Advil Liqui-Gels	Ibuprofen 200mg	**Adults & Peds ≥12 yrs:** 1-2 caps q4-6h. **Max:** 6 caps q24h.
Advil Migraine Capsules	Ibuprofen 200mg	**Adults:** 2 caps prn. **Max:** 2 caps q24h.
Advil Tablets	Ibuprofen 200mg	**Adults & Peds ≥12 yrs:** 1-2 tabs q4-6h. **Max:** 6 tabs q24h.
Aleve Caplets	Naproxen sodium 220mg	**Adults & Peds ≥12 yrs:** 1 tab q8-12h. May take 1 additional tab within 1h of first dose. **Max:** 2 tabs q8-12h or 3 tabs q24h.
Aleve Gelcaps	Naproxen sodium 220mg	**Adults & Peds ≥12 yrs:** 1 cap q8-12h. May take 1 additional cap within 1h of first dose. **Max:** 2 caps q8-12h or 3 caps q24h.
Aleve Liquid Gels	Naproxen sodium 220mg	**Adults & Peds ≥12 yrs:** 1 cap q8-12h. May take 1 additional cap within 1h of first dose. **Max:** 2 caps q8-12h or 3 caps q24h.
Aleve Tablets	Naproxen sodium 220mg	**Adults & Peds ≥12 yrs:** 1 tab q8-12h. May take 1 additional tab within 1h of first dose. **Max:** 2 tabs q8-12h or 3 tabs q24h.
Midol Liquid Gels	Ibuprofen 200mg	**Adults & Peds ≥12 yrs:** 1-2 caps q4-6h. **Max:** 6 caps q24h.
Midol Extended Relief Caplets	Naproxen sodium 220mg	**Adults & Peds ≥12 yrs:** 1-2 tabs q8-12h. **Max:** 2 tabs q8-12h or 3 tabs q24h.
Motrin Children's Suspension*	Ibuprofen 100mg/5mL	**Peds 2-3 yrs (24-35 lbs):** 1 tsp (5mL). **4-5 yrs (36-47 lbs):** 1.5 tsp (7.5mL). **6-8 yrs (48-59 lbs):** 2 tsp (10mL). **9-10 yrs (60-71 lbs):** 2.5 tsp (12.5mL). **11 yrs (72-95 lbs):** 3 tsp (15mL). May repeat q6-8h. **Max:** 4 doses q24h.

(Continued)

BRAND	INGREDIENTS/STRENGTH	DOSE
NSAIDs *(Continued)*		
Motrin IB Caplets	Ibuprofen 200mg	**Adults & Peds ≥12 yrs:** 1-2 tabs q4-6h. **Max:** 6 tabs q24h.
Motrin IB Tablets	Ibuprofen 200mg	**Adults & Peds ≥12 yrs:** 1-2 tabs q4-6h. **Max:** 6 tabs q24h.
Motrin Infants' Drops*	Ibuprofen 50mg/1.25mL	**Peds 6-11 months (12-17 lbs):** 1.25mL. **12-23 months (18-23 lbs):** 1.875mL. May repeat q6-8h. **Max:** 4 doses q24h.
Motrin Junior Strength Caplets*	Ibuprofen 100mg	**Peds 6-8 yrs (48-59 lbs):** 2 tabs. **9-10 yrs (60-71 lbs):** 2.5 tabs. **11 yrs (72-95 lbs):** 3 tabs. May repeat q6-8h. **Max:** 4 doses q24h.
Motrin Junior Strength Chewable Tablets*	Ibuprofen 100mg	**Peds 2-3 yrs (24-35 lbs):** 1 tab. **4-5 yrs (36-47 lbs):** 1.5 tabs. **6-8 yrs (48-59 lbs):** 2 tabs. **9-10 yrs (60-71 lbs):** 2.5 tabs. **11 yrs (72-95 lbs):** 3 tabs. May repeat q6-8h. **Max:** 4 doses q24h.
Pamprin All Day Caplets	Naproxen sodium 220mg	**Adults & Peds ≥12 yrs:** 1-2 tabs q8-12h. **Max:** 2 tabs q8-12h or 3 tabs q24h.
NSAID SLEEP AIDS		
Advil PM Caplets	Ibuprofen/Diphenhydramine citrate 200mg-38mg	**Adults & Peds ≥12 yrs:** 2 tabs qhs. **Max:** 2 tabs q24h.
Advil PM Liqui-Gels	Ibuprofen/Diphenhydramine 200mg-25mg	**Adults & Peds ≥12 yrs:** 2 caps qhs. **Max:** 2 caps q24h.
Motrin PM Caplets	Ibuprofen/Diphenhydramine citrate 200mg-38mg	**Adults & Peds ≥12 yrs:** 2 tabs qhs. **Max:** 2 tabs q24h.
SALICYLATES		
Bayer Aspirin Extra Strength Caplets	Aspirin 500mg	**Adults & Peds ≥12 yrs:** 1-2 tabs q4-6h. **Max:** 8 tabs q24h.
Bayer Aspirin Safety Coated Caplets	Aspirin 325mg	**Adults & Peds ≥12 yrs:** 1-2 tabs q4h. **Max:** 12 tabs q24h.
Bayer Low Dose Aspirin Chewable Tablets†	Aspirin 81mg	**Adults & Peds ≥12 yrs:** 4-8 tabs q4h. **Max:** 48 tabs q24h.
Bayer Low Dose Aspirin Safety Coated Tablets	Aspirin 81mg	**Adults & Peds ≥12 yrs:** 4-8 tabs q4h. **Max:** 48 tabs q24h.
Bayer Genuine Aspirin Tablets	Aspirin 325mg	**Adults & Peds ≥12 yrs:** 1-2 tabs q4h or 3 tabs q6h. **Max:** 12 tabs q24h.
Doan's Extra Strength Caplets	Magnesium salicylate tetrahydrate 580mg	**Adults & Peds ≥12 yrs:** 2 tabs q6h. **Max:** 8 tabs q24h.
Ecotrin Low Strength Tablets	Aspirin 81mg	**Adults:** 4-8 tabs q4h. **Max:** 48 tabs q24h.
Ecotrin Regular Strength Tablets	Aspirin 325mg	**Adults & Peds ≥12 yrs:** 1-2 tabs q4h. **Max:** 12 tabs q24h.
Halfprin 162mg Tablets	Aspirin 162mg	**Adults & Peds ≥12 yrs:** 2-4 tabs q4h. **Max:** 24 tabs q24h.
Halfprin 81mg Tablets	Aspirin 81mg	**Adults & Peds ≥12 yrs:** 4-8 tabs q4h. **Max:** 48 tabs q24h.
St. Joseph Chewable Aspirin Tablets	Aspirin 81mg	**Adults & Peds ≥12 yrs:** 4-8 tabs q4h. **Max:** 48 tabs q24h.
St. Joseph Enteric Safety-Coated Tablets	Aspirin 81mg	**Adults & Peds ≥12 yrs:** 4-8 tabs q4h. **Max:** 48 tabs q24h.
SALICYLATES, BUFFERED		
Alka-Seltzer Lemon-Lime Tablets	Aspirin/Citric acid/Sodium bicarbonate 325mg-1000mg-1700mg	**Adults & Peds ≥12 yrs:** 2 tabs q4h. **Max:** 8 tabs q24h. **≥60 yrs: Max:** 4 tabs q24h.

BRAND	INGREDIENTS/STRENGTH	DOSE
SALICYLATES, BUFFERED *(Continued)*		
Alka-Seltzer Original Effervescent Tablets	Aspirin/Citric acid/Sodium bicarbonate 325mg-1000mg-1916mg	**Adults & Peds ≥12 yrs:** 2 tabs q4h. **Max:** 8 tabs q24h. **≥60 yrs: Max:** 4 tabs q24h.
Alka-Seltzer Extra Strength Effervescent Tablets	Aspirin/Citric acid/Sodium bicarbonate 500mg-1000mg-1985mg	**Adults & Peds ≥12 yrs:** 2 tabs q6h. **Max:** 7 tabs q24h. **≥60 yrs: Max:** 3 tabs q24h.
Ascriptin Maximum Strength Tablets	Aspirin 500mg buffered with aluminum hydroxide/Calcium carbonate/ Magnesium hydroxide	**Adults:** 2 tabs q6h. **Max:** 8 tabs q24h.
Ascriptin Regular Strength Tablets	Aspirin 325mg buffered with aluminum hydroxide/Calcium carbonate/ Magnesium hydroxide	**Adults:** 2 tabs q4h. **Max:** 12 tabs q24h.
Bayer Extra Strength Plus Caplets	Aspirin 500mg buffered with calcium carbonate	**Adults & Peds ≥12 yrs:** 1-2 tabs q4-6h. **Max:** 8 tabs q24h.
Bayer Women's Low Dose Aspirin Caplets	Aspirin 81mg buffered with calcium carbonate 777mg	**Adults & Peds ≥12 yrs:** 4-8 tabs q4h. **Max:** 10 tabs q24h.
Bufferin Extra Strength Tablets*	Aspirin 500mg buffered with calcium carbonate/Magnesium oxide/Magnesium carbonate	**Adults & Peds ≥12 yrs:** 2 tabs q6h. **Max:** 8 tabs q24h.
Bufferin Low Dose Tablets*	Aspirin 81mg buffered with calcium carbonate/Magnesium carbonate/ Magnesium oxide	**Adults & Peds ≥12 yrs:** 4-8 tabs q4h. **Max:** 48 tabs q24h.
Bufferin Tablets*	Aspirin 325mg buffered with benzoic acid/Citric acid	**Adults & Peds ≥12 yrs:** 2 tabs q4h. **Max:** 12 tabs q24h.
SALICYLATE COMBINATIONS		
Anacin Max Strength Tablets	Aspirin/Caffeine 500mg-32mg	**Adults & Peds ≥12 yrs:** 2 tabs q6h. **Max:** 8 tabs q24h.
Anacin Regular Strength Caplets	Aspirin/Caffeine 400mg-32mg	**Adults & Peds ≥12 yrs:** 2 tabs q6h. **Max:** 8 tabs q24h.
Anacin Tablets	Aspirin/Caffeine 400mg-32mg	**Adults & Peds ≥12 yrs:** 2 tabs q6h. **Max:** 8 tabs q24h.
Bayer Back & Body Pain Caplets	Aspirin/Caffeine 500mg-32.5mg	**Adults & Peds ≥12 yrs:** 2 tabs q6h. **Max:** 8 tabs q24h.
Bayer AM Extra Strength Tablets	Aspirin/Caffeine 500mg-65mg	**Adults & Peds ≥12 yrs:** 2 tabs q6h. **Max:** 8 tabs q24h.
BC Arthritis Strength Powders	Aspirin/Caffeine 1000mg-65mg	**Adults & Peds ≥12 yrs:** 1 powder q6h. **Max:** 4 powders q24h.
BC Original Formula Powders	Aspirin/Caffeine 845mg-65mg	**Adults & Peds ≥12 yrs:** 1 powder q6h. **Max:** 4 powders q24h.
SALICYLATE/SLEEP AID		
Bayer PM Caplets	Aspirin/Diphenhydramine citrate 500mg-38.3mg	**Adults & Peds ≥12 yrs:** 2 tabs qhs prn.

*Currently on recall; generics may be available.
†Multiple flavors available.

COMMONLY USED HERBAL PRODUCTS

NAME	ACCEPTED USES	UNPROVEN USES	INTERACTIONS
Aloe vera	**Topical:** Resolution of psoriatic plaques, reduce desquamation, erythema, and infiltration. **Oral:** Constipation.	**Topical:** Burns, wounds, skin infections, frostbite, herpes simplex, psoriasis, pressure ulcers, wound healing. **Oral:** Heartburn, AIDS, arthritis, asthma, cancer, diabetes, ulcers, hyperlipidemia.	Antidiabetics, digoxin, diuretics, sevoflurane, stimulant laxatives, warfarin
Black cohosh	Menopausal symptoms (eg, hot flashes).	Labor induction, osteoporosis.	Atorvastatin, cisplatin, drugs metabolized by the liver (CYP450 2D6 substrates), hepatotoxic drugs
Black psyllium	Constipation, hypercholesterolemia.	Cancer, diarrhea, irritable bowel syndrome.	Antidiabetics, carbamazepine, digoxin, lithium
Capsicum (red/chili pepper)	**Topical:** Pain, fibromyalgia, prurigo nodularis. **Intranasal:** Cluster headache, perennial rhinitis (nonallergic, noninfectious).	**Oral:** Allergic rhinitis, dyspepsia, irritable bowel syndrome, peptic ulcers, swallowing dysfunction. **Intranasal:** Migraine headaches, sinonasal polyposis.	Cocaine, ACE inhibitors, anticoagulants, antiplatelets, theophylline, coca
Chamomile	Colic, dyspepsia, oral mucositis, coughs, bronchitis, fevers, colds, inflammation of the skin, mouth, pharynx, infection, wounds, burns.	Tension, anxiety, insomnia, perimenopausal and menopausal symptoms, diarrhea, dermatitis, fibromyalgia.	Anticoagulants, benzodiazepines, CNS depressants, contraceptives, drugs metabolized by the liver (CYP1A2, CYP3A4 substrates), estrogens, tamoxifen
Cranberry	Urinary tract infections.	Benign prostatic hyperplasia, urine deodorant, antioxidant.	Drugs metabolized by the liver (CYP2C9), warfarin
Echinacea	**Oral:** Common cold, flu-like symptoms, fever, chronic respiratory tract infections, urinary tract infections, vaginal candidiasis, inflammation of the mouth and pharynx. **Topical:** Superficial wounds, burns.	Influenza, leukopenia.	Anticancer drugs, caffeine, drugs metabolized by the liver (CYP1A2, CYP3A4 substrates), immunosuppressants, midazolam
Eucalyptus		Asthma, upper respiratory tract inflammation, wounds, burns, congestion, ulcers, acne, bleeding gums, bladder disease, diabetes, fever, flu, loss of appetite, arthritis pain, liver/gallbladder problems.	Drugs metabolized by the liver (CYP1A2, CYP2C19, CYP2C9, CYP3A4 substrates), antidiabetics, herbs that contain hepatotoxic pyrrolizidine alkaloids
Evening primrose oil	**Oral:** Mastalgia, osteoporosis.	Rheumatoid arthritis, breast cancer, Raynaud's syndrome, diabetic neuropathy, atopic dermatitis, ADHD, PMS, Sjogren's syndrome.	Anesthesia, anticoagulants, anticonvulsants, antiplatelets, phenothiazines
Feverfew	Migraine headaches.	Fever, menstrual irregularities, arthritis, psoriasis, allergies, asthma, dizziness, nausea, vomiting, earache, cancer, common cold.	Drugs metabolized by the liver (CYP1A2, CYP2C19, CYP2C9, CYP3A4 substrates) anticoagulants, antiplatelets
Flaxseed	Diabetes, hypercholesterolemia, menopausal symptoms, systemic lupus erythematosus nephritis.	Breast cancer, cardiovascular disease, colorectal cancer, constipation, endometrial cancer, lung cancer, mastalgia, prostate cancer.	Acetaminophen, antibiotics, anticoagulants, antiplatelets, antidiabetics, estrogens, furosemide, ketoprofen, metoprolol, decreased absorption of oral medications

(Continued)

NAME	ACCEPTED USES	UNPROVEN USES	INTERACTIONS
Garlic	**Oral:** Atherosclerosis, colorectal cancer, gastric cancer, hypertension, tick bites. **Topical:** tinea corporis (ringworm), tinea cruris (jock itch), tinea pedis (athlete's foot).	Benign prostatic hyperplasia, common cold, corns, preeclampsia, prostate cancer, warts.	Anticoagulants, antiplatelets, contraceptives, cyclosporine, drugs metabolized by the liver (CYP2E1, CYP3A4 substrates), isoniazid, non-nucleoside reverse transcriptase inhibitors, saquinavir
Ginger	Dysmenorrhea, morning sickness, osteoarthritis, postoperative nausea and vomiting, vertigo.	Chemotherapy-induced nausea and vomiting, migraine headache, myalgia, rheumatoid arthritis.	Anticoagulants, antiplatelets, antidiabetics, calcium channel blockers, phenprocoumon
Ginkgo	Age-related memory impairment, cognitive function, dementia, diabetic retinopathy, glaucoma, peripheral vascular disease, premenstrual syndrome, Raynaud's syndrome, vertigo.	Age-related macular degeneration, anxiety, ADHD, colorectal cancer, fibromyalgia, hearing loss, ovarian cancer, radiation exposure, schizophrenia, stroke, vitiligo.	Alprazolam, anticoagulants, antiplatelets, anticonvulsants, antidiabetics, buspirone, drugs metabolized by the liver (CYP1A2, CYP2C19, CYP2C9, CYP2D6, CYP3A4 substrates), efavirenz, fluoxetine, hydrochlorothiazide, ibuprofen, omeprazole, seizure threshold-lowering drugs, trazodone, St. John's wort
Ginseng	Diabetes, respiratory tract infections, fatigue, debility, declining concentration, use during convalescence, hyperlipidemia.	Improved endurance, stamina, and mental ability; ADHD, breast cancer, postmenopausal symptoms.	Albendazole, anticoagulants, antidiabetics, drugs metabolized by the liver (CYP3A4 substrates), estrogen, loop diuretics, monoamine oxidase inhibitors, nifedipine, opioid analgesics
Licorice	Dyspepsia.	Atopic dermatitis, hepatitis, muscle cramps, peptic ulcers, weight loss.	Cardiac glycoside-containing herbs (eg, digitalis), stimulant laxative herbs (eg, aloe), antihypertensives, corticosteroids, drugs metabolized by the liver (CYP2B6, CYP2C9, CYP3A4 substrates), digoxin, diuretics, estrogens, ethacrynic acid, furosemide, warfarin, grapefruit juice, salt
Milk thistle	Diabetes, dyspepsia, toxic liver damage, hepatic cirrhosis, chronic inflammatory liver disease.	Alcohol-related liver disease, *amanita* mushroom poisoning, hepatitis B or C, toxin-induced liver damage, gallstone prevention.	Drugs metabolized by the liver (CYP2C9 substrates), estrogens, drugs that undergo glucuronidation (eg, metronidazole), HMG-CoA reductase inhibitors ("statins"), tamoxifen
Peppermint	Barium enema-related colonic spasm, dyspepsia, irritable bowel syndrome, tension headache.	**Topical:** Postherpetic neuralgia.	Antacids, cyclosporine, drugs metabolized by the liver (CYP1A2, CYP2C19, CYP2C9, CYP3A4 substrates), H_2-blockers, proton pump inhibitors
Saw palmetto	Benign prostatic hyperplasia.	Androgenic alopecia, androgenic acne, chronic cystitis, prostate cancer, prostatitis and chronic pelvic pain syndrome, transurethral resection of the prostate.	Anticoagulants, antiplatelets, contraceptives, estrogens

NAME	ACCEPTED USES	UNPROVEN USES	INTERACTIONS
Senna	Constipation, bowel preparation.	Hemorrhoids, irritable bowel disease, weight loss.	Digoxin, diuretics, warfarin, horsetail, licorice, stimulant laxatives
St. John's wort	**Topical:** Acute injuries, bruises, myalgias, first-degree burns. **Oral:** Depression, menopausal symptoms, somatization disorder, wound healing.	Obsessive-compulsive disorder, premenstrual syndrome, seasonal affective disorder, smoking cessation, antiviral, antibacterial, acute otitis media (eardrops), obesity, fatigue, menopausal syndrome, improved sleep quality, and cognitive function.	St. John's wort interacts with numerous medications. Consult your physician prior to using this product.
Valerian	Insomnia.	Anxiety, dyssomnia, depression, convulsions, mild tremors, epilepsy, ADHD, chronic fatigue syndrome, muscle and joint pain, headache, upset stomach, menstrual pain, menopausal symptoms.	Alcohol, alprazolam, drugs metabolized by the liver (CYP3A4 substrates), benzodiazepines, CNS depressants
Source: Natural Medicines Comprehensive Database.			

ACE Inhibitors*

GENERIC (BRAND)	PEAK PLASMA LEVEL	FOOD EFFECT ON AMOUNT ABSORBED	HYPERTENSION DOSING†	HEART FAILURE DOSING	RENAL DOSE ADJUSTMENT
Benazepril (Lotensin)	1-2 hrs (fasting‡); 2-4 hrs (non-fasting‡)	None	Initial: 10mg qd. Usual: 20-40mg/day given qd-bid. Max: 80mg/day.§	Not FDA approved	CrCl <30mL/min/1.73m²: Initial: 5mg qd. Max: 40mg/day.
Captopril (Capoten)¶	1 hr	Reduced**	Initial: 25mg bid-tid. Usual: 25-150mg bid-tid. Max: 450mg/day.	Initial: 25mg tid. Usual: 50-100mg tid. Max: 450mg/day.	Significant Renal Dysfunction: Lower initial dose and titrate slowly.
Enalapril (Vasotec)¶	3-4 hrs‡	None	Initial: 5mg qd. Usual: 10-40mg/day given qd-bid.§	Initial: 2.5mg qd. Usual: 2.5-20mg given bid. Max: 40mg/day.	HTN: CrCl ≤30mL/min: Initial: 2.5mg/day. Max: 40mg/day. Dialysis: 2.5mg/day on dialysis day. HF: SrCr >1.6mg/dL: Initial: 2.5mg qd. Max: 40mg/day.
Fosinopril	3 hrs‡	None	Initial: 10mg qd. Usual: 20-40mg/day. Max: 80mg/day.§	Initial: 10mg qd. Usual: 20-40mg qd. Max: 40mg/day.	HTN: No dosage adjustment needed. HF: Moderate to severe renal failure/vigorous diuresis: Initial: 5mg qd.
Lisinopril (Prinivil, Zestril)¶	7 hrs	None	Initial: 10mg qd. Usual: 20-40mg/day qd. Max: 80mg/day.§	(Prinivil) Initial: 5mg qd. Usual: 5-20mg qd. (Zestril) Initial: 5mg qd. Usual: 5-40mg qd. Max: 40mg/day.	HTN: CrCl 10-30mL/min: Initial: 5mg qd. Max: 40mg/day. CrCl <10mL/min: Initial: 2.5mg qd. Max: 40mg/day. HF: CrCl ≤30mL/min: Initial: 2.5mg qd.
Moexipril (Univasc)	1.5 hrs‡	Reduced**	Initial: 7.5mg qd. Usual: 7.5-30mg/day given qd-bid. Max: 60mg/day.	Not FDA approved	CrCl ≤40mL/min/1.73m²: Initial: 3.75mg qd. Max: 15mg/day.
Perindopril (Aceon)¶	3-7 hrs‡	None	Initial: 4mg qd. Usual: 4-8mg/day given qd-bid. Max: 16mg/day.	Not FDA approved	CrCl ≥30mL/min: Initial: 2mg qd. Max: 8mg/day.
Quinapril (Accupril)	2 hrs‡	Reduced (after high-fat meals)	Initial: 10-20mg qd. Usual: 20-80mg/day given qd-bid.	Initial: 5mg bid. Usual: 20-40mg bid.	CrCl 30mL-60mL/min: Initial: 5mg/day. CrCl 10-30mL/min: Initial: 2.5mg/day.
Ramipril (Altace)¶	2-4 hrs‡	None	Initial: 2.5mg qd. Usual: 2.5-20mg/day given qd-bid.	Post MI: Initial: 2.5mg bid; 1.25mg bid if hypotensive. Titrate to 5mg bid.	HTN: Initial: 1.25mg qd. Max: 5mg/day. Post MI: Initial: 1.25mg/day. Max: 2.5mg bid.
Trandolapril (Mavik)¶	4-10 hrs‡	None	Initial: 1mg qd in non-black patients. 2mg qd in black patients. Usual: 2-4mg/day given qd. Max: 8mg/day.	Post MI: Initial: 1mg qd. Titrate to 4mg qd if tolerated.	CrCl <30mL/min: Initial: 0.5mg qd. Titrate slowly.

*Boxed Warning: D/C ACE Inhibitors as soon as pregnancy is detected.
†Note: Dosages may need to be adjusted when used in combination with other antihypertensives (ie, diuretics). Monitor patient closely. For more information, refer to monograph listings or drug's FDA-approved labeling.
‡Peak effect of active metabolite.
§Refer to monograph for pediatric dosing.
¶There are additional indications found in the FDA-approved labeling.
**Administer 1 hour before meals.

ANTIARRHYTHMIC AGENTS

GENERIC (BRAND)	HOW SUPPLIED	INDICATION	DOSAGE	HEPATIC/RENAL DOSE ADJUSTMENT*
CLASS IA ANTIARRHYTHMICS				
Disopyramide (Norpace, Norpace CR)	**Cap:** (Norpace) 100mg, 150mg; **Cap, ER** (Norpace CR) 100mg, 150mg	Treatment of documented life-threatening VT.	**Adults: Usual:** 400-800mg/day in divided dose. **Recommended:** 150mg q6h immediate-release (IR) or 300mg q12h extended-release (CR). Adjust dose with anticholinergic effects. **Rapid Control of VT: LD:** 300mg IR (200mg if <110 lbs). Follow with maint dose. **Cardiomyopathy/Cardiac Decompensation: Initial:** 100mg q6-8h IR. Adjust gradually. See labeling if no response or toxicity occurs. **Elderly:** Start at low end of dosing range.	**Weight <110 lbs/Moderate Hepatic or Renal Insufficiency (CrCl >40mL/min):** 100mg q6h IR or 200mg q12h CR. **Severe Renal Insufficiency (with or without initial 150mg LD (CrCl 30-40mL/min):** 100mg q8h IR. **CrCl 30-15mL/min:** 100mg q12h IR. **CrCl <15mL/min:** 100mg q24h IR.
Procainamide	**Inj:** 100mg/mL, 500mg/mL	Treatment of documented life-threatening VT.	**Adults: IM: Initial:** 50mg/kg/day. Divide into fractional doses of $\frac{1}{8}$-$\frac{1}{4}$ to be injected q3-6h until PO therapy is possible. If >3 doses given, assess patient factors and adjust dose for individual. **Arrhythmias Associated with Anesthesia/Surgical Operation:** 100-500mg IM. **IV:** 100mg q5min until arrhythmia suppressed or 500mg administered. Wait ≥10 min before resuming. **Max:** 50mg/min. **Alternate Regimen: LD:** 20mg/mL at 1mL/min for 25-30 min to deliver 500-600mg. **Max:** 1g. **Maint:** 2mg/mL at 1-3mL/min. **Limited Daily Total Fluid Intake:** 4mg/mL at 0.5-1.5mL/min to deliver 2-6mg/min.	May need dose adjustment for hepatic/renal impairment.
Quinidine gluconate	**Tab, ER:** 324mg; **Inj:** 80mg/mL	Conversion of symptomatic A-Fib/Flutter to normal SR, and suppression of VT. **(Tab)** Reduction of relapse frequency into A-Fib/Flutter.	**Adults: A-Fib/Flutter Conversion: Initial:** 2 tabs q8h. **Titrate:** Increase cautiously if no effect after 3-4 doses. **Alternate Regimen:** 1 tab q8h for 2 days, then 2 tabs q12h for 2 days, then 2 tabs q8h up to 4 days. **A-Fib/ Flutter Relapse Reduction:** 1 tab q8-12h. **Titrate:** Increase cautiously if needed.† May break tab in half. Do not chew or crush. **IV: A-Fib/Flutter:** 0.25mg/kg/min. **Max:** 5-10mg/kg.* Consider alternate therapy if conversion to SR not achieved. **Elderly:** Start at low end of dosing range.	**Renal/Hepatic Impairment or CHF:** Reduce dose.

(Continued)

GENERIC (BRAND)	HOW SUPPLIED	INDICATION	DOSAGE	HEPATIC/RENAL DOSE ADJUSTMENT†
CLASS IA ANTIARRHYTHMICS *(Continued)*				
Quinidine sulfate	**Tab:** 200mg, 300mg; **(ER)** 300mg	Conversion of symptomatic A-Fib/Flutter to normal SR, reduction of relapse frequency into A-Fib/Flutter, and suppression of VT.	**Adults: A-Fib/Flutter Conversion: Initial:** 400mg q6h. **Titrate:** Increase cautiously if no effect after 4-5 doses. **(ER):** 300mg q8-12h. **Titrate:** Increase dose cautiously if needed. **A-Fib/Flutter Relapse Reduction: Initial:** 200mg q6h. **(ER)** 300mg q8-12h. **Titrate:** Increase cautiously if needed.†	**Renal/Hepatic Impairment or CHF:** Reduce dose.
CLASS IB ANTIARRHYTHMICS				
Lidocaine and dextrose	**Inj:** 0.4%-5%, 0.8%-5%	Acute management of VT occurring during cardiac manipulations and life-threatening arrhythmias which are ventricular in origin.	**Adults: Initial:** 50-100mg IV bolus of lidocaine injection. If arrhythmias recur or incapable of receiving oral antiarrhythmics, continue with 1-4mg/min IV infusion of lidocaine and dextrose (0.4% sol given at 15-60mL/hr; 0.8% sol given at 7.5-30mL/hr). Determine dose by patient response. Reduce rate of infusion of lidocaine by 50% after 1st 24 hrs.	
Mexiletine	**Cap:** 150mg, 200mg, 250mg	Treatment of life-threatening VT.	**Adults: Initial:** 200mg q8h when rapid control is not essential. **Titrate:** Adjust by 50-100mg, not less than every 2-3 days. **Usual:** 200-300mg q8h. **Max:** 1200mg/day. If control with ≤300mg q8h, then may divide daily dose and give q12h. **Max:** 450mg q12h. **For Rapid Control: LD:** 400mg, then 200mg in 8 hrs. **Transfer from Class I Oral Agents: Initial:** 200mg and titrate as above. Refer to monograph for wait time between previous oral agent and mexiletine.	**Severe Hepatic Disease:** May need lower dose.
CLASS IC ANTIARRHYTHMICS				
Flecainide (Tambocor)	**Tab:** 50mg, 100mg*, 150mg*	Prevention PSVT, PAF associated with disabling symptoms in patients without structural heart disease. Prevention of life-threatening VT.	**Adults: PSVT/PAF: Initial:** 50mg q12h. **Titrate:** May increase by 50mg bid every 4 days. **Max:** 300mg/day. **Sustained VT: Initial:** 100mg q12h. **Titrate:** May increase by 50mg bid every 4 days. **Max:** 400mg/day. Reduce dose by 50% with amiodarone.	**CrCl ≤35mL/min: Initial:** 100mg qd or 50mg bid. **Less Severe Renal Disease: Initial:** 100mg q12h.

GENERIC (BRAND)	HOW SUPPLIED	INDICATION	DOSAGE	HEPATIC/RENAL DOSE ADJUSTMENT†
CLASS IC ANTIARRHYTHMICS *(Continued)*				
Propafenone (Generic, Rythmol SR)	**Tab:** 150mg*, 225mg*, 300mg*; (SR) **Cap, ER:** 225mg, 325mg, 425mg	To prolong the time to recurrence of PAF/Flutter and PSVT associated with disabling symptoms in patients without structural heart disease. Treatment of life-threatening documented VT. (SR) To prolong time to recurrence of symptomatic A-Fib in patients with episodic A-Fib without structural heart disease.	**Adults: Initial:** 150mg q8h. **Titrate:** May increase at minimum 3-4 day intervals to 225mg q8h, then to 300mg q8h if needed. **Max:** 900mg/day. **Elderly/Marked Myocardial Damage:** Increase more gradually during initial phase. **SR: Adults: Initial:** 225mg q12h. **Titrate:** May increase at minimum 5-day intervals to 325mg q12h, then to 425mg q12h if needed. **QRS Widening/2nd- or 3rd-degree AV Block:** Reduce dose.	**Hepatic Dysfunction:** Give 20-30% of normal dosage. **(SR) Hepatic Impairment:** Reduce dose.
CLASS II ANTIARRHYTHMICS (BETA-BLOCKERS)				
Acebutolol (Sectral)	**Cap:** 200mg, 400mg	Management of hypertension and ventricular premature beats.	**Adults: VT: Initial:** 200mg bid. **Maint:** Increase gradually to 600-1200mg/day. **Elderly:** Lower daily doses. **Max:** 800mg/day.	**CrCl <50mL/min:** Decrease daily dose by 50%. **CrCl <25mL/min:** Decrease daily dose by 75%.
Esmolol (Brevibloc)	**Inj:** 10mg/mL, 20mg/mL	For rapid control of ventricular rate in A-Fib/Flutter in perioperative, postoperative, or other emergent circumstances. For noncompensatory sinus tachycardia.	**Adults: Supraventricular Tachycardia:** Titrate dose based on ventricular rate. **LD:** 0.5mg/kg over 1 min. **Maint:** 0.05mg/kg/min for next 4 min. May continue at 0.05mg/kg/min or increase stepwise with each step maintained for ≥4 min to max 0.2mg/kg/min. **Rapid Slowing of Ventricular Response:** Repeat 0.5mg/kg LD over 1 min, then 0.1mg/kg/min for 4 min. If needed, another (final) LD of 0.5mg/kg over 1 min, then 0.15mg/kg/min for 4 min then up to 0.2mg/kg/min if needed. May continue infusions for 24hrs. **Intraoperative/Postoperative Tachycardia: Immediate Control: Initial:** 80mg bolus over 30 seconds. **Maint:** 0.15mg/kg/min. May titrate up to 0.3mg/kg/min. **Gradual Control: Initial:** 0.5mg/kg/min over 1 min. **Maint:** 0.05mg/kg/min for 4 min. Then, if needed, may repeat LD and increase maintenance infusion to 0.1mg/kg/min.	

(Continued)

GENERIC (BRAND)	HOW SUPPLIED	INDICATION	DOSAGE	HEPATIC/RENAL DOSE ADJUSTMENT[†]
CLASS II ANTIARRHYTHMICS (BETA-BLOCKERS) *(Continued)*				
Propranolol	**Inj:** 1mg/mL; **Tab:** 10mg*, 20mg*, 40mg*, 60mg*, 80mg*	**Inj:** For cardiac arrhythmias (supraventricular, ventricular tachycardia, tachyarrhythmia of digitalis intoxication, resistant tachyarrhythmia). **Tab:** To control ventricular rate in patients with A-Fib and a rapid ventricular response.	**Adults:** (Inj) 1-3mg IV at 1mg/min. May give 2nd dose after 2 min, subsequent doses ≥4 hrs later. **A-Fib:** (Tab) 10-30mg PO tid-qid ac and hs.	Hepatic insufficiency: May need to lower dose.
Sotalol (Betapace)[‡]	**Tab:** 80mg*, 120mg*, 160mg*	Treatment of documented life-threatening VT.	**Adults: Initial:** 80mg bid. **Titrate:** Increase to 120-160mg bid if needed. Allow 3 days between dose increments. **Usual:** 160-320mg/day given bid-tid. **Refractory Patients:** 480-640mg/day.	**CrCl 30-59mL/min:** Dose q24h. **CrCl 10-29mL/min:** Dose q36-48h. **CrCl <10mL/min:** Individualize dose. May increase dose with renal impairment after at least 5-6 doses at appropriate intervals.
Sotalol (Betapace AF)[‡]	**Tab:** 80mg*, 120mg*, 160mg*	Maintenance of normal sinus rhythm with symptomatic A-Fib/Flutter in patients who are currently in sinus rhythm.	**Adults:** Initiate with continuous ECG monitoring. Give dose qd for CrCl 40-60mL/min and bid for CrCl >60mL/min. **Initial:** 80mg. Monitor QT 2-4 hrs after each dose. Reduce dose or d/c if QT >500msec. If QT <500msec after 3 days (after 5th or 6th dose if receiving qd dosing), discharge on current treatment. Alternately, may increase dose to 120mg during hospitalization and follow for 3 days with bid dose and for 5 or 6 doses if receiving qd dose. **Max:** 160mg qd or bid depending on CrCl.	Renal Impairment: Reduce dose or increase interval.
CLASS III ANTIARRHYTHMICS				
Amiodarone (Cordarone, Nexterone, Pacerone)	**Tab:** 100mg, 200mg*, (generic) 400mg*; **Inj:** 1.5mg/mL, 1.8mg/mL, 50mg/mL	Treatment and prophylaxis (Inj) of documented, life-threatening recurrent VT and recurrent hemodynamically unstable ventricular tachycardia.	**Adults:** Give LD in hospital. **LD:** 800-1600mg/day for 1-3 weeks. Give in divided doses with meals for total daily dose ≥1000mg or if GI intolerance occurs. After control is achieved, then 600-800mg/day for 1 month. **Maint:** 400mg/day; up to 600mg/day if needed. Use lowest effective dose. Take consistently with regard to meals. **Elderly:** Start at low end of dosing range. **IV: Adults: LD:** 150mg over 1st 10 min (15mg/min), then 540mg over remaining 18 hrs (0.5mg/min). **Maint:** 0.5mg/min for 2-3 weeks. **Breakthrough Ventricular Tachycardia/ Ventricular Fibrillation:** 150mg supplement IV over 10 min. Increase rate to achieve suppression. **Max Infusion Rate:** 30mg/min (initial); 2mg/mL (>1 hr, unless central venous catheter used). See PI for transition to oral amiodarone. **Elderly:** Start at low end of dosing range.	

GENERIC (BRAND)	HOW SUPPLIED	INDICATION	DOSAGE	HEPATIC/RENAL DOSE ADJUSTMENT†
CLASS III ANTIARRHYTHMICS *(Continued)*				
Dofetilide (Tikosyn)	**Cap:** 125mcg, 250mcg, 500mcg	Conversion to and maintenance of normal SR in A-Fib/Flutter.	**Adults:** Refer to monograph for individualized dosing based on CrCl and QTc.	**CrCl 40-60mL/min:** 250mcg bid. **CrCl 20-<40mL/min:** 125mcg bid. **CrCl <20mL/min:** Do not use. Monitor ECG.
Dronedarone (Multaq)§	**Tab:** 400mg	Reduces risk of cardiovascular hospitalization with paroxysmal or persistent A-Fib/Flutter with a recent episode of A-Fib/Flutter and associated cardiovascular risk factors, in patients who are in SR or who will be cardioverted.	**Adults:** 400mg bid (with am and pm meals).	
Ibutilide (Corvert)	**Inj:** 0.1mg/mL	For rapid conversion of A-Fib/Flutter of recent onset to SR.	**Adults: ≥60kg:** 1 mg over 10 min. **<60kg:** 0.01mg/kg over 10 min. If arrhythmia still present within 10 min after completion of 1st infusion. Continuous ECG monitoring for 4 hrs after infusion or until QTc returns to baseline.	
CLASS IV ANTIARRHYTHMICS (CALCIUM CHANNEL BLOCKERS)				
Diltiazem Injection	**Inj:** 5mg/mL	Temporary control of rapid ventricular rate in A-Fib/Flutter. Rapid conversion of PSVT to SR.	**Adults: Bolus:** 0.25mg/kg IV over 2 min. If no response after 15 minutes, may give 2nd dose of 0.35mg/kg over 2 min. **Continuous Infusion:** 0.25-0.35mg/kg IV bolus, then 10mg/hr. **Titrate:** Increase by 5mg/hr. **Max:** 15mg/hr and duration up to 24 hrs.	
Verapamil (Calan)	**Tab:** 40mg, 80mg*, 120mg*; **Inj:** 2.5mg/mL (generic)	**Tab:** With digitalis, for control of ventricular rate at rest and during stress in patients with chronic AFL and/or A-Fib and prophylaxis of repetitive PSVT. **Inj:** Rapid conversion of PSVT to SR, including those as-sociated with accessory bypass tracts and temporary control of rapid ventricular rate in A-Fib/Flutter except when associated with accessory bypass tracts.	**Adults: A-Fib (Digitalized): Usual:** 240-320mg/day PO given tid-qid. **PSVT Prophylaxis (Non-Digitalized):** 240-480mg/day PO given tid-qid. Max 480mg/day. (Inj): **Adults:** Initial: 5-10mg IV bolus over 2 min. If first dose not adequate, repeat 10mg over 2 min 30 min after first dose. **Elderly:** Administer dose over at least 3 min.	Severe Hepatic Dysfunction: (Tab) Give 30% of normal dose.

(Continued)

A117

GENERIC (BRAND)	HOW SUPPLIED	INDICATION	DOSAGE	HEPATIC/RENAL DOSE ADJUSTMENT†
CLASS V ANTIARRHYTHMICS				
Adenosine (Adenocard)	**Inj:** 3mg/mL	Conversion of PSVT (including that associated with accessory bypass tracts) to SR.	**Adults:** 6mg rapid IV bolus over 1-2 sec. If not converted to SR within 1-2 min, give 12mg rapid IV bolus; may give second 12mg dose if needed. **Max:** 12mg/dose.	
Digoxin (Lanoxin)	**Inj:** (Pediatric Inj) 0.1mg/mL, 0.25mg/mL; **Sol:** (generic) 0.05mg/mL; **Tab:** 0.125mg*, 0.25mg*	Treatment of mild-to-moderate heart failure and to control ventricular response rate with chronic A-Fib.	**Adults: Rapid Digitalization: LD:** (Inj) 0.4-0.6mg IV single dose or (Tab) 0.5-0.75mg PO, may give additional (Inj) 0.1-0.3mg or (Tab) 0.125-0.375mg at 6-8 hr intervals until clinical effect. **Maint:** (Tab) 0.125-0.5mg qd. **A-Fib:** Titrate to minimum effective dose for desired response. (Sol) **Initial:** 3mcg/kg/day. Refer to PI for details.	**Elderly (>70 yrs)/Renal Dysfunction: Initial:** 0.125mg qd. **Marked Renal Dysfunction: Initial:** 0.0625mg qd. **Titrate:** Increase every 2 weeks based on response.

Abbreviations:

A-Fib = Atrial fibrillation

A-Fib/Flutter = Atrial fibrillation/Flutter

AFL = Atrial flutter

ER = Extended-release

PAF = Paroxysmal atrial fibrillation/flutter

PSVT = Paroxysmal atrial supraventricular tachycardias

SR = Sinus rhythm

VT = Ventricular arrhythmia

*Scored.

†Ventricular Arrhythmia: Dosing regimens not adequately studied. Generally similar to A-Fib/Flutter.

‡Also has Class III properties.

§Has antiarrhythmic properties of all four classes.

Please refer to individual monograph for pediatric dosing.

ARBs* AND COMBINATIONS

GENERIC (BRAND)	USUAL ADULT HTN† DOSAGE RANGE	HOW SUPPLIED
ANGIOTENSIN II RECEPTOR BLOCKERS		
Azilsartan	40-80mg/day	**Tab:** 40mg, 80mg
Candesartan (Atacand)	8-32mg/day‡	**Tab:** 4mg, 8mg, 16mg, 32mg
Eprosartan (Teveten)	400-800mg/day	**Tab:** 400mg, 600mg
Irbesartan (Avapro)	150-300mg/day	**Tab:** 75mg, 150mg, 300mg
Losartan (Cozaar)	25-100mg/day‡	**Tab:** 25mg, 50mg, 100mg
Olmesartan (Benicar)	20-40mg/day‡	**Tab:** 5mg, 20mg, 40mg
Telmisartan (Micardis)	20-80mg/day	**Tab:** 20mg, 40mg, 80mg
Valsartan (Diovan)	80-320mg/day‡	**Tab:** 40mg, 80mg, 160mg, 320mg
COMBINATIONS		
Azilsartan-Chlorthalidone	40/12.5-40/25mg/day	**Tab:** 40mg-12.5mg, 40mg-25mg
Candesartan-Hydrochlorothiazide (Atacand HCT)	16/12.5-32/25mg/day	**Tab:** 16mg-12.5mg, 32mg-12.5mg, 32mg-25mg
Eprosartan-Hydrochlorothiazide (Teveten HCT)	600/12.5-600/25mg/day	**Tab:** 600mg-12.5mg, 600mg-25mg
Irbesartan-Hydrochlorothiazide (Avalide)	150/12.5-300/25mg/day	**Tab:** 150mg-12.5mg, 300mg-12.5mg
Losartan-Hydrochlorothiazide (Hyzaar)	50/12.5-100/25mg/day	**Tab:** 50mg-12.5mg, 100mg-12.5mg, 100 mg-25mg
Olmesartan-Amlodipine (Azor)	20/5-40/10mg/day	**Tab:** 20mg-5mg, 20mg-10mg, 40mg-5mg, 40mg-10mg
Olmesartan-Amlodipine-Hydrochlorothiazide (Tribenzor)	Individualize dose up to 40/10/25mg/day§	**Tab:** 20mg-5mg-12.5mg, 40mg-5mg-12.5mg, 40mg-5mg-25mg, 40mg-10mg-12.5mg, 40mg-10mg-25mg
Olmesartan-Hydrochlorothiazide (Benicar HCT)	20/12.5-40/25mg/day	**Tab:** 20mg-12.5mg, 40mg-12.5mg, 40mg-25mg
Telmisartan-Amlodipine (Twynsta)	40/5-80/10mg/day	**Tab:** 40mg-5mg, 40mg-10mg, 80mg-5mg, 80mg-10mg
Telmisartan-Hydrochlorothiazide (Micardis HCT)	40/12.5-160/25mg/day	**Tab:** 40mg-12.5mg, 80mg-12.5mg, 80mg-25mg
Valsartan-Amlodipine (Exforge)	160/5-320/10mg/day	**Tab:** 160mg-5mg, 160mg-10mg, 320mg-5mg, 320mg-10mg
Valsartan-Amlodipine-Hydrochlorothiazide (Exforge HCT)	Individualize dose up to 320/10/25mg/day§	**Tab:** 160mg-5mg-12.5mg, 160mg-5mg-25mg, 160mg-10mg-12.5mg, 160mg-10mg-25mg, 320mg-10mg-25mg
Valsartan-Hydrochlorothiazide (Diovan HCT)	160/12.5-320/25mg/day	**Tab:** 80mg-12.5mg, 160mg-12.5mg, 160mg-25mg, 320mg-12.5mg, 320mg-25mg

*ARBs: angiotensin II receptor blockers.

†HTN: hypertension.

‡Refer to monograph for pediatric dosing.

§Exforge HCT and Tribenzor are not indicated for initial therapy of hypertension unless determined by a physican. May be used for patients not adequately controlled on any two of the following antihypertensive classes: calcium channel blockers, angiotensin receptor blockers, and diuretics.

Boxed Warning for ARBs: Drugs that act directly on the renin-angiotensin system can cause injury and death to the developing fetus. Discontinue ARBs as soon as possible once pregnancy is detected.

BETA-BLOCKERS

GENERIC	BRAND	HOW SUPPLIED	HYPERTENSION DOSING	ANGINA DOSING	POST-MI DOSING
NONSELECTIVE BETA-BLOCKERS					
Nadolol	Corgard	**Tab:** 20mg, 40mg, 80mg	**Initial:** 40mg qd. **Usual:** 40mg-80mg qd. **Max:** 320mg/day.	**Initial:** 40mg qd. **Usual:** 40mg-80mg qd. **Max:** 240mg/day.	Not FDA approved
Penbutolol sulfate	Levatol	**Tab:** 20mg	**Initial and Usual:** 20mg qd.	Not FDA approved	Not FDA approved
Pindolol	Various generics	**Tab:** 5mg, 10mg	**Initial:** 5mg bid. **Max:** 60mg/day.	Not FDA approved	Not FDA approved
Propranolol HCl*	Various generics†	**Tab:** 10mg, 20mg, 40mg, 60mg, 80mg	**Initial:** 40mg bid. **Usual:** 120mg-240mg/day. **Max:** 640mg/day.	**Usual:** 80mg-320mg/day.	**Initial:** 40mg tid. **Usual:** 180mg-240mg/day. **Max:** 240mg/day.
	Inderal LA†	**Cap, LA:** 60mg, 80mg, 120mg, 160mg **Cap, ER** (Generic): 60mg, 80mg, 120mg, 160mg	**Initial:** 80mg qd. **Usual:** 120mg-160mg qd. **Max:** 640mg/day.	**Initial:** 80mg qd. **Usual:** 160mg qd. **Max:** 320mg qd.	Not FDA approved
	Innopran XL	**Cap, ER:** 80mg, 120mg	**Initial:** 80mg qhs. **Max:** 120mg qhs.	Not FDA approved	Not FDA approved
Timolol maleate	Various generics	**Tab:** 5mg, 10mg, 20mg	**Initial:** 10mg bid. **Usual:** 20mg-40mg/day. **Max:** 60mg/day.	Not FDA approved	**Usual:** 10mg bid (post acute MI)
SELECTIVE BETA$_1$-BLOCKERS					
Acebutolol	Sectral†	**Cap:** 200mg, 400mg	**Initial:** 400mg qd or in divided doses. **Usual:** 400mg-800mg/day. **Max:** 1200mg/day.	Not FDA approved	Not FDA approved
Atenolol	Tenormin	**Tab:** 25mg, 50mg, 100mg	**Initial:** 50mg qd. **Max:** 100mg qd.	**Initial:** 50mg qd. **Usual:** 100mg qd. **Max:** 200mg qd.	**Usual:** 50mg bid or 100mg qd for 6-9 days post MI.
Betaxolol HCl	Various generics	**Tab:** 10mg, 20mg	**Initial:** 10mg qd. **Max:** 20-40mg qd.	Not FDA approved	Not FDA approved
Bisoprolol fumarate	Zebeta	**Tab:** 5mg, 10mg	**Initial:** 2.5mg-5mg qd. **Usual:** 5mg-20mg qd. **Max:** 20mg qd.	Not FDA approved	Not FDA approved
Esmolol	Brevibloc†	**Inj:** 10mg/mL, 20mg/mL	**Immediate Control: Initial:** 80mg bolus over 30 sec. **Maint:** 0.15mg/kg/min. May titrate up to 0.3mg/kg/min. **Gradual Control: Initial:** 0.5mg/kg/min over 1 min. **Maint:** 0.05mg/kg/min for 4 min. If needed, may repeat loading dose. **Maint:** follow with increase to 0.1mg/kg/min.‡	Not FDA approved	Not FDA approved

GENERIC	BRAND	HOW SUPPLIED	HYPERTENSION DOSING	ANGINA DOSING	POST-MI DOSING
SELECTIVE BETA₁-BLOCKERS (Continued)					
Metoprolol succinate	Toprol-XL†	**Tab, XL:** 25mg, 50mg, 100mg, 200mg	**Initial:** 25mg-100mg qd. **Max:** 400mg/day.	**Initial:** 100mg qd. **Max:** 400mg/day.	Not FDA approved
Metoprolol tartrate*	Lopressor	**Tab:** 50mg, 100mg	**Initial:** 100mg qd or in divided doses. **Usual:** 100mg-450mg/day. **Max:** 450mg/day.	**Initial:** 50mg bid. **Usual:** 100mg-400mg/day. **Max:** 400mg/day.	**Usual Maint:** 100mg bid for at least 3 months.
	Various generics	**Tab:** 25mg, 50mg, 100mg	**Initial:** 100mg qd or in divided doses. **Usual:** 100mg-450mg/day. **Max:** 450mg/day.	**Initial:** 50mg bid. **Usual:** 100mg-400mg/day. **Max:** 400mg/day.	**Usual Maint:** 100mg bid for at least 3 months.
Nebivolol	Bystolic	**Tab:** 2.5mg, 5mg, 10mg, 20mg	**Initial:** 5mg qd. **Titrate:** May increase dose if needed at 2-week intervals. **Max:** 40mg.	Not FDA approved	Not FDA approved
MIXED ALPHA- AND BETA- BLOCKERS					
Carvedilol	Coreg†	**Tab:** 3.125mg, 6.25mg, 12.5mg, 25mg	**Initial:** 6.25mg bid. **Max:** 50mg/day.	Not FDA approved	**Left Ventricular Dysfunction post MI: Initial:** 6.25mg bid, then increase to 12.5mg bid after 3-10 days. **Usual Target:** 25mg bid.
	Coreg CR†	**Cap, ER:** 10mg, 20mg, 40mg, 80mg	**Initial:** 20mg qd. **Max:** 80mg/day.	Not FDA approved	**Left Ventricular Dysfunction post MI: Initial:** 10mg-20mg qd. **Usual:** 80mg qd.
Labetalol HCl*	Trandate	**Tab:** 100mg, 200mg, 300mg	**Initial:** 100mg bid. **Usual:** 200mg-400mg bid.	Not FDA approved	Not FDA approved
COMBINATIONS					
Atenolol/ Chlorthalidone	Tenoretic	**Tab:** 50mg/25mg, 100mg/25mg	**Initial:** 50mg/25mg qd. **Max:** 100mg/25mg/day.	Not FDA approved	Not FDA approved
Nadolol/ Bendroflumethiazide	Corzide	**Tab:** 40mg/5mg, 80mg/5mg	**Initial:** 40mg/5mg qd. **Max:** 80mg/5mg/day.	Not FDA approved	Not FDA approved
Bisoprolol/ fumarate/HCTZ§	Ziac	**Tab:** 2.5mg/6.25mg, 5mg/6.25mg, 10mg/6.25mg	**Initial:** 2.5mg/6.25mg qd. **Max:** 20mg/12.5mg/day.	Not FDA approved	Not FDA approved

GENERIC	BRAND	HOW SUPPLIED	HYPERTENSION DOSING	ANGINA DOSING	POST-MI DOSING
COMBINATIONS *(Continued)*					
Metoprolol tartrate/ HCTZ§	Lopressor HCT	**Tab:** 50mg/25mg, 100mg/25mg, (generic) 100mg/50mg	Individualize dose. **Lopressor Usual Initial:** 100mg/day qd or in divided doses. **Lopressor Max:** 450mg/ day. **HCTZ Usual:** 12.5mg-50mg/ day. HCTZ dose >50mg/day not recommended.	Not FDA approved	Not FDA approved
Propranolol/HCTZ§	Various generics	**Tab:** 40mg/25mg, 80mg/25mg	Individualize dose. **Propranolol Alone Initial:** 80mg/day. **Usual:** 160mg-480mg/day. **HCTZ Use Alone:** 12.5mg-50mg/day. **Inderide Max Dose:** 160mg/50mg.	Not FDA approved	Not FDA approved

*For additional dosage forms, refer to FDA-approved labeling.
†For additional indications, refer to FDA-approved labeling.
‡Brevibloc is used for the treatment of tachycardia and hypertension that occur during induction and tracheal intubation, during surgery, on emergence from anesthesia, and in the postoperative period.
§Hydrochlorothiazide.

Note: Sotalol (Betapace) is indicated for ventricular arrhythmia. Refer to FDA-approved labeling for dosing and additional information.

Source: FDA-approved labeling.

CALCIUM CHANNEL BLOCKERS

GENERIC	BRAND	HOW SUPPLIED	HYPERTENSION DOSING*	ANGINA DOSING*
DIHYDROPYRIDINES				
Amlodipine besylate	Norvasc	**Tab:** 2.5mg, 5mg, 10mg	**Initial:** 5mg qd. **Max:** 10 mg qd.	**Usual:** 5-10mg qd.
Clevidipine butyrate	Cleviprex	**Inj:** 0.5mg/mL	**Initial:** 1-2mg/hr. **Maint:** 4-6mg/hr. **Max:** 21mg/hr or 1000mL per 24 hrs.	Not FDA approved
Felodipine	Generic	**Tab, ER:** 2.5mg, 5mg, 10mg	**Initial:** 5mg qd. **Usual:** 2.5-10mg qd.	Not FDA approved
Isradipine	DynaCirc CR, Generic	**Tab, CR:** 5mg, 10mg; **Cap:** 2.5mg, 5mg	**Initial: Cap:** 2.5mg bid or (CR): 5mg qd. **Max:** 20mg/day.	Not FDA approved
Nicardipine HCl†	Generic	**Cap:** 20mg, 30mg	**Initial:** 20mg tid. **Usual:** 20-40mg tid.	**Initial:** 20mg tid. **Usual:** 20-40mg tid.
	Cardene SR	**Cap, ER:** 30mg, 45mg, 60mg	**Initial:** 30mg bid. **Usual:** 30-60mg bid.	Not FDA approved
Nifedipine	Adalat CC	**Tab, ER:** 30mg, 60mg, 90mg	**Initial:** 30mg qd. **Usual:** 30-60mg qd. **Max:** 90mg/day.	Not FDA approved
	Afeditab CR, Nifediac CC	**Tab, ER:** 30mg, (Afeditab CR) 60mg	**Initial:** 30mg qd. **Usual:** 30-60mg qd. **Max:** 90mg/day.	Not FDA approved
	Procardia	**Cap:** 10mg	Not FDA approved	**Initial:** 10mg tid. **Usual:** 10-20mg tid. **Max:** 180mg/day.
	Procardia XL	**Tab, ER:** 30mg, 60mg, 90mg	**Initial:** 30-60mg qd. **Max:** 120mg qd.	**Initial:** 30-60mg qd. **Max:** 120mg/day.
Nisoldipine	Generic	**Tab, ER:** 20mg, 30mg, 40mg; 8.5mg, 17mg, 25.5mg, 34mg	**Initial:** 20mg qd. **Usual:** 20-40mg qd. **Max:** 60mg/day. *OR* **Initial:** 17mg qd. **Usual:** 17-34mg qd. **Max:** 34mg/day.	Not FDA approved
	Sular	**Tab, ER:** 8.5mg, 17mg, 25.5mg, 34mg	**Initial:** 17mg qd. **Usual:** 17-34mg qd. **Max:** 34mg/day.	Not FDA approved
NON-DIHYDROPYRIDINES				
Diltiazem HCl†	Cardizem	**Tab:** 30mg, 60mg, 90mg, 120mg	Not FDA approved	**Initial:** 30mg qid. **Usual:** 180-360mg/day.
	Cardizem CD, Cartia XT, Dilt-CD	**Cap, ER:** 120mg, 180mg, 240mg, 300mg (Cardizem CD) 360mg	**Initial:** 180-240mg qd. **Usual:** 240-360mg qd. **Max:** 480mg qd.	**Initial:** 120mg-180mg qd. **Max:** 480mg/day.
	Cardizem LA	**Tab, ER:** 120mg, 180mg, 240mg, 300mg, 360mg, 420mg	**Initial:** 180-240mg qd. **Max:** 540mg/day.	**Initial:** 180mg qd. **Max:** 360mg/day.
	Dilacor XR, Diltia XT	**Cap, ER:** 120mg, 180mg, 240mg	**Initial:** 180-240mg qd. **Usual:** 180-480mg qd. **Max:** 540mg qd.	**Initial:** 120mg qd. **Max:** 480mg/day.
	Diltzac, Tiazac, Taztia XT	**Cap, ER:** 120mg, 180mg, 240mg, 300mg, 360mg, (Tiazac) 420mg	**Initial:** 120-240mg qd. **Usual:** 120-540mg qd. **Max:** 540mg qd.	**Initial:** 120-180mg qd. **Max:** 540mg/day.

(Continued)

GENERIC	BRAND	HOW SUPPLIED	HYPERTENSION DOSING*	ANGINA DOSING*
Verapamil HCl†	Calan‡	**Tab:** 40mg, 80mg, 120mg	**Initial:** 80mg tid. **Usual:** 360-480mg/day.	**Usual:** 80-120mg tid. **Max:** 480mg/day.
	Calan SR	**Cap, ER:** 120mg, 180mg, 240mg	**Initial:** 180mg qam. **Max:** 480mg/day.	Not FDA approved
	Covera HS	**Tab, ER:** 180mg, 240mg,	**Initial:** 180mg qhs. **Max:** 480mg qhs.	**Initial:** 180mg qhs. **Max:** 480mg qhs.
	Isoptin SR	**Tab, ER:** 120mg, 180mg, 240mg	**Initial:** 180mg qam. **Max:** 480mg/day.	Not FDA approved
	Verelan	**Cap, ER:** 120mg, 180mg, 240mg, 360mg	**Initial:** 240mg qam. **Max:** 480mg qam.	Not FDA approved
	Verelan PM	**Cap, ER:** 100mg, 200mg, 300mg	**Initial:** 200mg qhs. **Max:** 400mg qhs.	Not FDA approved

*NOTE: Adult dosing shown is for monotherapy. Dosage needs to be adjusted by titration to individual patient needs. Dosages may need to be reduced in the elderly, or in patients with renal/hepatic impairment. When used in combination with other antihypertensives, the dosage of the calcium channel blocker or the concomitant antihypertensive agent may need to be adjusted due to possible additive effects. Monitor the patient closely. For more information, refer to the monograph listings or the drug's FDA-approved labeling.

†For additional dosage forms, refer to the monograph listings or the drug's FDA-approved labeling.

‡For additional indications, refer to the monograph listings or the drug's FDA-approved labeling.

CHOLESTEROL-LOWERING AGENTS

GENERIC (BRAND)	HOW SUPPLIED (MG)*	USUAL DOSAGE RANGE†	T-CHOL (% DECREASE)	LDL (% DECREASE)	HDL (% INCREASE)	TG (% DECREASE)
HMG-COA REDUCTASE INHIBITORS (STATINS)						
Atorvastatin (Lipitor)	**Tab:** 10, 20, 40, 80	10-80mg/day	29 to 45	39 to 60	5 to 9	19 to 37
Fluvastatin (Lescol)	**Cap:** 20, 40	20-80mg/day	17 to 27	22 to 36	3 to 6	12 to 18
Fluvastatin (Lescol XL)	**Tab, ER:** 80	80mg/day	25	35	7	19
Lovastatin (Altoprev)	**Tab, ER:** 20, 40, 60	20-60mg/day	17.9 to 29.2	23.8 to 40.8	9.4 to 13.1	9.9 to 25.1
Lovastatin (Mevacor)	**Tab:** 20, 40	10-80mg/day	17 to 29	24 to 40	6.6 to 9.5	10 to 19
Pitavastatin (Livalo)	**Tab:** 1, 2, 4	1-4mg/day	23 to 31	32 to 43	5 to 8	15 to 19
Pravastatin (Pravachol)	**Tab:** 10, 20, 40, 80	40-80mg/day	16 to 27	22 to 37	2 to 12	11 to 24
Rosuvastatin (Crestor)	**Tab:** 5, 10, 20, 40	5-40mg/day	33 to 46	45 to 63	8 to 14	10 to 35
Simvastatin (Zocor)	**Tab:** 5, 10, 20, 40, 80	5-40mg/day	19 to 36	26 to 47	8 to 16	12 to 33
FIBRATES‡						
Fenofibrate (Antara)	**Cap:** 43, 130	43-130mg/day	16.8 to 22.4	20.1 to 31.4	9.8 to 14.6	23.5 to 35.9
Fenofibrate (Fenoglide)	**Tab:** 40, 120	40-120mg/day	16.8 to 22.4	20.1 to 31.4	9.8 to 14.6	23.5 to 35.9
Fenofibrate (Lipofen)	**Cap:** 50, 150	50-150mg/day	16.8 to 22.4	20.1 to 31.4	9.8 to 14.6	23.5 to 35.9
Fenofibrate (Lofibra)	**Tab:** 54, 160; **Cap:** 67, 134, 200	54-160mg/day, 67-200mg/day	16.8 to 22.4	20.1 to 31.4	9.8 to 14.6	23.5 to 35.9
Fenofibrate (Tricor)	**Tab:** 48, 145	48-145mg/day	16.8 to 22.4	20.1 to 31.4	9.8 to 14.6	23.5 to 35.9
Fenofibrate (Triglide)	**Tab:** 50, 160	50-160mg/day	16.8 to 22.4	20.1 to 31.4	9.8 to 14.6	23.5 to 35.9
Fenofibric Acid (Fibricor)	**Tab:** 35, 105	35-105mg/day	16.8 to 22.4	20.1 to 31.4	9.8 to 14.6	23.5 to 35.9
Fenofibric Acid (Trilipix)	**Cap, Delayed-Release:** 45, 135	45-135mg/day	16.8 to 22.4	20.1 to 31.4	9.8 to 14.6	23.5 to 35.9
Gemfibrozil (Lopid)	**Tab:** 600	1200mg/day in divided doses	Moderate reduction	4.1	12.6	Significant reduction
BILE-ACID SEQUESTRANTS						
Cholestyramine (Prevalite)	**Powder for Oral Suspension:** 4g/packet or level scoopful	2-6 packets or level scoopfuls (8-24g)/day	7.2	10.4	N/A	N/A
Colesevelam HCl (Welchol)	**Tab:** 625; **Powder for Oral Suspension:** 3.75g packet, 1.875g packet	3750mg/day	7	15	3	+10

(Continued)

GENERIC (BRAND)	HOW SUPPLIED (MG)*	USUAL DOSAGE RANGE†	T-CHOL (% DECREASE)	LDL (% DECREASE)	HDL (% INCREASE)	TG (% DECREASE)
BILE-ACID SEQUESTRANTS *(Continued)*						
Colestipol (Colestid)	**Granules for Suspension:** 5g/packet or level scoopful; **Tab:** 1000	**Granules for Suspension:** 1-6 packets or level scoopfuls/ day; **Tab:** 2-16g/day	N/A	N/A	N/A	N/A
CHOLESTEROL ABSORPTION INHIBITOR						
Ezetimibe (Zetia)	**Tab:** 10	10mg/day	13	18	1	8
NICOTINIC ACID DERIVATIVE						
Niacin, ER (Niaspan)	**Tab, ER:** 500, 750, 1000	500-2000mg/ day	3 to 10	5 to 14	18 to 22	13 to 28
LIPID-REGULATING AGENT						
Omega-3-Acid Ethyl Esters (Lovaza)	**Cap:** 1000	4g/day	9.7	+44.5	9.1	44.9
COMBINATIONS						
Amlodipine/ Atorvastatin (Caduet)	**Tab:** 2.5/10, 2.5/20, 2.5/40, 5/10, 5/20, 5/40, 5/80, 10/10, 10/20, 10/40, 10/80	5/10mg – 10/80mg /day	N/A	36.6 to 49.1	N/A	N/A
Ezetimibe/ Simvastatin (Vytorin)	**Tab:** 10/10, 10/20, 10/40, 10/80	10/10 mg – 10/80mg /day	31 to 43	45 to 60	6 to 10	23 to 31
Niacin ER/ Lovastatin (Advicor)	**Tab, ER:** 500/20, 750/20, 1000/20, 1000/40	500/20mg – 2000/40mg/day	N/A	30 to 42	20 to 30	32 to 44
Niacin ER/ Simvastatin (Simcor)	**Tab, ER:** 500/20, 500/40, 750/20, 1000/20, 1000/40	500/20mg – 2000/40mg/day	1.6 to 11.1	5.1 to 14.3	15.4 to 29	22.8 to 38.0
Sitagliptin/ Simvastatin (Juvisync)	**Tab:** 100/10, 100/20, 100/40	100/10 – 100/40/day	23 to 31	29 to 41	8 to 13	15 to 28

Abbreviations: ER, extended-release; N/A, not applicable.

*Unless otherwise indicated.

† NOTE: Usual Dosage Range shown is for adults and may need to be adjusted to individual patient needs. For specific dosing and administration information including pediatric, geriatric, and renal/hepatic impairment dosing please refer to the individual monograph listing or the drug's FDA-approved labeling. According to NCEP-ATP III guidelines, lipid-altering agents should be used in addition to a diet restricted in saturated fat and cholesterol only when the response to diet and other nonpharmacological measures has been inadequate.

‡ Refer to the drug's FDA-approved labeling for the lipid parameter changes observed for the treatment of hypertriglyceridemia; LDL increases reported.

Major Contraindications (refer to the FDA-approved labeling for a complete list of warnings and precautions).

Statins: Active liver disease or unexplained persistent elevations of hepatic transaminase levels; women who are pregnant or may become pregnant; nursing mothers.

Fibrates: Severe renal dysfunction (including patients receiving dialysis), active liver disease, gallbladder disease, nursing mothers.

Bile-acid sequestrants: History of bowel obstruction; serum triglycerides >500mg/dL; history of hypertriglyceridemia-induced pancreatitis.

Cholesterol absorption inhibitors: Statin contraindications apply when used with a statin: active liver disease or unexplained persistent elevations in hepatic transaminase levels, women who are pregnant or may become pregnant, nursing mothers.

Nicotinic acid derivatives: Active liver disease or unexplained persistent elevations in hepatic transaminases; active peptic ulcer disease; arterial bleeding.

Combinations: Refer to individual therapeutic class contraindications.

COAGULATION MODIFIERS[†]

GENERIC (BRAND)	HOW SUPPLIED	INDICATIONS	DOSAGE	HEPATIC/RENAL IMPAIRMENT
THROMBOLYTICS				
Alteplase (Activase)	**Inj:** 50mg, 100mg [vials]	Management of acute myocardial infarction (AMI) in adults for the improvement of ventricular function following AMI, the reduction of the incidence of congestive heart failure, and the reduction of mortality associated with AMI. Management of acute ischemic stroke in adults for improving neurological recovery and reducing the incidence of disability. Management of acute massive pulmonary embolism (PE) in adults.	**AMI:** Administer as soon as possible after the onset of symptoms. **Accelerated Infusion:** Recommended total dose is based on patient weight, not to exceed 100mg. **Patients weighing >67kg:** 100mg as a 15mg IV bolus, followed by 50mg infused over next 30 min, and then 35mg infused over next 60 min. **Patients weighing ≤67kg:** 15mg IV bolus, followed by 0.75mg/kg infused over next 30 min (not to exceed 50mg), then 0.50mg/kg over the next 60 min (not to exceed 35mg). **3-hour Infusion:** 100mg administered as 60mg in the first hour (of which 6-10mg is administered as a bolus), then 20mg over second hour, and 20mg over third hour. **Smaller patients (<65kg):** 1.25mg/kg over 3 hrs as described above may be used. **Acute Ischemic Stroke:** 0.9mg/kg IV over 60 min with 10% of the total dose administered as an initial IV bolus over 1 min (total dose should not exceed 90mg). **PE:** 100mg by IV infusion over 2 hrs. Heparin therapy should be instituted or reinstituted near the end or immediately after infusion when partial thromboplastin time or thrombin time returns to twice normal or less.	
Reteplase (Retavase)	**Inj:** 10.4 U [vials] Kit, Half-Kit	Management of AMI in adults for the improvement of ventricular function following AMI, the reduction of the incidence of congestive heart failure, and the reduction of mortality associated with AMI.	Administered as a 10 + 10 unit double bolus injection. Each bolus is administered as an IV injection over 2 min. The second bolus is given 30 min after initiation of the first bolus injection.	
Tenecteplase (TNKase)	**Inj:** 50mg [vial]	Reduction of mortality associated with AMI.	IV administration only. A single bolus dose should be administered over 5 seconds based on patient weight (see PI for detailed dosage information). The recommended total dose should not exceed 50mg. Treatment should be initiated as soon as possible after the onset of AMI symptoms.	

(Continued)

GENERIC (BRAND)	HOW SUPPLIED	INDICATIONS	DOSAGE	HEPATIC/RENAL IMPAIRMENT
PLATELET AGGREGATION INHIBITORS				
Abciximab (ReoPro)	**Inj:** 2mg/mL [5mL vial]	Adjunct to percutaneous coronary intervention (PCI) for the prevention of cardiac ischemic complications in patients undergoing PCI and in patients with unstable angina not responding to conventional medical therapy when PCI is planned within 24 hrs. Abciximab is intended for use with aspirin and heparin.	Recommended dose in adults is a 0.25mg/kg IV bolus given 10-60 min before the start of PCI, followed by a continuous IV infusion of 0.125mcg/kg/min (to a maximum of 10mcg/min) for 12 hrs. Patients with unstable angina may be treated with 0.25mg/kg IV bolus followed by an 18- to 24-hr IV infusion of 10mcg/min, concluding 1 hr after the PCI.	
Anagrelide HCl (Agrylin)	**Cap:** 0.5mg, (generic) 1mg	Treatment of patients with thrombocythemia, secondary to myeloproliferative disorders, to reduce the elevated platelet count and the risk of thrombosis and to ameliorate associated symptoms, including thrombo-hemorrhagic events.	Recommended starting dosage for adults is 0.5mg qid or 1mg bid for at least 1 wk. Recommended starting dose for pediatric patients is 0.5mg per day. Doses should be adjusted in both adult and pediatric patients to the lowest effective dosage required to reduce and maintain platelet count below 600,000/µL, and ideally to normal range. The dosage should be increased by not more than 0.5mg/day in any one week. Maintenance dosing is not expected to differ between adult and pediatric patients. Dosage should not exceed 10mg/day or 2.5mg in a single dose. Platelet counts should be preformed every 2 days during first week of treatment, and at least weekly thereafter until maintenance dose is reached.	**Moderate Hepatic Impairment: Initial:** 0.5mg/day for at least 1 wk with careful monitoring of cardiovascular effects. Increase by no more than 0.5mg/day in any 1 wk. Use in patients with severe hepatic impairment is contraindicated.
Cilostazol (Pleta)	**Tab:** 50mg, 100mg	The reduction of symptoms of intermittent claudication, as indicated by an increased walking distance.	100mg bid, taken at least half an hour before or 2 hrs after breakfast and dinner. A dose of 50mg bid should be considered during coadministration of such inhibitors of CYP3A4 and CYP2C19.	Special caution is advised when used in patients with moderate-severe hepatic impairment and in patients with severe renal impairment (CrCl <25mL/min).
Clopidogrel (Plavix)	**Tab:** 75mg, 300mg	Reduction of combined endpoint of new ischemic stroke, new MI, and other vascular death in patients with a history of recent MI, recent stroke, or established peripheral artery disease (PAD). **Acute Coronary Syndrome (ACS):** Patients with non-ST-segment elevation ACS [unstable angina (UA)/non-ST-elevation MI (NSTEMI)]; and patients with ST-elevation myocardial infarction (STEMI).	**Recent MI, Recent Stroke or Established PAD:** 75mg once daily. **Acute Coronary Syndrome: Non-ST segment elevation ACS (UA/ NSTEMI):** 300mg loading dose, followed by 75mg once daily in combination with 75-325mg aspirin once daily. **STEMI:** 75mg once daily in combination with aspirin 75-325mg once daily, with or without a LD and w or w/o thrombolytics.	

GENERIC (BRAND)	HOW SUPPLIED	INDICATIONS	DOSAGE	HEPATIC/RENAL IMPAIRMENT
PLATELET AGGREGATION INHIBITORS *(Continued)*				
Dipyridamole (Persantine)	**Tab:** 25mg, 50mg, 75mg	Adjunct to coumarin anticoagulants for prevention of postoperative thrombo-embolic complications of cardiac valve replacement.	75-100mg qid as an adjunct to the usual warfarin therapy.	
Dipyridamole and aspirin (Aggrenox)	**Cap:** (Dipyridamole Extended-Release/ Aspirin) 200mg-25mg	Reduce the risk of stroke in patients who have had transient ischemia of the brain or completed ischemic stroke due to thrombosis.	1 cap bid (morning and evening). In case of intolerable headaches during initial treatment, switch to 1 capsule at bedtime and low-dose aspirin in the AM; resume bid dosing within 1 wk.	Avoid using aspirin-containing products, including Aggrenox, in patients with severe hepatic or severe renal dysfunction (glomerular filtration rate <10mL/min).
Eptifibatide (Integrilin)	**Inj:** 0.75mg/mL [100mL vial], 2mg/mL [10mL vial, 100mL vial]	Treatment of patients with acute coronary syndrome (ACS) (unstable angina/non-ST-segment elevation myocardial infarction), including patients who are to be managed medically and those undergoing percutaneous coronary intervention (PCI). Treatment of patients undergoing PCI, including those undergoing intracoronary stenting.	**ACS:** Recommended adult dosage is 180mcg/kg IV bolus ASAP following diagnosis, followed by a continuous infusion of 2mcg/kg/min until hospital discharge or initiation of CABG surgery, up to 72 hrs. If patient is to undergo a PCI, the infusion should be continued up to a hospital discharge, or up to 18-24 hrs post-procedure, whichever comes first, allowing for up to 96 hrs of therapy. **PCI:** Recommended adult dosage is 180mcg/kg IV bolus immediately before the initiation of PCI, followed by a continuous infusion of 2mcg/kg/min and a second bolus of 180mcg/kg 10 min after first bolus. Infusion should be continued until hospital discharge or for up to 18-24 hrs, whichever comes first. A minimum of 12 hrs of infusion recommended. See PI for concomitant aspirin and heparin doses.	**ACS (Nondialysis-dependent patients w/ CrCl <50mL/min):** 180mcg/kg IV bolus ASAP following diagnosis, immediately followed by a continuous infusion of 1mcg/kg/min. **PCI (Non-dialysis-dependent patients w/ CrCl <50mL/min):** 180mcg/kg IV bolus immediately before PCI, immediately followed by a continuous infusion of 1mcg/kg/min and a second bolus of 180mcg/kg administered 10 min after the first.
Prasugrel HCl (Effient)	**Tab:** 5mg, 10mg	Reduction of thrombotic cardiovascular events (including stent thrombosis) in patients with acute coronary syndrome (ACS) who are being managed with percutaneous coronary intervention (PCI). Patients with unstable angina (UA) or non-ST-elevation myocardial infarction (NSTEMI) and patients with ST-elevation myocardial infarction (STEMI) when managed with primary or delayed PCI.	Initiate treatment as a single loading dose of 60mg. Then continue at 10mg once daily. Patients should also take aspirin 75mg-325mg qd. Maintenance dosage of 5mg daily should be considered in low-weight patients (<60kg).	Patients with severe hepatic disease are generally at higher risk of bleeding.

(Continued)

GENERIC (BRAND)	HOW SUPPLIED	INDICATIONS	DOSAGE	HEPATIC/RENAL IMPAIRMENT
PLATELET AGGREGATION INHIBITORS *(Continued)*				
Ticlopidine HCl (Ticlid)	**Tab:** 250mg	To reduce the risk of thrombotic stroke in patients who have experienced stroke precursors, and in patients who have had a complete thrombotic stroke (should be reserved for patients who are intolerant or allergic to aspirin therapy or who have failed aspirin therapy). Adjunctive therapy with aspirin to reduce the incidence of subacute stent thrombosis in patients undergoing successful coronary stent implantation.	Take with food. **Stroke:** 250mg bid. **Coronary Artery Stenting:** 250mg bid with antiplatelet doses of aspirin for up to 30 days of therapy following successful stent implantation.	May need dose adjustment with hepatic/renal impairment.
Tirofiban HCl (Aggrastat)	**Inj:** 50mcg/mL premixed (100mL, 250mL vials); 250mcg/mL (50mL vials)	In combination with heparin for the treatment of acute coronary syndrome, including patients who are to be managed medically and those undergoing PTCA or atherectomy.	In most patients, Aggrastat should be administered IV at a rate of 0.4mcg/kg/min for 30 min and then continued at 0.1mcg/kg/min. The infusion should be continued through angiography and for 12-24 hrs after angioplasty or atherectomy. Prior to use, Aggrastat injection (250mcg/mL) must be diluted to the same strength as the premixed injection (50mcg/mL).	Patients with severe renal insufficiency (CrCl <30mL/min) should receive half the usual rate of infusion. See PI for detailed information.
COAGULATION FACTOR INHIBITORS				
Dalteparin sodium (Fragmin)	**Inj:** Single-dose prefilled syringe: 2500 IU/0.2mL, 5000 IU/0.2mL, 7500 IU/0.3mL, 10,000 IU/0.4mL, 12,500 IU/0.5mL, 15,000 IU/0.6mL, 18,000 IU/0.72mL. Single-dose graduated syringe: 10,000 IU/ 1mL. **Multiple-Dose Vials:** 25,000 IU/mL [3.8mL], 10,000 IU/ mL [9.5mL]	Prophylaxis of ischemic complications in unstable angina and non-Q-wave myocardial infarction when concurrently administered with aspirin therapy. Prophylaxis of deep vein thrombosis (DVT) which may lead to pulmonary embolism (PE) in patients undergoing hip replacement surgery, abdominal surgery (who are at high risk for thromboembolic complications), and for those medical patients who are at risk for thromboembolic complications due to severely restricted mobility during acute illness. Extended treatment of symptomatic venous thromboembolism (VTE; proximal DVT and/or PE), to reduce the recurrence of VTE in patients with cancer.	Administer SQ. **Unstable Angina/Non-Q-wave MI:** 120 IU/kg of body weight (not more than 10,000 IU) q12h with concurrent oral aspirin (75-165mg once daily) therapy. Treatment should be continued until patient is stabilized (usually 5-8 days). See PI for dosing options (the usual duration is 5-10 days after surgery). **Prophylaxis of VTE Following Hip Replacement Surgery:** See PI for dosing options (the usual duration is 5-10 days after surgery). **Prophylaxis of VTE Following Abdominal Surgery:** Patients with a risk of thromboembolic complications, 2500 IU once daily starting 1-2 hrs prior to surgery and repeated once daily post-op (usual duration is 5-10 days). Patients undergoing surgery associated with a high risk of thromboembolic complications (eg, malignant disorder), 5000 IU the evening before surgery, then once daily postoperatively (usual duration is 5-10 days). In patients with malignancy, 2500 IU administered 1-2 hrs before surgery followed by 2500 IU 12 hrs later, and then 5000 IU once daily post-op (usual duration is 5-10 days). **Medical Patients with Severely Restricted Mobility During Acute Illness:** 5000 IU once daily (usual duration is 12-14 days). **Extended Treatment of Symptomatic VTE in Cancer Patients:** 200 IU/kg once daily for first 30 days, then 150 IU/kg once daily for months 2-6. Total daily dose should not exceed 18,000 IU/day. See full PI for dose reductions for thrombocytopenia.	Dose reductions for renal insufficiency in extended treatment of acute symptomatic VTE in patients with cancer: Severe renal impairment (CrCl <30mL/min): Monitoring for anti-Xa levels is recommended to determine appropriate dose. Target range: 0.5-1.5 IU/mL. Sampling should be performed 4-6 hrs after dosing and only after 3-4 doses.

GENERIC (BRAND)	HOW SUPPLIED	INDICATIONS	DOSAGE	HEPATIC/RENAL IMPAIRMENT
COAGULATION FACTOR INHIBITORS *(Continued)*				
Enoxaparin sodium (Lovenox)	**Inj 100mg/mL:** (MDV: 300mg/3mL); (prefilled syringe: 30mg/0.3mL, 40mg/0.4mL, 60mg/0.6mL, 80mg/0.8mL, 100mg/mL) **150 mg/mL:** (prefilled syringe: 120mg/0.8mL, 150mg/mL)	Prophylaxis of deep vein thrombosis (DVT) in hip or knee replacement surgery, abdominal surgery, or medical patients with severely restricted mobility during acute illness. In conjunction with warfarin sodium, inpatient treatment of acute DVT with or without pulmonary embolism (PE) and outpatient treatment of DVT without PE. Prophylaxis of ischemic complications of unstable angina and non-Q-wave myocardial infarction (MI) when concurrently administered with aspirin. Treatment of acute ST-segment elevation MI (STEMI) in patients receiving thrombolysis and being managed medically or with percutaneous coronary intervention (PCI) when administered concurrently with aspirin.	See full prescribing information for detailed dosing. **Abdominal Surgery:** 40mg SQ once daily. **Knee Replacement Surgery:** 30mg SQ q12h. **Hip Replacement Surgery:** 30mg SQ q12h or 40mg SQ once daily. **Medical Patients:** 40mg SQ once daily. **Inpatient Acute DVT with or without PE :** 1mg/kg SQ q12h or 1.5mg/kg SQ once daily for a minimum of 5 days until therapeutic oral anticoagulant effect is achieved. Warfarin therapy should be started when appropriate(usually within 72 hrs). **Outpatient Acute DVT Without PE:** 1mg/kg SQ q12h for a minimum of 5 days until therapeutic oral anticoagulant effect is achieved. Warfarin therapy should be started when appropriate (usually within 72 hrs). **Unstable Angina/ Non-Q-Wave MI:** 1mg/kg SQ q12h with aspirin 100-325mg once daily. Treatment should be prescribed for a minimum of 2 days and continued until stabilization. **Acute STEMI Patients <75 yrs old:** 30mg single IV bolus plus a 1mg/kg SQ dose followed by 1mg/kg SQ q12h (Max: 100mg for first 2 doses only)with aspirin (75mg-325mg once daily). **Patients ≥75 yrs old:** 0.75mg/kg SQ q12h (no bolus: max 75mg for first 2 doses only) with aspirin (75mg-325mg once daily). When given with thrombolytic, enoxaparin dose should be given between 15 min before and 30 min after start of fibrinolytic therapy. With PCI, if last enoxaparin SQ dose was given >8 hrs before balloon inflation, an IV bolus of 0.3mg/kg of enoxaparin should be administered.	**Severe Renal Impairment (CrCl <30mL/min):** See full prescribing information for detailed dosage adjustments.
Fondaparinux sodium (Arixtra)	**Inj:** (prefilled syringe): 2.5mg/0.5mL, 5mg/0.4mL, 7.5mg/0.6mL, 10mg/0.8mL	Prophylaxis of deep vein thrombosis (DVT) in patients undergoing hip fracture surgery (including extended prophylaxis); hip replacement surgery; knee replacement surgery and patients undergoing abdominal surgery who are at risk for thromboembolic complications. Treatment of DVT or acute pulmonary embolism (PE) when administered with warfarin.	**DVT Prophylaxis:** 2.5mg SQ once daily after hemostasis has been established; initial dose should be given no earlier than 6-8 hrs post-op and continued for 5-9 days. Extended prophylaxis for hip fracture surgery patients up to 24 additional days is recommended. **DVT/PE Treatment: Patients <50kg:** 5mg SQ once daily; **Patients 50-100kg:** 7.5mg SQ once daily; **Patients >100kg:** 10mg SQ once daily. Initiate concomitant treatment with warfarin ASAP (usually within 72 hrs). Continue treatment for at least 5 days until a therapeutic effect is established (INR 2-3).	**Severe Renal Impairment (CrCl <30mL/min):** Avoid use.

(Continued)

A133

GENERIC (BRAND)	HOW SUPPLIED	INDICATIONS	DOSAGE	HEPATIC/RENAL IMPAIRMENT
COAGULATION FACTOR INHIBITORS *(Continued)*				
Heparin sodium	**Inj:** 1000 U/mL, 5000 U/mL, 10,000 U/mL, 20,000 U/mL	Anticoagulant therapy in prophylaxis and treatment of venous thrombosis and its extension. Prophylaxis and treatment of pulmonary embolism (PE). Atrial fibrillation with embolization. Low-dose regimen for prevention of postoperative deep vein thrombosis (DVT) and PE in at-risk patients undergoing major abdominothoracic surgery. Diagnosis and treatment of acute and chronic consumptive coagulopathies. Prevention of clotting in arterial and cardiac surgery. Prophylaxis and treatment of peripheral arterial embolism. Employed as an anticoagulant in blood transfusions, extracorporeal circulation, dialysis procedures, and in blood samples for labs.	Dosage should be based on patient's coagulation test results. The following dosage schedules may be used as guidelines based on a 68kg (150 lb) patient: **Deep SQ (Intrafat) Injection: Initial Dose:** 5000 U by IV injection, followed by 10,000-20,000 U of a concentrated solution SQ, followed by 8,000-10,000 U of a concentrated solution q8h or 15,000-20,000 U of a concentrated solution q12h. **Intermittent IV Injection: Initial Dose:** 10,000 U (either undiluted or in 50-100mL of 0.9% sodium chloride injection), followed by 5,000-10,000 U (undiluted or in 50-100mL of 0.9% sodium chloride injection) q4-6h. **IV Infusion: Initial Dose:** 5000 U by IV injection, followed by continuous dose of 20,000-40,000 U/24 hrs in 1000mL of 0.9% sodium chloride injection (or any compatible solution) for infusion. See PI for details in specific conditions. **Pediatrics: The following dosage schedule may be used as a guideline: Initial Dose:** 50 U/kg (IV, infusion). **Maintenance Dose:** 100 U/kg (IV, infusion) q4h or 20,000 U/m²/24 hrs continuously.	
Protein C concentrate, human (Ceprotin)	**Inj:** 500 IU, 1000 IU [vials]	In patients with severe congenital protein C deficiency for the prevention and treatment of venous thrombosis and purpura fulminans. Indicated as a replacement therapy for pediatric and adult patients.	The dose regimen should be adjusted according to the pharmacokinetic profile for each individual patient. Administer by IV injection. **Acute Episodes/Short-Term Prophylaxis: Initial Dose:** 100-120 IU/kg. **Subsequent 3 Doses:** 60-80 IU/kg q6h. **Maintenance dose:** 45-60 IU/kg q6h or q12h. Adjust dose to maintain target peak protein C activity of 100%. After resolution of acute episode, continue patient on same dose to maintain trough protein C activity level above 25% for duration of treatment. **Long-Term Prophylaxis: Maintenance Dose:** 45-60 IU/kg q12h. Higher peak protein C activity levels may be warranted in situations of increased risk of thrombosis. Maintenance of trough protein C activity levels above 25% is recommended.	
Tinzaparin sodium (Innohep)	**Inj:** 20,000 anti-Xa IU/mL [2mL multiple-dose vial]	Treatment of acute symptomatic deep vein thrombosis (DVT) with or without pulmonary embolism (PE) when administered in conjunction with warfarin sodium.	175 anti-Xa IU/kg SQ once daily for at least 6 days and until the patient is adequately anticoagulated with warfarin (INR at least 2.0 for 2 consecutive days). Warfarin therapy should be initiated when appropriate (usually within 1-3 days of Innohep initiation).	A reduction in tinzaparin sodium clearance was observed in patients with moderate (CrCl 30-50mL/min) to severe (<30mL/min) renal impairment.

GENERIC (BRAND)	HOW SUPPLIED	INDICATIONS	DOSAGE	HEPATIC/RENAL IMPAIRMENT
COAGULATION FACTOR INHIBITORS *(Continued)*				
Warfarin sodium (Coumadin, Jantoven)	**Inj:** (Coumadin) 5mg [vial]; **Tab:** (Coumadin, Jantoven) 1mg*, 2mg*, 2.5mg*, 3mg*, 4mg*, 5mg*, 6mg*, 7.5mg*, 10mg*. *scored	Prophylaxis and treatment of venous thrombosis and its extension, pulmonary embolism (PE). Prophylaxis and treatment of thromboembolic complications associated with atrial fibrillation and/or cardiac valve replacement. Reduction in the risk of death, recurrent myocardial infarction (MI), and thromboembolic events such as stroke or systemic embolization after MI.	Individualize dosing regimen for each patient and adjust based on INR response. Adjust dose based on INR and condition treated. Knowledge of genotype can inform initial dosage selection. Obtain daily INR determinations upon initiation until stable in the therapeutic range. Obtain subsequent INR determinations every 1-4 wks. Review conversion instructions from other anticoagulants. Consult the latest evidence-based clinical practice guidelines from the American College of Chest Physicians (ACCP) to assist in the determination of duration and intensity of anticoagulation. See full PI for detailed dosage information.	Hepatic impairment can potentiate the response of warfarin through impaired synthesis of clotting factors and decreased metabolism of warfarin. Use with caution in these patients.
THROMBIN INHIBITORS				
Antithrombin (recombinant) (ATryn)	**Inj:** 1750 IU [single-dose vial]	Prevention of perioperative and peripartum thromboembolic events in hereditary antithrombin-deficient patients.	Dosage is to be individualized based on patient's pretreatment functional AT level, body weight, and using therapeutic drug monitoring. The goal of treatment is to restore and maintain functional AT activity levels between 80-120% of normal (0.8-1.2 IU/mL). Treatment should be initiated prior to delivery or approximately 24 hrs prior to surgery. AT activity monitoring is required for proper treatment. Administer loading dose as a 15 min IV infusion, followed by continuous infusion of the maintenance dose. Continue administration until adequate follow-on anticoagulation has been established. Refer to PI for dosing formula and monitoring/dose adjustment information.	
Antithrombin III (human) (Thrombate III)	**Inj:** 500 IU [single-dose vial]	Treatment of patients with hereditary antithrombin III deficiency in connection with surgical or obstetrical procedures or when they suffer from thromboembolism.	Exact loading dose, maintenance dose and dosing intervals should be individualized for each patient based on the individual clinical conditions, response to therapy, and actual plasma AT-III levels achieved. Dosage should be determined on an individual basis based on pretherapy plasma antithrombin III (AT-III) level, in order to increase levels to those found in normal human plasma (100%). Must be administered IV and may be infused over 10-20 min. See PI for dosing formula guide, patient monitoring, and additional information.	

(Continued)

GENERIC (BRAND)	HOW SUPPLIED	INDICATIONS	DOSAGE	HEPATIC/RENAL IMPAIRMENT
THROMBIN INHIBITORS *(Continued)*				
Argatroban	Inj: 100mg/mL [2.5mL single-use vial]	As an anticoagulant for prophylaxis or treatment of thrombosis in patients with heparin-induced thrombocytopenia. As an anticoagulant in patients with or at risk for heparin-induced thrombocytopenia who are undergoing percutaneous coronary intervention (PCI).	**HIT/HITTS:** Discontinue heparin therapy and obtain baseline aPTT before administration. The recommended initial dose for adults without hepatic impairment is 2mcg/kg/min as a continuous infusion. Check the aPTT 2 hrs after initiation of therapy and any dose change. Dose can be adjusted as clinically indicated (not to exceed 10mcg/kg/min) until the steady state aPTT is 1.5-3 times the initial baseline value (not to exceed 100 seconds). **PCI in HIT/HITTS Patients:** Infusion should be started at 25mcg/kg/min and a bolus of 350mcg/kg administered via a large bore IV line over 3-5 min. Activated clotting time (ACT) should be checked 5-10 min after the bolus dose is completed. The procedure may proceed if the ACT is >300 seconds. See PI for detailed information, including dose adjustment, therapy monitoring/conversion, and dosing in special populations.	**Hepatic Impairment in Adult Patients With Heparin-Induced Thrombocytopenia:** The initial dose should be reduced (0.5mcg/kg/min is recommended) in patients with moderate hepatic impairment. The aPTT should be monitored closely and dosage adjusted as clinically indicated. **Hepatic Impairment in HIT/HITTS Patients Undergoing PCI:** Carefully titrate until desired level of anticoagulation is achieved.
Bivalirudin (Angiomax)	Inj: 250mg [single-use vial]	Intended for use with aspirin as an anticoagulant in patients with unstable angina who are undergoing percutaneous transluminal coronary angioplasty (PTCA); patients undergoing percutaneous coronary intervention (PCI); and in patients with or at risk of heparin-induced thrombocytopenia (HIT) or heparin-induced thrombocytopenia and thrombosis syndrome (HITTS) who are undergoing PCI.	IV administration only. Intended for use with aspirin 300-325mg daily. **Patients Without HIT/HITTS:** 0.75mg/kg IV bolus, followed by an infusion of 1.75mg/kg/hr for duration of PCI/PTCA procedure. An activated clotting time (ACT) should be performed 5 minutes after the bolus dose. An additional bolus of 0.3mg/kg can be given if needed. **Patients With HIT/HITTS Undergoing PCI:** 0.75mg/kg IV bolus, followed by a continuous infusion of 1.75mg/kg/hr for the duration of the procedure. **Post-Procedure Treatment:** Continuation of infusion following PCI/PTCA for up to 4 hrs is optional. After 4 hrs, an additional IV infusion may be initiated at 0.2mg/kg/hr (low-rate infusion) for up to 20 hrs if needed.	**Renal Impairment:** No reduction in bolus dose needed. The infusion dose may need to be reduced and anticoagulant status monitored. **CrCl <30mL/min:** Consider 1mg/kg/min infusion. The infusion rate should be reduced in patients on hemodialysis to 0.25mg/kg/hr.
Dabigatran etexilate mesylate (Pradaxa)	Cap: 75mg, 150mg	To reduce the risk of stroke and systemic embolism in patients with non-valvular atrial fibrillation.	Assess renal function prior to initiation of treatment. Periodically assess renal function as clinically indicated and adjust therapy accordingly. **Patients with CrCl >30mL/min:** 150mg bid. Refer to PI for detailed information, including surgery/interventions dosing and conversions to/from warfarin and parenteral anticoagulants.	**Severe Renal Impairment (CrCl 15-30mL/min):** 75mg bid.

GENERIC (BRAND)	HOW SUPPLIED	INDICATIONS	DOSAGE	HEPATIC/RENAL IMPAIRMENT
THROMBIN INHIBITORS (Continued)				
Lepirudin (Refludan)	**Inj:** 50mg [vial]	Anticoagulation in patients with heparin-induced thrombocytopenia (HIT) and associated thromboembolic disease to prevent further thromboembolic complications.	0.4mg/kg body weight (up to 110kg) slow IV (over 15-20 seconds) as a bolus dose followed by 0.15mg/kg (up to 110kg/hr) as a continuous IV infusion for 2-10 days or longer if needed. Maximal initial bolus dose (44mg) and infusion dose (16.5mg/hr). Therapy should be monitored and adjusted using the aPTT ratio (1.5-2.5 target range during treatment). A baseline aPTT should be determined prior to therapy (should not start in patients with a ratio of 2.5 or more). **Concomitant Use w/ Thrombolytic Therapy:** 0.2mg/kg Initial IV bolus and 0.1mg/kg continuous IV infusion. Refer to PI for detailed information, including monitoring and therapy adjustments/conversions.	**Renal Impairment:** The bolus dose and the infusion rate must be reduced in case of known or suspected renal insufficiency (CrCl <60mL/min or serum creatinine >1.5mg/dL). Additional aPTT monitoring is highly recommended. The bolus dose is to be reduced to 0.2mg/kg in all patients with renal insufficiency. Refer to PI for detailed information including the reduction of infusion rate.

†Refer to full FDA-approved Prescribing Information for details.

DIURETICS

GENERIC	BRAND	USUAL HYPERTENSION DOSAGE RANGE	HOW SUPPLIED
ALDOSTERONE-RECEPTOR BLOCKERS			
Eplerenone	Inspra	50mg qd or bid	**Tab:** 25mg, 50mg
Spironolactone	Aldactone	50mg-100mg/day	**Tab:** 25mg, 50mg, 100mg
LOOP DIURETICS			
Bumetanide*	N/A	†	**Tab:** 0.5mg, 1mg, 2mg
Furosemide*	Lasix	40mg bid§	**Tab:** 20mg, 40mg, 80mg
Torsemide*	Demadex	5mg-10mg qd	**Tab:** 5mg, 10mg, 20mg, 100mg
POTASSIUM-SPARING DIURETICS			
Amiloride	Midamor	5mg-10mg qd	**Tab:** 5mg
Triamterene	Dyrenium	†	**Cap:** 50mg, 100mg
THIAZIDE DIURETICS			
Chlorothiazide*	Diuril	**Sus:** 0.5-1g/day§	**Sus:** 250mg/5mL
	Various Generics	**Tab:** 0.5g-1g/day§	**Tab:** 250mg, 500mg
Chlorthalidone	Thalitone	15mg-50mg qd	**Tab:** 15mg
	Various Generics	25mg-100mg qd	**Tab:** 25mg, 50mg
Hydrochlorothiazide	Microzide	12.5mg-50mg qd	**Cap:** 12.5mg
	Various Generics	12.5mg-50mg qd§	**Cap:** 12.5mg; **Tab:** 12.5mg, 25mg, 50mg
Indapamide	Various Generics	1.25mg-5mg qd	**Tab:** 1.25mg, 2.5mg
Methyclothiazide	N/A	2.5-5mg qd	**Tab:** 5mg
QUINAZOLINE DIURETIC			
Metolazone	Zaroxolyn	2.5-5mg qd	**Tab:** 2.5mg, 5mg, 10mg
COMBINATION DIURETICS‡			
Amiloride-Hydrochlorothiazide	Various Generics	1-2 tabs qd (5/50mg-10/100mg/day)	**Tab:** 5/50mg
Spironolactone-Hydrochlorothiazide	Aldactazide	50/50mg-100/100mg/day	**Tab:** 25/25mg, 50/50mg
Triamterene-Hydrochlorothiazide	Dyazide, Maxzide	37.5/25mg-75/50mg/day	**Cap:** 37.5/25mg; **Tab:** 37.5/25mg, 75/50mg

Abbreviation: N/A, not applicable.

* For additional dosage forms refer to monograph listings or drug's FDA-approved labeling.

† Not indicated for hypertension. For other indications refer to monograph listings or drug's FDA-approved labeling.

§ Pediatric dosing available.

‡ Fixed combination drugs are indicated for the treatment of hypertension in patients who develop hypokalemia on hydrochlorothiazide alone.

PSORIASIS MANAGEMENT: SYSTEMIC THERAPIES*

GENERIC (BRAND)	HOW SUPPLIED	DOSAGE	FREQUENT SIDE EFFECTS
ANTIMETABOLITE			
Methotrexate	**Inj:** 10mg/mL, 25mg/mL; **Tab:** 2.5mg	Weekly single oral, IM, or IV starting dosage schedule is 10-25mg/wk until response is achieved. Divided oral starting dose schedule is 2.5mg at 12-hr intervals x 3 doses. Doses may be gradually adjusted to achieve optimal response. **Max:** 30 mg/wk. Once optimal response is achieved, dosage schedule should be reduced to the lowest possible amount of drug and the longest possible rest period.	Ulcerative stomatitis, leukopenia, nausea, abdominal distress, malaise, undue fatigue, chills, fever, dizziness, decreased resistance to infection
IMMUNOSUPPRESSIVES			
Alefacept (Amevive)	**Inj:** 15mg/vial	15mg IM once weekly for 12 wks. Monitor CD4+ T lymphocyte counts every 2 wks during dosing period. If counts are <250 cells/μL, withhold dosing and monitor weekly. D/C therapy if counts remain <250 cells/μL for 1 month. An additional 12-wk course may be initiated if ≥12 wks have passed since previous course and CD4+ T lymphocyte counts are normal.	Pharyngitis, dizziness, increased cough, nausea, pruritus, myalgia, chills, injection-site pain/inflammation, accidental injury
Cyclosporine (Gengraf, Neoral)	**Cap:** 25mg, 100mg; **Sol:** 100mg/mL [50mL]	**Initial:** 1.25mg/kg bid for ≥4 wks, barring adverse events. If significant improvement has not occurred, dosage should be increased at 2-wk intervals. Based on patient response, dose increases of approximately 0.5mg/kg/day should be made to a max of 4mg/kg/day.	Renal dysfunction, headache, hypertension, hypertriglyceridemia, hirsutism/hypertrichosis, paresthesia or hyperesthesia, influenza-like symptoms, nausea/vomiting, diarrhea, abdominal discomfort, lethargy, musculoskeletal or joint pain
MONOCLONAL ANTIBODY			
Ustekinumab (Stelara)	**Inj:** 45mg/0.5mL, 90mg/1mL	Patients weighing ≤100 kg (220 lbs): 45mg SQ initially and 4 wks later, followed by 45mg q12 wks. Patients weighing >100 kg (220 lbs): 90mg SQ initially and 4 wks later, followed by 90mg q12 wks.	Nasopharyngitis, upper respiratory infection, headache, fatigue
MONOCLONAL ANTIBODIES/TNF BLOCKERS			
Adalimumab (Humira)	**Inj:** 20mg/0.4mL, 40mg/0.8mL	**Initial:** 80mg; **Maint:** 40mg every other wk starting 1 wk after initial dose.	Infections (eg, upper respiratory, sinusitis), injection-site reactions, headache, and rash
Infliximab (Remicade)	**Inj:** 100mg	Administer by IV infusion over a period of not less than 2 hrs: 5mg/kg at 0, 2, and 6 wks, then every 8 wks as directed.	Infections (eg, upper respiratory, sinusitis, pharyngitis), infusion-related reactions, headache, and abdominal pain
PSORALENS			
Methoxsalen† (8-Mop, Oxsoralen-Ultra)	**Cap:** 10mg	Take 2 hrs before UVA exposure with some food or milk. Dosing is based on patient's weight as follows: 10mg if <30 kg (66 lbs); 20mg if 30-50 kg (66-110 lbs); 30mg if 51-65 kg (112-143 lbs); 40mg if 66-80 kg (146-176 lbs); 50mg if 81-90 kg (179-198 lbs); 60mg if 91-115 kg (201-254 lbs); 70 mg if >115 kg (254 lbs). Dosage may be increased by 10mg after the 15th treatment under certain conditions as directed. Treatments should not be given more often than once every other day.	Nausea, nervousness, insomnia, depression, pruritis, erythema

(Continued)

GENERIC (BRAND)	HOW SUPPLIED	DOSAGE	FREQUENT SIDE EFFECTS
RETINOID			
Acitretin (Soriatane)	**Cap:** 10mg, 17.5mg, 25mg	**Initial:** 25-50mg per day as a single dose with the main meal. **Maint:** 25 to 50mg/day may be given dependent upon patient response to initial treatment. Relapses may be treated as outlined for initial therapy. When used with phytotherapy, prescriber should decrease the phytotherapy dose, dependent upon the patient's individual response, as directed.	Cheilitis, rhinitis, dry mouth, epistaxis, alopecia, dry skin, rash, skin peeling, nail disorder, pruritus, paresthesia, paronychia, skin atrophy, sticky skin, xerophthalmia, arthralgia, rigors, spinal hyperostosis, hyperesthesia
TNF-BLOCKING AGENT			
Etanercept (Enbrel)	**Inj:** 25mg [vial and prefilled syringe]; 50mg [prefilled syringe and autoinjector]	**Initial:** 50mg SQ twice weekly for 3 months. **Maint:** 50mg once weekly.	Infections and injection-site reactions

*Refer to full FDA Prescribing Information for details.

†Oxsoralen-Ultra and 8-MOP are not interchangeable due to significantly greater bioavailability and earlier photosensitization onset time of Oxsoralen-Ultra.

Source: FDA-approved product labeling.

PSORIASIS MANAGEMENT: TOPICAL THERAPIES

GENERIC (BRAND)	HOW SUPPLIED*	USUAL DOSAGE*	COMMON SIDE EFFECTS*
TOPICAL IMMUNOSUPPRESSANT			
Pimecrolimus (Elidel)	**Cre:** 1% [30g, 60g, 100g]	Apply a thin layer to affected skin bid.	Application-site burning and reaction, bronchitis, cough, upper respiratory tract infection, pyrexia, nasopharyngitis, influenza, headache
TOPICAL STEROIDS			
Betamethasone valerate (Luxiq)	(Generic) **Cre:** 0.1% [15g, 45g], **Oint:** 0.1% [15g, 45g], **Lot:** 0.1% [60mL]; (Luxiq) **Aerosol Foam:** 0.12% [50g, 100g]	**Cre, Oint:** Apply a thin layer to affected areas 1-3 times a day. **Lot:** Apply a few drops to the affected area bid in the am and hs ud. **Aerosol Foam:** Apply to scalp bid, am and hs ud.	Application-site burning, itching, irritation, stinging, dryness
Clobetasol propionate (Temovate, Temovate-E, Temovate Scalp Application, Clobex, Olux, Olux-E)	(Temovate) **Cre, Oint:** 0.05% [15g, 30g, 45g, 60g]; **Gel:** 0.05% [15g, 30g, 60g]; (Temovate Scalp Application) **Sol:** 0.05% [50mL]; (Temovate-E) **Cre:** 0.05% [60g]; (Clobex): **Lot:** 0.05% [59mL, 118mL]; **Shampoo:** 0.05% [118mL]; **Spray:** 0.05% [2oz, 4.25oz,]; (Olux) **Foam:** 0.05% [50g, 100g]; (Olux-E) **Foam:** 0.05% [50g, 100g]	**Cre, Gel, Oint, Lot:** Apply to affected areas bid. **Sol:** Apply bid am and pm; limit treatment to 2 consecutive wks. **Shampoo:** Apply to affected areas of scalp once a day ud. **Spray:** Spray directly onto affected areas bid. Do not exceed 50g/wk or 26 sprays/application or 52 sprays/day. (Olux) **Foam:** Apply to affected area bid am and hs; do not use more than 1½ capfuls per application. (Olux-E) **Foam:** Apply to affected areas bid, am and pm x 2 consecutive wks. Max wkly dose is 50g.	Application-site reactions, burning/stinging sensation and pruritus
Fluocinolone acetonide	**Cre:** 0.01%, 0.025% [15g, 60g]; **Oint:** 0.025% [15g, 60g]; **Sol:** 0.01% [60mL]	Apply a thin film to affected area bid-qid ud.	Burning, itching, irritation dryness, folliculitis, skin atrophy
Fluocinonide (Vanos)	(Generic) **Cre:** 0.05% [15g, 30g, 60g, 120g]; **Cre (Emulsified base):** 0.05% [15g, 30g, 60g]; **Gel:** 0.05% [15g, 30g, 60g]; **Oint:** 0.05% [15g, 30g, 60g]; **Sol:** 0.05% [20mL, 60mL]; (Vanos) **Cre:** 0.1% [30mg, 60mg, 120mg]	(Generic) **Cre, Cre (Emulsified base), Gel, Oint, Sol:** Apply a thin film to affected area bid-qid ud. (Vanos) **Cre:** Apply a thin layer to affected areas once or twice daily.	Burning, itching, irritation, dryness, folliculitis, headache, nasopharyngitis, nasal congestion
Halcinonide (Halog)	**Cre:** 0.1% [30g, 60g, 216g]; **Oint:** 0.1% [30g, 60g]	Apply to the affected area bid-tid.	Burning, itching, irritation, dryness, folliculitis, hypopigmentation, allergic contact dermatitis
Hydrocortisone (Anusol-HC, Locoid, Locoid Lipocream, Pandel, Proctocort, Westcort)	(Anusol-HC) **Cre:** 2.5% [30g]; (Locoid) 0.1% **Cre, Oint:** [15g, 45g]; **Sol:** [20mL, 60mL]; (Locoid Lipocream) **Cre:** 0.1% [15g, 45g, 60g]; (Pandel) **Cre:** 0.1% [15g, 45g, 80g]; (Proctocort) **Cre:** 1% [1oz]; (Westcort) **Cre, Oint:** 0.2% [15g, 45g, 60g]	(Anusol-HC) Apply to affected area bid-qid. (Locoid, Locoid Lipocream, Westcort) Apply a thin film to affected areas bid-tid. (Pandel) Apply a thin film to affected area once or twice a day. (Proctocort) Apply a thin film to affected area bid-qid.	Application-site reactions, burning, stinging, itching, dryness, folliculitis, hypopigmentation, skin atrophy, HPA axis suppression

(Continued)

GENERIC (BRAND)	HOW SUPPLIED*	USUAL DOSAGE*	COMMON SIDE EFFECTS*
Hydrocortisone acetate-pramoxine HCl (Epifoam, Novacort, Pramosone)	(Epifoam) **Foam:** 1%-1% [10g]; (Novacort) **Gel:** 2%-1% [29g]; (Pramosone) **Cre:** 1%-1%, 2.5%-1% [1oz, 2oz]; **Lot:** 1%-1% [60mL, 120mL, 240mL], 2.5%-1% [60mL, 120mL]; **Oint:** 1%-1%, 2.5%-1% [1oz]	Apply to affected area tid-qid ud.	Burning, itching, irritation, dryness, folliculitis
Mometasone furoate (Elocon)	**Cre, Oint:** 0.1% [15g, 45g]; **Lot:** 0.1% [30mL, 60mL]	**Cre, Oint:** Apply a thin film to the affected areas once daily. **Lot:** Apply a few drops to the affected areas once daily.	Burning, pruritus, skin atrophy, rosacea, acneiform reaction, tingling, stinging, furunculosis, folliculitis
Prednicarbate (Dermatop)	**Cre, Oint:** 0.1% [15g, 60g]	Apply a thin film to the affected areas bid. Rub in gently.	Burning, pruritus, irritant dermatitis, drying, scaling, cracking/pain, skin atrophy
Triamcinolone acetonide (Kenalog)	**Cre, Oint:** 0.025% [15g, 80g], 0.1% [15g, 80g, 454g], 0.5% [15g]; **Lot:** 0.025%, 0.1% [60mL]; **Spray:** 0.147mg/g [63g,100g]	**Cre, Lot, Oint:** 0.025%: Apply to the affected area bid-qid ud. 0.1% or 0.5%: Apply to the affected area bid-tid ud. **Spray:** Apply tid-qid ud.	Burning, itching, irritation, dryness, folliculitis, hypopigmentation, allergic contact dermatitis
Tazarotene (Tazorac)	**Cre:** 0.05%, 0.1% [30g, 60g]; **Gel:** 0.05%, 0.1% [30g, 100g]	Apply a thin film to lesions once a day in the evening ud.	Pruritus, burning/stinging, erythema, irritation, dry skin, rash
VITAMIN D DERIVATIVES & COMBINATIONS			
Calcitrol (Vectical)	**Oint:** 3mcg/g [5g, 100g]	Apply to affected area(s) bid, morning and evening. Max wkly dose should not exceed 200g.	Skin discomfort, pruritus, hypercalcemia, laboratory test abnormality, urine abnormality
Calcipotriene (Dovonex, Dovonex Scalp, Sorilux)	(Dovonex) **Cre:** 0.005% [60g, 120g]; (Dovonex Scalp) **Sol:** 0.005% [60mL]; (Sorilux) **Foam:** 0.005% [60g, 120g]	Apply to affected areas bid; rub in gently and completely ud.	Skin irritation, rash, pruritus, burning, stinging, tingling
Calcipotriene-betamethasone dipropionate (Taclonex, Taclonex Scalp)	**Oint:** 0.005%-0.064% [60g, 100g]; **Sus:** 50mcg-0.643mg/g [30g, 60g]	**Oint:** Apply to affected areas qd for up to 4 wks. Max wkly dose should not exceed 100g; **Sus:** Apply to affected areas once daily for 2 wks or until cleared (up to 8 wks). Max wkly dose should not exceed 100g.	Pruritus, burning sensation, folliculitis, scaly rash
MISCELLANEOUS AGENTS			
Anthralin (Dritho-Crème, Zithranol-RR)	(Dritho-Crème) **Cre:** 1% [50g]; (Zithranol-RR) **Cre:** 1.2% [15g, 45g]	Apply once a day ud.	Transient primary irritation, staining (skin and fabric), temporary discoloration of hair and fingernails
Urea	**Gel:** 40% [15mL]; **Lot:** 40% [236.6mL]	Apply to affected areas bid ud.	Transient stinging, burning, itching, irritation

Source: FDA-approved drug labeling.
*Refer to full FDA-approved prescribing information for details.

TOPICAL CORTICOSTEROIDS

STEROID	DOSAGE FORM(S)	STRENGTH (%)	POTENCY	FREQUENCY
Alclometasone dipropionate (Aclovate)	Cre, Oint	0.05	Low-Medium	bid/tid
Amcinonide	Lot	0.1	Medium*	bid/tid
	Cre, Oint	0.1	High*	bid/tid
Augmented betamethasone dipropionate (Diprolene, Diprolene AF)	Lot, Oint	0.05	Super High	qd/bid
	Cre	0.05	High	qd/bid
Betamethasone dipropionate	Cre, Lot	0.05	Medium*	qd/bid
	Oint	0.05	High	qd/bid
Betamethasone valerate (Luxiq)	Cre, Oint	0.1	Medium*	qd/tid
	Foam (Luxiq)	0.12	Medium	bid
	Lot	0.1	Low*	bid
Clobetasol propionate (Clobex, Cormax, Olux, Olux E, Temovate, Temovate-E)	Cre (Temovate), Foam (Olux, Olux-E), Gel, Lotion (Clobex), Oint (Cormax), Shampoo (Clobex), Sol (Cormax, Temovate Scalp Application)	0.05	Super High	**Cre, Foam, Lotion, Sol, Gel, Oint:** bid **Shampoo:** qd
Clocortolone pivalate (Cloderm)	Cre	0.1	Medium	tid
Desonide (Desonate, DesOwen, Verdeso)	Cre/Lot/Oint (Desowen), Foam (Verdeso), Gel (Desonate)	0.05	Low-Medium	**Foam/Gel:** bid; **Cre/Lot/Oint:** bid-tid
Desoximetasone (Topicort, Topicort LP)	Cre (Topicort LP)	0.05	Medium*	bid
	Gel (Topicort LP)	0.05	High*	bid
	Cre, Oint (Topicort)	0.25	High*	bid
Diflorasone diacetate (ApexiCon, Florone, Psorcon, Psorcon E)	Cre (ApexiCon E, Florone, Psorcon, Psorcon E), Oint (ApexiCon, Psorcon, Psorcon E)	0.05	High-Super High*	**Apexicon, Apexicon E, Psorcon Oint, Psorcon E Cre:** qd/tid; **Psorcon Cre:** bid; **Florone, Psorcon E Oint:** qd/qid
Fluocinolone acetonide (Capex, Derma-Smoothe/FS)	Cre, Oint	0.025	Medium	tid/qid
	Cre, Sol	0.01	Low*	tid/qid
	Oil (Derma-Smoothe/FS)	0.01	Low-Medium	**Adult:** tid; **Peds:** bid
	Shampoo (Capex)	0.01	Low-Medium	qd
Fluocinonide (Vanos)	Cre, Gel, Oint, Sol	0.05	High*	bid/qid
	Cre (Vanos)	0.1	Super High	qd/bid
Flurandrenolide (Cordran, Cordran SP)	Cre (Cordran SP) Oint (Cordran)	0.025	Medium*	bid/tid
	Cre (Cordran SP) Lot, Oint (Cordran)	0.05	Medium*	bid/tid
	Tape (Cordran)	4mcg/cm^2	Super High†	qd/bid
Fluticasone propionate (Cutivate)	Cre	0.05	Medium	qd/bid
	Lot	0.05	Medium‡	qd
	Oint	0.005	Medium	bid
Halcinonide (Halog)	Cre, Oint	0.1	High‡	bid/tid

(Continued)

STEROID	DOSAGE FORM(S)	STRENGTH (%)	POTENCY	FREQUENCY
Halobetasol propionate (Ultravate)	Cre, Oint	0.05	Super High	qd/bid
Hydrocortisone (Anusol HC, Ala Cort)	Cre	1	Low*	bid/tid
	Cre (Ala Cort)	1	Low*	bid/qid
	Oint	1	Low*	tid/qid
	Cre, Lot, Oint	2.5	Low*	bid/qid
Hydrocortisone acetate (U-cort)	Cre (U-cort)	1	Low	bid/qid
	Gel	2	Low	tid/qid
Hydrocortisone butyrate (Locoid, Locoid Lipocream)	Cre, Oint, Sol	0.1	Medium‡	bid/tid
	Lot	0.1	Medium‡	bid
Hydrocortisone probutate (Pandel)	Cre	0.1	Medium	qd/bid
Hydrocortisone valerate (Westcort)	Cre, Oint	0.2	Medium	bid/tid
Mometasone furoate (Elocon)	Cre, Lot, Oint	0.1	Medium	qd
Prednicarbate (Dermatop)	Cre, Oint	0.1	Medium	bid
Triamcinolone acetonide (Kenalog, Triderm)	Cre, Lot, Oint	0.025	Medium*	bid/qid
	Cre, Lot, Oint	0.1	Medium*	bid/tid
	Cre, Oint	0.5	Medium*	bid/tid
	Spray	0.147mg/g	Medium	tid/qid

†Refer to the full FDA prescribing information for details.

* **Source:** Fougera & Co. website: Available at: www.fougera.com/knowledge_center/steroid potency.asp.

† **Source:** www.cordrantape.com/hcp-about.asp.

‡ **Source:** Topical steroid potency chart–National Psoriasis Foundation www.psoriasis.org.

INSULIN FORMULATIONS

TYPE OF INSULIN*	BRAND	ONSET†	PEAK†	DURATION†
Rapid-acting				
Insulin glulisine	Apidra	5-15 mins	0.5 to 1.5 hrs	<5 hrs
Insulin lispro	Humalog	5-15 mins	2.4 hrs	
Insulin aspart	NovoLog	10-20 mins	40-50 mins	
Short-acting				
Regular insulin	Humulin R‡	<30-45 mins	4.4 (4.0-5.5) hrs	6-11.5 hrs
	Novolin R	30 mins	1.5-2 hrs	Up to 8 hrs
Immediate-acting				
NPH (isophane)	Humulin N		5.5 (3.5-9.5) hrs	
	Novolin N	1.8 hrs	4-12 hrs	Up to 24 hrs
Long-acting				
Insulin glargine	Lantus	1 hrs	Peakless	Up to 24 hrs
Insulin detemir	Levemir	1.6 hrs	Peakless	Up to 24 hrs
Combinations				
Isophane insulin suspension (70%)/ regular insulin (30%)	Humulin 70/30		4.4 (1.5-16) hrs	
	Novolin 70/30	30 mins	4.2 hrs	Up to 24 hrs
Insulin aspart protamine (70%)/insulin aspart (30%)	NovoLog Mix 70/30	10-20 mins	2.4 hrs	Up to 24 hrs
Insulin lispro protamine (50%)/insulin lispro (50%)	Humalog Mix 50/50	5-15 mins	0.75-2 hrs	10-16 hrs
Insulin lispro protamine (75%)/insulin lispro (25%)	Humalog Mix 75/25	5-15 mins	Dual	10-16 hrs

*Dose regimens of all insulins will vary among patients and should be determined by the healthcare professional familiar with the patient's metabolic needs, eating habits, and other lifestyle variables.

†Assumes 0.1-0.3 units/kg/injection. Onset and duration may vary by injection site.

‡Also available as 500 U/mL for insulin-resistant patients (rapid onset; up to 24-hr duration).

Niswender K. Early and aggressive initiation of insulin therapy for type 2 diabetes: what is the evidence? *Clin Diabetes.* 2009;27:60-68.

National Diabetes Information Clearinghouse (NDIC). Types of Insulin. http://diabetes.niddk.nih.gov/dm/pubs/medicines_ez/insert_C.aspx. Accessed March 20, 2012.

ORAL ANTIDIABETIC AGENTS

BRAND (GENERIC)	HOW SUPPLIED	INITIAL* & (MAX) DOSE	USUAL DOSE RANGE*	PROPERTIES
BIGUANIDES				
Fortamet† (Metformin HCl)	Tab: ER: 500mg, 1000mg	1000mg qd with evening meal (2500mg/day)	500mg-2500mg/day	Mechanism: Activates AMP-Kinase Action(s): Hepatic glucose production ↓, intestinal glucose absorption ↓, insulin action ↑ Advantages: No weight gain, no hypoglycemia, reduction in cardiovascular events and mortality Disadvantages: GI side effects (diarrhea, abdominal cramping), lactic acidosis (rare), vitamin B₁₂ deficiency, Contraindications: Reduced kidney function
Glumetza† (Metformin HCl)	Tab: ER: 500mg, 1000mg	Metformin-Naïve: 500mg qd with evening meal (2000mg/day)	500mg-2000mg/day	
Glucophage†, Riomet† (Metformin HCl)	Tab: 500mg, 850 mg, 1000mg Sol: 500mg/5mL	500mg bid or 850mg qd with meals (2550mg/day)	850mg-2000mg/day	
Glucophage XR† (Metformin HCl)	Tab: ER: 500mg, 750mg	500mg qd with evening meal (2000mg/day)	500mg-2000mg qd or divided doses	
BILE-ACID SEQUESTRANT				
Welchol (Colesevelam HCl)	Tab: 625mg; Sus: 3.75g, 1.875g [pkt]	Tab: 1875mg bid or 3750 qd; Sus: 1.875g pkt bid or 3.75g pkt qd	3750mg/day	Mechanism: Binds bile acids/cholesterol Action(s): Unknown Advantages: No hypoglycemia, LDL cholesterol ↓ Disadvantages: Constipation, triglycerides ↑, may interfere with absorption of other medications
DIPEPTIDYL PEPTIDASE-4 INHIBITORS				
Tradjenta (Linagliptin)	Tab: 5mg	5mg qd	5mg/day	Mechanism: Inhibits DPP-4 activity, prolongs survival of endogenously released incretin hormones Action(s): Active GLP-1 concentration ↑, active GIP concentration ↑, insulin secretion ↑, glucagon secretion ↓ Advantages: No hypoglycemia, weight "neutrality" Disadvantages: Occasional reports of urticaria/angioedema, cases of pancreatitis observed, long-term safety unknown
Onglyza (Saxagliptin)	Tab: 2.5mg, 5mg	2.5-5mg qd	2.5-5mg/day	
Januvia (Sitagliptin)	Tab: 25mg, 50mg, 100mg	100mg qd	100mg/day	
GLUCOSIDASE INHIBITORS				
Precose (Acarbose)	Tab: 25mg, 50mg, 100mg	25mg tid at start of each meal (≤60kg: 50mg tid, >60kg: 100mg tid)	50-100mg tid	Mechanism: Inhibits intestinal α-glucosidase Action(s): Intestinal carbohydrate digestion (and, consecutively, absorption) slowed Advantages: Nonsystemic medication, postprandial glucose ↓ Disadvantages: GI side effects (gas, flatulence, diarrhea), dosing frequency
Glyset (Miglitol)	Tab: 25mg, 50mg, 100mg	25mg tid at start of each meal (300mg/day)	50-100mg tid	

(Continued)

BRAND (GENERIC)	HOW SUPPLIED	INITIAL* & (MAX) DOSE	USUAL DOSE RANGE*	PROPERTIES
MEGLITINIDES				
Starlix (Nateglinide)	**Tab:** 60mg, 120mg	120mg tid before meals	120mg tid	**Mechanism:** Closes K_{ATP} channels on β-cell plasma membranes **Action(s):** Insulin secretion ↑ **Advantages:** Accentuated effects around meal ingestion **Disadvantages:** Hypoglycemia, weight gain, may blunt myocardial ischemic preconditioning, dosing frequency
Prandin (Repaglinide)	**Tab:** 0.5mg, 1mg, 2mg	0.5-2mg with each meal (16mg/day)	0.5-4mg with each meal	
SULFONYLUREAS				
Diabinese (Chlorpropamide)	**Tab:** 100mg, 250mg	Initial: 250mg qd. **Elderly:** 100-125mg qd (750mg/day)	<100-500mg qd. Most patients controlled with 250mg qd	**Mechanism:** Closes K_{ATP} channels on β-cell plasma membranes **Action(s):** Insulin secretion ↑ **Advantages:** Generally well tolerated, reduction in CV events and mortality **Disadvantages:** Relatively glucose-independent stimulation of insulin secretion: hypoglycemia, including episodes necessitating hospital admission and causing death; weight gain; may blunt myocardial ischemic preconditioning; low "durability"
Amaryl (Glimepiride)	**Tab:** 1mg, 2mg, 4mg	1-2mg qd w/breakfast or first main meal (8mg/day)	1-8mg/day	
Glucotrol (Glipizide)	**Tab:** 5mg, 10mg	5mg qd before breakfast (40mg/day)	5-40mg; divided doses if >15mg/day	
Glucotrol XL (Glipizide)	**Tab: ER:** 2.5mg, 5mg, 10mg	5mg qd w/break-fast (20mg/day)	5-10mg	
Diabeta (Glyburide)	**Tab:** 1.25mg, 2.5mg, 5mg	2.5-5mg qd w/ breakfast or first main meal (20mg/day)	1.25-20mg in single or divided doses	
Glynase PresTab (Glyburide Micronized)	**Tab:** 1.5mg, 3mg, 6mg	1.5-3mg qd w/ breakfast or first main meal (12mg/day)	0.75-12mg in single or divided doses	
Tolazamide	**Tab:** 250mg, 500mg	100-250mg qd with breakfast or first main meal (1000mg/day)	100-1000mg; divided doses if >500mg/day	
Tolbutamide	**Tab:** 500mg	1000-2000mg qd or divided doses (3000mg/day)	250-3000mg in single or divided doses	
THIAZOLIDINEDIONES				
Actos‡ (Pioglitazone HCl)	**Tab:** 15mg, 30mg, 45mg	15-30mg qd (45mg/day)	15-45mg	**Mechanism:** Activates the nuclear transcription factor PPAR-γ **Action(s):** Peripheral insulin sensitivity ↑ **Advantages:** No hypoglycemia; (Actos) HDL cholesterol ↑, triglycerides ↓ **Disadvantages:** Weight gain, edema, heart failure, bone fractures; (Avandia) LDL cholesterol ↑, increased CV events (mixed evidence), FDA warnings on CV safety, contraindicated in patients with heart disease
Avandia‡ (Rosiglitazone maleate)	**Tab:** 2mg, 4mg, 8mg	2mg bid or 4mg qd (8mg/day)	4-8mg/day	

BRAND (GENERIC)	HOW SUPPLIED	INITIAL* & (MAX) DOSE	USUAL DOSE RANGE*	PROPERTIES
COMBINATIONS				
(Glipizide/ Metformin HCl)	**Tab:** 2.5mg/250mg, 2.5mg/500mg, 5mg/500mg	2.5mg/250mg qd w/meals or 2.5mg/500mg bid (20mg/2000mg/day)	2.5mg/250mg qd-5mg/500mg bid	
Glucovance† (Glyburide/ Metformin HCl)	**Tab:** 1.25mg/250mg, 2.5mg/500mg, 5mg/500mg	1.25mg/250mg qd or bid with meals (20mg/2000mg/day)	1.25mg/250mg qd-5mg/500mg bid	
Jentadueto† (Linagliptin/ Metformin HCl)	**Tab:** 2.5mg/500mg, 2.5mg/850mg, 2.5mg/1000mg	2.5mg/500mg bid with meals (5mg/2000mg/day)	2.5mg/500mg-2.5mg/1000mg bid	
Duetact (Pioglitazone/ Glimepiride)	**Tab:** 30mg/2mg, 30mg/4mg	30mg/2mg or 30mg/4mg qd with first meal (45mg/8mg/day)	30mg/2mg-30mg/4mg/day	
Actoplus Met†,‡ (Pioglitazone/ Metformin HCl)	**Tab:** 15mg/500mg, 15mg/850mg	15mg/500mg or 15mg/850mg qd-bid with food (45mg/2550mg/day)	15/500mg qd-15/850mg bid/day	
Actoplus Met XR†,‡ (Pioglitazone/ Metformin HCl)	**Tab: ER:** 15mg/1000mg, 30mg/1000mg	15mg/1000mg or 30mg/1000mg qd with evening meal (45mg/2000mg/day)	15mg/1000mg-30mg/1000mg/day	
PrandiMet‡ (Repaglinide/ Metformin HCl)	**Tab:** 1mg/500mg, 2mg/500mg	1mg/500mg bid before meals (10mg/2500/day)	1mg/1500mg bid-2mg/1500mg tid	
Avandaryl‡ (Rosiglitazone/ Glimepiride)	**Tab:** 4mg/1mg, 4mg/2mg, 4mg/4mg, 8mg/2mg, 8mg/4mg	4mg/1mg qd or 4mg/2mg qd w/first meal (8mg/4mg/day)	1 tab qd	
Avandamet†,‡ (Rosiglitazone/ Metformin HCl)	**Tab:** 2mg/500mg, 4mg/500mg, 2mg/1000mg, 4mg/1000mg	Individualize: 2mg/500mg bid w/meals (8mg/2000mg/day)	1 tab bid	
Kombiglyze XR† (Saxagliptin/ Metformin HCl)	**Tab: ER:** 5mg/500mg, 5mg/1000mg, 2.5/1000mg	5mg/500mg or 2.5mg/1000mg qd with evening meal (5mg/2000mg/day)	1 tab qd	
Janumet† (Sitagliptin/ Metformin)	**Tab:** 50mg/500mg, 50mg/1000mg	50mg/500mg or 50mg/1000mg bid w/meals (100mg/2000mg/day)	50mg/500mg-50mg/1000mg bid	

*Usual dose ranges are derived from the drug's FDA-approved labeling. There is no fixed dosage regimen for the management of diabetes mellitus with any hypoglycemic agent. The initial and maintenance dosing should be conservative, depending on the patient's individual needs, especially in elderly, debilitated, or malnourished patients, and with impaired renal or hepatic function. Management of type 2 diabetes should include blood glucose and HbA1c monitoring, nutritional counseling, exercise, and weight reduction as needed. For more detailed information, refer to the individual monograph listings or the drug's FDA-approved labeling.

†**BOXED WARNING:** Products containing metformin may cause lactic acidosis due to metformin accumulation. Refer to package insert for more details.

‡**BOXED WARNING:** Products containing thiazolidinediones, including pioglitazone or rosiglitazone, may cause or exacerbate congestive heart failure in some patients. Refer to package insert for more details regarding this warning.

Source: Standards of Medical Care in Diabetes—2012. *Diabetes Care.* 2012;35(Suppl 1):S11-S49.

ANTIEMETICS

GENERIC (BRAND)	INDICATIONS	HOW SUPPLIED	ADULT DOSAGE	PEDIATRIC DOSAGE
ANTICHOLINERGIC AGENT				
Scopolamine (Transderm Scop)	Prevention of N/V associated with motion sickness or recovery from anesthesia and PONV.	**Patch:** 1mg/72 hrs [4S]	**PONV:** Apply 1 patch the evening before surgery or 1 hr prior to cesarean section. Keep in place for 24 hrs following surgery. **Motion Sickness:** Apply patch to a hairless area behind the ear at least 4 hrs before needed. Do not cut patch in half.	
ANTIHISTAMINES				
Dimenhydrinate	Prevention and treatment of nausea, vomiting, or vertigo caused by motion sickness.	**Inj:** 50mg/mL	(Inj) 50mg q4h, may increase to 100mg q4h if drowsiness is desirable. For IV administration, dilute each mL of solution in 10mL of 0.9% sodium chloride and inject over 2 min. IM injection is administered undiluted.	(IM) 1.25mg/kg or 37.5mg/m² body surface area qid. Max: 300mg/day.
Meclizine HCl (Antivert)	Management of nausea, vomiting, and dizziness associated with motion sickness.	**Tab:** 12.5mg, 25mg, 50mg* *scored	Motion Sickness: 25-50mg 1 hr prior to trip/ departure; repeat q24h prn.	≥12 yrs: Motion Sickness: 25-50mg 1 hr prior to trip/departure; repeat q24h prn.
Promethazine HCl (Promethegan)	Prevention and control of N/V associated with certain types of anesthesia and surgery. Active and prophylactic treatment of motion sickness. Postoperative antiemetic therapy.	**Sup:** 50mg (Generic): 12.5mg, 25mg; **Liq:** 6.25/5mL [118mL, 473mL]; **Tab:** 12.5mg, 25mg, 50mg; **Inj:** 25mg/mL, 50mg/mL	**N/V:** 12.5-25mg q4-6h. Do not give IV administration >25mg/mL and at a rate >25mg/min. **Motion Sickness:** 25mg 0.5-1 h prior to trip/departure, repeat after 8-12 hrs if needed. Maint: 25mg bid.	≥2 yrs: Motion Sickness: 12.5-25mg bid. N/V: 12.5-25mg may be repeated at 4-6 hr intervals. Usual: 0.5mg/lb: adjust for patient's age and weight and condition severity. Dose should not exceed half of the adult dose. Do not give IV administration >25mg/mL and at a rate >25mg/min.
CANNABINOIDS				
Dronabinol (Marinol)	Treatment of N/V associated with chemotherapy when conventional treatment has failed.	**Cap:** 2.5mg, 5mg, 10mg	**Initial:** 5mg/m² given 1-3 hrs before chemotherapy, then q2-4h after chemotherapy, up to 4-6 doses/day. **Titrate:** May increase by 2.5mg/m² increments. **Max:** 15mg/m²/dose.	**Initial:** 5mg/m² given 1-3 hrs before chemotherapy, then q2-4h after chemotherapy, up to 4-6 doses/day. **Titrate:** May increase by 2.5mg/m² increments. **Max:** 15mg/m²/dose. Use caution because of psychoactive effects.

(Continued)

GENERIC (BRAND)	INDICATIONS	HOW SUPPLIED	ADULT DOSAGE	PEDIATRIC DOSAGE
CANNABINOIDS *(Continued)*				
Nabilone (Cesamet)	Treatment of N/V associated with chemotherapy when conventional treatment has failed.	**Cap:** 1mg	**Usual:** 1 or 2mg bid. Give initial dose 1-3 hrs before chemotherapy. A dose of 1 or 2mg the night before may be useful. May be given bid-tid during chemotherapy cycle and, if needed, for 48 hrs after the last dose of each cycle. **Max:** 6mg/day given in divided doses tid.	
5-HT₃ ANTAGONISTS				
Dolasetron mesylate (Anzemet)	(Inj) Prevention and treatment of PONV. (Tab) Prevention of N/V associated with moderately emetogenic cancer chemotherapy and prevention of PONV.	**Inj:** 20mg/mL; **Tab:** 50mg, 100mg	(Inj) **Prevention/Treatment of PONV:** 12.5mg IV single dose 15 min before cessation of anesthesia or as soon as N/V presents. (Tab) **Prevention of Chemotherapy-Induced Nausea/Vomiting (CINV):** 100mg PO within 1 hr before chemotherapy. **Prevention of PONV:** 100mg PO within 2 hrs before surgery.	**2-16 yrs:** (Inj) **Prevention/Treatment of PONV:** 0.35mg/kg IV single dose 15 min before cessation of anesthesia or as soon as nausea/vomiting presents. Max: 12.5mg single dose. May mix 1.2mg/kg inj in apple or apple-grape juice and take orally within 2 hrs before surgery. Max: 100mg/dose. (Tab) **Prevention of CINV:** 1.8mg/kg PO within 1 hr before chemotherapy. Max: 100mg. **Prevention of PONV:** 1.2mg/kg PO within 2 hrs before surgery. Max: 100mg.
Granisetron HCl (Kytril)	(Inj, Sol, Tab) Prevention of CINV, including high-dose cisplatin. (Sol, Tab) Prevention of nausea and vomiting associated with radiation. (Inj) Prevention and treatment of PONV.	**Inj:** 0.1mg/mL, 1mg/mL; **Sol:** 2mg/10mL [30mL]; **Tab:** 1mg	(Sol/Tab) **Prevention of CINV:** 2mg qd up to 1 hr before chemotherapy or 1mg bid (given up to 1 hr before chemotherapy and 12 hrs later). (Inj) 10mcg/kg within 30 min before chemotherapy. **Prevention with Radiation:** (Sol/Tab) 2mg within 1 hr of radiation. **Prevention and Treatment of PONV:** (Inj) Administer 1mg over 30 sec before induction of anesthesia or immediately before anesthesia reversal.	**2-16 yrs: Prevention of CINV:** 10mcg/kg IV within 30 min before chemotherapy.

GENERIC (BRAND)	INDICATIONS	HOW SUPPLIED	ADULT DOSAGE	PEDIATRIC DOSAGE
5-HT₃ ANTAGONISTS (Continued)				
Granisetron transdermal system (Sancuso)	Prevention of N/V in patients receiving moderately and/or highly emetogenic chemotherapy regimens of up to 5 consecutive days duration.	**Patch:** 3.1mg/24 hrs [1⁵]	Apply patch to upper outer arm 24 hrs prior to chemotherapy. The patch may be applied up to a maximum of 48 hrs before chemotherapy. Remove patch a minimum of 24 hrs after completion of chemotherapy. Patch can be worn for up to 7 days depending on duration of chemotherapy regimen.	
Ondansetron (Zuplenz)	Prevention of N/V associated with: Highly emetogenic cancer chemotherapy, including cisplatin ≥50mg/m²; moderately emetogenic cancer chemotherapy with initial and repeat courses; radiotherapy in patients receiving either total body irradiation, single high-dose fraction to abdomen, or daily fractions to the abdomen. Prevention of PONV.	**Film, Oral:** 4mg, 8mg	**Prevention of N/V Associated with Highly Emetogenic Chemotherapy:** 24mg 30 min before chemotherapy. **Prevention of N/V Associated with Moderately Emetogenic Chemotherapy:** 8mg bid; give first dose 30 min before chemotherapy, then 8 hrs later, then bid (q12h) for 1-2 days after completion of chemotherapy. **Prevention of N/V Associated with Radiotherapy:** 8mg tid. **Total Body Irradiation:** 8mg 1-2 hrs before each fraction of radiotherapy administered each day. **Single High-Dose Fraction Radiotherapy to Abdomen:** 8mg 1-2 hrs before therapy then q8h after first dose for 1-2 days after completion of therapy. **Daily Fractionated Radiotherapy to Abdomen:** 8mg 1-2 hrs before therapy then q8h after first dose for each day radiotherapy is given. **Prevention of PONV:** 16mg 1 hr before induction of anesthesia. **Severe Hepatic Dysfunction (Child-Pugh ≥10): Max:** 8mg/day.	**≥12 yrs: Prevention of N/V Associated with Moderately Emetogenic Chemotherapy:** 8mg bid; give first dose 30 min before chemotherapy, then 8 hrs later, then bid (q12h) for 1-2 days after completion of chemotherapy. **4-11 years:** 4mg tid; give first dose 30 min before chemotherapy, then 4 and 8 hrs later, then tid (q8h) for 1-2 days after completion of chemotherapy. **Severe Hepatic Dysfunction (Child-Pugh ≥10): Max:** 8mg/day.

(Continued)

GENERIC (BRAND)	INDICATIONS	HOW SUPPLIED	ADULT DOSAGE	PEDIATRIC DOSAGE
5-HT₃ ANTAGONISTS *(Continued)*				
Ondansetron HCI (Zofran)	(Inj) Prevention of N/V associated with initial and repeat courses of emetogenic cancer chemotherapy, including high-dose cisplatin. Prevention of PONV. (Sol/Tab) Prevention of N/V associated with highly emetogenic cancer chemotherapy, including cisplatin ≥50mg/m²: initial and repeat courses of moderately emetogenic cancer chemotherapy; and radiotherapy in patients receiving either total body irradiation, single high-dose fraction to the abdomen, or daily fractions to the abdomen. Prevention of PONV.	**Inj:** 2mg/mL; **Sol:** 4mg/5mL [50mL]; **Tab:** 4mg, 8mg; **Tab, Disintegrating:** 4mg, 8mg	**Prevention of CINV:** (Inj) 32mg single dose or three 0.15mg/kg doses; give first dose (over 15 min) 30 min before chemotherapy. For three-dose regimen, give subsequent two doses 4 and 8 hrs after first dose. **Prevention of CINV, Highly Emetogenic Therapy:** (Tab) 24mg given as three 8mg tablets administered 30 min before chemotherapy. **Prevention of CINV, Moderately Emetogenic Therapy:** (Sol/Tab) 8mg bid, first dose 30 min before chemotherapy, then 8 hrs later, then bid for 1-2 days after chemotherapy. **Prevention of PONV:** (Inj) 4mg undiluted IM/IV immediately before anesthesia or post-op if nausea or vomiting occurs; as IV, infuse over 2-5 min. (Sol/Tab) 16mg 1 hr before anesthesia. **Prevention of N/V Associated with Radiation Therapy:** (Sol/Tab) Usual: 8mg tid. **Total Body Irradiation:** 8mg 1-2 hrs before each fraction of therapy daily. **Single High-Dose Therapy to Abdomen:** 8mg 1-2 hrs before therapy then q8h after first dose for 1-2 days after completion of therapy. **Daily Fractionated Therapy to Abdomen:** 8mg 1-2 hrs before therapy then q8h after first dose for each day radiotherapy is given. **Severe Hepatic Dysfunction (Child-Pugh ≥10): Max:** 8mg/day IV single dose infused over 15 min; start 30 min before chemotherapy or 8mg/day PO.	**Prevention of CINV:** (Inj) **6 months-18 yrs:** Three 0.15mg/kg doses, first dose 30 min before chemotherapy, then 4 and 8 hrs after the first dose. Infuse over 15 min. (Sol/Tab) **Prevention of CINV, Moderately Emetogenic Therapy: ≥12 yrs:** 8mg bid, first dose 30 min before chemotherapy, then 8mg 8 hrs later, then bid for 1-2 days after chemotherapy. **4-11 yrs:** 4mg tid, first dose 30 min before chemotherapy, then 4 and 8 hrs after first dose, then tid for 1-2 days after chemotherapy. **Prevention of PONV:** (Inj) **1 month-12 yrs: ≤40kg:** 0.1mg/kg single dose. **>40kg:** 4mg single dose. Infuse over 2-5 min immediately before or after anesthesia induction or post-op if N/V occurs. **Severe Hepatic Dysfunction: Max:** 8mg/day IV single dose infused over 15 min, start 30 min before chemotherapy or 8mg/day PO.	
Palonosetron HCI (Aloxi)	(Inj) Prevention of acute and delayed N/V associated with initial and repeat courses of moderately emetogenic cancer chemotherapy and prevention of acute N/V associated with initial and repeat courses of highly emetogenic cancer chemotherapy. Prevention of PONV for up to 24 hrs following surgery.	**Inj:** 0.25mg/5mL, 0.075mg/1.5mL	**Chemo-Induced N/V:** 0.25mg IV single dose over 30 sec, 30 min before start of chemotherapy. **PONV:** 0.075mg IV single dose 10 sec before induction of anesthesia.	

GENERIC (BRAND)	INDICATIONS	HOW SUPPLIED	ADULT DOSAGE	PEDIATRIC DOSAGE
MISCELLANEOUS				
Droperidol	To reduce incidence of N/V associated with surgical and diagnostic procedures.	**Inj:** 2.5mg/mL	Initial (Max): 2.5mg IM/IV. May give additional 1.25mg cautiously to achieve desired effect. Lower initial doses in elderly, debilitated, poor-risk patients.	**2-12 yrs:** Initial (Max): 0.1 mg/kg IM/IV. May give additional dose cautiously. Lower initial doses in debilitated, poor-risk patients.
Metoclopramide (Reglan)	Prevention of PONV or CINV.	**Inj:** 5mg/mL	**PONV:** 10-20mg IM near end of surgery. **CINV:** 1-2mg/kg IV over not less than 15 min, 30 min before chemotherapy then q2h for 2 doses, then q3h for 3 doses. Give 2mg/kg for highly emetogenic drugs for initial 2 doses. For CrCl <40mL/min: Give approx. half the recommended dosage.	
Trimethobenzamide HCl (Tigan)	Treatment of PONV and for nausea associated with gastroenteritis.	**Cap:** 300mg; **Inj:** 100mg/mL	(Cap) 300mg tid-qid. (Inj) 200mg IM tid-qid. **Renal Impairment (CrCl ≤70mL/min/1.73m²):** Reduce dose or increase dosing interval.	
PHENOTHIAZINE DERIVATIVE				
Prochlorperazine (Compro)	Control of severe N/V.	**Inj:** (Edisylate) 5mg/mL; **Supp:** (Compro) 25mg; **Tab:** (Maleate) 5mg, 10mg	**N/V:** (Tab) Usual: 5-10mg tid-qid. >40mg/day only in resistant cases. (Supp) 25mg bid. (IM) 5-10mg IM q3-4h prn. Max: 40mg/day. (IV) 2.5-10mg IV (not bolus) at rate ≤5mg/min. Max: 10mg single dose and 40mg/day. **N/V with Surgery:** 5-10mg IM 1-2 hrs or 5-10mg IV (not bolus) at rate ≤5mg/min 15-30 min before anesthesia (repeat once in 30 min if needed for IM), or to control acute symptoms during or after surgery; repeat once if needed. Max: 10mg single dose and 40mg/day.	**N/V: Tab: 20-29 lbs:** Usual: 2.5mg qd-bid. Max: 7.5mg/day. **30-39 lbs:** 2.5mg bid-tid. Max: 10mg/day. **40-85 lbs:** 2.5mg tid or 5 mg bid. Max: 15mg/day. (IM) 0.06mg/lb, usually single dose for control.

(Continued)

GENERIC (BRAND)	INDICATIONS	HOW SUPPLIED	ADULT DOSAGE	PEDIATRIC DOSAGE
SUBSTANCE P/NEUROKININ₁ RECEPTOR ANTAGONISTS				
Aprepitant (Emend)	In combination with other antiemetics for prevention of acute and delayed N/V associated with initial and repeat courses of highly emetogenic cancer chemotherapy (eg, high-dose cisplatin) or moderately emetogenic cancer chemotherapy. For the prevention of PONV.	**Cap:** 40mg, 80mg, 125mg; **Tri-Pak:** (one 125mg & two 80mg caps)	**Prevention of CINV: Day 1:** 125mg 1 hr prior to chemotherapy. Days 2 and 3: 80mg qam. Regimen should include a corticosteroid and a 5-HT₃ antagonist. **Prevention of PONV:** 40mg within 3 hrs prior to induction of anesthesia.	
Fosaprepitant dimeglumine (Emend for injection)	In combination with other antiemetics for prevention of acute and delayed N/V associated with initial and repeat courses of highly emetogenic cancer chemotherapy (eg, high-dose cisplatin) or moderately emetogenic cancer chemotherapy.	**Powder (Vial):** 115mg, 150mg	**Prevention of Highly Emetogenic CINV: 3-Day Dosing Regimen:** 115mg IV over 15 min initiated 30 min prior to chemotherapy on day 1 only of a 3-day regimen, in addition to corticosteroid and 5-HT₃ antagonist. **Single-Dose Regimen:** 150mg IV over 20-30 min initiated 30 min prior to chemotherapy, in addition to a corticosteroid and 5-HT₃ antagonist. **Prevention of Moderately Emetogenic CINV: 3-Day Dosing Regimen:** 115mg IV over 15 min 30 min prior to chemotherapy on day 1 only of a 3-day regimen, in addition to corticosteroid and 5-HT₃ antagonist.	

Abbreviations: CINV = chemotherapy-induced nausea and vomiting; N/V = nausea and vomiting; PONV = post-op nausea and vomiting

H₂ Antagonists And PPI Comparison*

	DRUG	HOW SUPPLIED	Heartburn	PUD	GERD	Esophagitis	Zollinger-Ellison	H. pylori	NSAID† Induced	Upper GI‡ Bleeding	Duodenal Ulcer
H₂ ANTAGONISTS	**CIMETIDINE**										
	Generic	Inj: 150mg/mL,		X			X			X	X
		Sol: 300mg/5mL§		X	X	X	X				X
		Tab: 200mg, 300mg, 400mg, 800mg§	X	X	X	X	X				X
	FAMOTIDINE										
	Pepcid	Inj: 10mg/mL§		X	X	X	X				X
		Sus: 40mg/5mL	X	X	X	X	X				X
		Tab: 20mg, 40mg	X	X	X	X	X				X
	NIZATIDINE										
	Axid	Cap: 150mg, 300mg§ Sol: 15mg/mL	X	X	X	X					X
	RANITIDINE										
	Zantac	Inj: 1mg/mL, 25mg/mL Syrup: 15mg/1mL Tab: 150mg, 300mg Tab, Effervescent: 25mg	X	X	X	X	X				X
PROTON PUMP INHIBITORS	**DEXLANSOPRAZOLE**										
	Dexilant	Cap, DR: 30mg, 60mg	X		X	X					
	ESOMEPRAZOLE										
	Nexium	Cap, DR: 20mg, 40mg	X		X	X	X	X	X		
		Sus, DR: 2.5 mg, 5mg, 10mg, 20mg, 40mg (granules/packet)	X		X	X	X	X	X		
		Inj: 20mg, 40mg			X	X					
	Vimovo	Tab, DR: (Esomeprazole Magnesium-Naproxen) 20mg-375mg, 20mg-500mg							X		
	LANSOPRAZOLE										
	Prevacid	Cap, DR: 15mg, 30mg Tab, Disintegrating: 15mg, 30mg	X	X	X	X	X	X	X		X
	Prevpac	Cap: (Amoxicillin) 500mg Tab: (Clarithromycin) 500mg Cap, DR: (Lansoprazole) 30mg						X			X
	OMEPRAZOLE										
	Prilosec	Cap, DR: 10mg, 20mg, 40mg Sus, DR: 2.5mg, 10mg (granules/packet)	X	X	X	X	X	X			X

(Continued)

	DRUG	HOW SUPPLIED	INDICATIONS								
			Heartburn	PUD	GERD	Esophagitis	Zollinger-Ellison	H. pylori	NSAID† Induced	Upper GI‡ Bleeding	Duodenal Ulcer
PROTON PUMP INHIBITORS	Zegerid	(Omeprazole-Sodium bicarbonate); **Cap:** 20mg-1100mg, 40mg-1100mg	X	X	X	X				X	X
		Pow: 20mg-1680mg/packet, 40mg-1680mg/packet									
	PANTOPRAZOLE										
	Protonix	**Inj:** 40mg **Tab, DR:** 20mg, 40mg **Sus, DR:** 40mg (granules/packet)	X		X	X	X				
	RABEPRAZOLE										
	Aciphex	**Tab, DR:** 20mg	X	X	X			X	X		X

Abbreviations: DR = delayed-release; GERD = gastroesophageal reflux disease; GI = gastrointestinal; NSAID = non-steroidal antiinflammatory drug; PUD = peptic ulcer disease.

*Rx products only. For OTC products, refer to Antacid and Heartburn Products on page XXX.

†Prevention of NSAID-induced gastric ulcers.

‡Prevention of upper GI bleeding in critically ill patients.

§Product available generically only.

DRUG TREATMENTS FOR COMMON STDs*

DISEASE	DRUG	RECOMMENDED DOSAGE
BACTERIAL VAGINOSIS		
Nonpregnant Women	Metronidazole *OR*	500mg PO bid x 7d.
	Clindamycin cre *OR*	2%, 1 full applicator intravaginally qhs x 7d.
	Metronidazole gel	0.75%, 1 full applicator intravaginally qd x 5d.
Alternative Regimens Nonpregnant Women	Clindamycin *OR*	300mg PO bid x 7d.
	Clindamycin ovules	100mg intravaginally qhs x 3d.
	Tinidazole	2g PO qd x 3d OR 1g PO qd x 5d.
Pregnant Women	Metronidazole *OR*	250mg PO tid x 7d OR 500mg PO bid x 7d.
	Clindamycin	300mg PO bid x 7d.
CHANCROID		
	Azithromycin *OR*	1g PO single dose.
	Ceftriaxone *OR*	250mg IM single dose.
	Ciprofloxacin *OR*	500mg PO bid x 3d.
	Erythromycin base	500mg PO tid x 7d.
CHLAMYDIAL INFECTION		
Nonpregnant Women	Azithromycin *OR*	1g PO single dose.
	Doxycycline	100mg PO bid x 7d.
Pregnant Women	Azithromycin *OR*	1g PO single dose.
	Amoxicillin	500mg PO tid x 7d.
Alternative Regimens Nonpregnant Women	Erythromycin base *OR*	500mg PO qid x 7d
	Erythromycin ethylsuccinate *OR*	800mg PO qid x 7d
	Ofloxacin *OR*	300mg PO bid x 7d.
	Levofloxacin	500mg PO qd x 7d.
Pregnant Women	Erythromycin base *OR*	250mg PO qid x 14d
	Erythromycin ethylsuccinate	400mg PO qid x 14d.
EPIDIDYMITIS		
Gonococcal OR Chlamydial Infection	Ceftriaxone *plus*	250mg IM single dose.
	Doxycycline	100mg PO bid x 10d.
Acute Epididimitis Most Likely Caused by Enteric ORganisms	Ofloxacin *OR*	300mg PO bid x 10d.
	Levofloxacin	500mg PO qd x 10d.
GRANULOMA INGUINALE		
	Doxycycline	100mg PO bid for at least 3 weeks and until all lesions have completely healed.
Alternative Regimens	Ciprofloxacin *OR*	750mg PO bid for at least 3 weeks and until all lesions have completely healed.
	Erythromycin base (during pregnancy) *OR*	500mg PO qid for at least 3 weeks and until all lesions have completely healed.
	Azithromycin *OR*	1g PO once weekly for at least 3 weeks and until all lesions have completely healed.
	Trimethoprim/Sulfamethoxazole *plus*	1 tab (DS) PO bid for at least 3 weeks and until all lesions have completely healed.
	Aminoglycoside (ie, gentamicin) if improvement is not evident within the first few days.	1mg/kg IV q8h.
HERPES SIMPLEX VIRUS (HSV)		
First Episode	Acyclovir *OR*	400mg PO tid x 7-10d OR 200mg PO 5x/d x 7-10d.
	Famciclovir *OR*	250mg PO tid x 7-10d.
	Valacyclovir	1g PO bid x 7-10d.

DISEASE	DRUG	RECOMMENDED DOSAGE
HERPES SIMPLEX VIRUS (HSV) *(Continued)*		
Episodic Therapy for Recurrent Genital Herpes	Acyclovir *OR*	400mg PO tid x 5d OR 800mg PO bid x 5d OR 800mg PO tid x 2d.
	Famciclovir *OR*	1g bid x 1d OR 125mg PO bid x 5d OR 500mg once followed by 250mg bid x 2d.
	Valacyclovir	500mg PO bid x 3d OR 1g PO qd x 5d.
Suppressive Therapy for Recurrent Genital Herpes	Acyclovir *OR*	400mg PO bid.
	Famciclovir *OR*	250mg PO bid.
	Valacyclovir	500mg PO qd (<10 episodes/yr) OR 1g PO qd.
HUMAN PAPILLOMAVIRUS (HPV) INFECTION		
External Genital Area	Podofilox *OR*	0.5% sol OR gel (patient-applied) bid x 3d, wait 4d, repeat as necessary x 4 cycles. Limit application to 0.5mL/day and to <10cm² wart area.
	Imiquimod	5% cre (patient-applied) hs, 3 times a wk for up to 16 wks.
	Sinecatechins	15% oint tid (0.5cm strand/wart) x ≤16 wks.
	Cryotherapy *OR*	Physician-applied every 1-2 wks.
	Podophyllin resin	10-25% (physician-applied) qwk if necessary. Limit application to <0.5mL and to <10cm² wart area per session. Do not apply to area with open lesions OR wounds.
	Trichloroacetic acid *OR*	80-90% (physician-applied) qwk if necessary.
	Bichloroacetic acid *OR*	80-90% (physician-applied) qwk if necessary.
	Surgical removal	
Alternative Regimens	Intralesional interferon *OR* Photodynamic therapy *OR* Topical cidofovir	
Vaginal Warts	Cryotherapy *OR*	With liquid nitrogen.
	Trichloroacetic acid *OR*	80-90% (physician-applied) qwk if necessary.
	Bichloroacetic acid	80-90% (physician-applied) qwk if necessary.
Urethral Meatus Warts	Cryotherapy *OR*	With liquid nitrogen.
	Podophyllum	10-25% (physician-applied) qwk if necessary.
Anal Warts	Cryotherapy *OR*	With liquid nitrogen.
	Trichloroacetic acid *OR*	80-90% (physician-applied) qwk if necessary.
	Bichloroacetic acid *OR*	80-90% (physician-applied) qwk if necessary.
	Surgical removal	
LYMPHOGRANULOMA VENEREUM		
	Doxycycline	100mg PO bid x 21d.
Alternative Regimens (including pregnancy)	Erythromycin base	500mg PO qid x 21d.
NONGONOCOCCAL URETHRITIS		
	Azithromycin *OR*	1g PO single dose.
	Doxycycline	100mg PO bid x 7d.
Alternative Regimens	Erythromycin base *OR*	500mg PO qid x 7d.
	Erythromycin ethylsuccinate *OR*	800mg PO qid x 7d.
	Ofloxacin *OR*	300mg PO bid x 7d.
	Levofloxacin	500mg PO qd x 7d.
Recurrent and Persistent Urethritis	Metronidazole *OR*	2g PO single dose.
	Tinidazole *plus*	2g PO single dose.
	Azithromycin	1g PO single dose (if not used for initial episodes).

DISEASE	DRUG	RECOMMENDED DOSAGE
PEDICULOSIS PUBIS		
	Permethrin cre *OR* Pyrethrins with piperonyl butoxide	1% cre: Apply to affected area & wash off after 10 min. Apply to affected area and wash off after 10 min.
Alternative Regimens	Malathion *OR* Ivermectin	0.5% lot: Apply for 8-12 hours and wash off. 250µg/kg repeat in 2 weeks.
PELVIC INFLAMMATORY DISEASE		
Parenteral Regimen A	Cefotetan *OR* Cefoxitin *plus* Doxycycline	2g IV q12h. 2g IV q6h. 100mg IV q12h.
Parenteral Regimen B	Clindamycin *plus* Gentamicin	900mg IV q8h. LD: 2mg/kg IM/IV. MD: 1.5mg/kg IM/IV q8h. May substitute with 3-5 mg/kg IM/IV single daily dose.
Alternative Regimen	Ampicillin/Sulbactam *plus* Doxycycline	3g IV q6h. 100mg PO/IV q12h.
Oral Regimen	Ceftriaxone *plus* Doxycycline *w/ or w/o* Metronidazole *OR*	250mg IM single dose. 100mg PO bid x 14d. 500mg PO bid x 14d.
	Cefoxitin with probenecid *plus* Doxycycline *w/ or w/o* Metronidazole *OR*	2mg IM single dose with probenecid 1g PO single dose. 100mg PO bid x 14d. 500mg PO bid x 14d.
	3rd Gen Cephalosporin *plus* Doxycycline *w/ or w/o* Metronidazole	Given IV/IM 100mg PO bid x 14d. 500mg PO bid x 14d.
Alternative Oral Regimen (Use only if negative NAAT test OR negative gonococcal culture)	Levofloxacin *OR* Ofloxacin *w/ or w/o* Metronidazole	500mg PO qd x 14d. 400mg PO bid x 14d. 500mg PO bid x 14d.
PROCTITIS, PROCTOCOLITIS, & ENTERITIS		
	Ceftriaxone *plus* Doxycycline	250mg IM. 100mg PO bid x 7d.
SCABIES		
	Permethrin cre *OR* Ivermectin	5% cre: Apply to body from the neck down & wash off after 8-14h. 200mcg/kg PO; repeat in 2 weeks.
Alternative Regimen	Lindane	1% lot or cre: Apply 1oz lot or 30g cre to body from the neck down & wash off after 8h (not recommended in people with extensive dermatitis, pregnancy, lactating women, or children <2 yrs).
SYPHILIS		
Primary & Secondary Disease	Benzathine penicillin G	**Adults:** 2.4 MU IM single dose. **Peds ≥1 mo:** 50,000 U/kg IM single dose. **Max:** 2.4 MU/single dose.
Penicillin Allergy	Doxycycline *OR* Tetracycline	100mg PO bid x 14d. 500mg PO qid x 14d.
Early Latent Disease	Benzathine penicillin G	**Adults:** 2.4 MU IM single dose. **Peds:** 50,000 U/kg IM single dose. **Max:** 2.4 MU/dose.

(Continued)

DISEASE	DRUG	RECOMMENDED DOSAGE
SYPHILIS *(Continued)*		
Late Latent, Unknown Duration	Benzathine penicillin G	**Adults:** 2.4 MU IM single dose. **Pediatrics ≥1 mo:** 50,000 U/kg IM single dose. **Max:** 2.4 MU/single dose.
Tertiary Disease	Benzathine penicillin G	2.4 MU IM qwk x 3 doses.
Neurosyphilis	Aqueous crystalline penicillin G	3-4 MU IV q4h OR continuous infusion x 10-14d.
Alternative Regimen	Procaine penicillin *plus*	2.4 MU IM qd x 10-14d.
	Probenecid	500mg PO qid x 10-14d.
TRICHOMONIASIS		
	Metronidazole	2g PO single dose.
	Tinidazole	2g PO single dose.
Alternative Regimen	Metronidazole	500mg PO bid x 7d.
Pregnant Women	Metronidazole	2g PO single dose.
UNCOMPLICATED GONOCOCCAL INFECTIONS		
Cervix, Urethra, and Rectum *Recommended Regimens*	Ceftriaxone *OR*	250mg IM single dose.
	Cefixime *OR*	400mg PO single dose.
	Single-dose injectable cephalosporin regimens:	
	Ceftizoxime *OR*	500mg IM single dose.
	Cefotaxime *OR*	500mg IM single dose.
	Cefoxitin with probenecid *plus*	2g IM with probenecid 1g PO.
	Azithromycin *OR*	1g PO single dose.
	Doxycycline	100mg PO qd x 7d.
Alternative Regimens	Cefpodoxime	400mg PO.
	Cefuroxime axetil	1g PO.
	Azithromycin	2g PO.
Pharynx *Recommended Regimens*	Ceftriaxone *plus*	250mg IM single dose.
	Azithromycin *OR*	1g PO single dose.
	Doxycycline	100mg PO qd x 7d.
VULVOVAGINAL CANDIDIASIS		
Intravaginal Agents	Butoconazole *OR*	2% cre, 5g intravaginally x 3d. (OTC)
	Butoconazole *OR*	2% cre, 5g intravaginally single dose. (Rx)
	Clotrimazole *OR*	1% cre, 5g intravaginally x 7-14d.
	Clotrimazole *OR*	2% cre, 5g intravaginally x 3d.
	Miconazole *OR*	2% cre, 5g intravaginally x 7d.
	Miconazole *OR*	4% cre, 5g intravaginally x 3d.
	Miconazole *OR*	200mg vaginal supp x 3d.
	Miconazole *OR*	100mg vaginal supp x 7d.
	Miconazole *OR*	1200mg vaginal supp single dose.
	Nystatin *OR*	100,000-U vaginal tab x 14d.
	Tioconazole *OR*	6.5% oint, 5g intravaginally single dose.
	Terconazole *OR*	0.4% cre, 5g intravaginally x 7d.
	Terconazole *OR*	0.8% cre, 5g intravaginally x 3d.
	Terconazole *OR*	80mg vaginal supp x 3d.
Oral Agent	Fluconazole	150mg tab PO single dose.

*Adapted from: Centers for Disease Control and Prevention. Sexually Transmitted Diseases Treatment Guidelines 2010. *MMWR*. 2010;59(No. RR-12):1-109.

HIV/AIDS PHARMACOTHERAPY

GENERIC [BRAND]	HOW SUPPLIED	USUAL DOSAGE	PEDIATRIC DOSAGE	FOOD EFFECT	BOXED WARNING*
CCR5 ANTAGONIST					
Maraviroc (MVC) [Selzentry]	**Tab:** 150mg, 300mg	**Adults ≥16 yrs:** Give in combination with other anti-retroviral medications. With Strong CYP3A Inhibitors (with or without CYP3A inducers) Including PIs (except tipranavir/ritonavir), Delavirdine, Ketoconazole, Itraconazole, Clarithromycin, Others (eg, nefazodone, telithromycin): 150mg bid. With NRTIs, Tipranavir/Ritonavir, Nevirapine, Raltegravir, Enfuvirtide, Other Drugs That Are Not Strong CYP3A Inhibitors/Inducers: 300mg bid. With Strong CYP3A Inducers (without strong CYP3A inhibitor) Including Efavirenz, Rifampin, Etravirine, Carbamazepine, Phenobarbital, Phenytoin: 600mg bid.		Take without regard to meals.	Hepatotoxicity
HIV INTEGRASE STRAND TRANSFER INHIBITOR					
Raltegravir [Isentress]	**Tab:** 400mg	**Adults:** 400mg bid. **With Rifampin:** 800mg bid.	Check PI for age/weight based dosing.	Take without regard to meals.	
NUCLEOSIDE REVERSE TRANSCRIPTASE INHIBITORS (NRTIs)					
Abacavir (ABC) [Ziagen]	**Sol:** 20mg/mL [240mL]; **Tab:** 300mg	**Adults:** 300mg bid or 600mg qd.	**Peds ≥3 mos:** 8mg/kg bid. **Max:** 300mg bid.	Take without regard to meals.	Hypersensitivity reactions/lactic acidosis/severe hepatomegaly
Didanosine (ddI) [Videx Powder for Oral Sol; Videx EC]	**Powder for Sol:** 10mg/mL [2g, 4g]; **Cap, Delayed Release:** (Videx EC) 125mg, 200mg, 250mg, 400mg	**Adults ≥60kg:** (Cap) 400mg qd; (Sol) 200mg bid or 400mg qd. **With TDF:** 250mg qd or 200mg qd if <60kg. **<60kg:** (Sol) 125mg bid or 250mg qd. (Cap) 250mg qd. **20-25kg:** (Cap) 200mg qd.	**Peds 2 wks-8 mos:** (Sol) 100mg/m² bid. **>8 mos:** 120mg/m² bid.	Take on empty stomach at least 30 minutes before or 2 hrs after meals. Swallow caps whole.	Pancreatitis/lactic acidosis/hepatomegaly with steatosis
Emtricitabine (FTC) [Emtriva]	**Cap:** 200mg; **Sol:** 10mg/mL [170mL]	**Adults ≥18 yrs:** (Cap) 200mg qd; (Sol) 240mg (24mL) qd.	**Peds 0-3 mos:** 3mg/kg qd. **3 mos-17 yrs:** (Cap) **≥33kg:** 200mg qd. (Sol) 6mg/kg qd. **Max:** 240mg (24mL) qd.	Take without regard to meals.	Lactic acidosis/severe hepatomegaly with steatosis/posttreatment exacerbation of hepatitis B

(Continued)

GENERIC [BRAND]	HOW SUPPLIED	USUAL DOSAGE	PEDIATRIC DOSAGE	FOOD EFFECT	BOXED WARNING*
NUCLEOSIDE REVERSE TRANSCRIPTASE INHIBITORS (NRTIs) *(Continued)*					
Lamivudine [Epivir]	**Sol:** 10mg/mL [240mL]; **Tab:** 150mg, 300mg	**Adults >16 yrs:** 150mg bid or 300mg qd.	**Peds 3 mos-16 yrs:** 4mg/kg bid. **Max:** 150mg bid.	Take without regard to meals.	Lactic acidosis/posttreatment exacerbations of hepatitis B in co-infected patients/different formulations of Epivir
Stavudine (d4T) [Zerit]	**Cap:** 15mg, 20mg, 30mg, 40mg; **Sol:** 1mg/mL [200mL]	**Adults ≥60kg:** 40mg q12h. **<60kg:** 30mg q12h.	Check PI for age/weight based dosing.	Take without regard to meals.	Lactic acidosis/hepatomegaly with steatosis/pancreatitis
Tenofovir disoproxil fumarate (TDF) [Viread]	**Tab:** 300mg	**Adults:** 300mg qd.	**Peds ≥12 yrs: ≥35kg:** 300mg qd	Take without regard to meals.	Lactic acidosis/severe hepatomegaly with steatosis/ posttreatment exacerbation of hepatitis B
Zidovudine (AZT, ZDV) [Retrovir]	**Cap:** 100mg; **Inj:** 10mg/mL; **Syrup:** 50mg/5mL [240mL]; **Tab:** 300mg	**Adults:** (Cap, Tab, Syrup) 600mg/day in divided doses (300mg bid or 200mg tid). (Inj) 1mg/kg IV over 1 hr 5-6 times/day.	Check PI for age/weight based dosing.	Take without regard to meals.	Risk of hematological toxicity/ myopathy/lactic acidosis
NON-NUCLEOSIDE REVERSE TRANSCRIPTASE INHIBITORS (NNRTIs)					
Delavirdine (DLV) [Rescriptor]	**Tab:** 100mg, 200mg	**Adults: Usual:** 400mg tid.	**Peds ≥16 yrs: Usual:** 400mg tid.	Take without regard to meals. Separate doses from antacids by 1 hr.	
Efavirenz (EFV) [Sustiva]	**Cap:** 50mg, 200mg; **Tab:** 600mg	**Adults: Initial:** 600mg qd at bedtime.	Check PI for age/weight based dosing.	Take on an empty stomach, preferably at bedtime.	
Etravirine (ETR) [Intelence]	**Tab:** 100mg, 200mg	**Adults:** 200mg bid.		Take following a meal.	
Nevirapine (NVP) [Viramune]	**Sus:** 50mg/5mL [240mL]; **Tab:** 200mg*; **XR Tab:** 400mg	**Adults ≥16 yrs:** 200mg qd for 14 days (lead-in period), then 200mg bid. **Adults ≥16 yrs: XR Tab Therapy-Naive:** One 200mg immediate-release tab qd for 14 days followed by one 400 mg XR tab qd.	**Peds >15 days:** 150mg/m² qd for 14 days, then 150mg/ m² bid. **Max:** 400mg/day.	Take without regard to meals or antacid.	Life-threatening hepatotoxicity/skin reactions
Rilpivirine [Edurant]	**Tab:** 25 mg	**Adults:** 25mg tab qd.		Take with meals.	

GENERIC [BRAND]	HOW SUPPLIED	USUAL DOSAGE	PEDIATRIC DOSAGE	FOOD EFFECT	BOXED WARNING*
PROTEASE INHIBITORS (PIs)					
Atazanavir (ATV) [Reyataz]	**Cap:** 100mg, 150mg, 200mg, 300mg	**Adults: Therapy-Naïve:** 400mg qd or (ATV 300mg + RTV 100mg) qd. **With EFV:** (ATV 400mg + RTV 100mg) qd. **Therapy-Experienced:** (ATV 300mg + RTV 100mg) qd.	Check PI for age/weight based dosing.	Take with food. If you are taking antacids, take atazanavir 2 hr before or 1 hr after.	
Darunavir (DRV) [Prezista]	**Tab:** 75mg, 150mg, 400mg, 600mg; **Sus:** 100 mg/mL	**Adults: Therapy-Naïve or Therapy-Experienced With No DRV Resistance Associated Mutations:** (DRV 800mg + RTV 100mg) qd. **Therapy-Experienced Patients With at Least 1 DRV Mutation:** (DRV 600mg + RTV 100mg) bid.	Check PI for age/weight based dosing.	Take with food. (Sus) 8mL doses should be taken as two 4mL administrations with supplied oral dosing syringe.	
Fosamprenavir (FPV) [Lexiva]	**Tab:** 700mg; **Sus:** 50mg/mL [225mL]	**Adults: Therapy-Naïve:** FPV 1400mg bid OR FPV 1400mg qd + RTV 200mg qd OR FPV 1400mg qd + RTV 100mg qd OR FPV 700mg bid + RTV 100mg bid. **PI-Experienced:** FPV 700mg bid + RTV 100mg bid.	Check PI for age/weight based dosing.	(Tab) Take w/o regard to meals (if not boosted with RTV tab). (Sus) **Adults:** Take w/o food. **Peds:** Take with food. (FPV with RTV Tab) Take with meals.	
Indinavir (IDV) [Crixivan]	**Cap:** 100mg, 200mg, 400mg	**Adults:** 800mg q8h. **RTV Boost:** (IDV 800mg + RTV 100mg or 200mg) q12h.		Take 1 hr before or 2 hr after meals; may take with skim milk or low-fat meal. (RTV Boost) Take w/o regard to meals.	
Nelfinavir (NFV) [Viracept]	**Sus:** (powder) 50mg/g [144g]; **Tab:** 250g, 625mg	**Adults:** 1250mg bid or 750mg tid.	Check PI for age/weight based dosing.	Take with meals.	
Ritonavir (RTV) [Norvir]	**Cap, Tab:** 100mg; **Sol:** 80mg/mL [240mL]	**Adults: Initial:** 300mg bid. **Titrate:** Increase every 2-3 days by 100mg bid. **Maint:** 600mg bid.	**Peds >1 mo:** Initial: 250mg/m² bid. **Titrate:** Increase by 50mg/m² bid every 2-3 days. **Maint:** 350-400mg/m² bid or highest tolerated dose. **Max:** 600mg bid.	(Cap, Sol) Take with food, may improve tolerability. (Tab) Take with food.	Coadministration with hypnotics, antiarrhythmics, or ergot alkaloid preparations
Saquinavir (SQV) [Invirase]	**Cap:** 200mg; **Tab:** 500mg	**Adults >16 yrs:** 1000mg bid with RTV 100mg bid OR 1000mg bid with LPV/RTV 400mg/100mg bid (no additional RTV).		Take within 2 hrs after a meal when taken with RTV.	

(Continued)

GENERIC [BRAND]	HOW SUPPLIED	USUAL DOSAGE	PEDIATRIC DOSAGE	FOOD EFFECT	BOXED WARNING*
PROTEASE INHIBITORS (PIs) *(Continued)*					
Tipranavir (TPV) [Aptivus]	**Cap:** 250mg; **Sol:** 100mg/mL	**Adults:** (500mg + RTV 200mg) bid.	**Peds ≥2-18 yrs:** 14mg/kg + RTV 6mg/kg (or 375mg/m² + RTV 150mg/m²) bid. **Max:** (500mg + RTV 200mg) bid.	(TPV taken with RTV tab) Take with meals. (TPV taken with RTV cap or sol) Take w/o regard to meals.	
FUSION INHIBITOR					
Enfuvirtide (T20) [Fuzeon]	108mg/vial	**Adults:** 90mg SQ bid.	Check PI for age/weight based dosing.		
COMBINATIONS					
EFV/FTC/TDF [Atripla]	**Tab:** (Efavirenz-Emtricitabine-Tenofovir DF) 600mg-200mg-300mg	**Adults ≥18 yrs:** 1 tab qd, preferably at bedtime. Do not give if CrCl <50mL/min.		Take on empty stomach.	Lactic acidosis/severe hepatomegaly with steatosis/posttreatment exacerbation of hepatitis B
3TC/ZDV [Combivir]	**Tab:** (Lamivudine-Zidovudine) 150mg-300mg	**Adults/Pediatrics ≥30kg:** 1 tab bid. Do not give if CrCl <50mL/min or if <30kg weight.		Take without regard to meals.	Risk of hematological toxicity/myopathy/lactic acidosis/exacerbations of hepatitis B
ABC/3TC [Epzicom]	**Tab:** (Abacavir Sulfate-Lamivudine) 600mg-300mg	**Adults ≥18 yrs: CrCl ≥50mL/min:** 1 tab qd. Do not give if CrCl <50mL/mL.		Take without regard to meals.	Risk of hypersensitivity reactions/lactic acidosis/severe hepatomegaly/exacerbations of hepatitis B
LPV/RTV [Kaletra]	**Tab:** (Lopinavir-Ritonavir) 200mg-50mg; 100mg-25mg; **Sol:** (Lopinavir-Ritonavir) 80mg-20mg/mL [160mL]	**Adults:** 400mg/100mg bid or 800mg/200mg qd. **With EFV or NVP (PI-Naïve or PI-Experienced Patients):** 500mg/125mg tab bid or 533mg/133mg sol bid.	Check PI for age/weight based dosing.	(Tab) Take without regard to meals. (Sol) Take with meals.	
ABC/ZDV/3TC [Trizivir]	**Tab:** (Abacavir-Lamivudine-Zidovudine) 300mg-150mg-300mg	**Adults/Adolescents ≥40kg and CrCl ≥50mL/min:** 1 tab bid.		Take without regard to meals.	Risk of hypersensitivity reactions/hematologic toxicity/myopathy/lactic acidosis/severe hepatomegaly/exacerbations of hepatitis B

GENERIC [BRAND]	HOW SUPPLIED	USUAL DOSAGE	PEDIATRIC DOSAGE	FOOD EFFECT	BOXED WARNING*
COMBINATIONS (*Continued*)					
FTC/TDF [Truvada]	**Tab:** (Emtricitabine-Tenofovir Disoproxil Fumarate) 200mg-300mg	**Adults & Peds ≥12 yrs: ≥35 kg: CrCl ≥50 mL/min:** 1 tab qd. **CrCl 30-49 mL/min:** 1 tab q48h.		Take without regard to meals.	Lactic acidosis/severe hepatomegaly with steatosis/posttreatment acute exacerbation of hepatitis B
[Complera]	**Tab:** (Emtricitabine, Rilpivirine, and Tenofovir Disoproxil Fumarate) 200 mg-25mg-300 mg	**Adults ≥18 yrs: CrCl≥50 mL/min:** 1 tab qd.		Take with meals.	Lactic acidosis/severe hepatomegaly with steatosis/posttreatment acute exacerbation of hepatitis B

* Refer to monograph for full boxed warning and for detailed dosing information.

†Scored.

Sources: FDA-approved Labeling; Guidelines for the Use of Antiretroviral Agents in HIV-1-Infected Adults and Adolescents – October 14, 2011.

HIV/AIDS COMPLICATIONS THERAPY

HIV/AIDS DISEASE-RELATED COMPLICATIONS	GENERIC (BRAND)	RECOMMENDED DOSAGE
ASPERGILLOSIS, INVASIVE		
Recommended Treatment Regimen	**Voriconazole** (Vfend)*	Refer to *Systemic Antifungals* chart.
Alternative Treatment Regimen	**Amphotericin B Liposome** (AmBisome)	
	Amphotericin B (Amphotec)	
	Amphotericin B Lipid Complex (Abelcet)	
	Caspofungin (Cancidas)	
	Itraconazole (Sporanox)	
	Posaconazole (Noxafil)	
CANDIDIASIS		
Prevention/Treatment	**Amphotericin B Liposome** (AmBisome)	Refer to *Systemic Antifungals* chart.
	Amphotericin B Lipid Complex (Abelcet)	
	Anidulafungin (Eraxis)	
	Caspofungin (Cancidas)	
	Fluconazole (Diflucan)†	
	Itraconazole (Sporanox)	
	Micafungin (Mycamine)	
	Posaconazole (Noxafil)	
	Voriconazole (Vfend)*	
CMV RETINITIS		
Treatment	**Cidofovir** (Vistide)†	**Adults: Induction‡:** 5mg/kg IV infusion q1wk x 2 wks. **Maint:** 5mg/kg IV q2wk. Give at a constant rate over 1 hr.
	Foscarnet†	**Adults: Induction:** 90mg/kg over 1.5-2 hrs IV infusion q12h or 60mg/kg over 1 hr IV infusion q8h x 2-3 wks. **Maint:** 90-120mg/kg/d IV over 2 hrs.
	Ganciclovir (Cytovene)†	**Adults: Induction:** 5mg/kg IV infusion q12h x 14-21 days. **Maint:** 5mg/kg IV hr qd x 7 days/wk or 6mg/kg IV qd x 5 days/wk. Give at a constant rate over 1 hr.
	Ganciclovir (Vitrasert)	**Adults/Peds ≥9 yrs:** One implant q5-8 months.
	Valganciclovir (Valcyte)	**Adults: Induction:** 900mg PO bid x 21 days w/food. **Maint:** 900mg PO qd w/food.
CRYPTOCOCCAL MENINGITIS		
Treatment	**Amphotericin B Liposome** (AmBisome)	Refer to *Systemic Antifungals* chart.
	Fluconazole (Diflucan)	
HSV		
Recommended Regimen for Daily Suppressive Therapy	**Acyclovir** *or*	Refer to *Drug Treatments For Common STDs* chart.
	Famciclovir (Famvir) *or*	
	Valacyclovir	
Recommended Regimen for Episodic Infections	**Acyclovir** *or*	
	Famciclovir† *or*	
	Valacyclovir	

(Continued)

HIV/AIDS DISEASE-RELATED COMPLICATIONS	GENERIC (BRAND)	RECOMMENDED DOSAGE
KAPOSI'S SARCOMA		
Treatment	**Alitretinoin** (Panretin)	**0.1% gel: Adults: Initial:** Apply bid to lesions. May increase to tid-qid based on individual lesion tolerance. Temporarily discontinue if severe irritation occurs.
	Daunorubicin (DaunoXome)§	**Adults:** 40mg/m² IV over 60 min q2wk. Blood counts should be repeated prior to each dose. Hold dose if absolute granulocyte <750 cells/mm³.
	Doxorubicin (Doxil)	**Adults:** 20mg/m² IV q3wk. **Initial Rate:** 1mg/min. May be increased to administer over 1 hr if tolerated.
	Interferon alfa-2b (Intron A)†	**Adults:** 30 million IU/m²/dose SQ/IM tiw until disease progression or max response achieved after 16 wks.
	Paclitaxel (Taxol)	**Adults:** 135mg/m² IV over 3 hrs q3wk or 100mg/m² IV over 3 hrs q2wk. **Dose Intensity:** 45-50mg/m²/wk.
MAC		
Prevention/Treatment	**Azithromycin** (Zithromax)	**Adults: Prevention:** 1200mg once wkly. **Treatment:** 600mg PO qd with ethambutol 15mg/kg qd.
Prevention/Treatment	**Clarithromycin** (Biaxin)	**Prevention/Treatment: Adults:** 500mg PO bid. **Peds:** 7.5mg/kg bid up to 500mg bid.
Prevention	**Rifabutin** (Mycobutin)†	**Adults‡:** 300mg PO qd. **N/V/GI Upset:** 150mg bid w/food.
PCP		
Prevention/Treatment	**Atovaquone** (Mepron)	**Adults/Peds 13-16 yrs: Prevention:** 1500mg PO qd w/meals. **Adults/Peds 13-16 yrs: Treatment (mild-moderate):** 750mg PO bid w/meals x 21 days. **TDD:** 1500mg. Failure to administer Atovaquone with meals may result in lower drug plasma concentrations and may limit response to therapy.
	TMP/SMX (Bactrim)	**Adults/Peds: Treatment:** 15-20mg/kg/d TMP and 75-100mg/kg/d SMX in divided doses q6h x 14-21 days.
	TMP/SMX (Bactrim DS)	**Adults: Prevention:** 1 DS tab (160/800mg) qd. **Peds: Prevention:** 150mg/m²/d TMP with 750mg/m²/d SMX PO bid in equally divided doses on 3 consecutive days/wk. **Max TDD:** 1600mg SMX/320mg TMP.
VISCERAL LEISHMANIASIS		
Treatment	**Amphotericin B Liposome** (AmBisome)	Refer to *Systemic Antifungals* chart.
WEIGHT LOSS		
Anorexia	**Dronabinol** (Marinol)	**Adults‡:** 2.5mg PO bid; before lunch and supper. **Max:** 20mg/d in divided doses.
Anorexia, cachexia, unexplained weight loss	**Megestrol** (Megace)	**Adults: Initial:** 800mg/d. **Usual:** 400-800mg/d.
Cachexia/Wasting	**Somatropin** (Serostim)	**Adults:** >55kg: 6mg SQ qhs. **45-55kg:** 5mg SQ qhs. **35-45kg:** 4mg SQ qhs. **<35kg:** 0.1mg/kg SQ qhs. **Max:** 6mg/d.

Abbreviations: CMV=cytomegalovirus; HSV=herpes simplex virus; MAC=*Mycobacterium avium* complex; PCP=*Pneumocystis carinii* pneumonia.

*Use cautiously in patients on protease inhibitors and efavirenz.

†For dosing in special populations, see the complete prescribing information.

‡Check monograph for detailed dosing guidelines (CrCl, Urine Protein, SCr, etc.).

§Withhold therapy if the absolute granulocyte count is less than 750 cells/mm³.

Sources: Prescribing information; Guidelines for prevention and treatment of opportunistic infections in HIV-infected adults and adolescents. *MMWR.* 2009;Vol 59:No. RR-12.

MANAGEMENT OF HEPATITIS C*

BRAND (GENERIC)	HOW SUPPLIED	DOSAGE (ADULTS)	DOSAGE (PEDIATRICS)	COMMENTS
BIOLOGICAL RESPONSE MODIFIERS				
Infergen (Interferon alfacon-1)	**Inj:** 9mcg/0.3mL, 15mcg/0.5mL	**Adults ≥18 yrs: Monotherapy:** Initial treatment is 9mcg as a single SQ inj 3x/wk (tiw) for 24 wks. The dosage for patients who tolerated previous interferon therapy and did not respond or relapsed following discontinuation is 15mcg as a single SQ inj tiw for up to 48 wks. **Combination Treatment:** 15mcg daily as a single SQ injection in combination with weight-based ribavirin at 1000mg–1200mg orally in 2 divided doses for up to 48 wks.		Discontinue or modify dosage if a serious adverse reaction develops during treatment. **Monotherapy:** Dose reduction to 7.5mcg may be necessary following a serious adverse reaction. **Combination Therapy:** Stepwise dose reduction from 15mcg to 9mcg and from 9mcg to 6mcg may be necessary for serious adverse reactions. Infergen/ribavirin should not be used in patients with CrCl <50 mL/min.
Intron A (Interferon alfa-2b, recombinant)	**Inj:** [Powder 10 MIU, 18 MIU, 50 MIU]; [Multidose Pen 22.5 MIU/1.5mL, 37.5 MIU/1.5mL, 75 MIU/1.5mL]; [Sol 22.8 MIU/3.8mL, 32 MIU/3.2mL]	**Adults ≥18 yrs:** 3 million IU administered IM or SQ 3x/wk (tiw). Therapy should be extended to 18-24 months for patients tolerating therapy with normalization of ALT at 16 wks of treatment.		If severe adverse reactions or laboratory abnormalities develop during therapy, the dose should be modified (50% reduction) or discontinued if appropriate until adverse reactions abate. Therapy should be discontinued if intolerance persists after dose adjustment. Acetaminophen may be administered at the time of injection to reduce the incidence of certain adverse reactions.
NUCLEOSIDE ANALOGS				
Copegus (Ribavirin)	**Tab:** 200mg	**Monoinfection:** 800mg to 1200mg per day administered in two divided doses. Dose should be individualized depending on disease characteristics (genotype), response to treatment, and tolerability. **Genotypes 1, 4:** 1000mg (if <75kg) or 1200mg (≥75kg) daily along with 180mcg Pegasys SQ once wkly for 48 wks. **Genotypes 2, 3:** 800mg daily along with 180mcg Pegasys SQ once wkly for 24 wks. **HCV/HIV Co-Infection:** 800mg daily along with 180mcg Pegasys SQ once wkly for 48 wks regardless of genotype.	**Monoinfection in Pediatric Patients ≥5 yrs:** Recommended doses are approximately 15mg/kg/day based on patient body weight given daily in divided doses (AM and PM) in combination with Pegasys 180mcg/1.73m² × BSA SQ once wkly. Refer to the full PI for complete dosing recommendations schedule. Recommended treatment duration for genotype 2 or 3 is 24 wks (48 wks for other genotypes).	Take with food. Refer to dose modifications guidelines in PI for adverse reactions, lab abnormalities, and renal impairment. Should be given in combination with Pegasys and never be given as monotherapy.

(Continued)

BRAND (GENERIC)	HOW SUPPLIED	DOSAGE (ADULTS)	DOSAGE (PEDIATRICS)	COMMENTS
NUCLEOSIDE ANALOGS *(Continued)*				
Rebetol (Ribavirin)	**Cap:** 200mg; **Sol:** 40mg/mL	**In Combination with Intron A:** Daily dosage based on patient body weight. Patients ≤75kg: 400mg qam and 600mg qpm. Patients >75kg: 600mg qam and 600mg qpm. Treat for 24-48 wks in patients previously untreated with interferon and for 24 wks in patients who have relapsed following nonpegylated interferon monotherapy. **In Combination with PegIntron:** Daily doses of 800-1400mg orally in divided doses based on patient body weight. Treatment duration for genotype 1 is 48 wks. Genotypes 2 and 3 should be treated for 24 wks. Treatment duration for patients who previously failed therapy is 48 wks (regardless of genotype). See full PI for detailed dosage information.	**Pediatric Patients 3-17 yrs:** Dosage determined by patient body weight; 15mg/kg/day given in 2 divided doses qam and qpm. Treatment duration for genotype 1 is 48 wks. Treatment duration for genotypes 2 and 3 is 24 wks. See PI for detailed dosage information.	Monotherapy is not permitted. Take with food. Refer to dose modification and discontinuation guidelines in PI for adverse reactions, lab abnormalities, and renal impairment. Should not be used in patients with CrCl <50mL/min.
Ribasphere (Ribavirin)	**Tab:** 200mg, 400mg, 600mg; **Cap:** 200mg	**Tab:** Given in combination with peginterferon alfa-2a. Monotherapy: Dose is administered according to body weight and genotype and ranges from 800mg-1200mg/day in 2 divided doses. Dose should be individualized based on disease characteristics, response to therapy, and tolerability. Treatment duration for genotypes 1 and 4 is 48 wks. Treatment duration for genotypes 2 and 3 is 24 wks. See full PI for detailed dosage information. HCV/HIV Co-Infection: 800mg daily for 48 wks. **Cap:** Given in combination with interferon alfa-2b. Dose is administered according to body weight and ranges from 800mg-1400mg per day in 2 divided doses (AM and PM). Treatment duration for genotype 1 is 48 wks. Patients with genotypes 2 and 3 should be treated for 24 wks. See full PI for detailed dosage information.	**Pediatric Patients 3-17 yrs: Cap:** 15mg/kg/day in 2 divided doses (AM and PM) in combination with peginterferon alfa-2b. Treatment duration for patients with genotype 1 is 48 wks. Patients with genotypes 2 and 3 should be treated for 24 wks. See full PI for more detailed dosage information.	Refer to dose modification and discontinuation guidelines in PI for lab abnormalities, adverse reactions, and renal impairment. Take with food. Should not be used in patients with CrCl <50mL/min. Monotherapy is not permitted.

BRAND (GENERIC)	HOW SUPPLIED	DOSAGE (ADULTS)	DOSAGE (PEDIATRICS)	COMMENTS
PEGYLATED VIRUS PROLIFERATION INHIBITORS				
Pegasys (Peginterferon alfa-2a)	**Inj:** 180mcg/0.5mL [prefilled syringe]; 180mcg/mL [single-use vial]; 180mcg/0.5mL, 135mcg/ 0.5mL [Autoinjector]	**Adults ≥18 yrs:** Administered as SQ injection in abdomen or thigh. **Monotherapy:** 180mcg SQ once wkly for 48 wks. **Combination Therapy With Copegus:** 180mcg SQ once wkly for either 24 wks (genotypes 2 and 3) or 48 wks (genotypes 1 and 4). Daily dosage of Copegus ranges from 800-1200mg based on patient weight and genotype. **HCV/HIV Co-infection: Monotherapy:** 180mcg once wkly for 48 wks. **Combination Therapy with Copegus:** 180mcg once wkly and Copegus 800mg daily in 2 divided doses for 48 wks (regardless of genotype).	**Pediatric Patients 5-17 yrs: Combination Therapy with Copegus:** 180mcg/1.73m^2 x BSA as SQ injection once wkly (max 180mcg) in combination with Copegus at approximate dose of 15mg/kg/day. Treatment duration is 24 wks for genotypes 2 and 3, and 48 wks for other genotypes.	Refer to dose modification/discontinuation guidelines in PI for adverse reactions, lab abnormalities, and renal impairment.
PegIntron (Peginterferon alfa-2b)	**Inj:** [Vials: 50mcg/0.5mL, 80mcg/0.5mL, 120mcg/0.5mL, 150mcg/0.5mL], [REDIPEN 50mcg/0.5mL, 80mcg/0.5mL, 120mcg/0.5mL, 150mcg/0.5mL]	**Adults ≥18 yrs:** Administer by SQ injection. **Monotherapy:** 1mcg/kg/wk for 1 year administered on the same day of the wk. **Combination Therapy:** 1.5mcg/kg/wk plus Rebetol 800-1400mg/day based on patient's body weight. Duration of treatment is 48 wks for genotype 1 and 24 wks for genotypes 2 and 3.	**Pediatric Patients 3-17 yrs:** Dosing is determined by body surface area for PegIntron and body weight for Rebetol. **Combination Therapy:** 60mcg/m²/wk SQ along with Rebetol 15mg/kg/day in 2 divided doses. Duration of treatment is 48 wks for genotype 1 and 24 wks for genotypes 2 and 3.	Refer to dose modification and discontinuation guidelines in PI for adverse effects, lab abnormalities, and renal impairment
PROTEASE INHIBITORS				
Incivek (Telaprevir)	**Tab:** 375mg	**In Combination with Peginterferon Alfa and Ribavirin:** 750mg PO tid (7-9 hrs apart) with food (not low fat). Recommended treatment duration is 12 wks. Refer to PI for duration of dual therapy regimens with peginterferon alfa and ribavirin after completion of triple therapy.		HCV-RNA levels should be monitored at wks 4 and 12 to determine combination treatment duration and assess for treatment futility. Refer to PI for dose reduction and discontinuation information. Do not administer as monotherapy.
Victrelis (Boceprevir)	**Cap:** 200mg	**Adults ≥18 yrs: In Combination with Peginterferon Alfa and Ribavirin:** 800mg tid (every 7-9 hrs) with food (meal or light snack). Victrelis is added to regimen after 4 wks of peginterferon alfa and ribavirin therapy. Refer to Response-Guided Therapy (RGT) guidelines in PI to determine duration of treatment.		Must be administered in combination with peginterferon alfa and ribavirin. Dose reduction of Victrelis is not recommended. Refer to PI regarding dose modification and discontinuation information.

* Refer to full FDA-approved Prescribing Information for detailed information.

ORAL AND SYSTEMIC ANTIBIOTICS*

GENERIC (BRAND)	HOW SUPPLIED	INDICATIONS**
AMINOGLYCOSIDES		
Amikacin sulfate (Amikacin)	Inj: 50mg/mL, 250mg/mL	Short-term treatment of serious infections caused by gram-negative bacteria, such as septicemia, respiratory tract, bone and joint, CNS (including meningitis), skin and soft tissue, and intra-abdominal infections; burns and postoperative infections; complicated and recurrent UTIs; and staphylococcal disease. Concomitant therapy with a PCN-type drug as treatment of certain severe infections such as neonatal sepsis.
Gentamicin sulfate	Inj: 10mg/mL, 40mg/mL	Treatment of bacterial neonatal sepsis, bacterial septicemia, and serious bacterial infections of the CNS (meningitis), urinary tract, respiratory tract, GI tract (including peritonitis), skin, bone and soft tissue (including burns) and infections caused by susceptible strains of microorganisms.
Streptomycin sulfate	Inj: 1g	Treatment of moderate to severe infections such as *M. tuberculosis* and non-TB infections (eg, plague, tularemia, chancroid, brucella, donovanosis, granuloma inguinale, *H. influenzae* infections, *K. pneumoniae* pneumonia, UTI, gram-negative bacillary bacteremia, endocardial infections).
Tobramycin (TOBI)	Sol: 60mg/mL (300g/5mL ampule)	Management of cystic fibrosis patients with *P. aeruginosa.*
Tobramycin sulfate	Inj: 10mg/mL, 40mg/mL, 1.2g/vial	Treatment of serious infections, including: LRT, CNS (eg, meningitis), intra-abdominal, bone, SSSI, and complicated/recurrent UTIs; and septicemia caused by susceptible strains of microorganisms.
CARBAPENEMS		
Doripenem (Doribax)	Inj: 250mg, 500mg	Treatment of infections such as complicated intra-abdominal infections and UTIs, including pyelonephritis, caused by susceptible microorganisms.
Ertapenem sodium (Invanz)	Inj: 1g	Treatment of complicated intra-abdominal infections, SSSI (including diabetic foot infections without osteomyelitis), CAP, complicated UTI (including pyelonephritis), and acute pelvic infections (including postpartum endomyometritis, septic abortion, and postsurgical gynecologic infections); also used in prophylaxis of surgical-site infection following elective colorectal surgery.
Meropenem (Merrem)	Inj: 500mg, 1g	Treatment of intra-abdominal infections, bacterial meningitis (pediatric patients ≥3 months only), and complicated SSSI caused by susceptible strains of microorganisms in adults and pediatric patients ≥3 months.
CEPHALOSPORINS, FIRST-GENERATION		
Cefadroxil hemihydrate	Cap: 500mg; Sus: 125mg/5mL, 250mg/5mL, 500mg/5mL; Tab: 1g	Treatment of SSSI, UTI, pharyngitis, and tonsilitis.
Cefazolin sodium	Inj: 500mg, 1g, 10g, 20g	Treatment of RT, UTI, SSSI, biliary tract, bone and joint, and genital infections, septicemia, and endocarditis caused by susceptible strains of microorganisms. Perioperative prophylaxis for surgical procedures classified as contaminated or potentially contaminated.
Cephalexin (Keflex)	Cap: 250mg, 500mg, 750mg; (Generic) Sus: 125mg/5mL; 250mg/5mL Tab: 250mg, 500mg	Treatment of otitis media and SSSI; bone, GU tract, and RT infections.

(Continued)

GENERIC (BRAND)	HOW SUPPLIED	INDICATIONS**
CEPHALOSPORINS, SECOND-GENERATION		
Cefaclor	Cap: 250mg, 500mg; Sus: 125mg/5mL, 187mg/5mL, 250mg/5mL, 375mg/5mL	Treatment of otitis media, pharyngitis, tonsilitis, LRTI, UTI, and SSSI caused by susceptible strains of microorganisms.
Cefaclor ER	Tab, Extended-Release: 500mg	Treatment of ABECB, secondary bacterial infections of acute bronchitis, pharyngitis, tonsilitis, and uncomplicated SSSI caused by susceptible strains of microorganisms.
Cefotetan	Inj: 1g, 2g, 10g	Treatment of SSSI; UTI; LRTI; gynecologic, intra-abdominal, bone and joint infections; and surgical prophylaxis. May use with an aminoglycoside for sepsis or other serious infections in which causative organism has not been identified.
Cefoxitin sodium (Mefoxin)	Inj: 1g, 2g, 10g	Treatment of LRTI, UTI, intra-abdominal infection, gynecological infection, SSSI, bone and joint infections, and septicemia. For surgical prophylaxis.
Cefprozil	Sus: 125mg/5mL, 250mg/5mL; Tab: 250mg, 500mg	Mild to moderate pharyngitis/tonsilitis, otitis media, acute sinusitis, secondary bacterial infection of acute bronchitis, ABECB, and uncomplicated SSSI.
Cefuroxime (Zinacef)	Inj: 750mg, 1.5g, 7.5g, 750mg/50mL, 1.5g/50mL	Treatment of septicemia; meningitis; gonorrhea; LRTI, UTI, SSSI, and bone and joint infections caused by susceptible strains of microorganisms. For preoperative and perioperative surgical prophylaxis.
Cefuroxime axetil (Ceftin)	Sus: 125mg/5mL, 250mg/5mL; Tab: 250mg, 500mg	**Sus/Tab:** Pharyngitis/tonsilitis, acute bacterial otitis media. **Sus:** Impetigo. **Tab:** Uncomplicated SSSI and UTI, uncomplicated gonorrhea, early Lyme disease, acute bacterial maxillary sinusitis, ABECB, and secondary bacterial infections of acute bronchitis.
CEPHALOSPORINS, THIRD-GENERATION		
Cefdinir	Cap: 300mg; Sus: 125mg/5mL, 250mg/5mL	In adults and adolescents, used to treat CAP, ABECB, acute maxillary sinusitis, pharyngitis/tonsilitis, uncomplicated SSSI; in pediatric patients, used to treat acute bacterial otitis media, pharyngitis/tonsilitis, uncomplicated SSSI.
Cefditoren pivoxil (Spectracef)	Tab: 200mg, 400mg	Treatment of ABECB, pharyngitis/tonsilitis, CAP, and uncomplicated SSSI in adults and adolescents ≥12 yrs.
Cefixime (Suprax)	Sus: 100mg/5mL, 200mg/5mL; Tab: 400mg	**Sus/Tab:** Pharyngitis, tonsilitis, acute bronchitis, ABECB, uncomplicated UTIs, and uncomplicated cervical/urethral gonorrhea caused by susceptible strains. Otitis media should be treated with suspension.
Cefotaxime sodium (Claforan)	Inj: 500mg, 1g, 2g, 10g	Treatment of LRT, GU, gynecologic, intra-abdominal, skin and skin structure, bone and joint, and CNS infections (eg, meningitis), as well as bacteremia and septicemia; administered preoperatively to reduce incidence of certain infections from surgical procedures (abdominal hysterectomy, GI and GU tract surgery) that may be classified as contaminated/potentially contaminated; administered during cesarean section postoperatively and intraoperatively (after clamping the umbilical cord) to reduce certain postoperative infections.
Cefpodoxime proxetil (Vantin)	Sus: 50mg/5mL, 100mg/5mL; Tab: 100mg, 200mg	Acute otitis media, pharyngitis/tonsilitis, CAP, ABECB, acute uncomplicated urethral and cervical gonorrhea, acute uncomplicated ano-rectal infections in women, uncomplicated SSSI, acute maxillary sinusitis, uncomplicated UTI.
Ceftazidime (Tazicef)	Inj: 1g, 2g, 6g; (Generic) 500mg, 1g, 2g, 6g	Treatment of LRT (eg, pneumonia), skin and skin structure, bone and joint, gynecologic, CNS (eg, meningitis), and intra-abdominal infections, complicated and uncomplicated UTI, and bacterial septicemia. Treatment of sepsis.
Ceftazidime (Fortaz)	Inj: 500mg, 1g, 1g/50mL, 2g, 2g/50mL, 6g	Treatment of LRT (eg, pneumonia), skin and skin structure, bone and joint, gynecologic, CNS (eg, meningitis), and intra-abdominal infections, complicated and uncomplicated UTI, and bacterial septicemia. Treatment of sepsis.
Ceftibuten (Cedax)	Cap: 400mg; Sus: 90mg/5mL, 180mg/5mL	Treatment of individuals with mild to moderate infections caused by susceptible strains of the designated microorganisms in ABECB, acute bacterial otitis media, pharyngitis, and tonsilitis.

GENERIC (BRAND)	HOW SUPPLIED	INDICATIONS**
CEPHALOSPORINS, THIRD-GENERATION *(Continued)*		
Ceftriaxone sodium (Rocephin)	**Inj:** 500mg, 1g; (Generic) 250mg, 500mg, 1g, 2g, 10g	Treatment of LRTIs, SSSI, bone and joint infections, intra-abdominal infections, acute otitis media, uncomplicated gonorrhea, PID, complicated and uncomplicated UTI, bacterial septicemia, and meningitis. For surgical prophylaxis.
CEPHALOSPORIN, FOURTH-GENERATION		
Cefepime HCl (Maxipime)	**Inj:** 500mg, 1g, 2g	Treatment of uncomplicated/complicated UTI, uncomplicated SSSI, complicated intra-abdominal infections, and moderate to severe pneumonia. Empiric therapy for febrile neutropenia.
CEPHALOSPORIN, FIFTH-GENERATION		
Ceftaroline fosamil (Teflaro)	**Inj:** 400mg, 600mg	Treatment of acute bacterial SSSI and CABP caused by susceptible strains of microorganisms.
FLUOROQUINOLONES		
Ciprofloxacin HCl (Cipro)	**Sus:** 250mg/5mL, 500mg/5mL; **Tab:** 250mg, 500mg, 750mg	**Adults:** Treatment of LRT, complicated intra-abdominal, skin and skin structure, bone and joint infections, and UTI; ABECB, acute sinusitis, acute uncomplicated cystitis in females, chronic bacterial prostatitis, infectious diarrhea, typhoid fever, uncomplicated cervical and urethral gonorrhea; **Adults/Pediatrics:** Post-exposure inhalation anthrax; **Pediatrics:** Complicated UTIs and pyelonephritis.
Ciprofloxacin HCl (Proquin XR)	**Tab, Extended-Release:** 500mg	Treatment of uncomplicated UTIs (acute cystitis) caused by *E. coli* and *K. pneumoniae.*
Ciprofloxacin (Cipro IV)	**Inj:** 10mg/mL, 200mg/100mL, 400mg/200mL	**Adults:** Treatment of SSSI, bone and joint, and complicated intra-abdominal infections, LRTI, and UTI; nosocomial pneumonia, acute sinusitis, chronic bacterial prostatitis, and empirical therapy for febrile neutropenia; **Adults/Pediatrics:** Post-exposure inhalation anthrax; **Pediatrics:** Complicated UTIs and pyelonephritis.
Ciprofloxacin (Cipro XR)	**Tab, Extended-Release:** 500mg, 1000mg	Uncomplicated (acute cystitis) and complicated UTI, and acute uncomplicated pyelonephritis due to *E. coli.*
Gemifloxacin (Factive)	**Tab:** 320mg	Treatment of mild to moderate CAP, MDRSP, and ABECB.
Levofloxacin (Levaquin)	**Inj:** 5mg/mL, 25mg/mL; **Sol:** 25mg/mL; **Tab:** 250mg, 500mg, 750mg [Leva-pak]	Uncomplicated and complicated SSSI, uncomplicated and complicated UTI, acute bacterial sinusitis, ABECB, CAP, nosocomial pneumonia, chronic bacterial prostatitis, and acute pyelonephritis caused by susceptible strains of microorganisms. To reduce the incidence or progression of disease of inhalation anthrax following exposure to *B. anthracis.*
Moxifloxacin HCl (Avelox)	**Inj:** 400mg/250mL; **Tab:** 400mg	Acute bacterial sinusitis, ABECB, uncomplicated and complicated SSSI, cIAIs, and CAP (including multidrug-resistant *S. pneumoniae*).
Norfloxacin (Noroxin)	**Tab:** 400mg	Treatment of adults with uncomplicated (including cystitis) and complicated UTI, prostatitis, and uncomplicated cervical and urethral gonorrhea caused by susceptible strains of microorganisms.
Ofloxacin	**Tab:** 200mg, 300mg, 400mg	Treatment of complicated UTI and uncomplicated SSSI, ABECB, CAP, acute uncomplicated urethral and cervical gonorrhea, nongonococcal urethritis and cervicitis, mixed infections of the urethra and cervix, acute PID, uncomplicated cystitis and prostatitis.
MACROLIDES		
Azithromycin (Zithromax)	**Inj:** 500mg; **Sus:** 100mg/5mL, 200mg/5mL, 1g/pkt; **Tab:** 250mg [Z-Pak, 6 tabs], 500mg [Tri-Pak, 3 tabs], 600mg	**PO:** 600mg tab: Treatment of nongonococcal urethritis and cervicitis due to *C. trachomatis*, as well as prophylaxis (with or without rifabutin) and treatment (in combination with ethambutol) of disseminated MAC disease in advanced HIV infection. **Adults:** Treatment of acute bacterial exacerbations of COPD, acute bacterial sinusitis, CAP, pharyngitis/tonsillitis, uncomplicated SSSI, urethritis/cervicitis, genital ulcer disease (men); **Peds:** Acute otitis media, pharyngitis/tonsillitis, CAP. **IV:** Treatment of CAP and PID.

(Continued)

GENERIC (BRAND)	HOW SUPPLIED	INDICATIONS**
MACROLIDES (Continued)		
Azithromycin (Zmax)	**Sus, Extended-Release:** 2g	Treatment of mild to moderate acute bacterial sinusitis in adults and treatment of CAP in adults and pediatric patients (≥6 months) caused by susceptible strains of microorganisms.
Clarithromycin (Biaxin)	**Sus:** 125mg/5mL, 250mg/5mL; **Tab:** 250mg, 500mg	**Adults:** Pharyngitis/tonsilitis, acute maxillary sinusitis, ABECB, CAP, uncomplicated SSSI, disseminated mycobacterial infections. **Tab:** Combination therapy for *H. pylori* infection with duodenal ulcers; MAC prophylaxis in advanced HIV. **Peds:** Pharyngitis/tonsilitis, CAP, acute maxillary sinusitis, acute otitis media, uncomplicated SSSI, disseminated mycobacterial infections.
Clarithromycin (Biaxin XL)	**Tab, Extended-Release:** 500mg [PAC 14ˢ, 60ˢ, 100ˢ]	Treatment of acute maxillary sinusitis, CAP, and ABECB.
Erythromycin (ERYC)	**Cap, Delayed-Release:** 250mg	Mild to moderate URTI and LRTI, SSSI, listeriosis, pertussis, diptheria, erythrasma, intestinal amebiasis, acute PID (*N. gonorrhoeae*), primary syphilis (caused by *T. pallidum*) in PCN allergy, Legionnaires' disease, chlamydial infections (eg, newborn conjunctivitis, pneumonia of infancy, urogenital infections during pregnancy); uncomplicated urethral, endocervical, or rectal infections; and nongonococcal urethritis (caused by *U. urealyticum*). Used for prevention of initial and recurrent attacks of rheumatic fever with PCN allergy.
Erythromycin (Ery-Tab)	**Tab, Delayed-Release:** 250mg, 333mg, 500mg; **(Generic) Cap, Delayed Release:** 250mg	Mild to moderate URTI and LRTIs, SSSIs, listeriosis, pertussis, diptheria, erythrasma, intestinal amebiasis, acute PID (*N. gonorrhoeae*), primary syphilis in PCN allergy, Legionnaires' disease, chlamydial infections (eg, newborn conjunctivitis, pneumonia of infancy, urogenital infections during pregnancy); uncomplicated urethral, endocervical, rectal infections, and nongonococcal urethritis (when tetracyclines are contraindicated or not tolerated). Prevention of initial and recurrent attacks of rheumatic fever with PCN allergy.
Erythromycin (PCE)	**Tab:** 333mg, 500mg	Mild to moderate URTI and LRTIs, SSSIs, listeriosis, pertussis, diptheria, erythrasma, intestinal amebiasis, acute PID (*N. gonorrhoeae*), primary syphilis in PCN allergy, Legionnaires' disease, chlamydial infections (eg, newborn conjunctivitis, pneumonia of infancy, urogenital infections during pregnancy); uncomplicated urethral, endocervical, rectal infections, and nongonococcal urethritis (when tetracyclines are contraindicated or not tolerated). Prevention of initial and recurrent attacks of rheumatic fever with PCN allergy.
Erythromycin base	**Tab:** 250mg, 500mg	Mild to moderate URTI and LRTIs, SSSIs, listeriosis, pertussis, diptheria, erythrasma, intestinal amebiasis, acute PID (*N. gonorrhoeae*), primary syphilis in PCN allergy, Legionnaires' disease, chlamydial infections (eg, newborn conjunctivitis, pneumonia of infancy, urogenital infections during pregnancy); uncomplicated urethral, endocervical, and rectal infections, and nongonococcal urethritis (when tetracyclines are contraindicated or not tolerated). Prevention of initial and recurrent attacks of rheumatic fever with PCN allergy.
Erythromycin ethylsuccinate (E.E.S.)	**Sus (in liquid and granule premix form):** 200mg/5mL, 400mg/5mL; **Tab:** 400mg	Mild to moderate URTI and LRTIs, SSSIs, listeriosis, pertussis, diptheria, erythrasma, intestinal amebiasis, acute PID (*N. gonorrhoeae*), primary syphilis in PCN allergy, Legionnaires' disease, chlamydial infections (eg, newborn conjunctivitis, pneumonia of infancy, urogenital infections during pregnancy); uncomplicated urethral, endocervical, and rectal infections, and nongonococcal urethritis (when tetracyclines are contraindicated or not tolerated). Prevention of initial and recurrent attacks of rheumatic fever with PCN allergy.
Erythromycin ethylsuccinate (EryPed)	**Sus:** 200mg/5mL, 400mg/5mL; **(Drops):** 200mg/5mL	Mild to moderate URTI and LRTIs, SSSIs, listeriosis, pertussis, diptheria, erythrasma, intestinal amebiasis, acute PID (*N. gonorrhoeae*), primary syphilis in PCN allergy, Legionnaires' disease, chlamydial infections (eg, newborn conjunctivitis, pneumonia of infancy, urogenital infections during pregnancy); uncomplicated urethral, endocervical, and rectal infections, and nongonococcal urethritis (when tetracyclines are contraindicated or not tolerated). Prevention of initial and recurrent attacks of rheumatic fever with PCN allergy.

GENERIC (BRAND)	HOW SUPPLIED	INDICATIONS**
MACROLIDES *(Continued)*		
Erythromycin ethylsuccinate/ Sulfisoxazole acetyl	**Sus:** 200mg-600mg/5mL	For treatment of acute otitis media in children that is caused by susceptible strains of *H. influenzae.*
Erythromycin lactobionate (Erythrocin)	**Inj:** 500mg, 1g	Mild to moderate URTI and LRTIs, SSSI, diptheria, erythrasma, acute PID (*N. gonorrhoeae*), and Legionnaires' disease. Prevention of initial and recurrent attacks of rheumatic fever with PCN allergy. Prevention of bacterial endocarditis with PCN allergy.
Erythromycin stearate (Erythrocin)	**Tab:** 250mg	Mild to moderate URTI and LRTIs, SSSIs, listeriosis, pertussis, diptheria, erythrasma, intestinal amebiasis, acute PID (*N. gonorrhoeae*), primary syphilis in PCN allergy, Legionnaires' disease, chlamydial infections (eg, newborn conjunctivitis, pneumonia of infancy, urogenital infections during pregnancy) uncomplicated urethral, endocervical, and rectal infections, and nongonococcal urethritis (when tetracyclines are contraindicated or not tolerated). Prevention of initial and recurrent attacks of rheumatic fever with PCN allergy.
Fidaxomicin (Dificid)	**Tab:** 200mg	Treatment of *C. difficile*-associated diarrhea in adults (≥18 yrs).
MONOBACTAM		
Aztreonam (Azactam)	**Inj:** 1g, 2g, 1g/50mL, 2g/50mL	Treatment of septicemia and LRTIs (eg, pneumonia, bronchitis); SSSIs (eg, postoperative wounds, ulcers, burns); complicated/uncomplicated UTIs, including pyelonephritis and initial/recurrent cystitis; gynecologic infections (eg, endometritis, pelvic cellulitis); and intra-abdominal (eg, peritonitis) infections caused by susceptible microorganisms. Adjunct therapy to surgery for management of infections caused by susceptible microorganisms (eg, abscesses, hollow viscus perforation infections, cutaneous infections, infections of serous surfaces).
Aztreonam (Cayston)	**Sol (for inhalation):** 75mg/vial (lyophilized)	To improve respiratory symptoms in cystic fibrosis patients with *P. aeruginosa.*
PENICILLINS		
Amoxicillin	**Cap:** 250mg, 500mg; **Sus:** 125mg/mL, 200mg/5mL, 250mg/5mL, 400mg/5mL; **Tab:** 500mg, 875mg; **Tab, Chewable:** 125mg, 200mg, 250mg, 400mg; **Tab, Dispersible:** 200mg, 400mg, 600mg	Infections of the ear, nose, throat, GU tract, SSSI, and LRTI due to susceptible (beta-lactamase-negative) organisms, as well as gonorrhea (acute, uncomplicated). Also used in combination therapy for *H. pylori* eradication to reduce the risk of duodenal ulcer recurrence.
Amoxicillin (Moxatag)	**Tab, Extended-Release:** 775mg	Treatment of tonsilitis and/or pharyngitis secondary to *S. pyogenes* in adults and pediatric patients ≥12 yrs.
Amoxicillin-Clavulanate potassium (Augmentin)	**Sus:** 125-31.25mg/5mL, 200-28.5mg/5mL, 250-62.5mg/5mL, 400-57mg/5mL; **Tab:** 250-125mg, 500-125mg, 875-125mg; **Tab, Chewable:** 125-31.25mg, 200-28.5mg, 250-62.5mg 400-57mg	Treatment of LRTI, SSSI, and UTI, as well as otitis media and sinusitis.
Amoxicillin-Clavulanate potassium	**Sus:** 600mg-42.9mg/5mL	Treatment of pediatric patients with recurrent or persistent acute otitis media with the following risk factors: antibiotic exposure for acute otitis media within in the last 3 months and ≤2 yrs or daycare attendance.
Amoxicillin-Clavulanate potassium (Augmentin XR)	**Tab, Extended-Release:** 1000mg-62.5mg	Treatment of CAP or acute bacterial sinusitis due to confirmed or suspected β-lactamase-producing pathogens and *S. pneumoniae* with reduced susceptibility to PCN.

(Continued)

GENERIC (BRAND)	HOW SUPPLIED	INDICATIONS**
PENICILLINS (Continued)		
Ampicillin	**Cap:** 250mg, 500mg; **Sus:** 125mg/5mL, 250mg/5mL	Treatment of meningitis and infections of GU tract (including gonorrhea), RT, and GI tract caused by susceptible strains of microorganisms.
Ampicillin sodium (Ampicillin)	**Inj:** 125mg, 250mg, 500mg, 1g, 2g, 10g	Treatment of RT, UT, and GI infections, bacterial meningitis, septicemia, endocarditis.
Ampicillin sodium/ Sulbactam sodium (Unasyn)	**Inj:** 1g-0.5g, 2g-1g, 10g-5g	Treatment of SSSI, intra-abdominal, and gynecological infections caused by susceptible microorganisms.
Dicloxacillin sodium	**Cap:** 250mg, 500mg	Infections caused by penicillinase-producing staphylococci.
Penicillin G benzathine- Penicillin G procaine (Bicillin C-R)	**Inj:** 600,000-600,000 U/2mL	Treatment of moderately severe to severe URTI, SSSI, scarlet fever, and erysipelas due to streptococci. Treatment of moderately severe pneumonia and otitis media due to pneumococci.
Penicillin G benzathine- Penicillin G procaine (Bicillin C-R 900/300)	**Inj:** 900,000-300,000 U/2mL	Treatment of moderately severe to severe URTI, SSSI scarlet fever, and erysipelas due to streptococci. Treatment of moderately severe pneumonia and otitis media due to pneumococci.
Penicillin G benzathine (Bicillin L-A)	**Inj:** 600,000 U/mL, 1,200,000 U/2mL, 2,400,000 U/4mL	Treatment of mild to moderate URTI due to streptococci and venereal infections (eg, syphilis, yaws, bejel, pinta); prophylaxis to prevent recurrence of rheumatic fever or chorea. As follow-up prophylactic therapy for rheumatic heart disease and acute glomerulonephritis.
Penicillin G benzathine (Permapen)	**Inj:** 600,000 U/mL	Treatment of microorganisms susceptible to low and very prolonged serum levels in URTIs (streptococci group A, without bacteremia), syphilis, yaws, bejel, and pinta; prophylaxis for rheumatic fever and/ or chorea. Follow-up prophylactic therapy for rheumatic heart disease and acute glomerulonephritis.
Penicillin G potassium (Pfizerpen)	**Inj:** 5 MU, 20 MU	For therapy of severe infections when rapid and high blood levels of PCN required. Management of streptococcal, pneumococcal, staphylococcal, clostridial, fusospirochetal, listeria, gram-negative bacillary, and pasteurella infections. For anthrax, actinomycosis, diptheria, erysipeloid endocarditis, meningitis (including meningococci), endocarditis, bacteremia, rat-bite fever, syphilis, and gonorrheal endocarditis and arthritis; with combined oral therapy, prophylaxis against endocarditis in patients with congenital heart disease, rheumatic disease, or other acquired valvular heart disease undergoing dental procedures or surgical procedures of URT.
Penicillin V potassium (Penicillin VK)	**Sus:** 125mg/5mL, 250mg/5mL; **Tab:** 250mg, 500mg	Treatment of mild to moderately severe infections due to PCN G-sensitive microorganisms; mild to moderate URTI, scarlet fever, and mild erysipelas; mild to moderately severe RT and oropharynx infections; mild SSSI. Prevention of recurrence following rheumatic fever and/or chorea. May be useful as prophylaxis against bacterial endocarditis in patients with congenital heart disease or rheumatic or other acquired valvular heart disease who are undergoing dental procedures and surgical procedures of the URT.
Piperacillin	**Inj:** 2g, 3g, 4g, 40g	Treatment of serious intra-abdominal, UT, gynecologic, LRT, SSSI, bone and joint, and uncomplicated gonococcal infections, as well as septicemia. Prophylactic use in surgery.
Piperacillin sodium/ Tazobactam sodium (Zosyn)	**Inj:** 2g-0.25g, 3g-0.375g, 4g-0.5g, 2g-0.25g/50mL, 3g-0.375g/50mL, 4g-0.5g/100mL, 36g-4.5g	Treatment of appendicitis, peritonitis, uncomplicated/complicated SSSIs, postpartum endometritis, PID, moderately severe CAP, and moderate to severe nosocomial pneumonia.
Ticarcillin-Clavulanate potassium (Timentin)	**Inj:** 3g-100mg, 30g-1g	Treatment of LRT, bone and joint infections, SSSI, uncomplicated/ complicated UTI, gynecologic, and intra-abdominal infections (peritonitis), as well as septicemia.

GENERIC (BRAND)	HOW SUPPLIED	INDICATIONS**
TETRACYCLINES		
Demeclocycline HCl	**Tab:** 150mg, 300mg	Treatment of susceptible infections including illness due to *Rickettsiae*, respiratory infections, lymphogranuloma venereum, trachoma, inclusion conjunctivitis, psittacosis, nongonococcal urethritis, relapsing fever, chancroid, plague, tularemia, cholera, *C. fetus* infections, brucellosis, bartonellosis, and granuloma inguinale. Treatment of gram-negative infections (eg, respiratory, urinary tract) and gram-positive infections (eg, URT, and SSSI). When PCN is contraindicated, treatment of uncomplicated urethritis in men, uncomplicated gonococcal infections, syphilis, yaws, listeriosis, anthrax, Vincent's infection, actinomycosis, and clostridial disease. Adjunct therapy in acute intestinal amebiasis and severe acne.
Doxycycline (Oracea)	**Cap:** 40mg	Treatment of only inflammatory lesions (papules and pustules) of rosacea in adults.
Doxycycline (Vibramycin)	**Cap:** (Doxycycline hyclate) 50mg, 100mg; **Syrup:** (Doxycycline calcium) 50mg/5mL; **Sus:** (Doxycycline monohydrate) 25mg/5mL; **Tab:** 100mg	Treatment of susceptible infections, including respiratory, urinary, lymphogranuloma venereum, psittacosis, trachoma, inclusion conjunctivitis, uncomplicated urethral/endocervical/rectal infections, relapsing fever, nongonococcal urethritis, illnesses caused by *Rickettsiae*, chancroid, tularemia, plague, cholera, *C. fetus* infections, brucellosis, bartonellosis, and granuloma inguinale. Treatment of anthrax. When PCN is contraindicated, treatment of uncomplicated gonorrhea, syphilis, listeriosis, *Clostridium* species infections, actinomycosis, yaws, and Vincent's infection. Adjunct therapy for amebiasis (adjunct to amebicides) and severe acne. Prophylaxis of malaria.
Doxycycline hyclate	**Inj:** 100mg	Treatment of *Rickettsiae*, *M. pneumoniae*, psittacosis, ornithosis, lymphogranuloma venereum, granuloma inguinale, relapsing fever, chancroid, *P. pestis*, *P. tularensis*, *B. bacilliformis*, *Bacteroides* species, *V. comma*, *V. fetus*, *Brucella* species, *E. coli*, *E. aerogenes*, *Shigella* species, *Mima* species, *Herellea* species, *H. influenzae*, *Klebsiella* species, *Streptococcus* species, *D. pneumoniae*, *S. aureus*, anthrax, and trachoma. When PCN is contraindicated; treatment of *N. gonorrhoeae*, *N. meningitis*, syphilis, yaws, *L. monocytogenes*, *Clostridium* species, Vincent's infection, and *Actinomyces* species. Adjunct therapy for amebiasis.
Doxycycline hyclate (Doryx)	**Tab, Delayed-Release:** 75mg, 100mg, 150mg	Treatment of susceptible infections, including RTI, UTI, uncomplicated urethral/endocervical/rectal, lymphogranuloma venereum, psittacosis, trachoma, inclusion conjunctivitis, relapsing fever due to *B. recurrentis*, nongonococcal urethritis, *Rickettsiae*, plague, granuloma inguinale, cholera, brucellosis, bartonellosis, *C. fetus* infections, tularemia, inhalation anthrax (post-exposure). When PCN is contraindicated, treatment of syphilis, yaws, Vincent's infection, actinomycosis, and infections from *Clostridium* species. Adjunct therapy for amebiasis and severe acne. Prophylaxis of malaria.
Doxycycline hyclate (Periostat)	**Tab:** 20mg	Adjunct to scaling and root planing to promote attachment level gain and reduce pocket depth in patients with adult periodontitis.
Doxycycline monohydrate (Monodox)	**Cap:** 50mg, 75mg, 100mg	Treatment of RTI, UTI, and SSSIs, uncomplicated urethral/endocervical/rectal infection caused by *C. trachomatis*, illnesses due to *Rickettsiae*, relapsing fever, nongonococcal urethritis caused by *U. urealyticum*, lymphogranuloma venereum, psittacosis, trachoma & inclusion conjunctivitis caused by *C. trachomatis*, chancroid, plague, cholera, brucellosis, tularemia, *C. fetus* infections, bartonellosis, and granuloma inguinale. Treatment of anthrax. When PCN is contraindicated, treatment of uncomplicated gonorrhea, syphilis, listeriosis, *Clostridium* species infections, actinomycosis, Vincent's infection, and yaws. Adjunct therapy for amebicides (adjunct to amebicides) and severe acne.

(Continued)

GENERIC (BRAND)	HOW SUPPLIED	INDICATIONS**
TETRACYCLINES (Continued)		
Minocycline HCl (Dynacin)	**Tab:** 50mg, 75mg, 100mg	Treatment of RTI, UTI, and SSSIs, lymphogranuloma venereum, psittacosis, trachoma, endocervical/rectal infection, nongonococcal urethritis, chancroid, plague, tularemia, cholera, brucellosis, inclusion conjunctivitis, bartonellosis, *C. fetus* infections, granuloma inguinale, relapsing fever, and illness due to *Rickettsiae*. When PCN is contraindicated, treatment of urethritis in men, gonococcal infections, syphilis, listeriosis, anthrax, *Clostridium* species infections, yaws, Vincent's infection, actinomycosis. Adjunct therapy for amebicides (in acute intestinal amebiasis) and severe acne. Treatment of *M. marinum* and asymptomatic carriers of *N. meningitidis*.
Minocycline HCl (Minocin)	**Cap:** 50mg, 100mg; **Inj:** 100mg/vial	Treatment of inclusion conjunctivitis, trachoma, relapsing fever, lymphogranuloma venereum, *Rickettsiae*, plague, tularemia, cholera, *C. fetus* infections, brucellosis, bartonellosis, granuloma inguinale, nongonococcal urethritis, and other infections (eg, RT, endocervical, and rectal infections, UTI, SSSI) caused by susceptible strains of microorganisms. When PCN is contraindicated (PO, INJ), treatment of yaws, listeriosis, Vincent's infection, actinomycosis, syphilis, anthrax, and *Clostridium* species infections. Adjunctive therapy in acute intestinal amebiasis and severe acne. (PO) Treatment of *M. marinum* and asymptomatic carriers of *N. meningitidis*. Treatment of chancroid. When PCN is contraindicated, treatment of uncomplicated urethritis in men and infections in women caused by *N. gonorrhoeae* and other gonococcal infections. (Inj) When PCN is contraindicated, treatment of meningitis.
Minocycline HCl (Solodyn)	**Tab, Extended-Release:** 45mg, 55mg, 65mg, 80mg, 90mg, 105mg, 115mg, 135mg	Treatment of inflammatory lesions of non-nodular moderate to severe acne vulgaris in patients ≥12 yrs.
Tetracycline HCl	**Cap:** 250mg, 500mg, 100mg	Treatment of RTI, UTI, and SSSIs, lymphogranuloma venereum, psittacosis, trachoma, uncomplicated urethral/endocervical/rectal infection caused by *Chlamydia*, chancroid, plague, tularemia, cholera, brucellosis, inclusion conjunctivitis, bartonellosis, *C. fetus* infections, granuloma inguinale, relapsing fever, and illnesses due to *Rickettsiae*. When PCN is contraindicated, treatment of *N. gonorrhoeae* infections, syphilis, listeriosis, anthrax, *Clostridium* species infections, yaws, Vincent's infection, actinomycosis. Adjunct therapy for amebicides (in acute intestinal amebiasis) and severe acne.
MISCELLANEOUS		
Clindamycin HCL (Cleocin HCL)	**Cap:** (HCl) 75mg, 150mg, 300mg; **Pediatric Solution:** palmitate (HCl) 75mg/5mL	Serious infections caused by anaerobes, streptococci, pneumococci, and staphylococci. Reserve for PCN allergy or if PCN is inappropriate.
Clindamycin phosphate (Cleocin Phosphate)	**Inj:** 150mg/mL, 300mg/50mL, 600mg/50mL, 900mg/50mL	Serious infections caused by anaerobes, streptococci, pneumococci, and staphylococci. LRTIs, SSSI, gynecological, intra-abdominal, and bone and joint infections, and septicemia.
Colistimethate sodium (Coly-Mycin M)	**Inj:** 150mg	Treatment of acute or chronic infections due to certain gram-negative bacilli (eg, *P. aeruginosa, E. aerogenes, E. coli, K. pneumoniae*).
Dalfopristin-Quinupristin (Synercid)	**Inj:** 350mg-150mg per 500mg vial	Treatment of complicated SSSI caused by *S. aureus* (methicillin-susceptible) or *S. pyogenes*.
Dapsone (Dapsone)	**Tab:** 25mg, 100mg	Treatment of leprosy and dermatitis herpetiformis.
Daptomycin (Cubicin)	**Inj:** 500mg/vial	Susceptible complicated SSSI. *S. aureus* bloodstream infections (bacteremia), including those with right-sided infective endocarditis.
Fosfomycin tromethamine (Monurol)	**Pow:** 3g/sachet	Uncomplicated UTI (acute cystitis) in women due to susceptible strains of *E. coli* and *E. faecalis*.

GENERIC (BRAND)	HOW SUPPLIED	INDICATIONS**
MISCELLANEOUS		
Isoniazid-Rifampin (Rifamate)	**Cap:** 150mg-300mg	For pulmonary TB when patient has been titrated on the individual components and it has been established that fixed dosage is therapeutically effective. Not for initial therapy or prevention of TB.
Isoniazid-Rifampin-Pyrazinamide (Rifater)	**Tab:** 50mg-300mg-120mg	For initial phase of short-course treatment of pulmonary TB.
Lincomycin HCl (Lincocin)	**Inj:** 300mg/mL	Treatment of serious infections due to streptococci, pneumococci, and staphylococci. Reserve for PCN allergy or if PCN is inappropriate.
Linezolid (Zyvox)	**Inj:** 2mg/mL; **Sus:** 100mg/5mL; **Tab:** 600mg	Vancomycin-resistant *E. faecium* infections; nosocomial pneumonia caused by *S. aureus* (methicillin-susceptible and resistant strains) or *S. pneumoniae* (including drug-resistant strains [MDRSP]); complicated SSSI, including diabetic foot infections without concomitant osteomyelitis (caused by *S. aureus* [methicillin-susceptible and resistant strains], *S. pyogenes*, or *S. agalactiae*); uncomplicated SSSIs caused by *S. aureus* (methicillin-susceptible only) or *S. pyogenes*; CAP caused by *S. pneumoniae* (MDRSP) or *S. aureus* (methicillin-susceptible strains only).
Methenamine hippurate (Hiprex)	**Tab:** 1g	Prophylaxis or suppression of recurrent UTIs when long-term therapy is necessary. For use only after infection is eradicated by other appropriate antimicrobials.
Metronidazole (Flagyl)	**Cap:** 375mg; **Tab:** 250mg, 500mg	Treatment of symptomatic and asymptomatic trichomoniasis, asymptomatic consorts, amebiasis, and anaerobic bacterial infections (following IV metronidazole therapy for serious infections). Treatment of intra-abdominal, gynecologic, bone and joint, CNS (eg, meningitis and brain abscess) infections, SSSI, and LRTIs, as well as endocarditis and bacterial septicemia.
Metronidazole HCl (Flagyl IV)	**Inj:** 500mg/100mL	Treatment of anaerobic intra-abdominal, skin and skin structure, gynecologic, bone and joint, and CNS infections, and LRTIs, as well as endocarditis and bacterial septicemia. Prophylaxis preoperatively, intraoperatively, and postoperatively to reduce incidence of postoperative infection in patients undergoing contaminated or potentially contaminated elective colorectal surgery. Effective against *B. fragilis* infections resistant to clindamycin, chloramphenicol, and PCN.
Nitrofurantoin (Furadantin)	**Sus:** 25mg/5mL	Treatment of UTIs when due to susceptible strains of *E. coli*, enterococci, *S. aureus*, and certain susceptible strains of *Klebsiella* and *Enterobacter* species.
Nitrofurantoin macrocrystals (Macrodantin)	**Cap:** 25mg, 50mg, 100mg	Treatment of UTIs when due to susceptible strains of *E. coli*, enterococci, *S. aureus*, and certain susceptible strains of *Klebsiella* and *Enterobacter* species.
Nitrofurantoin macrocrystals/ Nitrofurantoin monohydrate (Macrobid)	**Cap:** 100mg	Treatment of acute uncomplicated UTIs (acute cystitis) caused by susceptible strains of *E. coli* or *S. saprophyticus*.
Rifampin (Rifadin)	**Cap:** 150mg, 300mg; **Inj:** 600mg	Treatment of all forms of TB. Treatment of asymptomatic carriers of *N. meningitidis* to eliminate *meningococci* from the nasopharynx. **Inj:** For initial treatment and retreatment of TB when drug cannot be taken by mouth.
Sulfamethoxazole-Trimethoprim (Bactrim), (Bactrim DS), (Septra), (Septra DS), (Sulfatrim)	**Inj:** 80mg-16mg/mL; **Sus:** 200mg-40mg/5mL; **Tab:** 400mg-80mg; **Tab, DS:** 800mg-160mg	Treatment of UTI, *P. carinii* pneumonia (PCP), enteritis caused by *Shigella*, AECB, travelers' diarrhea, and acute otitis media.
Telavancin (Vibativ)	**Inj:** 250mg, 750mg	Treatment of adult patients with complicated SSSI caused by susceptible gram-positive microorganisms.

(Continued)

GENERIC (BRAND)	HOW SUPPLIED	INDICATIONS**
MISCELLANEOUS		
Telithromycin (Ketek)	**Tab:** 300mg, 400mg	Treatment of mild to moderate CAP due to *S. pneumoniae* (including MDRSP), *H. influenzae*, *M. catarrhalis*, *C. pneumoniae*, or *M. pneumoniae* in patients ≥18 yrs.
Tigecycline (Tygacil)	**Inj:** 50mg/5mL, 50mg/10mL [vial]	Treatment of complicated SSSIs, cIAIs, and CABP caused by susceptible strains of indicated pathogens in patients ≥18 yrs.
Trimethoprim	**Tab:** 100mg, 200mg	Treatment of initial episodes of uncomplicated UTIs due to susceptible organisms.
Trimethoprim HCl (Primsol)	**Sol:** 50mg/5mL	Treatment of acute otitis media in pediatrics and UTI in adults.
Vancomycin HCl	**Inj:** 500mg/vial, 750mg/vial, 1g/vial, 5g/vial, 10g/vial	Treatment of severe infections caused by susceptible strains of methicillin-resistant staphylococci. Indicated for PCN-allergic patients, those who cannot receive or have failed to respond to other drugs, and for vancomycin-susceptible organisms that are resistant to other antimicrobials.
Vancomycin HCl (Vancocin)	**Cap:** 125mg, 150mg	Treatment of enterocolitis caused by *S. aureus* (including methicillin-resistant strains) and *C. difficile*-associated diarrhea.

*To reduce the development of drug-resistant bacteria and maintain the effectiveness of antibacterial drugs, antibiotics should be used only to treat or prevent infections that are proven or strongly suspected to be caused by susceptible bacteria.

**Refer to monograph or full FDA-approved prescribing information for more information on specific antibacterial coverage.

ABECB = acute bacterial exacerbation of chronic bronchitis

GI = gastrointestinal

PID = pelvic inflammatory disease

CABP = community-acquired bacterial pneumonia

GU = genitourinary

SSSI = skin and skin structure infection

CAP = community-acquired pneumonia

LRTI = lower respiratory tract infection

TB = tuberculosis

cIAIs = complicated intra-abdominal infections

MAC = *Mycobacterium avium* complex

URTI = upper respiratory tract infection

MDRSP = multidrug-resistant *Streptococcus pneumoniae*

UTI = urinary tract infection

PCN = penicillin

ORAL AND SYSTEMIC ANTIFUNGALS

GENERIC (BRAND)	INDICATION	DOSAGE FORM	DOSAGE*	ADDITIONAL COMMENTS
Amphotericin B	Progressive, potentially life-threatening fungal infections: Aspergillosis, cryptococcosis, North American blastomycosis, systemic candidiasis, coccidioidomycosis, histoplasmosis, zygomycosis, sporotrichosis, and infections due to *Conidiobolus* and *Basidiobolus* species. May be useful for treatment of American mucocutaneous leishmaniasis.	**Inj:** 50mg	**Initial:** 0.25mg/kg. **Titrate:** Increase by 5-10mg/day, depending on cardio-renal status, up to 0.5-0.7mg/kg/day. **Max:** 1mg/kg/day or 1.5mg/kg/day when given on alternate days.	**BW:** Used primarily to treat progressive and potentially life-threatening fungal infections. • Doses greater than 1.5mg/kg should not be given. • Verify product's name and dosage preadministration and use caution to prevent inadvertent overdosage which may result in cardiopulmonary arrest. • Administer by slow IV infusion.
Amphotericin B cholesteryl sulfate (Amphotec)	Treatment of invasive aspergillosis in patients with renal impairment, unacceptable toxicity, or previous failure to amphotericin B deoxycholate.	**Inj:** 50mg, 100mg	3-4mg/kg/day at 1mg/kg/hr.	• Infusion time may be shortened to a minimum of 2 hrs if no evidence of intolerance or infusion-related reactions. • If patient experiences acute reactions or cannot tolerate the infusion volume, the infusion time may be extended. • Administer IV.
Amphotericin B lipid complex injection (Abelcet)	Invasive fungal infections in patients who are refractory to or intolerant of conventional amphotericin B deoxycholate.	**Inj:** 5mg/mL	Single infusion 5mg/kg at 2.5mg/kg/hr.	• If the infusion time exceeds 2 hrs, mix the contents by shaking the infusion bag every 2 hrs. • Administer IV.
Amphotericin B liposome injection (AmBisome)	Treatment of patients with *Aspergillus* species, *Candida* species, and/or *Cryptococcus* species infections refractory to amphotericin B deoxycholate or in patients where renal impairment or unacceptable toxicity precludes the use of amphotericin B deoxycholate. Treatment of visceral leishmaniasis. Empirical therapy for presumed fungal infections in febrile neutropenic patients. Treatment of cryptococcal meningitis in HIV-infected patients.	**Inj:** 50mg	**Empiric Therapy:** 3mg/kg/day. **Systemic Infections** (*Aspergillus, Candida, Cryptococcus*): 3-5mg/kg/day. **Cryptococcal Meningitis in HIV:** 6mg/kg/day IV. **Visceral Leishmaniasis for Immunocompetent Patients:** 3mg/kg/day on Days 1-5 and Days 14, 21. **Visceral Leishmaniasis in Immunocompromised Patients:** 4mg/kg/day on Days 1-5 and Days 10, 17, 24, 31, 38.	• AmBisome should be administered by IV infusion using a controlled infusion device over a period of approximately 120 minutes. • Administer IV.
Anidulafungin (Eraxis)	Treatment of candidemia and other forms of *Candida* infections, esophageal candidiasis.	**Inj:** 50mg, 100mg	**Candidemia:** LD: 200mg on Day 1, followed by 100mg qd. Treat for at least 14 days after last positive culture. **Esophageal Candidiasis:** LD: 100mg qd x 1 day then 50mg qd. Treat for minimum of 14 days and for at least 7 days after symptoms resolve.	• The rate of infusion should not exceed 1.1mg/min. • Administer IV.

ORAL AND SYSTEMIC ANTIFUNGALS

GENERIC (BRAND)	INDICATION	DOSAGE FORM	DOSAGE*	ADDITIONAL COMMENTS
Caspofungin acetate (Cancidas)	Treatment of candidemia and the following *Candida* infections: intra-abdominal abscesses, peritonitis, and pleural space infections. Treatment of esophageal candidiasis. Treatment of invasive aspergillosis in patients who are refractory to or intolerant of other therapies. Empirical therapy for presumed fungal infections in febrile, neutropenic patients.	**Inj:** 50mg, 70mg	70mg LD on Day 1 and then 50mg qd. **Esophageal Candidiasis:** 50mg qd.	• Maximum loading dose and daily maintenance dose should not exceed 70mg, regardless of the patient's calculated dose. • Administer by slow IV infusion over approximately 1 hr.
Clotrimazole (Mycelex Troche)	Oropharyngeal candidiasis. To prevent oropharyngeal candidiasis in immunocompromised conditions.	**Loz/Troche:** 10mg	1 troche in mouth 5 times/day for 14 days. **Prophylaxis:** 1 troche tid for duration of chemotherapy or until steroids reduced to maintenance levels.	• Not indicated for treatment of systemic mycoses, including systemic candidiasis.
Fluconazole (Diflucan)	Treatment of vaginal, oropharyngeal and esophageal candidiasis. The treatment of *Candida* urinary tract infections, peritonitis, and systemic *Candida* infections, including candidemia, disseminated candidiasis, and pneumonia. Treatment of cryptococcal meningitis. Prophylaxis in patients undergoing bone marrow transplantation receiving chemotherapy and/or radiation therapy.	**Inj:** 200mg/100mL, 400mg/200mL; **Sus:** 350mg/35mL, 1400mg/35mL [35mL]; **Tab:** 50mg, 100mg, 150mg, 200mg	**Vaginal Candidiasis:** 150g PO single dose. **Cryptococcal Meningitis:** 400mg on Day 1, then 200mg qd. **Prophylaxis in Patients Undergoing Bone Marrow Transplantation:** 400mg qd. **Oropharyngeal Candidiasis:** 200mg on Day 1, then 100mg qd. **Esophageal Candidiasis:** 200mg on Day 1, then 100mg qd. **Max:** 400mg/day. **Systemic *Candida* Infections:** Up to 400mg/day. **UTI/Peritonitis:** 50-200mg/day.	• Diflucan may be administered orally or by IV infusion. • The IV infusion of diflucan should be administered at a maximum rate of approximately 200mg/hr as a continuous infusion.
Flucytosine (Ancobon)	Treatment of septicemia, endocarditis, and urinary tract infections caused by *Candida*. Treatment of meningitis and pulmonary infection caused by *Cryptococcus*.	**Cap:** 250mg, 500mg	50-150mg/kg/day given in divided doses q6h.	**BW:** Use with extreme caution in patients with impaired renal function; monitor hematologic, renal, and hepatic status. • Ancobon should be used in combination with amphotericin B for the treatment of systemic candidiasis and cryptococcosis because of the emergence of resistance.
Griseofulvin (Grifulvin V)	Treatment of ringworm.	**Sus:** 125mg/mL [120mL]	0.5-1g qd.	• Periodic monitoring of organ system function, including renal, hepatic and hematopoietic, should be done. • Medication must be continued until the infecting organism is completely eradicated as indicated by appropriate clinical or laboratory examination.

GENERIC (BRAND)	INDICATION	DOSAGE FORM	DOSAGE*	ADDITIONAL COMMENTS
Griseofulvin (Gris-PEG)	Treatment of ringworm.	**Tab:** (ultramicrosize): 125mg, 250mg	375mg as a single dose or in divided doses.	• Periodic monitoring of organ system function, including renal, hepatic and hematopoietic, should be done. • Medication must be continued until the infecting organism is completely eradicated as indicated by appropriate clinical or laboratory examination.
Itraconazole (Sporanox)	(Cap) Onychomycosis of the toenail and fingernail. Treatment of blastomycosis and histoplasmosis. Treatment of aspergillosis if refractory to or intolerant of amphotericin B. (Sol) Treatment of oropharyngeal and esophageal candidiasis.	**Cap:** 100mg; **Sol:** 10mg/mL [150mL]	**(Cap) Blastomycosis/ Histoplasmosis:** 200mg qd. **Titrate:** 100mg increments. **Max:** 400mg/day. **Aspergillosis:** 200-400mg/day. **Onychomycosis: Toenail:** 200mg qd for 12 weeks. **Fingernail:** 200mg bid for 1 week, skip 3 weeks, then repeat. **(Sol) Oropharyngeal Candidiasis:** 200mg/day for 1-2 weeks. Swish 10mL at a time for several sec and swallow. **Esophageal Candidiasis:** 100-200mg/ day for at least 3 weeks. Doses above 200mg should be given in two divided doses.	**BW:** Sporanox should not be administered for the treatment of onychomycosis in patients with evidence of ventricular dysfunction. Coadministration of cisapride, pimozide, quinidine, dofetilide, or levacetylmethadol is contraindicated. • Sporanox Capsules is a different preparation than Oral Solution; these should not be used interchangeably.
Ketoconazole (Nizoral)	Candidiasis, chronic mucocutaneous candidiasis, oral thrush, candiduria, blastomycosis, coccidioidomycosis, histoplasmosis, chromomycosis, and paracoccidioidomycosis. Treatment of patients with severe recalcitrant cutaneous dermatophyte infections not responsive to topical therapy or oral griseofulvin.	**Tab:** 200mg	200mg qd. **Max:** 400mg qd.	**BW:** Oral use of ketoconazole has been associated with hepatic toxicity. Coadministration of terfenadine, cisapride, and astemizole is contraindicated. Tablets should not be used for treatment of fungal meningitis.
Micafungin sodium (Mycamine)	Esophageal candidiasis and prophylaxis of *Candida* infection in HSCT patients. Treatment of candidemia, acute disseminated candidiasis, *Candida* peritonitis, and abscesses.	**Inj:** 50mg, 100mg	**Candidemia, Acute Disseminated Candidiasis, *Candida* Peritonitis, and Abscesses:** 100mg IV qd (usual range 10-47 days). **Esophageal Candidiasis:** 150mg/day (usual range 10-30 days). **Prophylaxis (HSCT):** 50mg IV qd (usual range 6-51 days).	• A loading dose is not required. • Infuse IV over 1 hour.
Miconazole (Oravig)	Local treatment of oropharyngeal candidiasis.	**Tab, Buccal:** 50mg	Apply 1 buccal tab to upper gum region qd for 14 days.	• Oravig should not be crushed, chewed, or swallowed.

(Continued)

GENERIC (BRAND)	INDICATION	DOSAGE FORM	DOSAGE*	ADDITIONAL COMMENTS
Nystatin	(Sus) Treatment of oral candidiasis. (Tab) Treatment of non-esophageal mucous membrane GI candidiasis.	**Sus:** 100,000 U/mL [60mL, 480mL]; **Tab:** 500,000 U	**(Sus) Oral Candidiasis:** 2-3mL in each side of mouth qid. Retain in mouth as long as possible before swallowing. **(Tab) Non-Esophageal GI Candidiasis:** 1-2 tab tid.	• Not indicated for treatment of systemic mycoses.
Posaconazole (Noxafil)	Prophylaxis of invasive *Aspergillus* and *Candida* infections. Treatment of oropharyngeal candidiasis, including oropharyngeal candidiasis refractory to itraconazole and/or fluco-nazole.	**Sus:** 40mg/mL [105mL]	**Prophylaxis:** 200mg tid. **Oropharyngeal Candidiasis:** 100mg bid x 1 day, 100mg qd x 13 days. **Oropharyngeal Candidiasis Refractory to Itraconazole and/or Fluconazole:** 400mg bid.	• Each dose of Noxafil should be administered during or immediately (ie, within 20 minutes) following a full meal. • In patients who cannot eat a full meal, each dose of Noxafil should be administered with a liquid nutritional supplement or an acidic carbonated beverage.
Terbinafine HCl (Lamisil)	(Tab): Onychomycosis of the toenail or fingernail. (Granules): Tinea capitis in patients ≥4 years old.	**Tab:** 250mg; **Granules:** 125mg/packet and 187.5mg/packet	**(Tab)** 250mg PO qd for 6 weeks for fingernail and 12 weeks for toenail. **(Gran)** <25kg: 125mg/day, 25-35kg: 187.5mg/day, >35kg: 250mg/day. Take for 6 weeks.	• Prior to initiating treatment, appropriate nail specimens for laboratory testing (KOH preparation, fungal culture, or nail biopsy) should be obtained to confirm the diagnosis of onychomycosis.
Voriconazole (Vfend)	Invasive aspergillosis, esophageal candidiasis, serious fungal infections caused by *Scedosporium apiospermum* and *Fusarium* spp. Including *Fusarium solani*, candidemia in non-neutropenic patients, and disseminated candidiasis.	**Inj:** 200mg; **Sus:** 40mg/mL; **Tab:** 50mg, 200mg	**IV LD:** 6mg/kg q12h for first 24h. **IV MD:** 3-4mg/kg q12h. **PO MD:** ≥40kg: 200mg q12h. May increase to 300mg q12h. **<40kg:** 100mg q12h. May increase to 150mg q12h.	• Vfend Tablets or Oral Suspension should be taken at least one hour before or after a meal. • Vfend IV for Injection requires reconstitution to 10mg/mL and subsequent dilution to 5mg/mL or less prior to administration as an infusion, at a maximum rate of 3mg/kg per hour over 1 to 2 hours. • Do not administer as an IV bolus injection.

Abbreviations: BW = Boxed Warning; LD = loading dose
*Refer to FDA-approved labeling for specific dosing information in Pediatrics, Special Populations, and for Duration of Treatment.

TREATMENT OF TUBERCULOSIS

TREATMENT ALGORITHM FOR TUBERCULOSIS

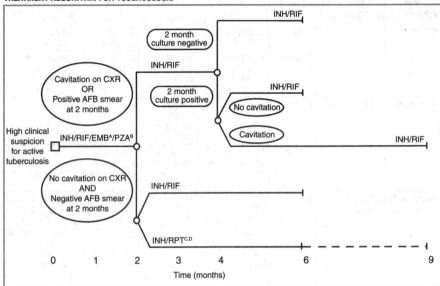

Abbreviations: CXR=chest radiograph; EMB=ethambutol; INH=isoniazid; PZA=pyrazinamide; RIF=rifampin; RPT=rifapentine.

A EMB may be discontinued when results of drug susceptibility testing indicate no drug resistance.

B PZA may be discontinued after it has been taken for 2 months (56 doses).

C RPT should not be used in HIV-infected patients with tuberculosis or in patients with extrapulmonary tuberculosis.

D Therapy should be extended to 9 months if 2-month culture is positive.

Source: Centers for Disease Control and Prevention. Treatment of Tuberculosis. American Thoracic Society, CDC, and Infectious Diseases Society of America. *MMWR.* 2003;52(No. RR-11).

DOSES* OF ANTITUBERCULOSIS DRUGS FOR ADULTS AND CHILDREN†

			DOSES			
DRUG	**PREPARATION**	**ADULTS/ CHILDREN**	**DAILY**	**1X/WK**	**2X/WK**	**3X/WK**
FIRST-LINE DRUGS						
Isoniazid	Tablets (50mg, 100mg, 300mg); elixir (50mg/5mL); aqueous solution (100mg/mL); for intravenous or intramuscular injection	Adults (max)	5mg/kg (300mg)	15mg/kg (900mg)	15mg/kg (900mg)	15mg/kg (900mg)
		Children (max)	10-15mg/kg (300mg)	—	20-30mg/kg (900mg)	—
Rifampin	Capsule (150mg, 300mg); powder may be sus- pended for oral administration; aqueous solution for intravenous injection	Adults‡ (max)	10mg/kg (600mg)	—	10mg/kg (600mg)	10mg/kg (600mg)
		Children (max)	10-20mg/kg (600mg)	—	10-20mg/kg (600mg)	—

(Continued)

DRUG	PREPARATION	ADULTS/ CHILDREN	DOSES			
			DAILY	1X/WK	2X/WK	3X/WK
FIRST-LINE DRUGS *(Continued)*						
Rifabutin	Capsule (150mg)	Adults[‡] (max)	5mg/kg (300mg)	—	5mg/kg (300mg)	5mg/kg (300mg)
		Children	Appropriate dosing for children is unknown	Appropriate dosing for children is unknown	Appropriate dosing for children is unknown	Appropriate dosing for children is unknown
Rifapentine	Tablet (150mg, film coated)	Adults	—	10mg/kg (continuation phase) (600mg)	—	—
		Children	The drug is not approved for use in children	The drug is not approved for use in children	The drug is not approved for use in children	The drug is not approved for use in children
Pyrazinamide	Tablet (500mg, scored)	Adults	40-55kg: 1000mg (18.2-25.0mg/kg); 56-75kg: 1500mg (20-26.8mg/kg); 76-90kg: 2000mg[¶] (22.5-26.3mg/kg)	—	40-55kg: 2000mg (36.4-50.0mg/kg); 56-75kg: 3000mg (40.0-53.6mg/kg); 76-90kg: 4000mg[¶] (44.4-52.6mg/kg)	40-55kg: 1500mg (27.3-37.5mg/kg); 56-75kg: 2500mg (33.3-44.6mg/kg); 76-90kg: 3000mg[¶] (33.3-39.5mg/kg)
		Children (max)	15-30mg/kg (2.0g)	—	50mg/kg (2g)	—
Ethambutol	Tablet (100mg, 400mg)	Adults	40-55kg: 800mg (14.5-20.0mg/kg); 56-75kg: 1200mg (16-21.4mg/kg); 76-90kg: 1600mg[¶] (17.8-21.1mg/kg)	—	40-55kg: 2000mg (36.4-50.0mg/kg); 56-75kg: 2800mg (37.3-50.0mg/kg); 76-90kg: 4000mg[¶] (44.4-52.6mg/kg)	40-55kg: 1200mg (21.8-30.0mg/kg); 56-75kg: 2000mg (26.7-35.7mg/kg); 76-90kg: 2400mg[¶] (26.7-31.6mg/kg)
		Children[§] (max)	15-20mg/kg daily (1.0g)	—	50mg/kg (2.5g)	—
SECOND-LINE DRUGS						
Cycloserine	Capsule (250mg)	Adults (max)	10-15mg/kg/d (1.0g in two doses), usually 500-750mg/d in two doses[¶]	There are no data to support intermittent administration	There are no data to support intermittent administration	There are no data to support intermittent administration
		Children (max)	10-15mg/kg/d (1.0g/d)	—	—	—

		ADULTS/	DOSES			
DRUG	PREPARATION	CHILDREN	DAILY	1X/WK	2X/WK	3X/WK
SECOND-LINE DRUGS *(Continued)*						
Ethionamide	Tablet (250mg)	Adults# (max)	15-20mg/kg/d (1.0g/d), usually 500-750mg/d in a single daily dose or two divided doses#	There are no data to support intermittent administration	There are no data to support intermittent administration	There are no data to support intermittent administration
		Children (max)	15-20mg/kg/d (1.0g/d)	There are no data to support intermittent administration	There are no data to support intermittent administration	There are no data to support intermittent administration
Streptomycin	Aqueous solution (1-g vials) for intravenous or intramuscular administration	Adults (max)	**	**	**	**
		Children (max)	20-40mg/kg/d (1g)	—	20mg/kg	—
Amikacin/ Kanamycin	Aqueous solution (500-mg and 1-g vials) for intravenous or intramuscular administration	Adults (max)	**	**	**	**
		Children (max)	15-30mg/kg/d (1g) intravenous or intramuscular as a single daily dose	—	15-30mg/kg	—
Capreomycin	Aqueous solution (1-g vials) for intravenous or intramuscular administration	Adults (max)	**	**	**	**
		Children (max)	15-30mg/kg/d (1g) as a single daily dose	—	15-30mg/kg	—
p-Aminosal-icylic Acid (PAS)	Granules (4-g packets) can be mixed with food; tablets (500mg) are still available in some countries, but not in the United States; a solution for intravenous administration is available in Europe	Adults	8-12g/d in two or three doses	There are no data to support intermittent administration	There are no data to support intermittent administration	There are no data to support intermittent administration
		Children	200-300mg/kg/d in two to four divided doses (10g)	There are no data to support intermittent administration	There are no data to support intermittent administration	There are no data to support intermittent administration
Levofloxacin	Tablets (250mg, 500mg, 750mg); aqueous solution (500-mg vials) for intravenous injection	Adults	500-1000mg daily	There are no data to support intermittent administration	There are no data to support intermittent administration	There are no data to support intermittent administration
		Children	††	††	††	††
Moxifloxacin	Tablets (400mg); aqueous solution (400mg/250mL) for intravenous injection	Adults	400mg daily	There are no data to support intermittent administration	There are no data to support intermittent administration	There are no data to support intermittent administration
		Children	‡‡	‡‡	‡‡	‡‡

(Continued)

			DOSES			
DRUG	PREPARATION	ADULTS/ CHILDREN	DAILY	1X/WK	2X/WK	3X/WK
SECOND-LINE DRUGS *(Continued)*						
Gatifloxacin	Tablets (400mg); aqueous solution (200mg/20mL; 400mg/40mL) for intravenous injection	Adults	400mg daily	There are no data to support intermittent administration	There are no data to support intermittent administration	There are no data to support intermittent administration
		Children	§§	§§	§§	§§

* Dose per weight is based on ideal body weight. Children weighing more than 40kg should be dosed as adults.

† For purposes of this document adult dosing begins at age 15 years.

‡ Dose may need to be adjusted when there is concomitant use of protease inhibitors or nonnucleoside reverse transcriptase inhibitors.

§ The drug can likely be used safely in older children but should be used with caution in children less than 5 years of age, in whom visual acuity cannot be monitored. In younger children EMB at the dose of 15mg/kg per day can be used if there is suspected or proven resistance to INH or RIF.

¶ It should be noted that, although this is the dose recommended generally, most clinicians with experience using cycloserine indicate that it is unusual for patients to be able to tolerate this amount. Serum concentration measurements are often useful in determining the optimal dose for a given patient.

⌐ The single daily dose can be given at bedtime or with the main meal.

** Dose: 15mg/kg per day (1g), and 10mg/kg in persons more than 59 years of age (750mg). Usual dose: 750-1000mg administered intramuscularly or intravenously, given as a single dose 5-7 days/week and reduced to two or three times per week after the first 2-4 months or after culture conversion, depending on the efficacy of the other drugs in the regimen.

†† The long-term (more than several weeks) use of levofloxacin in children and adolescents has not been approved because of concerns about effects on bone and cartilage growth. However, most experts agree that the drug should be considered for children with tuberculosis caused by organisms resistant to both INH and RIF. The optimal dose is not known.

‡‡ The long-term (more than several weeks) use of moxifloxacin in children and adolescents has not been approved because of concerns about effects on bone and cartilage growth. The optimal dose in unknown.

§§ The long-term (more than several weeks) use of gatifloxacin in children and adolescents has not been approved because of concerns about effects on bone and cartilage growth. The optimal dose in unknown.

¶¶ Maximum dose regardless of weight.

Source: Centers for Disease Control and Prevention. Treatment of Tuberculosis. American Thoracic Society, CDC, and Infectious Diseases Society of America. *MMWR.* 2003;52(No. RR-11).

ANKYLOSING SPONDYLITIS AGENTS

GENERIC (BRAND)	HOW SUPPLIED	DOSAGE	MAX DOSE
COX-2 INHIBITOR			
Celecoxib (Celebrex)	**Cap:** 50mg, 100mg, 200mg, 400mg	200mg qd or 100mg bid	400mg/day
MONOCLONAL ANTIBODIES/TNF-RECEPTOR BLOCKERS			
Adalimumab (Humira)	**Inj:** 20mg/0.4mL, 40mg/0.8mL	40mg SQ every other wk	NA
Golimumab (Simponi)	**Inj:** 50mg/0.5mL	50mg SQ every month	NA
Infliximab (Remicade)	**Inj:** 100mg/20mL	5mg/kg as IV infusion; repeat at 2 and 6 wks then q6wk thereafter*	NA
NSAIDs			
Diclofenac sodium	**Tab, Delayed-Release:** 25mg, 50mg, 75mg	25mg qid and 25mg qhs prn	NA
Indomethacin (Indocin)	**Sus:** 25mg/5mL [50mL, 237mL]; **Cap:** (generic) 25mg, 50mg; **Cap, Extended-Release:** (generic) 75mg; **Suppository:** (generic) 50mg	**Cap/Sus/Suppository:** 25mg bid-tid; may increase by 25-50mg/day at weekly intervals. **ER:** 75mg qd; may increase by 75mg/day	**Cap/Sus:** 150-200mg/day. **ER:** 150mg/day
Naproxen (EC-Naprosyn, Naprosyn)	**Sus:** 125mg/5mL [473mL]; **Tab:** 250mg, 375mg, 500mg; **Tab, Delayed-Release:** (generic) 375mg, 500mg	250mg, 375mg, or 500mg bid	1500mg/day
Naproxen sodium			
(Anaprox)	**Tab:** 275mg	275mg bid with food	1500mg/day
(Anaprox DS)	**Tab:** 550mg	550mg bid with food	1500mg/day
(Naprelan)	**Tab, Extended-Release:** 375mg, 500mg, 750mg	750mg-1g bid with food	1500mg/day
Sulindac (Clinoril)	**Tab:** 150mg, 200mg†	150mg-200mg bid with food	400mg/day with food
TNF-RECEPTOR BLOCKER			
Etanercept (Enbrel)	**Inj:** 25mg [vial]; 50mg/mL [syringe]	50mg SQ per wk	50mg/wk

*Doses >5mg/kg are contraindicated in patients with moderate to severe heart failure.
†Scored.

DIETARY CALCIUM INTAKE

RECOMMENDED CALCIUM INTAKES*

AGE	DAILY INTAKE (MG)
Birth-6 months	200
6 months-1 year	260
1-3 years	700
4-8 years	1000
9-18 years	1300
19-50 years	1000
51-70 years (male)	1000
51-70 years (female)	1200
>70 years	1200
PREGNANT OR LACTATING	
14-18 years	1300
19-50 years	1000

*Source: National Institute of Arthritis and Musculoskeletal and Skin Diseases (NIAMS), National Institutes of Health.

ESTIMATING DAILY DIETARY CALCIUM INTAKE

Step 1: Estimate calcium intake from calcium-rich foods.*

Product	Servings/Day	Calcium/Serving (mg)		Calcium (mg)
Milk (8 oz)	_____	x 300	=	_____
Yogurt (8 oz)	_____	x 300	=	_____
Cheese (1 oz, or 1 cubic inch)	_____	x 200	=	_____
Fortified foods or juices	_____	x 80-1000**	=	_____
Total Daily Calcium Intake in mg			=	_____

Step 2: List the estimated number of servings of each food item under "servings per day"

Step 3: Multiply the number of "servings per day" by the number of milligrams (mg) under "Calcium"

Step 4: Add the totals in the right hand column to get your Total Daily Calcium Intake. (Note: 250 mg of calcium is automatically added under estimated total from other foods)

Step 5: Subtract the final total daily calcium intake from the recommended amount of calcium you need each day. This number is the additional calcium you need each day. Get this by adding calcium rich foods to your diet and/or by taking a calcium supplement.

*About 75-80% of the calcium consumed in American diets is from dairy products.
**Calcium content of fortified foods varies.

FACTORS RELATED TO VITAMIN D THAT MAY AFFECT CALCIUM ABSORPTION:

- National Osteoporosis Foundation recommends an intake of 800 to 1000 International Units (IU) of vitamin D_3 per day for adults over age 50 and 400 to 800 IU of vitamin D_3 for <50 years of age

- There are 2 types of vitamin D supplements: vitamin D_2 (ergocalciferol) and vitamin D_3 (cholecalciferol); they are both equally good for bone health

- Desired level for the average adult's serum 25(OH)D concentration is 30 ng/mL (75 nmol/L) or higher

- Safe upper limit for vitamin D intake for normal adult population was set at 4000 IU per day

- Patients with malabsorption (eg, celiac disease) or chronic renal insufficiency, or those who are housebound, chronically ill, or have limited sun exposure, may need vitamin D supplements

Sources: National Institute of Arthritis and Musculoskeletal and Skin Diseases (NIAMS), National Institutes of Health; National Osteoporosis Foundation.

GOUT AGENTS

GENERIC (BRAND)	HOW SUPPLIED	USUAL DOSAGE RANGE	MAX DOSE
ALKALINIZING AGENTS			
Citric Acid/Potassium Citrate (Cytra-K Crystals)	(Citric Acid Monohydrate/ Potassium Citrate Monohydrate) 1002mg-3300mg/pack [100ˢ]	1 packet qid after meals and at bedtime. Reconstitute with at least 6 oz of cool water or juice.	
Citric Acid Monohydrate/Potassium Citrate Monohydrate/Sodium Citrate Dihydrate (Cytra-3 Syrup)	**Syr:** (Citric Acid Monohydrate-Potassium Citrate Monohydrate-Sodium Citrate Dihydrate) 334mg-550mg-500mg/5mL	15-30mL diluted with water, qid after meals and at bedtime.*	
Citric Acid Monohydrate/Potassium Citrate Monohydrate (Cytra-K Oral Solution)	(Citric Acid Monohydrate-Potassium Citrate Monohydrate) 334mg-1100mg/5mL	10-15mL diluted with a glassful of water, qid after meals and at bedtime.*	
CORTICOSTEROIDS			
Hydrocortisone Sodium Succinate (A-Hydrocort)	**Inj:** 100mg/2mL	**Acute Gout:** Individualized dosing. May repeat dose at intervals of 2, 4, or 6 hrs based on patient response.	
Hydrocortisone (Cortef)	**Tab:** 5mg, 10mg, 20mg	**Acute Gout:** Individualized dosing.	
Methylprednisolone (Medrol)	**Tab:** 4mg, 8mg, 16mg, 32mg	**Acute Gout:** Individualized dosing.	
Prednisone	**Tab:** 1mg, 2.5mg, 5mg, 10mg, 20mg, 50mg; **Sol:** 5mg/mL, 5mg/5mL	**Acute Gout:** Individualized dosing.	
NSAIDs			
Indomethacin (Indocin)	**Cap:** (Generic) 25mg, 50mg; **Supp:** 50mg; **Sus:** 25mg/5mL [237mL]	**Acute Gout:** 50mg tid until pain is tolerable, then d/c.	
Naproxen (Naprosyn)	**Sus:** 125mg/5mL [473mL]; **Tab:** 250mg†, 375mg, 500mg†	**Acute Gout:** 750mg followed by 250mg q8h until attack subsides.	
Naproxen Sodium (Anaprox)	**Tab:** 275mg	**Acute Gout:** 825mg followed by 275mg q8h until attack subsides.	
(Anaprox DS)	**Tab:** 550mg†	**Acute Gout:** 825mg followed by 275mg q8h until attack subsides.	
(Naprelan)	**Tab, Controlled-Release:** 375mg, 500mg, 750mg	**Acute Gout:** 1-1.5g qd on the first day, then 1g qd until attack subsides.	1.5g/day
Sulindac (Clinoril)	**Tab:** (Generic) 150mg; (Clinoril, Generic) 200mg†	**Acute Gout:** 200mg bid with food, usually for 7 days.	400mg/day
PHENANTHRENE DERIVATIVE			
Colchicine (Colcrys)	**Tab:** 0.6mg	**Acute Gout:** 1.2mg at first sign of flare, then 0.6mg 1 hr later. **Prophylaxis:** 0.6mg qd-bid.	**Acute Gout:** 1.8mg over 1 hr period. **Prophylaxis:** 1.2mg/day
RECOMBINANT URICASE			
Pegloticase (Krystexxa)	**Inj:** 8mg/mL	**Chronic Gout:** 8mg IV infusion q2wks.	

(Continued)

GENERIC (BRAND)	HOW SUPPLIED	USUAL DOSAGE RANGE	MAX DOSE
URICOSURIC AGENT			
Probenecid	**Tab:** 500mg	**Initial:** 250mg bid x 1 wk. **Maint:** 500mg bid. **Titrate:** May increase by 500mg every 4 wks.	2g/day
XANTHINE OXIDASE INHIBITORS			
Allopurinol (Zyloprim)	**Tab:** 100mg†, 300mg†	**Mild Gout:** 200-300mg/day. **Moderate-Severe Gout:** 400-600mg/day.	800mg/day
Febuxostat (Uloric)	**Tab:** 40mg, 80mg	**Initial:** 40mg qd. Increase to 80mg qd if serum uric acid ≥6mg/dL after 2 wks.	
COMBINATION			
Colchicine/Probenecid	**Tab:** (Colchicine-Probenecid) 0.5mg-500mg	1 tab qd x 1 wk, then 1 tab bid. **Titrate:** May increase by 1 tab/day q4wks.	4 tabs/day

*Check PI for pediatric dosing.
†Scored

OSTEOARTHRITIS AGENTS

GENERIC (BRAND)	HOW SUPPLIED	USUAL ADULT DOSE RANGE	MAX DOSE
COX-2 INHIBITOR			
Celecoxib (Celebrex)	**Cap:** 50mg, 100mg, 200mg, 400mg	200mg qd or 100mg bid	200mg/day
NSAIDs			
Diclofenac epolamine (Flector)	**Patch:** 1.3% (180mg)	Apply 1 patch to most painful area bid.	360mg/day
Diclofenac potassium (Cataflam)	**Tab:** 50mg	50mg bid-tid	150mg/day
Diclofenac sodium (Generic)	**Tab, Delayed-Release:** 25mg, 50mg, 75mg	50mg bid-tid or 75mg bid	150mg/day
(Voltaren-XR)	**Tab, Extended-Release:** 100mg	100mg qd	100mg/day
(Voltaren Gel)	**Gel:** 1% (10mg/g)	**Lower Extremities:** Apply 4g to affected area qid ud. **Upper Extremities:** Apply 2g to affected area qid ud.	**Lower Extremities:** 16g/day to any one affected joint. **Upper Extremities:** 8g/day to any one affected joint. Total dose should not exceed 32g/day over all affected joints.
(Pennsaid)	**Topical Sol:** 1.5% (16.05mg/mL)	40 drops on each painful knee qid.	
Diflunisal	**Tab:** 500mg	500mg-1000mg qd in two divided doses.	1500mg/day
Etodolac	**Cap:** 200mg, 300mg; **Tab:** 400mg, 500mg; **Tab, Extended-Release:** 400mg, 500mg, 600mg	300mg bid-tid or 400mg-500mg bid. Lower dosage of 600mg/day may suffice for long-term administration.	1000mg/day
Fenoprofen calcium (Nalfon)	**Cap:** (Nalfon) 200mg, 400mg; **Tab:** (Generic) 600mg	**Cap:** 400mg-600mg tid-qid; **Tab:** 300mg-600mg tid-qid	3200mg/day
Flurbiprofen (Ansaid)	**Tab:** 50mg, 100mg	200mg-300mg/day given bid, tid, or qid	Maximum single dose in a multiple-dose daily regimen is 100mg.
Ketoprofen	**Cap:** 50mg, 75mg; **Cap, Extended-Release:** 100mg, 150mg, 200mg	**Cap:** 75mg tid or 50mg qid; **Cap, Extended-Release:** 200mg qd	**Cap:** 300mg/day; **Cap, Extended-Release:** 200mg/day
Ibuprofen	**Sus:** 100mg/5mL	300mg qid or 400mg, 600mg, or 800mg tid-qid	3200mg/day
	Tab: 400mg, 600mg, 800mg	300mg qid or 400mg, 600mg, or 800mg tid-qid	3200mg/day
Indomethacin (Indocin)	**Cap:** (Generic) 25mg, 50mg; **Cap, Extended Release:** (Generic) 75mg; **Sus:** (Indocin) 25mg/5mL	**Cap/Sus:** 25mg bid-tid to start. May increase by 25mg-50mg at weekly intervals until satisfactory response or total daily dose of 150mg-200mg. **Cap, Extended Release:** 75mg qd to start. May increase up to 75mg bid.	**Cap/Sus:** 200mg/day. **Cap, Extended-Release:** 150mg/day
Meclofenamate sodium	**Cap:** 50mg, 100mg	200mg-400mg/day in 3-4 equal doses.	400mg/day
Meloxicam (Mobic)	**Sus:** 7.5mg/5mL; **Tab:** 7.5mg, 15mg	7.5mg qd to start. May increase to 15mg qd.	15mg/day

(Continued)

GENERIC (BRAND)	HOW SUPPLIED	USUAL ADULT DOSE RANGE	MAX DOSE
NSAIDs *(Continued)*			
Nabumetone	**Tab:** 500mg, 750mg	1000mg qd to start. Dose may be increased to 1500mg-2000mg per day either qd or bid.	2000mg/day
Naproxen (Naprosyn)	**Sus:** 125mg/5mL; **Tab:** 250mg, 375mg, 500mg	250mg, 375mg, or 500mg bid	1500mg/day
(EC-Naprosyn)	**Tab, Delayed-Release:** 375mg, 500mg	375mg or 500mg bid	1500mg/day
Naproxen sodium (Anaprox)	**Tab:** 275mg	275mg bid	1650mg/day
(Anaprox DS)	**Tab:** 550mg*	550mg bid	1650mg/day
(Naprelan)	**Tab, Extended-Release:** 375mg, 500mg, 750mg	750mg-1000mg qd	1500mg/day
Oxaprozin (Daypro)	**Tab:** 600mg*	1200mg qd	1800mg/day or 26mg/kg/day in divided doses, whichever is lower.
Piroxicam (Feldene)	**Cap:** 10mg, 20mg	20mg qd or 10mg bid	20mg/day
Sulindac (Clinoril)	**Tab:** (Generic) 150mg, (Clinoril, generic) 200mg*	150mg bid with food	400mg/day
Tolmetin sodium	**Cap:** 400mg; **Tab:** 200mg*, 600mg	200mg-600mg tid	1800mg/day
NSAID COMBINATION			
Diclofenac sodium/ Misoprostol (Arthrotec)	**Tab:** 50mg/200mcg, 75mg/200mcg	50mg/200mcg tid	**Diclofenac:** 150mg/day; **Misoprostol:** 200mcg/ dose, 800mcg/day
SALICYLATES			
Salsalate	**Tab:** 500mg, 750mg	3000mg daily (1500mg bid or 1000mg tid)	3000mg/day
MISCELLANEOUS			
Botanical/Mineral/Animal substances: Homeopathic Combination Drug (Traumeel Inj)	**Inj:** 2.2mL amps	1 amp qd for acute disorders, otherwise 1 amp 1-3 times per week IM/SC/IV/ID or periarticular ud.	N/A
Flavocoxid (Limbrel)	**Cap:** 250mg, 500mg	250mg-500mg q12h taken with or without zinc.	500mg-1000mg/day
Sodium hyaluronate (Euflexxa)	**Inj:** 1% (10mg/mL)	2mL injected into the knee joint once a week for a total of 3 injections.	2mL per week/total of 3 injections
(Hyalgan)	**Inj:** 10mg/mL	2mL by intra-articular injection once a week for 5 injections.	2mL per week/ total of 5 injections
(Supartz)	**Inj:** 10mg/mL	2.5mL by intra-articular injection once a week (one week apart) for a total of 5 injections.	2.5mL per week/total of 5 injections
Hyaluronan (Orthovisc)	**Inj:** 15mg/mL	2mL injected into the knee joint once a week (one week apart) for a total of 3 or 4 injections.	2mL per week/ total 3 or 4 injections
Hylan G-F 20 (Synvisc)	**Inj:** 8mg/mL	2mL by intra-articular injection once a week (one week apart) for a total of 3 injections.	2mL per week/ total of 3 injections
(Synvisc-One)	**Inj:** 48mg/6mL	Single intra-articular injection	1 injection
*Scored			

OSTEOPOROSIS DETECTION, PREVENTION, AND TREATMENT

OSTEOPOROSIS RISK FACTORS

NONMODIFIABLE RISK FACTORS

Gender	Women > men
Age	Older age > younger age
Body	Low body weight (small and thin) > high or overweight; broken bones or height loss during adult years
Ethnicity	Caucasian, Asian, or Hispanic/Latino descent > African heritage
Family history	History of fractures or osteoporosis
Sex hormones	Females: delayed puberty, amenorrhea, early menopause, removal of ovaries, low estrogen levels
	Males: low testosterone

MODIFIABLE RISK FACTORS

Lifestyle	Cigarette smoking, weight loss, excessive alcohol (>3 drinks/day), excessive caffeine and protein intake, high salt intake
Exercise	Inactive or bedridden
Diet	Low intake of calcium, vitamin D, phosphorous, magnesium, vitamin K, vitamin B_6, vitamin B_{12}

Drugs that may cause bone loss
- Aluminum-containing antacids
- Anticoagulants
- Antiseizure drugs
- Aromatase inhibitors
- Barbiturates
- Cancer chemotherapeutic drugs
- Cyclosporine A and tacrolimus
- Glucocorticoids (≥5 mg/d of prednisone or equivalent for ≥3 mo)
- Gonadotropin-releasing hormone agonists
- Heparin
- Lithium
- Medroxyprogesterone acetate for contraception
- Methotrexate
- Proton pump inhibitors
- Selective serotonin reuptake inhibitors
- Tamoxifen
- Thiazolidinediones
- Thyroid hormones in excess

Diseases/conditions that may cause bone loss
- AIDS/HIV
- Ankylosing spondylitis
- Blood and bone marrow disorders
- Breast cancer
- Chronic obstructive pulmonary disease (COPD), including emphysema
- Cushing's syndrome
- Depression
- Diabetes
- Eating disorders, especially anorexia nervosa
- Female athlete triad (includes loss of menstrual periods, an eating disorder, and excessive exercise)
- Gastrectomy
- Gastrointestinal bypass procedures
- Hyperparathyroidism
- Hyperthyroidism
- Inflammatory bowel disease, including Crohn's disease and ulcerative colitis
- Kidney disease that is chronic and long lasting
- Liver disease that is severe, including biliary cirrhosis
- Lupus

(Continued)

- Lymphoma and leukemia
- Malabsorption syndromes, including celiac disease
- Multiple myeloma
- Multiple sclerosis
- Organ transplants
- Parkinson's disease
- Polio and postpolio syndrome
- Poor diet, including malnutrition
- Premature menopause
- Prostate cancer
- Rheumatoid arthritis
- Scoliosis
- Spinal cord injuries
- Stroke
- Thalassemia
- Thyrotoxicosis
- Weight loss

Note: This list is not inclusive of all drugs, diseases/conditions that may increase the risk factors for osteoporosis.

Source: National Osteoporosis Foundation.

BONE MINERAL DENSITY CLASSIFICATION/TESTS

WORLD HEALTH ORGANIZATION (WHO) DEFINITION OF OSTEOPOROSIS

Normal	Bone mineral density within 1 standard deviation (SD) of the young adult mean (T-score ≥-1.0)
Osteopenia (low bone mass)	Bone mineral density between 1.0 and 2.5 SD below the young adult mean (-2.5 < T-score <-1.0)
Osteoporosis	Bone mineral density 2.5 SD or more below the young adult mean (T-score ≤-2.5)

Note: The definitions above should not be applied to premenopausal women, men <50 years of age, and children.

BONE MINERAL DENSITY (BMD) TESTS

- BMD tests provide a measurement of T-score for bone density at hip and spine to:

  — Establish and confirm a diagnosis of osteoporosis

  — Predict future fracture risk

  — Measure response to osteoporosis treatment

- BMD is measured in grams of mineral per square centimeter scanned (g/cm^2) and compared to the expected BMD for the patient's age and sex (Z-score) or compared with "normal adults" of the same sex (T-score).

- The difference between the patient's score and the optimal BMD is expressed in SD above and below the mean. Usually 1 SD equals about 10-15% of the bone density value in g/cm^2.

- Negative values for T-score, such as -1.5, -2, or -2.5, indicate low bone mass.

- The greater the negative score, the greater the risk of fracture.

PREVENTION STRATEGIES

A balanced diet rich in calcium and vitamin D along with exercise helps strengthen bone. This alone may not be enough to stop bone loss caused by lifestyle, medications, or menopause.

- The U.S. Preventive Services Task Force recommends routine osteoporosis screening for women ≥65 years.

- The task force recommends that screenings begin at 60 years in women at increased risk for osteoporotic fractures.

- Consider bone testing in patients taking glucocorticoid medications for 2 months or more and in those with conditions that place them at high risk for fracture.

OSTEOPOROSIS AGENTS

GENERIC (BRAND)	INDICATIONS	HOW SUPPLIED	DOSAGE
BIOPHOSPHONATES & COMBINATIONS			
Alendronate sodium (Fosamax)	Treatment and prevention of osteoporosis in postmenopausal women. Treatment to increase bone mass in men with osteoporosis. Treatment of glucocorticoid-induced osteoporosis.	**Sol:** 70mg [75mL]; **Tab:** 5mg, 10mg, 35mg, 40mg, 70mg	**Osteoporosis: Treatment:** 70mg once weekly or 10mg qd. **Prevention:** 35mg once weekly or 5mg qd. **Increase Bone Mass in Men with Osteoporosis:** 70mg once weekly or 10mg qd. **Glucocorticoid-Induced:** 5mg qd; 10mg qd for post-menopausal women not on estrogen. Take at least 30 min before the first food, beverage (other than plain water), or medication. Take tabs with 6-8 oz plain water or 2 oz with oral sol. Do not lie down for at least 30 min and until after 1st food of day.
Alendronate sodium/ Cholecalciferol (Fosamax Plus D)	Treatment of osteoporosis in postmenopausal women. Treatment to increase bone mass in men with osteoporosis.	**Tab:** (Alendronate sodium-Cholecalciferol) 70mg-2800 IU, 70mg-5600 IU	**Osteoporosis:** 1 tab (70mg/5600 IU or 70mg/2800 IU) once weekly. Take at least 30 min before the 1st food, beverage (other than plain water), or medication. Do not lie down for at least 30 min and until after 1st food of day.
Ibandronate sodium (Boniva)	(Inj) Treatment of osteoporosis in postmenopausal women. (PO) Treatment and prevention of postmenopausal osteoporosis.	**Inj:** 3mg/3mL; **Tab:** 150mg	**Inj:** 3mg IV over 15-30 sec every 3 months. **PO:** 150mg once monthly. Swallow whole with 6-8 oz plain water. Do not lie down for 60 min after dose. Take at least 60 min before 1st food, drink (other than plain water), medication, or supplement.
Risedronate sodium (Actonel)	Treatment and prevention of osteoporosis in postmenopausal women and glucocorticoid-induced osteoporosis in men and women. Treatment to increase bone mass in men with osteoporosis.	**Tab:** 5mg, 30mg, 35mg, 150mg	**Osteoporosis: Prevention/Treatment:** 5mg qd or 35mg once weekly or 150mg once a month. **Glucocorticoid-Induced:** 5mg qd. **Increase Bone Mass in Men with Osteoporosis:** 35mg once weekly. Take at least 30 min before the first food or drink of the day other than water. Swallow tab in upright position with 6-8 oz of plain water. Do not lie down for 30 min after dose.
Risedronate sodium (Atelvia)	Treatment of osteoporosis in postmenopausal women.	**Tab, Delayed-Release:** 35mg	**Osteoporosis: Treatment:** 35mg once weekly; take in am immediately after breakfast. Swallow tab in upright position with 4 oz of plain water. Do not lie down for 30 min after dose.
Zoledronic acid (Reclast)	Treatment and prevention of osteoporosis in postmenopausal women. Treatment to increase bone mass in men with osteoporosis. Treatment and prevention of glucocorticoid-induced osteoporosis in men and women.	**Sol:** 5mg/100mL [100mL]	**Osteoporosis: Treatment (Men and Postmenopausal Women):** 5mg IV once a year over >15 min at a constant infusion rate. **Prevention of Osteoporosis (Postmenopausal Women):** 5mg IV given every 2 yrs over >15 min at a constant infusion rate. **Treatment/ Prevention of Glucocorticoid-Induced Osteoporosis:** 5mg IV once a year over >15 min at a constant infusion rate.*
HORMONE THERAPY†‡			
Conjugated estrogens (Premarin Tabs)	Prevention of postmenopausal osteoporosis.	**Tab:** 0.3mg, 0.45mg, 0.625mg, 0.9mg, 1.25mg	**Prevention of Osteoporosis: Initial:** 0.3mg qd continuous or cyclically (eg, 25 days on, 5 days off). Re-evaluate periodically.

(Continued)

GENERIC (BRAND)	INDICATIONS	HOW SUPPLIED	DOSAGE
HORMONE THERAPY†,‡ *(Continued)*			
Conjugated estrogens/ Medroxyprogesterone acetate (Premphase)	Prevention of postmenopausal osteoporosis in women with intact uterus.	**Tab:** 0.625mg, (Estrogens, Conjugated) and 0.625mg-5mg (Estrogens, Conjugated-Medroxyprogesterone)	0.625mg tab qd on Days 1-14 and 0.625mg-5mg tab qd on Days 15-28. Re-evaluate periodically.
Conjugated estrogens/ Medroxyprogesterone acetate (Prempro)	Prevention of postmenopausal osteoporosis in women with intact uterus.	**Tab:** (Estrogens, Conjugated-Medroxyprogesterone) 0.3mg-1.5mg, 0.45mg-1.5mg, 0.625mg-2.5mg, 0.625mg-5 mg	Take 1 tab qd. Re-evaluate periodically.
Estradiol (Alora)	Prevention of postmenopausal osteoporosis.	**Patch:** 0.025mg/24 hrs, 0.05mg/24 hrs, 0.075mg/24 hrs, 0.1mg/24 hrs	Apply to lower abdomen, upper quadrant of the buttocks or the hip; avoid breasts and waistline. Rotate application sites. Allow 1 week between same site. **Osteoporosis:** Apply 0.025mg/day twice weekly. **Titrate:** May increase depending on bone mineral density and adverse events.
Estradiol (Climara)	Prevention of postmeno-pausal osteoporosis.	**Patch:** 0.025mg/day, 0.0375mg/day, 0.05mg/day, 0.06mg/day, 0.075mg/day, 0.1mg/day	Apply 1 patch weekly to lower abdomen or upper area of buttocks; avoid breasts and waistline. Rotate application sites. Allow 1 week between same site. **Minimum Effective Dose:** 0.025mg/day once weekly. Re-evaluate as clinically appropriate.
Estradiol (Estrace)	Prevention of osteoporosis.	**Tab:** 0.5mg§, 1mg§, 2mg§	Lowest effective dose has not been determined.
Estradiol (Estraderm)	Prevention of postmenopausal osteoporosis.	**Patch:** 0.05mg/24 hrs, 0.1mg/24 hrs	**Initial:** 0.05mg/day. May give continuously without intact uterus. May give cyclically (3 weeks on, 1 week off) with intact uterus. Dosage may be adjusted if necessary. Apply to clean, dry area on trunk of body. Do not apply to breast, waistline or a site exposed to sunlight. Replace twice weekly. Rotate application site. Allow 1 week between same site.
Estradiol (Menostar)	Prevention of postmenopausal osteoporosis.	**Patch:** 14mcg/day	Apply 1 patch weekly to lower abdomen; avoid breasts, waistline, and areas where sitting would dislodge the patch. Rotate application sites. Allow 1 week between same site.
Estradiol (Vivelle-Dot)	Prevention of postmenopausal osteoporosis.	0.025mg/day, 0.0375mg/day, 0.05mg/day, 0.075mg/day, 0.1mg/day [8§, 24§]	**Minimum Effective Dose:** 0.025mg/day twice weekly. Apply to clean, dry area of the trunk; avoid breasts and waistline. Rotate sites; allow 1 week between same site. Without intact uterus, may give continuously; with intact uterus, may give cyclically (3 weeks on, 1 week off) with a progestin.
Estradiol/ Levonorgestrel (Climara Pro)	Prevention of postmenopausal osteoporosis.	**Patch:** (Estradiol-Levonorgestrel): 0.045mg-0.015mg/day	Apply 1 patch weekly to lower abdomen; avoid breasts and waistline. Rotate application site; allow 1 week between same site. Re-evaluate periodically to determine if treatment is still necessary (3-6-month intervals).
Estradiol/ Norethindrone (Activella)	Prevention of postmenopausal osteoporosis in women with intact uterus.	**Tab:** (Estradiol-Norethindrone) 1mg-0.5mg, 0.5mg-0.1mg	1 tab qd. Re-evaluate periodically to determine if treatment is still necessary (3-6-month intervals).

GENERIC (BRAND)	INDICATIONS	HOW SUPPLIED	DOSAGE
HORMONE THERAPY†,‡ *(Continued)*			
Estradiol/ Norgestimate (Prefest)	Prevention of postmenopausal osteoporosis in women with intact uterus.	**Tab:** (Estradiol) 1mg and (Estradiol-Norgestimate) 1mg-0.09mg	1 estradiol (peach color) tab for three days followed by 1 estradiol-norgestimate (white color) tab for three days. Repeat regimen continuously.
Estropipate	Prevention of postmenopausal osteoporosis.	**Tab:** 0.75mg§, 1.5mg§, 3mg§, 6 mg§	0.75mg (as estropipate) qd for 25 days of 31-day cycle.
Ethinyl Estradiol/ Norethindrone (Femhrt)	Prevention of postmenopausal osteoporosis in women with intact uterus.	**Tab:** (Ethinyl Estradiol-Norethindrone) 2.5mcg-0.5mg, 5mcg-1mg	1 tab qd. Assess response by measuring bone mineral density. Re-evaluate periodically to determine if treatment is still necessary (3-6-month intervals).
MISCELLANEOUS			
Calcitonin-Salmon (Miacalcin)	Treatment of postmenopausal osteoporosis in females >5 yrs postmenopause in conjunction with an adequate calcium and vitamin D intake.	**Inj:** 200 IU/mL; **Nasal Spray:** 200 IU/inh	(Inj) 100 IU IM/SQ every other day. If >2mL, use IM injection. (Spray) 200 IU qd intranasally. Alternate nostrils daily. Take with supplemental calcium and vitamin D for postmenopausal osteoporosis.
Calcitonin-Salmon (Fortical)	Treatment of postmenopausal osteoporosis in females >5 yrs postmenopause in conjunction with an adequate calcium and vitamin D intake.	**Nasal Spray:** 200 IU/inh	200 IU qd intranasally. Alternate nostrils daily. Take with supplemental calcium and vitamin D for postmenopausal osteoporosis.
Denosumab (Prolia)	Treatment of postmenopausal women with osteoporosis at high risk for fracture (eg, history of osteoporotic fracture, multiple risk factors for fracture) or patients who have failed or cannot tolerate other available osteoporosis therapy.	**Inj:** 60mg/mL	60mg as single SQ injection once q6 months. Administer in the upper arm, upper thigh, or abdomen. All patients should receive calcium 1000mg and at least 400 IU vitamin D qd.
Raloxifene† (Evista)	Treatment and prevention of osteoporosis in postmenopausal women.	**Tab:** 60mg	60mg qd without regard to meals.
Teriparatide† (Forteo)	Treatment of postmenopausal women with osteoporosis at high risk for fracture. To increase bone mass in men with primary or hypogonadal osteoporosis at high risk for fracture. Treatment of men and women with glucocorticoid-induced osteoporosis at high risk for fracture.	**Inj:** 600mcg/2.4mL [2.4mL pen]	20mcg qd SQ into thigh or abdominal wall. Administer initially under circumstances where patient can sit or lie down if symptoms of orthostatic hypotension occur. Discard pen after 28 days. Use of the drug for more than 2 years during a patient's lifetime is not recommended.

*Patients on Reclast must be adequately supplemented with calcium and vitamin D if dietary intake is not sufficient. An average of at least 1200mg calcium and 800-1000 IU vitamin D daily is recommended.

†Check PI for important Boxed Warnings.

‡When prescribing solely for the prevention of postmenopausal osteoporosis, therapy should be considered only for women at significant risk for osteoporosis; non-estrogen medications should be carefully considered.

§Scored.

RHEUMATOID ARTHRITIS AGENTS

GENERIC (BRAND)	HOW SUPPLIED	USUAL DOSAGE RANGE	MAX DOSE
5-AMINOSALICYLIC ACID DERIVATIVE			
Sulfasalazine (Azulfidine EN)	**Tab, Delayed-Release:** 500mg	1g bid.	3g/day.
COPPER CHELATING AGENT			
Penicillamine (Cuprimine, Depen)	**Cap:** (Cuprimine) 250mg; **Tab:** (Depen) 250mg*	**Initial:** 125-250mg/day. **Maint:** 500-750mg/day.	1.5g/day.
COX-2 INHIBITOR			
Celecoxib (Celebrex)	**Cap:** 50mg, 100mg, 200mg, 400mg	100-200mg bid.	
DIHYDROFOLIC ACID REDUCTASE INHIBITOR			
Methotrexate sodium (Trexall)	**Inj:** (Generic) 25mg/mL, 10mg/mL; **Tab:** (Generic) 2.5mg, (Trexall) 5mg, 7.5mg, 10mg, 15mg	7.5mg once weekly or 2.5mg q12h for a total of 3 doses weekly.	20mg/wk.
GOLD AGENT			
Auranofin (Ridaura)	**Cap:** 3mg	6mg qd or 3mg bid.	9mg/day.
IMMUNOSUPPRESSANTS			
Azathioprine (Imuran)	**Tab:** 50mg*; **Inj:** (Generic) 100mg/20mL	**Initial:** 1mg/kg/day given qd-bid. **Titrate:** May increase by 0.5mg/kg/day after 6-8 wks, then at 4-wk intervals.	2.5mg/kg/day.
Cyclosporine (Neoral)	**Cap:** 25mg, 100mg; **Sol:** 100mg/mL [50mL]	**Initial:** 2.5mg/kg/day given bid. **Titrate:** May increase by 0.5-0.75mg/kg/day after 8 wks and again after 12 wks. D/C if no benefit by wk 16.	4mg/kg/day.
INTERLEUKIN-1 RECEPTOR ANTAGONIST			
Anakinra (Kineret)	**Inj:** 100mg/0.67mL	100mg SQ qd.	
INTERLEUKIN-6 RECEPTOR ANTAGONIST			
Tocilizumab (Actemra)	**Inj:** 20mg/mL [80mg/4mL, 200mg/10mL, 400mg/20mL]	**Monotherapy or in Combination with MTX: Initial:** 4mg/kg every 4 wks as 60 min infusion. **Titrate:** Increase to 8mg/kg based on response.	800mg/infusion.
MONOCLONAL ANTIBODIES/CD20-BLOCKER			
Rituximab (Rituxan)	**Inj:** 10mg/mL	Two 1000mg IV infusions separated by 2 wks, with MTX. Give subsequent courses every 24 wks or based on clinical evaluation, but not sooner than every 16 wks. See PI for premedication.	
MONOCLONAL ANTIBODIES/TNF-BLOCKERS			
Adalimumab (Humira)	**Inj:** 20mg/0.4mL, 40mg/0.8mL [Prefilled Glass Syringe], 40mg/0.8mL [Prefilled Pen]	40mg SQ every other wk.	Consider 40mg every wk when taken w/o MTX.
Golimumab (Simponi)	**Inj:** 50mg/0.5mL [Prefilled Glass Syringe]	50mg SQ once a month. Give with MTX.	

(Continued)

GENERIC (BRAND)	HOW SUPPLIED	USUAL DOSAGE RANGE	MAX DOSE
MONOCLONAL ANTIBODIES/TNF-BLOCKERS *(Continued)*			
Infliximab (Remicade)	**Inj:** 100mg	**Induction:** 3mg/kg IV infusion w/ MTX, then repeat at 2 and 6 wks. **Maint:** 3mg/kg every 8 wks, starting at 14 wks.	10mg/kg or every 4 wks.
NONSTEROIDAL ANTI-INFLAMMATORY DRUGS (NSAIDs)			
Diclofenac potassium (Cataflam)	**Tab:** 50mg	50mg tid-qid.	
Diclofenac sodium (Voltaren XR)	**Tab, Delayed-Release:** 25mg, 50mg, 75mg **Tab, Extended-Release:** 100mg	50mg tid-qid or 75mg bid. 100mg qd-bid.	
Diflunisal	**Tab:** 500mg	500mg-1g/day in two divided doses.	1500mg/day.
Etodolac	**Cap:** 200mg, 300mg; **Tab:** 400mg, 500mg **Tab, Extended-Release:** 400mg, 500mg, 600mg	300mg bid-tid or 400-500mg bid. **ER Tabs:** 400-1000mg qd. 400-1000mg qd.	1000mg/day. 1000mg/day.
Fenoprofen calcium (Nalfon)	**Cap:** (Nalfon) 200mg, 400mg; **Tab:** (Generic) 600mg	400-600mg tid-qid; 300-600mg tid-qid	3200mg/day. 3200mg/day.
Flurbiprofen (Ansaid)	**Tab:** 50mg, 100mg	200-300mg/day given bid, tid, or qid.	100mg/dose.
Ibuprofen	**Sus:** 100mg/5mL [120mL, 473mL] **Tab:** 400mg, 600mg, 800mg	300mg qid or 400mg, 600mg, or 800mg tid-qid. 1200-3200mg/day given 400mg, 600mg, or 800mg tid-qid.	3200mg/day. 3200mg/day.
Indomethacin (Indocin)	**Cap:** (Generic) 25mg, 50mg; **Cap, Extended-Release:** (Generic) 75mg; **Sus:** (Indocin) 25mg/5mL [50mL, 237 mL]	**Initial:** 25mg bid-tid. **Titrate:** Increase by 25mg or 50mg at weekly intervals until reach satisfactory response. **ER: Initial:** 75mg qd. **Titrate:** May increase to 75mg bid.	200mg/day.
Ketoprofen	**Cap:** 50mg, 75mg; **Cap, Extended-Release:** 100mg, 150mg, 200mg	75mg tid or 50mg qid. **ER:** 200mg qd.	300mg/day. **ER:** 200mg/day.
Meclofenamate sodium	**Cap:** 50mg, 100mg	200-400mg/day in 3-4 divided doses.	400mg/day.
Meloxicam (Mobic)	**Sus:** 7.5mg/5mL; **Tab:** 7.5mg, 15mg	7.5mg qd.	15mg/day.
Nabumetone	**Tab:** 500mg, 750mg	1000mg qd or divided bid	2000mg/day.
Naproxen (Naprosyn) (EC-Naprosyn)	**Sus:** 125mg/5mL; **Tab:** 250mg, 375mg, 500mg **Tab, Delayed-Release:** 375mg, 500mg	250mg, 375mg, or 500mg bid. 375mg or 500mg bid.	1500mg/day. 1500mg/day.
Naproxen sodium (Anaprox) (Anaprox DS) (Naprelan)	**Tab:** 275mg **Tab:** 550mg* **Tab, Extended-Release:** 375mg, 500mg, 750mg	275mg bid. 550mg bid. 750mg-1g qd.	1500mg/day. 1500mg/day. 1500mg/day.
Oxaprozin (Daypro)	**Tab:** 600mg*	1200mg qd.	1800mg/day or 26mg/kg/day in divided doses (whichever is lower).

GENERIC (BRAND)	HOW SUPPLIED	USUAL DOSAGE RANGE	MAX DOSE
NONSTEROIDAL ANTI-INFLAMMATORY DRUGS (NSAIDs) *(Continued)*			
Piroxicam (Feldene)	**Cap:** 10mg, 20mg	20mg qd or 10mg bid.	
Sulindac (Clinoril)	**Tab:** 200mg*, (Generic) 150mg	150mg-200mg bid with food.	400mg/day with food.
Tolmetin	**Cap:** 400mg; **Tab:** 200mg*, 600mg	200-600mg tid.	1800mg/day.
NSAID/PROSTAGLANDIN E₁ ANALOGUE			
Diclofenac sodium/ **Misoprostol** (Arthrotec)	**Tab:** 50mg-200mcg, 75mg-200mcg	50mg tid-qid.	**Diclofenac:** 225mg/day; **Misoprostol:** 200mcg/dose, 800mcg/day.
PYRIMIDINE SYNTHESIS INHIBITOR			
Leflunomide (Arava)	**Tab:** 10mg, 20mg, 100mg	**LD:** 100mg qd x 3 days. **Maint:** 10mg-20mg/day.	
SALICYLATE			
Salsalate	**Tab:** 500mg, 750mg	3000mg daily, given as 1500mg bid or 1000mg tid.	
SELECTIVE COSTIMULATION MODULATOR			
Abatacept (Orencia)	**Inj:** 250mg	**Initial:** IV:<60kg: 500mg; 60-100kg: 750mg; >100kg: 1g. Give at 2 and 4 wks after initial infusion, then q4 wks thereafter. Following IV loading dose, give 125mcg SQ within a day, then weekly.	
TNF-RECEPTOR BLOCKERS			
Certolizumab pegol (Cimzia)	**Inj:** 200mg/mL	**Initial:** 400mg SQ initially and at wks 2 and 4, followed by 200mg every other wk. **Maint:** 400mg SQ every 4 wks can be considered.	
Etanercept (Enbrel)	**Inj:** 25mg [vial], 50mg/mL [syringe]	50mg SQ per wk.	50mg/wk.
MISCELLANEOUS			
Hydroxychloroquine (Plaquenil)	**Tab:** 200mg	**Initial:** 400-600mg qd. **Maint:** When good response is obtained (usually in 4-12 wks), 200-400mg qd with meal or milk.	

*Scored

Some of these products are also indicated for juvenile rheumatoid arthritis; refer to individual PI for detailed dosing.

ADHD AGENTS

BRAND (GENERIC)	HOW SUPPLIED	ADULT DOSE	PEDIATRIC DOSE
(Amphetamine plus dextroamphetamine)	**Tab:** 5mg, 7.5mg, 10mg, 12.5mg, 15mg, 20mg, 30mg		**3-5 yrs: Initial:** 2.5mg qd. **Titrate:** May increase by 2.5mg weekly. **≥6 yrs: Initial:** 5mg qd-bid. May increase by 5mg weekly. Give first dose upon awakening and add'l doses q4-6h. **Max (Usual):** 40mg/day.
Adderall XR* (Amphetamine salt combo)	**Cap:** 5mg, 10mg, 15mg, 20mg, 25mg, 30mg	20mg qam	**Ages 6-17:** 10mg qam. **6-12 yrs: Max:** 30mg qd.
Concerta† (Methylphenidate HCl)	**Tab, ER:** 18mg, 27mg, 36mg, 54mg	**Methylphenidate-Naïve: Initial:** 18mg or 36mg qam. Dosage may be increased by 18mg/day at weekly intervals. **Max:** 72mg/day	**Methylphenidate-Naïve Children and Adolescents:** 18mg qam. Dosage may be increased by 18mg/day at weekly intervals. **Max for Children:** 54mg/day. **Max for Adolescents:** 72mg/day.
Daytrana (Methylphenidate transdermal system)	**Patch:** 10mg/9 hrs, 15mg/9 hrs, 20mg/9 hrs, 30mg/9 hrs	Individualize dose. Apply to hip area 2 hrs before effect is needed and remove 9 hrs after application. **Recommended Titration Schedule: Week 1:** 10mg/9 hrs. **Week 2:** 15mg/9 hrs. **Week 3:** 20mg/9 hrs. **Week 4:** 30mg/9 hrs.	≥6 yrs: Individualize dose. Apply to hip area 2 hrs before effect is needed and remove 9 hrs after application. **Recommended Titration Schedule: Week 1:** 10mg/9 hrs. **Week 2:** 15mg/9 hrs. **Week 3:** 20mg/9 hrs. **Week 4:** 30mg/9 hrs.
Desoxyn (Methamphetamine HCl)	**Tab:** 5mg		**≥6 yrs: Initial:** 5mg qd-bid. **Titrate:** May increase weekly by 5mg/day until optimum response. **Usual:** 20-25mg/day; may be given in 2 divided doses.
Dexedrine (Dextroamphetamine sulfate)	**Cap, ER:** (Spansules) 5mg, 10mg, 15mg		**≥6 yrs:** 5mg qd-bid. **Titrate:** May increase weekly by 5mg/day. **Max (Usual):** 40mg/day.
(Dextroamphetamine sulfate)	**Tab:** 5mg, 10mg		**3-5 yrs: Initial:** 2.5mg/day. **Titrate:** May increase weekly by 2.5mg/day until optimum response. **≥6 yrs: Initial:** 5mg qd-bid. **Titrate:** May increase weekly by 5mg/day until optimum response. Give first dose upon awakening, and additional doses q4-6h. **Max (Usual):** 40mg/day.
Focalin (Dexmethylphenidate HCl)	**Tab:** 2.5mg, 5mg, 10mg	Take bid at least 4 hrs apart. **Methylphenidate-Naïve: Initial:** 2.5mg bid. **Titrate:** May increase weekly by 2.5-5mg/day. **Max:** 20mg/day. **Currently on Methylphenidate: Initial:** Take ½ of methylphenidate dose. **Max:** 20mg/day. Reduce or d/c if paradoxical aggravation of symptoms occurs. D/C if no improvement after appropriate dosage adjustments over 1 month.	≥6 yrs: Take bid at least 4 hrs apart. **Methylphenidate-Naïve: Initial:** 2.5mg bid. **Titrate:** Increase weekly by 2.5-5mg/day. **Max:** 20mg/day. **Currently on Methylphenidate: Initial:** Take ½ of methylphenidate dose. **Max:** 20mg/day. Reduce or d/c if paradoxical aggravation of symptoms occurs. D/C if no improvement after appropriate dosage adjustments over 1 month.

(Continued)

BRAND (GENERIC)	HOW SUPPLIED	ADULT DOSE	PEDIATRIC DOSE
Focalin XR* (Dexmethylphenidate HCl)	Cap, ER: 5mg, 10mg, 15mg, 20mg, 25mg, 30mg, 35mg, 40mg	**Methylphenidate-Naïve: Initial:** 10mg/day. **Titrate:** May adjust weekly by 10mg/day. **Max:** 40mg/day. **Currently on Methylphenidate: Initial:** Take ½ of methylphenidate dose. **Max:** 40mg/day. **Currently on Focalin:** May switch to same daily dose of Focalin XR. Reduce or d/c if paradoxical aggravation of symptoms occurs. D/C if no improvement after appropriate dosage adjustments after 1 month.	**≥6 yrs: Methylphenidate-Naïve: Initial:** 5mg/day. **Titrate:** May adjust weekly by 5mg/day. **Max:** 30mg/day. **Currently on Methylphenidate: Initial:** Take ½ of methylphenidate dose. **Max:** 30mg/day. **Currently on Focalin:** May switch to same daily dose of Focalin XR. Reduce or d/c if paradoxical aggravation of symptoms occurs. D/C if no improvement after appropriate dosage adjustments over 1 month.
Intuniv† (Guanfacine)	Tab, ER: 1mg, 2mg, 3mg, 4mg		**6-17 yrs: Initial:** 1mg/day. **Titrate:** Adjust dose by increments of ≤1mg/week. **Maint:** 1-4mg/day based on clinical response and tolerability. **Dosing based on mg/kg: Range:** 0.05-0.08mg/kg/day. If well tolerated, doses up to 0.12mg/kg/day may provide additional benefit. **Max:** 4mg/day. D/C in decrements of no more than 1mg every 3-7 days. **Reinitiation:** Consider titration based on tolerability. Renal/Hepatic Impairment: Consider dose adjustment.
Kapvay† (Clonidine HCl)	Tab, ER: 0.1mg, 0.2mg		**6-17 yrs: Initial:** 0.1mg hs. **Titrate:** Adjust in increments of 0.1mg/day at weekly intervals until desired response is achieved. **Max:** 0.4mg/day. D/C in decrements of no more than 0.1mg every 3-7 days. Doses should be taken bid with equal or higher split dose given hs.
Metadate CD* (Methylphenidate HCl)	Cap, ER: 10mg, 20mg, 30mg, 40mg, 50mg, 60mg	**Usual:** 20mg qam before breakfast. **Titrate:** May adjust weekly by 10-20mg depending on tolerability/efficacy. **Max:** 60mg/day. Reduce dose or d/c if paradoxical aggravation of symptoms occurs. D/C if no improvement after appropriate dose adjustments over 1 month.	**≥6 yrs: Usual:** 20mg qam before breakfast. **Titrate:** May adjust weekly by 10-20mg depending on tolerability/efficacy. **Max:** 60mg/day. Reduce dose or d/c if paradoxical aggravation of symptoms occurs. D/C if no improvement after appropriate dose adjustments over 1 month.
Metadate ER† (Methylphenidate HCl)	Tab, ER: 20mg	(Immediate-Release Methylphenidate) 10-60mg/day given bid-tid 30-45 min ac. If insomnia occurs, take last dose before 6 pm.‡	**≥6 yrs: (Immediate-Release Methylphenidate) Initial:** 5mg bid before breakfast and lunch. **Titrate:** Increase gradually by 5-10mg weekly. **Max:** 60mg/day. Reduce dose or d/c if paradoxical aggravation of symptoms occurs. D/C if no improvement after appropriate dose adjustment over 1 month.‡
Methylin† (Methylphenidate HCl)	Sol: 5mg/mL [500mL]; 10mg/5mL [500mL]; Tab: 5mg, 10mg, 20mg; Chewable: 2.5mg, 5mg, 10mg; Tab, ER: 10mg, 20mg	(Sol/Tab/Tab, Chewable) 10-60mg/day given bid-tid 30-45 min ac. If insomnia occurs, take last dose before 6 pm.‡	**≥6 yrs: (Sol/Tab/Tab, Chewable) Initial:** 5mg bid before breakfast and lunch. **Titrate:** Increase gradually by 5-10mg weekly. **Max:** 60mg/day. Reduce dose or d/c if paradoxical aggravation of symptoms occurs. D/C if no improvement after appropriate dose adjustment over 1 month.‡

BRAND (GENERIC)	HOW SUPPLIED	ADULT DOSE	PEDIATRIC DOSE
Ritalin, Ritalin LA*, Ritalin SR† (Methylphenidate HCl)	Cap, ER (Ritalin LA): 10mg, 20mg, 30mg, 40mg; Tab (Ritalin): 5mg, 10mg, 20mg; Tab, ER (Ritalin SR): 20mg	(Tab) 10-60mg/day given bid-tid 30-45 min ac. Take last dose before 6 pm if insomnia occurs. (Cap, ER) Initial: 20mg qam. Max: 60mg qam.‡ Previous Methylphenidate Use: Refer to PI. Reduce dose or d/c if paradoxical aggravation of symptoms occurs. D/C if no improvement after appropriate dose adjustment over 1 month.‡	≥6 yrs: (Tab) Initial: 5mg bid before breakfast and lunch. Titrate: Increase gradually by 5-10mg weekly. Max: 60mg/day. (Cap, ER) Initial: 20mg qam. Titrate: Adjust weekly by 10mg. Max: 60mg qam. Previous Methylphenidate Use: Refer to PI. Reduce dose or d/c if paradoxical aggravation of symptoms occurs. D/C if no improvement after appropriate dose adjustment over 1 month.‡
Strattera (Atomoxetine HCl)	Cap: 10mg, 18mg, 25mg, 40mg, 60mg, 80mg, 100mg	Initial: 40mg/day given qam or evenly divided doses in the am and late afternoon/early evening. Titrate: Increase after minimum of 3 days to target dose of about 80mg/day. After 2-4 weeks, may increase to max of 100mg/day. Max: 100mg/day. Dose adjust in hepatic insufficiency and when used with concomitant CYP450 2D6 inhibitors. See PI for detailed dosing information.	≥6 yrs: ≤70kg: Initial: 0.5mg/kg/day given qam or evenly divided doses in the am and late afternoon or early evening. Titrate: Increase after minimum of 3 days to target dose of about 1.2mg/kg/day. Max: 1.4mg/kg/day or 100mg, whichever is less. >70kg: Refer to adult dosing.
Vyvanse (Lisdexamfetamine dimesylate)	Cap: 20mg, 30mg, 40mg, 50mg, 60mg, 70mg	Individualize dose. Initial: 30mg qam. Titrate: If needed, may increase in increments of 10mg or 20mg at weekly intervals. Max: 70mg/day. Swallow caps or dissolve contents in glass of water; do not store once dissolved. Re-evaluate periodically.	Individualize dose. 6-17 yrs: Initial: 30mg qam. Titrate: If needed, may increase in increments of 10mg or 20mg at weekly intervals. Max: 70mg/day. Swallow caps or dissolve contents in glass of water; do not store once dissolved. Re-evaluate periodically.

Abbreviations: ADHD = attention-deficit/hyperactivity disorder; ER = extended-release.

*Swallow cap whole or open cap and sprinkle contents on applesauce; do not chew beads.

†Swallow whole; do not chew, crush, or divide.

‡Tab, ER: May use in place of immediate-release tabs when the 8-hr dose corresponds to the titrated 8-hr immediate-release dose.

ALZHEIMER'S DISEASE AGENTS

GENERIC (BRAND)	INDICATIONS	HOW SUPPLIED	DOSAGE	SIDE EFFECTS
Donepezil HCl (Aricept)	Treatment of dementia of the Alzheimer's type.	**Tab:** 5mg, 10mg, 23mg; **Tab, Disintegrating:** 5mg, 10mg	**Mild to moderate: Initial:** 5mg qd. **Usual:** 5-10mg. **Titrate:** May increase to 10mg after 4-6 weeks. **Moderate to severe: Initial:** 5mg qd. **Usual:** 10-23mg qd. **Titrate:** May increase to 10mg after 4-6 weeks, then to 23mg after ≥3 months.	Nausea, diarrhea, insomnia, vomiting, muscle cramps, fatigue, anorexia, dizziness, pain, headache, ecchymosis
Ergoloid mesylates (Ergoloid mesylates)	Treatment of symptomatic decline in mental capacity of unknown etiology (eg, Alzheimer's dementia, multi-infarct dementia).	**Tab:** 1mg	**Usual:** 1mg tid.	Transient nausea, gastric disturbances
Galantamine HBr (Razadyne, Razadyne ER)	Treatment of mild to moderate dementia of the Alzheimer's type.	**Sol:** (Razadyne) 4mg/mL [100mL]; **Tab:** (Razadyne) 4mg, 8mg, 12mg; **Cap, Extended-Release:** (Razadyne ER) 8mg, 16mg, 24mg	(Sol, Tab) **Initial:** 4mg bid with am and pm meals. **Titrate:** Increase to 8mg bid after 4 weeks if tolerated, then increase to 12mg bid after 4 weeks if tolerated. **Usual:** 16-24mg/day. (Cap, ER) **Initial:** 8mg qd with am meal. **Titrate:** Increase to 16mg qd after 4 weeks, then increase to 24mg qd after 4 weeks if tolerated. **Usual:** 16-24mg/day. See PI for dose modification in moderate renal/hepatic impairment.	Nausea, vomiting, diarrhea, anorexia, weight loss, fatigue, dizziness, headache, depression, insomnia, abdominal pain, dyspepsia, UTI
Memantine HCl (Namenda, Namenda XR)	Treatment of moderate to severe dementia of the Alzheimer's type.	**Sol:** 2mg/mL [360 mL]; **Tab:** 5mg, 10mg; Titration-Pak: 5mg [28ˢ], 10mg [21ˢ]; **Cap, Extended-Release:** (Namenda XR) 7mg, 14mg, 21mg, 28mg; Titration-Pak: 7mg[7ˢ], 14mg[7ˢ], 21mg[7ˢ], 28mg[7ˢ]	(Sol/Tab) **Initial:** 5mg qd. **Titrate:** Increase at intervals of at least one week to 5mg bid, then 5mg and 10mg as separate doses, then to 10mg bid. (Cap, ER) **Initial:** 7mg qd. **Titrate:** Increase at intervals of at least 1 week in 7mg increments to 28mg qd. **Max:** 28mg qd. See PI for switching from Namenda to Namenda XR or for Severe Renal Impairment dosing.	Dizziness, confusion, headache, constipation, coughing, HTN, pain, vomiting, somnolence, hallucinations
Rivastigmine tartrate (Exelon)	Treatment of mild to moderate dementia of the Alzheimer's type.	**Cap:** 1.5mg, 3mg, 4.5mg, 6mg; **Sol:** 2mg/mL [120mL]; **Patch:** 4.6mg/24hrs, 9.5mg/24hrs/[30ˢ]	(Cap) **Initial:** 1.5mg bid. **Titrate:** May increase by increments of 1.5mg bid every 2 weeks. **Max:** 12mg/day. If not tolerating, suspend therapy for several doses and restart at same or next lower dose. If interrupted longer than several days, reinitiate with lowest daily dose and titrate as above. (Patch) **Initial:** Apply 4.6mg/24hrs patch qd to clean, dry, hairless, intact skin. **Maint:** 9.5mg/24hrs. Increase dose after minimum of 4 weeks. **Max:** 9.5mg/24hrs if well tolerated. Switching from Capsules/Oral Sol: Refer to PI.	Nausea, vomiting, abdominal pain, dyspepsia, anorexia/decreased appetite, weight decrease, asthenia, headache, dizziness, fatigue, diarrhea, depression, anxiety, insomnia, UTI

ANTIPARKINSON AGENTS

GENERIC (BRAND)	INDICATIONS	HOW SUPPLIED	DOSAGE	SIDE EFFECTS
Amantadine HCl	Treatment of idiopathic Parkinson's disease (paralysis agitans), postencephalitic parkinsonism, and symptomatic parkinsonism. Treatment of drug-induced extrapyramidal reactions.	**Cap, Tab:** 100mg; **Syr:** 50mg/5mL	**Parkinsonism: Initial:** 100mg bid. **Serious Associated Illness/Concomitant High-Dose Antiparkinson Agent: Initial:** 100mg qd. **Titrate:** May increase to 100mg bid after 1 to several weeks. **Max:** 400mg/day. Drug-induced extrapyramidal reactions: 100mg bid. **Max:** 300mg/day. **Renal Impairment:** Check PI for dosing adjustments.	Nausea, dizziness, insomnia, depression, anxiety and irritability, hallucinations, confusion, anorexia, dry mouth, constipation, ataxia, livedo reticularis, peripheral edema, orthostatic hypotension, headache, somnolence, nervousness, dream abnormality, agitation, dry nose, diarrhea, fatigue
Apomorphine HCl (Apokyn)	Indicated for the acute, intermittent treatment of hypomobility, "off" episodes ("end-of-dose wearing off" and unpredictable "on/off" episode) associated with advanced Parkinson's disease. Apokyn has been studied as an adjunct to other medications.	**Inj:** 10mg/mL	**Test dose:** 0.2mL (0.2 mg); SQ assess efficacy/tolerability. See PI for details. **Max:** 0.6mL (6mg)/dose. **Renal Impairment: Test Dose/Initial:** 0.1mL.	Yawning, dyskinesias, nausea, vomiting, drowsiness, somnolence, dizziness, rhinorrhea, hallucinations, edema, chest pain/pressure/angina, hallucination, confusion
Benztropine mesylate (Cogentin)	Adjunct in all forms of parkinsonism. Control of drug-induced extrapyramidal disorders.	**Inj:** 1mg/mL; (Generic) **Tab:** 0.5mg, 1mg, 2mg	**Idiopathic Parkinsonism: Initial:** 0.5-1mg PO or IV/IM qhs. **Postencephalitic Parkinsonism: Initial:** 2mg/day PO or IV/IM given in 1 or more doses. **Titrate:** May increase every 5-6 days by 0.5mg. **Usual:** 1-2mg PO or IV/IM qhs. **Max:** 6mg/day. **Drug-Induced Extrapyramidal Disorders: Recommended Dose:** 1-4mg qd or bid. Dosing must be individualized and periodically withdrawn to reassess symptoms.	Tachycardia, paralytic ileus, constipation, vomiting, nausea, dry mouth, confusion, blurred vision, urinary retention, heat stroke, hyperthermia, fever
Bromocriptine mesylate (Parlodel)	Treatment of signs and symptoms of idiopathic or postencephalitic Parkinson's disease. May provide additional therapeutic benefits as adjunctive treatment to levodopa.	**Tab, Snap:** 2.5mg*; **Cap:** 5mg	**Initial:** 1.25mg bid. **Titrate:** If needed, increase by 2.5mg/day q2-4 weeks. **Max:** 100mg/day. Take with food. Assess need for medication at 2-week intervals.	Dizziness, insomnia, hallucinations, abnormal involuntary movements, depression, visual disturbance, asthenia, nausea, confusion, "on-off" phenomenon, drowsiness, faintness/fainting, vomiting, abdominal discomfort, ataxia, hypotension, constipation, vertigo

(Continued)

GENERIC (BRAND)	INDICATIONS	HOW SUPPLIED	DOSAGE	SIDE EFFECTS
Carbidopa (Lodosyn)	For use with Sinemet or levodopa in treatment of symptoms of idiopathic Parkinson's disease, postencephalitic parkinsonism, and symptomatic parkinsonism. For use in patients for whom the dosage of Sinemet provides less than adequate daily dosage (usually 70mg daily) of carbidopa. For use with levodopa in the patient whose dosage requirement of carbidopa and levodopa necessitates separate titration of each entity. Use with Sinemet or levodopa to permit the administration of lower doses of levodopa with reduced nausea and vomiting, more rapid dosage titration, and with a somewhat smoother response.	**Tab:** 25mg*	**With Sinemet or levodopa:** Determine dose by careful titration. Most patients respond to a 1:10 proportion of carbidopa: levodopa provided carbidopa dose is ≥70mg/day. **Max:** 200mg/day. Consider amount of carbidopa in Sinemet when calculating dose. See PI for detailed dosing information.	Dyskinesias (choreiform, dystonic, and other involuntary movements), psychotic episodes, delusions, hallucinations, paranoid ideation, depression with or without suicidal tendencies, dementia, convulsions
Carbidopa/Levodopa (Parcopa)	Treatment of symptoms of idiopathic Parkinson's disease, postencephalitic parkinsonism, and symptomatic parkinsonism.	**Tab, Disintegrating:** (Carbidopa-Levodopa) 10mg-100mg*, 25mg-100mg*, 25mg-250mg*	**25mg-100mg Tab: Initial:** 1 tab tid. **Titrate:** Increase by 1 tab qd or qod up to 8 tabs/day. **10mg-100mg Tab: Initial:** 1 tab tid-qid. **Titrate:** Increase by 1 tab qd or qod up to 2 tabs qid. 70-100mg/day carbidopa required. **Max:** 200mg/day carbidopa. Conversion from levodopa: See PI.	Dyskinesia (choreiform, dystonic, and other involuntary movements), nausea. Check PI for a more comprehensive list of adverse reactions
Carbidopa/Levodopa (Sinemet, Sinemet CR)	Treatment of symptoms of idiopathic Parkinson's disease, postencephalitic parkinsonism, and symptomatic parkinsonism.	**Tab:** (Carbidopa-Levodopa) 10mg-100mg, 25mg-100mg, 25mg-250mg; **Tab, Extended-Release:** 25mg-100mg, 50mg-200mg	(Tab) **25mg-100mg Tab: Initial:** 1 tab tid. **Titrate:** Increase by 1 tab qd or qod up to 8 tabs/day. **10mg-100mg Tab: Initial:** 1 tab tid-qid. **Titrate:** May increase by 1 tab qd or qod up to 2 tabs qid. 70-100mg/day carbidopa required. **Max:** 200mg/day carbidopa. Conversion from levodopa: See PI. (Tab, Extended-Release) **No Prior Levodopa Use: Initial:** One 50mg-200mg tab bid at intervals ≥6 hrs. **Titrate:** Increase or decrease dose or interval accordingly. Adjust dose at interval of ≥3 days. **Usual:** 400-1600mg/day levodopa, given in 4-8 hr intervals while awake. **Conversion to Extended-Release Tabs:** See PI.	Dyskinesia (choreiform, dystonic, and other involuntary movements), nausea. Check PI for a more comprehensive list of adverse reactions

GENERIC (BRAND)	INDICATIONS	HOW SUPPLIED	DOSAGE	SIDE EFFECTS
Carbidopa/Levodopa/ Entacapone (Stalevo)	Treatment of idiopathic Parkinson's disease to substitute for equivalent doses of immediate-release carbidopa/levodopa and entacapone previously administered as individual products, or to replace immediate-release carbidopa/levodopa (without entacapone) for those experiencing signs and symptoms of end-of-dose "wearing off" and taking up to 600mg/day levodopa without experiencing dyskinesias.	**Tab:** (Carbidopa/ Levodopa/ Entacapone): Stalevo 50: 12.5mg/ 50mg/200mg; Stalevo 75: 18.75mg/75mg/ 200mg; Stalevo 100: 25mg/100mg/ 200mg; Stalevo 125: 31.25mg/125mg/ 200mg; Stalevo 150: 37.5mg/ 150mg/200mg; Stalevo 200: 50mg/ 200mg/200mg	**Currently Taking Carbidopa/Levodopa and Entacapone:** May switch directly to corresponding strength of levodopa/carbidopa/ entacapone. **Currently Taking Carbidopa/Levodopa, but not Entacapone:** First, titrate individually with carbidopa/levodopa product and entacapone product, then transfer to corresponding dose. **Max:** 8 tabs/day except Stalevo 200. **Stalevo 200 Max:** 6 tabs/day.	Dyskinesia, (choreiform, dystonic, and other involuntary movements), nausea. Check PI for a more comprehensive list of adverse reactions
Diphenhydramine HCl Injection	For parkinsonism when oral therapy is not possible or is contraindicated, as follows: elderly who are unable to tolerate more potent agents, mild cases of parkinsonism in other age groups, and in combination with centrally acting anticholinergic agents.	**Inj:** 50mg/mL	**Usual:** 10-50mg IV at ≤25mg/min or up to 100mg IM if needed. **Max:** 400mg/day.	Sedation, sleepiness, drowsiness, dizziness, disturbed coordination, epigastric distress, thickening of bronchial secretions
Entacapone (Comtan)	Adjunct to levodopa/carbidopa for treatment of idiopathic Parkinson's disease if experience signs and symptoms of end-of-dose "wearing-off."	**Tab:** 200mg	**200mg with Each Levodopa/Carbidopa Dose: Max:** 1600mg/day. Withdraw slowly for discontinuation.	Dyskinesia, hyperkinesia, hypokinesia, dizziness, nausea, diarrhea, abdominal pain, constipation, urine discoloration, fatigue
Hyoscyamine sulfate (Levsin, Levbid)	To reduce rigidity and tremors of Parkinson's disease and to control associated sialorrhea and hyperhidrosis.	(Levbid) **Tab, Extended-Release:** 0.375mg. (Levsin) **Tab:** 0.125mg. **Tab, Sublingual:** 0.125mg; **Drops:** 0.125mg/mL; **Elixir:** 0.125mg/5mL	May chew or swallow SL tab. May also place on tongue and disintegrate chewable tab. Levsin: 0.125-0.25mg q4h or prn. **Max:** 1.5mg/24 hrs. Levbid: 0.375-0.75mg q12h. **Max:** 1.5mg/24 hrs. Do not crush or chew.	Anticholinergic effects, drowsiness, headache, nervousness

(Continued)

GENERIC (BRAND)	INDICATIONS	HOW SUPPLIED	DOSAGE	SIDE EFFECTS
Pramipexole dihydrochloride (Mirapex)	Treatment of signs and symptoms of idiopathic Parkinson's disease.	**Tab:** 0.125mg, 0.25mg*, 0.5mg*, 0.75mg*, 1mg*, 1.5mg*	**Initial:** 0.125mg tid. **Titrate:** May increase every 5-7 days (eg, Week 2: 0.25mg tid; Week 3: 0.5mg tid; Week 4: 0.75mg tid; Week 5: 1mg tid; Week 6: 1.25mg tid; Week 7: 1.5mg tid). **Maint:** 0.5-1.5mg tid. **Max:** 1.5mg tid.[†]	Nausea, dizziness, somnolence, constipation, asthenia, hallucinations, vision abnormalities, general and peripheral edema, insomnia, confusion, amnesia, hypoesthesia
(Mirapex ER)		**(Tab, ER):** 0.375mg, 0.75mg, 1.5mg, 2.25mg, 3mg, 3.75mg, 4.5mg	**(Tab, ER) Initial:** 0.375mg qd. **Titrate:** May increase gradually not more frequently than q5-7 days, first to 0.75mg/day and then by 0.75mg increments based on efficacy and tolerability. **Max:** 4.5mg/day. Refer to PI for more detailed dosing information.[†]	**(Tab, ER)** Somnolence, nausea, constipation, dizziness, fatigue, hallucinations, dry mouth, muscle spasms, peripheral edema
Rasagiline mesylate (Azilect)	Treatment of signs and symptoms of idiopathic Parkinson's disease as initial monotherapy and adjunct therapy to levodopa.	**Tab:** 0.5mg, 1mg	**Monotherapy:** 1mg qd. **Adjunctive Therapy: Initial:** 0.5mg qd. **Titrate:** May increase to 1mg qd. Adjust dose of levodopa with concomitant use. **Concomitant Ciprofloxacin or Other CYP1A2 Inhibitors/Mild Hepatic Impairment:** 0.5mg qd.	Headache, accidental injury, arthralgia, depression, fall, flu syndrome, dyskinesia, nausea, weight loss, constipation, postural hypotension, vomiting, dry mouth, rash, somnolence
Rivastigmine (Exelon)	Treatment of mild-to-moderate dementia associated with Parkinson's disease.	**Cap:** 1.5mg, 3mg, 4.5mg, 6mg; **Patch:** 4.6mg/24h, 9.5mg/24h; **Sol:** 2mg/mL	**(Cap, Sol): Initial:** 1.5mg bid with meals in am and pm. **Titrate:** May increase at 4-week intervals to 3mg bid, then 4.5mg bid, and 6mg bid if tolerable. **Usual:** 1.5-6mg bid. **Patch: Initial:** 4.6mg/24h. **Titrate:** After 4 weeks, may increase to 9.5mg/24h if tolerated. **Max:** 9.5mg/24h.	Nausea, vomiting, anorexia, tremor, dizziness, diarrhea
Ropinirole HCl (Requip, Requip XL)	Treatment of signs and symptoms of idiopathic Parkinson's disease.	**Tab:** 0.25mg, 0.5mg, 1mg, 2mg, 3mg, 4mg, 5mg; **Tab, ER:** 2mg, 4mg, 6mg, 8mg, 12mg	**Initial:** 0.25mg tid. **Titrate:** May increase weekly by 0.25mg tid (0.75mg/day) for 4 weeks. After Week 4, may increase weekly by 1.5mg/day up to 9mg/day, then by 3mg/day weekly to 24mg/day. **Max:** 24mg/day. **Withdrawal:** Decrease dose to bid for 4 days, then qd for 3 days. (Requip XL) **Tab, Extended-Release: Initial:** 2mg qd for 1-2 weeks. Swallow whole. **Titrate:** May increase at ≥1-week intervals by 2mg/day. **Max:** 24mg/day. **Switching from IR to ER:** Closely match total daily IR dose with initial extended-release dose. See PI for detailed information.	Hallucinations, somnolence, vomiting, headache, constipation, dyspepsia, abdominal pain, pharyngitis, UTI, increased sweating, asthenia, edema, fatigue, syncope, orthostatic symptoms, dizziness, nausea, viral infection, confusion, abnormal vision
Selegiline HCl (Eldepryl)	Adjunct in the management of Parkinsonian patients being treated with levodopa/carbidopa who exhibit deterioration in the quality of their response to this therapy.	**Cap:** 5mg; (Generic) **Tab:** 5mg	5mg bid at breakfast and lunch. **Max:** 10mg/day. May attempt to reduce levodopa/carbidopa by 10-30% after 2-3 days of therapy. May reduce further with continued therapy.	Nausea, dizziness, lightheadedness, fainting, abdominal pain, confusion, hallucinations, dry mouth

GENERIC (BRAND)	INDICATIONS	HOW SUPPLIED	DOSAGE	SIDE EFFECTS
Selegiline (Zelapar)	Adjunct in the management of patients with Parkinson's disease being treated with levodopa/carbidopa who exhibit deterioration in the quality of their response to this therapy.	**Tab, Orally Disintegrating:** 1.25mg	1.25mg qd for ≥6 weeks. **Titrate:** After 6 weeks, may increase to 2.5mg qd if the desired benefit is not achieved and patient can tolerate it. **Max:** 2.5mg/day.	Nausea, dizziness, pain, headache, insomnia, rhinitis, skin disorders, dyskinesia, backache, dyspepsia, stomatitis, constipation, hallucinations, pharyngitis, rash
Tolcapone (Tasmar)	Adjunct to levodopa/carbidopa for the treatment of the signs and symptoms of idiopathic Parkinson's disease.	**Tab:** 100mg, 200mg	**Initial:** 100mg tid. Use 200mg tid only if clinical benefit is justified. May need to decrease levodopa dose.	Dyskinesia, nausea, sleep disorder, dystonia, excessive dreaming, anorexia, muscle cramps, orthostatic complaints, somnolence, diarrhea, confusion, dizziness, headache, hallucination, vomiting, constipation, fatigue, upper respiratory tract infection, falling, increased sweating, UTI, xerostomia, abdominal pain, urine discoloration, hepatotoxicity
Trihexyphenidyl HCl	Adjunct treatment for all forms of parkinsonism (postencephalitic, arteriosclerotic, and idiopathic). For control of extrapyramidal disorders caused by CNS drugs.	**Sol:** 2mg/5mL; **Tab:** 2mg*, 5mg*	**Idiopathic Parkinsonism:** 1mg on Day 1. **Titrate:** Increase by 2mg q3-5 days. **Usual:** 6-10mg/day. **Max:** 15mg/day. **Drug-Induced Parkinsonism: Initial:** 1mg. If extrapyramidal manifestations not controlled in a few hrs, increase dose until control is achieved. **Usual:** 5-15mg/day. **Concomitant Levodopa or Other Parasympathetic Inhibitors:** See PI.	Dry mouth, blurred vision, dizziness, nausea, nervousness, constipation, drowsiness, urinary hesitancy/retention, tachycardia, pupil dilation, increased intraocular tension, vomiting, weakness, headache

*Scored.
†Refer to full prescribing information for dosing instructions in renally compromised patients.

OPIOID PRODUCTS

GENERIC	BRAND	DOSAGE FORMS	USUAL ADULT DOSE	MAX DOSE	INDICATION	DEA SCHEDULE
MILD TO MODERATELY SEVERE PAIN						
Codeine sulfate		**Tab:** 15mg, 30mg, 60mg; **Sol:** 30mg/5mL	PO, IM, SQ 15-60mg up to q4h prn.	360mg/24hrs.	Relief of mild to moderately severe pain.	Schedule II
Codeine phosphate/ Acetaminophen		**Elixir:** 12mg-120mg/5mL	15mL q4h prn.	**Codeine:** 360mg/day. **APAP:** 4g/day.	Relief of mild to moderately severe pain.	Schedule V
		Tab: 15mg-300mg	15-60mg codeine/dose and 300-1000mg APAP. Doses may be repeated q4h.			Schedule III
	Tylenol #3	**Tab:** 30mg-300mg				Schedule III
	Tylenol #4	**Tab:** 60mg-300mg				Schedule III
MODERATE TO MODERATELY SEVERE PAIN						
Dihydrocodeine bitartrate/ Aspirin/Caffeine	Synalgos-DC	**Cap:** 16mg-356.4mg-30mg	2 caps q4h prn.		Relief of moderate to moderately severe pain.	Schedule III
Hydrocodone bitartrate/ Acetaminophen	Generic	**Tab:** 5mg-325mg, 7.5mg-325mg, 2.5mg-500mg, 5mg-500mg, 7.5mg-500mg, 7.5mg-650mg	**(5/325, 2.5/500, 5/500):** 1-2 tabs q4-6h prn. **(7.5/325, 7.5/500, 7.5/650):** 1 tab q4-6h prn.	**(5/325, 2.5/500, 5/500):** 8 tabs/day. **(7.5/325, 7.5/500, 7.5/650):** 6 tabs/ day.	Relief of moderate to moderately severe pain.	Schedule III
		Cap: 5mg-500mg	1-2 caps q4-6h prn.	8 caps/day.		
	Co-gesic	**Tab:** 5mg-500mg	1-2 tab q4-6h prn.	8 tab(s)/day.		
	Hycet	**Sol:** 7.5mg-325mg/15mL	1 tbsp q4-6h prn.	6 tbsp/day.		
	Lorcet Plus, Lorcet 10/650	**Tab:** (Plus) 7.5mg-650mg, (10/650) 10mg-650mg	1 tab q4-6h prn.	6 tabs/day.		
	Lortab Elixir, Lortab	**Sol:** 7.5mg-500mg/15mL	**(Sol):** 1 tbsp q4-6h prn.	**(Sol):** 6 tbsp/day.		
		Tab: 5mg-500mg, 10mg-500mg	**(5/500):** 1-2 tabs q4-6h prn. **(10/500):** 1 tab q4-6h prn.	**(5/500):** 8 tabs/day. **(10/500):** 6 tabs/day.		
	Norco	**Tab:** 5mg-325mg, 7.5mg-325mg, 10mg-325mg	**(5/325):** 1-2 tabs q4-6h prn. **(7.5/325, 10/325):** 1 tab q4-6h prn.	**(5/325):** 8 tabs/day. **(7.5/325):** 6 tabs/day. **(10/325):** 6 tabs/day.		
	Vicodin	**Tab:** 5mg-500mg	1-2 tabs q4-6h prn.	8 tabs/day.		
	Vicodin ES	**Tab:** 7.5mg-750mg	1 tab q4-6h prn.	5 tabs/day.		

(Continued)

GENERIC	BRAND	DOSAGE FORMS	USUAL ADULT DOSE	MAX DOSE	INDICATION	DEA SCHEDULE
MODERATE TO MODERATELY SEVERE PAIN *(Continued)*						
Hydrocodone bitartrate/ Acetaminophen *(Continued)*	Vicodin HP	**Tab:** 10mg-660mg	1 tab q4-6h prn.	6 tabs/day.		
	Zydone	**Tab:** 5mg-400mg, 7.5mg-400mg, 10mg-400mg	**(5/400):** 1-2 tabs q4-6h prn. **(7.5/400, 10/400):** 1 tab q4-6h prn.	**(5/400):** 8 tabs/day. **(7.5/400, 10/400):** 6 tabs/day.	Short-term (generally <10 days) management of acute pain.	Schedule III
Hydrocodone bitartrate/ Ibuprofen	Reprexain	**Tab:** 2.5mg-200mg, 5mg-200mg, 10mg-200mg	1 tab q4-6h prn.	5 tabs/day.		
	Vicoprofen	**Tab:** 7.5-200mg	1 tab q4-6h prn.	5 tabs/day.		
Oxycodone/Acetaminophen	Percocet	**Tab:** 2.5mg-325mg, 5mg-325mg, 7.5mg-325mg, 7.5mg-500mg, 10mg-325mg, 10mg-650mg	**(2.5/325):** 1-2 tabs q6h. **(5/325):** 1 tab q6h prn. **(7.5/500):** 1 tab q6h prn. **(10/650):** 1 tab q6h prn. **(7.5/325):** 1 tab q6h prn. **(10/325):** 1 tab q6h prn.	**(2.5/325):** 12 tabs/day. **(5/325):** 12 tabs/days. **(7.5/500):** 8 tabs/day. **(10/650):** 6 tabs/day. **(7.5/325):** 8 tabs/day. **(10/325):** 6 tabs/day.	Relief of moderate to moderately severe pain.	Schedule II
	Roxicet	**Tab:** 5mg-325mg, 5mg-500mg; **Sol:** 5mg-325mg/5mL	**Tab:** 1 tab q6h prn. **Sol:** 5 mL q6h prn.	**Tab: (5/325):** 12 tabs/day. **(5/500):** 8 tabs/day. **Sol:** 60mL/day. **APAP:** 4g/day		
	Tylox	**Cap:** 5mg-500mg	1 cap q6h prn.	**APAP:** 4g/day.		
Oxycodone HCl/Aspirin	Percodan	**Tab:** 4.8355mg-325mg	1 tab q6h prn.	12 tabs/day or ASA 4g/day.	Management of moderate to moderately severe pain.	Schedule II
MODERATE TO SEVERE OR CHRONIC PAIN						
Buprenorphine	Butrans	**Patch:** 5mcg/hr, 10mcg/hr, 20mcg/hr	5mcg/hr for 7 days/patch if opioid-naive. See PI for instructions if already receiving opioids. Individually titrate after a minimum of 72 hours.	20mcg/hr.	Management of moderate to severe chronic pain in patients requiring a continuous, around-the-clock opioid for an extended period of time.	Schedule III

GENERIC	BRAND	DOSAGE FORMS	USUAL ADULT DOSE	MAX DOSE	INDICATION	DEA SCHEDULE
MODERATE TO SEVERE OR CHRONIC PAIN *(Continued)*						
Fentanyl	Duragesic	**Patch:** 12mcg/hr, 25mcg/hr, 50mcg/hr, 75mcg/hr, 100mcg/hr	**Initia:** 25mcg/hr for 72 hrs. Individualize dose.		Management of persistent moderate to severe chronic pain that requires continuous, around-the-clock opioid administration for an extended period of time, and cannot be managed by other means such as nonsteroidal analgesics, opioid combination products, or immediate-release opioids.	Schedule II
Hydromorphone HCl	Dilaudid, Dilaudid-HP	**Tab:** 2mg, 4mg, 8mg; **Sol:** 1mg/mL; **Inj:** 1 mg/mL, 2mg/mL, 4mg/mL; **HP: Inj:** 10mg/mL [10mg, 50mg, 250mg, 500mg]	**Tab:** 2-4mg PO q4-6h. **Sol:** 2.5-10mL q3-6h as directed. **Inj:** 1-2mg IM/SQ q2-3h prn; 0.2-2mg IV q2-3h over ≥2-3 min. **HP:** Individualized dose for each patient.		Management of pain where an opioid is appropriate. **HP:** Relief of moderate to severe pain in opioid-tolerant patients requiring higher than usual doses of opioids to provide adequate pain relief.	Schedule II
	Exalgo	**Tab, ER:** 8mg, 12mg, 16mg	**Dose range:** 8-64mg. Administer once q24h. Individualize dose.		Management of moderate to severe pain in opioid-tolerant patients requiring continuous, around-the-clock opioid analgesia for an extended period of time.	Schedule II
Levorphanol tartrate		**Tab:** 2mg	**Initia:** 2mg PO q6-8h. Titrate to 3mg or higher q6-8h if needed.		Management of moderate to severe pain where an opioid is appropriate.	Schedule II
Meperidine HCl		**Syr:** 25mg/mL, 50mg/mL, 75mg/mL, 100mg/mL	See dosage for Demerol.		Moderate to severe pain.	Schedule II

(Continued)

A227

GENERIC	BRAND	DOSAGE FORMS	USUAL ADULT DOSE	MAX DOSE	INDICATION	DEA SCHEDULE
MODERATE TO SEVERE OR CHRONIC PAIN *(Continued)*						
Meperidine HCl *(Continued)*	Demerol	**Tab:** 50mg, 100mg; **Inj:** 25mg/mL, 50mg/mL, 75mg/mL, 100mg/mL	**Tab:** 50-150mg q3-4h prn. **Inj:** 50-150mg IM/SQ q3-4h prn; 50-100mg IM/SQ 30-90 min prior to anesthesia for pre-op use or at 1- to 3-hr intervals during obstetrical analgesia. Individualize dose for anesthesia support.		Relief of moderate to severe pain. **Inj:** Also for preoperative medication, anesthesia support, and obstetrical analgesia.	
Methadone HCl	Dolophine, Methadose	**Inj:** 10mg/mL	**Pain:** 2.5-10mg q8-12h, slowly titrated to effect.		To treat moderate to severe pain not responsive to non-narcotic analgesics.	Schedule II
		Tab: 5mg, 10mg; **Sol:** 10mg/mL				
Morphine sulfate/ Naltrexone HCl	Embeda	**Cap, ER:** 20mg-0.8mg, 30mg-1.2mg, 50mg-2mg, 60mg-2.4mg, 80mg-3.2mg, 100mg-4mg	**First opioid analgesic:** May be administered qd or bid. The lowest dose should be used. Titrate no more frequently than qod. **Conversion from oral morphine formulation:** 50% of daily oral morphine dose q12h or 100% of daily oral morphine dose q24h.		Management of moderate to severe pain when a continuous around-the-clock opioid analgesic is needed for an extended period of time.	Schedule II
Morphine sulfate	Astramorph PF	**Inj:** 0.5mg/mL, 1mg/mL	**IV:** 2-10mg/70kg of body weight. **Epidural: Initial:** 5mg. **Titrate:** If inadequate pain relief in 1 hr, administer incremental doses of 1-2mg at intervals sufficient to assess effectiveness. **Continuous Infusion:** 2-4mg/24 hrs. **IT:** 0.2-1mg single dose. If pain recurs with IT, consider alternative routes of administration.	**Epidural:** 10mg/24h.	Management of pain not responsive to non-narcotic analgesics.	Schedule II
	Avinza	**Cap, ER:** 30mg, 45mg, 60mg, 75mg, 90mg, 120mg	**Opioid-naïve: Initial:** 30mg q24h. **Titrate:** Increase by ≤30mg every 4 days. Individualize dose.	1600mg/day.	Relief of moderate to severe pain requiring continuous, around-the-clock opioid therapy for an extended period of time.	
	Infumorph	**Inj:** 10mg/mL (200mg), 25mg/mL (500mg)	**IT:** 0.2-10mg/day. **Epidural:** 3.5-30mg/day. Individualize dose.		Treatment of intractable chronic pain for use in microinfusion devices.	

GENERIC	BRAND	DOSAGE FORMS	USUAL ADULT DOSE	MAX DOSE	INDICATION	DEA SCHEDULE
MODERATE TO SEVERE OR CHRONIC PAIN *(Continued)*						
Morphine sulfate *(Continued)*	Kadian	**Cap, ER:** 10mg, 20mg, 30mg, 50mg, 60mg, 80mg, 100mg, 200mg	Give 50% of daily oral morphine dose q12h or give 100% oral morphine dose q24h.	Do not give more frequently than q12h.	Management of moderate to severe pain when a continuous, around-the-clock opioid analgesic is needed for an extended period of time.	
	MS Contin	**Tab, ER:** 15mg, 30mg, 60mg, 100mg, 200mg	Give 50% of patient's 24-hr immediate-release oral morphine requirement q12h or ⅓ of patient's 24-hr requirement q8h.		Management of moderate to severe pain when a continuous, around-the-clock analgesic is needed for an extended period of time.	
Oxycodone HCl		**Cap, IR:** 5mg	5-15mg q4-6h prn. Individualized based on previous analgesic treatment.		Management of moderate to severe acute and chronic pain where the use of an opioid analgesic is appropriate.	Schedule II
		Sol: 1mg/mL	5-15mg q4-6h prn. Individualized based on previous analgesic treatment.		Management of moderate to severe acute and chronic pain where the use of an opioid analgesic is appropriate.	Schedule II
		Sol: 20mg/mL			Management of moderate to severe acute and chronic pain in opioid-tolerant patients.	Schedule II
	Oxecta	**Tab:** 5mg, 7.5mg	**Initial:** 5-15mg q4-6h prn if opioid-naive; may need to dose at lowest dosage level that achieves acceptable analgesia.		Management of acute and chronic moderate to severe pain where the use of an opioid is appropriate.	Schedule II
	Roxicodone	**Tab:** 5mg, 15mg, 30mg	**Tab:** 5-15mg q4-6h prn. Individualized based on previous analgesic response.		Management of moderate to severe pain where the use of an opioid analgesic is appropriate.	Schedule II

(Continued)

GENERIC	BRAND	DOSAGE FORMS	USUAL ADULT DOSE	MAX DOSE	INDICATION	DEA SCHEDULE
MODERATE TO SEVERE OR CHRONIC PAIN *(Continued)*						
Oxycodone HCl *(Continued)*	OxyContin	**Tab, ER:** 10mg, 15mg, 20mg, 30mg, 40mg, 60mg, 80mg	Individualize dosing for each patient. **Opioid-naive:** 10mg q12h. **Opioid-experienced:** 1/2 the total daily immediate release oxycodone dose given q12h. May increase the total daily dose by 25-50% of the current dose every 1-2 days prn.		Management of moderate to severe pain when a continuous, around-the-clock opioid analgesic is needed for an extended period. Postoperative use only in patients already receiving the drug before surgery or those expected to have moderate-severe postoperative pain for an extended period of time.	Schedule II
Oxymorphone HCl	Opana	**Inj:** 1mg/mL; **Tab:** 5mg, 10mg	**Inj: SQ/IM:** 1-1.5mg q4-6h prn, IV: **Initial:** 0.5mg. Individually titrate. **Labor Analgesia:** 0.5-1mg IM. **Tab:** 10-20mg PO q4-6h.		**(Inj):** Relief of moderate to severe acute pain. For preoperative medication, for support of anesthesia, for obstetrical analgesia, and for relief of anxiety in patients with dyspnea associated with pulmonary edema secondary to acute left ventricular dysfunction. **(Tab):** Relief of moderate to severe acute pain.	Schedule II
	Opana ER	**Tab, ER:** 5mg, 7.5mg, 10mg, 15mg, 20mg, 30mg, 40mg	**Opioid-naive:** 5mg q12h ≥1 hr prior to or 2 hr after eating. Titrate individually at increments of 5-10mg q12h every 3-7 days. **Opioid-experienced:** 1/2 the total daily oral immediate-release oxymorphone dose q12h.		Relief of moderate to severe pain in patients requiring continuous, around-the-clock opioid treatment for an extended period of time.	Schedule II
Tapentadol	Nucynta	**Tab:** 50mg, 75mg, 100mg	50mg, 75mg, or 100mg q4-6 hrs depending upon pain intensity. On the first day only, a second dose may be given 1 hr after first dose if inadequate pain relief.	700 mg/day on first day of therapy; 600 mg/day on subsequent days of therapy.	Relief of moderate to severe acute pain in patients ≥18 yrs.	Schedule II

GENERIC	BRAND	DOSAGE FORMS	USUAL ADULT DOSE	MAX DOSE	INDICATION	DEA SCHEDULE
MODERATE TO SEVERE OR CHRONIC PAIN *(Continued)*						
Tapentadol *(Continued)*	Nucynta ER	**Tab:** 50mg, 100mg, 150mg, 200mg, 250mg	50mg q12h if not currently taking opioids or 1/2 the total daily imme-diate-release tapentadol dose q12h. Individually titrate by increments of 50mg bid every 3 days to 100-250mg q12h.	500mg/day.	Management of moderate to severe chronic pain in adults when a continuous, around-the-clock opioid analgesic is needed for an extended period of time.	Schedule II
BREAKTHROUGH PAIN						
Fentanyl	Abstral	**Tab, SL:** 100mcg, 200mcg, 300mcg, 400mcg, 600mcg, 800mcg	**Initial:** 100mcg. Individually titrate.	2 doses/episode of breakthrough pain separated by 30 min. Wait 2 hrs between episodes.	Management of breakthrough pain in cancer patients ≥18 years who are already receiving, and who are tolerant to, opioid therapy for their underlying persistent cancer pain.	Schedule II
	Lazanda	**Nasal:** 100mcg/spr, 400mcg/spr	**Initial:** 100mcg. Individually titrate.	2 doses/episode of breakthrough pain separated by 30 min. Wait ≥2 hrs between episodes.	Management of breakthrough pain in cancer patients ≥18 years who are already receiving, and who are tolerant to, opioid therapy for their underlying persistent cancer pain.	Schedule II
	Subsys	**Spr, SL:** 100mcg/spr, 200mcg/spr, 400mcg/spr, 600mcg/spr, 800mcg/spr	**Initial:** 100mcg. Individually titrate.	2 doses/episode of breakthrough pain separated by 30 min. Wait ≥4 hrs between episodes.	Management of breakthrough pain in cancer patients ≥18 years who are already receiving, and who are tolerant to, opioid therapy for their underlying persistent cancer pain.	Schedule II

(Continued)

GENERIC	BRAND	DOSAGE FORMS	USUAL ADULT DOSE	MAX DOSE	INDICATION	DEA SCHEDULE
BREAKTHROUGH PAIN *(Continued)*						
Fentanyl *(Continued)*	Actiq	**Loz:** 200mcg, 400mcg, 600mcg, 800mcg, 1200 mcg, 1600 mcg	200mcg. Dispense no more than 6 units. Individually titrate.	2 doses/episode of breakthrough pain separated by 15 min (30 min after start of dose). Wait 4 hrs between episodes. 4 units/day.	Management of breakthrough pain in patients ≥16 yrs who are already receiving and are tolerant to around-the-clock opioid therapy for their underlying persistent cancer pain.	Schedule II
Fentanyl citrate	Fentora	**Tab, Buccal:** 100mcg, 200mcg, 400mcg, 600mcg, 800mcg	**Initial:** 100mcg. **Converting from Actiq doses ≥600mcg:** 200mcg; proceed using multiples of this strength. **Titrate: If 100mcg Initial Dose:** Give two 100-mcg tabs (one on each side of mouth); may increase to four 100-mcg tabs (two on each side of mouth). Use multiples of 200mcg tabs for doses >400mcg.	2 doses/episode of breakthrough pain separated by 30 min. Wait 4 hrs between episodes. Not more than 4 tabs simultaneously.	Management of breakthrough pain in patients ≥18 yrs who are already receiving, and are tolerant to, around-the-clock opioid therapy for their underlying persistent cancer pain.	Schedule II
	Onsolis	**Film, Buccal:** 200mcg, 400mcg, 600mcg, 800mcg, 1200mcg	**Initial:** 200mcg. **Titrate:** Use multiples of 200mcg films. Increase by 200mcg per subsequent episode until effect.	Not more than four 200mcg films simultaneously. If no adequate pain relief and tolerant to 800mcg, give one 1200mcg film. Single doses are given 2 hrs apart; use once per breakthrough pain episode.	Management of breakthrough pain in patients ≥18 yrs who are already receiving and are tolerant to opioid therapy for their underlying persistent cancer pain.	
MISCELLANEOUS						
Morphine sulfate	Oramorph SR	**Tab, SR:** 15mg, 30mg, 60mg, 100mg	Give 1/2 of daily oral morphine requirement q12h.		Relief of pain in patients who require opioid analgesics for more than a few days.	Schedule II
	Depodur	**Inj:** 10mg/mL	**Epidural:** 10-15mg.		Treatment of pain following major surgery.	Schedule II

GENERIC	BRAND	DOSAGE FORMS	USUAL ADULT DOSE	MAX DOSE	INDICATION	DEA SCHEDULE
MISCELLANEOUS *(Continued)*						
Morphine sulfate *(Continued)*	Duramorph	**Inj:** 0.5mg/mL, 1mg/mL	**IV:** 2-10mg/70kg of body weight. **Epidural: Initial:** 5mg. **Titrate:** If inadequate pain relief in 1 hr, administer incremental doses of 1-2mg at intervals sufficient to assess effectiveness. **IT:** 0.2-1mg single dose. If pain recurs with IT, consider alternative routes of administration.	**Epidural:** 10mg/24h.	Management of pain not responsive to non-narcotic analgesics.	Schedule II

*Other formulations are available.
***IM.
Refer to full FDA-approved prescribing information for more detailed dosing.

ORAL ANTICONVULSANTS

GENERIC (BRAND)	USUAL ADULT DOSE*	THERAPEUTIC SERUM LEVELS	INDICATIONS							
			SEIZURE DISORDERS					NEUROPATHIC PAIN	LENNOX-GASTAUT SYNDROME	
			ABSENCE	AKINETIC	MYOCLONIC	PARTIAL	TONIC-CLONIC			
BARBITURATES										
Phenobarbital†	60-200mg/day	10-40mcg/mL			X	X	X			
Primidone (Mysoline)	750-2000mg/day	5-12mcg/mL				X	X		X	
BENZODIAZEPINES										
Clonazepam (Klonopin)	1.5-20mg/day	N/A	X	X	X					
Clorazepate dipotassium (Tranxene T-Tab)	22.5-90mg/day	N/A				X				
Diazepam (Valium)‡	4-40mg/day	N/A								
HYDANTOINS										
Ethotoin (Peganone)	2000-3000mg/day	N/A				X	X			
Phenytoin (Dilantin, Phenytek)	300-600mg/day (Suspension: 375-625mg/day)	10-20mcg/mL				X	X			
SUCCINIMIDES										
Ethosuximide (Zarontin)	500-1500mg/day	40-100mcg/mL	X							
Methsuximide (Celontin)	300-1200mg/day	N/A	X							
MISCELLANEOUS										
Carbamazepine (Carbatrol, Tegretol)	800-1200mg/day	4-12mcg/mL				X	X	X		
Divalproex sodium§ (Depakote, Depakote ER, Depakote Sprinkles)	10-60mg/kg/day	50-100mcg/mL	X		X	X	X			
Valproic acid§ (Depakene, Stavzor)			X		X	X	X			
Felbamate† (Felbatol)	2400-3600mg/day	N/A				X			X	
Gabapentin (Neurontin)	900-1800mg/day	N/A				X		X		

(Continued)

A235

GENERIC (BRAND)	USUAL ADULT DOSE*	THERAPEUTIC SERUM LEVELS	INDICATIONS						NEUROPATHIC PAIN	LENNOX-GASTAUT SYNDROME
			SEIZURE DISORDERS							
			ABSENCE	AKINETIC	MYOCLONIC	PARTIAL	TONIC-CLONIC			
MISCELLANEOUS *(Continued)*										
Lacosamide (Vimpat)	200-400mg/day	N/A				X				
Lamotrigine (Lamictal, Lamictal CD, Lamictal ODT, Lamictal XR)	100-500mg/day (Lamictal XR: 200-600mg/day)	N/A				X	X			X
Levetiracetam (Keppra, Keppra XR)	1000-3000mg/day	N/A			X	X	X			
Oxcarbazepine (Trileptal)	1200-2400mg/day	N/A				X				
Pregabalin (Lyrica)	150-600mg/day	N/A				X			X	
Rufinamide (Banzel)	3200mg/day	N/A								X
Tiagabine HCl (Gabitril)	32-56mg/day	N/A				X				
Topiramate (Topamax, Topamax Sprinkle)	200-400mg/day	N/A				X	X			X
Vigabatrin (Sabril)	3g/day	N/A				X				
Zonisamide (Zonegran)	100-400mg/day	N/A				X				

Abbreviation: N/A, not applicable.

* Refer to complete monograph for full dosing information including pediatric dosing.

† Phenobarbital is also indicated in generalized seizures.

‡ Oral Valium may be used adjunctively in convulsive disorders, although it has not proved useful as the sole therapy.

§ Divalproex sodium and Valproic acid are also indicated as adjuncts in mutiple seizure types.

¶ For severe epilepsy refractory to other treatment where the risk of aplastic anemia and/or liver failure is deemed acceptable. Fully advise patient and obtain written, informed consent before treatment. Closely monitor patient.

TRIPTANS FOR ACUTE MIGRAINE

GENERIC	BRAND	HOW SUPPLIED	INITIAL & (MAX) DOSE*	HEPATIC/RENAL DOSE ADJUSTMENT*
Almotriptan malate	Axert	**Tab:** 6.25mg, 12.5mg	6.25-12.5mg. May repeat after 2 hrs (25mg/24 hrs)	**Initial:** 6.25mg; **Max:** 12.5mg/24 hrs
Eletriptan HBr	Relpax	**Tab:** 20mg, 40mg	20-40mg. May repeat after 2 hrs (40mg/dose or 80mg/day)	**Severe Hepatic Impairment:** Avoid use
Frovatriptan succinate	Frova	**Tab:** 2.5mg	2.5mg. May repeat after 2 hrs (7.5mg/day)	No adjustment
Naratriptan HCl	Amerge	**Tab:** 1mg, 2.5mg	1-2.5mg. May repeat after 4 hrs (5mg/24 hrs)	**Severe Renal/Hepatic Impairment:** Avoid use **Mild-Moderate Renal/Hepatic Impairment:** Use lower dose; **Max:** 2.5mg/24 hrs
Rizatriptan benzoate	Maxalt	**Tab:** 5mg, 10mg	5-10mg. May repeat after 2 hrs (30mg/24 hrs)	No adjustment
	Maxalt-MLT	**Tab, Disintegrating:** 5mg, 10mg	5-10mg. May repeat after 2 hrs (30mg/24 hrs)	No adjustment
Sumatriptan	Alsuma, Imitrex, Sumavel DosePro	(Alsuma, Imitrex, Sumavel DosePro) **Inj†:** 6mg/0.5mL; (Imitrex) **Inj†, stat dose system:** 4mg, 6mg	(Alsuma, Imitrex, Sumavel DosePro) 6mg SQ. May repeat after 1 hr (6mg/dose or 12mg/24 hrs)	(Imitrex) **Severe Hepatic Impairment:** Avoid use
		Nasal Spray: 5mg, 20mg	5mg, 10mg, or 20mg single dose into 1 nostril. May repeat after 2 hrs (40mg/24 hrs)	**Severe Hepatic Impairment:** Avoid use
		Tab: 25mg, 50mg, 100mg	25-100mg. May repeat after 2 hrs (200mg/24 hrs)	**Severe Hepatic Impairment:** Avoid use; **Hepatic Disease: Max:** 50mg/single dose
Zolmitriptan	Zomig	**Nasal Spray:** 5mg	5mg. May repeat after 2 hrs (10mg/24 hrs)	**Hepatic Impairment:** Use doses <2.5mg of alternate formulation
		Tab: 2.5mg, 5mg	2.5mg or lower. May repeat after 2 hrs (10mg/24 hrs)	**Hepatic Impairment:** Use lower dose
	Zomig-ZMT	**Tab, Disintegrating:** 2.5mg, 5mg	2.5mg. May repeat after 2 hrs (10mg/24 hrs)	**Hepatic Impairment:** Use lower dose
COMBINATION DRUG				
Naproxen-Sumatriptan	Treximet	**Tab:** (Naproxen-Sumatriptan): 500mg/85mg [9ˢ]	1 tab; may repeat after 2 hrs (2 tabs/24 hrs). Do not split, crush, or chew	**Hepatic Impairment/Advanced Renal Disease (CrCl <30mL/min):** Avoid use.

*Dosages shown are for adults ≥18 yrs. For more detailed information, refer to the individual monograph or the drug's FDA-approved labeling.
†Also indicated for acute treatment of cluster headaches.

FERTILITY AGENTS*

GENERIC (BRAND)	INDICATIONS	HOW SUPPLIED	DOSAGE†
Cetrorelix acetate (Cetrotide)	For the inhibition of premature LH surges in women undergoing controlled ovarian stimulation.	**Inj:** 0.25mg, 3mg [packaged trays]	**Multiple-Dose Regimen:** 0.25mg SQ once daily; start either on stimulation Day 5 (AM or evening) or Day 6 (AM). Continue daily until hCG administration day. **Single-Dose Regimen:** 3mg SQ when serum estradiol level indicates appropriate stimulation response, usually on stimulation Day 7 (range: Day 5-9). If hCG was not given within 4 days after Cetrotide 3mg injection, Cetrotide 0.25mg should be given SQ once daily until the day of hCG administration.
Choriogonadotropin alfa (Ovidrel)	For the induction of final follicular maturation and early luteinization in infertile women who have undergone pituitary desensitization and have been appropriately pretreated with follicle-stimulating hormones as part of an assisted reproductive technology (ART) program such as in vitro fertilization and embryo transfer. Also indicated for the induction of ovulation (OI) and pregnancy in anovulatory infertile patients in whom the cause of infertility is functional and is not due to primary ovarian failure.	**Inj:** 250µg/0.5mL [prefilled syringe]	250µg SQ one day following the last dose of the follicle-stimulating agent. Do not administer until adequate follicular development is indicated by serum estradiol and vaginal ultrasonography. Administration should be withheld in situations where there is an excessive ovarian response.
Chorionic gonadotropin (Novarel, Pregnyl)	Induction of ovulation and pregnancy in the anovulatory, infertile woman in whom the cause of anovulation is secondary and not due to primary ovarian failure, and who has been appropriately pretreated with human menotropins.	**Inj:** 10,000 USP Units	5000-10,000 USP Units IM one day following the last dose of menotropins.
Clomiphene citrate (Clomid, Serophene)	Treatment of ovulatory dysfunction in women desiring pregnancy.	**Tab:** 50mg (scored)	Treatment should begin with a low dose, 50mg/day for 5 days. Therapy may be started any time in patients without recent uterine bleeding. If progestin-induced bleeding is intended, or if spontaneous bleeding occurs prior to therapy, start on or about the fifth day of the cycle. If ovulation does not appear to occur after the first course of therapy, a second course of 100mg as a single daily dose for 5 days should be given. This course may be started as early as 30 days after previous dose, after presence of pregnancy has been excluded. Increases in dosage or duration beyond 100mg/day for 5 days is not recommended. Further treatment is not recommended beyond 3 courses or 3 ovulatory responses without pregnancy. Long-term cyclic therapy is not recommended beyond a total of about 6 cycles. Patients should be evaluated to exclude pregnancy, ovarian enlargement, or ovarian cyst formation between each treatment cycle.

(Continued)

GENERIC (BRAND)	INDICATIONS	HOW SUPPLIED	DOSAGE†
Follitropin alfa (Gonal-f)	**Women:** For the development of multiple follicles in the ovulatory patient participating in an assisted reproductive technology (ART) program. Also, for the induction of ovulation and pregnancy in the anovulatory infertile patient in whom the cause of infertility is functional and not due to primary ovarian failure. **Men:** For the induction of spermatogenesis in men with primary and secondary hypogonadotropic hypogonadism in whom the cause of infertility is not due to primary testicular failure.	**Inj:** 450 IU, 1050 IU [multiple-dose vials]	Dosage must be individualized for each patient. **Infertile Patients with Oligo-Anovulation: Initial:** 75 IU/day SQ. **Titrate:** May consider an incremental adjustment in dose of up to 37.5 IU after 14 days. Further dose increases of same magnitude could be made if necessary every 7 days. Treatment should not exceed 35 days of therapy unless an E2 rise indicates imminent follicular development. To complete follicular development and effect ovulation in the absence of endogenous LH surge, hCG 5000 Units should be given 1 day after the last dose. Doses larger than 300 IU/day are not routinely recommended. **ART:** Therapy should be initiated in the early follicular phase (cycle day 2 or 3) at a dose of 150 IU/day until sufficient follicular development is attained. In most cases, therapy should not exceed 10 days. If patient's endogenous gonadotropin levels are suppressed, initiate therapy at 225 IU/day. Treatment should be continued until adequate follicular development is indicated. Adjustments to dose may be considered after 5 days based on patient's response; subsequently, dosage should be adjusted no more frequently than every 3-5 days and by no more than 75-150 IU additionally per adjustment. Doses greater than 450 IU/day are not recommended. Once follicular development is evident, hCG 5000-10,000 Units should be given to induce maturation in preparation for oocyte retrieval. Withhold hCG if ovaries are abnormally enlarged on the last day of therapy. **Hypogonadotropic Hypogonadism:** Must be given in conjunction with hCG. Pretreatment with hCG alone 1000-2250 U 2-3x/week is required. After normal serum testosterone levels are reached, the recommended dosage is 150 IU SQ 3x/week and hCG 1000 units (or dose needed to maintain normal serum testosterone levels) 3x/week. Dose of Gonal-f may be increased to a maximum dose of 300 IU 3x/week prn. Treatment may be needed for up to 18 months.
Follitropin alfa (Gonal-f RFF)	For development of multiple follicles in the ovulatory patient participating in an assisted reproductive technology (ART) program. Also for the induction of ovulation and pregnancy in the oligo-anovulatory infertile patient in whom the cause of infertility is functional and not due to primary ovarian failure.	**Inj:** [vial] 75 IU [prefilled pen] 300 IU/0.5mL, 450 IU/0.75mL, 900 IU/1.5mL	Dosage must be individualized for each patient. **Infertile Patients with Oligo-Anovulation:** Recommended initial dose for the first cycle is 75 IU/day SQ. Incremental adjustment in dose of up to 37.5 IU may be considered after 14 days. Further dose increases of the same magnitude could be made every 7 days if needed. Duration should not exceed 35 days of therapy unless an E2 rise indicates imminent follicular development. To complete follicular development and effect ovulation in the absence of endogenous LH surge, hCG should be given after the last dose. Doses larger than 300 IU/day are not routinely recommended. **ART:** Therapy should be initiated in the early follicular phase (cycle day 2 or 3) at a dose of 150 IU/day SQ until sufficient follicular development (usually not >10 days). If endogenous gonadotropin levels are suppressed, initiate at 150 IU/day for patients <35 yrs of age and 225 IU/day for patients ≥35 years of age. Treatment should be continued until adequate follicular development is indicated. Adjustments to dose may be considered after 5 days based on patient response; subsequent adjustments should be made no more than every 3-5 days and not more than 75-150 IU additionally at each adjustment. Doses greater than 450 IU per day are not recommended. hCG should be administered if adequate follicular development is evident to induce maturation and prepare for oocyte retrieval. Withhold hCG if ovaries are abnormally enlarged on the last day of therapy.

GENERIC (BRAND)	INDICATIONS	HOW SUPPLIED	DOSAGE†
Follitropin beta (Follistim AQ)	**Women: (Cartridge and Inj)** For the induction of ovulation and pregnancy in anovulatory infertile patients in whom the cause of infertility is functional and not due to primary ovarian failure. **(Inj)** For the development of multiple follicles in ovulatory women participating in an assisted reproductive technology (ART) program. **(Cartridge)** For pregnancy in normal ovulatory women undergoing controlled ovarian stimulation as part of an in vitro fertilization (IVF) or intracytoplasmic sperm injection (ICSI) cycle. **Men: (Cartridge and Inj)** For the induction of spermatogenesis in men with primary and secondary hypogonadotropic hypogonadism in whom the cause of infertility is not due to primary testicular failure.	**Cartridge:** 175 IU/0.210 mL, 350 IU/0.420mL, 650 IU/0.780mL, 975 IU/1.170 mL. **Inj:** 75 IU/0.5mL, 150 IU/0.5mL	Dosing scheme is stepwise and individualized for each woman. **Ovulation Induction (Cartridge):** Starting daily dose of 50 IU SQ qd for at least 7 days. Subsequent dosage adjustments are made at weekly intervals based on ovarian response. Increases should be made by 25 or 50 IUs per week until adequate ovarian response. Maximum daily dose is 250 IU. **(Inj):** Starting daily dose of 75 IU IM or SQ for at least the first 7 days of treatment. Dose is increased by 25-50 IU at weekly intervals until adequate response is indicated. The maximum daily dose is 300 IU. **(Cartridge/Inj):** hCG 5000-10,000 IU is administered to achieve final oocyte maturation when acceptable preovulatory state conditions are achieved. **Controlled Ovarian Stimulation (Cartridge):** Starting dose of 200 IU SQ qd for at least the first 7 days. **Titrate:** Adjust dose (down or up) based on ovarian response. Maximum daily dose is 500 IU. When a sufficient number of follicles of adequate size are present, dosing is stopped and final oocyte maturation is induced by administering hCG 5000-10,000 IU. Oocyte retrieval should be performed 34-36 hours after hCG. **ART (Inj):** Starting dose of 150-225 IU SQ/IM qd for at least the first 4 days of treatment. Dosage adjustments are based upon ovarian response. Maximum daily dose is 600 IU. Final oocyte maturation is induced with a dose of hCG 5000-10,000 IU. Oocyte retrieval is performed 34-36 hours later. **Induction of Spermatogenesis (Cartridge/Inj):** Pretreatment with hCG alone (1500 IU 2×/week) is required. hCG may be increased to 3000 IU 2×/week if serum testosterone levels have not normalized after 8 weeks of treatment. After normalization, administer Follistim AQ 450 IU/week SQ (either 225 IU 2×/week or 150 IU 3×/week) with the same pretreatment hCG dose used to normalize testosterone levels. May consider a lower dose with cartridge. Concomitant therapy should be continued for at least 3-4 months.
Ganirelix acetate	For inhibition of premature LH surges in women undergoing controlled ovarian hyperstimulation.	**Inj:** 250µg/0.5mL [prefilled syringe]	After initiating FSH therapy on Day 2 or 3 of the cycle, give 250µg SQ once daily during the mid-to-late portion of the follicular phase. Should be continued daily until the day of hCG administration.
Lutropin alfa (Luveris)	Concomitantly administered with Gonal-f (follitropin alfa) for stimulation of follicular development in infertile hypogonadotropic hypogonadal women with profound LH deficiency (LH<1.2 IU/L).	**Inj:** 75 IU	75 IU concomitantly administered SQ with 75-150 IU of Gonal-f daily as two separate injections in the initial treatment cycle. Treatment duration should not normally exceed 14 days of therapy unless signs of imminent follicular development are present. hCG should be given 1 day after the last dose. Doses administered in subsequent cycles should be individualized based on prior response. Doses of Gonal-f greater than 225 IU/day are not routinely recommended.

(Continued)

GENERIC (BRAND)	INDICATIONS	HOW SUPPLIED	DOSAGE†
Menotropins (Repronex)	In conjunction with hCG, for multiple follicular development (controlled ovarian stimulation) and ovulation induction in patients who have previously received pituitary suppression.	**Inj:** (FSH-LH) 75 IU-75 IU, 150 IU-150 IU	**Infertile Patients with Oligo-Anovulation:** Dose must be individualized for each patient. The recommended initial dose for patients who have received GnRH agonist or antagonist pituitary suppression is 150 IU daily SQ/IM for the first 5 days of treatment. Based on clinical monitoring, subsequent dosing should be based on patient response. Adjustments in dose should not be made more frequently than once every 2 days and should not exceed more than 75 to 150 IU per adjustment. Maximum daily dosage should not exceed 450 IU/day and dosing beyond 12 days is not recommended. If patient response is appropriate, 5000-10,000 U hCG should be given 1 day following the last dose. Patients should be followed closely for 2 weeks after hCG administration. May repeat course if necessary. **ART:** The recommended initial dose for patients who have received GnRH agonist or antagonist pituitary suppression is 225 IU SQ/IM. Based on clinical monitoring, subsequent dosing should be based on individual response. Adjustments should not be made more frequently than once every 2 days and not exceed 75-150 IU/adjustment. Maximum daily dose should not exceed 450 IU. Dosing >12 days is not recommended. Once adequate follicular development is evident, 5000-10,000 U hCG should be administered to induce maturation in preparation for oocyte retrieval.
Menotropins (Menopur)	Development of multiple follicles and pregnancy in ovulatory patients participating in an assisted reproductive technology (ART) program.	**Inj:** (FHS-LH) 75 IU-75 IU	Recommended initial dose for patients who have received a GnRH agonist for pituitary suppression is 225 IU SQ. Subsequent dosing based on clinical monitoring should be adjusted according to individual response and not made more frequently than once every 2 days (should not exceed 150 IU/adjustment). The maximum daily dose is 450 IU/day. Dosing beyond 20 days is not recommended. hCG should be administered once adequate follicular development is evident.
Progesterone (Crinone, Prochieve)	Progesterone replacement or supplementation as part of an assisted reproductive technology (ART) treatment for infertile women with progesterone deficiency.	**Gel:** 8% [90mg] single-use prefilled vaginal applicators	**ART:** 90mg vaginally once daily in women who require progesterone supplementation. The dosage for women with partial or complete ovarian failure who require progesterone replacement is 90mg vaginally bid. If pregnancy occurs, treatment may be continued until placental autonomy is achieved, up to 10-12 weeks.
Progesterone (Endometrin)	To support embryo implantation and early pregnancy by supplementation of corpus luteal function as part of an assisted reproductive technology (ART) treatment program for infertile women.	**Vaginal Insert:** 100mg [21s]	100mg vaginally bid or tid starting the day after oocyte retrieval and continuing for up to 10 weeks total duration.

GENERIC (BRAND)	INDICATIONS	HOW SUPPLIED	DOSAGE†
Urofollitropin (Bravelle)	**Ovulation Induction:** Administered SQ or IM in conjunction with hCG in patients who have previously received pituitary suppression. **Multifollicular Development during ART:** Administered SQ in conjunction with hCG, for multiple follicular development (controlled ovarian stimulation) during assisted reproductive technology (ART) cycles in patients who previously received pituitary suppression.	**Inj:** 75 IU	**Infertile Patients with Oligo-Anovulation:** Dose must be individualized for each patient. The recommended initial dose for patients who have received GnRH agonist or antagonist pituitary suppression is 150 IU daily SQ/IM for the first 5 days of treatment. Subsequent dosing is based on clinical monitoring and should be adjusted to individual response. Dose adjustments should not be made more frequently than once every 2 days and should not exceed more than 75-150 IU/adjustment. The maximum daily dose should not exceed 450 IU/day. In most cases, dosing beyond 12 days is not recommended. If patient response is appropriate, hCG 5000-10,000 U should be given 1 day following the last dose of Bravelle. Patients should be followed closely for at least 2 weeks following hCG administration. May repeat course if inadequate follicle development or ovulation without pregnancy occurs. **ART:** The recommended initial dose for patients undergoing IVF and donor egg patients who have received GnRH agonist or antagonist pituitary suppression is 225 IU SQ qd for the first 5 days of treatment. Adjust subsequent doses to individual response based on clinical monitoring at intervals not more frequently than every 2 days (should not exceed 75-150 IU/adjustment). Maximum daily dose should not exceed 450 IU/day. In most cases, dosing beyond 12 days is not recommended. Once adequate follicular development is evident; hCG 5000-10,000 IU should be administered to induce maturation in preparation for oocyte retrieval.

*Refer to full FDA-approved prescribing information for details.

†Do not administer hCG if ovaries are abnormally enlarged or excessive estradiol production has occurred on the last day of therapy.

GYNECOLOGICAL ANTI-INFECTIVES

DRUG	CLASS	FORMULATION	ROUTE	RECOMMENDED DOSAGE
ANTIBACTERIALS				
Clindamycin				
Cleocin Vaginal	RX	**Cre:** 2%	Vaginal	**Bacterial Vaginosis: Adults:** 1 applicatorful qhs x 3-7 days (nonpregnant) or x 7 days (2nd or 3rd trimester).
Cleocin Vaginal Ovules	RX	**Sup:** 100mg	Vaginal	**Bacterial Vaginosis: Adults:** 1 sup qhs x 3 days (nonpregnant).
Clindesse	RX	**Cre:** 2%	Vaginal	**Bacterial Vaginosis: Adults:** 1 applicatorful once (nonpregnant).
Metronidazole				
Flagyl*	RX	**Cap:** 375mg; **Tab:** 250mg, 500mg	Oral	**Trichomoniasis: Adults:** (Cap) 375mg bid; (Tab) 250mg tid x 7 days. **Alternate regimen (Tab):** If nonpregnant, 2g as single or divided dose.
Flagyl ER*	RX	**Tab, ER:** 750mg	Oral	**Bacterial Vaginosis: Adults:** 750mg qd x 7 days.
MetroGel Vaginal	RX	**Gel:** 0.75%	Vaginal	**Bacterial Vaginosis: Adults:** 1 applicatorful qd-bid x 5 days. For qd dosing, administer qhs.
Vandazole	RX	**Gel:** 0.75%	Vaginal	**Bacterial Vaginosis: Adults:** 1 applicatorful qhs x 5 days (nonpregnant).
MISCELLANEOUS				
Tindamax	RX	**Tab:** 250mg, 500mg	Oral	**Bacterial Vaginosis:** 2g qd for 2 days or 1g qd for 5 days (nonpregnant). **Trichomoniasis:** 2g single dose. Treat sexual partner with same dose and at same time.
ANTIFUNGALS: CANDIDIASIS TREATMENT				
Butoconazole				
Gynazole-1	RX	**Cre:** 2%	Vaginal	**Adults:** 1 applicatorful single dose.
Clotrimazole				
Gyne-Lotrimin 3	OTC	**Cre:** 2%	Vaginal	**Adults/Peds ≥12 yrs:** 1 applicatorful qhs x 3 days.
Gyne-Lotrimin 7	OTC	**Cre:** 1%	Vaginal	**Adults/Peds ≥12 yrs:** 1 applicatorful qhs x 7 days.
Fluconazole				
Diflucan	RX	**Tab:** 150mg	Oral	**Adults:** 150mg single dose.
Miconazole				
Monistat 1 Combination Pack	OTC	**External Cre:** 2% + **Ovule Insert:** 1200mg	Vaginal	**Adults/Peds ≥12 yrs:** 1 sup single dose hs. Apply cream externally bid up to 7 days prn.
Monistat 3	OTC	**Cre:** 4%	Vaginal	**Adults/Peds ≥12 yrs:** 1 applicatorful qhs x 3 days.
Monistat 3 Combination Pack	OTC	**External Cre:** 2% + **Ovule Insert:** 200mg or **Cre:** 4%	Vaginal	**Adults/Peds ≥12 yrs:** 1 sup or applicatorful qhs x 3 days. Apply cream bid externally up to 7 days prn.
Monistat 7	OTC	**Cre:** 2%	Vaginal	**Adults/Peds ≥12 yrs:** 1 applicatorful qhs x 7 days. Apply cream bid externally up to 7 days prn.
Monistat 7 Combination Pack	OTC	**Cre:** 2% + **External Cre:** 2%	Vaginal	**Adults/Peds ≥12 yrs:** 1 applicatorful qhs x 7 days. **(External Cream)** Apply cream bid externally up to 7 days prn.

DRUG	CLASS	FORMULATION	ROUTE	RECOMMENDED DOSAGE
ANTIFUNGALS: CANDIDIASIS TREATMENT *(Continued)*				
Sulfanilamide				
AVC	RX	**Cre:** 15%	Vaginal	**Adults:** 1 applicatorful qd-bid x 30 days.
Terconazole				
Terazol 3	RX	**Cre:** 0.8%; **Sup:** 80mg	Vaginal	**Adults:** 1 applicatorful or 1 sup qhs x 3 days.
Terazol 7	RX	**Cre:** 0.4%	Vaginal	**Adults:** 1 applicatorful qhs x 7 days.
Tioconazole				
Monistat 1, Vagistat 1	OTC	**Oint:** 6.5%	Vaginal	**Adults/Peds ≥12 yrs:** 1 applicatorful single dose hs.
*Contraindicated in first trimester.				

HORMONE THERAPY

GENERIC	BRAND	STRENGTH (MG)*
INTRAMUSCULAR ESTROGEN PRODUCTS		
Estradiol valerate	Delestrogen	10mg/mL, 20mg/mL, 40mg/mL
Estradiol cypionate	Depo-Estradiol	5mg/mL
ORAL ESTROGEN PRODUCT		
Conjugated estrogens	Premarin	0.3, 0.45, 0.625, 0.9, 1.25
ORAL SYNTHETIC CONJUGATED ESTROGEN PRODUCTS		
Estradiol acetate	Femtrace	0.45, 0.9, 1.8
Synthetic conjugated estrogens	Cenestin	0.3, 0.45, 0.625, 0.9, 1.25
	Enjuvia	0.3, 0.45, 0.625, 0.9, 1.25
Esterified estrogens	Menest	0.3, 0.625, 1.25, 2.5
Micronized 17β-estradiol	Estrace	0.5, 1, 2
Estropipate	(Generic)	0.75 (0.625), 1.5 (1.25), 3 (2.5), 6 (5)
TRANSDERMAL ESTROGEN PRODUCTS		
17β-estradiol matrix patch	Alora	0.025, 0.05, 0.075, 0.1
	Climara	0.025, 0.0375, 0.05, 0.06, 0.075, 0.1
	Vivelle, Vivelle-Dot	(Vivelle) 0.05, 0.1; (Vivelle-Dot) 0.025, 0.0375, 0.05, 0.075, 0.1
17β-estradiol	Divigel	0.1% gel
17β-estradiol reservoir patch	Estraderm	0.05, 0.1
17β-estradiol	Elestrin	0.06% gel
17β-estradiol	Estrogel	0.06% gel
17β-estradiol hemihydrate	Estrasorb	(emulsion): 4.35mg/1.74g
17β-estradiol	Evamist	(spray): 1.53mg/spray
VAGINAL ESTROGEN PRODUCTS		
VAGINAL CREAMS		
17β-estradiol	Estrace Vaginal Cream	0.01%
Conjugated estrogens	Premarin Vaginal Cream	0.625mg/g
Estropipate	Ogen Vaginal Cream	1.5mg/g
VAGINAL RING		
17β-estradiol	Estring	2mg
	Femring	0.05 or 0.1mg/day
VAGINAL TABLET		
Estradiol hemihydrate	Vagifem	10mcg
ORAL PROGESTOGEN-ONLY PRODUCTS		
Medroxyprogesterone acetate	Provera	2.5, 5, 10
Norethindrone acetate	Aygestin	5
Progesterone USP (in peanut oil)	Prometrium	100, 200
ESTROGEN + PROGESTOGEN COMBINATIONS		
ORAL CONTINUOUS-CYCLIC REGIMEN		
Conjugated estrogens (E) + Medroxyprogesterone acetate (P)	Premphase	0.625mg (E), 0.625mg (E) + 5mg (P)
17β-estradiol (E) + Norgestimate (P)	Prefest	1mg (E), 0.09mg (P)+ 1mg (E)

(Continued)

GENERIC	BRAND	STRENGTH (MG)*
ESTROGEN + PROGESTOGEN COMBINATIONS *(Continued)*		
ORAL CONTINUOUS-COMBINED REGIMEN		
Conjugated equine estrogens (E) + Medroxyprogesterone (P)	Prempro	0.3mg (E) + 1.5mg (P); 0.45mg (E) + 1.5mg (P); 0.625mg + 2.5 or 5mg (P)
Estradiol (E) + Drospirenone (P)	Angeliq	0.5mg (E) + 0.25 (P); 1mg (E) + 0.5mg (P)
Ethinyl estradiol (E) + Norethindrone acetate (P)	Femhrt	2.5mcg (E) + 0.5mg (P); 5mcg (E) + 1mg (P)
17β-estradiol (E) + Norethindrone acetate (P)	Activella	1mg (E) + 0.5mg (P); 0.5mg (E) + 0.1mg (P)
TRANSDERMAL CONTINUOUS-CYCLIC OR CONTINUOUS-COMBINED REGIMEN		
17β-estradiol (E) + Norethindrone acetate (P)	CombiPatch	0.05mg/day (E) + 0.14 or 0.25mg/day (P)
Estradiol (E) + Levonorgestrel (P)	Climara Pro	0.045mg/day (E) + 0.015mg/day (P)

NOTE: This list is not inclusive of all estrogen and progestogen products available. Indications vary among the different products. For more detailed information, please refer to the individual monograph listings or the drug's FDA-approved labeling. Unopposed estrogen replacement therapy (ERT) is for use in women without an intact uterus. For women with an intact uterus, progestin must be added to the ERT for protection against estrogen-induced endometrial cancer. As with any therapy, the lowest possible effective dosage should be used. Re-evaluate periodically.

*Units are in mg unless otherwise stated.

ORAL CONTRACEPTIVES

DRUG	ESTROGEN	PROGESTIN	STRENGTH (ESTROGEN/PROGESTIN)
MONOPHASIC			
[Aviane 28, Lessina 28, Lutera, Orsythia, Sronyx 28]*	Ethinyl estradiol	Levonorgestrel	20mcg/0.1mg
Beyaz†, YAZ [Gianvi, Loryna, Vestura]*	Ethinyl estradiol	Drospirenone	20mcg/3mg
Brevicon, Modicon [Necon 0.5/35, Nortrel 0.5/35]*	Ethinyl estradiol	Norethindrone	35mcg/0.5mg
Desogen [Apri, Emoquette, Reclipsen, Solia]*	Ethinyl estradiol	Desogestrel	30mcg/0.15mg
Femcon Fe, Ovcon 35 [Balziva, Briellyn, Philith, Zenchent, Zenchent Fe]*	Ethinyl estradiol	Norethindrone	35mcg/0.4mg
Loestrin 21 1/20, Loestrin Fe 1/20 [Gildess Fe 1/20, Junel 1/20, Junel Fe 1/20, Microgestin 1/20, Microgestin Fe 1/20]* Loestrin 24 Fe	Ethinyl estradiol	Norethindrone acetate	20mcg/1mg
Loestrin 21 1.5/30, Loestrin Fe 1.5/30 [Gildess 1.5/30, Junel 1.5/30, Junel Fe 1.5/30, Microgestin 1.5/30, Microgestin Fe 1.5/30]*	Ethinyl estradiol	Norethindrone acetate	30mcg/1.5mg
Lo/Ovral [Cryselle, Low-Ogestrel-28]*	Ethinyl estradiol	Norgestrel	30mcg/0.3mg
Lybrel [Amethyst]*	Ethinyl estradiol	Levonorgestrel	20mcg/0.09mg
Nordette-28 [Altavera, Levora, Marlissa, Portia 28]*	Ethinyl estradiol	Levonorgestrel	30mcg/0.15mg
Norinyl 1/35, Ortho-Novum 1/35 [Alyacen 1/35, Cyclafem 1/35, Dasetta 1/35, Necon 1/35, Norethin 1/35E, Nortrel 1/35]*	Ethinyl estradiol	Norethindrone	35mcg/1mg
[Norinyl 1/50, Necon 1/50]*	Mestranol	Norethindrone	50mcg/1mg
Ortho-Cyclen [MonoNessa, Previfem, Sprintec]*	Ethinyl estradiol	Norgestimate	35mcg/0.25mg
Ovcon 50‡	Ethinyl estradiol	Norethindrone	50mcg/1mg
Ogestrel 28˙	Ethinyl estradiol	Norgestrel	50mcg/0.5mg
Safyral†, Yasmin [Ocella, Syeda, Zarah]*	Ethinyl estradiol	Drospirenone	30mcg/3mg
Seasonale [Jolessa, Introvale, Quasense]*	Ethinyl estradiol	Levonorgestrel	30mcg/0.15mg
Zovia 1/35E [Kelnor]*	Ethinyl estradiol	Ethynodiol diacetate	35mcg/1mg
Zovia 1/50E*	Ethinyl estradiol	Ethynodiol diacetate	50mcg/1mg
BIPHASIC			
Mircette [Azurette, Kariva]*	Ethinyl estradiol	Desogestrel	**Phase 1:** 20mcg/0.15mg **Phase 2:** 10mcg/NONE
Lo Loestrin Fe‡	Ethinyl estradiol	Norethindrone acetate	**Phase 1:** 10mcg/1mg **Phase 2:** 10mcg/NONE
Loseasonique [Amethia Lo]*	Ethinyl estradiol	Levonorgestrel	**Phase 1:** 20mcg/0.1mg **Phase 2:** 10mcg/NONE
Necon 10/11*	Ethinyl estradiol	Norethindrone	**Phase 1:** 35mcg/0.5mg **Phase 2:** 35mcg/1mg

(Continued)

DRUG	ESTROGEN	PROGESTIN	STRENGTH (ESTROGEN/PROGESTIN)
BIPHASIC *(Continued)*			
Seasonique (Amethia, Camrese)*	Ethinyl estradiol	Levonorgestrel	**Phase 1:** 30mcg/0.15mg **Phase 2:** 10mcg/NONE
TRIPHASIC			
Cyclessa (Caziant, Cesia, Velivet)*	Ethinyl estradiol	Desogestrel	**Phase 1:** 25mcg/0.1mg **Phase 2:** 25mcg/0.125mg **Phase 3:** 25mcg/0.15mg
Estrostep Fe (Tilia Fe, Tri-legest Fe)*	Ethinyl estradiol	Norethindrone acetate	**Phase 1:** 20mcg/1mg **Phase 2:** 30mcg/1mg **Phase 3:** 35mcg/1mg
Ortho Novum 7/7/7 [Alyacen 7/7/7, Cyclafem 7/7/7, Dasetta 7/7/7, Nortel 7/7/7]*	Ethinyl estradiol	Norethindrone	**Phase 1:** 35mcg/0.5mg **Phase 2:** 35mcg/0.75mg **Phase 3:** 35mcg/1mg
Ortho Tri-Cyclen [Tri-Previfem, Trinessa, Tri-Sprintec]*	Ethinyl estradiol	Norgestimate	**Phase 1:** 35mcg/0.18mg **Phase 2:** 35mcg/0.215mg **Phase 3:** 35mcg/0.25mg
Ortho Tri-Cyclen Lo (Tri Lo Sprintec)*	Ethinyl estradiol	Norgestimate	**Phase 1:** 25mcg/0.18mg **Phase 2:** 25mcg/0.215mg **Phase 3:** 25mcg/0.25mg
[Trivora 28, Enpresse 28, Levonest]*	Ethinyl estradiol	Levonorgestrel	**Phase 1:** 30mcg/0.05mg **Phase 2:** 40mcg/0.075mg **Phase 3:** 30mcg/0.125mg
Tri-Norinyl (Aranelle, Leena)*	Ethinyl estradiol	Norethindrone	**Phase 1:** 35mcg/0.5mg **Phase 2:** 35mcg/1mg **Phase 3:** 35mcg/0.5mg
FOUR-PHASE			
Natazia‡	Ethinyl valerate	Dienogest	**Phase 1:** 3mg/NONE **Phase 2:** 2mg/2mg **Phase 3:** 2mg/3mg **Phase 4:** 1mg/NONE
PROGESTIN-ONLY			
Nor-Q.D, Ortho-Micronor [Camila, Errin, Heather, Jolivette, Nora-BE]*		Norethindrone	0.35mg
Plan B [Next Choice]*		Levonorgestrel	0.75mg
Plan B One Step		Levonorgestrel	1.5mg
MISCELLANEOUS			
Ella§		Ulipristal acetate (progestin agonist/antagonist)	30mg

*Branded generics.
†Also contains levomefolate calcium.
‡Currently NO generics available.
§Selective progesterone receptor modulator.

BREAST CANCER RISK FACTORS

UNMODIFIABLE RISK FACTORS	
Gender	Women > Men
Age	1 out of 8 breast cancer diagnoses are in women <45 yrs, while about 2 out of 3 occur in women ≥55 yrs
Genetic	BRCA1 and BRCA2 gene mutations, single ATM gene mutation, CHEK2 gene mutation, TP53 tumor suppressor gene mutation, PTEN gene mutations, CDH1 gene mutation, STK11 gene mutation
Race	Whites > African Americans. Women <45 yrs: African Americans > Whites
Family history	Having a first-degree relative with breast cancer doubles risk; having 2 first-degree relatives increases risk about 3-fold. <15% of women with breast cancer have a significant family history of breast cancer
Personal history of breast cancer	Women with cancer in one breast have a 3- to 4-fold increased risk of developing a new cancer in another area of the same breast or in the opposite breast
Abnormal breast biopsy	Nonproliferative lesions, proliferative lesions with or without atypia. Women with a family history of breast cancer and hyperplasia or atypical hyperplasia have an even greater risk
Early menarche	Women who started menstruating at an early age (<12 yrs)
Age at menopause	Women who went through menopause at a late age (>55 yrs)
Personal history of breast abnormalities	Women with lobular carcinoma in situ (LCIS) have a 7- to 11-fold increased risk of developing cancer in either breast
Earlier breast radiation exposure	Women <40 who had radiation therapy to the chest area as treatment for another cancer
Breast density	Women with a higher proportion of dense breast tissue (eg, connective and milk duct tissue)

Lifestyle factors associated with increased risk of breast cancer

- Alcohol (2-5 drinks/day)
- High body mass index
- Not having children or having them when >30 yrs
- Lack of physical activity
- Not breastfeeding

Drugs associated with increased risk of breast cancer

- Oral contraceptives
- DES (diethylstilbestrol)
- Postmenopausal hormone therapy or hormone replacement therapy

Uncertain risk factors

- Antiperspirants
- Bras
- Breast implants
- High-fat diets
- Induced abortion
- Miscarriages
- Night work
- Pollution (chemicals)
- Smoking (active or passive)

Sources: American Cancer Society and National Cancer Institute.

BREAST CANCER TREATMENT OPTIONS

GENERIC (BRAND)	INDICATIONS	HOW SUPPLIED	DOSAGE‡
ANDROGENS			
Fluoxymesterone (Androxy)	Secondarily used in women with advancing inoperable metastatic (skeletal) mammary cancer who are 1-5 yrs postmenopausal.	**Tab:** 10mg* *scored	10-40mg/day in divided doses. Continue therapy for at least 3 months for objective response. **Advanced Mammary Carcinoma:** Duration depends on response and appearance of adverse effects.
Methyltestosterone (Testred)	Secondarily used in women with advancing inoperable metastatic (skeletal) mammary cancer who are 1-5 yrs postmenopausal.	**Cap:** 10mg	50-200mg/day.
Testosterone (Delatestryl)	Secondarily used in women with advancing inoperable metastatic (skeletal) mammary cancer who are 1-5 yrs postmenopausal.	**Inj:** 200mg/mL [5mL]	200-400mg IM every 2-4 weeks.
ANTIESTROGEN			
Fulvestrant (Faslodex)	Treatment of hormone receptor-positive metastatic breast cancer in postmenopausal women with disease progression following anti-estrogen therapy.	**Inj:** 50mg/mL [5mL]	500mg IM into the buttocks slowly (1-2 min/inj) as two 5mL injections, one in each buttock, on Days 1, 15, 29, and once monthly thereafter.
ESTROGENS			
Conjugated estrogens (Premarin Tablets)	Palliative treatment of breast cancer in selected patients with metastatic disease.	**Tab:** 0.3mg, 0.45mg, 0.625mg, 0.9mg, 1.25mg	10mg tid for at least 3 months.
Esterified estrogens (Menest)	Palliative therapy of breast cancer in selected patients with metastatic disease.	**Tab:** 0.3mg, 0.625mg, 1.25mg, 2.5mg	10mg tid for at least 3 months.
Estradiol (Estrace)	Palliative treatment of breast cancer in selected patients with metastatic disease.	**Tab:** 0.5mg*, 1mg*, 2mg* *scored	10mg tid for at least 3 months.
LHRH AGONIST			
Goserelin (Zoladex 1-Month)	Palliative treatment of advanced breast cancer in pre- and perimenopausal women.	**Implant:** 3.6mg	3.6mg SQ every 28 days into anterior abdominal wall below navel line.
PROGESTIN			
Megestrol acetate	Palliative treatment of advanced breast carcinoma (eg, recurrent, inoperable, or metastatic disease).	**Tab:** 20mg*, 40mg* *scored	40mg qid for at least 2 months.
SELECTIVE ESTROGEN RECEPTOR MODULATORS			
Raloxifene (Evista)	Reduction in risk of invasive breast cancer in postmenopausal women with osteoporosis or at high risk for invasive breast cancer.	**Tab:** 60mg	60mg qd. Optimum duration of treatment is not known.
Tamoxifen citrate	Treatment of metastatic breast cancer in women and men. Treatment of node-positive (in postmenopausal women) and axillary node-negative breast cancer in women following mastectomy, axillary dissection, and breast irradiation. To reduce risk of invasive breast cancer in women with DCIS (ductal carcinoma in-situ) following breast surgery and radiation. Reduction of breast cancer incidence in high-risk women (at least 35 yrs of age with a 5-year predicted risk of breast cancer ≥1.67%; refer to PI for more details).	**Tab:** 10mg, 20mg	20-40mg qd for 5 yrs. Divide dosages >20mg into AM and PM doses. **Risk Reduction/DCIS:** 20mg qd for 5 yrs.

(Continued)

GENERIC (BRAND)	INDICATIONS	HOW SUPPLIED	DOSAGE‡
SELECTIVE ESTROGEN RECEPTOR MODULATORS *(Continued)*			
Toremifene (Fareston)	Treatment of metastatic breast cancer in postmenopausal women with estrogen receptor-positive or unknown tumors.	**Tab:** 60mg	60mg qd. Take until disease progression is evident.
SELECTIVE NONSTEROIDAL AROMATASE INHIBITORS (POSTMENOPAUSAL WOMEN ONLY)			
Anastrozole (Arimidex)	Adjuvant treatment of postmenopausal women with hormone receptor-positive early breast cancer. First-line treatment of postmenopausal women with hormone receptor-positive or hormone receptor-unknown locally advanced or metastatic breast cancer. Second-line treatment of advanced breast cancer in postmenopausal women with disease progression following tamoxifen therapy.	**Tab:** 1mg	1mg qd. Continue until tumor progression with advanced breast cancer.
Letrozole (Femara)	Adjuvant treatment of postmenopausal women with hormone receptor-positive early breast cancer. Extended adjuvant treatment of early breast cancer in post-menopausal women who have received 5 yrs of adjuvant tamoxifen therapy. First-line treatment of hormone receptor-positive or unknown locally advanced or metastatic breast cancer in postmenopausal women. Treatment of advanced breast cancer with disease progression following antiestrogen therapy in postmenopausal women.	**Tab:** 2.5mg	2.5mg qd. **First-Line Treatment:** Continue until tumor progression is evident. **Cirrhosis/Severe Liver Dysfunction:** 2.5mg every other day.
ANTHRACYCLINES			
Doxorubicin (Adriamycin)	To produce regression in disseminated neoplastic conditions such as breast carcinoma. Adjuvant therapy in women with evidence of axillary lymph node involvement following resection of primary breast cancer.	**Inj:** (2mg/mL) 10mg, 20mg, 50mg, 200mg	**Monotherapy:** 60-75mg/m² IV every 21 days. Use the lower dose with inadequate bone marrow reserves due to old age, prior therapy, or neoplastic marrow infiltration. **Concomitant Chemotherapy:** 40-60mg/m² IV every 21-28 days.
Epirubicin (Ellence)	Adjuvant treatment in patients with evidence of axillary node tumor involvement following resection of primary breast cancer.	**Inj:** 2mg/mL [25mL, 100mL]	**Initial:** 100-120mg/m² IV infusion, repeat at 3-4 week cycles. May give total dose on Day 1 of each cycle or divide equally on Days 1 and 8. **Bone Marrow Dysfunction: Initial:** 75-90mg/m².
ANTIMICROTUBULE AGENTS			
Eribulin (Halaven)	Treatment of metastatic breast cancer in patients who have previously received ≥2 chemotherapeutic regimens (should have included an anthracycline and a taxane in either the adjuvant or metastatic setting).	**Inj:** 0.5mg/mL [2mL]	Administer 1.4mg/m² IV over 2-5 min on Days 1 and 8 of a 21-day cycle.
Ixabepilone (Ixempra)	In combination with capecitabine for treatment of patients with metastatic or locally advanced breast cancer resistant to treatment with an anthracycline and a taxane, or whose cancer is taxane-resistant and for whom further anthracycline therapy is contraindicated. As monotherapy for treatment of metastatic or locally advanced breast cancer in patients whose tumors are resistant or refractory to anthracyclines, taxanes, and capecitabine.	**Inj:** 15mg, 45mg	40mg/m² IV infusion over 3 hrs every 3 weeks.

GENERIC (BRAND)	INDICATIONS	HOW SUPPLIED	DOSAGE‡
KINASE INHIBITOR			
Lapatinib (Tykerb)	Treatment of patients with advanced or metastatic breast cancer, in combination with capecitabine, whose tumors overexpress HER2 and who received prior therapy including an anthracycline, a taxane, and trastuzumab. In combination with letrozole for treatment of postmenopausal women with hormone receptor-positive metastatic breast cancer overexpressing HER2 receptor, for whom hormone therapy is indicated.	**Tab:** 250mg	Give at least 1 hr before or 1 hr after a meal. **HER2-Positive Metastatic Breast Cancer: Usual:** 1250mg qd on Days 1-21 with capecitabine 2000mg/m²/day (2 doses 12 hrs apart with food) on Days 1-14 in a repeating 21-day cycle. **Hormone Receptor-Positive, HER2-Positive Metastatic Breast Cancer:** 1500mg qd with letrozole 2.5mg.
MISCELLANEOUS			
Capecitabine (Xeloda)	Treatment of metastatic breast cancer in combination with docetaxel after failure of prior anthracycline-containing chemotherapy. Treatment of metastatic breast cancer in patients resistant to paclitaxel and anthracycline-containing chemotherapy or resistant to paclitaxel and for whom further anthracycline therapy is not indicated.	**Tab:** 150mg, 500mg	Take with water within 30 min after a meal. **Usual:** 1250mg/m² bid for 2 weeks, then 1 week off. Give as 3-week cycles. **Combination with Docetaxel: Usual:** 1250mg/m² bid for 2 weeks followed by 1-week rest period, combined with docetaxel 75mg/m² as 1 hr IV infusion q3 weeks.
Cyclophosphamide	Treatment of breast carcinoma.	**Inj:** 500mg, 1g, 2g; **Tab:** 25mg, 50mg	**Malignant Diseases (Without Hematologic Deficiency): Monotherapy: Initial:** 40-50mg/kg IV in divided doses over 2-5 days, or 10-15mg/kg IV given every 7-10 days, or 3-5mg/kg twice weekly. **Oral Dosing: Initial/Maint:** 1-5mg/kg/day PO. Adjust dose according to antitumor activity and/or leukopenia. May need to reduce dose when combined with other cytotoxic drugs.
Dexrazoxane (Zinecard)	To reduce the incidence and severity of cardiomyopathy associated with doxorubicin in women with metastatic breast cancer who received a cumulative doxorubicin dose of 300mg/m² and who will continue doxorubicin therapy to maintain tumor control.	**Inj:** 250mg, 500mg	**IV:** 10:1 ratio of Zinecard: doxorubicin (eg, 500mg/m² Zinecard: 50mg/m² doxorubicin). Give doxorubicin within 30 min after the start of infusion. Do not administer via IV push. **Hepatic Impairment:** Reduce dose proportionally. If CrCl <40 mL/min, the recommended dosage ration is 5:1 (Zinecard: doxorubicin).

(Continued)

GENERIC (BRAND)	INDICATIONS	HOW SUPPLIED	DOSAGE‡
MISCELLANEOUS *(Continued)*			
Fluorouracil	Palliative management of breast carcinoma.	**Inj:** 50mg/mL [10mL, 20mL, 50mL, 100mL]	12mg/kg IV qd for 4 days. **Max:** 800mg/day. If no toxicity, give 6mg/kg IV on 6th, 8th, 10th, and 12th days. Skip Days 5, 7, 9, and 11. Discontinue therapy at the end of Day 12. **Inadequate Nutritional State:** 6mg/kg IV for 3 days. If no toxicity, give 3mg/kg IV on 5th, 7th, and 9th days. **Max:** 400mg/day. Skip Days 4, 6, and 8. **Maint (Use Schedule 1 or Schedule 2):** Schedule 1: If no toxicity, repeat 1st course every 30 days after last day of previous course. Schedule 2: When toxic signs from initial course subside, give 10-15mg/kg/week IV single dose; do not exceed 1g/week.
Methotrexate	Alone or in combination with other anticancer agents in treatment of breast cancer.	**Inj:** 25mg/mL, 10mg/mL, **Tab:** 2.5mg†	Oral administration in tablet form is often preferred when low doses are being administered since absorption is rapid and effective serum levels are obtained. Methotrexate injection may be given by the intramuscular, intravenous, or intra-arterial route. Refer to PI for more information.
MONOCLONAL ANTIBODY/HER2 BLOCKER			
Trastuzumab (Herceptin)	Adjuvant treatment of HER2-overexpressing node-positive/negative breast cancer. 1st-line treatment of HER2-overexpressing metastatic breast cancer in combination with paclitaxel. Single agent for treatment of HER2-overexpressing breast cancer in patients who received 1 or more chemotherapy regimens for metastatic disease.	**Inj:** 440mg	**Adjuvant Treatment: During and Following Paclitaxel, Docetaxel, or Docetaxel/Carboplatin for 52 Weeks Total: Initial:** 4mg/kg IV infusion over 90 min. **Maint:** 2mg/kg IV infusion over 30 min weekly during chemotherapy for the first 12 weeks (paclitaxel or docetaxel) or 18 weeks (docetaxel/carboplatin). **1 Week Following the Last Weekly Dose of Herceptin:** 6mg/kg IV infusion over 30-90 min every 3 weeks. **Following Completion of Multimodality, Anthracycline-Based Regimen as a Single Agent: Initial:** 8mg/kg IV infusion over 90 min. **Maint:** 6mg/kg over 30-90 min every 3 weeks. **Metastatic Breast Cancer: Alone or with Paclitaxel:** Initial: 4mg/kg IV infusion over 90 min, then 2mg/kg IV infusion weekly over 30 min until disease progression.

GENERIC (BRAND)	INDICATIONS	HOW SUPPLIED	DOSAGE‡
NUCLEOSIDE ANALOGUE/ANTIMETABOLITE			
Gemcitabine (Gemzar)	Adjunct with paclitaxel for 1st-line treatment of metastatic breast cancer after failure of prior anthracycline-containing adjuvant chemotherapy, unless anthracyclines were clinically contraindicated.	**Inj:** 200mg, 1g	1250mg/m² IV over 30 min on Days 1 and 8 of each 21-day cycle. Give paclitaxel 175mg/m² as a 3-hr IV infusion on Day 1 before gemcitabine. Adjust dose based on hematologic toxicity.
TAXANES			
Docetaxel (Taxotere)	Treatment of locally advanced or metastatic breast cancer after failure of prior chemotherapy. In combination with doxorubicin and cyclophosphamide for the adjuvant treatment of operable, node-positive breast cancer.	**Inj:** 20mg/0.5mL, 80mg/2mL; (Generic) 20mg/2mL, 80mg/8mL, 160mg/16mL	**For Locally Advanced or Metastatic Breast Cancer:** 60-100mg/m² IV over 1 hr every 3 weeks. **Adjuvant Treatment of Operable Node-Positive Breast CA:** 75mg/m² 1 hr after doxorubicin 50mg/m² and cyclophosphamide 500mg/m² every 3 weeks for 6 courses.
Paclitaxel	Treatment of breast cancer after failure with combination chemotherapy for metastatic disease or relapse within 6 months of adjuvant chemotherapy; prior therapy should have included an anthracycline unless clinically contraindicated. Adjuvant treatment of node-positive breast cancer administered sequentially to doxorubicin-containing chemotherapy.	**Inj:** 6mg/mL	**Adjuvant Treatment of Node-Positive:** 175mg/m² IV over 3 hrs every 3 weeks for 4 courses given sequentially to doxorubicin-containing chemotherapy. Failure of initial chemotherapy for metastatic disease or relapse: 175mg/m² over 3 hrs every 3 weeks.
Paclitaxel protein-bound particle for injectable suspension (Abraxane)	Treatment of breast cancer after failure of combination chemotherapy for metastatic disease or relapse within 6 months of adjuvant chemotherapy. Prior therapy should have included an anthracycline unless clinically contraindicated.	**Inj:** 100mg	260mg/m² IV over 30 min every 3 weeks.
VINCA ALKALOID			
Vinblastine	Palliative treatment of breast carcinoma unresponsive to appropriate endocrine surgery and hormonal therapy.	**Inj:** 1mg/mL [10mL]	Dose at intervals of ≥7 days. **1st Dose:** 3.7mg/m². **2nd Dose:** 5.5mg/m². **3rd Dose:** 7.4mg/m². **4th Dose:** 9.25mg/m². **5th Dose:** 11.1mg/m². Max: 18.5mg/m². Do not increase dose after that dose which reduces WBC to 3000 cells/mm³. **Maint:** Use dose of 1 increment smaller than this dose at weekly intervals. Only dose if WBC ≥4000 cell/mm³.

For additional information, refer to the National Comprehensive Cancer Clinical Practice (NCCN) Guideline in Oncology, 2011.

‡Refer to complete prescribing information for premedication guidelines in regard to severe hypersensitivity reactions and for dosage adjustment.

CHEMOTHERAPY REGIMENS*†

CANCER TYPE	PREFERRED THERAPIES	ALTERNATIVE REGIMENS
BLADDER		
	Neoadjuvant, adjuvant, and metastatic: • Gemcitabine/cisplatin (preferred); or • Methotrexate/vinblastine/doxorubicin/cisplatin (MVAC)	**Neoadjuvant, adjuvant, and metastatic:** Carboplatin and taxane-based therapy or single-agent therapy
	Adjuvant intravesical treatment: Bacillus Calmette-Guerin (BCG)	**Adjuvant intravesical treatment:** Mitomycin C (MMC)
BREAST		
Adjuvant (trastuzumab-containing)	• Doxorubicin/cyclophosphamide followed by paclitaxel + trastuzumab (AC → T + trastuzumab) • Docetaxel, carboplatin, trastuzumab (TCH)	• Docetaxel + trastuzumab → fluorouracil/epirubicin/cyclophosphamide (FEC) • Chemotherapy followed by trastuzumab sequentially • (AC) → docetaxel + trastuzumab
Neoadjuvant (trastuzumab-containing)	• Paclitaxel + trastuzumab followed by cyclophosphamide/epirubicin/fluorouracil + trastuzumab (T + trastuzumab → CEF + trastuzumab)	
Adjuvant (non-trastuzumab containing)	• Docetaxel/doxorubicin/cyclophosphamide (TAC) • Dose-dense AC → paclitaxel every 2 weeks • (AC) → weekly paclitaxel • Docetaxel and cyclophosphamide (TC)	• Doxorubicin/cyclophosphamide (AC) • Fluorouracil/doxorubicin/cyclophosphamide (FAC/CAF) • Cyclophosphamide/epirubicin/fluorouracil (FEC/CEF) • Cyclophosphamide/methotrexate/fluorouracil (CMF) • (AC) → docetaxel every 3 weeks • Epirubicin/cyclophosphamide (EC) • Doxorubicin followed by paclitaxel followed by cyclophosphamide (every 2-week regimen) with filgrastim support (A → T → C) • Fluorouracil/epirubicin/cyclophosphamide followed by docetaxel (FEC → T) • Fluorouracil/epirubicin/cyclophosphamide followed by weekly paclitaxel (FEC → T)
Recurrent or metastatic	**Single agents:** • Anthracyclines: Doxorubicin, epirubicin, pegylated liposomal doxorubicin • Taxanes: paclitaxel, docetaxel, albumin-bound paclitaxel • Antimetabolites: capecitabine, gemcitabine • Other microtubule inhibitors: vinorelbine, eribulin	**Other single agents:** Cyclophosphamide, mitoxantrone, cisplatin, etoposide (PO), vinblastine, fluorouracil CI, ixabepilone
	Combinations: • Cyclophosphamide/doxorubicin/fluorouracil (CAF/FAC) • Fluorouracil/epirubicin/cyclophosphamide (FEC) • Doxorubicin/cyclophosphamide (AC) • Epirubicin/cyclophosphamide (EC); Doxorubicin/docetaxel • Doxorubicin/paclitaxel (AT) • Cyclophosphamide/methotrexate/fluorouracil (CMF) • Docetaxel/capecitabine • Gemcitabine/paclitaxel (GT)	**Other combinations:** Ixabepilone + capecitabine

(Continued)

CANCER TYPE	PREFERRED THERAPIES	ALTERNATIVE REGIMENS
BREAST *(Continued)*		
HER2-positive metastatic disease	**Trastuzumab with:** • Paclitaxel ± carboplatin • Docetaxel • Vinorelbine • Capecitabine **Trastuzumab-exposed** • Lapatinib + capecitabine • Trastuzumab + (other first-line agents) • Capecitabine or lapatinib (without cytotoxic therapy)	
COLORECTAL		
	High-risk Stage II/Adjuvant Stage III: • 5-FU/LV/oxaliplatin (mFOLFOX6) or • Bolus 5-FU/LV/oxaliplatin or • Capecitabine/oxaliplatin (CapeOx) **Advanced or metastatic disease:** (Intensive therapy appropriate) *Initial Therapy:* • (FOLFOX) ± bevacizumab or • CapeOX ± bevacizumab or • FOLFOX ± panitumumab (KRAS wild-type [WT] gene only) or • Irinotecan + LV + 5-FU (FOLFIRI) + bevacizumab or • FOLFIRI ± cetuximab or panitumumab (KRAS WT gene only) or • 5-FU/LV or capecitabine ± bevacizumab or • Irinotecan + LV + 5-FU + oxaliplatin (FOLFOXIRI). *Refer to NCCN guidelines for therapy after first and second progression and for nonintensive-therapy appropriate patients.*	**High-risk Stage II/Adjuvant Stage III:** • Single-agent capecitabine or • 5-FU/LV in patients felt to be inappropriate for oxaliplatin therapy
ESOPHAGEAL		
Definitive chemoradiation	• Cisplatin + fluoropyrimidine (5-FU or capecitabine) • Oxaliplatin + fluoropyrimidine (5-FU or capecitabine) • Paclitaxel and carboplatin • Docetaxel or paclitaxel + fluoropyrimidine • Oxaliplatin, docetaxel, and capecitabine	
Locally advanced or metastatic (chemoradiation not indicated)	• Trastuzumab (HER2-neu overexpressing adenocarcinoma) + cisplatin + fluoropyrimidine • Docetaxel/cisplatin/5-FU (DCF) • Epirubicin/cisplatin/5-FU (ECF) • Fluoropyrimidine (5-FU or capecitabine) + cisplatin	**DCF modifications:** • Docetaxel/5-FU + oxaliplatin or carboplatin **ECF modifications:** • Epirubicin + oxaliplatin/5-FU or • Cisplatin/capecitabine or • Oxaliplatin/capecitabine • Fluoropyrimidine + oxaliplatin or irinotecan • Paclitaxel with cisplatin or carboplatin • Docetaxel with cisplatin or irinotecan • Fluoropyrimidine (5-FU or capecitabine) • Docetaxel or paclitaxel • Trastuzumab + other chemotherapy agents <u>except</u> anthracyclines • Irinotecan and cisplatin or fluoropyrimidine, or docetaxel, or mitomycin

CANCER TYPE	PREFERRED THERAPIES	ALTERNATIVE REGIMENS
LEUKEMIA		
Acute lymphocytic leukemia (ALL)—Adults	**Induction:** • Vincristine + anthracycline + prednisone ± asparaginase ± cyclophosphamide** **Postremission therapy:** • Chemotherapy, ongoing treatment with a Bcr-abl tyrosine kinase inhibitor such as imatinib, nilotinib, or dasatinib	**Induction:** • Imatinib mesylate (Philadelphia [Ph1] positive ALL) **Recurrent:** • Dasatinib (imatinib-resistant BCR/ABL mutations or imatinib intolerance)
Acute myeloid leukemia (AML)	**Induction (pt <60):** • Standard-dose cytarabine + daunorubicin or idarubicin **Induction (pt ≥60):** • Standard-dose cytarabine + idarubicin or daunorubicin or mitoxantrone **Post-induction (after standard dose cytarabine induction):** • (pt <60): High-dose _or_ standard-dose cytarabine + idarubicin or daunorubicin (unless hypoplasia; see induction-failure therapy); followed by induction-failure therapy, if incomplete response (see induction-failure therapy) **Post-Induction:** • (pt ≥60): Induction-failure therapy (significant residual blasts only), standard-dose cytarabine + idarubicin or daunorubicin or mitoxantrone (significant cytoreduction + low % residual blasts after induction only), or post-remission therapy (hypoplasia after induction therapy); followed by post-remission therapy (cytoreduction + low % residual blasts only) _Refer to guidelines for post-remission therapy._	**Induction:** • (pt <60) High-dose cytarabine (HiDAC) + idarubicin or daunorubicin **Induction:** • (pt ≥60) Low-intensity therapy: subQ cytarabine + 5-azacytidine + decitabine; or intermediate-intensity therapy: clofarabine; or best supportive care (hydroxyurea) **Induction-failure therapy:** • (pt <60) High-dose cytarabine ± daunorubicin or idarubicin (unless complete response to induction/post-induction therapy) • (pt ≥60) Supportive care **Post-induction: (pt ≥60):** • Low-intensity SQ cytarabine, 5-azacytidine, decitabine • Intermediate-intensity therapy (clofarabine) or • Best supportive care (hydroxyurea, transfusion support)
Acute promyelocytic leukemia (APL)	**Induction:** • _Able to tolerate anthracyclines:_ All-trans retinoic acid (ATRA) + daunorubicin/cytarabine or idarubicin • _Not able to tolerate anthracyclines:_ ATRA + arsenic trioxide **Post-remission/First relapse:** • Arsenic trioxide ± ATRA	_Refer to guidelines for consolidation and post-consolidation therapy._
Chronic lymphocytic leukemia (CLL)	**First-line therapy (without 17p del or del 11q):** (pt ≥70 or younger pts with comorbidities) • Chlorambucil ± rituximab • Bendamustine, rituximab (BR) • Cyclophosphamide, prednisone ± rituximab • Alemtuzumab • Rituximab • Fludarabine ± rituximab • Cladribine (Pt <70 or older pts without significant comorbidities) • Fludarabine cyclophosphamide, rituximab (FCR) • Fludarabine, rituximab (FR) • Pentostatin, cyclophosphamide, rituximab (PCR) • Bendamustine, rituximab (BR) _Refer to guidelines for relapsed/refractory therapy._	**First-line therapy (with 17p del):** • FCR; FR; high-dose methylprednisolone (HDMP) + rituximab; alemtuzumab ± rituximab **(with 11q): (pt ≥70 or younger pts with comorbidities):** • Chlorambucil ± rituximab; BR; cyclophosphamide, prednisone ± rituximab; reduced-dose FCR; alemtuzumab; rituximab **(with 11q): (pt <70 or older pts without significant comorbidities)** • FCR; BR; PCR _Refer to guidelines for relapsed/refractory therapy._

CANCER TYPE	PREFERRED THERAPIES	ALTERNATIVE REGIMENS
LEUKEMIA *(Continued)*		
Chronic myelogenous leukemia (CML)	**Primary treatment:** Imatinib 400mg or nilotinib 300mg bid or dasatinib 100mg qd	**Follow-up therapy:** (3-months) Continue same dose if complete hematologic response • Nilotinib 400mg bid or dasatinib 100mg qd for incomplete hematologic response • (6-months) continue same dose if complete/partial cytogenetic response; continue same dose of nilotinib/dasatinib or increase imatinib to 800mg (max dose) if minor cytogenetic response; dasatinib 100mg qd or nilotinib 400mg bid if no cytogenetic response • (12-months) Continue same dose for complete cytogenetic response; continue same dose of nilotinib/dasatinib or increase imatinib to 800mg for partial cytogenetic response; dasatinib 100mg qd or nilotinib 400mg bid for minor/no cytogenetic response; dasatinib 100mg qd, nilotinib 400mg bid, or imatinib 800mg for cytogenetic relapse
Hairy cell leukemia	**Initial:** Purine analog (cladribine or pentostatin). *Incomplete response or relapse <1 year:* • Alternate purine analog (cladribine or pentostatin) ± rituximab, interferon α, or rituximab alone • **Relapse ≥1 year:** Purine analog ± rituximab	Interferon alfa
LIVER		
(Hepatocellular carcinoma)	**Unresectable, metastatic, or inoperable by performance status or comorbidity, local disease, or local disease with minimal extrahepatic disease:** • Sorafenib (Child-Pugh Class A [category 1] or B)	
LUNG		
Non-small cell	**Advanced disease:** *First-line:* • Chemotherapy ± bevacizumab *Second-line:* • Docetaxel, pemetrexed, or erlotinib *Third-line:* • Erlotinib	**First-line:** • Cetuximab + vinorelbine/cisplatin • Cisplatin/pemetrexed for nonsquamous • Cisplatin/gemcitabine if squamous • Erlotinib for EGFR mutation positive • Crizotinib if ALK positive • Cisplatin or carboplatin with either paclitaxel, docetaxel, gemcitabine, etoposide, vinblastine, vinorelbine, or pemetrexed • Gemcitabine with docetaxel or vinorelbine
Small cell	**Limited stage:** • Cisplatin or carboplatin with etoposide **Extensive stage:** • Cisplatin or carboplatin with etoposide or irinotecan *Refer to guidelines for subsequent chemotherapy for relapses.*	

CANCER TYPE	PREFERRED THERAPIES	ALTERNATIVE REGIMENS
LYMPHOMA		
HODGKIN'S DISEASE		
Lymphoma	**Classical:** • Doxorubicin/bleomycin/vinblastine/ dacarbazine (ABVD) ± RT • Doxorubicin/vinblastine/mechlorethamine/ etoposide/vincristine/bleomycin/prednisone (Stanford V)	• Bleomycin/etoposide/doxorubicin/ cyclophosphamide/vincristine/ procarbazine/prednisone (BEACOPP)
	Lymphocyte-predominant: • ABVD ± rituximab or cyclophosphamide/ doxorubicin/vincristine/prednisone ± rituximab (CHOP) ± rituximab	• Cyclophosphamide/vincristine/prednisone (CVP) ± rituximab or • Cyclophosphamide/doxorubicin/etoposide/ vincristine/prednisone (EPOCH) ± rituximab or rituximab (monotherapy)
NON-HODGKIN'S LYMPHOMA		
Follicular lymphoma	**First-line:** • Rituximab ± bendamustine • Rituximab, cyclophosphamide, doxorubicin, vincristine, prednisone (RCHOP) • Rituximab, cyclophosphamide, vincristine, prednisone (RCVP) **Second-line:** • Bendamustine, bortezomib, rituximab (BVR) • Fludarabine, cyclophosphamide, mitoxan-trone, rituximab (FCMR) • Fludarabine + rituximab	**First-line:** • Bendamustine + rituximab • Rituximab, fludarabine, mitoxantrone, dexamethasone (RFND) • Rituximab (monotherapy preferred for elderly or infirm) • Radioimmunotherapy • Chlorambucil or cyclophosphamide ± rituximab (elderly or infirm only)
Mantle cell lymphoma	**Aggressive therapy:** • HyperCVAD (cyclophosphamide, vincristine, doxorubicin, dexamethasone alternating with high-dose methotrexate + cytarabine) + rituximab • NORDIC (rituximab/cyclophosphamide/ vincristine/doxorubicin/prednisone [maxi-CHOP] alternating with rituximab + high-dose cytarabine) • CALGB (rituximab + methotrexate with augmented CHOP [see above]) • Sequential RCHOP/RICE (rituximab/ cyclophosphamide/doxorubicin/vincristine + prednisone)/(rituximab/ifosfamide/ carboplatin/etoposide) • Alternating RCHOP/RDHAP (RCHOP; see above)/(rituximab/dexamethasone/cisplatin/ cytarabine) **Less aggressive therapy:** • Bendamustine + rituximab • CHOP + rituximab • Cladribine + rituximab • CVP (cyclophosphamide/vincristine/ prednisone) + rituximab • Dose-adjusted EPOCH (etoposide/prednisone/ vincristine/ cyclophosphamide, doxorubicin) + rituximab • Modified rituximab-HyperCVAD (see Aggressive therapy) with rituximab maintenance in pts >65	**Second-line therapy:** • Bendamustine ± rituximab • Bortezomib ± rituximab • Cladribine ± rituximab • FC (fludarabine, cyclophosphamide) ± rituximab • FCMR (fludarabine, cyclophosphamide, mitoxantrone, rituximab) • FMR (fludarabine, mitoxantrone, rituximab); Lenalidomide ± rituximab) • PCR (pentostatin, cyclophosphamide, rituximab) • PEPC (prednisone, etoposide, procarbazine, cyclophosphamide) ± rituximab

(Continued)

CANCER TYPE	PREFERRED THERAPIES	ALTERNATIVE REGIMENS
LYMPHOMA *(Continued)*		
NON-HODGKIN'S LYMPHOMA *(Continued)*		
Diffuse large B-cell	**First-line:** • Rituximab, cyclophosphamide, doxorubicin, vincristine, prednisone (RCHOP) *Refer to guidelines for first-line therapy with poor left ventricular function.*	**First-line:** • Dose-dense RCHOP • Dose-adjusted EPOCH (etoposide, prednisone, vincristine, cyclophosphamide, doxorubicin) + rituximab **Second-line:** • DHAP (dexamethasone/cisplatin/ cytarabine) ± rituximab • ESHAP (etoposide/methylprednisolone/ cytarabine/cisplatin) ± rituximab • GDP (gemcitabine/dexamethasone/ [cisplatin or carboplatin]) ± rituximab • GemOx (gemcitabine/oxaliplatin) ± rituximab • ICE (ifosfamide/carboplatin/etoposide) ± rituximab • MINE (mesna/ifosfamide/mitoxantrone/ etoposide) ± rituximab *Refer to guidelines for non-candidates for high-dose second-line therapy.*
Burkitt's	**Low-risk combination:** CALGB 10002 regimen: • Cyclophosphamide + prednisone → ifosfamide or cyclophosphamide; high-dose methotrexate, LV, vincristine, dexamethasone, and doxorubicin or etoposide or cytarabine; or intrathecal triple therapy (methotrexate, cytarabine, hydrocortisone) + rituximab • CODOX-M: Cyclophosphamide, vincristine, doxorubicin, intrathecal methotrexate + cytarabine → high-dose systemic methotrexate ± rituximab • Dose-adjusted EPOCH: (etoposide, prednisone, vincristine, cyclophosphamide, doxorubicin) + rituximab (min 3 cycles plus one additional beyond CR) + intrathecal methotrexate • (HyperCVAD) (see Mantle cell lymphoma) alternating with high-dose methotrexate + cytarabine + rituximab **High-risk combination:** • CALGB 10002 regimen (see Low-risk combination above) + prophylactic CNS irradiation in select pts + rituximab • (CODOX-M) alternating with IVAC (ifosfamide, etoposide, cytarabine, intrathecal methotrexate ± rituximab • Dose-adjusted EPOCH (see Low-risk combination above) + rituximab • (HyperCVAD) alternating with high-dose methotrexate and cytarabine + rituximab	**Second-line therapy:** • Dose-adjusted EPOCH + rituximab • RICE (rituximab, ifosfamide, cytarabine, etoposide) + intrathecal methotrexate (if not received previously) • RIVAC (rituximab, ifosfamide, cytarabine, etoposide) + intrathecal methotrexate (if not received previously) • RGDP (rituximab, gemcitabine, dexametha-sone, cisplatin) • HDAC (high-dose cytarabine)
Lymphoblastic	• Standard BFM (Berlin-Frankfurt-Munster) regimen • Augmented BFM regimen • CALGB ALL regimen • HyperCVAD regimen • LMB-86 regimen • Maintenance chemotherapy *Refer to guidelines for specific information on each regimen.*	

CANCER TYPE	PREFERRED THERAPIES	ALTERNATIVE REGIMENS
LYMPHOMA (Continued)		
NON-HODGKIN'S LYMPHOMA (Continued)		
Peripheral T-cell	**First-line:** ALCL, ALK+ histology: • Cyclophosphamide, doxorubicin, vincristine, prednisone (CHOP-21) • (CHOP-21) ± etoposide (CHOEP-21) Other histologies: • CHOEP • CHOP-14 • CHOP-21 • CHOP → ICE (ifosfamide, carboplatin, etoposide) • CHOP → IVE (ifosfamide, etoposide, epirubicin) alternating with intermediate dose methotrexate, or • HyperCVAD with alternating high-dose methotrexate + cytarabine *Refer to guidelines for first-line consolidation therapy.*	**Second-line:** Brentuximab vedotin for Nodal ALCL (excluding cutaneous ALCL) • Dexamethasone, cisplatin, cytarabine (DHAP) • Etoposide, methylprednisolone, cytarabine, cisplatin (ESHAP) • Gemcitabine, dexamethasone, cisplatin (GDP) • Gemcitabine, oxaliplatin (GemOX) • ICE (ifosfamide, carboplatin, etoposide) • Mesna, ifosfamide, mitoxantrone/etoposide (MINE) • Pralatrexate or Romidepsin *Refer to guidelines for regimens in noncandidates for transplant.*
OVARIAN		
	Primary chemotherapy/Adjuvant: Paclitaxel/carboplatin **Secondary chemotherapy/Adjuvant:** Paclitaxel	Docetaxel/carboplatin, paclitaxel/cisplatin
Germ cell tumor	Bleomycin/etoposide/cisplatin (BEP)	Recurrent/persistent: Paclitaxel/ifosfamide/cisplatin (TIP)
PANCREATIC		
	Locally advanced unresectable or metastatic: • 5-FU, LV, irinotecan, oxaliplatin (FOLFIRINOX) • Gemcitabine ± erlotinib **Salvage therapy:** Gemcitabine or fluoropyrimidine-based therapy (alternative to initial)	Gemcitabine- or fluoropyrimidine-based therapy or Capecitabine
PROSTATE		
	Docetaxel/prednisone *Refer to guidelines for androgen-deprivation therapy.*	Mitoxantrone/prednisone

Abbreviations: MTX = methotrexate; 5-FU = 5-fluorouracil; LV = leucovorin; pt(s) = patient(s).
* Selected cancers. For more detailed information, refer to the individual monograph listings or the drug's FDA-approved labeling.
**Refer to www.cancer.gov for more information, such as therapies for CNS prophylaxis.
†**Source:** National Comprehensive Cancer Network (NCCN) Clinical Practice Guidelines in Oncology, 2011.

COLORECTAL CANCER TREATMENT OPTIONS*

GENERIC (BRAND)	INDICATIONS	HOW SUPPLIED	DOSAGE	SPECIAL INSTRUCTIONS
Bevacizumab (Avastin)	First- or second-line treatment of patients with metastatic carcinoma of the colon or rectum in combination with intravenous (IV) 5-fluorouracil (5-FU)-based chemotherapy.	**Inj:** 100mg/4mL, 400mg/16mL [single-use vials]	5mg/kg or 10mg/kg every 2 wks when used in combination with IV 5-FU-based chemotherapy. Administer 5mg/kg when used in combination with bolus-IFL. Administer 10mg/kg when used in combination with FOLFOX4.	Administer only as an IV infusion. Administer 1st IV infusion over 90 min. If 1st infusion is tolerated, give 2nd infusion over 60 min and all subsequent infusions over 30 min if tolerated.
Capecitabine (Xeloda)	First-line treatment of patients with metastatic colorectal carcinoma when treatment with fluoropyrimidine therapy alone is preferred. Adjuvant treatment as a single agent in patients with Dukes' C colon cancer who have undergone complete resection of the primary tumor when treatment with fluoropyrimidine therapy alone is preferred.	**Tab:** 150mg, 500mg	**Standard Starting Dose Monotherapy:** 1250mg/m^2 bid (morning and evening) for 2 wks followed by 1-wk rest period given as 3-wk cycles. Take with water within 30 min after a meal. Adjuvant treatment in patients with Dukes' C colon cancer is recommended for a total of 6 months, given as 3-wk cycles for a total of 8 cycles (24 wks).	Dosage may need to be individualized to optimize patient management. Toxicity may be managed by symptomatic treat-ment, dose interruptions, and dose adjustments (refer to PI for details). A dose reduction to 75% of the starting dose is recommended in patients with moderate renal impairment.
Cetuximab (Erbitux)	As a single agent for the treatment of epidermal growth factor receptor (EGFR)-expressing metastatic colorectal cancer after failure of both irinotecan- and oxaliplatin-based regimens. Treatment of EGFR-expressing metastatic colorectal cancer in patients intolerant to irinotecan-based regimens. In combination with irinotecan for the treatment of EGFR-expressing metastatic colorectal carcinoma in patients who are refractory to irinotecan-based chemotherapy.	**Inj:** 2mg/mL [50mL, 100mL single-use vials]	**Recommended Initial Dose, Either as Monotherapy or in Combination with Irinotecan:** 400mg/m^2 administered as a 120-minute IV infusion (maximum infusion rate: 10 mg/min). Recommended subsequent wkly dose, either as monotherapy or in combination with irinotecan, is 250mg/m^2 IV infused over 60 min (maximum infusion rate 10mg/min) until disease progression or unacceptable toxicity.	Premedication with H$_1$ antagonist (eg, diphenhydramine 50mg) IV 30-60 min prior to first dose is recommended. Refer to PI for dose modifications regarding infusion reactions and dermatologic toxicity.

(Continued)

GENERIC (BRAND)	INDICATIONS	HOW SUPPLIED	DOSAGE	SPECIAL INSTRUCTIONS
Fluorouracil	Palliative management of carcinomas of the colon and rectum.	**Inj:** 50mg/mL [10mL, 20mL, 50mL, 100mL]	12mg/kg IV qd for 4 successive days. The daily dose should not exceed 800mg. If no toxicity is observed, 6mg/kg are given on the 6th, 8th, 10th, and 12th days unless toxicity occurs. No therapy is given on the 5th, 7th, 9th, and 11th days. D/C therapy at the end of Day 12. **Poor Risk Patients/Inadequate Nutritional State:** 6mg/kg/day for 3 days. If no toxicity is observed, 3mg/kg may be given on the 5th, 7th, and 9th days unless toxicity occurs. No therapy is given on the 4th, 6th, or 8th days. The daily dose should not exceed 400mg. **For Maintenance Therapy in instances where toxicity has not been a problem, it is recommended to continue therapy using either of the following schedules:** 1) Repeat dosage of first course every 30 days after the last day of the previous course of treatment. 2) When toxic signs from the initial course of therapy subside, give a maintenance dosage of 10-15mg/kg/wk as a single dose; do not exceed 1g/wk.	Patients should be carefully evaluated prior to treatment to accurately estimate the optimum initial dosage. Administer only IV.
Irinotecan hydrochloride (Camptosar)	A component of first-line therapy in combination with 5-FU and leucovorin (LV) for patients with metastatic carcinoma of the colon or rectum. Also for patients with metastatic carcinoma of the colon or rectum whose disease has recurred or progressed following initial 5-FU-based therapy.	**Inj:** 20mg/mL [2mL, 5mL, 15mL single-use vials]	**Combination Agent Dosing:** Administer Irinotecan as an IV infusion over 90 min; the dose of LV should be administered immediately after Irinotecan with the administration of 5-FU immediately after LV. Refer to PI for recommended regimens and dose modifications. **Single-Agent Dosage Schedule:** Administer as an IV infusion over 90 min for both the wkly and once-every-three-wk dosage schedules.	It is recommended that patients receive premedication with antiemetic agents. Refer to PI for recommended regimens and dose modifications.

GENERIC (BRAND)	INDICATIONS	HOW SUPPLIED	DOSAGE	SPECIAL INSTRUCTIONS
Leucovorin calcium	In combination with 5-FU to prolong survival in the palliative treatment of patients with advanced colorectal cancer.	**Inj:** 10mg/mL [50mg, 100mg, 200mg, 350mg, 500mg single-use vials]	Either of the following two regimens is recommended: 1) Administer at 200mg/m² slow IV injection over a minimum of 3 min followed by 5-FU IV injection at 370mg/m² or 2) 20mg/m² IV injection followed by 5-FU at 425mg/m² by IV injection. Treatment is repeated daily for 5 days. This course may be repeated at 4-week (28-day) intervals for 2 courses and then repeated at 4- to 5-week (28-35 day) intervals if patient has completely recovered from toxic effects of prior treatment course. Dosage should be adjusted based on patient tolerance of the prior treatment course.	Refer to PI for detailed dosage and administration information. LV and 5-FU should be administered separately.
Oxaliplatin (Eloxatin)	In combination with infusional 5-FU/LV for treatment of advanced colorectal cancer and adjuvant treatment of Stage III colon cancer in patients who have undergone complete resection of the primary tumor.	**Inj:** 50mg, 100mg, 50mg/10mL, 100mg/20mL [single-use vials]	**Day 1:** 85mg/m² IV infusion in 250-500mL 5% Dextrose Injection, USP and LV 200mg/m² IV infusion in 5% Dextrose Injection, USP, both given over 120 min at same time in separate bags using a Y-line, followed by 5-FU 400mg/m² IV bolus over 2 to 4 min, followed by 5-FU 600mg/m² IV infusion in 500mL Dextrose Injection, USP as a 22-hour continuous infusion. **Day 2:** LV 200mg/m² IV infusion over 120 min, followed by 5-FU 400mg/m² IV bolus over 2-4 min, followed by 5-FU 600mg/m² IV infusion in 500mL 5% Dextrose Injection, USP as a 22-hr continuous infusion.	Administer in combination with 5-FU/LV every 2 wks. For advanced disease, treatment is recommended until disease progression or unacceptable toxicity. For adjuvant use, treatment is recommended for a total of 6 months (12 cycles). Refer to PI for dose modification recommendations. Premedication with antiemetics is recommended.
Panitumumab (Vectibix)	As a single agent for the treatment of EGFR-expressing, metastatic colorectal carcinoma with disease progression on or following fluoropyrimidine-, oxaliplatin-, and irinotecan-containing chemotherapy regimens.	**Inj:** 20mg/mL [5mL, 10mL, 20mL single-use vials]	6mg/kg as an IV infusion over 60 min every 14 days. Doses higher than 1000mg should be administered over 90 min.	Do not administer as IV push or bolus. Refer to PI for dose modifications for infusion reactions and dermatologic toxicities.

Premedication with an antihistamine, corticosteroid, or an H_2 antagonist may be required for chemotherapy regimens. Refer to PI for details and for dose modifications following adverse effects, toxicities, and renal/hepatic impairment.

Sources: FDA-approved product labeling.

*Refer to the full FDA-approved prescribing information for additional details.

LUNG CANCER TREATMENT OPTIONS

GENERIC (BRAND)	INDICATIONS	HOW SUPPLIED	DOSAGE
ANTIMICROTUBULE AGENTS			
Docetaxel (Taxotere)	Treatment of locally advanced or metastatic NSCLC after failure of prior platinum-based chemotherapy. In combination with cisplatin for treatment of unresectable, locally advanced or metastatic NSCLC patients who have not previously received chemotherapy for this condition.	**Inj:** 20mg/0.5mL, 80mg/2mL	NSCLC: After platinum therapy failure: 75mg/m^2 IV over 1 hr q3wk. For chemotherapy-naïve patients: 75mg/m^2 IV over 1 hr followed by cisplatin 75mg/m^2 q3wk.
Paclitaxel	First-line treatment of NSCLC in combination with cisplatin in patients who are not candidates for potentially curative surgery and/or radiation therapy.	**Inj:** 30mg/5mL, 100mg/16.7mL, 150mg/25mL, 300mg/50mL	NSCLC: 135mg/m^2 IV over 24 hrs q3wk followed by cisplatin 75mg/m^2.
PODOPHYLLOTOXIN DERIVATIVES			
Etoposide phosphate (Etopophos)	First-line combination therapy for treatment of SCLC.	**Inj:** 100mg	SCLC: (Range) 35mg/m^2/day for 4 days to 50mg/m^2/day for 5 days.
Etoposide	First-line combination therapy for treatment of SCLC.	**Cap:** 50mg	SCLC: 2x the IV dose rounded to nearest 50mg; eg, 2 x 35mg/m^2/day IV for 4 days to 50mg/m^2/day for 5 days.
VINCA ALKALOID			
Vinorelbine tartrate (Navelbine)	Single agent or in combination with cisplatin for first-line treatment of unresectable, advanced NSCLC, including Stage IV NSCLC. For use in combination with cisplatin for Stage III NSCLC.	**Inj:** 10mg/mL	Single-agent: 30mg/m^2 IV weekly over 6-10 min. With cisplatin: 25mg/m^2 weekly with cisplatin 100mg/m^2 q4wk, or 30mg/m^2 weekly with cisplatin 120mg/m^2 on Days 1 and 29, then q6wk.
DIHYDROFOLIC ACID REDUCTASE INHIBITOR			
Methotrexate sodium	Treatment of lung cancer as a single agent or as combination therapy.	**Inj:** 10mg/mL, 25mg/mL; **Tab:** 2.5mg* *scored	Oral administration in tablet form is often preferred when low doses are being administered since absorption is rapid and effective serum levels are attained. Methotrexate injection may be given by the intramuscular, intravenous, or intra-arterial route. Refer to PI for more information.
NUCLEOSIDE ANALOGUE METABOLITE			
Gemcitabine HCl (Gemzar)	Combination with cisplatin for first-line treatment of inoperable, locally advanced (Stage IIIA or IIIB), or metastatic (Stage IV) NSCLC.	**Inj:** 200mg, 1g	4-Week schedule: 1000mg/m^2 IV over 30 min on Days 1; 8, and 15 of each 28-day cycle. Give cisplatin 100mg/m^2 IV on Day 1 after gemcitabine HCl infusion. 3-Week schedule: 1250mg/m^2 IV over 30 min on Days 1 and 8 of each 21-day cycle. Give cisplatin 100mg/m^2 IV on Day 1 after gemcitabine HCl infusion.
NITROGEN MUSTARD ALKYLATING AGENT			
Mechlorethamine HCl (Mustargen)	(IV) Palliative treatment of bronchogenic carcinoma.	**Inj:** 10mg	IV: 0.4mg/kg/course given as a single dose or in divided doses of 0.1-0.2mg/kg/day.
ANTHRACYCLINE			
Doxorubicin HCl	To produce regression in disseminated neoplastic conditions such as bronchogenic carcinoma.	**Inj:** 10mg, 20mg, 50mg, 2mg/mL	Monotherapy: 60-75mg/m^2 IV q21d. Concomitant chemotherapy: 40-60mg/m^2 IV q21-28d. Refer to PI for studied doses.

(Continued)

GENERIC (BRAND)	INDICATIONS	HOW SUPPLIED	DOSAGE
PHOTOSENSITIZER			
Porfimer sodium (Photofrin)	Reduction of obstruction and palliation of symptoms in patients with completely or partially obstructive endobronchial NSCLC. Treatment of microinvasive endobronchial NSCLC in patients for whom surgery and radiotherapy are not indicated.	**Inj:** (powder) 75mg	Photodynamic therapy (PDT) for endobronchial cancer: 2mg/kg IV over 3-5 min. Deliver laser light therapy (refer to PI for details) 40-50 hrs following injection. A second laser light treatment may be given 96-120 hrs following injection. Max: 3 courses of PDT separated by 30-days.
TOPOISOMERASE I INHIBITORS			
Topotecan HCl (Hycamtin injection)	Treatment of SCLC-sensitive disease after first-line chemotherapy failure.	**Inj:** 4mg	SCLC: $1.5mg/m^2$ IV qd over 30 min for 5 days, starting on Day 1 of 21-day course. Minimum of 4 courses recommended in absence of tumor progression.
Topotecan HCl (Hycamtin capsules)	Treatment of relapsed SCLC patients with a prior complete or partial response and who are at least 45 days from the end of first-line chemotherapy.	**Cap:** 0.25mg, 1mg	SCLC: $2.3mg/m^2$/day PO qd for 5 consecutive days, repeated every 21 days. Round calculated dose to nearest 0.25mg and give minimum number of 1mg and 0.25mg caps.
ANTIFOLATE			
Pemetrexed disodium (Alimta)	In combination with cisplatin for the initial treatment of locally advanced or metastatic nonsquamous NSCLC. Maintenance treatment in patients with locally advanced or metastatic nonsquamous NSCLC whose disease has not progressed after 4 cycles of platinum-based first-line chemotherapy. Single agent for the treatment of patients with locally advanced or metastatic nonsquamous NSCLC after prior chemotherapy. In combination with cisplatin for the treatment of patients with malignant pleural mesothelioma whose disease is unresectable or who are otherwise not candidates for curative surgery.	**Inj:** 100mg, 500mg	Combination with cisplatin: Nonsquamous NSCLC/mesothelioma: $500mg/m^2$ IV infused over 10 min on Day 1 of each 21-day cycle. Give cisplatin $75mg/m^2$ infused over 2 hrs beginning 30 min after the end of administration. Patient should receive appropriate hydration prior to and/or after receiving cisplatin. Single agent: Nonsquamous NSCLC: $500mg/m^2$ IV infused over 10 min on Day 1 of each 21-day cycle. Refer to PI for dose adjustments for hematologic, nonhematologic, and neurotoxicities. Give premedications (eg, dexamethasone, folic acid) as necessary.
VASCULAR ENDOTHELIAL GROWTH FACTOR INHIBITOR			
Bevacizumab (Avastin)	First-line treatment of unresectable, locally advanced, recurrent, or metastatic nonsquamous NSCLC, in combination with carboplatin and paclitaxel.	**Inj:** 100mg, 400mg	NSCLC: 15mg/kg q3wk (in combination with carboplatin/paclitaxel).
EPIDERMAL GROWTH FACTOR TYROSINE KINASE INHIBITOR			
Erlotinib HCl (Tarceva)	Treatment of locally advanced or metastatic NSCLC after failure of at least one prior chemotherapy regimen. Maintenance treatment of locally advanced or metastatic NSCLC in patients whose disease has not progressed after 4 cycles of platinum-based first-line chemotherapy.	**Tab:** 25mg, 100mg, 150mg	NSCLC: 150mg/qd.

Abbreviations: NSCLC=non-small cell lung cancer; SCLC=small cell lung cancer.

PROSTATE CANCER TREATMENT OPTIONS

GENERIC (BRAND)	INDICATIONS	HOW SUPPLIED	DOSAGE
BISPHOSPHONATE			
Zoledronic acid (Zometa)	Treatment of documented bone metastases from solid tumors (prostate cancer that progressed after treatment with one hormonal therapy), in conjunction with standard antineoplastic therapy.	**Inj:** 4mg/5mL	4mg as a single-dose IV infusion over ≥15 min q3-4wks with CrCl >60mL/min. Coadminister oral calcium 500mg and vitamin D 400 IU daily.
CHEMOTHERAPY AGENTS			
Cabazitaxel (Jevtana)	In combination with prednisone for the treatment of patients with hormone-refractory metastatic prostate cancer previously treated with a docetaxel-containing treatment regimen.	**Inj:** 60mg/1.5mL	$25mg/m^2$ administered as a 1-hr IV infusion q3wk in combination with prednisone 10mg PO administered qd throughout treatment.
Docetaxel (Taxotere)	In combination with prednisone for the treatment of androgen-independent (hormone-refractory) metastatic prostate cancer.	**Inj:** 20mg/0.5mL, 80mg/2mL	**Usual:** $75mg/m^2$ q3wk IV infusion over 1 hr; administer with prednisone 5mg bid continuously.
Estramustine phosphate sodium (Emcyt)	Palliative treatment of metastatic and/or progressive prostate carcinoma.	**Cap:** 140mg	**Usual:** 14mg/kg/d given tid-qid. Take with water at least 1 hr before or 2 hrs after meals. Treat for 30-90 days before determining possible benefits of continued therapy.
Mitoxantrone (Novantrone)	In combination with corticosteroids for the initial treatment of patients with pain related to advanced hormone-refractory prostate cancer.	**Inj:** 2mg/mL	$12\text{-}14mg/m^2/d$ IV q21d.
Sipuleucel-T (Provenge)	Treatment of asymptomatic or minimally symptomatic metastatic castrate-resistant (hormone-refractory) prostate cancer.	**Sus:** 250mL	Infuse 250mL over 60 min q2wk for 3 doses. Premedicate with oral acetaminophen and an antihistamine 30 min prior to administration.
ESTROGENS			
Conjugated estrogens tablets (Premarin)	Palliative treatment of advanced androgen-dependent prostatic carcinoma.	**Tab:** 0.3mg, 0.45mg, 0.625mg, 0.9mg, 1.25mg	1.25-2.5mg tid. Effectiveness of therapy judged by phosphatase determinations and symptomatic improvement.
Esterified estrogens tablets (Menest)	Palliative therapy for advanced prostatic carcinoma.	**Tab:** 0.3mg, 0.625mg, 1.25mg, 2.5mg	1.25-2.5 mg tid. Effectiveness of therapy judged by phosphatase determinations and symptomatic improvement.
Estradiol tablets (Estrace)	Palliative treatment of advanced androgen-dependent prostatic carcinoma.	**Tab:** 0.5mg*, 1mg*, 2mg* *scored	1-2 mg tid. Effectiveness of therapy judged by phosphatase determinations and symptomatic improvement.
Estradiol valerate injection (Delestrogen)	Palliative treatment of advanced androgen-dependent prostatic carcinoma.	**Inj:** 10mg/mL, 20mg/mL, 40mg/mL	30mg or more every 1 or 2 weeks.
GNRH ANALOGUES			
Goserelin acetate implant (Zoladex 3.6mg)	Palliative treatment of advanced prostatic carcinoma. Management of locally confined Stage T2b-T4 (Stage B2-C) prostate cancer in combination with flutamide.	**Implant:** 3.6mg	Inject SQ into anterior abdominal wall below navel line. **Advanced Prostatic Carcinoma:** 3.6mg every 28 days. **Stage B2-C Prostatic Carcinoma:** 3.6mg starting 8 weeks before radiotherapy, then 10.8mg depot formulation 28 days after 1st injection, or 4 doses of 3.6mg at 28-day intervals (2 before and 2 during radiotherapy).

(Continued)

GENERIC (BRAND)	INDICATIONS	HOW SUPPLIED	DOSAGE
GNRH ANALOGUES *(Continued)*			
Goserelin acetate implant (Zoladex 10.8mg)	Palliative treatment of advanced prostatic carcinoma. Management of locally confined Stage T2b-T4 (Stage B2-C) prostate cancer in combination with flutamide.	**Implant:** 10.8mg	Inject SQ into anterior abdominal wall below navel line. **Advanced Prostatic Carcinoma:** 10.8mg every 12 weeks. **Stage B2-C Prostatic Carcinoma:** 3.6mg depot formulation 8 weeks before radiotherapy, followed by 10.8mg 28 days after 1st injection.
GNRH ANTAGONIST			
Degarelix for injection (Firmagon)	Treatment of advanced prostate cancer.	**Inj:** 80mg, 120mg	**Initial:** 240mg (given as 2 SQ injections of 120mg) at 40mg/mL concentration. **Maint:** 80mg SQ every 28 days at 20mg/mL concentration.
LHRH AGONISTS			
Histrelin implant (Vantas)	Palliative treatment of advanced prostate cancer.	**Implant:** 50mg	50mg (1 Implant) every 12 months. Insert SQ in the inner aspect of upper arm.
Leuprolide acetate (Eligard)	Palliative treatment of advanced prostate cancer.	**Inj:** 7.5mg, 22.5mg, 30mg, 45mg	7.5mg SQ monthly, 22.5mg SQ every 3 months, 30mg SQ every 4 months, or 45mg SQ every 6 months. Rotate injection sites.
Leuprolide acetate	Palliative treatment of advanced prostate cancer.	**Inj:** 1mg/0.2mL	1mg SQ qd. Rotate injection sites.
Leuprolide acetate (Lupron Depot)	Palliative treatment of advanced prostate cancer.	**Inj:** 7.5mg, 22.5mg, 30mg, 45mg	7.5mg single IM monthly, 22.5mg IM every 12 weeks, 30mg IM every 16 weeks, or 45mg IM dose every 24 weeks. Give as single IM injection; rotate injection sites.
Triptorelin pamoate (Trelstar)	Palliative treatment of advanced prostate cancer.	**Inj:** 3.75mg, 11.25mg, 22.5mg	3.75mg IM q4wk or 11.25mg IM q12wk or 22.5mg IM q24wk.
NONSTEROIDAL ANTIANDROGENS			
Bicalutamide (Casodex)	Treatment of Stage D2 metastatic carcinoma of the prostate in combination with an LHRH analogue.	**Tab:** 50mg	50mg (1 tab) qd at same time each day (morning or evening). Initiate simultaneously with an LHRH analogue.
Flutamide	Treatment of locally confined Stage B2-C and Stage D2 metastatic carcinoma of the prostate in combination with an LHRH analogue.	**Cap:** 125mg	250mg q8h. **Max:** 750mg/d.
Nilutamide (Nilandron)	Treatment of Stage D2 metastatic prostatic cancer in combination with surgical castration.	**Tab:** 150mg	**Initial:** 300mg qd for 30 days beginning on the day of, or on the day after, surgical castration. **Maint:** 150mg qd.

Abbreviations: LHRH=luteinizing hormone-releasing hormone; GnRH=gonadotropin-releasing hormone.

Sources: FDA-approved product labeling.

National Comprehensive Cancer Network Clinical Practice Guidelines in Oncology; Prostate Cancer. Version 1.2010.

Note: Premedication with an antihistamine, corticosteroid, or H_2 antagonist may be required for chemotherapy regimens. Refer to PI for details and for dose modifications following adverse effects, toxicities, and renal/hepatic impairment.

ANTIDEPRESSANTS

GENERIC (BRAND)	HOW SUPPLIED	ADULT DAILY DOSE INITIAL (I), USUAL (U), MAX (M)	TITRATE‡
AMINOKETONES			
Bupropion HCl (Wellbutrin)	**Tab:** 75mg, 100mg	**(I)**200mg **(U)**300mg **(M)**450mg	Increase in dose should not exceed 100mg/d q3d.
(Wellbutrin SR)	**Tab, SR:** 100mg, 150mg, 200mg	**(I)**150mg **(U)**300mg **(M)**400mg	May increase to 300mg/d as early as Day 4 of dosing if tolerated. May increase to 400mg/d after several wks if no clinical improvement. Allow at least 8 hrs between doses.
(Wellbutrin XL)	**Tab, ER:** 150mg, 300mg	**(I)**150mg **(U)**300mg **(M)**450mg	May increase to 300mg/d as early as Day 4 of dosing if tolerated. May increase to 450mg/d after several wks if no clinical improvement. Allow at least 24 hrs between doses.
Bupropion HBr (Aplenzin)	**Tab, ER:** 174mg, 348mg, 522mg	**(I)**174mg **(U)**348mg **(M)**522mg	May increase to 348mg/d as early as Day 4 of dosing if tolerated. May increase to 522mg/d after several wks if no clinical improvement. Allow at least 24 hrs between doses.
MONOAMINE OXIDASE INHIBITORS			
Isocarboxazid (Marplan)	**Tab:** 10mg*	**(I)**20mg **(M)**60mg	May increase by 10mg q2-4d to 40mg/d by end of first wk if tolerated, then increase by increments of up to 20mg/wk if needed and tolerated to 60mg/d.
Phenelzine sulfate (Nardil)	**Tab:** 15mg	**(I)**45mg **(U)**15mg qd or qod **(M)**90mg	Dosage should be increased to at least 60mg/d at a fairly rapid pace if tolerated. May need to be increased up to 90mg/d.
Selegiline (Emsam)	**Patch:** 6mg/24 hr, 9mg/24 hr, 12mg/24 hr	**(I,U)**6mg/24 hr **(M)**12mg/24 hr	May increase by 3mg/24 hrs at intervals of no less than 2 wks.
Tranylcypromine sulfate (Parnate)	**Tab:** 10mg	**(I,U)**30mg **(M)**60mg	May increase by 10mg/d at intervals of 1-3 wks.
PHENYLPIPERAZINE			
Nefazodone HCl	**Tab:** 50mg, 100mg*, 150mg*, 200mg, 250mg	**(I)**200mg **(U)**300-600mg **(M)**600mg	Increases should occur in increments of 100-200mg/d at intervals of no less than 1 wk.
SELECTIVE SEROTONIN NOREPINEPHRINE REUPTAKE INHIBITORS			
Desvenlafaxine (Pristiq)	**Tab, ER:** 50mg, 100mg	**(I,U)**50mg **(M)**400mg	N/A
Duloxetine HCl (Cymbalta)	**Cap, DR:** 20mg, 30mg, 60mg	**(I)**40-60mg **(U)** 60mg **(M)**120mg	N/A
Venlafaxine HCl (Effexor)	**Tab:** 25mg*, 37.5mg*, 50mg*, 75mg*, 100mg*	**(I)**75mg **(U)**75-225mg **(M)**375mg	Doses may be increased in increments up to 75mg/d if needed and should be made at intervals of no less than 4 days.
(Effexor XR)	**Cap, ER:** 37.5mg, 75mg, 150mg	**(I)**37.5-75mg **(U)**75-225mg **(M)**225mg	Doses may be increased in increments up to 75mg/d if needed and should be made at intervals of no less than 4 days.
Venlafaxine	**Tab, ER;** 37.5mg, 75mg, 150mg, 225mg		

(Continued)

GENERIC (BRAND)	HOW SUPPLIED	ADULT DAILY DOSE INITIAL (I), USUAL (U), MAX (M)	TITRATE‡
SELECTIVE SEROTONIN REUPTAKE INHIBITOR/5-HT1A PARTIAL AGONIST			
Vilazodone HCl (Viibryd)	**Tab:** 10mg, 20mg, 40mg	**(I)**10mg/d **(U,M)**40mg	Initial dose of 10mg/d for 7 days. Increase to 20mg/d for an additional 7 days, then increase to 40mg/d.
SELECTIVE SEROTONIN REUPTAKE INHIBITORS			
Citalopram HBr (Celexa)	**Sol:** 10mg/5mL; **Tab:** 10mg, 20mg*, 40mg*	**(I)**20mg **(U,M)**40mg	Dose increase should usually occur in increments of 20mg at intervals of no less than 1 wk.
Escitalopram oxalate (Lexapro)	**Sol:** 1mg/mL; **Tab:** 5mg, 10mg*, 20mg*	**(I,U)**10mg **(M)**20mg	If the dose is increased to 20mg/d, it should occur after a minimum of 1 wk.
Fluoxetine HCl (Prozac)	**Cap:** 10mg, 20mg, 40mg; **Sol:** (generic) 20mg/5mL **Tab:** (generic) 10mg*, 20mg*, 60mg*	**(I)**20mg **(U)**20-80mg **(M)**80mg	Dose increase may be considered after several weeks if insufficient clinical improvement is observed.
(Prozac Weekly)	**Cap, DR:** 90mg	**(I,U,M)** 90mg	Weekly dosing is recommended to be initiated 7 days after the last daily dose of Prozac 20mg ud.
Paroxetine HCl (Paxil)	**Sus:** 10mg/5mL; **Tab:** 10mg*, 20mg*, 30mg, 40mg	**(I)**20mg **(U)**20-50mg **(M)**50mg	Some patients not responding to 20mg dose may benefit from dose increases in 10mg/d increments up to 50mg/d. Dose changes should occur at intervals of at least 1 wk.
(Paxil CR)	**Tab, CR:** 12.5mg, 25mg, 37.5mg	**(I)**25mg **(U)**25mg-62.5mg **(M)**62.5mg	Some patients not responding to the 25mg dose may benefit from dose increases in 12.5mg/d increments up to a maximum of 62.5mg/d. Dose changes should occur at intervals of at least 1 wk.
Paroxetine mesylate (Pexeva)	**Tab:** 10mg, 20mg*, 30mg, 40mg	**(I)**20mg **(U)**20-50mg **(M)**50mg	Some patients not responding to a 20mg dose may benefit from dose increases in 10mg/d increments up to 50mg/d. Dose changes should occur at intervals of at least 1 wk.
Sertraline HCl (Zoloft)	**Sol:** 20mg/mL; **Tab:** 25mg*, 50mg*, 100mg*	**(I)**50mg **(U)**50-200mg **(M)**200mg	Patients not responding to a 50mg dose may benefit from dose increases up to a max of 200mg/d. Dose changes should not occur at intervals of less than 1 wk.
TETRACYCLICS			
Maprotiline HCl	**Tab:** 25mg*, 50mg*, 75mg*	**(I)**OP: 25mg-75mg **IP:** 100mg-150mg **(U)**OP: 150mg; **IP:** 150mg-225mg **(M)**OP: 150mg-225mg; **IP:** 225mg	Initial dosages should be maintained for 2 wks. Dosages may then be increased gradually in 25mg increments as required and tolerated. Most severely depressed patients may be gradually increased to a max daily dosage of 225mg.
Mirtazapine (Remeron, Remeron SolTab)	**Tab:** 15mg*, 30mg*, 45mg*; **Tab, Disintegrating:** 15mg, 30mg, 45mg	**(I)**15mg **(U)**15mg-45mg **(M)**45mg	Dose changes should not be made at intervals of less than 1 to 2 wks.

GENERIC (BRAND)	HOW SUPPLIED	ADULT DAILY DOSE INITIAL (I), USUAL (U), MAX (M)	TITRATE‡
TRIAZOLOPYRIDINE			
Trazodone HCl	**Tab:** 50mg*, 100mg*, 150mg*, 300mg*	**(I)**150mg **(M)OP:** 400mg; **IP:** 600mg	Dose may be increased by 50mg/d q3-4d as directed.
(Oleptro)	**Tab ER:** 150mg*, 300mg*	**(I)**150mg **(M)**375mg	Dose may be increased by 75mg/d q3d as directed.
TRICYCLICS			
Amitriptyline HCl	**Tab:** 10mg, 25mg, 50mg, 75mg, 100mg, 150mg	**(I)OP:** 50-100mg, **IP:**100mg **(U)OP:**75-150mg **IP:**100-200mg **(M)OP:** 150mg, **IP:** 300mg	**OP:** Dosage may be increased by 25-50mg/d at bedtime as needed. **IP:** Dosages should be increased gradually. In some patients, 40mg/d is a sufficient maintenance dose.
Amoxapine	**Tab:** 25mg*, 50mg*, 100mg*, 150mg*	**(I)**100-150mg **(U)**200-300mg **(M)OP:** 400mg, **IP:** 600mg	Initial dose may be increased to 200-300mg by the end of the first wk ud. If no response is seen after treatment of 300mg/d for at least 2 wks, dosages may be increased to 400mg/d (IP) or 600mg/d (IP) prn as directed.
Clomipramine HCl (Anafranil)	**Cap:** 25mg, 50mg, 75mg	**(I)**25mg **(U)**100-250mg **(M)**250mg	Initial dose should be gradually increased as tolerated over the first 2 wks to approximately 100mg/d. Thereafter, dose may be increased gradually over the next several wks up to a maximum of 250mg/d.
Desipramine HCl (Norpramin)	**Tab:** 10mg, 25mg, 50mg, 75mg, 100mg, 150mg	**(U)**100-200mg **(M)**300mg	Dosage should be initiated at a lower level and increased according to tolerance and clinical response. Treatment of patients requiring as much as 300mg should generally be initiated in hospitals.
Doxepin HCl	**Cap:** 10mg, 25mg, 50mg, 75mg, 100mg, 150mg; **Sol:** 10mg/mL	**(I)**75mg **(U)**75-150mg **(M)**300mg	Severely ill patients may require doses with gradual increases to 300mg/d. Patients with mild symptoms may require doses as low as 25-50mg/d. The 150mg capsule is intended for maintenance therapy only.
Imipramine HCl (Tofranil)	**Tab:** 10mg, 25mg, 50mg	**(I)OP:** 75mg, **IP:** 100mg **(U)OP:** 50-150mg, **IP:** 200mg **(M)OP:** 200mg, **IP:**250-300mg	**IP:** Gradually increase initial dose to 200mg/d as required. May increase to 250-300mg/d if no response after 2 wks. **OP:** Initially, 75mg/d increased to 150mg/d ud.
Imipramine pamoate (Tofranil PM)	**Cap:** 75mg, 100mg, 125mg, 150mg	**(I)OP:** 75mg, **IP:** 100-150mg **(U)**75-150mg **(M)OP:** 200mg, **IP:** 250-300mg	**OP:** Initial dose may be increased to 150mg/d and then increased to 200mg/d prn ud. **IP:** Initial dose may be increased to 200mg/d and, if no response after 2 wks, should be increased to 250-300mg/d ud.
Nortriptyline HCl (Pamelor)	**Cap:** 10mg, 25mg, 50mg, 75mg; **Sol:** 10mg/5mL	**(U)**75-100mg **(M)**150mg	Dosage should begin at a low level and be increased as required.
Protriptyline HCl (Vivactil)	**Tab:** 5mg, 10mg	**(U)**15-40mg **(M)**60mg	Dosage should be initiated at a low level and increased gradually, noting clinical response and tolerance. Dosage may be increased to 60mg/d if necessary. Increases should be made in the AM dose.

(Continued)

GENERIC (BRAND)	HOW SUPPLIED	ADULT DAILY DOSE INITIAL (I), USUAL (U), MAX (M)	TITRATE‡
TRICYCLICS (CONTINUED)			
Trimipramine maleate (Surmontil)	**Cap:** 25mg, 50mg, 100mg	**(I)OP:** 75mg, **IP:** 100mg **(U)** 50-150mg **(M)OP:** 200mg, **IP:** 250-300mg	Dosage should be initiated at a low level and increased gradually, noting clinical response and tolerance. **OP:** Initial dose increases to 150mg/d ud. **IP:** Initial dose may be increased gradually in a few days to 200mg/d and, if no response after 2-3 wks, may be increased to 250-300mg/d ud.

Abbreviations: IP=inpatient; OP=outpatient

*Scored

‡Titration dosing refers to upward titration only.

Refer to full product labeling for discontinuation of treatment, as a gradual reduction in dose may be required.

For dosing in hepatic/renal Impairment or geriatric or adolescent patients, see individual PI.

ANTIPSYCHOTIC AGENTS FOR SCHIZOPHRENIA TREATMENT

GENERIC (BRAND)	HOW SUPPLIED	INITIAL & (MAX) DOSE*	USUAL DOSE RANGE*
ATYPICAL			
Aripiprazole (Abilify)	**Tab:** 2mg, 5mg, 10mg, 15mg, 20mg, 30mg	10-15mg qd (30mg/day)	10-15mg qd
	Sol: 1mg/mL		
	Inj: 7.5mg/mL		
(Abilify Discmelt)	**Tab, Orally Disintegrating:** (Discmelt) 10mg, 15mg	10-15mg qd (30mg/day)	10-15mg qd
Asenapine (Saphris)	**Tab, SL:** 5mg, 10mg	5mg bid (20mg/day)	5-10mg bid
Clozapine			
(Clozaril)	**Tab:** 12.5mg†, 25mg, 50mg†, 100mg, 200mg†	12.5mg qd-bid (900mg/day)	100-900mg/day given tid
(Fazaclo)	**Tab, Orally Disintegrating:** 12.5mg, 25mg, 100mg, 150mg, 200mg	12.5mg qd-bid (900mg/day)	100-900mg/day given tid
Iloperidone (Fanapt)	**Tab:** 1mg, 2mg, 4mg, 6mg, 8mg, 10mg, 12mg,	**Schizophrenia: Initial:** 1mg bid. **Titrate:** Must titrate dose slowly to avoid orthostatic hypotension. **Day 2:** 2mg bid. **Day 3:** 4mg bid. **Day 4:** 6mg bid. **Day 5:** 8mg bid. **Day 6:** 10mg bid. **Day 7:** 12mg bid. **Max:** 12mg bid (24mg/day)	6-12mg bid
Lurasidone HCl (Latuda)	**Tab:** 20mg, 40mg, 80mg	40mg qd (80mg/day)	40-80mg qd
Olanzapine			
(Zyprexa)	**Tab:** 2.5mg, 5mg, 7.5mg, 10mg, 15mg, 20mg	**Schizophrenia:** 5-10mg qd (20mg/day)	**Schizophrenia:** 10-20mg qd
(Zyprexa Zydis)	**Tab, Orally Disintegrating:** 5mg, 10mg, 15mg, 20mg		
(Zyprexa IntraMuscular)	**Inj:** 10mg/vial	**Agitation:** 10mg IM (3 doses 2-4 hrs apart)	**Agitation:** 2.5-10mg IM
(Zyprexa Relprevv)	**Inj, Extended-Release:** 210mg, 300mg, 405mg	Establish tolerability with oral olanzapine prior to initiating treatment. (405mg q4wk or 300mg q2wk)	150-300mg q2wk or 405mg q4wk
Paliperidone			
(Invega)	**Tab, Extended-Release:** 1.5mg, 3mg, 6mg, 9mg	6mg qd (12mg/day)	3-12mg/day
(Invega Sustenna)	**Inj, Extended-Release:** 39mg, 78mg, 117mg, 156mg, 234mg	234mg IM on treatment Day 1 and 156mg IM after 1 week (234mg IM)	39-234mg IM
Quetiapine fumarate			
(Seroquel)	**Tab:** 25mg, 50mg, 100mg, 200mg, 300mg, 400mg	**Schizophrenia:** 25mg bid (800mg/day)	**Schizophrenia:** 150-750mg/day
(Seroquel XR)	**Tab, Extended-Release:** 50mg, 150mg, 200mg, 300mg, 400mg	**Initial:** 300mg/day (800mg/day)	400-800mg/day
Risperidone			
(Risperdal)	**Sol:** 1mg/mL	**Schizophrenia:** 2mg/day given qd-bid (16mg/day)	**Schizophrenia:** 4-8mg/day
	Tab: 0.25mg, 0.5mg, 1mg, 2mg, 3mg, 4mg		
(Risperdal M-Tab)	**Tab, Orally Disintegrating:** 0.5mg, 1mg, 2mg, 3mg, 4mg		
(Risperdal Consta)	**Inj:** 12.5mg, 25mg, 37.5mg, 50mg	**Schizophrenia:** 25mg IM q2wk (50mg q2wk)	**Schizophrenia:** 25-50mg IM q2wk

(Continued)

GENERIC (BRAND)	HOW SUPPLIED	INITIAL & (MAX) DOSE*	USUAL DOSE RANGE*
ATYPICAL (Continued)			
Ziprasidone HCl (Geodon)	**Cap:** 20mg, 40mg, 60mg, 80mg	**Schizophrenia:** 20mg bid (80mg bid)	**Schizophrenia:** 20-80mg bid
Ziprasidone mesylate (Geodon for Injection)	**Inj:** 20mg/mL	**Agitation:** 10mg IM q2h or 20mg IM q4h (40mg/day)	Switch to oral for long-term therapy.
CONVENTIONAL			
Chlorpromazine†	**Inj:** 25mg/mL	10mg tid-qid or 25mg bid-tid or 25mg IM (1000mg/day PO)	PO: 30-800mg/day
	Tab: 10mg, 25mg, 50mg, 100mg, 200mg		IM: Additional 25-50mg IM in 1 hr. Increase subsequent doses over several days until patient is controlled.‡ Switch to PO when controlled.
Fluphenazine HCl†	**Elixir:** 2.5mg/5mL	2.5-10mg/day in divided doses q6-8h (40mg/day)	1-5mg qd
	Sol, Conc: 5mg/mL		
	Tab: 1mg, 2.5mg, 5mg, 10mg		
	Inj: 2.5mg/mL	2.5-10mg/day IM in divided doses q6-8h (10mg/day)	Individualize to patient. Switch to PO when controlled.
Fluphenazine decanoate†	**Inj:** 25mg/mL	12.5-25mg IM/SQ (100mg/dose)	Individualize to patient.
Haloperidol†	**Sol, Conc:** 2mg/mL	**Moderate:** 0.5-2mg bid-tid	Reduce to minimum effective dose.
	Tab: 0.5mg, 1mg, 2mg, 5mg, 10mg, 20mg	**Sev/Resist:** 3-5mg bid-tid (100mg/day)	
Haloperidol lactate (Haldol)	**Inj:** 5mg/mL	2-5mg IM q4-8h or hourly if needed	Individualize to patient. Switch to PO when controlled.
Haloperidol decanoate (Haldol decanoate)	**Inj:** 50mg/mL, 100mg/mL	10-20x daily oral dose up to 100mg/dose (450mg/month)	10-15x daily oral dose depending on the clinical response of the patient.
Loxapine succinate†	**Cap:** 5mg, 10mg, 25mg, 50mg	10mg bid up to 50mg/day (250mg/day)	60-100mg/day
Perphenazine†	**Tab:** 2mg, 4mg, 8mg, 16mg	**Nonhospitalized:** 4-8mg tid. **Hospitalized:** 8-16mg bid-qid (64mg/day)	Reduce dose as soon as possible to minimum effective dose.
Prochlorperazine edisylate†	**Inj:** 5mg/mL	10-20mg IM q2-4h or hourly if needed	Switch to PO when controlled.
Prochlorperazine maleate†	**Tab:** 5mg, 10mg	**Mild:** 5mg tid-qid (20mg x 12wks). **Moderate/Severe (Hospitalized):** 10mg tid-qid.	**Mild:** 5-10mg tid-qid. **Moderate/Severe (Hospitalized):** 50-150mg/day **Severe:** 100-150mg/day
Thioridazine HCl†	**Tab:** 10mg, 25mg, 50mg, 100mg	50-100mg tid (800mg/day)	200-800mg/day given bid-qid
Thiothixene (Navane)	**Cap:** 1mg, 2mg, 5mg, 10mg, 20mg	**Mild:** 2mg tid **Severe:** 5mg bid (60mg/day)	20-30mg/day. 60mg/day is often effective in some patients.
Trifluoperazine HCl†	**Tab:** 1mg, 2mg, 5mg, 10mg	2-5mg bid	15-20mg/day

Note: This list is not inclusive of all antipsychotic agents. Indications may vary among the different products.

*Doses shown are for adults. For pediatric dosing and additional information, please refer to the individual monograph listings or the drug's FDA-approved labeling. Dosages need to be adjusted by titration to individual patient needs and may need to be reduced in the elderly, debilitated, or patients with renal/hepatic impairment. Periodically reassess to determine the need for maintenance treatment.

†Available only in generic forms.

‡Severe cases may require up to 2g/day or 400mg/dose IM.

BIPOLAR DISORDER PHARMACOTHERAPY

GENERIC (BRAND)	INDICATIONS	HOW SUPPLIED	USUAL DOSAGE	COMMENTS
MOOD STABILIZERS				
Lithium	Treatment of manic episodes in bipolar disorder and maintenance treatment of bipolar disorder.	**Cap:** 150mg, 300mg, 600mg; **Tab:** 300mg; **Sol:** 8mEq/5mL	**Adults/Pediatrics ≥12 yrs: Acute Mania:** 600mg or 10mL tid to achieve effective serum levels of 1-1.5mEq/L; monitor levels twice a week until stabilized. **Maint:** 300mg or 5mL tid-qid to maintain serum levels of 0.6-1.2 mEq/L; monitor levels every 2 months.	**Elderly:** Start at lower end of dosing range.
Lithium ER (Lithobid)	Treatment of manic episodes in bipolar disorder and maintenance treatment of bipolar disorder.	**Tab, Extended-Release:** 300mg, (generic) 450mg	**Adults/Pediatrics ≥12 yrs: Acute Mania:** 1800mg/day given in divided doses bid-tid to achieve effective serum levels of 1-1.5mEq/L; monitor levels twice a week until stabilized. **Maint:** 900-1200mg/d given in divided doses bid-tid to maintain serum levels of 0.6-1.2 mEq/L; monitor levels every 2 months.	**Elderly:** Start at lower end of dosing range. Do not crush or chew tab.
ANTICONVULSANTS				
Carbamazepine (Equetro)	Treatment of acute manic and mixed episodes associated with bipolar I disorder.	**Cap, Extended-Release:** 100mg, 200mg, 300mg	**Adults: Initial:** 400mg/day given in divided doses bid. **Titrate:** Adjust in increments of 200mg/day. **Max:** 1600mg/day.	Do not crush or chew.
Divalproex sodium (Depakote ER, Depakote)	Acute manic or mixed episodes associated with bipolar disorder.	**Tab, Extended-Release:** 250mg, 500mg	**Adults: Mania: Initial:** 25mg/kg/day given once daily. **Titrate:** Increase rapidly to lowest therapeutic dose producing the desired clinical effect or plasma concentration. **Max:** 60mg/kg/day. Conversion from Depakote: Refer to PI.	**Elderly:** Give lower initial dose and titrate slowly. Decrease dose or d/c if decreased food or fluid intake or if excessive somnolence occurs. Swallow whole; do not crush or chew.
	Treatment of manic episodes associated with bipolar disorder.	**Tab, Delayed-Release:** 125mg, 250mg, 500mg	**Adults: Mania:** 750mg daily in divided doses. **Titrate:** Increase rapidly to lowest therapeutic dose producing the desired clinical effect or plasma concentration. **Max:** 60mg/kg/day.	**Elderly:** Give lower initial dose and titrate slowly. Decrease dose or d/c if decreased food or fluid intake or if excessive somnolence occurs.

(Continued)

GENERIC (BRAND)	INDICATIONS	HOW SUPPLIED	USUAL DOSAGE	COMMENTS
ANTICONVULSANTS *(Continued)*				
Lamotrigine (Lamictal)	Maintenance treatment of bipolar I disorder to delay the time to occurrence of mood episodes (depression, mania, hypomania, mixed episodes) in adults (≥18 yrs) treated for acute mood episodes with standard therapy.	**Tab:** 25mg*, 100mg*, 150mg*, 200mg*, *scored **Tab, Chewable:** (Lamictal CD) 2mg, 5mg, 25mg **Tab, Disintegrating:** (Lamictal ODT) 25mg, 50mg, 100mg, 200mg	**Adults: Bipolar Disorder: Patients not Taking Carbam-azepine, Other Enzyme-Inducing Drugs (EIDs), or VPA:** Weeks 1 and 2: 25mg qd. Weeks 3 and 4: 50mg qd. Week 5: 100mg qd. Weeks 6 and 7: 200mg qd. **Patients Taking VPA:** Weeks 1 and 2: 25mg every other day. Weeks 3 and 4: 25mg qd. Week 5: 50mg qd. Weeks 6 and 7: 100mg qd. **Patients Taking Carbamazepine (or other EIDs) and not Taking VPA:** Weeks 1 and 2: 50mg qd. Weeks 3 and 4: 100mg qd (divided doses). Week 5: 200mg qd (divided doses). Week 6: 300mg qd (divided doses). Week 7: Up to 400mg qd (divided doses). **After Discontinuation of Psychotropic Drugs Excluding VPA, Carbamazepine, or Other EIDs:** Maintain current dose. **After Discontinuation of VPA and Current Lamotrigine Dose of 100mg qd:** Week 1: 150mg qd. Week 2 and onward: 200mg qd. **After Discontinuation of Carbamazepine or Other EIDs and Current Lamotrigine Dose of 400mg qd:** Week 1: 400mg qd. Week 2: 300mg qd. Week 3 and onward: 200mg qd.	Refer to PI for additional dosing information.
Valproic acid (Stavzor)	Treatment of manic episodes associated with bipolar disorder.	**Cap, Delayed Release:** 125mg, 250mg, 500mg	**Adults: Mania: Initial:** 750mg daily in divided doses. **Titrate:** Increase dose rapidly to lowest therapeutic dose producing the desired clinical effect or plasma concentration (Trough: 50-125mcg/mL). **Max:** 60mg/kg/day.	
CONVENTIONAL ANTIPSYCHOTIC				
Chlorpromazine HCl	Control manifestations of manic type of manic-depressive illness.	**Inj:** 25mg/mL; **Tab:** 10mg, 25mg, 50mg, 100mg, 200mg	**Adults: Inpatient: Acute Schizophrenic/Manic State:** 25mg IM then 25-50mg IM in 1 hr if needed. **Titrate:** Increase over several days up to 400mg q4-6h until controlled then switch to PO. **Usual:** 500mg/day PO. **Max:** 1000mg/day PO (gradual increases to 2000mg/day or more may be necessary). **Less Acutely Disturbed:** 25mg PO tid. **Titrate:** Increase gradually to 400mg/day. Outpatient: 10mg PO tid-qid or 25mg PO bid-tid. **More Severe:** 25mg PO tid. **Titrate:** After 1-2 days, increase by 20-50mg semiweekly until calm. **Prompt Control of Severe Symptoms:** 25mg IM, may repeat in 1 hr then 25-50mg PO tid.	

GENERIC (BRAND)	INDICATIONS	HOW SUPPLIED	USUAL DOSAGE	COMMENTS
ATYPICAL ANTIPSYCHOTICS				
Aripiprazole (Abilify)	(PO) Acute and maintenance treatment of manic and mixed episodes associated with bipolar I disorder, both as monotherapy and as an adjunct to lithium or valproate, in adults and pediatrics aged 10-17 yrs. (Inj) Acute treatment of agitation associated with bipolar disorder, manic or mixed, in adults.	**Tab:** 2mg, 5mg, 10mg, 15mg, 20mg, 30mg; **Tab, Disintegrating** (Discmelt): 10mg, 15mg; **Sol:** 1mg/mL [150mL]; **Inj:** 7.5mg/mL	**Adults:** (PO) **Bipolar Disorder Monotherapy: Initial:** 15mg/day. **Adjunct:** 10-15mg qd. **Target:** 15mg/day. **Max:** 30mg/day. (Inj) **Agitation:** 9.75mg IM. **Range:** 5.25-15mg IM. **Max:** 30mg/day; initiate PO therapy as soon as possible. **Pediatrics: Bipolar Disorder (Monotherapy or Adjunct) 10-17 yrs: Initial:** 2mg/day. **Titrate:** 5mg/day after 2 days. **Target:** 10mg/day after 2 additional days. May adjust dose in 5mg/day increments.	Periodically reassess need for maintenance therapy. Refer to PI for detailed dosage adjustments in special populations or in concomitant therapies.
Asenapine (Saphris)	As monotherapy or adjunctive therapy with either lithium or valproate for the acute treatment of manic or mixed episodes associated with bipolar I disorder.	**Tab, SL:** 5mg, 10mg	**Adults: Monotherapy: Initial/Usual/Max:** 10mg bid SL. May decrease to 5mg bid if needed. **Adjunctive Therapy (with lithium/valproate): Initial:** 5mg bid SL. **Titrate:** May increase to 10mg bid based on response and tolerability. **Max:** 10mg bid. Recommend to continue treatment beyond acute response.	
Olanzapine (Zyprexa, Zyprexa Zydis)	Acute treatment of manic or mixed episodes associated with bipolar I disorder and maintenance treatment of bipolar I disorder in adults and adolescent patients (ages 13-17 yrs). Adjunct to lithium or valproate for the treatment of manic episodes or mixed episodes associated with bipolar I disorder in adults. For depressive episodes associated with bipolar I disorder in combination with fluoxetine. (Inj) Treatment of acute agitation associated with bipolar I mania.	**Inj:** 10mg; **Tab:** 2.5mg, 5mg, 7.5mg, 10mg, 15mg, 20mg; **Tab, Disintegrating** (Zydis) 5mg, 10mg, 15mg, 20mg	**Adults: Bipolar I Disorder (Manic or Mixed Episodes): Initial:** 10-15mg qd. **Titrate:** May increase/decrease dose by 5mg daily at intervals of not less than 24 hrs. **Maint:** 5-20mg/day. Periodically re-evaluate. **Max:** 20mg/day. **With Lithium or Valproate: Initial/Usual:** 10mg qd. **Max:** 20mg/day. **Depressive Episodes Associated with Bipolar I Disorder: Initial:** 5mg with 20mg fluoxetine qd in the pm. **Titrate:** Adjust dose based on efficacy and tolerability. **Usual:** 5-12.5mg with 20-50mg fluoxetine. **Max:** 18mg with fluoxetine 75mg. **Agitation: Initial:** 10mg IM. **Usual:** 2.5-10mg IM. Assess for orthostatic hypotension prior to subsequent dosing. **Max:** 30mg/day or 3 doses of 10mg IM q2-4h.	Refer to PI for detailed dosage adjustments in special populations or in concomitant therapies.
Olanzapine-Fluoxetine (Symbyax)	Acute treatment of depressive episodes associated with bipolar I disorder in adults.	**Cap:** (Olanzapine-Fluoxetine): 3-25mg, 6-25mg, 6-50mg, 12-25mg, 12-50mg	**Initial:** 6-25mg qd in the evening. **Range:** 6-12mg (olanzapine)-25-50mg (fluoxetine). Adjust dose based on efficacy and tolerability. **Max:** 18-75mg/day. Re-examine the need for continued pharmacotherapy periodically.	Refer to PI for detailed dosage adjustments in special populations or in concomitant therapies.

(Continued)

GENERIC (BRAND)	INDICATIONS	HOW SUPPLIED	USUAL DOSAGE	COMMENTS
ATYPICAL ANTIPSYCHOTICS *(Continued)*				
Quetiapine (Seroquel, Seroquel XR)	Acute treatment of manic episodes associated with bipolar I disorder, both as monotherapy and as an adjunct therapy to lithium or divalproex in adults and pediatrics (10-17 yrs). Monotherapy for acute treatment of depressive episodes associated with bipolar disorder in adults. Maintenance treatment of bipolar I disorder as adjunct therapy to lithium or divalproex.	**Tab:** 25mg, 50mg, 100mg, 200mg, 300mg, 400mg	**Adults: Bipolar I Disorder: Manic Episodes: Monotherapy/ Adjunct:** Give bid. Day 1: 100mg/day, increase to 400mg/day on Day 4 in increments of up to 100mg/day and further adjust up to 800mg/day by Day 6 in increments of ≤200mg/day. **Max:** 800mg/day. **Depressive Episodes:** Give qd at hs. Day 1: 50mg/day. Day 2: 100mg/day. Day 3: 200mg/day. Day 4: 300mg/day. **Maint (Bipolar I Disorder):** 400-800mg/day given bid as adjunct therapy to lithium or divalproex. **Pediatrics: Bipolar I Disorder: Manic Episodes: 10-17 yrs:** Administer bid or tid based on response and tolerability. Day 1: 50mg/day. Day 2: 100mg/day. Day 3: 200mg/day. Day 4: 300mg/day. Day 5: 400mg/day. After Day 5, adjust dose based on response and tolerability within recommended range of 400-600mg/day with increments of ≤100mg/day. **Max:** 600mg/day.	Refer to PI for detailed dosage adjustments in special populations or concomitant therapies.
	Acute treatment of manic or mixed episodes associated with bipolar I disorder, both as monotherapy and as an adjunct to lithium or divalproex. Acute treatment of depressive episodes associated with bipolar disorder. Maintenance treatment of bipolar disorder as adjunct therapy to lithium or divalproex.	**Tab, Extended Release:** 50mg, 150mg, 200mg, 300mg, 400mg	**Adults: Bipolar Disorder: Bipolar Mania: Monotherapy/ Adjunct:** Give qd in pm. Day 1: 300mg/day. Day 2: 600mg/day. **Titrate:** May adjust dose between 400-800mg beginning on Day 3 depending on response and tolerance. **Depressive Episodes:** Give qd in pm. Day 1: 50mg/day. Day 2: 100mg/day. Day 3: 200mg/day. Day 4: 300mg/day. **Maint (Bipolar I Disorder):** 400-800mg/day as adjunct therapy to lithium or divalproex. Periodically reassess the need for maintenance treatment and the appropriate dose.	Refer to PI for detailed dosage adjustments in special populations or in concomitant therapies.
Risperidone (Risperdal)	Short-term treatment of acute manic or mixed episodes associated with bipolar I disorder as monotherapy (adults and pediatrics 10-17 yrs) or in combination with lithium or valproate (adults). **Inj:** Maintenance treatment of bipolar I disorder as monotherapy or in combination with lithium or valproate.	**Sol:** 1mg/mL [30mL]; **Tab:** 0.25mg, 0.5mg, 1mg, 2mg, 3mg, 4mg; **Tab, Disintegrating:** (M-Tab) 0.5mg, 1mg, 2mg, 3mg, 4mg; **Inj:** (Risperdal Consta) 12.5mg, 25mg, 37.5mg, 50mg	**Adults: Bipolar Mania: Initial:** 2-3mg qd. **Titrate:** Adjust dose at intervals not <24 hrs and in increments/decrements of 1mg/day. Range: 1-6mg/day. **Max:** 6mg/day. **Pediatrics: 10-17 yrs: Bipolar Mania: Initial:** 0.5mg qd in morning or evening. **Titrate:** Adjust dose, if needed, in increments of 0.5 or 1mg/day and at intervals not <24 hrs, as tolerated, to recommended dose of 2.5mg/day. **Max:** 6mg/day. Periodically reassess to determine maintenance treatment. **Inj:** Establish PO tolerability prior to IM treatment. Give 1st inj with PO risperidone or other antipsychotic, continue for 3 weeks, then d/c PO therapy. **Usual:** 25mg IM q2wk. **Titrate:** Upward dose adjustment should not be more frequent than q4 weeks. **Max:** 50mg IM q2wk.	Refer to PI for detailed dosage adjustments in special populations or in concomitant therapies.

GENERIC (BRAND)	INDICATIONS	HOW SUPPLIED	USUAL DOSAGE	COMMENTS
ATYPICAL ANTIPSYCHOTICS *(Continued)*				
Ziprasidone (Geodon)	Monotherapy for acute treatment of manic or mixed episodes associated with bipolar I disorder. Adjunct to lithium or valproate for the maintenance treatment of bipolar I disorder.	**Cap:** 20mg, 40mg, 60mg, 80mg	**Adults: Initial:** 40mg bid with food. **Titrate:** Increase to 60-80mg bid on 2nd day of treatment, then adjust dose based on tolerance and efficacy. **Maint:** 40-80mg bid.	

Source: FDA-approved labeling.
Refer to complete prescribing information for detailed dosage adjustments in special populations or concomitant therapies.

ASTHMA AND COPD MANAGEMENT

GENERIC (BRAND)	DOSAGE FORM	ADULT DOSAGE	CHILD DOSAGE
ANTICHOLINERGICS			
Ipratropium (Atrovent HFA)†	**MDI:** 0.017mg/inh	2 inh qid. **Max:** 12 inh/24 hrs	
Tiotropium (Spiriva)†	**Cap, Inh:** 18mcg	2 inh of contents of 1 cap qd	
COMBINATION AGENTS			
Budesonide/Formoterol (Symbicort)*‡	**MDI:** (Budesonide-Formoterol) 80mcg-4.5mcg/inh, 160mcg-4.5mcg/inh	**Asthma: Initial:** 2 inh bid (am/pm q12h). Starting dose is based on asthma severity. **Max:** 160mcg-4.5mcg bid. **COPD:** 2 inh of 160mcg-4.5mcg bid	**≥12 yrs:** 2 inh bid (am/pm q12h). **Max:** 160mcg-4.5mcg bid
Fluticasone/Salmeterol (Advair Diskus)*‡	**DPI:** (Fluticasone-Salmeterol) 100mcg-50mcg/inh, 250mcg-50mcg/inh, 500mcg-50mcg/inh	**Asthma:** 1 inh bid (am/pm q12h). Starting dose is based on asthma severity. **Max:** 500mcg-50mcg bid. **COPD:** 1 inh of 250mcg-50mcg bid (am/pm q12h)	**≥12 yrs:** 1 inh bid (am/pm q12h). **Max:** 500mcg-50mcg bid. **4-11 yrs:** 1 inh of 100mcg-50mcg bid (am/pm q12h)
Fluticasone/Salmeterol (Advair HFA)‡	**MDI:** (Fluticasone-Salmeterol) 45mcg-21mcg/inh, 115mcg-21mcg/inh, 230mcg-21mcg/inh	**Initial:** 2 inh bid (am/pm q12h). Recommended starting dosages are based upon patient's current therapy. **Max:** 2 inh of 230mcg-21mcg bid	**≥12 yrs: Initial:** 2 inh bid (am/pm q12h). **Max:** 2 inh of 230mcg-21mcg bid
Ipratropium/Albuterol (Combivent)†	**MDI:** (Albuterol-Ipratropium) 0.09mg-0.018mg/inh	2 inh qid. **Max:** 12 inh/24 hrs	
Ipratropium/Albuterol (Duoneb)†	**Sol, Inh:** (Albuterol-Ipratropium) 3mg-0.5mg/3mL	3mL qid via nebulizer with up to 2 additional 3mL doses/day	
Mometasone/Formoterol (Dulera)‡	**MDI:** (Mometasone-Formoterol) 100mcg-5mcg/inh, 200mcg-5mcg/inh	**≥12 yrs:** 2 inh bid (am/pm). Starting dosage is based on prior therapy.** **Previous Corticosteroid Therapy: Inhaled Medium-Dose Corticosteroids: Initial:** 2 inh of 100mcg-5mcg bid. **Max:** 400mcg-20mcg/day. **Inhaled High-Dose Corticosteroids: Initial:** 2 inh of 200mcg-5mcg bid. **Max:** 800mcg-20mcg/day	Refer to adult dosing.
COMBINATION AGENT—MISCELLANEOUS			
Dyphylline/Guaifenesin (Lufyllin-GG)	**Sol:** (Dyphylline-Guaifenesin) 100mg-100mg/15mL	30mL qid	**>6 yrs:** 15-30mL tid-qid
CORTICOSTEROIDS			
Beclomethasone dipropionate HFA (QVAR)	**MDI:** 40mcg/inh, 80mcg/inh	**Initial:** 40-160mcg bid. **Max:** 320mcg bid. Dosage based on prior therapy**	**Adolescents: Initial:** 40-160mcg bid. **Max:** 320mcg bid. **5-11 yrs: Initial:** 40mcg bid. **Max:** 80mcg bid
Budesonide DPI (Pulmicort Flexhaler)	**DPI:** 90mcg/inh, 180mcg/inh	**Initial:** 180-360mcg bid. **Max:** 720mcg bid	**6-17 yrs: Initial:** 180-360mcg bid. **Max:** 360mcg bid

(Continued)

GENERIC (BRAND)	DOSAGE FORM	ADULT DOSAGE	CHILD DOSAGE
CORTICOSTEROIDS *(continued)*			
Budesonide neb (Pulmicort Respules)	**Sus, Inh:** 0.25mg/2mL, 0.5mg/2mL, 1mg/2mL		**12 months-8 yrs: Initial:** 0.25mg/day-1mg/day via nebulizer. **Max:** 0.5-1mg/day. Dosage based on prior therapy
Ciclesonide (Alvesco)	**MDI:** 80mcg/inh, 160mcg/inh	**Initial:** 80mcg bid-320mcg bid. **Max:** 160mcg bid-320mcg bid. Dosage based on prior therapy**	Refer to adult dosing
Flunisolide (Aeropsan)	**MDI:** 78mcg/inh	**Initial:** 160mcg bid. **Max:** 320mcg bid	**≥12 yrs: Initial:** 160mcg bid. **Max:** 320mcg bid. **6-11 yrs: Initial:** 80mcg bid. **Max:** 160mcg bid
Fluticasone propionate (Flovent Diskus)	**DPI:** 50mcg/inh, 100mcg/inh, 250mcg/inh	**Initial:** 100mcg bid-1000mcg bid. **Max:** 500mcg bid-1000mcg bid. Dosage based on prior therapy**	**≥12 yrs: Initial:** 100mcg-1000mcg bid. **Max:** 500mcg bid-1000mcg bid. **4-11 yrs: Initial:** 50mcg bid. **Max:** 100mcg bid
Fluticasone propionate (Flovent HFA)	**MDI:** 44mcg/inh, 110mcg/inh, 220mcg/inh	**Initial:** 88mcg bid-440mcg bid. **Max:** 440mcg bid-880mcg bid. Dosage based on prior therapy**	**≥12 yrs: Initial:** 88mcg bid-440mcg bid. **Max:** 440mcg bid-880mcg/day. **4-11 yrs: Initial/Max:** 88mcg bid
Mometasone furoate (Asmanex Twisthaler)	**DPI:** 110mcg/inh, 220mcg/inh	**Initial:** 220mcg qd hs-440mcg bid. **Max:** 440-880mcg/day. Dosage based on prior therapy**	**≥12 yrs: Initial:** 220mcg qd hs-440mcg bid. **Max:** 440mcg-880mcg/day. **4-11 yrs: Initial/Max:** 110mcg qd hs.
Triamcinolone Acetonide (Azmacort)	**MDI:** 75mcg/inh	**Initial:** 150mcg tid-qid or 300mcg bid. **Max:** 1200mcg/day	**6-12 yrs: Initial:** 75-150mcg tid-qid or 150mcg-300mcg bid. **Max:** 900mcg/day
MAST CELL STABILIZER			
Cromolyn	**Sol, Inh:** 10mg/mL	20mg nebulized qid	**≥2 yrs:** 20mg nebulized qid
LEUKOTRIENE MODIFIERS			
Montelukast (Singulair)	**Tab:** 10mg; **Tab, Chewable:** 4mg, 5mg; **Granules:** 4mg	10mg qpm	**≥15 yrs:** 10mg qpm. **6-14 yrs:** 5mg chewable tab qpm. **2-5 yrs:** 4mg chewable tab or 4mg oral granules pkt qpm. **12-23 months:** 4mg oral granules pkt qpm
Zafirlukast (Accolate)	**Tab:** 10mg, 20mg	20mg bid. Take at least 1 hour before or 2 hours after meals	**≥12 yrs:** 20mg bid. **5-11 yrs:** 10mg bid
Zileuton (Zyflo, Zyflo CR)	**Tab:** 600mg; **Tab, Extended-Release:** 600mg	**Tab:** 600mg qid. **Max:** 2400mg/day. (Tab, Extended-Release) 1200mg bid. **Max:** 2400mg/day	Refer to adult dosing
LONG-ACTING β₂-AGONISTS			
Arformoterol (Brovana)†	**Sol, Inh:** 15mcg/2mL	15mcg bid via nebulizer. **Max:** 30mcg/day	
Formoterol (Foradil)*‡	**Cap, Inh:** 12mcg	1 cap (inh) q12h. **Max:** 24mcg/day	**≥5 yrs:** Refer to adult dosing
Formoterol (Perforomist)†‡	**Sol, Inh:** 20mcg/2mL	2mL q12h via nebulizer. **Max:** 40mcg/day	

GENERIC (BRAND)	DOSAGE FORM	ADULT DOSAGE	CHILD DOSAGE
LONG-ACTING β₂-AGONISTS *(continued)*			
Metaproterenol	**Syrup:** 10mg/5mL; **Tab:** 10mg, 20mg; **Sol, Inh:** 0.4%, 0.6%	20mg tid-qid **(Sol)** one vial per nebulization tid-qid	**6-9 yrs or <60 lbs:** 10mg tid-qid. **>9 yrs or >60 lbs:** 20mg tid-qid. **(Sol) ≥12 yrs:** 1 vial per nebulization tid-qid
Salmeterol (Serevent)*‡	**DPI:** 50mcg/inh	1 inh q12h. **Max:** 24mcg/day	**≥4 yrs:** 1 inh q12h
Terbutaline	**Tab:** 2.5mg, 5mg; **Inj:** 1mg/mL	**(PO)** 2.5-5mg q6h tid. **Max:** 15mg/day. (Inj) 0.25mg SQ into the lateral deltoid area. May repeat in 15-30 min if no improvement. **Max:** 0.5mg/4h	**(PO) 12-15 yrs:** 2.5mg tid. **Max:** 7.5mg/day. **(Inj) ≥12 yrs:** 0.25mg SQ. May repeat in 15-30 min if no improvement. **Max:** 0.5mg/4 h
METHYLXANTHINE			
Theophylline (Elixophyllin)§	**Elixir:** 80mg/15mL	**Adults & Children >45 kg: Initial:** 300mg/day divided q6-8h. **After 3 days if tolerated:** 400mg/day divided q6-8h. **After 3 more days if tolerated:** 600mg/day divided q6-8h	**1-15 yrs (<45 kg): Initial:** 12-14mg/kg/day. **Max:** 300mg/day divided q4-6h. **After 3 days if tolerated:** 16mg/kg/day. **Max:** 400mg/day divided q4-6h. After 3 more days if tolerated: 20mg/kg/day. **Max:** 600mg/day divided q4-6h. See PI for infant dose
Theophylline (Theo-24)§	**Cap, Extended-Release:** 100mg, 200mg, 300mg, 400mg	**Adults & Children >45 kg: Initial:** 300-400mg/day q24h. **After 3 days if tolerated:** 400-600mg/day q24h. **After 3 more days if tolerated and needed:** Doses >600mg should be titrated according to blood levels (see PI)	**12-15 yrs (<45 kg): Initial:** 12-14mg/kg/day. **Max:** 300mg/day q24h. **After 3 days if tolerated:** 16mg/kg/day. **Max:** 400mg/day q24h. **After 3 more days if tolerated and needed:** 20mg/kg/day. **Max:** 600mg/day q24h
Theophylline (Generic)	**Tab, Extended-Release:** 400mg, 600mg	**Adults & Children >45 kg: Initial:** 300-400mg/day. **After 3 days if tolerated:** 400-600mg/day. **After 3 more days if tolerated and needed:** Doses >600mg should be titrated according to blood levels (see PI)	**12-15 yrs (<45 kg): Initial:** 12-14mg/kg/day. **Max:** 300mg/day. **After 3 days if tolerated:** 16mg/kg/day. **Max:** 400mg/day. **After 3 more days if tolerated and needed:** 20mg/kg/day. **Max:** 600mg/day
MONOCLONAL ANTIBODY/IgE-BLOCKER			
Omalizumab (Xolair)‡	**Inj:** 150mg	150-375mg SQ q2 or 4 weeks. Determine dose and dosing frequency by serum total IgE level (IU/mL), measured before the start of treatment, and body weight (kg). See PI for dose determination charts	**≥12 yrs:** Refer to adult dosing
PHOSPHODIESTERASE₄ INHIBITOR			
Roflumilast (Daliresp)†	**Tab:** 500mcg	500mcg qd	

(Continued)

GENERIC (BRAND)	DOSAGE FORM	ADULT DOSAGE	CHILD DOSAGE
SHORT-ACTING β₂-AGONISTS			
Albuterol	**Sol, Inh:** 0.083%, 0.5%; **Syrup:** 2mg/5mL; **Tab (scored):** 2mg, 4mg; **Tab, Extended-Release:** 4mg, 8mg	**(Tab, Extended-Release) Initial:** 4-8mg q12h. **Max:** 32mg/day. **(Sol)** 2.5mg tid-qid via nebulizer. **(Syrup, Tab):** 2-4mg tid-qid. **Max:** 8mg qid	**>14 yrs: (Syrup) Initial:** 2-4mg tid-qid. **Max:** 8mg qid. **>12 yrs: (Tab) Initial:** 2-4mg tid-qid. **Max:** 8mg qid. **(Tab, Extended-Release) Initial:** 4-8mg q12h. **Max:** 32mg/day. **6-14 yrs: (Syrup) Initial:** 2mg tid-qid. **Max:** 24mg/day. **6-12 yrs: (Tab, Extended-Release) Initial:** 4mg q12h. **Max:** 24mg/day. **(Tabs) Initial:** 2mg tid-qid. **Max:** 24mg/day. **2-12 yrs: (Sol) ≥15 kg:** 2.5mg tid-qid via nebulizer. **10-15 kg:** 1.25mg tid-qid. Use 0.5% solution for 1.25mg/dose. **2-5 yrs: (Syrup) Initial:** 0.1mg/kg tid (not to exceed 2mg tid). **Titrate:** May increase to 0.2mg/kg tid. **Max:** 4mg tid
Albuterol Sulfate (AccuNeb)	**Sol, Inh:** 0.63mg/3mL, 1.25mg/3mL		**2-12 yrs:** 0.63mg or 1.25mg tid-qid via nebulizer
Albuterol Sulfate (ProAir HFA, Proventil HFA, Ventolin HFA)	**MDI:** 90mcg/inh	**Treatment:** 2 inh q4-6h or 1 inh q4h. **Prevention of exercise-induced bronchospasm:** 2 inh 15-30 min before exercise	**≥4 yrs:** Refer to adult dosing
Levalbuterol (Xopenex, Xopenex HFA)	**Sol, Inh:** 0.31mg/3mL, 0.63mg/3mL, 1.25mg/3mL (HFA) 45mcg/inh	0.63-1.25mg tid q6-8h via nebulizer. (HFA) 2 inh (90mcg) q4-6h or 1 inh (45mcg) q4h. Dosage based on severity of asthma	**≥12 yrs:** Refer to adult dosing. **6-11 yrs:** 0.31mg tid **Max:** 0.63mg tid. **≥4 yrs:** (HFA) 2 inh (90mcg) q4-6h or 1 inh (45mcg) q4h
Pirbuterol (Maxair)	**MDI:** 0.2mg/inh	1-2 inh q4-6h. **Max:** 12 inh/day	**≥12 yrs:** Refer to adult dosing
SYSTEMIC CORTICOSTEROIDS			
Methylprednisolone	**Tab:** 2mg, 4mg, 8mg, 16mg, 32mg	**Initial:** 5-60mg. Dosage must be individualized based on the disease state and patient response	
Prednisolone	**Tab:** 5mg; **Liq:** 5mg/5mL, 15mg/5mL		
Prednisone	**Tab:** 1mg, 2.5mg, 5mg, 10mg, 20mg, 50mg; **Liq:** 5mg/5mL, 15mg/5mL		

MDI = metered-dose inhaler; DPI = dry-powder inhaler

†Indicated for COPD only.

*Indicated for asthma & COPD.

**Check monograph for detailed dosing guidelines.

§The dose of theophylline must be individualized based on peak serum theophylline concentrations.

‡Check monograph for important Boxed Warnings.

Adapted from: The NAEPP Expert Panel Report: Guidelines for the Diagnosis and Management of Asthma—Update on Selected Topics 2007. http://www.nhlbi.nih.gov/guidelines/asthma/asthsumm.htm

ASTHMA TREATMENT PLAN*

CLASSIFICATION	LUNG FUNCTION	STEPWISE APPROACH TO THERAPY IN PATIENTS ≥12 YEARS OF AGE
Intermittent • Symptoms ≤2 days/wk • Short-acting β_2-agonist use for symptom control ≤2 days/wk • Nighttime awakenings ≤2 times/month • Interference with normal activity—none	• Normal FEV_1 b/w exacerbations • FEV_1 >80% predicted • FEV_1/FVC—normal	**Step 1** • **Short-acting inhaled β_2-agonists as needed** • Severe exacerbations may occur, separated by long periods of normal lung function and no symptoms; a course of systemic corticosteroids is recommended.
Mild persistent • Symptoms >2 days/wk but not daily • Short-acting β_2-agonist use for symptom control >2 days/wk but not daily, and not more than 1x on any day • Nighttime awakenings 3-4x/month • Interference with normal activity—minor limitation	• FEV_1 >80% predicted • FEV_1/FVC—normal	**Step 2** • **Low-dose ICS** • **Short-acting inhaled β_2-agonists as needed** ALTERNATIVE TREATMENT: • Cromolyn, LTRA, nedocromil OR theophylline
Moderate persistent • Daily symptoms • Short acting β_2-agonist use for symptom control daily • Nighttime awakening >1x/wk but not nightly • Interference with normal activity—some limitation	• FEV_1 >60% but <80% predicted • FEV_1/FVC reduced 5%	**Step 3** • **Low-dose ICS + LABA or medium-dose ICS** AND • **Short-acting inhaled β_2-agonists as needed** ALTERNATIVE TREATMENT: • Low-dose ICS + either LTRA, theophylline, or zileuton
Severe persistent • Symptoms throughout the day • Short-acting β_2-agonist use for symptoms several times per day • Nighttime awakenings often >7x/wk • Interference with normal activity—extreme limitation	• FEV_1 <60% predicted • FEV_1/FVC reduced >5%	**Step 4** • **Medium-dose ICS + LABA (Step 4)** or • **High-dose ICS + LABA (Step 5)** or • **High-dose ICS + LABA + oral corticosteroid (Step 6)** AND • Consider omalizumab for patients who have allergies (Steps 5 and 6) • **Short-acting inhaled β_2-agonists as needed** ALTERNATIVE TREATMENT: • Medium-dose ICS + either LTRA, theophylline, or zileuton (Step 4)

Note: Preferred treatments are in bold.

Key Points:

Stepwise approach presents general guidelines. Review treatment every 1-6 months to maintain control. A gradual reduction in treatment may be possible if well controlled for at least 3 months. If control is not maintained, consider step up and re-evaluate in 2-6 weeks.

The presence of one of the features of severity is sufficient to place a patient in that category. An individual should be assigned to the most severe grade in which any feature occurs (PEF is % of personal best; FEV is % predicted).

Short-acting β_2-agonists as needed for symptomatic relief for all patients. Intensity of treatment will depend on severity of exacerbation; up to 3 treatments at 20-minute intervals as needed. Course of systemic corticosteroids may be needed.

Use of short-acting β_2-agonists >2 days/wk for symptom relief generally indicates inadequate control and the need to step up treatment.

Airflow obstruction is indicated by reduced FEV_1 and FEV_1/FVC values relative to reference or predicted values.

Abnormalities of lung function are categorized as restrictive and obstructive defects. A reduced ratio of FEV_1/FVC (eg, <65%) indicates obstruction to the flow of air from the lungs, whereas a reduced FVC with a normal or increased FEV_1/FVC ratio suggests a restrictive pattern.

Abbreviations: FEV_1=forced expiratory volume in one second; FVC=forced vital capacity; ICS=inhaled corticosteroid; LABA=long-acting inhaled β_2-agonist; LTRA=leukotriene receptor antagonist.

*Adapted from *Expert Panel Report 3: Guidelines for the Diagnosis and Management of Asthma. Full Report 2007*. National Heart, Lung, and Blood Institute, National Asthma Education and Prevention Program, U.S. Department of Health and Human Services.

ERECTILE DYSFUNCTION TREATMENT

GENERIC (BRAND)	HOW SUPPLIED	DOSAGE
PROSTAGLANDINS		
Alprostadil (Edex, Caverject, Caverject Impulse)	**Edex: Inj:** 10, 20, 40mcg (sterile powder) **Caverject: Inj:** 5, 10, 20, 40mcg (sterile powder); **Inj:** 10, 20mcg (Impulse)	**Vasculogenic, Psychogenic, or Mixed Etiology: Initiate:** 2.5mcg. Increase to 5mcg, then by 5-10mcg based on response until erection of 1 hr max duration. **No Response to 2.5mcg: Initiate:** 7.5mcg, followed by 5-10mcg increments. **Pure Neurogenic Etiology (Spinal Cord Injury):** Initiate: 1.25mcg. Increase to 2.5mcg, followed by a 5mcg dose, then increase by 5mcg increments until erection of 1 hr max duration. Patient must stay in physician's office until complete detumescence. If no response, give next higher dose within 1 hr. If response, min 24 hrs before next dose. Dose range: 1-40mcg. Give injection over 5-10 second interval. **Maint:** Give no more than 3 times weekly; allow 24 hrs between doses. (Caverject) **Max:** 60mcg/ dose.
Alprostadil (Muse)	**Suppositories, Urethral:** 125, 250, 500, 1000mcg	**Initial:** 125-250mcg. **Titration:** Increase or decrease dose based on individual response. **Max:** 2 administrations within 24 hrs.
PHOSPHODIESTERASE INHIBITORS		
Sildenafil (Viagra)	**Tablets:** 25, 50, 100mg	**Usual:** 50mg prn 1 hr prior to sexual activity. **Titration:** Increase to 100mg qd or decrease to 25mg qd based on efficacy/tolerability. **Max:** 1 dose qd.
Tadalafil (Cialis)	**Tablets:** 2.5, 5, 10, 20mg	**PRN use: Initial:** 10mg prior to sexual activity qd. **Titration:** Increase to 20mg qd or decrease to 5mg qd based on efficacy/tolerability. QD use: 2.5mg qd. **Titration:** Increase to 5mg qd based on efficacy/ tolerability. **Max:** 1 dose qd.
Vardenafil (Levitra)	**Tablets:** 2.5, 5, 10, 20mg	**Usual:** 10mg 1 hr prior to sexual activity qd. **Titration:** Increase to 20mg qd or decrease to 5mg qd based on efficacy/tolerability. **Max:** 1 dose qd.
Vardenafil (Staxyn)	**Tab, Disintegrating:** 10mg	10mg 1 hr prior to sexual activity prn. **Max:** 1 tab qd. Place on tongue to disintegrate. Take without liquid.

UROLOGICAL THERAPIES

OVERACTIVE BLADDER AGENTS

GENERIC	BRAND	HOW SUPPLIED	DOSAGE	COMMENTS
Darifenacin	Enablex	**Tab, ER:** 7.5mg, 15mg	**Initial:** 7.5mg qd. **Max:** 15mg qd.	Swallow whole. Moderate Hepatic Impairment/Concomitant Potent CYP3A4 Inhibitors: Do not exceed 7.5mg/day. Severe Hepatic Impairment: Avoid use.
Fesoterodine	Toviaz	**Tab, ER:** 4mg, 8mg	**Initial:** 4mg qd. **Max:** 8mg/day.	Swallow whole. CrCl <30mL/min/Concomitant Potent CYP3A4 Inhibitors: Do not exceed 4mg/day. Severe Hepatic Impairment: Avoid use.
Oxybutynin	Ditropan	**(Generic) Syrup:** 1mg/1mL; **Tab:** 5mg	**Usual:** 5mg bid-tid. **Max:** 5mg qid.	A lower starting dose of 2.5mg bid-tid is recommended for elderly patients. **Pediatrics >5 yrs:** 5mg bid. **Max:** 5mg tid.
	Ditropan XL	**Tab, ER:** 5mg, 10mg, 15mg	**Initial:** 5mg or 10mg qd. **Max:** 30mg/day.	Swallow whole. Increase dose by 5mg weekly if needed. **Pediatrics ≥6 yrs:** 5mg qd. **Max:** 20mg/day.
	Gelnique	**Gel:** 10% (1g/pkt)	Apply contents of 1 pkt qd to dry skin on abdomen, upper arms/shoulders, or thighs.	Rotate application sites.
	Oxytrol	**Patch:** 3.9mg/day	**Usual:** Apply 1 patch twice weekly (every 3-4 days).	Rotate application sites.
Solifenacin	VESIcare	**Tab:** 5mg, 10mg	**Usual:** 5mg qd. **Max:** 10mg qd.	Swallow whole. Renal (CrCl <30mL/min)/Moderate Hepatic Impairment/Concomitant Potent CYP3A4 Inhibitors: Do not exceed 5mg/day. Severe Hepatic Impairment: Avoid use.
Tolterodine	Detrol	**Tab:** 1mg, 2mg	**Initial:** 2mg bid.	Decrease dose to 1mg bid if needed. Significant Hepatic/Renal Dysfunction/Concomitant Potent CYP3A4 Inhibitors: 1mg bid.
	Detrol LA	**Cap, ER:** 2mg, 4mg	**Initial:** 4mg qd.	Swallow whole. Decrease dose to 2mg qd if needed. Mild-Moderate Hepatic/Severe Renal Dysfunction (CrCl 10-30 mL/min)/Concomitant Potent CYP3A4 Inhibitors: 2mg qd. Severe Hepatic Impairment/CrCl <10mL/min: Avoid use.
Trospium	Sanctura	**Tab:** 20mg	**Usual:** 20mg bid.	Take 1 hr before meals or on empty stomach. CrCl <30mL/min: 20mg qhs. **Elderly ≥75 yrs:** May titrate to 20mg qd based on tolerability.
	Sanctura XR	**Cap, ER:** 60mg	**Usual:** 60mg qam.	Take on empty stomach 1 hr before meal. CrCl <30mL/min: Avoid use.

(Continued)

BENIGN PROSTATIC HYPERTROPHY AGENTS

GENERIC	BRAND	HOW SUPPLIED	DOSAGE	COMMENTS
ALPHA-BLOCKERS				
Alfuzosin	Uroxatral	**Tab, ER:** 10mg	**Usual:** 10mg qd.	Take dose immediately with the same meal each day. Swallow whole. Moderate to Severe Hepatic Impairment/Potent CYP3A4 Inhibitors: Contraindicated.
Doxazosin	Cardura	**Tab:** 1mg, 2mg, 4mg, 8mg	**Initial:** 1mg qd. **Max:** 8mg/day.	Stepwise titration every 1-2 weeks if needed.
	Cardura XL	**Tab, ER:** 4mg, 8mg	**Initial:** 4mg qd. **Max:** 8mg qd.	Take with breakfast. Swallow whole. Titrate after 3-4 weeks if needed.
Silodosin	Rapaflo	**Cap:** 4mg, 8mg	**Usual:** 8mg qd.	Take with food. CrCl 30-50mL/min: 4mg qd. Severe Renal Impairment (CrCl <30mL/min)/ Severe Hepatic Impairment: Contraindicated.
Tamsulosin	Flomax	**Cap:** 0.4mg	**Initial:** 0.4mg qd. **Max:** 0.8mg qd.	Take dose 30 min after the same meal each day. Titrate after 2-4 weeks if needed. Restart at initial dose if therapy is interrupted. Do not use in combination with strong CYP3A4 inhibitors.
Terazosin	Hytrin	**Tab, Cap:** 1mg, 2mg, 5mg, 10mg	**Initial:** 1mg qhs. **Usual:** 10mg/day. **Max:** 20mg/day.	Increase stepwise as needed. Restart at initial dose if therapy is interrupted.
5-ALPHA-REDUCTASE INHIBITORS				
Dutasteride	Avodart	**Cap:** 0.5mg	**Usual:** 0.5mg qd.	Swallow whole. May be administered with tamsulosin.
Finasteride	Proscar	**Tab:** 5mg	**Usual:** 5mg qd.	May be administered with doxazosin with or without meals.
COMBINATION				
Dutasteride/ Tamsulosin	Jalyn	**Cap:** 0.5mg/0.4mg	**Usual:** 1 cap qd.	Swallow whole. Take dose 30 min after the same meal each day. Do not use in combination with strong CYP3A4 inhibitors.

RECOMMENDED IMMUNIZATION SCHEDULE FOR PERSONS AGED 0-6 YEARS—UNITED STATES, 2012

Vaccine ▼ Age ►	Birth	1 month	2 months	4 months	6 months	9 months	12 months	15 months	18 months	19–23 years	2–3 years	4–6 years
Hepatitis B[1]	Hep B	HepB					HepB					
Rotavirus[2]			RV	RV	RV[2]							
Diphtheria, tetanus, pertussis[3]			DTaP	DTaP	DTaP		see footnote[3]	DTaP				DTaP
Haemophilus influenzae type b[4]			Hib	Hib	Hib[4]		Hib					
Pneumococcal[5]			PCV	PCV	PCV		PCV					PPSV
Inactivated poliovirus[6]			IPV	IPV			IPV					IPV
Influenza[7]							Influenza (Yearly)					
Measles, mumps, rubella[8]							MMR		see footnote[8]			MMR
Varicella[9]							Varicella		see footnote[9]			Varicella
Hepatitis A[10]							Dose 1[10]				HepA Series	
Meningococcal[11]							MCV4 — see footnote[11]					

Range of recommended ages for all children   Range of recommended ages for certain high-risk groups   ///// Range of recommended ages for all children and certain high-risk groups

This schedule includes recommendations in effect as of December 23, 2011. Any dose not administered at the recommended age should be administered at a subsequent visit, when indicated and feasible. The use of a combination vaccine generally is preferred over separate injections of its equivalent component vaccines. Vaccination providers should consult the relevant Advisory Committee on Immunization Practices (ACIP) statement for detailed recommendations, available online at http://www.cdc.gov/vaccines/pubs/acip-list.htm. Clinically significant adverse events that follow vaccination should be reported to the Vaccine Adverse Event Reporting System (VAERS) online (http://www.vaers.hhs.gov) or by telephone (800-822-7967).

1. Hepatitis B (HepB) vaccine. (Minimum age: birth)
At birth:
- Administer monovalent HepB vaccine to all newborns before hospital discharge.
- For infants born to hepatitis B surface antigen (HBsAg)–positive mothers, administer HepB vaccine and 0.5 mL of hepatitis B immune globulin (HBIG) within 12 hours of birth. These infants should be tested for HBsAg and antibody to HBsAg (anti-HBs) 1 to 2 months after receiving the last dose of the series.
- If mother's HBsAg status is unknown, within 12 hours of birth administer HepB vaccine for infants weighing ≥2000 grams, and HepB vaccine plus HBIG for infants weighing <2000 grams. Determine mother's HBsAg status as soon as possible and, if she is HBsAg-positive, administer HBIG for infants weighing ≥2000 grams (no later than age 1 week).

Doses after the birth dose:
- The second dose should be administered at age 1 to 2 months. Monovalent HepB vaccine should be used for doses administered before age 6 weeks.
- Administration of a total of 4 doses of HepB vaccine is permissible when a combination vaccine containing HepB is administered after the birth dose.
- Infants who did not receive a birth dose should receive 3 doses of a HepB-containing vaccine starting as soon as feasible (see the *Catch-Up Immunization Schedule*).
- The minimum interval between dose 1 and dose 2 is 4 weeks, and between dose 2 and 3 is 8 weeks. The final (third or fourth) dose in the HepB vaccine series should be administered no earlier than age 24 weeks and at least 16 weeks after the first dose.

2. Rotavirus (RV) vaccines. (Minimum age: 6 weeks for both RV-1 [Rotarix] and RV-5 [Rota Teq])

- The maximum age for the first dose in the series is 14 weeks, 6 days; and 8 months, 0 days for the final dose in the series. Vaccination should not be initiated for infants aged 15 weeks, 0 days or older.
- If RV-1 (Rotarix) is administered at ages 2 and 4 months, a dose at 6 months is not indicated.

3. Diphtheria and tetanus toxoids and acellular pertussis (DTaP) vaccine. (Minimum age: 6 weeks)
- The fourth dose may be administered as early as age 12 months, provided at least 6 months have elapsed since the third dose.

4. Haemophilus influenzae type b (Hib) conjugate vaccine. (Minimum age: 6 weeks)
- If PRP-OMP (PedvaxHIB or Comvax [HepB-Hib]) is administered at ages 2 and 4 months, a dose at age 6 months is not indicated.
- Hiberix should only be used for the booster (final) dose in children aged 12 months through 4 years.

5. Pneumococcal vaccines. (Minimum age: 6 weeks for pneumococcal conjugate vaccine [PCV]; 2 years for pneumococcal polysaccharide vaccine [PPSV])
- Administer 1 dose of PCV to all healthy children aged 24 through 59 months who are not completely vaccinated for their age.
- For children who have received an age-appropriate series of 7-valent PCV (PCV7), a single supplemental dose of 13-valent PCV (PCV13) is recommended for:
  — All children aged 14 through 59 months
  — Children aged 60 through 71 months with underlying medical conditions.
- Administer PPSV at least 8 weeks after last dose of PCV to children aged 2 years or older with certain underlying medical conditions, including a cochlear

(Continued)

implant. See *MMWR* 2010:59(No. RR-11), available at http://www.cdc.gov/mmwr/pdf/rr/rr5911.pdf.

6. Inactivated poliovirus vaccine (IPV). (Minimum age: 6 weeks)
- If 4 or more doses are administered before age 4 years, an additional dose should be administered at age 4 through 6 years.
- The final dose in the series should be administered on or after the fourth birthday and at least 6 months after the previous dose.

7. Influenza vaccines. (Minimum age: 6 months for trivalent inactivated influenza vaccine [TIV]; 2 years for live, attenuated influenza vaccine [LAIV])
- For most healthy children aged 2 years and older, either LAIV or TIV may be used. However, LAIV should not be administered to some children, including 1) children with asthma, 2) children 2 through 4 years who had wheezing in the past 12 months, or 3) children who have any other underlying medical conditions that predispose them to influenza complications. For all other contraindications to use of LAIV, see *MMWR* 2010;59(No. RR-8), available at http://www.cdc.gov/mmwr/pdf/rr/rr5908.pdf.
- For children aged 6 months through 8 years:
  — For the 2011–12 season, administer 2 doses (separated by at least 4 weeks) to those who did not receive at least 1 dose of the 2010–11 vaccine. Those who received at least 1 dose of the 2010–11 vaccine require 1 dose for the 2011–12 season.
  — For the 2012–13 season, follow dosing guidelines in the 2012 ACIP influenza vaccine recommendations.

8. Measles, mumps, and rubella (MMR) vaccine. (Minimum age: 12 months)
- The second dose may be administered before age 4 years, provided at least 4 weeks have elapsed since the first dose.
- Administer MMR vaccine to infants aged 6 through 11 months who are traveling internationally. These children should be revaccinated with 2 doses of MMR vaccine, the first at ages 12 through 15 months and at least 4 weeks after the previous dose, and the second at ages 4 through 6 years.

9. Varicella (VAR) vaccine. (Minimum age: 12 months)
- The second dose may be administered before age

4 years, provided at least 3 months have elapsed since the first dose.
- For children aged 12 months through 12 years, the recommended minimum interval between doses is 3 months. However, if the second dose was administered at least 4 weeks after the first dose, it can be accepted as valid.

10. Hepatitis A (HepA) vaccine. (Minimum age: 12 months)
- Administer the second (final) dose 6 to 18 months after the first.
- Unvaccinated children 24 months and older at high risk should be vaccinated. See *MMWR* 2006;55(No. RR-7), available at http://www.cdc.gov/mmwr/pdf/rr/rr5507.pdf.
- A 2-dose HepA vaccine series is recommended for anyone aged 24 months and older, previously unvaccinated, for whom immunity against hepatitis A virus infection is desired.

11. Meningococcal conjugate vaccines, quadrivalent (MCV4). (Minimum age: 9 months for Menactra [MCV4-D], 2 years for Menveo [MCV4-CRM])
- For children aged 9 through 23 months 1) with persistent complement component deficiency; 2) who are residents of or travelers to countries with hyperendemic or epidemic disease; or 3) who are present during outbreaks caused by a vaccine serogroup, administer 2 primary doses of MCV4-D, ideally at ages 9 months and 12 months or at least 8 weeks apart.
- For children aged 24 months and older with 1) persistent complement component deficiency who have not been previously vaccinated; or 2) anatomic/functional asplenia, administer 2 primary doses of either MCV4 at least 8 weeks apart.
- For children with anatomic/functional asplenia, if MCV4-D (Menactra) is used, administer at a minimum age of 2 years and at least 4 weeks after completion of all PCV doses.
- See *MMWR* 2011;60:72–76, available at http://www.cdc.gov/mmwr/pdf/wk/mm6003. pdf, and Vaccines for Children Program resolution No. 6/11-1, available at http://www. cdc.gov/vaccines/programs/vfc/downloads/resolutions/06-11mening-mcv.pdf, and *MMWR* 2011;60:1391–2, available at http://www.cdc. gov/mmwr/pdf/wk/mm6040. pdf, for further guidance, including revaccination guidelines.

RECOMMENDED IMMUNIZATION SCHEDULE FOR PERSONS AGED 7-18 YEARS—UNITED STATES, 2012

Vaccine ▼ Age ►	7–10 years	11–12 years	13–18 years
Tetanus, diphtheria, pertussis[1]	1 dose (if indicated)	1 dose	1 dose (if indicated)
Human papillomavirus[2]	see footnote[2]	3 doses	Complete 3-dose series
Meningococcal[3]	See footnote[3]	Dose 1	Booster at 18 years old
Influenza[4]	Influenza (yearly)		
Pneumococcal[5]	See footnote[5]		
Hepatitis A[6]	Complete 2-dose series		
Hepatitis B[7]	Complete 3-dose series		
Inactivated poliovirus[8]	Complete 3-dose series		
Measles, mumps, rubella[9]	Complete 2-dose series		
Varicella[10]	Complete 2-dose series		

Range of recommended ages for all children   Range of recommended ages for catch-up immunization   Range of recommended ages for certain high-risk groups

This schedule includes recommendations in effect as of December 23, 2011. Any dose not administered at the recommended age should be administered at a subsequent visit, when indicated and feasible. The use of a combination vaccine generally is preferred over separate injections of its equivalent component vaccines. Vaccination providers should consult the relevant Advisory Committee on Immunization Practices (ACIP) statement for detailed recommendations, available online at http://www.cdc.gov/vaccines/pubs/acip-list.htm. Clinically significant adverse events that follow vaccination should be reported to the Vaccine Adverse Event Reporting System (VAERS) online (http://www.vaers.hhs.gov) or by telephone (800-822-7967).

1. **Tetanus and diphtheria toxoids and acellular pertussis (Tdap) vaccine.** (Minimum age: 10 years for Boostrix and 11 years for Adacel)
   - Persons aged 11 through 18 years who have not received Tdap vaccine should receive a dose followed by tetanus and diphtheria toxoids (Td) booster doses every 10 years thereafter.
   - Tdap vaccine should be substituted for a single dose of Td in the catch-up series for children aged 7 through 10 years. Refer to the *Catch-Up Schedule* if additional doses of tetanus and diphtheria toxoid–containing vaccine are needed.
   - Tdap vaccine can be administered regardless of the interval since the last tetanus and diphtheria toxoid–containing vaccine.

2. **Human papillomavirus (HPV) vaccines (HPV4 [Gardasil] and HPV2 [Cervarix]).** (Minimum age: 9 years)
   - Either HPV4 or HPV2 is recommended in a 3-dose series for females aged 11 or 12 years. HPV4 is recommended in a 3-dose series for males aged 11 or 12 years.
   - The vaccine series can be started beginning at age 9 years.
   - Administer the second dose 1 to 2 months after the first dose and the third dose 6 months after the first dose (at least 24 weeks after the first dose).
   - See *MMWR* 2010;59:626–632, available at http://www.cdc.gov/mmwr/pdf/wk/mm5920.pdf.

3. **Meningococcal conjugate vaccines, quadrivalent (MCV4).**
   - Administer MCV4 at age 11 through 12 years with a booster dose at age 16 years.
   - Administer MCV4 at age 13 through 18 years if patient is not previously vaccinated.

   - If the first dose is administered at age 13 through 15 years, a booster dose should be administered at age 16 through 18 years with a minimum interval of at least 8 weeks after the preceding dose.
   - If the first dose is administered at age 16 years or older, a booster dose is not needed.
   - Administer 2 primary doses at least 8 weeks apart to previously unvaccinated persons with persistent complement component deficiency or anatomic/functional asplenia, and 1 dose every 5 years thereafter.
   - Adolescents aged 11 through 18 years with human immunodeficiency virus (HIV) infection should receive a 2-dose primary series of MCV4, at least 8 weeks apart.
   - See *MMWR* 2011;60:72–76, available at http://www.cdc.gov/mmwr/pdf/wk/mm6003.pdf, and Vaccines for Children Program resolution No. 6/11-1, available at http://www.cdc.gov/vaccines/programs/vfc/downloads/resolutions/06-11mening-mcv.pdf, for further guidelines.

4. **Influenza vaccines (trivalent inactivated influenza vaccine [TIV] and live, attenuated influenza vaccine [LAIV]).**
   - For most healthy, nonpregnant persons, either LAIV or TIV may be used, except LAIV should not be used for some persons, including those with asthma or any other underlying medical conditions that predispose them to influenza complications. For all other contraindications to use of LAIV, see *MMWR* 2010;59(No.RR-8), available at http://www.cdc.gov/mmwr/pdf/rr/rr5908.pdf.
   - Administer 1 dose to persons aged 9 years and older.
   - For children aged 6 months through 8 years:
     — For the 2011–12 season, administer 2 doses (separated by at least 4 weeks) to those who did

(Continued)

not receive at least 1 dose of the 2010–11 vaccine. Those who received at least 1 dose of the 2010–11 vaccine require 1 dose for the 2011–12 season.

— For the 2012–13 season, follow dosing guidelines in the 2012 ACIP influenza vaccine recommendations.

5. Pneumococcal vaccines (pneumococcal conjugate vaccine [PCV] and pneumococcal polysaccharide vaccine [PPSV]).

• A single dose of PCV may be administered to children aged 6 through 18 years who have anatomic/functional asplenia, HIV infection or other immunocompromising condition, cochlear implant, or cerebral spinal fluid leak. See *MMWR* 2010:59(No. RR-11), available at http://www.cdc.gov/mmwr/pdf/rr/rr5911.pdf.

• Administer PPSV at least 8 weeks after the last dose of PCV to children aged 2 years or older with certain underlying medical conditions, including a cochlear implant. A single revaccination should be administered after 5 years to children with anatomic/functional asplenia or an immunocompromising condition.

6. Hepatitis A (HepA) vaccine.

• HepA vaccine is recommended for children older than 23 months who live in areas where vaccination programs target older children, who are at increased risk for infection, or for whom immunity against hepatitis A virus infection is desired. See *MMWR* 2006;55(No. RR-7), available at http://www.cdc.gov/mmwr/pdf/rr/rr5507.pdf.

• Administer 2 doses at least 6 months apart to unvaccinated persons.

7. Hepatitis B (HepB) vaccine.

• Administer the 3-dose series to those not previously vaccinated.

• For those with incomplete vaccination, follow the catch-up recommendations.

• A 2-dose series (doses separated by at least 4 months) of adult formulation Recombivax HB is licensed for use in children aged 11 through 15 years.

8. Inactivated poliovirus vaccine (IPV).

• The final dose in the series should be administered at least 6 months after the previous dose.

• If both OPV and IPV were administered as part of a series, a total of 4 doses should be administered, regardless of the child's current age.

• IPV is not routinely recommended for U.S. residents aged 18 years or older.

9. Measles, mumps, and rubella (MMR) vaccine.

• The minimum interval between the 2 doses of MMR vaccine is 4 weeks.

10. Varicella (VAR) vaccine.

• For persons without evidence of immunity (see *MMWR* 2007;56[No. RR-4], available at http://www.cdc.gov/mmwr/pdf/rr/rr5604.pdf), administer 2 doses if not previously vaccinated or the second dose if only 1 dose has been administered.

• For persons aged 7 through 12 years, the recommended minimum interval between doses is 3 months. However, if the second dose was administered at least 4 weeks after the first dose, it can be accepted as valid.

• For persons aged 13 years and older, the minimum interval between doses is 4 weeks.

CATCH-UP IMMUNIZATION SCHEDULE FOR PERSONS AGED 4 MONTHS THROUGH 18 YEARS WHO START LATE OR WHO ARE MORE THAN 1 MONTH BEHIND—UNITED STATES, 2012

Vaccine	Minimum Age for Dose 1	Minimum Interval Between Doses			
		Persons aged 4 months through 6 years			
		Dose 1 to dose 2	Dose 2 to dose 3	Dose 3 to dose 4	Dose 4 to dose 5
Hepatitis B[1]	Birth	4 weeks	8 weeks and at least 16 weeks after first dose; minimum age for the final dose is 24 weeks		
Rotavirus[1]	6 weeks	4 weeks	4 weeks[1]		
Diphtheria, tetanus, pertussis[2]	6 weeks	4 weeks	4 weeks	6 months	6 months[2]
Haemophilus influenzae type b[3]	6 weeks	4 weeks if first dose administered at younger than age 12 months / 8 weeks (as final dose) if first dose administered at age 12–14 months / No further doses needed if first dose administered at age 15 months or older	4 weeks[3] if current age is younger than 12 months / 8 weeks (as final dose)[3] if current age is 12 months or older and first dose administered at younger than age 12 months and second dose administered at younger than 15 months / No further doses needed if previous dose administered at age 15 months or older	8 weeks (as final dose) This dose only necessary for children aged 12 months through 59 months who received 3 doses before age 12 months	
Pneumococcal[4]	6 weeks	4 weeks if first dose administered at younger than age 12 months / 8 weeks (as final dose for healthy children) if first dose administered at age 12 months or older or current age 24 through 59 months / No further doses needed for healthy children if first dose administered at age 24 months or older	4 weeks if current age is younger than 12 months / 8 weeks (as final dose for healthy children) if current age is 12 months or older / No further doses needed for healthy children if previous dose administered at age 24 months or older	8 weeks (as final dose) This dose only necessary for children aged 12 months through 59 months who received 3 doses before age 12 months or for children at high risk who received 3 doses at any age	
Inactivated poliovirus[5]	6 weeks	4 weeks	4 weeks	6 months[5] minimum age 4 years for final dose	
Meningococcal[6]	9 months	8 weeks[6]			
Measles, mumps, rubella[7]	12 months	4 weeks			
Varicella[8]	12 months	3 months			
Hepatitis A	12 months	6 months			
		Persons aged 7 through 18 years			
Tetanus, diphtheria/ tetanus, diphtheria, pertussis[9]	7 years[9]	4 weeks	4 weeks if first dose administered at younger than age 12 months / 6 months if first dose administered at 12 months or older	6 months if first dose administered at younger than age 12 months	
Human papillomavirus[10]	9 years	Routine dosing intervals are recommended[10]			
Hepatitis A	12 months	6 months			
Hepatitis B	Birth	4 weeks	8 weeks (and at least 16 weeks after first dose)		
Inactivated poliovirus[5]	6 weeks	4 weeks	4 weeks[5]	6 months[5]	
Meningococcal[6]	6 months	8 weeks[6]			
Measles, mumps, rubella[7]	12 months	4 weeks			
Varicella[8]	12 months	3 months if person is younger than age 13 years / 4 weeks if person is aged 13 years or older			

The figure below provides catch-up schedules and minimum intervals between doses for children whose vaccinations have been delayed. A vaccine series does not need to be restarted, regardless of the time that has elapsed between doses. Use the section appropriate for the child's age. Always use this table in conjunction with the accompanying childhood and adolescent immunization schedules (Figures 1 and 2) and their respective footnotes.

1. **Rotavirus (RV) vaccines (RV-1 [Rotarix] and RV-5 [Rota Teq]).**
   - The maximum age for the first dose in the series is 14 weeks, 6 days; and 8 months, 0 days for the final dose in the series. Vaccination should not be initiated for infants aged 15 weeks, 0 days or older.
   - If RV-1 was administered for the first and second doses, a third dose is not indicated.

2. **Diphtheria and tetanus toxoids and acellular pertussis (DTaP) vaccine.**
   - The fifth dose is not necessary if the fourth dose was administered at age 4 years or older.

3. **Haemophilus influenzae type b (Hib) conjugate vaccine.**
   - Hib vaccine should be considered for unvaccinated persons aged 5 years or older who have sickle cell disease, leukemia, human immunodeficiency virus (HIV) infection, or anatomic/functional asplenia.
   - If the first 2 doses were PRP-OMP (PedvaxHIB or Comvax) and were administered at age 11 months or younger, the third (and final) dose should be administered at age 12 through 15 months and at least 8 weeks after the second dose.

   - If the first dose was administered at age 7 through 11 months, administer the second dose at least 4 weeks later and a final dose at age 12 through 15 months.

4. **Pneumococcal vaccines.** (Minimum age: 6 weeks for pneumococcal conjugate vaccine [PCV]; 2 years for pneumococcal polysaccharide vaccine [PPSV])
   - For children aged 24 through 71 months with underlying medical conditions, administer 1 dose of PCV if 3 doses of PCV were received previously, or administer 2 doses of PCV at least 8 weeks apart if fewer than 3 doses of PCV were received previously.
   - A single dose of PCV may be administered to certain children aged 6 through 18 years with underlying medical conditions. See age-specific schedules for details.
   - Administer PPSV to children aged 2 years or older with certain underlying medical conditions. See *MMWR* 2010:59(No. RR-11), available at http://www.cdc.gov/mmwr/pdf/rr/rr5911.pdf.

5. **Inactivated poliovirus vaccine (IPV).**
   - A fourth dose is not necessary if the third dose was administered at age 4 years or older and at least 6 months after the previous dose.

- In the first 6 months of life, minimum age and minimum intervals are only recommended if the person is at risk for imminent exposure to circulating poliovirus (ie, travel to a polio-endemic region or during an outbreak).
- IPV is not routinely recommended for U.S. residents aged 18 years or older.

6. **Meningococcal conjugate vaccines, quadrivalent (MCV4).** (Minimum age: 9 months for Menactra [MCV4-D]; 2 years for Menveo [MCV4-CRM])
   - See *Recommended Immunization Schedule for Persons Aged 0 through 6 Years* and *Recommended Immunization Schedule for Persons Aged 7 through 18 Years* for further guidance.

7. **Measles, mumps, and rubella (MMR) vaccine.**
   - Administer the second dose routinely at age 4 through 6 years.

8. **Varicella (VAR) vaccine.**
   - Administer the second dose routinely at age 4 through 6 years. If the second dose was administered at least 4 weeks after the first dose, it can be accepted as valid.

9. **Tetanus and diphtheria toxoids (Td) and tetanus and diphtheria toxoids and acellular pertussis (Tdap) vaccines.**
   - For children aged 7 through 10 years who are not fully immunized with the childhood DTaP vaccine series, Tdap vaccine should be substituted for a single dose of Td vaccine in the catch-up series; if additional doses are needed, use Td vaccine. For these children, an adolescent Tdap vaccine dose should not be given.
   - An inadvertent dose of DTaP vaccine administered to children aged 7 through 10 years can count as part of the catch-up series. This dose can count as the adolescent Tdap dose, or the child can later receive a Tdap booster dose at age 11–12 years.

10. **Human papillomavirus (HPV) vaccines (HPV4 [Gardasil] and HPV2 [Cervarix]).**
    - Administer the vaccine series to females (either HPV2 or HPV4) and males (HPV4) at age 13 through 18 years if patient is not previously vaccinated.
    - Use recommended routine dosing intervals for vaccine series cacth-up; see *Recommended Immunization Schedule for Persons Aged 7 through 18 Years.*

Clinically significant adverse events that follow vaccination should be reported to the Vaccine Adverse Event Reporting System (VAERS) online (http://www.vaers.hhs.gov) or by telephone (800-822-7967). Suspected cases of vaccine-preventable diseases should be reported to the state or local health department. Additional information, including precautions and contraindications for vaccination, is available from CDC online (http://www.cdc.gov/vaccines) or by telephone (800-CDC-INFO [800-232-4636]).

RECOMMENDED ADULT IMMUNIZATION SCHEDULE

Recommended adult immunization schedule, by vaccine and age group[1] — United States, 2012

VACCINE ▼ AGE GROUP►	19–21 years	22–26 years	27–49 years	50–59 years	60–64 years	≥65 years
Influenza[2,*]	1 dose annually					
Tetanus, diphtheria, pertussis (Td/Tdap)[3,*]	Substitute 1-time dose of Tdap for Td booster; then boost with Td every 10 years					////// Td/Tdap[3] //////
Varicella[4,*]	2 doses					
Human papillomavirus (HPV)[5,*] Female	3 doses					
Human papillomavirus (HPV)[5,*] Male	3 doses					
Zoster[6]					1 dose	
Measles, mumps, rubella (MMR)[7,*]	1 or 2 doses				1 dose	
Pneumococcal (polysaccharide)[8,9]			1 or 2 doses			1 dose
Meningococcal[10,*]	1 or more doses					
Hepatitis A[11,*]	2 doses					
Hepatitis B[12,*]	3 doses					

* Covered by the Vaccine Injury Compensation Program

| | For all persons in this category who meet the age requirements and who lack documentation of vaccination or have no evidence of previous infection | | Recommended if some other risk factor is present (e.g., on the basis of medical, occupational, lifestyle, or other indications) | ////// | Tdap recommended for ≥65 if contact with <12 month old child. Either Td or Tdap can be used if no infant contact | | No recommendation |

Vaccines that might be indicated for adults, based on medical and other conditions[1] — United States, 2012

INDICATION► VACCINE ▼	Pregnancy	Immunocompromising conditions (excluding human immunodeficiency virus [HIV])[4,6,7,14]	HIV infection[4,2,13,14] CD4+ T lymphocyte count		Men who have sex with men (MSM)	Heart disease, chronic lung disease, chronic alcoholism	Asplenia[13] (including elective splenectomy and persistent complement component deficiencies)	Chronic liver disease	Diabetes, kidney failure, end-stage renal disease, receipt of hemodialysis	Health-care personnel
			<200 cells/μL	≥200 cells/μL						
Influenza[2,*]	1 dose TIV annually				1 dose TIV or LAIV annually	1 dose TIV annually				1 dose TIV or LAIV annually
Tetanus, diphtheria, pertussis (Td/Tdap)[3,*]	Substitute 1-time dose of Tdap for Td booster; then boost with Td every 10 years									
Varicella[4,*]	Contraindicated				2 doses					
Human papillomavirus (HPV)[5,*] Female	3 doses through age 26 years				3 doses through age 26 years					
Human papillomavirus (HPV)[5,*] Male	3 doses through age 26 years				3 doses through age 21 years					
Zoster[6]	Contraindicated				1 dose					
Measles, mumps, rubella[7,*]	Contraindicated				1 or 2 doses					
Pneumococcal (polysaccharide)[8,9]	1 or 2 doses									
Meningococcal[10,*]	1 or more doses									
Hepatitis A[11,*]	2 doses									
Hepatitis B[12,*]	3 doses									

* Covered by the Vaccine Injury Compensation Program

| | For all persons in this category who meet the age requirements and who lack documentation of vaccination or have no evidence of previous infection | | Recommended if some other risk factor is present (e.g., on the basis of medical, occupational, lifestyle, or other indications) | | Contraindicated | | No recommendation |

1. Additional information

- Advisory Committee on Immunization Practices (ACIP) vaccine recommendations and additional information are available at: http://www.cdc.gov/vaccines/pubs/acip-list.htm
- Information on travel vaccine requirements and recommendations (eg, for hepatitis A and B, meningococcal, and other vaccines) available at http://wwwnc.cdc.gov/travel/page/vaccinations.htm

2. Influenza vaccination

- Annual vaccination against influenza is recommended for all persons 6 months of age and older.
- Persons 6 months of age and older, including pregnant women, can receive the trivalent inactivated vaccine (TIV).
- Healthy, nonpregnant adults younger than age 50 years without high-risk medical conditions can receive either intranasally administered live, attenuated influenza vaccine (LAIV) (FluMist), or TIV. Healthcare personnel (HCP) who care for severely immunocompromised persons (ie, those who require care in a protected environment) should receive TIV rather than LAIV. Other persons should receive TIV.
- The intramuscular or intradermal administered TIV are options for adults aged 18-64 years.
- Adults aged 65 years and older can receive the standard dose TIV or the high-dose TIV (Fluzone High-Dose).

3. Tetanus, diphtheria, and acellular pertussis (Td/Tdap) vaccination

- Administer a one-time dose of Tdap to adults younger than age 65 years who have not received Tdap previously or for whom vaccine status is unknown to replace one of the 10-year Td boosters.

- Tdap is specifically recommended for the following persons:
  - pregnant women more than 20 weeks' gestation,
  - adults, regardless of age, who are close contacts of infants younger than age 12 months (eg, parents, grandparents, or child care providers), and
  - HCP.
- Tdap can be administered regardless of interval since the most recent tetanus or diphtheria-containing vaccine.
- Pregnant women not vaccinated during pregnancy should receive Tdap immediately postpartum.
- Adults 65 years and older may receive Tdap.
- Adults with unknown or incomplete history of completing a 3-dose primary vaccination series with Td-containing vaccines should begin or complete a primary vaccination series. Tdap should be substituted for a single dose of Td in the vaccination series with Tdap preferred as the first dose.
- For unvaccinated adults, administer the first 2 doses at least 4 weeks apart and the third dose 6-12 months after the second.
- If incompletely vaccinated (ie, less than 3 doses), administer remaining doses. Refer to the ACIP statement for recommendations for administering Td/Tdap as prophylaxis in wound management.*

4. Varicella vaccination

- All adults without evidence of immunity to varicella (as defined below) should receive 2 doses of single-antigen varicella vaccine or a second dose if they have received only 1 dose.
- Special consideration for vaccination should be given to those who
  - have close contact with persons at high risk for severe disease (eg, HCP and family contacts of persons with immunocompromising conditions) or
  - are at high risk for exposure or transmission (eg, teachers; child care employees; residents and staff members of institutional settings, including correctional institutions; college students; military personnel; adolescents and adults living in households with children; nonpregnant women of childbearing age; and international travelers).
- Pregnant women should be assessed for evidence of varicella immunity. Women who do not have evidence of immunity should receive the first dose of varicella vaccine upon completion or termination of pregnancy and before discharge from the healthcare facility. The second dose should be administered 4-8 weeks after the first dose.
- Evidence of immunity to varicella in adults includes any of the following:
  - documentation of 2 doses of varicella vaccine at least 4 weeks apart;
  - U.S.-born before 1980 (although for HCP and pregnant women, birth before 1980 should not be considered evidence of immunity);
  - history of varicella based on diagnosis or

verification of varicella by a healthcare provider (for a patient reporting a history of or having an atypical case, a mild case, or both, healthcare providers should seek either an epidemiologic link to a typical varicella case or to a laboratory-confirmed case or evidence of laboratory confirmation, if it was performed at the time of acute disease);
  - history of herpes zoster based on diagnosis or verification of herpes zoster by a healthcare provider; or
  - laboratory evidence of immunity or laboratory confirmation of disease.

5. Human papillomavirus (HPV) vaccination

- Two vaccines are licensed for use in females, bivalent HPV vaccine (HPV2) and quadrivalent HPV vaccine (HPV4), and one HPV vaccine for use in males (HPV4).
- For females, either HPV4 or HPV2 is recommended in a 3-dose series for routine vaccination at 11 or 12 years of age, and for those 13 through 26 years of age, if not previously vaccinated.
- For males, HPV4 is recommended in a 3-dose series for routine vaccination at 11 or 12 years of age, and for those 13 through 21 years of age, if not previously vaccinated. Males 22 through 26 years of age may be vaccinated.
- HPV vaccines are not live vaccines and can be administered to persons who are immunocompromised as a result of infection (including HIV infection), disease, or medications. Vaccine is recommended for immunocompromised persons through age 26 years who did not get any or all doses when they were younger. The immune response and vaccine efficacy might be less than that in immunocompetent persons.
- Men who have sex with men might especially benefit from vaccination to prevent condyloma and anal cancer. HPV4 is recommended for men who have sex with men through age 26 years who did not get any or all doses when they were younger.
- Ideally, vaccine should be administered before potential exposure to HPV through sexual activity; however, persons who are sexually active should still be vaccinated consistent with age-based recommendations. HPV vaccine can be administered to persons with a history of genital warts, abnormal Papanicolaou test, or positive HPV DNA test.
- A complete series for either HPV4 or HPV2 consists of 3 doses. The second dose should be administered 1-2 months after the first dose; the third dose should be administered 6 months after the first dose (at least 24 weeks after the first dose).
- Although HPV vaccination is not specifically recommended for HCP based on their occupation, HCP should receive the HPV vaccine if they are in the recommended age group.

6. Zoster vaccination

- A single dose of zoster vaccine is recommended for adults 60 years of age and older regardless of whether they report a prior episode of herpes zoster. Although the vaccine is licensed by the Food and Drug Administration (FDA) for use among and can be administered to persons 50 years and older, ACIP recommends that vaccination begins at 60 years of age.

- Persons with chronic medical conditions may be vaccinated unless their condition constitutes a contraindication, such as pregnancy or severe immunodeficiency.
- Although zoster vaccination is not specifically recommended for HCP, HCP should receive the vaccine if they are in the recommended age group.

7. Measles, mumps, rubella (MMR) vaccination

- Adults born before 1957 generally are considered immune to measles and mumps. All adults born in 1957 or later should have documentation of 1 or more doses of MMR vaccine unless they have a medical contraindication to the vaccine, laboratory evidence of immunity to each of the three diseases, or documentation of provider-diagnosed measles or mumps disease. For rubella, documentation of provider-diagnosed disease is not considered acceptable evidence of immunity.

Measles component:

- A routine second dose of MMR vaccine, administered a minimum of 28 days after the first dose, is recommended for adults who
  — are students in postsecondary educational institutions;
  — work in a healthcare facility; or
  — plan to travel internationally.
- Persons who received inactivated (killed) measles vaccine or measles vaccine of unknown type from 1963 to 1967 should be revaccinated with 2 doses of MMR vaccine.

Mumps component:

- A routine second dose of MMR vaccine, administered a minimum of 28 days after the first dose, is recommended for adults who
  — are students in postsecondary educational institutions;
  — work in a healthcare facility; or
  — plan to travel internationally.
- Persons vaccinated before 1979 with either killed mumps vaccine or mumps vaccine of unknown type who are at high risk for mumps infection (eg, persons who are working in a healthcare facility) should be considered for revaccination with 2 doses of MMR vaccine.

Rubella component:

- For women of childbearing age, regardless of birth year, rubella immunity should be determined. If there is no evidence of immunity, women who are not pregnant should be vaccinated. Pregnant women who do not have evidence of immunity should receive MMR vaccine upon completion or termination of pregnancy and before discharge from the healthcare facility.

HCP born before 1957:

- For unvaccinated HCP born before 1957 who lack laboratory evidence of measles, mumps, and/or rubella immunity or laboratory confirmation of disease, healthcare facilities should consider routinely vaccinating personnel with 2 doses of MMR vaccine at

the appropriate interval for measles and mumps or 1 dose of MMR vaccine for rubella.

8. Pneumococcal polysaccharide (PPSV) vaccination

- Vaccinate all persons with the following indications:
  — age 65 years and older without a history of PPSV vaccination;
  — adults younger than 65 years with chronic lung disease (including chronic obstructive pulmonary disease, emphysema, and asthma); chronic cardiovascular diseases; diabetes mellitus; chronic liver disease (including cirrhosis); alcoholism; cochlear implants; cerebrospinal fluid leaks; immunocompromising conditions; and functional or anatomic asplenia (eg, sickle cell disease and other hemoglobinopathies, congenital or acquired asplenia, splenic dysfunction, or splenectomy [if elective splenectomy is planned, vaccinate at least 2 weeks before surgery]);
  — residents of nursing homes or long-term care facilities; and
  — adults who smoke cigarettes.
- Persons with asymptomatic or symptomatic HIV infection should be vaccinated as soon as possible after their diagnosis.
- When cancer chemotherapy or other immunosuppressive therapy is being considered, the interval between vaccination and initiation of immunosuppressive therapy should be at least 2 weeks. Vaccination during chemotherapy or radiation therapy should be avoided.
- Routine use of PPSV is not recommended for American Indians/Alaska Natives or other persons younger than 65 years of age unless they have underlying medical conditions that are PPSV indications. However, public health authorities may consider recommending PPSV for American Indians/Alaska Natives who are living in areas where the risk for invasive pneumococcal disease is increased.

9. Revaccination with PPSV

- One-time revaccination 5 years after the first dose is recommended for persons 19 through 64 years of age with chronic renal failure or nephrotic syndrome; functional or anatomic asplenia (eg, sickle cell disease or splenectomy); and for persons with immunocompromising conditions.
- Persons who received PPSV before age 65 years for any indication should receive another dose of the vaccine at age 65 years or later if at least 5 years have passed since their previous dose.
- No further doses are needed for persons vaccinated with PPSV at or after age 65 years.

10. Meningococcal vaccination

- Administer 2 doses of meningococcal conjugate vaccine quadrivalent (MCV4) at least 2 months apart to adults with functional asplenia or persistent complement component deficiencies.
- HIV-infected persons who are vaccinated should also receive 2 doses.
- Administer a single dose of meningococcal vaccine to microbiologists routinely exposed to isolates of *Neisseria meningitidis*, military recruits, and persons

(Continued)

who travel to or live in countries in which meningococcal disease is hyperendemic or epidemic.

- First-year college students up through age 21 years who are living in residence halls should be vaccinated if they have not received a dose on or after their 16th birthday.
- MCV4 is preferred for adults with any of the preceding indications who are 55 years old and younger; meningococcal polysaccharide vaccine (MPSV4) is preferred for adults 56 years and older.
- Revaccination with MCV4 every 5 years is recommended for adults previously vaccinated with MCV4 or MPSV4 who remain at increased risk for infection (eg, adults with anatomic or functional asplenia or persistent complement component deficiencies).

11. Hepatitis A vaccination
- Vaccinate any person seeking protection from hepatitis A virus (HAV) infection and persons with any of the following indications:
  - men who have sex with men and persons who use injection drugs;
  - persons working with HAV-infected primates or with HAV in a research laboratory setting;
  - persons with chronic liver disease and persons who receive clotting factor concentrates;
  - persons traveling to or working in countries that have high or intermediate endemicity of hepatitis A; and
  - unvaccinated persons who anticipate close personal contact (eg, household or regular babysitting) with an international adoptee during the first 60 days after arrival in the United States from a country with high or intermediate endemicity.* The first dose of the 2-dose hepatitis A vaccine series should be administered as soon as adoption is planned, ideally 2 or more weeks before the arrival of the adoptee.
- Single-antigen vaccine formulations should be administered in a 2-dose schedule at either 0 and 6-12 months (Havrix), or 0 and 6-18 months (Vaqta). If the combined hepatitis A and hepatitis B vaccine (Twinrix) is used, administer 3 doses at 0, 1, and 6 months; alternatively, a 4-dose schedule may be used, administered on days 0, 7, and 21-30 followed by a booster dose at month 12.

12. Hepatitis B vaccination
- Vaccinate persons with any of the following indications and any person seeking protection from hepatitis B virus (HBV) infection:
  - sexually active persons who are not in a long-term, mutually monogamous relationship (eg, persons with more than one sex partner during the previous 6 months); persons seeking evaluation or treatment for a sexually transmitted disease (STD); current or recent injection-drug users; and men who have sex with men;
  - HCP and public safety workers who are exposed to blood or other potentially infectious body fluids;

- persons with diabetes younger than 60 years as soon as feasible after diagnosis; persons with diabetes who are 60 years or older at the discretion of the treating clinician based on increased need for assisted blood glucose monitoring in long-term care facilities, likelihood of acquiring hepatitis B infection, its complications or chronic sequelae, and likelihood of immune response to vaccination;
- persons with end-stage renal disease, including patients receiving hemodialysis; persons with HIV infection; and persons with chronic liver disease;
- household contacts and sex partners of persons with chronic HBV infection; clients and staff members of institutions for persons with developmental disabilities; and international travelers to countries with high or intermediate prevalence of chronic HBV infection; and
- all adults in the following settings: STD treatment facilities; HIV testing and treatment facilities; facilities providing drug-abuse treatment and prevention services; healthcare settings targeting services to injection-drug users or men who have sex with men; correctional facilities; end-stage renal disease programs and facilities for chronic hemodialysis patients; and institutions and nonresidential daycare facilities for persons with developmental disabilities.

- Administer missing doses to complete a 3-dose series of hepatitis B vaccine to those persons not vaccinated or not completely vaccinated. The second dose should be administered 1 month after the first dose; the third dose should be given at least 2 months after the second dose (and at least 4 months after the first dose). If the combined hepatitis A and hepatitis B vaccine (Twinrix) is used, give 3 doses at 0, 1, and 6 months; alternatively, a 4-dose Twinrix schedule, administered on days 0, 7, and 21-30 followed by a booster dose at month 12 may be used.
- Adult patients receiving hemodialysis or with other immunocompromising conditions should receive 1 dose of 40 μg/mL (Recombivax HB) administered on a 3-dose schedule or 2 doses of 20 μg/mL (Engerix-B) administered simultaneously on a 4-dose schedule at 0, 1, 2, and 6 months.

13. Selected conditions for which *Haemophilus influenzae* type b (Hib) vaccine may be used
- 1 dose of Hib vaccine should be considered for persons who have sickle cell disease, leukemia, or HIV infection, or who have anatomic or functional asplenia if they have not previously received Hib vaccine.

14. Immunocompromising conditions
- Inactivated vaccines generally are acceptable (eg, pneumococcal, meningococcal, and influenza [inactivated influenza vaccine]), and live vaccines generally are avoided in persons with immune deficiencies or immunocompromising conditions. Information on specific conditions is available at http://www.cdc.gov/vaccines/pubs/acip-list.htm

*These schedules indicate the recommended age groups and medical indications for which administration of currently licensed vaccines is commonly indicated for adults ages 19 years and older, as of January 1, 2012. For all vaccines being recommended on the adult immunization schedule: a vaccine series does not need to be restarted, regardless of the time that has elapsed between doses. Licensed combination vaccines may be used whenever any components of the combination are indicated and when the vaccine's other components are not contraindicated. For detailed recommendations on all vaccines, including those used primarily for travelers or that are issued during the year, consult the manufacturers' package inserts and the complete statements from the Advisory Committee on Immunization Practices (http://www.cdc.gov/vaccines/pubs/acip-list.htm).

Report all clinically significant postvaccination reactions to the Vaccine Adverse Event Reporting System (VAERS). Reporting forms and instructions on filing a VAERS report are available at http://www.vaers.hhs.gov or by telephone, 800-822-7967.

Information on how to file a Vaccine Injury Compensation Program claim is available at http://www.hrsa.gov/vaccinecompensation or by telephone, 800-338-2382. Information about filing a claim for vaccine injury is available through the U.S. Court of Federal Claims, 717 Madison Place, N.W., Washington, D.C. 20005; telephone, 202-357-6400.

Additional information about the vaccines in this schedule, extent of available data, and contraindications for vaccination also is available at http://www.cdc.gov/vaccines or from the CDC-INFO Contact Center at 800-CDC-INFO (800-232-4636) in English and Spanish, 8:00 a.m. to 8:00 p.m., Monday through Friday, excluding holidays.

Use of trade names and commercial sources is for identification only and does not imply endorsement by the U.S. Department of Health and Human Services.

ALCOHOL-FREE PRODUCTS

The following is a selection of alcohol-free products grouped by therapeutic category. This list is not comprehensive. Generic and alternate brands may be available. Always check product labeling for definitive information on specific ingredients.

Analgesics

Advil Children's Suspension	Pfizer Consumer
Advil Infant's Suspension	Pfizer Consumer
APAP Elixir	Bio-Pharm
Motrin Children's Suspension	McNeil Consumer
Motrin Infants' Suspension	McNeil Consumer
Silapap Children's Liquid	Silarx
Silapap Infant's Drops	Silarx
Tylenol Children's Suspension	McNeil Consumer
Tylenol Infant's Suspension	McNeil Consumer

Anticonvulsant

Zarontin Syrup	Pfizer

Antiviral Agent

Epivir Oral Solution	ViiV

Cough/Cold/Allergy Preparations

Banophen Elixir	Major
Benadryl Allergy Solution	McNeil Consumer
Benadryl-D Allergy & Sinus Children's Liquid	McNeil Consumer
Bromphenex DM Solution	Breckenridge
Bromplex DM Solution	Prasco
Bromtuss DM Solution	Breckenridge
Broncotron Liquid	Seyer Pharmatec
Broncotron-D Suspension	Seyer Pharmatec
Carbaphen 12 Ped Suspension	Gil
Carbaphen 12 Suspension	Gil
Carbatuss Liquid	GM
Carbatuss-12 Suspension	GM
Carbetaplex TS Suspension	Breckenridge
Children's Dimetapp Cold & Allergy Solution	Pfizer Consumer
Children's Dimetapp Long Acting Cough Plus Cold Solution	Pfizer Consumer
Children's Dimetapp Multi-Symptom Cold & Flu Solution	Pfizer Consumer
Children's Dimetapp Nighttime Cold & Congestion Solution	Pfizer Consumer
Children's Dimetapp Nighttime Flu Syrup	Pfizer Consumer
Children's Dimetapp DM Cold & Cough Solution	Pfizer Consumer
Children's Mucinex Cold Solution	Reckitt Benckiser
Children's Mucinex Cough Syrup	Reckitt Benckiser
Children's Mucinex Syrup	Reckitt Benckiser
Children's Sudafed Nasal Decongestant	McNeil Consumer
Children's Sudafed PE Cold & Cough Liquid	McNeil Consumer
Children's Sudafed PE Nasal Decongestant	McNeil Consumer
Coughtuss Solution	Breckenridge
Crantex HC Syrup	Breckenridge
Crantex Syrup	Breckenridge
Creomulsion Cough Syrup	Summit Industries
Creomulsion for Children Syrup	Summit Industries
Dacex-DM Solution	Cypress
Dallergy Solution	Laser
De-Chlor DR Solution	Cypress
Dehistine Syrup	Cypress
Despec Liquid	International Ethical
Diabetic Siltussin DAS-Na	Silarx
Diabetic Siltussin-DM DAS-Na	Silarx
Diabetic Tussin Cough Lozenges	Health Care Products
Diabetic Tussin Night Time Formula Solution	Health Care Products
Diabetic Tussin Solution	Health Care Products
Diabetic Tussin DM Solution	Health Care Products
Diabetic Tussin DM Maximum Strength Liquid	Health Care Products
Donatussin Solution	Laser
Donatussin DC Syrup	Laser
Donatussin DM Syrup	Laser
Double-Tussin DM Liquid	Reese
Dynatuss HC Solution	Breckenridge
Father John's Medicine Plus Drops	Oakhurst
Giltuss Liquid	Gil
Giltuss Ped-C Solution	Gil
H-C Tussive Syrup	Bryant Ranch
Histinex HC Syrup	Ethex
Histinex PV Syrup	Ethex
Hydramine Elixir	Quality Care Products
Hydro-Tussin HC Syrup	Ethex
Hydro-Tussin HD Liquid	Ethex
Hydro-Tussin XP Syrup	Ethex
Lohist D Syrup	Larken
Motrin Cold Children's Suspension	McNeil Consumer
Myhist-PD Solution	Larken
Neo AC Syrup	Laser
Neo DM Drops	Laser
Neo DM Suspension	Laser
Neo DM Syrup	Laser
Neotuss S/F Liquid	A.G. Marin
Neotuss-D Liquid	A.G. Marin
PediaCare Allergy Liquid	Prestige
PediaCare Allergy & Cold Liquid	Prestige
PediaCare Children's Fever Reducer & Pain Reliever Liquid	Prestige
PediaCare Cough & Congestion Liquid	Prestige

(Continued)

Cough/Cold/Allergy Preparations *(Continued)*

PediaCare Decongestant Liquid	Prestige
PediaCare Fever Reducer Plus Cough & Runny Nose Liquid	Prestige
PediaCare Fever Reducer Plus Cough & Sore Throat Liquid	Prestige
PediaCare Fever Reducer Plus Flu Liquid	Prestige
PediaCare Fever Reducer Plus Multi-Symptom Cold Liquid	Prestige
PediaCare Infant's Fever Reducer & Pain Reliever Liquid	Prestige
PediaCare Multi-Symptom Cold Liquid	Prestige
Pedia-Relief Liquid	Major
Phena-HC Solution	GM
Phena-S Liquid	GM
Poly Hist HC Solution	Poly
Poly Hist PD Solution	Poly
Poly-Tussin Solution	Poly
Poly-Tussin AC	Poly
Poly-Tussin DHC	Poly
Poly-Tussin HD Syrup	Poly
Poly-Tussin XP Solution	Poly
Q-Tussin Liquid	Qualitest
Rescon-DM Liquid	Capellon
Rescon-GG Liquid	Capellon
Rindal HD Liquid	Breckenridge
Rindal HD Plus Solution	Breckenridge
Robitussin Children's Cough & Cold CF Solution	Pfizer Consumer
Robitussin Children's Cough & Cold Long-Acting Solution	Pfizer Consumer
Robitussin Children's Cough Long-Acting Liquid	Pfizer Consumer
Robitussin Cough & Chest Congestion DM Liquid	Pfizer Consumer
Robitussin Cough & Chest Congestion DM Max Liquid	Pfizer Consumer
Robitussin Cough & Chest Congestion DM Sugar-Free Liquid	Pfizer Consumer
Robitussin Multi-Symptom Cold Liquid	Pfizer Consumer
Robitussin Long-Acting Cough Liquid	Pfizer Consumer
Robitussin Maximum Strength Multi-Symptom Cold Liquid	Pfizer Consumer
Robitussin Nighttime Multi-Symptom Cold Liquid	Pfizer Consumer
Scot-Tussin Diabetes CF Liquid	Scot-Tussin
Scot-Tussin DM Solution	Scot-Tussin
Scot-Tussin Expectorant Solution	Scot-Tussin
Scot-Tussin Senior Solution	Scot-Tussin
Siladryl Allergy Solution	Silarx
Siltussin DAS Liquid	Silarx
Siltussin DM DAS Cough Formula Syrup	Silarx
Siltussin SA Syrup	Silarx
Theracof Plus	Reese
Tussi-Pres Liquid	Kramer-Novis
Tussi-Pres Pediatric Solution	Kramer-Novis
Tylenol Children's Liquid	McNeil Consumer
Tylenol Cold & Cough Daytime Liquid	McNeil Consumer
Tylenol Cold & Cough Nighttime Liquid	McNeil Consumer
Tylenol Cold & Flu Severe Liquid	McNeil Consumer
Tylenol Cold Sore Throat Liquid	McNeil Consumer
Tylenol Infants' Concentrated Drops	McNeil Consumer
Tylenol Plus Multi-Symptom Cold Children's Liquid	McNeil Consumer
Tylenol Plus Cold & Allergy Children's Liquid	McNeil Consumer
Tylenol Plus Cold & Cough Children's Suspension	McNeil Consumer
Tylenol Plus Cough & Runny Nose Children's Liquid	McNeil Consumer
Tylenol Plus Cough & Sore Throat Children's Liquid	McNeil Consumer
Tylenol Plus Cold & Stuffy Nose Children's Liquid	McNeil Consumer
Tylenol Plus Cold Children's Liquid	McNeil Consumer
Tylenol Plus Flu Children's Liquid	McNeil Consumer
Vazol Solution	Wraser Pharm
Vicks 44 Custom Care Chesty Cough Liquid	Procter & Gamble
Vicks 44 Custom Care Congestion Liquid	Procter & Gamble
Vicks 44 Custom Care Cough & Cold PM Liquid	Procter & Gamble
Vicks 44 Custom Care Dry Cough Suppressant Liquid	Procter & Gamble
Vicks Dayquil Cold & Flu Relief Liquid	Procter & Gamble
Vicks Dayquil Cough Liquid	Procter & Gamble
Vicks Dayquil Mucus Control Liquid	Procter & Gamble
Vicks Dayquil Mucus Control DM Liquid	Procter & Gamble
Vicks Nyquil Children's Liquid	Procter & Gamble
Z-Tuss AC Liquid	Magna

Ear/Nose/Throat Products

4-Way Saline Moisturizing Mist Spray	Bristol-Myers
Ayr Baby Saline Spray	Ascher
Bucalsep Solution	Gil
Bucalsep Spray	Gil
Cheracol Sore Throat Spray	Lee
Fresh N Free Solution	Geritrex
Gly-Oxide Solution	GlaxoSmithKline
Listermint Solution	McNeil Consumer
Nasal Moist Gel	Blairex
Orajel Baby Naturals Gel	Del
Orajel Baby Nighttime Teething Pain Medicine Gel	Del

OraMagic Plus Powder	MPM Medical
OraMagicRx Powder	MPM Medical
Tanac Liquid	Del
Throto-Ceptic Spray	S.S.S.
Vicks Sinex 12 Hour Spray	Procter & Gamble
Zilactin Tooth and Gum	Blairex
Instant Pain Reliever,	
Maximum Strength	

Gastrointestinal Agents

Axid Solution	Braintree
Colace Syrup	Purdue
Imogen Liquid	PGD
Mylicon Infants' Drops	Johnson & Johnson/
	Merck
PediaCare Infants' Gas Relief Drops	Prestige

Topical Products

Dermatone Lips N Face	Dermatone
Protector Ointment	
Dermatone	Dermatone
Sunblock Cream	
Dermatone Skin Protector	Dermatone
Cream	
Handclens Solution	Woodward
Neutrogena Acne Wash Liquid	Neutrogena
Neutrogena Toner Solution	Neutrogena
Sea Breeze Foaming	Clairol
Face Wash Gel	

Sportz Bloc Cream	Med-Derm
Tiger Balm Arthritis Rub Lotion	Prince of Peace

Vitamins/Minerals/Supplements

Adaptosode For Stress Liquid	HVS
Adaptosode R+R	HVS
For Acute Stress Liquid	
Apetigen Elixir	Kramer-Novis
Biosode Liquid	HVS
Detoxosode Products Liquid	HVS
Multi-Delyn Liquid	Silarx
Multi-Delyn w/Iron Liquid	Silarx
Nutrivit Solution	Llorens
Poly-Vi-Sol Drops	Mead Johnson
Poly-Vi-Sol w/Iron Drops	Mead Johnson
Protect Plus Liquid	Gil
Strovite Forte Syrup	Everett
Supervite Liquid	Seyer Pharmatec
Tri-Vi-Sol w/Iron Drops	Mead Johnson
Vitafol Syrup	Everett

Miscellaneous

Cytra-2 Solution	Cypress
Cytra-K Solution	Cypress
Fluorinse Solution	Oral B
Namenda Solution	Forest
Primsol Solution	FSC

CYTOCHROME P450 ENZYMES: INDUCERS, INHIBITORS, AND SUBSTRATES

CYP1A2 INDUCERS

Broccoli
Brussel sprouts
Carbamazepine
Charbroiled food
Citalopram hydrobromide
Diltiazem HCl
Diltiazem maleate
Erythromycin
Esomeprazole sodium
Fluvoxamine
Fluvoxamine maleate
Hypericum perforatum
Insulin
Lansoprazole
Nafcillin sodium
Nicotine
Omeprazole
Phenobarbital
Phenytoin
Primidone
Rifampicin
Rifampin
Ritonavir
Tobacco

CYP1A2 INHIBITORS

Alatrofloxacin mesylate
Amiodarone HCl
Anastrozole
Cimetidine
Ciprofloxacin
Clarithromycin
Desogestrel
Enoxacin
Ethinyl estradiol
Fluvoxamine
Gatifloxacin
Gemifloxacin mesylate
Grapefruit
Grepafloxacin HCl
Isoniazid
Ketoconazole
Levofloxacin

Levonorgestrel
Lomefloxacin HCl
Mestranol
Methoxsalen
Mexiletine HCl
Mibefradil DiHCl
Moxifloxacin HCl
Nalidixic acid
Norethindrone
Norfloxacin
Norgestrel
Ofloxacin
Omeprazole
Paroxetine
Ranitidine HCl
Ritonavir
Sildenafil citrate
Sparfloxacin
Tacrine HCl
Ticlopidine HCl
Troleandomycin
Trovafloxacin mesylate
Vardenafil HCl
Zileuton

CYP1A2 SUBSTRATES

Acetaminophen
Alatrofloxacin mesylate
Aminophylline
Amiodarone HCl
Amitriptyline HCl
Amoxapine
Anagrelide HCl
Caffeine
Chlordiazepoxide
Cimetidine HCl
Ciprofloxacin
Clomipramine HCl
Clopidogrel bisulfate
Clozapine
Cyclobenzaprine
Desipramine HCl
Diazepam
Diltiazem HCl

Doxepin HCl
Enoxacin
Erythromycin
Estradiol
Ethinyl estradiol
Flutamide
Fluticasone propionate
Fluvoxamine
Grepafloxacin HCl
Haloperidol
Imipramine HCl
Levobupivacaine HCl
Lomefloxacin HCl
Maprotiline HCl
Methadone HCl
Mexiletine HCl
Mirtazapine
Moxifloxacin HCl
Nafcillin sodium
Naproxen
Nicotine
Norethindrone
Norfloxacin
Nortriptyline HCl
Ofloxacin
Olanzapine
Ondansetron
Phenobarbital
Phenytoin
Propafenone HCl
Propranolol HCl
Protriptyline HCl
Riluzole
Ritonavir
Ropinirole HCl
Ropivacaine HCl
Tacrine HCl
Tamoxifen citrate
Theobromine
Tizanidine
Tizanidine HCl
Trimethaphan camsylate
Trimipramine maleate
Trovafloxacin mesylate

Verapamil HCl
Warfarin sodium
Zileuton
Zolmitriptan

CYP2C6 SUBSTRATES

Acetaminophen
Anisindione
Dicumarol
Halothane
Nicotine
Warfarin sodium

CYP2B6 INDUCERS

Carbamazepine
Fosphenytoin
Mephenytoin
Nevirapine
Phenobarbital
Phenytoin
Primidone
Rifampin

CYP2B6 INHIBITORS

Amiodarone HCl
Amlodipine besylate
Azelastine HCl
Citalopram hydrobromide
Clopidogrel bisulfate
Clopidogrel hydrogen sulfate
Clotrimazole
Desipramine HCl
Desvenlafaxine
Disulfiram
Doxorubicin HCl
Escitalopram oxalate
Ethinyl estradiol
Fluoxetine
Fluvoxamine
Fluvoxamine maleate
Isoflurane
Ketoconazole
Methimazole
Miconazole
Nateglinide
Nelfinavir mesylate
Norfluoxetine
Orphenadrine citrate

Orphenadrine HCl
Paroxetine
Paroxetine mesylate
Sertraline HCl
Tamoxifen citrate
Thiotepa
Ticlopidine HCl
Venlafaxine HCl

CYP2B6 SUBSTRATES

Amitriptyline HCl
Bupropion
Cisapride
Cyclophosphamide
Diazepam
Diclofenac
Disulfiram
Divalproex sodium
Efavirenz
Erythromycin
Estradiol
Estrogen
Estrone
Estropipate
Ethinyl estradiol
Fluoxetine
Halothane
Ifosfamide
Imipramine HCl
Imipramine pamoate
Irinotecan HCl
Isotretinoin
Ketamine
Lidocaine
Meperidine HCl
Mephenytoin
Mephobarbital
Methadone HCl
Methyltestosterone
Midazolam HCl
Nevirapine
Nicotine
Orphenadrine citrate
Orphenadrine HCl
Polyestradiol phosphate
Promethazine
Promethazine HCl

Propofol
Ritonavir
Ropivacaine HCl
Selegiline
Sertraline HCl
Sevoflurane
Tamoxifen citrate
Temazepam
Testosterone
Tretinoin
Trimipramine maleate
Valproate sodium
Valproic acid
Verapamil HCl

CYP2C18 INHIBITORS

Cimetidine

CYP2C18 SUBSTRATES

Naproxen
Omeprazole
Piroxicam
Propranolol HCl
Tretinoin
Warfarin sodium

CYP2C19 INDUCERS

Carbamazepine
Norethindrone
Phenobarbital
Phenytoin
Prednisone
Rifampin

CYP2C19 INHIBITORS

Cimetidine
Citalopram hydrobromide
Delavirdine
Delavirdine mesylate
Desogestrel
Efavirenz
Esomeprazole magnesium
Esomeprazole sodium
Ethinyl estradiol
Ethynodiol diacetate
Felbamate
Fluoxetine
Fluvastatin sodium
Fluvoxamine

Indomethacin
Isoniazid
Ketoconazole
Lansoprazole
Letrozole
Levonorgestrel
Mestranol
Modafinil
Norethindrone
Norethynodrel
Norgestimate
Norgestrel
Omeprazole
Oxcarbazepine
Paroxetine
Quinidine
Ritonavir
Sertraline HCl
Sildenafil citrate
Sulfaphenazole
Telmisartan
Ticlopidine HCl
Tolbutamide
Tolbutamide sodium
Topiramate
Tranylcypromine sulfate
Vardenafil HCl
Voriconazole

CYP2C19 SUBSTRATES

Amitriptyline HCl
Amoxapine
Carisoprodol
Cilostazol
Citalopram hydrobromide
Clomipramine HCl
Cyclophosphamide
Desipramine HCl
Dextromethorphan
Diazepam
Divalproex sodium
Doxepin HCl
Esomeprazole
Ethosuximide
Ethotoin
Felbamate
Formoterol fumarate

Fosphenytoin
Gabapentin
Imipramine
Indomethacin
Lamotrigine
Lansoprazole
Levetiracetam
Maprotiline HCl
Mephenytoin
Mephobarbital
Meprobamate
Methsuximide
Midazolam HCl
Nelfinavir mesylate
Nilutamide
Nortriptyline HCl
Omeprazole
Oxcarbazepine
Pantoprazole sodium
Paramethadione
Pentamidine isethionate
Phenacemide
Phenobarbital
Phensuximide
Phenytoin
Primidone
Progesterone
Proguanil HCl
Propranolol HCl
Protriptyline HCl
Rabeprazole sodium
Sertraline HCl
Teniposide
Thioridazine
Tiagabine HCl
Tolbutamide
Topiramate
Trimethadione
Trimipramine maleate
Valproate sodium
Valproic acid
Voriconazole
Warfarin sodium
Zonisamide

CYP2C8 INDUCERS

Carbamazepine

Phenobarbital
Primidone
Rifabutin
Rifampin

CYP2C8 INHIBITORS

Anastrozole
Cimetidine
Gemfibrozil
Nicardipine
Omeprazole
Quercetin
Sulfaphenazole
Sulfinpyrazone
Trimethoprim

CYP2C8 SUBSTRATES

Amiodarone HCl
Amitriptyline HCl
Amoxapine
Benzphetamine HCl
Carbamazepine
Clomipramine HCl
Desipramine HCl
Diazepam
Diclofenac
Docetaxel
Doxepin HCl
Fluvastatin sodium
Imipramine
Isotretinoin
Maprotiline HCl
Mephobarbital
Nortriptyline HCl
Omeprazole
Paclitaxel
Phenytoin
Pioglitazone HCl
Protriptyline HCl
Repaglinide
Rosiglitazone
Rosiglitazone/Metformin
Tolbutamide
Tretinoin
Trimipramine maleate
Verapamil HCl
Vitamin A
Warfarin sodium
Zopiclone

CYP2C9 INDUCERS

Aprepitant
Carbamazepine
Dexamethasone
Phenobarbital
Phenytoin
Primidone
Rifampin
Rifapentine
Secobarbital sodium

CYP2C9 INHIBITORS

Amiodarone HCl
Anastrozole
Bendroflumethiazide
Chloramphenicol
Chlorothiazide
Chlorpropamide
Cimetidine
Clopidogrel bisulfate
Clotrimazole
Diclofenac
Disulfiram
Efavirenz
Fenofibrate
Fluconazole
Fluorouracil
Fluoxetine
Fluoxetine HCl
Flurbiprofen
Fluvastatin sodium
Fluvoxamine
Gemfibrozil
Glipizide
Glyburide
Hydrochlorothiazide
Hydroflumethiazide
Imatinib mesylate
Isoniazid
Itraconazole
Ketoconazole
Ketoprofen
Leflunomide
Lovastatin
Methyclothiazide
Metronidazole
Miconazole

Miconazole nitrate
Modafinil
Nifedipine
Omeprazole
Omeprazole magnesium
Oxiconazole nitrate
Paroxetine
Phenylbutazone
Polythiazide
Ritonavir
Sertraline HCl
Sildenafil citrate
Sulfacytine
Sulfamethizole
Sulfamethoxazole
Sulfasalazine
Sulfinpyrazone
Sulfisoxazole acetyl
Terconazole
Ticlopidine HCl
Tolazamide
Tolbutamide
Troglitazone
Vardenafil HCl
Voriconazole
Zafirlukast

CYP2C9 SUBSTRATES

Acarbose
Amitriptyline HCl
Candesartan cilexetil
Carbamazepine
Carvedilol
Celecoxib
Chlorpropamide
Clomipramine HCl
Desogestrel
Dextromethorphan
Diazepam
Diclofenac
Dronabinol
Eprosartan mesylate
Etodolac
Fenoprofen calcium
Fluoxetine
Flurbiprofen

Fluvastatin sodium
Glimepiride
Glipizide
Ibuprofen
Imipramine
Indomethacin
Irbesartan
Ketoprofen
Ketorolac tromethamine
Lansoprazole
Losartan potassium
Meclofenamate sodium
Mefenamic acid
Meloxicam
Metformin HCl
Miglitol
Mirtazapine
Montelukast sodium
Nabumetone
Naproxen
Naproxen sodium
Nateglinide
Nifedipine
Omeprazole
Oxaprozin
Phenylbutazone
Phenytoin
Phenytoin sodium
Pioglitazone HCl
Piroxicam
Repaglinide
Rofecoxib
Rosiglitazone
Sildenafil citrate
Sulfamethoxazole
Sulindac
Suprofen
Tamoxifen citrate
Telmisartan
Tolazamide
Tolbutamide
Tolmetin sodium
Torsemide
Troglitazone
Valdecoxib

Valsartan
Vardenafil HCl
Verapamil HCl
Voriconazole
Warfarin sodium
Zafirlukast
Zileuton

CYP2D6 INDUCERS

Carbamazepine
Ethanol
Hypericum
Phenobarbital
Phenytoin
Primidone
Rifampin
Ritonavir

CYP2D6 INHIBITORS

Amiodarone HCl
Amitriptyline HCl
Amoxapine
Bupropion HCl
Celecoxib
Chloroquine
Chlorpheniramine
Cimetidine
Citalopram hydrobromide
Clomipramine HCl
Cocaine HCl
Desipramine HCl
Diphenhydramine
Doxepin HCl
Escitalopram oxalate
Fluoxetine
Fluphenazine
Fluvoxamine
Halofantrine HCl
Haloperidol
Hydroxychloroquine sulfate
Imatinib mesylate
Imipramine
Maprotiline HCl
Methadone HCl
Mibefradil DiHCl
Moclobemide
Nortriptyline HCl
Paroxetine

Perphenazine
Propafenone HCl
Propoxyphene
Protriptyline HCl
Quinacrine HCl
Quinidine
Ranitidine
Ritonavir
Sertraline HCl
Sildenafil citrate
Terbinafine HCl
Thioridazine
Trimipramine maleate
Vardenafil HCl

CYP2D6 SUBSTRATES

Amitriptyline HCl
Amphetamine aspartate
Amphetamine resins
Amphetamine sulfate
Atomoxetine HCl
Bisoprolol fumarate
Captopril
Carvedilol
Cevimeline HCl
Chlorpromazine
Chlorpropamide
Clomipramine HCl
Clozapine
Codeine
Cyclobenzaprine
Debrisoquine
Desipramine HCl
Dexfenfluramine HCl
Dextroamphetamine
Dextromethorphan
Dolasetron mesylate
Donepezil HCl
Doxepin HCl
Encainide HCl
Esomeprazole
Fentanyl
Flecainide acetate
Fluoxetine
Fluoxetine HCl
Fluphenazine
Fluvoxamine

Formoterol fumarate
Galantamine hydrobromide
Haloperidol
Hydrocodone bitartrate
Imipramine
Indoramin HCl
Labetalol HCl
Lidocaine
Maprotiline HCl
Meperidine HCl
Methadone HCl
Methamphetamine HCl
Methoxyphenamine
Metoprolol
Mexiletine HCl
Mirtazapine
Morphine sulfate
Nelfinavir mesylate
Nortriptyline HCl
Olanzapine
Omeprazole
Ondansetron
Oxyoodone HCl
Paroxetine HCl
Pindolol
Propafenone HCl
Propoxyphene
Propranolol HCl
Quetiapine fumarate
Quinidine
Risperidone
Ritonavir
Tamoxifen citrate
Teniposide
Testosterone
Thioridazine
Timolol maleate
Tolterodine tartrate
Tramadol HCl
Trazodone HCl
Triazolam
Trimipramine maleate
Venlafaxine HCl
Vinblastine sulfate
Zonisamide

CYTOCHROME P450 ENZYMES

CYP3A4 INDUCERS

Allium sativum
Aminoglutethimide
Aprepitant
Betamethasone
Bosentan
Carbamazepine
Ciprofloxacin
Cisplatin
Cortisone acetate
Dexamethasone
Doxorubicin HCl
Efavirenz
Ethosuximide
Felbamate
Fludrocortisone acetate
Fosphenytoin
Garlic
Hydrocortisone
Hypericum
Mephenytoin
Methsuximide
Methylprednisolone
Modafinil
Nafcillin sodium
Nevirapine
Oxcarbazepine
Phenobarbital
Phenytoin
Prednisolone
Prednisone
Primidone
Rifabutin
Rifampicin
Rifampin
Rifapentine
Sulfinpyrazone
Theophyllinate
Theophylline
Triamcinolone
Troglitazone

CYP3A4 INHIBITORS

Acetazolamide
Amiodarone HCl
Amprenavir
Anastrozole

Aprepitant
Atazanavir
Cimetidine
Ciprofloxacin
Clarithromycin
Clotrimazole
Conivaptan HCl
Cyclosporine
Dalfopristin
Danazol
Darunavir
Dasatinib
Delavirdine
Desloratadine
Diltiazem HCl
Diltiazem maleate
Efavirenz
Erythromycin
Fluconazole
Fluoxetine
Fluvoxamine
Fluvoxamine maleate
Fosamprenavir calcium
Grapefruit
Imatinib mesylate
Indinavir sulfate
Isoniazid
Itraconazole
Ketoconazole
Lapatinib
Lopinavir
Loratadine
Metronidazole
Miconazole
Miconazole nitrate
Mifepristone
Nefazodone HCl
Nelfinavir mesylate
Nevirapine
Niacin
Niacinamide
Niacinamide hydroiodide
Nicotinamide
Nifedipine
Norfloxacin
Omeprazole
Paroxetine

Posaconazole
Propoxyphene
Quinidine
Quinine
Quinupristin
Ranitidine
Ritonavir
Saquinavir
Sertraline HCl
Sildenafil citrate
Telithromycin
Troglitazone
Troleandomycin
Valproate sodium
Vardenafil HCl
Verapamil HCl
Voriconazole
Zafirlukast
Zileuton

CYP3A4 POTENT INHIBITORS

Amprenavir
Atazanavir
Clarithromycin
Delavirdine
Fosamprenavir calcium
Indinavir sulfate
Itraconazole
Ketoconazole
Lopinavir
Nefazodone HCl
Nelfinavir mesylate
Posaconazole
Ritonavir
Saquinavir
Telithromycin
Troleandomycin
Voriconazole

CYP3A4 SUBSTRATES

Alfentanil HCl
Alprazolam
Amiodarone HCl
Amitriptyline HCl
Amlodipine besylate
Aprepitant
Astemizole
Atorvastatin calcium

Belladonna ergotamine
Buspirone HCl
Busulfan
Carbamazepine
Cerivastatin sodium
Chlorpheniramine
Cisapride
Clarithromycin
Cyclosporine
Dapsone
Desogestrel
Diazepam
Dihydroergotamine mesylate
Diltiazem
Disopyramide
Disulfiram
Doxorubicin HCl
Dronabinol
Ergonovine maleate
Ergotamine tartrate
Erythromycin
Esomeprazole
Estradiol
Ethinyl estradiol
Ethosuximide
Ethynodiol diacetate
Etoposide
Felodipine
Fentanyl
Haloperidol
Indinavir sulfate
Isradipine
Itraconazole
Ixabepilone
Ketoconazole
Levonorgestrel
Lidocaine
Lovastatin
Mestranol
Methadone HCl
Midazolam HCl
Nefazodone HCl
Nelfinavir mesylate
Nicardipine
Nifedipine
Nimodipine
Nisoldipine

Nitrendipine
Norethindrone
Norgestrel
Omeprazole
Ondansetron
Paclitaxel
Pimozide
Polyestradiol phosphate
Quinidine
Quinine
Rifabutin
Ritonavir
Saquinavir
Saquinavir mesylate
Sertraline HCl
Sildenafil citrate
Simvastatin
Sirolimus
Tacrolimus
Tadalafil
Tamoxifen citrate
Terfenadine
Theophylline
Tiagabine HCl
Tolterodine tartrate
Trazodone HCl
Triazolam
Vardenafil HCl
Verapamil HCl
Vinblastine sulfate
Vincristine sulfate
Warfarin sodium

CYP3A INDUCERS
Allium sativum
Aprepitant
Carbamazepine
Dexamethasone
Efavirenz
Ethosuximide
Hypericum
Modafinil
Nevirapine
Phenobarbital
Phenytoin
Rifabutin
Rifampicin

Rifampin
Rifapentine

CYP3A INHIBITORS
Amiodarone HCl
Amprenavir
Aprepitant
Atazanavir
Atazanavir sulfate
Cimetidine
Ciprofloxacin
Clarithromycin
Cyclosporine
Delavirdine
Diltiazem
Efavirenz
Erythromycin
Fluconazole
Fluoxetine
Fluvoxamine
Fosamprenavir calcium
Grapefruit
Indinavir sulfate
Isoniazid
Itraconazole
Ketoconazole
Lopinavir
Metronidazole
Miconazole
Nefazodone HCl
Nelfinavir mesylate
Nifedipine
Norfloxacin
Paroxetine
Quinine
Ritonavir
Saquinavir
Sertraline HCl
Troleandomycin
Venlafaxine HCl
Verapamil HCl
Voriconazole
Zafirlukast
Zileuton

CYP3A SUBSTRATES
Alfentanil HCl
Alprazolam

Cytochrome P450 Enzymes

Aminophylline
Amitriptyline HCl
Amlodipine besylate
Aprepitant
Astemizole
Atorvastatin calcium
Bromocriptine mesylate
Buspirone HCl
Busulfan
Carbamazepine
Cerivastatin sodium
Chlorpheniramine
Cilostazol
Cisapride
Clarithromycin
Cyclosporine
Desogestrel
Dexamethasone
Diazepam
Dihydroergotamine mesylate
Diltiazem
Disopyramide
Disopyramide phosphate
Doxorubicin HCl
Dronabinol
Dyphylline
Ergotamine tartrate
Erythromycin
Estrogen
Ethinyl estradiol
Ethosuximide
Ethynodiol diacetate
Etoposide
Felodipine
Fentanyl
Glyburide
Haloperidol
Indinavir sulfate
Isradipine
Itraconazole
Ketoconazole
Levonorgestrel
Lidocaine
Lidocaine HCl
Lovastatin
Mestranol

Methadone HCl
Methylprednisolone
Midazolam HCl
Nefazodone HCl
Nelfinavir mesylate
Nicardipine
Nicardipine HCl
Nifedipine
Nimodipine
Nisoldipine
Norethindrone
Norgestrel
Ondansetron
Paclitaxel
Pimozide
Quinidine
Quinine
Rifabutin
Ritonavir
Saquinavir
Sertraline HCl
Sildenafil citrate
Simvastatin
Sirolimus
Tacrolimus
Tamoxifen citrate
Terfenadine
Testosterone
Theophylline
Tiagabine HCl
Tolterodine tartrate
Trazodone HCl
Triazolam
Venlafaxine HCl
Verapamil HCl
Vinblastine sulfate
Vincristine sulfate
Warfarin sodium

CYP450 INDUCERS

Allium
Aminoglutethimide
Aprepitant
Betamethasone
Bosentan
Broccoli

Brussel sprouts
Carbamazepine
Charbroiled food
Ciprofloxacin
Cisplatin
Citalopram hydrobromide
Cortisone acetate
Dexamethasone
Diltiazem
Doxorubicin HCl
Efavirenz
Erythromycin
Escitalopram oxalate
Esomeprazole sodium
Ethanol
Ethosuximide
Felbamate
Fludrocortisone acetate
Fluvoxamine
Fosphenytoin
Garlic extract
Garlic oil
Hydrocortisone
Hypericum
Insulin
Lansoprazole
Mephenytoin
Methsuximide
Methylprednisolone
Modafinil
Nafcillin sodium
Nevirapine
Nicotine
Norethindrone
Omeprazole
Oxcarbazepine
Phenobarbital
Phenytoin
Prednisolone
Prednisone
Primidone
Rifabutin
Rifampicin
Rifampin
Rifapentine
Ritonavir
Secobarbital sodium

Sulfinpyrazone
Theophyllinate
Theophylline
Tobacco
Triamcinolone
Troglitazone

CYP450 INHIBITORS

Acetazolamide
Alatrofloxacin mesylate
Amiodarone HCl
Amitriptyline HCl
Amoxapine
Amprenavir
Anastrozole
Aprepitant
Atazanavir
Atazanavir sulfate
Azosulfisoxazole
Bendroflumethiazide
Bupropion HCl
Celecoxib
Chloramphenicol
Chloroquine
Chlorothiazide
Chlorpheniramine
Chlorpropamide
Cimetidine
Ciprofloxacin
Citalopram hydrobromide
Clarithromycin
Clomipramine HCl
Clopidogrel
Clotrimazole
Cocaine HCl
Conivaptan HCl
Cyclosporine
Dalfopristin
Danazol
Darunavir
Dasatinib
Delavirdine
Desipramine HCl
Desloratadine
Desogestrel
Diclofenac

Diltiazem
Diphenhydramine
Disulfiram
Doxepin HCl
Efavirenz
Enoxacin
Erythromycin
Escitalopram oxalate
Esomeprazole
Ethinyl estradiol
Ethynodiol diacetate
Felbamate
Fenofibrate
Fluconazole
Fluorouracil
Fluoxetine
Fluphenazine
Flurbiprofen
Fluvastatin sodium
Fluvoxamine
Fosamprenavir calcium
Gatifloxacin
Gemfibrozil
Gemifloxacin mesylate
Glipizide
Glyburide
Grapefruit
Grepafloxacin HCl
Halofantrine HCl
Haloperidol
Hydrochlorothiazide
Hydroflumethiazide
Hydroxychloroquine sulfate
Imatinib mesylate
Imipramine
Indinavir sulfate
Indomethacin
Isoniazid
Itraconazole
Ketoconazole
Ketoprofen
Lansoprazole
Lapatinib
Leflunomide
Letrozole
Levofloxacin
Levonorgestrel

Lomefloxacin HCl
Lopinavir
Loratadine
Lovastatin
Maprotiline HCl
Mestranol
Methadone HCl
Methoxsalen
Methyclothiazide
Metronidazole
Mexiletine HCl
Mibefradil DiHCl
Miconazole
Mifepristone
Moclobemide
Modafinil
Moxifloxacin HCl
Nalidixic acid
Nefazodone HCl
Nelfinavir mesylate
Nevirapine
Niacinamide
Nicardipine
Nicotinamide
Nifedipine
Norethindrone
Norethynodrel
Norfloxacin
Norgestimate
Norgestrel
Nortriptyline HCl
Ofloxacin
Omeprazole
Oxcarbazepine
Oxiconazole nitrate
Paroxetine
Perphenazine
Phenylbutazone
Polythiazide
Posaconazole
Propafenone HCl
Propoxyphene
Protriptyline HCl
Quercetin
Quinacrine HCl
Quinidine
Quinine

CYTOCHROME P450 ENZYMES

Quinupristin
Ranitidine
Ritonavir
Saquinavir
Sertraline HCl
Sildenafil citrate
Sparfloxacin
Sulfacytine
Sulfamethizole
Sulfamethoxazole
Sulfaphenazole
Sulfasalazine
Sulfinpyrazone

Sulfisoxazole acetyl
Sulfisoxazole diolamine
Tacrine HCl
Telithromycin
Telmisartan
Terbinafine HCl
Terconazole
Thioridazine HCl
Ticlopidine HCl
Tolazamide
Tolbutamide
Topiramate
Trimethoprim

Trimipramine maleate
Troglitazone
Troleandomycin
Trovafloxacin mesylate
Valproate sodium
Vardenafil HCl
Venlafaxine HCl
Verapamil HCl
Voriconazole
Zafirlukast
Zileuton

DRUGS EXCRETED IN BREAST MILK

The following list is not comprehensive; generic forms and alternate brands of some products may be available. When recommending drugs to pregnant or nursing patients, always check labeling for specific precautions.

Abstral
Accolate
Accupril
Accuretic
Acetaminophen/Codeine
Aclovate
Actiq
Activella
Acyclovir
Adalat CC
Adderall XR
Advicor
Aggrenox
Aldactazide
Aldactone
Allegra-D
Aloprim
Alora
Altace
Ambien
Ambien CR
Amcinonide
Amiloride/HCTZ
Amitriptyline
Amoxapine
Amoxicillin
Ampicillin
Amturnide
Anafranil
Analpram-HC
Angeliq
Ansaid
Anusol-HC Cream
Aplenzin
Apriso
Armour Thyroid
Arthrotec
Asacol
Astramorph PF
Atacand HCT
ATryn
Atuss DS
Augmentin
Augmentin ES-600
Augmentin XR
Avalide
AVC
Avelox
Aviane
Avinza
Aygestin
Azactam
Azasan
Azulfidine
Azulfidine EN
Bactrim
Banzel
Benicar HCT
Bentyl
BenzaClin
Benzamycin
Betamethasone Dipropionate

Betamethasone Valerate
Betapace
Betapace AF
Beyaz
Bicillin C-R
Bicillin L-A
Biltricide
Buprenex
Butisol
Butorphanol
Butrans
Calan
Calan SR
Capex
Carbatrol
Cardene IV
Cardizem
Cardizem CD
Catapres
Cefaclor ER
Cefazolin
Cefotetan
Cefoxitin
Cefpodoxime
Cefprozil
Ceftin
Ceftriaxone
Celebrex
Celestone
Celexa
Cenestin
Cephadyn
Cephalexin
Ceredase
Chloral Hydrate
Chlorothiazide
Chlorpromazine
Chlorthalidone
Cipro
Cipro XR
Cisplatin
Claforan
Clarinex
Clarinex-D
Clenia
Cleocin
Cleocin T
Climara
Climara Pro
Clindagel
Clindamax
Clobex
Cloderm
Co-Gesic
Colcrys
CombiPatch
Combivir
Compro
Cordarone
Cordran
Corgard
Cortifoam

Cortisporin
Corzide
Cosopt
Covera-HS
Crinone
Cutivate
Cyclessa
Cyklokapron
Cymbalta
Cytomel
Cytotec
Dantrium IV
Dapsone
Daraprim
Delestrogen
Demeclocycline HCl
Demerol
Depacon
Depakote
Depakote ER
DepoDur
Depo-Estradiol
Depo-Provera
depo-subQ provera 104
Derma-Smoothe/FS
Dermatop
DermOtic Oil
Desonate
Dexamethasone
Dexedrine Spansules
Dexferrum
Dextroamphetamine Sulfate
Diabinese
Dicloxacillin
Didrex
Diethylpropion
Diflorasone
Diflucan
Diflunisal
Dilacor XR
Dilantin
Dilaudid
Diltiazem
Diovan HCT
Dipentum
Diprivan
Diprolene
Dipyridamole
Divigel
Dolophine
Doral
Doryx
Doxorubicin HCl
Droxia
Duac
Duexis
Duragesic
Duramorph
Dyazide
Dynacin
E.E.S.
Effexor XR

Elestrin
Elixophyllin
Elocon
Embeda
EMLA
Enalapril/HCTZ
Enalaprilat
Endometrin
Enjuvia
Epifoam
Epivir
Epivir-HBV
Epzicom
Equetro
Ergomar
ERYC
EryPed
Ery-Tab
Erythrocin
Erythrocin Lactobionate
Erythromycin
Erythromycin Ethylsuccinate
    and Sulfisoxazole Acetyl
Esgic
Esgic-Plus
Estrace
Estraderm
Estradiol
Estrasorb
Estring
EstroGel
Estropipate
Estrostep Fe
Evamist
Evoclin
Exalgo
Exforge HCT
Exparel
Famotidine
Felbatol
Feldene
femhrt
Femring
Femtrace
Fentora
Fioricet
Fioricet with Codeine
Fiorinal
Fiorinal with Codeine
Flagyl
Flagyl ER
Flagyl IV
Fleet Enema
Flo-Pred
Fludrocortisone
Fluocinolone Acetonide
Fluocinonide
Fluorescite
Fluoxetine
Fluvoxamine
Folic Acid
Forfivo XL

(Continued)

DRUGS EXCRETED IN BREAST MILK

Fortaz
Fosamax Plus D
Fosinopril/HCTZ
Fragmin
Furosemide
Gablofen
Gadavist
Gengraf Capsules
Gleevec
Glyset
Gralise
Guanidine HCl
Haldol Decanoate
Halog
Haloperidol
Helidac
Hydrea
Hydrochlorothiazide
Hyzaar
Ifex
Imitrex
Implanon
Imuran
Inderal LA
Indomethacin
INFeD
Infumorph
InnoPran XL
Intermezzo
Invanz
Invega
Invega Sustenna
Isoniazid
Isoptin SR
Jenloga
Kadian
Kapvay ER
Kenalog
Keppra
Keppra XR
Ketoconazole
Ketorolac
Labetalol
Lamictal
Lamictal XR
Lamisil
Lanoxin
Lazanda
Levaquin
Levbid
Levoxyl
Levsin
Lexapro
Lialda
Lidocaine Cream
Lidoderm Patch
Lindane
Lioresal
Lipitor
Lithium
Lithium ER
Lo Loestrin Fe
Lo/Ovral
Locoid
Loestrin 21
Loestrin 24 Fe
Loestrin Fe
Lopressor

Lorcet
Lortab
Loseasonique
Lotensin
Lotensin HCT
Lotrel
Lusedra
Luvox CR
Luxiq
Lysteda
Magnevist
Makena
Maprotiline
Marcaine
Marcaine Spinal
Marinol
Maxipime
Maxitrol Ointment
Maxzide
MDP-25
Meclofenamate
Mefloquine
Menest
Menostar
Meperidine
Meprobamate
Meruvax II
Methadone
Methadose
Methotrexate
Methyclothiazide
Methyldopa
Methyldopa/HCTZ
Methyldopate
Metoclopramide
Metoprolol/HCTZ
Metozolv ODT
MetroGel-Vaginal
Mexiletine
Micardis HCT
Microzide
Midazolam
Minipress
Minoxidil
Mircette
Mirena
M-M-R II
Modicon
Monodox
Monopril
Morphine
Moxeza
MS Contin
Myambutol
Myochrysine
Mysoline
Nafcillin Sodium
Nalbuphine
Naprelan
Naprosyn
Natazia
Nature-Throid
Necon 10/11
Nembutal Sodium Solution
Neomycin/Polymyxin B/
  Dexamethasone
Neoral
Neurontin

Nexiclon XR
Nexplanon
Nexterone
Niaspan
Nicotrol Nasal Spray
Niravam
Nizatidine
Norco
Nordette-28
Norinyl 1/50
Noritate
Nor-QD
Novacort
Novantrone
NuvaRing
Ofirmev
Ofloxacin
Olux-E
Onfi
Onsolis
Oracea
Orapred
Oraqix
Ortho Evra
Ortho Micronor
Ortho Tri-Cyclen
Ortho Tri-Cyclen Lo
Ortho-Cept
Ortho-Cyclen
Ortho-Novum 1/35
Ortho-Novum 7/7/7
Ovcon-35
Oxecta
Oxistat
Oxycodone IR
OxyContin
Pandel
Paxil
Paxil CR
PCE
Pediapred
Peganone
Penicillin G Potassium
Penicillin G Procaine
Pentasa
Percocet
Percodan
Periostat
Persantine
Pexeva
Pfizerpen
Phenobarbital
Phoslyra
Phrenilin Forte
Plexion
Poly-Pred
Ponstel
Pramosone
Pravachol
Prefest
Premarin
Premphase
Prevpac
Prilosec
Primsol
Prinivide
Prinzide
Pristiq
Proctocort Cream

ProctoFoam-HC
Progesterone
Prograf
Promethazine VC/Codeine
Promethazine w/Codeine
Prometrium
Propranolol
Propranolol/HCTZ
Propylthiouracil
Proquin XR
Prosed EC
Protonix
Protopic
Provera
Prozac
Pulmicort
Pylera
Pyrazinamide
Qualaquin
Quinidine Gluconate
Quinidine Sulfate
Quixin
Qvar
Reserpine
Restasis
Retrovir
Rezira
Rhinocort Aqua
Rifater
Risperdal
Risperdal Consta
Robaxin
Rocaltrol
Rosac
Roxicet
Roxicodone
Rybix ODT
Rythmol SR
Sabril
Safyral
Salsalate
Sandimmune
Sarafem
Seasonale
Seconal Sodium
Sectral
Semprex-D
Sensorcaine-MPF
Septra
Seromycin
Seroquel
Seroquel XR
Silenor
Simcor
Sinemet CR
Solodyn
Solu-Cortef
Solu-Medrol
Soma
Soma Cmpd/Codeine
Soma Compound
Soriatane
Spectracef
Sporanox
Sprix
SSKI
St. Joseph 81 mg Aspirin
Stavzor

Stelara	Transderm Scop	Valtrex	Xyzal
Streptomycin	Tranxene T-Tab	Vandazole	Yasmin
Stromectol	Trental	Vanos	YAZ
Suboxone Sublingual Film	Treximet	Vasotec	Zanaflex
Subsys	Triamcinolone	Venlafaxine	Zantac
Sumycin	Tribenzor	Verapamil	Zarah
Symbyax	Trileptal	Verdeso	Zarontin
Synthroid	Tri-Luma	Verelan	Zebutal
Taclonex	Trimethoprim	Verelan PM	Zegerid
Tambocor	Triphasil	Vibramycin	Zestoretic
Tapazole	Trisenox	Vicodin	Zevalin
Tarka	Trivora	Vigamox	Ziac
Tazicef	Trizivir	Vimovo	Ziana
Tegretol	Tysabri	Viramune	Zinacef
Tekturna HCT	Ultane	Viread	Zolpimist
Tenoretic	Ultracet	Visudyne	Zonalon
Tenormin	Ultravate	Vivelle-Dot	Zonegran
Teveten HCT	Unasyn	Vivitrol	Zosyn
Theo-24	Uniretic	Vyvanse	Zovia
Theophylline	Unithroid	Wellbutrin SR	Zovirax Oral
Thyrolar	Urex	Wellbutrin XL	Zyban
Tiazac	Urogesic Blue	Westcort	Zydone
Tilia Fe	UTA	Westhroid	Zyprexa
Timoptic	Utira-C	Xanax	Zyprexa Relprevv
Tindamax	Vagifem	Xanax XR	
Toprol-XL	Valium	Xylocaine Jelly	

Abbreviation: HCTZ, hydrochlorothiazide

DRUGS THAT MAY CAUSE PHOTOSENSITIVITY

The drugs in this table are known to cause photosensitivity in some individuals. Effects can range from itching, scaling, rash, and swelling to skin cancer, premature skin aging, skin and eye burns, cataracts, reduced immunity, blood vessel damage, and allergic reactions. The list is not all-inclusive, and shows only representative brands of each generic. When in doubt, always check specific product labeling. Individuals should be advised to wear protective clothing and to apply sunscreen while taking the medications listed below.

GENERIC NAME	BRAND NAME
Acamprosate calcium	Campral
Acetazolamide	Diamox Sequels
Acitretin	Soriatane
Acyclovir	Zovirax
Alendronate sodium	Fosamax
Alendronate sodium/ Cholecalciferol	Fosamax Plus D
Aliskiren hemifumarate/ Amlodipine besylate/HCTZ	Amturnide
Aliskiren/HCTZ	Tekturna HCT
Almotriptan malate	Axert
Amiloride HCl/HCTZ	
Aminolevulinic acid HCl	Levulan Kerastick
Amiodarone HCl	Cordarone, Pacerone
Amitriptyline HCl	
Amitriptyline HCl/ Chlordiazepoxide	Limbitrol, Limbitrol DS
Amitryptyline HCl/ Perphenazine	
Amlodipine/HCTZ/ Olmesartan medoxomil	Tribenzor
Amlodipine besylate HCTZ/ Valsartan	Exforge HCT
Amoxapine	
Amphetamine aspartate/ Amphetamine sulfate/ Dextroamphetamine saccharate/ Dextroamphetamine sulfate	Adderall XR
Anagrelide HCl	Agrylin
Aprepitant	Emend Injection
Aripiprazole	Abilify
Atenolol/Chlorthalidone	Tenoretic
Atovaquone/Proguanil HCl	Malarone
Azithromycin	Zithromax, Zmax
Benazepril HCl	Lotensin
Benazepril HCl/HCTZ	Lotensin HCT
Benzoyl peroxide/Erythromycin	Benzamycin Pak
Bexarotene	Targretin
Bismuth subcitrate potassium/ Metronidazole/Tetracycline HCl	Pylera
Bismuth subsalicylate/ Metronidazole/Tetracycline HCl	Helidac Therapy

GENERIC NAME	BRAND NAME
Bisoprolol fumarate/HCTZ	Ziac
Bupropion HBr	Aplenzin
Bupropion HCl	Budeprion SR, Budeprion XL, Buproban, Wellbutrin SR, Wellbutrin XL, Zyban
Candesartan cilexetil/HCTZ	Atacand HCT
Capecitabine	Xeloda
Captopril	Capoten
Captopril/HCTZ	Capozide
Carbamazepine	Carbatrol, Epitol, Tegretol, Tegretol-XR
Carvedilol	Coreg
Carvedilol phosphate	Coreg CR
Celecoxib	Celebrex
Cevimeline HCl	Evoxac
Chloroquine phosphate	Aralen
Chlorothiazide	Diuril
Chlorpheniramine maleate/ Dextromethorphan HBr/ Pseudoephedrine HCl	Dicel DM
Chlorpheniramine maleate/ Pseudoephedrine HCl	Sudal-12 Tannate
Chlorpromazine HCl	
Chlorthalidone	Thalitone
Chlorthalidone/Clonidine HCl	Clorpres
Cidofovir	Vistide
Ciprofloxacin	Cipro XR
Ciprofloxacin HCl	Proquin XR
Citalopram HBr	Celexa
Clemastine fumarate	
Clindamycin phosphate	Clindagel
Clomipramine HCl	Anafranil
Clonidine HCl/Chlorthalidone	Clorpres
Clozapine	Clozaril, FazaClo
Cromolyn sodium	Gastrocrom
Cyclobenzaprine HCl	Flexeril
Cyproheptadine HCl	
Dacarbazine	
Dasatinib	Sprycel

(Continued)

Drugs That May Cause Photosensitivity

GENERIC NAME	BRAND NAME	GENERIC NAME	BRAND NAME
Demeclocycline HCl	Declomycin	Etodolac	Lodine, Lodine XL
Desipramine HCl	Norpramin	Ezetimibe/Simvastatin	Vytorin
Desvenlafaxine	Pristiq	Febuxostat	Uloric
Dextromethorphan HBr/ Promethazine HCl	Promethazine DM	Fenofibrate	Lofibra
		Floxuridine	
Dextromethorphan HBr/ Pseudoephedrine HCl/ Chlorpheniramine maleate	Atuss DS Tannate	Flucytosine	Ancobon
		Fluorouracil	Adrucil, Carac, Efudex, Flouroplex
Dextromethorphan HBr/ Quinidine sulfate	Nuedexta	Fluoxetine HCl/Olanzapine	Symbyax
		Fluphenazine decanoate	
Diclofenac potassium	Cambia, Cataflam, Zipsor	Fluphenazine HCl	Prolixin
		Flurbiprofen	Ansaid
Diclofenac sodium	Solaraze Gel, Voltaren-XR	Flutamide	Eulexin
		Fluvoxamine maleate	Luvox CR
Diclofenac sodium/Misoprostol	Arthrotec	Fluvastatin sodium	Lescol, Lescol XL
Diflunisal	Dolobid	Fosinopril sodium	Monopril
Diltiazem HCl	Cardizem, Cardizem CD, Cardizem LA, Cartia XT, Tiazac	Fosinopril sodium/HCTZ	Monopril HCT
		Fosphenytoin sodium	Cerebyx
		Furosemide	Lasix
Diphenhydramine HCl	Benadryl Injection	Gabapentin	Neurontin
Dipivefrin HCl	Propine Ophthalmic Solution	Gemfibrozil	Lopid
		Gemifloxacin mesylate	Factive
Divalproex sodium	Depakote, Depakote ER, Depakote Sprinkle	Glimepiride	Amaryl
		Glimepiride/Pioglitazone HCl	Duetact
Doxepin HCl	Silenor, Sinequan, Zonalon	Glimepiride/Rosiglitazone maleate	Avandaryl
Doxorubicin HCl	Adriamycin	Glipizide	Glucotrol
Doxycycline	Monodox, Oracea	Glyburide	Glynase PresTab, Diabeta
Doxycycline calcium	Vibramycin		
Doxycycline hyclate	Atridox, Doryx, PerioStat, Vibra-Tabs	Griseofulvin	Grifulvin V, Gris-PEG
		Haloperidol decanoate	Haldol Decanoate
Duloxetine HCl	Cymbalta	Haloperidol lactate	Haldol
Enalapril maleate	Vasotec	HCTZ	Microzide
Enalapril maleate/HCTZ	Vaseretic	HCTZ/Irbesartan	Avalide
Enalaprilat		HCTZ/Lisinopril	Prinzide, Zestoretic
Epirubicin HCl	Ellence	HCTZ/Losartan potassium	Hyzaar
Eprosartan mesylate/HCTZ	Teveten HCT	HCTZ/Methyldopa	
Erythromycin ethylsuccinate/ Sulfisoxazole acetyl	Eryzole, Pediazole	HCTZ/Metoprolol tartrate	Lopressor HCT
		HCTZ/Moexipril HCl	Uniretic
Escitalopram oxalate	Lexapro	HCTZ/Olmesartan medoxomil	Benicar HCT
Esomeprazole magnesium	Nexium	HCTZ/Propranolol HCl	
Esomeprazole magnesium/ Naproxen	Vimovo	HCTZ/Quinapril HCl	Accuretic
		HCTZ/Spironolactone	Aldactazide
Estazolam	Prosom	HCTZ/Telmisartan	Micardis HCT
Estradiol cypionate	Depo-Estradiol	HCTZ/Triamterene	Dyazide, Maxzide
Eszopiclone	Lunesta	HCTZ/Valsartan	Diovan HCT
Ethinyl estradiol/ Norelgestromin	Ortho Evra		
Ethionamide	Trecator		

GENERIC NAME	BRAND NAME
Hexachlorophene	pHisoHex
Hydroxocobalamin	Cyanokit
Hydroxychloroquine sulfate	Plaquenil
Imipramine HCl	Tofranil
Imipramine pamoate	Tofranil-PM
Indapamide	Lozol
Interferon alfa-2b	Intron A
Interferon alfa-N3	Alferon N
Irbesartan/HCTZ	Avalide
Isocarboxazid	Marplan
Isoniazid/Pyrazinamide/ Rifampin	Rifater
Isotretinoin	Amnesteem, Claravis, Sotret
Itraconazole	Sporanox
Ketoprofen	
Ketorolac tromethamine	Toradol
Lamotrigine	Lamictal
Leuprolide acetate	Lupron, Lupron Depot
Levofloxacin	Levaquin
Lisinopril	Prinivil, Zestril
Losartan potassium	Cozaar
Lovastatin	Altoprev, Mevacor
Maprotiline HCl	
Mefenamic acid	Ponstel
Meloxicam	Mobic
Mesalamine	Pentasa
Methotrexate	
Methyclothiazide	
Methyl aminolevulinate HCl	Metvixia Cream
Metolazone	Zaroxolyn
Metoprolol succinate	Toprol-XL
Metoprolol tartrate	Lopressor
Minocycline HCl	Arestin, Dynacin, Minocin, Solodyn
Mirtazapine	Remeron, RemeronSolTab
Moexipril HCl	Univasc
Moxifloxacin HCl	Avelox
Nabilone	Cesamet
Nabumetone	
Naproxen	EC-Naprosyn, Naprosyn
Naproxen sodium	Anaprox, Anaprox DS, Naprelan
Nadolol/Bendroflumethiazide	Corzide
Naratriptan HCl	Amerge

GENERIC NAME	BRAND NAME
Niacin/Lovastatin	Advicor
Nifedipine	Adalat CC, Nifediac CC, Nifedical XL, Procardia, Procardia XL
Nilotinib	Tasigna
Nisoldipine	Sular
Norfloxacin	Noroxin
Nortriptyline HCl	Pamelor
Ofloxacin	Floxin
Olanzapine	Zyprexa, Zyprexa Zydis
Olsalazine sodium	Dipentum
Omeprazole magnesium	Prilosec
Omeprazole/Sodium bicarbonate	Zegerid
Oxaprozin	Daypro
Oxaprozin potassium	Daypro Alta
Oxcarbazepine	Trileptal
Oxycodone HCl	Roxicodone
Paclitaxel	Abraxane
Panitumumab	Vectibix
Pantoprazole	Protonix
Paroxetine HCl	Paxil, Paxil CR
Paroxetine mesylate	Pexeva
Pentosan polysulfate sodium	Elmiron
Perphenazine	
Perphenazine/Amitriptyline HCl	
Pilocarpine HCl	Salagen
Piroxicam	Feldene
Polymyxin B sulfate/ Trimethoprim sulfate	Polytrim
Porfimer sodium	Photofrin
Pravastatin sodium	Pravachol
Pregabalin	Lyrica
Prochlorperazine	Compro
Prochlorperazine maleate	
Promethazine HCl	Phenadoz, Phenergan, Promethegan, Vivactil
Promethazine HCl/Codeine phosphate	
Promethazine HCl/ Phenylephrine HCl	Phenergan VC
Promethazine HCl/ Phenylephrine HCl/ Codeine phosphate	Phenergan VC with Codeine
Protriptyline HCl	Vivactil
Pyrazinamide	
Quetiapine fumarate	Seroquel, Seroquel XR

(Continued)

GENERIC NAME	BRAND NAME	GENERIC NAME	BRAND NAME
Quinidine gluconate		Thalidomide	Thalomid
Quinidine sulfate	Qualaquin	Thioridazine HCl	
Ramipril	Altace	Thiothixene	Navane
Rosagiline mesylate	Azilect	Tigecycline	Tygacil
Riluzole	Rilutek	Tipranavir	Aptivus
Ritonavir	Norvir	Tolbutamide	
Rizatriptan benzoate	Maxalt	Topiramate	Topamax
Selegiline HCl	Eldepryl	Triamcinolone acetonide	Azmacort
Sertraline HCl	Zoloft	Triamterene	Dyrenium
Sildenafil citrate	Viagra	Trifluoperazine HCl	
Simvastatin	Zocor	Trimipramine maleate	Surmontil
Simvastatin/Niacin	Simcor	Valacyclovir HCl	Valtrex
Sitagliptin/Simvastatin	Juvisync	Valproate sodium	Depacon
Sotalol HCl	Betapace, Betapace AF	Valproic acid	Depakene, Stavzor
Sulfamethoxazole/Trimethoprim	Bactrim, Bactrim DS, Septra, Septra DS, Sulfatrim	Varenicline	Chantix
		Vemurafenib	Zelboraf
		Venlafaxine HCl	Effexor XR
Sulfasalazine	Azulfidine, Azulfidine EN-tabs	Verteporfin	Visudyne
		Voriconazole	Vfend
Sulindac	Clinoril	Zaleplon	Sonata
Sumatriptan	Sumavel DosePro	Zolmitriptan	Zomig
Sumatriptan succinate	Alsuma, Imitrex	Zolpidem tartrate	Ambien, Ambien CR, Edluar, Zolpimist
Tacrolimus	Prograf		
Tetracycline HCl	Sumycin		

Abbreviations: HCTZ = hydrochlorothiazide; HCl = hydrochloride

DRUGS THAT MAY CAUSE QT PROLONGATION

BRAND	GENERIC
Abilify	Aripiprazole
Ablavar	Gadofosveset trisodium
AccuNeb	Albuterol sulfate
Advair Diskus, Advair HFA	Fluticasone propionate/Salmeterol
Albuterol sulfate ER	Albuterol sulfate
Aloxi	Palonosetron HCl
Alsuma	Sumatriptan
Amerge	Naratriptan HCl
Anzemet	Dolasetron mesylate
Apokyn	Apomorphine HCl
Arcapta Neohaler	Indacaterol
Avelox	Moxifloxacin HCl
Betapace, Betapace AF	Sotalol HCl
Biaxin, Biaxin XL	Clarithromycin
Brovana	Arformoterol tartrate
Butrans	Buprenorphine
Caprelsa	Vandetanib
Cardene SR	Nicardipine HCl
Celexa	Citalopram HBr
Cerebyx	Fosphenytoin sodium
Coartem	Artemether/Lumefantrine
Combivent	Ipratropium bromide/Albuterol sulfate
Cordarone	Amiodarone HCl
Corvert	Ibutilide fumarate
Definity	Perflutren, lipid
Detrol, Detrol LA	Tolterodine tartrate
Diflucan	Fluconazole
Ditropan, Ditropan XL	Oxybutynin Cl
Dolophine HCl	
Droperidol	Droperidol
Dulera	Formoterol fumarate dihydrate/Mometasone
DuoNeb	Albuterol sulfate/Ipratropium bromide
E.E.S. Granules, EryPed	Erythromycin ethylsuccinate
Effexor XR	Venlafaxine HCl
Eraxis	Anidulafungin
Eryc, Ery-Tab, PCE Dispertab	Erythromycin
PCE Dispertab	Erythromycin lactobionate
Erythrocin stearate	Erythromycin stearate
Exelon	Rivastigmine tartrate
Factive	Gemifloxacin mesylate

(Continued)

BRAND	GENERIC
Fanapt	Iloperidone
Fareston	Toremifene citrate
Firmagon	Degarelix
Fleet	Dibasic/Monobasic sodium phosphate
Foradil	Formoterol fumarate
Foscarnet sodium	
Geodon	Ziprasidone HCl
Granisetron HCl	
Granisol	Granisetron HCl
Halaven	Eribulin mesylate
Haldol	Haloperidol decanoate
Haloperidol	
Imitrex	Sumatriptan succinate
Intuniv	Guanfacine
Invega	Paliperidone
Invega Sustenna	Paliperidone palmitate
Invirase	Saquinavir mesylate
Isradipine	Isradipine
Istodax	Romidepsin
Kaletra	Lopinavir/Ritonavir
Kapvay	Clonidine HCl
Kayexalate Powder, Kionex	Sodium polystyrene sulfonate
Ketek	Telithromycin
Levaquin	Levofloxacin
Levatol	Penbutolol sulfate
Levitra	Vardenafil HCl
Lexapro	Escitalopram oxalate
Lupron Depot	Leuprolide acetate
Maxair Autohaler	Pirbuterol acetate
Mefloquine HCl	
Methadone HCl	
Methadose	Methadone HCl
Multaq	Dronedarone
MultiHance	Gadobenate dimeglumine
Namenda, Namenda XR	Memantine HCl
Nexterone	Amiodarone HCl
Noroxin	Norfloxacin
Norpace CR	Disopyramide phosphate
Noxafil Oral Suspension	Posaconazole
Nuedexta	Dextromethorphan HBr/Quinidine sulfate
Ofloxacin	
Oleptro	Trazodone HCl
Orap	Pimozide

BRAND	GENERIC
OsmoPrep	Dibasic/Monobasic sodium phosphate
Pepcid	Famotidine
Perforomist	Formoterol fumarate
Pletal	Cilostazol
PrevPAC	Amoxicillin/Clarithromycin/Lanzoprazole
ProAir HFA	Albuterol sulfate
Prograf	Tacrolimus
Proventil HFA	Albuterol sulfate
Prozac	Fluoxetine HCl
Qualaquin USP	Quinine sulfate
Quinidine gluconate	
Quinidine sulfate	
Ranexa	Ranolazine
Razadyne	Galantamine HBr
Reyataz	Atazanavir sulfate
Risperdal, Risperdal Consta	Risperidone
Rythmol SR	Propafenone HCl
Sancuso	Granisetron HCl
Sandostatin, Sandostatin LAR	Octreotide acetate
Saphris	Asenapine
Sarafem	Fluoxetine HCl
Serevent Diskus	Salmeterol xinafoate
Seroquel, Seroquel XR	Quetiapine fumarate
Sprycel	Dasatinib
Staxyn	Vardenafil HCl
Strattera	Atomoxetine HCl
Sumavel DosePro	Sumatriptan
Sutent	Sunitinib malate
Symbicort	Budesonide/Formoterol fumarate dihydrate
Symbyax	Fluoxetine/Olanzapine
Tambocor	Flecainide acetate
Tasigna	Nilotinib
Terbutaline sulfate	
Thioridazine HCl	
Tikosyn	Dofetilide
Toviaz	Fesoterodine fumarate
Trisenox	Arsenic trioxide
Tykerb	Lapatinib
Uniretic	Moexipril/HCTZ
Velcade	Bortezomib
Venlafaxine	
Ventolin HFA	Albuterol sulfate
VESIcare	Solifenacin succinate

(Continued)

BRAND	GENERIC
VFEND	Voriconazole
Vibativ	Telavancin
Viracept	Nelfinavir mesylate
Visicol	Monobasic/Dibasic sodium phosphate
Votrient	Pazopanib
Xalkori	Crizotinib
Xenazine	Tetrabenazine
Xopenex HFA	Levalbuterol tartrate
Xopenex	Levalbuterol HCl
Zelboraf	Vemurafenib
Zithromax, Zmax	Azithromycin
Zofran	Ondansetron HCl
Zoloft	Sertraline HCl
Zomig	Zolmitriptan
Zuplenz	Ondansetron
Zyprexa Relprevv	Olanzapine
Zytiga	Abiraterone acetate

NOTE: This list does not include all of the drugs that may cause QT disturbance. For more information, please refer to the specific product's full Prescribing Information.

DRUGS THAT SHOULD NOT BE CRUSHED

Listed below are various slow-release as well as enteric-coated products that should not be crushed or chewed. Slow-release (sr) represents products that are controlled-release, extended-release, long-acting, or timed-release. Enteric-coated (ec) represents products that are delayed release.

In general, capsules containing slow-release or enteric-coated particles may be opened and their contents administered on a spoonful of soft food. Instruct patients not to chew particles, though. (Patients should, in fact, be discouraged from chewing any medication unless it is specifically formulated for that purpose.)

This list should not be considered all-inclusive. Generic and alternate brands of some products may exist. Tablets intended for sublingual or buccal administration (not included in this list) should be administered only as intended, in an intact form.

DRUG	MANUFACTURER	FORM	DRUG	MANUFACTURER	FORM
AcipHex	Eisai	ec	Budeprion XL	Teva	sr
Actoplus Met XR	Takeda	sr	Buproban	Teva	sr
Adalat CC	Bayer Healthcare	sr	Calan SR	Pfizer	sr
Adderall XR	Shire U.S.	sr	Campral	Forest	ec
Adenovirus Type 4 and Type 7 Vaccine	Teva Women's Health, Inc.	ec	Carbatrol	Shire U.S.	sr
			Cardene SR	EKR Therapeutics	sr
Advicor	Abbott	sr	Cardizem CD	Biovail	sr
Afeditab CR	Watson	sr	Cardizem LA	Abbott	sr
Aggrenox	Boehringer Ingelheim	sr	Cardura XL	Pfizer	sr
Aleve Cold & Sinus	Bayer Healthcare	sr	Cartia XL	Watson	sr
Aleve Sinus & Headache	Bayer Healthcare	sr	Cemill 500	Miller	sr
Allegra-D 12 Hour	sanofi-aventis	sr	Cemill 1000	Miller	sr
Allegra-D 24 Hour	sanofi-aventis	sr	Certuss-D	Capellon	sr
Allerx	Cornerstone	sr	Chlorex-A	Cypress	sr
Allfen	MCR American	sr	Chlor-Phen	Truxton	sr
Allfen-DM	MCR American	sr	Chlor-Trimeton Allergy	Schering Plough	sr
Alophen	Numark	ec	Cipro XR	Schering Plough	sr
Altoprev	Watson	sr	Clarinex-D 24 Hour	Schering Plough	sr
Ambien CR	sanofi-aventis	sr	Claritin-D	Schering	sr
Ampyra ER	Acorda Therapeutics	sr	Claritin-D 12 Hour	Schering	sr
Amrix	Cephalon	sr	Claritin-D 24 Hour	Schering	sr
Aplenzin	sanofi-aventis	sr	Concerta	Ortho-McNeil-Janssen	sr
Apriso	Salix	sr	Contac 12-Hour	GlaxoSmithKline	sr
Arthrotec	Pfizer	ec	Correctol	Schering Plough	ec
Asacol	Procter & Gamble	ec	Coreg CR	GlaxoSmithKline	sr
Asacol HD	Procter & Gamble	ec	Covera-HS	Pfizer	sr
Ascriptin Enteric	Novartis Consumer	ec	CPM 8/PE 20/MSC 1.25	Cypress	sr
Augmentin XR	GlaxoSmithKline	sr	Creon 5	Solvay	ec
Avinza	King	sr	Creon 10	Solvay	ec
Azulfidine Entabs	Pfizer	ec	Creon 20	Solvay	ec
Bayer Aspirin Regimen	Bayer Healthcare	ec	Cymbalta	Eli Lilly	ec
Biaxin XL	Abbott	sr	Dairycare	Plainview	ec
Bidex-A	SJ Pharmaceuticals	sr	Deconsal II	Cornerstone	sr
Blanex-A	Blansett	sr	Deconex DM	Poly	sr
Bontril Slow-Release	Valeant	sr	Depakote	Abbott	ec
Bromfed-PD	Victory	sr	Depakote ER	Abbott	sr
Bromfenex PD	Quality Care	sr	Depakote Sprinkles	Abbott	ec
Budeprion SR	Teva	sr	Despec SR	International Ethical	sr

Enteric-coated = ec

Slow-released = sr

(Continued)

DRUG	MANUFACTURER	FORM	DRUG	MANUFACTURER	FORM
Detrol LA	Pfizer	sr	Flagyl ER	Pharmacia	sr
Dexedrine Spansules	GlaxoSmithKline	sr	Fleet Bisacodyl	Fleet, C.B.	ec
Dexilant	Takeda	sr	Focalin XR	Novartis	sr
Diamox Sequels	Duramed	sr	Folitab 500	Rising	sr
Dilacor XR	Watson	sr	Fortamet	Shionogi Pharma	sr
Dilantin	Pfizer	sr	Forfivo XL	IntelGenx	sr
Dilantin Kapseals	Pfizer	sr	Fumatinic	Laser	sr
Dilatrate-SR	UCB	sr	Genacote	Teva	ec
Diltia XT	Watson	sr	GFN 600/	Cypress	sr
Dilt-CD	Apotex	sr	Phenylephrine 20		
Ditropan XL	Ortho-McNeil Janssen	sr	Gilphex TR	Gil	sr
Donnatal Extentabs	PBM	sr	Glucophage XR	Bristol-Myers-Squibb	sr
Doryx	Warner Chilcott	ec	Glucotrol XL	Pfizer	sr
D-Phen 1000	Midlothian	sr	Glumetza	Depomed	sr
Dulcolax	Boehringer Ingelheim	ec	Guaifenex GP	Ethex	sr
Duomax	Capellon	sr	Guaifenex PSE 60	Ethex	sr
Duratuss	Physicians Total Care	sr	Guaifenex PSE 80	Ethex	sr
Duratuss DA	Victory	sr	Guaifenex PSE 85	Ethex	sr
Dynacirc CR	GlaxoSmithKline	sr	Guaifenex PSE 120	Ethex	sr
Dynex LA	Athlon	sr	Halfprin	Kramer	ec
Dynex VR	Athlon	sr	Hemax	Pronova	sr
Dytan-CS	Hawthorn	sr	Histacol LA	Breckenridge	sr
Easprin	Rosedale	ec	Horizant	GlaxoSmithKline	sr
EC Naprosyn	Genentech	ec	Iberet-500	Abbott	sr
Ecotrin	GlaxoSmithKline	ec	Iberet-Folic-500	Abbott	sr
Ecotrin Adult Low Strength	GlaxoSmithKline	ec	Icar-C Plus SR	Hawthorn	sr
			Inderal LA	Akrimax	sr
Ecotrin Maximum Strength	GlaxoSmithKline	ec	Indocin SR	Forte Pharma	sr
			Innopran XL	GlaxoSmithKline	sr
Ecpirin	Prime Marketing	ec	Intuniv	Shire	sr
Ed A-Hist	Edwards	sr	Invega	Ortho-McNeil-Janssen	sr
Effexor-XR	Wyeth	sr	Isochron	Forest	sr
Embeda	King	sr	Isoptin SR	Ranbaxy	sr
Enablex	Novartis Consumer	sr	Janumet XR	Merck Sharp & Dohme Corp.	sr
Entercote	Global Source	ec			
Entocort EC	Prometheus	ec	Kadian	Actavis	sr
Equetro	Validus	sr	Kapvay ER	Shionogi	sr
ERYC	Warner Chilcott	sr	Kaon-Cl 10	Savage	sr
Ery-Tab	Abbott	ec	Keppra XR	UCB	sr
Exalgo	Mallinckrodt	sr	Klor-Con 8	Upsher-Smith	sr
Extress-30	Key	sr	Klor-Con 10	Upsher-Smith	sr
Extress-60	Key	sr	Klor-Con M10	Upsher-Smith	sr
Feen-A-Mint	Schering Plough	ec	Klor-Con M15	Upsher-Smith	sr
Femilax	G & W	ec	Klor-Con M20	Upsher-Smith	sr
Fero-Folic-500	Abbott	sr	Kombiglyze ER	BMS/AstraZeneca	sr
Fero-Grad-500	Abbott	sr	K-Tab	Abbott	sr
Ferro-Sequels	Inverness Medical	sr	K-Tan	Prasco	sr
Ferrous Fumarate DS	Vita-Rx	sr	Lamictal XR	GlaxoSmithKline	sr
Fetrin	Lunsco	sr	Lescol XL	Novartis	sr

DRUG	MANUFACTURER	FORM	DRUG	MANUFACTURER	FORM
Levall G	Auriga	sr	Norel SR	U.S. Pharmaceutical	sr
Levbid	Alaven	sr	Norpace CR	Pfizer	sr
Levsinex	Alaven	sr	Nucynta ER	Janssen	sr
Lialda	Shire	ec	Obstetrix EC	Seyer Pharmatec	ec
Lipram 4500	Global	ec	Oleptro	LaboPharm	sr
Lipram-PN10	Global	ec	Opana ER	Endo	sr
Lipram-PN16	Global	ec	Oramorph SR	Xanodyne	sr
Lipram-PN20	Global	ec	Oracea	Galderma	sr
Liquibid-D	Capellon	sr	Oxecta	King Pharmaceuticals	sr
Liquibid-D 1200	Capellon	sr	Oxycontin	Purdue	sr
Lithobid	Noven Therapeutics	sr	Palcaps 10	Breckenridge	ec
Lohist-12	Larken	sr	Palcaps 20	Breckenridge	ec
Luvox CR	Jazz Pharmaceuticals	sr	Pancreaze	Ortho-McNeil-Janssen	ec
Mag Delay	Major	ec	Pancrecarb MS-4	Digestive Care	ec
Mag64	Rising	ec	Pancrecarb MS-8	Digestive Care	ec
Mag-Tab SR	Niche	sr	Pancrecarb MS-16	Digestive Care	ec
Maxifed	MCR American	sr	Pangestyme CN-10	Ethex	ec
Maxifed DM	MCR American	sr	Pangestyme CN-20	Ethex	ec
Maxifed DMX	MCR American	sr	Pangestyme EC	Ethex	ec
Maxifed-G	MCR American	sr	Pangestyme MT16	Ethex	ec
Medent PE	SJ Pharmaceuticals	sr	Pangestyme UL12	Ethex	ec
Mega-C	Merit	sr	Pangestyme UL18	Ethex	ec
Menopause Trio	Mason Vitamins	sr	Pangestyme UL20	Ethex	ec
Mestinon Timespan	Valeant	sr	Panocaps	Breckenridge	ec
Metadate CD	UCB	sr	Panocaps MT 16	Breckenridge	ec
Metadate ER	UCB	sr	Panocaps MT 20	Breckenridge	ec
Methylin ER	Mallinckrodt	sr	Paser	Jacobus	sr
Micro-K	Ther-Rx	sr	Pavacot	Truxton	sr
Micro-K 10	Ther-Rx	sr	Paxil CR	GlaxoSmithKline	sr
Mild-C	Carlson, J.R.	sr	PCE Dispertab	Abbott	sr
Mirapex ER	Boehringer Ingelheim	sr	PCM LA	Cypress	sr
Moxatag	Victory	sr	Pendex	Cypress	sr
MS Contin	Purdue	sr	Pentasa	Shire U.S.	sr
Mucinex	Reckitt Benckiser	sr	Pentoxil	Upsher-Smith	sr
Mucinex D	Reckitt Benckiser	sr	Phenavent D	Ethex	sr
Mucinex DM	Reckitt Benckiser	sr	Phenytek	Mylan	sr
Mydocs	Centurion	sr	Phlemex-PE	Cypress	sr
Myfortic	Novartis	ec	Poly Hist Forte	Poly	sr
Nalex-A	Blansett	sr	Poly-Vent	Poly	sr
Namenda XR	Forest	sr	Prehist D	Marnel	sr
Naprelan	Victory	sr	Prevacid	Takeda	ec
New Ami-Tex LA	Actavis	sr	Prilosec	AstraZeneca	ec
Nexium	AstraZeneca	ec	Prilosec OTC	Procter & Gamble	sr
Nexiclon XR	Next Wave	sr	Pristiq	Wyeth	sr
Niaspan	Abbott	sr	Procardia XL	Pfizer	sr
Nifediac CC	Teva	sr	Prolex PD	Blansett	sr
Nifedical XL	Teva	sr	Prolex-D	Blansett	sr
Nitro-Time	Time-Cap	sr	Proquin XR	Depomed	sr

(Continued)

DRUG	MANUFACTURER	FORM	DRUG	MANUFACTURER	FORM
Protid	Lunsco	sr	Taztia XT	Watson	sr
Protonix	Wyeth	ec	Tegretol-XR	Novartis	sr
Prozac Weekly	Eli Lilly	ec	Theo-24	UCB	sr
Pseudocot-C	Truxton	sr	Theocron	Carac	sr
Pseudocot-G	Truxton	sr	Theo-Time	Major	sr
Pseudovent DM	Ethex	sr	Tiazac	Forest	sr
Ralix	Cypress	sr	Toprol XL	AstraZeneca	sr
Ranexa	Gilead	sr	Totalday	National Vitamin	sr
Razadyne ER	Ortho-McNeil-Janssen	sr	Toviaz	Pfizer	sr
Requip XL	GlaxoSmithKline	sr	Trental	sanofi-aventis	sr
Rescon-Jr	Capellon	sr	Treximet	GlaxoSmithKline	ec
Respa-AR	Respa	sr	Trilipix	Abbott	ec
Respa-BR	Respa	sr	Tussicaps	Mallinckrodt	sr
Respaire-120 SR	Laser	sr	Tylenol Arthritis	McNeil Consumer	sr
Rhinacon A	Breckenridge	sr	Ultram ER	Valeant	sr
Ritalin LA	Novartis	sr	Urocit-K 5	Mission	sr
Ritalin-SR	Novartis	sr	Urocit-K 10	Mission	sr
Rodex Forte	Legere	sr	Uroxatral	sanofi-aventis	sr
Ru-Tuss	Carwin	sr	Utira	Hawthorn	sr
Rythmol SR	GlaxoSmithKline	sr	Veracolate	Numark	ec
Ryzolt	Purdue	sr	Verelan	UCB	sr
SAM-e	Pharmavite	ec	Verelan PM	UCB	sr
Sanctura XR	Allergan	sr	Videx EC	Bristol-Myers-Squibb	ec
Seroquel XR	AstraZeneca	sr	Vimovo	AstraZeneca	ec
Simcor	Abbott	sr	Vivitrol	Alkermes	sr
Sinemet CR	Bristol-Myers Squibb	sr	Voltaren-XR	Novartis	sr
Slo-Niacin	Upsher-Smith	sr	Vospire ER	Dava	sr
Slow Fe	Novartis Consumer	sr	Votrient	GlaxoSmithKline	ec
Slow Fe With Folic Acid	Novartis Consumer	sr	Wellbutrin SR	GlaxoSmithKline	sr
Slow-Mag	Purdue	ec	Wellbutrin XL	GlaxoSmithKline	sr
Solodyn	Medicis	sr	Wobenzym N	Marlyn	ec
St. Joseph Pain Reliever	McNeil Consumer	ec	Xanax ER	Pfizer	sr
Stahist	Magna	sr	Xedec II	Cypress	sr
Stavzor	Noven	sr	Xpect-AT	Hawthorn	sr
Sudafed 12 hour	McNeil Consumer	sr	Xpect-HC	Hawthorn	sr
Sudafed 24 hour	McNeil Consumer	sr	Xpect-PE	Hawthorn	sr
Sular	Shionogi Pharma	sr	Zenpep	Eurand	ec
Sulfazine EC	Qualitest	ec	Zmax	Pfizer	sr
Symax Duotab	Capellon	sr	Zyban	GlaxoSmithKline	sr
Symax-SR	Capellon	sr	Zyflo CR	Cornerstone	sr
Tarka	Abbott	sr	Zyrtec-D	McNeil Consumer	sr

DRUGS THAT SHOULD NOT BE USED IN PREGNANCY

Abiraterone acetate
Acitretin
Ambrisentan
Amlodipine besylate/Atorvastatin calcium
Anastrozole
Aspirin
Atorvastatin calcium
Benzphetamine hydrochloride
Bexarotene
Bicalutamide
Boceprevir
Bosentan
Caffeine
Cetrorelix acetate
Chenodiol
Cholecalciferol
Choriogonadotropin alfa
Chorionic gonadotropin
Clomiphene citrate
Danazol
Degarelix
Desogestrel/Ethinyl estradiol
Diclofenac sodium
Dienogest/Estradiol valerate
Dihydroergotamine mesylate
Dronedarone
Drospirenone/Ethinyl estradiol
Dutasteride
Dutasteride/Tamsulosin hydrochloride
Ergotamine tartrate
Estazolam
Estradiol
Estrogens, Conjugated, Synthetic B
Estropipate
Ethinyl estradiol/Ethynodiol diacetate

Ethinyl estradiol/Etonogestrel
Ethinyl estradiol/Ferrous fumarate/ Norethindrone
Ethinyl estradiol/Levonorgestrel
Ethinyl estradiol/Norelgestromin
Ethinyl estradiol/Norethindrone acetate
Ethinyl estradiol/Norgestimate
Ethynodiol diacetate
Exemestane
Ezetimibe
Ezetimibe/Simvastatin
Finasteride
Fluorouracil
Fluoxymesterone
Fluvastatin sodium
Follitropin alfa
Follitropin beta
Ganirelix acetate
Genistein aglycone
Goserelin acetate
Histrelin acetate
Iodine I 131 tositumomab
Isotretinoin
Leflunomide
Lenalidomide
Letrozole
Leuprolide acetate
Levonorgestrel
Lovastatin
Lovastatin/Niacin
Lutropin alfa
Medroxyprogesterone acetate
Megestrol acetate
Menotropins
Meprobamate
Mequinol/Tretinoin

Mestranol/Norethindrone
Methotrexate
Methyltestosterone
Mifepristone
Miglustat
Misoprostol
Nafarelin acetate
Niacin
Norethindrone acetate
Oxandrolone
Pitavastatin
Pravastatin sodium
Quazepam
Raloxifene hydrochloride
Ribavirin
Rosuvastatin calcium
Simvastatin
Simvastatin/Sitagliptin
Tamsulosin
Tazarotene
Telaprevir
Temazepam
Tesamorelin
Testosterone
Testosterone cypionate
Testosterone enanthate
Thalidomide
Tositumomab
Tretinoin
Triptorelin pamoate
Ulipristal acetate
Urofollitropin
Vitamin A palmitate
Warfarin sodium
Zinc bisglycinate

PREGNANCY CATEGORY X

Studies in animals or humans, or investigational or postmarketing reports, have demonstrated fetal risk, which clearly outweighs any possible benefit to the patient.

LACTOSE- AND GALACTOSE-FREE DRUGS

The following is a selection of lactose- and galactose-free products. The list is not comprehensive. Generic and alternate brands may exist. Always check product labeling for definitive information on specific ingredients.

TRADE NAME (OTC)	FORM
Advil	Tablets, Caplets, Gel Caplets, Liquigels
Advil PM	Liquigels
Advil Cold and Sinus	Caplets, Liquigels
Aleve	Tablets
Aleve Smooth Gels	Gel Tablets
Alka-Seltzer	Effervescent Tablets
Alka-Seltzer Plus Cold	Effervescent Tablets, Softgels
Alka-Seltzer Plus Cold and Cough Formula	Effervescent Tablets, Liquigels
Alka-Seltzer Plus Day and Night Cold Formula	Effervescent Tablets, Liquigels
Alka-Seltzer Plus Flu Formula	Effervescent Tablets
Alka-Seltzer Plus Mucus and Congestion	Liquigels
Alka-Seltzer Plus Night Cold Formula	Effervescent Tablets, Liquigels
Alka-Seltzer Plus Sinus Formula	Effervescent Tablets
Ascriptin	Tablets
Axid	Tablets
Axid AR	Tablets
Benadryl	Liquid
Benadryl Allergy Plus Cold	Kapgels
Benadryl Dye-Free Allergy	Liquigels
Benadryl Allergy Ultratab	Tablets
Benadryl Quick Dissolve Strips	Oral Films
Benadryl Allergy Kapgels	Capsules
Benadryl Allergy Plus Sinus	Caplets
Benadryl D Allergy Plus Sinus	Tablets
Benadryl Severe Allergy Plus Sinus Headache	Caplets
Benadryl Children's Perfect Measure	Liquid
Benadryl Children's Allergy	Liquid
Benadryl Children's Dye-Free Allergy	Liquid
Benadryl-D Children's Allergy and Sinus	Liquid
Caltrate 600	Tablets
Caltrate 600 PLUS	Tablets
Caltrate 600+D Plus Minerals	Tablets, Chewables
Claritin-D 24	Tablets
Claritin Reditabs	Tablets (disintegrating)
Colace	Capsules
Dramamine Chewable	Tablets

TRADE NAME (OTC)	FORM
Elecare	Powder
Enfamil ProSobee	Liquid, Powder
Ensure	Liquid, Powder
Ensure Bone Health	Liquid
Ensure Clinical Strength	Liquid
Ensure Fiber	Liquid
Ensure High Calcium	Liquid
Ensure High Protein	Liquid
Ensure Immune Health	Liquid
Ensure Muscle Health	Liquid
Ensure Plus	Liquid
Excedrin Extra-Strength	Caplets, Capsules, Tablets
Excedrin Migraine	Capsules, Tablets, Gel Tablets
Excedrin Menstrual Complete	Capsules
Excedrin Tension Headache	Caplets, Capsules, Tablets
Excedrin Back and Body	Caplets
Excedrin PM	Caplets, Gel Tablets
Ex-Lax Maximum Strength	Tablets
Ex-Lax Regular Strength	Tablets
Fergon	Tablets
Gaviscon Regular Strength	Tablets
Imodium A-D	Liquid, Tablets
Jevity	Liquid
Kaopectate Cherry	Liquid
Kaopectate Peppermint	Liquid
Kaopectate Advanced Formula	Suspension
Kaopectate Vanilla	Liquid
Konsyl	Powder
Konsyl Bladder Control	Capsules
Lactaid	Tablets
Lactaid Fast Act	Caplets, Chewables
MCT Oil	Oil
Medi-Lyte	Tablets
Metamucil	Capsules, Powder, Wafers
Motrin Children's	Suspension
Motrin IB	Tablets
Motrin Infants'	Drops
Motrin Junior Strength	Caplets, Tablets
Mylanta Gas Maximum Strength	Softgels
Mylanta Maximum Strength	Tablets, Chewables
Mylanta Regular Strength	Liquid

(Continued)

TRADE NAME (OTC)	FORM
Mylanta Supreme	Liquid
Mylanta Ultimate Strength	Liquid
Mylicon Infants'	Drops
Ocuvite Vitamin and Mineral Supplement	Tablets
One-A-Day Cholesterol Plus	Tablets
One-A-Day Energy	Tablets
One-A-Day Essential	Tablets
One-A-Day VitaCraves Gummies	Gummies
One-A-Day Maximum	Tablets
One-A-Day Men's	Tablets
One-A-Day Men's Health Formula	Tablets
One-A-Day Men's 50+ Advantage	Tablets
One-A-Day Men's Pro Edge	Tablets
One-A-Day Menopause Formula	Tablets
One-A-Day Teen Advantage	Tablets
One-A-Day Women's	Tablets
One-A-Day Women's 50+ Advantage	Tablets
One-A-Day Women's Active Mind & Body	Tablets
One-A-Day Women's Active Metabolism	Tablets
One-A-Day Women's Prenatal	Tablets
Pepto-Bismol	Suspension, Caplets
Pepto-Bismol Instacool Chewable	Tablets
Pepto-Bismol Max. Strength	Suspension
Pepto Children's Chewable	Tablets
Percy Medicine	Suspension
Polycose	Liquid, Powder
Prilosec OTC	Tablets
Promote	Liquid
Promote with Fiber	Liquid
Pulmocare	Liquid
RCF	Liquid
Simply Sleep	Caplets
St. Joseph Adult Low Strength Aspirin	Tablets
Sucrets Children's	Lozenges
Sucrets Complete	Lozenges
Sucrets Cough	Lozenges
Sucrets Herbal	Lozenges
Sucrets Liquid	Liquid
Sucrets Maximum Strength	Lozenges
Sudafed	Tablets
Sudafed 12 Hour	Tablets
Sudafed 24 Hour	Tablets
Sudafed Children's	Liquid
Sudafed Congestion	Tablets
Sudafed OM Sinus Congestion Spray	Liquid

TRADE NAME (OTC)	FORM
Sudafed PE Cold and Cough	Caplets
Sudafed PE Sinus and Allergy	Tablets
Sudafed PE Day and Night Cold	Caplets
Sudafed PE Day and Night Congestion	Tablets
Sudafed PE Congestion	Tablets
Sudafed PE Non-Drying Sinus	Caplets
Sudafed PE Pressure and Pain	Caplets
Sudafed PE Severe Cold Formula	Caplets
Sudafed PE Triple Action	Caplets
Sudafed PE Sinus and Allergy	Tablets
Sudafed Triple Action	Caplets
Titralac	Tablets
Titralac Plus	Tablets
Tums	Tablets
Tums E-X 750	Tablets
Tums E-X- Sugar Free	Tablets
Tums Kids	Tablets
Tums Ultra 1000	Tablets
Tylenol	Tablets
Tylenol Children's Plus Cold	Liquid
Tylenol Children's Plus Cold & Allergy	Liquid
Tylenol Children's Plus Cold & Cough	Liquid
Tylenol Children's Plus Cold & Stuffy Nose	Liquid
Tylenol Children's Plus Cough & Runny Nose	Liquid
Tylenol Children's Plus Cough & Sore Throat	Liquid
Tylenol Children's Plus Flu	Liquid
Tylenol Children's Plus Multi-Symptom Cold	Suspension
Tylenol Infants'	Suspension
Tylenol Meltaways Jr.	Tablets
Unisom SleepTabs	Gels, Melts, Tablets
Unisom PM Pain SleepCaps	Caplets
Zantac 75	Tablets
Zantac 150	Tablets
Zantac 150 Cool Mint	Tablets

TRADE NAME (Rx)	FORM
Actigall	Capsules
Advicor	Tablets
Aldactazide	Tablets
Aldactone	Tablets
Allegra Children's Oral	Suspension
Allegra	Suspension, Tablets
Allegra-D 12 Hr, 24 Hr	Tablets
Altace	Capsules

TRADE NAME (Rx)	FORM	TRADE NAME (Rx)	FORM
Amicar	Solution, Tablets	Esgic-Plus	Capsules, Tablets
Amnesteem	Capsules	Exelon	Capsules, Solution
Antivert	Tablets	Exforge HCT	Tablets
Aplenzin	Tablets	Exforge	Tablets
Apriso	Capsules	Fibricor (fenofibric acid)	Tablets
Aromasin	Tablets	Fioricet	Tablets
Augmentin Chewable	Tablets	Fioricet with Codeine	Capsules
Augmentin ES 600	Powder	Flomax	Capsules
Augmentin XR	Tablets	Gleevec	Tablets
Augmentin	Suspension, Tablets	Glucotrol XL	Tablets
Axid	Solution	Glucovance	Tablets
Bactrim	Tablets	Glyset	Tablets
Bactrim DS	Tablets	GoLYTELY	Powder
Biaxin Granules	Suspension	Grifulvin V	Suspension, Tablets
Biaxin Filmtab	Tablets	Inderal LA	Capsules
Calan SR	Tablets	Isoptin SR	Tablets
Cambia	Solution	Kaletra	Solution, Tablets
Carafate	Suspension, Tablets	Kapidex	Capsules
Cardizem CD	Capsules	Keppra	Solution, Tablets
Cardizem LA	Tablets	K-Lor	Powder
Ceftin	Suspension, Tablets	K-Phos Neutral	Tablets
Cefzil	Suspension, Tablets	K-Phos Original Formula	Tablets
Cipro XR	Tablets	K-Tab	Tablets
Cipro	Suspension, Tablets	Lamisil	Tablets, Oral Granules
Citranatal RX	Tablets		
Clinoril	Tablets	Lescol	Capsules
Coartem	Tablets	Lescol XL	Tablets
Combivir	Tablets	Levaquin	Solution, Tablets
Comtan	Tablets	Levothroid	Tablets
Covera-HS	Tablets	Levoxyl	Tablets
Creon	Capsules	Lexapro	Solution, Tablets
Cytotec	Tablets	Lomotil	Tablets
Daypro	Tablets	Lopid	Tablets
Demerol	Tablets	Lysteda	Tablets
Depakene	Capsules, Solution	Malarone	Tablets
Depakote	Tablets	Malarone Pediatric	Tablets
Depakote Sprinkle	Capsules	Maxzide	Tablets
Detrol	Tablets	Methylin ER	Tablets
Detrol LA	Capsules	Micardis	Tablets
DiaBeta	Tablets	Micro-K	Capsules
Diovan HCT	Tablets	Micronase	Tablets
Diovan	Tablets	Minipress	Capsules
E.E.S	Suspension, Tablets	Minocin	Capsules
Edluar	Tablets	Moxatag	Tablets
Embeda	Capsules	Niaspan	Tablets
Entereg	Capsules	Norpramin	Tablets
Epivir	Solution, Tablets	Norvasc	Tablets
Epivir-HBV	Solution, Tablets	Omnicef	Capsules, Suspension
Ery-Tab	Tablets		

(Continued)

TRADE NAME (Rx)	FORM	TRADE NAME (Rx)	FORM
Onsolis	Buccal Film	Tikosyn	Capsules
Pamelor	Capsules	Tofranil	Tablets
Pamine Forte	Tablets	Tofranil-PM	Capsules
Patanase	Liquid	Toprol-XL	Tablets
Paxil	Suspension, Tablets	Treanda	Powder
Pepcid	Suspension, Tablets	Trental	Tablets
Percocet	Tablets	Treximet	Tablets
Percodan	Tablets	Trileptal	Suspension, Tablets
Plaquenil	Tablets	Trilipix	Capsules
Pletal	Tablets	Trizivir	Tablets
PrandiMet	Tablets	Twynsta	Tablets
Prandin	Tablets	Tyvaso	Liquid
Precose	Tablets	Uniphyl	Tablets
Prevacid	Capsules	Urex	Tablets
Prinivil	Tablets	Valcyte	Solution, Tablets
Pristiq	Tablets	Valtrex	Caplets
Procardia	Capsules	Valturna	Tablets
Procardia XL	Tablets	Vibramycin Hyclate	Capsules, Suspension
Promacta	Tablets	Vicodin	Tablets
Prometrium	Capsules	Vicodin ES	Tablets
Protonix	Suspension, Tablets	Vicodin HP	Tablets
Prozac	Capsules	Vicoprofen	Tablets
Qualaquin	Capsules	Videx EC	Capsules, Delayed Release Tablets
Questran	Powder	Vimpat	Solution, Tablets
Questran Light	Powder	Visicol	Tablets
Rapaflo	Capsules	Vistaril	Capsules
Remeron SolTab	Tablets	Votrient	Tablets
Rifadin	Capsules, Solution	Welchol	Suspension, Tablets
Robaxin	Tablets	Wellbutrin	Tablets
Ryzolt	Tablets	Wellbutrin SR	Tablets
Sabril	Solution, Tablets	Wellbutrin XL	Tablets
Saphris	Tablets	Xenical	Capsules
Sarafem	Tablets	Zantac	Efferdose Tablets, Syrup, Tablets
Savella	Tablets	Zarontin	Capsules, Solution
Sectral	Capsules	Zebeta	Tablets
Sinemet	Tablets	Zenpep	Capsules
Sinemet CR	Tablets	Zestril	Tablets
Soma	Tablets	Ziac	Tablets
Stalevo	Tablets	Ziagen	Solution, Tablets
Stavzor	Capsules	Zipsor	Capsules
Sucraid	Solution	Zofran	Solution
Tamiflu	Capsules, Suspension	Zoloft	Oral Concentrate, Tablets
Tegretol/Tegretol-XR	Suspension, Tablets	Zonegran	Capsules
Tenoretic	Tablets	Zyban	Tablets
Tenormin	Tablets	Zyvox	Suspension, Tablets
Tessalon	Capsules		
Tiazac	Capsules		
Ticlid	Tablets		

FDA-APPROVED NEW DRUG PRODUCTS

BRAND NAME	GENERIC NAME	INDICATION
Abstral	Fentanyl	Management of breakthrough cancer pain in opioid-tolerant patients.
Adcetris	Brentuximab vedotin	Treatment of Hodgkin's lymphoma and systemic anaplastic large cell lymphoma (ALCL).
Amturnide	Aliskiren hemifumarate/ Amlodipine besylate/ Hydrochlorothiazide	Treatment of hypertension.
Anascorp	Centruroides [scorpion] Immune F(ab')2 [equine]	Treatment of clinical signs of scorpion envenomation.
Arcapta Neohaler	Indacaterol inhalation powder	Long-term, once-daily maintenance bronchodilator treatment of airflow obstruction in people with chronic obstructive pulmonary disease (COPD).
Benlysta	Belimumab	Treatment of active, autoantibody-positive lupus (systemic lupus erythematosus) who are receiving standard therapy, including corticosteroids, antimalarials, immunosuppressives, and nonsteroidal anti-inflammatory drugs.
Brilinta	Ticagrelor	To reduce cardiovascular death and heart attack in patients with acute coronary syndromes (ACS).
Butrans	Buprenorphine	Treatment of moderate-to-severe chronic pain when continuous opioid analgesia is needed for extended time period.
Caprelsa	Vandetanib	Treatment of metastatic medullary thyroid cancer in patients who are ineligible for surgery and who have disease that is metastatic or symptomatic.
Complera	Emtricitabine/Rilpivirine/ Tenofovir disoproxil fumarate	Treatment of HIV-1.
Corifact	Factor XIII concentrate [human]	Routine prophylactic treatment of congenital Factor XIII deficiency.
Daliresp	Roflumilast	To decrease the frequency of flare-ups or worsening of symptoms from severe COPD.
DaTscan	Ioflupane i-123	Brain imaging solution to assist in the evaluation of adult patients with suspected Parkinsonian syndrome.
Dificid	Fidaxomicin	Treatment of *Clostridium difficile*-associated diarrhea (CDAD).
Edarbi	Azilsartan medoxomil	Treatment of hypertension.
Edurant	Rilpivirine	Treatment of HIV-1.
Ella	Ulipristal acetate	Prevention of pregnancy.
Firazyr	Icatibant	Prevention of acute attacks of a rare condition called hereditary angioedema (HAE).
Fortesta	Testosterone	Treatment of primary hypogonadism/hypogonadotropic hypogonadism.
Gadavist	Gadobutrol	Contrast agent to help detect lesions in patients undergoing magnetic resonance imaging (MRI) of the central nervous system.
Gralise	Gabapentin	Treatment of postherpetic neuralgia.
Horizant	Gabapentin enacarbil	Treatment of moderate-to-severe primary restless legs syndrome (RLS) in adults.
Incivek	Telaprevir	For treatment of certain adults with chronic hepatitis C infection.
Juvisync	Sitagliptin/Simvastatin	Sitagliptin: management of type 2 diabetes; Simvastatin: treatment of hyperlipidemia and secondary prevention of cardiovascular events.
Kapvay	Clonidine hydrochloride	Management of attention-deficit hyperactivity disorder (ADHD).

(Continued)

BRAND NAME	GENERIC NAME	INDICATION
Kombiglyze XR	Saxagliptin/Metformin HCl	Treatment of type 2 diabetes when treatment with both saxagliptin and metformin is appropriate.
Latuda	Lurasidone HCl	Treatment of schizophrenia.
LaViv	Azficel-T	Treatment to improve the appearance of moderate-to-severe nasolabial fold wrinkles.
Lazanda	Fentanyl	Management of breakthrough pain in opioid-tolerant patients already receiving therapy and who are tolerant to continuous opioid therapy for underlying persistent cancer pain.
Makena	Hydroxyprogesterone caproate	To reduce risk of preterm birth in women with a singleton pregnancy who have a history of singleton spontaneous preterm birth.
Natroba	Spinosad	Treatment of head lice infestation.
Nuedexta	Dextromethorphan HBr/Quinidine sulfate	Treatment of pseudobulbar affect (PBA).
Nulojix	Belatacept	Prevention of organ rejection in adult patients who have had a kidney transplant, in combination with other immunosuppressants.
Potiga	Ezogabine	Add-on medication to treat seizures associated with epilepsy in adults.
Safyral	Drospirenone/Ethinyl estradiol/ Levomefolate calcium tablets and Levomefolate calcium	Prevention of pregnancy and to raise folate levels in women who choose to use an OC.
Solesta		Fecal incontinence in patients who have failed conservative therapy (eg, diet, fiber therapy, antimotiltiy drugs).
Teflaro	Ceftaroline fosamil	Treatment of acute bacterial skin and skin-structure infections and community acquired bacterial pneumonia.
Tradjenta	Linagliptin	Treatment of type 2 diabetes.
Victrelis	Boceprevir	Management of chronic hepatitis C infection.
Viibryd	Vilazodone	Treatment of major depressive disorder (MDD).
Xalkori	Crizotinib	Treatment of late stage (locally advanced or metastatic), non–small cell lung cancers (NSCLC) who express the abnormal anaplastic lymphoma kinase (ALK) gene.
Xarelto	Rivaroxaban	To reduce the risk of blood clots, deep vein thrombosis (DVT), and pulmonary embolism (PE) following knee or hip replacement surgery.
Xerese	Acyclovir/Hydrocortisone	Treatment of recurrent herpes labialis to reduce the likelihood of ulcerative cold sores and to shorten the lesion healing time.
Yervoy	Ipilimumab	Treatment of metastatic melanoma.
Zelboraf	Vemuranfenib	Treatment of metastatic or unresected melanoma in patients whose tumors express a gene mutation called BRAF V600E.
Zytiga	Albiraterone acetate	For use in combination with prednisone to treat patients with metastatic, castration-resistant prostate cancer who have received prior docetaxel.

Note: This list is not comprehensive. For a complete listing, please refer to the FDA website at: www.fda.gov/Drugs.

OBESITY TREATMENT GUIDELINES

ADULTS

Overweight or obese patients are at an increased risk for developing cardiometabolic complications, including cardiovascular diseases, type 2 diabetes, dyslipidemia, hypertension, and conditions like osteoarthritis, obstructive sleep apnea, hepatobiliary disease, and some cancers.

ASSESSMENT:
A. Body mass index
- Body mass index (BMI) is integral in classifying a patient into an overweight or obese category.
- Calculate BMI: weight (kg)/height (m²). Overweight is defined as a BMI of 25-29.9 kg/m². Obesity is defined as an excess of total body fat that is documented by BMI ≥30 kg/m². [**See table.**]

B. Degree of abdominal fat
- Excess fat in the abdomen is an independent predictor of risk factors and morbidity.
- Waist circumference measurement can assess a patient's abdominal fat content before and during weight loss treatment. [**See table.**]
  – High risk = Men >102 cm (>40 in)
  – High risk = Women >88 cm (>35 in)
- High waist circumference is associated with an increased risk for type 2 diabetes, dyslipidemia, hypertension, and CVD in patients with BMI in a range of 25-34.9 kg/m².

C. Risk status
- Identify patients at very high *absolute* risk.
  – Establish coronary heart disease [CHD] (history of coronary artery surgery, angina pectoris [stable or unstable], coronary artery surgery, coronary artery procedures), presence of atherosclerotic diseases (peripheral arterial disease, abdominal aortic aneurysm, symptomatic carotid artery disease), type 2 diabetes, sleep apnea.
- Identify obesity-associated disease (require appropriate assessment and management).
  – Gynecological abnormalities, osteoarthritis, gallstones and their complications, stress incontinence.
- Identify cardiovascular risk factors that impart a high absolute risk.
  – Overweight patients require equal emphasis on weight loss therapy and control of cardiovascular risk factors.
  – Patients can be classified as being at high absolute risk for obesity-related disorders if they have three or more of the following risk factors:
    ○ Cigarette smoking; hypertension; high-risk low-density lipoprotein cholesterol (LDL >160 mg/dL); low high-density lipoprotein cholesterol (HDL <35 mg/dL); impaired fasting glucose; family history of premature CHD; age: male ≥45 years, female ≥55 years (postmenopausal); lack of physical activity; high triglycerides.

CLASSIFICATION OF OVERWEIGHT AND OBESITY BY BMI, WAIST CIRCUMFERENCE, AND ASSOCIATED DISEASE RISK*				
			DISEASE RISK* RELATIVE TO NORMAL WEIGHT AND WAIST CIRCUMFERENCE†	
	BMI (kg/m²)	Obesity Class	Men ≤102 cm (≤40 in) Women ≤88 cm (≤35 in)	Men >102 cm (>40 in) Women >88 cm (>35 in)
Underweight	<18.5			
Normal	18.5 - 24.9			
Overweight	25.0 - 29.9		Increased	High
Obesity	30.0 - 34.9	I	High	Very High
	35.0 - 39.9	II	Very High	Very High
Extreme Obesity	≥40	III	Extremely High	Extremely High

*Disease risk (relative risk, not absolute risk) for type 2 diabetes, hypertension, and CVD.

†Increased waist circumference can also be a marker for increased risk even in persons of normal weight.

Source: Adapted from Preventing and Managing the Global Epidemic of Obesity. Report of the World Health Organization Consultation of Obesity. WHO, Geneva, June 1997.

GOALS: *(Based on NHLBI guidelines unless otherwise indicated)*
A. Weight loss
- Initial goal of weight-loss therapy should be to reduce body weight by approximately 10% from baseline.
- Weight loss should be about 1 to 2 lbs/week (resulting from a calorie deficit of 500 to 1000 kcal/day) for a period of 6 months, with the subsequent strategy based on the amount of weight loss.
- Further weight loss considered after initial goal is achieved and maintained (1 year or longer).

More recent American College of Physicians recommendation: Weight loss should be based on the patient's individual risk factors and may include not only weight loss but other parameters like reducing blood pressure or fasting blood glucose. The goal is the reduction of abdominal fat content and amelioration of obesity-related health risks.

B. Maintain a lower body weight over the long term
- Maintenance program should be a priority after initial 6 months.
- Maintain a lower body weight over the long term; successful weight maintenance is defined as a weight regain of <3 kg (6.6 lb) in 2 years and a sustained reduction in waist circumference of at least 4 cm.
- Maintenance is enhanced with dietary therapy, physical activity, and behavioral therapy (continue this indefinitely). May also initiate drug therapy.

C. Prevent further weight gain

TREATMENT:
Each treatment plan should be tailored to the individual patient based on his or her psychobehavioral characteristics, past attempts at weight loss, financial considerations, age, degree of obesity, gender, and ability to exercise, individual health risks, or patient motivation.

Nonpharmacological
A. Dietary management
- All obese patients with BMI ≥30 kg/m^2 on lifestyle and behavioral modifications (diet, exercise); patient goals for weight loss individually determined.
- Low-calorie diets reduce body weight by an average of 8% and reduce abdominal fat content over a period of approximately 6 months.
- Reduced calorie intake:
  - Women: 1000 to 1200 kcal/day
  - Men: 1200 to 1500 kcal/day
- Total fat intake: ≤30% of total calories.

B. Physical activity
- Physical activity independently reduces CVD risk factors and improves cardiorespiratory fitness.
- Initiate activity slowly (eg, walking, swimming 30 to 45 minutes, 3 to 5 days per week).
- Long-term goal: Moderate-intensity physical activity ≥30 minutes most or all days per week.

C. Behavioral therapy
- Self-monitoring (eg, keeping food and activity logs), stimulus control (ie, controlling cues associated with eating), stress management, nutrition education, slower eating habits, physical activity, problem solving, rewarding changes in behavior, social support, relapse preventions.

D. Smoking cessation

Pharmacological
Weight loss drugs may be used only as part of a comprehensive weight loss program that includes diet and physical activity for patients with a BMI of ≥30 with no concomitant obesity-related risk factors or diseases, or for patients with a BMI of ≥27 with concomitant obesity-related risk factors or disease.

MEDICATIONS APPROVED FOR WEIGHT LOSS			
DRUG	**TREATMENT PERIOD**	**DOSE**	**SIDE EFFECTS**
Diethylpropion	Approved for short-term use (ie, 12 weeks in a 12-month period) Sympathomimetic amine; acts as a centrally acting appetite suppressant	**IM:** 25mg TID-QID, 1 hr before meals and mid-evening **CR:** 75mg QD	Withdrawal, arrhythmias, increased blood pressure, seizures, tremor, headache, GI complaints, bone marrow suppression
Phentermine		18.75-37.5mg before breakfast or 2 hours after breakfast or 18.75mg BID or 15-30mg 2 hours after breakfast	Withdrawal, arrhythmias, increased blood pressure, seizures, tremor, headache, GI complaints
Orlistat [Alli (OTC), Xenical]	Approved for long-term (>12 weeks) use for weight loss and weight maintenance Lipase inhibitor; acts peripherally to reduce absorption of dietary fat in the gut	**Alli:** 60mg up to TID with each fat-containing meal **Xenical:** 120mg TID with fat-containing meal	Gas, oily spotting, fecal incontinence, urgency or frequency, oily or fatty stool, abdominal or rectal pain, nausea, hepatitis, pancreatitis

Surgery
Bariatric surgery
- An option for weight reduction for patients with severe and resistant obesity.
- GI surgery or gastric bypass is an available option for motivated patients with a BMI ≥40 or ≥35 (who have comorbid conditions) and acceptable operative risks.
- Only recommended for those who have failed to lose weight after lifestyle modification failure of at least 6 to 12 months and who have failed exercise and diet (with or without drug therapy).
- Also recommended for those ≥65 years to improve quality of life.

CHILDREN

Intervention in overweight and obese children and adolescents can prevent obesity-related comorbidities (eg, glucose intolerance, type 2 diabetes, metabolic syndrome, dyslipidemia, and hypertension).

ASSESSMENT:
A. BMI
- Diagnosis of a patient is dependent on BMI as well as CDC growth charts, gender, age, risk factors, and ethnicity.
- Considered overweight if BMI of at least in the 85th percentile but less than the 95th percentile for age and sex.
- Considered obese if the BMI is at least in the 95th percentile for age and sex.
- Children with a BMI in at least the 85th percentile should be evaluated for comorbidities and complications.

B. Risk status
- Cardiovascular risk factors
  - Hypertriglyceridemia, high LDL, low HDL, hyperinsulinemia, and hypertension.
- Comorbidities
  - Glucose intolerance, type 2 diabetes, metabolic syndrome, dyslipidemia, and hypertension.

TREATMENT:

Nonpharmacological
A. Dietary management
- Avoid consumption of calorie-dense, nutrient-poor foods (eg, sweetened beverages, sports drinks, fruit drinks and juices, most fast-food and calorie-dense snacks).
- Portion control.
- Reduce saturated dietary fat intake for children older than 2 years of age.
- Increase intake of dietary fiber, fruits, and vegetables.
- Eat timely, regular meals.

B. Physical activity
- 60 minutes of daily moderate-to-vigorous physical activity.
- Sedentary activity (eg, watching television, playing video games, or using computers for recreation) should be limited to 1 to 2 hours per day.

C. Behavioral therapy
- Educate parents about the need for healthy rearing patterns related to diet and activity (eg, avoid overly strict dieting and using food as a reward or punishment, set limits of acceptable behaviors).

Pharmacological
In combination with lifestyle modification, pharmacotherapy can be considered in:
- Obese children only after failure of a formal program of intensive lifestyle modification.
- Overweight children only if severe comorbidities persist despite intensive lifestyle modification (strong family history of type 2 diabetes, or premature CV disease).

Pharmacotherapy should be provided only by clinicians who are experienced in the use of antiobesity agents and aware of the potential for adverse reactions.

Surgery
Bariatric Surgery
- Indicated for adolescents with a BMI >50 kg/m² or BMI >40kg/m² with severe comorbidities in whom lifestyle modifications and/or pharmacotherapy have failed.
- Must be psychologically stable and capable of adhering to lifestyle modifications.
- Not recommended for preadolescent children, pregnant or breastfeeding adolescents, or those who have not mastered principles of healthy eating and physical activity, are planning to become pregnant within 2 years of surgery, have an unresolved eating disorder, or who have an untreated psychiatric disorder or Prader-Willi syndrome.

(Continued)

REFERENCES:

1. Cannon C, Kumar A. Treatment of overweight and obesity: Lifestyle, pharmacologic, and surgical options. *Clin Cornerstone.* 2009;9(4):55-71.

2. Centers for Disease Control and Prevention (CDC). *Healthy weight—it's not a diet, it's a lifestyle!* Available at: http://www.cdc.gov/healthyweight/index.html. Accessed on February 15, 2012.

3. National Heart, Lung, and Blood Institute Obesity Education Initiative. *Clinical Guidelines on the Identification, Evaluation, and Treatment of Overweight and Obesity in Adults. The Evidence Report.* U.S. Department of Health and Human Services, Public Health Service, National Institutes of Health, National Heart, Lung and Blood Institute; 1998.

4. Alli [package insert]. Moon Township, PA: GlaxoSmithKline Consumer Healthcare LP; 2011.

5. Diethylpropion [package insert]. Corona, CA: Watson Laboratories, Inc.; 2007.

6. Phentermine [package insert]. Various manufacturers.

7. Xenical [package insert]. South San Francisco, CA: Genentech; 2012.

8. Snow V, Barry P, Fitterman N, et al. Pharmacologic and surgical management of obesity in primary care: A clinical practice guideline from the American College of Physicians. *Ann Intern Med.* 2005;142(7):525-531.

9. August GP, Caprio S, Fennoy I, et al. Prevention and treatment of pediatric obesity: An Endocrine Society clinical practice guideline based on expert opinion. *J Clin Endocrinol Metab.* 2008;93(12):4576-4599.

POISON ANTIDOTE CHART

Warning: While every effort has been made to ensure the accuracy of this chart, it is not intended to serve as the sole source of information on antidotes. Guidelines may need to be adjusted based on factors such as anticipated usage in the hospital's local area, the nearest alternate sources of antidotes, and distance to tertiary care institutions. Contact your nearest regional poison control center (1-800-222-1222) for treatment information regarding any exposure, including indications for use of antidote therapy. Directions in this chart assume that all basic life support and decontamination measures have been initiated as needed.

ANTIDOTE	POISON DRUG/TOXIN	SUGGESTED MINIMUM STOCK QUANTITY	RATIONALE/COMMENTS
N-Acetylcysteine [NAC] (Mucomyst, Acetadote)	Acetaminophen Carbon tetrachloride Other hepatotoxins	IV: 150 mL Acetadote PO: 8 x 30 mL of 20% NAC This would be enough to treat one 100-kg patient x 24 hours	Acetaminophen is the most common drug involved in intentional and unintentional poisonings. 600 mL (120 g) of the oral product provides enough to treat an adult for an entire 3-day course of therapy, or enough to treat 3 adults for 24 h. Several vials may be stocked in the ED to provide a loading dose and the remaining vials in the pharmacy for the q4h maintenance doses. 150 mL (30 g) of IV product will treat one 100-kg adult patient for an entire 21-hour IV protocol. Note: While controversial, IV NAC may be preferable in patients who have hepatic encephalopathy or are pregnant.
Amyl nitrite, sodium nitrite, and sodium thiosulfate (Cyanide antidote kit)	Acetonitrile Acrylonitrile Bromates (thiosulfate only) Chlorates (thiosulfate only) Cyanide (eg, HCN, KCN, and NaCN) Cyanogen chloride Cyanogen glycoside natural sources (eg, apricot pits and peach pits) Hydrogen sulfide (nitrites only) Laetrile Mustard agents (thiosulfate only) Nitroprusside (thiosulfate only) Smoke inhalation (combustion of synthetic materials)	1-2 kits Each kit contains: 12 x 30 mL amyl nitrite ampules 2 vials 3% sodium nitrite, 10 mL each 2 vials 25% sodium thio-sulfate, 50 mL each	Stock 1 kit in the ED. Consider also stocking 1 kit in the pharmacy. Note: This kit has a short shelf life of 24 months. Stocking this kit may be unnecessary if an adequate supply of hydroxocobalamin HCl is available. Significant adverse reactions include methemoglobinemia and hypotension. For smoke inhalation victims, thiosulfate, without the use of nitrites, may be considered.
Antivenin, *Crotalidae* Polyvalent (Equine Origin)	Pit viper envenomation (eg, rattlesnakes, cottonmouths, and copperheads)	None	As of March 31, 2007, this product is no longer available from the manufacturer. However, some supplies may still be available. See Antivenin, *Crotalidae* Polyvalent Immune Fab–Ovine in this chart.

This chart is adapted from material furnished by the Illinois Poison Center, a program of the Metropolitan Chicago Healthcare Council.

(Continued)

ANTIDOTE	POISON DRUG/TOXIN	SUGGESTED MINIMUM STOCK QUANTITY	RATIONALE/COMMENTS
Antivenin, *Crotalidae*, Polyvalent Fab–Ovine (CroFab)	Pit viper envenomation (eg, rattlesnakes, cottonmouths, and copperheads)	12-18 vials	Advised in geographic areas with endemic populations of copperhead, water moccasin, eastern massasauga, or timber rattlesnake. In low-risk areas, know nearest alternate source of antivenin. This product has a lower risk of hypersensitivity reaction than previously marketed equine product. Average dose in premarketing trials was 12 vials but more may be needed. 12 vials will cover 8 hours of treatment, while 18 vials will cover 24 hours of treatment. Stock in pharmacy. Store in refrigerator. Equine product is no longer available after March 31, 2007.
Antivenin, *Latrodectus mactans* (Black widow spider)	Black widow spider envenomation	0-1 vial	This product is only used for severe envenomations. Antivenin must be given in a critical care setting since it is an equine-derived product which may cause anaphylaxis. Stock in pharmacy. Product must be refrigerated at all times. Know the nearest source of antidote.
Atropine sulfate	Alpha$_2$ agonists (eg, clonidine, guanabenz, and guanfacine) Alzheimer drugs (eg, donezepil, galantamine, rivastigmine, tacrine) Antimyesthenic agents (eg, pyridostigmine) Bradyarrhythmia-producing agents (eg, beta-blockers, calcium channel blockers, and digitalis glycosides) Cholinergic agonists (eg, bethanechol) Muscarine-containing mushrooms (eg, *Clitocybe* and *Inocybe*) Nerve agents (eg, sarin, soman, tabun, and VX) Organophosphate and carbamate insecticides	175 mg or greater Available in various formulations: 0.4 mg/mL (1 mL, 0.4 mg ampules) 0.4 mg/mL (20 mL, 8 mg vials) 0.1 mg/mL (10 mL, 1 mg ampules) Atropine sulfate military-style auto-injectors: (Atropen): 2mg/0.7 mL, 1 mg/0.7 mL, 0.5 mg/0.7 mL, 0.25 mg/0.3 mL Atropine sulfate 2.1 mg/0.7 mL with Pralidoxime chloride 600 mg/2 mL (DuoDote)	The product should be immediately available in the ED. Some also may be stored in the pharmacy or other hospital sites, but should be easily mobilized if a severely poisoned patients needs treatment. Note: Product is necessary to be adequately prepared for WMD incidents; the suggested amount may not be sufficient for mass casualty events. Auto-injectors are available from Bound Tree Medical, Inc. Drug stocked in chempack containers is intended only for use in mass casualty events.
Botulinum antitoxin As of March 13, 2010, the only botulinum antitoxin available is HBAT (heptavalent types A-G). This product replaces bivalent antitoxins type AB and antitoxin type E. Baby Botulism Immune Globulin (BIG)	Food-borne botulism Wound botulism Botulism as a biological weapon Note: Heptavalent antitoxin is not currently recommended for infant botulism	None Product is stored at 9 CDC regional centers (including the Chicago Quarantine). To obtain antitoxin, hospitals must call the Illinois Department of Public Health which contacts the CDC in Atlanta. The CDC emergency operation center can be reached at 770-488-7100.	Antitoxin must be given in a critical care setting since it is an equine-derived product. Note: Product must be refrigerated at all times. Heptavalent antitoxin is stored in the CDC SNS. BabyBIG is available for infant botulism types A and B, through the Infant Botulism Treatment and Prevention Program, sponsored by the California Department of Public Health, telephone: 510-231-7600, http://www.infantbotulism.org/physician/obtain.php

ANTIDOTE	POISON DRUG/TOXIN	SUGGESTED MINIMUM STOCK QUANTITY	RATIONALE/COMMENTS
Calcium disodium EDTA (Versenate)	Lead Zinc salts (eg, zinc chloride)	2 x 5 mL amp (200 mg/mL)	One vial provides 1 day of therapy for a child. 2-4 g per 24 hours may be necessary in adult patients. Stock in pharmacy. Important note: Edetate disodium (Endrate) is not the same as calcium disodium EDTA, and is used primarily as an IV chelator for emergent treatment of hypercalcemia, etc.
Calcium chloride and Calcium gluconate	Calcium channel blockers Fluoride salts (eg, NaF) Hydrofluoric acid (HF) Hyperkalemia (not digoxin-induced) Hypermagnesemia	10% calcium chloride: 10 x 10 mL vials 10% calcium gluconate: 30 x 10 mL vials	Many ampules of calcium chloride may be necessary in life-threatening calcium channel blocker or HF poisoning. Stock in ED. More may be stocked in pharmacy. The chloride salt provides 3 x more calcium than the gluconate salt. Calcium chloride is very irritating and administration through a central line is preferable. Topical calcium gluconate or carbonate gels may be extemporaneously prepared by the pharmacy. Calgonate (calcium gluconate 2.5% gel) is not FDA-approved but is manufactured in an FDA-GMP approved facility and is distributed by Calgonate Corp in Port St. Lucie, Florida.
Deferoxamine mesylate (Desferal)	Iron	12-36 g (Available in 500 mg and 2 g vials)	Quantity recommended supplies 8-24 hours of therapy for a 100-kg adult. Per package insert, the maximum daily dose is 6g (12 vials). However, this dose may be exceeded in serious acute iron poisonings. Stock in pharmacy.
Digoxin immune Fab (Digibind, DigiFab)	Cardiac glycoside-containing plants (eg, foxglove and oleander) Digitoxin Digoxin	15 vials Each vial (38 mg) neutralizes 0.5 mg of digoxin	An initial dose of 2-3 vials for chronic poisoning or 10 vials for acute poisoning may be given to a digoxin-poisoned patient in whom the digoxin level is unknown. More may be necessary in severe intoxications. 15 vials would effectively neutralize a steady-state digoxin level of 15 ng/mL in a 100-kg patients. Know nearest source of additional supply. Stock in ED or pharmacy.
Dimercaprol (BAL in oil)	Arsenic Copper Gold Lead Lewisite Mercury	2 x 3 mL ampules (100 mg/mL)	This amount provides 2 doses of 3-5 mg/kg/dose given q4h to treat 1 seriously poisoned adult or provides enough to treat a 15-kg child for 24 h. Stock in pharmacy.
DMPS (2,3-dimercaptopro-panol-sulfonic acid, Dimaval, Unithiol)	Arsenic Bismuth Lead Mercury	None (Available as 50 mg/mL vials from McGuff Pharmacy)	DMPS is a water-soluble analog of BAL. Unlike BAL, it does not have a potential risk of redistributing metals to the CNS. Also has a more favorable side effect profile, though further study is needed to fully elucidate advantages/disadvantages compared to other chelators.

(Continued)

A353

ANTIDOTE	POISON DRUG/TOXIN	SUGGESTED MINIMUM STOCK QUANTITY	RATIONALE/COMMENTS
Ethanol	Ethylene glycol Methanol	Consider stocking 180-360 g in the form of 95% ethanol or equivalents. 10% alcohol in D5W was discontinued in 2004; 5% alcohol in D5W was discontinued in 2007. However, 10% alcohol can be prepared from dehydrated alcohol and D5W. Consult PCC.	180 g provides loading and maintenance doses for a 100-kg adult for 8-24 h. More alcohol or fomepizole will be needed during dialysis or prolonged treatment. 95% or 40% alcohol diluted in juice may be given PO if IV alcohol is unavailable. Stock in pharmacy. Note: Ethanol is unnecessary if adequate amounts of fomepizole are stocked. See also fomepizole in this chart. May cause hypotension or metabolic abnormalities (eg, hypoglycemia) esp. in pediatric patients.
Fat emulsion (Intralipid, Liposyn II, Liposyn III)	Local anesthetics and possibly other cardiac toxins (eg, bupropion, calcium channel blockers, cocaine, beta blockers, tricyclic antidepressants)	Quantity determined by institution. Available in 100 mL of 20% emulsion.	Fat emulsion is an experimental therapy showing promise in the reverse of cardiac toxicity induced by local anesthetics and other cardiac toxins. The evidence for the efficacy of fat emulsion therapy is solely based on animal studies and human case reports, and its safety has not yet been established. Consultation with a regional PCC toxicologist is advised. Initial dose: 1.5 mL/kg IV over 1 min. Follow with infusion of 0.25 mL/kg/min over 30 min. Loading dose may be repeated once. Rate may be increased to 0.5 mL/kg/min for 60 min if blood pressure drops. Maximum total dose is 8 mL/kg. Consider storage in pharmacy, ED, and possibly surgical units.
Flumazenil (Romazicon)	Benzodiazepines Zaleplon Zolpidem	Total 6-12 mg Available in 5 and 10 mL vials (0.1 mg/mL)	Due to risk of seizures, use with extreme caution, if at all, in poisoned patients. More may be stocked in the pharmacy for use in reversal of conscious sedation. Stock in ED, pharmacy, and any unit where procedural sedation is performed.
Folic acid and Folinic acid (Leucovorin)	Formaldehyde/Formic acid Methanol Methotrexate, Trimetrexate Pyrimethamine Trimethoprim	Folic acid: 3 x 50 mg vials Folinic acid: 1 x 50 mg vial	For adjunctive treatment of methanol-poisoned patients with an acidosis, give 50 mg folinic acid initially, then 50 mg of folic acid q4h for 6 doses. For methotrexate-poisoned patients, administer folinic acid only. Stock in pharmacy.
Fomepizole (Antizol) 4-methylpyrazole (4-MP)	Ethylene glycol Methanol	1 to 2 x 1.5 g vials Note: Available in a kit of 4 x 1.5 g vials	One 1.5 g vial provides an initial dose of 15 mg/kg/12 h to an adult weighing up to 100 kg. Hospitals with critical care and hemodialysis capabilities should consider stocking 1 kit of 4 vials or more. More frequent dosing (ie, q4h) is required if the patient is dialyzed. Note: Product has a 2-year shelf life; however, the manufacturer offers a credit for unused, expired product. Ethanol is unnecessary if adequate supply of fomepizole is stocked. Fomepizole is preferred to ethanol because of ease of use, fewer adverse effects, simplicity of dosing, less need for close monitoring. Stock in pharmacy. Know where nearest alternate supply is located.

ANTIDOTE	POISON DRUG/TOXIN	SUGGESTED MINIMUM STOCK QUANTITY	RATIONALE/COMMENTS
Glucagon HCl	Beta blockers Calcium channel blockers Hypoglycemia Hypoglycemic agents	50 to 90 x 1 mg vials	This quantity provides 4-8 hours of maximum dosing, ie, a 10 mg IV bolus dose followed by 10 mg/h. More may be necessary. Know where the nearest alternate supply is located. Stock 30 mg in ED and remainder in pharmacy.
Hydroxocobalamin HCl (Cyanokit)	Acetonitrile Acrylonitrile Cyanide (eg, HCN, KCN, and NaCN) Cyanogen chloride Cyanogenic glycoside natural sources (eg, apricot pits and peach pits) Laetrile Nitroprusside Smoke inhalation (combustion of synthetic materials)	2-4 kits Each kit contains 2 x 2.5 g vials Note: Diluent is not included in the kit.	Seriously poisoned cyanide patients may require 5-10 g (1 or 2 kits). Stock 2 kits in ED. Consider also stocking 2 kits in the pharmacy. The product has a shelf-life of 30 months post-manufacture.
Hyperbaric oxygen (HBO)	Carbon monoxide and possibly the following: Carbon tetrachloride Cyanide Hydrogen sulfide Methemoglobinemia	Post the location and phone number of nearest HBO chamber in the ED.	Consult PPC to determine if HBO treatment is indicated.
Insulin and dextrose	Calcium channel blockers (diltiazem, nifedipine, verapamil) and possibly beta blockers	Quantity determined by institution. Humulin R is available as 100 units/mL in a 1.5 mL cartridge and a 10 mL bottle. Dextrose 50% in water is available in 50 mL ampules and syringes. Dextrose 25% is available in 10 mL vials and syringes for pediatric use.	High dose insulin and dextrose therapy has reversed cardiovascular toxicity associated with calcium channel blocker overdose. Begin with 10 units to 1 unit/kg regular insulin IV bolus (with 1 amp D50), then start a drip at 0.5 units/kg/h (consider addition of D10 drip with insulin drip) and titrate upward until hypotension improves. Stock in ED and pharmacy.
Methylene blue	Methemoglobin-inducing agents including: Aniline dyes Dapsone Dinitrophenol Local anesthetics (eg, benzocaine) Metoclopramide Monomethylhydrazine-containing mushrooms (eg, Gyromitra) Naphthalene Nitrates and nitrites Nitrobenzene Phenazopyridine	6 x 10 mL ampules (10 mg/mL)	The usual dose is 1-2 mg/kg IV (0.1-0.2 mL/kg). A second dose may be given in 1 hour. More may be necessary. 6 ampules provides 3 doses of 2 mg/kg for a 100-kg adult. Stock in pharmacy.

(Continued)

ANTIDOTE	POISON DRUG/TOXIN	SUGGESTED MINIMUM STOCK QUANTITY	RATIONALE/COMMENTS
Naloxone (Narcan)	Alpha$_2$ agonists (eg, clonidine, guanabenz, and guanfacine) Unknown poisoning with mental status depression Opioids (eg, codeine, diphenoxylate, fentanyl, heroin, meperidine, morphine, and propoxyphene)	Naloxone: total 40 mg, any combination of 0.4 mg, 1 mg, and 2 mg ampules	Stock 20 mg naloxone in the ED and 20 mg elsewhere in the institution. Note: Nalmefene (Revex), a longer-acting opioid antagonist, was discontinued by the manufacturer in July 2008.
Octreotide acetate (Sandostatin)	Sulfonylurea hypoglycemic agents (eg, glipizide, glyburide)	225 mcg Available in 1 mL ampules (0.05 mg/mL, 0.1 mg/mL, and 0.5 mg/mL) and 5 mL multidose vials (0.2 and 1 mg/mL)	Octreotide acetate blocks the release of insulin from pancreatic beta cells that along with IV dextrose can reverse sulfonylurea-induced hypoglycemia. The usual adult dose is 50-100 mcg IV or SC q6-12h. The usual pediatric dose is 1-1.5 mcg/kg IV or SC q6-12h. 225 mcg provides 4 x 75 mcg adult doses. Stock in pharmacy.
D-Penicillamine (Cuprimine)	Arsenic Copper Lead Mercury	None required as an antidote Available in bottles of 100 capsules (125 mg or 250 mg/capsule)	D-Penicillamine is no longer considered the drug of choice for heavy metal poisonings. It may be stocked in the pharmacy for other indications such as Wilson's disease or rheumatoid arthritis.
Physostigmine salicylate (Antilirium)	Anticholinergic alkaloid-containing plants (eg, deadly nightshade and jimson weed) Antihistamines Atropine and other anticholinergic agents	2 x 2 mL ampules (1 mg/mL)	Usual adult dose is 1-2 mg slow IV push. Note: Duration of effect is 30-60 min. Stock in ED or pharmacy.
Phytonadione (Vitamin K1) (AquaME-PHYTON, Mephyton)	Indandione derivatives Long-acting anticoagulant rodenticides (eg, brodifacoum and bromadiolone) Warfarin	100 mg injectable; 100 mg oral Available as: 0.5 mL ampules (2 mg/mL) and 1 mL ampules (10 mg/mL) 5 mg tablets in packages of 10, 12, and 100	Patients who are poisoned by long-acting anticoagulant rodenticides may require 50-100 mg/day or more for weeks to months to maintain normal INRs. An oral suspension for pediatric patients may be extemporaneously prepared by the pharmacy. Stock in pharmacy.
Pralidoxime chloride (2-PAM) (Protopam)	Organophosphate insecticides (OPI) Nerve agents (eg, sarin, soman, tabun, and VX) And possibly: Antimyesthenic agents (eg, pyridostigmine) Tacrine	18 x 1 g vials Also available as: Pralidoxime chloride military-style auto-injectors: 600 mg/2 mL Atropine sulfate 2.1 mg/0.7 mL with Pralidoxime chloride 600 mg/2 mL (DuoDote)	18 g provides an adult dose of 750 mg/h for 24 h. More may be needed in severe poisoning. Healthcare facilities located in agricultural areas where OPIs are used should maintain adequate supplies. Product is necessary to be adequately prepared for WMD incidents; the suggested amount may not be sufficient for mass casualty events. Auto-injectors are available from Bound Tree Medical, Inc. The drug stocked in chempack containers is intended for use in mass casualty events only. Stock in ED or pharmacy.
Protamine sulfate	Heparin Low molecular weight heparins (eg, enoxaparin, dalteparin, tinzaparin)	Variable, consider recommendation of hospital P&T Committee Available as 5 mL ampules (10 mg/mL) and 25 mL vials (250 mg/25 mL)	The usual dose is 1-1.5 mg for each 100 units of heparin. Stock in pharmacy in refrigerator. Preservative-free formulation does not require refrigeration.

ANTIDOTE	POISON DRUG/TOXIN	SUGGESTED MINIMUM STOCK QUANTITY	RATIONALE/COMMENTS
Pyridoxine hydrochloride (Vitamin B$_6$)	Acrylamide Ethylene glycol Hydrazine Hydrazine MAOIs (isocarboxazid, phenelzine) Isoniazid (INH) Monomethylhydrazine-containing mushrooms (eg, Gyromitra)	10 g (100 vials) Available as 1 mL vials (100 mg/mL)	Usual dose is 1 g of pyridoxine HCl for each g of INH ingested. If amount ingested is unknown, give 5 g of pyridoxine. Repeat 5 g dose if seizures are uncontrolled. More may be necessary. Know nearest source of additional supply. For ethylene glycol, a dose of 100 mg/day may enhance the clearance of toxic metabolite. Stock in ED or pharmacy.
Silibinin (Legalon-SIL)	Cyclopeptide-containing mushrooms (eg, *Amanita phalloides, Amanita verna, Amanita virosa, Galerina autumnalis, Lepiota josserabdi*, and others)	None 350 mg/vial	Silibinin is a water-soluble preparation of silymarin, a flavolignone extracted from the milk thistle plant. It inhibits uptake of cyclopeptides in hepatocytes. These hepatotoxins are responsible for high morbidity and mortality following ingestion of these mushrooms. Silibinin is manufactured by Madaus, Inc. in Germany, and has been widely used in Europe since 1984. The initial adult loading dose consists of a 1 h infusion of 5 mg/kg via continuous IV infusion. Product is now available in the U.S. under an open-treatment IND. Physicians can obtain the product free-of-charge by contacting the primary investigator at 866-520-4412.
Sodium bicarbonate	Chlorine gas Hyperkalemia (not digoxin-induced) Serum alkalinization: Agents producing a quinidine-like effect as noted by widened QRS complex on EKG (eg, amantadine, carbamazepine, chloroquine, cocaine, diphenhydramine, flecainide, propafenone, propoxyphene, tricyclic antidepressants, quinidine and related agents) Urine alkalinization: Weakly acidic agents (eg, chlorophenoxy herbicides, chlorpropamide, methotrexate, phenobarbital, and salicylates)	20 to 25 x 50 mL vials of either 84% (50 mEq/50 mL) or 7.5% (44 mEq/50 mL). Consider stocking 4.2% (5 mEq/10 mL) for pediatric patients.	Stock 20 vials in ED and remainder in pharmacy. Nebulized 2.5-5% sodium bicarbonate has been demonstrated in anecdotal case reports to provide symptomatic relief for chlorine gas inhalation.

(Continued)

ANTIDOTE	POISON DRUG/TOXIN	SUGGESTED MINIMUM STOCK QUANTITY	RATIONALE/COMMENTS
Succimer (Chemet) Dimercaptosuccinic acid (DMSA)	Arsenic Lead Lewisite Mercury	0-10 capsules Available in bottles of 100 capsules (100 mg/capsule)	Initial treatment of severely symptomatic heavy metal poisoning consists of parenterally administered chelators (eg, BAL, Ca, Na$_2$EDTA). Patients who markedly improve may eventually be started on oral DMSA. Asymptomatic or minimally symptomatic patients do not require parenteral therapy and are often treated as outpatients with an oral chelator. FDA approved only for pediatric lead poisoning, however it has shown efficacy for other heavy metal poisonings. 10 capsules represent an initial dose of 10 mg/kg in a 100-kg adult. Stock in pharmacy.

ADJUNCTIVE AGENTS

ADJUNCTIVE AGENT	POISON/DRUG/TOXIN	SUGGESTED MINIMUM STOCK QUANTITY	RATIONALE/COMMENTS
Benztropine mesylate (Cogentin)	Medications causing a dystonic reaction or other EPS	Quantity determined by institution. Available in tablets of 0.5 mg, 1 mg, 2 mg (bottles of 100 or 1000) and in 2 mg/mL injectable ampules.	Maximum daily adult dose is 6 mg/d. Stock some in ED and some in pharmacy. See diphenhydramine also.
Bromocriptine mesylate (Parlodel)	Medications causing NMS	Quantity determined by institution. Available in 2.5 mg tablets or 5 mg capsules (bottles of 30 or 100).	Dose for NMS is 2.5-10 mg every 6-8 hours. Bromocriptine is a centrally acting dopamine agonist that reverses excessive dopamine blockade. Use with caution as this may worsen serotonin syndrome. Stock in pharmacy.
Centruroides Immune F(ab)$_2$ - Equine (Anascorp)	Scorpion envenomation by *Centruroides sculpturatus*, the most venomous scorpion in the U.S. Note: It is found in southeastern California, Arizona, Nevada, southern Utah, and southwestern New Mexico.	None	This product is manufactured in Mexico by the Instituto Bioclon. In the U.S., it is marketed by Rare Disease Therapeutics, Inc. in Nashville, Tennessee. It is not FDA-approved; however, it is available as an investigational new drug. Currently, the product is distributed to zoos and venom banks only. Usual dose: 1-3 vials.
L-Carnitine (Carnitor)	Valproic acid	Quantity determined by institution. Available as 330 mg and 500 mg tablets, 250 mg and 300 mg capsules, 200 mg/mL IV solution, and 100 mg/mL PO solution.	L-Carnitine may be considered in valproate intoxication associated with elevated serum ammonia levels and/or hepatotoxicity. Doses of 100 mg/kg/d up to 2 g a day PO divided into 3 doses, or 150-500 mg/kg/d IVS (maximum 3 g daily) in 3 or 4 divided doses are recommended for a period of 3-4 days or until clinical improvement. Stock in pharmacy.
Cyproheptadine HCL (Periactin)	Medications causing serotonin syndrome	Quantity determined by institution. Available in 4 mg tablets (bottles of 100, 250, 500, and 1000) and 2 mg/5 mL PO solution.	Cyproheptadine HCl is a nonspecific 5-HT antagonist that has been used in the treatment of serotonin syndrome. Adult dose is 4-8 mg PO repeated every 1-4 h until therapeutic effect is observed or maximum of 32 mg administered. Stock in pharmacy.

ADJUNCTIVE AGENT	POISON/DRUG/TOXIN	SUGGESTED MINIMUM STOCK QUANTITY	RATIONALE/COMMENTS
Dantrolene sodium (Dantrium)	Medications causing NMS Medications causing malignant hyperthermia	Quantity determined by institution. Available in 25, 50, and 100 mg capsules (bottles of 100 or 500) and injectable 20 mg/vial form.	The recommended dose for NMS is 1 mg/kg IV; may repeat as needed every 5-10 min for a maximum of 10 mg/kg. Dantrolene sodium inhibits calcium release from the sarcoplasmic reticulum of skeletal muscle and thereby reduces rigidity. Stock in pharmacy. Any hospital using inhalational anesthetics should strongly consider stocking dantrolene for treatment of malignant hyperthermia.
Diazepam (Valium)	Chloroquine and related antimalarial drugs NMS Serotonin syndrome Severe agitation from any toxic exposure/overdose (eg, cocaine, PCP, methamphetamine)	Quantity determined by institution. Available as 5 mg/mL injectables in 2 mL ampules, 2 mL disposable syringes, and 10 mL multidose vials. Diazepam military-style auto-injectors for nerve agent-induced seizures: 10 mg/2 mL.	Diazepam is used in conjunction with epinephrine for patients with chloroquine toxicity (seizures, dysrhythmias, hypotension) or if the amount ingested is more than 5 g. Intravenous loading dose of 2 mg/kg over 30 min. Maintenance dose of 1-2 mg/kg/day for 2-4 days. Diazepam and other benzodiazepines are also used in poisoned and nonpoisoned patients as an anticonvulsant, muscle relaxant, and antianxiety agent. They are usually the first-line therapy for drug-induced agitation, tachycardia, and hypertension. Benzodiazepines are a mainstay in the treatment of NMS and serotonin syndrome. Stock in ED and pharmacy. Adequate supply is necessary to be prepared for WMD incidents. Auto-injectors are available from Bound Tree Medical, Inc.
Diphenhydramine HCl (Benadryl)	Medications causing a dystonic reaction or other EPS	Quantity determined by institution. Available in 25 and 50 mg capsules (bottles of 30, 100, or 1000). Also in oral liquid formulation of 12.5 mg/5 mL (4 ounce bottle) and 50 mg/mL injectable syringes.	In addition to its use as an anticholinergic agent, diphenhydramine is a widely used antihistamine in the management of minor or severe allergic reactions. Stock in ED and pharmacy.
Glycopyrrolate bromide (Robinul)	OPIs Nerve agents	Quantity determined by institution. Available as 0.2 mg/mL in vials of 1 mL, 2 mL, 5 mL, and 20 mL.	The dose of glycopyrrolate for OPI poisoning is 0.01-0.02 mg/kg IV. Glycopyrrolate is a quaternary ammonium antimuscarinic agent which may assist in the control of hypersecretions caused by acetylcholinesterase inhibition. This agent produces less tachycardia and CNS effects than atropine. Stock in ED and pharmacy.
Phentolamine mesylate (Regitine)	Catecholamine extravasation Intradigital epinephrine injection	Quantity determined by institution. Available as a 5 mg/vial powder with 1 mL diluent.	Phentolamine is an alpha adrenergic antagonist which will reverse vasoconstriction and peripheral ischemia associated with extravasation of adrenergic agents. When phentolamine is not available, consider using subcutaneous terbutaline sulfate (Brethine). Phentolamine also offers an additional option in the management of drug-induced hypertension. Stock in ED and pharmacy.

(Continued)

ADJUNCTIVE AGENT	POISON/DRUG/TOXIN	SUGGESTED MINIMUM STOCK QUANTITY	RATIONALE/COMMENTS
Sodium nitrite	Hydrogen sulfide (H_2S)	0-1 vial Available as 3% sodium nitrite in 10 mL vial	Nitrite therapy for H_2S poisoning is controversial. Seriously poisoned patients should receive nitrites within 1 hour of exposure. Sodium thiosulfate is not administered in H_2S poisoning. The product is available from Hope Pharmaceuticals in Scottsdale, Arizona. If the amyl nitrite/sodium nitrite/sodium thiosulfate CN antidote kits are stocked, additional sodium nitrite vials may not be necessary. Stock in pharmacy.
Sodium thiosulfate	Bromates (thiosulfate only) Chlorates (thiosulfate only) Mustard agents Nitroprusside Smoke inhalation	Quantity determined by institution Available in 100 mg/mL, 10 mL vials and 250 mg/mL, 50 mL vials	Sodium thiosulfate (without nitrites) has been advocated in the treatment of smoke inhalation related to CN exposure; however, it would not be necessary if hydroxocobalamin is available. Sodium thiosulfate may be used in conjunction with cisplatin to reduce toxicity of this chemotherapy agent. Sodium thiosulfate is found in the amyl nitrite/sodium nitrite/sodium thiosulfate CN antidote kits; however, additional vials may be stocked. Stock in pharmacy.
Thiamine	Ethanol Ethylene glycol	Quantity determined by institution Available as 100 mg/mL in 2 mL vials	Parenteral thiamine precedes IV dextrose in patients with chronic ethanol abuse. Thiamine 100 mg every 6 hours enhances clearance of toxic metabolites of ethylene glycol. Stock in ED and pharmacy.
AGENTS FOR RADIOLOGICAL EXPOSURES			
Calcium-diethylene-triamine pentaacetic acid (Ca-DTPA; Pentetate calcium trisodium injection) Zinc-diethylene-triamine pentaacetic acid (Zn-DTPA; Pentetate zinc trisodium injection)	Internal contamination with transuranium elements: americium, curium, plutonium	Quantity determined by institution Supplied as 200 mg/mL, 5 mL ampules for IV or inhalation administration. The product is sponsored through Hameln Pharmaceuticals, GmbH, of Hameln, Germany. Distributed in the United States by Akorn, Inc.	1 ampule provides the usual adult dose of 1 g q24h. More would be necessary in a mass casualty event. Ca-DTPA and Zn-DTPA are available through the SNS and REAC/TS, Oak Ridge, Tennessee, at 865-576-3131 (business hours) or 865-576-1005 (after hours).
Potassium iodide, KI tablets (Iostat, Thyrosafe) KI liquid (Thyroshield, SSKI)	Prevents thyroid uptake of radioactive iodine (I-131).	Quantity determined by institution Available in 130 mg and 65 mg tablets, and PO solutions: 65 mg/mL (30 mL bottle) and 1 g/mL (30 mL and 240 mL bottle)	One 130 mg tablet represents the initial daily adult dose. More would be necessary in a mass casualty event. KI tablets and oral solution are non-prescription. The Illinois Department of Nuclear Safety makes KI tablets available to healthcare facilities and the general public located near nuclear reactors.

ADJUNCTIVE AGENT	POISON/DRUG/TOXIN	SUGGESTED MINIMUM STOCK QUANTITY	RATIONALE/COMMENTS
Prussian blue, ferric hexacyanoferrate (Radiogardase)	Radioactive cesium (Cs-137), radioactive thallium (TI-201), and non-radioactive thallium.	None recommended at the present time Available in bottles of 30 capsules (500 mg/capsule)	The usual oral adult dose is 3 g, 3 times a day. The product is manufactured by Haupt Pharma Berlin GmbH for distribution by HEYL Chemisch-pharmazeutische Fabrik GmbH & Co. KG, Berlin, Germany, and is available in the U.S. from Heyltex Corporation. Prussian Blue is also available through the SNS and REAC/TS, Oak Ridge, Tennessee, at 865-576-3131 (business hours) or 865-576-1005 (after hours).

Abbreviations: BAL = British anti-Lewisite; CDC = Centers for Disease Control and Prevention; CN = cyanide; ED = emergency department; EDTA = ethylenediaminetetraacetic acid; EPS = extrapyramidal symptom; FDA = Food and Drug Administration; HCl = hydrochloride; IV = intravenous; MAOI = monoamine oxidase inhibitor; NMS = neuroleptic malignant syndrome; OPI = organophosphate insecticide; P&T = pharmacy and therapeutics; PCC = poison control center; PO = oral; REAC/TS = radiation emergency assistance center/training site; SNS = Strategic National Stockpile; WMD = weapons of mass destruction

APPROVED RISK EVALUATION/MITIGATION STRATEGIES (REMS)

The Food and Drug Administration Amendments Act of 2007 gave FDA the authority to require a Risk Evaluation and Mitigation Strategy (REMS) from manufacturers to ensure that the benefits of a drug or biological product outweigh its risks. The table below provides a list of products for which current REMS have been approved by FDA, as of publication.

DRUG NAME (generic name)	DRUG NAME (generic name)
Abstral (fentanyl)	Forteo (teriparatide [rDNA origin])
Actemra (tocilizumab)	Fortesta (testosterone)
Actiq (fentanyl citrate)	Gilenya (fingolimod)
Actoplus Met (pioglitazone hydrochloride/metformin hydrochloride)	H.P. Acthar Gel (repository corticotropin)
Actoplus Met XR (pioglitazone/metformin)	Isotretinoin Capsules
Actos (pioglitazone hydrochloride)	Kalbitor (ecallentide)
Advair Diskus (fluticasone propionate/salmeterol xinafoate inhalation powder)	Krystexxa (pegloticase)
	Lazanda (fentanyl)
Advair HFA (fluticasone propionate/salmeterol xinafoate inhalation powder)	Letairis (ambrisentan)
	Levaquin (levofloxacin)
Ampyra (dalfampridine)	Lotronex (alosetron hydrochloride)
Androgel (testosterone) Gel	Lumizyme (alglucosidase alfa)
Androgel (testosterone) 1.62% Gel	Meridia (subutramine hydrochloride)
Aranesp (darbepoetin alfa)	Metoclopramide Oral Solution
Arcapta Neohaler (indacaterol maleate)	Mifeprex (mifepristone)
Avandamet (rosiglitazone maleate/metformin hydrochloride)	Multaq (dronedarone)
	Myobloc (rimabotulinumtoxinB)
Avandaryl (rosiglitazone maleate/glimepiride)	Nplate (romiplostim)
Avandia (rosiglitazone maleate)	Nucynta ER (tapentadol)
Axiron (testosterone)	Nulojix (belatacept)
Botox/Botox Cosmetic (onabotulinumtoxinA)	Onsolis (fentanyl buccal soluble film)
Brilinta (ticagrelor)	Opana ER (oxymorphone hydrochloride)
Brovana (arformoterol tartrate)	Oxycodone Hydrochloride Oral Solution
Butrans (buprenorphine)	Oxycontin (oxycodone hydrochloride)
Bydureon (exenatide)	PegIntron Rebetol Combopack (Peginterferon alfa-2b, Redipen Single-dose Delivery System, and Rebetol Ribavirin)
Caprelsa (vandetanib)	
Chantix (varenicline)	Perforomist (formoterol fumarate)
Darvon Capsules, Darvon-N Tablets, and Darvocet-N (propoxyphene)	Potiga (ezogabine)
	Prolia (denosumab)
Duetact (pioglitazone hydrochloride/glimepiride)	Promacta (eltrombopag)
Dulera (mometasone furoate/formoterol fumarate)	Qualaquin (quinine sulfate)
Dysport (abobotulinumtoxinA)	Revlimid (lenalidomide)
Effient (prasugrel)	Sabril (vigabatrin)
Embeda (morphine sulfate/naltrexone hydrochloride)	Samsca (tolvaptan)
Entereg (alvimopan)	Serevent Diskus (salmeterol xinafoate)
Epogen/Procrit (epoetin alfa)	Soliris (eculizumab)
Exalgo (hydromorphone hydrochloride)	Stelara (ustekinumab)
Extraneal (icodextrin)	Suboxone (buprenorphine/naloxone) Sublingual Film
Fentanyl Citrate Transmucosal Lozenge	Suboxone (buprenorphine/naloxone) Sublingual Tablets
Fentora (fentanyl citrate)	Subsys (fentanyl)
Foradil (formoterol fumarate)	Subutex (buprenorphine)

Approved Risk Evaluation/Mitigation Strategies (REMS)

Symbicort (budesonide/formoterol)

Tapentadol Tablets

Tasigna (nilotinib)

Testim (testosterone)

Thalomid (thalidomide)

Tikosyn (dofetilide)

Tracleer (bosentan)

Trileptal (oxcarbazepine)

Tysabri (natalizumab)

Vandetanib (vandetanib)

Venlafaxine hydrochloride

Vibativ (telavancin)

Victoza (liraglutide)

Vivitrol (naltrexone)

Wellbutrin, Wellbutrin SR (bupropion hydrochloride)

Wellbutrin XL (bupropion hydrochloride)

Xenazine (tetrabenazine)

Xeomin (incobotulinumtoxinA)

Xiaflex (collagenase clostridium histolyticum)

Yervoy (ipilimumab)

Zortress (everolimus)

Zyban (bupropion hydrochloride)

Zyprexa Relprevv (olanzapine)

SCREENING AND DIAGNOSIS OF GESTATIONAL DIABETES MELLITUS

TIMELINE*	SCREENING	DIAGNOSTIC CRITERIA	DIAGNOSIS
1st prenatal visit	Screen for undiagnosed type 2 diabetes mellitus in those with risk factors	Following 75g 2-hr OGTT, one or more of the following blood glucose levels must be found: • A1C ≥6.5% • FPG ≥126 mg/dL OR 2-hr PG ≥200 mg/dL during an OGTT • Random PG ≥200 mg/dL[†]	Women with a positive diagnosis of diabetes, receive a diagnosis of overt, not gestational, diabetes
24 to 28 weeks' gestation	Screen all women not previously known to have diabetes at 24 to 28 weeks	Diagnosis of GDM is made when any of the following PG values are exceeded[‡]: • Fasting ≥92 mg/dL • 1 h ≥180 mg/dL • 2 h ≥153 mg/dL	Women who test positive for GDM will need to screen for persistent diabetes at 6-12 weeks' postpartum
HISTORY OF GESTATIONAL DIABETES MELLITUS			
6 to 12 weeks' postpartum	Any history of GDM warrants lifelong screening for development of diabetes or prediabetes at least every 3 years	Use of A1C is not recommended for diagnosis of persistent diabetes at postpartum visits	Women with a history of GDM and who develop prediabetes, should be offered lifestyle interventions or metformin

Abbreviations: FPG, fasting plasma glucose; GDM, gestational diabetes mellitus; OGTT, oral glucose tolerance test; PG, plasma glucose.

*According to the American Diabetes Association guidelines, pregnant women are to be screened for type 2 diabetes at their first prenatal visit and screened for GDM 24-28 weeks into pregnancy.

[†]In the absence of hyperglycemia, results should be confirmed by repeat testing.

[‡]Perform 75g OGTT, with plasma glucose measurement fasting and at 1 and 2 hours, at 24 to 28 weeks' gestation in women not previously diagnosed with overt diabetes. This OGTT should be performed in the morning after an overnight fast of at least 8 hours.

CRITERIA FOR TESTING FOR DIABETES IN ALL ASYMPTOMATIC ADULT INDIVIDUALS

Testing should be considered in all adults of any age who are overweight (BMI ≥25 kg/m^2) or obese and who have one or more additional risk factors:

• Physical inactivity

• First-degree relative with diabetes

• High-risk race/ethnicity (eg, African Americans, Latino, Native American, Asian American, Pacific Islander)

• Women who delivered a baby weighing >9 lbs or who were diagnosed with GDM

• Hypertension (blood pressure ≥140/90 mmHg or on therapy for hypertension)

• HDL cholesterol level <35 mg/dL and/or a triglyceride level >250 mg/dL

• Women with polycystic ovary syndrome

• A1C ≥5.7%; IGT or IFG on previous testing

• Other clinical conditions associated with insulin resistance (eg, severe obesity, acanthosis nigricans)

• History of CVD

In the absence of the above criteria, testing for diabetes should begin at age 45 yrs.

If results are normal, testing should be repeated at least at 3-year intervals, with consideration of more frequent testing depending on initial results (eg, those with prediabetes should be tested yearly) and risk status.

Abbreviations: CVD, cardiovascular disease; IFG, impaired fasting glucose (FPG levels 100mg/dL-125mg/dL); IGT, impaired glucose tolerance (2-hr values in the OGTT of 140mg/dL-199mg/dL).

Source: Standards of Medical Care in Diabetes—2012. *Diabetes Care.* 2012;35(Suppl 1):S11-S49.

SUGAR-FREE PRODUCTS

The following is a selection of sugar-free products grouped by therapeutic category. When recommending these products to diabetic patients, keep in mind that many may contain sorbitol, alcohol, or other sources of carbohydrates. This list is not comprehensive. Generic and alternate brands may be available. Check product labeling for a current listing of inactive ingredients.

Analgesics

Addaprin Tablets	Dover
Aminofen Tablets	Dover
Back Pain-Off Tablets ‡	Medique
I-Prin Tablets ‡	Medique
Medi-Seltzer Effervescent Tablets	Medique
Methadose Sugar Free Oral Concentrate	Covidien
Ms.-Aid Tablets ‡	Medique
Children's Silapap Liquid	Silarx

Antacids/Antiflatulants

Alcalak Chewable Tablets*† ‡ §	Medique
Diotame Chewable Tablets*† ‡ §	Medique
Pepto-Bismol Caplets † ‡	Procter & Gamble
Tums Extra Sugar Free Tablets* §	GlaxoSmithKline Consumer

Anti-asthmatic/Respiratory Agent

Jay-Phyl Syrup	JayMac

Antidiarrheal

Imogen Liquid	Pharm Generic

Blood Modifier/Iron Preparation

I.L.X. B-12 Elixir	Kenwood

Corticosteroid

Pediapred Solution* §	UCB

Cough/Cold/Allergy Preparations

Bromhist-DM Solution	Cypress
Bromhist Pediatric Solution	Cypress
Bromphenex DM Solution*† §	Breckenridge
Bromplex DM Solution*† §	Prasco
Broncotron Liquid	Seyer Pharmatec
Broncotron-D Suspension	Seyer Pharmatec
Carbaphen 12 Ped Suspension	Gil
Carbaphen 12 Suspension	Gil
Carbatuss-12 Suspension	GM
Carbatuss-CL Solution	GM
Cetafen Cough & Cold Tablets ‡	Hart Health and Safety
Cetafen Cold Tablets ‡	Hart Health and Safety
Cheratussin DAC Liquid	Qualitest
Coldcough PD Syrup* §	Breckenridge
Coldcough Syrup* §	Breckenridge
Coldonyl Tablets	Medique
Corfen DM Solution	Cypress
Crantex Syrup	Breckenridge
De-Chlor DM Solution	Cypress
Despec Liquid	International Ethical
Despec-SF Liquid	International Ethical
Diabetic Tussin	Health Care Products
Diabetic Tussin DM Liquid §	Health Care Products
Diabetic Tussin Solution§	Health Care Products
Diabetic Siltussin DAS-Na	Silarx
Diabetic Siltussin-DM DAS-Na	Silarx
Diphen Capsules ‡	Medique
Double Tussin DM Liquid	Reese
Dytan-CS Tablets	Hawthorn
Emagrin Forte Tablets	Medique
Gilphex TR Tablets	Gil
Giltuss Ped-C Solution§	Gil
Neo DM Syrup*† §	Laser
Neotuss-D Liquid † §	A.G. Marin
Neotuss S/F Liquid † §	A.G. Marin
Phena-HC Solution	GM
Phena-S 12 Suspension	GM
Phena-S Liquid	GM
Poly Hist PD Solution	Poly
Scot-Tussin Diabetes CF Liquid	Scot-Tussin
Scot-Tussin Expectorant Solution	Scot-Tussin
Scot-Tussin Senior Solution	Scot-Tussin
Siladryl Allergy Solution* §	Silarx
Siltussin DAS Liquid*† §	Silarx
Siltussin DM DAS Cough Formula Syrup*† §	Silarx
Siltussin SA Liquid*† §	Silarx
Children's Sudafed PE Cough & Cold Liquid*† §	McNeil Consumer
Children's Sudafed Nasal	McNeil Consumer
Supress DX Pediatric Drops † §	Kramer-Novis
Suttar-SF Syrup	Gil
Vazol Solution	Wraser

* Contains sorbitol.
† May contain other sugar alcohols (eg, glycerol, isomalt, maltitol, mannitol, xylitol).
‡ May contain other sources of carbohydrates (eg, cellulose, lactose, maltodextrin, polydextrose, starch).
§ May contain natural or artificial flavors.

(Continued)

Cough/Cold/Allergy Preparations *(Continued)*

Z-Tuss DM Syrup † §	Magna
Z-Tuss Expectorant Solution † §	Magna

Fluoride Preparations

Fluor-A-Day Liquid	Arbor
Fluor-A-Day Tablets*† §	Arbor
Sensodyne with Fluoride Cool Gel*† ‡ §	GlaxoSmithKline Consumer
Sensodyne Tartar Control with Whitening † ‡ §	GlaxoSmithKline Consumer
Sensodyne w/Fluoride Toothpaste Original Flavor*† ‡ §	GlaxoSmithKline Consumer

Laxatives

Benefiber Powder	Novartis
Citrucel Powder ‡ §	GlaxoSmithKline Consumer
Colace Solution	Purdue Products
Fiber Choice Tablets* ‡ §	GlaxoSmithKline Consumer
Fibro-XL Capsules	Key
Konsyl Easy Mix Formula Powder ‡	Konsyl
Konsyl Orange Powder ‡ §	Konsyl
Konsyl Powder ‡	Konsyl
Metamucil Smooth Texture Powder ‡	Procter & Gamble
Reguloid Powder Regular Flavor ‡	Rugby
Reguloid Powder Orange Flavor ‡ §	Rugby

Mouth/Throat Preparations

Cepacol Dual Relief Sore Throat Spray † §	Combe
Cepacol Sore Throat + Coating Relief Lozenge † §	Combe
Cepacol Sore Throat Lozenges † §	Combe
Cheracol Sore Throat Spray †	Lee
Chloraseptic Spray*† §	Prestige
Diabetic Tussin Cough Drops † §	Health Care Products
Fisherman's Friend Sugar Free Mint Lozenges*	Lofthouse of Fleetwood
Fresh N Free Liquid	Geritrex
Listerine Pocketpaks Film ‡ §	Johnson & Johnson
Luden's Sugar Free & Wild Cherry Throat Drops † §	McNeil Consumer
Medikoff Sugar Free Drops †	Medique

N'ice Lozenges* §	Heritage/Insight
Oragesic Solution* §	Parnell
Oragel Dry Mouth Moisturizing Gel*† ‡ §	Del
Orajel Dry Mouth Moisturizing Spray † ‡ §	Del
Sepasoothe Lozenges* ‡ §	Medique

Vitamins/Minerals/Supplements

Adaptosode For Stress Liquid	HVS
Adaptosode R+R For Acute Stress Liquid	HVS
Alamag Tablets*† ‡ §	Medique
Alcalak Tablets*† ‡	Medique
Apetigen Elixir*†	Kramer-Novis
Apptrim Capsules	Physician Therapeutics
Apptrim-D Capsules	Physician Therapeutics
Bevitamel Tablets	Westlake
Biosode Liquid	HVS
Bugs Bunny Complete	Bayer
C&M Caps-375 Capsules	Key
Cal-Cee Tablets	Key
Calcet Plus Tablets	Mission Pharmacal
Calcimin-300 Tablets	Key
Cerefolin NAC Tablets	Pamlab
Chromacaps ‡	Key
Delta D3 Tablets ‡	Freeda Vitamins
Detoxosode Liquids	HVS
DHEA Capsules	ADH Health Products
Diatx ZN Tablets ‡	Centrix
Diucaps Capsules	Legere
DL-Phen-500 Capsules	Key
Enterex Diabetic Liquid ‡	Victus
Evening Primrose Oil Capsules †	Nature's Bounty
Ex-L Tablets ‡	Key
Extress Tablets	Key
Eyetamins Tablets ‡	Rexall Consumer
Fem-Cal Citrate Tablets ‡	Freeda Vitamins
Fem-Cal Tablets ‡	Freeda Vitamins
Fem-Cal Plus Tablets	Freeda Vitamins
Ferrocite Plus Tablets ‡	Breckenridge
Folacin-800 Tablets ‡	Key
Folbee Plus Tablets ‡	Breckenridge
Folbee Tablets ‡	Breckenridge
Folplex 2.2 Tablets ‡	Breckenridge
Foltx Tablets ‡	Pamlab
Gabadone Capsules	Physician Therapeutics
Gram-O-Leci Tablets*† ‡	Freeda Vitamins
Herbal Slim Complex Capsules	ADH Health Products
Hypertensa Capsules ‡	Physician Therapeutics
Lynae Calcium/Vitamin C Chewable Tablets	Boscogen
Lynae Chondroitin/ Glucosamine Capsules	Boscogen

---

* Contains sorbitol.
† May contain other sugar alcohols (eg, glycerol, isomalt, maltitol, mannitol, xylitol).
‡ May contain other sources of carbohydrates (eg, cellulose, lactose, maltodextrin, polydextrose, starch).
§ May contain natural or artificial flavors.

Lynae Ginse-Cool Chewable Tablets	Boscogen
Magimin Tablets ‡	Key
Magnacaps Capsules ‡	Key
Mag-Ox 400 Tablets	Health Care Products
Medi-Lyte Tablets ‡	Medique
Metanx Tablets ‡	Pamlab
Multi-Delyn with Iron Liquid †	Silarx
New Life Hair Tablets ‡	Rexall Consumer
Niferex Elixir* ‡ §	Ther-Rx
Nutrisure OTC Tablets	Westlake
Nutrivit Solution*† §	Llorens
Ob Complete Tablets	Vertical
O-Cal Fa Tablets ‡	Pharmics
Os-Cal 500 + D Tablets ‡	GlaxoSmithKline Consumer
Powervites Tablets ‡	Green Turtle Bay Vitamin
Prostaplex Herbal Complex Capsules	ADH Health Products
Protect Plus Liquid	Gil
Protect Plus Liquid NR Softgels	Gil
Pulmona Capsules	Physician Therapeutics
Quintabs-M Tablets ‡	Freeda Vitamins
Replace w/o Iron Capsules ‡	Key
Samolinic Softgels †	Key
Sea Omega 30 Softgels †	Rugby
Sea Omega 50 Softgels †	Rugby
Sentra AM Capsules	Physician Therapeutics
Sentra PM Capsules	Physician Therapeutics
Soy Care for Menopause Capsules	Inverness Medical

Span C Tablets ‡	Freeda Vitamins
Strovite Forte Syrup	Everett
Sunnie Tablets	Green Turtle Bay Vitamin
Sunvite Tablets † ‡	Rexall Naturalist
Super Dec B100 Tablets ‡	Freeda Vitamins
Super Quints B-50 Tablets ‡	Freeda Vitamins
Supervite Liquid	Seyer Pharmatec
Theramine Capsules	Physician Therapeutics
Triamin Tablets	Key
Triamino Tablets* ‡	Freeda Vitamins
Ultramino Powder	Freeda Vitamins
Uro-Mag Capsules ‡	Health Care Products
Vitafol Tablets † ‡	Everett
Vitamin C/Rose Hips Tablets	ADH Health Products
Xtramins Tablets	Key
Ze Plus Softgels	Everett

Miscellaneous

Acidoll Capsules	Key
Alka-Gest Tablets	Key
Cafergot Tablets ‡	Sandoz
Cytra-2 Solution* §	Cypress
Cytra-K Solution* §	Cypress
Cytra-K Crystals	Cypress
Melatin Tablets ‡	Mason Vitamins
Namenda Solution*† §	Forest
Prosed/DS Tablets ‡	Ferring
Questran Light Powder ‡ §	Par

BRAND/GENERIC INDEX

Organized alphabetically, this index includes the brand and generic names of each drug in the Product Information section. Brand-name drug entries are capitalized; generic names are not. If more than one brand name is associated with a generic, each brand can be found under the generic entry.

THERAPEUTIC CLASS INDEX

Organized alphabetically, this index includes the therapeutic class of each drug in the Product Information section. Therapeutic class headings are based on information provided in the drug monographs. The drug entries listed under each bold therapeutic class are organized alphabetically by brand name or monograph title (shown in capitalized letters), followed by the generic name in parentheses.

F

G

ISONICOTINIC ACID HYDRAZIDE
  ISONIAZID
  (isoniazid) 504

ISONICOTINIC ACID HYDRAZIDE/RIFAMYCIN DERIVATIVE
  RIFAMATE
  (rifampin-isoniazid).....................................836

ISONICOTINIC ACID HYDRAZIDE/RIFAMYCIN DERIVATIVE/NICOTINAMIDE ANALOGUE
  RIFATER
  (rifampin-isoniazid-pyrazinamide) 837

K

K⁺ SUPPLEMENT
  K-DUR
  (potassium chloride) 519
  KLOR-CON M
  (potassium chloride) 527
  K-TAB
  (potassium chloride) 530
  MICRO-K
  (potassium chloride) 620

K⁺-SPARING DIURETIC
  DYRENIUM
  (triamterene) 332

K⁺-SPARING DIURETIC/THIAZIDE DIURETIC
  ALDACTAZIDE
  (hydrochlorothiazide-spironolactone)........... 46
  DYAZIDE
  (triamterene-hydrochlorothiazide)...............330
  MAXZIDE
  (triamterene-hydrochlorothiazide)............. 600

KERATINOCYTE GROWTH FACTOR
  KEPIVANCE
  (palifermin)..520

KETOLIDE ANTIBIOTIC
  KETEK
  (telithromycin) 523

KINASE INHIBITOR
  AFINITOR
  (everolimus)..38
  CAPRELSA
  (vandetanib) 185
  SPRYCEL
  (dasatinib) 892
  TASIGNA
  (nilotinib)..923
  TYKERB
  (lapatinib)..985
  ZELBORAF
  (vemurafenib) 1086

L

LEUKOTRIENE RECEPTOR ANTAGONIST
  ACCOLATE
  (zafirlukast) 6
  SINGULAIR
  (montelukast sodium).................................. 879
  ZYFLO CR
  (zileuton)...1122

LINCOMYCIN DERIVATIVE
  CLEOCIN
  (clindamycin)... 228
  CLINDAGEL
  (clindamycin phosphate) 231
  CLINDESSE
  (clindamycin phosphate) 232
  EVOCLIN
  (clindamycin phosphate) 383

LINCOSAMIDE DERIVATIVE/RETINOID
  VELTIN GEL
  (clindamycin phosphate-tretinoin) 1013
  ZIANA
  (clindamycin phosphate-tretinoin) 1097

LIPASE INHIBITOR
  XENICAL
  (orlistat) 1064

LIPID-REGULATING AGENT
  LOVAZA
  (omega-3-acid ethyl esters).........................580

LOCAL ANESTHETIC
  XYLOCAINE INJECTION
  (lidocaine HCl)... 1071

LOOP DIURETIC
  BUMETANIDE
  (bumetanide)...167
  FUROSEMIDE
  (furosemide)...436
  TORSEMIDE
  (torsemide)..959

LOW MOLECULAR WEIGHT HEPARIN
  FRAGMIN
  (dalteparin sodium).....................................434
  INNOHEP
  (tinzaparin sodium).................................... 491
  LOVENOX
  (enoxaparin sodium) 580

M

MACROCYCLIC LACTONE IMMUNOSUPPRESSANT
  RAPAMUNE
  (sirolimus)... 809

MACROLACTAM ASCOMYCIN DERIVATIVE
  ELIDEL
  (pimecrolimus)..341

MACROLIDE
  AZASITE
  (azithromycin)..133
  BIAXIN
  (clarithromycin) 158
  DIFICID
  (fidaxomicin) 299
  ERY-TAB
  (erythromycin)..371
  ZITHROMAX
  (azithromycin)... 1101
  ZMAX
  (azithromycin)... 1102

MACROLIDE IMMUNOSUPPRESSANT
  PROTOPIC
  (tacrolimus) 795

Visual Identification Guide

VISUAL IDENTIFICATION GUIDE*

ABILIFY

RX

(aripiprazole)
BRISTOL-MYERS SQUIBB/OTSUKA

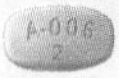

2 mg

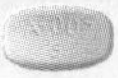

5 mg

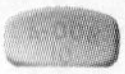

10 mg

15 mg

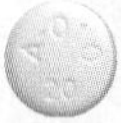

20 mg

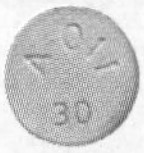

30 mg

Also available in an oral solution.

ABILIFY DISCMELT

RX

(aripiprazole)
BRISTOL-MYERS SQUIBB/OTSUKA

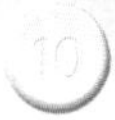

10 mg

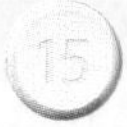

15 mg

Orally Disintegrating Tablets

ABILIFY INJECTION

RX

(aripiprazole)
BRISTOL-MYERS SQUIBB/OTSUKA

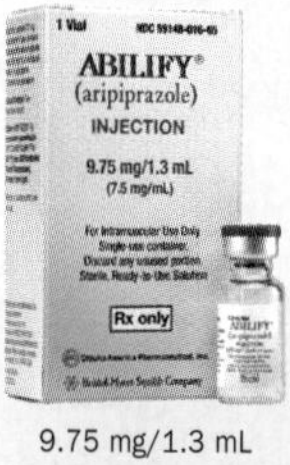

9.75 mg/1.3 mL

ACTOS

RX

(pioglitazone HCl)
TAKEDA

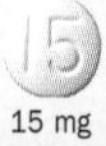

15 mg

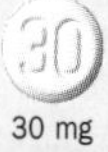

30 mg

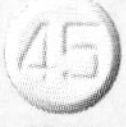

45 mg

ACTOPLUS MET XR

RX

(pioglitazone HCl/metformin HCl)
TAKEDA

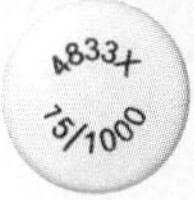

15 mg/1000 mg

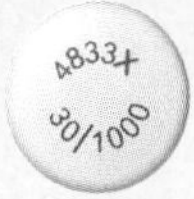

30 mg/1000 mg

Extended-Release Tablets

ADDERALL XR

CII

(dextroamphetamine sulfate, dextroamphetamine saccharate,
amphetamine aspartate monohydrate, amphetamine sulfate)
SHIRE

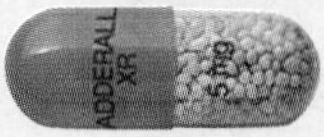

5 mg

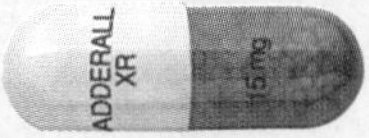

15 mg

Also available in 10 mg, 20 mg, 25 mg, and 30 mg capsules.

ADVICOR

RX

(niacin extended-release/lovastatin tablets)
ABBOTT

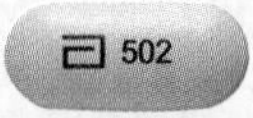

502

500 mg/20 mg

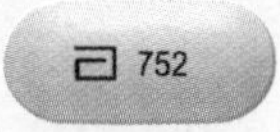

752

750 mg/20 mg

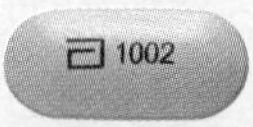

1002

1000 mg/20 mg

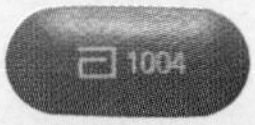

1004

1000 mg/40 mg

AFINITOR

RX

(everolimus)
NOVARTIS

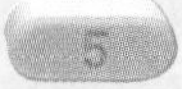

5

5 mg

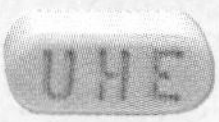

U H E

10 mg

Also available in 2.5 mg and 7.5 mg tablets.

Other dosage forms and strengths may be available.

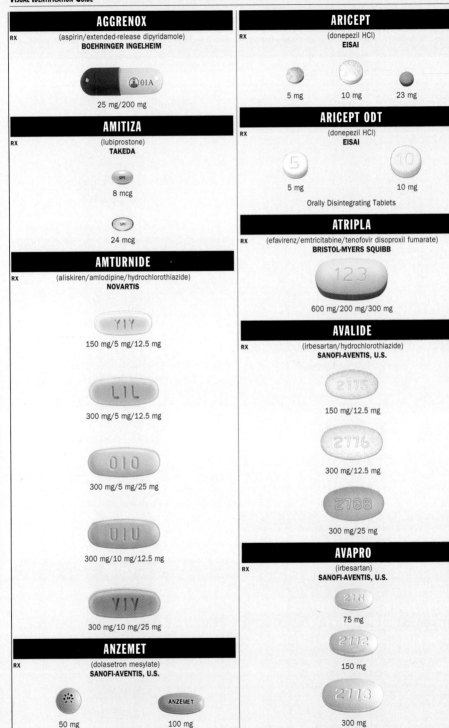

AGGRENOX
RX
(aspirin/extended-release dipyridamole)
BOEHRINGER INGELHEIM

25 mg/200 mg

AMITIZA
RX
(lubiprostone)
TAKEDA

8 mcg

24 mcg

AMTURNIDE
RX
(aliskiren/amlodipine/hydrochlorothiazide)
NOVARTIS

150 mg/5 mg/12.5 mg

300 mg/5 mg/12.5 mg

300 mg/5 mg/25 mg

300 mg/10 mg/12.5 mg

300 mg/10 mg/25 mg

ANZEMET
RX
(dolasetron mesylate)
SANOFI-AVENTIS, U.S.

50 mg

100 mg

ARICEPT
RX
(donepezil HCl)
EISAI

5 mg

10 mg

23 mg

ARICEPT ODT
RX
(donepezil HCl)
EISAI

5 mg

10 mg

Orally Disintegrating Tablets

ATRIPLA
RX
(efavirenz/emtricitabine/tenofovir disoproxil fumarate)
BRISTOL-MYERS SQUIBB

600 mg/200 mg/300 mg

AVALIDE
RX
(irbesartan/hydrochlorothiazide)
SANOFI-AVENTIS, U.S.

150 mg/12.5 mg

300 mg/12.5 mg

300 mg/25 mg

AVAPRO
RX
(irbesartan)
SANOFI-AVENTIS, U.S.

75 mg

150 mg

300 mg

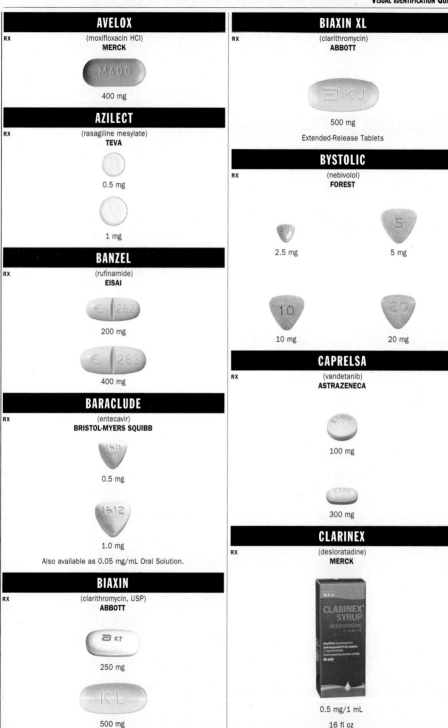

AVELOX
RX
(moxifloxacin HCl)
MERCK

M400

400 mg

AZILECT
RX
(rasagiline mesylate)
TEVA

0.5 mg

1 mg

BANZEL
RX
(rufinamide)
EISAI

€ 262

200 mg

€ 263

400 mg

BARACLUDE
RX
(entecavir)
BRISTOL-MYERS SQUIBB

1611

0.5 mg

1612

1.0 mg

Also available as 0.05 mg/mL Oral Solution.

BIAXIN
RX
(clarithromycin, USP)
ABBOTT

a kt

250 mg

KL

500 mg

BIAXIN XL
RX
(clarithromycin)
ABBOTT

a KJ

500 mg

Extended-Release Tablets

BYSTOLIC
RX
(nebivolol)
FOREST

2½

2.5 mg

5

5 mg

10

10 mg

20

20 mg

CAPRELSA
RX
(vandetanib)
ASTRAZENECA

100 mg

300 mg

CLARINEX
RX
(desloratadine)
MERCK

16 fl oz
**CLARINEX®
SYRUP**
(desloratadine)
0.5 mg per 1 mL

Rx only

0.5 mg/1 mL

16 fl oz

V3

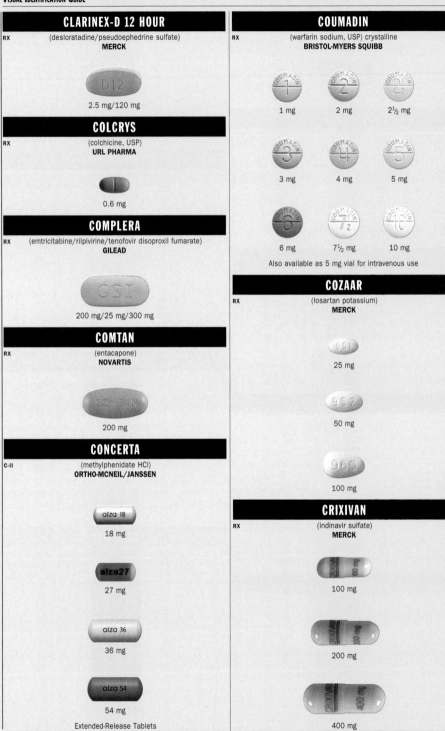

CLARINEX-D 12 HOUR

RX (desloratadine/pseudoephedrine sulfate)
MERCK

2.5 mg/120 mg

COLCRYS

RX (colchicine, USP)
URL PHARMA

0.6 mg

COMPLERA

RX (emtricitabine/rilpivirine/tenofovir disoproxil fumarate)
GILEAD

200 mg/25 mg/300 mg

COMTAN

RX (entacapone)
NOVARTIS

200 mg

CONCERTA

C-II (methylphenidate HCl)
ORTHO-MCNEIL/JANSSEN

alza 18
18 mg

alza27
27 mg

alza 36
36 mg

alza 54
54 mg

Extended-Release Tablets

COUMADIN

RX (warfarin sodium, USP) crystalline
BRISTOL-MYERS SQUIBB

1 mg

2 mg

2½ mg

3 mg

4 mg

5 mg

6 mg

7½ mg

10 mg

Also available as 5 mg vial for intravenous use

COZAAR

RX (losartan potassium)
MERCK

25 mg

50 mg

100 mg

CRIXIVAN

RX (indinavir sulfate)
MERCK

100 mg

200 mg

400 mg

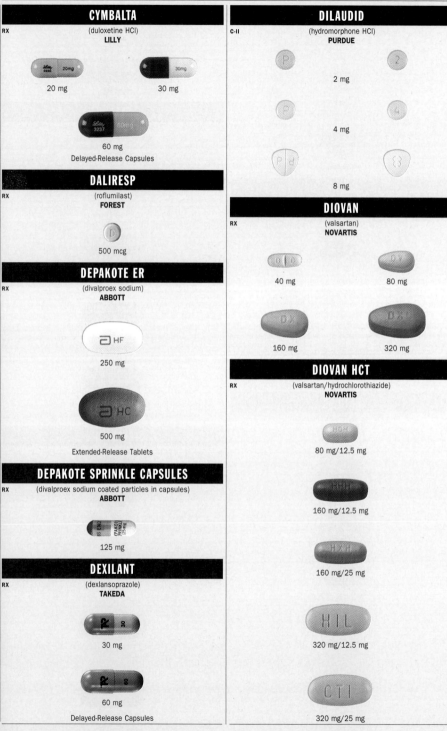

CYMBALTA

RX

(duloxetine HCl)
LILLY

20 mg

30 mg

60 mg
Delayed-Release Capsules

DALIRESP

RX

(roflumilast)
FOREST

500 mcg

DEPAKOTE ER

RX

(divalproex sodium)
ABBOTT

250 mg

500 mg

Extended-Release Tablets

DEPAKOTE SPRINKLE CAPSULES

RX

(divalproex sodium coated particles in capsules)
ABBOTT

125 mg

DEXILANT

RX

(dexlansoprazole)
TAKEDA

30 mg

60 mg

Delayed-Release Capsules

DILAUDID

C-II

(hydromorphone HCl)
PURDUE

2 mg

4 mg

8 mg

DIOVAN

RX

(valsartan)
NOVARTIS

40 mg

80 mg

160 mg

320 mg

DIOVAN HCT

RX

(valsartan/hydrochlorothiazide)
NOVARTIS

80 mg/12.5 mg

160 mg/12.5 mg

160 mg/25 mg

320 mg/12.5 mg

320 mg/25 mg

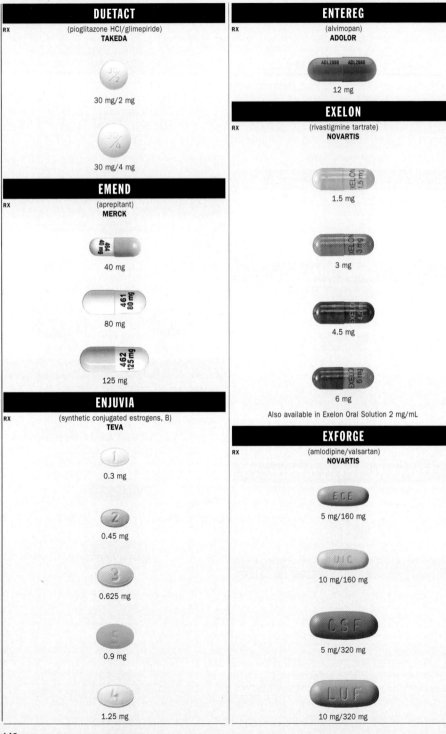

DUETACT

RX

(pioglitazone HCl/glimepiride)
TAKEDA

30 mg/2 mg

30 mg/4 mg

EMEND

RX

(aprepitant)
MERCK

40 mg

80 mg

125 mg

ENJUVIA

RX

(synthetic conjugated estrogens, B)
TEVA

0.3 mg

0.45 mg

0.625 mg

0.9 mg

1.25 mg

ENTEREG

RX

(alvimopan)
ADOLOR

12 mg

EXELON

RX

(rivastigmine tartrate)
NOVARTIS

1.5 mg

3 mg

4.5 mg

6 mg

Also available in Exelon Oral Solution 2 mg/mL

EXFORGE

RX

(amlodipine/valsartan)
NOVARTIS

5 mg/160 mg

10 mg/160 mg

5 mg/320 mg

10 mg/320 mg

EXFORGE HCT

RX

(amlodipine/valsartan/hydrochlorothiazide)
NOVARTIS

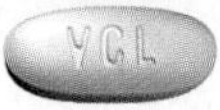

YGL
5 mg/160 mg/12.5 mg

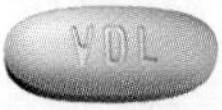

YDL
10 mg/160 mg/12.5 mg

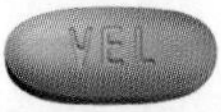

YEL
5 mg/160 mg/25 mg

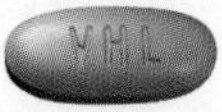

YHL
10 mg/160 mg/25 mg

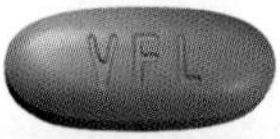

YFL
10 mg/320 mg/25 mg

FANAPT

RX

(iloperidone)
NOVARTIS

1 — 1 mg   2 — 2 mg

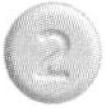

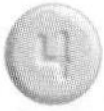

4 — 4 mg   6 — 6 mg

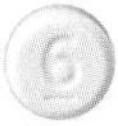

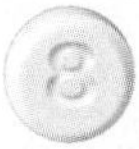

8 — 8 mg   10 — 10 mg

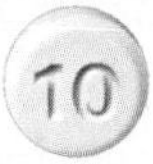

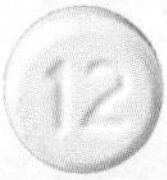

12 — 12 mg

FEMARA

RX

(letrozole)
NOVARTIS

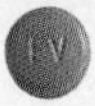

LV
2.5 mg

FOCALIN XR

C-II

(dexmethylphenidate HCl)
NOVARTIS

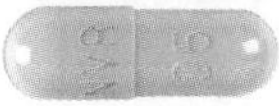

NVR D5
5 mg

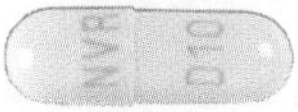

NVR D10
10 mg

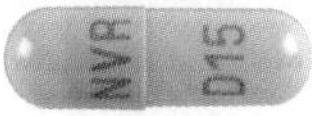

NVR D15
15 mg

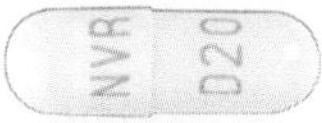

NVR D20
20 mg

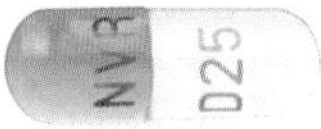

NVR D25
25 mg

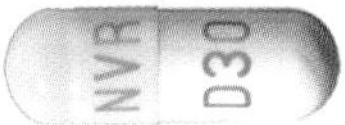

NVR D30
30 mg

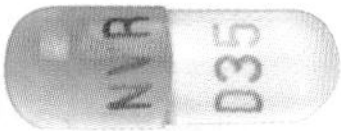

NVR D35
35 mg

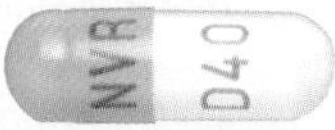

NVR D40
40 mg

Extended-Release Capsules

FOSAMAX

RX

(alendronate sodium)
MERCK

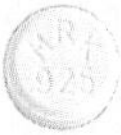

MRK 925 — 5 mg   936 — 10 mg   77 — 35 mg

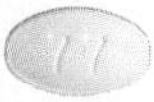

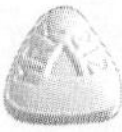

A 40 mg 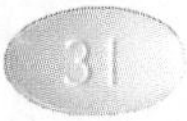   31 — 70 mg

V7

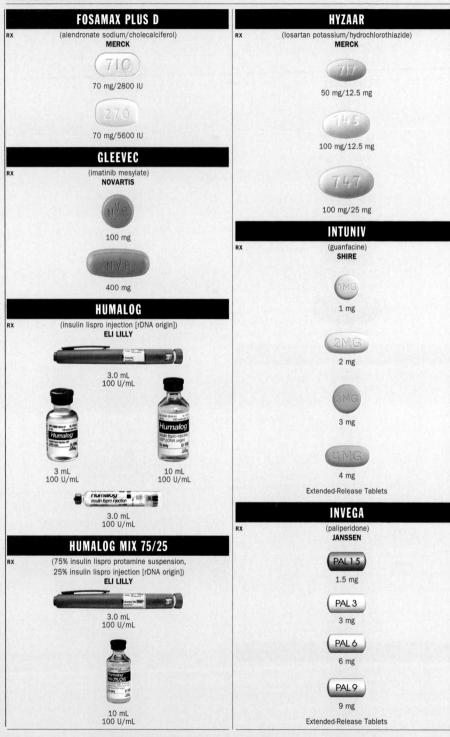

FOSAMAX PLUS D

RX

(alendronate sodium/cholecalciferol)
MERCK

710

70 mg/2800 IU

270

70 mg/5600 IU

GLEEVEC

RX

(imatinib mesylate)
NOVARTIS

N V R

100 mg

N V R

400 mg

HUMALOG

RX

(insulin lispro injection [rDNA origin])
ELI LILLY

3.0 mL
100 U/mL

3 mL
100 U/mL

10 mL
100 U/mL

3.0 mL
100 U/mL

HUMALOG MIX 75/25

RX

(75% insulin lispro protamine suspension,
25% insulin lispro injection [rDNA origin])
ELI LILLY

3.0 mL
100 U/mL

10 mL
100 U/mL

HYZAAR

RX

(losartan potassium/hydrochlorothiazide)
MERCK

717

50 mg/12.5 mg

145

100 mg/12.5 mg

747

100 mg/25 mg

INTUNIV

RX

(guanfacine)
SHIRE

1MG

1 mg

2MG

2 mg

3MG

3 mg

4MG

4 mg

Extended-Release Tablets

INVEGA

RX

(paliperidone)
JANSSEN

PAL 1.5

1.5 mg

PAL 3

3 mg

PAL 6

6 mg

PAL 9

9 mg

Extended-Release Tablets

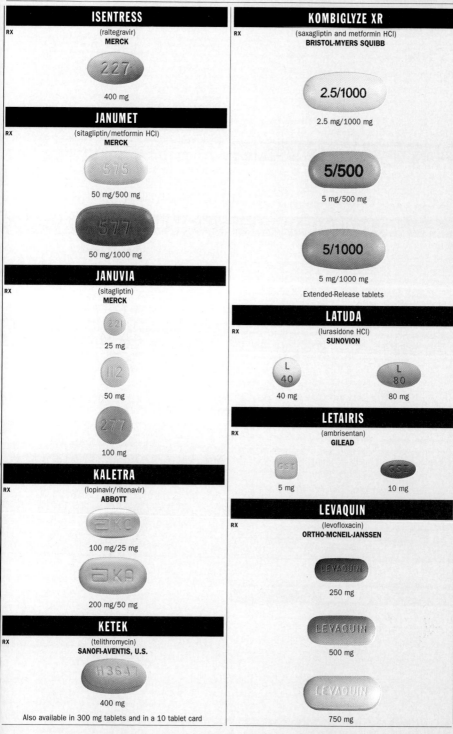

ISENTRESS

RX

(raltegravir)
MERCK

400 mg

JANUMET

RX

(sitagliptin/metformin HCl)
MERCK

50 mg/500 mg

50 mg/1000 mg

JANUVIA

RX

(sitagliptin)
MERCK

25 mg

50 mg

100 mg

KALETRA

RX

(lopinavir/ritonavir)
ABBOTT

100 mg/25 mg

200 mg/50 mg

KETEK

RX

(telithromycin)
SANOFI-AVENTIS, U.S.

400 mg

Also available in 300 mg tablets and in a 10 tablet card

KOMBIGLYZE XR

RX

(saxagliptin and metformin HCl)
BRISTOL-MYERS SQUIBB

2.5/1000

2.5 mg/1000 mg

5/500

5 mg/500 mg

5/1000

5 mg/1000 mg

Extended-Release tablets

LATUDA

RX

(lurasidone HCl)
SUNOVION

L 40

40 mg

L 80

80 mg

LETAIRIS

RX

(ambrisentan)
GILEAD

5 mg

10 mg

LEVAQUIN

RX

(levofloxacin)
ORTHO-MCNEIL-JANSSEN

250 mg

500 mg

750 mg

V9

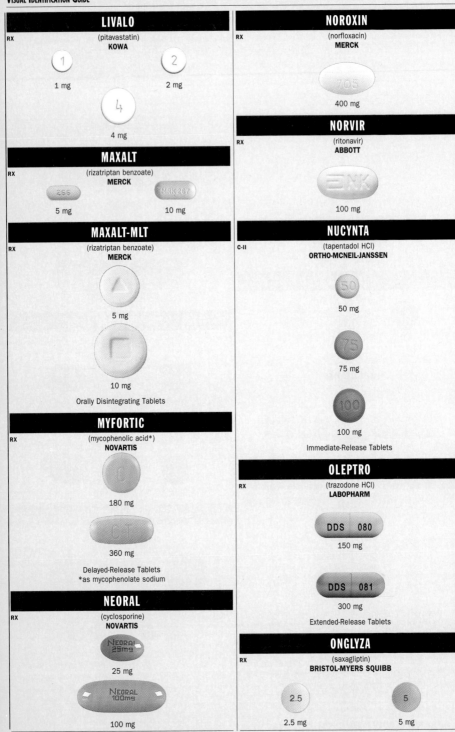

LIVALO
RX
(pitavastatin)
KOWA

1 — 1 mg
2 — 2 mg
4 — 4 mg

MAXALT
RX
(rizatriptan benzoate)
MERCK

266 — 5 mg
MRK 267 — 10 mg

MAXALT-MLT
RX
(rizatriptan benzoate)
MERCK

5 mg

10 mg

Orally Disintegrating Tablets

MYFORTIC
RX
(mycophenolic acid*)
NOVARTIS

180 mg

360 mg

Delayed-Release Tablets
*as mycophenolate sodium

NEORAL
RX
(cyclosporine)
NOVARTIS

Neoral 25mg — 25 mg

Neoral 100mg — 100 mg

NOROXIN
RX
(norfloxacin)
MERCK

705 — 400 mg

NORVIR
RX
(ritonavir)
ABBOTT

100 mg

NUCYNTA
C-II
(tapentadol HCl)
ORTHO-MCNEIL-JANSSEN

50 — 50 mg
75 — 75 mg
100 — 100 mg

Immediate-Release Tablets

OLEPTRO
RX
(trazodone HCl)
LABOPHARM

DDS | 080 — 150 mg

DDS | 081 — 300 mg

Extended-Release Tablets

ONGLYZA
RX
(saxagliptin)
BRISTOL-MYERS SQUIBB

2.5 — 2.5 mg
5 — 5 mg

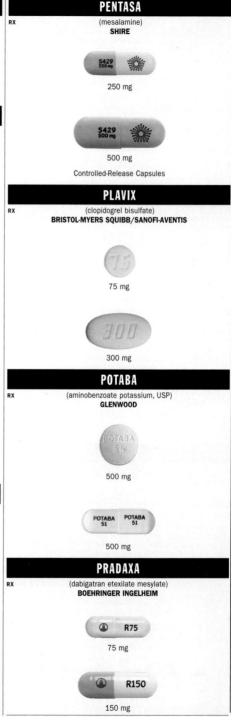

OSMOPREP

RX (sodium phosphate monobasic monohydrate, USP, and sodium phosphate dibasic anhydrous, USP)
SALIX

1.5 g

OXYCONTIN

C-II (oxycodone HCl)
PURDUE

10 mg

15 mg

20 mg

30 mg

40 mg

60 mg

80 mg

Controlled-Release Tablets

PANCREAZE

RX (pancrelipase)
JANSSEN

4,200 Lipase Units

10,500 Lipase Units

16,800 Lipase Units

21,000 Lipase Units

Delayed-Release Capsules

PENTASA

RX (mesalamine)
SHIRE

250 mg

500 mg

Controlled-Release Capsules

PLAVIX

RX (clopidogrel bisulfate)
BRISTOL-MYERS SQUIBB/SANOFI-AVENTIS

75 mg

300 mg

POTABA

RX (aminobenzoate potassium, USP)
GLENWOOD

500 mg

500 mg

PRADAXA

RX (dabigatran etexilate mesylate)
BOEHRINGER INGELHEIM

75 mg

150 mg

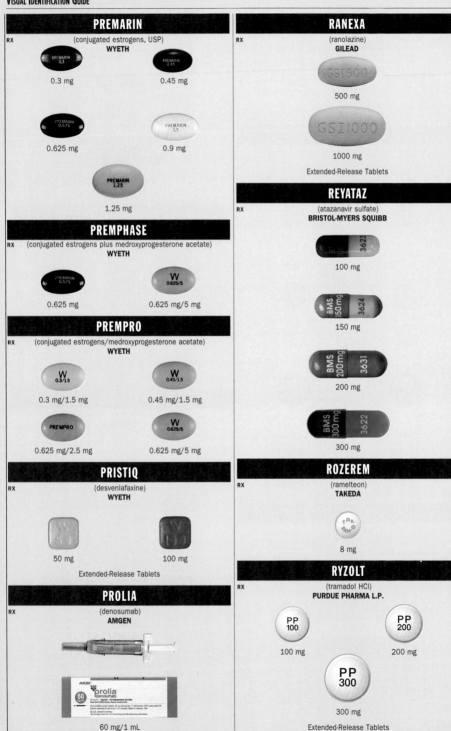

PREMARIN
RX (conjugated estrogens, USP)
WYETH

0.3 mg 0.45 mg

0.625 mg 0.9 mg

1.25 mg

PREMPHASE
RX (conjugated estrogens plus medroxyprogesterone acetate)
WYETH

0.625 mg 0.625 mg/5 mg

PREMPRO
RX (conjugated estrogens/medroxyprogesterone acetate)
WYETH

0.3 mg/1.5 mg 0.45 mg/1.5 mg

0.625 mg/2.5 mg 0.625 mg/5 mg

PRISTIQ
RX (desvenlafaxine)
WYETH

50 mg 100 mg

Extended-Release Tablets

PROLIA
RX (denosumab)
AMGEN

60 mg/1 mL

RANEXA
RX (ranolazine)
GILEAD

500 mg

1000 mg

Extended-Release Tablets

REYATAZ
RX (atazanavir sulfate)
BRISTOL-MYERS SQUIBB

100 mg

150 mg

200 mg

300 mg

ROZEREM
RX (ramelteon)
TAKEDA

8 mg

RYZOLT
RX (tramadol HCl)
PURDUE PHARMA L.P.

100 mg 200 mg

300 mg

Extended-Release Tablets

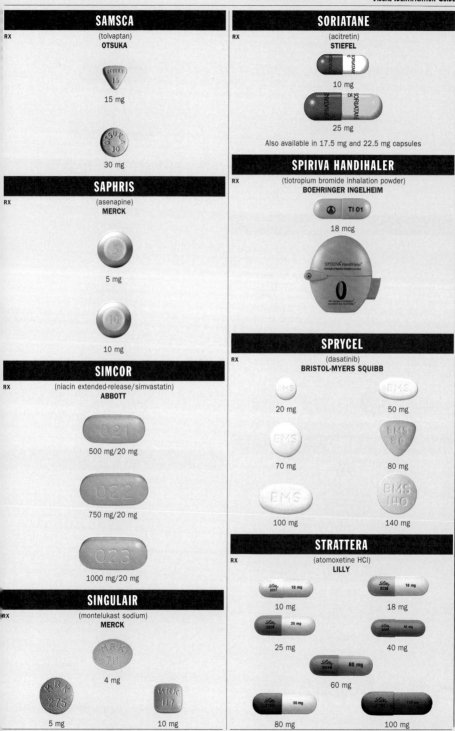

SAMSCA

RX

(tolvaptan)
OTSUKA

15 mg

30 mg

SAPHRIS

RX

(asenapine)
MERCK

5 mg

10 mg

SIMCOR

RX

(niacin extended-release/simvastatin)
ABBOTT

500 mg/20 mg

750 mg/20 mg

1000 mg/20 mg

SINGULAIR

RX

(montelukast sodium)
MERCK

4 mg

5 mg

10 mg

SORIATANE

RX

(acitretin)
STIEFEL

10 mg

25 mg

Also available in 17.5 and 22.5 mg capsules

SPIRIVA HANDIHALER

RX

(tiotropium bromide inhalation powder)
BOEHRINGER INGELHEIM

18 mcg

SPRYCEL

RX

(dasatinib)
BRISTOL-MYERS SQUIBB

20 mg

50 mg

70 mg

80 mg

100 mg

140 mg

STRATTERA

RX

(atomoxetine HCl)
LILLY

10 mg

18 mg

25 mg

40 mg

60 mg

80 mg

100 mg

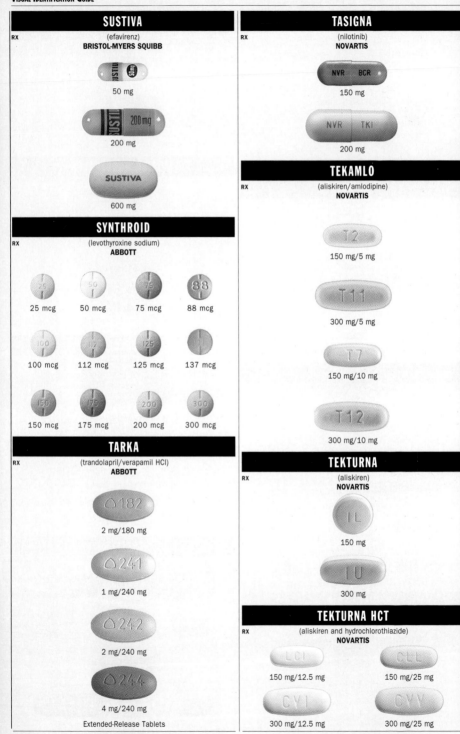

SUSTIVA
RX
(efavirenz)
BRISTOL-MYERS SQUIBB

50 mg

200 mg

600 mg

SYNTHROID
RX
(levothyroxine sodium)
ABBOTT

25 mcg 50 mcg 75 mcg 88 mcg

100 mcg 112 mcg 125 mcg 137 mcg

150 mcg 175 mcg 200 mcg 300 mcg

TARKA
RX
(trandolapril/verapamil HCl)
ABBOTT

182 — 2 mg/180 mg

241 — 1 mg/240 mg

242 — 2 mg/240 mg

244 — 4 mg/240 mg

Extended-Release Tablets

TASIGNA
RX
(nilotinib)
NOVARTIS

NVR BCR — 150 mg

NVR TKI — 200 mg

TEKAMLO
RX
(aliskiren/amlodipine)
NOVARTIS

T2 — 150 mg/5 mg

T11 — 300 mg/5 mg

T7 — 150 mg/10 mg

T12 — 300 mg/10 mg

TEKTURNA
RX
(aliskiren)
NOVARTIS

IL — 150 mg

IU — 300 mg

TEKTURNA HCT
RX
(aliskiren and hydrochlorothiazide)
NOVARTIS

LCI — 150 mg/12.5 mg   CLL — 150 mg/25 mg

CVI — 300 mg/12.5 mg   CVV — 300 mg/25 mg